Staff Library
Education Centre
Royal Liverpool University Hospital
Prescot Street
LIVERPOOL
L7 8XP

Colon and Rectal Surgery

Fifth Edition

Colon and Rectal Surgery

Fifth Edition

Marvin L. Corman, M.D.
Professor of Surgery
State University of New York at Stony Brook
Stony Brook, NY
Professor of Surgery
Albert Einstein College of Medicine
New York, NY

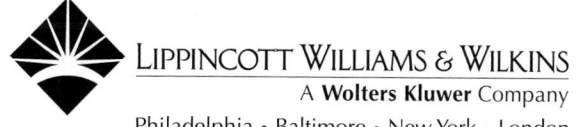

LIPPINCOTT WILLIAMS & WILKINS
A **Wolters Kluwer** Company

Philadelphia • Baltimore • New York • London
Buenos Aires • Hong Kong • Sydney • Tokyo

Acquisitions Editor: Brian Brown
Managing Editors: Erin McMullan and Michelle M. LaPlante
Project Manager: Fran Gunning
Manufacturing Manager: Ben Rivera
Marketing Manager: Adam Glazer
Production Services: Print Matters, Inc.
Compositor: Compset, Inc.
Printer: Edwards Brothers

© 2005 by LIPPINCOTT WILLIAMS & WILKINS
530 Walnut Street
Philadelphia, PA 19106 USA
LWW.com

Printed in the USA

Library of Congress Cataloging-in-Publication Data
Corman, Marvin L., 1939–
    Colon and rectal surgery / Marvin L. Corman. — 5th ed.
      p. ; cm.
    Includes bibliographical references and index.
    ISBN 0-7817-4043-6 (HC)
    1. Colon (Anatomy)—Surgery. 2. Rectum—Surgery. I. Title.
Edgar D. III. Ultrasound for the surgeon.
    [DNLM: 1. Rectal Diseases—surgery. 2. Colonic Diseases—surgery. WI 650 C811c 2004]
RD544.C67 2004
617.5′547—dc22
                                                                                    2004048792

10 9 8 7 6 5 4 3 2

To My Grandchildren
Ben, Max, Charlie, Sami and Harry

GUEST CONTRIBUTORS

Alan V. Abrams, M.D.
Assistant Clinical Professor of Surgery
Weill Medical College
Cornell University
New York, NY

Homayoon Akbari, M.D.
Assistant Professor
Department of Surgery
Attending Surgeon
Thomas Jefferson University Hospital
Philadelphia, PA

Frank H. Chae, M.D.
Assistant Professor of Surgery
University of Colorado Health Sciences Center
Boulder, CO

John A. Coller, M.D.
Director, Endoscopy and Anorectal Physiology Laboratories
Lahey Clinic Medical Center

Eric J. Daniels, M.D.
Resident in Surgery
University of California, Los Angeles
Los Angeles, CA

Herbert M. Dean
Assistant Professor of Medicine
University of Massachusetts Medical School
Worcester, MA

Victor W. Fazio, M.D.
Professor of Surgery
Lerner College of Medicine of Case Western Reserve
    University
Rupert Turnbull Jr. Chairman
Department of Colorectal Surgery
Cleveland Clinic
Cleveland, OH

Susan Feldman, R.N., E.T.
Enterostomal Therapist
Long Island Jewish Medical Center
New Hyde Park, NY

Robert Gilliland, M.D.
Consultant, General and Colorectal Surgeon
Londonderry, Northern Ireland

Anthony A. Goodman, M.D.
Adjunct Professor of Medicine
W.W.A.M.I. Department of Medical Sciences
Montana State University
Bozeman, MT

Lester Gottesman, M.D.
Associate Professor of Clinical Surgery
Columbia University
College of Physicians and Surgeons
Director
Division of Colon and Rectal Surgery
St. Luke's-Roosevelt Hospital Center
New York, NY

José Marcio Neves Jorge, M.D.
Associate Professor of Coloproctology
Director, Anorectal Physiology Laboratory
University of São Paulo
Hospital das Clinicas
São Paulo, Brazil

Marc Levitt, M.D.
Pediatric Surgeon
Schneider Children's Hospital
Long Island Jewish Medical Center
New Hyde Park, NY

Alberto Peña, M.D.
Chief, Division of Pediatric Surgery
Schneider Children's Hospital
Long Island Jewish Medical Center
New Hyde Park, NY

John L. Petrini, M.D.
Chief, Department of Gastroenterology
Sansum Medical Clinic
Santa Barbara, CA

Daniel Rosenthal, M.D.
The Michael E. DeBakey International Professor of Surgery
Department of Surgery
Uniformed Services University of the Health Sciences
Brooke Army Medical Center
Bethesda, MD

Jonathan M. Sackier, M.D.
Professor, Department of Surgery
George Washington University Medical Center
Washington, DC

T. Cristina Sardinha, M.D.
Attending Colon and Rectal Surgeon
Long Island Jewish Medical Center
New Hyde Park, NY

Ronald M. Stewart, M.D.
Director, Trauma and Emergency Surgery
University of Texas Health Sciences Center
San Antonio, TX

Paula Erwin-Toth, R.N., E.T.
Director of Enterostomal Therapy Education Program
Manager of Enterostomal Therapy Nursing
Cleveland ClinicFoundation
Cleveland, OH

Steven D. Wexner, M.D.
Chairman, Department of Colorectal Surgery
Cleveland Clinic Florida
Weston, FL

FOREWORD TO THE SECOND EDITION

I have reproduced the Foreword to the Second Edition of this text as a memorial tribute to John Cedric Goligher, my mentor, my role model, and my treasured friend.

MLC
April 1, 1998

To be asked by a colleague to write a foreword for one of his literary works is always a considerable compliment and honor. But Marvin Corman's invitation to contribute such an introduction to the second edition of his *Colon and Rectal Surgery* has afforded me special pleasure for a very personal reason. I recognize full well that most of his surgical knowledge and expertise has been derived from his training at the University of Pennsylvania and The Harvard Surgical Service at Boston City Hospital, and from his years of practice at the Lahey Clinic in Boston and the Sansum Clinic in Santa Barbara. But I believe it would be fair to claim that his first really intensive exposure to colorectal surgery was obtained whilst he was doing a 12-month overseas assignment as an assistant with me in Leeds in 1968, and that that experience influenced him considerably in deciding subsequently to concentrate his efforts on this field of surgical endeavour. Naturally, therefore, it has been with much interest and no small measure of pride that I have followed the gradual evolution over the years of this talented young trainee into the present immensely experienced and successful colorectal surgeon, now in an extremely busy middle period of this career.

As I see it, the traditional role of an independent foreword is twofold—to say something by way of introduction about the author, especially when he happens to be relatively little known, and to offer some words of explanation and commendation about the book itself (all these remarks, needless to say, being couched in as favorable terms as possible). But on this occasion there can be little excuse for indulging in such ritual praises and platitudes, for Marvin Corman already enjoys a truly international reputation in colorectal surgery, and the uniformly favorable reviews accorded to the first edition of his book (including First Prize of The American Medical Writers Association) and the large readership that it has since acquired have established beyond question its great merits and rendered inappropriate any further exercises in unalloyed eulogy. What then can one say? Well, it might be interesting and even useful to try to identify those factors that may have helped to secure the outstanding success of this work. Perhaps the best way to do so would be,

first of all, to itemize the features that appear, at any rate to me, especially necessary in any text that aims to cover an area of surgical practice and to be available for consultation, not merely in hospital or medical school libraries, but also and more importantly in the surgeon's own office or study, and then to see how well Marvin Corman's book satisfies those postulated requirements.

I consider one of the most desirable attributes to be *really comprehensive coverage of the subject matter,* so that the readers can feel confident that in turning to it they will, as a rule, be able to obtain good advice and not too often encounter disconcerting hiatuses. To be able to offer such an assurance involves a thorough analysis of current knowledge, including an up-to-date review of the relevant literature. Naturally the author's own personal experience and his favored concepts on controversial issues and preferred methods of treatment of various conditions may receive some special attention, but this should not be at the expense of independent essays on selected subtopics, however authoritatively written and valuable for library reading, leaves too many gaps to be an adequate substitute for a well-integrated, relatively unbiased text as a personal reference volume.

An equally important requirement is a book of this kind is a *high quality of illustrations*. As is generally agreed, good illustrations are a considerable help in imparting knowledge on many subjects, but they become well-nigh indispensable when expounding on operative techniques. Indeed, trying to describe surgical operations without the aid of a good illustrative material is about as difficult as attempting to perform these very procedures with one arm tied behind one's back! A few well-executed sketches can enormously clarify and shorten accounts of operative maneuvers.

The *relative merits of single and multiple authorship* have been much debated. Multiple authorship has the advantage of making it possible to allocate to different writers subjects in which they have a special interest and experience. But, even with firm editorship, this arrangement affords a much less even literary format and incurs a greater risk of creating defects or overlaps in coverage. A single authorship has the great merit of presenting a uniform and more agreeable literary style. Moreover, I feel compelled to say that, when writing on a fairly limited theme, such as diseases of the colon and rectum, it ought in my opinion to be possible for one experienced and determined writer to circumscribe the whole field with adequate authority entirely by himself, with perhaps a little assistance from one or two colleagues on slightly more esoteric or specialized aspects of the subject.

Turning now to Marvin Corman's Colon and Rectal Surgery, I feel that it warrants high ratings on each of these three important points. It unquestionably provides good or very adequate coverage on all major issues. The illustrations, particularly those of operative techniques, are quite superb and represent one of the most attractive features of the works. The text is essentially by one author, insofar as Dr. Corman himself has been responsible for all of it except for that part pertaining to pediatric conditions, which are dealt with very effectively by the well-known pediatric surgeon, Dr. Alberto Peña. Dr. Corman writes clearly and attractively, making for easy reading and ready understanding. the outcome is a most handsome and helpful volume, which it is a pleasure to consult.

In conclusion and at the risk of exposing myself to a charge of conceit, I should like to point out that for most of the past three decades the need of surgeons for a comprehensive, consistently updated text, covering the whole field of colorectal surgery with some thoroughness, has been met mainly—and, for a considerable part of that time, solely—by my *Surgery of the Anus, Rectum and Colon* (London: Baillière-Tindall, 1st ed, 1961; 5th ed, 1984 [editor's note: newly revised by Keighley and Williams in 1999]). But in more recent years several other books on this subject (or on selected parts of it) have emerged—and, if rumor is to be believed, two more are due to appear in the near future—so that a steadily increasing number of alternative texts is becoming available. Doubtless each of these volumes will suit different surgical tastes and needs. He would be a brave man who would attempt any sort of objective assessment of their relative merits, and certainly this is not the place in which to undertake such an adjudication. All I would like to say in this connection is that in my opinion one of these works, the second edition of Corman's *Colon and Rectal Surgery*, is certainly a very good substitute for mine, and I have no hesitation in recommending it strongly as a reliable guide to the sound practice of contemporary colorectal surgery.

John Goligher
Emeritus Professor of Surgery,
University of Leeds, England;
Consulting Surgeon,
St. Mark's Hospital for Diseases of the Rectum and Colon,
London, England
June 1, 1988

PREFACE

Why does someone elect to author a medical book? It has been said that writing and publishing may be the safest means for achieving fame or at least some level of eminence. The alternative avenues for comparable recognition were for me either impossible or unacceptable, such as becoming a surrealistic poet, dying in battle, obtaining entrée into the Encyclopedia Britannica, facing capital punishment for apostasy, or going on an ill-fated expedition—just to name a few options. No, I'll just rewrite my text. But it is not a labor of love. To quote that extraordinary statesman and prolific author, Winston Churchill, "A book is an unforgiving mistress." When asked by a reporter to describe the playwright's profession, the late Herb Gardner replied: "How do you ask a kamikaze pilot if his work is going well?"

I am fortunate again to have the opportunity of changing my mind, of clarifying confusion and my confused thinking, of correcting misstatements, and of remaining contemporary. Frankly, I am embarrassed by previous inaccuracies. Still, it is better to recant than to be accused of having a pertinacious little mind. With this version I hope to have deracinated all that is incorrect or irrelevant. In other words, I think with the fifth edition I finally got it right.

Why should one revise a text approximately every five years? What is so special about this interval that motivates authors and publishers to rejuvenate their interest in such an endeavor? Laënnec encouraged one not to fear to repeat that which has already been said. "People need truth dinned into their ears many times from all sides." He wrote that the first rumor makes them prick up their ears, the second registers, and the third enters.

And what of the fourth or even the fifth—overkill, redundant, unnecessary? I think not. Every chapter has been rewritten, new references added, and art expanded. Areas of management no longer considered applicable have been deleted. The fact is, as George Pickering implied, that within 30 to 40 years, 50 percent of medical writing will be wrong or obsolete. The question, of course, is: "Which 50 percent?"

Henry Bowditch stated in 1887 that the accumulated literature in medicine is already so enormous and is increasing at such a rapid rate that "any association or individual undertaking to contribute thereto should do so only under a sense of grave moral responsibility." This comment is even more applicable today. I take this responsibility very seriously. If I fail, I expect the reader to hold me to task.

I try to be a conveyor of knowledge, not a hoarder. This is indeed the role of someone who writes. One will note, however, that this is a rather opinionated text, frequently interspersed with my views and commentaries. The purpose, however, is not to be peremptory. These thoughts should serve simply as a focus for stimulating reasoned discussion, not to preclude debate or to limit the expression of alternative perspectives. I have strived, whenever possible, to vivify the experience and to relieve the triteness and the boredom usually associated with this kind of reading.

I have become increasingly aware that my book has been inappropriately used as an "authoritative" treatise, at least in the United States, by members of the legal profession through our tort system. How one defines the word, authoritative, is of no mean consequence on the witness stand. I wish to state for the record that herein there are no sacred truths, no dicta, only personal opinion and the perspectives and reflections of clinical and laboratory investigators, especially those of highly experienced surgeons. One may rely on the integrity of the process, but clearly I do not agree with all of the comments and opinions that are expressed within these pages. Moreover, I acknowledge that every reasonable surgeon has the right to harbor heterodox beliefs. On this subject, I have added another chapter to this edition, that of the medical-legal aspects of colon and rectal surgery.

Because of my particular interest in the history of medicine, specifically colon and rectal surgery, I have expanded the *biographic sketches* considerably. In *Eccliasticus* it is said: "All these were honored in their generations, and were the glory of their times." Not knowing from where we have come causes us to lose perspective as to where we are going. I have encouraged a number of students and residents in surgery to undertake the task of providing much of this additional material. Where these contributions appear the individuals are recognized. These wonderful people have been the greatest source of joy (and occasional tribulation) for me. As a surgeon who has devoted his life to teaching I take great pride in their accomplishments.

Da Costa commented that to write a book is to reveal oneself. Such an endeavor is, in a sense, somewhat like an autobiography. For me it is more analogous to appearing naked before one's peers. Laënnec further stated that he risked his life, but he hoped that the book he was going to publish would be useful enough sooner or later to be worth the life of a man. Having completed four editions I had previously decided that the process had been all too consuming of my life, that I no longer required the scratch of a pen to address the itch of writing, nor did I feel, having tasted type for many years, that I would return to this old indulgence. I wished those that succeeded me Godspeed, for critical writing

had never been more important to the health of the medical profession. I still believe this is true, and so I changed my mind once again. Whether this will be my final edition will be a decision made by the three goddesses of destiny. While I offer no apologia for the book's contents, I would value the opinions, criticisms and suggestions of the reader. After all, I am still in the process of learning.

Marvin L. Corman
September, 2004

ACKNOWLEDGMENTS

There are so many individuals whom I would like to thank for their help in the completion of this text. In addition to the contributors, who I recognize individually in their chapters, I am, of course, indebted to Lois Barnes, a medical illustrator of international repute. She was required to provide illustrative consistency by rendering all of the art of the contributors. She did so with remarkable patience, grace, compulsivity, and her usual professionalism. I am certain that the reader will recognize the exceptional quality of her work.

Although I risk omitting someone, I want to acknowledge a number of individuals who offered special help in the completion of this book: the librarians at the Long Island Jewish Medical Center, the Wellcome Trust Medical Library, and my friends and colleagues, Herand Abcarian, Clive Bartram, Robert Beart, John Bookwalter, Herbert Dean, Theodore Eisenstat, Victor Fazio, James Fleshman, Gary Gecelter, Stanley Goldberg, Jose Guillem, Anthony Goodman, Barton Hoexter, Rolland Parc, David Rothenberger, Marc Sher, and Douglas Wong. I want to express my sincerest appreciation to three dear and special friends: Elliot Prager, Edouard Seroussi, and David Wanicur. They were important counselors to me during this ordeal. Special recognition must be given to my long-suffering administrative assistant, Joyce Owsinski, and to my nurse, Linda Israeli. Both were forced to accept the whims associated with a haphazard schedule in order to accommodate my needs and those of my patients. Moreover, I want to express my appreciation to Barbara Craig and to Ariana Saunders for their help and their special facility with the computer. During the year it took me to re-write this little vade mecum, my wife, Claudia, had to endure my seclusion. She represents the epitome of patience, kindness, and generosity.

I wish also to thank my publisher, Lippincott Williams & Wilkins, for its support, especially that of my editors, Craig Percy, Lisa McAllister, Erin McMullan and Michelle LaPlante. I want also to thank Frances Lennie, who did such a compulsive and superb job on the indexing of the fourth edition and made herself available again this time.

CONTENTS

Anatomy and Embryology of the Anus, Rectum, and Colon

Guest Contributors: Steven D. Wexner and J. Marcio N. Jorge

I have asked Drs. Wexner and Jorge to contribute this chapter because of their extensive knowledge of this topic, and I respect very much their expertise in this regard. Dr. Wexner is Chairman, Department of Colorectal Surgery, Cleveland Clinic Florida, Weston, Florida. Dr. Jorge is Associated Professor of Coloproctology and Director of the Anorectal Physiology Laboratory, University of São Paulo, Hospital das Clinicas, São Paulo, Brazil.

MLC

In anatomy,
it is better to have learned and lost
than never to have learned at all.
W. Somerset Maugham—*Of Human Bondage*

Although the need for an understanding of colonic, anorectal, and pelvic anatomy is consistent with the objective of a comprehensive textbook on colon and rectal surgery, little emphasis is placed on these subjects in training programs today. The most comprehensive observations had been made as early as 1543 by Andreas Vesalius through anatomic dissections. Several aspects, however, remain controversial. Anatomy of this region, especially that of the rectum and anal canal, is so intrinsically related to its physiology that much can be appreciated only in the living. Therefore, it is a region in which the colorectal surgeon has an advantage over the anatomist through *in vivo* dissection, physiologic investigation, and endoscopic examination. More recently, the accumulated experience with diverse operative techniques has added to advances in physiologic testing and has demanded more in-depth knowledge of the anatomy of the large intestine.[33,50,51,56,121-123] Dissection of both humans and animals, sometimes associated with physiologic evaluation, observations *in vivo*, and historical reviews, has been revived, and in fact some concepts of the anatomy, especially of the rectum and anal canal, have been challenged.[20,38,59,60,65,68,71,104,110,113]

EMBRYOLOGY

The primitive gut tube develops from the endodermal roof of the yolk sac. At the beginning of the third week of development, it can be divided into three regions: the foregut in the head fold, the hindgut with its ventral allantoic outgrowth in the smaller tail fold, and, between these two portions, the midgut, which at this stage opens ventrally into the yolk sac (Figure 1-1). After the stages of physiologic herniation, return to the abdomen, and fixation, the midgut progresses below the major pancreatic papilla to form the small intestine, the ascending colon, and the proximal two thirds of the transverse colon. This segment is supplied by the midgut (superior mesenteric) artery, with corresponding venous and lymphatic drainage.[106] The sympathetic innervation of the midgut and likewise the hindgut originates from T-8 to L-2, via splanchnic nerves and the autonomic abdominopelvic plexuses. The parasympathetic outflow to the midgut is derived from the tenth cranial nerve (vagus) with preganglionic cell bodies in the brainstem.

The distal colon (distal third of the transverse colon), the rectum, and the anal canal above the dentate line are all derived from the hindgut. Therefore, this segment is supplied by the hindgut (inferior mesenteric) artery with corresponding venous and lymphatic drainage. Its parasympathetic outflow comes from S-2, S-3, and S-4 via splanchnic nerves.

The dentate line marks the fusion between endodermal and ectodermal tubes, where the terminal portion of the hindgut or cloaca fuses with the proctodeum, an ingrowth from the anal pit. The cloaca originates at the portion of the rectum below the pubococcygeal line, whereas the hindgut originates above it. Before the fifth week of development, the intestinal and urogenital tracts terminate in conjunction with the cloaca. At the sixth week, the urorectal septum migrates caudally, and the

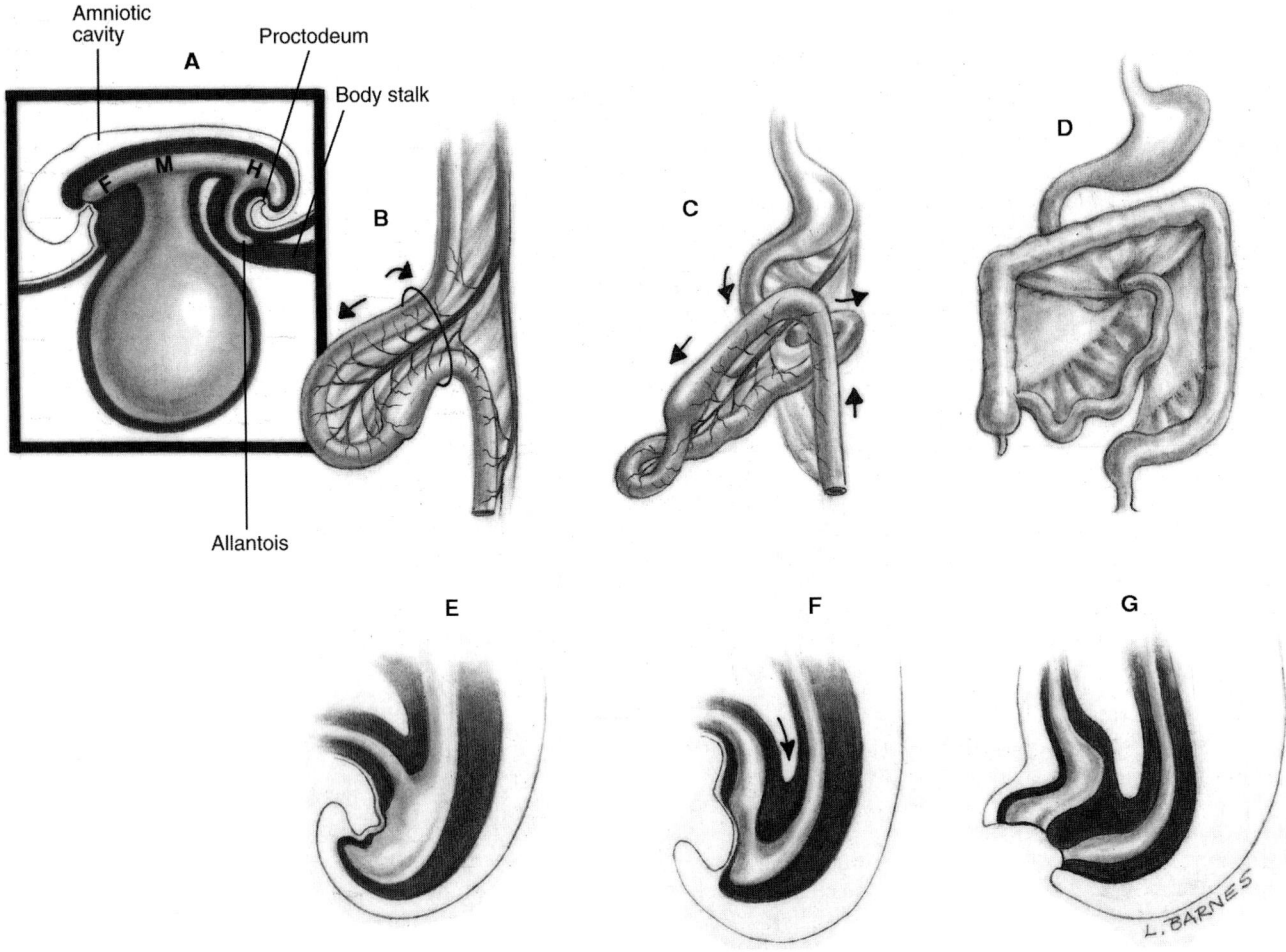

FIGURE 1-1. Embryology of the large intestine. **(A)** At the third week of development, the primitive tube can be divided into three regions: the foregut in the head fold, the hindgut with its ventral allantoic outgrowth in the smaller tail fold, and the midgut between these two portions. Stages of development of the midgut are shown. **(B)** Physiologic herniation. **(C)** Return to the abdomen. **(D)** Fixation. **(E)** At the sixth week, the urogenital septum migrates caudally and separates the intestinal and urogenital tracts **(F,G)**.

two tracts are separated. The cloacal part of the anal canal, which has both endodermal and ectodermal elements, forms the anal transitional zone after breakdown of the anal membrane.[106] During the tenth week, the anal tubercles, a pair of ectodermal swellings around the proctodeal pit, fuse dorsally to form a horseshoe-shaped structure and anteriorly to create the perineal body. The cloacal sphincter is separated by the perineal body into urogenital and anal portions [external anal sphincter (EAS)]. The internal anal sphincter (IAS) is formed later (sixth to twelfth week) from enlarging fibers of the circular layer of the rectum.[65,86] The sphincters apparently migrate during their development; the external sphincter grows cephalad, and the internal sphincter moves caudally. Concomitantly, the longitudinal muscle descends into the intersphincteric plane.[65,127]

ANATOMY OF THE COLON

The colon, so named from the Greek *koluein* ("to retard"), is a capacious tube described in humans to be somewhere between the short, straight type with a rudimentary cecum, such as that of the carnivores, and a long sacculated colon with a capacious cecum, such as that of the herbivores. The colon roughly surrounds the loops of small intestine as an arch. Its length in the adult is variable, averaging approximately 150 cm, about one fourth the length of the small intestine. Its diameter, which can be substantially augmented by distension, gradually decreases from 7.5 cm at the cecum to 2.5 cm at the sigmoid.

Anatomic differences between the small and large intestines include position, caliber, degree of fixation, and, in the colon, the presence of three distinct characteris-

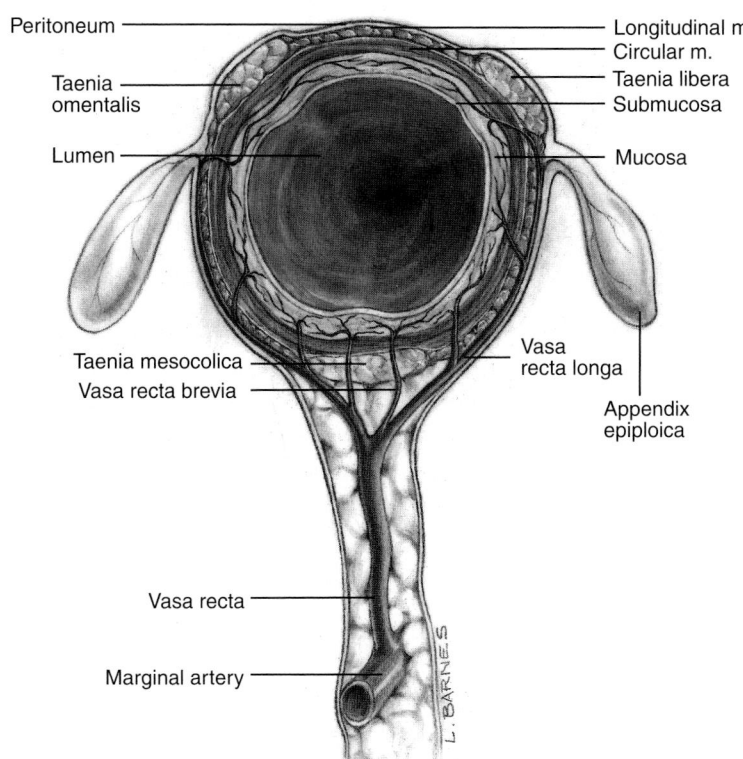

Peritoneum

Taenia
omentalis

Lumen

Taenia mesocolica
Vasa recta brevia

Vasa recta

Marginal artery

Longitudinal m.
Circular m.
Taenia libera
Submucosa

Mucosa

Vasa
recta longa

Appendix
epiploica

L. BARNES

FIGURE 1-2. Cross-section of the colon and meso-colon demonstrates the arrangement of the vasa recta and their branches.

tics: the taeniae coli, the haustra, and the appendices epi-ploicae. The three taeniae coli, anterior (taenia libera), posteromedial (taenia mesocolica), and posterolateral (taenia omentalis), represent bands of the outer longitudinal coat of muscle that traverse the colon from the base of the appendix to the rectosigmoid junction, where they merge. The muscular longitudinal layer is actually a complete coat around the colon, although it is considerably thicker at the taeniae.[35] The haustra or haustral sacculations are outpouchings of bowel wall between the taeniae; they are caused by the relative shortness of the taeniae, about one sixth shorter than the length of bowel wall.[82] The haustra are separated by the plicae semilunares or crescentic folds of the bowel wall, which give the colon its characteristic radiographic appearance when filled with air or barium. The appendices epiploicae are small appendages of fat that protrude from the serosal aspect of the colon (Figure 1-2).

Cecum

The cecum is the segment of the large bowel that projects downward as a blind pouch (Latin *caecus,* "blind") below the entrance of the ileum. It is a sacculated organ of 6 to 8 cm in both length and breadth, usually situated in the right iliac fossa. The cecum is almost entirely, or at least in its lower half, invested with peritoneum. How-

ever, its mobility is usually limited by a small mesocecum. In approximately 5% of individuals, the peritoneal covering is absent posteriorly; it then rests directly on the iliacus and psoas major muscles.[41] Alternatively, an abnormally mobile cecum-ascending colon, resulting from an anomaly of fixation, can be found in 10% to 22% of individuals.[98] In this case, a long mesentery is present, and the cecum may assume varied positions. This lack of fixation may predispose to the development of volvulus (see Chapter 28).

The ileum terminates in the posteromedial aspect of the cecum; the angulation between these two structures is maintained by the superior and inferior ileocecal ligaments. These ligaments, along with the mesentery of the appendix, form three pericecal recesses or fossae: superior ileocecal, inferior ileocecal, and retrocecal (Figure 1-3). Viewed from the cecal lumen, the ileocecal junction is represented by a narrow, transversely situated, slitlike opening known as the ileocecal valve or the valve de Bauhin. At either end, the two prominent semilunar lips of the valve fuse and continue as a single frenulum of mucosa. A circular sphincter, the ileocecal sphincter, originates from a slight thickening of the muscular layer of the terminal ileum. A competent ileocecal valve is related to the critical closed-loop type of colonic obstruction. However, ileocecal competence is not always demonstrated on barium enema studies. Instead of preventing

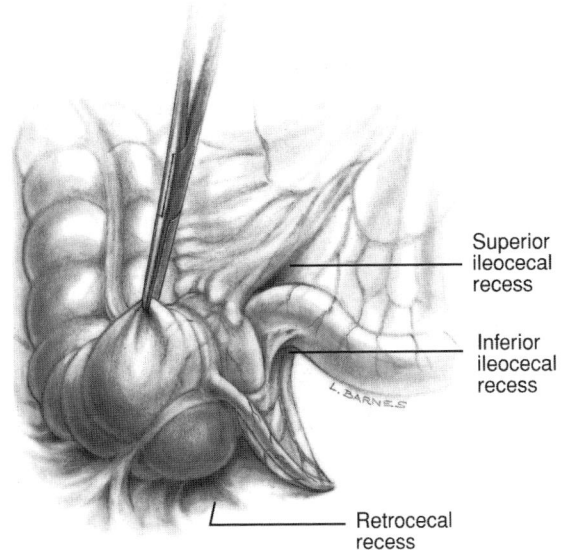

FIGURE 1-3. Ileocecal region. The superior ileorectal, inferior ileocecal, and rectocecal recesses are shown.

reflux of colonic contents into the ileum, the ileocecal valve regulates ileal emptying. The ileocecal sphincter seems to relax in response to the entrance of food into the stomach.[47]

As in the gastroesophageal junction, extrasphincteric factors apparently play a role in the prevention of reflux from the colon to the ileum. The ileocecal angulation has been emphasized by Kumar and Phillips.[60] They filled the ascending colon with saline solution in a retrograde fashion and found that the ileocecal junction was competent to pressures up to 80 mm Hg in 12 of 14 human autopsy specimens. In this group, removal of mucosa at the ileocecal junction or a strip of circular muscle did not impair competence to pressures above 40 mm Hg, but division of the superior and inferior ileocecal ligaments rendered the junction incompetent in all specimens. Furthermore, surgical reconstruction of the ileocecal angle restored competence in four of them.

Appendix

The vermiform appendix is an elongated diverticulum that arises from the posteromedial aspect of the cecum about 3 cm below the ileocecal junction. Its length varies from 2 to 20 cm (mean, 8 to 10 cm), and it is approximately 5 mm in diameter. The confluence of the three taeniae is a useful guide in locating the base of the appendix. The appendix, because of its great mobility, may occupy a variety of positions, possibly at different times in the same individual: retrocecal (65%), pelvic (31%), subcecal (2.3%), preileal (1.0%), and retroileal (0.4%) (Figure 1-4).[116] Some authors have found, however, that in 85% to 95% it lies posteromedial on the cecum toward

the ileum.[106] The mesoappendix, a triangular fold attached to the posterior leaf of the mesentery of the terminal ileum, usually contains the appendicular vessels close to its free edge.

Ascending Colon

The ascending colon, extending from the level of the ileocecal junction to the right colic or hepatic flexure, is approximately 15 cm long. It ascends laterally to the psoas muscle and anteriorly to the iliacus, the quadratus lumborum, and the lower pole of the right kidney. The ascending colon is covered with peritoneum anteriorly and on both sides. In addition, fragile adhesions between the right abdominal wall and its anterior aspect, known as Jackson's membrane, may be present.[85] Like the descending colon on its posterior surface, the ascending colon is devoid of peritoneum, which is instead replaced by an areolar tissue (fascia of Toldt) resulting from an embryologic process of fusion or coalescence of the mesentery to the posterior parietal peritoneum.[106] In the lateral peritoneal reflection, this process is represented by the white line of Toldt, which is more evident at the descending-sigmoid junction. This line serves as a guide for the surgeon when the ascending, descending, or sigmoid colon is mobilized.

At the visceral surface of the right lobe of the liver and lateral to the gallbladder, the ascending colon turns

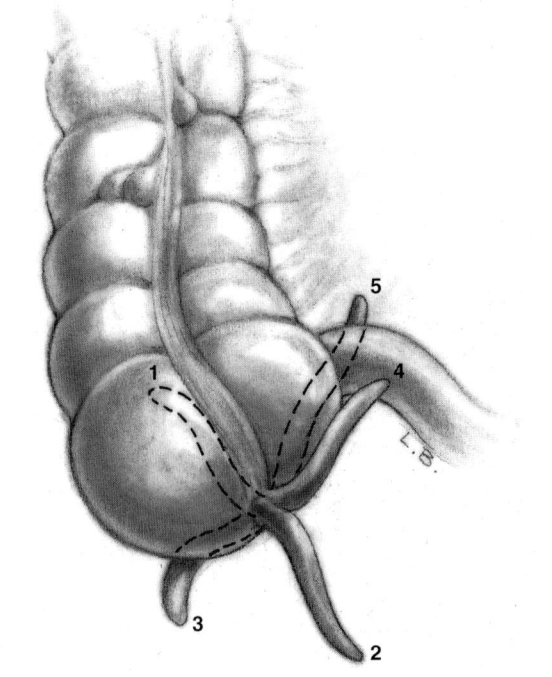

FIGURE 1-4. Vermiform appendix. The five most common variations in its position are shown in order of frequency.

sharply medially and slightly caudad and ventrally to form the right colic (hepatic) flexure (see Figure 22-36). This flexure is supported by the nephrocolic ligament and lies immediately ventral to the lower part of the right kidney and over the descending duodenum.

Relationship to Ureters

In resections of the right and left colon, identification of the ureters is usually necessary to avoid injury to their abdominal or pelvic portions.[73] On both sides, the ureters rest on the psoas muscle in their inferomedial course; they are crossed obliquely by the spermatic vessels anteriorly and the genitofemoral nerve posteriorly. The right ureter lies lateral to the inferior vena cava and is crossed anteriorly by the right colic and ileocolic arteries, the root of the mesentery, and the terminal ileum. In its pelvic portion, the ureter crosses the pelvic brim in front of or a little lateral to the bifurcation of the common iliac artery, and it descends abruptly between the peritoneum and the internal iliac artery. Before entering the bladder in the male, the vas deferens crosses lateromedially on its superior aspect. In the female, as the ureter traverses the posterior layer of the broad ligament and the parametrium close to the side of the neck of the uterus and upper part of the vagina, it is enveloped by the vesical and vaginal venous plexuses and is crossed above and lateromedially by the uterine artery.

Transverse Colon

The transverse colon is the longest segment of the large bowel (45 cm long). It crosses the abdomen, usually with an inferior curve immediately caudad to the greater curvature of the stomach. The transverse colon is relatively fixed at each flexure. In between, it is completely invested with peritoneum and suspended by a transverse mesocolon having an average width of 10 to 15 cm and providing variable mobility; the nadir of the transverse colon may reach the hypogastrium. The greater omentum is fused on the anterosuperior aspect of the transverse colon. Therefore, an intercoloepiploic dissection is necessary to mobilize this portion of the colon or to enter the lesser sac of the peritoneum. The left colic (splenic) flexure is situated beneath the lower angle of the spleen and firmly attached to the diaphragm by the phrenocolic ligament, which also forms a shelf to support the spleen (see Figure 22-47). Because of the risk for hemorrhage, mobilization of the splenic flexure should be approached with great care, preceded by dissection upward along the descending colon and medially to laterally along the transverse colon toward the splenic flexure (see Chapter 22). This flexure, when compared with the hepatic flexure, is more acute, higher, and more deeply situated.

Descending Colon

This segment of the large intestine courses downward from the splenic flexure to the brim of the true pelvis, a distance of approximately 25 cm. The segment of descending colon between the iliac crest and the brim of the true pelvis is also known as the iliac colon.[41] Like the ascending colon, the descending colon is covered by peritoneum only on its anterior and lateral aspects. Posteriorly, it rests directly against the left kidney and the quadratus lumborum and transversus abdominis muscles. However, the descending colon is narrower and more dorsally situated than the ascending colon.

Sigmoid Colon

The sigmoid colon, extending from the lower end of the descending colon at the pelvic brim to the proximal limit of the rectum, varies dramatically in length (15 to 50 cm; mean, 38 cm) and configuration. More commonly, the sigmoid colon is a mobile, ω-shaped loop completely invested by peritoneum. The mesosigmoid is attached to the pelvic walls in an inverted-V shape, resting in a recess known as the intersigmoid fossa. The left ureter lies immediately underneath this fossa and is crossed on its anterior surface by the spermatic, left colic, and sigmoid vessels.

Rectosigmoid Junction

Both the anatomy and function of the rectosigmoid junction have been matters of substantial controversy. O'Beirne postulated that because the rectum is usually emptied and contracted, the sigmoid plays a role in continence as the fecal reservoir.[87] Subsequently, a thickening of the circular muscular layer between the rectum and sigmoid was described and diversely termed the sphincter ani tertius,[53] rectosigmoid sphincter,[72] and pylorus sigmoidorectalis,[16] and it has probably been mistaken for one of the transverse folds of the rectum.[52,90] Balli considered the rectosigmoid junction to be one of the functional sphincters of the colon.[5] The rectosigmoid junction has been considered, at least externally, an indistinct zone, a region that to some surgeons comprises the last 5 to 8 cm of sigmoid and the uppermost 5 cm of the rectum.[31,41] However, surgeons as well as anatomists have divergent opinions. Others have considered it a clearly defined segment, because it is the narrowest portion of the large intestine; in fact, it is usually characterized endoscopically as a narrow and sharply angulated segment.[14,105] Stoss, in a study of 39 human cadavers, found the rectosigmoid junction situated 6 to 7 cm below the sacral promontory.[110] Macroscopically, it has been identified as the point where the taenia libera and the taenia omentalis fuse to form a single anterior taenia and where both haustra and mesocolon terminate. With microdissection, this segment is characterized by conspicuous strands of longitudinal muscle fibers that are more prominent than in the sigmoid and less so than in the rectum. Additionally, curved interconnecting fibers between the longitudinal and circular muscle layers have been noted, resulting in a delicate syncytium of smooth muscle that allows synergistic interplay between the two layers. Stoss concluded, based on the anatomic definition of a sphincter as "a band of thickened circular muscle that closes the lumen by contraction and of a longitudinal muscle that dilates it," that the rectosigmoid cannot be considered as such.[66,110] Still, this segment

may be regarded as a functional sphincter because mechanisms of active dilation and passive "kinking" occlusion do exist.[108]

Rectum

The rectum is believed to be 12 to 15 cm in length, but both the proximal and distal limits are debatable (Figure 1-5).[127] For example, the rectosigmoid junction is considered to be at the level of the third sacral vertebra by anatomists but at the sacral promontory by surgeons. Likewise, the distal limit is regarded to be the muscular anorectal ring by surgeons and the dentate

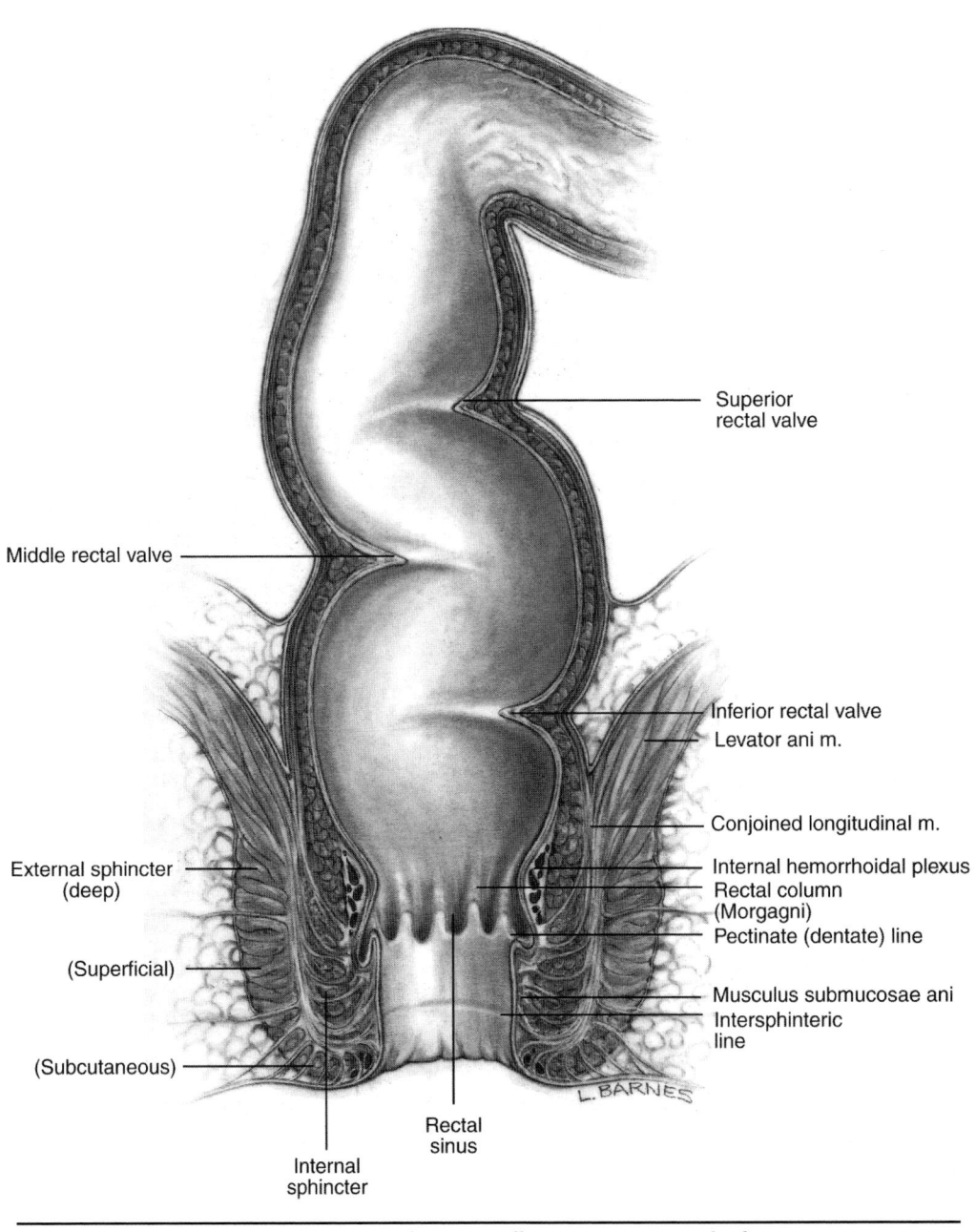

FIGURE 1-5. Anorectal anatomy illustrating curves and valves.

line by anatomists. The rectum occupies the sacral concavity and ends 2 to 3 cm anteroinferiorly from the tip of the coccyx. At this point, it angulates backward sharply to pass through the levators and becomes the anal canal. Posterior to the rectum lie the median sacral vessels and the roots of the sacral nerve plexus. Anteriorly, in women, the rectum is closely related to the uterine cervix and posterior vaginal wall; in men, it lies behind the bladder, vas deferens, seminal vesicles, and prostate.

The nonmobilized rectum has three lateral curves: the upper and lower are convex to the right, and the middle is convex to the left (Figure 1-5). These curves correspond intraluminally to the folds or valves of Houston.[2,52] The two left-sided folds are usually noted at 7 to 8 cm and at 12 to 13 cm, respectively, and the one on the right is generally at 9 to 11 cm. The middle valve is the most consistent in presence and location (also known as Kohlrausch's plica) and corresponds to the level of the anterior peritoneal reflection. The rectal valves do not contain all the muscle wall layers and do not have a specific function. However, from a clinical point of view, they are an excellent location for performing a rectal biopsy, as they are readily accessible with minimal risk for perforation.[85] The valves of Houston must be negotiated during proctosigmoidoscopy. However, they are not present after mobilization of the rectum; this is attributed to the 5-cm length gained following complete surgical dissection.

The rectum is characterized by the absence of taeniae, epiploic appendices, haustra, or a well-defined mesentery. The prefix "meso," in gross anatomy, refers to two layers of peritoneum that suspend an organ. Normally, the rectum is not suspended but entirely extraperitoneal on its posterior aspect and close to the sacral hollow. Consequently, the term mesorectum is anatomically inappropriate.[18,80] An exception, however, is that a peritonealized mesorectum may be noted in patients with procidentia. Nonetheless, the term mesorectum has gained widespread popularity among surgeons to address the perirectal areolar tissue, which is thicker posteriorly, containing terminal branches of the inferior mesenteric artery and enclosed by the fascia propria (Figure 1-6).[17,51,58] The mesorectum may be a metastatic site for rectal cancer and is removed during surgery for rectal cancer (see Chapter 23). Its removal is undertaken without clinical sequelae because no functionally

significant nerves pass through it.[51] The upper third of the rectum is anteriorly and laterally invested by peritoneum; the middle third is covered by peritoneum on its anterior aspect only. Finally, the lower third of the rectum is entirely extraperitoneal because the anterior peritoneal reflection occurs at 9.0 to 7.0 cm from the anal verge in men and at 7.5 to 5.0 cm from the anal verge in women.

The rectum has a wide, easily distensible lumen. The rectal mucosa is smooth, pink, and transparent, which allows visualization of small and large submucosal vessels. This characteristic vascular pattern disappears in inflammatory conditions and in melanosis coli.

Fascial Relationship of the Rectum

The walls and floor of the pelvis are lined by the parietal *endopelvic fascia*, which continues on the internal organs as a visceral pelvic fascia. The fascia propria of the rectum is therefore an extension of the pelvic fascia, enclosing the rectum, fat, nerves, and the blood and lymphatic vessels. It is present mainly in the lateral and posterior extraperitoneal portion of the rectum. Distal condensations of this fascia form the lateral ligaments or lateral stalks of the rectum. These are described by Goligher as a roughly triangular structure with a base on the lateral pelvic wall and an apex attached to the lateral aspect of the rectum[41]. As pointed out by Church and colleagues, these ligaments have been the subject of anatomic confusion and misconception.[20] One such misconception is that they are composed essentially of connective tissue and nerves, and that the middle rectal artery does not traverse the lateral stalks of the rectum. Minor branches, however, course through in approximately 25% of cases.[13,126] Consequently, division of the lateral stalks during rectal mobilization is associated with a 25% risk for bleeding. Although the lateral stalks do not contain important structures, the middle rectal artery and the pelvic plexus are both closely related, coursing at different angles beneath them in various patients.[84] One theoretical concern in ligation of the stalks is leaving behind lateral mesorectal tissue, which may limit adequate lateral or mesorectal margins during cancer surgery (Figure 1-7).[17,51,97]

The *presacral fascia* is a thickened part of the parietal endopelvic fascia that covers the concavity of the sacrum and coccyx, nerves, the middle sacral artery, and pre-

---

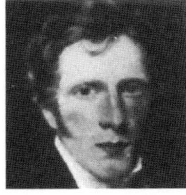
John Houston (1802–1845) Born in the north of Ireland, Houston was adopted by a physician uncle. He attached himself to one of the first native Dublin anatomists and became a curator of the museum of the Royal College of Surgeons in Ireland in 1824. In 1826, he received his medical degree from Edinburgh University. On the establishment of the City of Dublin Hospital in 1832, Houston became one of its surgeons. He was regarded as an acute observer of disease and an excellent clinical surgeon. In 1830, he published the report in which he described the valves that bear his name. He died while lecturing, presumably of complications of an intracranial hemorrhage. (Houston J. Observations of the mucous membrane of the rectum. *Dublin Hosp Rep Communications Med Surg* 1830;5:158.)

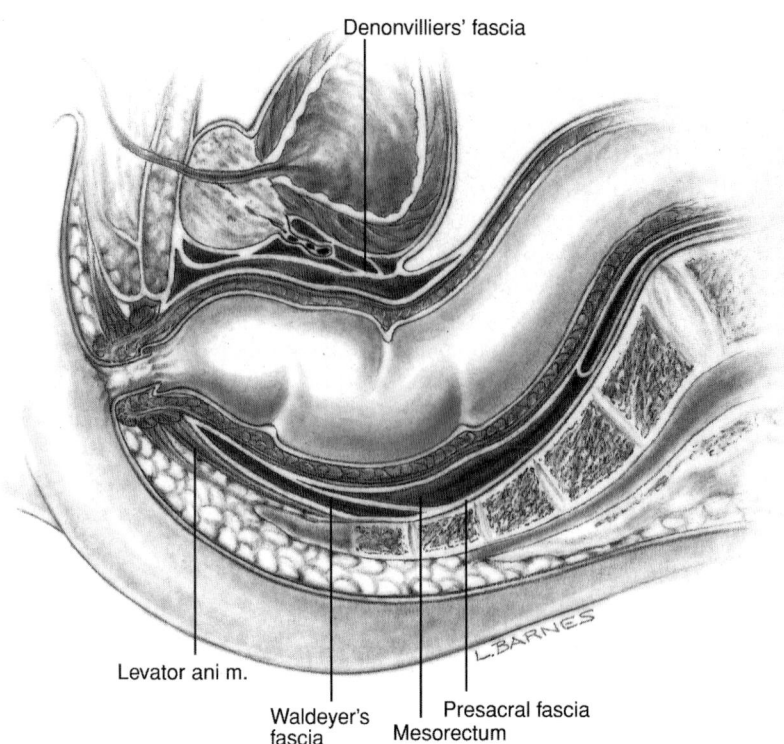

FIGURE 1-6. Lateral view of the male rectum illustrating the mesorectum and its relationship with other pelvic structures.

sacral veins (Figure 1-8). Operative dissection deep to the presacral fascia may cause troublesome bleeding from the underlying presacral veins. The incidence of such hemorrhage has been cited to be as high as 4.6% to 7.0% of resections for rectal neoplasms.[56,118,128] These veins are avalvular and communicate via the basivertebral veins with the internal vertebral venous system (Figure 1-8).

With the patient in the lithotomy position, this system can attain hydrostatic pressures of 17 to 23 cm H_2O, two to three times the normal pressure of the inferior vena cava.[118] The adventitia of the basivertebral veins adheres firmly to the sacral periosteum at the level of the ostia of the sacral foramina (mainly at the level of S3–4).[118] Despite its venous nature, presacral hemorrhage can be

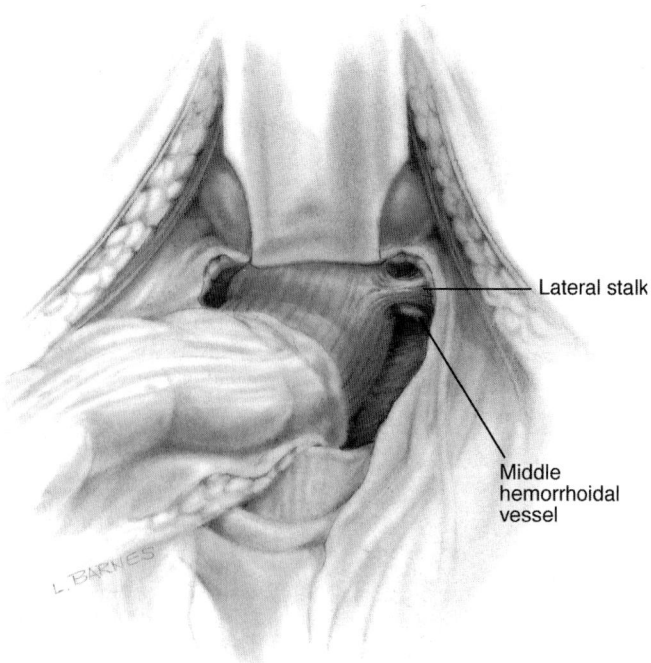

FIGURE 1-7. The right lateral stalk with associated middle hemorrhoidal artery is seen.

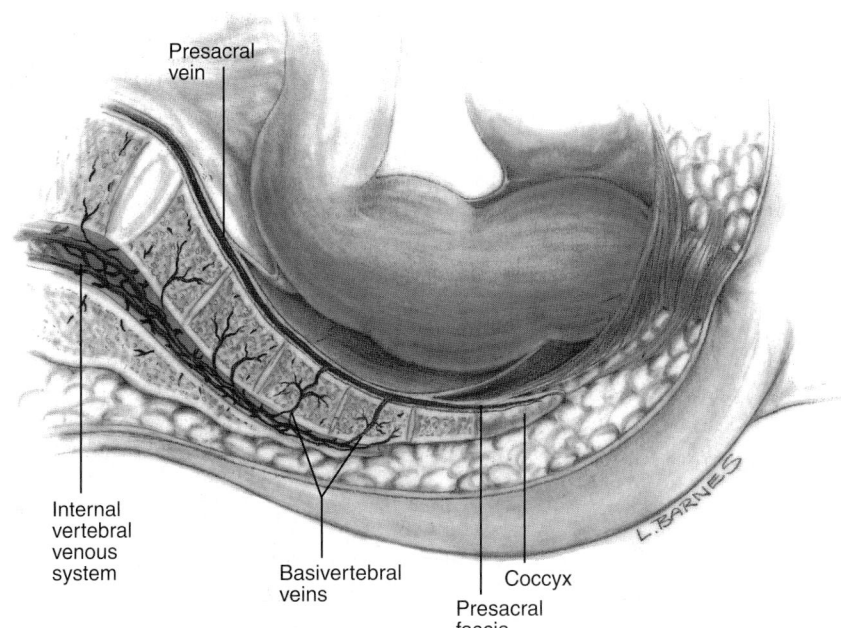

Presacral
vein

Internal
vertebral
venous
system

Basivertebral
veins

Coccyx

Presacral
fascia

FIGURE 1-8. Sagittal section of the pelvis showing the fascial relationships of the rectum and the presacral and vertebral venous system.

life-threatening. This is a consequence of the high hydrostatic pressure and the difficulty in securing control because of retraction of the vascular stump into the sacral foramen.

The *rectosacral fascia* is an anteroinferiorly directed thick fascial reflection from the presacral fascia at the S-4 level to the fascia propria of the rectum just above the anorectal ring.[23] The rectosacral fascia, an important landmark during posterior rectal dissection, is classically known as the fascia of Waldeyer, but this is a misnomer because Wilhelm Waldeyer first described all of the pelvic fascia, not particularly emphasizing the rectosacral fascia.[20,23] Anteriorly, the extraperitoneal rectum is separated from the prostate and seminal vesicles or vagina by a tough fascial investment, the visceral pelvic fascia of Denonvilliers.[114] Therefore, three structures lie between the anterior rectal wall and the seminal vesicles and prostate: the anterior mesorectum, the fascia propria of the rectum,

and Denonvilliers' fascia (Fig.1-6). A general consensus has been reached regarding the anatomic plane of posterior and lateral rectal dissection. However, anteriorly the matter is more controversial. The anterior plane of rectal dissection may not necessarily follow the same plane as that of posterior and lateral dissection. Therefore, the use of the terms close rectal, mesorectal, and extramesorectal have been suggested to describe the anterior planes.[68] The close rectal plane, also known as the perimuscular plane, lies immediately on the rectal musculature, inside the fascia propria of the rectum. However, it is more difficult to navigate and bloodier than the mesorectal plane and consequently is not considered a true anatomic plane. The mesorectal plane represents the continuation of the same plane of posterior and lateral dissection of the rectum. It is the appropriate anterior plane for most rectal cancers, a natural anatomic plane that is familiar to colorectal surgeons. Finally, the extramesorectal plane involves resec-

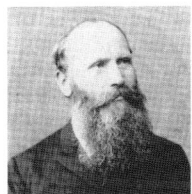
Heinrich Wilhelm Gottfried von Waldeyer-Hartz (1836–1921) Waldeyer was born on October 6, 1836 in Helen an der Weser, Germany, the son of an estate manager and a school teacher. He received his early education at Paderborn. In 1856, he entered the University of Göttingen to study mathematics and natural sciences. However, through his acquaintance with the anatomist Friedrich Henle, whose lectures he attended, he began the study of medicine. Waldeyer attended the University of Göttingen from 1856 to 1859. As a Prussian, he could not complete his studies, and he transferred to Greifswald, where he became an assistant in the Anatomical Institute. He then moved on to Berlin to pursue his great interest in anatomy, obtaining his doctorate in 1861. There followed a series of appointments to the University of Königsberg and the University of Breslau. In 1868, at the age of 32, he was appointed to the Chair of Pathology at Breslau. His work at this time was chiefly concentrated on the diagnosis of early cancer. In 1887, he was one of the German doctors called upon to diagnose Emperor Frederick III's vocal cord tumor. In 1872, Waldeyer went to the University of Strasbourg as Chair of Anatomy. He remained there for 11 years, returning in 1883 to Berlin, where he eventually taught anatomy to more than 20,000 students. He published numerous papers on a wide variety of anatomic subjects, including studies of the urogenital system, anthropology, and topographical observations of the pelvis (Waldeyer's fascia). Today, Wilhelm von Waldeyer-Hartz is remembered as the founder of the neurone theory, coining the term "neurone" to describe the cellular unit of the nervous system (1891). He also coined the term "chromosome" (1888) to describe the bodies in the nucleus of cells. Waldeyer remained at the University of Berlin until he was 80 years old. He died in Berlin on January 23, 1921. (With appreciation to Faisal Aziz, M.D. Figure courtesy of the National Library of Medicine.)

tion of Denonvilliers' fascia, with exposure of the prostate and seminal vesicles. This plane is associated with a high risk of both parasympathetic and sympathetic injury to the periprostatic plexus. In addition, dissection in this plane generally predisposes to an increased risk of intraoperative hemorrhage.

Anal Canal

Although representing a relatively small segment of the digestive tract, the anal canal is anatomically unique, with a complex physiology that accounts for both its vital role in continence and its susceptibility to a variety of diseases. In the literature, two definitions are found to describe the anal canal. The "surgical" or "functional" anal canal extends for approximately 4 cm from the anal verge to the anorectal ring. This definition correlates with both digital and sonographic assessment, but it does not correspond to either the embryologic or histologic architecture of the anal canal. The "anatomic" or "embryologic" anal canal is shorter (2 cm), extending from the anal verge to the dentate line. The latter is the level that corresponds to the procotodeal membrane (see Figure 8-2).[86,127]

The anus or anal orifice is an anteroposterior cutaneous slit that, along with the anal canal, remains virtually closed at rest. This is the result of tonic circumferential contraction of both the sphincters and the anal cushions. Posteriorly, the anal canal is related to the coccyx, and anteriorly to the urethra (in the male) and to the perineal body and the lowest part of the posterior vaginal wall (in the female). Laterally, the ischiorectal fossa is situated on either side. The fossa contains fat and the inferior rectal vessels and nerves, which cross it to enter the wall of the anal canal.

Epithelium

The lining of the anal canal consists of an upper mucosal and a lower cutaneous segment. The dentate (pectinate) line describes the "saw-toothed" junction of the ectoderm and the endoderm. It therefore represents an important landmark between two distinct origins of venous and lymphatic drainage, nerve supply, and epithelial lining.[125] Above the dentate line, the intestine is innervated by the sympathetic and parasympathetic systems, with venous, arterial, and lymphatic drainage to and from the hypogastric vessels. Distal to the dentate line, the anal canal is innervated by the somatic nervous system, with blood supply and drainage from the inferior hemorrhoidal system. These differences are important when the classification and treatment of hemorrhoids are considered.

The pectinate or dentate line corresponds to a line of anal valves that represent remnants of the proctodeal membrane. Above each valve, there is a little pocket known as an anal sinus or crypt. These crypts are connected to a variable number of glands, with an average of six (range, three to 12 crypts per patient [see Figs. 24-1 and 24-2]).[43,67] The anal glands are more concentrated in the posterior quadrants. More than one gland may open into the same crypt, whereas half the crypts have no communication. The anal gland ducts enter the submucosa in an outward and downward route; two thirds enter the IAS, and half of them terminate in the intersphincteric plane (see Figs. 24-3 and 10-1).[67] The anal glands were first described by Chiari in 1878, but it was not until 1961 that Parks addressed their role in the pathogenesis of fistulous abscess[19,92] (see Chapters 10 and 11). Obstruction of these ducts, presumably by accumulation of foreign material in the crypts, may lead to abscesses and fistula.[92]

Cephalad to the dentate line, eight to 14 longitudinal folds, known as the rectal columns (columns of Morgagni), have their bases connected in pairs to each valve at the dentate line (see Figure 8-2). At the lower end of the columns are the anal papillae. The mucosa in the area of the columns consists of several layers of cuboidal cells. The lining exhibits a deep purple color because of the underlying internal hemorrhoidal plexus. The 0.5- to 1.0-cm strip of mucosa above the dentate line is known as the anal transitional or cloacogenic zone and represents the site and source of certain anal tumors (see Chapter 24). Cephalad to this area, the epithelium changes to a single

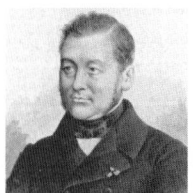

Charles Pierre Denonvilliers (1808–1872)   Son of a landlord, Denonvilliers was born in Paris on February 4, 1808. He studied medicine at the Paris Faculty, from which he graduated in 1835. His first post was that of surgeon to the Bureau Central (1840). In 1842, he became Chief of the School of Practical Anatomy of the Hôtel-Dieu, and in 1856 he achieved the position as Professor of Surgery at the same institution. Denonvilliers' interests resided more in anatomy than in surgery. Through the years, he made numerous and varied contributions to the field, including a description of the fascia for which he achieved eponymous immortality. In 1836, Denonvilliers reported to the Société Anatomique concerning an "aponeurosis" as follows: "Behind the prostate and between the seminal vesicles and the rectum, there is a distinct membranous layer, which I call prostatoperitoneal." In 1858, Denonvilliers was awarded the important position of Inspector-General of Public Instruction for Medicine. Through this role, he has been credited with modernizing the French medical curriculum by the development of new concepts in the teaching of physiology, pathology, and surgery. His extensive work in the field of descriptive and surgical anatomy led to the publication of numerous articles and textbooks as well as to the elaboration of innovative surgical techniques, particularly in the field of reconstructive plastic surgery. His professional activity ceased in 1864 with the death of his prematurely born son, a tragedy from which he never fully recovered. Thought to be a great loss to the field of medical science by his contemporaries, Denonvilliers died of a stroke on July 5, 1872. (With appreciation to Keith P. Meslin, M.D.)

layer of columnar cells, macroscopically acquiring the characteristic pink color of the rectal mucosa.

The cutaneous part of the anal canal consists of modified squamous epithelium—thin, smooth, pale, stretched, and devoid of hair and glands. The terms *pecten* and *pecten band* have been used to define this segment.[1] However, as pointed out by Goligher, the round band of fibrous tissue called pecten band, which is divided in the case of anal fissure (pectenotomy), probably represents a spastic IAS.[41,42] The anal verge (anocutaneous line of Hilton; see biography, Chapter 9) marks the lowermost edge of the anal canal and is sometimes the level of reference for measurements taken during colonoscopy or surgery.[30,32] Others favor the dentate line as a landmark because it is more precise.[14] The difference between the two can be as great as 1 to 2 cm. Distal to the anal verge, the lining becomes thicker and pigmented and is arranged in radiating folds around the anus. The epithelium then acquires hair follicles, glands (including apocrine glands), and other features of normal skin. For this reason, perianal hidradenitis suppurativa, inflammation of the apocrine glands, may be excised with preservation of the anal canal (see Chapter 19).

Anal Canal and Pelvic Floor Musculature

The muscles within the pelvis can be divided into three categories: the anal sphincter complex; the pelvic floor muscles, and the muscles that line the sidewalls of the osseous pelvis.[58] This last category forms the external boundary of the pelvis and includes the obturator internus and piriform muscles. These muscles, compared with the other two groups, lack clinical relevance to anorectal diseases; however, they do provide open communication to allow pelvic infection to reach extrapelvic spaces. For example, infection from the deep postanal space originating from the posterior midline glands can track along the obturator internus fascia and reach the ischiorectal fossa.

The anal sphincter and pelvic floor muscles, based on phylogenetic studies, are derived from two embryonic cloaca groups, sphincter and lateral compressor, respectively.[120] The sphincteric group is present in almost all animals. In mammals, this group is divided into ventral (urogenital) and dorsal (anal) components.[91] In primates, the latter forms the EAS. The lateral compressor or pelvicaudal group connects the rudimentary pelvis to the caudal end of the vertebral column. This group is more differentiated and subdivided into lateral and medial compartments only in reptiles and mammals. The homologue of the lateral compartment is the ischiococcygeus, and of the medial pelvicaudal compartment, the pubococcygeus and ileococcygeus. In addition, most primates possess a variably sized group of muscle fibers close to the inner border of the medial pelvicaudal muscle, which attaches the rectum to the pubis. In humans, the fibers are more distinct and are known as the puborectalis muscle.

Internal Anal Sphincter

The IAS represents the distal (2.5 to 4.0 cm) condensation of the circular muscle layer of the rectum (see Figure 8-2). As a smooth muscle in a state of continuous maxi-

---

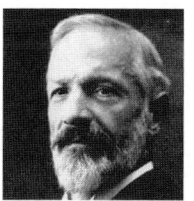

Hans Chiari (1851–1916) Hans Chiari was born in Vienna on September 4, 1851, ultimately studying medicine in that city. From 1874–1875, he served as assistant to the famous pathologist, Karl Freiherr von Rokitansky (1804–1878). His other influential mentor was Richard Ladislaus Heschl (1824–1881), for whom he served as assistant from 1876 until 1879. Chiari was appointed that year professor in pathologic anatomy at the German University of Prague and the following year became superintendent of the pathologic-anatomic museum. In 1906, he was appointed director of pathologic anatomy in Strassbourg, where he remained until his death in 1916. During the years 1876 to 1916, Chiari published more than 175 papers. The majority of his work concerned systematic postmortem examinations. He was in constant search of new and interesting material, because of his academic interests but also for the museum. Out of his many investigations, his work on glands, neural deformities, large vessels, and the heart are considered of special importance. He first described the concept of autodigestion of the pancreas gland. In 1891, he reported the first case of herniation of the cerebellar hemispheres and the medulla oblongata into the spinal canal, now named Arnold-Chiari syndrome. He described additional cases and identified the distinction between deformities of the brainstem and the cerebellum. In 1898, he reported on liver infarction due to thrombosis of the hepatic veins, a condition now known by the eponym Budd-Chiari syndrome. Other work concerned atherosclerotic lesions of the carotid arteries wherein he suggested an association with cerebral emboli. (With appreciation to Udo Rudloff, M.D.)

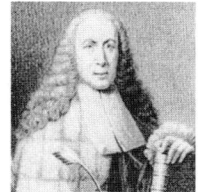

Giovanni Battista Morgagni (1682–1771) Giovanni Battista Morgagni was born in Bologna, Italy and studied medicine at the University of Bologna, graduating with degrees in philosophy and medicine at the age of 19. In 1706, he succeeded Valsalva in his position as anatomic demonstrator, and in 1715 he was appointed to the first chair of anatomy at the university of Padua, a tenure that he held with distinction for the rest of his life. His work, *Adversaria Anatomica* (1706–1719), is a series of researches into anatomy, an effort that secured his reputation. Morgagni's studies produced new information about the larynx, trachea, and glottal regions, the male urethra, and the female genitalia. He also described the fine vertical folds in the mucous membrane of the upper half of the rectum, still known as the columns of Morgagni. His most important work, *Seats and Causes of Disease Investigated by Means of Anatomy*, was published in 1761. In this work, one of the most fundamentally important works in the history of medicine, he reports in precise detail his findings in 640 autopsy dissections. He was the first to describe cerebral gumma, diseases of heart valves, heart block, Fallot's tetralogy, aortic coarctation, and pneumonia with consolidation. The Royal Society of England elected him a fellow in 1724, the Academy of Sciences of Paris made him a member in 1731, the Imperial Academy of St. Petersburg in 1735, and the Academy of Berlin in 1754. (Courtesy of University of Virginia Health Sciences Library and with appreciation to Yossef Yonatan Nasseri, M.D.)

mal contraction, the IAS is a natural barrier to the involuntary loss of stool and gas.[94] This is a consequence of both intrinsic myogenic and extrinsic autonomic neurogenic properties. The IAS is responsible for 50% to 85% of the resting tone, the EAS accounts for 25% to 30%, and the remaining 15% is attributed to expansion of the anal cushions.[36,40,64]

The lower, rounded edge of the IAS can be felt on physical examination, about 1.2 cm distal to the dentate line. The groove between it and the EAS, the intersphincteric sulcus, can be visualized or easily palpated. The different echogenic patterns of the anal sphincters facilitate their visualization during endosonography (see Fig. 6-22). The IAS is a 2- to 3-mm-thick circular band exhibiting a uniform hypoechogenicity. The puborectalis and the EAS, despite their mixed linear echogenicity, are both predominantly hyperechogenic, with a mean thickness of 6 mm (range, 5 to 8 mm). Distinction is made by position, shape, and topography.[24,113] Both anal endosonography and endocoil magnetic resonance imaging have been used to detail the anal sphincter complex in living healthy subjects (Figure 1-9).[12,37,81,124] These tests provide a three-dimensional mapping of the anal sphincter; furthermore, they help to identify gender differences in the anatomic arrangement of the EAS as well as to uncover any sphincter disruption or defect during vaginal deliveries.

Conjoined Longitudinal Muscle

Whereas the inner circular layer of the rectum gives rise to the IAS, the outer longitudinal layer, at the level of the anorectal ring, mixes with fibers of the levator ani muscle to form the conjoined longitudinal muscle (CLM [see Figure 8-2]). This muscle descends between the IAS and the EAS, and ultimately some of its fibers (referred to as the corrugator cutis ani muscle) traverse the lowermost part of the EAS to insert into the perianal skin.

Lunniss and Phillips, in a comprehensive review of the CLM, explored the controversy and speculation of both the anatomy and physiology of this muscle.[71] Other sources for the striated component of the CLM include the puborectalis and deep EAS,[78] the pubococcygeus and top loop of the EAS,[103] and the lower fibers of the puborectalis.[62] In its descending course, the CLM may give rise to medial extensions that cross the IAS to contribute the smooth muscle of the submucosa (musculus canalis ani, sustentator tunicae mucosae, Treitz muscle, musculus submucosae ani).[99] Others describe outward filamentous extensions of the CLM crossing the whole length of the EAS to enter the fat of the ischiorectal fossa.[22] Possible functions of the CLM include attaching the anorectum to the pelvis and acting as a skeleton that supports and binds the IAS and EAS complex together.[22] Shafik consid-

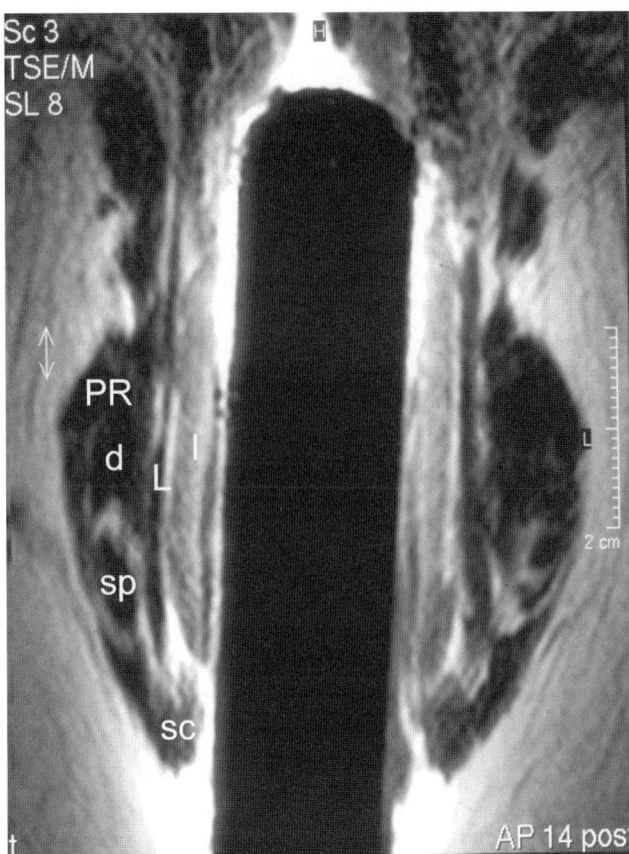

FIGURE 1-9. An endocoil magnetic resonance image of the anal canal in the coronal plane view. *I*, internal anal sphincter (moderate signal); *L*, longitudinal muscle (low signal); *PR*, puborectalis, with *d*, deep part of the external sphincter; *sp*, superficial part; and *sc*, subcutaneous part. All the striated muscle is of low signal. The high signal on either side of the longitudinal muscle indicates a thin layer of fat. (Courtesy of Professor Clive Bartram, Clinical Director of St. Mark's Hospital, Northwick Park, United Kingdom.)

ers only a minimal role for the CLM in the maintenance of continence, and that is specifically to potentiate the action of the base loop in maintaining an anal seal.[103] He ascribes its primary responsibility during defecation as causing shortening and widening of the anal canal as well as eversion of the anal orifice. Shafik has proposed the term, "evertor ani muscle," for the CLM. Haas and Fox consider that the meshwork formed by the CLM may minimize functional deterioration of the sphincters after surgical division and act as a support to prevent hemorrhoidal and rectal prolapse.[48] Finally, the CLM and its extensions to the intersphincteric plane divide the adjacent tissues into subspaces and may actually play a role in the containment of sepsis.[71] They also are responsible for the septation of thrombosed external hemorrhoids. Therefore, cure of such a thrombus requires excision of this septated region rather than simply an incision between fibers of a single clot.

External Anal Sphincter

The EAS is the elliptical cylinder of striated muscle that envelops the entire length of the inner tube of smooth muscle, but it ends slightly more distal to the terminus of the IAS (see Figure 8-2). The EAS was initially described as encompassing three divisions: subcutaneous, superficial, and deep.[78] However, Goligher and colleagues described the EAS as a simple, continuous sheet that forms, along with the puborectalis and levator ani, one funnel-shaped skeletal muscle.[42] The deepest part of the EAS is intimately related with the puborectalis muscle; they opine that the latter is actually considered a component of both the levator ani and the EAS muscle complexes. Others consider the EAS as being composed of a deep compartment (deep sphincter and puborectalis) and a superficial compartment (subcutaneous and superficial sphincter).[38,85] Oh and Kark noted differences in the arrangement of the EAS between the sexes.[88] In the male, the upper half of the EAS is enveloped anteriorly by the CLM, whereas the lower half is crossed by it. In the female, the entire EAS is encapsulated by a mixture of fibers derived from both longitudinal and IAS muscles. Based on embryologic study, the EAS also seems to be subdivided into two parts, superficial and deep, neither having any connection with the puborectalis.[65] Shafik proposed the concept of a three-U–shaped loop system in which each loop is a separate sphincter with distinct attachments, muscle bundle directions, and innervations; each loop complements the others to help maintain continence (Figure 1-10).[101,104] However, clinical experience has not supported Shafik's three-part schema. The EAS is, in fact, more likely to be one muscle unit, attached by the anococcygeal ligament posteriorly to the coccyx and anteriorly to the perineal body, not divided into layers or laminae.[4] However, there is some degree of anatomic asymmetry of the EAS, which accounts for both radial and longitudinal functional asymmetry observed during anal manometry.[55]

The EAS, along with the pelvic floor muscles, unlike other skeletal muscles that are usually inactive at rest, maintains unconscious resting electrical tone through a reflex arc at the cauda equina level. Histologic studies have shown that the EAS, puborectalis, and levator ani muscles have a predominance of type I fibers, which are a peculiarity of skeletal muscles that produce tonic contractile activity.[112] In response to conditions of threatened incontinence, such as increased intraabdominal pressure and rectal distension, the EAS and puborectalis reflexively or voluntarily contract further to prevent fecal leakage. Because of muscular fatigue, maximal voluntary contraction of the EAS can be sustained for only 30 to 60 seconds. The automatic continence mechanism is then formed by the resting tone, maintained by the IAS, and magnified by reflex EAS contraction.[57] Garavoglia and coworkers suggest three types of striated muscular function as the mechanism for continence: lateral compression from the pubococcygeus, circumferential closure from the deep EAS, and angulation from the puborectalis.[38]

Levator Ani

Figure 1-11 illustrates the male perineal muscle at three different levels. The levator ani muscle, or pelvic diaphragm, comprises the major component of the pelvic floor (Figure 1-11C). It is a pair of broad, symmetric sheets composed of three striated muscles: iliococcygeus, pubococcygeus, and puborectalis (Figure 1-12). A variable fourth co mponent, the ischiococcygeus or coccygeus, is rudimentary in humans and represented by only a few muscle fibers on the surface of the

(text continues on page 16)

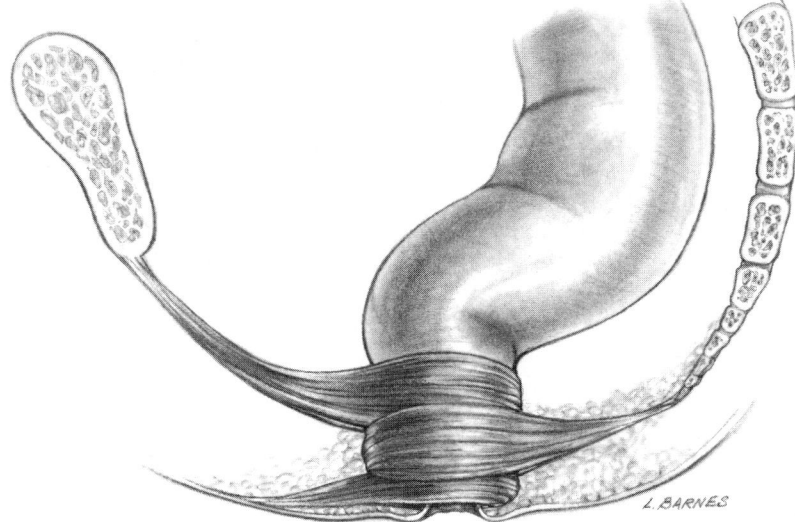

FIGURE 1-10. Triple-loop system of Shafik.[101] The top loop arises and inserts on the pubis and is made up of the deep external sphincter and puborectalis. The middle loop attaches to the coccyx (superficial external sphincter). The lower loop inserts in the anterior perianal skin (subcutaneous external sphincter).

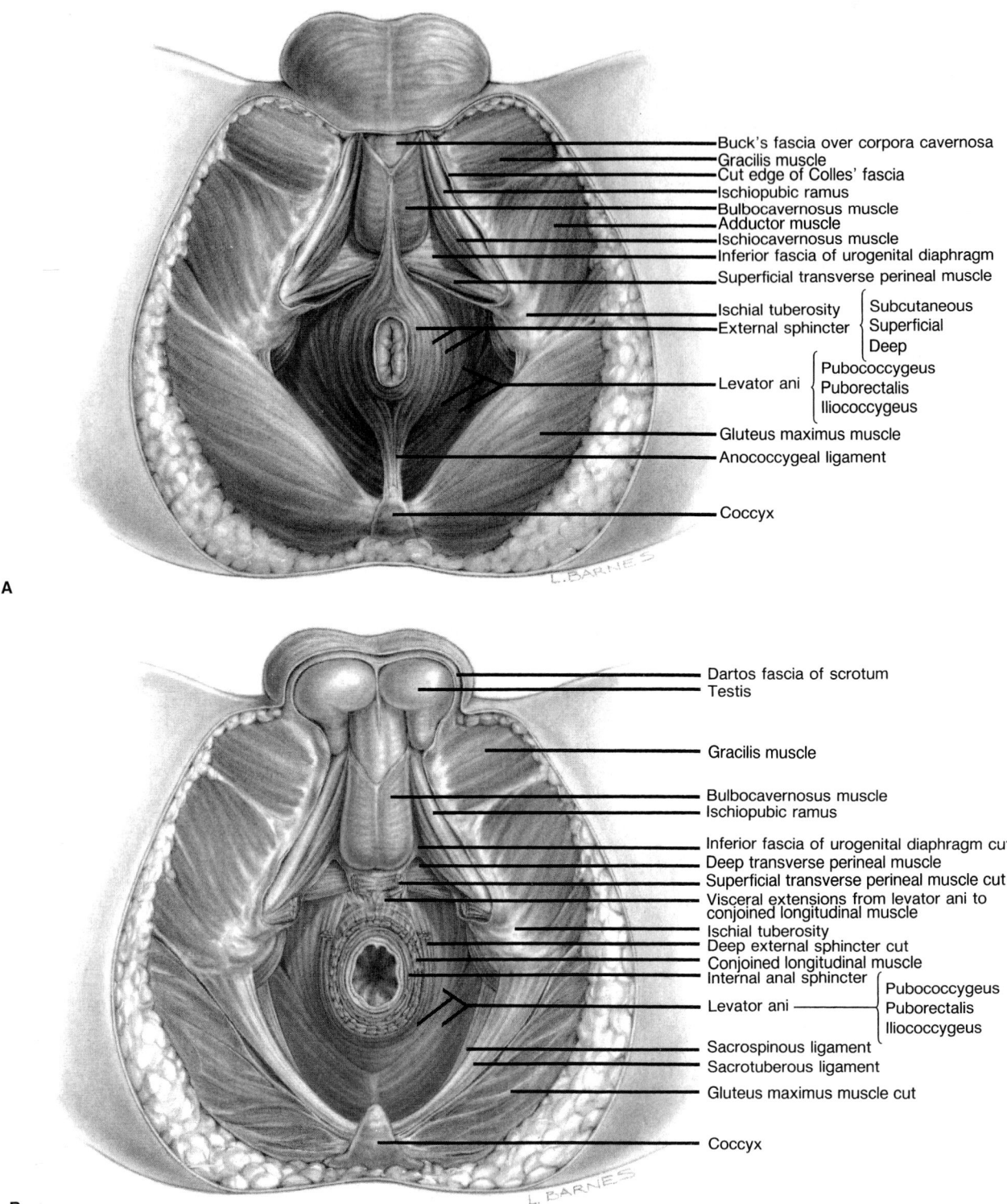

A

- Buck's fascia over corpora cavernosa
- Gracilis muscle
- Cut edge of Colles' fascia
- Ischiopubic ramus
- Bulbocavernosus muscle
- Adductor muscle
- Ischiocavernosus muscle
- Inferior fascia of urogenital diaphragm
- Superficial transverse perineal muscle
- Ischial tuberosity
- External sphincter { Subcutaneous / Superficial / Deep
- Levator ani { Pubococcygeus / Puborectalis / Iliococcygeus
- Gluteus maximus muscle
- Anococcygeal ligament
- Coccyx

B

- Dartos fascia of scrotum
- Testis
- Gracilis muscle
- Bulbocavernosus muscle
- Ischiopubic ramus
- Inferior fascia of urogenital diaphragm cut
- Deep transverse perineal muscle
- Superficial transverse perineal muscle cut
- Visceral extensions from levator ani to conjoined longitudinal muscle
- Ischial tuberosity
- Deep external sphincter cut
- Conjoined longitudinal muscle
- Internal anal sphincter
- Levator ani { Pubococcygeus / Puborectalis / Iliococcygeus
- Sacrospinous ligament
- Sacrotuberous ligament
- Gluteus maximus muscle cut
- Coccyx

FIGURE 1-11. Male perineal musculature. **(A)** Inferior view of the male perineum at a superficial level with the skin and subcutaneous tissue removed. **(B)** The male perineum at the level of the midanal canal. **(C)** The male perineum at the level of the lower rectum.

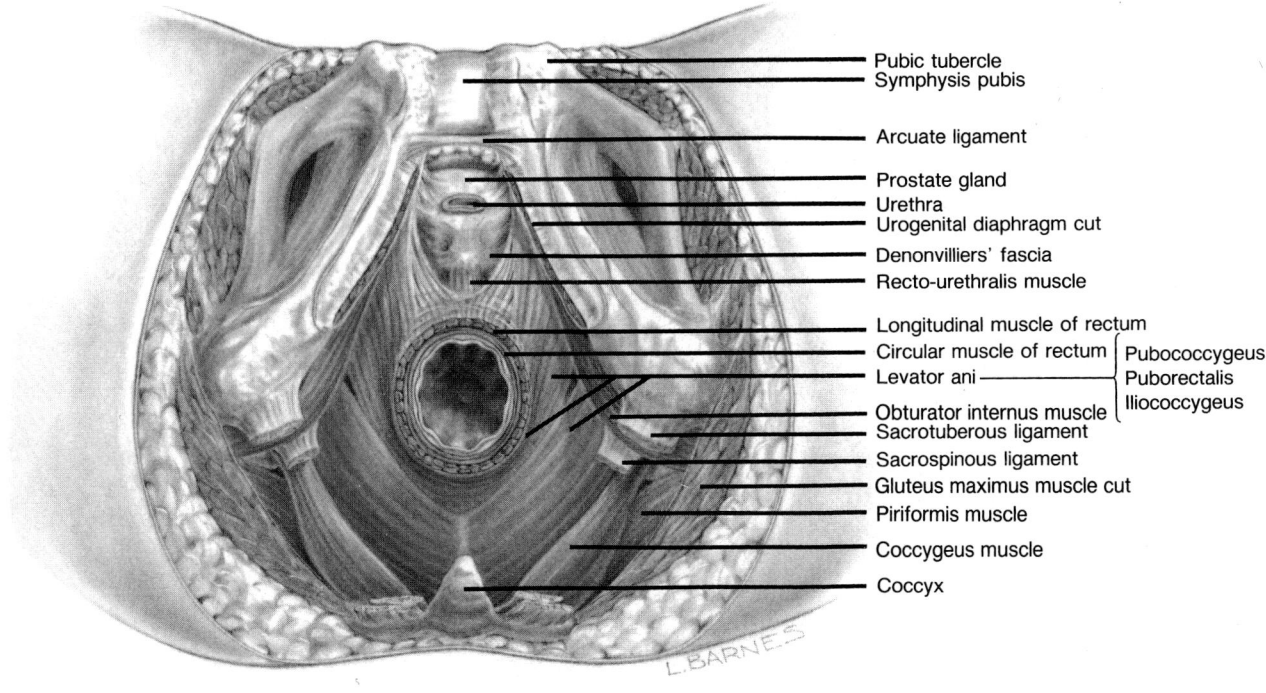

c

FIGURE 1-11. *(Continued)*

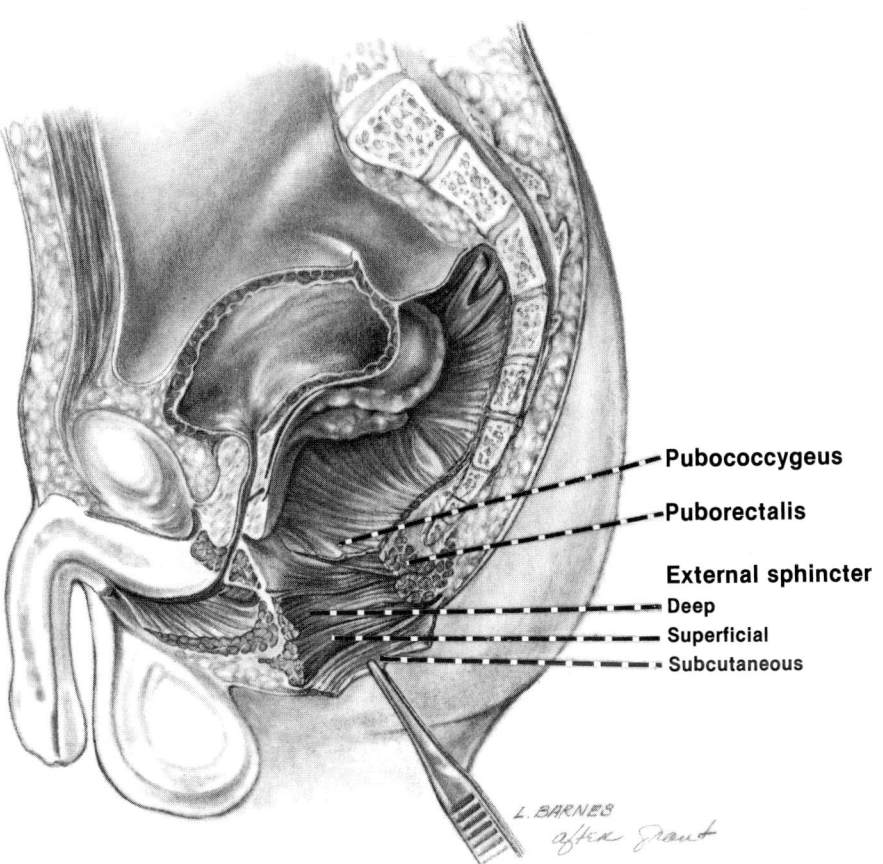

FIGURE 1-12. Muscles of the pelvic floor.

sacrospinous ligament.[125] Ileococcygeus fibers arise from the ischial spine and posterior part of the obturator fascia and course inferiorly and medially. They insert into the lateral aspects of S-3 and S-4, the coccyx, and the anococcygeal raphe. The pubococcygeus arises from the posterior aspect of the pubis and the anterior part of the obturator fascia. It runs dorsally alongside the anorectal junction to decussate with fibers of the opposite side at the anococcygeal raphe, inserting into the anterior surface of the fourth sacral and first coccygeal segments.

The pelvic floor is "defective" in the midline where the lower rectum, urethra, and either the dorsal vein of the penis in men, or the vagina in women, pass through it. This defect is called the levator hiatus; this consists of an elliptical space situated between the two pubococcygeus muscles.[100] The hiatal ligament, originating from the pelvic fascia, keeps the intrahiatal viscera together and prevents their constriction during contraction of the levator ani. A dilator function has been attributed to the anococcygeal raphe because of its criss-cross arrangement.[102]

The puborectalis muscle is a strong, U-shaped loop of striated muscle that slings the anorectal junction to the posterior aspect of the pubis. The puborectalis is the most medial portion of the levator ani muscle. It is situated immediately cephalad to the deep component of the external sphincter. Because the junction between the two muscles is indistinct, and they have similar innervation (pudendal nerve), the puborectalis has been regarded by some authors as a part of the EAS and not of the levator ani complex.[88,102] Anatomic and phylogenetic studies suggest that the puborectalis may be a part of the levator ani[91] or of the EAS.[62,120] Based on microscopic examinations in 18 human embryos, Levi and colleagues have observed that the puborectalis has a common primordium with the ileococcygeus and pubococcygeus muscles, and that in different stages of development it is never connected with the EAS.[65] Additionally, neurophysiologic studies have implied that the innervation of these muscles may not be the same, because stimulation of the sacral nerves results in electromyographic activity in the ipsilateral puborectalis muscle, but not in the EAS.[95] However, one can appreciate that this is a controversial issue, and as a consequence the puborectalis is currently considered to belong to both muscular groups, the EAS and the levator ani.[100]

Two anatomic structures of the junction of the rectum and anal canal are related to the puborectalis muscle: the anorectal ring and the anorectal angle (Figure 1-13). The anorectal ring, a term coined by Milligan and Morgan, is a strong muscular ring that represents the upper end of the sphincter (more precisely the puborectalis) and the upper border of the IAS, around the anorectal junction.[78]

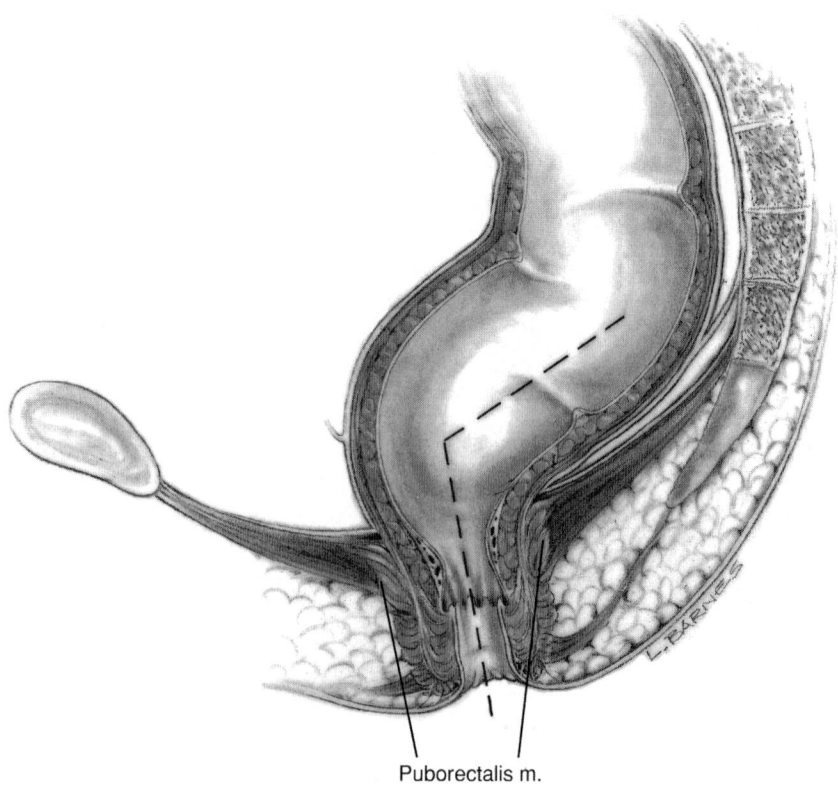

FIGURE 1-13. The anteriorly directed pull of the puborectalis contributes to the angulation between the rectum and anal canal, the anorectal angle (*dashed line*).

Puborectalis m.

Despite its lack of embryologic significance, it is an easily recognized boundary of the anal canal that can be appreciated on physical examination. It is of particular clinical relevance because division of this structure during surgery for abscess or fistula inevitably results in fecal incontinence. The anorectal angle is thought to be the result of the anatomic configuration of the U-shaped sling of puborectalis muscle around the anorectal junction. Whereas the anal sphincters are responsible for closure of the anal canal to retain gas and liquid stool, the puborectalis muscle and the anorectal angle are designed to maintain gross fecal continence. Different theories have been postulated to explain the importance of the puborectalis and the anorectal angle in the maintenance of fecal continence. Parks and coworkers opined that increasing intraabdominal pressure forces the anterior rectal wall down into the upper anal canal, occluding it by a type of flap-valve mechanism that creates an effective seal.[93] Subsequently, it has been demonstrated that the flap mechanism does not occur. Instead, a continuous sphincteric occlusion-like activity that is attributed to the puborectalis has been observed.[7,8]

Para-anal and Para-rectal Spaces

Potential spaces of clinical significance in the anorectal region include the following: ischiorectal, perianal, intersphincteric, submucous, superficial postanal, deep postanal, supralevator, and retrorectal (Figure 1-14).

The ischiorectal fossa is subdivided by a thin horizontal fascia into two spaces: the perianal and ischiorectal. The ischiorectal space comprises the upper two thirds of the ischiorectal fossa. It is pyramidal in shape and is situated on both sides between the anal canal and the lower part of the rectum medially and the sidewall of the pelvis laterally. Some authors consider the term ischiorectal fossa misleading and prefer to use the expression ischioanal fossa because its medial limit is at the level of the anal canal rather than the rectum.[58] The apex is at the origin of the levator ani muscle from the obturator fascia; the base is the perianal space. Anteriorly, the fossa is bounded by the urogenital diaphragm and the transversus perinei muscle. Posterior to the ischiorectal fossa is the sacrotuberous ligament and the inferior border of the gluteus maximus. On the superolateral wall, the pudendal nerve and the internal pudendal vessels run in the pudendal canal (Alcock's canal). The ischiorectal fossa contains fat and the inferior rectal vessels and nerves.

The perianal space surrounds the lower part of the anal canal. It is continuous with the subcutaneous fat of the buttocks laterally and extends into the intersphincteric space medially. The external hemorrhoidal plexus lies in the perianal space and communicates with the internal hemorrhoidal plexus at the dentate line. This space is the typical site of anal hematomas, perianal abscesses, and anal fistula tracts. The perianal space also encloses the subcutaneous part of the EAS, the lowest part of the IAS, and fibers of the longitudinal muscle. These fibers function as septa, dividing the space into a compact arrangement, which may account for the severe pain caused by a perianal hematoma or abscess.

The intersphincteric space is a potential space between the IAS and the EAS. It is important in the genesis of perianal abscess, because most of the anal glands end in this space. The submucous space is situated between the IAS and the mucocutaneous lining of the anal canal. This space contains the internal hemorrhoidal plexus and the muscularis submucosae ani. Above, it is continuous with the submucous layer of the rectum, and inferiorly it ends at the level of the dentate line.

The superficial postanal space is interposed between the anococcygeal ligament and the skin. The deep postanal space, also known as the retrosphincteric space of Courtney, is situated between the anococcygeal ligament and the anococcygeal raphe.[21] Both postanal spaces communicate posteriorly with the ischiorectal fossa and are the sites of horseshoe abscesses.

The supralevator spaces are situated between the peritoneum superiorly and the levator ani inferiorly. Medially, these bilateral spaces are limited by the rectum, and, laterally, by the obturator fascia. Supralevator abscesses may occur as a result of upward extension of a cryptoglandular infection or develop from a pelvic origin. The retrorectal space is located between the fascia propria of the rectum anteriorly and the presacral fascia posteriorly. Laterally are found the lateral rectal ligaments and inferiorly the rectosacral ligament; the space above is continuous with the retroperitoneum. The retrorectal space is a frequent site for embryologic remnants and rare presacral tumors (see Chapter 25).

Arterial Supply

Two of the three major gut vessels, the superior and inferior mesenteric arteries, nourish the entire large intestine (Figure 1-15). The limit between the two territories is the junction between the proximal two thirds and the distal third of the transverse colon. This represents the embryologic division between the midgut and the hindgut. Collateral circulation between these two arteries is formed by a "continuous" communicating arcade along the mesenteric border of the colon, the marginal artery, from which the vasa recta supply the bowel. The colon is much less vascular and consequently more vulnerable to necrosis than is the small bowel, because communications be-

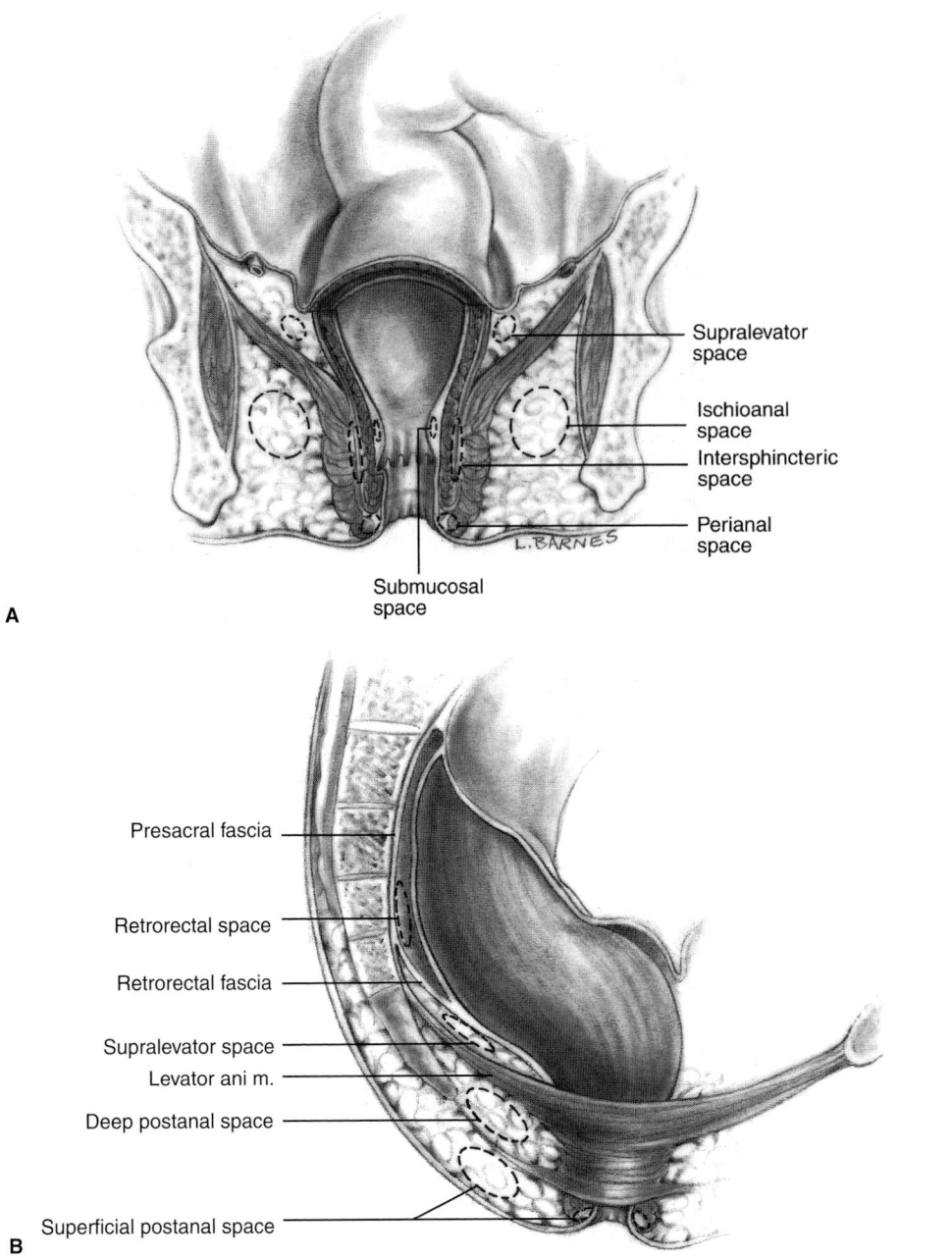

FIGURE 1-14. Para-anal and para-rectal spaces. **(A)** Frontal view. **(B)** Lateral view.

tween both adjacent and opposite-sided vasa recta are few. The anorectum is, in addition, supplied by the internal iliac arteries.

Superior Mesenteric Artery

The superior mesenteric artery originates from the aorta behind the superior border of the pancreas at L-1, supplying the cecum, appendix, ascending colon, and most

of the transverse colon. Additionally, the superior mesenteric artery supplies the entire small bowel, the pancreas, and occasionally the liver. After passing behind the neck of the pancreas and anteromedial to the uncinate process, the superior mesenteric artery crosses the third part of the duodenum, continuing downward and to the right, along the base of the mesentery. From its left side arises a series of 12 to 20 jejunal and ileal branches. From its right side arise the colic branches: middle, right, and ileo-

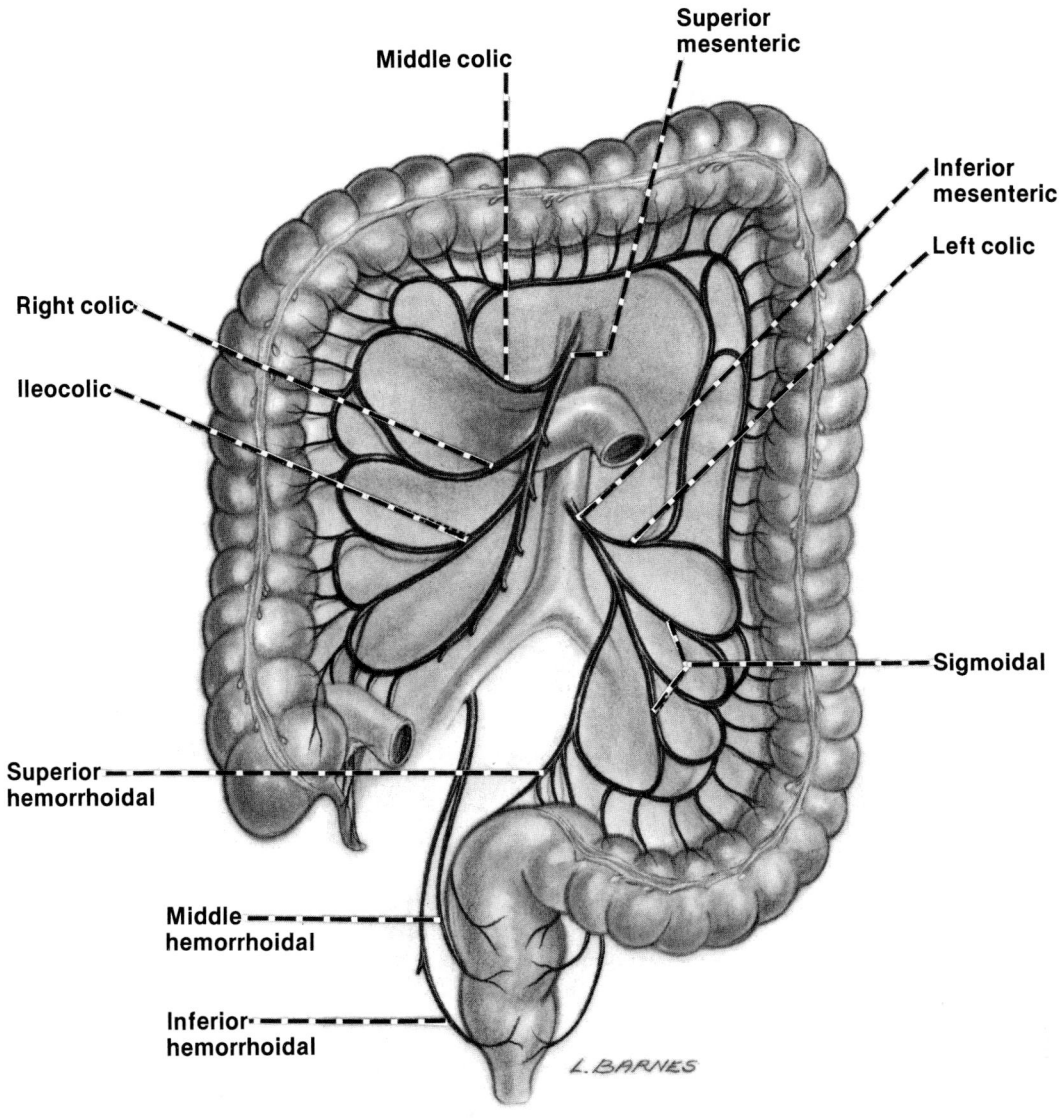

FIGURE 1-15. The blood supply to the colon originates from the superior and inferior mesenteric arteries.

colic arteries. The ileocolic is the most constant of these vessels, being present in all 600 specimens studied by Sonneland and coworkers.[107] It bifurcates into a superior or ascending branch, which communicates with the descending branch of the right colic artery, and an inferior or descending branch, which gives off the anterior cecal, posterior cecal, and appendicular divisions. Finally, it supplies the distal small bowel mesentery as the ileal branch.

The right colic artery may also arise from the ileocolic or middle colic arteries; it is absent in 2% to 18% of specimens.[76,107,109] This vessel supplies the ascending colon and hepatic flexure through its ascending and descend-

ing branches, both of which join with neighboring vessels to contribute to the marginal artery.

The middle colic artery is the highest of the three colic branches of the superior mesenteric artery, arising close to the inferior border of the pancreas. Its right branch supplies the right transverse colon and hepatic flexure, anastomosing with the ascending branch of the right colic artery. Its left branch supplies the distal half of the transverse colon. Anatomic variations of this artery include absence in 4% to 20% of cases and the presence of an accessory middle colic artery in 10%; the middle colic artery is the main supply to the splenic flexure in about one third of individuals.[44,107]

Inferior Mesenteric Artery

The inferior mesenteric artery originates from the left anterior surface of the aorta, 3 to 4 cm above its bifurcation at the level of L2–3, and runs downward and to the left to enter the pelvis. Within the abdomen, the inferior mesenteric artery branches into the left colic artery and two to six sigmoidal arteries. After crossing the left common iliac artery, it acquires the name, superior hemorrhoidal artery (superior rectal artery is generally not preferred [Figure 1-15]).

The left colic artery, the highest branch of the inferior mesenteric artery, bifurcates into an ascending branch, which runs upward to the splenic flexure to contribute to the arcade of Riolan, and a descending branch, which supplies most of the descending colon. The sigmoidal arteries form arcades within the sigmoid mesocolon, resembling the small bowel vasculature, and anastomose with branches of the left colic artery proximally and with the superior hemorrhoidal artery distally. The marginal artery terminates within the arcade of sigmoidal arteries. The superior hemorrhoidal artery is the continuation of the inferior mesenteric artery once it crosses the left iliac vessels. The artery descends in the sigmoid mesocolon to the level of S-3 and then to the posterior aspect of the rectum. In 80% of cases, it bifurcates into right (usually wider) and left terminal branches; multiple branches are present in 17% of patients[76] These divisions, once within the submucosa of the rectum, run straight downward to supply the lower rectum and anal canal. The branches that reach the level of the rectal columns (approximately five) condensate in capillary plexuses, mostly at the right posterior, right anterior, and left lateral positions; these branches correspond to the location of the major internal hemorrhoid groups.

The major blood supply to the anorectum is represented by the superior and inferior hemorrhoidal arteries. The contribution of the middle hemorrhoidal artery varies with the size of the superior hemorrhoidal artery; this may explain its controversial anatomy. Some authors report absence of the middle hemorrhoidal artery in 40% to 88%,[3,27] whereas others identify it in 94% to 100% of specimen.[47,76] This vessel originates more commonly from the anterior division of the internal iliac or the pudendal arteries and reaches the rectum. The middle hemorrhoidal artery reaches the lower third of the rectum anterolaterally, close to the level of the pelvic floor and deep to the levator fascia. Contrary to popular misconception, it therefore does not run in the lateral ligaments (inclined posterolaterally).[20,84] The middle hemorrhoidal artery is more prone to be injured during low anterior resection, when anterolateral dissection of the rectum is performed close to the pelvic floor, and the prostate and seminal vesicles or upper part of the vagina are being separated.[84] The anorectum

has a profuse intramural anastomotic network, which probably accounts for the fact that division of both superior and middle hemorrhoidal arteries does not result in necrosis of the rectum. This tenet is fundamental to ileoanal reservoir surgery and restorative proctocolectomy.

The paired inferior hemorrhoidal arteries are branches of the internal pudendal artery, which, in turn, is a branch of the internal iliac artery. The inferior hemorrhoidal artery arises within the pudendal canal and is throughout its course entirely extrapelvic. It traverses the obturator fascia, the ischiorectal fossa, and the EAS to reach the submucosa of the anal canal, ultimately ascending in this plane. The inferior rectal artery needs to be ligated during the perineal stage of abdominoperineal resection. Klosterhalfen and coworkers performed postmortem angiographic, manual, and histologic evaluations, identifying two topographic variants of this vessel.[59] In the so-called type I, the most common type (85%), the posterior commissure was less well perfused than were the other sections of the anal canal. In addition, the blood supply could be jeopardized by contusion of the vessels passing vertically through the muscle fibers of the IAS when sphincter tone was increased. These authors postulated that in a pathogenetic model of primary anal fissure, the resulting decreased blood supply may lead to ischemia at the posterior commissure.

Collateral Circulation

In spite of the fact that prior to the seventeenth century, anatomy of the mesenteric circulation was a source of concern, this subject still has not been clarified in most textbooks. This, in part, may be attributed to the inherent confusion in the use of eponyms. A central anastomotic artery that connects all colonic mesenteric branches was initially described by von Haller in 1786.[49] Later it became known as the marginal artery of Drummond, because it was he, in 1913, who first demonstrated its surgical significance. Drummond proved that the sigmoidal vessels could be filled with contrast material following injection of the ileocolic artery and ligation of the right, middle, and left colic arteries at their origin.[28,29] Subsequent examiners have demonstrated discontinuity of the marginal artery at the lower ascending colon and especially at the splenic flexure and sigmoid colon. This theoretically hypovascular area is a potential source of concern during colonic resection.[125] The splenic flexure comprises the watershed between midgut and hindgut blood supply (Griffiths' critical point); this anastomosis is of variable significance, and in fact it may be absent in about 50% of cases.[75] For this reason, ischemic colitis usually affects or is most severe near the splenic flexure.[26] Despite this logic, a predilection for the right colon has been found by several investigators.[46,61,70] Sudeck's critical point, an area of discontinuity of the marginal artery between the distal sigmoid and the superior hemorrhoidal arteries, may be unnecessarily emphasized.[111] Surgical experience and radiologic studies have both demonstrated adequate communication between these vessels.[44,115] Furthermore, anastomosis between the superior and middle hemorrhoidal arteries, commonly observed with aortography, may prevent gangrene of the pelvis and even the lower extremities wherein the distal aorta is occluded. This can be attributed to the collateral network involving middle hemorrhoidal, internal iliac, and external iliac arteries.[45,69]

Jean Riolan (1580–1657) was the first to describe the communication between the superior and inferior mesenteric arteries, and the term arc of Riolan was vaguely defined in the author's original work. Later, the eponym, marginal artery of Drummond, confused the subject.[34] In 1964, Moskowitz and coworkers proposed another term, meandering mesenteric artery, and differentiated it from the marginal artery of Drummond.[83] The meandering mesenteric artery is a thick and tortuous vessel that makes a crucial communication between the middle colic artery and the ascending branch of the left colic artery, especially in advanced atherosclerotic disease. Fisher and Fry claimed that the meandering mesenteric artery could be easily recognized either preoperatively by arteriography (because of its size, tortuosity, and uniform caliber), or intraoperatively (by palpation, because of its promi-

nent arterial pulsations flow).[34] The presence of the meandering mesenteric artery indicates severe stenosis of either the superior mesenteric artery (retrograde flow) or inferior mesenteric artery (antegrade flow). If during a left colon operation the meandering mesenteric artery is divided, vascular compromise may ensue, depending on the direction of the flow. Necrosis of the right colon and entire small bowel may occur if the flow is retrograde, and necrosis of the sigmoid colon and upper rectum, as well as vascular insufficiency in the lower extremity, may occur if the flow is antegrade.

Venous Drainage

The venous drainage of the large intestine basically follows its arterial supply (Figure 1-16). Blood from the right colon, via the superior mesenteric vein, and from left colon and rectum, via the inferior mesenteric vein, reaches the intrahepatic capillary bed through the portal vein. The anorectum also drains, via middle and inferior hemorrhoidal veins, to the internal iliac vein and then to the inferior vena cava. Although it is still a controversial subject, the presence of communications among these three venous systems may explain the lack of correlation between portal hypertension and hemorrhoids.[10]

The paired inferior and middle hemorrhoidal veins and the single superior hemorrhoidal vein originate from three anorectal arteriovenous plexuses (Figure 1-17). The external hemorrhoidal plexus, situated subcutaneously around the anal canal below the dentate line, constitutes

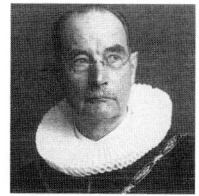

Paul Hermann Martin Sudeck (1866–1945) Paul Sudeck was born in 1866 in Pinneberg/Holstein/Germany, the son of an attorney. Despite his father's wishes, he entered the study of medicine at the Universities of Tübingen, Kiel, and Würzburg. In 1890, he earned his doctorate at the Pathological Institute of the University of Würzburg, after which he became an assistant at the Eppendorf Hospital in Hamburg. It was there that he spent his entire career. Sudeck became Professor of Surgery in 1919 and was named the first Director and Chairman of the Department in 1923 at the new University of Hamburg. His primary contributions to medicine were in anesthesia and orthopedics. He was responsible for reintroducing inhalational anesthesia into Germany, using ether and chloroform. In 1901, he developed a new anesthetic mask (the Sudeck-Inhalator), which contained an exhalation valve that avoided the accumulation of toxic gas. He recognized reflex sympathetic dystrophy, a debilitating soft tissue atrophy following bony fractures, which now bears his name (Sudeck's dystrophy). He emphasized that there is a failure of the marginal artery circulation between the lowest sigmoid artery and the branches of the superior hemorrhoidal artery (Sudeck's point). He had a strong interest in biomechanics and made many contributions to the rehabilitation of trauma victims. Sudeck died in Hamburg, September 28, 1945. (With appreciation to Ali Khoynezhad, M.D. and Udo Rudloff, M.D.)

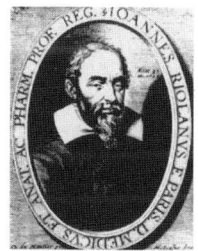

Jean Riolan (1577–1657) Riolan was born in Paris, France, the son of a physician and leading member of the Paris Medical Faculty. His mother's family also played a prominent role in Parisian medicine during the sixteenth and seventeenth centuries. He studied chiefly under his uncle and received his doctorate in medicine in 1604. Riolan was also named archdeacon of schools, a position that placed him in charge of the material for anatomy courses.

He became a trained anatomist and dissector and advocated active anatomic observation in preference to long reading and meditation. He was also a staunch defender of traditional medicine and considered himself an enemy of chemical healers. A violent adversary of Harvey, he maintained that if dissections no longer agreed with those of Galen, it should be attributed to the fact that Nature had changed since Galen's time. He believed that one should never admit that Galen was incorrect. Despite his reactionary opinions, Riolan distinguished himself through a series of textbooks, including *Anthropographia* in 1626 and *Encheiridium* in 1648. From 1604 to 1640, he was Professor of Anatomy and Botany at the University of Paris and Professor of Medicine at the College Royal, as well as Dean of the Royal College from 1640 to 1657. Riolan also served as physician to Henry IV and Louis XIII. He died at the age of 77 in Paris. (With appreciation to the Galileo Project Files, Rice University, and Michael Eng, M.D.)

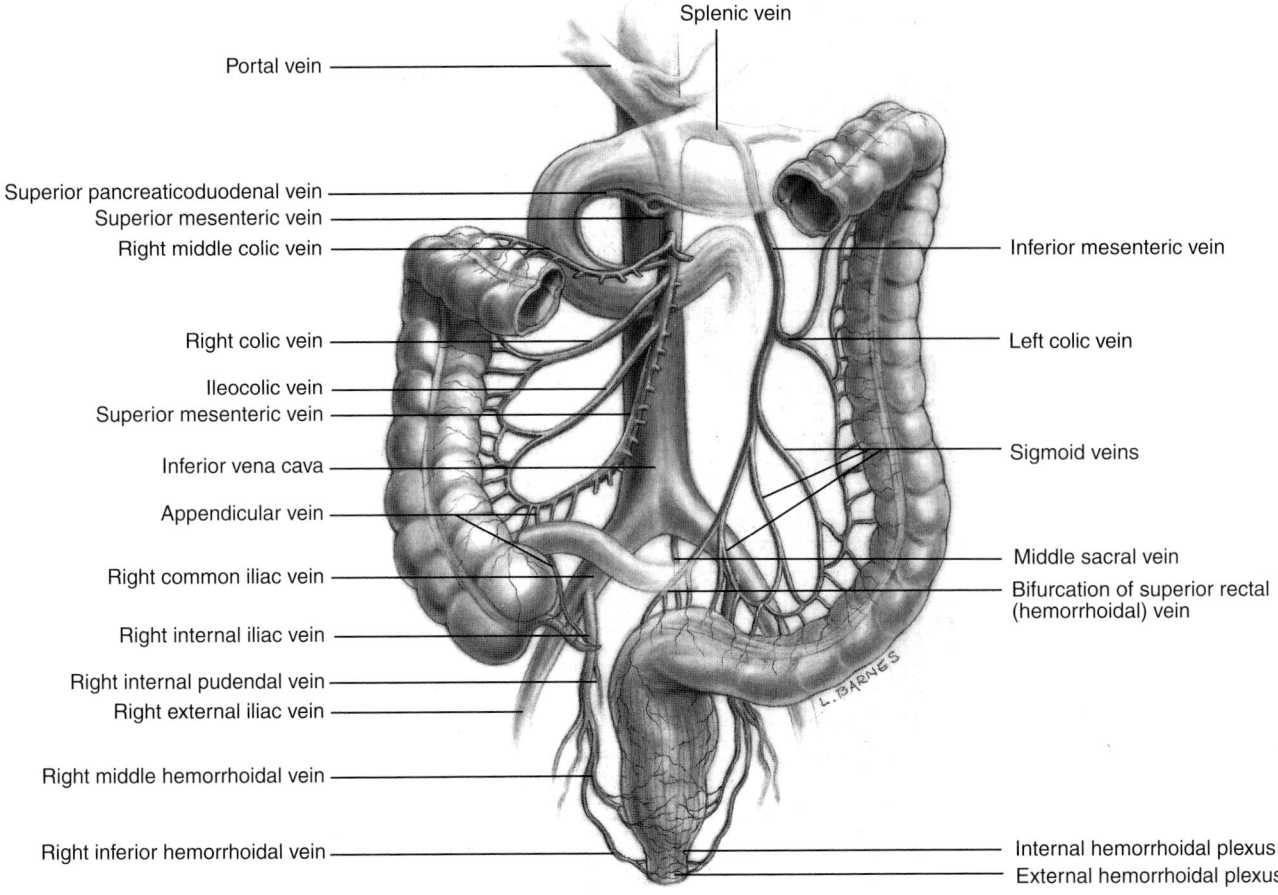

FIGURE 1-16. Venous drainage of the colon.

the external hemorrhoids when it is dilated. The internal hemorrhoidal plexus is situated submucosally, around the upper anal canal and above the dentate line. The internal hemorrhoids originate from this plexus. The perirectal or perimuscular rectal plexus drains to the middle and inferior hemorrhoidal veins.

Lymphatic Drainage

The lymphatic drainage from all parts of the colon follows its vascular supply. The submucous and subserous layers of the colon and rectum have a rich network of lymphatic plexuses, which drain into an extramural system of lymph channels and nodes.[11] Colorectal lymph nodes are classically divided into four groups: epiploic, paracolic, intermediate, and principal (Figure 1-18).[54] The epicolic group lies on the bowel wall under the peritoneum and in the appendices epiploicae; they are more numerous in the sigmoid and are known in the rectum as the nodules of Gerota. The paracolic nodes are situated along the marginal artery and on the arcades; they are considered to have the most numerous filters. The inter-

mediate nodes are situated on the primary colic vessels, and the main or principal nodes are situated on the superior and inferior mesenteric vessels. The lymph then drains to the cisterna chyli via the paraortic chain of nodes. Colorectal carcinoma staging systems are based on the neoplastic involvement of these various lymph node groups.

Lymph from the upper two thirds of the rectum drains exclusively upward to the inferior mesenteric nodes and then to the paraaortic nodes (Figure 1-19). Lymphatic drainage from the lower third of the rectum occurs, not only cephalad along the superior hemorrhoidal and inferior mesentery arteries, but also laterally, along the middle hemorrhoidal vessels to the internal iliac nodes. Studies using lymphoscintigraphy have failed to demonstrate communications between inferior mesenteric and internal iliac lymphatics.[79] In the anal canal, the dentate line is the landmark for two different systems of lymphatic drainage: above, to the inferior mesenteric and internal iliac nodes, and below, along the inferior rectal lymphatics to the superficial inguinal nodes, or less frequently along the inferior hemorrhoidal artery. Block and Enquist injected dye 5 cm above the anal verge in the female and

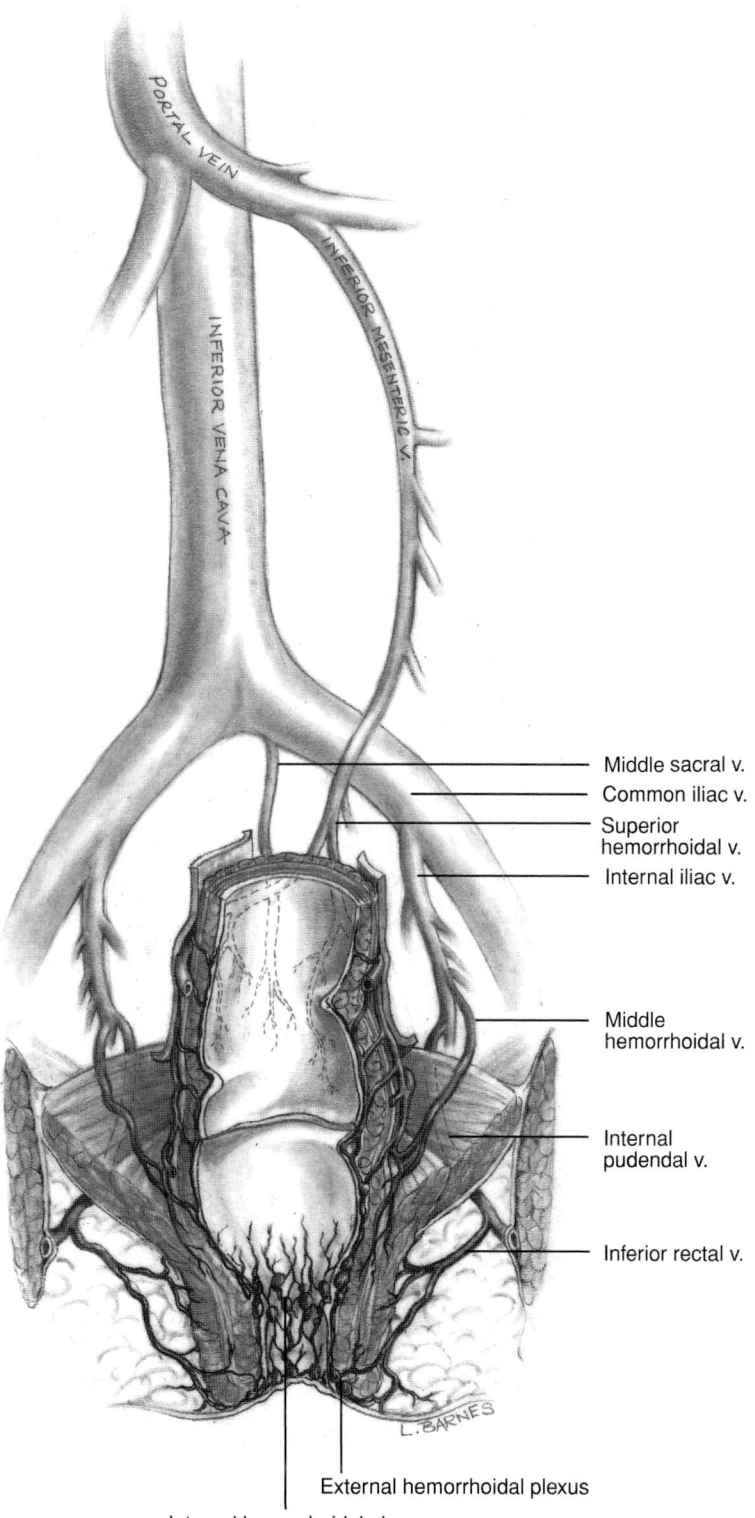

Middle sacral v.
Common iliac v.
Superior
hemorrhoidal v.
Internal iliac v.

Middle
hemorrhoidal v.

Internal
pudendal v.

Inferior rectal v.

External hemorrhoidal plexus

Internal hemorrhoidal plexus

FIGURE 1-17. Venous drainage of the colon.

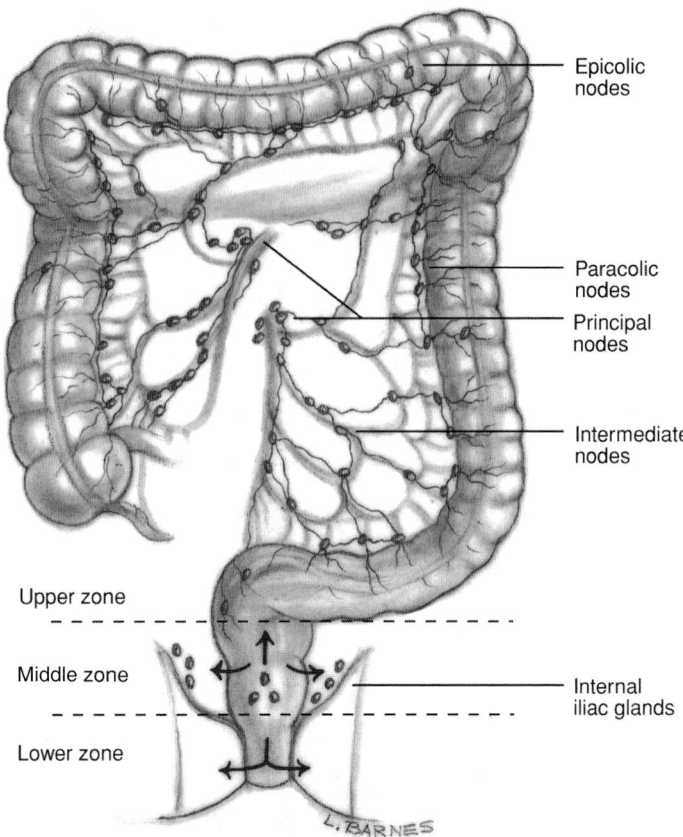

FIGURE 1-18. Lymphatic drainage of the colon.

demonstrated that lymphatic drainage may also spread to the posterior vaginal wall, uterus, cervix, broad ligament, fallopian tubes, ovaries, and cul-de-sac.[11] After injection of dye at 10 cm above the anal verge, spread occurred only to the broad ligament and cul-de-sac, and at the 15-cm level, no spread to the genitals was seen.

Innervation

The sympathetic and parasympathetic components of the autonomic innervation of the large intestine closely follow the blood supply.

Right Colon

The sympathetic supply originates from the lower six thoracic segments. These thoracic splanchnic nerves reach the celiac, preaortic, and superior mesenteric ganglia, where they synapse. The postganglionic fibers then course along the superior mesenteric artery to the small bowel and right colon. The parasympathetic supply comes from the right (posterior) vagus nerve and celiac plexus. The fibers travel along the superior mesenteric artery and finally synapse with cells in the autonomic plexuses within the bowel wall.

Left Colon and Rectum

The sympathetic supply arises from L-1, L-2, and L-3. Preganglionic fibers, via lumbar sympathetic nerves, synapse in the preaortic plexus, and the postganglionic fibers follow the branches of the inferior mesenteric artery and superior rectal artery to the left colon and upper rectum. The lower rectum is innervated by the presacral nerves, which are formed by fusion of the aortic plexus and lumbar splanchnic nerves. Just below the sacral promontory, the presacral nerves form the hypogastric plexus (or superior hypogastric plexus). Two main hypogastric nerves, on either side of the rectum, carry sympathetic innervation from the hypogastric plexus to the pelvic plexus. The pelvic plexus lies on the lateral side of the pelvis at the level of the lower third of the rectum, adjacent to the lateral stalks. The term inferior hypogastric plexus has been used to mean the hypogastric nerves or the pelvic plexus; therefore, it is inaccurate.[20]

The parasympathetic supply derives from S-2, S-3, and S-4 (Figure 1-20). These fibers emerge through the sacral foramen and are called the *nervi erigentes*. They pass laterally, forward, and upward to join the sympathetic hypogastric nerves at the pelvic plexus. From the pelvic plexus, combined postganglionic parasympathetic

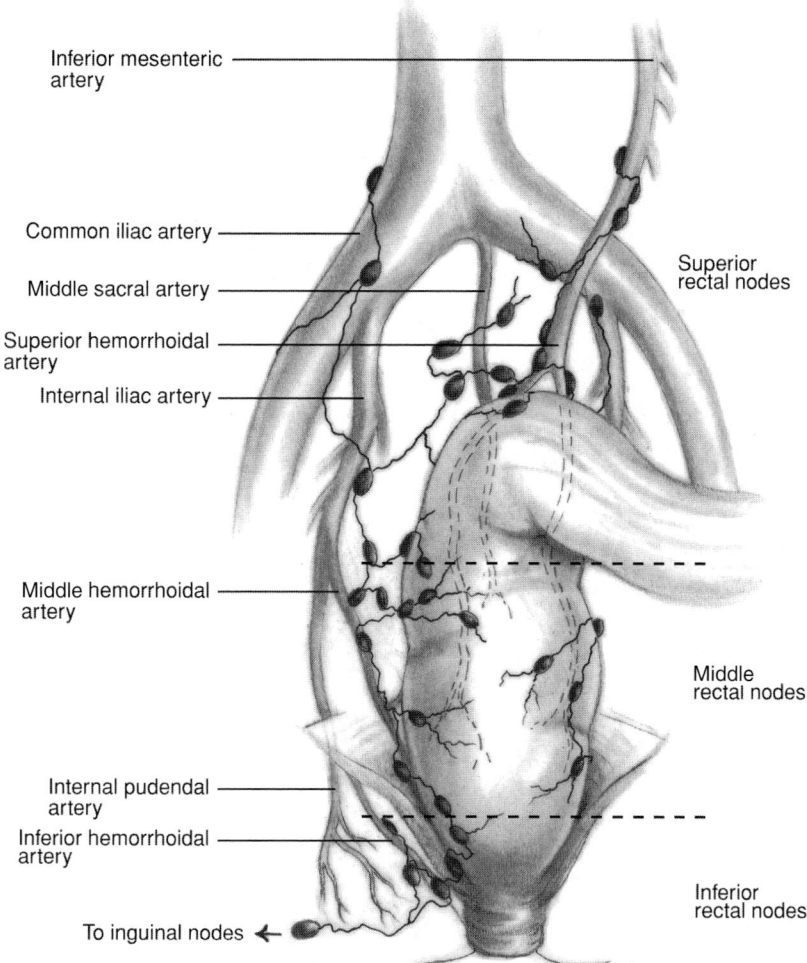

Inferior mesenteric artery

Common iliac artery

Middle sacral artery

Superior hemorrhoidal artery

Internal iliac artery

Middle hemorrhoidal artery

Internal pudendal artery

Inferior hemorrhoidal artery

To inguinal nodes ←

Superior rectal nodes

Middle rectal nodes

Inferior rectal nodes

L. BARNES

FIGURE 1-19. Lymphatic drainage of the colon.

and sympathetic fibers are distributed to the left colon and upper rectum via the inferior mesenteric plexus and directly to the lower rectum and upper anal canal. The periprostatic plexus, a subdivision of the pelvic plexus situated on Denonvilliers' fascia, supplies the prostate, seminal vesicles, corpora cavernosa, vas deferens, urethra, ejaculatory ducts, and bulbourethral glands.

Sexual function is regulated by cerebrospinal, sympathetic, and parasympathetic components. Erection of the penis is mediated by both parasympathetic (arteriolar vasodilation) and sympathetic inflow (inhibition of vasoconstriction). Urinary and sexual dysfunctions are commonly seen after a variety of pelvic surgical procedures, including low anterior resection and abdominoperineal resection. Permanent bladder paresis occurs in 7% to 59% of patients after abdominoperineal resection of the rectum[39]; the incidence of impotence is reported to range from 15% to 45% and that of ejaculatory dysfunction from 32% to 42%.[89] The overall incidence of sexual dysfunction after proctectomy may reach 100% when the

procedure is performed for malignant disease[6,25,119]; however, these rates are much lower for benign conditions, such as inflammatory bowel disease (0% to 6%).[6,9,25,117] This may be a consequence of the fact that dissections performed for benign conditions are undertaken closer to the bowel wall, thus reducing the possibility of nerve injury.[63] A more likely reason, however, is the age of the patient and the preoperative libido.

All pelvic nerves lie in the plane between the peritoneum and the endopelvic fascia and are in danger of injury during rectal dissection. Trauma to the autonomic nerves may occur at several points. During high ligation of the inferior mesenteric artery, close to the aorta, the sympathetic preaortic nerves may be injured. Division of both superior hypogastric plexus and hypogastric nerves may occur also during dissection at the level of the sacral promontory or in the presacral region. In such circumstances, sympathetic denervation with intact nervi erigentes results in retrograde ejaculation and bladder dysfunction. The nervi erigentes are located

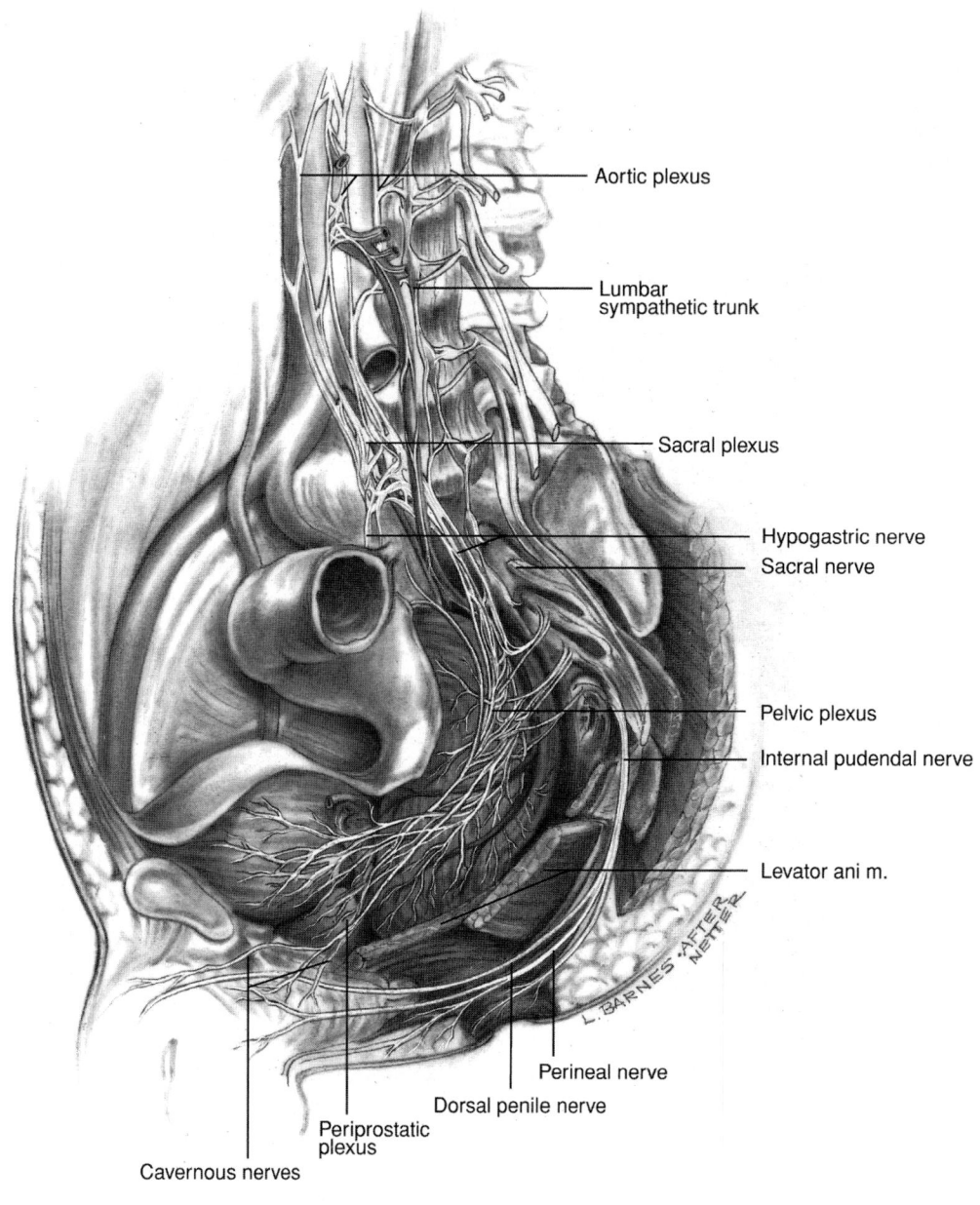

FIGURE 1-20. Innervation of the rectum and sphincters.

in the posterolateral aspect of the pelvis and at the point of fusion with the sympathetic nerves are closely related to the middle hemorrhoidal artery. An isolated injury to these nerves will completely abolish erectile function.[9] The pelvic plexus may be damaged either by excessive traction on the rectum, particularly laterally, or during division of the lateral stalks when this is performed close to the lateral pelvic wall. Finally, dissection near the seminal vesicles and prostate may damage the periprostatic plexus, leading to a mixed parasympathetic and sympathetic injury. This can result in erectile impotence as well as a flaccid, neurogenic bladder. Sexual complications after rectal surgery are readily evident in men but are probably underdiagnosed in women.[74] Following proctocolectomy in female patients, some discomfort during intercourse is reported in 30%,[15] with dyspareunia occurring in 10%.[96] Some investigators believe that sexual function in women is primarily mediated by cerebral centers and impulses carried by the pudendal nerves.[9] Parenthetically, the pudendal nerves are covered by dense endopelvic fascia and are therefore more protected from operative injury. Their function is completely independent of the more easily damaged nervi erigentes.

Anal Canal

Motor Innervation

The IAS is supplied by the sympathetic (L-5) and parasympathetic nerves (S-2, S-3, and S-4); these nerves follow the same route as those leading to the rectum. The levator ani is supplied by sacral roots on its pelvic surface (S-2, S-3, and S-4) as well as the perineal branch of the pudendal nerve on its inferior surface. The puborectalis muscle receives additional innervation from the inferior rectal nerves. The EAS is innervated on each side by the inferior rectal branch of the pudendal nerve (S-2 and S-3) and by the perineal branch of S-4. Despite the fact that the puborectalis and EAS have somewhat different innervations, these muscles seem to act as an indivisible unit.[101,102] After unilateral transection of a pudendal nerve, EAS function is still preserved because of the crossover of the fibers at the spinal cord level.

Sensory Innervation

The upper anal canal contains a rich profusion of both free and organized sensory nerve endings, especially in the vicinity of the anal valves.[30] Organized nerve endings include Meissner's corpuscles (touch), Krause's bulbs (cold), Golgi-Mazzoni bodies (pressure), and genital corpuscles (friction). Anal sensation is carried in the inferior rectal branch of the pudendal nerve and is thought to play a role in maintenance of fecal continence.[77]

SUMMARY

In this chapter, one has attempted not merely to present a description of the anatomy of the colon, rectum, and anus, but also to provide clinical correlation wherever appropriate or helpful. Knowledge of colon and rectal anatomy, blood supply, lymphatic drainage, innervation, and muscle function and distribution are all extremely important in order to minimize complications represented by the host of surgical challenges that are discussed in subsequent chapters.

REFERENCES

1. Abel AL. The pecten band: pectenosis and pectenectomy. *Lancet* 1932;1:714–718.
2. Abramson DJ. The valves of Houston in adults. *Am J Surg* 1978;136:334–336.
3. Ayoub SF. Arterial supply of the human rectum. *Acta Anat* 1978;100:317–327.
4. Ayoub SF. Anatomy of the external anal sphincter in man. *Acta Anat* 1979;105:25–36.
5. Balli R. The sphincters of the colon. *Radiology* 1939;33:372–376.
6. Balslev I, Harling H. Sexual dysfunction following operation for carcinoma of the rectum. *Dis Colon Rectum* 1983;26:785.
7. Bannister JJ, Gibbons C, Read NW. Preservation of faecal continence during rises in intra-abdominal pressure: is there a role for the flap valve? *Gut* 1987;28:1242–1245.
8. Bartolo DCC, Roe AM, Locke-Edmunds JC, et al. Flap-valve theory of anorectal continence. *Br J Surg* 1986;73: 1012–1014.
9. Bauer JJ, Gerlent IM, Salky B, et al. Sexual dysfunction following proctectomy for benign disease of the colon and rectum. *Ann Surg* 1983;197:363–367.
10. Bernstein WC. What are hemorrhoids and what is their relationship to the portal venous system? *Dis Colon Rectum* 1983;26:829–834.
11. Block IR, Enquist IF. Studies pertaining to local spread of carcinoma of the rectum in females. *Surg Gynecol Obstet* 1961;112:41–46.
12. Bollard RC, Gardiner A, Lindow S, et al. Normal female anal sphincter: difficulties in interpretation explained. *Dis Colon Rectum* 2002;45:171–175.
13. Boxall TA, Smart PJG, Griffiths JD. The blood-supply of the distal segment of the rectum in anterior resection. *Br J Surg* 1963;50:399–404.
14. Brauss H, Elze C. *Anatomie des Menschen*, 3rd ed. Berlin: Springer, 1956.
15. Burnham WR, Lennard-Jones JE, Brooke BN. Sexual problems among married ileostomists. *Gut* 1977;18:673–677.
16. Cantlie J. The sigmoid flexure in health and disease. *J Trop Med Hyg* 1915;18:1–7.
17. Cawthorn SJ, Parums DV, Gibbs NM, et al. Extent of mesorectal spread and involvement of lateral resection margin as prognostic factors after surgery for rectal cancer. *Lancet* 1990;335:1055–1059.
18. Chapuis P, Bokey L, Fahrer M, et al. Mobilization of the rectum: anatomic concepts and the bookshelf revisited. *Dis Colon Rectum* 2002;45:1–9.
19. Chiari H. Über die Nalen Divertik Fel der Rectum-schleimhaut und Ihre Beziehung zu den anal fisteln. *Wien Med Press* 1878;19:1482.
20. Church JM, Raudkivi PJ, Hill GL. The surgical anatomy of the rectum: a review with particular relevance to the hazards of rectal mobilisation. *Int J Colorectal Dis* 1987;2: 158–166.
21. Courtney H. Posterior subsphincteric space: its relation to posterior horseshoe fistula. *Surg Gynecol Obste* 1949;89: 222–226.
22. Courtney H. Anatomy of the pelvic diaphragm and anorectal musculature as related to sphincter preservation in anorectal surgery. *Am J Surg* 1950;79:155–173.
23. Crapp AR, Cuthbertson AM. William Waldeyer and the rectosacral fascia. *Surg Gynecol Obstet* 1974;138:252–256.
24. Cuesta MA, Meijer S, Derksen EJ, et al. Anal sphincter imaging in fecal incontinence using endosonography. *Dis Colon Rectum* 1992;35:59–63.
25. Danzi M, Ferulano GP, Abate S, et al. Male sexual function after abdominoperineal resection for rectal cancer. *Dis Colon Rectum* 1983;26:665–668.
26. Dickstein G, Boley SJ. Colonic ischemia. In: Zuidema GD, ed. *Shackelford's surgery of the alimentary tract*. Philadelphia: WB Saunders, 1991:84–94.
27. Didio LJA, Diaz-Franco C, Schemainda R, et al. Morphology of the middle rectal arteries: a study of 30 cadaveric dissections. *Surg Radiol Anat* 1986;8:229–236.
28. Drummond H. Some points relating to the surgical anatomy of the arterial supply of the large intestine. *Proc R Soc Med (Proctol)*1913;7:185–193.
29. Drummond H. The arterial supply of the rectum and pelvic colon. *Br J Surg* 1914;1:677–685.
30. Duthie HL, Gairns FW. Sensory nerve endings and sensation in the anal region in man. *Br J Surg* 1960;47:585–595.
31. Ewing MR. The significance of the level of the peritoneal reflection in the surgery of rectal cancer. *Br J Surg* 1952;39:495–5000.
32. Ewing MR. The white line of Hilton. *Proc R Soc Med* 1954;47:525–530.

33. Farouk R, Duthie GS, Bartolo DCG. Functional anorectal disorders and physiological evaluation. In: Beck DE, Wexner SD, eds. *Fundamentals of anorectal surgery*. New York: McGraw-Hill, 1992:68–88.

34. Fisher DF, Fry WI. Collateral mesenteric circulation. *Surg Gynecol Obstet* 1987;164:487–492.

35. Fraser ID, Condon RE, Schulte WJ, et al. Longitudinal muscle of muscularis externa in human and nonhuman primate colon. *Arch Surg* 1981;116:61–63.

36. Frenckner B, Euler CHRV. Influence of pudendal block on the function of the anal sphincters. *Gut* 1975;16:482–489.

37. Fritsch H, Brenner E, Lienemann A, et al. Anal sphincter complex: reinterpreted morphology and its clinical relevance. *Dis Colon Rectum* 2002;45:188–194.

38. Garavoglia M, Borghi F, Levi AC. Arrangement of the anal striated musculature. *Dis Colon Rectum* 1993;36:10–15.

39. Gerstenberg TC, Nielsen ML, Clausen S, et al. Bladder function after abdominoperineal resection of the rectum for anorectal cancer. *Am J Surg* 1980;91:81–86.

40. Gibbons CP, Trowbridge EA, Bannister JJ, et al. Role of anal cushions in maintaining continence. *Lancet* 1986;1:886–887.

41. Goligher J. *Surgery of the anus, rectum and colon*. London: Baillière Tindall, 1984:1–47.

42. Goligher JC, Leacock AG, Brossy JJ. The surgical anatomy of the anal canal. *Br J Surg* 1955;43:51–61.

43. Gordon PH. Anorectal anatomy and physiology. *Gastroenterol Clin North Am* 2001;30:1–13.

44. Griffiths JD. Surgical anatomy of the blood supply of the distal colon. *Ann R Coll Surg Engl* 1956;19:241–256.

45. Griffiths JD. Extramural and intramural blood supply of the colon. *BMJ* 1961;1:322–326.

46. Guttmorson NL, Bubrick MP. Mortality from ischemic colitis. *Dis Colon Rectum* 1989;32:469–472.

47. Guyton AC, ed. *Textbook of medical physiology*. Philadelphia: WB Saunders, 1986:754–769.

48. Haas PA, Fox TA. The importance of the perianal connective tissue in the surgical anatomy and function of the anus. *Dis Colon Rectum* 1977;20:303–313.

49. Haller A. The large intestine. In: Cullen W, ed. *First lines of physiology*. [Reprint of the 1786 edition.] Sources of Science 32. New York: Johnson Reprint Corporation, 1966:139–140.

50. Harnsberger AM, Vernava AM III, Longo WE, et al. The utility of the anorectal physiology lab in influencing clinical decision making. *Dis Colon Rectum* 1993;36:11–12.

51. Heald RJ, Husband EM, Ryall RD. The mesorectum in rectal cancer surgery: the clue to pelvic recurrence? *Br J Surg* 1982;69:613–616.

52. Houston J. Observation on the mucous membrane of the rectum. *Dublin Hosp Rep Communications Med Surg* 1830;5:158–165.

53. Hyrtl J. *Handbuch der topographischen Anatomie und ihrer praktisch medicinisch-chirurgischen Anwendungen*, 4th ed, 2 vols. Wien: Braumüller, 1860.

54. Jameson JK, Dobson JF. The lymphatics of the colon. *Proc R Soc Med* 1909;2:149–172.

55. Jorge JMN, Habr-Gama A. The value of sphincter asymmetry index in anal incontinence. *Int J Colorectal Dis* 2000;15:303–310.

56. Jorge JMN, Habr-Gama A, Souza AS Jr, et al. Rectal surgery complicated by massive presacral hemorrhage. *Arq Bras Circ Dig* 1990;5:92–95.

57. Jorge JMN, Wexner SD. Etiology and management of fecal incontinence. *Dis Colon Rectum* 1993;36:77–97.

58. Kaiser AM, Ortega AE. Anorectal anatomy. *Surg Clin North Am* 2002;82:1125–1138.

59. Klosterhalfen B, Vogel P, Rixen H, et al. Topography of the inferior rectal artery: a possible cause of chronic, primary anal fissure. *Dis Colon Rectum* 1989;32:43–52.

60. Kumar D, Phillips SF. The contribution of external ligamentous attachments to function of the ileocecal junction. *Dis Colon Rectum* 1987;30:410–416.

61. Landreneau RJ, Fry WJ. The right colon as a target organ of non-occlusive mesenteric ischemia. *Arch Surg* 1990;125:591–594.

62. Lawson JON. Pelvic anatomy II. Anal canal and associated sphincters. *Ann R Coll Surg Engl* 1974;54:288–300.

63. Lee ECG, Dowling BL. Perimuscular excision of the rectum for Crohn's disease and ulcerative colitis: a conservative technique. *Br J Surg* 1972;59:29–32.

64. Lestar B, Penninckx F, Kerremans R. The composition of anal basal pressure: an in vivo and in vitro study in man. *Int J Colorectal Dis* 1989;4:118–122.

65. Levi AC, Borghi F, Garavoglia M. Development of the anal canal muscles. *Dis Colon Rectum* 1991;34:262–266.

66. Liebermann-Meffert D. Anatomie des gastrooesophagealen Verschluborgans. In: Blum AL, Siewert JR, eds. *Refluxtherapie*. New York: Springer, 1981.

67. Lilius HG. Investigation of human fetal anal ducts and intramuscular glands and a clinical study of 150 patients. *Acta Chir Scand Suppl* 1968;383:1–88.

68. Lindsey I, Guy RJ, Warren BF, et al. Anatomy of Denonvilliers'fascia and pelvic nerves, impotence, and implications for the colorectal surgeon. *Br J Surg* 2000;87:1288–1299.

69. Lindstrom BL. The value of the collateral circulation from the inferior mesenteric artery in obliteration of the lower abdominal aorta. *Acta Chir Scand* 1950;1:677–685.

70. Longo WE, Ballantyne GH, Gursberg RJ. Ischemic colitis: patterns and prognosis. *Dis Colon Rectum* 1992;35:726–730.

71. Lunniss PJ, Phillips RKS. Anatomy and function of the anal longitudinal muscle. *Br J Surg* 1992;79:882–884.

72. Mayo WJ. A study of the rectosigmoid. *Surg Gynecol Obstet* 1917;25:616–621.

73. McVay CB. *Anson and McVay surgical anatomy*. Philadelphia: WB Saunders, 1984:565–777.

74. Metcalf AM, Dozois RR, Kelly KA. Sexual function in women after proctocolectomy. *Ann Surg* 1986;204:624–627.

75. Meyers CB. Griffiths' point: critical anastomosis at the splenic flexure. *AJR Am J Roentgenol* 1976;126:77.

76. Michels NA, Siddharth P, Kornblith PL, et al, The variant blood supply to the small and large intestines: its importance in regional resections: a new anatomic study based on four hundred dissections with a complete review of the literature. *J Int Colorectal Surg* 1963;39:127–170.

77. Miller R, Bartolo DCC, Cervero F, et al. Anorectal sampling: a comparison of normal and incontinent patients. *Br J Surg* 1988;75:44–47.

78. Milligan ETC, Morgan CN. Surgical anatomy of the anal canal: with special reference to anorectal fistulae. *Lancet* 1934;2:1150–1156.

79. Miscusi G, Masoni L, Dell'Anna A, et al. Normal lymphatic drainage of the rectum and the anal canal revealed by lymphoscintigraphy. *Coloproctology* 1987;9:171–174.

80. Morgado PJ. Total mesorectal excision: a misnomer for a sound surgical approach. *Dis Colon Rectum* 1998;41:120–121.

81. Morren GL, Beets-Tan RGH, van Engelshoven JMA. Anatomy of the anal canal and perianal structures as defined by phased-array magnetic resonance imaging. *Br J Surg* 2001;88:1506–1512.

82. Morson BC, Dawson IMP. *Gastrointestinal pathology*. Oxford: Blackwell Scientific Publications, 1972:603–606.

83. Moskowitz M, Zimmerman H, Felson H. The meandering mesenteric artery of the colon. *AJR Am J Roentgenol* 1964;92:1088–1099.

84. Nano M, Dal Corso HM, Lanfranco G, et al. Contribution to the surgical anatomy of the ligaments of the rectum. *Dis Colon Rectum* 2000;43:1592–1598.

85. Nivatvongs S, Gordon PH. Surgical anatomy. In: Gordon PH, Nivatvongs S, eds. *Principle and practice of surgery for the colon, rectum and anus*. St. Louis, MO: Quality Medical Publishing, 1992:3–37.

86. Nobles VP. The development of the human anal canal. *J Anat* 1984;138:575.

87. O'Beirne J, ed. *New views of the process of defecation and their application to the pathology and treatment of diseases of the stomach, bowels and other organs.* Dublin: Hodges and Smith, 1833.
88. Oh C, Kark AE. Anatomy of the external anal sphincter. *Br J Surg* 1972;59:717–723.
89. Orkin BA. Rectal carcinoma: treatment. In: Beck DE, Wexner SD, eds. *Fundamentals of anorectal surgery.* New York: McGraw-Hill, 1992:260–369.
90. Otis WJ. Some observations on the structure of the rectum. *J Anat Physiol* 1898;32:59–63.
91. Paramore RH. The Hunterian lectures on the evolution of the pelvic floor in non-mammalian vertebrates and pronograde mammals. *Lancet* 1910;1:1393–1399, 1459–1467.
92. Parks AG. Pathogenesis and treatment of fistula-in-ano. *BMJ* 1961;1:463–469.
93. Parks AG, Porter NH, Hardcastle J. The syndrome of the descending perineum. *Proc R Soc Med* 1966;59:477–482.
94. Pemberton JH. Anatomy and physiology of the anus and rectum. In: Zuidema GD, ed. *Shackelford's surgery of the alimentary tract.* Philadelphia: WB Saunders, 1991:242–273.
95. Percy JP, Swash M, Neill ME, et al. Electrophysiological study of motor nerve supply of pelvic floor. *Lancet* 1981;1:16–17.
96. Petter O, Gruner N, Reidar N, et al. Marital status and sexual adjustment after colectomy. *Scand J Gastroenterol* 1977;12:193–197.
97. Quirke P, Durdey P, Dixon MF, et al. Local recurrence of rectal adenocarcinoma due to inadequate surgical resection: histopathological study of lateral tumour spread and surgical excision. *Lancet* 1986;1:996–998.
98. Romolo JL. Congenital lesions: intussusception and volvulus. In: Zuidema GD, ed. *Shackelford's surgery of the alimentary tract.* Philadelphia: WB Saunders, 1991:45–51.
99. Roux C. Contribution to the knowledge of the anal muscles in man. *Arch Mikr Anat* 1881;19:721–723.
100. Russell KP. Anatomy of the pelvic floor, rectum and anal canal. In: Smith LE, ed. *Practical guide to anorectal testing.* New York: Igaku-Shoin Medical Publishers, 1991:744–747.
101. Shafik A. A new concept of the anatomy of the anal sphincter mechanism and the physiology of defecation: the external anal sphincter: a triple loop system. *Invest Urol* 1975;12:412.
102. Shafik A. A new concept of the anatomy of the anal sphincter mechanism and the physiology of defecation. II. Anatomy of the levator ani muscle with special reference to puborectalis. *Invest Urol* 1975;12:175–182.
103. Shafik A. A new concept of the anatomy of the anal sphincter mechanism and the physiology of defecation. III. The longitudinal anal muscle: anatomy and role in sphincter mechanism. *Invest Urol* 1976;13:271–277.
104. Shafik A. A concept of the anatomy of the anal sphincter mechanism and the physiology of defecation. Dis Colon Rectum 1987;30:970–982.
105. Sieglbauer F. *Lehrbuch der normalen Anatomie des Menschen,* 9th ed. Wien: Urban und Schwartzenberg, 1963.
106. Skandalakis JE, Gray SW, Ricketts R. The colon and rectum. In: Skandalakis JE, Gray SW, eds. *Embryology for surgeons: the embryological basis for the treatment of congenital anomalies.* Baltimore: Williams & Wilkins, 1994:242–281.
107. Sonneland J, Anson BJ, Beaton LE. Surgical anatomy of the arterial supply to the colon from the superior mesenteric artery based upon a study of 600 specimens. *Surg Gynecol Obstet* 1958;106:385–398.
108. Stelzner F. Die Verschlubsysteme am Magen-Darm-Kanal und ihre chirurgische Bedeutung. *Acta Chir Aust* 1987;19:565–569.
109. Steward JA, Rankin FW. Blood supply of the large intestine: its surgical considerations. *Arch Surg* 1933;26:843–891.
110. Stoss F. Investigations of the muscular architecture of the rectosigmoid junction in humans. *Dis Colon Rectum* 1990;33:378–383.
111. Sudeck P. Über die Gefassversorgung des Mastdarmes in Hinsicht auf die Operative Gangran. *Munch Med Wochenschr* 1907;54:1314.
112. Swash M. Histopathology of pelvic floor muscles in pelvic floor disorders. In: Henry MM, Swash M, eds. *Coloproctology and the pelvic floor.* London: Butterworth-Heinemann, 1992:173–183.
113. Tjandra JJ, Milsom JW, Stolfi VM, et al. Endoluminal ultrasound defines anatomy of the anal canal and pelvic floor. *Dis Colon Rectum* 1992;35:465–470.
114. Tobin CE, Benjamin JA. Anatomical and surgical restudy of Denonvilliers' fascia. *Surg Gynecol Obstet* 1945;80:373–388.
115. Torsoli A, Ramorino ML, Crucioli V. The relationships between anatomy and motor activity of the colon. *Am J Dig Dis* 1968;13:462–467.
116. Wakeley CPG. The position of the vermiform appendix as ascertained by an analysis of 10,000 cases. *J Anat* 1983;67:277–283.
117. Walsh PC, Schlegel PN. Radical pelvic surgery with preservation of sexual function. *Ann Surg* 1988;208:391–400.
118. Wang Q, Shi W, Zhao Y, et al. New concepts in severe presacral hemorrhage during proctectomy. *Arch Surg* 1985;120:1013–1020.
119. Weinstein M, Roberts M. Sexual potency following surgery for rectal carcinoma: a follow-up of 44 patients. *Ann Surg* 1977;185:295–300.
120. Wendell-Smith CP. Studies on the morphology of the pelvic floor. Ph.D. thesis, University of London, 1967.
121. Wexner SD, Cheape JD, Jorge JMN, et al. Prospective assessment of biofeedback for the treatment of paradoxical puborectalis contraction syndrome. *Dis Colon Rectum* 1992;35:145–150.
122. Wexner SD, Daniel N, Jagelman DG. Colectomy for constipation: physiologic investigation is the key to success. *Dis Colon Rectum* 1991;34:851–856.
123. Wexner SD, Jorge JMN, Nogueras JJ, et al. Colorectal physiological tests: use or abuse of technology? *Eur J Surg* 1994;160:167–174.
124. Williams AB, Bartram CI, Halligan S, et al. Endosonographic anatomy of the normal anal compared with endocoil magnetic resonance imaging. *Dis Colon Rectum* 2002;45:176–183.
125. Williamson RCN, Mortensen NJMcC. Anatomy of the large intestine. In: Kirsner JB, Shorter RG, eds. *Diseases of the colon, rectum and anal canal.* Baltimore: Williams & Wilkins, 1987:1–22.
126. Wilson PM. Anchoring mechanisms of the anorectal region. *S Afr Med J* 1967;141:1138–1143.
127. Wood BA, Kelly AJ. Anatomy of the anal sphincters and pelvic floor. In: Henry MM, Swash M, eds. *Coloproctology and the pelvic floor.* London: Butterworth-Heinemann, 1992:3–19.
128. Zama N, Fazio VW, Jagelman DG, et al. Efficacy of pelvic packing in maintaining hemostasis after rectal excision for cancer. *Dis Colon Rectum* 1988;31:923–928.

Physiology of the Colon

Guest Contributor: Eric J. Daniels

Eric Daniels is a general surgery resident at the University of California, Los Angeles. I am delighted to include his contribution, which provides an overview of this often poorly understood subject. Physiology of the rectum and anus is also addressed in individual chapters as part of each pathologic process. Additionally, the reader is referred to Chapters 4 and 6 for further discussion concerning evaluation and physiologic studies.

MLC

> Man and the animals are merely
> a passage and channel for food,
> a tomb for other animals,
> a haven for the dead,
> giving life by the death of others,
> a coffer full of corruption.
>
> Leonardo da Vinci: *Codice Atlantico,* 76

The study of large bowel physiology has historically been overshadowed by concerted efforts to comprehend the workings of the stomach and small intestine. Despite this indifference, which is perhaps in part a consequence of the knowledge that human beings can thrive in the absence of a colon, we have become aware that the large intestine is responsible for maintaining important homeostatic functions. The primary physiologic purposes of the large bowel include the following: further breakdown of ingested materials by microfloral metabolism, absorption of water and electrolytes, secretion of electrolytes and mucus, storage of semisolid matter, and propulsion of feces toward the rectum and anus. These colonic functions act in concert to respond to the needs of the body while concomitantly producing fecal material suitable for evacuation. For example, although the digestive functions of the large bowel are dwarfed by the contributions of the small intestine, the absorptive and secretory capacities of the colonic mucosa are critical for regulating the intraluminal fluid volume and contributing to serum electrolyte balance. In addition, the role of the colon in intermittent storage and propulsion of semisolid matter is central to normal defecation and is the consequence of complex neural and hormonal interactions. The purpose of this chapter is to present a current, general view of normal large bowel physiology

to facilitate the discussion of colonic pathophysiologic processes presented subsequently.

FUNCTIONAL CLASSIFICATION

The large bowel is approximately 150 cm (5 ft) in length and consists of the vermiform appendix, cecum, colon (ascending, transverse, descending, sigmoid), and rectum. This somewhat arbitrary segmentation of the large bowel is not strictly anatomic, because it is now widely appreciated that the large intestine is a heterogeneous organ with regional, biochemical, pharmacologic, and thus functional differences.

Cecum and Ascending Colon (Right Colon)

Digested material entering the large intestine at the ileocecal junction remains in the cecum and right colon for an extended period of time. Here the resting propulsion rate is only 1 cm/hour.[96] This retention and mixing of ileal effluent permit aerobic and anaerobic metabolism of residual carbohydrate and protein by the intestinal flora, thereby producing multiple byproducts, most of which are then absorbed through the remaining colon. In addition to being the primary site for bacterial fermentation, the ascending colon (along with the transverse colon) is involved in regulating intraluminal fluid volume as well as sodium and water absorption.[37,38] The importance of these colonic functions can be appreciated by reviewing recorded motility patterns, which demonstrate frequent retropulsive waves extending from the transverse colon back toward the cecum.[15,96]

Transverse Colon

The transverse colon is generally believed to serve as a rapid conduit between the proximal (right) and distal (left) components of the large bowel. This belief is supported by the finding that the basal electrical rhythm and muscle-generated pressure waves in this segment occur with a greater frequency than is identified in the right colon. This observation suggests a rapid, propulsive function.[19,118,122] As mentioned previously, the transverse colon is also an important site for sodium and water absorption, a function that is critical to volume regulation.

Left Colon

The left colon is the site for final modulation of intraluminal contents before evacuation. The diminished rate of fluid and electrolyte transfer seen in the descending colon is ultimately a result of distinct protein ion channels in the luminal (apical) and serosal (basolateral) membranes of mucosal cells, which exhibit different biochemical and pharmacologic properties when compared with those of the ascending colon. The distal large intestine also is thought to exhibit a reservoir function or storage capacity, which some believe is important in maintaining anal continence. Although the concept is somewhat controversial, it theoretically relies on the physical barrier of the sigmoid angulations and myoelectrical differences between the sigmoid colon and rectum. This is discussed later. With respect to the rectum, *in vitro* studies have demonstrated that little or no net absorption occurs there.[37,38]

DIGESTION

Digestion within the large bowel is an often overlooked issue, given the enormous capacity of the small intestine in this regard. However, despite its poorly recognized participation in the breakdown of foodstuffs to fulfill energy requirements, the healthy colon is capable of salvaging calories from poorly absorbed carbohydrates and proteins.

Flora of the Large Intestine

The digestive processes of the colon are a consequence of the microorganisms that colonize the bowel and thereby participate in a symbiotic relationship with the host. Whereas yeast and other fungi are normally present in very small numbers,[30] bacteria clearly dominate the lumen. In humans, the large intestine is the primary site of bacterial colonization, with more than 400 different species of bacteria identified[46] Bacterial colonization begins in infancy and occurs predominantly in the cecum and right colon. Studies reveal up to 10^{12} bacteria per gram of wet fece[103] Given this amount, it is not surprising that bacteria make up 40% to 55% of fecal solids in individuals consuming a typical Western die.[113]

The primary tasks of gut flora can be divided into metabolic, trophic, and protective functions. Metabolic functions include fermentation of nondigestible dietary residue and endogenous mucus, production of short-chain fatty acids (SCFAs), and production of vitamin K. Trophic functions comprise controlling epithelial cell proliferation and differentiation as well as homoeostasis of the immune system. The protective activity of the colonic flora stems from the ability to serve as a barrier of colonization against pathogens. Although these functions are robust in healthy individuals, a breakdown of the dynamic relationship between the gut flora and its host may lead to disease states.

Guarner and Malagedlada reviewed the role of gut flora health and disease.[58] The authors note that a dysfunction in the barrier activity of gut flora can result in the translocation of many viable microorganisms, particularly the gram-negative aerobic genera. Once beyond the epithelial reef, the organisms can travel to extraintestinal organs via the lymphatic highway.[58] Dissemination of enteric bacteria can lead to sepsis, shock, multisystem organ failure, and ultimately death for the patient. The rates of positive blood cultures are significantly higher in individuals with conditions such as intestinal obstruction and inflammatory bowel disease.[74] O'Boyle and colleagues reported that bacterial translocation is associated with an increase in postoperative sepsis.[88] In addition to transocation of bacteria, gut flora have been implicated to play an active role in carcinogenesis and inflammatory bowel disease. Bacteria belonging to the *Bacteroides* and *Clostridium* genera have been shown to increase the incidence of tumor formation in laboratory animals.[65] In patients with Crohn's disease and ulcerative colitis, there is increased secretion of immunoglobulin G, a class of antibody that can damage intestinal mucosa through activation of the complement cascade.[12,77]

Within the complex ecosystem of the large intestine, certain groups of bacteria thrive over others. In principle, those able to transform variable amounts and types of substrate into energy are likely to be present in large proportions. Although *Bacteroides* organisms (gram-negative rods) are most commonly identified, the gram-positive *Eubacterium* and *Bifidobacterium* are also present in large numbers, along with several gram-positive cocci and *Clostridium* species.[30,46,84] It is axiomatic that the surgeon's knowledge of normal colonic flora is paramount to proper antibiotic management for both prophylactic and postoperative situations.

Substrates for Fermentation

Nondigestible Starch

To appreciate the end products of bacterial fermentation, one must first look at the substrate that passes through the ileocecal junction and is presented to the microorganisms. Quantitatively, the most important is nonhydrolyzed or resistant starch. Christl and colleagues performed breath hydrogen and methane studies using whole-body calorimetry to measure undigested polysaccharide reaching the large intestine.[23] The authors noted that starch is to some degree incompletely digested in the small bowel and is passed onto the ascending colon. Others have confirmed this observation.[44,73] Generally, it is accepted that approximately 10% of ingested starch will elude small bowel digestion to reach the colon and be available for fermentation in individuals consuming a Western diet.[30]

Nonstarch Polysaccharides

Nonstarch polysaccharides represent another class of substrate available for bacterial metabolism. These molecules are the derivatives of plant material and include cellulose as well as noncellulose substrates. The degree of nonstarch polysaccharide metabolism is dependent on several physiologic circumstances. For example, the smaller and more hydrophilic the substrate, the more readily digestible it is.[62,112] This and other physiologic variables, such as transit time, ultimately determine the extent of cellulose and noncellulose breakdown by the resident flora. Topping and Clifton contrasted the role of resistant starch and nondigestible starch in human colonic function.[102] The authors viewed the actions of resistant starch and nondigestible starch in the context of a balance between luminal passage and fermentation. Fiber-rich foods, with a high content of insoluble nonstarch polysaccharides, are not as fermentable by microflora. As such, fiber-rich foods serve well as laxatives. On the other hand, most resistant starches are readily fermentable by large bowel microflora, giving rise to the SCFAs discussed later. Topping and Clifton state that the greatest difference between resistant starches and nonstarch polysaccharides lies in relation to cancer risk.[117] The authors report that whereas the protective effect of resistant starches to chemically induced cancers is inconsistent in small animals,[7,61] there exist strong epidemiologic data pointing to a negative relationship between total starch consumption and large bowel neoplasms.[111,116] However, evidence of a discrete benefit for fiber is not as strong, with several low-risk populations ingesting little fiber.[63,71,89] The authors conclude that although the protective effect of resistant starch is encouraging, the limitations of methodology and small animal models cannot justify a recommendation to increase dietary levels at this time.

Other Substrates

Although most of the substrate made available to the colonic bacteria consists of the starch and nonstarch polysaccharides mentioned earlier, other substances do pass into the cecum and are subsequently metabolized. For example, sugar and sugar alcohols, such as lactose, raffinose, lactulose, and sorbitol, are readily metabolized by the bowel microorganisms.[30,114] In addition to polysaccharides, various peptide substrates are made available for bacterial digestion. Poorly absorbed protein sources include elastin, collagen, and albumins, and most abundant are the pancreas-derived proteases.[30] In contrast, urea and ammonia are not generally available as nitrogen sources for the colonic flora.[48] Overall, the daily ileal effluent will make available 6 to 18 g of nitrogen-containing compounds for bacterial fermentation, compared with 8 to 40 g of carbohydrate.[30]

Products of Bacterial Metabolism

The principal products of microorganism fermentation of polysaccharides in the large bowel are SCFAs or volatile fatty acids. The production of SCFAs decreases from the proximal to the distal colon, an observation that can be most likely attributed to the different bacterial populations in these regions. These fatty acids contain from one to six carbons and are the predominant colonic anions. The three most abundant are acetate, propionate, and butyrate, with their production accounting for to 95% of total SCFA generation.[30]

It has long been thought that dietary intake should have profound effects on fermentation products. However, several investigators have noted that variations in diet have only a minimal effect on SCFA production. Saunders and Wiggins employed three different sugars—mannitol, lactulose, and raffinose—and measured SCFA production.[107] They found no significant variability among the different sugar substrates. This finding has been confirmed by others through a variety of fermentation substrates, including wheat bran.[29] On the basis of these metabolic studies, it has been calculated that the conversion for the amount of SCFAs produced per unit weight of carbohydrate is 50%.

Short-Chain Fatty Acid Absorption

More than 90% of SCFAs produced by bacterial fermentation are taken up by the colonic mucosal cells.[81,95] In small animal models, approximately 60% of the uptake is by simple diffusion of protonated, neutral SCFA. The remainder of uptake (ionized SCFA) occurs by active, cellular uptake.[47] However, the mechanism for uptake by the colonic epithelium remains unresolved. It is clear, however, that the absorption mechanism differs from that of the long-chain fatty acids absorbed in the small intestine. For example, long-chain fatty acids require emulsification with bile salts.

Experimental models have been used to attempt to clarify the transport mechanisms involved. A large body of evidence exists pointing to the passive diffusion of these fatty acids toward the serosa.[24,105] As mentioned earlier, SCFAs are weak acids with negative logs of dissociation constant ranging from 4.75 to 4.87, and most of these molecules exist in their ionized form at a pH higher than 5. As charged species, the SCFAs would be unable to traverse the hydrophobic environment of the apical membrane. However, studies of the mammalian gastrointestinal tract have shown SCFAs to be absorbed rapidly at a pH of 7.[2] In light of this apparent contradiction, some investigators have pursued the possible protonization (binding of a hydrogen ion) of the anionic form of the SCFA, rendering the molecule neutral and thus better able to cross the lipophilic membrane. One proposed mechanism is that protons are generated from the conversion of carbon dioxide and water by intramucosal carbonic anhydrase. This would account for the accumulation of bicarbonate seen with SCFA absorption.[4,104] An additional source of protons may be found in the presence of a sodium ion-proton antiport (exchange), an idea supported by the fact that SCFA absorption has been reported to increase sodium and water absorption.[105] Using *in situ* perfusion of guinea pig colon, Oltmer and von Engelhardt reported that inhibition of the apical proton antiport and carbonic anhydrase systems resulted in decreased SCFA absorption.[90] Although neither of these mechanisms can completely explain SCFA absorption, their existence is consistent with the fact that SCFA transport is associated with increased luminal pH, increased bicarbonate ion concentration, and enhanced sodium absorption.[60]

Outside of the passive mechanisms discussed earlier, the presence of an apical, carrier-mediated anionic exchange involving SCFAs and bicarbonate ion has been suggested.[79,121] Harig and colleagues used human luminal vesicles to investigate the transport of *N*-butyrate.[60] The authors found that butyrate transport was minimal in the presence of an inward pH gradient but significantly increased by an outward bicarbonate ion gradient. Furthermore, the effects of sodium and chloride on transport were negligible. The authors concluded that the primary mechanism for butyrate transport appears to be through a bicarbonate-SCFA antiport system independent of sodium transport or bicarbonate-chloride anion exchange. As more becomes known about the mechanisms of SCFA transport, it is increasingly clear that this function is a heterogeneous one, with observed segmental differences.[86,110]

Additional investigations are being conducted on the transport mechanisms responsible for SCFA absorption. This interest is being stimulated by the potential utility of such knowledge in clinical situations, such as promoting caloric intake in patients with short-bowel syndrome, developing SCFA enemas for patients with ulcerative colitis, and understanding mechanisms underlying diarrhea and even colonic neoplasms.

Physiologic Actions of Short-Chain Fatty Acids

The SCFAs produced as a result of bacterial fermentation of poorly absorbed polysaccharides play several important roles in large bowel function. SCFAs are relatively weak acids. Therefore, higher concentrations of SCFAs lower the luminal pH. Lower pH values can alter the growth profiles of pH-sensitive pathogenic bacteria such as *Escherichia coli* and *Salmonella*.[20] As such, SCFAs have been shown to assist in the treatment of infectious diarrhea. Furthermore, elevation of fecal SCFAs has been shown to diminish the fluid loss and speed of remission during the active phase of cholera.[94]

These acids are readily absorbed by the columnar epithelium, as discussed earlier.[13,27,28] Once absorbed, the SCFAs have been reported to contribute up to 7% of the basal metabolic requirements of humans.[28] In fact, the colonic epithelium derives almost 75% of its energy needs from these fatty acids through metabolism to carbon dioxide, ketone bodies, and lipid precursors.[100,101] In addition to luminal nutrition, SCFAs have been investigated for their antiinflammatory properties as well as their antitumor effects.[1] They have also been shown to increase regional blood flow and have a demonstrable effect upon gastrointestinal muscular activity. Rectal infusion of SCFA into human surgical patients leads to a 1.5- to 5-fold increase in splanchnic blood flow as well as to a decrease in gastric tone leading to volume expansion.[85,102] Additionally, the absorption of SCFAs is tied closely to the transport of bicarbonate, sodium, and water, thus providing a mechanism for the regulation of intraluminal volume.[82,108]

Other Products of Noncarbohydrate Fermentation

The fermentation of peptides by microorganisms results in substances such as SCFAs, branched-chain fatty acids, isobutyrate, and methylbutyrate. However, not all end products of peptide metabolism are of benefit to the organism. For example, the deamination of amino acids gives rise to ammonia, which has been demonstrated to have toxic effects on colonic epithelium by altering normal cell metabolism.[123,127] In addition, the catabolism of amino acids results in the production of phenols, indoles, and amines, which have been implicated in disease states such as hepatic coma and colorectal cancer.[39,40,91]

Conclusion

The digestive processes that take place in the large bowel are clearly focused on the activities of the colonic flora. The surgeon's interest in these normal metabolic processes is obvious, because disruption of this otherwise stable community by either pathologic or surgical intervention may lead to disease states discussed later in this text.

COLONIC ABSORPTION AND SECRETION

The absorption and secretion of water, mucus, and electrolytes, particularly sodium, are complex and central processes of normal colonic activity. These processes determine the electrolyte and volume content of feces. However, the capacity of the colon to absorb and digest material is not uniform, with the proximal mucosa exhibiting different properties from its distal counterpart. Although colonic epithelium does not participate in active glucose or amino acid absorption,[9] as occurs in the small intestine, the mechanistic and functional segmental differences of these cells are of importance to the surgeon, because the diverse colonic resection procedures have various consequences. As with the evaluation of absorption and secretion in other organs, such as the small intestine and kidney, study of transport in the colon is directed toward an understanding of the epithelial phenomena.

Sodium Absorption

Animal studies have demonstrated that sodium movement across the colonic wall involves overcoming two opposing forces. First, a formidable concentration gradient opposes the movement of sodium. This is a consequence of the higher sodium concentration of plasma in comparison with the colonic lumen.[126] In addition to the uphill concentration gradient, measurement of the transmural potential differences reveals an electronegative lumen (5 to 15 mV), which serves to retard the movement of sodium across the membrane.[31] Despite these two forces, measurements of normal daily fecal water show 1 to 5 mEq of sodium, representing more than 90% absorption of the 200 mEq of sodium found in the ileal effluent.[95,108] One must conclude from these perfusion studies that sodium transport is an active process.

Transport Mechanisms

Electrogenic Transport

The movement of sodium across a membrane resulting in a separation of charge is a common method of so-dium transport widely known to be active in small intestine and kidney epithelia. This type of transport has also been reported to be present in the distal human colon.[26,57] The mechanism involves the movement of sodium from the lumen into the mucosal cell down an electrochemical gradient. The sodium ions, unable to permeate the phospholipid membrane, pass through protein channels characterized by their sensitivity to amiloride, a sodium transport blocker and aldosterone antagonist.[125] These amiloride-sensitive epithelial sodium channels consist of three homologous subunits—α, β, and γ—with a small unitary conductance of approximately 5 picosiemens (pS).[75] The permeability of sodium across the apical membrane is dependent on several physiologic factors. One is the intracellular sodium concentration, shown to be inversely related to apical membrane sodium permeability.[120] In order to ensure an adequate concentration difference, this value must be kept relatively low compared with the luminal sodium concentration. This challenge is met by the sodium/potassium-adenosine triphosphatase (ATPase) located on the basolateral aspect of the colonic epithelial cells. Therefore, the net movement of sodium across the colonic wall through this active mechanism is a combination of both apical and basolateral membrane activities. Thus, regulation of this method of transport can be targeted to either apical or basolateral processes.

Electroneutral Absorption

Bulk transport of sodium chloride in colonic epithelium is secondary to electroneutral absorption. Several lines of experimental evidence support the belief that this electroneutral process occurs primarily through the coupling of parallel, apical sodium-hydrogen and chloride-bicarbonate ion exchanges.[11] For example, the addition of a carbonic anhydrase inhibitor blocks the net flux of sodium and chloride, presumably by inhibiting the intracellular production of necessary protons and bicarbonate ions.[10] Further studies have indicated the existence of several types of sodium-hydrgen as well as chloride-bicarbonate exchanges, all having an impact on the electroneutral absorption of sodium chloride and mucosal pH in the colonic epithelium.[70]

Effects of Aldosterone

For decades, aldosterone has been known to have marked effects on epithelial transport activities, including but not limited to acceleration of sodium absorption and sodium/potassium-ATPase rates.[18,51,119,124] These effects are believed to be brought about primarily through stimulation of sodium absorption by the electrogenic mechanism discussed earlier. This belief coincides well with the fact that aldosterone has been repeatedly shown to increase the colonic transpotential differences.[41]

As a steroid hormone, aldosterone crosses the cell membrane and binds to an intracellular receptor. This ligand-receptor interaction eventually leads to the events seen empirically. In the distal colon of animals treated with mineralocorticoids, a large increase in the β and γ subunits of amiloride-sensitive sodium channels is observed.[75] This upregulation of electoneutral sodium absorption is paralleled by downregulation of electrogenic absorption, shedding light on why no significant electrogenic sodium absorption is seen in the proximal colon, despite the presence of aldosterone receptors. Although much emphasis has been placed on the ability of aldosterone to augment sodium permeability and to increase the rate of ATPase activity, the specific roles played by aldosterone in mammalian tissue remain undefined.[80]

Segmental Heterogeneity

As stressed earlier in this chapter, the colon is anatomically and functionally segmented. The aforementioned mechanisms of sodium absorption and the effects of aldosterone on these actions have been elucidated primarily from studies of mammalian distal bowel. Investigations focused on mammalian proximal colon reveal differing modes of transport and regulation. For instance, studies of rat proximal colocytes using voltage clamp techniques have demonstrated that sodium absorption is electroneutral, yet no net chloride movement is measured.[49] In addition, the application of aldosterone upregulates sodium-chloride electroneutral absorption, in clear contrast to the electrogenic induction seen in the distal colon.[49] These unique features, along with distinct mechanisms of transport seen in the rabbit proximal colon,[109] naturally raise many unanswered questions and underscore the lack of definitive sodium transport characterization. Consequently, the continuing investigation of colonic (specifically cecal) sodium transport is undoubtedly warranted.

Chloride Ion Absorption

The mechanism of chloride ion transport across the human colonic apical membrane remains without clear definition, appearing to result from several processes. Chloride absorption in the colon is generally accepted to occur by means of an energy-independent, passive mechanism. This process relies on the negative charge of the ion and the diffusion potential generated by electrogenic sodium absorption. The presence of the chloride ion in an environment where the gastrointestinal lumen is electronegative establishes a force driving chloride across the apical membrane. Davis and coworkers, investigating human colon *in vivo*, opined that upward of 75% of total chloride absorption occurs via this favorable electrochemical gradient.[32] These authors believe that the remaining 25% occurs through an active, apical chloride-bicarbonate antiport. Additional evidence for the existence of this active antiport comes from multiple investigative approaches. These include perfusion studies demonstrating that filling the luminal space with a chloride solution results in a decrease in chloride ion concentration, with a concomitant increase in luminal bicarbonate ion concentration.[8] Furthermore, Mahajan and colleagues used a rapid millipore filtration system to study the uptake of $^{36}Cl^-$ in human proximal colonic apical vesicles.[78] They found that luminally directed bicarbonate gradients stimulated the uptake of chloride ions and concluded that an electroneutral chloride-bicarbonate transport contributes to the primary mechanism of sodium chloride absorption in the human proximal colon. In rat distal colon, Rajendran and Binder described two distinct ion exchanges (chloride-bicarbonate and chloride-hydroxyl) as the mechanism responsible for chloride uptake.[93] The authors postulated that these two ion channels possess unique functional features, with one involved in chloride transcellular transport and the other concerned with intracellular pH maintenance.[93] Additional studies are needed to explore the detailed mechanism, regulation, and relative contributions of both active and passive chloride transport.

With respect to colonic chloride secretion, the cystic fibrosis transmembrane conductance regulator (CFTR) (mutated in patients with CF) is primarily responsible.[1] Numerous studies have demonstrated that CFTR is the primary chloride channel in airways, sweat ducts, and the colon. As such, patients with CF have mutations in CFTR and have impaired secretion of chloride as well as diminished absorption of sodium in the colon through modulation of the sodium electroneutral absorption mechanism.

Water Movement

One of the central functions of the large intestine is to control the level of fecal water. Average ileocecal flow for a healthy individual is approximately 1,500 to 2,000 mL/day.[33] Of this amount, only 100 to 150 mL of water appears in the stool. The colon harbors a tremendous reserve transport capacity and is capable of absorbing as much as 5 to 6 L over a 24-hour period if challenged.[33] Whereas water absorption is affected by the volume and flow of luminal contents, it is generally believed to follow the osmotic gradient established by the absorption of electrolytes.[33] For example, if the gastrointestinal lumen is perfused with a hypertonic mannitol solution, water will flow into the lumen, lending support to its passive movement.[8] Evidence suggests that intestinal aquaporin channels, as well as CFTR, may play a role in colonic fluid absorption and fecal dehydration.[1,68] Ultimately, regulating the amount of water absorption is accomplished by any mediator of luminal flow, fluid composition, or net electrolyte transport. A basic appreciation of colonic water-absorbing capacity is fundamental to the understanding of the possible causes of diarrhea.[92]

Bicarbonate Transport

As previously indicated in the discussion of sodium and chloride absorption, transport of bicarbonate ion across the apical membrane of colonic epithelium is generally considered a secretory process involving a chloride-bicarbonate ion antiport. To appreciate the mechanism of this system, the transmural potential difference and charged nature of the ion species must be considered. However, the measured intraluminal bicarbonate ion concentration is higher than can be generated by the available electrochemical forces under physiologic conditions. This suggests an energy-requiring secretory process.[80] Evidence for this active transport mechanism comes from experiments in which a significant reduction of chloride within the gastrointestinal lumen results in a reduced rate of bicarbonate secretion.[54] Clearly, the most likely source of the intracellular bicarbonate ion is the conversion of carbon dioxide and water by carbonic anhydrase, whose levels have been found to be elevated in colonic mucosal cells.[17]

Potassium Transport

The mechanisms of colonic potassium transport have historically been poorly defined and confusing. For example, perfusion studies have pointed to the passive absorption and secretion of potassium,[36,56] whereas other *in vivo* reports using small intraluminal dialysis bags found evidence against diffusion and in support of active mechanisms. However, since the mid-1990s, numerous efforts have been successfully undertaken to elucidate better the mechanisms involved in the movement of potassium. As with other colonic functions, the transport mechanisms associated with potassium transport have been found to be segmental, with proximal mucosal cells behaving distinctly from their distal counterparts.[25] Binder and Sandle have used this point to explain the inconsistency of previous *in vivo* perfusion studies, postulating that experiments not targeted to specific segments of the colon can provide at best only limited data.[11]

Foster and coworkers, measuring potassium currents in isolated segments of proximal rat colon, demonstrated a net potassium secretion.[50] The authors found that this secretory mechanism was abolished by sodium removal, stimulated by aldosterone, not inhibited by amiloride, and probably electrogenic. Additional ion flux studies have shown potassium secretion to be abolished by the addition of ouabain, an inhibitor of the sodium/ potassium-ATPase pump.[59,80] These results, and similar studies, point to a secretory mechanism in which energy is used to drive a basolateral sodium/potassium or sodium/ potassium/chloride pump, which, in turn, promotes the diffusion of potassium ions down an electrochemical gradient into the lumen through apical, potassium-permeable ion channels. Other investigators have confirmed this mechanism.[34]

The same methods used to ascertain the mechanism for potassium secretion have been applied to discern the mechanisms for absorption. McCabe and colleagues measured ion fluxes in 16 pairs of rabbit descending colon tissue.[80] Through the addition of ouabain and 2,4-dinitrophenol, the authors found that the distal colon was able both to absorb and to secrete potassium. In a similar study by Halm and Frizzell, potassium absorption was inhibited by the addition of barium to the serosal surface.[59] The authors concluded that these findings were consistent with an energy-dependent apical uptake of potassium, with potassium exit occurring through a basolateral, barium-sensitive ion channel. Others have proposed a similar mechanism.[35] As a result of these and other studies, potassium absorption is believed to be predominantly a phenomenon of the distal colon that is electroneutral, sodium independent, and mediated through an apical potassium/hydrogen-ATPase and a basolateral potassium ion channel.

However, not all data are consistent with these findings.[25] Feldman and Ickes reported their experience using ion-specific electrodes to measure ion fluxes in segments of rat distal colon.[45] The authors applied various chemical mediators and were unable to correlate proton and potassium ion fluxes. The authors postulated that these currents occur through separate pathways. Because the maintenance of potassium levels is critical to proper cell and body function, continuing interest in colonic regulation of this ion is of obvious importance.

COLONIC MOTILITY

The phenomenon of gastrointestinal motility integrates numerous complex tissue functions, including smooth muscle electrical activity, contractile activity, intraluminal pressure, and both extrinsic and intrinsic neural coordination. However, a clear understanding of the normal function, underlying motility, and regulatory patterns is often unappreciated.

The failure to comprehend the intricacies of colonic motility can be attributed to the following circumstances:

- Intermittent and irregular nature of activity
- Absence of a reliable, consistent animal model
- Lack of ready accessibility to the entire organ
- Heterogeneity of colonic function

In the face of these limitations, certain techniques have been employed to study colonic motility. Three methods of measurement have been employed—colonic manometry, radiographic observation (i.e., radiopaque markers, fluoroscopy, defecography), and scintigraphy.[53,99] Through these modalities, investigators have reported macroscopic patterns of motility that can be seen in numerous mammalian species. For the practicing surgeon, an understanding of basic patterns of motility can lead to an enhanced appreciation of the functional gastrointestinal disorders, including functional dyspepsia, irritable bowel syndrome, and constipation.

Patterns of Motility

It is well known that patterns of motility illustrate considerable variability from one segment of bowel to another. Early investigators, by using contrast radiography and by direct observation in animals, observed a unique antiperistaltic pattern of ring contractions in the right colon.[15,43] From these findings and other studies, it has been proposed that this retrograde movement serves to retard the progression of contents, in order to encourage thorough mixing, microbial metabolism, and absorption of substances.[96] Although investigations have shown that segmental movements of the ascending bowel promote mixing and absorption, the presence of a retrograde pattern of motility in the *human* proximal colon has not been definitively demonstrated.[42] Furthermore, Krevsky and colleagues, through the use of colonic transit scintigraphy in seven normal volunteers, showed that the cecum and ascending colon empty rapidly and suggested that the transverse colon may be the site of colonic storage.[69]

An additional pattern observed by early investigators[15,43] and confirmed by others[98] is described by intermittent, contractile waves that result in a segmented appearance of the colon. These tonic or rhythmic contractions have been observed to move luminal contents slowly in an aboral direction. In addition, these contractions propel material in a back-and-forth pattern over short distances, thereby encouraging mixing and kneading of fecal matter.

The smooth muscle wall of the large intestine has also been shown to generate strong, propulsive, contractile movements over a large area. These forceful waves of contraction have been termed mass movement. Because these waves are infrequent, it is only through recent technical developments, permitting prolonged recording of myoelectrical and contractile activity, that this phenomenon has been observed and studied.[6] Increased electrical activity and mass propulsion are initiated at the transverse colon and seem to occur primarily after awakening or following the intake of food.[52,64,97] Narducci and coworkers reported their experience with 14 healthy individuals in whom motor activity of the transverse, descending, and sigmoid colon was recorded for 24 hours by means of colonoscopically positioned catheters.[87] The authors reported that all but two of the patients demonstrated isolated, high-amplitude (200 mm Hg) contractions at 1 cm/sec that propagated over long distances. In agreement with the findings of other investigations, the majority of these contractions occurred after awakening and were associated with the urge to defecate.

Regulation of Motility

Myogenic Regulation

Electrical slow waves are the result of the rhythmic alterations in smooth muscle membrane potentials as recorded on electromyogram studies. In the colon, these slow waves are of variable amplitude and frequency but do not necessarily correlate with the contraction of muscle fibers.[53] Contraction of the muscle occurs only with those slow waves that carry a strong initiating depolarization or spike. Christensen characterizes the slow wave as a mechanism to fix muscular contraction to a given time and place, and, as such, the slow wave regulates this contractility.[21] The cells responsible for production of slow waves are known as the pacemaker cells of the colon. Studies using mammalian models have demonstrated the origin of these pacemaker cells to be in the circular muscle layer of the colonic wall.[16] Using phase-contrast microscopy and patch clamp techniques, which allow for the detailed study of electrical properties of isolated cell membranes, Langton and coworkers provided evidence that the interstitial cells of Cajal are the actual, spontaneous pacesetters of the colon.[72] The same authors propose that the mechanism for spontaneous depolarization appears to be sodium-independent but does require calcium.[72] Camilleri, in his review of functional disorders, points out evidence that the interstitial cells of Cajal are involved in the pathophysiology underlying constipation, both in acquired slow-transit constipation without colonic dilatation to megacolon and in neonatal colonic pseudoobstruction.[14]

Electromyographic studies have been undertaken in several mammalian models, particularly the cat, to correlate the observed macroscopic patterns of contraction with the underlying myoelectrical activity. Investigations of this type have demonstrated a frequency gradient of slow waves generated by a single, variably placed pacemaker in the transverse colon.[22] In this model, slow waves propagated toward the cecum (away from the pacemaker), whereas migrating spike bursts moved toward the rectum.

Additional myoelectrical studies have been conducted in the human colon in an effort to discover similar patterns of muscle activity. In most of these investigations, slow-wave activity has been demonstrated to be intermittent. Some of these, through the use of both electrodes and intraluminal probes, have demonstrated the presence of contractile activity in the low-frequency range.[52,106] It has been suggested that this type of electrical activity produces the observed colonic segmentation that may be attributed to these short, bidirectional contractions.[66] Continued investigation of myoelectrical behavior in the human colon has revealed migrating bursts of contractions occurring over long lengths of colon that are likely associated with mass movements.[52,55] These studies have provided insight into *in vivo* colonic motility. Some authors, however, express caution regarding the interpretation of such studies because of a lack of *in vitro* evidence, variability of recording sites, and segmental heterogeneity of the colon.[21]

Neural Regulation

From numerous pharmacologic and histologic studies, four types of external nerves have been found to be active in colonic muscle.[21] They are cholinergic and noncholinergic *excitatory* nerves and adrenergic and nonadrenergic *inhibitory* nerves.[15] As with so many colonic functions, a clear understanding of the nerves involved and of their mechanisms of action is thus far an unattained ideal.

Cholinergic innervation of the large bowel is provided by the vagus and the sacral nerves. The main parasympathetic supply arises from the second and third sacral roots, innervating the distal colon and rectum. The vagus nerve, carrying cranial parasympathetic supply, is generally believed to innervate the ascending colon. An important component of this nerve carries the afferent supply from the colon. In fact, the afferent supply is reported to contain ten times as many fibers as the efferent.[55] In addition, animal studies have shown that afferent fibers of the vagus nerve contain the following neuropeptides: substance P, somatostatin, gastrin, cholecystokinin, and vasoactive inhibitory peptide.[76]

Vagal innervation of the myenteric plexus, which controls the intrinsic neural regulation of motility, is believed to contain two types of neurons.[3] In addition to the well-characterized preganglionic cholinergic nerve, the vagus supply to the colon is believed to contain a preganglionic, noncholinergic, nonadrenergic neuron. This type of neuron is believed to synapse with inhibitory neurons of the myenteric plexus and use vasoactive inhibitory peptide as a neurotransmitter. It is worth mentioning that several pharmacologic agents have been reported to improve postoperative ileus by increasing parasympathetic activity.[115] The best known of these, cisapride, which promotes the release of acetylcholine at the mesenteric plexus, was removed from the United States market secondary to several instances of cardiac arrhythmias.[83]

Sympathetic innervation of the colon begins with cell bodies located in the dorsal horn of the lumbar spinal cord. The axons from these nerves course through several pathways to synapse with postganglionic adrenergic neurons found in the celiac, superior, and inferior mesenteric ganglia. Most of these fibers find their way to the array of ganglia making up the inferior mesenteric plexus.[55,67] Large numbers of postganglionic nerves arise from the inferior mesenteric ganglia and pass on to innervate the colon as the lumbar colonic nerves. Segmental organization of these nerves has been reported.[66] Cell bodies in T-10 to T-12 supply the proximal colon, those in L-1 to L-2 supply the distal colon, and cell bodies in T-12 to L-1 innervate the midcolon.

The sympathetic nervous system is well known to exhibit an inhibitory influence on the colon, as evidenced by the fact that disruption of pelvic sympathetic flow results in colonic contraction. In addition to efferent adrenergic nerves, the sympathetic neurons of the inferior mesenteric ganglia receive input from neurons whose cell bodies are in the colon wall as well as in other abdominal viscera.[66] The neurotransmitters in these ganglion cells are the same neuropeptides seen mediating parasympathetic function as well as numerous other activities unrelated to motility. Continued interest in and study of these neuropeptides will undoubtedly reveal important new information regarding the mechanisms of colonic function.

CONCLUSION

The three central functions of the normal, healthy colon are digestion, motility, and transport. All are important components of human physiology. Unfortunately, they have not only been poorly understood but also inadequately studied. This is changing, however. From the information provided in this chapter, one can appreciate that the mechanisms of colonic function are an active topic of research, which in time may lead to the introduction of new treatments for a host of conditions that affect the large bowel.

REFERENCES

1. Andoh A, Tsujikawa T, Fujiyama Y. Role of dietary fiber and short-chain fatty acids in the colon. *Curr Pharm Des* 2003;9:347.
2. Argenzio RA, Southworth M. Sites of organic acid production and absorption in the gastrointestinal tract of the pig. *Am J Physiol* 1974;228:454.
3. Armstrong DN, Ballantyne GH. Physiology of the small and large intestines. In: Mazier WP, Levien DH, Luchtefeld MA, et al, eds. *Surgery of the colon, rectum, and anus.* Philadelphia: WB Saunders, 1995:40.
4. Ash RW, Dobson A. The effect of absorption on the acidity of rumen contents. *J Physiol (Lond)* 1963;169:39.

5. Barrett KE, Keely SJ. Chloride secretion by the intestinal epithelium: molecular basis and regulatory aspects. *Annu Rev Physiol* 2000;62:535.
6. Bassotti G, Crowell MD, Whitehead WE. Contractile activity of the human colon: lessons from 24-hour studies. *Gut* 1993;34:129.
7. Bauer HG, Asp NG, Dahlqvist A, et al. Effect of two kinds of pectin and guar gum on 1,2-dimethylhydrazine initiation of colon tumors and on fecal beta-glucoronidase activity in the rat. *Cancer Res* 1981;41:2518.
8. Billich CO, Levitan R. Effect of sodium concentration and osmolality on water and electrolyte absorption from the intact human colon. *J Clin Invest* 1969;48:1336.
9. Binder HJ. Amino acid absorption from the mammalian colon. *Biochim Biophys Acta* 1970;219:503.
10. Binder HJ, Foster E, Budinger ME, et al. Mechanism of electroneutral sodium-chloride absorption in distal colon of the rat. *Gastroenterology* 1987;93:449.
11. Binder HJ, Sandle GI. Electrolyte transport in the mammalian colon. In: Johnson LR, ed. *Physiology of the gastrointestinal tract*, 3rd ed. New York: Raven Press, 1994: 2133.
12. Brandtzaeg P, Halstensen TS, Kett K, et al. Immunobiology and immuno-pathology of human gut mucosa: humoral immunity and intraepithelial lymphocytes. *Gastroenterology* 1989;97:1562.
13. Bugaut M. Occurrence, absorption, and metabolism of short-chain fatty acids in the digestive tract of mammals. *Comp Biochem Physiol* 1987;86:439.
14. Camilleri M. Dyspepsia, irritable bowel syndrome, and constipation: review and what's new. *Rev Gastroenterol Disord* 2001;1:2.
15. Cannon WB. The movements of the intestines studied by means of the roentgen rays. *Am J Physiol* 1902;6:251.
16. Caprilli R, Onori L. Origin, transmission and ionic dependence of colonic electrical slow waves. *Scand J Gastroenterol* 1972;7:65.
17. Carter MJ, Parsons DS. The isoenzymes of carbonic anhydrase: tissue, subcellular distribution and functional significance, with particular reference to the intestinal tract. *J Physiol (Lond)* 1971;215:71.
18. Charney AN, Kinsey MD, Myers L, et al. Na⁺-K⁺-activated adenosine triphosphate and intestinal electrolyte transport: effect of adrenal steroids. *J Clin Invest* 1975;56:653.
19. Chauve A, Devroede G, Bastin E. Intraluminal pressure during perfusion of the human colon in situ. *Gastroenterology* 1976;70:336.
20. Cherrington CA, Hinton M, Pearson GR, et al. Short-chain organic acids at pH 5.0 kill *Escherichia coli* and *Salmonella* species without causing membrane perturbation. *J Appl Bacteriol* 1991;70:161.
21. Christensen J. The motility of the colon. In: Johnson LR, ed. *Physiology of the gastrointestinal tract*, 3rd ed. New York: Raven Press, 1994:991.
22. Christensen J, Anuras S, Hauser RL. Migrating spike bursts and electrical slow waves in the cat colon: effect of sectioning. *Gastroenterology* 1974;66:240.
23. Christl S, Murgatroyd PR, Gibson GR, et al. Total hydrogen and methane production from fermentation in man measured in a whole body calorimeter. *Gastroenterology* 1992;102:1269.
24. Clarkson TW, Rothstein A, Cross A. Transport of monovalent anions by isolated small intestine of the rat. *Am J Physiol* 1961;200:781.
25. Clauss W, Hornicke H. Segmental differences in potassium transport across rabbit proximal and distal colon *in vivo* and *in vitro*. *Comp Biochem Physiol* 1984;79A:267.
26. Cremashi D, Ferguson DR, Henin S, et al. Postnatal development of amiloride-sensitive sodium transport in pig distal colon. *J Physiol (Lond)* 1979;292:481.
27. Cummings JH. Dietary fibre. *Br Med Bull* 1981;37:65.
28. Cummings JH. Short-chain fatty acids in the human colon. *Gut* 1981;22:763.
29. Cummings JH, Hill MJ, Jenkins DJA, et al. Changes in faecal composition and colonic function due to cereal fiber. *Am J Clin Nutr* 1976;29:1468.
30. Cummings JH, Macfarlane GT. The control and consequences of bacterial fermentation in the human colon. *J Appl Bacteriol* 1991;70:443.
31. Curran PF, Schwartz GF. Na, Cl and water transport by rat colon. *J Gen Physiol* 1960;43:555.
32. Davis G, Morawski S, Santa Ana C, et al. Evaluation of chloride/bicarbonate exchange in the human colon *in vivo*. *J Clin Invest* 1983;71:201.
33. Debongnie JC, Phillips SF. Capacity of the human colon to absorb fluid. *Gastroenterology* 1978;74:698.
34. Del Castillo JR, Sepulveda FV. Activation of a sodium/potassium/chloride cotransport system by phosphorylation in crypt cells isolated from guinea pig distal colon. *Gastroenterology* 1995;109:387.
35. Del Castillo JR, Sulbaran-Carrasco MC, Burguillos L. Potassium transport in isolated guinea pig colonocytes: evidence for sodium-independent ouabain-sensitive potassium pump. *Am J Physiol* 1994;266:G1083.
36. Devroede GJ, Phillips SF. Conservation of sodium, chloride, and water by the human colon. *Gastroenterology* 1969;56:101.
37. Devroede GJ, Phillips SF. Failure of the human rectum to absorb electrolyte and water. *Gut* 1970;11:438.
38. Devroede GJ, Phillips SF, Code CF, et al. Regional differences in rates of insorption of sodium and water from the human large intestine. *Can J Physiol Pharmacol* 1971;49:1023.
39. Drasar BS, Hill MJ. *Human intestinal flora*. London: Academic Press, 1974.
40. Dunning WT, Curtis MR, Mann ME. The effect of added dietary tryptophane on the occurrence of 2-acetylaminofluorescence–induced liver and bladder cancer in rats. *Cancer Res* 1950;10:454.
41. Edmonds CJ, Marriott JC. The effect of aldosterone and adrenalectomy on the electrical potential difference of rat colon and on the transport of sodium, potassium, chloride and bicarbonate. *J Endocrinol* 1967;39:517.
42. Edwards DAW, Beck ER. Fecal flow, mixing, and consistency. *Am J Dig Dis* 1971;16:708.
43. Elliot TR, Barclay-Smith E. Antiperistalsis and other muscular activities of the colon. *J Physiol (Lond)* 1904;31:272.
44. Englyst HN, Cummings JH. Digestion of polysaccharides of potato in the human small intestine. *Am J Clin Nutr* 1987;45:423.
45. Feldman GM, Ickes JW Jr. Net proton and potassium fluxes across the apical surface of rat distal colon. *Am J Physiol* 1997;272:G54.
46. Finegold SM, Sutter VL, Mathisen GE. Normal indigenous intestinal flora. In: Hentges DJ, ed. *Human intestinal microflora in heath and disease*. London: Academic Press, 1983:3.
47. Fleming SE, Choi YS, Fitch DM. Absorption of short-chain fatty acids from the rat cecum *in vivo*. *J Nutr* 1991;121:1787.
48. Florin THJ, Neale G, Cummings JH. The effect of dietary nitrate on nitrate and nitrite excretion in ileal effluent and urine in man. *Br J Nutr* 1990;64:387.
49. Foster ES, Budinger ME, Hayslett JP, et al. Ion exchange in the rat proximal colon: sodium depletion stimulates neutral sodium chloride absorption. *J Clin Invest* 1986;77:228.
50. Foster ES, Hayslett JP, Binder HJ. Mechanism of active potassium absorption and secretion in the rat colon. *Am J Physiol* 1984;246:G611.
51. Foster ES, Zimmerman TW, Hayslett JP, et al. Corticosteroid alternation of active electrolyte transport in rat distal colon. *Am J Physiol* 1983;245:G668.

52. Frexinos J, Bueno L, Fioramonti J. Diurnal changes in myo-electric spiking activity of the human colon. *Gastroenterology* 1985;88:1104.

53. Frexinos J, Delvaux M. Colonic motility. In: Kumar D, Wingate D, eds. *An illustrated guide to gastrointestinal motility.* New York: Churchill Livingstone, 1993:427.

54. Frizzell RA, Koch MJ, Schultz SG. Ion transport by rabbit colon. I. Active and passive components. *J Membr Biol* 1976;27:297.

55. Gabella G. *Structure of the autonomic nervous system.* New York: John Wiley & Sons, 1976.

56. Giller J, Phillips SF. Electrolyte absorption and secretion in the human colon. *Am J Dig Dis* 1972;17:1003.

57. Grady GF, Duhamel RC, Moore EW. Active transport of sodium by human colon in vitro. *Gastroenterology* 1970;59:583.

58. Guarner F, Malagedlada J-R. Gut flora in health and disease. *Lancet* 2003;361:512.

59. Halm DR, Frizzell RA. Active potassium transport across rabbit distal colon: relation to sodium absorption and chloride secretion. *Am J Physiol* 1986;251:C252.

60. Harig JM, Ng EK, Dudeja PK, et al. Transport of N-butyrate into human colonic luminal membrane vesicles. *Am J Physiol* 1996;271:G415.

61. Heitman DW, Hardman WE, Cameron IL. Dietary supplementation with pectin and guar gum on 1,2-dimethylhydrazine–induced colon carcinogenesis in rats. *Carcinogenesis* 1992;13:815.

62. Heller SN, Hackler LR, Rivers JM, et al. Dietary fiber: the effect of particle size of wheat bran on colonic function in young adult men. *Am J Clin Nutr* 1980;34:1734.

63. Hill MJ. Cereals, cereal fibre and colorectal cancer risk. *Eur J Cancer Prev* 1997;6:219.

64. Holdstock DJ, Misiewicz JJ, Smith T, et al. Propulsion (mass movements) in the human colon and its relationship to meals and somatic activity. *Gut* 1970;11:91.

65. Horie H, Kanazawa K, Okada M, et al. Effects of intestinal bacteria on the development of colonic neoplasm: an experimental study. *Eur J Cancer Prev* 1999;8:237.

66. Huizinga JD, Daniel EE. Motor functions of the colon. In: Phillips SF, Pemberton JH, Shorter RG, eds. *The large intestine: physiology, pathophysiology, and disease.* New York: Raven Press, 1991:93.

67. Hultén L. Extrinsic nervous control of colonic motility and blood flow. *Acta Physiol Scand* 1969;S335:1.

68. Koyama Y, Yamamoto T, Tani T, et al. Expression and localization of aquaporins in rat gastrointestinal tract. *Am J Physiol* 1999;276:C1294.

69. Krevsky B, Malmud LS, D'Ercole F, et al. Colonic transit scintigraphy: a physiologic approach to the quantitative measurement of colonic transit in humans. *Gastroenterology* 1986;91:1102.

70. Kunzelmann K, Mall M. Electrolyte transport in the mammalian colon: mechanisms and implications for disease. *Physiol Rev* 2002;82:245.

71. Kuratsune M, Honda T, Englyst HN, et al. Dietary fiber in the Japanese diet as investigated in connection with colon cancer risk. *Jpn J Cancer Res* 1986;77:736.

72. Langton P, Ward SM, Carl A, et al. Spontaneous electrical activity of interstitial cells of Cajal isolated from canine proximal colon. *Proc Natl Acad Sci U S A* 1989;86:7280.

73. Levitt MD, Hirsch P, Fetzer CA, et al. Hydrogen excretion after ingestion of complex carbohydrates. *Gastroenterology* 1987;92:383.

74. Lichtman SM. Bacterial translocation in humans. *J Pediatr Gastroenterol Nutr* 2001;33:1.

75. Linguelglia E, Voilley N, Lazdunski M, et al. Molecular biology of the amiloride-sensitive epithelial sodium channel. *Exp Physiol* 1996;81:483.

76. Lundberg JM, Hökfelt T, Nilsson G, et al. Peptide neurons in the vagus, splanchnic and sciatic nerves. *Acta Physiol Scand* 1978;104:499.

77. Macpherson A, Khoo UY, Forgacs I, et al. Mucosal antibodies in inflammatory bowel disease are directed against intestinal bacteria. *Gut* 1996;38:365.

78. Mahajan RJ, Baldwin ML, Harig JM, et al. Chloride transport in human proximal colonic apical membrane vesicles. *Biochim Biophys Acta* 1996;1280:12.

79. Mascola N, Rajendran VM, Binder HJ. Mechanism of short-chain fatty acid uptake by apical membrane vesicles of rat distal colon. *Gastroenterology* 1991;101:331.

80. McCabe R, Cooke HJ, Sullivan LP. Potassium transport by rabbit descending colon. *Am J Physiol* 1982;242:C81.

81. McNeil NI. Human large-intestinal absorption of SCFAs. In: Kasper H, Goebel H, eds. *Colon and nutrition.* Boston: MTP Press, 1982:55.

82. McNeil NI, Cummings JH, James WPT. Rectal absorption of short-chain fatty acids in the absence of chloride. *Gut* 1979;20:400.

83. Miedema BW, Johnson JO. Methods for decreasing postoperative gut dysmotility. *Lancet Oncol* 2003;4:365.

84. Moore WEC, Holdeman LV. Human fecal flora: the normal flora of 20 Japanese Hawaiians. *Appl Microbiol* 1974;27:961.

85. Mortensen FV, Hessov I, Birke H, et al. Microcirculatory and trophic effects of short chain fatty acids in the human rectum after Hartmann's procedure. *Br J Surg* 1991;78:1208.

86. Mortensen PB, Clausen MR. Short-chain fatty acids in the human colon: relation to gastrointestinal health and disease. *Scand J Gastroenterol* 1996;S216:132.

87. Narducci F, Bassotti G, Gaburri M, et al. Twenty-four-hour manometric recording of colonic motor activity in healthy man. *Gut* 1987;28:17.

88. O'Boyle CJ, MacFie J, Mitchell CJ, et al. Microbiology of bacterial translocation in humans. *Gut* 1998;42:29.

89. O'Keefe SJ, Kidd M, Espitalier-Noel G, et al. Rarity of colon cancer in Africans is associated with low animal product consumption, not fiber. *Am J Gastroenterol* 1999;94:1373.

90. Oltmer S, von Engelhardt W. Absorption of short-chain fatty acids from the in situ-perfused caecum and colon of the guinea pig. *Scand J Gastroenterol* 1994;29:1009.

91. Phear EA, Ruebner B. The *in vitro* production of ammonium and amines by intestinal bacteria in relation to nitrogen toxicity as a factor in hepatic coma. *Br J Exp Pathol* 1956;37:253.

92. Phillips SF, Giller J. The contribution of the colon to electrolyte and water conservation in man. *J Lab Clin Med* 1973;81:733.

93. Rajendran VM, Binder HJ. Cl-HCO$_3$ and Cl-OH exchanges mediate Cl uptake in apical membrane vesicles of rat distal colon. *Am J Physiol* 1993;264:G874.

94. Ramakrishna BS, Benkataraman S, Srinivasan S, et al. Amylase-resistant starch plus oral rehydration solution for cholera. *N Engl J Med* 2000;342:308.

95. Rechkemmer G, Ronnau K, von Engelhardt W. Fermentation of polysaccharides and absorption of short-chain fatty acids in the mammalian hindgut. *Comp Biochem Physiol* 1988;90A:563.

96. Ritchie JA. Colonic motor activity and bowel function. I. Normal movement of contents. *Gut* 1968;9:442.

97. Ritchie JA. Colonic motor activity and bowel function. II. Distribution and incidence of motor activity at rest and after food and carbachol. *Gut* 1968;9:502.

98. Ritchie JA. Movement of segmental constrictions in the human colon. *Gut* 1971;12:350.

99. Ritchie JA. Mass peristalsis in human colon after contact with oxyphenisatin. *Gut* 1972;13:211.

100. Roediger WEW. Role of anaerobic bacteria in the metabolic welfare of the colonic mucosa of man. *Gut* 1980;21:793.

101. Roediger WEW. Short-chain fatty acids as metabolic regulators of ion absorption in the colon. *Acta Vet Scand* 1989;S86:116.

102. Ropert A, Cherbut C, Roze C, et al. Colonic fermentation and gastric tone in humans. *Gastroenterology* 1996;111: 289.
103. Rosebury T. *Microorganisms indigenous to man.* New York: McGraw-Hill, 1962:435.
104. Rübsamen K, von Engelhardt W. Bicarbonate secretion and solute absorption in forestomach of the llama. *Am J Physiol* 1978;235:E1–E6.
105. Ruppin H, Bar-Meir S, Soergel K-H, et al. Absorption of SCFA by the colon. *Gastroenterology* 1980;78:1500.
106. Sarna SK. Colonic motor activity. *Surg Clin North Am* 1993;73:1201.
107. Saunders DR, Wiggins HS. Conservation of mannitol, lactulose and raffinose by the human colon. *Am J Physiol* 1981;241:G397–G401.
108. Schultz SG. Ion transport by mammalian large intestine. In: Johnson LR, ed. *Physiology of the gastrointestinal tract.* New York: Raven Press, 1981:991.
109. Sellin J, DeSoignie R. Rabbit proximal colon: a distinct transport epithelium. *Am J Physiol* 1984;246:G603.
110. Sellin JH, DeSoignie R, Burlingame S. Segmental differences in short-chain fatty acid transport in rabbit colon: effect of pH and sodium. *J Membr Biol* 1993;136: 147.
111. Steinmetz K, Potter JD. Vegetables, fruit, and cancer. I. Epidemiology. *Cancer Causes Control* 1991;2:325.
112. Stephens AM, Cummings JH. Water holding by dietary fibre in vitro and its relationship to faecal output in man. *Gut* 1979;20:722.
113. Stephens AM, Cummings JH. The microbial contribution to human fecal mass. *J Med Microbiol* 1980;13:45.
114. Tadesse K, Smith D, Eastwood MA. Breath hydrogen (H_2) and methane (CH_4) excretion patterns in normal man in clinical practice. *Q J Exp Physiol* 1980;65:85.
115. Thompson JS, Quigley EMM. Prokinetic agents in the surgical patient. *Am J Surg* 1999;177:508.
116. Thun MJ, Calle EE, Namboodiri MM, et al. Risk factors for fatal colon cancer in a large prospective study. *J Natl Cancer Inst* 1992;84:1491.
117. Topping DL, Clifton PM. Short-chain fatty acids and human colonic function: roles of resistant starch and nonstarch polysaccharides. *Physiol Rev* 2001;81:1031.
118. Torsoli A, Ramorino ML, Crucioli V. The relationships between anatomy and motor activity of the colon. *Am J Dig Dis* 1968;13:462.
119. Turnamian SG, Binder HJ. Regulation of active sodium and potassium transport in the distal colon of the rat: role of the aldosterone and glucocorticoid receptors. *J Clin Invest* 1989;84:1924.
120. Turnheim K, Thompson SM, Schultz SG. Relation between intracellular sodium and active sodium transport across rabbit colon *in vitro*. *J Membr Biol* 1983;76:299.
121. Umesaki Y, Yajima T, Yokokura T, et al. Effect of organic acid absorption on bicarbonate transport in rat colon. *Pflugers Arch* 1979;379:43.
122. Vanasin B, Ustach TJ, Schuster MM. Electrical and motor activity of human and dog colon in vitro. *Johns Hopkins Med J* 1974;134:201.
123. Visek WJ. Diet and cell growth modulation by ammonia. *Am J Clin Nutr* 1978;31:S216.
124. Will PC, Lebovitz FL, Hopfer U. Induction of amiloride-sensitive sodium transport in the rat colon by mineralocorticoids. *Am J Physiol* 1980;238:F261.
125. Wils NK, Alles WP, Sandle GI, et al. Apical membrane properties and amiloride-binding kinetics of the human descending colon. *Am J Physiol* 1984;247:G749.
126. Wong O, Metcalfe-Gibson A, Morrison RBI, et al. *in vivo* dialysis of faeces as a method of stool analysis. I. Techniques and results in normal subjects. *Clin Sci* 1965;28:1965.
127. Wrong OM, Vince AJ, Waterlow JC. The contribution of endogenous urea to faecal ammonia in man, determined by ^{15}N labelling of plasma urea. *Clin Sci* 1985;68:193.

Diet and Drugs in Colorectal Surgery

Guest Contributor: John L. Petrini

I have asked a former colleague, John Petrini, to provide this contribution to the fifth edition of this book. Dr. Petrini is Chief of the Department of Gastroenterology at the Sansum Medical Clinic in Santa Barbara, California. During our 12 years of association, I have relied on him for his expertise and insight into the management of some of the difficult conditions that colon and rectal surgeons face. I believe that a chapter on diet and drugs for the benefit of general surgeons, as well as colon and rectal surgeons, should be a useful addition to this text.

MLC

A drug is a substance that,
when injected into a rat,
produces a scientific paper.

Anonymous

The role of diet in a healthy bowel has been a stimulating and controversial subject for two millennia. There are data to support numerous statements and recommendations, but controlled clinical trials defining the benefits of various foods and therapies are quite limited. In general, diets high in fiber and roughage help facilitate the normal passage of stool. In addition, they may be beneficial to the overall health of an individual by reducing cholesterol, maintaining blood sugar in the normal range, and decreasing the incidence of diverticulosis. Cruciferous plants also contain anticarcinogens that may reduce the incidence of colonic neoplasms. Furthermore, aspirin and other nonsteroidal antiinflammatory drugs (NSAIDs) appear to reduce the incidence of colon cancer. Other ideas—for example, that cow's milk and dairy products may be harmful for young children and most adults—have some validity. There are a host of other claims, but the data in support of them are very weak.

Patients may solicit the opinion of a physician for concerns that do not necessarily require surgical intervention, or they may experience gastrointestinal symptoms that are consequences of an operation. For many, dietary manipulations and medical therapy may provide relief of the discomfort and disability. Initial therapy for most disorders of the colon and rectum is usually dietary adjustment. This approach is often instituted by the patient himself or herself. The symptoms of certain conditions, such as irritable bowel syndrome (IBS), inflammatory bowel disease, diverticulitis, diarrhea, and constipation, can often be ameliorated by dietary manipulation, even though the cause of the disorder may not be related to a specific food. The addition of medication, either for symptomatic relief or to treat the specific disease state, may also contribute to the relief of a patient's symptoms. It is important, however, to understand the pathophysiology underlying the bowel symptoms in order to offer the appropriate treatment. Unfortunately, there is a paucity of information available for many disorders affecting the gastrointestinal tract that may aid the physician in appropriate therapeutic decision making. This chapter focuses on some of the more common symptoms and conditions for which patients seek the attention of physicians trained in gastrointestinal disease and gastrointestinal surgery.

BOWEL MANAGEMENT PROBLEMS

Constipation

Constipation can be defined as either a decrease in the frequency of stools or an increase in the difficulty of passage of stool. Patients may also complain of hard bowel movements, small actions, inability to evacuate, or the sensation of incomplete evacuation. Some studies have demonstrated that 95% of healthy adults will have a minimum of three bowel movements per week.[25,33] Those with fewer than three stools a week are considered to have "constipation," but they may not be truly symptomatic or seek medical attention. Those who do request help usually complain of either decreased frequency or difficulty in passing stool. Therapy is therefore directed at either increasing the water content (i.e., softening the stool) or increasing the frequency of bowel movements.

History

In order to make a recommendation concerning therapy, a carefully obtained history is essential. This should include the duration of the complaints, dietary habits, the use of medications, and lifestyle. These often provide the information necessary to arrive at the source of the patient's complaints. It is not within the purview of this chapter to present a complete discussion of all the disease states, endocrine abnormalities, medications, neurologic disorders, and dietary issues that are associated with constipation. However, it is important to note the more common endocrine conditions that may affect the bowels and that should be considered: hypothyroidism, diabetes mellitus, and hyperparathyroidism. Other diseases that predispose to constipation include uremia, porphyria, amyloidosis, and short-segment Hirschsprung's disease.

As mentioned, medications are a frequent cause of constipation, so it is important to obtain a history of all medications used, including those available over the counter. Although the list is extensive, the more common ones to consider include the opiate/analgesics, antipsychotics (particularly the monoamine oxidase inhibitors and tricyclic antidepressants), anticholinergics, iron and other heavy metals, antacids, anticonvulsants, calcium channel blockers, and diuretics.

Evaluation

The perineum should be carefully inspected for obvious pathologic entities that may impede the passage of stool. Instrument examination, contrast studies, transit studies, gynecologic examination, ultrasonography, computed tomography, and physiologic studies may be required in selected patients. Certainly, gastrointestinal evaluation at some point must be accomplished to rule out the presence of a specific etiologic factor. These are discussed in the following chapters.

Treatment

The standard treatment of nonspecific constipation begins with dietary manipulation, usually through increasing dietary fiber and fluid intake. In addition, several classes of medication are available to increase stool water or stool frequency. These include bulk laxatives, stool softeners, osmotic or saline laxatives, cathartics, and motility-enhancing drugs (prokinetics).

Those who have constipation usually benefit from increasing the water content of the stool by increasing their intake of fiber and water. It is well known that individuals who live in so-called developing countries consume a large amount of unprocessed fiber. However, the diet in most developed countries contains inadequate roughage or unprocessed dietary fiber.[6,18] Dietary fiber consists of plant products that are not digested or absorbed by the small intestine. These include cellulose, lignin, gums, pectins, hemicelluloses, and polysaccharides. Increasing fluid intake without adding fiber to the diet is usually ineffective for correcting constipation.

▶ **TABLE 3-1 Fiber Content of Selected Dietary Items**

Food Group	Low Fiber	High Fiber
Fruits	Apples (cooked)	Prunes (stewed)
	Oranges	Raspberries
	Pears	Apples (with peel)
	Bananas	Dates (dried)
	Grapes	
	Fruit juices	
Vegetables	Cabbage	Spinach
	Celery	Sweet potato
	Lettuce	Corn
	Summer squash	Broccoli
	Vegetable juices	Turnips
	Eggplant	Greens
Starches	Bagel	Lentils
	White bread	Bran
	Flour, white	Barley
	Potato (mashed, chips)	Kidney beans
	Pasta	Peas
	Popcorn	Brown rice
		Granola
		Flour, whole wheat
Other	Meats, seafood	
	Dairy products, eggs	
	Nuts and seeds	
	Oils	

Fiber, however, will improve stool consistency irrespective of the water intake.[45] Interestingly, fiber with small amounts of water can be used to treat diarrhea. Some foods, particularly dairy products, actually decrease stool water content and contribute to constipation. Good sources of dietary fiber include fresh fruits and vegetables, whole grain cereals, and unprocessed carbohydrates such as bran, whole wheat, and brown rice (Table 3-1). Total daily fiber intake should be adjusted to approximately 30 g or more.

Fiber Products

Those individuals whose diet remains inadequate in fiber can increase stool water-carrying capacity by adding a fiber-containing bulk laxative. Psyllium husk, either as powder or granules, is obtained from various species of plantain. Bran is a product of the milling of wheat. Either, when taken with adequate dietary water, will provide additional bulk to the stool and increase the water content, trapping it in a mucin within the stool.

Other bulk laxatives utilize hydrophilic substances, such as polycarbophil and powdered karaya (sterculia) gum. The amount of bulking agents can be adjusted to what is required to alleviate the patient's constipation. This range is usually between 4 and 10 g/day, with the administration divided if a higher dose is required.

The major disadvantage of bulking agents is the bloating and gas commonly associated with the cellulose and lignin-based products. Fiber products with a base of hemicellulose or pectin seem to reduce these side effects, as does the use of the polycarbophil bulk agents. However, patients seem to require higher doses of the latter than of the cellulose-based products in order for similar results to be achieved. One of the side benefits of the use of bulk agents is the lowering of serum cholesterol. This is probably effected through the binding of bile salts and reducing their reabsorption, so that the bile salt pool is lowered. Problems associated with the use of bulking agents include intestinal obstruction and fecal impaction, particularly if there is an underlying pathologic entity. Additionally, allergic reactions have been reported.

Stool Softeners

Patients who are resistant to the bulking agents alone can increase the water content further with stool softeners or emollients. The principal agent is docusate (dioctyl sulfosuccinate), which is available as the sodium, calcium, or potassium salt. These products inhibit the normal water-absorptive capacity of the colon while producing only a minimal decrease in the transit of fecal contents. Once one of these products has been administered, it may take 1 to 3 days to see an effect. In essence, they act to soften the stool but do not promote defecation. The usual adult does is from 50 to 250 mg/day. Ducosate should not be given with mineral oil because absorption of the oil as well as other medications is enhanced.

Osmotic and Saline Laxatives

Should bulking agents and surfactants fail to enhance the passage of stool, the next preferred step would be to employ an osmotic or saline laxative. Magnesium phosphate, sodium sulfate, and potassium tartrate are poorly absorbed chemicals. Ingestion increases the stool water content through an osmotic effect. Surgeons are familiar with the use of saline laxatives for bowel preparations before operative or diagnostic procedures. In smaller doses, they can be utilized for their cathartic effect. However, they should be used only intermittently. Certain antacid products contain magnesium, and it is this agent that produces the side effect of diarrhea. There is, furthermore, some evidence that magnesium may actually increase motility of the small intestine through stimulation the release of cholecystokinin from the duodenum.[16] The phosphate-containing solutions may cause a high serum phosphate level and impair cardiac contractility. They should therefore be used with caution in individuals with renal, cardiac, or hepatic disease. Dehydration can also be a consequence of the use of saline laxatives. Patients should be cautioned to take adequate fluids when using these agents.

Modified doses of colonic purgatives used to clear the colon prior to surgery and gastrointestinal procedures are also available to treat constipation.[10] Miralax provides increased water to the colon by adding an osmotically neutral fluid to the gastrointestinal tract. The osmotically nonabsorbed, active agents, polyethylene glycol and a mixture of sodium and potassium sulfate, are not absorbed. The usual dose is 17 g mixed with water; it can be given on a daily basis. There is minimal fluid or electrolyte shift, and side effects are rare.

Polysaccharides

Some carbohydrates are also poorly absorbed. This results in an osmotic effect that leads to enhanced water in the stool. These products include lactose, lactulose, and sorbitol. Lactulose has been particularly useful in the treatment of hepatic encephalopathy, but lower doses (30 to 60 mL/day) can be an effective laxative for patients with chronic constipation. Side effects include gas, bloating, cramps, flatulence, and, of course, fluid loss at high doses.

Lubricants

Mineral oil, a petroleum distillate, has been employed for the treatment of constipation. The mechanism of action appears to be penetration of the stool by the oil with resulting softening. However, because of the potential for complications, long-term use should be avoided. These include decreased absorption of fat-soluble vitamins and essential fatty acids. Furthermore, penetration of the mucosa can occur, and a foreign-body reaction in the mesenteric lymph nodes, mucosa, and spleen has been reported. As previously mentioned, mineral oil should not be used with surfactants, because there is the potential for increased absorption of the mineral oil.

Stimulant Laxatives

What rhubarb, senna or what purgative drug, would scour these English hence?
William Shakespeare: *Macbeth* V, iii, 55

Cathartic laxatives are mucosally active agents that reduce net water and electrolyte absorption in addition to increasing bowel motility. The most frequently employed substances include phenolphthalein and the anthraquinone cathartics (senna, cascara sagrada, danthron). These drugs act primarily to increase periodic mass movements within the colon and to decrease the segmental contractions that slow bowel activity. Generally, they become effective in 4 to 6 hours. The primary side effect, in addition to diarrhea, is that of cramping. Another drug, bisacodyl (Dulcolax), is a synthetic diphenylmethane that is similar to phenolphthalein. However, it is available not only available for oral administration but also for rectal use. Because of the problem of gastric irritation, it is enteric coated. The standard adult dose is 10 to 15 mg.

Senna is an anthraquinone cathartic obtained from *Cassia acutifolia* or *Cassia angustifolia*. Preparations of the whole plant, leaflets, pods, and extracts are commercially available. Cascara sagrada is another anthraquinone; it is obtained from the bark of the buckthorn tree. Like all cathartics, these are variously effective depending on the dosage but can cause a problem with cramping. Furthermore, melanosis coli, a dark pigmentation of the colon mucosa, may be a consequence of long-term use of senna and cascara (see Color Figure 16-11).

Another cathartic, castor oil, a triglyceride of ricinoleic acid, acts in the small intestine by pancreatic hydrolysis, thereby decreasing water and electrolyte absorption and decreasing transit time. Because it is quite potent, it should be employed with special care. Long-term use should be avoided.

Motility Agents

Three agents are currently available that decrease transit time through acceleration of the muscular activity of the bowel. Gastrointestinal motility can be enhanced through the use of metoclopramide, erythromycin, and tegaserod. Another agent, the subject of considerable investigational effort, is cisapride, but it has been taken off the market in the United States. Metoclopraminde and erythromycin have little or no effect on the colon, but tegaserod has been shown to increase bowel activity and ease constipation in those patients with IBS in whom constipation predominates.[22] Tegaserod is a partial agonist of the type 4 serotonin receptor (5-HT$_4$) with high binding affinity and little or no affinity for other serotonin receptors. It appears to enhance motor activity in the colon and elsewhere in the gastrointestinal tract by normalizing motility and stimulating intestinal secretion. Another beneficial effect in patients with IBS appears to be reduction in visceral sensitivity, thus ameliorating abdominal pain. Tegaserod is approved for oral administration, 6 mg twice daily, before meals for 4 to 6 weeks, with another 6-week course if needed.

Summary

Long-term use of intestinal stimulants and cathartics can lead to fluid and electrolyte disturbances, including dehydration, hypokalemia, hyponatremia, hypoalbuminemia, steatorrhea, protein-losing enteropathy, and secondary hyperaldosteronism. Furthermore, patients may become dependent upon laxatives, and what is known as a "cathartic colon," or a chronically flaccid colon, may develop. A good general principle is that if laxatives are to be used, the lowest effective dose should be given. Long-term use should be discouraged. Most individuals will benefit from a program of increasing fiber and water content of the stool, with the addition of laxatives intermittently as needed to produce at least two or three bowel movements per week. The application of surgical intervention as a treatment for constipation should be offered only after an adequate trial of medical therapy and appropriate evaluation of the gastrointestinal tract (see Chapter 16).

Diarrhea

Diarrhea is a common complaint in numerous disorders, most of which are not attributable to colonic sources. A host of etiologic factors may produce an increase in stool water or stool frequency, including medications, infection, the consequences of radiation, hepatic or biliary disease, pancreatic insufficiency, intolerance to ingested food components, infiltration of the mucosa or submucosa with lymphocytes or eosinophils, neoplasm, inflammatory bowel disease, and IBS. It is beyond the scope of this chapter to offer a comprehensive discussion on the etiology and treatment of all the possible conditions that can lead to the symptom of diarrhea.

The most common presentation is that of increased stool water. This leads to loose stools, watery stools, and increased stool volume and/or frequency. The maximum number of bowel movements that is still considered within normal range is three per day, assuming that this does not represent a change in the individual's normal bowel habits. By definition, diarrhea is classified as acute until symptoms have been present for more than 6 weeks. After this time, it is considered chronic.

Acute Diarrhea

Acute diarrhea is often caused by medication or an infectious process, including bacterial enteritis, toxin ingestion, and infestation by the common intestinal parasites (e.g., *Giardia, Cryptosporidium, Isospora*). A discussion of the infectious and noninfectious colitides can be found in Chapter 33. The use of broad-spectrum antibiotics with resultant infection by *Clostridium difficile* is a frequent source of acute diarrheal illness (see also Chapter 33).

Principles of Management

Treatment for acute diarrhea involves identification of the offending agent and initiation of whatever specific measures are necessary to eliminate the source or eradicate the organism. The use of medications that decrease gastrointestinal motility in acute, febrile diarrheal illnesses should be avoided, because prolonged contact time can enhance the likelihood of transmucosal migration of the organism and systemic infection. A better alternative is the use of pectin or bismuth compounds, such as kaolin-pectin or bismuth subcitrate. These products bind shiga toxins and other cyclic guanosine monophosphate–stimulatory toxins associated with bacterial infection and decrease the net water and chloride secretion by the small bowel. If systemic signs and symptoms of infection are not present, the use of opiates to increase transit time and slow stool frequency offers symptomatic relief. By prolonging contact time with the intestinal tract, fluid and electrolyte absorption will be enhanced.

Chronic Diarrhea

Chronic diarrheal illnesses may be caused by a wide variety of disorders that affect the hepatobiliary system, pancreas, and small or large bowel. Individuals with chronic diarrhea present a challenge in differential diagnosis. This inevitably may lead to an extensive and expensive workup. Assuming that such an evaluation fails to establish a specific cause for the patient's symptoms, the most likely disorder is the so-called IBS. Treatment for this complaint is to reduce the volume and frequency of bowel movements, so that the patient's lifestyle can be improved.

Treatment

The approach to the management of patients with chronic diarrhea without a definable cause begins with a carefully taken dietary history. An offending food or substance may be found in the patient's intake that increases the frequency of bowel action. For example, lactose-containing diary products may induce symptoms of cramping or diarrhea in up to 65% of the adult population. Furthermore, caffeine-containing beverages may increase bowel activity and stool output. Additionally, sugarless candies, sodas, and fruits high in fructose or sorbitol may lead to symptoms of diarrhea. Therefore, removing the offending agent will usually improve symptoms.

Medical therapy encompasses a wide number of options. The following discussion focuses on those agents used specifically to treat diarrhea.

The fiber-containing bulk agents previously alluded to decrease stool water when they are given with less than the recommended volume of liquid. Any of the bulk agents taken under these circumstances decreases the absorption of water through the gastrointestinal tract. However, there are the side effects of bloating, gas, and cramping. Another means for binding stool water is through the use of bile salt resins, such as cholestyramine. Bile salt resins are the preferred drugs for the management of diarrhea associates with ileal resection.

Kaolin, a dehydrated aluminum silicate, and pectin, a carbohydrate (polygalacturonic acid), can also be used as adsorbents to treat diarrhea. Bismuth subcitrate may also be employed to bind stool water and ameliorate diarrheal symptoms, but these agents are less effective than are the opiates. The most efficacious

use of these products may be to prevent or to treat traveler's diarrhea.

The opiates are the most effective form of therapy in the management of diarrheal illnesses. These are usually given in the form of diphenoxylate or loperamide, but they are available in many other substances, including codeine phosphate and tincture of opium (paregoric). Opiates are habit-forming, but this risk is much less when they are taken orally. Still, loperamide, which fails to cross the blood-brain barrier, should be the initial choice. Studies have shown it to be comparable to diphenoxylate (Lomotil), which can cause euphoria in high doses. A patient whose diarrhea fails to resolve with the foregoing measures requires further evaluation.

Irritable Bowel Syndrome

IBS is defined as abdominal pain with or without alterations in bowel habits and with no evidence of abnormality on diagnostic testing. Patients may present with a wide variety of complaints, but more than 90% will have two or more of the following: visible abdominal distension, increased frequency of bowel movements with the onset of pain, looser stools with the onset of pain, and relief of pain with defecation.[24] Most individuals typically complain of crampy, diffuse abdominal pains that are associated with alternating constipation and diarrhea. A consensus conference led to the publishing of the "Rome II" criteria for establishing the diagnosis of IBS.[11] These include 12 weeks or more of abdominal discomfort within the preceding 12 months or pain that consists of two out of three features:

- Discomfort relieved by defecation
- Onset associated with a change in frequency of stools
- Onset associated with a change in stool form (appearance)

The 12 weeks do not need to be consecutive. One assumes that evaluation for other disorders is negative.

Etiology and Pathogenesis

The etiology of IBS is unknown. However, there is considerable evidence to implicate the roles of stress and psychiatric illness in the pathogenesis of this condition. Various psychiatric abnormalities can be seen in the majority of individuals with IBS. In 85% of these, psychiatric symptoms either preceded or occurred coincidentally with the onset of the abdominal complaints.[8,19,41] The condition is clearly associated with stress and emotional disturbances. Individuals frequently report exacerbation of their symptoms under these conditions. It has been shown that persons with IBS have a higher incidence of psychiatric illness when compared with those who do not or with those harboring other gastrointestinal disorders.[43] Finally, there is emerging evidence to suggest that a history of physical or sexual abuse may be associated with IBS.[12,42]

Numerous abnormalities have been implicated in the pathogenesis of IBS. Patients with this condition have been demonstrated to exhibit altered colonic motility in response to meals when compared with subjects without IBS. Balloon distension studies suggest that these individuals have an increased rectal sensitivity to pressure.[27] Further studies of the myoelectrical activity of the bowel suggest that approximately 40% of patients have abnormalities or alterations. For example, a decrease is observed in the normal six cycles per minute of basic electrical rhythm to three cycles per minute. This decrease may persist despite treatment that effectively controls IBS symptoms.[37] Discomfort following distension of the ileum and the rectum is also increased in patients with IBS when compared with controls.[21,44] It is interesting that the perception of pain does not appear to be increased elsewhere in the body.

Treatment

The lack of a definable abnormality in patients with IBS contributes to our inability to correct the patients' symptoms in a uniformly effective manner. For the most part, IBS is a lifelong illness, with periods of health punctuated by episodes of symptoms. The approach to management begins with evaluation of the potential contributing factors, primarily emotional and dietary. If the patient's emotional or psychological history is probed in a careful and sensitive manner, the physician can often identify a source for the discomfort for which the patient has been unaware.

The use of psychiatric therapy in this condition has been the subject of numerous studies. Hypnotherapy, stress reduction psychotherapy, dynamic psychotherapy, and relaxation techniques have all been successfully employed. Unfortunately, when one reviews these approaches, there is a consensus that the trials are plagued with poor methodology. As a consequence, there is no general acceptance of any specific technique.[39] Still, these studies do suggest a role for psychotherapy for those who are willing to consider this approach to treatment.

There is no doubt that dietary factors can play a role in IBS and lead to increased abdominal cramping or pain. Patients with diarrhea should be counseled with respect to foods that are likely to increase stool water and frequency. These include fiber, nonabsorbed carbohydrates, caffeine, and lactose. If constipation is the primary symptom, increased fiber and water intake may help reduce the difficulty in passing stools, but the consequences of bloating, cramps, and abdominal pain may make the use of this approach counterproductive.

For the majority of patients, crampy abdominal pain is the major reason for seeking medical care. The pain is often difficult to characterize but is usually diffuse, intermittent, and frequently localized to the left lower quadrant of the abdomen. The pain may be exacerbated by meals and relieved somewhat by defecation or the passage of flatus. Because the regulation of bowel movements may offer some relief from the discomfort, it should be part of the treatment for all patients with IBS. Although elimination of pain may not be successfully accomplished in everyone, a graduated approach provides the best chance of alleviating symptoms.

The current first line of medications is the anticholinergic class of drugs.[34] Anticholinergics can reduce the rate of spike activity, thereby decreasing tonic contractions in the colon. This may lead to decreased cramping and bloating. Anticholinergics may be administered alone or in combination with other sedative/hypnotic medications, such as atropine, scopolamine, hyoscyamine, and phenobarbital in combination (Donnatal) and a combination of clinidium and chlordiazepoxide (Librax). The addition of these drugs may also be useful for those patients in whom anxiety contributes to the symptoms. Short-acting anticholinergics can be administered sublingually or orally and can be used to suppress symptoms when they occur. Long-acting preparations may be helpful for the management of chronic symptoms.

Antidepressants have also been shown to provide relief from the pain of IBS, often at doses far lower than those used to achieve an antidepressant effect. Furthermore, this is seen at doses at which the anticholinergic effects are negligible. Imipramine, amitriptyline, or nortriptyline given at a starting dose of 10 mg at bedtime, will often reduce or eliminate the abdominal pain associated with IBS. The dose can be increased, but at higher doses side effects are common. One side effect of the tricyclic class of antidepressants is constipation. Of course, this may help in those individuals who have diarrhea as a major component of their IBS, but it will certainly exacerbate symptoms for those whose primary complaint is constipation. In this latter group of patients, one may address this concern by switching to the selective serotonin reuptake inhibitors (SSRIs): fluoxetine (Prozac), paroxetine (Paxil), or sertraline (Zoloft), again at low doses. Although the SSRIs are less likely to be associated with constipation as a side effect, diarrhea may be aggravated. One must appreciate the importance of titration of the various medication choices in trying to identify the appropriate approach to the management of a given individual.

Various other medications have been used to treat the symptoms of IBS, but the data are preliminary, and the studies have been undertaken with only small groups of selected individuals.[23] Fedotozine, a gut κ receptor agonist, appears to decrease visceral sensitivity in animals. One study suggested improvement in the symptoms of bloating and abdominal pain when this drug was given during a 6-week trial.[9] Leuprolide, a gonadotropin-releasing hormone agonist, has been demonstrated to improve the symptoms of nausea, vomiting, bloating, abdominal pain, and early satiety in a group of women with functional gastrointestinal symptoms.[26] Octreotide has also been shown to improve the visceral perception of pain in patients with IBS without affecting the small intestinal muscle tone.[5,17] Cholecystokinin analogues have been demonstrated to offer some relief from the discomfort of IBS, but they are currently unavailable for use in the United States. Cromolyn sulfate has been shown in one study to improve the symptoms of IBS.[38] Patients were selected for diarrhea-predominant IBS, and the drug was compared with an elimination diet. Both groups showed similar improvement. In addition, and as mentioned previously, tegaserod, a 5-HT$_4$ agonist, may be useful for patients with constipation-predominant IBS.

NSAIDs appear to have little role in the treatment of the pain of IBS, and there is absolutely no place for stronger pain medications such as opiates or narcotics. Obviously, it is essential to avoid potentially addictive psychotropic medications in those individuals whose disease state often has such a strong emotional component.

Short Bowel Syndrome

Patients who have undergone resection of the small intestine, particularly the distal ileum, may present with symptoms of urgency and diarrhea (especially after meals), weight loss, or dehydration. When an extensive portion of the small intestine has been resected, there may be insufficient surface area available for absorption of nutrients. It has been estimated that the minimal length of small intestine necessary to sustain adequate enteral nutrition is approximately 1 m, although the presence of the colon my reduce that requirement. Preservation of the proximal bowel (duodenum and jejunum) appears more likely to facilitate nutrient absorption than does the presence of ileum, with the exception of certain specific nutrients, such as vitamin B$_{12}$. Those individuals who are unable to achieve adequate enteral nutrition require parenteral hyperalimentation (see Chapter 30).

Studies have demonstrated that the colon actually is able to absorb a reasonable amount of calories, largely in the form of short-chain fatty acids.[30] In addition to providing nutrient value to the cells of the colonic mucosa itself, 500 kcal/day may actually be absorbed into the systemic circulation.

It has been demonstrated by utilizing growth hormone and glutamine, with a diet of increased carbohydrates and decreased fat, that this combination is associated with an increase in the absorption of protein and a decrease in stool output.[7] In some individuals with small intestine too limited to provide adequate absorptive area, this regimen has been able to decrease or completely eliminate the need for parenteral hyperalimentation.

The proximal duodenum is the most efficient area of absorption of most nutrients, but jejunum and ileum can adapt and increase absorption. This has been demonstrated following duodenal resection or bypass, provided there is adequate time for mixing of bile and pancreatic secretions with the ingested food. The distal ileum is the primary absorptive area for bile salts and vitamin B$_{12}$, so that removal of this area can result in cholerrheic diarrhea and vitamin B$_{12}$ deficiency.

Those individuals who have undergone small bowel resection but still have adequate surface area for absorption may initially experience symptoms of rapid transit and diarrhea. In most cases, the remaining bowel can adapt to allow adequate nutrition, although a period of adjustment may be necessary. As previously suggested, patients with 100 cm of small bowel remaining should be able to subsist on an elemental diet, but the palatability of predigested food is very poor. Only very highly motivated individuals can tolerate oral elemental feedings, so usually a nasogastric tube, gastrostomy, or jejunostomy tube is required to achieve adequate caloric intake. With this regimen, patients often suffer an initial period of frequency, bloating, and loose stools. These symptoms gradually improve with time. Supplemental liquid nutrition given between meals may help maintain body weight. Additional therapy, including bile salt–binding resins and loperamide or diphenoxylate, will slow transit and should help improve absorption. The typical patient will initially suffer weight loss, but ultimately achieve a new steady state at lower body mass. With this type of patient, oral intake is usually adequate to maintain metabolic balance. It is rare that parenteral nutrition will be required, and with appropriate management, individuals should be able to maintain a positive metabolic balance. However, those who have an inadequate small bowel surface area for absorption of nutrients will require some form of supplementation or parenteral nutrition.

Cholerrheic Diarrhea

Individuals who have undergone resection of the distal ileum, particularly if the ileocecal valve is removed, may exhibit symptoms of cramping, bloating, and diarrhea, often accompanying intake of food. The etiology of these complaints is not clear, but it appears to be related to deconjugation of nonabsorbed bile salts by the colonic bacteria. Deconjugated bile salts are toxic to the lining of the colon; they initiate fluid and electrolyte secretion and lead to symptoms of cramping and diarrhea (cholerrheic diarrhea). This theory is supported by the observation that bile salt–binding medications, such as cholestyramine, often ameliorate the symptoms associated with distal ileal resection and cholerrheic diarrhea. The dosage can be adjusted to achieve normal bowel movements without induction of constipation. Additional reduction in diarrhea can be afforded by the use of loperamide or diphenoxylate in those individuals whose diarrhea persists despite bile salt–binding medications.

Postoperative Ileus

Ileus is a common consequence of any abdominal operation and, obviously, of any operation on the intestinal tract. It may occur after minor surgical procedures, even those outside the abdomen, but it is clearly related to intraabdominal surgery.[3] Why this occurs is not entirely clear, but it is thought to be due to the effects of the anesthetic, manipulation of the bowel, a generalized increase in sympathetic tone, or the opiates that may be used to control postoperative pain.[29] The effects of bowel manipulation are controversial, but it appears that less invasive surgical procedures are associated with less severe postoperative ileus. This, of course, is a contention of the advantage of minimally invasive surgery (see Chapter 27). The effects of the ileus appear most pronounced on the colon, with the small bowel and the stomach recovering function earlier.

Treatment

I do not presume to tell surgeons how to manage patients who have postoperative ileus. However, certain points are worth emphasizing, at least from the perspective of a gastroenterologist. Studies evaluating the efficacy of prokinetic agents (erythromycin, metoclopramide, and cisapride) have failed to generate consistent results that could suggest a reduced duration of postoperative ileus.[4,20,35,40] This lack of an effective medical approach mandates modification of oral intake following surgery. Most surgeons wait for evidence of bowel activity (the passage of flatus, the presence of bowel sounds, or a bowel movement) before resuming oral feedings. However, recent evidence suggests that one may, with caution, commence oral intake a lot sooner than had been previously recommended. This is based to some extent on the evidence gleaned from early alimentation following laparoscopic procedures.

There is no evidence that nasogastric tube suction in the absence of vomiting provides any benefit, but patients with distension and vomiting will have these symptoms ameliorated by gastric suction (see Chapter 22). With a nasogastric tube in place, the volume of aspirate can be ascertained, and this can be utilized as a guide for the initiation of oral feedings. Although there is a reasonable difference of opinion concerning when to remove the tube, the volume should be less than 50 mL/hr before it is eliminated. Alternatively, clamping the tube for several hours or overnight and measuring the residual gas-

tric fluid comprise a useful guide. If the residual is less than 100 mL after clamping for 4 hours, bowel activity may be presumed to have developed.

Clear liquids are usually offered initially, although the rationale for this concept remains murky. For example, there is no evidence to suggest that a regular diet should be initially avoided. This may be largely a consequence of the fact that it is easier to aspirate gastric retention if there is no residual solid material present. Diet is then advanced as tolerated, usually to a full liquid diet and then to a selected diet. However, certain clear liquids may produce untoward symptoms. For example, fruit juices that contain poorly absorbed carbohydrates, especially fructose, may lead to distension, bloating, and diarrhea. Apple juice, a staple in the clear liquid diet, is a particularly offending agent. Caffeine is a well-known gastric irritant. This may lead to substernal burning and to nausea. Full liquid diets may be high in dairy products and lactose. As mentioned, 65% of adults have varying degrees of intolerance to these substances.

A similar approach to avoiding items that may lead to dietary intolerance should be employed when enteral tube feedings are used. Tube feedings occasionally can cause diarrhea, possibly from the high osmolality of the feedings or to rapid feedings. However, the etiology of diarrhea is multifactorial and in the postoperative patient may include antibiotic use, the vehicles used to make medication soluble, the fact that it may be delivered by a tube, particularly sorbitol,[14] intraabdominal infection, and the consequences of an anastomosis. Avoiding poorly tolerated carbohydrates, including fructose, lactose, lactulose, and sorbitol, can minimize the bowel discomfort often experienced by patients in the postoperative period.

Diverticular Disease

Diverticular disease is a frequently encountered condition in developed countries. The prevalence appears to be over 30% in adults over the age of 50 and rises with advancing age.[32] The presence of the mucosal herniations thorough the bowel wall is thought to be a consequence of decreased dietary fiber, a finding supported by epidemiologic data (see the discussion on diet in Chapter 26). In countries where the intake of dietary fiber is five to ten times that of the United States, diverticular disease is a rare finding.[6,30] Patients with diverticulosis are usually asymptomatic, but abdominal pain has been attributed to spasm often seen in the presence of diverticula. Because IBS is found in approximately 12% of adults in the United States, it is not clear whether diverticulosis or IBS is responsible for the cramping abdominal pain in these individuals.[31] In one study, the poorly absorbed oral antibiotic, rifaximin, when given with fiber supplementation, reduced the discomfort of diverticular disease.[31]

Increasing dietary fiber is associated with an increase in the water content of stool and may ease its passage through the colon. If the theory that diverticula are more likely to occur in the setting of increased intraluminal pressure is correct, increased fiber should reduce the likelihood of new diverticula forming, but not eliminate the diverticula already present. Despite conventional wisdom, there is no evidence to suggest that seeds, nuts, popcorn husks, and other small, sharp, or firm food contents are responsible for acute attacks of diverticulitis. Furthermore, eliminating these products from the diet does not confer protection from future attacks.

When patients are experiencing the symptoms of diverticulitis, luminal narrowing is associated with distension, bloating, and alterations in bowel habits. With acute diverticulitis, reducing stool volume should decrease discomfort associated with the partial blockage of the bowel. Dietary therapy consists of clear liquid diet until normal fecal flow is established, followed by resumption of a high-fiber diet (if tolerated) once the inflammation has subsided. These measures are used to reduce bloating and distension, but the treatment of the acute episode remains broad-spectrum antibiotics.[13] Any one of a number of antibiotics is useful in this acute inflammatory condition, with surgery required for complications (see Chapter 26).

Chemoprophylaxis

Recent studies have renewed one's interest in probiotics, minerals, and NSAIDs in the prevention of gastrointestinal problems. Some of the more definitive therapies are discussed in the next sections.

Pouchitis

Patients who have undergone proctocolectomy with reservoir-anal procedures or continent pouches often present with inflammatory changes in the reservoir, a consequence of what has been attributed to bacterial overgrowth (see Chapter 29). Successful treatment usually consists of antibiotics such as metronidazole, 250 mg three times daily, or ciprofloxacin, 500 mg twice daily. However, some patients experience recurrent bouts of pouchitis that may be difficult to control. Studies using a probiotic, VSL-3, have suggested a prolonged remission from pouchitis with this combination of bacteria.[15] The preparation contains multiple strains of bacteria that, theoretically, replenish the gut flora consortium that help to preserve a healthy colon mucosa. The medication is available online at www.questcor.com.

Colon Polyps and Cancer Prevention

Anecdotal reports and case-control studies suggest that patients taking aspirin, fiber, and vitamins and who consume vegetarian and low-fat diets have a reduced incidence of colon polyps. This has spurred interest in polyp chemoprevention. However, initial studies failed to demonstrate benefit with supplementary vitamins E, C, and β-carotene, as well as with fiber supplementation. A randomized, controlled trial found a reduction in new polyp formation though the use of calcium supplements.[1] Patients were given 1,200 mg of elemental calcium. Those so treated had an adjusted risk ratio for the formation of new polyps of 0.85 compared with the placebo-treated population.

Reports that sulindac reduced the development of adenomatous polyps in familial adenomatous polyposis syndrome, as well as case-control studies in aspirin users, further stimulated interest in the use of NSAIDs to reduce new polyp formation. Prospective, randomized, controlled studies have suggested a reduction in the formation of new neoplastic polyps in patients with prior colorectal cancer or adenomas through the use of aspirin. Patients with previous colorectal cancer were placed on 325 mg of aspirin daily. They had an adjusted relative risk of forming new polyps of 0.65 compared with placebo-treated patients.[2] In the second study, two doses of aspirin, 325 mg or 81 mg, were compared with a placebo in preventing new polyps in patients with prior adenomas. Low-dose aspirin was associated with a modest risk reduction (0.81) compared with a placebo, but the regular aspirin tablet was no better than a placebo.[36] These studies suggest a modest effect of NSAIDs in reducing the formation of new polyps in patients prone to development of adenomas. However, the high rate of upper gastrointestinal complications associated with the use of NSAIDs, coupled with only a modest reduction in new polyp incidence, makes it difficult for one to advocate aspirin therapy at this time for this indication.

REFERENCES

1. Baron JA, Beach M, Mandel JS, et al. Calcium supplements for the prevention of colorectal adenomas. *N Engl J Med* 1999;340:101–107.
2. Baron JA, Cole BF, Sandler RS. A randomized trial of aspirin to prevent colorectal adenomas. *N Engl J Med* 2003;248:891–899.
3. Benson MJ, Roberts JP, Wingate DL, et al. Small-bowel motility following major intra-abdominal surgery: the effects of opiates and rectal cisapride. *Gastroenterology* 1994;106:924–936.
4. Bonacini M, Quiason S, Reynolds M, et al. Effects of intravenous erythromycin on postoperative ileus. *Am J Gastroenterol* 1993;88:208–211.
5. Bradette M, Delvaux M, Staumont G, et al. Octreotide increases thresholds of colonic visceral perception in IBS patients without modifying muscle tone. *Dig Dis Sci* 1994;39:1171–1178.
6. Burkitt DP, Walker ARP, Painter NS. Effect of dietary fibre on stools and transit times, and its role in the causation of disease. *Lancet* 1972;2:1408–1412.
7. Byrne TA, Persinger RL, Young LS, et al. A new treatment for patients with short-bowel syndrome: growth hormone, glutamine, and a modified diet. *Ann Surg* 1995;222:243–254.

8. Creed F, Guthrie E. Psychological factors in the irritable bowel syndrome. *Gut* 1987;28:1307–1318.
9. Dapoigny M, Abitbol J-L, Fraitag B. Efficacy of peripheral kappa agonist fedotozine versus placebo in treatment of irritable bowel syndrome. *Dig Dis Sci* 1995;40:2244–2248.
10. Di Palma JA, De Ridder PH, Orlando RC, et al. A randomized, placebo-controlled, multicenter study of the safety and efficacy of a new polyethylene glycol laxative. *Am J Gastroenterol* 2000;95:446–450.
11. Drossman D. Rome II critera. *Am J Gastroenterol* 1999;94:2912–2917.
12. Drossman DA, Leserman J, Nachman G, et al. Sexual and physical abuse in women with functional or organic gastrointestinal disease. *Ann Intern Med* 1900;113:828–833.
13. Duma RJ, Kellum JM. Colonic diverticulitis: microbiologic, diagnostic and therapeutic considerations. *Curr Clin Topics Infect Dis* 1991;11:218–247.
14. Edes TE, Walk BE, Austin JL. Diarrhea in tube-fed patients: feeding formula not necessarily the cause. *Am J Med* 1990;88:91–93.
15. Giondretti P, Rizzello F, Venturi A, et al. Oral bacteriotherapy as maintenance treatment in patients with chronic pouchitis: a double-blind, placebo-controlled trial. *Gastroenterology* 2000;119:305–309.
16. Harvey RF, Read AE. Mode of action of the saline purgatives. *Am Heart J* 1975;89:810–212.
17. Hasler WL, Soudah HC, Owyang C. Somatostatin analog inhibits afferent response to rectal distention in diarrhea-predominant irritable bowel patients. *J Pharmacol Exp Ther* 1994;268:1206–1211.
18. Heller SN, Hackler LR. Changes in the crude fiber content of the American diet. *Am J Clin Nutr* 1978;31:1510–1514.
19. Hislop IG. Psychological significance of the irritable colon syndrome. *Gut* 1971;12:452–457.
20. Jepson S, Klaerke A, Nielsen PH, et al. Negative effect of metoclopramide in postoperative adynamic ileus: a prospective, randomized, double-blind study. *Br J Surg* 1986;73:290–291.
21. Kellow JE, Phillips SF. Altered small-bowel motility in irritable bowel syndrome is correlated with symptoms. *Gastroenterology* 1987;92:1885–1893.
22. Lacy BE, Yu S. Tegaserod: a new 5-HT4 agonist. *J Clin Gastroenterol* 2002;34:27–33.
23. Longo WE, Vernava AM III. Prokinetic agents for lower gastrointestinal motility disorders. *Dis Colon Rectum* 1993;36:696.
24. Manning AP, Thompson WG, Heaton KW, et al. Towards positive diagnosis of the irritable bowel. *BMJ* 1978;2:653–654.
25. Martelli H, Duguay C, Devroede G, et al. Some parameters of large bowel function in man. *Gastroenterology* 1978;75:612–618.
26. Mathias JR, Clench MH, Reeves-Darby VG, et al. Effect of leuprolide acetate in patients with moderate to severe functional bowel disease. *Dig Dis Sci* 1994;39:1155–1162.
27. Munakata J, Naliboff B, Harraf F, et al. Repetitive sigmoid stimulation induces rectal hyperalgesia in patients with irritable bowel syndrome. *Gastroenterology* 1997;112:55–63.
28. Nordgaard I, Nortensen PB. Digestive processes in the human colon. *Nutrition* 1995;12:35–45.
29. Ogilvy AJ, Smith G. The gastrointestinal tract after anesthesia. *Eur J Anaesthesiol Suppl* 1995;10:35–42.
30. Painter NS, Burkitt DP. Diverticular disease of the colon: a deficiency disease of Western civilization. *BMJ* 1971;2:450–454.
31. Papi C, Ciaco A, Koch M, et al. Efficacy of rifaximin in the treatment of symptomatic diverticular disease of the colon: a multicentre double-blind placebo-controlled trial. *Aliment Pharmacol Ther* 1995;9:33–39.
32. Parks TC. Natural history of diverticular disease of the colon. *Clin Gastroenterol* 1975;4:53–69.
33. Rendtdorff RC, Kashgarian M. Stool patterns of healthy adult males. *Dis Colon Rectum* 1967;10:222–228.
34. Ritchie JA, Truelove SC. Treatment of irritable bowel syndrome with lorazepam, hyoscine butylbromide and ispaghula husk. *BMJ* 1979;1:376–378.
35. Roberts JP, Benson MJ, Rogers J, et al. Effect of cisapride on distal colonic motility in the early postoperative period following left colonic anastamosis. *Dis Colon Rectum* 1995;38:139–145.
36. Sandler RS, Halabi S, Baron JA, et al. A randomized trial of aspirin to prevent colorectal adenomas in patients with previous colorectal cancer. *N Engl J Med* 2003;348:883–889.
37. Snape WJ Jr, Carlson GM, Cohen D. Colonic myoelectrical activity in the irritable bowel syndrome. *Gastroenterology* 1976;70:326–330.
38. Stefanini GF, Saggioro A, Alvisi V, et al. Oral cromolyn sodium in comparison with elimination diet in the irritable bowel syndrome, diarrheic type. *Scand J Gastoenterol* 1995;30:535–541.
39. Talley NJ, Owen BK, Boyce P, et al. Psychological treatments for irritable bowel syndrome: a critique of controlled treatment trials. *Am J Gastroenterol* 1996;91:277–286.
40. Verlinden M, Michiels G, Boghaert A, et al. Treatment of postoperative gastrointestinal atony. *Br J Surg* 1987;74:614–617.
41. Walker EA, Byrne PP, Katon WJ. Irritable bowel syndrome and psychiatric illness. *Am J Psychiatry* 1990;147:565–572.
42. Walker EA, Katon WJ, Roy-Byrne PP, et al. Histories of sexual victimization in patients with irritable bowel syndrome or inflammatory bowel disease. *Am J Psychiatry* 1993;150:1502–1506.
43. Walker EA, Roy-Byrne PP, Katon WJ, et al. Psychiatric illness and irritable bowel syndrome: a comparison with inflammatory bowel disease. *Am J Psychiatry* 1990;147:1656–1661.
44. Whitehead WE, Holtkotter B, Enck P, et al. Tolerance for recto-sigmoid distention in irritable bowel syndrome. *Gastroenterology* 1990;98:1187–1192.
45. Zieghagen DJ, Tewinkel G, Kruis W, et al. Adding more fluid to wheat bran has no significant effects on intestinal functions of healthy subjects. *J Clin Gastroenterol* 1991;13:525–530.

Chapter 4

Evaluation and Diagnostic Techniques

Come, come, and sit you down. You shall not budge!
You go not till I set you up a glass
Where you may see the inmost part of you.
                William Shakespeare: *Hamlet* III, iv, 18

This chapter addresses the evaluation of the symptoms frequently associated with diseases of the anus, rectum, and colon. In addition, the instrumentation, the studies, and the tests available for the diagnosis of these conditions are presented. Flexible sigmoidoscopy and colonoscopy are discussed, however, in Chapter 5. General principles of history taking and physical examination are introduced, but the reader is advised to consult the appropriate chapter for evaluation of a particular disease or condition.

HISTORY

As in all fields of medicine, the patient's history is the single most important piece of information that the physician can obtain. A carefully obtained interview will in all probability either establish the diagnosis or at least suggest it. In consideration of the pathologic conditions affecting the anus, rectum, and colon, there are a limited number of issues and questions that are pertinent.

Bleeding

Bleeding from the rectum has long been accepted as an important warning sign of bowel cancer, yet cancer is not the most likely cause of hematochezia. Blood may be pink, bright red, mahogany, black, or inapparent (i.e., occult). It may be noticed on the toilet paper, in the toilet bowl, or both. None of these manifestations of blood loss is specifically diagnostic of the location or type of pathologic process; thus it is import to keep an open mind. That stated, blood that appears solely on the toilet paper is suggestive of a distal cause (e.g., hemorrhoids, fissure). Altered (i.e., dark) blood suggests a more proximal lesion (e.g., carcinoma of the cecum). Blood found in the toilet bowl may or may not indicate a greater blood loss. One drop of blood will turn the water pink, and a few drops

will turn it red. Blood that is not observed by the patient but is revealed through guaiac or orthotoluidine testing (see Occult Blood Determination of Stool) requires comprehensive gastrointestinal (GI) evaluation.

Rectal bleeding may not be an isolated symptom. When associated with a painful lump and unrelated to defecation, it is usually the result of a thrombosed hemorrhoid. When related to defecation and associated with pain, it is often the result of an anal fissure, the most common cause of bleeding in the infant. When bleeding accompanies diarrhea, inflammatory bowel disease must be considered.

The physician must have a reasonable index of suspicion, as well as competent clinical judgment, before embarking on additional studies to evaluate the cause of rectal bleeding. In exercising this judgment, it is proper to withhold radiologic studies and defer additional diagnostic procedures if the bleeding is from a readily apparent cause. However, bleeding is an important symptom not to have. If it is believed to be caused by hemorrhoids, appropriate treatment should be instituted to control the symptoms. If bleeding persists despite an attempt at treatment, it is the responsibility of the physician to order or to perform the studies necessary to establish a diagnosis or exclude within the limitations of the state of medical knowledge the presence of significant pathologic features.

Pain

Anorectal pain is a frequent complaint, one that can be most disabling to the patient. If it is continuous, unrelated to defecation, and associated with a lump, a thrombosed hemorrhoid is the probable diagnosis. An anorectal abscess is another possibility. If the pain is exacerbated during and following defecation, examination will usually reveal the presence of an anal fissure. If the pain is deep seated, intermittent, and unrelated to defecation, the patient is probably experiencing proctalgia fugax (i.e., levator spasm). If related to the coccyx and worsened by moving from a sitting to a standing position, coccygodynia is the probable cause. Incidentally, for the reader, that is the correct spelling. Anorectal pain is rarely associated with a tumor unless the lesion invades the anal canal or internal sphincter to produce tenesmus—a painful, ineffective desire to defecate.

Abdominal pain, if colicky in nature, may be caused by bowel obstruction but most commonly can be attributed to the irritable bowel syndrome. Physical examination and plain abdominal films readily distinguish the two entities. When abdominal pain is continuous, it may be a consequence of peritoneal irritation from any of a number of sources. Here again, physical examination and determination of the presence or absence of peritoneal signs will lead the physician to pursue the appropriate diagnostic and therapeutic course.

Anal and Perianal Masses

The differential diagnosis of an anal or perianal lump involves a spectrum of benign and malignant lesions as well as a host of dermatologic conditions. Probably the most common causes are a thrombosed hemorrhoid and a skin tag. Other frequently observed lumps include sebaceous cysts, lipomas, hypertrophied anal papillae, and condylomata. Protrusion or prolapse of hemorrhoids that reduces spontaneously or requires manual reduction may also be the cause of the mass. Uncommonly, rectal prolapse (i.e., procidentia) may present as a rectal mass. With lesions of uncertain nature, biopsy is mandatory.

Rectal Discharge

Mucous discharge and soiling of the underclothes are frequent complaints in the experience of most colon and rectal surgeons. The patient may have undergone prior anal surgery with resultant deformity and scarring or may have sustained sphincter injury from surgical, accidental, or obstetric trauma. Again, it is important to obtain an accurate history. Systemic disease (e.g., diabetes mellitus) or neurologic conditions may also be factors. Of course, when purulent discharge is accompanied by a painful swelling, the patient usually has an anal or perianal abscess.

Rectal discharge, however, is usually not related to the presence of a specific pathologic entity. Most individuals experience the difficulty because of dietary indiscretion or too vigorous attention to anal hygiene. Appropriate dietary and hygiene counseling may be all the treatment that is required (see Chapter 19). In patients with a lax anus, perineal strengthening exercises may be helpful (see Chapter 13).

Incontinence

Fecal incontinence is defined by most colon and rectal surgeons in accordance with the presenting complaint(s): incontinence of gas, soiling of the underclothes, incontinence for loose stool, incontinence for formed stool, and the requirement for the use of a pad. The condition may be caused by anorectal disease, fecal impaction, laxative abuse, neurologic disease, and trauma (surgical, obstetric, blunt and sharp). The complaint of fecal incontinence requires at least a minimal neurologic examination (e.g., sensory evaluation of the perianal area)[22]: Repair or reconstruction is usually advocated for incontinence secondary to trauma or to congenital anomaly (see Chapter 13).

Change in Bowel Habits

The impression by the patient that the bowels have changed may have great significance. It is one of the symptoms suggestive of colonic neoplasm and almost always requires endoscopic or radiologic investigation for adequate assessment.

A change in bowel habits may be as obvious as diarrhea when the patient has had a long history of constipation or as subtle as the development of normal, easy bowel movements after many years of a difficult or irregular pattern. The presence of bleeding with a change in bowel habits increases exponentially the likelihood of the presence of a malignant neoplasm.

PHYSICAL EXAMINATION

A general physical examination of the patient with a colorectal complaint is usually an unrewarding exercise. If the physician practices "chief complaint" medicine, nothing is improper in limiting the examination to the abdomen, which is also usually nonproductive, and to the rectum. Conversely, to embark on endoscopic or radiologic investigation without performing a complete rectal examination is inappropriate and inadequate.

The standard approaches to evaluation of the anus, rectum and colon include the following:

- Inspection
- Palpation
- Anoscopy
- Proctosigmoidoscopy or flexible sigmoidoscopy
- Colonoscopy or barium enema (with or without air)

Generally, the term *proctosigmoidoscopy* is used interchangeably with the words *procto* and *sigmoidoscopy*. All three imply the use of the 25-cm rigid instrument.

Positioning the Patient for Rigid Sigmoidoscopy

It is regrettable that the technique for performing rigid sigmoidoscopy is becoming an art that may be rele-

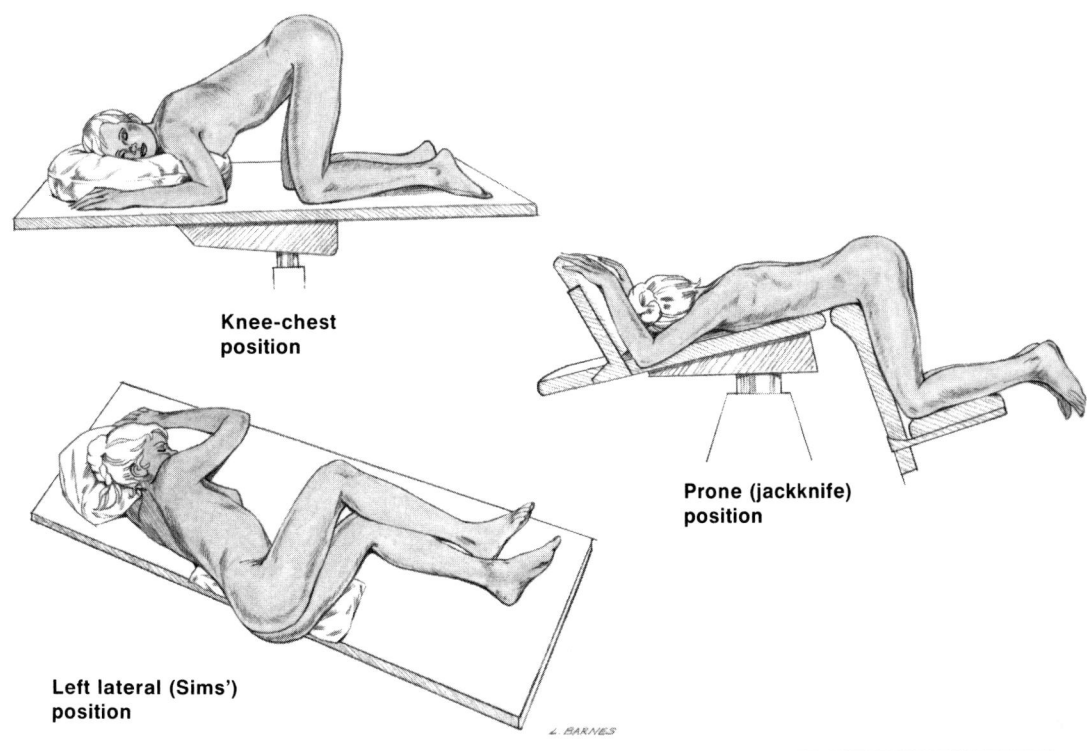

Knee-chest position

Prone (jackknife) position

Left lateral (Sims') position

L. BARNES

FIGURE 4-1. Positions commonly used for performing sigmoidoscopy are the knee-chest, prone, and left lateral.

gated to the status of historical curiosity. This is particularly unfortunate because there are circumstances for which the rigid approach is preferred, and flexible sigmoidoscopy and colonoscopy are limiting. For example, ironing out the rectal valves can be more readily accomplished with a rigid instrument. Therefore, a better visualization of areas that are potentially awkward to view may be achieved. In addition, the rigid instrument permits accurate measurement of the level of a lesion. Very often, the flexible instrument results in a measurement that is falsely higher than is truly the case. The three commonly used patient positions for performing sigmoidoscopy are the prone, the left lateral, and the knee-chest (Figure 4-1).

The prone jackknife position requires a special table that tilts the patient's head down (Figure 4-2). The table is expensive, but it provides the easiest access and the best view for the examiner. It is the least comfortable position, however, for the patient.

The most comfortable position for an individual undergoing this examination is the left lateral (i.e., Sims') position. The patient lies on the left side on the examining table or bed with the buttocks protruding over the edge, hips flexed, knees slightly extended, and right shoulder rotated anteriorly. The examiner may sit or stand depending on the height of the table or bed. Although

this position is the easiest of the three for the patient, it is not as convenient for the examiner as is the prone position.

The knee-chest position is probably somewhat more comfortable for the patient than the prone, but it is the

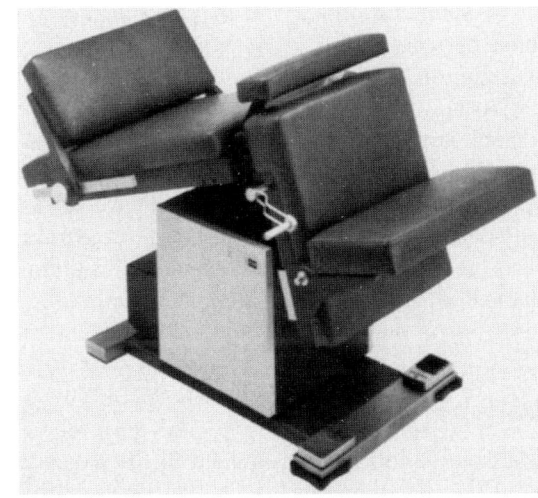

FIGURE 4-2. The Ritter table is used for examination in the prone jackknife position. (Courtesy of Sybron Corporation, Evanston, IL.)

most awkward of all for the physician. In my opinion, the knee-chest position should be abandoned.

Some physicians believe that the sigmoidoscope can be inserted farther when an individual is in one position rather than another, but there is no evidence to suggest that position either interferes with or facilitates insertion of the instrument to its full length.

If one is to perform a satisfactory and reasonably comfortable examination and obtain all necessary information, it is essential to inform the patient continually what is to be expected and what is happening. Rectal examination may be a frustratingly unsuccessful experience for both the physician and the patient if proper concern is not demonstrated for the patient's understandable reluctance to submit to such an unpleasant intrusion of the intestinal tract. Warm hands and a reassuring demeanor are most helpful. Additionally, a relaxed and supportive attitude with due consideration for the patient's modesty is suggested, as is limiting the number of observers to no more than two.[32]

Inspection

Inspection of the anal area may reveal hemorrhoids, skin tags, a sentinel pile indicative of an underlying anal fissure, dermatologic problems, including pruritic changes, an abscess, a fistula, a scar, or a deformity. Evaluation of the sacrococcygeal region may disclose a laminectomy scar, possibly suggesting a neurologic cause for any incontinence symptoms.[101] Pain on spreading the buttocks may indicate the presence of an anal fissure.

In addition to mere inspection of the perianal skin, evaluation of the resting state of the anal opening is possible. A patulous anal orifice may be seen. This may be due to a concomitant rectal prolapse, neurologic abnormality, or sphincter injury, or it may be a sign of an ano-receptive person.[113]

By asking the patient to strain, additional valuable information may be obtained. A rectal prolapse, hypertrophied anal papilla, or, most commonly, hemorrhoids may protrude. It should be remembered, however, that the prone jack-knife position is least conducive to demonstrating conditions that tend to prolapse. If the physician suspects procidentia, then the examination should be conducted while the patient sits and attempts to strain while sitting on the toilet.

Palpation

A water-soluble lubricant is applied to the gloved index finger. Although some physicians prefer to use a finger cot, a disposable latex glove is ideal for rectal examination. The patient is informed that a finger will be passed into the rectum and that this will make him or her feel as if the bowels will move. Again, it is imperative to inform,

distract, and reassure the patient continually. The physician should examine the rectum and its surrounding structures in an organized approach. Assessment of sphincter tone and contractility is an important part of the rectal examination, and these should be noted routinely whenever a patient complains of problems with fecal control or discharge.

In the male patient, the prostate is felt anteriorly. It should be assessed for hypertrophy, nodularity, and firmness.

In the female patient, the cervix can be palpated, unless it is surgically absent. The uterine body may be felt to be displaced posteriorly, and the presence of fibroid tumors may be noted. The uninitiated examiner may misinterpret the uterus or cervix as being an intrarectal tumor. Another common error of rectal palpation in women is to misjudge a vaginal tampon for a rectal wall lesion. With experience, however, there should be no confusion. A posteriorly displaced uterus may serve to warn the examiner that rigid proctosigmoidoscopy to the full length of the instrument may not be possible. Bidigital examination (i.e., one finger in the rectum and the other in the vagina) will readily distinguish any anatomic or pathologic variations.

The physician should then sweep the examining finger from anterior to posterior and back again, *consciously* thinking of a possible lesion that could be present. The conscious thought process is emphasized, because all too often this phase of the examination is performed reflexively, with the assumption that any lesion will be identified by the instrument if it is not perceived by the examining finger. However, a submucosal rectal nodule may not be visible and would otherwise go undiagnosed if direct visualization alone were employed. It may even be possible to feel a tumor in the sigmoid colon or a diverticular mass. Asking the patient to strain down (i.e., Valsalva's maneuver) will sometimes reveal a lesion in the upper rectum or rectosigmoid that otherwise would not be palpable. Examination above the prostate in the male patient or in the cul-de-sac in the female patient may reveal Blumer's shelf, a hard mass on the anterior rectal wall caused by metastatic tumor, usually of gastric or pancreatic origin. Attention to the presacral area may reveal an extrinsic mass (e.g., cyst, tumor, or sacrococcygeal chordoma).

Finally, as the finger is withdrawn, the presence of anal disease is noted (e.g., hypertrophied papilla, thrombosed hemorrhoid, stenosis, scarring). It is well recognized that digital examination of the anal canal is the most accurate means of diagnosing Crohn's disease in this area.

Prostate Evaluation

There are three methods available for diagnosing prostatic carcinoma:

- Digital rectal examination
- Measurement of prostate-specific antigen (PSA)
- Transrectal ultrasonography (TRUS) and biopsy

Although digital examination should be considered the most important of these methods, it is accurate in detecting only 60% of prostatic carcinomas. As a consequence, it is recommended that all men 50 years of age or older undergo serum PSA determination on an annual basis, ideally with blood drawn before digital rectal manipulation. TRUS is not yet believed to be sufficiently accurate to be used as a diagnostic screening test for prostatic carcinoma. This study should be reserved for those individuals with subtle or irregular prostatic abnormalities identified on digital examination or for those who demonstrate an elevated PSA determination. A positive family history of prostatic cancer is another rationale for ordering a screening ultrasonogram. Certainly, all patients who harbor suspect prostatic abnormalities should undergo TRUS, because this provides the most accurate method for evaluation, with biopsy performed if indicated.

Anoscopy

Anoscopic examination unfortunately may be employed as an alternative to proctosigmoidoscopy by some physicians who do not have a sigmoidoscope available in the office. A barium enema study may then be performed. Sadly, with this type of workup, a rectal lesion can be overlooked. Conversely, when proctosigmoidoscopy is performed, anoscopy is often omitted. The anoscope is not a substitute for the sigmoidoscope, nor is sigmoidoscopy an effective replacement for anoscopy. Anoscopy offers the best means to evaluate hemorrhoids, fissures, papillae, or other lesions of the anal canal. It is the requisite instrument if the physician is to perform an anal procedure or to treat a condition of the anal canal.

Numerous anoscopes and specula are available (Figure 4-3), but the one I prefer is the Hirschman. The physician can purchase either reusable or disposable fiberoptic modifications to the Hirschman anoscope; some have a light source that fits into the instrument (Electro Surgical Instrument Co., Rochester, NY; WelchAllyn, Inc., Skaneateles Falls, NY; Figure 4-4). Although relatively ex-

pensive, lighted anoscopes are ideal for diagnostic purposes. However, they may be somewhat limiting when a procedure is attempted through the instrument. Still, the choice of instrument and whether a light source is an intrinsic component are variables that are decided on the basis of an individual's training, experience, and personal preference. A fiberoptic, malleable light source can also be used (Figure 4-5), but a simple gooseneck lamp works reasonably well. Even a hand-held light may be adequate, although it is somewhat cumbersome. I personally find that side-view instruments fail to give a proper perspective of anal canal anatomy and of anal pathology, but many qualified surgeons will disagree. If a side view is required for performing an office procedure (e.g., sphincterotomy) a narrow (i.e., 2.2-cm) Hill-Ferguson retractor is very useful (Figure 4-6). When rotating the anoscope around the anal canal circumference, it is helpful to reinsert the obturator to turn the instrument. By doing so, the tendency to drag or pinch the anal canal or perianal skin is minimized.

Finally, when pathologic features are noted or treated, the site should be recorded as follows: right anterior, left lateral, and so forth. The use of o'clock descriptions should be abandoned, because it requires a known patient position, and this may differ from one examination or examiner to another. Left posterior is left posterior even if the patient is hanging from a chandelier!

Rigid Proctosigmoidoscopy

The sigmoidoscope is one of our most valuable diagnostic tools, perhaps even more useful than the stethoscope. The stethoscope is not likely to identify a cardiac, pulmonary, or abdominal abnormality that is not already evident from a carefully taken history. Also, stethoscopic findings almost always require confirmation by roentgenography or electrocardiography. I do not expect physicians to discard the traditional auscultatory tool and begin carrying a sigmoidoscope in a hip holster to undertake the procedure on every patient they see. However, because colorectal cancer is the second most common visceral malignancy in the United States today, it is a pity that more physicians do not perform sigmoidoscopy.

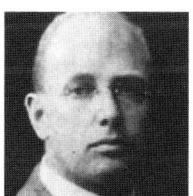

George Blumer (1872–1962) Blumer was born in England and later moved with his family to California. As a house officer at Johns Hopkins Hospital in Baltimore, he worked under Halsted, Osler, Thayer, Welch, and Flexner. Blumer became director of the Bender Hygienic Laboratory in Albany, New York, and then accepted successive appointments to the Albany Medical College, Cooper Medical College, University of California Medical School, and Yale University Medical School. In 1910, he became dean of the medical faculty at Yale. He was a prolific writer and wrote a three-volume text on bedside diagnosis. (Blumer G. The rectal shelf: a neglected rectal sign of value in the diagnosis and prognosis of obscure malignant and inflammatory disease within the abdomen. *Albany Med Ann* 1909;30:361.)

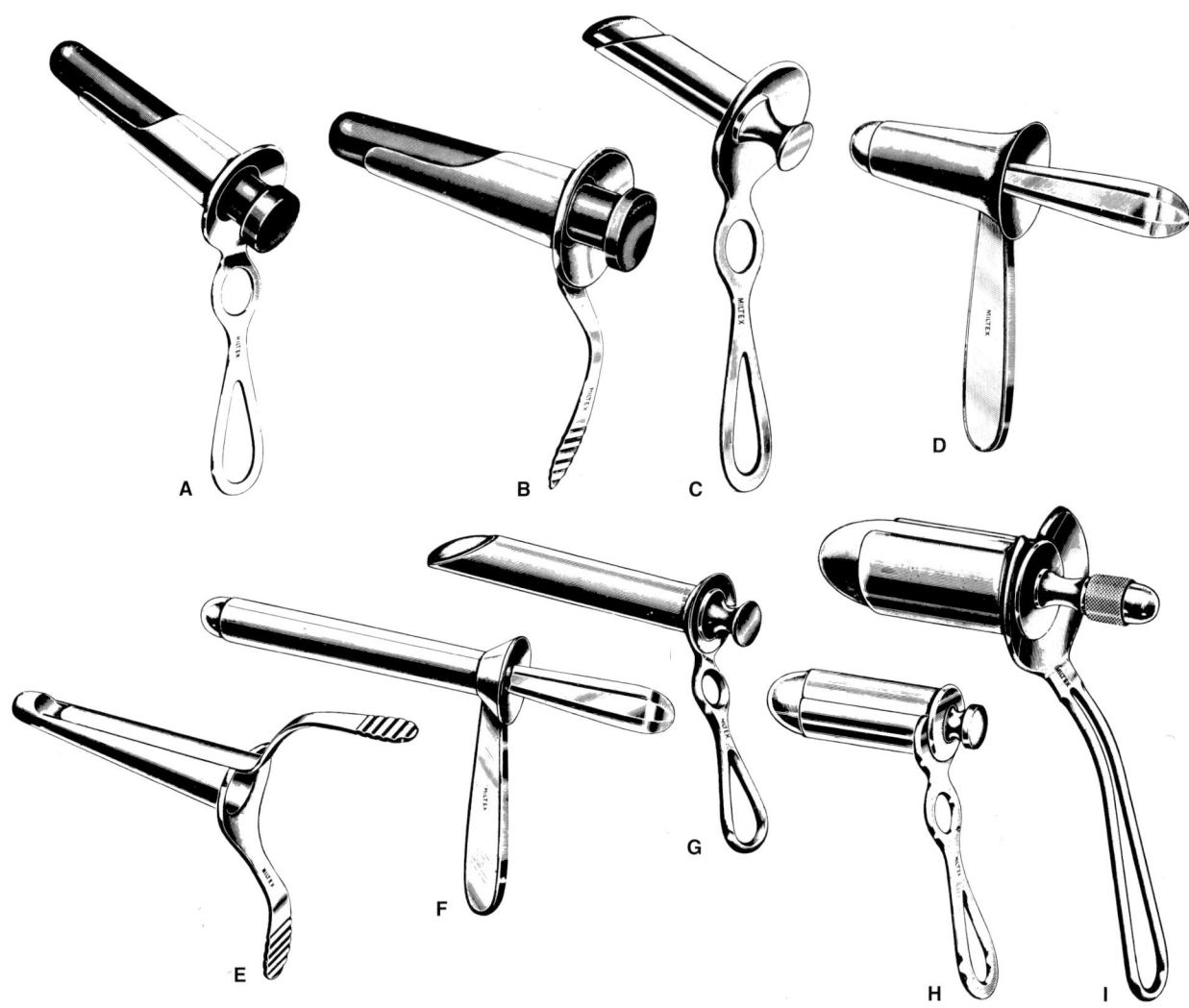

FIGURE 4-3. Anoscopes. **(A)** Pennington. **(B)** Fansler-Ives. **(C)** Hirschman, available in three diameters: 7/8 inch (2.2 cm), 11/16 inch (1.75 cm), and 9/16 inch (1.43 cm). **(D)** Kelly. **(E)** Brinkerhoff. **(F)** Kelly proctoscope. **(G)** Hirschman proctoscope. **(H)** Chelsea Eaton. **(I)** Fansler operating speculum. (Courtesy of Miltex Instrument Co., Inc, York, PA.)

Ideally, every individual should undergo this procedure at the same time as one has a complete medical examination, although for screening purposes the longer, flexible instrument is obviously preferred. In a perfect world, an initial sigmoidoscopic examination should be accomplished when a patient is in the late teens to detect any tendency to form polyps. Investigators have confirmed a relatively high yield of asymptomatic polyps when proctosigmoidoscopy is performed as part of a complete physical examination. Swinton reported an incidence of 5% in a series of 3,000 routine examinations.[118] Portes and Majarakis noted almost an 8% incidence in 50,000 asymptomatic patients.[92] In our experience, approximately 9% of patients were found to have benign lesions.[17] After a negative result on initial examination, sig-

moidoscopy is not necessary as a routine diagnostic test for asymptomatic patients until they are 50 years of age, and every 2 years thereafter. Of course, anyone, regardless of age, who has symptoms such as rectal bleeding or a change in bowel habit should undergo the appropriate investigational procedures.

As previously mentioned, the rigid sigmoidoscope is the optimal instrument for evaluation of the rectum. Barium enema study is a poor technique for diagnosing rectal disease, and even flexible sigmoidoscopy and colonoscopy are not as satisfactory as rigid sigmoidoscopy for evaluating ampullary lesions, unless a retroflexion maneuver is performed (see Chapter 5). Examination with the sigmoidoscope may reveal mucosal excrescences, polypoid lesions, cancer, inflammatory changes, stricture, vas-

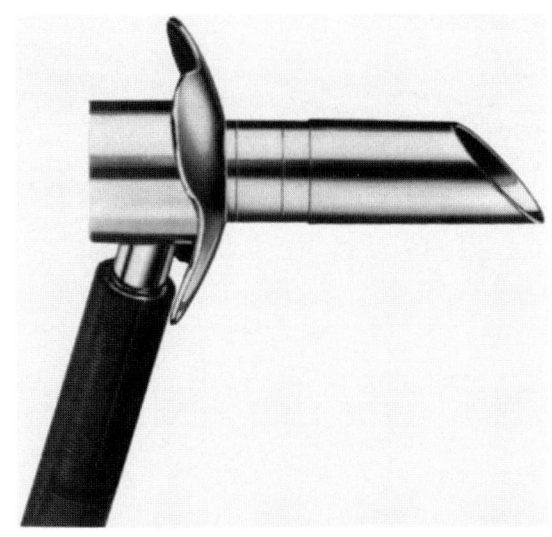

FIGURE 4-4. The fiberoptic anoscope (obturator not shown) is available in three diameters: 2.7, 2.3, and 1.9 cm. (Courtesy of WelchAllyn, Inc., Skaneateles Falls, NY.)

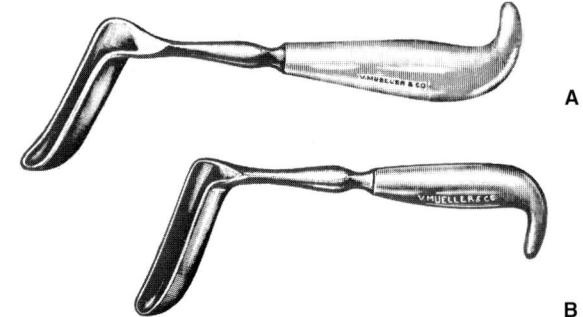

FIGURE 4-6. Anorectal retractors. **(A)** The Ferguson-Moon rectal retractor is available in two depths and widths. **(B)** The Hill-Ferguson rectal retractor is available in three depths and widths. (Courtesy of V. Mueller, McGraw Park, IL.)

cular malformation, or anatomic distortion from extraluminal masses. It may also detect anal conditions, but, as mentioned, it should not replace the anoscope for this purpose.

Equipment

Numerous reusable or disposable rigid sigmoidoscopes are available, with proximal or distal lighting, and with or without fiberoptics (Figs. 4-7, 4-8, and 4-9). Reusable instruments require care and cleansing, with the need for sterilization equipment and with the burden of governmental regulations concerning ventilation and the use of hazardous materials (at least in the United States). Disposable ones are obviously discarded. If only a few examinations a day are performed, the reusable instrument may be more appropriate. If many examinations are undertaken every day, then the disposable instrument is usually preferred, unless the physician can afford the luxury of having a number of instruments and can justify the expense and inconvenience of cleansing them.

Reusable instruments are available in several diameters, ranging from 1.1 to 2.7 cm. The medium or 1.9-cm instrument is an excellent compromise that offers the physician the ability both to screen the patient and to perform procedures. The large-bore instrument is less useful for screening because of greater patient discomfort but may be invaluable for removing a large polyp. The narrow sigmoidoscope (1.1 cm) is a good screening tool and is particularly useful if an anal stricture precludes the use of the larger-diameter instrument. It is very limiting, however, if one attempts to perform procedures with it. Unfortunately, as of this writing, disposable sigmoidoscopes are only available in one diameter (1.9 cm).

In addition to the speculum tube, the instrumentation includes a light source, a proximal magnifying lens, and

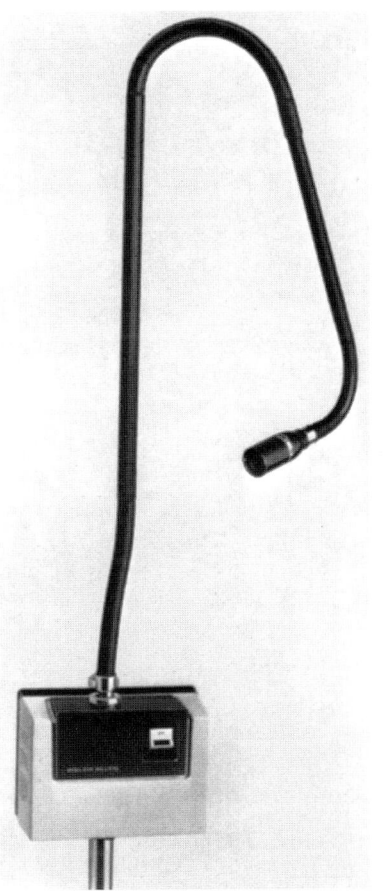

FIGURE 4-5. Fiberoptic malleable halogen examination light. (Courtesy of WelchAllyn, Inc., Skaneateles Falls, NY.)

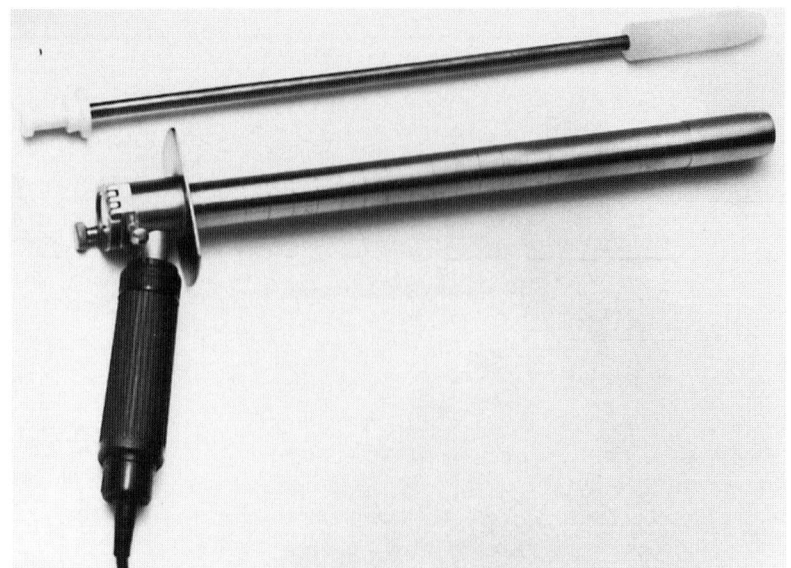

FIGURE 4-7. This reusable and autoclavable fiberoptic sigmoidoscope measures 1.9 cm in diameter and 25 cm in length. (Courtesy of Welch-Allyn, Inc., Skaneateles Falls, NY.)

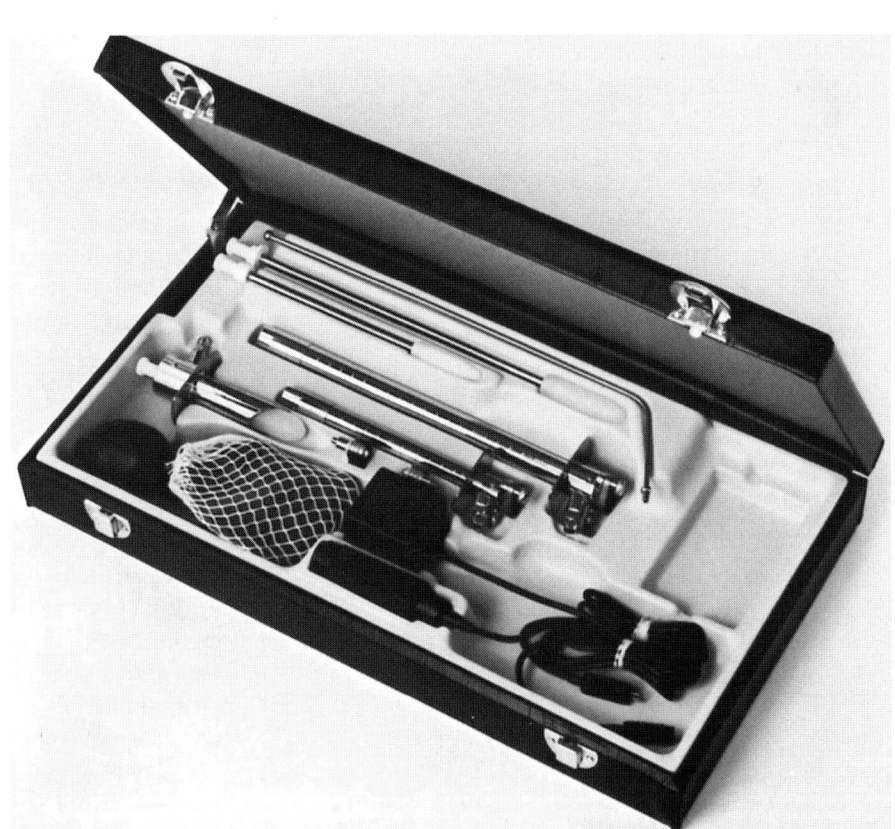

FIGURE 4-8. Fiberoptic endoscopic set, including pediatric proctoscope. (Courtesy of WelchAllyn, Inc., Skaneateles Falls, NY.)

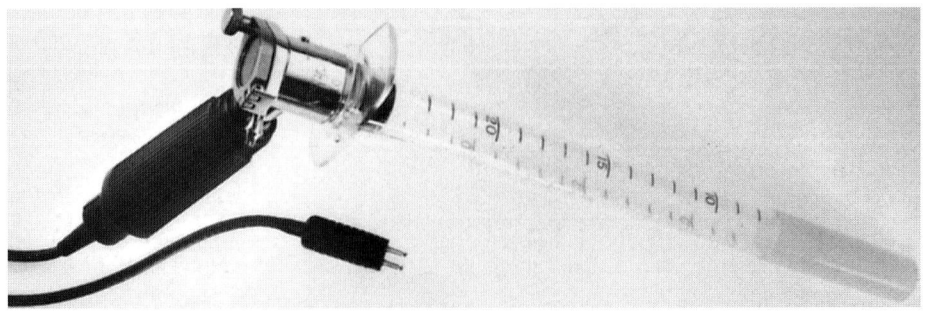

FIGURE 4-9. Disposable fiberoptic sigmoidoscope. (Courtesy of WelchAllyn, Inc., Skaneateles Falls, NY.)

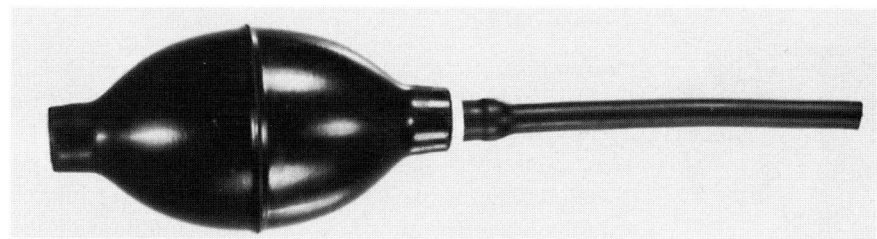

FIGURE 4-10. Insufflation bulb without reservoir. (Courtesy of Cameron-Miller, Inc., Chicago, IL.)

an attachment for the insufflation of air. There is a mistaken concept that the reservoir is an important piece of equipment. However, its presence creates a cumbersome and inconvenient apparatus. The first action the physician should take after purchasing new equipment is to remove the reservoir and attach the bulb to the eyepiece by the shortest length of tubing possible (Figure 4-10). Another important detail is adequate provision for suction. This can be accomplished by attachment to a vacuum pump or a water tap. Long swabs (i.e., chimney sweeps) are also helpful (Figure 4-11).

Preparation

Adequate preparation of the distal bowel is a *sine qua non* for a complete and satisfactory examination. A small-volume enema (e.g., Fleet) is advised prior to the procedure unless the patient has a history suggestive of inflammatory bowel disease. Vigorous catharsis the day before the examination and dietary restrictions are unnecessary.

Technique

There are five principles that should be adhered to if the physician is to conduct a safe, competent sigmoidoscopic examination:

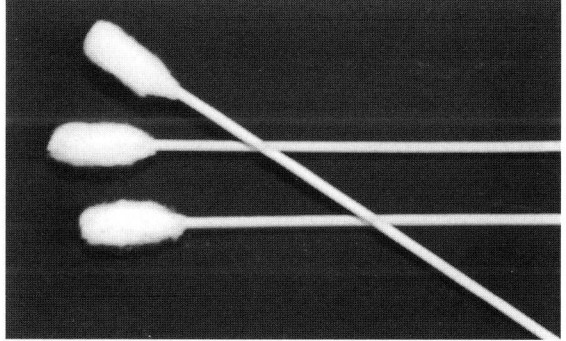

FIGURE 4-11. Chimney sweeps are long cotton-tip applicators useful for removing small amounts of stool.

- Be expeditious.
- Insufflate minimal air.
- Always have a nurse or assistant available.
- Keep talking to the patient: explain, reassure, distract.
- Do no harm.

As mentioned earlier, a digital rectal examination should always precede instrumentation. In addition to providing valuable information, this procedure permits the sphincter to relax sufficiently to accept an instrument. The well-lubricated, warmed sigmoidoscope is then inserted and passed to the maximal height as quickly as possible while causing minimal discomfort to the patient.

Air insufflation is of value in demonstrating the lumen of the bowel and is of even greater benefit in visualizing the mucosa when the instrument is withdrawn. Air insufflation should, however, be kept to a minimum, because it tends to cause abdominal cramping that may persist for many hours. The novice should not pass the sigmoidoscope without clearly observing the lumen. However, as skill develops, the physician can determine the amount of gentle pressure that can be safely exerted as long as the mucosa is seen to be sliding past. When an obstacle is reached, the instrument is withdrawn slightly and redirected to view the lumen again; it is then readvanced.

The physician should withdraw in a rotating fashion, carefully viewing the entire circumference of the bowel wall and ironing out mucosal folds to be certain that no small lesion is missed. Several lateral folds are often encountered in the rectum, the so-called valves of Houston (see Biography, Chapter 1). Usually, three folds can be identified: the upper and lower are convex to the right, and the middle one is convex to the left (Figure 4-12). The valves can serve as useful sites for performing rectal biopsy when the mucosa is grossly normal, because of technical ease as well as the limited risk for perforation. Particular care should be taken to view the posterior wall that sits in the hollow of the sacrum. This may necessitate the awkward placement of the examiner's head behind the patient's knees.

Successful insertion of the sigmoidoscope requires familiarity with the anatomy of the rectum and sigmoid colon. Knowing where the lumen probably is located without actually visualizing it permits the examiner considerable freedom in passing the instrument. When the

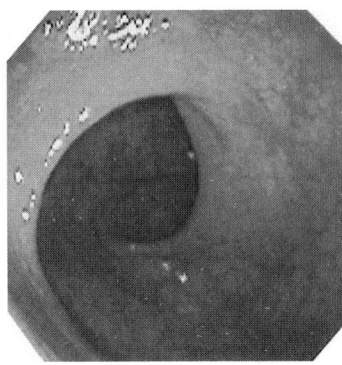

FIGURE 4-12. The middle and upper rectal valves of Houston. (See Color Fig. 4-12.)

sigmoidoscope is inserted, the low rectal and midrectal areas are midline structures. As the upper rectum is reached, the bowel bends slightly to the left. At the rectosigmoid junction, the tendency is for the instrument to turn to the right and ventrally. Therefore, if difficulty is encountered at the level of 15 or 16 cm, a maneuver to the left may reveal the proximal bowel. At a level of 18 or 19 cm, a more vigorous maneuver to the right and ventrally may permit the proximal colon to be entered.

In my experience, the average length that one can insert the instrument is 20 cm.[17] In a report from the Mayo Clinic in Rochester, Minnesota, 25% of patients could not be examined beyond this point.[104] Nivatvongs and Fryd reported the average depth of insertion to be 19.5 cm .[83] The two structures that may preclude complete (to 25 cm) examination are the uterus and the prostate gland. An enlarged prostate, a uterus containing fibroid tumors, or a uterus that is displaced posteriorly may make it impossible to pass the instrument beyond the 14- or 15-cm level. Persistence in attempting to achieve a higher penetration is usually unrewarding and may be dangerous, and it is most uncomfortable for the patient. As mentioned previously, the potential for encountering this difficulty can often be predicted by careful digital examination.

Men are examined to the full length of the instrument much more often than women. Even when the uterus is surgically absent, fixation of the bowel in the pelvis may preclude further passage. A careful history will alert the examiner, thereby expediting the procedure and minimizing further discomfort.

Younger individuals are often more difficult to examine than older patients; because they usually have better sphincter tone, insertion of the instrument may cause more discomfort. The discomfort leads to apprehension and a tendency to bear down, making the examination more tedious. Also, pelvic organs are less lax in younger than in older women, causing it to be somewhat more difficult to displace the uterus and allow passage of the sigmoidoscope.

Complications

Perforation

The physician must take care when passing the instrument without visualizing the lumen. Fortunately, perforation from rigid sigmoidoscopy is extremely unusual. Swinton reported two such occurrences in almost 100,000 examinations (Swinton NW, personal communication). Gilbertsen reported five perforations in 103,000 examinations,[43] and Nelson and colleagues noted two in more than 16,000 proctosigmoidoscopies.[82]

I have not experienced this occurrence in more than 75,000 examinations, but one death has occurred as a consequence of ventricular fibrillation. My own feeling is that perforation of the normal rectum or sigmoid colon should not occur from the instrument alone, but attempting to pass the rigid sigmoidoscope in a patient with inflammatory bowel disease, diverticulitis, radiation proctitis, or cancer can sometimes be a hazardous undertaking. Air insufflation can cause perforation of a diverticulum or of a walled-off abscess, and obviously such procedures as biopsy and electrocoagulation can result in perforation.

Bacteremia and Antibiotic Prophylaxis

Bacteremia can be associated with all endoscopic procedures.[1,23,61,65,69,100] Even rectal examination itself may predispose to such an occurrence, but there is some difference of opinion concerning the incidence (0% to approximately 25%) and significance of a transient nonfebrile episode.[57] Durack reported the following rates of bacteremia for a number of invasive colorectal procedures[26]:

Rates of Bacteremia

Procedure	*Incidence (Range), %*
Barium enema	10 (5–11)
Colonoscopy	5 (0–5)
Flexible sigmoidoscopy	0
Rigid sigmoidoscopy	5 (0–13)

Note that in this study, brushing teeth had an incidence of 40% (range, 7%–50%).[26]

In 1992, the Standards Task Force of the American Society of Colon and Rectal Surgeons published practice parameters for antibiotic prophylaxis during colon and rectal endoscopy.[3] These recommendations were updated in the year 2000.[115] Prophylactic antibiotic therapy is advised for those individuals at high risk, in accordance with the recommendations of the American Heart Association.[20] These recommendations are made for patients who undergo proctosigmoidoscopy with biopsy, flexible sigmoidoscopy with biopsy, colonoscopy, or an anal procedure (e.g., rubber ring ligation of hemorrhoids), even though invasive procedures are not the cause of most instances of endocarditis.[109,115] The following list illustrates the conditions for which endocarditis prophylaxis is necessary:[115]

High-Risk Conditions Associated with Endocarditis

Prosthetic cardiac valves, including bioprosthetic and homograft valves
History of endocarditis
Surgically constructed systemic-pulmonary shunts
Complex cyanotic congenital heart disease
Vascular grafts (within 6 months of implantation)
Previous bacterial endocarditis, even in the absence of heart disease

Because these patients are at high risk for the development of endocarditis, it is probably prudent to employ antibiotics even for minor intrusions of the GI tract (e.g., proctoscopy alone or barium enema). Postoperative coronary artery bypass graft surgery is not believed to require prophylactic antibiotic therapy, nor is such a protocol recommended for individuals who have cardiac pacemakers, implanted defibrillators, or physiologic, functional, or innocent heart murmurs.

Enterococci are the organisms most commonly associated with endocarditis, even though the physician is usually most concerned about gram-negative bacteria in the colonic flora. The following regimens are recommended:[115]

Prophylactic Antibiotic Regimens

Ampicillin/ gentamicin/ amoxicillin	Ampicillin, 2 g (50 mg/kg for children) intramuscularly or intravenously, plus gentamicin, 1.5 mg/kg (not to exceed 120 mg) intramuscularly or intravenously; both administered half an hour before the procedure, followed by amoxicillin (1 g) orally, intravenous or intramuscular 6 hours after initial dose

Patients Allergic to Ampicillin/Amoxicillin/Penicillin

Vancomycin and gentamicin	Intravenous vancomycin (1.0 g) given slowly over 1 to 2 hours, plus intravenous or intramuscular gentamicin, 1.5 mg/kg (not to exceed 120 mg); complete infusion within 30 minutes of starting procedure

Procedures Performed through the Sigmoidoscope

Three procedures are frequently performed through the rigid proctosigmoidoscope:

- Biopsy
- Electrocoagulation
- Snare excision

Gear and Dobbins have published a comprehensive review of the diagnostic usefulness of rectal biopsy, to which is appended an extensive bibliography.[39] It is interesting to note, however, the virtual absence of writings on rigid sigmoidoscopic procedures since the 1980s, owing to the fact that the technique has been virtually replaced by the flexible instruments (see Chapter 5). This is unfortunate indeed, because many diagnostic and therapeutic procedures are preferably performed through the rigid sigmoidoscope or via a transanal approach, an observation that needs to be reinforced time and again to gastroenterologists.

Instruments and Methods

Biopsy forceps are available with various biting tips (Figure 4-13). I prefer the Buie instrument (Figure 4-14), because I consider it the most responsive and have had less success with the others. Some instruments are electrified for biopsy and coagulation, but this is an unnecessary encumbrance in my opinion. Rarely is bleeding a problem when a biopsy is taken from an obvious lesion (see Complications of Procedures). Biopsy of the mucosa when a lesion is not present, such as is undertaken for amyloid, should always be performed on the posterior wall or on a valve of Houston. The valves are only mucosal structures, so perforation is virtually impossible. Conversely, biopsy of this area is not advisable if the physician wishes to obtain a sample of muscularis propria.

Electrocoagulation obviously requires familiarity with electrosurgical equipment. Most surgeons find the instrument setting that works well for the procedure performed, but the same maneuvers carried out in the hospital, with similar or different equipment, may produce inadequate or too vigorous electrocoagulation. The physician is advised to test any unfamiliar equipment on a bar of soap, adjusting the setting for the appropriate conditions.

My experience has been primarily with the suction-fulgurating unit made by Cameron-Miller (Chicago, IL: 773-523-6360; Figs. 4-15 and 4-16). This type of electrode removes gas, smoke, liquid stool, and blood during electrocoagulation. Other companies make comparable electrosurgical equipment (e.g., Elmed, Inc., Addison, IL: 708-543-2792; Valley Lab, Inc., Boulder, CO: 800-255-8522; Circon ACMI, Santa Barbara, CA: 805-961-1661). Although it is helpful to know that a

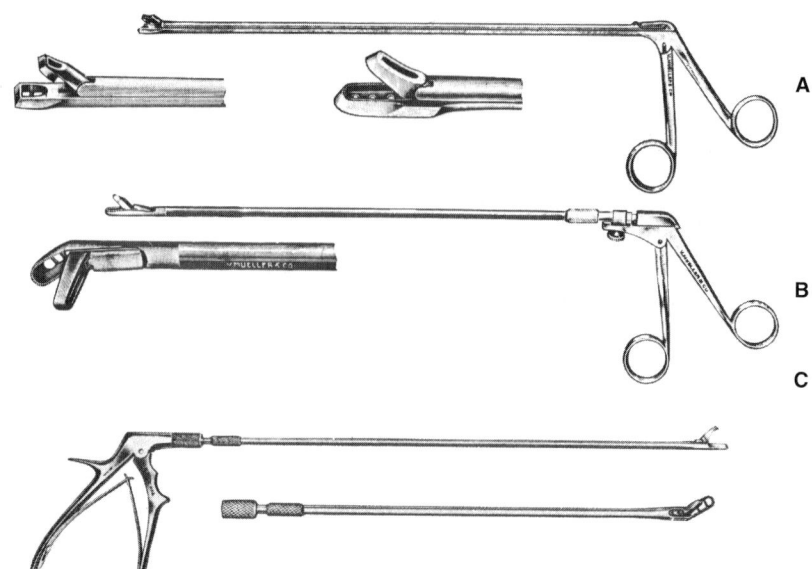

A

B

C

FIGURE 4-13. Rectal biopsy forceps. **(A)** V. Mueller forceps (bite, 3.5 mm × 5.5 mm). **(B)** Yeoman forceps (bite, 4 mm × 10 mm). **(C)** Turell angulated specimen forceps. **(D)** Biopsy forceps. The curved upper jaw has a 360-degree rotation feature. (Courtesy of V. Mueller, McGraw Park, IL.)

D

FIGURE 4-14. Buie rectal biopsy forceps. (Courtesy of V. Mueller, McGraw Park, IL.)

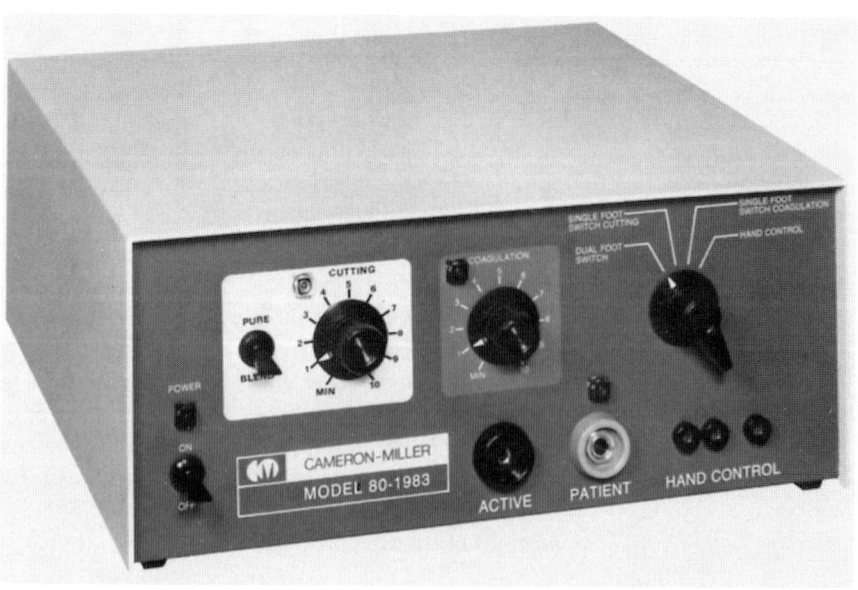

FIGURE 4-15. Cameron-Miller electrosurgery unit. (Courtesy of Cameron-Miller, Inc., Chicago, IL.)

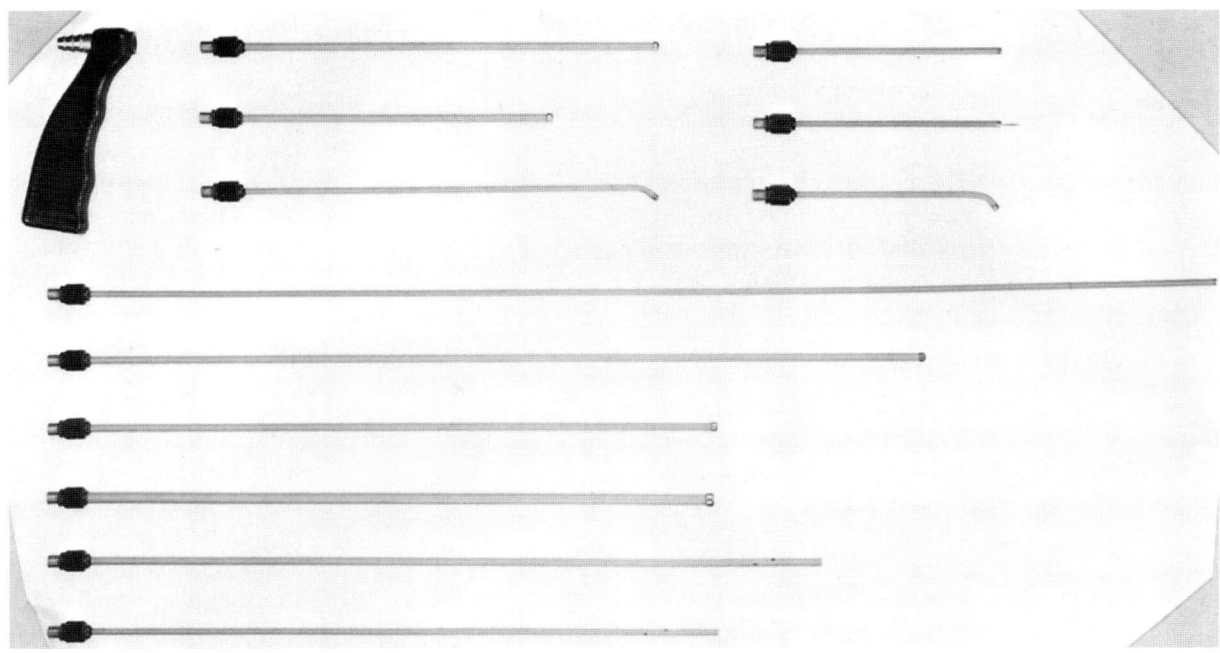

FIGURE 4-16. Suction coagulation electrodes. (Courtesy of Cameron-Miller, Inc., Chicago, IL.)

small lesion is a neoplasm (e.g., polypoid adenoma rather than a hyperplastic polyp), biopsy of every mucosal excrescence is meddlesome and unnecessary (see Chapter 21). The physician can feel content to fulgurate lesions smaller than 5 mm without biopsy. However, for larger tumors, it is preferable for one to obtain pathologic confirmation through either a biopsy or a snare excision.

Use of the *wire loop snare* (Figure 4-17) requires considerably more skill than fulguration alone. The technique usually permits complete excision with one application, although sometimes multiple snarings are required to remove larger growths (see Chapters 5 and 21). This is still an office procedure if the surgeon has the appropriate equipment.

The snare is passed around the polyp and the wire loop slowly closed; the instrument is jiggled as the wire tightens the base. This maneuver permits adjacent mucosa to escape and minimizes the risk of burning the bowel wall. Coagulation rather than cutting current is preferred for snare excision because greater control of the speed of cutting through tissue can be exerted. If a thick pedicle is present,

the physician may take several minutes to excise the specimen. After the polyp is removed, it is helpful to have long alligator or biopsy forceps to retrieve it.

Principles of Electrosurgery

I believe it is useful, especially for the resident who may not be familiar with electrosurgical equipment, to pen a few words about electrosurgical principles. The reader is encouraged to read a monograph on this subject that has been made available to members of the profession by Valley Lab, a division of Tyco Healthcare (see earlier address). The following glossary of definitions and principles is useful:

Electrocautery	Direct current (electrons flow in one direction). Current does not enter the patient's body.
Electrosurgery	The patient is included in the circuit; current enters the patient's body.

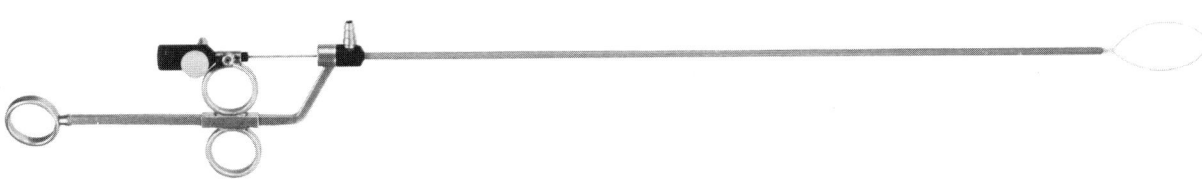

FIGURE 4-17. A wire loop snare and handle are used for polyp removal. (Courtesy of Cameron-Miller, Inc., Chicago, IL.)

Circuit	Pathway for the uninterrupted flow of electrons. The circuit is composed of the generator, active electrode, patient, and patient return electrode.
Ground	The position or portion of an electrical circuit that is at zero potential with respect to the earth; that is, a conducting connection to such a position. Pathways to ground may include the operating room table, surgeon, and equipment.
Voltage	Force pushing current through resistance, measured in volts.
Current	Flow of electrons during a period of time, measured in amperes.
Resistance	Obstacle to the flow of current, synonymous with impedance, measured in ohms. The patient's tissue provides the impedance. This produces heat as the electrons overcome this resistance.
Generator	A unit that converts 60 cycle current to more than 200,000 cycles per second. At this frequency, electrosurgical energy can pass through the patient with minimal neuromuscular electrostimulation and with no risk of electrocution.
Patient return electrode	Removes current from the patient safely. A burn occurs when the heat produced is not dissipated by its size or conductivity. Placing electrode over well-vascularized muscle mass is critical.
Bipolar electrosurgery	Both the active electrode and return electrode functions are performed at the site of the surgery, for example, two tines of a forceps in which only the tissue is grasped. No patient return electrode is necessary.
Monopolar electrosurgery	The most common modality. The active electrode is in the patient; the return electrode is attached somewhere else on the patient. Current flow is through the patient to the patient return electrode.
Coagulation current	The generator setting that produces an intermittent waveform. This will produce less heat. Instead of tissue vaporization, a coagulum is produced. Cutting with the coagulation current can be accomplished by touching the tissue and adjusting the power settings.
Cutting current	The generator setting that produces a constant waveform. Tissue is vaporized or "cut" without hemostasis. Cutting with the "cut current" uses less voltage, an important consideration when performing laparoscopy (see Chapter 27). One may also coagulate with the cutting current.
Blended current	A modification of the duty cycle, not a mixture of cutting and coagulation. A lower blend vaporizes tissue with minimal hemostasis, whereas a higher blend produces maximum hemostasis with less effective cutting.
Electrosurgical cutting	Dividing tissue with electrical sparks that focus intense heat at the surgical site. By withdrawing the electrode slightly away from the tissue, a spark is created that produces a large amount of heat to vaporize the tissue.
Fulguration	Accomplished by sparking with the coagulation waveform. The result is a coagulum rather than vaporization. This modality is useful for electrocoagulation of rectal cancer (see Chapter 23).
Desiccation	Direct application of the electrode to the tissue, more efficiently achieved with cutting current. Less heat is generated, and no cutting occurs.

Complications of Procedures

Bleeding I have previously stated that bleeding is an unusual concern indeed if a biopsy is taken from a lesion, benign or malignant. The occasional incident of bleeding usually occurs when a specimen is obtained from a

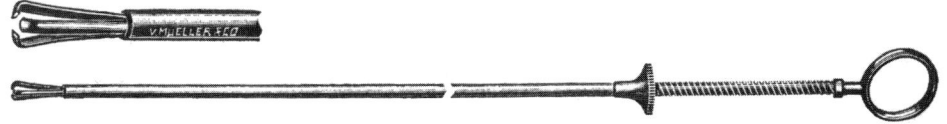

FIGURE 4-18. Frankfeldt forceps. (Courtesy of V. Mueller, McGraw Park, IL.)

normal-appearing rectum, that is, when the physician is seeking a diagnosis of conditions such as Hirschsprung's disease or amyloidosis. Unless the bleeding is pulsatile, I rarely prolong the examination to await complete hemostasis. If persistent bleeding occurs, it may be treated by applying direct pressure with an epinephrine-soaked, cotton-tipped stick (i.e., a chimney sweep) or by saturation with the styptic, Monsel's solution, rather than by electrocoagulation. Electrocoagulating a bleeding area when a biopsy specimen has been taken from a grossly normal rectum may lead to perforation.[36]

If bleeding occurs from the pedicle of a snared polyp, it may be secured by fulguration, by application of pressure with an epinephrine-soaked chimney sweep, or by the use of a long-armed (i.e., extended) rubber ring ligator (see Chapter 8). By grabbing the pedicle with alligator forceps, rubber ring ligation can be performed to establish hemostasis. This technique, however, is obviously not applicable to a sessile area of bleeding. Another method that has been advocated is the use of a "plumber's helper," or Frankfeldt forceps (Figure 4-18), to grasp and twist the bleeding area.[5] This instrument may be secured to the patient for up to 24 hours.

Explosion In contrast to closed-system flexible endoscopy, electrocoagulation or snare excision with the open-ended sigmoidoscope does not require a full bowel preparation. Under these circumstances, an explosive gas mixture may be present. However, there are no adverse consequences because venting is sufficient to prevent proximal bowel injury. Although the "popping sound" or "firecracker-sounding explosion" may be quite disconcerting, no harm will ensue, at least for the patient.

Perforation Bowel perforation from a biopsy, with or without electrocoagulation, or snare excision is a potential hazard that can lead to perforation. However, this is extremely uncommon for two reasons. First, the surgeon limits biopsy of grossly normal bowel to the area below the peritoneal reflection. Even a transmural injury at this location is generally harmless. Second, colonoscopy has supplanted polypectomy through the rigid sigmoidoscope. When a lesion is found within range of the short instrument, the patient is inevitably and appropriately submitted to complete colon evaluation.

As with colonoscopy perforation, the patient may develop signs and symptoms of bowel perforation within a few minutes of electrocoagulation, polyp excision, or biopsy, or septic problems may develop as long as 10 days later. Anyone complaining of abdominal pain who has undergone such a procedure within that interval requires reevaluation and examination. The presence of free intra-abdominal or retroperitoneal gas establishes the diagnosis of a perforated viscus, but in the absence of obvious peritonitis, treatment may consist of in-hospital observation, restriction of oral intake, intravenous fluid replacement, and broad-spectrum antibiotics. Fever or leukocytosis is not necessarily an indication for surgical intervention. Each clinical situation must be addressed individually. In an equivocal circumstance, the physician may consider a water-soluble enema study (i.e., Gastrografin; see Alternatives to the Use of Barium). No one should be critical of the surgeon who performs a negative exploratory laparotomy in an individual whose abdominal signs and symptoms are increasing in severity or who continues to manifest fever and leukocytosis. If patients are going to improve on conservative treatment, they almost always will do so within 24 hours. The principles of management are similar to those described for perforation following colonoscopy (see Chapter 5).

BARIUM ENEMA

Walter B. Cannon is credited with the development of the contrast study of the GI tract through the use of bismuth. Until the advent of colonoscopy, the barium enema had been the standard procedure for evaluation

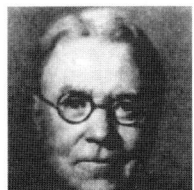

Walter Bradford Cannon (1871–1945) Born in Prairie du Chien, Wisconsin, Cannon was granted a scholarship to Harvard University, graduating *summa cum laude* in 1896. As a medical student at Harvard, he used the newly discovered roentgen ray to study the process of digestion in animals. His initial observations were made after administering mush mixed with bismuth to a goose. Following these studies, he focused his attention on gastrointestinal motility, tracing on toilet paper the fluoroscopic appearance of the gut. Cannon's ring was described as the tonic contraction often seen radiologically in the right transverse colon. He is credited with discovering sympathin E (i.e., the excitor factor) and sympathin I (i.e., the inhibitor), terms that have been replaced by epinephrine and norepinephrine. He discovered the chemical mediation of nerve impulses and coined the word *homeostasis*. Even though he established the principle of lining the fluoroscopy tube with lead to limit scattered radiation, he became a martyr to his work with x-rays, dying of complications of lymphoma. (Cannon WB. The movements of the intestines studied by means of the Roentgen rays. *Am J Physiol* 1901/1902;6:251.)

of any mucosal abnormality.[12–14] Furthermore, with the development of computed tomography (CT), the barium enema study has been virtually replaced for extramucosal pathologic features as well. So infrequent are contrast studies of the GI tract requested today, that in the United States it is virtually impossible to recruit a GI radiologist. They simply do not exist. This is a pity. Barium enema is, in fact, an ideal study for demonstrating colonic anatomy (dolichocolon, redundancy, extrinsic compression, narrowing, intramural mass, incomplete rotation, etc.). At the very least, barium enema complements other investigations, facilitates the correct diagnosis, and thereby permits the implementation of proper treatment. It is a relatively simple examination to perform, it is time and cost efficient, and generally is well tolerated by patients.[44]

Indications

Evaluation of the colon by barium enema is the most cost-effective means of identifying colon disorders (e.g., benign and malignant lesions, diverticular disease, inflammatory conditions, congenital anomalies, intrinsic and extrinsic abnormalities; Figure 4-19).[62,77] It can be usefully employed in urgent or emergency circumstances to differentiate among small and large bowel obstruction,

acute appendicitis, and periappendiceal abscess. It also has been successfully used in the therapeutic setting to reduce volvulus and intussusception.

However, as a screening tool for neoplasms in an asymptomatic patient with no preexisting history of polypoid disease or cancer, it cannot be recommended. Benjamin and Todd performed barium enema examinations on 8,420 asymptomatic patients and found that only 45 had evidence suggestive of neoplasm, an incidence of 0.5%.[10] Gianturco and Miller reported a 2.3% incidence of polyps in 35,000 asymptomatic patients who underwent air-contrast barium enema studies.[42] It appears, then, that if the physician is to use barium enema for screening (a doubtful indication), the preferred approach is the air-contrast technique.

In patients with known, asymptomatic rectal polyps, Drexler reported proximal lesions in 4.7%.[25] Our experience in 200 such individuals revealed an incidence of only 2.5%.[18] However, when the rectal polyp initially identified was pedunculated, 13% of the patients had a proximal lesion, compared with approximately 1% with a sessile rectal polyp ($p = .01$)).[18] One criticism of this study, however, is that not all rectal polyps had pathologic confirmation; some may have been hyperplastic and not true neoplasms.

Preparation

The procedure is essentially a meaningless exercise if the preparation has been inadequate. Without proper cleansing, it may be difficult to distinguish tumor from stool and impossible to exclude the presence of small neoplasms (Figure 4-20). Sands was inspired to write the following ode to the subject:

> O for a colon that's pure and untrammeled,
> O for a colon that's clean.
> You may have a heart that's as pure as the snow,
> And still have a bowel that's obscene.[105]

Numerous bowel preparations have been recommended, but basically they consist of some dietary restrictions the day before the procedure (e.g., a low-residue diet with a clear-liquid supper), a vigorous laxative, and perhaps a suppository or enema the day of the examination. Many studies have been performed concerning the optimal bowel preparation. Dodds and colleagues, in a controlled evaluation, demonstrated that regimens using magnesium citrate and bisacodyl were superior to those using castor oil, both in terms of cleansing efficacy and of patient complaints.[24] Other commercial preparations contain senna or cascara sagrada.

Another technique involves the oral administration—or more commonly, nasogastric tube instillation—of Ringer's lactate or another saline solution.[56,111] This preparation

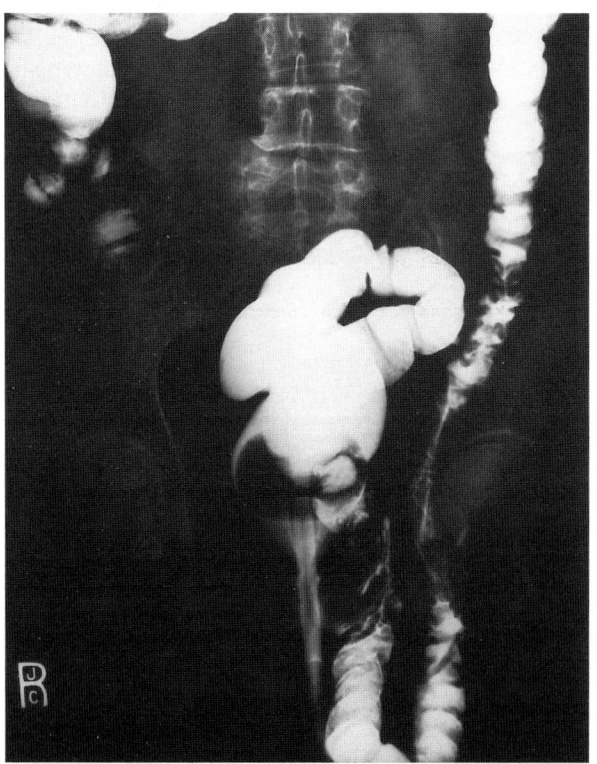

FIGURE 4-19. Barium enema demonstrates sigmoid colon in large scrotal hernia.

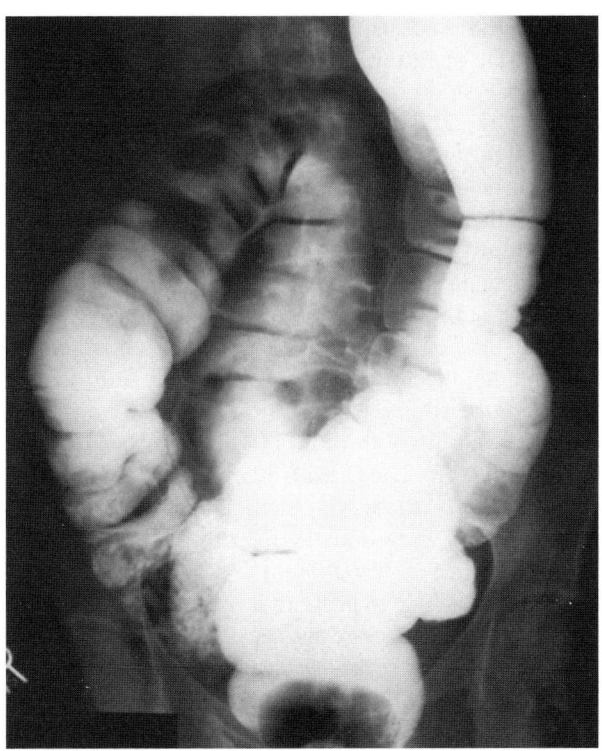

FIGURE 4-20. Barium enema with a large amount of retained stool makes diagnosis of an intraluminal lesion virtually impossible.

has also been advocated for colon cleansing before colonoscopy and bowel resection (i.e., Crapp prep).[19] Four liters are generally required, and evacuation may be complete in as little as 2 to as many as 6 hours.

It is important to maintain adequate hydration if a stimulant laxative preparation is used. Many of the individuals who require this procedure are elderly, and a barium enema study requires a considerable catharsis. This, in turn, can lead to renal, cardiac, and electrolyte problems. By encouraging the patient to drink water frequently, in addition to clear juice and bouillon, these complications can be avoided. Cardiovascular and renal problems are more likely to occur with the gastric intubation technique. This method therefore is relatively contraindicated in elderly patients and in those with renal or cardiovascular diseases. Morbidity can be reduced, however, by intravenous hydration. I continue to favor either Fleet Phospho-Soda or magnesium citrate with a supplemental small-volume enema the morning of the study.

Technique of Examination Using a Single-Contrast Barium Enema

The colon is not the easiest organ to examine. To evaluate all of the twists, turns, and redundancies, it is inappropriate simply to instill a measured amount of barium

and shoot a film with the patient lying supine on the table. Radiologists believe that 90% of the information from the study is gleaned during the fluoroscopic part of the examination. The final films are really a modus for creating a permanent record for future reference and comparison.

Cannon first instilled contrast material into the GI tract using bismuth subnitrate.[12] Shortly thereafter, barium began to be used because of its radiopacity, lack of absorption, ease of preparation, and low cost. Unfortunately, USP barium sulfate tends to settle and flocculate, and it is composed of varying-sized particles. Present preparations, however, are micronized with standard, small particles in a suspending agent containing a measured amount of tannic acid. Barium is commercially available in a disposable bag, prepared for the addition of a specified amount of water. High voltage (approximately 100 kV) is used to ensure sufficient penetration of the barium column.

It is important to realize that administration of an opaque material within a hollow viscus does not fill the organ. What is seen is the contrast material against one wall of the colon with the nondependent wall not identified because it is not filled. That is why radiologists perform fluoroscopy with the patient in the supine position to evaluate the posterior wall of the bowel and make the overhead radiographs with the individual in the prone position to evaluate the anterior wall of the bowel. Questionable areas on the anterior wall then necessitate returning the patient to the x-ray table for fluoroscopy and respotting with the patient in the prone position.

Preliminary films of the abdomen (i.e., kidney, ureter, and bladder) are obtained to identify areas of calcification, the presence of air- or fluid-filled loops of intestine, residual fecal material, or barium from previous contrast studies, and any soft tissue or bony abnormalities.

By means of an appropriate catheter, the barium-water mixture is inserted into the colon with the patient in the prone position until the column of barium reaches the splenic flexure. The tubing and tip must be of sufficient caliber to allow free flow of the contrast medium. A smooth enema tip with both end- and side-hole openings is preferred. For those individuals who have difficulty retaining an enema, it is helpful to use a tip with an inflatable cuff (Figure 4-21). It should be remembered, however, that an inflated balloon in the rectum will obscure the bowel wall. The barium enema is therefore inadequate for evaluation of the rectum or for identifying a lesion in this location. Endoscopic examination of the rectum should routinely be employed before this radiologic study.

As the barium flows, the radiologist looks for distensibility and interruption or deviation of the flow. Sometimes it is difficult to determine whether certain areas

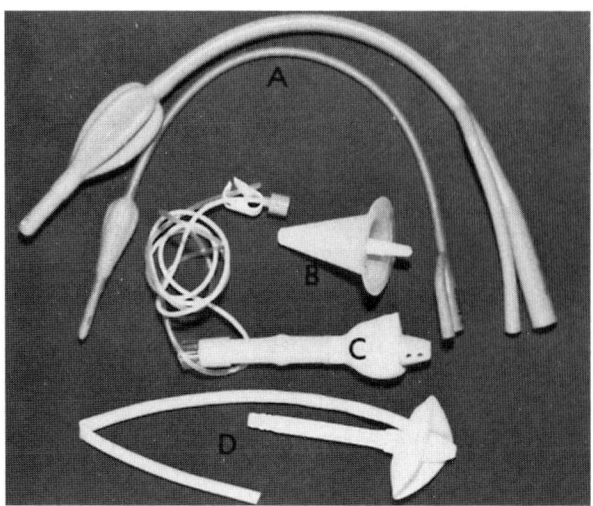

FIGURE 4-21. Barium enema catheter tips. **(A)** Bardex retention balloon catheters (pediatric and adult). **(B)** Colostotip for irrigating or performing contrast studies through a stoma. **(C)** Catheter for air-contrast enema. **(D)** Argyle retention cuff catheter.

represent a fixed or anatomic narrowing or whether the narrowing is physiologic (i.e., spasm). Many patients have been submitted to exploratory laparotomy for a suspected neoplasm because of this kind of misinterpretation (Figure 4-22). Anticholinergic agents have been employed to prevent spasm, but because of side effects they are no longer recommended and have been abandoned

by most physicians. Glucagon (1 to 2 mg) given by the intramuscular or intravenous route has been shown to be an effective smooth muscle relaxant when administered parenterally.[78] It is as efficacious as anticholinergic drugs and has fewer side effects. Relaxation of the colon with reduction of discomfort allows the radiologist to perform a more satisfactory examination.

Spot films are usually taken of the rectosigmoid, hepatic flexure, splenic flexure, and cecum (Figure 4-23). Compression spot films are useful to identify small polyps (Figure 4-24). Angled views of the sigmoid colon (right anterior oblique in the prone position and left posterior oblique in the supine position) are most helpful in delineating this portion of the bowel for more thorough evaluation (Figure 4-25). The Chassard-Lapiné view (Figure 4-26) may be helpful in identifying sigmoid and rectosigmoid lesions, but it is hazardous in the reproductive years because of the increased radiation exposure.[27] Spot films of the cecum are made to prove that this area is indeed filled with barium, not necessarily because of difficulties with overlapping bowel. Peristalsis usually begins in the cecum, so that this area is frequently contracted or empty by the time the overhead films are taken.

How does the radiologist know that the cecum has been filled? Ideally, if the appendix fills or if reflux is seen in the terminal ileum, this would solve the issue, but the former is noted in only 30% of cases, and the latter no more than half the time. However, there are certain characteristics of the cecum to look for, such as the largest haustral marking and the ileocecal valve.

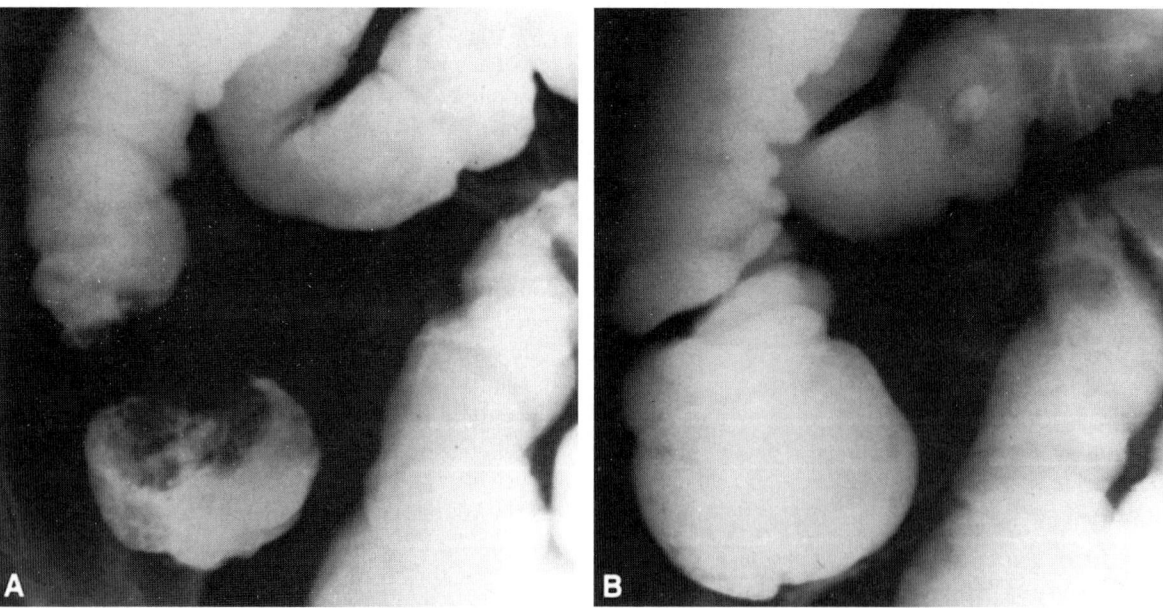

FIGURE 4-22. (A) Barium enema study reveals an apparent mass in the cecum. **(B)** A later film following administration of glucagon reveals no abnormality.

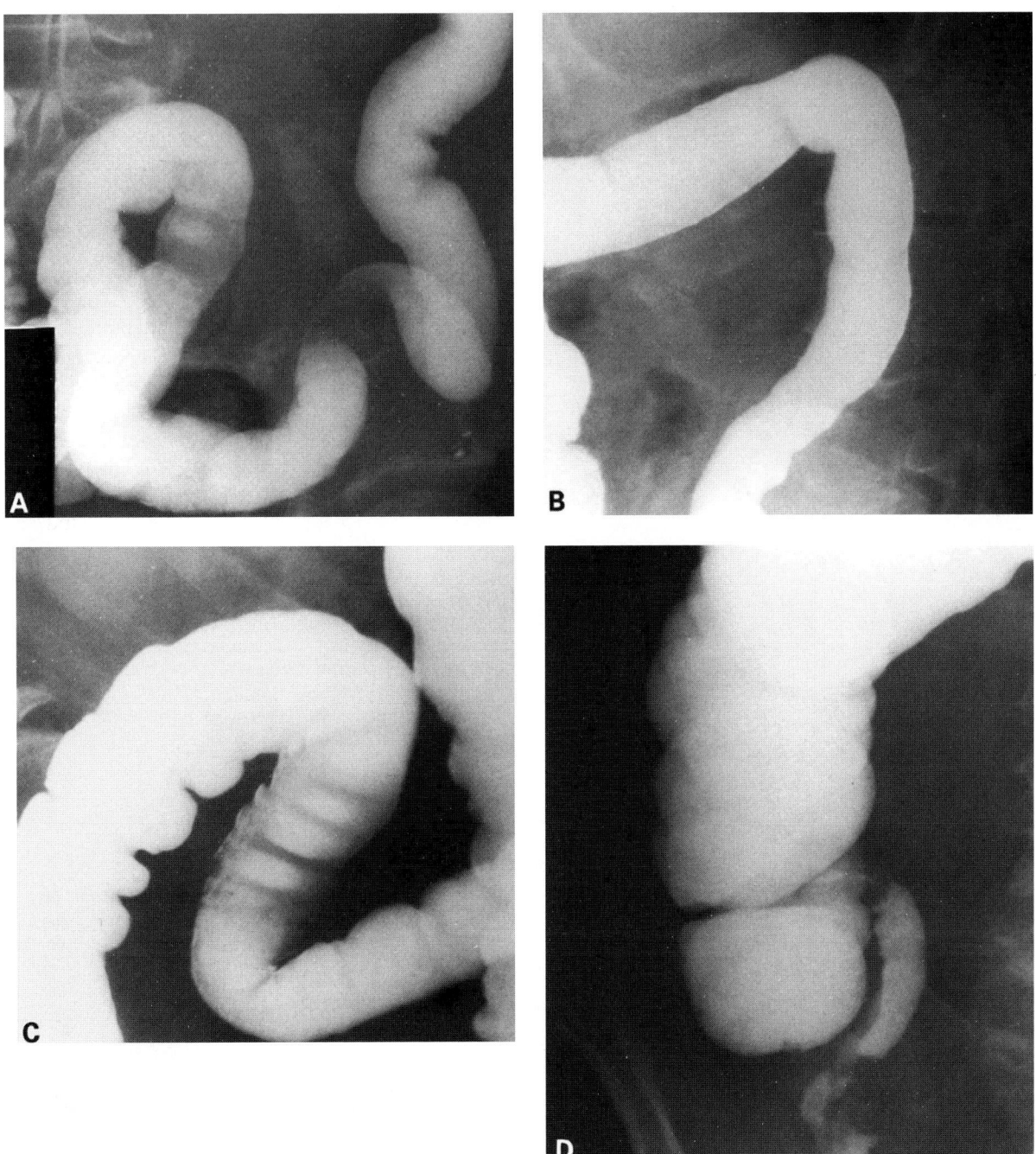

FIGURE 4-23. Spot films taken following barium enema of the **(A)** rectosigmoid, **(B)** splenic flexure, **(C)** hepatic flexure, and **(D)** cecum.

The rectum also requires special radiologic views. The radiologist is constantly endeavoring to move and massage the colon, to empty it and fill it. The rectum, however, is the only area of the bowel that the radiologist cannot manipulate by abdominal pressure. A lateral view must be obtained to visualize anterior and posterior wall lesions and to be certain that the rectum lies well back in the hollow of the sacrum (Figure 4-27) and is not displaced forward by retrorectal inflammation or tumor (Figure 4-28).

Although the identification of intrinsic lesions of the colon is the primary purpose of the barium enema study, it is important to recognize that some organs, normal and abnormal, may be visualized by the defect produced

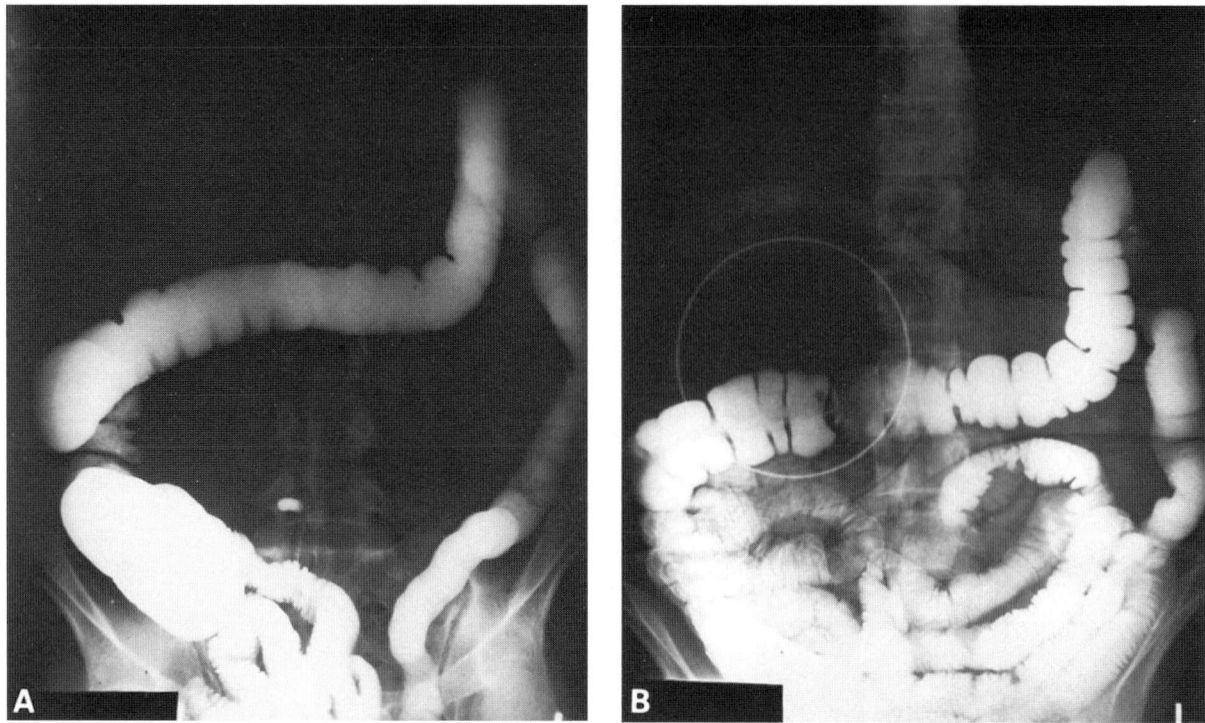

FIGURE 4-24. (A) This transverse colon polyp is poorly seen after barium enema. **(B)** A compression spot film demonstrates a small polyp.

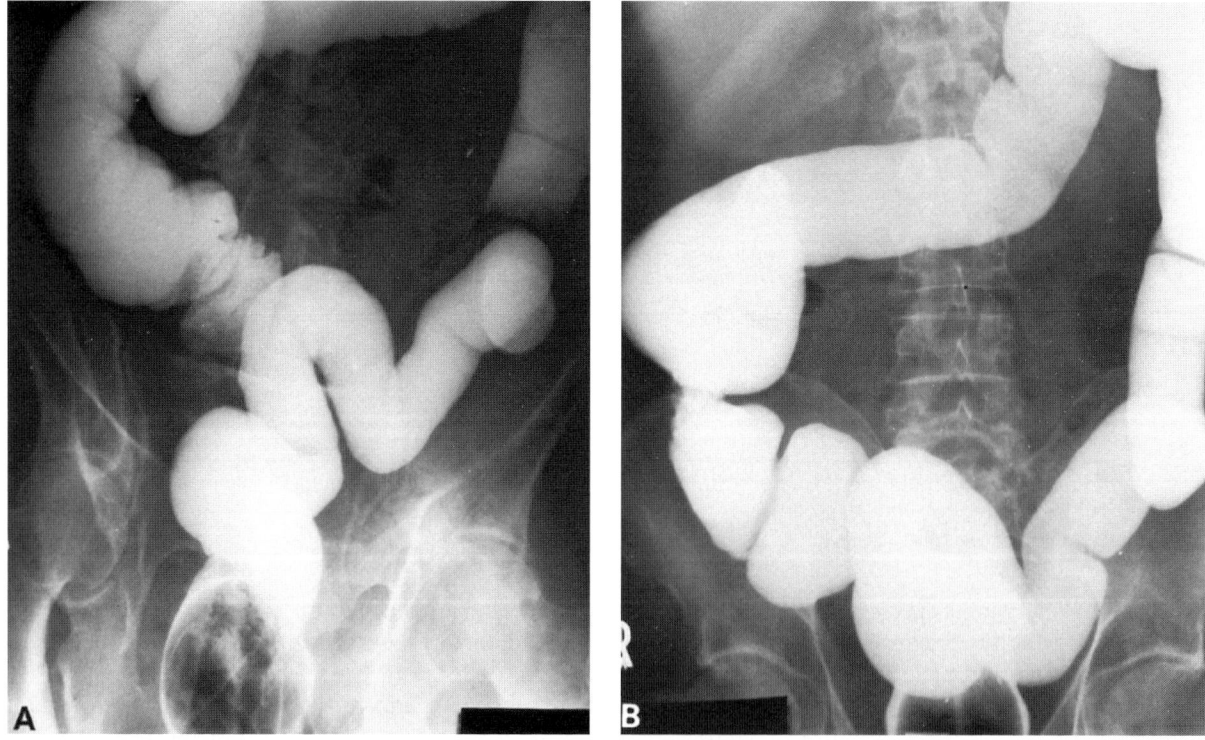

FIGURE 4-25. Barium enema. **(A)** An oblique view of the sigmoid colon permits better evaluation. **(B)** In the posteroanterior projection, the area would be obscured.

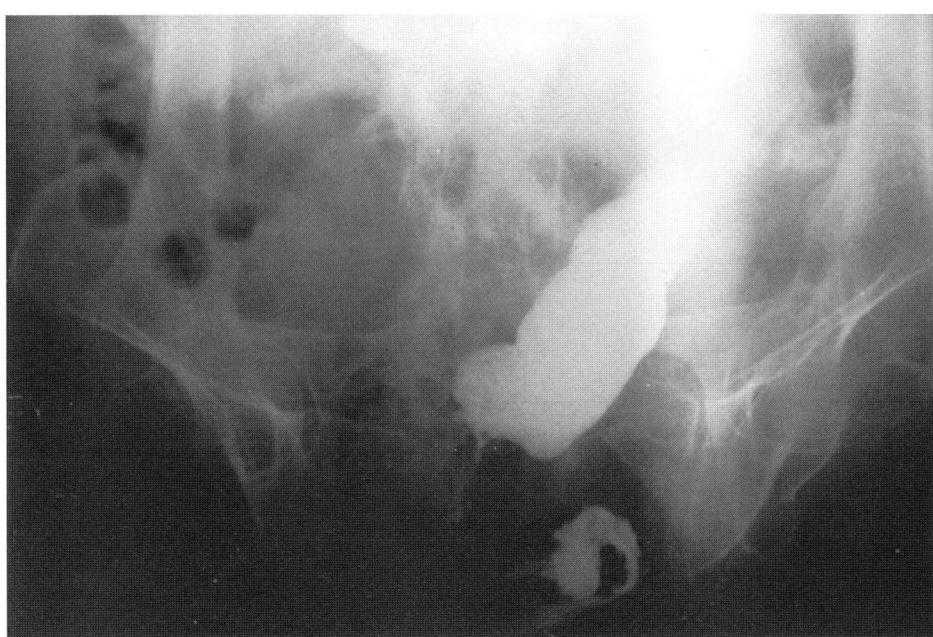

FIGURE 4-26. The Chassard-Lapiné view may be useful to demonstrate lesions in a redundant sigmoid colon. In this patient, an annular carcinoma is seen.

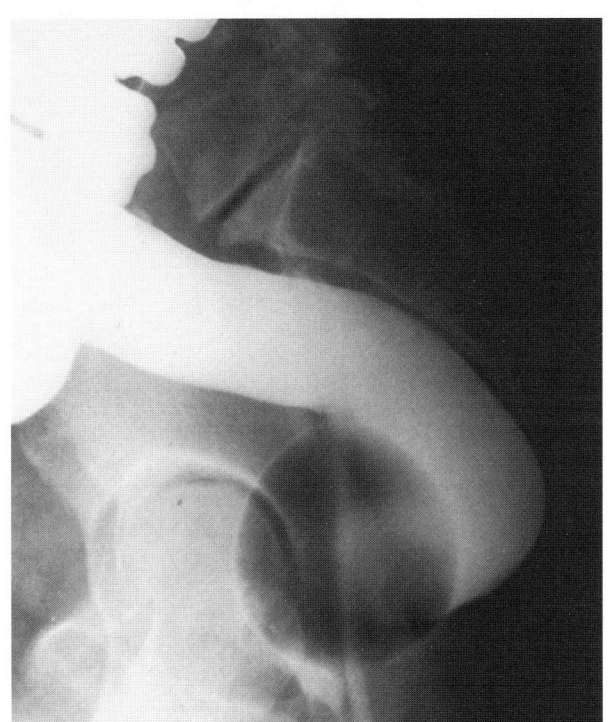

FIGURE 4-27. Normal lateral view of rectum taken after barium enema.

through extrinsic compression (Figure 4-29). Probably the most important permanent film of the single-contrast barium enema is the postevacuation study (Figure 4-30). If there has been good evacuation, it is the one time when all the walls of the colon are demonstrated. With a completely collapsed bowel, the physician can identify the mucosal pattern or lesions that disturb or destroy it.

To cover the colon satisfactorily, a small amount of tannic acid is added to the barium. This substance stimulates the bowel to empty more completely and effectively and causes the barium to contact the mucosa despite mucous secretion. Tannic acid is relatively contraindicated in patients with inflammatory bowel disease and in other ulcerative or inflammatory colon conditions because of the possibility of absorption and subsequent hepatic injury.

Alternatives to the Use of Barium

Barium is a substance that is potentially dangerous when used in a patient with a suspected bowel perforation. Barium peritonitis is often a lethal complication; that is why relative contraindications to barium enema include toxic megacolon, peritonitis, and biopsy or snare excision of a polyp within 24 hours. However, if the biopsy has been performed for an exophytic lesion, I believe the barium enema need not be deferred. Some radiologists are concerned about the difficulty of interpreting the finding of a rectal ulcer when a barium study is performed within a few days of the biopsy, and that this may lead to the performance of inappropriate follow-up studies.[79] Obviously, communication with the radiologist is suggested if a contrast study is requested within a few days following a rectal biopsy.

An alternative to barium is one of the water-soluble solutions of diatrizoate sodium (e.g., Hypaque, Gastrografin). These solutions provide reasonable radiopacity,

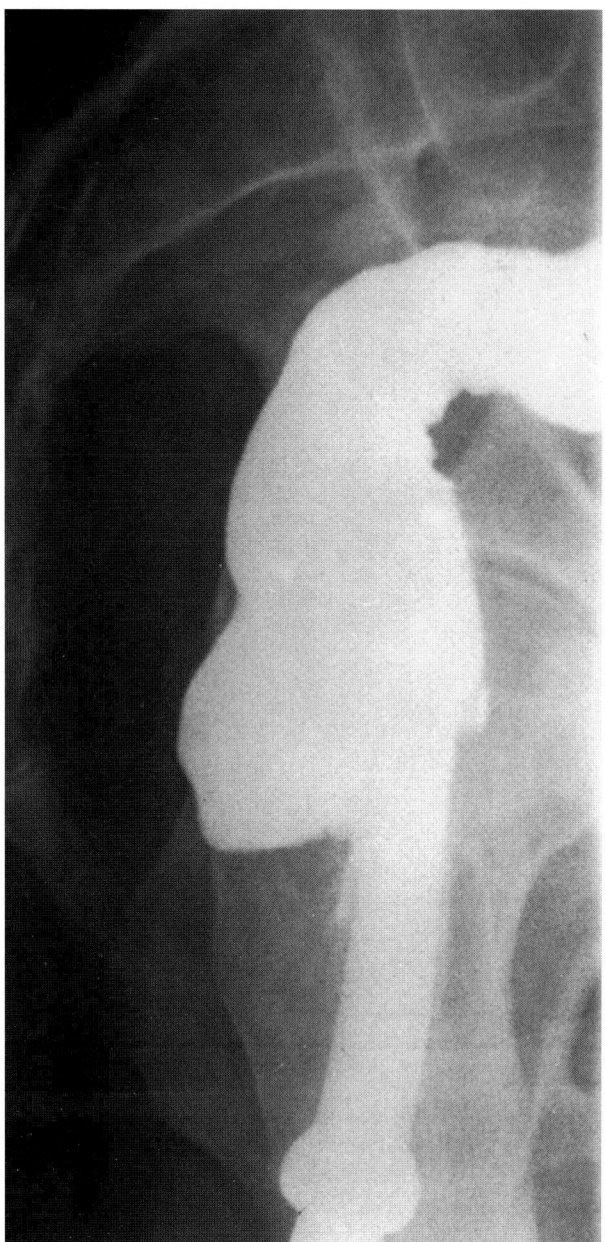

FIGURE 4-28. On lateral projection after barium enema, anterior displacement of the rectum from recurrent tumor is evident. Note the increased distance from the sacrum when compared with the normal position in Figure 4-27.

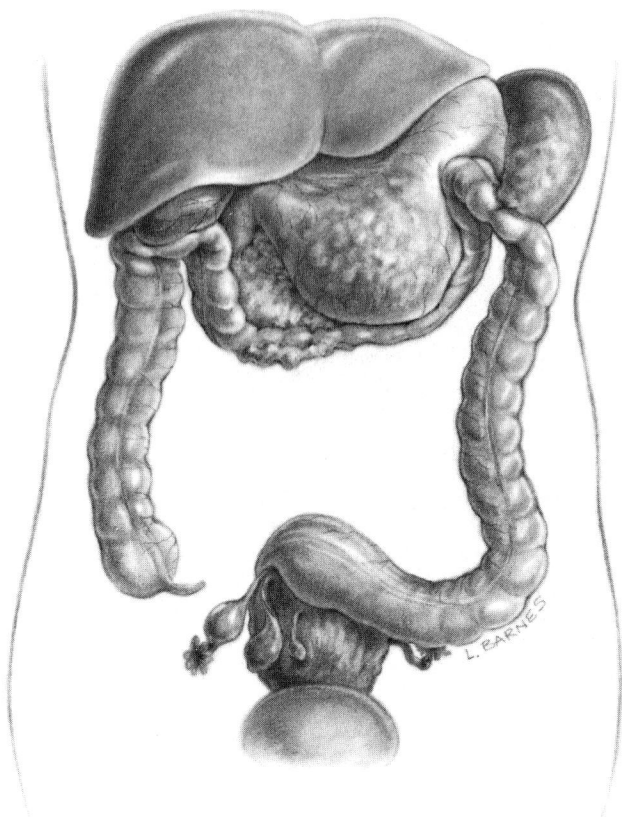

FIGURE 4-29. The colon and rectum can be deviated, distorted, compressed, or invaded as a consequence of problems in other organs, especially the spleen, pancreas, stomach, liver, gallbladder, uterus, ovaries, and prostate.

are nonirritating, and are relatively well tolerated if accidentally introduced into the peritoneal cavity. Because they are hypertonic with respect to plasma, they can act as saline cathartics and may be of value for this reason in the diagnosis and management of acute, partial large bowel obstruction.[116] The result is a rapid dilution of the opacity, but because of the cathartic effect they may be of benefit in the immediate preoperative situation.

There are, however, certain disadvantages of diatrizoate sodium. The major limitation is that because of reduced opacification, visualization is sometimes less than adequate. In essence, there is no postevacuation residual. Hypertonicity is a hazard in another respect; significant alteration in serum electrolytes can occur, especially in children and elderly patients. Individuals with cardiac or renal disease are also at increased risk when these agents are employed. Finally, the cost of the Gastrografin is approximately $50 per bottle (five or more may be required), compared with $4 for the barium preparation. Parenthetically, Hypaque is also very inexpensive.

Double-Contrast or Air-Contrast Barium Enema

The double-contrast (i.e., air-contrast) barium enema study has been advocated as an improved means of evaluating the colon, identifying small mucosal lesions, and diagnosing inflammatory bowel disease.[67,68,125,126] Others suggest that either study may be optimal under a given circumstance.[41,75]

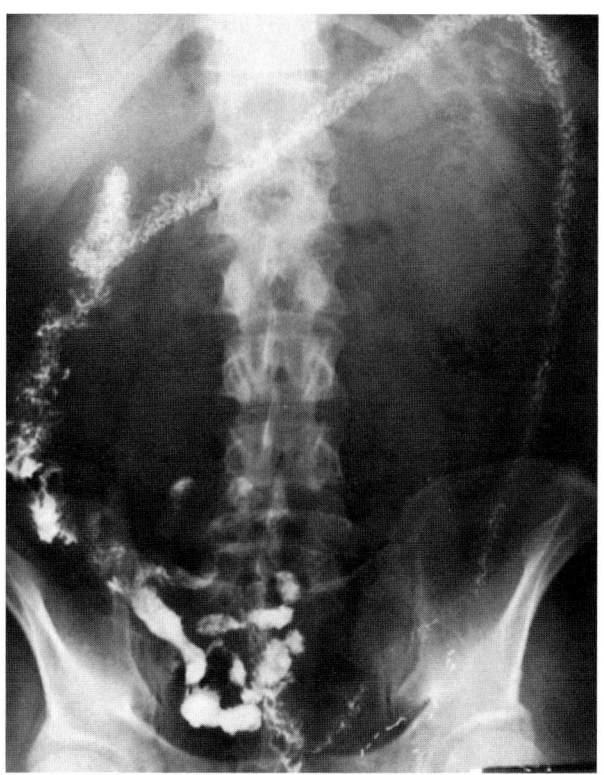

FIGURE 4-30. A postevacuation film following barium enema clearly demonstrates the normal mucosal pattern.

With the double-contrast examination, an attempt is made to coat the colon with a thin layer of contrast material and distend the bowel with air so that the entire mucosal circumference is visualized (Figure 4-31). The barium used is a heavy-density, viscous material. To deliver this, a large-caliber enema tube is required. This has a soft tip and an inflatable cuff and uses a system that delivers air and barium separately (Figure 4-21C).

There are several disadvantages to the air-contrast enema. First, the study inevitably results in considerably more radiation exposure. An adequate examination necessitates ten or 12 overhead films plus several spot films. Second, it requires a cooperative patient who is able to roll around, support his or her own weight, and comprehend instructions. A third relative disadvantage is that fluoroscopy has a lesser role in the course of the examination. The radiologist endeavors to move the viscous barium around the colon as expeditiously as possible and then depends largely on the permanent films for diagnosis. However, despite the foregoing concerns, with appropriate care, air-contrast enema can be accomplished in virtually all individuals.

Air-contrast enema has become the routine study for evaluation of the bowel because very small lesions and ulcers are seen to advantage with this technique. In a prospective study of single- and double-contrast methods, de Roos and colleagues demonstrated that the latter procedure is superior when screening for polyps, but that single-contrast is particularly useful for problem areas such as the sigmoid and rectum.[21] There is a theoretical disadvantage of the air-contrast technique when a large lesion or a pedunculated polyp is present, but as with any other aspect of medicine, skill and experience are the most important requisites. I am impressed by the studies, particularly those from the Department of Radiology at the Mayo Clinic, which indicate that careful single-contrast barium enema with fluoroscopy is as sensitive a study as can be performed with the x-ray, but theirs is a minority opinion.[58,121] The point is moot, however. Rather than elect the double-contrast approach for neoplasm screening, virtually all physicians, irrespective of specialty, employ colonoscopy, with barium enema or air-contrast enema reserved for an individual whose examination was incomplete or inadequate.

Complications of Barium Enema Examination

Complications of barium enema examination are fortunately rare. However, when they occur, they can be of catastrophic consequence. Numerous complications have been reported, as listed here:

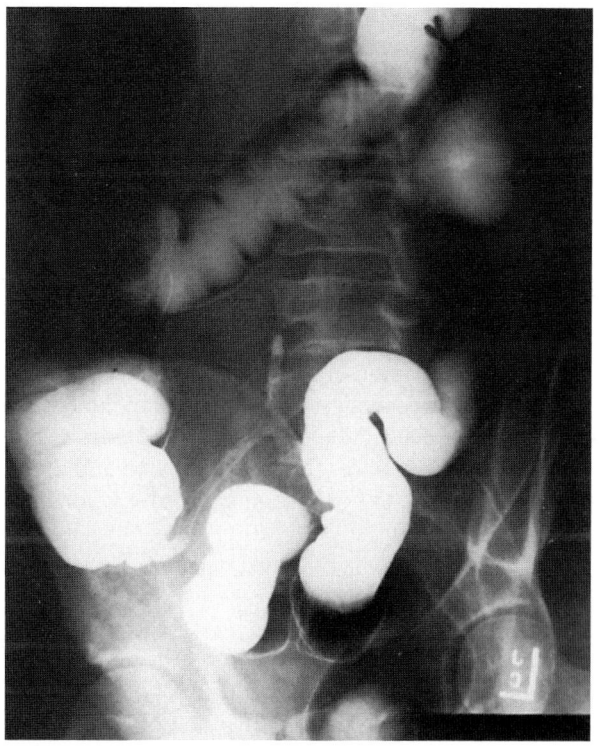

FIGURE 4-31. This double-contrast (air-contrast) barium enema study demonstrates a normal colon.

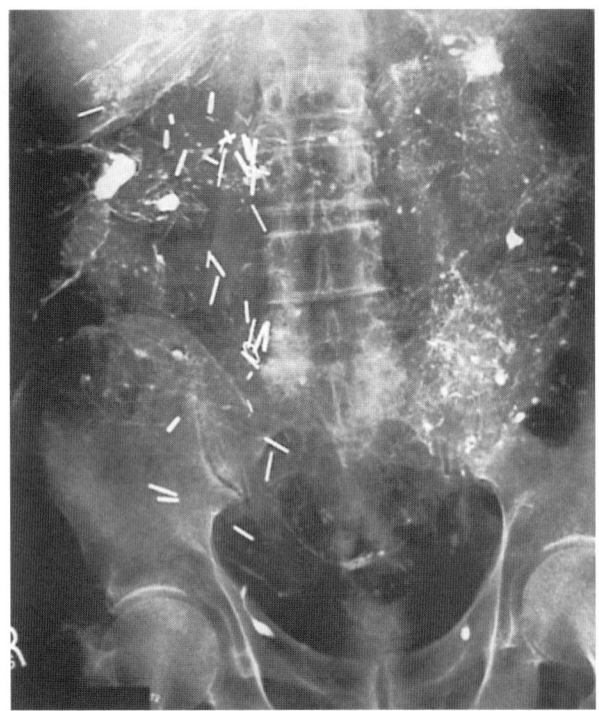

FIGURE 4-32. Barium peritonitis. Single view of the abdomen (kidneys, ureters, bladder) demonstrates extravasated barium. Note the dispersed appearance, with the barium outlining the inferior margin of the liver.

Rectal perforation from enema tip or excessive balloon
    inflation
Rectal tear or hemorrhage
Colonic perforation
Barium peritonitis
Barium submucosal granuloma
Toxic megacolon
Septicemia
Venous barium embolism
Retrograde GI filling with vomiting and aspiration in
    infants

In 1988, perforation of the colon or rectum during the course of barium enema study was estimated to occur in approximately 500 patients in the United States annually,[16] but certainly many fewer now may be anticipated, with the decreased use of barium studies for colon evaluation. Rectal tearing or perforation is usually caused by trauma when the enema tip is inserted or by overinflation of a balloon catheter.[34,108] The tip or balloon can also lacerate the rectal wall and produce rectal bleeding. Use of a balloon for barium enema through a colostomy can produce colonic perforation at and below the stoma. This technique should never be employed; a Colostotip, catheter, or cone should be substituted (Figure 4-21*B*).

Colonic perforation with barium peritonitis has historically been associated with at least a 50% mortality

rate (Figure 4-32; see Figure 28-29), although there is a suggestion the rate has fallen considerably since the availability of more effective antibiotics and early surgical intervention.[16,47,48] The mortality rate is influenced to a great extent by the volume of the extravasated barium. Although perforation at the site of tumor, diverticulitis, ischemic colitis, and nonspecific inflammatory bowel disease are the usual associated circumstances, perforation can occur in an otherwise normal bowel.[60,132] As implied, those who undergo barium contrast studies through stomas are at particular risk.

Idiopathic perforation has been reported to occur in one of 5,000 barium enema studies, usually in the right colon because of the lower bursting pressure in this area.[50] Between 1977 and 1996 at the Mayo Medical Center, 13,000 barium enema studies were performed.[48] Colorectal perforation occurred in five patients (incidence, 0.04%). Barloon and Schumway presented an interesting study on medical malpractice involving radiologic colon examinations.[8] The distribution of 18 cases of colon perforation in this group of litigious patients was as follows: cecum, onw; transverse colon, one; extraperitoneal rectum, seven; rectosigmoid, one; colostomy stoma, two; unspecified, six.

It may be suspected that the term idiopathic is a euphemism for overfilling the colon or employing a high hydrostatic pressure. Fry and colleagues noted that five of 2,200 such studies were associated with perforation of the rectum or sigmoid colon, but only one bowel was considered normal.[37] The authors further observed the pressures created by a standard barium delivery set by using 1-m columns of water, 25% diatrizoate sodium (Hypaque), 20% barium, and 80% barium. The columns generated pressures of 70, 85, 95, and 120 mm Hg, respectively. They suggested the following options should be considered to reduce the incidence of perforation:[37]

Perform proctoscopy before barium enema study.
Avoid the use of a rectal balloon, especially with a known
    or suspected rectal lesion.
Avoid barium study in patients with active colitis.
Avoid generation of pressure greater than that created by
    a column of barium suspension of 1 m.
Use a lower concentration of barium whenever possible.

As previously mentioned, the timing of a barium enema examination following biopsy of the rectum or colon has been the subject of considerable debate. Is there truly an increased risk for perforation? Many radiologists will not perform barium studies within 24 hours of such a procedure. Some insist on 48 hours and others on a delay of up to 1 week. On the basis of clinical studies and animal experiments, Harned and his associates suggest that a small biopsy with colonoscopic forceps requires no waiting period before a barium enema study is performed.[53] Conversely, the authors recommend deferring the examination for 1 week if proctoscopic forceps are used. My own approach would be to carry on without delay if the biopsy is of an exophytic lesion in order to avoid subsequent reexamination. Otherwise, the biopsy is performed after the x-ray study. This discussion, however, is meaningless because virtually all physicians will go directly to colonoscopy for proximal bowel evaluation in these circumstances.

Barium submucosal dissection with subsequent granuloma formation is very rarely seen today because of the infrequency of a barium enema study (see Chapter 25).[11,72] The resultant lesion may be attributed to healing of an ulcer or injury with entrapment of contrast material or to the performance of a barium study right after biopsy. The barium poses no threat, but the differential diagnosis of a yellow, submucosal rectal nodule includes a carcinoid tumor. It is therefore important to limit the possibility of this complication, a circumstance that would otherwise necessitate a diagnostic biopsy or excision.

Management of Barium Enema Perforation

When free perforation is recognized, emergency surgical intervention is required. At laparotomy, it is necessary to remove as much of the contaminant as possible, an extremely tedious if not impossible task because of the pastelike consistency of the barium. Wiping the serosal surface with a moistened sponge or pad is a frustratingly unsuccessful exercise. Yamamura and colleagues describe the technique of irrigating the peritoneal cavity with a concentrated solution of urokinase (72,000 IU in 500 mL of normal saline solution).[129] With irrigation and mechanical wiping, this approach almost completely removed the barium from the surface of the peritoneum in their experience. I have not used this technique, but if confronted today with such a catastrophic complication, I would be motivated to try it. Obviously, resection of the perforated segment and a diversionary procedure are mandatory.

Barium and feces produce a severe exudative peritonitis. Large fluid and protein losses occur almost immediately. If the patient is fortunate enough to survive the initial hospitalization, there is grave risk for the development of intestinal obstruction because of the dense adhesions that form.

Management of the patient with a rectal tear through which barium has extravasated poses a less clear-cut problem. Ultimately, a diversionary procedure may be required, but, depending on the extent of the injury, medical management should be considered, at least initially. This should consist of vigorous intravenous fluid replacement, antibiotics, and dietary restriction. Three rectal perforations were managed conservatively in two individuals and by proximal diversion in one in the Mayo Clinic report.[48] All patients recovered. The authors opined that

a localized, contained extraperitoneal rectal perforation can be managed conservatively in selected patients.

Perforation of the rectum or colon may also occur as a consequence of the double-contrast examination, with extravasation of air, but not necessarily of barium. Because clinical signs of peritonitis may not be evident, it has been suggested that asymptomatic patients with radiographic findings of perirectal, mediastinal, or cervical emphysema be managed in the hospital with close observation, rather than having to undergo immediate laparotomy.[37,88] The success achieved with this approach may be attributable to the fact that the patients generally have undergone a complete bowel cleansing. The risk for gross fecal contamination is therefore minimized. Parapharyngeal emphysema has been reported to cause a voice change, which may be the earliest recognizable symptom of the perforation.[94] Finally, approximately 12 cases of portal venous intravasation of contrast have been observed following barium enema study, a potentially devastating complication.[127] Virtually all these patients harbored a condition that disrupted mucosal integrity, such as inflammatory bowel disease or diverticulitis.

DEFECOGRAPHY

Defecography is a radiologic technique whereby the lower bowel is examined with the patient in the sitting or squatting position in the act of eliminating the barium. It has been recommended in the evaluation of individuals with irritable bowel syndrome, solitary rectal ulcer, rectal prolapse, proctalgia fugax, constipation, obstructed defecation, and internal procidentia (i.e., the preprolapse condition).[9,31,64] It is for the last two conditions, however, that the technique is most usefully employed.

The procedure can be performed using a cineradiographic technique or simply by obtaining lateral spot films at different times during evacuation. Ekberg and colleagues reported 90 examinations performed on 83 patients with defecatory problems.[31] Whereas results of approximately one third of the studies were normal, abnormalities such as intussusception, enterocele, proctocele, and fecal retention were clearly appreciated. I believe that this can be a valuable adjunctive study for assessing patients with defecation problems and should be included in the evaluation of these individuals before relegating them to the all-encompassing category of irritable bowel syndrome. However, confusion concerning interpretation and the significance of observed abnormalities still exists. In fact, there is a tendency to overinterpret every finding. This can lead to inappropriate treatment and unnecessary or unhelpful surgery. The technique and clinical applications of defecography are discussed in Chapters 6, 16, and 17.

ULTRASOUND

Ultrasound of the abdomen has been reported to be a helpful and a reasonably accurate diagnostic modality for a number of conditions affecting the bowel: Crohn's disease, cancer, diverticulitis, and intestinal obstruction.[99] Clearly, the technique is very much operator dependent. For practical purposes, however, despite the fact that it is noninvasive and well tolerated by patients, it is unlikely to replace or even to supplement barium enema, CT, or colonoscopy for any colonic condition. There are, however, specific ultrasound applications that are especially valuable for colon and rectal and general surgeons. These include intraoperative ultrasound (see Chapter 22), endorectal ultrasound (see Chapters 6 and 23), and endoanal ultrasound (see Chapters 6, 11, 13, and 24). These are discussed with respect to each pathologic entity.

COMPUTED TOMOGRAPHY

CT has become the radiologic "gold standard" for a host of conditions affecting the GI tract, both for diagnostic purposes and when performed with an interventional technique. Clearly, the diagnosis of diverticulitis is optimally made with CT. Metastatic cancer evaluation always includes CT. With the use of oral contrast, the site of a bowel obstruction may be identified, and the differential between partial and complete obstruction may be elucidated. Intravenous contrast CT allows for an accurate assessment of the urinary tract. Important technical details in the performance of the examination include the following[4]:

- Fasting for 12 hours is preferred (although not always possible). Bowel cleansing limits interference by fecal residue.
- Induction of intestinal hypomobility [0.1 mg of glucagon or 0.2 mg of scopolamine (Buscopan)] avoids peristaltic artifact and permits distension.
- Intravenous contrast enhancement is used.
- Adequate distension of the bowel with iodinated or hypodense (air, water, methylcellulose) contrast media introduced orally or rectally is ensured.

The possibilities for application of CT touch every aspect of the surgeon's art. Each will be discussed in the relevant chapter.

VIRTUAL COLONOSCOPY

Virtual colonoscopy (VC) or CT colonography (CTC) was first introduced by Vining and colleagues in 1994.[123,124] Because the x-ray tube is continuously rotating while the patient moves through the scanner, the beam describes a spiral pathway through the body,

hence the term spiral CT.[49] Using a conventional workstation and a dynamic display of images, the radiologist can simulate an examination of the colon in much the same way as an endoscopist. The effect is to create images that are not dissimilar to those that are observed with optical colonoscopy (Figure 4-33). By the use of both two-dimensional and three-dimensional images, CTC has advantages over other imaging methods. It is able to examine the entire bowel wall as well as extracolonic organs. Furthermore, it can demonstrate tissue density, a singularly valuable asset in helping to characterize the nature of the lesion.

As with colonoscopy the technique requires the patient to undergo a full bowel preparation. An intravenous smooth muscle relaxant may be administered, and the colon is insufflated with air until fully distended.[33] Intravenous contrast may also supplement the examination if indicated. If one is seeking a large or obvious lesion in a frail or elderly patient, the examination may be undertaken without a bowel cleansing.[49] There is also the potential for a limited bowl preparation with stool tagging to reduce patient discomfort.[90]

Published reports indicate that VC affords great accuracy in the detection of colon polyps that exceed or are equal to 5 mm.[15,49,130] It is a relatively safe procedure without the risk of sedation or anesthesia and essentially without risk of perforation.[40] CTC has gained acceptance after failed colonoscopy, as an alternative to optical colonoscopy for infirm individuals, and for those who fear optical colonoscopy.[73]

Although it is certain that a complete examination will be obtained by this technique, sensitivity and specificity issues are genuine concerns. Radiation exposure, especially if regular follow-up examinations are required, is also potentially worrisome.

The following comment with respect to VC and the denial of insurance coverage by Aetna Insurance Company as published on its website is worth reproducing here:

. . . . This method is being promoted by some as a noninvasive screening test for colorectal neoplasia. The current cost of [VC] probably prohibits its use as a screening tool . . . . To be economically feasible . . . , the cost would need to drop below the cost of conventional colonoscopy, since [VC] is only a screening test. An appreciable number of patients would need a subsequent colonoscopy and biopsy to confirm the diagnosis and to resect polyps. The need for a follow-up colonoscopy must be included in any cost-effectiveness analysis of screening with [VC]. The relatively low specificity of [VC] in most series (i.e., the many false positive results) reduces its cost-effectiveness, because falsely positive results lead to many unnecessary follow-up conventional colonoscopies. More clinical trials need to be conducted to assess the cost-effectiveness and efficacy of [VC] in comparison with conventional colonoscopy and sigmoidoscopy.

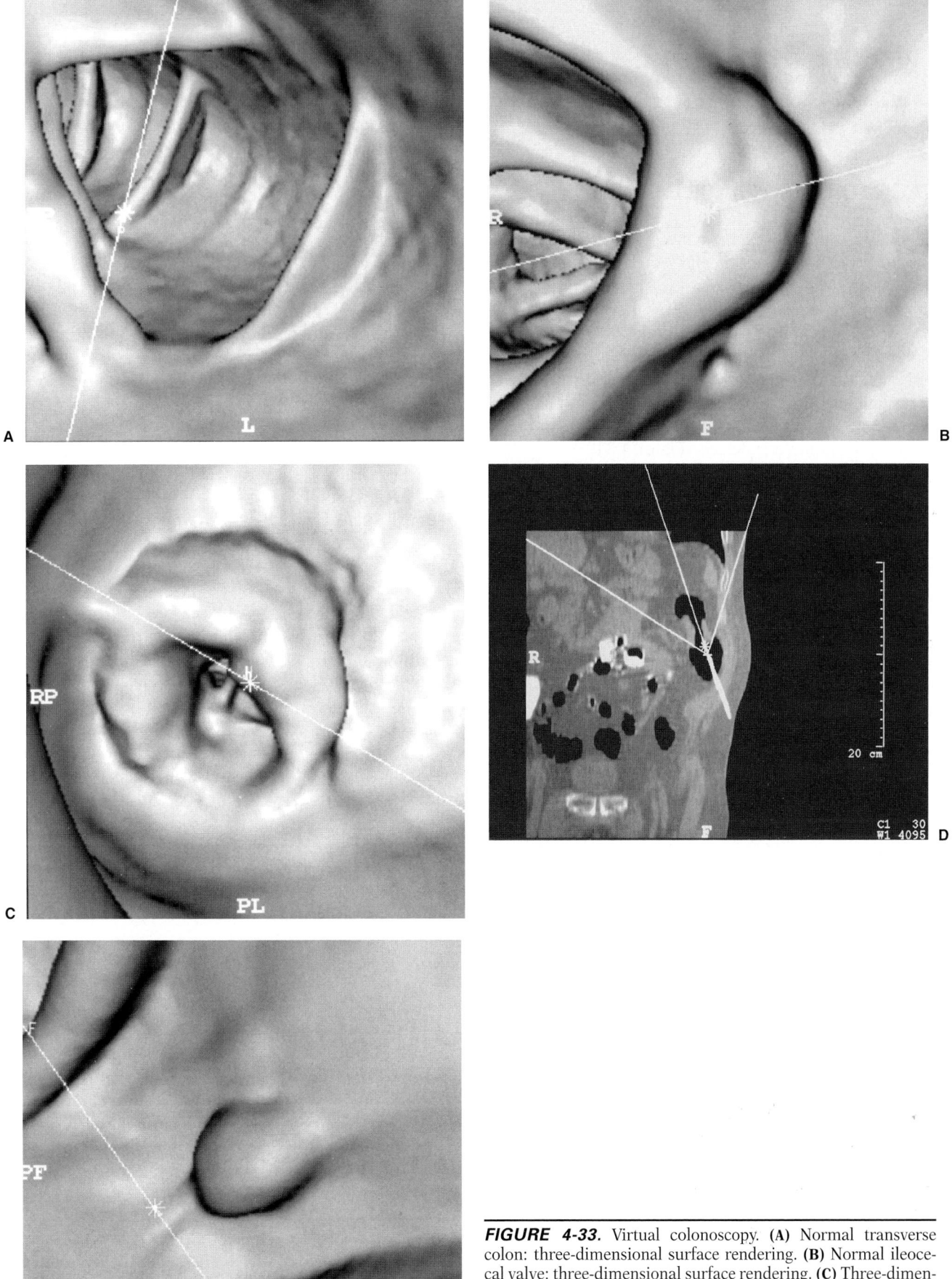

FIGURE 4-33. Virtual colonoscopy. **(A)** Normal transverse colon: three-dimensional surface rendering. **(B)** Normal ileocecal valve: three-dimensional surface rendering. **(C)** Three-dimensional surface rendering of an annular carcinoma near the splenic flexure. **(D)** Coronal view of annular carcinoma. **(E)** Colonic polyp: three-dimensional surface rendering. (Courtesy of Victor J. Scarmato, M.D.)

VC as of this writing is primarily of value for those individuals who are unable to undergo colonoscopy or who underwent an incomplete examination. Still, future improvements in CTC may result in an increased role.

MAGNETIC RESONANCE IMAGING

Magnetic resonance imaging is becoming a very important diagnostic tool for colon and rectal conditions, especially for imaging the pelvis and for identifying normal and pathologic anorectal anatomy. As with endosonography, special application has been found for this modality in the evaluation of anorectal disease. Magnetic resonance imaging with endorectal coils can provide excellent imaging for anal and rectal cancer staging (including lymph nodes), fistula tracts, fluid collection and abscesses, and sphincteric defects (Figure 4-34).[117]

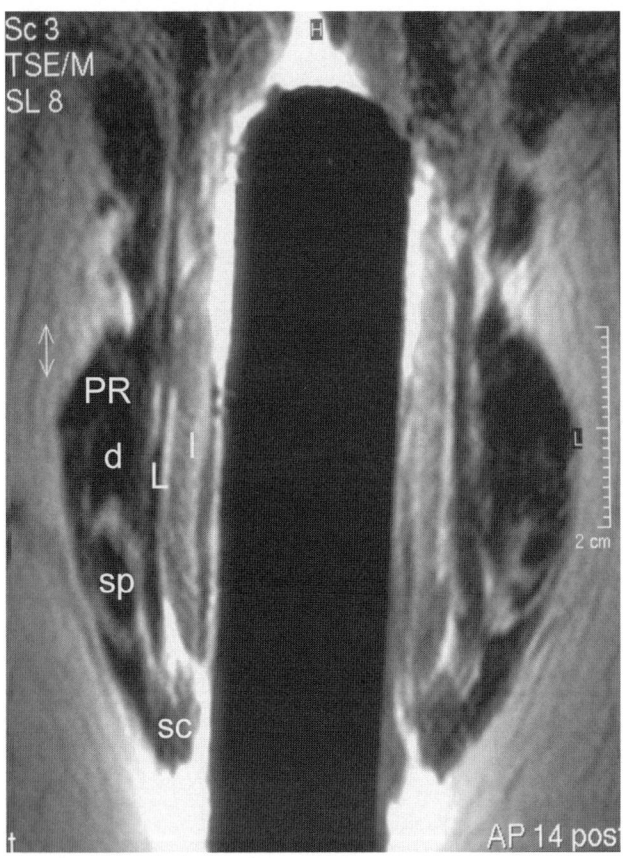

FIGURE 4-34. Endocoil magnetic resonance image of the anal canal in the coronal plane view. *I,* internal anal sphincter (moderate signal); *L,* longitudinal muscle (low signal); *PR,* puborectalis with *d,* deep part of the external anal sphincter; *sp,* superficial part; and *sc,* subcutaneous part. All the striated muscle is of low signal. The high signal on either side of the longitudinal muscle indicates a thin layer of fat. (Courtesy of Professor Clive Bartram, Harrow, United Kingdom.)

POSITRON EMISSION TOMOGRAPHY

The application of positron emission tomography (PET) for colorectal cancer was defined in 1982 and is based on the finding that the tracer 2-[^{18}F]fluoro-2-deoxy-D-glucose concentrates in malignant tissue as a consequence of increased glycolysis compared with the normal.[6,131] Whereas CT provides information on anatomy, PET specifically addresses metabolic or physiologic data. However, when PET is combined with CT, the study affords an assessment of metabolic activity as well as spatial and anatomic relationships. PET is a very expensive modality, with systems costing in the United States from $800,000 to 2.5 million and a cost per examination in the range of $2,000 (2001 figures).[6] The PET scan has its primary usefulness in the assessment of recurrent or metastatic colorectal cancer (see Chapter 22).[59]

RADIOLOGY OF THE SMALL INTESTINE

Although the small bowel represents 75% of the length and 90% of the mucosal surface of the alimentary tract, the incidence of small bowel disease is low.[74] For one to undertake a small bowel examination in every individual with complaints referable to the abdomen is generally a fruitless exercise. Even with a clear indication, a small bowel series is less than an ideal investigation for evaluating such a long section of the intestinal tract (when compared with contrast studies in other organs). The following conditions, however, often require this study:

Crohnease
Polyposis
Unexplained iron-deficiency anemia
Unexplained GI bleeding
Diarrhea or steatorrhea
Unexplained abdominal pain
Fever of unknown origin

Technique

This evaluation is undertaken following an overnight fast. The most important characteristic of a proper contrast material for the small bowel study is a barium that suspends easily and does not flocculate, precipitate, or settle.[76] The small bowel is examined following administration of a mixture that is half barium sulfate and half water. A large volume of barium is especially helpful in interpretation of diffuse lesions of the small bowel. Compression studies are used whenever necessary for better delineation of a lesion, and they are routinely employed in demonstrating the ter-

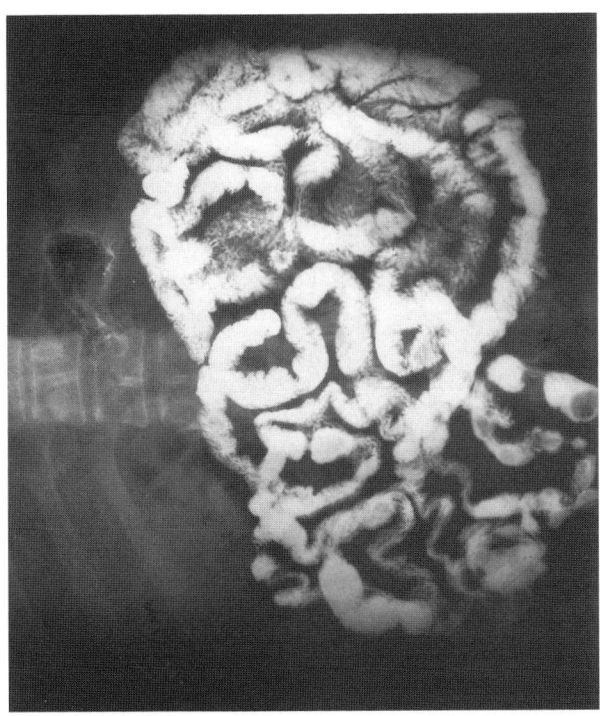

FIGURE 4-35. Small bowel series demonstrates normal mucosal pattern throughout. This is a study at 1.5 hours. The colon has not yet filled.

minal ileum.[76] Initially the patient is examined fluoroscopically, and if the barium meal has progressed sufficiently, a film is taken. Further filming depends on the rate of passage of the barium and is usually performed once every 30 to 60 minutes until the material has reached the colon. In physiologically normal persons, the barium column may take from 2 hours to as long as 6 hours (Figure 4-35). The terminal ileum must always be compressed. This segment of bowel tends to be hidden by overlapping loops in the pelvis, and because it is the most frequent site of small bowel disease, special study is required. This is obviously particularly true in cases of Crohn's disease.

Enteroclysis

Enteroclysis involves the use of 250 mL of high-density barium. This is supplemented by methylcellulose, which acts to distend the small intestine. The material is inserted through a nasogastric tube with the tip of the small bowel ideally located at the ligament of Treitz. This permits a study equivalent to that of an air-contrast enema performed in the colon.

Enteroclysis is the most accurate available technique for contrast examination of the small intestine. Its main advantage is that intubation beyond the pylorus bypasses its sphincteric restriction and makes possible the infu-

sion of contrast material at a required rate.[54] There is the obvious disadvantage, however, of the need for intubation. The technique involves the infusion of a methylcellulose solution that follows the introduction of barium. The demonstration of small bowel detail is possible during single-contrast and double-contrast stages.[54] It should be remembered, however, that this technique is not the best method for evaluation of a problem related to the terminal ileal area.

Capsule Endoscopy

As implied, diseases affecting the small intestine are often difficult to diagnose because the traditional methods of radiology and endoscopy fail to provide a complete and accurate assessment of the entire organ. A new and different concept has been developed to address this problem, that of capsule endoscopy. Introduced in 1998, the M2A Capsule Endoscopy Given Diagnostic System (Given Imaging Ltd., New Industrial Park, 2 Hacarmel St, Yoqneam 20692 Israel; info@givenimaging.com) is a noninvasive diagnostic imaging device (Figure 4-36). The capsule is swallowed and traverses the entire GI tract, transmitting color videos during its passage. The patient is fully ambulating and continues normal daily activities throughout the "endoscopic" examination.

Method

A 10-hour fast is required prior to the procedure. The capsule is then swallowed with a small amount of water. Images and data are acquired as the capsule passes through the digestive system. This information is then transmitted via an array of sensors secured to the abdomen to the DataRecorder affixed to a belt worn around the patient's waist. The duration of the examination is about 8 hours.

The patient returns the DataRecorder for processing on the RAPID workstation. Images can then be analyzed and saved. The capsule is eliminated as a one-time use device. Figure 4-37 illustrates three lesions within the small intestinal that were successfully identified by this means. Numerous publications testify to the fact that capsule endoscopy is a valuable diagnostic tool for identifying Crohn's disease and bleeding lesions within the small bowel that cannot be visualized by conventional imaging techniques.[30,35,55,71,106]

EXFOLIATIVE CYTOLOGY

Exfoliative cytology has been recommended as a screening technique for the evaluation of iron-deficiency anemia, for early detection of colonic neoplasms, and to ascertain whether known lesions as determined by colonoscopy or

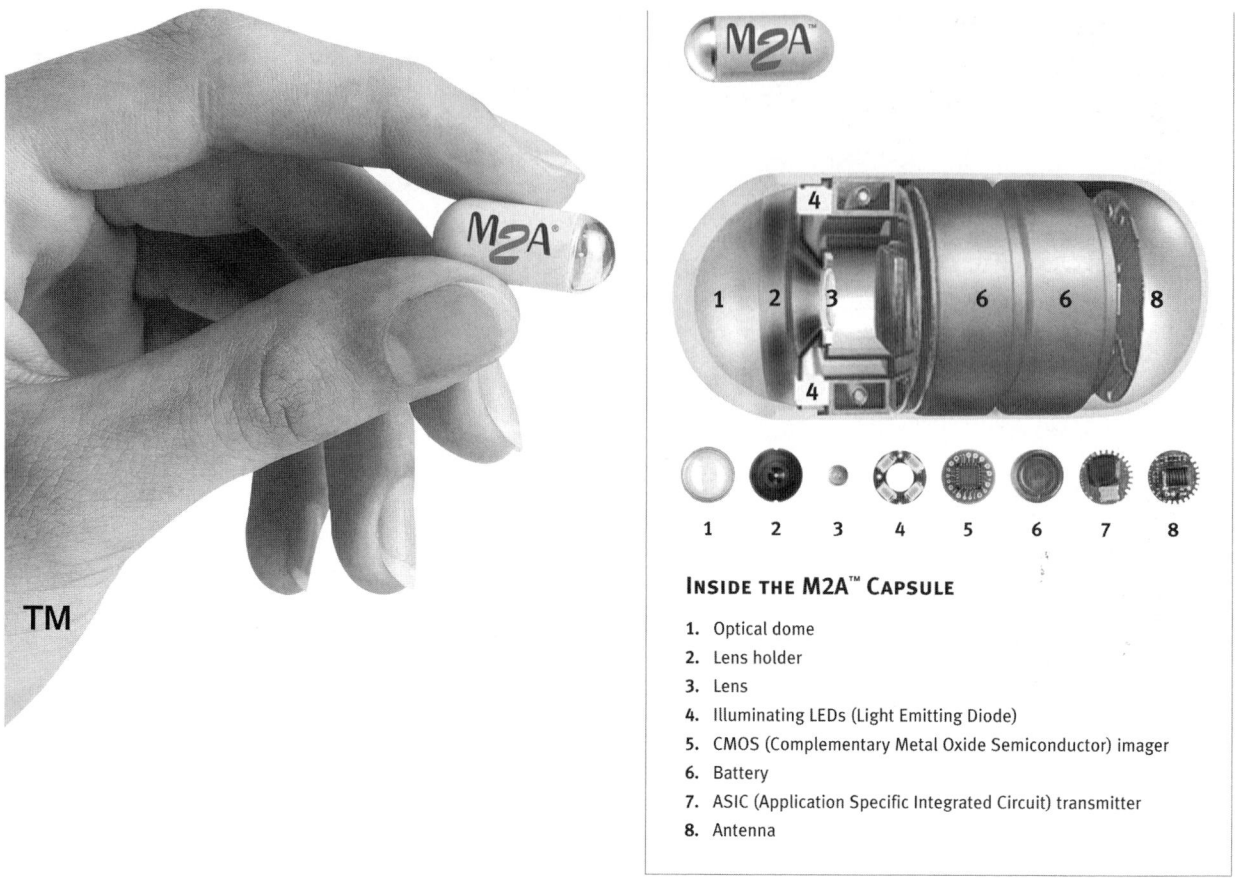

A **B**

FIGURE 4-36. (A) Given Imaging Capsule as held in the fingers. (B) Capsule components. (Courtesy of Given Imaging, Yoqneam, Israel.)

roentgenography are benign or malignant.[96] The procedure involves a vigorous bowel cleansing.[7,28,85,96] Raskin and Pleticka advocate in-hospital evaluation to ensure such thoroughness.[97] Through a sigmoidoscope, a large-diameter rubber catheter is inserted and the instrument withdrawn. Irrigation is then carried out, usually by a trained technician, and slides are collected and reviewed by a pathologist (Figure 4-38).

Exfoliative cytology has never gained much acceptance, primarily because of the cumbersome methodology and the fact that colonoscopy is far superior for evaluation of the entire bowel. Unless it can be simplified and the results interpreted with accuracy, the procedure will become obsolete.

OCCULT BLOOD DETERMINATION OF STOOL

Colorectal cancer is the fourth most common noncutaneous malignancy in the United States and is the second leading cause of cancer mortality. In 2003, the American Cancer Society estimated that there would be 147,500

new cases diagnosed. Prostate cancer is the most common (2003 estimate, 220,900), followed by breast cancer (2003 estimate, 212,600) and cancer of the lung and bronchus (2003 estimate, 171,900). Inarguably the least expensive mass-screening technique available for detection of GI disease is the occult blood determination.[110,128] The value of this procedure is particularly enhanced because of evidence that colorectal cancer appears increasingly to be affecting the bowel in a more proximal location (see Chapter 22).

Materials and Methods

Guaiac is a chemical test for peroxidase activity that is present in both hemoglobin and certain foods.[102] The commercially available guaiac-impregnated slide (Hemoccult II, Beckman-Coulter, Inc., Fullerton, CA) has come to be used as the primary resource for this screening study. A newer modification is the Hemoccult II SENSA test from the same manufacturer. Seracult is another commercially available fecal occult blood test (Propper Manufacturing Co., Inc., Long Island City, NY).

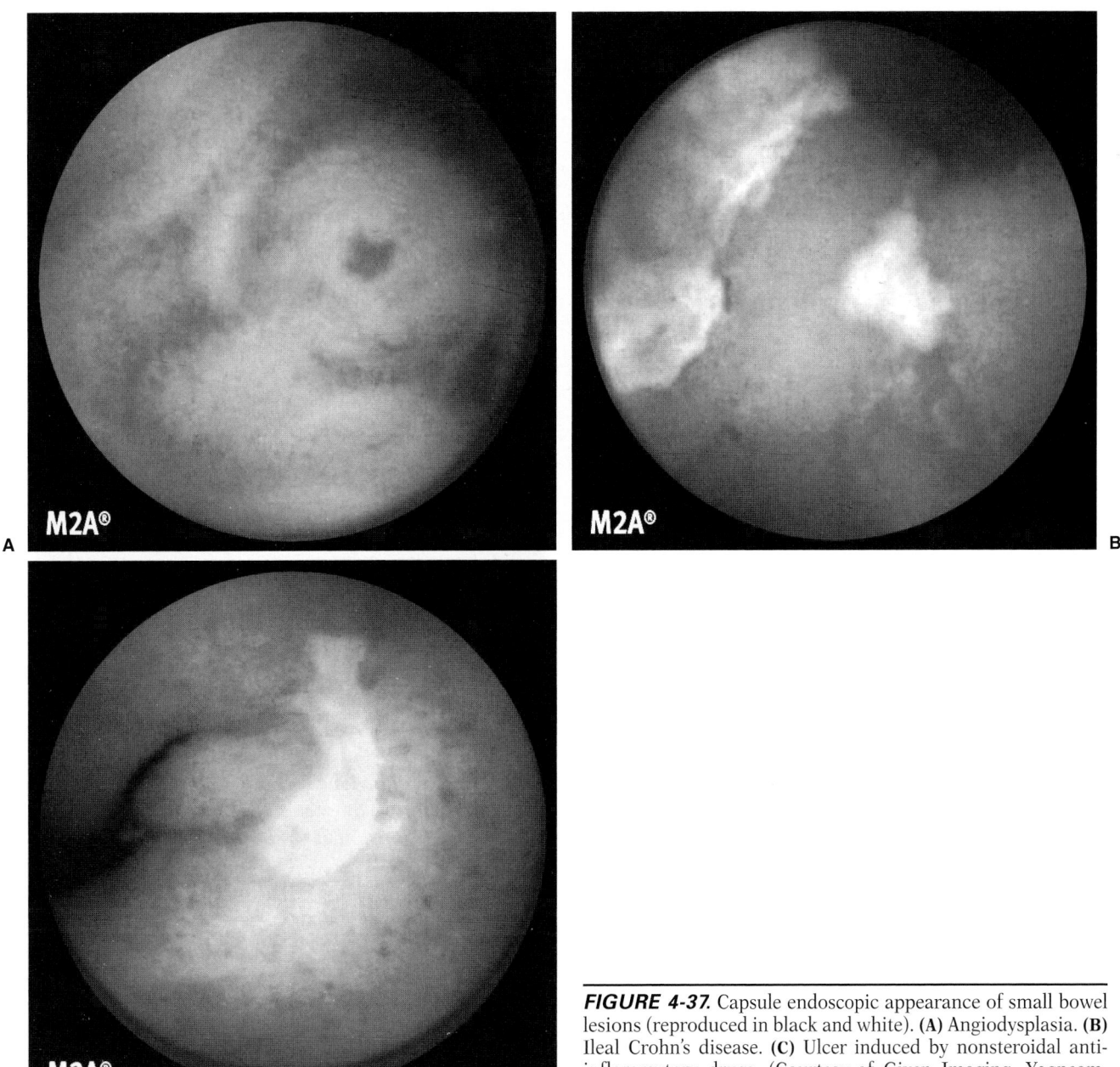

FIGURE 4-37. Capsule endoscopic appearance of small bowel lesions (reproduced in black and white). **(A)** Angiodysplasia. **(B)** Ileal Crohn's disease. **(C)** Ulcer induced by nonsteroidal antiinflammatory drugs. (Courtesy of Given Imaging, Yoqneam, Israel.)

Occult blood determination, however, is generally believed to be a suboptimal exercise unless strict dietary instructions are adhered to. The real question is whether one wishes to substitute increased sensitivity for increased specificity. Interestingly, it has been shown that the method of stool collection affects the outcome of fecal occult blood testing. Stool obtained by digital rectal examination has a poorer positive predictive value for cancer and for polyps than stool obtained through routine screening.[80]

For at least 48 hours prior to the collection of the first stool specimen, rare meat, turnips, melons, horseradish, salmon, and sardines should be avoided to reduce the likelihood of false-positive determinations. A high-fiber diet is usually advised, but concern has been expressed that the increased fecal weight significantly lowers fecal hemoglobin concentration, with the implication of a false-negative result.[112] Medications such as aspirin and vitamin preparations, especially vitamin C (ascorbic acid) in excess of 250 mg/day, are excluded. Aspirin or other nonsteroidal antiinflammatory drugs should be avoided for 7 days before and during the test period.

An immunochemical test for occult stool human hemoglobin is also available (FlexSure OBT, Beckman-

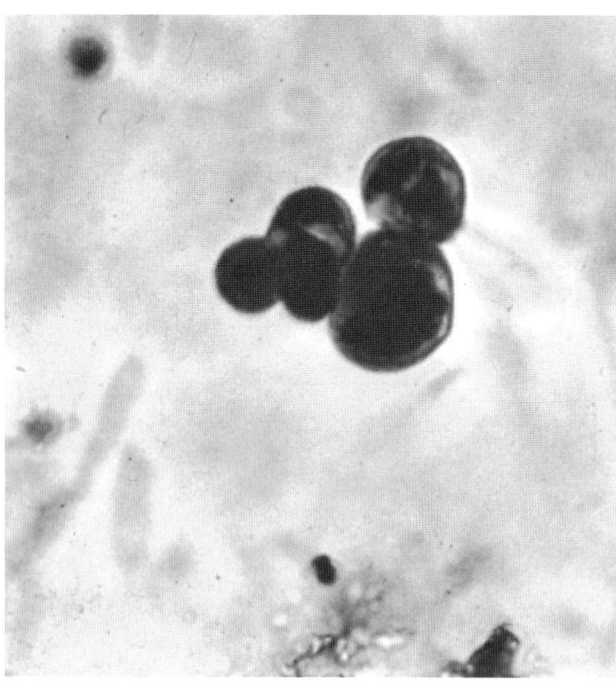

FIGURE 4-38. Exfoliative cytology demonstrates cancer cells in colonic washings (original magnification × 600). (Courtesy of Rudolf Garret, M.D.)

Coulter, Inc.). Both this method and Hemoccult SENSA were compared in an endoscopic study by Rozen and colleagues to determine which to recommend for a population screening program.[102] Hemoccult SENSA had greater sensitivity, but FlexSure OBT had significantly greater specificity.

The test is commenced on the third day, with the patient taking a sample from the stool and smearing it on the card. Samples from three consecutive bowel movements are suggested. In interpreting results, the American Cancer Society recommends that doubtful readings should be recorded as negative and trace readings as positive.[29] A single positive slide is understood to mean that all determinations are positive. With such a conclusion, the physician is obligated to perform in sequential order, a digital rectal examination, proctosigmoidoscopy or flexible sigmoidoscopy, and colonoscopy; if results of the colonoscopy are normal, upper GI roentgenography and a small bowel series should follow.[122] Some have recommended that the physician should go immediately to colonoscopy, because this procedure is inevitably required for completeness. In one study, the higher cost of this examination was offset by its greater sensitivity as well as its capacity for biopsy and therapy.[66]

Problems with patient compliance and the high cost of false-positive results have stimulated the development of

alternative screening approaches by other pharmaceutical companies. HemoQuant (Smith Kline Diagnostics, Sunnyvale, CA) requires 2 to 3 g of feces but allegedly is more sensitive and requires fewer dietary restrictions. ColoCare (Helena Laboratories, Claremont, Ontario, Canada), and EZ Detect™ (Biomerica, Inc., Newport Beach, CA.) are home-detection products whose efficacy has not been clearly established. These generally involve placement of a specially prepared, chemically impregnated, biodegradable paper in the toilet bowl. The individual then observes the paper for a color change following defecation.

Results

Numerous reports of the beneficial results and cost-effectiveness of mass screening for colorectal cancer have been published (see Chapter 22).[38,45,46,51,52,63,81,84,89,103,114,120] Those patients found to harbor a malignant lesion usually have a much earlier-stage tumor. Schnell and coworkers studied almost 30,000 individuals who returned their fecal blood test cards.[107] Eighty-two percent of all colorectal cancers that were detected by fecal occult blood testing were diagnosed at a favorable stage. However, the majority of known, advanced tumors (62%) escaped early detection by this method. The authors concluded that utilizing this test alone may provide a false sense of security, especially in those individuals with advanced left-sided colorectal cancer.[107] Hardcastle and associates recruited approximately 75,000 individuals in a screening group and the same number as controls.[51] Of 893 cancers (20% stage Dukes' A) diagnosed in participants in the screening group, 26.4% were detected by fecal occult blood screening, 27.9% presented after a negative result on occult blood testing or investigation, and 44.8% presented in nonresponders. The incidence of cancer in the control group was 1.44 per 1,000 person-years. Three hundred sixty people died of colorectal cancer in the screening group, compared with 420 in the control group, a 15% reduction in cumulative colorectal cancer mortality by screening.[51] Likewise, others have shown that screening by means of fecal occult blood testing can reduce colorectal cancer mortality.[63]

Reilly and colleagues have shown the obvious, that colonoscopy is superior to occult blood testing as a screening test for detecting neoplastic disease, but the question is whether the cost can be justified.[98] In a study by Sontag and associates, there was a 5% incidence of positive results using occult blood determination, much less than with colonoscopy.[114] Of those who completed the GI workup, 48% were found to have neoplastic lesions, almost one third of which were malignant. Leicester and colleagues studied 802 symptomatic patients with suspected colorectal disease.[70] There was good compliance (92.5%), and a high specificity for colorectal cancer was noted (85.4%). The false-positive rate was 8.6%, but the false-negative rate for rectal cancer was unacceptably high (45.4%). Of course, in these symptomatic patients, it is expected that at least a proctosigmoidoscopy would have been performed.

A contrary assessment on the place of this screening modality has been offered by Ransohoff and Lang.[95] They conclude that there is no justification for performing such testing on asymptomatic persons with no risk factors. Others have demonstrated that most known, advanced cases of colorectal cancer (62%) escape early detection with fecal occult testing.[107] Conversely, 82% of all colorectal cancers that were detected by this screening method were diagnosed at a favorable stage. The problem, of course, is that the test may provide a false sense of security.[107] Ahlquist and colleagues performed a prospective study using occult blood testing in two groups of patients: those undergoing surveillance following curative resection of a colorectal tumor and relatives of patients with colorectal cancer who were at least 50 years of age.[2] They observed that most cancers and polyps were missed and concluded that fecal occult blood appears to be a very poor marker for colorectal neoplasms. Others agree and suggest that although there is no requirement for a new strategy, there is a need for new markers.[86] Such a recommendation implies that efforts be made to search for more potent genetic and biochemical markers, such as "ectopic proteins" other than blood.

Regardless of criticisms, most investigators and clinicians believe that there is ample evidence to suggest that occult blood determination of the stool should be an integral part of a complete physical examination, but by how much screening reduces mortality is still an unanswered question.

Conclusion

The concept of the cost-benefit analysis of the various methods of screening for colorectal cancer is subject to debate. This is also true in other areas, medical and nonmedical. For example, the number of lives saved and injuries prevented by means of seat belts and air bags in automobiles, as well as the use of seat belts in airplanes, have not been satisfactorily analyzed. The value of earthquake retrofitting is another controversial subject. The critical question, of course, is how much is a human life worth? I do not pretend to know the answer to that conundrum.

FECES COLLECTION

The frequent complaint of diarrhea in the experience of every surgeon and the differential diagnosis of infectious enteritis require that one be familiar with at least the fundamentals of stool collection and its purpose.

Collecting Stool for Culture

The stool sample should arrive in the laboratory within half an hour of having been taken unless it is placed in a transport medium. Refrigeration is contraindicated. Swabs should not be used for collection.

Stool cultures are made by placing a sterile swab into the specimen and streaking a portion of several agar plates containing various inhibitory and noninhibitory agents in order to allow the recovery of both intestinal flora and pathogenic organisms (e.g., *Salmonella*, *Shigella*, *Campylobacter*; see Chapter 33). The plates are examined at 24 hours, and suspect colonies are inoculated into identification media. If *Salmonella* or *Shigella* species are found, a subculture is sent for serologic typing or confirmation.

Certain organisms are somewhat unusual and difficult to identify in a stool specimen. A specific request is usually necessary for their culture because they require special techniques. These organisms include fungi (the test is generally limited to screening for *Candida*), *Mycobacterium*, pathogenic *Vibrio* (i.e., cholera), *Campylobacter*, and *Yersinia*. The discovery of certain organisms mandates reporting to the local public health authority.

Collecting Stool for Examination for Ova and Parasites

The specimen must be less than 1 hour old when received by the laboratory. Three specimens are recommended for screening over a 5-day period. Collection can be made by using a warm saline solution or Fleet enema. Bismuth, mineral oil, castor oil, psyllium, and magnesium compounds used as laxatives produce specimens that are unsatisfactory for evaluation. Also, stools should not be collected if a barium study has been performed within 1 week.

Stool specimens for parasites are examined macroscopically for color and appearance (e.g., formed or liquid, with mucus or blood). They are also checked for adult worms or tapeworm proglottids (see Chapter 33).

A wet-mount preparation of stool on a glass slide with a drop each of saline solution and iodine is coverslipped and examined microscopically for evidence of parasites (e.g., eggs, cysts, larvae) as well as for fecal leukocytes. A small portion of the specimen is also treated to concentrate the eggs and cysts and later examined microscopically with wet mounts. Finally, a slide is streaked, trichrome stained, and examined histologically with the oil immersion lens. For the diagnosis and treatment of a specific pathologic organism and disease, see the Index.

INTRAVENOUS PYELOGRAPHY AND UROLOGIC EVALUATION

The routine assessment of the urinary tract prior to major colon and especially rectal surgery has been strongly recommended by many surgeons. Although intravenous pyelogram had been for many years the principal investigation for accomplishing this objective, it has been virtually completely replaced today by CT. Furthermore, there is an inherent risk to intravenous pyelography, especially for those allergic to the intravenous dye. What abnormalities may be anticipated was reported by Prager and colleagues in a review of our experience with intravenous pyelography in 180 patients.[93] Seventy-eight (43%) were found to have abnormalities. Table 4-1 illustrates those that were believed to be related to the primary disease, and Table 4-2 summarizes the unexpected findings.

Conditions such as inflammatory bowel disease, diverticulitis, and carcinoma of the rectum or rectosigmoid frequently are associated with urinary symptoms because of the proximity of the bowel to the adjacent bladder or ureter.

The concept of having a road map of the urinary tract before surgical intervention is supported by the high frequency of symptoms and associated abnormalities. Tank and colleagues, for example, noted that among 150 patients who underwent abdominoperineal resection, postoperative voiding difficulties developed in 30%.[119] Peel and coworkers, in a prospective series of 176 individuals who underwent surgery for carcinoma or diverticular disease, noted urologic symptoms in almost one third.[87A] As may be anticipated, the incidence of pyelogram abnormalities is much higher in symptomatic patients than in those without complaints. The coincidental discovery of such conditions as ureteric duplication and unilateral

kidney and the risk for intraoperative injury to the urinary tract strongly support the routine preoperative assessment of urologic anatomy in all patients who are to undergo bowel surgery, especially those individuals who have undergone radiation treatment, who have urinary tract symptoms, and who are to undergo repeat pelvic surgery (see Chapters 22 and 23). However, with the frequent preoperative use of CT the point may be moot, because the presence of an abnormality of the urinary tract is usually appreciated.

FLEXIBLE SIGMOIDOSCOPY AND COLONOSCOPY

See Chapter 5.

PHYSIOLOGIC STUDIES

See Chapter 6.

REFERENCES

1. Adami B, Eckardt VF, Suermann RB, et al. Bacteremia after proctoscopy and hemorrhoidal injection sclerotherapy. *Dis Colon Rectum* 1981;24:373.
2. Ahlquist DA, Wieand HS, Moertel CG, et al. Accuracy of fecal occult blood screening for colorectal neoplasia: a prospective study using Hemoccult and HemoQuant tests. *JAMA* 1993;269:1262.

▶ **TABLE 4-2** Abnormal or Coincidental Intravenous Pyelogram Findings

Abnormality	Number
Ureteric duplication	4
Unilateral kidney	1
Ptotic kidney	1
Atrophic pyelonephritis	1
Bilateral sponge kidney	1
Bladder carcinoma	1
Neurogenic bladder	1
Poor visualization, both kidneys	1
Malrotated kidney	1
Renal carcinoma	1
Displaced kidney (secondary hypersplenism)	1
Caliectasis	4
Calyceal diverticulum	4
Renal pelvic cyst	1
Renal pelvic papilloma	2

From Prager E, Swinton NW, Corman ML, Veidenheimer MC. Intravenous pyelography in colorectal surgery. *Dis Colon Rectum* 1973;16:479, with permission.

▶ **TABLE 4-1** Abnormal Intravenous Pyelogram Findings Presumed Secondary to Primary Colon Disease

Abnormality	Number
Hydroureter	6
Bilateral hydroureter and hydronephrosis	2
Unilateral hydronephrosis	3
Ureteric deviation	3
Extrinsic pressure on bladder	7
Urinary tract calculi	8
Postvoiding residual	
Modest	22
Marked	5

From Prager E, Swinton NW, Corman ML, Veidenheimer MC. Intravenous pyelography in colorectal surgery. *Dis Colon Rectum* 1973;16:479, with permission.

3. American Society of Colon and Rectal Surgeons. Practice parameters for antibiotic prophylaxis to prevent infective endocarditis or infected prosthesis during colon and rectal endoscopy. *Dis Colon Rectum* 1992;35:277.

4. Angelelli G, Ianora AA, Scardapane A, et al. Role of computerized tomography in the staging of gastrointestinal neoplasms. *Semin Surg Oncol* 2001;20:109–121.

5. Anseline PF, Fazio VW. Management of massive postpolypectomy hemorrhage. *Dis Colon Rectum* 1982;25:251.

6. Arulampalam THA, Costa DC, Loizidou M, et al. Positron emission tomography and colorectal cancer. *Br J Surg* 2001;88:176–89.

7. Bader GM, Papanicolaou G. The application of cytology in the diagnosis of cancer of the rectum, sigmoid and descending colon. *Cancer* 1952;5:307.

8. Barloon TJ, Shumway J. Medical malpractice involving radiologic colon examinations: a review of 38 recent cases. *AJR Am J Roentgenol* 1995;165:343.

9. Bartolo DCC, Roe AM, Virjee J, et al. Evacuation proctography in obstructed defaecation and rectal intussusception. *Br J Surg* 1985;72[Suppl]:111.

10. Benjamin HG, Todd JD. Routine roentgenologic examination of the colon in patients with anorectal complaints. *Dis Colon Rectum* 1959;2:196.

11. Burnikel RH. Barium granuloma. *Dis Colon Rectum* 1962; 5:224.

12. Cannon WB. The movements of the stomach studied by means of the Röntgen rays. *Am J Physiol* 1898;1:360.

13. Cannon WB. The movements of the intestines studied by means of the Röntgen rays. *Am J Physiol* 1901/1902;6:251.

14. Cannon WB, Moser A. The movements of the food in the esophagus. *Am J Physiol* 1898;1:435.

15. Carrascosa P, Castiglioni R. Virtual colonoscopy: experience after 350 studies. *Dis Colon Rectum* 2001;44:A5–A26.

16. Cordone RP, Brandeis SZ, Richman H. Rectal perforation during barium enema: report of a case. *Dis Colon Rectum* 1988;31:563.

17. Corman ML, Coller JA, Veidenheimer MC. Proctosigmoidoscopy: age criteria for examination in the asymptomatic patient. *CA* 1975;25:286.

18. Corman ML, Veidenheimer MC, Coller JA. Barium-enema study findings in asymptomatic patients with rectal polyps. *Dis Colon Rectum* 1974;17:325.

19. Crapp AR, Powis SJA, Tillotson P, et al. Preparation of the bowel by whole-gut irrigation. *Lancet* 1975;2:1239.

20. Dajani AS, Bisno AL, Chung KJ, et al. Prevention of bacterial endocarditis: recommendations by the American Heart Association. *JAMA* 1990;264:2929.

21. de Roos A, Hermans J, Shaw PC, et al. Colon polyps and carcinomas: prospective comparison of the single- and double-contrast examination in the same patients. *Radiology* 1985;154:11.

22. Dickinson VA. Maintenance of anal continence: a review of pelvic floor physiology. *Gut* 1978;19:1163.

23. Dickman MD, Farrell R, Higgs RH, et al. Colonoscopy associated bacteremia. *Surg Gynecol Obstet* 1976;142:173.

24. Dodds WJ, Scanlon GT, Shaw DK, et al. An evaluation of colon cleansing regimens. *AJR Am J Roentgenol* 1977;128:57.

25. Drexler J. Asymptomatic polyps of the colon and rectum. III. Proximal and distal polyp relationships. *Arch Intern Med* 1971;127:466.

26. Durack DT. Prevention of infective endocarditis. *N Engl J Med* 1995;332:38–44.

27. Dysart DN. Angled sigmoid view. In: Greenbaum EI, ed. *Radiographic atlas of colon disease.* Chicago: Year Book, 1980:31.

28. Ebeling CE, Little JW. The demonstration of malignant cells exfoliated from the proximal colon. *Ann Intern Med* 1957;46:21.

29. Eddy D. Cancer of the colon and rectum. *CA* 1980;30:208.

30. Eliakim R, Fischer D, Suissa A, et al. Wireless capsule video endoscopy in a superior diagnostic tool in comparison to barium follow-through and computerized tomography in patients with suspected Crohn's disease. *Eur J Gastroenterol Hepatol* 2003;15:363.

31. Ekberg O, Nylander, G, Fork F-T. Defecography. *Radiology* 1985;155:45.

32. Farmer KCR, Church JM. Open sesame: tips for traversing the anal canal. *Dis Colon Rectum* 1992;35:1092.

33. Fenlon HM. Virtual colonoscopy. *Br J Surg* 2002;89:1–3.

34. Fielding J, Lumsden K. Large-bowel perforations in patients undergoing sigmoidoscopy and barium enema. *BMJ* 1973;1:471.

35. Fireman Z, Mahajna E, Broide E, et al. Diagnosing small bowel Crohn's disease with wireless capsule endoscopy. *Gut* 2003;52:390.

36. Frühmorgen P, Bodem F, Reidenbach HD, et al. Endoscopic laser coagulation of bleeding gastrointestinal lesions with report of the first therapeutic application in men. *Gastrointest Endosc* 1976;23:73.

37. Fry RD, Shemesh EI, Kodner IJ, et al. Perforation of the rectum and sigmoid colon during barium-enema examination: management and prevention. *Dis Colon Rectum* 1989; 32:759.

38. Fujita M, Sugiyama R, Kumanishi Y, et al. Evaluation of effectiveness of mass screening for colorectal cancer. *World J Surg* 1990;14:648.

39. Gear EV, Dobbins WO. Rectal biopsy. *Gastroenterology* 1968;55:522.

40. Gelfand DW, Chen MY, Ott DJ. Preparing the colon for the barium enema examination. *Radiology* 1991;178:609.

41. Gelfand DW, Ott DJ. Single vs. double-contrast gastrointestinal studies: critical analysis of reported statistics. *AJR Am J Roentgenol* 1981;137:523.

42. Gianturco C, Miller GA. Routine search for colonic polyps by high-voltage radiography. *Radiology* 1953;60:496.

43. Gilbertsen VA. Proctosigmoidoscopy and polypectomy in reducing the incidence of rectal cancer. *Cancer* 1974; 34[Suppl]:936.

44. Gourtsoyiannis N, Grammatikakis J, Prassopoulos P. Role of conventional radiology in the diagnosis and staging of gastrointestinal tract neoplasms. *Semin Surg Oncol* 2001;20:91–108.

45. Greegor DH. Occult blood testing for detection of asymptomatic colon cancer. *Cancer* 1971;28:131.

46. Greegor DH. Detection of colorectal cancer using guaiac slides. *CA* 1972;22:361.

47. Grobmyer AJ III, Kerlan RA, Peterson CM, et al. Barium peritonitis. *Am Surg* 1984;50:116.

48. Hakim NS, Sarr MG, Bender CE, et al. Management of barium enema-induced colorectal perforation. *Am Surg* 1992; 58:673.

49. Halligan S, Fenlon HM. Virtual colonoscopy. *BMJ* 1999; 319:1249–52.

50. Han SY, Tishler JM. Perforation of the colon above the peritoneal reflection during the barium-enema examination. *Radiology* 1982;144:253.

51. Hardcastle JD, Chamberlain JO, Robinson MHE, et al. Randomised controlled trial of faecal-occult-blood screening for colorectal cancer. *Lancet* 1996;348:1472.

52. Hardcastle JD, Thomas WM, Chamberlain J, et al. Randomised, controlled trial of faecal occult blood screening for colorectal cancer: results for first 107,349 subjects. *Lancet* 1989;1:1160.

53. Harned RK, Consigny PM, Cooper NB, et al. Barium enema examination following biopsy of the rectum or colon. *Radiology* 1982;145:11.

54. Herlinger H. Guide to imaging of the small bowel. *Gastroenterol Clin North Am* 1995;24:309.

55. Herrerías JM, Caunedo A, Rodríguez-Téllez M, et al. Capsule endoscopy in patients with suspected Crohn's disease and negative endoscopy. *Endoscopy* 2003;35:564.

56. Hewitt J, Reeve J, Rigby J, et al. Whole-gut irrigation in preparation for large-bowel surgery. *Lancet* 1973;2:337.

57. Hoffman BI, Kobasa W, Kaye D. Bacteremia after rectal examination. *Ann Intern Med* 1978;88:658.

58. Johnson CD, Carlson HC, Taylor WF, et al. Barium enemas of the colon: sensitivity of double- and single-contrast studies. *AJR Am J Roentgenol* 1983;140:1143.

59. Johnson K, Bakhsh A, Young D, et al. Correlating computed tomography and positron emission tomography scan with operative findings in metastatic colorectal cancer. *Dis Colon Rectum* 2001;44:354.

60. Kahn SP, Lindenauer SM, Wojtalik RS. Perforation of the normal colon during barium contrast examination. *Am Surg* 1976;42:789.

61. Kelley CJ, Ingoldby CJH, Blenkharn JI, et al. Colonoscopy related endotoxemia. *Surg Gynecol Obstet* 1985;161:332.

62. Knutson CO, Williams HC, Max MH. Detection of intracolonic lesion by barium contrast enema. *JAMA* 1979;242: 2206.

63. Kronborg O, Fenger C, Olsen J, et al. Randomised study of screening for colorectal cancer with faecal-occult-blood test. *Lancet* 1996;348:1467.

64. Kuijpers HC, Bleijenberg G. The spastic pelvic floor syndrome: a cause of constipation. *Dis Colon Rectum* 1985; 28:669.

65. Kumar S, Abcarian H, Prasad ML, et al. Bacteremia associated with lower gastrointestinal endoscopy, fact of fiction? *Dis Colon Rectum* 1982;25:131.

66. Lashner BA, Silverstein MD. Evaluation and therapy of the patient with fecal occult blood loss: a decision analysis. *Am J Gastroenterol* 1990;85:1088.

67. Laufer I. The radiologic demonstration of early changes in ulcerative colitis by double contrast technique. *J Can Assoc Radiol* 1975;26:116.

68. Laufer I, Mullens JE, Hamilton J. Correlation of endoscopy and double-contrast radiography in the early stages of ulcerative and granulomatous colitis. *Radiology* 1976;118:1.

69. LeFrock JL, Ellis CA, Turchik JB, et al. Transient bacteremia associated with sigmoidoscopy. *N Engl J Med* 1973; 289:467.

70. Leicester RJ, Lightfoot A, Millar J, et al. Accuracy and value of the Hemoccult test in symptomatic patients. *BMJ* 1983;286:673.

71. Liangpunsakul S, Chadalawada V, Rex DK, et al. Wireless capsule endoscopy detects small bowel ulcers in patients with normal results from state of the art enteroclysis. *Am J Gastroenterol* 2003;98:1295.

72. Lull GF Jr, Byrne JP, Sanowski RA. Barium sulfate granuloma of the rectum. *JAMA* 1971;217:1102.

73. Macari M, Berman P, Dicker M, et al. Usefulness of CT colonography in patients with incomplete colonoscopy. *AJR Am J Roentgenol* 1999;173:561.

74. Maglinte DDT, Kelvin FM, O'Connor K, et al. Current status of small bowel radiography. *Abdom Imaging* 1996;21: 247.

75. Margulis AR. Is double-contrast examination of the colon the only acceptable radiographic examination? *Radiology* 1976;119:741.

76. Marshak RH, Lindner AE. *Radiology of small intestine.* Philadelphia: WB Saunders, 1978:1–8.

77. Martel W, Robins JM. The barium enema: technique, value and limitations. *Cancer* 1971;28:137.

78. Miller RE, Chernish SM, Skucas J, et al. Hypotonic colon examination with glucagon. *Radiology* 1974;113:555.

79. Millward SF, Chapman A, Somers S, et al. Rectal biopsy as a cause of rectal ulceration. *Radiology* 1985;156:42.

80. Nakama H, Zhang B, Fattah ASM, et al. Does stool collection method affect outcomes in immunochemical fecal occult blood testing? *Dis Colon Rectum* 2001;44:871–5.

81. Nakama H, Zhang B, Zhang X, et al. Age-related cancer detection rate and costs for one cancer detected in one screening by immunochemical fecal occult blood test. *Dis Colon Rectum* 2001;44:1696–1699.

82. Nelson RL, Abcarian H, Prasad ML. Iatrogenic perforation of the colon and rectum. *Dis Colon Rectum* 1982;25:305.

83. Nivatvongs S, Fryd DS. How far does the proctosigmoidoscope reach? *N Engl J Med* 1980;303:380.

84. Nivatvongs S, Gilbertsen VA, Goldberg SM, et al. Distribution of large-bowel cancers detected by occult blood test in asymptomatic patients. *Dis Colon Rectum* 1982;25:420.

85. Oakland DJ. The diagnosis of carcinoma of the colon by exfoliative cytology. *Proc R Soc Med* 1964;57:279.

86. Otto S, Eckhardt S. Early detection for colorectal cancer: new aspects in fecal occult blood screening. *J Surg Oncol* 2000;75:2206.

87. Peel ALG, Benyon L, Grace RH. The value of routine preoperative urological assessment in patients undergoing elective surgery for diverticular disease or carcinoma of the large bowel. *Br J Surg* 1980;67:42.

88. Peterson N, Rohrmann CA Jr, Lennard ES. Diagnosis and treatment of retroperitoneal perforation complicating the double-contrast barium-enema examination. *Radiology* 1982;144:249.

89. Petrelli NJ, Palmer M, Michalek A, et al. Massive screening for colorectal cancer: a single institution's public commitment. *Arch Surg* 1990;125:1049.

90. Pickhardt PJ, Choi JH. Electronic cleansing and stool tagging in CT colonography: advantages and pitfalls with primary three-dimensional evaluation. *AJR Am J Roentgenol* 2003;181:799.

91. Pineau BC, Paskett ED, Chen GJ, et al. Virtual colonoscopy using oral contrast compared with colonoscopy for the detection of patients with colorectal polyps. *Gastroenterology* 2003;125:608.

92. Portes C, Majarakis JD. Proctosigmoidoscopy: incidence of polyps in 50,000 examinations. *JAMA* 1957;163:411.

93. Prager E, Swinton NW, Corman ML, et al. Intravenous pyelography in colorectal surgery. *Dis Colon Rectum* 1973;16:479.

94. Rabin DN, Smith C, Witt TR, et al. Voice change after barium enema: a clinical sign of extraperitoneal colon perforation. *AJR Am J Roentgenol* 1987;148:145.

95. Ransohoff DF, Lang CA. Screening for colorectal cancer. *N Engl J Med* 1991;325:37.

96. Raskin HF, Palmer WL, Kirsner JB. Exfoliative cytology in diagnosis of cancer of the colon. *Dis Colon Rectum* 1959;2:46.

97. Raskin HF, Pleticka S. Exfoliative cytology of the colon. *Cancer* 1971;28:127.

98. Reilly JM, Ballantyne GH, Fleming FX, et al. Evaluation of the occult blood test in screening for colorectal neoplasms: a prospective study using flexible endoscopy. *Am Surg* 1990;56:119.

99. Richardson NGB, Heriot AG, Kumar D, et al. Abdominal ultrasonography in the diagnosis of colonic cancer. *Br J Surg* 1998;85:530–3.

100. Rodriguez W, Levine JS. Enterococcal endocarditis following flexible sigmoidoscopy. *West J Med* 1984;140:951.

101. Rosen L. Physical examination of the anorectum: a systematic technique. *Dis Colon Rectum* 1990;33:439.

102. Rozen P, Knaani J, Samuel Z. Comparative screening with a sensitive guaiac and specific immunochemical occult blood test in an endoscopic study. *Cancer* 2000;89:46–52.

103. Saito H. Screening for colorectal cancer: current status in Japan. *Dis Colon Rectum* 2000;43[Suppl]:S78–S84.

104. Salazar M, Jackman RJ. Reasons for incomplete proctoscopy. *Dis Colon Rectum* 1969;12:19.

105. Sands J. Quoted by Masel H, Masel JP, Casey KV. A survey of colon examination techniques in Australia and New Zealand, with a review of complications. *Australas Radiol* 1971;15:140.

106. Scapa E, Jacob H, Lewkowicz S, et al. Initial experience of wireless-capsule endoscopy for evaluating occult gastrointestinal bleeding and suspected small bowel pathology. *Am J Gastroenterol* 2002;97: 2776.

107. Schnell T, Aranha G, Sontag SJ, et al. Fecal occult blood testing: a false sense of security? *Surgery* 1994;116:798.

108. Seaman WB, Wells J. Complications of the barium enema. *Gastroenterology* 1965;48:728.
109. Shulman ST, Amren DP, Bisno AL, et al. Prevention of bacterial endocarditis: a statement for health professionals by the Committee on Rheumatic Fever and Infective Endocarditis of the Council on Cardiovascular Disease in the Young. *Circulation* 1984;70:1123.
110. Simon JB. Occult blood screening for colorectal carcinoma: a critical review. *Gastroenterology* 1985;88:820.
111. Skucas J, Cutcliff W, Fischer HW. Whole-gut irrigation as a means of cleaning the colon. *Radiology* 1976;121:303.
112. Slavin JL, Melcher EA, Sundeen M, et al. Effects of high-fiber diet on fecal blood content (HemoQuant assay) in healthy subjects. *Dig Dis Sci* 1991;36:929.
113. Sohn N, Robilotti JA. The gay bowel syndrome. *Am J Gastroenterol* 1977;67:478.
114. Sontag SJ, Durczak C, Aranha GV, et al. Fecal occult blood screening for colorectal cancer in a Veterans Administration hospital. *Am J Surg* 1983;145:89.
115. Standards Task Force, American Society of Colon and Rectal Surgeons. Practice parameters for antibiotic prophylaxis to prevent infective endocarditis or infected prosthesis during colon and rectal endoscopy. *Dis Colon Rectum* 2000;43:1193–1200.
116. Stewart J, Finan PJ, Courtney DF, et al. Does a water-soluble contrast enema assist in the management of acute large-bowel obstruction? A prospective study of 117 cases. *Br J Surg* 1984;71:799.
117. Stoker J, Rociu E, Wiersma TG, et al. Imaging of anorectal disease. *Br J Surg* 2000;87:10–27.
118. Swinton NW. Polyps of rectum and colon. *JAMA* 1954; 154:658.
119. Tank ES, Ernst CB, Woolston ST, et al. Urinary tract complications of anorectal surgery. *Am J Surg* 1972;123:118.
120. Tate JJT, Northway J, Royle GT, et al. Faecal occult blood testing in symptomatic patients: comparison of three tests. *Br J Surg* 1990;77:523.
121. Teefey SA, Carlson *HC. The fluoroscopic barium enema in colonic polyp detection. AJR Am J Roentgenol* 1983;141: 1279.
122. Thomas WM, Hardcastle JD. Role of upper gastrointestinal investigations in a screening study for colorectal neoplasia. *Gut* 1990;31:1294.
123. Vining D, Gelfand D. Noninvasive colonoscopy using helical CT scanning, 3D reconstruction and virtual reality. Paper presented at the meeting of the Society of Gastrointestinal Radiologists, February 13–18, 1994, Maui, Hawaii.
124. Vining D, Gelfand D, Bechtold R. Technical feasibility of colon imaging with helical CT and virtual reality. *AJR Am J Roentgenol* 1994;162[Suppl]:104.
125. Welin S. Results of the Malmö technique of colon examination. *JAMA* 1967;199:119.
126. Welin S. Newer diagnostic techniques: the superiority of double-contrast roentgenology. *Dis Colon Rectum* 1974; 17:13.
127. Wheatley MJ, Eckhauser FE. Portal venous barium intravasation complicating barium enema examination. *Surgery* 1991;109:788.
128. Winawer S, Schottenfeld D, Sherlock P. Screening for colorectal cancer: the issues [Editorial]. *Gastroenterology* 1985;88:841.
129. Yamamura M, Nishi M, Furubayashi H, et al. Barium peritonitis: report of a case and review of the literature. *Dis Colon Rectum* 1985;28:347.
130. Yee J, Akerkar GA, Hung RK, et al. Colorectal neoplasia: performance characteristics of CT colonography for detection in 300 patients. *Radiology* 2001;219:685.
131. Yonekura Y, Benua RS, Brill AB, et al. Increased accumulation of 2-deoxy-2[^{18}F] fluoro-D-glucose in liver metastases from colon carcinoma. *J Nucl Med* 1982;23: 1133.
132. Yudis M, Cohen A, Pearce AE. Perforation of the transverse colon during barium enema and air-contrast studies. *Am Surg* 1968;34:334.

Flexible Sigmoidoscopy and Colonoscopy

One look is worth a thousand listens.

Aphorism

The ability to visualize the colon, rectum, and anus has essentially paralleled the precision with which the surgeon has been able to diagnose and treat individuals with diseases of this area of the digestive tract. In the midnineteenth century, visualization was accomplished by means of a hollow tube illuminated by a candle and focused with a parabolic mirror. However, examination of the entire colon had not been possible prior to the introduction of x-rays (see Chapter 4). Although improved radiologic techniques facilitated the accuracy of colonic diagnoses, distal bowel visualization was limited to that which could be accomplished with the rigid proctosigmoidoscope. Illumination was provided by a lightbulb within the instrument or directed to the tip by means of straight fibers (see Chapter 4).

The origin of flexible endoscopy of the colon began with the introduction of semirigid and then flexible upper gastrointestinal instruments (esophogogastroscopy). Hopkins and Kapany are generally credited with describing the initial flexible fiberscope, in 1954.[98] Subsequently, a major improvement in the quality of light transmission was made with the establishment of a glass-coated fiber that permitted the transmission of illumination along nonlinear paths. When combined with a similar fiber bundle whose orientation was preserved, the illuminated image could be transmitted back to the observer. Initially, the technology was applied to the stomach, but this was quickly adapted to the colon. Short, flexible fiberoptic instrument examinations of the rectum and distal colon were performed, but soon longer instruments were developed, usually with the use of gastroscopes applied to the bowel. It came to be appreciated, however, that successful colonic examination often required more forceful manipulation than was necessary for upper gastrointestinal endoscopy. Consequently, the later versions of the colonoscope that evolved were longer and more robust (see later).

A later advance in instrumentation has been the introduction of videoendoscopy. The image-transmitting fiberoptic bundle has been replaced by a charged coupled device that provides an electronic image of the field of view. The examiner no longer has to contend with broken fiber bundles and progressive degradation of the endoscopic picture. Furthermore, the endoscopist no longer needs to squint into the lens at the end of the instrument, but can instead work directly from a high-resolution monitor. In addition, the digitized image can be handled like any electronic file: stored, printed, and annotated. This has proved to be a clearly superior method of record keeping and documentation.

FLEXIBLE FIBEROPTIC SIGMOIDOSCOPY AND VIDEOENDOSCOPY

The term endoscope is derived from two Greek words: *endon*, meaning within, and *skopein*, to view. With the fiberoptic sigmoidoscope, the diameters of the individual glass fibers in the image-conveying aligned bundles are similar, ranging from 9 to 12 μm.[59] The individual fibers are bound together at their ends, while the rest of the fibers remain loose and flexible. The fiberoptic endoscope can be made as long as necessary because light loss is negligible over several meters.[59]

There is no doubt that flexible sigmoidoscopy (FS) inspects more bowel surface area than is possible with the rigid proctosigmoidoscope. Marks and associates reached 50 cm or more in approximately two thirds of their patients.[123] The overall yield of pathology was more than three times greater with the flexible instrument. Wherry and Thomas recruited more than 4,000 asymptomatic patients in a screening program utilizing FS.[194] Eleven carcinomas were detected, an overall rate of 3.2 per 1,000 subjects screened. Others also report considerable satisfaction in this regard,[17,25,69,152,197] but the length of bowel examined is often considerably less than it might appear.

For example, Lehman and colleagues determined the anatomic extent of insertion by placing a clip on the bowel mucosa and subsequently identifying that point on a barium enema study.[116] A so-called 60-cm examination viewed the entire sigmoid in only 81% of patients. It is also important to recognize that if an individual were to undergo subsequent barium enema study, regardless of the endoscopic findings, there would be no appreciable difference between rigid proctosigmoidoscopy and FS in the incidence of detection of neoplasms.[173] This presupposes, of course, that the barium enema examination is of optimal quality (see Chapter 4).

FS is not a simple examination to master. The most difficult part of colonoscopy is negotiation of the sigmoid colon, and this problem pertains equally to FS; the only difference perhaps is that the physician does not usually employ various straightening maneuvers, although this can be accomplished if necessary (see Colonoscopy). The examination requires skill and patience, and there is no substitute for experience. To paraphrase Hedberg, if only we could omit the first 100 endoscopies and begin with number 101, a more comprehensive examination would be obtained, and we would experience very few complications indeed (Hedberg SE, personal communication).

In addressing the assertion that the procedure is more comfortable than rigid proctosigmoidoscopy, this may be more a reflection of patient position than of the examination. As mentioned in Chapter 4, the lateral Sims' position is preferred for patient comfort, and this is the recommended approach for FS. The examination does, however, take longer; approximately one half of the procedures took more than 5 minutes in a series by Marks and associates, and my experience has been similar, especially with women.[123] It has been shown, in fact, that women who have undergone hysterectomy have more difficult, painful, and more limited examinations (4). Analgesia (i.e., conscious sedation) should perhaps be considered in this group of patients. With air insufflation, gas cramping tends to persist for a much longer period of time following FS. The list here illustrates some real and theoretical disadvantages to this examination:

Cost
  Capital expense and repairs
  Personnel time for enema administration, cleansing
  Duration
Communicable disease
Complications
  Perforation
  Hemorrhage with concomitant procedure
  Explosion with electrocautery
  Compromise of adequate colon examination when
    colonoscopy is indicated

The first and most often quoted criticism of the technique is the cost of the equipment, which may exceed $15,000, including light source and accessories. In addition to the outlay for the capital expense and repairs, there are the costs of personnel (e.g., longer time for examination, need for cleansing the instrument, patient preparation). Of course, a critical consideration is the cost to the patient. In polling numerous medical centers and physicians, the fee for the examination ranged from a minimum of 25% more than for rigid proctosigmoidoscopy to as much as 200% more.

It is essential to know whether the patient has a communicable disease when a reusable instrument, such as a fiberoptic or videoendoscope, is to be employed. The physician therefore must be circumspect in the performance of routine screening tests or pay special attention to sterilization when he or she examines an individual who has had a history of hepatitis, anal condylomata, and other infectious or communicable conditions (see Sterilization of Equipment).[25] It is to address this concern that a sheath (Vision Sciences, Inc., 6 Strathmore Rd., Natick, MA 01760; 800–874–9975) system has been developed to provide a barrier for patient and staff protection (Figure 5-1). The concept has several practical advantages:

- It reduces instrument inventory.
- It reduces instrument repairs.
- It eliminates the requirement for instrument washers.
- It reduces personnel time.
- It provides a sterile covering for each procedure.

Sardinha and coworkers demonstrated an almost tenfold difference in the time saved by using the sheathed FS system when compared with the conventional flexible in-

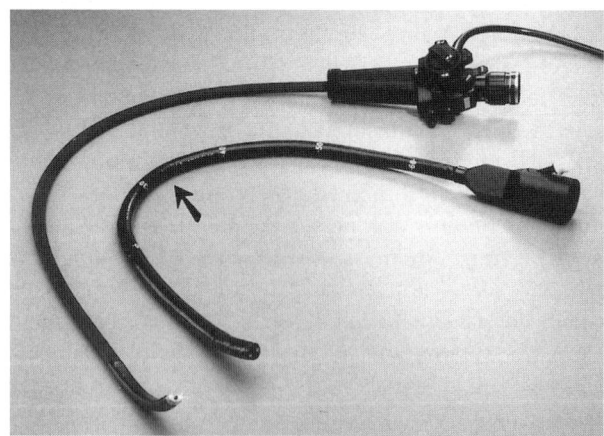

FIGURE 5-1. The Vision System instrument is composed of a disposable sterile EndoSheath that fits over the endoscope, containing all of the hard-to-clean air/water and biopsy/suction channels, so that when the sheath is discarded at the end of the procedure, all body fluids are disposed of along with it. (Courtesy of Vision Sciences, Inc., Natick, MA.)

strument.[160] This was accomplished through reduced endoscope turnover time, as well as reduction or elimination of the need for washers and backup instruments. The concept certainly allows for optimal use of the nursing staff.

FS is an advance over rigid proctosigmoidoscopy as a screening tool, but it is not a substitute for colonic assessment. When a complete evaluation of the colon is indicated, such as when occult blood is present or when polyps have been documented, colonoscopy is the requisite procedure. There is, however, a place for rigid sigmoidoscopy. This technique is often preferred when large a biopsy is required, when a distal anastomosis needs to be visualized, when a culture needs to be obtained, or when inflammatory disease is confined to the rectum.

FS is indicated in the following situations:

■ As a substitute for rigid proctosigmoidoscopy in screening, in evaluation of gastrointestinal complaints, and in interim polyp and cancer surveillance between colonoscopic examinations for distal disease
■ For evaluation of questionable radiologic findings in the sigmoid colon
■ For confirmation of radiographic findings within range of the instrument
■ For diagnostic and follow-up evaluation of a patient with inflammatory bowel disease, especially if the disease is confined to the left or distal colon
■ For inspection of colon anastomosis when it is within range of the instrument

Therapeutically, FS may be employed to reduce sigmoid volvulus and in combination with the snare to remove a foreign body. Absolute contraindications to this examination include fulminant colitis, toxic megacolon, peritonitis, and acute diverticulitis. A poorly prepared bowel and an uncooperative patient are certainly limiting factors.

Instrumentation

The flexible fiberoptic sigmoidoscope is available in the United States through several companies [Olympus America (Melville, NY), Pentax (Orangeburg, NY), Fujinon (Wayne, NJ), and Vision Sciences (Natick, MA)]. The specifications of the instruments vary somewhat among the manufacturers. Generally, the channel size ranges between 2.6 and 3.8 mm, the instrument diameter varies from 12.2 to 14.0 mm, and lengths range from 60 to 71 cm. Figure 5-2 illustrates a flexible fiberoptic sigmoidoscope, and a close-up view of the bending section is shown in Figure 5-3. Biopsy forceps, a cytology brush, or a snare and electrocautery may be passed through the

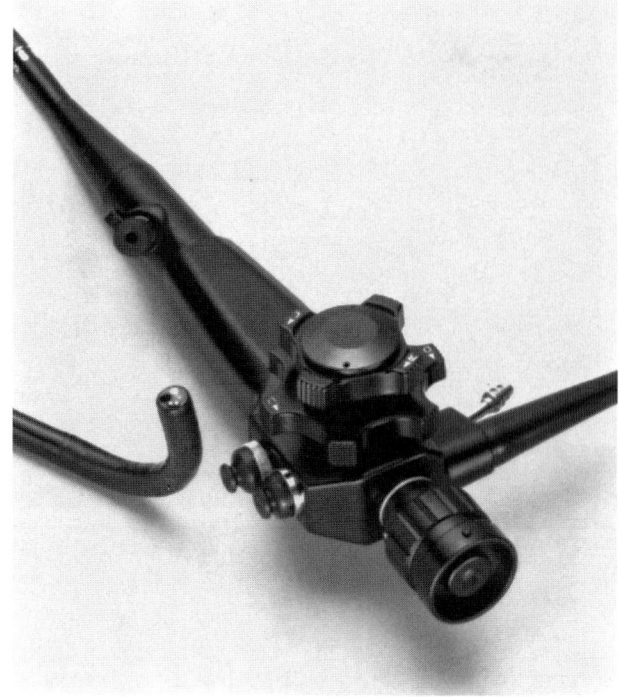

FIGURE 5-2. Pentax slim model (11.5-mm diameter) fiberoptic sigmoidoscope (model FS-34P2) with 70-cm working length. (Courtesy of Pentax Precision Instrument Corp., Orangeburg, NY.)

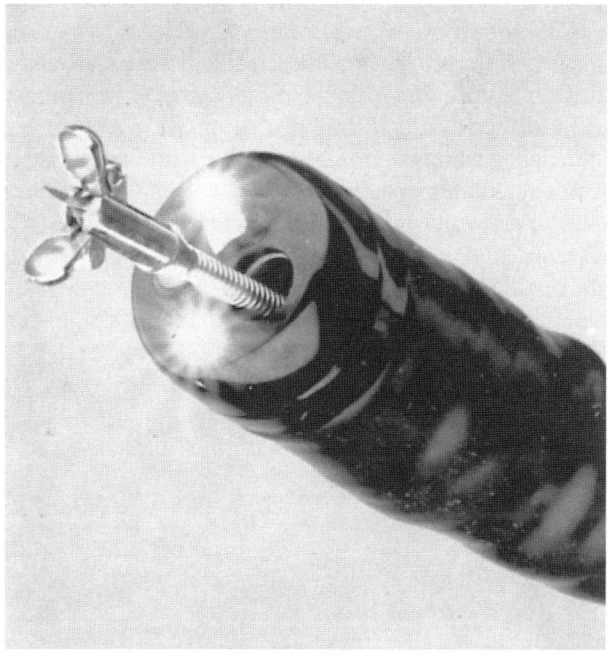

FIGURE 5-3. Close-up of the bending section with biopsy forceps of a fiberoptic sigmoidoscope (model CF-P20S). Channel size is 3.2 mm; diameter is 12.20 mm. (Courtesy of Olympus America, Melville, NY.)

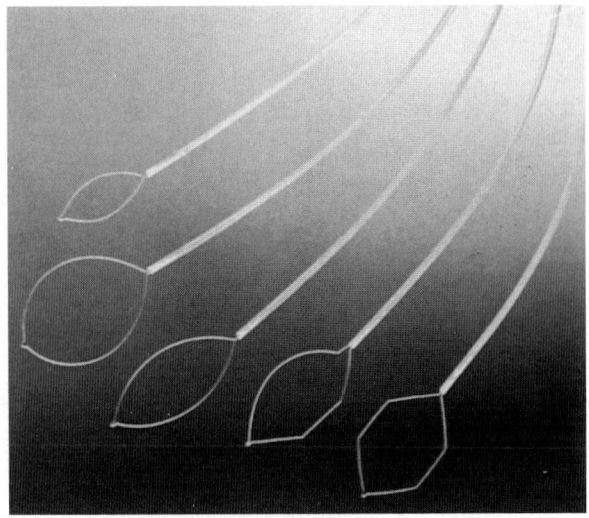

FIGURE 5-4. Variety of Captivator snares. (Courtesy of Microvasive, Boston Scientific Corp., Watertown, MA.)

working channel (Figure 5-4). The tip of the instrument is deflected by rotation of the larger dial in each direction (Figure 5-5). The smaller dial deflects the tip from side to side. If both dials are turned maximally, it produces a tight bend that causes the instrument to double back and impede further passage. When passing the instrument, it is advantageous to keep the dials in the neutral position as much as possible (see Colonoscopy).

The 35-cm flexible instrument should be mentioned, especially regarding the relative merits of this shorter diagnostic endoscope. As a tool for screening, there seems to be little difference between the two fiberoptic instruments with respect to identification of neoplasms.[57,86] Furthermore, patients report that examination with the shorter instrument is, not surprisingly, more comfortable. I see, however, no great advantage in limiting the area of colon to be screened, and, in fact, with increased experience of the examiner, the length of time to perform the procedure should not be significantly different. The 35-cm flexible sigmoido-

scope will in all probability be employed almost exclusively by the nonsurgeon and nonspecialist endoscopist.

Preparation

The use of FS requires only a limited bowel preparation. Two small enemas (e.g., Fleet) are given separately, the second approximately 10 minutes after the first has been eliminated. Dietary restrictions and oral laxatives are unnecessary.

Technique

The patient is placed in the left lateral (Sims' position) on a relatively high examining table. The patient's right leg is flexed more than the left, and the right shoulder is rotated anteriorly. It is usually easier for the physician to stand than to sit. Some physicians prefer a two-person team approach, one to handle the dials and the other to advance the instrument. Members of this school believe that in this way the procedure can be carried out much more expeditiously. This approach requires the use of a fiberoptic teaching attachment or videoendoscope (Figure 5-6). Conversely, most individuals believe that a single person can maneuver the dials with one hand and guide the instrument with the other, thereby permitting a more facile straightening maneuver. As a consequence, this may offer a more comfortable experience for the patient. The concept of discomfort has been addressed in a paper by Palakanis and colleagues on the effect of music therapy with individuals undergoing FS.[148] Not surprisingly, the authors discovered that those who listened to self-selected music tapes during the procedure had significantly decreased anxiety inventory measurements (State-Trait Anxiety Inventory). Furthermore, they had statistically significantly reduced heart rates and decreased arterial blood pressures in comparison with control subjects. The authors concluded that music is a very effective anxiolytic for the patient who undergoes FS.[148]

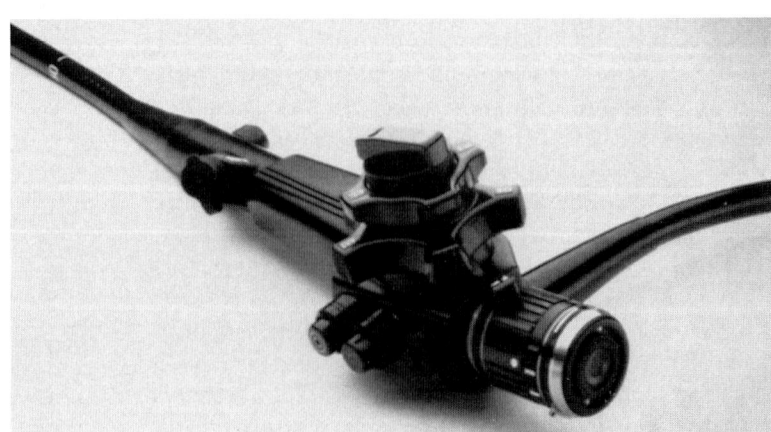

FIGURE 5-5. The control unit of the CF-P20S model fiberoptic sigmoidoscope has a maximum tip deflection of 180 degrees vertically, 160 degrees horizontally. (Courtesy of Olympus America, Melville, NY.)

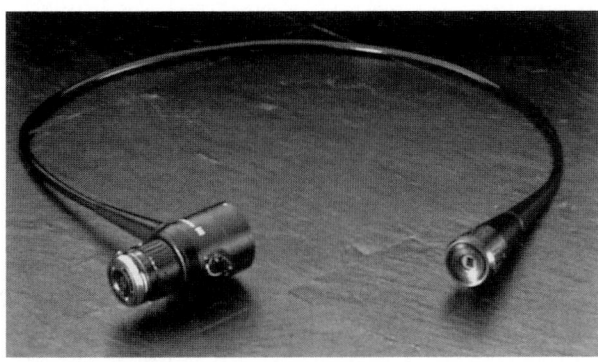

FIGURE 5-6. Fiberoptic teaching attachment, model LS-10. (Courtesy of Olympus America, Melville, NY.)

A well-lubricated finger is passed into the rectum, and then the instrument is inserted. Passing the blunt-ended endoscope through the anal canal without prior digital examination is difficult to accomplish and leads to considerable apprehension and discomfort for the patient.

What is usually encountered initially is a dull pink or orange haze, perhaps with some fecal debris or retained enema fluid. While insufflating air rather than redirecting the tip, the examiner passes the instrument to a depth of 10 or 12 cm. This will permit visualization of the rectal ampulla. If a two-team approach is used, the person who advances the instrument has greater control of the course of the examination than the individual handling the dials. In training an assistant or a resident to do FS, I prefer to insert the instrument until the assistant has become competent with the proximal end before reversing roles. In any surgical procedure, the assistant can either impede or expedite the operation, making the surgeon appear incompetent or highly experienced. In the former circumstance, the assistant has often been referred to as "the enemy." Alternatively, the skilled surgeon acting as a first assistant can orchestrate the procedure so effectively that the trainee can scarcely believe how talented he or she has become.

The instrument is passed with the lumen seen either under direct visualization or with the mucosa seen sliding past. Again, the person on the distal end can judge how firmly to push while watching the mucosa rush by. This approach is quite similar to that applicable to rigid proctosigmoidoscopy, but this maneuver is not preferable to luminal visualization and must be undertaken with great caution.

If further passage is impeded, the instrument is withdrawn slightly, the lumen is searched out by dial manipulation and rotation, and the instrument is advanced again. Coller has described in detail various methods helpful in advancing the instrument. He calls them torquing, dithering, and dither-torquing (i.e., accordionization; see later.[38]

By using the approach of dithering—the principle by which a person sitting on a chair with feet raised can move it across the floor through abrupt, jerking motions of the body—staccato movements of the instrument forward and backward may permit the bowel virtually to intubate itself onto the instrument.[38]

Negotiation of the sigmoid colon is the most difficult part of the procedure. With an intended limited examination, straightening the sigmoid is, perhaps, of less importance than it is with colonoscopy. If all the physician accomplishes, however, is to stretch the colon through attempts at advancement, another maneuver must be tried. Counterclockwise rotation of the instrument produces the alpha loop (Figure 5-7). Clockwise rotation results in relative straightening of the sigmoid and the opportunity to advance the instrument into the descending colon. Sedation may be required to accomplish this, but this is usually not available for office examination. Another means of proceeding into the descending colon when the sigmoid loop has already been traversed is to withdraw the instrument while rotating it clockwise.

After the instrument has been passed to its full length or as far as is possible, it is carefully and slowly withdrawn. Suction, irrigation, and air insufflation are alternately employed as indicated to obtain clear visualization of the entire mucosa. Biopsy without electrocoagulation or brush cytology is obtained if appropriate, and the instrument is removed. It is important to remember that FS and colonoscopy are suboptimal tools for evaluation of ampullary or distal rectal disorders. Particular care is required for examination of this area, and retroflexion is strongly recommended as the ultimate maneuver (Figure 5-8).

Rectal Retroflexion

The importance of rectal retroflexion (RR) has been emphasized by Hanson and colleagues.[90] They compared 480 patients who had undergone FS without RR with a subsequent examination wherein RR was employed routinely. Discomfort precluded completion of this maneuver in 3.5%. There was a 1% increased yield of identifiable adenomas when RR was performed.[90]

The technique for accomplishing RR has been well described[90]:

- Advance the shaft approximately 10 cm above the mucocutaneous junction.
- Maximally deflect the shaft upward.
- Advance the instrument an additional 5 to 10 cm against the rectal fold.
- Rotate the retroflexed shaft to view the circumference of the anorectal junction.

Finally, the physician must not forget why the examination was being performed in the first instance. If bleed-

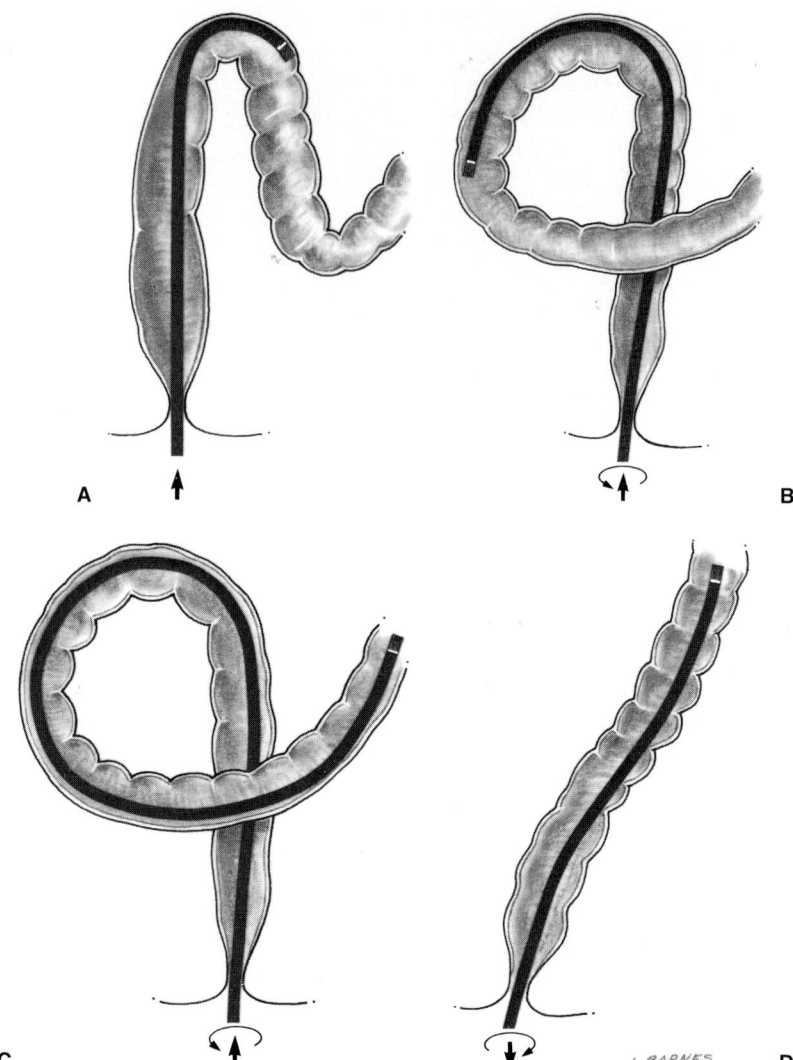

FIGURE 5-7. Alpha loop maneuver. **(A)** The instrument is advanced into the sigmoid colon. **(B)** Counter-clockwise rotation during advancement results in the loop. **(C)** The sigmoidoscope enters the descending colon. **(D)** Clockwise torque during withdrawal permits straightening of the sigmoid colon.

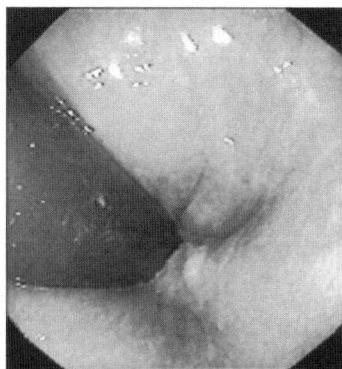

FIGURE 5-8. Retroflexion of the flexible sigmoidoscope. (See Color Fig. 5-8.)

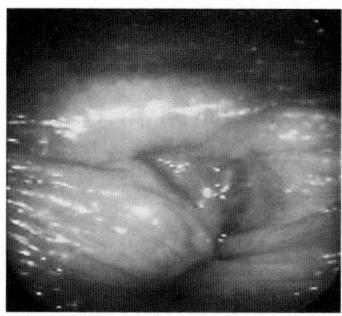

FIGURE 5-9. Anal fissure can be seen with the flexible sigmoidoscope. However, this is not the optimal way for making the diagnosis. (See Color Fig. 5-9.)

ing was the indication, it is not sufficient to reassure the patient that FS was normal. Furthermore, the flexible sigmoidoscope is not the optimal tool for diagnosing pruritus ani, hemorrhoids, or fissure and obviously is not the ideal instrument for evaluating the anal canal (Figure 5-9). Anoscopy and additional studies may be required. Gastroenterologists, however, because they do not generally perform anoscopy, seem quite comfortable with using FS and colonoscopy with RR as a diagnostic instrument for anal disorders. Although this is the standard of care for this specialty, I am convinced that anal lesions can be missed or misinterpreted if anoscopy is not performed when an anal problem is suspected.

Videoendoscopy

In 1983, the WelchAllyn Corporation (Skaneateles Falls, NY) introduced a special feature for viewing the gastrointestinal tract, the videoendoscope. The endoscopic images are transmitted by a small electronic chip known as a charged coupled device.[162] Other companies have since entered the field, each producing video screen imagery with the ability to videotape examinations, to produce remote hard copy, and, of course, to serve as an excellent teaching modality (Figure 5-10). Information can be displayed on the monitor (i.e., patient's name, physician's name, pertinent history) to create a useful database for retrieval purposes.[168] Figure 5-11 shows the basic equipment. With the cost in excess of $25,000, this method is employed primarily in teaching centers and in endoscopy units, especially wherein there are numbers of patients sufficient to justify a considerable capital investment. An attachment for converting the fiberoptic output to a video screen is also available (Figure 5-12). There principles of

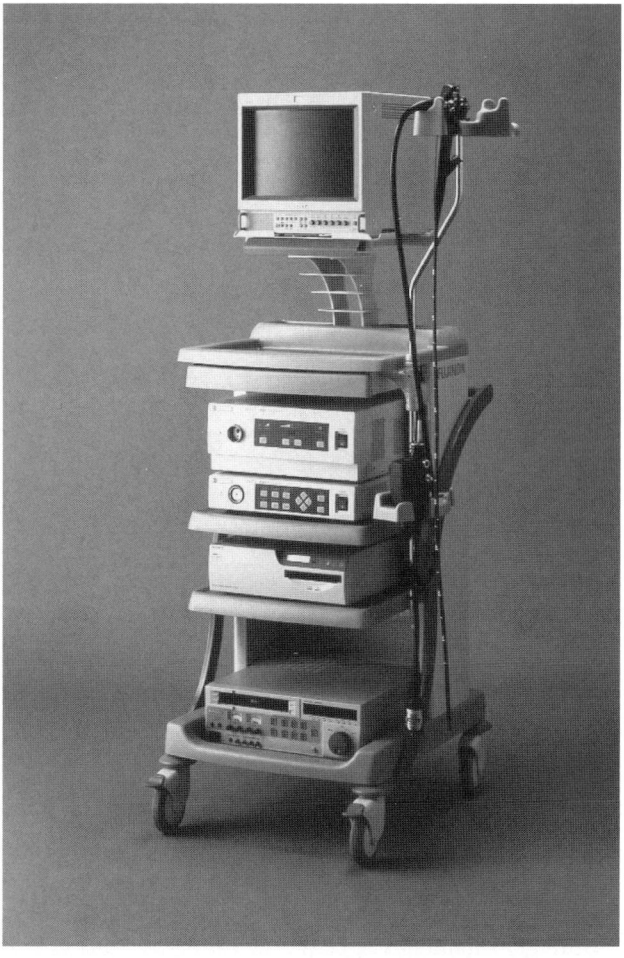

FIGURE 5-11. Videoendoscope system with colonoscope, light source, processor, and monitor. Remote switching gives the endoscopist the power to freeze images and to activate a number of hard copy devices. (Courtesy of Olympus America, Melville, NY.)

passage are identical to those of FS with the fiberoptic instrument.

Complications of Flexible Sigmoidoscopy

Complications such as hemorrhage or perforation should not occur with any greater frequency with a flexible instrument than with the rigid, especially if the examiner does not force its passage—at least there are no randomized, clinical trials that demonstrate a difference. However, if an alpha or a straightening maneuver is undertaken, it is possible for the sigmoid colon to be torn and a perforation to occur. Attention to limiting patient discomfort is therefore an important concern. Furthermore, caution is obviously required whenever the procedure is undertaken in the presence of bowel disease. Depending on the acuteness of the process, especially with active in-

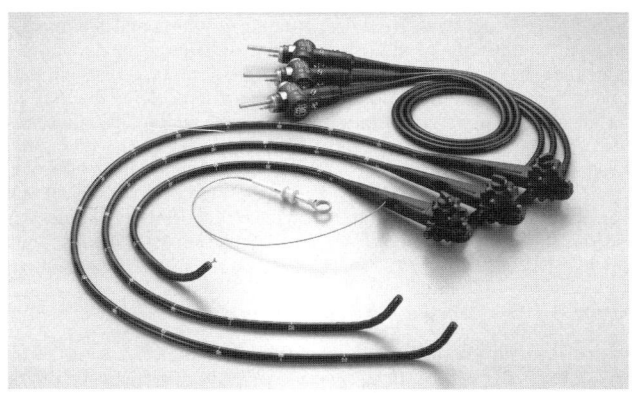

FIGURE 5-10. Videosigmoidoscope [73 cm (Model CF-Q160S)] and videocolonoscopes [in two lengths: 133 cm (Model CF-Q1601) and 168 cm (Model CF-Q160L)]. (Courtesy of Olympus America, Melville, NY.)

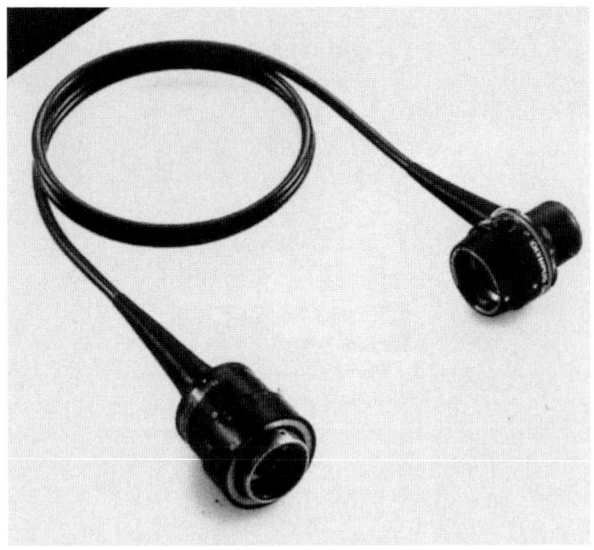

FIGURE 5-12. A direct video converter will convert standard endoscopic images for video-monitor viewing. (Courtesy of Olympus America, Melville, NY.)

flammation, diverticulitis, or ischemia, FS may be contraindicated. Minimal air should be used when inflammation is present. Care should also be observed, especially with respect to insufflation of air, when an individual has a known inguinal hernia. Incarceration and obstruction of a herniated sigmoid colon from overdistension has been reported.[195] Explosions should not occur, because electrocautery should not be employed for biopsy or snare excision with this instrument unless a full bowel preparation has been used. The limited bowel preparation that is

usually employed, combined with a closed system, presents a potential hazard for the presence of an explosive gas mixture. Biopsies should be carried out only with "cold" forceps. Brush cytology may, of course, be safely employed.

COLONOSCOPY

In 1969, fiberoptic colonoscopy was introduced as a means of directly visualizing the colon and rectum, and, in many instances, even the terminal ileum. Within a few years, Wolff and Shinya demonstrated that by using a wire loop snare and electrocautery, polyps could be removed through the instrument, thus virtually rendering colotomy and polypectomy obsolete.[198]

Instrumentation

As mentioned earlier, there are numerous suppliers of colonoscopes in the United States, most of which use similar optical or video structures. The instruments vary mainly in length, total diameter, and maneuverability and have a number of accessories. Working lengths vary from approximately 115 cm to almost 180 cm. They are forward viewing and may offer a field of view up to 140 degrees (Figure 5-13). Some individuals prefer a two-channel system in order to use two accessories for treatment, including that of polypectomy (Figure 5-14). As with FS, four-way angulation of the distal end is achieved from approximately 180 degrees up or down and 160 degrees right and left by manipulating the control knobs (Figure 5-5). Additional features include an air outlet, a forward water jet channel, and

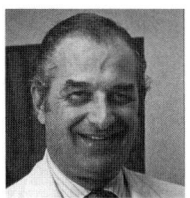

William I. Wolff (1916–Present) William Wolff was born in New York City and attended the University of Maryland School of Medicine, where he received the Prize Gold Medal. He then entered the Cornell and Columbia residency program at Bellevue Hospital in New York, with his training interrupted by World War II. While serving in a field hospital in Belgium after the Normandy invasion, he barely escaped capture during the Battle of the Bulge. After the war, he completed his residency at the Bronx Veterans Hospital in New York. As an attending surgeon at Cornell Division at Bellevue, he developed a research facility and an open heart surgery program. In 1962, he became the first full-time Director of Surgery at the Beth Israel Medical Center in New York and Professor of Surgery at the then new Mount Sinai School of Medicine. In the mid-1960s, he and his young associate, Hiromi Shinya, established an upper gastrointestinal fiberoptic endoscopic laboratory and clinical facility. Their work led to the development of the first flexible instruments for evaluating the entire colon. After a successful study, the era of colonoscopy and colonoscopic polypectomy was born. Their efforts resulted in what Francis Moore described as a "quantum advance in surgery." Their article was, in fact, selected by members of the American Society of Colon and Rectal Surgeons as among the top 11 literature contributions to twentieth century colon and rectal surgery (42). A founding member of the Society of American Gastrointestinal Endoscopic Surgeons, Wolff received the highest award given to an alumnus of his alma mater, the University of Maryland, for "outstanding contributions to medicine and distinguished service to mankind."

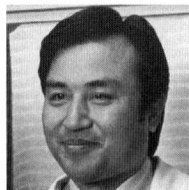

Hiromi Shinya (1935–Present) Hiromi Shinya was born in Yanagawa, Fukuoka prefecture, Japan, and completed his medical studies in 1960 at Tokyo's Jutendo University. After his internship at the United States Naval Hospital in Yokosuka, he arrived in New York City to begin his general surgical residency at the Beth Israel Medical Center. In 1967, while still in his residency, he became interested in the newly evolving instrumentation for upper gastrointestinal endoscopy. As a consequence of this experience, he moved on to develop the technique for examination of the colon, devising many of the accessories, such as the snare-cautery. In 1969, with the support and encouragement of his chief, William Wolff, he began a series of successful polypectomy procedures. Because of his unique experience and abilities, he received a special visa waiver by order of the President of the United States to remain in the country and to continue his work. His colonoscopy experience to date exceeds 250,000 patients.

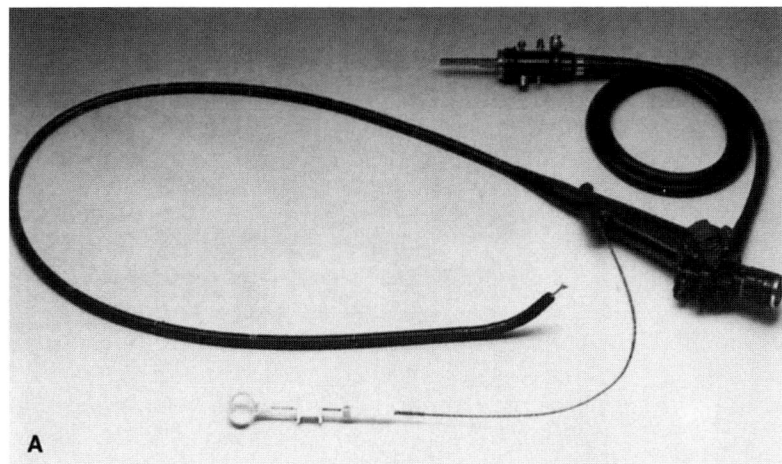

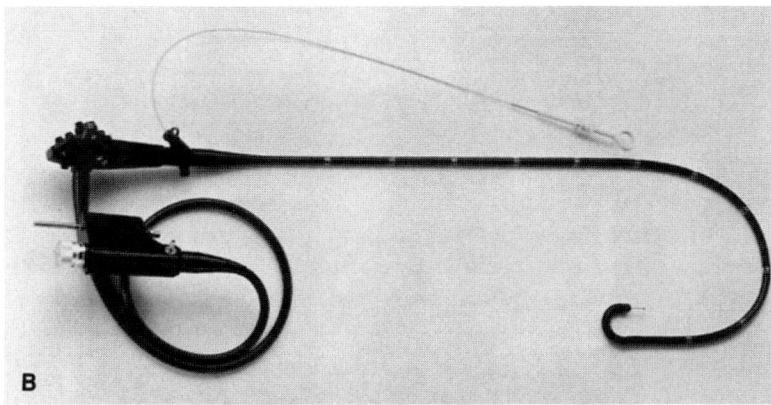

FIGURE 5-13. Colonoscopes. **(A)** The fiberoptic colonoscope, model PCF-10 with biopsy instrument, is a 133-cm instrument. (Courtesy of Olympus America, Melville, NY.) **(B)** Slim video colonoscope, model EC-3400. (Courtesy of Pentax Precision Instrument Corp., Orangeburg, NY.)

a suction/forceps channel. Air or carbon dioxide can be insufflated and liquid debris removed during the procedure. Accessories include a halogen light source (Figure 5-15) and an electrosurgical unit (Figure 5-16), as well as photographic equipment. Requisite items for procedures include biopsy forceps, a diathermy snare, and grasping forceps, in addition to an instrument for brush cytology.

Cost is also a major concern when contemplating the purchase of a colonoscope. The cost of a video colonoscope approximates $13,000. With all the accessories, the comprehensive unit could cost three times that amount. Repairs and the limited life expectancy of the instruments also must be considered in assessing the expense. However, there is universal agreement that, with the plethora of colon disorders in Western countries, especially neoplasms, colonoscopy and colonoscopy-polypectomy are among the most important advances for diagnosis and treatment to become available since the late 1960s.

Indications

It is generally agreed that colonoscopy supplements but does not necessarily replace the barium enema in the evaluation of colon disorders. (1) The list here summarizes the indications for this procedure:

Confirmation or refutation of suspected or equivocal radiologic abnormality [e.g., filling defects, narrowing (intrinsic versus extrinsic lesion), polyps]

Evaluation and follow-up of inflammatory bowel disease (e.g., dysplasia)

Differential diagnosis of diverticular disease and malignancy

Presence of a rectal polyp with or without barium enema abnormality (e.g., synchronous lesions)

Gastrointestinal symptoms (e.g., bleeding, abdominal pain, iron-deficiency anemia) with or without radiologic investigation failing to reveal the source

Follow-up evaluation of patient with prior colon surgery

Cancer screening

Acute lower gastrointestinal bleeding

Clinically significant diarrhea of unexplained origin

Endoscopic polypectomy

Reduction of sigmoid volvulus

Decompression of dilated colon (e.g., Ogilvie's syndrome)

Intraoperative colonoscopy; confirmation of location of lesion at time of laparotomy or during laparoscopic procedures

Colonoscopic percutaneous colostomy

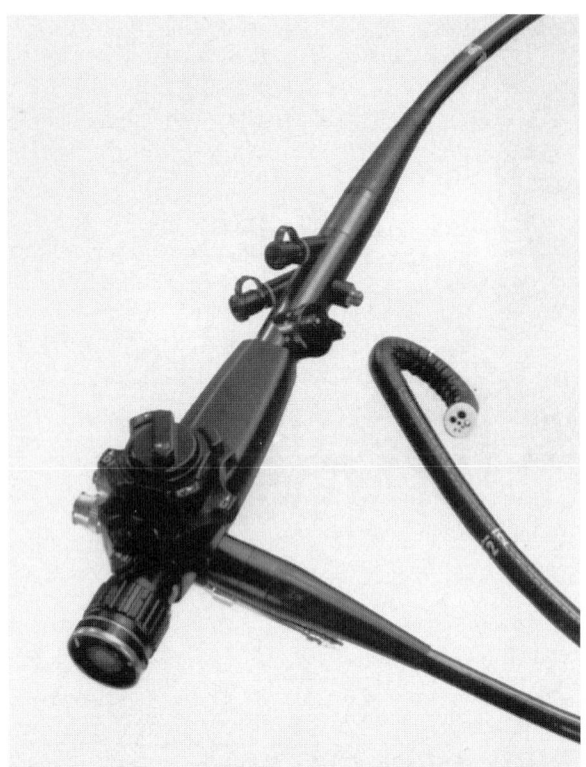

FIGURE 5-14. Two-channel therapeutic colonofiberscope (model FC-38TLH) features water jet. (Courtesy of Pentax Precision Instrument Corp., Orangeburg, NY.)

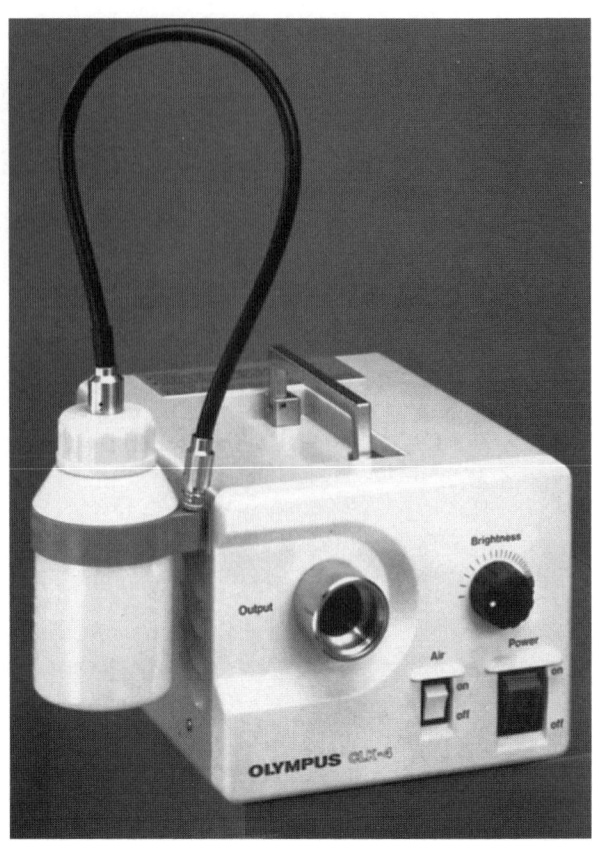

FIGURE 5-15. This simplified 150-watt halogen light source includes an air pump and water container with pipe. (Courtesy of Olympus America, Melville, NY.)

In some instances, the procedure is employed either because the barium enema study or virtual colonoscopy demonstrates a possible abnormality or because other investigations fail to indicate or identify the source when symptoms suggest colonic disease.[40] In two reports analyzing the results of unexplained rectal bleeding, 30% of the patients were found to have significant lesions in spite of a normal barium enema examination.[19,181] Needless to state, however, that colonoscopic procedures are usually carried out without the patient having undergone a prior contrast study.

Colonoscopy has been demonstrated to be of diagnostic usefulness in a host of clinical situations (e.g., screening for colorectal cancer, diverticular disease, inflammatory bowel disease, ischemic colitis, pseudomembranous colitis, and unexplained rectal bleeding, to name only a few; see endoscopic photographs that appear throughout this text).[16,19,20,49,52,68,71,77,88,97,113,119,128,135, 169,177,180,181,187] Other conditions for which diagnosis has been confirmed or expedited by colonoscopy include amebic colitis, intestinal tuberculosis, pneumatosis cystoides intestinalis, radiation colitis, and, by exclusion, irritable bowel syndrome.[40,51,174]

Diagnostic colonoscopy is generally not appropriate for chronic, stable, irritable bowel complaints, in acute

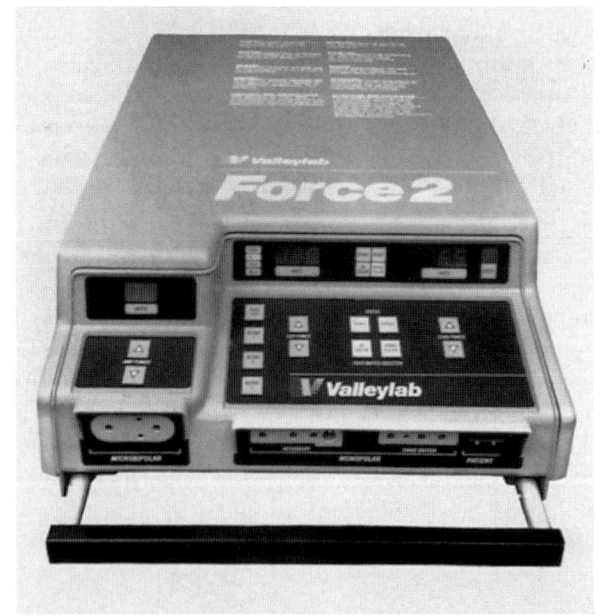

FIGURE 5-16. Electrosurgery generator. This unit has simultaneous independent coagulation ability, microbipolar mode, and handswitching and footswitching controls. (Courtesy of Tyco Valleylab, Inc., Boulder, CO.)

limited diarrhea, when bleeding is readily observed to come from an obvious source (e.g., fissure, hemorrhoids, peptic ulcer), when patient management would be unaffected by the findings (e.g., metastatic carcinoma in the absence of bowel symptoms), and routine screening in someone who is not at an increased risk for malignancy.

Contraindications and Concerns

Absolute contraindications to this examination are essentially limited to those patients with an acute cardiovascular problem (e.g., unstable angina, myocardial infarction) and those with an acute abdominal inflammation (e.g., peritonitis), acute diverticulitis, fulminant colitis, bowel perforation, and toxic megacolon. Relative contraindications include the last two trimesters of pregnancy, pregnancy at any stage if fluoroscopy is to be employed, marked splenomegaly, and an abdominal aortic aneurysm.[39]

Aspirin

Traditional teaching is to withhold aspirin 7 days prior to colonoscopy because of the concern for bleeding. Ker and colleagues challenged this concept by prospectively randomizing 205 patients to receive 650 mg of aspirin for 10 days prior to colonoscopy with biopsy or polypectomy or not to receive the drug.[110] The bleeding time was marginally prolonged in the former group, the platelet count was not affected, and there was no increased incidence of bleeding. The authors concluded that aspirin can be safely continued in preparation for colonoscopy.[110]

Anticoagulation

Patients who may be anemic or at a risk for bleeding because of a possible blood dyscrasia should undergo coagulation studies prior to colonoscopy. Those receiving the anticoagulant sodium warfarin (Coumadin) should ideally have the medication discontinued prior to the procedure.[39] Caliendo and coworkers performed a retrospective review of their patients with respect to anticoagulation.[23] They observed that colonoscopy without polypectomy may be performed safely without discontinuing therapy. However, resuming antiplatelet treatment immediately after colonoscopy-polypectomy was associated with a high risk of bleeding. There were no thromboembolic complications. Timothy and colleagues, also in a retrospective review involving 94 patients (109 examinations) on warfarin, noted that colonoscopy could be performed safely, but that there was a slightly increased incidence of hemorrhagic complications with biopsy or snare excision.[183] Their recommended approach to the patient on warfarin who can tolerate a "period" of "normal" coagulation is as follows[183]:

- Stop warfarin for 3 days.
- Obtain the prothrombin time/INR (international normalized ratio) prior to the procedure.
- If the INR is less than 2, proceed with colonoscopy and restart warfarin (using prior dosage) on the first postoperative day.
- If the INR is 2 or greater, postpone the procedure for 1 to 2 days or, alternatively, perform the diagnostic procedure and postpone restarting warfarin for 2 to 3 days if a therapeutic procedure is contemplated.
- If a diagnostic procedure is performed, restart warfarin at the prior dose on postprocedure day 1.

Privileging and Credentialing

Wexner, Eisen, and Simmang, in 2002, prepared a consensus document concerning endoscopic privileging and credentialing that has been endorsed by the Society of American Gastrointestinal Endoscopic Surgeons, the American Society for Gastrointestinal Endoscopy, and the American Society of Colon and Rectal Surgeons.[193] They emphasized that the credentialing structure and process are the responsibility of the health care facility, and that uniform standards should be developed for performing specific endoscopic procedures regardless of the specialty in which an individual physician practices. Training may be accomplished through a formal surgery or gastroenterology residency program or through an equivalent "certification of experience by a skilled endoscopic practitioner." Determination of competence requires the following:

- Completion of a residency program with structured, documented experience in gastrointestinal endoscopy, or
- Demonstrated proficiency in technique and clinical judgment equivalent to that which is obtained in a residency program, and
- Confirmation in writing from the endoscopic director as to the applicant's training, experience, and observed level of competency

The consensus document also incorporates statements on training in new techniques, proctoring of applicants for privileges, criteria for competency, monitoring of performance, requirement for continuing medical education, and the renewal of privileges.[193]

Preparation of the Patient

As with barium enema examination, the importance of an adequately cleansed colon cannot be overemphasized.[178] There are two reasons for requiring a clean colon before proceeding with colonscopic examination: safety and accuracy. The danger of causing injury when trying to intubate a feces-laden bowel is appreciable. The presence of formed stool may obscure the lumen and lead the endoscopist to apply forces in dangerous ways. Even a minor amount of stool can lead to confusion and misinterpretation. For example, a piece of stool that is firmly adherent to the lens may require removal of the instrument blindly and the necessity of starting all over again. When residual fecal matter is encountered, it is important to irrigate it free before passing on to other areas.

For most ambulatory patients, a vigorous cathartic followed by colonic irrigation or a small-volume enema (i.e., Fleet) along with appropriate dietary restriction is generally satisfactory and can be commenced in the morning for an afternoon examination or in the evening prior to a morning endoscopy. However, sedentary or frail individuals may require several days to prepare the bowel adequately, especially if a less vigorous cleansing regimen is adopted. Care must be taken to maintain adequate fluid intake and to avoid electrolyte abnormalities, because fluid loss may cause patients to lose as much as 7 pounds (3.2 kg).[22,194] This is of particular concern in individuals with cardiovascular or renal disease. Those taking diuretic medications should undergo serum electrolyte determination prior to initiating cathartics, and supplementary potassium may be administered during the course of the preparation if necessary. A synthetic amino acid diet may facilitate bowel cleansing, and if hydration is maintained, the osmotic catharsis will help in removing the fecal matter; however, it tends to be rather unpalatable and is quite expensive.[40]

In patients with ulcerative colitis, there is concern about exacerbating the condition when total colonoscopy is performed for dysplasia screening (see Chapter 29). Gould and Williams found that both castor oil (30 mL) and senna tablets (Senokot 75-mg sennosides) followed by two tap-water enemas produced equally satisfactory preparations in a prospective trial.[84] Neither group of patients developed a serious exacerbation of colitis. As previously mentioned, fulminant ulcerative colitis and toxic megacolon are contraindications to this procedure.

The nonabsorbed oligosaccharide, mannitol, has been advocated for colon preparation prior to barium enema examination and to colonoscopy.[109] In a study by Newstead and Morgan, during the afternoon of the day prior to the examination, patients consumed 500 mL of a 10% or 20% solution; the mean number of bowel actions was seven.[139] When using mannitol, additional oral fluid intake should be encouraged. Again, care must be taken when using this technique in the elderly or the infirm. However, reports of fatal explosions after mannitol administration and colonoscopy-polypectomy have dampened most physicians' ardor for this preparation.[15,140] Hydrogen and methane produced by bacterial degradation of the mannitol have been suggested as causative factors.

The preparation developed by Crapp and associates (whole-gut irrigation) has been recommended as an effective, well-tolerated alternative to standard oral cathartics and enemas for colonoscopy and barium enema examination.[46] Minervini and associates compared three methods of whole bowel irrigation: nasogastric saline solution alone, the solution with oral mannitol, and oral mannitol alone.[134] The best preparation was the combined approach, but patients and nursing staff preferred the oral mannitol alone.

Davis and colleagues devised an electrolyte solution containing primarily sodium sulfate with polyethylene glycol (PEG) as an additional osmotic agent (i.e., Golytely).[48] Studies have been published that verify the safety and efficacy of this lavage method in preparation for colonoscopy and for barium enema examination, especially if bisacodyl (Dulcolax) is added to ensure evacuation of residual fluid.[54,60,80,81] It has become, at least for endoscopists, if not for patients, the most popular preparation in the United States for colonoscopy.

The preparation can be administered orally or by tube feedings. A dose of 4 L is usually sufficient to produce adequate cleansing. If the patient drinks the solution at a rate of 230 mL (8 oz) every 10 minutes, ingestion of the entire 4-L dose will evacuate the gastrointestinal tract in approximately 3.5 hours. The most frequent complaint about this method of cleansing the bowel and the primary drawback are the discomfort and distaste associated with consumption of such a large quantity of fluid. "The preparation was worse than the procedure" is a frequently voiced statement. Another PEG preparation, Colyte, has been made available in various flavors to deal with the difficulties associated with poor patient compliance.[126] However, to quote some of my patients: "a flavored disgusting drink is still disgusting."

It is because of patient complaints that I prefer to apply another colon cleansing technique in most individuals. It is not applicable for those with the following conditions: renal failure, ascites, congestive heart failure, a diversionary stoma, a history of myocardial infarction within 6 months, or those taking a calcium channel blocker such as nifedipine (Procardia) or verapamil (Calan). A case of hyperphosphatemia and hypocalcemic tetany in an individual with renal insufficiency has been reported.[185] Besides the usual clear liquid diet commencing at 2 P.M. the day prior to the examination, the patient drinks 480 mL of clear fluids every hour for the ensuing 4 hours. At 6 P.M., he or she consumes one 45-mL (1.5 oz.) bottle of Fleet Phospho-Soda (active ingredient, sodium phosphate), diluting it in an equal volume of water. At 6 A.M. the following morning, the regimen is repeated. This completes the preparation, and the expectation is that a vigorous catharsis will result.

Barclay and coworkers, concerned about intravascular volume contraction when this regimen is employed, prospectively randomized patients to receive a balanced carbohydrate-electrolyte rehydration solution (Gatorade) with that of ordinary clear fluids in patients preparing for colonoscopy.[12] They found a significant reduction in the amount of volume contraction with the Gatorade-treated patients as well as improved bowel cleansing.

Results of Studies of Preparations

Studies have been published that compare the various methods for bowel preparation prior to colonoscopy. Vanner and colleagues compared Phospho-Soda with that of the standard Golytely method in a randomized, prospective fashion.[184] They found that the former was less expensive, more effective, safer, and better tolerated. There may be more residual fluid in the bowel, but this can readily be aspirated. Kolts and colleagues randomized individuals to receive Fleet Phospho-Soda lemon-flavored castor oil, or the PEG solution.[111] As one could anticipate, the PEG preparation was least likely to be completed. Scores for cleansing the colon as determined by endoscopists who were blinded to the cathartic agent were highest in those receiving Fleet Phospho-Soda. The authors concluded that this agent is a cost-effective preparation that is better tolerated and more effective than the PEG lavage solution or castor oil.[111] Similarly, Golub and coworkers randomized patients to use three different bowel preparation regimens: PEG, PEG with oral metoclopramide, and oral Fleet Phospho-Soda.[82] They observed that all regimens were found to be equally effective. However, the Phospho-Soda was better tolerated and more likely to be completed than either of the other preparations. Others confirm the foregoing conclusion.[5,37,102]

Sedation and Monitoring

Sedation with monitoring is usually employed whenever total colonoscopy is undertaken. The insufflation of air or carbon dioxide—the latter is more rapidly absorbed—and traction on the bowel from the instrument may cause considerable discomfort and anxiety. Complete anesthesia, however, is contraindicated except for special circumstances. It is important for the examiner to be aware of any excessive discomfort that the patient is experiencing in order to avoid possible injury to the bowel wall, mesentery, or adjoining structures. The need for routine administration of sedatives or analgesics has been questioned[26]; at least 80% of patients can undergo a complete examination without such procedures.[94] However, "vocal anesthesia" is not considered acceptable.

Certain combinations of medications have been advised to reduce discomfort, including sodium pentobarbital (Nembutal), meperidine hydrochloride (Demerol),

hydroxyzine hydrochloride (Vistaril), diazepam (Valium), and midazolam (Versed).[40] Irrespective of the choice of medication, a heparin lock is recommended for intravenous access and is generally required by standardized conscious sedation regulations. Several publications have appeared cautioning as to the risks of oversedation and the requirement for continuous monitoring, including electrocardiogram, blood pressure, pulse oximetry, nasal air flow by thermistor probe, and impedance pneumography.[92] Care should be taken to avoid respiratory depression and hypotension; elderly patients and those with respiratory and pulmonary difficulties are at particular risk. The most frequently employed monitoring device is the pulse oximeter, a method that provides continuous noninvasive measurement of arterial hemoglobin and oxygen saturation.

One of the real concerns about monitoring has been the cost. A manual sphygmomanometer is about $150; an automatic pressure monitor, $3,000; electrocardiographic monitoring systems, $5,000 to $6,000; and pulse oximeters, $2,000 to $5,000.[65] Some recommendations concerning monitoring for conscious sedation have been offered by Fleisher.[65] However, there are no controlled studies that address the question of whether noninvasive monitoring decreases the incidence of complications. These guidelines have been fairly standardized and established at all hospitals and endoscopy centers. They generally include the following[65]:

- Monitoring should be part of the overall quality assurance program for the endoscopy unit.
- A competent assistant is the most important part of the monitoring process.
- The amount of monitoring should be proportional to the risk of the procedure for that individual.
- Minimal monitoring should include heart rate, blood pressure, and respiratory rate prior to, during, and immediately after the procedure and when the individual is about to leave the room.
- The requirement for sedation or analgesic medication must, perforce, be related to the technical facility of the examiner.

The American Society for Gastrointestinal Endoscopy has published a protocol for sedation and monitoring of patients undergoing endoscopic procedures. This is perhaps worth quoting:

> Every available means to ensure the safety of patients during endoscopic procedures is mandatory. This begins with a fully trained and knowledgeable endoscopist, thorough preparation of the unit to handle endoscopic procedures and potential adverse outcomes, appropriate patient preparation, skilled assistants, and monitoring of the patient's well-being before, during and after the procedure.

The relative risks involved can be estimated from patient and procedural factors and should be determined for each examination. The level and type of monitoring during endoscopic procedures are dependent upon a thorough understanding and assessment of the risk to the patient.

Monitoring of patients undergoing endoscopic procedures is mandatory and prudent. The ultimate responsibility for protecting the patient rests with the endoscopist and cannot be assigned to an assistant or to an electronic monitoring device. However, both may greatly improve the ability to detect patient distress at a time when intervention will prevent an otherwise adverse outcome.

Antibiotic Prophylaxis

The risk of infective endocarditis or other infectious complications from colonoscopy is quite low. Still, there is indeed a risk.[155] Recommendations for antibiotic prophylaxis are discussed in Chapter 4 and are equally applicable to colonoscopy and FS.

Technique of Examination: General Principles

If you don't know where you are going, all roads will get you there.

Koran

I have asked a former colleague, John A. Coller, staff surgeon in the Department of Colon and Rectal Surgery at the Lahey Clinic in Burlington, Massachusetts, to contribute his wise counsel on the technique of colonoscopy. Dr. Coller has had much experience with endoscopy and was instrumental in creating one of the early devices for performing polypectomy. He is currently Chairman of the Technology Committee of the American Society of Colon and Rectal Surgeons. For many years he has been on the Board of Governors of the Society of American Gastrointestinal Endoscopic Surgeons and has served in many capacities, including President. I am indeed grateful to Dr. Coller for his willingness to contribute to this text.

MLC

Colonoscopic examination is often viewed by the uninitiated as the process of pushing a tube up into the colon until the cecum is reached. On occasion, particularly if there has been a prior sigmoid resection, it may be almost that simple. However, most examinations require at least a modest amount of manipulation, and many are truly challenging. It is particularly important that the endoscopist has a thorough understanding of the interaction between a relatively unforgiving instrument and the variably compliant colon. Furthermore, a clear understanding of colonic anatomy is essential. For example, it is fixed at the rectum and is usually attached to the retroperitoneum at the descending, cecal, and ascending portions. Others areas, such as the hepatic and splenic flexures, although not fixed in the abdominal cavity, are intimately related to adjacent structures. Certain parts, notably the sigmoid and transverse colon, may have considerable mobility, being tethered only by the mesentery. Each portion of the colon has its own individual compliance. Successful intubation is in great part dependent upon taking advantage of this compliance as well as overcoming the varied obstacles to passage.

There are certain properties of the colonoscope and maneuvers that must be employed in order to accomplish successful intubation. These include tip deflection, shaft torquing, and shaft dithering. These physical movements of the instrument are combined with air insufflation, deflation, patient positioning, and abdominal pressure.

Tip Deflection

The articulating deflection tip is the most critical element in the design of the colonoscope. The ability to move the viewing tip off center by more than 180 degrees in any direction enables the examiner to have active control of what happens at the far end of the instrument. Deflection permits the endoscopist to look around a bend or fold in order to see in just which direction one needs to proceed. Folds can be pressed against the wall so that small lesions which would otherwise stay hidden are exposed. This articulation is essential during therapeutic maneuvers in order to aim a snare or biopsy forceps in the proper direction. In selected instances, the deflection tip may be retroflexed in order to obtain a clearer view of an obscured area such as the top of the anal canal (Figure 5-8) or the cecal side of the ileocecal valve (Figs. 5-22 and 5-23 later).

The articulating deflection tip, as essential as it is to facilitating intubation, may at the same time be the single greatest impediment to successful passage, at least for the novice colonoscopist. It also represents that part of the instrument most responsible for injury. As the tip is deflected from the straight position, a gentle curve forms along the distal 10 to 12 cm. With a relatively modest bend of 30 to 45 degrees, advancement of the instrument shaft will not distort the contour of the colon. However, when one attempts to increase the deflection to more than 90 degrees, in an effort to see around a curve or angle of the bowel, the distribution of forces against the colon wall changes profoundly. In the latter situation, a greater proportion of the advancing force is distributed against the sidewall of the bowel rather than in the forward direction of the lumen. In addition, the application of extreme deflection to both knob controls further deviates force distribution and precludes all attempts at advancement. Longitudinal advancement of the scope no longer follows the tip of the instrument. Instead, the deflection bend now becomes the leading edge of the instrument, with forward force transmitted directly to the wall of the colon. As a consequence, blunt or tearing trauma can easily occur. This can take the form of splitting of the fibers of the muscle wall or frank perforation. The operator can avoid this complication by simply recognizing that extreme deflection is being employed, and that with attempted instrument advancement the bowel under view seems to be getting further away rather than closer. Occasionally, extreme deflection is required in order to find the lumen. But once identified, the deflection should be eased, preferably to less than 90 degrees before attempting further advancement of the scope.

In summary, the least amount of deflection that is necessary in order to acquire the desired view is preferred. Limiting deflection to the use of the up-down dial only, while abjuring the simultaneous application of both controls, is helpful for minimizing inappropriate deflection.

Shaft Torquing

Torquing is an essential maneuver for effective intubation as well as for optimal surface visualization during extubation. Shaft torquing can produce three major effects. When left-handed or counterclockwise torque is applied, there is a tendency to produce a loop in the redundant sigmoid colon. Second, if clockwise torque is applied, the sigmoid colon tends to straighten. The third effect is produced at the tip of the scope. When the shaft is torqued in either direction in the presence of modest tip deflection, strong leverage is transmitted toward the entrance to the more proximal bowel. Using torque with modest tip deflection is generally more effective in locating an elusive proximal segment, as opposed to holding the shaft rigid while manipulating the deflection tip alone.

As more instrument is introduced, the response to torquing becomes more complex. If the scope is relatively straight, the torque will transmit nearly one to one to the viewing lens of the instrument. The field of view will simply be rotated; this facilitates identification of lesions or positioning of snares. However, if the scope shaft is within one or more loops, the results of torquing will have a much more profound effect on the bowel than on what is perceived through the viewing end of the instrument. If there is a so-called alpha loop present in the sigmoid colon, the effect of clockwise torquing (especially when combined with shaft withdrawal) is to reduce that loop by accordionizing the bowel onto the scope. This occurs without loss of intubation distance. However, once reduced, the sigmoid loop will have a tendency to form again, particularly if counterclockwise torque is applied during subsequent scope advancement. Therefore, in order to maintain reduction of a redundant sigmoid loop, one must advance the instrument while maintaining clockwise torque. The examiner can readily perceive this tendency to form the loop again by applying clockwise torque; the scope will appear to advance. Counterclockwise movement will reveal that the scope tends to lose ground.

Occasionally, an extremely redundant sigmoid colon will develop two complete loops during intubation. Nearly always, both are reducible. However, unlike the single loop configuration, the first loop is removed by counterclockwise rotation and the second by clockwise rotation. Removing both loops is usually essential before proximal passage into the descending colon can be accomplished. After both loops have been straightened, the sigmoid colon is once again most likely to remain in this position only if clockwise torque is continued during further intubation.

Torque is also a very important maneuver in manipulations in the area of the hepatic flexure. If the transverse colon is held in the upper abdomen, the scope takes a straight line to the hepatic flexure. At this point, clockwise torque is usually beneficial as the gently deflected tip is directed down the ascending colon. Conversely, if the transverse colon is redundant, stretching down toward the pelvis, the hepatic flexure is then approached from below. When the ascending colon is viewed in this situation, there is a rather sharp deflection of the tip. Once again, gentle scope withdrawal along with clockwise torquing, as well as intermittent desufflation, all combine to broaden the hepatic flexure and to drop the instrument down into the ascending colon and cecum.

During extubation, torquing is an extremely important manipulation for efficient and thorough examination of the colon surface. As the instrument is withdrawn, the right hand is maintained on the shaft to apply torque. The left hand supports the scope head with the thumb free to move the up-down control. By combining back-and-forth torque with simultaneous small tip deflections, one can continuously examine the colon surface with minimal risk of overlooking lesions. This permits the colon that has been accordionized onto the scope to be dropped off, a bit at a time. If, rather than torquing, one simply withdraws while using both hands of the dial controls, the view behind prominent folds is likely to be inadequate. Furthermore, if the colon is redundant, the bowel will likely fly off the scope at an uncontrollable rate.

Advancement/Withdrawal ("Dithering")

Colonoscopic intubation would be a simple matter if the colon were a noncompliant tube without redundancy or irregularity. The procedure would be nothing more than an effortless advancement of the instrument. On occasion, especially after sigmoid colon resection, colonoscopic intubation may be no more demanding than this. However, under most circumstances, the in-and-out movements of the shaft are only effective when combined with appropriate tip deflection and torquing. There is a tendency for the inexperienced endoscopist to resist losing ground even though it is unclear in which direction the scope should be advanced. Almost always, when anatomy is unclear or visualization is difficult, it is best and certainly safest to withdraw rather than to continue blind manipulation or advancement.[192] The simple process of limited withdrawal is most likely to reveal the proper direction in which to proceed.

When progression of the instrument is not impeded by severe tip deflection, redundant colon can be encouraged to accordionize along its length. This is most likely to occur if the scope is repeatedly advanced and withdrawn, a process referred to as "dithering." When combined with torquing in the sigmoid/descending colon, short dithering strokes can often reduce sigmoid redundancy as the scope is advanced, thereby avoiding the creation of a full loop. In less tethered segments, such as with a redundant transverse colon, it is often advantageous to perform long (30- to 50-cm) dithering strokes in order to accordionize the excess bowel onto a limited segment of instrument.

Gas Insufflation

Insufflation of gas is essential for effective visualization during colonoscopy. However, insufflation should be used sparingly. Excess gas can lead to abdominal distension that results in severe discomfort and a possible vasovagal reaction. Unfortunately, the design of the insufflation mechanism contributes to the possibility of inadvertent administration of unnecessary gas. This occurs because air is constantly being pumped to the insufflation trumpet valve on the control unit of the colonoscope. By simply covering the vent hole with a finger, one diverts a large volume of air into the colon. Depression of the trumpet valve diverts the air stream to the much smaller-volume flow of the lens cleaning system. Consequently, if one develops the habit of resting the finger on part or all of the trumpet valve, colonic distension will inevitably result. If intubation of the distal ileum is performed, only a limited insufflation may lead to the accumulation of considerable small bowel gas.

Excessive intraluminal gas often works against the process of intubation, particularly at a flexure or when a redundant loop is being negotiated. Gas distension pushes the proximal end of the loop or flexure away from the end of the scope. As a consequence, the angle becomes more acute and therefore more difficult to pass. This is most evident at the hepatic flexure when the tip deflection is sharply angulated into the distal ascending colon. As air is introduced, the ileocecal valve is seen in the distance to move still further away. Conversely, when air is aspirated, the cecal area is observed to be almost sucked into the scope. This manuever is facilitated by concomitant torquing.

Patient Position and Abdominal Pressure

Although there is no single position that is ideal, the construction of most endoscopes and the right-handedness of most physicians tend to favor the patient's assuming the left lateral position. Patients with a colostomy or ileostomy may be more comfortable in either the lateral or supine position. In patients with poor abdominal wall muscle tone (e.g., paraplegia, large hernia, prior dehiscence), examination in the prone position may be helpful. An elastic abdominal binder will provide an artificial abdominal wall resistance.

Changing positions during the examination when forward progress becomes stalled is often very beneficial. Rotating the patient 90 degrees to the left is analogous to torquing the scope 90 degrees to the right. Changing the patient position not only alters the relationship of the instrument to the colon, it also redistributes organ pressures within the abdominal cavity. Not infrequently, when one negotiates a difficult splenic flexure, the proximal bowel comes easily into view during the process of changing patient position. With the individual in the prone position, pressure in the abdominal cavity is increased. Once an excessively redundant sigmoid loop has been reduced, the broad pressure afforded by the prone position will discourage its reformation. To this one can add focal pressure by having an assistant push down on the abdomen in order to maintain straightening of the instrument.[191] Pressure from just to the right of the umbilicus and directed toward the left iliac fossa will discourage sigmoid looping. Similarly, central abdominal pressure will help keep the redundant transverse colon from dropping deeply into the pelvis.

If there is difficulty with entry into the ascending colon, the patient is rotated onto the right lateral decubitus position. This is an important and helpful maneuver when one must deal with a recalcitrant hepatic flexure. One presumes that pressure from the liver in this position flattens the flexure sufficiently to allow the scope to slip down the ascending colon.

Many endoscopists prefer to perform much of the examination with the patient in the supine position.[99, 147, 186] However, there are difficulties with this. If the scope is brought out between the patient's legs, there is minimal working room between the anus and the bed or gurney to allow adequate manipulation. If the instrument is brought out beneath the raised right leg, one must continually reposition the leg or utilize an assistant to attend to this.

General Preparations

Before actually starting the procedure, it is important to check that the instrument is in proper working order. This includes such basic maneuvers as switching on the suction and ensuring that the line is attached. Air insufflation and lens washing are tested. The deflection tip should be maximally flexed and examined for both the degree of deflection and integrity of the covering surface.

Some endoscopists prefer to use a two-person approach to colonoscopy. One handles the dial-control housing while an assistant advances and torques the shaft. In my opinion, this team method is very difficult to coordinate, because it is virtually impossible for each individual to have a sense of what the other is doing. Although it is helpful to have the assistant stabilize the shaft when positioning a snare onto a difficult polyp, it is strongly suggested that both shaft and dial controls be under the direction of a single mind.

The expert colonoscopist should be able to perform an expeditious and thorough examination by avoiding the formation of bowel loops that interfere with advancement. When loop formation is a problem, one should be able to widen the loop radius to facilitate intubation. The colonoscopist can detect the subtle clues that indicate a loop is starting to form: the loss of the one-to-one correspondence of instrument insertion to image movement; a gradual increase in resistance to forward motion, and signs of patient discomfort. As mentioned previously, instrument withdrawal often facilitates subsequent passage. Advancement of the scope should nearly always be under direct vision. The "slide-by" technique, whereby the viewing tip is partially buried in the colon wall, should be avoided. Although it is often necessary to accept less than a totally clear view, insertion when one is blind to lumen orientation is strongly discouraged. One should be concerned of the possibility of causing injury if the colonic mucosa blanches or if the patient experiences pain.

There is always the desire not to lose ground, especially after spending considerable time reaching an area during a difficult colonoscopy. The endoscopist may be very reluctant to give up what has been accomplished even if there is no apparent outlet. This attitude will most likely impede passage rather than preserve it. By "periscoping" the deflection tip and stretching the colon, one inevitably embeds the instrument in a self-made recess, the consequence of an abrupt bend in the next segment. At the risk of redundancy, I cannot overemphasize the requirement for one to withdraw shaft length whenever progress is arrested. Withdrawal is often the only means for visualizing the direction of the next segment of colon.

Fluoroscopy

Although not required for most examinations, the availability of fluoroscopy can be invaluable for difficult cases. When previous examinations have been inadequate or confusion as to the anatomy and lesion location exists, fluroscopic guidance should be considered. In addition, fluoroscopy is especially useful in training. How one perceives the configuration of the scope as compared with how it really exists in the bowel can be easily shown with fluoroscopic confirmation. A survey of members of the Society of American Gastrointestinal Endoscopic Surgeons and the American Society of Colon and Rectal Surgeons was undertaken to quantify the use of fluoroscopy

and to elicit impressions regarding its capabilities, indications, and usefulness.[153] Seventy-five percent never used this modality, the most frequent reason being lack of need or inaccessibility of the equipment. Ninety-two percent of the frequent users reported that they would feel significantly impaired without having the capability of performing fluoroscopy.

Electronic Imaging

Real-time electromagnetic imaging has been applied as an aid for the performance of colonoscopy.[161] By this means, three sets of generator coils are placed beneath the endoscopy table, producing pulsed, low-strength electromagnetic fields outside of the patient. These fields are detected by a series of sensor coils positioned at 12-cm intervals along the length of a catheter that is inserted down the biopsy channel of the colonoscope. From the electrical signal produced in the sensor coil, the exact position and orientation of each can be calculated. In a controlled trial from the United Kingdom, Saunders and coworkers determined that there was no significant difference in intubation time and duration of loop formation. However, the number of attempts taken to straighten the colonoscope was less when the endoscopist was able to see the imager view.[161] Another study by Adam and colleagues in 2001 compared the amount of colon actually seen as assessed with this imaging technique with how far the endoscopists thought they had reached.[3] In 119 patients, clinical assessment was correct in only 92 (77%). When the endoscopist reported that cecal landmarks had been visualized, the instrument was found to be distal to the cecum in 8.2%. Without identification of cecal landmarks, the endoscopist was accurate in only 41%. The consequences of this report are particularly disturbing, especially in the circumstances when colonoscopy is being performed for occult blood positivity or for equivocal findings on radiologic study.

High-Magnification Chromoscopic Colonoscopy

The concept of trying to find small or flat cancers of the colon has led the Japanese to develop methods for early identification of cancer through magnification chromoscopy.[75] The technique involves the use of one of two stains, either indigo carmine (preferred) or crystal violet. The solution is flushed through the biopsy channel of the colonoscope. Subtle endoscopic changes, such as pallor, erythema, unevenness, and superficial elevated lesions, may prompt the examiner to use a localized dye spraying or chromoscopy to aid in visualization.[101] Patterns of mucosal appearance suggestive of minute cancers or of an "invasive pit pattern" may lead one to consider a local treatment or a more radical one. The implication of detecting these lesions is potentially significant, but more study needs to be accomplished before the technique is applied routinely.

Sedation

Without sedation, colonoscopy of the entire colon may be an intolerably painful experience, thereby precluding a comprehensive evaluation. Although it has been demonstrated that some patients can undergo colonoscopy without sedation,[26] I prefer to initiate the examination after administering a small intravenous dose of meperidine (Demerol) and midazolam (Versed). This regimen may be supplemented, if necessary, depending on the patient's sensory and physiologic reactions. One should not strive to avoid medication but rather to provide a safe and reasonably comfortable examination for the patient (see previous discussion).

Performing the Examination

Rectal Examination

A digital rectal examination is a requisite initial step for every patient. As discussed in Chapter 4, it is not unusual to find important pathologic features, such as large hemorrhoids, an anal fissure, a prostatic nodule, or an anorectal mass. Furthermore, extrarectal lesions cannot be identified by the instrument alone. Digital examination also permits one to gauge anal sphincter tone. Knowing that an individual has poor tone will alert the examiner that it will be difficult for the patient to retain insufflated air. Alternatively, a tight or strictured anus may require gentle dilatation in order to accommodate the instrument. Finally, the examiner's finger prepares the patient for the subsequent insertion of the instrument.

Anorectal Intubation

Because the anus has been prelubricated with jelly during the digital examination, only a light coating need be placed along the shaft. Care should be taken to avoid the application of lubricant to the lens because it is not easily removed with the cleansing water jet. The scope should not be introduced end-on. Instead, the tip should be gently guided through the anal canal at an angle by using the index finger to support the flexible end. This will keep the tip from buckling during anal canal entry. Once inside the rectum, anatomic and technical factors may preclude clear visualization of the rectal ampulla during intubation. While the anal canal is oriented in the direction of the umbilicus, it joins the rectal ampulla, whose access is directed posteriorly toward the sacrum. The tip deflection mechanism responds poorly at this level because much of the deflection system still remains outside the

anus. It is not until the deflecting section has completely traversed the sphincter that the examiner may begin to have control of tip deflection. Once the tip of the scope has been inserted approximately 10 cm above the anal verge, tip deflection will respond properly, and the middle and upper rectum can be readily visualized. The most frequently cause of poor visualization in the middle and upper rectum is not disease, but rather the failure to provide adequate insufflation.

I prefer to perform the intubation portion of the examination with minimal attention to any intended therapy. There is often liquid residue from the preparation that must be aspirated. This liquid will pool in dependent areas of the colon and may obscure rather significant lesions. If one waits until extubation to clear this material, one needs to continually collapse the bowel, losing visualization, when all effort should be made to perform an uninterrupted assessment.

Sigmoid Intubation

Once the rectosigmoid has been reached, the stage is set for the technique of sigmoid intubation. With the instrument tip positioned in the rectosigmoid, one should take the control section with one's left hand while the right hand is positioned on the shaft. Throughout the remainder of the examination, this hand placement is the basic posture that will be employed. Both dial controls are maintained in the unlocked position. Tip deflection is managed virtually exclusively by rotation of the larger up-down control, using the thumb from beneath the control housing. This keeps the index or middle finger free to operate the suction or air insufflation.

Sigmoid-Descending Colon Intubation

As previously mentioned, proper and efficient negotiation of the sigmoid is often the most challenging aspect of colonoscopy, frequently determining the success of the entire procedure. Avoidance of bowel loop formation is not only more comfortable for the patient, but it also permits a more expeditious and more complete examination with a shorter length of instrument. While holding the control housing with the left hand, the right hand firmly grasps the shaft no more than 10 to 15 cm from the anus. A conscious effort is made to avoid bringing the right hand up to the dial controls. If one uses both hands simultaneously on the dial controls to periscope the deflection tip, although occasionally necessary, it usually results in overdeflection. Furthermore, this prevents one from using the very effective maneuver of simultaneous deflection and torquing. By keeping the hand on the shaft close to the anus, there is better control of the instrument and less tendency simply to push excess scope into the colon.

The three methods of traversing the sigmoid colon are intubation by elongation, by looping (alpha maneuver), and by accordionization (dither-torquing).[188] Although distinctly different techniques, they are not mutually exclusive solutions to the same problem. By utilizing these principles, the operator can more deliberately and effectively control the process of intubation.

Intubation by Elongation

Intubation by elongation merely refers to the process by which the instrument is inserted until either there is no apparent place to go or there is no more scope left. Indeed, this is probably the most commonly used approach when one performs FS. No fancy maneuvers: just advance the shaft, and periscope the deflection tip to find the luminal direction. If the sigmoid is minimally redundant, there may be a reasonably straight shot through the sigmoid and descending colon to the level of the splenic flexure. Unfortunately, more often this technique merely stretches a redundant sigmoid until the sigmoid-descending colon junction is reached, if it is reached at all. At this point, entry into the descending colon is associated with an increased angle to 180 degrees. This angle at the deflection tip is too sharp to permit passage to progress. Additional shaft advancement therefore merely stretches the sigmoid further.

Intubation by Looping (Alpha Maneuver)

The relatively mobile sigmoid colon is fixed proximally at the descending colon junction and distally at the rectum. The best means to appreciate the varied configurations that can develop during sigmoid manipulation is to view the examination under fluoroscopic control (see earlier). In contrast to simple advancement, counterclockwise torque with gentle tip deflection stretches the midsigmoid, first in a ventral direction, and then toward the right lower quadrant of the abdomen (Figure 5-7). As the scope is advanced utilizing continuous counterclockwise torque, it courses back across the upper pelvis to the sigmoid-descending colon junction. Fluoroscopic examination will demonstrate a loop that resembles the Greek letter alpha (α). This intentionally created, broad curve flattens the angle at the sigmoid-descending colon junction into a gentle curve. Once the tip of the scope has passed to the level of the middescending colon, reduction can be undertaken. In order to remove the loop, the instrument is simultaneously withdrawn while clockwise torque is applied (Figure 5-7). It is evident that derotation is being accomplished when the endoscopist observes the advancement of the image in spite of the fact that the instrument is being withdrawn. Once the loop has been reduced, the scope can be readily advanced to the splenic flexure by maintaining clockwise torque during advancement of the shaft (Figure 5-9). This is quite an efficient technique for negotiating a moderately redundant sigmoid colon if multiple tightly adherent loops are absent. However, if several adherent loops are present, this method cannot be successfully employed and only increases the level of discomfort for the patient. If the sigmoid loop is extremely large, it may not be able to be reduced by derotation until the proximal end of the instrument has been passed well into the transverse colon. The loop should be reduced either before the tip reaches the splenic flexure or after it has passed the distal transverse colon. A word of caution! Derotation with the deflection tip sharply angulated at the splenic flexure invites traction trauma to attachments that exist between the colon and the spleen (see Complications).

Intubation by Accordionization ("Dither-Torquing")

When the colon segment to be intubated is not a straight shot or when one is not able to create a large, gentle loop, it is often best to use a dither-torquing approach. This method attempts to straighten a tightly nested colon as the scope is advanced. In this approach, one is trying to accordionize as much colon as possible onto a limited length of instrument.

The technique employs simultaneous application of both dithering and torquing. Dithering refers to the repeated in-and-out movement of the instrument shaft. While the shaft is being advanced proximally 6 to 10 cm, a small amount of counterclockwise torque of about 45 to 60 degrees is applied. The process is reversed by using clockwise torque during simultaneous withdrawal of the scope for the same length. This cycle is repeated in a rhythmic fashion at a rate of about 1 to 2 cycles/second, taking care to avoid net advancement of the shaft. The shaft is gripped with the right hand close to the anus in order to minimize premature advancement of the scope. Only after the lumen appears to be straight ahead with minimal tip deflection should one regrasp the shaft to a new position. If this precaution is not heeded, it is likely that the shaft will be inappropriately advanced, leading to the development of a large loop. Although the first few dither-torquing cycles may appear to accomplish little, by rhythmically continuing this motion one will enable the bowel to accordionize onto the scope, straightening the colon as the examination proceeds. With experience, it becomes apparent that the cyclic rhythm, amount of torque, degree of tip deflection, and shaft advancement distance are all variables that can be altered to achieve the maximal effect. If successful, the descending colon as far as the splenic flexure may be intubated through the application of clockwise torque during shaft advancement with minimal deflection of the tip. In more proximal segments, such as in the transverse colon, the same dither-torquing maneuver may be utilized. Here, however, dithering can be extended to 50 to 60 cm at a time.

Splenic Flexure and Transverse Colon Intubation

If the sigmoid colon has been accordionized onto the scope and is straightened into a gentle, smooth curve, negotiation of the splenic flexure is usually not difficult. Even if the flexure is quite high and sharply angulated, the deflection tip can be rotated into the distal transverse colon without much problem. It is at this point that one must remember the hazard of creating an excessive deflection bend. As soon as there is visual acquisition of the distal transverse colon lumen, the degree of the deflection should be eased in order to provide a gentle bend of less than 90 degrees. In order to achieve this less acute angle, one must course along the outside curve of the colon wall rather than view the center of the lumen. Although the lumen may be partially obscured by the outside wall, it should not be entirely lost. In fewer than 5% of patients, the splenic flexure must be intubated in essentially a reverse fashion, with the deflection tip stretching and coursing the flexure to the left and caudad, before proceeding into the transverse colon. Once the instrument has been passed to the level of the midtransverse colon, this splenic flexure loop can generally be removed with a counterclockwise rotation (Figure 5-17).

Advancing the colonoscope through the transverse colon is usually uneventful. This part of the colon is distinguished by its well-defined triangular appearance (Figure 5-18). If the transverse colon is without redundancy, the intubation will proceed directly across the upper abdomen to the hepatic flexure (Figure 5-19). This redundancy can consume a considerable amount of scope length. When combined with a persistent sigmoid loop, there may be insufficient instrument left to complete the exam-

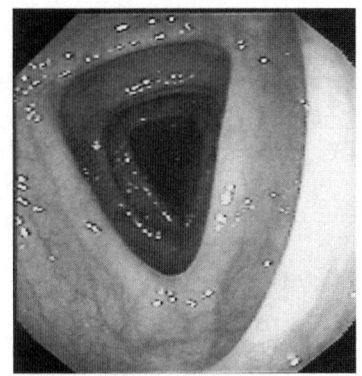

FIGURE 5-18. Normal transverse colon. (See Color Fig. 5-18.)

ination. Redundancy of the transverse colon may result in a loop that has the configuration of the Greek letter gamma (γ) when viewed by fluoroscopy. This loop is optimally removed by clockwise rotation of the shaft before attempting to proceed into the ascending colon. Once this has been accomplished, it will usually stay derotated. However, if it does tend to reform, external pressure at the umbilicus will often prevent this. If the transverse colon is redundant, one can also use the dither-torquing technique when progress is impeded. In this area, the dither-torquing maneuver is often best performed with longer, 30- to 60-cm strokes, rather than the short ones used in the sigmoid colon.

Hepatic Flexure and Ascending Colon Intubation

The hepatic flexure is often recognized by a bluish discoloration of the wall where the liver is in close proximity

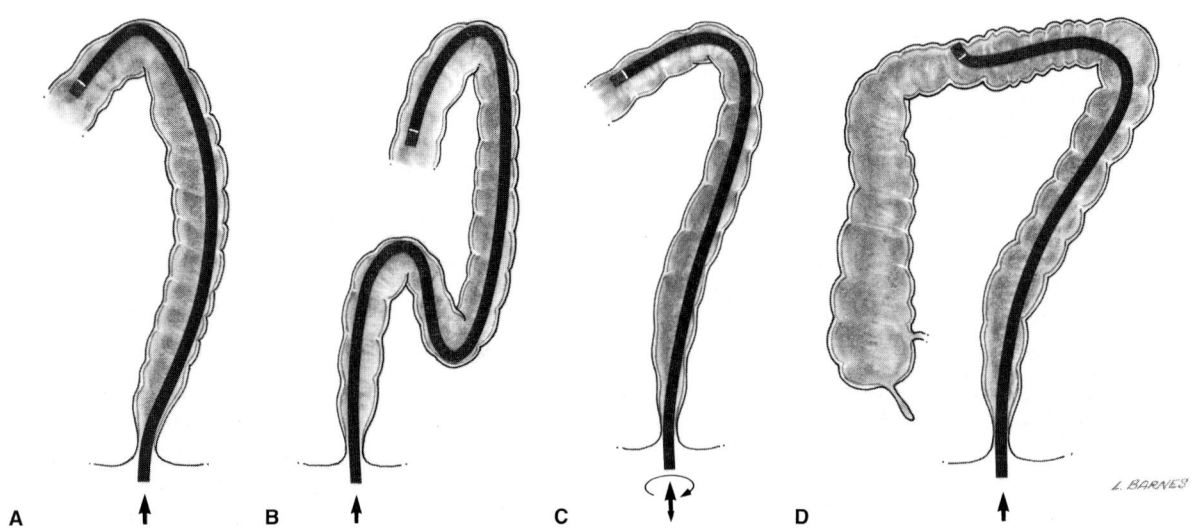

FIGURE 5-17. The colonoscope is maneuvered into the transverse colon by the following steps. **(A)** "Hooking" the splenic flexure. **(B)** Advancing the instrument. **(C)** Withdrawing and straightening the tip while maintaining clockwise torque. **(D)** Negotiating the transverse colon by hooking the bowel wall.

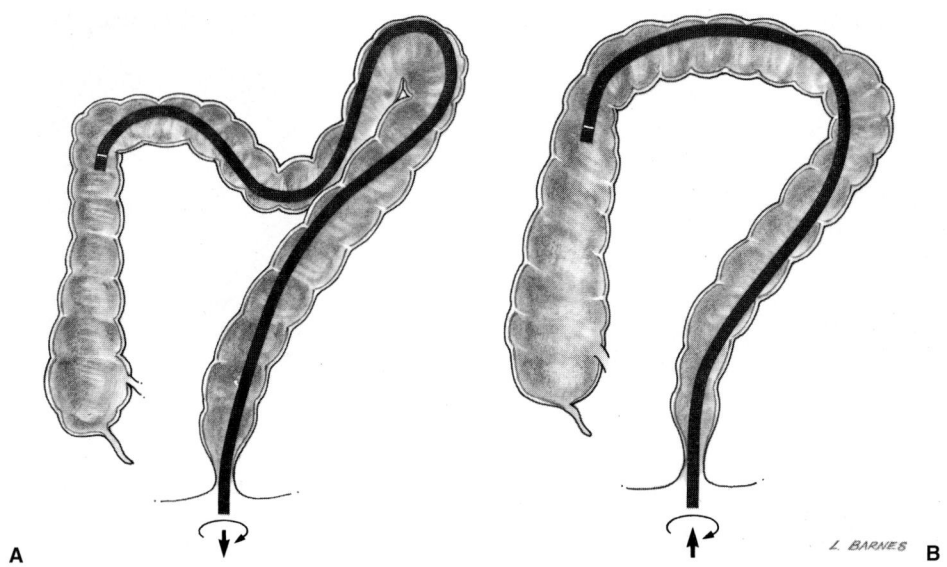

FIGURE 5-19. The colonoscope negotiates the ascending colon through the following steps. **(A)** The tip is directed to visualize the ascending colon. **(B)** Withdrawal produces advancement; this is expedited by the use of suction.

(Figure 5-20). Not infrequently, however, the hepatic flexure is not immediately evident because of acute angulation. The deflection tip may be sharply flexed with bowel lumen distorted by stretching. This often gives the endoscopist a false sense of accomplishment, leading him or her to believe that the cecum has been reached because there is apparently no colon left. If most of the colonoscope has been used and the specific cecal landmarks have not been identified, one is most likely at the hepatic flexure—not yet at the cecum. The true location is unlikely to be revealed until the shaft is withdrawn and torqued clockwise to bring the distal ascending colon into view.

If the transverse colon has been able to be negotiated straight across, or straight down from a high splenic flexure, then intubation into the ascending colon is usually accomplished by clockwise torque, flattening of the deflection tip, and simultaneous gas aspiration. These three

mechanisms combine to drop the scope into the cecum. If the transverse colon is excessively redundant, it may not be able to be maintained in the upper abdomen, even if abdominal pressure is applied. The instrument therefore approaches the hepatic flexure from below rather than from across. Inevitably, the deflection tip will require a 180-degree bend to negotiate this area. Once again, clockwise torque, flattening deflection, and gas aspiration, combined with what may be considerable shaft withdrawal, permit entry into the ascending colon. However, it is unlikely that the scope will drop into the ascending colon with a first attempt at torquing, flattening, and aspiration. Repeated efforts will usually be required to gather more colon progressively onto the instrument. Still, the maneuver that will finally drop the scope into the ascending colon and cecum will be the combination of clockwise torque, tip flattening, and gas aspiration (Figure 5-19).

Finally, if negotiation of the hepatic flexure continues to be a problem, changing the position is often beneficial. Initially, the patient should be rotated to the prone position. If this is not helpful, the right lateral decubitus position should be attempted. The liver may have a flattening effect on the flexure in this position, thus permitting further passage.

Cecum and Distal Ileum Intubation

The most reliable landmarks for visual confirmation of reaching the cecum are as follows:

- Appendiceal orifice (Figure 5-21)
- Ileocecal valve (Figs. 5-22 and 5-23)
- Triangulation of the tinea (5-24)
- Intubation of the distal ileum (Figure 5-25)

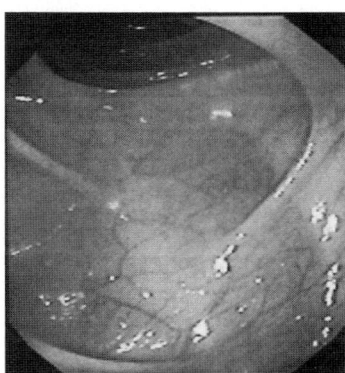

FIGURE 5-20. Hepatic flexure. (See Color Fig. 5-20.)

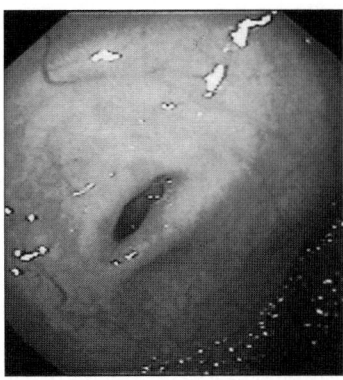

FIGURE 5-21. The appendiceal orifice. (See Color Fig. 5-21.)

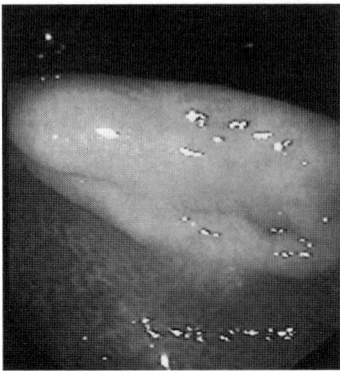

FIGURE 5-22. The ileocecal valve seen from a retroflexed instrument position. (See Color Fig. 5-22.)

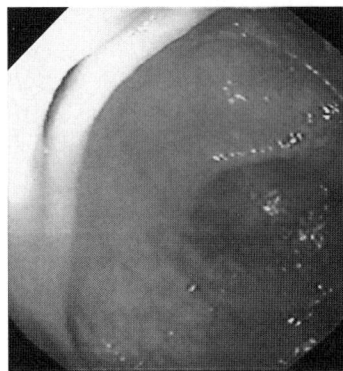

FIGURE 5-23. The ileocecal valve as is appears entering the cecum. (See Color Fig. 5-23.)

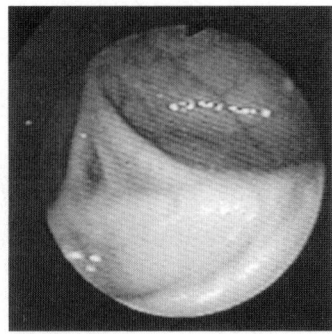

FIGURE 5-24. Normal cecal base with triangulation of the tinea. (See Color Fig. 5-24.)

roscopy as mentioned is helpful, but it must be kept in mind that the cecum is not always in the right iliac fossa. The same holds true if a plain abdominal film is completed at the end of the evaluation (Figure 5-26). Most newer equipment has a transillumination setting on the light source. However, the amount of interposing tissue can confuse interpretation, and difficulty with directing the light limits its applicability. Furthermore, a redundant transverse colon that extends into the right lower quadrant may mimic complete intubation if one were to rely on indirect criteria. Clearly, the least reliable indicator that the cecum has been reached is the impression that there is no remaining colon. If the usual landmarks of an ileocecal location are not present and there seems to be no remaining colon, the endoscopist has probably stretched a more proximal segment into a blind recess (e.g., the proximal transverse colon). Fleshner and colleagues suggest that there are mucosal spots or "freckles" that correlate microscopically with subepithelial and submucosal lymphoid follicles, an endoscopic feature of the cecum seen in approximately one third of individuals.[66] Most experienced endoscopists can achieve the cecum more than 95% of the time.[190]

Sometimes it is important to intubate the distal ileum, especially for the evaluation of an individual with inflammatory bowel disease (Figure 5-25). The success rate for

Cirocco and Rusin believe that the ileocecal valve is the most reliable cecal landmark and is invariably visualized even when all other landmarks are obscure.[35] Palpation of the right lower quadrant with concomitant movement of the colon endoscopically and transillumination of the abdominal wall in the right iliac fossa are less dependable signs. When compressing the right lower quadrant, visual evidence of scope movement may be seen even if the viewing tip is at a considerable distance. Fluo-

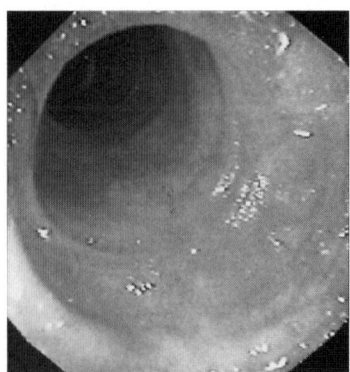

FIGURE 5-25. Normal terminal ileum. (See Color Fig. 5-25.)

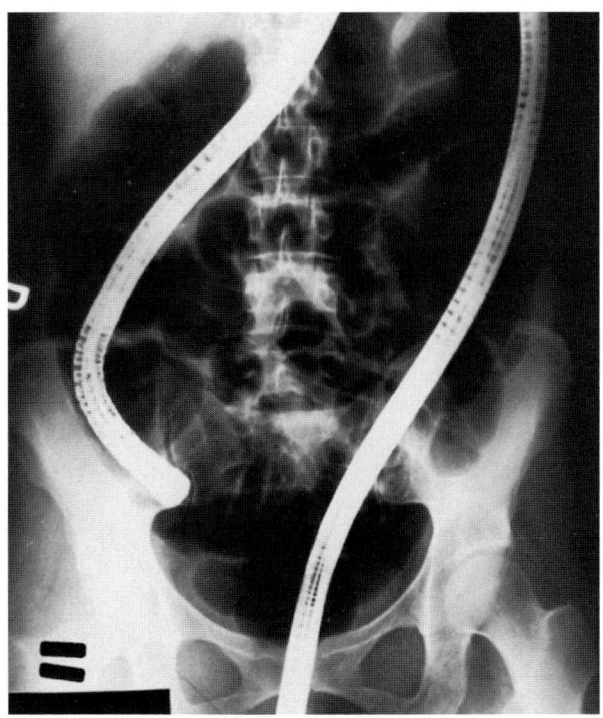

FIGURE 5-26. Plain abdominal film demonstrates a colonoscope that has reached the cecum.

accomplishing this maneuver increases with experience and is generally reported to be in the range of 80%.[18] Petrini visualized the ileum in 91% of the 97% in whom the cecum was reached (116 consecutive patients.[150] Muscular thickening of some ileocecal valves as well as the flutterlike configuration of others preclude a higher rate of intubation. My own preference is not to attempt ileocecal intubation on a routine basis because there is no clinical benefit. Furthermore, when one attempts to distend the valve, considerable air may be introduced into the ileum. The small bowel offers little resistance to the retrograde accumulation of air. Because it is not readily evacuated, it may lead to considerable postexamination discomfort.

When intubation of the distal ileum is indicated, one must recognize that the entrance is at an angle that is less than 90 degrees to the axis of the ascending colon. This angle is made even more acute because of the caudad displacement of the cecum produced by air insufflation when complete colon intubation has been accomplished. As viewed from the proximal ascending colon, only the prominent bilobar-shaped distal lip of the valve is in view (Figure 5-22). The tip of the instrument must be positioned on the cecal side of the valve. The deflection tip is then angled toward the valve, prying the orifice open as the shaft is slightly withdrawn. A combination of torquing and suction will usually direct the scope into the terminal ileum. Others have developed their own methods for successful intubation.[27] The mucosal surface is recognized by its roughened, ground-glass appearance. This is in con-

trast to the smooth texture of the distended, adjacent cecum.

Withdrawal and Examination

Inspection of the colon should be a smooth and continuous process. If the instrument is simply withdrawn, the accordionized colon will fly off the end of the scope in an uncontrolled fashion at various points along the way. Hidden areas behind folds will go unexamined. In some instances, even long segments will evade adequate assessment. Expeditious withdrawal therefore usually results in poor evaluation of the colon.

Inspection of the mucosa for abnormalities will be facilitated if residual debris from the preparation has been removed during intubation. Conversely, if there is foreign material present, the endoscopist will have to aspirate frequently, collapsing the bowel lumen and interrupting the process of visual examination. Distension of the lumen will once again have to be established before inspection can proceed. When fluid must be removed, it is advantageous to position it at about five o'clock with respect to the viewing lens. This will permit removal without having to collapse the field from view completely. Sometimes muscular spasm or irritability of the colon interferes with optimal withdrawal visualization. This problem can sometimes be ameliorated by administering glucagon, 1 mg, intravenously. However, this is not effective when the underlying impediment is due to a fibrotic stricture or bowel wall thickening associated with diverticulitis.

Examination of the colon during extubation is most efficiently performed by keeping the right hand on the shaft while controlling tip deflection with the left hand. The view of the lumen can be continuously readjusted while the shaft is being withdrawn. When there has been considerable redundancy and a substantial length of colon has been accordionized onto the scope, the instrument should be withdrawn by small amounts. My preference is to withdraw 5 to 15 cm and then push the instrument back in. The excessive colon is released from the shaft, bit by bit. One must be particularly attentive at the flexures. The inner aspects of the proximal sides of both the hepatic and splenic flexures are areas that must be dropped from the scope very carefully in order to avoid missing what can be rather large lesions.

Cleansing the Instrument

The concern for transmitting disease may be exaggerated, but the fear of contracting hepatitis and acquired immunodeficiency syndrome (AIDS) has led to the marketing of numerous products for cleansing endoscopic equipment. Actually, the most common agents of infection transmitted by gastrointestinal endoscopy are *Salmonella* species and *Pseudomonas aeruginosa*.[172] In the United States, government regulation through the

Centers for Disease Control and Prevention have produced numerous recommendations. Vigorous mechanical cleansing and the use of an enzymatic detergent immediately after the procedure, followed by a disinfectant and thorough rinsing, have been considered the most effective.[62,93,106,127,166] The channels should be likewise cleansed and air dried. Gas sterilization is very effective but shortens the useful life of these very expensive instruments. Ultrasonic sterilizers, scope washers, and automatic computer-programmed disinfectors have been developed to reduce the possibility of toxic effects to the patient and to the personnel who handle the chemicals. Such products and companies are becoming numerous, and concepts are continuing to evolve in this area. In fact, as previously mentioned, a sheathed fiberoptic sigmoidoscope is now available to reduce or perhaps eliminate the need for backup instruments and scope washers and to provide, theoretically, improved patient safety (Figure 5-1).

Although it is true that, in principle, all patients should be considered infected, and cleansing methods should be consistently applied, it is important to mention that special consideration should be given to the high-risk individuals, those who are suspected of harboring the hepatitis B virus and those with AIDS. These patients should undergo endoscopy at the end of the daily schedule. Ethylene oxide gas sterilization of instruments and accessories has been recommended by some,[14] but others stipulate that the human immunodeficiency virus can be eliminated after 10 minutes of cleansing with standard 2% alkaline glutaraldehyde (Cidex, Surgikos, Arlington, TX).[91] Alternatively, soaking in 70% ethyl alcohol for at least 4 minutes is acceptable as a second-line disinfectant (67). It should be remembered that the endoscope control head represents a potential source of cross-infection and should not be neglected in any cleansing procedure.[171] Severely neutropenic or immunocompromised individuals should be examined with recently sterilized instruments.[14]

It is important to note that following disinfecting the instruments should be thoroughly washed with plain water. A type of chemical colitis has been observed in a some individuals, a complication believed to be due to contamination of the air-water channel with potentially toxic cleansing chemicals.[105]

Therapeutic Colonoscopy

Biopsy

Biopsy devices are available for sampling colonic mucosa and lesions. For reasons of reliability and the potential for contamination, these instruments are often disposable. Multiple specimens can be gathered within the cups of a large biopsy forceps, especially if a central spike is present to hold them (Figure 5-3). This is particularly

useful when gathering a large number of samples for dysplasia surveillance in chronic ulcerative colitis (see Chapter 29). Hot biopsy forceps are insulated and can be connected to a monopolar generator. This is particularly helpful for the management of small mucosal polyps. These lesions, which are usually not sufficiently defined to enable safe snare excision, can be grasped with a forceps and removed during simultaneous electrocoagulation. With the polyp tented into the lumen, brief spurts of coagulation are applied until there is the first appearance of a whitish coagulum at the base of the forceps. Because the small surface area of contact results in a relatively high current density, electrocoagulation should be limited. Excessive or prolonged burning can result in full-thickness bowel injury. It is because of this concern that some endoscopists utilize a "cold biopsy" technique. The forceps will not sever the tissue in a scissorslike fashion; the instrument therefore must be abruptly pulled from the bowel wall. The specimen within the biopsy cut will be relatively unaffected by the coagulation current. Unlike a cold biopsy, the foregoing method will usually destroy any surrounding adenomatous tissue, thereby resulting in definitive treatment of small neoplastic polyps.

Blood vessel lesions, such as vascular ectasias (see Color Figure 28-1), are optimally treated by using a bipolar electrode. Complete destruction can be accomplished with minimal risk of bowel injury (see Chapter 28).

Snare Polypectomy

One of the most important advances in colon surgery during the past few decades has been the development of endoscopic polypectomy. The contrast between a 1-week hospitalization for an open colotomy-polypectomy and that of an outpatient colonoscopy-polypectomy performed in less than 1 hour is dramatic. The concept of following a polyp observed on barium enema examination to avoid a laparotomy, colotomy, and polypectomy is no longer valid (see Chapter 22). Using colonoscopy, most polyps can be removed or at least examined by biopsy. Patients who harbor a colon or rectal polyp require an aggressive approach to diagnosis and treatment.[41]

Equipment

As mentioned earlier, performance of polypectomy requires an electrical generating power source that, for endoscopic use, is transmitted by means of a wire loop snare or coagulating electrode. Polypectomy is undertaken through the accessory channel of the instrument. Most commercially available high-frequency units permit tube or cutting current and a spark gap current, which produce coagulation or a blend of the two (Figure 5-16 and Chapter 4).[72]

Gas insufflation during polypectomy is a matter of particular concern because of the potential hazard of an explosive mixture's being present.[10] The necessity for adequate bowel preparation has been discussed previously. The use of an inert gas—most commonly carbon dioxide—has been recommended, particularly if mannitol has been used as a bowel preparation. However, the requirements of tank storage and accessories have made this a rather impractical and, in the opinion of many, unnecessary alternative when other cathartic regimens are employed. Frühmorgen reported no instance of gas explosion using standard methods of bowel preparation in more than 2700 colonoscopy-polypectomy procedures.[72] With respect to insufflation of air as a source of discomfort during colonoscopy, Church and Delaney performed a randomized trial with the use of air in one half of patients and carbon dioxide in the other half.[34] There were 124 in the air group and 123 in the carbon dioxide group. There were no differences with respect to sedation/analgesia requirements during the procedure, but there was significantly less abdominal pain noted 10 minutes after conclusion of the examination when carbon dioxide was employed.

In addition to the previously mentioned equipment, many cold and hot biopsy forceps, snares, baskets, and hooks for retrieval are commercially available. Shapes include oval, eccentric, and hexagonal. I prefer to use a hexagonal snare for most polyps. This configuration seems to hold its shape during difficult positioning or if multiple excisions are required. For polyps that are too large for hot biopsy excision, it is best to use a minisize snare. Milsom and Gottesman advise removing the snare wire and applying suction through the sheath for the removal of small polyps, especially from the right side of the colon.[132]

In 1976, Frühmorgen and others introduced the concept of applying the argon laser to the endoscopic treatment of a bleeding lesion.[74] The laser, an acronym for light amplification by stimulated emission of radiation, produces an intense monochromatic light which can destroy tissue to varying depths of penetration. The argon laser is considered to be most useful for treating mucosal lesions, because energy from this source penetrates only l mm of tissue; the neodymium:yttrium-aluminum;garnet laser is better for deep and exophytic lesions, because it penetrates 3 to 4 mm of tissue.[45] Optical fibers have been produced to fit through the open channel of most endoscopic instruments. Lasers have been used most effectively in the treatment of angiodysplastic lesions, but they have also been applied to benign and malignant tumors, as well as to a variety of anatomic abnormalities.[64,100,125]

Indications

The primary indications for the use of colonoscopy as a therapeutic tool are polypectomy and biopsy. Therapeutic colonoscopy is also indicated for treatment of bleed-

ing lesions such as vascular anomalies, ulcerations, tumors, and those at the polypectomy site. Additional applications include decompression of cecal and sigmoid volvulus, colonic decompression in Ogilvie's syndrome, foreign body removal, balloon dilatation of stricture, and palliative treatment of stenosing or bleeding malignant lesions.

Technique

The technique for removal of a polyp is not dissimilar to that employed with the rigid sigmoidoscope, but maintaining adequate visualization and holding instrument position obviously pose more of a problem. The distal orifice for the snare exits the scope at the five o'clock position relative to the luminal view. If the polyp is on the opposite side (11 o'clock), the view will be lost when the snare is passed over the polyp. Consequently, whenever possible, it is best to rotate the scope so that the base of the polyp is located at the five o'clock position. This will ensure that the polyp remains in view while the snare loop is positioned.

The two-team approach or the presence of an assistant is a requisite. Usually, the polyp is visualized 2 or 3 cm distal to the endoscope. By maneuvering the tip of the colonoscope and sometimes the patient, the wire loop is advanced and the head of the polyp encircled (Figure 5-27). Small lesions can be removed simply with the biopsy instrument (Figure 5-28). The loop is drawn down to the pedicle until the latter is secured. The endoscope is then maneuvered to hold the polyp away from the bowel wall to avoid injury and possible perforation. The current is then applied and the polyp excised. It can then be removed using forceps, a hook or basket, or the suction device. When other polyps are present, they may be removed individually or collected by straining the stool following the procedure (Figure 5-29). Pathologic confirmation is, of course, required.

Large polyps (i.e., those greater than 2.5 cm) can be removed by the foregoing technique if adequate visualization of the pedicle is possible and the head can be ensnared. Failing this, however, it can be removed piecemeal, and the specimens collected as described. The expertise of the endoscopist determines the size and the nature of lesion one is willing to approach. Sessile and even submucosal lesions can be removed by endoscopy, but ulcerating tumors should not be.[29,30] Care must be taken to elevate the mucosa as the snare is tightened. Stripping the mucosa and submucosa is safe, but the physician must endeavor to leave intact the muscularis propria (Figs. 5-30 through 5-32). Obviously, the risk of bowel perforation is increased when the physician attempts to remove such lesions.

A sessile polyp, however, may not permit adequate viewing of the entire lesion when the snare is applied. Under these circumstances, removal is accomplished in a

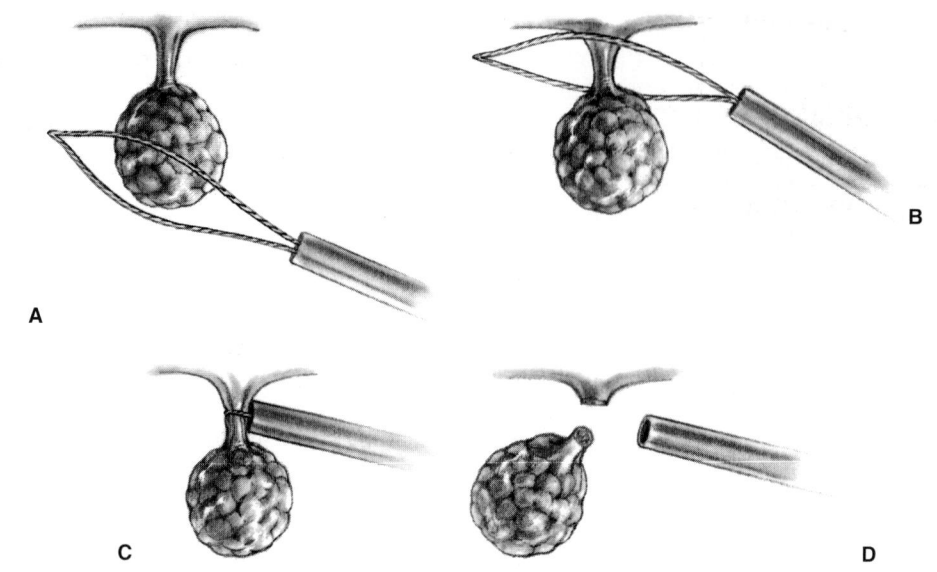

FIGURE 5-27. Techniques involved in polypectomy. **(A,B)** The polyp is ensnared. **(C)** Loop tightening results in coagulation and strangulation. **(D)** The polyp is removed.

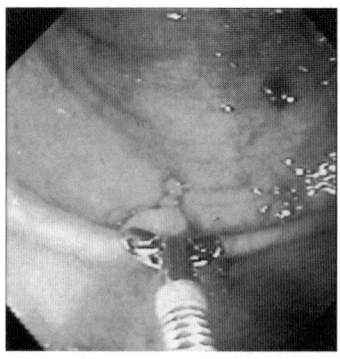

FIGURE 5-28. A small polyp is removed with biopsy forceps. (See Color Fig. 5-28.)

piecemeal fashion so that each lobule that is excised can be clearly seen (Figure 5-33).

Several techniques may be used for removing larger sessile lesions. A two-channel scope permits the endoscopist to employ both a snare and a grasper to manipulate the polyp. The snare is passed through the one chan-nel, and a grasper or large biopsy forceps is placed in the second. The latter is then passed out through the open loop of the snare. In this fashion, the polyp can be manip-ulated into the snare. Sometimes it is helpful to elevate a sessile polyp above the plane of the colon wall by inject-ing saline into the submucosa. This provides greater sep-aration between the muscularis propria and the polyp base. In addition, the improved tissue hydration facili-tates the electrocoagulation.

The proper application of electrocautery is essential for safe and effective polypectomy (see Chapter 4). There is no single combination of cutting and coagulation cur-rent or wattage that must be used or is preferred. A colono-scopist gradually develops confidence in his or her own electrosurgical method. What is remarkable is how var-ied these techniques may be. The general approach that many have employed utilizes short bursts of monopolar, blended, cutting current while one squeezes the snare. By using intermittent bursts, deep tissue cooling is permit-ted, thereby minimizing the likelihood of a full-thickness burn. Whenever possible, the polyp is suspended within

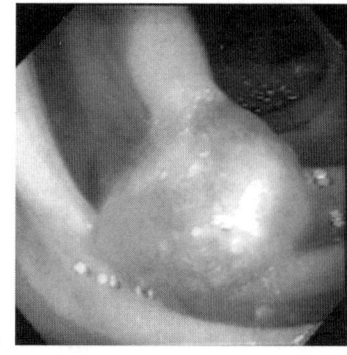
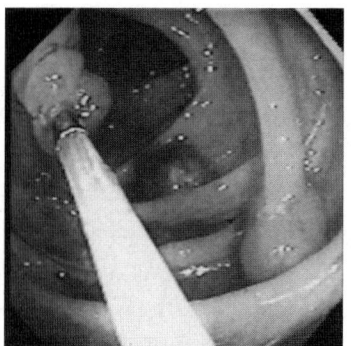

FIGURE 5-29. Technique of snare polypectomy. (See Color Fig. 5-29.) **(A)** A polyp on a stalk is seen in the midsigmoid colon. **(B)** The snare encom-passes the head of the polyp; an adjacent peduncu-lated polyp can be seen.

A   B

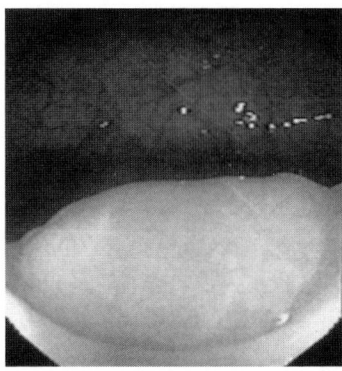

FIGURE 5-30. Sessile polypoid tumor of the rectosigmoid. (See Color Fig. 5-30.)

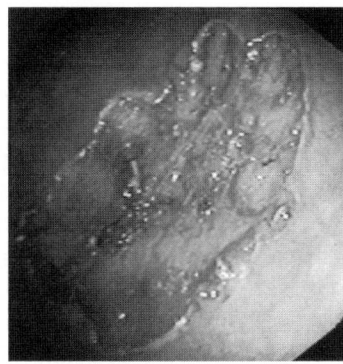

FIGURE 5-31. Removal of a tumor has been effected with snare cautery. (See Color Fig. 5-31.)

the lumen to avoid adjacent tissue injury. If the polyp is too large to avoid touching the wall, then surface contact should intentionally be maximized in order to avoid pinpoint areas of high current density.

Although inpatient observation for 24 to 48 hours has been recommended in the past, the physician may feel confident in outpatient treatment, provided the patient is informed of the potential hazards and remains relatively close to the area for a day or so. At our institution, virtually all patients are managed on an ambulatory basis.

Malignant polyps, even if technically removable at colonoscopy, may require a subsequent resection (see

Chapter 22). Such lesions are unlikely to be palpable at the time of operation. Accurate localization is important, particularly if intraluminal landmarks are absent and fluoroscopic control is unavailable. Some have advised the performance of a localizing preoperative barium enema (70). Another alternative is to place a clip on the lesion (e.g., HX-2U Clip-Fixing Device, Olympus America, Melville, NY) using a plain abdominal radiograph for localization.[176] An injection of particulate India ink or charcoal suspension, applied submucosally with a sclerotherapy needle, will persist indefinitely and allow identification of the dye on the serosal aspect at the time of laparotomy.[103,136,165] This technique is not without complications, however. Fat necrosis with inflammatory pseudotumor as well as colonic abscess and focal peritonitis have been reported secondary to India ink tattooing of the colon.[43,149]

Comment on Polypectomy (MLC)

The foregoing represents John Coller's thoughts about colonoscopy and colonoscopy polypectomy. I wanted to provide a personal comment, however, about the issue of one's willingness to attempt removal of large polyps. Referral to a specialist endoscopist will certainly increase the likelihood that a large or sessile polyp will be removed or at least removal will be attempted.[21,50] This is even more apt to occur when the specialist is a surgeon, as opposed to a gastroenterologist. The surgeon's ability to deal with his or her own endoscopic complication, without the need for additional consultation, emboldens one. Conversely, even the most experienced gastroenterologist is less likely to expose the patient and himself (herself) to a high-risk procedure when the potential complication will require involvement of a surgeon. In an ideal world, especially in the practice of medicine, ego should not be an issue, but even if it were not, there is a greater willingness on the part of surgeons to attempt to accomplish a more invasive procedure—that is perhaps one reason why they are surgeons. And then there is the issue of politics. How does a surgeon reconcile his or her conflict when the patient is referred by a gastroenterologist to undergo a laparotomy for a polyp that could not be removed

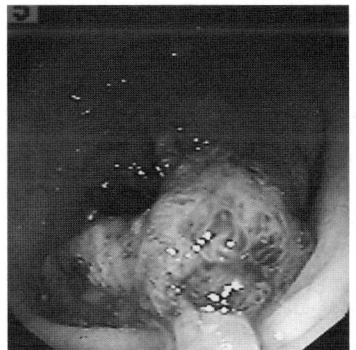
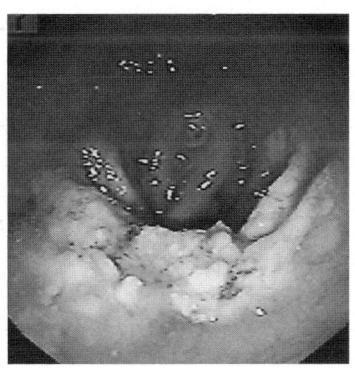

A   B

FIGURE 5-32. Snare excision of large polyp. **(A)** Snare is passed around polypoid lesion. **(B)** Coagulum appears at the site of polyp removal. (See Color Fig. 5-32.)

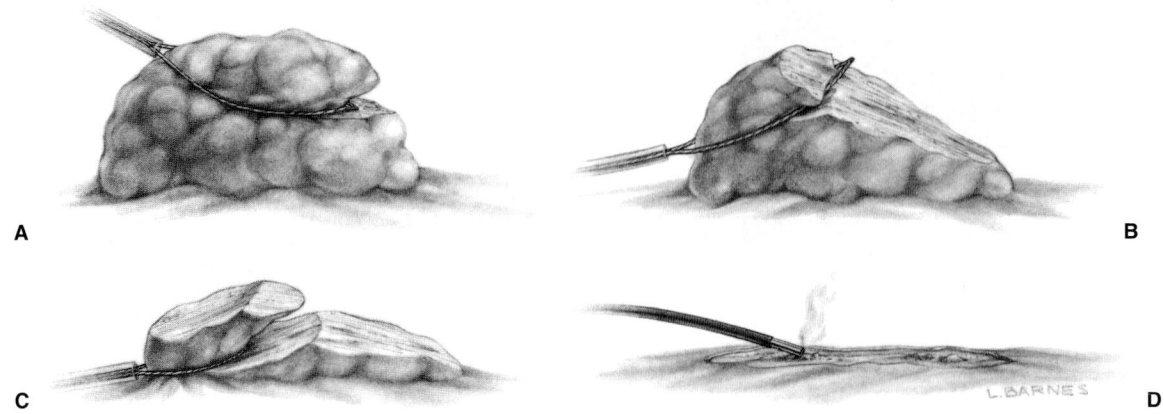

FIGURE 5-33. Technique for removal of a sessile polyp. **(A)** The polyp is ensnared. **(B)** The mucosa is elevated. **(C)** Excision is done piecemeal. **(D)** The residual polyp is removed and its base electrocoagulated.

endoscopically by the gastroenterologist, but could be successfully removed by the surgeon? Even with the increased possibility of perforation, a properly informed patient may be well served by colonoscopy-polypectomy even if operative intervention occasionally is required for a complication (see Complications). The bowel is well prepared, and morbidity and mortality should be very low indeed.

Results

Coller and colleagues reported colonoscopy on 146 patients with radiographically suspected polyps.[41] Of the 110 individuals found to have a neoplastic lesion, 62 were found to have an additional neoplasm (56%). It is because of this association that total colonoscopy is recommended for a patient found to harbor a colorectal neoplasm. Removing the lesion without such a complete evaluation is believed to be inadequate management.

Shinya and Wolff reported their experience of 7,000 polyps removed endoscopically.[167] There was no mortality. Most series, and the publications are numerous, report approximately two thirds of the lesions to be adenomatous polyps (i.e., tubular adenomas), a few as villous adenomas, and the remainder as malignant tumors, other benign neoplasms, and nonneoplastic conditions. The significance of polyps, their distribution, and the follow-up of patients are discussed in Chapter 21.

Complications

The sheer volume of examinations that have been performed since the introducion of colonoscopy has resulted in a broad spectrum of complications from both diagnostic as well as therapeutic endeavors. The frequency of complications, however, has remained fairly constant since the mid-1970s.

There are numerous complications that are associated with colonoscopy and colonoscopy-polypectomy. Generally, they may be attributed to certain predisposing causes: bowel preparation and medication, equipment misuse or malfunction, patient factors (e.g., communicable disease, underlying cardiocerebral-pulmonary-renal disease), and factors related to trauma coincident with the procedure.[85,122,156,158,164]

The following list shows the complications of colonoscopy and colonoscopy-polypectomy:

Hemorrhage due to intraluminal or mesenteric injury, seromuscular tear, splenic trauma
Perforation
Retroperitoneal abscess
Retroperitoneal and mediastinal emphysema
Vertebral venous air embolism
Pneumoscrotum
Pneumothorax
Explosion
Postcolonoscopy distension
Postpolypectomy coagulation syndrome
Colonic obstruction
Loss of polyp
Volvulus
Internal hernia
Bacteremia
Infections
Medical problems (e.g., pulmonary, cardiovascular, renal)
Mechanical failure

In 1976, Smith polled members of the American Society of Colon and Rectal Surgeons.[170] He learned from the 162 respondents that over 20,000 colonoscopies were performed. The overall complication rate was 0.4% for diagnostic colonoscopy and 1.8% for polypectomy. In like manner, Berci and colleagues questioned members of the Southern California Society for Gastrointestinal Endoscopy in 1974.[13] The incidence of perforation following colonoscopy and polypectomy (901 procedures) was 0.33%, whereas that following colonoscopy alone (3,850 procedures) was 0.25%. There was one death (0.02%). Bleeding occurred in 0.66% of polypectomized patients. Nivatvongs reported 19 complications following removal of 1,555 polyps, an incidence of 1.2%.[140] Bleeding was the most frequent problem. In these and in other studies, it becomes readily apparent that the incidence of complications decreases considerably as the examiner becomes more experienced. In the experience of the Ochsner Clinic group, in New Orleans, LA, over a 30-year period, more than 34,000 colonoscopies resulted in 31 perforations (0.09%).[9] It is probably axiomatic that therapeutic colonoscopy should not be performed until one achieves at least 50 diagnostic procedures.

Hemorrhage

Bleeding is the most common complication following polypectomy, representing 53% of all complications in the experience of Nivatvongs.[141] Hemorrhage can also be due to biopsy, laceration of the mucosa by the instrument, or tearing of the mesentery or the splenic capsule.[8,18,133,145] As previously suggested, those patients who are at an increased risk for bleeding must be identified and appropriate measures taken. Obtaining an adequate history before performing endoscopic procedures is therefore essential. Familiarity with the electrical equipment and use of coagulating current and the endoscopist's clinical experience reduce the risk of this complication (see Chapter 4). Inevitably, if the physician performs a sufficient number of examinations and procedures, bleeding will be encountered. Special caution should be employed when the endoscopist attempts removal of a polyp with a thick pedicle. Blended current is suggested by many experienced endoscopists under these circumstances. Intermittent application offers the best control and will most likely avoid precipitous transection. By alternately loosening and tightening the snare during the course of application of the current, a controlled division of the pedicle can be achieved more effectively.

The decision of how to manage the problem of bleeding depends on the magnitude of the hemorrhage. If bleeding is recognized at the time of polypectomy, the area should be resnared (if the pedicle is still apparent) and strangulated for at least 5 minutes. Electrocautery should not be used, especially if no pedicle is present. If the area is within reach of the rigid proctosigmoidoscope, it may be controlled by one of the means suggested in Chapter 4. In-hospital observation is mandatory if control has not been established with reasonable certainty, and operative intervention may be necessary if bleeding persists. This is particularly true if bleeding is secondary to a mesenteric tear or to splenic injury, both of which may not be readily apparent for several hours. Symptoms include the usual signs of hemorrhage (i.e., weakness, syncope, pallor, hypotension, and tachycardia), but abdominal pain and distension as well as left shoulder pain may also be observed. A falling hematocrit is obviously ominous. Although computed tomography (CT) may be helpful, the greatest aid to an early diagnosis is the knowledge that this complication may indeed occur.[55,83] A splenic subcapsular hematoma may be observed by means of CT as long as 10 days after colonoscopy.[131,179]

Gibbs and colleagues reported the Ochsner Clinic experience with postpolypectomy colonic hemorrhage.[79] During a 5-year period, more than 12,000 colonoscopies were performed at that institution, of which approximately one half required polypectomy or biopsy. The incidence of lower intestinal hemorrhage was 0.2% for individuals requiring hospitalization (13 patients). All episodes of bleeding occurred within 12 days following the procedure. Technetium-tagged red blood cell scintigraphy (see Chapter 28) was performed in all but one patient and was successful in localizing the bleeding in four (31%). In those with normal scintigrams, hemorrhage did not recur. Arteriography was performed in five individuals (38%), two of four with positive scintigrams; bleeding was controlled with selective vasopressin infusion. The fifth patient underwent vasopressin infusion without prior diagnostic study. In summary, of the 13 patients with hemorrhage, cessation occurred with rest and hydration in nine (69%), selective vasopressin infusion in three (23%), and endoscopic cautery in one (8%). No individual required surgical intervention. The authors concluded that technetium-tagged red blood cell scintigraphy identifies those individuals who have ongoing bleeding and in whom additional invasive procedures, such as arteriography or repeat endoscopy, are warranted.[79] I believe that this is an excellent algorithm for the management of postpolypectomy hemorrhage.

Perforation

Perforation of the colon with pneumoperitoneum usually becomes manifest almost immediately or within a few hours following the procedure. The incidence of perforation has been reported to range from 0.03% to 0.65% for diagnostic colonoscopies and from 0.07% to 2.1% for therapeutic endoscopies.[47,104,137] Perforation is usually due to polypectomy, to disease in the colon (e.g., diverticulitis), or to vigorous manipulation, rotation, or angulation of the instrument. Overdistension with air or gas can also precipitate a perforation. The embarrassing observation of an appendix epiploica during colonoscopy establishes the diagnosis with certainty. Ileal perforation following colonoscopy has also been reported.[138] This has been attributed to the rigidity of the small intestine that may be produced by prior abdominal surgery or by adhesions.

The classic presentations of transmural burn are fever, localized abdominal pain, tenderness, focal peritoneal signs, distension, and leukocytosis.[141] Again, inpatient treatment is required. Occasionally the patient's symptoms may be minimal relative to the amount of gas that is apparent on abdominal roentgenogram. In selected cases in which the bowel has been well prepared, cautious continued observation may be considered.[2] This is particularly true if the patient presents many hours or a day or two after the procedure. Nonsurgical management may be considered reasonable under the following circumstances[9,24,31,89,96]:

- Stable condition
- Late diagnosis
- Good bowel preparation
- Pneumoperitoneum not expanding
- No evidence for peritonitis
- No distal obstruction
- Improvement with supportive care
- Absence of underlying pathologic features that would ultimately require resection

Frequent follow-up evaluation is, of course, required. Oral intake should be withheld, and intravenous fluid replacement with broad-spectrum antibiotics is advisable. A limited water-soluble (Gastrografin) enema may also be considered in the equivocal situation (see Chapter 4). The sigmoid colon is the most common site of perforation. This may be because it is the area of greatest difficulty to negotiate and the most frequent location for pathologic findings (e.g., polyp, diverticulitis).

Laparotomy should be undertaken if the patient exhibits signs and symptoms of peritonitis. Furthermore, surgery is most definitely indicated in the presence of a large perforation demonstrated either colonoscopically or radiographically and in the setting of generalized peritonitis or ongoing sepsis.[47] The presence of concomitant pathologic features at the time of the perforation, such as a large sessile polyp that may be malignant, intractable colitis, or a perforation proximal to a colonic lesion that will inevitably require surgery, generally mandates that the physician proceed to immediate operation.[47] Fever and leukocytosis alone or in combination are not necessarily absolute indications for surgical intervention, but the burden of responsibility falls on the surgeon for unwarranted delay. A perforation that has sealed or even a negative laparotomy should not evoke criticism.

When a perforation is recognized shortly following the endoscopy, the hole or tear usually can be closed primarily without the need for a diversionary procedure if the bowel has been well prepared. If a resection is considered advisable, it can be safely undertaken without the need

for proximal colostomy or ileostomy unless sepsis or gross contamination is observed. Most surgeons and endoscopists agree that selective management of colonoscopic perforations is appropriate. It is recognized that perforations from therapeutic colonoscopy occur by a different mechanism than that from diagnostic colonoscopy and may be selectively managed without an operation.[9,107,120] Usually, perforations from diagnostic colonoscopy result in larger defects, and these are much more likely to require operative management.

As with prevention of hemorrhage, the risk of perforation is greatly reduced if intermittent bursts of current are applied. This reduces the likelihood of more extensive tissue injury, a consequence of transfer of heat into the deeper tissues or of contact of the polyp head with the bowel wall. When possible, an attempt should be made to suspend the polyp within the intestinal lumen during electrosurgical removal.[39]

Rectal perforation as a consequence of colonoscopy is extremely unusual; only one case has been reported, in which the patient developed a retroperitoneal abscess 1 month after the procedure.[146] The site of injury to the rectum was still evident at the time of presentation. One could expect that the frequency of this complication is higher than that reported in the literature, especially with the recommendation to employ RR routinely.

Subcutaneous, retroperitoneal, and mediastinal emphysema after colonoscopy have been reported, as well as pneumoscrotum, pneumothorax, and vertebral venous air embolism6,.[28,63,117,163,200] These presentations do not necessarily constitute indications for surgical exploration because free perforation of the colon is not implied. It is therefore important to distinguish between retroperitoneal and intraperitoneal gas. In the former situation, nonsurgical treatment should be the initial approach (see Figure 29-37). In fact, as stated earlier, close observation with antibiotic administration may be considered reasonable even with a pneumoperitoneum.

Comment

Perforations occurring in the course of diagnostic colonoscopy are most frequently located in the sigmoid colon and appear to be a consequence of manipulation and intubation. Twisting and stretching a redundant, narrow, or diverticular-loaded sigmoid colon represent particular areas of relative difficulty. Consequently, when trauma ensues, it is more likely to be a broader injury. A sharp bend in the deflection tip provides the potential for hidden injury, causing a longitudinal tear along the bowel wall, especially on the antimesenteric surface. Such defects, once created, are most likely to persist and require surgical intervention. A particularly jagged, broad defect usually requires resection. Conversely, perforation associated with polypectomy, hot biopsy excision, or laser therapy is usually a fairly discrete lesion that may seal rapidly.

Under these circumstances, the perforation may be treated nonoperatively through bowel rest and antibiotics. In any case, the decision of whether to operate is based upon clinical observation and a surgeon's good judgment.

Explosion

Explosion should not occur in a well-prepared colon, although as mentioned previously, the use of mannitol as a bowel preparation has been implicated as a causative factor. The use of an inert gas, such as carbon dioxide, has been advocated by some, but is probably an unnecessary caution (see previous discussion).[15] It should be remembered, however, that with an essentially closed system such as is present when colonoscopy-polypectomy is performed, there is no means for gas to escape once ignited. This is not true for the open-ended rigid proctosigmoidoscope. The examiner should be wary of using electric current if dissatisfied with the adequacy of the bowel preparation.

Postcolonoscopy Distension

A postcolonoscopy syndrome has been described, manifested by abdominal distension, discomfort, and dilated loops of bowel on the roentgenogram.[130,148] Patients do not exhibit signs of peritonitis. This is probably secondary to air insufflation, especially in a patient with an incompetent ileocecal valve. Treatment consists of observation and medical management.

Postpolypectomy Coagulation Syndrome

The postpolypectomy coagulation syndrome was described by Waye in 1981.[189] The patient may develop localized signs of peritonitis—pain, fever, and leukocytosis—without evidence of perforation on radiologic examination. The condition is believed to be due to transmural thermal injury of the bowel at the site of the polypectomy.[36,189] Treatment may require inpatient observation, intravenous fluid therapy, and broad-spectrum antibiotics.

Obstruction and Incarcerated Hernia and Internal Hernia

Colonic obstruction can be precipitated by colonoscopy, usually at the site of underlying sigmoid disease. Volvulus has also been reported, possibly secondary to the alpha maneuver or to overinsufflation of air. Incarceration of the colonoscope in an inguinal hernia that does not permit reduction of the hernia nor removal of the instrument has been reported, along with the technique for extraction.[112,196] An acute small bowel obstruction has been described as a consequence of a rent in the mesentery caused by a diagnostic colonoscopy.[32]

Loss of Polyp

All removed polyps should be submitted to histologic examination. Those less than 8 mm in diameter may be suctioned through the accessory channel of the colonoscope with the aid of a mucus trap.[36] If the polyp cannot be removed by the standard methods of suctioning onto the tip of the instrument or snare recapture, an enema is administered. The polyp is then evacuated with the fluid into a bedpan. Unfortunately, despite all reasonable efforts, a polyp is sometimes not recovered.

Bacteremia

Bacteremia has been reported to be associated with colonoscopy, but other studies have failed to confirm this observation.[44,53,114,143,144] Routine antibiotic prophylaxis is indicated for the high-risk patient (e.g., valvular heart disease, valve prosthesis; see Chapter 4).

Medical Problems

Hypotension, bradycardia, tachycardia, and myocardial infarction have all been observed during and after colonoscopy. Electrocardiogram monitoring with the addition of oxygen for patients at increased risk is worthy of consideration. Individuals with pacemakers may require a fixed rate if electrocoagulation is employed, even though there may be proper grounding and adequate shielding of the pacemaker. Herman and colleagues observed 233 consecutive patients who underwent colonoscopy for evidence of diaphoresis, bradycardia, or hypotension.[95] Of the 37 (16.5%) who demonstrated a vasovagal response, there was no difference with respect to the variables of examination difficulty, colon preparation, cardiopulmonary disease, or medications. However, there was a significantly greater dose of midazolam utilized in the vasovagal-response group. Furthermore, diverticulosis was more frequently observed in these patients.

Mechanical Failure

Numerous problems can develop from malfunction of the instruments and accessories (e.g., breakage of the colonoscope with entrapment of the instrument). Defective electrical equipment and inexperience with its use are two of the most common reasons for polypectomy hemorrhage and bowel wall necrosis. The snare wire can break or become fused with the polyp. Incomplete division of the pedicle can occur with the snare completely closed.

Conclusion

Despite the long list of complications, colonoscopy and colonoscopy-polypectomy can be undertaken with very low morbidity and very rare mortality—certainly lower mortality than may be anticipated after operative intervention.

Special Situations

Foreign Body Removal

The problems of removal of foreign bodies inserted into the rectum as well as ingested foreign bodies are addressed in Chapter 15. The colonoscope has been successfully employed for such extractions. For example, Frühmorgen removed a dental prosthesis as well as intestinal tubes by using this instrument (see Chapter 15).[73]

Volvulus

Colonoscopy has been successfully applied to the treatment of sigmoid volvulus.[78,159,175] Although rigid proctosigmoidoscopy is more readily available and easier to employ, there is the occasional situation when an attempt at reduction with a colonoscope may be indicated, especially when it involves more proximal bowel. The diagnosis and therapy of volvulus are discussed in Chapter 28.

Intraoperative Colonoscopy

Intraoperative colonoscopy may be considered in several situations:

When prior conventional colonoscopy has been unsuccessful
To evaluate the remainder of the colon when a partial resection is contemplated
To avoid contamination when an unsuspected polyp is found during a "clean" operation
To localize the site of a lesion or prior excision site, including with laparoscopic surgery
To complement arteriography in the diagnosis of the source of gastrointestinal hemorrhage[58,61,124,130,157]

The patient ideally is placed in the perineolithotomy position (see Figure 23-13) as if for combined abdominoperineal resection of the rectum. The abdominal surgeon guides the instrument through the bowel, thus expediting the procedure.

Comment

Although the application of this technique is limited, it may become of greater value in the diagnosis and treatment of lower gastrointestinal hemorrhage with improved methods for clearing liquid and clotted blood through the colonoscope.

Unfortunately, the requirement for intraoperative colonoscopy is often the result of failure to consider tat-tooing of the site of prior polyp removal or the willingness on the part of the surgeon to accept the information from the gastroenterologist as to the location of the lesion. The apothegm, "Don't let the enemy choose the territory!" is well advised when it comes to surgery for a small malignant tumor or a benign one. The surgeon must be circumspect or even a bit cynical when informed as to the location of such a lesion. Too often, a tumor that is proximal to the rectum is in "no man's land." One that is thought to be at 50 cm could be in the right or transverse colon, or even distal sigmoid. A straightforward operation then becomes an exercise in tedium and frustration, a situation that can usually be avoided. It would be imprudent and inappropriate indeed if a surgeon were to embark on a proposed low anterior resection without personally confirming the location of the lesion. With a more proximal tumor, however, the surgeon should at least feel reasonably confident that he or she knows exactly where that lesion is or, alternatively, expects to have no difficulty in finding it.

Pediatric Colonoscopy

Pediatric colonoscopy can be performed with a narrow-caliber endoscope or with the standard instrument, depending on the age of the patient. A general anesthetic is usually recommended for infants and young children. Preparation in infants usually consists of a clear liquid diet for 24 hours, but a laxative is usually advised for older children. Evaluation of rectal bleeding, suspicion of polyps, inflammatory bowel disease, and congenital anomalies are the most common indications for the procedure.[76,87,151,195] Colonoscopy is not useful in the evaluation of children with constipation and isolated recurrent abdominal pain.[108]

The technique for performing colonoscopy is somewhat modified when examination is undertaken in children, minimizing loop formation in order to provide greater comfort. Emphasis is made on intubating the terminal ileum as a standard part of pediatric colonoscopy because of its importance in the evaluation of Crohn's disease.[108] Obviously, children require close monitoring for respiratory depression, and resuscitation equipment with appropriate pediatric dosages should be readily available.

BARIUM ENEMA AND VIRTUAL COLONOSCOPY VERSUS COLONOSCOPY

There is no disagreement that colonoscopy is more likely to detect small excrescences than will a barium enema examination, even with an optimal preparation and double-contrast technique.[53,56,111,182,199] It is fallacious to assume, however, that the radiologist can determine whether a polyp is benign or malignant. This is a distinction that must be made by histologic examination. Virtual CT colonography has a diagnostic sensitivity similar to that of standard colonoscopy for lesions at least 5 or 6 mm in diameter,[115] but as with barium enema, any polyp that is identified will require a repeat examination and procedure with the colonoscope (see Chapter 4).

Anderson and colleagues reviewed the radiographs and clinical records of 26 patients with colorectal cancer missed on barium enema study and subsequently detected by colonoscopy.[7] More than one half were in the sigmoid colon and 8% in the rectum. In 76%, the cancer could be seen in retrospect. The most frequent error was caused by missing the lesion in a pool of barium, although the usual contributing factors, such as overlapping loops, were also observed. The authors advise double reporting of all barium enemas to improve detection rates.

For screening purposes, barium enema has historically been considered the procedure of choice, but the question is—screening for what population? Certainly, if it has been determined that the patient is in a higher risk group for the development of a neoplasm, periodic colonoscopy should be the diagnostic study employed (see Chapter 21). Furthermore, colonoscopy is recommended as the primary colonic evaluation for individuals with occult or obvious blood in the stool.[169] It has also been suggested by some investigators that colonoscopy be employed for asymptomatic, hemoccult-negative men older than 50 years of age, as part of a complete physical examination.[118,119] Others suggest that because of the low yield, the procedure should be limited to individuals who are at least 60 years of age.[154]

Any polyp discovered at the time of sigmoidoscopy requires the patient to undergo total colonoscopy rather than to employ barium enema or air-contrast enema. The need for a "road map" of the colon prior to colonoscopy is an outdated concept that is mentioned here only to refute it. Protocols have been developed for follow-up evaluation of patients with rectal polyps (see Chapter 21), all involving the use of colonoscopy. In my opinion, the primary benefit of barium enema is for evaluation of patients on whom a neoplasm is not suspected (e.g., extrinsic lesion or compression, diverticular disease, as part of physiologic assessment, or concomitant with defecography).

With respect to colonoscopic screening of individuals with a family history of colon cancer, the recommendation is less clear. According to Luchtefeld and colleagues, little rationale could be offered for the advisability of such screening in this group of family members.[121] Others, however, recommend colonoscopy in those older than 60 years of age with a family history of colon cancer.[11] In the evaluation of patients with chronic or occult gastrointestinal bleeding, colonoscopy is associated with fewer inconclusive examinations and more positive correct findings to explain the cause of bleeding than is barium enema.[129,142] Although the initial selection of lower gastrointestinal radiologic investigation for this indication cannot be criticized, studies suggest that colonoscopy in the first instance is the more pragmatic alternative, irrespective of the pattern of bleeding presentation.[33]

Opinion (John A. Coller, M.D.)

As improvements have been made in large bowel endoscopic visualization, so too have contrast radiologic examinations of the colon become more reliable. Depending upon the circumstances, colonoscopy and air-contrast barium enema may be either complementary or a duplication. Patients who are anemic, who have a positive occult blood determination, or who are bleeding should undergo colonoscopy as the primary evaluation of the colon. Certainly, if a contrast enema is performed and no lesion is found, colonoscopy would be mandatory. Additionally, if the contrast enema demonstrated a polyp or an equivocal lesion, a colonoscopy is required to remove the polyp or to resolve the ambiguous finding. The only reasons for reversing the order—that is, performing a barium enema after a colonoscopy—would be if the cecum were not achieved or if a nearly obstructing lesion prevented more proximal colonic evaluation.

REFERENCES

1. Abrams JS. A hard look at colonoscopy. *Am J Surg* 1977; 133:111.
2. Adair HM, Hishon S. The management of colonoscopic and sigmoidoscopic perforation of the large bowel. *Br J Surg* 1981;68:415.
3. Adam IJ, Ali Z, Shorthouse AJ. Inadequacy of colonoscopy revealed by three-dimensional electromagnetic imaging. *Dis Colon Rectum* 2001;44:978.
4. Adams, C, Atkin W, Cook C, et al. Past hysterectomy reduces completion rate and polyp detection rate at flexible sigmoidoscopy. *Dis Colon Rectum* 2002;45:A16.
5. Afridi SA, Barthel JS, King PD, et al. Prospective, randomized trial comparing a new sodium phosphate-bisacodyl regimen with conventional PEG-ES lavage for outpatient colonoscopy preparation. *Gastrointest Endosc* 1995;41:485.
6. Amshel AL, Shonberg IL, Gopal KA. Retroperitoneal and mediastinal emphysema as a complication of colonoscopy. *Dis Colon Rectum* 1982;25:167.
7. Anderson N, Cook HB, Coates R. Colonoscopically detected colorectal cancer missed on barium enema. *Gastrointest Radiol* 1991;16:123.
8. Anseline PF, Fazio VW. Management of massive postpolypectomy hemorrhage. *Dis Colon Rectum* 1982;25:251.
9. Araghizadeh FY, Timmcke A, Opelka FG, et al. Colonoscopic perforations. *Dis Colon Rectum* 2001;44:713.
10. Avgerinos A, Kalantzis N, Rekoumis G, et al. Bowel preparation and the risk of explosion during colonoscopic polypectomy. *Gut* 1984;25:361.
11. Baker JW, Gathright JB Jr, Timmcke AE, et al. Colonoscopic screening of asymptomatic patients with a family history of colon cancer. *Dis Colon Rectum* 1990;33:926.
12. Barclay RL, Depew WT, Vanner SJ. Carbohydrate-electrolyte rehydration protects against intravascular volume

contraction during colonic cleansing with orally administered sodium phosphate. *Gastrointest Endosc* 2002;56:633.

13. Berci G, Panish JF, Schapiro M, et al. Complications of colonoscopy and polypectomy. *Gastroenterology* 1974;67:584.

14. Berkowitz D. Disinfection and sterilization: recommended practices. *Endosc Rev* 1984;1:29.

15. Bigard MA, Gaucher P, Lassalle C. Fatal colonic explosion during colonoscopic polypectomy. *Gastroenterology* 1979;77:1307.

16. Blackstone MO, Riddell RH, Rogers BHG, et al. Dysplasia-associated lesion or mass (DALM) detected by colonoscopy in long-standing ulcerative colitis: an indication for colectomy. *Gastroenterology* 1981;80:366.

17. Bohlman TW, Katon RM, Lipshutz GR, et al. Fiberoptic pansigmoidoscopy: an evaluation and comparison with rigid sigmoidoscopy. *Gastroenterology* 1977;72:644.

18. Borsch G, Schmidt G. Endoscopy of the terminal ileum: diagnostic yield in 400 consecutive examinations. *Dis Colon Rectum* 1985;28:499.

19. Brand EJ, Sullivan BH, Sivak MV, et al. Colonoscopy in the diagnosis of unexplained rectal bleeding. *Ann Surg* 1980;192:111.

20. Breiter JR, Hajjar JJ. Segmental tuberculosis of the colon diagnosed by colonoscopy. *Am J Gastroenterol* 1981;76:369.

21. Brooker JC, Saunders BP, Shah SG, et al. Endoscopic resection of large sessile colonic polyps by specialist and non-specialist endoscopists. *Br J Surg* 2002;89:1020.

22. Burbige E, Bourke E, Tarder G. Effect of preparation for colonoscopy on fluid and electrolyte balance. *Gastrointest Endosc* 1978;24:286.

23. Caliendo F, Eisenstat T, Oliver G, et al. Anticoagulants: do they need to be held in preparation for colonoscopy? *Dis Colon Rectum* 2001;44:A5.

24. Carpio G, Albu E, Gumbs MA, et al. Management of colonic perforation after colonoscopy: report of three cases. *Dis Colon Rectum* 1989;32:624.

25. Carter HG. Short flexible fiberoptic colonoscopy in routine office examinations. *Dis Colon Rectum* 1981;24:17.

26. Cataldo PA. Colonoscopy without sedation: a viable alternative. *Dis Colon Rectum* 1996;39:257.

27. Chen M, Khanduja KS. Intubation of the ileocecal valve made easy. *Dis Colon Rectum* 1997;40:494.

28. Chorost MI, Wu JT, Webb H, et al. Vertebral venous air embolism: an unusual complication following colonoscopy. *Dis Colon Rectum* 2003;46:1138.

29. Christie JP. Colonoscopic excision of sessile polyps. *Am J Gastroenterol* 1976;66:23.

30. Christie JP. Colonoscopic excision of large sessile polyps. *Am J Gastroenterol* 1977;67:430.

31. Christie JP, Marazzo J III. "Miniperforation" of the colon: not all postpolypectomy perforations require laparotomy. *Dis Colon Rectum* 1991;34:132.

32. Chung H, Yuschak JV, Kukora JS. Internal hernia as a complication of colonoscopy: report of a case. *Dis Colon Rectum* 2003;46:1416.

33. Church JM. Analysis of the colonoscopic findings in patients with rectal bleeding according to the pattern of their presenting symptoms. *Dis Colon Rectum* 1991;34:391.

34. Church J, Delaney C. Randomized, controlled trial of CO_2 insufflation during colonoscopy. *Dis Colon Rectum* 2003;46:322.

35. Cirocco WC, Rusin LC. Confirmation of cecal intubation during colonoscopy. *Dis Colon Rectum* 1995;38:402.

36. Cohen LB, Waye JD. Treatment of colonic polyps: practical considerations. *Clin Gastroenterol* 1986;15:359.

37. Cohen SM, Wexner SD, Binderow SR, et al. Prospective, randomized endoscopic-blinded trial comparing precolonoscopy bowel cleansing methods. *Dis Colon Rectum* 1994;37:689.

38. Coller JA. Technique of flexible fiberoptic sigmoidoscopy. *Surg Clin North Am* 1980;60:465.

39. Coller JA. Complications of endoscopy of the colon and rectum. In: Ferrari BT, Ray JE, Gathright JB, eds. *Complications of colon and rectal surgery*. Philadelphia: WB Saunders, 1985;69.

40. Coller JA, Corman ML, Veidenheimer MC. Diagnostic and therapeutic applications of fiberoptic colonoscopy. *Geriatrics* 1974;29:67.

41. Coller JA, Corman ML, Veidenheimer MC. Colonic polypoid disease: need for total colonoscopy. *Am J Surg* 1976;131:490.

42. Corman ML. Landmark articles of the 20th century. *Semin Colon Rectal Surg* 1999;10:247–252.

43. Coman E, Brandt LJ, Brenner S, et al. Fat necrosis and inflammatory pseudotumor due to endoscopic tattooing of the colon with India ink. *Gastrointest Endosc* 1991;37:65.

44. Coughlin GP, Butler MHA, Grant AK. Colonoscopy and bacteraemia. *Gut* 1977;18:678.

45. Council on Scientific Affairs. Council report: lasers in medicine and surgery. *JAMA* 1986;256:900.

46. Crapp AR, Powis SJA, Tillotson P, et al. Preparation of the bowel by whole-gut irrigation. *Lancet* 1975;2:1239.

47. Damore LJ, Rantis PC, Vernava AM, et al. Colonoscopic perforations: etiology, diagnosis, and management. *Dis Colon Rectum* 1996;39:1308.

48. Davis GR, Santa Ana CA, Morawski SG, et al. Development of a lavage solution associated with minimal water and electrolyte absorption or secretion. *Gastroenterology* 1980;78:991.

49. Dean ACB, Newell JP. Colonoscopy in the differential diagnosis of carcinoma from diverticulitis of the sigmoid colon. *Br J Surg* 1973;60:633.

50. Dell'Abate P, Iosca A, Galimberti A, et al. Endoscopic treatment of colorectal benign-appearing lesions 3 cm or larger: techniques and outcome. *Dis Colon Rectum* 2001;44:112.

51. Desbaillets LG, Mangla JC. Pneumatosis cystoides intestinalis diagnosed by colonoscopy. *Gastrointest Endosc* 1974;20:126.

52. Dickinson RJ, Dixon MF, Axon ATR. Colonoscopy and the detection of dysplasia in patients with longstanding ulcerative colitis. *Lancet* 1980;2:620.

53. Dickman MD, Farrell R, Higgs RH, et al. Colonoscopy associated bacteremia. *Surg Gynecol Obstet* 1976;142:173.

54. DiPalma JA, Brady CE III, Stewart DL, et al. Comparison of colon cleansing methods in preparation for colonoscopy. *Gastroenterology* 1984;86:856.

55. Doctor NM, Monteleone F, Zarmakoupis C, et al. Splenic injury as a complication of colonoscopy and polypectomy: report of a case and review of the literature. *Dis Colon Rectum* 1987;30:967.

56. Dodds WJ, Stewart ET, Hogan WJ. Role of colonoscopy and roentgenology in the detection of polypoid colonic lesions. *Dig Dis Sci* 1977;22:646.

57. Dubow RA, Katon RM, Benner KG, et al. Short (35-cm) versus long (60-cm) flexible sigmoidoscopy: a comparison of findings and tolerance in asymptomatic patients screened for colorectal neoplasia. *Gastrointest Endosc* 1985;31:305.

58. Eisenberg HW. Fiberoptic colonoscopy: intraoperative colonoscopy. *Dis Colon Rectum* 1976;19:405.

59. Epstein M. Endoscopy: developments in optical instrumentation. *Science* 1980;210:280.

60. Ernstoff JJ, DeGrasia AH, Howard JBM, et al. A randomized blinded clinical trial of a rapid colonic lavage solution (Golytely) compared with standard preparation for colonoscopy and barium enema. *Gastroenterology* 1983;84:1512.

61. Farinon AM, Vadora E. Endometriosis of the colon and rectum: an indication for preoperative coloscopy. *Endoscopy* 1980;12:136.

62. Favero MS. Strategies for disinfection and sterilization of endoscopes: the gap between basic principles and actual practice. *Control Hosp Epidemiol* 1991;12:279.

63. Fishman EK, Goldman SM. Pneumoscrotum after colonoscopy. *Urology* 1981;18:171.
64. Fleischer D. Lasers and colon polyps. Technology and pathology: the courtship continues [Editorial]. *Gastroenterology* 1986;90:2024.
65. Fleischer D. Monitoring the patient receiving conscious sedation for gastrointestinal endoscopy: issues and guidelines. *Gastrointest Endosc* 1989;35:262.
66. Fleshner PR, Ackroyd FW, Shellito PC. The freckle sign: an endoscopic feature of the cecum. *Dis Colon Rectum* 1990;33:836.
67. Fong T-L, Valenzuela JE. Prevention of transmission of human immunodeficiency virus. *Practical Gastroenterol* 1990;14:12.
68. Forde KA, Lebwohl O, Wolff M, et al. Reversible ischemic colitis: correlation of colonoscopic and pathologic changes. *Am J Gastroenterol* 1979;72:182.
69. Foster GE, Vellacott KD, Balfour TW, et al. Outpatient flexible fiberoptic sigmoidoscopy, diagnostic yield and the value of glucagon. *Br J Surg* 1981;68:463.
70. Frager DH, Frager JD, Wolf EL, et al. Problems in the colonoscopic localization of tumors: continued value of the barium enema. *Gastrointest Radiol* 1987;12:343.
71. Franklin GO, Mohapatra M, Perrillo RP. Colonic tuberculosis diagnosed by colonoscopic biopsy. *Gastroenterology* 1979;76:362.
72. Frühmorgen P. Therapeutic colonoscopy. In: Hunt RH, Waye JD, eds. *Colonoscopy: techniques, clinical practice and colour atlas.* London: Chapman and Hall, 1981:199.
73. Frühmorgen P. Therapeutic colonoscopy. In: Hunt RH, Waye JD, eds. *Colonoscopy: techniques, clinical practice and colour atlas.* London: Chapman and Hall, 1981:222.
74. Frühmorgen P, Bodem F, Reidenbach HD, et al. Endoscopic laser coagulation of bleeding gastrointestinal lesions with report of the first therapeutic application in man. *Gastrointest Endosc* 1976;23:73.
75. Fujii T, Hasegawa RT, Saitoh Y, et al. Chromoscopy during colonoscopy. *Endoscopy* 2001;33:1036.
76. Gans SL. A new look at pediatric endoscopy. *Postgrad Med* 1977;61:91.
77. Geboes K, Vantrappen G. The value of colonoscopy in the diagnosis of Crohn's disease. *Gastrointest Endosc* 1975;22:18.
78. Ghazi A, Shinya H, Wolff WI. Treatment of volvulus of the colon by colonoscopy. *Ann Surg* 1976;183:263.
79. Gibbs DH, Opelka FG, Beck DE, et al. Postpolypectomy colonic hemorrhage. *Dis Colon Rectum* 1996;39:806.
80. Girard CM, Rugh KS, DiPalma JA, et al. Comparison of Golytely lavage with standard diet/cathartic preparation for double contrast barium enema. *AJR Am J Roentgenol* 1984;142:1147.
81. Goldman J, Reichelderfer M. Evaluation of rapid colonoscopy preparation using a new gut lavage solution. *Gastrointest Endosc* 1982;28:9.
82. Golub RW, Kerner BA, Wise WE Jr, et al. Colonoscopic bowel preparations: which one? A blinded, prospective, randomized trial. *Dis Colon Rectum* 1995;38:594.
83. Gores PF, Simon LA. Splenic injury during colonoscopy. *Arch Surg* 1989;124:1342.
84. Gould SR, Williams CB. Castor oil or senna preparation before colonoscopy for inactive chronic ulcerative colitis. *Gastrointest Endosc* 1982;28:6.
85. Graham J, Eusebio EB. Complications of colonoscopy. *IMJ* 1977;152:39.
86. Griffin JW Jr. Flexible fiberoptic sigmoidoscopy: longer may not be better for the "nonendoscopist" [Editorial]. *Gastrointest Endosc* 1985;31:347.
87. Habr-Gama A, Alves PRA, Gama-Rodrigues JJ, et al. Pediatric colonoscopy. *Dis Colon Rectum* 1979;22:530.
88. Hagihara PF, Ernst CB, Griffen WO. Incidence of ischemic colitis following abdominal aortic reconstruction. *Surg Gynecol Obstet* 1979;149:571.
89. Hall C, Dorricott NJ, Donovan IA, et al. Colon perforation during colonoscopy: surgical versus conservative management. *Br J Surg* 1991;78:542.
90. Hanson JM, Atkin WS, Cunliffe WJ, et al. Rectal retroflexion: an essential part of lower gastrointestinal endoscopic examination. *Dis Colon Rectum* 2001;44:1706.
91. Hanson PJV, Gor D, Jeffries DJ, et al. Elimination of high titre HIV from fibreoptic endoscopes. *Gut* 1990;31:657.
92. Hartke RH Jr, Gonzalez-Rothi RJ, Abbey NC. Midazolam-associated alterations in cardiorespiratory function during colonoscopy. *Gastrointest Endosc* 1989;35:232.
93. Hedrick E. Guidelines for cleaning and disinfection of flexible fiberoptic endoscopes (FFE) used in GI endoscopy. *J Am Pract Infect Control* 1978;6:8.
94. Herman FN. Avoidance of sedation during total colonoscopy. *Dis Colon Rectum* 1990;33:70.
95. Herman LL, Kurtz RC, McKee KJ, et al. Risk factors associated with vasovagal reactions during colonoscopy. *Gastrointest Endosc* 1993;39:388.
96. Ho HC, Burchell S, Morris P, et al. Colon perforation, bilateral pneumothoraces, pneumopericardium, pneumomediastinum, and subcutaneous emphysema complicating endoscopic polypectomy: anatomic and management considerations. *Ann Surg* 1996;62:770.
97. Hogan WJ, Hensley GT, Greenen JE. Endoscopic evaluation of inflammatory bowel disease. *Med Clin North Am* 1980;64:1083.
98. Hopkins HH, Kapany NS. A flexible fiberscope using static scanning. *Nature* 1954;173:39.
99. Hunt RH, Waye JD, eds. *Colonoscopy: techniques, clinical practice and colour atlas.* London: Chapman and Hall, 1981.
100. Hunter JG, Bowers, Burt RW, et al. Lasers in endoscopic gastrointestinal surgery. *Am J Surg* 1984;148:736.
101. Hurlstone DP, Fujii T, Lobo AJ. Early detection of colorectal cancer using high-magnification chromoscopic colonoscopy. *Br J Surg* 2002;89:272.
102. Huynh T, Vanner S, Paterson W. Safety profile of 5-h oral sodium phosphate regimen for colonoscopy cleansing: lack of clinically significant hypocalcemia or hypovolemia. *Am J Gastroenterol* 1995;90:104.
103. Hyman N, Waye JD. Endoscopic four quadrant tattoo for the identification of colonic lesions at surgery. *Gastrointest Endosc* 1991;37:56.
104. Jentschura D, Raute M, Winter J, et al. Complications in endoscopy of the lower gastrointestinal tract: therapy and prognosis. *Surg Endosc* 1994;8:672.
105. Jonas G, Mahoney A, Murray J, et al. Chemical colitis due to endoscope cleaning solutions: a mimic of pseudomembranous colitis. *Gastroenterology* 1988;95:1403.
106. Kaczmarek RG, Moore RM, McCrohan J, et al. Multi-state investigation of the actual disinfection/sterilization of endoscopes in health care facilities. *Am J Med* 1992;92:257.
107. Kavin H, Sinicrope F, Esker AH. Management of perforation of the colon at colonoscopy. *Am J Gastroenterol* 1992;87: 161.
108. Kay M, Wylie R. Pediatric colonoscopy. *Practical Gastroenterol* 1997;26:7.
109. Kelley CJ, Ingoldby CJH, Blenkharn JI, et al. Colonoscopy related endotoxemia. *Surg Gynecol Obstet* 1985;161:332.
110. Ker T, Run J, Beart R. Aspirin can be safely continued in preparation of colonoscopy. *Dis Colon Rectum* 2002;45: A16.
111. Kolts BE, Lyles WE, Achem SR, et al. A comparison of the effectiveness and patient tolerance of oral sodium phosphate, castor oil, and standard electrolyte lavage for colonoscopy or sigmoidoscopy preparation. *Am J Gastroenterol* 1993;88:1218.
112. Koltun WA, Coller JA. Incarceration of colonoscope in an inguinal hernia: "pulley" technique of removal. *Dis Colon Rectum* 1991;34:191.
113. Koo J, Ho J, Ong GB. The value of colonoscopy in the diagnosis of ileo-caecal tuberculosis. *Endoscopy* 1982;14:48.

114. Kumar S, Abcarian H, Prasad ML, et al. Bacteremia associated with lower gastrointestinal endoscopy, fact or fiction? *Dis Colon Rectum* 1982;25:131.

115. Laghi A, Iannaccone R, Carbone I, et al. Detection of colorectal lesions with virtual computed tomographic colonography. *Am J Surg* 2002; 183:124.

116. Lehman GA, Buchner DM, Lappas JC. Anatomical extent of fiberoptic sigmoidoscopy. *Gastroenterology* 1983;84:803.

117. Lezak MB, Goldhamer M. Retroperitoneal emphysema after colonoscopy. *Gastroenterology* 1974;66:118.

118. Lieberman DA, Smith FW. Screening for colon malignancy with colonoscopy. *Am J Gastroenterol* 1991;86:946.

119. Liebermna DA, Weiss DG, Bond JH, et al. Use of colonoscopy to screen asymptomatic adults for colorectal cancer. *N Engl J Med* 2000;343:162.

120. Lo AY, Beaton HL. Selective management of colonic perforations. *J Am Coll Surg* 1994;179:333.

121. Luchtefeld MA, Syverson D, Solfelt M, et al. Is colonoscopic screening appropriate in asymptomatic patients with family history of colon cancer? *Dis Colon Rectum* 1991;34:763.

122. Marino AWM. Complications of colonoscopy. *Dis Colon Rectum* 1979;21:15.

123. Marks G, Boggs HW, Castro AF, et al. Sigmoidoscopic examinations with rigid and flexible fiberoptic sigmoidoscopes in the surgeon's office. *Dis Colon Rectum* 1979;22:162.

124. Martin PJ, Forde KA. Intraoperative colonoscopy: preliminary report. *Dis Colon Rectum* 1979;22:234–237.

125. Mathus-Vliegen EMH, Tytgat GNJ. Nd:YAG laser photocoagulation in colorectal adenoma: evaluation of its safety, usefulness, and efficacy. *Gastroenterology* 1986;90:1865.

126. Matter SE, Rice PS, Campbell DR. Colonic lavage solutions: plain versus flavored. *Am J Gastroenterol* 1993;88:49.

127. Matteucci DJ, Organ CH Jr, Dykstra M, et al. Efficacy of a simplified lower gastrointestinal flexible endoscope cleaning method. *Dis Colon Rectum* 1985;28:653.

128. Max MH, Knutson CO. Colonoscopy in patients with inflammatory colonic strictures. *Surgery* 1978;84:551.

129. Maxfield RG. Colonoscopy as a primary diagnostic procedure in chronic gastrointestinal bleeding. *Arch Surg* 1986; 121:401.

130. Mendoza CB, Watne AL. Value of intraoperative colonoscopy in vascular ectasia of the colon. *Am Surg* 1982;48: 153.

131. Merchant AA, Cheng EH. Delayed splenic rupture after colonoscopy. *Am J Gastroenterol* 1990;85:906.

132. Milsom JW, Gottesman L. A suction retriever to expedite recovery of colonic polyps. *Dis Colon Rectum* 1987;30:644.

133. Millward SF, Chapman A, Somers S, et al. Rectal biopsy as a cause of rectal ulceration. *Radiology* 1985;156:42.

134. Minervini S, Alexander-Williams J, Donovan IA, et al. Comparison of three methods of whole bowel irrigation. *Am J Surg* 1980;140:400.

135. Myren J, Serck-Hanssen A, Solberg L. Routine and blind histological diagnoses on colonoscopic biopsies compared to clinical-colonoscopic observations in patients without and with colitis. *Scand J Gastroenterol* 1976;11:135.

136. Naveau S, Bonhomme L, Preaux N, et al. A pure charcoal suspension for colonoscopic tattoo. *Gastrointest Endosc* 1991;37:624.

137. Nelson RL, Abcarian H, Prasad ML. Iatrogenic perforation of the colon and rectum. *Dis Colon Rectum* 1982;25:305.

138. Nemeh HW, Ranzinger MR, Dutro JA. Mid-ileal perforation secondary to colonoscopy. *Am Surg* 1994;60:228.

139. Newstead GL, Morgan BP. Bowel preparation with mannitol. *Med J Aust* 1979;2:582.

140. Nivatvongs S. Complications in colonoscopic polypectomy: an experience with 1555 polypectomies. *Dis Colon Rectum* 1986;29:825.

141. Nivatvongs S. Complications in colonoscopic polypectomy: lessons to learn from an experience of 1576 polyps. *Am Surg* 1988;54:61.

142. Nord HJ. The workup of a patient with a positive fecal occult blood test: one procedure? Two procedures? *Am J Gastroenterol* 1991;86:542.

143. Norfleet RG, Mitchell PD, Mulholland DD. Does bacteremia follow colonoscopy? II. *Gastrointest Endosc* 1976;23: 31.

144. Norfleet RG, Mulholland DD, Mitchell PD, et al. Does bacteremia follow colonoscopy? *Gastroenterology* 1976;70:20.

145. Ong E, Böhmler U, Wurbs D. Splenic injury as a complication of endoscopy: two case reports and a literature review. *Endoscopy* 1991;23:302.

146. Ostyn B, Bercoff E, Manchon ND, et al. Retroperitoneal abscess complicating colonoscopy polypectomy. *Dis Colon Rectum* 1987;30:201.

147. Overholt BF. Colonoscopy: a review. *Gastroenterology* 1975; 68:1308.

148. Palakanis KC, DeNobile JW, Sweeney WB, et al. Effect of music therapy on state anxiety in patients undergoing flexible sigmoidoscopy. *Dis Colon Rectum* 1994;37:478.

149. Park SI, Genta RS, Romeo DP, et al. Colonic abscess and focal peritonitis secondary to India ink tattooing of the colon. *Gastrointest Endosc* 1991;37:68.

150. Petrini JL Jr. Terminal ileal intubation at colonoscopy. *Gastrointest Endosc* 1989;35:182(abst 133).

151. Plucnar BJ. Colonoscopy in infancy and childhood with special regard to patient preparation and examination technique. *Endoscopy* 1981;13:14.

152. Ransohoff DF, Lang CA. Sigmoidoscopic screening in the 1990s. *JAMA* 1993;269:1278.

153. Rauh SM, Coller JA, Schoetz DJ Jr. Fluoroscopy in colonoscopy: who is using it and why? *Am Surg* 1989;55:669.

154. Rex DK, Lehman GA, Hawes RH, et al. Screening colonoscopy in asymptomatic average-risk persons with negative fecal occult blood tests. *Gastroenterology* 1991;100:64.

155. Rodriguez W, Levine JS. Enterococcal endocarditis following flexible sigmoidoscopy. *West J Med* 1984;140:951.

156. Rogers BHG, Silvis SE, Nebel OT, et al. Complications of flexible fiberoptic colonoscopy and polypectomy. *Gastrointest Endosc* 1975;22:73.

157. Saclarides TJ, Wolff BG, Pemberton JH, et al. Clean sweep of the colon: the use of intraoperative colonoscopy. *Dis Colon Rectum* 1989;32:864.

158. Sands J. Quoted by Masel H, Masel JP, Casey KV. A survey of colon examination techniques in Australia and New Zealand, with a review of complications. *Australas Radiol* 1971;15:140.

159. Sanner CJ, Saltzman DA. Detorsion of sigmoid volvulus by colonoscopy. *Gastrointest Endosc* 1977;23:212.

160. Sardinha TC, Wexner SD, Gilliland J, et al. Efficiency and productivity of a sheathed fiberoptic sigmoidoscope compared with a conventional sigmoidoscope. *Dis Colon Rectum* 1997;40:1248.

161. Saunders BP, Bell GD, Williams CB, et al. First clinical results with a real time, electronic imager as an aid to colonoscopy. *Gut* 1995;36:913.

162. Schapiro M. Electronic video endoscopy: a comprehensive review of the newest technology and techniques. *Practical Gastroenterol* 1986;10:8.

163. Schmidt G, Börsch G, Wegener M. Subcutaneous emphysema and pneumothorax complicating diagnostic colonoscopy. *Dis Colon Rectum* 1986;29:136.

164. Schwesinger WH, Levine BA, Ramos R. Complications of colonoscopy. *Surg Gynecol Obstet* 1979;148:270.

165. Shatz BA, Thavorides V. Colonic tattoo for follow-up of endoscopic sessile polypectomy. *Gastrointest Endosc* 1991;37: 59.

166. Shields N. A survey of the costs of flexible endoscope cleaning and disinfection. *Gastroenterol Nurs* 1993;16:53.

167. Shinya H, Wolff WI. Morphology, anatomic distribution and cancer potential of colonic polyps. *Ann Surg* 1979; 190:679.

168. Sivak MV. Video endoscopy. *Clin Gastroenterol* 1986;15:205.

169. Smith GA, Oien KA, O'Dwyer PJ. Frequency of early colorectal cancer in patients undergoing colonoscopy. *Br J Surg* 1999;86:1328.
170. Smith LE. Fiberoptic colonoscopy: complications of colonoscopy and polypectomy. *Dis Colon Rectum* 1976;19:407.
171. Sobala GM, Lincoln C, Axon ATR. Does the endoscope control head need to be disinfected between examinations? *Endoscopy* 1989;21:19.
172. Spach DH, Silverstein FE, Stamm WE. Transmission of infection by gastrointestinal endoscopy and bronchoscopy. *Ann Intern Med* 1993;118:117.
173. Spencer RJ, Wolff BG, Ready RL. Comparison of the rigid sigmoidoscope and the flexible sigmoidoscope in conjunction with colon x-ray for detection of lesions of the colon and rectum. *Dis Colon Rectum* 1983;26:653.
174. Stevens AF. Colonoscopy in the irritable bowel syndrome. *Gut* 1973;14:432.
175. Sugarbaker PH, Vineyard GC, Lewicki AM, et al. Colonoscopy in the management of diseases of the colon and rectum. *Surg Gynecol Obstet* 1974;139:341.
176. Tabibian N, Michaletz PA, Schwartz JT, et al. Use of an endoscopically placed clip can avoid diagnostic errors in colonoscopy. *Gastrointest Endosc* 1988;34:262.
177. Tawile NT, Priest RJ, Schuman BM. Colonoscopy in inflammatory bowel disease. *Gastrointest Endosc* 1975;22:11.
178. Taylor EW, Bentley S, Youngs S, et al. Bowel preparation and the safety of colonoscopic polypectomy. *Gastroenterology* 1981;81:1.
179. Taylor FC, Frankl HD, Riemer KD. Late presentation of splenic trauma after routine colonoscopy. *Am J Gastroenterol* 1989;84:442.
180. Tedesco FJ. Antibiotic associated pseudomembranous colitis with negative proctosigmoidoscopy. *Gastroenterology* 1979;77:295.
181. Tedesco FJ, Pickens CA, Griffin JW, et al. Role of colonoscopy in patients with unexplained melena: analysis of 53 patients. *Gastrointest Endosc* 1981;27:221.
182. Thoeni RF, Menuck L. Comparison of barium enema and colonoscopy in the detection of small colonic polyps. *Radiology* 1977;124:631.
183. Timothy SKC, Hicks TC, Opelka FG, et al. Colonoscopy in the patient requiring anticoagulation. *Dis Colon Rectum* 2001;44:1845.
184. Vanner SJ, MacDonald PH, Paterson WG, et al. A randomized prospective trial comparing oral sodium phosphate with standard polyethylene glycol–based lavage solution (Golytely) in the preparation of patients for colonoscopy. *Am J Gastroenterol* 1990;85:422.
185. Vukasin P, Weston LA, Beart RW. Oral Fleet Phospho-Soda laxative-induced hyperphosphatemia and hypocalcemia tetany in an adult: report of a case. *Dis Colon Rectum* 1997;40:497.
186. Waye JD. Colonoscopy: a clinical view. *Mt Sinai J Med* 1975;42:1.
187. Waye JD. Colitis, cancer and colonoscopy. *Med Clin North Am* 1978;62:211.
188. Waye JD. Colonoscopy intubation techniques without fluoroscopy. In: Hunt RH, Waye JD, eds. *Colonoscopy: techniques, clinical practice and colour atlas.* London: Chapman and Hall, 1981:170.
189. Waye JD. The postpolypectomy coagulation syndrome. *Gastrointest Endosc* 1981;27:184.
190. Waye JD, Bashkoff E. Total colonoscopy: is it always possible? *Gastrointest Endosc* 1991;37:152.
191. Waye JD, Yessayan SA, Lewis BS, et al. The technique of abdominal pressure in total colonoscopy. *Gastrointest Endosc* 1991;37:147.
192. Webb WA. Colonoscoping the "difficult" colon. *Am Surg* 1991;57:178.
193. Wexner SD, Eisen GM, Simmang C. Principles of privileging and credentialing for endoscopy and colonoscopy. *Dis Colon Rectum* 2002;45:161.
194. Wherry DC, Thomas WM. The yield of flexible fiberoptic sigmoidoscopy in the detection of asymptomatic colorectal neoplasia. *Surg Endosc* 1994;8:393.
195. Williams CB, Laage NJ, Campbell CA, et al. Total colonoscopy in children. *Arch Dis Child* 1982;57:49.
196. Williard W, Satava R. Inguinal hernia complicating flexible sigmoidoscopy. *Am Surg* 1990;56:800.
197. Winnan G, Berci G, Panish J, et al. Superiority of the flexible to the rigid sigmoidoscope in routine proctosigmoidoscopy. *N Engl J Med* 1980;302:1011.
198. Wolff WI, Shinya H. Polypectomy via the fiberoptic colonoscope: removal of neoplasms beyond the reach of the sigmoidoscope. *N Engl J Med* 1973;288:329.
199. Wolff WI, Shinya H, Geffen A, et al. Comparison of colonoscopy and the contrast enema in five hundred patients with colorectal disease. *Am J Surg* 1975;129:181.
200. Yassinger S, Midgley RC, Cantor DS, et al. Retroperitoneal emphysema after colonoscopic polypectomy. *West J Med* 1978;128:347.

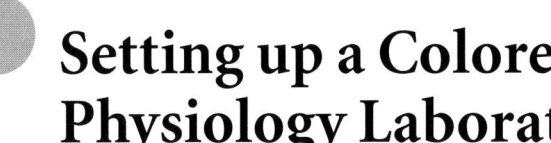

Chapter 6

Setting up a Colorectal Physiology Laboratory

Guest Contributors: Steven D. Wexner, T. Cristina Sardinha, and Robert Gilliland

It has been recognized that the colorectal physiology laboratory at the Cleveland Clinic, Florida is one of the premier centers in the world for these investigative efforts. Dr. Wexner is Chairman of the Department, Dr. Sardinha at the time of this writing was a Resident in Colon and Rectal Surgery, and Dr. Gilliland is now a Consultant General and Colorectal Surgeon in Londonderry, Northern Ireland. I am delighted that this chapter has been contributed by such authorities.

MLC

Pathology is the accomplished tragedy; physiology is the basis on which our treatment rests.

Samuel Butler

Since the mid-1980s, evaluation of the physiology of the anus, rectum, and colon has become an increasingly important concept in the management of the conditions affecting this area.[88,137,216] Such testing has not only advanced our understanding of the physiologic processes but has also provided requisite information for optimal treatment.[158,211] A search for an understanding of the pathophysiology of disorders of evacuation, constipation, incontinence, and rectal prolapse has stimulated many clinicians and institutions to establish their own physiology laboratories. Indeed the presence of an active anorectal physiology laboratory has become a requisite for training in colorectal surgery in the United States and in the United Kingdom. Some of these tests provide important diagnostic information and are available in most laboratories. Other investigations are predominantly research tools that are used when one has a basic science interest or when there is a mission to develop new technologies. In this chapter, most of the currently available tests are discussed along with their applicability to both clinical practice and research. However, methodologic details about the performance of all procedures are not necessarily described. The primary purpose of this chapter is to outline the available choices and to discuss the relative merits of each, in order to enable a clinician to make informed decisions concerning which equipment

to purchase when setting up his or her own laboratory. Fine books and monographs are available that provide a more extensive discussion on this subject.[25,215,241]

No single test can adequately define the status of the anorectum either in health or when diseased. Accurate diagnosis depends on the integration of an adequate history and clinical examination along with several physiologic investigations. Thus any functioning laboratory must have the resources, space, and personnel to perform several different physiologic studies. Setting up a new laboratory is an expensive venture, and administrative authorities may understandably require a cost-benefit analysis or business plan in this new cost center. Required data include anticipated case volumes and reimbursements.

Still, much of the capital outlay can be minimized if intradepartmental arrangements can be made to share rooms, equipment, and ancillary personnel. For example, the computer hardware equipment, which can be used for both esophageal and anorectal manometry, can be purchased jointly by gastroenterology and colorectal departments. Specific software packages and catheters can then be acquired. Similarly, an ultrasound scanner can be shared among gynecologists, urologists, and colorectal surgeons, with each using a specific probe. Defecography can be performed in a standard fluoroscopy suite, and electromyography (EMG) equipment can be shared with the neurology department.

Ideally, the various tests should be available in close proximity so that they can be performed in a relatively short time and with minimal inconvenience to the patient. The number of required personnel is dependent on the volume of tests undertaken each day. Many units have specifically trained nursing staff to perform these tests under appropriate supervision. The same nurses who perform a given procedure for one department can also perform the analogous procedure for the department sharing the equipment.

MANOMETRY

Anorectal manometry is an objective method of assessing anal muscular tone, rectal compliance, and anorectal sensation and of verifying the integrity of the rectoanal inhibitory reflex (RAIR). Unfortunately, there is no standardized methodology for obtaining and analyzing this information. Therefore, because no single method is universally accepted, manometric data from different institutions are difficult to compare. Available techniques include water- or air-filled balloons, sleeve catheters, pressure tranducers, and water-filled catheters.[10] Regardless of the method chosen, it is imperative that manometry be performed in a precise and reproducible manner and that measured parameters are clearly defined. Furthermore, each individual laboratory must ascertain the range of normal values in its specific population.

Indications

Manometry has been widely used in the investigation of patients with fecal incontinence to identify the presence of sensory or muscular defects as well as to define functional weakness of the internal and/or external anal sphincter. Patients with fecal incontinence or proctitis may present with significant loss of the ability to sense rectal distension.[228] A maximal tolerable volume less than 100 ml may indicate visceral hypersensitivity, poor compliance, or rectal irritability. Manometry is also used to document sphincter function before procedures that may affect continence or require optimal continence (e.g., colonic or ileal pouch-anal anastomosis).[160] Manometry may be helpful in the evaluation of chronic constipation, especially in children, young adults, and those with a lifelong history.[135] This diagnostic modality has also been of great value in assessing patients with Hirschsprung's and Chagas' disease by demonstrating the absence of the RAIR.[160] Manometry, although not a first-line investigation, has been used in the evaluation of may other anal and colorectal conditions.[17,65,88,82,187]

Patient Preparation

The following comments are applicable to the performance of all static manometric examinations. The use of enemas to empty the rectum before examination is somewhat controversial. Some believe that measurements should be taken in the normal or "as is" state. Other physicians contend that reproducible results require some element of uniformity, and that the presence of a variable amount of stool within the rectum may affect the validity of the data, especially the sensory threshold and maximal tolerable volume. These authors recommend the use of one or more sodium phosphate enemas (C.B. Fleet Co., Inc. Lynchburg, VA) to clear the rectum

adequately. The enemas should be taken at least 2 hours before the procedure because they may alter sphincter tone and motility patterns.[83,156] For similar reasons, if same-day endoscopy is planned, it should be performed *after* rather than before manometry.

The purpose and nature of the procedure should be explained to the patient in order to allay any anxiety. It should be emphasized that anorectal manometry is painless. If a water perfusion system is being used, the person should be warned that he or she may experience some leakage onto the buttocks. Furthermore, one may experience some fullness and perhaps the need to evacuate during the elicitation of the RAIR as well as the testing of sensation, capacity, and compliance. In the past, patients were positioned on an examination couch that was capable of being raised or lowered so that the water-perfused catheters were at the same level as the transducers. However, most current software programs have the capacity to reset the baseline regardless of the level of the patient. Examinations should be performed in the left lateral, decubitus position with the patient's hips flexed to as near 90 degrees as is comfortable. During the acquisition of the data, the individual should be discouraged from excessive talking or motion because this may introduce artifact into the recording.

Anorectal Manometry Systems

There are three basic types of systems used for performing manometric examinations: air- or water-filled balloon systems, water perfusion systems and solidstate microtransducer systems.

Air-Water-Filled Balloon Systems

In these systems, fluid- or air-filled balloons are placed within the anus and rectum and are connected to transducers via small catheters. One of the early designs was that of Schuster and colleagues.[205] This device consists of a hollow metal tube 4 inches in length surrounded by a latex balloon tied in such a way so as to create two separate compartments. Each balloon communicates with a pressure transducer via two plastic catheters. A further balloon can be placed into the rectum via the metal tube. The apparatus is placed in the rectum so that the internal balloon is surround by the internal sphincter and the external balloon is encircled by the superficial fibers of the external anal sphincter (Figure 6-1).[206] The device is set by inflating the rectal balloon to elicit the RAIR, which automatically seats the catheter in position. Thereafter, mean resting and squeeze pressures, the presence of the RAIR, rectal sensitivity, and compliance can all be assessed.

Theoretically, this device should be able to assess pressures from the internal and external anal sphincter sepa-

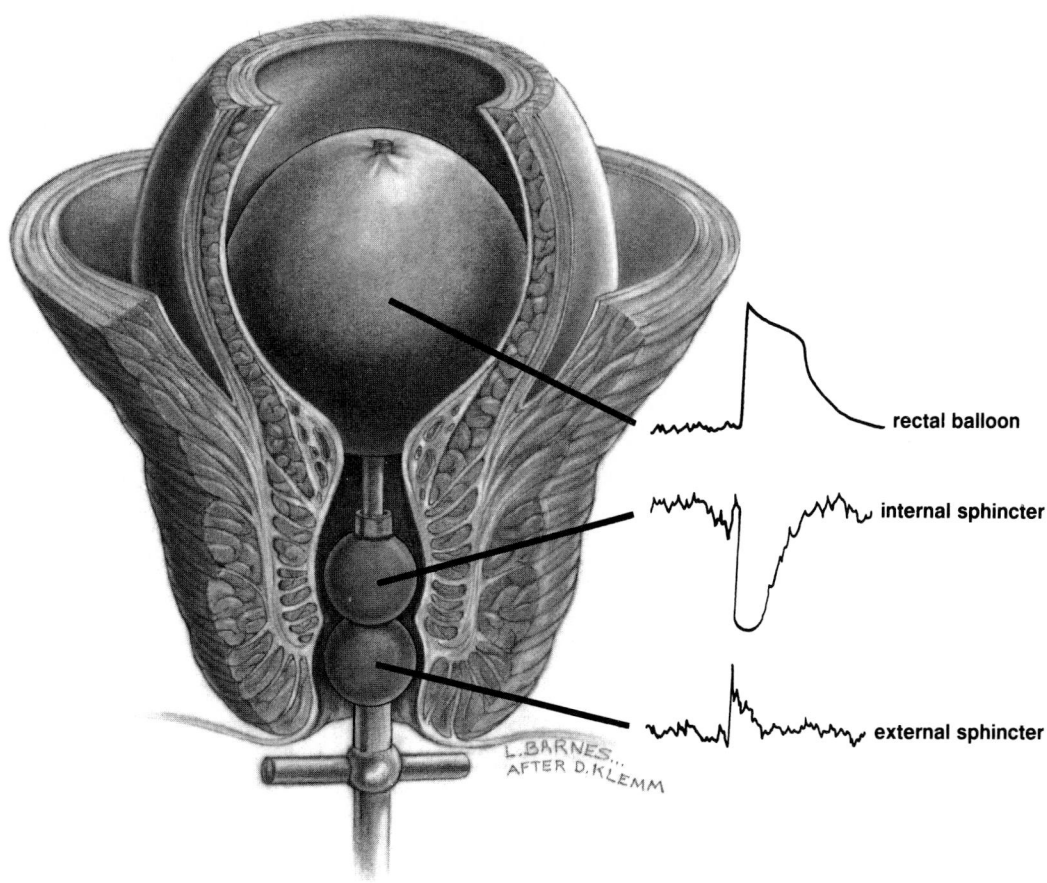

rectal balloon

internal sphincter

external sphincter

L. BARNES
AFTER D. KLEMM

FIGURE 6-1. Anorectal manometric tracings indicate the pressure changes at each level after distension of the balloon in the ampulla. (Adapted from Rosen LS, Khubchandani IT, Sheets JA, et al. Management of anal incontinence. *J Am Fam Pract* 1986;33:129, with permission.)

rately, but in practice the overlap of these two muscles is too great to allow differentiation.[205] Furthermore, because pressures within the anus are in part influenced by the distortion of the anal canal, a probe with a large balloon yields a greater pressure than does one with a smaller balloon in the same subject.[79,227] In addition, rapid distension of the balloon will generate a higher pressure.[79,227] One final area for confusion with this method is that air is compressible, and the pressures recorded may be somewhat lower than the true values.

These disadvantages prompted the development of another balloon system that uses smaller, water-filled balloons (Marquat Company, Boissy-Saint-Léger Cedex, France).[79] However, although accurate assessments can be performed with these catheters, they permit measurement of only a limited area of the anal canal.[90]

Both these systems are relatively simple, and once placed they do not require further movement. Investigations, therefore, can be performed by one operator. However, the information ascertainable from these systems is relatively limited because the pressure measured is the sum of all forces acting upon the balloon. Thus, only deter-

minations of the global resting and squeeze pressures of the anal canal can be obtained. Indeed, because as implied, larger balloons produce more distortion of the anal canal, basal pressure measurements may be unreliable, with only the changes in pressure being reproducible.[79] The presence of the RAIR and information on rectal sensitivity and compliance can be obtained using either system.

Water-Perfused Systems

Water-perfused systems were developed by Arndorfer and colleagues and are the most widely used for performing manometry in the United States.[7] These systems function by creating an artificial cavity between the anus and the catheter. As perfusion continues, the full capacity is reached. Thereafter, fluid leaks into the rectal ampulla or out of the anus. The pressure required to overcome initial resistance after the space is filled is termed the *yield pressure*.[84,111] As the pressure in the anal canal increases, the mucosa will be brought into contact with the catheter ports, thereby impeding the flow of water. The yield pressure then becomes the pressure required to overcome

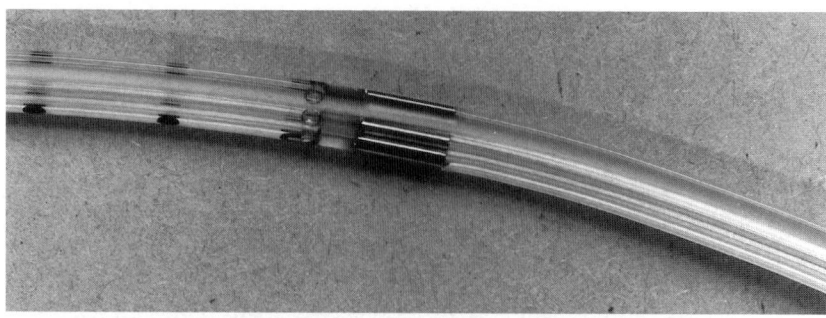

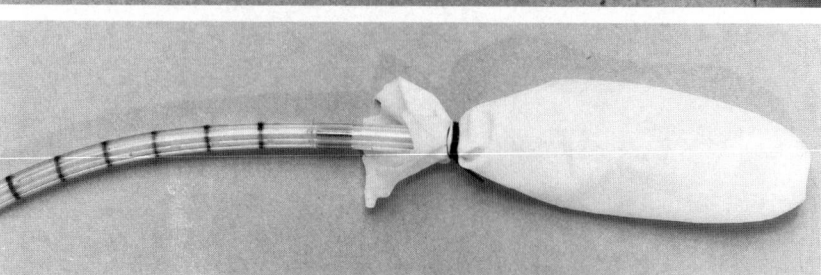

FIGURE 6-2. Water-perfused anorectal manometry catheters. **(A)** Eight-channel radial catheter suitable for vector volume analysis. (Courtesy of Synectics Medical, Irving, TX.) **(B)** Custom-built four-channel radial catheter with two intra-balloon channels. (Courtesy of Arndorfer, Inc., Greendale, WI.)

this obstruction. This information is then transmitted via nondistensible capillary tubing to transducers that convert this pressure to electrical signals.

Equipment

Catheters Catheters vary according to rigidity, diameter, and number and location of the ports. Rigid catheters tend to be easier to insert, but more flexible catheters cause less artifact and are, therefore, often preferred. The external diameter should be 4 to 8 mm in order to minimize distortion of the anal canal.[66,151] The number of lumina and ports ranges from 2 to 8 and may be arranged either radially or longitudinally in a spiral fashion at 5- to 8-mm intervals (Figure 6-2A). Additional ports for assessment of pressures inside rectal balloons can also be included (Figure 6-2B). Distal balloons may come preattached, but many investigators prefer to use either condoms or latex balloons made of a thinner and more compliant material. Radial catheters are used for assessment of the pressure profile of the anal canal, whereas spiral catheters are often preferred for elicitation of the RAIR. Many catheter varieties are available from a host of manufacturers (Table 6-1). These are multiuse catheters with a life span of 1 to 2 years, depending on the number of evaluations performed. Satisfactory cleansing is therefore a priority. This can be accomplished by using activated dialdehyde solution (Cidex, Johnson & Johnson Medical, Inc., Arlington, TX). Proper facilities for the use of this chemical, especially adequate ventilation, are required.

Withdrawal Motor Unlike balloon catheters, these devices are designed to measure pressures along the whole length of the anal canal. Some investigators prefer a manual pull-through technique that can be performed by a skilled technician. However, the rate of retraction is more easily standardized by using a withdrawal motor

▶ **TABLE 6-1 Manometry Catheters**

Manufacturer	Telephone	Water Perfused	Solid State
Arndorfer, Inc., Greendale, WI 53129, USA	414-425-1661	X	
Dantec Electronics, Bristol, UK	44-12-753-75333	X	
Gaeltec Ltd., Isle of Skye, UK	44-14-705-21385		X
Konigsberg Instruments, Pasadena, CA 91107, USA	818-449-0016		X
Millar Instruments, Houston, TX 77023, USA	1-800-669-2343		X
	713-923-9171		
MUI Scientific, Ontario, Canada	1-800-303-6611	X	
	905-890-5525		
Synectics Medical, Irving, TX 75038, USA	1-800-227-3191	X	
	214-518-0518		
Synectics Medical AB, Stockholm, S-116 28, Sweden	46-8640-23-50	X	

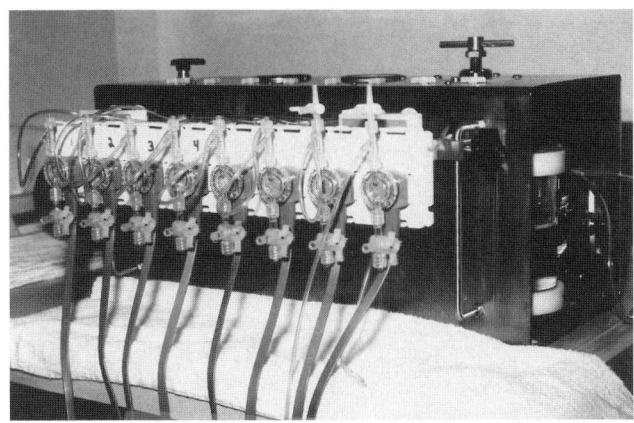

FIGURE 6-3. Eight-channel hydraulic capillary infusion system. (Courtesy of Arndorfer, Inc., Greendale, WI.)

that can be controlled by computer software (Narco Bio-Systems, Austin, TX).

Perfusion Apparatus Hydraulic capillary infusion systems use nitrogen gas or compressed air to force water from a reservoir through small capillary tubes, thereby allowing perfusion of each transducer and catheter channel separately (Figure 6-3).[7] The number of channels required is dependent on the type of catheter used. An apparatus with four, eight, and 12 channels is available (Table 6-2). Other similar options are also manufactured (International Biomedical, Austin, TX) but are sold only in conjunction with complete motility and analysis systems (Narco Bio-Systems, Austin, TX). Figure 6-4 shows an integrated computerized manometry biofeedback pudendal nerve terminal motor latency system.

Transducers The number required depends on the number of channels within the catheter.

Recording Apparatus Previously most recordings were made on paper or smoked polygraph drums. Although real-time chart recording is available (MMS-200, Narco Bio-Systems, Austin, TX), computers have surpassed this method of data collection for a number of reasons (Figure 6-5). For example, menu-driven software programs can be specially created that contain fixed pro-

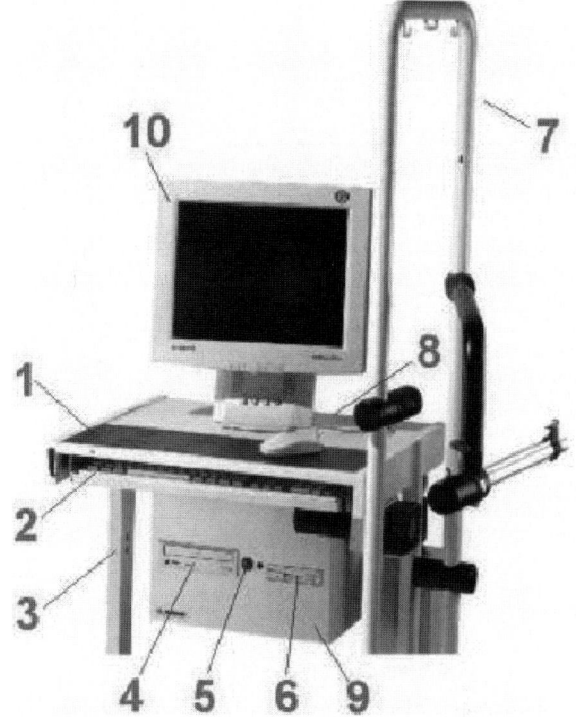

1.	Dedicated Keyboard	2.	PC Keyboard
3.	Trolley	4.	CD-ROM Drive
5.	Standby /Power ON	6.	Disk Drive
7.	Infusion Pole	8.	Rear Panel
9.	Control Unit	10.	Color Monitor (optional)

FIGURE 6-4. Medtronic Duet Logic Manometry/Biofeedback/Pudendal Nerve Terminal Motor Latency integrated computerized system. (Courtesy of Medtronic Functional Diagnostics, Shoreview, MN.)

tocols with instructions and prompts for performing various manometric investigations.[39,203,204] Software may also contain the mathematical algorithms for calculating pressure changes. Now more complex programs are being created that automatically calculate many manometric parameters. Three-dimensional reconstruction of the pressure profile of the anal sphincter can

TABLE 6-2 Capillary Infusion Systems

Manufacturer	Telephone	Gas	Channels
Arndorfer, Inc., Greendale, WI 53129, USA	414-425-1661	Nitrogen	4, 8, 12
International Biomedical, Austin, TX	1-800-433-5615	Nitrogen	4, 8
Mui Scientific, Mississauga, Ontario, Canada	1-800-303-6611 905-890-5525	Nitrogen/air compression	4, 6, 8, 12, 16

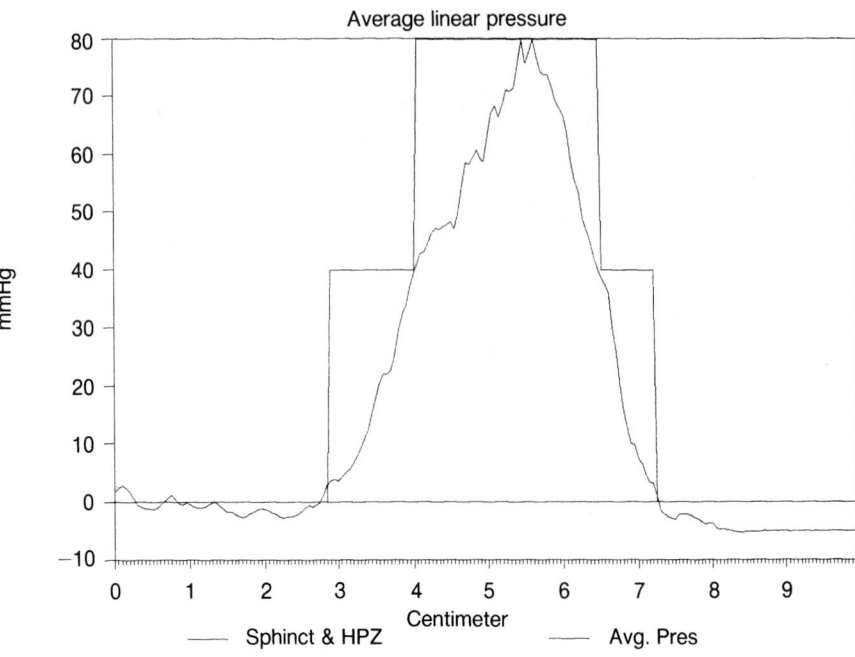

FIGURE 6-5. Normal longitudinal pressure profile of the anal sphincter provided by the Narco Bio-Systems MMS-200 physiologic recorder. The graph is made by pulling a radial catheter through the anal canal by computer control at the rate of 1 mm/second. Pressures are simultaneously acquired by eight radially positioned orifices; the average pressure is displayed in the graph. All pressures are referenced to a rectal pressure of zero so that atmospheric pressure will be a negative number. The maximum average resting pressure of the sphincter is approximately 80 mm Hg, and the sphincter length is 4.4 cm. (Courtesy of Narco Biosystems, Austin, TX, and John A. Coller, M.D.)

demonstrate sphincter asymmetry and the presence of defects (Figs. 6-6 through 6-8). Several systems now have the capability of integrating and displaying dynamic radiologic investigations with simultaneous motility studies. In addition, computers can also operate accessory equipment such as probe withdrawal motors and are excellent for storing data so that tests can be recalled and reviewed. Several manufacturers provide integrated hardware and software systems, some of which can also be used in combination with solid-state catheters (Table 6-3).

In summary, water-perfusion systems provide a large amount of reproducible data about the status of the anal sphincters and rectum. The one limitation is that they require the patient to be in the lateral decubitus position, thereby precluding ambulatory study.

Solid-State Noninfusion Catheters

Noninfusion transducer catheters usually contain three or more pressure channels. Although not as versatile as infusion catheters, they eliminate concerns about positioning

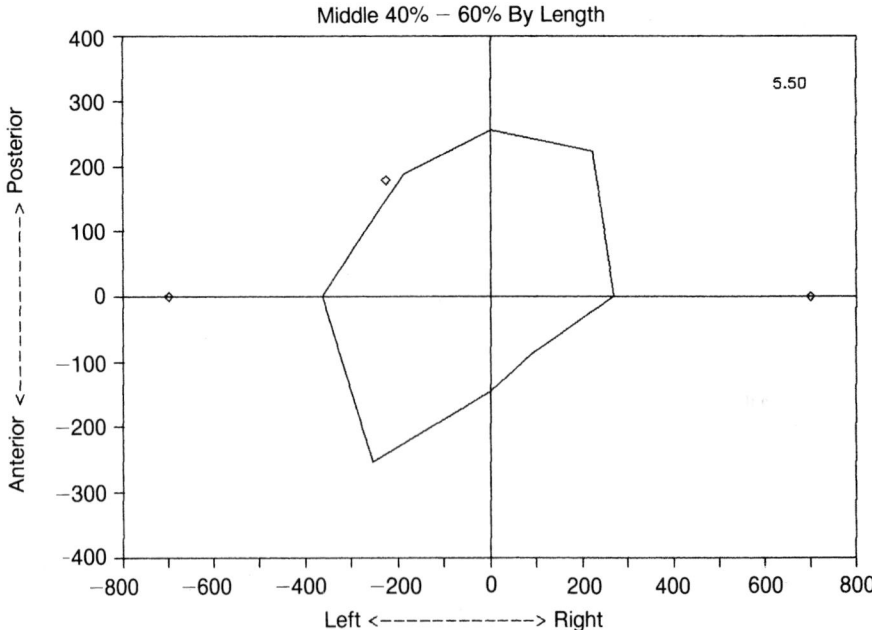

FIGURE 6-6. Cross-sectional analysis of pressures in the midportion of an anal sphincter that has been damaged as a consequence of an obstetric injury. Note that anteriorly, especially in the right anterior position, pressures are considerably reduced when compared with those posteriorly. (Courtesy of John A. Coller, M.D.)

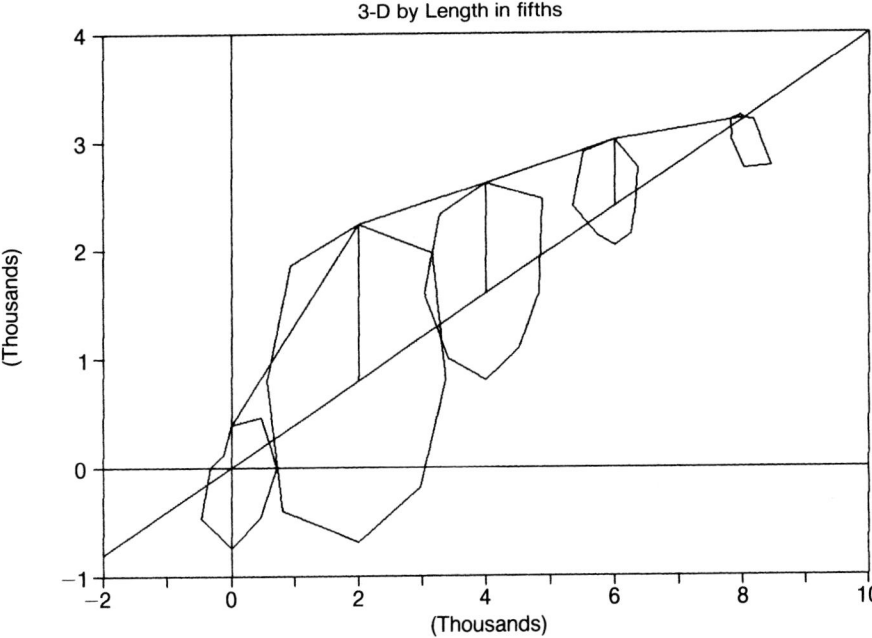

FIGURE 6-7. In this simple cross-sectional, computer-generated representation of the sphincter, there is a posterior predominance in the proximal portion of the anal canal and an anterior predominance in the distal portion. (Courtesy of John A. Coller, M.D.)

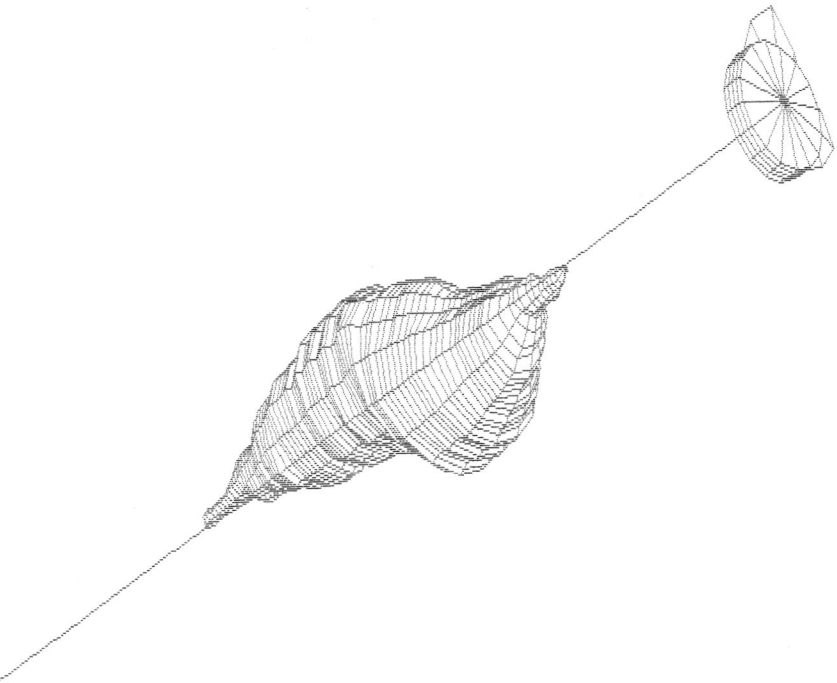

FIGURE 6-8. Three-dimensional reconstruction of same patient illustrated in Fig. 6-7 using computer-aided design program. (Courtesy of John A. Coller, M.D.)

▶ **TABLE 6-3 Manometry Systems**

Manufacturer	Telephone	System	Compatibility	
			Water Perfused	Solid State
Medical Management Systems, Enschede, Holland	31-534-308-803			X
Medtronic Functional Diagnostics, Shoreview, MN 55126 USA	1-800-328-0810	X	X	
Narco Bio-Systems, Austin, TX 78754, USA	1-800-433-5615 512-873-0033	MMS-200	X	X
Sandhill Scientific, Highlands Ranch, CO 80126, USA	1-800-468-4556 303-470-7020	BioLAB		X
Synectics Medical, Irving, TX 75038, USA	1-800-227-3191 214-518-0518	PC Polygraph	X	X
Synectics Medical AB, Stockholm, S-116 28, Sweden	46-8640-23-50		X	X

so that recordings can be made with patients sitting, the preferred physiologic condition.[11,195,245] Furthermore, these catheters can be used for ambulatory recordings. Several manufacturers produce suitable equipment (Table 6-1).

Technique of Manometric Evaluation

Our preference is to perform a station pull-through technique using a custom-built 4.8-mm diameter polypropylene flexible catheter with four radial ports located 8.5 cm from the tip (Arndorfer, Inc., Greendale, WI).[105,106] A further two ports are positioned 2 cm from the end of the catheter and are enclosed within a thin latex rubber balloon fashioned from the finger of an examination glove (Floor/exam latex glove no. 8857, Baxter Health Care Corporation, Valencia, CA). This balloon is tied at 3 cm from the tip of the catheter using a 2–0 silk ligature. An eight-channel hydraulic capillary infusion system (Arndorfer, Inc., Greendale, WI) is used with Medex transducers (M6677, Medex, Inc., Hilliard, OH). Mechanical pressures are transmitted to a PC Polygraf HR (Synectics Medical, Inc., Irving, TX). The resulting electrical impulses are displayed on an IBM-compatible computer with a Pentium 90-MHz coprocessor, 16 MB RAM, and a VGA 800 × 600 color monitor (Dell Computer Corp., Austin, TX) using Polygram V6.4 software (Synectics Medical, Inc., Irving, TX).

With the patient in the left lateral decubitus position, the catheter is inserted to 6 cm, and 20 to 30 seconds are allowed for the sphincter to recover from this insult and for the pressures to equilibrate. It is important to permit adequate time for the small cavity between the rectal wall and the catheter to fill with perfusate so that the yield pressure is reached.

Following this period of equilibration, various wave patterns may emerge that demonstrate the presence of intrinsic cyclic activity attributable primarily to the internal sphincter.[239] Three basic patterns are observed. *Slow waves* are the most frequently encountered. These vary in frequency from 10 to 20 cycles/minute with an amplitude from just above physiologic baseline noise to 15 mm Hg (Figure 6-9).[203] They can most often be observed in the region between the proximal border of the sphincter and the area of the maximal average resting pressure.[39,179] The clinical significance of these waves is unknown.

Ultraslow waves are the second most common wave forms recorded. They have a frequency of 0.5 to 1.5 cycles/minute and are of large amplitude (up to 100 mm Hg).[203] They are found more frequently in patients with high resting anal pressures,[85] such as in those individuals with an anal fissure,[82] hemorrhoids,[81] or primary anal sphincter hypertonia. They are seen most commonly in the region of maximal average resting pressure.

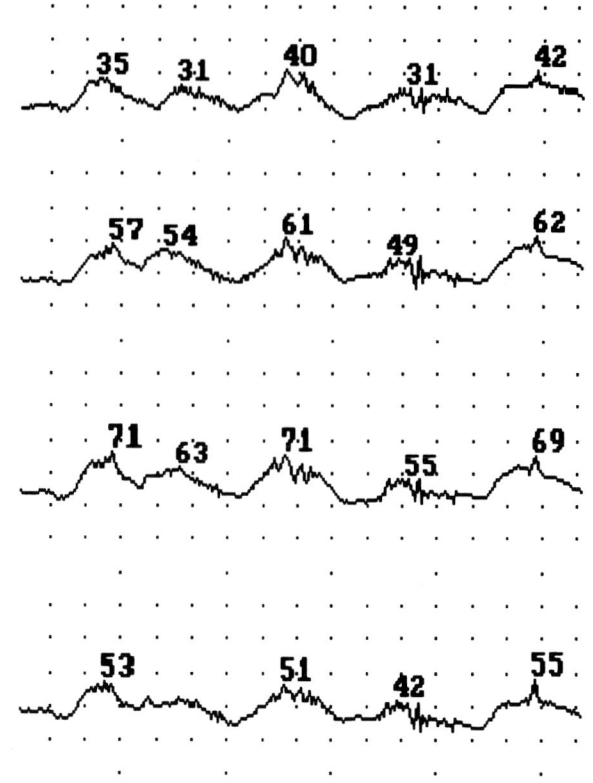

FIGURE 6-9. Slow waves noted in the region of the high-pressure zone. (Polygram software; courtesy of Synectics Medical, Irving, TX.)

The *intermediate wave* is the least frequently observed type of oscillation (frequency, 4 to 8 cycles/minute). They are most often noted in patients with neurogenic fecal incontinence or following ileal pouch-anal anastomosis (Figure 6-10).[225] When present, they make interpretation of resting and squeeze pressures more difficult. *Resting pressure* should be assumed to be the mean of the peak and trough pressures at rest.

Following equilibration of the pressures, the patient is asked to perform a single maximum squeeze effort followed by a period of rest, and then a maximal push effort (Figure 6-11). These measurements are repeated at a further five stations separated by 1-cm intervals as the catheter is progressively moved caudally. Thus, the rest and squeeze pressures over the entire length of the anal canal can be measured, and the mean resting and squeeze pressures over the *high-pressure zone* (HPZ) can be calculated. The HPZ is defined as that length of the anal canal through which pressures are greater than 50% of the average maximum pressure. This definition is similar to that used when a continuous pull-through technique is used. Alternatively, the HPZ can be defined as that zone bounded caudally by a rise in pressure of 20 mm Hg and cephalad by a fall in pressure of 20 mm Hg in at least

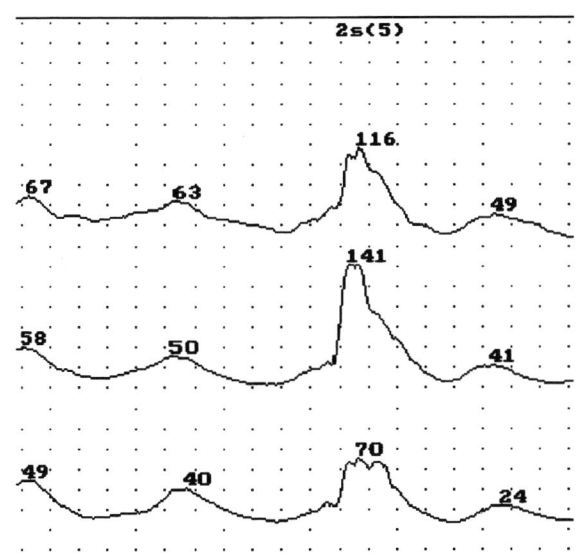

FIGURE 6-10. Intermediate waves in a patient following colonic pouch-anal anastomosis. (Polygram software; courtesy of Synectics Medical, Irving, TX.)

50% of the channels. This latter definition may present a more accurate picture of the sphincters in incontinent patients because pressures are so low that there is no true HPZ. However, using the former definition, the HPZ will always be at least 1 cm, but this may be an inaccurate value in a patient with a patulous anus.

The catheter is then reinserted to a distance of 2 cm from the anal verge, and the latex balloon is insufflated with 40 mL of air over 2 to 3 seconds and kept inflated for 20 seconds in order to elicit the RAIR. In response to distension of the lower rectum and upper anal canal, external sphincter contraction is followed by internal sphincter relaxation (Figure 6-12). If the reflex is not present, it is important to repeat the test with increased insufflation. Some patients, especially those with neurogenic fecal incontinence, decreased anal sensation, or megarectum, may respond only at a higher volume. The air is removed and the balloon reinflated with 50 or 60 mL until a reflex is observed. If the reflex is still undetectable, the catheter is inserted to 3 cm and repeat insufflations are

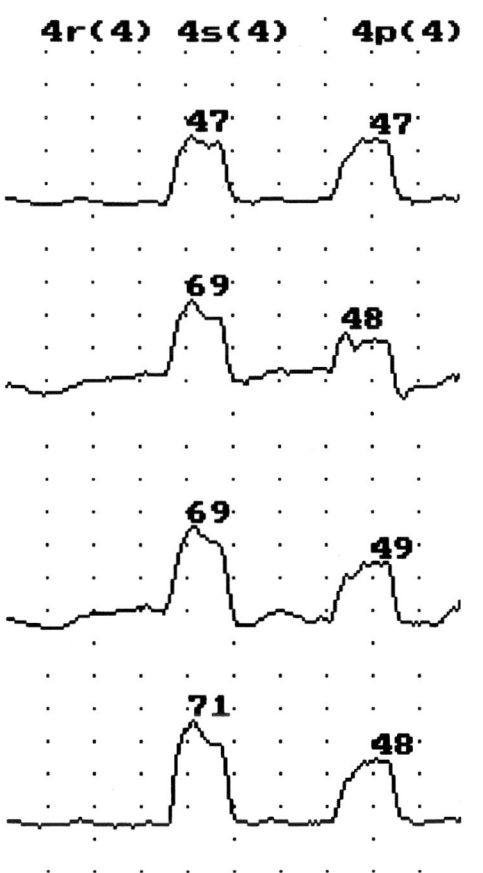

FIGURE 6-11. Rest, squeeze, and push phases of station pull-through manometry recorded at 4 cm from the anal verge. (Polygram software; courtesy of Synectics Medical, Irving, TX.)

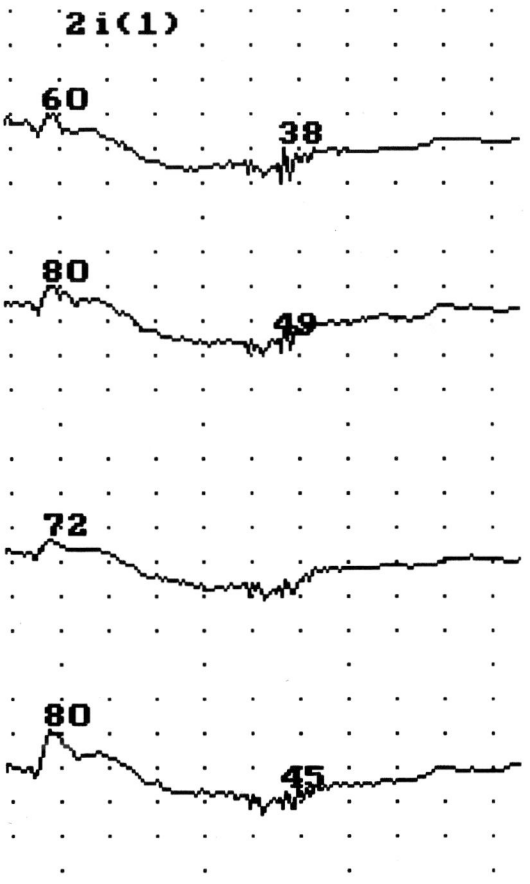

FIGURE 6-12. Rectoanal inhibitory reflex recorded at 2 cm from the anal verge in response to distension of the rectal balloon with 40 mL of air. (Polygram software; courtesy of Synectics Medical, Irving, TX.)

performed. In our laboratory we record only the presence or absence of the reflex. Some software programs contain the algorithms for calculating various reflex parameters, including duration, percentage of excitation, and excitation latency. Although some authors suggest that delayed, diminutive or absent excitation, or excitation only in response to large volumes may be used as a crude indicator of pudendal neuropathy, the clinical implications of these values are problematic.[204] Some prefer a spiral catheter to detect the presence of the RAIR over the entire length of the anal canal. However, the use of a radial catheter at the two stations where the reflex is most likely to be detected avoids this requirement for each investigation. In rare instances in which a reflex cannot be elicited and there is no evidence of megarectum, the spiral catheter may be useful. The most common reasons for absence of the RAIR are megarectum and a prior ileoanal or coloanal anastomosis.

The catheter is then inserted to a distance of 6 cm from the anal verge, positioning the balloon in the rectal ampulla. The balloon is then slowly filled with core temperature water at a rate of approximately 1 mL/second. The first sensation perceived by the patient is noted as the minimal sensory volume, and the mean intraballoon pressure is noted. Thereafter, balloon filling is continued until the maximum tolerable volume is reached, and again the intraballoon pressure is noted. Using these values, rectal compliance can be calculated from the formula $\Delta V/\Delta P$.[105] Thus, with a large balloon volume and only a small increase in rectal pressure, the rectum is considered very compliant. In patients suffering from ulcerative colitis, Crohn's proctitis, or radiation proctitis, the rectum may be poorly compliant in that a small increase in volume will result in a large increase in pressure. When one uses this technique it is important to know the compliance of the balloon at various stages of insufflation so that it can be subtracted from the pressure measured via the intraballoon ports. Latex balloons may deform along the longitudinal axis with increased infusion of water. This may give a false impression of high rectal compliance.[142] As a consequence, some clinicians prefer to use barostat equipment to calculate this param-

eter, using a noncompliant balloon that does not deform with increasing pressure.

The measurement of *compliance* is not a diagnostic test but supplements other investigations for evaluating the pathophysiology of anorectal disease. It is of particular value in patients with proctitis and incontinence through ascertaining whether the incontinence is due to lack of rectal reservoir function or diminished anal sphincter tone. Similarly, in some constipated patients, compliance may be abnormally high. This can reflect overaccommodation and, therefore, a sensory contribution to the outlet obstruction.

MANOVOLUMETRY

Although the ability of the rectum to accommodate to increasing volumes may play some role in the maintenance of continence, the function of the anal sphincter mechanism is of greater import.[94] Nonetheless, rectal compliance is responsible for the degree of urgency to evacuate. Therefore, assessment of rectal compliance by the previously mentioned techniques is a useful investigation. Limitations, however, include the dependency on the subject's perception of the rectal balloon. Accordingly, psychological factors may influence the patient's interpretation of the sensory threshold and maximal tolerable volume and lead to variation in results. Second, as already alluded to, the use of deformable balloons may lead to inaccuracy. The velocity of water infusion into the balloon may also affect the sensitivity of this test.[10] Therefore, the injection of water should be gentle and continuous. Moreover, the patient must be well informed about the technique and what to expect with the filling of the balloon in the rectum. The technique of manovolumetry avoids these pitfalls and may provide a more objective measurement of compliance.[80]

Equipment

Manovolumetry equipment was initially designed for the investigation of hollow organs other than the rectum[148] but was modified for anorectal studies (Figure 6-13).[3,173]

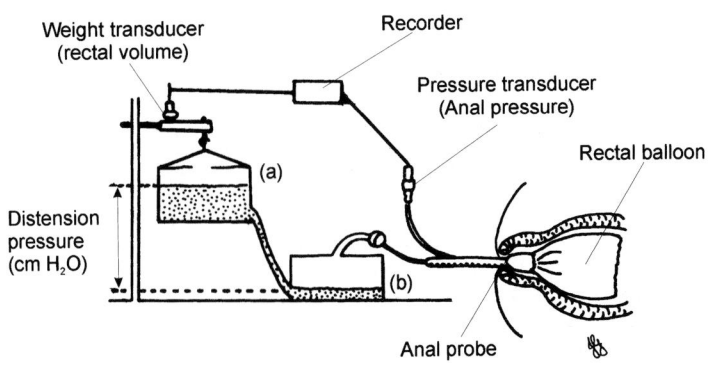

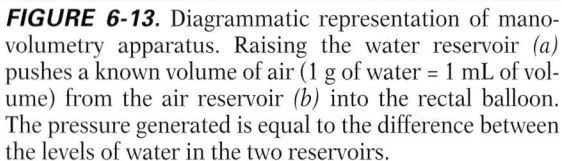

FIGURE 6-13. Diagrammatic representation of manovolumetry apparatus. Raising the water reservoir *(a)* pushes a known volume of air (1 g of water = 1 mL of volume) from the air reservoir *(b)* into the rectal balloon. The pressure generated is equal to the difference between the levels of water in the two reservoirs.

A wide-diameter, water-filled, cylindric vessel, open to the air, is suspended from a strain gauge. This is in continuity via a nondistensible plastic tube with a similar water-filled vessel that is sealed from the atmosphere. The top of a second reservoir is connected by means of a plastic tube to a thin-walled, highly compliant, disposable polyethylene bag (maximal capacity of 500 to 600 ml). The bag is placed within the rectum. An intraanal manometry catheter may also be positioned for measuring anal pressures and for identifying the RAIR. Raising the water reservoir increases the pressure within the air reservoir, which is automatically transmitted to the intrarectal bag. The pressure generated is equal to the difference between the levels of water in the two reservoirs. The quantity of water that flows into the air reservoir is measured as a weight reduction (1 g of water = 1 ml volume).

Procedure

Following emptying of the rectum with one or two Fleet's enemas, the patient is placed in the left lateral decubitus position. After insertion of the catheters, a series of distensions is commenced, beginning at a pressure of 5 cm of water and increasing stepwise by increments of 5 cm of water, emptying the balloon between each distension. Each distension lasts for at least 1 minute.

A graph of volume (ml) versus distension pressure (cm water) can be plotted and compared to the graph of normal controls. The compliance of the rectum can be determined at defined distension/pressure intervals, yielding reliable interpatient comparisons.

DEFECOGRAPHY (EVACUATION PROCTOGRAPHY)

Defecography is the fluoroscopic examination of the act of rectal expulsion. The term evacuation proctography may be preferred given that this study is not a true representation of the act of defecation, because of the nature of the rectal contents and the semipublic atmosphere in which the examination is performed.[14] This dynamic investigation of the mechanism of defecation has become an increasingly popular investigation since it was described by Walldén in 1952[238] and Burhenne in 1964.[29] Improvements in the technique, such as cinedefecography and videoproctography, have led to a better understanding of the evacuation process, thereby facilitating the identification of conditions that disturb the physiology of rectal emptying. Whereas balloon expulsion from the rectum tests motor function as well as coordination of the process of evacuation, cinedefecography, performed with barium paste injected into the rectum, seems better to mimic the mechanism by simulating stool consistency.[160] Nonetheless, the evaluation of the mechanism of

rectal emptying by means of defecography may require additional physiologic tests to increase diagnostic capability further.[27] The newly available digital radiographic imagery has further improved the potential utility of the technique.[60]

Indications

Defecography not only affords one the ability to measure the anorectal angle, but also permits evaluation of the position of the pelvic floor through the determination of the presence of perineal descent during rest and straining. This technique is often used in the investigation of evacuatory complaints, particularly constipation and outlet obstructive symptoms, as well as rectocele and perineal descent.[37] Agachan and colleagues reported the incidence and clinical significance of defecographic findings in patients with evacuation complaints.[2] Twelve percent of the 744 patients reviewed had normal findings, 8% were found to have rectal prolapse, 26% rectocele, 11% sigmoidocele, 13% intussusception, and 30% had a combination of findings.

Patients with colonic inertia often undergo defecography before colectomy in order to exclude pelvic floor dysfunction. The procedure may also be indicated for the investigation of individuals with solitary rectal ulcer syndrome or rectal pain.[71,123,144] With respect to evaluation of patients with fecal incontinence, the role of defecography is less clear, because information relative to the anorectal angle and its role in maintaining bowel control is a subject of controversy.[54,55,73]

Equipment

Imaging

The procedure can be carried out in a standard fluoroscopic suite, with a table capable of supine and erect positioning (see Figure 17-11). A videocassette recorder can be connected to the video output of the fluoroscopic system to record the procedure. Some radiologists prefer to take rapid sequence pictures at 1 to 2 frames/second.[11,130,143] Others utilize digital subtraction to remove bone and soft tissue images and to enhance the contrast-filled structures.[19] Digital imagery is now frequently employed to process, store, share, and capture images. A standard examination will deliver 0.02 to 0.66 cGy to the skin of the right hip and 0.036 to 0.053 cGy to the ovaries.[14]

Commode

Almost all investigators perform this procedure with the patient in the seated position. A chair or commode is, therefore, required, some of which are commercially available, such as the Brunswick chair (E-Z-EM, Inc.,

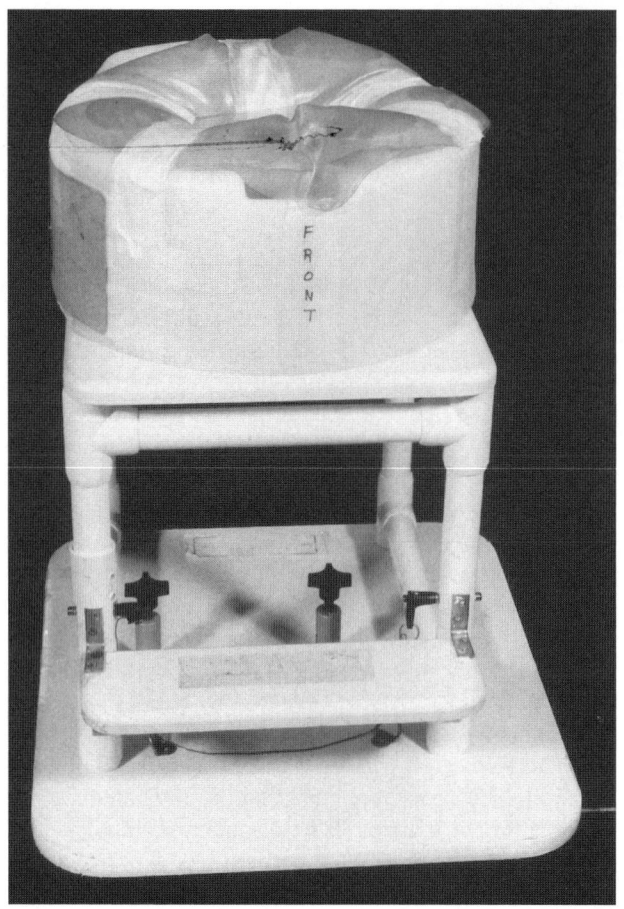

FIGURE 6-14. Defecography commode with modifications. The so-called blooming effect is diminished by the use of a water-filled rubber-ring seat. (Courtesy of the Cleveland Clinic Florida, Weston, FL).

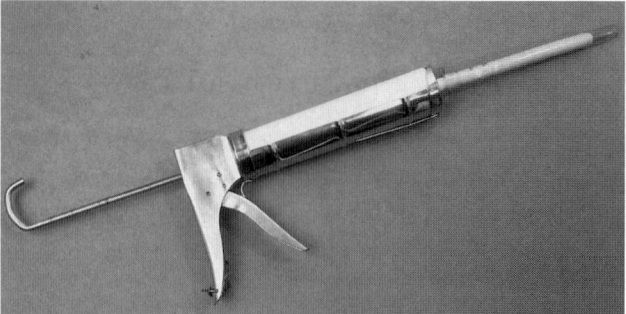

FIGURE 6-15. Standard caulking gun with barium paste.

Westbury, NY) (see Figure 17-10) and Portapotti (Figure 6-14), but several individuals have developed their own modifications. With the pelvis examined in profile, x-rays must pass through much tissue, thereby creating considerable absorption of the beam. Movement of the beam caudally, in order to examine anal movement during evacuation or to delineate rectoanal intussusception further, causes x-rays to pass through subcutaneous fat or air. This loss of tissue density and its resultant lack of absorption cause an excessive "flare" or "blooming," seriously detracting from the quality of the image. Various methods have been developed to address this problem, including the use of one or more water-filled rubber rings,[58] specifically designed Perspex water-filled commodes,[11] different thickness of leaded plexiglass,[189] and the use of carefully positioned copper or lead plates.[19]

Contrast Media

A varying amount of liquid barium of the type used for double contrast enemas [58% weight/weight (wt/wt) barium sultate suspension] can be administered using a standard enema-tipped catheter. In addition, most investigators use a high-density, high-viscosity barium paste to simulate stool. Many investigators have prepared "home" recipes that involve thickening barium sulfate with methyl cellulose, porridge oats, potato starch, or Maizena.[11,131,143,195,209] It is much easier, though, to use a preloaded commercially available caulking tube for administration and a standard caulking gun (Evacu-paste, E-Z-EM Inc., Westbury, NY; Anatrast, Lafayette Pharmaceuticals, Inc., Lafayette, IN; Figure 6-15).

Modified Techniques

The standard procedure has been outlined by Mahieu and colleagues.[143] Some investigators prefer to prepare the rectum before investigation, whereas others perform the examination in the "as is" state.[58] Some physicians use liquid barium alone,[124,183,208] but most authors stress the need for a semisolid contrast medium to simulate feces, hence the use of barium paste (see previous discussion).[124,183] Other investigators use a mixture of these media, such as using a small quantity of liquid barium, to outline the rectum followed by the installation of a larger volume of rectal paste.[11,103,105] Careful explanation of the entire procedure is necessary in order to allay anxieties concerning the public performance of a normally private act. The contrast medium is introduced into the rectum with the patient in the left lateral position.

Some authors have made refinements to this basic rectal evacuation technique in an attempt to visualize the entire pelvic floor.[4] For example, the bladder can be outlined by introducing water-soluble contrast media through a urinary catheter.[131] Additionally, a barium-soaked tampon or compress can be placed into the posterior fornix of the vagina in order to delineate the vagina and to help assess for the possible interposition of abdominal contents (e.g., enterocele or sigmoidocele).[93,143,213] Oral contrast in the form of barium sulfate suspension, 40 wt/wt, or a mixture of liquid barium and a hyperosmolar water-soluble contrast, such as diatrizoate sodium (Hypaque, Nycomed, Inc., New York, NY), can be used to outline the small bowel.[25,70,131] As an alternative to oral contrast to delineate an enterocele, some authors prefer to use nonionic water-soluble contrast injected intraperitoneally (Omnipaque, Nycomed, Inc., New York, NY; Renograffin-60, Squibb Diagnostics, Princeton, NJ).[26,209] In addition to the standard lateral views, anteroposterior images may also be obtained and may potentially reveal additional details.

Defecography has been combined with simultaneous manometric and EMG assessment of the anorectum,[11,195,245] but because of its complexity this technique has not been widely employed.[58] Other investigators have combined defecography with simultaneous cystometrography in patients with combined proctologic and urologic symptoms.[231] As of this writing, this dual evaluation has not gained general acceptance.

Author's Preferred Technique

Because most of our patients have several physiologic investigations performed on the same day, bowel preparation by means of a Fleet enema is usually performed before manometry. With the patient in the left lateral decubitus position, a digital rectal examination is performed to lubricate the anal canal, to ascertain the presence of any pathologic abnormality, and to ensure that the patient understands the instructions of how to squeeze and to push. Through an enema-tipped catheter, 50 mL of liquid barium (58% wt/wt barium sulfate suspension, Polybar) is introduced into the rectum followed by the insufflation of a small quantity of air to coat the mucosa of the sigmoid colon. Barium paste is then introduced into the rectum using the caulking gun until the patient experiences a feeling of fullness. Finally, a small quantity of paste is inserted into the anus as the gun is removed in order to outline the anal canal. The patient is then turned to the right lateral position, and the table is slowly brought to the erect position. This enables one to slide down the table and to sit on the commode. The fluoroscopy tube is positioned so that the coccyx and the symphysis pubis are both visible on screening. Still pictures (*proctograms*) are taken at rest and at maximal squeeze before starting the video recording (Figure 6-16). At the

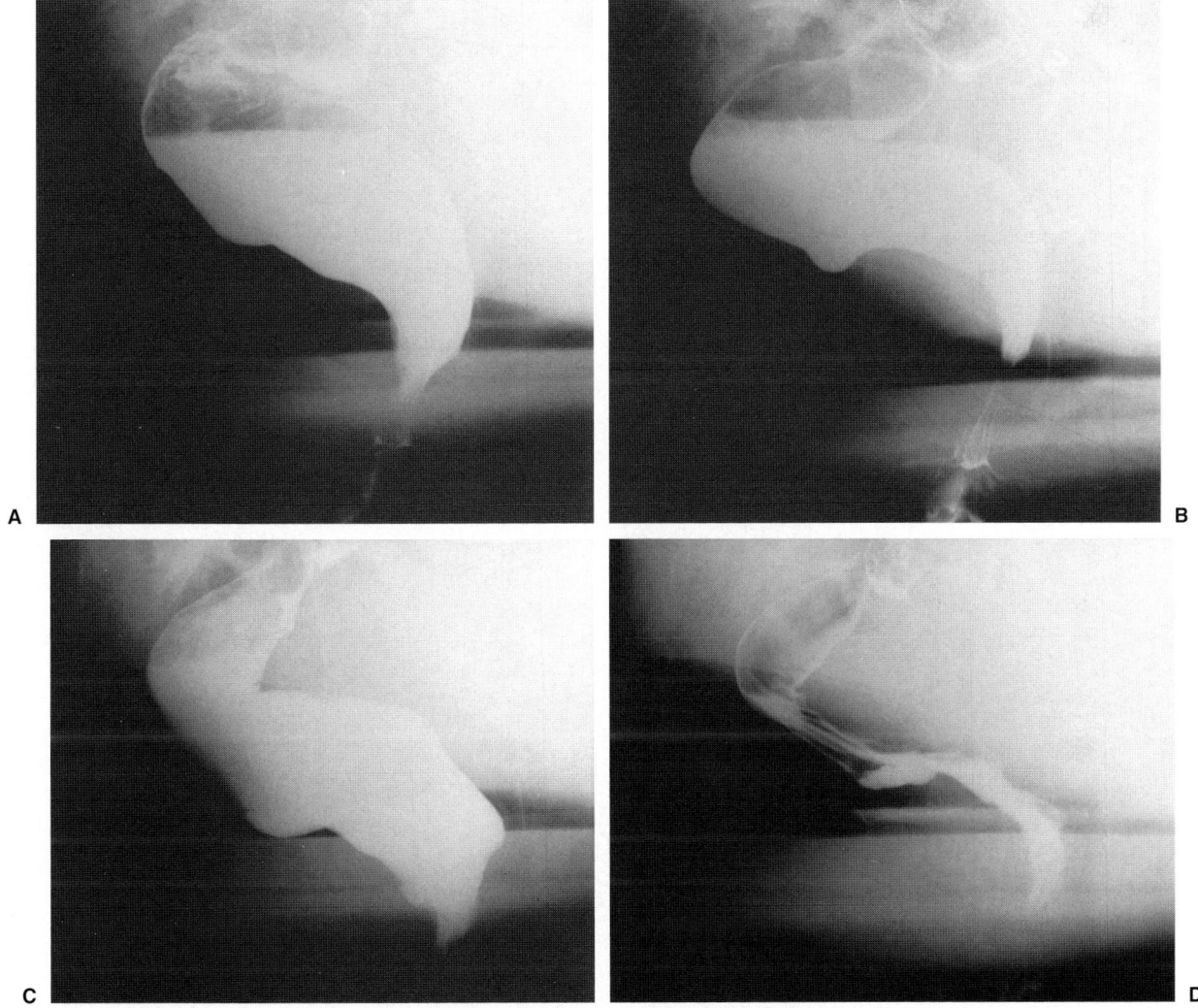

FIGURE 6-16. Proctogram series. **(A)** Rest. **(B)** Squeeze. **(C)** Push. **(D)** Postevacuation.

commencement of the video, the patients are asked to squeeze, to relax, and then to try to commence evacuation. As elimination starts, a further still picture is taken. Following evacuation, the recording is recommended while the patient squeezes and pushes, in order to check for the presence of an intussusception or nonemptying rectocele. A single still image of the evacuated rectum at rest is also obtained (Figure 6-16D). We do not use contrast media to outline other structures. Although these methods provide additional information, the impact of the data on clinical decision making has not been demonstrably useful.[4,25] Therefore, the added cost and invasive nature of these procedures do not justify routine application.

With completion of the study, three lines of reference are drawn, so that the anorectal angle, puborectalis length, and extent of perineal descent can be assessed on the proctograms. First, a line is drawn between the tip of the coccyx and the anterosuperior surface of the symphysis pubis. Lines are also drawn along the axis of the midanal canal and along the posterior rectal wall (Figure 6-17).[104] A

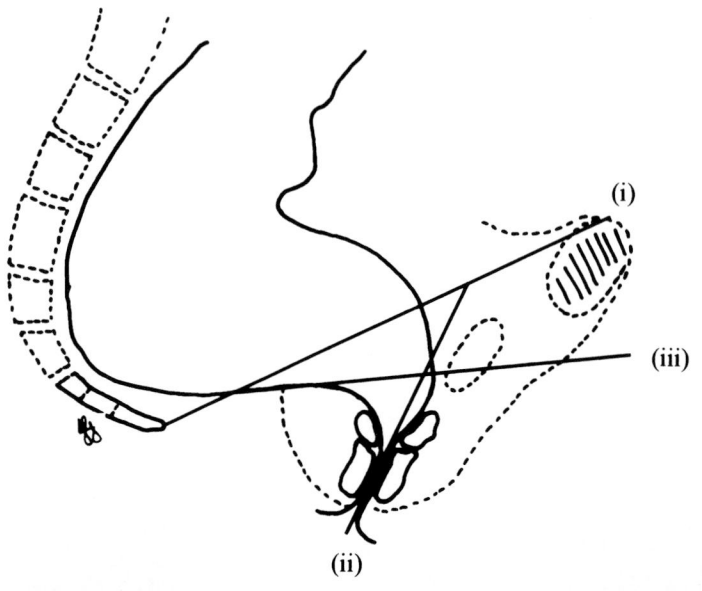

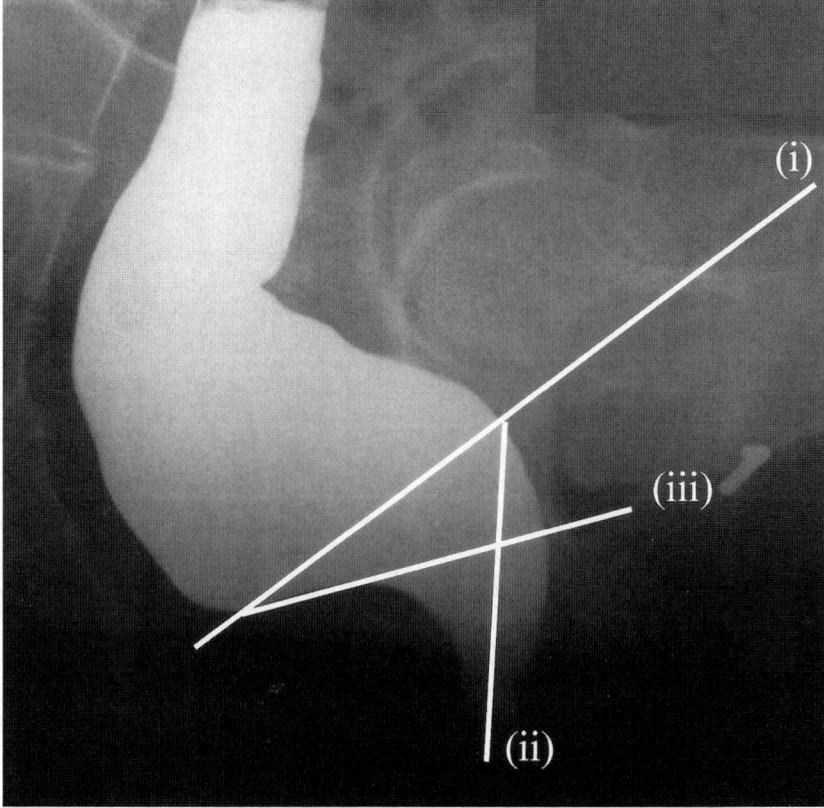

FIGURE 6-17. Lines of reference for analysis of proctograms. **(A)** Diagrammatic representation of *(i)* pubococcygeal line; *(ii)* midanal line; and *(iii)* posterior rectal line. **(B)** Resting proctogram with lines demonstrated.

midrectal or anterior rectal line is not used because its position depends on rectal filling.[12,49,100,125] However, the axis of the midrectal line is often a useful guide to the orientation of the posterior rectal wall. This can be confusing, especially in the presence of a posterior rectocele, perineal hernia, or double puborectalis impression.[104]

Anorectal Angle

Much attention has been directed to the *anorectal angle* since Parks first proposed its role in maintaining fecal continence.[177] The anorectal angle is the angle formed by the axis of the posterior rectal wall and the axis formed by the anal canal; it is usually 70 to 140 degrees at rest.[72,143,234,236] This angle becomes more acute during the squeeze phase (75 to 90 degrees) and becomes more obtuse during evacuation (100 to 180 degrees at maximum strain).[55,104] Some investigators have reported greater anorectal angles in men,[214] but most clinicians believe that it is not affected by gender.[9,54,72] The wide variation in observed normal values is probably due to differences in interpretation.[55,73,179,213] It has even been suggested that a normal range is impossible to define.[214] Therefore, the change in angle seen during the squeeze and push phases is more important than the actual measurement.

Puborectalis Length and Perineal Descent

The *puborectalis length* is measured as the minimal distance between the anterosuperior aspect of the symphysis pubis and the puborectalis notch. This ranges between 14 and 16 cm in the rest position, shortens to between 12 and 15 cm during the squeezing phase, and is elongated to 15 to 18 cm during the push phase.[104] As with the anorectal angle determination, the change in these parameters is more important than their definitive value.

Perineal descent is assessed as the length of a perpendicular dropped from the pubococcygeal line to the anorectal junction. Perineal descent of either more than 3 cm in the rest phase or a further increase of 3 cm in the push phase is considered abnormal.

Interpretation

A normal defecogram should demonstrate relaxation of the puborectalis as indicated by (a) an increase in the anorectal angle, (b) lengthening of the puborectalis, and (c) a blunting of the puborectalis notch. These changes should be accompanied by symmetric opening of the anal canal to form a cone that is wider cephalad than it is caudad. This process takes approximately 4 to 5 seconds. Contrast material in the upper rectum should subsequently be passed into the lower rectum and out the anus by rectal contraction, a process that may be facilitated by Valsalva's maneuver, squeezing the rectum onto the levator plate.[140,212] Complete evacuation takes about 10 to 12 seconds when thickened contrast medium is used but is more rapid (8 to 9 seconds) when the mixture is more fluid.[13,125]

In up to 50% of anatomically normal patients, some folding in of the mucosa on the posterior wall of the rectum is a common finding during evacuation (approximately 3 to 7 cm proximal to the anal canal).[213] If these folds become circumferential and form a ring pocket, then an intussusception is truly present. Obviously, if this intussusception is extruded outside the anal canal, then it is termed a rectal prolapse or procidentia. However, one should not need the radiologist to tell the clinician that a procidentia is present.

Bulging of the anterior or posterior wall of the rectum is a relatively common finding on defecography, particularly in women.[125] In female patients, an anterior *rectocele* 2 cm in size that empties on evacuation is considered within normal limits. The presence of a nonemptying rectocele may be considered pathologic, but this finding should be interpreted in accordance with the patient's symptoms. The presence of a *sigmoidocele* is assessed during the maximum straining phase. The presence of a first-degree sigmoidocele (a sigmoid loop that is present within the true pelvis but does not reach or cross the pubococcygeal line) is considered a normal finding. A second-degree sigmoidocele, one that extends to or below the pubococcygeal line, is considered abnormal. However, it may not be clinically significant. A sigmoid loop that extends below a line drawn between the coccyx and the ischial tuberosities is an uncommon finding and is termed a third-degree sigmoidocele (Figure 6-18).[107]

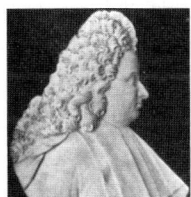

Antonio Maria Valsalva Bas-relief in the library of Imola, Italy

Antonio Maria Valsalva (1666–1723) Valsalva was born in Imola, Italy on January 17, 1666, the son of a merchant and aristocrat. He was educated by the Jesuits and achieved his MD and PhD in 1687 from the University of Bologna. Upon graduation he was appointed Inspector of Public Health in Bologna. He was a pupil of Malpighi and teacher of Morgagni. Valsalva was a brilliant anatomist and became well recognized for his studies on the anatomy and physiology of the ear, a fact that culminated in the publication of his book, *De aure humana* (1704). His contributions to our understanding of a host of conditions were myriad. His name is eponymously associated with the outpouching of the noncoronary sinus (aneurysm of the sinus of Valsalva), Valsalva's antrum, V's dysphagia, V's methods, V's muscle, V's ligaments, and of course, V's maneuver—the increase of intrapulmonic (and intraabdominal) pressure caused by forcible exhalation against the closed glottis—thereby facilitating pelvic floor descent and defecation. He wrote, "If the glottis be closed after a deep inspiration, and a strenuous and prolonged expiratory effort be then made, such pressure can be exerted upon the heart and intrathoracic vessels that the movement and flow of the blood are temporarily arrested." In 1705, Valsalva was appointed Lecturer and Demonstrator in Anatomy at the university, a position he retained for the remainder of his life.

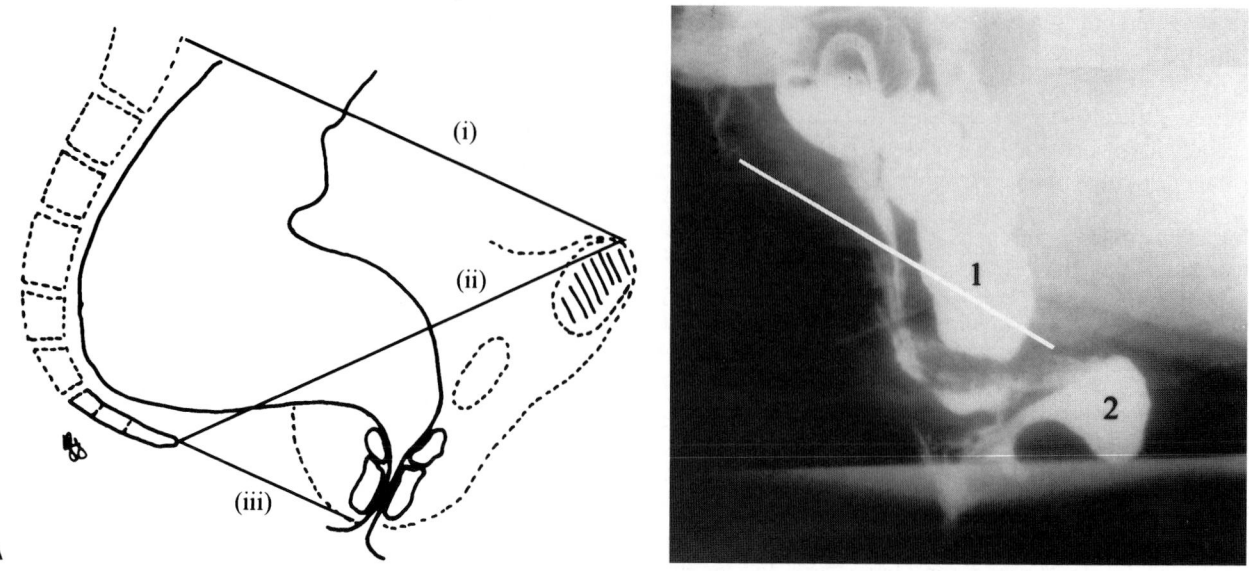

FIGURE 6-18. Lines of reference for classification of sigmoidoceles. **(A)** Diagrammatic representation of *(i)* the pubosacral line; *(ii)* the pubococcygeal line; and *(iii)* the ischiococcygeal line. **(B)** Evacuation proctogram demonstrating *(1)* a third-degree sigmoidocele with *(2)* a concomitant anterior rectocele. (From Jorge JMN, Yang YK, Wexner SD. Incidence and clinical significance of sigmoidoceles as determined by a new classification system. *Dis Colon Rectum* 1993;37:1112–1117, with permission.)

Obstructed Defecation

In constipated patients, failure to evacuate or delayed evacuation of the rectal contents is a common finding. This inability is most frequently the result of inappropriate puborectalis or external sphincter contraction.[101,103] This observation is known by a number of terms, including anismus,[185] obstructed defecation, spastic pelvic floor syndrome,[122] nonrelaxing puborectalis,[103] and paradoxical puborectalis syndrome (see Chapter 16).[101] However, it remains unclear whether these findings seen in a defecogram are truly representative of a diseased state because similar features have been described inphysiologically normal individuals.[101] Some physicians prefer to treat only those patients who have outlet obstruction confirmed by other physiologic tests, such as EMG or colonic transit study.[242] Although paradoxical puborectalis contraction may be found in asymptomatic individuals, when it is identified in those with otherwise normal evaluations and who complain of inability to complete an evacuation, it should be regarded as the cause of the problem.

EMPTYING STUDIES

The ability to evacuate normally and with equanimity in the presence of an audience is not a facility that all patients possess. Consequently, unsuccessful elimination may lead one to make a false-positive diagnosis of outlet obstruction. In order to overcome understandable patient inhibition, numerous emptying methods have been designed. These have the advantage of maintaining patient privacy, because evacuation can take place in an ordinary toilet. Furthermore, x-ray visualization is not required. However, the disadvantage is that other pathologic parameters cannot be evaluated. The options range from fairly simple tests in which evacuation is described as complete or incomplete to more sophisticated evaluations that attempt to quantify the completeness of the evacuation.

The simplest of these involves the installation of 300 mL of porridge into the rectum, following which the patient evacuates in privacy. The completeness of evacuation is then confirmed by the investigator's measurement.[22] Alternatively, a balloon proctogram can be performed in which an intrarectal balloon is distended with water via a double-lumen catheter until a call to stool is appreciated.[184] Patients are again asked to evacuate in privacy.

Scintigraphy

Several investigators have used radioactive isotopes and scintigraphy to perform a quantitative assessment of evacuation.[169,226] This technique involves the rectal introduction of a semisolid material similar in consistency to that of stool [e.g., oat porridge or scrambled eggs prelabeled with technetium-99m (^{99m}Tc)]. A standard gamma camera is used to obtain images before and after the patient has evacuated in private. The percentage of emptying can be calculated using the equation:

$$\% \text{ evacuation} = 100 \times \frac{\text{preevacuation count} - \text{postevacuation count}}{\text{postevacuation count}}$$

Some investigators have assessed the *dynamics* of evacuation using a similar technique.[99,176] Although this test provides good quantitative information about the percentage of rectal contents evacuated per unit time, it has the disadvantages of requiring the patient to perform in public and provides no information about intussusception or other anatomic abnormalities.

Fecoflowmetry

This test assesses not only the completeness of evacuation, but also the rate at which the evacuation occurs. After emptying the rectum, the patient assumes the left lateral decubitus position. A known quantity of water or barium paste is then instilled. He or she is then asked to walk until the desire to defecate is appreciated. The individual is then seated on the commode of a fecoflowmeter and is left to evacuate in private. This device consists of a weight transducer connected to an amplifier and an oscilloscope.[210] The rate and extent to which the rectal contents are evacuated are calculated from the changing weight within the fecoflowmeter. Plotting weight against time results in a defecation flow curve. In constipated patients, two separate patterns are observed: one representing nonobstructed and the other, obstructed defecation.[211]

This technique may be of value in the detection of neurogenic disturbances of the anorectum in patients, such as in those with tethered spinal cord syndrome.[113] The significance of the results as well as whether the knowledge gleaned can influence treatment are unknown. Thus, the test is not widely used.

PERINEOGRAPHY

Simultaneous dynamic proctography and peritoneography may provide additional information in the identification of both rectal and pelvic floor pathologies. The method described by Sentovich and colleagues consists of the injection of nonionic contrast material into the peritoneal cavity by using fluoroscopy.[209] Anteroposterior and lateral pelvic radiographs are obtained during the Valsalva maneuver. A barium paste enema consisting of 100 to 120 mL is administered, in addition to vaginal insertion of 20 to 50 mL of liquid barium. The patient is placed on a commode, and lateral radiographs are again obtained during rest and with maximal anal squeeze. Patients are then asked to evacuate the rectal contrast material, which is observed on videotape using fluoroscopy. A final radiograph is taken while the patient strains to evacuate.

This technique can help determine the anorectal angle and perineal descent while rectocele, enterocele, and rectal prolapse can be identified during the evacuation phase. Enterocele is diagnosed if peritoneal contrast separates the rectum from the vagina. Peritoneography, however, has yet to be widely accepted because of the invasive nature of the intraperitoneal injection.[166]

PERINEOMETRY

An alternative and simpler method to the previously mentioned calculations for assessing perineal descent is to use a device known as a St. Mark's perineometer (Figure 6-19).[87] This consists of a steel frame with two metal bars fashioned to rest against the ischial tuberosities. The patient is examined in the left lateral position. The central graduated latex cylinder is capable of free movement within the frame and is brought into contact with the perianal skin. Measurements of the perineal plane in relation to the ischial tuberosities are then made at rest and during maximal straining.[172] The normal value at rest is 2.5±0.6 cm above the ischial tuberosity. On maximal straining, the normal perineum descends to 0.9±1.0 cm above the tuberosities.[86] Although a simple test, perineometry has little to add over defecography and is of limited value in patient assessment.[110] As of this writing, we are unaware of any colorectal physiology unit in the United States employing this technique.

ENDOLUMINAL ULTRASOUND

Anal ultrasonography is a very important tool for the evaluation and quantification of anatomic defects of the sphincteric complex. Moreover, *anorectal* ultrasonography is currently the most accurate and most cost-effective imaging modality used to stage rectal cancer.[33,74,118,199] Pulsed sound waves of a specific frequency are emitted from a transducer. As they traverse tissue planes, some of

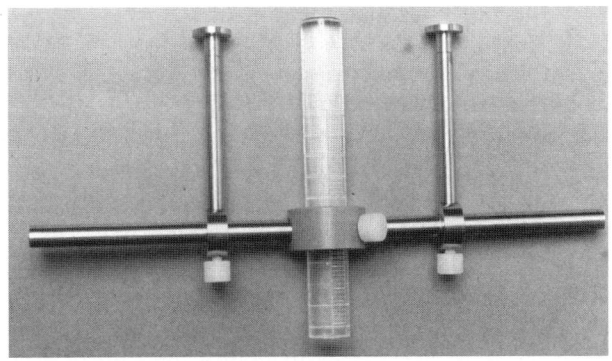

FIGURE 6-19. St. Mark's perineometer.

the sound waves are reflected back toward the transducer. The quantity reflected is dependent on the acoustic impedance of the different tissue densities An image is generated by the digital sequential processing of these sound waves based on the time difference between sound transmission and reception of the echo.

Ultrasonography is a safe test, without the risk of radiation exposure. Therefore, it is ideal for children and for pregnant women.[199] Limitations of anorectal ultrasonography are few and include obstructing anal or rectal lesions that limit insertion of the proctoscope and transducer and painful anal conditions, such as fissure or abscess.[246] These last concerns may require sedation and analgesia in order to complete the examination. Generally, however, the study is easily performed without anesthesia in the office or outpatient setting, with the results immediately obtainable.

Indications

The usefulness of anorectal ultrasonography in the evaluation of many anorectal conditions has been demonstrated through numerous publications.[61,141,145,146,167,170,224,247,249] The procedure not only provides an accurate anatomic description of the anal sphincters, but can also determine the extent of any muscular defects. In addition to its role in the evaluation of fecal incontinence, anorectal ultrasonography is also an important tool in the assessment of occult perianal abscess, recurrent fistula, and certain patients with rectal pain.[149,199] Anorectal fistula is diagnosed as a hyperechoic tract representing surrounding inflammation. The occasional presence of beads of air within the tract may facilitate the diagnosis. Gentle pressure of the probe will displace the beads of air within the fistulous tract. Furthermore, injection of hydrogen peroxide through the external opening will also facilitate the delineation of the fistulous tract. Schwartz and colleagues demonstrated the accuracy of anorectal ultrasonography in the evaluation of perianal Crohn's disease to be 82% versus 24% for computed tomography.[207] Surgically confirmed findings were also compared with that of anorectal ultrasonography and magnetic resonance imaging (MRI); the former was accurate in 82% versus 50% in the latter.[206]

Potential options in the management of rectal cancer include radical resection and local excision. Furthermore, The National Institutes of Health Consensus Conference in 1990 recommended that a patient with locally invasive rectal cancer should be considered for neoadjuvant therapy.[163] The benefits of this approach to treatment were confirmed by the Swedish Rectal Cancer Trial.[128] Hence, the therapeutic approach and the prognosis for patients with rectal cancer lie in the ability of one to stage the tumor accurately. Therefore, the search for an accurate preoperative diagnostic modality of rectal cancer has been very important.

Endorectal ultrasonography not only has emerged as a superior method for pretreatment staging of rectal cancer when compared with computed tomography and MRI, but also is a more cost effective and safer technique. Endorectal ultrasonography can accurately determine the depth of invasion in 85% to 95% of rectal tumors. However, these results decrease to 60% to 85% when evaluating lymph node metastasis (see Chapter 23).[63,150,153,175,246] Preoperative radiotherapy will also decrease the accuracy of endorectal ultrasonography because of the increased echogenicity noted in the radiated rectal wall.[64,69,229] Still, endorectal ultrasonography is useful as a follow-up modality for determining local recurrence. When used alone, its accuracy in detecting local recurrence varies from 75% to 91%. However, with the addition of fine needle aspiration, the overall accuracy increases to 92% to 100%.[207] The specificity of this combined modality is 93% compared with 57% for computerized tomography. The problem of differentiating local recurrence from that of postoperative changes can be minimized by performing a baseline endorectal ultrasonography 3 months after surgery, by which time most acute inflammatory reaction has decreased.

Equipment

Numerous ultrasound scanners and probes are available (Figs. 6-20 and 6-21). Early versions did not have rotating transducer heads and could, therefore, only scan sectors of the anal canal ranging from 90 to 320 degrees. Even though accurate imaging was possible, it was difficult to ensure that pictures from different sectors were taken at the same level of the anus. Thus, it was problematic for the examiner to recreate the anatomy of the anal canal. This difficulty has been surmounted by the development of a 360-degree rotating transducer (Figure 6-21; Brüel and Kjaer, Naerum, Denmark and North Billerica, MA; Table 6-4). Transducers of differing frequencies have also been used. Early models employed 4- and 5-MHz transducers,[33,74] but owing to focal length deficiencies these probes have been superseded by 7- and 10-MHz endoprobes. However, some controversy exists as to whether a 10-MHz transducer (focal length 1 to 4 cm) gives a higher resolution of the anal sphincters than does the 7-MHz transducer (focal length 2 to 5 cm). Based on ultrasonographic physics, higher frequency (number of cycles per second) improves resolution. Meanwhile, wave length (distance traveled by the ultrasonic wave per cycle) decreases as frequency increases, thus allowing better resolution but poorer tissue penetration.[199]

The transducer head is covered by a sonolucent hard cone, 1.7 cm in external diameter (Figure 6-21). This cone is carefully filled with water to ensure that all air bubbles are excluded because they will produce artifacts. Some investigators do not believe that the use of a plastic

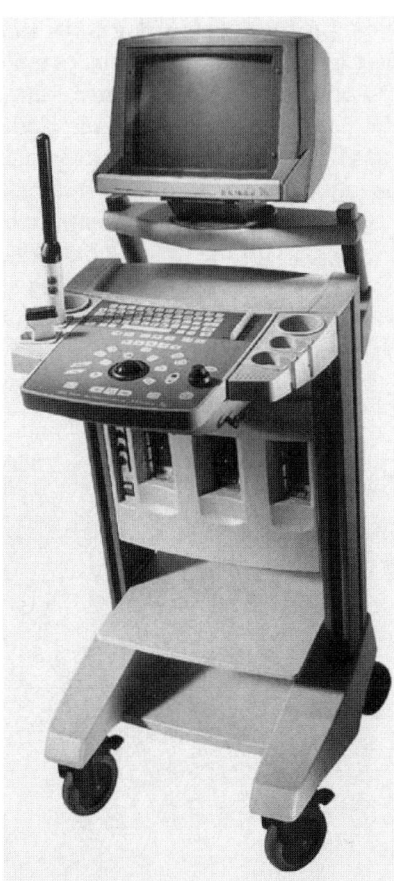

FIGURE 6-20. Falcon ultrasound scanner, probe and monitor. (Courtesy of Brüel & Kjaer Instruments, Inc., Billerica, MA.)

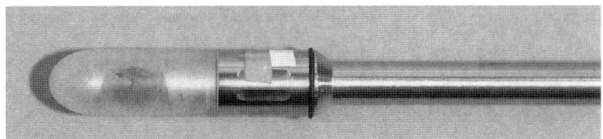

FIGURE 6-21. Transducer head of a 7-mHz rotating endoanal ultrasound probe (B & K 1850). (Courtesy of Brüel and Kjaer Instruments, Inc., Billerica, MA.)

output from the scanner can be connected to a video printer so that still pictures can be taken. The signal can be relayed through the printer to a standard VHS video recorder because real-time images are more informative than still pictures, especially when attempting to identify fistula tracts or abscess cavities.

Ultrasonic probes are available in combination with various endoscopes to allow simultaneous observation of ultrasonic and endoscopic images. This technology is expensive, but because these endoscopes are widely used in gastroenterologic practice, shared equipment should reduce capital outlay. Two designs are available. A convex, longitudinal scanning system is preferred by some manufacturers because of improved reliability and the ease of use of accessory tools, such as biopsy needles. These endoscopes also provide color Doppler facility but only permit scanning through a sector of 100 degrees. Other manufacturers prefer a 360-degree mechanical radial scanner (Table 6-4).

Interpretation

Examination takes place with the patient in the left lateral decubitus position, with the probe orientated so that the water spigot is in the upright position. Using this orientation, the anterior quadrant of the anal canal is seen in the superior aspect of the screen with the right quadrant seen on the left side of the screen. The different tissue densities and interfaces create a series of hyperechoic

cone is necessary and employ a latex balloon inflated with degassed water for acoustic couplings. They claim that good sonographic images with minimal anatomic distortion of the anal canal can be achieved by this means.[232]

A condom containing ultrasound gel is placed over the probe, and a water-soluble lubricant is applied. The video

▎ **TABLE 6-4 Ultrasound Equipment Suppliers**

Manufacturer	Telephone	Model	Type	Scanning System	Scanning Angle	Frequency
Bruel and Kjaer, North Billerica, MA 01862, USA	1-800-876-7226	Probe 1850 Scanner 1846	Rigid	Mechanical, radial	360 degrees	7 or 10 MHz
Bruel and Kjaer, Naerum, Denmark	45-45-97-01-00					
Olympus America Inc., Melville, NY 11747, USA	1-800-222-4554 516-844-5000	GF-UM20 gastroscope	Endoscopic	Mechanical, radial	360 degrees	7.5 or 12 MHz switchable
Olympus Keymed, Southport-on-Sea, SS2 5QH, UK	44-1702-616-333	CF-UM20 colonoscope	Endoscopic	Mechanical, radial	360 degrees	7.5 or 12 MHz
Pentax Precision Instrument Corp., Orangeburg, NY 10962, USA	1-800-431-5880 914-365-0700	FG-32UA	Endoscopic	Convex, longitudinal	100 degrees	5 or 7.5 MHz switchable
Pentax UK Ltd., Slough, SL3 8PN, UK	44-1753-792-723					

and hypoechoic images, corresponding to the different anatomic layers of the anal canal.[232] Using a 7-MHz probe, three distinct layers are seen. The mucosa/submucosa complex appears as a hyperechoic band surrounding the transducer. Outside this layer is a hypoechoic band that can be seen most clearly in the midanal canal; this represents the internal anal sphincter. The band has an average thickness of 2 to 4 mm. Parenthetically, it has been noted to increase with age.[30] The final layer is a thicker band of mixed echogenicity that represents the external anal sphincter. The junction between external sphincter and perirectal fat is not clearly defined, making

it difficult to measure the thickness of the sphincter clearly.[227] Average values of 4 to 8 mm are reported.

Using a 10-MHz probe, other observers have described six ultrasonic layers of the anal canal. They divide the first hyperechoic layer into three parts: a hypoechoic layer (representing the mucosa) is sandwiched between a superficial hyperechoic layer (representing the interface of the latex balloon with the tissues) and a deeper hyperechoic layer (representing subepithelial tissue). A further hyperechoic layer can be seen between the internal and external sphincter and is said to represent the longitudinal muscle of the intersphincteric plane.[13]

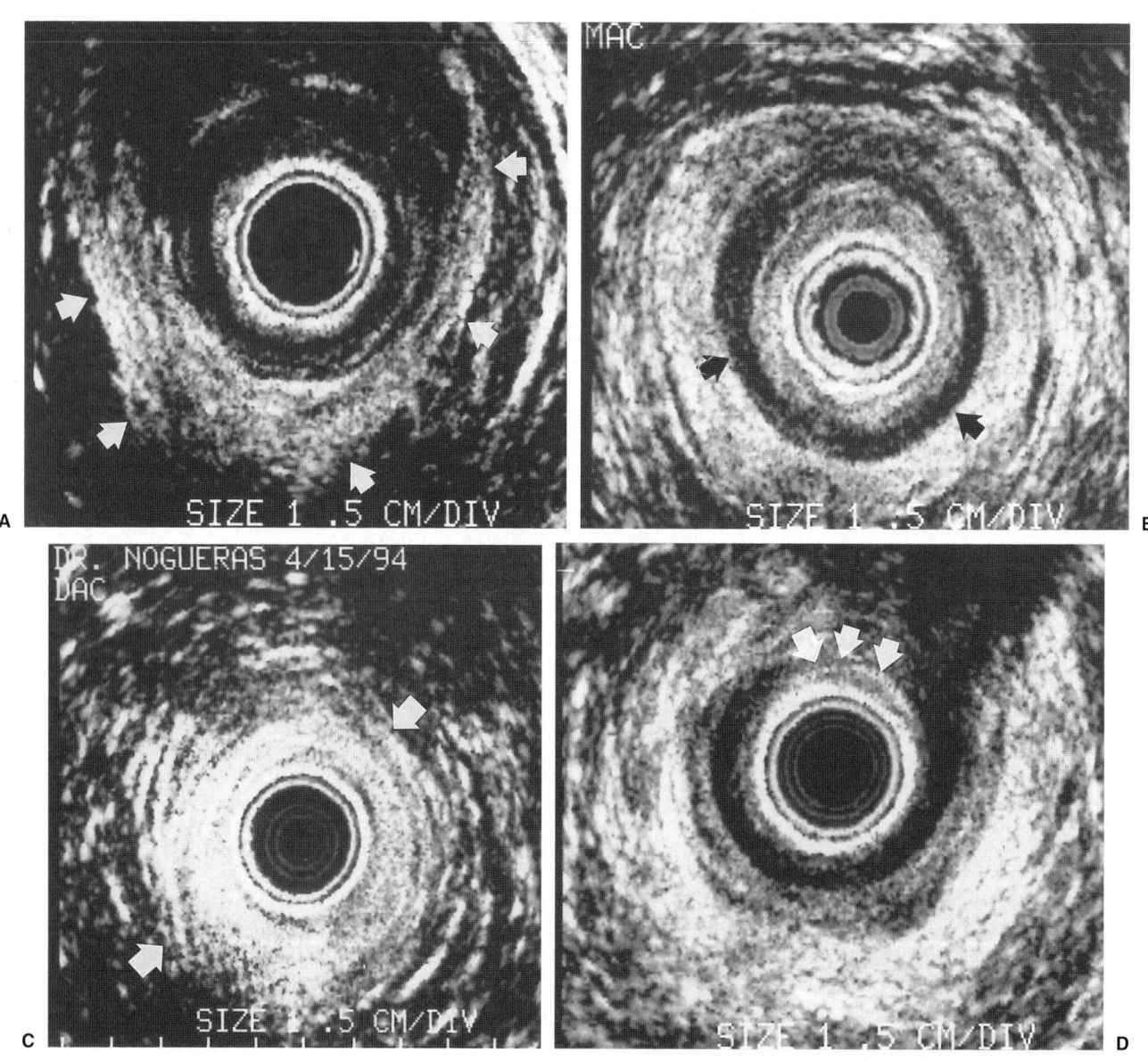

FIGURE 6-22. Endoanal ultrasound images. **(A)** Upper anal canal: puborectalis sling posteriorly *(arrows)*. **(B)** Middle anal canal: the hypoechoic internal sphincter *(arrows)* is at its maximum thickness. **(C)** Lower anal canal: the hypoechoic internal sphincter has disappeared and is replaced by hyperechoic external sphincter *(arrows)*. **(D)** Anterior sphincter defect in the midanal canal with absent external sphincter and scarring of the internal sphincter *(arrows)*.

Using these layers, one can divide the anal canal can into three regions. The start of the upper anal canal is marked by the puborectalis muscle. This appears as a U- or V-shaped band of mixed echogenicity passing behind the lumen of the anus (Figure 6-22*A*). Because of the lack of muscle anteriorly, especially in women, care must be taken not to interpret this area as a sphincteric defect. As the scanner is slowly withdrawn, the hypoechoic layer that represents the internal sphincter gradually increases in thickness, and the layer of mixed echogenicity meets anteriorly to form a continuous band of muscle. The point of maximum thickness of the internal anal sphincter marks the midanal canal (Figure 6-22*B*). As scanning continues distally, the internal sphincter gradually disappears to an almost imperceptibly thin strip. At this point, the hyperechoic superficial portion of the external anal sphincter at the level of the lower anal canal can be visualized (Figure 6-22*C*). Figure 6-22*D* illustrates a typical sphincteric disruption in a woman following obstetric injury.

Author's Technique

Bowel preparation is not required for endoanal ultrasonography. After careful explanation of the procedure, a digital rectal examination is performed to lubricate the anal canal, to assess any anatomic defects, and to ensure that the probe can be introduced into the anal canal easily and without discomfort. The probe (7-MHz, type 1850) is inserted into the lower rectum and then is gradually withdrawn until the puborectalis sling can be most clearly identified. Using a video copy processor (P40U, Mitsubishi Electric, Inc., Cypress, CA), one takes a still picture at this level. Scanning continues distally until the level of the midanal canal. At this point, a careful assessment is made of the continuity of both internal and external sphincters. The maximum thickness of both of these muscles is measured using the software accompanying the B & K scanner, and further still photographs are taken. A photograph of the lower anal canal is obtained before the probe is withdrawn.

Conclusions and Recommendations

Ultrasound has a number of advantages when compared with other physiologic and anatomic investigations. First, it is usually painless and is, therefore, preferable to concentric needle EMG for mapping sphincter defects. Thus, patient compliance with respect to follow-up is generally not a problem. Second, ultrasound is less expensive than is other imaging modalities such as computed tomography or MRI. It is also quicker to perform than these two techniques, and the patient is not exposed to radiation. Finally, because the equipment is portable it can be taken to the operating room or used in the clinician's examination room.

The question of who should perform endoanal ultrasonography remains somewhat controversial. This is often a turf issue and ultimately is resolved by who owns the equipment and where it is maintained. In our view, endoanal ultrasonography should be performed by the surgeon, because he or she understands the anatomy, is fully acquainted with the patient's history, and is responsible for making a recommendation based on the findings. There are no dicta regarding the length of time required to become skilled at performing and interpreting endoanal ultrasonography. However, endorectal ultrasonography is known to have a steep learning curve,[148] and our experience suggests that this is true. It is, therefore, preferable that the performance and interpretation of endoanal ultrasound be concentrated in the hands of limited numbers of individuals who have become familiar with the technique.

MAGNETIC RESONANCE IMAGING

The advent of MRI provided a new modality for the investigation of anorectal function. Some of the disadvantages and limitations associated with endoanal ultrasonography can be overcome using MRI in association with a surface or endoanal coil.[8,96] For instance, because endoanal ultrasonography is operator dependent and only axial images can be obtained, the complex anatomic relationships may be difficult to comprehend. Furthermore, the internal anal sphincter is the only structure consistently seen with endoanal ultrasound. Most probes make it difficult to visualize the longitudinal muscle, and the interface between the outer border of the external sphincter and the surrounding ischioanal spaces are often indistinct. The development of the endoanal coil, a device that has an increased signal-to-noise ratio, has resulted in the acquisition of high-quality images of the anal musculature.[44,45,96] These images may alter our perception of the anatomy of the sphincter apparatus and may prove to be of benefit in the assessment of sphincter injury before surgical intervention. Furthermore, the enhanced imaging of this area and its associated anatomic spaces, using either surface or endoanal coils, enhances the diagnosis and classification of anal fistula.[97,139,161] MRI, however, is considerably more expensive than ultrasonography and it is not widely available. Moreover, it is a problem for patients suffering from claustrophobia and cannot be undertaken when mechanical devices such as pacemakers or metallic prostheses are present.[60]

MRI has the advantage of being nonoperator dependent. Additionally, one can obtain images in either the sagittal or coronal planes. Although defecography remains the imaging modality of choice for the dynamic analysis of the anorectum, fast MRI has been introduced as an alternative.[121,248] This test is a noninvasive procedure requiring no special preparation, because, with the patient in the prone position, gas collects in the rectum and acts as a natural contrast medium. Images during rest, squeeze, and push phases can be obtained. In addition, dynamic MRI, in contrast to defecography, does not expose the patient to radiation. Initial reports have suggested that MRI is an excellent means for determining the size of the anorectal angle as well as the degree of perineal descent during simulated defecation.[121] The interobserver variation in the assessment of these parameters has been reported to be small.[121] However, although it is true that these anatomic parameters can be accurately defined, functional abnormalities occurring during defecation, such as intussusception, prolapse, and rectocele cannot be detected.[43,121] Furthermore, the equipment is vastly more expensive and requires greater capital for construction of a copper-lined room when compared with the standard lead-lined fluoroscopy suites. Additionally, the patient is deprived of the normal physiologic position for evacuation and is instead asked to relax and evacuate in the lateral position. Despite these disadvantages, Fletcher and associates described pelvic MRI as a comprehensive imaging modality to evaluate not only anatomic but also functional disorders of the pelvic floor.[60] They also were able to demonstrate that MRI with endorectal coil is comparable to anal ultrasonography in the evaluation of defects of the internal and external anal sphincters. However, only MRI could demonstrate atrophy of the anal sphincter muscles and puborectalis. In addition, the authors found that magnetic resonance fluoroscopy (dynamic pelvic MRI) is an excellent means for assessing the pelvic floor and pelvic organs during evacuation, rest, and squeeze maneuvers. However, the limited availability, cost, and reimbursement concerns in the United States have limited dynamic pelvic MRI to that of an investigational tool.

COLONIC TRANSIT STUDY

Although constipation is often the result of dietary issues or evacuation difficulties, some element of colonic inertia is not uncommon. A transit abnormality is noteworthy for resistance to standard medical treatment with dietary manipulation and cathartics. It is, therefore, important to be able to identify those who are suffering primarily from a disturbance in colonic motility (see Chapter 16).[181] Indeed, in a study conducted among colorectal surgeons in the United States and the United Kingdom, colonic transit studies were deemed to be the most helpful of all available physiology tests.[110]

Historically, intestinal transit was assessed by the ingestion of nonabsorbable colored glass or plastic beads that were then collected following defecation.[5] This process was obviously aesthetically unpleasant for both patient and investigator. Similarly, other clinicians have used colored powders, such as carmine and charcoal, or chemically detectable markers, such as chromium oxide and copper thiocyanate.[46,147,244] All of these methods have the same aesthetic and cumbersome disadvantages and are no longer used. At the present time, assessment of colonic transit is most commonly done through the use of either radiopaque markers or colonic scintigraphy.

Radiopaque Markers

In the initial use of this modality, radiopaque markers were ingested and their excretion in stool was monitored by serial radiographs of the feces.[92] Although this technique has the advantage of not exposing the patient to radiation, it is unpleasant for both the patient and the radiologist, and it gives no indication as to the anatomic distribution of markers over time. In 1981, Arhan and colleagues modified the procedure by taking serial x-ray studies of the abdomen every 24 hours for up to 7 days following ingestion of the markers.[6]

By using bony landmarks to divide the abdomen into three areas, some appreciation of segmental colonic transit can be obtained. For example, markers that are located to the right of the spinous processes of the vertebrae and above a line drawn from the fifth lumbar vertebra to the pelvic outlet are in the right colon. Markers to the left of the vertebral spinous processes and above a line from the fifth lumbar vertebra to the iliac crest are in the left colon. Markers below the line of the pelvic brim on the right and the iliac crest on the left are said to be in the rectosigmoid and rectum (Figure 6-23). If a single bolus of 20 markers is given and serial x-ray studies are taken every 24 hours, Arhan's initial formula for the calculation of mean transit time (hours) per segment can be simplified to

$$\text{mean transit} = 1.2 \, (n_1 + n_2 + n_3 + \cdots + n_j)$$

where n equals the number of markers present on each film and j is the total number of films.

The problem with this approach, however, is that daily x-ray studies will expose the patient to more radiation than is necessary. This can be reduced without compromising the quality of the information by employing the technique described by Hinton and Lennard-Jones.[91] They suggested ingestion of a single capsule of 20 radiopaque rings followed by daily abdominal roentgenographs (see Figs. 16-8 and 16-9). A normal study is one in which 16 or more of the markers have passed by the fifth postingestion day and all have been evacuated by the seventh day. Metcalf and co-workers modified the test by suggesting the use of three boluses of 20 markers each, ingested at 24-hour intervals, and then taking two plain abdominal radiographs at 24 and 96 hours following the ingestion of the third bolus.[154] The same formula noted earlier can be

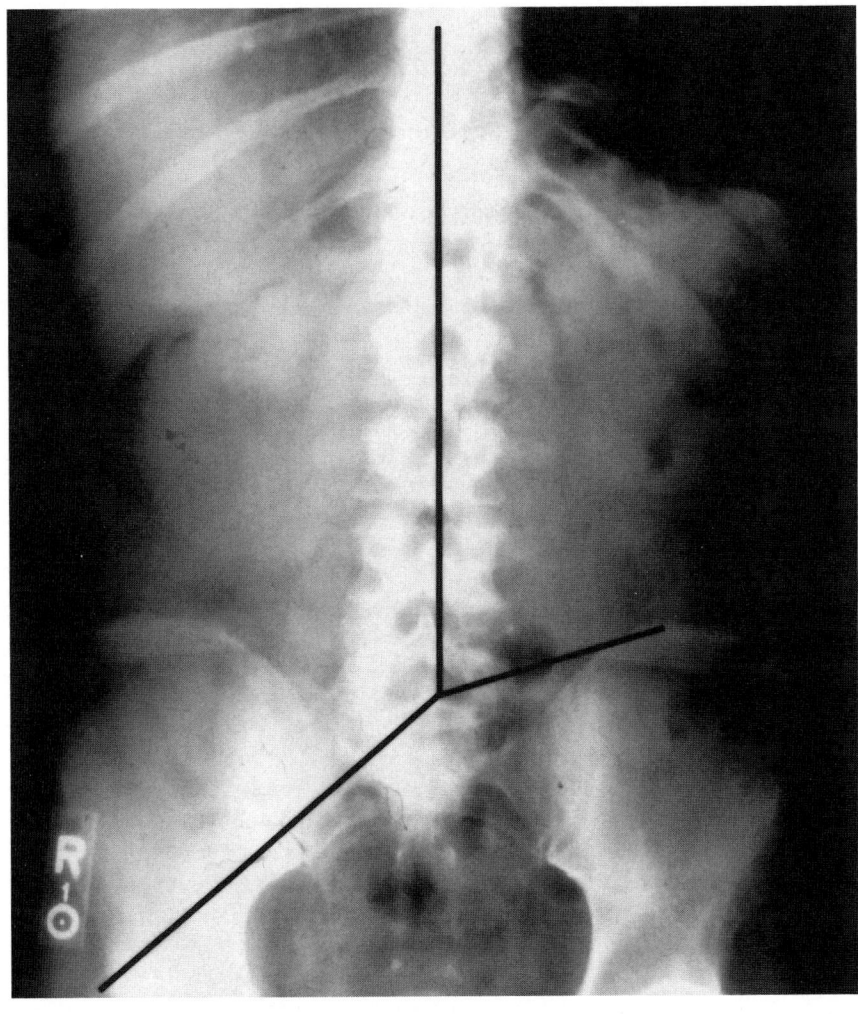

FIGURE 6-23. Plain abdominal x-ray study demonstrating lines of reference for segmental colonic transit marker studies.

used to calculate segmental transit time.[155] Using modifications of these methods, transit through the right colon has been estimated to be from 6.9 to 13 hours, transit through the left colon from 9.1 to 15 hours, and transit through the rectosigmoid from 11 to 18.4 hours.[6,36,154] Because the radiopaque marker study is simple, inexpensive, and reproducible, it is the most widely performed colonic transit evaluation.

Although it is certainly intellectually gratifying and potentially useful to know the segmental transit, there appears to be little clinical relevance based upon our current therapeutic algorithms.[138,182] Accordingly, the simple method upon which we have settled is for the patient to ingest a single capsule containing 24 commercially available rings (Sitz Marks, Konsyl Pharmaceuticals, Lafayette, TX). A single radiograph obtained 5 days after ingestion of the capsule can provide all of the necessary information. Specifically, retention of 20% or more of the markers can be interpreted as abnormal. There are three basic results to this single-capsule, single-radiograph study. First, if fewer than 20% of the markers are retained, this should be considered a "normal" study. Second, if 20% or more of the markers are retained in the rectosigmoid, a functional or anatomic pelvic outlet obstruction is thought to exist. Third, if 20% or more of the markers are retained and diffusely situated throughout the colon, this is suggestive of colonic inertia (see Chapter 16).

Colonic Scintigraphy

This procedure entails the tracking of a radionuclide-labeled bolus through the colon by using a gamma camera. It has been advocated as an accurate method of assessing colonic transit time, but has the inconvenience of requiring that the radionuclide bolus be delivered to the cecum. This can be accomplished by direct installation into the cecum through either orocecal intubation or via colonoscopy.[108,120] Both of these methods are obviously invasive, and colonoscopic installation requires bowel preparation, which may confuse interpretation of colonic transit results. As an alternative, polystyrene pellets or resin particles labeled with ^{99m}Tc or indium (^{111}In) can be incorporated into a gelatin capsule coated with a methacrylate polymer.[188] Following ingestion, this capsule will remain intact through the acid pH of the stomach and duodenum but will dissolve in the distal small bowel where the pH is typically between 7.2 and 7.4.[52,215] Multiple images can be obtained without increasing the radiation exposure over 3 consecutive days.[98] However, this type of intensive study makes considerable time demands on gamma camera use and is inconvenient for the patient. These difficulties can be ameliorated by limiting data acquisition to three times: 28 hours, 52 hours, and 60 hours following ingestion.[168]

Sequential transit times can be calculated as the time difference between the initial detection of activity in one region of interest and initial detection of activity in the adjacent region of interest. This provides information about the rate of transit of the head of the meal and may differ from the transit time of the bulk of the meal. Furthermore, identification of the time when the meal enters a particular region is subject to further error, depending on the frequency with which images are obtained. To further confuse matters, image resolution is not ideal. This leads to difficulty in interpreting the anatomic layout of the colon, loops of which may be superimposed or confused with small bowel.

Clearly, because of the complexity of this technique, it has limited clinical application. It does, however, remain as an investigational modality.

Recommendation

We prefer to use a modification of Hinton's and Lennard-Jones' original method.[91] No bowel preparation is carried out. The patient is given a single capsule containing 24 radiopaque markers (Sitzmarks, Konsyl Pharmaceuticals, Inc., Fort Worth, TX; see Figure 16-8). One is instructed to refrain from the use of laxatives or fiber products from the day before capsule ingestion until after completion of the study. Abdominal x-ray studies, which include the diaphragms and the pubis, are taken on days 3 and 5 following ingestion, and the total number of markers is counted on each film.[182] If most markers are delayed in the rectosigmoid area, outlet obstruction is probable.[242] The test is deemed to be normal if 80% of the markers have been evacuated by the fifth day.[6,92]

SMALL BOWEL TRANSIT

It has generally been believed that prolonged oroanal transit times reflect mainly colonic transit abnormality. However, many patients with delayed colonic transit times may have a generalized motility disturbance of the gastrointestinal tract. Thus, before submitting a patient to total colectomy, it may be advisable to obtain some measure of small bowel transit. Of course, an indication of small bowel transit time may be of benefit in the investigation of individuals with diarrhea, malabsorption,

or increased stool frequency following coloanal or ileal pouch-anal anastomosis.[24,119]

Breath Hydrogen Analysis

The investigation of small bowel transit time by the use of the breath hydrogen test was first described by Bond and colleagues in 1975.[24] Strictly speaking, it is a measure of orocecal transit. Following an overnight fast, the subject ingests a nonabsorbable carbohydrate such as lactulose (1,4-β-galactofructose), which providess a value for liquid transit,[133] or baked beans, which gives a figure for solid transit.[192] On entering the cecum, these substrates are metabolized by colonic bacteria to hydrogen and short-chain fatty acids. Hydrogen, which is highly diffusible and relatively insoluble in water, is rapidly absorbed into the blood, transported to the lungs, and exhaled.[133]

Although this is a relatively simple test, certain caveats may interfere with its interpretation. First, 5% to 20% of the population are so-called "nonfermenters"; they do not produce hydrogen.[21,22] In addition, oral bacteria may cause some breakdown of the substrate, but this can be easily overcome by the use of a mouthwash before the administration of the test meal.[230] Similarly, small intestinal bacterial overgrowth will result in early metabolism of the substrate.[41] This, unfortunately, is less easy to manage. Furthermore, antibiotics consumed within the prior 10 days may deplete the colonic flora and result in a falsely prolonged result. Smoking and vigorous exercise should also be avoided before the test because these factors may influence breath hydrogen. There may also be some difficulty in interpreting the first peak of breath hydrogen, thus making the results unreliable.[95]

Despite the limitations and the drawbacks, the breath hydrogen test has proven to be a simple, noninvasive technique to study small bowel transit time. Unfortunately, normal values often vary from center to center because of the different criteria used to identify the time of entry of the meal into the cecum. Certain investigators have used the first rise of breath hydrogen by 20 parts per million (ppm),[34] others 5 ppm,[200] still others 3 ppm,[10,102] or 2 ppm.[15] Some have calculated small bowel transit as the time from ingestion to maximal peak in breath hydrogen.[223]

Salicylazosulfapyridine

Another option for determining small bowel transit is this investigation. Following the oral administration of sulphasalazine (Azulfidine, Kabi Pharmacia, Piscataway, NJ), the azo-bond is hydrolyzed by colonic bacteria, releasing mesalazine and sulfapyridine. Sulfapyridine is absorbed and can be detected within the patient's blood. This test of orocecal transit has the disadvantage of requiring multiple blood samples; up to 300 mL of blood may be removed. This test also may be adversely affected

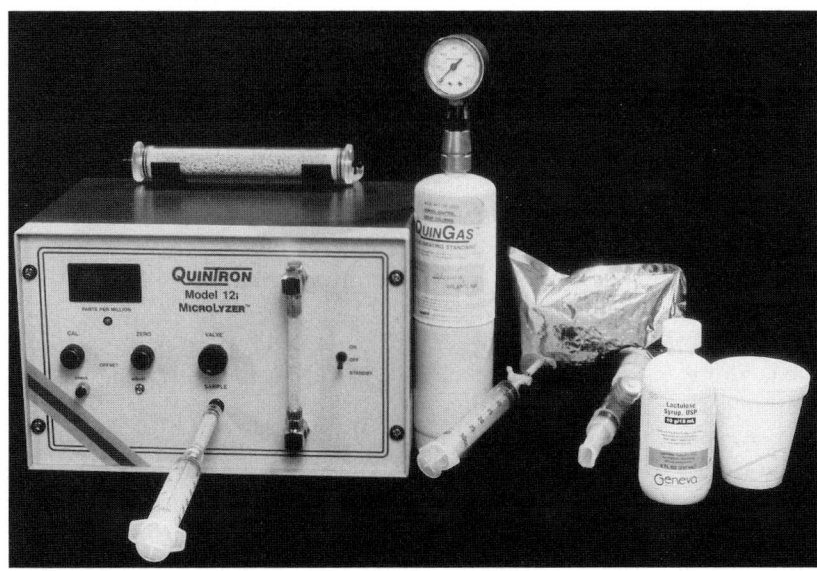

FIGURE 6-24. Microlyzer gas chromatograph analyzer. (model 12). (Courtesy of Quintron, Milwaukee, WI.)

by small bowel bacterial overgrowth or by antibiotic ingestion. Because of its cost and more invasive nature, it is not frequently utilized.

Small Intestinal Scintigraphy

Gastric emptying and small bowel transit time can be assessed by the ingestion of polystyrene pellets labeled with either ^{99m}Tc or ^{111}In or by labeling a meal of mashed potatoes with ^{99m}Tc sulfur colloid or diethylenetriaminepentaacetic acid (DTPA).[32,192] Some physicians prefer ^{99m}Tc-HIDA. This tracer given intravenously is excreted in the bile and delivered into the duodenum, thereby avoiding any influence of gastric emptying rate on small bowel results.[78] Methods using polystyrene pellets measure the small bowel transit of nondigestible solids, whereas the mashed potato meal is probably a measurement of liquid transit. Small bowel transit time is calculated to be the time taken for a fixed quantity of the isotope (e.g., 10% or 50%) to empty from the stomach and enter the colon.[32,76] As with colonic scintigraphy, these radioisotope techniques are unaffected by bacterial overgrowth or antibiotics but do expose patients to low radiation doses. Interpretation may be made difficult by small bowel loops overlying the cecum.[34] This can be clarified by allowing the test to continue so that accurate images of cecal filling can be obtained.

Recommendations

In our laboratory, small bowel transit is primarily used as an adjunct to colonic transit studies in order to identify individuals with generalized intestinal hypomotility.[18,235] We have found that measurements of orocecal transit using breath hydrogen are reliable, reproducible, and well tolerated.[102] After an overnight fast, patients are given

10 g/15 mL lactulose (UDL Laboratories, Inc., Rockford, IL) with 100 mL of water. This small dose produces values for orocecal transit that are more accurate; larger doses decrease transit times because of the osmotic effect.[24] Care is taken to ensure that the patient has refrained from antibiotics and bowel cleansing agents for the previous 7 days and from smoking on the morning of the test. End-expiratory breath samples (100 to 200 mL) are obtained every 15 minutes by having the patient exhale slowly into a 750-mL multipatient collection bag (QT 00841-P, Quintron, Milwaukee, WI). Samples are analysed using a Microlyzer gas chromatograph analyzer (model 12i, Quintron, Milwaukee, WI) (Figure 6-24), which is calibrated using an air/hydrogen mixture (98.2 parts per million hydrogen; Matheson Gas Products, Inc., Joliet, IL). Results are plotted as hydrogen (ppm) versus time (minutes), and sampling is continued for up to 3 hours or until the graph reaches a plateau, whichever is sooner.

In our laboratory, a rise of 3 ppm has been demonstrated to produce the lowest coefficient of variation between subjects and is, therefore, the value used to determine that the meal has reached the cecum.[102] Patients who fail to produce an appreciable rise (more than 2 ppm) or sustained rise (more than three consecutive measurements) in breath hydrogen within 3 hours of ingestion are assumed to be nonfermenters.[102]

SMALL BOWEL, COLONIC, AND RECTAL MOTILITY

Nonambulatory Studies

The relationship between the motor activity of the small bowel and the colon and rectum is not completely understood. Most studies have been performed on healthy volunteers, and the implications of abnormal activity in disease states, therefore, is uncertain. Although prolonged recordings using water-perfused manometric equipment have been performed in both small bowel and rectum, the use of solid-state transducer catheters is now more common and indeed may be more physiologic.[57,130,174,186,190] These catheters can be custom built to any length with the transducers placed at the areas of interest. They can be introduced under colonoscopic or sigmoidoscopic control, and their position can be verified fluoroscopically.[162,190,197,233] Small portable recorders are now available that can incorporate information from multiple channels for 24 hours or more (Gaeltec 7MPR, Gaeltec Ltd., Isle of Skye, UK).[194] The information gathered by these systems is complex, requiring computer analysis programs that have the ability to remove high-frequency, low-amplitude artifact.[57]

These studies have led to the identification of cyclical bursts of contractility within the rectum, known as rectal motor complexes.[127,174] These complexes appear to occur more frequently at night and during periods of fasting.[127,190] Furthermore, there seems to be a temporal relationship between colonic motility and the rectal motor complexes. Rao and Welcher found that 81% of nocturnal bursts of rectal motor activity occur within 5 minutes of a motor event in the more proximal colon.[190] Ferrara and colleagues noted that a rectal motor complex is always associated with a rise in mean anal canal pressure in order to maintain continence.[57] As yet there has been no relationship found between small intestinal migrating motor complex and rectal motor activity.[186] Because these investigations do not at present have a clear clinical implication in the management of patients, they are not performed in our laboratory.

Ambulatory Studies

Anally inserted manometric catheters usually require an empty colon. The laxative or enemas, themselves, are known to alter colonic motility. In addition, the subject lies on a couch during the investigation, not in the normal physiologic state. Information obtained from these tests may, therefore, deviate considerably from normal motility patterns. Two methods have been developed that permit ambulatory monitoring without a bowel preparation.[219]

Radiotelemetry

The use of a pressure sensing device that can be swallowed and continuously transmit signals via radio waves was initially described by Connell and co-workers in 1963.[40] Two different designs exist. In one, a metal diaphragm with attached ferrite disc is displaced inward in response to colonic pressure. Its movement changes the inductance of an oscillating circuit, causing a change in the frequency of the emitted radio signal. The signals are

sensed by three receivers attached to the patient's belt. The second design is considerably more expensive. It contains a pressure-sensitive transducer, the output of which is converted to a fixed-frequency pulsed radio signal.[28] Both these capsules can be placed inside a latex rubber sleeve to prevent contamination with feces. The device is usually swallowed at 10 A.M., migrating through the stomach and small intestine during the overnight fast. The 24-hour recording period starts at 9 A.M. the following morning.

Although the technique is well accepted by patients, retrieval of the capsule is somewhat unpleasant.[193] There are, however, two other disadvantages. First, pressures are recorded at only one site, and this is without investigator control. Furthermore, the capsule is likely to be propelled ahead of the pressure wave. Therefore, important pressure changes may not be ascertained.

Tube-Mounted Transducers

Some of the disadvantages previously cited may be overcome by this method. It allows the placement of solid-state transducers, mounted on a manometry catheter in specific sites, without the need for endoscopy or prior bowel cleansing. A fine tube with a balloon mounted at its tip is introduced through the patient's nostril. When the balloon enters the duodenum it is inflated. During the next 2 to 3 days, it will be propelled through the intestine until it emerges at the anus. A recording device (usually three, tube-mounted, solid-state transducers) is then attached to the tip of the tube and pulled through the intestine until the distal recording transducer reaches the rectum, at which point the traction tube is removed.[187] Although this method provides excellent data, it is cumbersome and may require several days to position the recording device. Thus, it has not been extensively utilized in clinical practice.

ELECTROMYOGRAPHY

EMG of the anal sphincter was first reported by Beck in 1930.[16] Anal EMG is a recording of the electrical activity from the muscle fibers of the external sphincter and puborectalis complex during rest, during maximum squeeze, during simulated defecation, and in response to various reflexes.

Electrical activity may be measured from individual fibers (fibrillation potentials). It is more common, however, to assess the summation of the electrical activity from a number of muscle fibers derived from a single motor unit. This activity forms a motor unit action potential. A motor unit is composed of an anterior horn cell, its axon and terminal branches, and the muscle fibers that it supplies. Depolarization of the motor end plate by the release of acetylcholine in response to a nerve impulse results in depolarization of the muscle fiber with resultant contraction. EMG records the change of electrical potential during muscle depolarization. Four techniques can be used to record this electrical activity: concentric needle EMG, monopolar wire electrode EMG, single-fiber EMG, and surface or anal plug electrode EMG. Anal EMG has been used for sphincter mapping in patients with fecal incontinence and is also of use in assessing the function of the pelvic floor in individuals with constipation.

Normal Anal Findings

At rest there is observed a constant baseline EMG activity that is constantly changing.[60] During maximum voluntary contraction the amplitude of the motor unit potential is, on average, 200 to 600 µV, with a maximum of 2 to 3 mV. However, amplitude depends on the number of fibers that discharge simultaneously. It also varies with the distance of the recording electrode from the motor unit. Amplitude values are, therefore, not useful for comparative purposes. Duration of the motor unit potential is more reproducible but has been noted to increase with age.[53] The mean duration of motor unit potentials of the adult anal sphincter during voluntary contraction is 5 to 7.5 milliseconds. Motor unit potentials are usually biphasic or triphasic. However, polyphasic potentials (with four or more phases) are observed in the normal external sphincter. Reported incidences vary between 7% and 25%.[52]

Abnormal Anal Findings

Damage to the anal sphincter often causes scarring resulting in a markedly decreased number of motor unit potentials at rest, during squeeze, and during reflex elicitation.[164] Damage to the nerve supply of a muscle will result in two different patterns of EMG activity, depending on the severity of the injury. In a severely injured sphincter, EMG activity is significantly decreased or even silenced. However, if the injury is incomplete, reinnervation will occur by either regrowth of the damaged axons or sprouting of unaffected axons into different muscle fibers. Sprouting will alter the distribution of muscle fibers within motor units, a process known as fiber type grouping. This results in motor potentials of increased amplitude and prolonged duration and an increase in the number of polyphasic potentials.[51,56,165,217] These immature nerve fibers cannot conduct the nerve impulses quickly, which results in prolongation of the action potential.

During evacuation, EMG activity of the external sphincter and puborectalis should be almost silent. However, in patients with paradoxical contraction or nonrelaxation of the puborectalis the EMG activity will increase or will remain unchanged during simulated defecation.[22,42,59,185,201] Fucini and colleagues evaluated patients with symptoms of obstructed defecation using EMG of the pelvic floor muscles.[62] They showed a lower frequency of pubococcygeal muscle inhibition in this specific study population.

Concentric Needle Electromyography

Adrian and Bronck designed the first concentric needle electrode in 1929.[1] This consisted of a bare-tipped steel wire, 0.1 mm in diameter, surrounded by a resin insulation. The needle can record electrical activity from a small area that includes a few motor units. Individual muscle fiber action potentials cannot be identified with this apparatus, however. The electrical activity is amplified and displayed using one of many recorders available from several commercial sources (Table 6-5). Concentric needle EMG provides data on sphincter damage and reinnervation, and is useful for sphincter mapping. However, it is painful, and patients will seldom be willing to undergo follow-up evaluation.

Single-Fiber Electromyography

A single-fiber EMG electrode consists of a needle slightly less than 0.1 mm in diameter that is filled with resin. A 25-µm diameter electrode projects through this needle. The cannula of the electrode acts as the reference electrode; a separate surface electrode to ground is also required. The single-fiber electrode measures electrical activity from a radius of 270 µm. An amplifier with a 500-Hz low-frequency filter setting and a trigger delay line are necessary, with the amplifier set at 2 to 5 milliseconds per division. Twenty different recordings are taken from each lateral hemisphere of the sphincter, and the fiber density is calculated as the mean number of single muscle fiber action potentials per position.[222] The

▎**TABLE 6-5 Neurophysiologic Equipment Suppliers**

Manufacturer	Telephone
Axon Systems Inc., Hauppauge, NY 11788, USA	516-436-5112
	1-800-888-2966
Clark Electromedical Instruments, Reading, UK	44-17-348-43888
Dantec Medical A/S, Skovlunde, Denmark	45-44-92-31-32
Dantec Medical Inc., Campbell, CA 95008, USA	408-374-1400
	1-800-222-0074
Medelec, Woking, UK	44-14-837-70331
Nicolet Medical Inc., Madison, WI 53744, USA	1-800-356-0007
Teca Corporation, Pleasantville, NY 10570, USA	914-769-5900
	1-800-438-8322
Telefactor, Conshohocken, PA 19428, USA	1-800-654-6754

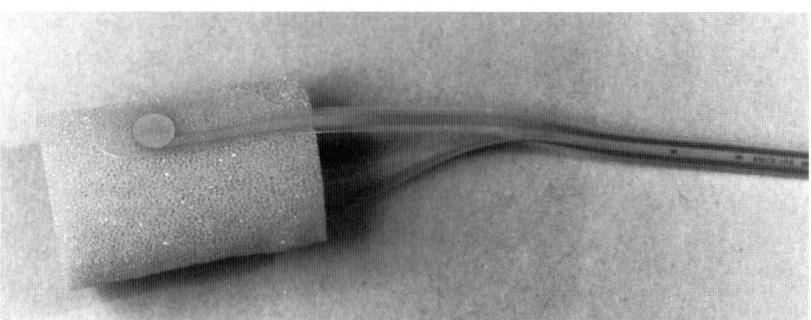

FIGURE 6-25. Intraanal sponge plug electrode (model 13L81). (Courtesy of Dantec Medical, Inc., Allendale, NJ.)

normal fiber density is 1.5±0.6.[165] The fiber density will increase during the period of reinnervation following nerve injury, because more fibers are innervated by an individual axon.

The time interval between action potentials is called neuromuscular jitter. This parameter is an indication of variability in the speed of the transmission of impulses across the neuromuscular junction, but its clinical relevance is uncertain. This also can be assessed by using a single-fiber EMG electrode in such a manner that when the electrode is placed it records two fibers from the same motor unit.[50]

Surface Anal Plug Electromyography

Surface electrodes have been used to record the electrical activity of the sphincter apparatus, but they have since been replaced through the development of intraanal plug EMG electrodes.[171] These plastic or sponge plugs have longitudinal or circular electrodes mounted on their surfaces and can be placed inside the anus with ease. Binnie and colleagues have demonstrated that longitudinal electrodes are superior to the circular design because they correlate with fine-wire electrodes.[20] Furthermore, they are much better tolerated but only provide crude global information about the sphincter. As such, although they are useful in evaluating those with constipation, they cannot be applied for sphincter mapping in incontinent patients. A study by Lopez and associates demonstrated a good correlation between sur-face electrodes and concentric needle electrodes in the diagnosis of paradoxical anal sphincter reaction.[136] EMG may also be an important adjunct to biofeedback in the management of patients with fecal incontinence and obstructed defecation.

Simultaneous Ambulatory Electromyography and Manometry

Twenty-four-hour monitoring of EMG and manometry activity of the sphincter mechanism has been performed in some centers.[126] However, it is technically difficult to accomplish and requires specialized equipment as well as a considerable learning curve. In addition, patients may be reluctant to have these electrodes placed for a prolonged period of time.

Equipment

Probe

EMG electrodes, pairs of fine-barbed bare steel wires, 0.13 mm in diameter, can be inserted through the use of a 19-gauge needle.

Manometry Catheters

Ambulatory manometry requires the use of solid-state microtransducer, pressure-sensitive catheters. The catheter most commonly employed has transducers mounted at 1 to 10 and 14 cm from the anal verge.

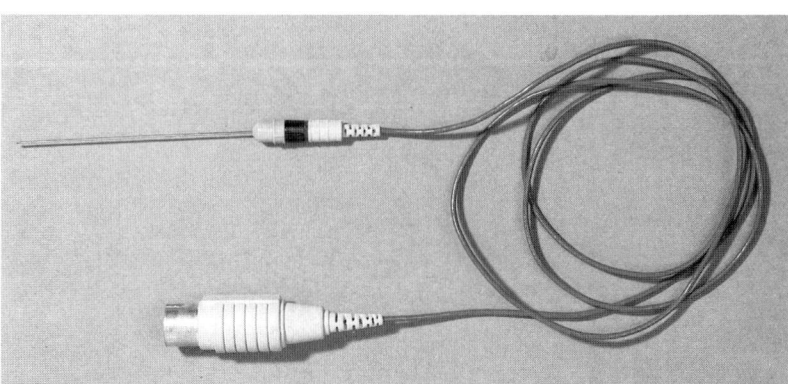

FIGURE 6-26. Bipolar concentric electromyographic needle (no. 53158). (Courtesy of Teca, Pleasantville, NY.)

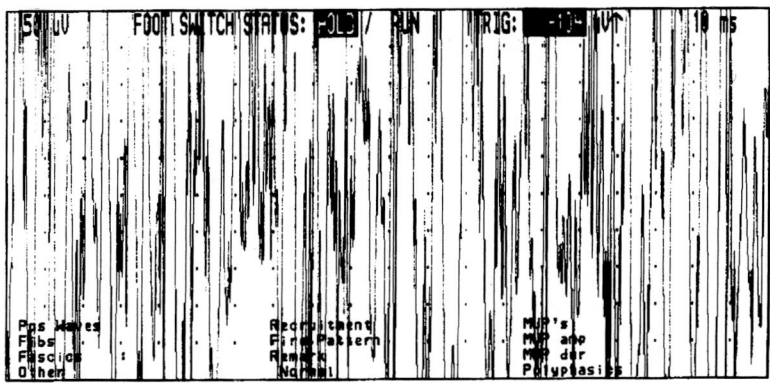

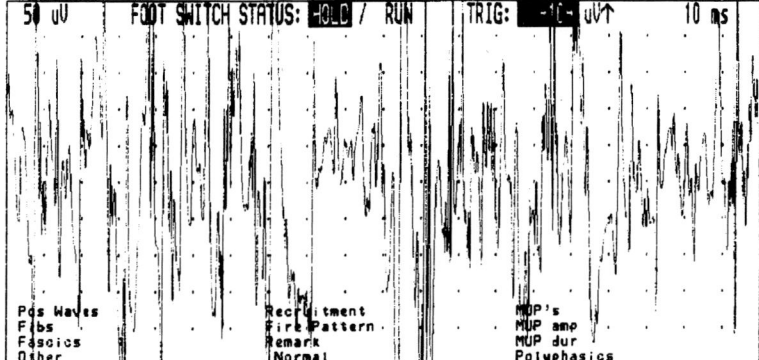

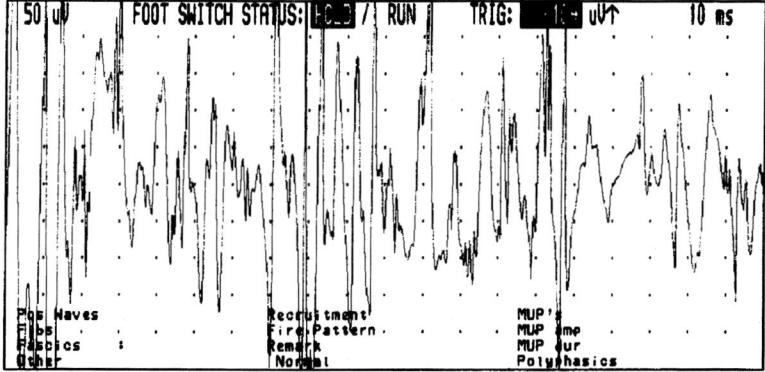

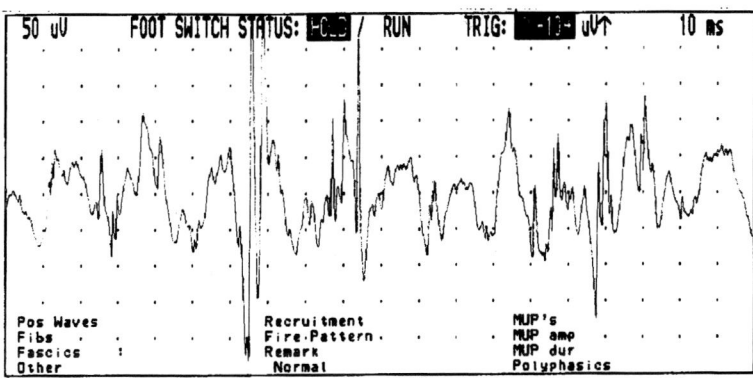

FIGURE 6-27. External anal sphincter electromyography during voluntary contraction. **Top to bottom:** Normal recruitment; mild decrease in recruitment; moderate decrease in recruitment; severe decrease in recruitment.

Recorder

A small portable recorder with a memory capacity capable of recording 24 hours of data is required. The 7MPR recorder (Gaeltec Ltd., Isle of Skye, UK) has a 512-kbyte capacity and can record seven separate channels at one time. Amplifiers for EMG recording must to be supplied separately (Gaeltec Ltd., Isle of Skye, UK).

Storage and Display

Information stored within the recorder can be downloaded for screen display and printout, using an Epson compatible screen dump.

Procedure

Following a 1-hour topical application of lidocaine cream, a pair of fine wire electrodes is inserted into the internal and external anal sphincters and the puborectalis muscle. The internal and external sphincters are identified by palpating the groove between the two muscles. The puborectalis is palpated at the level of the anorectal ring, and its position is confirmed by asking the patient to strain. After insertion, the wires are connected to the header amplifier board, and after positioning has been confirmed by the electrical tracings, the electrodes and amplifier are taped securely. The manometry probe is then inserted via a pediatric anoscope and the lower transducers positioned by continuous pull-through within the HPZ of the anal canal. The probe is also securely taped. Recordings can then be commenced. The patient utilizes a diary logbook to record events such as eating, bowel activity, and passage of flatus. The portable recording device has a button that the patient pushes in order to mark each event on the tracing.

Recommendations

Concentric needle EMG is the preferred method in our laboratory for mapping the electrical activity of the anal sphincter in incontinent patients.[38] However, if the patient's complaint is constipation, with symptoms suggestive of outlet obstruction, an intraanal sponge plug EMG is often used (Figure 6-25). Local anesthesia is not required for either technique. A four-quadrant examination is performed using a bipolar concentric, 0.64-mm diameter, 23-gauge, 50- to 75-mm-long needle (Figure 6-26). The recording apparatus (Nicolet Viking IIe, Nicolet Biomedical, Inc., Madison, WI) is attached to a speaker that provides an audible signal correlating with the level of EMG activity. Recordings are made during rest, voluntary contraction, involuntary contraction (cough) and simulated defecation. Reductions in MUP recruitment and/or increases in polyphasic waves are subjectively graded (Figure 6-27).

PUDENDAL NERVE TERMINAL MOTOR LATENCY

Because the external anal sphincter is innervated by the pudendal nerve, the quantitative assessment of the speed of impulse transmission along this pathway can provide useful information in patients with incontinence, rectal prolapse, and constipation.[101,164] Based on the technique of electroejaculation, Kiff and Swash developed a finger-stall device containing stimulating and recording electrodes that could be used intrarectally to stimulate the pudendal nerve and to record the impulse distally.[26,117] The time taken for the impulse to be transmitted is known as the pudendal nerve terminal motor latency (PNTML). A disposable electrode based on this original design was developed by Rogers and colleagues.[198] In addition to bowel management concerns, the PNTML can be used to assess perineal nerve function indirectly in patients with urinary incontinence. There is a linear relationship between the terminal motor latencies of the perineal and pudendal nerves, the perineal nerve latencies being slightly longer.

Equipment

Electrode

The Dantec St. Mark's pudendal nerve stimulating device is used at most centers. This consists of a thin strip of paper with adhesive on the surface to be placed on the gloved finger. There are two stimulating electrodes, a larger anode and a smaller cathode, 1 cm apart at the tip, and two recording electrodes at the base, 4 cm distal to the anode (Figure 6-28).

Electromyographic Equipment

A unit that can deliver a 50-V square-wave stimulus of 0.1 millisecond in duration and can record the resultant motor unit potential is required.

Recommendations

A single Fleet enema is used to empty the rectum before the examination. The patient is placed in the left lateral decubitus position. An electrode is secured on the volar aspect of the examiner's gloved index finger. Following the application of electrode gel to the electrodes, the examiner's index finger is inserted into the rectum until the coccyx is palpated posteriorly. The finger is then moved laterally to the left and the left ischial spine palpated. The EMG equipment (Nicolet Viking IIe, Nicolet Biomedical, Inc., Madison, WI) is set to deliver 22- to 35-mA impulses controlled by a foot switch as the finger is moved across the pelvic side wall in order to determine the optimal site

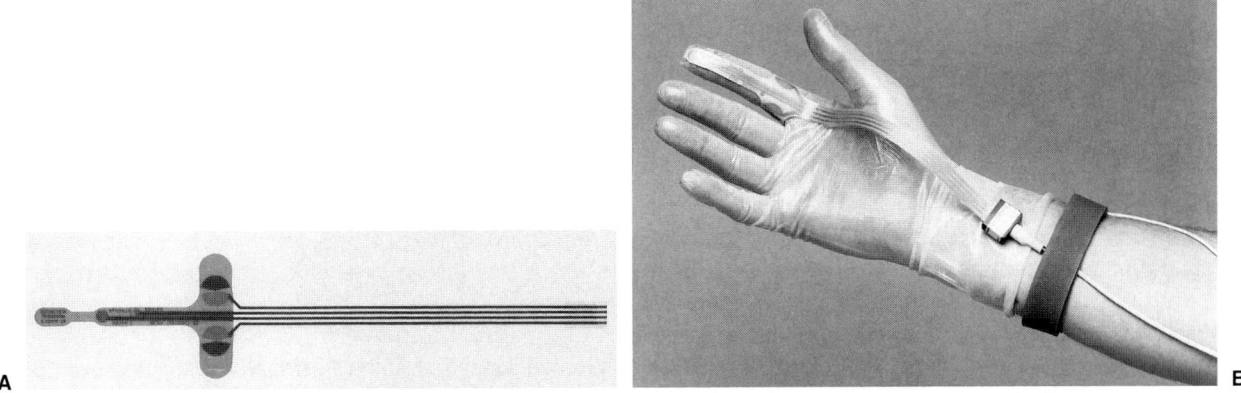

FIGURE 6-28. St. Mark's pudendal nerve stimulating device 13L40 showing arrangement of anode and cathode **(A)** and correct positioning for examination **(B)**. (Courtesy of Dantec Medical, Inc., Allendale, NJ.)

for assessing nerve latency. This point is recognized by a strong contraction of the external sphincter around the examiners finger and a coincident maximal amplitude motor unit potential of the recording apparatus (Figure 6-29). During recording, sensitivity is set at 50 µV, the low-frequency filter is set at 2 Hz, and the high-frequency filter is set at 5 kHz. The terminal motor latency is the time interval between the onset of the stimulus and the onset of the motor unit potential. Three values are taken from one nerve before rotating the finger and repeating the process on the contralateral nerve. The motor unit potential image will be inverted on this side. The normal value for PNTML in our laboratory is 2.0±0.2 milliseconds.[117,218,243] Along with anal ultrasonography, these tests are the most important in the evaluation of fecal incontinence.

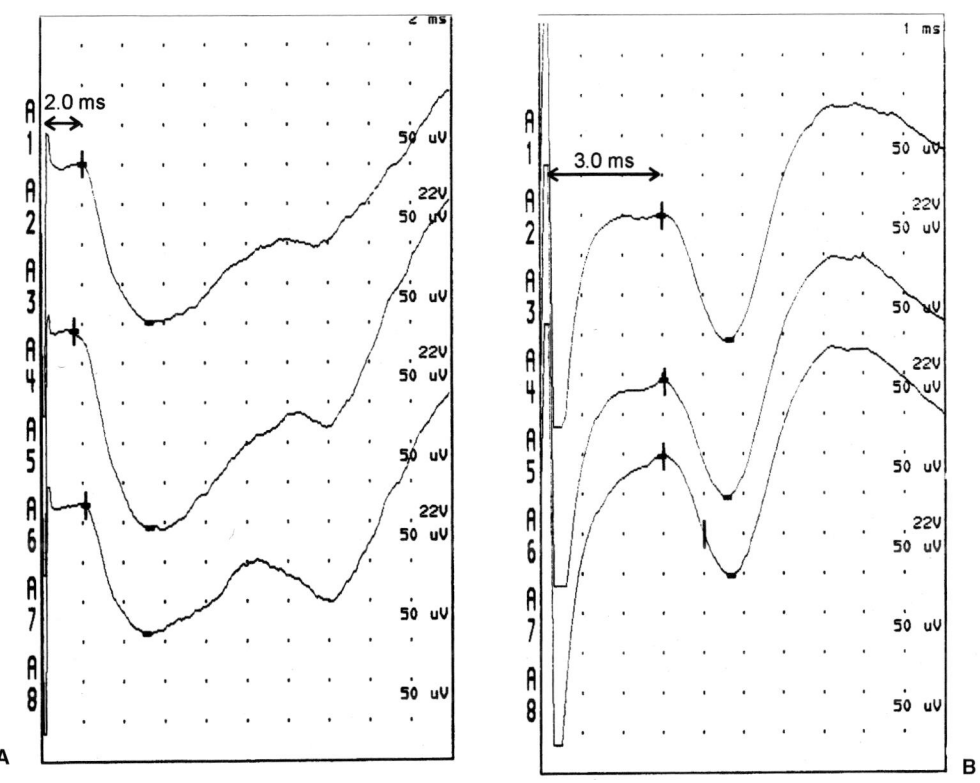

FIGURE 6-29. Pudendal nerve terminal motor latencies showing normal latency **(A)** and prolonged latency **(B)**.

ANORECTAL SENSATION

The maintenance of normal continence is in part the result of anorectal sensation. The anal canal is innervated by both free nerve endings and by sensory organs. The maximal density of free nerve endings is in the region of the anal crypts and the mucosa just cephalad to the crypts, that is, the anal transitional zone. Distal to this area, the anal epithelium is sensitive to pain, temperature, and touch. Proximally, there are no pain fibers, but there are numerous Golgi-Mazzoni bodies and pacinian corpuscles that are sensitive to pressure changes.

The rectum is not sensitive to pain but is sensitive to distension of its lumen, giving rise to a feeling of fullness. It has been hypothesized that this sensation is not perceived at the mucosal level because there are few nerve fibers, but it arises from stimulation of the pelvic floor muscles and receptors in surrounding structures.[75,129]

The precise role of sensation in the maintenance of continence is unclear. The sampling reflex, which is important in enabling individuals to discriminate among flatus, liquid, and solid stool, is usually ablated following ileoanal or coloanal anastomosis. However, these patients usually maintain continence. Furthermore, neither excision nor preservation of the anal transitional zone has led to a functionally different result following this type of surgery.[115] Furthermore, application of lidocaine gel into the rectum of normal subjects fails to produce incontinence to instilled liquids.[191] In spite of these findings there has been considerable interest in the investigation of the sensory component of the anal canal. In particular, two techniques have been described, mucosal electrosensitivity and temperature sensation.[157,196]

Mucosal Electrosensitivity

Although Duthie and Gairns measured anal canal electrosensitivity in 1960,[48] a more elegant technique has been developed by Roe and colleagues.[196] A specially constructed probe is required (Department of Clinical Medicine, Royal Devon and Exeter Hospital, Devon UK; Caesar, Valencia, Spain), which, after lubrication with conductive jelly, is inserted into the upper anal canal.[128,220] A constant current generator, which can produce a square-wave stimulus with a frequency of 5 Hz, is used to generate an electrical potential between the electrodes. This stimulus is gradually increased in 1-mA increments until the patient first feels a tingling sensation. This data is digitally recorded, and the mean of the readings is noted as the threshold of sensation. The probe is then moved to the middle and then the lower anal canal where the procedure is repeated.

More recently, *rectal* electrosensitivity testing has been developed and used in the investigation of patients with idiopathic or iatrogenic constipation.[109,220,221] It had been thought that rectal sensation is decreased in these patients, but that theory has recently been challenged. Meagher and co-workers suggest that this observation may be due to damage to the sensory innervation of the surrounding muscles or to feces preventing optimal mucosal contact.[152] This actually gives some credence to earlier theories about the origins of rectal sensation.[75,129]

Temperature Sensation

Rectal sensation has traditionally been measured by balloon distension or mucosal electrostimulation. There is some evidence that temperature appreciation may play a role in the ability to discriminate among flatus, liquid, and solid stool.[47] Miller and colleagues, using a water-perfused thermode, investigated the thermal sensitivity of the anorectum.[157] Water from three thermostatically controlled water baths can be selectively pumped through the thermode so that the temperature can be held at 37°C or increased and decreased rapidly by 4.5°C. The temperature at the thermode/mucosal interface is measured by a small thermocouple. At the point where the patient appreciates a temperature change, the temperature from the thermocouple is recorded. Thermal sensitivity is noted over four temperature ranges: normal to hot, hot to normal, normal to cold, and cold to normal. The median of these four measurements is recorded as the thermal sensitivity. The readings are taken in the upper, middle, and lower anal canal.

Chan and co-workers were able to demonstrate a repeatable sensory response to heat stimulation in normal subjects using their specially designed thermal probe.[35] There was a strong correlation between balloon distension to maximal tolerable volume and heat thresholds.

Opinion

Both of these modalities are largely investigational, with their role in the clinical management of patients unclear. Neither technique is used in our laboratory.

BIOFEEDBACK

Biofeedback, a treatment whereby patients are trained to be more aware of and responsive to biologic information provided to them, has been increasingly utilized in the management of functional pelvic floor disorders, such as fecal incontinence,[114,134] rectal pain,[67,77] and obstructed defecation.[22,59,68,242] Because many of the investigational modalities already discussed have the capability of being used to provide biofeedback, a brief discussion of the available techniques is warranted.

In the treatment of fecal incontinence, biofeedback attempts to improve both the patient's awareness of his or her sphincter mechanism and the muscular function of this apparatus. Similarly, in patients with obstructed defecation, biofeedback is used to heighten the patient's awareness of the sphincters so that they can be trained to consciously relax these muscles during evacuation. Hence, provision of visual or auditory feedback of the muscular tone within the external sphincter/puborectalis complex is of importance. This input is generally provided through the use of manometry,[114,116,237,240] balloon defecography,[23,59,132] surface EMG,[134,202] or intraanal EMG.[42,68] Intrarectal balloon sensation training can be used separately or in combination with muscular training, particularly in those with fecal incontinence. Some authors have found this last approach to be useful,[134,159,237] but this view has been challenged. Several investigators use home-training units,[11,112] but the benefits of this method have been questioned in a prospective randomized trial (Table 6-6).[89] Most of the aforementioned manometric programs have the capability for biofeedback, but some believe that EMG-based programs are preferable.[23] It has been shown that sphincter endurance and net strength of the sphincter muscles demonstrated by EMG significantly improves after using biofeedback in the management of patients with incontinence and constipation.[21,178]

Recommendation

At our institution, we prefer to use an intraanal plug EMG to provide biofeedback (Figure 6-30). The intraanal plug is equipped with longitudinal electrodes. Following insertion, the patient dresses. Biofeedback is carried out with the patient sitting on a chair. Sessions lasting 1 hour are scheduled regularly until the person has demonstrated control of the pelvic floor, and this has been accompanied by symptomatic improvement. We have not found the addition of balloon sensation training or home training to be helpful.[89]

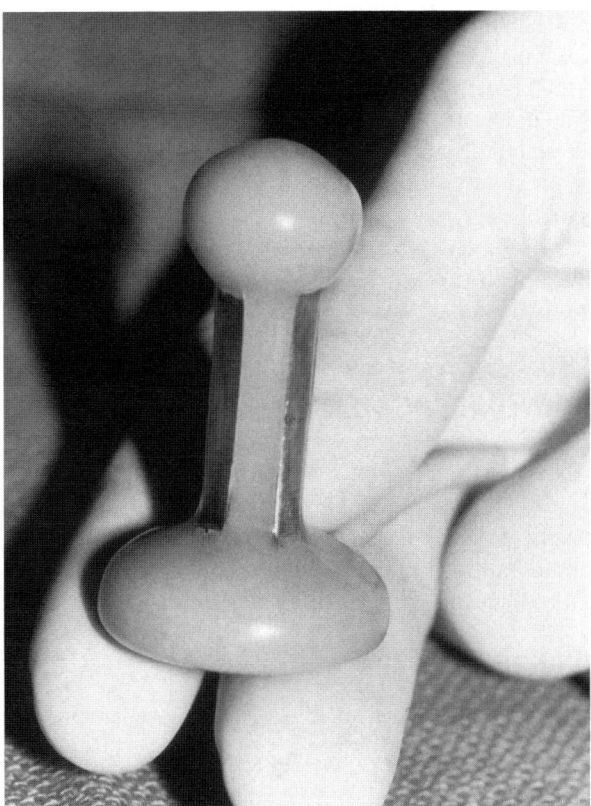

FIGURE 6-30. Perrymeter. (Courtesy of Synectics Medical, Irving, TX.)

CONCLUSIONS

Not very long ago, anorectal physiology was considered a conglomeration of interesting but impractical investigations that provide novel but clinically irrelevant information. Currently, anorectal physiology is not only familiar to all who perform colorectal surgery but is available to most practitioners. Viewed no longer as exclusively a research tool, anorectal physiology provides useful data for both clinical decision making and prognostic information. In

▶ **TABLE 6-6 Biofeedback Equipment**

Manufacturer	Telephone	Equipment	Type
Sandhill, Highlands Ranch, CO 80126, USA	1-800-468-4556	Orion	Anal plug EMG
	303-470-7020	Orion PC/4	Anal plug EMG
		Regain	Anal Plug EMG (home trainer)
Synectics Medical, Irving, TX 75038, USA	1-800-227-3191	Perrymeter	Anal plug EMG
	214-518-0518	Perrymeter	Anal plug EMG (home trainer)
Biosearch Medical, Somerville, NJ 08876, USA	1-800-326-5976	System 5, System 10 (home trainer)	Manometry
	908-722-5000		
Synectics Medical, Irving, TX 75038, USA	1-800-227-3191	Polygram	Manometry
	214-518-0518		

EMG, electromyography.

this chapter, we outline some of the more widely available physiologic investigations. We endeavor to provide a comprehensive list of the tools necessary to complete these evaluations. However, owing to space constraints we do not elaborate upon every facet of these studies. Instead, we provide resource tables so that individuals interested in obtaining more information can contact the manufacturer directly. In addition, we provide a detailed reference list so that further knowledge can be gleaned from the cited publications.

ACKNOWLEDGMENTS

We wish to thank all the manufacturers referenced in this chapter for their help in supplying current equipment specifications. We also wish to thank Robert Cravero (photography) and Janice Gilliland (illustrations).

REFERENCES

1. Adrian ED, Bronck DW. The discharge of impulses in motor nerve fibres. *J Physiol* 1929;67:119–151.
2. Agachan F, Pfeifer J, Wexner SD. Defecography and proctography: results of 744 patients. *Dis Colon Rectum* 1996; 39:899.
3. Åkervall S, Fasth S, Nordgren S, et al. Manovolumetry: a new method for investigation of anorectal function. *Gut* 1988;29:614–623.
4. Altringer WE, Saclarides TJ, Dominguez JM, et al. Four-contrast defecography: pelvic fluoroscopy. *Dis Colon Rectum* 1995;38:695–699.
5. Alvarez WC, Freedlander BL. The rate of progress of food residues through the bowel. *JAMA* 1924;83:576–580.
6. Arhan P, Devroede G, Jehannin B, et al. Segmental colonic transit time. *Dis Colon Rectum* 1981;24:625–629.
7. Arndorfer RC, Stef JJ, Dodds W, et al. Improved infusion system for intraluminal eosophageal manometry. *Gastroenterology* 1977;73:23–27.
8. Aronson MP, Lee RA, Berquist TH. Anatomy of anal sphincters and related structures in continent women studied with magnetic resonance imaging. *Obstet Gynecol* 1990; 76:846–851.
9. Bannister JJ, Abouzekry L, Read NW. Effect of aging on anorectal function. *Gut* 1987;28:353–357.
10. Barnett JL, Hasler WL, Camilleri M. American Gastroenterological Association medical position statement on anorectal testing techniques. *Gastroenterology* 1999;116: 732.
11. Bartolo DC, Read NW, Jarratt JA, et al. Differences in anal sphincter function and clinical presentation in patients with pelvic floor descent. *Gastroenterology* 1983;85:68–75.
12. Bartolo DC, Roe AM, Virjee J, et al. Evacuation proctography in obstructed defaecation and rectal intussusception. *Br J Surg* 1985;72:S111–S116.
13. Bartram CI, Burnett SJD. *Atlas of anal endosonography.* Oxford: Butterworth-Heinemann, 1991.
14. Bartram CI, Turnbull GK, Lennard-Jones JE. Evacuation proctography: an investigation of rectal expulsion in 20 subjects without defecatory disturbance. *Gastrointest Radiol* 1988;13:72–80.
15. Basilisco G, Bozzani A, Camboni G, et al. Effect of loperamide and naloxone on mouth-to-caecum transit time evaluated by lactulose hydrogen breath test. *Gut* 1985;26: 700–703.
16. Beck A. Electomyographische Untersuchungen am Sphinkter ani. *Arch Physiol* 1930;224:278–292.
17. Belliveau P, Thomson JP, Parks AG. Fistula-in-ano: a manometric study. *Dis Colon Rectum* 1983;26:152–154.
18. Berman IR, Manning DH, Harris MS. Streamlining the management of defecation disorders. *Dis Colon Rectum* 1990;33:778–785.
19. Bernier P, Stevenson GW, Shorvon P. Defecography commode. *Radiology* 1988;166:891–892.
20. Binnie NR, Kawimbe M, Papachrysostomou M, et al. The importance of the orientation of the electrode plates in recording the external anal sphincter EMG by non-invasive anal plug electrodes. *Int J Colorectal Dis* 1990;6:5–8.
21. Bjorneklett A, Jenssen E. Relationships between hydrogen (H_2) and methane (CH_4) production in man. *Scand J Gastroenterol* 1982;17:985–992.
22. Bleijenberg G, Kuijpers HC. Treatment of the spastic pelvic floor syndrome with biofeedback. *Dis Colon Rectum* 1987: 108–111.
23. Bleijenberg G, Kuijpers HC. Biofeedback treatment of constipation: a comparison of two methods. *Am J Gastroenterol* 1994;89:1021–1026.
24. Bond JH, Levitt MD, Prentiss R. Investigation of small bowel transit time in man utilizing pulmonary hydrogen (H_2) measurements. *J Lab Clin Med* 1975;85:546–555.
25. Bremmer S, Ahlbäck S-O, Udén R, et al. Simultaneous defecography and peritoneography in defecation disorders. *Dis Colon Rectum* 1995;38:969–973.
26. Brindley GS. Electroejaculation: its technique, neurological implications and uses. *J Neurol Neurosurg Psychiatry* 1981;44:9–18.
27. Broden B, Snellman B. Procidentia of the rectum studied with cineradiography: a contribution to the discussion of causative mechanism. *Dis Colon Rectum* 1968;11:330–347.
28. Browning C, Valori R, Wingate DL, et al. A new pressure-sensitive radio-telemetric capsule. *Lancet* 1981;2:504–505.
29. Burhenne HJ. Intestinal evacuation study: a new roentgenologic technique. *Radiol Clin North Am* 1964;33:79–84.
30. Burnett SJ, Bartram CI. Endosonographic variations in the normal internal anal sphincter. *Int J Colorectal Dis* 1991;6: 2–4.
31. Camboni G, Basilisco G, Bozzani A, et al. Repeatability of lactulose hydrogen breath test in subjects with normal or prolonged orocaecal transit. *Dig Dis Sci* 1988;33:1525–1527.
32. Camilleri M, Colemont LJ, Phillips SF, et al. Human gastric emptying and colonic filling of solids characterized by a new method. *Am J Physiol* 1989;257:G284–G290.
33. Cammarota T, Discalzo L. Corno F, et al. First experiences with trans-rectal echotomography in perianal abscess pathology. *Radiol Med* 1986;72:837–840.
34. Caride VJ, Prokop EK, Troncale FJ, et al. Scintigraphic determination of small intestinal transit time: comparison with the hydrogen breath technique. *Gastroenterology* 1984;86:714–720.
35. Chan CLH, Scott SM, Mirch MJ, et al. Rectal heat thresholds: a novel test of the sensory afferent pathway. *Dis Colon Rectum* 2003;46:590.
36. Chaussade S, Roche H, Khyari A, et al. Mesure du temps de transit colique (TTC): description et validation d'une nouvelle technique. *Gastroenterol Clin Biol* 1986;10:385–389.
37. Chen HH, Iroatulam A, Alabaz O, et al. Associations of defecography and physiologic findings in male patients with rectocele. *Tech Coloproctol* 2001;5:157–161.
38. Cheong DM, Vaccaro CA, Salanga VD, et al. Electrodiagnostic evaluation of fecal incontinence. *Muscle Nerve* 1995; 18:612–619.
39. Coller JA, Sangwan YP. Computerized anal sphincter manometry performance and analysis. In: Smith LE ed. *Practical guide to anorectal testing*, 2nd ed. New York: Igaku-Shoin, 1995:51–100.
40. Connell JM, McCall J, Misiewicz J, et al. Observations on the clinical use of radio pills. *BMJ* 1963;2:771–774.

41. Corazza GR, Menozzi MG, Strocchi A, et al. The diagnosis of small bowel bacterial overgrowth: reliability of jejunal culture and inadequacy of breath hydrogen testing. *Gastroenterology* 1990;98:302–309.

42. Dahl J, Lindquist BL, Tysk C, et al. Behavioral medicine treatment in chronic constipation with paradoxical anal sphincter contraction. *Dis Colon Rectum* 1991;34:769–776.

43. Delemarre JBVM, Kruyt RH, Doornbos J, et al. Anterior rectocele: assessment with radiographic defecography, dynamic magnetic resonance imaging, and physical examination. *Dis Colon Rectum* 1994;37:249–259.

44. deSouza NM, Kmiot WA, Puni R, et al. High resolution magnetic resonance imaging of the anal sphincter using an internal coil. *Gut* 1995;37:284–287.

45. deSouza NM, Puni R, Kmiot WA, et al. MRI of the anal sphincter. *J Comput Assist Tomogr* 1995;19:745–755.

46. Dick M. Use of cuprous thiocyanate as a short-term continuous marker for faeces. *Gut* 1969;10:408–412.

47. Duthie GS, Farouk R, Bartolo DCC. Anorectal sensation. In: Kuijpers HC, ed. *Colorectal physiology: fecal incontinence.* Boca Raton, FL: CRC Press, 1994:125–130.

48. Duthie HL, Gairns FW. Sensory nerves and sensation in the anal region of man. *Br J Surg* 1960;47:585–595.

49. Ekberg O, Nylander G, Fork FT. Defecography. *Radiology* 1985;155:45–48.

50. Ekstedt J. Human single muscle fibre action potentials. *Acta Physiol Scand* 1964;61:1–98.

51. Enck P, von Giensen HJ, Schafer A, et al. Comparison of anal sonography with conventional needle electromyography in the evaluation of anal sphincter defects. *Am J Surg* 1996;91:2539–2534.

52. Evans DF, Pye G, Bramley R, et al. Measurement of gastrointestinal pH profiles in normal ambulant human subjects. *Gut* 1988;29:1035–1041.

53. Farouk R. Electromyographic techniques. In: Smith LE, ed. *Practical guide to anorectal testing,* 2nd ed. New York: Igaku-Shoin, 1995:195–206.

54. Felt-Bersma RJ, Luth WJ, Janssen JJ, et al. Defecography in patients with anorectal disorders: which findings are clinically relevant? *Dis Colon Rectum* 1990;33:277–284.

55. Ferrante SL, Perry RE, Schreiman JS, et al. The reproducibility of measuring the anorectal angle in defecography. *Dis Colon Rectum* 1991;34:51–55.

56. Ferrara A, Lujan JH, Cebrian J, et al. Clinical, manometric, and EMG characteristics of patients with fecal incontinence. *Tech Coloproctol* 2001;5:13–18.

57. Ferrara A, Pemberton JH, Levin KE, et al. Relationship between anal canal tone and rectal motor activity. *Dis Colon Rectum* 1993;36:337–342.

58. Finlay IG, Bartolo DCC, Bartram CI, et al. Proctography. *Int J Colorectal Dis* 1988;3:67–89.

59. Fleshman JW, Dreznik Z, Meyer K, et al. Outpatient protocol for biofeedback therapy of pelvic floor outlet obstruction. *Dis Colon Rectum* 1992;35:1–7.

60. Fletcher JG, Busse RF, Riederer SJ, et al. Magnetic resonance imaging of anatomic and dynamic defects of the pelvic floor in defecatory disorders. *Am J Gastroenterol* 2003;98:399–411.

61. Floyd WF, Walls EW. Electromyography of the sphincter ani externus in a man. *J Physiol* 1953;122:500–609.

62. Fucini C, Ronchi O, Elbetti C. Electromyography of the pelvic floor musculature in the assessment of obstructed defection symptoms. *Dis Colon Rectum* 2001;44:1168–1175.

63. Garcia-Aguilar J, Pollack J, Lee SH, et al. Accuracy of endorectal ultrasonography in preoperative staging of rectal tumors. *Dis Colon Rectum* 2002;45:10–15.

64. Gavioli M, Bagni A, Piccagli I, et al. Usefulness of endorectal ultrasound after preoperative radiotherapy in rectal cancer. *Dis Colon Rectum* 2000;43:1075–1083.

65. Ger GC, Wexner SD, Jorge JMN, et al. Evaluation and treatment of chronic intractable rectal pain: a frustrating endeavor. *Dis Colon Rectum* 1993;36:139–145.

66. Gibbons CP, Read NW. Anal hypertonia in fissures: cause or effect? *Br J Surg* 1986;73:443–445.

67. Gilliland R, Heymen JS, Altomare DF, et al. Biofeedback for intractable rectal pain: outcome and predictors of success. *Dis Colon Rectum* 1997;40:190.

68. Gilliland R, Heymen S, Altomare DF, et al. Outcome and predictors of success of biofeedback for constipation. *Br J Surg* 1997;84:1123.

69. Glaser F, Kuntz C, Schlag P, et al. Endorectal ultrasound for control of preoperative radiotherapy of rectal cancer. *Ann Surg* 1993;217:64–71.

70. Glassman LM. Defecography. In: Smith LE, ed. *Practical guide to anorectal testing,* 2nd ed. New York: Igaku-Shoin, 1995:143–160.

71. Goei R, Baeten C, Arends JW. Solitary rectal ulcer syndrome: findings at barium enema study and defecography. *Radiology* 1988;168:303–306.

72. Goei R, van Engelshoven J, Schouten H, et al. Anorectal function: defecographic measurement in asymptomatic subjects. *Radiology* 1989;173:137–141.

73. Goei R. Anorectal function in patients with defecation disorders and asymptomatic subjects: evaluation with defecography. *Radiology* 1990;174:121–123.

74. Goldman S, Glimelius B, Norming L, et al. Transanorectal ultrasonography in anal canal carcinoma. *Acta Radiol* 1988;29:337–341.

75. Goligher JD, Hughes ES. Sensibility of the rectum and colon: its role in the mechanism of anal continence. *Lancet* 1951;1:543–548.

76. Greydanus MP, Camilleri M, Colemont LJ, et al. Ileocolonic transfer of solid chyme in small intestinal neuropathies and myopathies. *Gastroenterology* 1990;99:158–164.

77. Grimaud J-C, Bouvier M, Naudy B, et al. Manometric and radiologic investigations and biofeedback treatment of chronic idiopathic anal pain. *Dis Colon Rectum* 1991;34:690–695.

78. Gryback P, Jacobson H, Blomquist L, et al. Scintigraphy of the small intestine: a simplified standard for study of transit with reference to normal values. *Eur J Nucl Med Mol Imaging* 2002;29:39–45.

79. Hallböök O, Sjödahl R. Techniques of rectal compliance measurement. *Semin Colon Rect Surg* 1992;3:88–91.

80. Hémond M, Bédard G, Bouchard H, et al. Step-by-step anorectal manometry: small balloon tube. In: Smith LE ed. *Practical guide to anorectal testing,* 2nd ed. New York: Igaku-Shoin, 1995:101–142.

81. Hancock BD. Internal sphincter and the nature of haemorrhoids. *Gut* 1977;18:651–655.

82. Hancock BD. The internal sphincter and anal fissure. *Br J Surg* 1977;64:92–95.

83. Hardcastle JD, Mann CV. Study of large bowel peristalsis. *Gut* 1968;9:512–520.

84. Harris LD, Winans CS, Pope CE II. Determination of yield pressures: a method for measuring anal sphincter competence. *Gastroenterology* 1966;50:754–760.

85. Haynes WG, Read NW. Ano-rectal activity in man during rectal infusion of saline: a dynamic assessment of the anal continence mechanism. *J Physiol* 1982;330:45–56.

86. Henry M. In: Smith LE, ed. *Practical guide to anorectal testing,* 2nd ed. New York: Igaku-Shoin, 1995:185–188.

87. Henry MM, Parks AG, Swash M. The pelvic floor musculature in the descending perineum syndrome. *Br J Surg* 1982;69:470–472.

88. Henry MM, Swash M. *Coloproctology and the pelvic floor: pathophysiology and management.* London: Butterworth, 1985.

89. Heymen S, Vickers D, Weiss EG, et al. A prospective randomized trial comparing four biofeedback techniques for patients with constipation. *Gastroenterology* 1996;110:A678.

90. Hill JR, Kelley ML Jr, Schlegel JF, et al. Pressure profile of the rectum and anus of healthy persons. *Dis Colon Rectum* 1960;3:203–209.

91. Hinton JM, Lennard-Jones JE. Constipation: definition and classification. *Postgrad Med J* 1968;44:720–733.

92. Hinton JM, Lennard-Jones JE, Young AC. A new method for studying transit times using radiopaque markers. *Gut* 1969;10:842–847.

93. Hock D, Lombard R, Jehaes C, et al. Colpocystodefecography. *Dis Colon Rectum* 1993;36:1015–1021.

94. Holmberg A, Graf W, Österberg A, et al. Anorectal manovolumetry in the diagnosis of fecal incontinence. *Dis Colon Rectum* 1995;38:502–508.

95. Howard PJ, Lazarus C, Maisey MN, et al. Interpretation of postprandial breath hydrogen excretion in relation to small bowel transit and ileocecal flow patterns of a radiolabeled solid meal in man. *J Gastrointest Motil* 1990;2:194–201.

96. Hussain SM, Stoker J, Lameris JS. Anal sphincter complex: endoanal MR imaging of normal anatomy. *Radiology* 1995; 197:671–677.

97. Hussain SM, Stoker J, Schouten WR, et al. Fistula in ano: endoanal sonography versus endoanal MR imaging in classification. *Radiology* 1996;200:475–481.

98. Hutchinson R, Kumar D. Colonic and small bowel transit studies. In: Wexner SD, Bartolo DCC, eds. *Constipation: etiology, evaluation and management.* Oxford: Butterworth-Heinemann, 1995:52–62.

99. Hutchinson R, Mostafa AB, Grant EA, et al. Scintigraphic defecography: quantitative and dynamic assessment of anorectal function. *Dis Colon Rectum* 1993;36:1132–1138.

100. Infantino A, Masin A, Pianon P, et al. Role of proctography in severe constipation. *Dis Colon Rectum* 1990;33:707–712.

101. Jones PN, Lubowski DZ, Swash M, et al. Is paradoxical contraction of the puborectalis muscle of functional importance? *Dis Colon Rectum* 1987;30:667–670.

102. Jorge JMN, Wexner SD, Ehrenpreis ED. The lactulose hydrogen breath test as a measure of orocaecal transit time. *Eur J Surg* 1994;160:409–416.

103. Jorge JMN, Wexner SD, Ger GC, et al. Cinedefecography and electromyography in the diagnosis of nonrelaxing puborectalis syndrome. *Dis Colon Rectum* 1993;36:668–676.

104. Jorge JMN, Wexner SD, Marchetti F, et al. How reliable are currently available methods of measuring the anorectal angle? *Dis Colon Rectum* 1992;35:332–338.

105. Jorge JMN, Wexner SD. A practical guide to basic anorectal physiology investigations. *Contemp Surg* 1993;43:214–224.

106. Jorge JMN, Wexner SD. Anorectal manometry: techniques and clinical applications. *South Med J* 1993;86:924–931.

107. Jorge JMN, Yang Y-K, Wexner SD. Incidence and clinical significance of sigmoidoceles as determined by a new classification system. *Dis Colon Rectum* 1994;37:1112–1117.

108. Kamm MA, Lennard-Jones JE, Thompson DG, et al. Dynamic scanning defines a colonic defect in severe idiopathic constipation. *Gut* 1988;29:1085–1092.

109. Kamm MA, Lennard-Jones JE. Rectal mucosal electrosensory testing-evidence for a rectal sensory neuropathy in idiopathic constipation. *Dis Colon Rectum* 1990;33:419–423.

110. Karulf RE, Coller JA, Bartolo DCC, et al. Anorectal physiology testing: a survey of availability and use. *Dis Colon Rectum* 1991;34:464–468.

111. Katz LA, Kaufman HJ, Spiro HM. Anal sphincter pressure characteristics. *Gastroenterology* 1967;52:513–518.

112. Kawimbe BM, Papachrysostoman M, Binnie NR, et al. Outlet obstruction constipation (anismus) managed by biofeedback. *Gut* 1991;32:1175–1179.

113. Kayaba H, Hebiguchi T, Iloh Y, et al. Evaluation of anorectal function in patients with tethered cord syndrome: saline enema test and fecoflowmetry. *J Neurosurg* 2003;98[Suppl 3]:251–257.

114. Keck JO, Staniunas RJ, Coller JA, et al. Biofeedback training is useful in fecal incontinence but disappointing in constipation. *Dis Colon Rectum* 1994;37:1271–1276.

115. Keighley MR, Winslett MC, Yoshioka K, et al. Discrimination is not impaired by excision of the anal transition zone after restorative proctocolectomy. *Br J Surg* 1987;74:1118–1121.

116. Keren S, Wagner Y, Heldenberg D, et al. Studies of manometric abnormalities of the rectoanal region during defecation in constipated and soiling children: modification through biofeedback therapy. *Am J Gastroenterol* 1988;83:827–831.

117. Kiff ES, Swash M. Slowed conduction in the pudendal nerves in idiopathic (neurogenic) faecal incontinence. *Br J Surg* 1984;71:614–616.

118. Kim NK, Kim MJ, Yun SH, et al. Comparative study of transrectal ultrasonography, pelvic computerized tomography, and magnetic resonance imaging in preoperative staging of rectal cancer. *Dis Colon Rectum* 1992;42:770–775.

119. Kmiot WA, O Brien JD, Awad R, et al. Estimation of small bowel transit time following colectomy and ileal reservoir construction. *Br J Surg* 1992;79:697–700.

120. Krevsky B, Malmud LS, D'Ercole F, et al. Colonic transit scintigraphy: a physiologic approach to the quantitative measurement of colonic transit in humans. *Gastroenterology* 1986;91:1102–1112.

121. Kruyt RH, Delemarre JBVM, Doornbos J, et al. Normal anorectum: dynamic MR imaging anatomy. *Radiology* 1991;179:159–163.

122. Kuijpers HC, Bleijenberg G. The spastic pelvic floor syndrome: a cause of constipation. *Dis Colon Rectum* 1985;28:669–672.

123. Kuijpers HC, Schreve RH, Hoedemakers HTC. Diagnosis of functional disorders of defecation causing the solitary rectal ulcer syndrome. *Dis Colon Rectum* 1986;29:126–129.

124. Kuijpers HC, Strijk SP. Diagnosis of disturbances of continence and defecation. *Dis Colon Rectum* 1984;27:658–662.

125. Kuijpers HC. Defaecography. In: Wexner SD, Bartolo DCC, eds. *Constipation: etiology, evaluation and management.* Oxford: Butterworth-Heinemann, 1995:77–85.

126. Kumar D, Waldron D, Williams NS, et al. Prolonged anorectal manometry and external anal sphincter electromyography in ambulant human subjects. *Dig Dis Sci* 1990; 35:641–648.

127. Kumar D, Williams NS, Waldron D, et al. Prolonged manometric recording of anorectal motor activity in ambulant human subjects: evidence of periodic activity. *Gut* 1989;30:1007–1011.

128. Kumar D. Anal sensation. In: Smith LE ed. *Practical guide to anorectal testing,* 2nd ed. New York: Igaku-Shoin, 1995:235–241.

129. Lane RH, Parks AG. Function of the anal sphincters following colo-anal anastomosis. *Br J Surg* 1977;64:596–599.

130. Lesaffer LPA. The mechanism of expulsion during defecation. *Coloproctology* 1993;3:187–192.

131. Lesaffer LPA. Digital subtraction defecography. In: Smith LE, ed. *Practical guide to anorectal testing,* 2nd ed. New York: Igaku-Shoin, 1995:161–184.

132. Lestàr B, Penninckx F, Kerremans R. Biofeedback defecation training for anismus. *Int J Colorectal Dis* 1991;6:202–207.

133. Levitt MD. Production and excretion of hydrogen gas in man. *N Engl J Med* 1969;281:122–127.

134. Loening-Baucke V. Efficacy of biofeedback training in improving fecal incontinence and anorectal physiologic function. *Gut* 1990;31:1395–1402.

135. Loening-Baucke V. Modulation of abnormal defecation dynamics by biofeedback treatment in chronically constipated children with encopresis. *J Pediatr* 1990;116:214–222.

136. Lopez A, Nilsson BY, Mellgren A, et al. Electromyography of the external anal sphincter: comparison between needle and surface electrodes. *Dis Colon Rectum* 1999;42:482–485.

137. Lowry AC, Simmang CI, Boulos P, et al. Consensus statement of definitions for anorectal physiology and rectal cancer. July 2001. *http://www.farcs.org/dcr/0701.html.*

138. Ludin E, Karlbom U, Påhlman L, Graf W. Outcome of segmental colonic resection for slow transit constipation. *Br J Surg* 202;89:1270–1274.

139. Lunniss PJ, Armstrong P, Barker PG, et al. Magnetic resonance imaging of anal fistulae. *Lancet* 1992;340:394–396.

140. MacDonald A, Paterson PJ, Baxter JN, et al. Relationship between intra-abdominal and intrarectal pressure in the proctometrogram. *Br J Surg* 1993;80:1070–1071.

141. Mackay SG, Pager CK, Joseph D, et al. Assessment of the accuracy of transrectal ultrasonography in anorectal neoplasia. *Br J Surg* 2003;90:346–350.

142. Madoff RD, Orrom WJ, Rothenberger DA, et al. Rectal compliance: a critical reappraisal. *Int J Colorectal Dis* 1990; 5:37–40.

143. Mahieu P, Pringot J, Bodart P. Defecography: I. Description of a new procedure and results in normal patients. *Gastrointest Radiol* 1984;9:247–251.

144. Mahieu PH. Barium enema and defaecography in the diagnosis and evaluation of the solitary rectal ulcer syndrome. *Int J Colorectal Dis* 1986;1:85–90.

145. Malfair D, Brown JA, Phang TP. Preoperative rectal cancer imaging: endorectal ultrasound, magnetic resonance imaging, and CT imaging all have useful roles to play when assessing rectal cancer. *B C Med J* 2003;45:259–261.

146. Malouf AJ, Williams AB, Halligan S, et al. Prospective assessment of accuracy of endoanal MR imaging and endosonography in patients with fecal incontinence. *AJR Am J Roentgenol* 2000;175:741–745.

147. Manousos ON, Truelove SC, Lumsden K. Transit times of food in patients with diverticulosis or irritable colon syndrome and normal subjects. *BMJ* 1967;3:760–762.

148. Martinson J. Studies on afferent vagal control of the stomach. *Acta Physiol Scand* 1965;225:1–24.

149. Matamaros Jr A. Fecal incontinence? Use ultrasound. *Am J Gastroenterol* 2001;96:277–278.

150. Matsuoka H, Nakamura A, Masaki T, et al. Comparison between endorectal coil and pelvic phased-array coil magnetic resonance imaging in patients with anorectal tumor. *Am J Surg* 2003;185:328–332.

151. McHugh SM, Diamant NE. Effect of age, gender, and parity on anal canal pressures: contribution of impaired anal sphincter function to fecal incontinence. *Dig Dis Sci* 1987; 32:726–736.

152. Meagher AP, Kennedy ML, Lubowski DZ. Rectal mucosal electrosensitivity: what is being tested? *Int J Colorectal Dis* 1996;11:29–33.

153. Mellgren A, Sirivongs P, Rothenberger DA, et al. Is local excision adequate therapy for early rectal cancer? *Dis Colon Rectum* 2000;43:1064–1074.

154. Metcalf AM, Phillips SF, Zinsmeister AR, et al. Simplified assessment of segmental colonic transit. *Gastroenterology* 1987;92:40–47.

155. Metcalf AM. Transit time. In: Smith LE ed. *Practical guide to anorectal testing*, 2nd ed. New York: Igaku-Shoin, 1995: 17–21.

156. Meunier P, Marechal JM, de Beaujeu MJ. Rectoanal pressures and rectal sensitivity studies in chronic childhood constipation. *Gastroenterology* 1979;77:330–336.

157. Miller R, Bartolo DC, Cervero F, et al. Anorectal temperature sensation: a comparison of normal and incontinent patients. *Br J Surg* 1987;74:511–515.

158. Mills PM, Hosker GL, Phill M, et al. Strength during resting of the external anal sphincter in females with anorectal dysfunction. *Dis Colon Rectum* 2002;45:83–90.

159. Miner PB, Donnelly TC, Read NW. Investigation of mode of action of biofeedback in treatment of fecal incontinence. *Dig Dis Sci* 1990;35:1291–1298.

160. Moreira H Jr, Wexner SD. Anorectal Physiologic Testing. In: Beck DE, Wexner SD, eds. *Fundamental of anorectal surgery*, 2nd ed. London: WB Saunders, 1998:37–53.

161. Myhr GE, Myrvold HE, Nilsen G, et al. Perianal fistulas: use of MR imaging for diagnosis. *Radiology* 1994;191:545–549.

162. Narducci F, Bassoti G, Gabum M, et al. Twenty-four hour manometric recording of colonic motor activity in healthy man. *Gut* 1987;28:17–25.

163. National Cancer Institute. Benefits of adjuvant therapy for rectal cancer. March 1991. *http://www.nlm.gov/databases/alerts/rectal_cancer.html*.

164. Neill ME, Parks AG, Swash M. Physiological studies of the anal sphincter musculature in faecal incontinence and rectal prolapse. *Br J Surg* 1981;68:531–536.

165. Neill ME, Swash M. Increased motor unit fibre density in the external anal sphincter muscle in ano-rectal incontinence: a single fibre EMG study. *J Neurol Neurosurg Psychiatry* 1980;43:343–347.

166. Nivatvongs S. Diagnosis. In: Gordon PH, Nivatvongs S, eds. *Principles and practice of surgery for the colon, rectum, and anus.* St. Louis, MO: Quality Medical Publishers, 1999: 87–131.

167. Nogueras JJ. Endorectal ultrasonography: technique, image interpretation, and expanding indications in 1995. *Semin Colon Rectal Surg* 1995;6:70–77.

168. Notghi A, Hutchinson R, Kumar D, et al. Simplified method for the measurement of segmental colonic transit time. *Gut* 1994;35:976–981.

169. O'Connell PR, Pemberton JH, Brown ML, et al. Determinants of stool frequency after ileal pouch-anal anastomosis. *Am J Surg* 1987;153:157–164.

170. O'Connor JJ. Sonographic diagnosis of anorectal inflammatory disease. *http://csgen.it/medicina/961UCP/961_p006.htm.*

171. O'Donnell P, Beck C, Doyle R, et al. Surface electrodes in perineal electromyography. *Urology* 1988;32:375–379.

172. Oettle GJ, Roe AM, Bartolo DC, et al. What is the best way of measuring perineal descent? A comparison of radiographic and clinical methods. *Br J Surg* 1985;72:999–1001.

173. Öresland T, Fasth S, Åkervall S, et al. Manovolumetric and sensory characteristics of the ileoanal J pouch compared with healthy rectum. *Br J Surg* 1990;77:803–806.

174. Orkin AB, Hanson RB, Kelly KA. The rectal motor complex. *J Gastrointest Motil* 1989;1:5–8.

175. Orrom WJ, Wong WD, Rothenberger DA, et al. Endorectal ultrasound in the preoperative staging of rectal tumors: a learning experience. *Dis Colon Rectum* 1990;33:654–659.

176. Papachrysostomou M, Stevenson AJM, Ferrington C, et al. Evaluation of isotope proctography in constipated subjects. *Int J Colorectal Dis* 1993;8:18–22.

177. Parks AG. Anorectal incontinence. *J R Soc Med* 1975;68: 681–690.

178. Patankar SK, Ferrara A, Larach SW, et al. Electromyographic assessment of biofeedback training for fecal incontinence and chronic constipation. *Dis Colon Rectum* 1997;40:907–911.

179. Penninckx F, Debruyne C, Lestar B, et al. Observer variation in the radiological measurement of the anorectal angle. *Int J Colorectal Dis* 1990;5:94–97.

180. Penninckx F, Kerremans R, Beckers J. Pharmacological characteristics of the non-striated anorectal musculature in cats. *Gut* 1973;14:393–398.

181. Pfeifer J, Agachan F, Wexner SD. Surgery for constipation: a review. *Dis Colon Rectum* 1996;39:444–460.

182. Picirillo MF, Reissman P, Wexner SD. Colectomy as treatment for constipation in selected patients. *Br J Surg* 1995; 82:898–901.

183. Poon FW, Lauder JC, Finlay IG. Technical report: evacuating proctography: a simplified technique. *Clin Radiol* 1991; 44:113–116.

184. Preston DM, Lennard-Jones JE, Thomas BM. The balloon proctogram. *Br J Surg* 1984;71:29–32.

185. Preston DM, Lennard-Jones JE. Anismus in chronic constipation. *Dig Dis Sci* 1985;30:413–418.

186. Prior A, Fearn UJ, Read NW. Intermittent rectal motor activity: a rectal motor complex? *Gut* 1991;32:1360–1363.

187. Prior A, Maxton DG, Whorwell PJ. Anorectal manometry in irritable bowel syndrome: differences between diarrhoea and constipation predominant subjects. *Gut* 1990;31:458–462.

188. Proano M, Camilleri M, Phillips SF, et al. Unprepared human colon does not discriminate between solids and liquids. *Am J Physiol* 1991;260:G13–G16.

189. Rafert JA, Lappas JC, Wilkins W. Defecography: techniques for improved image quality. *Radiol Technol* 1990;61:368–373.

190. Rao SSC, Welcher K. Periodic rectal motor activity: the intrinsic colonic gatekeeper? *Am J Gastroenterol* 1996;91: 890–897.

191. Read MG, Read NW. Role of anorectal sensation in preserving continence. *Gut* 1982;23:345–347.

192. Read NW, Miles CA, Fisher D, et al. Transit of a meal through the stomach, small intestine, and colon in normal subjects and its role in the pathogenesis of diarrhea. *Gastroenterology* 1980;79:1276–1282.

193. Reynolds JR, Clark AG, Evans DF, et al. Investigations of the daily variation of colonic motor activity in man using a portable pressure recording system. *Dig Dis Sci* 1986;31: 414–415.

194. Roberts JP, Benson MJ, Rogers J, et al. Effect of cisapride on distal colonic motility in the early postoperative period following left colonic anastomosis. *Dis Colon Rectum* 1995; 38:139–145.

195. Roberts JP, Womack NR, Hallan RI, et al. Evidence from dynamic integrated proctography to redefine anismus. *Br J Surg* 1992;79:1213–1215.

196. Roe AM, Bartolo DC, Mortensen NJ. New method for assessment of anal sensation in various anorectal disorders. *Br J Surg* 1986;73:310–312.

197. Rogers JR, Henry M, Misiewicz JJ. Increased segmental activity and intraluminal pressures in the sigmoid colon of patients with the irritable bowel syndrome: a new manometric technique. *Gut* 1987;28:A1344.

198. Rogers J, Henry MM, Misiewiscz JJ. Disposable pudendal nerve stimulator: evaluation of the standard instrument and new device. *Gut* 1988;29:1131–1133.

199. Rozycki GS. Ultrasonography: surgical applications. In: *American College of Surgeons: principle and practice*. XXXX, XX: American College of Surgeons, 2003:1–15.

200. Rubinoff MJ, Piccione PR, Holt PR. Clonidine prolongs human small intestine transit time: use of the lactulose-breath hydrogen test. *Am J Gastroenterol* 1989;84:372–374.

201. Rutter KR. Electromyographic changes in certain pelvic floor abnormalities. *Proc R Soc Med* 1974;67:53–56.

202. Ryn AK, Morren GL, Hallbook O, et al. Long term results of electromyographic biofeedback training for fecal incontinence. *Dis Colon Rectum* 2000;43:1262–1266.

203. Sangwan YP, Coller JA, Schoetz DJ, et al. Relationship between manometric anal waves and fecal incontinence. *Dis Colon Rectum* 1995;38:370–374.

204. Sangwan YS, Coller JA, Barrett RC, et al. Distal rectoanal excitatory reflex: a reliable index of pudendal neuropathy? *Dis Colon Rectum* 1995;38:916–920.

205. Schuster MM, Hookman P, Hendrix TR, et al. Simultaneous manometric recording of the internal and external anal sphincter reflexes. *Bull Johns Hopkins Hosp* 1965;116: 79–88.

206. Schuster MM. Colon motility and anosphincteric manometric recordings by air-filled balloon technique. In: Smith LE, ed. *Practical guide to anorectal testing*, 2nd ed. New York: Igaku-Shoin, 1995:37–50.

207. Schwartz DA, Harewood GC, Wierma MJ. EUS for rectal disease. *Gastrointest Endosc* 2002;56:100.

208. Selvaggi F, Pesce G, Di Carlo ES, et al. Evaluation of normal subjects by defecographic technique. *Dis Colon Rectum* 1990;33:698–702.

209. Sentovich SM, Rivela LJ, Thorson AG, et al. Simultaneous dynamic proctography and peritoneography for pelvic floor disorders. *Dis Colon Rectum* 1995;38:912–915.

210. Shafik A, Abdel-Moneim K. Fecoflowmetry: a new parameter assessing rectal function. *Int Surg* 1992;77:190–194.

211. Shafik A, Abdel-Moneim K. Fecoflowmetry: a new parameter assessing rectal function in normal and constipated subjects. *Dis Colon Rectum* 1993;36:35–42.

212. Shafik A, El-Sibai O. Study of the levator ani muscle in the multipara: role of levator dysfunction in defecation disorders. *J Obstet Gynecol* 2002;22:187–192.

213. Shorvon PJ, McHugh S, Diamant NE, et al. Defecography in normal volunteers: results and implications. *Gut* 1989; 30:1737–1749.

214. Skomorowska E, Hegedus V. Sex differences in anorectal angle and perineal descent. *Gastrointest Radiol* 1987;12: 353–355.

215. Sladen GE. pH profile of *Gut* as measured by radiotelemetry capsule. *BMJ* 1972;2:104–106.

216. Smith LE, ed. *Practical guide to anorectal testing*, 2nd ed. New York: Igaku-Shoin, 1995.

217. Snooks SJ, Barnes PR, Swash M, et al. Damage to the innervation of the pelvic floor musculature in chronic constipation. *Gastroenterology* 1985;89:977–981.

218. Snooks SJ, Swash M. Nerve stimulation techniques. In: Henry MM, Swash M, eds. *Coloproctology and the pelvic floor: pathophysiology and management*. London: Butterworth, 1985:112–128.

219. Soffer EE, Wingate DL. Colonic motility: a new technique for prolonged ambulating recording. *Gastroenterology* 1988; 94:A435.

220. Solana A, Roig JV, Villoslada C, et al. Anorectal sensitivity in patients with obstructed defaecation. *Int J Colorectal Dis* 1996;11:65–70.

221. Speakman CT, Madden MV, Nicholls RJ, et al. Lateral ligament division during rectopexy causes constipation but prevents recurrence: results of a prospective randomised trial. *Br J Surg* 1991;78:1431–1433.

222. Stalberg E, Thiele B. Motor unit fibre density in the extensor digitorum communis muscle: single fibre electromyographic study in normal subjects at different ages. *J Neurol Neurosurg Psychiatry* 1975;38:874–880.

223. Staniforth DH, Rose D. Statistical analysis of the lactulose/breath hydrogen test in the measurement of orocaecal transit: its variability and predictive value in assessing drug action. *Gut* 1989;30:171–175.

224. Starck M, Bohe M, Simanaitis M, et al. Rectal endosonography can distinguish benign rectal lesions from invasive early rectal cancers. *Colorectal Dis* 2003;5:246–250.

225. Stein BL, Roberts PL. Manometry and the rectoanal inhibitory reflex. In: Wexner SD, Bartolo DCC, eds. *Constipation: etiology, evaluation and management*. Oxford: Butterworth-Heinemann, 1995.

226. Stivland T, Camilleri M, Vassallo M, et al. Scintigraphic measurement of regional *Gut* transit in idiopathic constipation. *Gastroenterology* 1991;101:107–115.

227. Sultan AH, Kamm MA, Talbot IC, et al. Anal endosonography for identifying external sphincter defects confirmed histologically. *Br J Surg* 1994;81:463–465.

228. Sun WM, Read NW, Prior A, et al. Sensory and motor responses to rectal distention vary according to rate and pattern of balloon inflation. *Gastroenterology* 1990;99:1008–1015.

229. Swedish Rectal Cancer Trial. Improved survival with preoperative radiotherapy in resectable rectal cancer. *N Engl J Med* 1997;336:980–987.

230. Thompson DG, Binfield P, De Belder A, et al. Extra intestinal influences on exhaled breath hydrogen measurements during the investigation of gastrointestinal disease. *Gut* 1985;26:1349–1352.

231. Thorpe AC, Williams NS, Badenoch DF, et al. Simultaneous dynamic electromyographic proctography and cystometrography. *Br J Surg* 1993;80:115–120.

232. Tjandra JJ, Milsom JW, Stolfi VM, et al. Endoluminal ultrasound defines anatomy of the anal canal and pelvic floor. *Dis Colon Rectum* 1992;35:465–470.

233. Trotman IF, Misiewicz JJ. Sigmoid motility in diverticular disease and the irritable bowel syndrome. *Gut* 1988;29: 218–222.

234. Turnbull GK, Bartram CI, Lennard-Jones JE. Radiologic studies of rectal evacuation in adults with idiopathic constipation. *Dis Colon Rectum* 1988;31:190–197.

235. Vasilevsky CA, Nemer FD, Balcos EG, et al. Is subtotal colectomy a viable option in the management of chronic constipation? *Dis Colon Rectum* 1988;31:679–681.

236. Wald A, Caruana BJ, Freimanis MG, et al. Contributions of evacuation proctography and anorectal manometry to evaluation of adults with constipation and defecatory difficulty. *Dig Dis Sci* 1990;35:481–487.

237. Wald A, Chandra R, Gabel S, et al. Evaluation of biofeedback in childhood encopresis. *J Pediatr Gastroenterol Nutr* 1987;6:554–558.

238. Walldén L. Defecation block in cases of deep rectogenital pouch. *Acta Chir Scand* 1952;165:1–22.

239. Wankling WJ, Brown BH, Collins CD, et al. Basal electrical activity in the anal canal in man. *Gut* 1968;9:457–460.

240. Weber J, Ducrotte PH, Touchais JY, et al. Biofeedback training for constipation in adults and children. *Dis Colon Rectum* 1987;30:844–846.

241. Wexner SD, Bartolo DCC, eds. *Constipation: etiology, evaluation and management.* Oxford: Butterworth-Heinemann, 1995.

242. Wexner SD, Cheape JD, Jorge JMN, et al. Prospective assessment of biofeedback for the treatment of paradoxical puborectalis syndrome. *Dis Colon Rectum* 1992;35:145–150.

243. Wexner SD, Marchetti F, Salanga VD, et al. Neurophysiologic assessment of the anal sphincters. *Dis Colon Rectum* 1991;34:606–612.

244. Whitby LG, Lang D. Experience with the chromic oxide method of fecal marking in metabolic balance investigations on humans. *J Clin Invest* 1960;39:854–863.

245. Womack NR, Williams NS, Holmfield JH, et al. New method for the dynamic assessment of anorectal function in constipation. *Br J Surg* 1985;72:994–998.

246. Wong WD, Bernick P. Preoperative staging investigations for rectal cancer. In: Seventeenth annual surgical update: rectal cancer. British Columbia Surgical Society. Vancouver, December 2, 2000. *http://www.bcss.ca/wong.html.*

247. Wong WD, Orrom WJ, Jensen LL. Preoperative staging of rectal cancer with endorectal ultrasonography. *Perspect Colon Rect Surg* 1990;3:315–334.

248. Yang A, Mostwin JL, Rosenhein NB, et al. Pelvic floor descent in women: dynamic evaluation with fast MR imaging and cinematic display. *Radiology* 1991;179:25–33.

249. Yang Y-K, Wexner SD, Nogueras JJ, et al. The role of anal ultrasound in the assessment of benign anorectal diseases. *Coloproctology* 1993;5:260–264.

Analgesia in Colon and Rectal Surgery

I am most grateful to Dr. Anthony M. Nyerges, an individual who has written extensively in his field, for helping to provide his thoughts about analgesia as applied to surgery of anus, rectum, and colon. Dr. Nyerges is Associate Professor of Anesthesia at the University of California, Los Angeles (UCLA) and Co-Director of the UCLA Pain Management Center.
MLC.

The art of life is the art of avoiding pain.
Thomas Jefferson (1743–1826)
Letter to Maria Cosway, October 12, 1786

With the exception of pudendal nerve block and local infiltration of the anal and perianal areas, there is no specific anesthetic situation that is unique to the field of colon and rectal surgery.[17,38,44] The method of performing a "field block" for hemorrhoidectomy is discussed in Chapter 8. Certainly, the principles and techniques of anesthetic induction and maintenance are of interest to any surgeon, but such a discussion is not within the purview of a text on colon and rectal surgery. However, the management of pain is a situation that every surgeon must confront and for which he or she must provide direction and care. It is in this area that I would like to review in this chapter.

The severity of postoperative pain encountered in the practice of all surgeons is often not adequately appreciated and, as a consequence, is often inadequately treated.[8] One method for analyzing the efficacy of pain control has been the development of a so-called visual analog pain score. If one assumes that a score of 3 for pain with movement is unacceptably high,[24] a multiinstitutional study demonstrated that more than 80% of individuals experienced more pain than was considered appropriate both with the use of epidural and with patient-controlled analgesia (PCA).[31]

The management of postoperative pain is often difficult not only because of the obvious variation in analgesic requirements, but also because of the variability of pathophysiologic interactions with different therapies and, of course, the individual's subjective pain experiences. Recent concepts in the management of postoperative pain utilize the assessment of pain in three situations: when moving (e.g., during physical therapy), when in bed, and the worst pain during a day.

There are obviously numerous approaches to controlling pain depending on the individual circumstances, each with varying degrees of effectiveness. For example, it has been demonstrated that epidural analgesia provides more effective pain relief than does either PCA or intramuscular drug administration.[47] It is not simply the route of administration that one must consider, however. Opiate tolerance effects, as manifested by comorbid preoperative use of these medications, certainly affect postoperative consumption.[46] Furthermore, preoperative pain and opiate use generally are associated with a greater degree of postoperative pain.[7]

OPIATES

Opiates affect neuronal activity at the pain control apparatus (substantia gelatinosa, spinal trigeminal nucleus, periaqueductal gray, medullary raphe nucleus, and hypothalamus). Receptors are present in the limbic system, thalamus, striatum, hypothalamus, midbrain, and spinal cord. These receptors have been given various Greek letter identifications based on their location. For example, the *mu receptor* is found in the pain control apparatus of the central nervous system (CNS) and spinal cord. The *kappa receptor* is found in the deep layers of the cerebral cortex. The *delta receptor* is localized to the limbic system. The *sigma receptor* is involved in the dysphoric (excessive pain; anguish; agitation) and dyschonimitic-stimulating effects of opiates. Agonist activity at the mu and kappa receptors produce analgesia, miosis, and increased body temperature. It is the mu receptor activity that is responsible for opiate dependency. Respiratory depression is, in all probability, mediated through the mu and kappa activity.

Actions and Effects

Opiates have profound and varied effects on the CNS. For example, large doses may induce excitation or seizures. Normeperidine, the principal metabolite of meperidine

(Demerol), is well known to induce "pseudoseizures" particularly in individuals who have renal insufficiency. This is because the metabolite is long-lived in these circumstances, accumulates, and is cleared slowly. Opiates also suppress the cough reflex by direct activity on the medulla. Furthermore, through a direct effect on the brain stem (pons, medulla), opiates alter respiratory rhythm and voluntary control as well as decrease responsiveness to carbon dioxide tension. Normally, as arteriole carbon dioxide tension rises, cerebrovascular dilatation occurs, with the resultant increase in cerebral blood flow and cerebrospinal fluid (CSF) pressure. This response is diminished with the use of opiates, an effect that is much more likely with intravenous administration.

Another effect is nausea, which develops as a consequence of orthostatic hypotension or by direct stimulation of a chemotactic trigger zone in the medulla oblongata. Orthostasis may occur as a result of vasodilatation from histamine release or from the suppression of sympathetic outflow from the vasomotor medullary center. The medullary nuclei may also be stimulated to cause bradycardia. The one exception to this phenomenon is the opiate meperidine, which is usually associated with tachycardia. Finally, there is increased vestibular activity observed with opiates as well.

As can be readily appreciated, there are numerous and profound effects produced by the administration of opiates. In addition to the foregoing, opiates increase smooth muscle tone throughout the gastrointestinal tract, including the gastric antrum, duodenum, large bowel, and the various gastrointestinal and biliary sphincters. When measured, the amplitude of nonpropulsive contractions is increased, but the intensity of propulsive contractions is decreased. The exception is meperidine. Whereas it does have some sympathomimetic (anticholinergic-like, atropine-like) effects, it may produce less smooth muscle spasm. Therefore, this drug should be considered the preferred opiate to use after bowel surgery because it is least likely to affect return of intestinal function. The effects are not always uniform with opiates, however. In other words, for example, biliary spasm does not always occur. Some individuals have no change in ductal diameter or pressure. The rank order for producing a spastic potential is: morphine → methadone → meperidine → codeine.

Another effect that opiates have is to increase the tone of the bladder sphincter, impeding urination. There is also an increased tone and contraction in the lower one third of the ureter. Furthermore, tone of the detrusor muscle is increased, which may result in urinary urgency. Finally, opiates may increase secretion of vasopressin, a consequence of which may be oliguria.

Opiates can also have a profound effect on the endocrine system. Inhibition of the release of thyrotropin from the adenohypophysis leads to a decrease in thyroid hormone. Opiates may also produce hyperglycemia by

▶ **TABLE 7-1 Potency of Opiates**

Analgesic	Equivalent Potency IM	Conversion	
		Oral (mg)	IV (mg)
Morphine	10	40–60	10
Codeine	130	200	—
Heroin	5	60	5
Hydromorphone	1.5	7.5	1.0
Levorphanol	2	4	1.5
Meperidine	75	400	75
Methadone	10	20	10
Oxycodone	15	30	—
Fentanyl	—	500 μg	100 μg

stimulating receptors near the foramen of Monro or by releasing epinephrine. This may be associated with a decrease in the metabolic rates by about 10% to 20%.

The relative potency of the various opiates is summarized in Table 7-1.

Metabolism

Opiates are primary metabolized by the microsomes in the endoplasmic reticulum of the liver. Additionally, metabolism also occurs in the CNS, kidneys, lungs, and placenta. This is accomplished by hydrolysis, oxidation, and conjugation with glucuronide.

Mechanism of Action

All opiate receptors appear to function primarily by exerting inhibitory modulation of transmission of synapses in the spinal cord, the myenteric plexus, and the CNS. When located at a presynaptic terminal, these receptors act to reduce neurotransmitter release and, therefore, to decrease conductance. All appear to be linked to guanine nucleotide-binding regulator proteins (G proteins). Opioids regulate the so-called transmembrane signaling system—adenylate cyclase activity, ion channel activity, and the activity of phospholysasis or phosphoinositol. So-called kappa agonistic activity inhibits N-type voltage-dependent calcium channels, specifically in the myenteric plexus and the dorsal root ganglia. Stimulation of mu receptors in the locus ceruleus produces membrane hyperpolarization by an inward potassium rectifying current. The opioid receptors on terminals of afferent nerves in the CNS and in the spinal cord mediate inhibition of the release of neurotransmitters, including substance P. Enhanced activity in descending aminergic bulbospinal pathways then exerts inhibitory effects on the processing of nociceptive information. Specifically, mu opioids in the ventral tegmentum activate certain dopaminergic and γ-aminobutyric acid–ergic neurons that project to the nucleus accumbens. This is the site that is postulated to be the central point producing opiate euphoria and the self-reinforcing effects well known to individuals familiar with addiction.[27]

Within the *intestinal tract*, enterocytes themselves may possess opioid receptors. As a consequence, opiates inhibit transfer of fluid and electrolytes into the intestinal lumen through their actions on the intestinal mucosa. Through effects on the submucosal plexus, there is a decrease in enterocyte basal secretion. Additionally, there is an inhibition of stimulatory effects of acetylcholine, prostaglandin E_2, and vasoactive intestinal peptides. The pressure of opiates at the periaqueductal gray or in the spinal cord will also inhibit gastrointestinal activity as long as the extrinsic innervation to the bowel is intact. This may explain why agents with poor penetration of the CNS (e.g., paregoric) can produce constipation at subanalgesic dosages.

Patient-Controlled Analgesia

In the postoperative setting, a PCA device is used primarily for the administration of opiates to alleviate pain. Usually, morphine, hydromorphone (Dilaudid), fentanyl, or meperidine is used. A PCA device can also be programmed for use with epidural infusions, patient-controlled epidural analgesia. As is well known to every surgeon, the goal of the PCA is to administer more timely drug doses and thereby to enhance patient satisfaction. Furthermore, it may decrease the amount of drug administered, because it is more closely matched to the painful activity or stimulus encountered.[48] If morphine is used, the dosage range is from 1 to 3 mg/hour following abdominal surgery. Self-reporting scales that have been assessed with this drug note effective analgesia.[48]

The choice of agent is often a determination made by the surgeon on the basis of his or her comfort level. Because of its roughly eightfold higher potency, faster onset, and greater lipid solubility (hence greater CNS penetration), hydromorphone (Dilaudid) is usually selected for more severe pain. Certainly, for those who require more close matching of drug delivery, time of onset, and proximity to painful stimulus, hydromorphone is a sound alternative. Owing to the accumulation of a normeperidine metabolite, meperidine (Demerol) at the usual clinical doses is recommended by many individuals familiar with pain control only when the specific advantages (sympathomimetic anticholinergic properties, known anaphylaxis to alternative opiates, etc.) outweigh this disadvantage. In the hands of most practitioners, the use of fentanyl in PCA should be approached with caution. Although its potency, speed of onset, and density of analgesic action are perhaps desirable, the likelihood of respiratory suppression, accumulation of drug-inhibiting gastrointestinal function, and sedation limit this opiate to management by only those specially qualified.

In initially programming a PCA device, a target hourly "safe" dose should be selected. Then, the "demand" and "interval time" can be set according to the half-life alpha distribution times and times to peak analgesia. Morphine is typically set at 1 mg every 8 minutes. This results in a maximum dose of 7 mg/hour. The peak effect of morphine occurs in about 10 minutes after intravenous administration. Less than 0.1% of intravenously administered morphine enters the CNS at the time of peak plasma concentrations.[33] Therefore, the demand interval is set slightly less than that. The peak effect of hydromorphone is approximately 5.5 minutes; its interval is set at about 3 to 4 minutes. The total analgesic administered per hour is dependent on the volume of distribution, acid-base status, plasma protein-binding capacity, ventilatory mechanics, cerebral blood flow patterns, and presence of metabolic abnormalities (e.g., hypothyroidism), as well as a number of other subtle factors.

One should certainly consider the use of basal infusions when using PCA. In monitored areas such as intensive care units or operating suites, errors or overdosing can be quickly observed and treated. Because basal (continuous) infusions are not patient regulated, sedation and other side effects may accumulate rapidly. Although one may achieve more "stable" pharmacologic plasma levels by the use of basal infusions, annoying pruritus, nausea, and prolonged ileus may result.

The choice of opiate depends on the volume and the route of administration, the side effects and toxicities, and the physiologic factors of the individual that affect drug excretion. For example, fentanyl has a membrane stabilizing influence that may potentiate the activity of local anesthetics. Alternatively, with respect to its anesthetic effectiveness, morphine may be more desirable when a greater spread involving more dermatomes is necessary. This is because of morphine's hydrophilicity and lack of segmental spinal cord binding (lipophilic binding). Ultimately, the surgeon uses whichever agent he or she feels most familiar with and most comfortable.

KETOROLAC

Ketorolac (Toradol) is a nonsteroidal antiinflammatory drug that is available or oral or for intravenous use. It possesses no sedative or anxiolytic properties and has its peak analgesic effect within 2 to 3 hours of administration. It is principally metabolized in the liver and excreted in the urine. In several prospective, randomized studies comparing it with morphine and meperidine, ketorolac has been shown to have a longer duration of efficacy. Furthermore, when given in combination with opioids, this drug significantly reduces the requirement for narcotics. The primary concern with the use of this agent is an increased risk of gastrointestinal bleeding, presumably because of its effect on platelet aggregation, especially in the elderly. Therefore, ketorolac is contraindicated in patients with a history of gastrointestinal bleeding and those with peptic ulcer disease. The combined duration for its use must not exceed 5 days.

Place and colleagues evaluated ketorolac in a prospective, randomized study in patients undergoing anorectal surgery.[35] They found that the addition of this drug (60 mg), either given intravenously or injected in combination with a local anesthetic, decreased the risk of urinary retention as well as that of analgesic requirements.

EPIDURAL ANALGESIS

In a busy postoperative acute pain service, continuous epidural infusions of local anesthetics at dilute concentrations, in combination with epidural opioids, are an effective means for treating pain.[11] However, in addition to providing pain relief, consideration has to be given to the outcome, cost, and length of hospital stay in determining the appropriate analgesic. All epidural opiates will achieve some plasma systemic levels. However, the use of epidural analgesia has a particular value in that it appears to be associated with faster resolution of postoperative ileus.[29,41] Another advantage is that epidural analgesia has been demonstrated to decrease the inflammatory sequelae in the perioperative period.[22] In a landmark study to assess the basis for using intensive postoperative analgesia, Mangano and colleagues studied coronary artery bypass graft patients and found intensive prolonged analgesia reduced the number and severity of postoperative ischemic episodes.[32]

Not only has postoperative morbidity from all causes been reduced through the use of epidural analgesia, but also the length of hospitalization has been demonstrated to be decreased.[14,49] Epidural analgesia appears to have the greatest potential to improve perioperative outcome and morbidity when high-risk patients undergo major operations. This has been demonstrated to be the case for perioperative cardiovascular morbidity, pulmonary complications, and infection.[14,45,49]

Epidural Opiates

Epidural opiates act both by venous absorption, thereby producing systemic plasma levels, and by dispersion to the CSF. Approximately 10% to 15% of epidural morphine reaches the CSF. Their activity may result from direct binding at the mu receptor complex in the substantia gelatinosa, direct binding onto nerve roots, or spread and assimilation of morphine through the CSF to the periaqueductal gray of the CNS. Despite their acknowledged efficacy, opiates alone are inadequate for complete intraoperative and postoperative pain relief. The local anesthetics are the agents responsible for affording anesthesia. However, by means of synergistic activity with opiates, the concentrations can be reduced, thereby minimizing motor blockade or total sensory blockade.

Epidural local anesthetic infusions in combination with opiates may inhibit efferent sympathetic pathways and neural reflex arcs.[4] Through this action, the incidence of perioperative increase in coagulation tendency can be reduced, with concomitant decrease in venous and arterial thrombosis.[43,45]

Cousins and colleagues studied selective spinal analgesia and demonstrated the difference between analgesia obtained with nonselective axonal conduction block by a local anesthetic and that of spinal opiates.[9] They observed that selective block of nociception through the use of opiates at the spinal cord does not cause sympathetic block or orthostasis. Furthermore, this selectivity permits ambulation without motor blockade. Additionally, it is not associated with seizures or hypotension. Spinal opiates, however, do cause both early and late respiratory depression. This is usually slow in onset and is augmented by parenteral sedative, hypnotic agents. Unique to spinal opiates is the fact that they cause pruritus and are more likely to be associated with nausea and vomiting. Still, they have about the same incidence of urinary retention as is associated with the use of local anesthetics.

Onset of epidural opiate analgesia is directly related to the lipid partition coefficient. The higher the lipid solubility, the more rapid the onset of analgesia. The duration of analgesia is inversely related to lipid solubility, but it is also influenced by the rate of dissociation from receptors and perhaps by the deposition in the lipid of the epidural space.

It has been demonstrated that if similar dosages of opiates are given intramuscularly and epidurally, blood concentrations are similar. However, analgesia is significantly greater for epidural opiates when compared with the intramuscular route.[19] This points to a central or spinal effect. It has also been shown that analgesia is longer lasting and denser when equivalent doses of fentanyl have been given epidurally rather than intramuscularly.[30] Others have demonstrated in a study of 14,000 patients given epidural morphine at a dose of 4 mg that delayed respiratory depression occurred at a rate of 1 in 1,000.[37] This compares with a rate for the intrathecal use of morphine (0.2 to 0.8 mg) of 1 in 275. Those patients who had never been exposed to opiates, and presumably having no tolerance, were found to have rare respiratory depression as long as no other opiates had been administered by other routes.[20] One must weigh the potential benefit of the superior analgesia obtained with epidural opiates against the greater invasiveness and the possible complications of respiratory depression, pruritus, nausea, and urinary retention. Alternatively, as discussed previously, infusions of opioids may provide similar analgesia, albeit not as satisfactory in some respects, but they do so less invasively and with a lower rate of complications.[40]

Complications

Clearly, as with all invasive techniques, complications can arise from their use. With respect to epidural analgesia, these include toxicity and seizures, urinary retention, epidural abscess, inadvertent dural puncture, backache, and nerve root injury. Two of these complications are discussed.

Epidural Abscess

Epidural abscess is a rare complication of epidural analgesia. Baker and colleagues reviewed a series of 39 abscesses and found that 38 were associated with simultaneous systemic infections.[1] The diagnosis was made on the basis of the patient complaining of severe back pain, local tenderness, and fever. Leukocytosis was also present. Subsequent myelography demonstrated obstruction to flow.

Epidural Hematoma

Epidural hematoma as a consequence of epidural anesthesia and analgesia is most probably the result of needle or catheter trauma to the epidural veins. Generally, in a hematologically normal patient, bleeding is minimal and ceases rapidly. There has only been one reported case of hematoma formation with the potential for neurologic compromise when the coagulation profile had been determined to be normal.[28] However, when anticoagulant therapy is administered (e.g., aspirin, heparin), an epidural hematoma may develop from catheter insertion or simply by the placement of a needle.[12,28] Still, there may be some confusion as to the cause because there have been more than 100 instances of hematoma formation spontaneously produced in this area and not associated with epidural management in patients who are on anticoagulants.[18] Interestingly, the risk of epidural hematoma or related neurologic injury is not increased by preoperative oral anticoagulation with warfarin (Coumadin)[21,34] or with intraoperative anticoagulation with heparin for patients undergoing regional blockade for major vascular surgery.[36] However, both these studies recommend against the use of regional anesthesia if thrombocytopenia is present, if antiplatelet agents are given, or if there is a qualitative defect in platelets (e.g., an abnormal bleeding time). If anticoagulation is continued in the postoperative period, the potential movement of the epidural catheter as a consequence of ambulation poses a

risk for venous trauma and hematoma formation. Consequently, anesthesiologists are opposed to the use of continuous catheter techniques in such instances.

Low-dose heparin therapy for deep venous thrombosis prophylaxis represents a controversial area for the use of epidural analgesia. Obviously, the risks and benefits of epidural blockade need to be weighed against the risks and benefits of deep venous thrombosis prophylaxis with heparin or enoxaprin. One should not consider epidural block if full-dose intravenous heparin administration has been previously given. Because there is a small chance of trauma and bleeding with an indwelling catheter, even with the patient receiving low-dose or mini-dose heparin, the anesthesiologist may well be advised to decline placement and/or continuation of this technique.

Duration of Catheter Placement

The duration for epidural catheter use is generally quite variable. There certainly is a response that takes place when a catheter is inserted. For example, a fibrous tissue reaction occurs at about 72 hours.[16] A distinct advantage of an epidural catheter, however, is that it does not break the protective barrier of the dura, thereby limiting the likelihood of an infection developing in the CSF. Furthermore, use of epidural catheters avoids the headache associated with puncture of the dura when intrathecal catheters are placed.

One study evaluated the use of percutaneous catheters on a long-term basis (72 days).[50] Complications included catheter dislodgement, obstruction, and localized site infection. There were two instances of nonfatal meningitis in a total of 139 patients. In another study involving 105 individuals in whom a total of 215 catheters were placed, no infectious complications were observed.[10] A Silastic catheter can be tunneled and left in place for more than 1 year, particularly if a silver-silver chloride cuff (VITA CUFF) is used at the exit site.[15] In most instances, however, an epidural catheter is left in place for about 7 days before a change of sites is recommended.

A very rare occurrence is the migration of the catheter into the intravascular, subdural, or subarachnoid space.[9] Vertebral column movement, ligamentum flavum movement, and respiratory-induced space pressure variations make epidural catheters mobile, but catheter tip design and integrity of dural arachnoid membrane generally prevent this from occurring.

Factors Affecting Epidural Blockade

With respect to adult body weight, there appears to be no correlation between this variable and the spread of the analgesia. As may be expected, blockade is most intense and has the most rapid onset close to the site of injection. Increasing spread of injection, however, has no effect on the spread of solutions in the epidural space. Studies by Bromage have demonstrated the mass of drug itself determines the spread of analgesia.[6] If one increases the dose or mass of the pharmacologic agent, the amount of sensory blockade and its duration are increased. In addition, by increasing the concentration of the drug, the onset time is reduced, and greater motor block is achieved. Furthermore, the intensity of sensory and motor blockade increases with subsequent injections. This intensification and deepening of blockade is important with the use of dilute local anesthetic solutions that are applied for differential postoperative blockade (sensory versusmotor).

An example of spread is as follows. The four-segment spread for 2% lidocaine is 15±5 minutes. This can be compared to 18±10 minutes for 0.5% bupivicaine. The two-segment repression time is 100±40 minutes, compared with 200±80 minutes (the "wear-off" time of the block).[5] The duration of the blockade is related to the commencement of the regression of the block. The onset time (four-segment spread) indicates that all blocks take time to establish. It requires the patience of all individuals involved while the local anesthetic "takes."

In summary, then, the use of epidural analgesics introduces risks that must be balanced against the benefits. That said, epidural analgesia has proven to be an extremely safe and effective technique.[14,39,42]

BALANCED ANALGESIA

Henrik Kehlet and his colleagues at Copenhagen University Hospital have been singularly important contributors to the concept of expediting the recovery process through what they have termed, "balanced analgesia".[2,3,23,25,26] This is defined as the achievement of optimal pain relief and return of normal function through a combination of different analgesics and methods of administration. It is, of course, well known that limiting factors for early discharge from the hospital (in addition to pain) include ileus, organ dysfunction, and fatigue.[26] By a multimodality program, including initially spinal-epidural anesthesia, postoperative epidural analgesia for 48 hours, and immediate oral nutrition and mobilization, Kehlet was able to discharge their patients following open sigmoid colectomy at a median of 2 days.[26] In another study involving patients who underwent restoration of continuity following Hartmann's operation, postoperative stay was reduced to 3 days through continuous epidural analgesia with local anesthetic, enforced oral nutrition and mobilization, a laxative, and a "planned 2-day hospital stay".[3] The same protocol with similar results was applied to abdominal rectopexy for prolapse.[2] In a prospective, randomized, controlled trial from the Cleveland Clinic (Ohio)

Group, 64 patients were evaluated who underwent intestinal or rectal resection.[13] The authors found through the application of a postoperative care pathway using controlled rehabilitation with early ambulation and diet (CREAD), *without epidural analgesia*, that patients had a shorter hospital stay with no adverse consequences. With increasing focus on cost containment and with limitation on hospital resources, it seems prudent for one to encourage surgeons to increase their collaboration with anesthesiologists, to minimize pain while preventing ileus and to improve patient outcome.[13,23,25]

REFERENCES

1. Baker AS, Ojemann RG, Swartz MN, et al. Spinal epidural abscess. *N Engl J Med* 1975;293:463.
2. Basse L, Billesbolle P, Kehlet H. Early recovery after abdominal rectopexy with multimodal rehabilitation. *Dis Colon Rectum* 2002;45:195.
3. Basse L, Jacobsen DH, Billesbolle P, et al. Colostomy closure after Hartmann's procedure with fast-track rehabilitation. *Dis Colon Rectum* 2002;45:1661.
4. Blomberg SG, Emanuelsson H, Kuist H, et al. Effects of thoracic epidural anesthesia on coronary arteries and arterioles in patients with coronary artery disease. *Anesthesiology* 1990;73:840.
5. Bromage PR. *Epidural analgesia.* Philadelphia: WB Saunders, 1978.
6. Bromage PR. Mechanism of action of extradural analgesia. *Br J Anaesth* 1975;47:199.
7. Burns JW, Hodsman NB, McLintock TC, et al. The influence of patients' characteristics on the requirements of postoperative analgesia. *Anaesthesia* 1989;44:2.
8. Cousins M. Acute and postoperative pain. In: Wall PD, Melzack R, eds. *Textbook of pain.* New York: Churchill Livingstone, 1994:357.
9. Cousins MJ, Glynn CJ, Wilson PR, et al. Epidural morphine. *Anaesth Intensive Care* 1980;8:217.
10. Crawford ME, Andersen HB, Augustenborg G, et al. Pain treatment on an outpatient basis utilizing extradural opiates: a Danish multicenter study comprising 105 patients. *Pain* 1983;16:41.
11. Dahl JB, Rosenberg, Hansen B, et al. Differential analgesic effects of low dose epidural morphine and morphine-bupivicaine at rest and during mobilization after major abdominal surgery. *Anesth Analg* 1992;74:362.
12. De Angelis J. Hazards of subdural and epidural anesthesia during anticoagulant therapy: a case report and review. *Anesth Analg* 1972;51:676.
13. Delaney CP, Zutshi M, Senagore AJ, et al. Prospective randomized, controlled trial between a pathway of controlled rehabilitation with early ambulation and diet and traditional postoperative care after laparotomy and intestinal resection. *Dis Colon Rectum* 2003;46:851.
14. DeLeon-Cassasola O, Parker B, Lema M, et al. Postoperative epidural bupivicaine-morphine therapy. *Anesthesiology* 1994;81:368.
15. Dupen SL. Silastic long term epidural catheters. *Anesthesiology* 1986;65:195.
16. Durant PA, Yaksh TL. Epidural injections of bupivicaine, morphine, fentanyl, lofentanil and DADC in chronically implanted rats: a pharmacological and pathological study. *Anesthesiology* 1986;64:43.
17. Gabrielli F, Chiarelli M, Cioffi U, et al. Day surgery for mucosal-hemorrhoidal prolapse using circular stapler and modified regional anesthesia. *Dis Colon Rectum* 2001;44:842.

18. Gingrich TF. Spinal epidural hematoma following continuous epidural anesthesia. *Anesthesiology* 1968;29:162.

19. Gustafsson LL, Johannisson J, Garle M. Extradural and parenteral pethidine as analgesia after total hip replacement: effect and kinetics: a controlled clinical study. *Eur J Clin Pharmacol* 1986;29:529.

20. Gustaffson LL, Schildt B, Jacobsen KJ. Adverse effects of extradural and intrathecal opiates: report of a nationwide survey in Sweden. *Br J Anaesth* 1982;54:479.

21. Harik SI, Raichle ME, Reis DJ. Spontaneously remitting spinal epidural hematoma in a patient on anticoagulants. *N Engl J Med* 1971;284:1355.

22. Hendolin H, Lahtinen J, Lansimies E, et al. The effect of thoracic epidural analgesia on postoperative stress and morbidity. *Ann Chir Gynaecol* 1987;76:234.

23. Holte K, Kehlet H. Postoperative ileus: a preventable event. *Br J Surg* 2000;87:1480.

24. Kehlet H. Postoperative pain relief: what is the issue? *Br J Anaesth* 1994;72:373.

25. Kehlet H. Balanced analgesia: a prerequisite for optimal recovery. *Br J Surg* 1998;85:3.

26. Kehlet H. Hospital stay of 2 days after open sigmoidectomy with a multimodal rehabilitation programme. *Br J Surg* 1999;86:227.

27. Koob GF, Bloom FE. Cellular and molecular mechanisms of drug dependence. *Science* 1988;242:715.

28. Lerner SM, Gutterman P, Jenkins F. Epidural hematoma and paraplegia after numerous lumbar punctures. *Anesthesiology* 1973;39:550.

29. Liu S, Carpenter R, Mackey D, et al. Effects of perioperative analgesic technique on rate of recovery after colon surgery. *Anesthesiology* 1995;83:757.

30. Lomessey A, Magnin C, Viale JP, et al. Clinical advantages of fentanyl given epidurally for postoperative analgesia. *Anesthesiology* 1984;61:466.

31. Lynch EP, Lazor MA, Gellis JE, et al. Patient experience of pain after elective noncardiac surgery. *Anesth Analg* 1997;85:117.

32. Mangano DT, Silicano D, Hollenberg M, et al. Postoperative myocardial ischemia. *Anesthesiology* 1992;72:342.

33. Mule SJ. Physiological dispositions of narcotic agonists and antagonists. In: Clouet DH, ed. *Narcotic drugs: biochemical pharmacology*. New York: Plenum Press, 1971.

34. Odoom JA, Sih IL. Epidural analgesia and anticoagulant therapy. *Anaesthesia* 1984;38:254.

35. Place RJ, Coloma M, White PF, et al. Ketorolac improves recovery after outpatient anorectal surgery. *Dis Colon Rectum* 2000;43:804.

36. Rao TK, Eletr A. Anticoagulation following placement of epidural and subarachnoid catheters: an evaluation of neurological sequelae. *Anesthesiology* 1981;55:618.

37. Rawal N, Arner S, Gustaffson L, et al. Present state of extradural and intrathecal opioid analgesia in Sweden: a nationwide follow-up survey. *Br J Anaesth* 1987;59:791.

38. Read TE, Henry SE, Hovis RM, et al. Prospective evaluation of anesthetic technique for anorectal surgery. *Dis Colon Rectum* 2002;45:1553.

39. Ready L, Loper K, Nessly M, et al. Postoperative epidural morphine is safe on surgical wards. *Anesthesiology* 1991;75:452.

40. Rosenberg PH, Heino A, Scheinin B. Comparison of intramuscular analgesia, intercostal block, epidural morphine and on demand IV fentanyl in the control of pain after abdominal surgery. *Acta Anaesthesiol Scand* 1984;28:603.

41. Scheinen B, Asantila R, Orko R. The effect of bupivicaine and morphine on pain and bowel function after colonic surgery. *Acta Anaesthesiol Scand* 1987;31:161.

42. Senagore AJ, Delaney CP, Mekhail N, et al. Randomized clinical trial comparing epidural *Anaesthesia* and patient-controlled analgesia after laparoscopic segmental colectomy. *Br J Surg* 2003;90:1195.

43. Sharrock N, Ranawat C, Urquhart B, et al. Factors influencing deep vein thrombosis following total hip arthroplasty under epidural anesthesia. *Anesth Analg* 1993;76:756.

44. Tan PY, Vukasin P, Chin ID, et al. The WAND local anesthetic delivery system: a more pleasant experience for anal anesthesia. *Dis Colon Rectum* 2001;44:686.

45. Tuman KJ, McCarthy RJ, March RJ, et al. Effects of epidural anesthesia and analgesia on coagulation and outcome after major vascular surgery. *Anesth Analg* 1991;73:696.

46. Voulgari A, Lykouras L, Papanikolaum, et al. Influence of psychological and clinical factors on postoperative pain and narcotic consumption. *Psychother Psychosom* 1991;55:191.

47. Weller R, Rosenblum M, Conard P, et al. Comparison of epidural and patient controlled intravenous morphine following joint replacement surgery. *Can J Anaesth* 1991;38:582.

48. White PF. Patient controlled analgesia: a new approach to the management of postoperative pain. *Semin Anesth* 1985;4:255.

49. Yeager MP, Glass DO, Neff RK, et al. Epidural anesthesia and analgesia in high risk surgical patients. *Anesthesiology* 1987;66:729.

50. Zenz M. Epidural opiates: long term experiences in cancer pain. *Klin Wochenschr* 1985;63:225.

Chapter 8

Hemorrhoids

And the men that died not were smitten
with the emerods; and the cry of the city went
up to heaven.

1 Samuel 5:12*

* It is always stimulating to receive comments from readers of prior editions, especially those that are not merely flattering but from which I may learn of mistakes and omissions. The following communication was received from Professor Samuel Argov in Haifa, Israel.

MLC

"I read the Bible in its original Hebrew, and, being a colorectal surgeon, I have investigated the story of the Holy Ark, the Philistines, and the Israelites, as narrated in Samuel 1, Chapters 5,6. It would appear that the Philistines were struck by an epidemic which is almost certainly bubonic plague, caused by *Yersinia pestis*. As is well-known, the disease is transmitted by mice and rats through their fleas. The epidemic swept quickly through the population (Samuel 1, Chapters 5,11,12). It is difficult to conceive of an epidemic of hemorrhoids. The fact that the Philistines gave an offering of five golden mice implies that they knew the pathogenesis of the plague (Samuel 1, Chapter 6, verse 4). This confusion of interpretation arises from an early incorrect translation of the Hebrew word *Tchorim* by the vulgata and later copiers to mean hemorrhoids. In actuality, the original Hebrew word *Tchorim* meant a ball or bubo. The mistake was carried forward into modern Hebrew. Even today in Israel, everyone uses the biblical term for the wrong disease."

Hemorrhoid disease affects more than 1 million Americans per year.[32] It has been estimated that over a period of 3 years, approximately 4.4% of the United States population will have symptoms attributed to hemorrhoids.[121] Although the condition is rarely life-threatening, the complications of therapy can be. This fact led to the beatification of St. Fiachre, the patron saint of gardeners and hemorrhoid sufferers.[211,239] From the patient's perspective, the complaint of "hemorrhoids" simply represents the diagnosis for a host of anal problems, including itching, a lump, pain, swelling, bleeding, and protrusion. In most physicians' office practices, it is as likely that an individual's symptoms will be attributable to another cause as they are to hemorrhoids.

Hemorrhoid complaints are one of the most common afflictions of Western civilization. The problem can occur at any age and can affect both sexes. It has been estimated that at least 50% of individuals over the age of 50 years have at some time experienced symptoms related to hemorrhoids. Johanson and Sonnenberg analyzed data from governmental sources and concluded that the prevalence rate in the United States is 4.4%.[121] In their study, whites were affected more frequently than African Americans, and there was an increased frequency in those of higher socioeconomic status. It is also more common in rural than in urban areas. Some reports have commented on the relative rarity of the condition in rural Africa.[37]

The following have been suggested as factors that contribute to the development of hemorrhoids:

- Heredity
- Anatomic features
- Nutrition
- Occupation
- Climate
- Psychological problems
- Senility
- Endocrine changes
- Food and drugs
- Infection
- Pregnancy
- Exercise
- Coughing
- Straining
- Vomiting
- Constrictive clothing
- Constipation[16,66]

Burkitt and Graham-Stewart refute most of these concepts and provide their own theories of pathogenesis (see the following section).[37] This report and those of others have clarified the anatomy and attempted to establish the etiology on a more scientific footing.

ETIOLOGY AND ANATOMY

In 1975, Thomson published his master's thesis based on anatomic and radiologic studies and introduced the term *vascular cushions*.[259] According to this theory, the submucosa does not form a continuous ring of thickened tissue in the anal canal, but rather a discontinuous series of cushions; the three main cushions are found in the left lateral, right anterior, and right posterior positions (Figure 8-1). The submucosal layer of each of these thicker regions

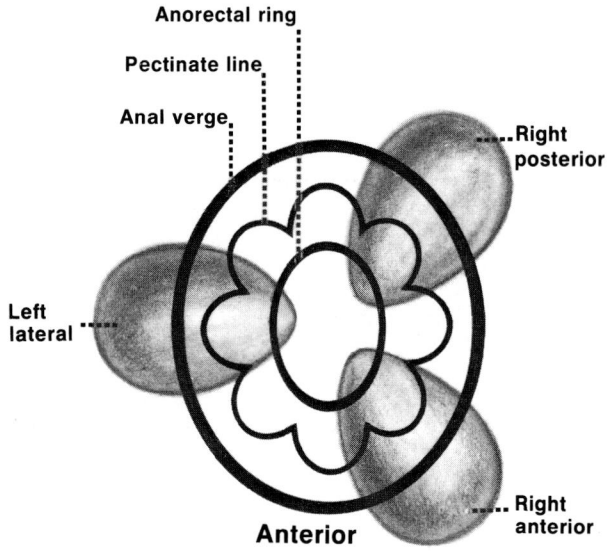

FIGURE 8-1. The three primary hemorrhoidal groups.

is rich with blood vessels and muscle fibers, the latter known as the muscularis submucosa (Figure 8-2).[199,280] These fibers, arising from the internal sphincter and from the conjoined longitudinal muscle, are important in maintaining adherence of mucosal and submucosal tissues to the underlying internal sphincter and in supporting the blood vessels of the submucosa. It is postulated that the cushions, by filling with blood during the act of defecation, protect the anal canal from injury. The muscularis

submucosa and its connective tissue fibers return the anal canal lining to its initial position after the temporary downward displacement that occurs during defecation.

The anal cushions receive their blood supply primarily from the terminal branches of the superior hemorrhoidal artery (i.e., superior rectal artery) and, to a lesser extent, from branches of the middle hemorrhoidal arteries.[28,199] These branches communicate with one another and with branches of the inferior hemorrhoidal arteries, which supply the lower portion of the anal canal. The superior, middle, and inferior hemorrhoidal veins, which drain blood from the tissues of the anal canal, correspond to each of the hemorrhoidal arteries.[28,106,199]

Anatomic studies by Haas and colleagues reveal that anchoring and supporting tissue deteriorates with aging, and that this phenomenon becomes apparent in the third decade of life (Figure 8-3).[104] This ultimately produces venous distension, erosion, bleeding, and thrombosis (Figure 8-4).

The following are the four major theories regarding the causes of hemorrhoids.

1. Abnormal dilatation of the veins of the internal hemorrhoidal venous plexus, a network of the tributaries of the superior and middle hemorrhoidal veins[37,197]
2. Abnormal distension of the arteriovenous anastomoses, which are in the same location as the anal cushions[106,107]
3. Downward displacement or prolapse of the anal cushions[64,258]
4. Destruction of the anchoring connective tissue system[104]

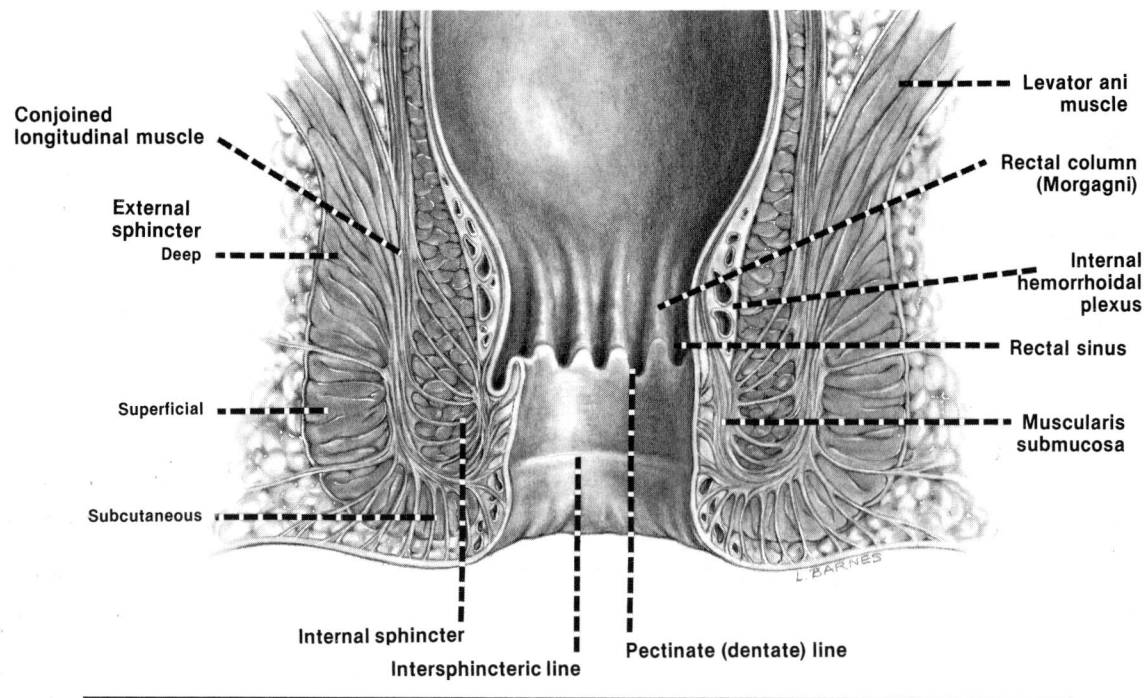

FIGURE 8-2. Anatomy of the anal region.

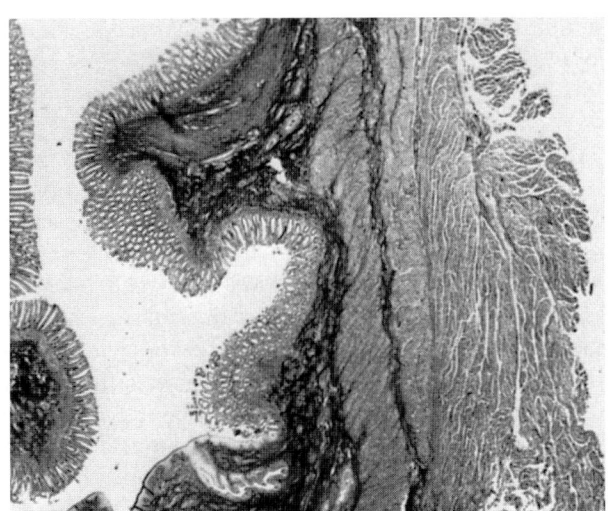

FIGURE 8-3. Longitudinal section through the anal canal of a newborn. Note the well-organized, firm connective tissue fibers that support the vessels within the hemorrhoidal pad and anchor them to the internal sphincter and conjoined longitudinal muscle. (Original magnification × 16; courtesy of Peter A. Haas, M.D.)

Other theories have been proposed to explain abnormal distension of hemorrhoidal vessels. For example, hemorrhoids may be caused by a backflow of venous blood from transient increases in intraabdominal pressure. It is this observation and the relative infrequency of the condition in rural Africa that caused Burkitt (see Biography, Chapter 26) and Graham-Stewart to assert the importance of crude fiber in the daily food intake to avoid

straining with defecation.[37] They even suggested that because Napoleon was troubled by hemorrhoids at Waterloo, the course of history could have been changed but for a few ounces of bran. However, others have called the presumption of causality between straining or constipation and hemorrhoids into question.[121]

Pressure exerted on the hemorrhoidal veins by a fetus explains the exacerbation of the condition in pregnant women.[155,200] Engorgement of vessels may result from a defect in venous drainage, which, in turn, may be caused by failure of the internal sphincter to relax as it should during defecation. Vascular distension may be attributed to augmented arterial flow; this would explain why people with hemorrhoids sometimes feel additional discomfort after a heavy meal. More blood is delivered to the digestive system through the mesenteric artery, of which the superior hemorrhoidal artery is a branch.[251] Hemorrhoids, however, are not varicose veins. They are structures that are normally present but do not produce symptoms until the fibromuscular supporting tissue above the cushions deteriorates.[30] This permits the cushions to slide, engorge, prolapse, and bleed.

Hemorrhoids may be caused by more than one factor. Although some evidence suggests that hemorrhoids are familial, it is not known whether this is caused by hereditary influences (e.g., weak-walled veins, atrophied or weakened fibrocollagenous supporting tissue) or environmental factors (e.g., family members may have similar dietary or bowel habits).

Despite a vast literature on the subject of hemorrhoids, the pathogenesis and even the function of this tis-

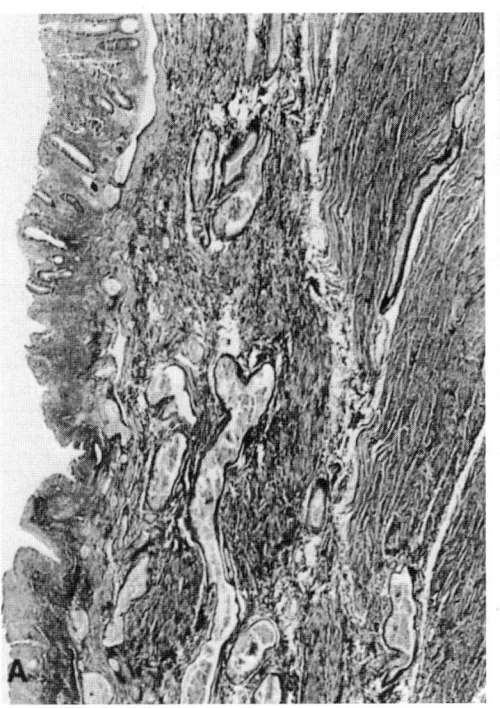

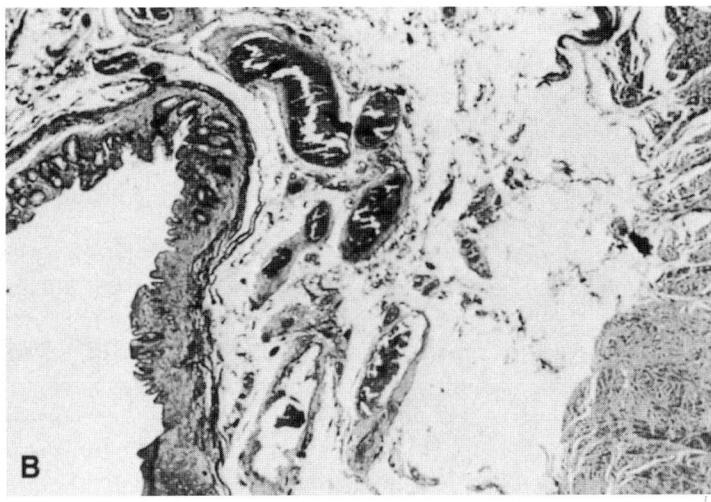

FIGURE 8-4. **(A)** Early disintegration of the connective tissue fibers. Venous sinuses in the submucosa have lost their support and are moderately distended. (Original magnification × 16.) **(B)** Complete breakdown of the anchoring and supporting connective tissue system. Mucosa and perianal skin are separated from the internal sphincter. (Original magnification × 20; courtesy of Peter A. Haas, M.D.)

sue remain controversial. Furthermore, there still exists a difference of opinion as to the definition of hemorrhoidal disease. The high prevalence of anoscopic evidence of this pathologic entity and its problematic relationship to symptoms suggests that perhaps these findings may be more a consequence of the aging process than truly a disease entity.[151]

Wexner and Baig opine, however, that hemorrhoidal tissue performs three main functions besides that of the veins providing drainage of blood from the area.[274] These functions theoretically include the following:

- Maintenance of continence through the filling of the vascular cushions (15% to 20% of resting anal pressures)
- "Protection" of the sphincter mechanism by providing a cushion
- Augmentation of the anal closure mechanism[274]

Portal Hypertension and Rectal Varices

What of the relationship of hemorrhoids to portal hypertension? The most common manifestation of hemorrhage in patients with liver disease is upper gastrointestinal bleeding, not lower gastrointestinal bleeding. Numerous studies have failed to demonstrate an increased incidence of hemorrhoids in this population. However, rectal varices may be seen as enlarged portal-systemic collateral veins in patients with portal hypertension.[272] This collateral circulation from the portal vein passes into the systemic circulation through the middle and inferior hemorrhoidal veins. In other words, hemorrhoids and rectal varices must be recognized as two separate entities. Hosking and colleagues evaluated 100 consecutive patients with cirrhosis and noted that 44% had anorectal varices.[114] Goenka and associates performed a prospective study to evaluate the prevalence of this finding in 75 individuals with known portal hypertension.[95] Sixty-seven (89.3%) were demonstrated to have lower gastrointestinal varices, the rectum being the most common site. There was no correlation, however, between the presence of these varices and the severity of esophagogastric mucosal changes of portal hypertension.

It is essential to differentiate anorectal varices from bleeding hemorrhoids, because the treatment is so obviously different. Endoscopic ultrasonography and magnetic resonance imaging are noninvasive modalities for diagnosis and control after treatment.[76]

Bleeding from varices may be treated by transanal suture technique, by trans-hepatic inferior mesenteric venography and embolization, or by any one of the methods of portal-systemic shunting and decompression.[76,115,181,272]

PHYSIOLOGY

The anal sphincters of many patients with hemorrhoids demonstrate an abnormal rhythm of contraction and exert a greater force of contraction than those of asymptomatic control subjects. Whether this sphincter abnormality is a cause or an effect of hemorrhoids is not known, but it may relate to any of the hypotheses outlined. An overactive sphincter could contribute to venous congestion, expose the anal cushions to greater shearing forces, or do both by constricting the anal canal.[11,105] Objective anorectal manometric studies reveal increased anal canal pressure in patients with symptomatic hemorrhoids when they are compared with control subjects.[73,109,254] Sun and colleagues performed a combined manometric and ultrasonographic study of the internal anal sphincter in 20 individuals with hemorrhoids and in 20 age-matched normal controls.[253] As expected, mean basal anal pressures were significantly higher in the patients with hemorrhoids than in the control patients. The mean maximal residual pressure was significantly higher in these individuals. Furthermore, direct pressure measurement in the anal canal cushions of the patients with hemorrhoids demonstrated abnormally high median pressure in comparison with that in controls. However, ultrasonographic study of the anal canal revealed a clear image of the internal sphincter that could easily be measured and was essentially no different from that of controls. The authors conclude that the absence of any significant differences in internal sphincter thickness between subjects without hemorrhoids and patients with hemorrhoids suggests that the high anal pressure observed in those with hemorrhoids is of a vascular origin.[253] This elevated pressure usually returns to normal levels following hemorrhoidectomy.

The hypothesis that this condition results from chronic constipation was investigated by Gibbons and colleagues, who studied bowel habits, anal pressure profiles, and anal compliance.[91] Hemorrhoids were associated with significantly longer anal high-pressure zones and significantly greater maximal resting pressures at all levels of anal distension. However, constipated women had normal pressure profiles and pressures. The study affirmed that patients with hemorrhoids are not necessarily constipated, and that chronically constipated individuals do not necessarily have hemorrhoids.

Other physiologic studies have been performed on patients with enlarged, symptomatic hemorrhoids. Various abnormalities have been reported, including increased electromyographic activity, increased external sphincter fiber density, prolonged pudendal nerve terminal motor latencies, reduced anal electrosensitivity, reduced temperature sensation, and reduced rectal compliance.[274]

CLASSIFICATION

Hemorrhoids are classified by location (i.e., external, internal, or mixed) or by degree (i.e., first, second, third, and fourth).[84] External hemorrhoids arise from the inferior hemorrhoidal plexus and are covered by modified squamous epithelium. They occur below the pectinate line and may become thrombotic and ulcerate. Internal hemorrhoids occur above the pectinate line. They may prolapse, ulcerate, bleed, and/or thrombose. They may be reducible or irreducible. Internal hemorrhoids arise from the superior hemorrhoidal plexus and are covered by mucosa. Mixed hemorrhoids (i.e., external-internal) may be prolapsed, irreducible, thrombosed, or ulcerated. They arise from the inferior and superior hemorrhoidal plexus and their anastomotic connections.

A grading system has been established for hemorrhoids, but this classification applies only to the internal variety. In first-degree hemorrhoids, the veins of the anal canal are increased in number and size, and they may bleed at the time of defecation. They do not prolapse but merely project into the lumen. Second-degree hemorrhoids present to the outside of the anal canal during defecation but return spontaneously to within the anal canal where they remain the rest of the time. Third-degree hemorrhoids protrude outside the anal canal and require manual reduction. Fourth-degree hemorrhoids are irreducible and constantly remain in the prolapsed state.

External Hemorrhoids

Two types of hemorrhoids are found at the external anal orifice. One occurs predominantly in the form of dilatation and engorgement of the veins beneath the skin, and the other is manifested as a thrombosis of these veins. When the clot forms, the patient becomes aware of its presence. The degree of pain depends on the size of the clot and the relationship it bears to the anal sphincters. A large clot will cause pain, but even if a clot is small, it can be quite uncomfortable if it lies within the anal musculature. Small, thrombosed hemorrhoids rarely ulcerate and bleed.

When the process spreads into external and internal tissue surrounding hemorrhoidal veins, considerable external swelling develops as edematous fluid fills the subcutaneous area at the anal margin. This may result in acute external and internal hemorrhoidal venous thrombosis and prolapse.

External Tags or Skin Tabs

External tags or skin tabs are deformities of the skin of the external anal margin and occur as redundant folds. These may be the residual of prior thrombosed hemorrhoids that have become organized into fibrous appendages. More than likely the patient will have no antecedent history that would suggest the origin of the tags. Women, however, will often state that the tags arose during pregnancy, especially during the third trimester, persisting following delivery.

The practice of removing hemorrhoids in three primary groups usually leaves bridges of tissue between the sites of the hemorrhoidal masses. When hemorrhoid disease is extensive, some of the diseased veins remain beneath these bridges of skin; these, too, may become fibrous skin tags after the wounds have healed (discussed later in the chapter).

Internal Hemorrhoids

The usual internal hemorrhoid is not evident on visual inspection of the anal area, especially if the patient is not bearing down. When an individual strains, a bulging mass may appear that involves all or part of the anal canal. The full extent of pressure is exerted on the anorectal outlet only during defecation or straining. Therefore, a truly reliable examination cannot be made with the patient in either the recumbent or the inverted jackknife position. Optimally, to assess the full extent of the process, examination with the patient seated on a commode is preferred.

Thrombosed Hemorrhoids

Thrombosed hemorrhoids (i.e., clotted hemorrhoids) are seen most often in patients who strain while defecating or when lifting heavy objects, those who have frequent bowel actions, such as occurs with inflammatory bowel disease or malabsorption, and those who sit for long periods of time (e.g., long-distance truck drivers, motorcycle policemen, airline pilots, operators of heavy construction equipment). Theoretically, direct trauma to the area creates an inflammatory response, which leads to thrombosis. Additionally, the Valsalva action during straining can lead to protrusion, which, if irreducible, can precipitate this complication. Stasis of the blood flow during straining is another possible explanation.

One of the most common etiologic associations of thrombosed hemorrhoids is the maintenance of a "library" in the toilet. Virtually every patient who experiences recurrent thromboses will harbor such a home resource.

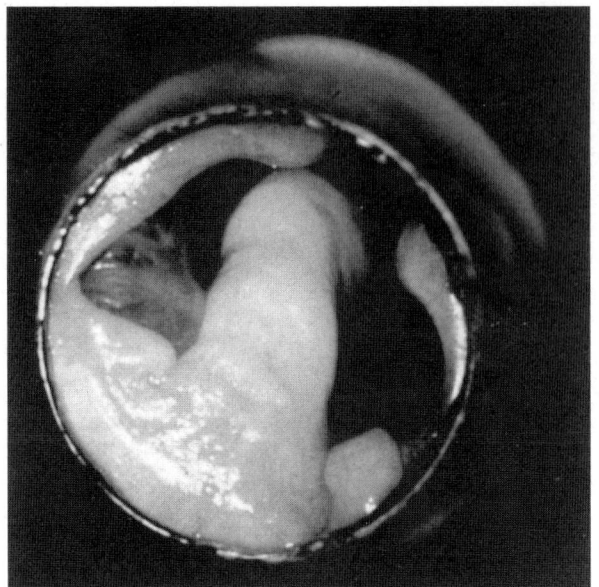

FIGURE 8-5. Anoscopic view of hypertrophied anal papilla. (Courtesy of Elliot D. Prager, M.D.)

DIFFERENTIAL DIAGNOSIS

Polyp, Adenoma, and Carcinoma

Sessile, polypoid masses (e.g., adenomas) and carcinomas, which are easily palpated or seen, should be readily differentiated from hemorrhoidal tissue. Internal hemorrhoids uncomplicated by thrombosis, edema, prolapse, or other factors are usually simple to diagnose. However, biopsy and microscopic study of any suspicious lesion are essential to establish the diagnosis with certainty. The old adage, "when in doubt, biopsy," is worth remembering.

Hypertrophied Anal Papilla

A firm mass that seems to arise from an attached pedicle in the region of the dentate line is most likely to represent a hypertrophied anal papilla (Figs. 8-5 and 8-6; see Figure 9-3). Ansocopy will clarify any confusion by revealing that the pedicle arises from the dentate margin and that the entire lesion is invested by skin.

Rectal Prolapse

Rectal prolapse may be either partial, involving only the mucosal layer of the rectal wall, or complete, involving the full thickness. Partial prolapse may affect either part or all of the circumference of the anal outlet. Differentiating prolapsed internal hemorrhoids from partial or mucosal prolapse may be somewhat confusing at times, but internal hemorrhoids are separated by sulci that radiate peripherally from the center of the anal outlet, whereas mucosal prolapse usually exhibits a more uniformly con-

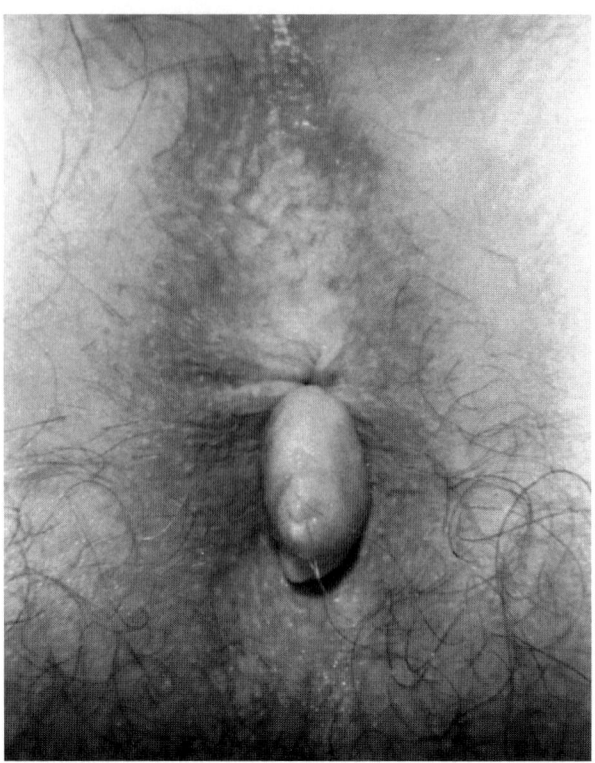

FIGURE 8-6. Prolapsed hypertrophied anal papilla. The fact that the lesion is covered by skin should eliminate confusion regarding the diagnosis.

centric protrusion. Often there is some element of mucosal prolapse when a circumferential rosette of hemorrhoids becomes irreducible and thrombosed (Figure 8-7). Complete rectal prolapse, however, should be readily distinguished by its concentrically arranged mucosal folds, which are strikingly different from the radiating sulci separating prolapsed internal hemorrhoids.

SIGNS AND SYMPTOMS

The most common presenting complaint of patients with hemorrhoids is bleeding. This usually occurs during or after defecation and is exacerbated by straining and by frequent bowel actions. Blood can be evident on the paper, in the toilet bowl, or both. Occasionally, blood loss may be severe enough to produce profound anemia. Pain is usually not caused by hemorrhoids, unless the hemorrhoidal vein is thrombosed, ulcerated, or gangrenous. The most common cause of anal pain is fissure. Prolapse, either with spontaneous return or requiring manual reduction, is a common presentation of hemorrhoids. The hemorrhoids may also be irreducible. Pruritus ani is often attributed to hemorrhoids, but frequently the examination fails to reveal significant hemorrhoidal disease. That is why, unfortunately, many patients who undergo operative hemorrhoidectomy discover that the pruritic symp-

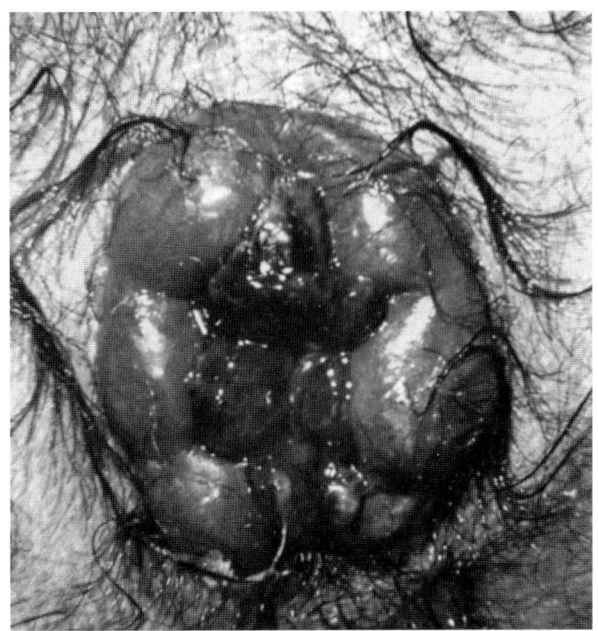

FIGURE 8-7. Prolapsed, thrombosed hemorrhoids. These are irreducible and have an element of mucosal prolapse.

toms persist. Pruritus ani is a condition whose treatment includes diet, bowel management, anal hygiene, and perhaps medication (see Chap. 19).

Constipation is not a symptom of hemorrhoids, but defecation may be difficult when thrombosis or gangrene produces pain. Patients tend to avoid the toilet if hemorrhoidal symptoms are exacerbated by defecation; this can lead to refusal of the urge to pass stool and can result in constipation or even obstipation.

EXAMINATION

Physical examination should include proctosigmoidoscopy and anoscopy. Colonoscopy or a barium enema study must be performed in all patients who have rectal bleeding when the source is not readily apparent from these examinations. In patients older than 50 years of age, an evaluation of the colon should be performed at some time, even if hemorrhoids are the apparent cause of the patient's symptoms. This may be deferred if an individual's symptoms or inconvenience preclude carrying out such studies at the time of the examination.

Kluiber and Wolff at the Mayo Clinic iin Rochester, Minnesota reviewed in a retrospective fashion the incidence of hemorrhoidal bleeding that produced anemia.[137] The incidence of bleeding attributed to hemorrhoids that caused anemia was found to be 0.5/100,000 population per year in Olmsted County, Minnesota from 1976 to 1990. The authors found that recovery from anemia after definitive treatment by means of hemorrhoidectomy was quite rapid. From a mean hemoglobin concentration be-

fore treatment of 9.4 g/dL, it was found that the hemoglobin concentration increased to 12.3 g/dL after 2 months. By 6 months, the mean hemoglobin concentration was 14.1 g/dL. The authors concluded that failure to recover hemoglobin concentration should prompt further or repeated evaluation for other causes of the anemia.[137]

GENERAL PRINCIPLES OF TREATMENT

Bleeding

Bleeding, if occasional and related to straining or to diarrhea, can often be managed without direct treatment of the hemorrhoids; in other words, treatment should be directed to the cause of the bleeding. Constipation may be controlled by appropriate dietary measures, a bowel-management program, stool softeners, laxatives, or a combination of these. Moesgaard and colleagues, in a prospective double-blind trial of a bulk agent (i.e., psyllium) versus a placebo in patients with bleeding and pain at defecation, noted a statistically significant difference in improvement of symptoms during a 6-week period ($p < .025$).[169] They recommended the use of a high-fiber diet as the initial approach to the treatment of patients with symptomatic hemorrhoids. Diarrhea or frequent defecation may be managed with antidiarrheal medications and diet. Attention should also be given to improvement of anal hygiene.

The use of commercial topical creams, lotions, and suppositories is worthy of comment. These preparations include Tucks pads and cream, Anusol cream and suppositories, Balneol lotion, Prax, ProctoFoam, and the most ubiquitous self-medication employed by the average American for "symptomatic hemorrhoids," Preparation H. Preparation H has been alleged in the past to contain shark liver oil as well as a "skin respiratory factor" of unknown formulation that is supposed to improve wound healing. Its active ingredient today is phenylephrine hydrochloride (0.25%), a vasoconstrictor that may lead to temporary relief of burning and itching. Subramanyam and colleagues created rectal ulcers by performing rectal biopsy on volunteer subjects, determined the speed of healing with use of this product in suppository form, and compared it with a placebo.[252] Although healing was quicker and more complete in the Preparation H group, the number of patients in the study was too small to achieve statistical significance. In my personal opinion, Preparation H acts essentially to soothe skin irritation and is as effective for this purpose as virtually any topical cream, lotion, or ointment. Symptoms of pruritus ani may be ameliorated, but there is no evidence that Preparation H causes hemorrhoids to shrink. There are also commercially available mechanical devices and products that are used to facilitate cleansing of the anus, such as mini-bidets, Shower Mini, and Water-pic.

Suppositories have been employed since the civilization of ancient Egypt for three basic reasons:

- To promote defecation
- To introduce medications into the body
- To treat anorectal disease[16]

It is difficult to assess the actual efficacy of suppositories with regard to this last condition. Because the anorectal disease is often self-limited, resolution may occur irrespective of this treatment. Furthermore, the physician cannot gainsay the psychological benefit that vigorous promotional effort of such products produces for the patient. Finally, the bullet-shaped suppository often used in the treatment of anal conditions cannot exert its primary benefit within the anal canal, because it must advance at least as far as the rectum. To be truly useful Banov suggests that the suppository be hourglass or collar button shaped to maintain effective contact with the anal mucosa.[19] Such a modification has yet to be produced.

If bleeding persists despite the foregoing approaches, some form of interventional treatment should be offered. If the patient believes that bleeding is caused by hemorrhoids and does not seek medical attention, or if the surgeon accepts this diagnosis without attempting to address the bleeding, a neoplasm may develop and go unrecognized. Such a situation could jeopardize the opportunity for early diagnosis and treatment.

Prolapse

Prolapsed hemorrhoids that return spontaneously or are manually reducible can usually be treated by a number of the office procedures discussed later. Attempting reduction is important, because persistent prolapse predisposes the patient to thrombosis and possibly even necrosis. If the prolapse is irreducible or if an external component is present, an excisional approach may be indicated.

Pain

If pain is caused by gangrenous, ulcerated, or thrombosed hemorrhoids, a surgical procedure is the best means of treatment. If symptomatic or extensive hemorrhoids are associated with an anal fissure, hemorrhoidectomy should be considered and the fissure treated by internal anal sphincterotomy (discussed later in chapter;

see also Chapter 9). A thrombosed external hemorrhoid that produces pain should be treated by local excision.

The physician should consider the value of sitz baths in the treatment of any anal problem. Subjectively, there is little question that pain is ameliorated by the application of heat. Studies suggest there may be an explanation for how heat contributes to this response. Dodi and colleagues performed anorectal manometry on volunteers and on patients with anorectal problems (e.g., hemorrhoids, anal fissure) and determined pressure changes after immersion in warm (40°C) and cold (5°C and 23°C) water.[70] In all subjects, a statistically significant decrease in resting pressure was observed after immersion in the warm water. No change was seen when patients were exposed to the colder temperatures. Because patients with certain anal conditions often have elevated pressures, the lowering of resting anal canal pressure probably produces the observed symptomatic improvement.

AMBULATORY TREATMENT

In 1993, practice parameters for ambulatory anorectal surgery were established by the Standards Task Force of the American Society of Colon and Rectal Surgeons.[249] These guidelines may have been prepared to deal with the threat of regulations from governmental and various insurance agencies. A disclaimer was incorporated recognizing that the guidelines were not inclusive of all proper methods and did not exclude other reasonable options. The subject of *parameters* and *guidelines* will be discussed in other chapters where such management issues are addressed.

Gastroenterologists, internists, and family practitioners have all invaded the hitherto sacrosanct domain of the surgeon through the invasive treatment of hemorrhoids. This contemporary change seems reasonable when specialized training that nonsurgeons may receive in the management of other invasive techniques is considered.[235] In fact, some of the tools that are advocated for the outpatient treatment of hemorrhoids are directly marketed to nonsurgeons by mail and at meetings and conventions. I believe that it is fitting and proper for any physician to perform many of the following discussed procedures, with the provision that they are held to the same standards of care that are demanded of surgeons.

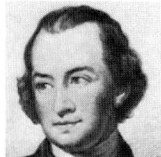

John Morgan (1820–1891)   Morgan was born in Bath, England, the son of a physician. After the death of his father, he moved to London and entered King's College. As was the custom of the day, he became apprenticed to a surgeon and attended lectures, especially at St. George's Hospital. He established himself as a surgeon in London in 1845 in the neighborhood of Hyde Park, the area being the "resort of the wealthy and successful." Little is known about how Morgan came to employ the technique of injection, but he did achieve a significant reputation in the medical community as an anatomist and surgeon. (Morgan J. Varicose state of saphenous haemorrhoids treated successfully by the injection of tincture of persulphate of iron. *Med Press Circular* 1869:29.)

Likewise, surgeons must be held to the very same criteria for competence as are gastroenterologists when they perform colonoscopy or colonoscopy-polypectomy.

Sclerotherapy: Injection Treatment of Hemorrhoids

The first attempt to obliterate hemorrhoids by means of injection was reported in 1869 by John Morgan. Morgan used iron persulfate to treat external hemorrhoids, varicose veins, and vascular lesions. In 1871, this unique form of therapy, using phenol and other chemical agents, was introduced into the United States. It was advertised as a "painless cure for piles without surgery."[9] Because specula were not available at that time, only prolapsed hemorrhoids were selected for treatment, with a single massive injection given to slough off the hemorrhoid. In 1879, Edmund Andrews, President of the Chicago Medical Society, presented a report of 3,295 patients, collected through correspondence, who had undergone injection therapy.[9] Many of the patients had been treated by itinerant charlatans and inadequately trained physicians. Numerous complications, including severe pain, sloughing, and even death (nine cases), were reported. Despite these problems, Andrews believed that cautious application of the procedure was appropriate if the following criteria were met: internal hemorrhoids were treated, the patient was kept at bed rest for at least 8 hours after the procedure, and carbolic acid in oil or glycerine was employed. At about this time, Kelsey in the United States and Edwards in England recognized that the injection method was beneficial and substituted a weaker solution of 5% to 7.5% carbolic acid in glycerine and water; this resulted in less sloughing.[71,129] Phenol (5%) in almond or vegetable oil is still the primary sclerosing agent used in Great Britain today; 3 ml is usually injected into each hemorrhoid site.

The combination of quinine and urea hydrochloride, widely used as a local anesthetic agent before the introduction of procaine, was associated with the development of fibrous tissue proliferation and sometimes sloughing at the site of injection.[257] In 1913, Terrell first used this substance in the injection treatment of internal hemorrhoids, with dramatic results. He concluded that a 5% solution was satisfactory from the standpoint of effectiveness and the patient's safety.[257] The historical implications of the development of the injection method are well described by Anderson in his 1924 review.[7] Sclerosants include sodium morrhuate and sodium tetradecyl sulfate (i.e., Sotradecol), but the safest continues to be phenol (5%) in vegetable oil. In essence, all the ambulatory, nonexcisional treatments of hemorrhoids produce fibrosis of the submucosa, thereby obliterating the redundant tissue.

Indications and Contraindications

The nonprolapsing internal hemorrhoid is most amenable to injection treatment. Sometimes, a large, slightly protruding hemorrhoid can be successfully treated in this manner. Injection usually affords only temporary relief of symptoms when hemorrhoids are voluminous, contain a

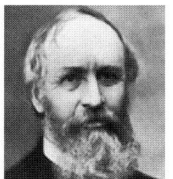

Edmund Andrews (1824–1904) Andrews was born in Putney, Vermont. At the age of 16, he moved to Detroit and completed his literary studies at the University of Michigan, graduating in 1849. He received his medical degree 3 years later from the same university. After several years on the faculty in the Department of Anatomy at the university, he joined the Department of Surgery at the Rush Medical College. In 1854, Andrews founded the Chicago Academy of Sciences. During the Civil War, he served as Chief of Surgery at one of the camp hospitals and directed mobile surgical units in Tennessee and Mississippi, with the responsibility for maintaining the records of surgery during the war. As Professor of Surgery at Rush, he ultimately became dissatisfied and severed his connections there. With several other well-recognized physicians in Chicago, Andrews established the Lind University Medical School, which eventually became the Medical School of Northwestern University; for 46 years he was Professor of Surgery. An innovative surgeon, Andrews developed many instruments, including braces for correction of spinal curvature, an appliance for trephining, and an early endoscope that paved the way for modern cystoscopy. Following a trip to England in 1867, he was the first surgeon in the West to use and promote Lister's antiseptic methods.

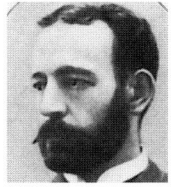

Charles Boyd Kelsey (1850–1917) Kelsey was born in Farmington, Connecticut, the son of a Protestant minister. He received his medical degree from the College of Physicians in New York in 1873 and became a house surgeon at St. Luke's Hospital in New York. There followed a period of 5 years in the Department of Anatomy at his alma mater as a demonstrator, during which time he developed a commitment to the treatment of anorectal diseases. In 1880, he was instrumental in the establishment of a hospital in New York that was "founded on the same general plan as St. Mark's Hospital in London." St. Paul's Infirmary for Hemorrhoids, Fistula, and Other Diseases of the Rectum survived for only a few years, but Kelsey became recognized as one of the leading authorities on rectal surgery in the United States. His books, *Surgery of the Rectum and Pelvis* and *Diseases of the Rectum and Anus: Their Pathology, Diagnosis and Treatment*, were considered the most authoritative texts in the United States at the time on the subject of rectal disease. Kelsey became Professor in the Department of Diseases of the Rectum at the University of Vermont in 1889 and 2 years later occupied the same chair at the New York Postgraduate School. (Kelsey CB. *Surgery of the rectum and pelvis*. New York: W. Wood, 1902; Kelsey CB. *Diseases of the rectum and anus: their pathology, diagnosis and treatment*. New York: W. Wood, 1890; Banov L Jr. St. Paul's infirmary for haemorrhoids, fistula, and other diseases of the rectum. *South Med J* 1978;71:1559.)

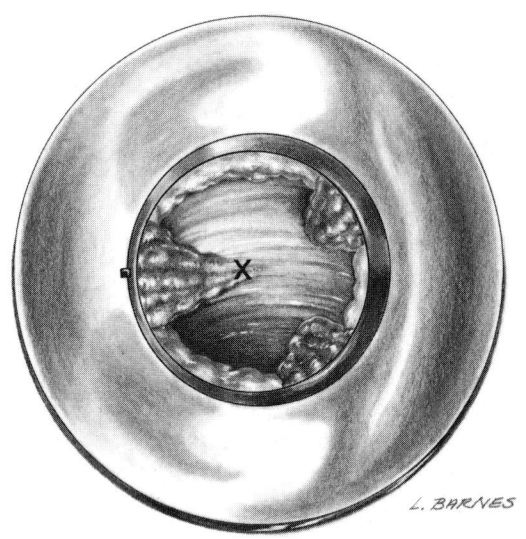

FIGURE 8-8. Hemorrhoids in commonly seen locations in the anal canal as viewed through the anoscope. The *X* indicates the planned site for injection of the left lateral pile, in an insensitive area of the anal canal.

great deal of fibrous tissue, or require digital replacement after defecation. External hemorrhoids should never be treated by injection. Internal hemorrhoids that are infected or contain thrombi likewise should not be injected. Hemorrhoids with evidence of inflammation, such as ulceration and gangrene, are also unsuitable for injection treatment. Tags, fistulas, tumors, and anal fissure are complicating conditions that contraindicate use of the injection method.

Technique

With the patient in the semiinverted jackknife or left lateral (i.e., Sims') position, an anoscope is inserted and the anal canal observed (Figure 8-8). The entire region is inspected so that, ideally, a diagram of the position of the hemorrhoids can be drawn on the patient's chart (Figure 8-1). This is especially useful when long intervals elapse between injections. The point at which each injection is

made, the amount of solution used, and the date of the injection should be recorded on the chart, or at least clearly documented in the notes. The term *o'clock* should not be used to describe the location of the treatment or the location of the hemorrhoids. Left lateral is left lateral whether the patient is in the prone jackknife position, in the lithotomy position, or hanging from the chandelier. The use of the word *o'clock* mandates that the position of the patient be described, and this is inevitably absent in most office notes and communications.

Figure 8-9 shows the syringe and long, angled needle used for sclerotherapy. Although this type of needle is very well known to head and neck surgeons, its value for the colon and rectal surgeons is not generally appreciated. More to the point, however, is the fact that standard, straight, disposable needles are a requisite for every physician's office. Still, the longer the needle that is used (e.g., a spinal needle), the better the visualization is of the pile site.

The needle is introduced through the mucous membrane into the center of the mass of veins (Figure 8-10). No antiseptic is necessary. Care must be taken to avoid bringing the point of the needle into contact with the sensitive margin of the pectinate line. Because of the extremely remote possibility that the needle could enter the lumen of a vein and that the solution could be injected into the circulation, some surgeons withdraw the plunger of the syringe to see whether blood appears. Unlike sclerotherapy for varicose veins, this technique requires that intraluminal injection be avoided, but in actuality it is virtually impossible to perform an intravenous injection.

After the needle is in position, 0.5 ml of sodium morrhuate, quinine, and urea hydrochloride, or Sotradecol is slowly injected submucosally into each pile site. Alternatively, the physician may employ a 5% solution of phenol in almond, vegetable, or arachis oil. A wheal should form, indicating that the injection was given in the proper plane. No more than 3 mL should be used in total if a commercial sclerosant is being used. Conversely, with the phenol in oil solution, 3 mL may be injected into each pile site. All hemorrhoids should be injected at the first treatment session.

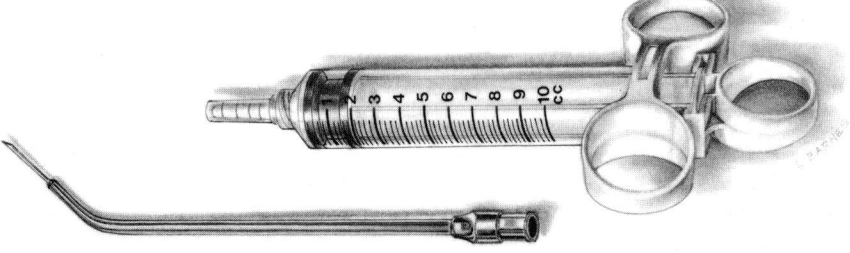

FIGURE 8-9. Syringe and angled hemorrhoid needle used for sclerotherapy. An angled needle permits better visualization than does a straight one. Alternatively, a fine-bore hypodermic needle can be employed.

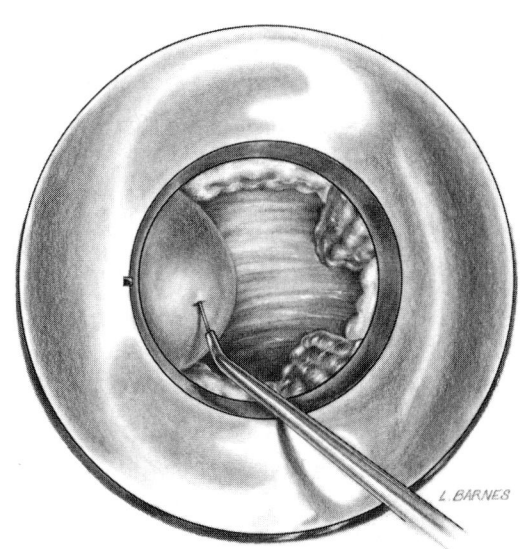

FIGURE 8-10. Sclerotherapy. If a wheal is not produced, the injection is too deep, and the needle should be withdrawn. An injection that is too superficial can cause necrosis of the lining of the anal canal.

A modification has been adopted by some gastroenterologists, that is, injection via a catheter passed through the channel of a colonoscope. Because gastroenterologists generally do not use anoscopy, they look at the anal canal (as best they can) through a retroflexed, long instrument. This technique is mentioned only to condemn it. However, having never attempted it, I can only imagine what a cumbersome exercise it must be to endeavor to perform sclerotherapy by this technique.

Complications

Sloughing

If sloughing follows the injection of a sclerosant, one or more of three errors are usually responsible:

- The injection was too superficial.
- Too much solution was injected into one area.
- A second injection was made into a hemorrhoid too soon after the first.

Expectant management usually results in resolution without long-term sequelae. However, anal stricture can be a consequence of extensive tissue destruction.[222]

Thrombosis and Necrosis (Sloughing)

Thrombosed hemorrhoids, whether internal, external, or both, are uncommon consequences of properly performed sclerotherapy. However, necrosis of anal mucosa or perianal skin is usually the result of too superficial an injection, the injection of too much sclerosant ,or the injection of overlapping areas. Generally, treatment is conservative and consists of sitz baths, analgesics, and topical anal creams. If scarring or stricture supervenes, an anoplasty should be considered (see later).

Burning

Burning in the anal canal is a late consequence of repeated sclerotherapy. The discomfort can in some patients be quite disabling, unremitting, and unresponsive to the usual local measures. Systemic pain medication may be the only effective therapy. I do not recommend repeated injections primarily because of my fear of this complication.

Local Abscess and Paraffinoma

Submucous abscess and paraffinoma (i.e., oleogranuloma) have been reported, the latter after the use of oil-based sclerosing agents (see Chapter 25).[69,176]

Bacteremia and Sepsis

Bacteremia following sclerotherapy has been reported in 8% of patients who undergo this procedure.[2] Although septicemia did not develop in any of the patients, antibiotic prophylaxis is recommended for those individuals at an increased risk (e.g., valvular heart disease; see Chapter 5). Other extremely rare reported complications include urologic sepsis, prostatic abscess, epididymitis, seminal vesicle abscess, urinary-perineal fistula, retroperitoneal sepsis, perineal and scrotal necrotizing fasciitis, septic shock, and rectal perforation with retroperitoneal abscess.[102,216] In the era of human immunodeficiency virus (HIV) and the immunocompromised patient, one must be sensitive to the potential for an increased risk of septic complications in these individuals.

Results

Few reports of sclerotherapy have been published in contemporary English language publications. Khoury and colleagues conducted a randomized trial that compared single versus multiple phenol injections in the treatment of hemorrhoids.[131] Results were assessed up to 1 year later. Most patients fell into the category of mild to moderate hemorrhoid disease. The authors demonstrated that a single session of injection treatment using "adequate doses of sclerosant" (i.e., 3 to 5 mL) was as effective as multiple treatments. Dencker and colleagues reported on the comparative results obtained from three forms of treatment of internal hemorrhoids—ligation, operation according to Milligan, and injection—and concluded that the results obtained with injection were poor.[65] Only 21% of patients were well at the time of review. Santos and co-workers assessed the outcome following single-session sclerotherapy with 5% phenol in almond oil in 189 patients.[231] With a 4-year follow-up, the authors concluded that this approach to the management of hemorrhoids provided only short-term benefit for the majority of individuals. Additional studies demonstrate sclerosant therapy to be less effective than a number of other options.[5,87,147,242)] Because other methods afforded Dencker and colleagues better results, they did not think that injection treatment should be used routinely for internal hemorrhoids.

Alexander-Williams and Crapp, in a report on conservative management of hemorrhoids, stated that they had used sclerotherapy extensively in the past and as part of clinical comparative trials. They found that it gave satisfactory short-term results, particularly in the treatment of patients with first-degree hemorrhoids.[3]

Opinion

I believe injection treatment is a reasonable option for the treatment of a limited number of individuals who have symptomatic hemorrhoids, especially bleeding, and in whom rubber band ligation cannot be tolerated (see next section). Because of my concern for the complication of intractable burning and discomfort from multiple injections, only one treatment of all pile sites is advisable. If symptoms persist, an alternative approach should be offered.

Rubber Ring Ligation

Tissue necrosis and fixation can also be produced by rubber ring ligation.[67,68] In 1954, Blaisdell described an instrument for ligation of internal hemorrhoids as an outpatient procedure.[31] In 1962, Barron modified this instrument and presented two series reporting excellent results (Figure 8-11).[21,22] The results of the ligation technique have been so gratifying that this approach has replaced surgical hemorrhoidectomy for approximately 80% of my patients.[57]

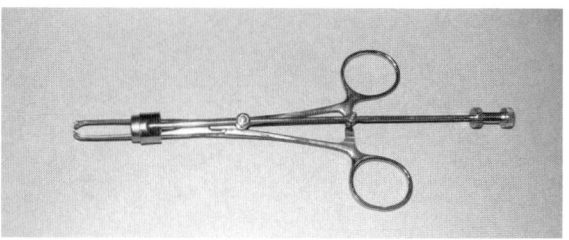

FIGURE 8-11. Original Barron hemorrhoid ligator. (Courtesy of Theodore E. Eisenstat, M.D.)

Any individual who has hemorrhoids manifested by bleeding, prolapse, or both is a candidate for this procedure. No anesthetic is required, but the rubber rings must be placed on an insensitive area, usually at or just above the dentate line. Skin tags or hypertrophied anal papillae cannot be treated by ligation because the patient would experience too much discomfort.

After a small cleansing enema has been given, proctosigmoidoscopy and anoscopy are performed. If the patient's history is suggestive of colonic disease, colonoscopy or barium enema examination is completed before any treatment of the hemorrhoids is considered. Several treatments, spaced over 3- to 4-week intervals, may be required, depending on how many pile sites must be eliminated to alleviate the symptoms. Generally, I do not recommend multiple bandings in the first treatment session. I make exceptions to this policy on the basis of patient insistence or convenience, lack of discomfort with a past treatment, or the necessity of the patient to travel a considerable distance for subsequent therapy. However, multiple bandings are offered or routinely employed by some physicians.

Technique

Figure 8-12 shows the McGivney ligator; I prefer this instrument to the Barron ligator. It has a much more secure shaft, which may be rotated in a 360-degree arc to facilitate placement. All nonsuction instruments have the relative disadvantage of requiring two people to perform the procedure: one to maintain the anoscope or retractor in position and the other to hold the ligator and grasping

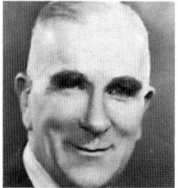

Edward Thomas Campbell Milligan (1886–1972)   Milligan was born at Waterloo, near Ballarat, Victoria, Australia, the son of a gold miner. He attended Ballarat College and received his medical training at Melbourne University, graduating with honors in 1910. In 1914, he went to France with the Australian Expeditionary Force and distinguished himself by the application of the radical exploration and debridement of wounds. At the conclusion of the war, he received the Order of the British Empire and settled in London to become a consultant to a number of hospitals, including St. Mark's. He developed an interest in anal diseases and became extremely adept in performing a combined abdominoperineal resection. It was said that he was a "master of surgical planes and deft atraumatic dissection, and even after the most major procedures his patients looked undisturbed." One of his outstanding achievements was the work that he and his junior colleagues prepared on the detailed anatomy of the pelvis, the sphincter mechanism, and the treatment of hemorrhoids. (Milligan ETC, Morgan CN, Jones LE, et al. Surgical anatomy of the anal canal, and the operative treatment of haemorrhoids. *Lancet* 1937;233:1119.)

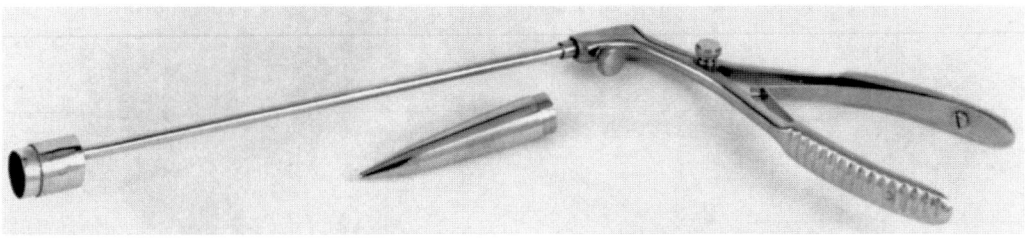

FIGURE 8-12. McGivney hemorrhoid ligator. This improved model has an offset handle for better vision; working length is 7 in. There are two thumb screws: one to assemble and secure the handle on the shaft and the other to permit rotation of the shaft in a 360-degree arc to facilitate placement on to the pile. (Courtesy of Miltex Instrument Co., Lake Success, NY.)

forceps. Alternatively, the physician may use a suction hemorrhoidal ligator such as the Lurz-Goltner (Figure 8-13) or the McGown ligator (Figure 8-14). These instruments draw the hemorrhoid into the cup through suction and therefore do not require a grasping forceps. Because the Lurz-Goltner ligator is a side-application device, maneuvering the ligator onto the pile is quite easy. An end-suction instrument, such as the McGown ligator, is also very simple to use, but it requires slightly more manipulation to fit it onto the hemorrhoid. Conversely, the disadvantage of the side-suction ligator is that mechanical problems often prevent the instrument from working optimally. Treatment with a suction ligator seems to be associated with less patient discomfort, but this is perhaps because the drum incorporates a smaller volume of tissue. This factor, of course, is a potential disadvantage, because the open-barrel device can permit incorporation of very large hemorrhoids and even redundant rectal mucosa.

Figure 8-15 shows an anal canal in which the ligator and alligator forceps have been inserted. I personally prefer to use the long alligator forceps because they securely grab the tissue, but more importantly they facilitate clear visualization of the site to be treated. However, most surgeons are familiar with and use Allis forceps. This short instrument is less than ideal because one's hand is often in the way, but the angled Allis forceps help somewhat in ameliorating this difficulty.

The most prominent hemorrhoid is treated first. It is grasped with the forceps as illustrated in Figure 8-16A and pulled up through the drum of the ligator (Figure 8-16B). If the patient experiences pain, a slightly more proximal point is selected, and this step is repeated. If the patient is still very uncomfortable, the wise course is to abandon this method of treatment and consider one of the alternatives. The tissue is drawn into the drum until it is taut, and the trigger is released, expelling two rubber rings (Figure 8-16C). Two rings are advised in case one breaks; there is considerable variation in the form and force of the rubber rings available on the market.[126] When the rings are in place, the anoscope is withdrawn (Figure 8-16D). As previ-

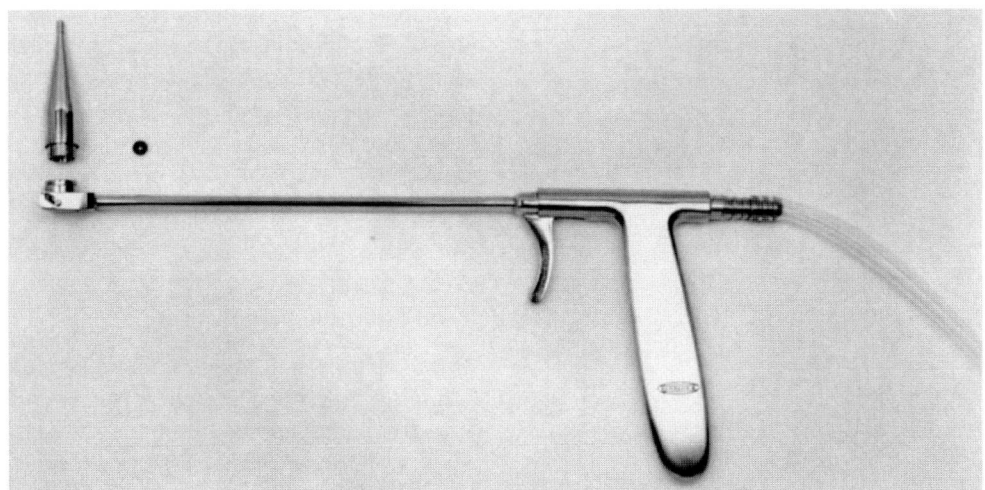

FIGURE 8-13. Lurz-Goltner suction hemorrhoidal ligator. (Courtesy of Scanlan International, St. Paul, MN.)

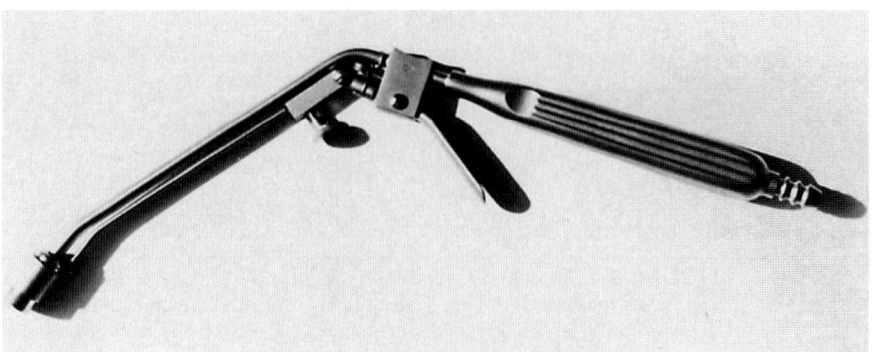

FIGURE 8-14. McGown one-hand hemorrhoidal ligator. This instrument has two interchangeable heads and a thumb suction activator. (Courtesy of George P. McGown, M.D.)

ously mentioned, if the physician uses the suction ligator, no grasping instrument is required.

The patient rarely experiences pain so severe that removal of the rings is necessary, but if required, this can be done by interposing the end of a conventional dispos-

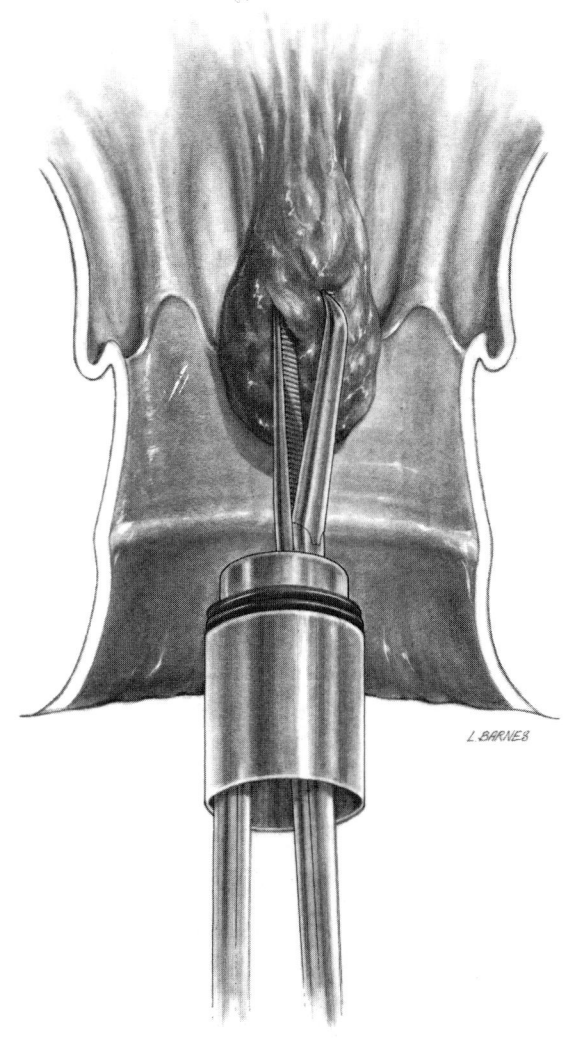

FIGURE 8-15. Rubber ring ligation. Alligator forceps are used to grasp the hemorrhoid. The forceps pass through the drum of the ligator.

able suture-removal scissors or the application of a crochet hook. George McGown (Pembroke Pines, FL) has designed a cutting hook for this sole purpose (Figure 8-17). Other methods for removing the rings, such as cutting with a scalpel, tend to precipitate bleeding. Removal of the rubber rings can be accomplished with minimal trauma within a few minutes after application. However, if the patient returns at a later time because of pain, the associated edema precludes the possibility of safe removal. Adequate analgesic medication, therefore, is the preferred option. This presupposes that sepsis is not the cause (see Complications).

A newer modification of a rubber band ligator has been developed, that of a disposable instrument, the O'Regan System (Figs. 8-18 and 8-19). This device is a self-contained syringe-like instrument that eliminates the need for wall suction and tubing. As with the reusable instrument, it requires only one person, but clearly the primary advantage is that of disposability. In an era of concern for reprocessing costs, occupational health issues, and the risks of cross-contamination, this alternative has real merit. The technique is illustrated in Figure 8-20.

Armstrong has developed a modified anoscope with lateral aperatures at the left lateral, right anterior, and right posterior quadrants, in order to enable synchronous exposure and concomitant multiple hemorrhoidal ligations (Figs. 8-21 and 8-22).[13] Another innovation that facilitates the performance of multiple ligations in one sitting is a multiple-banding instrument, the ShortShot Saeed Hemorrhoidal Multi-Band Ligator (Figure 8-23). This is a suction ligating device that permits up to four bandings with the one instrument.

Care Following Treatment

Bowel actions should be maintained without the patient straining. Appropriate dietary instructions, bulk agents, or a stool softener should be considered. The individual should be forewarned that some bleeding may be noted initially and again when the rubber rings are dislodged.

One of the major advantages of rubber ring ligation is its convenience. The patient need not return at fixed intervals for further ligation. Nothing is lost if one chooses

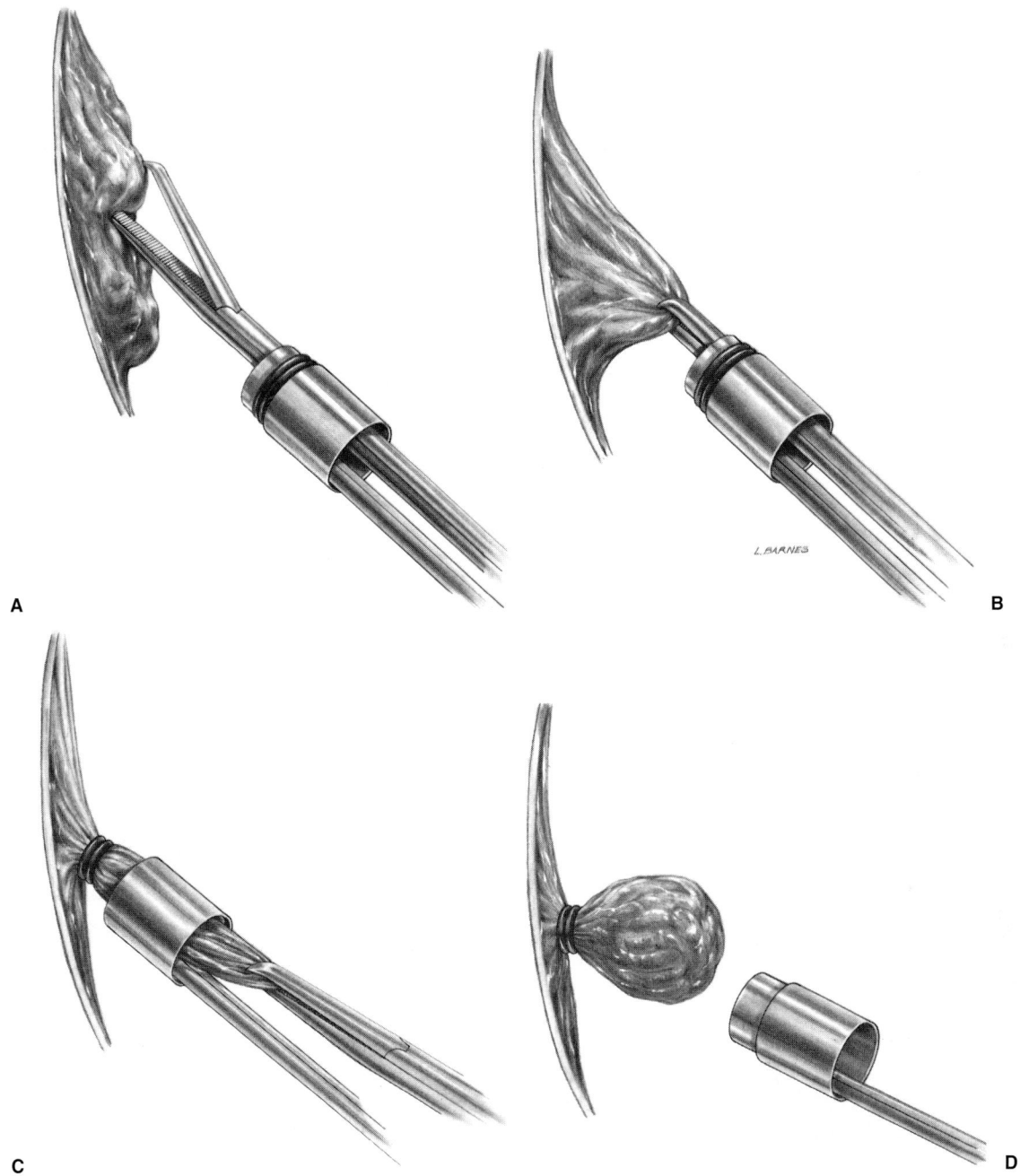

FIGURE 8-16. Rubber ring ligation. **(A,B)** The hemorrhoid is grasped and firmly tethered. **(C)** The tissue is drawn int o the drum. If the patient tolerates the maneuver, ligation can be performed with minimal or no discomfort. **(D)** The two rubber rings are released.

to return 3 months, 6 months, or even years later. Other areas subsequently can be treated equally well despite such delays. However, the patient should realize that if symptoms are not completely relieved, it is probably because other hemorrhoidal areas need to be addressed, assuming of course that there is no other explanation for the bleeding. Conversely, if the individual experiences complete relief after the initial ligation, there is no need to continue therapy. Under these circumstances, the patient is advised to return if and when symptoms recur.

Complications

A moderate sense of discomfort or fullness in the rectum can be anticipated for a few days following the procedure, but complaints are usually minimal and can often be relieved by sitz baths and mild analgesics. Complications are occasionally seen after rubber ring ligation and may include the following:

- Delayed hemorrhage
- Severe pain

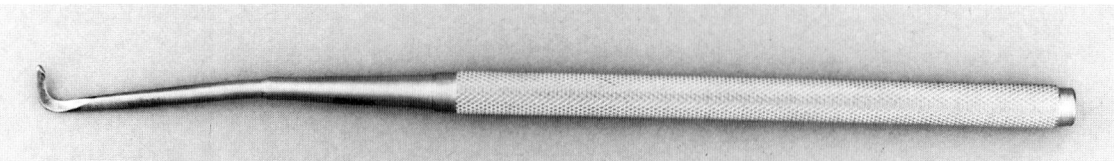

FIGURE 8-17. Rubber band cutter (model 30020). (Courtesy of George P. McGown, M.D.)

- External hemorrhoidal thrombosis
- Ulceration
- Slippage of the ligature
- Fulminant sepsis

Delayed Hemorrhage

Late hemorrhage (i.e., 1 to 2 weeks after treatment) following rubber ring ligation occurs in approximately 1% of patients. As with late hemorrhage after surgical hemorrhoidectomy (see later), this may be attributed to sepsis in the pedicle or to early cutting through of the tissue.

Significant bleeding, as determined by the presence of clots or by the passage of blood without stool, requires urgent assessment, even emergency management. Patients may be evaluated in the emergency department or, if convenient, in the surgeon's office. Anoscopic examination is mandatory. If the patient is unstable, hypotensive, or tachycardic, hospitalization is required. It must be remembered that individuals who have undergone rubber ring ligation can bleed massively. Transfusion may be necessary. Usually a local anesthetic, field block (see later), or general or spinal anesthetic is required. If the bleeding site is identified, suture ligation is performed. If the facilities are unsatisfactory for adequate visualization and suturing, packing the anus with gauze and with a hemostatic agent such as Surgicel, Gelfoam, or Avitene may

be effective on a temporary basis. The use of a Foley catheter with a 30-mL balloon has also been suggested as a useful means for tamponading the bleeding. Often, however, no active bleeding site is appreciated at the time of assessment. Under these circumstances, the use of a hemostatic agent may be reassuring, in addition to hospital admission and observation. It is because of the risk of late hemorrhage that rubber ring ligation is absolutely contraindicated for individuals who are taking anticoagulants. An excisional option, sclerotherapy, infrared coagulation, or one of the other alternatives may be considered, unless the anticoagulant can be discontinued.

Pain

Pain requiring removal of the rings and measures to alleviate discomfort have been mentioned previously. Tchirkow and colleagues recommend injection of a local anesthetic solution into the hemorrhoid bundle.[256] In my experience, however, in most patients who complain of pain, this symptom develops after the anesthetic effect would have dissipated. However, a local anesthetic at the time of treatment may be a valuable adjunct if the patient is particularly apprehensive.

In my opinion, pain is much more likely to be a source of concern if multiple bandings are attempted. Although this statement is not supported by controlled studies, it

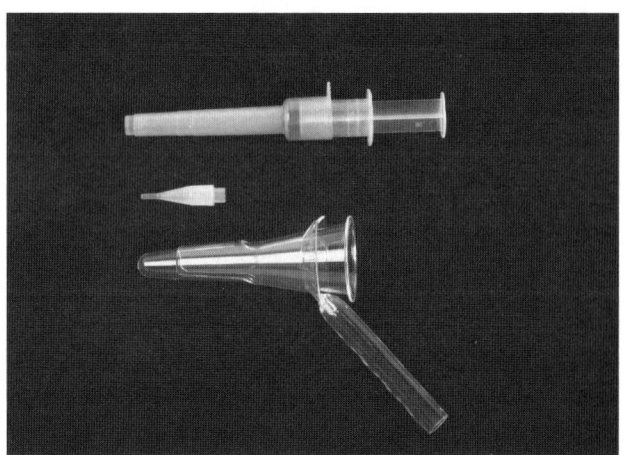

FIGURE 8-18. O'Regan Disposable Banding System. This includes (from **top**): suction-ligating syringe with band pusher; rubber band applicator; and slotted anoscope with obturator. (Courtesy of Medsurge Medical Products Corp., North Vancouver, Canada.)

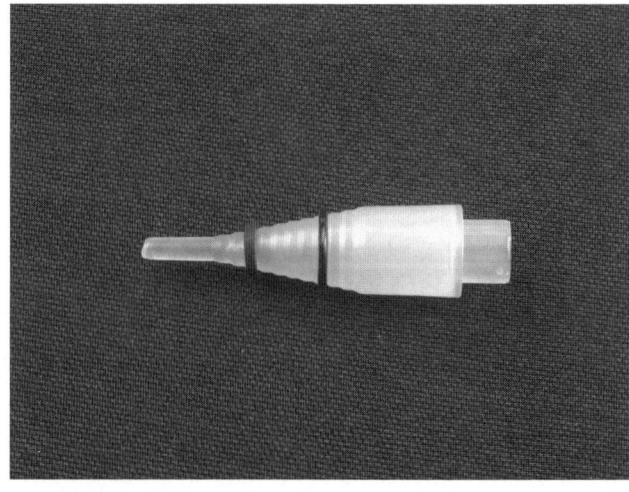

FIGURE 8-19. O'Regan Disposable Banding System. Rubber band applicator with rings. (Courtesy of Medsurge Medical Products Corp., North Vancouver, Canada.)

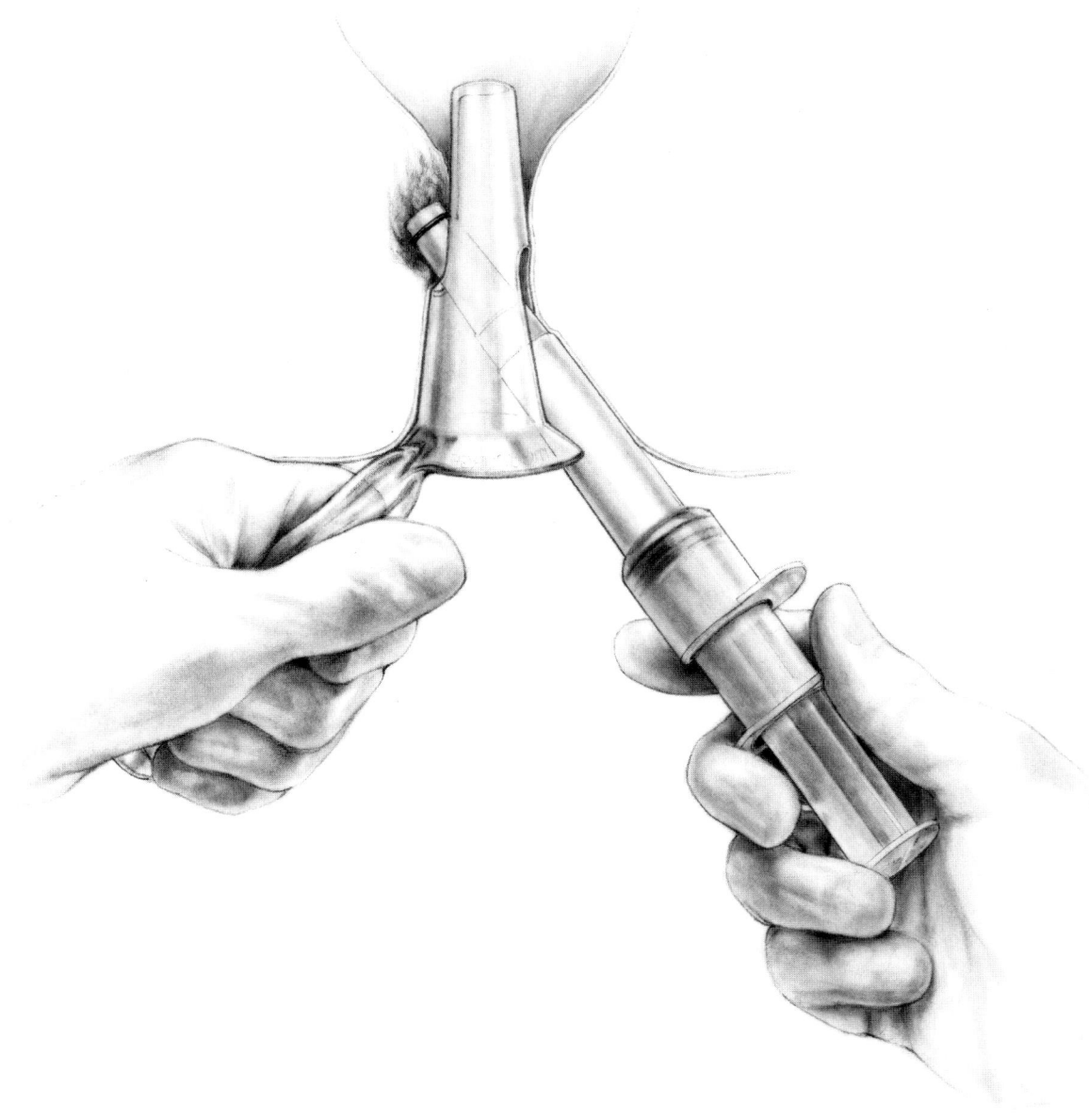

A

FIGURE 8-20. Technique of ligation using the O'Regan Ligating System. Ligator positioned through lateral slot of anoscope **(A)**. plunger withdrawn and locked in first position to effect initial suction. *(continued)*.

seems reasonable to conclude that the simultaneous ligation of three pile sites will inevitably lead to three times the risk of discomfort. Pain that seems to worsen a few days following treatment merits reevaluation of the patient, especially if fever supervenes or if a problem with micturition develops. Anal and perineal sepsis can lead to gangrene and result in death (see Sepsis).

In the usual scenario, however, sitz baths and an over-the-counter or nonnarcotic prescription pain medication should be sufficient to relieve discomfort associated with rubber ring ligation. If the patient returns within a few hours of banding with exquisite pain, attempt at removal of the rubber rings is generally a bloody, unhappy exercise for

both patient and surgeon. It is better to offer a stronger, even a narcotic prescription, rather than to struggle trying to remove the rings. Removal, if advisable, should only be performed, in my opinion, soon after banding (see Technique). With respect to subsequent management, it seems reasonable to conclude that if the patient tolerated the initial ligation poorly, an alternative approach should be considered should additional treatment be required.

Thrombosis

With ligation of internal hemorrhoids, the risk for subsequent thrombosis of corresponding external hemorrhoids is 2% to 3%. If thrombosis occurs, sitz baths

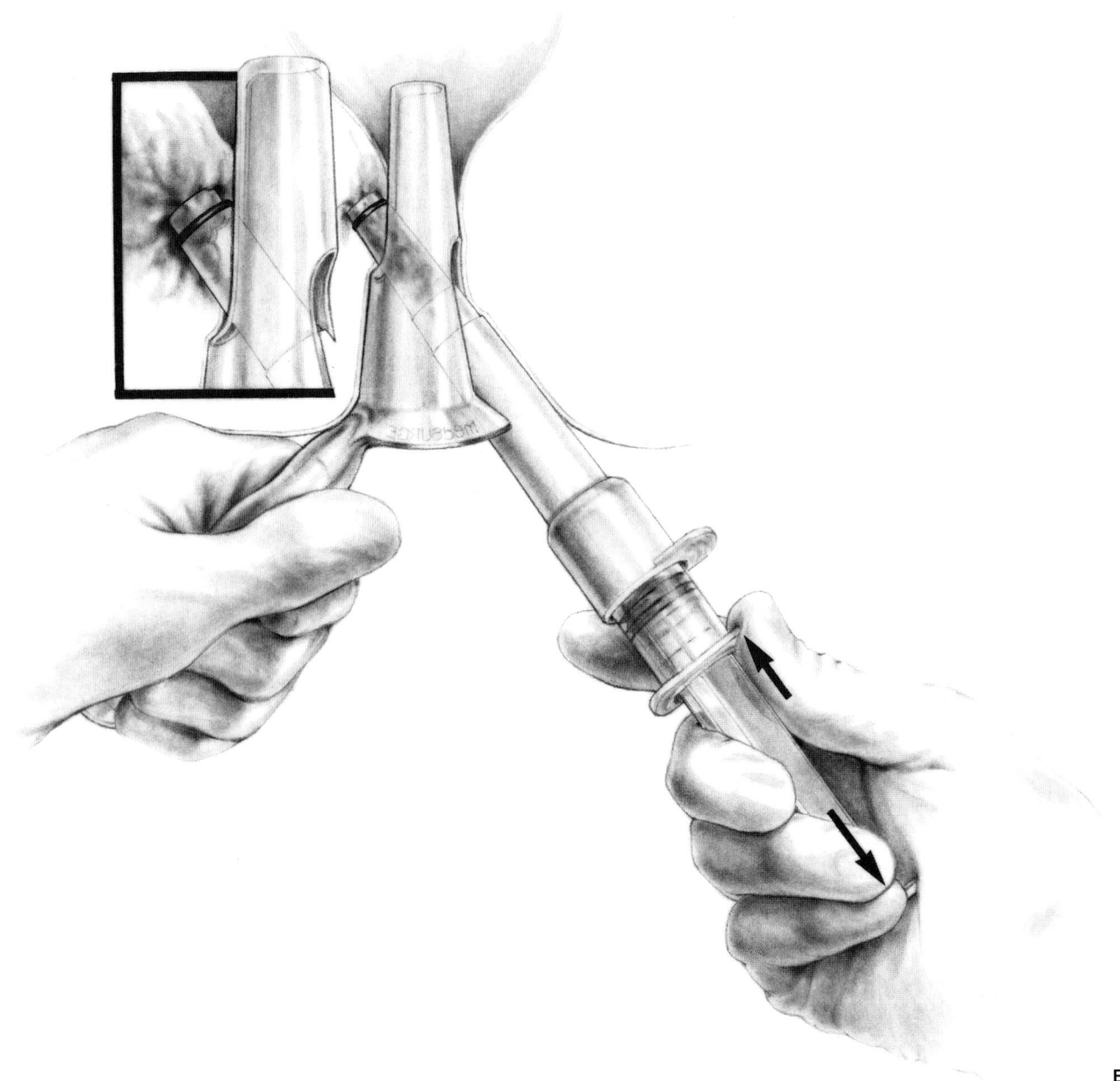

FIGURE 8-20. *(continued)* **(B)**; plunger withdrawn to second position to create maximum suction **(C)**; the pusher is advanced to release rings. The **inset** shows a ligated hemorrhoid pedicle.

and stool softeners are recommended. Occasionally, excision of the thrombosed hemorrhoid is required (see later).

Ulceration

Anal ulceration is a normal consequence of ligation. The rubber rings cause tissue necrosis, and they generally fall off in 2 to 5 days, leaving an ulcerated area. On rare occasions, a large ulcer, sometimes associated with a fissure, may be a troublesome complication. Treatment consists of sitz baths and perhaps a topical cortisone preparation, but if the fissure persists, internal anal sphincterotomy should be considered (see Chapter 9).

Slippage

The rubber rings can slip or break at any time, but this usually happens after the initial bowel movement. Breakage may be caused by a defective rubber ring, hence, the reason I prefer to use two. A more likely explanation is that it is a consequence of tension produced by a large bulk of tissue that has been ligated. The use of a mild laxative, bulking agent, or stool softener can help prevent

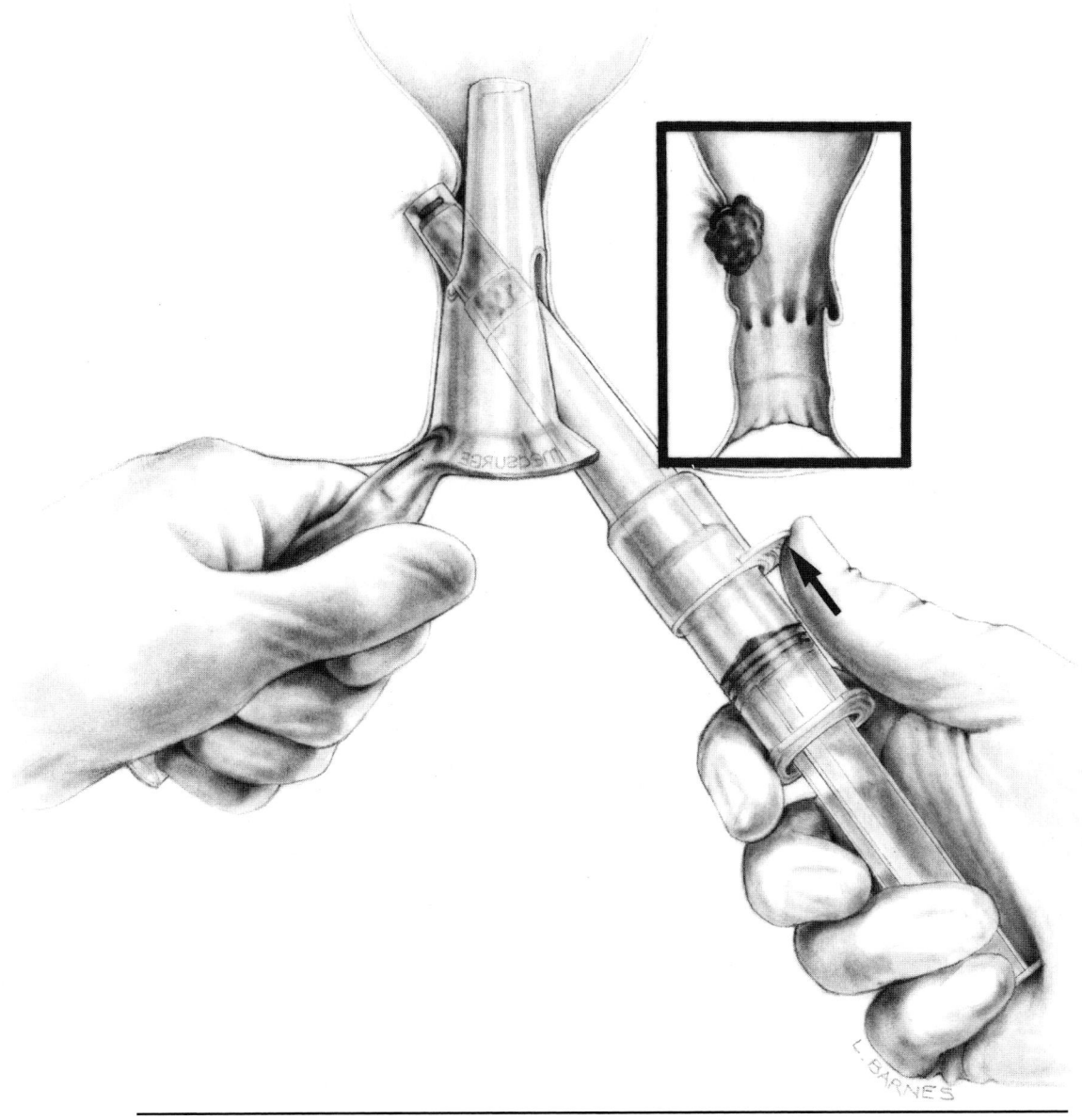

FIGURE 8-20. (*continued*).

the passage of a hard stool and, it is hoped, avoid precipitous dislodgement of the rings. If necessary, a repeat ligation of the same pile site can be reasonably performed 3 to 4 weeks after the initial procedure.

Sepsis

Aside from the normal sloughing that occurs from necrosis of tissue, sepsis following rubber ring ligation had been unknown for more than 20 years since rubber ring ligation had been generally available. A case of tetanus was reported as a possible consequence of treatment in 1978,[176] but the first reported incident of a profound infection was reported by O'Hara in 1980, that of a patient who developed fatal clostridial sepsis following rubber ring ligation.[190] Since the latter observation, others have described the same or a similar complication.[51,210,224,234,245,271] There seems to be a characteristic scenario of events. Young male patients seem to be at the greatest risk. A complaint of increasing anorectal pain, perineal pain, scrotal swelling, or difficulty urinating mandates emergency evaluation. So horrendous is this complication that I specifically inform all young male patients to be aware of the warning signs.

The origin of this potentially devastating complication is unclear, but some have suggested that many of these individuals may actually be in an immunocompromised state. For example, the initial reports of this complication

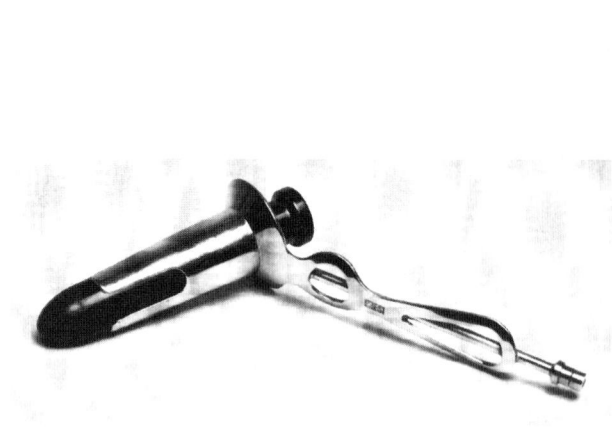

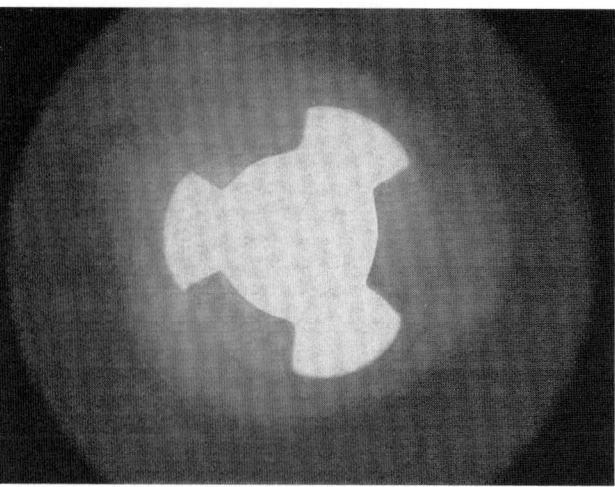

A

B

FIGURE 8-21. Armstrong anoscope for synchronous hemorrhoidal ligation. (Courtesy of David N. Armstrong, M.D.) **(A)** With obturator in place. **(B)** End view without obturator. Note the lateral apertures.

originated from the San Francisco Bay area before the recogniztion of HIV, in a community with a large gay population. However, Moore and Fleshner report that rubber band ligation can be safely performed in select HIV-positive patients.[171] Another possible explanation is that the physician failed to recognize a septic process as the cause of the patient's so-called "hemorrhoid" complaints. Obviously, the physician should vigorously seek alternative causes of anorectal complaints, especially pain, before embarking on rubber ring ligation.[242] Still, there are highly experienced colon and rectal surgeons who have had the rare patient develop this complication and for whom there has been no satisfactory explanation.

Findings on physical examination may include fever, perineal edema, scrotal edema, perineal ulceration, cellulitis, or frank gangrene. Rectal examination usually demonstrates a boggy, edematous anal canal that is exquisitely tender. Computed tomography and magnetic resonance imaging of the pelvis are useful, especially to identify thickening of the rectal wall, gas within the wall of the bowel or within the pelvis, a pelvic fluid collection, or any other extrarectal disorder.[234]

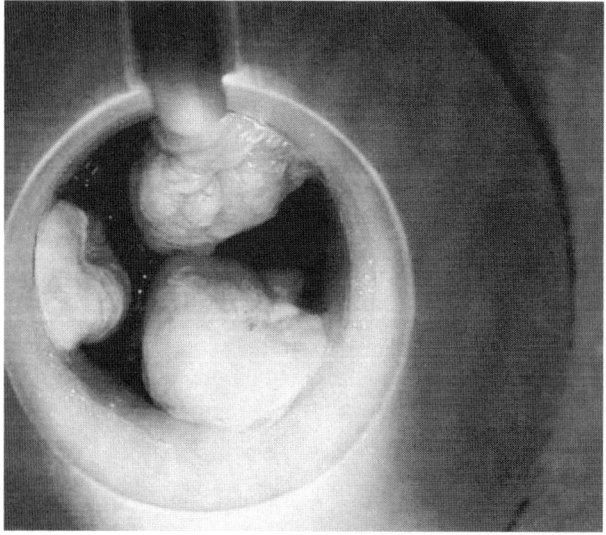

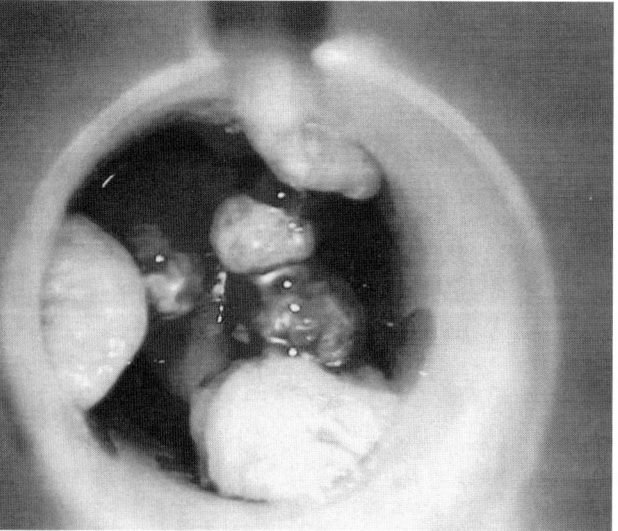

A

B

FIGURE 8-22. Multiple hemorrhoid ligations. Appearance of internal hemorrhoids prior to synchronous ligation **(A)** and following ligations **(B)**. (Courtesy of David N. Armstrong, M.D.)

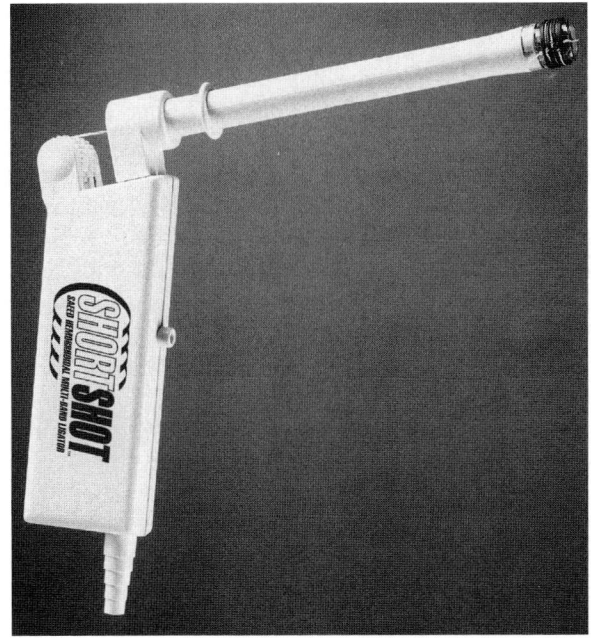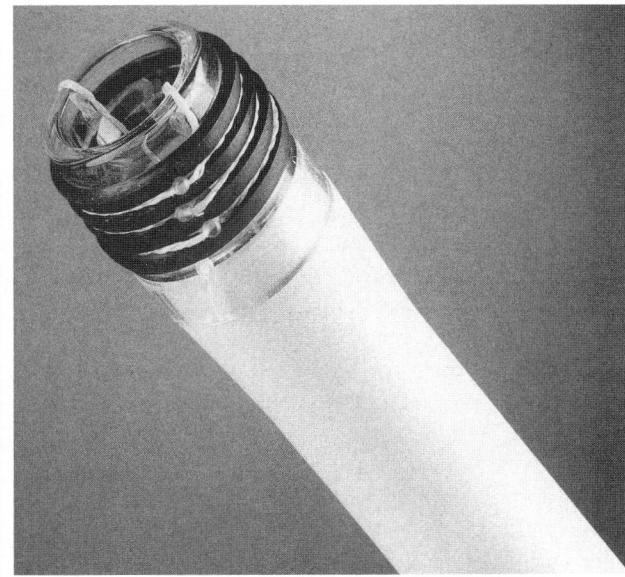

A
B

FIGURE 8-23. ShortShot Saeed Hemorrhoidal Multi-Band Ligator. **(A)** Suction instrument. **(B)** Close-up view of the instrument head shows the four rubber bands in place. (Courtesy of Wilson-Cook Medical GI Endoscopy, Winston-Salem, NC.)

Treatment requires massive antibiotic therapy, vigorous debridement, and possibly hyperbaric oxygen treatment. A colostomy may be necessary. Survival is problematic in the advanced case; those who recovered were inevitably recognized early and treated aggressively. Suggestions for prevention have included using prebanding enemas, prophylactic antibiotics, and even meticulous sterile technique (whatever that may be).[127] I believe that such measures are neither appropriate nor helpful. However, I routinely administer a small-volume Fleet enema before all anorectal procedures, primarily for aesthetic purposes (I simply do not enjoy the presence of stool in the field) and the fact that usually the patient need not be concerned about defecating for the remainder of the day.

Error in Diagnosis

A theoretical disadvantage of rubber ring ligation and all the nonexcisional methods for treating hemorrhoids is that no pathologic specimen is obtained. Invasive epidermoid carcinoma or other tumor occasionally has been reported in an excised hemorrhoid specimen (perhaps in less than 1% of cases). In the rare instance of its occurrence, such a lesion will obviously be missed. However, the physician should not condemn the procedure and limit its application because of an apparently reasonable, albeit truly unwarranted, concern. One must be mindful of the fact that the standard of care no longer requires submission of a pathologic specimen even when a surgical hemorrhoidectomy is performed. Cataldo and Mac-

Keigan reviewed more than 20,000 hemorrhoid operations over a 20-year period.[39] Only one example of an unsuspected carcinoma of the anus was diagnosed solely by microscopic analysis. The authors conclude that selective rather than routine pathologic evaluation of hemorrhoidectomy specimens should be the policy. I concur. As stated previously, however, if there is any doubt or concern about the presence of a lesion or the possibility of an underlying malignancy, biopsy should be performed.

Results

In 1977, Bartizal and Slosberg published a retrospective review of the records of 670 patients who underwent 3,208 rubber ring ligations for internal hemorrhoids.[23] The degree of discomfort after banding and the presence and amount of rectal bleeding were assessed. All were followed for a minimum of 1 month after the completion of banding.

Complications were confined to pain and bleeding. Only 21 patients (4%) had any pain. Mild pain was defined as that which did not require treatment; moderate pain required analgesics, and severe pain caused limitation of activities. No bleeding at all was reported by 642 (96%). Bleeding to a slight degree was noted by 19 (3%) but required no specific treatment. Bleeding to a significant degree occurred in nine patients (1%). Most were treated successfully with bed rest, but two required hospitalization. When those patients who had moderate and severe pain were combined with those who had severe bleeding, only 13 (2% of all patients treated) had complications severe enough to interfere with daily activity.

Bat and co-workers performed a prospective study involving in excess of 500 patients who underwent rubber band ligation.[25] The hospitalization rate was 2.5%, with approximately half of these admissions based on delayed massive rectal bleeding. There was no incident of overwhelming sepsis. An additional 4.6% suffered minor complications, including thrombosed hemorrhoids, mild bleeding, and urinary retention.

Steinberg and colleagues, by means of a questionnaire answered by 125 of 147 patients, conducted a long-term assessment (mean, 4.8 years) of the value of rubber ring ligation as a treatment for hemorrhoids.[250] Most (89%) considered themselves cured or greatly improved; however, only 44% were completely free of symptoms. Intermittent mild discomfort, occasional spotting of blood, and an awareness of lumps at the anus were the principal residual symptoms. Nevertheless, many were reportedly happier with this condition than with their state before treatment. Patients who suffered persistent or severe recurrent symptoms after rubber ring ligation were treated by further conservative measures. Fifteen patients (12%) had another rubber ring ligation, anal dilatation, or lateral sphincterotomy.

My colleagues and I reported our long-term results with rubber ring ligation (mean, 60 months).[286] Of 352 patients who were sent a questionnaire, 266 (76%) responded. Although many continued to have some symptoms, the condition of 80% of the respondents was improved by the procedure. The best results were obtained in patients who had grade I hemorrhoids. Patients with grade IV hemorrhoids were less likely to have had a good result ($p < .02$). The effectiveness of treatment did not depend on the number of hemorrhoids ligated. Those who had a single pile site treated were as likely to have had a good result as those in whom two or more bands were applied. Perhaps the most meaningful conclusion of our study is that a single treatment can achieve satisfactory results.[286] If more than three sessions are required to control symptoms, the procedure should probably be abandoned and hemorrhoidectomy performed.

The Cleveland Clinic group reported that 77% of their patients were asymptomatic following treatment.[89] Their technique differed in that approximately 90% of patients were treated by multiple ligations in a single session. Although the long-term results indicated fewer symptoms, pain after treatment was more frequently observed and was more severe.

Lau and colleagues performed rubber ring ligation on all three primary hemorrhoids at each single outpatient session.[143] Good to excellent results were noted in 91%, but moderate to severe pain was reported by 58 patients (29%). Although the authors strongly endorsed this approach, their rate of complications (i.e., hemor-

rhage, urinary retention, anal stenosis) was 3.5%. Khubchandani conducted a controlled study of single, double, and triple bandings.[132] There was no significant difference in the incidence of complaints of bleeding or pain following any of these three approaches; however, some patients had to have the rubber bands removed because of discomfort. Poon and colleagues compared single versus multiple ligations in a prospective, randomized trial.[208] Both methods were effective, and the incidence of complications and complaints was similar. The authors recommend multiple ligations—the patients are less inconvenienced, and they anticipated there should be some cost savings. The Mayo Clinic experience also reflects an acceptably low rate of complications.[144]

Other studies have demonstrated that rubber ring ligation is far superior to sclerosing agents.[87,242] Better long-term results, significantly more effective management of symptoms of protrusion, and greater likelihood of control of bleeding symptoms can be anticipated with this method of treatment. Chew and colleagues, however, recommend combining sclerotherapy with rubber band ligation.[43]

In order to compare this modality with surgical hemorrhoidectomy, Murie and colleagues randomly allocated 80 patients to ligation or to surgery.[175] Follow-up results at varying intervals for up to 3 years revealed no significant difference in the frequency of amelioration of symptoms, although it was not clear to me whether patients with more severe hemorrhoidal manifestations were excluded.

Comment

Rubber ring ligation is an excellent alternative to surgical hemorrhoidectomy for most patients. However, one must understand that the results may not equal those that can be achieved by surgery. Nevertheless, because of the limited morbidity, adequate long-term effectiveness, convenience, and patient acceptability, I recommend this procedure as the primary outpatient therapy for bleeding and for reducible hemorrhoid prolapse. However, in the presence of an external component, hypertrophied anal papilla, associated fissure, or large (grade IV) hemorrhoids, surgical treatment is unquestionably more effective.

Cryosurgery

Cryosurgery is based on the concept of cellular destruction through rapid freezing followed by rapid thawing. The treatment of hemorrhoids by this technique had been advocated by Lewis and colleagues and by others as painless, effective, and especially recommended for those patients who are medically unable to undergo general anesthesia.[52,92,150,275,277] The principle of cryosurgery is well described in these cited articles.

Technique

The following protocol has been recommended by most authors:

■ The procedure is explained, and the patient is advised of the probability of profuse drainage and considerable swelling. If necessary, an intravenous injection of a sedative is administered, and a local anesthetic is usually recommended.

■ The patient is placed in either the left lateral or prone jackknife position. The surgeon's fingers, a plastic vaginal speculum, or a modified plastic proctoscope are used to isolate one primary hemorrhoidal plexus at a time. A metal instrument is not employed because it would conduct cold, and a water-soluble jelly is used to achieve good contact between the cryoprobe and the hemorrhoid.

■ The cryoprobe is applied. The tissue freezes around the tip. Thus, the distance between the tip and the outer border of the ice ball equals the depth of the ice ball. This allows the surgeon to determine visually how much tissue is being destroyed. Only that tissue encompassed within the ice ball allegedly will undergo irreversible cellular destruction. Changes at the boundary between the ice ball and normal tissue are reversible, and theoretically, no true cellular destruction occurs.

Theoretically, both internal and external hemorrhoids can be treated in one operation. The tip of the cryoprobe is placed in the center of either the internal or external hemorrhoidal plexus and remains there until the tissue to be destroyed is enveloped by the ice ball (Figure 8-24). The period of freezing varies according to the cooling power of the probe. With a liquid nitrogen probe at −196°C or a liquid nitrous oxide probe at −89°C, the application time is about 2 minutes per hemorrhoid area. The greater the vascularity of the hemorrhoid, the greater is the cooling power required to freeze it. Therefore, the liquid nitrogen probe is more effective for large hemorrhoids than is the nitrous oxide probe. When an adequate amount of tissue has been frozen, the probe is switched off, rewarmed, and detached from the hemorrhoid; each plexus in turn is treated the same way.

Care After Treatment

Considerable swelling and edema occur within 24 hours of the procedure, but generally these effects do not interfere with normal bowel function and elimination. Drainage usually starts several hours later; it is fairly

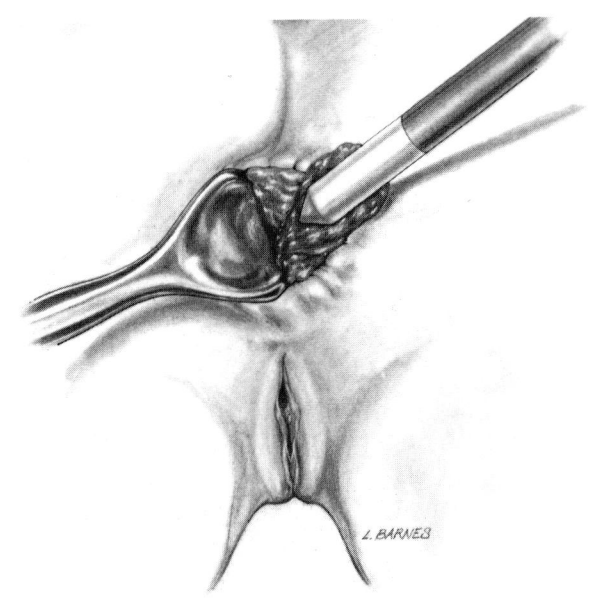

FIGURE 8-24. Cryosurgical destruction. The cryoprobe is applied to a combined internal-external hemorrhoid.

heavy for the first 3 to 4 days but decreases during the following 2 to 3 weeks. Patients are instructed to use some form of sterile pad and to change the pad several times a day during the first 3 to 4 days.

Two to 3 hours after freezing, the tissue becomes swollen and erythematous. Within 72 hours, pale spots appear on the surface, and these coalesce to form irregular patches by the fourth day. By the fifth or sixth day, the whole hemorrhoidal area is pale; black, gangrenous areas may then appear. Necrosis is usually complete between postoperative days 7 and 9. Thereafter, the hemorrhoid begins to disintegrate and should come away completely by the eighteenth postoperative day, leaving, it is hoped, a normal-appearing anus.

Results

Wilson and Schofield reported 100 consecutive cases of hemorrhoids treated by cryosurgery.[278] All were managed on an ambulatory basis, usually without an anesthetic. A nitrous oxide cryoprobe was used. Watery discharge has been said to occur in all patients, but in this study many did not notice a discharge at all, and only one complained that the discharge was a nuisance. Four patients experienced immediate pain during the freezing process; three required a general anesthetic. An additional six patients underwent elective general anesthesia. Only one complained of pain during the first 5 days after treatment, and many returned to work the following day. No major hemorrhages were encountered, although the watery discharge was sanguineous in some. The patients were assessed at 6 weeks and 3 months, with satisfactory results obtained in 94%.

Savin reported 444 operations performed with a nitrous oxide probe.[233] Excellent results were obtained, according to the author, in that all hemorrhoidal tissue and symptoms were eliminated in 431 of 434 patients. Ten patients were lost to follow-up study, and three patients had some residual hemorrhoidal tissue. Additionally, cryosurgery was successful in removing 97% of the concomitant pathologic conditions treated, such as anal fissure, anal fistula, hypertrophied anal papilla, condyloma acuminatum, and mucosal prolapse. Of 155 patients evaluated 1 to 2 years after operation, 151 were graded as having excellent results; three had small, asymptomatic internal hemorrhoids; one had an external hemorrhoid; three were found to have hypertrophied anal papillae not present before; and two patients still had persistent hypertrophied anal papillae.

O'Connor reported results of nitrous oxide cryohemorrhoidectomy in 117 patients.[184] Skin tags larger than those the patients had before the procedure were found in four; five had persistence of internal hemorrhoids. Three of the five complained of bleeding with bowel movements and were subsequently treated by ligation. The major complications after cryosurgery were pain, bleeding, and fecal impaction. Six patients complained of pain lasting longer than 2 days, two of them experiencing discomfort for as long as 14 days. Bleeding necessitating hospitalization occurred in three patients, and fecal impaction also developed in three individuals. No urinary retention, ulceration, stenosis, or incontinence was reported. The average time lost from work was 2 days, with a range of none to 14 days. O'Connor concluded that internal hemorrhoids were easily treated by cryosurgery, and that thrombosed and edematous hemorrhoids should be managed by methods other than cryosurgery. He further advised that thick skin tags and large prolapsing hemorrhoids should be treated by excisional surgery. It would appear from the author's subsequent report, however, that he had abandoned this method for the indications outlined in favor of infrared coagulation (see Infrared Coagulation).

Oh initially reviewed 100 patients who had undergone cryohemorrhoidectomy, and he subsequently reported on 1,000 of these individuals.[187,188] In his initial report, two thirds experienced pain, two suffered massive hemorrhage, and five encountered urinary difficulties. Effectiveness of cryotherapy was 90%, similar to that for rubber ring ligation, but the discomfort, prolonged drainage, and prolonged recovery were believed to be distinct disadvantages when cryohemorrhoidectomy was compared with ligation. MacLeod, in his report on 528 patients treated by cryotherapy, recommended that this modality be used only on internal hemorrhoids and that the treatments be staged.[156]

Traynor and Carter reported a prospective study on the treatment of second- and third-degree hemorrhoids by cryotherapy.[260] Approximately half of the 125 patients analyzed were hospitalized for less than 24 hours. Profuse serous discharge was reported by two thirds; more than 90% returned to work within 3 weeks. The principal long-term disadvantage appeared to be the failure to eliminate skin tags.

Smith and colleagues reported a study in which closed hemorrhoidectomy and cryotherapy were performed on 26 patients.[247] One side of the anus was designated at random for surgery and the other for cryotherapy. Although pain was initially less after cryosurgery (only one patient noted severe pain on the cryotherapy side), 12 had pain for more than 2 weeks on the cryotherapy side, compared with only three patients who experienced pain after 2 weeks on the surgical side. Interestingly, patients could determine which side had been surgically treated and which side had been "frozen." Of 24 patients examined 1 year after treatment, 13 had residual hemorrhoids, 12 of which were at the cryosurgical site. Six of these 13 patients requested further treatment. When patient opinion was ascertained, 65% said they preferred operative hemorrhoidectomy and 35% said they preferred cryosurgery.

Comment

When cryosurgical hemorrhoidectomy was first introduced, it was claimed to be painless, anesthetic-free, and effective for external tags and hypertrophied papillae. Since that time, reports have confirmed that it is not painless—local or general anesthetic has been suggested by almost all observers—and that it is less effective, and in many ways ineffective, for the treatment of hypertrophied anal papillae and skin tags. For internal hemorrhoids, rubber ring ligation is superior to cryosurgery. It is quicker and cheaper and requires no anesthetic. For the external component or hypertrophied papilla, excision after local infiltration rapidly removes the offending tissue. Complete healing takes place in 7 to 10 days. Cryosurgical destruction requires the use of relatively expensive equipment and is time-consuming to perform—some authors recommend hospitalization or an outpatient setting. In addition, it results in profuse drainage and sometimes delayed healing. True, the initial postanesthetic pain may be somewhat less than with surgical hemorrhoidectomy, but this pain usually can be controlled with a mild analgesic (see later).

In my opinion, cryosurgery adds nothing to the treatment of hemorrhoids that is not available by other means at lower cost, at greater efficiency, with fewer complications, and with as good if not better results. Others must agree, because I have not been able to identify more re-

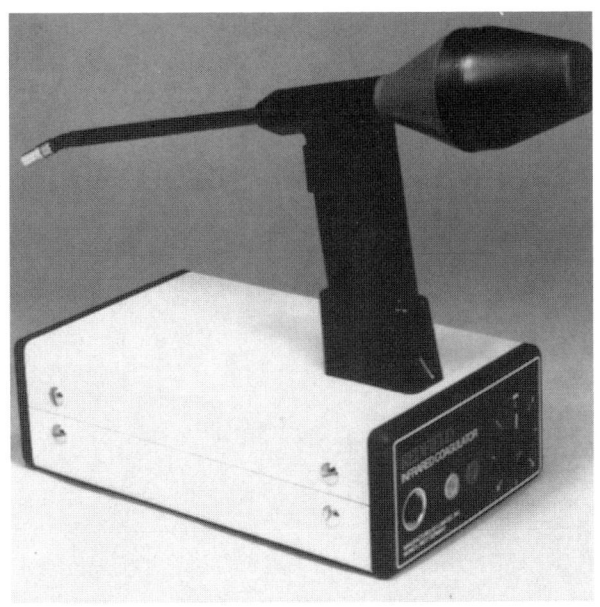

FIGURE 8-25. Infrared coagulator: power supply unit and applicator. (Courtesy of Redfield Corporation, Montvale, NJ.)

cent references in peer-reviewed publications with this technique since the second edition of this text (1989).

Infrared Coagulation

In 1979, Neiger described a method for the treatment of hemorrhoids using infrared coagulation.[177] Leicester and associates reported a prospective, randomized trial using this technique and found that it compared favorably with injection sclerotherapy and rubber ring ligation, except perhaps for the management of prolapse.[147,148]

The apparatus produces infrared radiation and is focused by a photoconductor (Figure 8-25). It was developed as an offshoot of laser technology, but it is not a laser (see Laser Surgery). Infrared light penetrates the tissue to a predetermined level at the speed of light and is converted to heat.[185] The amount of tissue destruction can be regulated by direct visualization and by adjusting the pulse setting on the instrument.

Technique

The procedure is relatively simple and easy to learn. A sterile, disposable sheath is placed over the lightguide. An anoscope is inserted, and the lightguide is placed in direct contact with the mucosa at the base of the hemorrhoid. A 1- or 1.5-second pulse is usually used in the treatment of hemorrhoids, with the probe applied at the same site where the physician would normally inject. The radiation causes protein coagulation 3 mm wide and 3 mm deep. The manufacturer recommends the applica-

tion of three to five pulses.[193] Following coagulation, the tissue appears as a whitish, circular eschar. Over the following week, a dark eschar forms, ultimately leaving a slightly puckered, pink to red scar.[185] The physician may elect to treat one area at a time or ablate all evident hemorrhoids. Additional treatments may be repeated every 2 or 3 weeks if necessary. Although some authors can perform the procedure without a local anesthetic, particularly if the coagulator is applied above the pectinate line, infiltrating the area with 0.5% bupivacaine (Marcaine) is often recommended. Of course, if an external tag is to be treated, a local anesthetic is required.

Results

Infrared coagulation of hemorrhoids has an excellent record of safety with minor bleeding and some discomfort occasionally observed. There have been no reported incidents of sepsis or stricture. Ambrose and colleagues compared photocoagulation and rubber ring ligation in the treatment of hemorrhoids by means of a randomized controlled study of 268 patients.[4] There was no difference in the symptomatic outcome between these two groups up to 1 year following the procedure. A higher incidence of bleeding and pain was noted following banding that was statistically significant, but additional outpatient procedures were more frequently encountered with photocoagulation. Another study from the same surgical unit compared photocoagulation with injection sclerotherapy.[5] The results were considered comparable, although the injection group required fewer additional treatments. Weinstein and colleagues noted a different result in their prospective, randomized trial of rubber ring ligation and infrared coagulation.[273] A significantly better result at 1 month and at 6 months was achieved by the former method. There was no difference with respect to pain, although banding was associated with two complications: thrombosed hemorrhoids and delayed bleeding. In the manufacturer's rebuttal to this article, Osur noted that the infrared coagulator was not designed to achieve optimal results in a single treatment session.[193] In their survey, only 3.7% of users employed just one session.

Comparison studies of the use of infrared coagulation and of bipolar diathermy (BICAP; see Bipolar Diathermy) revealed no significant difference in rate of complications and number of treatments required.[69] In a three-armed report involving the infrared technique, the heater probe, and the Ultroid device (Microvasive, Watertown, MA; see later), it was concluded that all three methods are effective modalities for first- and second-degree hemorrhoids, but that the Ultroid was associated with less discomfort and fewer complications.[289] Furthermore, the authors believed that this last method may be more applicable for larger piles.

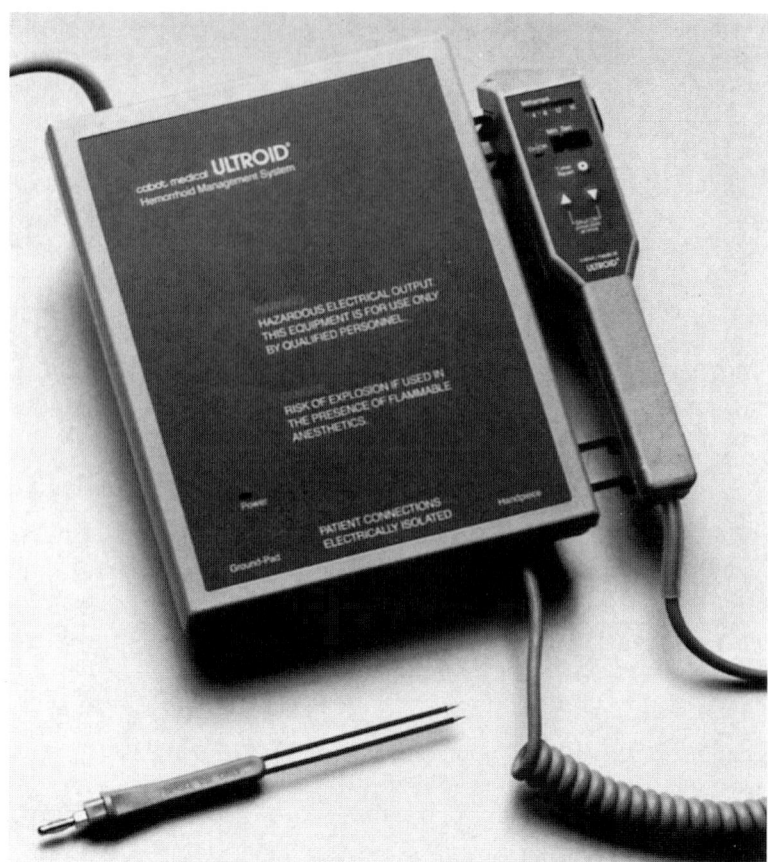

FIGURE 8-26. This Ultroid device with a generator source and handle uses disposable probes. (Courtesy of Microvasive, Watertown, MA.)

Comment

I believe that infrared coagulation has rung the death knell for cryosurgery; the most outspoken enthusiasts for cryosurgery seem now to prefer photocoagulation. It is as if the option of freezing hemorrhoids is no longer available, if the apparent void in journal articles is any indication. However, the equipment is expensive, and rubber rings are not. Moreover, even the manufacturer concurs that the technique is not recommended for the management of prolapsing hemorrhoids.

My own approach is to use infrared coagulation as the preferred alternative to injection therapy. Symptomatic hemorrhoids that are too small to band are optimally treated by this technique. I also occasionally offer it to patients for treatment of the external component (with a local anesthetic) when I do not wish to employ excisional therapy.

Ultroid

The Ultroid device is another tool for the ambulatory treatment of hemorrhoids. It is a monopolar, low-voltage instrument that includes a generator unit, an attachable handle, single-use sterile probes, a grounding pad, and a nonconductive anoscope (Figure 8-26). Some have commented that it is confusing to have two electrodes, yet the instrument is not bipolar.[68] The company contends that the mode of action of this device is not thermal but rather is a consequence of the production of sodium hydroxide at the negative electrode. It strains credulity that this is the mechanism, but as I am not a biophysicist, I can merely offer healthy skepticism.

Technique

By means of the nonconductive anoscope, the probe tip is placed at the apex of the hemorrhoid, above the dentate line. The amperage is slowly increased to the level of patient tolerance as the probe is inserted into the hemorrhoid. The usual treatment range is 6 to 16 mA. The probe is left in position for approximately 10 minutes, or until the "popping" sounds cease. Once the treatment has been completed, the current is gradually decreased to zero. Failure to do this will result in pain on removal of the probe. One site is usually treated per session, usually because of time constraints and the fact that the patient does not usually appreciate a prolonged anoscopy.

Results

Norman and colleagues reported the application of this technique in 120 patients.[182] Ablation of the hemorrhoids was directly correlated with the amount of current employed and the duration of the treatment. The procedure was completely successful, according to the authors in every patient (i.e., all became asymptomatic), and there were no complications. Most hemorrhoid disease (78%) was successfully treated with one application of direct current. The group included 46 individuals with grade III hemorrhoids and 37 with grade IV, a most remarkable accomplishment indeed.

Dennison and colleagues comment that they achieved results comparable with those of other techniques in their 25 patients, but the time required for treatment was a particular disadvantage.[68] In addition, the operator is required to hold the probe quite still for a period of time.[67] Zinberg and colleagues noted good results in 85% of those with grade III hemorrhoids, but none of four persons with grade IV disease could be classified as having good results.[289] As previously stated, Zinberg and colleagues affirmed that Ultroid therapy was associated with less discomfort and fewer complications than either infrared coagulation or heater probe coagulation therapy. Hinton and Morris observed that the technique was effective in 26 patients, including those with large, prolapsing piles.[110] Wright and co-workers reported a prospective study from the Division of Gastroenterology at the University of Louisville, Kentucky, comparing direct current electrotherapy with standard medical therapy for symptomatic hemorrhoidal disease.[285] Those who did not respond to initial treatment were crossed over at 8 weeks, receiving alternate therapy twice. The authors concluded that no difference could be found between the standard medical therapy and that of direct current electrotherapy. The obvious extension of this conclusion is that because direct current electrotherapy is no better than standard medical treatment, it cannot be recommended for the management of symptomatic hemorrhoid disease.[285]

Comment

There is a paucity of articles in the surgical literature on the Ultroid device, perhaps because the device is also marketed to family practitioners and gastroenterologists. Personally, I am skeptical that this approach will be high on the list of options for surgeons in the ambulatory management of hemorrhoids. Most surgeons have neither the time nor the patience to stand around holding the probe for more than 10 minutes. Given the choice, it is unlikely that patients themselves will elect to have a "poker" in their anus for any more time than is necessary to get the job done.

Bipolar Diathermy

Like photocoagulation, BICAP is a method of treating hemorrhoids that is designed to produce tissue destruction, ulceration, and fibrosis by the local application of heat.[68]

The diathermy system was originally developed for the treatment of bleeding peptic ulcers and was later employed to palliate esophageal and rectal carcinomas.[67] The disposable Circon ACMI BICAP hemorrhoid probe uses bipolar RF current to coagulate the blood vessels (Figure 8-27). The principle of action is the passage of current through tissue as it travels between adjacent electrodes located at the tip of the probe. The espoused, perhaps theoretical, advantage of this technique over other methods such as monopolar coagulation, laser coagulation, or photocoagulation is that the BICAP device maintains a short current path, thereby producing a limited depth of penetration even after multiple applications.

Technique

With the use of a disposable, nonconductive anoscope, the side of the probe tip is applied directly and firmly to the hemorrhoid above the dentate line.[67] The generator is used on the infinity setting and is activated by a foot switch. A white coagulum approximately 3 mm deep is produced. All hemorrhoids are treated in one session, and no local anesthetic is usually required.

Results

Numerous controlled trials have been published comparing BICAP with other ambulatory methods in the management of hemorrhoids. Hinton and Morris randomly allocated patients with third-degree hemorrhoids to either this technique or to the Ultroid.[110] Both were believed to be effective, essentially equally so. There were no particular complications in either group, but the time advantage, and therefore better patient acceptability, was enjoyed by BICAP. Dennison and colleagues compared BICAP with infrared photocoagulation.[69] The authors opined that BICAP permits multiple applications to the same site without producing excessive tissue penetration, whereas infrared photocoagulation produces further penetration under these circumstances. Overheating and breakdown were problems more frequently encountered with the infrared coagulator. Griffith and colleagues randomized 110 patients to receive either BICAP or rubber ring ligation.[101] There were no substantive differences in the results when the two methods were compared.

Randall and co-workers compared direct current (Ultroid) and bipolar electrocoagulation (BICAP).[214] There were no statistically significant differences with respect to the two modalities, but because of the speed of the latter technique, the authors recommended it. Yang and others concurred with the issue of pain in their randomly assigned study with direct current versus bipolar electrocoagulation.[287] In addition, however, there was a statistically significantly increased incidence of pain with the Ultroid device.

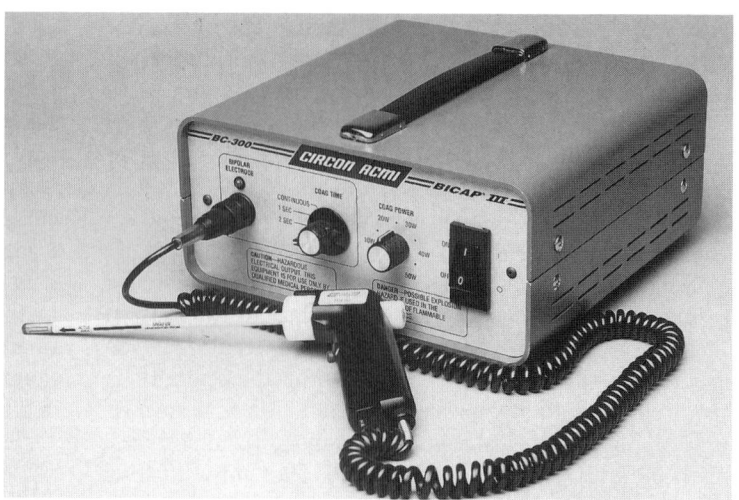

FIGURE 8-27. Bipolar diathermy (BICAP) hemorrhoid probe and generator. (Courtesy of Circon ACMI, Santa Barbara, CA.)

Ultrasonic Doppler-Guided Transanal Hemorrhoidal Ligation (Dearterialization)

In 1995, Morinaga and colleagues suggested another method of treatment of hemorrhoids by means of identification of the hemorrhoidal arteries through the use of a Doppler transducer.[173] A modified proctoscope with built-in ultrasound transducer, light, and special window Echo sounder (KM-25, VaiDan Medical Corporation, St. Petersburg, FL) is inserted and rotated to locate the artery to be ligated. The arterial sound is clearly audible when the Doppler transducer is directly over the hemorrhoidal artery. The vessel is then suture ligated.

Results

In 2001, Sohn and co-workers reported their experience with the technique in 60 patients.[248] Eight percent experienced sufficient pain to lose 2 or more days from work. Residual prolapse developed in 7%, and 3% required subsequent hemorrhoidectomy. They concluded that the procedure is an effective alternative to hemorrhoidectomy.

Opinion

The primary advantage of this technique is that there is no cutting; hence, there is less discomfort. Historically, however, the concept of hemorrhoid ligation without excision was associated with a high rate of persistent symptoms, and, as a consequence, the procedure fell into disrepute. However, perhaps the ability to clearly identify and ligate the arteries will permit long-term benefit. Longer follow-up is required before one can adequately assess the merits of this new approach.

Lord's Dilatation

In addition to the nonexcisional methods of treatment for hemorrhoids that have been discussed, another procedure, that of anal dilatation, should be included in this category. In 1968, Lord reported a method he had devised for the treatment of hemorrhoids.[153] He based his approach on the hypothesis that increased anal canal pressure contributes to the hemorrhoid problem, and that dilatation reduces this pressure, thereby ameliorating the condition. Although this method requires a general or spinal anesthetic, hospitalization can often be limited to a 1-day stay, or the patient can be discharged from an ambulatory care facility or similar surgical center.

Technique

Lord stated, "The procedure takes a little less time to perform than to describe."[154] The instruments are not sterile. The patient is placed on the left side and given an intravenous anesthetic. A constriction to the outlet, which Lord believes is present in all patients with third-degree hemorrhoids, is identified.

Two fingers of one hand are pulled upward, and the index finger of the other hand presses downward to feel the constriction. The aim is to dilate the lower part of the rectum and anal canal gently and firmly until no constrictions remain. It is an "ironing out" process that is carried out by a circular movement through all four quadrants. Tearing should be avoided. During the procedure, eight fingers are inserted as high as they will reach, actually dilating not only the anal canal, but also the rectal ampulla. Not all patients can be dilated safely to this extent, and Lord cautions that it is much better to do too little than too much.

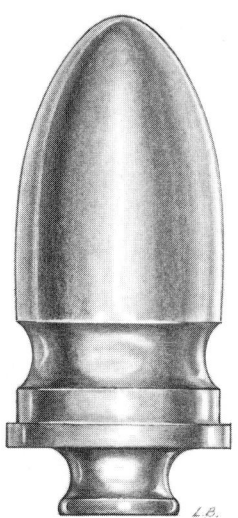

FIGURE 8-28. Lord's dilator.

As dilatation is achieved, an assistant inserts a sponge, usually by means of ring forceps. The sponge presses on the walls of the lower part of the rectum and anal canal and is apparently used to reduce the risk for postoperative hematoma formation. The sponge is left in place for 1 hour, and the patient is discharged when alert.

Postoperative Care

The patient is instructed on the insertion of a dilating cone (Figure 8-28), which can be used as required for anal symptoms, but even Lord wondered whether it is vital to the success of the method. Vellacott and Hardcastle randomly allocated one group of patients to a bulk laxative and the other to a dilator.[265] Because there was no difference in results, they concluded that an anal dilator was not necessary. However, Greca and colleagues reported the opposite to be true.[100] The patient is advised to take 2 or 3 days off from work and be seen after 2 weeks. If free of symptoms at that time, the patient is discharged.

Results

Lord claimed that less pain and postoperative morbidity occur after dilatation than after hemorrhoidectomy. He states that his method does not cause urinary retention, deep vein thrombosis, postoperative bleeding, or fecal impaction. The patients are free of pain during defecation, operating room time is saved, and the hospital stay is greatly shortened. Still, in Lord's opinion, rubber ring ligation is the treatment of choice for most hemorrhoid problems, and dilatation should be used as an alternative to surgical hemorrhoidectomy. However, he suggests that hemorrhoidectomy should be considered when hypertrophied papillae and external tags are present.

Creve and Hubens noted the effect of the procedure on anal pressure.[61] They found a significant lowering of pressure following dilatation compared with that occurring after conventional hemorrhoidectomy. Keighley and colleagues, in a prospective trial, compared dilatation, sphincterotomy, and a high-fiber diet in patients classified into two groups: those with low maximal resting anal pressure and those with elevated maximal resting anal pressure.[128] They concluded that Lord's procedure significantly lowered resting anal pressure, but it should be the treatment of choice in those patients with a preoperative elevation in pressure.

A 5-year follow-up study of 100 patients who underwent Lord's dilatation for hemorrhoids was reported by Walls and Ruckley.[267] Hemorrhoids were first-degree lesions in 15 patients, second-degree in 48, and third-degree in 37. Seventy-five patients were free of symptoms or greatly improved following dilatation, but the treatment was unsuccessful in 22. All except one of these patients reported failure within 3 months, and 19 were subsequently treated by hemorrhoidectomy.

A prospective study was carried out by McCaffrey on 50 patients with hemorrhoids treated by the Lord method and followed for at least 4 years.[161] Of 36 individuals who were free of symptoms, 19 still had evidence of anal congestion but no distinct hemorrhoids, and four subsequently underwent a standard hemorrhoid operation for persistent prolapse and bleeding.

Jones compared three different methods of treatment (i.e., surgical hemorrhoidectomy, rubber ring ligation, and maximal anal dilatation) used successively, with 100 patients in each group.[123] Follow-up was obtained at 4 weeks and at 6 months. The author believed that a reasonable effort should be made to avoid excisional surgery except when one of the other methods fails to relieve symptoms. Older patients who underwent anal dilatation occasionally reported control problems, so Jones recommends that Lord's procedure be limited to those younger than 55 years of age. Twenty (40%) of McCaffrey's patients had mild incontinence from 4 to 26 days after operation.[161] The problem was primarily limited to flatus and mucus, with minimal impairment of control of feces.

Lewis and colleagues randomly allocated 112 patients with prolapsing hemorrhoids to maximal anal dilatation, rubber ring ligation, cryosurgery, and hemorrhoidectomy.[149] Five weeks after treatment, anal dilatation was found to be as effective as surgical removal in control of symptoms, but residual hemorrhoids were more evident after Lord's procedure. The other methods were less successful. Follow-up as long as 5 years revealed that surgical hemorrhoidectomy offered the best results for this group of patients.

In the most recent published paper (2000), Konsten and Baeten followed patients for a median of 17 years in a prospective, randomized trial of hemorrhoidectomy versus Lord's method.[138] Recurrent hemorrhoids were noted in 26% of patients who underwent hemorrhoidectomy but in 46% with the operative dilation (with the postoperative dilation program). Interestingly, those who were not dilating postoperatively did better (39% recurrence). Fifty-two percent of those who underwent Lord's procedure experienced incontinence symptoms. The authors concluded that the procedure should be abandoned.

Opinion

When one performs this maneuver it has been facetiously remarked that the surgeon (or more likely the patient) will chant, "Lord, Lord!" I do not recommend Lord's dilatation for the treatment of hemorrhoids. Failure to deal with tags and papillae, as well as the risk of incontinence, especially in patients older than 60 years of age, should preclude the application of this technique. The physician must recognize that sphincter stretch inevitably must attenuate the external sphincter as well as the internal. With the plethora of innovations for the treatment of hemorrhoids, excisional and nonexcisional, I expect that the procedure inevitably will be referred to as a historical curiosity.

Internal Anal Sphincterotomy

Using the principle that many patients who harbor hemorrhoids have elevated anal canal pressure, Schouten and van Vroonhoven selected those with such elevations for sphincterotomy as the primary treatment of symptomatic hemorrhoids.[236] For a discussion of the techniques and indications for internal anal sphincterotomy, see Chapter 9. Individuals with normal or low anal pressures were treated by rubber ring ligation or hemorrhoidectomy. About 75% of patients who were managed by sphincterotomy alone were considered successfully treated. The authors suggest that this procedure is a good alternative in selected patients.

Opinion

Seventy-five percent is usually considered a passing grade in an examination, not for a surgical procedure. There is a real morbidity associated with internal anal sphincterotomy (see Chapter 9). Sphincterotomy alone

for the primary treatment of hemorrhoids should not be done—full stop.

TREATMENT OF THROMBOSED HEMORRHOIDS

External Hemorrhoids

The patient with thrombosed external hemorrhoids usually presents with a painful, tender mass (Figure 8-29) and may report that the lump appeared following a bout of constipation or diarrhea. If one or the other is a frequent occurrence, appropriate counseling needs to be implemented. An important predisposing factor for the development of recurrent thrombosed hemorrhoids is spending too much time on the toilet. Counseling should also include the suggestion of removing the library from the bathroom as a prophylactic measure.

If the problem has been present for more than 2 or 3 days, the discomfort usually has begun to subside. Under these circumstances, medical management should be offered. This consists of appropriate counseling in the use of sitz baths and stool softeners. A mild analgesic may be

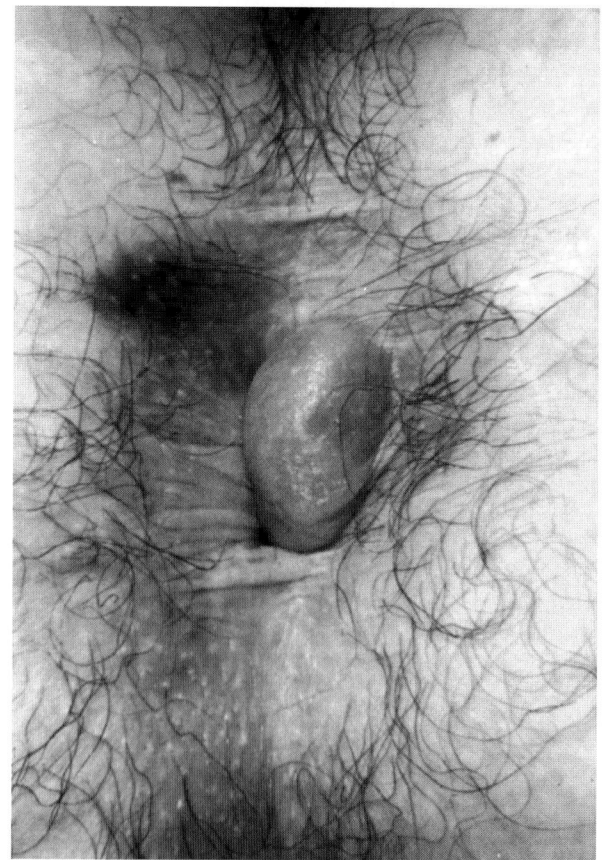

FIGURE 8-29. A thrombosed external hemorrhoid.

recommended. Topical nifedipine (0.3% nifedipine and 1.5% lidocaine ointment, every 12 hours), a calcium channel antagonist, has also been demonstrated to afford excellent pain relief in a prospective, randomized clinical trial.[204] The control group received only the lidocaine.

The mass will usually resolve in 7 to 10 days, especially if the patient makes a vigorous effort to apply heat to the area. If the area involved corresponds to the location where the patient reports a tendency for prolapse, rubber ring ligation should be considered following resolution of symptoms. If ulceration or rupture has occurred, or if the patient is seen within 48 hours, it is usually advisable to excise the lesion. Certainly, if the pain is severe, excision is preferred.

Technique

The hemorrhoid should be excised, not incised. Making a small incision and shelling the clot out like a pea from a pod often results in recurrent hemorrhage into the subcutaneous tissue and clot reaccumulation. Simple incision often produces more swelling and pain with recurrent bleeding than did the original thrombosis. This necessitates a visit to the emergency facility with the inevitable consequence of an angry patient.

Figure 8-30 demonstrates the proper technique for performing the excision, albeit with a bit of artistic license and exaggeration of the size of the defect to make a point. The principle is to leave the wound open a bit to permit drainage. The area is infiltrated with a local anesthetic of choice [e.g., a solution of 0.5% bupivacaine (Marcaine) in 1:200,000 epinephrine]. The bupivacaine solution as commercially prepared is quite acidic and is often associated with extreme burning pain upon injection[55]; however, pH adjustment through increased alkalinization ameliorates this problem considerably.[163,164,172,191,198] The alkalinization of bupivacaine has been said to be difficult because precipitation occurs rapidly, thus limiting the increase in pH.[34] Because epinephrine is unstable in alkaline solution, it is important that administration take place within 6 hours after alkalinization. It is therefore recommended that 1 ml of 8.4% sodium bicarbonate solution, USP, be added to 9 ml of bupivacaine with epinephrine. This markedly improves the discomfort associated with the injection. We have also had a favorable experience with the WAND local anesthetic delivery system (Milestone Scientific, Inc., Livingston, NJ).[255] This foot pedal-controlled, computer-automated apparatus allows precise delivery of anesthesia at a constant flow rate. As such it is quite effective in providing a more comfortable experience for the patient.

The underlying hemorrhoid is excised, as is a wedge of skin (Figure 8-30). Bleeding is controlled with pressure,

topically applied epinephrine, or electrocautery.[124] Another option is Monsel's solution, a chemical styptic agent (ferric subsulfate).[120] A pressure dressing is used.

Postoperative Care

The patient is instructed to maintain the pressure dressing in place for a few hours. By this time there is usually some discomfort, and the dressing is then removed. Sitz baths are then commenced. If bleeding occurs, it can usually be controlled by the application of direct pressure on the wound with a cloth or compress. A small dressing or pad can be used to avoid soiling clothing. Twice-daily sitz baths are recommended until the wound heals (i.e., 7 to 10 days). A mild analgesic and a topical anesthetic cream are usually salutary.

Internal Hemorrhoids

In addition to the previously mentioned factors that may cause thrombosis of external hemorrhoids, prolapse with inadequate reduction may cause thrombosis of internal hemorrhoids. As a result, stasis develops within the vein and thrombosis occurs.

The treatment of thrombosed internal hemorrhoids is not as straightforward as that for external hemorrhoids. Fortunately, however, pain is not as frequent a complaint. Excision of a thrombosed internal hemorrhoid, however, requires instrumentation and a more extensive local infiltration or field block. Suturing within the anal canal is always necessary to maintain hemostasis, simply because the application of adequate direct pressure is virtually impossible.

Because operative intervention for the acute problem is rarely indicated, sitz baths are recommended, as well as a mild systemic analgesic and a topical anesthetic cream or suppository. A stool softener is also advisable. If the patient has concurrent extensive hemorrhoids, tags, hypertrophied papillae, or associated anal fissure, a surgical approach is usually advocated.

GANGRENOUS, PROLAPSED, EDEMATOUS HEMORRHOIDS

The patient who presents with severely disabling, irreducibly prolapsed, gangrenous hemorrhoids requires emergency medical measures and, ideally, some form of surgical intervention. A carefully conceived hemorrhoidectomy within 24 hours is the preferred approach if convenient for the patient, but there are other options. Pain,

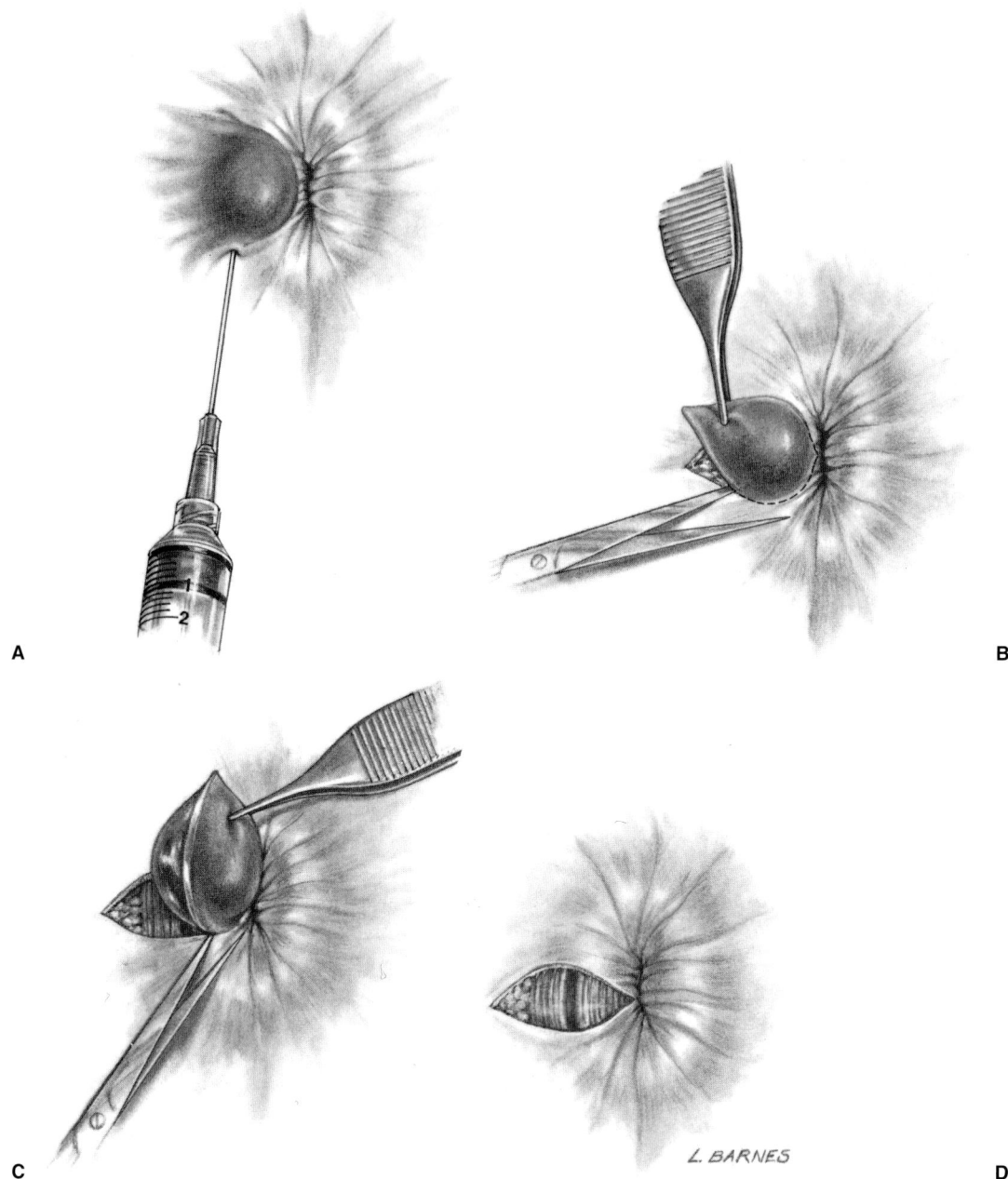

FIGURE 8-30. Excision of a thrombosed hemorrhoid. **(A)** The area is infiltrated with 0.5% bupivacaine in 1:200, epinephrine. **(B,C)** The thrombosis is excised with the underlying vein and with a wedge of skin. **(D)** Skin edges are sufficiently separate to permit adequate drainage, thereby preventing reaccumulation of a clot.

swelling, bleeding, foul-smelling discharge, and difficulty defecating are common presenting complaints. Of prior hemorrhoidal difficulties, prolapse is the most frequent. Proctosigmoidoscopic and anoscopic examination reveal edematous, thrombosed, irreducible hemorrhoids (Figs. 8-7 and 8-31).

Nonoperative alternatives consist of warm sitz baths, analgesics, stool softeners, creams, lotions, and supposi-

tories. Ice packs and bed rest with the legs elevated have also been recommended, but confining a patient under such circumstances suggests to me nineteenth-century medicine rather than twenty-first, especially because the end point may not be reached for 2 or 3 weeks. Other options include reduction of the mass by means of a field block (see later) followed by the application of pressure, the injection of hyaluronidase to dissipate the edema,

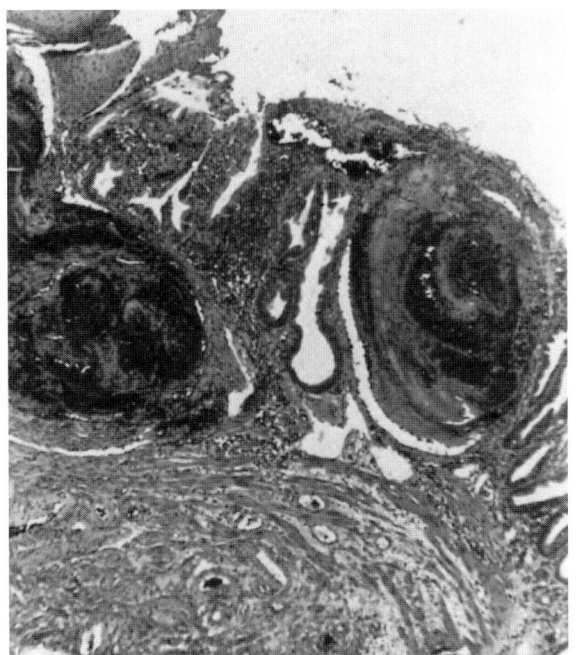

FIGURE 8-31. Hemorrhoidal tissue with hemorrhage is seen in a patient who underwent urgent hemorrhoidectomy. Note the dilated veins close to the surface containing recent blood clots. (Original magnification × 180.)

and evacuation of the clots, with or without concomitant rubber band ligations.

Technique of Creating a Field Block

A perianal field block is established by using a local anesthetic solution. My own preference is to employ an alkalinized solution of 0.5% bupivacaine (Marcaine) with 1:200,000 epinephrine, and ideally adding to this two 1 mm ampules of hyaluronidase [300 NF units of hyaluronidase (Wydase)]. Unfortunately, the availability of hyaluronidase in the United States has been called into question. A subcutaneous circumanal wheal is infiltrated in the edematous hemorrhoidal tissue (Figure 8-32). Four deep injections are made in the intersphincteric groove in each quadrant to effect paralysis of the sphincter mechanism and to create total perianal anesthesia. The finger may be inserted into the rectum during introduction of the needle to avoid penetrating the lumen of the bowel, but this is unlikely to occur. Care should also be taken to avoid entering the vagina, prostate, or urethra anteriorly. After a few minutes, in order to allow the medication to take effect, direct massaging pressure is applied with a sterile pad to reduce the hemorrhoidal mass. A pressure dressing is used, and the buttocks are taped if no further intervention is planned at the time. Alternatively, one may elect to evacuate the clots and even to per-

form multiple rubber band ligations, as has been advocated by some surgeons.

My personal approach is, ideally, to admit the patient to the hospital on an emergency basis, and a hemorrhoidectomy is performed the same day or the following. With reduction maintained, one is usually quite comfortable, and an adequate, safe operation can be performed with less edema than would be present without reduction (see Surgical Hemorrhoidectomy).

Results of Emergency Surgery

Historically, the concept of surgical hemorrhoidectomy in the presence of thrombosed, ulcerated, gangrenous hemorrhoids was considered unwise because of the risks for pyelophlebitis, perianal sepsis, hemorrhage, and the subsequent development of anal stricture. However, with the application of proper surgical technique, the complication rate should be minimal. Ackland reported 25 patients with prolapsed and strangulated hemorrhoids who underwent emergency operations.[1] The results were compared with those in a similar group who had elective surgery for chronic hemorrhoids. According to this study, operation for prolapsed and strangulated hemorrhoids in the acute stage was safe and effective, comparable to that of elective operation for chronic hemorrhoidal complaints. Postoperative pain was not significantly different. Anal stenosis, however, developed in one individual. Shieh and Gennaro reported 23 patients who underwent "semiemergency" hemorrhoidectomy 12 to 24 hours after manual reduction by a method similar to that described earlier.[243] Early hemorrhage developed in one person, and an episode of late bleeding in another, but there were no other complications, save urinary retention, that could be directly attributed to the procedure. Others have also reported success with this management.[74,108] Eisenstat and colleagues used the aforementioned field block and then performed multiple rubber ring ligations, incising any thromboses, rather than performing a surgical hemorrhoidectomy.[72] They reported gratifying results without significant complication.

Comment

As suggested, because conservative treatment of strangulated hemorrhoids (i.e., sitz baths, analgesics, and stool softeners) entails the prolongation of disability and perhaps financial hardship, urgent operation is advised for all such individuals. It must be remembered, however, that the patient may harbor colonic pathology (e.g., inflammatory bowel disease or neoplasm) that may be the predisposing factor for the hemorrhoid problem. At minimum, a proctosigmoidoscopic examination should be performed before hemorrhoidectomy. The decision

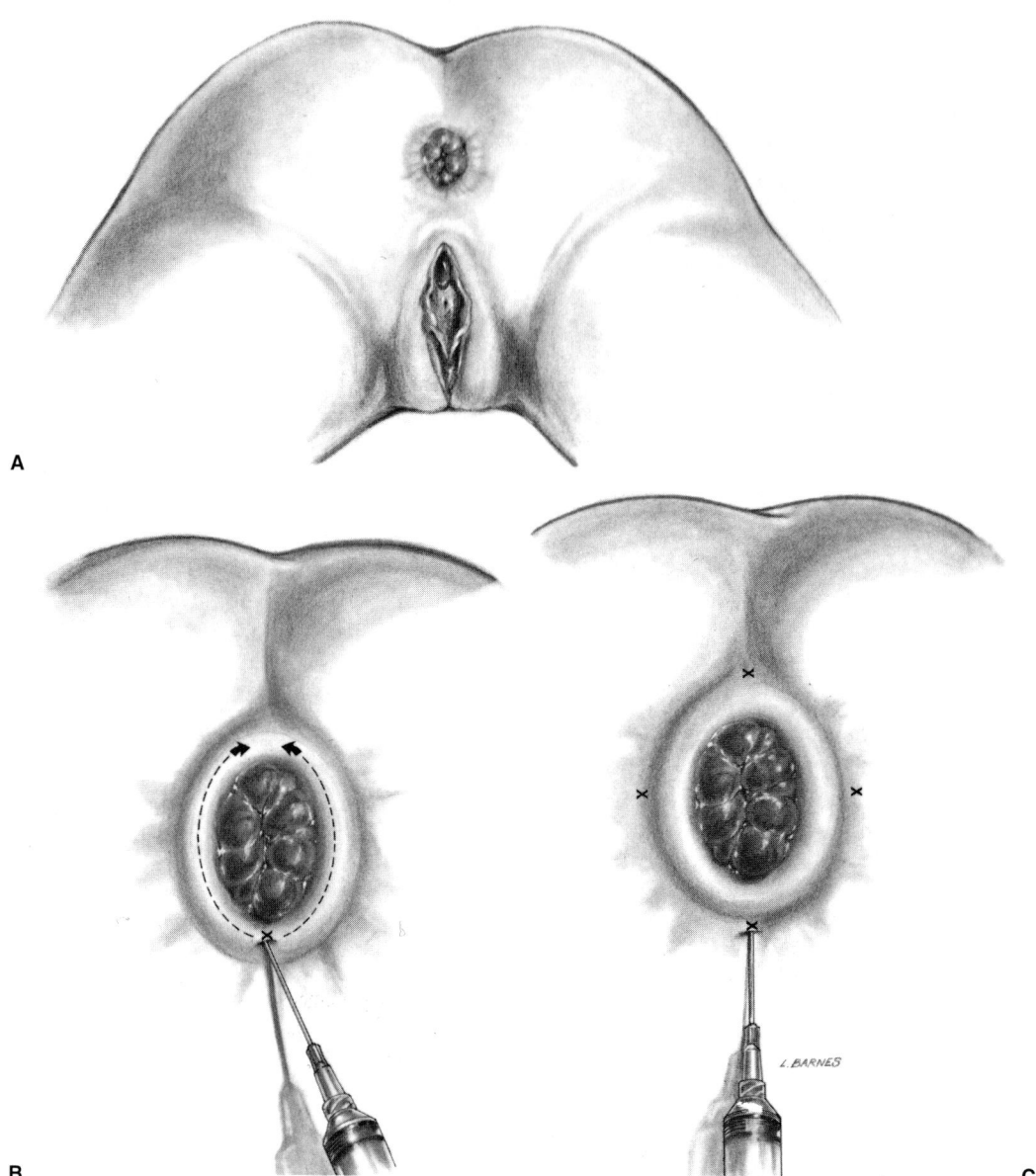

FIGURE 8-32. Method of establishing perianal field block. **(A)** The patient is placed in the prone (i.e., jackknife) position. **(B)** A subcutaneous perianal wheal is raised. **(C)** Deep injections are made at four sites to effect further anesthesia and paralysis of sphincter muscles.

whether to embark on a more extensive evaluation before or after the operation should rest on the surgeon's judgment in the individual case.

OPERATIVE APPROACHES TO THE TREATMENT OF HEMORRHOIDS

Surgical hemorrhoidectomy should be considered when the anorectal architecture has been severely compromised (e.g., with an external component, ulceration, gangrene, extensive thrombosis, hypertrophied papillae, or associated fissure). In 1993, the previously mentioned Standards Task Force of the American Society of Colon and Rectal Surgeons stipulated that excision of a "solitary external hemorrhoid can be performed as an outpatient procedure. For the satisfactory surgical treatment of internal hemorrhoids, with or without external hemorrhoids, ambulatory or inpatient stay is determined by the operating surgeon based on the preoperative clinical findings or the pathologic findings at surgery".[249] In 2003, Practice Parameters for Ambulatory Anorectal Surgery were published by the Standards Task Force.[6] The following were some of the conclusions:

- Anorectal surgery may be safely and cost-effectively performed in an ambulatory surgery center.
- Approximately 90% of anorectal cases may be suitable for ambulatory surgery.
- Patients with American Society of Anesthesiology classifications I and II are generally considered suitable; selected category III patients may also be appropriate candidates.
- The choice of preoperative investigations should be determined by the history and physical examination.
- Most anorectal surgery may be safely and cost-effectively performed with a local anesthesic; regional and general anesthesia can be used depending upon physician and patient preference.

One should add, however, that in the United States, the decisions on the facility for undertaking the procedure (hospital, ambulatory surgery facility, or office) and whether hospitalization is optimal for the patient are always determined by a third-party payer. The likelihood that the patient will be permitted hospitalization beyond what is termed, "a 23-hour stay" is virtually nonexistent.

Preoperative, Intraoperative, and Postoperative General Principles

The most useful preoperative measure, in my opinion, is a small-volume enema (e.g., Fleet) the morning of operation. Vigorous mechanical cleansing by means of laxatives is counterproductive. The patient should be able to defecate as soon as possible after the operation and yet be empty of stool that could be a nuisance to the surgeon during the procedure.

No antibiotics are indicated, absent those conditions that always require prophylaxis (see Chapter 4). Minimal intravenous fluids should be administered before and during the anesthesia, and the patient should be encouraged to void following the procedure. However, I do not increase fluid intake in the recovery room in order to stimulate urinating and have no aversion about overrul-

ing hospital policy that mandates voiding before discharge (see Complications, Urinary Retention). Patients do better in the peacefulness of their own familiar environment when compared with the public performance that is sometimes demanded in the recovery area. A small area may be shaved in the operating room if the situation warrants.

Surgical Approaches

Ideally, the goal of conventional hemorhoidectomy is to excise completely all the hemorrhoidal tissue without postoperative complication. Unfortunately, this is sometimes an unrealized objective. Part of the failure could be attributed to the low priority that operations in the anal area command in most general surgery residency training programs, at least in the United States. As a consequence, the performance of surgical hemorrhoidectomy too frequently involves instruction of the surgical resident by an inexperienced surgeon. No less an authority than the late John Goligher stated, "Anal surgery is usually a matter of the novice being taught by the incompetent."

Hemorrhoidectomy should be planned at the operating table and should proceed according to the dictates of the individual case. Inserting a dry sponge into the rectum and withdrawing it is an excellent way to demonstrate hemorrhoidal tissue, tags, papillae, and the extent of redundant mucosa. Not every patient will have hemorrhoids in the classical three-quadrant distribution previously mentioned. The surgeon should, therefore, be prepared to excise any and all hemorrhoidal disease and redundant mucosa, irrespective of the location within and outside the anal canal. However, a bridge of intact skin and mucosa should be left between excised hemorrhoidal sites to avoid subsequent stricture formation (see Complications). This is particularly important when operating for acute, edematous, or gangrenous hemorrhoids.

Numerous approaches have been used for the surgical removal of hemorrhoids. Some eponymous operations include those of Buie, Fansler, Ferguson, Milligan-Morgan, Parks, Salmon, and Whitehead and their col-

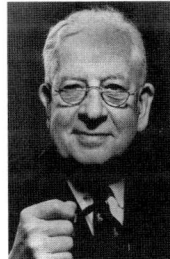

Clifford Naunton Morgan (1901–1986) Naunton Morgan was born in Penygraig, Glamorgan, Wales on December 20, 1901. He was educated at the Royal Masonic School, Bushey, and at University College Cardiff, Wales, before entering St. Bartholomew's Hospital Medical College. Having received his Fellowship in the Royal College of Surgeons in 1927, he subsequently became an anatomy demonstrator at St. Bartholomew's. Following several years initially as assistant surgeon and then as chief assistant to Charles Gordon-Watson, he ultimately was appointed surgeon to St. Mark's Hospital as well as Assistant Director of the Professorial Surgical Unit at St. Bartholomew's Hospital. Following the outbreak of World War II, Naunton Morgan joined the Royal Army Medical Corps and was appointed officer-in-charge of a surgical division with the rank of Lieutenant Colonel, ultimately achieving the rank of Brigadier to the East African Command. He remained a consultant surgeon to the Navy, Army, and Air Force until his retirement. Naunton Morgan contributed numerous articles and chapters in colon and rectal surgery, receiving many awards and recognitions, including Honorary Fellow of the American College of Surgeons, President of the Association of Surgeons of Great Britain and Ireland, and President of the Section of Proctology of the Royal Society of Medicine. He died February 24, 1986 at the age of 84. (Photograph, Courtesy of St. Mark's Hospital, Harrow, UK)

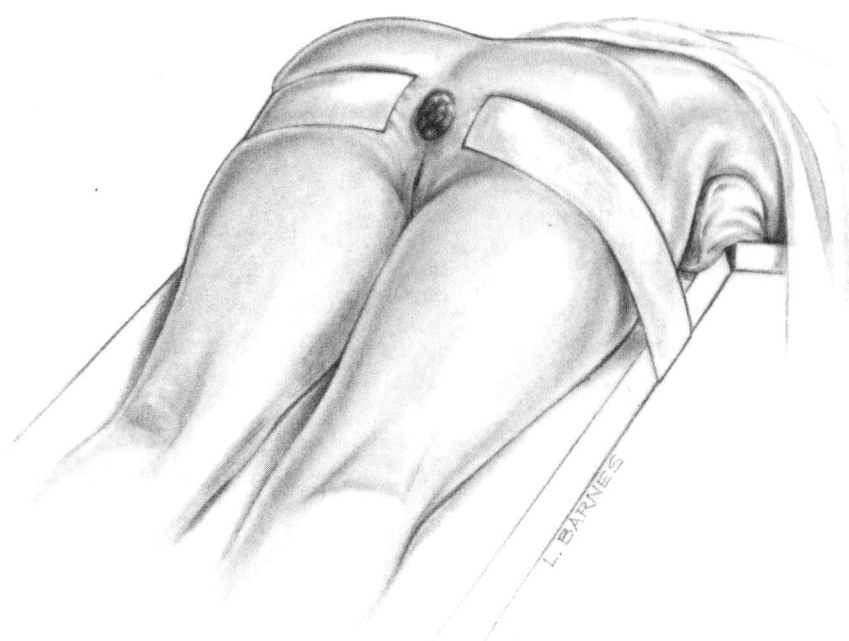

FIGURE 8-33. Position of the patient for hemorrhoidectomy. Local anesthesia with intravenous sedation is ideal. However, spinal, caudal, or general endotracheal anesthesia is frequently employed.

leagues.[36,75,80,167,197,228,276] The procedure that I favor is a modification of Ferguson's or closed hemorrhoidectomy.

Closed (Ferguson's) Hemorrhoidectomy

Anesthesia and Patient Position

The patient is placed in the prone jackknife position with the buttocks taped apart (Figure 8-33). Having the patient in the lithotomy position is awkward for the assistant, because a moderate amount of suturing is required when the primary closure technique is used. However, many surgeons in the United Kingdom prefer lithotomy, although this is changing. Often the choice of position is dictated by demands made by the anesthesiologist, especially if the patient is obese or has breathing problems. Given the opportunity, most anesthesiologists would never elect to place the patient in the prone jackknife position because of airway concerns, but with reasoned communication between congenial colleagues the optimal solution can usually be achieved, even though our compatriots at the head of the table always manage to contain their enthusiasm. Having

had considerable experience with both approaches, in Britain as a senior registrar and in the United States, I think there is no comparison between the two. Admittedly, however, if one leaves the wounds open, the difference in patient position is less evident. The lateral decubitus position has been recommended for many years by the Ferguson Clinic Group and their disciples, a compromise between the other two alternatives. In my opinion, this position is also very inconvenient for the assistant.

Read and colleagues prospectively analyzed anesthetic technique for anorectal surgery on 413 consecutive patients.[215] Most underwent their procedures in the prone position (389 patients). Two thirds of these patients received intravenous sedation with local anesthesia (260 patients). All but one of the others received a caudal or epidural anesthetic. Although patients were obviously not randomized to one or the other position, and the study does imply a certain selectivity bias, two conclusions could be reached. First, only two patients (0.8%) of the 260 patients required turning to the supine position before completion of the surgery, and second, discharge

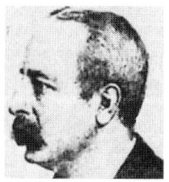

Walter Whitehead (1840–1913) Whitehead was born at Haslem Hey, Bury, England, where his father's family had resided for more than 200 years. At the age of 19, he decided to study medicine and practiced initially in Mansfield, where he organized a small cottage hospital. In 1867, he was appointed to the St. Mary's Hospital for Women and Children in Manchester. He became involved in a number of charitable organizations and was instrumental in the introduction of a bill before the House of Commons on the protection of infant life. In 1885, he was elected President of the Manchester Medical Society, and at his inaugural address he attracted much attention for initially recognizing the increased incidence of cancer. Whitehead's operative technique seemed to be characterized by originality as well as by a certain simplified approach. Two operations bear his name: his method of excising the tongue and his method of hemorrhoidectomy. This latter operation was severely criticized even in his own day because of the "deformity," perhaps in some cases the result of misapplication of "drawing down the divided surface of mucous membrane and attaching [it] by several fine silk sutures to the denuded border at the verge of the anus." (Whitehead W. The surgical treatment of haemorrhoids. *BMJ* 1882;1:148.)

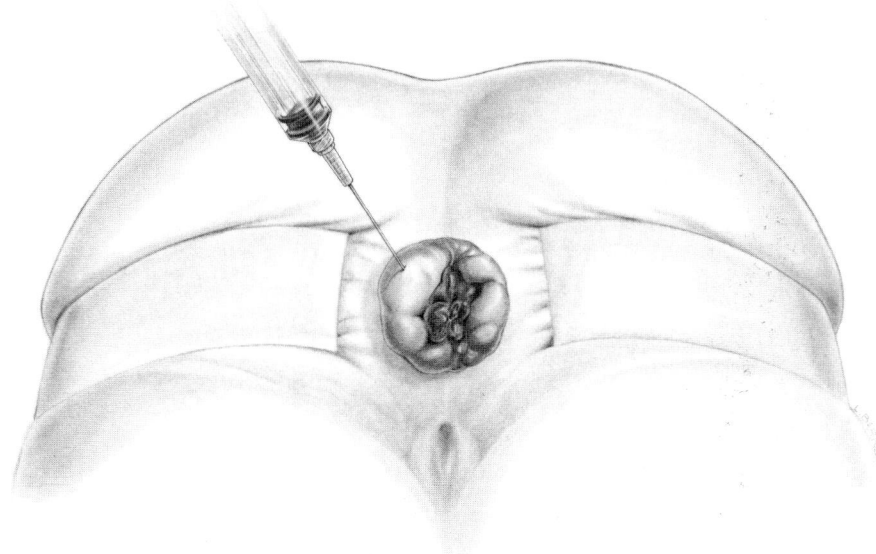

FIGURE 8-34. In preparation for hemorrhoidectomy, the anus is infiltrated with a local anesthetic of bupivacaine in epinephrine.

from recovery was much sooner when compared with those undergoing regional anesthesia.

The anus is infiltrated with a solution of approximately 20 ml of 0.5% bupivacaine in 1:200,000 epinephrine (Figure 8-34). This low dose usually does not affect the heart rate or the blood pressure. The infiltration technique minimizes bleeding, and the anatomic plane between the hemorrhoidal masses and the underlying internal sphincter muscle is clearly delineated. Furthermore, by using local anesthesia and the previously discussed field block technique, often with supplementary intravenous sedation while the medication is administered, no additional anesthesia is necessary. As mentioned, a general, caudal, or spinal anesthetic may be used.

Technique

A Hill-Ferguson retractor (see Figure 4-6) placed in the anal canal reveals the extent of the hemorrhoids. Alternatively, there are many other rectal specula and retractors that a surgeon may prefer (Figure 8-35). For a right-handed surgeon, it is usually best to deal with the more difficult pile first—the one in the right posterior quadrant (if it is to be excised). Alternatively, one may elect to switch sides, depending on the hemorrhoid side one is treating, and the comfort and handedness of the surgeon. Some surgeons like to place an anchoring suture in the distal rectum corresponding to the site of the hemorrhoid, but I prefer placing only a clamp that incorporates the skin tag and hemorrhoid that will be excised (Figure 8-36). The reason for doing this is that the suture tends to limit the dissection, and there is no chance of cutting a stitch out that has *not* been placed. Excision can be performed with a knife, scissors, electrocautery, laser,

or with the Harmonic scalpel.[14] There has not been good evidence to indicate an advantage of one cutting method over another. However, in a prospective, randomized trial comparing the Harmonic scalpel, bipolar scissors, and ordinary scissors in hemorrhoidectomy, Chung and colleagues found the Harmonic scalpel to be superior because less pain was associated with it.[47] The observed benefits were small and did not affect time off from work and other activities.

A recent approach to hemorrhoid excision is the use of the Ligasure device (Valleylab, Boulder, CO). Having been designed primarily for abdominal surgery, it can seal vessels up to 7 mm in diameter; it has also found some acceptance for the treatment of hemorrhoids.[48,82,166,194] Historically, this is not dissimilar to that of the old "clamp and cautery" method.

The incision should be carried well beyond the anal verge, removing the external hemorrhoidal plexus and exposing the subcutaneous portion of the external sphincter muscle (Figure 8-37). The incision is then carried into the anal canal; the internal sphincter muscle is carefully dropped away from the plane of dissection. Bleeding is avoided when the dissection is outside the hemorrhoid and medial to the internal sphincter. When the entire hemorrhoid pedicle has been mobilized, a suture ligature is placed using absorbable material (2–0 or 3–0 chromic catgut, 3–0, 4–0 or 5–0 Dexon or Vicryl). A 5/8 circle needle is ideal for suturing within the anal canal. The pedicle is suture-ligated, and the hemorrhoid is excised (Figure 8-38). Any residual small internal or external hemorrhoids should be removed by means of Allis forceps and fine scissors (Figure 8-39). By undermining the mucosa or skin for a short distance and removing the veins, one can limit the likelihood of later symptoms

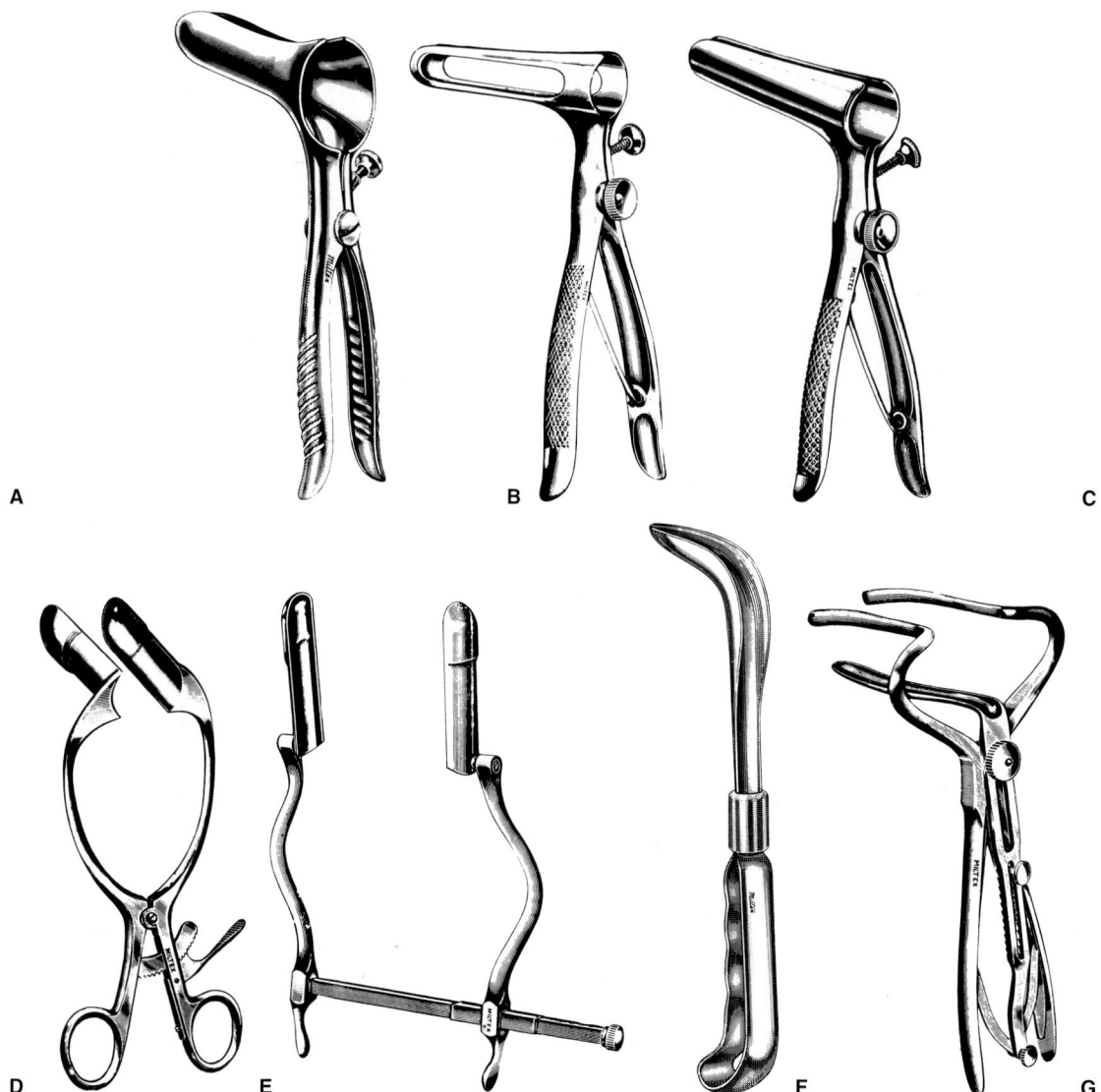

FIGURE 8-35. Rectal retractors. **(A)** Pratt. **(B)** Sims. **(C)** Bodenhammer. **(D)** Barr. **(E)** Smith (or Buie). **(F)** Sawyer. **(G)** Cook. (Courtesy of Miltex Instrument Co., Lake Success, NY.)

from hemorrhoidal veins that have been left behind. Hemostasis can be achieved with electrocautery.

The wound is closed completely with a continuous suture, using the same stitch that was employed to ligate the hemorrhoid pedicle (Figure 8-40). When the mucocutaneous junction is reached, the skin is closed in either a subcuticular fashion or by a continuous simple suture. In like manner, the remaining pile sites are excised, ligated, and primarily closed (Figure 8-41). Aside from the cosmetic appearance of the wounds, the fact that the physician is able to close all incisions and maintain the retractor in place as is illustrated implies that the anal canal opening is adequate. The physician need not be concerned about the subsequent development of a stricture under these circumstances.

The wounds are cleansed, and povidone-iodine (Betadine) ointment and a small dressing are applied. A bulky pressure dressing is avoided; no packing is necessary. Packing or anything else placed within the anal canal is undercomfortable. If the surgeon is concerned about hemostasis, he or she should take a few extra moments to ensure that it has been established.

Hemorrhoidectomy and Sphincterotomy

If a fissure is present, usually in the posterior position, an internal anal sphincterotomy is undertaken in the lateral pile site by dividing the lower one-third of the internal anal sphincter (Figure 8-42). Even in the absence of anal fissure some surgeons believe that this procedure re-

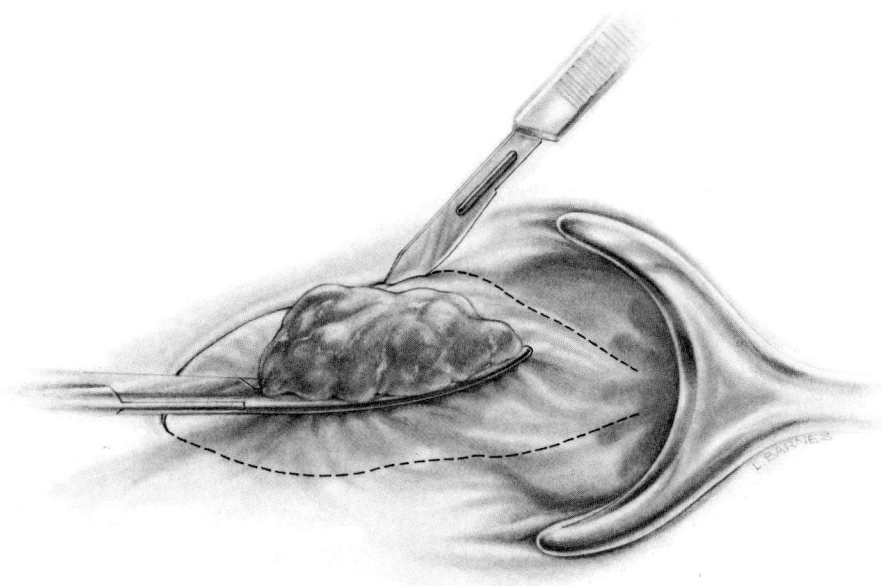

FIGURE 8-36. The hemorrhoid is identified and grasped with a clamp. The area for excision is outlined by a broken line.

duces complaints of pain. Khubchandani undertook a prospective, randomized, controlled study involving 42 patients, half of whom underwent concomitant sphincterotomy with their hemorrhoidectomies and half did not.[134] There was no difference in the perception of pain when the two groups were compared. Asfar and colleagues compared anal stretch and sphincterotomy in a prospective randomized fashion in more than 250 patients who underwent operative hemorrhoidectomy.[15] The sphincterotomy was undertaken usually at one of the lateral hemorrhoidectomy sites. Only 18.4% of those who underwent concomitant sphincterotomy required narcotics for pain, compared with 100% of those who underwent sphincter stretch. Additionally, urinary retention and fecal soilage were much more frequently observed in those who underwent the latter procedure.

Opinion

I do not employ sphincterotomy in the absence of a fissure. It is meddlesome, does not ameliorate the pain of hemorrhoidectomy, and may result in morbidity—infection, fistula, and some degree of impairment for bowel control (see Chapter 9).

Open Hemorrhoidectomy

Modifications of a closed or open hemorrhoidectomy are myriad. In the previous procedure, the wounds are completely closed. When hemorrhoids are gangrenous or circumferential, or when closure of wounds cannot be carried out with even a narrow retractor in place (generally a technical judgmental error), an open approach at one, two, or all of the pile sites may be indicated. Certainly,

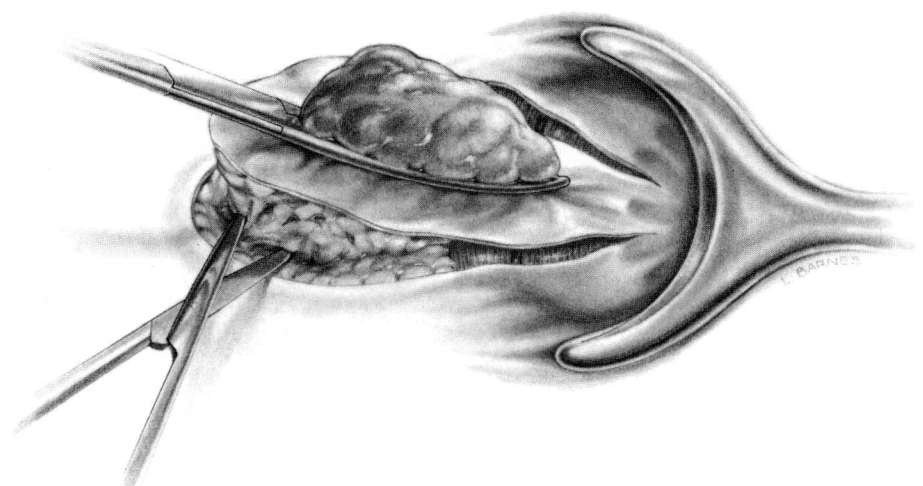

FIGURE 8-37. After the area for excision is outlined, the hemorrhoidal plexus is removed from the underlying subcutaneous portion of the external and internal sphincters.

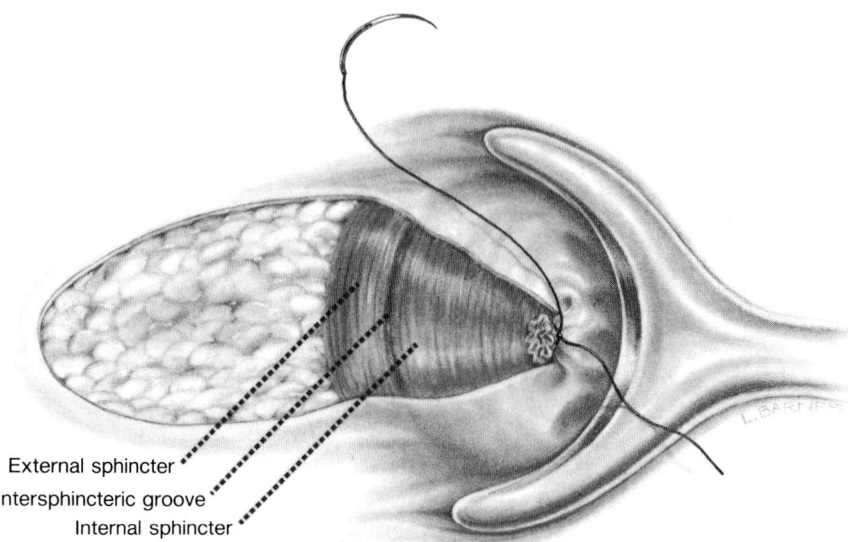

External sphincter
Intersphincteric groove
Internal sphincter

FIGURE 8-38. Open wound after excision of the hemorrhoid. No external or internal veins remain.

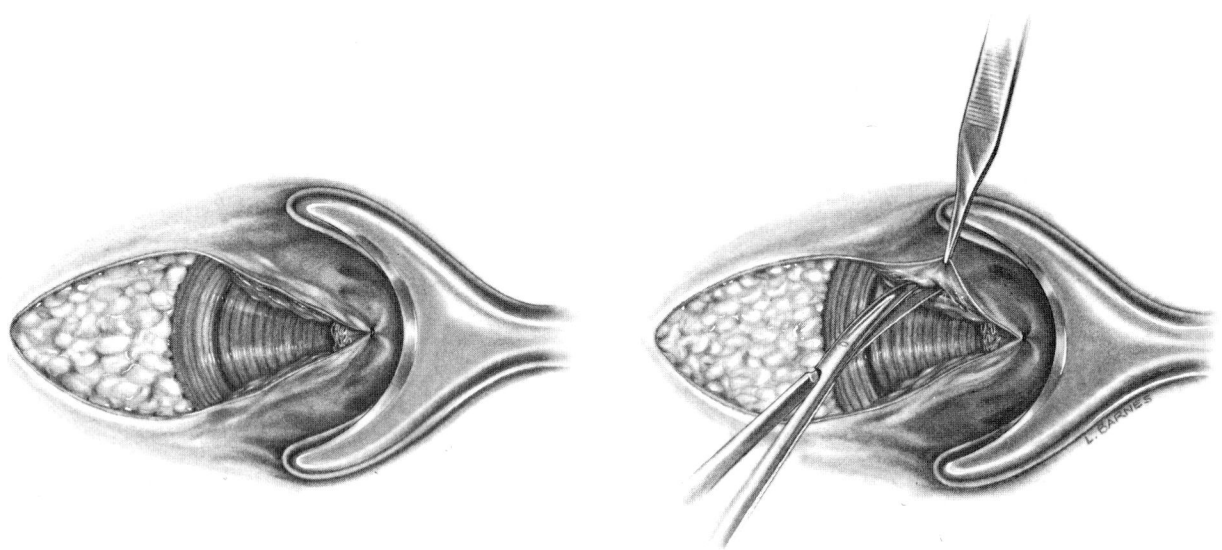

FIGURE 8-39. Residual hemorrhoids are removed by undermining the mucosa.

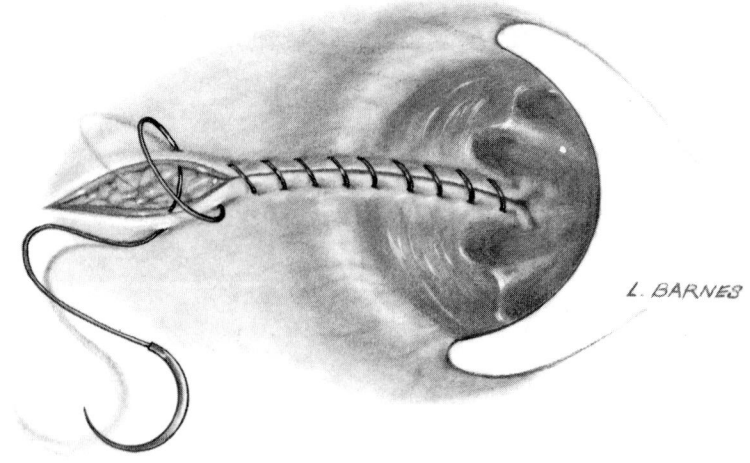

FIGURE 8-40. The wound is primarily closed.

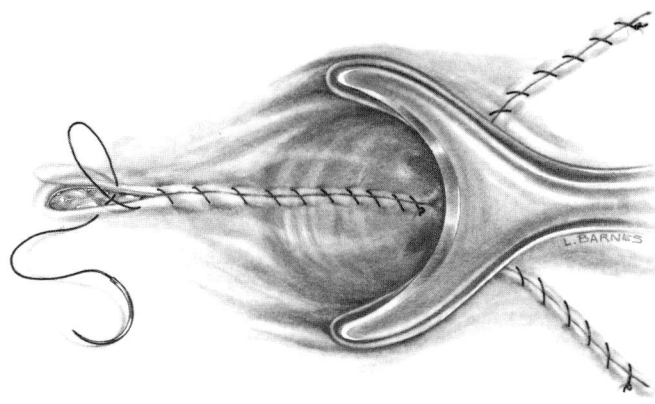

FIGURE 8-41. Completed closed (i.e., Ferguson) hemorrhoidectomy. With a Hill-Ferguson retractor in place, there can be no anal canal narrowing.

the open hemorrhoidectomy is quicker to accomplish and in any event may ultimately be the appearance of closed hemorrhoidectomy a few days following the operation for many patients.

With an open technique, the procedure is identical to that described for Ferguson's operation, with suture ligation of the hemorrhoidal pedicles, except that the operation ends at this point (Figs. 8-43 and 8-44). Additional hemostasis can be established with electrocautery. The aesthetic appearance of the result is reflected by the

aphorism, "If it looks like a clover, the operation is over; if it looks like a dahlia, it's a failure." Alternatively, one or two sites may be left open, closed, or partially closed, depending on the circumstances and the surgeon's preference. Good results are possible with a combination of open and closed approaches to each pile site.

Submucosal Hemorrhoidectomy or Parks' Hemorrhoidectomy

In the submucosal hemorrhoidectomy described by Parks, the mucosa of the anal canal and rectum is incised, and the hemorrhoidal tissue beneath is removed.[196] The mucosa is then reapproximated. The goal of this method is to excise all the hemorrhoidal tissue without injuring the overlying squamous and columnar epithelium. The advantage of this procedure is that the wounds allegedly heal more quickly, with reduced induration and scarring and less likelihood of the development of a stricture.

Technique

A self-retaining anal (i.e., Parks) retractor is usually recommended, primarily by United Kingdom surgeons; however, virtually any conventional anal retractor may be used. A solution of 0.5% bupivacaine or lidocaine in 1:200,000 epinephrine is injected into the submucosa and the hemorrhoidal mass (Figure 8-45A). The skin incision starts outside the anus and is carried around the forceps holding the anal skin, removing a minimal amount of anal canal mucosa (Figure 8-45B). The anal canal is undermined by scissor dissection to expose the hemorrhoidal tissue. The mucosa is elevated off of the hemorrhoidal vessels (Figure 8-45C). The upper limit of the dissection should be about 4 cm above the mucocutaneous junction. The external and internal sphincters are identified as the hemorrhoidal mass is elevated and stripped off the internal sphincter to what is considered an adequate level (Figure 8-45D). The hemorrhoidal mass

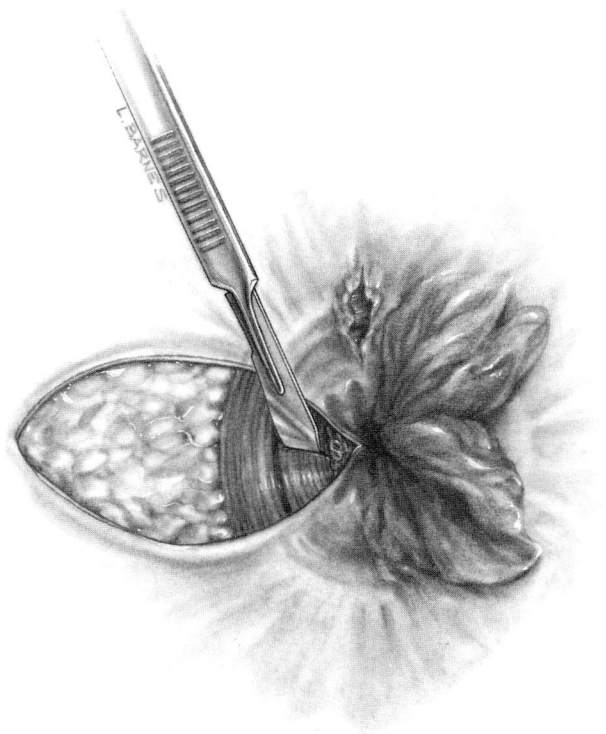

FIGURE 8-42. An internal anal sphincterotomy is performed at the site of excision of a left lateral pile in a patient with anal fissure.

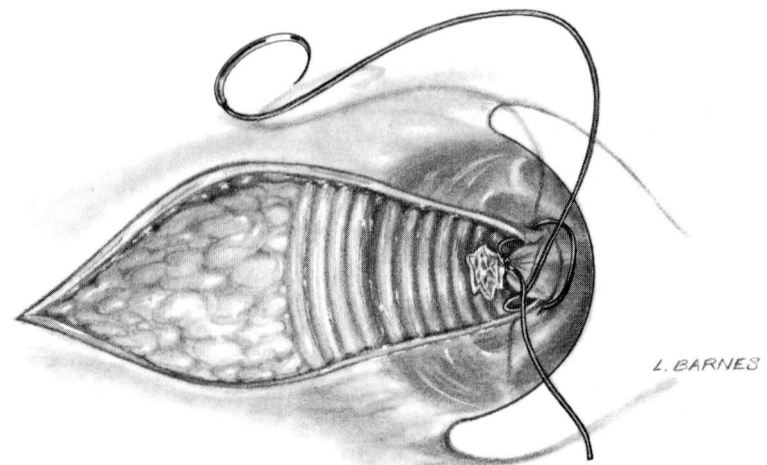

FIGURE 8-43. Open hemorrhoidectomy: technique of burying the hemorrhoidal pedicle.

is transfixed (Figure 8-45*E*), and the hemorrhoid is excised. The flaps of the mobilized anal canal mucosa are reapproximated, and the underlying internal sphincter is incorporated with the sutures to prevent dislodgement (Figure 8-45*F*). The skin may be left open or closed.

A modification of the Parks operation has been offered by Selvaggi and colleagues.[238] They describe a technique that allegedly permits excision of circumferential hemorrhoids and grafting via an open technique (Figure 8-46).

Opinion

The Parks hemorrhoidectomy is an elegant approach that minimizes tissue loss, but, as described, does not deal with the external component, hypertrophied anal papillae, or redundant mucosa. The development of a stricture is virtually impossible unless the overlying mucosa has been devascularized. However, I do not feel that the effort required for one to accomplish the procedure is justified. In my opinion, it should be relegated to that of historic interest except to emphasize and to illustrate the value of submucosal dissection in removing residual hemorrhoidal veins.

Whitehead's Hemorrhoidectomy

As previously suggested, Whitehead's hemorrhoidectomy is very rarely employed by surgeons today because of the complications of stricture and ectropion, but the procedure that frequently results in these complications is not truly the one that was described by the author.[276] As originally recommended by Whitehead, the mucosa was sutured to the anal canal above the level of the pectinate line, but later surgeons misinterpreted this description and anchored the mucosa to the skin at the anal verge (Figure 8-47). All too often, the suture line dehisced, and the wound was left to granulate and heal by second intention. More commonly, a mucosal ectropion, the so-called wet anus or Whitehead deformity, was the consequence (Figure 8-48). Poor Dr. Whitehead was tarred with this same brush, achieving eponymous immortality for a complication for which he was not responsible.

Results

Although favorable results have been reported with a modified Whitehead procedure, it is my impression that the authors are merely performing a variation of an open

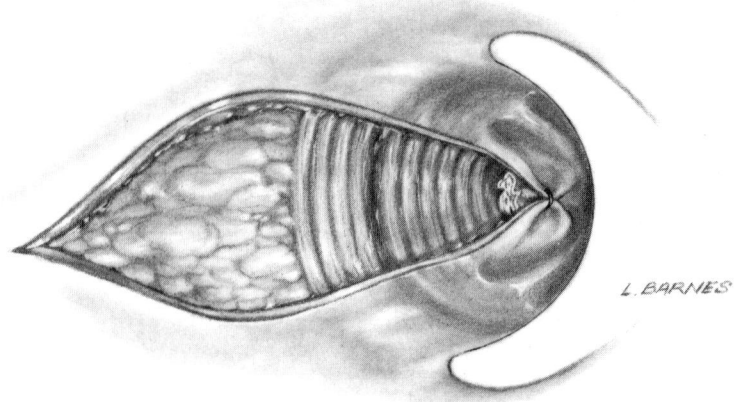

FIGURE 8-44. Completed open hemorrhoidectomy. Partial closure to the mucocutaneous junction is another option.

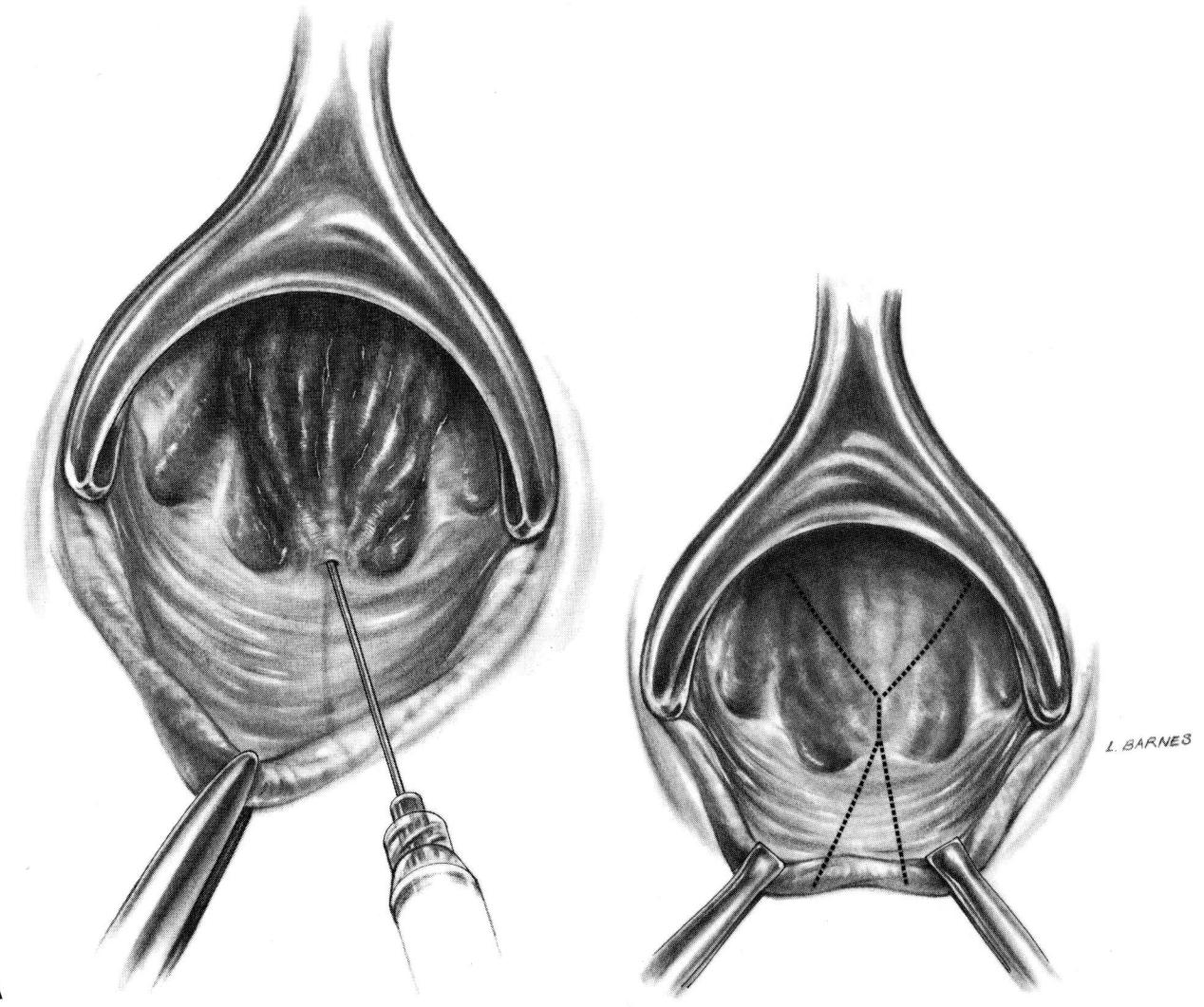

A   B

FIGURE 8-45. Parks' hemorrhoidectomy. **(A)** Epinephrine is injected for hemostasis and clarification of planes of dissection. **(B)** The incision is essentially cruciate. Two limbs of the V-shaped incision meet at the mucocutaneous junction and split again approximately 1 cm above this point. (*continued*)

hemorrhoidectomy.[33,282] In other words, whether the physician simply anchors the cut edge of the rectum to the underlying internal sphincter or combines an amputative hemorrhoidectomy with advancement of the perianal skin into the anal canal, the results should be quite satisfactory. Clearly, the mucosa should never be anchored to the skin outside the anus.

Barrios and Khubchandani related their experience with a modified Whitehead operation.[20] Their modification involved removal of the entire anoderm, but the perianal skin was preserved and the edges of the anal mucosa were sutured to the subcutaneous tissue, not to the skin. Although reporting satisfactory results in 41 patients, they noted a 32% incidence of urinary retention, a 5% inci-

dence of hemorrhage, and a 10% incidence of late complications (i.e., stenosis, ectropion, and incontinence). A later report from one of the authors on the results of Whitehead's operation on 84 patients revealed late complications in 13%.[135] Among these were varying problems with continence in three patients and the development of anal strictures in three. There was no instance of ectropion.

Ligasure Hemorrhoidectomy

The newer approach of sealing the pedicle by meals of the application of a bipolar electrothermal device has been mentioned previously. I suggested that this tech-

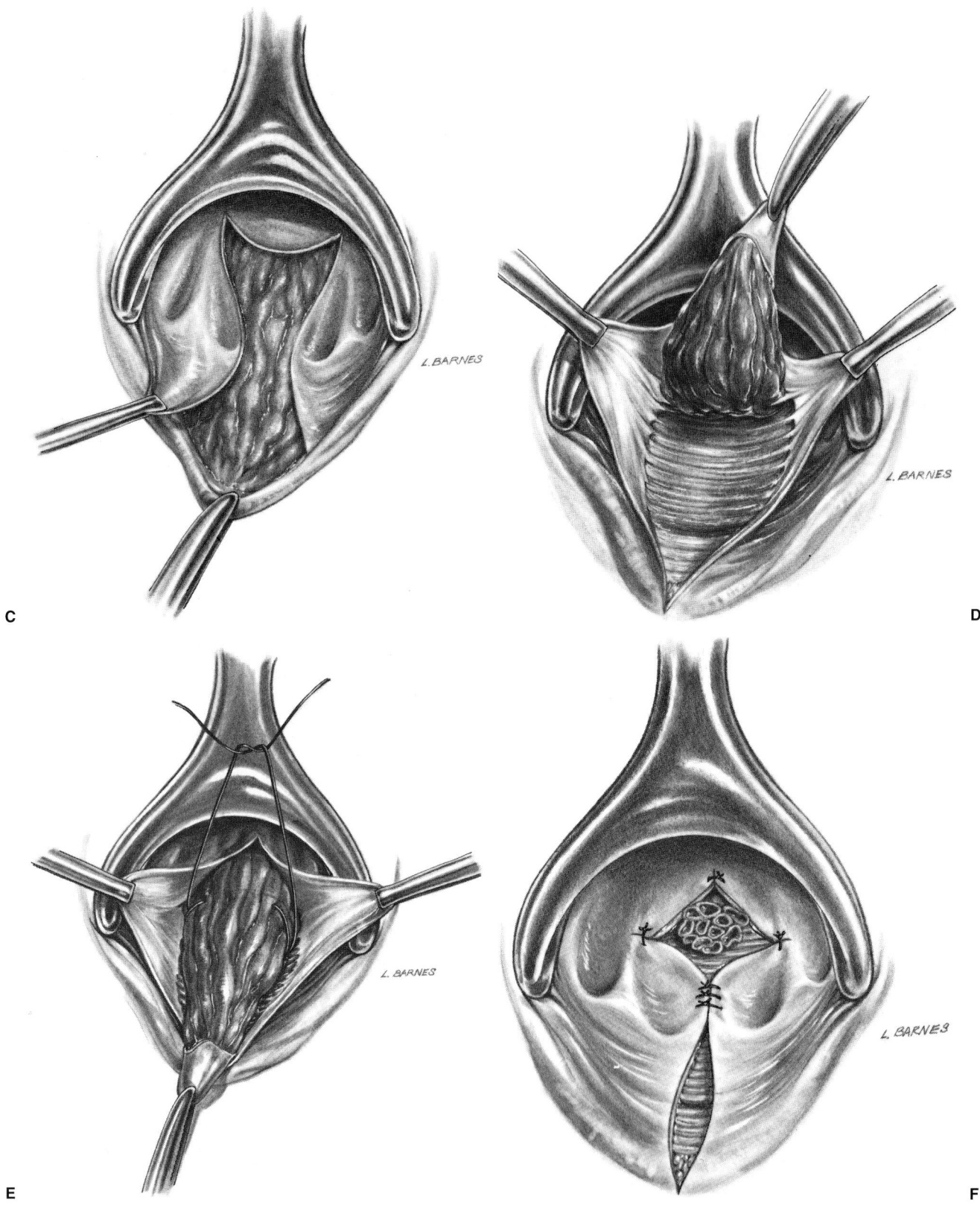

C

D

E

F

FIGURE 8-45. (*continued*) **(C)** The mucosa is elevated from the underlying hemorrhoidal mass by scissors dissection. **(D)** The hemorrhoid mass is elevated from the underlying internal anal sphincter. **(E)** Suture ligation of the hemorrhoid. **(F)** The anal mucosa is partially closed and the skin left open.

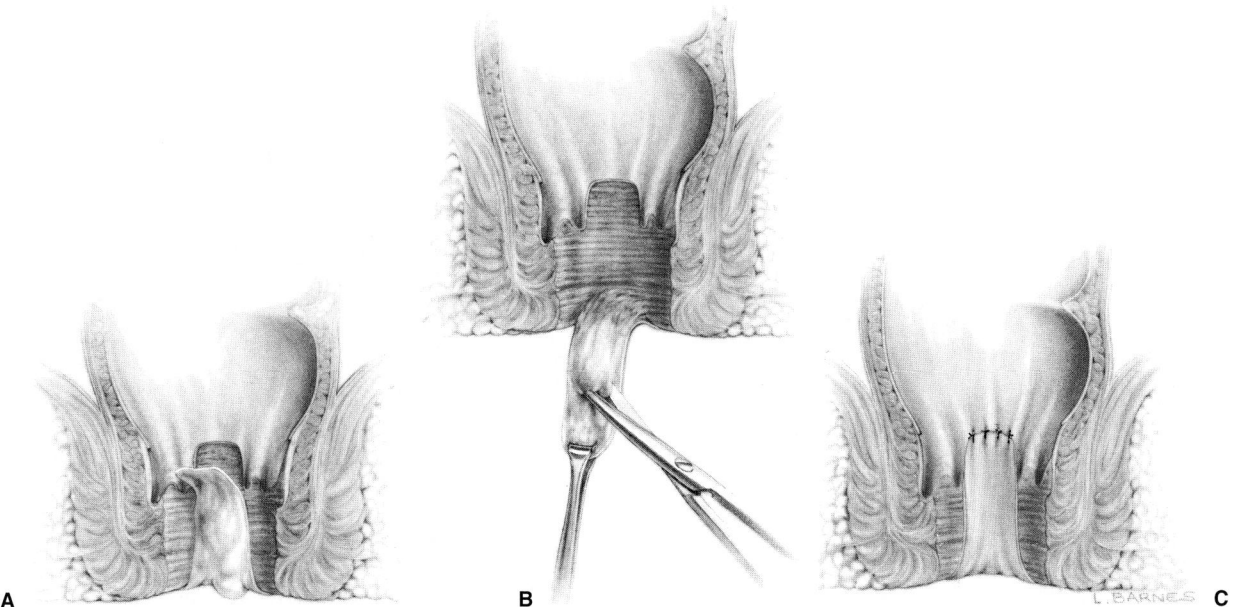

FIGURE 8-46. Submucosal hemorrhoidectomy as advocated by Selvaggi and colleagues. **(A)** If large residual hemorrhoids are identified, a transverse incision is made above the apex. **(B)** Allis forceps are used to apply tension to the anodermal flap, and the submucosal plexus is removed. **(C)** Absorbable sutures are used to reanchor the flap to the cut edge of the rectum and the underlying internal sphincter.

nique is analygous to that of the outmoded clamp and cautery method.

Results

Several prospective, randomized trials have been published in which Ligasure was compared with other alternatives. Jayne and colleagues compared this approach with that of diathermy hemorrhoidectomy.[118] They noted a shorter operative time and a higher frequency of hospital discharge the day of surgery. However, there was no difference with respect to pain, complications, or patient satisfaction. Milito and co-workers compared this approach in a randomized trial with open diathermy hemorrhoidectomy.[166] A statistically significant advantage was observed with respect to operative time, pain medication requirements, time to return to work, and wound healing. Others report advantages when compared with open hemorrhoidectomy.[194]

Opinion

The Ligasure method of performing a hemorrhoidectomy is qualitatively and quantitatively different from that of conventional hemorrhoidectomy. For example, the amount of tissue actually removed is inevitably much less

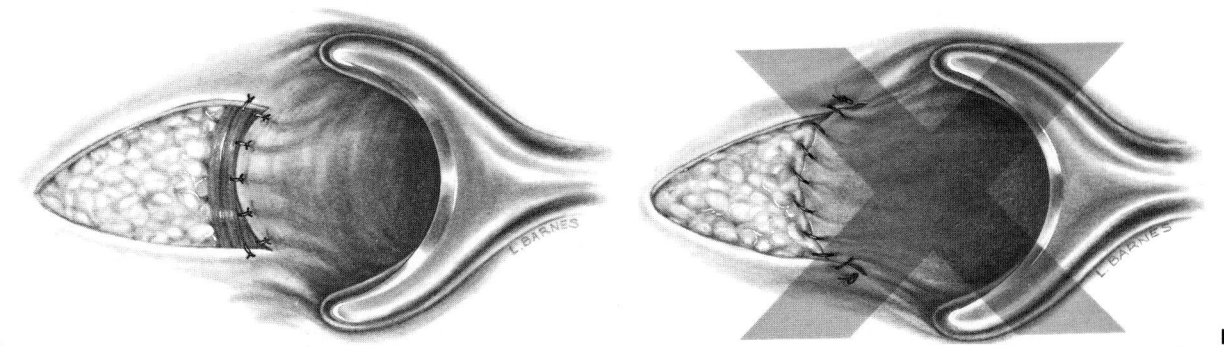

FIGURE 8-47. Whitehead's hemorrhoidectomy. **(A)** Proper mucosal anchoring to the underlying internal sphincter. **(B)** Improper anchoring may lead to ectropion.

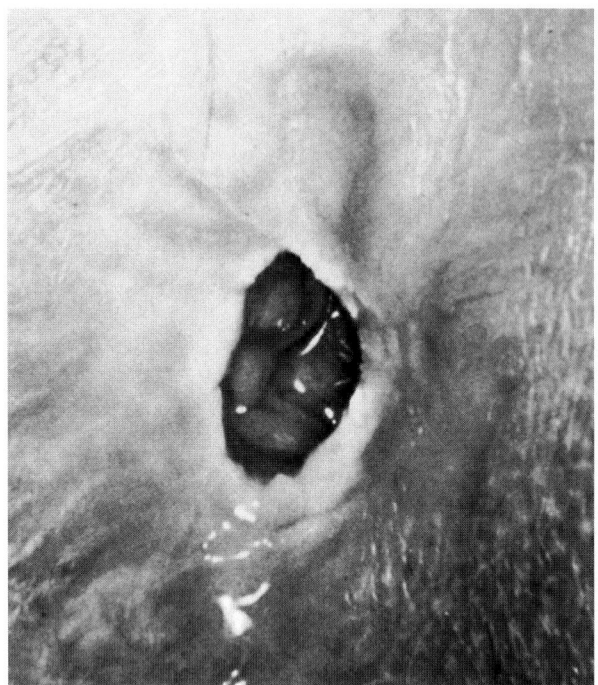

FIGURE 8-48. Whitehead's deformity. Note the mucosal ectropion that developed after excision of all of the anal canal, the characteristic "wet anus."

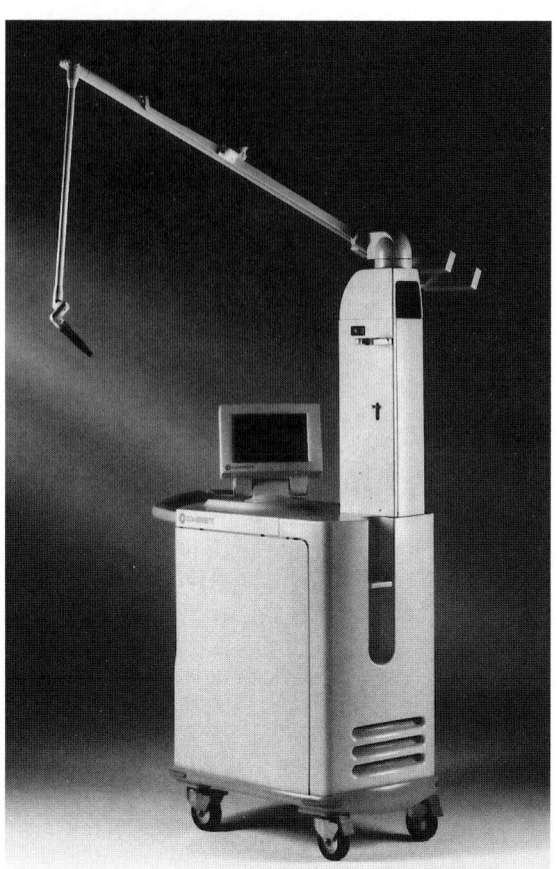

FIGURE 8-49. UltraPulse carbon dioxide laser system with a computerized pattern generator. (Courtesy of Coherent, Palo Alto, CA.)

with the former approach. Furthermore, it is not clear what (if anything) is being done with the external component. The length of follow-up is relatively short—a few months (if it is mentioned at all). For me, before considering the possibility of adopting this alternative, I would require a randomized trial that compares it with rubber band ligation.

Laser Surgery

As discussed in Chapter 5, the laser has been applied to the treatment of polyps and other lesions. It has also been advocated in the management of hemorrhoids (Figure 8-49). The three most common surgical lasers are the carbon dioxide, argon, and neodymium:yttrium-aluminum garnet (YAG). The different wavelengths of their light produce characteristic tissue effects that determine their usefulness in surgery. The carbon dioxide laser primarily cuts and is awkward to use endoscopically. Conversely, the argon laser coagulates surface vessels quite well, whereas the noncontact Nd:YAG can be used with deep vessels. Both, however, are limited by their unsatisfactory cutting qualities. A distinct advantage is the fact that Nd:YAG light will pass through optical fibers and can, therefore, be used through the operating channel of most endoscopy equipment.

Technique

Use of the laser requires special training and precautions. Because the light is invisible, the operator must wear goggles to protect the eyes. Yu and Eddy reported the results of treatment of 134 patients using the Nd:YAG laser to perform hemorrhoidectomies.[288] After administration of a local anesthetic, with the patient in the prone position and with a Hill-Ferguson retractor in place, the laser beam is aimed directly onto the surface of the pile. Iwagaki and colleagues believe that the carbon dioxide laser is suitable for hemorrhoidectomy because of the predictable biologic effects, minimal damage to adjacent normal tissue, good hemostasis, and precision of technique.[117] A red pilot light, provided by low-power laser, permits precise focusing of the therapeutic beam. The handle is moved while the laser beam destroys the tissue until the area is covered by a white membrane. Internal and external hemorrhoids are treated similarly. The authors required 30 to 45 minutes for each operation, and the patients were discharged the same day but were followed daily in the office for the first week. Sankar and Joffe suggest that large hemorrhoids may be treated by a submucosal technique.[230] It is therefore essentially Parks' hemorrhoidectomy, except that the laser augments the suturing for controlling blood loss.

Results

Narcotic pain medication is necessary for the first few days according to Yu and Eddy, and usually, healing was accomplished in about 1 month.[288] The early and late complication rates were not significantly different from those of conventional surgical hemorrhoidectomy, although an anal stenosis developed in three patients. Other physicians have also reported a favorable experience with laser hemorrhoidectomy.[117]

Wang and colleagues performed a randomized trial of hemorrhoidectomy either by means of Nd:YAG laser phototherapy or Ferguson's technique in 88 patients.[268] There was a statistically significant difference in the need for narcotic medication (laser, 11%; Ferguson, 56%); additionally, postoperative urinary retention was much less frequent when the laser was used (7% versus 39%). Postoperative stay was also much shorter with the laser hemorrhoidectomy. Conversely, Nicholson and colleagues noted no advantage in using the sapphire-tip Nd:YAG laser in treating grade III or IV hemorrhoids.[179] When they compared this approach with closed hemorrhoidectomy in a randomized, controlled way, they observed no differences in the duration of hospitalization, requirement for catheterization, operative time, blood loss, or narcotic use. Wound healing was also similar in both methods.

Chia and co-workers randomized 28 patients to either receive carbon dioxide laser hemorrhoidectomy or the conventional surgical approach.[44] The laser group required less postoperative pain medication. They were also able to demonstrate that the carbon dioxide laser did not cause any alteration in anorectal physiology. Others have concluded that laser hemorrhoidectomy compares favorably.[112]

Leff performed a prospective study that compared hemorrhoidectomy by means of a carbon dioxide laser (170 patients) with conventional, closed hemorrhoidectomy (56 patients).[145] The author observed no differences with respect to pain, wound healing, or complication rate. Similarly, Senagore and colleagues performed a prospective, randomized trial comparing sharp dissection using a scalpel with that of the contact Nd:YAG laser.[240] Both techniques involved the standard, Ferguson-closed hemorrhoidectomy in a total of 86 patients. There were no significant differences between the groups, except that there was actually more inflammation and a greater incidence of dehiscence with the laser procedure. Because of the increased cost for the laser group, there was a significant price differential also. The authors concluded that the therapeutic efficacy and cost-benefit ratio with the application of lasers to the treatment of hemorrhoids could not be supported.

Comment

In some of the earlier writing on the application of lasers, those who have had the most experience with laser hemorrhoidectomy seem to be the same people who previously had been the enthusiastic advocates of cryosurgery. I do not mean to imply criticism, merely skepticism. It is alleged to be less painful, but there is little documentation to support this claim. It assuredly requires specialized, expensive equipment that mandates a period of education and is not without unique risk. As with all laser applications, safety is an important concern. In light of the dearth of recent publications on this subject, I am not motivated to abandon the technique that has served me, most other surgeons, and patients so effectively—that is, conventional excisional (scissors or knife) hemorrhoidectomy—although stapled hemorrhoidopexy is now quite tempting (see the following).

Stapled Hemorrhoidopexy

There has truly been a renascent interest in surgical hemorrhoidectomy since the introduction of the circular stapling device for the treatment of hemorrhoid prolapse by Longo in 1998.[152] A plethora of publications have appeared in the past few years on this approach, primarily from Europe and Asia, but more recently in the United States.[26,59,77,86,111,130,165,192,203,205,223,246,270]

In accordance with recommendations proposed in the 1993 by the Standards Task Force of the American Society of Colon and Rectal Surgeons on the treatment of hemorrhoids,[249] as well as the reported complications,[42,50,103,159,160,170,218] it was thought prudent to examine this new modality in light of the publicity, both within the profession and in the lay press. An international working party was convened in July, 2001. This consisted of 11 individuals with experience in the performance of the hemorrhoid operation by means of the circular stapler (Figure 8-50), the so-called "stapled hemorrhoidectomy." The conference resulted in the development of a consensus paper to establish the criteria for performing this procedure.[56] The following were the recommendations:

Name of Procedure

■ Stapled hemorrhoidopexy

The panel believed that the operation is *not* a hemorrhoidectomy. Neither anal mucosa nor hemorrhoidal tissue is removed in a properly performed procedure.

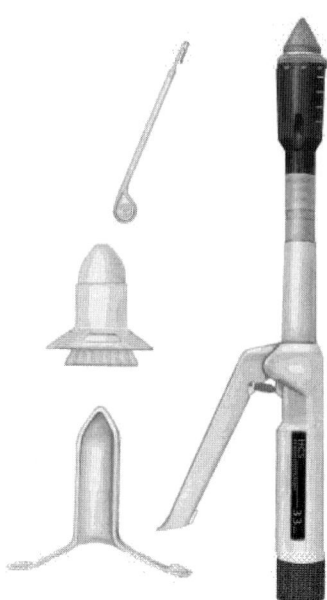

FIGURE 8-50. Proximate HCS procedure for prolapse and hemorrhoids (PPH) set with hemorrhoid circular stapler (HCS33), circular anal dilator (CAD33), purse-string suture anoscope, and suture threader (ST100). (Courtesy of Ethicon Endo-Surgery, Inc., Cincinnati, OH.)

Therefore, the term, "stapled hemorrhoidectomy," should not be applied.

Indications

- Prolapsing hemorrhoids requiring manual reduction (grade III)
- Uncomplicated hemorrhoids, irreducible by the patient but reducible at surgery (grade IV)
- Irreducible hemorrhoids at surgery but by a modified surgical technique (see later)
- Selected prolapsing hemorrhoids with spontaneous reduction (grade II)
- Failure to alleviate hemorrhoidal symptoms by other methods (e.g., rubber band ligation)

Issues and Concerns (Different from Those of Conventional Hemorrhoidectomy)

- Anal intercourse (male or female)
- Anal fissure
- Anal fistula
- Skin tags
- Hypertrophied anal papillae
- Thrombosis
- Preexisting sphincter injury or loss
- Excessive rectal mucosal prolapse

Anal intercourse is a unique concern. Although the staples generally slough out or ultimately become completely buried within the mucosa and submucosa, there still remains a small risk of penile injury with anal inter-

course during the first several months following operation. *Anal fissure* is traditionally managed at the time of conventional hemorrhoidectomy by sphincterotomy at one of the pile sites. Because no wound is created within the anal canal by stapled hemorrhoidopexy, a concomitant or independent procedure would be necessary (if indicated). As with anal fissure, concomitant *anal fistula* requires a procedure that could not be performed at the site of hemorrhoid removal. The surgeon is advised to use his or her good judgment as to the appropriateness of concomitant stapled hemorrhoidopexy when this condition is present. *Skin tags* and *hypertrophied papillae* need to be managed individually (if indicated).

The presence of *acute thrombosis* is a very real concern if a stapled hemorrhoidopexy is to be performed. It is strongly recommended that the thrombotic area be incised and removed if this procedure is to be undertaken.

Preexisting sphincter injury or loss and *anal incontinence* were considered by the panel to be very real concerns if stapled hemorrhoidopexy is to be performed. The reason is that the operation requires the insertion of a relatively large circular anal dilator [CAD (33 mm)]. The stretching associated with the placement of this instrument can lead to further impairment of bowel control. Finally, *excessive mucosal prolapse* is considered a concern because of the inability of the instrument to adequately encompass all of the redundant tissue (see later).

Contraindications

- Abscess
- Gangrene
- Anal stenosis
- Full-thickness rectal prolapse

Performance of stapled hemorrhoidopexy in the presence of *gangrenous* or *infected tissue* is absolutely contraindicated because the operation fails to remove the source of sepsis. Furthermore, opening additional tissue planes may expose the patient to pelvic sepsis and to the possibility of Fournier's gangrene (see later). The presence of *anal stenosis* is a contraindication because of one's inability to insert the CAD. *Full-thickness rectal prolapse* is not appropriately treated by this operation. There is no evidence, even anecdotal, that the operation can ameliorate true procidentia.

Informed Consent (Unique to the Procedure)

- Urgency and rectal irritation
- Pain and swelling (thrombosis of residual hemorrhoids)
- Anastomotic stenosis
- Anal intercourse

Because the procedure is undertaken within the rectum, itself, and in effect is associated with a staple line that is somewhat analogous to that of a distal rectal anastomosis, patients may experience *urgency* to defecate and may have transient problems with *discharge* and *irritation*. With respect to *pain* and *swelling*, especially as a consequence of thrombosed hemorrhoids that develop during the postoperative period, this must be considered a complication of the procedure. Because the dissection is not undertaken within the anal canal and hemorrhoidal veins are *not* removed, stapled hemorrhoidopexy can lead to this complication in the occasional patient. *Anastomotic stenosis* has been reported but should be quite unusual with the PPH instrument, given its relatively large diameter. The major precaution is that the surgeon must create the staple line *above the anal canal* (see later).

Patient Position (Surgeon's Preference)

Surgeons should choose the position with which they are most comfortable as if conventional hemorrhoidectomy were to be performed.

Anesthesia (Surgeon's Preference)

■ Local (conscious sedation is required)
■ Regional
■ General

If local anesthesia is elected, conscious sedation is strongly recommended. Placement of the purse-string suture into the rectal mucosa can be associated with discomfort that would not necessarily be adequately controlled by means of a local anesthetic alone.

Technique

The hemorrhoids are assessed, and the CAD is inserted and anchored to the skin by means of a heavy suture on a cutting needle; the procedure is aborted if stenosis precludes passage (Figure 8-51). Countertraction is applied to the skin to facilitate insertion. It is important to reduce the external component as much as possible manually. The purse-string suture anoscope is introduced through the CAD. Its rotation allows the placement of a circumferential pursestring at the correct height (3 to 4 cm above the dentate line) and depth (only mucosa and submucosa). Small bites placed close together are advised. A 2–0 monofilament suture on a 25- to 30-mm curved needle is used (Figure 8-52). One must confirm the completeness of the purse-string to ensure that there are no gaps or "dog ears" present. The fully opened stapler head is then inserted through the purse-string (Figure 8-53). The purse-string is then tied with just one throw knot. One then draws the two tails of the suture through the lateral channels in the head of the anvil with the suture threader (Figure 8-53). The purse-string is secured under direct visualization. The tails are knotted externally or clamped with a forceps Figure 8-54). The sta-

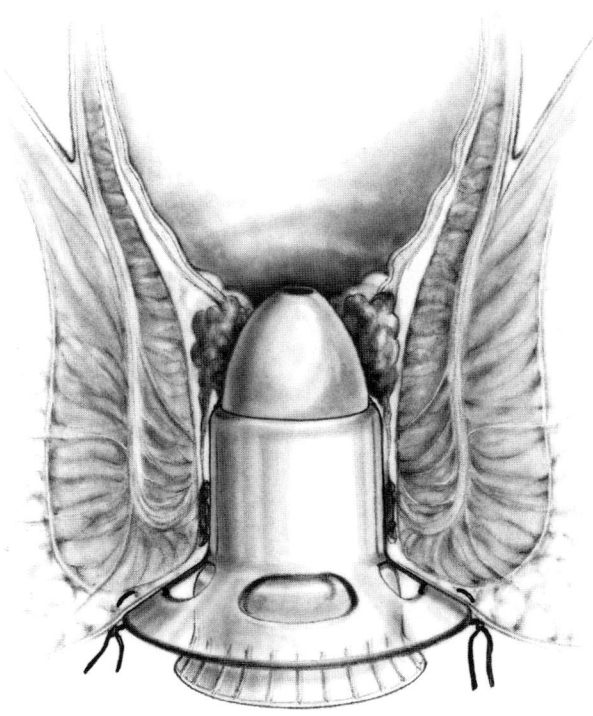

FIGURE 8-51. The circular anal dilator (CAD33) is inserted, and the obturator is removed. The prolapse is reduced and the dentate line identified. The device should remain in position throughout the procedure and may be secured to the skin with sutures.

pler is aligned along the axis of the anal canal and closed while maintaining moderate downward tension on the purse-string (Figure 8-55). At the end of the closure the 4-cm mark should be at the level of the anal verge. If the patient is a woman, it is advisable to pass a finger into the vagina, checking the posterior vaginal wall to be certain that it has not been incorporated. The stapler is then fired. The head is then opened and the stapler removed. At this point one should carefully inspect the staple line for bleeding and reinforce with absorbable sutures if necessary (Figure 8-56). It is not unusual that a suture or two may be required (at least 50% of cases). Electrocoagulation should be used only with caution because of the presence of the staples The anal mucosa with both internal and even external hemorrhoids is pulled cephalad. The mucosal sleeve should be inspected to confirm that the technique has been properly performed. The specimen may be submitted for pathologic evaluation if judged necessary or if required by departmental or hospital policy.

Because no procedure is performed within the anal canal with the stapled hemorrhoidopexy, concomitant ex-

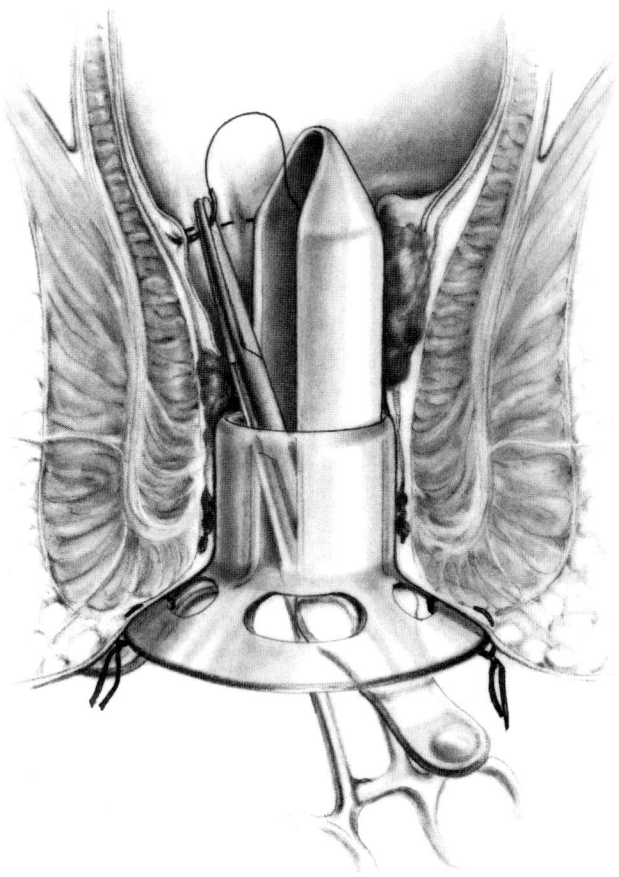

FIGURE 8-52. Placement of the purse-string suture 3 to 4 cm above the dentate line.

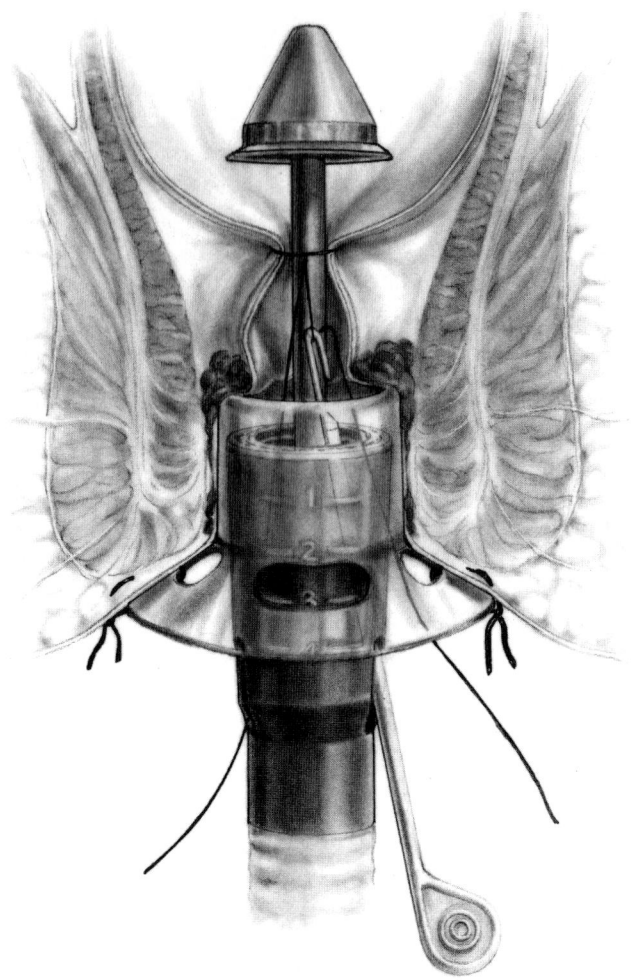

FIGURE 8-53. The circular stapler (HCS33) is fully opened prior to insertion. One throw knot secures the purse-string suture. By using the suture threader, the tails are drawn through the lateral channels.

cision may be indicated for skin tags, papillae, or thrombosis (see previous discussion). An internal anal sphincterotomy would, of necessity, require either an open or closed procedure in accordance with the surgeon's personal preference.

Credentialing

Since the 1970s, numerous innovations have been developed in the field of colon and rectal surgery alone. Examples are colonoscopy and colonoscopy/polypectomy, stapled anastomotic techniques, intestinal reservoirs, and laparoscopic colectomy. There is ample precedent for determining the means for proper introduction of new technology. The following represents the consensus of the Working Party as minimal requirements. These are not meant to be standards but recommended guidelines.

- Experience with anorectal surgery and an understanding of anorectal anatomy should be a requisite.
- Experience with circular stapling devices is essential.
- The surgeon should attend a formal course—including lectures, videos, the application of the instrument in models, and observation of the operation performed by a surgeon recognized by his or her peers—leading

ultimately to undertaking the procedure while being observed by an experienced surgeon. Following satisfactory completion of the foregoing, independent responsibility should be determined by each individual's surgical department.

Complications

There have been some disconcerting complications that are unique to the procedure of stapled hemorrhoidopexy as well as a suggestion of an increased risk of septic complications. These include rectal perforation, retropneumoperitoneum, and pneumomediastinum,[218] pelvic sepsis,[160,170] persistent severe pain and fecal urgency,[42] rectal perforation,[284] rectal stricture,[206] rectal obstruction,[50] and rectovaginal fistula. Sepsis has been recognized, albeit rarely, as a complication of conventional hemorrhoidectomy, however. An increased incidence of inconsequential bacteremia has been reported in a prospective, randomized trial.[159] Some have recommended the routine application of pro-

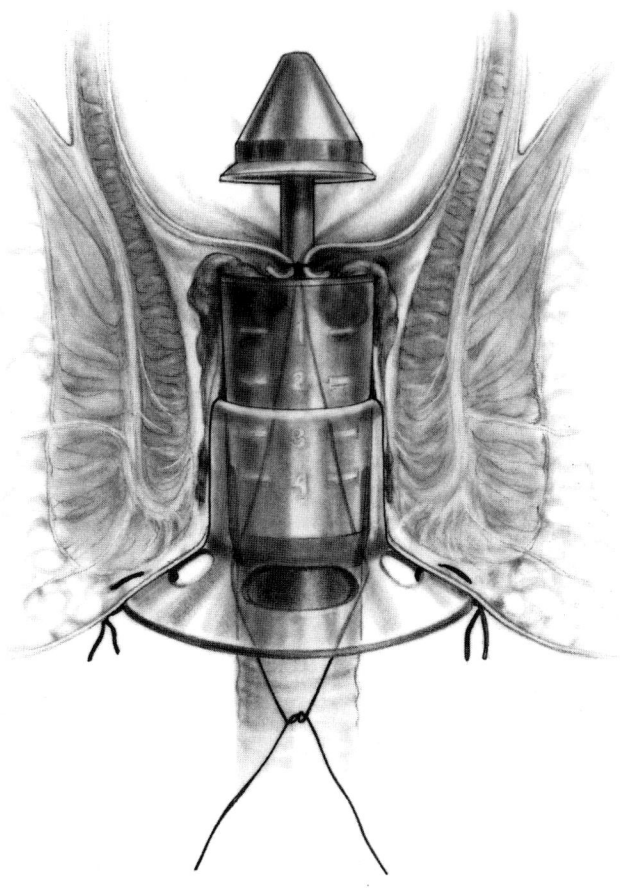

FIGURE 8-54. External knotting or clamping of suture tails.

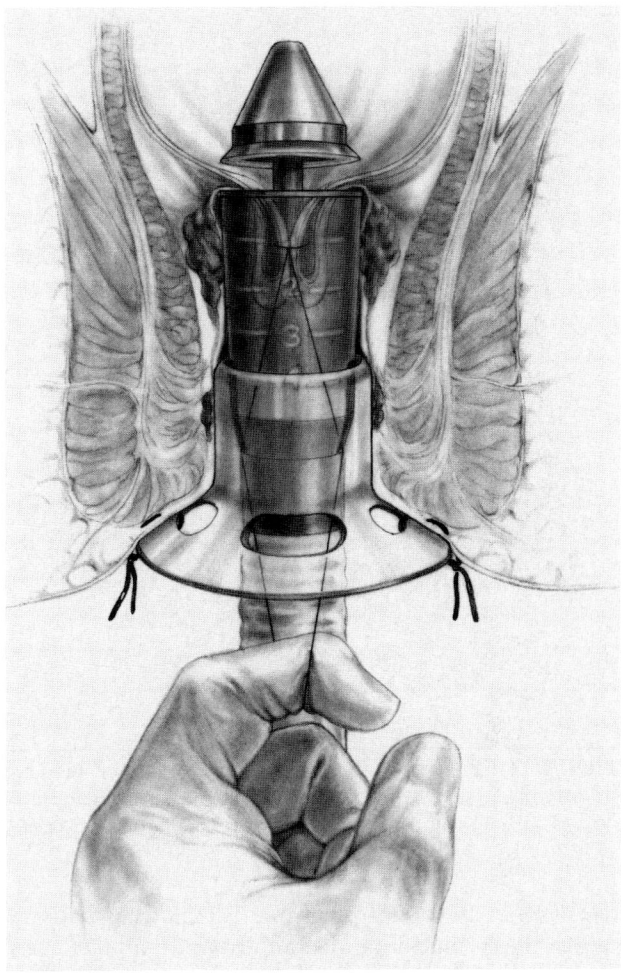

FIGURE 8-55. The instrument is closed and fired with continued downward traction on the purse-string suture. This draws the mucosa into the head of the stapler.

phylactic antibiotics, but there is no evidence to suggest that this is appropriate or likely to be helpful. It has become abundantly clear that this procedure should be performed only by surgeons experienced with the technique and who are truly mindful of the potential complications.

Results

There have been many published studies, often prospectively randomized, that are worthy of mentioning. In every study comparing this approach with hemorrhoidectomy by any method, there is a highly significant reduction in postoperative pain.[59,86,111,125,130,165,192,223] This also translates to earlier return to normal activity and to greater patient satisfaction.[223,246] This is not surprising in light of the fact that there is no "cutting" within the anal canal or in perianal skin. What is being excised is a circumferential column of mucosa and submucosa above the anal canal. There may, however, be an increased risk of postoperative bleeding according to some investigators.[279] Others opine that there should be no such concern.[111,223] There is also some reports of fecal urgency, late-onset pain, and the possibility of having to undergo a secondary procedure at a later date, especially because of a sympto-

matic external component[41] or recurrent prolapse.[192] Short and intermediate follow-up studies (up to 1 year) are favorable,[26,86,203] but long-term results are truly needed.

Care Following Hemorrhoidectomy (An Opinion)

Each surgeon has his or her personal preference as to the follow-up management after any surgical procedure. Hemorrhoid operations are no exceptions. Rather than express the whole range of options, I will simply provide my personal preferences. The reader should understand, however, that surgeons who are otherwise quite objective, sensitive, and reasonable and who are worthy of great respect become quite exorcised over this issue. They will vigorously defend their personal approaches to postoperative management, virtually unto death. Nevertheless, I shall charge on.

Anal dressings are indeed painful. I try to avoid them and simply use a pad or panty liner for the expected

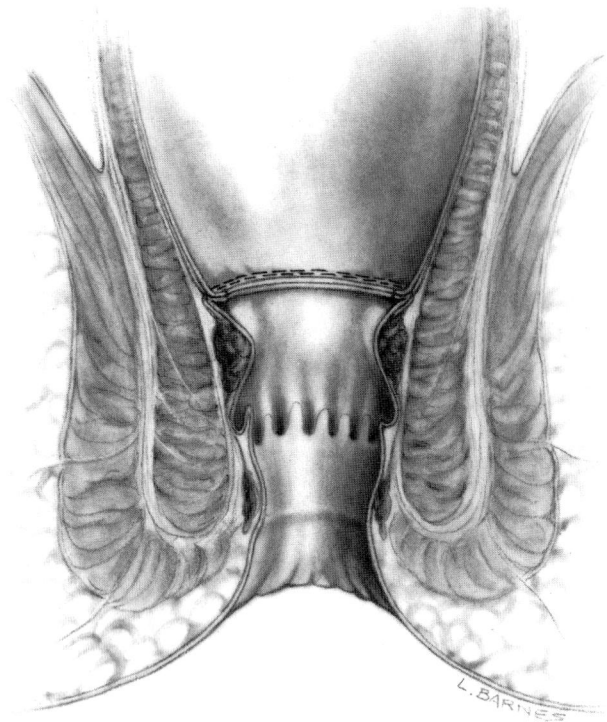

FIGURE 8-56. A strip of mucosa above the hemorrhoids has been removed with resultant "anal lifting." The circular staple line, ideally at least 2 cm proximal to the dentate line, is evident.

discharge. Any dressing, however, should ideally be removed the evening of the operation, and 20-minute warm sitz baths can be commenced. A warm water bath, three or four times a day, is probably the most salutary experience possible for an individual who has undergone anal surgery. A topical cream or lotion, such as Tucks, Balneol, Proctodon, Anusol, Analpram, or Prax (among others) may be applied. I avoid local anesthetic creams unless the patient is obstreperous, but ointments should not be used. They are too painful to remove. The cream should be left at the bedside, used liberally and applied frequently. A small dressing such as a Tucks pad, also kept at the bedside, helps to prevent soiling of sheets and garments. Tape should be avoided. Medications include a prescription analgesic (ideally a nonconstipating agent), a bulking agent (I prefer Konsyl), a stool softener or a stimulant laxative if necessary.

The patient is not seen until 3 or 4 weeks after discharge, at which time the wounds are usually healed. By delaying a follow-up visit until this time, one is protected from much complaining. It is much more pleasant to talk with a grateful patient who has hopefully suppressed the memory of any suffering. To undertake a digital examination at an earlier time in order to evaluate the possibility of a stricture, or worse, to dilate the anus, is cruel and inhuman punishment. A properly performed operation is

not likely to result in stricture formation; thus, weekly digital examinations are not necessary and merely serve to cause a mass exodus from one's waiting area.

Complications of Surgical Hemorrhoidectomy

To avoid the pitfalls of hemorrhoid surgery, conscientious effort is required—not only with respect to meticulous surgical technique, but also with regard to a compulsive approach to postoperative management. The following is a partial list of the potential problems of surgical hemorrhoidectomy:

- Pain
- Urinary retention
- Urinary tract infection
- Constipation
- Fecal impaction
- Hemorrhage
- Infection and sepsis
- Anal tags
- Mucosal prolapse
- Mucosal ectropion
- Rectal stricture
- Anal stenosis
- Anal fissure
- Pseudopolyps
- Epidermal cysts
- Anal fistula
- Pruritus ani
- Fecal incontinence
- Recurrent hemorrhoids

Pain

Although pain is not actually a complication of surgery but is an anticipated consequence, it is nonetheless the single most important reason that patients avoid hemorrhoidectomy. I am certain that it is because of this fear that so few surgeons elect the operation for themselves, often despite having a severe hemorrhoid problem. It has been mentioned previously that internal anal sphincterotomy or sphincter stretch concomitant with hemorrhoidectomy had been thought by some to ameliorate this concern, but I believe that this has been disproved to most surgeons' satisfaction. Sphincter stretch, particularly in the older patient, may be associated with the complications of soilage and incontinence. Internal anal sphincterotomy likewise can cause similar problems (see Chapter 9). Mortensen and colleagues performed a randomized study comparing surgical hemorrhoidectomy with and without anal dilatation.[174] They concluded that the combination did not improve cure rates compared with hemorrhoidectomy alone, but the addition of a sphincter stretch increased the risk for continence disturbances.[174] As mentioned previously, in the absence of a fissure or some other pathologic condition, I do not advocate either of these additional procedures.

A great deal of emphasis has been given to the management of pain in the posthemorrhoidectomy patient, not only because of the pain itself, but because of the role it plays in causing urinary complications (see the following section). Recent literature abounds with newer alternatives in the management of discomfort. Epidural morphine has been employed for analgesia after hemorrhoidectomy at some centers,[141] but with the requirement for early discharge, this approach has become a moot issue except for the individual who remains in the hospital. An ambulatory alternative that has been promoted is the STA Cath attachable infusion catheter. This consists of a special catheter that is sutured into the anal canal. A topical anesthetic medication is delivered to the affected area by means of an infusion pump (Advanced Infusion, Inc., Tempe, AZ). Injection of a long-acting local anesthetic (ropivacaine) has also been proved effective in at least one prospective, randomized, double-blind study.[266]

Goldstein and colleagues have employed a subcutaneous morphine pump in postoperative pain management.[96] Although this was not a controlled study in the true sense, the authors concluded that the combination of *outpatient hemorrhoidectomy* and the pump was cost-effective when compared with the inpatient stay.

Chiu and co-workers performed a prospective, randomized trial using transcutaneous electrical nerve stimulation in one arm of the study.[45] They found a statistically significant improvement in pain relief and in the frequency of urinary retention when compared with individuals receiving a more conventional pain management alternative.

Ketorolac tromethamine (Toradol) has also been advocated following anal surgery.[186,217] Many surgeons believe this is the most effective medication alternative for the posthemorrhoidectomy patient. One option is to inject 60 mg (2 ml) directly into the anal sphincter musculature at the time of its exposure. Studies suggest that there is a much reduced incidence not only of pain, but also of urinary retention.[186,217] Oral ketorolac is also quite effective following discharge when administered orally for pain control.

Another pain management option is the application of transdermal fentanyl (Duragesic).[136] Fentanyl has been recommended as an effective analgesic alternative that essentially improves the transition to outpatient management with a nonnarcotic pain medication. In a letter to the editor, however, criticism was expressed for encouraging the use of a "contraindicated" medication.[29] It was believed that there is an unacceptably high incidence of hypoventilation with possible respiratory depression. In fact, recommendations against this use have been included with the package insert by the manufacturer. Metronidazole (Flagyl) has been recommended as an effective medication for pain following hemorrhoidectomy, but a randomized, double-blind trial failed to support this conclusion.[18] Nitroglycerin ointment (0.2%) and Nitroderm TTS band application have been demonstrated in prospective, randomized trials, to reduce pain after hemorrhoidectomy.[60,270] Headache, however, is a potential problem. Finally, Davies and colleagues undertook a double-blind study of 50 consecutive patients who underwent Milligan-Morgan hemorrhoidectomy and assigned an internal sphincter injection of 0.4 mL of a solution containing either botulinum toxin (20 U; Botox) or normal saline.[63] Those who received the toxin injection had a significant pain reduction.

Opinion

It is my opinion that a simple and reasonably effective pain management approach is either ketorolac (Toradol) or an oral narcotic analgesic medication, administered in adequate doses and given frequently, such as oxycodone (Percocet) or hydrocodone (Vicodin). I fully recognize that the latter medications are quite constipating. Therefore, it is very important to provide a laxative to deal with this expected consequence.

Urinary Retention

Urinary retention is the most common complication following hemorrhoidectomy. Bleday and co-workers reported a 20% incidence of postoperative urinary complications.[32] Factors often held responsible include the following:

- Fluid overload
- Spinal anesthesia
- Rectal pain and spasm
- High ligation of the hemorrhoidal pedicle
- Rough handling of tissue
- Heavy suture material
- Numerous sutures
- Rectal packing
- Tight, bulky dressings
- Anticholinergics
- Narcotics[62,139,178,229]

Bailey and Ferguson demonstrated the effectiveness of fluid restriction in a carefully controlled, prospective randomized study of 500 patients.[17] One group was given free access to oral fluids after the operation. The other was permitted neither coffee nor tea, and oral fluids were limited to 250 mL until voiding was spontaneous or until a catheter was inserted. Both groups were treated identically in all respects except for the postoperative fluid intake. Each patient was instructed to empty the bladder before going to the operating room. Anesthesiologists were asked to limit intravenous fluids to the amount they considered a safe minimum. Patients were not routinely catheterized; this was carried out only in the case of bladder distension diagnosed by a physician.

Only 3.5% of the patients in the group having limited fluids required catheterization, versus 14.9% with unlimited fluids. No recognized postoperative complication was attributable to fluid restriction. The authors concluded that the postoperative catheterization rate was dramatically reduced by restricting fluids and delaying catheterization until the bladder was distended.

Scoma reported a similar study in an effort to eliminate this common postoperative complication.[237] The charts of 100 patients who underwent hemorrhoidectomy before the trial were reviewed. A second group consisted of 100 consecutive patients undergoing hemorrhoidectomy procedures performed by the author using local anesthesia (i.e., bupivacaine hydrochloride with epinephrine and hyaluronidase). None received atropine or scopolamine. The anesthesiologist was asked to give diazepam (Valium) intravenously with small doses of thiopental sodium (Pentothal), if necessary, at the beginning of the local infiltration. Amounts of intraoperative fluids were limited to 200 mL, and the infusion was terminated as the dressings were being applied.

Postoperatively, 100 mg of meperidine hydrochloride (Demerol) was given intramuscularly 4 hours after hemorrhoidectomy was completed and every 2 hours thereafter as needed. Patients were told to take only sips of water until they voided. Nurses catheterized the patient only after approval by the physician and were instructed not to urge the patient to void. The morning after operation, the patient sat in a bath of hot water and was encouraged to void. Those who did not urinate immediately in the bath stood under a hot shower to encourage voiding.

In the first group, 52% of the patients were catheterized, and in the second group, no one was catheterized. Of those in the second group, 86% voided before they took the hot bath, and the remaining voided in the bath or shower.

The incidence of urinary retention is not generally believed to be altered by the prophylactic administration of bethanechol chloride (Urecholine).[35] However, Gottesman and colleagues found that this drug, given in a dose of 10 mg subcutaneously, significantly lowered the incidence of postoperative urinary retention after anorectal surgery.[98] Prophylactic α-adrenergic blockade has failed to prevent this complication, as has the administration of anxiolytic agents.[40,98]

It is important to recognize that all reports indicate that with the promotion of ambulatory anorectal surgery the incidence of urinary retention is significantly lower than that of the historical in-hospital rate. It has also been observed that the use of local anesthesia is associated with a significantly lower incidence of urinary retention when compared with spinal anesthesia.[81] Hoff and colleagues noted that only one of their 190 patients required catheterization following ambulatory surgical hemorrhoidectomy.[113]

Comment

Pain and fluid overload are the primary factors that cause urinary retention. If pain medication is inadequate, the patient cannot relax the sphincter mechanism sufficiently to urinate—it simply hurts too much. Clearly, one must limit fluid intake. This requires education of the anesthesiologist, the nurses, and the house officers. Threatening the patient with a catheter or leaving standing orders for catheterization is a self-fulfilling prophesy for its subsequent insertion. The minimal intravenous infusion necessary is given during the operation, and the infusion is terminated in the recovery room. If hospital regulations require that an intravenous line must be maintained, a heparin lock will suffice. Oral fluids are restricted until the following morning. Finally, patients are not routinely catheterized; this is undertaken only when the bladder is distended or if the patient complains, and then only after examination by a physician.

The policy in many ambulatory surgical facilities is that the patient must void before discharge. I overrule any such dictum and mandate that the nurses not even ask about urinating, much less insist upon it. Later that day or evening, or the following morning, with the commencement of sitz baths or hot showers, virtually every patient will void. Once the nursing service (and the patient) has been educated, the incidence of retention and the associated complication of urinary tract infection will be virtually eliminated. However, if urinary retention does develop, the inconvenience, discomfort and anxiety are, for the patient, not inconsiderable.

If catheterization becomes necessary (in the hospital, in the emergency room, at the patient's home, or in the physician's office), it should be performed with a balloon catheter. If the residual urine is determined to be greater than 500 mL, the catheter should be left in place for 24 hours because it is unlikely that the patient will be able to void subsequently. Conversely, with a residual of less than 500 mL, the catheter can be removed with the reasonable expectation that spontaneous urination will occur.

Urinary Tract Infection

Urinary tract infection is usually a direct consequence of catheterization for urinary retention. The most common offending organisms are coliform bacteria. Appropriate antibiotics and catheter removal usually result in rapid resolution, but chronic infection, cystitis, and pyelonephritis can be late sequelae. Here again, the value of avoiding urinary retention cannot be overestimated.

Constipation

Patients who undergo hemorrhoidectomy await their postoperative bowel evacuation less than enthusiastically and always view the possibility of an enema intended to facilitate this function with apprehension. Constipation after anorectal surgery must be either relieved effectively or prevented, because if it is untreated, it may lead to fecal impaction—a matter of special concern in this group of patients. Despite awareness of this possibility, as long as 72 hours may elapse before one considers the value of administering a laxative agent.[178,262] Factors that contribute to this delay include the effects of analgesic medications given before or after the operation, the consequences of the anesthetic, itself, and local physiologic dysfunction resulting from surgical manipulation, as well as the tendency for the patient not to ambulate and the fear of painful defecation. A history of irregular bowel function and colonic hypomotility may complicate the problem further.

Johnson and colleagues prospectively randomized 30 hemorrhoidectomy patients into two groups: one received wheat fiber and the other a laxative regimen of sterculia, magnesium sulfate, and mineral oil.[122] Those who received the fiber had a significantly shorter hospital stay, less painful bowel actions, and less discharge and soiling.

I evaluated the efficacy of senna (Senokot S) tablets in a prospective fashion on 50 patients who underwent anal operations in an in-hospital setting.[53] Patients took two tablets with a full glass of water on the evening of the first day after operation. If no bowel movement occurred by the evening of the second day, the dose was changed to two tablets at bedtime and two tablets the following morning. If no stool was passed by the evening of the third day of treatment, the dose at bedtime was increased to three tablets. Enemas or other suitable forms of treatment were administered if function of the bowel was not restored by the evening of the fourth day. One of the options was to increase the dose of the test medication to a maximum of four tablets. No other laxatives or stool modifiers were taken during the trial period. The test preparation was administered for a maximum of 4 days. All patients achieved bowel movements during the study, and none required enemas. None passed hard stools on the day of release from the hospital.

Comment

As with the management of urinary retention, the patient can no longer be permitted the luxury of remaining in the hospital to await the first bowel action. Discharge instructions should include a bowel management program conducive to satisfactory bowel evacuation (e.g., a bulk laxative and a stimulant laxative). I believe that a

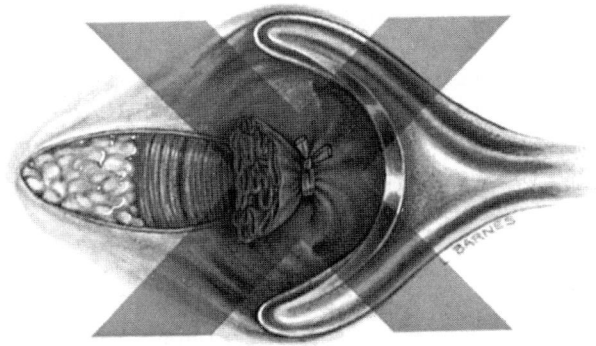

FIGURE 8-57. Incorrect mass ligation technique of the hemorrhoid pedicle. The pedicle must be suture ligated to limit the risk for early postoperative hemorrhage.

stimulant laxative should be given on the evening of the operation and continued in increasing doses until defecation occurs, as described above. By the third postoperative day with no bowel action, a vigorous laxative, such as Fleet phospho-soda or magnesium citrate, should be considered. If no bowel movement occurs by the fourth day, a gentle enema may be administered. If this fails to be rewarding, the patient will require reevaluation for the possibility of fecal impaction.

Hemorrhage

Massive hemorrhage that occurs in the recovery room is always the result of a technical error and can usually be attributed to improper or inadequate ligation of the hemorrhoid pedicle. This most commonly occurs if the pedicle is simply hand-tied rather than suture-ligated (Figure 8-57). Such a complication requires emergency surgical intervention. This should be quite unusual when Ferguson's hemorrhoidectomy is performed, because care is taken in closing the wounds. Although management of active bleeding soon after hemorrhoidectomy may include submucosal injection with 1 to 2 ml of 1:100,000 epinephrine, direct pressure with a finger or gauze, and the use of topical epinephrine, returning the patient promptly to the operating room for direct visualization of the operative site with suture ligation is the most effective, most reassuring, and the safest alternative.[183]

Delayed hemorrhage (i.e., 3 to 14 days postoperatively) is probably the result of sepsis in the pedicle or erosion of the suture. This occurs in approximately 2% of hemorrhoidectomies.[32] Patients may experience renewed slight bleeding, the passage of clots, or massive hemorrhage. Bleeding 1 week or longer following surgery, when the patient has previously ceased bleeding, warrants examination. Treatment varies from expectant management to in-hospital observation, transfusion, and resuture. Rosen and colleagues identified 27 patients with the complication of delayed hemorrhage over an 8-year period (1983 to 1990), an incidence of 0.8%.[221] The mean interval from the operation to hemorrhage was 6 days. Three fourths of the patients were treated by bedside anal packing, 18% by observation alone, and two individuals required suture ligation. Although initial packing was successful in all those so treated, 15% required repeated operation because of rebleeding. The packing material employed was a rolled, slightly moistened, absorbable gelatin sponge (Gelfoam). Basso and Pescatori observed an incidence of delayed bleeding of approximately 2%, with a mean interval from the operation to hemorrhage of 4 days.[24] They employed a Foley catheter technique for tamponade of the bleeding point, with complete success in all five individuals so treated. In my opinion, delayed hemorrhage usually is not a preventable complication.

Local Infection and Overwhelming Sepsis

It seems surprising that, because hemorrhoidectomy is carried out in a field with numerous and varied bacterial organisms present, there is not a higher incidence of septic complications following the operation. As Lal and Levitan have pointed out, hemorrhoidectomy may be followed by transient bacteremia and low-grade fever as a result of the relatively constant release of bacteria into the bloodstream from a feeding focus.[142] For example, an 8.5% rate of bacteremia has been reported following proctoscopic examination of patients with no evidence of lower intestinal disease.[146] However, despite the presence of potentially virulent organisms (e.g., clostridia, anaerobic streptococci, bacteroides, *Escherichia coli*), local infection and more generalized septic problems are indeed extremely rare.

It has been hypothesized that the major venous drainage of the rectum, by passing through the superior hemorrhoidal veins into the portal system, is cleared of organisms by the reticuloendothelial system of the liver.[146] This hepatic clearance, by effectively removing the bacteria released into the circulation, may be important in minimizing the impact of rectal colonic flora in the systemic circulation and may be the reason that infection is so uncommon, although liver abscess following hemorrhoidectomy has been reported.[195] Guy and Seow-Choen performed a Medline search to identify septic complications after surgical hemorrhoidectomy.[102] As opposed to the case reports of sepsis following stapled mucosectomy and rubber band ligation, there simply is a dearth of reported cases of overwhelming sepsis with conventional hemorrhoidectomy despite the well-recognized transient bacteremia. There have been, however, isolated reports of Fournier's gangrene as a consequence of this operation, but this complication appears to be associated with individuals who are in an immunocompromised state.[49]

Comment

Because sitz baths are a routine part of the postoperative management, most skin problems (e.g., cellulitis, abscess) theoretically might be treated in an essentially prophylactic manner. In an experience of more than 1,000 hemorrhoidectomies, I cannot recall ever seeing even cellulitis, much less draining an abscess. However, one must be circumspect if surgery on the anus is contemplated in an indivudal with acquired immunodeficiency syndrome (AIDS) or with leukemia, or in someone with agranulocytosis, receiving chemotherapy, or is immunocompromised.

Anal Tag

Anal tags, which can interfere with proper cleansing of the anus and thus lead to skin irritation, can usually be avoided by excising redundant skin at the time of operation. I suspect, however, that tags more often than not are the result of the manner in which the wounds heal, perhaps analogous to keloid formation in other incision sites. Bothersome tags can be excised as an office procedure if symptoms warrant.

Mucosal Prolapse

Inadequate removal of redundant or mobile rectal mucosa at the time of hemorrhoidectomy may result in mucosal prolapse. Patients may complain of a lump that requires manual reduction. Problems with mucous discharge and pruritic symptoms are common.

Treatment usually consists of rubber ring ligation of the prolapsed mucosa. If there seems to be extensive or circumferential involvement, the surgeon should conduct the examination while the patient strains on the toilet in order to look for procidentia.

Prevention of this complication requires that the surgeon remove any redundant mucosa at the time of hemorrhoidectomy. It will be interesting to note whether there is an increased incidence of recurrent prolapse following stapled hemorrhoidopexy.

Ectropion

Because the mucosa is more mobile than the perianal skin, the tendency for mucosal descent is greater than the likelihood of the skin ascending to reline the denuded anal canal (Figure 8-48). If redundant mucosa above the site of the excised hemorrhoid tissue is not properly anchored to the underlying internal sphincter, the mucosa

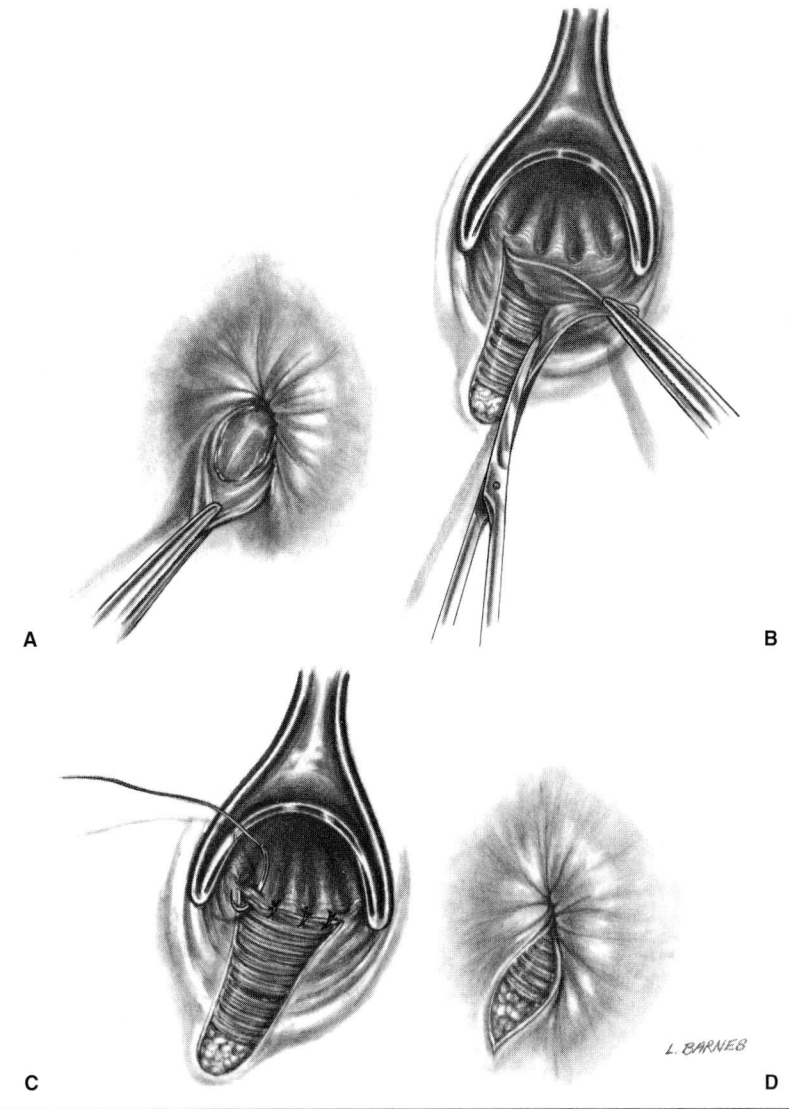

FIGURE 8-58. Treatment of mucosal ectropion. **(A)** The mucosa projects in one quadrant. **(B)** The mucosa is excised. **(C)** The edge of the rectum is sutured to the underlying internal sphincter. **(D)** The wound is left open to granulate.

can heal outside the anal verge (Figure 8-47). If the entire anal canal is removed, and the cut edge of the rectum is sutured to the perianal skin, characteristic Whitehead's deformity may be produced. If the surgeon anchors the mucosa to the skin in one or more quadrants, a partial ectropion may result. Interestingly, Khubchandani has reported treatment of anal stenosis by doing just what has been condemned—advancing the mucosa, albeit not beyond the anal verge.[133] Ectropion can lead to mucous discharge, skin irritation, and pruritus ani.[22,99] Prevention requires excising the redundant mucosa and anchoring the cut edge as described.

Treatment of an ectropion that is evident in only one quadrant is shown in Figure 8-58. As long as no stricture is present, a simple excision and transverse suture of the rectum to the underlying internal anal sphincter will suffice. The open wound should heal without the mucosal extrusion. An alternative approach is to perform an anoplasty (discussed later).

Anal Stricture

A considerable area of mucosa and anoderm may be denuded when the physician attempts to remove extensive, encircling hemorrhoids. If hemorrhoids are present in many areas, only minimal sections of intact, elastic anal tissue may be left following excision. With progressive

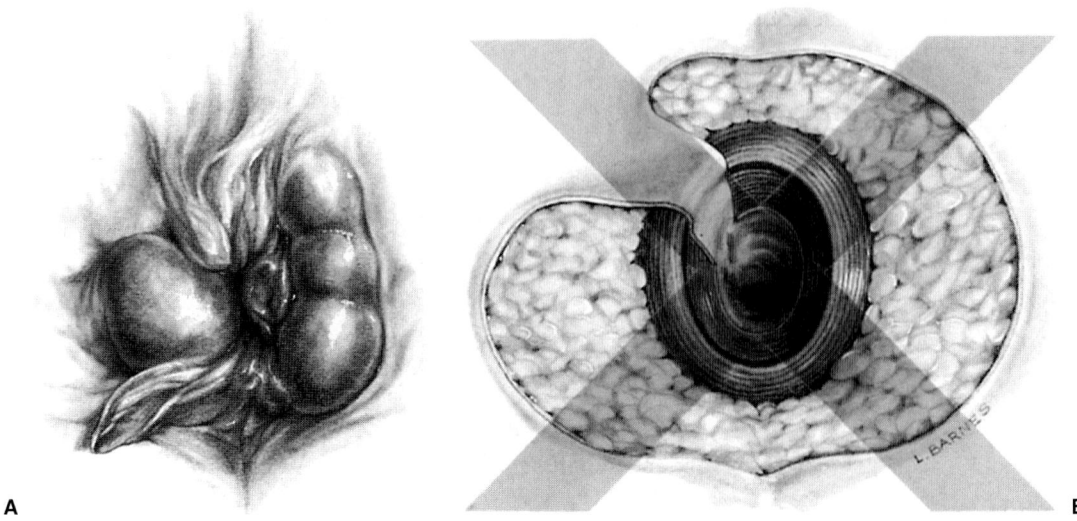

FIGURE 8-59. (**A**) Artist's conception of extensive circumferential hemorrhoids. (**B**) Virtual complete removal of the hemorrhoids with an inadequate attempt to preserve a mucocutaneous bridge.

healing, fibrous scar tissue may proliferate and contract the anorectal outlet.[269] When healing is complete, a narrow, foreshortened stenotic orifice may remain.

As with ectropion, anal stenosis is a preventable complication. If adequate skin bridges are preserved, the risk for reducing the circumference of the anal canal is minimized. However, in the presence of gangrenous hemorrhoids, distortion of the anal canal, fibrosis, chronic fissure, external tags, and hypertrophied anal papillae, extensive removal of the anal canal is often necessary to accomplish an adequate hemorrhoidectomy. Under these circumstances, the surgeon has two options: either compromise on the amount of tissue removed and accept the consequences of patient complaints of residual disease or consider the possibility of performing an anoplasty at the time of hemorrhoidectomy.

The physician must attempt to preserve skin bridges; even one bridge is better than none (Figure 8-59). If because of sepsis, sloughing, or radical surgery, the potential for stricture formation becomes evident, digital examination of the rectum is advisable. This is an exception to my approach of not performing rectal examinations on posthemorrhoidectomy patients. It is probably worthwhile to advise insertion of a dilator two or three times daily in patients at risk for stricture (Figure 8-60). Weekly office visits are also suggested. Prevention of anal stricture when there is legitimate justification for concern is, in my opinion, the only indication for frequent digital examinations and the use of a dilator. If the wound heals without a stricture, digital examination and the use of a dilator can be discontinued, usually within 6 to 8 weeks. However, if a healed, fixed stricture develops, I prefer to perform an anoplasty rather than to have the patient use a dilator indefinitely.

Anoplasty

Anoplasty is a procedure whereby perianal skin is moved to cover a defect in the anal canal. This defect is usually the result of an operative procedure, such as excision of a portion or all of the anal canal, hemorrhoidectomy, excision of an anal fissure, or excision of a lesion of the anal canal. Anoplasty may be performed to correct an anal stenosis or coincidentally with repair of a rectovaginal fistula or with sphincteroplasty for sphincteric injury.[54,58,79,116,158,180,189,213,232] The following list summarizes the indications for this procedure:

Indications

Anal stricture
Congenital
Inflammatory (e.g., fistula, abscess)
Trauma
  Operative (e.g., hemorrhoidectomy, fissurectomy, pull-through procedure, excisional procedures)
  Accidental

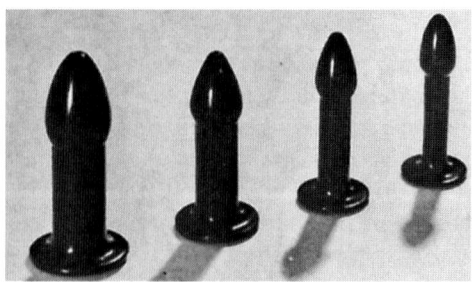

FIGURE 8-60. Young's Bakelite rectal dilators in a set of four adult sizes. (F.E. Young & Co., Highland Park, IL.)

Disuse caused by laxatives, enemas, chronic diarrhea
Coincident with excision of anal lesions
Ulcer
Concomitant with reconstructive anorectal operations
Rectovaginal fistula repair
Anterior fistula in women
Sphincter repair
Congenital anomaly (e.g., imperforate anus, ectopic anus)
Tumor excision

Anal stricture can be one of the most disabling complications of anal surgery or of anal disease. Stenosis can occur as a consequence of numerous conditions:

- Benign and malignant tumors
- Inflammations, especially Crohn's disease
- Congenital anomalies (e.g., ectopic anus and imperforate anus)
- Abuse of laxatives
- Trauma, especially surgical trauma

However, overzealous hemorrhoidectomy continues to be the most common reason that patients require an anoplasty. In the experience of Milsom and Mazier, 88% of 212 patients treated for anal stenosis had a history of prior hemorrhoidectomy.[168]

Symptoms, Findings, and Differential Diagnosis

The most troublesome complaint of patients with anal stenosis is difficulty with defecation. Constipation, obstipation, painful bowel movements, narrow caliber of the stool, abdominal cramping, and bleeding are frequently associated symptoms. The fear of fecal impaction or pain usually causes the patient to rely on daily laxatives or enemas.

Physical examination readily reveals the problem. It may be impossible to perform a digital examination, or only the small finger may be tolerated. Proctosigmoidoscopy and anoscopy require narrow-caliber instruments. If there is any question concerning the etiology of the stenosis or the possibility of a proximal lesion, a barium enema or colonoscopy should be performed, if such examinations are technically possible. Sometimes, it is difficult to distinguish true stenosis with tissue loss from the sphincter spasm associated with an anal fissure. Administration of a local anesthetic may be helpful, but on occasion a general anesthetic may be required. The anesthetic abolishes the spasm associated with an acute fissure but will not produce an increased luminal diameter in a patient with true stenosis.[263]

It is important to ascertain the cause of the stricture in order to determine proper therapy. Anal Crohn's disease is an absolute contraindication to anoplasty, and obviously a malignant process must be treated by excision or resection. Perhaps the most useful diagnostic tool is an accurate history. If the patient associates the onset of the problem with prior hemorrhoidectomy or with electrocoagulation of anal condylomata, for example, the condition may be appropriately treated by an anoplasty. Conversely, with no such history, such as in someone with long-term laxative use, correction of the stricture may produce anal incontinence. This problem occurs when sphincter muscle wasting accompanies an anal stricture, a consequence of passing small, narrow bowel actions over many years. Mineral oil is notorious for leading to stenosis, probably because the lubricated stool fails to dilate the anal canal.

Symptoms present from birth imply a congenital origin. Most common is an anteriorly situated ectopic anus, usually at the orifice introitus in female patients.[27] A hooded anus (see Figure 18-10) and anorectal atresia are also congenital lesions that may be associated with stenosis despite treatment early in life.

Medical Treatment

As mentioned, the conservative management of anal stenosis includes laxatives, suppositories, dilatation, and enemas. These approaches may effect defecation, but they do not specifically treat the cause of the problem, a narrow diameter of the anal canal. A dilator may tear the canal. In fact, a complication from its use may itself precipitate the need for surgical intervention.[261]

Surgical Treatment

Excision of Eschar and Sphincterotomy The classic surgical treatment of anal stricture is lysis of the stricture and excision of the eschar, ideally transverse suture of the rectal mucosa to the underlying internal sphincter, and sphincterotomy—the same procedure described for the treatment by excision of chronic anal fissure (see Figure 9-21). Although the results have been reported as excellent (i.e., several hundred patients of Pope, more than 200 patients of Turell and Gelernt, 17 patients of Shropshear, and 224 patients of Malgieri),[158,209,244,264] it is difficult to interpret whether the patients had significant narrowing or merely spasm associated with an anal fissure. Furthermore, the term *anoplasty* should be limited, in my opinion, to those procedures that actually replace the anal canal with new tissue.

TECHNIQUE An artist's conception of a deformed, narrowed anal orifice that does not admit the index finger is shown in Figure 8-61. When the stricture is excised or lysed, a 29-mm (medium-size) Hill-Ferguson retractor is inserted. The cut edge of the rectum can be sutured to the underlying internal anal sphincter in a transverse fashion, thereby widening the anal canal (Figure 8-62A,B). If

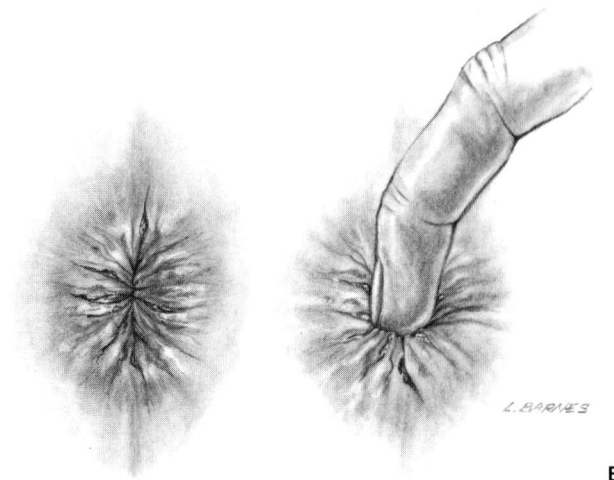

FIGURE 8-61. (**A**) Anal deformity with stricture. (**B**) This stricture does not permit digital examination.

the lumen is still inadequate, the same maneuver can be performed on the opposite side (Figure 8-62*C*).

This is a perfectly acceptable technique that will yield satisfactory results if sufficient skin bridges remain. However, if this is not the case, frequent digital examinations must be performed or dilators employed to prevent restricture. As with sphincterotomy or sphincter stretch (see Chapter 9), this operation does not create a new anal canal lining with sensory-bearing mucosa. However, this procedure, or even sphincterotomy alone, may be quite adequate for a patient with a mild degree of narrowing. For more profound stenosis, a formal anoplasty should

be performed to treat the basic problem—that is, loss of anal canal tissue.

Anoplasty for Minimal Stenosis Esoteric anoplastic maneuvers should be reserved for loss of anal canal tissue, but even mild anal stenosis can be treated by skin replacement. A small advancement flap (Y-V) may be useful for stenosis accompanying chronic posterior anal fissure.

PREOPERATIVE MANAGEMENT How aggressive should a bowel preparation be when the physician performs an anoplastic procedure? Probably all that is necessary is a

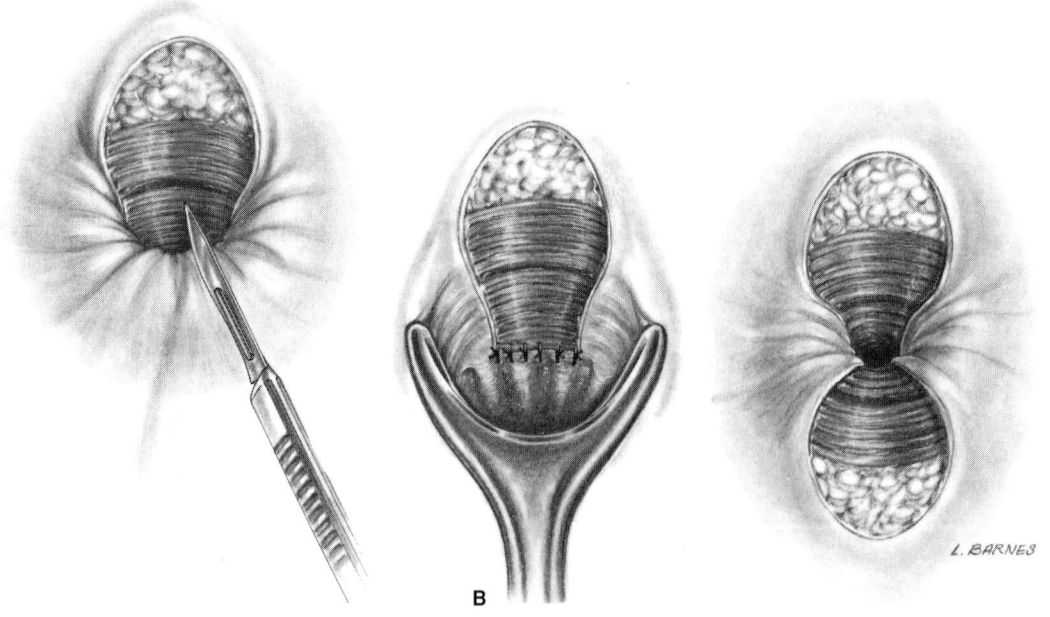

FIGURE 8-62. (**A**) Lysis of the anal stricture permits insertion of a 29-mm Hill-Ferguson retractor. (**B**) The rectum is sutured to the underlying internal anal sphincter. (**C**) When further widening is required, this can be done on the opposite side.

mechanical bowel preparation, but broad-spectrum, perioperative, systemic antibiotics are also suggested. The more extensive the skin mobilization, the more concerned I am about the possibility of sepsis. A cleansing enema before surgery is probably the most important. One does not wish to deal with stool in the field if performing skin grafting.

OPERATIVE TECHNIQUE The patient is placed in the prone jackknife position with the buttocks taped apart. Spinal, caudal, general endotracheal, or local anesthesia may be employed. The stricture is incised (Figure 8-63*A*), and an internal anal sphincterotomy may be performed, if indicated (Figure 8-63*B*). A full-thickness flap of skin is elevated in the posterior midline (Figure 8-63*C*). A 29-mm Hill-Ferguson retractor is kept in place for the entire operation to maintain the adequacy of the lumen. If the canal can be reconstructed with the retractor in place, the anal opening will inevitably be adequate.

Incisions are carried proximally for 5 to 8 cm. Care must be taken to avoid creating a narrow pedicle that could compromise the blood supply to the apex of the flap. Mobilization over the sacrum is unnecessary for this degree of anal canal defect. The full thickness of the skin is sutured to the rectal mucosa and to the underlying internal anal sphincter with interrupted long-term absorbable sutures. The completed repair is shown in Figure 8-63*D*. The external aspect may be left open if tension is produced by closure, or the entire wound may be closed primarily. The final, healed wounds can be seen in Figure 8-64 in a patient who underwent the operation for mild anal stenosis.

This technique is simple and quite useful for stricture associated with an anal fissure. However, if more than 25% of the circumference of the anal canal needs to be covered, another anoplastic approach is indicated.

A so-called V-Y or island flap anoplasty is another option for the management of mild anal stenosis or the treatment of a limited mucosal ectropion.[38,219] The full thickness of perianal skin is mobilized and advanced into the anal canal to create a new lining (Figure 8-65). Care must be taken to preserve the blood supply to the graft. A similar modification has been termed the house advancement flap.[46] Its theoretical advantages are that (a) it provides a broad skin flap for the entire length of the entire anal canal and (b) it allows for primary closure of the donor site. The word *house* denotes the schematic representation of a house in terms of the way the flap is created. The technique is illustrated in Figure 8-66.

POSTOPERATIVE MANAGEMENT The postoperative care of any patient who undergoes some type of anorectal reconstruction—that is, using skin or muscle—is the subject of much debate. There are no prospective, randomized trials with bowel confining regimens or with antibiotics (neither type nor duration). Therefore, one must resort to discuss-

ing *art*, not *science*. In all operations involving an anoplasty, an antibiotic, usually a cephalosporin, is given perioperatively. Whether it is continued postoperatively, orally or parenterally, for 1, 2, or more days, depends on the extent of the reconstruction and the surgeon's personal preference. Again, the decision of whether to prevent bowel action postoperatively is also surgeon's choice. Generally, however, because only a small graft is created in an anoplasty for mild stenosis, confining the bowels is unnecessary. Furthermore, the more vigorous the postoperative regimen, the longer one tends to stay in the hospital. Without a bowel-confining regimen, the patient is permitted a regular diet supplemented by a bulk laxative containing psyllium or a stool softener. Showers are permitted, but sitz baths are not recommended. Simple cleansing of the wound is all that is required. Rarely is it necessary to probe under the skin flap to evacuate a hematoma or purulent collection, but even under these circumstances the viability of the graft is usually not compromised. The patient is discharged when a bowel movement occurs (insurance company permitting), and is then seen weekly or every 2 weeks until the wounds heal, usually in 5 to 6 weeks.

Anoplasty for Moderate Stenosis When a greater area needs to be covered than can be accomplished with a single advancement flap, sufficient skin can often be obtained by performing bilateral advancements in the right lateral and left lateral positions. This will permit resurfacing of up to 50% of the anal canal circumference.

OPERATIVE TECHNIQUE The patient is placed in the prone jackknife position with the buttocks taped apart. A local anesthetic is not advised because of the extensive infiltration required and its associated discomfort. Figure 8-67 illustrates the technique. The full thickness of the skin is sutured to the cut edge of the rectum and the underlying internal sphincter with long-term absorbable sutures. This effectively increases the diameter of the anal canal.

POSTOPERATIVE MANAGEMENT It is usually advisable to confine the bowels after this procedure because of the extent of the skin coverage attempted. This is accomplished with diphenoxylate hydrochloride (Lomotil), up to eight tablets a day; codeine, up to 240 mg daily; and deodorized tincture of opium, up to 80 drops a day. As with all skin grafts, sitz baths are withheld. The wounds are cleansed with an antiseptic such as hydrogen peroxide or povidone-iodine four times daily.

My own, frequently changing preference is to discontinue the medications after 3 days. A regular diet is instituted, supplemented with a bulk laxative and a stool softener. Some small separation of the wound may occur, but satisfactory healing with an adequate anal opening may be anticipated. The patient is ideally discharged when bowel function has returned or at the

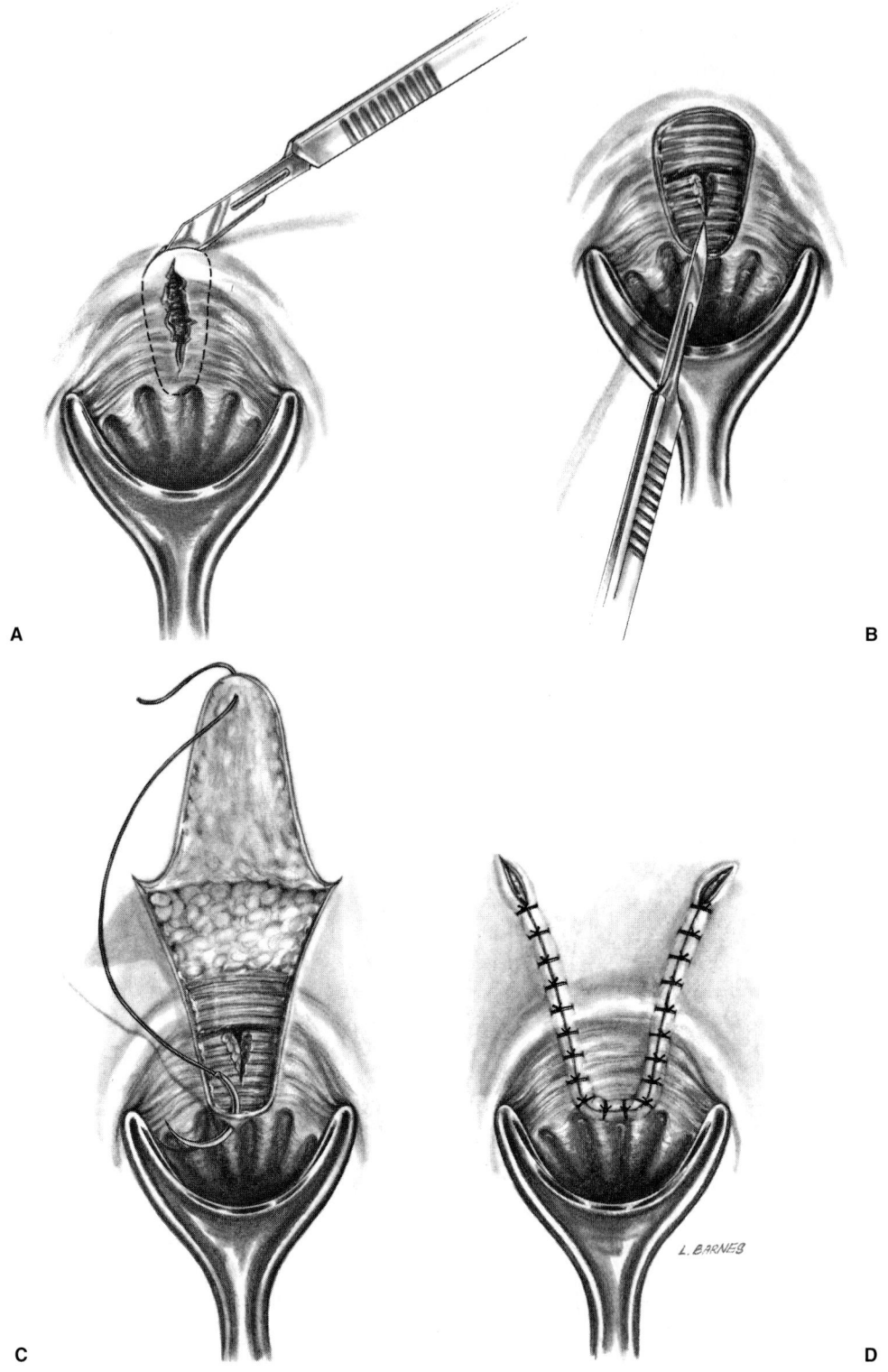

A

B

C

D

FIGURE 8-63. Anoplasty for chronic anal fissure with minimal stenosis. **(A)** The *dashed line* shows the planned incision. **(B)** An internal anal sphincterotomy is performed. **(C)** The skin flap is elevated. **(D)** The flap is advanced and sutured to the rectum.

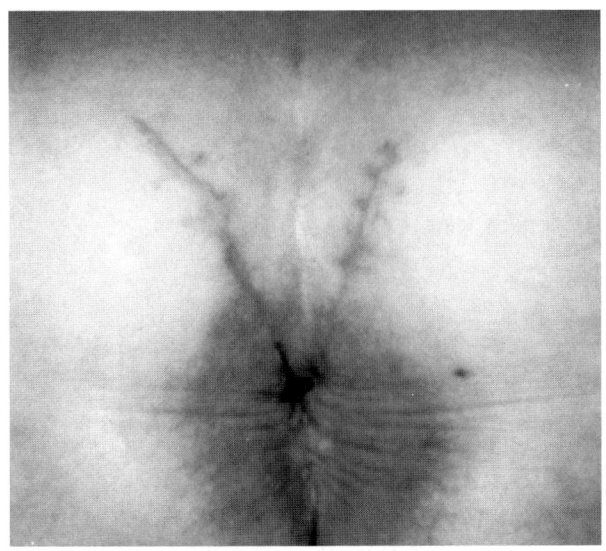

FIGURE 8-64. Postoperative appearance of Y-V anoplasty at 8 weeks.

insistence of the low dull normal bureaucrats who determine how one should practice medicine. The patient is seen usually every 10 to 14 days until complete healing has taken place.

Anoplasty for Severe Stenosis or for Major Coverage of the Anal Canal The plastic maneuvers previously described are useful for minimal or moderate problems of skin coverage. However, if 50% or more of the anal canal needs to be reconstructed, a rotation flap of skin should be considered. The reason for using this type of graft is that rotation flaps can cover a greater surface area without tension and with less concern for viability than can advancement flaps. Conditions that may necessitate this maneuver include stricture secondary to radical hemorrhoidectomy, concomitant tissue loss with excision of an

anal canal lesion, and mucosal ectropion. This last problem may be seen not only following the so-called Whitehead hemorrhoidectomy (Figure 8-48), but also after an abdominal-anal pull-through procedure or after any operation for imperforate anus. Another indication for this operation is to correct the "keyhole" deformity that may be a consequence of excision of an anal fissure or excision of an anal fistula.

OPERATIVE TECHNIQUE The patient is placed in the prone jackknife position, and the buttocks are taped apart. In most instances, a single rotation flap will provide adequate skin coverage (Figure 8-68). Figure 8-69 illustrates a keyhole deformity in the posterior midline, a consequence of excisional fissure surgery. After excision of the scar, an outline of the incision is made, the flap is elevated and rotated medially, and the wound is closed, primarily with interrupted, long-term absorbable sutures (Figure 8-70).

In the correction of Whitehead's deformity or when the entire anal canal must be replaced, a bilateral rotation flap (S-plasty) should be performed. Spinal, caudal, or general endotracheal anesthesia is employed; a locally administered anesthetic is not advised. The anal canal is incised posteriorly, and the lower portion of the internal sphincter is divided. The anal canal is incised farther to permit insertion of a Hill-Ferguson retractor.

A full-thickness flap of skin is elevated, and the incision is begun in the midline and carried laterally in a curvilinear fashion for approximately 8 to 10 cm. A longer length can be obtained by incising farther laterally and, eventually, somewhat medially. Care should be taken to avoid necrosis; a thick flap that includes subcutaneous tissue is preferred. As mentioned, more than one flap is rarely required, because a new anal canal along one half of the circumference is more than adequate. However, if the entire anal canal needs to be reconstructed, as has been mentioned with Whitehead's deformity or ectropion

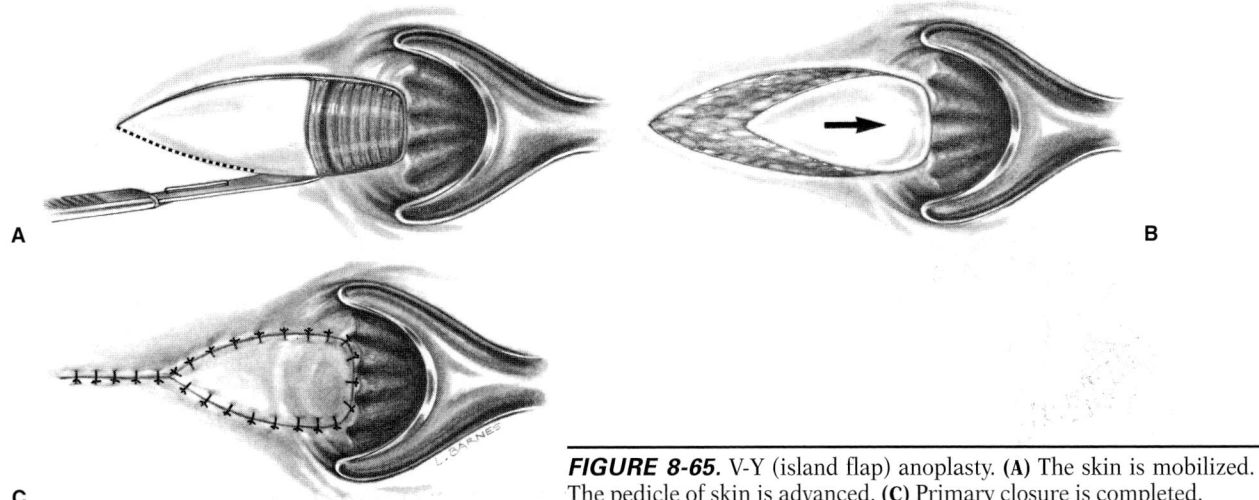

FIGURE 8-65. V-Y (island flap) anoplasty. **(A)** The skin is mobilized. **(B)** The pedicle of skin is advanced. **(C)** Primary closure is completed.

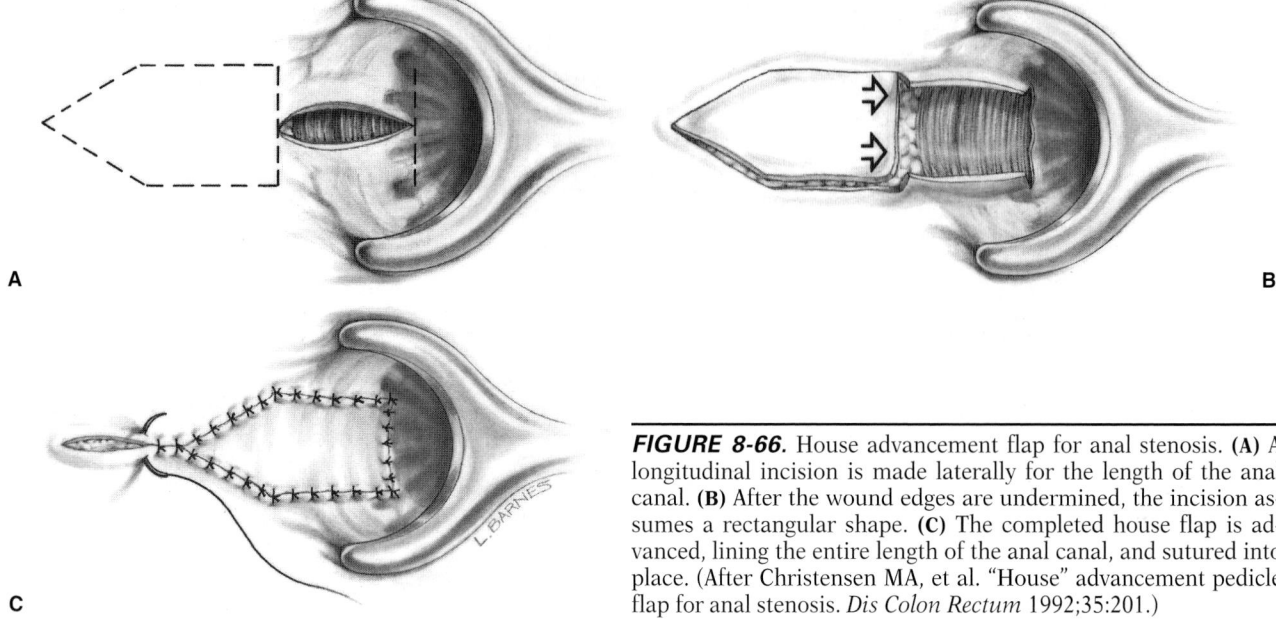

A

B

C

FIGURE 8-66. House advancement flap for anal stenosis. **(A)** A longitudinal incision is made laterally for the length of the anal canal. **(B)** After the wound edges are undermined, the incision assumes a rectangular shape. **(C)** The completed house flap is advanced, lining the entire length of the anal canal, and sutured into place. (After Christensen MA, et al. "House" advancement pedicle flap for anal stenosis. *Dis Colon Rectum* 1992;35:201.)

associated with surgery for imperforate anus (in which all the mucosa must be excised completely, thereby denuding the anal canal), a similar incision is performed on the opposite side. Hemostasis is effected with electrocautery. The wound is irrigated with saline solution, and the skin is rotated medially and sutured to the rectum and to the underlying internal sphincter with long-term absorbable sutures (Figure 8-71). Because there is a greater tendency for the mucosa to be mobile and to protrude quite readily, it is important to excise any redundant rectal mucosa. After the new mucocutaneous junction has been completed, continuous subcuticular 3–0 long-term absorbable or interrupted simple sutures of similar material are used, and the wounds are closed completely by mobilizing a full-thickness flap of skin cephalad and laterally (Figure 8-72). If there still is too much tension, the easiest alternative is to leave the lateral aspect open to granulate. If there is a very large defect, one may apply a split-thickness skin graft from the thigh, but this is rarely indicated.

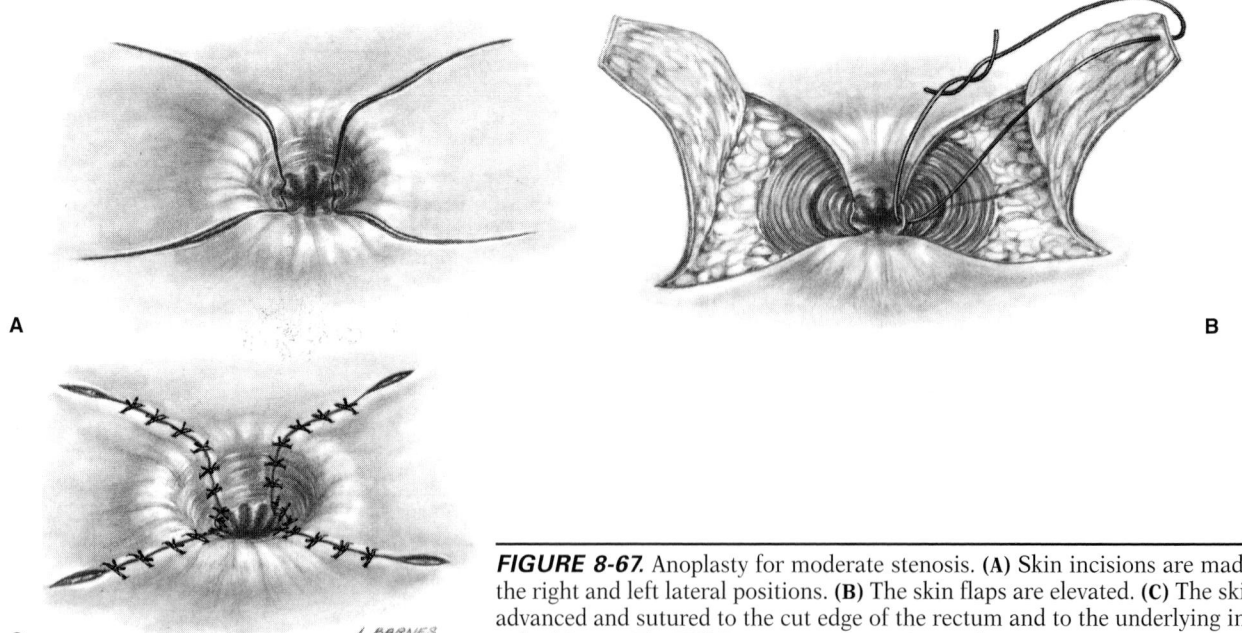

A

B

C

FIGURE 8-67. Anoplasty for moderate stenosis. **(A)** Skin incisions are made in the right and left lateral positions. **(B)** The skin flaps are elevated. **(C)** The skin is advanced and sutured to the cut edge of the rectum and to the underlying internal sphincter. The Hill-Ferguson retractor is not shown.

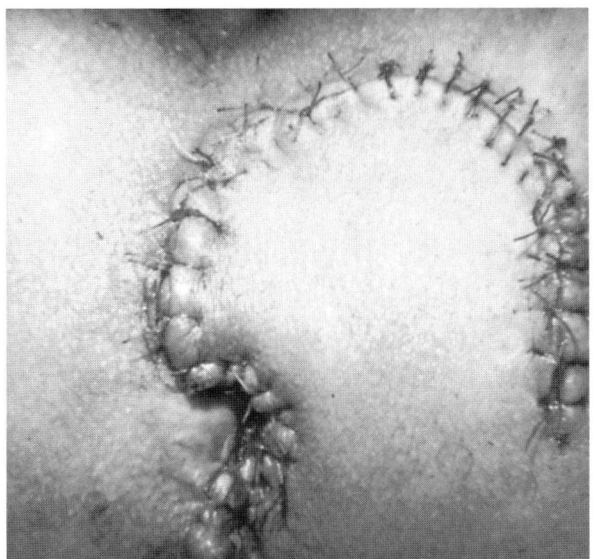

FIGURE 8-68. Immediate postoperative appearance of rotation skin flap repair for severe anal stenosis.

POSTOPERATIVE MANAGEMENT The bowel-confining regimen that has been described previously is carried out for 3 days. Systemic antibiotic coverage is continued during this time. Rarely, a hematoma or an abscess will develop underneath one of the flaps. By insertion of a hemostat between the sutures, evacuation of the collection usually can be achieved without compromising the graft.

An anal stenosis of long duration or Whitehead's deformity usually results in an attenuated sphincter mechanism. With a widely patent anal orifice, discharge of mucus and incontinence for flatus or even for feces may occur during the initial few weeks after operation. It is

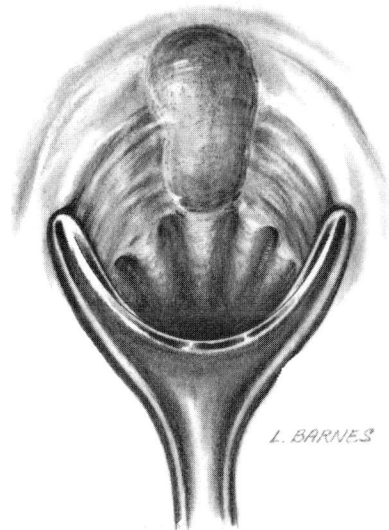

L. BARNES

FIGURE 8-69. Artist's conception of a keyhole deformity, a consequence of excision of an anal fissure in the posterior midline.

therefore advisable to start a regimen of perineal strengthening exercises (see Chapter 13), to be performed 10 to 15 times a day. Significant improvement in control may take many weeks, but relatively normal continence should be achievable except in the patient who has an anal stenosis with an atrophied sphincter. These individuals should be carefully selected before an anoplastic operation is considered. If surgery is believed to be advisable, a less-than-generous opening should be created. The patient needs to be forewarned that incontinence is a possibility.

Lateral Mucosal Advancement Anoplasty Another approach to the treatment of anal stricture that has been recommended is to advance the rectal mucosa downward, but only to the level of the intersphincteric groove (Figure 8-47A).[212] As previously discussed, this risks the possibility of creating a mucosal ectropion, but if performed carefully (with limited mucosal mobilization and excision of any mucosal redundancy) there may be selective application of this alternative.

Internal Pudendal Flap Anoplasty Another option for reconstructing the anal canal is the internal pudendal flap anoplasty.[226] This solitary case report was applied when extensive coverage was required concomitant with excision of Paget's disease of the anus. This flap is based on the terminal branches of the internal pudendal vessels. Because in my opinion one is most likely to require the services of a plastic surgeon, I have not included illustrations for this approach.

Foreskin Anoplasty An interesting operation has been described by Freeman for the treatment of mucosal ectropion—the foreskin anoplasty.[83] The procedure, which obviously implies that a prepuce to present and suitable, uses the foreskin to provide a full-thickness skin graft to the anal canal. The technique is shown in Figure 8-73. Freeman reported his experience with six children in 1984,[83] but no further publications have been noted since this initial report.

Anoplasty with Sphincteroplasty for Ectopic Anus, Perineal Body Reconstruction, and Management of Rectovaginal Fistulas and Obstetric Injury In restorative procedures of the anal sphincter mechanism as described in Chapter 13, the skin often must be mobilized concomitantly to effect an adequate repair. The anoplasty described in that chapter (see Figs. 13-26 through 13-39) is most useful in women with ectopic anus, rectovaginal fistula, or sphincter injury.

Results of Anoplasty It is extremely difficult to interpret the results of the various anoplastic maneuvers in the literature for the obvious reason that prospective trials do

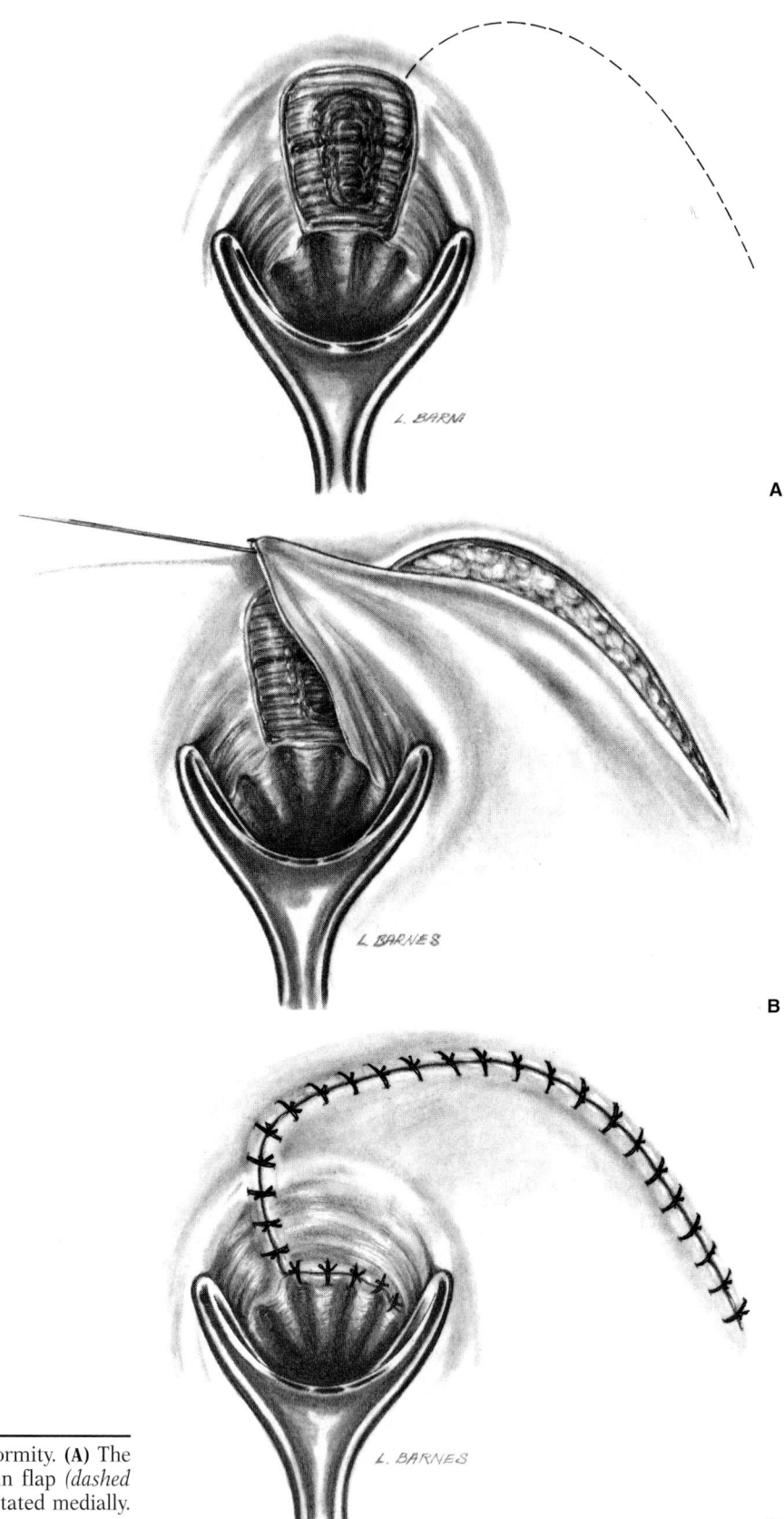

FIGURE 8-70. Correction of keyhole deformity. **(A)** The scar is excised; note the outline of the skin flap *(dashed line)*. **(B)** The skin flap is mobilized and rotated medially. **(C)** The wound is primarily closed.

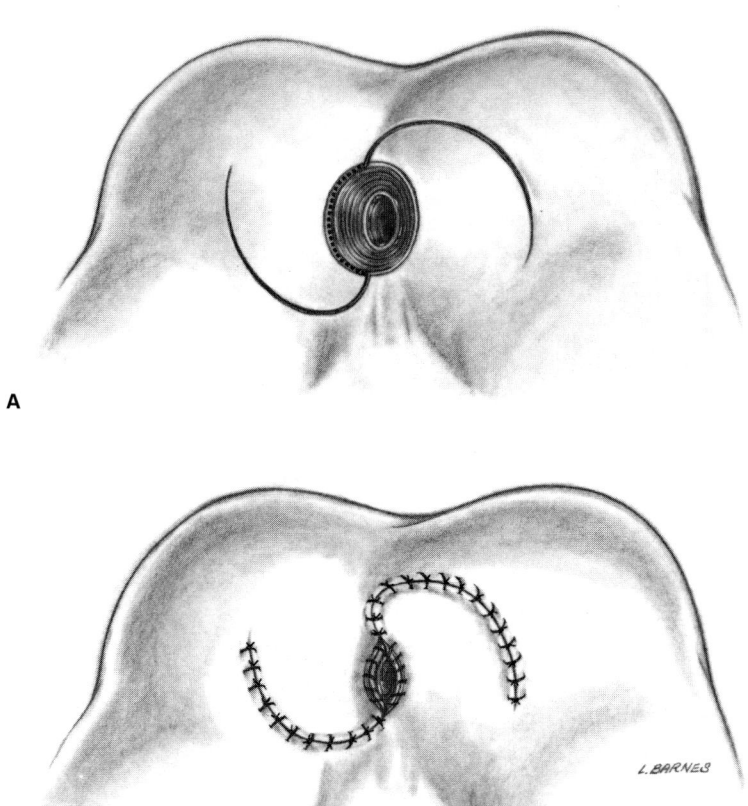

A

B

L. BARNES

FIGURE 8-71. Anoplasty is used for severe anal stenosis or for significant loss of anal canal tissue. **(A)** The skin flaps are outlined; the eschar has been excised. **(B)** The flaps are rotated and sutured to the rectum and underlying internal sphincter. The Hill-Ferguson retractor is not shown.

not exist. Sarner reported 21 patients who underwent one to four advancement flaps for symptomatic anal stenosis.[232] He stated, "Adequate relief was achieved in all cases".[232] Others have noted satisfaction with advancement flaps.[94,158,168,213,220] Ferguson and others have had an equally gratifying experience by using rotation flaps.[79,189] Pearl and colleagues reported 20 patients with benign anal strictures and five with mucosal ectropion treated

by means of either a U- or diamond-shaped island flap anoplasty.[210] There were two failures, neither attributable to lack of viability of the flaps. Pidala and co-workers reviewed 28 patients who underwent island flap anoplasty for mucosal ectropion and anal stenosis.[207] In those individuals available for follow-up, 91% judged their symptoms to be improved. In reality, every publication reflects contentment and success on the part of all authors.[10,97]

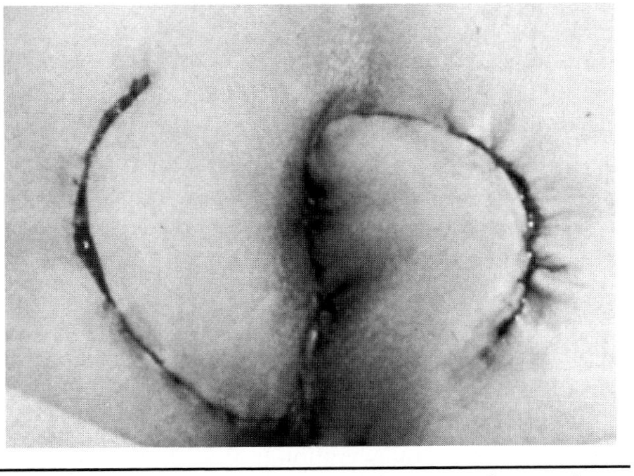

Comment There are no controlled studies on the comparative advantages and disadvantages of the various anoplastic procedures; however, almost any approach will at least improve the patient's symptoms. Certainly, in my experience of more than 250 anoplasties, no patient failed to have the condition ameliorated. Interestingly, stenosis following hemorrhoidectomy has become a rare indication for anoplasty. This is either a tribute to improvement in surgical technique or, more likely, to the much reduced application of surgical hemorrhoidectomy (at least in the United States).

The methods described for plastic reconstruction of the anal canal and perianal skin should be employed only in selected individuals. Routine application for the uncomplicated hemorrhoidectomy, fissure operation, or fistula repair is inappropriate. However, with anal stenosis, mucosal ectropion, sphincter injury, rectovaginal fistula,

FIGURE 8-72. S-plasty with bilateral rotation flaps is shown immediately after correction of a Whitehead deformity.

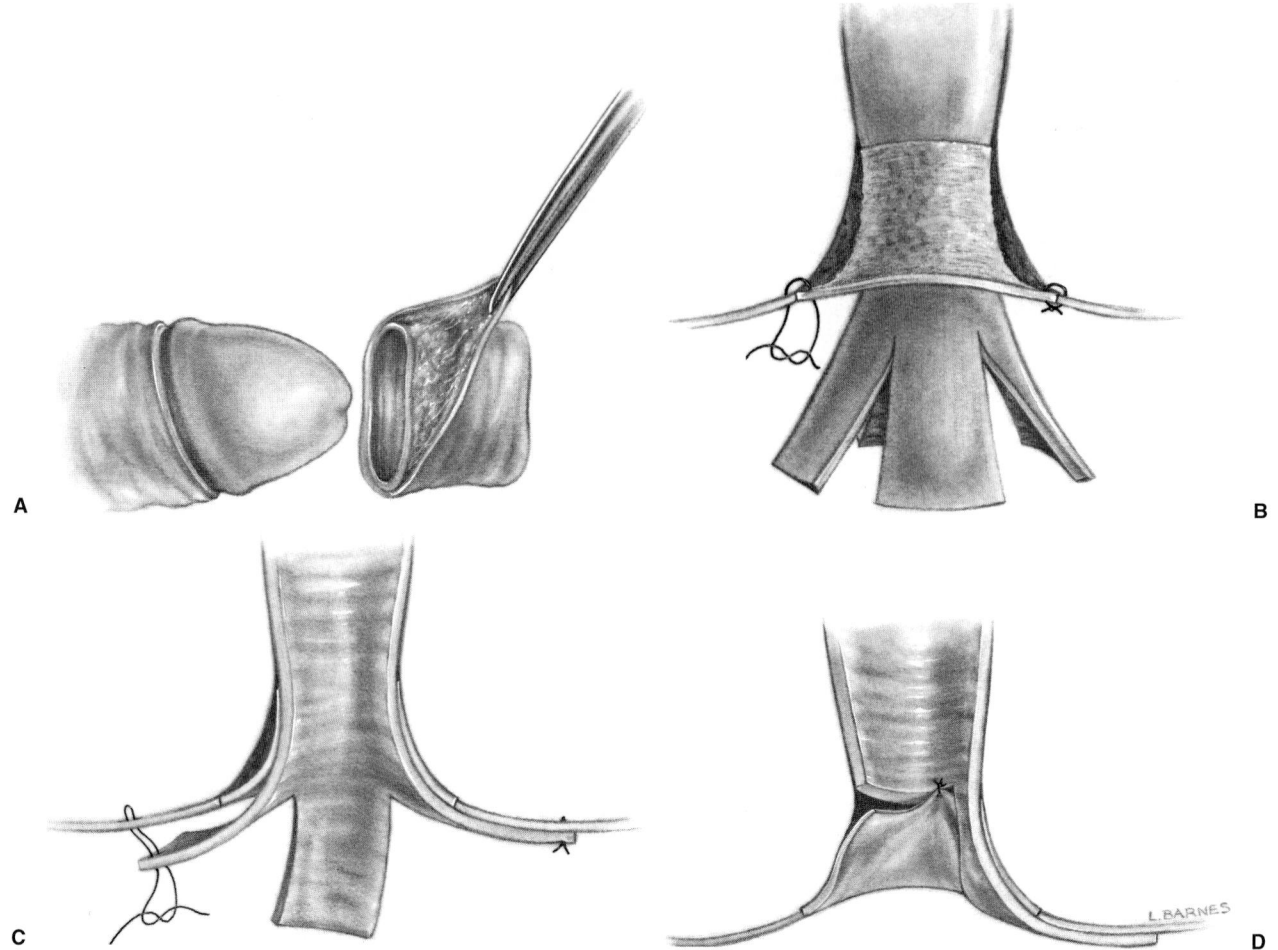

FIGURE 8-73. Foreskin anoplasty. **(A)** Circumcision is performed, and the two layers of foreskin are unfolded into a cylinder, with the raw surface exposed externally. **(B)** The caudal end of the cylinder is sutured at the anal verge. The rest of the graft lies against the rectum; the latter is split into quadrants. **(C)** The split bowel compresses the graft into its new position. **(D)** Redundant bowel is freed by removing stay sutures, cutting off the rectum deep within the anal canal, and suturing the proximal end to the foreskin. (Adapted from Freeman NV. The foreskin anoplasty. *Dis Colon Rectum* 1984;27:309, with permission.)

obstetric injury, or tissue loss from any reason, one of these procedures should be extremely effective in ensuring a successful result.

Rectal Stricture

Stricture of the rectum is a rare sequela of hemorrhoidectomy and usually is misdiagnosed as an anal stricture. The complication is caused by vigorous high ligation of the hemorrhoid pedicles that may strip the rectal mucosa in several areas or even circumferentially (Figure 8-74). This is most likely to occur if the patient has an element of prolapse or a laxity of the rectal mucosa. As with virtually all complications, prevention is the best approach. Care must be taken to avoid gathering a mass of rectal lining into the ligatures.

Management of this complication may require dilatation, either with Young's dilators (Figure 8-60) if the stricture is distal, or a Hegar dilator (see Figure 23-117) if the stricture is higher. Operative lysis may be necessary, possibly including either advancement of the rectal mucosa or proctoplasty (see Figure 23-119).

Fissure or Ulcer

An anal fissure may develop in a patient who has a contracted anorectal outlet after hemorrhoidectomy. Usually, the fissure is situated posteriorly. Repeated trauma from defecation results in laceration of the eschar, which may become a chronic, painful anal ulcer. Such postoperative fissures may respond to conservative management (e.g., laxatives, enemas, suppositories, topical creams such as

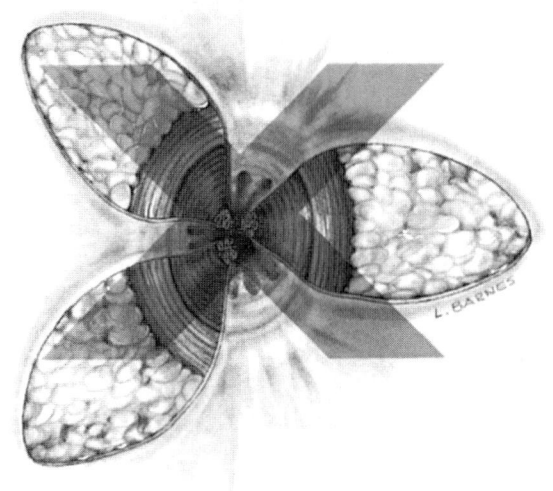

FIGURE 8-74. High ligation of rectal mucosa in an effort to remove mucosal redundancy or prolapse can result in stricture of the rectum.

cortisone) and dilatation. However, often an additional procedure is required, most commonly an internal anal sphincterotomy (see Chapter 9). Excision of the ulcer concomitant with the sphincterotomy may be of benefit, but some form of anoplasty may ultimately be required to increase anal canal circumference.

Pseudopolyps

Hemorrhoidectomy usually requires ligation of the stump of the hemorrhoid. Tissue strangulation will take place at the site of ligation, resulting in sloughing of the stump. This leaves a defect that heals by granulation, the end result of which may be a pseudopolyp. Another possible contributing factor is a foreign body granuloma, which may be a consequence of the prolonged presence of suture material.[88,93] This may be manifested by an edematous, polypoid, or sessile tumor at the site of the suture. Pseudopolyps can be excised with a local anesthetic or be electrocoagulated.

Epidermal Cyst

In rare instances, some months after hemorrhoidectomy, asymptomatic inclusion cysts may appear in the anal canal or in the immediate perianal region. Their origin has been attributed to retention of keratin elements, hair particles, or exfoliated squamous epithelial cells in the wound.[156] If these cysts are bothersome, they can be removed by local excision.

Anal Fistula

Anal fistula is an unusual complication of hemorrhoidectomy, occurring in approximately 1% of patients. It is allegedly more common after the closed operation than the open, but the incidence is so low that this observation is probably more theoretical than factual. The fistula is inevitably low and subcutaneous, not transsphincteric or even intersphincteric unless the finding is coincidental. Fistulotomy is the appropriate treatment and can often be accomplished in the office.

Pruritus Ani

Most causes of pruritus ani are related to diet or are caused by overaggressive attention to anal hygiene (see Chapter 19). However, pruritic symptoms following hemorrhoidectomy are not unusual and may actually have an anatomic basis. A mucosal ectropion or Whitehead's deformity, for example, can produce mucous discharge, which can contribute to the pruritus. With a specific anatomic abnormality, anoplasty may be advisable. The medical management of pruritus ani is discussed in Chapter 19.

Fecal Incontinence

Fecal soilage or incontinence following hemorrhoidectomy, although infrequent, is not as rare as the physician would expect. A possible explanation is the loss of anal canal sensation resulting from removal of sensory-bearing tissue and its replacement by scar. I do not subscribe to such a theory.

Almost all patients who have impairment of fecal control following hemorrhoidectomy are elderly. If the physician takes a careful history, it will probably be discovered that many of these individuals have experienced some soilage before the operation, although the procedure may have exacerbated the problem. This is often the case when the patient has some degree of mucosal or rectal prolapse, and it is a particular concern in women. Special care should be taken when performing this operation in the older age group; it is important to avoid unnecessary sphincter stretch or sphincterotomy. As previously mentioned, many surgeons are fond of sphincterotomy, because they believe it ameliorates the postoperative pain problem. When it is performed at the posterior pile site, a keyhole deformity can result. It is a potentially hazardous maneuver in an individual without a concomitant fissure and should be avoided, especially in someone older than 60 years of age.

Recurrence

Most patients who complain of recurrent hemorrhoids usually are describing skin tags or have pruritic symptoms. However, in some cases true hemorrhoidal veins have developed that have become symptomatic after an assumed complete hemorrhoidectomy. "Doctor, I had the operation 10 years ago, and now the hemorrhoids are back," is usually the expressed observation. However, piles that have been removed cannot recur. The "recurrence" consists of veins that, either because of their normal appearance at the time of hemorrhoidectomy or in an effort to preserve adequate mucosal bridges, were left undisturbed. With increased ingorgement, collateral circulation, or cushion laxity developing over the years, symptomatic hemorrhoids result.

Because of this potential problem, ideally all hemorrhoidal veins should be removed at the time of the surgical procedure. Tunneling out small vessels from the underlying mucosa and debriding all veins over the external sphincter are important prophylactic maneuvers (Figure 8-39). When recurrent piles become symptomatic, treatment can usually be accomplished by one of the office procedures, especially rubber ring ligation or office excision.

Retroperitoneal Air

A solitary case of retroperitoneal air following hemorrhoidectomy was reported by Kriss and colleagues.[140] The patient had been receiving steroids for rheumatoid arthritis, so this medication may have played some part in its occurrence. The authors suggest that air was introduced either during the dissection or subsequently, when the patient coughed or strained. A third explanation, not offered by the authors, is the possibility that this complication was unrelated to the operation. The patient responded well to nonoperative management.

Results of Surgical Hemorrhoidectomy

Few contemporary studies evaluate the results of hemorrhoidectomy, and those published reports that attempt to address the issue with long-term follow-up are subject to a number of criticisms. There are very few prospective studies, and retrospective interpretations tend to be rather self-serving. Simply stated, every surgeon who has made the effort to submit the results for publication is satisfied with the procedure. In 1971, Ganchrow and colleagues published the results of a retrospective study of 2,038 consecutive hemorrhoidectomies employing the Ferguson technique, together with 5-year follow-up results.[85] Eighty-two patients (4%) had postoperative complications; 40 patients (2%) had minimal bleeding; 27 patients (1.3%) needed subsequent suture ligation; and two postoperative deaths occurred (0.1%). One patient died at home 10 days after the operation following an uneventful course; postmortem examination was not performed. The other patient died of gram-negative sepsis secondary to a urinary tract infection 37 days after operation.

Between the fifth and seventh postoperative days, 700 patients (34.3%) were discharged from the hospital; 524 (26%) were discharged on the eighth postoperative day, and 770 were discharged after the eighth day. Fortunately or unfortunately, we shall never see reports of postoperative in-hospital recoveries of that duration again.

Questionnaires were returned by 1,018 persons (50%). Of the responses, 970 patients (95%) answered that they had relief of symptoms, 892 patients (88%) answered that they had satisfactory bowel movements since the operation, 732 (72%) had no rectal complaints whatsoever during the 5 years, and 293 (28%) had some complaints, of which pruritus was the most common.

McConnell and Khubchandani evaluated by questionnaire and by examination 441 patients who had undergone closed hemorrhoidectomy up to 7 years previously.[162] One patient required another hemorrhoidectomy. Residual hemorrhoid problems required treatment in 34 individuals (7.7%). Interestingly, of those responding to the questionnaire, 7.3% were dissatisfied with the results, and an additional 4.7% would not recommend the procedure. The authors state that the dissatisfaction was the result of failure to treat the preoperative complaints adequately. The implication, however, is that the indications for surgery may not have been sufficiently restrictive.

Wolf and colleagues sent a questionnaire to members of the American Society of Colon and Rectal Surgeons in 1979.[281] There was no statistically significant difference among the various techniques employed with respect to pain, complications, and length of hospital stay. However, the open technique was believed to have a slightly more rapid healing time and was associated with a lower incidence of stenosis in this flawed study.

Andrews and co-workers randomly allocated 20 consecutive patients to either diathermy hemorrhoidectomy or scissors dissection using the open technique (Milligan-Morgan).[8] There was no statistically significant difference between the two groups with respect to pain, length of hospitalization, or frequency of bowel movement. Others, in a prospective, pundomized study combining open and closed techniques opine that despite the longer healing time, pain is less when the operation is performed open.[90]

Eu and associates compared emergency and elective hemorrhoidectomy in a total of 704 patients.[74] Five hundred underwent an elective operation. They observed after the elective operation a 5.4% incidence of secondary hemorrhage, a very high incidence. After emergency surgery, secondary hemorrhage developed in 4.9%, also very high. There was also no statistically significant difference with respect to the other variables: incontinence (5.2% versus 4.4%), anal stenosis (5.9% versus 3.0%), and recurrent hemorrhoids (7.6% versus 6.9%).

Arbman and associates compared closed (Ferguson's) hemorrhoidectomy with open (Milligan-Morgan) hemorrhoidectomy in a prospective, randomized trial involving 77 patients.[12] No statistically significant differences in the incidence of complications were found between the two methods, except with respect to wound healing. At 3 weeks, 86% of the Ferguson patients were healed but only 18% of the Milligan-Morgan.

Peng and co-workers randomized 55 patients with grade III and "small" grade IV hemorrhoids to either rubber band ligation or stapled hemorrhoidopexy.[202] Statistically significantly increased pain was noted with an increased analgesia requirement in the latter group. The complication rate was also significantly increased.

Felt-Bersma and colleagues revealed unsuspected sphincteric defects following anorectal surgery by means of anal endosonography.[78] This observation is not unusual after fistula operations, but it is certainly a potential source of concern in the occasional patient following hemorrhoidectomy.

MacRae and McLeod performed a metaanalysis involving a total of 18 trials to assess whether any method of hemorrhoid treatment has been demonstrably superior.[157] The following were their conclusions:

- Hemorrhoidectomy was found to be significantly more effective than manual dilation, with less need for further therapy.
- No significant difference was observed in the incidence of complications.
- Hemorrhoidectomy was found to be associated with significantly more pain.
- Patients undergoing hemorrhoidectomy had a better response to treatment than those treated with rubber band ligation.
- Hemorrhoidectomy was associated with more complications than rubber band ligation.
- Rubber band ligation was better than sclerotherapy in the treatment of all grades of hemorrhoids.

Comment

Although I have not reviewed my experience with Ferguson's hemorrhoidectomy I have been very pleased with the technical aspects and the results of this operation. I, therefore, have used this technique almost exclusively in all individuals who have been candidates for the surgical removal of hemorrhoids. Usually, the patient's only regret is inappropriate procrastination before permitting operative intervention. With respect to stapled hemorrhoidopexy, I must confess that I initially was extremely skeptical about its value and its efficacy. Now that I have had a moderate experience (60 procedures as of this writing), I have been converted. This is truly an exciting concept. No, it is not a hemorrhoidectomy, but it may prove to be a preferable way of addressing the physiologic and anatomic problems that result in hemorrhoidal complaints. The fact is that it works, patients usually have little discomfort, it is technically relatively straightforward, and it is associated with minimal morbidity. However, the reported (albeit rare) complications are so devastating (rectovaginal fistula, overwhelming sepsis), that one still must be wary of becoming too much the enthusiast. And equally important, long-term follow-up as well as prospective trials with other methods of hemorrhoidectomy are awaited.

HEMORRHOIDS IN INFLAMMATORY BOWEL DISEASE

Exacerbation of hemorrhoidal complaints is not at all uncommon in patients with inflammatory bowel disease, or for that matter, with any of the infectious or noninfectious colitides. Jeffery and associates reported a retrospective review of 42 patients with ulcerative colitis and 20 with Crohn's disease who were treated for hemorrhoids and inflammatory bowel disease between 1935 and 1975.[119] Both surgical and conservative treatment of hemorrhoids in those with ulcerative colitis had low complication rates (i.e., four complications after 50 courses of treatment). In Crohn's disease, the complication rate was high, 11 complications after 26 courses of treatment. One of the 42 patients with ulcerative colitis and six of the 20 with Crohn's disease required rectal excision for complications apparently dating from the treatment of hemorrhoids. Wolkomir and Luchtefeld performed surgical hemorrhoidectomy on 17 patients with known Crohn's disease.[283] All but two healed without complication. Although no individual had acutely active disease, four had inflammatory changes in the rectum.

Comment

Despite the foregoing observation, in my opinion, any procedure performed on the anus or perianal skin in patients with inflammatory bowel disease should be limited to the minimal maneuvers that will effectively treat the patient's complaint. Definitive or extensive surgical treatment of any anorectal problem in such individuals could result in delayed healing or nonhealing, with greater disability to the patient than before the operation (see Chapters 11 and 30; see Figure 11-44). Occasionally, when disease is quiescent and sepsis, fistula formation, and scarring are not present, bleeding or protrusion of hemorrhoids may reasonably be treated by rubber ring ligation.

HEMORRHOIDECTOMY IN THE HIV-POSITIVE PATIENT

One of the most remarkable characteristics of the anus and rectum is the extraordinary resistance to infection in that area. This feature permits a successful outcome following a plethora of surgical procedures.[225] Safavi and colleagues presented a series of 75 consecutive surgical procedures on 40 HIV-positive individuals and 22 patients with AIDS.[225] Only those with the hemorrhoid manifestation of thrombosis were surgically treated, however. This represented four patients, three of whom healed; one obtained no relief.

Although not clearly documented by statistics in the literature, definitive surgical hemorrhoidectomy in HIV-positive patients is probably contraindicated (see also Chapter 20).

HEMORRHOIDECTOMY DURING PREGNANCY

As mentioned earlier in this chapter, women are often troubled by hemorrhoidal complaints during the latter part of pregnancy. Most such problems can be treated adequately by bowel management (e.g., laxatives, stool softeners) and by sitz baths. A thrombosed hemorrhoid can be excised in the usual way. There is no clear-cut answer to the question of what should be done when a woman has a sufficiently profound complication that surgical hemorrhoidectomy appears to be the best recourse.

Saleeby and colleagues performed operative hemorrhoidectomies on 25 of 12,455 pregnant women (0.2%) who delivered in their institution.[227] All but three were in their third trimester. The operations were of the closed type and were accomplished with a local anesthetic. Other than one instance of postoperative hemorrhage, there were no other maternal or fetal complications.

REFERENCES

1. Ackland TH. The treatment of prolapsed gangrenous hemorrhoids. *Aust N Z J Surg* 1961;30:201.
2. Adami B, Eckardt VF, Suermann, RB, et al. Bacteremia after proctoscopy and hemorrhoid injection sclerotherapy. *Dis Colon Rectum* 1981;24:373.
3. Alexander-Williams J, Crapp AR. Conservative management of haemorrhoids. Part I: injection, freezing and ligation. *Clin Gastroenterol* 1975;4:595.
4. Ambrose NS, Hares MM, Alexander-Williams J, et al. Prospective randomised comparison of photocoagulation and rubber band ligation in treatment of haemorrhoids. *BMJ* 1983;286:1389.
5. Ambrose NS, Morris D, Alexander-Williams J, et al. A randomized trial of photocoagulation or injection sclerotherapy for the treatment of first- and second-degree hemorrhoids. *Dis Colon Rectum* 1985;28:238.
6. Standards Task Force, American Society of Colon and Rectal Surgeons. Practice parameters for ambulatory anorectal surgery. *Dis Colon Rectum* 2003;46:573–576.
7. Anderson HG. The "injection" method for the treatment of haemorrhoids. *Practitioner* 1924;113:399.
8. Andrews BT, Layer GT, Jackson BT, et al. Randomized trial comparing diathermy hemorrhoidectomy with the scissor dissection Milligan-Morgan operation. *Dis Colon Rectum* 1993;36:580.
9. Andrews E. The treatment of hemorrhoids by injection. *Med Rec* 1879;15:451.
10. Angelchik PD, Harms BA, Starling JR. Repair of anal stricture and mucosal ectropion with y-v or pedicle flap anoplasty. *Am J Surg* 1993;166:55.
11. Arabi Y, Alexander-Williams J, Keighley MRB. Anal pressures in hemorrhoids and anal fissure. *Am J Surg* 1977;134:608.
12. Arbman G, Krook H, Haapaniemi S. Closed vs. open hemorrhoidectomy: is there a difference? *Dis Colon Rectum* 2000;43:31–34.
13. Armstrong DN: Multiple hemorrhoidal ligation: a prospective, randomized trial evaluating a new technique. *Dis Colon Rectum* 2003;46:179.
14. Armstrong DN, Frankum C, Schertzer ME, et al. Harmonic scalpel hemorrhoidectomy. Five hundred consecutive cases. *Dis Colon Rectum* 2002;45:354–359.
15. Asfar SK, Juma TH, Ala-Edeen T. Hemorrhoidectomy and sphincterotomy: a prospective study comparing the effectiveness of anal stretch and sphincterotomy in reducing pain after hemorrhoidectomy. *Dis Colon Rectum* 1988;31:181.
16. Bacon HE. *Anus, rectum and sigmoid colon,* 3rd ed, vol 1. Philadelphia: JB Lippincott, 1949:453.
17. Bailey HR, Ferguson JA. Prevention of urinary retention by fluid restriction following anorectal operations. *Dis Colon Rectum* 1976;19:250.
18. Balfour L, Stojkovic SG, Botterill ID, et al. A randomized, double-blind trial of the effect of metronidazole on pain after closed hemorrhoidectomy. *Dis Colon Rectum* 2002;45:1186–1190.
19. Banov J Jr. Suppositories: are they effective? *J S C Med Assoc* 1985;10:407.
20. Barrios G, Khubchandani M. Whitehead operation revisited. *Dis Colon Rectum* 1979;22:330.
21. Barron J. Office ligation of internal hemorrhoids. *Am J Surg* 1963;105:563.
22. Barron J. Office ligation treatment of hemorrhoids. *Dis Colon Rectum* 1963;6:109.
23. Bartizal J, Slosberg P. An alternative to hemorrhoidectomy. *Arch Surg* 1977;112:534.
24. Basso L, Pescatori M. Outcome of delayed hemorrhage following surgical hemorrhoidectomy [Letter]. *Dis Colon Rectum* 1994;37:288.
25. Bat L, Melzer E, Koler M, et al. Complications of rubber band ligation of symptomatic internal hemorrhoids. *Dis Colon Rectum* 1993;36:287.
26. Beattie GC, Loudon MA. Follow-up confirms sustained benefit of circumferential stapled anoplasty in the management of prolapsing haemorrhoids. *Br J Surg* 2001;88:850
27. Bentley JFR. Developmental anomalies and other diseases in children. In: Morson BC, ed. *Diseases of the colon, rectum and anus.* New York: Appleton-Century-Crofts, 1969:64.
28. Bernard A, Parnaud E, Guntz M, et al. Radioanatomie normale du réseau vasculaire hémorrhoidal. (Note préalable à propos d'une étude portant sur 15 cas). *Ann Radiol (Paris)* 1977;20:483.
29. Bernstein KJ, Klausner MA. Potential dangers related to transdermal fentanyl (Duragesic) when used for postoperative pain [Letter]. *Dis Colon Rectum* 1994;37:1339.
30. Bernstein WC. What are hemorrhoids and what is their relationship to the portal venous system? [Editorial] *Dis Colon Rectum* 1983;26:829.
31. Blaisdell PC. Prevention of massive hemorrhage secondary to hemorrhoidectomy. *Surg Gynecol Obstet* 1958;106:485.
32. Bleday R, Pena JP, Rothenberger DA, et al. Symptomatic hemorrhoids: current incidence and complications of operative therapy. *Dis Colon Rectum* 1992;35:477.
33. Bonello JC. Who's afraid of the dentate line? The Whitehead hemorrhoidectomy. *Am J Surg* 1988;156:182.
34. Bonhomme L, Benhamou D, Martre H, et al. Chemical stability of bupivacaine and epinephrine in pH-adjusted solutions. *Anesthesiology* 1987;37:279(abst).
35. Bowers FJ, Hartmann R, Khanduja KS, et al. Urecholine prophylaxis for urinary retention in anorectal surgery. *Dis Colon Rectum* 1987;30:41.
36. Buie LA. *Practical proctology.* Philadelphia: WB Saunders, 1937.
37. Burkitt DP, Graham-Stewart CW. Haemorrhoids: postulated pathogenesis and proposed prevention. *Postgrad Med J* 1975;51:631.

38. Caplin DA, Kodner IJ. Repair of anal stricture and mucosal ectropion by simple flap procedures. *Dis Colon Rectum* 1986;29:92.

39. Cataldo PA, MacKeigan JM. The necessity of routine pathologic evaluation of hemorrhoidectomy specimens. *Surg Gynecol Obstet* 1992;174:302.

40. Cataldo PA, Senagore AJ. Does alpha sympathetic blockade prevent urinary retention following anorectal surgery? *Dis Colon Rectum* 1991;34:1113.

41. Cheetham MJ, Cohen CRG, Kamm MA, et al. A randomized, controlled trial of diathermy hemorrhoidectomy vs. stapled hemorrhoidectomy in an intended day-care setting with longer-term follow-up. *Dis Colon Rectum* 2003;46:491–497.

42. Cheetham MJ, Mortensen NJM, Nystrom P-O, et al. Persistent pain and fecal urgency after stapled haemorrhoidectomy. *Lancet* 2000;356:730.

43. Chew SSB, Marshall L, Kalish L, et al. Short-term and long-term results of combined sclerotherapy and rubber band ligation of hemorrhoids and mucosal prolapse. *Dis Colon Rectum* 2003;46:1232.

44. Chia YW, Darzi A, Speakman CTM, et al. CO₂ laser haemorrhoidectomy: does it alter anorectal function or decrease pain compared to conventional haemorrhoidectomy? *Int J Colorectal Dis* 1995;10:22.

45. Chiu J-H, Chen W-S, Chen C-H, et al. Effect of transcutaneous electrical nerve stimulation for pain relief on patients undergoing hemorrhoidectomy: prospective, randomized, controlled trial. *Dis Colon Rectum* 1999;42:180–185.

46. Christensen MA, Pitsch RM Jr, Cali RL, et al. House advancement pedicle flap for anal stenosis. *Dis Colon Rectum* 1992;35:201.

47. Chung CC, Ha JPY, Tai YP, et al. Double-blind, randomized trial comparing Harmonic scalpel hemorrhoidectomy, bipolar scissors hemorrhoidectomy, and scissors excision: ligation technique. *Dis Colon Rectum* 2002;45:789–794.

48. Chung Y-C, Wu H-J. Clinical experience of sutureless closed hemorrhoidectomy with Ligasure. *Dis Colon Rectum* 2003;46:87–92.

49. Cihan A, Mentes BB, Sucak G, et al. Fournier's gangrene after hemorrhoidectomy: association with drug-induced agranulocytosis. *Dis Colon Rectum* 1999;42:1644–1648.

50. Cipriani S, Pescatori M. Acute rectal obstruction after PPH stapled hemorrhoidectomy. *Colorectal Dis* 2002;4:367–370.

51. Clay LD III, White JJ Jr, Davidson JT, et al. Early recognition and successful management of pelvic cellulitis following hemorrhoidal banding. *Dis Colon Rectum* 1986;29:579.

52. Cooper IS, Lee AS. Cryostatic congelation: a system for producing a limited, controlled region of cooling or freezing of biologic tissues. *J Nerv Ment Dis* 1961;133:259.

53. Corman ML. Management of postoperative constipation in anorectal surgery. *Dis Colon Rectum* 1979;22:149.

54. Corman ML. Anoplasty. In: Maingot R, ed. *Abdominal operations*, 7th ed. New York: Appleton-Century-Crofts, 1980:2367.

55. Corman ML. pH of local anesthetic solutions. *Dis Colon Rectum* 1990;23:166.

56. Corman ML, Gravié J-F, Hager T, et al. Stapled hemorrhoidopexy: a consensus position paper by an international working party—indications, contra-indications and technique. *Colorectal Dis* 2003;5:304–310.

57. Corman ML, Veidenheimer MC. The new hemorrhoidectomy. *Surg Clin North Am* 1973;53:417.

58. Corman ML, Veidenheimer MC, Coller JA. Anoplasty for anal stricture. *Surg Clin North Am* 1976;56:727.

59. Correa-Rovelo JM, Tellez O, Obregón L, et al. Stapled rectal mucosectomy vs. closed hemorrhoidectomy: a randomized clinical trial. *Dis Colon Rectum* 2002;45:1367.

60. Coskun A, Duzgun SA, Uzunkoy A, et al. Nitroderm TTS band application for pain after hemorrhoidectomy. *Dis Colon Rectum* 2001;44:680–685.

61. Creve U, Hubens A. The effect of Lord's procedure on anal pressure. *Dis Colon Rectum* 1979;22:483.

62. Crystal RF, Hopping RA. Early postoperative complications of anorectal surgery. *Dis Colon Rectum* 1974;17:336.

63. Davies J, Duffy D, Boyt N, et al. Botulinum toxin (Botox) reduces pain after hemorrhoidectomy: results of a double-blind, randomized study. *Dis Colon Rectum* 2003;46:1097.

64. Davy A, Duval C. Modifications macroscopiques et microscopiques du réseau vasculaire hémorrhoidal dans la maladie hémorrhoidaire. *Arch Fr Mal Appar Dig* 1976;65:515.

65. Dencker H, Hjorth N, Norryd C, et al. Comparison of results with different methods of treatment of internal haemorrhoids. *Acta Chir Scand* 1973;139:742.

66. Denis J. Étude numérique de quelques facteurs étiopathogéniques des troubles hémorrhoidaires de l'adulte. *Arch Fr Mal Appar Dig* 1976;65:529.

67. Dennison AR, Wherry DC, Morris DL. Hemorrhoids: non-operative management. *Surg Clin North Am* 1988;68:1401.

68. Dennison AR, Whiston RJ, Rooney S, et al. The management of hemorrhoids. *Am J Gastroenterol* 1989;84:475.

69. Dennison A, Whiston RJ, Rooney S, et al. A randomized comparison of infrared photocoagulation with bipolar diathermy for the outpatient treatment of hemorrhoids. *Dis Colon Rectum* 1990;33:32.

70. Dodi G, Bogoni F, Infantino A, et al. Hot or cold in anal pain? A study of the changes in internal anal sphincter pressure profiles. *Dis Colon Rectum* 1986;29:248.

71. Edwards FS. The treatment of piles by injection. *BMJ* 1888;2:815.

72. Eisenstat T, Salvati EP, Rubin RJ. The outpatient management of acute hemorrhoidal disease. *Dis Colon Rectum* 1979;22:315.

73. El-Gendi MA, Abdel-Baky N. Anorectal pressure in patients with symptomatic hemorrhoids. *Dis Colon Rectum* 1986;29:388.

74. Eu KW, Seow-Choen F, Goh HS. Comparison of emergency and elective hemorrhoidectomy. *Br J Surg* 1994;81:308.

75. Fansler WA, Anderson JK. A plastic operation for certain types of hemorrhoids. *JAMA* 1933;101:1064.

76. Fantin AC, Zala G, Risti B, et al. Bleeding anorectal varices: successful treatment with transjugular intrahepatic portosystemic shunting (TIPS). *Gut* 1996;38:932.

77. Fazio VW. Early promise of stapling technique for haemorrhoidectomy. *Lancet* 2000;355:768.

78. Felt-Bersma RJF, van Baren R, Koorevaar M, et al. Unsuspected sphincter defects shown by anal endosonography after anorectal surgery: a prospective study. *Dis Colon Rectum* 1995;38:249.

79. Ferguson JA. Repair of "Whitehead deformity" of the anus. *Surg Gynecol Obstet* 1959;108:115.

80. Ferguson JA, Heaton JR. Closed hemorrhoidectomy. *Dis Colon Rectum* 1959;2:176.

81. Fleischer M, Marini CP, Statman R, et al. Local anesthesia is superior to spinal anesthesia for anorectal surgical procedures. *Am Surg* 1994;60:812.

82. Franklin EJ, Seetharam S, Lowney J, et al. Randomized, clinical trial of Ligasure vs. conventional diathermy in hemorrhoidectomy. *Dis Colon Rectum* 2003;46:1380.

83. Freeman NV. The foreskin anoplasty. *Dis Colon Rectum* 1984;27:309.

84. Gabriel WB. *The principles and practice of rectal surgery*, 4th ed. London: HK Lewis, 1948.

85. Ganchrow MI, Mazier WP, Friend WG, et al. Hemorrhoidectomy revisited: a computer analysis of 2,038 cases. *Dis Colon Rectum* 1971;14:128.

86. Ganio E, Altomare DF, Gabrielli F, et al. Prospective randomized multicentre trial comparing stapled with open haemorrhoidectomy. *Br J Surg* 2001;88:669.

87. Gartell PC, Sheridan RJ, McGinn FP. Outpatient treatment of haemorrhoids: a randomized clinical trial to compare rubber band ligation with phenol injection. *Br J Surg* 1985;72:478.

88. Gaskin ER, Childer MD Jr. Increased granuloma formation from absorbable sutures. *JAMA* 1963;185:212.

89. Gehamy RA, Weakley FL. Internal hemorrhoidectomy by elastic ligation. *Dis Colon Rectum* 1974;17:347.

90. Gençosamoglu R, Sad O, Koç D, et al. Hemorrhoidectomy: open or closed technique? A prospective randomized clinical trial. *Dis Colon Rectum* 2002;45:70–75.

91. Gibbons CP, Bannster JJ, Read NW. Role of constipation and anal hypertonia in the pathogenesis of hemorrhoids. *Br J Surg* 1988;75:656.

92. Gill W, Fraser J, Da Costa J, et al. The cryosurgical lesion. *Am Surg* 1970;36:437.

93. Gillman T, Penn J, Bronks D, Roux M, et al. Reactions of healing wounds and granulation tissue in man to auto-Thiersch, autodermal, and homodermal grafts: with an analysis of implications of phenomena encountered for understanding of behaviour of grafted tissue and genesis of scars, keloids, skin carcinomata, and other cutaneous lesions. *Br J Plast Surg* 1953;6:153.

94. Gingold BS, Arvanitis M. Y-V anoplasty for treatment of anal stricture. *Surg Gynecol Obstet* 1986;162:241.

95. Goenka M, Kochhar R, Nagi B, et al. Rectosigmoid varices and other mucosal changes in patients with portal hypertension. *Am J Gastroenterol* 1991;86:1185.

96. Goldstein ET, Williamson PR, Larach SW. Subcutaneous morphine pump for postoperative hemorrhoidectomy pain management. *Dis Colon Rectum* 1993;36:439.

97. González AR, Oliveira OD Jr, Verzaro R, et al. Anoplasty for stenosis and other anorectal defects. *Am Surg* 1995; 61:526.

98. Gottesman L, Milsom JW, Mazier WP. The use of anxiolytic and parasympathomimetic agents in the treatment of postoperative urinary retention following anorectal surgery: a prospective, randomized double-blind study. *Dis Colon Rectum* 1989;32:867.

99. Granet E. Hemorrhoidectomy failures: causes, prevention and management. *Dis Colon Rectum* 1968;11:45.

100. Greca F, Hares M, Keighley MRB. Anal dilatation [Letter]. *Br J Surg* 1981;68:141.

101. Griffith CDM, Morris DL, Wherry DC, et al. Outpatient treatment of haemorrhoids: a randomised trial comparing contact bipolar diathermy with rubber ring ligation. *Coloproctology* 1987;9:332.

102. Guy RJ, Seow-Choen F. Septic complications after treatment of haemorrhoids. *Br J Surg* 2003;90:147.

103. Gy R, Seow-Choen F. Septic complications after treatment of haemorrhoids. *Br J Surg* 2003;90:147–156.

104. Haas PA, Fox TA Jr, Haas GP. The pathogenesis of hemorrhoids. *Dis Colon Rectum* 1984;27:442.

105. Hancock BD. Internal sphincter and the nature of hemorrhoids. *Gut* 1977;18:651.

106. Hansen HH. Neue Aspekte zur Pathogeneses und Therapie des Hämorrhoidalleidens. *Dtsch Med Wochenschr* 1977; 102:1244.

107. Hansen HH. Pathomorphologie und Therapie des Hämorrhoidalleidens. *Hautartz* 1977;28:364.

108. Heald RJ, Gudgeon AM. Limited haemorrhoidectomy in the treatment of acute strangulated haemorrhoids. *Br J Surg* 1986;73:1002.

109. Hiltunen K-M, Matikainen M. Anal manometric findings in symptomatic hemorrhoids. *Dis Colon Rectum* 1985;28:807.

110. Hinton CP, Morris DL. A randomized trial comparing direct current therapy and bipolar diathermy in the outpatient treatment of third-degree hemorrhoids. *Dis Colon Rectum* 1990;33:931.

111. Ho Y-H, Cheong W-K, Tsang C, et al. Stapled hemorrhoidectomy: cost and effectiveness. Randomized, controlled trial including incontinence scoring, anorectal manometry, and endoanal ultrasound assessments at up to three months. *Dis Colon Rectum* 2000;43:1666.

112. Hodgson WJB, Morgan J. Ambulatory hemorrhoidectomy with CO_2 laser. *Dis Colon Rectum* 1995;38:1265.

113. Hoff SD, Bailey HR, Butts DR, et al. Ambulatory surgical hemorrhoidectomy: a solution to postoperative urinary retention? *Dis Colon Rectum* 1994;37:1242.

114. Hosking SW, Smart HL, Johnson AG, et al. Anorectal varices, haemorrhoids, and portal hypertension. *Lancet* 1989; 1:349.

115. Hsieh J-S, Huang C-J, Huang Y-S, et al. Demonstration of rectal varices by transhepatic inferior mesenteric venography. *Dis Colon Rectum* 1986;29:459.

116. Hudson AT. S-plasty repair of Whitehead deformity of the anus. *Dis Colon Rectum* 1967;10:57.

117. Iwagaki H, Higuchi Y, Fuchimoto S, et al. The laser treatment of hemorrhoids: results of a study on 1816 patients. *Jpn J Surg* 1989;19:658.

118. Jayne DG, Botterill I, Ambrose NS, et al. Randomized clinical trial of Ligasure versus conventional diathermy for day-case haemorrhoidectomy. *Br J Surg* 2002;89:428.

119. Jeffery PJ, Ritchie JK, Parks AG. Treatment of hemorrhoids in patients with inflammatory bowel disease. *Lancet* 1977; 1:1084.

120. Jetmore AB, Heryer JW, Conner WE. Monsel's solution: a kinder, gentler hemostatic. *Dis Colon Rectum* 1993;36:866.

121. Johanson JF, Sonnenberg A. The prevalence of hemorrhoids and chronic constipation: an epidemologic study. *Gastroenterology* 1990;98:380.

122. Johnson CD, Budd J, Ward AJ. Laxatives after hemorrhoidectomy. *Dis Colon Rectum* 1987;30:780.

123. Jones CB. A comparative study of the methods of treatment for haemorrhoids. *Proc R Soc Med* 1974;67:51.

124. Jongen J, Bach S, Stübinger SH, et al. Excision of thrombosed external hemorrhoid under local anesthesia. *Dis Colon Rectum* 2003;46:1226.

125. Kairaluoma M, Nuorva K, Kellokumpu I. Day-case stapled (circular) vs. diathermy hemorrhoidectomy. *Dis Colon Rectum* 2003;46:93–99.

126. Katchian A. Hemorrhoids: measuring the constrictive force of rubber bands. *Dis Colon Rectum* 1984;27:471.

127. Katchian A. Rubber band ligation [Letter]. *Dis Colon Rectum* 1985;28:759.

128. Keighley MRB, Buchmann P, Minervini S, et al. Prospective trials of minor surgical procedures and high-fibre diet for hemorrhoids. *BMJ* 1979;2:967.

129. Kelsey CB. How to treat haemorrhoids by injections of carbolic acid. *N Y Med J* 1885;42:545.

130. Khalil KH, O'Bichere A, Sellu D. Randomized clinical trial of sutured versus stapled closed haemorrhoidectomy. *Br J Surg* 2000;87:1352.

131. Khoury GA, Lake SP, Lewis MCA, et al. A randomized trial to compare single with multiple phenol injection treatment for haemorrhoids. *Br J Surg* 1985;72:741.

132. Khubchandani IT. A randomized comparison of single and multiple rubber band ligations. *Dis Colon Rectum* 1983;26: 705.

133. Khubchandani IT. Mucosal advancement anoplasty. *Dis Colon Rectum* 1985;28:194.

134. Khubchandani IT. Internal sphincterotomy with hemorrhoidectomy does not relieve pain: a prospective, randomized study. *Dis Colon Rectum* 2002;45:1452.

135. Khubchandani M. Results of Whitehead operation. *Dis Colon Rectum* 1984;27:730.

136. Kilbride M, Morse M, Senagore A. Transdermal fentanyl improves management of postoperative hemorrhoidectomy pain. *Dis Colon Rectum* 1994;37:1070.

137. Kluiber RM, Wolff BG. Evaluation of anemia caused by hemorrhoidal bleeding. *Dis Colon Rectum* 1994;37:1006.

138. Konsten J, Baeten CGMI. Hemorrhoidectomy vs. Lord's method: 17-year follow-up of a prospective, randomized trial. *Dis Colon Rectum* 2000;43:503–506.

139. Kratzer GL. Local anesthesia in anorectal surgery. *Dis Colon Rectum* 1965;8:441.

140. Kriss BD, Porter JA, Slezak FA. Retroperitoneal air after routine hemorrhoidectomy: report of a case. *Dis Colon Rectum* 1990;33:971.

141. Kuo R-J. Epidural morphine for post-hemorrhoidectomy analgesia. *Dis Colon Rectum* 1984;27:529.

141. Lal D, Levitan R. Bacteremia following proctoscopic biopsy of a rectal polyp. *Arch Intern Med* 1972;130:127.

143. Lau WY, Chow HP, Poon GP, et al. Rubber band ligation of three primary hemorrhoids in a single session. *Dis Colon Rectum* 1982;25:336.

144. Lee HH, Spencer RJ, Beart RW Jr. Multiple hemorrhoidal bandings in a single session. *Dis Colon Rectum* 1994;37:37.

145. Leff EI. Hemorrhoidectomy: laser versus non-laser: outpatient surgical experience. *Dis Colon Rectum* 1992:35:743.

146. LeFrock JL, Ellis CA, Turchik JB, et al. Transient bacteremia associated with sigmoidoscopy. *N Engl J Med* 1973; 289:467.

147. Leicester RJ, Nicholls RJ, Mann CV. Comparison of infrared coagulation with conventional methods and the treatment of hemorrhoids. *Coloproctology* 1981;5:313.

148. Leicester RJ, Nicholls RJ, Mann CV. Infrared coagulation: a new treatment for hemorrhoids. *Dis Colon Rectum* 1981; 24:602.

149. Lewis AAM, Rogers HS, Leighton M. Trial of maximal anal dilatation, cryotherapy and elastic band ligation as alternatives to haemorrhoidectomy in the treatment of large prolapsing haemorrhoids. *Br J Surg* 1983;70:54.

150. Lewis MI. Cryosurgical hemorrhoidectomy: a follow-up report. *Dis Colon Rectum* 1972;15:128.

151. Loder PB, Kamm MA, Nicholls RJ, et al. Haemorrhoids: pathology, pathophysiology, and aetiology. *Br J Surg* 1994; 81:946.

152. Longo A. Treatment of hemorrhoid disease by reduction of mucosa and hemorrhoid prolapse with a circular-suturing device: a new procedure. In: *Proceedings of the Sixth World Congress of Endoscopic Surgery*. Rome: 1998: 777–784.

153. Lord PH. A new regime for the treatment of hemorrhoids. *Proc R Soc Med* 1968;61:935.

154. Lord PH. Diverse methods of managing hemorrhoids: dilatation. *Dis Colon Rectum* 1973;16:180.

155. Lurz KH, Göltner E. Hämorrhoiden in Schwanger-schaft und Wochenbett. *Munch Med Wochenschr* 1977;119:1551.

156. MacLeod JH. In defense of cryotherapy for hemorrhoids: a modified method. *Dis Colon Rectum* 1982;25:332.

157. MacRae HM, McLeod RS. Comparison of hemorrhoidal treatment modalities: a meta-analysis. *Dis Colon Rectum* 1995;38:687.

158. Malgieri JA. Anoplasty to correct anal stricture. *Dis Colon Rectum* 1961;4:289.

159. Maw A, Concepcion R, Eu KW, et al. Prospective randomized study of bacteraemia in diathermy and stapled haemorrhoidectomy. *Br J Surg* 2003;90:222.

160. Maw A, Eu K-W, Seow-Choen F. Retroperitoneal sepsis complicating stapled hemorrhoidectomy: report of a case and review of the literature. *Dis Colon Rectum* 2002;45: 826.

161. McCaffrey J. Lord treatment of haemorrhoids: four-year follow-up of fifty patients. *Lancet* 1975;1:133.

162. McConnell JC, Khubchandani IT. Long-term follow-up of closed hemorrhoidectomy. *Dis Colon Rectum* 1983;26:797.

163. McKay W, Morris R, Mushlin P. Sodium bicarbonate attenuates pain on skin infiltration with lidocaine, with or without epinephrine. *Anesth Analg* 1987;66:572.

164. McLeskey CH. pH of local anesthetic solutions. *Anesth Analg* 1980;59:892.

165. Mehigan BJ, Monson JRT, Hartley JE. Stapling procedures for haemorrhoids versus Milligan-Morgan haemorrhoidectomy: randomised controlled trial. *Lancet* 2000: 355:779.

166. Milito G, Gargiani M, Cortese F. Randomised trial comparing LigaSure haemorrhoidectomy with the diathermy dissection operation. *Tech Coloproctol* 2002;6:171.

167. Milligan ETC, Morgan CN, Jones LE, et al. Surgical anatomy of the anal canal, and operative treatment of haemorrhoids. *Lancet* 1937;2:1119.

168. Milsom JW, Mazier WP. Classification and management of postsurgical anal stenosis. *Surg Gynecol Obstet* 1986; 163:60.

169. Moesgaard F, Nielsen ML, Hansen JB, et al. High-fiber diet reduces bleeding and pain in patients with hemorrhoids. *Dis Colon Rectum* 1982;25:454.

170. Molloy RG, Kingsmore D. Life threatening pelvic sepsis after stapled haemorrhoidectomy. *Lancet* 2000;355:810.

171. Moore BA, Fleshner PR. Rubber band ligation for hemorrhoid disease can be safely performed in select HIV-positive patients. *Dis Colon Rectum* 2001;44:1079–1082.

172. Moore DC. The pH of local anesthetic solutions. *Anesth Analg* 1981;60:833.

173. Morinaga K, Hasuda K, Ikeda T. A novel therapy for internal hemorrhoids: ligation of the hemorrhoidal artery with a newly devised instrument (Moricorn) in conjunction with a Doppler flow meter. *Am J Gastroenterol* 1995;90: 610–613.

174. Mortensen PE, Olsen J, Pedersen IK, et al. A randomized study on hemorrhoidectomy combined with anal dilatation. *Dis Colon Rectum* 1987;30:755.

175. Murie JA, Sim AJW, Mackenzie I. Rubber band ligation versus haemorrhoidectomy for prolapsing haemorrhoids: a long-term prospective clinical trial. *Br J Surg* 1982;69:536.

176. Murphy KJ. Tetanus after rubber-band ligation of haemorrhoids. *BMJ* 1978;1:1590.

177. Neiger A. Hemorrhoids in everyday practice. *Proctology* 1979;2:22.

178. Nesselrod JP. *Clinical proctology*, 3rd ed. Philadelphia; WB Saunders, 1964.

179. Nicholson JD, Halleran DR, Trivisonno DP, et al. The efficacy of the contact sapphire tip Nd:YAG laser hemorrhoidectomy. Poster presentation at the 89th annual meeting of the American Society of Colon and Rectal Surgeons, St. Louis, April 29–May 4, 1990.

180. Nickell WB, Woodward ER. Advancement flaps for treatment of anal stricture. *Arch Surg* 1972;104:223.

181. Nivatvongs S. Suture of massive hemorrhoidal bleeding in portal hypertension. *Dis Colon Rectum* 1985;28:878.

182. Norman DA, Newton R, Nicholas GV. Direct current electrotherapy of internal hemorrhoids: an effective, safe, and painless outpatient approach. *Am J Gastroenterol* 1989; 84:482.

183. Nyam DCNK, Seow-Choen F, Ho YH. Submucosal adrenaline injection for posthemorrhoidectomy hemorrhage. *Dis Colon Rectum* 1995;38:776.

184. O'Connor JJ. Cryohemorrhoidectomy: indications and complications. *Dis Colon Rectum* 1976;19:41.

185. O'Connor JJ. Infrared coagulation of hemorrhoids. *Pract Gastroenterol* 1986;10:8.

186. O'Donovan S, Ferrara A, Larach S, et al. Intraoperative use of Toradol facilitates outpatient hemorrhoidectomy. *Dis Colon Rectum* 1994;37:793.

187. Oh C. The role of cryosurgery in management of anorectal disease: cryohemorrhoidectomy evaluated. *Dis Colon Rectum* 1975;18:289.

188. Oh C. One thousand cryohemorrhoidectomies: an overview. *Dis Colon Rectum* 1981;24:613.

189. Oh C, Zinberg J. Anoplasty for anal stricture. *Dis Colon Rectum* 1982;25:809.

190. O'Hara VS. Fatal clostridial infection following hemorrhoidal banding. *Dis Colon Rectum* 1980;23:570.

191. Okamura RK, Reisner LS, Kalichman MW. Effects of pH-adjusted lidocaine solutions on the compound action potential in intact rat sciatic nerves. *Anesthesiology* 1987;37: 281(abst).

192. Ortiz H, Marzo J, Armendariz P. Randomized clinical trial of stapled haemorrhoidectomy versus conventional diathermy haemorrhoidectomy. *Br J Surg* 2002;89:1376.

193. Osur D. [Letter.] *Surg Gynecol Obstet* 1988;167:148.

194. Palazzo FF, Francis DL, Clifton MA. Randomized clinical trial of Ligasure versus open haemorrhoidectomy. *Br J Surg* 2002;89:154–157.

195. Parikh SR, Molinelli B, Dailey TH. Liver abscess after hemorrhoidectomy: report of two cases. *Dis Colon Rectum* 1994;37:185.

196. Parks AG. Surgical treatment of haemorrhoids. *Br J Surg* 1956;43:337.

197. Parks AG. Hemorrhoidectomy. *Adv Surg* 1971;5:1.

198. Parnass SM, Baughman VL, Miletich DJ, et al. The effects of pH on the oxidation rate of epinephrine. *Anesthesiology* 1987;37:A280(abst).

199. Parnaud E, Guntz M, Bernard A, et al. Anatomie normale macroscopique et microscopique du réseau vasculaire hémorrhoidal. *Arch Fr Mal Appar Dig* 1976;65:501.

200. Parturier-Albot M, Rouzette P, Elizalde N. Hémorrhoides et vue génitale de la femme. *Arch Fr Mal Appar Dig* 1976; 65:537.

201. Pearl RK, Hooks VH III, Abcarian H, et al. Island flap anoplasty for the treatment of anal stricture and mucosal ectropion. *Dis Colon Rectum* 1990;33:581.

202. Peng BC, Jayne DG, Ho Y-H. Randomized trial of rubber band ligation vs. stapled hemorrhoidectomy for prolapsed piles. *Dis Colon Rectum* 2003; 46:291–297.

203. Pernice LM, BartalucciB, Bencini L, et al. Early and late (ten years) experience with circular stapler hemorrhoidectomy. *Dis Colon Rectum* 2001;44:836.

204. Perrotti P, Antropoli C, Molino D, et al. Conservative treatment of acute thrombosed external hemorrhoids with nifedipine. *Dis Colon Rectum* 2001;44:405–409.

205. Pescatori M. Stapled rectal prolapsectomy [Letter]. *Dis Colon Rectum* 2000;43:876–877.

206. Pescatori M. Management of post-anopexy rectal stricture. *Tech Coloproctol* 2002;6:125–126.

207. Pidala MJ, Slezak FA, Porter JA. Island flap anoplasty for anal canal stenosis and mucosal ectropion. *Am Surg* 1994; 60:194.

208. Poon GP, Chu KW, Lau WY, et al. Conventional versus triple rubber band ligation for hemorrhoids: a prospective, randomized trial. *Dis Colon Rectum* 1986;29:836.

209. Pope CE. An anorectal plastic operation for fissure and stenosis and its surgical principles. *Surg Gynecol Obstet* 1959;108:249.

210. Quevado-Bonilla G, Farkas AM, Abcarian H, et al. Septic complications of hemorrhoidal banding. *Arch Surg* 1988; 123:650.

211. Rachochot JE, Petourand CH, Riovoire JO. Saint Fiacre: the healer of hemorrhoids and patron saint of proctology. *Am J Proctol* 1971;22:175–177.

212. Rakhmanine M, Rosen L, Khubchandani I, et al. Lateral mucosal advancement anoplasty for anal stricture. *Br J Surg* 2002;89:1423.

213. Rand AA. The sliding skin-flap graft operation for hemorrhoids: a modification of the Whitehead procedure. *Dis Colon Rectum* 1969;12:265.

214. Randall GM, Jensen DM, Machicado GA, et al. Prospective randomized comparative study of bipolar versus direct current electrocoagulation for treatment of bleeding internal hemorrhoids. *Gastrointest Endosc* 1994;40: 403.

215. Read TE, Henry SC, Hovis RM, et al. Prospective evaluation of anesthetic technique for anorectal surgery. *Dis Colon Rectum* 2002;45:1553.

216. Ribbans WJ, Radcliffe AG. Retroperitoneal abscess following sclerotherapy for hemorrhoids. *Dis Colon Rectum* 1985; 28:188.

217. Richman IM. Use of Toradol in anorectal surgery. *Dis Colon Rectum* 1993;36:295.

218. Ripetti V, Caricato M, Arullani A. Rectal perforation, retropneumoperitoneum, and pneumomediastinum after stapling procedure for prolapsed hemorrhoids: report of a case and subsequent considerations. *Dis Colon Rectum* 2002;45:268.

219. Rosen L. Y-V advancement for anal ectropion. *Dis Colon Rectum* 1986;29:596.

220. Rosen L. Anoplasty. *Surg Clin North Am* 1988;68:1441.

221. Rosen L, Sipe P, Stasik JJ, et al. Outcome of delayed hemorrhage following surgical hemorrhoidectomy. *Dis Colon Rectum* 1993;36:743.

222. Rosser C. Chemical rectal stricture. *JAMA* 1931;96:1762.

223. Rowsell M, Bello M, Hemingway DM. Circumferential mucosectomy (stapled hemorrhoidectomy) versus conventional haemorrhoidectomy: randomised controlled trial. *Lancet* 2000;355:779.

224. Russell TR, Donohue JH. Hemorrhoidal banding: a warning. *Dis Colon Rectum* 1985;28:291.

225. Safavi A, Gottesman L, Dailey TH. Anorectal surgery in the HIV+ patient: update. *Dis Colon Rectum* 1991;34:299.

226. Saldana E, Paletta C, Gupta N, et al. Internal pudendal flap anoplasty for severe anal stenosis. *Dis Colon Rectum* 1996; 39:350.

227. Saleeby RG Jr, Rosen L, Stasik JJ, et al. Hemorrhoidectomy during pregnancy: risk or relief? *Dis Colon Rectum* 1991; 34:260.

228. Salmon F. *A practical essay on stricture of the rectum illustrated by cases, showing the connexion of that disease, with affections of the urinary organs and the uterus, with piles and various constitutional complaints*, 3rd ed. London: Whitaker, Treacher & Arnot, 1829:208.

229. Salvati EP. Urinary retention in anorectal and colonic surgery. *Am J Surg* 1957;94:114.

230. Sankar MY, Joffe SN. Technique of contact laser hemorrhoidectomy: an ambulatory surgical procedure. *Contemp Surg* 1987;30:9.

231. Santos G, Novell JR, Chir M, et al. Long-term results of large-dose, single-session phenol injection sclerotherapy for hemorrhoids. *Dis Colon Rectum* 1993;36:958.

232. Sarner JB. Plastic relief of anal stenosis. *Dis Colon Rectum* 1969;12:277.

233. Savin S. Hemorrhoidectomy: how I do it? Results of 444 cryoabdirectoryectal surgical operations. *Dis Colon Rectum* 1977;20:189.

234. Scarpa FJ, Hillis W, Sabetta JR. Pelvic cellulitis: a life-threatening complication of hemorrhoidal banding. *Surgery* 1988;103:383.

235. Schapiro M. The gastroenterologist and the treatment of hemorrhoids: is it about time? *Am J Gastroenterol* 1989; 84:493.

236. Schouten WR, van Vroonhoven TJ. Lateral internal sphincterotomy in the treatment of hemorrhoids: a clinical and manometric study. *Dis Colon Rectum* 1986;29:869.

237. Scoma JA. Hemorrhoidectomy without urinary retention and catheterization. *Conn Med* 1976;40:751.

238. Selvaggi F, Scotto di Carlo E, Silvestri A, et al. Surgical treatment of circumferential hemorrhoids. *Dis Colon Rectum* 1990;33:903.

239. Senagore AJ. Surgical management of hemorrhoids. *J Gastrointest Surg* 2002; 6:295–298.

240. Senagore A, Mazier WP, Luchtefeld MA, et al. Treatment of advanced hemorrhoidal disease: a prospective, randomized comparison of cold scalpel versus contact Nd:YAG laser. *Dis Colon Rectum* 1993;36:1042.

241. Seow-Choen F. Stapled haemorrhoidectomy: pain or gain. *Br J Surg* 2001;88:1.

242. Shemesh EI, Kodner IJ, Fry RD, et al. Severe complication of rubber band ligation of internal hemorrhoids. *Dis Colon Rectum* 1987;30:199.

243. Shieh CJ, Gennaro A. Treatment of acute prolapsed hemorrhoids: manual reduction followed by semi-emergent hemorrhoidectomy. *Am J Proctol Gastroenterol Colon Rectal Surg* 1985;36:12.

244. Shropshear G. Posterior and anterior anal proctotomy: a simplified technique for postoperative anal stenosis. *Dis Colon Rectum* 1971;14:62.

245. Sim AJW, Murie JA, Mackenzie I. Three-year follow-up study on the treatment of first- and second-degree hemorrhoids by sclerosant injection or rubber band ligation. *Surg Gynecol Obstet* 1983;157:534.

246. Singer MA, Cintron JR, Fleshman JW, et al. Early experience with stapled hemorrhoidectomy in the United States. *Dis Colon Rectum* 2002;45:360.

247. Smith LE, Goodreau JJ, Fouty J. Management of hemorrhoids: operative hemorrhoidectomy versus cryosurgery. *Dis Colon Rectum* 1979;22:10.

248. Sohn N, Aronoff JS, Cohen FS, et al. Transanal hemorrhoidal dearterialization is an alternative to operative hemorrhoidectomy. *Am J Surg* 2001;182:515–519.

249. Standards Task Force, American Society of Colon and Rectal Surgeons. Practice parameters for the treatment of hemorrhoids. *Dis Colon Rectum* 1993;36:1118.

250. Steinberg DM, Liegois H, Alexander-Williams J. Long-term review of the results of rubber band ligation of haemorrhoids. *Br J Surg* 1975;62:144.

251. Stelzner F, Staubesand J, Machleidt H. The corpus cavernosum recti: basis of internal hemorrhoids. *Langenbecks Chir Arch* 1962;299:302.

252. Subramanyam K, Patterson M, Gourley WK. Effects of Preparation H on wound healing in the rectum of man. *Dig Dis Sci* 1984;29:829.

253. Sun WM, Peck RJ, Shorthouse AJ, et al. Haemorrhoids are associated not with hypertrophy of the internal anal sphincter, but with hypertension of the anal cushions. *Br J Surg* 1992;79:592.

254. Sun WM, Read NW, Shorthouse AJ. Hypertensive anal cushions as a cause of the high anal canal pressures in patients with haemorrhoids. *Br J Surg* 1990;77:458.

255. Tan PY, Vukasin P, Chin ID, et al. The WAND local anesthetic delivery system: a more pleasant experience for anal anesthesia. *Dis Colon Rectum* 2001;44:686.

256. Tchirkow G, Haas PA, Fox TA. Injection of a local anesthetic solution into hemorrhoidal bundles following rubber band ligation. *Dis Colon Rectum* 1982;25:62.

257. Terrell EH. The treatment of hemorrhoids by a new method. *Trans Am Proctol Soc* 1916:65.

258. Thomson H. A new look at hemorrhoids. *Med Times* 1976; 04:116.

259. Thomson WHF. The nature of haemorrhoids. *Br J Surg* 1975;62:542.

260. Traynor OJ, Carter AE. Cryotherapy for advanced haemorrhoids: a prospective evaluation with 2-year follow-up. *Br J Surg* 1984;71:287.

261. Turell R. Postoperative anal stenosis. *Surg Gynecol Obstet* 1950;90:231.

262. Turell R. Preoperative and postoperative management in anorectal surgery. In: Turell R, ed. *Diseases of the colon and anorectum,* 2nd ed, vol 2. Philadelphia: WB Saunders, 1969:883.

263. Turell R, Gelernt IM. Anal stenosis. In: Turell R, ed. *Diseases of the colon and anorectum,* 2nd ed, vol 2. Philadelphia: WB Saunders, 1969:1046.

264. Turell R, Gelernt IM. Anal stenosis. In: Turell R, ed. *Diseases of the colon and anorectum,* 2nd ed, vol 2. Philadelphia: WB Saunders, 1969:1051.

265. Vellacott KD, Hardcastle JD. Is continued anal dilatation necessary after a Lord's procedure for hemorrhoids? *Br J Surg* 1980;67:658.

266. Vinson-Bonnet B, Coltat JC, Fingerhut A, et al. Local infiltration with ropivacaine improves immediate postoperative pain control after hemorrhoid surgery. *Dis Colon Rectum* 2002;45:104–108.

267. Walls ADF, Ruckley CV. A five-year follow-up of Lord's dilatation for haemorrhoids. *Lancet* 1976;1:1212.

268. Wang JY, Chang-Chien CR, Chen J-S, et al. The role of lasers in hemorrhoidectomy. *Dis Colon Rectum* 1991;34:78.

269. Watts JM, Bennett RC, Duthie HL, et al. Healing and pain after hemorrhoidectomy. *Br J Surg* 1964;51:808.

270. Wasvary HJ, Hain J, Mosed-Vogel M, et al. Randomized, prospective, double-blind, placebo-controlled trial of effect of nitroglycerine ointment on pain after hemorrhoidectomy. *Dis Colon Rectum* 2001;44:1069–1073.

271. Wechter DG, Luna GK. An unusual complication of rubber band ligation of hemorrhoids. *Dis Colon Rectum* 1987; 30:137.

272. Weinshel E, Chen W, Falkenstein DB, et al. Hemorrhoids or rectal varices: defining the cause of massive rectal hemorrhage in patients with portal hypertension. *Gastroenterology* 1986;90:744.

273. Weinstein SJ, Rypins EB, Houck J, et al. Single-session treatment for bleeding hemorrhoids. *Surg Gynecol Obstet* 1987;165:479.

274. Wexner SD, Baig K: The evaluation and physiologic assessment of hemorrhoidal disease: a review. *Tech Coloproctol* 2001;5:165–168.

275. White AC. Liquid air: its application in medicine and surgery. *Med Rec* 1899;56:109.

276. Whitehead W. The surgical treatment of haemorrhoids. *BMJ* 1882;1:148.

277. Williams KL, Haq IU, Elem B. Cryodestruction of haemorrhoids. *BMJ* 1973;1:666.

278. Wilson MC, Schofield P. Cryosurgical haemorrhoidectomy. *Br J Surg* 1976;63:497.

279. Wilson MS, Pope V, Doran HE, et al. Objective comparison of stapled anopexy and open hemorrhoidectomy: a randomized, controlled trial. *Dis Colon Rectum* 2002;45:1437.

280. Wilson PM. Anorectal closing mechanisms. *S Afr Med J* 1977;51:802.

281. Wolf JS, Munoz JJ, Rosin JD. Survey of hemorrhoidectomy practices: open versus closed techniques. *Dis Colon Rectum* 1979;22:536.

282. Wolff BG, Culp CE. The Whitehead hemorrhoidectomy: an unjustly maligned procedure. *Dis Colon Rectum* 1988;31: 587.

283. Wolkomir AF, Luchtefeld MA. Surgery for symptomatic hemorrhoids and anal fissures in Crohn's disease. *Dis Colon Rectum* 1993;36:545.

284. Wong L-Y, Jiang J-K, Chang S-C, et al. Rectal perforation: a life-threatening complication of stapled hemorrhoidectomy: report of a case. *Dis Colon Rectum* 2003;46: 116–117.

285. Wright RA, Kranz KR, Kirby SL. A prospective crossover trial of direct current electrotherapy in symptomatic hemorrhoidal disease. *Gastointest Endosc* 1991;37:621.

286. Wrobleski DE, Corman ML, Veidenheimer MC, et al. Long-term evaluation of rubber ring ligation in hemorrhoidal disease. *Dis Colon Rectum* 1980;23:478.

287. Yang R, Migikovsky B, Peicher J, et al. Randomized, prospective trial of direct current versus bipolar electrocoagulation for bleeding internal hemorrhoids. *Gastrointest Endosc* 1993;39:766.

288. Yu JC, Eddy HJ Jr. Laser, a new modality for hemorrhoidectomy. *Am J Proctol Gastroenterol Colon Rectal Surg* 1985;36:9.

289. Zinberg SS, Stern DH, Furman DS, et al. A personal experience in comparing three nonoperative techniques for treating internal hemorrhoids. *Am J Gastroenterol* 1989; 84:488.

Anal Fissure

Anal fissure (fissure-in-ano) is a common anorectal condition. It can be a very troubling condition because, if acute, the severity of patient discomfort and extent of disability far exceed that which would be expected from a seemingly trivial lesion.

An anal fissure is a cut or crack in the anal canal or anal verge that may extend from the mucocutaneous junction to the dentate line. It can be acute or chronic. It may occur at any age (it is the most common cause of rectal bleeding in infants) but is usually a condition of young adults. Both sexes are affected equally. However, an anterior fissure is much more likely to develop in women than in men (only 1% of those in men are located anteriorly). Still, fully 90% of fissures are found posteriorly in women.[37] Abramowitz and colleagues prospectively studied 165 consecutive women during their last 3 months of pregnancy and after delivery and noted that one third develop thrombosed external hemorrhoids or anal fissures.[3] They attribute the most important predisposing factor to dyschezia (difficult or painful evacuation).

ETIOLOGY AND PATHOGENESIS

Generally, anal fissure has been attributed to constipation or to straining at stool; theoretically, the hard fecal bolus is thought to crack the anal canal. To identify risk factors for the development of the condition, Jensen studied 174 patients with chronic anal fissure and compared them with controls as to diet, beverage consumption, occupational exposures, and medical/surgical history.[46] A decreased risk was associated with increased consumption of raw fruits, vegetables, and whole-grain bread. Significantly increased risk was noted with frequent consumption of white bread, sauces thickened with a roux, bacon, and sausage. Risk was not related to consumption of coffee, tea, or alcohol.

Anal fissure can also be a consequence of frequent defecation and diarrhea. It may be associated with nonspecific inflammatory bowel disease and must be considered in the differential diagnosis of certain specific inflammatory conditions (e.g., syphilis, tuberculosis, gonorrhea, chlamydial infection, herpes, acquired immunodeficiency syndrome, and others). If there is cause for concern as to the true nature of the ulcer or fissure, biopsy, stool culture, serology, and gastrointestinal evaluation may be indicated. When anal fissure occurs in an unusual location, especially laterally, the physician must entertain the possibility that the patient has ulcerative colitis or, more commonly, Crohn's disease (see Chapter 30).

Why the fissure is most commonly located in the posterior anal canal is a subject of some controversy. Lockhart-Mummery believed that the explanation can be found in the structure of the external sphincter.[61] The lower portion of this muscle is not truly circular, but rather consists of a band of muscle fibers that pass from posterior to anterior and split around the anus. He postulated that the anal mucosa is, therefore, best supported laterally and is weakest posteriorly. The decreased anterior support in women accounts for the greater occurrence in this location than in men. Additional evidence reinforcing the Lockhart-Mummery concept may be apparent when the physician inserts an anal retractor too vigorously at the time of hemorrhoid surgery. The split that may occur is almost invariably located posteriorly. Likewise, if the sphincter is stretched in the cadaver, tearing almost always occurs posteriorly.[62]

Another theory that has been suggested is related to the blood supply to the area. Klosterhalfen and colleagues visualized the inferior rectal artery by means of postmortem angiography, by manual preparations, and by histologic study following vascular injection.[54] They determined that in 85% of specimens, the posterior commissure is less well perfused than other areas of the anal canal. Hence, ischemia may be an important etiologic factor in causing anal fissure, especially in the posterior location. The authors further suggest that the blood supply, which is already tenuous, may be further compromised by compression and contusion as the branch of the inferior rectal artery passes

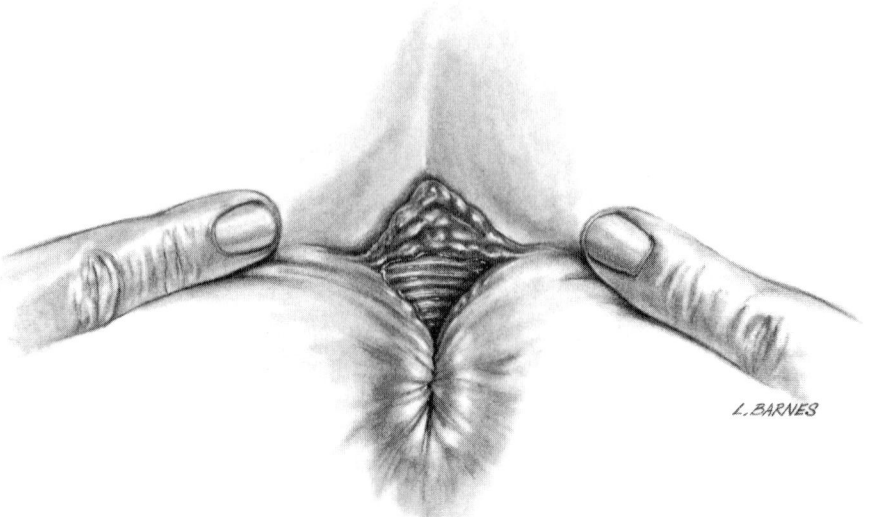

FIGURE 9-1. "Sentinel pile," or skin tab, at the lower edge of an anal fissure. This can easily be recognized without instrumentation.

through the internal anal sphincter. Others have confirmed in cadaveric studies that there is a significant trend to an increasing number of arterioles from posterior to anterior in the subanodermal space at all levels.[65]

Schouten and colleagues assessed microvascular perfusion of the anoderm by means of Doppler flowmetry in 27 patients.[95] Anodermal blood flow at the fissure site was significantly lower than at the posterior commissure of the controls. Reduction of anal pressure by sphincterotomy improved anodermal blood flow, resulting in healing of the fissure. These observations lend further support to the concept that ischemia is the etiologic factor that contributes to the development of fissure disease. A later study by the same authors, this time involving 178 subjects, confirmed that anodermal blood flow was less in the posterior midline than in other segments of the anal canal.[96]

Why some fissures heal spontaneously and others become chronic is an unresolved question. Ischemia, infection, or lymphatic obstruction secondary to persistent inflammation may be responsible. A characteristic skin tag (i.e., a sentinel pile) may develop distally, whereas proximally, a hypertrophied anal papilla may be seen (Figs. 9-1 through 9-3). If one wishes to at-

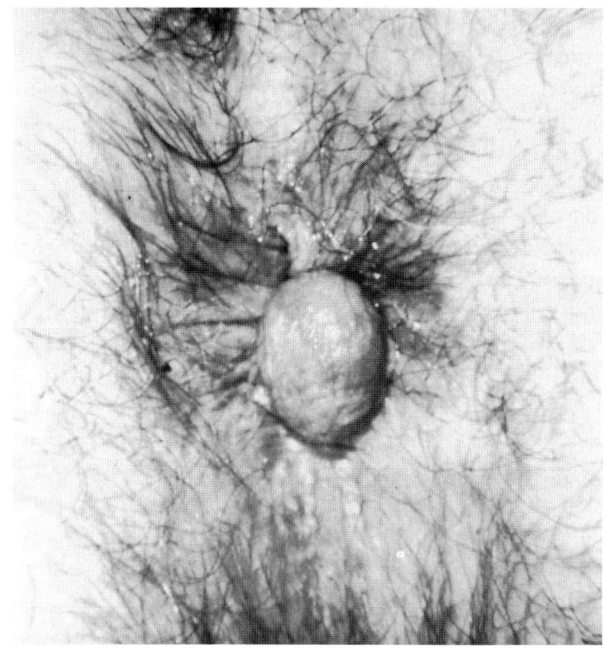

FIGURE 9-2. Prolapsed hypertrophied anal papilla associated with anal fissure. This condition must be distinguished from an external hemorrhoid in order to provide the appropriate treatment.

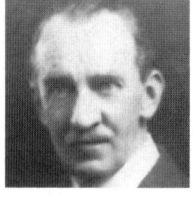

John Percy Lockhart-Mummery (1875–1957) Lockhart-Mummery was born at Islips Manor, Northolt, England, the eldest son of a distinguished dental surgeon. He was educated at Leys School and Caius College, Cambridge. He was an outstanding student and in 1897 was appointed an assistant demonstrator in anatomy at his alma mater. In 1900, he became a Fellow of the Royal College of Surgeons and subsequently received several hospital appointments. In 1903, having developed a special interest in proctology, he was appointed assistant surgeon at St. Mark's Hospital. In 1904, he was Hunterian Professor at the Royal College of Surgeons, and in 1909, he was Jacksonian prize winner at the college. He contributed extensively to the literature throughout his career. Among his writings were six books on colorectal surgery, in addition to two collections of essays on nonmedical subjects. He was a very energetic man, even "hopping up the steps to the hospital"—a rather relevant observation, as while a student at Cambridge, he had undergone a leg amputation for sarcoma by Lord Lister himself. He was the first secretary of the British Proctological Society and was instrumental in establishing it as an independent section of the Royal Society of Medicine. In 1937, he was elected a Fellow of the American College of Surgeons. In 1940, after 37 years at St. Mark's Hospital, Lockhart-Mummery was made an Honorary Consulting Surgeon. (Lockhart-Mummery P. Fissure-in-ano. In: *Diseases of the rectum and anus: a practical handbook.* New York: William Wood, 1944:169.)

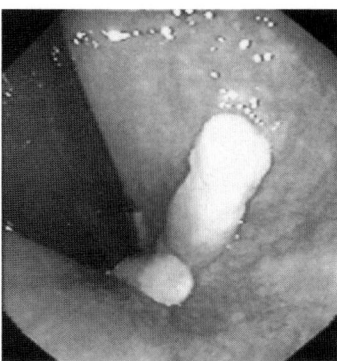

FIGURE 9-3. Hypertrophied anal papillae are seen through a retroflexed video-endoscope in a patient with a chronic anal fissure. (See Color Fig. 9-3.)

tempt an anthropomorphic explanation for the occurrence of skin tags and papillae, it is as if healing cannot take place across the defect produced by the fissure, so the body attempts to heal it through overgrowth on the proximal and distal ends of the defect. One often observes that the internal anal sphincter muscle fibers can be seen at the base of the open wound (Figure 9-4).

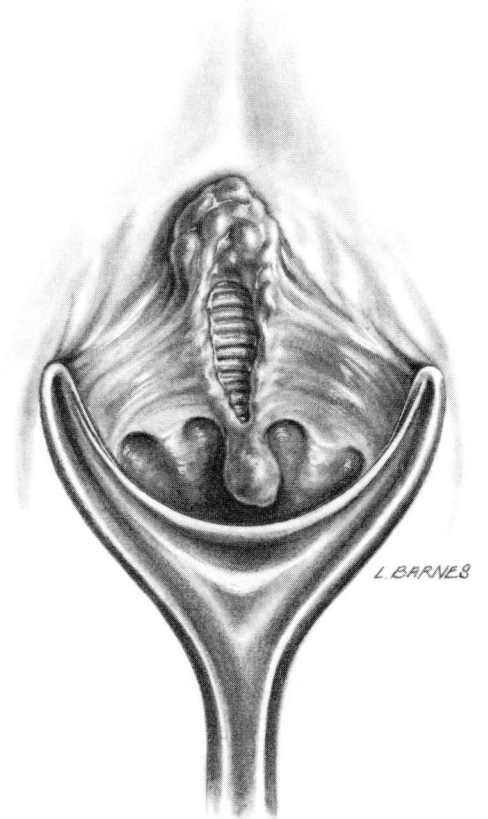

FIGURE 9-4. Chronic posterior anal fissure with skin tag and hypertrophied anal papilla. Note fibers of the internal anal sphincter at the base of the wound.

PHYSIOLOGIC STUDIES

Anal manometric pressure studies in patients with anal fissure have interested investigators for some time. Duthie and Bennett in 1964 were among the earliest who measured anal canal pressures. They used an open-ended tube connected to a recording device by a strain gauge.[22] Although all patients had demonstrable spasm of the sphincter on the basis of digital examination, no increase in the resting pressure was found when they were compared with control subjects. When sphincter stretch was performed, a moderate fall in pressure was noted, but it returned virtually to normal by the eighth postoperative day. It appeared to the authors that the therapeutic effect of sphincter stretch was not related so much to reduction in anal pressure as to prevention of the spasm.[22] Others have observed a similar pattern, in which the pressure falls after internal anal sphincterotomy.[7,15,40,96]

However, Gibbons and Read employed perfusion probes of varying diameters in patients with chronic anal fissure.[34] Resting pressures were *elevated* in all subjects when compared with controls, irrespective of probe size. They, therefore, postulated that resting pressures are indeed elevated in individuals with an anal fissure and that this observed phenomenon is not caused by spasm. They postulated that ischemia of the anal canal mucosa may be the cause of the pain and the failure of fissures to heal.

Nothmann and Schuster performed balloon rectosphincteric manometry on patients with anal fissure.[80] Resting pressures were twice as high as those measured in control subjects. Technique is important, however. One must recognize that resting pressures measured with an open-tipped tube in patients with anal fissure may be normal, whereas those measured by balloon catheter are usually elevated.[97] Following distension of the rectum by the balloon, there is the expected internal sphincter relaxation, but this is followed by a *marked and prolonged contraction above the initial baseline*, termed the "overshoot" phenomenon.[80] Nothmann and Schuster concluded that this reflexively stimulated sphincter spasm is involved in the etiology of the condition.[80]

Keck and colleagues examined manometric findings in patients with anal fissure by the use of a computer-assisted system.[51] They concluded that the primary abnormality in fissure is persistent hypertonia affecting the entire internal sphincter.

One can add another possibility to the theories and observations of the ameliorative effect of sphincterotomy. Abcarian and associates, by their manometric evaluation of patients with anal fissure, concluded that the benefit is really the consequence of an anatomic widening of the anal canal that occurs during sphincterotomy.[2]

Roe and colleagues have described a technique for quantifying anal canal sensation by means of two platinum electrodes placed 1 cm apart and connected to copper wires passed to a constant current generator.[90]

Patients with acute anal fissure exhibited a lower threshold of sensation at the site of the fissure. The authors propose that the findings may reflect stimulation of exposed nerve endings at the base of the fissure rather than actual heightened sensory awareness in this group of patients. The value of this experimental modality in the diagnosis and therapy of patients with anorectal disorders, particularly incontinence, has yet to be determined.

Another potentially useful investigative study is that of anal canal ultrasonography. Reissman believes that this investigation may be important in identifying unrecognized obstetrically related sphincteric injuries before performance of internal anal sphincterotomy.[88] Although it is recognized that anal ultrasound may be rather difficult to perform in the presence of an acute, painful fissure, one could consider the advisability of identifying such at-risk individuals.

HISTOPATHOLOGY

Nothing in particular is histologically diagnostic of an anal fissure (Figure 9-5). If the lesion is excised and submitted for pathologic examination, usually typical nonspecific inflammatory changes are observed. Brown and colleagues prospectively studied 18 consecutive patients who underwent internal anal sphincterotomy for chronic anal fissure and took a biopsy specimen from the base and also from the muscle before division.[14] Histologic evaluation confirmed the presence of fibrosis throughout the internal sphincter, but no such finding was identified in controls.

SYMPTOMS

The characteristic complaints of a patient with an acute anal fissure are pain and bleeding. The pain usually occurs with and immediately after defecation. Often, the pain ceases in a few minutes, but occasionally it may persist for hours. The patient often relates that constipation is the antecedent event, but once pain develops, the fear of the act of defecation and refusal of the call to stool can exacerbate this problem. This anxiety leads to fecal impaction, particularly in children and in the elderly. Bleeding is usually minimal and frequently occurs only on the toilet paper, but sometimes blood will be seen in the toilet bowl. It is not uncommon for patients to report no evidence of bleeding.

The pain of anal fissure can be differentiated from that of proctalgia fugax (see Chapter 16) in that the latter condition produces discomfort that is usually not related to bowel action. In addition, the patient with a fissure feels the discomfort in the anal area; the pain of proctalgia fugax is higher and more deep-seated. The other anal condition that commonly produces pain is a thrombosed hemorrhoid (see Chapter 8), but with this complaint, the patient also reports feeling a lump. This will not be present if an acute anal fissure is the cause of the pain.

Patients with a long-standing (i.e., chronic) anal fissure will present with a different symptom complex. They

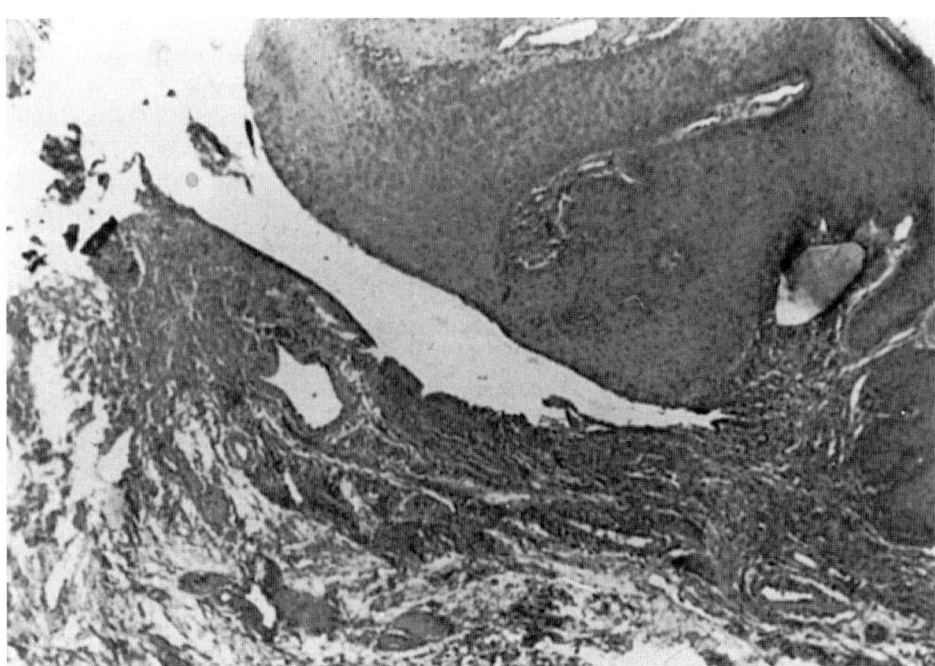

FIGURE 9-5. This anal fissure is an elongated defect surrounded by granulation tissue on one side and acanthotic squamous epithelium on the other. (Original magnification × 180.)

may complain of a lump representing the sentinel tag, drainage or discharge from the open wound, pruritus, or a combination of several symptoms. Bleeding may or may not be present, and pain is usually mild and frequently absent. Problems with micturition (e.g., retention, urgency, frequency) and dyspareunia occasionally accompany the symptoms of both acute and chronic fissure.

EXAMINATION

Acute Fissure

As suggested, the patient's history is usually so characteristic that the diagnosis can be easily established. By mere inspection or gentle retraction of the perianal skin, the open wound often can be seen (Figure 9-1). If the physician is unable to pry the buttocks apart to view the area, the presence of an acute anal fissure is a virtual certainty. Under such circumstances, to attempt digital examination or to insert an instrument is an unnecessary, counterproductive, inhumane exercise. Appropriate treatment should be initiated without more specific confirmatory evidence.

Examination may still be possible if the examiner is so committed and the patient is forbearing. A topical anesthetic jelly may be usefully employed if the physician is willing to wait a few minutes for it to take effect. Palpation will usually demonstrate a spastic anal sphincter or tight anal canal and will exacerbate the patient's discomfort. The open wound is often not appreciated by the examining finger in a patient with an acute anal fissure. Because the cut is relatively superficial, there is usually no fibrosis.

Anoscopic examination, if possible, confirms the location of the fissure. The ability to perform this examination, however, may reflect the chronicity of the problem. Ideally, proctosigmoidoscopic examination should be carried out before any surgical procedure to establish that the rectum, at least, is not involved by inflammatory bowel disease or other pathologic entity. However, the clinical picture is usually so characteristic that most physicians appropriately tend to omit or defer this examination. However, if anoscopy and sigmoidoscopy are to be attempted, it is suggested that narrow-caliber instruments be used.

Chronic Fissure

There is no real agreement as to what constitutes a chronic anal fissure.[84] One definition is that a fissure is chronic when it has become a clearly recognized, well-circumscribed ulcer.[79] Others suggest that it is a fissure that has been present for at least 2 months. I and perhaps others apply a similar rationale to that of the United States Supreme Court justice, Potter Stewart, when he offered the following opinion with regard to a ruling on pornography: " . . . [in certain cases one is] faced with the task of trying to define what may be indefinable. . . . But I know it when I see it." For chronic anal fissure, surgeons also seem to know it when they see it.

Examination of the patient with a chronic anal fissure often reveals the characteristic sentinel pile. This can at times become rather large (i.e., 3 to 4 cm). Digital examination characteristically permits palpation of the fissure, the open wound, induration, and fibrosis. A hypertrophied anal papilla often can be felt at the apex of the ulcer; sometimes it may be mistaken for a tumor (Figs. 9-2 through 9-4).

Because pain and tenderness are generally minimal or absent, anoscopy frequently can be accomplished without difficulty. However, scarring may result in some degree of narrowing of the anal canal, and it may be necessary to use a narrow-diameter anoscope. Characteristically, the internal anal sphincter fibers are clearly seen at the base of a chronic anal fissure. Proctosigmoidoscopy or flexible sigmoidoscopy should be performed to rule out the possibility of a concurrent tumor or distal inflammatory bowel disease.

Occasionally, the base of the fissure may become infected and form an abscess that may discharge as a fistula (Figure 9-6; see Chapter 10). When it occurs, the fistula is inevitably superficial—in fact, truly subcutaneous. Examination may reveal an external opening, virtually always in the midline, usually no more than 1 or 2 cm distal to the skin tag. Purulent material may be noted. A probe passed from the external opening emerges at the distal end of the fissure; usually, the internal anal sphincter is not traversed.

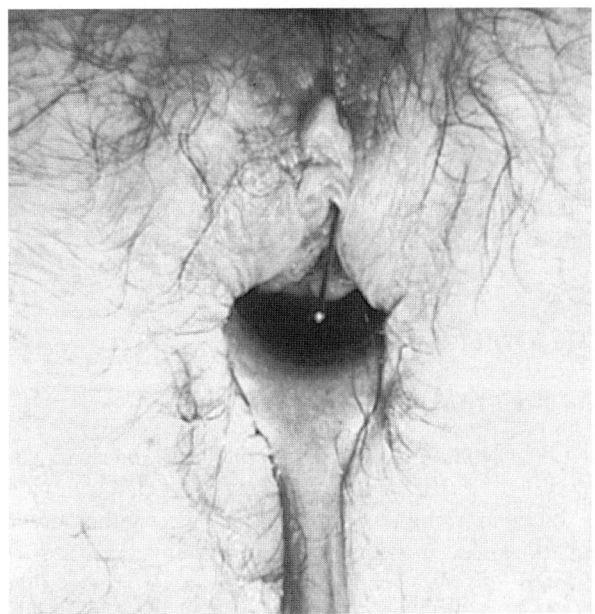

FIGURE 9-6. Anal fissure with associated fistula-in-ano. (Courtesy of Daniel Rosenthal, M.D.)

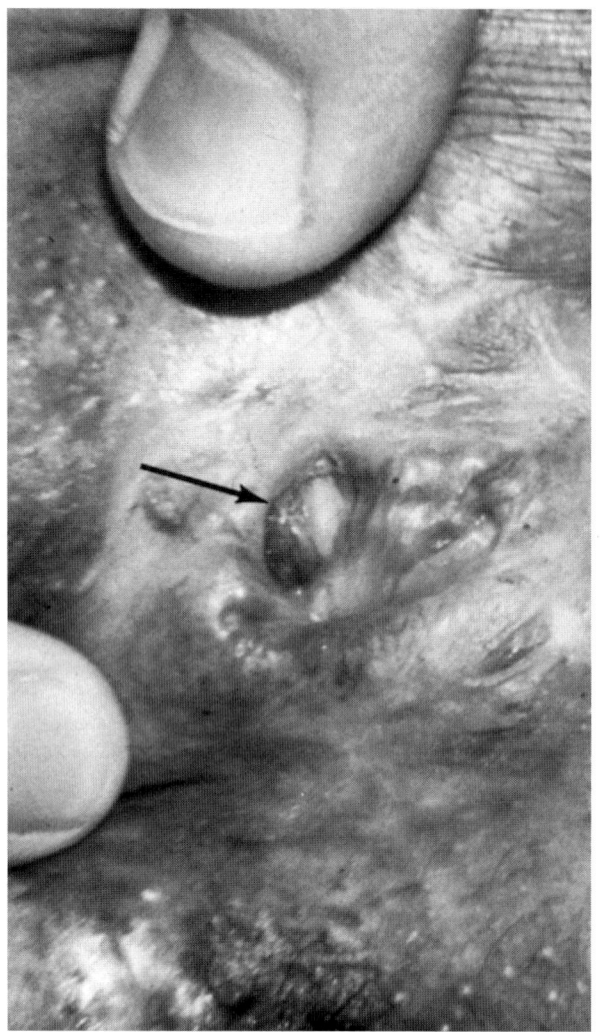

FIGURE 9-7. An anal fissure *(arrow)* resulting from stenosis following hemorrhoidectomy. (Courtesy of Daniel Rosenthal, M.D.)

As suggested, chronic anal fissure may sometimes be associated with anal stenosis, particularly if the fissure is the result of prior anal surgery (e.g., hemorrhoidectomy [Figure 9-7]). Under this circumstance, treatment may require an anoplasty (see Chapter 8).

TREATMENT

Medical Management

In 1992, the Standards Task Force of the American Society of Colon and Rectal Surgeons published guidelines for the management of anal fissure.[92] The statement cautioned, however, that ultimate judgment regarding the propriety of any procedure must be made by the physician based on all the circumstances presented by each individual patient. Those with a history suggestive of anal fissure of relatively recent onset are usually successfully treated by conservative measures, such as stool softeners (e.g., dioctyl sodium sulfosuccinate), bulking agents (e.g., psyllium), a high-fiber diet, and sitz baths. Preparations containing mineral oil are not advised because of difficulty in cleansing the area following defecation. Suppositories also are not recommended, because they do not act effectively within the anal canal. Inserting any one of several proprietary creams and ointments in the area, with or without a local anesthetic, may offer some transient relief. To prevent recurrence, the patient should be encouraged to continue with the diet, perhaps also with the addition of a bulk laxative agent, even after symptoms have resolved.

Topical anesthetic creams that are applied just before defecation and/or afterward may offer transient relief of pain. My own preference is lidocaine 5% anorectal cream (ela-Max5). Injection of a long-acting local anesthetic may also afford temporary relief and may permit examination, but its use on an ambulatory basis is impractical. Anal dilators should not be employed, and the application of silver nitrate without a local anesthetic will usually succeed in clearing the physician's waiting room, so dramatic is the patient's response.

Sclerotherapy

Periodic reports have surfaced in the literature concerning the use of sclerotherapy with that of a local anesthetic. In a nonrandomized, noncontrolled study, Antebi and colleagues treated acute anal fissure by injection of Sotradecol (i.e., sodium tetradecyl sulfate) directly into the fissure (6)[4] In 96 patients with a 1-year follow-up, 80% were free of symptoms and had no evidence of fissure. These investigators recommended the technique for those individuals who fail to respond to conservative management.

Solcoderm

Chen and co-workers reported the topical use of Solcoderm (Solco, Basel, Switzerland) in the treatment of anal fissure.[16] The product has been employed for the management of a variety of skin diseases. In a controlled study involving 25 patients in each group, a statistically significantly better healing rate was shown with the drug at 1 month (84% versus 28%) and at 1 year (84% versus 44%).

Hyperbaric Oxygen

On the theory that hypoxia is an important factor in leading to the development of an anal fissure, Cundall and colleagues treated eight patients in whom conservative treatment, including glyceryl trinitrate (GTN) ointment (see later), had failed.[21] Each patient received

15 hyperbaric treatments over 3 weeks. This consisted of 90 minutes of breathing 100% oxygen at 2.3 atmospheres. At the end of 3 months, five had healed. There were no side effects.

Glyceryl Trinitrate Ointment

The concept of a "chemical sphincterotomy" through the use of a nitric acid donor, GTN, has been the subject of numerous articles and considerable debate in both the medical literature and the lay press in recent years.[39,45,63,64,66,69,104] Nitric oxide is a neurotransmitter that leads to relaxation of the internal sphincter. When applied topically to the anal canal, GTN diffuses across the mucosa causing a reduction in internal anal sphincter pressure.[69] This leads to improvement of anal blood flow with the consequence of increased likelihood for healing of the fissure.

McLeod and Evans, in an article published in 2002, identified a total of nine randomized controlled trials in which the efficacy of GTN was studied.[69] Lund and Scholefield randomized 80 consecutive patients to receive treatments with topical 0.2% GTN ointment or a placebo.[66] After 8 weeks, healing was observed in 26 of the 38 patients treated with GTN (68%) but in only three of 39 treated with the placebo (8%). These differences were highly significant. The authors concluded that topical GTN provides rapid, sustained relief of pain in individuals with anal fissure. A multiinstitutional investigation was conducted in 17 centers with the aim of determining the optimal dosage and dosing interval for the use of GTN.[8] There were no significant differences observed in fissure healing among any of the treatment groups, but those who received 0.4% (1.5 mg) GTN ointment had a statistically significant decrease in pain intensity. The primary side effect was headache. Pitt and colleagues treated 1998 patients with 0.2% GTN ointment.[85] They found that the presence of a sentinel pile adversely affected the outcome. To put it another way, the longer the fissure is present, the less likely GTN will be helpful. Others have opined that GTN (0.2%), on the basis of their randomized, placebo-controlled, double-blind trial, fails to demonstrate any advantage despite demonstrable increased anal canal blood flow and reduced anal pressures.[4]

Botulinum Toxin

In 1993, Jost and Schimrigk, in a letter to the editor, originally reported the injection of botulinum toxin (BNT) into the anal sphincter as a new mode of treatment for anal fissure.[49] In a subsequent report involving 12 patients, two doses (each consisting of 0.1 mL of diluted toxin corresponding to 2.5 E BoTox; BoTox Allergan, Irvine, CA) were injected into the external anal sphincter on both sides lateral to the fissure.[50] Maria and co-workers conducted a double-blind, placebo-controlled study in 30 patients, with the use of saline injections for the control group.[67] They used 20 U of botulinum A for the treatment group. After 2 months, 11 individuals in the treated group had healed, whereas only 2 in the control group were healed ($p = .003$).

BNT is a powerful poison that inhibits neuromuscular transmission. While acting through a different mechanism than GTN, its beneficial effect should be to increase blood flow to the area. Some have warned that this drug needs greater regulation, with a careful review of the risks and benefits.[13] Although not common, side effects of its various applications have included increased urinary residual volume, heart block, skin and allergic reactions, muscle weakness, postural hypotension, and changes in heart rate and blood pressure.[13] Certainly, transient incontinence for flatus is not unusual.

Lindsey and colleagues employed BNT in a high-concentration, low-volume solution in the treatment of patients in whom GTN therapy had failed.[60] Two milliliters of 0.9% saline were injected into a 100-U vial of BNT and a 0.4-mL aliquot was drawn into a 1-mL syringe. With the use of a 27-gauge needle, a solution of 0.2 mL was injected into the internal sphincter on either side of but at some distance from the fissure.[60] With this "second-line therapy," approximately one half of the fissures healed. The authors concluded as follows: "A policy of first line GTN and second line BNT . . . avoids surgical sphincterotomy and its risks *in the short term* [italics mine] in almost 90 percent of cases".[60] Others have concluded that although GTN and BNT have negligible side effects, the success rates are no better than 80% initially, dropping to 55% with longer-term follow-up.[33]

Nifedipine

Calcium ions are important for smooth muscle contraction. It has, therefore, been suggested that calcium channel blockers may be an effective treatment for anal fissure. This represents a third method for relaxing the internal anal sphincter. Nifedipine has been shown to be an effected calcium channel antagonist. Cook and co-workers undertook a study with oral nifedipine on healthy volunteers and in 15 patients with chronic anal fissure.[19] A highly significant decrease in maximum resting pressure was observed along with a reduction in pain scores. Nine patients experienced complete healing after 8 weeks. Side effects included flushing and mild headache. Perotti and colleagues employed topical nifedipine (0.3%) with lidocaine ointment (1.5%) every 12 hours for 6 weeks in a prospective, randomized, double-blind study, with the control group receiving topical lidocaine ointment (1.5%) with hydrocortisone acetate (1%) in 110 patients with chronic anal fissure.[83] They found a 94.5% incidence of healing in the nifedipine group, but only 16.4% of the controls had healed.

Diltiazem

Diltiazem (DTZ) is another calcium channel blocker that has been proffered as an alternative for the treatment of chronic anal fissure. In a prospective assessment of 71 such patients, Knight and co-workers found a rate of healing of 75%.[55] They concluded that topical 2% DTZ has a high success rate. Jonas and colleagues employed DTZ in patients in whom GTN had failed.[48] Thirty-nine individuals were so treated, with 49% healing within 8 weeks. Side effects included headache, drowsiness, mood swings, and perianal itching. The same group compared oral versus topical DTZ and noted that the topical application is more effective and is associated with fewer side effects.[47] Kocher and associates performed a randomized trial in which the side effects of GTN were compared with those of DTZ.[56] These investigators found no difference in healing rates, but because of much fewer side effects associated with DTZ (especially headache), they opined that DTZ "may be the preferred first-line treatment for chronic anal fissure"[56]

Comment on Chemical Sphincterotomy

Clearly, there is inconsistency in the literature about the relative efficacy and benefit of the number of agents available for performing so-called chemical sphincterotomy in the treatment of anal fissure. There is also confusion with respect to interpretation of the published articles, for example, management of the acute condition versus that of chronic anal fissure. Furthermore, long-term follow-up is lacking. However, one issue appears certain—there are side effects, headache being the most common complaint. In 2001, Helton published a consensus statement on the treatment of anal fissure on behalf of a panel representing three organizations: the Society for Surgery of the Alimentary Tract, the American Gastroenterological Association, and the American Society for Gastrointestinal Endoscopy.[42] Among the panel's conclusions was the following statement:

> . . . . Currently, the available data suggest that the first-line treatment is GTN. However, the side effect profile limits its usefulness, making newer topical agents potentially more attractive. Pharmacologic treatment should balance efficacy, short- and long-term side effects, convenience, and expense. These data will permit the informed patient to make a choice.[42]

Irrespective of the approach to treatment, every patient, physician and surgeon should accept the validity of the concept that when pain resulting from anal fissure is intolerable, when the fissure has been unresponsive to nonoperative management, when the fissure has been present for a long time, or when the fissure recurs following medical treatment, an operative approach is not only reasonable, but indicated. Therefore, my practice is to offer the patient a choice of medical measures or of proceeding directly to internal anal sphincterotomy. The amount of discomfort with the condition versus the fear of the procedure will usually determine the patient's course of action. As of this writing, medical measures, for the individuals under my care, do *not* include the treatments that may lead to a chemical sphincterotomy.

Surgical Management

In 1991, a set of practice parameters devoted to the broad spectrum of ambulatory anorectal surgery was published by the Standards Task Force of the American Society of Colon and Rectal Surgeons and included that of anal fissure.[5] Recognizing that the ultimate judgment regarding "the propriety of any specific procedure" must rest with the surgeon, it may be useful to quote the entire recommendation:

> The treatment for fissure-in-ano refractory to nonoperative therapy is internal anal sphincterotomy. Both closed and open techniques are suitable in an outpatient setting with either general, regional, or local anesthesia. More extensive procedures, including but not limited to anoplasties (*i.e.*, Y-V, V-Y, S), or associated anorectal pathology that requires hemorrhoidectomy, fistulectomy, etc., may warrant an inpatient stay.[5]

The choice of operative approach to the treatment of anal fissure depends on the duration of symptoms and on the physical findings. For an acute anal fissure without a tag, hypertrophied papilla, or significant hemorrhoids, the two procedures that have historically been advocated are sphincter stretch and internal anal sphincterotomy. For chronic anal fissure with an external component, or when the condition is associated with symptomatic large hemorrhoids, at least partial excisional therapy with sphincterotomy is the preferred option.

Sphincter Stretch

Sphincter stretch was originally described by Récamier in 1838 for the treatment of proctalgia fugax and for anal fissure. The procedure can be carried out with a local infiltration, but a brief general anesthetic is preferable. An ambulatory surgical facility is ideal. The patient is placed in the lithotomy position; sterile draping is unnecessary. There are incorrect (Figure 9-8) and

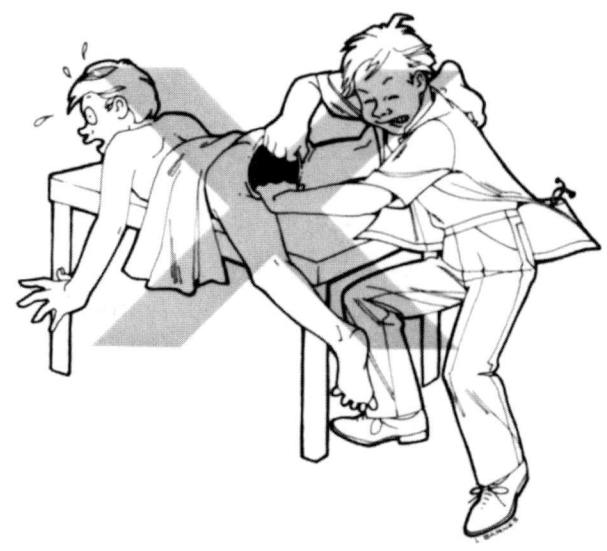

FIGURE 9-8. Incorrect technique for performing a sphincter stretch. A meticulous routine is required, not merely avulsion or distraction of the anal outlet.

correct methods (Figure 9-9) for performing sphincter stretch. The index finger of one hand is inserted into the rectum, followed by the index finger of the opposite hand. Gentle lateral retraction with each finger commences for approximately 30 seconds. The long finger is inserted and then the other long finger. With four fingers in place, the anal canal is stretched (massaged) cautiously for 4 minutes. In men, it is easier to stretch the sphincter in the anteroposterior plane because of the narrowness of the pelvic outlet. Sphincter stretch in women, however, should always be performed in the transverse plane (if undertaken at all). Narrowness is not a concern, but disruption of anterior sphincteric support is a real possibility.

Results

Sphincter stretch is a reasonably effective procedure for the symptomatic relief of anal fissure. In recent years, however, there has been an absence of reports on the results of treatment. This is undoubtedly because

the procedure has been supplanted by internal anal sphincterotomy.

Watts and associates (1964) performed sphincter stretch for anal fissure in 99 patients.[105] All were followed for at least 5 months. Three fourths of the patients achieved symptomatic relief within 48 hours; pain was resolved within 2 weeks in 20%. Six patients continued to have a fissure, although two were free of pain, and in five others recurrent discomfort developed without evidence of fissure. The most troublesome complication in this series was related to control, usually for flatus alone but occasionally for feces. Some swelling was also reported. Twenty-eight percent were noted to have at least one of these complaints.

Sohn and colleagues in 1992 precisely performed anorectal sphincter dilatation with a Parks retractor opened to 4.8 cm or with a 40-mm balloon.[98] The dilatations were sustained for exactly 5 minutes. The cure rates were 93% and 94%, respectively. There was no incident of incontinence in the latter group (66 patients). Two of 105 with the Parks dilatation noted incontinence.

Sphincter injury after anal dilatation has been assessed by anal endosonography.[75,100] In those individuals complaining of fecal incontinence, fragmentation or disruption of the internal sphincter is usually observed, in addition to defects in the external sphincter[100] (Figure 9-10). Sphincteric defects were found in 11 of 18 incontinent patients in a University of Copenhagen study.[75]

As discussed in Chapter 5, antibiotic prophylaxis should be considered with any patient who cannot afford an infection. Goldman and colleagues evaluated 100 patients who underwent anal dilatation for fissure and noted positive blood cultures in 8%.[36] There appeared to be some correlation with the extent of trauma as determined by the levels of elevation of serum muscle enzymes.

Opinion

I have found sphincter stretch to be a very effective treatment for cure, but have abandoned the procedure in favor of lateral internal anal sphincterotomy. If the surgeon

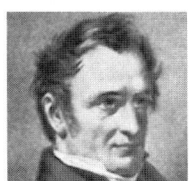

Jean-Claude-Anthelme Récamier (1774–1852) Récamier was born at Rochefort-en-Bugey to a well-educated, important local family. He studied medicine at the Belley Hospital and then at Bourg, where he was called for military service. In 1797, he went to Paris, and in 1806, at the age of 33, he became chief physician at the Hôtel-Dieu. He became interested in diseases of women and is considered a pioneer in gynecologic surgery, inventing the cylindric vaginal speculum and the bivalve speculum. His interest in uterine cancer led him to perform the first culpohysterectomy in 1829. He introduced the curette in the treatment of endometritis and incised pelvic abscesses through the posterior cul-de-sac. He is also recognized as the first person to apply forcible dilatation in the treatment of anal fissure. Récamier was named as one of the original members of the Académie de Médecine when it was founded in 1820. He was later appointed Professor in the Faculty of Medicine, and in 1826, he succeeded Laennec to the Chair of the College of France. He died of apoplexy. (Récamier JCA. Extension, massage et percussion cadencée dans le traitement des contractures musculaires. *Rev Med Fr* 1838;1:74. For translation, see *Dis Colon Rectum* 1980;23:362.)

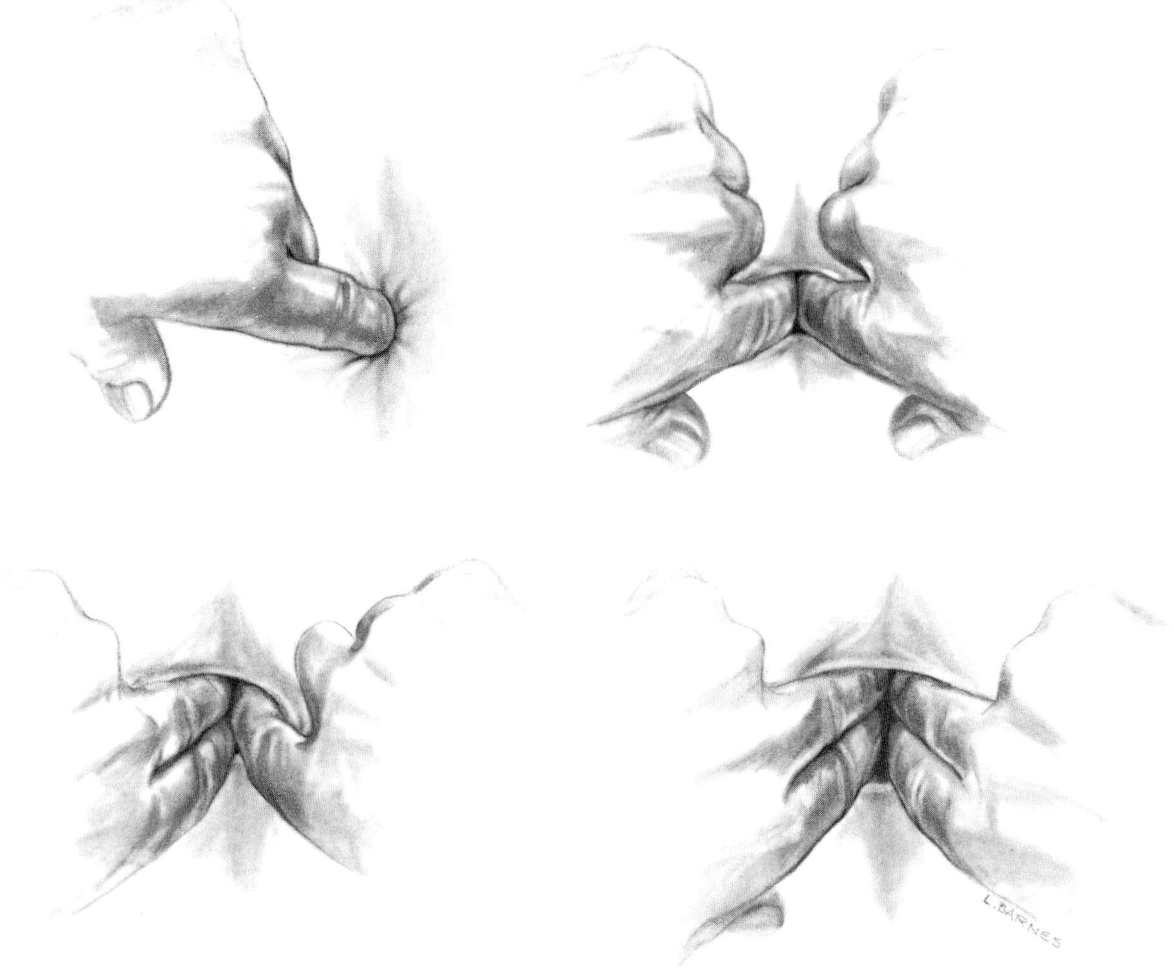

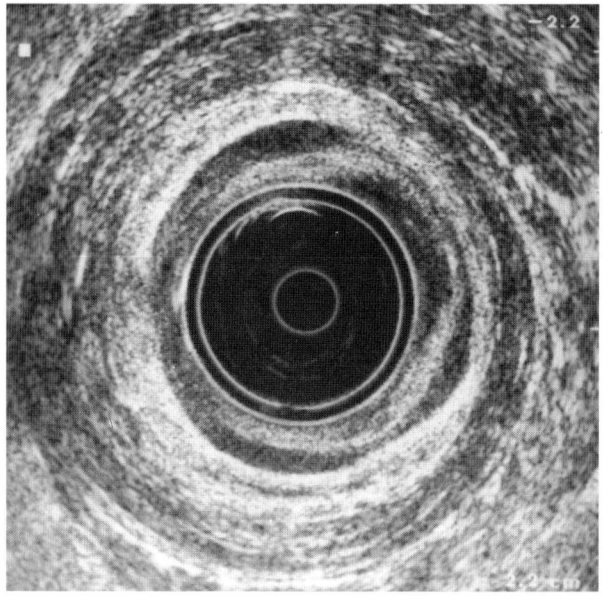

FIGURE 9-9. Proper approach to performing a sphincter stretch. Male patients may require an anteroposterior stretch, because of the limitations of a narrow outlet and close approximation of the ischial spines. Female patients should always undergo a lateral stretch.

FIGURE 9-10. A fragmented internal anal sphincter can be appreciated in this endorectal ultrasonogram. (Courtesy of C. I. Bartram, M.D., Department of Radiology, St. Mark's Hospital, Harrow, UK.)

elects sphincter stretch for the management of anal fissure, it should be applied to younger patients, and then limited to men only. In my opinion, it is contraindicated in individuals older than 60 years of age because of the increased likelihood of incontinence problems. Sphincter stretch that is performed in a woman is an invitation to disaster, especially for the patient. Furthermore, it could well be an opportunity to test one's skills in the legal arena. One must remember that sphincter stretch attenuates the external sphincter *pari passu*. Impairment for voluntary control is, therefore, a real possibility. Unless one makes an effort to quantitatively perform the stretch by using such criteria as have been described by Sohn and colleagues,[98] it is not a question of whether impairment for control will be a consequence, but how severe it will be.

Internal Anal Sphincterotomy

In 1839, Brodie was the first person to perform an anal sphincterotomy. He advocated the operation for "preternatural contraction of the anal sphincter." In

1863, Hilton also suggested that the treatment for anal ulcer should be sphincterotomy. However, Miles (see Biography, Chapter 23) is usually credited as the surgeon who gave the operation real credence, although Miles believed that he was dividing what he called "the pecten band".[38,72] In 1951, Eisenhammer was the first person to advocate internal anal sphincterotomy for anal fissure and to truly understand which muscle he was dividing.[23]

The internal anal sphincter is the continuation of the distal portion of the circular muscle of the rectum (see Figure 8-2). Its length is essentially equal to that of the anal canal. Distally, it can usually be felt medial to the intersphincteric groove outside the anal verge. The subcutaneous portion of the external sphincter is lateral to the groove.

The internal sphincter maintains the anal canal in the closed position; action is involuntary. The external sphincter is a striated muscle. The external sphincter and the levator ani are the muscles involved in voluntary control. Complete division of the internal anal sphincter is possible without creating significant impairment of fecal continence.[24] The reader is referred to Chapters 1, 2, and 13 for further discussion on the anatomy and physiology of the sphincter mechanism.

Technique

The procedure of internal anal sphincterotomy has classically been performed in the posterior midline. Although this approach usually cures the condition, it is associated with the complication of the so-called keyhole deformity (see Complications). Bennett and Goligher reported a high incidence of impairment for flatus with posterior internal anal sphincterotomy (34%) and a 15% incidence of difficulty controlling feces.[10] After a period of time, however, further improvement was evident, with a cure rate of 93%, but an appreciable morbidity rate remained.

Eisenhammer advocated the lateral position for sphincterotomy, dividing one half of the muscle in an open fashion.[24] In 1969, Notaras reported a technique

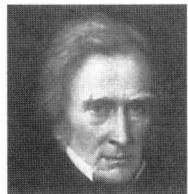

Benjamin Collins Brodie (1783–1862) Brodie was the son of a clergyman in Winterslow, Wiltshire, England. In 1798, when only 15 years old, he fought against Napoleon. In 1801, he decided to pursue a career in medicine, eventually becoming house surgeon at St. George's Hospital in 1822. In 1810, he was elected Fellow of the Royal Society after presenting a paper entitled "Dissection of a Fetus." It was because of this presentation that he began to achieve a considerable reputation, not only as a surgical anatomist but also as a writer and speaker. In 1813, Brodie described the joint disease that was later to bear his name. So universal were his writings that he seemed as comfortable discussing the subject of the influence of the nervous system on the production of animal heat as describing the pathology of anal fissure. In 1828, he became surgeon to King George IV. He held many prestigious positions, including President of the Medico-Chirurgical Society and President of the General Medical Council. He was the first surgeon to hold the position of President of the Royal Society. He died of a malignant disease, probably sarcoma, that originated in his shoulder. (Brodie BC. Preternatural contraction of the sphincter ani. *London Med Gazette* 1835;16:26.)

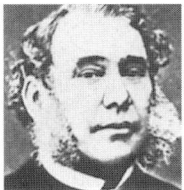

John Hilton (1805–1878) Hilton was born in the village of Sible Hedlingham in Essex, England. He was accepted at Guy's Hospital and after completing his studies was appointed a demonstrator in anatomy. During this period, he recognized that an inflamed joint not only referred pain to the skin over it but also caused muscle spasms that immobilized and protected the joint from further injury; this phenomenon became known as Hilton's Law. In 1844, Hilton was appointed assistant surgeon at Guy's Hospital and was promoted to full surgeon in 1849. He was one of the first surgeons to advocate a lumbar colostomy, and in 1846, he performed one of the first recorded operations for the relief of strangulated hernia. In 1860, Hilton was appointed Professor of Anatomy and Surgery at the Royal College of Surgeons. In 1863, he presented 18 lectures, including one on the treatment of anal ulcer in which he mentions that the internal sphincter can be transected safely using the whitish area over the groove between the internal and external sphincters as a landmark (i.e., the white line of Hilton). Unfortunately, this incorrectly became synonymous with the mucocutaneous junction. (Hilton J. *On the influence of mechanical and physiological rest in the treatment of accidents and surgical diseases, and the diagnostic value of pain.* London: Bell & Daldy, 1863:279. Reprinted in part by Bonello JC. *Dis Colon Rectum* 1987;30:304.)

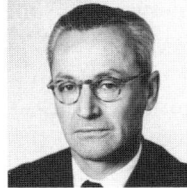

Stephen Eisenhammer (1906–1995) Eisenhammer was born in Middleburg, Cape Province, South Africa of parents of Viennese descent and grew up on a farm in what was then Southern Rhodesia. He began his medical studies at the University of Cape Town before moving to the University of Edinburgh, Scotland, from which he graduated in 1930. After various surgical appointments he became House Surgeon and Resident Surgical Officer at St Mark's Hospital. At the outbreak of World War II, he joined the London Emergency Medical War Services before returning to South Africa, where in 1942 he joined the South African Medical Corps, seeing service in Madagascar. In 1944, he started private practice in Johannesburg with the decision to specialize in proctology. In spite of not having a teaching appointment at any hospital or medical school, he proved to be a prolific researcher and writer in his chosen field. Beginning in the 1950s, he began to make notable contributions to a better understanding of hemorrhoids, anal fistula, anal abscess, and the application of internal anal sphincterotomy for fissure. In 1962, he was elected an Honorary Member of the Section of Proctology of the Royal Society of Medicine. He continued researching and publishing into the mid-1980s, by which time he was well into his 70s. (Photograph and biographic information courtesy of John Eisenhammer and with special appreciation to Gary R. Gecelter, MD.)

using a narrow-bladed scalpel to perform an internal anal sphincterotomy in a closed fashion in the lateral position.[76] In 66 patients so treated, he reported a 6% incidence of fecal soiling. Notaras subsequently described his procedure in detail by a technique in which he employed a scalpel used for cataract surgery.[77,78] His method involved submucosal insertion of a knife, followed by an outward incision to the intersphincteric groove. This has the advantage of minimizing the risk of mucosal injury, but it has at least the theoretical disadvantage of one not knowing how deep to cut, risking injury to the external sphincter. My own preference is to insert the knife into the groove and incising medially.

The procedure can be performed in the office using a local anesthetic [e.g., 0.5% bupivacaine (Marcaine) in 1:200,000 epinephrine] or in an ambulatory surgical facility, using a short-acting general anesthetic or local with conscious sedation. If the former method is used, the patient may be placed in stirrups, in the left lateral position, or in the prone jackknife position, depending on the surgeon's preference and the availability of the appropriate table. Women are obviously more accustomed to the lithotomy stirrups and are more tolerant of assuming that position. Men, however, are usually quite self-conscious, if not downright obstreperous, in the lithotomy position. Young men, in my experience, are preferably treated with an anesthesiologist's support.

In the office the fissure is infiltrated, as well as the site for insertion of the knife—either the right lateral or left lateral position. A narrow anal retractor (e.g., Hill-Ferguson) is employed. As previously suggested, in men I prefer to perform the procedure with a general anesthetic in the outpatient surgical setting, but both men and women are offered the choice between the two options. The intersphincteric groove is usually easily felt (Figure 9-11), and the knife blade is inserted into the left lateral aspect (Figure 9-12A). Some surgeons use a No. 11 blade, scissors (by the open technique; see later), or a hooked knife, but a Beaver (catalog no. 375220, Becton Dickinson and Company, Franklin Lakes, NJ) cataract blade (size 25.5 × 2.2 mm) is preferable. The knife is used as a stiletto and creates a very small wound. For a left-handed surgeon, operating on the right lateral aspect is easier. There is a theoretical advantage in cutting on the right side, because the hemorrhoid sites are usually in the anterior and posterior positions, but it requires a right-handed surgeon to operate backhanded, depending on the patient's position, of course. Therefore, I perform the sphincterotomy on the patient's left and accept the increased risk for a hematoma if the left lateral pile is lacerated. The foregoing admonitions refer to a patient placed in the lithotomy position.

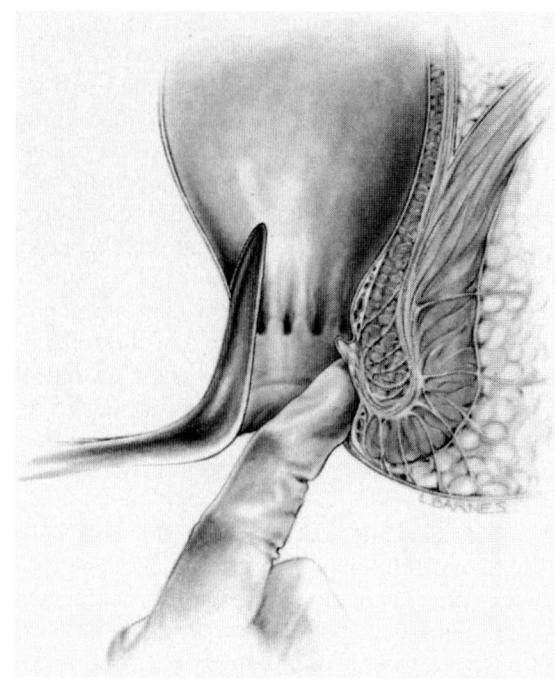

FIGURE 9-11. Digital examination to identify the intersphincteric groove. The novice should practice palpating the groove on numerous asymptomatic patients before embarking on closed sphincterotomy. The location of the groove can be quite variable. The finger may be used to protect the external sphincter as the knife blade is inserted.

The tip of the blade is angled medially (Figure 9-12B), pointing just above the dentate line, and the lower one third to one half of the internal anal sphincter is divided. When the knife is seen beneath the intact anal mucosa, it is withdrawn. The side of the finger is then used to break any residual sphincter fibers (Figure 9-12C). If the physician pushes with the fingertip, there is a tendency to tear the mucosa, which may then lead to bleeding and possibly the subsequent development of a fistula. If bleeding occurs at the wound puncture site, it can be readily controlled by a few moments of direct pressure. If a tag or papilla is present, it can be removed by excision with scissors or electrocautery. No dressings are required, and the patient is discharged when alert.

An alternative approach is to undertake the operation without a retractor in place. The index finger senses the knife blade beneath the anal mucosa, and the residual internal anal sphincter fibers are broken by the side of the finger (Figure 9-13).

Another variation of the lateral sphincterotomy is the open technique. This, too, can be performed either in the office or in the hospital. The disadvantages are that it takes longer to perform and usually requires suturing. Many surgeons prefer this approach to visualize the internal and the external sphincter directly.

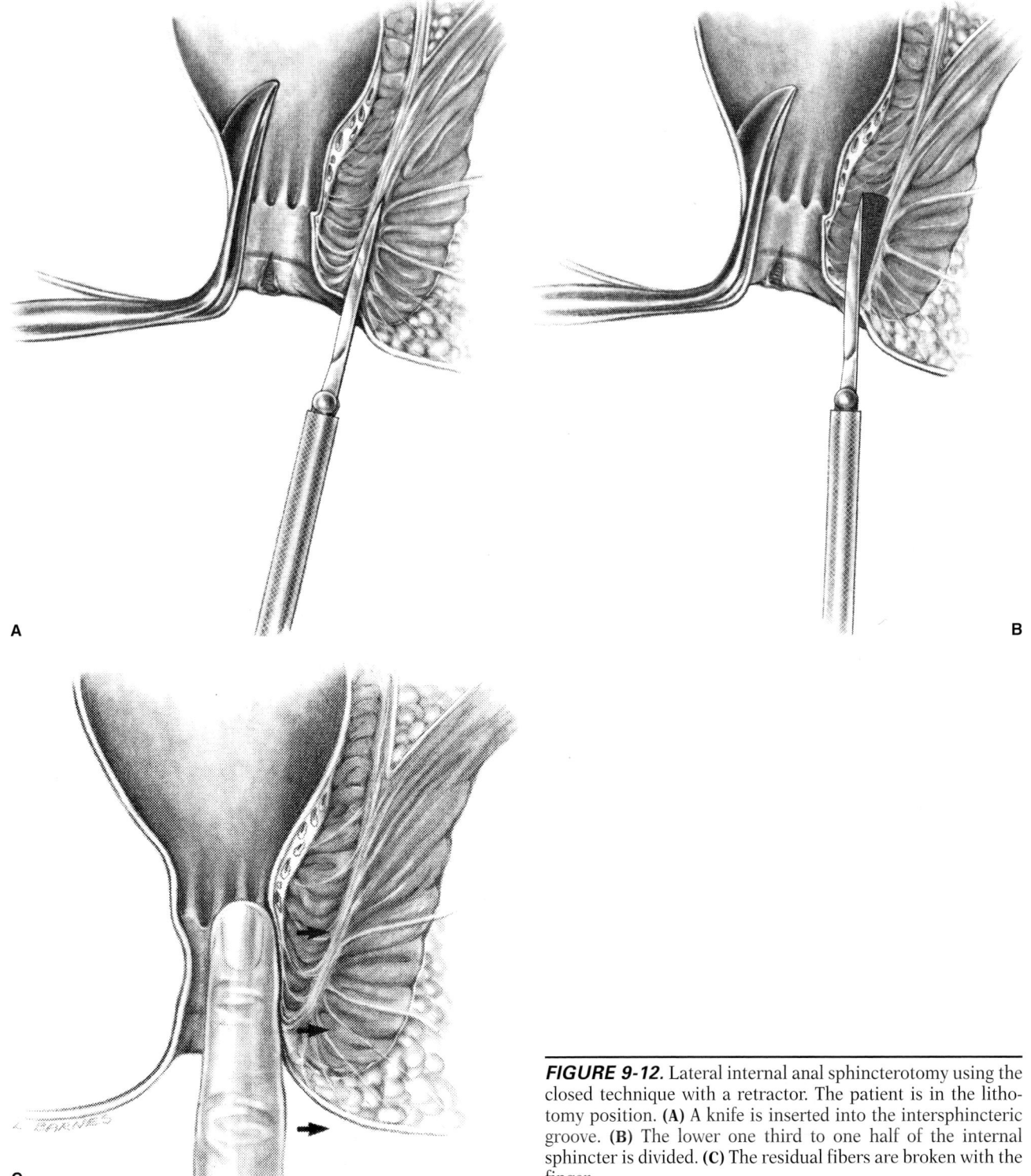

A

B

C

FIGURE 9-12. Lateral internal anal sphincterotomy using the closed technique with a retractor. The patient is in the lithotomy position. **(A)** A knife is inserted into the intersphincteric groove. **(B)** The lower one third to one half of the internal sphincter is divided. **(C)** The residual fibers are broken with the finger.

A small, radial incision is made laterally at the lower border of the internal sphincter and continued into the intersphincteric groove (Figure 9-14). Alternatively, a curvilinear incision outside the anal verge can be used. Because of the open wound and the possibility of bleeding, it is helpful to infiltrate the area with a local anesthetic containing epinephrine solution. The distal internal sphincter is grasped with forceps and bluntly freed. The lower one third to one half is divided with scissors. The wound is closed with absorbable suture material, and a small dressing is applied.

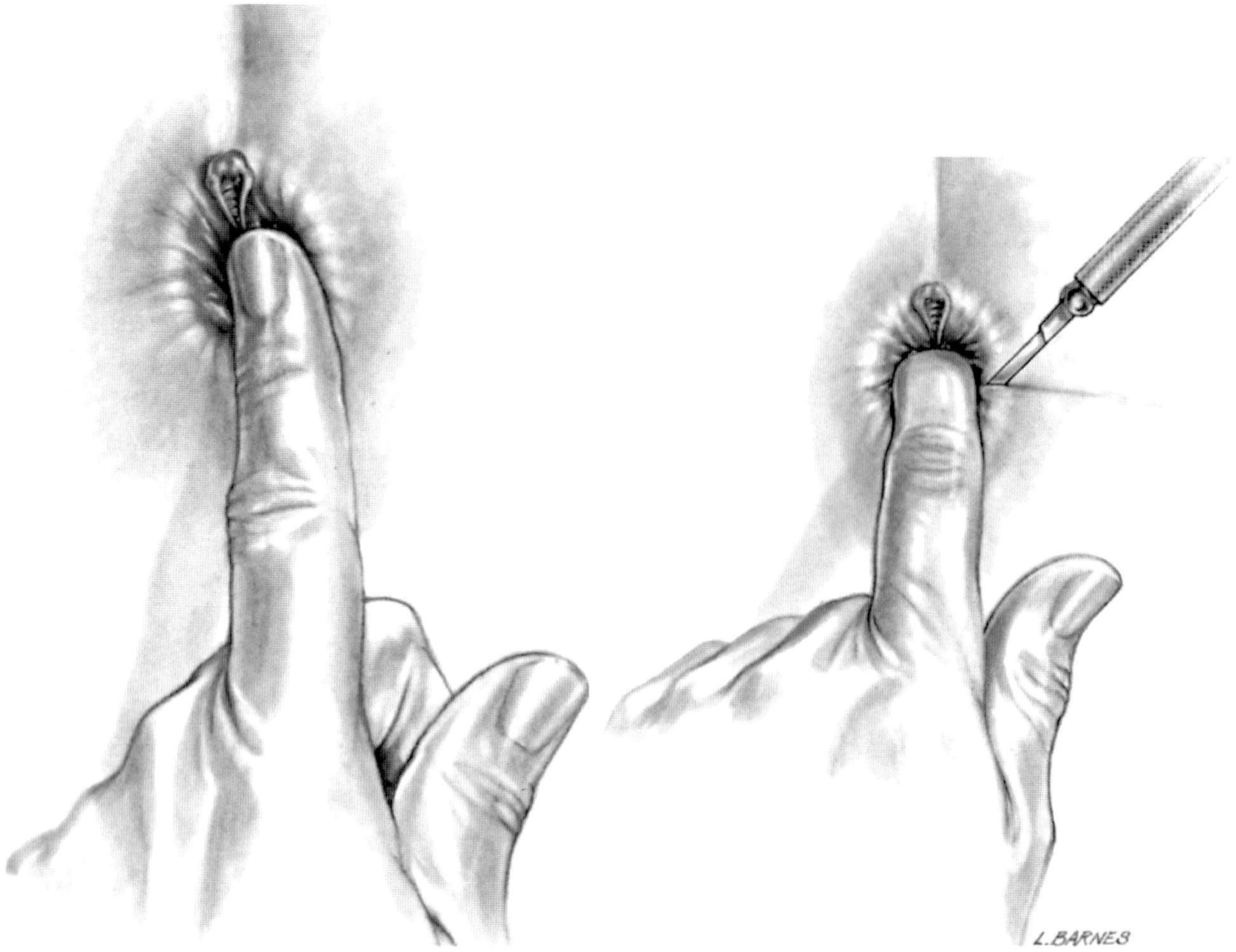

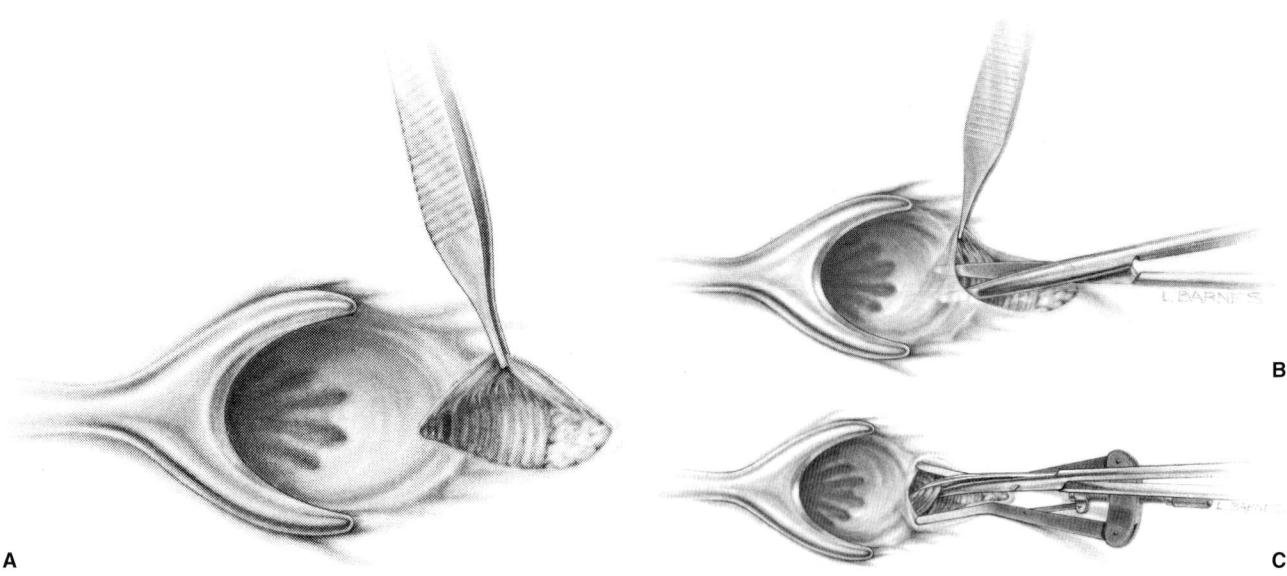

FIGURE 9-13. Lateral internal anal sphincterotomy using the closed technique, no retractor, and a local anesthetic. **(A)** A finger is inserted into the anal canal after anesthesia is established. **(B)** The sphincterotomy is performed with the finger in place.

FIGURE 9-14. Lateral internal anal sphincterotomy using the open technique with the patient placed in the lateral or the prone (i.e., jackknife) position. **(A)** A radial incision is made across the intersphincteric groove. A narrow Hill-Ferguson retractor is in place. **(B)** The internal sphincter is separated from the anoderm by blunt dissection. **(C)** The internal sphincter is divided. The wound may be closed or left open.

Postoperative Care

Sitz baths and a mild analgesic are the only postoperative measures advised. Pain is often less than that experienced preoperatively, and most patients resume their normal activities within 48 hours.

Complications

Surgery for anal fissure is associated with numerous complications, most of which are preventable by the application of judicious surgical technique and, of course, by familiarity with anorectal anatomy.

Ecchymosis is frequently noted around the entrance wound if the closed technique is used, but this is of no concern. A *hematoma* is rare and usually the result of failure to apply adequate pressure to the site. Likewise, *hemorrhage* is extremely unusual by either the closed or open method, but is much more likely to occur with the open procedure. Suture ligation may be required.

Perianal *abscess* occurs after 1% of closed internal anal sphincterotomies. It is virtually always associated with an anal fistula. This presumably is the result of penetration of the mucosa of the anal canal by the knife blade (Figure 9-15). It is surprising that this complication is not seen more frequently, because the anal canal mucosa must be breached more often than is suspected. Treatment requires drainage of the abscess, identification of an internal opening if present, and fistulotomy (see Chapter 11). Fortunately, the fistula is always low and submucosal or intersphincteric, provided the sphincterotomy was carried out by dividing only the internal anal sphincter.

True *fecal incontinence* following a properly performed internal anal sphincterotomy should be extraordinarily rare. However, as is discussed later, it is not that unusual for a patient to experience *soiling* of underclothes and *incontinence for flatus*. This is a particular problem in some women. Sultan and colleagues note that the performance of an internal anal sphincterotomy frequently divides more sphincter in women than it does in men.[101] They attribute this to the shorter anal canal of women. Particular caution should be exercised in patients with prior obstetric trauma and in those women with an ectopic anus (see Chapter 13).

Figure 9-16 illustrates the defect produced by lateral internal anal sphincterotomy through the means of endoanal ultrasonography. Garcia-Aguilar and co-workers studied the anatomic and functional consequences of lateral internal anal sphincterotomy in 13 patients with incontinence and 13 who had no such symptoms.[31] The only significant difference was that incontinent patients had undergone longer sphincterotomies. The fact that the external sphincter was also thinner in the incontinent patients suggests that a preoperative abnormality predisposed some of these patients to an increased risk of fecal incontinence, a problem that became unmasked by the addition of internal anal sphincterotomy. One wonders whether endoanal ultrasound should be performed before sphincterotomy to assess whether a patient could be at an

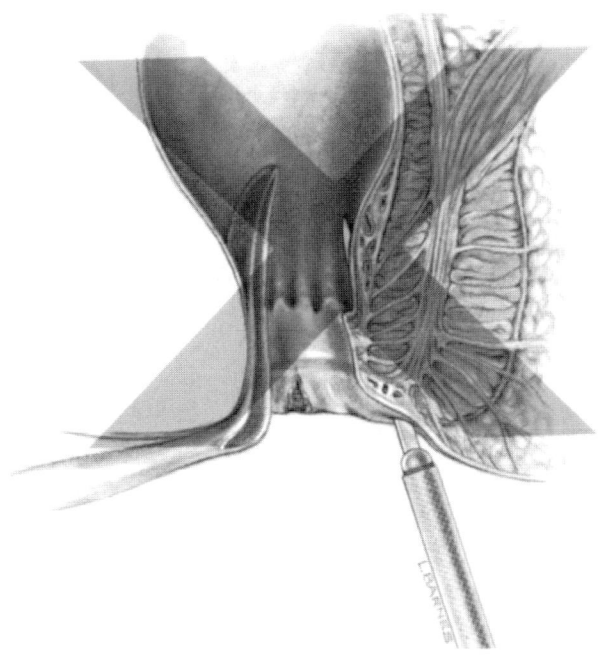

FIGURE 9-15. Sphincterotomy that penetrates through the anal mucosa may result in anal abscess and fistula.

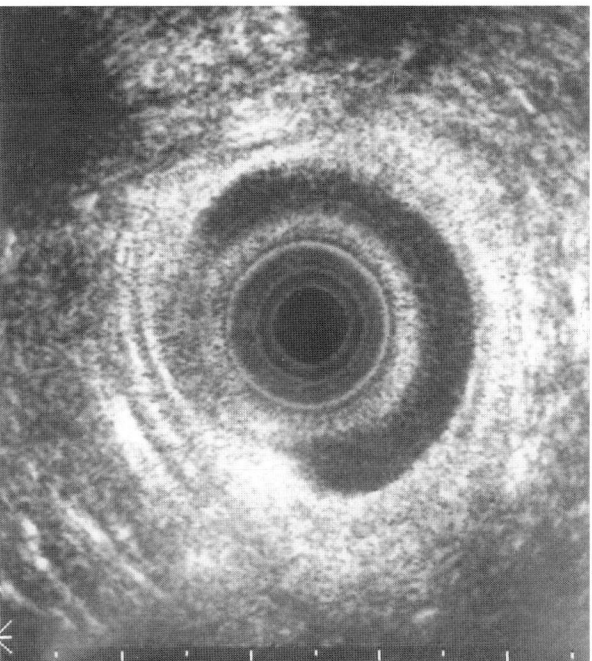

FIGURE 9-16. Ultrasonography demonstrates internal sphincter defect following sphincterotomy. (Courtesy of C. I. Bartram, M.D., Department of Radiology, St. Mark's Hospital, Harrow, UK.)

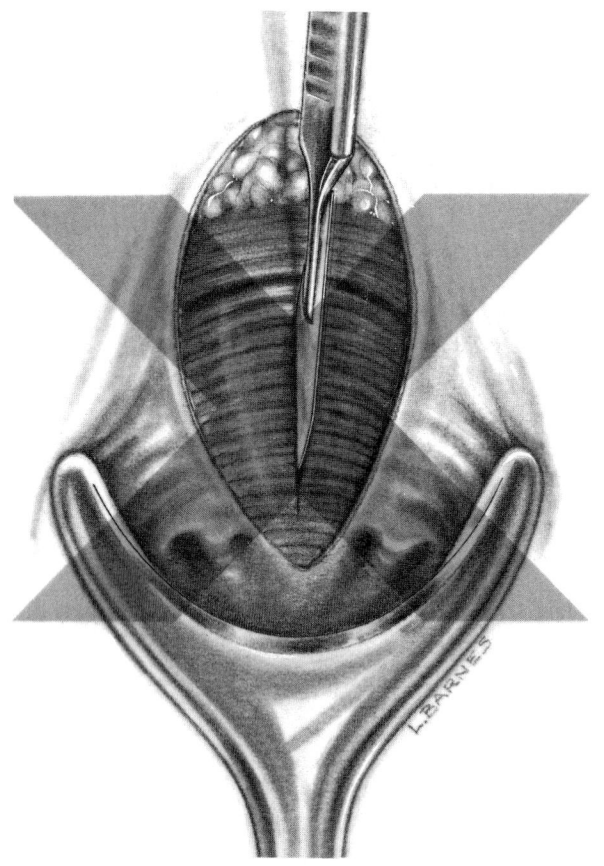

FIGURE 9-17. Excision of a fissure with posterior internal anal sphincterotomy is not a recommended technique.

increased risk for the development of this complication. However, the pain attendant with this study may preclude this investigation. Still, this concept merits further study.

A *keyhole deformity* is a troublesome consequence of fissure excision or internal anal sphincterotomy performed in the posterior midline (see Figure 8-53). The resultant defect may produce symptoms of mucous discharge, pruritus, and soiling of undergarments. Excision of an uncomplicated acute fissure with a posterior midline sphincterotomy should never be undertaken in my opinion (Figure 9-17). With persistent symptoms despite an appropriate bowel management program and cleansing methods, the deformity may be treated by anoplasty (see Chapter 8).

Results

Infection The primary initial concern following sphincterotomy is the risk of infection. We reported 350 patients who underwent open or closed lateral internal anal sphincterotomy for acute or chronic anal fissure.[59] Postoperative infections requiring drainage developed in eight patients (2.3%); one half of these were associated with a fistula.

The two concerning issues with respect to long-term results are incontinence and recurrent or persistent fissure.

Incontinence Complete fecal incontinence (i.e., the total loss of bowel control) should not occur following sphincterotomy because the internal anal sphincter plays very little role in maintaining anal continence. As mentioned previously there is a not surprising relationship between the length of the sphincterotomy and the risk of subsequent incontinence problems.[31] Notaras described 73 patients who underwent this procedure and found four who experienced soiling of the underclothes, two who had imperfect control of flatus, and one who had occasional fecal soilage.[77] This last patient was thought to have been a poor candidate for the procedure. Millar reported either a mucous discharge or flatus-control problems in three of 99 patients so treated.[73] Hoffmann and Goligher noted that 12 of 99 patients had some minor deficiency of anal control.[43] Pernikoff and colleagues reviewed 500 patients who underwent internal anal sphincterotomy and identified fecal incontinence in 8%.[82] In our experience, 60 individuals (17%) complained of incontinence for flatus or for stool, but for two thirds this was transient.[59]

It is probably wise to record the patient's preoperative bowel control status, especially if there is some degree of impairment reported during the preoperative interview. However, if significant incontinence does supervene, it is most likely the result of inadvertent or inappropriate division of a portion of the external sphincter. This may occur with the closed technique (Figure 9-18) or with the open method (Figure 9-19). If symptoms warrant, apposition or overlapping of the divided muscle will usually ameliorate the problem (see Chapter 13).

Recurrence The incidence of delayed healing or recurrence is the standard of measurement for the success or failure of the operation. Millar reported that 88% of patients were healed at 2 weeks, and 100% healed eventually.[73] Hoffman and Goligher noted that 2% were unhealed at 9 months.[43] Notaras and Ray and colleagues had an astounding rate of healing of 100%.[77,87] Marya and colleagues reported a 2% incidence of nonhealing, and Gilgold noted a rate of approximately 4%.[35,68] Rudd evaluated 200 patients and found only one unhealed; Crohn's disease subsequently developed in that person.[93] In the experience of Pernikoff and co-workers, 1% failed to heal.[82]

If the fissure persists despite conservative therapy (e.g., sitz baths, stool softeners), repeat sphincterotomy, during which a more generous portion of the internal sphincter is divided, is the appropriate treatment (Figure 9-20). If healing still does not take place, the patient should undergo gastrointestinal investigation to seek for the possibility of concurrent inflammatory bowel dis-

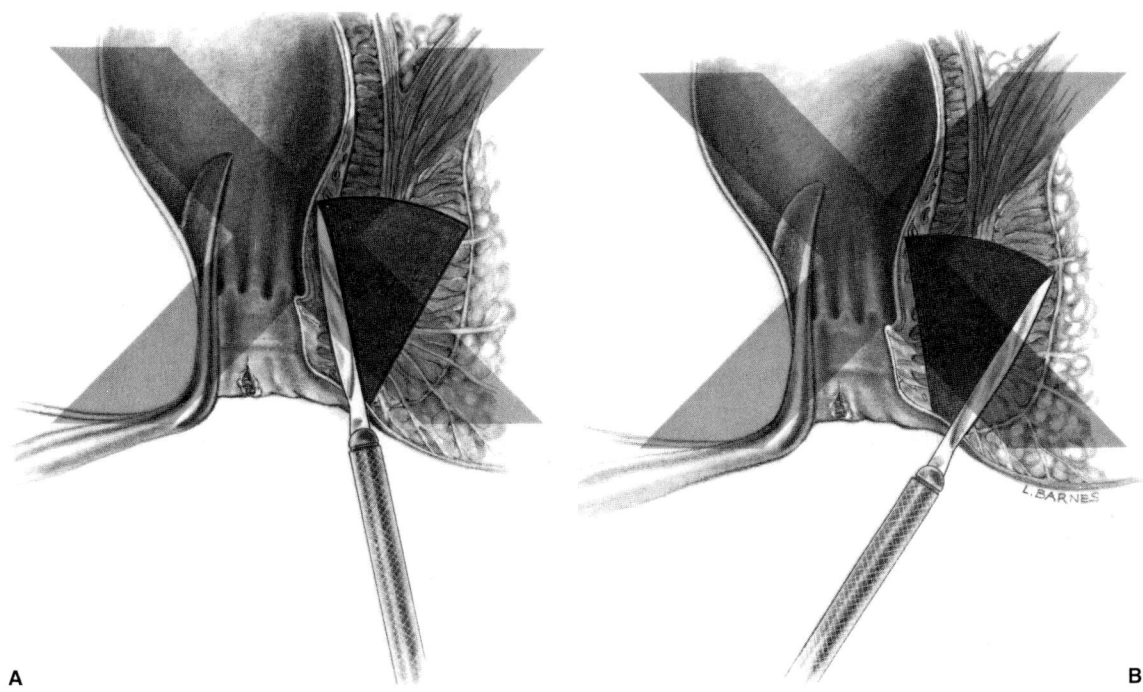

A **B**

FIGURE 9-18. Incorrect closed internal anal sphincterotomy. **(A)** The external sphincter can be divided inadvertently if the incision is made toward the anal canal. **(B)** The risk for injury is even greater with a lateral incision.

ease, assuming that this had not been accomplished previously (see Anal Fissure and Crohn's Disease).

Open versus Closed Walker and colleagues reviewed their experience with lateral internal anal sphincterotomy for anal fissure and stenosis in more than 300 patients.[103] Sphincterotomy was performed by several techniques (open, closed, multiple) and under diverse circumstances, so it is difficult to interpret the results.

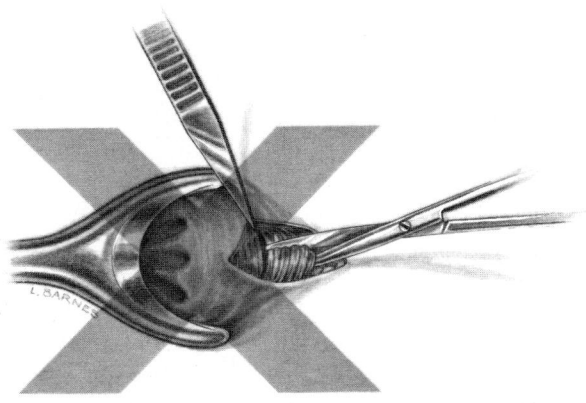

FIGURE 9-19. Improper open "external" anal sphincterotomy. Simply opening the area to visualize the site for sphincterotomy does not guarantee the absence of complications. Knowledge of the anatomy is still a requisite.

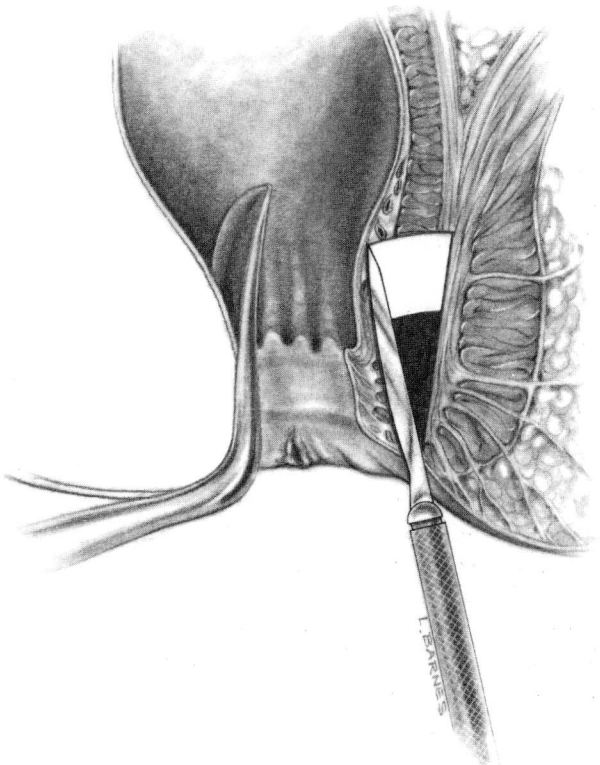

FIGURE 9-20. An anal fissure that fails to heal within a reasonable time may be treated by a more generous internal anal sphincterotomy.

It is apparent, however, that complications were lowest after the closed procedure (20%) and highest for open sphincterotomy (55%). Anal fistula occurred in three patients (l%). In the entire series, 15% reported various control difficulties, and when very strict criteria for evaluation of morbidity were used, minor complications occurred in 36%.

In our reported experience mentioned earlier, 21 of 350 patients (6%) failed to heal or had a recurrence during the follow-up period (mean, 14 months).[59] Five subsequently were found to have Crohn's disease. Excluding these individuals, the incidence of nonhealing was 4.6%. There was no statistically significant difference in healing rate or morbidity when the open was compared with the closed method.

Nelson undertook an analysis of nineteen publications encompassing 3,083 patients to determine whether a preferred technique could be identified.[74] He concluded as follows:

- Anal stretch is associated with a higher risk of persistent fissure.
- Anal stretch has a higher risk for minor incontinence.
- There is no difference in complication rate between open and closed sphincterotomy.
- Open and closed sphincterotomies are equally efficacious in curing anal fissure.

Anesthetic Type Keighley and associates compared lateral sphincterotomy performed with a local anesthetic versus lateral sphincterotomy performed with a general anesthetic.[52] They found a 50% incidence of delayed healing with a local and a 3% incidence after a general anesthetic. They concluded that the operation should not be performed with local infiltration.

Sphincterotomy versus Nitroglycerin A randomized, controlled trial was undertaken by the Canadian Colorectal Surgical Trials Group.[89] This involved 82 patients who were assessed at 6 weeks and 6 months. The study concluded that internal anal sphincterotomy is superior to topical TNG (0.25%), with a high rate of healing, few side effects, and low risk for early incontinence.[89] In another prospective trial from Australia involving 65 patients, the results and the recommendations were similar.[26] Although TNG paste healed the majority of anal fissures, many patients experienced little improvement or developed side effects that required subsequent sphincterotomy. Some fissures recurred after initially healing with TNG.

Sphincterotomy versus Botulinum Toxin Mentes and colleagues undertook a prospective, randomized trial in which internal anal sphincterotomy was compared with BNT.[71] In the BNT group (n = 61), a single injection re-sulted in complete healing in 74% of patients at the second month. A second injection, in those willing to undergo it, resulted in an overall healing rate at 6 months of 87%. At 1 year, the success rate fell to 75%. In the sphincterotomy group (n = 50), the success rate was 82% at 1 month and 98% at the second month. Sphincterotomy was associated with a significantly higher complication rate, specifically incontinence.

Physiologic Studies McNamara and colleagues performed a prospective, anorectal, manometric evaluation on 13 patients before and after closed internal anal sphincterotomy.[70] As expected, the resting pressure fell to normal levels following successful operation, which suggests that it is the internal anal sphincter that is responsible for the preoperative resting pressure elevation. Many investigators have concluded that healing of the anal fissure is a consequence of reduced anal pressure.[96]

Garcia-Granero and associates used anal endosonography to evaluate the extent of internal anal sphincter division following closed sphincterotomy to determine its role with respect to recurrence and incontinence.[32] They found that significant symptomatic recurrence was associated with an incomplete sphincterotomy.

Children Cohen and Dehn performed lateral subcutaneous sphincterotomy on 23 *children* (between the ages of 8 and 168 months).[18] All were healed by 8 weeks.

CHRONIC ANAL FISSURE

Chronic anal fissure usually produces symptoms of pain and bleeding, but the pain is not as severe as that with an acute fissure. Frequently, the patient's symptoms are attributable to secondary changes, such as the presence of a lump. Other common complaints include mucous discharge, soiling of the underclothes, and pruritus. If the patient is concerned primarily with the pruritic symptoms, cleansing the area with warm water following defecation is usually quite helpful. Many patients believe that itching is caused by a lack of cleanliness, and they vigorously scrub the area with soap and water; this only serves to exacerbate the problem. The patient should be cautioned not to use soap in the perianal area; this is not an area that requires sterilization. Avoiding coffee, alcoholic beverages, smoking, and spicy foods will also have an ameliorative effect (see Chapter 19). If discharge is a problem and surgery is not considered appropriate, or if the patient refuses surgery, a ball of cotton can be placed at the anal opening and changed as necessary to avoid soiling underclothes and exacerbating pruritic symptoms.

Surgical Treatment

The classic operative approach for chronic anal fissure is excision and internal anal sphincterotomy in the posterior position. This removes the eschar, skin tag, and papilla, but it may produce the complication of the previously mentioned keyhole deformity. This concern is probably exaggerated. Excision of the annoying tag and papilla is helpful, but in my opinion, the sphincterotomy should still be accomplished in the lateral position. Unless the edges of the fissure are very fibrotic, removal of the tag and papilla by snipping with scissors should suffice. However, a more formal excision can be accomplished if the surgeon prefers (Figure 9-21). In my opinion, the underlying internal anal sphincter should not be incised. As mentioned, the sphincterotomy can then be performed at a lateral site by one of the methods described previously.

Results

I have already alluded to the fact that there is confusion in the literature with respect to interpretation of the results of surgery for chronic anal fissure. It is often not clear whether patients truly fulfill the criteria, such as

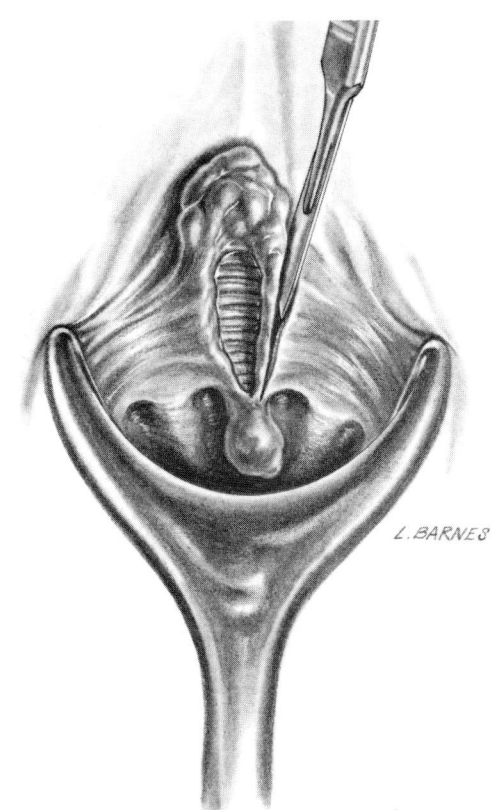

FIGURE 9-21. Chronic anal fissure is treated by excision of the fibrous tissue skin tag and hypertrophied anal papilla. Sphincterotomy should not be performed at this site.

a sentinel tag, hypertrophied anal papilla, and thickened, fibrotic appearance. That stated, reports of the treatment of chronic anal fissure by lateral internal anal sphincterotomy have been quite enthusiastic.[57] Bell noted one failure in 56 patients.[9] Ravikumar and colleagues reported all fissures healed by 5 weeks, and all but two within 3 weeks.[86] Kortbeek and associates, in a controlled study, found that healing was similar for the subcutaneous (96.6%) and open (94.4%) groups.[57] Anal canal pressure studies have repeatedly demonstrated that pressure reduction occurs and is maintained in patients who undergo open or closed lateral internal anal sphincterotomy for chronic anal fissure.[12,17,91]

Abcarian retrospectively analyzed 300 patients, one half of whom underwent lateral internal anal sphincterotomy, and the other half underwent fissurectomy and midline sphincterotomy.[1] Although both groups had the same incidence of delayed healing (two patients), no one experienced fecal soilage in the former group. Five percent noted this problem after the latter operation. Bode and colleagues performed fissurectomy with "superficial" midline sphincterotomy in 121 individuals.[11] No patient was found to have a keyhole deformity during a mean follow-up of more than 8 years. The recurrence rate was approximately 5%. Garcia-Aguilar and co-workers, in a retrospective analysis, found that closed sphincterotomy was preferable to open because it was associated with a similar rate of cure and fewer control complaints.[30]

Hawley reported a prospective study of three methods of treatment of chronic anal fissure: sphincter stretch, posterior sphincterotomy, and lateral sphincterotomy.[41] He found that lateral internal anal sphincterotomy was the preferred operation because it resulted in earlier wound healing, less postoperative discomfort, and fewer problems with soiling. Hsu and MacKeigan reported the treatment of more than 1,700 patients with chronic anal fissure by five different methods.[44] Fewer complications were noted with lateral sphincterotomy in comparison with excision and sphincterotomy. Conversely, Khubchandani and Reed noted no significant differences in patient satisfaction or functional results in more than 1,000 patients, irrespective of the method of treatment, whether lateral sphincterotomy, bilateral sphincterotomy, or posterior midline sphincterotomy.[53] However, the incidence of complications was relatively high: flatus control problems occurred in 35%, soiling in 22%, and "accidents" in 5%.

Engel and associates performed fissurectomy without sphincterotomy in 17 consecutive patients who did not respond to conservative measures using the nitric oxide donor, isosorbide dinitrate cream postoperatively.[25] All wounds healed within 10 weeks, with no recurrence at a median follow-up of 29 months. The authors concluded that one should consider this approach as a sphincter-sparing technique to minimize the risk of impairment for bowel control.

Chronic Anal Fissure with Stenosis

Difficulty with defecation secondary to narrowing of the anal canal from chronic fissure can occasionally occur. The problem is more commonly seen, however, when excess anal canal mucosa is removed at the time of hemorrhoidectomy. Stenosis and fissure may supervene. Conservative medical management with stool softeners and a dilator is often advised, but an anoplasty as recommended by Ferguson is the approach that I prefer (see Chapter 8).[20,27]

Even in the absence of stenosis, concomitant anoplasty has been recommended. Leong and Seow-Choen randomized 40 patients with chronic anal fissure to lateral sphincterotomy or to anal advancement flap.[58] This is an interesting conclusion because all healed with the former operation, and 15% failed to heal with the flap. Nyam and colleagues advise an island advancement flap as an alternative when resting or squeeze pressures are reduced or when there is increased risk by performing a "sphincter-weakening procedure".[81]

Anal Fissure and Hemorrhoids

When a patient harbors an anal fissure as well as a hemorrhoid problem sufficient to warrant surgical treatment, a hemorrhoidectomy with sphincterotomy should be performed concurrently (Figure 9-22; see Chapter 8). The

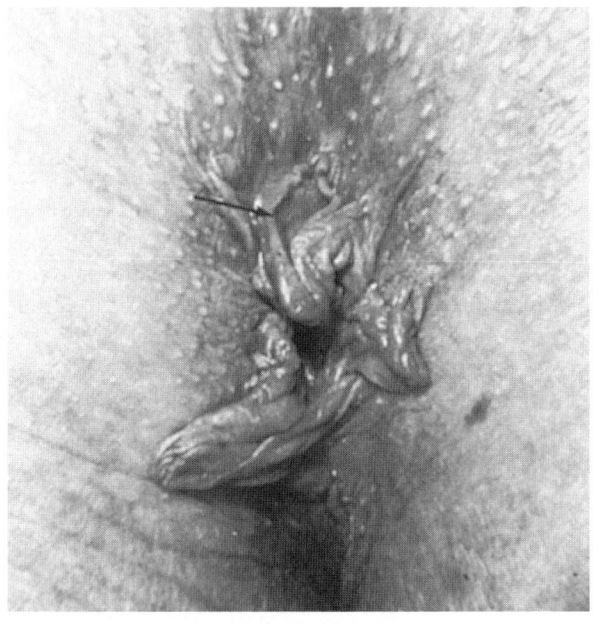

FIGURE 9-22. Hemorrhoids with an associated posterior anal fissure *(arrow)*. This problem is optimally treated by hemorrhoidectomy and lateral internal anal sphincterotomy.

sphincterotomy should be carried out laterally, usually at the site of the left lateral pile (see Figure 8-34).

Anal Fissure and Crohn's Disease

If the fissure is ectopic, extends proximal to the dentate line, is particularly broad-based, or is especially purulent, the association with underlying inflammatory bowel disease must be considered (see Chapters 11 and 30). A history of diarrhea or abdominal pain is highly suggestive. Fielding reported in a prospective study of 153 patients with Crohn's disease that more than one half had anal fissures, most of which were asymptomatic.[28] When doubt exists about the cause of the condition, intestinal evaluation, including small bowel roentgenography and colonoscopy (or barium enema), should be performed before a definitive surgical procedure is undertaken. It may be worthwhile to perform a small biopsy of the anal area, possibly to demonstrate a characteristic granuloma of Crohn's disease. Other conditions may produce an anal fissure or ulcer, but the differential diagnosis usually poses little problem. Anal canal carcinoma, carcinoma of the anal margin, and tuberculosis all exhibit more extensive changes than a solitary anal fissure. Conservative (i.e., medical) treatment is the prudent course. If a surgical procedure is undertaken, the resultant wound often tends to be indolent and leads to more symptoms than did the original condition. Furthermore, the patient's condition may be so debilitating that the need for a diversionary procedure may be precipitated. Still, some published studies have testified to a high rate of healing when internal anal sphincterotomy is performed, even in the presence of active Crohn's disease.[29,99,106] Certainly, the physician should consider the possibility of underlying inflammatory bowel disease in any patient whose fissure fails to heal following surgery.

Anal Fissure in the Homosexual Population

Anal fissures are common among male homosexuals, presumably as a consequence of traumatic anal intercourse.[94] However, numerous anal and perianal ulcers occur in these individuals that may pose a problem in differential diagnosis. Certainly, a primary syphilitic chancre may be confused with anal fissure (see Figure 19-38). Because a high index of suspicion is necessary for diagnosis of these conditions, any fissure or perianal ulcer should be cultured and a biopsy performed in this group of patients.[94] Besides syphilis, the causes of such lesions have been reported to include *Chlamydia, Haemophilus ducreyi,* cytomegalovirus, herpes simplex virus, human immunodeficiency virus (HIV) (see Chapters 19, 20, and 33), and neoplasms (e.g., squamous cell carcinoma, non-Hodgkin's lymphoma, and Kaposi's sarcoma; see Chapters 24 and 25).[94] Those HIV-positive individuals with no identifiable associated cause may be helped with aggressive debridement or intralesional steroid therapy.[102] Sphincterotomy for uncomplicated fissure can be performed with the expectation of healing if symptoms warrant and if medical management has been unsuccessful.[94]

REFERENCES

1. Abcarian H. Surgical correction of chronic anal fissure: results of lateral internal sphincterotomy versus fissurectomy-midline sphincterotomy. *Dis Colon Rectum* 1980; 23:31.
2. Abcarian H, Lakshmanan S, Read DR, et al. The role of internal sphincter in chronic anal fissures. *Dis Colon Rectum* 1982;25:525.
3. Abramowitz L, Sobhani I, Benifla JL, et al. Anal fissure and thrombosed external hemorrhoids before and after delivery. *Dis Colon Rectum* 2002;45:650.
4. Altomare DF, Rinaldi M, Milito G, et al.Glyceryl trinitrate for chronic anal fissure: healing or headache? Results of a multicenter, randomized placebo-controlled, double-blind trial. *Dis Colon Rectum* 2000;43:174.
5. Standards Task Force, American Society of Colon and Rectal Surgeons. Practice parameters for ambulatory anorectal surgery. *Dis Colon Rectum* 1991;34:285.
6. Antebi E, Schwartz P, Gilon E. Sclerotherapy for the treatment of fissure in ano. *Surg Gynecol Obstet* 1985; 160:204.
7. Arabi Y, Alexander-Williams J, Keighley MRB. Anal pressures in hemorrhoids and anal fissure. *Am J Surg* 1977;134:608.
8. Bailey HR, Beck DE, Billingham RP, et al. A study to determine the nitroglycerine ointment dose and dosing interval that best promote the healing of chronic anal fissures. *Dis Colon Rectum* 2002;45:1192.
9. Bell GA. Lateral internal sphincterotomy in chronic anal fissure: a surgical technique. *Am Surg* 1980;46:572.
10. Bennett RC, Goligher JC. Results of internal sphincterotomy for anal fissure. *BMJ* 1962;2:1500.
11. Bode WE, Culp CE, Spencer RJ, et al. Fissurectomy with superficial midline sphincterotomy: a viable alternative for the surgical correction of chronic fissure/ulcer-in-ano. *Dis Colon Rectum* 1984;27:93.
12. Boulos PB, Araujo JGC. Adequate internal sphincterotomy for anal fissure: subcutaneous or open technique? *Br J Surg* 1984;71:360.
13. Brisinda D, Maria G, Fenici R, et al. Safety of botulinum neurotoxin treatment in patients with chronic anal fissure. *Dis Colon Rectum* 2003;46:419.
14. Brown AC, Sumfest JM, Rozwadowski JV. Histopathology of the internal anal sphincter in chronic anal fissure. *Dis Colon Rectum* 1989;32:680.
15. Cerdàn FJ, deLion AR, Azpiroz F, et al. Anal sphincteric pressure in fissure-in-ano before and after lateral internal sphincterotomy. *Dis Colon Rectum* 1982;25:198.
16. Chen J, Michowitz M, Bawnik JB. Solcoderm as alternative conservative treatment for acute anal fissure: a controlled clinical study. *Am Surg* 1992;58:705.
17. Chowcat NL, Araujo JGC, Boulos PB. Internal sphincterotomy for chronic anal fissure: long-term effects on anal pressure. *Br J Surg* 1986;73:915.
18. Cohen A, Dehn TCB. Lateral subcutaneous sphincterotomy for treatment of anal fissure in children. *Br J Surg* 1995;82:1341.
19. Cook TA, Smilgin Humpreys MM, Mortensen NJMcC. Oral nifedipine reduces resting anal pressure and heals chronic anal fissure. *Br J Surg* 1999;86:1269.
20. Crapp AR, Alexander-Williams J. Fissure-in-ano and anal stenosis. Part I: conservative management. *Clin Gastroenterol* 1975;4:619.
21. Cundall JD, Gardiner A, Laden G, et al. Use of hyperbaric oxygen to treat chronic anal fissure. *Br J Surg* 2003;90:452.
22. Duthie HL, Bennett RC. Anal sphincteric pressure in fissure-in-ano. *Surg Gynecol Obstet* 1964;119:19.
23. Eisenhammer S. The surgical correction of chronic internal anal (sphincteric) contracture. *S Afr Med J* 1951;25:486.
24. Eisenhammer S. The evaluation of the internal anal sphincterotomy operation with special reference to anal fissure. *Surg Gynecol Obstet* 1959;109:583.
25. Engel AF, Eijsbouts QAJ, Balk AG. Fissurectomy and isosorbide dinitrate for chronic fissure *in* ano not responding to conservative treatment. *Br J Surg* 2002;89:79.
26. Evans J, Luck A, Hewett P. Glyceryl trinitrate vs. lateral sphincterotomy for chronic anal fissure: prospective, randomized trial. *Dis Colon Rectum* 2001;44:93.
27. Ferguson JA. Fissure-in-ano and anal stenosis. Part II: radical surgical managements. *Clin Gastroenterol* 1975;4:629.
28. Fielding JF. An enquiry into certain aspects of regional enteritis. M.D. thesis, National University of Ireland, 1967.
29. Fleshner PR, Schoetz DJ Jr, Roberts PL, et al. Anal fissure in Crohn's disease: a plea for aggressive management. *Dis Colon Rectum* 1995;38:1137.
30. Garcia-Aguilar J, Belmonte C, Wong WD, et al. Open versus closed sphincterotomy for chronic anal fissure: long-term results. *Dis Colon Rectum* 1996;39:440.
31. Garcia-Aguilar J, Montes CB, Perez JJ, et al. Incontinence after lateral internal sphincterotomy. *Dis Colon Rectum* 1998; 41:423.
32. Garcia-Granero E, Sanahuja A, Garcia-Armengol J, et al. Anal endosonographic evaluation after closed lateral subcutaneous sphincterotomy. *Dis Colon Rectum* 1998;41:598.
33. Gecim I. Comparison of glyceryl trinitrate and botulinum toxin A in treatment of chronic anal fissure: a prospective, randomized study. *Dis Colon Rectum* 2001;44:A5.
34. Gibbons CP, Read NW. Anal hypertonia in fissures: cause or effect? *Br J Surg* 1986;73:443.
35. Gilgold BS. Simple in-office sphincterotomy with partial fissurectomy for chronic anal fissure. *Surg Gynecol Obstet* 1987;165:46.
36. Goldman G, Zilberman M, Werbin N. Bacteremia in anal dilatation. *Dis Colon Rectum* 1986;29:304.
37. Goligher JC. *Surgery of the anus, rectum and colon,* 4th ed. New York: Macmillan, 1980:136.
38. Goligher JC. *Surgery of the anus, rectum and colon,* 4th ed. New York: Macmillan, 1980:147.
39. Gorfine SR. Treatment of benign anal disease with topical nitroglycerin. *Dis Colon Rectum* 1995;38:453.
40. Hancock BD. The internal sphincter and anal fissure. *Br J Surg* 1977;64:92.
41. Hawley PR. The treatment of chronic fissure-in-ano: a trial of methods. *Br J Surg* 1969;56:915.
42. Helton WS. 2001 consensus statement on benign anorectal disease. *J Gastrointest Surg* 2002;6:302.
43. Hoffmann DC, Goligher JC. Lateral subcutaneous internal sphincterotomy in treatment of anal fissure. *BMJ* 1970;3:673.
44. Hsu T-C, MacKeigan JM. Surgical treatment of chronic anal fissure: a retrospective study of 1753 cases. *Dis Colon Rectum* 1984;27:475.
45. Hyman NH, Cataldo PA. Nitroglycerine ointment for anal fissures: effective treatment or just a headache? *Dis Colon Rectum* 1999;42:383.
46. Jensen SL. Diet and other risk factors for fissure-in-ano: prospective case-control study. *Dis Colon Rectum* 1988;31:770.
47. Jonas M, Neal KR, Abercrombie JF, et al. A randomized trial of oral vs. topical diltiazem for chronic anal fissures. *Dis Colon Rectum* 2001;44:1074.
48. Jonas M, Speake W, Scholefield JH. Diltiazem heals glyceryl trinitrate-resistant chronic anal fissures: a prospective study. *Dis Colon Rectum* 2002;45:1091.

49. Jost WH, Schimrigk K. Use of botulinum toxin in anal fissure [Letter]. *Dis Colon Rectum* 1993;36:974.

50. Jost WH, Schimrigk K. Therapy of anal fissure using botulin toxin. *Dis Colon Rectum* 1994;37:1321.

51. Keck JO, Staniunas RJ, Coller JA, et al. Computer-generated profiles of the anal canal in patients with anal fissure. *Dis Colon Rectum* 1995;38:72.

52. Keighley MRB, Greca F, Nevah E, et al. Treatment of anal fissure by lateral subcutaneous sphincterotomy should be under general anesthesia. *Br J Surg* 1981;68:400.

53. Khubchandani IT, Reed JF. Sequelae of internal sphincterotomy for chronic fissure-in-ano. *Br J Surg* 1989;76:431.

54. Klosterhalfen B, Vogel P, Rixen H, et al. Topography of the inferior rectal artery: a possible cause of chronic, primary anal fissure. *Dis Colon Rectum* 1989;32:43.

55. Knight JS, Birks M, Farouk R. Topical diltiazem ointment in the treatment of chronic anal fissure. *Br J Surg* 2001;88:553.

56. Kocher HM, Steward M, Leather AJM, et al. Randomized clinical trial assessing the side-effects of glyceryl trinitrate and diltiazem hydrochloride in the treatment of chronic anal fissure. *Br J Surg* 2002;89:413.

57. Kortbeek JB, Langevin JM, Khoo REH, et al. Chronic fissure-in-ano: a randomized study comparing open and subcutaneous lateral internal sphincterotomy. *Dis Colon Rectum* 1992;35:835.

58. Leong AFPK, Seow-Choen F. Lateral sphincterotomy compared with anal advancement flap for chronic anal fissure. *Dis Colon Rectum* 1995;38:69.

59. Lewis TH, Corman ML, Prager ED, et al. Long-term results of open and closed sphincterotomy for anal fissure. *Dis Colon Rectum* 1988;31:368.

60. Lindsey I, Jones OM, Cunningham C, et al. Botulinum toxin as second-line therapy for chronic anal fissure failing 0.2 percent glyceryl trinitrate. *Dis Colon Rectum* 2003;46:361.

61. Lockhart-Mummery P. *Diseases of the rectum and anus.* New York: William Wood, 1914:169.

62. Lockhart-Mummery P. *Diseases of the rectum and anus.* New York: William Wood, 1914:171.

63. Loder PB, Kamm MA, Nicholls RJ, et al. Reversible chemical sphincterotomy by local application of glyceryl trinitrate. *Br J Surg* 1994;81:1386.

64. Lund JN, Armitage NC, Scholefield JH. Use of glyceryl trinitrate ointment in the treatment of anal fissure. *Br J Surg* 1996;83:776.

65. Lund JN, Binch C, McGrath J, et al. Topographical distribution of blood supply to the anal canal. *Br J Surg* 1999;86:496.

66. Lund JN, Scholefield JH. A randomised, prospective, double-blind, placebo-controlled trial of glyceryl trinitrate ointment in treatment of anal fissure. *Lancet* 1997;349:11.

67. Maria G, Cassetta E, Gui D, et al. A comparison of botulinum toxin and saline for the treatment of chronic anal fissure. *N Engl J Med* 1998;338:217.

68. Marya SK, Mittal SS, Singla S. Lateral subcutaneous internal sphincterotomy for acute fissure-in-ano. *Br J Surg* 1980;67:299.

69. McLeod RS, Evans J. Symptomatic care and nitroglycerin in the management of anal fissure. *J Gastrointest Surg* 2002;6:278.

70. McNamara MJ, Percy JP, Fielding IR. A manometric study of anal fissure treated by subcutaneous lateral internal sphincterotomy. *Ann Surg* 1990;211:235.

71. Mentes BB, Irkörücü O, Akin M, et al. Comparison of botulinum toxin injection and lateral internal sphincterotomy for the treatment of chronic anal fissure. *Dis Colon Rectum* 2003;46:232.

72. Miles WE. *Rectal surgery.* London: Cassell & Co, 1939.

73. Millar DM. Subcutaneous lateral internal anal sphincterotomy for anal fissure. *Br J Surg* 1971;58:737.

74. Nelson RL. A review of operative procedures for anal fissure. *J Gastrointest Surg* 2002;6:284.

75. Nielsen MB, Rasmussen O, Pedersen JF, et al. Risk of sphincter damage and anal incontinence after anal dilatation for fissure-in-ano: an endosonographic study. *Dis Colon Rectum* 1993;36:677.

76. Notaras MJ. Lateral subcutaneous sphincterotomy for anal fissure: a new technique. *Proc R Soc Med* 1969;62:713.

77. Notaras MJ. The treatment of anal fissure by lateral subcutaneous internal sphincterotomy: a technique and results. *Br J Surg* 1971;58:96.

78. Notaras MJ. Fissure-in-ano: lateral subcutaneous internal anal sphincterotomy. In: Todd IP, ed. *Colon, rectum, and anus,* 3rd ed. London: Butterworth, 1977:354 (Operative surgery series).

79. Notaras MJ. Anal fissure and stenosis. *Surg Clin North Am* 1988;68:1427.

80. Nothmann BJ, Schuster MM. Internal anal sphincter derangement with anal fissures. *Gastroenterology* 1974;67:216.

81. Nyam DCNK, Wilson RG, Stewart KJ, et al. Island advancement flaps in the management of anal fissures. *Br J Surg* 1995;82:326.

82. Pernikoff BJ, Eisenstat TE, Rubin RJ, et al. Reappraisal of partial lateral internal sphincterotomy. *Dis Colon Rectum* 1994;37:1291.

83. Perrotti P, Bove B, Antropoli C, et al. Topical nifedipine with lidocaine ointment vs. active control for treatment of chronic anal fissure: results of a prospective, randomized, double-blind study. *Dis Colon Rectum* 2002;45:1468.

84. Phillips R. Pharmacologic treatment of anal fissure with botoxin, diltiazem, or bethanechol. *J Gastrointest Surg* 2002;6:281.

85. Pitt J, Williams S, Dawson PM. Reasons for failure of glyceryl trinitrate treatment of chronic fissure-in-ano. *Dis Colon Rectum* 2001;44:864.

86. Ravikumar TS, Sridhar S, Rao RN. Subcutaneous lateral internal sphincterotomy for chronic fissure-in-ano. *Dis Colon Rectum* 1982;25:798.

87. Ray JE, Penfold JCB, Gathright JB, et al. Lateral subcutaneous internal anal sphincterotomy for anal fissure. *Dis Colon Rectum* 1974;17:139.

88. Reissman P. Significance of anal canal ultrasound before sphincterotomy in multiparous women with anal fissure [Letter]. *Dis Colon Rectum* 1996;39:1060.

89. Richard CS, Gregoire R, Plewes EA, et al. Internal sphincterotomy is superior to topical nitroglycerin in the treatment of chronic anal fissure: results of a randomized, controlled trial by the Canadian Colorectal Surgical Trials Group. *Dis Colon Rectum* 2000;43:1048.

90. Roe AM, Bartolo DCC, Mortensen NJMcC. New method for assessment of anal sensation in various anorectal disorders. *Br J Surg* 1986;73:310.

91. Romano G, Rotondano G, Santangelo M, et al. A critical appraisal of pathogenesis and morbidity of surgical treatment of chronic anal fissure. *J Am Coll Surg* 1994;178:600.

92. Rosen L, Abel ME, Gordon PH, et al. Practice parameters for the management of anal fissure. *Dis Colon Rectum* 1992;35:206.

93. Rudd WWH. Lateral subcutaneous internal sphincterotomy for chronic anal fissure, an outpatient procedure. *Dis Colon Rectum* 1975;18:319.

94. Safavi A, Gottesman L, Dailey TH. Anorectal surgery in the HIV+ patient: update. *Dis Colon Rectum* 1991;34:299.

95. Schouten WR, Briel JW, Auwerda JJA. Relationship between anal pressure and anodermal blood flow: the vascular pathogenesis of anal fissures. *Dis Colon Rectum* 1994;37:664.

96. Schouten WR, Briel JW, Auwerda JJA, et al. Ischaemic nature of anal fissure. *Br J Surg* 1996;83:63.

97. Schuster MM. The riddle of the sphincters. *Gastroenterology* 1975;69:249.

98. Sohn N, Eisenberg MM, Weinstein MA, et al. Precise anorectal sphincter dilatation: its role in the therapy of anal fissures. *Dis Colon Rectum* 1992;35:322.

99. Sohn N, Korelitz BI. Local operative treatment of anorectal Crohn's disease. *J Clin Gastroenterol* 1982;4:395.

100. Speakman CTM, Burnett SJD, Kamm MA, et al. Sphincter injury after anal dilatation demonstrated by anal endosonography. *Br J Surg* 1991;78:1429.

101. Sultan AH, Kamm MA, Nicholls RJ, et al. Prospective study of the extent of internal anal sphincter division during lateral sphincterotomy. *Dis Colon Rectum* 1994;37:1031.

102. Viamonte M, Dailey TH, Gottesman L. Ulcerative disease of the anorectum in the HIV+ patient. *Dis Colon Rectum* 1993;36:801.

103. Walker WA, Rothenberger DA, Goldberg SM. Morbidity of internal sphincterotomy for anal fissure and stenosis. *Dis Colon Rectum* 1985;28:832.

104. Watson SJ, Kamm MA, Nicholls RJ, et al. Topical glyceryl trinitrate in the treatment of chronic anal fissure. *Br J Surg* 1996;83:771.

105. Watts JM, Bennett RC, Goligher JC. Stretching of anal sphincters in treatment of fissure-in-ano. *BMJ* 1964;2:342.

106. Wolkomir AF, Luchtefeld MA. Surgery for symptomatic hemorrhoids and anal fissures in Crohn's disease. *Dis Colon Rectum* 1993;36:545.

Chapter 10

Anorectal Abscess

Staphylococcus Aureus
By Gram and Koch he swore
He would invade new regions
Unconquered heretofore—
By Gram and Koch he swore it,
To take a patient's life,
And called the Cocci, young and old,
From all his colonies of gold
To aid him in the strife
St. Bartholomew's Hospital Journal 1909;17:13
—"The Battle of Furunculus"

ETIOLOGY AND PATHOGENESIS

Anorectal abscess is an acute inflammatory process that often is the initial manifestation of an underlying anal fistula. An abscess in this area may also be a consequence of other causes and associations. These include the following:

- Foreign body intrusion
- Trauma
- Malignancy
- Radiation
- Immunocompromised state [e.g., leukemia, acquired immunodeficiency syndrome (AIDS)]
- Infectious dermatitides (e.g., suppurative hidradenitis)
- Tuberculosis
- Actinomycosis
- Crohn's disease
- Anal fissure[3,35]

Additionally, anorectal abscess may develop as a complication of anal operations, such as hemorrhoidectomy (rarely—see Chapter 8) and internal anal sphincterotomy (see Chapter 9).

The cause of nonspecific anorectal abscess and fistula is believed to be plugging of the anal ducts; this is known as the cryptoglandular theory. Credit for introducing the concept of gland infection in the pathogenesis of anal fistula is generally attributed to Chiari (1878)[14] and

to Herrmann and Desfosses (1880).[32] Klosterhalfen and colleagues examined 62 autopsy specimens by means of conventional and special immunohistologic staining methods and confirmed that anal intramuscular glands should be the anatomic correlate of anal fistulas.[37] Between six and ten of these glands and ducts are located around the anal canal and enter at the base of the crypts (see Figure 8-2). Parks (see Biography, Chapter 29) demonstrated by meticulous histologic review that one half of all crypts are not entered by glands, that the ducts usually end blindly, and that the most common direction of spread is downward into the submucosa.[48] Of particular interest is his observation that in two thirds of the specimens, one or more branches enter the sphincter, and in one half, the branches cross the internal sphincter completely to end in the longitudinal layer (Figure 10-1). In his study, however, no branches crossed into the external sphincter. The implication is that plugging or infection of the duct can result in an abscess that can spread in a several directions that may ultimately lead to the development of an anal fistula. In theory, therefore, an intersphincteric fistula may develop when the duct traverses the internal sphincter, and a transsphincteric fistula may be a consequence of the duct's traversing the external sphincter.

Shafer and colleagues performed surgery for anal fistula in 52 infants and noted a markedly irregular, thickened dentate line.[60] They attributed the condition to a defect in the dorsal portion of the cloacal membrane, which fuses with the hindgut during week 7 of gestation. In essence, then, contemporary theory implies that fistula-in-ano is the result of a congenital anomaly or predisposition.[16]

Further support for the proposition of a congenital origin, albeit by different mechanisms, has been offered by several authors. One theory holds that an excess of androgens may lead to the formation of abnormal glands *in utero* and that these abnormal glands are predisposed to infection.[22] Pople and Ralphs postulated that the "inappropriate" presence of columnar and transitional epithelium along the length of the excised fistula tracts of four

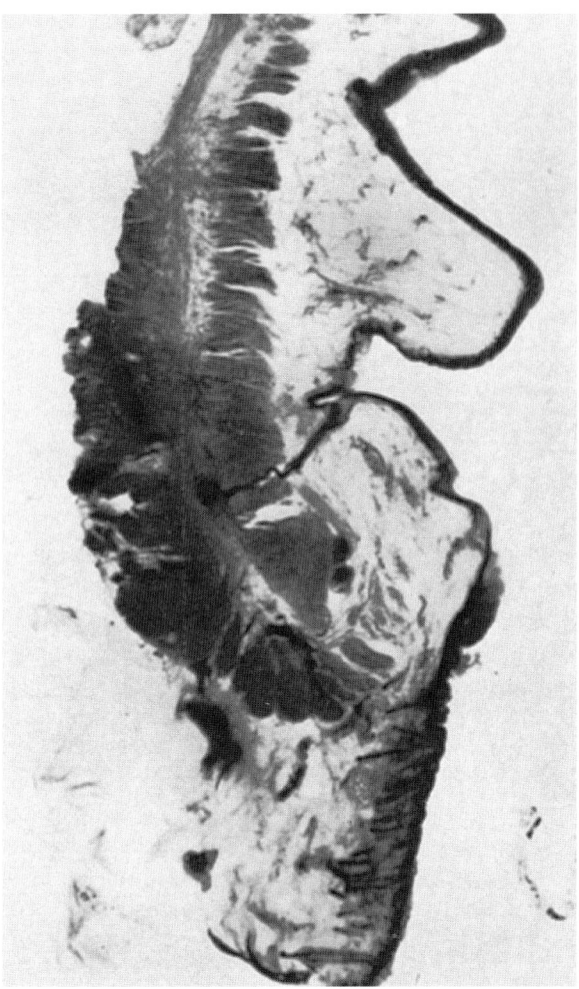

FIGURE 10-1. This thick section through the anal canal shows an anal gland penetrating the internal sphincter, terminating in the longitudinal layer. (From Parks AG. Fistula-in-ano. In: Morson BC, ed. *Diseases of the colon, rectum and anus.* New York: Appleton-Century-Crofts, 1969:277, with permission.)

infants is further evidence of a congenital abnormality presenting in the first few months of life.[53] They suggest that migratory cells from the urogenital sinus of the primitive hindgut become locally displaced and entrapped. Because fusion in females is less extensive, this could explain, according to the authors, the higher incidence of fistula in males.

AGE AND SEX

Abscess and fistula occur more commonly in men than in women. McElwain and colleagues reported a ratio of three men to one woman, whereas two large series from Cook County Hospital in Chicago were noted to have a two-to-one ratio.[44,55,56] At the time of presentation, two thirds of patients are in the third or fourth decade of

life.[44,55] There seems to be a seasonal occurrence for the condition, with the highest incidence in the spring and summer.

Hill reported a personal experience of 626 patients;[34] the youngest was 2 months of age, and the oldest was 79 years. The number of male patients was almost twice the number of female patients. In his experience, symptoms developed in most in the fourth, fifth, and sixth decades.

Infants younger than 2 years of age represent a different spectrum of the disease when compared with older children and adults. There is an overwhelming male predominance with abscess and with concomitant anal fistula, in excess of 85%.[1,37,52] However, the distribution in older children tends to resemble that seen in adults.

TYPES OF ABSCESS

Four presentations of anorectal abscess have been described:

- Perianal
- Ischiorectal
- Intersphincteric (also known as submucosal)
- Supralevator

These are illustrated in Figure 10-2. It is important to distinguish among these presentations, because the etiology, therapy, and implications for the presence or subsequent development of anal fistula are different for each.

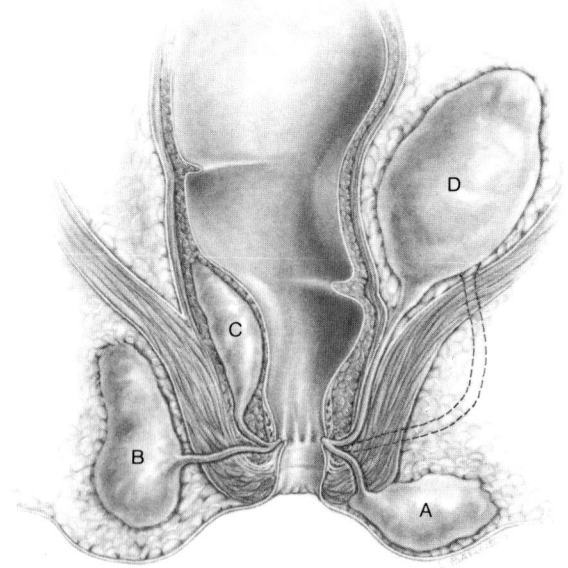

FIGURE 10-2. Infection of the anal duct can present as an abscess in a number of locations. *A,* Perianal. *B,* Ischiorectal. *C,* Intersphincteric. *D,* Supralevator.

Perianal Abscess

Perianal (or perirectal) abscess is identified as a superficial, tender mass outside the anal verge (Figure 10-3). It is arguably the most common type of anorectal abscess, occurring in perhaps 40% to 45% of cases, but this relatively high incidence may be a reflection of the nature of one's practice. The patient usually presents with a relatively short history of painful swelling that may be exacerbated by defecation and by sitting. Fever and leukocytosis are uncommon.

Physical examination reveals an area of erythema, induration, or fluctuance. Proctosigmoidoscopic examination may be difficult to perform because of pain, but even when it can be accomplished, it is usually unrewarding. Occasionally, however, anoscopic examination demonstrates pus exuding from the base of a crypt or at the site of a chronic anal fissure.

Treatment

As mentioned in other chapters, the American Society of Colon and Rectal Surgeons has established guidelines for the treatment of numerous conditions. These include the parameters for the treatment of abscess and anal fistula.[62] The society's recommendations are worth quoting:

Acute Suppuration (Abscess)

Presentation and Management An abscess should be drained in a timely manner; lack of fluctuance is not a reason for delay in treatment. If the abscess is superficial, it may be drained in the office setting using a local anesthetic. If the patient is too tender to permit examination and drainage, then these measures should be undertaken in the operating room. Antibiotics may have a role as adjunctive therapy in special circumstances, including valvular heart disease, immunosuppression, extensive cellulitis, or diabetes. Location of the abscess should be documented. If possible, anoscopy should be performed to reveal the primary site of infection. Patients should notify the physician if pain recurs after abscess drainage.

The following comments represent my own thoughts, but I believe they are consistent with the parameters established by the society:

When only erythema is present with no apparent mass, the surgeon may be misled into believing that incision and drainage will not be beneficial. Under such circumstances, the patient may be instructed to take sitz baths or may be given a broad-spectrum antibiotic and advised to return in 24 to 48 hours. Despite the absence of fluctuation or significant induration, an abscess is usually present. A patient who is dismissed without undergoing drainage may return a few hours or days later, distressed that spontaneous discharge has taken place, even though the discomfort may have been ameliorated. There is no place for antibiotics alone in the management of anorectal abscess. As I. J. Kodner has stated in numerous panel discussions on the subject, "The presence of pain suggests the need to drain."

The procedure is usually readily performed in the office with a local anesthetic. Alternatively, an emergency department setting or ambulatory surgical facility may be preferred. A large-bore hypodermic needle inserted into the region of induration is a simple diagnostic test. If purulence is present, a small incision is made using a local anesthetic. The pus is drained, a small gauze wick is inserted, and a dressing is applied. The patient is instructed to remove the dressing and the drain in 24 hours while taking a sitz bath. Baths three times daily are advised, and the patient is reexamined in 7 to 10 days. At this time, proctosigmoidoscopic and anoscopic examinations are performed. If an external opening persists and a fistula tract is identified, a definitive procedure is indicated (see Chapter 11, Anal Fistula).

Postoperative Antibiotics The value of postoperative antibiotics for someone who has undergone incision and drainage is open to question. However, those at an

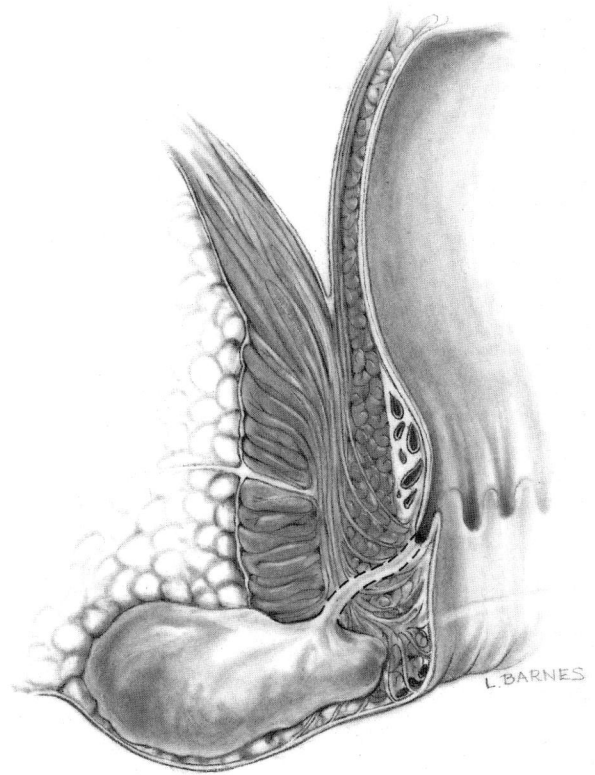

FIGURE 10-3. Perianal abscess. Only a few of these lesions are associated with an underlying fistula. The *dashed lines* illustrate the possible course of a fistula tract if it is present.

increased risk based on the criteria outlined in Chapter 4 should be so treated.

Microbiology The purpose of culturing the pus following drainage of a perianal or ischiorectal abscess is also a subject of some interest. Usually, the physician performs a culture to determine the appropriate antibiotic for treatment. As previously mentioned, however, antibiotics are usually unnecessary, but culture does have some benefit in determining the likelihood for the subsequent development of a fistula. If the culture demonstrates no bowel-derived organisms (i.e., skin bacteria), the chance of a subsequent fistula is virtually nil.[26,31] Conversely, if enteric organisms are identified, the probability of the presence of a fistula is increased. Lunniss and Phillips, in a prospective trial involving 22 patients, found culture of gut organisms to be quite sensitive for detecting an underlying fistula, but not particularly specific (80%).[41] Conversely, when an infection was present in the anorectal space, culture was 100% sensitive and 100% specific for the detection of an underlying fistula. Certainly, in this group of patients, surgical assessment is a better predictor of the subsequent development or presence of a fistula than is culture.

Study of the bacteriology of perirectal abscess in *children*, as in adults, has demonstrated that anaerobic organisms are the predominant isolates, although *Staphylococcus aureus* is frequently found.[9,39] Although no studies have been performed in children concerning the implication of the different culture results, it is reasonable to assume that the principle is identical.

Synchronous Fistulotomy

A fistula with an internal opening may be seen at the time that the abscess is drained. The incidence as reported from numerous centers is somewhat variable. This may be attributed to the variable aggressiveness of examiners in attempting to identify a fistula and perhaps also to demographic factors. Vasilevsky and Gordon reported recurrent abscess or the development of an anal fistula in 48% of patients who underwent drainage of a perianal or ischiorectal abscess.[65] Table 10-1 illustrates the results from the Cook County Hospital.

If the internal opening is low lying, the surgeon may elect to perform fistulotomy at the same time the abscess is drained to avoid the need for a second procedure. However, the literature is rather contradictory on this point, because it is not always clear from the article what type of fistula or abscess the author is treating. A recurrence rate of a mere 3.4% was reported by McElwain and colleagues following initial drainage and fistulotomy.[43] Their subsequent report demonstrated the rate of recurrence of abscess, fistula reformation, or both to be 3.6%, which compared quite favorably with their own recurrence rate of 6% when an established fistula was excised.[44] Waggener also recommends primary fistulotomy.[66]

Scoma and colleagues reported a retrospective review of 232 patients with anal abscess who underwent initial office drainage only.[58] A fistula subsequently developed in two thirds. Unfortunately, the authors failed to break down the incidence of fistula according to the type of abscess. They recommended that fistulotomy be delayed until the fistula becomes manifest. Others concur, although it is not always clear whether a vigorous attempt was made to identify a fistula at the initial procedure.[28] Tang and co-workers compared incision and drainage alone with concurrent fistulotomy for perianal abscess with a demonstrated internal opening in a prospective, randomized study involving 45 patients.[63] They concluded that incision with drainage alone was not associated with a statistically significantly higher incidence of recurrence of anal fistula when compared with concomitant fistulotomy. Therefore, a simple drainage procedure was essentially as good as a definitive fistula operation.

Opinion

In my own experience, an anal fistula is usually not recognized at the time of drainage of a perianal abscess. However, if a low-lying fistula is encountered, I recommend incision of the tract if it can be easily accomplished at that time. In accordance with my own preference, the patient usually undergoes drainage as an office procedure. Therefore, discomfort often precludes a more thorough evaluation, the identification of a fistula tract (if present), and the ability to perform definitive fistulotomy. Certainly, if an individual is to undergo a regional or general anesthetic, concurrent fistulotomy is a reasonable plan.

▶ **TABLE 10-1** Incidence of Fistula in Various Types of Anorectal Abscess

Type of Abscess	Number of Abscesses	Number with Fistulas	Percentage (%)
Perianal	437	151	34.5
Ischiorectal	233	59	25.3
Intersphincteric	219	104	47.4
Supralevator	75	32	42.6
Submucous of intermuscular	59	9	15.2

From Ramanujam PS, Prasad ML, Abcarian H, et al. Perianal abscesses and fistulas: a study of 1023 patients. *Dis Colon Rectum* 1984;27:593, with permission.

Ischiorectal Abscess

Ischiorectal abscess may present as a large, erythematous, indurated, tender mass of the buttock or may be virtually unapparent, the patient complaining only of severe pain (Figure 10-4). This type of abscess is seen in 20% to 25% of patients. Pus is almost always present. Waiting for the abscess to "mature" causes the patient to suffer needlessly. As with other suspected abscesses, needle aspiration will usually resolve the issue. Proctosigmoidoscopy and anoscopy are usually deferred because of the patient's discomfort, although the physician should keep in mind the possibility of rectal or anal cancer or other colorectal condition producing this manifestation.[3] Therefore, a thorough rectal evaluation at some point is mandatory.

Techniques of Drainage

Drainage of an ischiorectal abscess requires some planning, because the condition may well be associated with the subsequent development of a transsphincteric fistula (see Chapter 11). In fact, most patients with this type of abscess will require a subsequent fistula procedure. It is important, therefore, to drain the abscess by creating an external opening as close to the anal verge as is possible (Figure 10-5). If this is not considered, the subsequent fistulotomy may result in a large wound that requires a long time to heal (Figure 10-6). The abscess cavity can be readily entered and adequate drainage established without "attacking" the point of presentation or the most indurated or fluctuant area.

The technique for drainage of a large ischiorectal abscess is little different from that of a small perianal abscess. Neither necessarily requires a general anesthetic or vigorous operative manipulation. After administration of a local anesthetic, a small incision is made and the pus is evacuated. The cavity is irrigated, and a small gauze wick is inserted (not vigorously packed in). The concept of creating a large, cruciate incision and breaking up loculations is unnecessary and extremely uncomfortable. All one needs to accomplish is to establish adequate external drainage. Any residual pus will quickly drain if a small skin opening is maintained with gauze or some form of drain. A dressing is applied, and the patient is instructed to take warm sitz baths. The patient removes the drain in 48 to 72 hours and is seen again in 1 week, at which time probing of the external opening, proctosigmoidoscopy, and anoscopic examinations are performed.

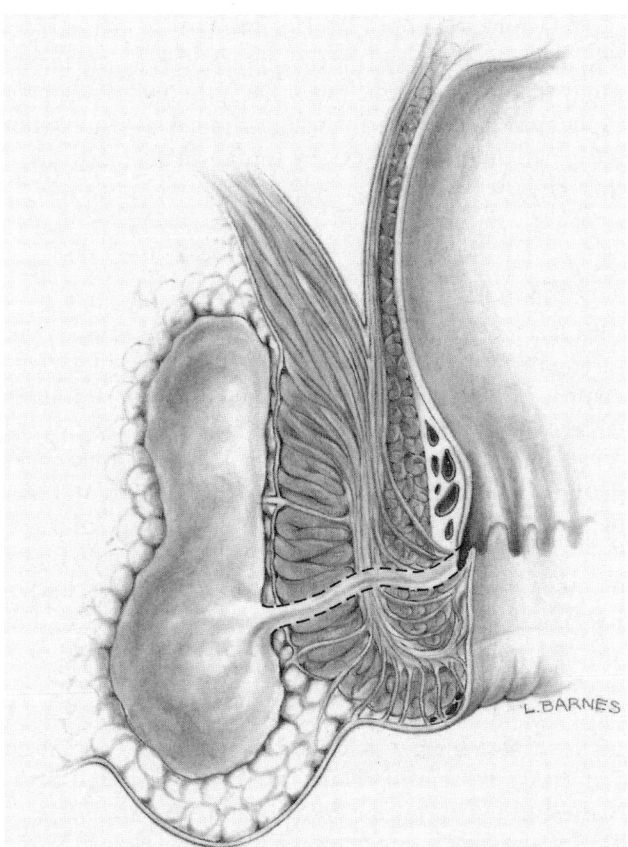

FIGURE 10-4. Ischiorectal abscess. This type of presentation often is inapparent on physical examination. One must maintain a high index of suspicion. The *dashed lines* illustrate the possible course of a fistula tract if it is present.

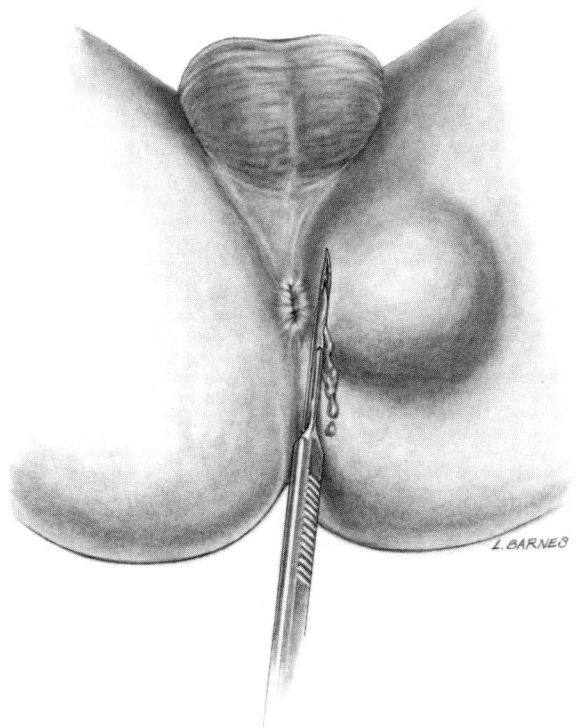

FIGURE 10-5. Proper drainage of an ischiorectal abscess requires that the incision be made as medially as possible, not necessarily at the point of maximal fluctuance. This enables the surgeon to avoid a subsequent long fistulotomy incision.

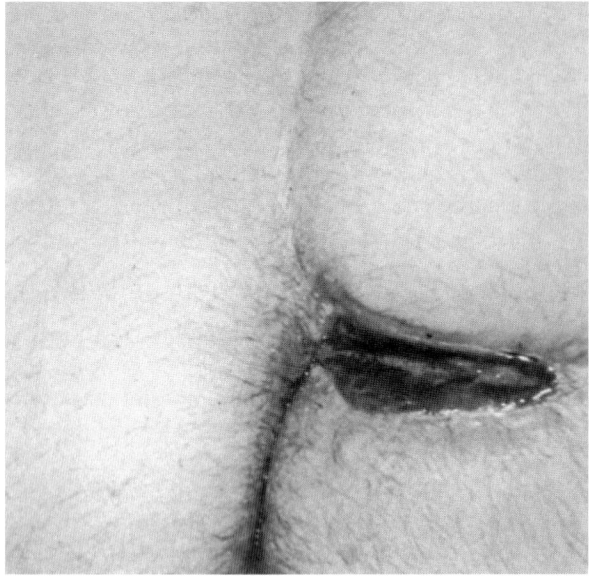

FIGURE 10-6. Drainage of a buttock abscess too far laterally results in a long fistula wound that requires a prolonged healing time.

In-Hospital Drainage

Several factors may contraindicate drainage of an ischiorectal abscess in the office. First, a general, spinal, or caudal anesthetic may be required because of patient insistence or because the patient is unable to tolerate the manipulation associated with a local procedure. Second, the surgeon may not have ideal space or office facilities. Contamination of the floor, walls, countertops, and instruments will certainly limit the use of the examining room for a time. Third, an ischiorectal abscess should not be drained in the office when the patient's condition is septic, except as a preamble to hospitalization. Other patients who are at particular risk for exclusively ambulatory treatment are those with insulin-dependent diabetes and those who are immunocompromised. Systemic antibiotics and more vigorous irrigations than are possible with an office procedure may be advisable.

In-hospital drainage follows essentially the same procedure advocated for office treatment. The incision should be minimal and medial. Irrigation with saline or an antiseptic solution is followed by insertion of a small drain or wick. Administration of an anesthetic also permits proctosigmoidoscopy and anoscopy, which may help to identify a specific cause for the abscess and localize an internal opening.

A simple method for determining whether an internal opening is present is to pass an anoscope while compressing the mass before drainage. Pus may be seen to exude from a crypt. If an opening is identified, its presence is noted for subsequent definitive treatment, usually after 2 weeks. I do not advocate fistulotomy of a transsphinc-

teric fistula synchronously with drainage of an ischiorectal abscess if for no other reason than providing adequate *informed consent* (see Chapter 11).

Once started, antibiotics are usually continued for 48 hours. As previously implied, although a culture of the pus may be taken in the operating room, it is rarely of use in treatment, except in predicting the possibility of a fistula. Drainage is the definitive therapy, and the patient almost invariably becomes afebrile within a short time following the procedure.

Intraanal Ultrasonography

The use of intraoperative ultrasonography for the evaluation of anorectal abscess and fistula has been a subject of some interest in the last few years. Cataldo and colleagues published their experience in 24 individuals with suspected perianal abscess and fistula.[13] All 19 patients subsequently were proved to harbor an abscess that was correctly identified preoperatively by intraanal ultrasonography. Furthermore, the technique helped to determine the relationship between the abscess and the sphincter muscles in approximately two thirds of the cases. However, whereas internal openings of fistula tracts were surgically found in 14 of 19 individuals, in only 28% were they identified by intraanal ultrasonography. The authors concluded that intraanal ultrasonography may be of value in certain clinical situations, but most patients with abscesses can be managed without this modality.

Primary Closure

Ellis has advocated incision, curettage, and primary suture with antibiotic coverage in the treatment of anorectal abscess.[20,21] Although he reported excellent results, in which primary healing took place in the vast majority of cases, one wonders about the likelihood of subsequent fistula development. Wilson reported on 100 of 120 patients so treated and followed for an average of more than 2 years.[69] Approximately two thirds initially had a perianal abscess; the remainder had an ischiorectal abscess. The overall recurrence rate was 22% (15.6% following perianal abscess and 33.3% following ischiorectal abscess). He too noted that recurrence was much more likely if the culture initially revealed predominantly *Escherichia coli* than if it yielded *S. aureus.* Mortensen and colleagues enrolled 107 patients in a study of primary suture with intraoperative parenteral antibiotics.[46] The incidence of recurrence was about the same, approximately 20%, in the two groups.

Goligher reported a prospective trial of conventional laying open versus incision, curettage, and suture.[24] Patients identified as having an internal opening at the time of drainage were excluded from the study. Healing occurred in more than 90% of those treated by primary suture. Because the follow-up period was less than 1 year, the rate of recurrence is difficult to judge.

Opinion

While it is true that I have had no experience with this technique, I can see no advantage in adopting it. Since I advocate minimal manipulation to effect drainage, the wound is inevitably quite small.

Deep Postanal Abscess

A transsphincteric fistula may present as an abscess in the deep postanal space (Figure 10-7). This space is deep to the external sphincter and inferior to the levator ani muscle. The patient will usually complain of severe rectal discomfort, often with radiation to the sacrum, coccyx, or buttock or will display a sciatic distribution. It may be exacerbated by sitting, defecation may be impaired, and a fecal impaction may be present. Symptoms may mimic proctalgia fugax, coccygodynia, or lumbosacral strain. A helpful finding that implies the true nature of the problem is that the patient is frequently febrile. Someone with posterior rectal pain and rectal tenderness of relatively short duration (i.e., less than 48 hours), wherein the pain is continuous rather than intermittent and is not affected by position, must be suspected of harboring an infection in the deep postanal space.

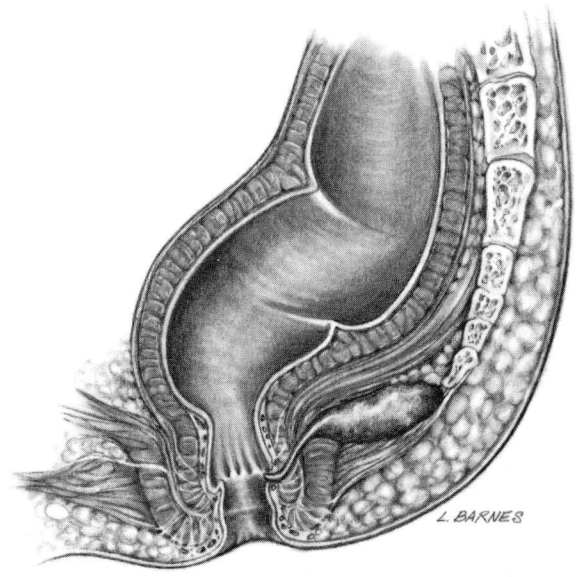

FIGURE 10-7. Deep postanal abscess originating from a posterior crypt. Drainage is effected through an incision from the internal opening to the coccyx.

Examination

Physical examination may be unrevealing except for exquisite posterior rectal tenderness. Very often, the diagnosis is missed, and the patient is sent home with instructions concerning warm sitz baths and perineal exercises and told to take an analgesic medication. Eventually, the abscess will usually present at the skin or drain spontaneously through the rectum. There is, however, the risk of sepsis and even Fournier's gangrene (see Chapter 19) if the condition is unrecognized and treatment is delayed. A high degree of suspicion, therefore, may be required if appropriate management is to be initiated. An attempt at aspiration between the rectum and coccyx in the midline will prove diagnostic. If an extrarectal mass is felt, the differential diagnosis includes presacral cyst, presacral lipoma, teratoma, chordoma, and a host of unusual retrorectal conditions, but these are all rarely tender. The physician must also be aware of the fact that postanal infections often communicate with the ischiorectal fossae on either side. The presentation may, therefore, be that of bilateral ischiorectal abscesses, also known as a horseshoe abscess.

Treatment

Management requires drainage of the deep postanal space, a procedure that cannot be accomplished adequately in the office with only a local anesthetic. Almost inevitably an internal opening in the posterior midline is identified at the time of drainage.

The best access to the deep postanal space to effect drainage was initially described by Hanley (see Chapter 11).[30] He advocated placing a probe in the primary opening in the posterior midline and making an incision over the probe toward the tip of the coccyx. This incision divides the internal sphincter and the superficial and subcutaneous portions of the external sphincter in order to enter and to decompress the cavity. Counterincisions may be made to drain the ischiorectal fossae if necessary (e.g., horseshoe abscess). Packing is advised and should be left in place for 24 to 48 hours (see Figure 11-25). By today's standards there is no other appropriate method for establishing drainage with this condition.[1,29]

Intersphincteric Abscess

Intersphincteric abscess was initially described by Eisenhammer and subsequently subdivided by him into a high type and a low type.[17,18] The condition arises from an infected crypt in the anal canal, but in this situation the infection usually burrows cephalad to present as a mass within the lower part of the rectum. It dissects in the intersphincteric plane, not under the mucosa, although it is frequently mistakenly called a "submucous" abscess (Figure

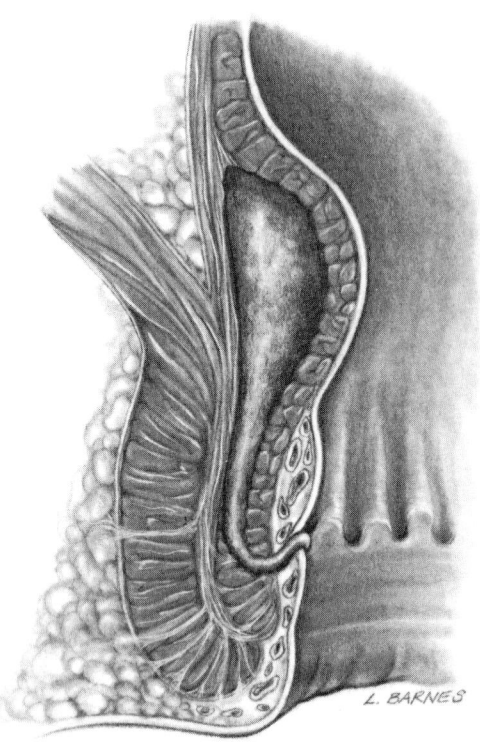

FIGURE 10-8. Intersphincteric abscess. The internal opening is at the level of the crypt with extension cephalad in the intermuscular plane.

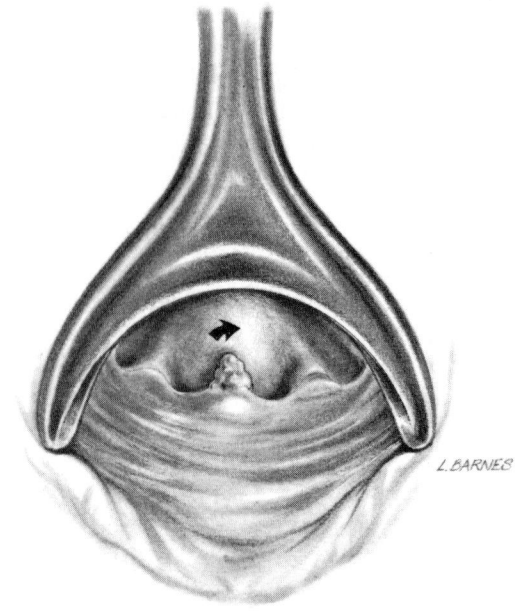

FIGURE 10-9. Opening of an intersphincteric abscess at the level of the crypt. Induration *(arrow)* is usually present proximal to this point.

10-8). Intersphincteric abscess is also sometimes classified as a submucous fistula, but this is an improper term because the condition does not fulfill the criterion for the definition of a fistula: a tract between two epithelial surfaces. Intersphincteric abscess represents between 2% and 5% of perirectal abscesses.

The patient usually complains of rectal or anal discomfort, which may be exacerbated by defecation. A sense of fullness in the rectum is often felt. Pus or mucous discharge may be noted. The individual may or may not be febrile.

Rectal examination may reveal a tender submucosal mass, which may not be readily apparent by anoscopy or proctosigmoidoscopy. The condition can be confused through palpation alone with a thrombosed internal hemorrhoid, but visual examination should distinguish the deep purple hemorrhoid from an abscess. The surface is edematous and indurated. An anal fissure is associated with the abscess in about 25% of patients.[50] Pus from the associated crypt should leave no doubt as to the nature of the lesion (Figure 10-9).

Treatment

Treatment usually requires a general, caudal, or spinal anesthetic, but a field block with conscious sedation may be attempted. However, this is *not* an office procedure. A

Hill-Ferguson retractor or other appropriate anal retractor is inserted. The abscess is excised through the internal sphincter, removing the associated crypt-bearing area (Figure 10-10). Finally, the cut edge of the rectum and the underlying internal sphincter can be sutured for hemostasis, leaving the wound open for drainage (Figure 10-11). No packing is required. The patient is discharged

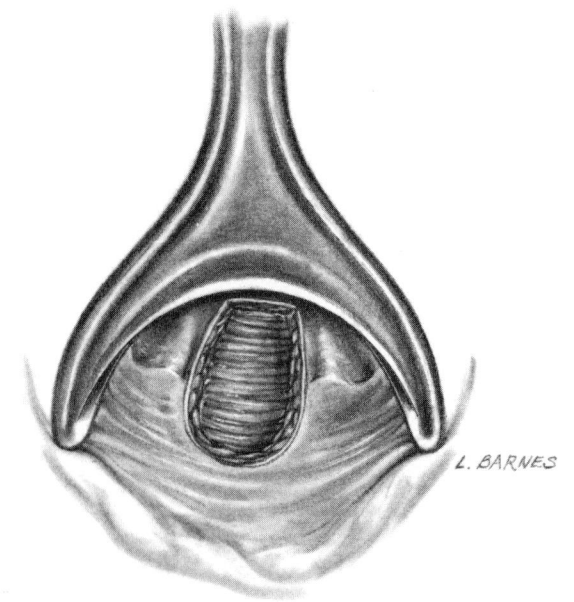

FIGURE 10-10. Intersphincteric abscess. The mucosa and the underlying internal sphincter are excised.

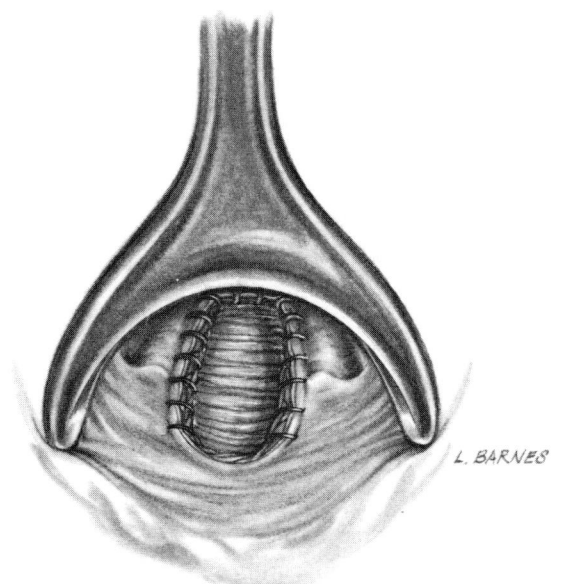

FIGURE 10-11. Intersphincteric abscess. The cut mucosal edge with the internal anal sphincter is sutured for hemostasis.

and advised to take a stool softener and warm sitz baths. Healing usually takes place within 3 to 4 weeks; no further procedure is required.

Supralevator Abscess

Supralevator abscesses are relatively rare, comprising fewer than 2.5% of abscesses in most series (Figure 10-12).[5,10,25,36] However, Goldenberg and Prasad and colleagues reviewed the Cook County Hospital experience and found the incidence to be 7.5% and 9.1%, respectively.[23,54] It is difficult to explain this variation in incidence; however, these reporters attribute their large experience to the low socioeconomic status of the patients, although I do not fully understand why this should be a factor. Obesity and diabetes mellitus were considered important contributing factors; one or the other was observed in 23% of patients. Perianal and buttock pain are the most common presenting complaints. Most patients are febrile and demonstrate leukocytosis.

Comment

In my experience, most individuals who present with a supralevator abscess have a characteristic history—namely, an underlying pelvic inflammatory process, prior recent abdominal surgery, or Crohn's disease. Parks and Gordon reported a number of cases of perineal fistula that developed secondary to an intraabdominal process.[49] Supralevator abscess may also occur as an in-continuity cephalad extension of a transsphincteric or rarely an intersphincteric abscess (Figure 10-2).

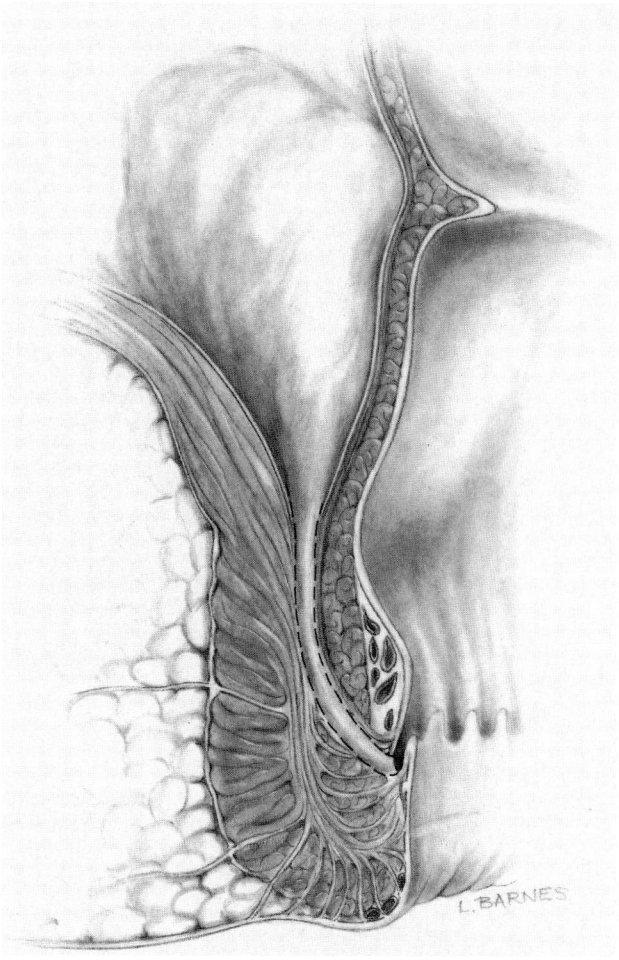

FIGURE 10-12. Supralevator abscess. As implied and as illustrated, the abscess is located in the space above the levators and adjacent to the rectum. The *dashed lines* illustrate the possible course of a fistula tract if it is present.

Treatment

The cause of the abscess determines the therapy: transrectal or transvaginal drainage for abscess caused by pelvic sepsis and external drainage for abscess secondary to transsphincteric fistula. To perform transrectal drainage when an internal opening is present at the level of the crypt is an invitation to disaster. Similarly, to drain an abscess to the perineum when a communication is present above the levators may result in a high extrasphincteric fistula. Management of this unfortunate sequela is notably highly complicated (see Chapter 11).

Effective treatment therefore mandates an understanding of the etiology of the septic process. To accomplish this, an appreciation of the history is very helpful (e.g., knowledge that the patient has Crohn's disease or has recently undergone abdominal surgery). More important, however, is to evaluate the situation by using an anesthetic and to attempt to identify an internal opening at the level

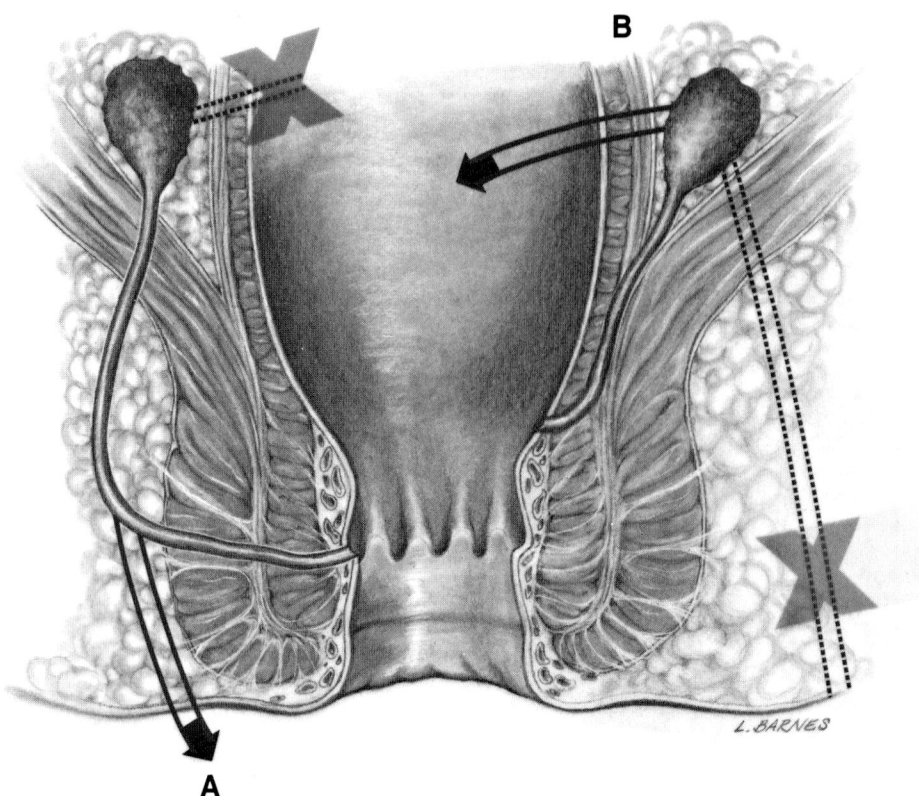

FIGURE 10-13. Methods of drainage for supralevator abscess. *(A)* Perineal drainage secondary to transsphincteric fistula. *(B)* Transrectal drainage from pelvic sepsis. Unfortunately, the clearly defined possible scenarios illustrated do not necessarily facilitate decision making in individual cases.

of the crypt. If such an opening is found, the drainage procedure should be external; if absent, drainage probably should be internal (Figure 10-13).

Internal Drainage
For *internal drainage,* the patient is optimally placed in the prone position if the abscess is located anteriorly or in the lithotomy position if the abscess is situated posteriorly. However, because the drainage procedure can be performed relatively quickly and anesthesiologists are rather disinclined to place patients face down, the lithotomy position is generally favored.

After aspiration, an incision is made into the cavity, either sharply with a knife or bluntly with a curved clamp (Figure 10-14). A de Pezzer (i.e., mushroom), Malecot, or Foley catheter is inserted into the cavity and delivered through the anal verge. The opening is made small enough for the catheter to remain in position without the need for suturing (Figure 10-15). Other modifications of this technique include placing a cut piece of rubber catheter through the tip of another to hold it in place or using a T tube. The drain is removed in 24 to 48 hours.

In women, whenever possible, an anterior abscess should be drained transvaginally through the posterior cul-de-sac (Figure 10-16). Drainage is technically easier to perform, and the patient is more comfortable if the intact anal sphincter is avoided.

Comment in Drains Despite the foregoing suggestions and admonitions, the physician may credibly argue that drains are probably unnecessary. Once the abscess has been effectively evacuated, the cavity usually collapses and heals rather quickly. Regardless of the technique, most drains fall out within a short time in any event.

External Drainage
If *external drainage* is deemed appropriate, the patient is placed in the prone jackknife position. A larger external wound is required than for other abscesses because it is imperative to drain the supralevator collection adequately. The location of the incision should be as medial as possible. The supralevator space may be packed, or a Foley, de Pezzer (i.e., mushroom), or Malecot catheter can be placed in the cavity and left for 24 to 48 hours (Figure 10-17). Irrigation through the catheter may also be considered.

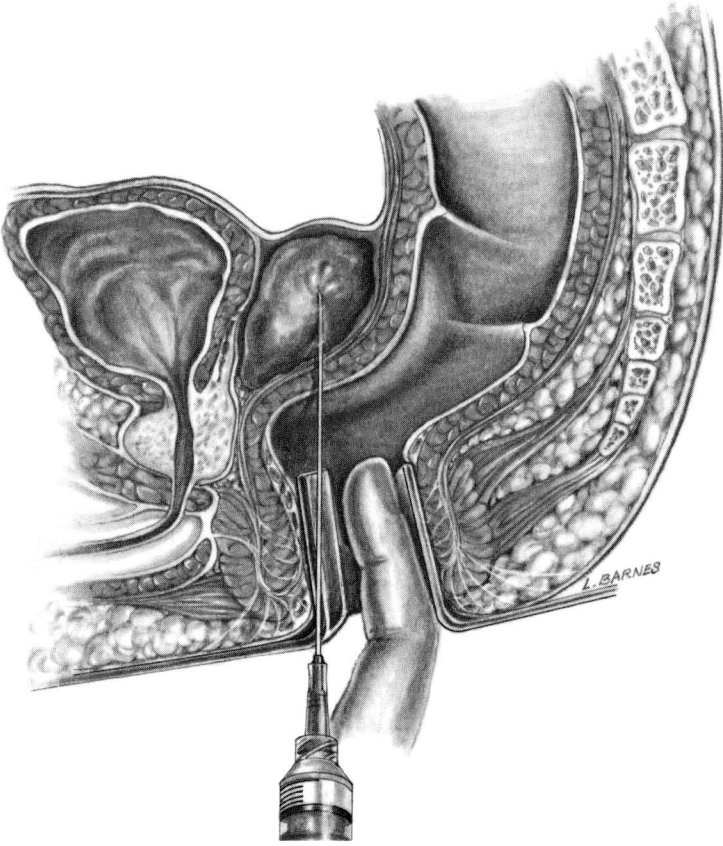

FIGURE 10-14. Aspiration of a supralevator abscess confirms the location for drainage and may be performed with a retractor in position or by manual assessment.

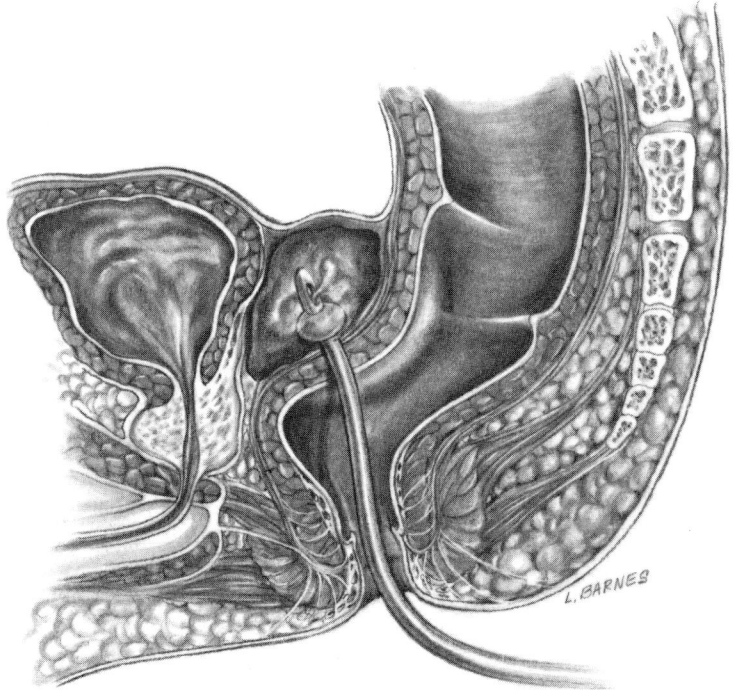

FIGURE 10-15. A catheter is inserted into the supralevator abscess cavity to maintain adequate drainage.

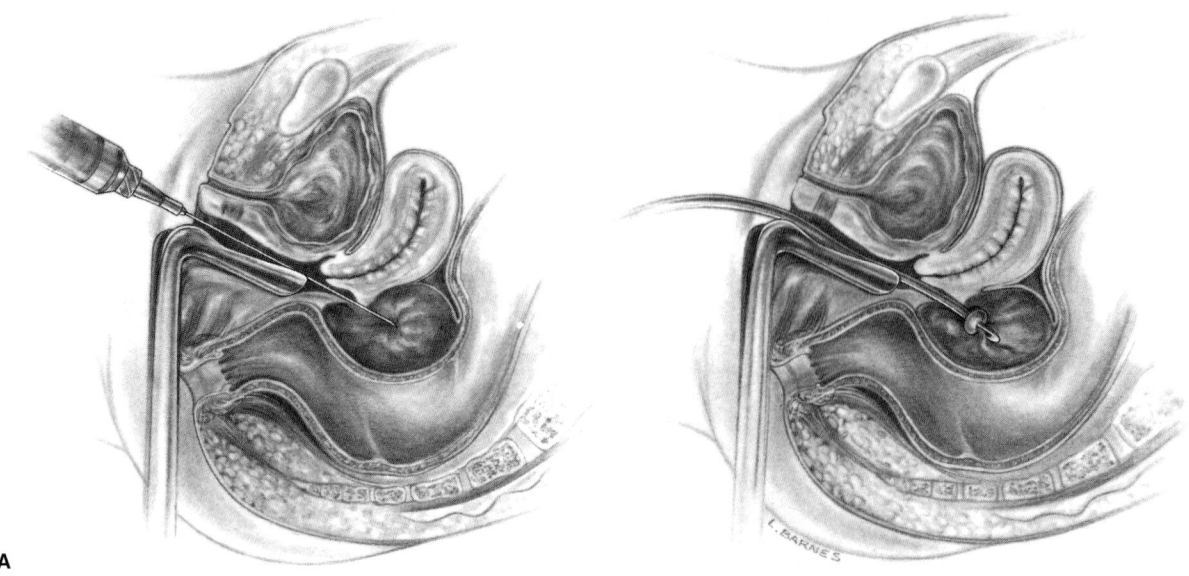

A   B

FIGURE 10-16. Drainage of pelvic abscess is performed transvaginally. **(A)** Needle aspiration. **(B)** Insertion of a catheter into the cavity.

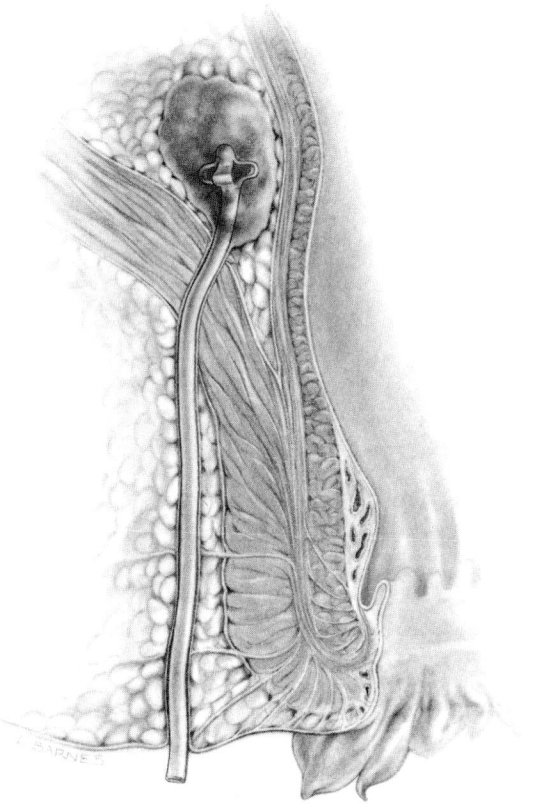

FIGURE 10-17. External drainage of a supralevator abscess with insertion of a catheter. This rather unusual approach is often undertaken in individuals whose complication is secondary to Crohn's disease. Long-term drainage is often necessary.

Results

It is essentially impossible to find any meaningful data in the literature on the results of surgery following drainage of supralevator abscesses. In the series of Prasad and associates, primary fistulotomy was performed in two thirds of patients who were found to have concurrent fistulas.[54] In my opinion, however, definitive fistula surgery should be undertaken during a subsequent hospitalization.

COMPLICATIONS AND OTHER CAUSES OF PERIANAL INFECTIONS

Necrotizing Infection

Necrotizing infection (i.e., Fournier's gangrene; see Chapter 19) can be a consequence of anorectal abscess.[5,8,42] Because diabetes mellitus is so frequently associated with the disease, it truly merits etiologic status.[19] This is why I feel so strongly about diabetic patients who develop perianal infections and the need for treatment within a hospital setting. *Tetanus* following drainage of anorectal abscess has also been reported.[40,47] Delay in diagnosis and treatment—a week or more in most cases—as well as associated conditions (diabetes, obesity, malignancy, AIDS, tuberculosis, and the immunocompromised state) are contributing factors (Figure 10-18 and Chapter 20).[2,45,67,70] Treatment requires antibiotics, nutritional support, wide debridement, adequate drainage, and usually proximal diversion.

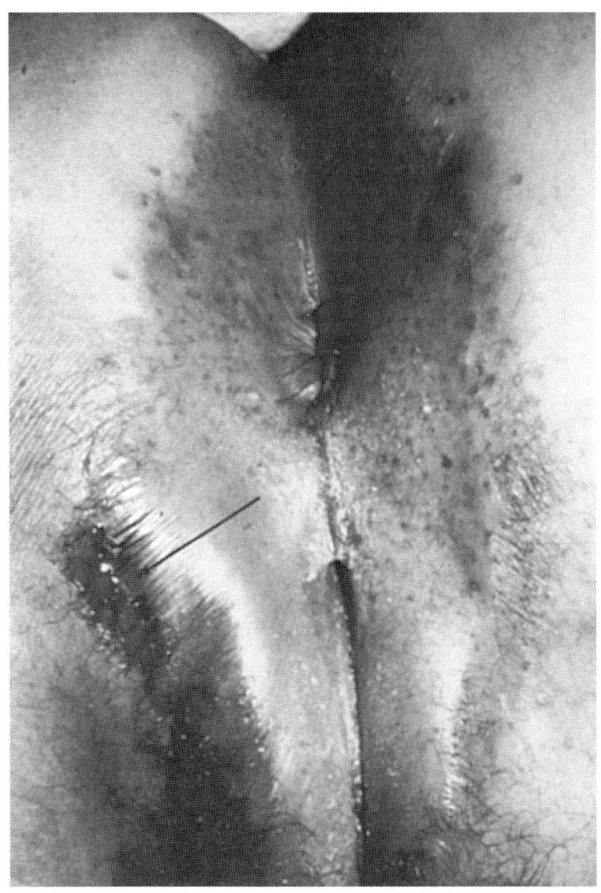

FIGURE 10-18. Anal fistula *(arrow)* in a patient with diabetes. Note the severe pruritic changes. (Courtesy of Daniel Rosenthal, M.D.)

Hematologic Disease

Abscess, fistula, and perirectal infections are commonly seen in patients with hematologic abnormalities (e.g., leukemia, granulocytopenia, lymphoma; see Chapter 19). These problems represent 3% to 8% of hematology admissions.[6,9,10,12,27,33,38,39,57,59,64] In the experience from one center in Turkey, the incidence of perianal infections was found to be 7.3% in 259 patients with acute leukemia, but only 1% in patients with chronic leukemia.[11] In another study of more than 200 individuals with acute leukemia, perianal infections developed in 7.9%.[4] The incidence in granulocytopenia, defined as a polymorphonuclear neutrophil count of less than 500/mm^3, has been reported to be 11%.[64] One half of the patients die within 1 month of diagnosis, most of septic complications.

Symptoms and Findings

Patients usually present with anal pain, but fever, septicemia, and shock may also be evident. Often, neither fluctuation nor pus is present. Urinary retention, peri-

toneal signs, and infection of the genitalia are common.[4] Of interest is the fact that cultured organisms may be quite different from those usually identified with uncomplicated perirectal septic processes.[33]

Treatment and Results

The prognosis is closely correlated with the response to management of the underlying hematologic disorder. Conservative treatment (e.g., antibiotics, warm sitz baths, granulocyte infusions) and perhaps radiotherapy are advised for those with leukemia if the disease is under poor control. Surgical drainage under such circumstances may result in fulminant sepsis and death. Shaked and Freund showed that patients with agranulocytosis who underwent operative intervention had slow wound healing, prolonged hospitalization, and a higher mortality rate when compared with the group that received antibiotics alone.[61] The authors believed that drainage may be performed, however, if the patient's disease is in relative remission.

In a retrospective review, Carlson and colleagues identified 20 patients with severe granulocytopenia and perianal infection.[12] Eleven were managed medically, and nine underwent operative drainage. With the exception of a higher frequency of positive blood cultures in those who had surgery, the two groups were similar. Mortality was 44.4% in the surgical versus 9% in the medical group. The authors concluded that operative drainage did not increase survival or decrease morbidity in those with severe granulocytopenia. Grewal and co-workers reported the experience of anorectal disease in neutropenic leukemia patients from the Memorial Sloan-Kettering Cancer Center in New York.[27] Because they did not observe excessive morbidity or mortality when comparing operated neutropenic leukemic patients with nonoperated patients (20% versus 18%), they concluded that selected individuals should not be denied anorectal surgery if indicated.

Hiatt and colleagues support the concept of an aggressive approach, stating that hemodynamic instability should be regarded as an indication for surgical intervention rather than a contraindication.[33] In addition to broad-spectrum antibiotic coverage, they advise wide debridement and end-sigmoid colostomy with closure of the distal rectum. Some advise a drainage procedure if there is persistent fever and the lesions fail to drain spontaneously.[4] Others recommend sitz baths, suppositories, antibiotics, and judicious surgical drainage.[7] Even abdominoperineal resection has been performed in a patient with extensive perirectal sepsis.[51] Although it is obvious that controversy exists concerning management options in these patients, a nonoperative approach is generally recommended, especially for the neutropenic individual. In others words, treatment should be directed to restoring the granulocyte count in these situations. The neutrophil count and its course during the infection are the most significant variables with respect to the evolution of perianal lesions and the ultimate prognosis.[11] However, with appropriate support, and with an adequate neutrophil count, perianal septic problems can reasonably be treated surgically.

Bone Marrow Transplantation

Perianal infection is a rare complication of bone marrow transplantation. Cohen and colleagues performed a retrospective review over a 10-year period that involved almost 1,000 patients who had undergone bone marrow transplantation at the City of Hope National Medical Center near Los Angeles.[15] Twenty-four were diagnosed with perianal infections following transplants (2.5%). The authors concluded that the management of this complication is essentially the same as that described for patients with hematologic diseases. In general, perianal wound healing is not prolonged in those undergoing surgical drainage for infection following bone marrow transplantation.[15]

Acquired Immunodeficiency Syndrome

Patients with acquired AIDS are extremely susceptible to opportunistic infections in the anorectal area. Wexner and colleagues reported their experience with 340 such patients from the St. Luke's–Roosevelt Hospital in New York City.[68] The incidence of anorectal disease, most commonly abscess and fistula, was 34%. The reader is referred to a discussion of the colorectal manifestations of AIDS in Chapter 20.

Anal Crohn's Disease

See Chapter 11.

Tuberculous Anal Sepsis

See Chapter 19.

Perianal Actinomycosis

See Chapter 19.

REFERENCES

1. Abcarian H. Surgical management of recurrent anorectal abscesses. *Contemp Surg* 1982;21:85.
2. Allen-Mersh TG. Symposium: the management of anorectal disease in HIV-positive patients. *Int J Colorectal Dis* 1990; 5:61.
3. Avill R. The management of carcinoma of the rectum presenting as an ischiorectal abscess. *Br J Surg* 1984;71:665.
4. Barnes SG, Sattler FR, Ballard JO. Perirectal infections in acute leukemia. *Ann Intern Med* 1984;100:515.
5. Bevans DW Jr, Westbrook KC, Thompson BW, et al. Perirectal abscess: a potentially fatal illness. *Am J Surg* 1973;126: 765.
6. Black WA. Anorectal complications in leukemia. *Am J Surg* 1955;90:738.
7. Boddie AW Jr, Bines SD. Management of acute rectal problems in leukemic patients. *J Surg Oncol* 1986;33:53.
8. Bode WE, Ramos R, Page CP. Invasive necrotizing infection secondary to anorectal abscess. *Dis Colon Rectum* 1982;25: 416.
9. Brook I, Martin WJ. Aerobic and anaerobic bacteriology of perirectal abscess in children. *Pediatrics* 1980;66:282.
10. Buchan R, Grace RH. Anorectal suppuration: the results of treatment and the factors influencing the recurrence rate. *Br J Surg* 1973;60:537.
11. Büyükasik Y, Özcebe OI, Sayinalp N, et al. Perianal infections in patients with leukemia: importance of the course of neutophil count. *Dis Colon Rectum* 1998;41:81–85.
12. Carlson GW, Ferguson CM, Amerson JR. Perianal infections in acute leukemia. *Am Surg* 1988;54:693.
13. Cataldo PA, Senagore A, Luchtefeld MA. Intrarectal ultrasound in the evaluation of perirectal abscesses. *Dis Colon Rectum* 1993;36:554.
14. Chiari H. Ueber die analen Divertikel der Rectumsschleimhaut und ihre Beziehung zu den Analfisteln. *Med Jahr* 1878; 8:419.
15. Cohen JS, Paz IB, O'Donnell MR, et al. Treatment of perianal infection following bone marrow transplantation. *Dis Colon Rectum* 1996;39:981.
16. Duhamel J. Anal fistulae in childhood. *Am J Proctol* 1975; 26:40.
17. Eisenhammer S. The internal anal sphincter; its surgical importance. *S Afr Med J* 1953;27:266.
18. Eisenhammer S. The internal anal sphincter and the anorectal abscess. *Surg Gynecol Obstet* 1956;103:501.
19. Eke N. Fournier's gangrene: a review of 1726 cases. *Br J Surg* 2000;87:718--728.
20. Ellis M. The use of penicillin and sulphonamides in the treatment of suppuration. *Lancet* 1951;1:774.
21. Ellis M. Recurrence of infection following treatment of anorectal abscesses by primary suture. *Proc R Soc Med* 1962; 55:757.
22. Fitzgerald RJ, Harding B, Ryan W. Fistula-in-ano in childhood: a congenital etiology. *J Pediatr Surg* 1985;20:80.
23. Goldenberg HS. Supralevator abscess diagnosis and treatment. *Surgery* 1982;91:164.
24. Goligher JC. Fistula-in-ano: management of perianal suppuration. *Dis Colon Rectum* 1976;19:516.
25. Goligher JC. *Surgery of the anus, rectum and colon,* 4th ed. New York: Macmillan, 1980:156.
26. Grace RH, Harper IA, Thompson RG. Anorectal sepsis: microbiology in relation to fistula-in-ano. *Br J Surg* 1982;69: 401.
27. Grewal H, Guillem JG, Quan SHQ, et al. Anorectal disease in neutropenic leukemic patients: operative versus nonoperative management. *Dis Colon Rectum* 1994;37:1095.
28. Hämäläinen K-PJ, Sainio AP. Incidence of fistulas after drainage of acute anorectal abscesses. *Dis Colon Rectum* 1998;41:1357.
29. Hamilton CH. Anorectal problems: the deep postanal space: surgical significance in horseshoe fistula and abscess. *Dis Colon Rectum* 1975;18:642.
30. Hanley PH. Conservative surgical correction of horseshoe abscess and fistula. *Dis Colon Rectum* 1965;8:364.
31. Henrichsen S, Christiansen J. Incidence of fistula-in-ano complicating anorectal sepsis: a prospective study. *Br J Surg* 1986;73:371.
32. Herrmann G, Desfosses L. Sur la muqueuse de la région cloacale du rectum. *C R Acad Sci* 1880;90:1301.

33. Hiatt JR, Kuchenbecker SL, Winston DJ. Perineal gangrene in the patient with granulocytopenia: the importance of early diverting colostomy. *Surgery* 1986;100:912.
34. Hill JR. Fistulas and fistulous abscesses in the anorectal region: personal experience in management. *Dis Colon Rectum* 1967;10:421.
35. Jackman RJ, Buie LA. Tuberculosis and anal fistula. *JAMA* 1946;130:630.
36. Kline RJ, Spencer RJ, Harrison EG Jr. Carcinoma associated with fistula-in-ano. *Arch Surg* 1964;89:989.
37. Klosterhalfen B, Offner F, Vogel P, et al. Anatomic nature and surgical significance of anal sinus and anal intramuscular glands. *Dis Colon Rectum* 1991;34:156.
38. Kott I, Urca I. Perianal abscess as a presenting sign of leukemia. *Dis Colon Rectum* 1969;12:338.
39. Krieger RW, Chusid MJ. Perirectal abscess in childhood. *Am J Dis Child* 1979;133:411.
40. Lichtenstein D, Stavorovsky M, Irge D. Fournier's gangrene complicating perianal abscess: report of two cases. *Dis Colon Rectum* 1978;21:377.
41. Lunniss PJ, Phillips RKS. Surgical assessment of acute anorectal sepsis is a better predictor of fistula than microbiological analysis. *Br J Surg* 1994;81:368.
42. Marks G, Chase WV, Mervine TB. The fatal potential of fistula-in-ano with abscess: analysis of 11 deaths. *Dis Colon Rectum* 1973;16:224.
43. McElwain JW, Alexander RM, MacLean MD. Primary fistulectomy for anorectal abscesses: clinical study of 500 cases. *Dis Colon Rectum* 1966;9:181.
44. McElwain JW, MacLean MD, Alexander RM, et al. Anorectal problems: experience with primary fistulectomy for anorectal abscess. A report of 1000 cases. *Dis Colon Rectum* 1975; 18:646.
45. Miles AJG, Mellor CH, Gazzard B, et al. Surgical management of anorectal disease in HIV-positive homosexuals. *Br J Surg* 1990;77:869.
46. Mortensen J, Kraglund K, Klaerke M, et al. Primary suture of anorectal abscess: a randomized study comparing treatment with clindamycin versus clindamycin and Gentacoll. *Dis Colon Rectum* 1995;38:398.
47. Myers KJ, Heppell J, Bode WE, et al. Tetanus after anorectal abscess. *Mayo Clin Proc* 1984;59:429.
48. Parks AG. Pathogenesis and treatment of fistula-in-ano. *BMJ* 1961;1:463.
49. Parks AG, Gordon PH. Perineal fistula of intra-abdominal or intrapelvic origin simulating fistula-in-ano: report of seven cases. *Dis Colon Rectum* 1976;19:500.
50. Parks AG, Thomson JP. Intersphincteric abscess. *BMJ* 1973; 2:537.
51. Paterson FWN, Wonke B, Piper JV. Abdominoperineal resection in acute myeloblastic leukemia. *BMJ* 1976;1:1124
52. Piazza DJ, Radhakrishnan J. Perianal abscess and fistula-in-ano in children. *Dis Colon Rectum* 1990;33:1014.
53. Pople IK, Ralphs DNL. An aetiology for fistula in ano. *Br J Surg* 1988;75:904.
54. Prasad ML, Read DR, Abcarian H. Supralevator abscess: diagnosis and treatment. *Dis Colon Rectum* 1981;24:456.
55. Ramanujam PS, Prasad ML, Abcarian H, et al. Perianal abscesses and fistulas: a study of 1023 patients. *Dis Colon Rectum* 1984;27:593.
56. Read DR, Abcarian H. A prospective survey of 474 patients with anorectal abscess. *Dis Colon Rectum* 1979;22: 566.
57. Schimpff SC, Wiernik PH, Block JB. Rectal abscesses in cancer patients. *Lancet* 1972;2:844.
58. Scoma JA, Salvati EP, Rubin RJ. Incidence of fistulas subsequent to anal abscesses. *Dis Colon Rectum* 1974;17:357.
59. Sehdev MK, Dowling MD, Seal SH, et al. Perianal and anorectal complications in leukemia. *Cancer* 1973;31:149.
60. Shafer AD, McGlone TP, Flanagan RA. Abnormal crypts of Morgagni: the cause of perianal abscess and fistula-in-ano. *J Pediatr Surg* 1987;22:203.
61. Shaked AA, Freund H. Managing the granulocytopenic patient with acute perianal inflammatory disease. *Am J Surg* 1986;152:510.
62. Standards Task Force, American Society of Colon and Rectal Surgeons. Practice parameters for treatment of fistula-in-ano. *Dis Colon Rectum* 1996;39:1361.
63. Tang C-L, Chew S-P, Seow-Choen F. Prospective randomized trial of drainage alone versus drainage and fistulotomy for acute perianal abscesses with proven internal opening. *Dis Colon Rectum* 1996;39:1415.
64. Vanheuverzwyn R, Delannoy A, Michaux JL, et al. Anal lesions in hematologic diseases. *Dis Colon Rectum* 1980;23: 310.
65. Vasilevsky C-A, Gordon PH. The incidence of recurrent abscesses or fistula-in-ano following anorectal suppuration. *Dis Colon Rectum* 1984;27:126.
66. Waggener HU. Immediate fistulotomy in the treatment of perianal abscess. *Surg Clin North Am* 1969;49:1227.
67. Wexner SD. Managing common anorectal sexually transmitted diseases. *Infect Surg* 1990;9:9.
68. Wexner SD, Smithy WB, Milsom JW, et al. The surgical management of anorectal diseases in AIDS and pre-AIDS patients. *Dis Colon Rectum* 1986;29:719.
69. Wilson DH. The late results of anorectal abscess treated by incision, curettage, and primary suture under antibiotic cover. *Br J Surg* 1964;51:828.
70. Wolkomir AF, Barone JE, Hardy HW III, et al. Abdominal and anorectal surgery and the acquired immune deficiency syndrome in heterosexual intravenous drug users. *Dis Colon Rectum* 1990;33:267.

Chapter 11

Anal Fistula

Bertram: What is it, my good lord,
       the King languishes of?
Lafew: A fistula, my lord.
   William Shakespeare: *All's Well That Ends Well,* I.1.37

A fascinating narrative of Shakespeare and the literary history of anal fistula has been written by Cosman.[32]

Anal fistula is a condition that has been described virtually from the beginning of medical history. Hippocrates, in about 430 B.C., suggested that the disease was caused by "contusions and tubercles occasioned by rowing or riding on horseback."[3] He was the first person to advocate the use of a seton (from the Latin *seta,* a bristle) in treatment by "taking a very slender thread of raw lint, uniting it into five folds of the length of a span, and wrapping them round with a horse hair."[3] The fascination with anal fistula for more than 2,000 years is manifested by the numerous papers and books on the subject. In fact, Salmon established a hospital in London devoted to the treatment of anal fistula and other rectal conditions—St. Mark's.

It has been said that more surgeons' reputations have been impugned because of the consequences of fistula operations than from any other operative procedure. Complications of fistula surgery are myriad and include fecal soilage, mucous discharge, varying degrees of incontinence (gas and/or stool), and recurrent abscess and fistula. In the United States, impairment for bowel control from even a properly performed operation for anal fistula is one of the most frequent reasons in the field of colon and rectal surgery for a patient to pay a visit to an attorney. It is for this reason that the prescient surgeon will make a special effort to explain in detail the attendant risks of the procedure. The fact is that no one goes whole to the grave with perfect anal control following surgery if an anal fistula traversed a significant portion of the external sphincter. Clearly, the surgeon who is fortunate enough to have the opportunity to treat the patient initially is the one most likely to effect a cure, to limit morbidity, and to minimize disability.

SYMPTOMS

The most frequent presenting complaints of patients with an anal fistula are swelling, pain, and discharge. The former two symptoms usually are associated with an abscess when the external or secondary opening has closed or has failed to develop. Discharge may be from the external opening or may be reported by the patient as mucus or pus mixed with the stool. Most patients with an overt fistula have an antecedent history of abscess that drained spontaneously or for which surgical drainage had been performed.

Anal fistula may be confused with suppurative hidradenitis and pilonidal sinus (see Chapter 19), may be secondary to anal or rectal carcinoma, or may be associated with specific and nonspecific inflammatory bowel disease (see later and Chapter 30).

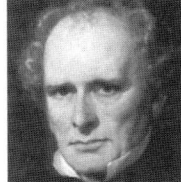

Frederick Salmon (1796–1868) Salmon was born in Bath, England. He received his medical education at St. Bartholomew's Hospital and became a member of the Royal College of Surgeons in 1818. After several years in the General Dispensary, Aldersgate Street, Salmon resigned his position, and in 1835 he opened an institution that was named "The Infirmary for the Relief of the Poor, Afflicted With Fistula and Other Diseases of the Rectum." After relocation two additional times, it was reopened on April 25, 1854 (St. Mark's Day)—hence, the adoption of the name St. Mark's Hospital. Salmon seemed to have more than his share of critics; the following is a quote from an obituary statement that appeared in the *British Medical Journal:* "How far the course which he took was prompted by difficulties in pursuing an useful and honourable career in a general hospital, where his labours would have been more useful and more instructive, it is now difficult to say. It was, we fully believe, contrary to the best interests both of the profession and of the public; and the success of St. Mark's Hospital was of unfortunate omen, and has since borne bad fruit in encouraging similar enterprises."

295

CLASSIFICATION

Parks and colleagues are credited with proposing the following somewhat complicated but extremely thorough classification[102]:

Classification of Fistula-in-Ano

Intersphincteric
  Simple low track
  High blind track
  High track with opening into rectum
  High fistula without a perineal opening
  High fistula with extrarectal or pelvic extension
  Fistula from pelvic disease
Transsphincteric
  Uncomplicated
  High blind track
Suprasphincteric
  Uncomplicated
  High blind tract
Extrasphincteric
  Secondary to transsphincteric fistula
  Secondary to trauma
  Secondary to anorectal disease (e.g., Crohn's)
  Secondary to pelvic inflammation
Combined
Horseshoe
  Intersphincteric
  Transsphincteric

"Complex fistula" is not a term included in the foregoing classification, but it has been applied to a number of articles on fistula. Simply stated, complex fistulas are those other than intersphincteric and low extrasphincteric fistulas. The implication is, obviously, that they are more difficult to treat than conventional fistulas and, in addition, are associated with increased risk of recurrence as well as a greater likelihood for impairment of control. The word "problematic" has also been used to describe the same perception.[1,121] Frentzel proposes a simplified classification based on the level of the fistula: low, mid-, and high/complex.[41] He hypothesizes that such a system will be more useful for determining the appropriate treatment and predicting long-term outcome.

Five types of fistulas are generally described by most authors:

- Submucous
- Intersphincteric (Figure 11-1)
- Transsphincteric (Figure 11-2)
- Suprasphincteric (Figure 11-3)
- Extrasphincteric (Figure 11-4)

The *submucous fistula* is a misnomer. See the discussion in Chapter 10.

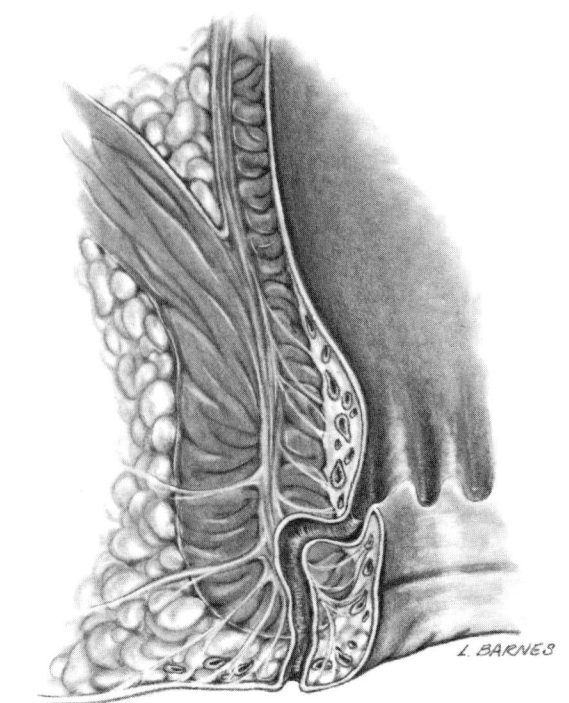

FIGURE 11-1. Intersphincteric fistula. The tract passes through the internal sphincter and in the intersphincteric plane.

An *intersphincteric fistula* passes through the internal sphincter, thence through the intersphincteric plane to the skin. Occasionally, an extension may be observed to proceed cephalad in the intersphincteric plain (i.e., high blind tract), but this is of no consequence in the therapeutic decision. It has also been reported to extend

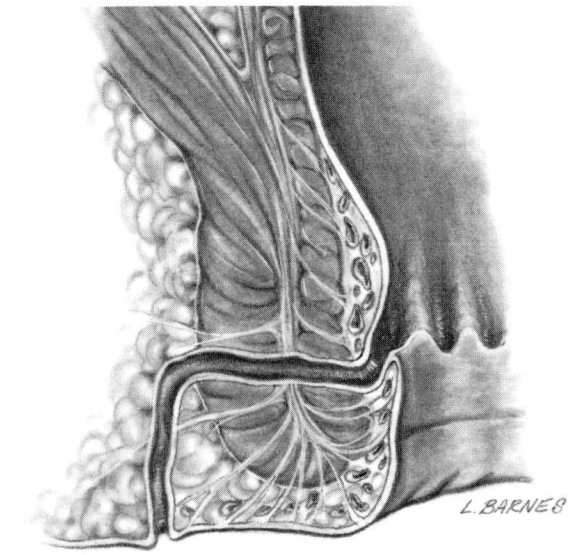

FIGURE 11-2. Transsphincteric fistula. The tract passes through both the internal and external sphincters, into the ischiorectal fossa, and to the skin.

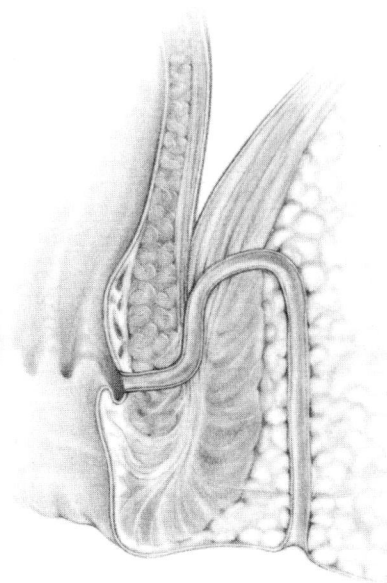

FIGURE 11-3. Suprasphincteric fistula. The tract courses above the puborectalis muscle after initially passing cephalad as an intersphincteric fistula. It then traverses downward through the ischiorectal fossa to the skin.

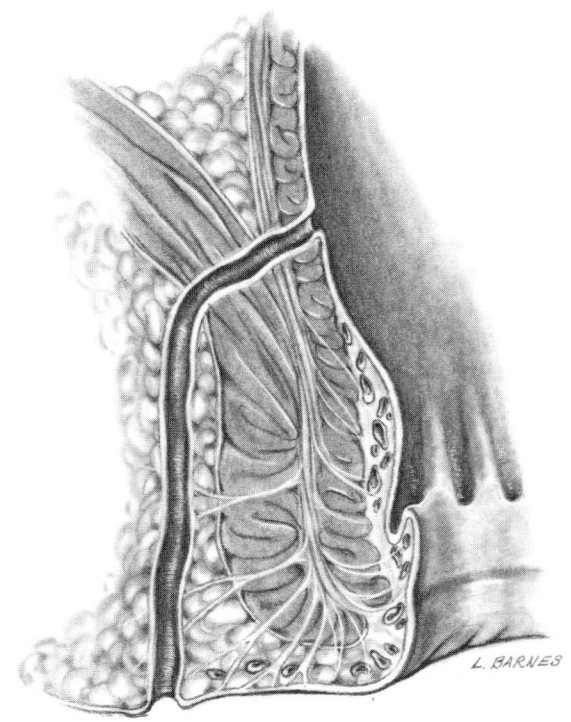

FIGURE 11-4. Extrasphincteric fistula. The internal opening is above the level of the levator ani muscle, and the tract passes to the skin deep to the external sphincter in the ischiorectal space.

cephalad and present with another opening in the rectum.[102] I have never seen this variation; I suspect it occurs as a result of the inappropriate creation of an artificial opening (see later). Only the most superficial or subcutaneous portions of the external sphincter may be divided when a fistulotomy is undertaken. The incidence of this fistula when compared with the others varies between 55% and 70%, depending on whom one reads. It is the most common of the fistula manifestations.

A *transsphincteric fistula* passes through both the internal and external sphincters before exiting to the skin. The level of the tract determines how much sphincter will, of necessity, be divided, and, therefore, the risk of impairment for bowel control. It may, as a consequence, alter the therapeutic approach. This type of fistula is observed in 20% to 25% of most series. Occasionally, a supralevator extension of a transsphincteric fistula is identified (Figure 11-5). Treatment requires recognition of this condition, curettage, irrigation, and packing of the supralevator extension. Under no circumstances should the extension be drained into the rectum.

A *suprasphincteric fistula* was noted by Parks and colleagues to comprise 20% of their series.[102] This seems to be an extraordinarily high incidence, certainly not consistent with all other published articles. In fact, suprasphincteric fistula is mentioned rarely, if at all, by other contributors. A more realistic incidence is probably in the range of 1% to 3%. The fistula is described as starting in the intersphincteric plane, passing to a supralevator location, and ultimately tracking between

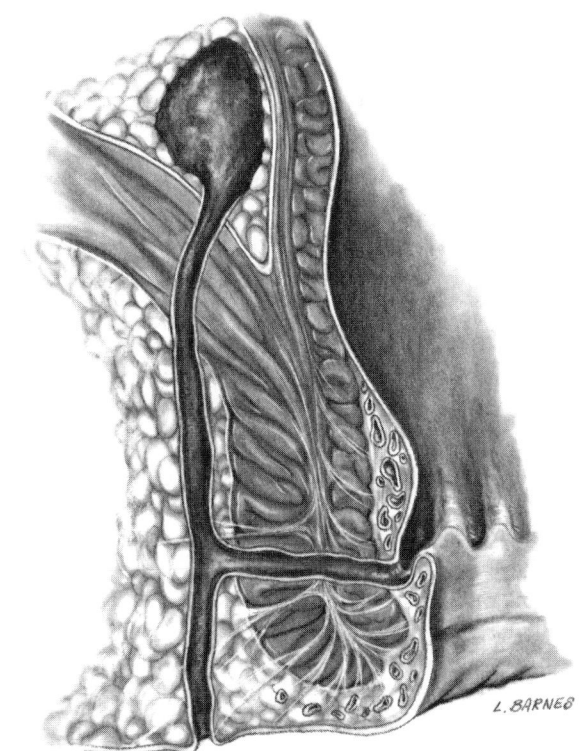

FIGURE 11-5. Transsphincteric fistula with supralevator extension. Drainage of the extension into the rectum is contraindicated.

the puborectalis and the levator ani muscles to end in the ischiorectal fossa.[102]

The *extrasphincteric fistula* is described by a supralevator internal opening with a tract that passes through the entire sphincter mechanism as it exits at the skin. It is usually a consequence of trauma (e.g., foreign body, surgical manipulation, impalement), Crohn's disease, or pelvic inflammatory disease. It can also develop when a supralevator abscess or transsphincteric fistula with supralevator extension ruptures spontaneously into the rectum. This type of fistula represents approximately 2% to 3% of fistulas, but if the physician's practice encompasses many individuals with inflammatory bowel disease, the incidence could be higher.

PRACTICE PARAMETERS FOR TREATMENT

As has been mentioned in prior chapters, practice parameters for the treatment of a number of colorectal conditions have been established by the Standards Practice Task Force of the American Society of Colon and Rectal Surgeons. These recommendations have also been established for the evaluation and treatment of fistula-in-ano.[127] Although I obviously believe that all of the subsequent descriptions and recommendations are consistent with those parameters, the reader is advised to review the Society's guidelines with respect to evaluation and treatment of this condition.

IDENTIFICATION OF THE FISTULA TRACT

How does the physician identify the type of fistula, the course of the tract, and the location of the internal opening? Numerous methods can be employed, the basic principles and procedures of which include the application of Goodsall's rule,[49] careful physical examination, probing of the tract, and a variety of injection and radiologic techniques.

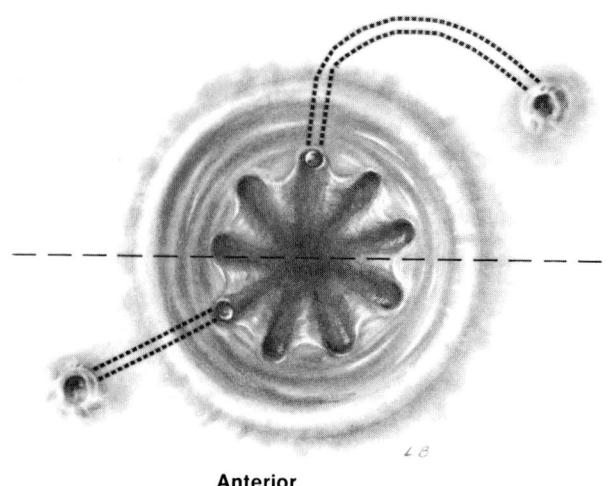

Anterior

FIGURE 11-6. Typical courses of fistula tracts according to Goodsall's rule.

Goodsall's Rule

When the external opening lies anterior to the transverse plane, the internal opening tends to be located radially. Conversely, when the external opening lies posterior to the plane, the internal opening is usually (but not always) located in the posterior midline (Figure 11-6). One must remember that this is a "rule," not a "law." There *are* exceptions to "rules."

There is some controversy over the reasons for the disparate manifestations. However, the reason for this eventuality probably lies with the fact that the posterior course is the result of a defect in fusion of the longitudinal muscle and the external sphincter in the posterior midline. A transsphincteric fistula is, therefore, more likely to occur in this position; the tract can then dissect into one or both ischiorectal fossae.

Cirocco and Reilly analyzed the predictive accuracy of this rule by reviewing 216 patients who underwent fistula surgery.[29] Only 49% of those who harbored an external opening anterior to the transverse plane had radially directed fistulas, but the accuracy rate of Goodsall's rule regarding posterior secondary openings was much greater.

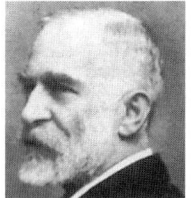

David Henry Goodsall (1843–1906)   Goodsall was born in Gravesend, England. His father had decided on medicine as a career. While performing a postmortem examination as a student at St. Bartholomew's Hospital, the elder Goodsall injured his hand and subsequently died, presumably because of sepsis. In 1865, the young Goodsall entered that same institution, his fees having been waived because of his father's tragic death. In 1870, he was appointed house surgeon to St. Mark's Hospital and he became full surgeon in 1888. It was there that he developed his lifelong interest in rectal surgery. He contributed many articles to the surgical literature, including reports on foreign bodies of the rectum, pilonidal sinus, colostomy, and anal fissure. However, his best-remembered work was accomplished in concert with W. Ernest Miles, a book entitled *Diseases of the Anus and Rectum*. In Goodsall's chapter on anal fistula, the rule is espoused that has become eponymously associated with Goodsall. He is thought to have died of a myocardial infarction. (Goodsall DH. Ano-rectal fistula. In: Goodsall DH, Miles WE, eds. *Diseases of the anus and rectum*. London: Longmans, Green & Co., 1900:92.)

Essentially, the rule should merely be used as a guide to help the surgeon find the tract when it may not be apparent. It is not a substitute for meticulous technique, clear identification of the direction of the tract, and location of the internal opening.

Usually, there is only one external or secondary opening. Most commonly, fistulas pass in the intersphincteric plane, but with transsphincteric fistulas, multiple openings can develop from communication with the deep postanal space and from the ischiorectal fossa; this is the origin of the so-called transsphincteric horseshoe fistula (see later).

Physical Examination and Endoscopy

Careful palpation may reveal the thickened tract proceeding into the anal canal if the fistula assumes a relatively superficial position. This finding is most characteristic of an intersphincteric fistula. Bidigital examination, placing the thumb on the outside and the index finger within the anal canal, may also help to reveal the course of the tract. Failure to identify the tract by palpation implies that it is deep and, therefore, more likely to be a transsphincteric fistula. Anoscopic examination may demonstrate purulent material exuding from the base of the crypt. By gentle probing with a crypt hook or malleable probe (Figure 11-7), the presence of the tract may be confirmed. This maneuver is easier to accomplish for a radially located fistula than for one that opens in the posterior midline. Occasionally, the tract will pass subcutaneously for a considerable distance and end in the perineum, scrotum, labia, or thigh (Figure 11-8). Failure to identify the internal opening does not mean that it has closed, however. Angulation or narrowing of the tract may preclude the possibility of adequate evaluation by probing, and excessive manipulation will certainly lead to considerable discomfort for the patient. Under these circumstances, examination under an anesthetic may be required to adequately delineate the course of the tract unless one wishes to perform special studies.

Passing a Probe

As implied, passage of a probe can be attempted from both the external and the internal openings. Sometimes it is easier to identify the tract from the internal opening, but probing through the external one will usually reveal the course more readily. Simultaneous passage of two probes, from the internal and the external openings, may confirm the tract's location if the tips of the probes touch. A stenotic or sharply angulated area within the tract may preclude complete passage from either end. The probe should never be forced, merely gently maneuvered (Figure 11-9).

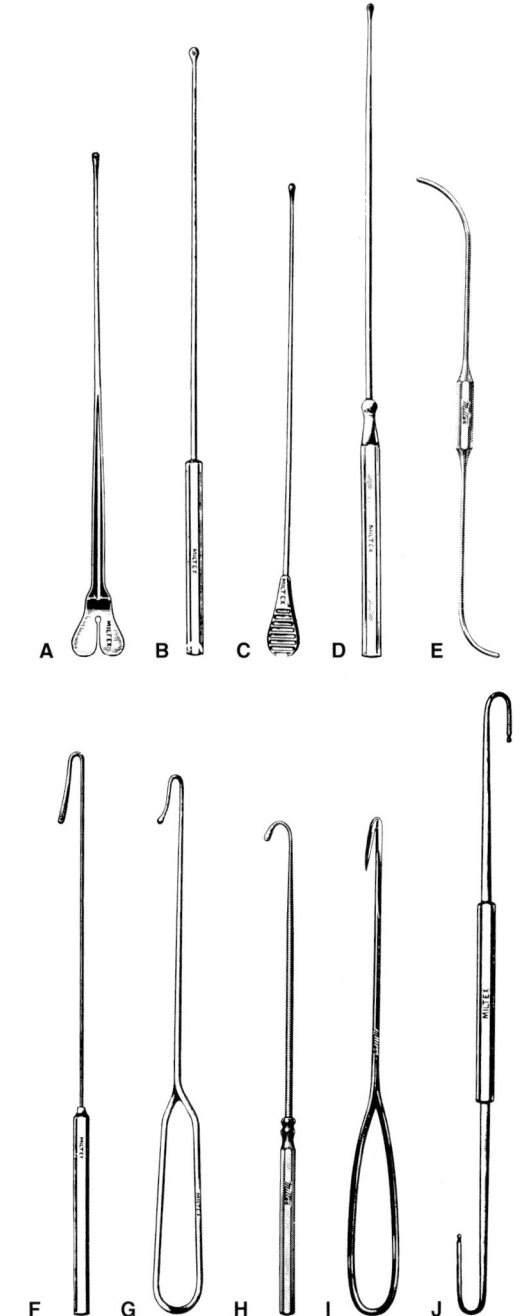

FIGURE 11-7. Anorectal probes. **(A)** Larry. **(B)** Barr. **(C)** Buie. **(D)** Pratt. **(E)** Barr double-ended. **(F)** Pratt crypt hook. **(G)** Stewart crypt hook. **(H)** Rosser crypt hook. **(I)** Blanchard cryptotome. **(J)** Barr crypt hook.

Traction on the Tract

Theoretically, if the physician mobilizes a small portion of the tract from the secondary (i.e., external) opening and applies traction, an indentation or dimpling will be evident at the level of the crypt—the site of the internal opening (Figure 11-10). With the exception of the most

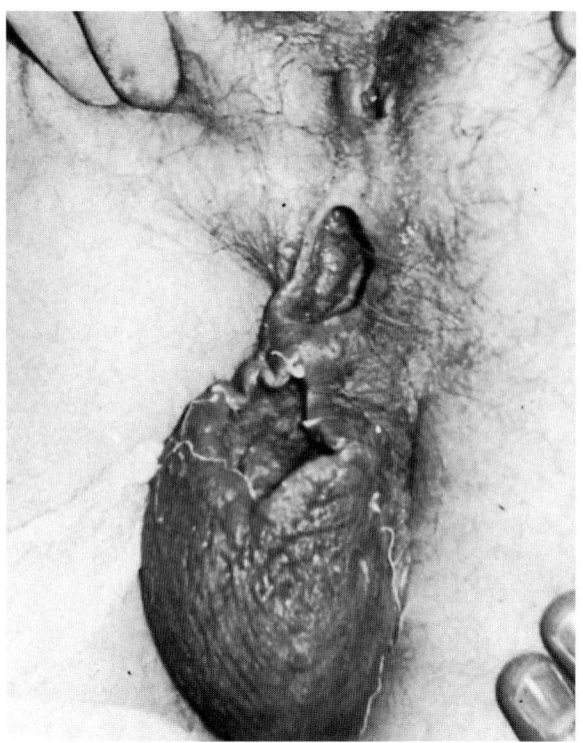

FIGURE 11-8. Scrotal fistula. The multiple openings are due to extensive subcutaneous tracking. Although on cursory examination the fistula may appear to be difficult to treat, the tract is usually quite superficial.

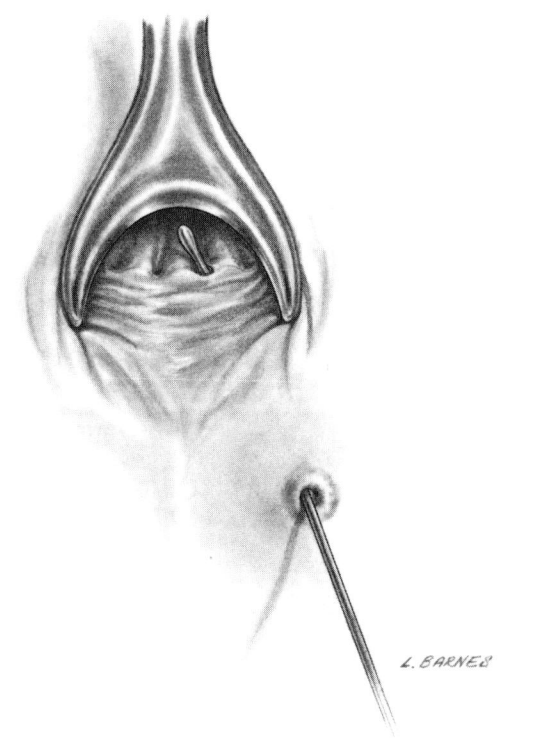

FIGURE 11-9. A malleable probe is passed from the external to the internal openings to confirm the course of the tract.

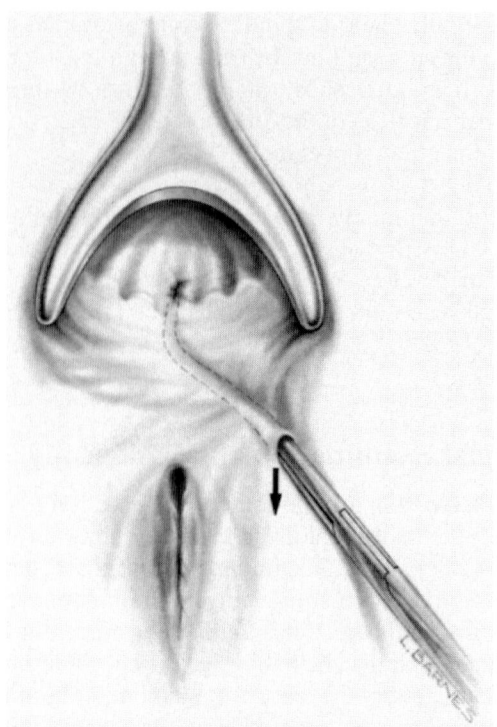

FIGURE 11-10. Attempt at identification of the primary (i.e., internal) opening by pulling on the epithelialized tract with a clamp. This may create a "dimpling" at the internal opening because of the tethering, indicating where the opening should be. This approach is unlikely to be successful unless the tract is radially located.

simple, radially directed tracts, I have not found this particular maneuver to be helpful. The variable and often curvilinear course of more complex fistulas lessens the potential benefit of this method for tract identification.

Injection Techniques

Dye

If a substance such as methylene blue or indigo carmine is injected through the tract, the dye may appear in the rectum, confirming the patency of the tract and its communication with an internal opening. The problem with such agents is that the surgeon may have only one opportunity to visualize the internal opening before the material stains the entire mucosa. It has been said that it would be as sensible to pour ink on a newspaper in order to facilitate reading.[38] I do not like this approach for that reason.

Milk

Milk can also be used to identify the tract and the internal opening; sterility is not required. A DeBakey olive-end needle may be used to inject the milk while an anoscope is in position in the rectum (Figure 11-11). Alternatively,

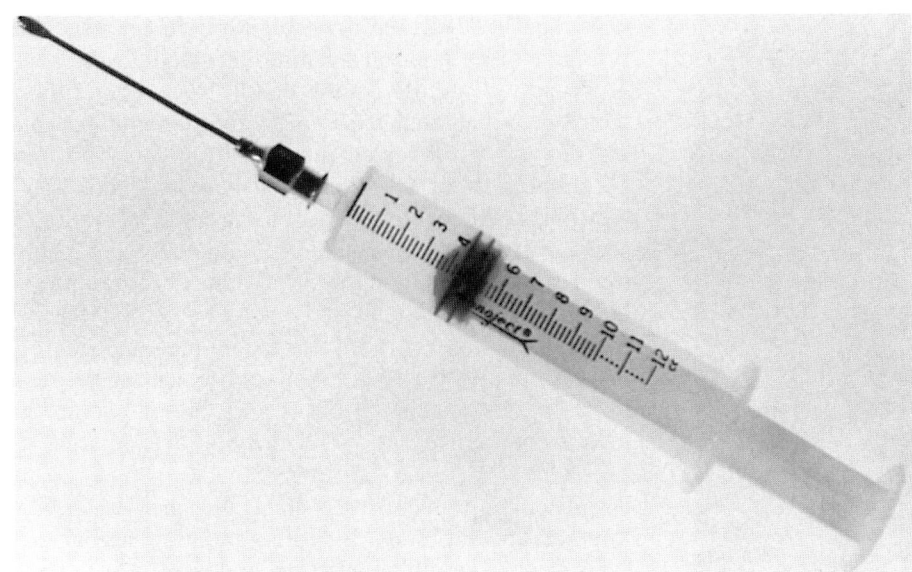

FIGURE 11-11. A DeBakey olive-end needle has a bulbous tip that permits insertion into the external opening without penetrating the wall of the tract.

an ordinary polyethylene intravenous catheter is equally effective. The milk can be wiped away without staining the tissue, permitting repeated attempts to inspect the internal opening. Failure to demonstrate communication with the internal opening implies stenosis of the tract, but if the milk is seen in the submucosa of the anal canal, even without escaping into the lumen, the associated crypt-bearing area should be excised with the presumption that the internal opening has closed.

Hydrogen Peroxide

Hydrogen peroxide injection is probably the ideal means for identifying the internal opening and is the method that I prefer. The liberated oxygen may be seen to bubble through the internal opening. The pressure created by the gas may be sufficient to penetrate even a stenotic tract and pass into the anal canal. Obviously, staining of the tissue does not occur.

Fistulography

Fistulography, the radiologic delineation of a fistula tract with a water-soluble contrast agent, is thought generally to be of limited value, having essentially been completely replaced by endoluminal sonography and magnetic resonance imaging (MRI).[128] However, the technique is quite simple to perform. The patient is placed on the x-ray table, usually in the left lateral position, and a small-bore catheter is inserted into the external opening. A few milliliters of water-soluble contrast material are injected, and films are taken in several projections (Figs. 11-12 and 11-13).

Kuijpers and Schulpen reviewed 25 patients for detection of extensions of the fistula and the presence of inter-

nal openings.[68] When compared with the subsequent surgical findings, the authors noted that the fistulograms were correct in only 16%, and false-positive results were identified in 10%. Weisman and colleagues undertook a retrospective review of 27 patients who underwent anal fistulography and arrived at a different conclusion.[138] Although the individuals were not randomly selected for the procedure, 48% were found to harbor unexpected pathologic features that led to an alternative surgical

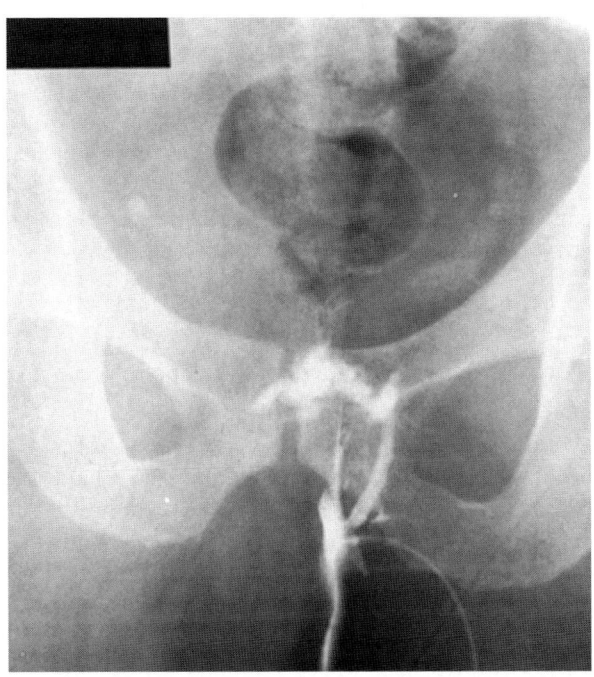

FIGURE 11-12. Fistulogram with water-soluble contrast material demonstrates the course of a transsphincteric fistula with an internal opening at the level of the anorectal ring.

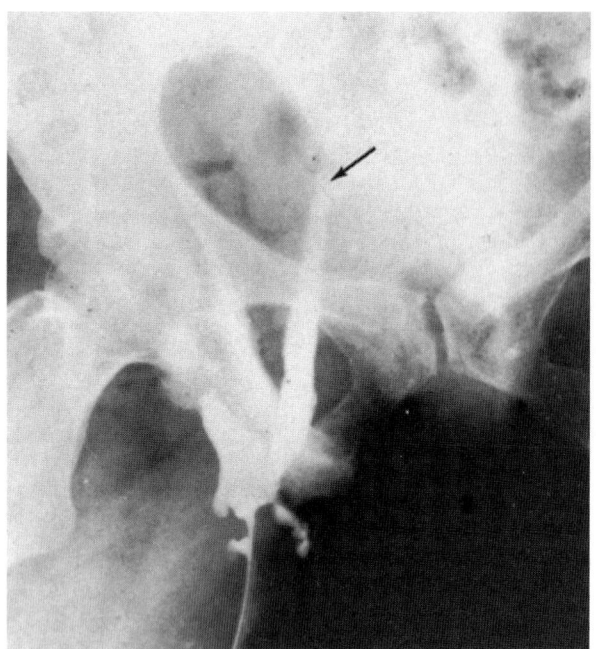

FIGURE 11-13. Fistulogram of an extrasphincteric fistula. The tract enters the rectum at the level of the *arrow*.

treatment. In a prospective study of 50 unselected patients, Ani and Lagundoye believed that the information gleaned was generally helpful.[8]

Comment

I believe that fistulography may be of value in those selected individuals with no identifiable internal opening, those with suspected or known Crohn's disease (see later), and for those who have undergone a prior unsuccessful fistula operation. Unfortunately, many of the patients in this last category will not benefit from the procedure because no internal opening will be evident.

Anal Endosonography

As with ultrasonography in the evaluation of rectal cancer (see Chapter 23), endoanal ultrasound has been recommended for imaging pathologic abnormalities in the anal canal and perianal region (see Chapter 6). Cammarota and colleagues used transrectal ultrasound to examine patients who had perianal abscesses and, in some instances, fistulas.[22] Law and colleagues initially reported the St. Mark's Hospital experience by using a specially designed, hard plastic cone attached to a rotating 7-MHz probe.[74] They evaluated 22 patients with recurrent perianal sepsis or anal fistula and compared the sonographic findings with those identified at sur-

gery. Specific features that were sought included the presence of an internal opening, muscle defect, or abscess, as well as the course of the tract. The authors concluded that anal endosonography should be considered as part of the evaluation of patients with anal fistula because of what they considered "excellent correlation" with the operative findings. For example, all seven of the fistulas considered "complex" were identified preoperatively, and there was good correlation with identifying horseshoe extensions and detecting foreign bodies. Others concur that this technique is an accurate and minimally invasive method for delineating the relationship between fistula tracts and the anal sphincter mechanism as well as for identifying deeper areas of sepsis.[34]

Particular problem areas, however, include specific internal opening sites and differentiation among abscess cavities, granulating tracts, and scars. Cheong and co-workers attempted to address this concern by accentuating tissue interface layers through the introduction of hydrogen peroxide into the fistula tract through the external opening in two individuals with recurrent anal fistula.[24] They concluded that hydrogen peroxide enhances the contrast and is a simple, effective, and safe method for improving the accuracy of endoanal ultrasound assessment for this condition.

Choen and colleagues undertook a prospective trial comparing the accuracy of digital examination and anal endosonography in defining the anatomy of anal fistulas.[25] Before surgery, 38 consecutive patients were assessed by the consultant surgeon, a research fellow, and two radiologists using anal endosonography. Clinical evaluation was found to be clearly superior to that of ultrasonography when the operative findings were compared.

Comment

There has been a great interest, especially in the radiologic literature, about endoanal ultrasound for identifying fistula tracts. Sensitivity and specificity rates are presented with the implication that the radiologist's interpretation is the accurate one, and the burden, therefore, must fall on the surgeon to support the findings. Such reasoning is clearly counterintuitive. More important, however, is that irrespective of the findings on anal ultrasound, it is up to the *surgeon* to find the internal opening—full stop. There is no benefit (except for research and publication) in performing this investigation for an uncomplicated, primary fistula. However, in my opinion, anal ultrasound *may* have some applicability in the evaluation of anal fistula disease under limited circumstances. For example:

- A fistula is suspected but no internal opening is found.
- The patient has had prior fistula surgery and has recurrence or persistence.
- The patient has underlying Crohn's disease.
- The fistula manifestations are highly complicated.

Magnetic Resonance Imaging

In order to avoid the consequences of a missed internal opening at the time of surgery, MRI has been advocated by many investigators, primarily nonsurgeons. Lunnis and co-workers evaluated 35 patients with anal fistula, using MRI on everyone, and comparing 20 of them with anal endosonography.[80] The authors concluded that MRI was superior to anal endosonography and actually demonstrated pathologic features that were missed at surgery. There was agreement between scan interpretation and operative findings with respect to the course of the primary tract in 30 of the 35 individuals. Buchanan and colleagues performed a prospective study involving 30 patients with suspected primary anal fistulas to determine the effect on outcome 1 year following surgery.[19] These investigators opined that MRI has a therapeutic impact of 10% for primary disease. In another study, the same investigators opined that preoperative MRI could alert surgeons to the potential hazard of fistulotomy's being more extensive than anticipated.[20]

Beckingham and colleagues compared digital rectal examination in a prospective fashion with dynamic contrast-enhanced MRI (DCEMRI) and surgical exploration.[11] The authors concluded that DCEMRI had a sensitivity of 97% and a specificity of 100% in the detection of anal fistulas. Furthermore, DCEMRI was able to identify more secondary tracts and was more accurate in identifying complex fistulas than either rectal examination alone or surgical exploration. Others have demonstrated that endoanal MRI provides high-resolution images of the relationship of collections and tracts and recommend this technique for the evaluation primarily of complex or recurrent fistulas and perianal septic conditions.[128,139,147]

Orsoni and associates compared the results of anal endosonography, MRI and surgical evaluation in the assessment of anorectal abscess and fistula in Crohn's disease.[99] They found that ultrasound provides more accurate information.

Opinion

At the risk of being a nihilist, I have a real problem with the results, recommendations, and conclusions of individuals who may be described as exhibiting the classic "valor of the noncombatant." The burden of proof for identifying the true nature of the pathology still must rest with the surgeon. Irrespective of the beautiful images conveyed through ultrasound or MRI, one must ultimately resort to identifying the condition *in vivo*. Unfortunately, converting the information to practical treatment remains, at least for me, an unachieved ideal. That said, imaging studies do have a role. At the very least, endosonography and MRI may explain why one fails to correct complex or recurrent anal fistulas surgically.

Additional Gastrointestinal Studies

Gastrointestinal evaluation in addition to rigid or flexible sigmoidoscopy is generally unnecessary for patients with conventional anal fistula. However, in the presence of known or suspected inflammatory bowel disease, colonoscopic examination and a small bowel series are strongly encouraged.

PRINCIPLES OF SURGICAL TREATMENT

The management of anal fistula by division or "laying open" the tract was initially described by John of Arderne in the fourteenth century.[9] With minor variations, this is the same method that is most commonly employed today.

John Arderne (1307–1380?) Arderne, or de Arderne, claimed descent from Saxon times. His family was one of the first to assume a surname in imitation of the Normans. He stated that he was 70 in the first year of the reign of Richard II (i.e., 1377), hence our ability to deduce the year of his birth. He was a surgeon of the pre-Renaissance period and quite well educated, but little is known about him except for information that was gleaned from autobiographic details in some of his manuscripts. Scholars surmise that he was educated at Montpellier and served on the English side in France during the early period of the One Hundred Years War. He treated patients in Newark, Nottinghamshire, from 1349 to 1370 and then came to London. In 1376, Arderne issued his *Treatise on Fistula-in-ano.* A prolific writer in colloquial Latin, he was soon translated into English. Although he was apparently a brilliant surgeon, he still adhered to and promulgated astrology, keeping his medicaments and plasters secret. In fact, his fame as a pharmacist was said to have long outlasted his reputation as a surgeon. (Arderne J. *Treatises of fistula-in-ano, hemorrhoids and clysters.* From an early fifteenth century manuscript translation by D'Arcy Power. London: Kegan Paul, Trench, Trubner, 1910.)

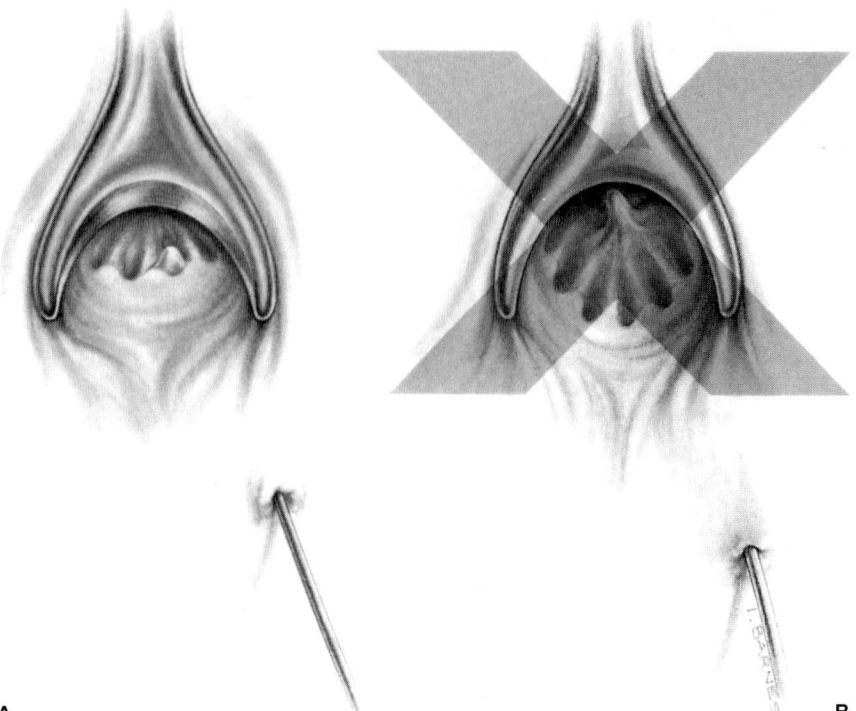

FIGURE 11-14. Probing the tract may reveal that the internal opening has sealed. **(A)** If the tip of the probe can be appreciated at the level of the crypt, a fistulotomy may be undertaken with safety. **(B)** However, creating an "artificial" internal opening is contraindicated at a higher level. **A**   **B**

Percivall Pott suggested that there are essentially three means for cure: caustic, ligature, and incision.

As previously mentioned, the surgeon who first treats the patient has the best opportunity to identify the tract, find the internal opening, and effect a cure. When this is not accomplished in the first instance, further surgery may be more complex, and the patient will be subjected to an increased risk of complication.

Failure to cure the patient is usually the result of either *timorousness* or *temerity*. If the surgeon traces the tract from the external opening to the level of the crypt but cannot pass the probe into the anal canal and subsequently desists from excising the crypt-bearing area, one is being too timid. In this situation, it is reasonable to assume that the crypt opening has sealed and that it is, indeed, the source of the fistula (Figure 11-14A). Likewise, if the surgeon identifies the internal opening of a "virgin fistula" but is reluctant to lay it open because of fear that

the opening is too high, that decision may jeopardize the opportunity of curing the patient. The fistula will inevitably persist, and the subsequent procedure will be performed without the security of knowing that the observed internal opening occurred as a natural consequence. With few exceptions (e.g., Crohn's disease, a history of trauma), the surgeon should be able to open the tract at the time of the initial operation without fear of causing significant impairment for bowel control. If there is concern about the safety of dividing at the internal opening, a seton can be temporarily employed (see later).

Conversely, if the tract is identified only partially (i.e., not to the level of the crypt), and the surgeon elects to guess or to assume where the opening should be, thereby creating an "artificial" internal opening, one is being too aggressive (Figure 11-14B). The actual opening and the tract have not been appreciated. When the surgeon is subsequently confronted with a persistent fistula after

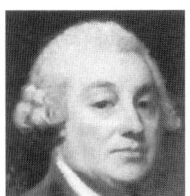

Percivall Pott (1714–1788)   Pott was born in London, the son of a scrivener, in a house on Threadneedle Street at which location now sits the Bank of England. With the assistance of a relation, the Bishop of Rochester, Pott was able to attend a private school in Kent. At the age of 16 he demonstrated an interest in surgery and was apprenticed to Edward Nourse, an assistant surgeon at St. Bartholomew's Hospital. It was Pott's responsibility to prepare anatomic subjects for Nourse's lectures. In 1736, Pott received his diploma and was admitted to the Company of Barber-Surgeons. Following dissolution of the company in 1745, Pott allied himself with the surgeons, having been appointed assistant surgeon at St. Bartholomew's. In his *Treatise on Fistula*, Pott stressed the advisability of minimal dissection, that is, the performance of limited fistulotomy. In 1756, Pott was thrown from his horse and suffered a compound fracture of the ankle. Despite having been advised to undergo amputation, he successfully managed to preserve the limb. The term Pott's fracture is still used to describe this particular injury. In 1786, the Royal College of Surgeons at Edinburgh elected Pott an Honorary Fellow, the first gentleman of the faculty to whom this honor was given. He served St. Bartholomew's Hospital for one half a century, and when he died the place in the Court of Assistants of the Surgeon's Company was filled by his eminent pupil, John Hunter. (Pott P. *The chirurgical works*, vols 1–3. London: J Johnson, 1808; adapted from Parks AG, Gordon PH, Hardcastle JD. A classification of fistula-in-ano. *Br J Surg* 1976;63:1.)

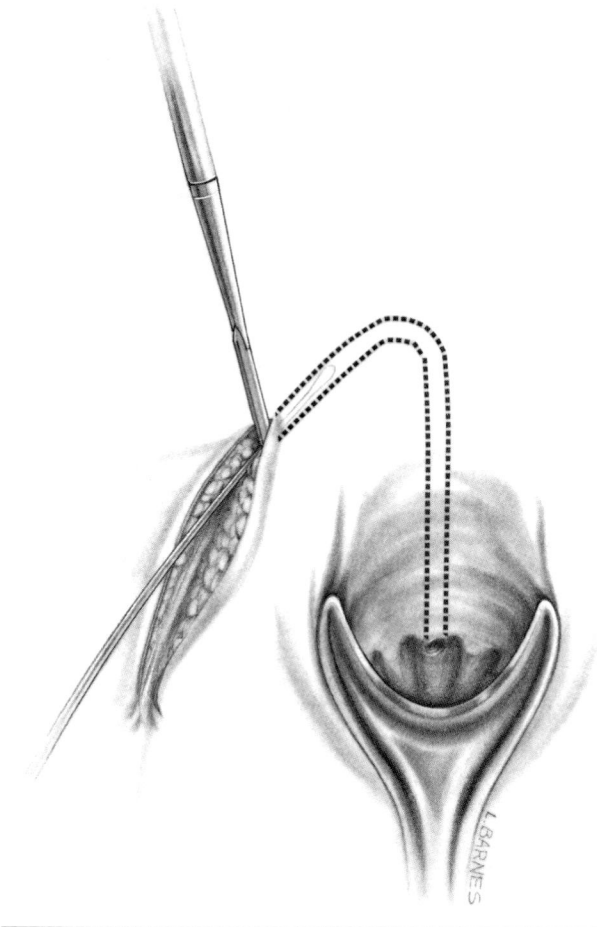

FIGURE 11-15. Progressive unroofing of a fistula with electrocautery, following the tract with the aid of a probe.

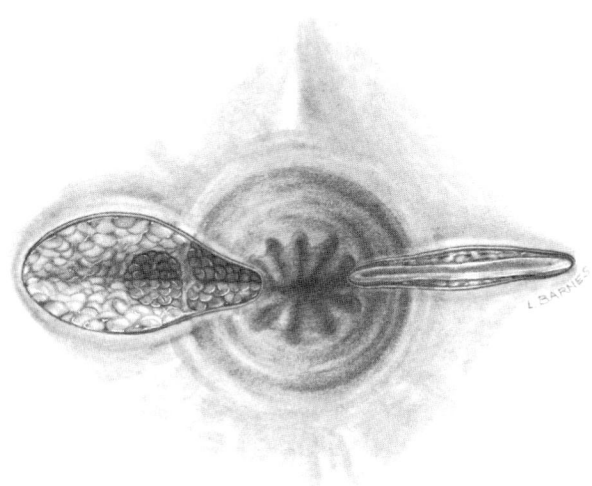

FIGURE 11-16. Fistulectomy versus fistulotomy, a matter of prolonged wound healing.

such an ill-conceived maneuver, both the natural and the artificial internal openings must be considered.

The previously mentioned injection techniques may confirm the presence of the fistula and the internal opening. They do not, however, identify the course of the tract. If a probe can be passed, it is only necessary to incise down onto it. However, if this cannot be accomplished, should a fistulotomy be elected, the dissection must be carried out slowly and meticulously, following the epithelialized tract until it communicates with the anal canal (Figure 11-15).

A fistula operation should always be performed with electrocautery. Identification of the tract requires a dry operative field. In such a vascular area, no better means exists for maintaining hemostasis than this tool.

Fistulotomy versus Fistulectomy

Another source of controversy has been whether to perform fistulectomy or fistulotomy. Kronborg randomly allocated patients with anal fistula to either an incisional or an excisional approach.[67] Times of healing were signif-

icantly shorter when the fistula was laid open in comparison with excision, whereas recurrence rates were comparable. Fistulotomy is certainly preferable in my experience because of the prolonged healing time associated with excisional techniques (Figs. 11-16 and 11-17). However, a small portion of the tract may be removed for pathologic examination, especially if there is a concern about the possibility of Crohn's disease (see later).

Office Fistulotomy

Office fistulotomy may be undertaken synchronously with drainage of an abscess if the internal opening is low or of the intersphincteric type. It may also be performed in the office as an interval procedure following abscess drainage. Local anesthesia or a field block is usually quite adequate (see Chapters 7 and 8). For the majority of patients, however, definitive fistula surgery should be performed in the operating room with a general, spinal, or caudal anesthetic under optimal conditions. A local anesthetic with conscious sedation may also be used in selected individuals. With the exception of certain complex fistulas or those in whom concomitant sphincter repair is undertaken, the operation can usually be undertaken on an ambulatory basis. This is also in accordance with the recommendations of the Standards Task Force of the American Society of Colon and Rectal Surgeons.[6] Their conclusions were as follows:

- A fistula, fistula with abscess, or a fistula associated with limited anorectal pathology may be treated on an outpatient basis if, in the judgment of the operating surgeon, it is safe to do so.
- Fistulas involving adjacent organs or structures (i.e., rectovaginal, rectourethral, or horseshoe) often require

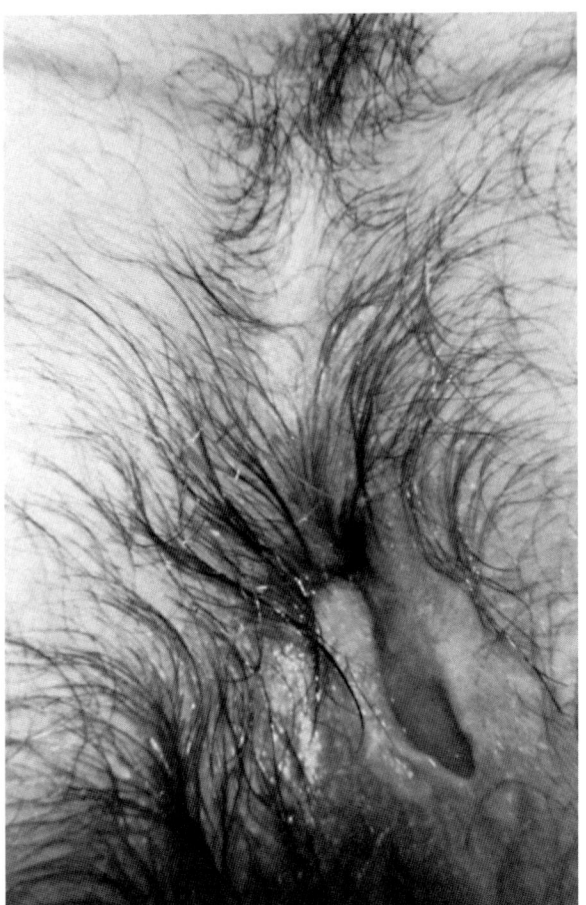

FIGURE 11-17. Anal fistulectomy may require prolonged healing time. This wound is still open 6 weeks after the operation.

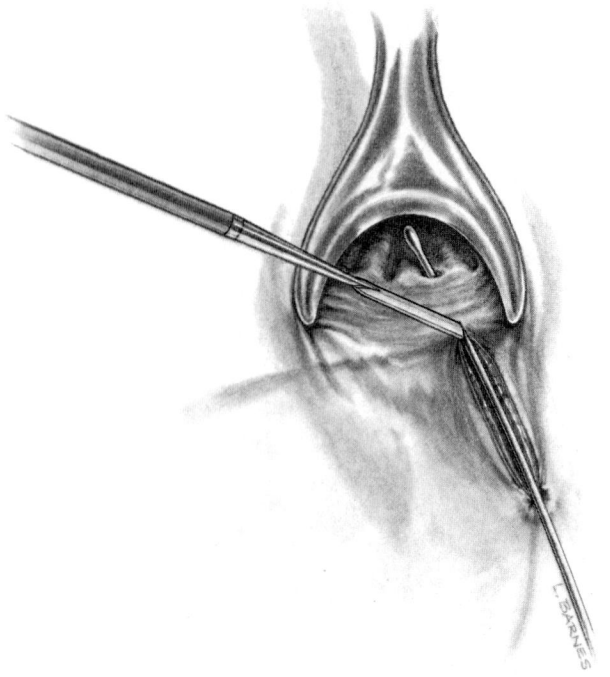

FIGURE 11-18. Conventional fistulotomy. With the use of electrocautery, the tract is laid open between the internal and external openings.

more extensive surgery, and inpatient postoperative care is usually needed.

■ Fistulas associated with extensive cellulitis or abscess or additional anorectal disease may require inpatient care, especially if intravenous antibiotics are necessary.[6]

SURGICAL APPROACHES

Treatment of Conventional Fistula

After the external and internal openings have been identified by one of the means mentioned, the tract is incised (Figure 11-18). Continuity of the epithelial lining confirms the completeness of the operation, and granulation tissue is removed by curettage. A portion of the tract may be excised and sent for pathologic examination. The external portion of the incision may be widened relative to the size of the opening in the anal canal, because skin tends to heal more rapidly than does the anal mucosa. If this procedure is not performed, delayed healing within the anal canal may result. The cut edges of the anal mucosa and the underlying internal anal sphincter can be oversewn with absorbable suture for hemostasis (Figure 11-19). The wound

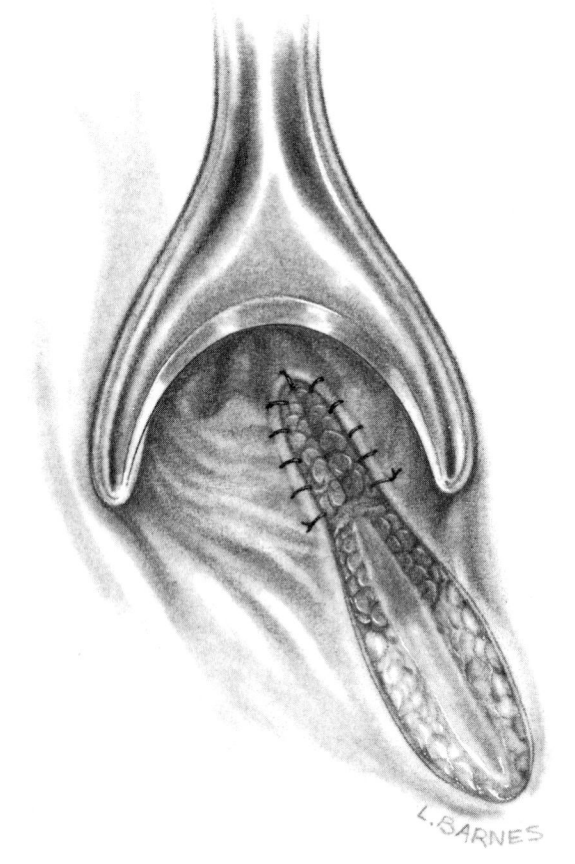

FIGURE 11-19. Conventional fistulotomy. The anal opening with the underlying internal sphincter is sutured for hemostasis.

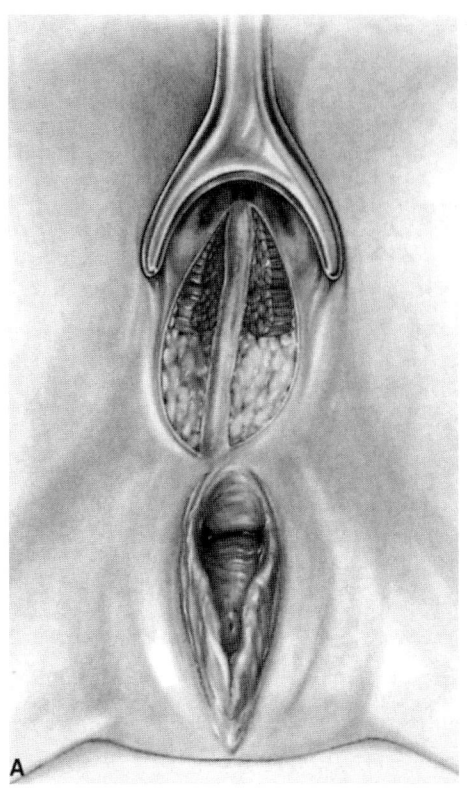 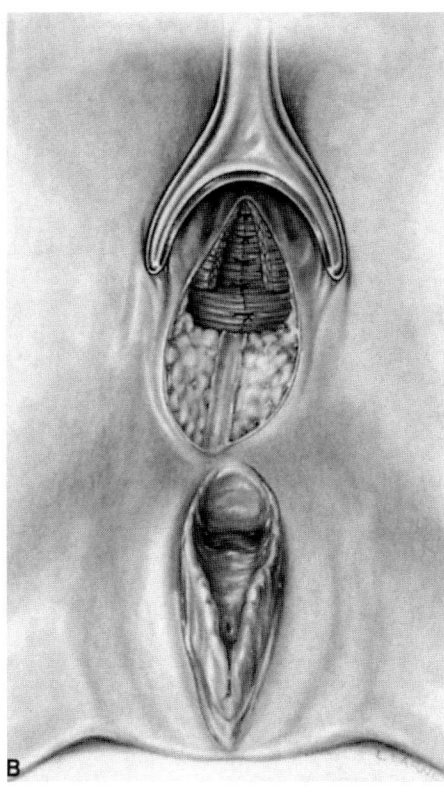

FIGURE 11-20. Anterior fistula in a female patient may be treated by repair of the external sphincter. **(A)** Fistulotomy divides a portion of the external sphincter. **(B)** Repair of the sphincter is effected, and the wound is left open.

is otherwise left open and gently packed. Petroleum-jelly gauze is preferred by some surgeons, because subsequent removal is less likely to induce bleeding. Others endorse the use of iodoform gauze, Surgicel, Telfa, or simply a gauze sponge.

To reiterate, my personal preference concerning the principles of operative treatment are as follows:

- Identify the tract.
- Incise the tract.
- Excise a portion for biopsy material (if considered potentially useful).
- Widen the external wound.
- Suture the cut edge of the anal canal.

The dressing is removed that evening or the next day, and sitz baths are commenced. Vigorous mechanical cleansing of the wound is encouraged, either by means of a washcloth or with a gauze pad. The use of a Water-Pic device or comparable irrigating equipment has definite merit in postoperative wound management. One should be as vigorous as possible, maintaining the wound in a well-debrided and clean state. An office visit is recommended approximately 10 days later, and usually every 1 to 2 weeks thereafter until healing has taken place. Less frequent appointments may be appropriate for individuals with straightforward fistulas if the patient understands the need for and is committed to vigorous cleansing.

If a large portion of the external sphincter must be divided, consideration should be given to primary sphinc-

ter repair or possibly to seton division (see later discussion). There is one situation, however, which should always be considered for either reconstruction or another alternative to limit sphincter injury—an anterior fistula in a woman (Figure 11-20). When a fistula occurs anterior to the transverse plane in a woman, surgical treatment inevitably will create some degree of impairment for control. To minimize the disability, sphincter reconstruction should be attempted at the time of fistulotomy. Another alternative for managing such a problem is to use a seton or to perform a closure of the internal opening with a sliding endorectal flap, such as that which may be recommended for rectovaginal fistula repair and high transsphincteric anal fistulas.

Horseshoe Fistula

Horseshoe fistula may be intersphincteric but is much more frequently transsphincteric. It is so called because it is composed of multiple external openings joined by a subcutaneous communication in a U or horseshoe shape (Figure 11-21). The arms of the U are almost always directed anteriorly, and the internal opening is in the posterior midline. Rarely, a horseshoe fistula may present with the opposite configuration; that is, the internal opening is in the anterior midline, and the arms of the U are directed posteriorly.

Treatment of this condition has evolved to be much less radical than has often been described. The classic

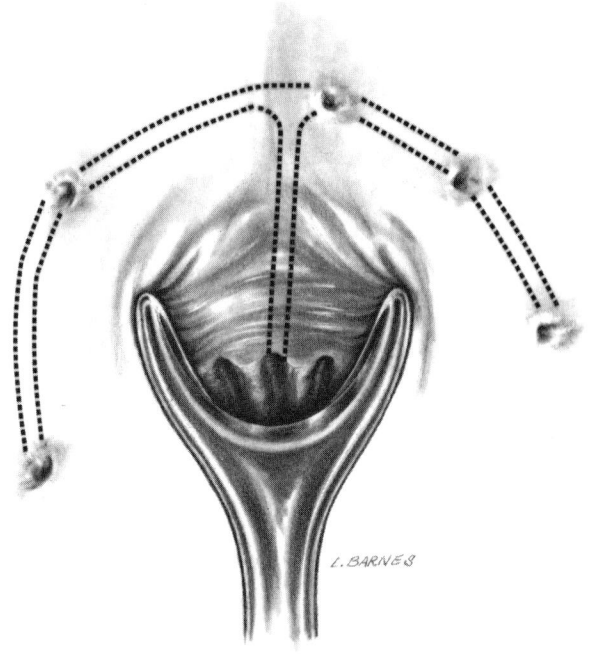

FIGURE 11-21. Diagrammatic representation of a horseshoe anal fistula. The internal opening is in the posterior midline.

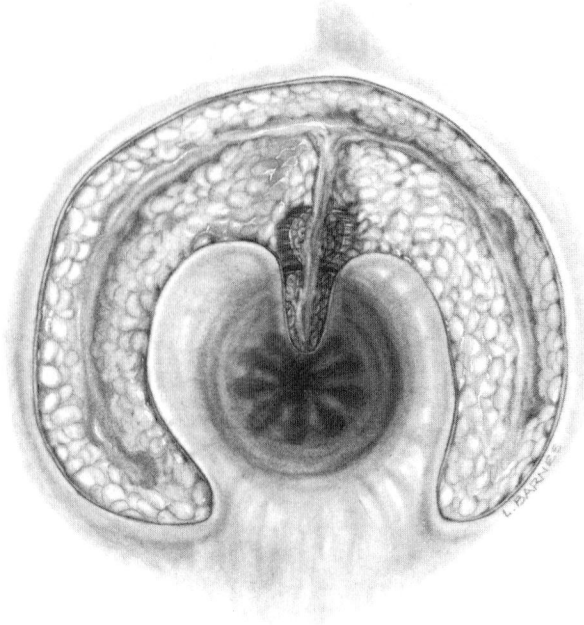

FIGURE 11-22. Classic treatment of horseshoe fistula requires excision of all openings.

procedure required identification of the tracts and internal opening and unroofing or excision of each of them (Figure 11-22). This inevitably resulted in a huge, gaping wound, which required a prolonged healing time (Figure 11-23). Disability after this operation can last for many months.

In 1965, Hanley described a rather conservative approach to the management of horseshoe fistula that limits the number and extent of the incisions.[53] It is self-evident that regardless of the number of tracts and external openings, they communicate. Because the most important aspect of the operation is to eliminate the internal opening, he and others suggested that this approach, along with the establishment of adequate external drainage, should cure the condition.[42,53] If the internal opening has been removed, the external openings will close. Most surgeons have successfully adopted this approach to the treatment of horseshoe anal fistula.

The deep postanal space must be entered, curetted, and irrigated if the fistula is of the transsphincteric type (Figure 11-24). This involves incision of both the internal sphincter and a portion of the external sphincter. It is then necessary only to unroof the external openings, curette the tracts, and drain the wounds (Figure 11-25). The cut edges of the anal canal and underlying internal sphincter are sutured for hemostasis. The deep postanal space is packed, usually with iodoform gauze, and a dressing is applied.

When the fistula is approached in this way, healing is generally rapid, and the risk of functional impairment to the anus from scarring and deformity is lessened considerably. Duration of disability is also markedly reduced.

Postoperatively, the packing is removed in 24 to 48 hours, and the patient is begun on sitz baths. Weekly office visits are recommended until the wounds have healed.

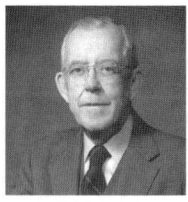

Courtesy Ochsner Clinic Foundation, New Orleans, Louisiana

Patrick H. Hanley (1909–1994) Patrick Hanley was born February 2, 1909, in Lockport, Louisiana. He graduated from Southwestern Louisiana Institute in 1929 and received his medical degree from Tulane University School of Medicine in 1933. He completed his surgical residency at Charity Hospital in New Orleans under the guidance of Alton Ochsner. During World War II, he served as a lieutenant commander in Bahia, Brazil, where he devoted himself to communicable disease prevention and to health education. After the war he returned to New Orleans and to the Ochsner Clinic, at which institution he developed a training program in colon and rectal surgery. He ultimately was promoted to Professor of Surgery at Tulane. Hanley supervised the training of 40 fellows in colon and rectal surgery. He wrote extensively and was especially recognized for his video presentations at national meetings in which he illustrated his surgical techniques. He was considered a pioneer in the use of this modality as a teaching tool. His major contributions included investigation of perineal and perianal anatomy and the relationship of anatomic structures to fistula disease. He was elected President of the American Society of Colon and Rectal Surgeons and of the International Society of University Colon and Rectal Surgeons. Patrick Hanley died on March 27, 1994. (With appreciation to David E. Beck, MD, Chairman, Department of Colon and Rectal Surgery, Ochsner Clinic Foundation, New Orleans, LA.)

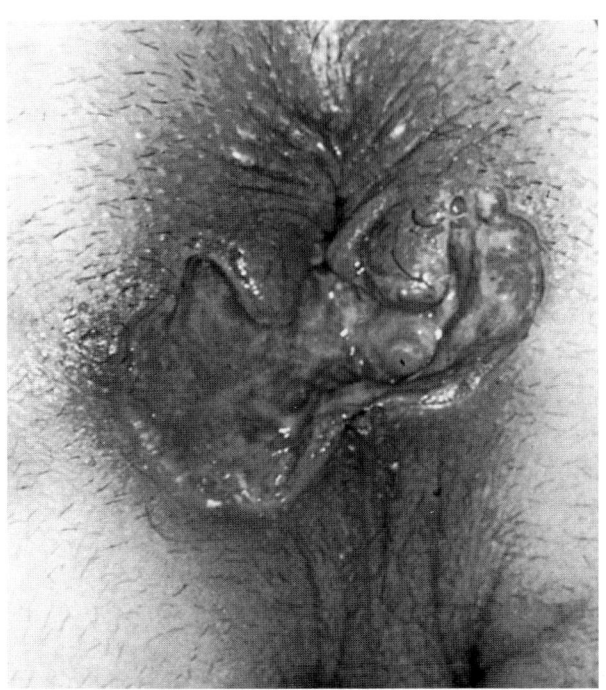

FIGURE 11-23. Treatment of an anterior horseshoe fistula by the classic technique leaves a large, gaping wound that requires prolonged healing time.

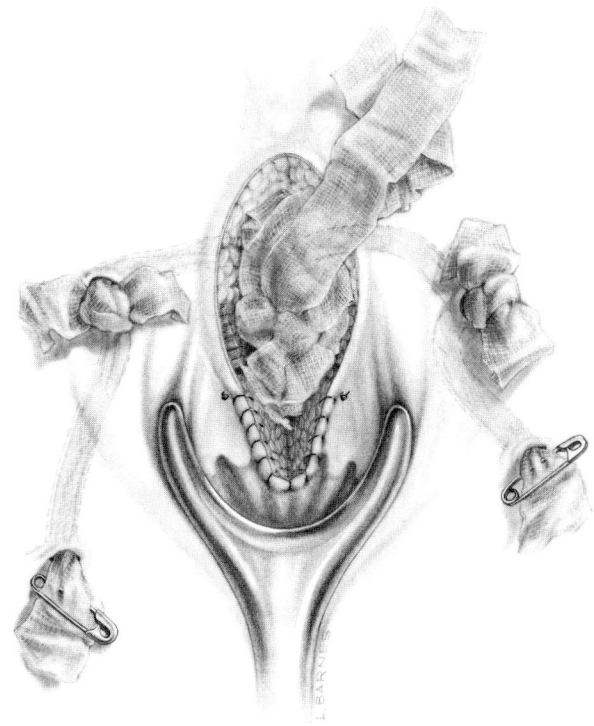

FIGURE 11-25. Treatment of horseshoe fistula-in-ano requires unroofing in the posterior midline to drain the deep postanal space adequately. The external openings are individually drained, with curettage only of the underlying tracts. Packing is placed through each opening and in the deep postanal space.

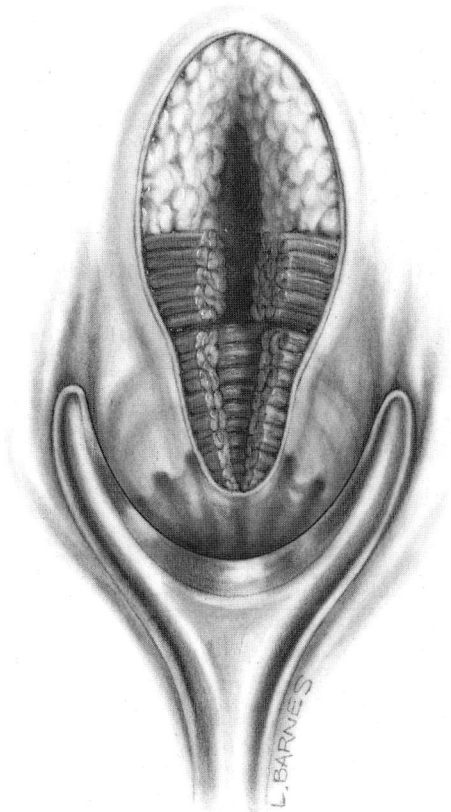

FIGURE 11-24. Successful management of a typical posterior horseshoe fistula requires entrance of the deep postanal space even though a portion of the internal and external sphincter must be divided.

Treatment of Suprasphincteric Fistula

With this manifestation, the management of suprasphincteric fistula is comparable to that of other complex fistulas and includes endorectal advancement flap, primary closure and drainage, and seton division. In general, once the fistula has been recognized as such, fistulotomy can be accomplished distal to the internal opening by dividing the lower portion of the internal and external sphincters (Figure 11-26). The cephalad component, including the internal opening, is treated by means of seton division (see later).

Treatment of Extrasphincteric Fistula

When the internal opening is thought to lie above the levators, division of the tract may result in fecal incontinence. If the puborectalis sling is completely divided, anal incontinence will surely ensue. When doubt exists as to the level of the internal opening, a seton can be employed as a diagnostic tool. This involves placing a heavy suture through the tract and out the anal canal. This can be facilitated by passing the suture material through the eye of a probe. The suture is loosely tied, and no further procedure is undertaken at that time.

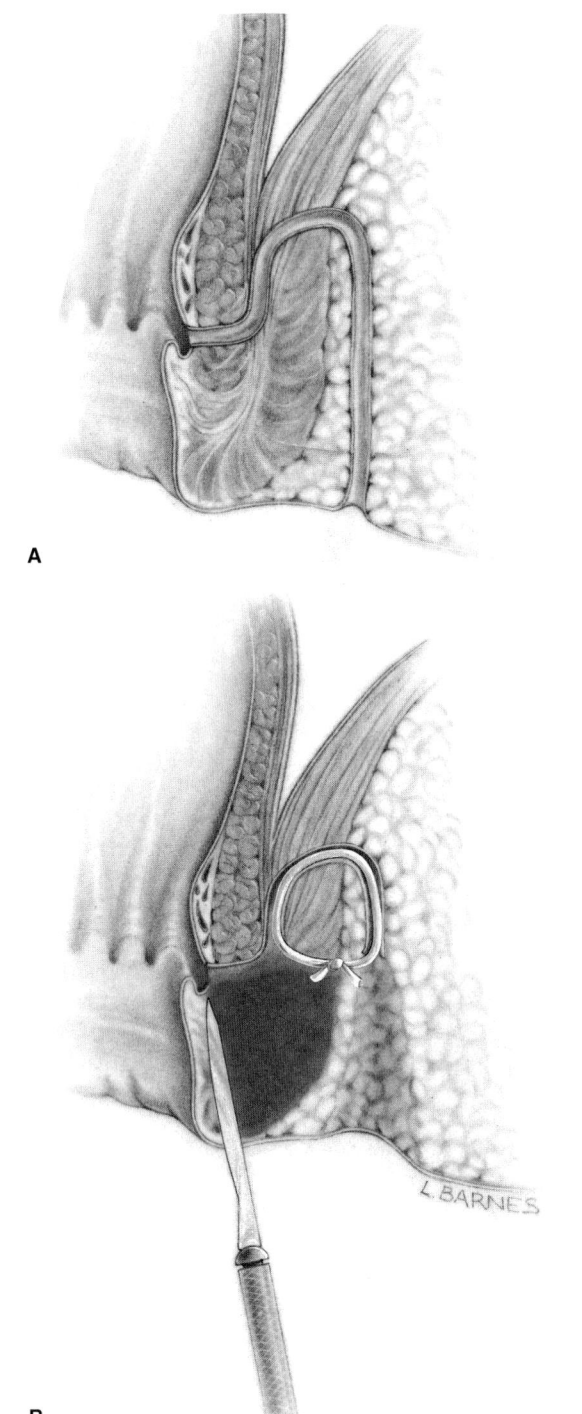

A

B

FIGURE 11-26. Suprasphincteric fistula. **(A)** The tract courses above the levatores, passing through to the skin in the ischiorectal fossa. **(B)** The internal and external sphincters have been incised, but the high opening is treated by seton division to minimize the risk of fecal incontinence.

When the patient is alert, rectal examination is performed. While he or she alternately tightens and relaxes the sphincter, the seton can be felt to lie above or below the levatores (Figure 11-27). If it is below, a fistulotomy can be performed safely. Conversely, if the internal open-

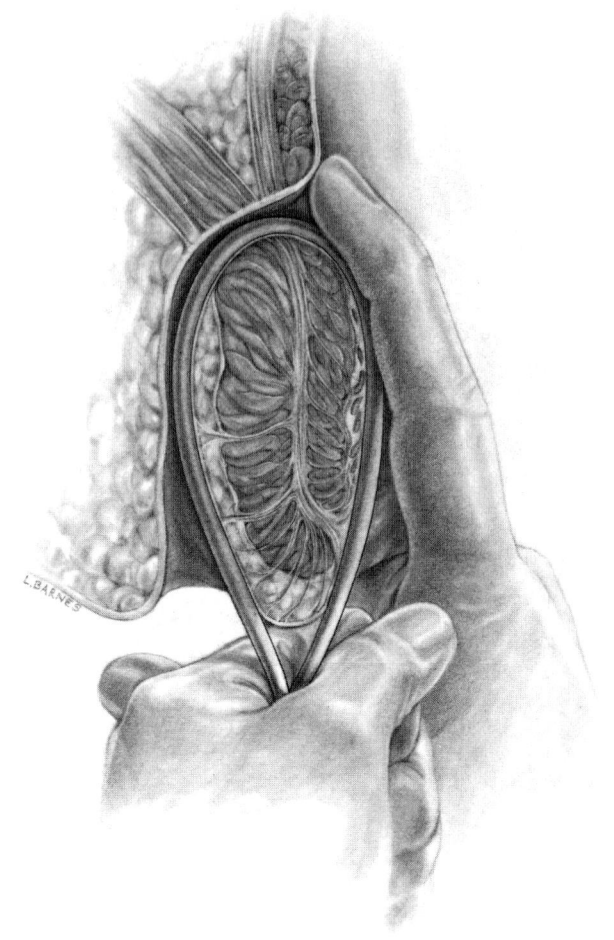

FIGURE 11-27. A seton is used to evaluate the level of the internal opening.

ing is above the level of the levatores, an alternative procedure must be undertaken. Several possible operative approaches exist for the treatment of extrasphincteric fistula.

Seton Division

Seton division was described by Hippocrates in the fifth century B.C., in his medical works known as the *Hippocratic Collection*.[3] His concepts are still applicable today for the management of difficult fistula problems. It is certainly the simplest of the methods available for the treatment of extrasphincteric fistula and probably produces results comparable to the more esoteric approaches, at least with respect to cure rate.[26,71,110] Bowel control, however, may be less satisfactory when compared with other options.

The principle involved in the use of the seton as a therapeutic tool is analogous to that of a wire cutting through a block of ice. The ice is still adherent after division by the wire. Theoretically, by tightening the suture and permitting it to cut through over a number of days or weeks,

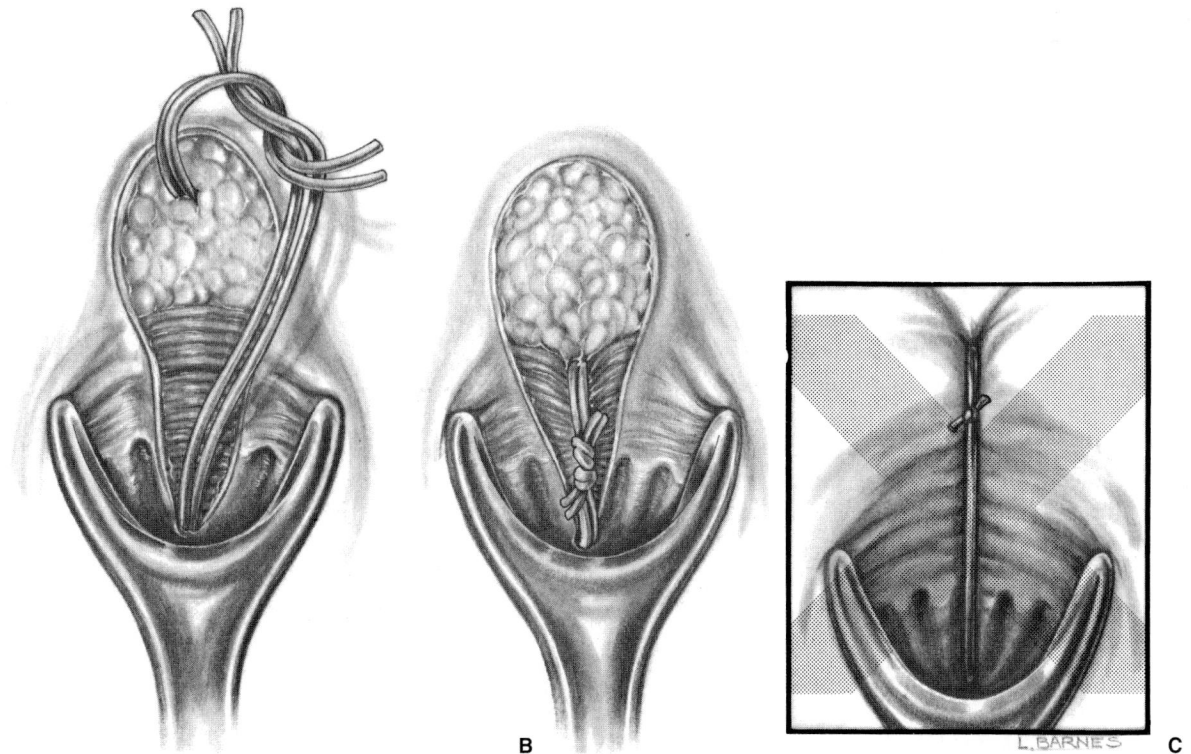

A   B   C

FIGURE 11-28. Application of a seton in the treatment of extrasphincteric fistula. **(A)** Doubled heavy sutures (silk is preferred) are passed through the external and internal openings. **(B)** The sutures are firmly secured. **(C)** The skin must be divided.

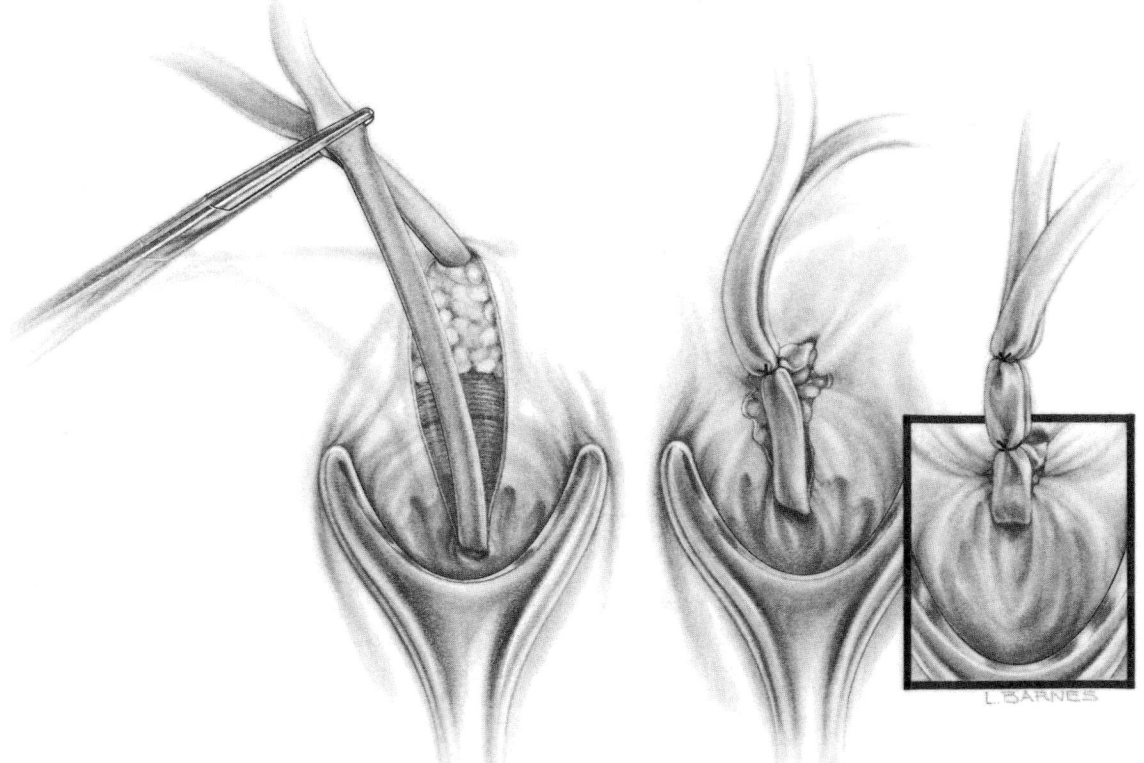

FIGURE 11-29. A ¼-inch Penrose drain is used to effect seton division. The inset demonstrates subsequent ligation of the drain at a higher level. (Adapted from Culp CE. Use of Penrose drains to treat certain anal fistulas: a primary operative seton. *Mayo Clin Proc* 1984;59:613, with permission.)

the resultant inflammatory response keeps the sphincter muscle from retracting and separating.

If a seton is employed, the skin and anal canal mucosa between the openings must be initially incised. Then the suture is passed (Figure 11-28A). Some surgeons prefer doubled No. 2 silk, but other alternatives include elastic bands (e.g., vessel loops) or a ¼-inch Penrose drain (Figure 11-29).[33] The seton is securely tied, usually with moderate tension (Figure 11-28B). Using a rubber band technique has been suggested to subsequently tighten the ligature (Figure 11-30).[30] Another method of securing and tightening the seton involves the use of a so-called hangman's knot (Figure 11-31).[79] Still another alternative is to insert multiple setons initially, securing only one.[47] As

each cuts through, another one is tied. If an elastic band, vessel loop (my preference), or Penrose drain is used, one secures the drain to itself with a ligature, thereby creating some compression of the tissue (Figure 11-32).

The patient is usually discharged the same day and is reexamined 1 week later. By this time, the suture has either loosened or, if minimal tissue has been incorporated, passed by necrosing through the residual muscle. Following injection of a local anesthetic into the sphincter, a second suture can be used. If some type of elastic band has been employed, it can be stretched and religated at a higher level (Figure 11-33). Two weeks later, the seton may have eroded through, depending on how much tissue needed to be divided. If not and there is minimal

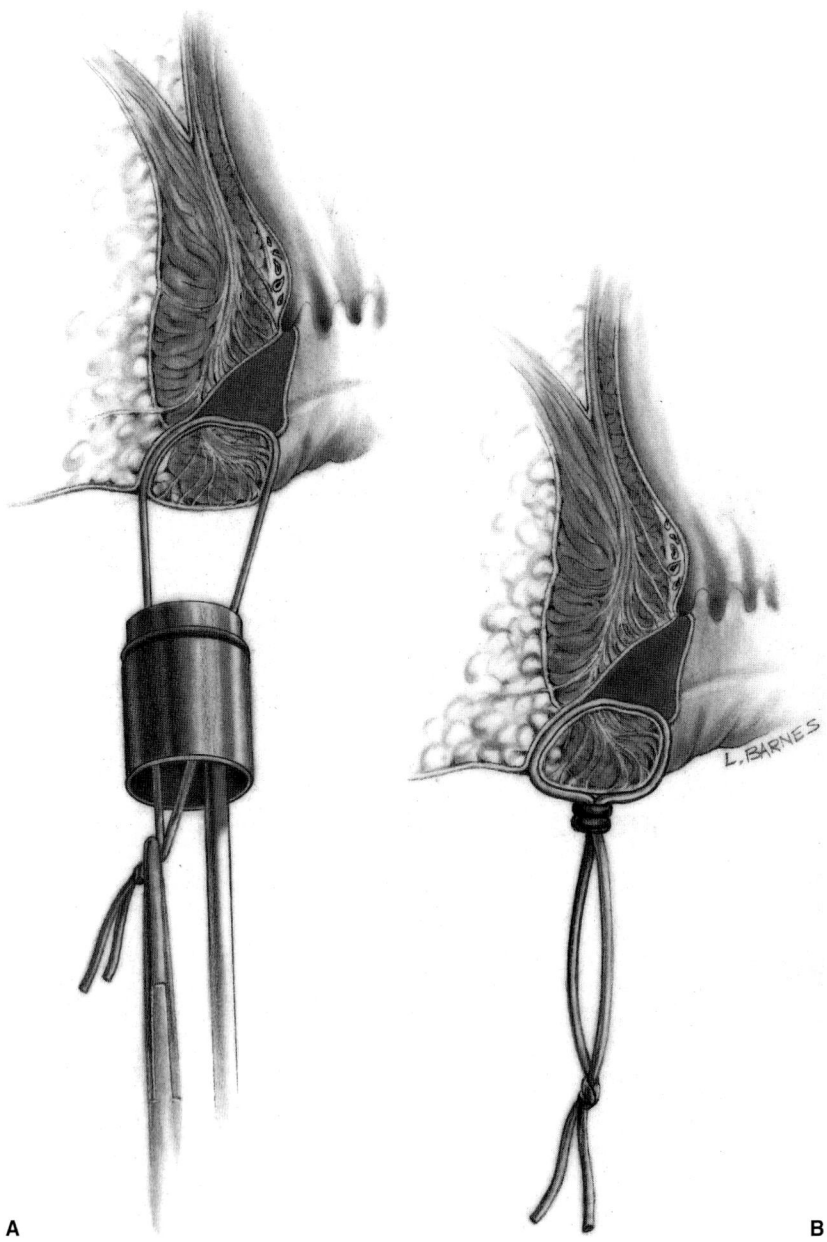

FIGURE 11-30. Seton fistulotomy utilizing elastic bands applied by rubber ring ligator as suggested by Cirocco and Rusin.[30] **(A)** A rubber band ligator is introduced. **(B)** Rubber bands are secured.

A

B

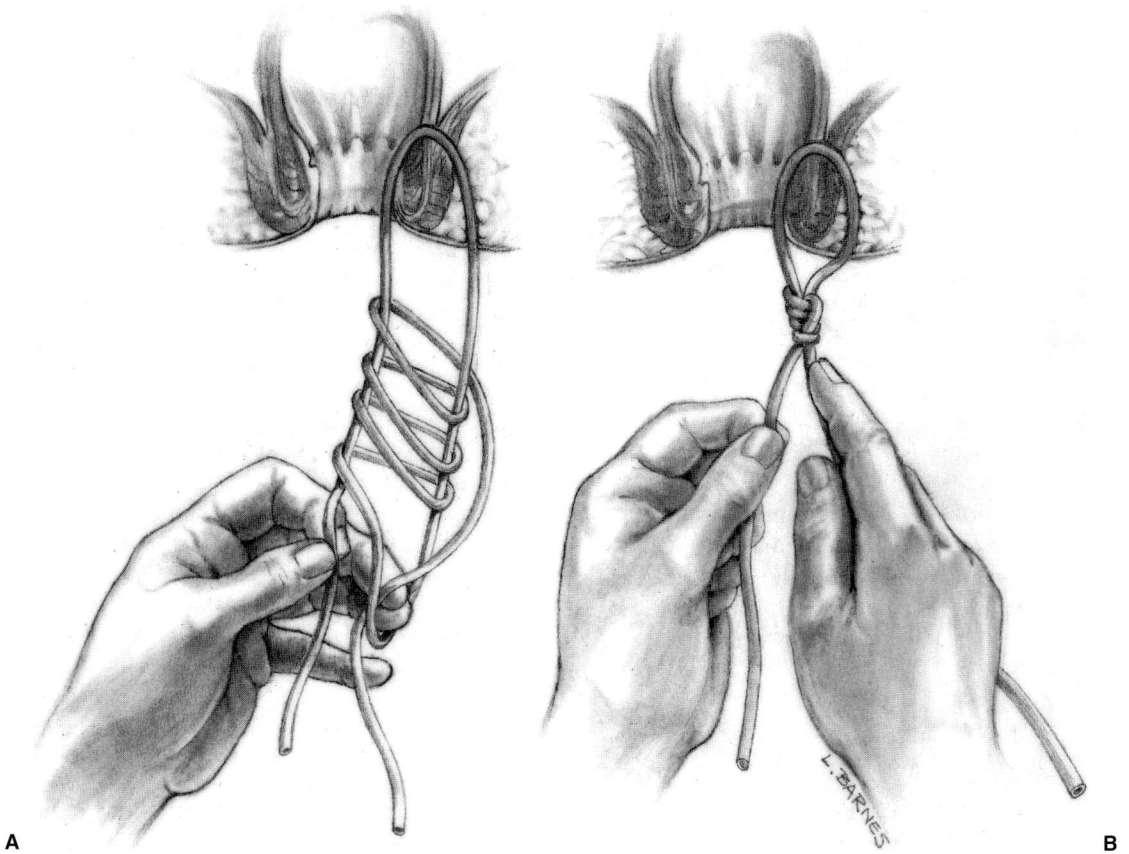

A   B

FIGURE 11-31. Securing the seton in such a matter that it permits tightening utilizing a hangman's tie. (Adapted from Loberman Z, Har-Shai Y, Schein M, et al. Hangman's tie simplifies seton management of anal fistulas. *Surg Gynecol Obstet* 1993;177:413, with permission.)

residual tissue, the fistulotomy can be completed in the office. However, if the surgeon prefers, a third tightening or even more can be performed, if indicated.

Thompson and colleagues suggest the use of a seton technique that can apply varying amounts of tension to accomplish sphincter division.[129] This approach has two theoretical advantages. First, pain, a consequence of tissue ischemia and necrosis, is a well-recognized problem

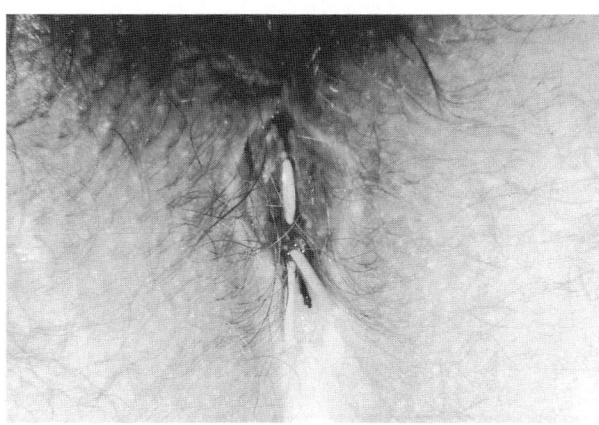

FIGURE 11-32. Seton fistulotomy by means of vessel retractor tape has been secured with a ligature in a woman with an anterior fistula.

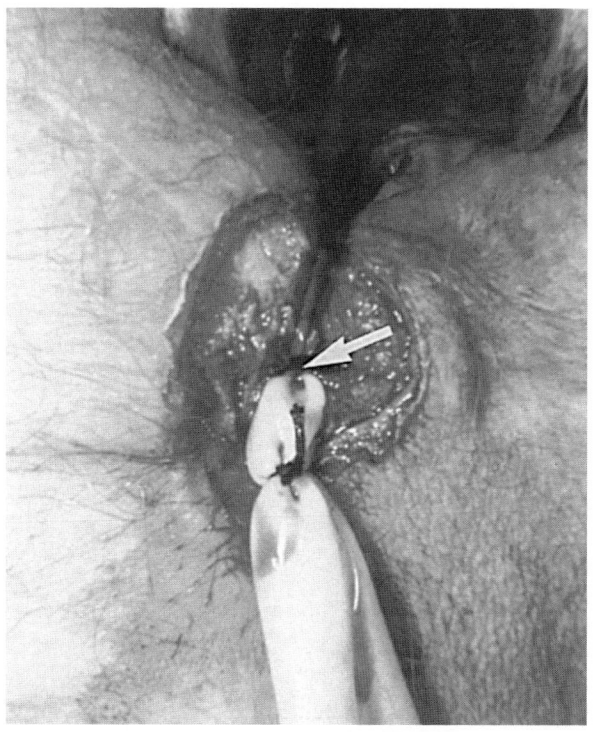

FIGURE 11-33. Seton division by means of a Penrose drain. Note that a second ligature *(arrow)* was added approximately 2 weeks following the initial procedure.

with seton division. Using a system that permits the patients to adjust the tension for minimal discomfort would certainly appear to be reasonable, provided, of course, it was effective. Second, this seton technique is, in essence, a one-stage procedure.

Technique
A No. 1 nylon or polypropylene suture is threaded around the sphincter in the usual way and tied loosely. A heavy elastic band is secured to the suture, and a safety pin is attached. The pin is then taped to the thigh with a small amount of tension, and the patient is instructed to adjust the amount that will produce minimal discomfort until the seton has cut through (Figure 11-34A). The authors offer another method of accomplishing patient-controlled seton division—tightening the noose by means of an adjustable tourniquet (Figure 11-34B).[92]

Long-Term Seton Drainage
The concept of seton drainage without definitive fistulotomy has been applied to the management of extrasphincteric fistulas, especially those associated with Crohn's disease (see later).[113,122] However, some surgeons have used this concept for the "therapeutic" management of low transsphincteric and intersphincteric anal fistulas.[75] In the experience of Lentner and Wienert, the suture

eventually either cut through the anal and perianal skin on its own, or the authors elected to perform fistulotomy at a subsequent operation.[75] The mean duration of the presence of the seton was in excess of 1 year. The recurrence rate was only 3.7%, and fewer than 1% experienced problems with bowel control. Still, the presence of a seton for a prolonged time is certainly a disadvantage in that the patient must contend with some discomfort, the presence of the foreign material, and the realization that there is no planned end point.

Comment
As long as the seton is in proper position, it will prevent an abscess from occurring. This should be the primary indication for long-term seton placement in my opinion—not to leave it in place until it gets caught on some object in the bathroom and performs an inadvertent fistulotomy. If the surgeon is uncomfortable about performing fistulotomy and elects to insert a seton, that is perfectly reasonable. What is not appropriate, however, is to fail to refer the patient to a specialist who is capable of eliminating the seton *and* the fistula. I have seen many patients who fit this description, having undergone seton insertion for uncomplicated transsphincteric fistula and having been told that the seton is permanent.

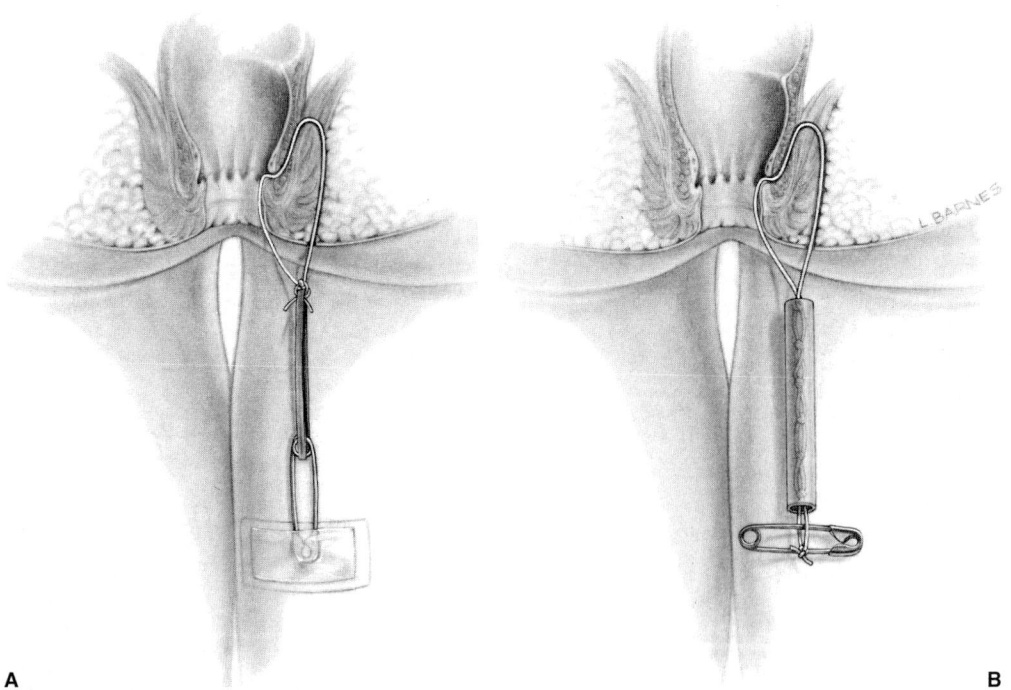

A   **B**

FIGURE 11-34. Adjustable seton in the management of a suprasphincteric anal fistula. **(A)** Variable tension is produced by the elastic secured to the thigh. **(B)** An adjustable tourniquet accomplishes the same ends. (Adapted from Thompson JE Jr, Bennion RS, Hilliard G. Adjustable seton in the management of complex anal fistula. *Surg Gynecol Obstet* 1989;169:551, with permission.)

Fistulotomy with Sphincter Repair

Complete division of an extrasphincteric fistula is a hazardous undertaking. Although direct repair can be performed immediately, breakdown is common. It should still be considered, however, to be an alternative technique for the treatment of high-level fistulas and, as has been mentioned previously, in the management of transsphincteric anterior fistulas in women.

Technique

The entire tract is divided. The epithelial lining is excised and the wound irrigated. A layered closure is performed using long-term absorbable sutures (e.g., 0 or 2–0 Vicryl), closing the rectal wall, and reconstructing the sphincter muscles. The ischiorectal fossa is widely drained externally. A protective colostomy is strongly suggested if fistulotomy with sphincter repair is contemplated for extrasphincteric fistula (Figure 11-35).

Comment

This operation is usually reserved for patients who have undergone multiple failed attempts to cure the fistula. The decision to embark on this approach should be made by someone who has specialized knowledge of anorectal anatomy and considerable experience with complex fistula surgery.

Closure of the Internal Opening and Drainage of the Extrasphincteric Tract

Closure of the internal opening and drainage of the extrasphincteric tract are less destructive of tissue than fistulotomy with sphincter repair, but the operation has a prohibitively high failure rate and, in my opinion, should be abandoned. It is included in this text simply because some surgeons selectively apply this approach in the unlikely event that it will heal. The procedure involves debridement and closure of the internal opening through a transanal operation. Adequate external drainage is established, and the supralevator area is vigorously curetted, irrigated, and packed (Figure 11-36). A concomitant colostomy should certainly be considered to enhance the possibility of a successful outcome.

Another option for conservation of the sphincter mechanism in high anal fistula is to perform the same operation with primary closure through the intersphincteric plane.

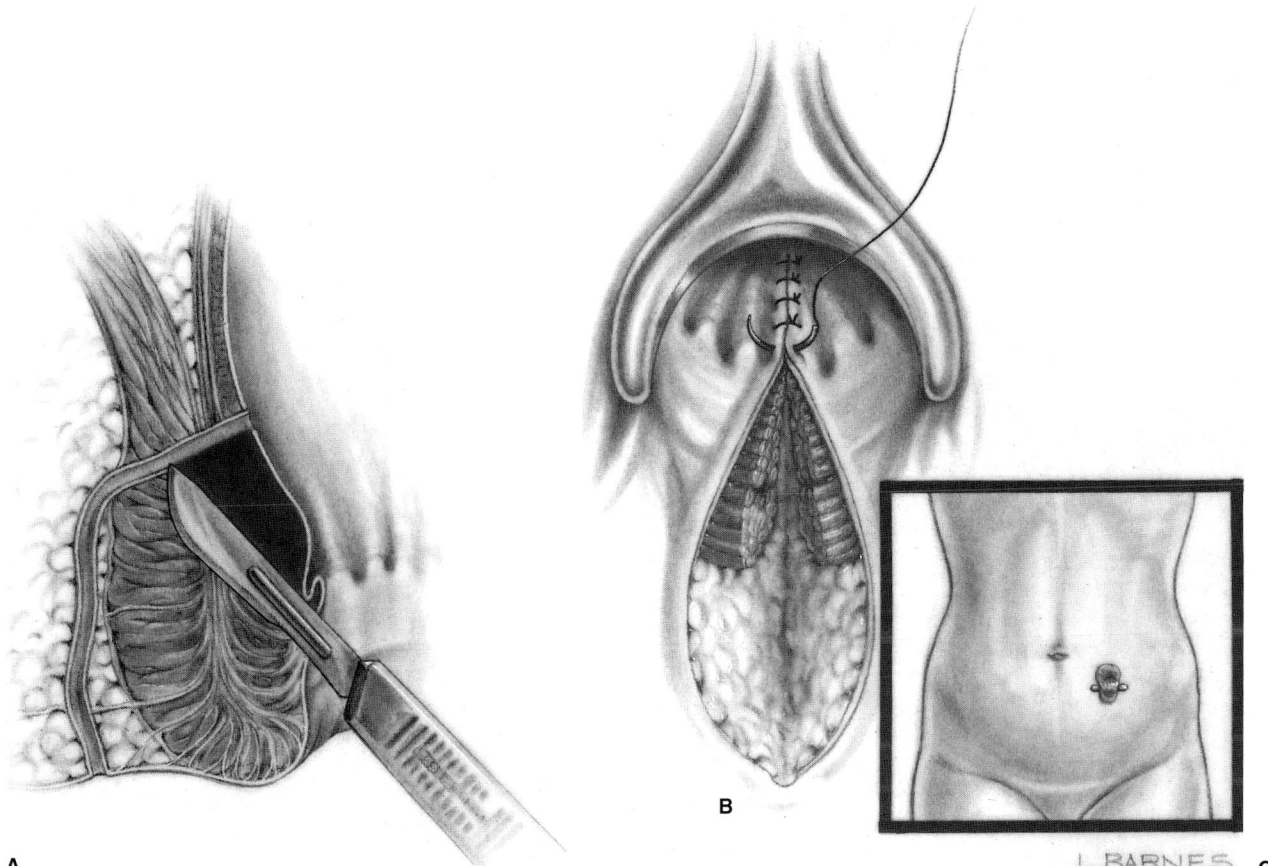

FIGURE 11-35. **(A)** Primary fistulotomy for extrasphincteric fistula. **(B)** Reconstruction is undertaken after excision of the tract. **(C)** A diverting colostomy is recommended for this approach.

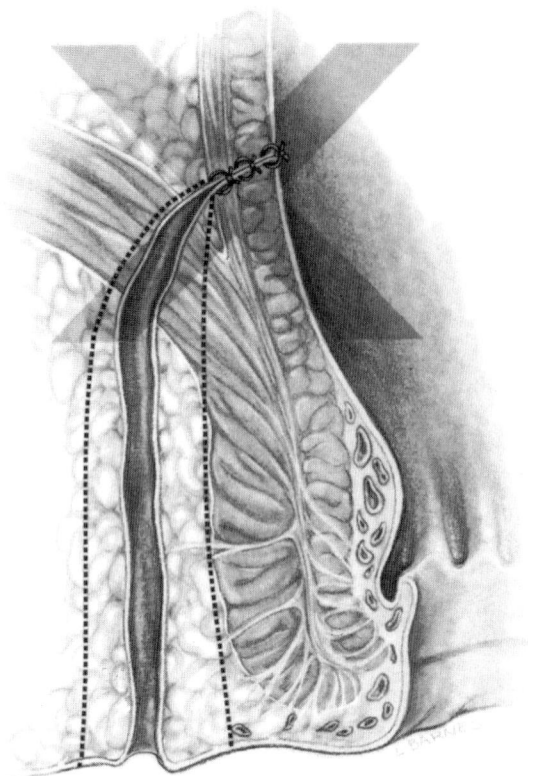

FIGURE 11-36. Treatment of extrasphincteric fistula by closure of the internal opening and wide drainage of the supralevator space and ischiorectal fossa *(broken line)*. The *X* indicates my feelings about the usefulness of this approach.

This has been described from the St. Mark's Hospital Group (Figure 11-37).[88] In their operation, the entire tract is excised through this approach, and the defects in the sphincter muscle that are produced as a consequence of tract removal are primarily closed. Although the authors report a failure rate of approximately 30%, they conclude that, if successful, continence is better than after other approaches.

Opinion

The St. Mark's procedure appears beautiful through the artist's eyes, but it seems technically impossible for me at least to accomplish the task. One sees the beautiful branched tract as the excised specimen, but it just does not represent a realistic procedure. Furthermore, I have seen no follow-up reports since the original publication. As opposed to fistulotomy with sphincter repair, closure of the internal opening and drainage of the extrasphincteric tract are unlikely harm to the patient. Regardless, I believe that the physician should initially attempt the following technique for this indication.

Endorectal Advancement Flap

Aguilar and colleagues have advocated preservation of the sphincter muscle by extrasphincteric fistulectomy, closure of the sphincteric defect, and endorectal mucosal advancement.[40] Their approach is a modification of the

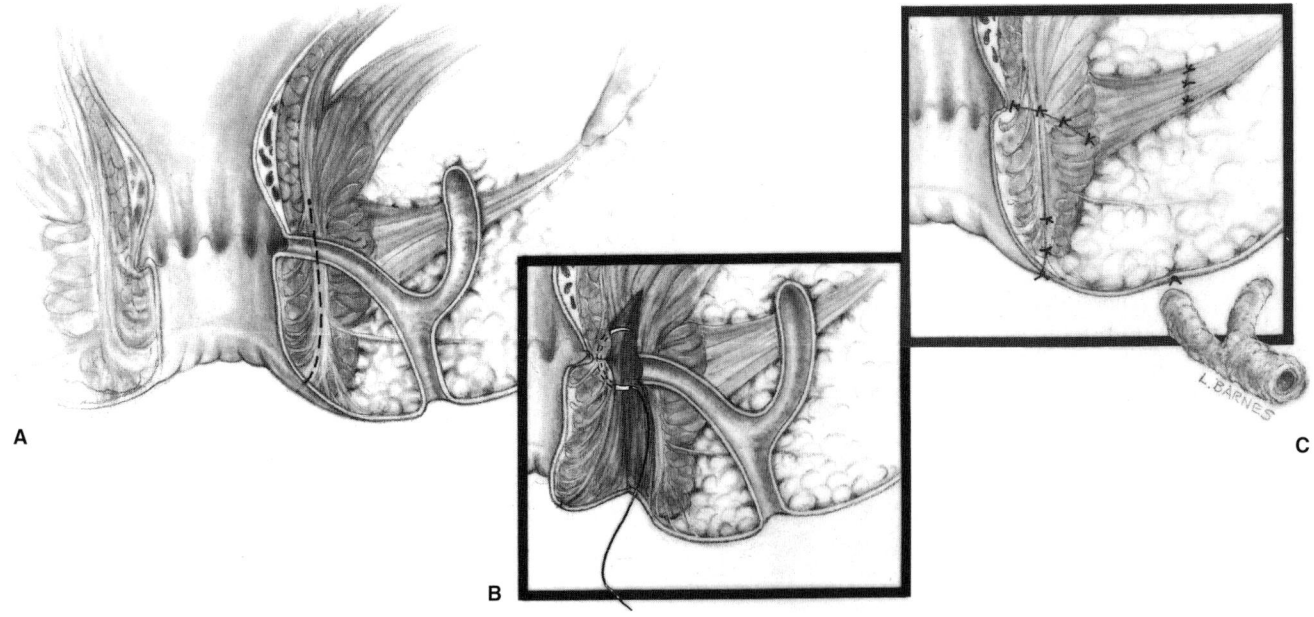

FIGURE 11-37. Total sphincter conservation in a high anal fistula. **(A)** A curvilinear incision is made over the intersphincteric groove between the external opening and the anus, deepening the incision in the intersphincteric space to divide the tract just deep to the internal opening. **(B)** The opening in the internal sphincter is oversewn with long-term absorbable sutures from within the intersphincteric space. **(C)** The tract outside the external sphincter is excised, and the defects in the muscle are repaired prior to primary wound closure. (Adapted from Matos D, Lunniss, Phillips RKS. Total sphincter conservation in high fistula in ano: results of a new approach. *Br J Surg* 1993;80:802, with permission.)

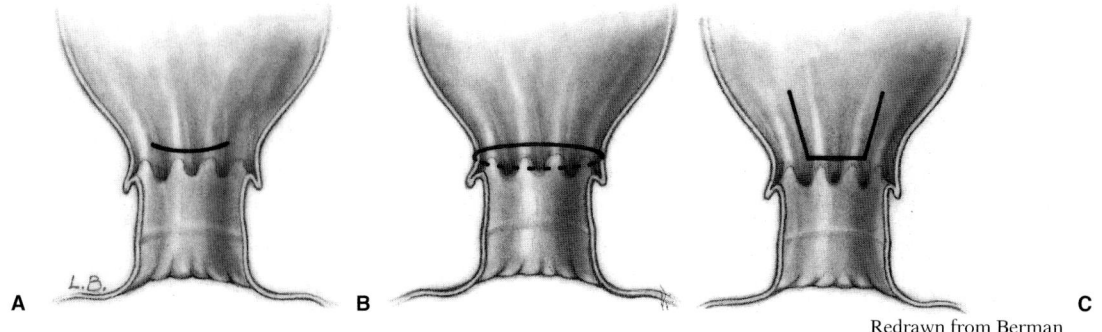

Redrawn from Berman

FIGURE 11-38. Endorectal mucosal advancement. **(A)** Semilunar flap. **(B)** Tubal or sleeve flap. **(C)** Vertical or tongue flap. (After Berman IR. Sleeve advancement anorectoplasty for complicated anorectal/vaginal fistula. *Dis Colon Rectum* 1991;34:1032, with permission.)

techniques described by Noble[97] and by Elting.[39] Berman states that the concept of endoanal or endorectal mucosal advancement has evolved into three principal methods: vertical tongue flaps, semilunar lip flaps, and circumferential tubal or sleeve flaps (Figure 11-38).[14] The concept of mucosal advancement may also be employed for the treatment of rectourethral fistula and selected rectovaginal fistulas (see Chapter 12).

Figure 11-39 describes the principles of the procedure. The incision begins *distal* to the internal opening, and the flap is mobilized, excising the scar. The method of flap construction is a matter of opinion. Some suggest an oblique incision, but this risks ischemic necrosis at the apex. Others prefer mobilization in a circumferential fashion, incorporating as much as 50% of the rectum. The dissection can be facilitated by means of infiltration with a dilute epinephrine solution. The *optimal depth* of the flap is another subject of dispute. It is the general contention that incorporating the mucosa alone is not adequate, and that part of the muscularis propria is also

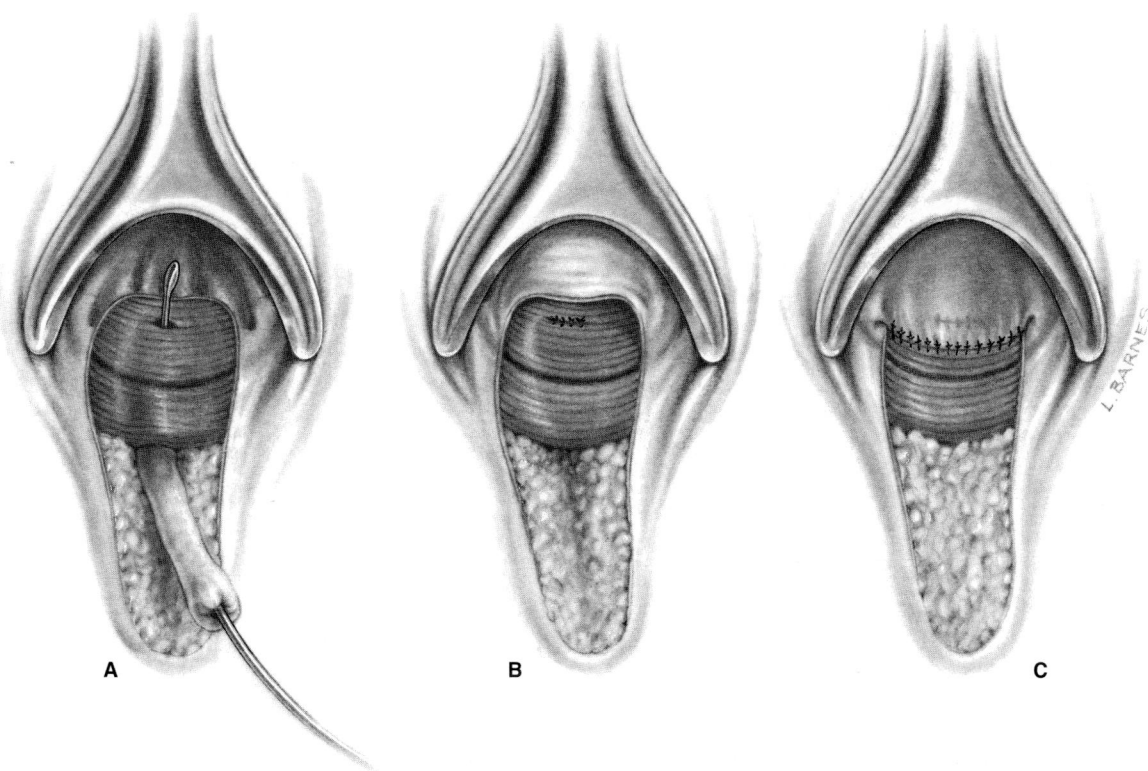

FIGURE 11-39. Mucosal advancement is performed by the following steps. **(A)** Excision of skin and mucosa with probe through fistula tract. **(B)** Repair of defect in sphincter. **(C)** Mucosa advanced and sutured over closed internal opening. (Adapted from Aguilar PS, Plasencia G, Hardy TG Jr, et al. Mucosal advancement in the treatment of anal fistula. *Dis Colon Rectum* 1985;28:496, with permission.)

required. Others believe that the flap should contain the full thickness of the rectal wall in order to limit the likelihood of dehiscence.[77] My own preference is to use at least part of the rectal wall, if not the full wall thickness, but *never* limiting it to the mucosa only. The internal opening is closed separately, perhaps in two layers.

Jun and Choi emphasize the important components of the procedure.[63] They are

- Excision of the internal opening
- Excision or curettage of the tract
- Closure of the internal opening by an anal, anorectal, rectal or anocutaneous flap
- External drainage

Realistically, the pathologic process that is illustrated in Figure 11-38 is more consistent with that of a high transsphincteric fistula than an extrasphincteric fistula. However, the principles outlined earlier are still relevant. The technique for accomplishing such a repair by means

of endorectal advancement is shown also in Figure 11-40, using the mucularis.

Management of the external portion of the tract is a matter of some controversy regarding "coring out" versus simple debridement. Because the former is often a technical *tour de force* and, in my opinion, unnecessary, I rely on debridement and gentle packing.

Berman also has suggested application of a sleeve advancement for individuals who have even more extensive fistula problems.[14] For example, a patient who has combined rectovaginal and cryptogenic fistulas may be managed by this approach. This is illustrated in Figure 11-41.

Transposition of the Fistula Tract

A unique concept in the management of extrasphincteric fistula has been proferred by Mann and Clifton. They advise rerouting the extrasphincteric portion of the tract

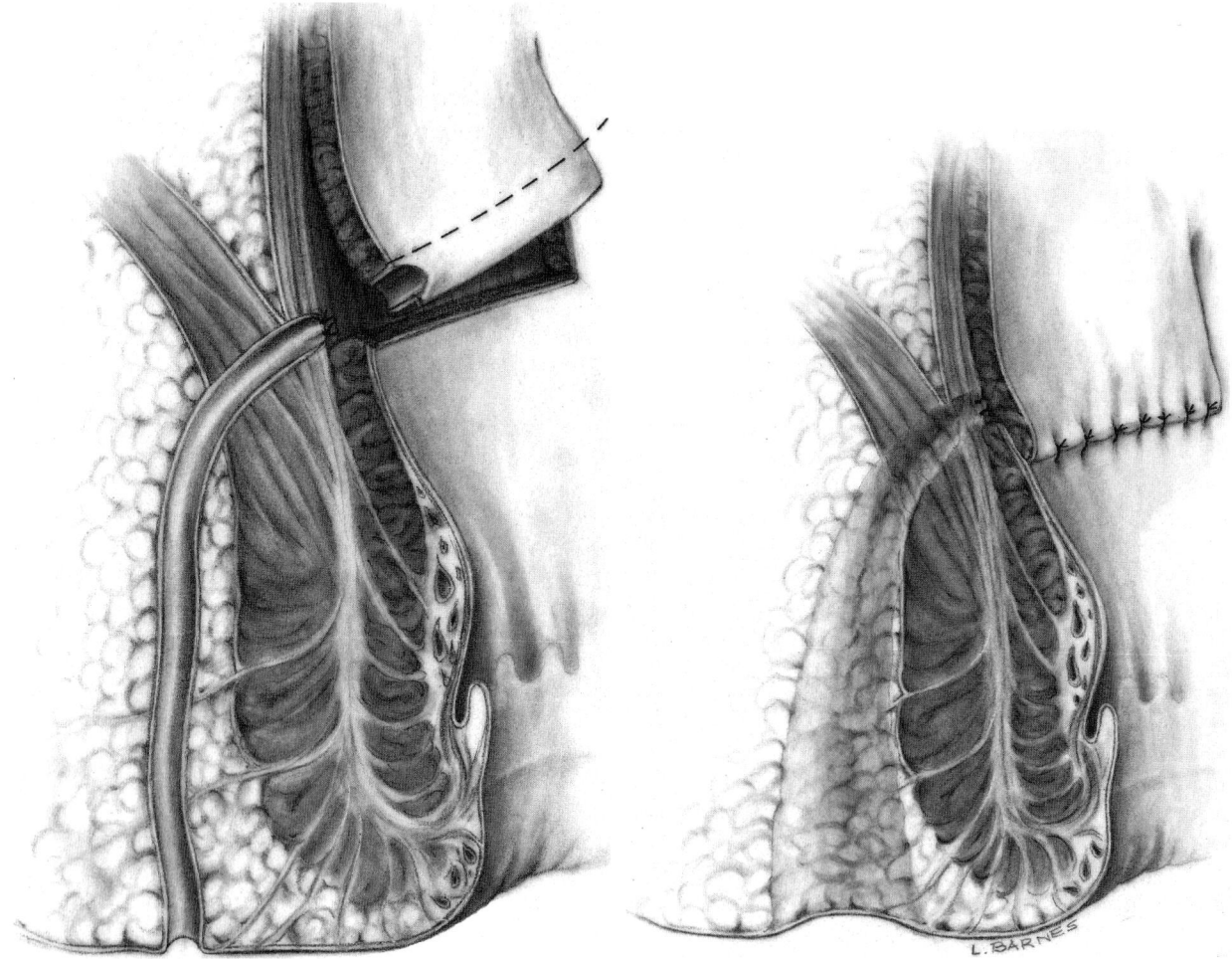

A   B

FIGURE 11-40. Extrasphincteric fistulectomy with endorectal flap advancement. A "mucosal" flap (including muscularis) is elevated, beginning distal to the opening. **(A)** The internal opening may be closed. **(B)** The "mucosa" is advanced and sutured distally. The external wound is then widely and adequately drained.

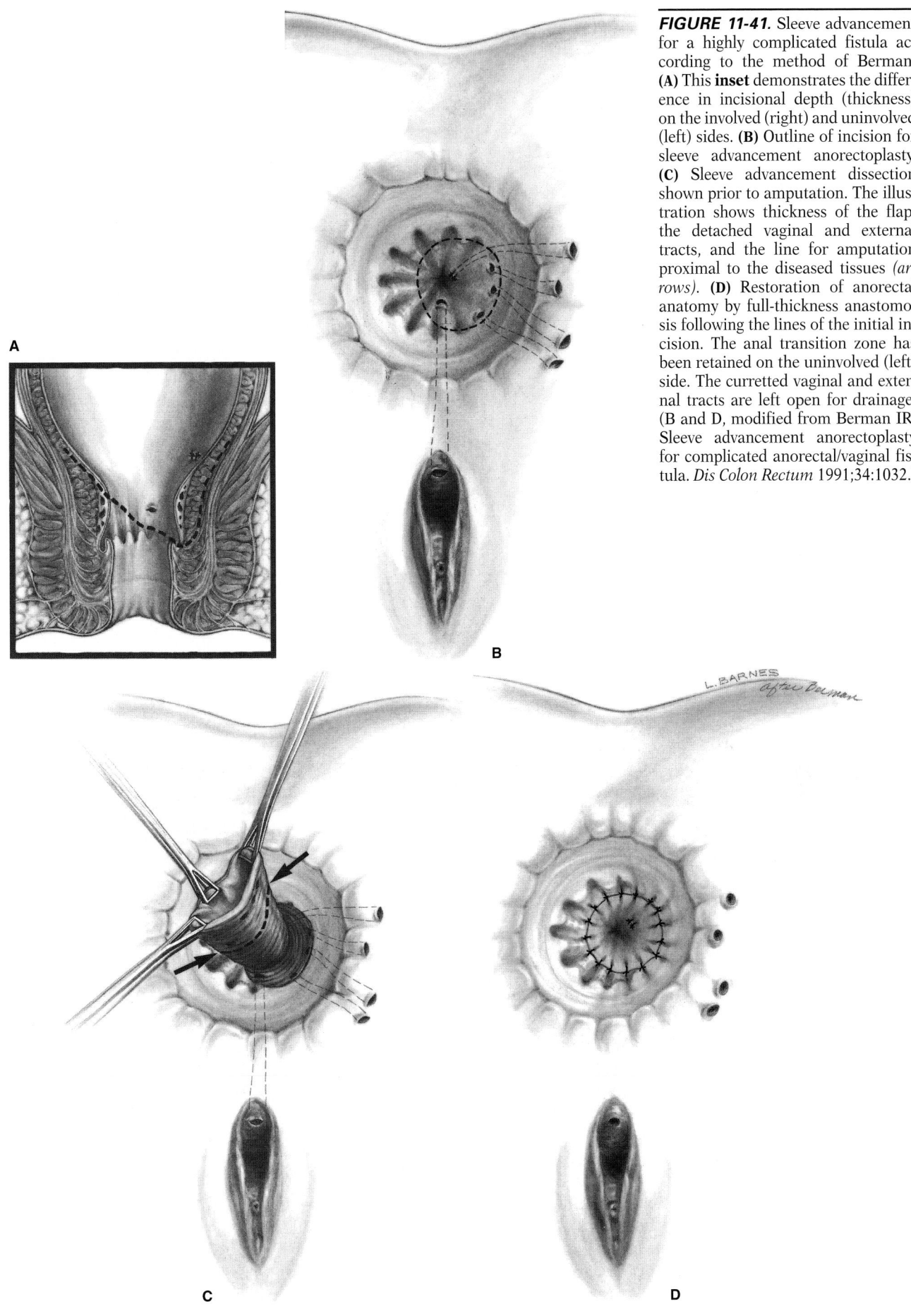

FIGURE 11-41. Sleeve advancement for a highly complicated fistula according to the method of Berman. **(A)** This **inset** demonstrates the difference in incisional depth (thickness) on the involved (right) and uninvolved (left) sides. **(B)** Outline of incision for sleeve advancement anorectoplasty. **(C)** Sleeve advancement dissection shown prior to amputation. The illustration shows thickness of the flap, the detached vaginal and external tracts, and the line for amputation proximal to the diseased tissues *(arrows)*. **(D)** Restoration of anorectal anatomy by full-thickness anastomosis following the lines of the initial incision. The anal transition zone has been retained on the uninvolved (left) side. The curretted vaginal and external tracts are left open for drainage. (B and D, modified from Berman IR. Sleeve advancement anorectoplasty for complicated anorectal/vaginal fistula. *Dis Colon Rectum* 1991;34:1032.)

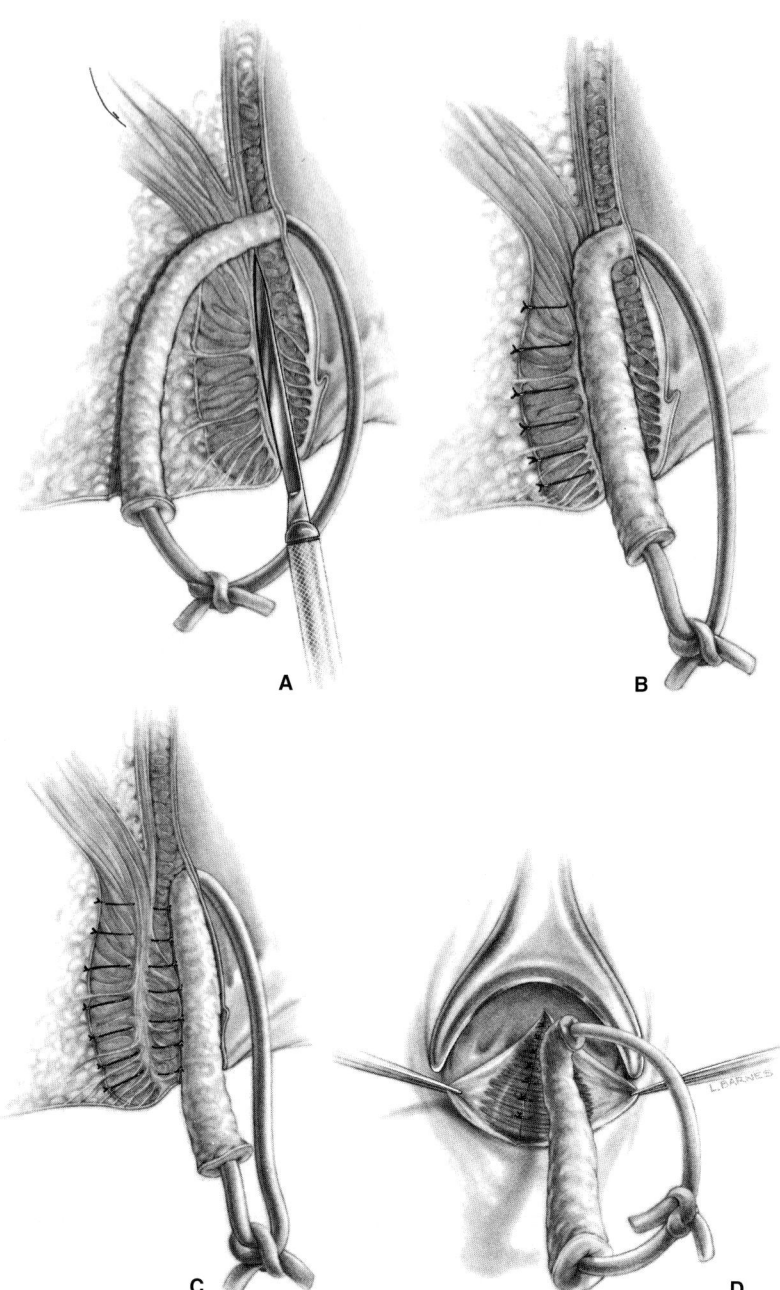

FIGURE 11-42. Transposition of the fistula tract. **(A)** Placement of a seton and division of the external sphincter. **(B)** Repair of the external sphincter with the tract now in the intersphincteric position. **(C)** The intersphincteric tract may be transposed by division and repair. **(D)** Completed fistula operation. (Adapted from Mann CV, Clifton MA. Re-routing of the track for the treatment of high and anorectal fistulae. *Br J Surg* 1985;72:134, with permission.)

into an intersphincteric position (Figure 11-42A).[85] The external sphincter is immediately repaired, and the newly positioned intersphincteric fistula is treated by a delayed procedure (Figure 11-42B). The intersphincteric tract may be further transposed at a later time into the submucous plane by division and immediate repair of the internal sphincter (Figure 11-42C). A third operation may be performed if it is elected to lay open the now submucosal fistula (Figure 11-42D). The authors reported five cases with complete healing and good functional results, but frankly it is difficult to comprehend not only how the procedure succeeds, but also how it is technically possible to accomplish. It is even more problematic than the

operation illustrated in Figure 11-37. The point is probably moot, however. There has been no further communication on this technique since the 1985 publication. One must assume that those involved have tempered their enthusiasm.

Use of Fibrin Glue

The concept of the use of fibrin as a surgical sealant of wounds and stimulant for fibroblast proliferation and collagen deposition dates back to the early 1940s. Although popular in Europe for years, it became approved in the United States only during the past decade.[136] Ini-

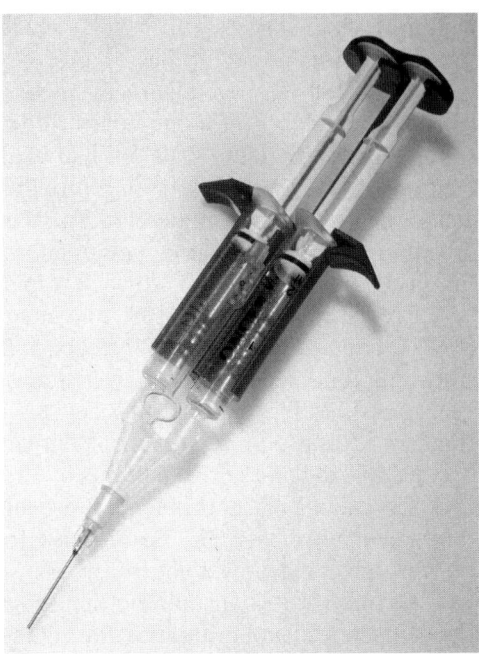

FIGURE 11-43. Tisseel Duploject System. This consists of a clip for two identical disposable syringes and a common plunger that ensures that equal volumes of the two components are fed through a common joining piece before mixing in the application needle and being ejected. (Courtesy of Baxter Healthcare Corporation, One Baxter Way, Glendale, CA.)

tially, autologous glue was formulated from the patient's own plasma or cryoprecipitate, which was then activated by mixing with thrombin.[150] The method of preparing the autologous fibrin tissue adhesive is well described by Cintron and colleagues.[27] Commercial preparations (e.g., Tisseel VH Fibrin Sealant) have since been developed that mix a fibrinogen solution with thrombin and calcium in a double syringe, in essence simulating the last stage of the clotting cascade (Figure 11-43). Fibrinolysis is inhibited by adding a specific factor.[150]

Technique

Numerous modifications for preparing the tract have been proposed. The principles (which are subject to individual variation) are as follows:

- Identify the internal and external openings of the fistula.
- Cleanse and debride the tract using a curette, gauze strip, or pipe cleaner.
- Inject the fibrin glue until it is seen exuding from the internal opening.
- Suture the internal opening closed (alternatively, Vaseline gauze compressed over each opening has also been recommended).

Sentovich recommends that a vessel loop be placed as a seton for 6 to 8 weeks before the fibrin glue treatment.[120]

Use of Polymethyl Methacrylate Beads

Kupferberg and colleagues reported the use of polymethyl methacrylate (PMMA) beads (Septopal) in the management of complex anal fistulas.[70] In five patients in whom more traditional approaches failed, all eventually healed by the gradual removal of the PMMA beads with closure of the internal opening. The bead material, used in the management of osteomyelitis, consists of a polymer impregnated with gentamicin sulfate and zirconium dioxide as a contrast medium. The authors theorize that an aseptic field that enhances wound healing is created. Further experience with the PMMA bead approach is awaited, although I have seen no further communications since this initial paper.

Other Techniques

Other approaches that can be used to manage an extrasphincteric fistula depend on its origin. These may include low anterior resection, coloanal pull-through, abdominosacral resection, and transsacral excision.[89] Rarely, a diverting colostomy alone will permit spontaneous healing, but it is reasonable to consider either a concomitant ileostomy or a colostomy when attempting a repair. This is especially true if a stoma is contemplated in the event of breakdown and recurrent fistula. When the patient has minimal symptoms, nonoperative management is a reasonable alternative (i.e., using a small dressing and sitz baths). In addition, draining an abscess if it occurs and inserting a small drain or seton in the tract may offer adequate palliation of symptoms (see later).

Results of Surgery for Anal Fistula

It is difficult to interpret the results of treatment for anal fistula for a number of reasons. One attempts to analyze variables that include an individual surgeon's personal operative preferences and technique, the type of fistula encountered, and the cause of the problem. Not only are the variables poorly defined in the numerous published papers, but also the clinical material often consists of a melange of fistula manifestations. Most important, there is a dearth of prospective, randomized trials.

The three primary criteria for determining success or failure of fistula surgery are the following:

- Recurrence
- Delayed healing
- Incontinence

A few generalizations can be made in attempting to interpret the published results:

- The more "complex" the fistula is, the higher the internal opening will be.

- The more sphincter that is divided, the longer it takes to heal, the greater the likelihood of recurrence, and the higher risk of fecal soiling.
- The most likely cause of recurrence is the failure to identify and adequately treat the internal opening.

Conventional Fistula

As mentioned, the results of surgery for anal fistula are extremely difficult to interpret from the published articles. Virtually all of the studies are retrospective and reflect the individual author's personal preference for management. Despite the fact that many of these series incorporate hundreds of patients, there is no consensus that can be derived. Generally, recurrence rates vary from 4% to 10%, with missed internal openings at the initial surgery accounting for the vast majority of such recurrences.[117] Certainly, those individuals with high openings, posterior openings, or fistula extensions are at increased risk to develop recurrence.[133] In the experience of the University of Minnesota Group, factors associated with recurrence included complex type of fistula, horseshoe extension, lack of identification or lateral location of the internal fistulous opening, prior fistula surgery, and even the variable of the surgeon.[45]

Besides the issue of recurrence, the other major concern is incontinence. This is reported to be noted in 10% to 50%. Again, from the Minnesota Group, greater than 50% complained of some degree of postoperative incontinence.[45] Articles have been published concerning manometric evaluation and anorectal function following fistula surgery.[12,114,116] The self-evident conclusion is that the more one divides or fails to preserve the sphincter, the lower the resting and squeeze pressures of the anal canal. Anorectal physiology and continence were assessed prospectively before and after surgery in 50 individuals with anal infection at St. Bartholomew's and St. Mark's Hospitals in London.[81] Functional deficit occurred in eight of 15 patients.

Parks and Stitz reviewed 158 patients treated by the senior author over a 15-year period.[103] Follow-up of at least one year was available in 142. There were 12 instances of recurrence (9%) and ten fistulas that remained unhealed (7%). The recurrences were noted with all types of fistulas, and all but two of the recurrent fistulas healed with reoperation. The authors also evaluated bowel control in their patients and found that 17% who had an intersphincteric fistula had difficulty with flatus control or occasional soiling. One third of those with transsphincteric fistulas reported one complaint or the other. It is worth recognizing, however, that, depending on the definition, no patient in either group became truly incontinent.

Hidaka and co-workers performed fistula operations on 2,242 patients, almost one half of whom underwent

"sphincter-preserving surgery."[57] They concluded that failure rates were similar and low (less than 5%).

Kuypers reported an overall recurrence rate of 4%, and a 10% incidence of some control difficulty.[72] Bennett noted in 114 patients that 12% had inadequate control for feces, 16% had poor flatus control, and 24% had frequent soiling of their underclothes.[13] Thirty-six percent of patients complained of one or more of the foregoing problems. Adams and Kovalcik reported an overall recurrence rate of 4% in 133 individuals.[2] Hill followed 476 patients for up to 20 years.[58] Delayed wound healing occurred in only seven; four experienced recurrence, and 19 had varying degrees of control difficulties. Results of treatment of fistula-in-ano were analyzed in 260 consecutive patients by Vasilevsky and Gordon.[135] Continence problems were observed in 6% and recurrence in 6.3%. Sainio and Husa reported minor defects in bowel control in 34% of their patients.[115] Of interest is their opinion that the amount of divided muscle did not influence the incidence of incontinence.

Extrasphincteric Fistula

It is virtually impossible to analyze the results of treatment for extrasphincteric fistula, because (absent Crohn's disease or a specific cause) the condition is extremely rare. Furthermore, those who do report some experience generally comingle the results or even confuse the condition with that of a high transsphincteric fistula. In the series of Parks and Stitz, only two of 13 patients who harbored extrasphincteric fistulas were incontinent. However, the method of treatment was not clearly stated.[103]

Cavanaugh and colleagues suggested that a more accurate interpretation of the functional results for fistula surgery (specifically fecal incontinence) could be achieved through the use of the Fecal Incontinence Severity Index (FISI, see Chapter 13).[23] The median score was 6, with 36% having a score of 0. As could be anticipated, direct correlation was identified with the amount of sphincter divided. Furthermore, there was an adverse effect upon quality-of-life issues (depression, embarrassment) that was directly proportional to a FISI score in excess of 30.[23]

Closure of the Internal Opening

Gustafsson and Graf reported their experience with the discredited operation of simple closure of the internal opening in 42 patients.[50] Core excision of the primary tract was performed with closure of the internal opening by suturing the internal sphincter and then mucosal layers. However, after eight cases, the authors switched to the advancement flap and combined the results.

Advancement Flap

As previously observed, one of the more popular methods for managing high anal and rectal (i.e., extrasphincteric) fistulas is the advancement flap.[35] Here again, however, the literature is confusing. Articles are published that mix extrasphincteric with transsphincteric fistulas. The advancement technique of Aguilar and colleagues was initially limited to transsphincteric horseshoe fistula, but subsequently was advocated for all fistulas when considerable sphincter muscle would otherwise be divided.[4] They noted three recurrences in 189 patients, but it is a potpourri of lesions. Wedell and colleagues employed a similar technique in 30 patients; no recurrence was observed, but one individual developed necrosis of the flap.[137] Reznick and Bailey reported seven individuals treated by this method with one recurrence (14%).[111] Oh noted that two of his 15 patients required reoperation for recurrence (13%).[98] Lewis and Bartolo applied this principle to eight people (six with Crohn's disease), all of whom had not been cured by prior fistula procedures.[77] One of the two patients without Crohn's disease experienced recurrence, as did one individual with the condition. The specific problem of fistulas in Crohn's disease is discussed later. The authors offer reasonable opinions—that healing seems more rapid than with the other methods, there is less tissue destruction, and postoperative discomfort is minimal. Certainly, bowel control should be optimal when compared with the other methods, and if recurrence develops, it is still possible to redo the repair without necessarily expecting deterioration of function.

The Cleveland Clinic group reported their experience with transanal advancement flap in the management of rectovaginal fistula and other complicated fistulas involving the anorectum.[101] There were 52 individuals with a rectovaginal fistula, 46 with anal/perineal fistulas, and three with rectourethral fistulas. Overall recurrence was seen in 29% (total 101 patients). The fact that a large percentage of these patients had Crohn's disease did not statistically affect the recurrence rates in this report.[101] Zimmerman and co-workers analyzed a consecutive series of 105 patients with respect to numerous variables that could affect the outcome.[149] These included age, sex, number of prior repair attempts, preoperative seton drainage, fistula type, presence of horseshoe extensions, location of the internal opening, postoperative drainage, body mass index, and the number of cigarettes smoked per day. Although patients with Crohn's disease were excluded from the study, the investigators found that only smoking affected the outcome of this operation.

Comment and Overview Advancement flap repair for anal fistula is today a very popular choice despite the fact that published results vary from the sublime to the woeful. The extraordinary success reported by some is especially curious because this approach is very often applied to the most complex fistula problems. For example, Jun and Choi treated 40 individuals with high transsphincteric or suprasphincteric fistulas, with only one failure.[63] Ortíz and Marzo reported a 98% success rate in 96 patients.[100] Amin and colleagues noted an 83% rate of success in their 18 patients.[7]

Sonoda and co-workers in 2001 expressed a cautionary tone with the following statement: "[While] mucosal advancement flap is effective for the treatment of fistula, . . . success may not be as optimistic as previously reported."[125] It turns out that their recurrence rate, as noted in a subsequent article, was 36%.[126] Kreis and associates were initially successful in curing 20 of 24 patients, but ultimately five more recurred, for an overall failure rate of 37.5%.[66] In all fairness to these investigators, some of the patients had Crohn's disease. Still, Zimmerman and associates reported success in only 12 of 26 patients (46%), all with high transsphincteric fistulas.[148] The Cleveland Clinic Florida group (total, 94 patients) noted a failure rate of 57% with fistulas in Crohn's disease and 33% without underlying disease, clearly a different experience from that of their Cleveland Clinic Ohio colleagues.[94]

I was pleased to read these more recent articles with the poorer results. I was beginning to think that something was wrong with my technique. My personal experience had led me to inform the patient that one in three operations will fail. In my opinion, that is simply not good enough, especially when fistulotomy (with or without a seton) will result in a 98% cure rate. However, there is a price that the patient may pay, and that is having some degree of impairment for bowel control. In my experience, it is the patient who requests an advancement flap—just like the individual who requests the tissue glue procedure. He or she has read about the alternatives and fears incontinence more than recurrence. As long as the patient is willing to trade one for the other I have no problem in attempting a less "invasive" approach. If it fails, one still has other options. As I stated out the outset, more surgeons' reputations have been impugned as a consequence of surgery for anal fistula than for any other single operation.

Seton Division

Kuypers reported his experience with the use of the seton in the treatment of extrasphincteric fistula.[71] No recurrences were observed in his ten patients; six experienced slight soiling, and one was incontinent. A more recent report from the same unit in the Netherlands included 34 patients.[134] Of the 29 patients available for follow-up, 12 had normal bowel control, five had no control for flatus, 11 were incontinent for liquid stool, and one had continued fecal leakage. The authors concluded that this technique is *not* recommended for fistulas with high openings.

Williams and colleagues reviewed their experience with 74 patients who underwent seton division of "high" anal fistulas by four techniques: staged fistulotomy, cutting seton, short-term drainage, and long-term drainage for Crohn's disease.[142] None who was treated with a cutting seton (13 patients) developed a recurrence. Minor instances of incontinence developed in 54% of those treated by two-stage fistulotomy or by cutting seton.

Pearl and colleagues, reporting from the Cook County Hospital in Chicago, accomplished seton fistulotomy in 116 patients.[104] Major fecal incontinence requiring the use of a pad occurred in 5%, with recurrent fistulas identified in 3%. The authors concluded that seton fistulotomy is a safe and effective method for treating high or complicated anorectal fistulas. García-Aguilar and co-workers retrospectively reviewed patients who were treated by seton fistulotomy or by placement of the seton to "stimulate fibrosis" and subsequent one-stage fistulotomy.[46] No difference was noted with respect to recurrence rates, incontinence, and incontinence scores. Other studies confirm the safety and efficacy of seton fistulotomy, although gas incontinence is a concern in up to 10%.[59,62,64,91]

Horseshoe Fistula

Hanley and colleagues reported their results in 41 patients with horseshoe fistula.[54] There was no problem with healing, recurrence, or incontinence using the technique previously described. Hamilton, using the same approach, reported four recurrences in 57 patients.[52] Held and colleagues noted a recurrence rate of 18% and advised more frequent use of a seton to promote drainage and to avoid premature closure.[55] Others have adopted a similar philosophy and used seton division with drainage in the management of this condition.[131] In 11 patients so treated, two developed recurrences (18.1%). Pezim also emphasized the importance deroofing the deep postanal space and achieved healing in 92% of his 24 patients.[106]

Fibrin Glue Treatment

Lindsey and colleagues randomly assigned patients to receive either fibrin glue or "conventional treatment."[78] Fibrin glue healed 50% of six individuals and 100% of those conventionally treated. Cintron and co-workers observed healing in their initial publication in 81% of their 26 patients.[27] However, long-term follow-up revealed a 46% failure rate in those who had undergone autologous fibrin tissue adhesive treatment with a 36% failure in those who received a commercially prepared fibrin sealant.[28] Sentovich reported 48 patients with a failure rate of 40%.[120] Retreatment led to healing in an additional 9%.

Buchanan and associates performed a prospective trial of healing following fibrin glue treatment, using clinical assessment and MRI to determine tract healing.[18] Twenty-two patients were followed for a median of 14 months. Despite skin healing in approximately three fourths of the patients at a median of 14 days following the procedure, only 14% remained healed at the conclusion of the study. The authors found that MRI could predict the outcome earlier than could physical examination.

Comment

I have previously commented on the issue of one's trading a higher recurrence rate for preservation of continence (see earlier). The same principle obtains for that of fibrin glue as it does for advancement flap. One who fails to comprehend the significance of these concerns to the patient does so at his or her own peril. At the risk of being redundant, this is such a litigious area, at least in the United States, that I am compelled to emphasize the potential consequences of a failure to appreciate fully the risks and alternatives in the treatment of this condition.

Special Situations

Management of Skin Defects

The use of skin grafting to treat defects in the skin that may occur following fistula operations was described rather unenthusiastically by Wilson.[145] I prefer to employ advancement or rotation flaps when scarring produces sufficient symptoms to warrant anoplasty (see Chapter 8). The methods of sphincter reconstruction to correct problems with fecal incontinence are discussed in Chapter 13.

Dual Anal Fistulas

Rarely, a patient may be found to have two anal fistulas, each with separate external and internal openings. Mazier noted an incidence of approximately 2% in 1,000 patients who presented with anal fistulas, and Hill reported a 4% incidence.[58,90]

Treatment of simultaneous low-lying fistulas consists of identifying the external and internal openings and performing fistulotomies in the standard fashion. However, consideration should certainly be given to preservation of the sphincter muscle through the use of an advancement flap or fibrin glue, because the risk of impairment for bowel control is theoretically doubled. This condition should be easily distinguished from horseshoe fistula, because the latter presentation is associated with only one internal opening.[93]

Tubercular Fistulas

Anorectal fistula on rare occasions may be a consequence of tubercular disease (see Chapter 19). Index of suspicion should be heightened in endemic countries and in patients with a history of a draining fistula for many years, the presence of multiple openings, the failure of a fistula wound to heal after 6 months following surgery, the presence of inguinal adenopathy, and the presence of caseation on histologic specimen. The diagnosis is usually established by microscopic evaluation using Ziehl-Neelsen stain and mycobacterial culture.[123]

Anal Fistula and Crohn's Disease

Fistula and abscess are among the most difficult manifestations of Crohn's disease to manage (see Chapter 30). In our experience, anal fissures, fistulas, and abscesses occurred as complications in 22% of 1,098 patients. This was more common with colonic inflammation (52%) than with small bowel involvement (14%).[141] The incidences in most other series are comparable.[21,56,68,87,144]

Clinical Features

Lesions in these patients tend to be chronic, indurated, and cyanotic, but they are often painless unless an abscess is present.[31] A typical perineum of an individual with anal Crohn's disease is shown in Figure 30-1. Alexander-Williams found that one half of his patients with anal fistula and Crohn's disease had no symptoms.[5] Skin irritation is frequently noted but may be due to diarrhea rather than to intrinsic disease of the anus. The fistula may be low lying, with an internal opening at the level of the crypt. More commonly, however, the fistula is associated with a deep ulcer, and the internal opening may either be inapparent or found in a supralevator location.

Indications and Treatment

The presence or absence of symptoms is the important criterion to determine therapy. Many individuals with fistulas are relatively asymptomatic; approximately 25% of patients in one series did not even require specific treatment.[132] At the Mayo Clinic in Rochester, Minnesota, 86 individuals were followed for a minimum of 10 years to determine the course of the disease.[146] The overall cumulative probability of avoiding proctectomy was 91.6% at 10 years and 82.5% at 20 years. Resection of all proximal Crohn's disease did not ameliorate the anorectal condition, except in those with all proximal disease removed previously *and* who had no recurrence.[146]

It has been suggested that metronidazole (Flagyl) may produce symptomatic improvement in some patients with perianal disease, but there is no irrefutable proof that fistulas are likely to close with continued therapy (see Chapter 30).[15,16]

When anal fistula occurs as a complication of the condition, it is important to distinguish between anal Crohn's disease with fistula and Crohn's disease of the intestinal tract and a coincidental fistula-in-ano. This distinction is critical, because the fistula procedure can be performed with relative safety in a patients with Crohn's

disease in whom the disease does not involve the anus, provided the abdominal condition is quiescent. A definitive fistula operation that is undertaken in the presence of active inflammatory bowel disease, however, is hazardous. The resulting wound may be a greater management problem than was the original condition (Figure 11-44). Alexander-Williams has stated that "incontinence in Crohn's disease is due to aggressive surgeons and not to progressive disease." Another important precaution is to evaluate the entire gastrointestinal tract before embarking on surgery for suspected anal Crohn's disease.

In the presence of known anal Crohn's disease, it may be possible to ameliorate the patient's condition and to relieve the discomfort associated with anal abscess and fistula without resorting to definitive fistulotomy. However, superficial fistulas of a cryptoglandular nature can be successfully treated by this method.[124]

Incision and drainage are obviously appropriate for treating perianal and ischiorectal abscesses. Makowiec and associates found that of 126 patients with Crohn's disease who were seen regularly at an outpatient clinic, almost one half developed at least one abscess during the mean follow-up period of 32 months.[84] As with abscess in the absence of Crohn's disease, the incision should be as medial as possible (see Management of Abscess in

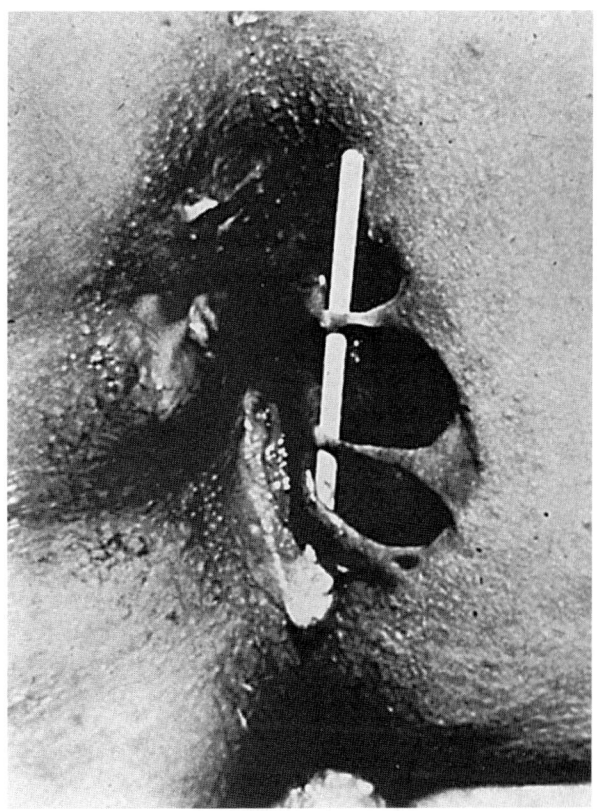

FIGURE 11-44. This indolent, ulcerating wound resulted from an ill-conceived fistulectomy in a patient with Crohn's disease. (Corman ML, et al. *Diseases of the anus, rectum and colon. Part II: inflammatory bowel disease.* New York: Medcom, 1976.)

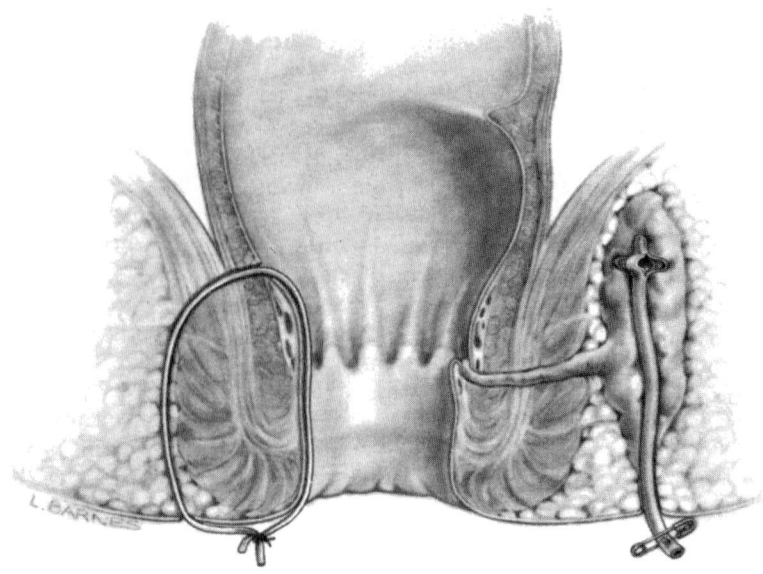

FIGURE 11-45. Sagittal view shows the seton drain in place on the **left,** with catheter drainage of the ischiorectal fossa on the **right.**

Chapter 10). Long-term, continuous drainage can be facilitated by insertion of a Pessar (i.e., mushroom) or Malecot catheter or by the application of seton drainage (Figs. 11-45 through 11-47). Another method of treating patients with Crohn's disease is to establish adequate drainage of the internal opening. This is best accomplished by excising the internal opening and the underlying internal anal sphincter in the same manner described for the treatment of intersphincteric abscess. The external opening can then be unroofed, and drainage can be established between the external sphincter and the external opening (Figure 11-48). This is not a conventional fistulotomy but is a complete drainage of the fistula on either side of the external sphincter. However, because this lesion frequently heralds the onset of intestinal manifestations, the most prudent course of action is to incise and drain the abscess when it becomes symptomatic.

A third alternative is to use a rectal mucosal advancement flap.[73] Fry and Kodner recommend placing a mushroom catheter through the external opening to permit adequate drainage (Figure 11-49).[43] If the physician wishes to attempt a definitive repair, this is the safest method for treating anterior fistulas in women, extrasphincteric fistulas, and high anal canal fistulas, especially in Crohn's disease. A fourth option, of course, is the use of fibrin glue.

Obviously, proctectomy will cure the fistula. Many individuals will be served best by removal of the rectum.

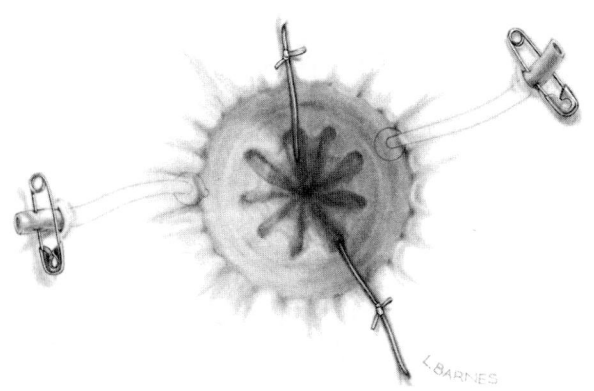

FIGURE 11-46. Seton drainage in combination with catheter drainage is an effective way to manage perineal septic problems in the patient with Crohn's disease.

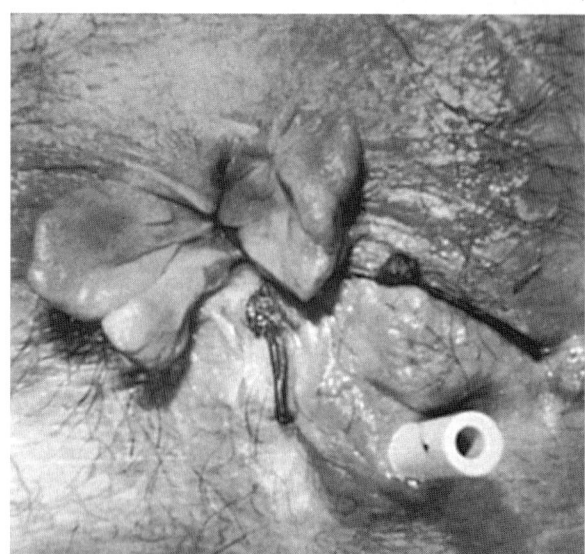

FIGURE 11-47. Perineum of a patient with Crohn's disease and multiple fistulas. Note the presence of two setons as well as a mushroom catheter to establish adequate drainage. This, one hopes, will maintain the patient in relative comfort and will obviate the need for more extensive surgical intervention.

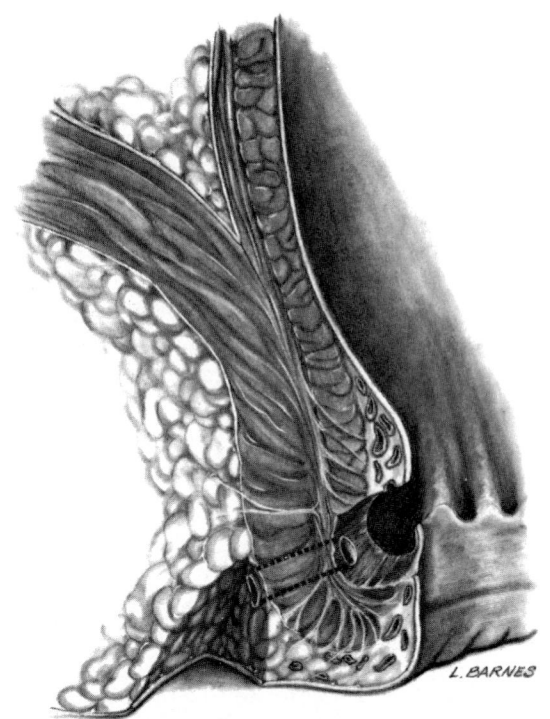

FIGURE 11-48. Treatment of a fistula in the presence of anal Crohn's disease. The internal opening and a portion of the internal sphincter are excised. The external opening has been adequately drained. A fistula tract through the external sphincter is indicated *(dotted lines);* this is not incised.

Results

Morrison and colleagues reviewed 35 patients with Crohn's disease operated on at the Ochsner Clinic in New Orleans, Louisiana.[95] With proper selection, more than 90% healed following definitive fistulotomy. Success correlated with absence of rectal disease and quiescence elsewhere in the gastrointestinal tract. The authors particularly counsel that primary fistulotomy should be avoided at the time of abscess drainage. Fry and colleagues evaluated 73 patients who underwent anorectal surgical procedures, with a mean follow-up of 4.6 years.[44] Nine healed after fecal diversion, and nine required proctectomy. Fry and others believe that anal and perianal suppurative disease can usually be managed by careful drainage, with the expectation that most can have their sphincters saved.[44,109]

Williams and colleagues reviewed the University of Minnesota experience with "aggressive" surgical treatment of anal fistula in Crohn's disease.[143] Forty-one fistulas in 33 patients were treated by conventional fistulotomy; only five of which were transsphincteric, and these were of the low variety. More than 90% were healed by 6 months, and three fourths were healed at 3 months. The authors advise that anal fistulas in Crohn's disease that involve minimal sphincter muscle can be successfully treated by definitive surgery. They further suggest that higher fistulas should be treated by seton drainage to limit symptoms and preserve function.[142,143] Topstad and co-workers used a regimen of

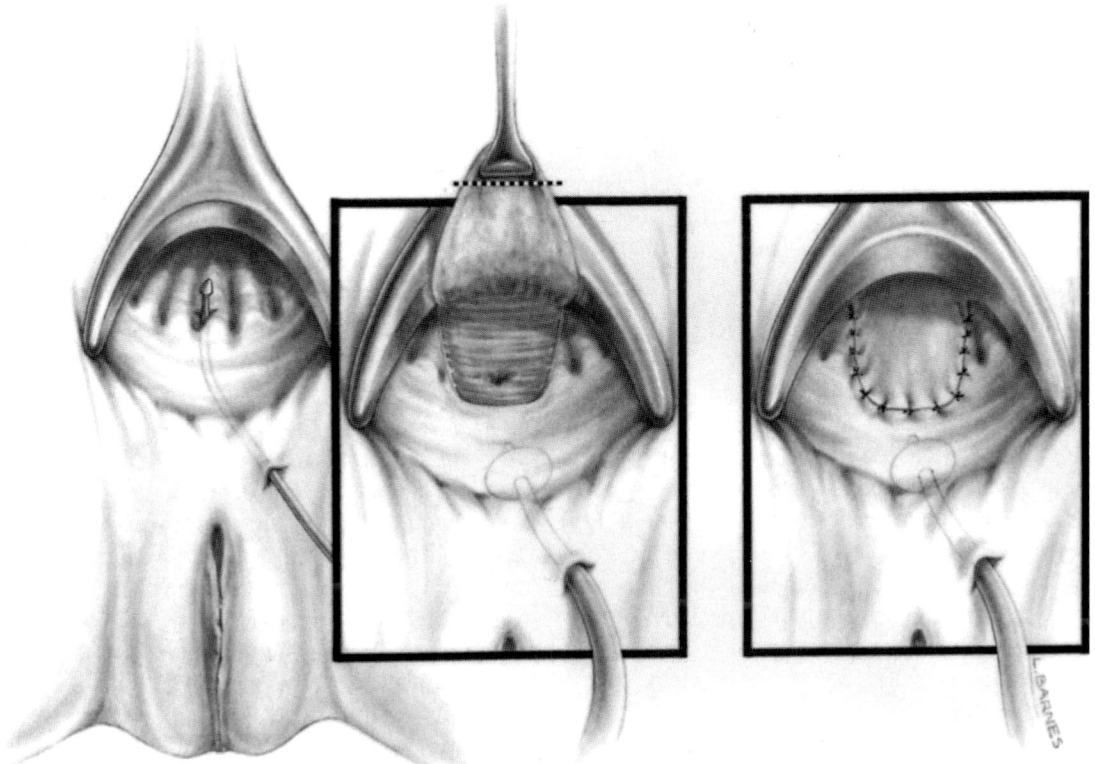

FIGURE 11-49. Advancement flap for anal fistula. This has been successfully used for fistulas in patients with Crohn's disease, with the addition of a mushroom catheter drain. The technique is otherwise comparable to the other advancement techniques. Amputation of the internal opening site is indicated *(dotted line).*

seton placement, infleximab infusion, and immunosuppresives and noted complete healing in two thirds of patients with anal fistula in Crohn's disease.[130]

With respect to advancement flap repairs for individuals with anal fistulas in association with Crohn's disease, Makowiec and colleagues reported their experience in 32 patients.[83] Of the 36 repairs performed on these individuals, four failed initially. In addition, 11 patients developed a recurrence after a median of 7 months, and a new fistula developed in six patients. Others concur, with the literature suggesting about a 50% "success rate," more or less.[86] This is true for advancement flap as well as for fibrin glue. It seems clear that the procedure is justifiable in this group of patients primarily by giving them short-term improvement without precipitating the need for more radical surgery and a permanent ostomy.

Medical treatment or a minimal surgical procedure is certainly preferred for complex fistulas, for high transsphincteric fistulas, or for extensive or active inflammatory bowel disease.[140] Proctectomy is ultimately the best option in this last group of patients. Conversely, most are willing to adopt the position that in carefully selected patients, definitive fistulotomy is a relatively safe procedure.[10,51,76,105,118,119]

Comment

In analyzing the results of treatment for anal fistulas associated with Crohn's disease, the physician is confronted with the same difficulties of interpretation that one experiences when attempting to review the literature of anal fistula in the absence of Crohn's disease. This, as well as the plethora of approaches employed and the varied presentations of the condition, may lead to confusion in the decision-making process. The following offers a reasonable starting point for developing some principles of management:

- Absence of symptoms: no treatment
- Active Crohn's disease: systemic treatment and surgical drainage, or long-term drainage only
- Quiescent Crohn's disease with anal and rectal sparing, and with superficial, intersphincteric, and low transsphincteric fistulas: definitive fistulotomy
- High transsphincter or complex fistulas: long-term drainage with consideration given to advancement flap or fibrin glue
- Low threshold for creating a "temporary" stoma concomitant with any definitive repair, especially an advancement flap

Anal Fistula and Carcinoma

Rarely, carcinoma can develop in a chronic anal fistula (Figs. 11-50 through 11-52). Getz and associates and others reported two cases and noted that there were fewer than 150 cases reported in the literature.[37,48,108] Ky and co-workers noted seven patients with carcinoma arising

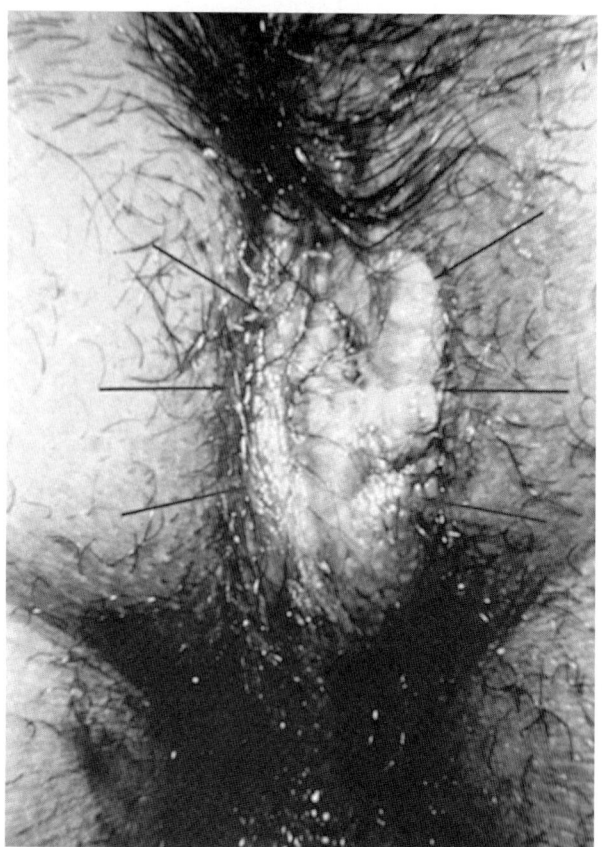

FIGURE 11-50. Adenocarcinoma *(arrows)* is seen arising in an anal fistula. (Courtesy of Daniel Rosenthal, M.D.)

in anorectal fistulas associated with Crohn's disease and identified 33 more in the literature.[73] Millar described three cases of villous tumors arising in anal fistulas.[92] Long-standing, chronic inflammation in the region of the anal glands is believed by some to lead to malignant degeneration. The presence of a tumor mass, bloody discharge, and mucin secretion are suggestive for the presence of an underlying tumor.[69] Delay in diagnosis, unfortunately, is not unusual.

Differential diagnosis includes anal canal carcinoma (e.g., epidermoid, cloacogenic) with fistula, carcinoma of the rectum with fistula, suppurative hidradenitis with malignant degeneration, and carcinoma arising in an anal duct.[40,48,96] Carcinoma of the colon has also been reported to seed into a preexisting fistula.[61,112] This observation certainly corroborates the opinion that the entire colon should be evaluated when a perianal malignancy is identified. Biopsy, especially of long-standing fistulas, is highly recommended. The importance of histologic examination of all tissues recovered from an anal fistula in an individual who is suspected of harboring a tumor is obviously extremely important.

Potentially curative treatment usually requires abdominoperineal resection, perhaps with preoperative chemoradiation therapy (see Chapters 23 and 24).

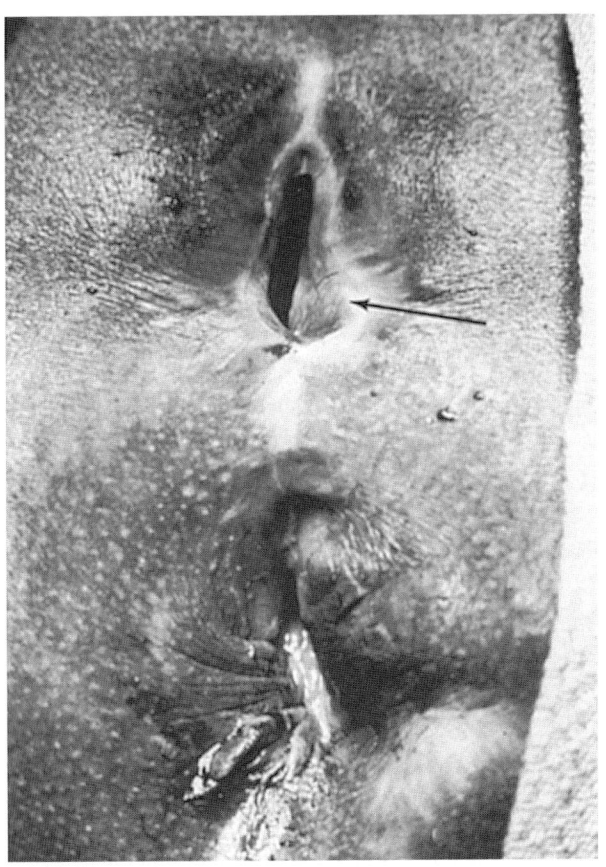

FIGURE 11-51. Squamous cell carcinoma *(arrow)* developed in a patient with a fistula that had been present for 4 years. (Courtesy of Daniel Rosenthal, M.D.)

Anal Fistula in Infants and Children

The anomaly of a congenital anal fistula without an imperforate anus is rare, representing fewer than 1% of anorectal malformations.[17] As mentioned in Chapter 10, there is an overwhelming male predominance in infants with abscess and concomitant anal fistula.[107] However, only 20% of abscesses are associated with the presence of a fistula.[82] The embryologic basis for this congenital malformation in a normally placed anus remains speculative and may not be the same for the two sexes.[17] In the experience of Duhamel, the onset of the condition in 70% was in the first 10 months of life, most arising in the first month (22%).[36] Presenting symptoms and signs include diarrhea, inguinal adenopathy, and proctitis. The fistula is usually simple, with a tract running directly between a crypt and the external opening.[36] In children, fistulas are almost always superficial and intersphincteric. Again, in the experience of Duhamel, multiple fistulas are fairly common, but these consist of separate tracts; he noted six double fistulas and four triple fistulas.[36]

Treatment consists of identification of the tract by one of the means described earlier and standard fistulotomy.[17,36,65] Recurrence or lack of healing after definitive fistulotomy should alert the physician to consider the possibility of Crohn's disease.[82]

REFERENCES

1. Abcarian H, Dodi G, Gironi J, et al. Symposium: fistula-in-ano. *Int J Colorectal Dis* 1987;2:51.
2. Adams D, Kovalcik PJ. Fistula in ano. *Surg Gynecol Obstet* 1981;153:731.

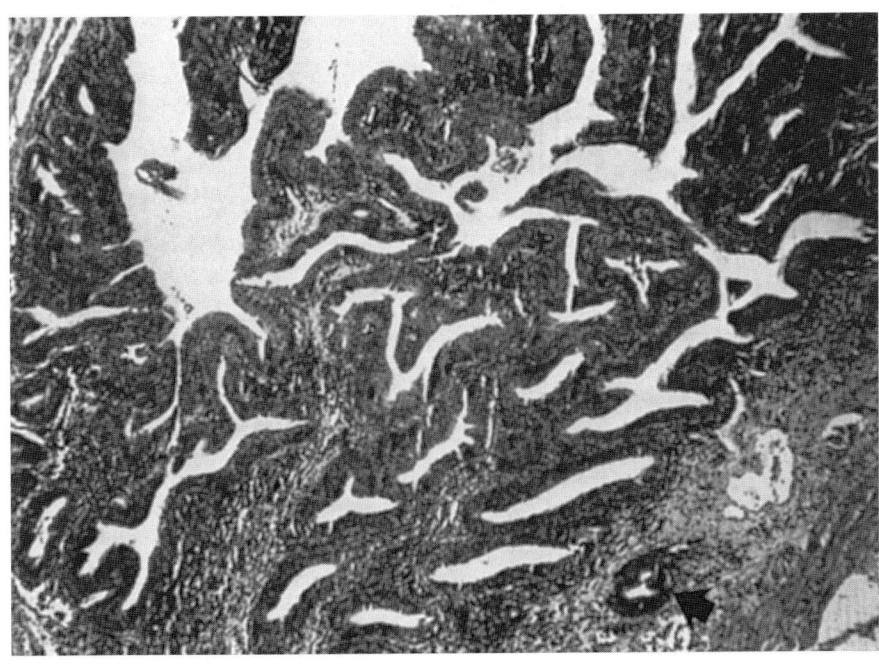

FIGURE 11-52. Adenocarcinoma arising in an anal fistula. Tortuous glandular structures are lined by proliferating epithelial cells. Note the infiltration of the wall of the fistula *(arrow)*. (Original magnification, ×260; courtesy of Rudolf Garret, M.D.)

3. Adams F. On fistulae. In: *The genuine works of Hippocrates translated from the Greek with a preliminary discourse and annotation.* New York: William Wood, 1849.

4. Aguilar PS, Plasencia G, Hardy TG Jr, et al. Mucosal advancement in the treatment of anal fistula. *Dis Colon Rectum* 1985;28:496.

5. Alexander-Williams J. Fistula-in-ano: management of Crohn's fistula. *Dis Colon Rectum* 1976;19:518.

6. Standards Task Force, American Society of Colon and Rectal Surgeons. Practice parameters for ambulatory anorectal surgery. *Dis Colon Rectum* 1991;34:285.

7. Amin SN, Tierney GM, Lund JN, et al. V-Y advancement flap for treatment of fistula in-ano. *Dis Colon Rectum* 2003; 46:540–543.

8. Ani AN, Lagundoye SB. Radiological evaluation of anal fistulae: a prospective study of fistulograms. *Clin Radiol* 1979; 30:21.

9. Arderne J. *Treatises of fistula-in-ano, hemorrhoids and clysters.* From an early fifteenth century manuscript translation as translated by D'Arcy Power. London: Kegan Paul, Trench, Trubner, 1910.

10. Bayer I, Gordon PH. Selected operative management of fistula-in-ano in Crohn's disease. *Dis Colon Rectum* 1994;37: 760.

11. Beckingham IJ, Spencer JA, Ward J, et al. Prospective evaluation of dynamic contrast enhanced magnetic resonance imaging in the evaluation of fistula in ano. *Br J Surg* 1996; 83:1396.

12. Belliveau P, Thomson JPS, Parks AG. Fistula-in-ano: a manometric study. *Dis Colon Rectum* 1983;26:152.

13. Bennett RC. A review of the results of orthodox treatment for anal fistulae. *Proc R Soc Med* 1962;55:756.

14. Berman IR. Sleeve advancement anorectoplasty for complicated anorectal/vaginal fistula. *Dis Colon Rectum* 1991; 34:1032.

15. Bernstein LH, Frank MS, Brandt LJ, et al. Healing of perineal Crohn's disease with metronidazole. *Gastroenterology* 1980;79:357.

16. Brandt LJ, Bernstein LH, Boley SJ, et al. Metronidazole therapy for perineal Crohn's disease: a follow-up study. *Gastroenterology* 1982;83:383.

17. Brem H, Guttman FM, LaBerge J-M, et al. Congenital anal fistula with normal anus. *J Pediatr Surg* 1989;24:183.

18. Buchanan GN, Bartram CI, Phillips RHK. Efficacy of fibrin sealant in the management of complex anal fistula: a prospective trial. *Dis Colon Rectum* 2003;46:1167.

19. Buchanan G, Halligan S, Williams A, et al. Magnetic resonance for primary fistula in ano. *Dis Colon Rectum* 2003; 90:877.

20. Buchanan GN, Williams AB, Bartram CI, et al. Potential clinical implications of direction of a trans-sphincteric anal fistula track. *Br J Surg* 2003;90:1250.

21. Buchmann P, Keighley MRB, Allan RN, et al. Natural history of perianal Crohn's disease. *Am J Surg* 1980;140:642.

22. Cammarota T, Discalzo L, Corno F, et al. Preliminary transrectal US experience in perianal abscesses [Italian]. *Radiol Med* 1986;72:837.

23. Cavanaugh M, Hyman N, Osler T. Fecal incontinence severity index after fistulotomy: a predictor of quality of life. *Dis Colon Rectum* 2002;45:349–353.

24. Cheong DMO, Nogueras JJ, Wexner SD, et al. Anal endosonography for recurrent anal fistulas: image enhancement with hydrogen peroxide. *Dis Colon Rectum* 1993;36: 1158.

25. Choen S, Burnett S, Bartram CI, et al. Comparison between anal endosonography and digital examination in the evaluation of anal fistulae. *Br J Surg* 1991;78:445.

26. Christensen A, Nilas L, Christiansen J. Treatment of transsphincteric anal fistulas by the seton technique. *Dis Colon Rectum* 1986;29:454.

27. Cintron JR, Park JJ, Orsay CP, et al. Repair of fistulas-in-ano using autologous fibrin tissue adhesive. *Dis Colon Rectum* 1999;42:607–613.

28. Cintron JR, Park JJ, Orsay CP, et al. Repair of fistulas-in-ano using autologous fibrin tissue adhesive: long-term follow-up. *Dis Colon Rectum* 2000;43:944–950.

29. Cirocco WC, Reilly JC. Challenging the predictive accuracy of Goodsall's rule for anal fistulae. *Dis Colon Rectum* 1992; 35:537.

30. Cirocco WC, Rusin LC. Simplified seton management for complex anal fistulas: a novel use for the rubber band ligator. *Dis Colon Rectum* 1991;34:1135.

31. Cohen Z, McLeod RS. Perianal Crohn's disease. *Gastroenterol Clin North Am* 1987;16:175.

32. Cosman, BC. All's well that ends well: Shakespeare's treatment of anal fistula. *Dis Colon Rectum* 1998;41:914.

33. Culp CE. Use of Penrose drains to treat certain anal fistulas: a primary operative seton. *Mayo Clin Proc* 1984;59: 613.

34. Keen KI, Williams JG, Hutchinson R, et al. Fistulas in ano: endoanal ultrasonographic assessment assists decision making for surgery. *Gut* 1994;35:391.

35. Del Pino A, Nelson RL, Pearl RK, et al. Island flap anoplasty for treatment of transsphincteric fistula-in-ano. *Dis Colon Rectum* 1996;39:224.

36. Duhamel J. Anal fistulae in childhood. *Am J Proctol* 1975; 26:40.

37. Dukes CE, Galvin C. Colloid carcinoma arising within fistulas in the ano-rectal region. *Ann R Coll Surg Engl* 1956; 18:246.

38. Dunphy JE, Pikula J. Fact and fancy about fistula-in-ano. *Surg Clin North Am* 1955;35:1469.

39. Elting AW. The treatment of fistula in ano. *Ann Surg* 1912; 5:744.

40. Fincato M, Corsi C, Perrone A, et al. Perianal fistulous abscesses and cloacogenic cancer. *Proctology* 1980;2:105.

41. Frenkel J. Fistula-in-ano: a new classification system for perirectal fistulas. *Dis Colon Rectum* 2002;45:A25-A28.

42. Friend WG. Anorectal problems: surgical incisions for complicated anal fistulas. *Dis Colon Rectum* 1975;18:652.

43. Fry RD, Kodner IJ. Management of anal and perineal Crohn's disease. *Infect Surg* 1989;June:209.

44. Fry RD, Shemesh EI, Kodner IJ, et al. Techniques and results in the management of anal and perianal Crohn's disease. *Surg Gynecol Obstet* 1989;168:42.

45. García-Aguilar J, Belmonte C, Wong DW, et al. Anal fistula surgery: factors associated with recurrence and incontinence. *Dis Colon Rectum* 1996;39:723.

46. García-Aguilar J, Belmonte C, Wong DW, et al. Cutting seton versus two-stage seton fistulotomy in the surgical management of high anal fistula. *Br J Surg* 1998;85:243–245.

47. García-Olmo D, Vázquez Aragón P, López Fando J. Multiple setons in the treatment of high perianal fistula. *Br J Surg* 1994;81:136.

48. Getz SB, Ough YD, Patterson RB, et al. Mucinous adenocarcinoma developing in chronic anal fistula: report of two cases and review of the literature. *Dis Colon Rectum* 1981; 24:562.

49. Goodsall DH. Anorectal fistula. In: Goodsall DH, Miles WE, eds. *Diseases of the anus and rectum,* part I. London: Longmans, Green & Co, 1900:92.

50. Gustafsson U-M, Graf W. Excision of anal fistula with closure of the internal opening: functional and manometric results. *Dis Colon Rectum* 2002;45:1672–1678.

51. Halme L, Sainio AP. Factors related to frequency, type, and outcome of anal fistulas in Crohn's Disease. *Dis Colon Rectum* 1995;38:55.

52. Hamilton CH. Anorectal problems: the deep postanal space: surgical significance in horseshoe fistula abscess: *Dis Colon Rectum* 1975;18:642.

53. Hanley PH. Conservative surgical correction of horseshoe abscess and fistula. *Dis Colon Rectum* 1965;8:364.

54. Hanley PH, Ray JE, Pennington EE, et al. Fistula-in-ano: a ten-year follow-up study of horseshoe abscess fistula-in-ano. *Dis Colon Rectum*; 1976;19:507.

55. Held D, Khubchandani I, Sheets J, et al. Management of anorectal horseshoe abscess and fistula. *Dis Colon Rectum* 1986;29:793.

56. Hellers G, Bergstrand O, Ewerth S, et al. Occurrence and outcome after primary treatment of anal fistulae in Crohn's disease. *Gut* 1980;21:525.

57. Hidaka H, Kuroki M, Hirokuni T, et al. Follow-up studies of sphincter-preserving operations for anal fistulas. *Dis Colon Rectum* 1997;40[Suppl]:107.

58. Hill JR. Fistulas and fistulous abscesses in the anorectal region: personal experience in management: *Dis Colon Rectum* 1967;10:421.

59. Ho KS, Tsang C, Seow-Choen F, et al. Prospective randomised trial comparing ayurvedic cutting seton and fistulotomy for low fistula-in-ano. *Tech Coloproctol* 2001;3:137–141.

60. Hobbiss JH, Schofield PF. Management of perianal Crohn's disease. *J R Soc Med* 1982;75:414.

61. Hyman N, Kida M. Adenocarcinoma of the sigmoid colon seeding a chronic anal fistula: report of a case. *Dis Colon Rectum* 2003;46:835–836.

62. Isbister WH, Al Sanea N. The cutting seton: an experience at King Faisal Specialist Hospital. *Dis Colon Rectum* 2001;44:722–727.

63. Jun SH, Choi GS. Anocutaneous advancement flap closure of high anal fistulas. *Br J Surg* 1999;86:490–492.

64. Kennedy M, Perera D, Sydney D. Fistula-in-ano: cutting seton in the management of fistula-in-ano. *Dis Colon Rectum* 2002;45:A25–A28.

65. Klingbeil JK, Toyama WM. Fistula-in-ano in infants and children. *Contemp Surg* 1995;46:133.

66. Kreis ME, Jehle EC, Ohlemann M, et al. Functional results after transanal rectal advancement flap repair of transsphincteric fistula. *Br J Surg* 1998;85:240–242.

67. Kronborg O. To lay open or excise a fistula-in-ano: a randomized trial. *Br J Surg* 1985;72:970

68. Kuijpers HC, Schulpen T. Fistulography for fistula-in-ano. *Dis Colon Rectum* 1985;28:103.

69. Kulaylat MN, Doerr RJ, Karamanoukian H, Barrios G. Basal cell carcinoma arising in a fistula-in-ano. *Am Surg* 1996;62:1000.

70. Kupferberg A, Zer M, Rabinson S. The use of PMMA beads in recurrent high anal fistula: a preliminary report. *World J Surg* 1984;8:970.

71. Kuypers HC. Use of the seton in the treatment of extrasphincteric anal fistula. *Dis Colon Rectum* 1984;27:109.

72. Kuypers JHC. Diagnosis and treatment of fistula-in-ano. *Neth J Surg* 1982;34:147.

73. Ky A, Sohn N, Weinstein MA, et al. Carcinoma arising in anorectal fistulas of Crohn's disease. *Dis Colon Rectum* 1998;41:992.

74. Law PJ, Talbot RW, Bartram CI, et al. Anal endosonography in the evaluation of perianal sepsis and fistula in ano. *Br J Surg* 1989;76:752.

75. Lenter A, Wienert V. Long-term, indwelling setons for low transsphincteric and intersphincteric anal fistulas: experience with 108 cases. *Dis Colon Rectum* 1996;39:1097.

76. Levien DH, Surrell J, Mazier WP. Surgical treatment of anorectal fistula in patients with Crohn's disease. *Surg Gynecol Obstet* 1989;169:133.

77. Lewis P, Bartolo DCC. Treatment of trans-sphincteric fistulae by full thickness anorectal advancement flaps. *Br J Surg* 1990;77:1187.

78. Lindsey I, Smilgin-Humphreys MM, Cunningham C, et al. A randomized, controlled trial of fibrin glue vs. conventional treatment for anal fistula. *Dis Colon Rectum* 2002;45:1608–1615.

79. Loberman Z, Har-Shai Y, Schein M, et al. Hangman's tie simplifies seton management of anal fistulas. *Surg Gynecol Obstet* 1993;177:413.

80. Lunniss PJ, Barker PG, Sultan AH, et al. Magnetic resonance imaging of fistula-in-ano. *Dis Colon Rectum* 1994;37:708.

81. Lunniss PJ, Kamm MA, Phillips RKS. Factors affecting continence after surgery for anal fistula. *Br J Surg* 1994;81:1382.

82. Macdonald A, Wilson-Storey D, Munro F. Treatment of perianal abscess and fistula-in-ano in children. *Br J Surg* 2003;90:220–221.

83. Makowiec F, Jehle EC, Becker H-D, et al. Clinical course after transanal advancement flap repair of perianal fistula in patients with Crohn's disease. *Br J Surg* 1995;82:603.

84. Makowiec F, Jehle EC, Becker H-D, et al. Perianal abscess in Crohn's disease. *Dis Colon Rectum* 1997;40:443.

85. Mann CV, Clifton MA. Re-routing of the track for the treatment of high anal and anorectal fistulae. *Br J Surg* 1985;72:134.

86. Marchesa P, Hull TL, Fazio VW. Advancement sleeve flaps for treatment of severe perianal Crohn's disease. *Br J Surg* 1998;85:1695.

87. Marks CG, Ritchie JK, Lockhart-Mummery HE. Anal fistulas in Crohn's disease. *Br J Surg* 1981;68:525.

88. Matos D, Lunniss PJ, Phillips RKS. Total sphincter conservation in high fistula in ano: results of a new approach. *Br J Surg* 1993;80:802.

89. Maxwell-Armstrong CA, Phillips RKS. Extrasphincteric rectal fistulas treated successfully by Soave's procedure despite marked local sepsis. *Br J Surg* 2003;90:237.

90. Mazier WP. The treatment and care of anal fistulas: a study of 1,000 patients. *Dis Colon Rectum* 1971;14:134.

91. McCourtney JS, Finlay IG. Cutting seton without preliminary internal sphincterotomy in management of complex high fistula-in-ano. *Dis Colon Rectum* 1996;39:55.

92. Millar DM. Villous neoplasms in anorectal fistulas. *Proctology* 1979;2:50.

93. Mirelman D, Corman ML. Dual anal fistulas: an uncommon manifestation of fistula-in-ano. *Dis Colon Rectum* 1978;21:54.

94. Mizrahi N, Wexner SD, Zmora O, et al. Endorectal advancement flap: are there predictors of failure? *Dis Colon Rectum* 2002;45:1616–1621.

95. Morrison JG, Gathright JB Jr, Ray JE, et al. Surgical management of anorectal fistulas in Crohn's disease. *Dis Colon Rectum* 1989;32:492.

96. Nelson RL, Prasad L, Abcarian H. Anal carcinoma presenting as a perirectal abscess or fistula. *Arch Surg* 1985;120:632.

97. Noble GH. A new operation for complete laceration of the perineum designed for the purpose of eliminating danger of infection from the rectum. *Trans Am Gynecol Soc* 1902;27:357.

98. Oh C. Management of high recurrent anal fistula. *Surgery* 1983;93:330.

99. Orsoni P, Barthet M, Portier F, et al. Prospective comparison of endosonography, magnetic resonance imaging and surgical findings in anorectal fistula and abscess complicating Crohn's disease. *Br J Surg* 1999;86:360–364.

100. Ortíz H, Marzo J. Endorectal flap advancement repair and fistulectomy for high trans-sphincteric and suprashpincteric fistulas. *Br J Surg* 2000;87:1680–1683.

101. Ozuner G, Hull TL, Cartmill J, et al. Long-term analysis of the use of transanal rectal advancement flaps for complicated anorectal/vaginal fistulas. *Dis Colon Rectum* 1996;39:10.

102. Parks AG, Gordon PH, Hardcastle JD. A classification of fistula-in-ano. *Br J Surg* 1976;63:1.

103. Parks AG, Stitz RW. The treatment of high fistula-in-ano. *Dis Colon Rectum* 1976;19:487.

104. Pearl RK, Andrews JR, Orsay CP, et al. Role of the seton in the management of anorectal fistulas. *Dis Colon Rectum* 1993;36:573.

105. Pescatori M, Interisano A, Basso L, et al. Management of perianal Crohn's disease. *Dis Colon Rectum* 1995;38:121.

106. Pezim ME. Successful treatment of horseshoe fistula requires deroofing of deep postanal space. *Am J Surg* 1994;167:513.

107. Piazza DJ, Radhakrishnan J. Perianal abscess and fistula-in-ano in children. *Dis Colon Rectum* 1990;33:1014.

108. Prioleau PG, Allen MS Jr, Roberts T. Perianal mucinous adenocarcinoma. *Cancer* 1977;39:1295.

109. Pritchard TJ, Schoetz DJ, Roberts PL, et al. Perirectal abscess in Crohn's disease: drainage and outcome. *Dis Colon Rectum* 1990;33:933.

110. Ramanujam PS, Prasad ML, Abcarian H. The role of seton in fistulotomy of the anus. *Surg Gynecol Obstet* 1983;157:419.

111. Reznick RK, Bailey HR. Closure of the internal opening for treatment of complex fistula-in-ano. *Dis Colon Rectum* 1988;31:116.

112. Rollinson PD, Dundas SAC. Adenocarcinoma of sigmoid colon seeding into pre-existing fistula. *Br J Surg* 1984;71:664.

113. Safavi A, Gottesman L, Dailey TH. Anorectal surgery in the HIV+ patient: update. *Dis Colon Rectum* 1991;34:299.

114. Sainio P. A manometric study of anorectal function after surgery for anal fistula, with special reference to incontinence. *Acta Chir Scand* 1985;151:695.

115. Sainio P, Husa A. Fistula-in-ano: clinical features and long-term results in 199 adults. *Acta Chir Scand* 1985;151:169.

116. Sainio P, Husa A. A prospective manometric study of the effect of anal fistula surgery on anorectal function. *Acta Chir Scand* 1985;151:279.

117. Sangwan YP, Rosen L, Riether RD, et al. Is simple fistula-in-ano simple? *Dis Colon Rectum* 1994;37:885.

118. Sangwan YP, Schoetz DJ Jr, Murray JJ, et al. Perianal Crohn's disease: results of local surgical treatment. *Dis Colon Rectum* 1996;39:529.

119. Scott HJ, Northover JMA. Evaluation of surgery for perianal Crohn's fistulas. *Dis Colon Rectum* 1996;39:1039.

120. Sentovich SM. Fibrin glue for anal fistulas: long-term results. *Dis Colon Rectum* 2003;46:498–502.

121. Seow-Choen, Phillips RKS. Insights gained from the management of problematical anal fistulae at St. Mark's Hospital, 1984–88. *Br J Surg* 1991;78:539.

122. Shah N, Remzi F, Massmann A, et al. Fistula-in-ano: management and treatment outcome of pouch-vaginal fistulas following restorative proctocolectomy. *Dis Colon Rectum* 2002;45:A25–A28.

123. Shan Y-S, Yan J-J, Sy ED, et al. Nested polymerase chain reaction in the diagnosis of nagative Ziehl-Neelsen stained *Mycobacterium tuberculosis* fistula-in-ano: report of four cases. *Dis Colon Rectum* 2002;45:1685–1688.

124. Sohn N, Korelitz BI, Weinstein MA. Anorectal Crohn's disease: definitive surgery for fistulas and recurrent abscesses. *Am J Surg* 1980;139:394.

125. Sonoda T, Hull T, Piedmonte M. Factors affecting successful repair of anal fistulas using mucosal advancement flap (MAF). *Dis Colon Rectum* 2001:44:A27–A59.

126. Sonoda T, Hull T, Piedmonte MR, et al. Outcomes of primary repair of anorectal and rectovaginal fistulas using the endorectal advancement flap. *Dis Colon Rectum* 2002;45:1622–1628.

127. Standards Practice Task Force, American Society of Colon and Rectal Surgeons. Practice parameters for treatment of fistula-in-ano. *Dis Colon Rectum* 1996;39:1361.

128. Stoker J, Rociu E, Wiersma TG, et al. Imaging of anorectal disease. *Br J Surg* 2000;87:10–27.

129. Thompson JE Jr, Bennion RS, Hilliard G. Adjustable seton in the management of complex anal fistula. *Surg Gynecol Obstet* 1989;169:551.

130. Topstad DR, Panaccione R, Heine JA, et al. Combined seton placement, infliximab infusion, and maintenance immunosuppressives improve healing rate in fistulizing anorectal crohn's disease: a single center experience. *Dis Colon Rectum* 2003;46:577–583.

131. Ustynoski K, Rosen L, Stasik J, et al. Horseshoe abscess fistula. *Dis Colon Rectum* 1990;33:602.

132. van Dongen LM, Lubbers E-JC. Perianal fistulas in patients with Crohn's disease. *Arch Surg* 1986;121:1187.

133. van Tets WF, Kuijpers HC. Continence disorders after anal fistulotomy. *Dis Colon Rectum* 1994;37:1194.

134. van Tets WF, Kuijpers JHC. Seton treatment of perianal fistula with high anal or rectal opening. *Br J Surg* 1995;82:895.

135. Vasilevsky C-A, Gordon PH. The incidence of recurrent abscesses or fistula-in-ano following anorectal suppuration. *Dis Colon Rectum* 1984;27:126.

136. Venkatesh KS, Ramanujam P. Fibrin glue application in the treatment of recurrent anorectal fistulas. *Dis Colon Rectum* 1999;42:1136.

137. Wedell J, Meier zu Eissen P, Banzhaf G, et al. Sliding flap advancement for the treatment of high level fistulae. *Br J Surg* 1987;74:390.

138. Weisman RI, Orsey CP, Pearl RK, et al. The role of fistulography in fistula-in-ano: report of five cases. *Dis Colon Rectum* 1991;34:181.

139. West RL, Zimmerman DDE, Dwarkasing S, et al. Prospective comparison of hydrogen peroxide-enhanced three dimensional endoanal endosonography and endoanal magnetic resonance imaging of perianal fistulas. *Dis Colon Rectum* 2003;46:1407.

140. White RA, Eisenstat TE, Rubin RJ, et al. Seton management of complex anorectal fistulas in patients with Crohn's disease. *Dis Colon Rectum* 1990;33:587.

141. Williams DR, Coller JA, Corman ML, et al. Anal complications in Crohn's disease. *Dis Colon Rectum* 1981;24:22.

142. Williams JG, MacLeod CA, Rothenberger DA, et al. Seton treatment of high anal fistulae. *Br J Surg* 1991;78:1159.

143. Williams JG, Rothenberger DA, Nemer FD, et al. Fistula-in-ano in Crohn's disease: results of aggressive surgical treatment. *Dis Colon Rectum* 1991;34:378.

144. Williams NS, MacFie J, Celestin LR. Anorectal Crohn's disease. *Br J Surg* 1979;66:743.

145. Wilson E. Skin grafts in surgery for anal fistula. *Dis Colon Rectum* 1969;12:327.

146. Wolff BG, Culp CE, Beart RW Jr, et al. Anorectal Crohn's disease: a long-term perspective. *Dis Colon Rectum* 1985;28:709.

147. Zbar AP, deSouza NM, Puni R, et al. Comparison of endoanal magnetic resonance imaging with surgical findings in perirectal sepsis. *Br J Surg* 1998;85:111–114.

148. Zimmerman DDE, Briel JW, Gosselink MP, et al. Anocutaneous advancement flap repair of transsphincteric fistulas. *Dis Colon Rectum* 2001:44:1474–1480.

149. Zimmerman DDE, Delemarre JBVM, Gosselink MP, et al. Smoking affects the outcome of transanal mucosal advancement flap repair of trans-sphincteric fistulas. *Br J Surg* 2003;90:351–354.

150. Zmora O, Mizrahi N, Rotholtz N, et al. Fibrin glue sealing in the treatment of perineal fistulas. *Dis Colon Rectum* 2003;46:584–589.

Rectovaginal and Rectourethral Fistulas

Mothers love their children more than fathers,
because parenthood costs the mothers more trouble.
Aristotle: *Nicomachean Ethics,* IX, vii

RECTOVAGINAL FISTULA

Anovaginal or rectovaginal fistula is not usually a manifestation of anal fistula, because it is rarely a consequence of cryptoglandular infection. The condition most commonly occurs following trauma, especially obstetric injury. Venkatesh and colleagues studied the incidence of complications following vaginal delivery in 20,500 women.[66] Five percent of all normal deliveries resulted in episiotomy-associated third- and fourth-degree lacerations. Of the fourth-degree lacerations, 10% disrupted after primary repair.

In addition to obstetrically related causes, other etiologic factors related to the development of rectovaginal fistula include the following:

- Inflammatory bowel disease—the second most frequent cause (Figure 12-1)
- Carcinoma
- Radiation
- Diverticulitis
- Foreign body
- Penetrating trauma
- Infectious processes
- Congenital anomalies
- Pelvic, perineal, and rectal surgery, especially vaginal hysterectomy and low anterior resection
- Anorectal eroticism
- Ergstnmine-induced[22]

Symptoms and Classification

Patients usually complain of passage of flatus, feces, or pus from the vagina. Depending on the etiology, location, extent, and associated injury, the woman may also have difficulty with the control of flatus and feces per rectum.

I prefer to categorize the fistula on the basis of its level in the anal or rectal opening, that is, anal, low rectal, or high rectal. The equivalent gynecologic classification is low vaginal, midvaginal, and high vaginal. The location of the fistula is important, because it will determine the operative approach.

A low fistula is usually readily apparent on inspection or upon anoscopy. One usually has little difficulty in identifying the tract and passing a probe, but careful assessment of the tone and contractility of the muscle above the fistula should be made. A midrectal (midvaginal) fistula is also relatively easy to visualize, particularly when one attempts to pass a probe from vagina to rectum. A high fistula may be quite difficult to diagnose, especially if the opening is small. This type is usually a complication of diverticulitis or of hysterectomy. It may also develop as a consequence of an anastomotic leak or staple injury following low anterior resection (Figure 12-2).

Evaluation

Physical examination should include both rectal and vaginal evaluations. Proctosigmoidoscopic examination and gastrointestinal contrast studies may be indicated, especially if there is doubt concerning the origin of the fistula. With high fistulas, proctosigmoidoscopic examination seldom will demonstrate the opening, but gentle probing at the apex of the vagina will often identify the defect. Barium enema examination may show opacification of the vagina (Figure 12-3). A biopsy should be performed if the fistula is secondary to radiation injury in order to determine the presence or absence of tumor.

If the patient's symptoms are characteristic, but the surgeon is unable to confirm a fistula by one of the foregoing means, there are two other approaches worth attempting. One procedure is to place the patient in the lithotomy position and insert a proctoscope in the rectum. With the woman in a slight Trendelenburg position, the vagina is filled with warm water. Air is then insufflated through the proctoscope; if bubbles are seen in the vagina, the diagnosis is confirmed. Another alternative is to give the patient a methylene blue small retention enema and leave a tampon in the vagina. The tampon is removed after 1 hour to see whether the blue color appears on it.

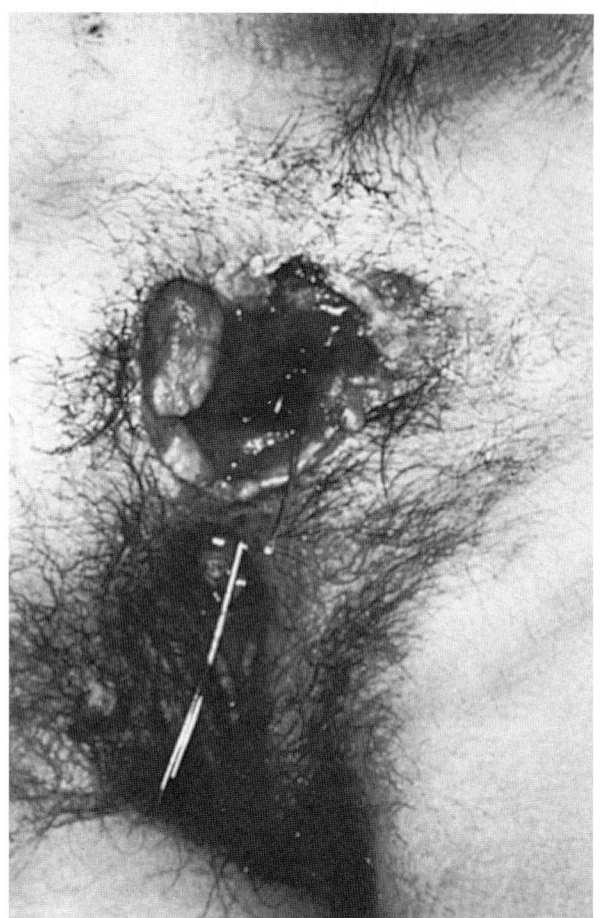

FIGURE 12-1. Rectovaginal fistula secondary to Crohn's disease. Note the marked disruption of the anal architecture.

Depending on the origin of the fistula, it may be appropriate to evaluate the proximal colon before definitive repair. This is usually readily accomplished by means of either colonoscopy or barium enema examination. Occasionally, however, it may be difficult to advance the endoscope above the fistula site, and contrast may preferentially pass completely out of the vagina. Under these circumstances, a combination of guidewire passage of the instrument and placement of a Foley catheter above the communication will facilitate proximal evaluation.[58]

Yee and co-workers reviewed their experience with endoanal ultrasound in patients with rectovaginal fistulas in order to define what role this modality has in preoperative assessment.[70] Although the authors believed that noncontrast ultrasound was not helpful for evaluation, they recommended its use in order to identify occult sphincter defects. The primary purpose, therefore, is to alert the surgeon to consider performing a sphincter reconstruction, but because I *always* undertake a sphincter repair whenever I treat the condition (with the exception of an advancement flap), the point for me is moot.

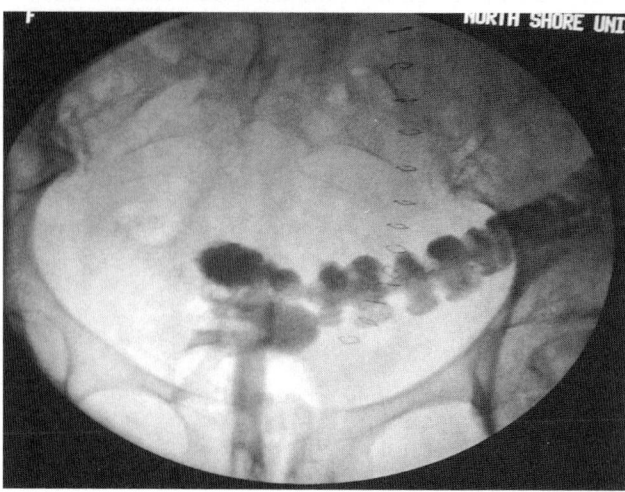

FIGURE 12-2. Barium enema reveals contrast material in the vagina as a consequence of the stapling device incorporating a portion of the posterior vaginal wall.

Treatment

As suggested, the treatment of rectovaginal fistula depends on the location and the cause. High rectovaginal fistulas are generally approached transabdominally and involve a bowel resection if colon or rectal disease precipitated the communication. If the fistula occurred secondary to hysterectomy, it may suffice to separate the bowel from the vagina, close the opening, and interpose omentum, a peritoneal flap, or fascia. For midvaginal and low rectovaginal fistulas, numerous operative approaches have been advocated, including transvaginal, perineal, transanal, and transsphincteric. One operation that should not be done, however, even for anovaginal or introital fistulas, is simple fistulotomy. Dividing the perineum, even for a relatively superficial fistula, will inevitably cause some degree of incontinence (see Chapter 11).[52] The following summarizes the various operative alternatives:

Operations for Rectovaginal Fistula

Perineal
    Fistulotomy alone
    Fistulotomy with muscle repair
       Anoplasty
    Interposition [e.g., bulbocavernosus-labial flap
       (Martius)
Transanal
    Repair in layers
    Repair in layers with sliding flap
       Anterior rectal wall
       Internal sphincter
Transsphincteric (Mason)

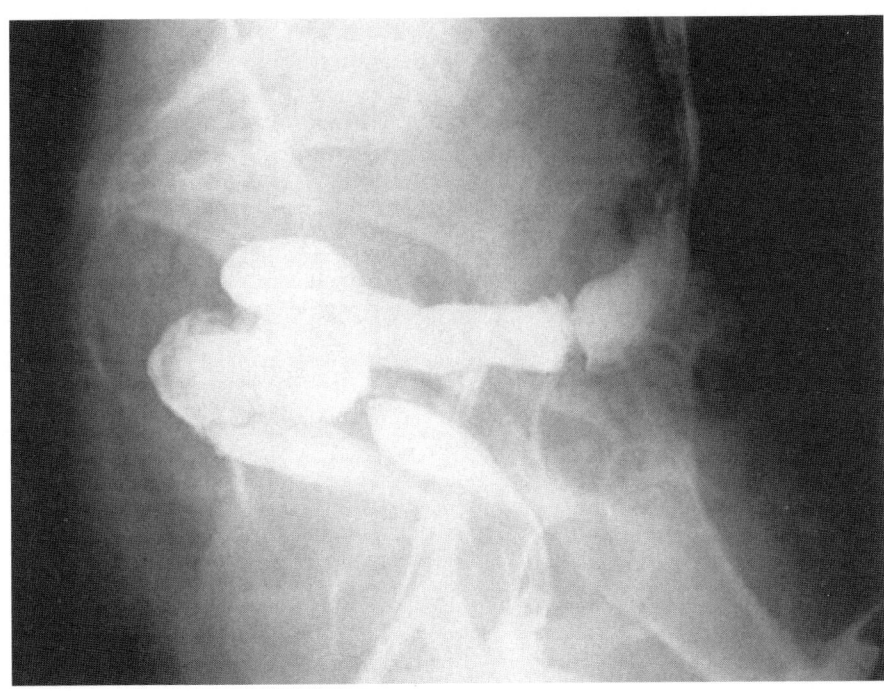

FIGURE 12-3. Rectovaginal fistula following hysterectomy. A barium enema demonstrates contrast material in the vagina.

Transvaginal
  Repair in layers
    With sliding vaginal flap (Warren)
    With interposition
Abdominal
  Simple closure
    With interposition
  Resection (low anterior, pull-through, abdominosacral, coloanal)
    With interposition
  Colostomy

The following discussion is confined to low-level and midlevel fistulas. Operations that require an abdominal approach are similar to those performed for other conditions; these are discussed in Chapters 22 and 23.

My own preference is to place the patient on a mechanical bowel preparation as if for colon resection. This includes a vigorous laxative 1 day before and a tap water enema the morning of surgery until the returns are clear. Others suggest that no cleanout is required, but even if there is no demonstrable increase in septic complications or breakdown of the repair, I personally do not enjoy wallowing in stool. Broad-spectrum intravenous antibiotics are also suggested within one half hour of incision time. A Foley catheter should be inserted before surgery and kept in place as long as is reasonable or convenient. Standard vaginal antiseptic preparation should be performed at the time of surgery.

Techniques for Repair of Anovaginal and Low Rectovaginal Fistulas

Any attempt at repair must primarily address the anal or rectal opening, even though the fistula may have arisen from a vaginal source (e.g., obstetric trauma). Many surgeons and all gynecologists prefer to repair a rectovaginal fistula using the transvaginal approach.[61] This is not recommended, because the high-pressure zone is in the rectum. If the repair of the rectal opening is satisfactorily accomplished, it is not even necessary to deal with the vagina. Conversely, no matter how meticulous the technique is when performed through the vagina, if the rectal closure does not remain secure, failure will result.

With an anal canal or low-rectal fistula occurring as a consequence of an obstetric injury, my preference is to perform a perineal operation with a concomitant anoplasty and sphincteroplasty (see Chapter 13). The reason I believe this to be necessary is that the condition is usually the result of an ectopic location—anterior displacement of the rectum (i.e., the anal opening is abnormally close to the vagina) (see Figs. 13-26 through 13-37). Many of these patients will have significant impairment for the control of feces even if they do not actually have a rectovaginal fistula. To effect a satisfactory repair, the surgeon should reconstruct the perineal body, and to accomplish this, an anoplasty is, in my opinion, preferred.[14,53] The operative technique for this procedure is discussed in Chapter 13.

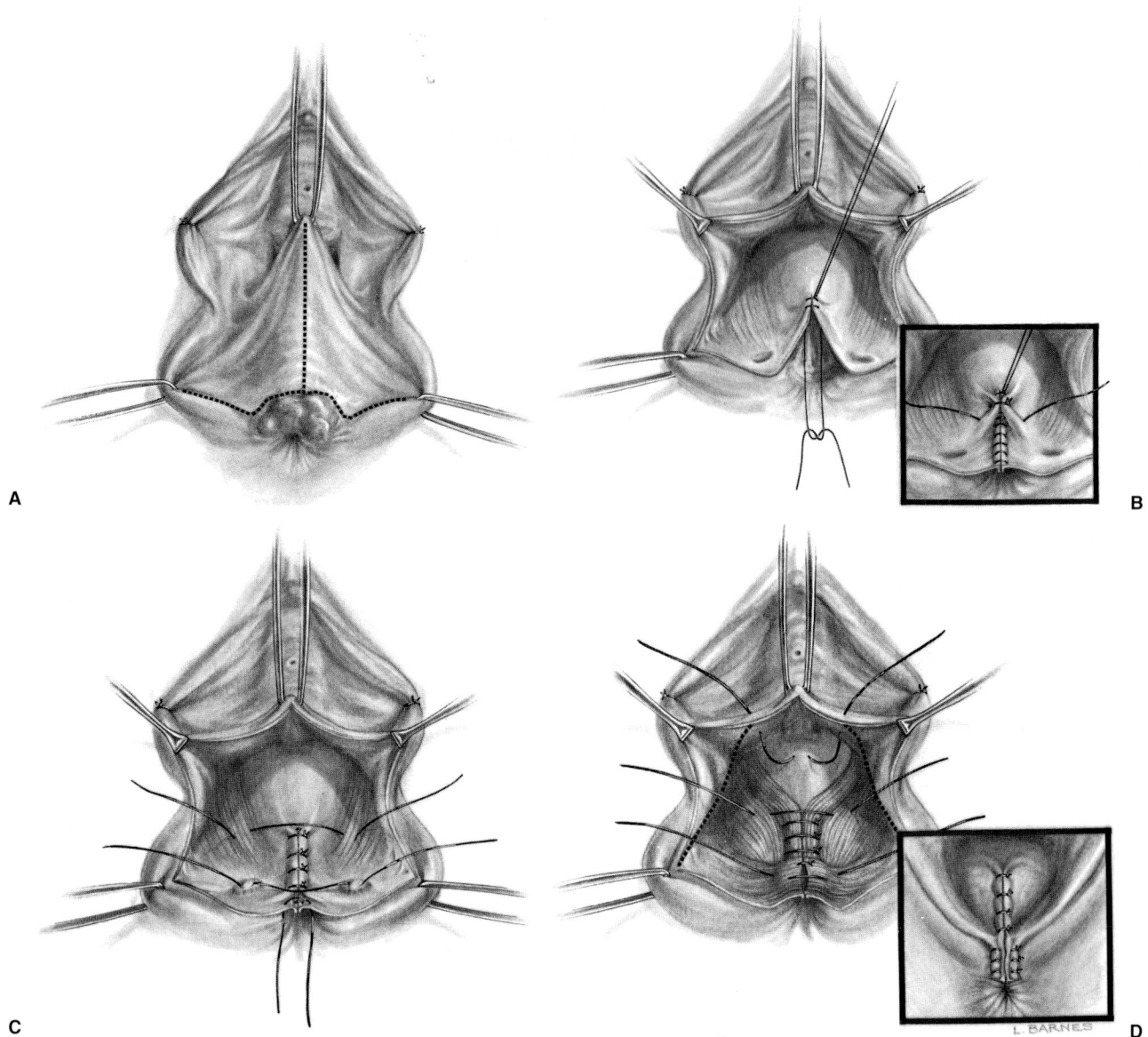

FIGURE 12-4. Repair of complete perineal body disruption with or without rectovaginal fistula. **(A)** Incisions in the posterior vaginal wall and perineum are indicated *(dotted lines).* **(B)** Repair of the anterior rectal wall. A second layer is placed through the muscularis **(inset)**. **(C,D)** The external sphincter and levator ani are sutured together. The wound is primarily closed **(inset)**. (Adapted from Howkins J, Hudson CN. *Shaw's textbook of operative gynaecology,* 4th ed. Edinburgh: Churchill Livingstone, 1977.)

Numerous other approaches to the management of this type of fistula have been described.[4,6,7,21,24,26,32,51,53] In general, gynecologists prefer a transvaginal repair—excising or dividing the fistula tract, closing the defects in the rectal and vaginal walls, and repairing the perineum. Three methods of transvaginal repair are illustrated in Figures 12-4 through 12-6.

General surgeons and colon and rectal surgeons in recent years have begun selectively to employ the *endorectal advancement flap* technique to repair anal and low-rectal fistulas.[31,60] This is the same principle described in Chapter 11 for fistula-in-ano. It is more likely to be successful for low rectovaginal fistulas than for anovaginal fistulas, however. Berman advocates a sleeve advancement technique for complicated anorectal and rectovaginal fistulas (see Figure 11-41).[6] This is believed to be particularly useful for individuals in whom the fistulas encompass an extensive portion of the anal or rectal wall or in those with multiple internal openings.

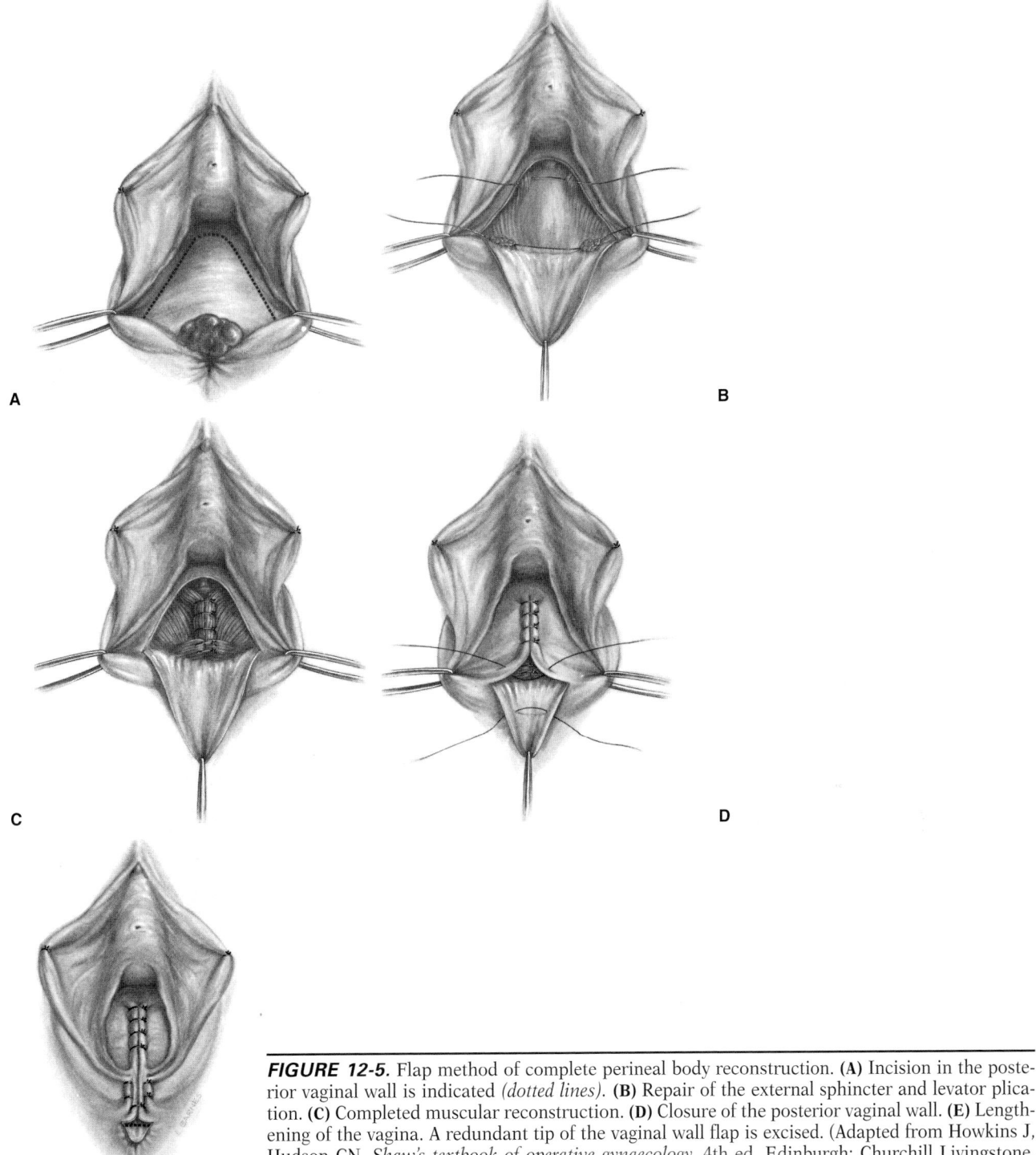

FIGURE 12-5. Flap method of complete perineal body reconstruction. **(A)** Incision in the posterior vaginal wall is indicated *(dotted lines)*. **(B)** Repair of the external sphincter and levator plication. **(C)** Completed muscular reconstruction. **(D)** Closure of the posterior vaginal wall. **(E)** Lengthening of the vagina. A redundant tip of the vaginal wall flap is excised. (Adapted from Howkins J, Hudson CN. *Shaw's textbook of operative gynaecology,* 4th ed. Edinburgh: Churchill Livingstone, 1977.)

Techniques for Repair of Midrectal Fistula

A midrectal (i.e., midvaginal) fistula is the most difficult type of gynecologic/intestinal fistula to repair satisfactorily. A theoretically simple approach would be to convert the fistula to that of a "fourth degree laceration." Fistula in this location is often a consequence of concomitant Crohn's disease, of tumor, of radiation injury, and of trauma (including obstetric and surgical). However, this would of necessity require division of the entire sphincter mechanism (see Figure 23-138). Although this can certainly be accomplished, and it will provide excellent

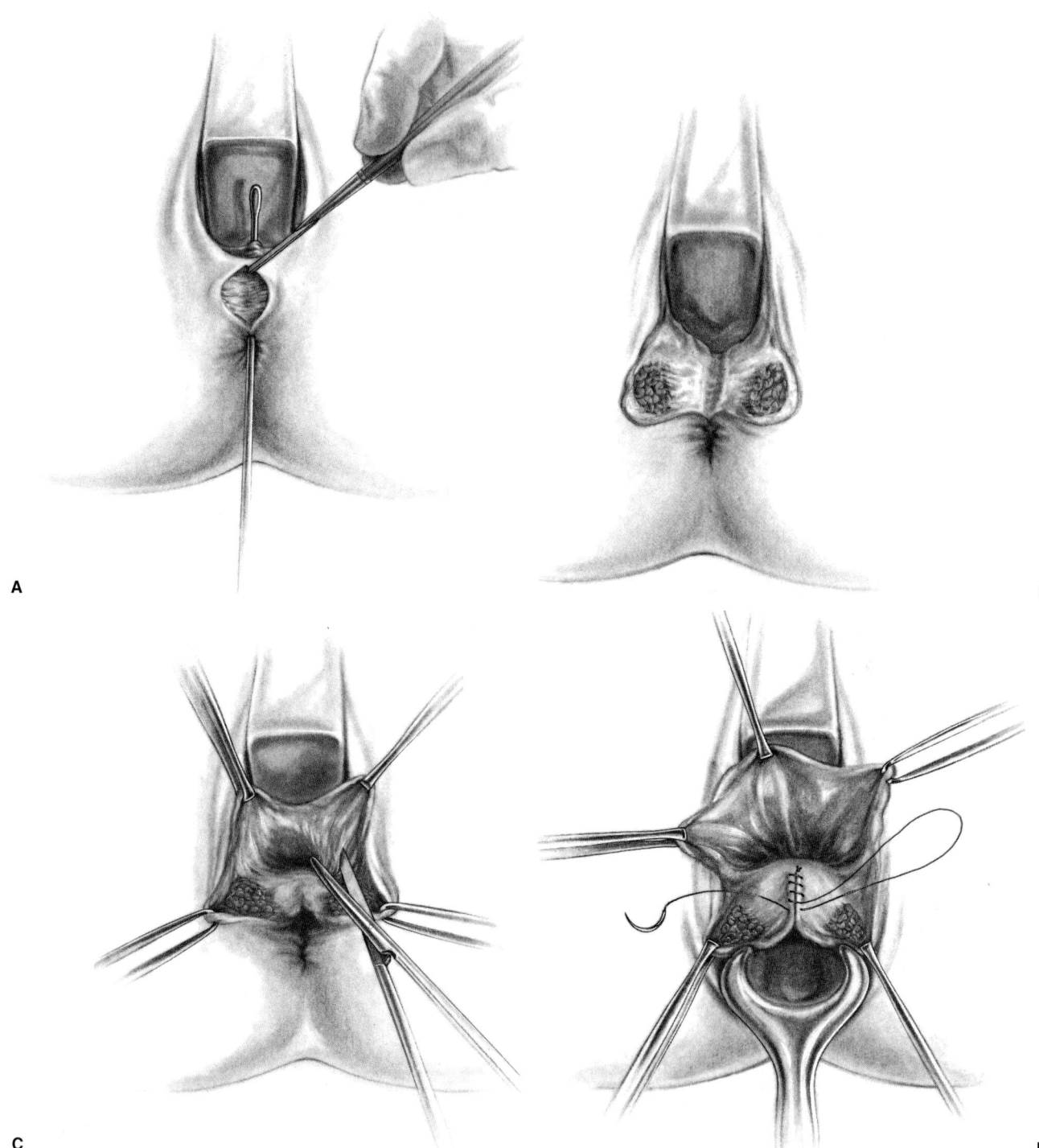

A

B

C

D

FIGURE 12-6. Transsphincteric rectovaginal fistula repair. **(A,B)** The fistula is divided. **(C)** Separation of the vagina from the rectum. **(D)** The rectal mucosa is closed. **(E)** Levator plication. **(F)** The external sphincter is repaired. **(G)** The perineal body is reconstructed by a layered closure. (Adapted courtesy of James A. Breen, M.D., and Caterina A. Gregori, M.D.)

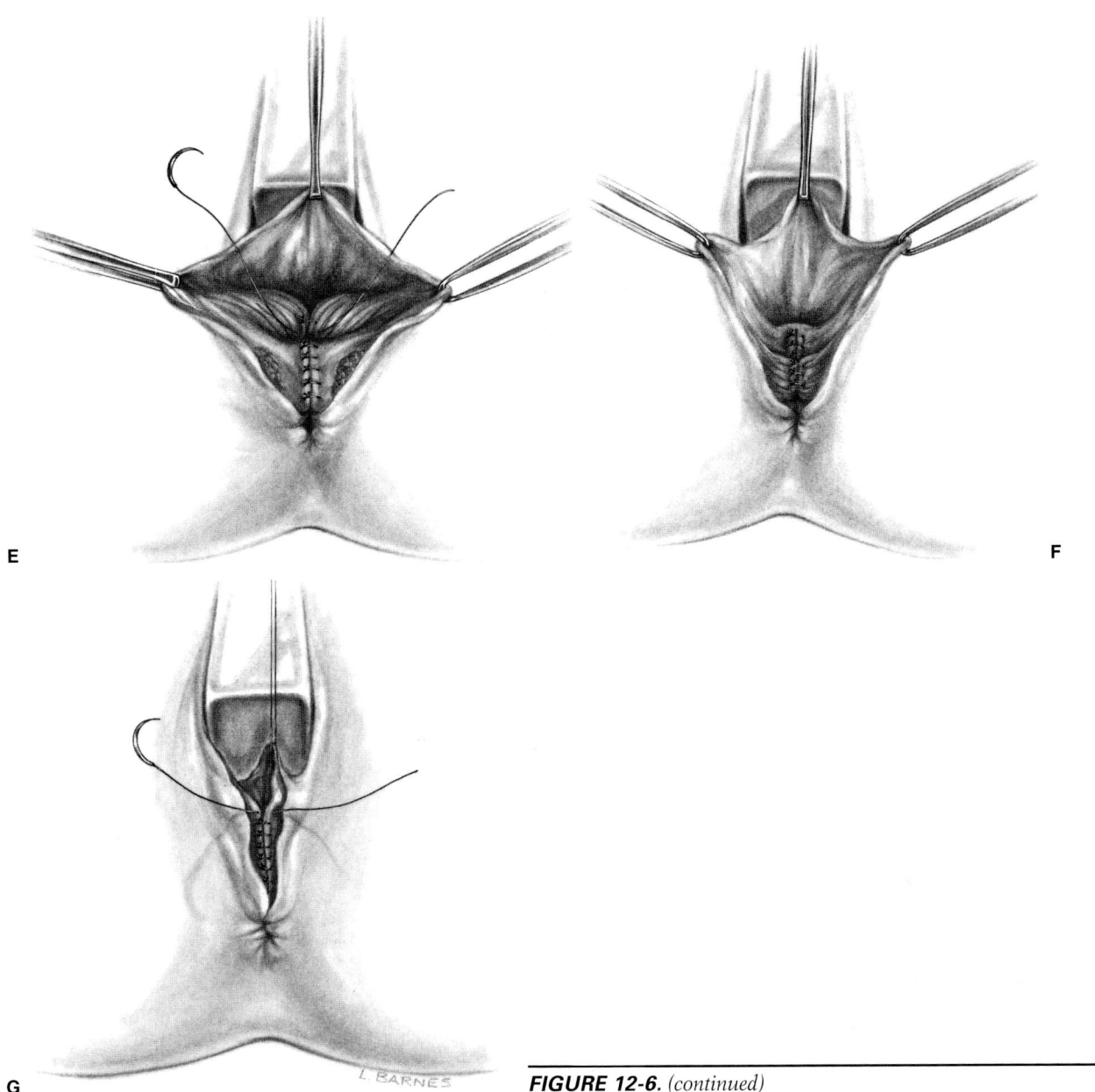

E

F

G

L. BARNES

FIGURE 12-6. *(continued)*

exposure indeed, the risk of breakdown and fecal incontinence should stay the surgeon's hand.

Simple Closure or Advancement Flap

This operation can readily be performed transvaginally, but a transanal or transcoccygeal approach is preferred (see earlier).[60] The principles of excision, layered closure, and endorectal advancement flaps are illustrated in Chapter 11 and Figure 12-7.

Transcoccygeal Repair

A transcoccygeal (or transsacral) alternative is shown in Figure 12-8. This approach is essentially the same as that described in Chapter 23 for the management of cer-

tain types of rectal tumors. It can also be very a very helpful exposure for closure of a rectourethral fistula (see later).

Use of Fibrin Glue

The use of fibrin to seal surgical openings has been applied for almost a century (see Chapter 11). With the development of microsurgical techniques, there has come into application, particularly in Europe, but more recently also in the United States, the use of a fibrin sealant system. It has been applied primarily in orthopedics but is finding use in other fields.[1] In spite of its relative success in the treatment of anal fistula, the failure rates for its use with rectovaginal fistula are prohibitively high.

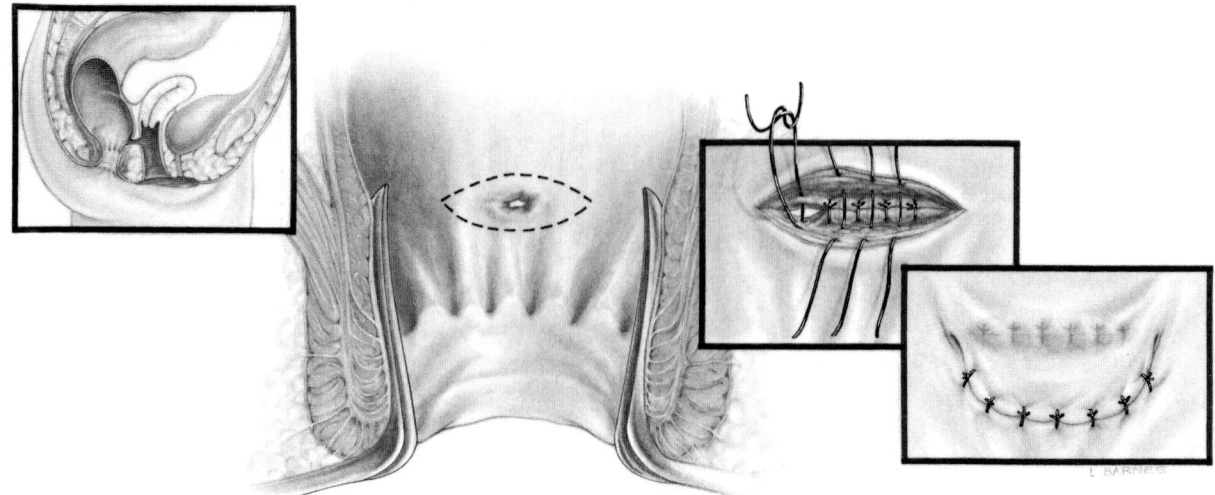

FIGURE 12-7. Transanal repair of a low to midrectovaginal fistula. The importance of the location is that it permits a layered closure with mucosal advancement. If the high-pressure zone in the rectum is successfully repaired, a vaginal approach or vaginal closure is unnecessary.

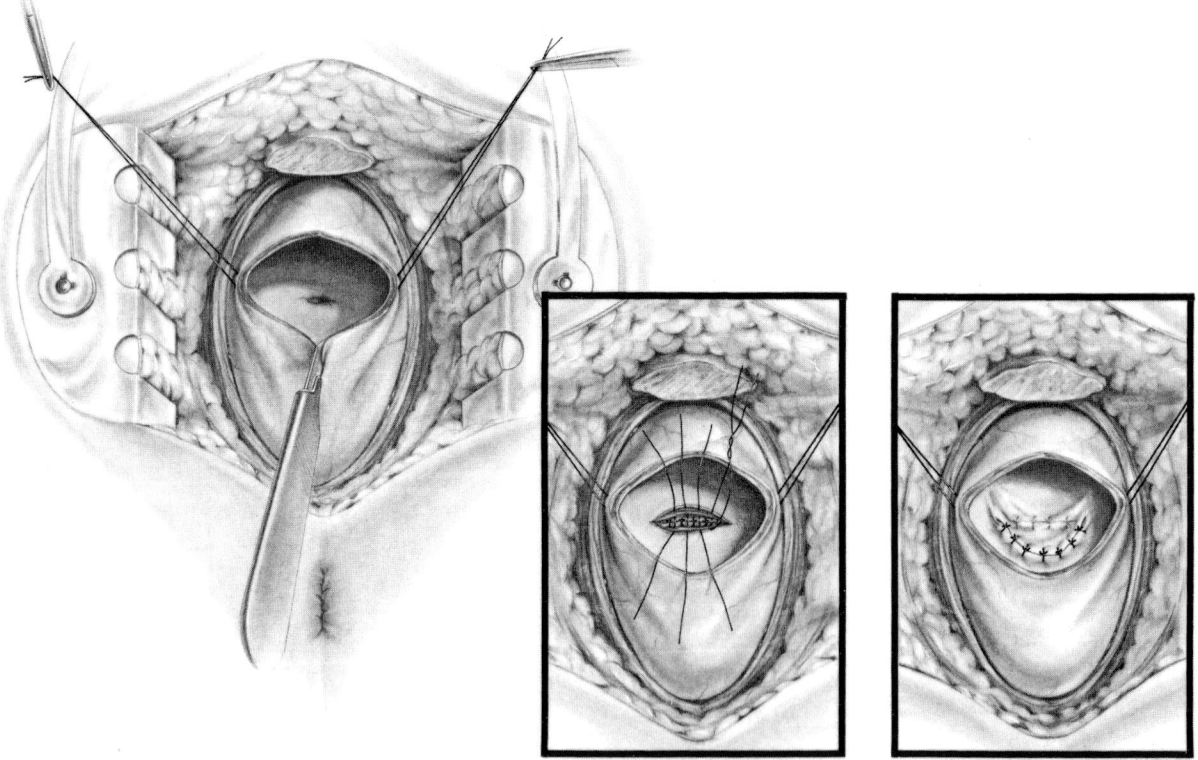

FIGURE 12-8. Transcoccygeal repair of rectovaginal or rectourethral fistula. The so-called Kraske operation permits excellent exposure for low or midrectal fistulas. Through a posterior proctotomy, the fistula site is identified and repaired by suture closure and mucosal advancement.

This, perhaps, is because the tract is too short to be filled by the sealant. In any event, its application for this fistula complication has been all but abandoned for that reason.

Other Options

Interposition of gracilis muscle, pudendal thigh, fascia lata, and fat has been advocated by various authors in order to minimize the likelihood of breakdown and recurrence.[11,35]

Results

Interpreting the results of various methods for repair of rectovaginal fistula in order to make a meaningful recommendation to the patient is a fruitless exercise. There are so many surgical options and causes of the fistulas that, at best, only generalizations can be made. Of course, it also depends on who is making the recommendation: gynecologist, general surgeon, or colon and rectal surgeon.

Given reported 32 operative repairs for rectovaginal fistula that were undertaken by 16 surgeons.[21] In ten cases, the entire perineal body was incised, converting the fistula into a complete laceration; this laceration was then repaired in layers. Primary healing took place in all patients. Other procedures were less successful, but the reasons may have had more to do with the level of the fistula and with the underlying pathology than with the method employed. Belt and Belt reported good results in all ten patients treated by dissecting and interposing the internal sphincter muscle.[5] Greenwald and Hoexter and their colleagues excised the fistula with a transanal approach and performed a layered closure; they reported 100% success in 35 patients.[24,28]

The transanal approach with endorectal advancement flap has become the most popular method for treating this complication today.[27,30,31,44,51,56] Kodner and colleagues reported their experience on 107 individuals who underwent this approach for rectovaginal and other complicated anorectal fistulas.[31] Their experience is summarized in Table 12-1.

Persistence of the fistula or recurrence developed in 17 patients (16%). Ultimately, the overall success rate in excess of 90% for this complicated group of patients, with the avoidance of fecal diversion, even on a temporary basis, is excellent.

The University of Minnesota Group initially reported 91% success with 35 patients.[51] However, a later publication involving 81 patients noted that this was reduced to 83%.[34] The Cleveland Clinic group observed a 77% success rate for this procedure.[30] The primary factor as noted in another publication from the same institution that adversely affected results was Crohn's disease.[60]

▶ **TABLE 12-1 Results of Endorectal Advancement Flap Repair of Fistulas According to Cause**

Cause	Healed Primarily (%)	Healed Including Further Treatment (%)
Obstetric injury	42/48 (88)	45/48[94]
Cryptoglandular	27/31 (87)	30/31[92]
Crohn's disease	17/24 (71)	22/24[92]
Trauma (two after sphincterotomy)	4/4 (100)	4/4[100]
Total	90/107[84]	101/107[93]

From Kodner IJ, Mazor A, Shemesh EI, et al. Endorectal advancement flap repair of rectovaginal and other complicated anorectal fistulas. *Surgery* 1993;114:682, with permission.

Wise and colleagues performed endorectal advancement flaps in 40 women, with the addition of sphincteroplasty or perineal body reconstruction in 15.[69] Those who underwent the combined procedures were continent, whereas seven of those who had not undergone either sphincteroplasty or perineal body reconstruction, in addition to the endorectal advancement flaps, reported impairment for control. It appears, therefore, that the importance of perineal body reconstitution is justified (see Chapter 13).

MacRae and co-workers, reporting from Toronto, caution that persistence of rectovaginal fistula after failed repair should not be managed by advancement flap.[35] In essence, they recommend (and I concur) that the patient has one shot at this approach. If it does indeed fail, another option should be selected. Watson and Phillips, reporting from St. Mark's Hospital in the United Kingdom, experienced overall success in all but three of their 26 patients with rectovaginal fistula.[68] However, the authors cautioned that this result obscures a high early failure rate in five of 12 patients having a transanal advancement flap. They also employed a temporary stoma in 11 individuals.

Lawson described a transvaginal approach to high rectovaginal fistulas that developed following obstetric injury.[32] This procedure involved incising the vagina, sometimes dividing the cervix, and opening the pouch of Douglas. As previously mentioned, it would seem that such a fistula could be more easily treated by an abdominal approach. Finally, the results of numerous transvaginal approaches are not summarized here. However, Tancer and colleagues, from the Department of Obstetrics and Gynecology, Maimonides Medical Center, Brooklyn, New York, reported 100% success in their 52 patients.[61]

Abel and colleagues applied this principle to the management of rectovaginal and complex anal fistulas.[1] In the ten individuals so treated, 60% reported complete healing with a follow-up of 3 to 12 months. Specifically, four of the five rectovaginal fistulas healed. Further clinical trials are awaited concerning the applicability of this new approach.

Rectovaginal Fistula in Crohn's Disease

One of the most challenging problems in patients with Crohn's disease is the management of rectovaginal fistula (see also Chapter 11).[2] At St. Mark's Hospital, one in ten women with the disease developed a rectovaginal fistula, a higher percentage than that usually reported by others.[50] The authors attributed this elevated rate to the theory that more patients attending St. Mark's have colorectal involvement. Certainly, rectovaginal fistula is more frequently associated with granulomatous colitis than with small bowel disease. This complication may ultimately require a diversionary procedure or a proctectomy; diversion alone, however, is unlikely to cure the condition. The endorectal advancement flap is probably the only definitive surgical option that the physician should consider if repair of the fistula is to be attempted. Besides the obvious, the major advantages of this approach are that no sphincter is divided, continence is not impaired, there is no perineal wound with which to contend, and rarely is the underlying condition exacerbated.

Technical considerations that should be implemented in the endorectal advancement flap advancement procedure include the following:

- Use the prone jackknife position.
- Ensure precise anatomic definition of the fistula.
- Infiltrate with epinephrine to facilitate dissection and minimize bleeding.
- Make the advancement flap quite thick; this may necessitate taking a portion of the internal sphincter for anovaginal fistulas.
- Mobilize without creating tension.
- Perform excision, curettage, and watertight closure, with closure of the defect in the muscularis.
- Strongly consider temporary fecal diversion.

Results

Several factors adversely influence the outcome of the advancement flap procedure:

- An internal opening higher than 2 cm from the dentate line
- Active Crohn's disease elsewhere
- Severe proctitis

- Persistent or undrained sepsis in the rectovaginal septum (long-term drainage should be performed initially).
- With proper patient selection, successful results are possible.[4,13,16,40,65]

Many patients with this complication are managed nonoperatively, whereas those who do come to the operating room are often submitted to proctectomy. More than one half of the patients with rectovaginal fistula from St. Mark's Hospital underwent rectal excision.[50] Scott and colleagues noted that only 13 of 38 women with perianal Crohn's disease without vaginal fistula required a stoma or proctectomy, whereas 18 of 29 with vaginal fistulization underwent one of these procedures.[55] These differences were statistically significant.

It should be kept in mind that rectovaginal fistula can, on occasion, be seen in individuals with *ulcerative colitis*. Froines and Palmer reported three patients who underwent ileoanal pouch procedures for this complication, with successful results.[19] However, for patients with Crohn's disease, the preferred method of repair is the endorectal advancement flap.[17,50] With this technique, the Cleveland Clinic group noted a rate of success of 60%.[30] A later report from the same institution revealed the recurrence rate to be only 29%.[42] They concluded that the failure rate was influenced only by the prior number of repairs. As noted from the earlier table, Kodner and co-workers experienced a 71% healing rate in individuals with Crohn's disease treated by endorectal advancement flap.[31] Bauer and Sher and their colleagues reported 14 patients from the Mount Sinai Hospital in New York who underwent a transvaginal operation, all with a diverting ostomy.[3,57] All but one healed. Follow-up ranged from 9 to 68 months. The authors emphasize that, in their opinion, success depends on the use of temporary fecal diversion.

Rectovaginal Fistula After Radiotherapy

Rectovaginal fistula after radiation therapy presents a particularly difficult problem in management (see Chapter 28). However, there are some patients for whom repair may produce quite satisfactory results.

Individuals with this condition often give a history of having undergone radiotherapy many years previously, usually for carcinoma of the cervix. In more recent, years such a complication may be the result of radiation treatment for cancer of the anal canal, rectum, or bladder. Most of these patients present with a fistula above the sphincters, usually in the midrectum or upper rectum.

With a history of prior malignancy, it is imperative to establish whether the patient has evidence of recurrent disease. Obviously, reconstruction is contraindicated under such circumstances. Complete evaluation by means of multiple biopsies, radiologic investigation, including computed tomography, and hematologic studies is required. The genitourinary tract should also be investigated.

Techniques and Results

Numerous operative approaches to the repair of radiation-induced rectovaginal fistula have been described.[9,10,23,36,45,62] Optimally, normal, nonradiated tissue should be brought to the area. This would involve a resection, such as the pull-through operation, coloanal anastomosis, bowel interposition, or the abdominosacral resection (see Chapter 23).[9,36,37,45,59,62]

Layered closure has also been used successfully, along with the sartorius muscle and the gracilis muscle interpositions.[10,23] The endorectal advancement flap is probably a poor choice, because radiated bowel inevitably would be used. There is genuine risk of the patient's developing an even more difficult management problem, that is, a bigger hole. Boronow reported his experience using a bulbocavernosus fat flap with transvaginal repair for radiation-induced fistulas.[8] Successful closure was effected in more than 80%. Although this is a relatively simple operation that could justifiably be applied as first-line therapy,[8] my own preference is to perform a colostomy at the time of the repair if a nonresection operation is carried out. Of course, if the patient is not a candidate for reconstruction, a diversionary procedure is indicated.

RECTOVAGINAL CYST

Benign cysts of the vagina, especially inclusion cysts, are quite common. These are usually located near the introitus or in episiotomy scars. Other cystic lesions that may appear in the area are Gartner's duct cysts, endometriosis, adenosis, and vaginitis emphysematosa.[54] Occasionally, an inclusion cyst can present in the rectovaginal septum. The lesion is often asymptomatic, but it may be associated with constipation, mucus discharge, and, if ulcerated, rectal bleeding. In the experience of Pradhan and Tobon with 41 patients, most complained of a swelling or mass in the vagina accompanied by stress incontinence in some, dyspareunia, dysfunctional uterine bleeding, or a history of episiotomy or vaginal lacerations.[48]

Physical examination usually reveals a mass in the rectovaginal septum, but endoscopy will fail to identify a mucosal abnormality. The size of the cyst may be quite variable (up to 7 cm in diameter), but most are smaller than 2 cm.[48]

Most of these lesions are simple inclusion cysts, but one third of the reported cases in one series were of müllerian origin.[15] However, others have reported a higher incidence of the müllerian type than the epidermal inclusion cyst. Other causes of the cyst include Gartner's duct type, Bartholin's duct type, and endometriotic type.

Most of these lesions can be excised transvaginally, but if the cyst seems to be extending into the submucosa of the rectum, transanal excision as described in Figure 12-9 is warranted.

RECTOURETHRAL FISTULA

Rectourethral fistula is, fortunately, a rare condition. It is seen as a complication of prostatectomy, especially when performed through the perineal route (see Figure 23-52). It may be seen as a consequence of radiation therapy for carcinoma of the bladder or prostate. Specifically, brachytherapy for prostatic cancer is probably the most common cause today. Trauma, infection, and Crohn's disease are more unusual causes. Even in the adult, a congenital anomaly may be the cause.[25]

Looser and colleagues reported the experience of colorectal–urinary tract fistulas at the Memorial Hospital in New York and found only two cases of rectourethral communication during a 17-year period.[33] One followed a low anterior rectal resection and the other a radical perineal prostatectomy. Thompson and colleagues reported the Mayo Clinic (Rochester, Minnesota) experience over a 30-year period.[63] There were 36 rectourethral fistulas. Fourteen followed prostatectomy, six occurred after trauma, three were associated with Crohn's disease, and four resulted from other causes. Nine patients had malignant fistulas. Although the authors did not distinguish between the symptoms of rectovesical and rectourethral fistulas, 90% had urinary tract infections, and 83% reported urine issuing from the rectum. More than one half of the patients noted pneumaturia and fecaluria. Bleeding through the rectum implied a malignant process. Cystoscopy established the diagnosis in 84%, and proctoscopy was of value in 70%.

Garofalo and colleagues reported the Cleveland Clinic (Ohio) experience with 23 men.[20] The cause was iatrogenic from prostatic or rectal surgery in ten patients, Crohn's disease in nine, and radiation in three. One patient developed a fistula following an automobile accident. The high incidence of fistula secondary to Crohn's disease is undoubtedly a reflection of the unique referral situation at that institution. Symptoms were multiple in 43%, urine per rectum in 39%, and pneumaturia in 9%, and one patient (5%) presented with fecaluria. Diagnosis was confirmed most frequently by cystoscopy, followed

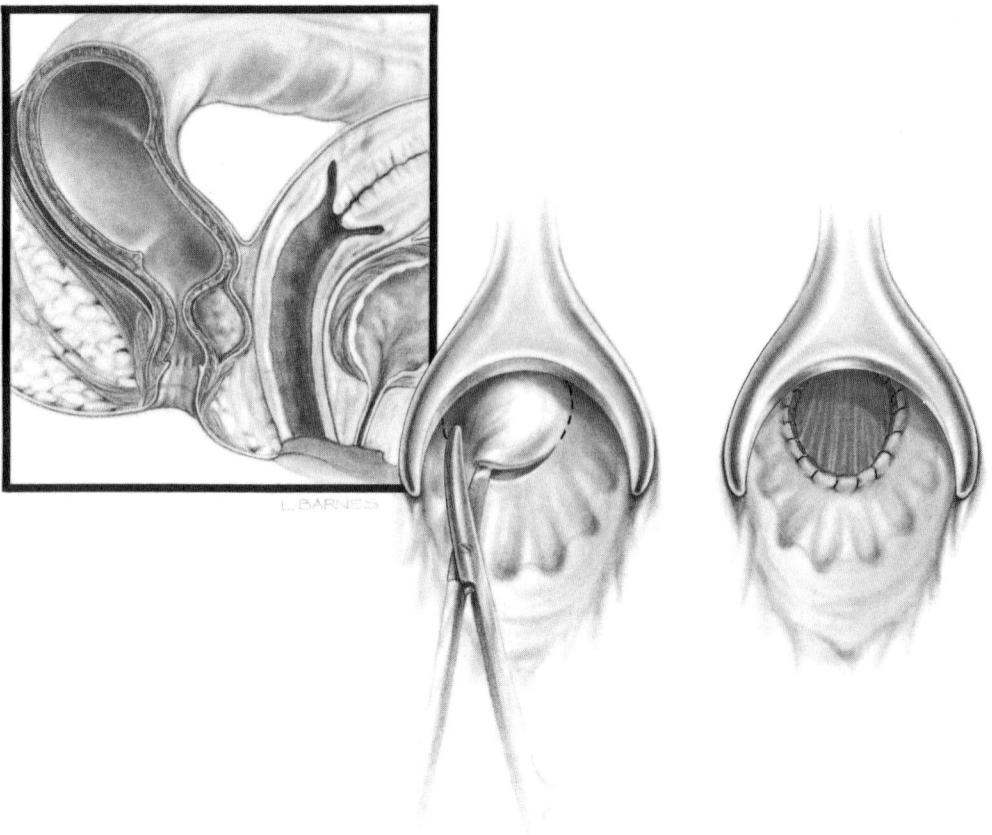

FIGURE 12-9. Transanal excision of a rectovaginal cyst. For a posterior presentation, the lesion is excised with care to avoid entering the vagina. The open wound is sutured for hemostasis but is left open to drain. Healing usually takes place within a few weeks.

by proctoscopy, cystography, and rectal contrast. The most sensitive test today, however, is computed tomography with rectal contrast.

Treatment and Results

Many approaches have been used to treat rectourethral fistula—transanal, transperineal, transcoccygeal (Figure 12-8), transabdominal (including pouch-anal anastomosis), with or without interposition of tissue, and with or without fecal and/or urinary diversion.[12,22,41,67] Hampton and Bacon favored abdominoanal pull-through with perineal repair.[25] Turner-Warwick preferred an abdominal operation with interposition of appropriately tailored omentum.[64] Others have interposed gracilis muscle.[71] Mason exposed the area by dividing the rectum and sphincters posteriorly; the fistula can then be closed in layers and the rectum reconstructed (see Figure 23-138).[38] Others have also recommended this technique.[49]

Transanal mucosal advancement has been strongly advocated, with or without fecal diversion.[18,29,30,46] In the Cleveland Clinic report, 12 men underwent this opera-

tion.[20] All seven patients whose fistulas were due to trauma healed successfully. The authors advocate this approach for all primary operations as well as repeat surgical procedures if this can be accomplished technically. They further advise that all patients undergo concomitant fecal diversion.

Zmora and co-workers reported the Cleveland Clinic (Florida) experience with the transperineal operation and gracilis muscle interposition.[71] Six patients had prior radiotherapy, and five others had failed repairs. Nine patients healed following this procedure. The authors emphasize the importance of obtaining pathologic material when there is a history of prior malignancy. In contrast to their northern colleagues, they consider this operation to be the procedure of choice. They also recommend fecal diversion. Likewise, the Mayo Clinic group concludes that patients with rectourethral fistula following prostatectomy or radiotherapy should undergo fecal (and urinary) diversion with muscle transposition.[41]

In those individuals with nonresectable malignant disease, a diversionary procedure is the treatment of choice. If the tumor *is* resectable, pelvic exenteration is the optimal course. When radiation injury is the causative factor or associated concern, hyperbaric oxygen treatment prior to reconstruction may have some value.[43] For benign conditions, successful repair generally requires long-term catheter or suprapubic drainage of the urinary tract.

In Goligher's hands, either the Mason approach or that of Turner-Warwick offered the best results.[22]

Opinion

This is a rare condition for me to treat. That is perhaps why I have not convinced myself that one technique is preferable. Alternatives that I believe are generally quite satisfactory for the nonirradiated patient are a transanal mucosal advancement, a transperineal approach with interposition of gracilis muscle, or a transcoccygeal operation with sliding rectal advancement flap. I strongly believe, however, in the importance of using the expertise of a urologist, ideally an individual who has special proficiency and interest in performing reconstructive urologic procedures.

ANTERIOR PERINEAL SINUS OR CYST

Congenital cysts of the genitoperineal raphe are extremely rare. Their initial description has been attributed to Mermet, who described the condition in 1895.[39] Two theories concerning their etiology have been proposed:

- Infolding of dermal elements at the time of closure of the genital folds
- Outgrowth of epithelial cells in the raphe after the genital folds have closed[42]
- Patients complain of perineal discharge, irritation, and pain; recurrent infection is quite common. Differential diagnoses include epidermal cyst, hidradenitis, and anal fistula.

Oliver and colleagues identified 31 patients from their practice during a 20-year period.[42] Male predominance (87%) and midlife presentation (mean age, 44 years) characterized these individuals. The lesions usually occurred along the median raphe. Treatment consisted of excision of any nodules with laying open of the sinus tracts. A recurrence rate of 15% was reported.

REFERENCES

1. Abel ME, Chiu YSY, Russell TR, et al. Autologous fibrin glue in the treatment of rectovaginal and complex fistulas. *Dis Colon Rectum* 1993;36:447.
2. Alexander-Williams J, Buchmann P. Perianal Crohn's disease. *World J Surg* 1980;4:203.
3. Bauer JJ, Sher ME, Jaffin H, et al. Transvaginal approach for repair of rectovaginal fistulae complicating Crohn's disease. *Ann Surg* 1991;213:151.
4. Beecham CT. Recurring rectovaginal fistula. *Obstet Gynecol* 1972;40:323.
5. Belt RL Jr, Belt RL. Repair of anorectal vaginal fistula utilizing segmental advancement of the internal sphincter muscle. *Dis Colon Rectum* 1969;12:99.
6. Berman IR. Sleeve advancement anorectoplasty for complicated anorectal/vaginal fistula. *Dis Colon Rectum* 1991;34:1032.
7. Block IR, Rodriguez S, Olivares AL. The Warren operation for anal incontinence caused by disruption of the anterior segment of the anal sphincter, perineal body, and rectovaginal septum. *Dis Colon Rectum* 1975;18:28.
8. Boronow RC. Repair of the radiation-induced vaginal fistula utilizing the Martius technique. *World J Surg* 1986;10:237.
9. Bricker EM, Johnston WD. Repair of post irradiation rectovaginal fistula and stricture. *Surg Gynecol Obstet* 1979;148:499.
10. Byron RL Jr, Ostergard DR. Sartorius muscle interposition for the treatment of the radiation-induced vaginal fistula. *Am J Obstet Gynecol* 1969;104:104.
11. Cardon A, Pattyn P, Monstrey S, et al. Use of a unilateral pudendal thigh flap in the treatment of complex rectovaginal fistula. *Br J Surg* 1999;86:645.
12. Celebrezze JP Jr, Medich DS. Rectal ulceration as a result of prostatic brachytherapy: a new clinical problem. Report of three cases. *Dis Colon Rectum* 2003;46:1277.
13. Cohen JL, Stricker JW, Schoetz DJ Jr, et al. Rectovaginal fistula in Crohn's disease. *Dis Colon Rectum* 1989;32:825.
14. Corman ML. Anal incontinence following obstetrical injury. *Dis Colon Rectum* 1985;28:86.
15. Deppisch LM. Cysts of the vagina: classification and clinical correlations. *Am J Obstet Gynecol* 1975;45:632.
16. Faulcolon HT, Muldoon JP. Rectovaginal fistula in patients with colitis. *Dis Colon Rectum* 1975;18:413.
17. Farkas AM, Gingold BS. Repair of rectovaginal fistula in Crohn's disease by rectal mucosal advancement flap. *Mt Sinai J Med* 1983;50:420.
18. Fazio VW, Jones IT, Jagelman DG, et al. Rectourethral fistulas in Crohn's disease. *Surg Gynecol Obstet* 1987;164:148.
19. Froines EJ, Palmer DL. Surgical therapy for rectovaginal fistulas in ulcerative colitis. *Dis Colon Rectum* 1991;34:925.
20. Garofalo TE, Delaney CP, Jones SM, et al. Rectal advancement flap repair of rectourethral fistula: a 20-year experience. *Dis Colon Rectum* 2003;46:762.
21. Given FT Jr. Rectovaginal fistula: a review of 20 years' experience in a community hospital. *Am J Obstet Gynecol* 1970;108:41.
22. Goligher JC. *Surgery of the anus, rectum and colon*, 4th ed. New York: Macmillan, 1980:193.
23. Graham JB. Vaginal fistulas following radiotherapy. *Surg Gynecol Obstet* 1965;120:1019.
24. Greenwald JC, Hoexter B. Repair of rectovaginal fistulas. *Surg Gynecol Obstet* 1978;146:443.
25. Hampton JM, Bacon HE. Diagnosis and surgical management of rectourethral fistulas. *Dis Colon Rectum* 1961;4:177.
26. Hibbard LT. Surgical management of rectovaginal fistulas and complete perineal tears. *Am J Obstet Gynecol* 1978;130:139.
27. Hilsabeck JR. Transanal advancement of the anterior rectal wall for vaginal fistulas involving the lower rectum. *Dis Colon Rectum* 1980;23:236.
28. Hoexter B, Labow SB, Moseson MD. Transanal rectovaginal fistula repair. *Dis Colon Rectum* 1985;28:572.
29. Johnson WR, Druitt DM, Masterson JP. Anterior rectal advancement flap in the repair of benign rectoprostatic fistula. *Aust N Z J Surg* 1981;51:383.
30. Jones IT, Fazio VW, Jagelman DG. The use of transanal rectal advancement flaps in the management of fistulas involving the anorectum. *Dis Colon Rectum* 1987;30:919.
31. Kodner IJ, Mazor A, Shemesh EI, et al. Endorectal advancement flap repair of rectovaginal and other complicated anorectal fistulas. *Surgery* 1993;114:682.

32. Lawson J. Rectovaginal fistulae following difficult labour. *Proc R Soc Med* 1972;65:283.
33. Looser KG, Quan SHQ, Clark DGC. Colo-urinary tract fistula in the cancer patient. *Dis Colon Rectum* 1979;22:143.
34. Lowry AC, Thorson AG, Rothenberger DA, et al. Repair of simple rectovaginal fistulas: influence of previous repairs. *Dis Colon Rectum* 1988;31:676.
35. MacRae HM, McLeod RS, Cohen Z, et al. Treatment of rectovaginal fistulas that has failed previous repair attempts. *Dis Colon Rectum* 1995;38:921.
36. Marks G. Combined abdominotranssacral reconstruction of the radiation-injured rectum. *Am J Surg* 1976;131:54.
37. Marks G, Mohiudden M. The surgical management of the radiation-injured intestine. *Surg Clin North Am* 1983;63:81.
38. Mason AY. The place of local resection in the treatment of rectal carcinoma. *Proc R Soc Med* 1970;63:1259.
39. Mermet P. Congenital cysts of the genitoperineal raphe. *Rev Chir* 1895;15:382.
40. Morrison JG, Gathright JB Jr, Ray JE, et al. Results of operation for rectovaginal in Crohn's disease. *Dis Colon Rectum* 1989;32:497.
41. Nyam DCNK, Pemberton JH. Management of iastrogenic rectourethral fistula. *Dis Colon Rectum* 1999;42:994.
42. Oliver GC, Rubin RJ, Salvati EP, et al. Anterior perineal sinus. *Dis Colon Rectum* 1991;34:777.
43. O'Reilly KJ, Hampson NB, Corman JM. Hyperbaric oxygen in urology. *AUA Update Series* 2001:21.
44. Ozuner G, Hull TL, Cartmill J, et al. Long-term analysis of the use of rectal advancement flaps for complicated anorectal/vaginal fistulas. *Dis Colon Rectum* 1996;39:10.
45. Parks AG, Allen CLO, Frank JD, et al. A method of treating post-irradiation rectovaginal fistulas. *Br J Surg* 1978;65:417.
46. Parks AG, Motson RW. Perianal repair of rectoprostatic fistula. *Br J Surg* 1983;70:725.
47. Pfeifer J, Reissman P, Wexner SD. Ergotamine-induced complex rectovaginal fistula: a report of a case. *Dis Colon Rectum* 1995;38:1224.
48. Pradhan S, Tobon H. Vaginal cysts: a clinicopathological study of 41 cases. *Int J Gynecol Pathol* 1986;5:35.
49. Prasad ML, Nelson R, Hambrick E, et al. York Mason procedure for repair of postoperative rectoprostatic urethral fistula. *Dis Colon Rectum* 1983;26:716.
50. Radcliffe AG, Ritchie JK, Hawley PR, et al. Anovaginal and rectovaginal fistulas in Crohn's disease. *Dis Colon Rectum* 1988;31:94.
51. Rothenberger DA, Christenson CE, Balcos EG, et al. Endorectal advancement flap for treatment of simple rectovaginal fistula. *Dis Colon Rectum* 1982;25:297.
52. Rothenberger DA, Goldberg SM. The management of rectovaginal fistulae. *Surg Clin North Am* 1983;63:61.
53. Russell TR, Gallagher DM. Low rectovaginal fistulas. *Am J Surg* 1977;134:13.
54. Scott JR, DiSaia PJ, Hammond CB, et al, eds. *Danforth's obstetrics and gynecology*, 6th ed. Philadelphia: JB Lippincott, 1990:967.
55. Scott NA, Nair A, Hughes LE. Anovaginal and rectovaginal fistula in patients with Crohn's disease. *Br J Surg* 1992;79:1379.
56. Shemesh EI, Kodner IJ, Fry RD, et al. Endorectal sliding flap repair of complicated anterior anoperineal fistulas. *Dis Colon Rectum* 1988;31:22.
57. Sher ME, Bauer JJ, Gelernt I. Surgical repair of rectovaginal fistulas in patients with Crohn's disease: transvaginal approach. *Dis Colon Rectum* 1991;34:641.
58. Silverman WB, Marmolya G. Endoscopic placement of a Foley catheter across a stricture and rectovaginal fistula to perform a barium enema. *Am J Gastroenterol* 1991;86:99.
59. Steichen FM, Barber HKR, Loubeau JM, et al. Bricker-Johnston sigmoid colon graft for repair of postradiation rectovaginal fistula and stricture performed with mechanical sutures. *Dis Colon Rectum* 1992;35:599.
60. Sonoda T, Hull T, Piedemonte MR, et al. Outcomes of primary repair of anorectal and rectovaginal fistulas using the endorectal advancement flap. *Dis Colon Rectum* 2002;45:1622.
61. Tancer ML, Lasser D, Rosenblum N. Rectovaginal fistula or perineal and anal sphincter disruption, or both, after vaginal delivery. *Surg Gynecol Obstet* 1990;171:43.
62. Thomford NR, Smith DE, Wilson WH. Pull-through operation for radiation-induced rectovaginal fistula. *Dis Colon Rectum* 1970;13:451.
63. Thompson JS, Engen DE, Beart RW Jr, et al. The management of acquired rectourinary fistula. *Dis Colon Rectum* 1982;25:689.
64. Turner-Warwick R. The use of pedicle grafts in the repair of urinary tract fistulae. *Br J Urol* 1972;44:644.
65. Tuxen PA, Castro AF. Rectovaginal fistula in Crohn's disease. *Dis Colon Rectum* 1979;22:58.
66. Venkatesh KS, Ramanujam PS, Larson DM, et al. Anorectal complications of vaginal delivery. *Dis Colon Rectum* 1989;32:1039.
67. Visser BC, McAninch JW, Welton ML. Rectourethral fistulae: the perineal approach. *J Am Coll Surg* 2002;195:138.
68. Watson SJ, Phillips RKS. Non-inflammatory rectovaginal fistula. *Br J Surg* 1995;82:1641.
69. Wise WE Jr, Aguilar PS, Padmanabhan A, et al. Surgical treatment of low rectovaginal fistulas. *Dis Colon Rectum* 1991;34:271.
70. Yee LF, Birnbaum EH, Read TE, et al. Use of endoanal ultrasound in patients with rectovaginal fistulas. *Dis Colon Rectum* 1999;42:1057.
71. Zmora O, Potenti FM, Wexner SD, et al. Gracilis muscle transposition for iatrogenic rectourethral fistula. *Ann Surg* 2003;237:483.

Anal Incontinence

My wind exploded like a thunder-clap
Iaso blushed a rosy red
And Panacea turned her head
Holding her nose:
My wind's not frankincense.

Aristophanes: Plutus

This chapter and Chapters 14 through 16 discuss conditions that are often interrelated—problems with incontinence, trauma, and foreign bodies, and those of disorders of defecation and the pelvic floor. These concerns often require similar techniques of evaluation, especially that of physiologic investigation. Furthermore, many patients who complain of problems with bowel control are, in reality, suffering the consequences of an elimination problem, especially constipation. To deal effectively with these conditions, it is essential for the physician to be aware of the potential of the various manifestations to affect adversely the results of his or her therapeutic efforts.

One of the concerns of interpreting the data from the numerous reports in the literature has been lack of a convenient classification system or grading and scoring system, defining the degree and type of anal incontinence. Pescatori and colleagues identified 13 classifications suggested by various authors, including one by myself.[265] Their suggestion takes into account both degree and frequency of symptoms in which A, B, and C reflect increasing problems with incontinence for stool and the number system indicates the frequency of the problem (occasional, weekly, and daily). In 1993, Jorge and Wexner proposed a continence grading scale that has come to be used by many investigators and termed the Cleveland Clinic Incontinence Score.[155] The following is the scale:

Type of Incontinence	Frequency				
	Never	Rarely	Sometimes	Usually	Always
Solid	0	1	2	3	4
Liquid	0	1	2	3	4
Gas	0	1	2	3	4
Wears pad	0	1	2	3	4
Lifestyle alteration	0	1	2	3	4

0 = Perfect
20 = Complete incontinence

Never = 0 (never)
Rarely = <1/month
Sometimes = <1/week, >1/month
Usually = <1/day, >1/week
Always = >1/day

The continence score is determined by adding points from this table, which takes into account the type and frequency of incontinence and the extent to which it alters the patient's life.[155]

There is always the attraction of a simplified classification, such as that of Lane.[185] He separates anal incontinence into three categories:

- True incontinence: passage of feces without the patient's knowledge, or without voluntary contraction, or both
- Partial incontinence: passage of flatus or mucus under the above circumstances
- Overflow incontinence: result of rectal distension with relaxation of the anal sphincters (e.g., fecal impaction)

Certainly, these scoring systems have considerable merit, but ideally what had been required was a consensus group, charged with determining a classification system that all would be willing to employ. This was in part addressed by a conference involving a number of individuals representing five well-recognized, academic Divisions of Colon and Rectal Surgery in the United States.[287] This culminated in the publication in 1999 of the *Fecal Incontinence Severity Index (FICI)*.[287] There are four incontinence events used to determine the FICI score—all calculated on the basis of frequency—gas, mucus, liquid stool, and solid stool. The type *x* matrix includes five frequencies: one to three times per month, once per week, twice per week, once per day, and twice per day.

The same group of individuals who proposed the FICI also turned their attention to the development of a health-related quality of life scale.[288] The questionnaire that the patient completes addresses four categories: lifestyle, coping/behavior, depression/self-perception, and embarrassment. Analysis is accomplished on the basis of the responses the patient supplies to a number of statements. Some investigators have commented on the import of referencing "quality of life" issues in the assessment of the success of a treatment for fecal incontinence.[43,295]

INCIDENCE

Anal incontinence may not be a life-threatening disease, but it is a traumatizing and often disabling condition. Many patients feel so inhibited and are so stigmatized by the affliction that they are reluctant to discuss the problem with a physician. There are limited reports of the incidence of incontinence, which may approximate 1% of individuals older than 65 years of age, but soiling of underclothes, incontinence for flatus, anal discharge, and even loss of fecal control are undoubtedly quite common complaints. Nelson and colleagues attempted to determine the prevalence and characteristics of anal incontinence in the general community.[238] A total of 2,570 households comprising almost 7,000 individuals were surveyed. The overall incidence of anal incontinence was 2.2%. Thirty percent were older than 65 years, and approximately two thirds were women. Of those with anal incontinence, 36% were incontinent for formed stool, 54% for liquid stool, and 60% for gas.

Fecal incontinence is particularly prevalent in the elderly and in those individuals in hospitals, psychiatric wards, and geriatric facilities. It is the second most common cause of institutionalization in the elderly, and it accounts for one half billion dollars per year in the United States for the equivalent of adult diapers.[155] Significant positive associations for fecal incontinence in the nursing home population include urinary incontinence, tube feeding, loss of activity, diarrhea, truncal restraints, pressure ulcers, dementia, impaired vision, fecal impaction, constipation, male gender, age, and increasing body mass index.[237] Bannister and co-workers measured anorectal function in 37 elderly patients and compared the results with 48 young, physiologically normal subjects.[13] Elderly individuals had lower anal pressures, required lower rectal volumes to inhibit anal sphincter tone, and had increased pressures as measured by balloon distension. These observations, as well as differences noted on defecation studies, appear to predispose older people to continence problems.[13] Some suggest that internal anal sphincter dysfunction may be the important criterion.[16] Others believe that, especially in women, the pudendal and somatic pelvic nerves are injured when there is perineal descent on straining. The effects of aging and a history of multiparity are, therefore, believed to be relevant.[186] Most specialists in geriatric medicine, however, believe that fecal incontinence is more likely due to a local cause (e.g., fecal impaction) than to senility, to menopause, or simply to old age.[211]

ETIOLOGY

Anal incontinence can result from a disturbance of any one or more of the mechanisms that normally ensure continence:

- Central nervous system damage
- Spinal cord damage
- Peripheral nerve injury and disease
- Loss of the afferent sensory component of the rectosphincteric reflex
- Diseases that impair smooth muscle (e.g., scleroderma)
- Diseases that impair striated muscle (e.g., polymyositis)
- Direct muscle damage that occurs with perianal disease or surgical trauma (see Causes of Fecal Incontinence).[3,311,313,379]

Causes of Fecal Incontinence

The causes of fecal incontinence are summarized as follows:

Trauma Surgical (e.g., fistulectomy, fistulotomy, hemorrhoidectomy, sphincterotomy, sphincter stretch, pull-through operations, low anastomoses)
    Obstetric
    Accidental (e.g., penetrating or avulsion injury, social injury)
Colorectal disease (e.g., hemorrhoids, rectal prolapse, inflammatory bowel disease, malignant tumors, radiation)
Congenital anomaly (e.g., spina bifida, myelomeningocele, imperforate anus, Hirschsprung's disease)
Neurologic disease
    Cerebral (e.g., tumor, vascular accident, dementia, trauma)
    Spinal
    Peripheral (e.g., diabetes mellitus, multiple sclerosis, pudendal nerve injury)
Miscellaneous conditions
    Laxative abuse
    Diarrheal conditions
    Fecal impaction
    Encopresis

Surgical Trauma

As discussed in Chapter 11, fistula surgery is the most common surgical cause of fecal incontinence (Figure 13-1).[26,27] Varying degrees of impairment for control are seen even after what is considered to be proper division of a portion of the sphincter muscle. Complete incontinence (for formed stool) that follows anorectal surgery is usually

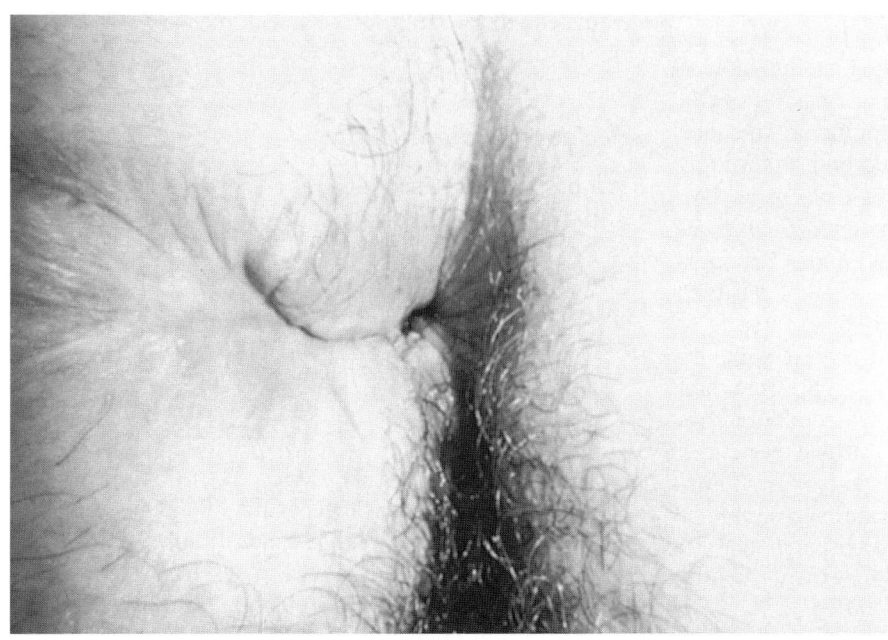

FIGURE 13-1. Scarring, deformity, and partial sphincter loss as a consequence of anal fistulectomy.

the result of inappropriate division of the anorectal ring. This is most likely to occur when a high-level fistula is laid open or an artificial internal opening is created.

Internal anal sphincterotomy when performed for anal fissure may produce some degree of impairment for bowel control (see Chapter 9). Symptoms may include soiling of the underclothes, leakage of gas and/or mucus, and perhaps urgency. Because the internal sphincter does not contribute to voluntary control, complete fecal incontinence should not occur. However, if the surgeon injudiciously divides a portion of the external sphincter, complaints may be more profound.

Sphincter stretch for anal fissure or manual dilatation as a treatment for hemorrhoids (e.g., Lord's procedure) may be associated with fecal incontinence, probably on the basis of injury to the external as well as the internal sphincter. Obviously, internal sphincter stretch, even when properly performed, must inevitably produce stretching of the external sphincter also. This procedure, therefore, should not be undertaken on patients older than 60 years of age. It is because of this complication, in fact, that I no longer employ manual dilatation (see Chapters 8 and 9).

Sphincter stretch to some degree is also achieved when a low anastomosis is effected, either by transanal stapling or by a transanal hand-sewn technique. Ho and colleagues performed a prospective, randomized study of patients who underwent transanal stapled anastomosis with those whose continuity was reestablished through the abdomen.[141] There was a statistically significant reduction in resting anal pressures. Endoanal ultrasound showed internal sphincter fragmentation as well as external sphincter defects when the stapler was used.

Partial incontinence may be a complication of hemorrhoidectomy. Removal of excessive mucosa of the anal canal, such as is performed during Whitehead's hemorrhoidectomy, may produce this distressing complication. Eschar may interfere with sphincter contraction, and rectal mucosa may prolapse through the cicatrix at the site of the excision. This may further impair closure of the canal and allow continuous discharge of mucus (see Chapter 8).[125]

Bowel resection designed to preserve the anal sphincter (e.g., low anterior resection, the various pull-through procedures, coloanal anastomosis, abdominosacral resection) frequently results in discharge of mucus or incontinence for flatus, possibly by interrupting the neural reflex.[125] Injury to the levator ani and external sphincter or to their innervation, and possibly the decreased capacity of the neorectum, may be contributing factors.[343]

Several misconceptions concerning sphincteric surgery should be mentioned if only to be refuted:

- Complete division of the muscles does not impair the sphincter's power of control provided there is no interference with its nerve supply.
- Dividing the sphincter in the posterior midline is safe.
- Dividing the sphincter transversely at right angles to the direction of the fibers, but not obliquely, is safe.
- Division of the muscle at several places instead of one will not lead to permanent loss of control.

Although some surgeons continue to believe some of these myths, the fact remains that if the sphincter muscle is divided through the puborectalis sling, the patient will be incontinent.

Obstetric Trauma

Anal incontinence from sphincter injury at the time of vaginal delivery is more common than had been thought. Although most injuries to the anal sphincter, so-called third-degree lacerations, are recognized and repaired by the obstetrician, adverse consequences can ensue. Pollack and colleagues prospectively evaluated 349 consecutive nulliparous patients before pregnancy and at 9 months and 5 years following delivery.[273] Thirty-eight suffered sphincter injury during the delivery (10.8%). In spite of the repair, almost half of the responders reported anal incontinence at 9 months, whereas slightly more than half noted incontinence at 5 years. If these women had a subsequent vaginal delivery, almost two thirds experienced incontinence symptoms. de Leeuw and co-workers found that 12 of their 34 patients (35%) who suffered sphincter injury at the time of delivery experienced bowel control difficulty.[77] Sphincter defects were demonstrated in the majority.

Fourth-degree perineal lacerations (i.e., into the rectum) can be treated with the expectation of healing. This, perhaps, is because the laxity of the pelvic floor and perineal musculature permits ready apposition without tension.[66] Occasionally, however, because of sepsis, hematoma, or suture breakage, the repair will separate. This occurrence not only may lead to impaired control for flatus or feces but also may be associated with a fistula between the anus or rectum and the vagina (see Chapter 12).

Even women without overt injury at the time of vaginal delivery are subject to an increased risk of subsequent impairment for fecal control. Physiologic studies on postpartum women have shown that multiparity, forceps delivery, increased duration of the second stage of labor, and high birth weight may lead to pudendal nerve damage and to sphincter atrophy.[336,337] Wynne and colleagues studied more than 1,200 mothers antenatally in order to determine the effects of vaginal delivery on the anal sphincter.[393] Approximately one half of them were also reassessed postnatally. All patients who had a vaginal delivery but not those you underwent cesarean section dropped their resting anal pressures from antenatal values ($p < .001$). The authors concluded that the first vaginal delivery causes a permanent lowering of resting anal pressures.[393] Others have shown a high prevalence of anal sphincter defects (up to 62%) as determined by ultrasound in a population of incontinent, parous women without a prior history of anal surgery.[73,234] Frudinger and associates found that anal continence deteriorated in 27.6% of women following delivery, 43.2% of whom had sonographic evidence of sphincter trauma.[107] Because of the relatively poor perineal support in women when compared with men, it may require only minimal injury to tip the balance toward impairment for control. This is especially true in the situation of an ectopic anus (see Obstetric Injuries).

Accidental Trauma

Trauma to the perineum can injure the sphincter mechanism (Figure 13-2). Impalement on a spike or pole as well as social injuries (e.g., fist fornication) may result in division of the sphincter and contamination of the extrarectal spaces.[41,70,203,247,382] Sepsis can supervene and lead to excessive scar formation with a resultant patulous anal canal and an incompetent sphincter (see also Chapters 14 and 15).

Colorectal Disease

Incontinence for flatus or feces may be associated with anorectal disease (e.g., hemorrhoids, fissure, fistula) even without surgical intervention. Prolapse of rectal mucosa or hemorrhoids and true procidentia may interfere with closure of the anal canal. With time, the protruding mass stretches the sphincter and may lead to further complaints of incontinence. Of course, attenuation of the pudendal nerve from the rectal prolapse may cause sphincter atrophy on a neurologic basis, or the neuropathy may precede the development of the prolapse. In the former situation, the incontinence is often ameliorated with definitive treatment of the prolapse (see Chapter 17).[302] Other conditions that may be associated with incontinence include nonspecific inflammatory bowel disease (ulcerative colitis and Crohn's disease), malignant conditions, and infectious and parasitic diseases.

Congenital Anomaly

Congenital incontinence may be caused by spina bifida, meningocele, myelomeningocele, aganglionic megacolon (i.e., Hirschsprung's disease), and surgery to correct anorectal malformations (e.g., imperforate anus; see Chapter 18) (Figure 13-3). Involvement of sensory or motor nerves may produce urinary and fecal incontinence and, ultimately, rectal prolapse, which will further exacerbate incontinence problems.

Neurologic Disease

Any neurologic disease may affect bowel control. Perhaps the most common condition that produces neuropathy is diabetes mellitus.[369] Patients may be particularly troubled both because of diarrhea from autonomic neuropathy and because of sphincter impairment. Schiller and colleagues, in their study on 16 such patients, concluded that incontinence in this group was due to internal anal sphincter dysfunction, and that diabetic patients without diarrhea have no impairment for fecal control.[309] Other

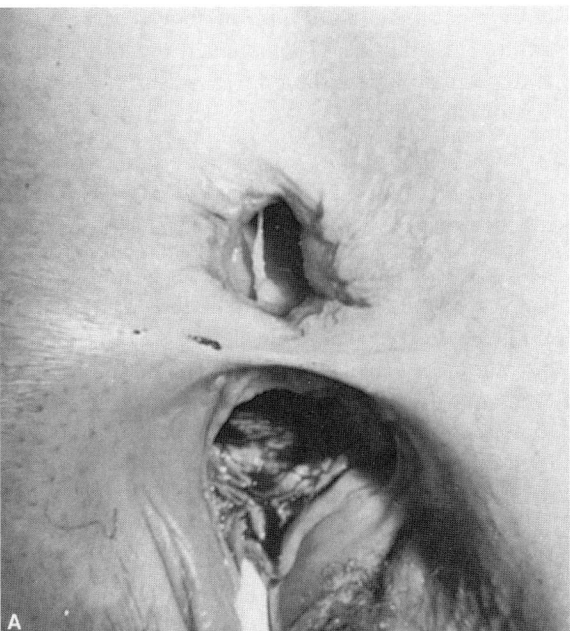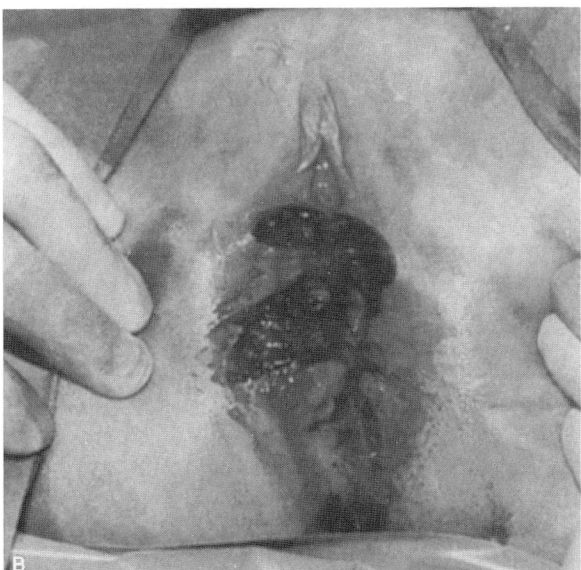

FIGURE 13-2. Perineal injuries as a consequence of accidental trauma. **(A)** Patulous anus with avulsed sphincter from impalement on a picket fence. **(B)** Severe perineal trauma from impalement on a bedpost as a consequence of jumping in bed.

conditions, such as progressive systemic sclerosis, may produce incontinence on either a neurologic or a myopathic basis.[50,152,196] Spinal cord injury, spinal cord tumor, and cauda equina lesions may produce incontinence by denervation of external sphincter and levator ani muscles (Figure 13-4).

Idiopathic incontinence is the term used to describe denervation injury to the sphincter muscle that occurs for no apparent cause. Habitual straining at defecation, nerve entrapment, the preprolapse state, and the syndrome of the descending perineum—all have been implicated.

Pelvic Radiotherapy

A history of prior pelvic radiotherapy as a cause of or an association with fecal incontinence presents a special management problem. Surgical options are limited, with every operative approach identified by a high complication and a high failure rate. Most patients are, therefore, usually managed conservatively (i.e., antidiarrheal agents and a bowel management program) or by fecal diversion.[132]

Laxative Use

One of the nonsurgical causes of fecal incontinence is laxative use and abuse. A notorious offender is mineral oil. The greasy, narrow stool that results from the use of

this substance slides through the sphincter without producing anal dilatation. Over a period of years, the muscle may atrophy because the sphincter is not stretched by a normal stool. Any attempt to repair the sphincter in a patient with such a history and origin of incontinence will be unsatisfactory.

Diarrhea

Diarrhea may be associated with fecal incontinence. Read and associates evaluated 29 patients with this symptom complex and determined the severity of the diarrhea by 72-hour stool collections.[282] They also studied anal manometry and continence for liquid, the latter by the patient's ability to retain a saline enema. Most, but not all, patients had low sphincter pressures and an impaired ability to retain the enema. This would suggest a defect in sphincteric function. However, some patients were found to have a normal sphincter mechanism. The implication is that a normal sphincter can be overwhelmed by a large volume of stool, especially if it is liquid.

Fecal Impaction

Fecal impaction frequently is associated with incontinence, presumably on an overflow basis. Patients with this problem are usually elderly and often suffer from diseases for which they may be taking constipating medications (see Chapter 3). For example, the medications

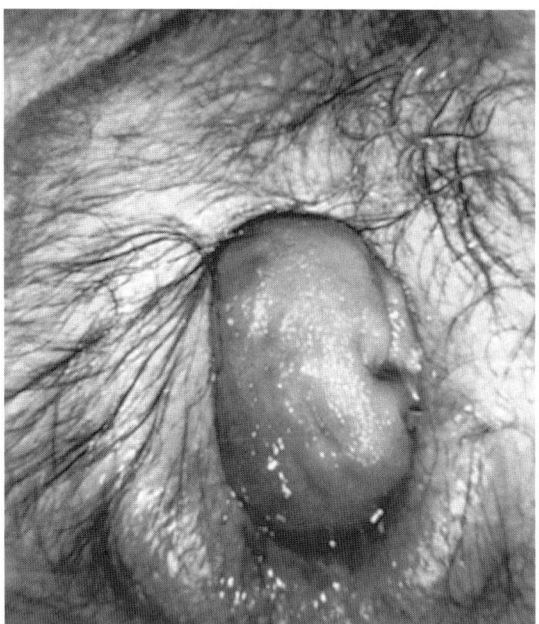

FIGURE 13-3. Anal incontinence following pull-through procedure for imperforate anus. Note mucosal prolapse and anal laxity.

often employed for treating parkinsonism are quite constipating; impaction is very common in these individuals.

Fecal impaction is also a troubling problem for the senile and the psychiatrically disturbed patient. Treatment may require manual disimpaction, enemas, and laxatives. After the impaction is cleared, prevention consists of the establishment of a proper bowel management program. This may be supplemented by colonic irrigations and perineal strengthening exercises (see Nonsurgical Treatment).

Encopresis

Encopresis, or psychogenic soiling, is defined as the passage of formed or semiformed stool in a child's underclothes (or other inappropriate places) that occurs regularly after the age of 4 years. It is essentially an involuntary evacuation of the bowel not caused by organic factors. Encopresis is at least four times more common in boys than in girls and is analogous to enuresis as it pertains to urinary incontinence.

The condition was first described by Weissenberg, who recognized that this form of fecal incontinence was associated with emotional disturbance.[373] Behavioral factors that may contribute to the problem include the following:

■ Excessive parental attention to toilet habits
■ Laxative use
■ Harsh or lax toilet training methods
■ Fear of the toilet or the loss of feces
■ Desire for attention
■ Family or personal stress[252]

In time, the increasing retention of feces leads to attenuation of the rectal wall, lax sphincter contractility, progressive constipation, obstipation, and fecal impaction.

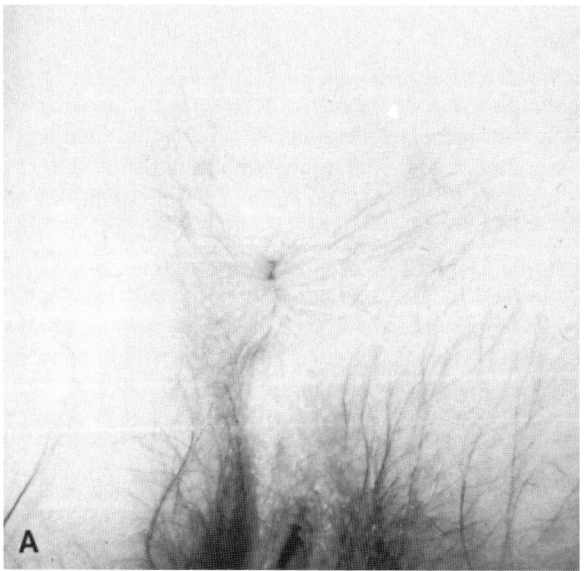
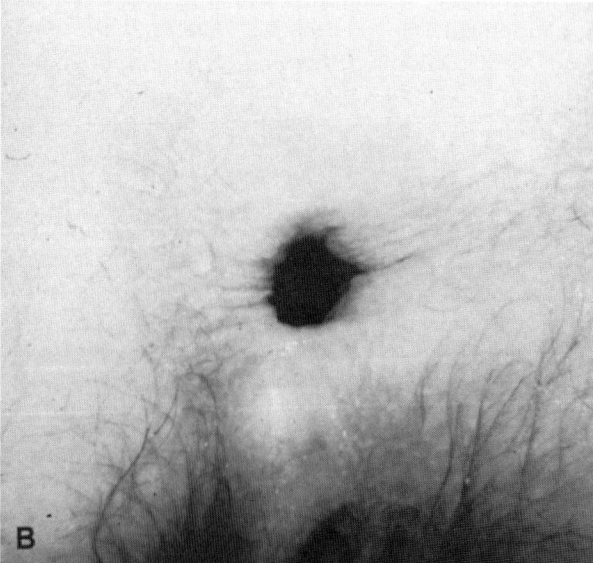

FIGURE 13-4. Anal incontinence secondary to spinal nerve injury. **(A)** Normal appearance of the anus. **(B)** The same patient with a patulous anus immediately after rectal examination.

Anal fissure and hemorrhoidal difficulties may develop. Loening-Baucke observed a common clinical history with children exhibiting chronic constipation and soiling, often many years of infrequent and abnormal stools, a dilated rectal ampulla, and the presence of an abdominal fecal mass.[201]

Treatment is usually directed toward bowel management, stress reduction, and child and family psychological counseling.[22,83,326] Laxatives, enemas, and dietary regimens are recommended, as well as encouraging the child to sit on the toilet for 10 minutes twice daily at the same time each day. The goal is to establish a practical time for defecation and, ultimately, a spontaneous bowel evacuation habit. Uridine-5-triphosphate has been suggested to have some limited success.[233] Although the mechanism of action of this drug has not been ascertained, it is believed to stimulate the cortical substance of the brain to make the child more aware of the need to defecate.

Loening-Baucke used anorectal manometry to evaluate 20 healthy children, 12 with constipation, and 20 with chronic constipation and encopresis.[201] Mean values for anal resting tone and anal pull-through pressure were lower in the constipated and the encopretic children than in the controls. The study was repeated up to 4 years after treatment for the condition; abnormal anorectal function was still apparent even years after cessation of treatment and apparent recovery. In a later study of 97 children, also by Loening-Baucke, the author reported that 57% had not recovered.[202] Using a host of training techniques, Loening-Baucke noted that there was no difference in recovery rates for boys and girls, and that the likelihood of success or failure could not be predicted *a priori*.

PHYSIOLOGIC AND ANATOMIC BASES OF CONTINENCE

The neuromuscular control for fecal continence has been the subject of considerable investigation and debate (see Chapter 6).[82,311,315,321] Continence is maintained partly under voluntary control by the striated muscles of the external sphincter and levator ani and partly through the autonomic nervous system by the smooth muscle of the internal sphincter. Levi colleagues studied the development of the anal canal muscles in 18 human embryos and noted a common origin of the puborectalis, ileococcygeus, and pubococcygeus muscles (see Chapter 1).[199] Their investigation appears to confirm that the puborectalis muscle is a portion of the levator ani rather than the external sphincter. They further demonstrated that both the external sphincter and the urogenital sphincter originate from the cloacal sphincter. Figure 1-10 illustrates the male per-

ineal musculature at three different levels. Understanding the complex anatomy of the area is of paramount importance if the physician is to embark on any reconstructive option. In essence, there are two concentric cylinders—an internal one composed of smooth muscle and an external one composed of striated muscle. The internal sphincter is the continuation of the distal portion of the circular muscle of the rectum (see Figure 8-2). This muscle appears later during embryologic development than does the striated musculature.[199] The internal sphincter is maintained in a state of near-maximal contraction at all times; its major reflex response to rectal distension is relaxation. Although the internal sphincter plays a less important role in maintenance of voluntary control, approximately 85% of the resting tone of the anal canal is contributed by this muscle.[340] For example, electromechanical dissociation with inappropriate relaxation of the internal sphincter is believed to be responsible for most cases of leakage and soilage.[94]

The external anal sphincter is part of a composite muscle encircling the anal canal that enables voluntary control of continence. It has been arbitrarily divided into three parts: subcutaneous, superficial, and deep (see Figure 1-11). The distinction between the three parts of the external sphincter is of little practical importance. Dalley recommends that "it be relegated to the junkyard of anatomic trivia where it may languish for the sake of the historical anatomist or the rare individual who spends time carving out the most meticulous of dissections".[72] There is considerable merit to this position, especially when reading other studies that hold that the external anal sphincter is formed by only two parts.[199]

The levator ani, arising from the bony pelvis and the obturator fascia, spreads out to form a muscular pelvic floor. The puborectalis muscle is the anteromedial portion of this diaphragm and, arising from the back of the symphysis, passes posteriorly around the lower part of the rectum, meeting fibers from the opposite side in a loop or U-shaped girdle. The puborectalis blends with the deep portion of the external sphincter, the longitudinal muscle, and the adjacent part of the internal sphincter to form the anorectal ring. Contraction of the levator ani with the puborectalis sling pulls the anorectal junction forward and upward, elongating the anal canal and increasing angulation between the anal canal and the rectum.[260] Contraction of the levator ani coordinated with that of the external anal sphincter results in effective closure of the anal canal.[109]

Another theory of pelvic muscle anatomy and function has been described by Shafik.[321] This involves a three-loop system with two U-shaped loops directed anteriorly and one posteriorly (see Figure 1-10). Although it is an interesting concept, this observation probably serves more to obfuscate than to clarify the issue of muscular control.

Another possible factor contributing to voluntary control is the angulation produced by contraction of the levator ani muscle. This has been said to cause the anterior wall of the rectum to cover the top of the closed anal canal like a flap valve, especially during straining (e.g., Valsalva's maneuver).[357] However, Bartolo and co-workers determined rectal and anal pressures with electromyography (EMG) and defecography simultaneously and found that the anterior rectal wall was always separated from the upper sphincter despite maximal effort by the patient.[19] This suggests that the puborectalis functions by occluding the anal canal. Bannister and associates believed, on the basis of their studies of physiologically normal subjects, that continence is normally maintained by a reflex contraction of the external anal sphincter.[14] However, those patients with idiopathic fecal incontinence fulfilled the criteria for a flap valve, albeit an incompetent one.

The practical importance of these two muscles in maintaining continence is that if the external anal sphincter is divided completely, satisfactory continence will be provided by the intact puborectalis muscle. If both the external sphincter and the puborectalis muscle are divided, the patient will be incontinent. Division of the puborectalis without division of the external sphincter may occur in infants during operation for high imperforate anus. These children are rendered incontinent despite having a normal, functioning external sphincter.[168]

Like the internal sphincter, the external sphincter is also in a state of contraction; however, its major reflex response to stimuli is contraction.[312] The degree of external sphincter contraction varies with alterations in intraabdominal pressure and posture.[313–315] As intraabdominal pressure is increased or as the patient rises to a more upright posture, electrical activity and tone increase gradually.[314] Resting activity may be supplemented by voluntary contraction, which is accompanied by a marked rise in electrical action potentials and a substantial increase in recorded intrasphincteric pressure.[316] Because of fatigue, maximal voluntary contraction can be maintained only for about 50 seconds.[316]

Response of the external sphincter can be produced by voluntary effort, postural change, rectal distension, increased intraabdominal pressure, and anal dilatation.[313–315] These responses involve several different neural pathways. Therefore, neurologic impairment can be differentiated from muscle disease if the sphincter responds to any one of these stimuli.[316] Failure to respond to all stimuli is indicative either of muscle disease or of a diffuse neurologic disorder.

The internal sphincter reflex is mainly initiated by rectal distension. The neural pathway for this response, however, is unknown. The internal sphincter has a dual innervation system that consists of a motor supply that travels through the hypogastric nerves from the sympathetic outflow tract and an inhibitory supply from the parasympathetic outflow tract (see Chapter 1).[124,204] The internal sphincter is also continuously active, with strips of the muscle demonstrating spontaneous contraction *in vitro*.[82] It has been shown that frequent abnormal episodes of internal anal sphincter relaxation may lead to stool leakage in those individuals with neurogenic fecal incontinence.[95]

Receptors for the external sphincter response must lie either in or near the rectal mucosa, because the reflex disappears after application of a topical anesthetic. The external sphincter is supplied only by somatic pudendal nerves, which arise from the second, third, and fourth sacral nerves. Because lesions of the cauda equina abolish the external sphincter reflex, it is evident that the reflex is mediated through the spinal cord.[25,274] This is not true of the internal sphincter response; this reflex can persist after transection of the lower spinal cord.[78,315]

Matzel and colleagues reported the results of their dissections of three male cadavers and traced the sacral nerves from their entrances into the pelvis, through the sacral foramina, to their final destinations.[216] They concluded that two different peripheral nerve supplies were responsible for anal continence. The levator ani and puborectalis muscles were found to be supplied by multiple direct branches recruited from the sacral nerves S2 to S4. The pudendal nerve supplies the external sphincter and is derived mainly from the second sacral nerve. The authors confirmed the accuracy of their observations by stimulating the nerves at different levels. Stimulation of the pudendal nerve increased anal canal pressure, whereas stimulation of S3 had the primary effect of decreasing the anorectal angle (see Postanal Pelvic Floor Repair or Parks' Repair).[257]

Comment

The foregoing discussion represents the thoughts and investigations of many distinguished individuals. Their opinions and conclusions are based on meticulous physiologic and anatomic studies. That stated, I cannot pretend to understand fully the mechanism for incontinence in many patients. Conversely, I do not always comprehend why certain individuals are indeed *continent* (see Physical Examination).

The factors responsible for *continence* are indeed complex. There may also be numerous contributions to the etiology of someone's *incontinence*. That is why it is so important to provide the patient with alternative treatments as well as to convey realistic expectations. So frustrating is the management for both patient and physician, it is not surprising that many colon and rectal surgeons choose to refer to someone with a compelling interest in this condition.

EVALUATION OF THE PATIENT

History

To determine the appropriate therapy for the patient with anal incontinence, probably the single most important criterion is the origin of the problem. Patients who have sustained loss of sphincter function through injury, whether surgical, obstetric, or accidental, are the most amenable to reconstructive efforts. However, those who are incontinent because of disease are generally poor candidates for an attempt at repair. In this group of patients, appropriate counseling (e.g., dietary, exercise, bowel management) may be the most efficacious mode of therapy (see later).

Requisite information should include an accurate bowel function history (onset, duration, contributing factors, frequency, medications), neurologic information including any sensory loss, obstetric history in female patients, and, of course, the degree of impairment for control—whether for flatus, loose stool, or formed movements.

Physical Examination

In the absence of a history of trauma, a comprehensive medical evaluation is frequently suggested but is rarely illuminating. Usually, inspection and palpation reveal the information that will dictate the therapy. By spreading the patient's buttocks, the physician will be able to determine whether there is a patulous anus, which implies either a loss of sphincter muscle or more likely neurologic impairment, evidence of a perineal tear or obstetric injury, or other scars or deformities. A mucosal ectropion or rectal prolapse may be noted, as may perineal descent, especially if the patient strains or is examined while sitting on the toilet (see Chapter 17). Spontaneous opening of the anal canal or sphincteric relaxation may be indicative of an anoreceptive individual or may suggest the possibility of neurologic impairment. It has also been thought to be a sign of sexual abuse in children.

Read and Sun studied the effect of parting the buttocks on anal function in normal subjects and in those with anorectal or spinal disease.[283] Normal subjects can consciously relax the external sphincter and even reduce anal canal pressure without the anal canal opening. Paraplegic patients who have lost conscious control of their external sphincters demonstrate anal gaping when the buttocks are parted.[283]

By means of palpation, the resting tone of the sphincter can be assessed, and by asking the patient to "tighten up," the degree of contractility can be evaluated. Asking the patient to pull the rectum up to the navel usually clarifies any confusion the patient may have as to what is meant. A defect in the sphincter muscle may also be perceived. In neurologic conditions, including lesions of the spinal cord and cauda equina, normal tone may be apparent. However, if gentle traction is applied to any segment of the anorectal ring, it is followed by gaping of the anal canal (Figure 13-4).[131] Even though this evaluation is relatively subjective, the information obtained, in my opinion, is often as valuable as so-called objective, investigative studies. In fact, Hill and colleagues performed a prospective study on 237 patients with idiopathic fecal incontinence.[138] This included obtaining a history, physical examination, and anorectal physiologic studies. The authors were able to demonstrate that an informed history and a digital examination can predict the manometric findings and specialized anorectal physiologic studies with a high degree of accuracy. In other words, history and examination, themselves, can give a reliable index of sphincter function in individuals with anal incontinence.

Sensory determination is also useful in examining a patient with anal incontinence. Impaired sensation to touch or to pinprick implies that the success of operative repair will be compromised.

The ability to retain a small-volume enema has been suggested as a means for evaluating incontinence.[339] Although retaining liquid implies good sphincter function, I have never found a truly incontinent patient able to perform this feat; therefore, I do not rely on this test. Although proctosigmoidoscopy, colonoscopy, and barium enema examinations are important studies in the evaluation of any patient with a colorectal problem, they are usually unrewarding in someone who complains of fecal incontinence. Conversely, defecography as it is used to diagnose the preprolapse condition may be helpful (see later and Chapters 6, 16, and 17).

Comment

In spite of the foregoing recommendations concerning the importance of obtaining an accurate history and of performing a comprehensive anorectal examination, I am often bewildered by the failure of patients to report impaired bowel control in spite of profound, objective weakness, deformity, or defect of the sphincter mechanism. When inquiring as to the status of the patient's continence under these circumstances, the physician is often met with a quizzical expression and an interrogatory, "Is there some problem, doctor?" Conversely, there are often circumstances when a patient complains bitterly of soilage or incontinence for flatus or feces, and yet there appears to be normal or near-normal anorectal anatomy, sphincter tone, and contractility that all but causes ischemic necrosis of the examining finger. I can only presume that in an individual without antecedent history suggestive of ego dysfunction, malingering, or hypochondriasis, this dichotomy is a result of our failure as physicians and surgeons to understand fully the complex mechanisms of defecation and continence.

Physiologic Studies

There has been a remarkable interest in recent years in physiologic evaluation of the gastrointestinal tract.[99] Many clinics and hospitals have established laboratories that promote these efforts, not only as research tools but also for application to the patient in a therapeutic setting. The American Board of Colon and Rectal Surgery encourages residents to obtain experience with anorectal physiologic testing as part of their training. The reader is referred to Chapters 2 and 6 for discussions on colorectal physiology and the setting up of such a laboratory. Still, some of the opinions and caveats are worth repeating here. This is not to say, however, that such investigations are always necessary, or that the results are always intelligible and have practical implications.

In 1988, some prominent investigators who have contributed extensively to the literature on anorectal physiology gathered to discuss methods and to identify areas of agreement with respect to determining indices of anorectal physiology.[161] Some of their conclusions are cited with each investigation as they are discussed and are referred to subsequently as the "working party."

The two primary studies for evaluating pelvic floor physiology are EMG and anorectal manometry, but there are a number of others (see Chapter 6). Cineradiography, defecography, and bowel transit time are also suggested, the first two particularly for those with suspected rectal prolapse or preprolapse (i.e., internal procidentia) and the last for those with defecatory disorders (e.g., constipation, fecal impaction).[33,82] The application of these methods is also discussed in Chapters 16 and 17. In addition to testing, if incontinence is believed to be a consequence of a neurologic problem, and that cause is by no means certain, evaluation by a neurologist is advisable.

Electromyography

EMG has been applied for evaluating the sphincter mechanism since the initial work of Beck in 1930 (see Chapter 6).[21] The investigation is believed to be an important tool for ascertaining the nature of neuromuscular dysfunction, whether secondary to disorders of the nervous system (e.g., spinal cord, spinal nerve roots, peripheral nerves) or to diseases of the muscle. The technique depends on the recording of electrical activity arising in muscle fibers dur-

ing voluntary contractility and at rest.[351] Unlike peripheral skeletal muscle, the external anal sphincter maintains its tone even when not voluntarily contracted.[170] The motor units fire at a low rate when the patient is at rest, and they vary with sleep and position changes. An absence of sphincter activity is noted only during attempted defecation, an observation which makes interpretation of EMG studies often quite difficult.[106,170,370] In fact, in my opinion the procedure is virtually always unreliable in patients who have sustained injury to the anal area, whether from direct trauma or because of prior anorectal surgery.[170,355] Furthermore, because of the activity normally seen even at rest, detection of spontaneous abnormal potentials may not be possible in the partially denervated muscle. This limits the benefit of the evaluation to those in whom the resting sphincter tone is absent or markedly reduced or to those without antecedent injury.[130] One final but not insignificant concern is that needle EMG is very uncomfortable for most patients, but there are EMG alternatives to this invasive technique.

Electrophysiologic tests have become even more specialized than the conventional needle EMG. Electrical activity can be recorded using surface electrodes, monopolar electrodes, or concentric needle electrodes. Additionally, a so-called single-fiber EMG can be employed that measures the number of muscle fibers innervated by a single motor axon.[350] This permits 20 consecutive recordings of the external anal sphincter or puborectalis muscle. Pinho and colleagues, responding to the concerns expressed by patients of the discomfort associated with conventional, invasive, needle EMG, evaluated intraanal EMG using an anal plug electrode.[270] A significant correlation was found between this technique and manometry. It was also noted to be reproducible when undertaken by two independent observers.

The previously mentioned working party concluded the following with respect to EMG:

> Fibre density or motor unit potential duration is the only objective assessment of denervation. Fine wire electrodes are optimal for monitoring electrical activity of all muscles of the pelvic floor, including that of the internal sphincter. EMG is useful for mapping a deficient or ectopic sphincter and for defining anismus (obstructed defecation).[161]

Applications

Henry and co-workers recorded the latency of the anal reflex in patients with fecal incontinence by means of EMG.[134] On the basis of 22 individuals with idiopathic fecal incontinence and no prior history of trauma, they concluded that a major cause of the incontinence was denervation of the sphincter musculature. The work of Bartolo and associates supports the suggestion that external sphincter neuropathy with idiopathic fecal incontinence is due to a stretch injury of the pudendal nerve.[18] Neill colleagues, in evaluating patients with fecal incontinence and rectal prolapse by means of EMG and anorectal manometry, demonstrated abnormal results in this group.[236]

Waylonis and Powers analyzed 184 pediatric and 81 adult patients, the former with suspected bowel and bladder dysfunction and the latter following abnormal EMG determinations.[371] Forty-nine of 54 children with myelomeningocele had reduced or absent external sphincter function. This implied the need for frequent urologic follow-up. Nineteen of 26 children who were incontinent following surgery for Hirschsprung's disease or imperforate anus had abnormal findings. The authors believed that EMG was particularly useful in determining either the presence and location or the absence of sphincter tissue in cases of imperforate anus. In adults with abnormal EMGs, 36% had abnormal spinal x-ray studies.

Another application for the EMG is in the investigation of patients with constipation (see Chapter 16). For example, Wexner and co-workers have shown that the most common EMG abnormality in constipated patients is paradoxical puborectalis contraction.[377]

Nerve Conduction Studies

Nerve conduction studies should be included as part of a comprehensive evaluation of the pelvic floor and sphincter mechanism. Pudendal and perineal nerve terminal motor latencies and spinal motor latencies can be assessed.[350] Pudendal and perineal nerve stimulation techniques evaluate the distal motor innervation of the external anal sphincter and periurethral striated sphincter muscles.[334] The method consists of stimulating the pudendal nerve on either side of the pelvis while measuring the latency until the onset of the electrical response in the muscle. This is usually accomplished by means of a gloved-finger having two metal stimulating electrodes at the tip and two surface-recording electrodes mounted at the base (see Chapter 6 and Figure 6-28). The working party that has been alluded to concluded with the following quotation with respect to nerve conduction studies:

> Measurement of pudendal nerve terminal motor latency is the most widely recognized and reproducible technique for detecting conduction defects in the terminal portion of the pudendal nerve.

Applications

The application of pudendal nerve terminal motor latency (PNTML) has been discussed in Chapter 6. It is generally considered one of the most useful of physiologic studies for evaluation of individuals with anal incontinence. This is because the investigation not only identifies any innervation abnormality, but it may be beneficial with respect to the prognosis following attempted repair of the sphincters.[139]

Yip and associates investigated the "learning curve" for a novice to perform PNTML.[395] Students tended to record longer latencies than the experienced investigator. This led to an increased rate of false-positive results. The authors concluded that, in order to master the test within a proper learning environment, approximately 40 patients or procedures are required.

Pudendal neuropathy is an etiologic or associated factor that may be present in patients with fecal incontinence under a number of circumstances. Roig and colleagues undertook a prospective study to determine the prevalence and association in 96 individuals with fecal incontinence.[292] Pudendal neuropathy (defined as a PNTML greater than 2.2 m/second) was found in 70% overall (75% in female and 50% in male patients). Neuropathy was also more frequent in patients with perineal descent or in those exhibiting risk factors, such as difficult labor or excessive defecatory straining. Others have compared measurement of the PNTML with anal manometry in patients with anal incontinence.[364] The conclusion is clear. Manometric evaluation alone is not helpful in identifying the neuropathic individual. Sangwan and co-workers undertook a study to determine the role of abnormal distal rectoanal excitatory reflex (RAER) as a marker of pudendal neuropathy and to compare the results with PNTML as well as with single-fiber density estimation.[306] Despite some slight discrepancy, the investigators believed that RAER compared favorably with PNTML in diagnosing pudendal neuropathy.

Another innovation for measuring the innervation of the pelvic floor electroneurographically is the use of magnetic stimulation.[157] This was accomplished by determining pudendal nerve motor latency of the overall distance by stimulation of nerve root S3 through the discharge of a magnetic coil. Using 18 volunteers, the investigators concluded that this method enabled precise diagnosis in pudendal neuropathies, more so than conventional electrical stimulation. However, the application of this particular test requires further exploration.

Anorectal Manometry

Anorectal manometry can be undertaken by numerous methods, such as open-tipped or closed-tipped catheters, perfused catheters, macroballoons, and microballoons (see Chapter 6). In the United States, the most common type is the open-tipped, perfused catheter, whereas in the United Kingdom the microballoon is preferred. The interpretation of anorectal manometric studies has been somewhat problematic because of the disparate results obtained when using catheters of different types, especially when comparing the open-tipped tube with the closed balloon system. Another source of debate has been the relative merit of an air-filled balloon as opposed to one that is water-filled.[223] In truth, all methods are essentially nonphysiologic because the tube, even if it is of very narrow caliber, creates its own artifact. Variations in recording instrument diameter consistently affect measurements of resting anal canal pressure and the maximum squeeze pressure (MSP).[219] Coller, in his review of the clinical applications of anorectal manometry, implies that much of the difficulty we have in interpreting data from physiologic studies is due to our failure to comprehend the physiology of defecation.[60] In order to obtain manometric values under physiologic conditions and to permit simultaneous registration of anal and rectal pressures for prolonged periods, ambulatory anorectal manometry has been developed.[9] Despite the myriad potential problems, anorectal manometry can measure the resting tone of the internal sphincter, the functional length of the anal canal, the anal reflex, and the voluntary contractility of the external sphincter.[357] Methods are discussed in Chapter 6.

An alternative to the conventional systems mentioned is the Millar microtip catheter pressure transducer (Millar, Houston, TX). This is a 120-cm long, woven-Dacron tube that contains a miniature silicone strain gauge at the tip.[310] The outside diameter is only 1.67 mm, so the confusion associated with interpretation of the results with a large-bore cannula is somewhat obviated. It is a simple technique that is well tolerated, even in pediatric patients.[213,294] Other modifications have been suggested, such as the air-filled microballoon (Dipped Latex Products, Gloucester, UK) and the Stryker 295–1 intracompartmental pressure monitor (Stryker Corp., Kalamazoo, MI).[224,227,249,250,386] Complete manometry, biofeedback, and PNTML systems are available in the United States through Sandhill Scientific and Medtronic (see Chapter 6).

Krogh, Pedersen, and Christiansen studied 78 healthy volunteers to determine the range of normal physiologic variations with anal manometry.[176] They found that the maximum intraindividual variations in the length of the anal high-pressure zone, the resting pressure, and the squeeze pressure were 10, 26, and 68 mm Hg, respectively. The median length of the pressure zone was 4 mm (14 mm Hg resting and 48 mm Hg squeeze). No gender difference was found in the length of the high-pressure zone, whereas resting pressure and squeeze pressure were higher in men than in women.[176] Interestingly, it has been shown that male patients with so-called "idiopathic" fecal seepage have a long anal sphincter with an abnormally high resting tone.[254] Generally, standard tests of anorectal sensorimotor function are repeatable by different investigators.[291] This suggests that comparison of data obtained from different institutions is probably valid, provided, of course, that the methods employed are clearly defined.

However, is anorectal manometry truly a more accurate technique for evaluation than the physician's index finger? Hallan and colleagues attempted to answer this question by assessing anal sphincter function by digital examination and by anal canal manometry in 66 patients and controls.[129] After analyzing the relative scores, the authors determined that the sensitivities and specificities of the two techniques in segregating continent and incontinent patients were similar. They concluded that digital estimation was of equal value in assessing anal sphincter function as anal canal manometry. Likewise, Kaushal and Goldner analyzed 27 patients with a spectrum of subjectively assessed sphincter tones.[159] In comparison with objective anal sphincter pressure measurements, an excellent correlation coefficient was revealed ($0.97; p < .05$).

The working party exhibited less of a consensus with the use of manometry than with EMG because there are so many different approaches. All affirmed, however, that whatever method was employed needed to be clearly identified (e.g., internal diameter of tubing, orientation of side holes, speed of withdrawal).[161] The following agreements were reached:

Anal pressures should be recorded in kilo Pascals (100 cm of water = 9.8 kPa); maximum resting anal pressure (MRP) should be used to denote the highest recorded pressure at any site in the anal canal at rest; and MSP should be used to denote the highest recorded pressure at any site in the anal canal during maximum pelvic floor contraction.[161]

Despite the recommendations concerning the use of the kilopascal as the unit of pressure measurement, the literature from the United States continues to be reported in millimeters of mercury.

Comment

The obvious question is, if one accepts the conclusions of the studies that manometry and subjective assessment by the physician are comparable, why do manometry? The answer lies with the nature of one's clinical practice. If the results of the manometric determination are not going to influence the treatment, then performance of the study is a waste of time and money. Conversely, if the results of manometry affect therapy, then the study is obviously worth obtaining. Finally, if one has an interest in publishing, having some method to objectify the clinical findings and the results is usually helpful.

Computerized Vector Manometry

Because conventional manometric techniques cannot ascertain the cause of the problem, whether diffuse or focal, a technique has been proposed to identify the specific quadrant of the injury or sphincter loss—three-dimensional computerized vector manometry.[31,264] Coller relates that there is nothing mystical about applying the computer to manometry, especially if it is used only to store data, but this technique offers a host of analytical functions.[61] The computer can construct a three-dimensional anal pressure vectorgram from the data obtained by manometry and allow the anus to be viewed from all perspectives (see Figs. 6-5 through 6-8). An injury may result in radial pressure asymmetry, an observation easily recognized on the vectorgram. Perry and colleagues believe that this technique can reveal occult anal sphincter injuries and may ultimately provide a means for selecting the most appropriate patients for sphincter repair.[264] The obvious question, therefore, is whether this very new modality, which provides a still more accurate assessment of the sphincter mechanism, will not merely permit better information, but lead to a more appropriate therapeutic approach in the individual patient.

Applications

Anorectal manometry has been found to be a useful tool for the preoperative and postoperative evaluation of patients who have problems with constipation or incontinence, whether the origin is any of the following:

- Hemorrhoids
- Anal fissure
- Anal fistula
- Rectal prolapse
- Perineal descent[259]
- Sigmoidorectal intussusception (i.e., the preprolapse condition)
- Procidentia
- Encopresis
- Sphincter-saving operations
- Obstetric injury
- Congenital anomalies (e.g., Hirschsprung's disease)[17, 42,59,101,143,150,230,246,279–281,332,388]

Additionally, the procedure is of value in assessing rectal compliance, information that is especially useful in those individuals who may be candidates for an ileorectal anastomosis in Crohn's disease.

Generally, patients suffering from problems with bowel control have lower anal canal pressures at rest and during maximum squeeze efforts than do those without continence difficulties. Kuijpers and Scheuer studied 208 patients with impaired control of feces: idiopathic (n = 107), iatrogenic (n = 57), and obstetric (n = 33).[177] However, many were found to have rectal prolapse. The authors concluded that although anal manometry provides useful information concerning anorectal physiology, there is considerable overlap in squeeze pressures between asymptomatic patients and those with impairment for bowel control. The authors postulate an explanation for this commonly observed phenomenon—that many factors contribute to the mechanism for continence and that

impairment for one may be compensated by the combined function of others.[177]

Keren and co-workers performed anorectal manometry on 12 physiologically normal children and 18 who suffered from constipation and soiling.[166] Although the study showed that the anal canal of all of the normal children relaxed during defecation, 78% of those who were constipated closed the canal by paradoxically contracting the anal sphincter. In this situation, biofeedback therapy is the appropriate treatment (see later).

Borden and associates developed an anorectal function profile by using pressure studies and the EMG.[30] They identified discrete defects in anorectal function, including high sensory threshold levels, discomfort with minimal rectal distension, persistence of external sphincter activity with maximum tolerable volume, and increasing rather than decreasing external sphincter activity with rectal distension. On the basis of these studies, they suggested that specific therapy may be selective (e.g., electrical stimulator for absent tonic external sphincter activity, biofeedback for abnormal external sphincter contraction reflex, rectal distension for high resting sphincter pressure, and bowel management for patients with high rectal volume and sensation thresholds).

Anal Sensation

The role of anal canal sensation in the maintenance of continence is an issue that has stimulated considerable debate. Roe and colleagues have reported a technique for quantifying the level of threshold sensation to electrical stimulation.[289] Objective measurements of a sensory deficit were noted in those patients with neuropathic incontinence. Variations in sensitivity were also seen in individuals with anal fissure or hemorrhoidal complaints. Others have supported the hypothesis that sensory function may be an independent factor contributing to continence.[18,23]

The working party opines that assessment of anal sensation is a research tool.[161] They affirm, however, that mucosal electrosensitivity is thought to provide objective assessment of denervation involving the afferent side of the reflex arc of the pudendal nerve.

It has also been shown that the normal anal canal is extremely sensitive to temperature. Furthermore, Miller and co-workers have been able to demonstrate that a temperature gradient exists between the rectum and the anal canal.[228] They established that the sphincter relaxes several times an hour, with concomitant equalization of rectal and anal pressures, permitting entry of rectal contents into the anal canal for evaluation. In another study, they evaluated the role of temperature sensation in 20 patients with idiopathic fecal incontinence and compared the findings with 33 normal subjects.[222] The temperature change was reported by the patient as the thermode temperature varied from 37°C to each extreme and on return to the baseline. At each level in the anal canal and lower rectum, the incontinent group was significantly less sensitive than the control. Another report from the same investigators involved patients with hemorrhoids, individuals with incontinence, and controls.[226] They ascertained that those patients with hemorrhoids have a mild sensory deficit, but not to the extent of that observed in those who were incontinent.

A contrary viewpoint was expressed in an article by Rogers and associates concerning the implication of a possible temperature gradient as a factor contributing to the continence mechanism.[290] In a study of 47 normal subjects, the maximum mean difference in temperature between the rectum and anal canal was 0.13°C and occurred 4 cm from the anal verge. The authors believed that this difference was too small to be detected by the anal canal mucosa, and they therefore concluded that, under normal circumstances, the conscious appreciation of temperature of feces passing from the rectum to the anal canal was impossible during the anorectal sampling reflex.

Rectal Sensation

Rectal sensation has been thought to play a part in the mechanism for maintaining bowel control, but it is poorly understood. The working party stipulated that testing can be effected by infusion or by incremental volumes of air introduced into a condom or into an ordinary balloon mounted on a catheter.[161] Rapid balloon distension of the rectum mimics the propulsion of feces or gas into the rectum and induces an involuntary rectal contraction, reflex relaxation of the internal sphincter, and a contraction of the external sphincter.[348] Impairment of this spinal reflex response, which can be considerably altered by conscious mechanisms, may lead to varying degrees of incontinence.

Chan and associates investigated the application to the rectum of a graded heat stimulus through the use of a thermal probe, in order to test the sensory afferent pathway.[48] Heat sensitivity was evaluated in 31 healthy subjects and compared with other standard physiologic measurements. A strong correlation was found between heat thresholds and balloon distension as well as defecatory desire. This suggests a common sensory afferent pathway and may be a comparable investigative tool to that of balloon distension or mucosal electrostimulation.

Applications

Sun and co-workers were able to demonstrate a close association between rectal distension and external sphincter contraction.[348] Fecal incontinence occurred in some

patients in their study as a result of delayed or absent external anal sphincter contraction when the internal sphincter relaxed. Bannister and colleagues analyzed the responses to rectal distension in 18 women with idiopathic fecal incontinence.[15] Two patterns were observed: one showed normal anal relaxation with reduced MSP; this implied weakness of the external sphincter. The other pattern exhibited lower resting pressures and showed only external sphincter contraction in response to rectal distension, with no internal sphincter relaxation. These diverse findings may ultimately suggest different modalities of therapy and prognoses. For example, it has been demonstrated that the mechanism of incontinence is different for those patients with seepage and soiling.[142] It is postulated that this involves a dyssynergy of rectal sensation and anal relaxation, which may be successfully managed through the use of stool bulking agents.

Proctometrography or Ampullometrography and Defecometry

A proctometrogram (i.e., ampullometrogram) is a procedure applied to the rectum that is analogous to the cystometrogram as used for evaluating bladder response to filling. Rectal distensibility, compliance, sensation threshold, and maximal tolerance can be determined by continuous controlled fluid inflation with a balloon probe or microtransducer in place.[37,362] It was agreed by the working party that this technique was the best method for measuring rectal compliance. The balloon should be perfused with water at 37°C using a constant infusion pump at the rate of 60 mL/minute. Compliance is recorded in milliliters per kilopascal over a range of volumes between zero and 1 L, depending on the patient's tolerance.[161]

A modification of this test uses the balloon with the subject in a sitting position. The patient is asked to retain the balloon as long as possible with increasing volume of fluid. This permits simultaneous assessment of the possibility to retain simulated stool, of the rectal sensation levels, and of the compliance values at each sensation level.[262] True compliance, however, is best measured in the reclining position, to limit the likelihood of balloon expulsion.

Another variation on this theme is the use of defecometry. Lestár and colleagues devised a balloon catheter device, which by connecting to pressure transducers, simultaneously records MRP and MSP.[198] The technique offers advantages over the simple balloon expulsion method, because it permits more adequate identification and characterization of the outlet obstruction and the constipation problem, as well as the analysis of sphincter activity during straining.

Applications

The role of abnormal or decreased rectal compliance in the cause of fecal incontinence is not always clear. Rasmussen and co-workers assessed this variable in physiologically normal individuals, those with incontinence, and a few with constipation.[278] Constipated patients had a higher constant defecation urge volume and maximal tolerable volume than controls. There was no difference in the parameters between patients with idiopathic fecal incontinence and those with incontinence caused by trauma.

Balloon Proctography or Topography

A balloon filled with barium or other radiopaque substance can be inserted into the rectum and used to evaluate pelvic floor and sphincter function during contraction and during straining.[184,276] This procedure is also known as balloon topography. One such modification balloon, the Lahr balloon (Sunburst Biomedical Corp., Belleville, IL) is commercially available (Figure 13-5). The device consists of a cylindric balloon connected by a hose to a bag of radiologic contrast material. Balloon fluid pressure inside the rectum can be controlled by raising or lowering the bag. Additionally, the shape of the flexible, contrast-filled balloon within the anal canal and rectum can be visualized flouroscopically. Pelvic anatomy can be defined at rest, during defecation, and during maximal squeeze efforts, and the results evaluated (see Chapter 17) (Figure 13-6). Lahr and co-workers reported the application of this technique on 280 patients.[183] They observed the method to be useful for identifying such specific problems as paradoxical puborectalis contraction, sphincter injury, and rectal prolapse, and for evaluating patients with incontinence and constipation (Figure 13-7).

The working party, however, believed that the Lahr balloon was unreliable and should not be used.[161] They agreed that proctography should be performed in the seated position on a water-filled apparatus to obtain lateral projections of the pelvis and perineum. Application of radiopaque markers to the vagina, anal canal, symphysis pubis, and perineal skin was believed to be important. In essence, they advocated defecography.

Defecography and Cineradiography or Videoproctography

Defecography is an excellent means for evaluating disorders of the lower bowel that would not be evident by direct visual examination. It is primarily a physiologic study, not simply an anatomic one. The rectosigmoid is filled with thickened barium suspension, and the patient is asked to defecate while sequential radiographs are

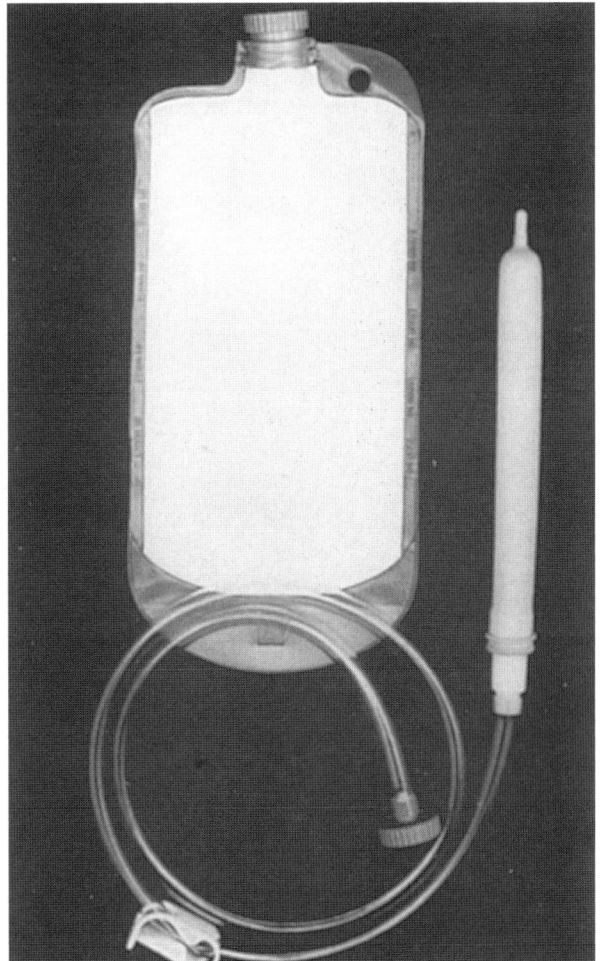

FIGURE 13-5. Lahr balloon. (Courtesy of Christopher J. Lahr, M.D.)

taken in the lateral projection. Fluoroscopic examination supplements the permanent films. Cinedefecography (i.e., video/proctography) provides a means for assessing the speed of evacuation as well as a dynamic recording for subsequent review and analysis. Both studies can illustrate functional disturbances of defecation such as may be seen in rectal prolapse, solitary rectal ulcer, and the preprolapse state (see Figs. 6-16 and 17-11 through 17-14). They have also been of demonstrable benefit in the postoperative review of children with anorectal malformations.[163] Additionally, the function of the pelvic floor muscles can be assessed by defecography to help determine the cause of fecal incontinence.[178] The applicability of this procedure for evaluating the preprolapse condition is discussed in Chapter 17. The investigation also enables the physician to observe the contractions of the rectum, the possible separation of the rectum from the sacrum, the descent of the pelvic floor, and the presence of a rectocele or of an intussusception. The working party cautions that there is a need for clear definitions of easily

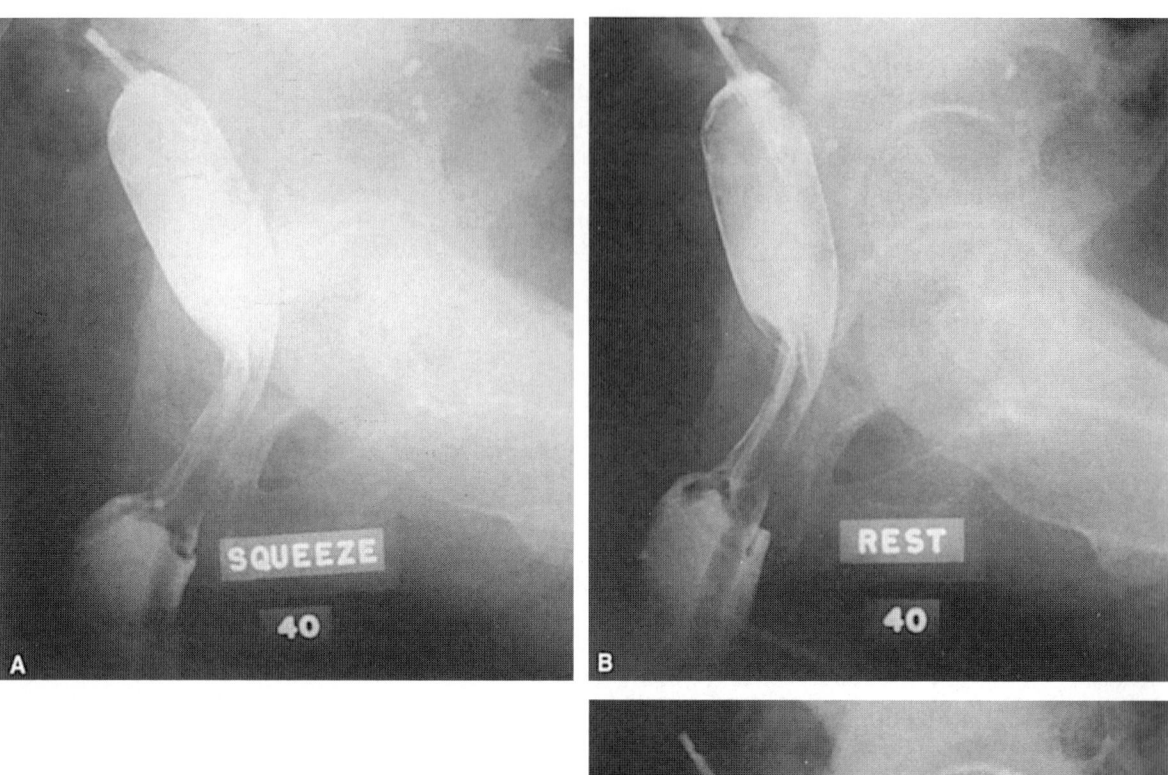

FIGURE 13-6. This Lahr balloon proctogram in a 67-year-old woman demonstrates **(A)** normal function of the pelvic floor during squeeze, **(B)** little change at rest (except the pubis-to-angle distance is somewhat longer), and **(C)** during push, the lengthening of the pubis-to-angle distance as the pelvic floor and puborectalis relax. (Courtesy of Christopher J. Lahr, M.D.)

misinterpreted abnormalities such as infoldings, rectal and anal intussusception, rectocele, and megarectum, because any and all of these may be observed in asymptomatic patients.[161]

Johansson and associates used a combined EMG/cineradiologic investigative approach in 20 patients with disorders of defecation.[154] They discovered that the procedures truly supplement each other and are of particular value in the assessment of obstructed defecation. Similarly, Jorge and colleagues from the Cleveland Clinic

compared two methods for measuring the anorectal angle: balloon proctography and cinedefecography.[156] In an evaluation of more than 100 patients with disorders of defecation, the investigators attempted to ascertain the reproducibility of the two studies at different times. Although there was a highly statistically significant disparity between the techniques, there was excellent correlation between the initial and subsequent measurements for each. The obvious query then becomes, what do the numbers truly imply? This remains an unanswered ques-

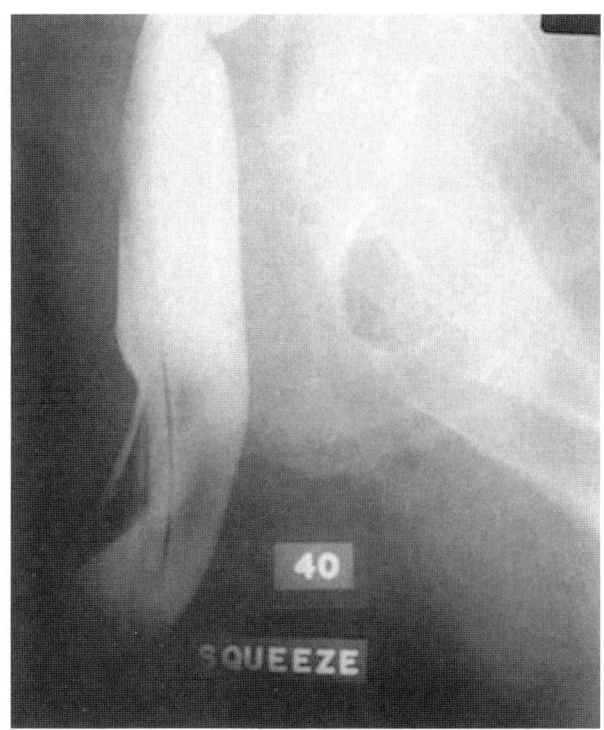

FIGURE 13-7. The Lahr balloon proctogram demonstrates weakness of external sphincter during maximum squeeze effort. This is demonstrated by the inability to collapse the balloon completely at 40 cm of barium-water mixture. (Courtesy of Christopher J. Lahr, M.D.)

tion. Yoshioka co-workers affirmed that there are essentially two methods for determining the anorectal angle: construction of a straight line along the lower border of the rectum or using the central longitudinal axis of the rectum.[399] They employed a computer program to derive the centroid of the rectum using the latter method. They concluded that, although the computer-derived data were more reliable for measuring the angles, a correction factor is required for rectocele in constipated patients and in controls.[399]

In order to assess pelvic floor physiology in a more comprehensive manner, numerous simultaneous investigations have been recommended, in addition to that of defecography. For example, Bremmer and co-workers utilized defecography and peritoneography in an effort to improve the diagnostic possibilities, particularly in the interpretation of enterocele.[32] By this method, peritoneal outlines and pouches can be studied directly during the act of defecation. They were able to observe three different types of peritoneocele: rectal, septal, and vaginal.

Sentovich and associates utilized simultaneous dynamic proctography and peritoneography.[320] They concluded that this methodology provides a qualitative assessment of pelvic floor disorders that which permits

better treatment planning in those selected individuals with obstructed defecation and pelvic descensus or prolapse.

In order to obtain a clearer analysis of pelvic floor relaxation disorders, Altringer and co-workers utilized oral, vaginal, bladder, and rectal contrast selectively and with the use of fluoroscopy.[7] They opine that four-contrast defecography improves diagnostic accuracy and helps to identify all pelvic floor defects before surgery. As with the other investigators, they believed that this approach helped in the planning of the correct operative approach.

Scintigraphic Defecography

Hutchinson and colleagues applied a method that had been utilized for evaluation of ileal pouch emptying for the quantitative and dynamic assessment of anorectal function/scintigraphic defecography.[148] Three radioactive technetium-99m (^{99m}Tc) markers were sited over the subject's pubis, lumbosacral junction, and coccyx. An artificial stool was made by adding water containing 100 MBq of ^{99m}Tc to oat-porridge to form a mixture of stool-like consistency. This was then introduced into the rectum. Dynamic images were then acquired every 5 seconds for 30 seconds during rest, and then the patients were instructed to evacuate with image acquisition continued every 5 seconds for up to 10 minutes. One of the advantages of the technique is that the patient is not subjected to the radiation exposure of conventional defecography.

The authors were able to demonstrate objective data on anorectal dynamics. Parameters such as anorectal angle, pelvic floor movement, and descent were measured and quantified. Pathologic entities, such as rectocele, could be clearly seen. The authors concluded that scintigraphic defecography is "the investigation of choice for objective assessment of anorectal function." Obviously, others need to corroborate this recommendation and opinion.

Anal Endosonography

In addition to Chapter 6, anal endosonography is discussed in Chapter 11 as it has been applied to the evaluation of patients with anal abscess and fistula. With this technique, high-resolution images of the sphincter muscles can be achieved. Defects appear as amorphous areas of varying echogenicity that interrupt the normal striated pattern.[190]

Numerous reports have emerged from the radiology department of St. Mark's Hospital in Harrow, United Kingdom, with respect to mapping of the external sphincter by anal endosonography (Figure 13-8).[189,190] The technique has also been compared with EMG findings in 15 women who sustained obstetric injuries.[189] Correlation

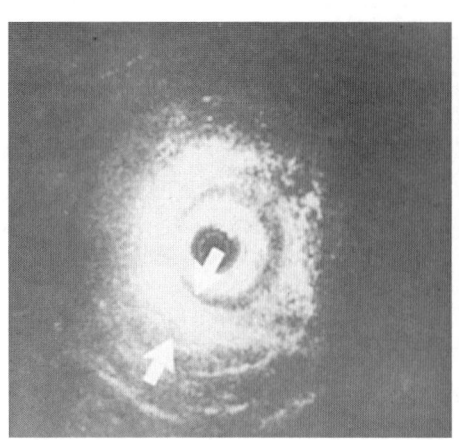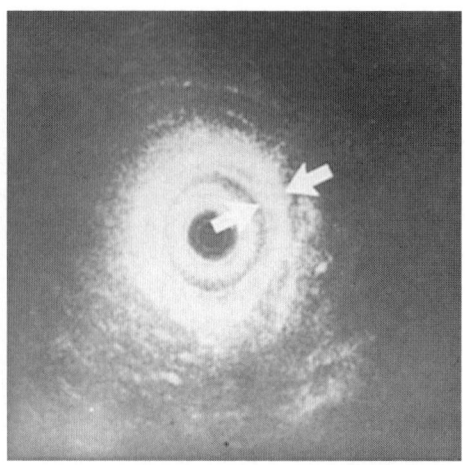

A   B

FIGURE 13-8. Anal endosonography scans in a normal 57-year-old woman. The patient is lying in the left lateral position and the scans are oriented in the same plane with the anterior on the right side of the film, posterior on the left, and the patient's right side uppermost. The upper scan is high in the anal canal with the deep part of the external sphincter forming a hyperechoic *(white)* U *(arrows)* and is contiguous with the puborectalis. Within this is the hypoechoic *(black)* ring of the internal sphincter. Note that the external sphincter is not a complete ring anteriorly at this level. In the lower scan, taken more caudally in the anal canal, the external sphincter is now a complete hyperechoic ring *(arrows)*. (Courtesy of Clive I. Bartram, Department of Radiology, St. Mark's Hospital, London.)

between the two methods was quite high, but anal endosonography was better tolerated by the patient. Another study, performed at the same institution, revealed significant abnormalities in most of 44 patients with incontinence.[190] Because the technique facilitated therapeutic decision making, the authors affirmed that this procedure fulfills a role complementary to that of anorectal physiologic studies (Figure 13-9). An additional publication from St. Mark's Hospital extols the virtues of the procedure by recommending that it be the initial investigation for locating sphincter defects.[39] Voyvodic and coworkers demonstrated a correlation between the presence or absence of sphincter injury and the manometry values.[366] Many others recommend endoanal ultrasound for all patients with fecal incontinence in order to detect occult sphincter defects.[71,75,76,85,87,92,98,285,346,359]

Sultan and colleagues have also utilized vaginal endosonography to image the anal sphincters.[347] The authors believe that there are potential applications for this imaging modality for a number of anorectal conditions, including tumors and anovaginal sepsis. Anterior internal and external sphincteric defects can be clearly identified with both techniques, but obviously vaginal endosonography is limited to the anterior sphincter.

Three-dimensional Endoanal Sonography

B-K Medical systems (Wilmington, MA) has introduced an anorectal transducer with built-in three-dimensional imaging capability (Figure 13-10). The scanning head is moved along a 60-mm distance inside a fully en-

capsulated probe by using two control buttons on the handle of the transducer.

Gold and co-workers at St. Mark's Hospital utilized this multiplanar imaging technique to reveal the length and radial extent of a sphincter tear.[120] Twenty controls and 24 patients with fecal incontinence were studied. They were also able to clearly demonstrate the sex differences in sphincter configuration. Bollard and associates attempted to quantify the nature, characteristics, and frequency of variations in female anal sphincter anatomy.[29] They observed that nulliparous women have a variable natural "defect" occurring along the anterior length of the sphincter, a factor that may contribute to overinterpretation of the existence of defects. Three-dimensional ultrasound imaging may ultimately prove to be the most useful diagnostic tool in the assessment of an individual with anal incontinence.

Magnetic Resonance Imaging

Magnetic resonance imaging (MRI) has been employed for a host of indications, including evaluation of sepsis and staging of tumors in the anus and rectum. The application of high-resolution imaging of the anal sphincter mechanism has been successfully achieved by means of an endoanal coil.[79] The St. Mark's Hospital group affirmed that an external sphincter injury can be readily assessed by means of endosonography, but endocoil MRI may be especially helpful in determining whether there is evidence of atrophy.[381] They also compared this tech-

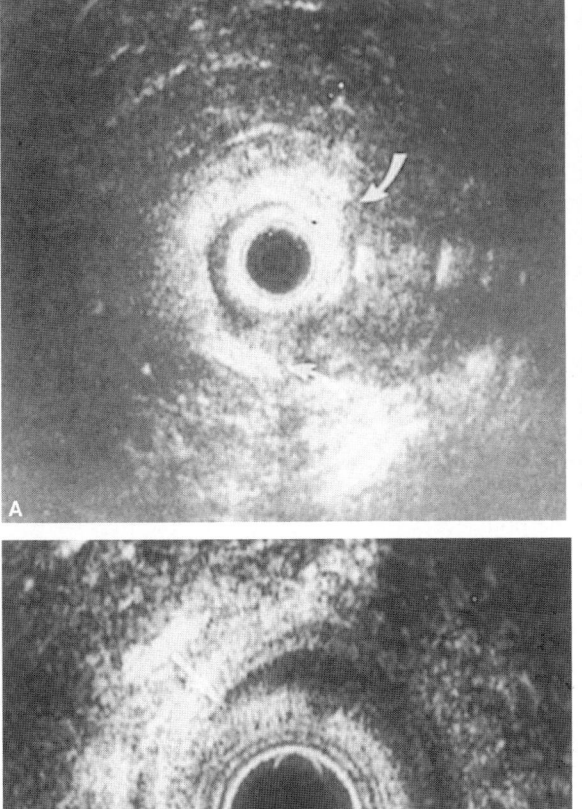

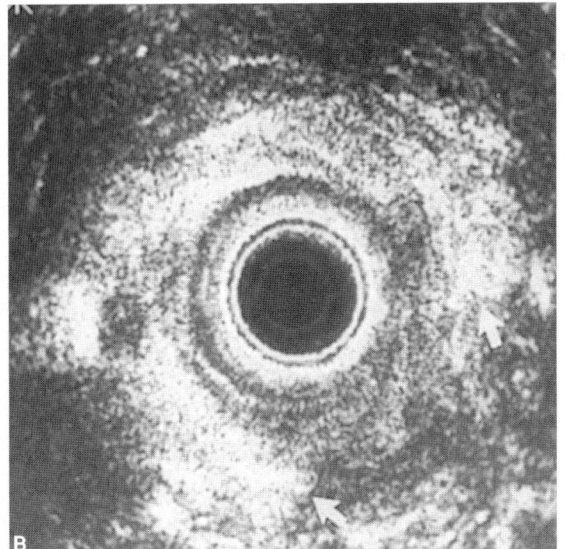

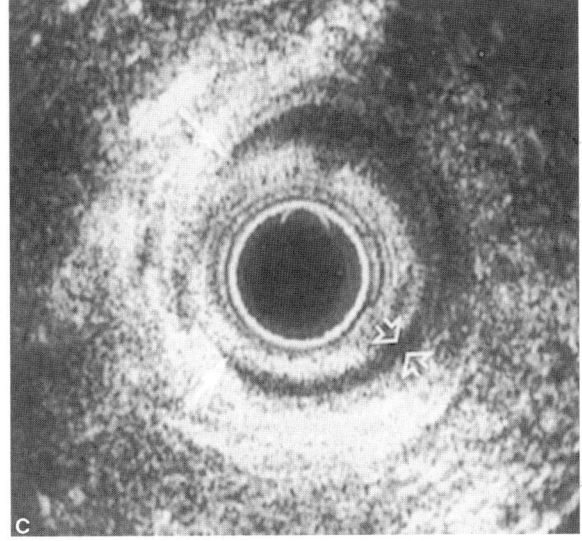

FIGURE 13-9. Anal endosonography. **(A)** Young woman with fecal incontinence following forceps delivery. A defect is noted in the anterior portion of the external sphincter *(between the arrows)*. There should be a continuous hyperechoic ring; there is a corresponding defect in the internal sphincter. **(B)** A male patient, age 47, became incontinent as a consequence of sphincter stretch. Note that there is fragmentation of the internal sphincter posteriorly *(open arrows)* and a defect between the closed arrows. **(C)** A 67-year-old woman who remained incontinent following a postanal repair. The internal sphincter is intact. There is deformity of the posterior aspect of the external sphincter consistent with the surgical repair, but there is an anterior defect in the external sphincter *between the two arrows*.

nique with that of three-dimensional endosonography, analyzing the anal anatomy at similar levels by a graphics-overlay technique.[380] The contributors believe that the overlay approach improves interpretation and that the two studies are indeed complimentary.[20] Certainly, valuable information can be ascertained in the preoperative assessment and surgical planning of patients by using either method.

Comment

Having stated that the history and physical examination are the most meaningful sources of information for determining the treatment in a patient with fecal incontinence, I believe that selective application of physiologic studies should be considered. For example, EMG may be very helpful in determining the presence and location of residual muscle in patients with congenital anomalies,

and Hirschsprung's disease can be definitively diagnosed by anorectal manometry. The value of PNTML is clear. It may serve as an important prognostic study prior to embarking on sphincter repair. It is helpful for a woman suffering from an obstetric injury to know in advance what the likelihood of alleviating symptoms following successful repair will be, because many of these patients suffer not only from the sphincter injury itself, but also from nerve injury as a consequence of prolonged labor or cephalopelvic disproportion.

Physiologic studies are useful as investigative tools, either used preoperatively or to quantify objectively the results of repair postoperatively. However, for practical purposes, the decision whether to operate and the choice of operation for individuals troubled by fecal incontinence are unlikely to be influenced by the knowledge gleaned from physiologic studies. The reason for this is that most patients, who have a defect that is amenable to

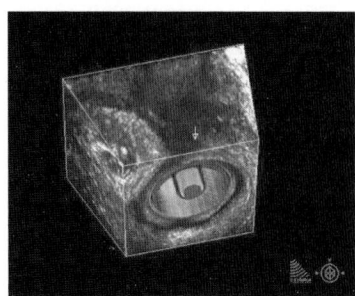

FIGURE 13-10. Three-dimensional anal ultrasound demonstrating anterior external sphincter defect *(arrow)* in a postpartum woman. (Courtesy of B & K Medical Systems, Inc., Wilmington, MA.)

reconstruction and in whom medical management has failed, are willing to embark on surgical repair in the hope that some improvement will result.

NONSURGICAL TREATMENT

The treatment of anal incontinence should always be directed to the cause. Patients who attribute their incontinence to trauma are the optimal candidates for repair. However, despite the potential appeal of surgical intervention, many individuals can be adequately managed by noninvasive means. Certainly, medical treatment should be offered those who have no antecedent history of trauma, those for whom the potential benefits are problematic, those who are believed to be at risk for surgery, and, obviously, those who decline an operation.

Bowel Management Program

The aim of a bowel management program is to establish a routine for defecation that is safe, convenient, and dependable. Ideally, the bowel can be reeducated to empty regularly and at a predictable time. This is the principle that permits patients with spinal cord injuries to avoid the need for fecal diversion. Of course, these individuals are often wheelchair-bound, so that the erect position does not exacerbate continence problems nor precipitate "accidents." Furthermore, neurologic problems are often associated with constipation, a factor that may be helpful in facilitating bowel training. Putting aside this clinical comparison, it is still usually possible through maintaining optimal fecal consistency, stimulating peristalsis, and controlling the time of evacuation, to establish an adequate, reflexive elimination pattern. Because individual patterns differ, it is not important that all patients defecate daily; a bowel action two or three times a week may be quite adequate as well as advantageous. The following

recommendations are made to help ensure that the patient will be clean and that minimal restrictions will be necessary because of the fear of loss of bowel control.

- Make certain that the patient has a well-balanced diet with sufficient fiber and an adequate fluid intake (2,500 to 3,000 mL/day).
- Establish a workable time for defecation. Ascertain the patient's prior bowel habit and plans for an optimal schedule. Take advantage of the gastrocolic reflex that occurs 20 to 30 minutes after meals to stimulate defecation.
- Start the training regimen after the rectum is empty; disimpact if necessary, and give enemas until the returns are clear.
- Insert a suppository, such as glycerine or bisacodyl (Dulcolax). The suppository should be inserted at the same hour every day or night during the first week of the program.
- Instruct the patient to massage the abdomen from right to left and top to bottom several times, beginning 15 to 20 minutes after insertion of the suppository; having the patient bend forward and strain may also be helpful.
- Stool softeners, constipating medications, bulk laxative preparations, or even stimulant cathartics may be given if required.

Perineal Exercises

In 1950, Kegel suggested an exercise regimen that appeared to be demonstrably beneficial in the medical treatment of both fecal and urinary incontinence.[160] Since that time, numerous articles have been published attesting to the validity of this method. Although it probably is not possible to increase internal anal sphincter tone by perineal strengthening exercises, muscle bulk and voluntary contractility of the external anal sphincter, puborectalis sling, and levatores may be improved by such a regimen. A simple exercise is to pretend to hold in a bowel movement and to count to 15. This can be performed 15 or 20 times a day, while walking down the street, riding in a car, or sitting in a chair—whenever the patient thinks of it. Bulging muscles should not be expected overnight, but, given sufficient time (i.e., several weeks to months), the patient may notice an improvement in voluntary control.

The following specific perineal strengthening exercise regimen is usually recommended:

- Lie on the back with knees bent, raise the head and reach the hands toward the knees. Raise the head and reach the right hand toward the left knee. Relax. Raise the head and reach the left hand toward right knee.

- Relax. Flatten the back. Pull the abdomen in and squeeze the buttocks together.
- While sitting, inhale deeply. Squeeze the buttocks together and tighten the anal sphincter. Relax.
- While standing, pull the abdomen in and squeeze the buttocks together. The knees should be relaxed.

Sometimes a patient does not understand how to undertake the exercises. Asking the person to pull the rectum up to the navel may clarify the issue somewhat. However, a more effective approach is to combine the exercise program with biofeedback, a method for reinforcement.

Operant Conditioning or Biofeedback

In 1974, an interesting observation on the value of exercise was made by Engel and colleagues in a report of six patients who had severe fecal incontinence from diverse causes.[90] These authors inserted a Miller-Abbott balloon with a 50-mL capacity into the rectum to record a measurable response to sphincter contractility on a polygraph. By positive or negative verbal reinforcement, each patient was able to sense the rectal distension and knew that this stimulus was the cue to initiate sphincter contractility. This technique is known as *biofeedback*, the use of visual, auditory or some other form of sensory reinforcement to clarify that what one is doing is correct and, hopefully, effective. During follow-up periods ranging from 6 months to 5 years, four patients remained completely continent and the other two were improved. One patient was able to relax the internal sphincter as well as to contract the external sphincter. It appears, then, at least in this individual, that autonomic regulation may be brought under voluntary control with operant conditioning. However, the success of this phenomenon needs additional substantiation.

Biofeedback training appears to be of specific value in the treatment of fecal incontinence in the elderly, as opposed to suboptimal results obtained by sphincter exercises without biofeedback.[378] Whitehead and co-workers employed behavioral modification in incontinent patients with spina bifida.[379] Using a bowel management program in addition to biofeedback, they reported improvement in 65%, with complete control in 30%. Maximum sphincter contraction and even the critical threshold for sensation of rectal distension have been demonstrated to improve with this technique.[4]

MacLeod reported the use of an intraanal plug, which adapts to an electromyometer.[206] The sphincter muscle contractions were converted to an audible sound to guide the patient in sphincter contraction. Weekly 20-minute sessions were carried out, and the patients were advised to perform frequent exercises in the interim. Ten of 17 individuals who were studied subjectively reported good to excellent results, but only three of them were shown to

have measurable improvement. A later report of more than 100 patients with a minimum 6-month follow-up revealed that 63% had at least a "90% decrease in the frequency of incontinence".[207] Interestingly, it has been demonstrated that improvement in continence may be independent of resting and squeeze pressures achieved after biofeedback therapy as determined by manometric evaluation.[305]

There have been numerous publications that attest to the success of biofeedback training for improving continence in both children and adults.[46,62,122,245,331,367-369] Biofeedback therapy has also been successfully applied to the management of refractory excessive stool frequency and/or incontinence following anterior resection and total colectomy.[140]

The results of biofeedback therapy on a long-term basis are somewhat problematic. In other words, it is generally believed that the initial good results may deteriorate over time.[102,126] It has been, therefore, suggested that it may be useful to reinitiate biofeedback therapy in some individuals, particularly if they report recurrence or deterioration of their situation. Others have noted that biofeedback training improves continence not only during treatment and in the first 2 years, but also for several years following therapy, provided patients are encouraged to continue their exercises.[88,253] Conversely, in a study undertaken to assess this method of treatment in individuals who were incontinent on a neurogenic basis, there was no improvement, and external sphincter function was not increased significantly.[361] Others have shown that incontinence associated with colonic and rectal resection or anal surgery responds significantly better to training than it does in those individuals whose etiology is neurogenic.[174] Heyman and associates reviewed the MEDLINE database from 1973 through 1999 and identified 35 published studies that involved biofeedback for fecal incontinence.[137] Although most articles reported positive results, these investigators concluded that "quality research is lacking." Their recommendations included improvement in experimental design, long-term follow-up data, and use of an adequate sample size that would permit meaningful statistical analysis.[137]

Several home biofeedback systems are available. One such option is the Orion/Perry EMG Continence System (Jeffers Health Systems, Inc., Lake Forest, CA), which uses the equivalent of a surface EMG response to give visual reinforcement.[263] Constantinides' device (Swan Attika, Ltd., Durban, Republic of South Africa) is battery operated with a control and display unit for visual confirmation of the success of the sphincter exercise. It comes equipped with adult and child balloon probes for rectal insertion (Figure 13-11).[62] Patients are encouraged to tighten the sphincter mechanism and to increase the arc of deflation registered on the meter. The specific meter readings, however, are not terribly relevant. Another such

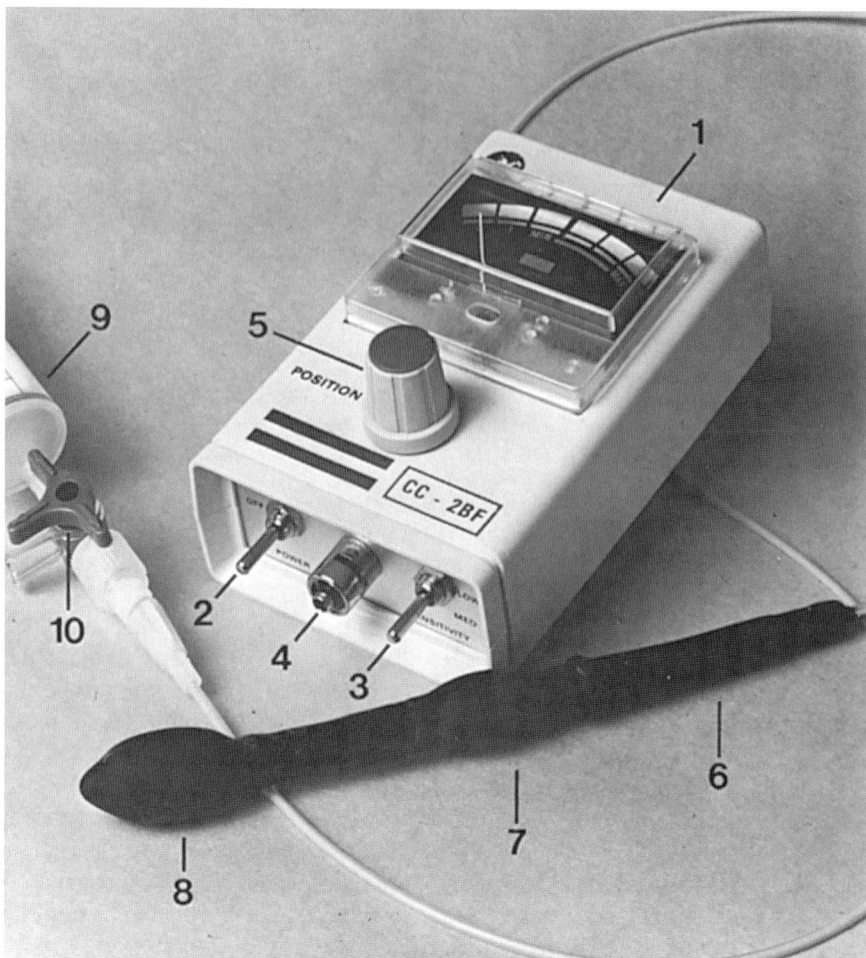

FIGURE 13-11. The CC-2BF anorectal biofeedback system is battery operated for home use: (1) control and display unit; (2) on/off battery check selector switch; (3) sensitivity selector switch; (4) probe input connector; (5) position adjustment knob; (6) anorectal probe; (7) anal air chamber; (8) replaceable rectal balloon; (9) rectal balloon insufflation syringe; (10) three-way stopcock. (Courtesy of Swan Attika, Durban, Republic of South Africa.)

device is the Dobbhoff Anorectal Biofeedback System (Biosearch Medical Products, Inc., Somerville, NJ) (Figure 13-12). This consists of a silicone anorectal probe and battery-charged monitor with color illumination to indicate the patient's response. I have found these last two units to be excellent tools for instructing patients on the correct method of performing perineal strengthening exercises as well as to use in the training of individuals troubled with obstructed defecation (see Chapter 16). I have had no personal experience with the Perry device.

Signaling Device

An interactive anal incontinence system has been submitted to preliminary clinical trials recently, the Procon system (Anatech, Inc. LLC, Houston, TX). A catheter with a balloon and sensor electrode is inserted into the rectum. A silent, vibrating signaling device is worn at the patient's waist, similar to a pager. The arrival of stool in the rectum theoretically alerts the patient to attend to this function. A preliminary report involving seven patients sug-

gests improvement in incontinence and quality of life scores.[116]

Anal Electrical Stimulation

Caldwell and colleagues and others reported success with electrical stimulation of the anal sphincter by means of an anal canal electrode.[44,118,144,145] The device applies a tetanizing stimulus to the anal sphincter and pelvic floor through a plug-shaped electrode (Figure 13-13). After the plug is inserted, the current is slowly increased until the patient is aware of a tingling sensation. This causes contraction of the anal musculature, possibly with the result of gradual buildup in sphincter tone and contractility. Pescatori and co-workers performed transanal electrostimulation on 15 individuals by means of a 10-second pulse.[266] The device was used for 30 minutes/day for 10 days. Two thirds of the patients noted improvement at the end of this time. Fynes and associates randomly assigned to receive "augmented biofeedback," which combined audiovisual biofeedback and electrical stimulation

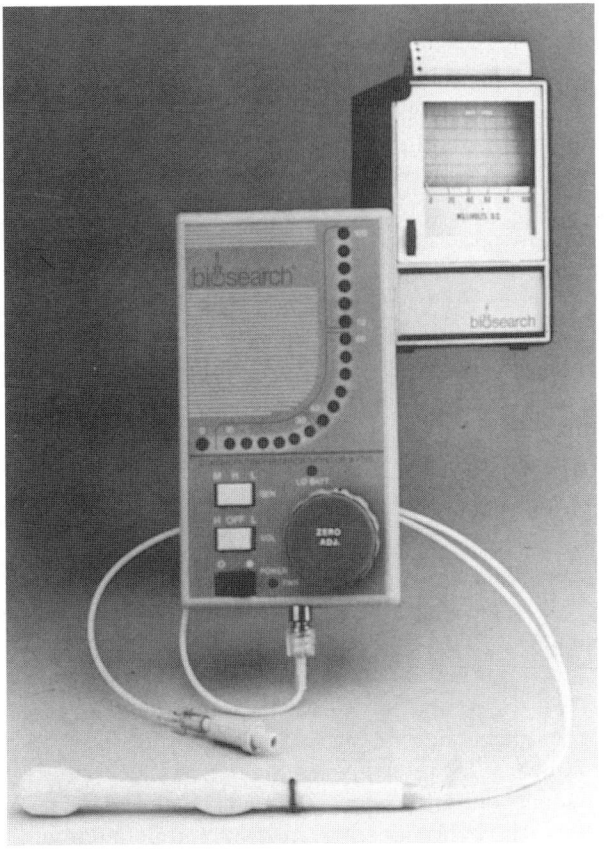

FIGURE 13-12. Dobbhoff anorectal biofeedback system demonstrating a silicone probe and battery-operated illuminated color display unit to indicate patient's biofeedback response. The strip chart recorder for creating a permanent record is optional. (Courtesy of Biosearch Medical Products, Inc., Somerville, NJ.)

using an Incare PRS 9300 endoanal probe system (Hollister, Inc., Libertyville, IL).[108] The electrical stimulation technique was compared with biofeedback alone. The investigators concluded that biofeedback augmented by electrical stimulation was more effective in the treatment of anal incontinence.

The electrogalvanic stimulator, which has been used in the management of levator spasm, may also be considered

for this purpose, but as of this writing no reports have emerged concerning this application (see Chapter 16).

Although perineal strengthening exercises would seem to accomplish the same goal as that of electrical stimulation, greater improvement in selected patients may be anticipated if one is unable to perform such exercises.

Perianal Injection

The concept of increasing the support around the anal canal to act as an artificial sphincter by a different mechanism than that of the various sling or Thiersch procedures (see later) may have some merit.[74] For example, collagen would seem to be a very appropriate agent for this purpose. However, there is a risk of inducing allergic reaction, and it is quite expensive, especially because injections have to be repeated.[322] Still, Kumar and associates treated 17 incontinent patients with collagen, all of whom had an intact external sphincter.[179] Eleven showed marked symptomatic improvement. The simplicity of the approach in these selected individuals is appealing, especially in the short term.

Shafik reported the use of two different approaches to supplement the sphincter through an injection technique—that of submucosal polytetrafluoroethylene and autologous fat.[322] Utilizing the latter approach, he performed this procedure on 14 individuals.[322] Fat was harvested by means of aspiration from the abdominal wall and injected into the submucosa. All patients were continent for the first 2 to 3 months. However, there was a tendency for this good result not to be maintained, but some of these outcomes could be salvaged by repeat injection.

Malouf and co-workers injected a silicone-based product, Bioplastique (Uroplasty, Ltd., Reading, UK), in ten patients with fecal incontinence.[210] Although the procedure was clinically effective over the short term, the benefit was maintained in only a few individuals. Feretis and associates reported the implantation of a microballoon composed of silicone and filled with a biocompatible hydrogel of polyvinyl pyrrolidone.[100] The material was inserted through a proctoscope into the submucosa of the

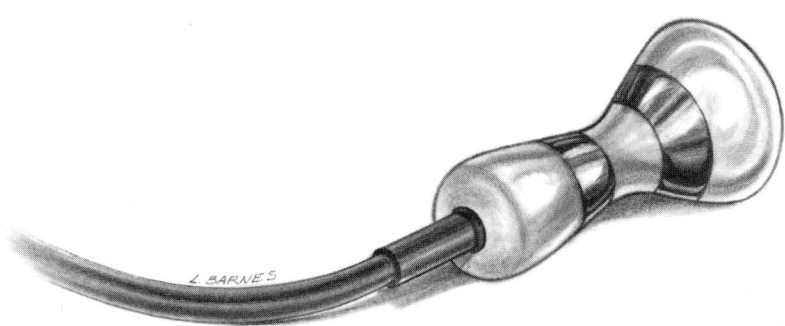

FIGURE 13-13. Birmingham continence aid. The anal canal electrode used for stimulating the sphincter mechanism is available in several diameters.

anal canal. The balloon itself is implanted by using the Self-Detachable Balloon System (Urosurge, Inc., Corallville, IA). Six patients were treated without adverse effects, and with all experiencing improvement in incontinence scores despite no change in the resting anal pressures.[100] Finally, Weiss and colleagues injected carbon-coated beads (ACYST, Carbon Medical Technologies, Inc., St. Paul, MN) into the submucosa in ten patients.[371] An overall 23% improvement in incontinence scores was noted in the responders at 6 months.

Nerve Stimulation

The concept of sacral spinal nerve stimulation has been developed to address the issue of anal incontinence when the nerves are ideally intact, but there is a functional deficit of the sphincter mechanism.[164,360] The method was developed for the treatment of urinary incontinence. Matzel and colleagues are credited with initially employing the technique for the treatment of fecal incontinence in 1995.[217] Percutaneous nerve stimulation of the S2, S3, and S4 nerve roots can be accomplished with the aid of a local anesthetic by employing a 20-gauge insulated spinal needle (Medtronic Model 041828–004, Minneapolis, MN) and an external neurostimulator (Medtronic Model 3625 Screener or Medtronic Model 3628 Dual Screener).[112] Stimulation of the S2 root produces movement of the perineum and contraction of the external sphincter with toe and foot contractions; stimulation of the S3 root produces elevation of the pelvic floor through external sphincter and levator contraction with plantar flexion of the great toe; and S4 stimulation causes sphincter contraction without leg movement.[112]

Ganio and colleagues performed short-term sacral nerve stimulation on 28 patients.[112] They concluded that the technique was quite useful as a diagnostic modality in order to assess the merit of long-term therapy by this approach. They subsequently demonstrated that these results could be reproduced when permanent implantation was undertaken.[111] They emphasize that an accurate preprocedural evaluation is critical, and that patients must be carefully selected to optimize outcome.[113]

Matzel and co-workers performed chronic spinal nerve stimulation in six patients with fecal incontinence either by the foregoing "closed" technique or through an "open" approach in which cuff electrodes are implanted at the time of a sacral laminectomy.[218] Incontinence improved in all patients, but two devices required removal because of intractable pain. Kenefick and associates initially undertook temporary stimulation with 15 individuals, and subsequently, permanent stimulation.[165] After up to 24 months, continence was determined to have improved in all. No implant required removal, and there were no complications. Others confirm the safety and efficacy of sacral nerve stimulation.[197]

Binnie and co-workers devised an electrical stimulator to treat neurogenic fecal incontinence caused by pudendal neuropathy.[24] Saline-soaked electrodes are applied to the skin, and the portable device, containing a rechargeable nickel cadmium battery power source, produces a stimulation voltage that causes a significant rise in EMG activity of the external sphincter. Treatment for 5 minutes, three times daily for 8 weeks, resulted in continence in seven of eight patients. However, others have demonstrated that electrostimulation does not improve internal or external sphincter function in patients with neurogenic fecal incontinence.[307]

Anal Plug

In 1983, Prager described a device for control of feces following abdominoperineal resection and sigmoid colostomy.[275] It was composed of two parts, a Dacron-impregnated silicone ring, and a silicone balloon plug of varying lengths. Because of problems associated with pressure necrosis, the continent colostomy device concept was discarded. However, the balloon has been shown to be of demonstrable benefit for selected patients with fecal incontinence, by inserting it into the rectum. (Prager E, personal communication). Through a simple valve mechanism, the balloon can be inflated and deflated with a 30-mL syringe (Figure 13-14).

Mortensen and Humphreys investigated the efficacy of three different designs of anal continence plugs in ten patients.[231] They were made of polyurethane sponge wrapped in a water-soluble coat to limit the size to that of a conventional suppository (Figure 13-15). The authors learned that the optimal design could be worn for a median of 12 hours and concluded that anal plugs may have a valid place in the treatment of selected patients with anal incontinence.

Although it is not truly a continent device, Kim and co-workers used their anal plug in 32 patients who were bedridden, with diarrhea and incontinence.[169] Their modification comprises an inner balloon surrounded by an outer balloon, both of which are mounted on a silicone tube containing a pair of air passages and an enema fluid inlet. The tube is designed to permit loose stool to drain through, thereby minimizing skin complications.

Rectal Dilation

Rectal dilation has been utilized in one patient with fecal incontinence and frequent bowel movements associated with low rectal compliance and capacity.[5] The patient regained complete fecal continence as a consequence of increased capacity, increased compliance, and increased cross-sectional area. This technique warrants further investigation, particularly in those individuals whose in-

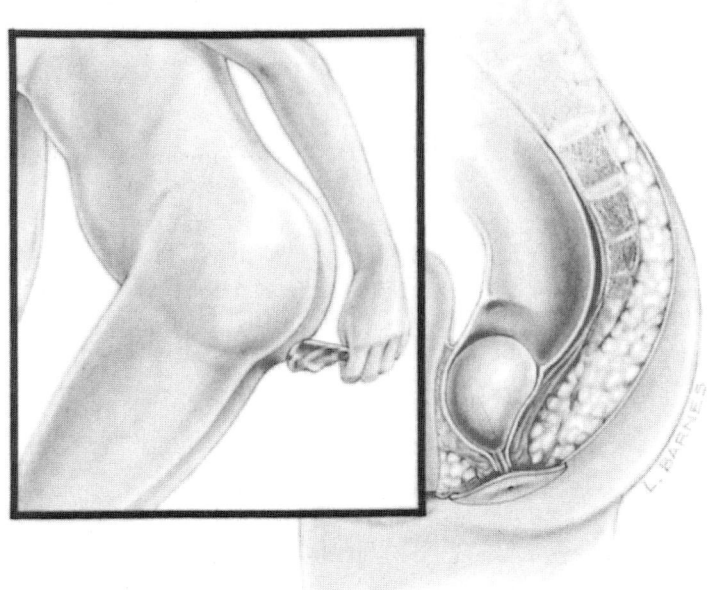

FIGURE 13-14. Prager Balloon Plug. Reasonable continence can be achieved by insertion and inflation of the balloon. Three different lengths and three different widths are available.

continence is on the basis of decreased rectal compliance and capacity.

Radiofrequency Energy Delivery for the Treatment of Fecal Incontinence (Secca Procedure)

Radiofrequency (RF) energy has been used for electro-surgery techniques (cutting and coagulation) since the 1920s. When delivered to tissue in the frequency range of 200 kHz to 3.3 MHz, RF energy results in vibration of water molecules and subsequent frictional heating. The Secca System (Curon Medical, Inc., Fremont, CA) is designed to deliver temperature-controlled RF energy to the muscle of the anal canal for the treatment of fecal incontinence. The RF energy handpiece is composed of a clear anoscopic barrel with four nickel-titanium curved needle electrodes (22 gauge, 6 mm in length; Figure 13-16). The needle electrodes are deployed through the mucosa of the anal canal and into the internal sphincter muscle. Upon deployment, there is a reduction in electrical impedance, indicating proper electrode penetration below the mucosal surface. Temperature is monitored automatically and processed by a temperature-control mechanism, which adjusts RF output to achieve a target temperature of 85°C at the tip of the needle electrode (Figure 13-17). Chilled water is perfused through the handpiece to cool the anoderm while the deeper tissue around the needle electrodes is heated. Anoderm temperature is continuously monitored, and energy delivery automatically ceases if anoderm temperatures exceed a preset limit of 42 degrees.

Technique

The procedure is undertaken on an outpatient basis, in an ambulatory surgical facility or endoscopy unit, using a local anesthetic field block and conscious sedation. The

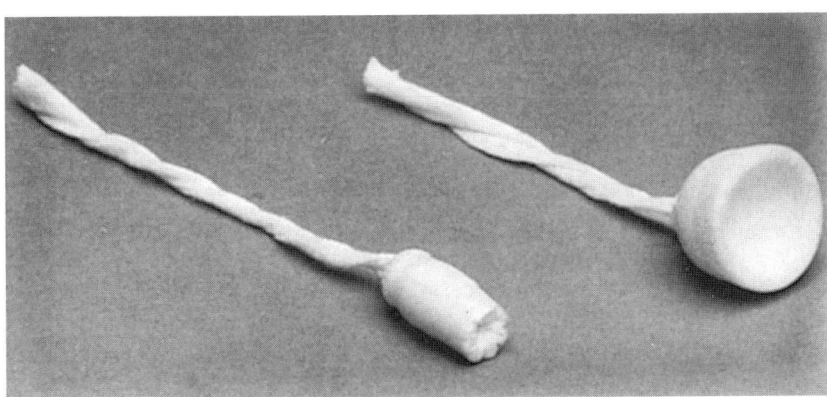

FIGURE 13-15. Prototype Conseal Anal Continence Plug. The plug is wrapped in a water-soluble coat **(left)** and is inserted like a suppository with the gauze tape outside the anal canal. The expanded plug sits in the upper portion of the anal canal to facilitate bowel control **(right)**. (Courtesy of Neil Mortensen, M.D., John Radcliffe Hospital, Oxford, U.K.)

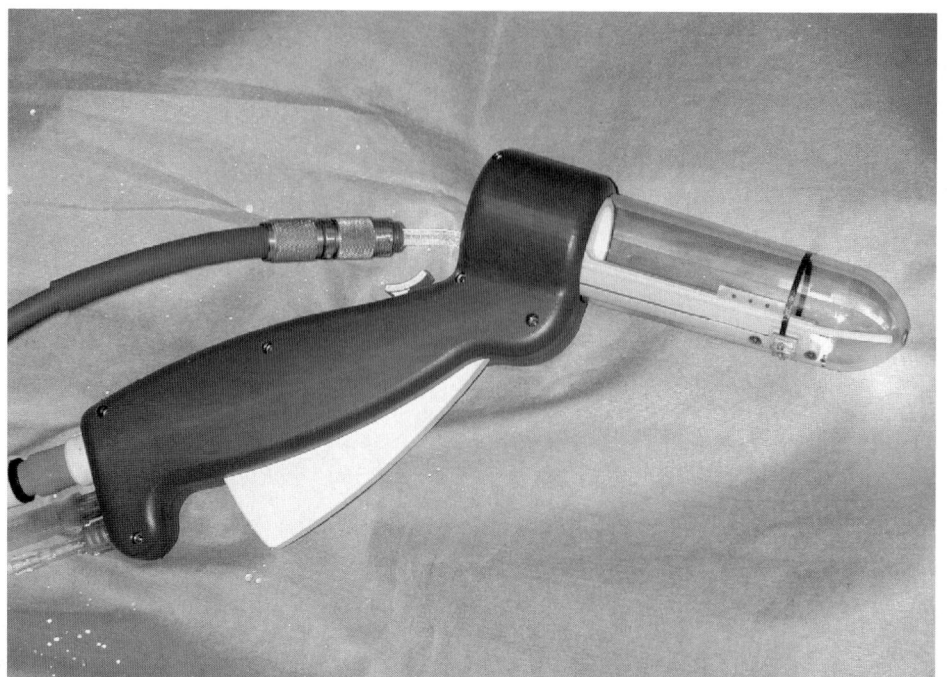

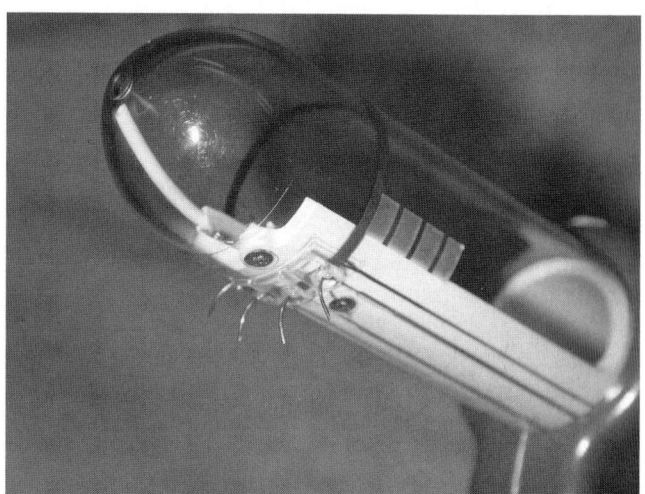

FIGURE 13-16. Secca handpiece. **(A)** Unit with handle/anoscope, light attachment, radiofrequency delivery connector, suction, and irrigation. **(B)** Close-up view with needles deployed. (Courtesy of Curon Medical, Fremont, CA.)

patient is placed in the prone jackknife position, and the handpiece is inserted and positioned with the needles 0.5 cm distal to the dentate line. The needles are then deployed into the tissue, and impedance is checked for proper tissue contact. Once appropriate tissue penetration is achieved, the operator initiates RF energy delivery, and the four-channel generator delivers this energy to all four electrodes to achieve a target temperature of 85°C. A 1-minute treatment is applied to each set. Ideally, 20 sets of four lesions each are created, beginning 5 mm distal to the dentate line and at 5-mm increments proximal to the original treatment site (Figure 13-18). Care must be taken during the anterior treatment in a woman to avoid penetrating the vagina. All four quadrants are treated in like manner, creating (if possible) 20 sets of lesions, each composed of four needle insertions. Depending on the number of sets, the procedure takes approximately 30

minutes. Patients are discharged in accordance with the criteria required for conscious sedation in an ambulatory setting.

Results

Takahashi and colleagues performed the initial clinical trial in which the feasibility, safety, and efficacy of the concept of RF energy delivery to the anal canal for the treatment of fecal incontinence was investigated.[353] Ten women, with incontinence of varying causes, were treated with this device. Median discomfort by a visual analog scale (0 to 10) was 3.8 during treatment and 0.9 2 hours following the procedure. Delayed bleeding (3 weeks after treatment) was a complication in four cases, three of which were self-limited and one of which required sutur-

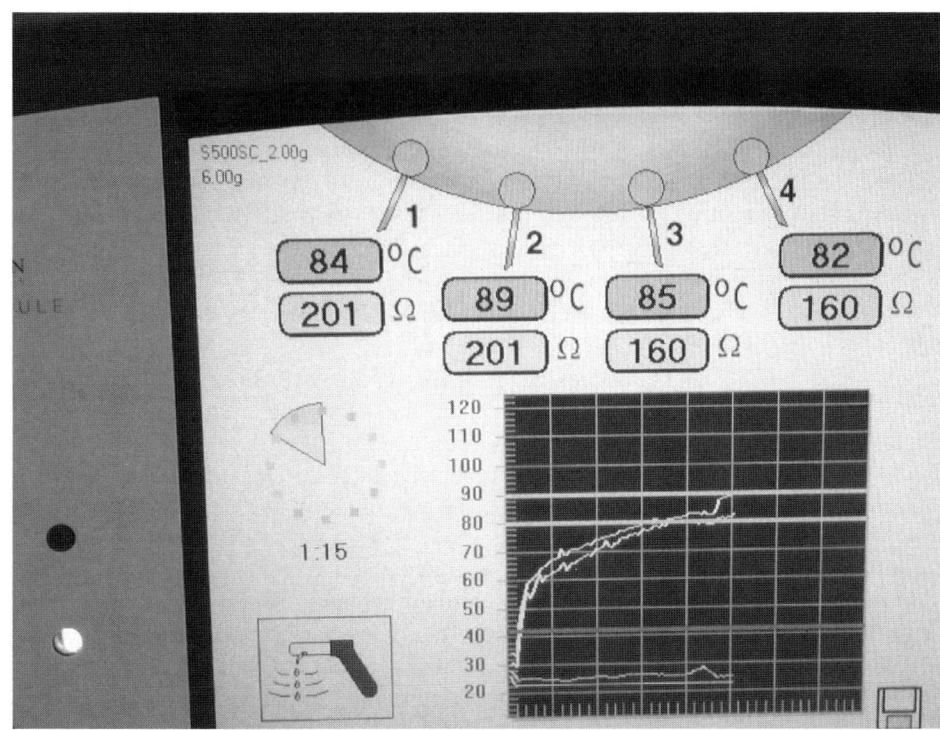

FIGURE 13-17. Monitor screen with schematically shown four electrodes with corresponding temperatures (84°C to 86°C) and impedances. Note that the temperature range over time is in the therapeutic range. Also note the flat two lines at the bottom of the graph showing cool surface temperatures. (Courtesy of Curon Medical, Fremont, CA.)

ing. All parameters of the fecal incontinence/quality of life index were improved—that is, lifestyle, coping, depression, and embarrassment. The only objective change was an improvement in both initial and maximal tolerable rectal distension volumes. A report of these individu-als at 2 years revealed a highly significant improvement in the mean Cleveland Clinic Florida Fecal Incontinence Score (CCF-FI) from 13.8 to 7.3 as well as a statistically significant improvement in the quality of life score (FIQL).[352] Of the seven women who required the use of a

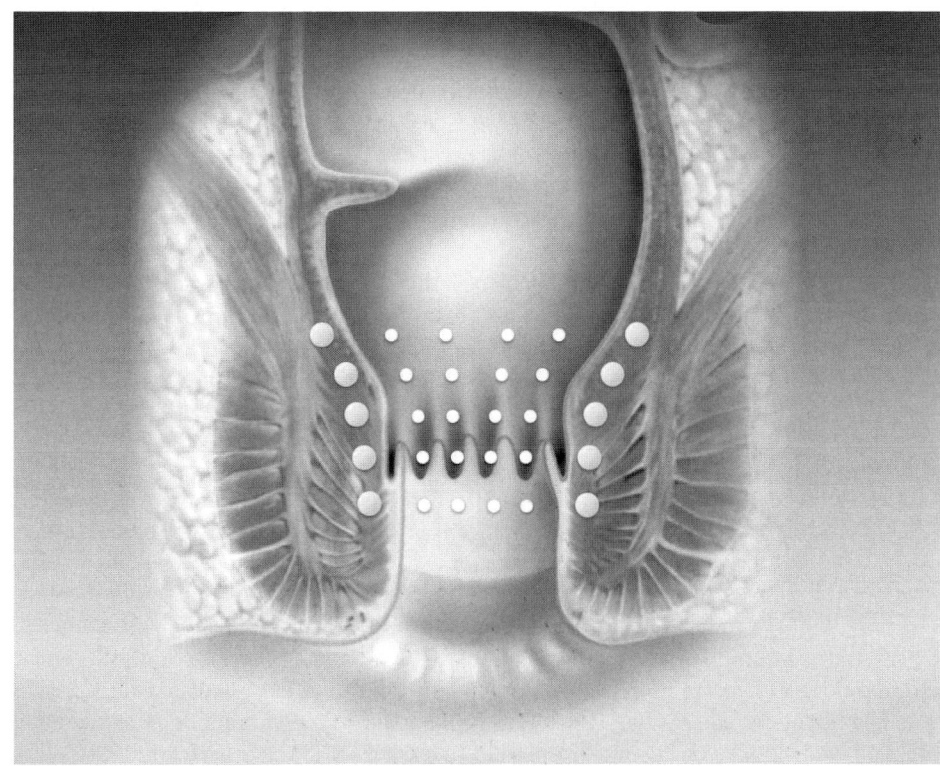

FIGURE 13-18. Schematic illustration of electrode deployment sites. Four quadrants are treated in a similar manner. (Courtesy of Curon Medical, Fremont, CA.)

protective pad, four were able to abandon this method of security.

A five-center study, in which I participated, involved 50 patients (43 women) with fecal incontinence, in all of whom medical or surgical management had failed.[86,103] Inclusion criteria included incontinence for stool as least once per week for 3 months. At baseline and at 6 months, the patients completed CCF-FI and the FIQL questionnaires as well as a social function questionnaire (SF-36). All subjects underwent anorectal manometry, PNTML, and anorectal ultrasound testing at baseline and 6 months. At 6 months, the mean CCF-FI score improved from 14.5 to 11.1 ($p < .0001$). All parameters in the FIQL were improved ($p < .001$). There was an overall statistically significant improvement in the days with fecal incontinence, the days with gas incontinence, the incidence of pad soiling, the days with urgency, and the days with fear of fecal incontinence. However, no objective changes were noted in physiologic studies with the exception that resting anal sphincter length increased by 25% ($p = .019$). Complications included mucosal ulceration (one superficial, one with underlying muscle injury) and one patient with delayed bleeding.

Comment

There is certainly a gap between nonoperative treatment of fecal incontinence, such as has been described in the preceding section, and that of surgery (see next section). The Secca procedure is intended to offer a less invasive option for the management of anal incontinence as compared with surgical alternatives. The Secca system received clearance from the United States Food and Drug Administration in early 2002 for the treatment of fecal incontinence. Although it is no longer considered an investigational approach, there is a unique study currently being undertaken—that of a prospective, randomized, *sham-controlled* United States trial in which the Secca procedure is compared with a placebo, anoscopic treatment. This is the first randomized sham-controlled clinical trial that will meaningfully assess the outcome of any of the interventional options for the treatment of fecal incontinence.

Regarding the Secca procedure and the currently available results, there is a favorable risk-to-benefit ratio when compared with alternative treatments. The Secca procedure is a minimally invasive, ambulatory procedure, and patients may return to normal activities within 48 hours. With respect to individuals who are potential candidates, it could be considered as first-line therapy for those with fecal incontinence because "no bridges are burned." That is not to say that someone with a reparable sphincter defect would be better served by RF treatment, simply that it is believed that this approach would not preclude a subsequent operation. It should also be considered following a procedure or a treatment that has been less than satisfactory or in someone who cannot tol-

erate an operation. Finally, it may certainly be offered as a "last resort" to a patient for whom there is no alternative except fecal diversion.

Issues that need to be understood are obviously the requirement for expensive equipment, the requisite training and familiarity with its use, and the fact that insurance reimbursement is problematic as of this writing.

SURGICAL TREATMENT

Successful surgical repair of incontinence requires an understanding of the underlying pathophysiology. Although a thorough examination may require an anesthetic, it is imperative to obtain as much information as possible with the patient fully awake in order to assess the voluntary and resting tone of the sphincter muscles as well as to identify any defect in the sphincter muscle.

The two primary methods of surgical treatment of anal incontinence are direct repair of a localized sphincter defect and repair designed to supplement the sphincter mechanism. A modified classification of the various methods of operative treatment, which was proposed by Hagihara and Griffen, is presented in the following list[128]:

Surgical Options in the Management of Incontinence

Anorectal muscle repairs
    Apposition of sphincter muscles
    Overlapping of sphincter muscles
    Plication (reefing) of sphincter muscles
    Postanal pelvic floor repair (i.e., Parks' procedure)
    Narrowing of the anal canal
    Use of perineal muscles other than the anal sphincter
Use of other muscles
    Gluteus
    Gracilis
Anal encirclement procedures
    Fascia lata
    "Thiersch operation," using Teflon, Marlex, catgut, Mersilene, Dacron-impregnated Silastic, to create an artificial sphincter
Antegrade colonic irrigation
Colostomy

Direct Sphincter Repair

Principles

As previously stated, the surgeon who has the initial opportunity to repair an injured sphincter has the best chance to obtain an optimal functional result. In the acute, emergency trauma situation, initial treatment usually consists of debridement of nonviable tissue, removal of foreign material, open drainage, and often proximal colostomy with distal washout (see Chapter 14). Depending on the extent of injury, especially that of associated trauma, reconstructive sphincteric surgery may be deferred. However, any attempt to appose the sphincter muscle, even in such adverse circumstances, should be ameliorative.

Direct repair of a localized sphincter defect may produce excellent results, but anatomic structures may be distorted or obliterated by scar. It may not be possible accurately to identify specific sphincter muscle, but even if this can be accomplished, the dissection may compromise viability of the tissue. The treatment approach should include excision of skin eschar and definition of the sphincter muscle with preservation of the fibrous ends for securing and suturing. If necessary, the cutaneous defect may be left open, partially closed, skin grafted, or ideally, covered with full-thickness skin.

There is no perfect incision for all sphincter repairs. A curvilinear incision outside the anal verge is commonly employed. This will usually provide adequate exposure of the underlying muscle if a direct repair is required. However, if additional skin coverage is needed to close a defect, a concomitant anoplasty may be necessary (see Chapter 8) (Figs. 13-19 and 13-20). In a woman, an important step after sphincter repair in my opinion is to maintain the increased distance between the anus and vagina. A cruciate incision with bilateral flap advancement is an effective way to accomplish this (see Obstetric Injuries).

The three standard operations for repairing the injured sphincter are apposition, overlapping, and plication or reefing. Each method has its advocates, but no one of these procedures can be consistently employed

with success. In principle, the surgeon usually attempts to repair the external sphincter muscle, puborectalis sling, or both. The internal sphincter is usually either unidentifiable or inadequate to contribute meaningfully to the result, although some surgeons make an effort to repair it as a separate entity if possible.

Identification of the residual sphincter for effecting a repair can often be accomplished by causing the muscle to contract with the use of electrocautery. Svenberg and Linderoth opine that, through the evoking of twitches in striated muscle with no reaction in smooth muscle, coagulating current facilitates identification and distinction between the internal and external sphincter.[349] Personally, I do not believe the distinction is important as long as the surgeon is certain to identify and suture the voluntary muscle.

A better tool for identification of the sphincter muscle is the Peña Muscle Stimulator (Radionics, Inc., Burlington, MA) (Figure 13-21). This is a portable, battery-operated instrument that permits precise location of muscle contraction; thus, it is especially valuable for anorectal reconstruction. Transcutaneous stimulation usually requires higher current intensities, in the range of 100 to 200 mA. Once the skin is incised, direct muscle stimulation can be achieved with a much lower current (20 to 80 mA). The use of muscle relaxants usually does not interfere with the response.

Repair of the sphincter in incontinent patients is most successfully undertaken after operative or nonoperative trauma and is best accomplished as soon as possible after the injury. The considerable success that gynecologists

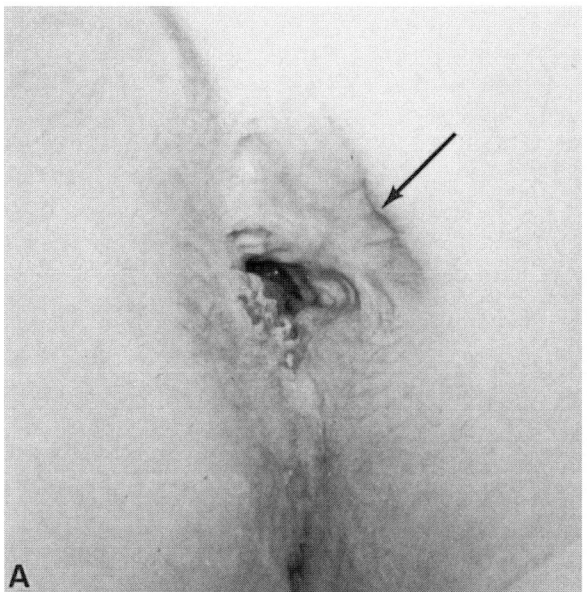

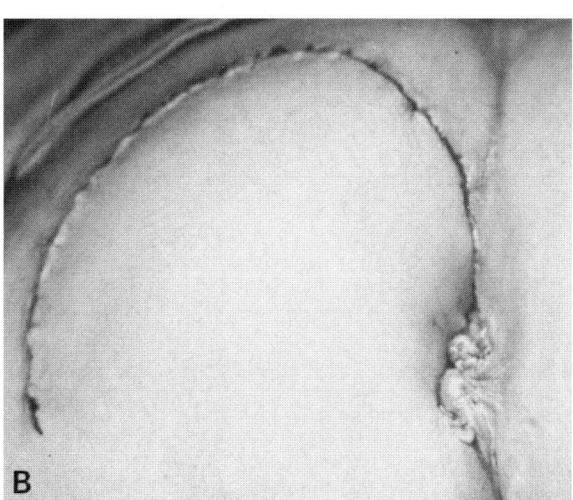

FIGURE 13-19. Fecal incontinence secondary to trauma with skin loss. **(A)** Considerable scarring and deformity are evident with a patulous anus *(arrow)* caused by an avulsion injury. **(B)** A rotation flap is used to cover the defect after sphincter repair has been completed.

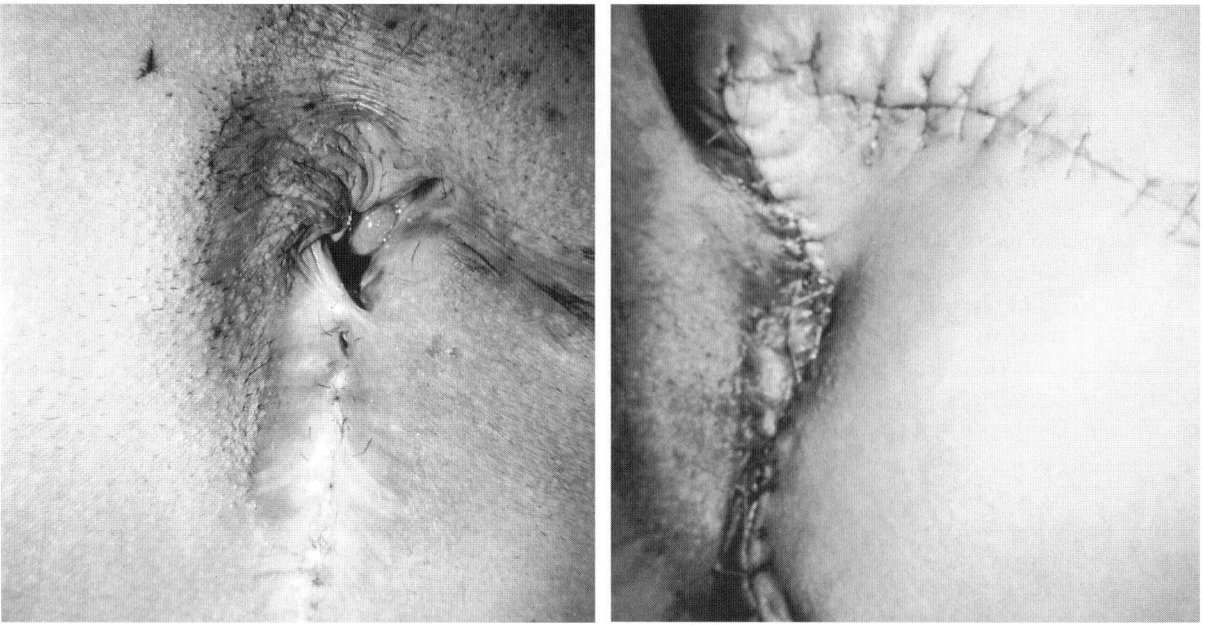

FIGURE 13-20. Anal incontinence secondary to fistulectomy. **(A)** Patulous anus is identified with scarring as a consequence of the fistulectomy. **(B)** Following anal sphincteroplasty, a rotation flap of full-thickness skin covers the defect.

have enjoyed by repairing the torn perineal musculature immediately after childbirth injury is a testament to this fact. However, repair can be carried out many months after the original trauma with the expectation of a good result. A point comes, however, when disuse, with its resultant loss of muscle tissue, takes its toll. An attenuated

muscle lacks holding power; sutures tend to cause necrosis and pull out easily. The surgeon who has the first opportunity to perform a direct sphincter repair has the best chance to effect a satisfactory outcome. If another operation becomes necessary, it may not be possible to use the patient's residual muscle, and another, perhaps

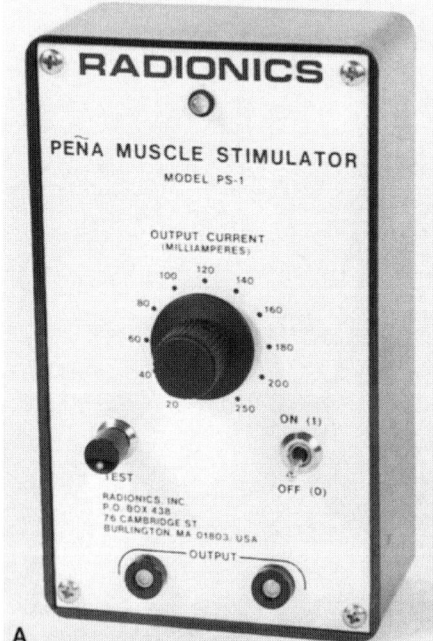

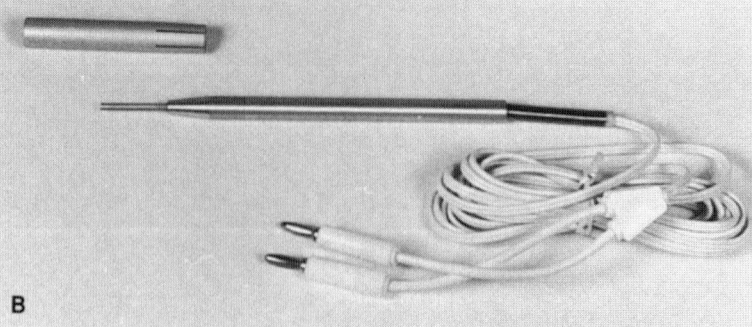

FIGURE 13-21. Peña Muscle Stimulator. **(A)** Portable battery-operated instrument designed initially for use by Peña for the technique of posterior sagittal anorectoplasty (see Chapter 18). **(B)** Bipolar probe. (Courtesy of Radionics, Inc., Burlington, MA.)

suboptimal alternative, such as that designed to supplement the sphincter, may be required.

Preoperative Preparation

All patients undergoing reconstructive anorectal surgical procedures should be prepared as if for colonic resection, that is, a vigorous oral cathartic regimen. However, there is no irrefragable evidence to suggest that this approach reduces the incidence of septic complications. Still, the thought of working up to one's elbows in stool is, at the very least, unaesthetic. The morning of operation, a small-volume or tap water enema may be given, but because these individuals often are not able to retain fluid, one should not rely on this preparation alone. The orally administered antibiotic regimen of erythromycin base and neomycin, as popularized by Nichols and colleagues, is not helpful.[240] A systemic, broad-spectrum antibiotic, such as a cephalosporin and metronidazole, should be administered not more than 1 hour before operation and for a varied duration postoperatively, depending on the nature of the procedure and the degree of contamination. This obviously is highly subjective advice.

Some patients undergoing anorectal surgery may already have a colostomy. The standard preoperative rectal irrigation can be undertaken, and if the stoma is fully diverting, no dietary restrictions need to be imposed. Under no circumstances should a colostomy be closed at the time of reconstruction. If the surgeon is so fortunate as to have it in place, it should be permitted to remain until the wounds are healed and the success of the repair can be judged. The advisability of creating a colostomy at the time of repair, however, is a matter of an individual surgeon's judgment. A generally safe rule may be this: the more extensive the reconstruction, the more one should consider a diversion. Certainly, no one can be critical of a desire to err on the side of conservatism.

An indwelling urinary catheter is always suggested for women. The advantages of the prone jackknife position have been discussed in previous chapters, and this recommendation is equally valid for any operation designed to repair the anal sphincter.

Techniques

Apposition

In Figure 13-22*A*, the appearance of a deformed anus after trauma is shown. In Figure 13-22*B*, the skin eschar has been excised, and the divided muscle ends with the attached fibrous scar are identified. For ease of visualization, an anal retractor (e.g., Hill-Ferguson; not shown)

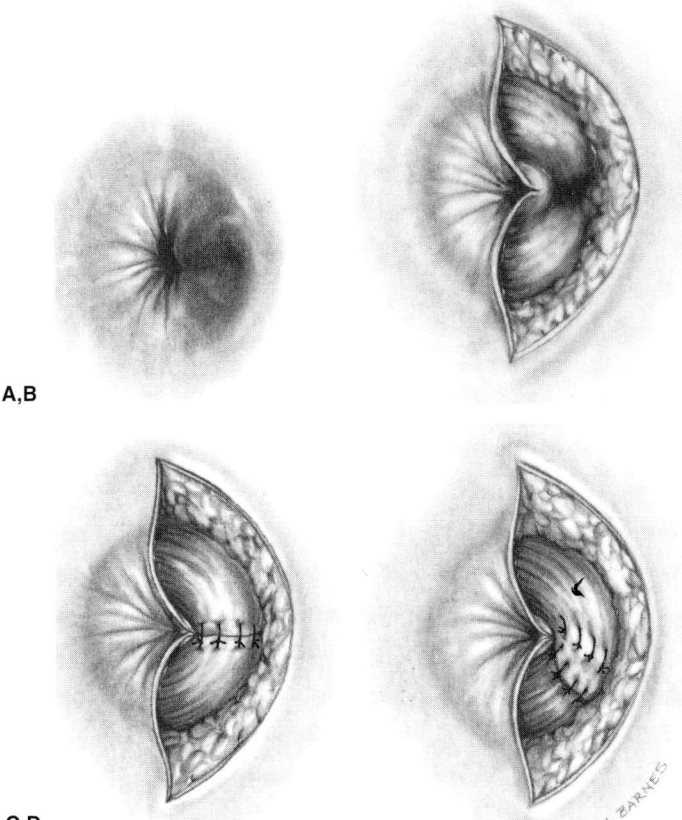

A,B

C,D

FIGURE 13-22. Technique of direct sphincter repair. **(A)** A defect on the right side as a consequence of tissue loss. **(B)** The ends of the divided sphincter are identified. Eschar is not debrided. **(C)** Technique of apposition. **(D)** Technique of overlapping.

should be used and kept in place for the entire operation to maintain the luminal diameter.

Numerous different suture materials have been suggested by various authors: monofilament nylon, pull-out wire, catgut, and silk. My own preference is to use No. 0 or 1, long-term absorbable material (i.e., Dexon or Vicryl), placed as simple, interrupted sutures. Repair of the sphincter muscle may be performed by the apposition technique (Figure 13-22C) or if sufficient residual muscle permits, by overlapping.

Overlapping

When adequate sphincter muscle remains or the defect is not excessive, an overlapping technique is preferred (Figure 13-22D). Greater length can be achieved by undermining the skin and by freeing the muscle for 1 or 2 cm at each end. With this technique, breakdown of the repair is less likely, and the results tend to be better. Of course, the more favorable outcome may be more a reflection of the magnitude of the sphincter loss than of the effect of this technique. That is to say, the procedure or the surgeon can hardly be blamed if there is insufficient tissue available to permit overlapping.

Unfortunately, the clearly illustrated problem shown in Figure 13-22 is not always the typical appearance found at the operating table. Often, only eschar and nonviable muscle remain. Under these circumstances, the surgeon may resort to suturing "stuff to stuff" in the hope of incorporating some tissue that will permit either improved voluntary control or will at least narrow the anal orifice. Such a frustrating operative session rarely produces significant improvement. It may be possible, however, to ameliorate the situation by extending the incision to or even beyond the midline anteriorly or posteriorly and by supplementing the repair with a reefing procedure.

As previously suggested, an important consideration at the completion of the repair is to establish proper skin coverage over the defect. If the loss has been minimal, primary closure is the most convenient method. With a wide skin defect, however, a new covering should be found. A split-thickness graft may be employed, but I prefer sensory-bearing, full-thickness skin, either advanced or rotated into position (Figs. 13-19, 13-20, and 13-23). Usually, drains are unnecessary, but if accumulation of fluid is a concern, a small, appropriately tailored, flat Silastic drain brought out through a counterincision may be advisable.

Reefing or Plication

Reefing, a procedure involving plication of the deep portion of the external sphincter and puborectalis sling, is the operation commonly employed transvaginally for posterior repair of rectocele. Its application in anovaginal reconstruction following obstetric injury is discussed later. Reefing may be performed anteriorly, as shown in Figure 13-24, or posteriorly, as shown in Figure 13-25.

In an anterior repair, the approach commonly employed in women, the vagina is mobilized and the external sphincter is divided. The levator ani muscle is plicated, and the puborectalis muscle and external sphincter are repaired. Care should be taken to avoid narrowing the anal orifice; a finger or retractor placed into the anal canal during the tying of the sutures minimizes this risk. The vagina

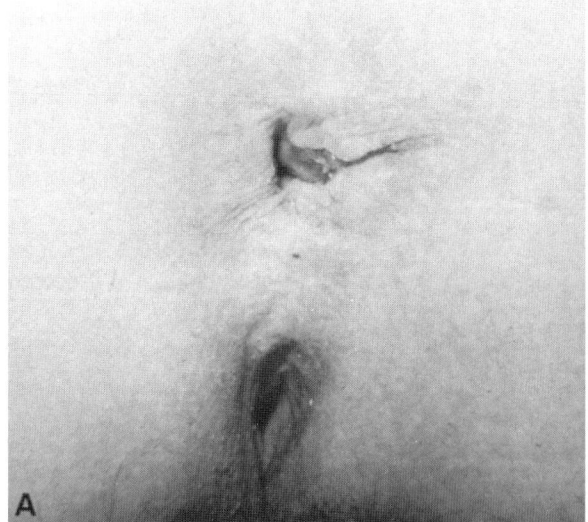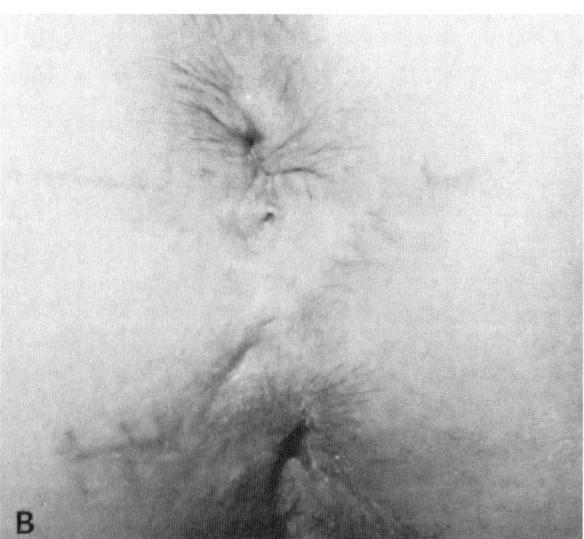

FIGURE 13-23. Sphincter injury following fistulectomy. **(A)** Preoperative appearance. **(B)** Appearance 3 months after surgery using overlapping repair and bilateral skin advancements in accordance with the method described later in this chapter for the management of obstetric injuries.

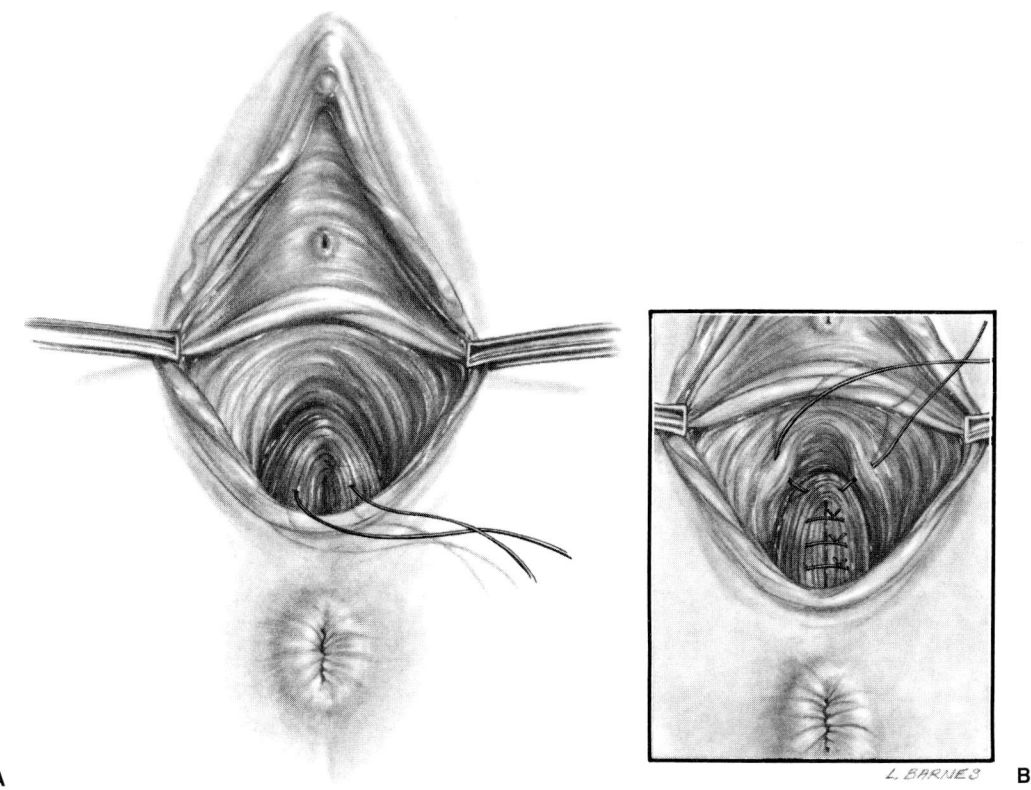

A   **B**

FIGURE 13-24. The reefing procedure as performed anteriorly in women. **(A)** The vaginal mucosa has been elevated and the sphincter identified. **(B)** The sphincter is reefed, and the perivaginal fascia is used to complete the repair.

is reapproximated with continuous or interrupted long-term absorbable sutures.

In the posterior plication (Figure 13-25), the external sphincter and levators are identified and sutured in the midline to narrow the anal orifice. Here, again, care must be taken to avoid too tight a closure. If it is not necessary to excise skin, the incision for this approach is often curvilinear. It should be made approximately 1 cm from the mucocutaneous junction and offers excellent exposure of the sphincter muscle.

Postoperative Care

Postoperatively, depending on the extent of the reconstruction and the risk of breakdown, the patient may be placed on a bowel-confining regimen. This consists of a

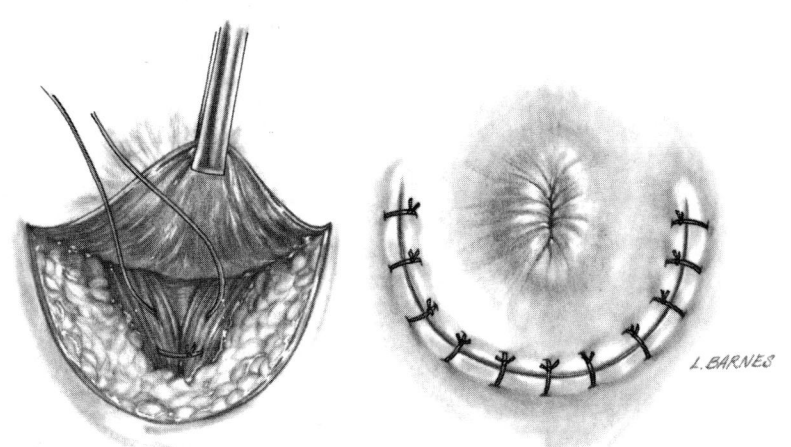

A   **B**

FIGURE 13-25. Posterior reefing procedure. **(A)** A curvilinear incision exposes the sphincter posteriorly. The sphincter is plicated posteriorly. **(B)** Closure should not be too tight.

clear liquid diet with the addition of the following medications: codeine (60 mg), diphenoxylate (Lomotil; 2 tablets), and deodorized tincture of opium (15 drops), each four times daily. The wounds are cleansed three times daily with a topical antiseptic solution. After 3 to 5 days, the medications are discontinued and a regular diet is instituted.

Nessim and co-workers (Cleveland Clinic Florida) conducted a prospective, randomized trial involving 54 patients, one half of whom received a bowel-confining regimen; the other half were fed a regular diet.[239] Thirty-two individuals underwent anal sphincter repairs. There were no differences observed between the two groups in the incidence of septic or urologic complications. The outcome was not adversely affected for those whose bowels were confined, and there were definite cost savings as a consequence of the reduced days in the hospital.

Results

It is very difficult to evaluate the relative merits of different operations for the treatment of fecal incontinence, particularly because of the rarity of prospective, randomized trials. Often the results of sphincter repair following obstetric injury are comingled with sphincter repair undertaken for other causes (e.g., anal fistula, trauma, perineal sepsis). Generally, the best results are obtained if direct sphincter repair is possible.[8,12,45,55,121,229,296,330] If there is little or no residual sphincter, an attempt at resuture is unlikely to be successful. Much, therefore, depends on the origin of the incontinence, the nature of the injury, the history of prior surgery, the physical findings, the degree of impairment, and, of course, the judgment of the surgeon. With respect to the value of certain preoperative physiologic studies, Buie and colleagues demonstrated that clinical rather than manometric assessment predicts continence after sphincter repair.[38] Unfortunately, not all of the foregoing variables are identified in the rather limited number of articles on the subject. Baig and Wexner opine as follows: "A common feature of all publications to date is that they are, to a degree, heterogeneous and subjective".[12] In recognizing these limitations, and with the understanding that there is indeed controversy, and that universal, definitive recommendations cannot be made, the following are a number of reports and opinions.

Goldberg and colleagues reviewed 47 cases treated by sphincteroplasty.[121] Almost one half of the patients had sustained obstetric or gynecologic trauma. The overall complication rate was 8.5%. An independent examiner found that 52% had excellent results, 37% good results, and 11% fair or poor results. In a later review from the same group in which 79 patients were studied, the authors advise that better results can be achieved *if the sphincter can be voluntarily contracted*, *if scar tissue is preserved on the muscle ends*, and *if a 3-month delay is elected after a failed attempt at repair.*[93]

Fleshman and co-workers performed overlapping sphincteroplasty in 55 women whose incontinence was primarily the result of obstetric injury.[105] No attempt was made to separate the vagina from the rectum by means of an anoplasty (see later). It was believed that the use of a perineal drain did not affect the functional results. The authors emphasized that, although the results were generally very good, complete continence was restored in only about one half of the patients. They concluded, first, that clinical assessment does not accurately reflect functional outcome, and, second, that it is important to ask the right questions of the patient if such evaluations are to be meaningful. In a later article from the same group, they note that the only factor that correlated with the return to normal sphincter function following overlapping sphincteroplasty was an increase in squeeze pressure.[127]

Rudd reported the treatment of 136 patients with anal incontinence.[296] Approximately one third were managed with exercises and bowel management and another one third with operant conditioning. Twenty-one underwent direct external sphincter repair, all but one of whom had good or excellent results. Of six patients requiring a puborectalis–external sphincter repair, five had good results.

The late Sir Alan Parks' personal experience with sphincter repair of 97 patients has been reported by others.[34,232] A high incidence of stricture was noted (16%), which the authors attributed to the use of wire. Fistulas occurred in seven patients. Those whose incontinence problems were the result of trauma had the best functional results (96% totally continent). In a report from the Mayo Clinic in Rochester, Minnesota, 62% of 40 patients were objectively evaluated to be improved following repair of divided sphincters, although more (85%) were subjectively better.[267] Halverson and Hull reported the Cleveland Clinic Ohio experience with long-term follow-up of overlapping sphincteroplasty.[130] Fifty-four percent were incontinent to liquid or solid stool.

Sitzler and Thomsom, reporting from St. Mark's Hospital, noted a successful outcome in 74.2% of their 31 patients.[328] In their postoperative assessment, they found that anal manometry was not discriminatory between successful and failed treatment. However, anal ultrasound appeared accurate in documenting residual sphincteric defects in those with a poor result. The use of a stoma in their experience was associated with fewer wound infections, but there was no statistically significant difference in success rate between those covered by a stoma and those not covered.[328] Anorectal ultrasound in the assessment of patients is discussed previously, and the use of this modality for postoperative evaluation has been increasingly applied. In the experience of Felt-Bersma and associates, 78% of individuals were shown to have diminution or disappearance of the sphincter defect that had been previously demonstrated endosonographically.[97] Likewise, Nielsen colleagues were able to explain the unsatisfactory results of surgery in some patients on the basis of endosonographic defects.[241] Giordano and co-workers comment that repeat anal sphincteroplasty that is undertaken in those persons who have had suboptimal functional results and in whom there is a residual defect may benefit from reoperative surgery.[117] The St. Mark's Hospital group concurs.[269]

Simmang and co-workers reviewed their experience with anal sphincter reconstruction in patients 55 years of age and older.[327] Their results were comparable to that achieved in younger patients for the same type of defect if they had normal pudendal nerve function.

Tjandra and colleagues, reporting from Melbourne, Australia, performed a study that is unique for this condition—a randomized, controlled trial. During a 5-year period, 23 patients were randomly assigned to direct end-to-end repair or to overlapping repair.[358] Both groups were comparable with respect to preoperative assessment. At a median follow-up of 18 months, the outcome was similar. There was no statistically significant association, but there was a tendency to an increased problem with bowel evacuation after the overlapping repair. This issue was mentioned previously as a potential concern if there is insufficient residual sphincter muscle present to permit this maneuver.

Sphincter Repair in Crohn's Disease

Despite the generally held admonition that reconstructive surgery for Crohn's disease should not be attempted, Scott and colleagues evaluated such repair efforts in a group of highly selected patients in whom the alternative would have been proctocolectomy.[317] All but one underwent successful repair, and, at the time of publication, only one had a permanent stoma. The authors do caution that temporary diversion is probably a prudent option.

Obstetric Injury

The incidence of anorectal complications following vaginal delivery has been reported to be approximately 5%.[363] Perhaps 10% of these repairs will fail at the time of delivery and require subsequent revision or reconstruction. In the experience of Fornell and colleagues from Linköping (Sweden), the overall incidence of sphincter rupture was 2.4%.[106]

Without doubt, the most common indication for one to perform an anal sphincter repair is prior obstetric injury. Sultan and colleagues sought to determine the incidence of damage to the anal sphincter and the relation of the injury to symptoms, physiologic function, and the

mode of delivery.[345] They analyzed 202 consecutive women 6 weeks before delivery, 150 of them 6 weeks after delivery, and 32 with abnormal findings 6 months following delivery. Thirteen percent of the primiparous women and 23% of the multiparous women who delivered vaginally had anal incontinence or urgency at the 6-week follow-up date. Thirty-five percent of the 79 primiparous women had a sphincter defect demonstrated on endoanal ultrasonography at 6 weeks; all who were followed at 6 months had a persistent defect. Of the 48 multiparous women, 40% had a sphincter defect prior to the surgery and 44% afterward. As may be expected, none of the 23 women who underwent cesarean section had a new sphincter defect following delivery. Eighty percent of the women who underwent forceps delivery were found to have sphincter defects, but none of the five women who underwent vacuum extractions were demonstrated to have such defects. It is evident from this study that occult sphincter defects are extremely common after vaginal delivery, especially if forceps are employed.

Ryhammer and co-workers demonstrated that women who have had one, two, and three vaginal deliveries developed permanent incontinence for flatus, 1.2%, 1.5%, and 8.3% of the time, respectively.[299,300] MacArthur and associates interviewed 906 women after childbirth (6 to 7 months following delivery) and identified 4% who developed fecal incontinence for the first time after the index birth.[205] Poen and co-workers evaluated 117 women who suffered third-degree lacerations at the time of delivery and noted that 40% complained of anal incontinence 5 years later.[272] Others confirm that fecal incontinence symptoms worsen with increased follow-up time, and that denervation injury is an independent risk factor for determining functional results.[235]

The timing of the repair following obstetric injury seems to be a crucial issue for gynecologists.[356] They generally believe that a 3- to 6-month waiting period is necessary to "achieve optimal tissue conditions." This seems to me to be a rather cavalier attitude, because it is the patient who must suffer the consequences of fecal soilage for this long interval. Most injuries to the sphincter, so-called third- and fourth-degree perineal lacerations (includes rectum), are recognized and satisfactorily repaired at the time of delivery. Perhaps this is due to laxity of the pelvic floor that permits apposition without tension. Still, my own experience supports the concept of repairing the injury at the convenience of the patient—that is, whenever the patient wishes to arrange for hospitalization.

A word of caution concerning episiotomy should be directed toward obstetricians, in the unlikely event they may read these comments. Although rectovaginal fistula and fourth-degree perineal injuries are infrequent complications of vaginal delivery, the physician should be wary of performing episiotomy in the midline, especially

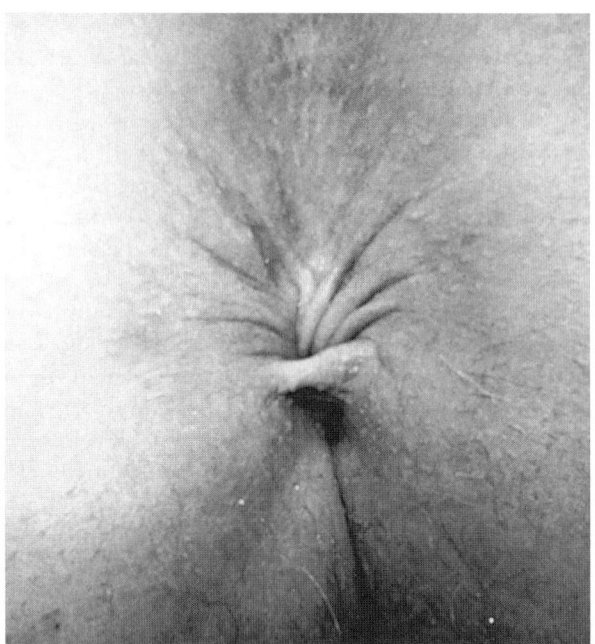

FIGURE 13-26. Ectopic anus. Anal opening is seen in close proximity to the vagina, a situation observed in 10% of women. This woman was completely asymptomatic.

if the woman is recognized to have an ectopic anus—that is, if the anus is anteriorly displaced toward the vagina (Figure 13-26).[284] This is a congenital variation seen in 10% of women.

Preoperative Assessment (Physiologic Studies)

An important observation concerning the nature and etiology of incontinence as a consequence of childbirth was reported by Snooks and co-workers.[338] Following studies on 71 women 2 to 3 days following delivery and again 2 months later, they found that in most cases the incontinence is caused by damage to the innervation of the pelvic floor muscles rather than by direct sphincter trauma.[338] There was a significantly prolonged mean PNTML, altered perineal position (i.e., descent) at rest and on straining, and reduced anal pressure on voluntary contraction. Patients who underwent cesarean section exhibited results essentially the same as that of controls. The authors concluded that unrecognized injury to pelvic floor innervation is responsible for what had previously been thought to be the inexplicably poor results of repair in some women. However, the results of surgical repair were excellent or good in eight of ten patients in whom there was no evidence of nerve injury, whereas this was the case in only one of nine when such damage occurred.[187] The authors suggested that pelvic floor surgery

may be required in addition to that of the sphincter repair.[333] They and others have since concluded that physiologic investigation, especially that of terminal motor nerve latency, should be considered because of the potential for effecting prognosis.[40]

Roberts and co-workers assessed nine patients with obstetric injuries by means of manometry, using a multilumen continuously perfused catheter.[286] Whereas an anterior defect should be expected, the authors discovered a global defect in five women. This suggests the possibility of a denervation injury, perhaps as a consequence of childbirth. Such an observation, if known prior to attempt at repair, may lead the surgeon to expect a less than perfect result. This is an area that deserves further exploration.

Other physiologic variables have been analyzed. For example, Cornes and associates assessed the effect of childbirth on anal canal sensation by means of mucosal electrosensitivity in 122 primiparous women in the immediate postpartum period and again 6 months later.[69] Sensation was impaired after both normal and forceps deliveries at all levels of the anal canal. However, with the exception of those who sustained sphincter injury, these values generally returned to normal by 6 months. Jacobs and colleagues performed EMG in patients who remained incontinent despite sphincteroplasty.[151] EMG demonstrated severe denervation, whereas sphincter mapping failed to identify any muscle discontinuity.

The previously mentioned study by Fleshman and co-workers involved the performance of anal manometry before and after surgical repair in 28 patients with obstetric injuries.[104] Complete bowel control could be achieved when the anal sphincter length, resting pressure, and especially squeeze pressure were returned to normal. Conversely, others have found that manometric assessment, in addition to single-needle EMG, were not useful in predicting continence, a fact perhaps attributable to pudendal nerve injury.[119] Especially with obstetric injury, objective physiologic improvement correlates well with subjective functional amelioration of incontinence.[376]

Technique of Repair

The patient is placed in the prone jackknife position. If the perineal body must be reconstituted, and/or it becomes necessary to find tissue to reconstruct the posterior vaginal wall and distal rectum, it is useful to perform bilateral advancement flaps. If one elects this approach, a cruciate incision is made across the perineal body, and full-thickness flaps of skin are developed as illustrated (Figure 13-27). However, if the perineal body is thought to be adequate, most surgeons prefer a curvilinear incision between the anus and the

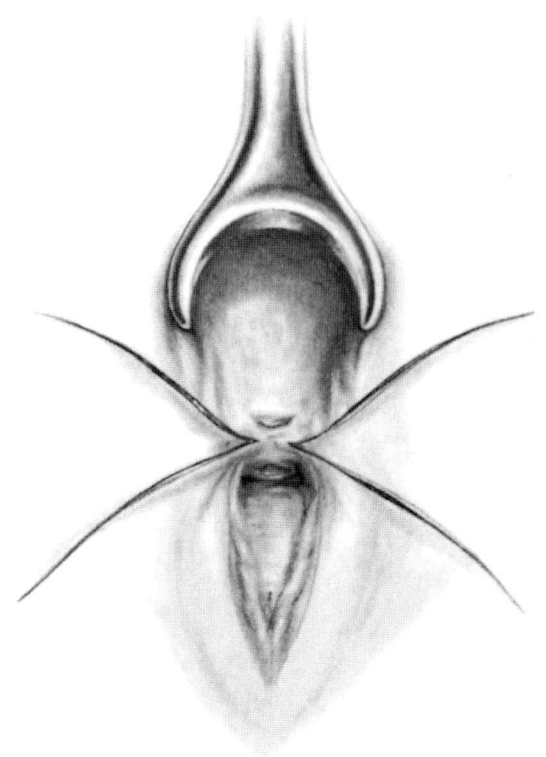

FIGURE 13-27. In anovaginal reconstruction, a cruciate incision is made across the perineal body. Note the close proximity between the anal verge and the introitus.

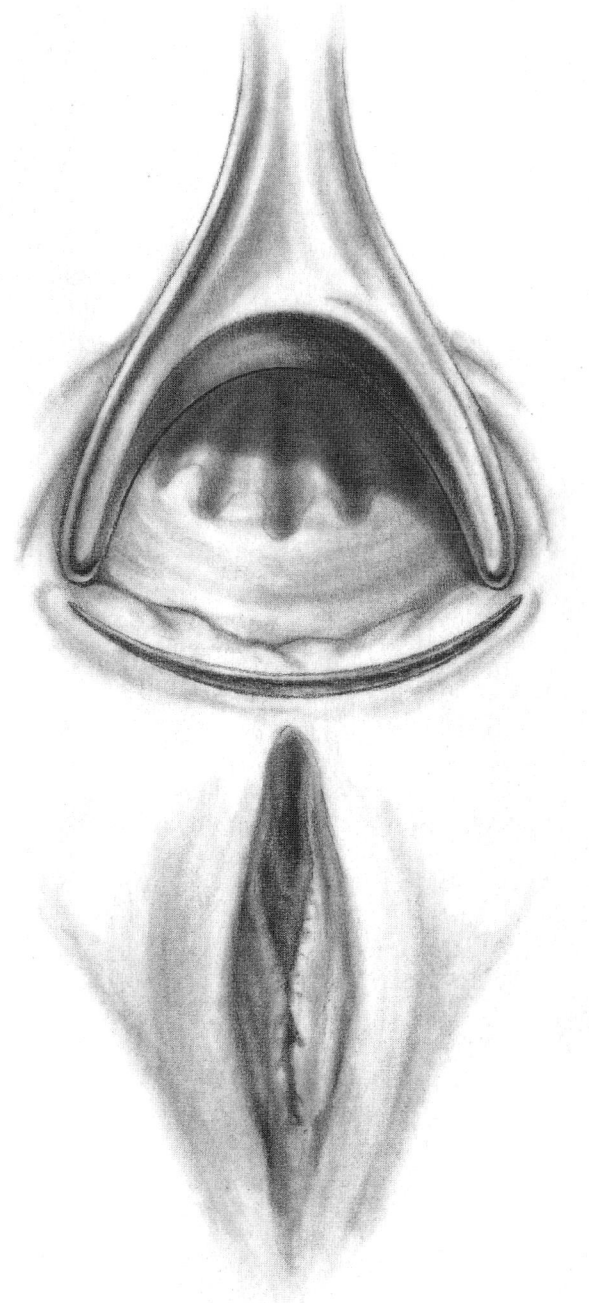

FIGURE 13-28. Standard transverse, curvilinear incision across the perineal body.

vagina (Figure 13-28). A Hill-Ferguson retractor is kept in the anal canal for the entire operation to maintain adequacy of the lumen while the muscle repair is completed. The rectovaginal septum is infiltrated with 0.5% bupivacaine (Marcaine) with 1:200,000 epinephrine (Figure 13-29). This aids in hemostasis and facilitates the dissection. The rectum is separated from the vagina, and any concomitant fistula tract, if present, is identified (Figure 13-30). The cephalad limit is reached, and plication of the levator ani muscle is carried out anterior to the rectum (Figure 13-31). This usually requires three or four long-term absorbable sutures (e.g., No. 0 or No. 1 Vicryl).

Often rectovaginal fistula repair requires a concomitant sphincter reconstruction (see Chapter 12). How the approach is effected depends upon the location of the openings and the origin of the problem. For a fistula between the vagina and the anal canal, my preference is to perform the repair through a transperineal approach, with a concomitant anoplasty. For a higher-level fistula, the option of mucosal advancement should be considered (see Chapter 12), although it may be possible to approach the fistula through the perineum. For still higher fistulas, either a mucosal advancement or an abdominal operation is suggested. As implied, most women with recto-

vaginal fistula as a consequence of an obstetric injury have an ectopic anus (Figure 13-26). To achieve the best functional results, in my opinion, reconstruction of the perineal body should also be undertaken in this group of patients.

The redundant mucosa, including any fistula, is excised from the vagina and the rectum (Figure 13-32). The external sphincter muscle is reapproximated in one

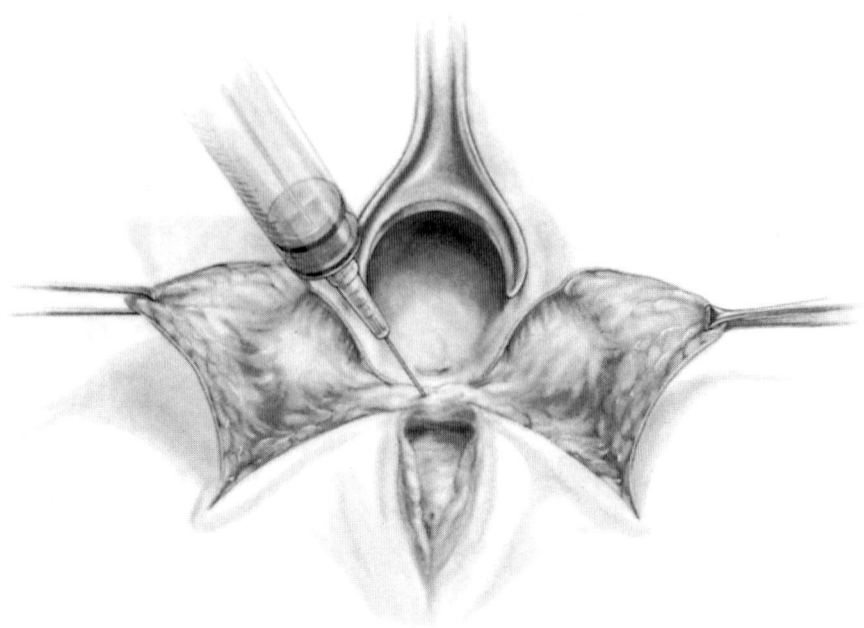

FIGURE 13-29. Anovaginal reconstruction: skin flaps are elevated, and a dilute epinephrine solution is injected into the rectovaginal septum to facilitate the dissection.

or two layers, using the same suture material (Figure 13-33). It may be rather difficult to identify the residual external sphincter, but the Peña stimulator can be used if there is a question. The final step in the operation is to advance and interdigitate the two triangular flaps of skin (Figure 13-34). The skin is sufficiently mobile so that in the midportion, the suture line will actually lie within the anal canal and vagina.

Robertson suggests a different method of covering the skin defect, that of advancing bilateral, full-thickness islands of skin (Figure 13-35).

A flat Silastic drain may be placed under the skin flaps and brought out through a stab wound in the buttock; it is then attached to continuous suction. The drain is removed in 48 to 72 hours. A firm pressure dressing is applied. A bowel-confining regimen is rec-

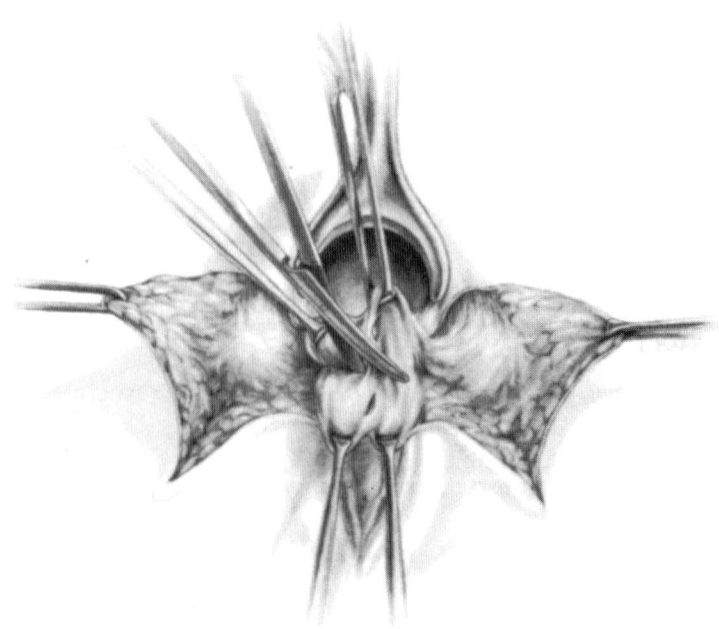

FIGURE 13-30. Anovaginal reconstruction: the rectum is separated from the vagina by careful sharp dissection.

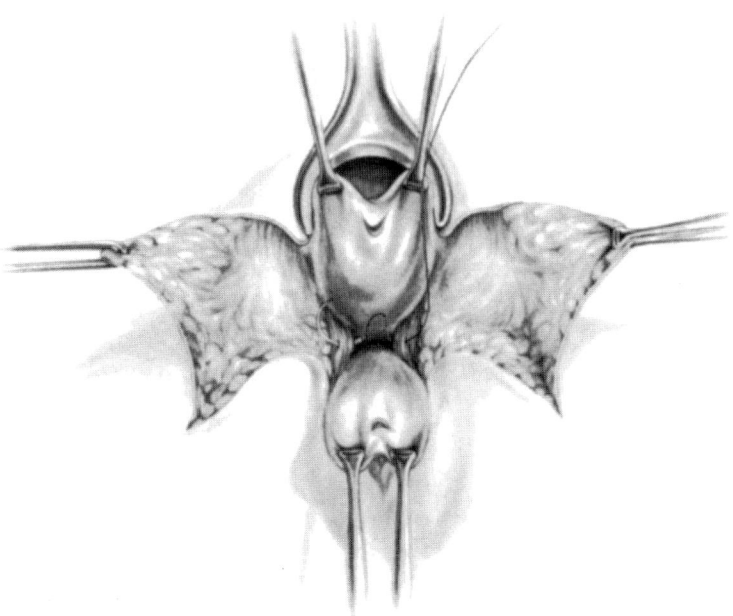

FIGURE 13-31. Anovaginal reconstruction: mobilization has been completed, and the levatores are now reefed. Three sutures of heavy, long-term absorbable material are recommended. Maintaining the retractor in place prevents the rectal lumen from being narrowed.

ommended postoperatively, especially when skin is mobilized. A protective colostomy is not necessary. Figures 13-36 and 13-37 show women who sustained obstetric trauma and who underwent this reconstructive approach. When a transverse incision is initially employed, the ultimate skin closure actually becomes longitudinal (Figure 13-38). This is a consequence of the muscle repair, bringing much more tissue into the midline to build up the perineal body. However, the midportion of the incision usually must be left open because of tension.

Results

I initially reported 28 women who underwent anovaginal reconstruction (i.e., sphincteroplasty and anoplasty) after sustaining obstetric injury.[66] All had varying degrees of incontinence for flatus or for feces, and most wore a

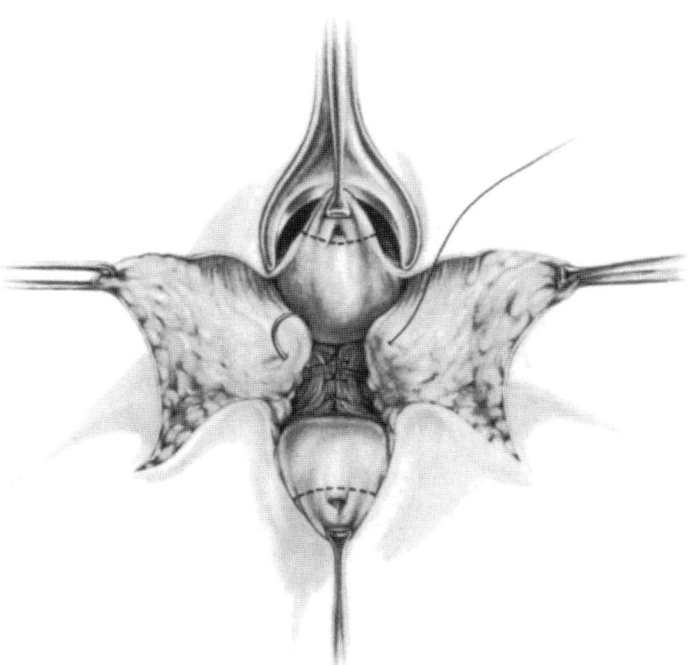

FIGURE 13-32. Anovaginal reconstruction: the fistula openings and redundant mucosa in both the rectum and vagina, if present, are excised *(dashed lines)*. The external sphincter repair is then begun.

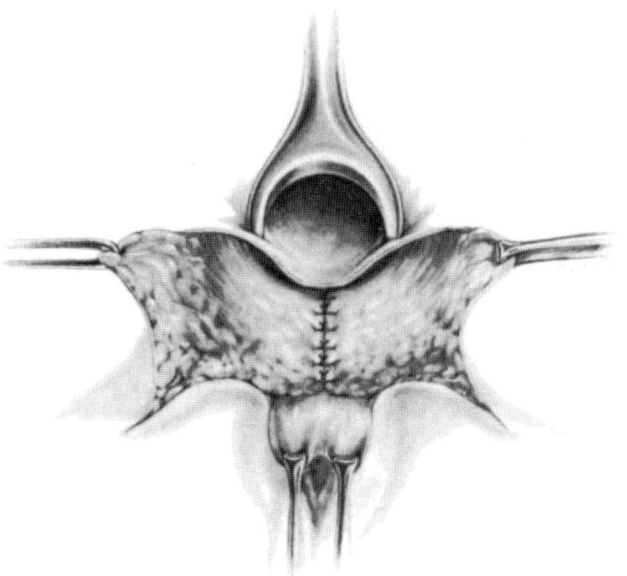

FIGURE 13-33. Anovaginal reconstruction: external sphincter repair has been completed in one or two layers.

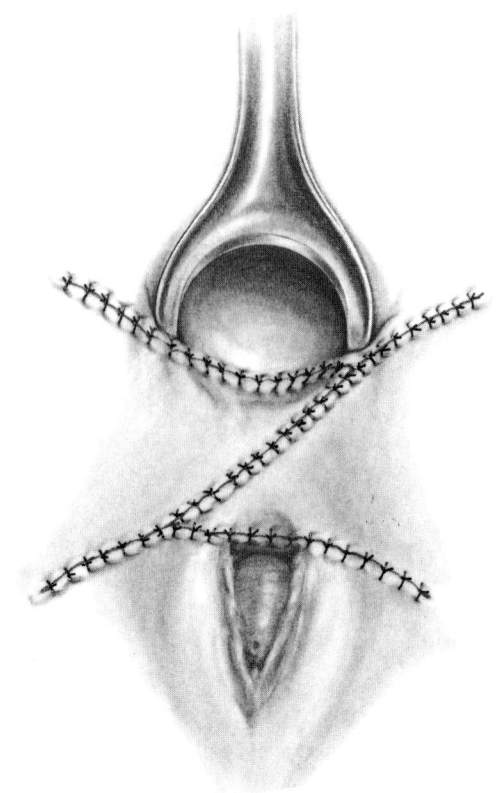

FIGURE 13-34. Anovaginal reconstruction: the skin flaps are advanced and interdigitated, thereby permitting the widened perineal body to be closed completely.

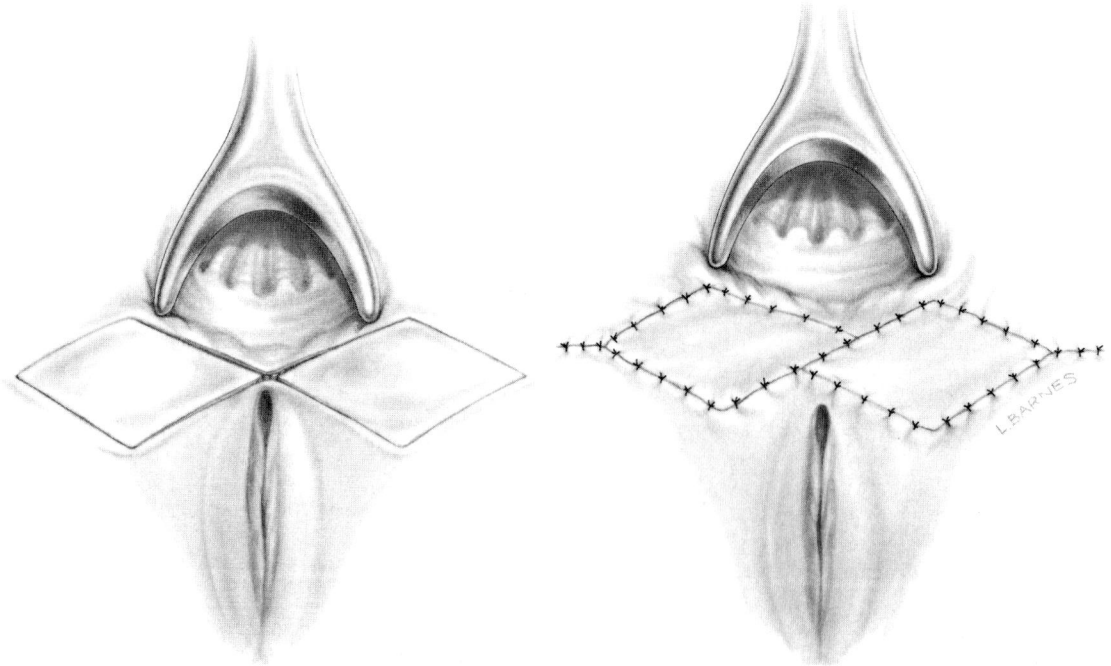

FIGURE 13-35. Anovaginal reconstruction: skin closure can also be effected by means of island flaps, as suggested by Robertson, the so-called Texas double-diamond.

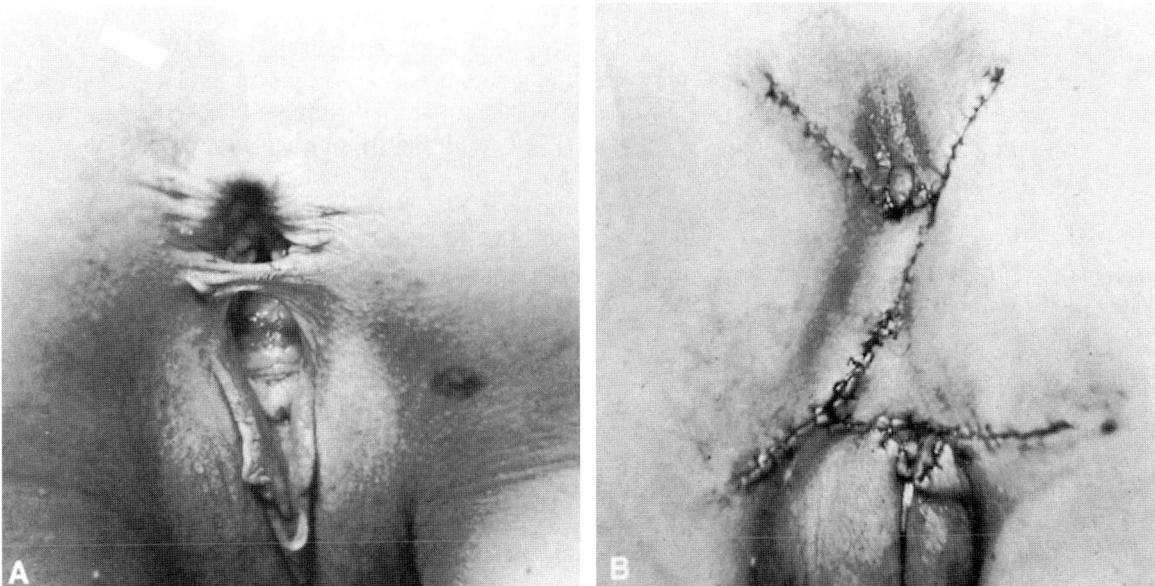

FIGURE 13-36. Rectovaginal fistula secondary to obstetric injury. **(A)** Note the ectopic (anterior) displacement of the anorectum. **(B)** Reconstruction completed by advancement of skin flaps. This distance between the anus and the vagina is normal.

pad. Twenty had undergone median (i.e., midline) episiotomy, and one had not. In the remaining seven, the type of episiotomy could not be ascertained. Approximately one half of the patients underwent prior attempts at repair; one patient had nine operations. All had anterior, ectopic displacement of the anus.

Following reconstruction, all patients experienced amelioration of their incontinence problems. All were continent for feces, but a recurrent fistula developed at a higher level in one woman, presumably secondary to rectal injury during the course of the dissection. This type of anovaginal construction has since been applied to 135

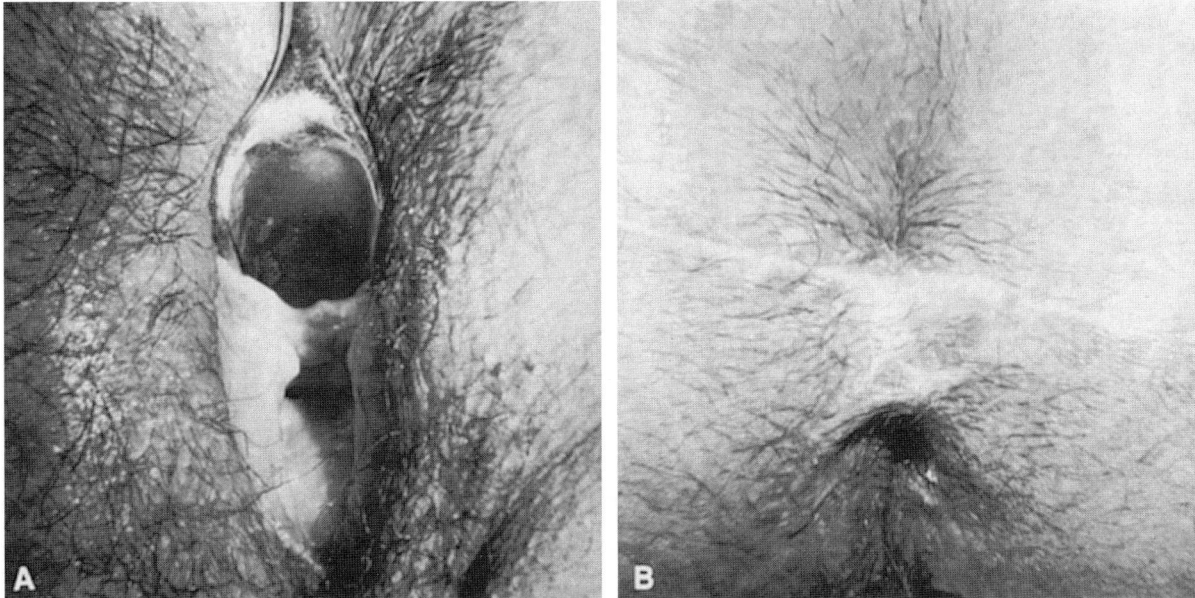

FIGURE 13-37. Anal incontinence secondary to obstetric injury. **(A)** Preoperative appearance. **(B)** Appearance 8 weeks following surgery.

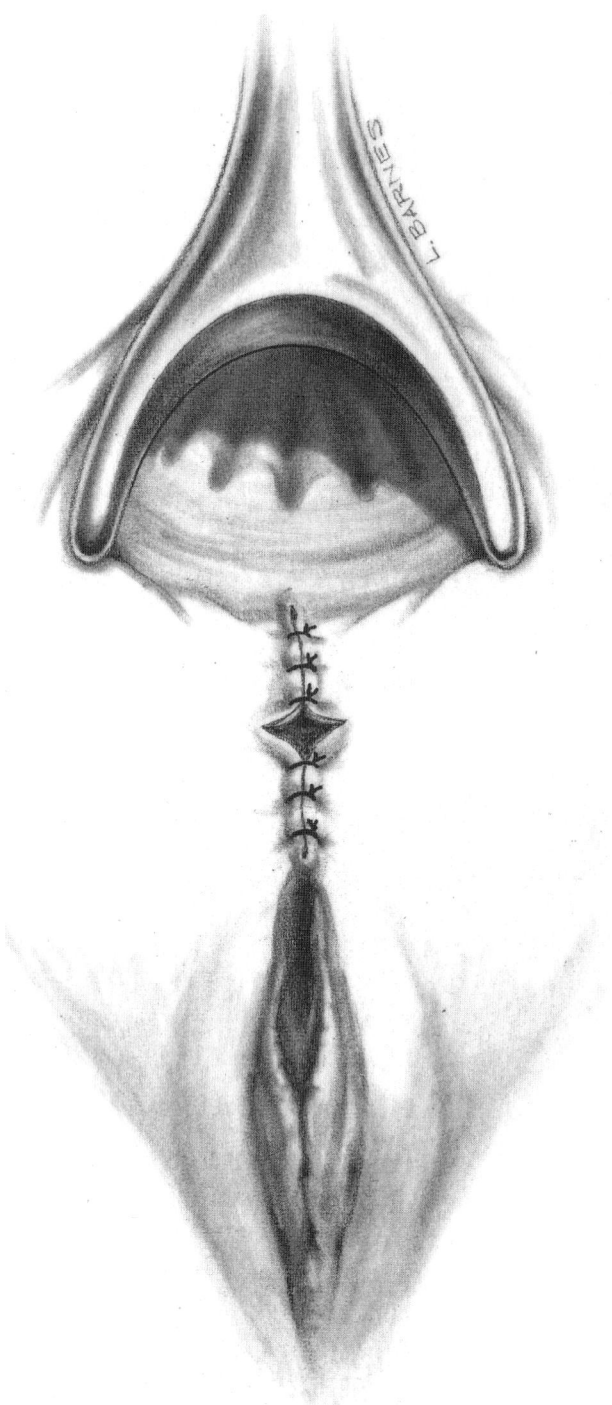

FIGURE 13-38. Following repair, the original transverse incision becomes longitudinal, further separating the anal verge from the introitus. Usually one cannot close the midportion of the wound.

patients as of this writing. Eight percent noted some degree of impairment, primarily that of incontinence for gas. Four of these patients stated that there was essentially no improvement compared with the preoperative status. All of these individuals had pudendal neuropathy. Ninety-two percent reported complete continence for loose stool.

Most authors have not given sufficient attention to the problem of reconstruction of the perineal body.[105,387] Unless the defect is corrected by early mobilization of skin flaps, as suggested by Russell and Gallagher, an optimal functional result may not be achieved.[298] The key to success for patients with an inadequate perineal body, in my opinion, is to begin the procedure by performing a cruciate incision. By applying this maneuver and the well-recognized principles of sphincter repair, excellent functional results can be anticipated, assuming there is no underlying neuropathy.

Abcarian and co-workers, however, are quite satisfied to accomplish the repair without moving skin.[1] They reported excellent anatomic and physiologic results in 43 patients who sustained injuries that created a cloacal defect. Others note generally satisfactory results with conventional sphincter repair for a host of anorectal complications associated with vaginal delivery, including sphincter disruption, rectovaginal fistula, cloacal defect, and fistula-in-ano.[105,344,363]

In spite of the foregoing recommended approaches, obstetricians and gynecologists, as well as some general surgeons, believe that good results may be anticipated, and, indeed, the repair is *best accomplished*, if a transvaginal technique is used.[28,354] For the reasons already mentioned, I disagree.

Khanduja and associates performed repair of obstetric injuries on 52 patients with a mean follow-up period of 16 months.[167] Perfect results in those individuals who sustained sphincteric injury were observed in 64%. Those with rectovaginal fistulas had a perfect result 56% of the time. Those with a combined fistula and incontinent anal sphincter also had a perfect result about two thirds of the time. No patient had a "poor result." Engel and colleagues undertook postoperative squeeze pressures and anal endosonography on 55 patients who sustained sphincteric injury.[89] The postoperative squeeze pressure was increased and the external sphincter was more frequently intact in those individuals who had a good outcome. The authors attributed the failure of repair to a persistent external sphincter defect. Furthermore, they opined that late-onset incontinence is usually associated with pudendal neuropathy and believed that this observation presages a poor outcome. In the experience of Sangalli and Marti with 36 sphincteroplasties, 78% were continent, 19% partially continent, and one totally incontinent.[304]

Comment

Generally, the results of anal sphincteroplasty with or without anoplasty in the delayed management of anal incontinence as a consequence of obstetric injury are quite good. The one exception appears to be those patients who harbor concomitant pudendal neuropathy. In order for the patient to make a reasoned decision and to have realistic expectations concerning the results of reconstructive surgery, PNTML is strongly recommended. It has been my experience, however, that irrespective of the results of this study, patients who have significant impairment for bowel control will opt for a repair, even though the prognosis may be ideal.

Postanal Pelvic Floor Repair or Parks' Repair

In 1975, the late Sir Alan Parks (see Biography, Chapter 29) emphasized the importance of levator plication in the procedure that he called a "postanal repair".[256] He believed that one of the major contributing factors for maintaining continence is the "valve effect caused by the double right-angle which normally exists between the anal canal, the lowermost rectum and the midrectum, although as previously mentioned this concept has not been supported by others".[256] He believed that the puborectalis muscle was the primary ingredient for establishing this angle. Because incontinence is often associated with loss of the normal angulation, Parks predicated his operative procedure on restoration of the anorectal angle.

The operation is usually advocated for those patients with incontinence associated with rectal prolapse, the descending perineum syndrome, and so-called idiopathic incontinence. Most of these patients have pudendal neuropathy. The procedure is not advised for the treatment of incontinence as a consequence of trauma.

Technique

The procedure is carried out in the intersphincteric plane (i.e., the plane between the internal and external sphincters). This is a relatively bloodless area through which dissection is less likely to cause nerve injury. The pelvic floor and sphincter muscles are approximated behind the anorectal junction, displacing them anteriorly and increasing the angulation.[258] It is believed that, by shortening the length of the puborectalis, those muscle fibers that are innervated and viable will function more effectively.[257,258]

As is often the custom with British surgeons and, of course, with the man who described the procedure, the lithotomy position is advised (although this belief is changing). However, as I have stated before, the prone position is infinitely more convenient, and so for the purpose of proselytism (and personal preference), the procedure has been illustrated in the optimal position for this text. The reader may choose to invert the pages if the lithotomy position is chosen.

The technique of the operation is essentially that which has been described by Parks in a number of publications.[256–258] A V-shaped incision is made approximately

6 cm posterior to the anal verge, a point emphasized because, ultimately, skin will be drawn into the anal canal (Figure 13-39A). An anterior skin flap is elevated until the lower borders of the internal and external anal sphincters are exposed (Figure 13-39B). Dissection is then carried out in the intersphincteric plane, displacing the posterior portion of the external sphincter through one half of its circumference (Figure 13-39C). The dissection proceeds cephalad by lifting the rectum off the upper part of the external sphincter. The internal sphincter becomes contiguous with the circular muscle of the rectum at about the level of the puborectalis muscle. Above the puborectalis, the fascia of Waldeyer is encountered, and the mesorectal fat and posterior rectal wall are exposed.

A deep retractor is inserted, displacing the rectum anteriorly. The levator ani muscle is exposed, and a lattice of monofilament nylon is constructed, either by continuous suture or with an interrupted technique (Figure 13-39D). The highest and most lateral point of the levators is identified close to the spines of the ischia (i.e., the ileococcygeus muscle). No attempt is made to approximate the muscle; even if it were possible to accomplish this, too much tension would be produced. The retractors are then somewhat withdrawn, and a second row of sutures is placed in either a continuous or interrupted fashion at about the level of the pubococcygeus muscle (Figure 13-39E). Because the anterior origin of this muscle is near the midline, it may be possible to approximate it at this location. Finally, a third row of sutures is placed into the puborectalis muscle (Figs. 13-39F and 13-39G). Apposition of this muscle is readily accomplished anteriorly, but care must be taken to avoid narrowing the rectum. Because the skin tends to be drawn into the anal canal, closure is usually effected in the shape of a Y (Figs. 13-39H and 13-39I). Drainage of the subcutaneous tissue is recommended.

Postoperative Care

As mentioned previously, the relative merits of a bowel-confining regimen have been the subject of debate. Despite the absence of evidence to support this restriction, my personal preference is that all patients who undergo reconstructive anorectal procedures involving repair of the sphincter, major replacement of skin, or both, should have a bowel-confining regimen in the postoperative period. With the aforementioned protocol, it is rare indeed for a patient to have a bowel movement. The duration of this program is even more subjective and depends on the extent of the reconstruction and may vary from as few as 2 to as many as 5 days. Unfortunately, it may not be possible to perform the optimal suggested regimen because of the constraints imposed by third-party insurance carriers. Still, when I communicate my concerns about ambulatory management of such a major reconstruction with an appropriately re-

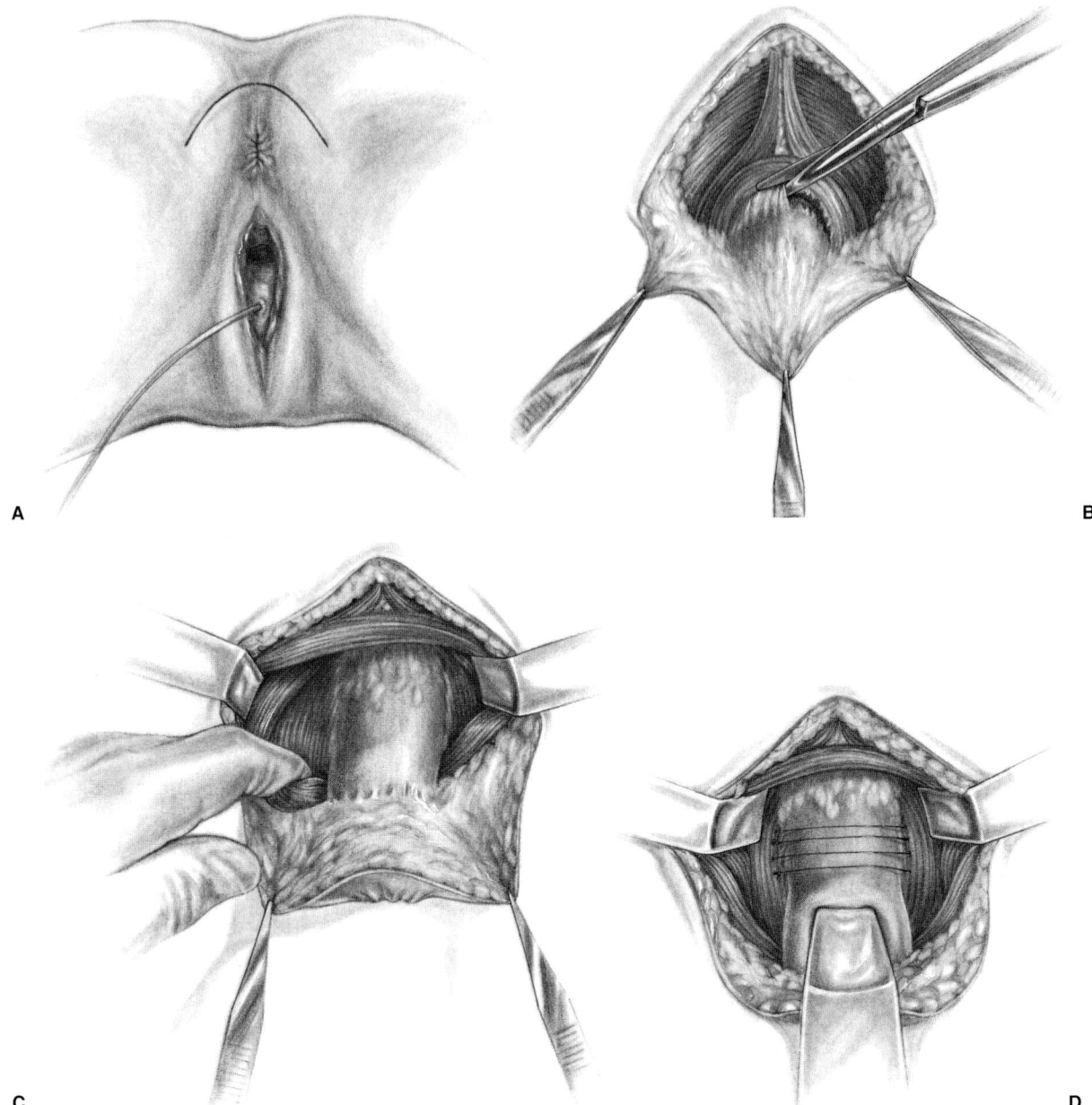

FIGURE 13-39. Parks' postanal pelvic floor repair. **(A)** V-shaped incision is made ~6 cm posterior to the anal verge. **(B)** The internal sphincter is separated from the external sphincter through one half of its circumference. **(C)** The rectum is lifted off the upper portion of the external sphincter reaching the puborectalis muscle. **(D)** Sutures of polypropylene are placed across the two limbs of the ileococcygeus muscle. Approximately three layers are placed at this topmost level and are tied loosely, without tension, to form a lattice across the pelvis. **(E)** The next layer is placed in the upper part of the pubococcygeus muscle as a lattice. The lower part, closer to the midline, can be approximated. **(F)** The puborectalis is now plicated. This is the strongest and thickest part and the muscle that is most easily visualized. **(G)** The external sphincter is sutured. **(H)** Repair results in the drawing forward of the anterior skin flap; simple reconstitution would be under tension. **(I)** Skin closure is Y-shaped. (Adapted from Parks AG, Percy J. Postanal pelvic floor repair for anorectal incontinence. In: Todd IP, Fielding LP, eds. *Operative surgery.* London: Butterworths, 1983:433, with permission.)

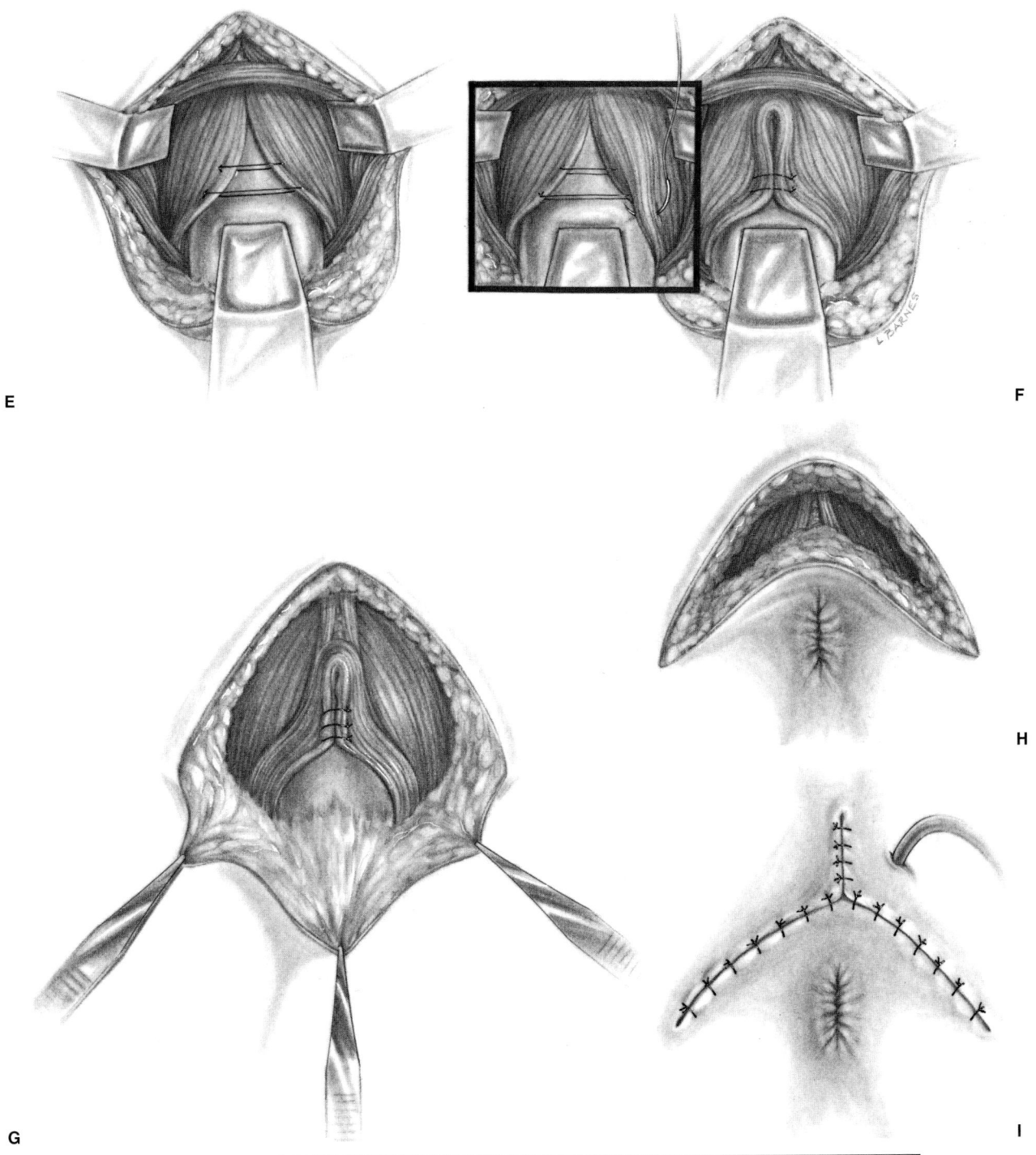

E

F

G

H

I

FIGURE 13-39. *(continued)*

sponsible individual, I seem to be successful. In women, an indwelling catheter is useful until defecation is permitted. Systemic antibiotics are suggested for from 2 to 5 days, depending on the amount of surgical manipulation and degree of contamination.

Local care includes gentle cleansing of the wound with an antiseptic solution (e.g., hydrogen peroxide)

three times daily and application of a topical antiseptic ointment, such as povidone-iodine (i.e., Betadine). Patients are encouraged to perform perineal strengthening exercises immediately after operation. When the person is able to resume a regular diet, a stool softener (e.g., dioctyl sodium sulfosuccinate) and a bulk laxative preparation containing psyllium (e.g., Konsyl) are often advisable. Following deep postanal repair, the necessity for avoiding straining to pass stool is very important.

Results

Parks reported 75 patients who underwent postanal repair, approximately two thirds of whom had a rectal prolapse.[256] Significantly, the best results were in the group *without* prolapse, the overall success rate being 83%. However, Keighley and Matheson have shown that rectopexy alone results in restoration of continence in 80% of procidentia patients following a definitive prolapse procedure.[162] Of those with persistent incontinence (four patients), postanal repair resulted in total bowel control in three patients and some improvement in the remaining one.

Henry and Simson reported the results of all postanal repairs performed by the surgical staff at St. Mark's Hospital during the period 1978 through 1983.[135] There were 242 patients, none of whom was incontinent as a result of trauma. The overall complication rate was approximately 20%, most of which was attributable to wound infection. A satisfactory result was achieved in almost 60%.

Yoshioka and Keighley evaluated 124 patients who underwent this procedure at the General Hospital, Birmingham, England.[398] Incontinence was improved in 81%, but 76% still leaked stool, and 52% required pads. These investigators concluded that the quality of continence after this operation is generally poor. The Lahey Clinic in Boston reported that of 14 patients, nine had initial improvement with two subsequent failures (i.e., a 50% success rate).[344] Jameson and colleagues, reporting from the Central Middlesex Hospital in London, evaluated 36 patients who underwent postanal repair at 6 months after operation.[153] By this time, 83% had obtained some benefit from the operation, but only approximately one half maintained this improvement.

In analyzing the reasons for failure of postanal repair in 20 patients, Snooks and associates performed electrophysiologic and manometric studies and concluded that progression of the neuropathic process was responsible.[335] It has also been suggested that the manipulation associated with the operation may predispose to further neurologic injury in some individuals.[188] It is interesting to note that many patients with subjective improvement in bowel control had no significant change in the anorectal angle.[248,389] Healy and colleagues, in fact, showed that there was no difference in static pelvic floor measurements when those remaining symptomatic after postanal repair were compared with those who had improved.[133] These investigators suggest that dynamic MRI may be able to explain the reasons for failure.

Miller and Orrom and their colleagues opined that successful outcome after any sphincter repair effort is most likely the result of improved sphincter pressures and anal sensation.[229,248] However, Yoshioka and Keighley observed that MRP and MSP did not change significantly after operation, irrespective of whether bowel control improved.[398] In another study, rectal compliance, rectal sensation, and emptying were not improved.[396] Scott and co-workers analyzed the results in 62 patients and attempted to relate clinical outcome to preoperative assessment of resting anal canal pressure, subjective evaluation of gape, and a combination of low pressure and gape.[318] None of these factors was believed to be predictive of a poor functional result. Others have demonstrated that resting and squeeze pressures improved with this operation.[225,308]

Yoshioka and associates studied 19 patients preoperatively and postoperatively in an attempt to determine who could benefit from repair.[396] None of the following pressures improved with surgery: low resting pressure, squeeze pressure, and strain anal pressure at 2 cm. Videoproctographic evidence of increased pelvic floor descent at rest, during contraction, and during straining also did not improve.[396] Scheuer and co-workers suggest that this operation "restores anatomy rather than function".[308]

One of the largest published series from the United States comes from the Cleveland Clinic Florida group.[214] Twenty-one patients underwent postanal repair between 1992 and 1998. None of the preoperative physiologic investigations was demonstrated to be predictive of outcome. The overall "success rate" was 35%. The authors conclude that in spite of the low success rate, the absence of mortality and the low morbidity should at least permit its application in selected instances.[214]

Opinion

Although I do not wish to appear insular, the postanal repair has not transplanted successfully to the United States. Although its proponents have been primarily British and continental Europeans, geography alone has not prevented other operations from being received enthusiastically in foreign countries. Whatever the explanation for its lack of application or success in the United States, I personally do not believe this procedure has a meaningful position in the management of patients with anal incontinence. It would be interesting to learn of a prospective, randomized, sham-controlled study with this operation. The effect of the unintended anoplasty, itself, may account for whatever is the observed success. However, one is not likely to read about this investigation anytime soon. Still, if the only option is a colostomy and the physician and patient are willing to accept the likelihood of failure, postanal repair may be considered as a possible option.

Operations for Supplementing the Sphincter Mechanism

When there is an adequate functioning residual sphincter, direct repair usually produces optimal results. However, if too much muscle tissue has been lost to effect reconstruction, whether as a result of trauma or disuse, such an approach is usually unsuccessful. In these instances, surgical reconstruction designed to create a supplementary sphincter may have some merit.[47]

Gracilis Muscle Transposition

In 1952, Pickrell and colleagues developed a procedure using the gracilis muscle as a substitute anal sphincter.[268] I have found this to be a very effective operation for selected patients when a supplementary sphincter is required or when multiple attempts at direct repair have been unsuccessful.[63,64,67] However, this operation is not for elderly patients who complain of soiling their underclothes. It is an esoteric sphincter-repairing approach to be used only in limited circumstances.

Indications

Gracilis muscle transposition (GMT) is a procedure so complex and technically difficult, with a high failure rate, that its application should be quite limited. The primary indication is obviously a patient with anal incontinence sufficiently severe that it cannot be controlled by nonoperative means, and in an individual whose sphincter either cannot be primarily repaired or whose sphincteroplasty has failed. Those most likely to benefit are young patients and those whose cause of incontinence is trauma or a congenital anomaly. The use of the gracilis muscle has also been applied for reconstruction of the anus after abdominoperineal resection and in the management of postirradiation necrosis (see later).[243,383]

Contraindications

Patients who have an irritable bowel, diarrhea, or intractable constipation are poor candidates. Those with healing problems, anal disease, radiated perineum, radiation proctitis, perineal thinning, obstetric injury as the cause of incontinence, concomitant neuropathy, older age or elderly status, will have suboptimal or poor results with this operation. This is *not* a pleasant walk in the noonday sun either for surgeon or for patient. It is an esoteric, sphincter-saving alternative, with myriad technical pitfalls and intraoperative and postoperative complications. Success depends on proper patient selection, the always expected, meticulous technique, and frankly, quite a bit of good luck.

Technique

The operation is undertaken with the patient in the perineolithotomy position in order to provide access to the thigh and to the proximal lower leg, groin, buttocks, and perineum. Although the presence of a colostomy has not been demonstrated to reduce the complication and failure rates, some surgeons prefer always to create one. I do not use a colostomy unless, of course, one is already present. A mechanical bowel preparation is advised along with perioperative systemic antibiotics.

The gracilis muscle, the most superficial muscle in the medial aspect of the thigh, is broad in the upper thigh, becomes narrow, and tapers to a tendon that inserts below the tibial tuberosity. The primary blood supply for this muscle almost always enters proximally. Therefore, division at the insertion with mobilization of the muscle to the proximal neurovascular bundle usually does not compromise viability. Unfortunately, on rare occasion there may be several anomalous vessels entering the muscle. One watches in dismay as the muscle changes color to an ominous deep purple as the vessels are ligated. When this is recognized, the operation can proceed only if the contralateral gracilis muscle is harvested. It is quite common, however, to note the presence of a solitary, distal perforating artery. Happily, ligating and dividing this structure do not compromise the muscle's viability.

The side selected for transposition is draped so that it can be removed easily from the stirrup. I prefer to use three incisions to mobilize the gracilis muscle—in the upper thigh, in the midthigh, and across the knee joint medially. The muscle can usually be located at the distance of two index finger-lengths from the anal verge. Although this is a somewhat arbitrary and unscientific measuring method, I have found it to be quite accurate. I believe it is easier to identify the muscle initially through the proximal incision, although some surgeons disagree. Distally, the gracilis tendon lies deep to the sartorius, an awkward initial exposure, at least for me.

A ¼-inch Penrose drain is passed under the muscle (Figure 13-40), and the dissection is carried cephalad to the neurovascular bundle (Figure 13-40, *inset*), which is the upper limit of the dissection. The muscle is mobilized to the tendinous insertion by incising the investing fascia and by blunt dissection beneath the skin bridges (Figure 13-41). Because the tendon of the gracilis muscle passes deep to the sartorius muscle, the latter muscle must be retracted anteriorly to identify the gracilis tendon. The dissection proceeds distally as far as possible, and the tendon is divided right off the bone (Figure 13-42). Every millimeter of tendon length is critical, because if there is inadequate muscle and tendon length to wrap around the anus and to properly attach it, the harvesting will be an exercise in futility. The two distal incisions are closed in two layers (i.e., subcutaneous tissue and skin), and the

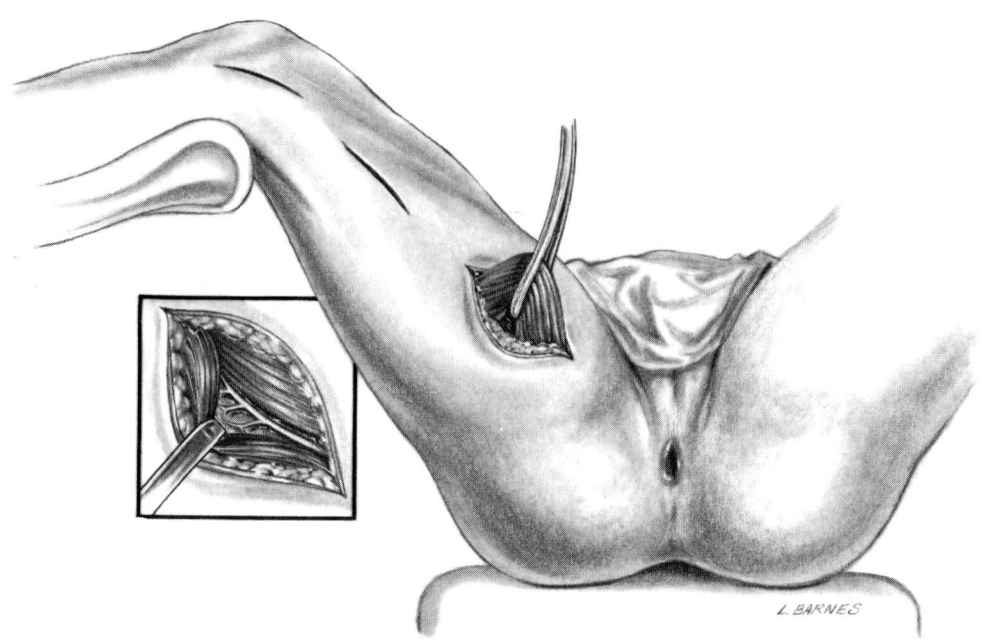

FIGURE 13-40. Gracilis muscle transposition: two incisions are made in the thigh and one across the knee joint for mobilizing the gracilis muscle. A Penrose drain is placed around the muscle proximally; this tethers the muscle and facilitates identification of the neurovascular bundle **(inset)**.

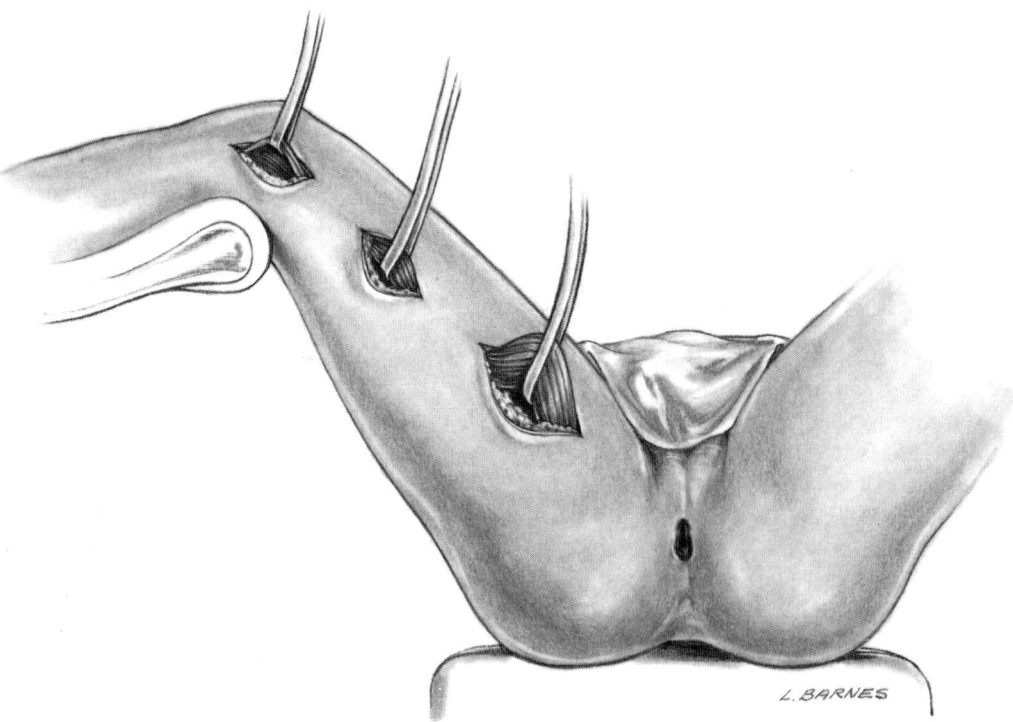

FIGURE 13-41. Gracilis muscle transposition: complete mobilization of muscle and tendon.

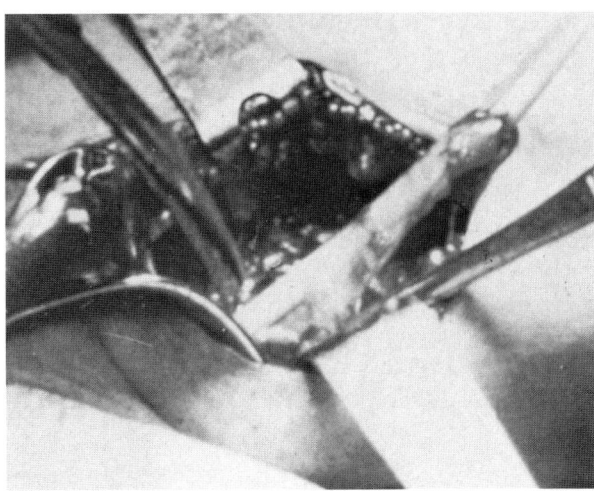

FIGURE 13-42. Gracilis muscle transposition: the muscle is fully mobilized to the tendinous insertion.

muscle is delivered through the proximal incision (Figure 13-43).

Attention is then turned to the perianal dissection. A curvilinear incision may be made approximately 1.5 cm from the anal verge anteriorly and posteriorly. If possible, an attempt should be made to preserve the raphes so that the muscle can be pulled around them as a pulley (Figure 13-44). The concept of the "pulleys" was Pickrell's idea. However, there is often no raphe to preserve when the

surgery is performed following a pull-through procedure for an imperforate anus or after surgical intervention for other conditions. One of the critical points in the operation is to cover the tendon under the incision adequately. If it becomes subsequently exposed, the repair will break down. We suggested a modification of the usual perianal approach, that is, the use of two incisions, anteriorly and posteriorly, preserving midline skin bridges (Figure 13-45).[158] This exposure permits improved access to the rectovaginal plane and to both ischiorectal fossae for circumferential passage of the muscle and tendon. This minimizes the risk of anterior and posterior skin breakdown with resultant tendon exposure, one of the most frequent causes of failure with this operation. (Note to reader: subsequent illustrations have not been redrawn to show this recommendation.)

A tunnel is developed between the proximal thigh incision and the anterior perianal incision. There requires a rather vigorous effort to break through the investing fascia in the thigh in order to enter the subcutaneous plane around the anus. Normally, a blunt, heavy clamp is needed and the opening enlarged to accommodate the muscle belly without constriction. The muscle is then pulled through (Figure 13-46).

A circumferential tunnel is developed in the ischiorectal fossa, on either side of the anal canal and in the deep postanal space. One must carefully separate the rectum from the vagina as cephalad as possible. It is easier and safer to perform this maneuver in the male patient. The

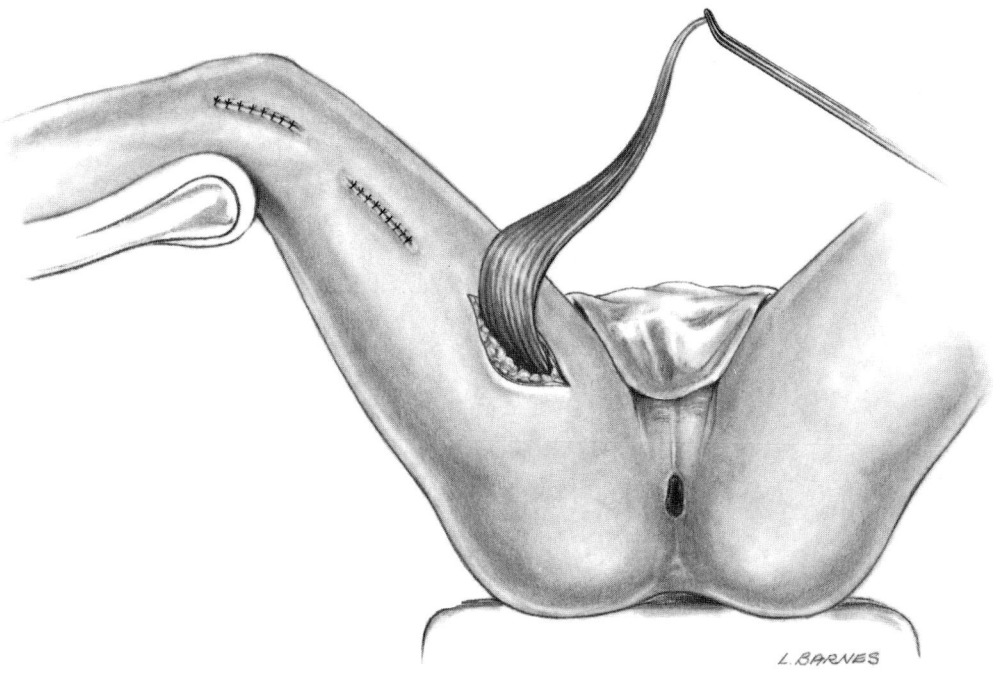

FIGURE 13-43. Gracilis muscle transposition: the muscle is delivered through the proximal incision.

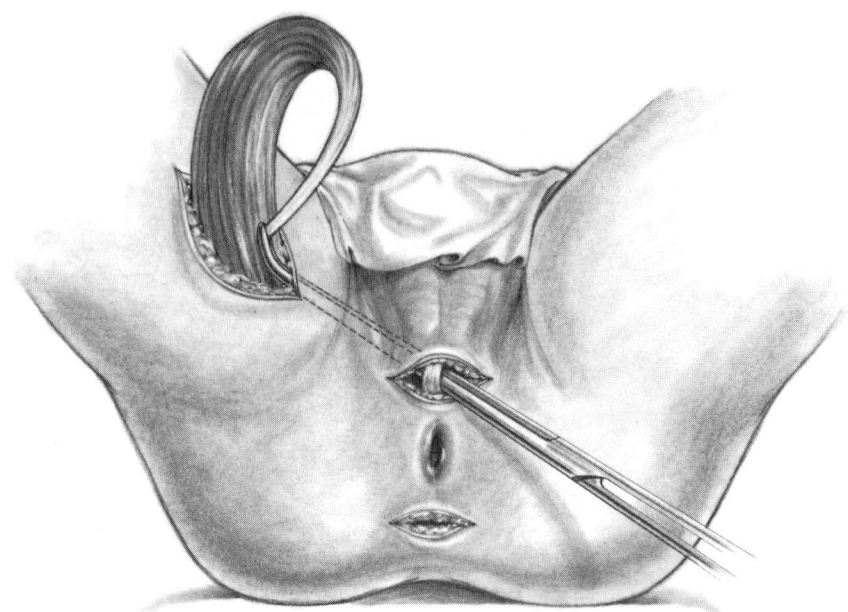

FIGURE 13-44. Gracilis muscle transposition: incisions are made anteriorly and posteriorly outside the anus, preserving the raphes. The placental forceps serve to deliver the tendon through the thigh tunnel.

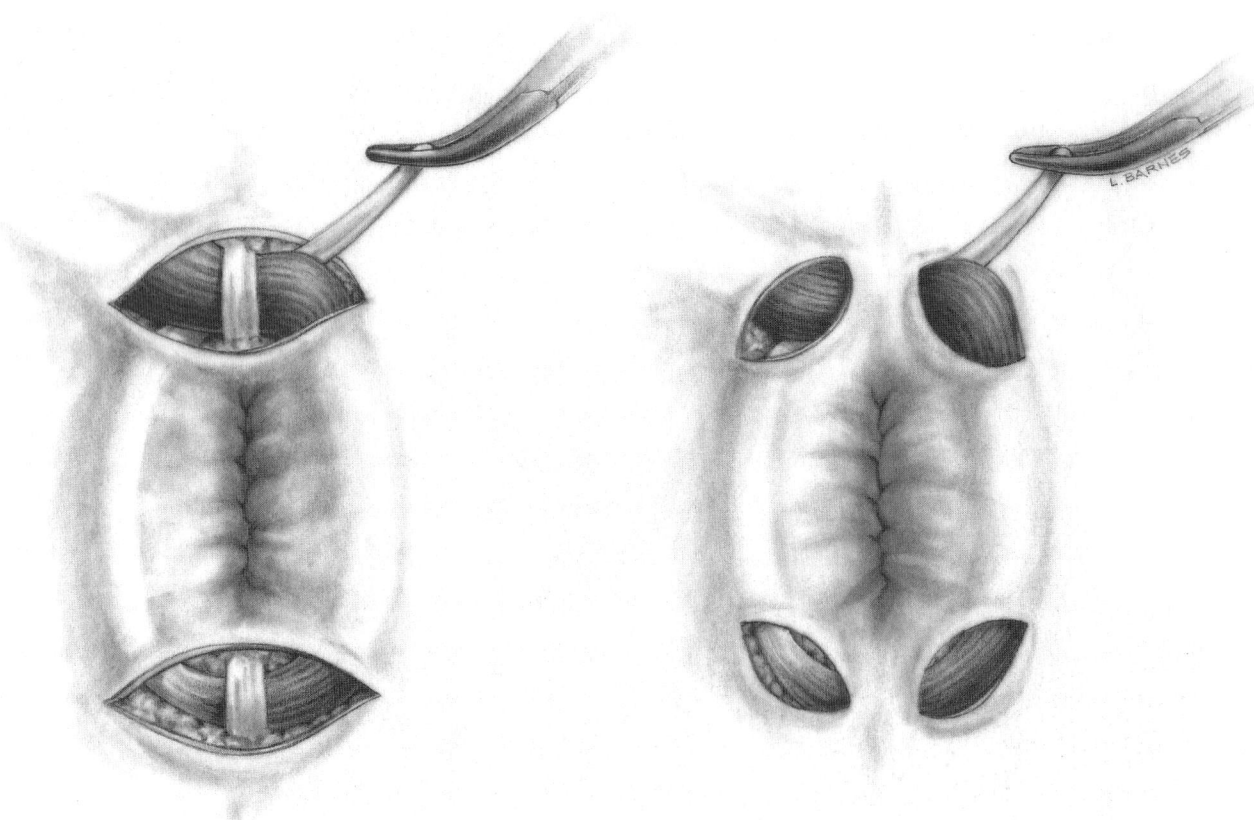

FIGURE 13-45. Gracilis muscle transposition. **(Left)** Conventional anterior and posterior incisions. Both raphes are preserved. **(Right)** Suggested perianal approach. Two anterior and posterior incisions are made, but the skin bridge in the middle is preserved. The raphes (if present) are, therefore, reinforced by the intact skin coverage. (From Kaiser AM, Corman ML. Modified perianal incisions in gracloplasty for fecal incontinence. *Dis Colon Rectum* 2002;45:703-704, with permission.)

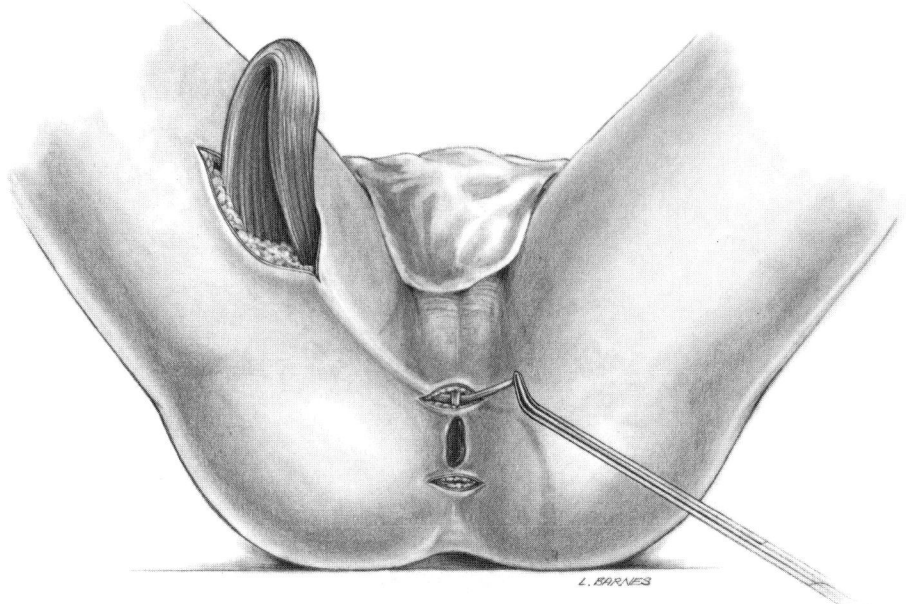

FIGURE 13-46. Gracilis muscle transposition: the tendon is delivered through the anterior perianal incision.

tendon is passed clockwise if the right gracilis muscle is being transposed or counterclockwise if the left gracilis muscle is used (Figure 13-47). The thigh incision can be closed when the tendon has been brought around one half of the circumference.

An incision is then made over the contralateral ischial tuberosity (i.e., the side opposite from which the gracilis muscle was taken). Three monofilament, nonabsorbable sutures (i.e., 00 Prolene) are placed into the periosteum of the ischium or into the gluteal fascia (Figure 13-48). Alternatively, a fascial stapler may be employed for anchoring. The tendon is passed 360 degrees and *behind* the muscle and is pulled through a tunnel developed between the ischial incision and the anterior perianal incision (Figure 13-49). At this point, the leg from which the gracilis muscle was taken is removed from the stirrup and

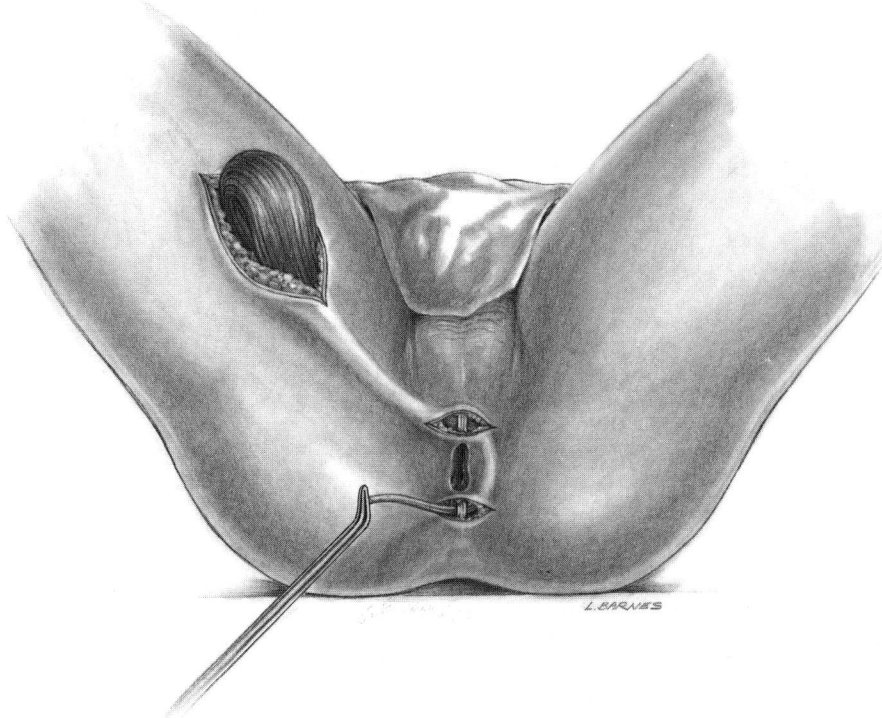

FIGURE 13-47. Gracilis muscle transposition: the tendon is brought out through the posterior incision.

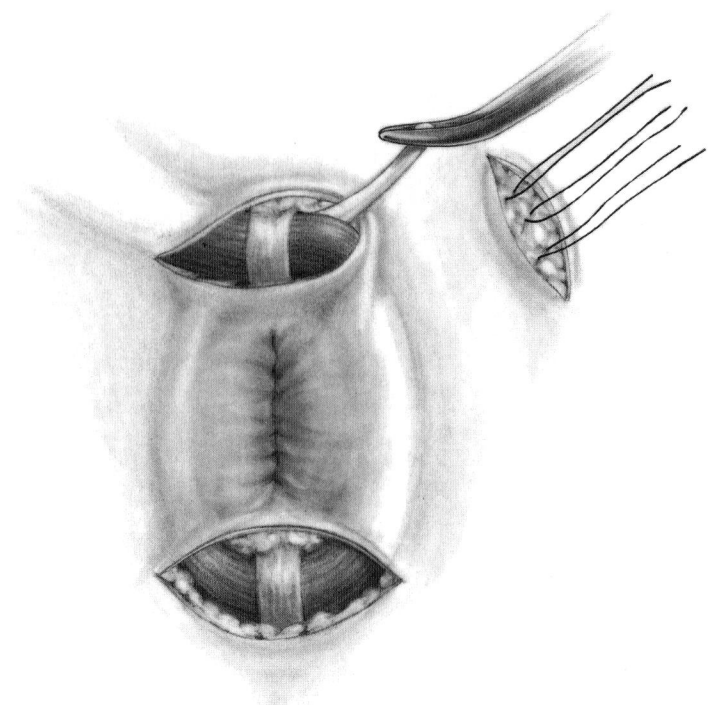

FIGURE 13-48. Gracilis muscle transposition: the tendon has encircled the anus. An incision is made over the contralateral ischial tuberosity, and sutures are placed in the gluteal fascia.

*ad*ducted (Figure 13-50). This is an extremely important maneuver because it releases some tension on the muscle. If the tendon were to be anchored without adduction, the substitute sphincter would be too loose, and the results would be unsatisfactory. When the leg is in maximal adduction, the surgeon pulls the tendon taut. It should be quite snug when a finger is inserted into the rectum. An anal orifice that is too tight may be corrected by dilatation. The sutures are placed through and around the tendon and secured. Three sutures are ideal. All incisions are closed, and no drains are employed (Figure 13-51). The new anatomic arrangement of the gracilis muscle is shown in Figure 13-52.

What should one do if there is insufficient length to anchor the tendon? This has been debated with neither consensus nor resolution. Because there are no prospective, randomized trials of the technique, one is left with more questions than answers, and ultimately a judgment decision has to be made. Is there any tissue one can use that will hold a suture? Shall the tendon be anchored to

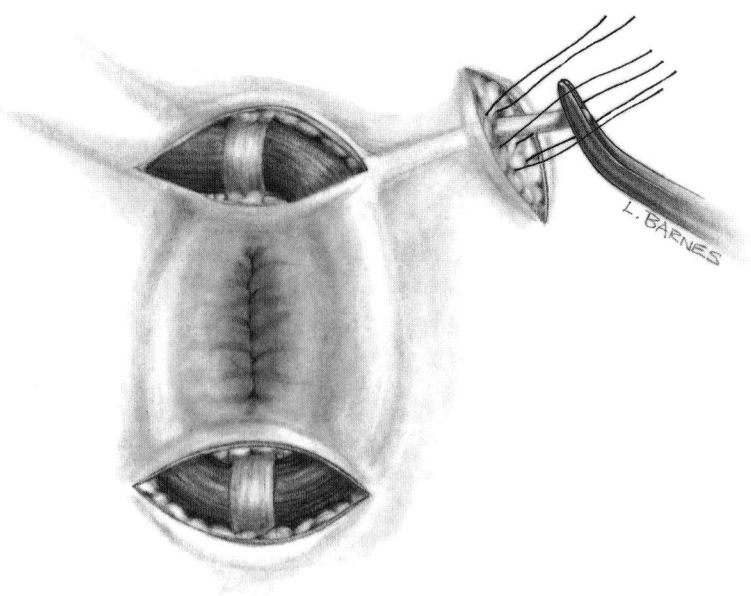

FIGURE 13-49. Gracilis muscle transposition: the tendon is brought out through the ischial tuberosity incision.

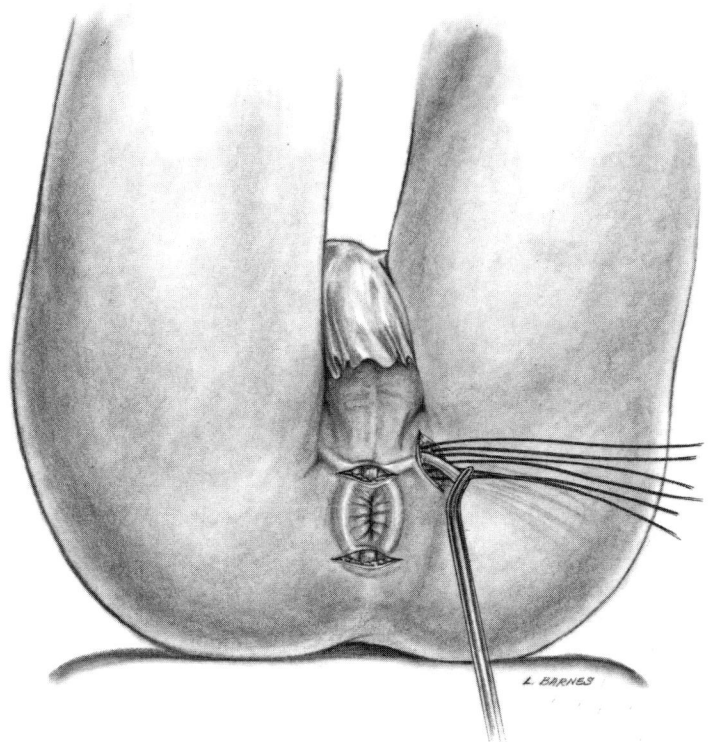

FIGURE 13-50. Gracilis muscle transposition: adduction of the thigh before the tendon is secured is an extremely important maneuver.

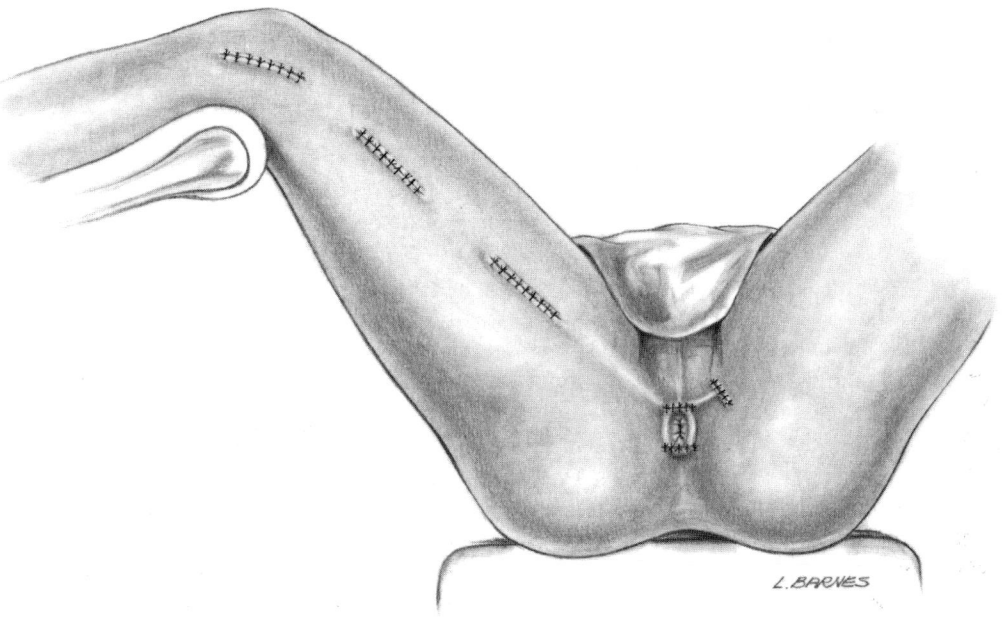

FIGURE 13-51. Gracilis muscle transposition: all wounds are primarily closed.

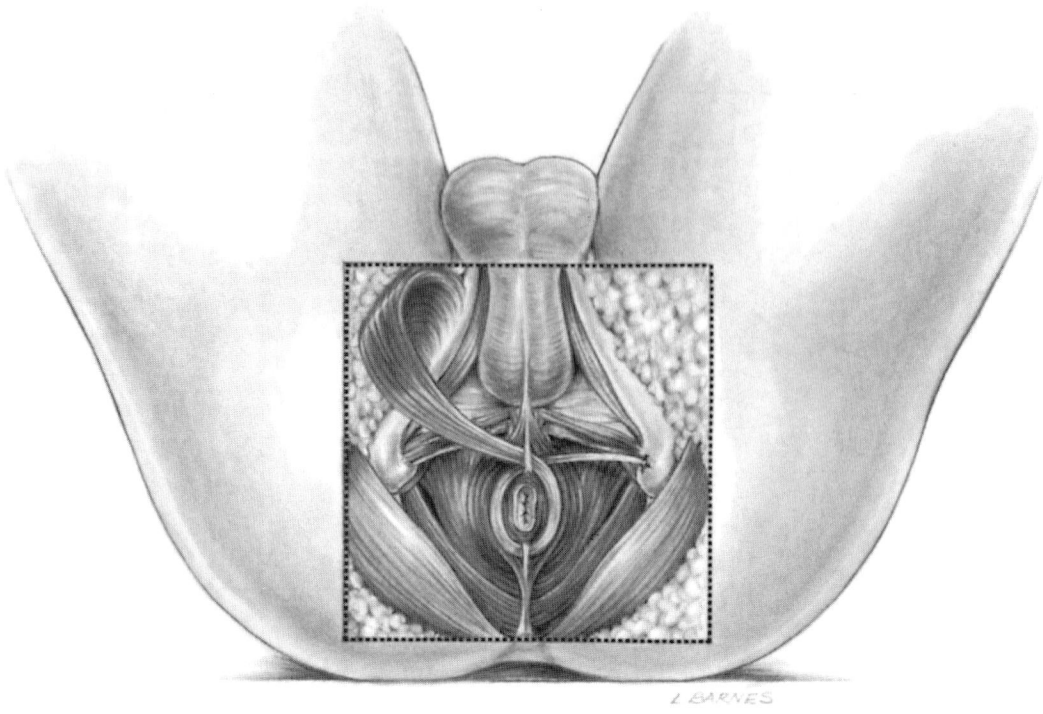

FIGURE 13-52. Gracilis muscle transposition: muscle is shown in its final position and site of insertion.

the ipsilateral tuberosity? Clearly, this is a shorter distance, but one must accept the fact that this will not be a circumferential implant. What about suturing the tendon to itself? Under these conditions, the GMT will be circumferential, but perhaps too tight or subject to an increased likelihood of necrosis. Should the contralateral muscle and tendon be harvested? And, of course, will any of these choices permit proper function even if it all heals? No one knows what is best. All have been tried and criticized in theory, except for harvesting the other muscle. This is why I have said fortune may play an important role in the ultimate success or failure of GMT.

Figure 13-53 illustrates the appearance before and after GMT in a young man who sustained severe perineal trauma from a motorcycle accident, rendering him completely incontinent. A concomitant anoplasty was required to create a new anal canal (see earlier discussions on the application of anoplasty and Chapter 8). Five years later, the patient experienced no difficulty with bowel control.

Postoperative Care

Postoperatively, ideally the bowels should be confined for 3 to 5 days. The patient is kept at bed rest for 72 hours in order to avoid undue manipulation of

the transplant, after which progressive ambulation is permitted. The perianal wounds are gently cleansed three times daily, and a topical antiseptic ointment is applied.

The postoperative management of these patients should be highly attentive. Lack of success with this procedure may be due to inadequate attention to this aspect of treatment. The repair is analogous to the Thiersch operation in that one narrows the anal orifice, except this circumanal implant is theoretically expandable and potentially dynamic. The anal canal can be stretched open; then it passively closes. Some surgeons believe that one can teach the patient to tighten and relax the muscle, but I harbor no such illusions. I do not pretend to understand the extraordinary capabilities of certain individuals to control their autonomic functions, and perhaps some can actually contract their gracilis in such a way that tightening and, therefore, voluntary control is effectuated, but I doubt it. I believe that a successful GMT results in anal continence by the simple expedient of a corklike effect, but a dynamic one at that. It can open when the patient squats—the position of maximal relaxation. It is maximally tight with the person in the upright posture—an ideal arrangement most of the time.

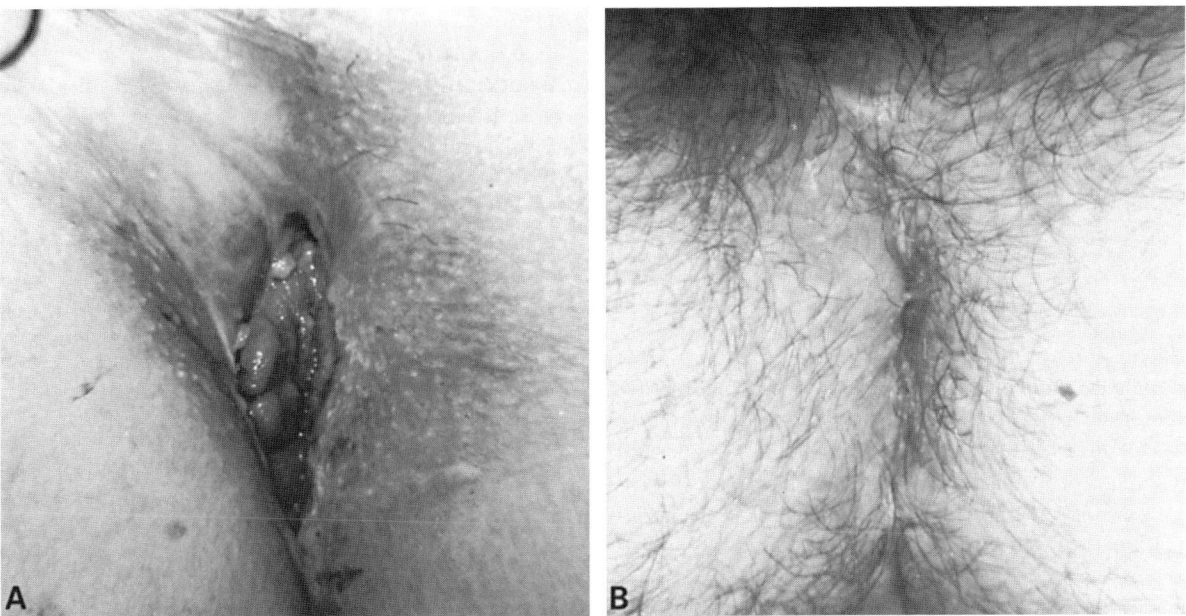

FIGURE 13-53. Severe anal trauma. **(A)** Preoperative appearance. **(B)** Appearance 6 months following gracilis muscle transposition with anoplasty.

The goal in the postoperative period is to establish a workable time for defecation (see Bowel Management Program). For most individuals, this time is in the morning. When the patient is eating a regular diet, a suppository, such as bisacodyl, is inserted immediately after breakfast. Ideally, the patient will defecate and remain clean until the next morning when the procedure is repeated. Ultimately, a pattern should be established that avoids the need for a suppository. Obviously, each patient must be treated individually. Some may require laxatives—others, slowing medications.

Results

I have reported my experience with patients who underwent GMT.[64,67] The procedure has been most efficacious for those who are incontinent as a result of trauma or as a consequence of a congenital anomaly, usually when other sphincteroplastic approaches have failed. As previously stated, patients who have a history of diarrhea are poor candidates, and those with neurologic impairment generally do less well. Individuals with bowel management problems are poorly suited for this procedure because it is difficult to train the bowel to defecate on command. Additionally, those whose incontinence is due to obstetric or gynecologic injury are optimally treated by an alternative method, usually an anovaginal reconstruction. Leguit and co-workers suggest that GMT is the procedure of choice for the management of total incontinence in individuals who have no functional anal sphincter.[191]

Yoshioka and Keighley reported their experience with six GMTs, all with poor results.[397] No objective improvement was seen, and every patient required a colostomy. It should be noted, however, that severe postoperative sepsis developed in all but one; this factor probably contributed to the failures. I have not experienced a single instance of a septic complication following this operation in 82 patients. Furthermore, every patient save one who has undergone GMT for sphincter loss as a consequence of trauma or who had a congenital anomaly as the cause noted improvement.

Christiansen and associates transposed the gracilis muscle in 13 patients.[58] All but three improved. Anal manometry in these individuals compared with anal manometry in a control group showed no alteration in resting anal pressure, whereas a statistically significant increase in MSP was demonstrated in those who underwent transposition. The authors concluded that, even though GMT does not result in normal bowel control, if careful attention is paid to the technical details and the postoperative management, successful results may be anticipated.

Faucheron and co-workers reviewed 22 patients who underwent GMT.[96] At 6 months, 18 were improved, but only one was fully continent. The authors concluded that GMT should be used initially, and then electrostimulation should be considered if the results are unsatisfactory (see Dynamic Graciloplasty). Eccersley and associates performed 12 GMTs and observed that their results were comparable to that reported for stimulated gaciloplasty.[84]

Bilateral Gracilis Muscle Transposition

Some investigators have advised simultaneous, bilateral GMT in the management of fecal incontinence.[180] Ten patients underwent this operation by Kumar and colleagues, all with a protective colostomy.[180] Every one was completely continent following stomal closure with a mean follow-up of 24 months. An illustration of the relative positions of the transplanted muscles is shown in Figure 13-54.

Opinion

In my experience, unilateral GMT has been eminently satisfactory in those patients for whom the procedure was performed with proper indications. I am concerned about using both muscles at once, because if there ultimately develops a perineal septic problem, there is no fallback position for the use of the other muscle. I have on two occasions returned to use the other muscle when one has failed.

Neuromuscular Stimulation of the Gracilis Muscle (Dynamic Grac\iloplasty)

Animal study by Salmons and Henriksson has demonstrated that so-called fast-twitch skeletal muscle, such as the gracilis, can be converted to a fatigue-resistant slow-twitch muscle by means of low-frequency electrical stimulation.[303] In 1988, Baeten and colleagues, from the Department of Surgery at Maastricht University Hospital in the Netherlands, reported a patient with a suboptimal GMT who underwent implantation of electrodes connected to a pulse generator (Itrel Model 7420, Medtronics, Minneapolis, MN).[10] Neuromuscular stimulation of the transposed muscle seemed to improve the function. Later, these investigators demonstrated histologic changes in the transposed muscle.[171] The mean percentage of type I slow-twitch, fatigue-resistant fibers in transposed gracilis muscle increased from 46% before electrical stimulation to 64% following stimulation. These differences were statistically significant. The external sphincters in cadavers were found to have a predominance of type I fibers (80%). Others have shown the same phenomenon.[115] Transposition of the gracilis muscle with chronic low-frequency electrical stimulation was associated with a shift in the frequency-response curve and a prolongation of the time course of individual muscle twitches, suggestive of transformation to a slow-twitch, fatigue-resistant type.[115]

Technique

The reader is referred to several articles that are referenced in this section describing the methods for implanting the stimulator, both epineurally and intramuscularly.[172]

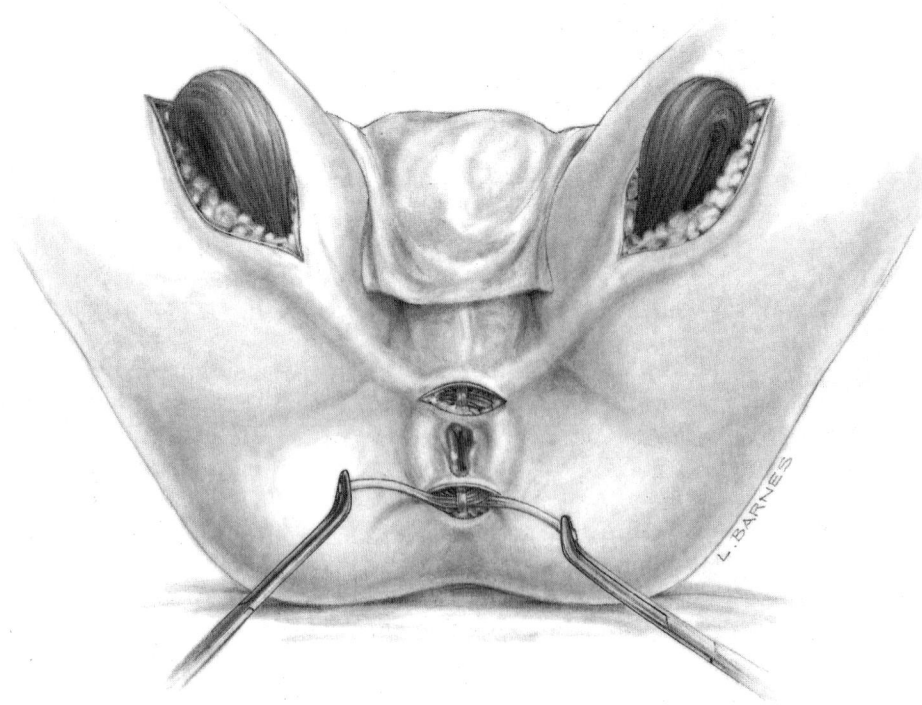

FIGURE 13-54. Representation of simultaneous, bilateral gracilis muscle transpositions.

Results

First, there are no prospective, randomized trials in which nonstimulated GMT is compared with dynamic gracilosplasty. The published systematic review by Chapman and colleagues implies that there is "no high-level evidence" for the benefit of this procedure over that of conventional GMT.[49] In 383 identified patients, there were 105 infections (28%) and 59 stimulator and lead faults (15%), including erosion, breakage, and displacement. Williams and associates transposed the gracilis muscle in six patients and applied chronic neurostimulation using an implanted electrical stimulator with an electrode plate positioned over the main trunk of the nerve and its branches (i.e., the proximal neurovascular bundle).[383] Successful conversion was achieved in all patients in that physiologic measurements identified that the neosphincter mounted a sustained contraction. Baeten's group published their large series in 1995 with stimulated gracilosplasty.[11] They treated 52 patients by this technique and evaluated them by interview, by anal manometry, and by enema testing. After a median follow-up of slightly more than 2 years, 73 persons were continent. At 1 year, the median frequency of defecation had been reduced from five to two times per day. Furthermore, the median time for defecation could be postponed from 9 seconds to 19 minutes, and the median time an enema could be retained from 0 to 180 seconds. All of these differences were highly statistically significant. In a still later report from the same group, now involving 67 patients, the authors reviewed their complications.[114] In total, 53 were identified in 36 patients. Failures were attributable to poor muscle contraction, perforation of the anal canal during stimulation, infection at the stimulator or lead site, and, of course, incontinence, soiling, and intractable constipation.[114] They concur with the observations that I made with respect with conventional GMT—that difficulties related to impaired sensation and/or motility are "impossible to treat," and careful patient selection is a requisite.

Williams and co-workers performed electrically stimulated gracilosplasty on 20 patients, 12 of whom were able to have functioning neosphincters.[385] Wexner and colleagues suggested a distal vascular delay in mobilizing the muscle to protect viability, as well as the creation of a temporary stoma.[375] Transposition of the muscle and implantation of the electrode is then accomplished as a second stage. They observed that the operation is associated with a very high morbidity, but 13 of the 15 eligible patients had their stomas reversed. Based on questionnaires, 60% reported improvement in continence and quality of life. However, one third used daily enemas to assist evacuation and to help with control. A less sanguine opinion was expressed by Korsgen and Keighley concerning this technique.[173] After procedures with four patients, they observed that three required permanent stomas. They concluded that the procedure requires a high motivation on the part of the patient (and perhaps the surgeon—MLC). In the multiinstitutional evaluation of 129 stimulated gracilosplasties, which included some of the aforementioned publications, Wexner and co-workers reported an overall success rate of 62%.[374]

The Maastricht (Netherlands) group evaluated their patients by means of defecography.[365] Of the 38 individuals with incapacitating fecal incontinence who underwent dynamic GMT, 24 achieved continence. This correlated quite well with defecographic evidence.[365] In a subsequent publication of 200 patients, the overall success rate was 72%, with an 82% success rate when the incontinence was the result of trauma.[293] Median survival of the implanted pulse generator until battery expiration was 405 weeks. They and others have shown significant improvement in resting pressures, pressure volume, and anal canal length.[215,394]

Rullier and co-workers had the temerity to embark upon double dynamic gracilosplasties in 15 patients.[297] Early and late morbidity were consequences in 11. These investigators concluded that this operation should *not* be performed.

Comment

The merit of dynamic gracilosplasty is essentially an academic issue, at least in the United States. The Food and Drug Administration has failed to approve the stimulator for implantation. It is, however, available for use in Europe and presumably in other countries outside of Europe. Regardless of availability, approval, or lack of approval, however, I remain unconvinced that the results are better than those that can be achieved without stimulation. At the very least, conventional GMT has the very real advantage of no special equipment to fail, to become infected, or to erode.

Gracilis Muscle Transposition Following Proctectomy

Mander and Williams and their colleagues employed the electrically stimulated neosphincter to supplement the sphincter muscle following restoration of intestinal continuity after abdominoperineal resection.[212,384,385] Seccia and co-workers reported an experience of 75 patients who underwent electrostimulated gracilosplasty following removal of the rectum for cancer.[319] Continence was achieved in 71%. This is certainly a remarkably good result for such an extensive operation. However, it is difficult to tell from their article the indications for the procedure with respect to the invasiveness of the primary tumor. Fully 30% of these patients were lost to follow-up or died.

Gluteus Maximus Transposition

In 1928, Stone reported the use of preserved fascia as a purse-string suture about the anus.[341] Although this did not permit voluntary control, it narrowed the anal outlet so that the patient had some degree of continence. The operation was subsequently extended and revised to encircle the fascia around the anus and to anchor the free ends to the gluteus maximus muscle on each side, a method popularized by Wreden.[342,392] The anal canal was thus enclosed in a fascial ring, which could theoretically be tightened by contraction of the gluteal muscle. Satisfactory results were reported in 30 patients, but no one seems to have reported this technique since 1941.[343] The gluteus, however, has been shown to be an effective substitute anal muscle through the experience in numerous case reports.[35,36,51,91,136,149,261]

Technique

The gluteus maximus is a broad, fan-shaped muscle with a wide origin from the ilium, sacrum, and coccyx and a narrow insertion along the iliotibial band of the lateral femur. The muscle is a strong thigh extensor and lateral hip rotator. Its blood supply originates from the superior and inferior gluteal arteries, supplemented by branches of the medial and lateral femoral circumflex arteries.[261] Motor innervation is from the inferior gluteal nerve (L5, S1,S2). Several modifications concerning harvesting the muscle, tunneling, and suturing have been described, but what follows represents the essentials common to all variations.[52,91,136,246, 261,277,329]

The patient is placed in the prone jackknife position. Two incisions are made in the lateral aspects outside of the anal verge. The skin is undermined to create a perianal, extrasphincteric tunnel, as described for the GMT. Another pair of incisions is made parallel to the caudal border of the gluteus maximus muscle, exposing the medial portion of the origin (Figure 13-55). Alternatively, the surgeon may consider using simply one long, curvilinear incision on each side. A portion of the muscle, including fascia, is then mobilized from the origin and freed distally as two strips, each approximately 2 cm wide (Figure 13-56). Care must be taken to preserve the neurovascular bundle, which usually arises near the ischial tuberosity. It is mandatory that sufficient length be achieved to effect a repair without tension. Hentz has demonstrated by means of cadaver studies that the muscle strip remains vascularized and innervated when each strip is prepared parallel with the fascicle direction to the length necessary for permitting rotation.[136]

A similar mobilization is then undertaken on the contralateral side. The muscle flaps are then brought through tunnels between the incisions and secured to its opposite member anteriorly and posteriorly—and ideally also to the ipsilateral slip—with long-term absorbable sutures (Figure 13-57).

Devesa co-workers caution that an end sigmoid colostomy should be performed at the time of reconstruction.[81] The authors emphasize the importance of the use of a nerve stimulator to monitor contractility, as well as of the placement of a tape around the neurovascular pedicle to keep it protected. They also express concern about the difficulty they have experienced with tension and necrosis when both sides are used. As a consequence, they now perform the procedure using only one side.

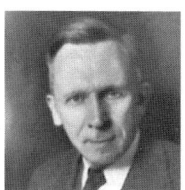

Harvey Brinton Stone (1882–1977)   Stone was born in Baltimore, Maryland, and graduated from Johns Hopkins University in 1902 and from the medical school in 1906. He completed his internship and residency also at Johns Hopkins. He then joined the faculty of the University of Virginia in Charlottesville, returning to Baltimore as Associate Professor of Surgery in 1908. In 1916, he published an article on the treatment of pruritus ani by alcohol injection, a method that was adopted by many proctologists for some years. Stone served in France during World War I, ultimately becoming the hospital base commander. He published approximately 100 articles, often on experimental surgery, and did some of the original work on endocrine gland transplantation. Stone was president of the Southern Surgical Association and the American Surgical Association. (Photograph courtesy of the Alan Mason Chesney Medical Archives of the Johns Hopkins Medical Institutions, Baltimore, MD.)

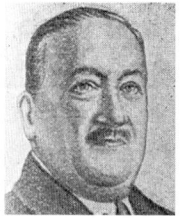

Roman R. Wreden (1867–1934)   Roman Wreden was a Russian surgeon who is known as the founder of Russian operative orthopedics. He graduated from the Military Medical Academy in 1890, completing his surgical training under Professor V. A. Ratimov. Wreden was awarded a Ph.D. in 1893 for his dissertation on cystitis. From 1893 to 1896, he was an Attending Surgeon in the Kiev Military Hospital. In 1896, Wreden became an Assistant Professor at the Military Medical Academy and Professor in 1900. Wreden organized and became head of the first Russian Orthopedic Institute in 1906, which he directed until his death. He published 80 scientific works, including a number of books. (Photograph courtesy of the Bakulev AN, ed. *Medical encyclopedia.* Moscow: Government Medical Publishing, 1958.)

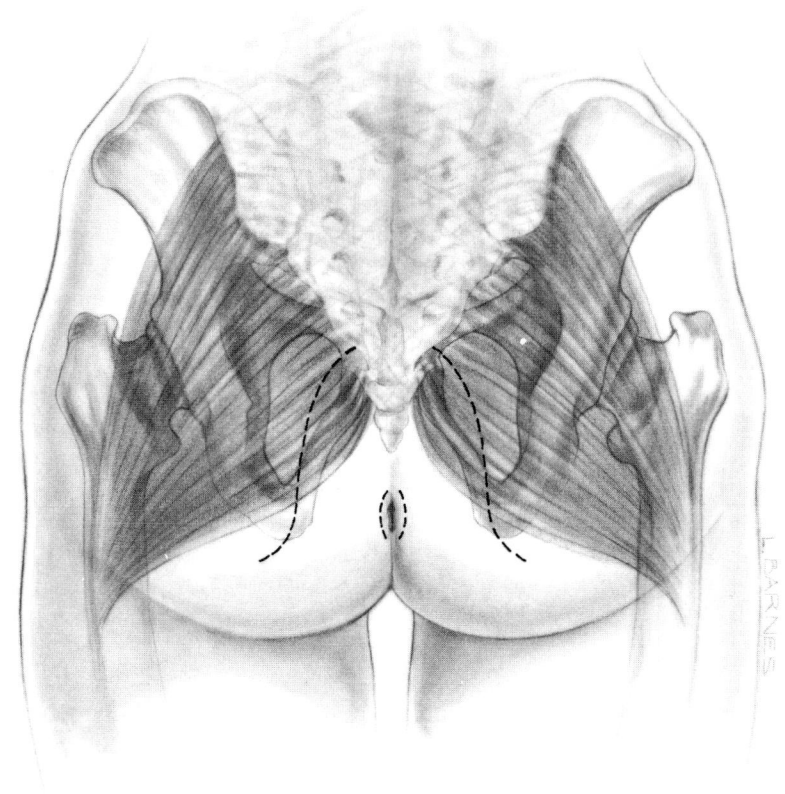

FIGURE 13-55. Gluteus maximus muscle transposition: a pair of lateral circumanal incisions are made to permit mobilization and suturing of the bifurcated ends of the transposed muscle. (Adapted from Hentz VR. Construction of a rectal sphincter using the origin of the gluteus maximus muscle. *Plast Reconstruct Surg* 1982;70:82; and Pearl RK, Prasad ML, Nelson RL, et al. Bilateral gluteus maximus transposition for anal incontinence. *Dis Colon Rectum* 1991;34:478, with permission.)

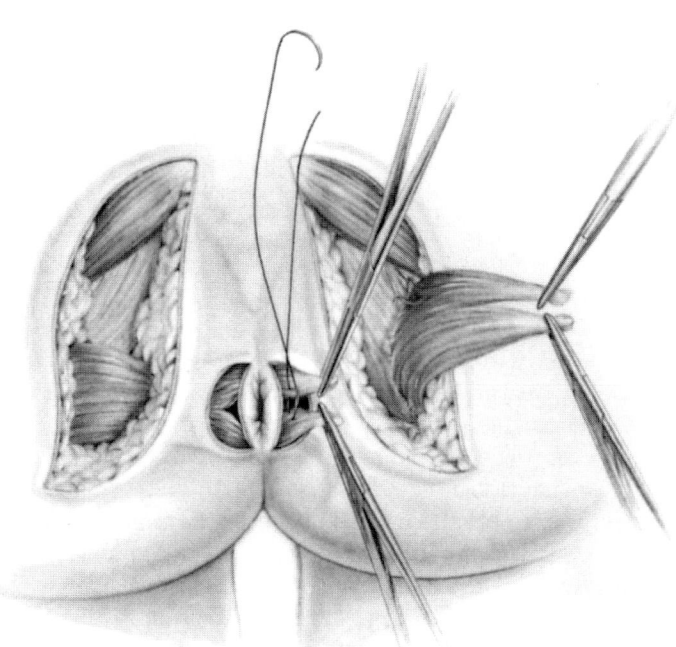

FIGURE 13-56. Gluteus maximus muscle transposition: a tunnel is created around the rectum. The freed muscle on each side is split to make two tails. Each side is passed anteriorly and posteriorly. (Adapted from Hentz VR. Construction of a rectal sphincter using the origin of the gluteus maximus muscle. *Plast Reconstruct Surg* 1982;70:82; and Pearl RK, Prasad ML, Nelson RL, et al. Bilateral gluteus maximus transposition for anal incontinence. *Dis Colon Rectum* 1991;34:478, with permission.)

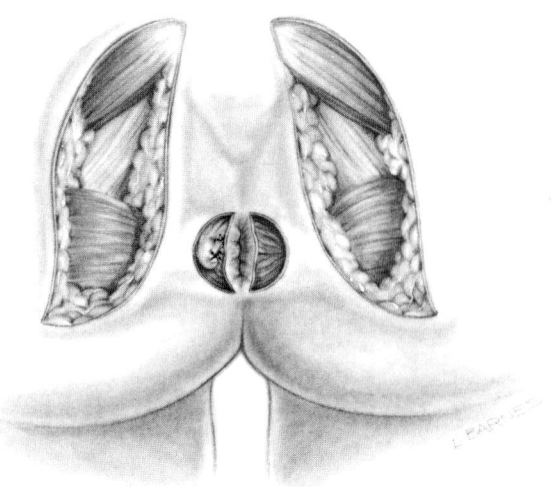

FIGURE 13-57. Gluteus maximus muscle transposition: the muscle tails from each side are secured to each other and to itself. All wounds are closed primarily. (Adapted from Hentz VR. Construction of a rectal sphincter using the origin of the gluteus maximus muscle. *Plast Reconstruct Surg* 1982;70:82; and Pearl RK, Prasad ML, Nelson RL, et al. Bilateral gluteus maximus transposition for anal incontinence. *Dis Colon Rectum* 1991;34:478, with permission.)

Postoperatively, a bowel-confining regimen is recommended. Subsequently, a vigorous bowel management program is instituted (see previous discussion).

Results

The obvious conceptual advantage of using the gluteus muscle for supplementing the anal sphincter is that contraction will more effectively result in closing of the anal orifice. In fact, the muscle normally acts as an accessory sphincter when impedance of elimination is desired.[136] Whether this is an effective response is doubtful, however. As with the GMT, narrowing of the anal orifice may also be a factor that contributes to improved function. These concepts are consistent with the observation that nighttime control is more likely to be impaired.[277]

There are few meaningful data concerning long-term functional results and morbidity of this procedure, because the literature, such as it is, essentially consists of articles noting one or two cases.[91,136,246,329] However, a few groups have a larger experience. Yuli and Xueheng performed the operation on six patients, two thirds of which procedures were "successful".[400] Prochiantz and Gross point out that a major difficulty with the technique involves obtaining sufficient length to encircle the rectum.[277] In four individuals, this could not be accomplished. In 11 others, an adequate repair was effected, but two early and two later failures occurred (overall failure rate, 36%). Pearl and colleagues at Cook County Hospital, Chicago, reported seven patients.[261] Indications were postfistulotomy status in four, pudendal nerve injury in

two, and imperforate anus in one. There was one failure, but only one patient maintained control for flatus. Although resting pressures were unchanged, voluntary squeeze pressures were markedly improved. Devesa and co-workers performed gluteus muscle transfer in ten patients using several different modifications of technique; their preferred method is to use only one side.[81] They believe that their approach is simpler and leads to a better, tension-free neosphincter. Assessment was obtained through manometry and EMG of the neosphincter and revealed subjective and objective improvement in all but one patient. Abou-Zeid and Marzouk noted improvement in all but two of their ten patients (one infection and one "bad selection").[2]

Christiansen and associates performed this operation on seven individuals for varying indications.[52] Five were women. Three experienced improved continence, but in four no change was observed. The authors concluded that gluteus maximus transposition offers no better improvement than that of nonstimulated graciloplasty.

Comment

As with all operations designed to supplement the sphincter mechanism, all authors counsel the importance of an aggressive training program. Optimal candidates are probably the same as those who are recommended for the GMT—patients with sphincter loss as a consequence of trauma or congenital anomaly. Those with a bowel management problem (i.e., constipation, diarrhea) or those with sensory impairment are poor individuals to select for reconstruction by this method. Such patients should be considered for one of the following approaches.

Artificial Sphincter Approaches

Anal Encircling Procedure or Thiersch Procedure

Anal encircling (i.e., Thiersch; see Biography in Chapter 17) procedures were originally advocated for the management of rectal prolapse (see Chapter 17), but Gabriel (see Biography in Chapter 23) recommended its application for the treatment of anal incontinence.[110] He reported good results in 11 patients with the use of silver wire. My own preference for such an approach to the treatment of rectal prolapse is to insert 5-mm Mersilene if mere circumanal suturing is appropriate. However, I have not found this material to be helpful in the management of anal incontinence.

A simple alternative to the transposition of the gracilis or gluteus muscle for supplementing the sphincter mechanism is to implant a *Dacron-impregnated Silastic sheet*, 501–7 (Dow-Corning, Midland, MI) as a prosthesis encircling the anus (Figure 13-58). Labow and colleagues originally described the use of this material as an alternative

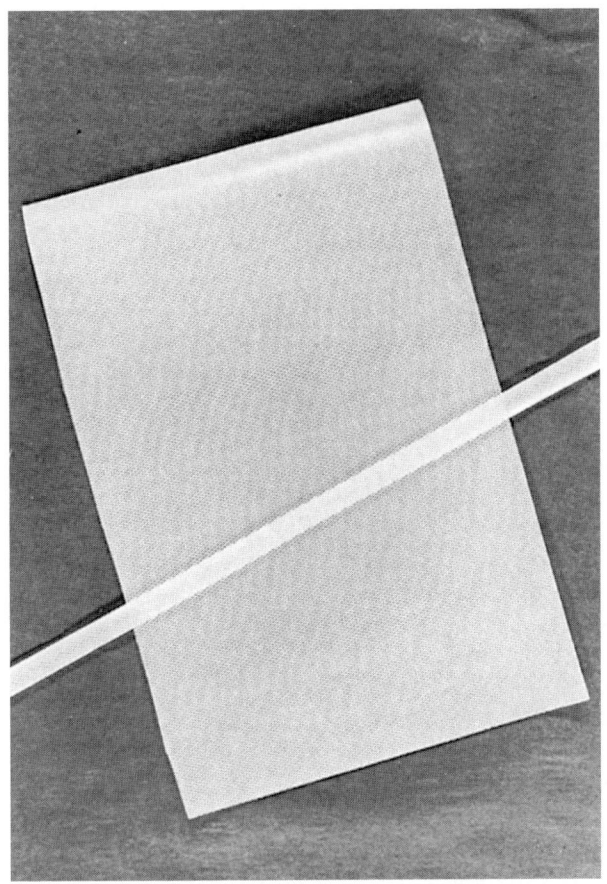

FIGURE 13-58. The elasticity of the 1.5-cm–wide strip can be readily appreciated. Care must be taken to trim the sheet along the proper axis.

to wire in the treatment of rectal prolapse.[182] Others, including myself, have found it to be an adequate substitute anal sphincter when implanted into some patients who have fecal incontinence.[65,68,146,181,344] Koplewitz simply uses a Silastic drain, because he is concerned about the lack of flexibility with the mesh and its tendency to erode (Koplewitz MJ, personal communication). It is his contention that this material is less traumatic to tissue.

Technique Two incisions are made, 3 cm on either side of the anal verge. The ischiorectal fossae are entered, and a tunnel is developed circumferentially around the anus. A 1.5-cm strip of mesh is cut in such a way that it is elastic along its longitudinal axis and inserted (Figure 13-59*A*). An overlap of approximately 1 cm is created with two straight clamps holding the mesh securely (Figure 13-59*B*). The implant is then replaced in the proper position (Figure 13-59*C*). The anal canal diameter is assessed for adequacy by digital examination and the mesh exteriorized. A linear stapler is then applied (Figure 13-59*D*). The suture line may be reinforced with interrupted nonabsorbable sutures, and all wounds are closed (Figs. 13-

59*E* and 13-59*F*). If the rectum is injured during the dissection, the procedure should be aborted. It is unlikely that the repair will heal in the presence of the foreign material, and the patient should, therefore, return on another day.

Because of the possibility of infection, the patient should undergo a mechanical bowel-cleansing regimen, and systemic perioperative antibiotics should be employed. The patient is ideally discharged in 2 or 3 days, ideally when bowel function has occurred.

The theoretical advantage of this material is that it can stretch, albeit only minimally. Thus, on rectal examination, it is difficult to distinguish the sensation of the sheet from that of a normal, intact anal sphincter. There is a tendency to make the anal canal diameter feel too perfect. The examining finger can stretch the material sufficiently to make it seem just that way. However, it is difficult for the patient to overcome even minimal resistance through defecation efforts. In fact, it is probably better to make the prosthesis a little too loose rather than risk the complication of fecal impaction or obstipation.

Results Figure 13-60 shows the preoperative and immediate postoperative appearance of the anus in a young man who suffered sphincter injury following a motorcycle accident and who was treated by this technique. Figure 13-61 illustrates the preoperative and later postoperative results in an older woman with presumed pudendal nerve injury as the cause of her incontinence.

I have used the Silastic sling in 52 patients as of this writing. My overall failure rate is approximately 40%, but others report good to excellent results in about 75% of patients.[146] The Lahey Clinic group emphasize that the sling should be positioned at least 2 cm from the anal verge to limit the likelihood of erosion and pain.[344] Sainio and colleagues performed anal encirclement with polypropylene mesh for rectal prolapse as well as for anal incontinence.[301] All three patients operated on for the latter indication improved. The authors caution that severe constipation is a relative contraindication to the procedure.

Complications of the procedure include infection, stricture, fecal impaction, persistent incontinence, and pain. It is primarily because of this last problem that removal of the sling becomes necessary. Additionally, migration and erosion are not uncommon, so Labow and colleagues have suggested affixing Dacron felt to the sheeting to prevent this complication.[181]

If symptoms warrant, removal of the sling can be accomplished with a local anesthetic as an office procedure. Interestingly, many patients experience amelioration of their symptoms when the mesh is removed. A probable explanation for this is that the subsequent scarring and capsule formation narrow the anal canal sufficiently to produce an effect comparable to that of the implant.

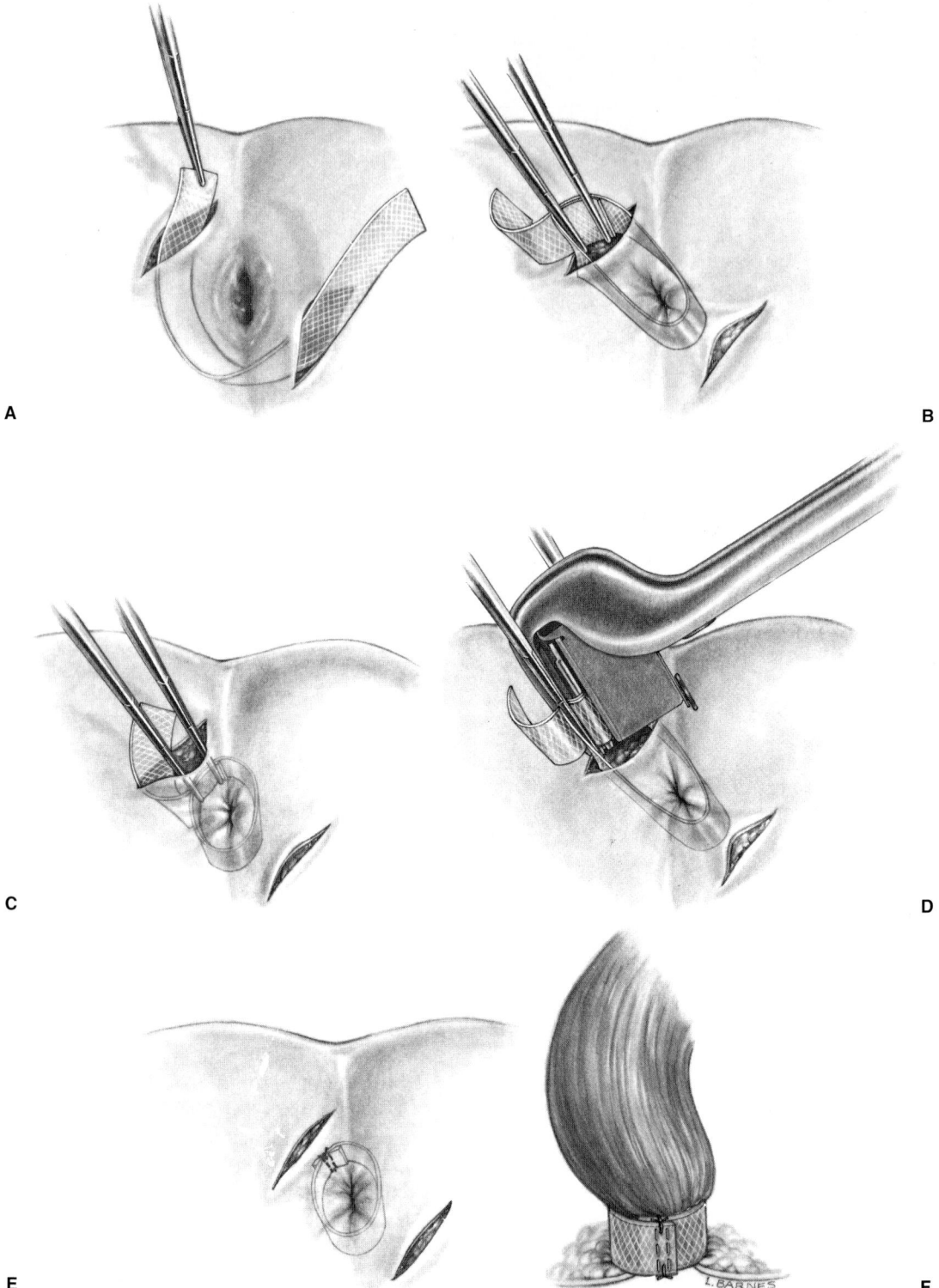

FIGURE 13-59. Silastic-Dacron implant. **(A)** Appropriately tailored sheet is passed circumferentially in the ischiorectal fossa. **(B)** Mesh is secured with paired straight clamps. **(C)** Implant is replaced and adequacy of the lumen determined by the index finger. **(D)** The ends are secured by stapling. **(E,F)** Final position of the implant.

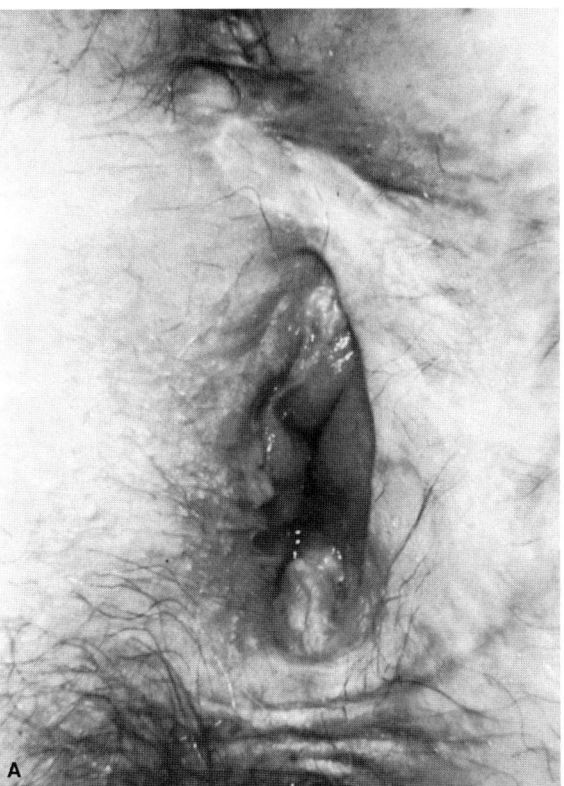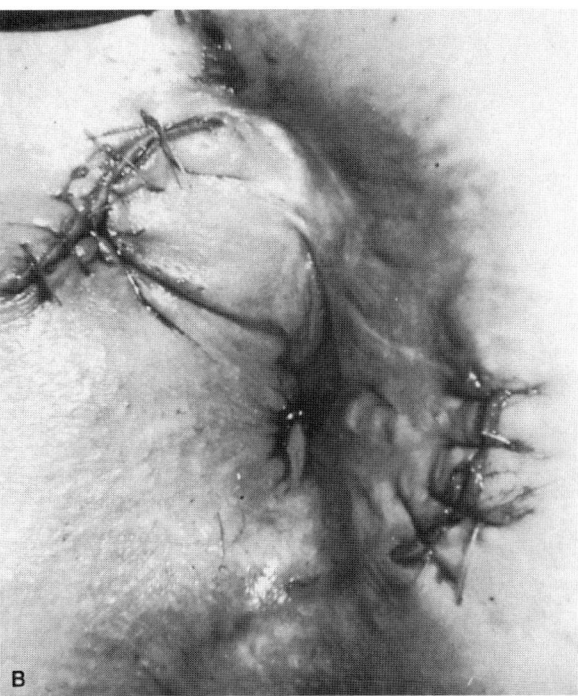

FIGURE 13-60. Incontinence following motorcycle trauma. **(A)** Note patulous anus. **(B)** Immediate postoperative appearance following elastic fabric sling.

Acticon (AMS) Device

The artificial urinary sphincter has been successfully employed for the treatment of urinary incontinence for many years, but its application to the management of anal incontinence has only relatively recently been suggested. In 1987, Christiansen and Lorentzen (Copenhagen) were the first to report the insertion of the AMS 800 Artificial Urinary Sphincter (American Medical Systems, Minnetonka, MN) for this indication.[53] A subsequent report involved five patients with presumed neuromuscular anal incontinence.[54] In a later publication involving 12 individuals, the authors noted no erosion through the anal canal.[57] Two experienced cuff-obstructed defecation. These investigators concluded that implantation of an artificial anal sphincter is a reasonable alternative to permanent colostomy. There have been articles from many investigators within the past few years, including a multicenter cohort study, in which the merits and problems associated with this unique device are evaluated.[6,56,80,192,208,220,242,251,390]

Indications and Contraindications It has been recommended by a group of colon and rectal surgical specialists that incontinent patients should be considered eligible for sphincter replacement only if they have severe incontinence that is not amenable to standard therapy or have failed prior surgical attempts.[208] In other words, this operation may be offered to the patient who has no other option except the *status quo* or a stoma.

Relative or absolute contraindications to undergoing implantation are those individuals whose healing potential may be impaired (e.g., radiation, steroids), those with local anal disease (e.g., anal fistula, Crohn's disease), those with severe diarrhea or irritable bowel, those with intractable constipation, those who have impairment in the use of their hands that would make them unable to use the pump (e.g., severe rheumatoid arthritis), and those who cannot be taught how to use the device (e.g., senility, mental retardation).

Preparation of the Patient It has been appropriately emphasized that strict attention to sterile technique and skin preparation and careful handling of the implants are requisites.[208] Furthermore, a mechanical bowel preparation and prophylactic intravenous antibiotics are mandatory. How long the antibiotics should be continued is a matter of opinion. A protective colostomy is not believed to be necessary, because no data exist to indicate that a two-stage operation reduces the risk of complications. However, no one would suggest that if a colostomy is present, it should be closed concomitant with the implant. That, in fact, would be foolish and probably contraindicated.

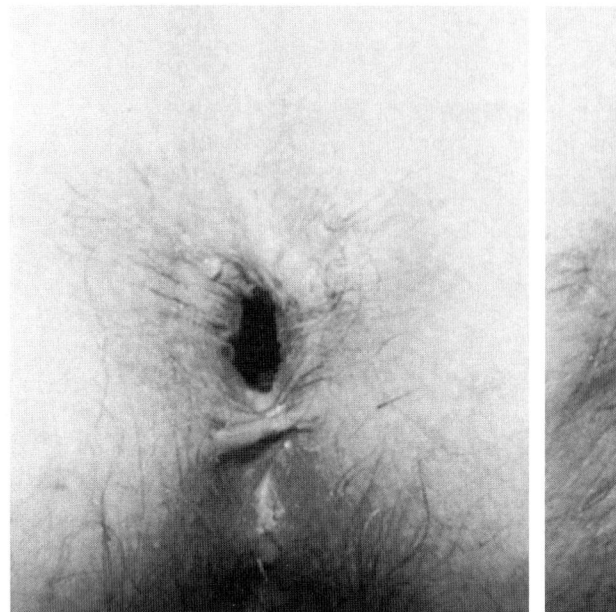
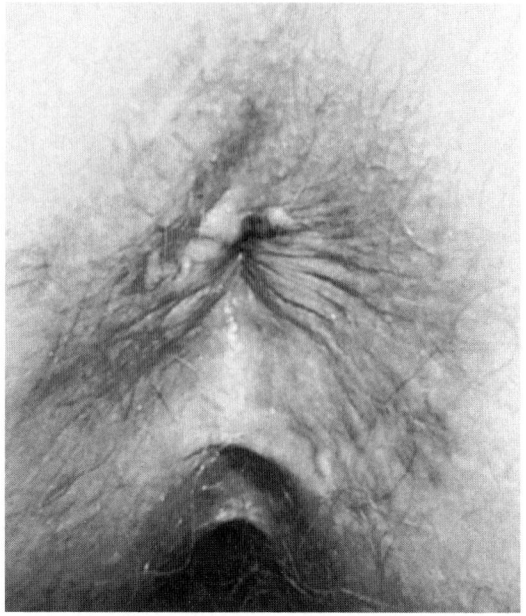

A

B

FIGURE 13-61. Incontinence of uncertain origin in an elderly woman presumably on the basis of pudendal nerve injury. **(A)** Patulous anus is evident on mere spreading of the buttocks. **(B)** Postoperative appearance 2 months following insertion of an elastic fabric sling.

Device Components The device consists of three Silastic components: an inflatable cuff, a pressure-regulating balloon, and a control pump that can be activated or deactivated. The cuff is available in different lengths and widths, and there are several pressure range balloons from 60 to 90 mm water.

Technique First, one must decide *a priori* whether to take advantage of the expertise of a urologist. I believe this concept is ideal. There are many specialists in urology who have considerable experience with the artificial urinary sphincter. Furthermore, the technical aspects of implantation of the reservoir and pump are identical to that required for implantation of the Acticon device. In addition, the operation can be undertaken as a two-team approach, with the abdominal surgeon implanting the reservoir, connecting the pump, and priming the tubing and connections. Still, if the surgeon is experienced and comfortable with performing all aspects of the operation, so be it. Regardless, the perineolithotomy position is required, and an indwelling catheter is placed.

The choice of incision is a matter of personal preference. There is certainly no standard. Some surgeons prefer to utilize two lateral incisions, because erosion is most likely to occur in the midline, especially in the perineum of a woman, in whom there often is limited tissue. Others utilize an anterior incision, rationalizing that this is the area where meticulous dissection is required. Still others opt for both anterior and posterior incisions in

order to minimize the technical difficulties associated with circumferential tunneling and the potential for injury to the posterior vaginal wall when the anterior tunnel is developed. My personal preference after trying all of the foregoing is a transverse perineal incision, dissecting proximally to the level of the levator ani muscle.

For the purpose of convenience and especially because the most patients who are potential candidates for the procedure are women, as well as because the hazards associated with the dissection are much greater in women, the illustrations are drawn in the female. The incision is deepened to separate the anterior rectal wall from the vagina. It is critically important with this exposure and is the main reason why I prefer it to deepen the plane of dissection for at least 5 cm. This will permit sufficient space to implant the cuff and to close the tissue deep to the skin in order to limit the risk of cuff erosion (Figure 13-62).

The ischiorectal fossae are then entered on each side, a blunt technique similar to that which has been illustrated for GMT. Finger dissection facilitates this maneuver. It is imperative that the tunnel be adequate to accommodate the cuff readily. The deep postanal space is traversed, thereby completing the tunnel dissection. At this point, a cuff-sizer (provided in the Acticon package) can be passed to determine the length of the cuff to be subsequently implanted. It is generally recommended that a cuff be selected for implantation that is 1 cm greater than that which is snugly measured

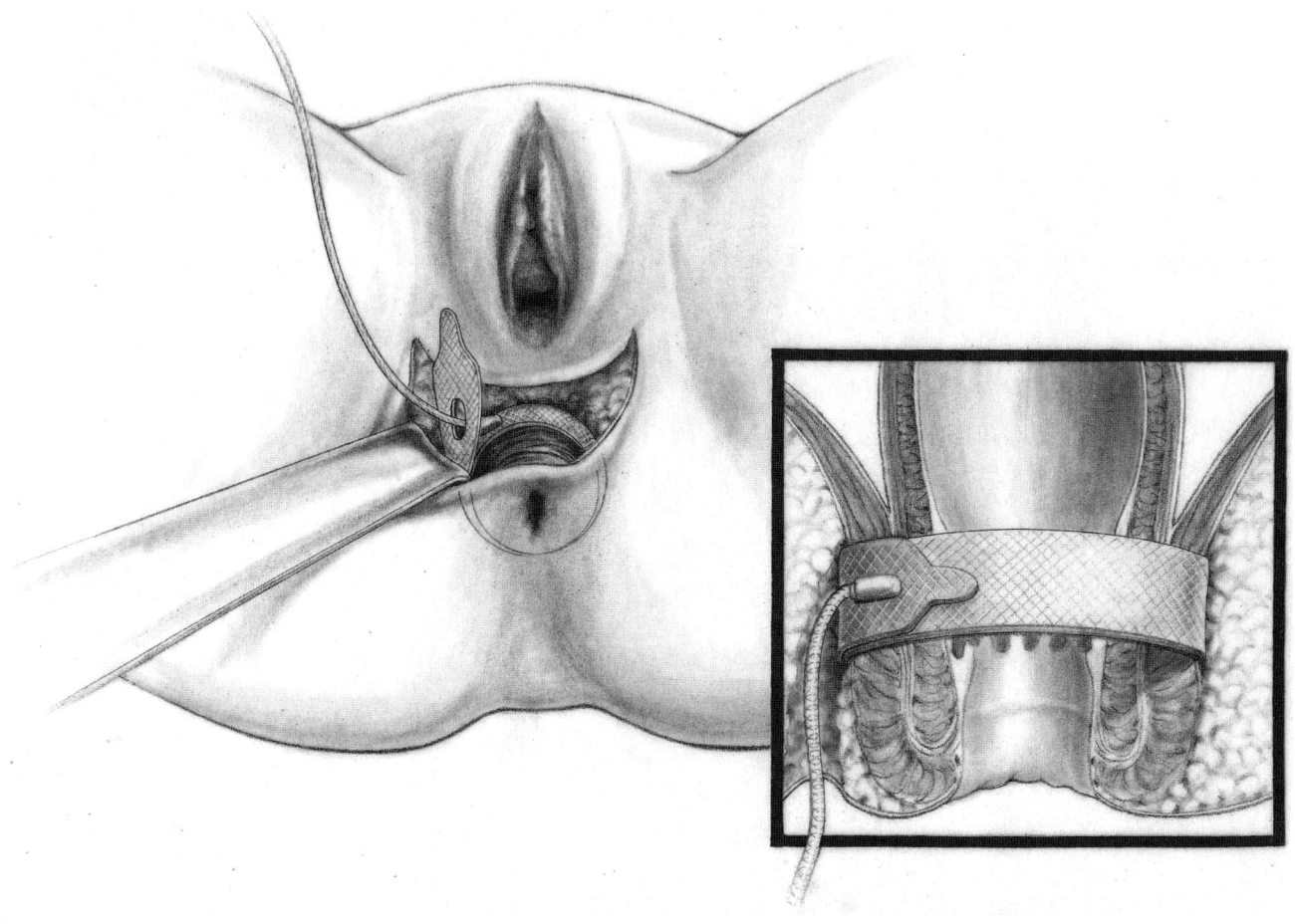

A   **B**

FIGURE 13-62. Artificial anal sphincter implantation. **(A)** The cuff is wrapped around the anorectum. **(B)** The cuff is secured by means of a knob and tab locking mechanism. The connecting tubing should be placed on either the right or left side, depending on which side of the groin will be dissected. All connections are completed. *(continued)*

with the sizer. Because this is an inexact science at best, my own preference is to make a subjective determination. Every patient is given a 12-cm–long cuff, except those with an obviously thickened rectal mesentery—they get a 13-cm implant. An truly thin rectal mesentery will accommodate an 11-cm implant. A sizer is also available to determine the ideal width for the implant—1.5 cm or 2.0 cm. My opinion—always use the 1.5 cm, and forget the measurement.

The abdominal operation is undertaken through a groin incision. Whether the left or right side is selected depends on the handedness of the patient (left side for right-handed and right side for left-handed patients) and to a lesser extent whether there is scarring or deformity on one or the other side. A muscle-splitting incision is performed and the space of Retzius is entered. A balloon that is calibrated to generate a pressure of between 81 and 90 cm of water is selected. The tubing from the cuff is attached to a trocar/tunneler and brought

into the groin incision. A tunnel is also developed between the groin incision and the medial aspect of the labium (or the most dependent part of the scotum in the male patient). Hegar dilators are ideal for this purpose. The pump is then implanted. The four tubes are then joined by the connectors that are provided. With meticulous hemostasis and following irrigation with an antiseptic solution, the wounds are closed in layers with absorbable suture material. The pump is deactivated in the operating room.

Postoperative Care and Subsequent Management The relative merit (or lack thereof) concerning a bowel-confining regimen has already been discussed and is equally applicable to implantation of the artificial anal sphincter. Systemic antibiotics are recommended, but the duration is a matter of personal preference and is more an emotional, feel-good issue, than one based on any meaningful data. The patient should be kept in the

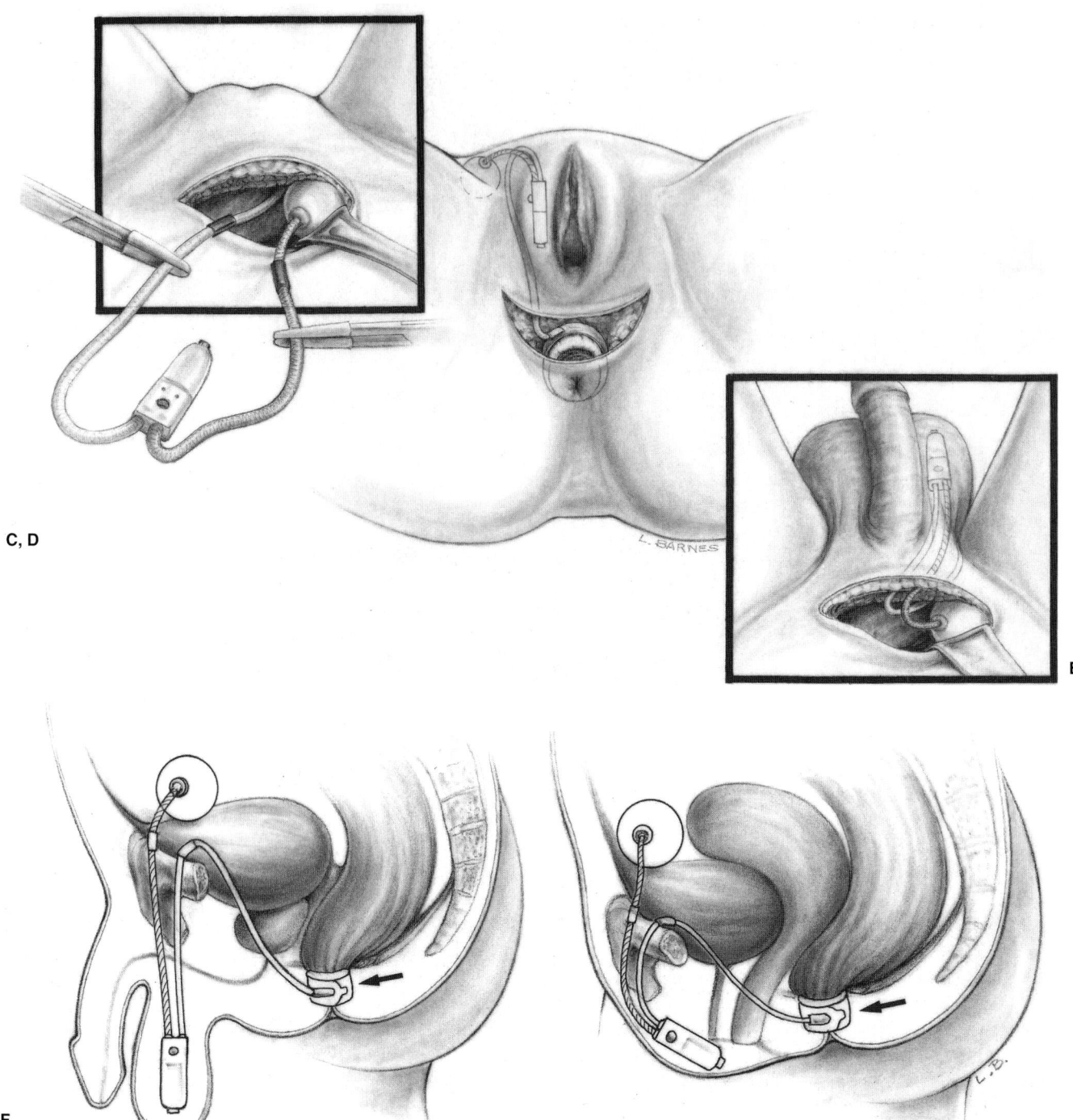

C, D

E

F

G

FIGURE 13-62. *(continued)* **(C)** The tubing to the cuff and the tubing to the balloon are each clamped with an atraumatic Silastic-shod mosquito clamp. The excess tubing is trimmed to the appropriate length so that the pump sits properly in the labium **(D)** or scrotum **(E)**. Schematic final position in the male **(F)** and in the female **(G)** patient.

hospital until bowel function has been restored unless a stoma is present.

Six weeks following implantation, the patient is taught how to activate the pump and to deactivate the device. If a stoma is present, one must make a decision whether to restore intestinal continuity. Criteria should be based simply on whether the wounds are healed and whether there is no evidence of erosion. Following ostomy closure, the patient can be instructed on activation while still recovering in the hospital.

Removal of the device is mandatory if infection supervenes or if erosion of the cuff occurs. There is absolutely no place for antibiotics in an attempt to save the implant. Conversely, it may be possible to preserve the pump and reservoir if the problem is limited to the cuff, but this is rarely successful. Mechanical problems, however, may be individually addressed with replacement and reconnection of the affected part. It is also possible to repressurize the system without removing all of the components.

Results Lehur and colleagues (Nantes, France) reported their initial results with implantation of the artificial sphincter in 13 patients.[193] Sepsis occurred in two, removal of the artificial sphincter and a colostomy was required in three, and one artificial sphincter cuff ruptured. After a median follow-up of 20 months, nine of ten individuals with a functioning sphincter were continent for stool, five being also continent for gas. Lehur's center has been in the forefront of investigators, developing greater experience, modifying their technique, and updating their results. After a median follow-up of 30 months, 11 patients had an active and functioning artificial sphincter, including two who underwent successful reimplantation.[192] In the year 2000, now with 24 patients, this group demonstrated a "high level of success" in 75%.[194] Others have also demonstrated that continence can be restored with an acceptable morbidity.[221,391]

Lehur's unit assessed the quality of life in 16 patients who underwent the Artificial Bowel Sphincter (ABS) procedure.[195] Significant improvement was noted in all domains. These results also correlated with both the clinical assessment and an increase in the MRP. Others have shown that manometric and defecographic studies seem to indicate that successful results may be attributable to maintenance of an acute anorectal angle, even during straining.[57] Most published reports present relatively short-term experience—up to 3 or 4 years. Generally, with this length of follow-up, failure is in the range of 25% to –50%.[80,244] The Minnesota group, in fact, quote a 50% failure rate to their prospective implant patients (personal communication). Their series of 45 patients was published in 2003.[255] They separated the patients based

on their initial experience: group I (10 patients—1989 to 1992) and group II (37 patients—1997 to 2001). In group I, four required explanation (two required stomas), and six had functioning artificial sphincters, two of which required replacement for fluid leaks. The overall failure rate in group II was 49%. Fecal incontinence and quality of life of life scores were significantly improved in those who were able to maintain the artificial sphincter. However, success rates in their experience had not improved despite their additional experience, with infection being the primary challenge.[255] Michot and colleagues implanted 37 patients, with a 58% failure rate in their initial 12.[220] Their subsequent failure rate was 20%. They attribute this improvement primarily to better patient selection—eliminating those with a severely scarred perineum, an irradiated perineum, and those with diarrhea. Altomare and associates performed 28 Acticon implants with a 75% success rate (median follow-up, 19 months).[6] Ortiz and colleagues inserted 24 artificial anal sphincter devices and calculated a cumulative probability of device explantation of 44% at 48 months.[251]

The safety and efficacy of the Acticon device were reported in a multicenter cohort study trial that was conducted with a common protocol.[390] Of the 112 patients who were enrolled, 73 required revision (46%). Seven underwent successful reimplantation, and a successful outcome was achieved in 85% of those individuals who had a functioning device. Christiansen's group reported 17 patients with long-term follow-up (at least 16 years).[56] Two died of unrelated causes, and three were explanted because of infection. Four required removal of the device because of malfunction. Therefore, approximately one half had a satisfactory long-term result.

Comment The foregoing results demonstrate that the artificial anal sphincter may play an important role in the treatment of individuals with fecal incontinence and in whom other less invasive procedures are not applicable or have failed. Regardless of the high complication rate, the artificial anal sphincter (Acticon) offers the best alternative for restoring continence, especially for those who have no other option except a stoma.

Standards for Anal Sphincter Replacement

In 2000, a working party, consisting of distinguished surgeons who are experienced with operations for fecal incontinence, prepared a report in which a review of the status of sphincter replacement surgery was presented.[208] Certain recommendations and conclusions evolved. They are as follows:

- Both electrically stimulated skeletal muscle neo-sphincter and artificial anal sphincter are options for patients with *end-stage* [italics mine] fecal incontinence. (Comment: The point made with respect to the former operation is moot, at least in the United States. The stimulator has not been approved by the Food and Drug Administration as of 2004—MLC.)
- Avoidance of complications requires strict attention to aseptic technique. Prophylactic antibiotics are required.
- Experience with the procedure is essential. These operations should, therefore, only be performed in a limited number of centers.

Nieriella and Deen in 2000 opined that because neo-anal sphincter operations are technically demanding and require a considerable learning experience, the proce-dures should be undertaken only at centers specializing in colorectal surgery.[242]

OTHER TREATMENT OPTIONS

Pudendal Neurolysis

Shafik has published several articles describing the treatment of anal incontinence by means of pudendal nerve decompression in those who have a pudendal nerve injury.[323-325] The technique involves a parasacral incision, division of the gluteus maximus muscle, exposure of the pudendal nerves, and tracking them down the pudendal canal. The procedure is undertaken bilaterally. The most recent report comprises 11 individuals. Following the procedure, the PNTML was significantly decreased in eight

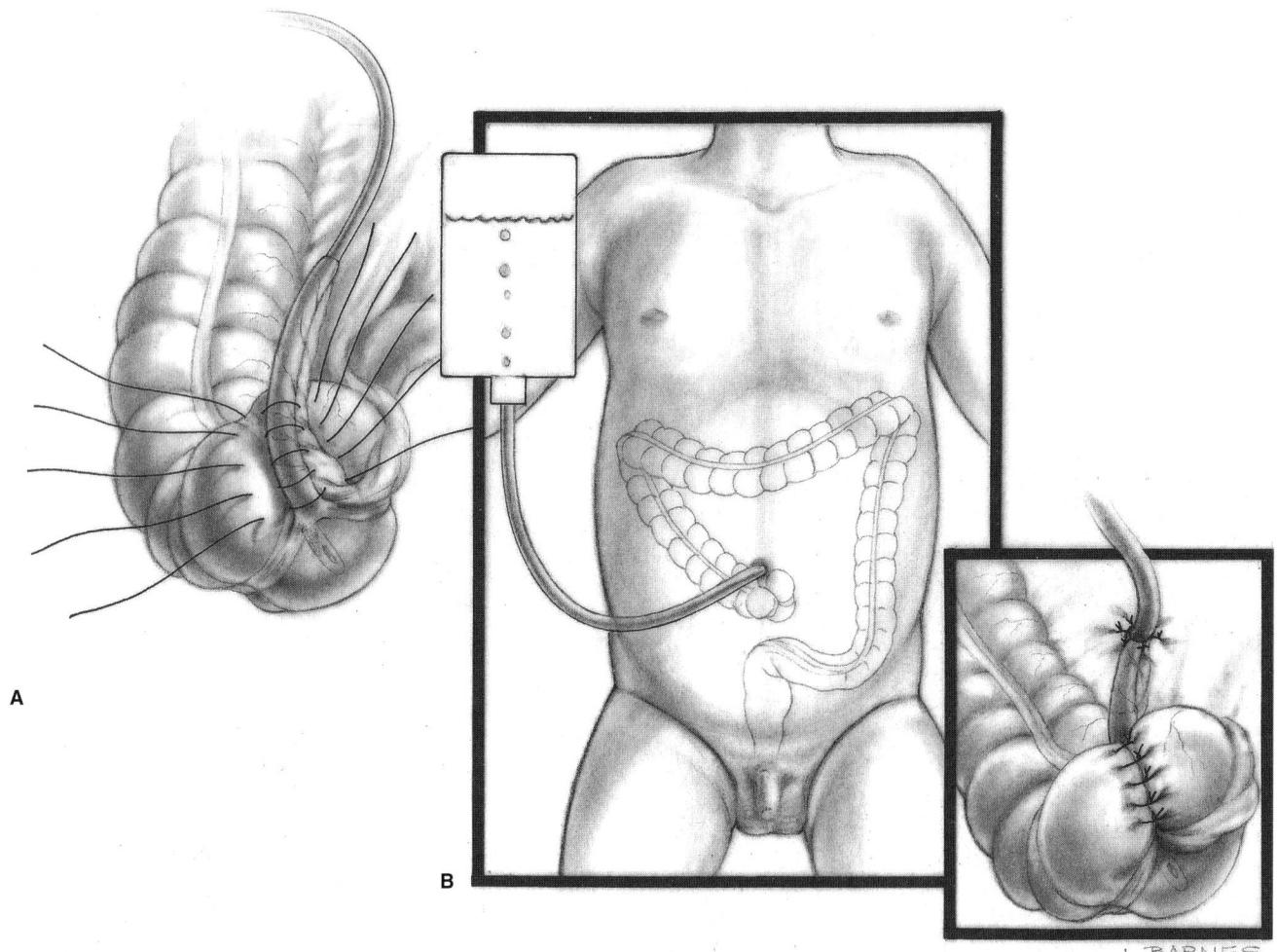

FIGURE 13-63. Appendicostomy. Cecal plication around the native appendix. **(A)** Appendix overlying cecum. **(B)** Administration of an enema through the umbilicus. **(C)** Completed plication. (From Levitt MA, Soffer SZ, Peña A. Continent appendicostomy in the bowel management of fecally incontinent children. *J Pediatr Surg* 1997; 32: 1630–1633, with permission.)

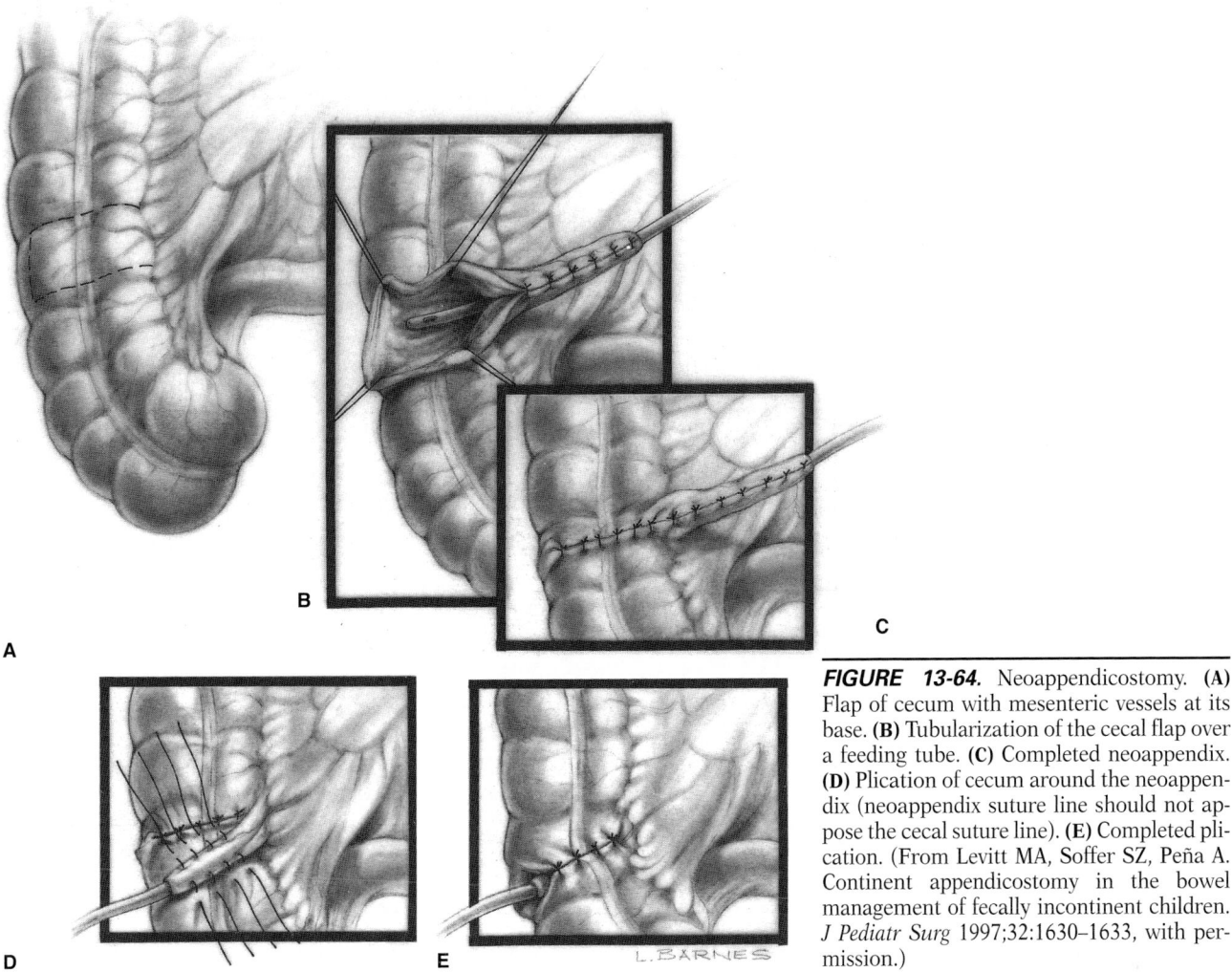

FIGURE 13-64. Neoappendicostomy. **(A)** Flap of cecum with mesenteric vessels at its base. **(B)** Tubularization of the cecal flap over a feeding tube. **(C)** Completed neoappendix. **(D)** Plication of cecum around the neoappendix (neoappendix suture line should not appose the cecal suture line). **(E)** Completed plication. (From Levitt MA, Soffer SZ, Peña A. Continent appendicostomy in the bowel management of fecally incontinent children. *J Pediatr Surg* 1997;32:1630–1633, with permission.)

of 11 patients. No improvement was noted in three. The author concluded that failure to improve may be ascribed to irreversible nerve damage.

This is a unique concept, and as of this writing there have been no reports from other individuals or institutions.

Fecal Diversion

The performance of a colostomy or ileostomy in a patient with fecal incontinence is thought generally to be an admission of failure, but it should not be regarded as such. Many individuals should not be submitted to the rigors of an esoteric sphincter-saving operation. For example, the likelihood of success in those who have severe neurologic deficit, who are retarded or senile, or who have profound bowel function problems is extremely limited. Fecal diversion is virtually often the optimal choice for a patient confined to a nursing home or to a convalescent facility. Irrespective of the method

of treatment, perhaps more frequently than any other condition discussed in this text, patients with fecal incontinence need to be willing partners in the decision-making process.

Antegrade Colonic Irrigation

In 1990, Malone and colleagues described an antegrade colonic irrigation technique for the management of anal incontinence through the creation of a tube-appendicostomy.[209] This procedure is occasionally applied to the treatment of defecatory disorders in children, especially those with intractable constipation and fecal incontinence. Levitt and colleagues developed a modification of this approach and reported their experience in 20 children with anal incontinence for whom bowel management with conventional enemas was unsuccessful (Figs. 13-63 and 13-64).[200] Krough and Laurberg reported 16 *adult* patients who underwent this approach

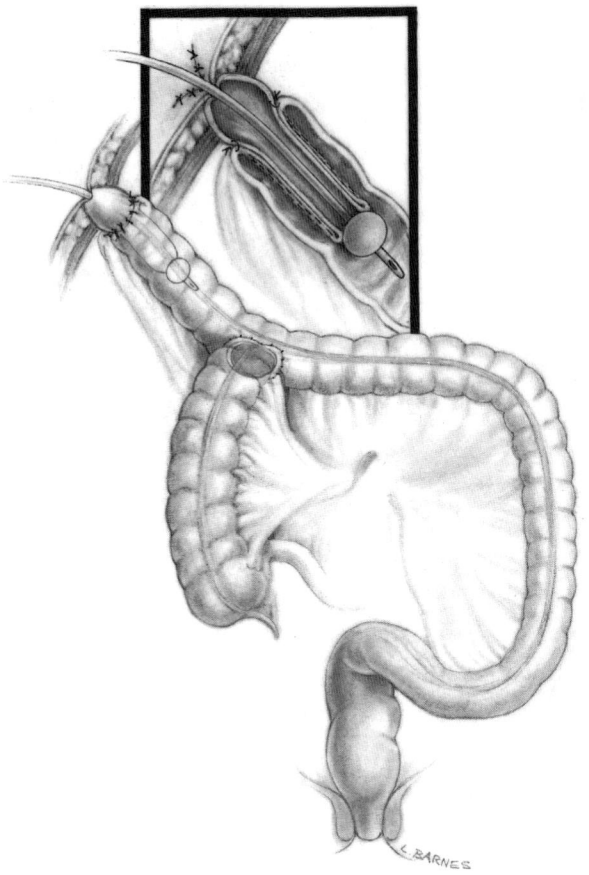

FIGURE 13-65. The colon is divided, and the proximal transverse colon is used to construct the conduit. An intussuscepting valve is created and fixed with sutures and staples. The conduit is exteriorized with skin flaps. (After Hughes SF, Williams NS. Continent colonic conduit for the treatment of faecal incontinence associated with disordered evacuation. *Br J Surg* 1995;82:1318.)

to management, ten of whom had fecal incontinence.[175] Marked improvement in incontinence was noted in eight, with all experiencing improvement in quality of life.

Hughes and Williams described a colonic conduit that incorporates an intussuscepting valve to manage fecal incontinence and disordered evacuation through an antegrade irrigation technique.[147] The procedure involves division of the bowel at the level of the proximal transverse colon with the creation of the conduit (Figure 13-65). In their experience, after 1 month there was no leakage of solid or liquid feces from the anus between irrigations, nor was there stool or irrigating fluid refluxing to the abdominal wall. No appliance was required.

CLOSING THE COLOSTOMY

When to close a colostomy that had been placed prior to reconstruction of the anal sphincter is often a difficult

decision. When making this decision, the physician may consider physiologic studies such as those discussed previously. Other options include encouraging the patient to hold an enema—a vigorous test for even a normal sphincter mechanism—or the use of a more formed substance that simulates feces (e.g., psyllium). This latter method has been advocated by Pittman and colleagues.[271] A mixture of psyllium and water is instilled through the distal limb of a loop stoma or through the mucous fistula.

From my experience and in my opinion, however, there is no satisfactory method for objectively assessing the prospects for continence prior to colostomy closure, because there are so many variables that contribute to bowel control. For example, in the barium enema study shown in Figure 13-66, the physician must consider that the long-disused rectum will certainly contribute to bowel management difficulties at least for a time. I, therefore, rely on physical examination, the presence of healed wounds, subjective estimation of the likelihood of success, and well-documented, informed consent.

CONCLUSIONS

The following recommendations are made for the surgical treatment of anal incontinence.

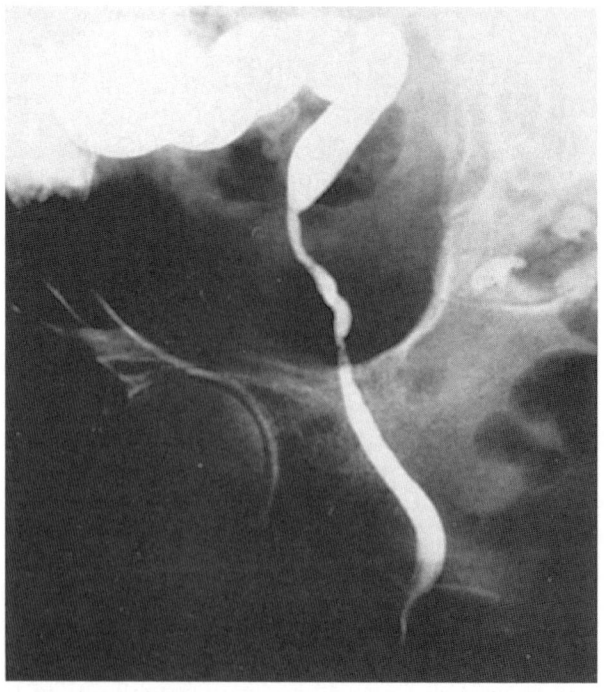

FIGURE 13-66. Barium study reveals an atrophic rectum, a consequence of disuse many years following the creation of a colostomy.

- Primary repair for reparable defects
- Artificial sphincter: when no reparable defect exists; good results anticipated when not complicated by erosion or sepsis (50% failure rate); ideal candidate is older, with neuropathy as the cause of the incontinence
- GMT: for sphincter loss secondary to trauma or congenital anomaly, in young patients, in the absence of diarrhea or irritable bowel
- Gluteus transposition: same as gracilis but higher failure rate
- Silastic-Dacron implant (Thiersch-type procedure): for elderly patients, neuropathic, with irritable bowel or diarrhea (50% report improvement)
- RF treatment (Secca): failure of above or first-line interventional procedure for elderly patients, those with neuropathy or with bowel management problem, as a salvage procedure, in patients unwilling or unable to undergo a more invasive option
- Antegrade colonic irrigation: alternative to stoma in a motivated patient, especially someone in whom one of the supplementary sphincter procedures has failed
- Stoma: last recourse; radiation injury, nursing management
- Sacral/pudendal nerve stimulation: investigational

REFERENCES

1. Abcarian H, Orsay CP, Pearl RK, et al. Traumatic cloaca. *Dis Colon Rectum* 1989;32:783.
2. Abou-Zeid AA, Marzouk DM. Gluteus maximus neosphincter is a viable option for patients with end-stage fecal incontinence. *Dis Colon Rectum* 2000;43:1635.
3. Ala J, Mendeloff AI, Hendrix TR, et al. Studies of fecal incontinence by combined manometric-electromyographic techniques. *Gastroenterology* 1965;48:863(abst).
4. Allen ML. Biofeedback for fecally incontinent children with repaired imperforate anus. *Pract Gastroenterol* 1990;14:53.
5. Alstrup NI, Rasmussen OED, Christiansen J. Effect of rectal dilation in rectal incontinence with low rectal compliance: report of a case. *Dis Colon Rectum* 1995;38:988.
6. Altomare DF, Dodi G, La Torre F, et al. Multicentre retrospective analysis of the outcome of artificial anal sphincter implantation for severe faecal incontinence. *Br J Surg* 2001;88:1481.
7. Altringer WE, Saclarides TJ, Dominguez JM, et al. Four-contrast defecography: pelvic "floor-oscopy." *Dis Colon Rectum* 1995;38:695.
8. Arnaud A, Sarles JC, Sielezneff I, et al. Sphincter repair without overlapping for fecal incontinence. *Dis Colon Rectum* 1991;34:744.
9. Auwerda JJA, Schouten WR. New device for adequate fixation of recording instruments in ambulant anorectal manometry. *Dis Colon Rectum* 1994;37:383.
10. Baeten C, Spaans F, Fluks A. An implanted neuromuscular stimulator for faecal continence. *Dis Colon Rectum* 1988;31:134.
11. Baeten CGMI, Geerdes B, Eddy MM, et al. Anal dynamic graciloplasty in the treatment of intractable fecal incontinence. *N Engl J Med* 1995;332:1600.
12. 9A.Baig MK, Wexner SD. Factors predictive of outcome after surgery for faecal incontinence. *Br J Surg* 2000;87:1316.
13. Bannister JJ, Abouzekry L, Read NW. Effect of aging on anorectal function. *Gut* 1987;28:353.
14. Bannister JJ, Gibbons C, Read NW. Preservation of faecal continence during rises in intra-abdominal pressure: is there a role for the flap valve? *Gut* 1987;28:1242.
15. Bannister JJ, Read NW, Donnelly TC, et al. External and internal anal sphincter responses to rectal distension in normal subjects and in patients with idiopathic faecal incontinence. *Br J Surg* 1989;76:617.
16. Barrett JA, Brocklehurst JC, Kiff ES, et al. Anal function in geriatric patients with faecal incontinence. *Gut* 1989;30:1244.
17. Bartolo DCC, Jarratt JA, Read MG, et al. The role of partial denervation of the puborectalis in idiopathic faecal incontinence. *Br J Surg* 1984;70:664.
18. Bartolo DCC, Jarratt JA, Read NW. The cutaneo-anal reflex: a useful index of neuropathy? *Br J Surg* 1983;70:660.
19. Bartolo DCC, Roe AM, Locke-Edmunds JC, et al. Flap-valve theory of anorectal continence. *Br J Surg* 1986;73:1012.
20. Bartram C, Halligan S. Endoanal MR is really complementary to endoanal US. *Radiology* 2000;216:918.
21. Beck A. Electromyographische Untersuchungen am Sphincter ani. *Pflugers Arch Ges Physiol* 1930;224:278.
22. Bellman M. Studies on encopresis. *Acta Paediatr Scand* 1966;170:1.
23. Bielefeldt K, Enck P, Erckenbrecht JF. Sensory and motor function in the maintenance of anal continence. *Dis Colon Rectum* 1990;33:674.
24. Binnie NR, Kawimbe BM, Papachrysostomou M, et al. Use of the pudendo-anal reflex in the treatment of neurogenic faecal incontinence. *Gut* 1990;31:1051.
25. Bishop B, Garry RC, Roberts TDM, et al. Control of the external sphincter of the anus in the cat. *J Physiol (Lond)* 1956;134:229.
26. Blaisdell PC. Repair of the incontinent sphincter ani. *Surg Gynecol Obstet* 1940;70:692.
27. Block IR. Repair of the incontinent sphincter ani following operative injury. *Surg Gynecol Obstet* 1959;109:111.
28. Block IR, Rodriguez S, Olivares AL. The Warren operation for anal incontinence caused by disruption of the anterior segment of the anal sphincter, perineal body, and rectovaginal septum. *Dis Colon Rectum* 1975;18:28.
29. Bollard RC, Gardiner A, Lindow S, et al. Normal female anal sphincter: difficulties in interpretation explained. *Dis Colon Rectum* 2002;45:171.
30. Borden EB, Sheran M, Sammartano RJ, et al. The complete anorectal function profile. *Gastroenterology* 1982;82:1023(abst).
31. Braun JC, Treutner KH, Dreuw B, et al. Vectormanometry for differential diagnosis of fecal incontinence. *Dis Colon Rectum* 1994;37:989.
32. Bremmer S, Ahlbäck S-O, Udén R, et al. Simultaneous defecography and peritoneography in defecation disorders. *Dis Colon Rectum* 1995;38:969.
33. Brocklehurst JC. Management of anal incontinence. *Clin Gastroenterol* 1975;4:479.
34. Browning GGP, Motson RW. Anal sphincter injury: management and results of Parks sphincter repair. *Ann Surg* 1984;199:351.
35. Bruining HA, Bos KE, Colthoff EG, et al. Creation of an anal sphincter mechanism by bilateral proximally based gluteal muscle transposition. *Plast Reconstr Surg* 1981;67:70.
36. Brummelkamp WH, Leguit P Jr, van Baal JG. Pedicle muscle grafts for rectal incontinence: a review. *Surg Rounds* 1986;9:66.
37. Bubrick MP, Godec CJ, Cass AS. Functional evaluation of the rectal ampulla with ampullometrogram. *J R Soc Med* 1980;73:234.
38. Buie WD, Lowry AC, Rothenberger DA, et al. Clinical rather than laboratory assessment predicts continence after anterior sphincteroplasty. *Dis Colon Rectum* 2001;44:1255.
39. Burnett SJD, Speakman CTM, Kamm MA, et al. Confirmation of endosonographic detection of external anal sphincter defects by simultaneous electromyographic mapping. *Br J Surg* 1991;78:448.

40. Burnett SJD, Spence-Jones C, Speakman CTM, et al. Unsuspected sphincter damage following childbirth revealed by anal endosonography. *Br J Radiol* 1991;64:225.
41. Busch DB, Starling JR. Rectal foreign bodies: case reports and a comprehensive review of the world's literature. *Surgery* 1986;100:512.
42. Buser WD, Miner PB Jr. Delayed rectal sensation with fecal incontinence: successful treatment using anorectal manometry. *Gastroenterology* 1986;91:1186.
43. Byrne CM, Pager CK, Rex J, et al. Assessment of quality of life in treatment of patients with neuropathic fecal incontinence. *Dis Colon Rectum* 2002;45:1431.
44. Caldwell KPS. The electrical control of sphincter incompetence. *Lancet* 1963;2:174.
45. Castro AF, Pittman RE. Repair of the incontinent sphincter. *Dis Colon Rectum* 1978;21:183.
46. Cerulli MA, Nikoomanesh P, Schuster MM. Progress in biofeedback conditioning for fecal incontinence. *Gastroenterology* 1979;76:742.
47. Chan C, Williams N, Tillin T, et al. Fecal incontinence: rectal augmentation. Evaluation of a novel surgical procedure for the management of severe faecal urgency. *Dis Colon Rectum* 2002;45:A34-A36.
48. Chan CLH, Scott SM, Birch MJ, et al. Rectal heat thresholds: a novel test of the sensory afferent pathway. *Dis Colon Rectum* 2003;46:590.
49. Chapman AE, Geerdes B, Hewett P, et al. Systematic review of dynamic graciloplasty in the treatment of faecal incontinence. *Br J Surg* 2002;89:138.
50. Chiou AW-H, Lin J-K, Wang F-M. Anorectal abnormalities in progressive systemic sclerosis. *Dis Colon Rectum* 1989;32:417.
51. Chittenden AS. Sphincter muscle and reconstruction. *Ann Surg* 1930;92:152.
52. Christiansen J, Hansen CR, Rasmussen O. Bilateral gluteus maximus transposition for anal incontinence. *Br J Surg* 1995;82:903.
53. Christiansen J, Lorentzen M. Implantation of artificial sphincter for anal incontinence. *Lancet* 1987;i:244.
54. Christiansen J, Lorentzen M. Implantation of artificial sphincter for anal incontinence: report of five cases. *Dis Colon Rectum* 1989;32:432.
55. Christiansen J, Pedersen IK. Traumatic anal incontinence: results of surgical repair. *Dis Colon Rectum* 1987;30:189.
56. Christiansen J, Rasmussen OO, Lindoff-Larsen K. Long-term results of artificial anal sphincter implantation for severe anal incontinence. *Ann Surg* 1999;230:45.
57. Christiansen J, Sparro B. Treatment of anal incontinence by an implantable prosthetic anal sphincter. *Ann Surg* 1992;215:383.
58. Christiansen J, Sorensen M, Rasmussen OO. Gracilis muscle transposition for faecal incontinence. *Br J Surg* 1990;77:1039.
59. Cohen M, Rosen L, Khubchandani I, et al. Rationale for medical or surgical therapy in anal incontinence. *Dis Colon Rectum* 1986;29:120.
60. Coller JA. Clinical application of anorectal manometry. *Gastroenterol Clin North Am* 1987;16:17.
61. Coller JA. Computerized anal sphincter manometry performance and analysis. In: Smith LE, ed. *Practical guide to anorectal testing*. New York: Igaku-Shoin, 1990:65.
62. Constantinides CG, Cywes S. Fecal incontinence: a simple pneumatic device for home biofeedback training. *J Pediatr Surg* 1983;18:276.
63. Corman ML. Gracilis muscle transposition. *Contemp Surg* 1978;13:9.
64. Corman ML. Follow-up evaluation of gracilis muscle transposition for fecal incontinence. *Dis Colon Rectum* 1980;23:552.
65. Corman ML. The management of anal incontinence. *Surg Clin North Am* 1983;63:177.
66. Corman ML. Anal incontinence following obstetrical injury. *Dis Colon Rectum* 1985;28:86.
67. Corman ML. Gracilis muscle transposition for anal incontinence: late results. *Br J Surg* 1985;72:21.
68. Corman ML. The treatment of anal incontinence. In: Cameron JL, ed. *Current surgical therapy: 2.* Toronto: BC Decker, 1986:144.
69. Cornes H, Bartolo DCC, Stirrat GM. Changes in anal canal sensation after childbirth. *Br J Surg* 1991;78:74.
70. Critchlow JF, Houlihan MJ, Landolt CC, et al. Primary sphincter repair in anorectal trauma. *Dis Colon Rectum* 1985;28:945.
71. Cuesta MA, Meijer S, Derksen EJ, et al. Anal sphincter imaging in fecal incontinence using endosonography. *Dis Colon Rectum* 1992;35:59.
72. Dalley AF II. The riddle of the sphincters: the morphophysiology of the anorectal mechanism reviewed. *Am Surg* 1987;53:298.
73. Damon H, Henry L, Barth X, et al. Fecal incontinence in females with a past history of vaginal delivery: significance of anal sphincter defects detected by ultrasound. *Dis Colon Rectum* 2002;45:1445.
74. Davis K, Kumar D. Fecal incontinence: clinical evaluation of an injectable anal sphincter bulking agent (Durasphere) in the management of patients with persistent faecal incontinence secondary to an internal anal sphincter defect. *Dis Colon Rectum* 2002;45:A34-A36.
75. Deen KI, Kumar D, Williams JG, et al. Anal sphincter defects: correlation between endoanal ultrasound and surgery. *Ann Surg* 1993;218:201.
76. Deen KI, Kumar D, Williams JG, et al. The prevalence of anal sphincter defects in faecal incontinence: a prospective endosonic study. *Gut* 1993;34:685.
77. de Leeuw J-W, Vierhout ME, Struijk PC, et al. Anal sphincter damage after vaginal delivery: relationship of anal endosonography and manometry to anorectal complaints. *Dis Colon Rectum* 2002;45:1004.
78. Denny-Brown D, Robertson EG. An investigation of the nervous control of defaecation. *Brain* 1935;58:256.
79. deSouza NM, Hall AS, Puni R, et al. High-resolution magnetic resonance imaging of the anal sphincter using a dedicated endoanal coil: comparison of magnetic resonance imaging with surgical findings. *Dis Colon Rectum* 1996;39:926.
80. Devesa JM, Rey A, Hervas PL, et al. Artificial anal sphincter: complications and functional results of a large personal series. *Dis Colon Rectum* 2002;45:1154.
81. Devesa JM, Vicente E, Enriquez JM, et al. Total fecal incontinence: a new method of gluteus maximus transposition. Preliminary results and report of previous experience with similar procedures. *Dis Colon Rectum* 1992;35:339.
82. Dickinson VA. Maintenance of anal continence: a review of pelvic floor physiology. *Gut* 1978;19:1163.
83. Easson WM. Encopresis: psychogenic soiling. *Can Med Assoc J* 1960;82:624.
84. Eccersley AJP, Lunniss PJ, Williams NS. Unstimulated graciloplasty in traumatic faecal incontinence. *Br J Surg* 1999;86;1071.
85. Eckardt VF, Jung B, Fischer B, et al. Anal endosonography in healthy subjects and patients with idiopathic fecal incontinence. *Dis Colon Rectum* 1994;37:235.
86. Efron JE, Corman ML, Fleshman J, et al. Safety and effectiveness of temperature-controlled radiofrequency energy delivery to the anal canal (Secca procedure) for the treatment of fecal incontinence. *Dis Colon Rectum* 2003;46:1600.
87. Emblem R, Dhaenens G, Stien R, et al. The importance of anal endosonography in the evaluation of idiopathic fecal incontinence. *Dis Colon Rectum* 1994;37:42.
88. Enck P, Däublin G, Lübke HJ, et al. Long-term efficacy of biofeedback training for fecal incontinence. *Dis Colon Rectum* 1994;37:997.
89. Engel AF, Kamm MA, Sultan AH, et al. Anterior anal sphincter repair in patients with obstetric trauma. *Br J Surg* 1994;81:1231.

90. Engel BT, Nikoomanesh P, Schuster MM. Operant conditioning of rectosphincteric responses in the treatment of fecal incontinence. *N Engl J Med* 1974;290:646.

91. Enriquez-Navascues JM, Devesa-Mugica JM. Traumatic anal incontinence: role of unilateral gluteus maximus transposition supplementing and supporting direct anal sphincteroplasty. *Dis Colon Rectum* 1994;37:766.

92. Falk PM, Blatchford GJ, Cali RL, et al. Transanal ultrasound and manometry in the evaluation of fecal incontinence. *Dis Colon Rectum* 1994;37:468.

93. Fang DT, Nivatvongs S, Vermeulen FD, et al. Overlapping sphincteroplasty for acquired anal incontinence. *Dis Colon Rectum* 1984;27:720.

94. Farouk R, Duthie GS, MacGregor AB, et al. Evidence of electromechanical dissociation of the internal anal sphincter in idiopathic fecal incontinence. *Dis Colon Rectum* 1994;37:595.

95. Farouk R, Duthie GS, Pryde A, et al. Internal anal sphincter dysfunction in neurogenic faecal incontinence. *Br J Surg* 1993;80:259.

96. Faucheron J-L, Hannoun L, Thome C, et al. Is fecal continence improved by nonstimulated gracilis muscle transposition? *Dis Colon Rectum* 1994;37:979.

97. Felt-Bersma RJF, Cuesta MA, Koorevaar M. Anal sphincter repair improves anorectal function and endosonographic image: a prospective clinical study. *Dis Colon Rectum* 1996;39:878.

98. Felt-Bersma RJF, Cuesta MA, Koorevaar M, et al. Anal endosonography: relationship with anal manometry and neurophysiologic tests. *Dis Colon Rectum* 1992;35:944.

99. Felt-Bersma RJF, Klinkenber-Knol EC, Meuwissen SGM. Anorectal function investigations in incontinent and continent patients. *Dis Colon Rectum* 1990;33:479.

100. Feretis C, Benakis P, Dailianas A, et al. Implantation of microballoons in the management of fecal incontinence. *Dis Colon Rectum* 2001;44:1605.

101. Ferguson EF. The Foley catheter in colon-rectal surgery. *Contemp Surg* 1983;22:43.

102. Ferrara A, De Jesus S, Gallagher JT, et al. Time-related decay of the benefits of biofeedback therapy. *Tech Coloproctol* 2001;5:131.

103. Fleshman J, Weston JE. Fecal incontinence: multicenter open label prospective trial evaluating the safety and effectiveness of temperature controlled radio-frequency energy delivery to the anal canal (Secca procedure) for treatment of fecal incontinence. *Dis Colon Rectum* 2002;45:A34–A36.

104. Fleshman JW, Dreznik Z, Fry RD, et al. Anal sphincter repair for obstetrical injury: manometric evaluation of functional results. *Dis Colon Rectum* 1991;34:1061.

105. Fleshman JW, Peters WR, Shemesh EI, et al. Anal sphincter reconstruction: anterior overlapping muscle repair. *Dis Colon Rectum* 1991;34:739.

106. Fornell EKU, Berg G, Hallböök O, et al. Clinical consequences of anal sphincter rupture during vaginal delivery. *J Am Coll Surg* 1996;183:553.

107. Frudinger A, Halligan S, Bartram CI, et al. Assessment of the predictive value of a bowel symptom questionnaire in identifying perianal and anal sphincter trauma after vaginal delivery. *Dis Colon Rectum* 2003;46:742.

108. Fynes MM, Marshall K, Cassidy M, et al. A prospective, randomized study comparing the effect of augmented biofeedback with sensory biofeedback alone on fecal incontinence after obstetric trauma. *Dis Colon Rectum* 1999; 42:753.

109. Gabriel WB. *The principles and practice of rectal surgery*, 5th ed. London: HK Lewis, 1963:18.

110. Gabriel WB. *The principles and practice of rectal surgery*, 5th ed. London: HK Lewis, 1963:106.

111. Ganio E, Luc AR, Clerico G, et al. Sacral nerve stimulation for treatment of fecal incontinence: a novel approach for intractable fecal incontinence. *Dis Colon Rectum* 2001; 44:619.

112. Ganio E, Masin A, Ratto C, et al. Short-term sacral nerve stimulation for functional anorectal and urinary disturbances: results in 40 patients: evaluation of a new option for anorectal functional disorders. *Dis Colon Rectum* 2001;44:1261.

113. Ganio E, Ratto C, Masin A, et al. Neuromodulation for fecal incontinence: outcome in 16 patients with definitive implant. The initial Italian Sacral Neurostimulation Group (GINS) experience. *Dis Colon Rectum* 2001;44:965.

114. Geerdes BP, Heinemen E, Konsten J, et al. Dynamic graciloplasty: complications and management. *Dis Colon Rectum* 1996;39:912.

115. George BD, Williams NS, Patel J, et al. Physiological and histochemical adaptation of the electrically stimulated gracilis muscle to neoanal sphincter function. *Br J Surg* 1993;80:1342.

116. Giamundo P, Wexner SD, Welber A, et al. Procon incontinence device: a prospective, non-randomized pilot study. *Am J Gastroenterol* 2002;97:2328.

117. Giordano P, Renzi A, Efron J, et al. Previous sphincter repair does not affect the outcome of repeat repair. *Dis Colon Rectum* 2002;45:635.

118. Glen ES. Effective and safe control of incontinence by the intra-anal plug electrode. *Br J Surg* 1971;58:249.

119. Go PMNYH, Dunselman GAJ. Anatomic and functional results of surgical repair after total perineal rupture at delivery. *Surg Gynecol Obstet* 1988;166:121.

120. Gold DM, Bartram CI, Halligan S, et al. Three-dimensional endoanal sonography in assessing anal canal injury. *Br J Surg* 1999;86:365.

121. Goldberg SM, Gordon PH, Nivatvongs S. *Essentials of anorectal surgery*. Philadelphia: JB Lippincott, 1980.

122. Goldenberg DA, Hodges K, Hersh T, et al. Biofeedback therapy for fecal incontinence. *Am J Gastroenterol* 1980; 74:342.

123. Goligher JC, Duthie HL, DeDombal FT, et al. Abdominoanal pull-through excision for tumours of the mid-third of the rectum: a comparison with low anterior resection. *Br J Surg* 1965;52:323.

124. Gorsch RV. *Proctologic anatomy*. Baltimore: Williams & Wilkins, 1955.

125. Granet E. Hemorrhoidectomy failures: causes, prevention and management. *Dis Colon Rectum* 1968;11:45.

126. Guillemot F, Bouche B, Gower-Rousseau C, et al. Biofeedback for the treatment of fecal incontinence: long-term clinical results. *Dis Colon Rectum* 1995;38:393.

127. Ha HT, Fleshman JW, Smith M, et al. Manometric squeeze pressure difference parallels functional outcome after overlapping sphincter reconstruction. *Dis Colon Rectum* 2001;44:655.

128. Hagihara PF, Griffen WO Jr. Delayed correction of anorectal incontinence due to anal sphincteral injury. *Arch Surg* 1976;111:63.

129. Hallan RI, Marzouk DEMM, Waldron DJ, et al. Comparison of digital and manometric assessment of anal sphincter function. *Br J Surg* 1989;76:973.

130. Halverson AL, Hull TL. Long-term outcome of overlapping anal sphincter repair. *Dis Colon Rectum* 2002;45:345.

131. Hardcastle JD, Porter NH. Anal continence. In: Morson BC, ed. *Diseases of the colon, rectum and anus*. New York: Appleton-Century-Crofts, 1969:251.

132. Hayne D, Vaizey CJ, Boulos PB. Anorectal injury following pelvic radiotherapy. *Br J Surg* 2001;88:1037.

133. Healy JC, Halligan S, Bartram CI, et al. Dynamic magnetic resonance imaging evaluation of the structural and functional results of postanal repair for neuropathic fecal incontinence. *Dis Colon Rectum* 2002;45:1629.

134. Henry MM, Parks AG, Swash M. The anal reflex in idiopathic faecal incontinence: an electrophysiologic study. *Br J Surg* 1980;67:781.

135. Henry MM, Simson JNL. Results of postanal repair: a retrospective study. *Br J Surg* 1985;72:S17.

136. Hentz VR. Construction of a rectal sphincter using the origin of the gluteus maximus muscle. *Plast Reconstr Surg* 1982;70:82.

137. Heyman S, Jones KR, Ringel Y, et al. Biofeedback treatment of fecal incontinence: a critical review. *Dis Colon Rectum* 2001;44:728.

138. Hill J, Corson RJ, Brandon H, et al. History and examination in the assessment of patients with idiopathic fecal incontinence. *Dis Colon Rectum* 1994;37:473.

139. Hill J, Hosker G, Kiff ES. Pudendal nerve terminal motor latency measurements: what they do and do not tell us. *Br J Surg* 2002;89:1268.

140. Ho Y-H, Chiang J-M, Tan M, et al. Biofeedback therapy for excessive stool frequency and incontinence following anterior resection or total colectomy. *Dis Colon Rectum* 1996; 39:1289.

141. Ho Y-H, Tsang C, Tang CL, et al. Anal sphincter injuries from stapling instruments introduced transanally: randomized, controlled study with endoanal ultrasound and anorectal manometry. *Dis Colon Rectum* 2000;43:169.

142. Hoffmann BA, Timmcke AE, Gathright JB, et al. Fecal seepage and soiling: a problem of rectal sensation. *Dis Colon Rectum* 1995;38:746.

143. Holmström B, Brodén G, Dolk A, et al. Increased anal resting pressure following the Ripstein operation: a contribution to continence? *Dis Colon Rectum* 1986;29:485.

144. Hopkinson BR, Lightwood R. Electrical treatment of anal incontinence. *Lancet* 1966;1:297.

145. Hopkinson BR, Lightwood R. Electrical treatment of incontinence. *Br J Surg* 1967;54:802.

146. Horn HR, Schoetz DJ Jr, Coller JA, et al. Sphincter repair with a silastic sling for anal incontinence and rectal procidentia. *Dis Colon Rectum* 1985;28:868.

147. Hughes SF, Williams NS. Continent colonic conduit for the treatment of faecal incontinence associated with disordered evacuation. *Br J Surg* 1995;82:1318.

148. Hutchinson R, Mostafa AB, Grant EA, et al. Scintigraphic defecography: quantitative and dynamic assessment of anorectal function. *Dis Colon Rectum* 1993;36:1132.

149. Iwai N, Kaneda H, Tsuto T, et al. Objective assessment of anorectal function after sphincter reconstruction using the gluteus maximus muscle. *Dis Colon Rectum* 1985;28:973.

150. Iwai N, Ogita S, Kida M, et al. A clinical and manometric correlation for assessment of postoperative continence in imperforate anus. *J Pediatr Surg* 1979;14:538.

151. Jacobs PPM, Scheuer M, Kuijpers JHC, et al. Obstetric fecal incontinence: role of pelvic floor denervation and results of delayed sphincter repair. *Dis Colon Rectum* 1990;33:494.

152. Jameson JS, Rogers J, Chia YW, et al. Pelvic floor function in multiple sclerosis. *Gut* 1994;35:388.

153. Jameson JS, Speakman CTM, Darzi A, et al. Audit of postanal repair in the treatment of fecal incontinence. *Dis Colon Rectum* 1994;37:369.

154. Johansson C, Ihre T, Holmstrom B, et al. A combined electromyographic and cineradiologic investigation in patients with defecation disorders. *Dis Colon Rectum* 1990; 33:1009.

155. Jorge JMN, Wexner SD. Etiology and management of fecal incontinence. *Dis Colon Rectum* 1993;36:77.

156. Jorge JMN, Wexner SD, Marchetti F, et al. How reliable are currently available methods of measuring the anorectal angle? *Dis Colon Rectum* 1992;35:332.

157. Jost WH, Schimrigk K. Magnetic stimulation of the pudendal nerve. *Dis Colon Rectum* 1994;37:697.

158. Kaiser AM, Corman ML. Modified perianal incisions in gracinloplasty for fecal incontinence. *Dis Colon Rectum* 2002;45:703.

159. Kaushal JN, Goldner F. Validation of the digital rectal examination as an estimate of anal sphincter squeeze pressure. *Am J Gastroenterol* 1991;86:886.

160. Kegel A. Active exercise of the pubococcygeus muscle. In: Meigs JV, Sturgis SH, eds. *Progress in gynecology.* New York: Grune and Stratton, 1950:778.

161. Keighley MRB, Henry MM, Bartolo DCC, Mortensen NJMC. Anorectal physiology measurement: report of a working party. *Br J Surg* 1989;76:356.

162. Keighley MRB, Matheson DM. Results of treatment for rectal prolapse and fecal incontinence. *Dis Colon Rectum* 1981;24:449.

163. Kelly JH. Cine radiography in anorectal malformations. *J Pediatr Surg* 1969;4:538.

164. Kenefick N, Vaizey C, Cohen R, et al. Fecal incontinence: a single-center experience of permanent sacral nerve neuromodulation for faecal incontinence. *Dis Colon Rectum* 2002;45:A34–A36.

165. Kenefick NJ, Vaizey CJ, Cohen RCG, et al. Medium-term results of permanent sacral nerve stimulation for faecal incontinence. *Br J Surg* 2002;89:896.

166. Keren S, Wagner Y, Heldenberg D, et al. Studies of manometric abnormalities of the rectoanal region during defecation in constipated and soiling children: modification through biofeedback therapy. *Am J Gastroenterol* 1988;83: 827.

167. Khanduja KS, Yamashita HJ, Wise WE Jr, et al. Delayed repair of obstetric injuries of the anorectum and vagina: a stratified surgical approach. *Dis Colon Rectum* 1994;37: 344.

168. Kiesewetter WB, Turner CR. Continence after surgery for imperforate anus: a critical analysis and preliminary experience with the sacroperineal pull-through. *Ann Surg* 1963;158:498.

169. Kim J, Shim M-C, Choi B-Y, et al. Clinical application of continent anal plug in bedridden patients with intractable diarrhea. *Dis Colon Rectum* 2001;44:1162.

170. Kimura J. *Electrodiagnosis in diseases of nerve and muscle: principles and practice.* Philadelphia: FA Davis, 1983:209.

171. Konsten J, Baeten CGMI, Havenith MG, et al. Morphology of dynamic graciloplasty compared with the anal sphincter. *Dis Colon Rectum* 1993;36:559.

172. Konsten J, Rongen MJ, Ogunbiyi OA, et al. Comparison of epineural or intramuscular nerve electrodes for stimulated graciloplasty. *Dis Colon Rectum* 2001;44:581.

173. Korsgen S, Keighley MRB. Stimulated gracilis neosphincter—not as good as previously thought: report of four cases. *Dis Colon Rectum* 1995;38:1331.

174. Kraemer M, Ho Y-H, Tan M. Effectiveness of anorectal biofeedback therapy for faecal incontinence: medium-term results. *Tech Coloproctol* 2001;5:125.

175. Krough K, Laurberg S. Malone antegrade continence enema for faecal incontinence and constipation in adults. *Br J Surg* 1998;85:974.

176. Krough K, Pedersen I, Christiansen J. A study of the physiological variation in anal manometry. *Br J Surg* 1989;76:69.

177. Kuijpers HC, Scheuer M. Disorders of impaired fecal control: a clinical and manometric study. *Dis Colon Rectum* 1990;33:207.

178. Kuijpers HC, Strijk SP. Diagnosis of disturbances of continence and defecation. *Dis Colon Rectum* 1984;27:658.

179. Kumar D, Benson MJ, Bland JE. Glutaraldehyde crosslinked collagen in the treatment of faecal incontinence. *Br J Surg* 1998;85:978.

180. Kumar D, Hutchinson R, Grant E. Bilateral gracilis neosphincter construction for treatment of faecal incontinence. *Br J Surg* 1995;82:1645.

181. Labow SB, Hoexter B, Moseson MD, et al. Modification of Silastic sling repair for rectal procidentia and anal incontinence. *Dis Colon Rectum* 1985;28:684.

182. Labow SB, Rubin RJ, Hoexter B, et al. Perineal repair of rectal procidentia with an elastic fabric sling. *Dis Colon Rectum* 1980;23:467.

183. Lahr CJ, Cherry DA, Jensen LL, et al. Balloon sphincterography: clinical findings after 200 patients. *Dis Colon Rectum* 1988;31:347.

184. Lahr CJ, Rothenberger DA, Jensen LL, et al. Balloon topography: a simple method of evaluating anal function. *Dis Colon Rectum* 1986;29:1.

185. Lane RH. Clinical application of anorectal physiology. *Proc R Soc Med* 1975;68:28.

186. Laurberg S, Swash M. Effects of aging on the anorectal sphincters and their innervation. *Dis Colon Rectum* 1989; 32:737.

187. Laurberg S, Swash M, Henry MM. Delayed external sphincter repair for obstetric tear. *Br J Surg* 1988;75: 786.

188. Laurberg S, Swash M, Henry MM. Effect of postanal repair on progress of neurogenic damage to the pelvic floor. *Br J Surg* 1990;77:519.

189. Law PJ, Kamm MA, Bartram CI. A comparison between electromyography and anal endosonography in mapping external anal sphincter defects. *Dis Colon Rectum* 1990; 33:370.

190. Law PJ, Kamm MA, Bartram CI. Anal endosonography in the investigation of faecal incontinence. *Br J Surg* 1991; 78:312.

191. Leguit P Jr, van Baal JG, Brummelkamp WH. Gracilis muscle transposition in the treatment of fecal incontinence. *Dis Colon Rectum* 1985;28:1.

192. Lehur P-A, Glemain P, des Varannes SB, et al. Outcome of patients with an implanted artificial anal sphincter for severe faecal incontinence: a single institution report. *Int J Colorectal Dis* 1998;13:88.

193. Lehur P-A, Michot F, Denis P, et al. Results of artificial sphincter in severe anal incontinence: report of 14 consecutive implantations. *Dis Colon Rectum* 1996;39:1352.

194. Lehur P-A, Roig JV, Duinslaeger M. Artificial anal sphincter: prospective clinical and manometric evaluation. *Dis Colon Rectum* 2000;43:1100.

195. Lehur P-A, Zerbib F, Neunlist M, et al. Comparison of quality of life and anorectal function after artificial sphincter implantation. *Dis Colon Rectum* 2002;45:508.

196. Leighton JA, Valdovinos MA, Pemberton JH, et al. Anorectal dysfunction and rectal prolapse in progressive systemic sclerosis. *Dis Colon Rectum* 1993;36:182.

197. Leroi A-M, Michot F, Grise P, et al. Effect of sacral nerve stimulation in patients with fecal and urinary incontinence. *Dis Colon Rectum* 2001;44:779.

198. Lestár B, Penninckx FM, Kerremans RP. Defecometry. a new method for determining the parameters of rectal evacuation. *Dis Colon Rectum* 1989;32:197.

199. Levi AC, Borghi F, Garavoglia M. Development of the anal canal muscles. *Dis Colon Rectum* 1991;34:262.

200. Levitt MA, Soffer SZ, Peña A. Continent appendicostomy in the bowel management of fecally incontinent children. *J Pediatr Surg* 1997;32:1630.

201. Loening-Baucke VA. Abnormal rectoanal function in children recovered from chronic constipation and encopresis. *Gastroenterology* 1984;87:1299.

202. Loening-Baucke V. Factors determining outcome in children with chronic constipation and faecal soiling. *Gut* 1989;30:999.

203. Lou MA, Johnson AP, Atik M, et al. Exteriorized repair in the management of colon injuries. *Arch Surg* 1981;116:926.

204. Louw JH. Congenital abnormalities of the rectum and anus. *Curr Probl Surg* 1965;May:1.

205. MacArthur C, Bick D, Keighley MRB. Incidence, morbidity, and obstetric factors in childbirth-related faecal incontinence. *Br J Surg* 1996;83[Suppl 1]:42.

206. MacLeod JH. Biofeedback in the management of partial anal incontinence: a preliminary report. *Dis Colon Rectum* 1979;22:169.

207. MacLeod JH. Management of anal incontinence by biofeedback. *Gastroenterology* 1987;93:291.

208. Madoff RD, Baeten CGMI, Christiansen J, et al. Standards for anal sphincter replacement. *Dis Colon Rectum* 1998;43: 135.

209. Malone PS, Ransley PG, Kiely EM. Preliminary report: the antegrade continence enema. *Lancet* 1990;336:1217.

210. Malouf AJ, Vaizey CJ, Norton CS, et al. Internal anal sphincter augmentation for fecal incontinence using injectable silicone biomaterial. *Dis Colon Rectum* 2001;44:595.

211. Mandelstam DA. Faecal incontinence: social and economic factors. In: Henry MM, Swash M, eds. *Coloproctology and the pelvic floor.* London: Butterworth, 1985:217.

212. Mander JB, Abercrombie JF, George BD, et al. The electrically stimulated gracilis neosphincter incorporated as part of total anorectal reconstruction after abdominoperineal excision of the rectum. *Ann Surg* 1996;224:702.

213. Mathias JR, Sninsky CA, Millar HD, et al. Development of an improved multi-pressure-sensor probe for recording muscle contraction in human intestine. *Dig Dis Sci* 1985; 30:119.

214. Matsuoka H, Mavrantonis C, Wexner SD, et al. Postanal repair for fecal incontinence: is it worthwhile? *Dis Colon Rectum* 2000;43:1561.

215. Matzel KE, Madoff RD, LaFontaine LJ, et al. Complications of dynamic graciloplasty: incidence, management, and impact on outcome. *Dis Colon Rectum* 2001;44:1427.

216. Matzel KE, Schmidt RA, Tanagho EA. Neuroanatomy of the striated muscular anal continence mechanism: implications for the use of neurostimulation. *Dis Colon Rectum* 1990;33:666.

217. Matzel KE, Stadelmaier U, Hohenfellner M, et al. Electrical stimulation of sacral nerves for treatment of faecal incontinence. *Lancet* 1995;346:1124.

218. Matzel KE, Stadelmaier U, Hohenfellner M, et al. Chronic sacral spinal nerve stimulation for fecal incontinence: long-term results with foramen and cuff electrodes. *Dis Colon Rectum* 2001;44:59.

219. McHugh SM, Diamant NE. Effect of age, gender, and parity on anal canal pressures: contribution of impaired anal sphincter function to fecal incontinence. *Dig Dis Sci* 1987; 32:726.

220. Michot F, Costaglioli B, Leroi A-M, et al. Artificial anal sphincter in severe fecal incontinence: outcome of prospective experience with 37 patients in one institution. *Ann Surg* 2003;237:52.

221. Michot F, Costaglioli B, Leroi AM, et al. Fecal incontinence: artificial anal sphincter in severe anal incontinence. Outcome of prospective experience with 42 patients in one institution. *Dis Colon Rectum* 2002;45:A34-A36.

222. Miller R, Bartolo DCC, Cervero F, et al. Anorectal temperature sensation: a comparison of normal and incontinent patients. *Br J Surg* 1987;74:511.

223. Miller R, Bartolo DCC, Cervero F, et al. Anorectal sampling: a comparison of normal and incontinent patients. *Br J Surg* 1988;75:44.

224. Miller R, Bartolo DCC, James D, et al. Air-filled microballoon manometry for use in anorectal physiology. *Br J Surg* 1989;76:72.

225. Miller R, Bartolo DCC, Locke-Edmunds JCC, et al. Prospective study of conservative and operative treatment for faecal incontinence. *Br J Surg* 1988;75:101.

226. Miller R, Bartolo DCC, Roe A, et al. Anal sensation and the continence mechanism. *Dis Colon Rectum* 1988;31:433.

227. Miller R, Bartolo DCC, Roe AM, et al. Assessment of microtransducers in anorectal manometry. *Br J Surg* 1988; 75:40.

228. Miller R, Lewis GT, Bartolo DCC, et al. Sensory discrimination and dynamic activity in the anorectum: evidence using a new ambulatory technique. *Br J Surg* 1988;75:1003.

229. Miller R, Orrom WJ, Cornes H, et al. Anterior sphincter plication and levatorplasty in the treatment of faecal incontinence. *Br J Surg* 1989;76:1058.

230. Molnar D, Taitz LS, Urwin OM, et al. Anorectal manometry results in defecation disorders. *Arch Dis Child* 1983;58:257.

231. Mortensen N, Humphreys MS. The anal continence plug: a disposable device for patients with anorectal incontinence. *Lancet* 1991;338:295.

232. Motson RW. Sphincter injuries: indications for, and results of sphincter repair. *Br J Surg* 1985;72:S19.

233. Musicco N. Encopresis: a good result in a boy with UTP (uridine-5-triphosphate). *Am J Proctol* 1977;28:43.

234. Nazir M, Carlsen E, Jacobsen AF, et al. Is there any correlation between objective anal testing, rupture grade, and bowel symptoms after primary repair of obstetric anal sphincter rupture: an observational cohort study. *Dis Colon Rectum* 2002;45:1325.

235. Nazir M, Stien R, Carlsen E. Early evaluation of bowel symptoms after primary repair of obstetric perineal rupture is misleading: an observational cohort study. *Dis Colon Rectum* 2003;46:1245.

236. Neill ME, Parks AG, Swash M. Physiological studies of the anal sphincter musculature in faecal incontinence and rectal prolapse. *Br J Surg* 1981;68:531.

237. Nelson R, Furner S, Jesudason V. Fecal incontinence in Wisconsin nursing homes: prevalence and associations. *Dis Colon Rectum* 1998;41:122.

238. Nelson R, Norton N, Cautley E, et al. Community-based prevalence of anal incontinence. *JAMA* 1995;274:559.

239. Nessim A, Wexner SD, Agachan F, et al. Is bowel confinement necessary after anorectal reconstructive surgery? A prospective, randomized, surgeon-blinded trial. *Dis Colon Rectum* 1999;42:16.

240. Nichols RL, Broido P, Condon RE, et al. Effect of preoperative neomycin-erythromycin intestinal preparation on the incidence of infectious complications following colon surgery. *Ann Surg* 1973;178:453.

241. Nielsen MB, Dammegaard L, Pedersen JF. Endosonographic assessment of the anal sphincter after surgical reconstruction. *Dis Colon Rectum* 1994;37:434.

242. Niriella DA, Deen KI. Neosphincters in the management of faecal incontinence. *Br J Surg* 2000;87:1617.

243. Nowacki MP, Towpik E. Reconstruction of the anus, rectovaginal septum, and distal part of the vagina after postirradiation necrosis: report of a unique case. *Dis Colon Rectum* 1988;31:632.

244. O'Brien PE, Skinner S. Restoring control: the Acticon neosphincter artificial bowel sphincter in the treatment of anal incontinence. *Dis Colon Rectum* 2000;43:1213.

245. Olness K, McFarland FA, Piper J. Biofeedback: a new modality in the management of children with fecal soiling. *J Pediatr* 1980;86:505.

246. Onishi K, Maruyama Y, Shiba T. A wrap-around procedure using the gluteus maximus muscle for the functional reconstruction of the sphincter in a case of anal incontinence. *Acta Chir Plast* 1989;31:56.

247. Oreskovich MR, Carrico CJ, Baker LW. Complications of penetrating colon injury. *Infect Surg* 1983;2:101.

248. Orrom WJ, Miller R, Cornes H, et al. Comparison of anterior sphincteroplasty and postanal repair in the treatment of idiopathic fecal incontinence. *Dis Colon Rectum* 1991;34:305.

249. Orrom WJ, Williams JG, Rothenberger DA, et al. Portable anorectal manometry. *Br J Surg* 1990;77:876.

250. Orrom WJ, Wong WD, Rothenberger DA, et al. Evaluation of an air-filled microballoon and mini-transducer in the clinical practice of anorectal manometry: preliminary communication. *Dis Colon Rectum* 1990;33:594.

251. Ortiz H, Armendariz P, DeMiguel M, et al. Complications and functional outcome following artificial anal sphincter implantation. *Br J Surg* 2002;89:877.

252. Owens-Stively J, McCain D, Wynne E. *Childhood constipation and soiling: a practical guide for parents and children.* Minneapolis, MN: Minneapolis Children's Medical Center, 1986.

253. Pager CK, Solomon MJ, Rex J, et al. Long-term outcomes of pelvic floor exercises and biofeedback treatment for patients with fecal incontinence. *Dis Colon Rectum* 2002;45:997.

254. Parellada CM, Miller AS, Williamson MER, et al. Paradoxical high anal resting pressures in men with idiopathic fecal seepage. *Dis Colon Rectum* 1998;41:593.

255. Parker SC, Spencer MP, Madoff RD, et al. Artificial bowel sphincter: long-term experience at a single institution. *Dis Colon Rectum* 2003;46:722.

256. Parks AG. Anorectal incontinence. *Proc R Soc Med* 1975; 68:681.

257. Parks AG. Postanal pelvic floor repair (and the treatment of anorectal incontinence). In: Todd IA, ed. *Operative surgery: fundamental international techniques.* London: Butterworth, 1977:249.

258. Parks AG, Percy J. Postanal pelvic floor repair for anorectal incontinence. In: Todd IP, Fielding LP, eds. *Rob and Smith's operative surgery.* London: Butterworth, 1983:433.

259. Parks AG, Porter NH, Hardcastle JD. The syndrome of the descending perineum. *Proc R Soc Med* 1966;59:477.

260. Parks AG, Porter NH, Melzak J. Experimental study of the reflex mechanism controlling the muscles of the pelvic floor. *Dis Colon Rectum* 1962;5:407.

261. Pearl RK, Prasad ML, Nelson RL, et al. Bilateral gluteus maximus transposition for anal incontinence. *Dis Colon Rectum* 1991;34:478.

262. Pennenckx FM, Lestár B, Kerremans RP. A new balloon-retaining test for evaluation of anorectal function in incontinent patients. *Dis Colon Rectum* 1989;32:202.

263. Perry JD, Hullett LT. The role of home trainers in Kegel's exercise program for the treatment of incontinence. *Ostomy Wound Manage* 1990;17:30.

264. Perry RE, Blatchford GJ, Christensen MA, et al. Manometric diagnosis of anal sphincter injuries. *Am J Surg* 1990; 159:112.

265. Pescatori M, Anastasio G, Bottini C, et al. New grading and scoring for anal incontinence: evaluation of 335 patients. *Dis Colon Rectum* 1992;35:482.

266. Pescatori M, Pavesio R, Anastasio G, et al. Transanal electrostimulation for fecal incontinence: clinical, psychologic, and manometric prospective study. *Dis Colon Rectum* 1991;34:540.

267. Pezim ME, Spencer RJ, Stanhope CR, et al. Sphincter repair for fecal incontinence after obstetrical or iatrogenic injury. *Dis Colon Rectum* 1987;30:521.

268. Pickrell KL, Broadbent TR, Masters FW, et al. Construction of a rectal sphincter and restoration of anal continence by transplanting gracilis muscle: report of four cases in children. *Ann Surg* 1952;135:853.

269. Pinedo G, Vaizey CJ, Nicholls RJ, et al. Results of repeat anal sphincter repair. *Br J Surg* 1999;86:66.

270. Pinho M, Hosie K, Bielecki K, et al. Assessment of noninvasive intra-anal electromyography to evaluate sphincter function. *Dis Colon Rectum* 1991;34:69.

271. Pittman RD, Medwell SJ, Friend WG. A method for determining fecal continence prior to closure of colostomy. *Surg Gynecol Obstet* 1985;161:389.

272. Poen AC, Felt-Bersma RJF, Strijers RLM, et al. Third-degree obstetric perineal tear: long-term clinical and functional results after primary repair. *Br J Surg* 1998; 85:1433.

273. Pollack J, Zetterström J, Lopez A, et al. Subsequent vaginal deliveries increase the risk for persistent anal incontinence after repair of sphincter injuries. *Dis Colon Rectum* 2001; 44:A27-A59.

274. Porter NH. A physiological study of the pelvic floor in rectal prolapse. *Ann R Coll Surg Engl* 1962;31:379.

275. Prager E. The continent colostomy. *Dis Colon Rectum* 1984;27:235.

276. Preston DM, Lennard-Jones JE, Thomas BM. The balloon proctogram. *Br J Surg* 1984;71:29.

277. Prochiantz A, Gross P. Gluteal myoplasty for sphincter replacement: principles, results and prospects. *J Pediatr Surg* 1982;17:25.

278. Rasmussen O, Christensen B, Srensen M, et al. Rectal compliance in the assessment of patients with fecal incontinence. *Dis Colon Rectum* 1990;33:650.

279. Read NW, Abouzekry L. Why do patients with faecal impaction have fecal incontinence? *Gut* 1986;27:283.

280. Read NW, Bartolo DCC, Read MG. Differences in anal function in patients with continence to solids and in patients with incontinence to liquids. *Br J Surg* 1984;71:39.

281. Read NW, Bartolo DCC, Read MG, et al. Differences in anorectal manometry between patients with haemorrhoids

and patients with descending perineum syndrome: implications for management. *Br J Surg* 1983;70:656.

282. Read NW, Harford WV, Schmulen AC, et al. A clinical study of patients with fecal incontinence and diarrhea. *Gastroenterology* 1979;76:747.

283. Read NW, Sun WM. Reflex anal dilatation: effect of parting the buttocks on anal function in normal subjects and patients with anorectal and spinal disease. *Gut* 1991;32:670.

284. Rex DK, Lappas JC, Popp B. Association of anterior ectopic anus and partial absence of musculature in a woman with impaired defecation: report of a case. *Dis Colon Rectum* 1990;33:974.

285. Rieger NA, Sweeney JL, Hoffmann DC, et al. Investigation of fecal incontinence with endoanal ultrasound. *Dis Colon Rectum* 1996;39:860.

286. Roberts PL, Coller JA, Schoetz DJJr, et al. Manometric assessment of patients with obstetric injuries and fecal incontinence. *Dis Colon Rectum* 1990;33:16.

287. Rockwood TH, Church JM, Fleshman JW, et al. Patient and surgeon ranking of the severity of symptoms associated with fecal incontinence: the Fecal Incontinence Severity Index. *Dis Colon Rectum* 1999;42:1525.

288. Rockwood TH, Church JM, Fleshman JW, et al. Fecal incontinence quality of life scale: quality of life instument for patients with fecal incontinence. *Dis Colon Rectum* 2000; 43:9.

289. Roe AM, Bartolo DCC, Mortensen NJMC. New method for assessment of anal sensation in various anorectal disorders. *Br J Surg* 1986;73:310.

290. Rogers J, Hayward MP, Henry MM, et al. Temperature gradient between the rectum and the anal canal: evidence against the role of temperature sensation as a sensory modality in the anal canal of normal subjects. *Br J Surg* 1988;75:1083.

291. Rogers J, Laurberg S, Misiewicz JJ, et al. Anorectal physiology validated: a repeatability study of the motor and sensory tests of anorectal function. *Br J Surg* 1989;76:607.

292. Roig JV, Villoslada C, Lledó S, et al. Prevalence of pudendal neuropathy in fecal incontinence: results of a prospective study. *Dis Colon Rectum* 1995;38:952.

293. Rongen M-J GM, Uludag O, Naggar KE, et al. Long-term follow-up of dynamic gracilloplasty for fecal incontinence. *Dis Colon Rectum* 2003;46:716.

294. Rosenberg AJ, Vela AR. A new simplified technique for pediatric anorectal manometry. *Pediatrics* 1983;71:240.

295. Rothbarth J, Bemelman WA, Meijerink WJHJ, et al. What is the impact of fecal incontinence on quality of life? *Dis Colon Rectum* 2001;44:67.

296. Rudd WWH. Anal incontinence [Symposium]. *Dis Colon Rectum* 1982;25:97.

297. Rullier E, Zerbib F, Laurent C, et al. Morbidity and functional outcome after double dynamic gracilloplasty for anorectal reconstruction. *Br J Surg* 2000;87:909.

298. Russell TR, Gallagher DM. Low rectovaginal fistulas. *Am J Surg* 1977;134:13.

299. Ryhammer AM, Bek KM, Laurberg S. Multiple vaginal deliveries increase the risk of permanent incontinence of flatus and urine in normal premenopausal women. *Dis Colon Rectum* 1995;38:1206.

300. Ryhammer AM, Laurberg S, Hermann AP. Long-term effect of vaginal deliveries on anorectal function in normal perimenopausal women. *Dis Colon Rectum* 1996;39:852.

301. Sainio AP, Halme LE, Husa AI. Anal encirclement with polypropylene mesh for rectal prolapse and incontinence. *Dis Colon Rectum* 1991;34:905.

302. Sainio AP, Voutilainen PE, Husa AI. Recovery of anal sphincter function following transabdominal repair of rectal prolapse: cause of improved continence? *Dis Colon Rectum* 1991;34:816.

303. Salmons S, Henriksson J. The adaptive response of skeletal muscle to increased use. *Muscle Nerve* 1981;4:94.

304. Sangalli MR, Marti MC. Results of sphincter repair in postobstetric fecal incontinence. *J Am Coll Surg* 1994;179:583.

305. Sangwan YP, Coller JA, Barrett RC, et al. Can manometric parameters predict response to biofeedback therapy in fecal incontinence? *Dis Colon Rectum* 1995;38:1021.

306. Sangwan YP, Coller JA, Barrett RC, et al. Prospective comparative study of abnormal distal rectoanal excitatory reflex, pudendal nerve terminal motor latency, and single fiber density as markers of pudendal neuropathy. *Dis Colon Rectum* 1996;39:794.

307. Scheur M, Kuijpers HC, Bleijenberg G. Effect of electrostimulation on sphincter function in neurogenic fecal continence. *Dis Colon Rectum* 1994;37:590.

308. Scheuer M, Kuijpers HC, Jacobs PP. Postanal repair restores anatomy rather than function. *Dis Colon Rectum* 1989;32:960.

309. Schiller LR, Santa Ana CA, Schumulen AC, et al. Pathogenesis of fecal incontinence in diabetes mellitus: evidence for internal-anal sphincter dysfunction. *N Engl J Med* 1982; 307:1666.

310. Schouten WR, van Vroonhoven TJ. A simple method of anorectal manometry. *Dis Colon Rectum* 1983;26:721.

311. Schuster MM. Clinical significance of motor disturbances of the enterocolonic segment. *Am J Dig Dis* 1966;11:320.

312. Schuster MM. Motor action of rectum and anal sphincters in continence and defecation. In: Code CR, ed. *Handbook of physiology: a critical, comprehensive presentation of physiological knowledge and concepts*, sect 6, vol. 4. Baltimore: Williams & Wilkins, 1968:2121.

313. Schuster MM. The riddle of the sphincters. *Gastroenterology* 1975;69:249.

314. Schuster MM, Mendeloff AI. Characteristics of rectosigmoid motor function: their relationship to continence, defecation and disease. In: Glass GBJ, ed. *Progress in gastroenterology*, vol. 2. New York: Grune and Stratton, 1970: 200.

315. Schuster MM, Hendrix TR, Mendeloff AI. The internal anal sphincter response: manometric studies on its normal physiology, neural pathways, and alteration in bowel disorders. *J Clin Invest* 1963;42:196.

316. Schuster MM, Hookman P, Hendrix TR, et al. Simultaneous manometric recording of internal and external anal sphincteric reflexes. *Bull Johns Hopkins Hosp* 1965;116:9.

317. Scott A, Hawley PR, Phillips RKS. Results of external sphincter repair in Crohn's disease. *Br J Surg* 1989;76:959.

318. Scott ADN, Henry MM, Phillips RKS. Clinical assessment and anorectal manometry before postanal repair: failure to predict outcome. *Br J Surg* 1990;77:629.

319. Seccia M, Menconi C, Balestri R, et al. Study protocols and functional results in 86 electrostimulated gracilloplasties. *Dis Colon Rectum* 1994;37:897.

320. Sentovich SM, Rivela LJ, Thorson AG, et al. Simultaneous dynamic proctography and peritoneography for pelvic floor disorders. *Dis Colon Rectum* 1995;38:912.

321. Shafik A. A new concept of the anatomy of the anal sphincter mechanism and the physiology of defecation: the external anal sphincter: a triple-loop system. *Invest Urol* 1975; 12:412.

322. Shafik A. Perineal injection of autologous fat for treatment of sphincteric incontinence. *Dis Colon Rectum* 1995;38: 583.

323. Shafik A. The posterior approach in the treatment of pudendal canal syndrome. *Coloproctology* 1992;5:310.

324. Shafik A. Pudendal canal decompression in the treatment of idiopathic fecal incontinence. *Dig Surg* 1992;9:265.

325. Shafik A. Pudendal canal syndrome: description of a new syndrome and its treatment: report of seven cases. *Coloproctology* 1991;2:102.

326. Silber DL. Encopresis: discussion of etiology and management. *Clin Pediatr* 1969;8:225.

327. Simmang C, Birnbaum EH, Kodner IJ, et al. Anal sphincter reconstruction in the elderly: does advancing age affect outcome. *Dis Colon Rectum* 1994;37:1065.

328. Sitzler PJ, Thomson JPS. Overlap repair of damaged anal sphincter: a single surgeon's series. *Dis Colon Rectum* 1996; 39:1356.

329. Skef Z, Radhakrishnan J, Reyes HM. Anorectal continence following sphincter reconstruction utilizing the gluteus maximus muscle: a case report. *J Pediatr Surg* 1983;18:779.

330. Slade MS, Goldberg SM, Schottler JL, et al. Sphincteroplasty for acquired anal incontinence. *Dis Colon Rectum* 1977;20:33.

331. Solomon MJ, Pager CK, Rex J, et al. Randomized, controlled trial of biofeedback with anal manometry, transanal ultrasound, or pelvic floor retraining with digital guidance alone in the treatment of mild to moderate fecal incontinence. *Dis Colon Rectum* 2003;46:703.

332. Snooks SJ, Henry MM, Swash M. Anorectal incontinence and rectal prolapse: differential assessment of the innervation to puborectalis and external anal sphincter muscles. *Gut* 1985;26:470.

333. Snooks SJ, Henry MM, Swash M. Faecal incontinence due to external anal sphincter division in childbirth is associated with damage to the innervation of the pelvic floor musculature: a double pathology. *Br J Obstet Gynaecol* 1985;92:824.

334. Snooks SJ, Swash M. Nerve stimulation techniques. In: Henry MM, Swash M, eds. *Coloproctology and the pelvic floor.* London: Butterworth, 1985:112.

335. Snooks SJ, Swash M, Henry M. Electrophysiologic and manometric assessment of failed postanal repair for anorectal incontinence. *Dis Colon Rectum* 1984;27:733.

336. Snooks SJ, Swash M, Henry MM. Risk factors in childbirth causing damage to the pelvic floor innervation. *Br J Surg* 1985;72:15.

337. Snooks SJ, Swash M, Henry MM, et al. Risk factors in childbirth causing damage to the pelvic floor innervation. *Int J Colorectal Dis* 1986;1:20.

338. Snooks SJ, Swash M, Setchell M, et al. Injury to innervation of pelvic floor sphincter musculature in childbirth. *Lancet* 1984;2:546.

339. Sørenson M, Tetzschner T, Rasmussen O, et al. Viscous fluid retention: a new method for evaluating anorectal function. *Dis Colon Rectum* 1992;35:357.

340. Speakman CTM, Kamm MA. The internal anal sphincter: new insights into faecal incontinence. *Gut* 1991;32:345.

341. Stone HB. Plastic operation for anal incontinence. *Trans South Surg Assoc* 1928;41:235.

342. Stone HB. Plastic operation for anal incontinence. *Arch Surg* 1929;18:845.

343. Stone HB, McLanahan S. Results with the fascia plastic operation for anal incontinence. *Ann Surg* 1941;114:73.

344. Stricker JW, Schoetz DJ, Jr, Coller JA, et al. Surgical correction of anal incontinence. *Dis Colon Rectum* 1988;31:533.

345. Sultan AH, Kamm MA, Hudson CN, et al. Anal-sphincter disruption during vaginal delivery. *N Engl J Med* 1993;329:1905.

346. Sultan AH, Kamm MA, Talbot IC, et al. Anal endosonography for identifying external sphincter defects confirmed histologically. *Br J Surg* 1994;81:463.

347. Sultan AH, Loder PB, Bartram CI, et al. Vaginal endosonography: new approach to image the undisturbed anal sphincter. *Dis Colon Rectum* 1994;37:1296.

348. Sun WM, Read NW, Miner PB. Relation between rectal sensation and anal function in normal subjects and patients with faecal incontinence. *Gut* 1990;31:1056.

349. Svenberg T, Linderoth B. Easy peroperative classification of perianal muscle as external or internal sphincter by means of diathermy. *Dis Colon Rectum* 1988;31:979.

350. Swash M. Anorectal incontinence: electrophysiological tests. *Br J Surg* 1985:14.

351. Swash M, Snooks SJ. Electromyography in pelvic floor disorders. In: Henry MM, Swash M, eds. *Coloproctology and the pelvic floor.* London: Butterworth, 1985:88.

352. Takahashi T, Garcia-Osogobio S, Valdovinos MA, et al. Extended two-year results of radio-frequency energy delivery for the treatment of fecal incontinence (the Secca procedure). *Dis Colon Rectum* 2003;46:711.

353. Takahashi T, Garcia-Osogobio S, Valdovinos MA, et al. Radio-frequency energy delivery to the anal canal for the treatment of fecal incontinence. *Dis Colon Rectum* 2002;45:915.

354. Tancer ML, Lasser D, Rosenblum N. Rectovaginal fistula or perineal and anal sphincter disruption, or both, after vaginal delivery. *Surg Gynecol Obstet* 1990;171:43.

355. Taverner D, Smiddy FG. An electromyographic study of the normal function of the external anal sphincter and pelvic diaphragm. *Dis Colon Rectum* 1959;2:153.

356. Tighe M, Taylor BA, Johnson MA. Fecal incontinence: emergency repair of obstetric injury to the anal sphincters: a role for the colorectal surgeon. *Dis Colon Rectum* 2002;45:A34-A36.

357. Thomson JPS. Anal sphincter incompetence. In: Russell RCG, ed. *Recent advances in surgery.* London: Churchill Livingstone, 1986:155.

358. Tjandra JJ, Han WR, Goh J, et al. Direct repair vs. overlapping sphincter repair: a randomized, controlled trial. *Dis Colon Rectum* 2003;46:937.

359. Tjandra JJ, Milsom JW, Schroeder T, et al. Endoluminal ultrasound is preferable to electromyography in mapping anal sphincteric defects. *Dis Colon Rectum* 1993;36:689.

360. Ulludag O, Dejong CHC, Maastricht CGMIB. Fecal incontinence: sacral neuromodulation for faecal incontinence. *Dis Colon Rectum* 2002;45:A34-A36.

361. van Tets WF, Kuijpers JHC, Bleijenberg G. Biofeedback treatment is ineffective in neurogenic fecal incontinence. *Dis Colon Rectum* 1996;39:992.

362. Varma JS, Smith AN. Reproducibility of the proctometrogram. *Gut* 1986;27:288.

363. Venkatesh KS, Ramanujam PS, Larson DM, et al. Anorectal complications of vaginal delivery. *Dis Colon Rectum* 1989;32:1039.

364. Vernava AM III, Longo WE, Daniel GL. Pudendal neuropathy and the importance of EMG evaluation of fecal incontinence. *Dis Colon Rectum* 1993;36:23.

365. Versluis PJ, Konsten J, Geerdes B, et al. Defecographic evaluation of dynamic graciloplasty for fecal incontinence. *Dis Colon Rectum* 1995;38:468.

366. Voyvodic F, Rieger NA, Skinner S, et al. Endosonographic imaging of anal sphincter injury: does the size of the tear correlate with the degree of dysfunction? *Dis Colon Rectum* 2003;46:735.

367. Wald A. Use of biofeedback in treatment of fecal incontinence in patients with meningomyelocele. *Pediatrics* 1981;68:45.

368. Wald A. Biofeedback therapy for fecal incontinence. *Ann Intern Med* 1981;95:146.

369. Wald A, Tunuguntla AK. Anorectal sensorimotor dysfunction in fecal incontinence and diabetes mellitus: modification with biofeedback therapy. *N Engl J Med* 1984;310:1282.

370. Waylonis GW, Krueger KC. Anal sphincter electromyography in adults. *Arch Phys Med Rehabil* 1970;51:409, 417.

371. Waylonis GW, Powers JJ. Clinical application of anal sphincter electromyography. *Surg Clin North Am* 1972;52:807.

372. Weiss EG, Efron JE, Nogueras JJ, et al. Submucosal injection of carbon coated beads is a successful and safe office-based treatment for fecal incontinence. *Dis Colon Rectum* 2002;45:A46(abst).

373. Weissenberg S. Encopresis. *Z Kinder* 1926;40:674.

374. Wexner SD, Baeten C, Bailey R, et al. Long-term efficacy of dynamic graciloplasty for fecal incontinence. *Dis Colon Rectum* 2002;45:809.

375. Wexner SD, Gonzalez-Padron A, Rius J, et al. Stimulated gracilis neosphincter operation: initial experience, pitfalls, and complications. *Dis Colon Rectum* 1996;39:957.

376. Wexner SD, Marchetti F, Jagelman DG. The role of sphincteroplasty for fecal incontinence reevaluated: a prospective physiologic and functional review. *Dis Colon Rectum* 1991;34:22.

377. Wexner SD, Marchetti F, Salanga VD, et al. Neurophysiologic assessment of the anal sphincters. *Dis Colon Rectum* 1991;34:606.

378. Whitehead WE, Burgio KL, Engel BT. Biofeedback treatment of fecal incontinence in geriatric patients. *J Am Geriatr Soc* 1985;33:320.

379. Whitehead WE, Parker L, Bosmajian LS, et al. Behavioral treatment of fecal incontinence secondary to spina bifida. *Gastroenterology* 1982;82:1209(abst).

380. Williams AB, Bartram CI, Halligan S, et al. Endosonographic anatomy of the normal anal canal compared with endocoil magnetic resonance imaging. *Dis Colon Rectum* 2002;45:176.

381. Williams AB, Bartram CI, Modhwadia D, et al. Endocoil mangetic resonance imaging quantification of external anal sphincter atrophy. *Br J Surg* 2001;88:853.

382. Williams L, Lewis E. Identification of small rectal perforations. *Surg Gynecol Obstet* 1987;164:475.

383. Williams NS, Hallan RI, Koeze TH, et al. Construction of a neoanal sphincter by transposition of the gracilis muscle and prolonged neuromuscular stimulation for the treatment of faecal incontinence. *Ann R Coll Surg Engl* 1990;72:108.

384. Williams NS, Hallan RI, Koeze TH, et al. Restoration of gastrointestinal continuity and continence after abdominoperineal excision of the rectum using an electrically stimulated neoanal sphincter. *Dis Colon Rectum* 1990;33:561.

385. Williams NS, Patel J, George BD, et al. Development of an electrically stimulated neoanal sphincter. *Lancet* 1991;338:1166.

386. Williamson JL, Nelson RL, Orsay C, et al. A comparison of simultaneous longitudinal and radial recordings of anal canal pressures. *Dis Colon Rectum* 1990;33:201.

387. Wise WE Jr, Aguilar PS, Padmanabhan A, et al. Surgical treatment of low rectovaginal fistulas. *Dis Colon Rectum* 1991;34:271.

388. Womack NR, Morrison JFB, Williams NS. The role of pelvic floor denervation in the aetiology of idiopathic faecal incontinence. *Br J Surg* 1986;73:404.

389. Womack NR, Morrison JFB, Williams NS. Prospective study of the effects of postanal repair in neurogenic faecal incontinence. *Br J Surg* 1988;75:48.

390. Wong WD, Congliosi SM, Spencer MP, et al. The safety and efficacy of the artificial bowel sphincter for fecal incontinence: results from a multicenter cohort study. *Dis Colon Rectum* 2002;45:1139.

391. Wong WD, Jensen LL, Bartolo DCC, et al. Artificial anal sphincter. *Dis Colon Rectum* 1996;39:1345.

392. Wreden RR. A method of reconstructing a voluntary sphincter ani. *Arch Surg* 1929;18:841.

393. Wynne JM, Myles JL, Jones I, et al. Disturbed anal sphincter function following vaginal delivery. *Gut* 1996;39:120.

394. Yip B, Barrett RC, Coller JA, et al. Linear pressure profiles and symmetric findings in the stimulated gracilis muscle. *Dis Colon Rectum* 2003;46:77.

395. Yip B, Barrett RC, Coller JA, et al. Pudendal nerve terminal motor latency testing: assessing the educational learning curve: can we teach our own? *Dis Colon Rectum* 2002;45:184.

396. Yoshioka K, Hyland G, Keighley MRB. Physiological changes after postanal repair and parameters predicting outcome. *Br J Surg* 1988;75:1220.

397. Yoshioka K, Keighley MRB. Clinical and manometric assessment of gracilis muscle transplant for fecal incontinence. *Dis Colon Rectum* 1988;31:767.

398. Yoshioka K, Keighley MRB. Critical assessment of the quality of continence after postanal repair for faecal incontinence. *Br J Surg* 1989;76:1054.

399. Yoshioka K, Pinho M, Ortiz J, et al. How reliable is measurement of the anorectal angle by videoproctography? *Dis Colon Rectum* 1991;34:1010.

400. Yuli C, Xueheng Z. Reconstruction of rectal sphincter by transposition of gluteus muscle for fecal incontinence. *J Pediatr Surg* 1987;22:62.

Colorectal Trauma

Guest Contributors: Ronald M. Stewart and Daniel Rosenthal

I have asked two distinguished colleagues to contribute this chapter on colorectal trauma, Drs. Ronald Stewart and Daniel Rosenthal. These two individuals have an enormous personal experience with this subject. Dr. Rosenthal is the Michael E. DeBakey International Professor of Surgery at the Uniformed Services University and Clinical Professor of Surgery at the University of Texas Health Sciences Center in San Antonio. He has been a consultant in colon and rectal surgery to the Surgeon General of the Army. Dr. Stewart is Director of Trauma and Emergency Surgery at the University of Texas Health Sciences Center in San Antonio, as well as Associate Professor of Surgery.

The profession of medicine, and surgery, must always rank as the most noble that men can adopt. The spectacle of a doctor in action among soldiers, in equal danger and with equal courage, saving life where all others are taking it, allaying pain where all others are causing it, is one which must always seem glorious, whether to God or man. It is impossible to imagine any situation from which a human being might better leave this world and embark on the hazards of the unknown.

Winston S. Churchill:
The Story of the Malakand Field Force

Since foemen learned to bare their weapons, the abdomen has always been a target of their murderous endeavors. In the book of Judges 3: 17–25,[1] we are told that Ehud, a man charged to bring Israel's tribute to the King of Moab, tricked the king into seeing him privately. Once alone with the king, in the privacy of the royal toilet, Ehud plunged a cubit-long dagger into the king's abdomen. The entire blade went in, and depending on which translation of the scripture one reads, stool came out of the wound. When the king's servants, worried about their master's absence, entered the "cold chamber," they found the king lying dead on the floor. Ehud's blade must have hit a major vessel causing the king to bleed to death. However, even if the king had been helped within moments of his wounding one can rest assured that no priest, soothsayer, or court physician would have been able to do anything to prevent the king's demise.

Hippocrates regarded all such wounds as deadly, and even Celsus advised that their cure be left to nature.[28] The injury may be caused by blunt or penetrating trauma of the abdomen or perineum. It may result in damage to the intraperitoneal or retroperitoneal bowel, or it may interrupt its blood supply. If the trauma is to the rectum or perineum, the sphincter mechanism may be injured, as may adjacent organs (e.g., bladder, urethra, and vagina).

Armies originally had both a physician general and a surgeon general, but because of the obvious inference concerning the importance of the latter in wartime, only this one term has survived.[112] It is self-evident that most of the literature on penetrating abdominal wounds in general, and colonic injury specifically, have come from experience on the battlefield. However, many of the classic dicta concerning management are not necessarily appropriate today, even with the high-velocity injuries that occur in the civilian population.

The colon is injured in 15% to 39% of penetrating abdominal wounds. It is expected that this will continue to be a pervasive problem in our society because of the frequency of motor vehicle accidents and the ready availability of firearms, especially in the United States. There still remains considerable controversy concerning the appropriate management of colorectal injuries. Therefore, all surgeons who deal with trauma victims should be familiar with the various options and issues in order to make reasoned, intelligent decisions. As with all aspects of the management of acute surgical illnesses, appropriate judgment, skill, and common sense are requisites. It is hoped that this chapter will provide supporting evidence-based guidelines for the diagnosis and treatment of colorectal injuries.

HISTORY

As previously mentioned, the first recorded injury to the colon was described in the Old Testament in the Book of Judges. For centuries, such injuries were untreatable and virtually always resulted in the victim's demise. The first instance of a successful repair of a musket ball injury to the colon was performed in 1831 by Lucien Baudens, a French military surgeon in Algeria.[5] Baudens digitally explored the wound and felt a loop of intestine seemingly hardened by the marked contraction of its muscle coat. Upon pulling his finger out, Baudens noticed that it was covered with feces. He enlarged the abdominal wound and asked the patient to cough. This resulted in a large expulsion of gas from within the peritoneal cavity and caused the injured segment of colon to protrude. The large intestine was noted to have a large, tangential laceration that he repaired with the use of Lembert sutures. The colon was replaced in the abdomen, the abdomen was closed, and the patient recovered. A second patient, operated for an apparently similar injury during the same campaign, died postoperatively. An autopsy revealed the presence of small bowel perforations that escaped Baudens' examination during the laparotomy.

During the American Civil War, penetrating abdominal injuries were treated nonoperatively and were thus associated with a 90% mortality rate. The decision about non-operative intervention was made simply because such injuries were virtually always fatal, regardless of the method of treatment. Furthermore, such a noninterventionist approach was probably based on the fact that surgeons at that time had no good idea of what to do when confronted with such a problem. Still, some military surgeons knew that if the stomach or intestines were divided, there could be no expectation that peritonitis could be averted unless by operative interference. Their recommendation, however, to enlarge the wound and cleanse the cavity to permit unity of the sections of discontinuity went virtually unheeded. In a publication based on the Civil War, one may find the following statement:

> . . . it may fairly be inferred that in all punctured and incised wounds of the intestinal canal attended with protrusion, the safest practice consists in closing the intestinal wound by suture and reducing the protruded viscus, unless its structure is irretrievably disorganized and the adoption of the alternative of establishing a preternatural anus is compulsory. In wounds of the intestine unattended by protrusion, when there is danger of extravasation, the external wound should be enlarged, and the wound and the intestine closed by suture.*

In fact, what usually doomed soldiers afflicted with intestinal perforations was the delay between the time of injury and the treatment, and, of course, the primitive status of visceral surgery.

Encouraged by the success of elective surgery following the introduction of anesthesia and of aseptic surgical technique, World War I surgeons began to operate on casualties suffering from abdominal wounds. The standard at that time was primary repair, a considerable improvement over nonoperative management, but the mortality rate was 60%.

With the advent of World War II came weapons with a much greater potential for creating massive intestinal in-

jury. Primary repair resulted in a prohibitively high rate of sepsis and death. As a consequence, Major General W. Heneage Ogilvie (see Biography, Chapter 16), senior surgical consultant for the British forces in the North African theater, mandated in 1942 that all colonic injuries should be exteriorized or treated with concomitant colostomies.[92] In 1943, the Surgeon General of the American forces in North Africa adopted the same policy.[91] This succeeded in lowering the mortality rate for colonic injury to 35%.

During the Korean conflict and the war in Vietnam, the mortality rate for colonic injuries was reduced still further, to 15% and 10%, respectively. This was largely attributed to the institution of a rapid evacuation system through the use of helicopters, the immediate availability of antibiotics and blood products, and improvement in methods of resuscitation. There was concern, however, about excessive reliance on modern medical technology, in that it appeared to lead to some reports of disastrous results. This led to the call for a return to a more "conservative" approach in the management of intestinal war injuries. For example, in 1970, the Commander-in-Chief of the Pacific (CINPAC) ordered the following:

> Previous recommendations for frequent use of the operation right colectomy and ileotransverse anastomosis for lesions of the right colon are withdrawn, and ileostomy with a distal mucous fistula is recommended. Holes 1 cm or smaller in diameter may be closed primarily.[99]

Following World War II, the combat-trained surgeon returned to civilian life and began to apply the principles of management that had been utilized for colon injuries experienced in warfare. Exteriorization of the injured segment, as well as the use of colostomy, became the standard treatment for all colorectal injuries. However, there was a significant difference in the nature of civilian penetrating injuries in that, at least in those early postwar years, the missiles were of low velocity. Some began to consider, because the injuries were not the same as those seen in war, in some circumstances primary repair could be an appropriate alternative. Numerous studies since the mid-1970s have demonstrated repeatedly that this form of treatment in selective instances may be quite safe.

Today in the United States, a victim of penetrating abdominal trauma is frequently transported to the hospital within a few minutes following injury. Sophisticated radiographic equipment is readily available, as well as intravenous fluids, blood, blood products, and antibiotics. Furthermore, a surgical team, even if not present, can be assembled in a relatively short period of time. Under these conditions, it is little wonder that the mortality rate for civilian colorectal injuries is now less than 5%.

A singular advance in the management of individuals with colonic injuries was made by Stone and Fabian in their 1979 publication in which they conducted a randomized trial of patients meeting so-called "good-risk" criteria.[122] Patients with colonic injuries who were believed to be good risks were randomly allocated to either undergo a primary repair or a colostomy. Fewer septic complications were observed in the former group. This study succeeded in inspiring others to implement primary repair more frequently. Numerous articles have since been published demonstrating the efficacy of primary repair, especially as applied to civilian trauma centers in the United States.[1,4,11,20,22,27,29,37,39,41–43,46,54,56,58,63,64, 74,77,85,88,106,113,114,123,125,132,136]

This trend continued into the 1990s, with numerous contributors advocating primary repair as the objective of management for both civilian and wartime colon injuries.[10,13,14,24,26,69,87,103,111] Furthermore, anastomotic failure rates have been quite low, reinforcing the fact that primary repair, at least today, is the ideal approach for the treatment of colonic injury.

ETIOLOGY AND EVALUATION

Penetrating Trauma

Most colon injuries result from penetrating wounds to the abdomen. Twenty percent of all such wounds are associated with injury to the large bowel. Septic morbidity is a real danger because of the combination of fecal spillage, soft tissue injury, and bleeding, all of which predispose to subsequent infection. Furthermore, gunshot wounds of the colon are typically associated with more tissue destruction and result in an increased number of associated injuries in comparison with stab wounds (Figs. 14-1 through 14-6).

With respect to etiology, it is generally self-evident as to the nature of the causative agent when one is confronted with a penetrating injury to the abdomen. However, how one proceeds with evaluation and treatment is subject to some controversy.

Because gunshot wounds to the abdomen are associated with intraabdominal injury in 95% of instances, there is little argument as to the requirement for laparotomy. This is in contrast to stab wounds of the abdomen, for which the associated intraabdominal injury rate is approximately 50%. Still, some presentations are quite clear. For example, all patients with signs of bleeding or shock or those with signs of peritoneal irritation should undergo laparotomy. Conversely, individuals who harbor wounds that do not penetrate the anterior fascia may be treated on an ambulatory basis. The real controversy, however, arises with respect to the management of stable patients without signs of peritoneal irritation and in whom the wound penetrates the anterior fascia or peritoneum. Under these circumstances, options include the following:

- Immediate exploratory laparotomy
- Diagnostic peritoneal lavage
- Close evaluation with serial abdominal examinations

Laparoscopy

Laparoscopy has also been suggested for the evaluation of patients with penetrating abdominal trauma.[32,35,53,66,108, 115,117,118,143] In stable individuals, laparoscopy is a highly sensitive test for determining peritoneal penetration. It can be particularly helpful for thoracoabdominal wounds in which local exploration may not be possible or may actually be contraindicated. In the intrathoracic abdomen, laparoscopy is sensitive for detecting a diaphragmatic wound, a situation in which observation, diagnostic peritoneal lavage or focused sonography may be wanting.[81] Although laparoscopy is sensitive for determining peritoneal penetration, it should be noted that this technique is not nearly as reliable for determining the presence of intraabdominal injury. Major trauma, particularly hollow viscus injuries, can be easily missed with laparoscopic exploration. Most investigators have cautioned against using laparoscopy for purposes other than determining peritoneal penetration. In summary, laparoscopy is useful in determining peritoneal penetration, particularly for stable patients with thoracoabdominal penetrating wounds and tangential gunshot wounds in whom the suspicion of intraperitoneal penetration is low.

Sonography and Focused Abdominal Sonographic Assessment for Trauma

Focused abdominal sonographic assessment for trauma (FAST) and high-resolution computed tomography (CT) scanning have both been employed as adjuncts to clinical assessment of the abdomen in stable patients with penetrating trauma. These techniques may be useful in the decision-making process as to the advisability of operative or nonoperative intervention in stable patients with penetrating wounds.[17,130]

Blunt Trauma

Blunt trauma to the abdomen is not usually associated with colonic injury; it occurs in fewer than 5% of these cases. Mobile segments of the colon (e.g., cecum, transverse colon, and sigmoid colon) are more susceptible to injury, although other areas of the bowel can be affected. Most perforations are found in the sigmoid colon, an observation that can be explained by its redundancy and tendency to form a closed loop. The right side of the colon, however, is the most common site for devascularizing injuries.[21] These patients are usually victims of motor vehicle accidents and, therefore, commonly have

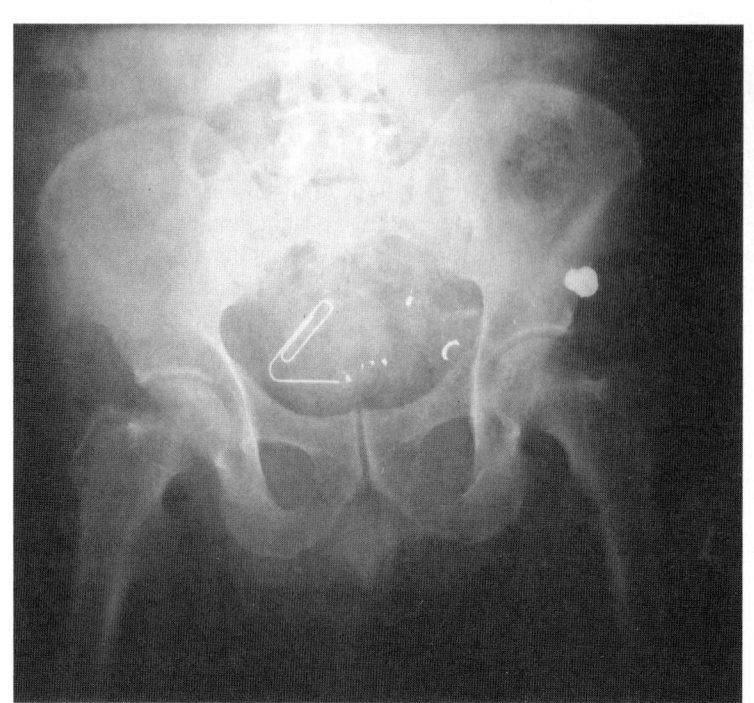

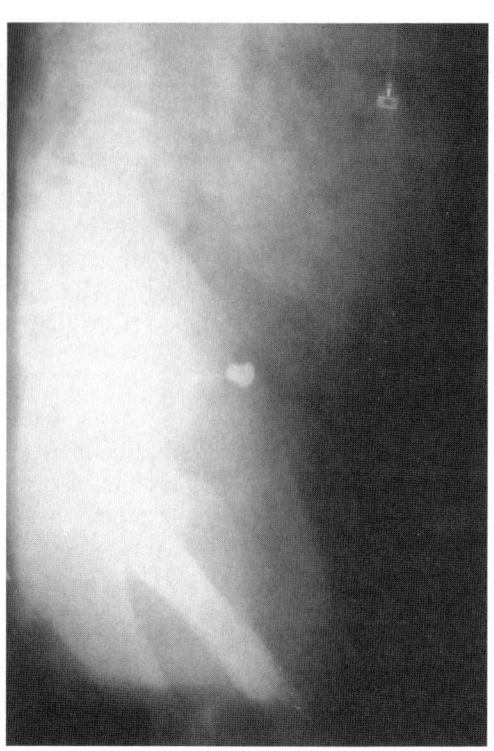

A   B

FIGURE 14-1. Bullet wound of the pelvis. **(A)** High-caliber bullet overlying the left ilium. Metallic fragments are consistent with striking bone. The tip of the paper clip indicates the entrance wound. The bullet traversed the sigmoid colon. **(B)** Lateral view in the same patient.

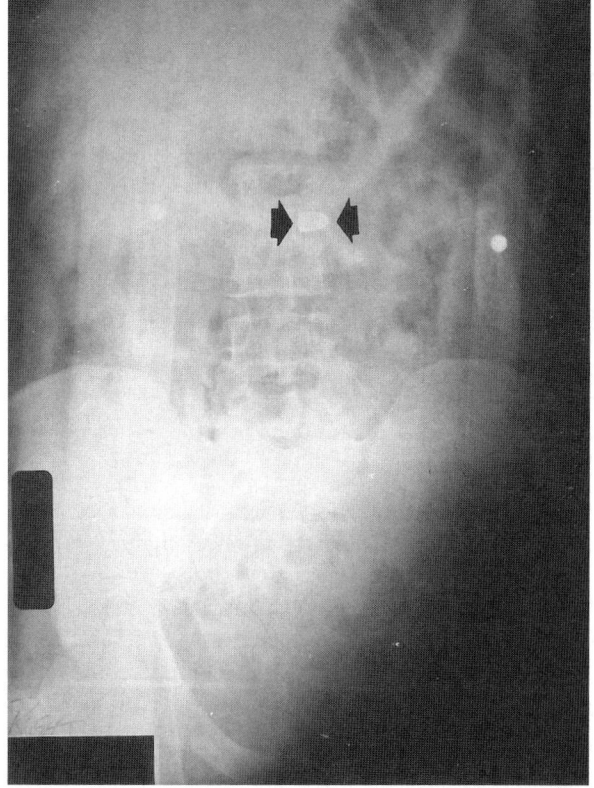

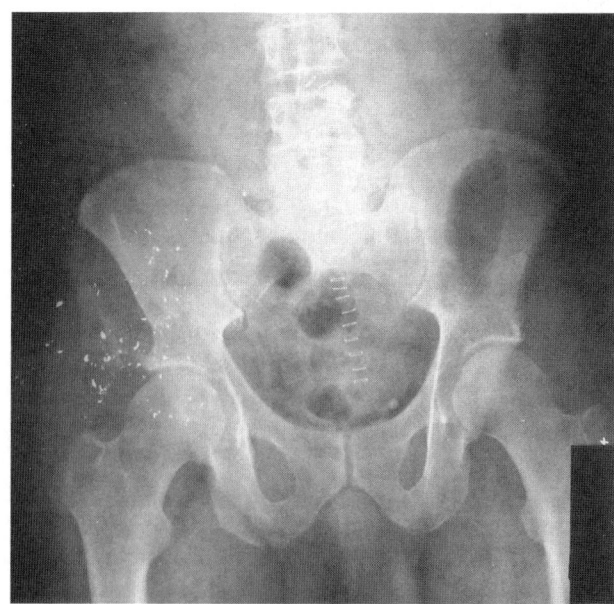

FIGURE 14-2. Bullet wound of the abdomen. The missile can be seen overlying the vertebra *(arrows)*. The missile traversed the transverse colon and the aorta. The patient survived this injury.

FIGURE 14-3. Metallic fragments overlying the right ilium imply that the missile struck bone. The distal small bowel and right colon were virtually vaporized.

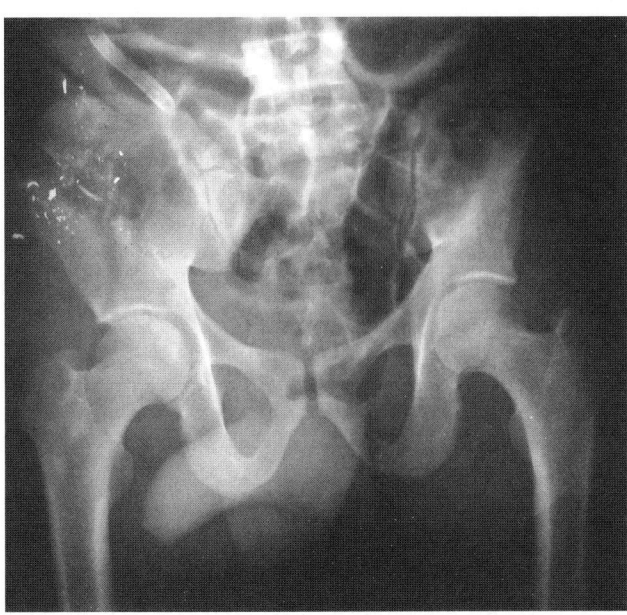

FIGURE 14-4. A similar injury was created from this bullet wound to that noted in Figure 14-3. However, note that the ilium was shattered. The patient also suffered major vessel injury to the right leg.

multisystem and multiorgan injuries (Figure 14-7).[15,21] The use of seat belts seems to be a predisposing factor.[2,6,47,96] Appleby and Nagy caution that a high degree of suspicion should be maintained in individuals who are found to have bruising of the abdominal wall as a consequence of the use of seat belts.[2] These individuals have a high incidence of gastrointestinal injuries and, in addition, associated lumbar spinal injuries.

Bubenik and colleagues describe three patients who sustained blunt colonic injury.[9] In their experience, a characteristic scenario was observed. Perforation was discovered 7 to 10 days following the incident and was indicated by findings suggestive of sepsis. A particularly prominent sign of occult infection was the syndrome of posttraumatic pulmonary insufficiency.

Wisner and co-workers identified 56 individuals who sustained blunt intestinal injury, but only six of these injuries were colonic.[138] As could be expected, most occurred at points of fixation in the proximal and distal small bowel, with devascularization most frequently seen in the ileum and in the sigmoid colon. The same principles of treatment as those discussed with respect to penetrating injuries apply here, but the authors caution that delay in diagnosis is one of the major concerns. They note further that CT was not especially helpful in the preoperative assessment.

Howell and colleagues identified 19 patients who sustained blunt trauma to the colon.[48] They advise that careful inspection of pericolic, subserosal, and mesenteric hematomas at the time of laparotomy is essential to the detection and management of such injuries. Unfortu-

nately, some individuals present many days following the initial injury and are found on exploratory laparotomy to have considerable contamination and sepsis. Under these circumstances, resection or exteriorization is indicated, in addition to a diversionary procedure (see later). As with other types of colonic trauma, infections are the major source of morbidity, but the nature of associated injuries is the principal determinant of survival.[48]

Diagnosis

Fortunately, blunt trauma to the abdomen rarely produces injury to the colon. However, when it occurs, the consequences can be devastating. Alterations in the patient's level of consciousness as well as the presence of associated injury present problems for diagnosis and therapeutic priorities. Peritoneal lavage, CT of the abdomen, and abdominal ultrasonography are all useful adjunctive measures for evaluating patients with such an injury. Of the three, peritoneal lavage is the most sensitive, particularly if it is performed more than 4 hours after the injury. Although the returns may be grossly positive, with stool or blood, or microscopically positive with blood, patients who have small perforations or mesenteric vascular injuries may not demonstrate an abnormality until a few hours following the injury.

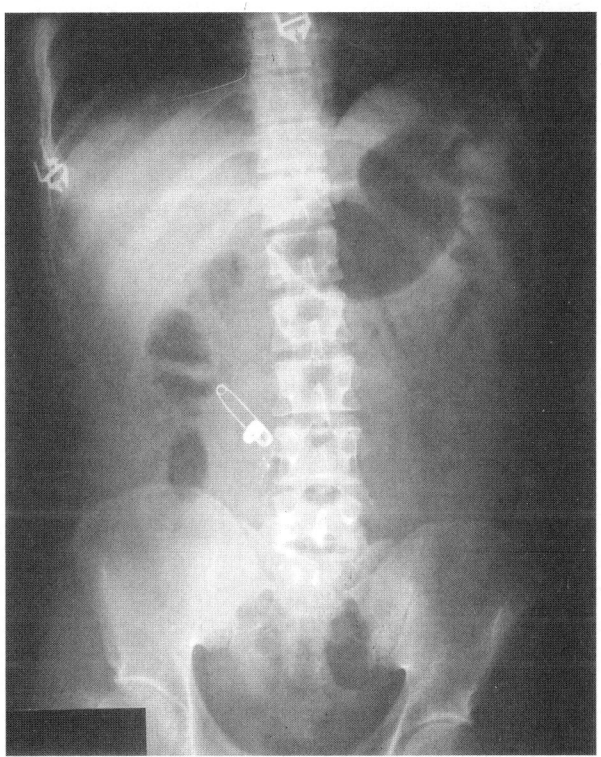

FIGURE 14-5. This bullet traversed the small bowel, the transverse colon, and the vena cava. The entrance wound is marked by a safety pin.

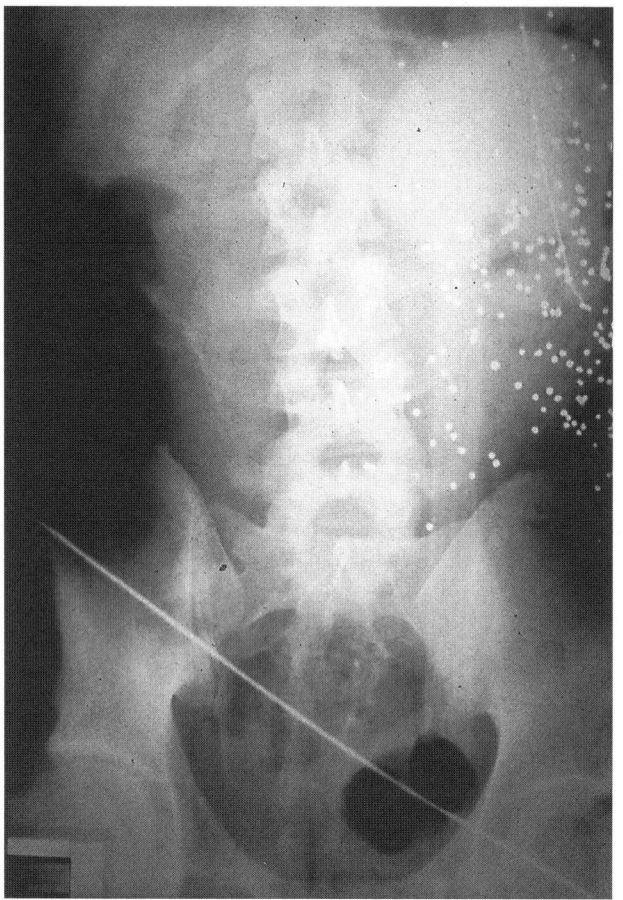

FIGURE 14-6. Shotgun wound to the left upper quadrant resulted in destruction of the splenic flexure, spleen, tail of pancreas, and kidney. Such low-velocity wounds can create devastating injury at close range.

Results of CT and ultrasonography may be difficult to interpret. Certainly, the presence of free fluid without liver and spleen injury is worrisome, as is the presence of mesenteric inflammatory change, edema, or hematoma. In blunt abdominal trauma, the presence of fluid in the peritoneal cavity when the solid organs appear intact on CT scan mandates laparotomy.

Abdominal ultrasonography will not detect an injury to the colon unless sufficient fluid or blood is present. Still, McElveen and Collin found an overall sensitivity of 88% and a 98% specificity when comparing this test with others in individuals with blunt abdominal trauma.[73] Originally very popular in Europe, FAST has gained much wider use in the United States since the mid-1990s, especially for determining the presence of a hemoperitoneum. This study is quite helpful when it is positive; the reported specificity rate is high for detecting hemoperitoneum (in the range of 95% to 100%). When the ultrasound scan is negative, the results are not as beneficial; the reported sensitivity rates range from 42% to 87%. The

wide discrepancy in sensitivities serves to emphasize another potential weakness of the ultrasound examination—that is, operator dependency. Taking this into consideration, the FAST examination is a useful adjunct for abdominal assessment during resuscitation for trauma. It is most helpful in patients with hemodynamic instability and in those who cannot readily be moved.

A large volume of literature supports the use of CT for patient assessment following abdominal trauma. CT scan has been shown to be highly sensitive and specific. However, the Achilles heel of CT scanning has been the presence of a mesenteric tear or an early hollow viscus injury. Still, the newer generation of CT scanners is more sensitive than prior technology, but such injuries can still be missed. A high degree of suspicion with appropriate clinical correlation improves the overall accuracy. Additional signs of colon or small bowel injury include mesenteric hematoma, edema, bowel wall thickening, and as mentioned, the presence of free fluid without evident solid organ injury. Nolan and colleagues opine that physicians should entertain the possibility of mesenteric injury in all patients presenting with blunt abdominal trauma, even if few clinical findings are initially present and/or CT fails to demonstrate a definitive abnormality or injury.[90] Blunt injury in particular requires a high degree of suspicion to minimize the likelihood of missing significant intra peritoneal trauma.

SURGICAL MANAGEMENT

General Principles

Once the decision has been made to perform an exploratory laparotomy, the abdomen is entered through a midline incision. As with all operations in the abdomen, a midline incision is recommended. It is important to preserve the area overlying the rectus muscles, in case a stoma should be required (see Chapter 31). Initial efforts are directed toward identifying and controlling any source of bleeding. An attempt should be made to contain spillage of intestinal contents by means of atraumatic clamps and sponges. Following control of hemorrhage and sources of contamination, a thorough search is made for all possible sites of injury. The entire gastrointestinal tract and mesentery are carefully inspected. Special attention should be given to the number and location of all wounds. Usually, there is an even number of openings in the bowel, compatible with a typical through-and-through injury pattern. However, when an odd number of wounds appears to be the case, the surgeon should make a great effort to look for the "missing hole." The bowel should be carefully reinspected, especially the region adjacent to the mesentery, where breaches of the bowel wall may be hidden. It is suggested that the entire gastroin-

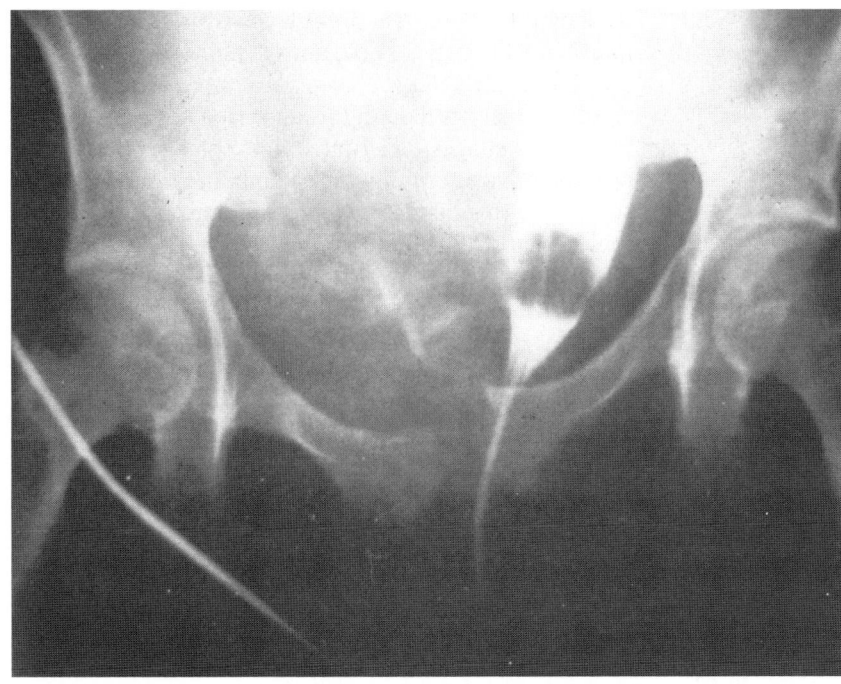

FIGURE 14-7. Motor vehicle accident causing severe blunt trauma resulted in a displaced pelvic fracture. The patient sustained bladder injury as well as major trauma to the sigmoid colon.

testinal tract be inspected twice, even when all wounds appear to be accounted for. Obviously, a missed visceral injury can have catastrophic consequences.

Once the injuries have been identified, the surgeon then proceeds with the repair. When primary repair is attempted, care must be taken to avoid narrowing the lumen; therefore, this is often accomplished in a transverse fashion (Figure 14-8). Whether a two-layer or a single-layer technique is employed is a matter of each individual surgeon's personal preference. When the colon is destroyed or its blood supply is compromised, resection is mandatory (Figure 14-9). If diversion of the fecal stream is required, either the injured segment is brought out to the abdominal wall or a proximal portion of bowel is selected as a colostomy or ileostomy. Meticulous attention should be given to creating a satisfactory stoma; some reports have suggested that complication rates for stomal construction in conditions of trauma are higher than those reported for elective surgery.[94,116,142] This may be attributed to the fact that sufficient attention is not paid to the creation of a satisfactory stoma when the surgeon is dealing with an emergency problem in a critically ill patient (see Chapter 31). It is generally advised that the skin wound be left open or sutures placed for delayed primary repair. Approximately 50% of all primarily closed wounds that are associated with emergency surgery for trauma become infected. Some are potentially life-threatening, necrotizing soft tissue infections. The presence of concomitant shock, soft tissue injury, and fecal contamination creates an environment unlike that of elective colon surgery, one that is much more conducive to the development of overwhelming sepsis.

Operative Alternatives for Treating Penetrating Colonic Injury

The choices of operations are summarized as follows:

Simple closure
Resection with primary anastomosis
Resection with proximal diversion
Exteriorization with repair
Exteriorization of injury site

Many different operative techniques are available for managing the injured colon. However, they can all be classified into one of three primary approaches: fecal diversion, primary repair, or exteriorization repair. Each approach has merit, with each having variable support in the literature. However, it should be noted that proximal diversion alone does not appear on this list. This approach is without merit because feces are likely to continue to contaminate the abdominal cavity through the open bowel wound (see also Chapter 26).

Exteriorization Repair

Exteriorization repair was initially suggested by Mason in 1945.[71] It is a hybrid of primary repair and fecal diversion in which the colon wound is repaired and brought out to the abdominal wall. Subsequently, if the enterotomy closure breaks down, it is then matured into a standard ostomy. However, if it heals, it is then replaced into the peritoneal cavity. Theoretically, exteriorization repair takes advantage of the benefits of the two approaches. It avoids a colostomy for those individuals whose repairs heal,

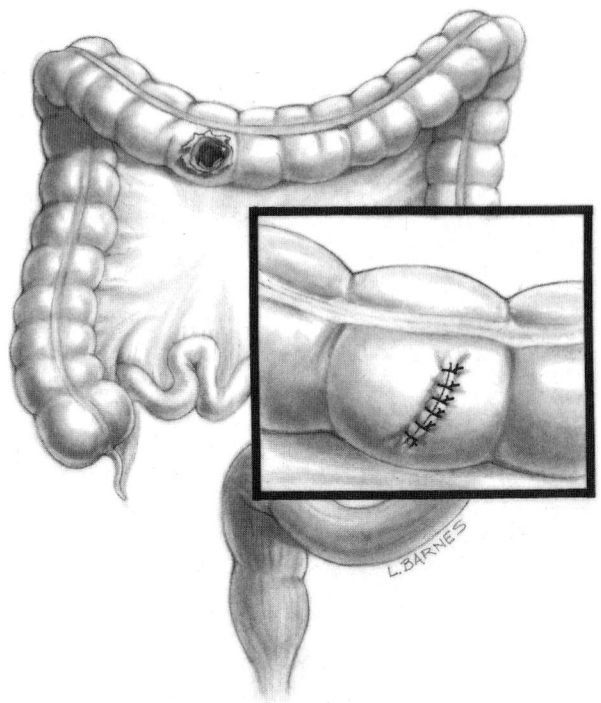

FIGURE 14-8. Artist's concept of a penetrating wound of the transverse colon that is treated by primary closure in a transverse fashion **(inset).**

while at the same time preventing contamination that could result in an anastomotic leak. Although some investigators have recommended this type of approach, conversion rates to an ostomy range between 21% and 50%.[80,127] This is considerably higher than the incidence of clinically significant leaks associated with primary repair.

Another concern is that the technique requires special postoperative management to prevent defecation. This problem leads to breakdown of the wound. Additionally, exteriorization repair does not preclude the possibility of

intraabdominal sepsis. Breakdown with abscess and/or fecal fistula is still possible once the bowel is returned to the abdomen.[64,83]

In summary, although this approach has certain theoretical advantages, exteriorization repair requires more postoperative attention than the other options and is associated with a higher complication rate. Most investigators have abandoned this approach, and, for the purposes of this discussion, it is not recommended.[69]

Fecal Diversion Versus Primary Repair

As mentioned, fecal diversion had been the mainstay of the management of civilian colonic injuries until relatively recently. Mandatory colostomy, even today, is conceptually attractive because it eliminates or at least minimizes the complications associated with the creation of an anastomosis. In 1951, Woodhall and Oschner suggested that primary repair could be appropriately applied to civilian practice.[140] Since that time, a vigorous debate has surrounded the management of colonic injuries. Variables that affect these decisions are summarized as follows:

Factors Predisposing to Increased Morbidity and Mortality

Increased age
Associated organ injury
Multiple blood transfusions
Left colon injury
Preoperative shock
Gross fecal contamination
Delay in initiating therapy
Extensive colonic injury
Questionable viability of the bowel
Requirement for more than one suture line to effect repair

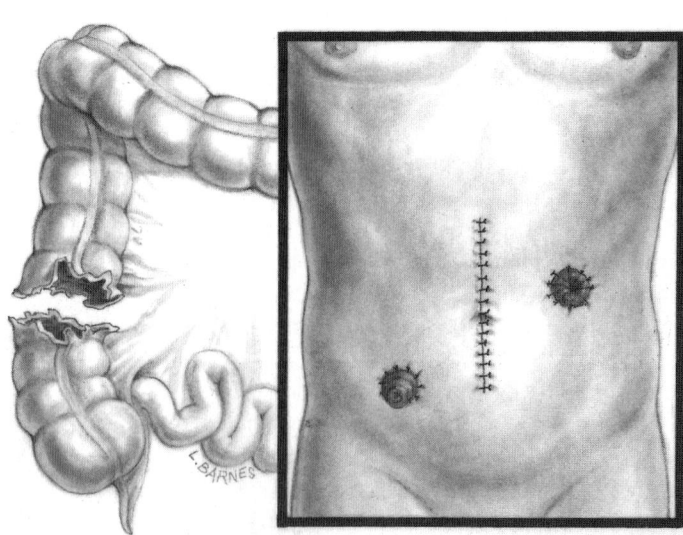

FIGURE 14-9. Artist's representation of a massive injury to the right colon requiring resection. This illustration demonstrates creation of an ileostomy with a mucous fistula.

▶ TABLE 14-1 Randomized Prospective Trials: Primary Repair Versus Colostomy

Article (ref.)	Primary Repairs	Resections and Anastomoses	Primary Repair Leaks	Resections and Anastomotic Leaks	Colostomy/ Exteriorization
Stone and Fabian[122]	67	0	1	—	72
Chappuis et al.[16]	17	11	0	0	28
Falcone et al.[34]	0	11	—	0	11
Sasaki et al.[110]	31	12	0	0	28
Gonzalez et al.[44]	51	5	0	1	53
Total	166	39	1 (0.6%)	1 (2.6%)	192

Table 14-1 illustrates five prospective, randomized trials that compare the two approaches.[16,34,44,109,122] In addition to these randomized studies, numerous large series have been reported that also compare these alternatives (Tables 14-2 and 14-3). These data provide very strong evidence to support the use of primary repair following colonic injury. In a metaanalysis of published randomized, controlled trials, Singer and Nelson found that primary repair was favored over fecal diversion for penetrating injuries.[114] All concluded that primary repair was safe and effective.

Retroperitoneal Trauma

Weil reported 66 patients who sustained retroperitoneal trauma to the colon and rectum.[134] These injuries usually affected both the intraperitoneal anterior and retroperitoneal posterior walls. The authors emphasize that the retroperitoneum must be inspected when an intraperitoneal hole is found or whenever the wound is in the flank or the back. Colostomy is always required for such an injury.

Strategies to Prevent Infection

As previously implied, the combination of soft tissue injury, hypotension, and fecal contamination provide all the elements necessary for infection (a nutritive medium,

a susceptible host, and the presence of bacteria). This triad is invariably present when the injury is caused by high-velocity missile or close-range shotgun wounds. Careful and vigorous debridement is mandatory. When the debridement has been completed, the remaining tissue should be uninjured, well vascularized, and clean. For major soft tissue injury, debridement should be succeeded by the use of a pressurized, pulsatile irrigation system. Such an approach is very effective for removing bacteria and microparticulate debris. In addition, planned reoperation for further debridement and irrigation must be considered.

Wounds should be managed either by delayed primary closure or by dressing changes, with healing to take place by secondary intention.

Antibiotics

It should be self-evident that antibiotics are considered an important part in the postoperative management of individuals with colonic trauma. No prospective, randomized clinical trial has compared the use of prophylactic antibiotics with that of a placebo following colonic injury. However, there are certainly data to support the use of such drugs in this circumstance.[40] Based simply on the principles of effective use of antibiotics in other clinical settings and the diverse colonic flora, a nontoxic drug directed at gram-negative aerobes and anaerobes should be administered as soon as possible after the injury. The tissue level should be high at the time the skin incision is

▶ TABLE 14-2 Colon Trauma: Prospectively Obtained Data

Article (ref.)	Primary Repairs	Resections and Anastomoses	Primary Repair Leaks	Resections and Anastomotic Leaks	Colostomy/ Exteriorization
George et al.[43]	83	12	0	1	7
Baker et al.[4]	172	0	1	—	217
Demetriades et al.[26]	76	0	2	—	24
Ivatury et al.[51]	159	26	0	2	67
Total	490	38	3 (0.6%)	3 (7.9%)	315

▶ **TABLE 14-3** Colon Trauma: Retrospective Data Collection

Article (ref.)	Primary Repairs	Resections and Anastomoses	Primary Repair Leaks	Resections and Anastomotic Leaks	Colostomy/ Exteriorization
Thigpen et al.[125]	35	0	U	—	37
Wiener et al.[136]	85	0	U	—	57
Dang et al.[20]	24	0	0	—	58
Karanfilian et al.[56]	17	9	0	3	106
Adkins et al.[1]	36	0	0	—	20
Cook et al.[18]	27	0	U	U	180
Nallathambi et al.[84]	43	16	0	0	77
Shannon and Moore[113]	80	30	1	0	118
Dawes et al.[22]	21	13	0	1	103
Miller et al.[74]	0	16	—	0	12
George et al.[42]	73	0	0	—	41
Frame et al.[39]	30	0	U	—	35
Nelken and Lewis[88]	34	3	1	0	39
Ridgeway et al.[101]	30	U	0	—	35
Orsay et al.[93]	1	2	U	U	230
Levison et al.[64]	98	8	1	0	133
Burch et al.[13]	564	50	9	4	344
Morgado et al.[78]	60	32	1	2	9
Schultz et al.[111]	40	17	0	0	43
Taheri et al.[124]	43	12	0	0	91
Sasaki et al.[110]	50	52	0	0	52
Bostick et al.[7]	59	U	2*	U	155
Stewart et al.[120]	0	43	—	6	7
Total	1,450	303	15 (1.0%)	16 (5.0%)	1982

U, unstated in article
*Combined primary repair and resection and anastomosis without stating numbers of each.
Modified from Timothy Fabian, M.D., with permission.

made to ensure maximum effectiveness. One trial concluded that aztreonam with clindamycin is superior to gentamicin and clindamycin in the prevention of infections following penetrating abdominal trauma.[33] Most surgeons treating trauma patients utilize either a broad-spectrum, second-generation cephalosporin (cefoxitin, cefotetan) or a broad-spectrum beta-lactam plus beta-lactamase inhibitor (ticarcillin-clavulanate, ampicillin-sulbactam, piperacillin-tazobactam). The use of second-generation cephalosporins has been associated with an increased incidence of enterococci as pathogens identified in superficial wound infections. However, no difference has been observed in deep infection rates.[133] Probably numerous antibiotic regimens and combinations are safe and effective for the management of patients who sustain colonic injury.

Generally, it is unnecessary to continue the antibiotics after 24 hours. Prospective, double-blind, randomized trials have demonstrated that 5 days of antibiotic therapy is not superior to 24 hours of therapy.[31] If intraoperative bleeding is a problem or the operation is longer than two drug half-lives, the antibiotics should be readministered intraoperatively. Prolonged use of antibiotics may be associated with superinfection, resistant organisms, and pseudomembranous colitis (see Chapter 33).

Nichols and colleagues demonstrated by logical regression analysis of 145 patients that a statistically significantly increased risk for infection was associated with increased age, injury to the left colon, the administration of a greater number of units of blood or blood products, and associated organ injury.[89] Others have confirmed the prognostic importance of these risk factors and advise colostomy as a minimal treatment if these are present.[22] Some antibiotic regimens have been employed that seem to be equally efficacious, but the single most important factor contributing to a low rate of infection is prompt surgical intervention.[23,89,105]

Hypothermia

Another factor that may be associated with an increased risk for the development of infection is hypothermia.[61] Therefore, avoidance of this complication should be added to adequate resuscitation in order to prevent infection during the intraoperative period.

Foreign Body

Another issue that has stimulated some interest is the presence of a retained foreign body—specifically the missile. Poret and colleagues reviewed a series of wounds, comparing patients who harbored missiles with those who did not.[97] They discovered that after the bullet passed through the colon, a retained foreign body was frequently the source of postoperative abscess. Others have reached a similar conclusion, but some have not been able to demonstrate an increased rate of infection.[25,38] Generally, removing the bullet is relatively easy to accomplish. Therefore, it is recommended that the surgeon take whatever additional time is reasonably necessary to remove the retained missile, especially if it has passed through the colon or rectum.

Nutrition

Another related issue concerning infection is the value of nutritional support. Two randomized trials have been published that report the use of jejunostomy followed by immediate enteral feeding.[59,75] Fewer abscesses and pulmonary infections have been noted in the enteral feeding groups. Another trial compared a standard elemental formula to one enhanced with arginine, omega-3 fatty acids, and glutamine (immune-enhancing diet).[76] The immune-enhancing regimen was associated with a statistically significantly reduced incidence of infections when compared with the standard regimen. The use of early enteral feeding is strongly recommended except in those individuals with severe hypotension or prolonged ileus. The placement of a small-bore feeding jejunostomy has itself been associated with a low complication rate.[82]

Results

As previously mentioned, Stone and Fabian performed a randomized controlled study of primary closure versus exteriorization in patients with perforating colon trauma (Table 14-1).[122] During a 44-month period, 268 individuals with colon wounds underwent operation. Excluded were those with profound preoperative shock, patients with blood loss in excess of 20% of estimated normal volume, those with more than two intraabdominal organ systems injured, those with significant fecal contamination, and patients in whom the surgery was begun more than 8 hours following the injury. Approximately one half of the patients had to be excluded because they did not

meet these criteria. The authors determined that morbidity for those who were randomized to have a colostomy was ten times as great as for those who underwent a primary closure. The average postoperative stay was 6 days longer if a colostomy had been created, not including the need for subsequent hospitalization for colostomy closure. The immediate mortality rates were identical, although one late death occurred following colostomy closure. The authors concluded that primary suture of colon wounds could be safely performed in selected patients if they met the criteria outlined.

Another randomized prospective study was undertaken by Chappuis and colleagues (Table 14-1).[16] This involved 56 patients who were managed either by primary repair or by resection in one group or diversion in the other. The authors concluded that independent of associated risk factors, the complication rates were similar. Falcone, Sasaki, and Gonzalez and their colleagues also conducted randomized, prospective trials that support the concept of primary repair of colon injuries (Table 14-1).[34,44,109] George and associates evaluated 102 individuals with penetrating wounds of the colon and concluded that nearly all such injuries can be repaired primarily or with resection and anastomosis, regardless of the risk factors.[42,43] However, many authors concur that increased penetrating abdominal trauma index (PATI) scores correlate with an increased incidence of septic complications, especially if the PATI score is greater than or equal to 25.[88,101]

Burch and colleagues reviewed more than 700 patients with civilian colon injuries.[11] They disagree with those who maintain that suture closure should not be performed in the presence of shock. They believe that simple suture of small wounds may be the most appropriate therapy to minimize blood loss and to save time. They believe that primary repair should be the benchmark for the treatment of most civilian injuries. Most concur that by judicious selection, trauma in this population can be treated by primary repair with debridement and closure or resection.[113]

Jacobson and co-workers evaluated the septic complications and leak rate in 58 consecutive patients with penetrating colon injuries managed exclusively by primary repair.[54] The incidence of complications was as follows:

- Intraabdominal abscess, 12.1%
- Bacteremia, 8.6%
- Fascial dehiscence, 13.8%
- Anastomotic leak (fistula), 0%
- Mortality, 0%

The authors observed that the presence of risk factors in accordance with the PATI score identified more severely injured patients and was associated with a higher incidence of intraabdominal abscess. They concluded that primary repair can safely be effected for virtually all penetrating colon injuries, even in those with "risk factors".[54] Durham and colleagues reached the same conclusion on the basis of their evaluation of 130 consecutive patients with colonic injuries.[29] By means of stepwise regression analysis of 13 factors, they ascertained that only "gross contamination" and PATI predicted the occurrence of intraabdominal complications.

Parks reported 106 patients who sustained colon injury as a consequence of the civil disturbances in Northern Ireland.[95] As would be expected, those whose injuries involved multiple organs had a much higher mortality rate. There were no deaths among patients who had isolated colonic or rectal injuries. Unfortunately, large bowel trauma tends to occur more often in association with injuries to other organs than it does in isolation. The author believed that primary closure of the wound should be considered in patients who had limited injury of less than 4 hours' duration, who had minimal peritoneal contamination, minimal blood loss, and little or no associated injury.

Wiener and associates, at the University of Texas in Galveston, reported their experience of 181 patients who sustained traumatic injury of the colon.[136] The authors emphasized that it is important to distinguish the treatment of colon injuries in civilian practice from the method of therapy commonly employed for war injuries. They believed that treatment must be individualized, with primary repair (i.e., debridement and suture or resection and anastomosis) possible in selected cases. In their experience, primary closure or resection resulted in a shorter hospital stay and lower morbidity. Exteriorization with a proximal colostomy was believed to be a reasonable alternative, but one that should be reserved for the more severely injured patients. Criteria for exteriorization in these authors' experience included extensive damage to the bowel wall, questionable viability of the bowel, difficult or insecure repair, severe associated injury, and an easily mobilized injured segment.

Lou and associates reported a successful experience of 50 patients treated by an exteriorization repair method.[67] There was no mortality and a relatively low complication rate (18%). The authors believed that this method should be employed for those patients who cannot be treated by another approach. Likewise, Dang and colleagues reported a favorable experience with exteriorization repair in 82 individuals.[20] Although the study was uncontrolled, the overall mortality rate was 2.4%, compared with no deaths in the patients who underwent an exteriorization repair. They concluded that this type of repair, with early "drop back," is safe and economical for most patients with moderate-risk injury and even for some selected patients who may be at greater risk.

Kirkpatrick and Rajpal reported their experience of 165 patients with colonic injuries.[57] Their results demonstrated that primary closure with exteriorization was a safe and reliable method of management if the patients were selected in accordance with a rigid protocol. They recommended that the procedure be performed in all patients with lesions above 18 cm requiring one suture line, provided the additional operating time of 20 minutes did not compromise the management of other injuries. These authors believed that if the patient could not fulfill these criteria, a colostomy should be performed. In their experience, it was possible to reduce the need for colostomy to approximately one half of those who sustained colonic injury.

Flint and colleagues reviewed their experience with colonic injury to ascertain whether their intraoperative classification could permit the assessment of patients and the determination of an appropriate choice of operative procedure.[37] Grade 1 injuries were characterized by minimal contamination and the absence of other organ involvement. These wounds were managed by primary closure, that is, suture closure of the perforation. Grade 2 injuries implied through-and-through perforation with moderate contamination, and grade 3 injury indicated severe tissue loss, devascularization, and considerable contamination. The authors advocated either exteriorization with or without colostomy or resection with colostomy for the last two groups. One of 25 patients classified as grade 1 died; there were no complications in this group of patients. In 116 patients with a grade 2 injury, the mortality rate was 2%, and the complication rate was 20%. With a grade 3 injury (16 patients), there were four deaths (25%) and a complication rate of 31%.

Carpenter and colleagues used the intracolonic bypass tube without concomitant colostomy in nine patients for whom they believed a fecal diversion would otherwise have been necessary.[14] All wounds healed without incident. However, the product is no longer available (ColoShield).

Right versus Left Colon Injuries

There is a controversy about whether penetrating injuries of the right colon should be treated differently from those of the left. This is because it has generally been believed that trauma to the right colon is usually associated with a more favorable result than trauma to the more distal portions of the bowel. Thompson and colleagues compared their experience in patients who sustained injury to the right colon with those who had left colon injury.[128] Both groups were similar with respect to the mechanism of injury, presence of shock at admission, degree of fecal contamination, severity of trauma, and frequency of associated intraabdominal problems. The number of patients managed by primary repair, resection, resection with exteriorization, and colostomy was comparable for right and left injuries, but it must be remembered that these were historical controls. The management of right colon injuries resulted in a morbidity rate of 32% and a mortality rate of 2%; left-sided injuries were found to have a 33% morbidity rate and a 4% mortality rate. Because of the comparable results, the authors concluded that penetrating trauma to the right and left colon should be managed similarly for the same degree of injury, contamination, and so forth. Stewart and colleagues also found no difference in leak or abscess rates in a group of severely injured patients with destructive colon wounds.[120] Similarly, Demetriades and colleagues stated that the clinical significance of the different anatomy, physiology, and bacteriology of the right and the left colon has been overemphasized.[27] They wrote that in most cases, primary repair can be safely performed irrespective of the location of the injury unless gross fecal contamination, extensive tissue destruction, or a considerable amount of retained feces is present. However, these and other studies have the drawback of being retrospective.[85] If extensive injury to the right colon necessitates a resection, and a primary anastomosis is not deemed advisable, Prasad and colleagues recommend that an ileostomy and mucous fistula be brought out through a common opening in the abdominal wall.[98] This minimizes inconvenience to the patient and simplifies the technique for the subsequent closure. Another approach that may be useful in selective circumstances is a primary repair followed by a proximal, protective loop ileostomy with distal irrigation of the protected segment. Thus if the anastomosis leaks, there is no fecal soilage.

Damage Control Procedures

The principles of management of severely injured patients have evolved considerably since the mid-1990s, but still the main determinant of survival is the extent of the initial injury. The triad of coagulopathy, acidosis, and hypothermia is a well-recognized harbinger of poor outcome. Strategies to control hemorrhage, minimize contamination, and reduce operative time are essential if one is to improve the prognosis. In a damage control approach, the goals are to minimize operative time while attempting to restore normal physiology. To meet these goals, the celiotomy must be abbreviated. Operative bleeding is controlled as rapidly as possible with the most expedient technique that is consistent with this objective. Visceral contamination is limited through the use of clamps followed by either an *expeditious* primary repair or resection with a stapling device. Alternatively, in the absence of special equipment, the bowel can be ligated with the use of an umbilical tape or equivalent and divided. No reconstruction is attempted during the initial stage of the damage control procedure. Once operative bleeding and visceral contamination are controlled, nonsurgically induced bleeding is controlled with packing. When possible, a nonadherent or hemostatic interface between the packing and the bleeding surface should be used in order to control hemorrhage better and to prevent rebleeding upon removal of the pack. The abdomen is then closed using a technique that does not injure the fascia. This usually entails either rapidly closing the skin or implanting a plastic prosthesis attached to the skin. Another popular technique involves placing a cover over the bowel and using a large Ioban drape or equivalent over the abdominal wall, with closed-suction drains placed underneath the Ioban drape to control drainage (vacuum-assisted drainage). Resuscitation to restore normal physiology is continued, with special attention to restoring adequate oxygen delivery, correcting any coagulopathy, and addressing hypothermia.

Following establishment of normal physiologic parameters, the patient is returned to the operating room, where the abdomen is reexplored. The packs are removed, hemostasis is secured, and hollow viscus reconstruction or an ostomy is performed. In general, restoration of small bowel continuity by performing a hand-sewn anastomosis is preferred (there are retrospective data that support a hand-sewn technique over staples because of the bowel edema). For colon injuries, one usually performs an ostomy by exteriorizing the stapled end while creating a mucous fistula. Alternatively, if the bowel appears healthy and viable, an anastomosis can be performed with a concomitant proximal ileostomy and with distal irrigation. This is an attractive approach because of the relative ease of performing the ileostomy closure. Care should be taken to allow sufficient distance between the stoma and the wound in order to avoid interference with subsequent reconstruction of the abdominal wall. Application of this alternative depends on the individual surgeon's personal preference.

At the second operation, appropriate drains and enteral tubes are placed. These may include closed-suction drains for liver, pancreatic or genitourinary injuries, and gastrostomy or jejunostomy tubes. If the abdomen cannot be closed primarily, numerous options are available. In general, we prefer to use an absorbable (Vicryl) mesh that is either sequentially tightened or allowed to reabsorb following skin graft application. A delayed abdominal wall reconstruction can then be undertaken.

Principles and Axioms for Surgery in Less Than Ideal Circumstances

Colon

Most abdominal injuries sustained in an armed conflict are of the penetrating type. This stated, there has been a marked decrease in the number of United States servicemen and servicewomen sustaining wounds of the torso. This is primarily because a soldier in a combat zone wears a protective vest that covers the torso, neck, and genitalia. Made of Kevlar, the vest is additionally reinforced with steel or ceramic plates that will stop high-velocity rifle bullets. However, blast injuries may be the cause of significant lung and intestinal injuries without external evidence of trauma. Blunt abdominal trauma is not uncommon in city "warfare" in which victims may be trapped under collapsed buildings. The niceties of debating the probabilities of penetration of an abdominal wound so common in civilian practice have no place in a combat zone or when one is faced with mass casualties. In the parlance of the card game, bridge, a peek is worth a hundred finesses.

A military physician close to a battlefield or a civilian surgeon far from a specialized trauma center could be faced with a mass casualty situation and have to treat colon injuries under less than optimal conditions. The following are principles of management under these circumstances.

When exploring the abdomen, colon wounds should be temporarily closed with clamps and the area of injury covered with gauze packs to minimize contamination.

War wounds of the colon, as a rule, should be treated by either exteriorization of the injury (as a colostomy) or by resection of the injured segment and exteriorization of both ends of the bowel. A small perforation of the colon can be managed by simple colorraphy, provided there are no other major intraabdominal injuries, and the repair is protected by an ileostomy. All stomas should be primarily matured. Although appealing in principle (see earlier discussion), *resection and ileocolic anastomosis should not be the treatment for war wounds of the right colon.* Instead, a right colectomy and a diverting ileostomy comprise the safer option. The open end of the transverse colon can either be delivered to the skin as a mucous fistula or tacked to the ileal mesentery close to the ileostomy in order to facilitate the subsequent reestablishment of intestinal continuity. Drains add little to the repair of bowel wounds; in fact, their use in these circumstances is contraindicated.

Most civilian colonic injuries today are closed primarily. Because the creation of a stoma is time-consuming and is associated with a not insignificant morbidity, there is a tendency among surgeons unfamiliar with war trauma to treat such injuries like those sustained in a civilian practice. *This is a mistake.* Abdominal war injuries are often multiple. Shock resulting from the severity of the injury (high-velocity missile) and delay in treatment are ever-present concerns. The close and intensive care available in metropolitan centers is an unachievable ideal near a battlefield or in a mass casualty situation. The concept of strict follow-up after surgery is also problematic when one is forced to accommodate the vagaries

of an evacuation system that, although well meaning, is often logistically stressed. Under these circumstances, the policy of eschewing primary colon repair is appropriate. Exteriorizing colon injuries in such a combat environment is safer and is logical. After all, this approach has been supported through extensive experience during World War II, in Korea, and in Vietnam by surgeons who have been involved in treating war injuries around the world.[3,49,70,91,92,99,135]

Some surgeons, however, claim that if one considers the advantages of a primary closure, even in the precarious situation when war surgery is often performed, the technique of primary repair merits consideration.[77] Many who work in developing countries may favor this approach when they are faced with gunshot wounds of the abdomen for several reasons. First, follow-up is practically impossible in many cases, and, therefore, leaving a patient with a stoma may not be an option. Second, stoma appliances are a luxury that may not be obtainable. Third, mortality and morbidity conferences are seldom held in the developing world during periods of conflict, either in the countryside or in urban areas. This last statement is not meant to imply justification for choosing a suboptimal operation—it is, however, the reality. Undoubtedly, in very specific instances (e.g., small fragment wounds of the bowel, the patient seen within a few hours of wounding, absence of other major intraabdominal injuries, absence of severe bleeding), such an attitude merits consideration, but it certainly should not stand as a matter of policy for dealing with war injuries of the colon.

Rectum

An extraperitoneal injury of the rectum, that is, below the rectovesical pouch, has few clinical signs, although blood may be seen on the examining glove. Victims of gunshot wounds of the buttocks and perineum and landmine casualties are prone to such injuries. It may be difficult to visualize the rectal tear because it can be very small. If such an injury is present, the abdomen should be explored and a colostomy performed. The rectum should be emptied and gently irrigated. Even a distal rectal injury may be difficult to repair. Two soft drains should be placed in the presacral space, with multiple perforations suggested. The space is entered by dividing the skin just anterior to the tip of the coccyx and by cutting the anococcygeal ligament. The injury will generally heal if the area is well drained and a colostomy is accomplished.

Intraperitoneal injuries of the rectum should be repaired from within the abdomen, and a proximal colostomy is then made. Occasionally, repair of the intraperitoneal rectum requires one to enter the presacral space. If bleeding is encountered, drainage of this space by means of sump drains brought out through the abdominal wall is advisable. If the pelvic bleeding associated with the rectal injury cannot be readily controlled, the presacral area should be packed with gauze and the area reexplored in 24 to 48 hours.

Damage Control Laparotomy

In a patient in shock and with multiple intraabdominal injuries, one may consider packing all four quadrants to control the bleeding and stapling the bowel ends closed or tying with umbilical tape proximal and distal to the sites of perforations. As previously noted, injured colon segments should be rapidly mobilized and exteriorized. The stomach should be drained by a nasogastric tube or preferably by a tube gastrostomy. The abdomen is then closed expeditiously or may be left open with the incision packed with gauze and covered with a plastic film. If this is not available and the abdominal closure seems to be under tension, a clean plastic intravenous fluid bag may be used to bridge the fascial gap and sutured to the fascia or skin. The patient is then supported and stabilized to the best of one's ability. If the patient survives, re-operation for the definitive care of the injuries is undertaken in 48 to 72 hours.[70,104]

Conclusions

Although we liberally apply the principle of primary repair for the management of colonic injuries, it is important to recognize that there are serious concerns if one forswears the use of colostomy. Patients who require colonic resection because of trauma to the bowel itself or because of disruption of the blood supply deserve special consideration. These individuals are at a high risk! Injuries are much more complex and frequently involve other organs. When the aforementioned prospective clinical trials were examined, the number of patients included in the so-called high-risk group was quite small. The total number of patients treated by primary resection and anastomosis in three trials was only 28.[1,27,37] The fact is that the randomized trials do not address a sufficient number of high-risk individuals to make possible clearcut recommendations. Stewart and colleagues expressed such a concern in their presentation.[120] They noted their experience at the Regional Trauma Center in Memphis, Tennessee, reviewing primary resection without a stoma, even in individuals with destructive or devitalized wounds. The leak rate in 43 patients so treated was 14%, much higher than had been anticipated. Specific risk factors that were identified by the investigators were multiple blood transfusions and preexisting medical illness.[120] The anastomotic breakdown rate in those without either risk factor was 3%, in comparison with 42% for those who had received greater than 6 units of transfused blood or had a preexisting medical condition. Interestingly, the amount of contamination or the presence of associated injury did not appear to increase the likelihood of breakdown. The leak rates and septic complication rates were identical when anastomosis between the ileum and the colon was compared with colocolonic anastomosis (see earlier discussion). The mortality rate for anastomotic breakdown was 40%.

A similar opinion was expressed by Ryan and associates.[107] They, too, concluded, on the basis of existing literature on primary repair of colon injuries, that pooling of the data contained in these three reports did not provide sufficient statistical power to support the superiority of this modality of treatment for all colon injuries. They concluded that to demonstrate a 5% difference between the two approaches, a prospective, randomized study consisting of 200 patients in each arm of the trial would be required.[107]

We and others have concluded that the physiologic status of the patient at the time of the anastomosis appears to be the best predictor for anastomotic success or failure. Therefore, colostomy is strongly recommended for high-risk patients with destructive colonic wounds. Figure 14-10 illustrates our algorithmic approach for the management of patients with colonic injuries.

On the basis of these studies, one may reasonably make certain recommendations. When contamination and associated organ injury are minimal, the surgeon may safely perform primary closure or resection and anastomosis. With extensive colonic trauma, vascular impairment, multiple organ involvement, gross contamination, and multiple blood transfusions, it is probably wiser to resect and to perform a diversionary procedure. Many factors, however, enter into decision making, so that despite the foregoing counsel and the various classifications that have been proposed to aid the surgeon, the choice of therapy will ultimately rest on the surgeon's personal experience and judgment.

Anorectal Trauma

Injuries to the anus and rectum may be the result of various surgical procedures (e.g., obstetric, gynecologic, and urologic), endoscopic procedures, ingestion of foreign bodies (see Chapter 15), and blunt and penetrating injuries to the perineum (Figs. 14-11 and 14-12). Additionally, trauma may be secondary to pneumatic injury, vacuum toilet, sexual assault, autoeroticism (e.g., "fist fornication," "handballing," "water sport"), insertion of enema nozzles and thermometers, bull horn injury, and even suicide attempts by rectal administration of corrosives.[19,30,50,65,79,86,139,141] In children, the most common cause is a fall astride an object, or impalement (see Figure 13-2). In the experience of Jones and Bass with 463 children younger than 13 years old, motor vehicle trauma and rape were responsible for the majority of severe perineal injuries.[55]

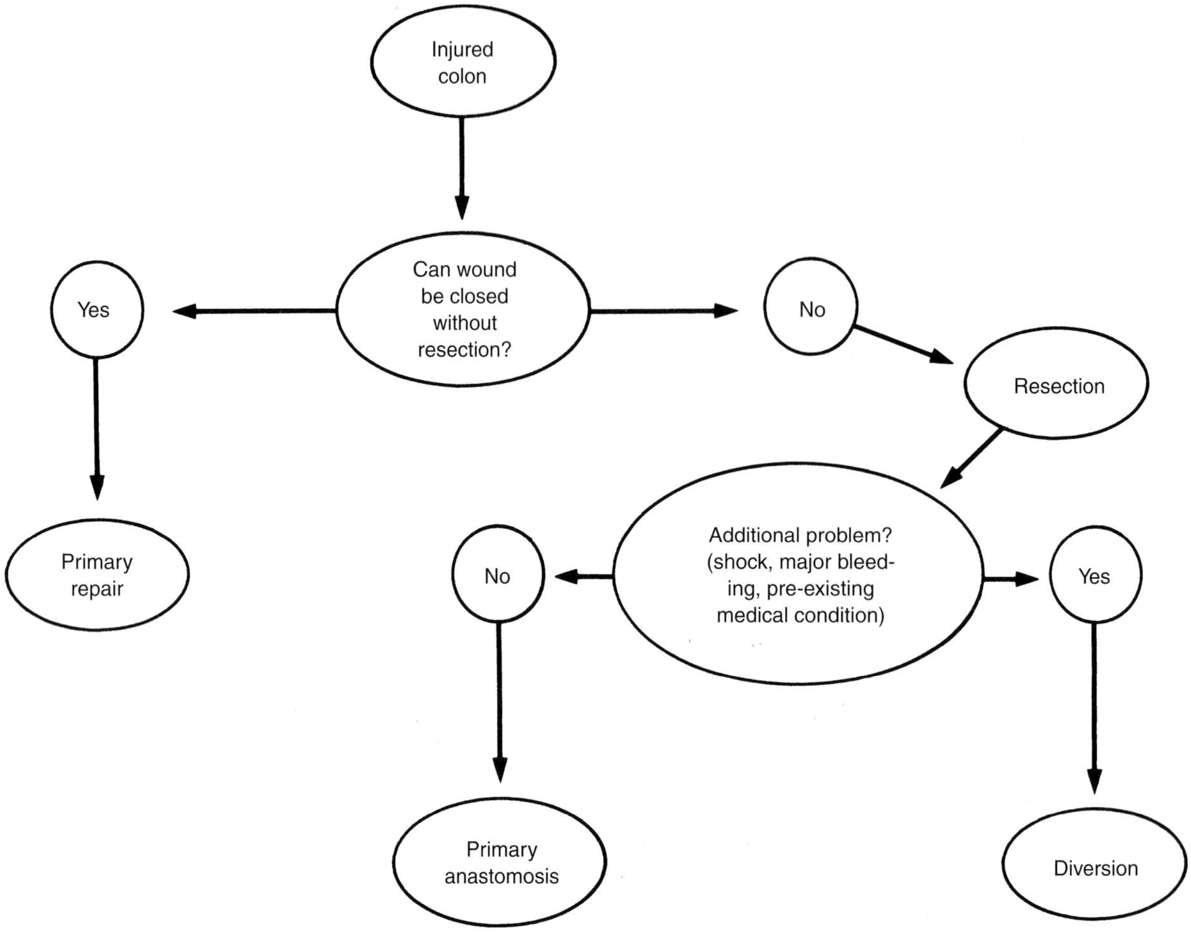

Injured
colon

Can wound
be closed
without
resection?

Yes

No

Resection

Primary
repair

No

Additional problem?
(shock, major bleed-
ing, pre-existing
medical condition)

Yes

Primary
anastomosis

Diversion

FIGURE 14-10. Algorithm for the patient who has sustained a colonic injury.

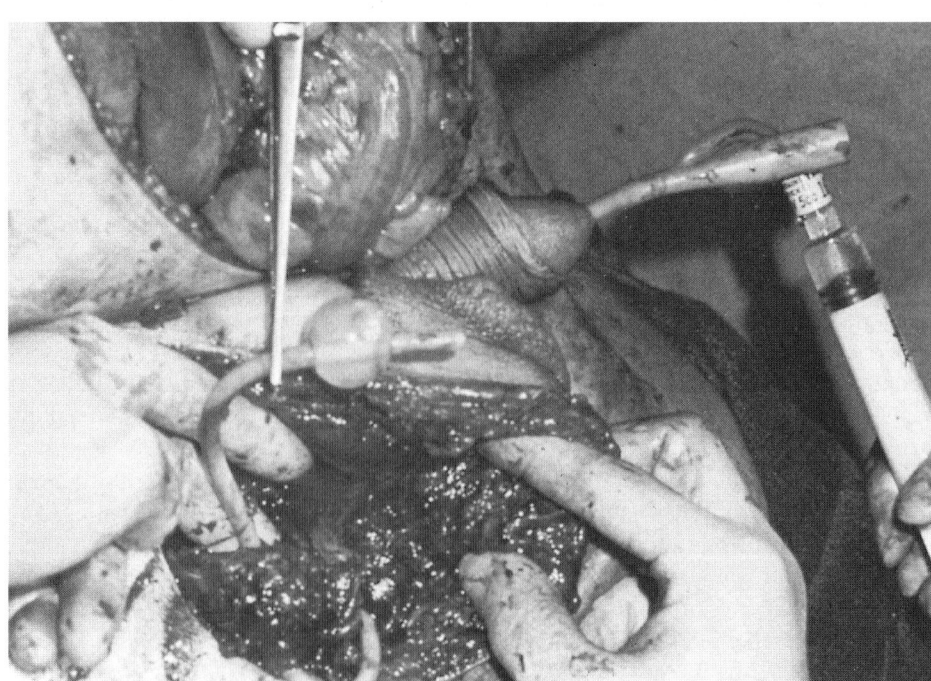

FIGURE 14-11. Perineal trauma. Severe avulsion injury from a motorcycle accident with laceration of the urethra and rectum. Note the Foley catheter emerging from the defect in the urethra.

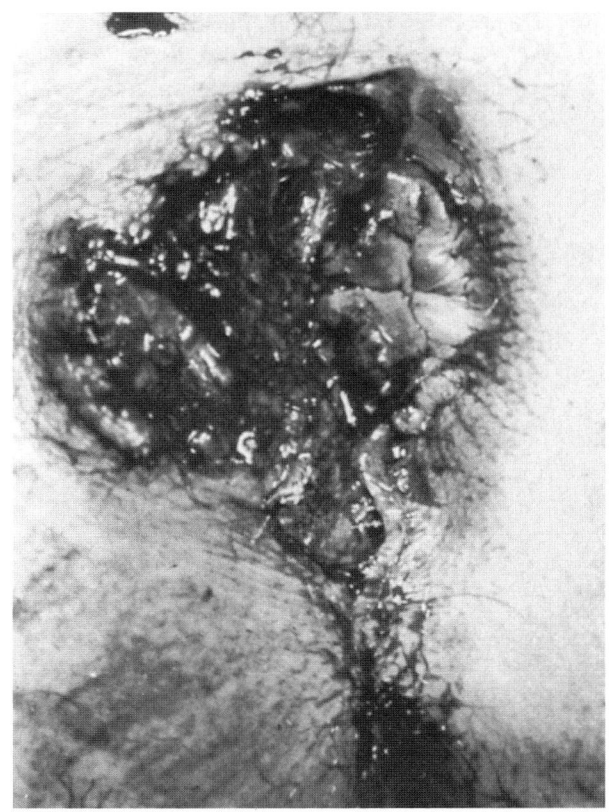

FIGURE 14-12. Anorectal impalement injury. The anus is displaced to the right side.

Haas and Fox described a wide variety of injuries and procedures used in treating the various types of anorectal trauma.[45] They classified the types of injury into the following groups:

- Intraperitoneal perforations
- Retroperitoneal perforations
- Subperitoneal perforations
- Incomplete perforations
- Perineal injuries

Sixty-two cases of rectal trauma between the sacral promontory and the anus were reviewed. The choice of therapy was dictated by the anatomic location, pathology, and etiology; the authors emphasized that there is no one "best treatment" for anorectal injury.[45]

Symptoms

In unsuspected rectal trauma, the usual complaint is rectal pain. This may be delayed for several hours to several days following the initial injury. Abdominal pain is an ominous sign because it implies peritonitis. Rectal bleeding with a history of trauma suggests a mucosal tear, at the minimum.

Examination

Physical examination should include digital rectal examination and careful palpation of the perineal area. In female patients, a vaginal examination should be performed. Asking the patient to "tighten up" will help evaluate the efficacy of the sphincteric mechanism and whether it is intact. Anoscopic and proctosigmoidoscopic examination should be performed, although care must be taken to avoid extending the injury. Rectal irrigation may be helpful in facilitating visualization.

Diagnostic Studies

Whenever there is a suggestion of anorectal trauma, the surgeon must take care not to underestimate the possible gravity of the injury. Usually, the diagnosis of rectal injury is not difficult to establish, because the history of trauma is self-evident. Occasionally, a high index of suspicion must be maintained if one is to determine the nature of the patient's complete injury and to initiate proper therapy. This is particularly true for avulsion injuries of the perineum and for gunshot wounds of the abdomen. The mortality rate can approach 100% if an untreated rectal injury continues to provide a source for sepsis. Barium enema examination is contraindicated if rectal injury is suspected; a water-soluble technique should be employed. Obviously, the presence of intraperitoneal gas implies a perforated viscus.

Urinalysis should be routinely obtained to detect the possible presence of hematuria. If blood is identified, a urethrocystogram should be obtained. It is also important to remember that failure to recognize an extraperitoneal perforation of the rectum is as potentially lethal as failure to identify an intraperitoneal perforation.

The place of peritoneal lavage was addressed by Robertson and colleagues through their experience with 36 patients who underwent treatment for rectal trauma.[102] The authors caution that although peritoneal lavage may be a useful diagnostic study in the evaluation of blunt abdominal trauma, it may give false-negative results in those who have sustained isolated rectal, retroperitoneal, or rectosigmoid perforation. As with colon trauma, the location, cause, length of time since the injury, and association with other organ system involvement dictate the appropriate treatment choice.

Treatment

If rectal injury is suspected, broad-spectrum antibiotic therapy should be initiated within as short a period of time as possible, preferably not longer than 6 hours after the incident. It has been demonstrated that the results of surgical treatment are improved if antibiotics are given as early as possible. It is often quite difficult to identify the site of injury to the rectum at the time of laparotomy.

A hematoma, if present, should be carefully assessed. Williams and Lewis suggest infusing methylene blue through a Foley catheter inserted into the rectum while the surgeon's fingers occlude the proximal bowel.[137] Minor to moderate injuries of the anus below the level of the levator ani muscle may be treated by debridement, suture, drainage, antibiotic therapy, tetanus prophylaxis, and close observation. Intravenous fluid replacement and restriction of oral intake are advised. An elemental diet may be implemented for several days until the patient's condition is believed to have stabilized.

Injuries above the levatores require a colostomy at the minimum. Ideally, the patient should be placed in the perineolithotomy position to gain effective access both to the rectal area and to the abdomen (see Chapter 23). Drainage, debridement, and distal washout of the rectum should be performed.[52,62,67,72,129] The surgeon who errs on the side of conservatism in the management of rectal trauma by performing a colostomy should not be criticized; conversely, the treatment of a rectal injury without a diversionary procedure is usually inconsistent with optimal care. That said, Thomas and colleagues believe that

a uniform approach for all such injuries may not be justified, and that perhaps a selective attitude concerning the physician's philosophy of management is more reasonable.[126] For example, Burch and associates found that the only statistically significant factor that increased the likelihood of septic complications was the failure to drain the presacral space (Figure 14-13).[12] Others report, however, that absence of drainage does not increase infectious complications in low-velocity rectal wounds.[119]

Whether to perform a direct sphincter repair as part of the initial management is a matter of some debate, because no meaningful statistics are available. Of course, every effort must initially be directed to saving the patient's life; therefore, it is not surprising that most articles place little or no emphasis on sphincter reconstruction. An important principle to remember, however, is that the surgeon should endeavor to preserve sphincter muscle if vigorous debridement of the perineum is required. Identification of the cut muscle can be subsequently facilitated by marking the ends with nonabsorbable sutures. Direct repair should also be performed at the time if prolonging the surgery does not compromise the patient's

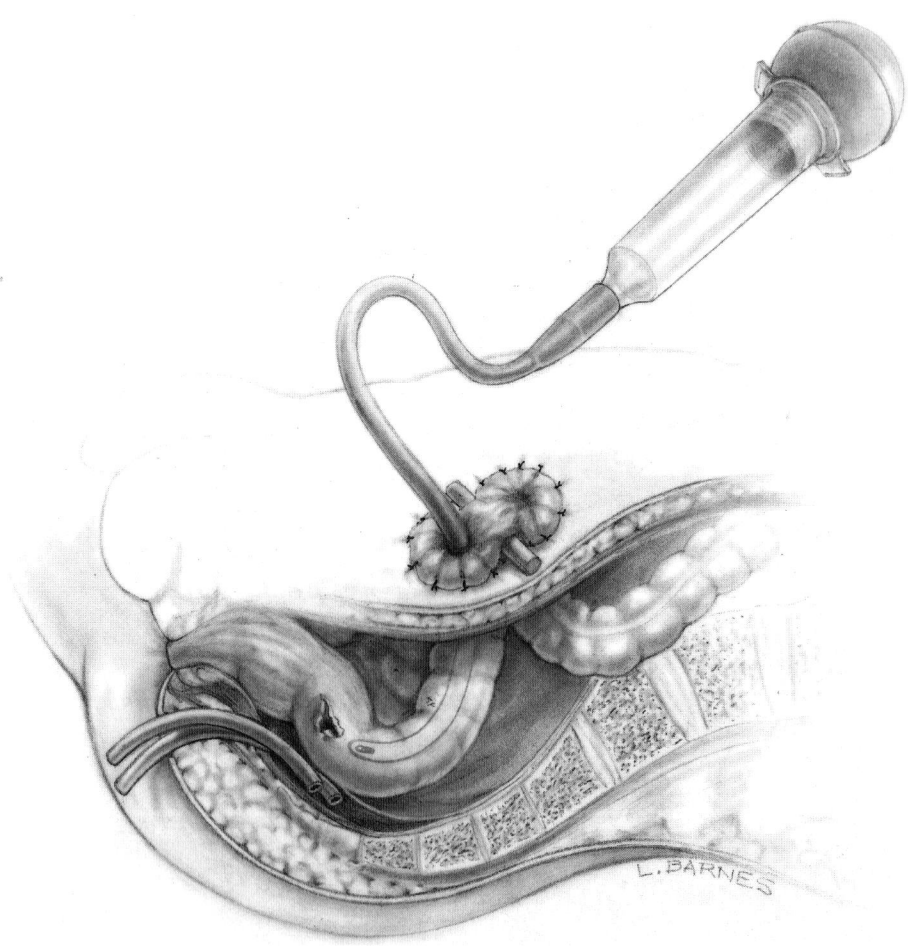

FIGURE 14-13. The concepts of the management of an extraperitoneal rectal injury can be appreciated. A colostomy is created; irrigation and presacral drainage are effected.

safety and if the surgeon is satisfied with the viability of the tissue. Delayed reconstruction should be considered in accordance with the principles outlined in Chapter 13. Finally, the likelihood of septic complications is reduced if perineal skin wounds are left open to heal by second intention or closed in accordance with a delayed primary repair technique.[50]

Principles of Managing Patients with Rectal Trauma

The principles of management are summarized as follows:

Perineolithotomy position
Management of concomitant injuries
Debridement
Proximal diversion
Removal of foreign body, if any
Drainage of presacral space
Distal rectal washout
Repair of rectal injury, if appropriate
Primary sphincter repair, if possible
External wound drainage
Broad-spectrum antibiotics
Skin left open

There are those who advocate selective use of primary repair without a diverting colostomy, but in the absence of a controlled trial, there are simply no adequate data to support this recommendation. As is illustrated in Figure 14-13, copious irrigation of the distal segment with normal saline solution is performed until the returns are clear. Drainage is established by entering the presacral space following division of the anococcygeal ligament. The principles of management are summarized by the mnemonic "three Ds"—diversion, distal irrigation, and drainage.

Most surgeons recommend closure of the stoma when the patient has completely recovered, usually in 3 to 4 months. However, Renz and colleagues prospectively studied the safety of same-admission colostomy closure in individuals who suffered rectal wounds.[100] In principle, all patients underwent a contrast enema on the tenth day following creation of the colostomy. Those who demonstrated no radiologic leakage, no infection, and no problem with bowel control underwent colostomy closure. Sixty percent with such injuries were considered candidates, 53% of whom were discharged with their colostomies closed. There were no rectal injury-related complications following colostomy closure.

In the absence of major bleeding from perineal and rectal lacerations, individuals with profound hypotension resistant to massive intravenous fluid and blood administration must be considered to have intraabdominal bleeding or an expanding pelvic hematoma.[8] For patients with persistent hypotension and a nondistended abdomen,

> ▶ **TABLE 14-4 Complex Perineal Wounds Management Guidelines**

- Resuscitation with hemorrhage control
- Identification and treatment of associated injuries
- Fecal diversion (consider feeding jejunostomy at same time)
- Urinary diversion for complex urologic injuries
- Aggressive initial debridement with pressurized pulsatile irrigation
- Immediate fracture fixation
- Early enteral nutrition
- Daily intraoperative debridement
- Wound coverage with skin graft as soon as feasible
- Deep venous thrombosis prophylaxis

pelvic arteriography and embolization of any bleeding vessel are recommended before a laparotomy is performed.[8] Ligation of the hypogastric arteries is no longer believed to be the optimal approach to the management of bleeding from pelvic fractures.

Complex Perineal Injuries

Complex wounds to the perineum with or without pelvic fracture present a considerable challenge to the surgeon.[60] Such injuries are usually the result of high-speed motor vehicle or motorcycle accidents and historically have been associated with a very high mortality rate (Figure 14-11). Early death is usually a consequence of bleeding and pelvic sepsis, whereas pulmonary embolism and multiple organ failure are the causes of late demise in these individuals. There is often associated extensive soft tissue injury. An organized approach is essential to prevent complications following these devastating wounds. The principles are summarized in Table 14-4.[121] As previously discussed, colostomy with distal irrigation is, of course, essential, as is aggressive soft tissue debridement, often by means of frequent examinations under anesthesia. This approach greatly reduces the incidence of pelvic sepsis. Although it is imperative to remove all nonviable tissue, every effort should be made to preserve the anal sphincter mechanism. Debridement of the muscle should be conservative. As stated earlier, repair should be delayed under these circumstances. One is advised to pay particular attention to the prevention of deep venous thrombosis, because pulmonary embolism is a frequent cause of morbidity and mortality, especially following pelvic injury with fracture.

Gunshot Wounds to the Buttocks

Gunshot wounds to the gluteal region warrant special consideration, because this type of injury often poses a challenging diagnostic and therapeutic dilemma. The question is whether it represents pure soft tissue injury—that is, injury unrelated to the colorectal area—or whether there is concern for associated bowel problems. Velmahos and colleagues identified 59 consecutive patients with wounds of the buttocks during a 1-year period at Los Angeles County, University of Southern California Medical Center.[132] The buttocks were defined as the body area confined between the posterior superior iliac spines superiorly, the gluteal folds inferiorly, and the projection of the midaxillary lines laterally. Superficial wounds and those tracking away from the retroperitoneum were excluded. The postulate in the study was the opinion of the investigators that clinical examination is a safe and reliable tool for triage in individuals with these types of injuries. In other words, it was believed that patients could be managed selectively on the basis of clinical findings alone. Based on these observations, approximately one third (19 patients) underwent surgery, with all but two individuals found to have significant intraabdominal injuries. The remaining 40 patients (two thirds) were successfully observed. There were no missed injuries or delays in diagnosis. The authors concluded that clinical examination is a safe method for selecting patients with gunshot wounds to the buttocks for nonoperative treatment.[132]

A particular caveat should be introduced, however, concerning the role of *sigmoidoscopy* in this situation. Ferraro and co-workers reviewed sigmoidoscopy in patients who sustained gunshot wounds to the buttocks.[36] Sixteen individuals underwent this examination, and a rectal injury was demonstrated in seven. There were no missed injuries and no morbidity in the remaining patients managed without sigmoidoscopy (an additional 52 patients). The authors concluded that sigmoidoscopy can be performed *selectively* in individuals who have sustained a gunshot wound to the buttocks when the possibility of involvement of the rectum is in doubt.[36] An abdominal pelvic CT scan may also help to determine the missile tract in these patients.

CONCLUSIONS AND RECOMMENDATIONS

The history of colorectal wound injuries and their management is fascinating, but it has often been surrounded by controversy. However, prospective, randomized, controlled trials have helped to clarify what should be the appropriate management for most patients. It is certainly clear that a reasonably consistent approach may be made for the treatment of nondestructive colon wounds. Unfortunately, the data are less conclusive for more extensive wounds and for rectal injuries.

In summary, all uncomplicated colon wounds (which represent 80% to 90% of all colon injuries) may be safely

managed by means of primary repair. Destructive or devitalized colonic injuries require resection and, perforce, have a higher leakage rate if an anastomosis is attempted. These should be selectively managed. Primary anastomosis without diversion should be reserved for *good-risk, healthy individuals who do not have associated significant hemorrhage.*

Extraperitoneal rectal injuries are managed preferentially by fecal diversion, distal irrigation, and presacral drainage. Although the data concerning drainage are somewhat less clear, this approach certainly minimizes the risk for pelvic sepsis and is associated with a very low morbidity rate.

REFERENCES

1. Adkins RB Jr, Zirkle PK, Waterhouse G. Penetrating colon trauma. *J Trauma* 1984;24:491.
2. Appleby JP, Nagy AG. Abdominal injuries associated with use of seat belts. *Am J Surg* 1989;157:457.
3. Artz CP. Battle casualties in Korea: studies of the surgical research team. In: *Battle wounds: clinical experiences*, vol 3. Washington, DC: Medical Service Graduate School, 1955.
4. Baker LW, Thomson SR, Chadwick SJ. Colon wound management and prograde colonic lavage in large-bowel trauma. *Br J Surg* 1990;77:872.
5. Baudens L. Clinique des plaies d'armes à feu (1836). Reported in: *Medical and surgical history of the war of rebellion*, part 2. Washington, DC: United States Government Printing Office, 1876:124.
6. Blumenberg RM. The seat belt syndrome: sigmoid colon perforation. *Ann Surg* 1967;165:637.
7. Bostick PJ, Heard JS, Islas JT, et al. Management of penetrating colon injuries. *J Natl Med Assoc* 1994;86:378.
8. Brunner RG, Shatney CH. Diagnostic and therapeutic aspects of rectal trauma: blunt versus penetrating. *Am Surg* 1987;53:215.
9. Bubenik O, Meakins JL, McLean APH. Delayed perforation of the colon in blunt abdominal trauma. *Can J Surg* 1980;23:473.
10. Bugis SP, Blair NP, Letwin ER. Management of blunt and penetrating colon injuries. *Am J Surg* 1992;163:547.
11. Burch JM, Brock JC, Gevirtzman L, et al. The injured colon. *Ann Surg* 1986;203:701.
12. Burch JM, Feliciano DV, Mattox KL. Colostomy and drainage for civilian rectal injuries: is that all? *Ann Surg* 1989;209:600.
13. Burch JM, Martin RR, Richardson RJ, et al. Evolution of the treatment of the injured colon in the 1980s. *Arch Surg* 1991;126:979.
14. Carpenter D, Bello J, Sokol TP, et al. The intracolonic bypass tube for left colon and rectal trauma: the avoidance of a colostomy. *Am Surg* 1990;56:769.
15. Carrillo EH, Somberg LB, Ceballos CE, et al. Blunt traumatic injuries to the colon and rectum. *J Am Coll Surg* 1996;183:548.
16. Chappuis CW, Frey DJ, Dietzen CD, et al. Management of penetrating colon injuries: a prospective randomized trial. *Ann Surg* 1991;213:492.
17. Chiu WC, Shanmuganathan K, Mirvis SE, et al. Determining the need for laparotomy in penetrating torso trauma: a prospective study using triple-contrast enhanced abdominopelvic computed tomography. *J Trauma* 2001;51:860.
18. Cook A, Levine BA, Rusing T, et al. Traditional treatment of colon injuries: an effective method. *Arch Surg* 1984;119:591.

19. Critchlow JF, Houlihan MJ, Landolt CC, et al. Primary sphincter repair in anorectal trauma. *Dis Colon Rectum* 1985;28:945.

20. Dang CV, Peter ET, Parks SN, et al. Trauma of the colon: early drop-back of exteriorized repair. *Arch Surg* 1982; 117:652.

21. Dauterive AH, Flancbaum L, Cox EF. Blunt intestinal trauma: a modern-day review. *Ann Surg* 1985;201:198.

22. Dawes LG, Aprahamian C, Condon RE, et al. The risk of infection after colon injury. *Surgery* 1986;100:796.

23. Dellinger EP, Wertz MJ, Lennard ES, et al. Efficacy of short-course antibiotic prophylaxis after penetrating intestinal injury: a prospective randomized trial. *Arch Surg* 1986;121:23.

24. Demetriades D. Penetrating injuries of the colon: changing perspectives. *S Afr J Surg* 1991;29:25.

25. Demetriades D, Charalambides D. Gunshot wounds of the colon: role of retained bullets in sepsis. *Br J Surg* 1993;80:772.

26. Demetriades D, Charalambides D, Pantanowitz D. Gunshot wounds of the colon: role of primary repair. *Ann R Coll Surg Engl* 1992;74:381.

27. Demetriades D, Rabinowitz B, Sofianos C, et al. The management of colon injuries by primary repair or colostomy. *Br J Surg* 1985;72:881.

28. Dinnick T. The origins and evolution of colostomy. *Br J Surg* 1934;22:142.

29. Durham RM, Pruitt C, Moran J, et al. Civilian colon trauma: factors that predict success by primary repair. *Dis Colon Rectum* 1997;40:685.

30. Engelberg M, Richter S. Self-induced recto-vesical injury due to auto-eroticism. *Am J Proctol Gastroenterol Colon Rectal Surg* 1983;34:8.

31. Fabian TC, Croce MA, Payne LW, et al. Duration of antibiotic therapy for penetrating abdominal trauma: a prospective trial. *Surgery* 1992;112:785.

32. Fabian TC, Croce M, Stewart RM. A prospective analysis of diagnostic laparoscopy in trauma. *Ann Surg* 1993;217:557.

33. Fabian TC, Hess MM, Croce MA, et al. Superiority of aztreonam/clindamycin compared with gentamicin/clindamycin in patients with penetrating abdominal trauma. *Am J Surg* 1994;167:291.

34. Falcone RE, Wanamaker SR, Santanello SA, et al. Colorectal trauma: primary repair or anastomosis with intracolonic bypass versus ostomy. *Dis Colon Rectum* 1992; 35:957.

35. Fernando HC, Alle KM, Chen J, et al. Triage by laparoscopy in patients with penetrating abdominal trauma. *Br J Surg* 1994;81:384.

36. Ferraro FJ, Livingston DH, Odom J, et al. The role of sigmoidoscopy in the management of gunshot wounds to the buttocks. *Am Surg* 1993;59:350.

37. Flint LM, Vitale GC, Richardson JD, et al. The injured colon: relationships of management to complications. *Ann Surg* 1981;193:619.

38. Flint LM Jr, Voyles CR, Richardson JD, et al. Missile tract infections after transcolonic gunshot wounds. *Arch Surg* 1978;113:727.

39. Frame SB, Ridgeway CA, Rice JC, et al. Penetrating injuries to the colon: analysis by anatomic region of injury. *South Med J* 1989;82:1099.

40. Fullen WD, Hunt J, Altemeir WA. Prophylactic antibiotics in penetrating wounds of the abdomen. *J Trauma* 1972;12:282.

41. Garrison RN, Shively EH, Baker C, et al. Evaluation of management of the emergency right hemicolectomy. *J Trauma* 1979;19:734.

42. George SM Jr, Fabian TC, Mangiante EC. Colon trauma: further support for primary repair. *Am J Surg* 1988;156:16.

43. George SM Jr, Fabian TC, Voeller GR, et al. Primary repair of colon wounds: a prospective trial in nonselected patients. *Ann Surg* 1989;209:728.

44. Gonzalez RP, Merlotti GJ, Holevar MR. Colostomy in penetrating colon injury: is it necessary? *J Trauma* 1996;41:271.

45. Haas PA, Fox TA Jr. Civilian injuries of the rectum and anus. *Dis Colon Rectum* 1979;22:17.

46. Hashmonai M, Torem S, Kam I, et al. Primary repair of colon injuries. *Isr J Med Sci* 1983;19:116.

47. Howdieshell TR, Delaurier G. An unusual injury of the sigmoid colon produced by seat belt trauma. *Am Surg* 1993;59:355.

48. Howell HS, Bartizal JF, Freeark RJ. Blunt trauma involving the colon and rectum. *J Trauma* 1976;16:624.

49. Husum H. *War surgery: field manual.* Penang, Malaysia: Third World Network,1995:383.

50. Idikula J, Moses BV, Sadhu D, et al. Bull horn injuries. *Surg Gynecol Obstet* 1991;172:220.

51. Ivatury RR, Gaudino J, Nallathambi MN, et al. Definitive treatment of colon injuries: a prospective study. *Am Surg* 1993;59:43.

52. Ivatury RR, Licata J, Gunduz Y, et al. Management options in penetrating rectal injuries. *Am Surg* 1991;57:50.

53. Ivatury RR, Simon RJ, Stahl WM. A critical evaluation of laparoscopy in penetrating abdominal trauma. *J Trauma* 1993;34:822.

54. Jacobson LE, Gomez GA, Broadie TA. Primary repair of 58 consecutive penetrating injuries of the colon: should colostomy be abandoned? *Am Surg* 1997;63:170.

55. Jones LW, Bass DH. Perineal injuries in children. *Br J Surg* 1991;78:1105.

56. Karanfilian RG, Ghuman SS, Pathak VB, et al. Penetrating injuries to the colon. *Am Surg* 1982;48:103.

57. Kirkpatrick JR, Rajpal SG. The injured colon: therapeutic considerations. *Am J Surg* 1975;129:187.

58. Komanov I, Kejla Z. Treatment of war injuries to the colon: primary resection and anastomosis without relieving colostomy. *Acta Med Croat* 1995;49:65.

59. Kudsk KA, Croce MA, Fabian TC, et al. Enteral versus parenteral feeding: effects on septic morbidity after blunt and penetrating abdominal trauma. *Ann Surg* 1992;215:503.

60. Kudsk KA, McQueen M, Voeller G, et al. Management of complex perineal soft tissue injuries. *J Trauma* 1990;30: 1155.

61. Kurz A, Sessler DI, Lenhardt R. Perioperative normothermia to reduce the incidence of surgical wound infection and shorten hospitalization: study of Wound Infection and Temperature Group. *N Engl J Med* 1996;334:1209.

62. Kusminsky RE, Shbeeb I, Makos G, et al. Blunt pelviperineal injuries: an expanded role for the diverting colostomy. *Dis Colon Rectum* 1982;25:787.

63. Leppaniemi A, Karppinen K, Haapiainen R. Stab wounds of the colon. *Ann Chir Gynaecol* 1994;83:26.

64. Levison MA, Thomas DD, Wiencek RG, et al. Management of the injured colon: evolving practice at an urban trauma center. *J Trauma* 1990;30:247.

65. Lischick WP, Knoll SM, Isaacson NH. Rectosigmoid perforations in homosexual patients. *Am Surg* 1985;51:602.

66. Livingston DH, Tortella BJ, Blackwood J, et al. The role of laparoscopy in abdominal trauma. *J Trauma* 1992;33:471.

67. Lou MA, Johnson AP, Atik M, et al. Exteriorized repair in the management of colon injuries. *Arch Surg* 1981;116:926.

68. Mangiante EC, Graham AD, Fabian TC. Rectal gunshot wounds: management of civilian injuries. *Am Surg* 1986; 52:37.

69. Martin RR, Burch JM, Richardson R, et al. Outcome for delayed operation of penetrating colon injuries. *J Trauma* 1991;31:1591.

70. Martin RR, Byrne M. Post-operative care and complication of damage control surgery. *Surg Clin North Am* 1997;77: 929.

71. Mason JM. Surgery of the colon in the forward battle area. *Surgery* 1945;18:534.

72. Maxwell TM. Rectal injuries. *Can J Surg* 1978;21:524.

73. McElveen TS, Collin GR. The role of ultrasonography in blunt abdominal trauma: a prospective study. *Am Surg* 1997;63:184.

74. Miller FB, Nikolov NR, Garrison RN. Emergency right colon resection. *Arch Surg* 1987;122:339.

75. Moore FA, Moore EE, Jones TN, et al. TEN versus TPN following major abdominal trauma: reduced septic morbidity with TEN. *J Trauma* 1989;29:916.

76. Moore FA, Moore EE, Kudsk KA, et al. Clinical benefits of an immune-enhancing diet for early post-injury enteral feeding. *J Trauma* 1994;37:607.

77. Moreels R, Pont M, Evan S, et al. Wartime colon injuries: primary repair or colostomy? *J R Soc Med* 1994;87:265.

78. Morgado PJ, Alfaro R, Morgado PJ Jr, et al. Colon trauma—clinical staging for surgical decision making: analysis of 119 cases. *Dis Colon Rectum* 1992;35:986.

79. Mortensen NJMcC, Irvin TT. Disembowelment per rectum: a fatal rectal injury. *Br J Surg* 1984;71:289.

80. Mulherin JL Jr, Sawyers JL. Evaluation of three methods for managing penetrating colon injuries. *J Trauma* 1975; 15:580.

81. Murray JA, Demetriades D, Cornwell EE 3rd, et al. Penetrating left thoracoabdominal trauma: the incidence and clinical presentation of diaphragm injuries. *J Trauma* 1997;43:624.

82. Myers J, Page CP, Stewart RM, et al. Complications of needle catheter jejunostomy in 2,022 consecutive applications. *Am J Surg* 1995;170:547.

83. Nallathambi MN, Ivatury RR, Rohman M, et al. Penetrating colon injuries: exteriorized repair versus loop colostomy. *J Trauma* 1987;27:876.

84. Nallathambi MN, Ivatury RR, Shah PM, et al. Aggressive definitive management of penetrating colon injuries: 136 cases with 3.7% mortality. *J Trauma* 1984;24:500.

85. Nallathambi MN, Ivatury RR, Shah PM, et al. Penetrating right colon trauma: the ever-diminishing role for colostomy. *Am Surg* 1987;53:209.

86. Nallathambi MN, Sleeper R, Smith M, et al. Acid burns of the rectum and colon: report of a case. *Dis Colon Rectum* 1987;30:469.

87. Naraynsingh V, Ariyanayagam D, Pooran S. Primary repair of colon injuries in a developing country. *Br J Surg* 1991; 78:319.

88. Nelken N, Lewis F. The influence of injury severity on complication rates after primary closure or colostomy for penetrating colon trauma. *Ann Surg* 1989;209:439.

89. Nichols RL, Smith JW, Klein DB, et al. Risk of infection after penetrating abdominal trauma. *N Engl J Med* 1984;311:1065.

90. Nolan BW, Gabram SGA, Schwartz RJ, et al. Mesenteric injury from blunt abdominal trauma. *Am Surg* 1995;61:501.

91. Office of the Surgeon General. Circular letter no. 178, October 23, 1943.

92. Ogilvie WH. Abdominal wounds in the western desert. *Surg Gynecol Obstet* 1944;78:225.

93. Orsay CP, Merlotti G, Abcarian H, et al. Colorectal trauma. *Dis Colon Rectum* 1989;21:188.

94. Pachter HL, Hoballah JJ, Corcoran TA, et al. The morbidity and financial impact of colostomy closure in trauma patients. *J Trauma* 1990;30:1510.

95. Parks TG. Surgical management of injuries of the large intestine. *Br J Surg* 1981;68:725.

96. Peterson-Brown S, Francis N, Whawell S, et al. Prediction of the delayed complications of intestinal and mesenteric injuries following experimental blunt abdominal trauma. *Br J Surg* 1990;77:648.

97. Poret H, Fabian TC, Croce MA, et al. Analysis of septic morbidity following gunshot wounds to the colon: the missile is an adjuvant for abscess. *J Trauma* 1991;31:1088.

98. Prasad ML, Pearl RK, Orsay CP, et al. End-loop ileocolostomy for massive trauma to the right side of the colon. *Arch Surg* 1984;119:975.

99. Proceedings of Commander-in-Chief of the Pacific 4th Conference on War Surgery, Tokyo 1970.

100. Renz BM, Feliciano DV, Sherman R. Same admission colostomy closure (SACC): a new approach to rectal wounds. A prospective study. *Ann Surg* 1993;218:279.

101. Ridgeway CA, Frame SB, Rice JC, et al. Primary repair versus colostomy for the treatment of penetrating colon injuries. *Dis Colon Rectum* 1989;32:1046.

102. Robertson HD, Ray JE, Ferrari BT, et al. Management of rectal trauma. *Surg Gynecol Obstet* 1982;154:161.

103. Ross SE, Cobean RA, Hoyt DB, et al. Blunt colonic injury: a multicenter review. *J Trauma* 1992;33:379.

104. Rotondo MF, Schwab CW, McGonigal MD, et al. Damage control: an approach for improved survival in exsanguinating penetrating abdominal injury. *J Trauma* 1993; 35:375.

105. Rowlands BJ, Ericsson CD. Comparative studies of antibiotic therapy after penetrating abdominal trauma. *Am J Surg* 1984;148:791.

106. Royle CA. Colonic trauma: modern civilian management and military surgical doctrine. *J R Soc Med* 1995;88:585P.

107. Ryan M, Dutta S, Masri L, et al. Fecal diversion for penetrating colon injuries: still the established treatment. *Dis Colon Rectum* 1995;38:264.

108. Salvino CK, Esposito TJ, Marshall WJ, et al. The role of diagnostic laparoscopy in the management of trauma patients: a preliminary assessment. *J Trauma* 1993;34:506.

109. Sasaki LS, Allaben RD, Golwala R, et al. Primary repair of colon injuries: a prospective randomized study. *J Trauma* 1996;39:895.

110. Sasaki LS, Mittal V, Allaben RD. Primary repair of colon injuries: a retrospective analysis. *Am Surg* 1994;60:522.

111. Schultz SC, Magnant CM, Richman MF, et al. Identifying the low-risk patient with penetrating colonic injury for selective use of primary repair. *Surg Gynecol Obstet* 1993; 177:237.

112. Shaftan GW. Abdominal trauma management in America. *ACS Bull* 1989;74:21.

113. Shannon FL, Moore EE. Primary repair of the colon: when is it a safe alternative? *Surgery* 1985;98:851.

114. Singer MA, Nelson RL. Primary repair of penetrating colon injuries: a systematic review. *Dis Colon Rectum* 2002; 45:1579.

115. Smith RS, Fry WR, Morabito DJ, et al. Therapeutic laparoscopy in trauma. *Am J Surg.* 1995;170:632.

116. Sola JE, Bender JS, Buchman TG. Morbidity and timing of colostomy closure in trauma patients. *Injury* 1993;24:438.

117. Sosa JL, Baker M, Puente I, et al. Negative laparotomy in abdominal gunshot wounds: potential impact of laparoscopy. *J Trauma* 1995;38:194.

118. Sosa JL, Puente I, Arrillaga A, et al. Laparoscopy in 121 consecutive patients with abdominal gunshot wounds. *J Trauma* 1995;39:501.

119. Steinig JP, Boyd CR. Presacral drainage in penetrating extraperitoneal rectal injuries: is it necessary? *Am Surg* 1996;62:765.

120. Stewart RM, Fabian TC, Croce MA, et al. Is resection with primary anastomosis following destructive colon wounds always safe? *Am J Surg* 1994;168:316.

121. Stewart RM, Kudsk KA. Perineal injuries. In: Maull K, Cleveland H, Feliciano D, et al, eds. *Advances in trauma and critical care*, vol 7. St. Louis, MO: CV Mosby, 1994: 175.

122. Stone HH, Fabian TC. Management of perforating colon trauma: randomization between primary closure and exteriorization. *Ann Surg* 1979;190:430.

123. Strada G, Raad L, Belloni G, et al. Large bowel perforations in war surgery: one-stage treatment in a field hospital. *Int J Colorectal Dis* 1993;8:213.

124. Taheri PA, Ferrara JJ, Johnson CE, et al. A convincing case for primary repair of penetrating colon injuries. *Am J Surg* 1993;166:39.

125. Thigpen JB Jr, Santelices AA, Hagan WV, et al. Current management of trauma to the colon. *Am Surg* 1980;46:108.

126. Thomas DD, Levison MA, Dykstra BJ, et al. Management of rectal injuries: dogma versus prejudice. *Am Surg* 1990;56: 507.

127. Thompson JS, Moore EE. Factors affecting the outcome of exteriorized colon repairs. *J Trauma* 1982;22:403.

128. Thompson JS, Moore EE, Moore JB. Comparison of penetrating injuries of the right and left colon. *Ann Surg* 1981;193:414.

129. Tuggle D, Huber PJ. Management of rectal trauma. *Am J Surg* 1984;148:806.

130. Udobi KF, Rodriguez A, Chiu WC, et al. Role of ultrasonography in penetrating abdominal trauma: a prospective clinical study. *J Trauma* 2001;50:475.

131. Velmahos GC, Demetriades D, Cornwell EE III, et al. Gunshot wounds to the buttocks: predicting the need for operation. *Dis Colon Rectum* 1997;40:307.

132. Velmahos GC, Souter I, Degiannis E, et al. Primary repair for colonic gunshot wounds. *Aust N Z J Surg* 1996;66:344.

133. Weigelt JA, Easley SM, Thal ER, et al. Abdominal surgical wound infection is lowered with improved perioperative enterococcus and bacteroides therapy. *J Trauma* 1993; 34:579.

134. Weil PH. Injuries of the retroperitoneal portions of the colon and rectum. *Dis Colon Rectum* 1983;26:19.

135. Whelan TJ Jr. Surgical lessons learned and relearned in Vietnam. *Surg Annu* 1975;7:1.

136. Wiener I, Rojas P, Wolma FJ. Traumatic colonic perforation: review of 16 years' experience. *Am J Surg* 1981; 142:717.

137. Williams L, Lewis E. Identification of small rectal perforations. *Surg Gynecol Obstet* 1987;164:475.

138. Wisner DH, Chun Y, Blaisdell FW. Blunt intestinal injury: keys to diagnosis and management. *Arch Surg* 1990;125: 1319.

139. Witz M, Shpitz B, Zager M, et al. Anal erotic instrumentation: a surgical problem. *Dis Colon Rectum* 1984;27:331.

140. Woodhall JP, Oschner A. The management of perforating injuries of the colon and rectum in civilian practice. *Surgery* 1951;29:305.

141. Wynne JB. Vacuum toilet evisceration. *JAMA* 1987;257: 1177.

142. Yajko RD, Norton LW, Bloemendal L, et al. Morbidity of colostomy closure. *Am J Surg* 1976;132:304.

143. Zantut LF, Ivatury RR, Smith RS. Diagnostic and therapeutic laparoscopy for penetrating abdominal trauma: a multicenter experience. *J Trauma* 1997;42:825.

Medical and surgical history of the war of rebellion, part 2, vol 1. Washington, DC: United States Government Printing Office, 1876:112.

Management of Foreign Bodies

Homo sum; humani nil a me alienum puto.
[I am a man, and nothing human is foreign to me.]
    Terence (185–159 B.C.): *Heauton Timorumenos*, Act I

In ancient times, it was customary to open the stomach to remove knives that had been accidentally swallowed, but it was not until 1807 that White excised a silver spoon from the intestines.[6,20] The ingestion of foreign materials may occur accidentally (e.g., swallowed dental bridge, nail, screw, paper clip, toothpick, chicken bone; Figs. 15-1 and 15-2), or it may be intentional (e.g., in psychiatric or prison populations).[16] Occasionally, a physician may be responsible for the introduction of a foreign body that requires special efforts to remove (Figure 15-3). Once an item passes beyond the pylorus, it usually can be eliminated without difficulty. One area of relative hindrance to passage, however, is the terminal ileum. Erosion can occur, which may lead to perforation, abscess, and fistula formation. For example, a case of aortocolic fistula caused by an ingested chicken bone has been reported.[5] Risk factors that increase the probability of foreign body perforation include inflammatory bowel disease, adhesions, diverticular disease, Meckel's diverticulum, tumors, and hernias.[14]

Schillingstad and colleagues categorize four groups of patients who are at risk for foreign body ingestion[18]:

- Children up to 5 years of age with accidental ingestion (e.g., buttons, coins)
- Adults who present with food impaction, often related to being edentulous
- Individuals who have accidentally or deliberately ingested a foreign body
- Individuals attempting to profit from drug smuggling (i.e., "mules"—also known as "body packers" or "body baggers"). Rupture or impaction can lead to fatal drug toxicity.

The list of objects that have been removed from the rectum is virtually endless (e.g., lightbulbs, catheters, pens and pencils, glass tubes, candles, vibrators, bottles, deceased gerbils, and jars; Figs. 15-4 through 15-9). Busch and Starling identified 182 cases from the world's literature and noted the recovery of objects from A (i.e., apple) to Z (i.e., zucchini).[4]

As can be appreciated, the variety of foreign bodies is limited only by one's imagination. Individuals may present with a host of complaints, including rectal bleeding, anorectal pain, and difficulty with micturition. Embarrassed, apprehensive, and uncomfortable, many deny the incident, often claiming to have fallen on the object, which miraculously disappeared beyond his or her reach.

EVALUATION

It is important to evaluate the patient's abdomen for signs and symptoms suggestive of peritoneal irritation. An indwelling catheter may be necessary if there is any concern about urinary retention. Inspection and palpation of the anal canal and rectum may reveal the foreign body. Note should be made of sphincter tone and contractility, especially if signs of anoreceptivity are evident. Such a situation may actually facilitate evaluation of the patient and extraction of the foreign body. An x-ray film of the pelvis will demonstrate the contours of any radiopaque foreign material. One should also seek to identify any unsuspected second foreign body.

PRINCIPLES OF MANAGEMENT

Extracting foreign bodies from the rectum has become virtually epidemic. The presence of these objects in the rectum or colon poses particular difficulty in management. The administration of glucagon, spinal anesthesia, or general anesthesia assists in relaxation of the sphincter, greatly facilitating removal of the object.[18] In general, foreign bodies located within the rectum can be extracted as an outpatient procedure or in the emergency department. Those positioned above the rectum should be removed in the operating room.

One may attempt extraction of colonic foreign bodies by means of the colonoscope, but if symptoms of peritoneal irritation develop, removal will require laparotomy and colotomy.[19] Removal by appendicostomy has also been suggested if the object is small.[15] Rocklin and Apelgren, in a literature review, found 29 instances of

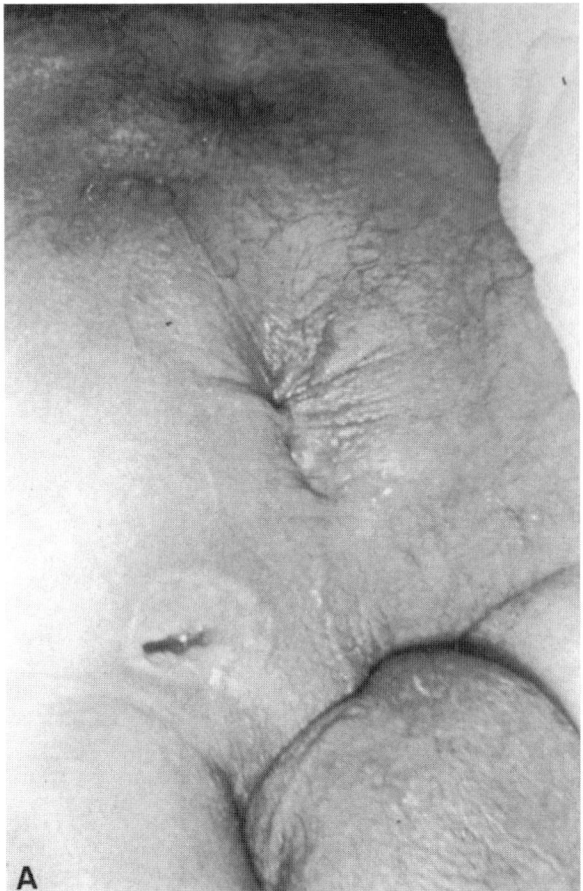

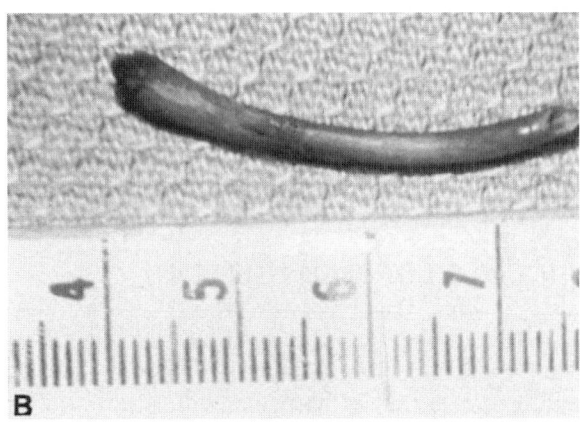

FIGURE 15-1. (A) Perforation of the rectum from an ingested foreign body that produced an ischiorectal abscess. (B) A chicken bone was the cause of the perforation. (Courtesy of Daniel Rosenthal, M.D.)

colonoscopic removal of a variety of objects reported in 14 publications.[17] Biopsy forceps, polypectomy snares, and stone-extracting baskets have all been successfully employed. The following protocol has been recommended for management of colon objects[17]:

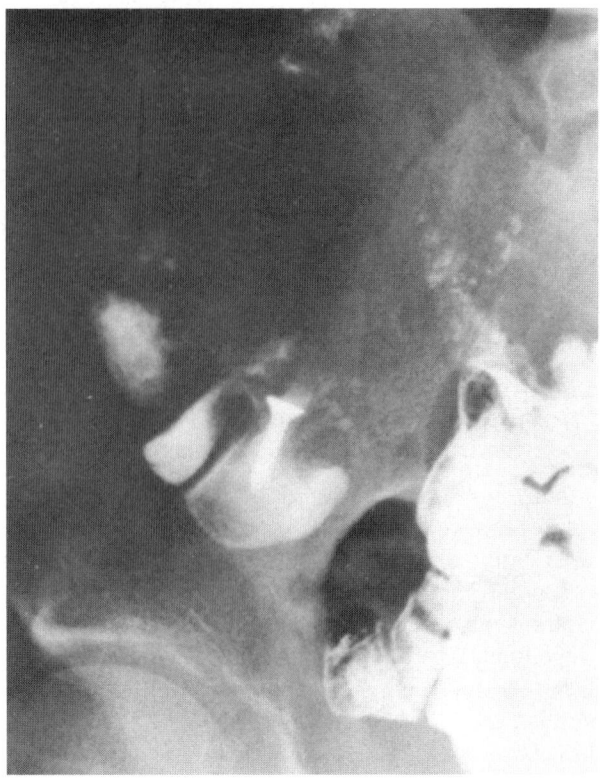

FIGURE 15-2. An accidentally swallowed wood screw is lodged in the cecum. Because of peritoneal signs, a laparotomy was undertaken. (Courtesy of Albert Medwid, M.D.)

- Plain abdominal radiograph for nature and location
- Immediate attempt at colonoscopic extraction if the foreign body is associated with bleeding or obstruction
- Barium enema for difficult-to-localize, suspected, or known radiolucent foreign body
- High-fiber diet, bulk laxative, mineral oil (no cathartics)
- Serial radiographs to follow progression
- Enemas before the procedure to enhance visualization
- Broad-spectrum antibiotics before the procedure
- Colonoscopic extraction if the object fails to progress on serial radiographs during 48 hours
- Observation for 24 hours after removal

Stewart (Stewart RM, personal communication, 1997) outlines the following principles of management of rectal foreign bodies:

- More damage is generally inflicted on the anorectum by a forceful attempt to remove a foreign body than by the original insertion.
- Never attempt to remove a foreign body unless the patient's anal sphincter is fully relaxed by local, spinal, or general anesthesia.

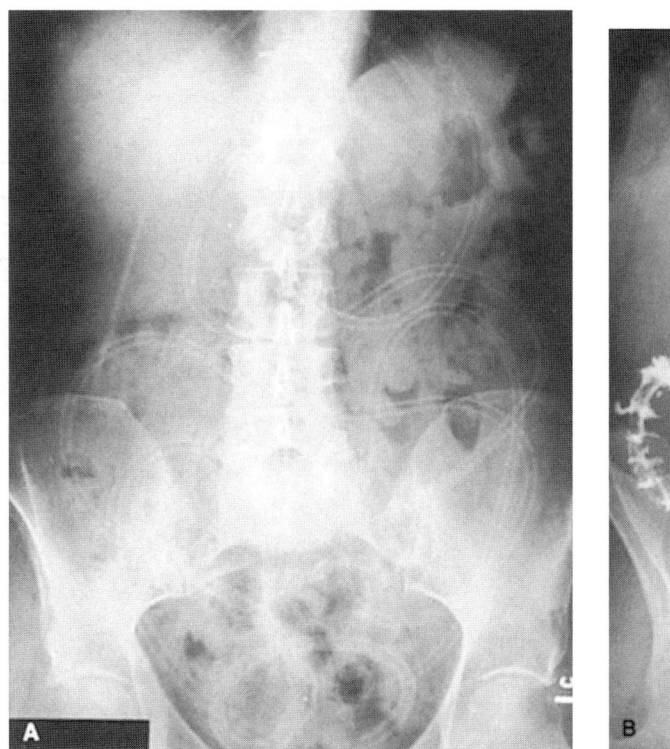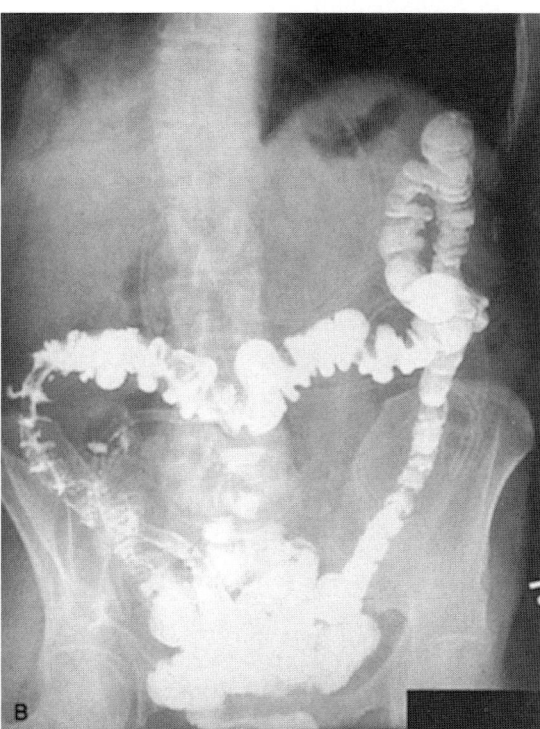

FIGURE 15-3. Miller-Abbott tube lodged in the intestine several years after it had been divided in the oropharynx with the expectation that it would pass **(A)**. Barium enema examination reveals that the distal end reaches the midtransverse colon **(B)**. Despite attempted removal via colonoscopy, a laparotomy was necessary.

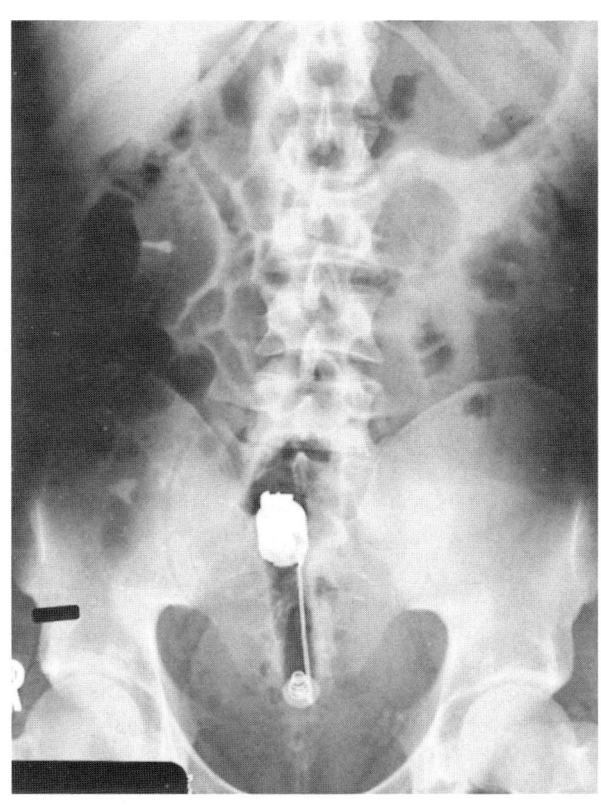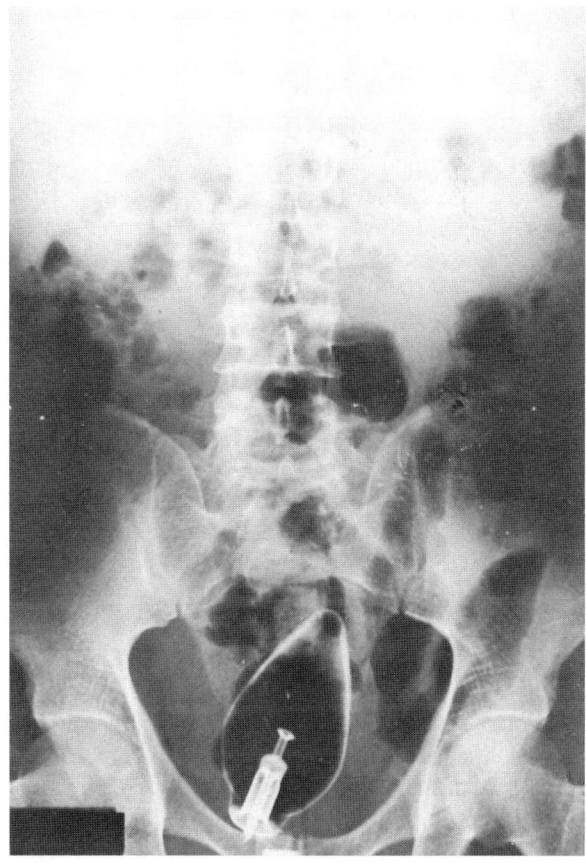

FIGURE 15-4. Foreign body: vibrator in the rectum.

FIGURE 15-5. Foreign body: lightbulb in the rectum.

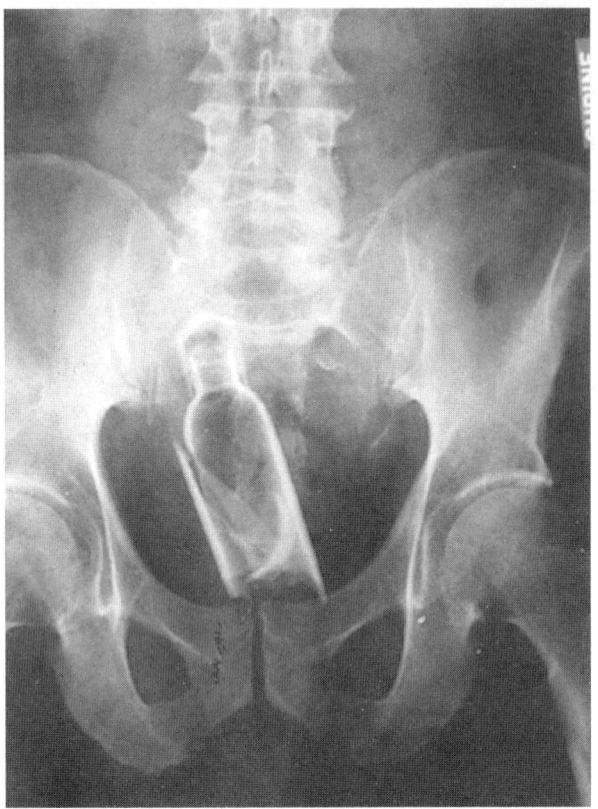

FIGURE 15-6. Foreign body. Extraction of broken bottle in the rectum presents a particularly challenging problem.

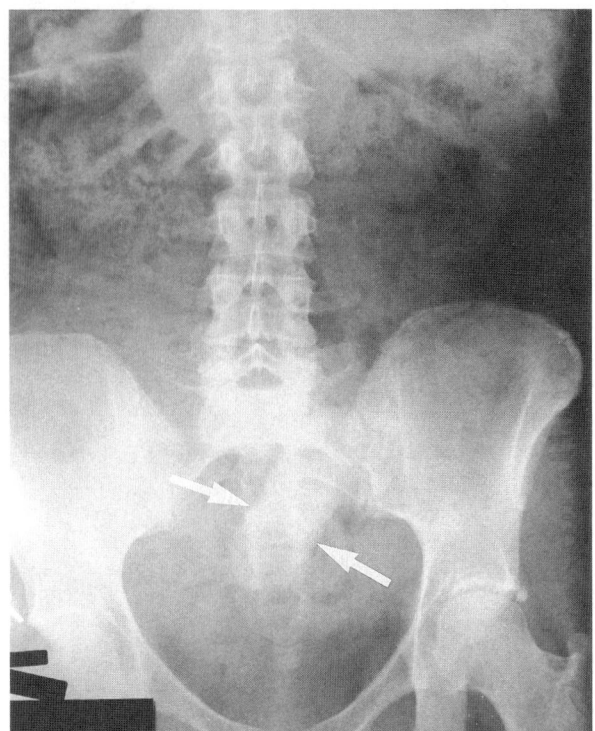

FIGURE 15-7. Foreign body: dildo in the rectum *(arrows)*.

- Never attempt to extract a foreign body using instruments in an uncooperative patient, because a sudden move can precipitate tearing or perforation.
- Large foreign bodies are preferentially removed in the operating room under a spinal or general anesthetic.
- Following retrieval of the object, meticulous endoscopic examination should be undertaken and repair effected for any associated lacerations.
- Rectal perforation, whether intraperitoneal or extraperitoneal, requires a diverting stoma.

Senile patients with a patulous anus can usually have foreign bodies removed without an anesthetic. Thermometers are the most frequently encountered foreign objects in this age group.

SPECIAL TECHNIQUES

Numerous techniques have been suggested to remove objects from the rectum, including the use of blunt hooks or sponge holders, bimanual manipulation, and the use of a nasogastric tube as a lasso.[9] A Foley catheter is particularly useful for a hollow body, such as a jar.[8,11] Drilling a hole in the bottom of a bottle or jar and inserting a Foley catheter is another means for removing such an item if the open end is directed cephalad. Garber and colleagues suggest using the more rigid endotracheal tube for such objects.[10] Foley catheters may be inserted above an object into the proximal bowel lumen. Gentle distal traction while inserting air above the object to break the vacuum often will result in successful extraction.[13] Aquino and Turner advise the use of three lubricated Tauber vaginal spatulas to break the suction and rock the object out.[1] Rubber-shod clamps may be employed to remove broken glass. Under these circumstances, with careful follow-up by means of computed tomography, looking for retroperitoneal air, an exploratory laparotomy may not be needed. Berci and Morgenstern describe use of an operating proctoscope and tenaculum for extraction of foreign bodies.[3] Johnson and Hartranft recommend the use of an obstetric vacuum extractor to remove glass foreign bodies.[12]

Eftaiha and colleagues reported their experience from the Cook County Hospital in Chicago with the removal of 31 objects from the rectum.[7] They employed the principles of biplane abdominal roentgenograms to identify the location, type, and number of foreign materials, and they emphasize the necessity of an anesthetic. It is crucial that once the presence of the foreign body has been deter-

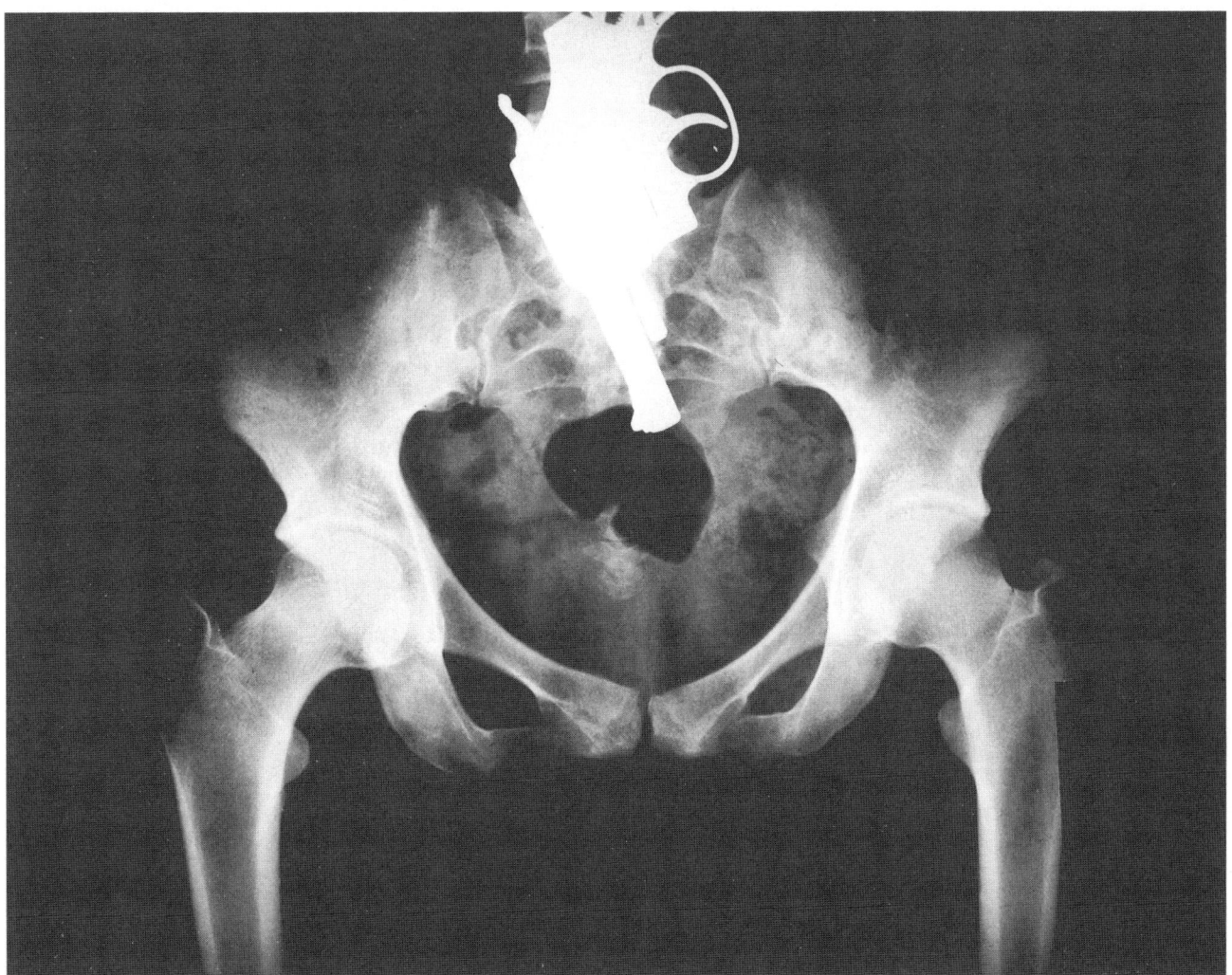

FIGURE 15-8. Foreign body: A pistol in the rectosigmoid gives a special meaning to the expression, "a shot in the dark." (Courtesy of Daniel Rosenthal, M.D.)

mined, it be removed while the patient is under adequate anesthesia to avoid the possibility of further injury. This is a particular concern if the object is glass. Whenever possible, transanal extraction should be used and laparotomy undertaken only as a last resort. Proctosigmoidoscopic examination should be performed after removal of the foreign body to be certain that no injury to the bowel has been sustained. It is also advisable to keep the patient in the hospital until a bowel movement has been achieved and the surgeon is convinced that sepsis or perforation is unlikely. A later report of 55 patients from the same institution confirms the wisdom of the policies stated earlier.[21] Conversely, in the experience of Barone and co-workers, of 112 patients who sustained trauma of the rectum or sigmoid from foreign bodies, most were able to have the foreign bodies removed on an outpatient basis.[2] These investigators do not believe that admission after removal is mandatory. Only one patient required a laparotomy, and this was performed because of signs and symptoms of peritonitis.

If a laparotomy is required, an attempt should be made to "milk" the foreign body down into the field of vision of the perineal operator; hence, the perineolithotomy position should be used. If injury to the rectum has occurred, the previously discussed principles apply. If the object cannot be removed transanally, a colotomy should be undertaken. In the controlled situation, without fecal contamination, no colostomy is performed.

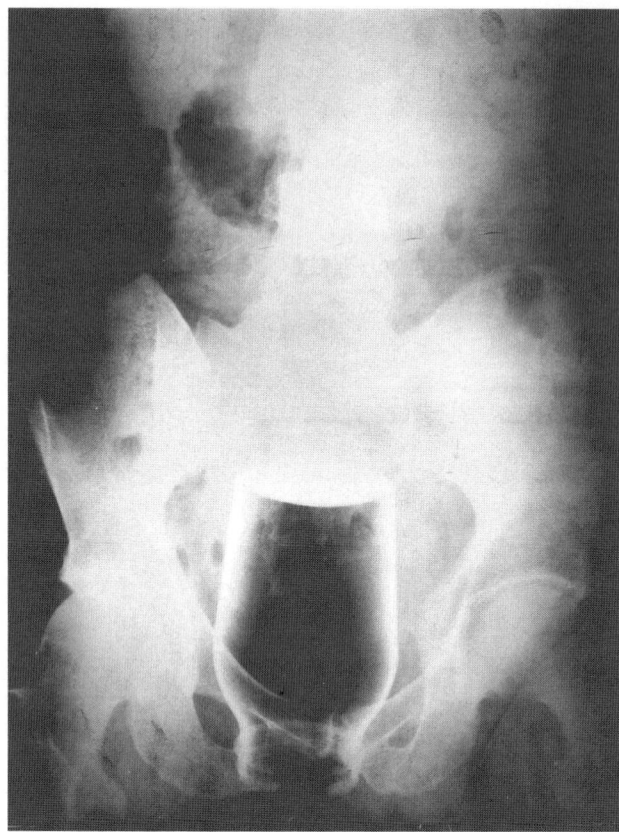

FIGURE 15-9. Foreign body: Bottle in the rectum.

REFERENCES

1. Aquino MM, Turner JW. A simple technique for removing an impacted aerosol-can cap from the rectum. *Dis Colon Rectum* 1986;29:675.

2. Barone JE, Yee J, Nealon TF Jr. Management of foreign bodies and trauma of the rectum. *Surg Gynecol Obstet* 1983; 156:453.

3. Berci G, Morgenstern L. An operative proctoscope for foreign-body extraction. *Dis Colon Rectum* 1983;26:193.

4. Busch DB, Starling JR. Rectal foreign bodies: case reports and a comprehensive review of the world's literature. *Surgery* 1986;100:512.

5. Caes F, Vierendeels T, Welch W, et al. Aortocolic fistula caused by an ingested chicken bone. *Surgery* 1988;103:481.

6. Dinnick T. The origins and evolution of colostomy. *Br J Surg* 1934;22:142.

7. Eftaiha M, Hambrick E, Abcarian H. Principles of management of colorectal foreign bodies. *Dis Colon Rectum* 1977; 112:691.

8. Floyd WF, Walls EW. Electromyography of the sphincter ani externus in man. *J Physiol (Lond)* 1953;122:599.

9. French GWG, Sherlock DJ, Holl-Allen RTJ. Problems with rectal foreign bodies. *Br J Surg* 1985;72:243.

10. Garber HI, Rubin RJ, Eisenstat TE. Removal of a glass foreign body from the rectum. *Dis Colon Rectum* 1981;24:323.

11. Hughes JP. Foreign body of the rectum removal. *Am J Proctol Gastroenterol Colon Rectal Surg* 1983;34:16.

12. Johnson SO, Hartranft TH. Nonsurgical removal of a rectal foreign body using a vacuum extractor: report of a case. *Dis Colon Rectum* 1996;39:935.

13. Kingsley AN, Abcarian H. Colorectal foreign bodies: management update. *Dis Colon Rectum* 1985;28:941.

14. McDowell GCII, Henry M, Ellison EC. Ingestion of sharpened pencils. *Surg Rounds* 1988;11:(12)77.

15. Mizrahi S, Eyal I, Shtamler B. Foreign body removal through an appendicostomy. *Dis Colon Rectum* 1990;33:902.

16. Mortensen NJMcC, Irvin TT. Disembowelment per rectum: a fatal rectal injury. *Br J Surg* 1984;71:289.

17. Rocklin MS, Apelgren KN. Colonoscopic extraction of foreign bodies from above the rectum. *Am Surg* 1989;55:119.

18. Shillingstad RB, Marks JM, Ponsky JL. Endoscopic management of gastrointestinal foreign bodies. *Contemp Surg* 1997;50:87.

19. Sorenson RM, Bond JH Jr. Colonoscopic removal of a foreign body from the cecum. *Gastrointest Endosc* 1975;21:134.

20. White SW. Remarkable case of the swallowing of a silver spoon and the excision of it from the intestinal canal with the recovery of the patient. *Med Repository* 1807;4:367.

21. Whitehead WE, Burgio KL, Engel BT. Biofeedback treatment of fecal incontinence in geriatric patients. *J Am Geriatr Soc* 1985;33:320.

Disorders of Defecation

Constipation, Melanosis Coli, Stercoral Ulcer, Obstructed Defecation (Anismus), Short-Segment Hirschsprung's Disease, Intestinal Pseudo-obstruction (Ogilvie's Syndrome), Proctalgia Fugax (Levator Spasm), Coccygodynia

I hav finally kum to the konklusion, that a good
reliable sett ov bowels iz wurth more tu a man,
than enny quantity of brains.
　　　Henry Wheeler Shaw (Josh Billings): *His Sayings*

This chapter addresses a number of conditions associated with bowel evacuation problems, the presenting complaint of which is often constipation.

CONSTIPATION

A man should always endeavor to keep his bowels lax;
they may even approach a diarrheal state. For this is a
leading rule in hygiene, as long as the bowels are constipated or when they act with difficulty, serious diseases ensue.
　　　Schulchan Aruch [*Code of Jewish Law*]

Chronic idiopathic constipation and abdominal pain are among the most common reasons for patients to solicit medical advice. Psychophysiologic gastrointestinal disorder, splenic flexure syndrome, and irritable bowel are just a few of the terms employed to describe these so-called "functional" complaints. In the United States alone, the cost of over-the-counter laxatives for 1991 was in excess of 400 million dollars. Constipation is more common in blacks (17%), in women (18%), in individuals older than 60 years of age (23%), and in those who are inactive, of low income, or who are poorly educated.[188]

Physiology

Motility

The two primary functions of the colon are absorption and propulsion (see Chapter 2). The bowel absorbs water, certain electrolytes, short-chain fatty acids, and bacterial metabolites. The basic motility activities of the colon are slow net distal propulsion, extensive kneading, and uniform exposure of its contents to the mucosal surface.[189] Material in the bowel is moved along a pressure gradient, with the rate and volume related to the pressure differential, the diameter of the tube, and the viscosity of the contents.[107] It may take only 1 or 2 hours for a meal to traverse the small intestine, but it may frequently take up to 30 hours to pass through the colon. The length and diameter of the colon tend to favor prolonged contact between the contents and the absorptive mucosa; this increases the amount of water removed and as a consequence may yield hard stools.[110] Additionally, widening of the rectosigmoid can produce a capacious distal reservoir; hence, a larger fecal mass is required to stimulate elimination.[110]

Three types of contractions are usually attributed to the colon (see also Chapters 2 and 6):

- Individual phasic contractions of short and long duration
- Organized groups of contractions
- Special propulsive contractions[189]

Individual phasic contraction is the basic unit of contractile activity throughout the gastrointestinal tract.[189] Short-duration contractions last less than 15 seconds, and long-duration contractions last 40 to 60 seconds. Individual phasic contractions are highly disorganized in time and in space; they are effective in mixing, in kneading, and in carrying out slow distal propulsion.[190] The special propulsive contractions (i.e., giant migrating contractions) provide the strong propulsive force required for defecation and for mass movements. Despite what may appear to be a straightforward concept, there is considerable controversy as to the relative merits of the physiologic techniques employed for assessment of the pathophysiology of the various processes and conditions. This is a consequence of several problems. First, the luminal contents vary considerably (fluid at one end and solid at the other); second, sampling is usually inadequate (so that characteristics are attributed to the entire colon when only the sigmoid has been evaluated); and third, the hypothesis that animal models are adequately representative of the human experience is probably erroneous.[107]

Even today, we do not fully understand how all the elements of the colon (i.e., morphology, innervation, function) integrate to produce organized movement of intestinal contents. Furthermore, both the normal range of colorectal motor activity and its variations in disease have yet to be clearly defined.[107] In fact, chronic constipation may be associated with either increased or decreased colonic motility. Perhaps in the future it will be advantageous if colonic motility can be combined with an isotopic assessment of rectosigmoid propulsive activity.[95]

The Defecation Process

The process of evacuation of feces consists of two stages. The first is involuntary, during which the contents are gradually propelled into the rectum. This is the total effect of short-duration, long-duration, and giant migrating contractions.[189] The second stage is the act of defecation, during which feces are expelled. When the process goes awry, the physician must have an organized approach to the evaluation and treatment of this extraordinarily commonplace symptom if appropriate therapy is to be instituted (Figs. 16-1 and 16-2). Certain specific studies, especially physiologic investigations, should be considered. Some of these are also discussed in Chapter 13. It may be useful to review the sections on physiologic studies in Chapters 2, 6, and 13 to obtain a better perspective of these two, often interrelated conditions.

Mechanical and physiologic retentive forces in the rectosigmoid normally maintain the distal rectum in an empty and collapsed state. The bends and folds of the rectosigmoid as well as the valves of Houston were originally believed to retard the material from entry into the rectum, but it is doubtful whether such a hypothesis is valid. The maintenance of continence and the mechanism of defecation depend on the interaction of neurosensory and neuromotor impulses. As feces accumulate in the rectum, the bowel wall muscle relaxes, allowing distension and accommodation of the enlarging fecal mass. Sensory receptors within the anal canal determine the nature of the luminal contents, whether flatus, liquid, or solid stool. Threshold stimulation of the afferent nerve endings is reached, and involuntary precipitation of the anal reflex occurs, enabling the rectum to empty. Successive functional segments of colon coordinate their activity to produce a mass peristaltic wave above the fecal mass. Concomitantly, the distal part of the intestine and the internal sphincter relax, and the external sphincter contracts. If elimination is to proceed, voluntary inhibition of external sphincter contraction occurs.

Distension of the rectum is the stimulus for defecation. As the stool enters the rectum, the internal sphincter relaxes and the external sphincter contracts. With voluntary inhibition of external sphincter contraction during a mass peristaltic propulsion, defecation will occur without effort, or gas will be passed selectively. With contraction of the external sphincter, accommodation occurs by relaxation of the rectal wall muscle. This, in a matter of seconds, will remove the urgency to defecate unless the volume is large or the individual has an impaired sphincter mechanism.

If a voluntary effort is required to defecate, intraabdominal pressure is increased by closure of the glottis

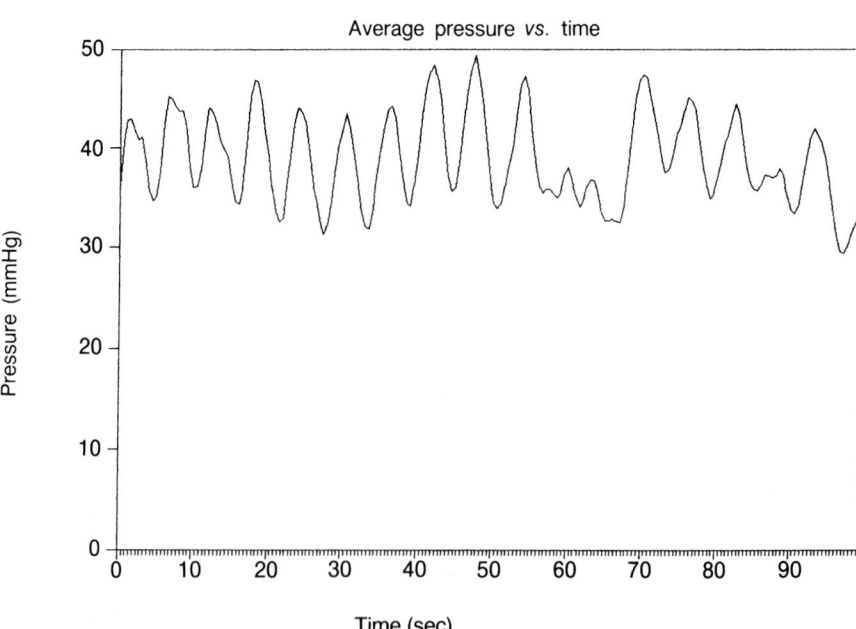

FIGURE 16-1. Evaluation of anal motility of a slow wave, which is usually found in the proximal portion of the anal sphincter. Typically, it has a frequency of approximately 10 to 14 cycles per minute and an average amplitude of 2 to 6 mm Hg. In this instance, an amplitude of 12 mm Hg has been recorded. (Courtesy of John A. Coller, M.D.)

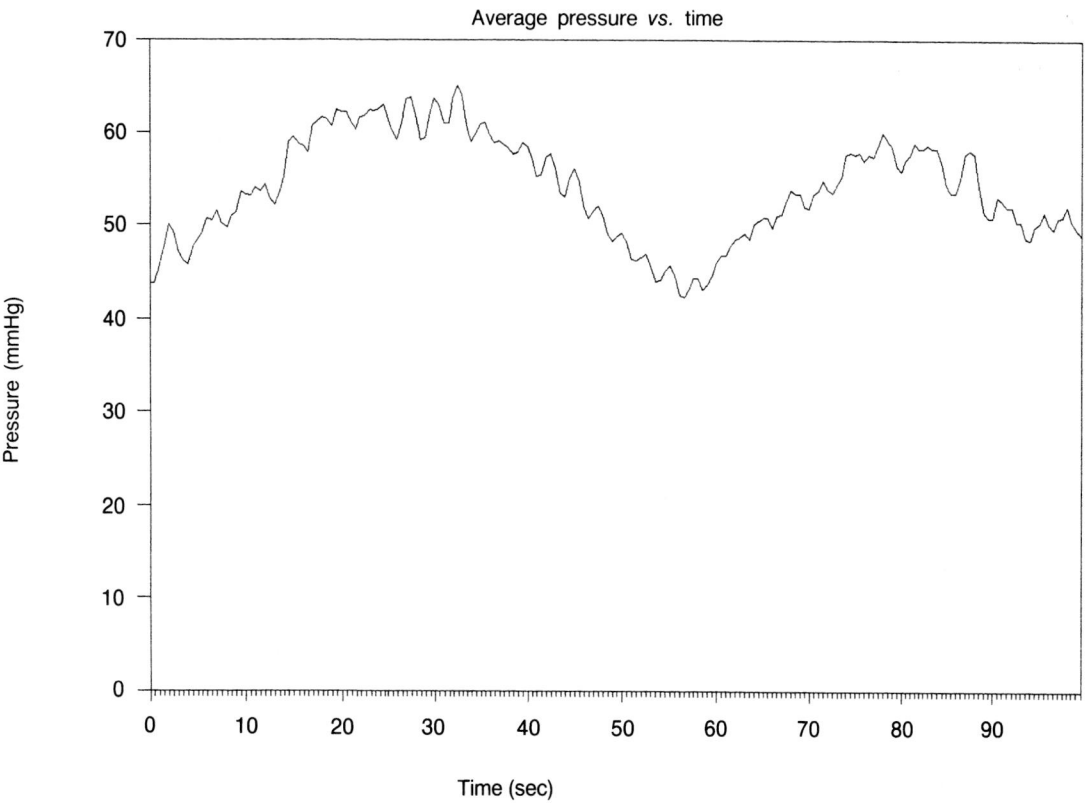

Average pressure *vs.* time

FIGURE 16-2. Evaluation of anal motility of an ultraslow wave, which usually has a frequency of one cycle every 50 to 70 seconds and an amplitude of 6 to 30 mm Hg. However, it may have an amplitude in excess of 60 mm Hg, and under such circumstances is often identified in the presence of sphincter hypertonia or obstructed defecation. (Courtesy of John A. Coller, M.D.)

and by contraction of the muscles of the pelvic floor (resisting the forward movement of stool and closing the lumen distally). The diaphragm descends, and the voluntary muscles of the abdominal wall are contracted, creating a closed system.[247] Relaxation of the pelvic muscles produces descent of the pelvic floor and straightening of the previously angulated rectum. Closure of the anal canal by the sphincters allows an increase of pressure within the rectum so that subsequent sphincteric inhibition results in expulsion of stool. When paradoxical contraction of the voluntary sphincter muscle occurs during attempts at evacuation, it is termed "obstructed defecation" or "anismus" (see later). The point at which complete inhibition of the external sphincter occurs can be demonstrated experimentally with an intrarectal balloon. When the volume reaches 150 to 200 mL of air, the intrarectal pressure achieves 45 to 55 mm Hg. At the end of defecation, when straining is discontinued, the pelvic floor rises to its normal position and again obliterates the lumen. A rebound contraction of the anal sphincter occurs; this has been termed the closing reflex.[165]

Berman and colleagues subdivide patients with disorders of defecation into three categories: those with motility (i.e., transit) problems, those with mural difficulties

(e.g., internal procidentia), and those with musculoskeletal problems (e.g., obstructed defecation).[16] Kuijpers applied the colorectal laboratory in the diagnosis of 74 patients with so-called functional constipation.[105] Outlet obstruction (see later) was noted in approximately three fourths, with abnormal transit times identified in two thirds. These results imply that only after evacuation studies have been proved to be normal should the physician embark on transit studies. Karasick and Ehrlich also suggested on the basis of their studies that constipation is often a disorder of defecation rather than an impairment of colonic motility.[90] However, Roe and colleagues believe that the most useful investigations are transit studies and defecography.[183] Grotz and co-workers performed a study to identify differences in rectal wall contractility between healthy volunteers and those with chronic severe constipation.[63] In response to feeding of a cholinergic agonist and a smooth-muscle relaxant, rectal wall contractility was decreased in constipated patients. The authors concluded that these findings suggest the presence of an abnormality of rectal muscular wall contractility in constipated patients.[63] To identify the optimal regimen for the management of intractable constipation, Wexner and Dailey offer an algorithmic approach.[240]

Etiology

Numerous diseases can be associated with chronic constipation and even megacolon. Some of these include various neurologic abnormalities (e.g., multiple sclerosis), diabetes mellitus, and connective tissue disorders (e.g., scleroderma).[28,54,125,186,198,205] Of course, the physician must establish whether the patient is taking any of a host of drugs that may produce constipation (see Chapter 3). The bowel symptoms and the radiologic findings of colonic dilatation may completely resolve after the medication has been discontinued.[25]

Another mechanism for producing intractable constipation or problems with elimination has been suggested by Kuijpers and Bleijenberg—the so-called spastic pelvic floor syndrome (i.e., anismus; see later).[106] This is described as a functional disorder of the pelvic floor muscle in which straining or attempting to eliminate leads to muscle contraction instead of relaxation, thereby causing a physiologic outlet obstruction and the inability to defecate.

One final cause of an evacuation problem is massive colonic dilatation suggesting an obstructed cause. Intestinal pseudo-obstruction (i.e., colonic ileus) has come to be known as Ogilvie's syndrome in recognition of the man who initially described the condition in 1948.[157] Ogilvie reported two patients who exhibited signs and symptoms of colonic obstruction without any evidence of an intrinsic or extrinsic lesion. He attributed the phenomenon to sympathetic deprivation caused by tumor elsewhere, which the patients did indeed harbor. The condition is discussed later in this chapter.

Causes of Constipation

An abbreviated summary of the causes of and conditions associated with constipation follows:

Dietary Causes
Low intake of fiber (consider poor dentition, poverty)
Poor intake of fluid

Functional Conditions
Depression
Confusion
Inadequate toilet facilities
Immobility
Psychosis
Encopresis

Medications
Anticholinergics
Antidepressants
Narcotics and opiates
Iron
Bismuth
Antiparkinsonians
Antacids (e.g., aluminum)
Antihypertensives (e.g., diuretics, ganglionic blockers, calcium channel blockers)
Anticonvulsants
Ion-exchange resins
Bulk laxatives without adequate hydration

Endocrine, Metabolic, and Collagen-Vascular Diseases
Hypothyroidism
Hypoparathyroidism
Diabetes mellitus
Hypokalemia
Chronic renal failure
Pregnancy
Hypopituitarism
Porphyria
Scleroderma
Amyloidosis
Hypercalcemia

Neuromuscular Disorders
Cerebral
    Cerebrovascular accident
    Parkinson's disease
    Intracranial tumor
Spinal
    Cauda equina lesion
    Myelomeningocele
    Trauma (e.g., spinal cord injury)
    Multiple sclerosis
    Tertiary syphilis
Peripheral
    Diabetes mellitus
    Autonomic neuropathy
    Chagas' disease
    Hirschsprung's disease
    von Recklinghausen's disease
    Stimulant laxative abuse
    Vincristine
Functional
    Outlet obstruction (i.e., anismus, obstructed defecation, spastic pelvic floor syndrome)

Colonic Inertia
Slow-transit constipation
Intestinal pseudo-obstruction (Ogilvie's syndrome)

Chronic severe constipation is usually defined as bowel movements less frequent than once in 5 days, with symptoms persisting longer than 18 months. Irrespective of the duration of symptoms, constipation is generally regarded as fewer than three bowel movements per week in an individual on a standard diet containing 19 g of fiber daily.[240] Among healthy elderly people, the incidence of constipation appears to increase with age, but fewer than 1% of individuals consuming a Western diet have fewer than three bowel movements per week.[248] There must be no evidence of intestinal obstruction, but there may be a prolonged intestinal transit time (see Bowel Transit Marker Study).

An important complication of constipation, especially in the elderly, is fecal impaction, but the proximate cause, complications, and diseases may be attributed to circumstances that are associated with the inability for a person to evacuate normally. A partial list of these includes the following conditions:

- Fecal incontinence
- Spurious diarrhea
- Urinary retention
- Mental disturbance and anxiety
- Rectal hyposensitivity[53]
- Arrhythmias
- Syncope
- Autonomic dysreflexia
- Pneumothorax
- Hypoxia
- Hypotension
- Dysfunctional labor
- Volvulus
- Stercoral ulceration
- Cecal perforation
- Hemorrhoids
- Anal fissure
- Rectal prolapse[240,248]

Clinical Presentations

There are a plethora of clinical presentations that encompass the broad clinical diagnosis attributed to the symptom of constipation. These may include such severe abdominal signs and symptoms as to mimic an acute abdominal catastrophe. Even hydronephrosis has been reported to be a consequence of a fecal impaction.[32] More commonly, however, patients simply complain of an inability to defecate. They may be free of pain and not even require a laxative, or they may report hard bowel movements and bloating with inadequate, incomplete, or infrequent evacuation. At least 80% are women.

The physician must be aware, however, of the paradoxical situation in which diarrhea or fecal incontinence supervenes, and the underlying problem is actually constipation with impaction. Although impaction as a cause of colonic obstruction is uncommon (1.3%), in selected populations (e.g., those in nursing homes or with spinal cord injuries), the incidence can approximate 50%.[248]

One group of patients, women with severe idiopathic constipation, is characterized by often extreme disability at a relatively young age and by severe abdominal pain and distension. The syndrome may commence in infancy or childhood but usually begins with menarche. Waldron and colleagues studied 44 such women along with 16 asymptomatic volunteers.[235] The constipated individuals

were found to require a greater volume and pressure of rectal distension for both sensation and sphincter relaxation, had diminished basal and postmorphine motility indices in the distal rectum, experienced delayed transit, and had an empty rectum even though severely constipated.[235] The authors postulated that a neural abnormality affecting afferent nerves may be present in these women.

It must be remembered that constipation is both a symptom and a disease. It may be a consequence of impaired colonic propulsion, which is a motility disorder, or of anal sphincter dysfunction, or it may be part of the clinical picture of the irritable bowel syndrome. Alternatively, the condition may be secondary to a host of underlying local or systemic disease processes.

Scoring System

In 1996, the Cleveland Clinic Group published their concept of a Constipation Scoring System.[2] This was based on the response to questions about symptoms. The authors observed that their proposed system correlated well with objective physiologic findings in individuals with constipation and allowed uniformity in the assessment of its severity. Knowles and colleagues presented their symptom scoring system and believe it may be useful in assisting in the diagnosis of constipation and in discriminating among pathophysiologic subgroups—the Knowles-Eccersley-Scott-Symptom (KESS) Questionnaire.[100]

Evaluation of the Constipated Patient

A thorough history of the constipated patient should be obtained, especially with regard to frequency of bowel actions, consistency of stools, and timing. It is important to note whether there is any associated pain, mucus, or blood, whether there is a sense of incomplete evacuation, and whether manual means are used to effect evacuation. Medical problems and medications must be identified (see earlier display and Chapter 3).

Physical Examination and Endoscopy

In a book limited to colon and rectal surgery, it would seem self-evident that digital rectal examination, anoscopy, and rigid or flexible sigmoidoscopy should be a routine part of the evaluation of anyone with bowel management complaints. As previously implied, constipation is one of the most common symptoms suggestive of underlying bowel disease. Anal fissure, rectal prolapse, hemorrhoids, benign and malignant neoplasms, diverticular disease, rectocele—in fact, virtually any disease that affects this area of the body—may at some time be associated with the symptom of constipation. Obviously, the surgeon must endeavor to eliminate a primary anal, rectal, or colon problem as the cause of this symptom. Although a special table and the use of the prone position with Trendelenburg tilt are convenient for the examiner, the presence of a prolapse may be masked (see Chapter 17). Asking the patient to strain or to bear down on the toilet is often quite revealing of unsuspected pathology. Subjective assessment of anal sphincter tone and contractility can be gleaned, and simple sensory evaluation by means of pinprick is also useful. Whether one wishes to embark on colonoscopy or barium enema study will depend on the patient's clinical history and findings and whether the physician is satisfied with the results of evaluation to that point.

Siproudhis and colleagues prospectively evaluated 50 individuals who complained of difficulty with defecation, in order to determine the accuracy of clinical examination in diagnosing and quantifying pelvic and rectal abnormalities.[201] These investigators concluded that clinical assessment is usually sufficient and accurate in most pelvirectal disorders encountered in patients complaining of elimination problems. They caution about the importance of identifying pelvic floor descent by asking the patient to strain down. They also concluded that certain physiologic studies, such as anorectal manometry and evacuation proctography, have a definite but limited place in the investigation of pelvirectal problems.[201]

Rectal Biopsy

See the discussion later in this chapter on short-segment Hirschsprung's disease.

Abdominal Radiography and Barium Enema

A plain film of the abdomen is a simple, highly useful study and should certainly be considered in any individual with abdominal distension. In a patient with colonic ileus, the cecum may be particularly dilated. This is a potentially dangerous consequence that may ultimately lead to perforation. Although this finding does not imply a specific origin for the problem, it indicates the magnitude of the anatomic abnormality and will inevitably influence the decision as to whether the patient is a candidate for surgical intervention. Meyers observed that massive cecal distension in colonic ileus may be horizontally oriented, a characteristic radiographic presentation (Figure 16-3).[137] Close observation by means of serial plain abdominal radiographs is required, similar to the evaluation of toxic dilatation in a patient with acute inflammatory bowel disease.

Barium enema in patients with constipation may reveal a hugely dilated colon with considerable fecal residue or a markedly redundant bowel (Figure 16-4). However,

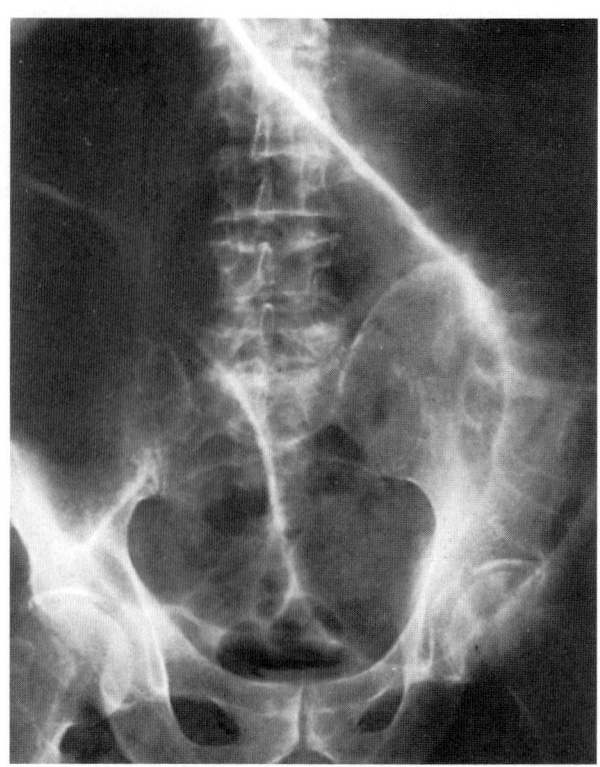

FIGURE 16-3. Pseudoobstruction of the colon (Ogilvie's syndrome) is assessed radiographically. This massively dilated colon is that of a patient with uncontrolled diabetes.

this study is not required to establish the diagnosis of colonic ileus and may be contraindicated. If the physician elects to undertake the procedure to rule out underlying colonic pathology in this condition, serious consideration should be given to performing the study with a water-soluble contrast agent.

Barium enema performed for suspected short-segment Hirschsprung's disease does not show the decompressed rectum seen with classic Hirschsprung's disease. On the contrary, the rectum is dilated to the level of the aganglionic segment (Figure 16-5).

Comment

One must recognize that barium enema is the preferred study for evaluating colonic anatomy—not colonoscopy. This, in combination with defecography (see Chapters 6 and 17), constitutes my preferred initial investigation once a neoplasm has been ruled out (see the following section). As discussed in prior chapters, colonoscopy is ideal for identifying mucosal lesions, but it is virtually useless for determining colonic redundancy, deformity, extrinsic compression, and a host of other problems. Sadly, a "normal" colonoscopy with reassurance is often the last "advice" given to someone with constipation. Yes, colonoscopy serves an important purpose, but the patient expects and

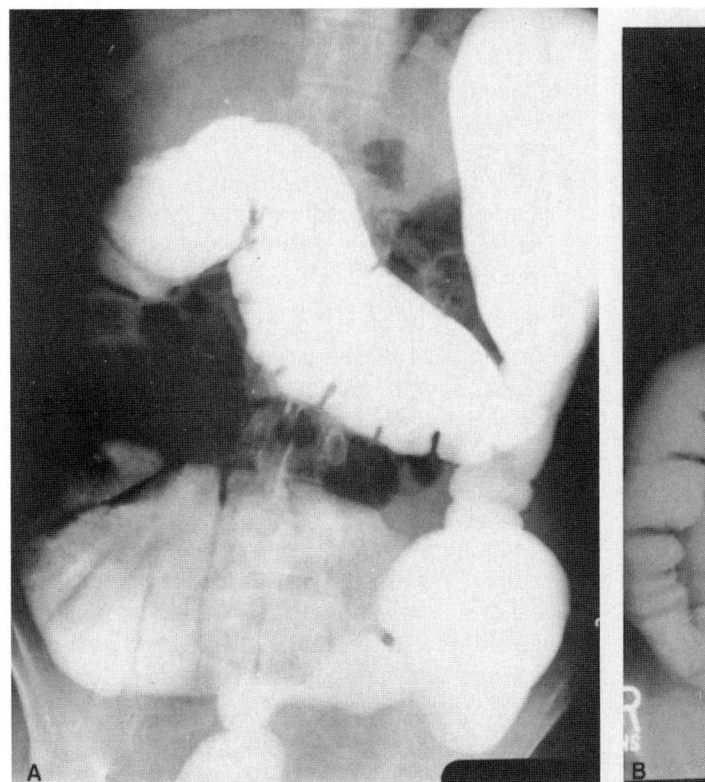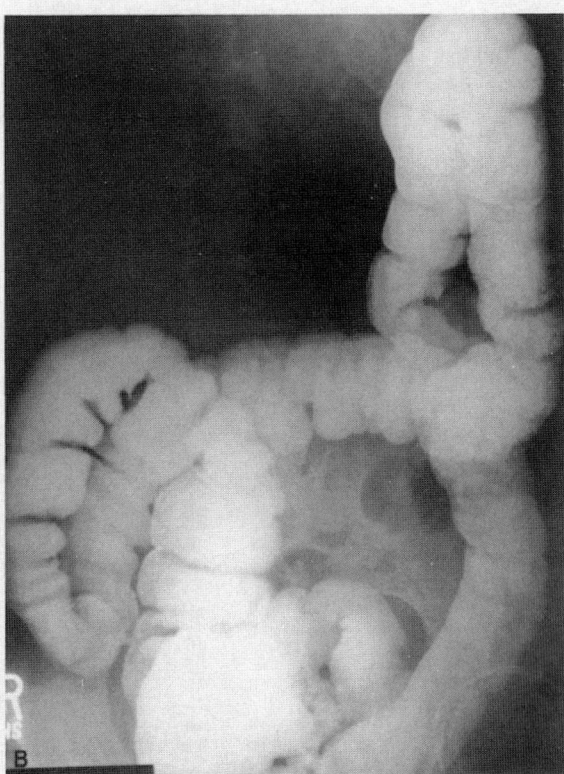

FIGURE 16-4. Barium enema studies of adult megacolon in patients with intractable constipation. **(A)** A large-caliber bowel is especially notable in the proximal right colon. The patient moved her bowels once in 2 weeks. **(B)** A markedly redundant colon leads to infrequent bowel action.

deserves more input and evaluation of his or her symptoms than a friendly pat on the back.

Defecography (Evacuation Proctography)

The method of performing defecography is discussed in Chapters 6 and 13 and is further addressed in Chapter 17. Ideally, the procedure should be performed with the patient in the seated position on a water-filled apparatus in order to obtain good lateral projections of the pelvis and perineum and to assess clearly anorectal angles and anterior displacement of the rectum.[95] Because interpretation is often subjective, it is important to evaluate the films oneself. Paradoxical puborectalis muscle contraction (anismus; obstructed defecation) can be appreciated during an attempt at eliminating the thickened barium (see later), or internal prolapse may be seen. The implication of the latter condition as a contributing factor to causing fecal incontinence is discussed in Chapter 13. Other observations may include the presence of an enterocele, a rectocele, perineal descent, and the possibility of unsuspected incontinence. The real concern is that there is often an absence of correlation between the results of this study and the clinical severity of the constipation.[81] In other words, one cannot use the defecogram alone in therapeutic decision making unless one of the specific conditions is unequivocally identified.[152,214]

Bowel Transit Marker Study

Although plain abdominal radiographs and barium enema evaluation are extremely useful in clarifying whether there is evidence of mechanical obstruction as a cause of the constipation, they do not present a physiologic or functional picture. In 1988, a working party of individuals, who have manifested particular interest in anorectal physiology and who have contributed considerably to the literature in the field, gathered to make recommendations concerning standardizing a number of investigations.[95] It was agreed that the most objective assessment of colonic transit was obtained by asking a patient to swallow three different types of radiopaque markers each morning for 3 days while taking no laxatives and being fully ambulatory. Another method for calculating colonic transit is discussed in Chapter 6.

A simple approach is to have the patient take a capsule containing 24 radiopaque rings (Konsyl Pharmaceuticals, Edison, NJ; Figure 16-6; also Figure 6-23). Laxatives must be avoided. A plain abdominal radiograph is taken on the fifth day after ingestion. Some suggest that the

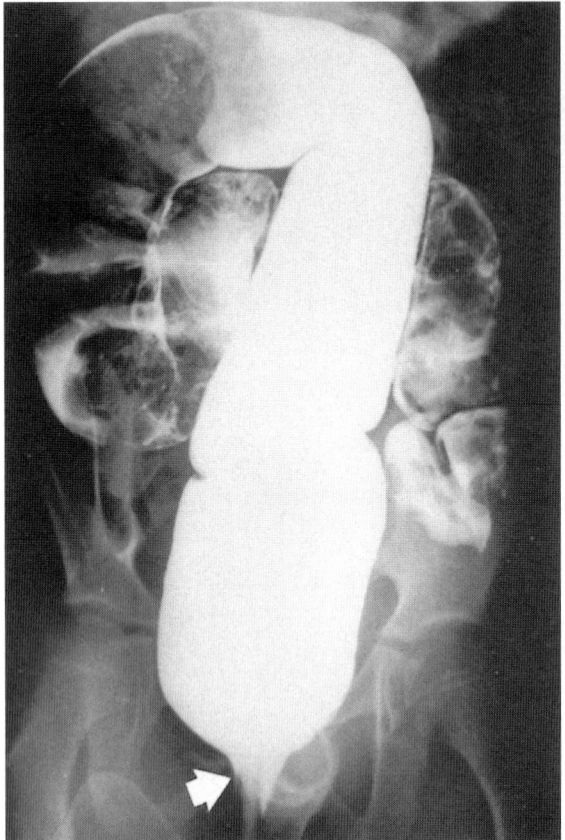

FIGURE 16-5. Short-segment Hirschsprung's disease is confirmed by the abrupt change in caliber from the normal-appearing distal rectum *(arrow)* to the dilated proximal bowel.

study be continued as long as the markers are present.[195] By the fifth day, 80% of the markers should have been eliminated, and all should be passed by the seventh day.

Schuster recognizes four categories of constipation[195]:

■ Hypotonic: This is often seen in the very young and in the elderly, and it shows radiographically dilated and flaccid colon and delayed transit time.

■ Spastic: This is commonly associated with irritable bowel syndrome and often responds to bulking agents and antispasmodics.
■ Colonic inertia: Radiopaque markers are delayed above the rectosigmoid area.
■ Outlet delay: This results in holdup of radiopaque markers in the rectum, and it indicates possible Hirschsprung's disease or obstructed defecation (anismus).

Figure 16-7 identifies three patterns of abnormal distribution of these markers, which serve to illustrate various pathophysiologic processes responsible for abnormalities of defecation. A typical hindgut inertia pattern is shown in Figure 16-8. Obviously, the results of the transit study must be correlated with other investigations.

Wald studied 21 patients with refractory idiopathic constipation by means of ingestion of radiopaque markers and daily abdominal radiographs to determine the value of this test in planning therapy and predicting clinical outcome.[232] Three transit patterns were observed: normal, colonic inertia, and distal slowing. Normal transit was interpreted by the author as evidence of psychosocial disturbance. Follow-up evaluation 2 years later revealed that six of eight patients with colonic inertia failed to improve, compared with only one of seven with distal slowing. Menardo and colleagues studied large-bowel transit times in patients with transection of the spinal cord above the lumbosacral parasympathetic outflow.[135] These investigators concluded that constipation, an inevitable consequence in this group of individuals, is caused by abnormal transit mainly at the level of the left colon and rectum.

Many studies have been undertaken to identify those individuals who have a specifically treatable situation, rather than an irritable bowel problem. Reynolds and colleagues evaluated 25 consecutive patients with severe constipation and found three patterns of abnormal motility in more than two thirds: isolated anal sphincter

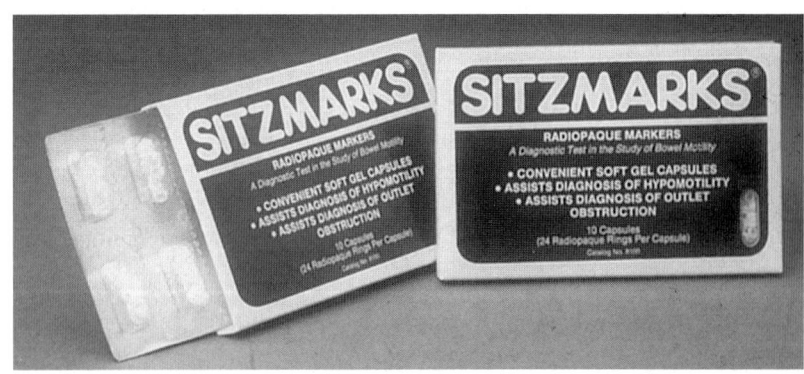
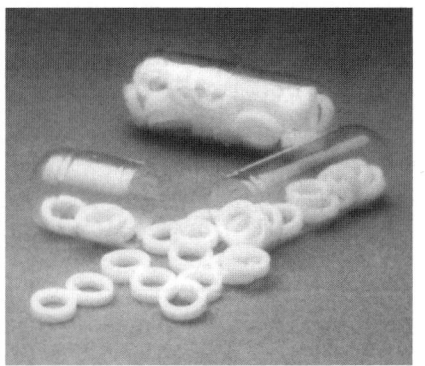

FIGURE 16-6. **(A)** Bowel transit markers are commercially available in gelatin capsules (Sitzmarks). **(B)** Each capsule contains 24 radiopaque markers.

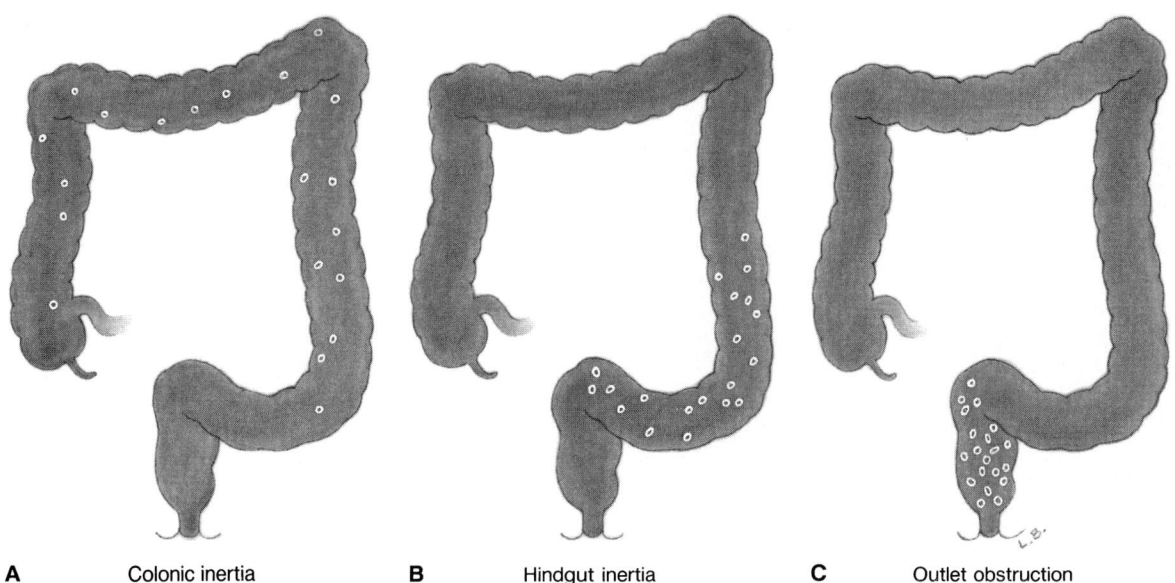

| A | Colonic inertia | B | Hindgut inertia | C | Outlet obstruction |

FIGURE 16-7. Artist's representation of three types of radiologic appearances that may be seen with radiopaque rings on the plain abdominal x-ray study. **(A)** Colonic inertia: typical pattern of distribution throughout the colon. **(B)** Hindgut inertia. Markers are clustered on the left side of the colon, but not limited to the rectum. **(C)** Outlet obstruction. Markers are clustered in the rectum, a classic pattern indicating obstructed defecation.

dysfunction (20%), generalized disorder of gastrointestinal motility (24%), and rectosigmoid dysfunction (24%).[178] Others have confirmed the importance of transit time study in the evaluation of patients with chronic constipation.[36,174,183,241]

Scintigraphic Study

Although radiopaque markers have been demonstrated to be highly useful in distinguishing patients with normal transit from those with slow intestinal transit, they are not especially helpful in identifying the precise region of delay. Esophageal transit scans and gastric emptying scans have been employed for some time, but small bowel and colonic transit scintigraphy is a newly emerging modality that has considerable promise. It has been specifically suggested that scintigraphic assessment may be used to evaluate intestinal transit in a quantitative, noninvasive manner.[153] For example, van der Sijp and colleagues compared the transit of a radioisotope-labeled meal with that of simultaneously ingested radiopaque markers in 12 healthy controls and 12 severely constipated women.[229] They concluded that radioisotope ingestion provides accurate information about the transit through individual colonic regions because of the possibility for frequent observations and the clear delineation of the entire colon.[229]

Notghi and co-workers measured segmental colonic transit in 101 patients with the use of indium-111 absorbed on resin pellets and encapsulated in an enteric-coated capsule.[155] Over the ensuing 3 days, these investigators were able to distinguish between patterns of transit (rapid, normal, and slow). Others have used the radioisotope technetium-99m liquid as well as indium-111 for evaluation of transit in both the upper and lower bowel.[47] An important variable to assess in some patients is transit through the small intestine. In such an individual, a panintestinal transit abnormality may account for the reason that symptoms are not ameliorated after removal of the colon.[69] Others have demonstrated the value of the technique for patients with colonic pseudo-obstruction. By using iodine-131 fiber, improved transit can be demonstrated with the prokinetic, cisapride.[153] Others have demonstrated that quantification of isotopic counts by means of resin pellets labeled with indium-111 provides an accurate summary of colonic transit with acceptable specificity at a high sensitivity in the detection of motility disorders of the colon.[24]

Anorectal Manometry

The value of anorectal manometry in the investigation of patients with fecal incontinence is discussed in Chapters 2, 6, and 13. Manometric studies have also been

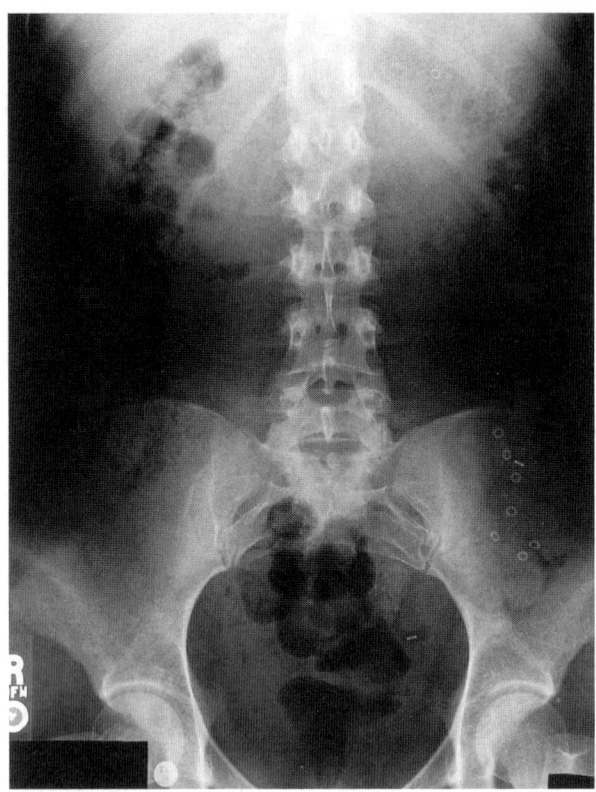

FIGURE 16-8. Plain abdominal radiograph showing radiopaque markers in the sigmoid colon, a distribution consistent with hindgut inertia.

demonstrated to be helpful for establishing the diagnosis of short-segment Hirschsprung's disease (see later). On inflation of a rectal balloon, a lack of the internal sphincter relaxation response, also known as the rectoanal inhibitory reflex (RAIR), is noted in this condition.[227] This physiologic finding, in addition to the characteristic history of the patient, has usually been believed to be pathognomonic for the disease. Others suggest that failure of relaxation of the internal sphincter is not necessarily diagnostic, especially in instances of severe, long-standing, idiopathic constipation.[139] The reflex may also be absent if resting anal canal pressures are low, as in some individuals with rectal prolapse and neurogenic fecal incontinence following low rectal excision.[95]

Waldron and colleagues demonstrated that a greater volume and pressure of rectal distension were required for both sensation and sphincter relaxation in a group of 44 severely constipated women. This led the authors to conclude that a neural abnormality affecting afferent nerves may be present in these individuals.[235]

Taylor and colleagues studied anorectal motility in the management of 19 patients with adult megacolon and compared the results with those in 12 anatomically normal subjects.[216] Adult Hirschsprung's disease was recognized by a lack of anal canal inhibition on rectal distension. Those patients with non-Hirschsprung's megacolon had an elevated anal canal pressure and were treated by repeated anal dilatation. Those with normal anal canal pressures were treated with enemas and suppositories but showed little improvement. The authors concluded that anorectal motility studies are useful in the evaluation and subsequent management of patients with adult megacolon.

Many studies of the problem of chronic constipation have been generated in Devroede's unit in Sherbrooke, Canada.[129,171] In those patients found to be negative for Hirschsprung's disease, manometric evaluation demonstrated decreased amplitude of the RAIR, a hypertonic anal canal that relaxed much more than is normal when rectal distension was performed, and a markedly unstable pressure in the upper anal canal. The authors emphasized that it is very important to ask patients about the onset of constipation. Those with a congenital type of constipation note problems from birth. In the adult with megacolon, difficulties with defecation usually are identified at a later time, most likely during adolescence. By using anorectal manometry as well as radiopaque markers, the authors attempted to identify those who would respond to a particular surgical procedure. Patients who failed to improve following myectomy seemed to suffer essentially from colorectal inertia. The authors found this to be particularly true when markers were present in the right colon a week or more after ingestion. They cautioned that histologic examination was of limited value in selecting constipated patients for surgery because the lack of ganglion cells did not necessarily predict the efficacy of surgical treatment.

Motility Studies

Ferrara and colleagues, reporting from the Mayo Clinic in Rochester, Minnesota, utilized ambulatory recordings of anorectal motility to compare control subjects with those having slow-transit constipation.[41] A motility index was calculated during fasting and after feeding. The authors determined that the rectal motility index and the frequency of anal canal contractions were lower in patients with constipation than in individuals in the control group. The differences were statistically significant (see also Chapter 6).

Electromyography

The role of electromyography (EMG) in the evaluation of patients with anal incontinence is discussed in Chapters

2, 6, and 15, but EMG of the external anal sphincter and puborectalis is another technique for establishing the diagnosis of paradoxical or inappropriate puborectalis contraction.[241,242] Failure of inhibition of electrical activity during the act of defecation is pathognomonic for anismus. Some believe that this study is preferable to defecography for establishing the diagnosis.

Waldron and colleagues evaluated eight patients with chronic intractable constipation by means of "prolonged ambulant manometry and electromyography".[236] External sphincter EMG activity did not differ from that of controls, but the study was able to identify reduced filling of the rectum, which suggested slow-transit constipation and a possible motor neuropathy.

Rectal Sensation

As mentioned in Chapter 15, rectal sensation is usually assessed by balloon distension. Kamm and Lennard-Jones applied a more precise technique, testing of rectal mucosal electrosensitivity by means of a bipolar ring electrode in 13 healthy women and in 26 with severe idiopathic constipation.[88] They observed a raised threshold to electrosensory testing that suggested the presence of a rectal sensory neuropathy in the severely constipated individuals. Others have investigated neuropathologic changes in the colonic wall of patients with slow-transit constipation by means of monoclonal antibodies raised against neurofilament.[194] Following colon resection, all specimens were investigated with the monoclonal antineurofilament antibody, NF_2F_{11}, and results were compared with those from control patients. In 29 of 39 individuals with idiopathic slow-transit constipation, the apparently normal axon bundles in the myenteric plexus stained markedly less than normal or failed to stain at all with the monoclonal antibody. The authors concluded that these findings indicate that visceral neuropathy seems to be present in most patients with slow-transit constipation.[194] How these observations will affect the subsequent therapeutic choices remains to be explored.

Analysis of Myoelectrical Activity

Myoelectrical activity of the colon can be assessed by means of sigmoidoscopic attachment of electrodes to the colorectal mucosa. Bassotti and colleagues recorded postprandial responses in volunteers and in patients with slow-transit constipation.[10] The constipated individuals failed to demonstrate an increase in spiking activity under these circumstances, which suggested the possibility of a neurogenic defect as the cause of this condition.

Pudendal Nerve Terminal Motor Latency

The importance of pudendal nerve terminal motor latency evaluation for patients with incontinence is discussed in Chapters 2, 6, and 13. Vaccaro and colleagues utilized this investigation to assess the incidence of pudendal neuropathy in constipated individuals.[228] They concluded that unsuspected neuropathy was present in 24% of patients. This finding correlated with age and with the presence of paradoxical puborectalis contraction but not with manometric anal pressures, motor unit potentials recruitment, or the presence of polyphasia.[228]

Psychological Profile

There has been some difference of opinion with respect to studies concerning the incidence of psychosocial disturbances in severely constipated women, especially those with slow-transit problems. Wald and colleagues prospectively evaluated such profiles and selected parameters of colonic and anorectal sensorimotor function in 25 patients with severe constipation.[234] A more recent study from the same group involved 38 patients with chronic, severe, idiopathic constipation who failed to respond to conventional therapy.[233] Subjects with normal-transit constipation demonstrated significantly higher scores for psychological distress than did those with slow-transit constipation and control subjects. The authors concluded that certain individuals may require a behavioral and psychological approach to the management of their constipation. In some centers, a standardized personality test [e.g., Beck Depression Inventory, Minnesota Multiphasic Personality Inventory (MMPI)] is administered to every patient for whom a surgical alternative is considered. Wald and colleagues believed that the Hopkins Symptom Checklist (SCL-90-R) is the preferred psychological instrument to evaluate patients with chronic severe constipation who fail to respond to conventional therapy.[233] Heyman and co-workers utilized the MMPI for psychological assessment and found that mean scores for hypochondriasis, depression, and hysteria were significantly elevated for those patients who had levator spasm.[71] A similar pattern was noted for the group with constipation, but those with fecal incontinence were within the normal range on all scales.

Comment

I agree that it is certainly appropriate to assess individually the psychosocial factors that may contribute to a given patient's complaint.[234] The fact is that many individuals with constipation problems who end up in the offices of surgeons, especially those with anismus and colonic transit abnormality, seem to have an inordinately high incidence of mental distress. As a nonpsychiatrist, I merely make this observation but offer no conclusions. Whether this phenomenon is a cause or a consequence of the bowel evacuation disorder I cannot state. Still, psychological evaluation and thyroid function tests are probably the most often omitted, yet potentially helpful, studies in the evaluation of patients with intractable constipation.

Dermatoglyphic Patterns

Gottlieb and Schuster in 1986, in an effort to determine whether congenital factors play a role, examined dermatoglyphic patterns (i.e., fingerprints) in 155 patients with gastrointestinal complaints.[60] Sixty-four percent who had reported constipation and abdominal pain before their tenth birthday had one or more digital arches, compared with 10% without such symptoms. Because these differences were statistically significant, the authors concluded that the presence of digital arches may help to differentiate a congenital organic syndrome from a functional disorder. The validity of this concept has not been confirmed by others.

Medical Management

Diet, Exercise, Laxatives, Enemas, and Suppositories

Usually, the treatment of constipation includes appropriate dietary counseling, a regimen of activity, and often the use of laxatives, enemas, or suppositories (see Chapter 3). When no organic pathologic process is present, or if the condition does not lend itself to management by means of specific medical or surgical measures, the initial approach to the treatment of uncomplicated constipation is usually directed toward dietary measures. Generally, this consists of increasing fiber intake, especially whole-grain cereals such as bran, fruits, and vegetables. An increase in the volume of fluid intake is also helpful.

Sedentary individuals are prone to constipation. Exercise is therefore added to the treatment regimen. Those who are confined to bed for prolonged periods of time are subject to the development of complications of constipation, such as fecal impaction (Figure 16-9).

Psychological stresses and the rapidly paced lives that many persons lead can have an adverse effect on bowel function. A busy individual may refuse the urge to pass stool because it is too inconvenient to stop work, but that call may not return for some time. When the person finally does try to eliminate, it may be difficult to do so.

Despite efforts at counseling constipated people to eat a proper diet, to exercise regularly, and not to disregard

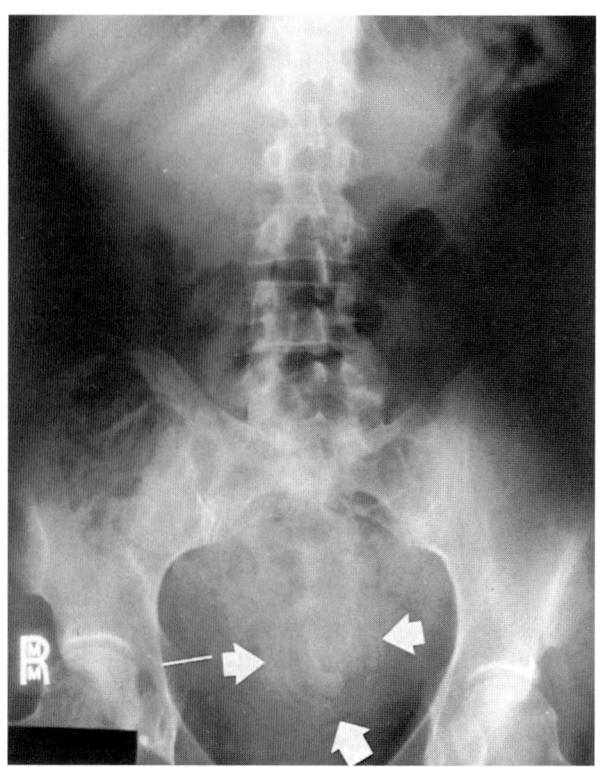

FIGURE 16-9. Fecal impaction. A large, laminated pelvic calcification *(arrows)* is indicative of a retained, massive fecaloma.

the urge to defecate, many believe that they require laxatives. Generally, surgeons prescribe cathartics only in the context of postoperative management. In fact, physicians often try to dissuade individuals from taking such drugs. Breaking the laxative habit is especially difficult because of advertisements implying that it is unhealthful not to have a daily bowel action. It has been virtually impossible for health professionals to alter this misconception. However, some people benefit from and indeed require cathartics (see also Chapter 3). For the physician to deny access to such agents in the truly needy patient, planting the fear of habituation and laxative-induced illness in a vulnerable person, is extreme. This is especially true when treating the elderly. Table 16-1 illustrates the classification of cathartics based on the mechanism of action of the drugs.

Stimulant Cathartics

Stimulant cathartics produce their effect by local irritation or by action on Auerbach's plexus, which results in increased motor activity of the intestine. The amount of cramping produced and the latent period for diarrhea vary from one drug to another and are dose dependent; therefore, these agents can be used interchangeably. As with all cathartics, stimulants are contraindicated in the presence of intestinal obstruction or peritonitis and in

▶ **TABLE 16-1 Classification of Cathartics**

Class	Drugs
Stimulant	Cascara sagrada
	Senna
	Danthron
	Phenolphthalein
	Acetphenolisatin
	Bisacodyl
	Castor oil
Saline	Magnesium sulfate
	Milk of magnesia
	Magnesium citrate
	Sodium sulfate
	Sodium phosphate
	Potassium phosphate
	Potassium sodium tartrate
Osmotic	Polyethylene glycol and electrolytes (i.e., Colyte, GoLytely)
Bulk-forming	Plantago (e.g., psyllium) seed
	Methylcellulose
	Sodium carboxymethylcellulose
	Agar
	Tragacanth
	Bran
Lubricant	Mineral oil
	Dioctyl sodium sulfosuccinate
	Calcium docusate

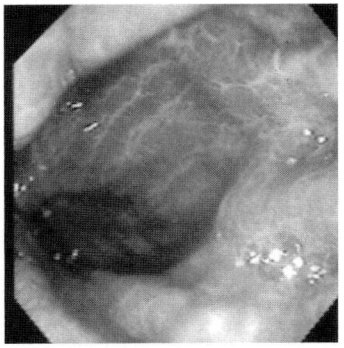

FIGURE 16-10. Colonoscopy demonstrates the typical cobblestone pattern of melanosis coli. (See Color Fig. 16-10.)

the postoperative period after laparotomy, especially after bowel resection.

Melanosis Coli Melanosis coli has been recognized since 1830, when it was described by Cruveilhier.[33] The anthraquinone cathartics, cascara sagrada and senna, are usually responsible. The pigment itself produces no symptoms. Proctosigmoidoscopic examination reveals the mucosa to be brown, deep purple, or black, broken into "small angular polyhedral designs by fine netlike striae of lighter shade, either yellow or brown" (Figs. 16-10 and 16-11).[20]

On careful inspection, the mucosa, although smooth, takes on a cobblestone appearance. It has variously been described, rather poetically in some instances, as having the appearance of a "toad's back" or a "cross-section of nutmeg," or looking like snake, crocodile, or tiger skin.[201]

Melanosis coli usually occurs in older age groups. Generally, it takes years of laxative use or abuse to produce color change of the mucosa. Wittoesch and associates reviewed 887 patients with this condition.[246] The overall incidence on routine proctosigmoidoscopic examination was approximately 1%. The greatest frequency was in the fifth, sixth, and seventh decades, and the youngest patient was 20 years old. Approximately three fourths were women, and virtually all were habitual users of laxatives. The incidence of this condition may be increasing because of the frequent use of cholagogues and slimming teas that contain anthraquinones, but it is still probably less than 5% for individuals older than 50 years of age.[5]

Biopsy of the rectum will reveal the presence of pigment-laden macrophages in the lamina propria; these are what give the mucosa its characteristic color (Figure 16-12). Electron microscopic evaluation has shown abnormalities of the absorptive epithelial cells in this condition.[6] The cells do not contain true melanin, and the lesion should not be confused with malignant melanoma

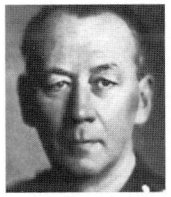

Léon Jean Baptiste Cruveilhier (1791–1874) Cruveilhier was the son of a military surgeon who had planned to enter the priesthood, but he was denied this course by his father who wanted him to become his successor. He attended the University at Limoges and in 1810 moved to Paris to study medicine under Guillaume Dupuytren, a friend of his father. Dupuytren made him his protégé and aroused his interest in pathology. Cruveilhier received his doctorate in medicine in 1816 with a dissertation on a new classification of organs according to their pathologic changes. Stung by failure to secure an appointment as surgeon in Limoges, he returned to Paris and, supported by Dupuytren, was appointed Professor Agrégé of Surgery at the Faculty of Medicine of Montpellier. In 1825, he accepted the position of Professor of Descriptive Anatomy in Paris and the following year was named Médecin des Hôpitaux. In 1836, he was elected to the Académie de Médecine and became President in 1839. In 1836, he was offered the first chair of pathologic anatomy, which had been established with funds from his teacher, Dupuytren. He remained in this position for more than 30 years. The vast material from the deadhouse of the Salpêtrière, the establishment of the Musée Dupuytren, and the lectureship in morbid anatomy provided the impetus for his prolific writings. His best-known work was *Anatomie pathologique du corps humain*, in which he reports the first pathologic account of disseminated sclerosis. Cruveilhier devoted himself to his enormous practice, following the rules of a very strict ethic that he condensed in his *Des devoirs et de la moralité du médecin* (1837). He died on his country estate in Sussac near Limoges, at the age of 83. (With appreciation to Faisal Aziz, M.D.)

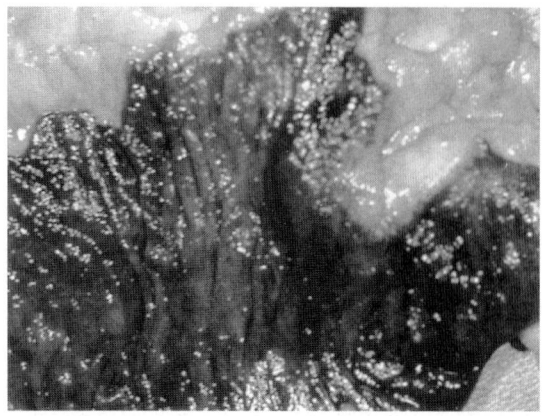

FIGURE 16-11. Note the dark black pigment characteristic of melanosis coli in a resected specimen. (See Color Fig. 16-11.)

(see Chapter 24). Melanosis coli has also led to confusion with respect to possible ischemic bowel when a heavily pigmented stoma has been created.[204] Although the occurrence of this condition is not increased in those who harbor a colorectal cancer, melanosis coli has been observed to be a useful marker in such individuals (Figure 16-13). Morgenstern and colleagues reported 30 patients with colorectal tumors and melanosis coli and found that the proliferating or neoplastic epithelium was notable by virtue of the absence of pigmentation.[142] Microscopically, this characteristic was a consequence of the lack or diminution of pigment-laden macrophages in the lamina propria underlying the lesions. When an individual ceases to take the anthracene laxative, the pigment often disappears within 3 to 6 months.[20,206]

Saline Cathartics

Saline cathartics achieve their effect on the intestinal tract by the osmotic activity of a slowly absorbed salt ion. Water is retained in the small intestine when salts that contain magnesium sulfate, phosphate, or tartrate are ingested. The increase in volume causes the intestine to contract and to expel the contents. The latency period for action depends on the dose and usually varies from 3 to 6 hours.

Although saline cathartics are relatively safe, some rather special problems are associated with their use. Individuals with renal disease may retain considerable amounts of magnesium if this type of saline cathartic is employed. This can cause central nervous system and neuromuscular depression. In addition, sodium-containing cathartics are relatively contraindicated in patients with cardiac problems or in those with inflammatory bowel disease.

Saline cathartics are of particular use as part of a bowel preparation for intestinal surgery or prior to a barium enema examination. However, dose for dose, they are not superior to stimulant cathartics. One particularly valuable application of such a cathartic, however, is as an enema. The osmotic effect of a relatively small quantity of concentrated salt solution can lead to rapid and fairly complete evacuation of the lower bowel. This is espe-

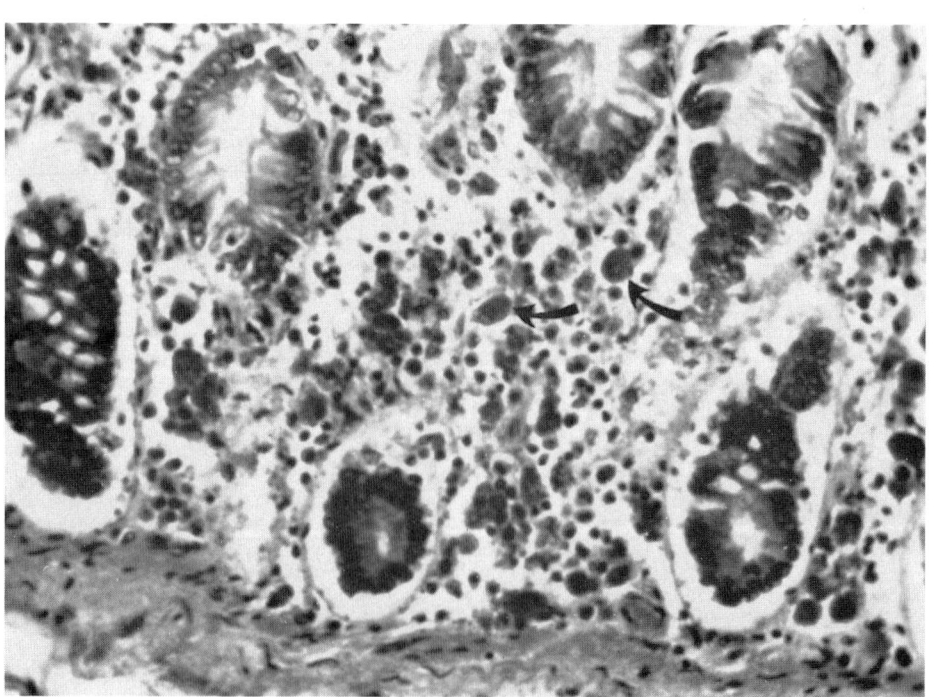

FIGURE 16-12. Melanosis coli. Pigmented macrophages *(arrows)* appear in the lamina propria. (Original magnification × 600; from Corman ML, Veidenheimer MC, Swinton NW. *Diseases of the anus, rectum and colon. Part I: neoplasms.* New York: Medcom, 1972.)

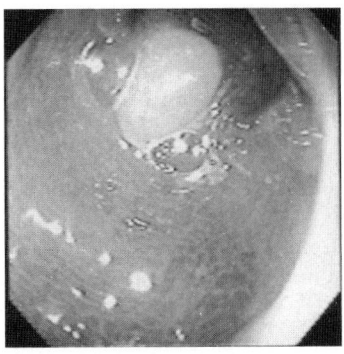

FIGURE 16-13. A polypoid lesion is clearly evident against the background of the darkly pigmented normal mucosa. (See Color Fig. 16-13.)

cially useful for preparation before proctosigmoidoscopy, flexible sigmoidoscopy, and anal operations. Therapeutically, it can be very effective for the treatment of a soft fecal impaction. Unfortunately, we still do not have an oral cathartic that can act on the descending colon, sigmoid colon, and rectum. That would be the ideal laxative indeed.

Osmotic Cathartics

Osmotic cathartics are usually orally administered electrolyte lavage preparations for the colon (e.g., GoLytely, Colyte) delivered in the form of water-soluble components for reconstitution. Despite the fact that they cleanse the colon rapidly and induce diarrhea, there is virtually no net ion absorption or loss even though large volumes of fluid are ingested. The major problems are the large volume, the time it takes to consume this large volume, and the salty, unpleasant taste. Even though some of the concerns can be ameliorated (e.g., administration through a nasogastric or feeding tube), patients commonly complain of nausea and bloating.

Osmotic cathartics are usually employed for bowel cleansing before colonoscopy, barium enema, or colon surgery. They are also useful in treating the severely constipated individual and are especially effective when combined with a volume enema.

Bulk-Forming Cathartics

Bulk-forming cathartics are composed of synthetic or natural polysaccharides and cellulose derivatives that swell or dissolve in the intestinal tract without being absorbed. They act primarily by adding bulk to the stool. Some form emollient gels, which lubricate the stool in its passage. These products may be considered to act in a more natural way than the saline or stimulant cathartics. Their effect is much less dramatic and may become ap-

parent 12 to 72 hours after administration. All bulk laxatives should be taken with adequate fluid. Although side effects are minimal, intestinal obstruction has been reported from improper use.

Lubricant Cathartics

Lubricant cathartics lubricate the feces without stimulating peristalsis. One such product is mineral oil, an indigestible petroleum product. Because it lubricates the stool, it is helpful in situations in which straining must be avoided (e.g., after hernia repair and for patients with coronary artery disease). However, mineral oil has many side effects and contraindications. For the person who has had anal surgery, mineral oil may cause severe irritation and pruritic symptoms. Granulomas may form at the site of the healing wounds. Aspiration of the ingested oil produces an often fatal lipoid pneumonia. If the oil is absorbed into the system, it may produce granulomas in the mesenteric lymph nodes, intestinal mucosa, liver, and spleen (see Figure 25-77). Finally, although mineral oil produces a lubricated stool, its prolonged use may lead to atrophy of the anorectal sphincter mechanism, because it is not stretched when a greasy stool is passed.

Digestible oils, such as olive oil, cottonseed oil, and corn oil, may also be used as lubricant cathartics. They do, however, increase caloric intake.

Dioctyl sodium sulfosuccinate and other emulsifying agents are considered lubricant cathartics. They have been widely used in industry to facilitate the mixture of water and fatty substances and are often prescribed as a stool softener after anal surgery.

Enemas

Enemas, although not truly laxatives, need to be considered as a therapeutic option in the management of the constipated patient. The many substances administered in this manner include tap water, soap suds, saline solution, vegetable oils, hydrogen peroxide, milk and molasses, and even champagne for certain special patients.

There are several specific indications for the use of enemas:

- To evacuate the bowel prior to surgery, childbirth, contrast radiologic study, or endoscopic examination
- To remove a fecal impaction, in conjunction with manual removal
- To rid the bowel of barium in order to prevent inspissation
- To stimulate bowel activity and evacuation after certain surgical procedures
- To relieve certain colonic obstructions, such as an impaction proximal to a carcinoma of the rectosigmoid colon
- To evacuate the bowel in patients with emptying problems, especially if caused by neurologic dysfunction

Suppositories

Suppositories may contain glycerin, bisacodyl, dioctyl sodium sulfosuccinate, or senna, or they may release carbon dioxide. They have been advocated by their manufacturers for use whenever an enema is considered, but the relative efficacy of enemas versus suppositories is open to question. Generally, a suppository is easier to administer. Thus, if the two are equally effective for a given patient, the suppository probably is a more acceptable bowel evacuant. Interestingly, there is a common misconception as to the proper method of insertion. Its "torpedo" shape should suggest that the proper method is apex-end first; in fact, the base should be inserted first. Abd-El-Maeboud and colleagues demonstrated in a series of more than 600 patients and medical personnel that insertion was easier and retention more effective when the latter technique was employed.[1]

Pharmacologic Therapy

Certain drugs have been demonstrated to have a profound effect on neurotransmission, but practical application of cholinomimetics (e.g., bethanechol) or narcotic antagonists (e.g., naloxone) in the management of patients with constipation has been illusory (see also Chapter 3). However, it is very appealing to have an agent that acts specifically to enhance propulsive activity rather than as an intestinal irritant. A newer class of drugs that augment intrinsic motor function of the gut are the *prokinetic agents*. The first was *metoclopramide* (Reglan), a substance that affects motility primarily in the upper gastrointestinal tract. Another prokinetic drug, *cisapride* (Propulsid), seemed to show considerable promise in the treatment of motility disorders affecting the hindgut. In a double-blind, randomized trial involving this drug and a placebo, cisapride increased spontaneous stool frequency from a mean of 1.1 to 3.0 times per week.[144] Staiano and colleagues evaluated the efficacy of this medication in 20 children with chronic idiopathic constipation.[208] Stool frequency was significantly increased in comparison with a placebo. Furthermore, anorectal manometry demonstrated that this drug significantly decreased the RAIR threshold and the conscious rectal sensitivity threshold. Despite the initial enthusiasm, the drug has not been available in the United States since Janssen Pharmaceutical pulled it from the market in 2000 because of problems associated with drug interaction and side effects.

Somatostatin has also been known to initiate a propagative pattern of motor stimulation of the gut. Soudah and colleagues related their experience with a somatostatin analogue, *octreotide*, in the management of intestinal motility problems in individuals with scleroderma.[205] These investigators demonstrated that migrating complexes propagated at the same velocity and had two thirds the amplitude of the spontaneous complexes in normal subjects. Abdominal symptoms such as nausea, bloating, and pain were much reduced. Further experience with this new agent is awaited.

Trimebutine maleate has also been used to treat manifestations of functional bowel disease, including abdominal pain and constipation.[192] The commercial name is Modulon or Dibridat. The chemical is believed to interact with various receptor subtypes in the gut that are responsible for both excitatory and inhibitory effects on motility. In a double-blind crossover study involving 24 patients, stool frequency, colonic transit time, and colonic electrical activity were measured.[192] The conclusion was that this drug may be of value in the treatment of patients with chronic idiopathic constipation, provided a careful pathophysiologic evaluation reveals a prolonged colonic transit time.

Related Disorders

Stercoral Ulcer

A hard, scybalous, inspissated fecal mass may produce an ulcerating lesion in the colon or rectum, which can then lead to perforation. The condition usually occurs in constipated, bedridden patients. It often presents as an isolated lesion in the rectosigmoid along the antimesenteric margin, but the lesions may be multiple.[98,131] It can also occur in a more proximal location and even in an unobstructed bowel.[118] In 1972, Bauer and colleagues identified 25 patients from the literature and described four of their own.[11] Since that time, numerous reviews have been published.[49,64,131,197,199]

The frequency of this complication is uncertain, but on the basis of postmortem examinations, the incidence may be greater than 5%.[199] Patients who harbor this condition and undergo an emergency operation for perforation may be labeled with the incorrect diagnosis of perforated diverticulitis (see Chapter 26). In fact, in one series, only 11% of patients were given a correct diagnosis regarding cause prior to operation.[199] A less common clinical manifestation is hemorrhage, but the true cause may not be apparent on the basis of the evaluation for lower gastrointestinal bleeding (see Chapter 28). It is certainly possible that a patient presumed to be bleeding from an angiodysplastic lesion could actually be bleeding as a consequence of a stercoral ulcer.

Maurer and co-workers undertook a study to determine the frequency of stercoral perforation of the colon and the criteria for establishment of the diagnosis.[132] In a 5-year period 1,295 patients underwent colonic surgical procedures, of which 44% were considered emergencies. Thirty-nine percent of the emergency colon operations were a consequence of perforation. Seven patients were thought to have stercoral perforations: 0.5% of all colon operations, 1.2% of all emergency colon surgeries, and 3.2% of all colonic perforations. All were left-sided or rec-

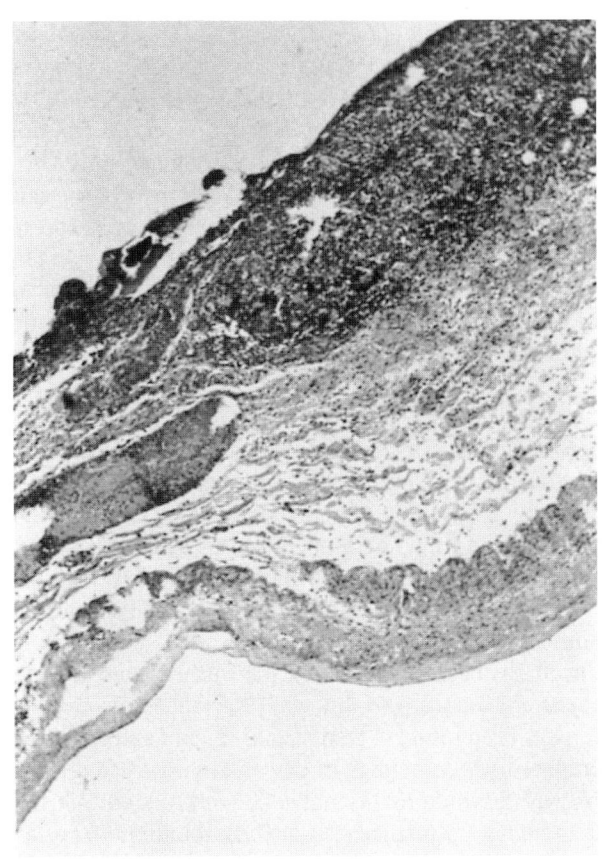

FIGURE 16-14. Stercoral ulcer, the floor of which is lined by inflammatory exudate. (See Color Fig. 16-14.) (Original magnification × 120; courtesy of Rudolf Garret, M.D.)

tal perforations. The authors opine that the diagnosis of stercoral perforation can be made if:

- The perforation is round or ovoid, exceeds 1 cm in diameter, and is in an antimesenteric position.
- "Fecalomas" are present within the colon, protruding though the perforation site, or lying within the abdominal cavity.
- Microscopic pressure necrosis, ulcer, or chronic inflammatory reaction is present.
- Other pathologic causes for the perforation have been excluded.

The investigators conclude that the incidence of stercoral perforation may be underestimated.[132]

Microscopically, the ulcer is essentially nonspecific (Figure 16-14). The epithelium is denuded over a variable area, depending on the size of the fecal mass.[131] With progressive penetration, the bowel wall may become necrotic and ultimately perforate. The diagnosis can be made with some degree of certainty if the physician can demonstrate a fecalith protruding through the site of a perforation or when the perforation is associated with a necrotic border.[49]

Treatment depends on the degree of contamination, the condition of the patient, and other factors discussed in subsequent chapters. In the absence of a perforation, an attempt to evacuate "fecalomas" from the colon should reduce the risk of pressure necrosis or ulceration.[15] As with perforation of the colon, irrespective of the origin, removal of the nidus of sepsis from the peritoneal cavity is essential. The involved bowel is resected, and the decision whether an anastomosis should be performed rests with the judgment of the surgeon (see Chapter 26).

In reviewing the literature, it is evident that the mortality rate associated with stercoral ulcer is very high. This can be attributed to several factors, not the least of which are the morbidity and mortality associated with colonic perforation and peritonitis. Additionally, these patients often are elderly and have major medical problems that place them at an increased risk. Serpell and Nicholls postulate that failure to resect as opposed to simple closure and proximal colostomy is responsible for the high mortality.[197] They emphasize that the disease involves a segment of colon and that merely addressing the focal point of perforation is inadequate.

Fecal Impaction

Fecal impaction is a common finding in surgical patients. The diagnosis is not usually difficult to make, unless the impaction is beyond the reach of the examining finger. Even under these circumstances, the patient's history and the plain abdominal radiograph are usually more than suggestive (Figure 16-9).

There are numerous complications of fecal impaction, the most common of which is incontinence. Other, more serious potential sequelae include the following:

- Stercoral ulceration (see earlier)
- Large bowel obstruction
- Perforation at some distance from the rectum, especially in the cecum
- Gangrene secondary to ischemia
- Autonomic dysreflexia
- Pneumothorax from straining
- Hypoxia
- Associated colorectal problems (e.g., hemorrhoids, rectal prolapse, volvulus)[196,248]

Treatment usually requires manual disimpaction, laxatives, and large-volume or retention enemas. In the interest of patient safety and comfort, manual disimpaction ideally should be undertaken in the operating room with intravenous sedation or a general, local, or regional anesthetic. Double gloves are recommended to minimize the retention of the odor on the physician's hands. A scissoring action will tend to fragment the stool, but in some cases, a large clamp may be necessary to accomplish this.

When the bulk of the mass has been removed, high colonic irrigation with isotonic salt solution is performed by means of a large-bore catheter. The use of the standard setup for cystoscopy irrigation is quite helpful. At the conclusion of the procedure, normal findings on sigmoidoscopic examination are most reassuring.

Kokoszka and colleagues reported the use of another means for treating fecal impaction—a pulsed irrigation-enhanced evacuation device.[102] This is a mobile unit that can be transported throughout the hospital. It consists of two components, the reservoir and irrigation/drainage system. The former serves as a storage compartment for the irrigant and has a capacity of 5 gallons. The latter consists of two tubes that are connected to the reservoir, the drainage bag, and a rectal speculum. In an experience with 14 individuals who had fecal impactions, the authors concluded that the pulsed irrigation technique is a simple, quick, and effective treatment for the management of severe fecal impaction.[102]

Spastic Pelvic Floor Syndrome (Obstructed Defecation; Anismus; Paradoxical Puborectalis Muscle Contraction)

Kuijpers and Bleijenberg evaluated 12 severely "constipated" individuals by means of defecography. They demonstrated that the anorectal angle did not increase during straining, but remained at 90 degrees (Figure 16-15).[106] EMG studies confirmed persistent contraction during defecation straining. This condition has been variously termed spastic pelvic floor syndrome, obstructed defeca-

tion, anismus, and paradoxical or inappropriate puborectalis (sphincter muscle) contraction. Other authors have demonstrated an abnormal increase in the activity of the sphincter mechanism during evacuation in this condition by means of defecography, simultaneous measurement of the intrarectal pressure, and electrical activity of the external anal sphincter.[247] Jones and colleagues have suggested that paradoxical contraction of the puborectalis muscle is not a specific finding.[83] In their EMG analyses, they observed this phenomenon in patients with solitary ulcer syndrome and in those with idiopathic perineal pain.

Pathophysiology

The pathophysiology of anismus is poorly understood. If one thinks psychometrically, it seems that the patient has simply forgotten how to poop. However, it clearly is more complex than this. There often appear to be predisposing or associated factors—physical and emotional stress, prior anal surgery, prior hysterectomy, and even sigmoidoscopy. Diminished rectal perception as determined by balloon distension has been reported, but the cause of this alteration in sensory response is unknown.[58] Rectal compliance, however, has been found to be normal.[57] Fucini and co-workers compared EMG findings in those with obstructed defecation with asymptomatic individuals and noted that there was a higher prevalence of coordinated inhibitory patterns in normal subjects and a lower frequency of pubococcygeus muscle inhibition in patients with anismus.[46]

Diagnosis

The diagnosis of the condition requires, at least initially, an index of suspicion. Most patients are women. The characteristic complaint is one of an inability to effect evacuation by straining, and yet the patient does not necessarily report that she or he is "constipated." Some have suggested that obstructed defecation may be diagnosed when two or more of the following symptoms are present: prolonged and unsuccessful straining at stool, a feeling of incomplete evacuation, the requirement for manual assistance, and the regular use of laxatives and enemas.[57]

Physical examination usually is unrewarding, but there may be an associated rectocele. Whether the presence of this anatomic abnormality predisposes to obstructed defecation is a matter of some debate. Regardless, with a history of manual means to effect evacuation and the presence of obstructed defecation, most surgeons would recommend rectocele repair if conventional treatment for symptoms fails (see Chapter 17).

The balloon expulsion test is a simple and inexpensive method to simulate a patient's ability to expel stool.[12,44] An ordinary latex toy balloon can be also used as well as a Foley catheter or one of the biofeedback devices mentioned in Chapter 13. As previously mentioned, cinedefecography (CD) and EMG have also been used to make the diagnosis of obstructed defecation.[85,182] Fleshman and colleagues compared balloon expulsion, defecogra-

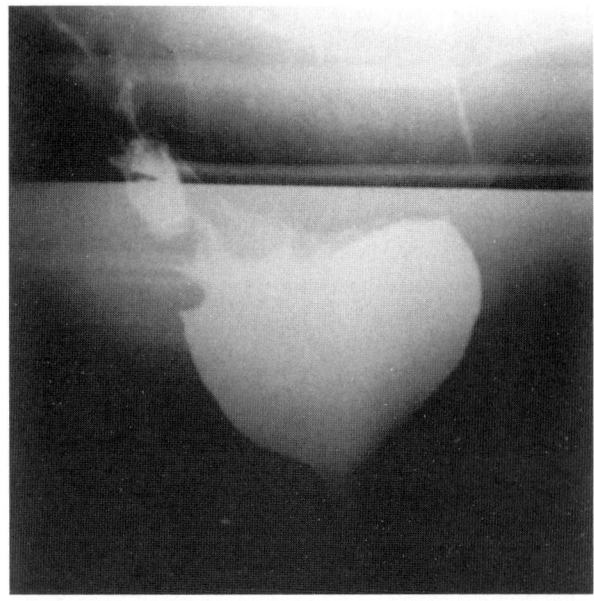

FIGURE 16-15. Obstructed defecation is demonstrated by defecogram. Note descent of the pelvic floor with a tight sphincter and no leakage of the thickened barium. (Courtesy of Christopher J. Lahr, M.D.)

phy, colonic transit times, anal manometry, and EMG in 21 individuals with severe constipation.[44] Twelve were unable to expel a balloon. These investigators concluded that balloon expulsion was the most reliable way to diagnose pelvic floor outlet obstruction resulting from nonrelaxation of the puborectalis muscle.

A prospective study was undertaken by Jorge and colleagues from the Cleveland Clinic Florida, who assessed the correlation between EMG and CD for the diagnosis of nonrelaxing puborectalis syndrome. Sensitivity, specificity, and predictive values of EMG and CD were considered suboptimal. The authors concluded that a combination of these two tests is suggested in order to make the diagnosis of anismus.[85] Roberts and co-workers believe that the definition of anismus should be based on three criteria: demonstration of puborectalis EMG recruitment of greater than 50%, evidence of an adequate level of intrarectal pressure on straining (greater than 50 cm H_2O), and the presence of defective evacuation.[182]

Comment In my experience, the diagnosis of obstructed defecation is not difficult to establish, provided, of course, that it is at least contemplated. The adage, "a diagnosis not considered is not made," is well applied to this condition. Although simple balloon expulsion is very useful, I prefer to objectify the findings through manometry and/or defecography. Figure 16-16 illustrates a manometry testing strip that shows paradoxical elevation of pressure when the patient tries to evacuate.

Treatment

OPERATIVE CONDITIONING (BIOFEEDBACK; BEHAVIORAL MEDICINE)
In Chapter 13, biofeedback is discussed as it applies to the management of individuals with fecal incontinence.

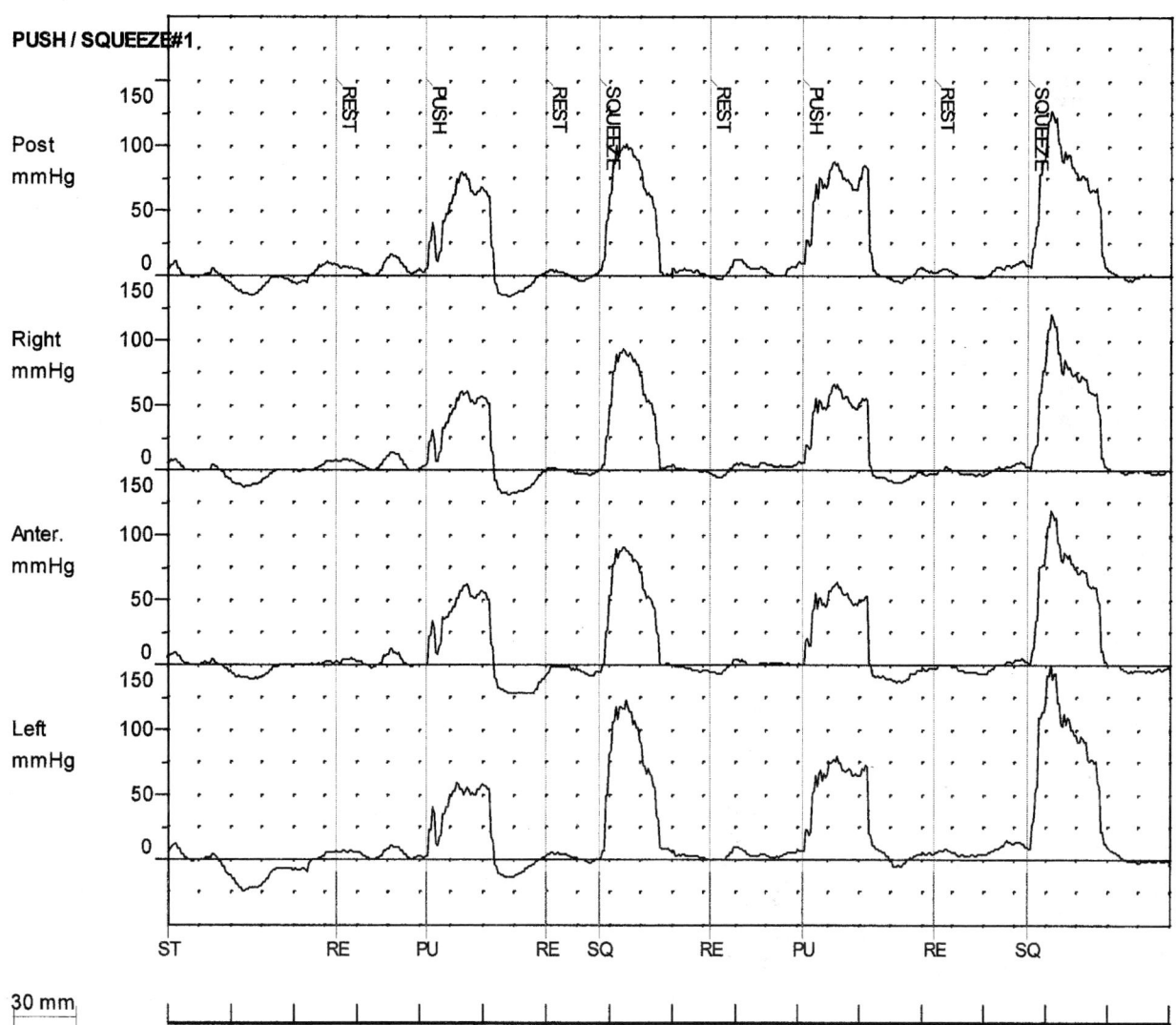

FIGURE 16-16. Paradoxical elevation of anal canal pressure when the patient tries to evacuate. Note that squeeze pressure and "push" pressures are quite similar.

By positive or negative verbal reinforcement or by the use of a variety of devices, bowel control may be improved. The same devices (see Figs. 13-11 and 13-12) can be used to train individuals who are constipated, especially those suffering from obstructed defecation.

BALLOON EXPULSION In biofeedback, patients watch a needle gauge or lights while trying to adjust their sphincter response to rectal balloon insufflation. In this way they can learn to relax the sphincteric mechanism in order to expel the balloon.

Ho and colleagues reported the results of biofeedback treatment utilizing the manometric biofeedback equipment described in Chapter 13.[75] Ninety percent of 56 patients were subjectively improved. Others have also demonstrated that biofeedback improves the defecation act in patients suffering from anismus.[161] However, Keck and colleagues, in their review of the results of biofeedback therapy at the Lahey Clinic in Boston, noted disappointing results in the management of constipation.[93] Among 12 patients with constipation, all could be taught to relax their sphincter in response to biofeedback, but only one reported resolution of symptoms. McKee and co-workers found that nine of their 30 patients improved on this regimen.[134]

ELECTROMYOGRAPHIC BIOFEEDBACK Bleijenberg and Kuijpers reported a treatment regimen of EMG biofeedback followed by simulation of the defecation process by rectal insertion of oatmeal porridge.[19] Seven of their ten patients achieved successful elimination by these techniques. Weber and colleagues also found that biofeedback training was quite useful by conditioning the sphincter to relax during the desire to defecate.[237] Dahl and colleagues treated nine women and five children by means of an EMG biofeedback device connected to an anal probe and had considerable success.[34] Kawimbe and colleagues used a self-applied biofeedback device that permitted EMG recording of the external anal sphincter.[92] Biofeedback training was maintained on a domiciliary basis for just over 3 weeks, with marked improvement noted. The clinical benefit persisted after a mean follow-up of more than 6 months. Wexner and colleagues performed a mean of 8.9 1-hour EMG-based biofeedback sessions on 18 patients.[239] They reported an 89% success rate at a mean length of follow-up of approximately 9 months. However, Loening-Baucke investigated the efficacy of biofeedback in 38 children with anismus and encopresis with somewhat disappointing results.[112] Biofeedback was completely unsuccessful in approximately 25%, and of the remainder, only half recovered from their constipation.

MANOMETRIC ANAL SPHINCTER PROBE FEEDBACK Turnbull and Ritvo used biofeedback from a manometric anal sphincter probe in their patients.[225] Follow-up of up to 4.5 years showed continued improvement in bowel function and abdominal symptoms.

OTHER METHODS Fleshman and colleagues used a fluctuating light bar or an auditory signal.[45] Each day, three training sessions were scheduled in the morning and three in the afternoon. By using an electrode plug, the patient records the muscular activity at rest, during squeeze, and during straining to expel the plug. Subsequent sessions are directed toward attempting to control the activity of the sphincter mechanism during straining. A final step is the instillation of 120 ml of psyllium slurry to simulate an actual bowel movement. The Cleveland Clinic Florida Group compared four methods of biofeedback: intraanal EMG, EMG plus intrarectal balloon, EMG plus home training, and EMG, balloon and home training.[72] All were associated with a significant improvement of outcome, but there was no significant difference in results regardless of the method. Heymen and co-workers performed a comprehensive review and meta-analysis of 38 studies in which biofeedback was used for the treatment of constipation.[73] They determined that there were no anatomic, physiologic, or demographic variables that could reasonably assist the physician in predicting success or failure.

COMMENT It is not clear how long and how often biofeedback sessions are necessary, but all investigators seem to agree that booster treatments are suggested in those individuals who have a relapse. Ideally, training should be performed several times a day for 10 or 15 minutes at a time, a recommendation that can be accomplished only with a home-training device. Unfortunately, despite establishment of the diagnosis with certainty and the availability of often elegant biofeedback alternatives, results are less than ideal. Hopefully at some point one will come to understand the underlying pathophysiology in order to direct an approach to management that will be more satisfactory.

Botulinum Toxin Joo and co-workers used botulinum toxin type A (BTX-A) for the treatment of anismus (see the discussion of botulinum toxin in Chapter 9).[84] Contingent on body mass, 6 to 15 units of BTX-A was injected bilaterally under EMG guidance into the external sphincter or the puborectalis muscle. Treatment was repeated as necessary for a maximum of three sessions during a 3-month period. Of four individuals who had failed to respond to conventional biofeedback, all improved with this treatment. There was no morbidity or mortality. The authors note, however, that longer-term results are only 50% successful. Maria and colleagues used this approach on four patients, one of whom was lost to follow-up.[127] The results were mixed. The investigators caution that repeated injections may be necessary if clinical improvement is to persist, because the drug effects wear off within 3 months.

Ron and associates report an overall satisfaction rate of 58% in their 25 patients but believe that there is a need for a prospective, double-blind study to determine the exact role of this approach to treatment.[184]

Surgical Approaches

RECTOPEXY With the physiologic abnormality described as the spastic pelvic floor syndrome, it would seem intuitively unlikely that colectomy or any other operative approach would be beneficial, unless the operation succeeds in overcoming the resistance of the spastic sphincters. Orrom and colleagues performed rectopexy in 17 patients with obstructed defecation.[160] No significant change was seen postoperatively in maximum resting pressure, maximum voluntary contraction, pelvic descent, or anorectal angle. After 30 months of follow-up, only two individuals (12%) were improved, and many reported a worsening of symptoms.

PUBORECTALIS MUSCLE DIVISION Barnes and colleagues offered what would seem to be a radical alternative in the treatment of anismus, posterior division of the puborectalis muscle.[8] Incontinence for solid stool was not reported, but only two of their nine patients were improved. Kamm and colleagues performed lateral division of the puborectalis muscle in 15 patients with severe idiopathic constipation and three with megarectum (12 unilateral and six bilateral).[87] The operation caused a marked reduction in voluntary squeeze pressure. However, only four patients experienced symptomatic improvement, and this did not correlate with the ability to expel a balloon; three experienced mild mucous or urgency incontinence. No one was incontinent for formed stool. I suggest that the surgeon await further reports of this procedure before embarking on such a potentially hazardous undertaking.

ANAL DILATION Maria and colleagues performed progressive anal dilation in 13 patients with anismus, by utilizing three dilators of 20, 23, and 27 mm in diameter.[126] These dilators were inserted every day for 30 minutes. At 6 months, there was significant improvement of weekly mean spontaneous bowel actions from zero to six, and the number of patients with a need for laxatives decreased from 12 (with a weekly mean of 4.6) to two (with a requirement of once per week). None was incontinent for formed stool, and none experienced mucous discharge or fecal urgency.

ANTEGRADE COLONIC IRRIGATION Heriot and associates describe one woman with a long history of obstructed defecation, in whom all treatment alternatives failed, who underwent percutaneous endoscopic colostomy and antegrade irrigation.[70] After 6 months, an improvement in the patient's quality of life was noted. The use of antegrade irrigation for constipation is discussed later in this chapter and in Chapter 13 for incontinence.

SACRAL NERVE STIMULATION Kenefick and colleagues have suggested that one may modify the neural control of the lower bowel and pelvic floor through sacral nerve stimulation, a technique that has been described for the treatment of anal incontinence (see Chapter 13).[96,97] A marked difference was found in bowel frequency in the same individuals who subsequently crossed over to nerve stimulation. Chronic sacral nerve stimulation continued to produce clinical benefit with an increased bowel frequency at 1 year after implantation.[97] The authors conclude that permanent sacral nerve stimulation can be used to treat patients with resistant idiopathic constipation.[96]

COMMENT The obvious questions are how aggressive should one be in the medical management of the individual with anismus, and at what point is surgical intervention warranted. Certainly, if the patient's symptoms are disabling or intractable despite the application of standard therapeutic measures, an alternative approach, possibly even somewhat radical, may be considered.

Constipation in Children

Constipation represents a common problem in children, with estimates varying from 0.3% of the pediatric population to as high as 8%.[113] It has been demonstrated that 85% of 1- to 4-year-old children pass stools once or twice a day, and 96% do so three times daily to once every other day. Loening-Baucke studied 174 children 4 years of age and younger who had chronic constipation and reported the long-term outcome in 90 of them.[113] Treatment consisted of education, disimpaction, and the promotion of regular bowel habits through the use of dietary fiber and milk of magnesia. The recovery rate of children 2 years of age or younger was significantly higher than in those older than 2 to 4 years. Constipation recurred as soon as laxatives were discontinued in 94% of them.

Hyman and co-workers assessed the response to cisapride in children with so-called chronic intestinal pseudo-obstruction.[79] This diagnosis was based on characteristic symptoms requiring special nutritional support and the absence of an anatomic obstruction. The most common complaints were abdominal pain, vomiting, and constipation or diarrhea, and the most common signs were abdominal distension and failure to thrive. Associated conditions included cystic fibrosis and gastroesophageal reflux. Children with a normal-diameter bowel responded more often than those with a dilated bowel. The response to cisapride was highly variable within the study group, but this could often be predicted by the presence or absence of bowel dilation and migrating motor complexes.[79] Cisapride, however, is not longer available in the United States.

Hirschsprung's Disease

Hirschsprung's disease occurs once in 5,000 births; it is seen four times more often in boys than in girls (see Chapter 18). The clinical picture is produced by a physiologic intestinal obstruction caused by lack of peristalsis in the aganglionic segment. Because of the failure to pass meconium in the first 24 to 48 hours of life, diagnosis is usually established within a relatively short time following birth. Depending on the level of the aganglionic segment, the infant may be initially treated by repeated digital examination, laxatives, and enemas. If the aganglionic segment is long, medical management is not possible.

Short-Segment, Adult, or Late-Onset Hirschsprung's Disease

Occasionally, a child may reach several years of age or even adulthood with a mild form of Hirschsprung's disease (i.e., short-segment involvement) that involves 2 or 3 cm of distal rectum. This manifestation, also known as adult or late-onset Hirschsprung's disease, can cause symptoms of severe constipation or the inability to eliminate except by means of rectal stimulation and enemas.

Manifestations

Udassin and associates reported 39 children who underwent treatment for a mild form of Hirschsprung's disease.[226] The authors distinguished the mild from the severe form on clinical grounds. In the former situation, patients were constipated, had abdominal distension, and exhibited soiling with stool in the rectum. The onset of symptoms tended to be late. In the severe form, the rectal ampulla was empty, soiling did not occur, and the onset of symptoms usually occurred within the first month of life.

Barnes and colleagues analyzed 65 patients and suggested that two subgroups of patients with Hirschsprung's disease can be distinguished: one with onset of symptoms in childhood and the other with complaints developing after 10 years of age and often in adulthood.[9] Distinguishing features, according to the authors, were that fecal soiling was virtually universal in the former but rare in the latter, and that medical treatment was successful in most patients with early onset but unsuccessful in those with development later in life.

Hirschsprung's disease in adults occurs presumably because some newborns have a milder form of the condition and are able, through the use of laxatives and enemas, to compensate for the distal, aganglionic rectum. Thus, they reach adulthood without a confirmatory diagnosis or definitive treatment. The condition may be confused with idiopathic megacolon (see later), but in the latter there is no aganglionic segment. Sometimes the patient will have undergone an unsuccessful surgical procedure during childhood.

Diagnostic Evaluation

The diagnosis is based on the clinical, radiographic, manometric, and histologic studies. Full-thickness rectal wall biopsy may be indicated if the surgeon suspects a form of Hirschsprung's disease. Classically, the lack of ganglion cells has been believed to be diagnostic of the condition (Figure 16-17; see also Color Figs. 18-1 and 18-2). It has been thought important to include the muscularis propria in order to obtain an adequate specimen for interpretation, but the major problem with such a biopsy for distal disease is that ganglion cells may be normally absent in this location. Ricciardi and colleagues have shown that the normal distance of aganglionic bowel wall is 2 cm or less above the dentate line.[179]

Acetylcholinesterase histochemistry has been shown to be highly accurate for the diagnosis of Hirschsprung's disease and can obviate the need for a *deep* rectal biopsy under a general anesthetic. Ikawa and colleagues achieved a 99% diagnostic accuracy, compared with a 61% accuracy using routine staining with hematoxylin and eosin staining.[80] A reliable diagnosis, even in adults, can be achieved by means of suction rectal biopsy and histochemical detection of acetylcholinesterase activity in the nerve fibers of the lamina propria and muscularis mucosae.[59]

Another excellent way of demonstrating the microinnervation of the bowel is to use a pair of immunocytochemical stains directed against the nervous system proteins, neuron-specific enolase and S-100 protein.[66] The former produces intense staining of the ganglion cell perikarya, facilitating recognition of small immature ganglion cells, and the latter highlights prominent, negatively stained ganglion cells surrounded by positive Schwann cells.[66] Still another technique is to use antibodies to neurofilament proteins to identify the heavily stained hyperplastic axon bundles.[99]

Nitric oxide synthase has gained increasing recognition in recent years as a candidate neurotransmitter responsible for relaxation of the internal anal sphincter.[141] The presence or absence of nitric oxide synthase-containing neurons is therefore important in the failure of internal anal sphincter relaxation that characterizes Hirschsprung's disease. Moore and colleagues utilized histologic and immunohistochemical evaluation in three cases of short-segment Hirschsprung's disease and in three normal controls, and they revealed the absence of nitric oxide synthase-containing neurons in two of the three patients with the disease.[141]

Evaluation by means of anorectal manometry has been believed to be a particularly reliable study for identifying patients with this condition. Failure of the internal sphincter to relax following balloon inflation, that is, the absence of the RAIR has been thought to be diagnostic. However, failure of relaxation of the internal sphincter is not necessarily diagnostic, especially in instances of severe, long-standing, idiopathic constipation.[139] The re-

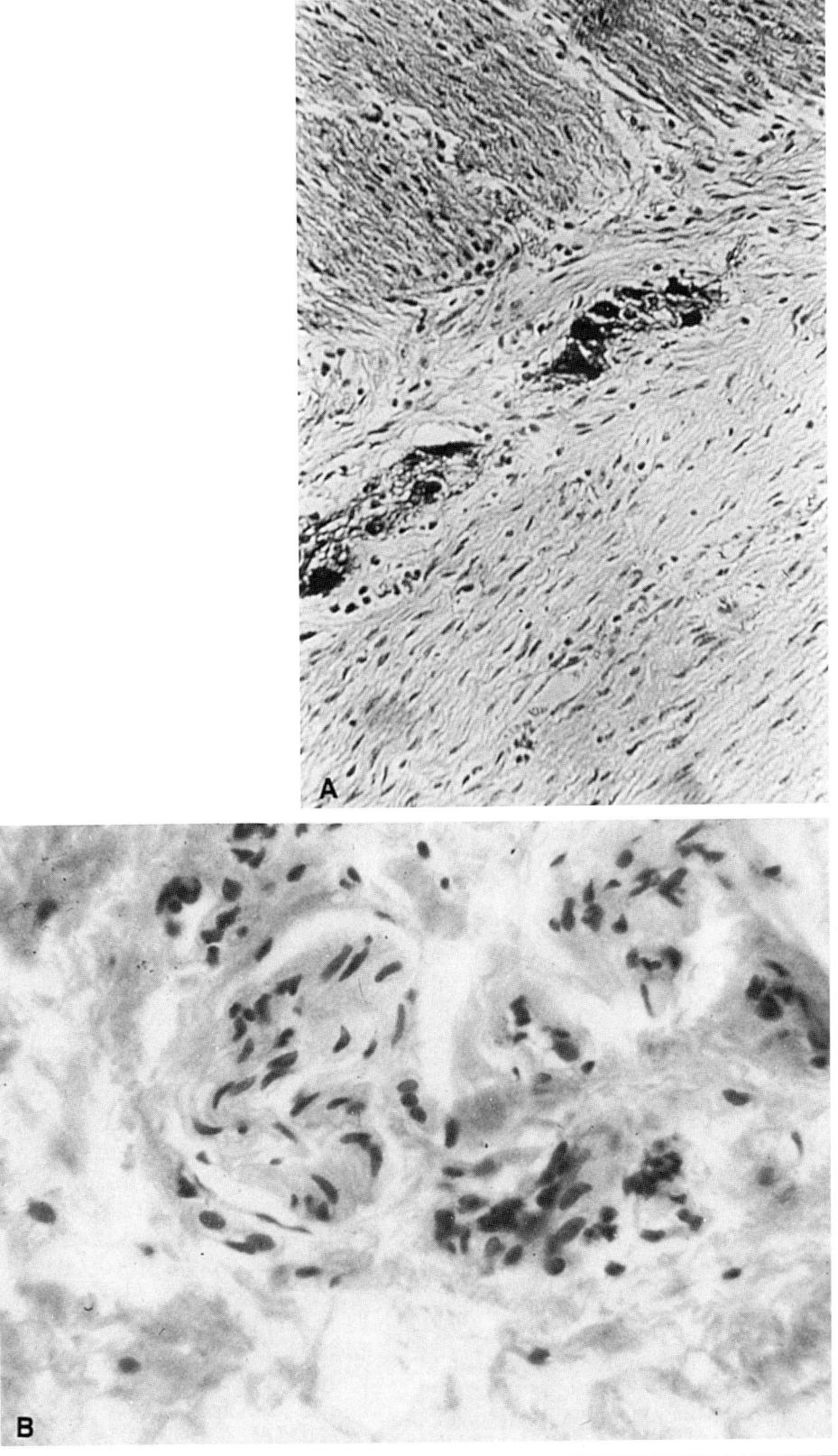

FIGURE 16-17. Diagnosis of Hirschsprung's disease is made by biopsy. **(A)** Normal ganglion cells in the submucosa are stained for acetylcholinesterase. (Original magnification × 200). **(B)** The nerve trunk in the submucosa of the bowel is without ganglion cells. (Original magnification × 600; courtesy of Rudolf Garret, M.D.)

flex may also be absent if resting anal canal pressures are low (see Anorectal Manometry earlier).

Treatment

The characteristic history, physical findings, radiologic picture, and manometric evaluation suggest that the same surgical procedures used in children may be of benefit in adults. *Anorectal myectomy* has been recommended for short-segment disease. Numerous reports have been published demonstrating that the technique can be safely and simply used in children, not only as a primary procedure for short-segment involvement, but also as a secondary operation after a failed low anterior resection or pull-through procedure. Anorectal myectomy is essentially an extensive internal anal sphincterectomy. The internal anal sphincter is divided—or, ideally, partially excised—in the lateral position from the level of the dentate line, incorporating the muscularis of the bowel wall for a distance of approximately 8 to 10 cm (Figure 16-18). Nissan and colleagues advise incising the mucosa transversely about 1 cm proximal to the mucocutaneous junction on the posterior wall of the anal canal.[154] Elevation of the mucosa is performed, and a strip of muscularis, including the internal sphincter, is excised as proximally as possible, including both muscle layers of the rectum. The authors estimate the length of muscle removed to be from 6 to 10 cm.

Once the colon has become very dilated, anorectal myectomy alone will probably fail to ameliorate the complaints adequately, even if the problem initially was a consequence of short-segment disease. Such an individual will usually require a more extensive resection. The enormous dilatation and lengthening of the proximal colon that may be encountered are a more serious concern in adults than it is in infants. Under such circumstances, some surgeons prefer to employ a modified *Duhamel procedure*, with or without a temporary proximal colostomy.[120,149,208] This is a particularly useful technique when a considerable discrepancy exists between the ganglionic and aganglionic segments.

Ricketts and Pettitt make several suggestions concerning technique with respect to the Duhamel operation in adolescents and in adults[180]:

The use of rectal tube decompression may facilitate bowel preparation.
If diversion is required, an ileostomy is advised to limit the risk for injury to the marginal artery. Several applications are required to divide the septum fully between the aganglionic rectum anteriorly and the normal colon posteriorly (see Figure 23-111).

Additional possibilities include the other pull-through procedures, such as Swenson's or Soave's, and low anterior resection with coloanal anastomosis, with or without

an intervening pouch.[207] An ileal pouch-anal anastomosis is another possibility. Finally, one may consider a perineal proctectomy (Altemeier) or Delorme procedure (see Chapter 17).

Results Udassin and colleagues described 30 children treated by a modification of internal anal sphincterectomy.[226] The mean age of the patients at diagnosis was approximately 6 years, and as would be expected, more than two thirds were boys. Four of the 30 patients subsequently had to undergo a Duhamel operation because of the failure of anal myectomy. Long-term follow-up results revealed that 27 patients were essentially without symptoms; seven had good results, and in one, the result was equivocal. Thomas and colleagues reported 11 patients with chronic constipation but without evidence of a long aganglionic segment on barium enema study.[222] These investigators performed a sphincterotomy and rectomyotomy through a posterior approach. Four of the 11 patients had previously undergone a Swenson procedure. The results were mixed and greatly depended on the length of the aganglionic segment; that is, the shorter the segment of involvement, the more successful the myotomy was in achieving a satisfactory result.

Lynn and Van Heerden reported the Mayo Clinic experience of 37 patients who underwent rectal myectomy for this condition.[121] Of the 28 for whom rectal myectomy was the definitive procedure, 20 had excellent results, six were improved, and two remained relatively unchanged. Of the four patients who underwent the procedure following a previous operation, three had excellent results and one was improved. Others have shown that rectal myectomy is an effective procedure for older children with Hirschsprung's disease.[191]

Yoshioka and Keighley reported 29 patients with chronic constipation who underwent anorectal myectomy for Hirschsprung's disease.[250] None had been able to defecate spontaneously more than once a week. All had two of three features suggesting a diagnosis of "outlet obstruction": failure to expel a balloon containing 80 mL of air from the rectum, increased electrical activity of the puborectalis on attempted defecation, and failure to evacuate contrast during proctography. Following anorectal myectomy, 62% were able to eliminate spontaneously more than three times per week. There was a significant fall in maximum resting anal pressure after operation in the patients who had a good result, whereas this was not observed in patients who had an unsatisfactory result. The authors also performed a randomized trial in constipated patients in which anorectal myectomy was compared with anal dilatation by means of a Parks' anal retractor.[251] No one was able to eliminate spontaneously before the procedure. Of the 13 who underwent myectomy, seven were able to defecate spontaneously more

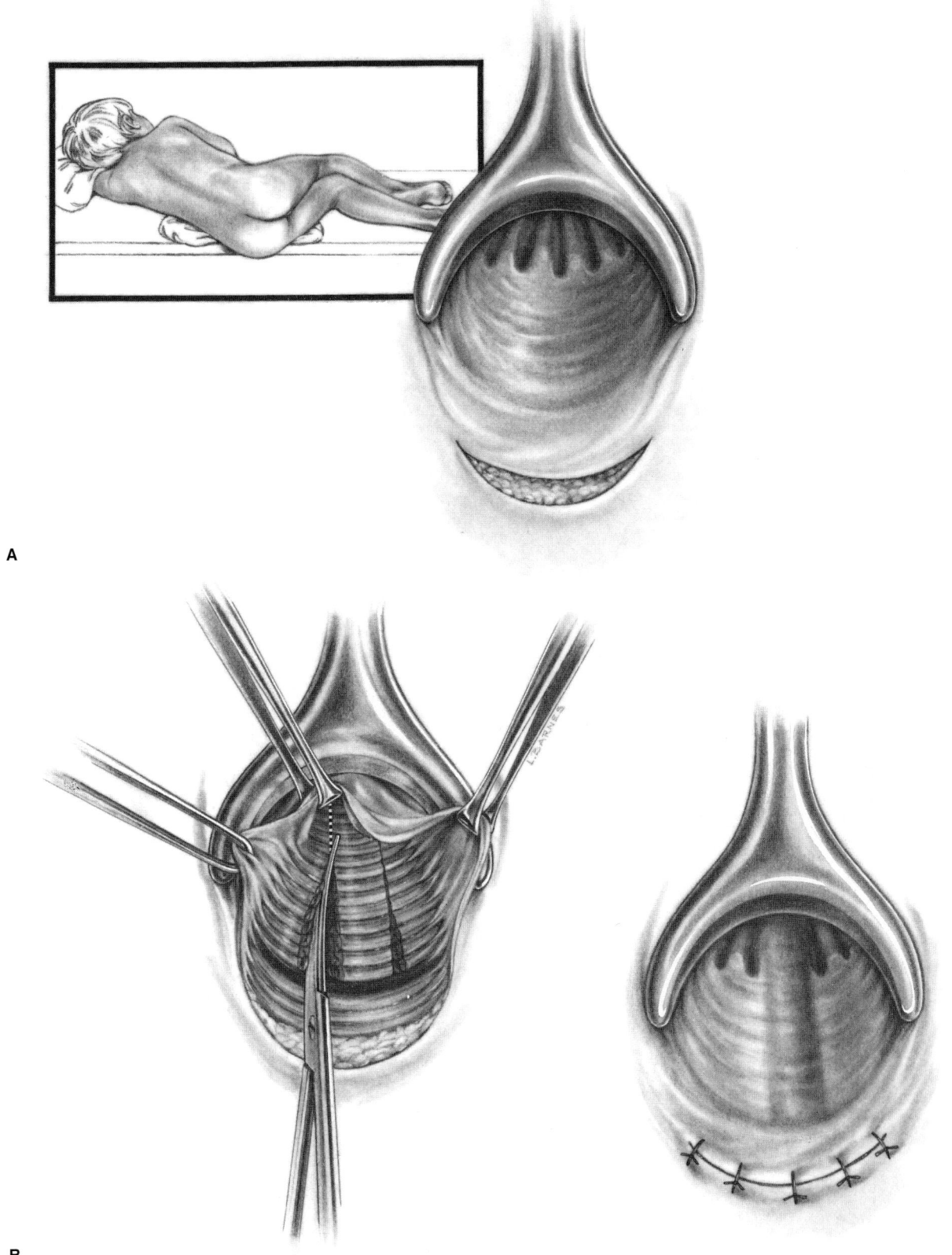

A

B

C

FIGURE 16-18. Treatment of short-segment Hirschsprung's disease by anorectal myectomy. **(A)** Child in the left lateral position with an incision made outside the anal verge. **(B)** Internal anal sphincterectomy performed for at least 8 cm, incorporating the muscularis propria of the rectum. **(C)** Primary wound closure.

than three times a week, compared with none after anal dilatation ($p < .05$). Another report from the same institution involving 63 patients revealed improvement in only 31%.[168,169] Results were independent of preoperative colonic transit or histologic evidence of aganglionosis.

Fishbein and colleagues presented a series of eight adult patients with lifelong refractory constipation successfully treated by rectal myectomy, alone or in combination with anterior resection.[42] Bowel resection was performed when there was a more extensive aganglionic section, but the sphincterectomy limited the amount of pelvic dissection. Elliot and Todd reviewed 39 adults with Hirschsprung's disease who were managed by the Duhamel procedure; all but two gave a history of constipation since birth.[40] Thirty-six (92%) were believed to have had an excellent functional result.

McCready and Beart reported the Mayo Clinic experience of surgery on 50 adult patients with so-called Hirschsprung's disease.[133] Numerous operations were employed, including the Swenson procedure, anorectal myectomy, and a variety of bowel resections. Although the morbidity rate was low, there was a high failure rate (38%). Because of the diverse treatments, however, it is difficult to interpret the results of this study. Wu and co-workers found that neither adult patient in their limited experience benefited from anorectal myectomy.[249] However, those who underwent resection, in which a conventional anastomosis to the anus was utilized, had an excellent functional improvement. Wheatley and colleagues reviewed the literature in 199 patients with adult Hirschsprung's disease.[243] Even with a comprehensive assessment of a relatively rare condition, no statistically significant differences could be determined because of the variety of procedures employed and the length of time encompassed by the study.

It is evident that there is no obvious best choice of operation for short-segment or adult Hirschsprung's disease, but anorectal myectomy, with or without low anterior resection, the endorectal pull-through, and the Duhamel procedure are all associated with relatively good long-term results.[243] Because untreated short-segment disease inevitably leads to intractable symptoms and to megacolon, it is wise to recommend surgery as soon as the diagnosis is confirmed.[120]

Idiopathic Megarectum and Megacolon

Megabowel is a rare condition. It is usually observed as a consequence of Hirschsprung's disease or Chagas' disease (see Chapter 33), and of course it may be seen with intestinal pseudo-obstruction (see later). Some opine that at least 50% of cases are idiopathic, that is, there appears to be no associated condition.[213] There may be a psychological association.[39] The condition may be found in individuals suffering from a panintestinal transit problem and has also been noted with pelvic floor disease, such as rectal prolapse and perineal descent. Surgical options include proctocolectomy and ileoanal reservoir (restorative proctocolectomy) or defunctioning stoma if medical treatment fails. Those with only megarectum may be treated with rectal resection and coloanal anastomosis, with or without colonic pouch.[213] Williams and colleagues described vertical reduction rectoplasty for megarectum in four patients and noted improvement in the frequency of bowel actions.[244]

Surgery in the Management of Constipation

> A large number of diseases, including diabetes and flat feet, are due to autointoxication arising from chronic sepsis in the intestinal cesspool.
>
> William Arbuthnot Lane (1900)

In 1908, Lane first offered a surgical alternative to the treatment of chronic constipation.[108] After initially performing ileocolonic bypass and then partial colectomy, he reported 38 patients who underwent subtotal colectomy for this complaint. However, it is only since the mid-1980s that publications have appeared to reconfirm the legitimacy of subtotal or total colectomy in the treatment of chronic constipation.[13,51,68,77,89,94,117,162,164,166,170,176,188,193,223,231,252,253]

The disease is of unknown etiology. Inevitably, despite all efforts to identify a histologic abnormality in the removed bowel, nothing is found when using conventional staining techniques. However, Park and associates (St. Mark's Hospital in the UK) employed quantitative immunohistochemistry in resected specimens from 14 patients with idiopathic chronic constipation, comparing them with 17 controls with obstructed cancer.[162] The

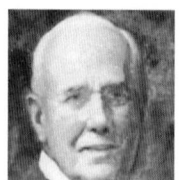

William Arbuthnot Lane (1856–1943)   Lane was born at Fort George, Inverness, Scotland, the eldest son of a military surgeon. As a youth, Lane moved frequently with his parents—to South Africa, Ceylon, Nova Scotia, Malta, and Ireland. He entered Guy's Hospital in London in 1872 and achieved his Fellowship of the Royal College of Surgeons in 1882. Following a period of travel in the Caribbean as a ship's surgeon, Lane was appointed to the staff of Guy's Hospital. He quickly became known as a master technician whose operations a patient could be expected to survive. There were three procedures for which he was renowned: the treatment of cleft palate, open reduction and internal fixation of fractures, and the surgical management of "chronic intestinal stasis." He wrote voluminously (313 articles) and produced a number of short books. During the First World War, Lane was consulting surgeon to the Aldershot Command, in addition to his responsibilities at Guy's Hospital and at the Hospital for Sick Children (Great Ormond Street). He received a baronetcy in 1913, and in 1917 he was named a Chevalier of the Legion of Honor. At the end of the war, he retired from Guy's, and shortly thereafter he extended his views from the hospital to the whole world. In 1925, he founded the New Health Society, an organization dedicated to social concerns in medicine. (Photo courtesy of Guy's Hospital, London.)

myenteric plexus appeared morphologically normal in all the patients with cancer, but there was an increased number of immunoreactive nerve fibers in the muscularis propria in constipated patients. These investigators concluded that intractably constipated patients have alterations in the neural composition of the colonic myenteric plexus and innervation of the circular muscle.[162] Wedel and associates obtained resected specimens from ten patients with slow-transit constipation and performed immunochemical analysis with the neuronal marker Protein Gene Product 9.5.[238] The total ganglionic area and neuronal number per intestinal length, as well as the mean neuronal content per ganglion, were significantly decreased within the myenteric and external submucous plexuses.[238] Tomita and colleagues found that colons in patients with slow-transit constipation were more strongly innervated by nonadrenergic, noncholinergic inhibitory nerves than normal bowel.[224] They suggested that an increase of nitric oxide at these sites plays a role in the dysmotility disorder.[224]

Clinical Characteristics, Evaluation, and Indications for Surgery

Characteristically, slow-transit constipation occurs primarily in young women. Onset is frequently at the time of the menarche, with worsening of symptoms during the teenage years. Most patients have seen their pediatricians, family practitioners, internists and gynecologists and have received the usual suggestions of diet, exercise, laxatives, enemas, and reassurance. It is the rare primary care doctor indeed who has even a remote concept of how to evaluate these unfortunate individuals. A recommendation for surgery is often condemned as typical surgical hubris. Thus, it is often difficult for the patient to accept the fact that the condition may be optimally treated by resection. Still, this is a major operation, with its attendant morbidity and even mortality; it is not a trivial concept, especially when one is dealing with a non–life-threatening ailment.

Patients complain of constipation, obstipation (patients may fail to eliminate for as much as 30 days), bloating, distension, and cramping abdominal pain. Although the condition is not exclusively found in young women, they represent the overwhelming preponderance of patients. So characteristic is the history that if a woman presents in her fifties with severe obstipation, symptoms are much less likely due to slow-transit problems than to obstructed defecation. The same is true for men.

The evaluation of patients with constipation, including slow-transit constipation, has been discussed earlier in this chapter. Once a person has been demonstrated to harbor the condition, one may reasonably recommend

operation. However, Nam and colleagues (Cleveland Clinic Florida) demonstrated that patients should have a repeat colonic transit study in order to improve patient selection for operation.[146] The reason is that there was a poor correlation coefficient in their experience for satisfactory functional results following operation when only one transit study was administered.

One recalls also that obstructed defecation may coexist with a transit abnormality. Ideally, the anismus should be addressed first, and then the colon can be removed. Unfortunately, some patients do not adequately respond to biofeedback. In this circumstance, the surgeon may be forced to press on with the operation despite someone's having both problems. Results are quite good under these circumstances (see Results).

Rarely, the transit abnormality affects the small intestine. Some physicians perform small bowel transit studies before embarking on colon surgery, but unless the radiopaque markers reside in the small intestine at 5 days, I do not pursue investigation of this area.

Surgery is advised when medical measures fail, when the symptoms are judged to be sufficiently severe, and when objective evidence demonstrates slow colonic transit. The surgeon should not accept a statement by the patient that she "miraculously" moved her bowels prior to the plain abdominal x-ray study. The study should be repeated with the reminder again to avoid laxatives, fiber products, enemas, suppositories, and herbs that promote defecation. In my opinion, if the patient "fails" two transit studies, one should not perform a resection but refer her elsewhere (to a nonsurgeon).

Total or Subtotal Colectomy

Despite contrary opinion, and that most often expressed by gastroenterologists and other nonsurgeons, if resection is to be performed as the definitive treatment for chronic idiopathic constipation, most or all of the colon must be removed. Where exactly to place the anastomosis and whether some of the rectum must be extirpated are unresolved issues. Certainly, to do so would inevitably result in diarrhea and the possibility of fecal incontinence. In the unusual circumstance of a megacolon and megarectum, some form of restorative operation (e.g., ileal pouch-anal anastomosis) would be appropriate. The technical aspects of all resective approaches are discussed elsewhere: subtotal and total colectomy in Chapter 22 and restorative proctocolectomy in Chapter 29.

Results

Pemberton and colleagues evaluated 277 patients who were referred to the Mayo Clinic for chronic intractable constipation.[163] These individuals underwent colon transit study, anorectal manometry, EMG, defecography, measurement of the anorectal angle, and a study of efficiency of evacuation by balloon expulsion. The authors were able to categorize patients as having slow-transit constipation, pelvic floor dysfunction, a combination of the two, or irritable bowel. By tailoring the treatment to the specific physiologic abnormality, they were able to select successfully those who would benefit from total colectomy and ileoproctostomy. A more recent report from the Mayo Clinic (1997) describes the long-term results of surgery for chronic constipation and compares preoperative colonic transit and pelvic floor function in an attempt to identify those individuals suitable for resective surgery.[156] Among the 1,009 patients studied, 52 were identified with slow-transit constipation and underwent colectomy and ileoproctostomy. An additional 22 had pelvic floor dysfunction as well as slow-transit constipation. Therefore, 74 underwent surgery and were followed for a mean of 56 months. There were no operative deaths; small bowel obstruction developed in 9% and a prolonged ileus in 12%. All were able to pass a stool spontaneously, and 97% were satisfied with the results of the surgery.[156] Interestingly, there was no difference in the outcome in those individuals who had slow-transit constipation alone compared with those who had concomitant pelvic floor dysfunction.

Belliveau and colleagues reported 48 patients treated for chronic, incapacitating constipation by resection, primarily subtotal colectomy.[14] More than 80% were women. The authors reported an overall success rate of approximately 80%, with a mean follow-up period of 5 years. Preston and colleagues found that colectomy with ileorectal or cecorectal anastomosis gave the best results in their patients.[173] Of the 16 so treated, ten subsequently experienced normal bowel function, and four were markedly improved. Roe and colleagues found that five of their seven patients achieved a successful result with this operation.[183] Leon and colleagues caution that although this procedure results in symptomatic improvement for most individuals, some complain of severe abdominal pain, diarrhea, and fecal incontinence.[111]

Yoshioka and Keighley performed subtotal colectomy on 40 patients with severe constipation.[252] Of these patients, 13% had a history of a serious psychiatric disorder, 40% had undergone a prior anorectal myectomy, and 15% (six patients) later underwent the ileal pouch-anal anastomosis procedure. Median bowel frequency increased from 0.3 times per week preoperatively to 21 postoperatively. Perhaps surprisingly, approximately one third of patients experienced incapacitating diarrhea. The authors caution that surgical therapy for constipation should be offered only to psychologically stable patients with an identifiable physiologic abnormality. Likewise, Pluta and co-workers observed that patients with a psychiatric history or physiologic evidence of an afferent

nerve defect had poorer results.[170] In the experience of Mollen and associates (the Netherlands) involving 21 patients who underwent colectomy and ileorectal anastomosis, morbidity was 33%, especially intestinal obstruction.[140] Although defecation frequency was increased in all, these investigators also noted that 17 patients continued to experience abdominal pain, and 13 still used laxatives and enemas.

Others also note a high morbidity rate after this procedure. Vasilevsky and colleagues found that small bowel obstruction developed in 36% of 52 individuals.[231] Kamm and colleagues, at St. Mark's Hospital, observed that abdominal pain persisted in 71% of patients postoperatively.[86] In addition, the preoperative abnormalities of paradoxical contraction of the pelvic floor during straining and impaired rectal evacuation of a water-filled balloon did not correlate with the clinical outcome. Lubowski and co-workers performed a total colectomy with ileorectal anastomosis in 59 consecutive patients who had severe slow-transit constipation.[117] Median bowel frequency was four times per 24 hours, with 10% using an antidiarrheal medicine regularly. Mean continence score was 1.8 (on a scale of 0 to 20); six patients were incontinent. In addition, 27% had difficulty with rectal evacuation. Although 52% had persistent abdominal pain, all reported improvement compared with their preoperative status. Piccirillo and co-workers, reporting from the Cleveland Clinic Florida, noted excellent or good results in 94% of their patients who underwent this operation.[166] A later experience identified 50 patients who underwent total colectomy for colonic inertia.[167] With a median follow-up of approximately 10 years, there was still a high level of patient satisfaction. In the experience of the Minnesota group involving 112 patients who underwent subtotal colectomy, 93% stated that given what they now know they would still undergo the operation again.[43]

Nicholls and Kamm performed rectal excision and an ileal reservoir with ileoanal anastomosis in two patients when intolerable constipation persisted after colectomy.[150] Both experienced symptomatic relief and were spared a permanent ileostomy. Hosie and colleagues identified 13 individuals who failed to achieve satisfactory functional results following a colectomy for slow-transit constipation; they subsequently underwent restorative proctocolectomy.[76] Nine (85%) were satisfied with the results of this procedure, but two were converted to a permanent stoma. Others opine that a completion proctectomy and an ileoanal pouch procedure may be a viable option in a highly select group of patients in whom subtotal or total colectomy has failed.[164]

Redmond and colleagues, reporting from Schuster's unit at the Johns Hopkins Medical Institutions in Baltimore, emphasized that one consider the condition affecting the entire intestinal tract (so-called generalized intestinal dysmotility).[176] Although 88% of patients with generalized intestinal dysmotility had initial improvement, only 13% had prolonged relief. The authors concluded that there are two distinct types of colonic dysmotility, with and without generalized disease. They emphasized the importance of upper gastrointestinal physiologic studies to identify those individuals who will have a poor long-term response to total colectomy.[176]

Comment

With proper evaluation and careful patient selection, subtotal or total colectomy virtually guarantees cure of the intractable symptoms associated with slow-transit constipation. Only those individuals with concurrent small bowel transit problems and the occasional patient with obstructed defecation who is unresponsive to treatment are less than delighted with the results. However, some patients will experience frequency to the point that "slowing medication" may be needed. Still, most patients will report bowel actions of from one to four times per day, without the requirement for a special diet and without medication. I have often said that these are my most grateful patients.

Partial Colectomy

Partial colon resection has been tried in the past with very limited success and has been fairly abandoned by the overwhelming majority of surgeons who evince an interest in this condition. Where long-term follow-up had been obtained, most of these patients underwent completion colectomy or lived with persistent or recurrent symptoms. Lundin and colleagues (Uppsala, Sweden) hypothesized that properly selected patients may achieve relief of their symptoms with a limited colectomy, thereby avoiding the potential for loose bowels.[119] They used scintigraphic assessment to evaluate segmental colonic transit, scanning at 1, 2, 3, 6 and 24 hours, and then every 24 hours until the radioactive markers had been evacuated. Patients were found to have marked delay in either the left or right colon with less impairment in the remaining segments.[119] Twenty-six left and two right hemicolectomies were performed, with 23 individuals satisfied with the results (82%). The authors recommend a prospective, randomized trial as well as long-term follow-up before one should replace subtotal (total) colectomy in the operative management of slow-transit constipation.

Antegrade Enema

Appendicostomy

The concept of antegrade continence enemas is discussed in Chapter 13. Operative techniques have been developed to facilitate the administration of antegrade washouts to empty the colon and to prevent soiling as well as to deal with constipation and the inability to evacuate.[35,74,104,124,185] This procedure usually involves the creation of an appendicocecostomy (see Fig. 13-63), which permits a channel that can be catheterized to allow colonic washouts. In the experience of Hill and colleagues at the Manchester Royal Infirmary, all six patients were able to initiate defecation and evacuate the colon within 1 hour of irrigation.[74] The procedure has also been employed successfully in children who have undergone pull-through procedures for Hirschsprung's disease or other anorectal malformations.[32]

Christensen and co-workers evaluated large bowel transport following antegrade colonic irrigation with a scintigraphic technique.[30] They found that this procedure induces highly effective emptying, especially of the rectosigmoid, descending colon and transverse colon.

Continent Colonic Conduit

This technique is of value when the appendix is not available (see Fig. 13-64). Williams and co-workers treated seven patients with evacuation disorders by means of this operation. There were two failures, and one patient required a temporary ileostomy.[245] A modification of this conduit was described for the transverse colon in nine patients (see Figure 13-65). Eccersley and colleagues (same group as Williams) suggest that the transverse colon offers better relief from constipation as a consequence of rectal evacuatory dysfunction than does the sigmoid colon.[38]

Comment

Idiopathic constipation may be attributable to several conditions: slow transit, rectal inertia, short-segment Hirschsprung's disease, and outlet dysfunction (i.e., obstructed defecation). Patients may exhibit characteristics of more than one of these conditions. For example, over the years, a profound degree of colonic dilatation is very likely to develop in a patient with short-segment Hirschsprung's disease. This individual is therefore unlikely to benefit from a surgical approach that addresses only the rectal disorder.

These patients must be sorted in an organized way according to cause of the condition. Specific investigations must include anorectal manometry or some means to determine whether a person is suffering from obstructed defecation. Manometry is also useful in establishing the diagnosis of Hirschsprung's disease, although biopsy with special staining techniques are at least as valuable. Alternatively, balloon expulsion, commercially available biofeedback devices, and defecography should be able to confirm or exclude anismus satisfactorily. Transit studies to determine the presence of slow-transit constipation and the primary area of involvement are mandatory.

My approach to treating the adult patient with megacolon in the absence of anorectal pathology is to perform a subtotal or total abdominal colectomy. Even if the rectum is abnormal, a dilated, atonic colon cannot be restored to normal function in these individuals. Unless there is a specific reason to do otherwise, if the rectum is normal, I place the anastomosis at approximately 15 to 18 cm from the anal verge. I believe that a lower anastomosis predisposes the patient to diarrhea and incontinence. Frankly, I have had no experience with the pouch procedures for this particular indication, but I would certainly consider this alternative in an individual with colonic ileus and evidence of short-segment Hirschsprung's disease. Using the criteria described, and applying the appropriate investigations in proper sequence, while performing strict preoperative selection, the physician can arrive at a suitable recommendation and embark on the treatment that is most likely to produce a satisfactory functional result.

INTESTINAL PSEUDO-OBSTRUCTION; OGILVIE'S SYNDROME

Ogilvie's syndrome (see Biography) and intestinal pseudo-obstruction are terms used to denote a condition in which patients appear to have signs and symptoms suggestive of intestinal obstruction without an evident mechanical source. As such, it is often seen in association with other diseases and occasionally complicates the postoperative course of patients who have undergone one of many operations, particularly abdominal surgery. The differential diagnosis includes Hirschsprung's disease, especially short-segment involvement, toxic megacolon in ulcerative colitis and Crohn's disease, volvulus, fecal impaction, and a distal obstructing lesion. Predisposing factors include a virtual textbook of medical and surgical ills, including the following:

- Scleroderma
- Dermatomyositis
- Systemic lupus erythematosus
- Periarteritis nodosa
- Chagas' disease
- Myotonic dystrophy

- Multiple sclerosis
- Familial visceral neuropathies
- Familial visceral myopathies
- Psychotic disorders
- Hypothyroidism
- Diabetes mellitus
- Hypoparathyroidism
- Renal failure
- Renal transplantation
- Blunt abdominal trauma
- Orthopedic procedures
- Porphyria
- Amyloidosis
- Congestive heart failure
- Hypoxia
- Sepsis
- Lead poisoning
- Electrolyte imbalance
- Cesarean section
- Radiotherapy
- Certain medications
- Drug abuse[4,5,7,55,115,137,147,158,175,210,215]

In recent years, the condition has been much more commonly recognized. For example, of renal transplant recipients alone, this complication develops in 10%, and up to 5% of these individuals progress to colonic perforation (see Chapter 26).[211]

In the United States, a support group has been established for adults with so-called chronic intestinal pseudo-obstruction (CIP). It is the American Society of Adults with Pseudo-obstruction (ASAP, Lexington, MA). Goals include education of the general public about the existence of the disease, provision of support for adults who are affected, and serving as a source of information for physicians.

Divining the etiology of colonic pseudo-obstruction is somewhat problematic. Many factors, including the underlying disease, contribute to the development of the dilatation. Impairment of electrical activity of the intestine as well as a defect in intestinal motility may be precipitated by numerous intrinsic and extrinsic agents, such as secretin, glucagon, epinephrine, anticholinergics, and prostaglandins. Ravo and associates believe that involvement of the sacral parasympathetic nerve supply to the

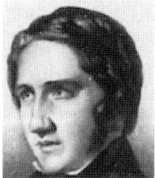

William Heneage Ogilvie (1887–1971) Ogilvie was born in Valparaiso, Chile; his father was an engineer from Dundee, Scotland, who had been in Chile for business reasons. He was educated at Clifton College and New College, Oxford, at which institution he gained first-class honors in physiology. He then entered Guy's Hospital in London for his medical training and obtained his Fellowship of the Royal College of Surgeons in 1920. He was one of the very few medical men of his generation who served in three wars—the Balkan War and the two World Wars. He rose to the rank of Major General and was the Consultant Surgeon to the East Africa Force in 1941. One of his most important admonitions was to require the performance of a colostomy for all wounds of the colon. It was for his military service that he was appointed Knight of the British Empire in 1946. He was considered a brilliant essayist and wrote several books, which provide some of the finest medical writing. He was also responsible for the first two editions of *Recent Advances in Surgery*. Ogilvie developed an international reputation, and many surgeons often visited his theater sessions. Among his many distinctions were honorary fellowships of the Royal College of Surgeons of Canada, the Royal Australasian College of Surgeons, and the American College of Surgeons. (Photograph courtesy of The Royal College of Surgeons of England.)

colon may be the explanation for the syndrome; this theoretical concept was based on their experience in pregnant women.[175]

In an attempt to identify the functional abnormalities in the bowel and in the anal canal, Loening-Baucke and colleagues compared measurements of motility and anorectal pressure in 11 patients with those in an equal number of control subjects.[114] As expected, lower-bowel motility was decreased and rectal wall elasticity was increased, but no specific neural or muscular morphologic defect was identified in colonic transmural pathologic sections in individuals without preexisting colonic disease. Krishnamurthy and co-workers analyzed the clinical, radiographic, manometric, and pathologic features of 26 women with severe idiopathic constipation.[103] They identified an abnormality of the myenteric plexus that could be distinguished from the one described in intestinal pseudo-obstruction. Koch and colleagues found that this condition is often associated with decreased colonic concentrations of vasoactive intestinal peptide.[101] This substance is identified in normal nerve fibers within the circular muscle of the colon.

Clinical Manifestations and Diagnosis

Presenting features of colonic ileus are abdominal distension, abdominal pain, constipation, and occasionally diarrhea. The surgeon must distinguish among severe idiopathic constipation, mechanical obstruction, and pseudo-obstruction. In the first situation, individuals usually have a flat abdomen with minimal gas in the colon, but there are many exceptions. Distinguishing between pseudo-obstruction and mechanical obstruction is usually fairly obvious if one accepts the tenet that the for-

mer is a "selective or disproportionate gaseous distension of the colon in the absence of mechanical obstruction".[202] In other words, pseudo-obstruction is basically a radiologic diagnosis (Figs. 16-3 and 16-19, and previous discussion). Computed tomography is usually unhelpful except to show the massively dilated bowel (Figure 16-19). Endoscopy and contrast studies may be necessary to confirm that there is no mechanical cause. Ogilvie's syndrome can usually be identified as a distinct clinical entity by the fact that the manifestation develops while the patient is in the hospital for another problem, whether surgical or nonsurgical. An antecedent history of colonic pseudo-obstruction is a helpful clue.

Chronic intestinal pseudo-obstruction is manifested, as may be suspected, by recurrent signs and symptoms. Patients are often cachectic, with hypoactive or absent bowel sounds, and have a mildly tender, distended abdomen.

Treatment and Results

Noninterventional Management

Initial management should include restriction of oral intake, nasogastric intubation, and correction of any fluid or electrolyte abnormalities. It is imperative that specific problems, such as infection, be treated if possible. Sloyer and colleagues reviewed the experience of 25 patients with Ogilvie's syndrome at the Memorial Sloan-Kettering Cancer Center in New York; all but one were treated conservatively.[202] This conservative treatment consisted of the foregoing measures of initial management plus gentle enemas, a rectal tube, and decreased narcotic dosage. There were no associated colonic perforations, nor were

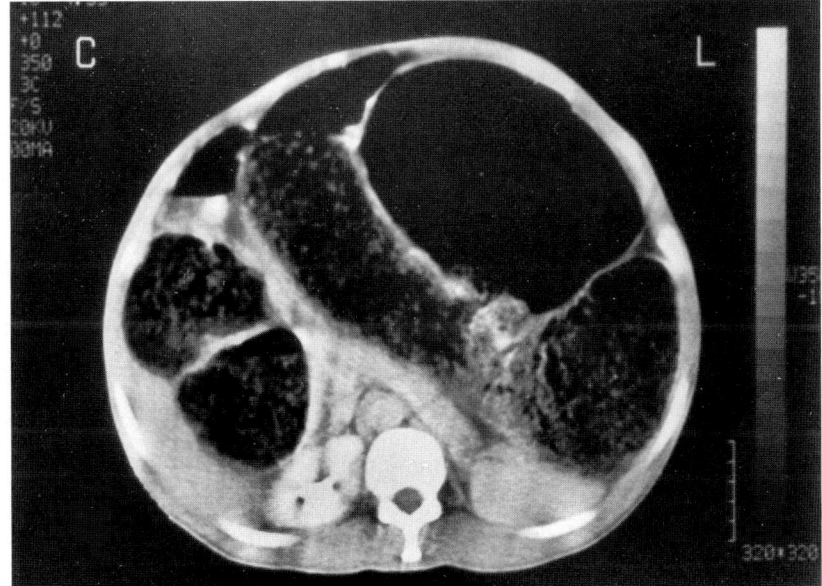

FIGURE 16-19. Computed tomography demonstrates a massively dilated colon. There is no evidence of perforation. Although not diagnostic, the radiologic picture is consistent with Ogilvie's syndrome.

there any obstruction-related deaths. Colonoscopy was not employed, and the authors questioned the appropriateness of this procedure or any surgical treatment in those with acute colonic ileus.

Colonoscopy

Despite the previous statement, colonic decompression by means of colonoscopy is thought to be the most effective therapeutic modality for selected patients with nonobstructive colonic dilatation.[21,22,48,56,130,143,181,212,230]

Care should be taken to visualize the lumen adequately and to insufflate minimal air. Safety and ease of passage may be facilitated by using carbon dioxide instead of air, or a water-instillation system instead of gas.[143,145] A tap water enema of about 1000 mL may be instilled before the procedure to allow the stool in the distal bowel to be aspirated.[145] Burke and Shellito advocate the use of a larger, flexible, fenestrated overtube (i.e., C tube), which permits continuous decompression after passage of a single-channel colonoscope.[23] This theoretically avoids the requirement for repeated colonoscopy for recurrent symptoms. Others have placed a catheter or have positioned a guidewire through the colonoscope and threaded the catheter over the guidewire.[17,31,136] Many endoscopists contend that the procedure is safer and easier than would be anticipated, perhaps because the colon is already filled with gas. This and greater wall compliance than that found in individuals with diverticular disease or toxic megacolon permit a certain margin of safety.[143] Most authors suggest that successful decompression should be verified by abdominal radiographs[165] and that unresolved cecal distension in excess of 12 cm warrants operative decompression to limit the risk for perforation.[130] In a review of 400 patients with this syndrome, Vanek and Al-Salti correlated increased age of the patient, maximal cecal diameter, and delay in initiating colonic decompression with increased mortality.[230]

Strodel and colleagues reviewed 44 patients who underwent 52 colonoscopic examinations for colonic ileus.[212] In approximately one fourth, the condition developed during convalescence from recent surgery, whereas two thirds had major systemic disorders. The mean cecal diameter before colonoscopy was approximately 13 cm. On the basis of radiographic or clinical criteria, 38 patients (86%) underwent successful decompression on the initial colonoscopic examination; perforation of the cecum occurred in one individual. The authors advocate at least an attempt at colonoscopic decompression before performing laparotomy or cecostomy. Vanek and Al-Salti performed colonoscopic decompression of 125 patients with a success rate of 82% and a recurrence rate of 22%.[230] Bode and colleagues decompressed the colon in 20 of 22 patients (91%) by this technique, although 18% experienced a recurrence.[21] Gosche and colleagues noted

an 89% rate of success, but 41% required repeated endoscopic decompression during their hospital stay.[56]

Epidural Anesthesia

On the theory that Ogilvie's syndrome is caused by excess sympathetic tone, Lee and colleagues performed splanchnic sympathetic blockade by means of epidural anesthesia in eight patients.[109] The epidural catheter was inserted in the T11–12 interspace and advanced cephalad; 0.25% bupivacaine was used with a loading dose of 5 to 10 mL, followed by continuous infusion at 3 mL/hour. Five of the patients (63%) were managed successfully. Whether this will ultimately prove to be a worthwhile therapeutic option remains to be determined.

Drug Therapy

Another possible method of treatment is the use of ceruletide, a synthetically produced decapeptide that has been demonstrated to stimulate intestinal motility. It is believed to act similarly to pancreatic extract, but it is not available in the United States as of this writing. Madsen and colleagues performed a double-blind clinical trial involving 18 patients and demonstrated a statistically significant effect on restoration of peristalsis in those who had intestinal paralysis following abdominal surgery.[123] An intramuscular injection of 0.3 μg/kg of body weight was given every 8 hours until passage of flatus or feces occurred or until three injections had been administered.

The use of the prokinetic agent cisapride has been mentioned previously. MacColl and colleagues evaluated its efficacy in the treatment of acute colonic pseudo-obstruction in one man who experienced complete resolution of symptoms.[122] However, this drug was withdrawn from the market in the United States.

Stephenson and co-workers undertook a study to determine the value of intravenous neostigmine in achieving adequate colonic decompression in patients with Ogilvie's syndrome.[210] Satisfactory decompression of large-bowel distension was achieved in 11 of 12 patients. This suggests that the syndrome is a consequence of excessive large-bowel parasympathetic suppression. Others have demonstrated this to be an effective alternative.

Surgery

In the patient with intestinal pseudo-obstruction, surgical intervention should not be performed unless there is a genuine fear of impending cecal perforation. This condition, in my opinion, is one of the few indications for performing a cecostomy. Generally, the operation is carried out by the standard open technique. Percutaneous cecostomy under computed tomographic guidance also has been successfully employed as an alternative to surgical cecostomy for decompressing a massively dilated cecum.[26] Another suggestion is to perform percutaneous colonoscopic cecostomy, a technique analogous to that of percutaneous gastrostomy.[172] Although the procedure may provide long-term decompression without the need for a laparotomy in patients with Ogilvie's syndrome, there is a risk of tearing the colonic wall, with resultant uncontrolled spillage into the peritoneal cavity. A technique of laparoscopically guided percutaneous cecostomy, using T fasteners to retract and anchor the cecum to the anterior abdominal wall, has been described.[37]

If the bowel is ischemic or perforated, resection with or without anastomosis is required in accordance with the principles discussed in Chapter 26. Results of resection are too apocryphal to submit here for comment.

CHRONIC IDIOPATHIC ANAL PAIN; PROCTALGIA FUGAX; LEVATOR SYNDROME; LEVATOR SPASM

Levator spasm (i.e., levator syndrome) was recognized as a clinical entity as early as 1841 by Hall,[14,148] but it was not until 1935 that the term proctalgia fugax was coined by Thaysen.[217] Hall's description was of a "peculiar and severe pain of the rectum, which comes on in paroxysms, generally during the first sleep".[65] This complaint is heard frequently, yet most physicians fail to recognize the entity and will often classify the patient as hysterical and prescribe various sedatives or tranquilizers as treatment.

The condition occurs predominantly in women. Characteristically, the patient complains of severe, episodic, often agonizing discomfort within the rectum. The location of the pain distinguishes proctalgia from a thrombosed hemorrhoid or an anal fissure, problems that are often localized to the anal or perianal area. The pain is often on the left side, may awaken the individual from sleep, and is usually unrelated to bowel activity, although sometimes it may be exacerbated by defecation. The discomfort usually lasts only a few moments but occasionally may persist for several hours. Patients will often sit on the toilet and strain, believing that this will cause the symptom to dissipate. In reality, this will more likely cause the discomfort to persist.

There is no unanimity of opinion as to the etiology of proctalgia fugax. Numerous causes have been suggested (e.g., neuralgia, neurosis, infection, allergy, vasospasm, venous stasis, mechanical factors), but none can be supported by conclusive evidence.[91] There is, however, general agreement that the specific problem is a muscle spasm of the levatores, analogous to a "charley horse" of the hamstring muscle. The condition often occurs in patients who spend a great deal of time on the toilet, whether straining, with diarrhea, or reading the newspaper. Other predisposing factors that have been suggested include trauma from riding a long distance, childbirth,

low anterior resection or pelvic surgery, anal surgery, spinal surgery, psychiatric disorders, irritable bowel syndrome, and the act of sexual intercourse.[50,187] A hereditary predisposition has also been reported.[27] The psychological aspects of proctalgia were examined by Renzi and Pescatori in 20 patients.[177] Interviews and personality testings demonstrated that patients showed elevated depression and anxiety levels as well as a "strong tendency to use primitive defense mechanisms and showed a lack of personality formation".[177] I do not know exactly what that all means, but if I felt the pain that many of these individuals perceive, the agony of the equivalent of a hot poker in the rectum all day, I suspect that I, too, would be a touch depressed and anxious.

Evaluation

Physical examination is usually unrewarding, but sometimes a tender, spastic puborectalis muscle may be felt, particularly on the left side. The characteristic discomfort may be duplicated when the physician presses on the sensitive area.

Christiansen and co-workers undertook a study to analyze whether anal ultrasound, physiologic evaluation, and histopathologic examination presented any specific abnormalities or common features.[29] None was found. However, Grimaud and colleagues studied 12 patients with proctalgia fugax by means of manometry and noted that the resting pressure in the anal canal of these individuals was significantly higher than that of controls.[62]

Treatment

Initial treatment should consist of instructions on bowel management and removing reading material from the toilet. Sitz baths may offer some relief, but often the pain will cease before the bath water can be drawn. Grant and colleagues believe that the syndrome is optimally treated by levator massage, with success reported in almost two thirds of their patients.[61] I have not found this approach helpful and recommend instead perineal strengthening exercises (see Chapter 13). With a vigorous exercise program and assurance that the pain is not caused by neurosis, the symptoms usually abate within a few days or weeks.

Grimaud's group assumed that their findings were caused by dysfunction of the external sphincter and observed that a biofeedback exercise regimen was very helpful in management.[62] Heah and co-workers studied the effects of biofeedback on pain relief in 16 consecutive patients with levator syndrome.[67] All underwent a course of biofeedback using a manometric balloon technique. After a mean follow-up of 1 year, all required fewer analgesics. Gilliland and colleagues utilized EMG-based biofeedback in 86 patients.[52] Thirty-four percent reported an improvement, with significant benefit observed in those individuals who completed the scheduled course of therapy and did not self-discharge.

In the intractable situation, muscle relaxants may be useful, but narcotic pain medication should not be given because of the risk for habituation. The teaching of self-hypnosis has been of benefit to some patients. Other alternatives that have been suggested are the administration of sublingual, topical, or controlled-release nitroglycerin and quinine sulfate.[116]

Idiopathic proctalgia is often associated with an irritable bowel. These individuals should receive appropriate medical management for this condition. Adequate control of the irritable bowel symptom complex often leads to amelioration of the proctalgia fugax, especially with the use of antispasmotic medication such as hyoscyamine (Levsin) and dicyclomine (Bentyl).

Another alternative in the treatment of the levator syndrome was reported initially by Sohn and colleagues—the use of electrogalvanic stimulation by means of a specially designed rectal probe (Electro-Med Health Industries, Miami, FL; 800–232-EMHI; Figure 16-20).[203] The negative electrode is used and the stimulator is set at 80 cycles per second. The machine is adjusted to deliver 150 to 400 V, depending on patient tolerance. The authors theorize that the technique may overstimulate and over-contract the levator muscle to fatigue it. They reported their results with 80 patients to be excellent in 69%, good in 21%, and poor in 10%. Nicosia and Abcarian treated 45 patients by this method for 20 minutes every other day.[151] On average, five sessions were required for complete pain relief. Excellent results (i.e., total pain relief) were obtained in 36 patients, good results in five, fair in two, and no relief in two. Other authors also report a favorable response to this modality in those individuals who failed to improve with conservative regimens.[159,187] Billingham and colleagues had less success, however.[18] In a follow-up survey of 20 patients, only five (20%) remained symptom-free. Hull and co-workers, reporting from the Cleveland Clinic, noted that only 19% had relief of symptoms with a mean follow-up of 28 months.[78] Partial relief was achieved in 24%, but 57% were unrelieved. When comparing three methods of treatment—electrogalvanic stimulation, biofeedback, and steroid caudal block—Ger and colleagues noted a success rate of 38%, 43%, and 18%, respectively.[50] More than half of the patients were refractory to all three therapeutic options.

A publication from Japan noted good or excellent results in 33 of 35 consecutive patients who complained of vague and deep pain in the anorectum treated by means of *linearly polarized near-infrared irradiation*.[138] This wavelength can penetrate the skin surface for a distance of more than 5 cm. Further experience and long-term follow-up are, of course, needed.

Comment

In my experience, approximately two thirds of patients seem to benefit from three or more electrogalvanic treatments of 1 hour each, spaced over weekly intervals. In an occasional individual, one session may suffice. About one third report no improvement. Unfortunately, the longer the patient has symptoms prior to implementation of this approach, the less likely will be the success. If all has been tried and these efforts fail, the surgeon's only recourse, in my opinion, is to refer the patient to a pain management center.

COCCYGODYNIA

The term coccygodynia was coined by Simpson in 1859, when he initially recognized this entity.[200] Because of the failure of standard pain medications to relieve the symptoms of coccygodynia, the author suggested that coccygectomy was the optimal treatment. Several comprehensive reviews of the subject have been published by Thiele.[218–221]

The condition is part of the levator syndrome, or another manifestation of proctalgia fugax, but the pain is directed to the coccyx. This is probably caused by spasm of the pubococcygeal portion of the levator ani muscle. Classically, the pain is exacerbated when the person rises from a sitting position.

Maroy reported a study analyzing the association between coccygodynia and depression.[128] A highly significant correlation was found between pain evoked by rectal digital examination and depressive status in patients without coccygodynia and between coccygodynia and evoked pain. Garnjobst editorializes in this article, reporting that although patients usually do not appear de-

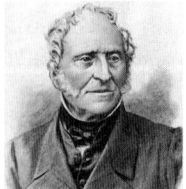

James Young Simpson (1811–1870)   Simpson was born in Bathgate, Scotland, the youngest of seven sons of the village baker. His mother died when he was quite young, but, because of James's obvious scholastic aptitude, his entire family agreed to do without to give him a higher education. Simpson entered Edinburgh University at the age of 14 and began his medical studies 2 years later, graduating with his M.D. in 1832. His extraordinary abilities were soon recognized. He was made President of the Royal Medical Society of Edinburgh in 1835 and was appointed to the Chair of Midwifery in 1839 at the age of 28. He was the first in Britain to employ ether as an anesthetic, and with his associates was the first to use chloroform as an anesthetic (1847). In addition to his achievements in the field of anesthesia, Simpson was responsible for laying a considerable part of the foundation of gynecology and obstetrics. He invented the uterine sound and the obstetric forceps. In 1866, Simpson was awarded a baronetcy, the first given to a doctor practicing in Scotland. When he died, his family declined the offer of a grave in Westminster Abbey, but a bust was placed there noting that to Simpson's "genius and benevolence the world owes the blessings derived from the use of chloroform for the relief of suffering." (Photo courtesy of the Royal College of Surgeons of England.)

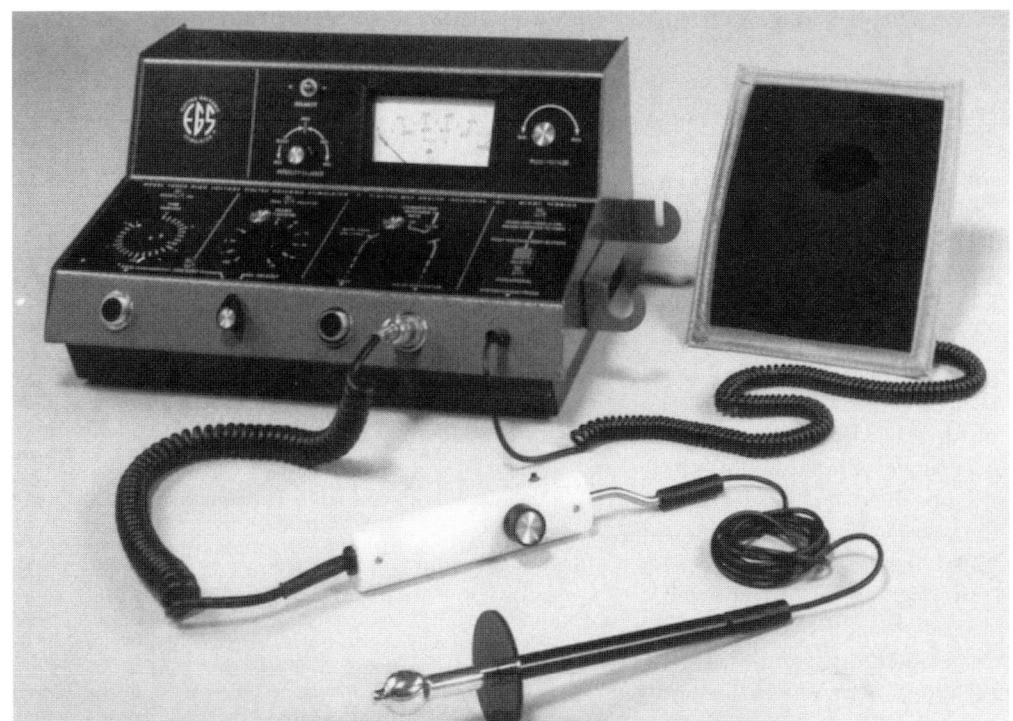

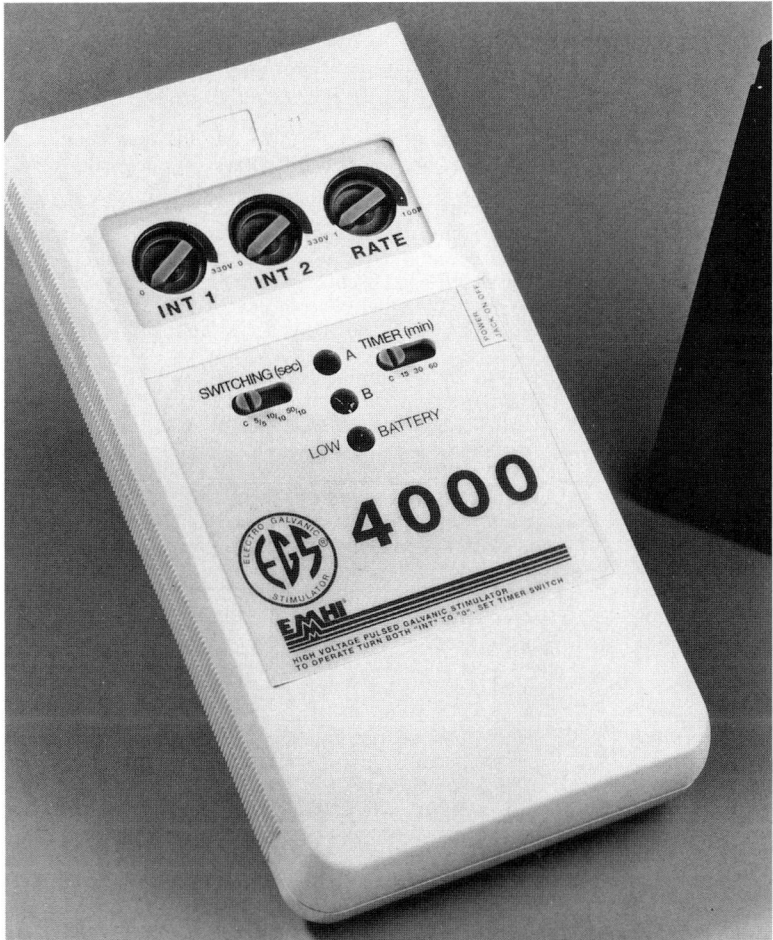

FIGURE 16-20. **(A)** An electrogalvanic stimulator (Model 100–2) with Sohn's electrode rectal probe. **(B)** EGS 4000 EGXtra-portable unit for home use. (Courtesy of Electro-Med Health Industries, Miami, FL.)

pressed initially, subsequent follow-up evaluation suggests that they are.[128]

To initiate proper therapy, it is important to recognize the clinical syndrome and the characteristic pain. Some authors advocate levator massage, but, as with proctalgia fugax, perineal strengthening exercises and appropriate bowel management are suggested. Electrogalvanic stimulation may be of value for selected individuals (see the discussion of proctalgia fugax).

Coccygectomy has been offered to treat coccygodynia, usually by orthopedic surgeons, but in my opinion, this operation should not be performed for this condition unless the coccyx has been injured or is dislocated. Even under these circumstances, coccygectomy rarely alleviates the pain. Johnson suggests that injection of a local anesthetic and cortisone may be beneficial; he cautions, however, that the relief is usually only temporary.[82] Albrektsson evaluated the long-term effects of sacral rhizotomy in 24 patients with coccygodynia.[3] Only six responded well to the procedure; serious complications occurred in 25%. I find it difficult to justify a surgical procedure of any kind in a patient with coccygodynia.

REFERENCES

1. Abd-El-Maeboud KH, El-Naggar T, el-Hawi EMM, et al. Rectal suppository: common sense and mode of insertion. *Lancet* 1991;338:798.
2. Agachan F, Chen T, Pfeifer J, et al. A constipation scoring system to simplify evaluation and management of constipated patients. *Dis Colon Rectum* 1996;39:681.
3. Albrektsson B. Sacral rhizotomy in cases of anococcygeal pain: a follow-up of 24 cases. *Acta Orthop Scand* 1981; 52:187.
4. Anuras S. Clinical presentation: chronic intestinal pseudo-obstuction. *Pract Gastroenterol* 1991;15:13.
5. Attiyeh FF, Knapper WH. Pseudo-obstruction of the colon (Ogilvie's syndrome). *Dis Colon Rectum* 1980;23:106.
6. Balazs M. Melanosis coli: ultrastructural study of 45 patients. *Dis Colon Rectum* 1986;29:839.
7. Bardsley D. Pseudo-obstruction of the large bowel. *Br J Surg* 1974;61:963.
8. Barnes PRH, Hawley PR, Preston DM, et al. Experience of posterior division of the puborectalis muscle in the management of chronic constipation. *Br J Surg* 1985;72:475.
9. Barnes PRH, Lennard-Jones JE, Hawley PR, et al. Hirschsprung's disease and idiopathic megacolon in adults and adolescents. *Gut* 1986;27:534.
10. Bassotti G, Morelli A, Whitehead WE. Abnormal rectosigmoid myoelectrical response to eating in patients with severe idiopathic constipation (slow-transit type). *Dis Colon Rectum* 1992;35:753.
11. Bauer JJ, Weiss M, Dreiling DA. Stercoraceous perforation of the colon. *Surg Clin North Am* 1972;52:1047.
12. Beck DE. Simplified balloon expulsion test. *Dis Colon Rectum* 1992;35:597.
13. Beck DE, Jagelman DG, Fazio VW. The surgery of idiopathic constipation. *Gastroenterol Clin North Am* 1987;16: 143.
14. Belliveau P, Goldberg SM, Rothenberger DA, et al. Idiopathic acquired megacolon: the value of subtotal colectomy. *Dis Colon Rectum* 1982;25:118.
15. Berardi RS, Lee S. Stercoraceous perforation of the colon: report of a case. *Dis Colon Rectum* 1983;26:283.
16. Berman IR, Manning DH, Harris MS. Streamlining the management of defecation disorders. *Dis Colon Rectum* 1990;33:778.
17. Bernton E, Myers R, Reyna T. Pseudo-obstruction of the colon. *Curr Surg* 1983;40:30.
18. Billingham RP, Isler JT, Friend WG, et al. Treatment of levator syndrome using high-voltage electrogalvanic stimulation. *Dis Colon Rectum* 1987;30:584.
19. Bleijenberg G, Kuijpers HC. Treatment of the spastic pelvic floor syndrome with biofeedback. *Dis Colon Rectum* 1987; 30:108.
20. Bockus HL, Willard JH, Bank J. Melanosis coli. The etiologic significance of the anthracene laxatives: a report of 41 cases. *JAMA* 1933;101:1.
21. Bode WE, Beart RW Jr, Spencer RJ, et al. Colonoscopic decompression for acute pseudo-obstruction of the colon (Ogilvie's syndrome): report of 22 cases and review of the literature. *Am J Surg* 1984;147:243.
22. Bullock PR, Thomas WEG. Acute pseudo-obstruction of the colon. *Ann R Coll Surg Engl* 1984;66:327.
23. Burke G, Shellito PC. Treatment of recurrent colonic pseudo-obstruction by endoscopic placement of a fenestrated overtube. *Dis Colon Rectum* 1987;30:615.
24. Camilleri M, Zinsmeister AR. Towards a relatively inexpensive, noninvasive, accurate test for colonic motility disorders. *Gastroenterology* 1992;103:36.
25. Campbell WL. Cathartic colon: reversibility of roentgen changes. *Dis Colon Rectum* 1983;26:445.
26. Casola G, Withers C, van Sonnenberg E, et al. Percutaneous cecostomy for decompression of the massively distended cecum. *Radiology* 1986;158:793.
27. Celik AF, Katsinelos P, Read NW, et al. Hereditary proctalgia fugax and constipation: report of a second family. *Gut* 1995;36:581.
28. Chiou AW-H, Lin J-K, Wang F-M. Anorectal abnormalities in progressive systemic sclerosis. *Dis Colon Rectum* 1989; 32:417.
29. Christiansen J, Bruun E, Skjoldbye B, et al. Chronic idiopathic anal pain: analysis of ultrasonography, pathology, and treatment. *Dis Colon Rectum* 2001;44:661.
30. Christensen P, Olsen N, Krogh K, et al. Scintigraphic assessment of antegrade colonic irrigation through an appendicostomy or a neoappendicostomy. *Br J Surg* 2002;89: 1275.
31. Chung RS. A technique for rapid intubation of the sigmoid and left colon. *Surg Gynecol Obstet* 1983;157:279.
32. Claffey KB, Patton ML, Haith LR, et al. Barium and fecal impaction: an unusual case of bilateral hydronephrosis. *Am Surg* 1995;61:709.
33. Cruveilhier J. *Anatomie pathologique du corps humain; ou, descriptions avec figures lithographiques et coloriées, des diverses altérations morbides dont le corps humain est susceptible.* Paris: JB Baillière, 1829–1842;19:6.
34. Dahl J, Lindquist BL, Tysk C, et al. Behavioral medicine treatment in chronic constipation with paradoxical anal sphincter contraction. *Dis Colon Rectum* 1991;34:769.
35. Dick AC, McCallion WA, Brown S, et al. Antegrade colonic enemas. *Br J Surg* 1996;83:642.
36. Ducrotte P, Rodomanska B, Weber J, et al. Colonic transit time of radiopaque markers and rectoanal manometry in patients complaining of constipation. *Dis Colon Rectum* 1986;29:630.
37. Duh Q-Y, Way LW. Diagnostic laparoscopy and laparoscopic cecostomy for colonic pseudo-obstruction. *Dis Colon Rectum* 1993;36:65.
38. Eccersley AJP, Maw A, Williams NS. Comparative study of two sites of colonic conduit placement in the treatment of constipation due to rectal evacuatory disorders. *Br J Surg* 1999;86:647.
39. Ehrentheil OF, Wells EP. Megacolon in psychotic patients: a clinical entity. *Gastroenterology* 1955;29:285.

40. Elliot MS, Todd IP. Adult Hirschsprung's disease: results of the Duhamel procedure. *Br J Surg* 1985;72:884.
41. Ferrara A, Pemberton JH, Grotz RL, et al. Prolonged ambulatory recording of anorectal motility in patients with slow-transit constipation. *Am J Surg* 1994;167:73.
42. Fishbein RH, Handelsman JC, Schuster MM. Surgical treatment of Hirschsprung's disease in adults. *Surg Gynecol Obstet* 1986;163:458.
43. FitzHarris GP, Garcia-Aguilar J, Parker SC, et al. Quality of life after subtotal colectomy for slow-transit constipation: both quality and quantity count. *Dis Colon Rectum* 2003;46:433.
44. Fleshman JW, Dreznik Z, Cohen E, et al. Balloon expulsion test facilitates diagnosis of pelvic floor outlet obstruction due to nonrelaxing puborectalis muscle. *Dis Colon Rectum* 1992;35:1019.
45. Fleshman JW, Dreznik Z, Meyer K, et al. Outpatient protocol for biofeedback therapy of pelvic floor outlet obstruction. *Dis Colon Rectum* 1992;35:1.
46. Fucini C, Ronchi O, Elbetti C. Electromyography of the pelvic floor musculature in the assessment of obstructed defecation symptoms. *Dis Colon Rectum* 2001;44:1168.
47. Gattuso JM, Phil M, Kamm MA, et al. Gastrointestinal transit in patients with idiopathic megarectum. *Dis Colon Rectum* 1996;39:1044.
48. Geelhoed GW. Colonic pseudo-obstruction in surgical patients. *Am J Surg* 1985;149:258.
49. Gekas P, Schuster MM. Stercoral perforation of the colon: case report and review of the literature. *Gastroenterology* 1981;80:1054.
50. Ger GC, Wexner SD, Jorge JMN, et al. Evaluation and treatment of chronic intractable rectal pain: a frustrating endeavor. *Dis Colon Rectum* 1993;36:139.
51. Gilbert KP, Lewis FG, Billingham RP, et al. Surgical treatment of constipation. *West J Med* 1984;140:569.
52. Gilliland R, Heyman JS, Altomare DF, et al. Biofeedback for intractable rectal pain: outcome and predictors of success. *Dis Colon Rectum* 1997;40:190.
53. Gladman MA, Scott SM, Chan CLH, et al. Rectal hyposensitivity: prevalence and clinical impact in patients with intractable constipation and fecal incontinence. *Dis Colon Rectum* 2003;46:238.
54. Glick ME, Meshkinpour H, Haldeman S, et al. Colonic dysfunction in multiple sclerosis. *Gastroenterology* 1982;83:1002.
55. Golladay ES, Byrne WJ. Intestinal pseudo-obstruction. *Surg Gynecol Obstet* 1981;153:257.
56. Gosche JR, Sharpe JN, Larson GM. Colonoscopic decompression for pseudo-obstruction of the colon. *Am Surg* 1989;55:111.
57. Gosselink MJ, Hop WCJ, Schouten WR. Rectal compliance in females with obstructed defecation. *Dis Colon Rectum* 2001;44:971.
58. Gosselink MJ, Schouten WR. Rectal sensory perception in females with obstructed defecation. *Dis Colon Rectum* 2001;44:1337.
59. Goto S, Ikeda K, Nagasaki A, et al. Hirschsprung's disease in an adult: special reference to histochemical determination of the acetylcholinesterase activity. *Dis Colon Rectum* 1984;27:319.
60. Gottlieb SH, Schuster MM. Dermatoglyphic (fingerprint) evidence for a congenital syndrome of early-onset constipation and abdominal pain. *Gastroenterology* 1986;91:428.
61. Grant SR, Salvati EP, Rubin RJ. Levator syndrome: an analysis of 316 cases. *Dis Colon Rectum* 1975;18:161.
62. Grimaud J-C, Bouvier M, Naudy B, et al. Manometric and radiologic investigations and biofeedback treatment of chronic idiopathic anal pain. *Dis Colon Rectum* 1991;34:690.
63. Grotz RL, Pemberton JH, Levin KE, et al. Rectal wall contractility in healthy subjects and in patients with chronic severe constipation. *Ann Surg* 1993;218:761.
64. Guyton DP, Evans D, Schreiber H. Stercoral perforation of the colon: concepts of operative management. *Am Surg* 1985;51:520.
65. Hall M. Severe pain of the rectum and its remedy. *Lancet* 1841;1:838, 854.
66. Hall CL, Lampert PW. Immunohistochemistry as an aid in the diagnosis of Hirschsprung's disease. *Am J Clin Pathol* 1985;83:177.
67. Heah S-M, Ho Y-H, Tan M, et al. Biofeedback is effective treatment for levator ani syndrome. *Dis Colon Rectum* 1997;40:187.
68. Heine JA, Wong WD, Goldberg SM. Surgical treatment for constipation. *Surg Gynecol Obstet* 1993;176:403.
69. Hemingway D, Neilly JB, Finlay IG. Biliary dyskinesia in idiopathic slow-transit constipation. *Dis Colon Rectum* 1996;39:1303.
70. Heriot AG, Tilney HS, Simon JNL. The application of percutaneous endoscopic colostomy to the management of obstructed defecation. *Dis Colon Rectum* 2002;45:700.
71. Heymen S, Wexner SD, Gulledge AD. MMPI assessment of patients with functional bowel disorders. *Dis Colon Rectum* 1993;36:593.
72. Heymen S, Wexner SD, Vickers D, et al. Prospective, randomized trial comparing four biofeedback techniques for patients with constipation. *Dis Colon Rectum* 1999;42:1388.
73. Heymen S, Jones KR, Scarlett Y, et al. Biofeedback treatment of constipation: a critical review. *Dis Colon Rectum* 2003;46:1208.
74. Hill J, Stott S, MacLennan I. Antegrade enemas for the treatment of severe idiopathic constipation. *Br J Surg* 1994;81:1490.
75. Ho Y-H, Tan M, Goh H-S. Clinical and physiologic effects of biofeedback in outlet obstruction constipation. *Dis Colon Rectum* 1996;39:520.
76. Hosie KB, Kmiot WA, Keighley MRB. Constipation: another indication for restorative proctocolectomy. *Br J Surg* 1990;77:801.
77. Hughes ESR, McDermott FT, Johnson WR, et al. Surgery for constipation. *Aust N Z J Surg* 1981;51:144.
78. Hull TL, Milsom JW, Church J, et al. Electrogalvanic stimulation for levator syndrome: how effective is it in the long term? *Dis Colon Rectum* 1993;36:731.
79. Hyman PE, Di Lorenzo C, McAdams L, et al. Predicting the clinical response to cisapride in children with chronic intestinal pseudo-obstruction. *Am J Gastroenterol* 1993;88:832.
80. Ikawa H, Kim SH, Hendren WH, et al. Acetylcholinesterase and manometry in the diagnosis of the constipated child. *Arch Surg* 1986;121:435.
81. Infantino A, Masin A, Pianon P, et al. Role of proctography in severe constipation. *Dis Colon Rectum* 1990;33:707.
82. Johnson PH. Coccygodynia. *J Ark Med Soc* 1981;77:421.
83. Jones PN, Lubowski DZ, Swash M, et al. Is paradoxical contraction of puborectalis muscle of functional importance? *Dis Colon Rectum* 1987;30:667.
84. Joo JS, Agachan F, Wolff B, et al. Initial North American experience with botulinum toxin type A for treatment of anismus. *Dis Colon Rectum* 1996;39:1107.
85. Jorge JMN, Wexner SD, Ger GC, et al. Cinedefecography and electromyography in the diagnosis of nonrelaxing puborectalis syndrome. *Dis Colon Rectum* 1993;36:668.
86. Kamm MA, Hawley PR, Lennard-Jones JE. Outcome of colectomy for severe idiopathic constipation. *Gut* 1988;29:969.
87. Kamm MA, Hawley PR, Lennard-Jones JE. Lateral division of the puborectalis muscle in the management of severe constipation. *Br J Surg* 1988;75:661.
88. Kamm MA, Lennard-Jones JE. Rectal mucosal electrosensory testing: evidence for a rectal sensory neuropathy in idiopathic constipation. *Dis Colon Rectum* 1990;33:419.
89. Kamm MA, Stabile G. Management of idiopathic megarectum and megacolon. *Br J Surg* 1991;78:899.

90. Karasick S, Ehrlich SM. Is constipation a disorder of defecation or impaired motility? Distinction based on defecography and colonic transit studies. *AJR Am J Roentgenol* 1996;166:63.
91. Karras JD, Angelo G. Proctalgia fugax. *Am J Surg* 1951; 82:616.
92. Kawimbe BM, Papachrysostomou M, Binnie NR, et al. Outlet obstruction constipation (anismus) managed by biofeedback. *Gut* 1991;32:1175.
93. Keck JO, Staniunas RJ, Coller JA, et al. Biofeedback training is useful in fecal incontinence but disappointing in constipation. *Dis Colon Rectum* 1994;37:1271.
94. Keighley MRB. Surgery for constipation. *Br J Surg* 1988; 75:625.
95. Keighley MRB, Henry MM, Bartolo DCC, et al. Anorectal physiology measurement: report of a working party. *Br J Surg* 1989;76:356.
96. Kenefick NJ, Nicholls RJ, Cohen RG, et al. Permanent sacral nerve stimulation for treatment of idiopathic constipation. *Br J Surg* 2002;89:882.
97. Kenefick NJ, Vaizey CJ, Cohen CRG, et al. Double-blind placebo-controlled crossover study of sacral nerve stimulation for idiopathic constipation. *Br J Surg* 2002;89:1570.
98. Kirshner R. Stercoraceous ulcer and perforation of the colon: a case report and review of the literature. *Contemp Surg* 1985;26:57.
99. Klück P, van Muijen GNP, van der Kamp AWM, et al. Hirschsprung's disease studied with monoclonal antineurofilament antibodies on tissue sections. *Lancet* 1984;1: 652.
100. Knowles CH, Eccersley AJ, Scott SM, et al. Linear discriminant analysis of symptoms in patients with chronic constipation): validation of a new scoring system (KESS). *Dis Colon Rectum* 2002;43:1419.
101. Koch TR, Carney JA, Go L, et al. Idiopathic chronic constipation is associated with decreased colonic vasoactive intestinal peptide. *Gastroenterology* 1988;94:300.
102. Kokoszka J, Nelson R, Falconio M, et al. Treatment of fecal impaction with pulsed irrigation-enhanced evacuation. *Dis Colon Rectum* 1994;37:161.
103. Krishnamurthy S, Schuffler MD, Rohrmann CA, et al. Severe idiopathic constipation is associated with a distinctive abnormality of the colonic myenteric plexus. *Gastroenterology* 1985;88:26.
104. Krogh K, Laurberg S. Malone antegrade continence enema for faecal incontinence and constipation in adults. *Br J Surg* 1998;85:974.
105. Kuijpers HC. Application of the colorectal laboratory in diagnosis and treatment of functional constipation. *Dis Colon Rectum* 1990;33:35.
106. Kuijpers HC, Bleijenberg G. The spastic pelvic floor syndrome: a cause of constipation. *Dis Colon Rectum* 1985; 28:669.
107. Kumar D, Wingae DL. Colorectal motility. In: Henry MM, Swash M, eds. *Coloproctology and the pelvic floor.* London: Butterworth, 1985:47.
108. Lane WA. Remarks on the results of the operative treatment of chronic constipation. *Br Med J* 1908;1:126.
109. Lee JT, Taylor BM, Singleton BC. Epidural anesthesia for acute pseudo-obstruction of the colon (Ogilvie's syndrome). *Dis Colon Rectum* 1988;31:686.
110. Lennard-Jones JE. Pathophysiology of constipation. *Br J Surg* 1985;72[Suppl]:7.
111. Leon SH, Krishnamurthy S, Schuffler MD. Subtotal colectomy for severe idiopathic constipation: a follow-up study of 13 patients. *Dig Dis Sci* 1987;32:1249.
112. Loening-Baucke V. Persistence of chronic constipation in children after biofeedback treatment. *Dig Dis Sci* 1991; 36:153.
113. Loening-Baucke V. Constipation in early childhood: patient characteristics, treatment, and long-term follow-up. *Gut* 1993;34:1400.
114. Loening-Baucke VA, Anuras S, Mitros FA. Changes in colorectal function in patients with chronic colonic pseudo-obstruction. *Dig Dis Sci* 1987;32:1104.
115. Lopez MJ, Memula N, Doss LL, et al. Pseudo-obstruction of the colon during pelvic radiotherapy. *Dis Colon Rectum* 1981;24:201.
116. Lowenstein B, Catlado PA. Treatment of prcotalgia fugax with topical nitroglycerin: report of a case. *Dis Colon Rectum* 1998;41:667.
117. Lubowski DZ, Chen FC, Kennedy ML, et al. Results of colectomy for severe slow-transit constipation. *Dis Colon Rectum* 1996;39:23.
118. Lui RC, Herz B, Plantilla E, et al. Stercoral perforation of the colon: report of a new location. *Am J Gastroenterol* 1988;83:457.
119. Lundin E, Karlborn U, Påhlman L, et al. Outcome of segmental colonic resection for slow-transit constipation. *Br J Surg* 2002;89:1270.
120. Luukkonen P, Heikkinen M, Huikuri K, et al. Adult Hirschsprung's disease: clinical features and functional outcome after surgery. *Dis Colon Rectum* 1990;33:65.
121. Lynn HB, Van Heerden JA. Rectal myectomy in Hirschsprung's disease: a decade of experience. *Arch Surg* 1975; 110:991.
122. MacColl C, MacCannell KL, Baylis B, et al. Treatment of acute colonic pseudo-obstruction (Ogilvie's syndrome) with cisapride. *Gastroenterology* 1990;98:773.
123. Madsen PV, Nielsen-Lykkegaard M, Nielsen OV. Ceruletide reduces postoperative intestinal paralysis: a double-blind, placebo-controlled trial. *Dis Colon Rectum* 1983;26:159.
124. Malone PS, Ransley PG, Kiely EM. Preliminary report: the antegrade continence enema. *Lancet* 1990;336:1217.
125. Mapp E. Colonic manifestations of the connective tissue disorders. *Am J Gastroenterol* 1981;75:386.
126. Maria G, Anastasio G, Brisinda G, et al. Treatment of puborectalis syndrome with progressive anal dilation. *Dis Colon Rectum* 1997;40:89.
127. Maria G, Brisinda G, Bentivoglio AR, et al. Botulinum toxin in the treatment of outlet obstruction constipation caused by puborectalis syndrome. *Dis Colon Rectum* 2000; 43:376.
128. Maroy B. Spontaneous and evoked coccygeal pain in depression. *Dis Colon Rectum* 1988;31:210.
129. Martelli H, Devroede G, Arhan P, et al. Mechanisms of idiopathic constipation: outlet obstruction. *Gastroenterology* 1978;75:623.
130. Martin FM, Robinson AM Jr, Thompson WR. Therapeutic colonoscopy in the treatment of colonic pseudo-obstruction. *Am Surg* 1988;54:519.
131. Maull KI, Kinning WK, Kay S. Stercoral ulceration. *Am Surg* 1982;48:20.
132. Maurer CA, Renzulli P, Mazzucchelli L, et al. Use of accurate diagnostic criteria may increase incidence of stercoral perforation of the colon. *Dis Colon Rectum* 2000;43:991.
133. McCready RA, Beart RW Jr. Adult Hirschsprung's disease: results of surgical treatment at the Mayo Clinic. *Dis Colon Rectum* 1980;23:401.
134. McKee RF, McEnroe L, Anderson JH, et al. Identification of patients likely to benefit from biofeedback for outlet obstruction constipation. *Br J Surg* 1999;86:355.
135. Menardo G, Bausano G, Corazziari E, et al. Large-bowel transit in paraplegic patients. *Dis Colon Rectum* 1987; 30:924.
136. Messmer JM, Wolper JC, Loewe CJ. Endoscopic-assisted tube placement for decompression of acute colonic pseudo-obstruction. *Endoscopy* 1984;16:135.
137. Meyers MA. Colonic ileus. In: Greenbaum EI, ed. *Radiographic atlas of colon disease.* Chicago: Year Book, 1980:95.
138. Mibu R, Hotokezaka M, Mihara S, et al. Results of linearly polarized near-infrared irradiation therapy in patients with intractable anorectal pain. *Dis Colon Rectum* 2003;46 [Suppl]: S50.

139. Mishalany HG, Woolley MG. Chronic constipation: manometric patterns and surgical considerations. *Arch Surg* 1984;119:1257.

140. Mollen RM, Kuijpers HC, Claassen AT. Colectomy for slow-transit constipation: preoperative functional evaluation is important but not a guarantee for a successful outcome. *Dis Colon Rectum* 2001;44:577.

141. Moore BG, Singaram C, Eckhoff DE, et al. Immunohistochemical evaluations of ultrashort-segment Hirschsprung's disease. *Dis Colon Rectum* 1996;39:817.

142. Morgenstern L, Shemen L, Allen W, et al. Melanosis coli: changes in appearance when associated with colonic neoplasia. *Arch Surg* 1983;118:62.

143. Morrisey KP, Cahan AC. Colonoscopic decompression for nonobstructed colonic dilatation. *Curr Concepts Gastroenterol* 1989;13:7.

144. Müller-Lissner SA, the Bavarian Constipation Study Group. Treatment of chronic constipation with cisapride and placebo. *Gut* 1987;28:1033.

145. Nakhgevany KB. Colonoscopic decompression of the colon in patients with Ogilvie's syndrome. *Am J Surg* 1984;148:317.

146. Nam Y-S, Pikarsky AJ, Wexner SD, et al. Reproducibility of colonic transit study in patients with chronic constipation. *Dis Colon Rectum* 2001;44:86.

147. Nanni G, Garbini A, Luchetti P, et al. Ogilvie's syndrome (acute colonic pseudo-obstruction): review of the literature (October 1948 to March 1980) and report of four additional cases. *Dis Colon Rectum* 1982;25:157.

148. Nathan BN. An early clinical account of proctalgia fugax. *Dis Colon Rectum* 1990;33:539.

149. Natsikas NB, Sbarounis CN. Adult Hirschsprung's disease: an experience with the Duhamel-Martin procedure with special reference to obstructed patients. *Dis Colon Rectum* 1987;30:204.

150. Nicholls RJ, Kamm MA. Proctocolectomy with restorative ileoanal reservoir for severe idiopathic constipation: report of two cases. *Dis Colon Rectum* 1988;31:968.

151. Nicosia JF, Abcarian H. Levator syndrome: a treatment that works. *Dis Colon Rectum* 1985;28:406.

152. Nielsen MB, Buron B, Christiansen J, et al. Defecographic findings in patients with anal incontinence and constipation and their relation to rectal emptying. *Dis Colon Rectum* 1993;36:806.

153. Niewiarowski T, Krevsky B. Radiologic and scintigraphic studies of chronic intestinal pseudo-obstruction. *Pract Gastroenterol* 1991;15:38.

154. Nissan S, Bar-Maor JA, Levy E. Anorectal myomectomy in the treatment of short-segment Hirschsprung's disease. *Ann Surg* 1969;170:969.

155. Notghi A, Hutchinson R, Kumar D, et al. Simplified method for the measurement of segmental colonic transit time. *Gut* 1994;35:976.

156. Nyam DCNK, Pemberton JH, Ilstrup DM, et al. Long-term results of surgery for chronic constipation. *Dis Colon Rectum* 1997;40:273.

157. Ogilvie H. Large-intestine colic due to sympathetic deprivation: a new clinical syndrome. *Br Med J* 1948;2:671.

158. Ohri SK, Patel T, Desa L, et al. Drug-induced colonic pseudo-obstruction. *Dis Colon Rectum* 1991;34:346.

159. Oliver GC, Rubin RJ, Salvati EP, et al. Electrogalvanic stimulation in the treatment of levator syndrome. *Dis Colon Rectum* 1985;28:662.

160. Orrom WJ, Bartolo DCC, Miller, et al. Rectopexy is an ineffective treatment for obstructed defecation. *Dis Colon Rectum* 1991;34:41.

161. Papachrysostomou M, Smith AN. Effects of biofeedback on obstructive defecation: reconditioning of the defecation reflex? *Gut* 1994;35:252.

162. Park HJ, Kamm MA, Abbasi AM, et al. Immunohistochemical study of the colonic muscle and innervation in idiopathic chronic constipation. *Dis Colon Rectum* 1995;38:509.

163. Pemberton JH, Rath DM, Ilstrup DM. Evaluation and surgical treatment of severe chronic constipation. *Ann Surg* 1991;214:403.

164. Pfeifer J, Agachan F, Wexner SD. Surgery for constipation: a review. *Dis Colon Rectum* 1996;39:444.

165. Pham TN, Cosman BC, Chu P, et al. Radiographic changes after colonoscopic decompression for acute pseudo-obstruction. *Dis Colon Rectum* 1999;42:1586.

166. Piccirillo MF, Reissman P, Wexner SD. Colectomy as treatment for constipation in selected patients. *Br J Surg* 1995;82:898.

167. Pikarsky AJ, Singh JJ, Weiss EG, et al. Long-term follow-up of patients undergoing colectomy for colonic inertia. *Dis Colon Rectum* 2001;44:179.

168. Pinho M, Yoshioka K, Keighley MRB. Long-term results of anorectal myectomy for chronic constipation. *Br J Surg* 1989;76:1163.

169. Pinho M, Yoshioka K, Keighley MRB. Long-term results of anorectal myectomy for chronic constipation. *Dis Colon Rectum* 1990;33:795.

170. Pluta H, Bowes KL, Jewell LD. Long-term results of total abdominal colectomy for chronic idiopathic constipation: value of preoperative assessment. *Dis Colon Rectum* 1996;39:160.

171. Poisson J, Devroede G. Severe chronic constipation as a surgical problem. *Surg Clin North Am* 1983;63:193.

172. Ponsky JL, Aszodi A, Perse D. Percutaneous endoscopic cecostomy: a new approach to nonobstructive colonic dilation. *Gastrointest Endosc* 1986;32:108.

173. Preston DM, Hawley PR, Lennard-Jones JE, et al. Results of colectomy for severe idiopathic constipation in women (Arbuthnot Lane's disease). *Br J Surg* 1984;71:547.

174. Preston DM, Lennard-Jones JE. Severe chronic constipation of young women: "idiopathic slow-transit constipation." *Gut* 1986;27:41.

175. Ravo B, Pollane M, Ger R. Pseudo-obstruction of the colon following caesarean section: a review. *Dis Colon Rectum* 1983;26:440.

176. Redmond JM, Smith GW, Barofsky I, et al. Physiological tests to predict long-term outcome of total abdominal colectomy for intractable constipation. *Am J Gastroenterol* 1995;90:748.

177. Renzi C, Pescatori M. Psychologic aspects in proctalgia. *Dis Colon Rectum* 2000;43:535.

178. Reynolds JC, Ouyang A, Lee CA, et al. Chronic severe constipation: prospective motility studies in 25 consecutive patients. *Gastroenterology* 1987;92:414.

179. Ricciardi R, Counihan TC, Banner BF, et al. What is the normal aganglionic segment of anorectum in adults? *Dis Colon Rectum* 1999;42:380.

180. Ricketts RR, Pettitt BJ. Management of Hirschsprung's disease in adolescents. *Am Surg* 1989;55:219.

181. Robbins RD, Schoen R, Sohn N, et al. Colonic decompression of massive cecal dilatation (Ogilvie's syndrome) secondary to caesarean section. *Am J Gastroenterol* 1982;77:231.

182. Roberts JP, Womack NR, Hallan RI, et al. Evidence from dynamic integrated proctography to redefine anismus. *Br J Surg* 1992;79:1213.

183. Roe AM, Bartolo DCC, Mortensen NJMcC. Diagnosis and surgical management of intractable constipation. *Br J Surg* 1986;73:854.

184. Ron Y, Avni Y, Lukovetski A, et al. Botulinum toxin type-A in therapy of patients with anismus. *Dis Colon Rectum* 2001;44:1821.

185. Rongen MJGM, van der Hoop AG, Baeten CGMI. Cecal access for antegrade colon enemas in medically refractory slow-transit constipation. *Dis Colon Rectum* 2001;44:1644.

186. Sacher P, Buchmann P, Burger H. Stenosis of the large intestine complicating scleroderma and mimicking a sigmoid carcinoma. *Dis Colon Rectum* 1983;26:347.

187. Salvati EP. The levator syndrome and its variant. *Gastroenterol Clin North Am* 1987;16:71.

188. Sandler RS, Jordan MC, Shelton BJ. Demographic and dietary determinants of constipation in the US population. *Am J Public Health* 1990;80:185.

189. Sarna SK. Physiology and pathophysiology of colonic motor activity: part one. *Dig Dis Sci* 1991;36:827.

190. Sarna SK. Physiology and pathophysiology of colonic motor activity: part two. *Dig Dis Sci* 1991;36:998.

191. Sawin R, Hatch E, Schaller R, et al. Limited surgery for lower-segment Hirschsprung's disease. *Arch Surg* 1994; 129:920.

192. Schang J-C, Devroede G, Pilote M. Effects of trimebutine on colonic function in patients with chronic idiopathic constipation: evidence for the need of a physiologic rather than clinical selection. *Dis Colon Rectum* 1993;36:330.

193. Schiller LR. Idiopathic constipation: to cut is to cure? *Gastroenterology* 1989;96:949.

194. Schouten WR, ten Kate FJW, de Graaf EJR, et al. Visceral neuropathy in slow-transit constipation: an immunohistochemical investigation with monoclonal antibodies against neurofilament. *Dis Colon Rectum* 1993;36:1112.

195. Schuster MM. Evaluation and treatment of constipation: the need for hard data about hard stools. *Pract Gastroenterol* 1986;10:15.

196. Senati A, Coen LD. Massive gangrene of the colon—a complication of fecal impaction: report of a case. *Dis Colon Rectum* 1989;32:146.

197. Serpell JW, Nicholls RJ. Stercoral perforation of the colon. *Br J Surg* 1990;77:1325.

198. Shamberger RC, Crawford JL, Kirkham SE. Progressive systemic sclerosis resulting in megacolon: a case report. *JAMA* 1983;250:1063.

199. Shatha AH, Ackerman NB. Stercoraceous ulcerations and perforations of the colon. *Dis Colon Rectum* 1977;20:524.

200. Simpson JY. Clinical lectures on the diseases of women. Lecture XVII. On coccygodynia, and the diseases and deformities of the coccyx. *Med Times Gaz* 1859;40:1.

201. Siproudhis L, Ropert A, Vilotte J, et al. How accurate is clinical examination in diagnosing and quantifying pelvirectal disorders? A prospective study in a group of 50 patients complaining of defecatory difficulties. *Dis Colon Rectum* 1993;36:430.

202. Sloyer AF, Panella VS, Demas BE, et al. Ogilvie's syndrome: successful management without colonoscopy. *Dig Dis Sci* 1988;33:1391.

203. Sohn N, Weinstein MA, Robbins RD. The levator syndrome and its treatment with high-voltage electrogalvanic stimulation. *Am J Surg* 1982;144:580.

204. Sosa JL, Cortes V, Zeppa R. Melanosis coli: a case report in a trauma patient and review of the literature. *Am Surg* 1991;57:378.

205. Soudah HC, Hasler WL, Owyang C. Effect of octreotide on intestinal motility and bacterial overgrowth in scleroderma. *N Engl J Med* 1991;325:1461.

206. Spiro HM. *Clinical gastroenterology*, 3rd ed. New York: Macmillan, 1983:729.

207. Stabile G, Kamm MA, Phillips RKS, et al. Partial colectomy and coloanal anastomosis for idiopathic megarectum and megacolon. *Dis Colon Rectum* 1992;35:158.

208. Staiano A, Cucchiara S, Andreotti MR, et al. Effect of cisapride on chronic idiopathic constipation in children. *Dig Dis Sci* 1991;36:733.

209. Starling JR, Croom RD III, Thomas CG Jr. Hirschsprung's disease in young adults. *Am J Surg* 1986;151:104.

210. Stephenson BM, Morgan AR, Salaman JR, et al. Ogilvie's syndrome: a new approach to an old problem. *Dis Colon Rectum* 1995;38:424.

211. Stratta RJ, Starling JR, D'Alessandro AM, et al. Acute colonic ileus (pseudo-obstruction) in renal transplant recipients. *Surgery* 1988;104:616.

212. Strodel WE, Nostrant TT, Eckhauser FE, et al. Therapeutic and diagnostic colonoscopy in nonobstructive colonic dilatation. *Ann Surg* 1983;197:416.

213. Súilleabháin CBÓ, Anderson JH, McKee RF, et al. Strategy for the surgical management of patients with idiopathic megarectum and megacolon. *Br J Surg* 2001;88:1392.

214. Sunderland GT, Poon FW, Lauder J, et al. Videoproctography in selecting patients with constipation for colectomy. *Dis Colon Rectum* 1992;35:235.

215. Tada S, Iida M, Yao T, et al. Intestinal pseudo-obstruction in patients with amyloidosis: clinicopathologic differences between chemical types of amyloid protein. *Gut* 1993;34: 1412.

216. Taylor I, Hammond P, Darby C. An assessment of anorectal motility in the management of adult megacolon. *Br J Surg* 1980;67:754.

217. Thaysen Th EH. Proctalgia fugax: a little-known form of pain in the rectum. *Lancet* 1935;2:243.

218. Thiele GH. Tonic spasm of the levator ani, coccygeus and piriformis muscles: its relationship to coccygodynia and pain in the region of the hip and down the leg. *Trans Am Proctol Soc* 1936;37:145.

219. Thiele GH. Coccygodynia and pain in the superior gluteal region and down the back of the thigh: causation by muscles and relief by massage of these muscles. *JAMA* 1937; 109:1271.

220. Thiele GH. Coccygodynia: the mechanism of its production and its relationship to anorectal disease. *Am J Surg* 1950;79:110.

221. Thiele GH. Coccygodynia: cause and treatment. *Dis Colon Rectum* 1963;6:422.

222. Thomas CG Jr, Bream CA, De Connick P. Posterior sphincterotomy and rectal myotomy in the management of Hirschsprung's disease. *Ann Surg* 1970;171:796.

223. Todd IP. Constipation: results of surgical treatment. *Br J Surg* 1985;72[Suppl]:S12.

224. Tomita R, Fujisaki S, Ikeda T, et al. Role of nitric oxide in the colon of patients with slow-transit constipation. *Dis Colon Rectum* 2002;45:593.

225. Turnbull GK, Ritvo PG. Anal sphincter biofeedback relaxation treatment for women with intractable constipation symptoms. *Dis Colon Rectum* 1992;35:530.

226. Udassin R, Nissan S, Lernau O, et al. The mild form of Hirschsprung's disease (short segment). *Ann Surg* 1981; 194:767.

227. Ustach TJ, Tobon F, Schuster MM. Simplified method for diagnosis of Hirschsprung's disease. *Arch Dis Child* 1969;44:964.

228. Vaccaro CA, Cheong DMO, Wexner SD, et al. Role of pudendal nerve terminal motor latency assessment in constipated patients. *Dis Colon Rectum* 1994;37:1250.

229. van der Sijp JRM, Kamm MA, Nightingale JMD, et al. Radioisotope determination of regional colonic transit in severe constipation: comparison with radio-opaque markers. *Gut* 1993;34:402.

230. Vanek VW, Al-Salti M. Acute pseudo-obstruction of the colon (Ogilvie's syndrome): an analysis of 400 cases. *Dis Colon Rectum* 1986;29:203.

231. Vasilevsky C-A, Nemer FD, Balcos EG, et al. Is subtotal colectomy a viable option in the management of chronic constipation? *Dis Colon Rectum* 1988;31:679.

232. Wald A. Colonic transit and anorectal manometry in chronic idiopathic constipation. *Arch Intern Med* 1986;146:1713.

233. Wald A, Burgio K, Holeva K, et al. Psychological evaluation of patients with severe idiopathic constipation: which instruments to use. *Am J Gastroenterol* 1992;87:977.

234. Wald A, Hinds JP, Caruana BJ. Psychological and physiological characteristics of patients with severe idiopathic constipation. *Gastroenterology* 1989;97:932.

235. Waldron D, Bowes KL, Kingma YJ, et al. Colonic and anorectal motility in young women with severe idiopathic constipation. *Gastroenterology* 1988;95:1388.

236. Waldron DJ, Kumar D, Hallan RI, et al. Evidence for motor neuropathy and reduced filling of the rectum in chronic intractable constipation. *Gut* 1990;31:1284.

237. Weber J, Ducrotte Ph, Touchais JY, et al. Biofeedback training for constipation in adults and children. *Dis Colon Rectum* 1987;30:844.

238. Wedel T, Roblick UJ, Ott V, et al. Oligoneuronal hypoganglionosis in patients with idiopathic slow-transit constipation. *Dis Colon Rectum* 2002;45:54.

239. Wexner SD, Cheape JD, Jorge JMN, et al. Prospective assessment of biofeedback for the treatment of paradoxical puborectalis contraction. *Dis Colon Rectum* 1992;35:145.

240. Wexner SD, Dailey TH. The diagnosis and surgical treatment of chronic constipation. *Contemp Surg* 1988;32:59.

241. Wexner SD, Daniel N, Jagelman DG. Colectomy for constipation: physiologic investigation is the key to success. *Dis Colon Rectum* 1991;34:851.

242. Wexner SD, Marchetti F, Salanga VD, et al. Neurophysiologic assessment of the anal sphincters. *Dis Colon Rectum* 1991;34:606.

243. Wheatley MJ, Wesley JR, Coran AG, et al. Hirschsprung's disease in adolescents and adults. *Dis Colon Rectum* 1990; 33:622.

244. Williams NS, Fajobi OA, Lunniss PJ, et al. Vertical reduction rectoplasty: a new treatment for idiopathic megarectum. *Br J Surg* 2000;87:1203.

245. Williams NS, Hughes SF, Stuchfield B. Continent colonic conduit for rectal evacuation in severe constipation. *Lancet* 1994;343:1321.

246. Wittoesch JH, Jackman RJ, McDonald JR. Melanosis coli: general review and a study of 887 cases. *Dis Colon Rectum* 1958;1:172.

247. Womack NR, Williams NS, Holmfield JHM, et al. New method for the dynamic assessment of anorectal function in constipation. *Br J Surg* 1985;72:994.

248. Wrenn K. Fecal impaction. *N Engl J Med* 1989;321:658.

249. Wu JS, Schoetz DJ Jr, Coller JA, et al. Treatment of Hirschsprung's disease in the adult: report of five cases. *Dis Colon Rectum* 1995;38:655.

250. Yoshioka K, Keighley MRB. Anorectal myectomy for outlet obstruction. *Br J Surg* 1987;74:373.

251. Yoshioka K, Keighley MRB. Randomized trial comparing anorectal myectomy and controlled anal dilatation for outlet obstruction. *Br J Surg* 1987;74:1125.

252. Yoshioka K, Keighley MRB. Clinical results of colectomy for severe constipation. *Br J Surg* 1989;76:600.

253. Zenilman ME, Dunnegan DL, Soper NJ, et al. Successful surgical treatment of idiopathic colonic dysmotility. *Arch Surg* 1989;124:947.

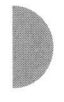 **C h a p t e r   1 7**

Rectal Prolapse, Solitary Rectal Ulcer, Syndrome of the Descending Perineum, and Rectocele

Man should always strive to have his intestines relaxed all the days of his life and that bowel function should approximate diarrhea. This is a fundamental principle in medicine, that whenever the stool is withheld or is extruded with difficulty, grave illnesses result.
Moses ben Maimon (Maimonides): *Mishneh Torah, Hilchoth De'oth, 4.13*

RECTAL PROLAPSE OR PROCIDENTIA

Rectal prolapse (i.e., procidentia) or "falling down of the hindgut" is an uncommon clinical entity that has long fascinated surgeons. It is a condition that was recognized in antiquity, having been described in the Ebers Papyrus of 1500 B.C.[149] It usually occurs in persons at the extremes of life. The two types of presentations are a complete or full-thickness involvement of the bowel and a partial or incomplete type involving prolapse of the mucosa only. The latter may be circumferential or may be limited to only a portion of the rectal mucosa.

Anatomy and Physiology

The precise cause of rectal prolapse is not thoroughly understood, but certain factors seem to be implicated in its development.[241] To understand the etiology, it is helpful to review the anatomy and the physiology. The normal spine with its vertebral curves and the tilt of the pelvis serve to shift the weight of the abdominal organs forward, away from the pelvic floor, and cause the rectum to follow a serpentine course through the pelvis.[181] The stability of the rectum is greatly aided by the support of the levator ani muscle. An extensive interweaving of the longitudinal fibers of the rectum with the levator fibers creates a stable attachment between the rectum and this muscle. This provides a firm fixation to the pelvic floor and is an important element in rectal stability; without it,

the rectum would slip down through the muscle during defecation (Figure 17-1).[34,181–183]

The puborectalis sling functions by elevating the lower end of the rectum and tilting it forward toward the pubis, creating an acute anorectal angle and compressing the structures in front of the rectum to decrease the opening of the pelvic floor. Relaxation of the puborectalis sling results in descent of the pelvic floor, obliterating the anorectal angle so that the rectum becomes more vertical.

During the act of defecation, intraabdominal pressure is increased by contraction of the abdominal wall musculature and the diaphragm. Contraction of the levator ani muscle is inhibited, the puborectalis sling lengthens, and the pelvic floor descends, thereby obliterating the anorectal angle. The external sphincter muscle, which functionally forms a single unit with the puborectalis sling, relaxes at the same time. The rectum now occupies a vertical position, and the fecal mass is expelled by the contraction of the circular muscle of the rectum combined with the pressure from above (see also Chapter 16, in the discussion on defecation). The rectum is held in place by fixation of the levator muscle anteriorly and by the various ligamentous structures laterally when the rectum is in a vertical position. The levator sling returns to its usual support position after defecation.

Etiology

The etiologic factors believed to produce rectal prolapse may be congenital or acquired.

Predisposing and Associated Factors for the Development of Procidentia

The following list summarizes possible predisposing influences and associated conditions:

Poor bowel habits, especially constipation

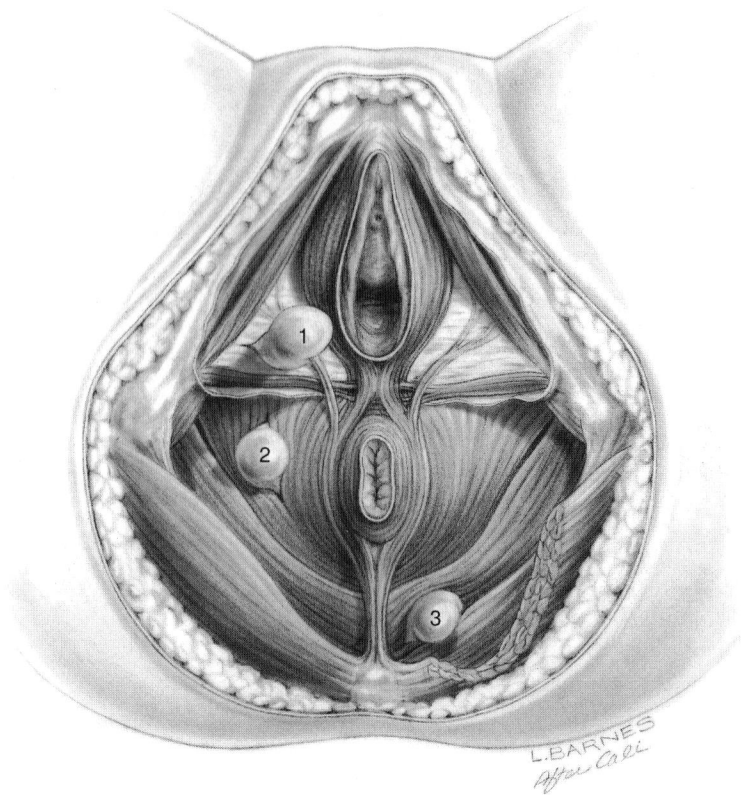

FIGURE 17-1. Muscles of the pelvic floor showing fixation of the rectum to the levator fibers. Weaknesses in the floor can lead to herniation as is illustrated in several locations: *(1)* anterior perineal hernia through the urogenital diaphragm; *(2)* posterior perineal hernia through the levator ani muscle; *(3)* posterior perineal hernia between the levator ani and coccygeus muscles. (Redrawn from Cali RL, Pitsch RM, Blatchford GJ, et al. Rare pelvic floor hernias: report of a case and review of the literature. *Dis Colon Rectum* 1992;35:604.)

Neurologic disease (e.g., congenital anomaly, cauda equina lesion, spinal cord injury, senility)
Female gender
Nulliparity
Redundant rectosigmoid
Deep pouch of Douglas
Patulous anus (i.e., weak internal sphincter)
Diastasis of levator ani muscle (i.e., defect in pelvic floor)
Lack of fixation of rectum to sacrum
Intussusception, possibly secondary to colon lesion
Operative procedure (e.g., hemorrhoidectomy, fistulectomy, abdominoanal pull-through)

The unique pelvic anatomy, especially as observed at the time of laparotomy, is thought to play an important role in the cause of prolapse. A redundant rectosigmoid is often seen, as is a deep pouch of Douglas (i.e., a deep rectovaginal or rectovesical pouch of peritoneum).[161] Whether these are truly causative factors or merely frequently associated anatomic variables has been a subject of considerable debate. Similarly, the patulous or weak sphincter mechanism, with diastasis of the levator ani muscle that produces a defect in the pelvic floor, seems more the *result* of the prolapse than its cause (Figure 17-2).

In infants, prolapse may be caused by a lack of skeletal support and by excessive intraabdominal pressures from above (see Rectal Prolapse in Children). In adults, pro-

lapse may result from incomplete skeletal development. A free mesentery to the entire colon and rectum is a congenital anomaly that may undermine the support mechanism. Because of the complicated development of the levator ani muscle and its fixation to the rectum, anomalies of this muscle, including tenuous fixation to the rectum, may occur more often than is realized and may also contribute to instability of the rectum.

After years of debate concerning the nature of procidentia, Ripstein and Lanter and others introduced the concept of intussusception as the primary cause.[52–54,197,200,233,241] What initiates the intussusception is not exactly clear, but, as demonstrated cineradiographically, over a period of time the intussusception pulls the rectum farther from the sacrum as it descends, and eventually the bowel presents at the anal verge.[32,198,233] Lack of fixation of the rectum to the sacrum can be observed both at the time of laparotomy and cineradiographically. When the act of defecation is viewed by this means or by defecography (see Defecography), the sequence of events is confirmed. A so-called colorectoanal intussusception may occur with a tumor acting as a lead point.[267]

Rectal prolapse may be a consequence of anorectal surgical procedures, but it is important from the perspective of treatment to distinguish between true procidentia and mucosal prolapse. An ectropion, sometimes referred to as a mucosal prolapse, is a frequent complication of

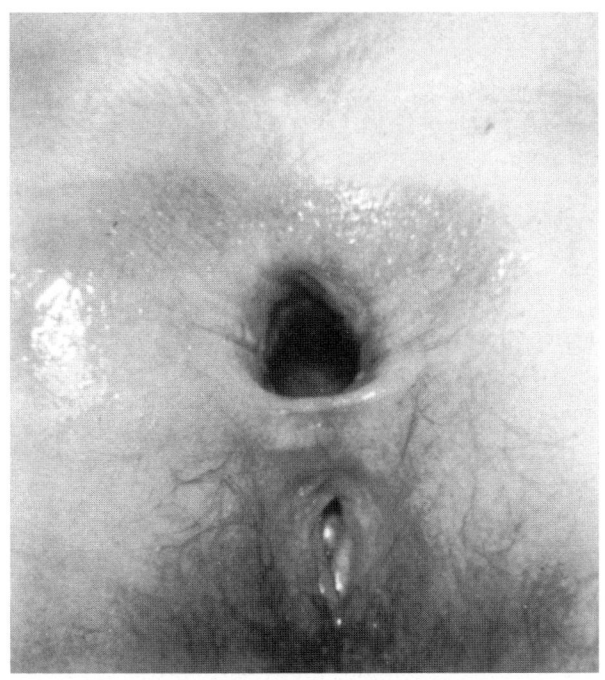

FIGURE 17-2. Patulous anus is seen after prolapse has been reduced. (From Corman ML, Veidenheimer MC, Coller JA. Managing rectal prolapse. *Geriatrics* 1974;29:87, with permission.)

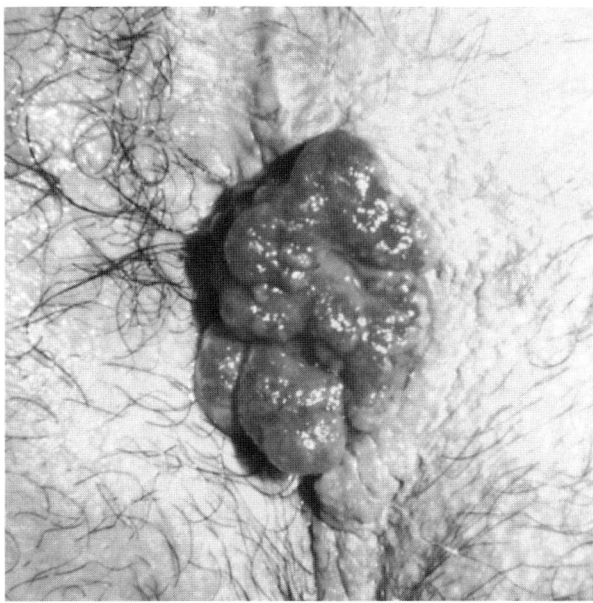

FIGURE 17-3. Incomplete prolapse following abdominoanal pull-through for imperforate anus.

the radical hemorrhoidectomy attributed to Whitehead (see Figure 8-47). Surgical injury to the puborectalis muscle, such as can occur after anal fistula procedures and pull-through operations, also may be a predisposing factor (Figs. 17-3 and 17-4). If a considerable portion of the sphincter has been divided, mucosal prolapse may be seen on the side of the injury.

Diseases of the nervous system and lesions of the cauda equina may lead to rectal prolapse. Excessive pressure on the pelvic floor, particularly when related to attenuated muscle, is another etiologic factor.[241]

Patients in psychiatric hospitals and nursing homes are occasionally afflicted with this otherwise rare condition. Goligher, as a nonpsychiatrist, described one third of his patients as being "rather odd," with approximately 3% "definitely psychotic."[78] Nearly one half of our patients demonstrated somewhat aberrant behavior.[114] The reason for the frequency of mental disturbance is not clearly understood, but it may have something to do with a systemic degenerative process.

In adults, patients with with rectal prolapse are women (90% in our experience and those of others).[114] The peak incidence occurs in the sixth decade. In the past, multiparity was sometimes mentioned as a possible etiologic factor, but in our experience, 40% were nulliparous.[114] Boutsis and Ellis reported that 58% of their patients with prolapse were childless, and Hughes reported an incidence of 39%.[30,102] Such rates of nulliparity are much higher than would be expected from the general population. With the frequent occurrence of bowel management problems in this disease, the most likely candidate for rectal prolapse is a neurotic, constipated, childless woman.

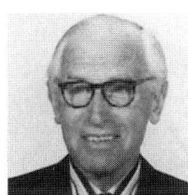

John Cedric Goligher (1912–1998) Goligher has been described as the preeminent clinical investigative surgeon in the world. He was born in Londonderry, Northern Ireland. He achieved his medical degree in 1934 from the University of Edinburgh, and after serving as a house officer at the Royal Infirmary in that city, took the post of Resident Surgical Officer at St. Mark's Hospital in London. Following a period as Senior Registrar at St. Mary's Hospital, he accepted a position as consultant surgeon to both St. Mary's and St. Mark's in 1947. In 1955, he assumed the Chair of the University of Leeds, Department of Surgery, and at the General Infirmary, achieving emeritus status in 1978. Professor Goligher's papers represent a spectrum of accomplishment that is unparalleled in contemporary surgery. His individually authored text, *Surgery of the Anus, Rectum and Colon,* has flourished through five editions. Others may attempt to imitate his mastery of the field, but none can equal it. He has been responsible for more than 15 named lectures and has been recognized through honorary fellowship in as many societies throughout the world, including that of the American Society of Colon and Rectal Surgeons. His theatres in Leeds have been the center for every surgeon pursuing an interest in gastrointestinal disease. I had the privilege of serving as his Senior Registrar for one memorable year. Professor Goligher is indeed the personification of the master surgeon.

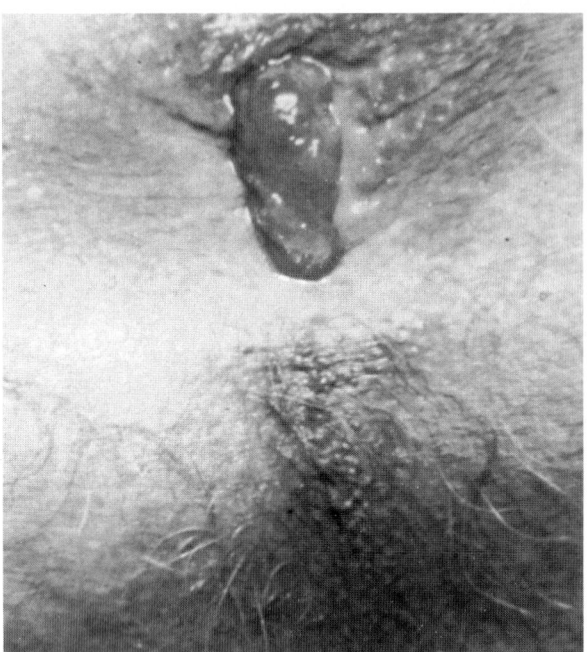

FIGURE 17-4. Mucosal prolapse (ectropion) caused by sphincteric defect following fistulectomy.

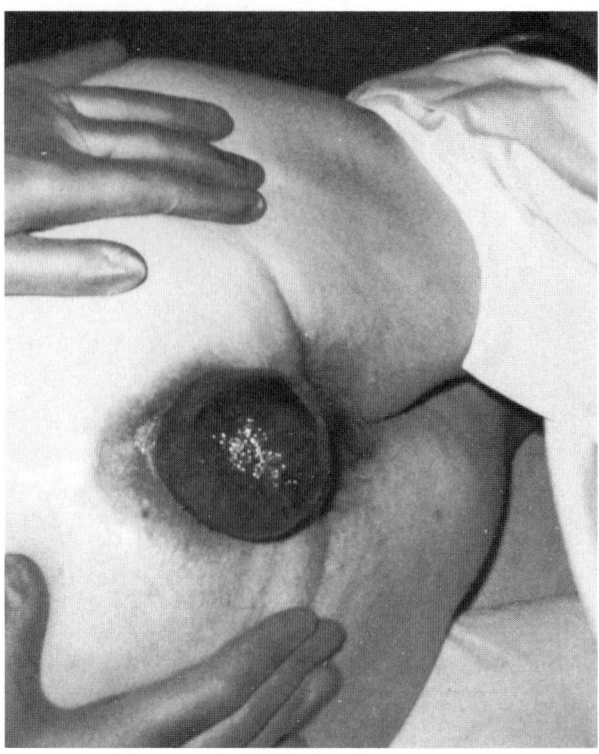

FIGURE 17-5. Standard, full-thickness rectal prolapse or procidentia. (From Corman ML, Veidenheimer MC, Coller JA. Managing rectal prolapse. *Geriatrics* 1974;29:87, with permission.)

Clinical Features and Examination

The most frequent primary complaint is referable to the prolapse itself: three fourths of patients report the protrusion. Problems with bowel regulation and incontinence are also common presenting features. Almost one half of our patients had a history of constipation.[114] Significant bleeding is rarely seen unless the prolapse is massive or irreducible.

Fecal incontinence associated with prolapse is a frequent complaint. Many reports have been published that confirm the association and utilize physiologic investigations, such as rectal sensation, manometry, electromyography (EMG), transit time, and defecography as part of the overall evaluation.[76,92,108,110,118,183,218,223,258] Parks and colleagues suggested that, because of stretch injury to pudendal and perineal nerves, loss of continence in individuals with rectal prolapse is secondary to prolonged protrusion (see Chapter 13).[186] They cite studies that demonstrate histologic abnormalities of small nerves supplying the anorectal musculature. Neill and associates reported EMG studies that showed reduced amplitude of action potentials in the external sphincter and puborectalis muscles in patients with fecal incontinence but not in those with rectal prolapse without incontinence.[167] These findings indicate that denervation causes pelvic floor weakness, with prolapse and incontinence in some patients; in others, however, prolapse occurs without detectable abnormality of the pelvic musculature.

Incontinence becomes more severe as the protrusion increases in degree. Dilatation of the canal by the mass results in further relaxation of the sphincter muscles and further prolapse.[210] Mucous discharge may also become a problem. Protrusion may occur when lifting or coughing, not necessarily solely on defecation. Manual replacement eventually becomes necessary, and ultimately, the mass may protrude from the anus most of the time. Infrequently, the prolapse may become incarcerated or even strangulated if it has occurred after excessive straining (Figure 17-21). Transanal evisceration of the small bowel through a rent in the protruding rectum has also been reported.[79]

The duration of symptoms before the patient seeks specialized attention is often quite prolonged. This may be a reflection of the patient's psyche, but too often it represents failure of the family physician to recognize the entity and to recommend appropriate consultation. Usually, the diagnosis of a full-thickness prolapse presents no problem (Figure 17-5). It may be associated with uterine descensus (Figure 17-6), uterine prolapse (Figure 17-7), or cystocele (Figure 17-8).[46]

When an individual's symptoms are suggestive of rectal prolapse, having the patient sit on the toilet and bear down may not be a particularly aesthetic experience for the patient or the surgeon, but it is often the only means by which rectal prolapse can be visualized. The least effective way of evaluating the condition is to place the pa-

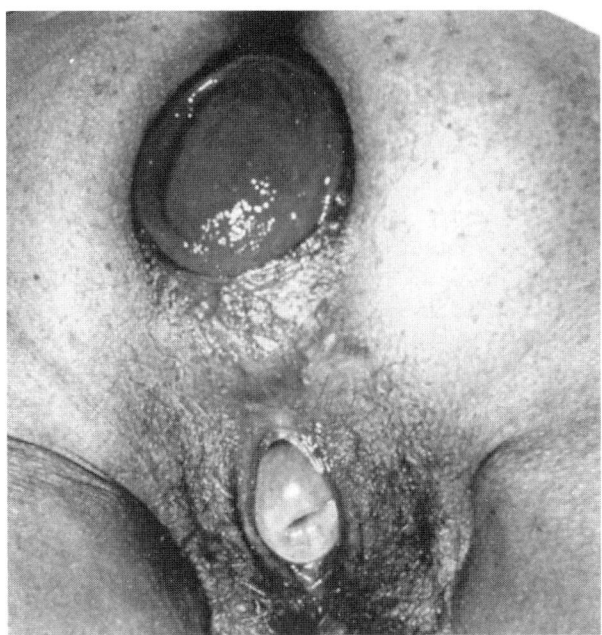

FIGURE 17-6. Rectal prolapse with uterine descensus. The cervical os appears at the introitus. (From Corman ML, Veidenheimer MC, Coller JA. Managing rectal prolapse. *Geriatrics* 1974;29:87, with permission.)

tient in the prone jackknife position on the examining table.

An important part of the examination is to determine the tone and contractility of the sphincter mechanism. If sphincter tone is poor and the anus patulous, and if the patient is unable to contract the puborectalis sling volun-

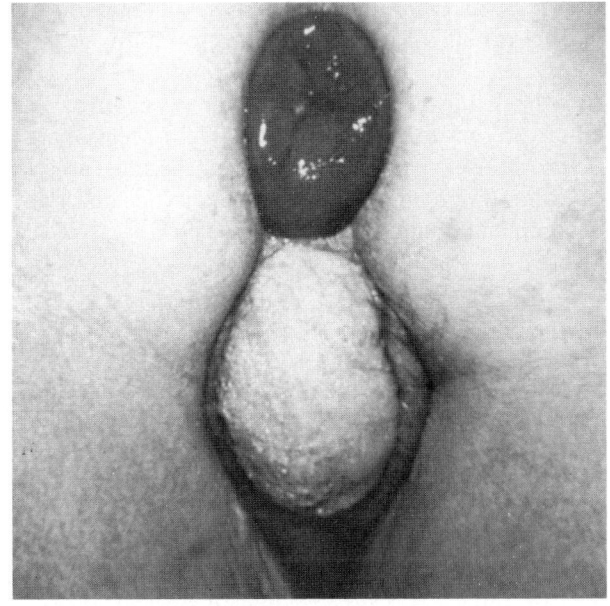

FIGURE 17-7. Rectal prolapse with uterine prolapse. (From Corman ML, Veidenheimer MC, Coller JA. Managing rectal prolapse. *Geriatrics* 1974;29:87, with permission.)

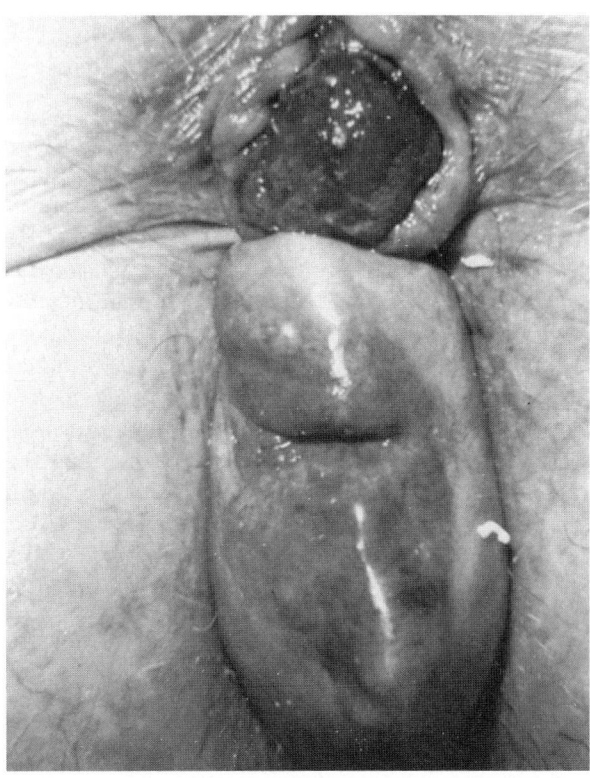

FIGURE 17-8. Rectal prolapse with fourth-degree cystocele. (From Corman ML, Veidenheimer MC, Coller JA. Managing rectal prolapse. *Geriatrics* 1974;29:87, with permission.)

tarily, functional results after repair of the prolapse may be suboptimal. Conversely, if the patient has relatively good sphincter tone and contractility, good bowel control can be anticipated following successful repair.

It is important to specify the degree of prolapse and whether it is full thickness or mucosal. A thorough endoscopic examination is necessary in individuals with any anorectal complaint, and this is especially true in patients with rectal prolapse. Occasionally, a polyp or carcinoma of the rectum or sigmoid colon may be the "lead point" for an intussusception. A high index of suspicion should be maintained, especially in a male patient who has no evidence of neurologic disease. Total colonic evaluation, either by means of barium enema or by colonoscopy, is mandatory. Unfortunately, patients with rectal prolapse often have considerable difficulty retaining the contrast material, and abundant fecal residue is the rule rather than the exception. Therefore, despite the patient's frail state, an adequate oral cathartic regimen must be administered. Hospitalization may be required to accomplish this in some individuals.

Flexible sigmoidoscopy or colonoscopy may reveal the straightened rectal segment and an intussusception if the examination is performed with the patient straining and in a sitting position.[199] Likewise, cinefluorography may be helpful if the diagnosis is in question.

Differential Diagnosis

The condition that most often misleads the examiner into believing he or she is dealing with procidentia is prolapsed hemorrhoids (see Figure 8-7). A protruding mass of hemorrhoidal tissue tends to be lobular; a definite sulcus or groove is present between the masses of tissue and the perianal skin. With very large hemorrhoids that have become edematous and thrombosed, the enlarged size frequently gives the incorrect impression that the entire rectal wall is protruding. However, with rectal prolapse, concentric rings of intact tissue are evident throughout the entire circumference.

Sometimes the differential diagnosis may include a large rectal polypoid lesion prolapsing through the anus. The physician should replace the mass and examine the rectum manually and endoscopically. A polypoid lesion is usually mobile and can be separated from the lower part of the rectum and anal canal by digital examination. Proctosigmoidoscopic examination should clarify any differential diagnostic problem.

As already mentioned, the anal deformities associated with radical hemorrhoidectomy, fistula surgery, and pull-through procedures may produce an ectropion or mucosal prolapse, but they should pose no difficulty in differential diagnosis. However, it is extremely important to distinguish full-thickness prolapse from mucosal prolapse because treatment of the two conditions is decidedly different. Many patients have undergone multiple anal operations because rectal prolapse has been mistaken for hemorrhoids.

Physiologic Studies

As mentioned, there is merit for performing certain physiologic studies, especially with respect to complaints of anal incontinence.[95,136] The various studies and techniques are discussed in Chapters 6 and 13. Sun and colleagues evaluated anorectal pressures at rest, during contraction, and during balloon distension of the rectum in individuals with full-thickness rectal prolapse, anterior mucosal prolapse, and solitary rectal ulcer.[230] When compared with control subjects, those with rectal prolapse, mucosal prolapse, and solitary rectal ulcer had lower anal pressures, demonstrated a higher incidence of repetitive rectal contractions, and required lower threshold volumes to cause a desire to defecate. The authors hypothesized that the similarity of these observations suggest that the three disease entities share a common pathophysiology. Solitary rectal ulcer is discussed later in this chapter (see Solitary Rectal Ulcer Syndrome).

The value of pudendal nerve terminal motor latency (PNTML) studies is also discussed in prior chapters. As in the evaluation of patients who have sustained obstetric injury and who are incontinent, this study should be considered for individuals with procidentia. When there is associated pudendal neuropathy, the prognosis for improved bowel control following surgical repair of the prolapse is not as good as when there is no conduction abnormality. Although the presence of pudendal neuropathy does not contraindicate repair, it is helpful to know this in advance in order to give the patient an understanding of the likelihood of resolution of the incontinence problem after cure of the prolapse. Still, I have been surprised at how well patients manage, even in the presence of profoundly abnormal PNTML studies when the prolapse has been repaired. Others report that the status of anal continence after surgical correction of the prolapse can be predicted by postoperative measurement of the PNTML.[26]

PREPROLAPSE (INTERNAL PROCIDENTIA, SIGMOIDORECTAL INTUSSUSCEPTION, INTERNAL INTUSSUSCEPTION OF THE RECTUM)

Preprolapse of the rectum was described by Asman in 1957 as a condition that precedes the development of true procidentia.[12] Since this initial report, numerous articles have appeared on the subject.[22,42,97,104,105,251] As with rectal prolapse, women are overwhelmingly affected.

The patient may complain of a feeling of fullness or a lump inside the rectum. Symptoms may be exacerbated by prolonged periods of standing or sitting. Often, one experiences the perception of an obstruction when attempting to pass flatus or to have a bowel movement. There may be a sensation of incomplete evacuation, and the application of manual pressure to eliminate is frequently reported. Some patients complain that something drops down and blocks the anal opening.[12] Pain may be present in the perineal area with occasional sciatic or obturator radiation. However, the most frequent indication for an operation, according to one observer, is the complaint of incontinence.[104]

Evaluation

Proctosigmoidoscopic examination by the inexperienced examiner may be singularly unrewarding, especially if the prone jackknife position is used. Careful inspection of the mucosa may reveal an area of hyperemia and edema from 8 to 15 cm, and the bowel wall may appear to be thickened. Occasionally, the physician may perceive an intussusception of the rectosigmoid. With this history and with the proctoscopic findings described, there is a strong likelihood of preprolapse. According to Thompson, the diagnosis of intussusception of the rectum can

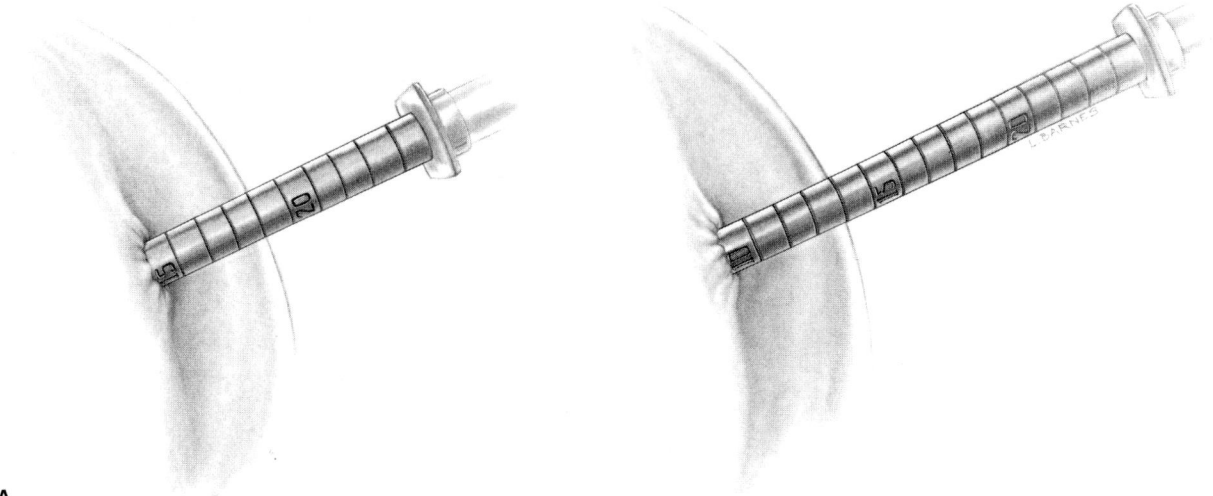

A   **B**

FIGURE 17-9. Diagnosis of the preprolapse condition (sigmoidorectal intussusception). **(A)** The sigmoidoscope in position with the level of insertion carefully identified. **(B)** Visualization is maintained at the same point on the mucosa. When the patient strains, the instrument is seen to move out.

be inferred by performing a simple maneuver with the sigmoidoscope.[236] If the examiner asks the patient to strain down while an area of mucosa is kept in sight, the instrument may be moved distally several centimeters or even out of the rectum (Figure 17-9). Personally, I have never found this method to be helpful.

Defecography

Radiologic study of the rectum by means of defecography is the most effective means for identifying the preprolapse condition and other defecatory disorders.[2,12,16,22,67,97,104,105,158] The technique of defecography obviously requires the cooperation of the radiology department and, ideally, a radiologist who is interested in developing expertise with the technique (see Chapter 6). A wide platform is constructed on the foot of the x-ray table on which a radiolucent commode can be placed.[22] This can be a commercially available product, such as the Brunswick Chair (E-Z-EM Co., Westbury, NY) (Figure 17-10), or an ordinary portable "potty" can be substituted (Figure 17-11). The barium can be thickened by means of carboxymethylcellulose in order to simulate fecal matter.[97] A commercially available product (i.e., Evacupaste) is also supplied by the E-Z-EM Company (Figure 17-12). Evacupaste is a barium sulfate paste containing gums and emulsifiers and is so thick and difficult to administer manually that it should be inserted with a standard caulking gun. Fluoroscopic and spot filming in the lateral projection is accomplished with the patient sitting and straining. Much of the physiologic nature of defecation is lost when the patient lies down, as it is when one performs a standard barium enema examination.[67,112]

Selvaggi and others have demonstrated the normal anorectal angle to be 90.00 ± 4.76 degrees at rest and to be 111.00 ± 5.02 degrees during straining,[212] but others suggest that this determination lacks clinical relevance.[69] Besides intussusception and increased distance between the rectum and sacrum, defecographic abnormalities that can be observed include the following:

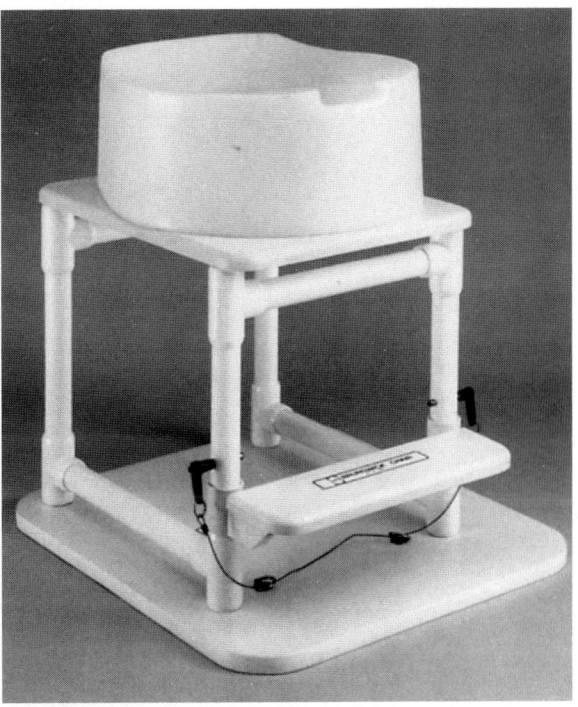

FIGURE 17-10. Brunswick defecography chair. (Courtesy of E-Z-EM, Inc., Westbury, NY.)

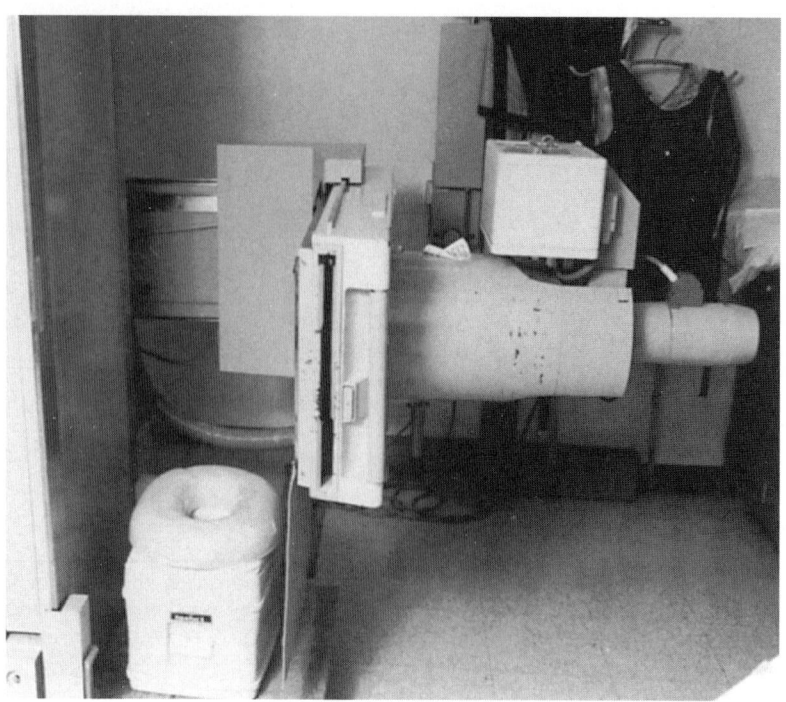

FIGURE 17-11. Defecogram unit in radiology suite using standard portable radiomscent toilet (Port-A-Potti).

- Megarectum
- Unsuspected incontinence
- Abnormal anorectal angle
- Nonrelaxing puborectalis (i.e., obstructed defecation; see Chapter 16)
- Abnormal perineal descent (i.e., less than 2.5 cm)
- Mucosal prolapse
- Solitary ulcer
- Rectocele (Figure 17-13)
- Enterocele[23,75]

Findings suggestive of preprolapse include funnel-shaped configuration of the rectum, lack of fixation of the rectum to the sacrum, excessive rectosigmoid mobility, the formation of a "ring pocket," and, of course, a demonstrable intussusception (Figs. 17-14 and 17-15).[67,97] As with typical rectal prolapse, a redundant sigmoid colon with a wide, deep pouch of Douglas may be seen. Irrespective of the radiologic findings, however, the physician must be circumspect and not attempt to overinterpret possible abnormalities. For example, Shorvon and col-

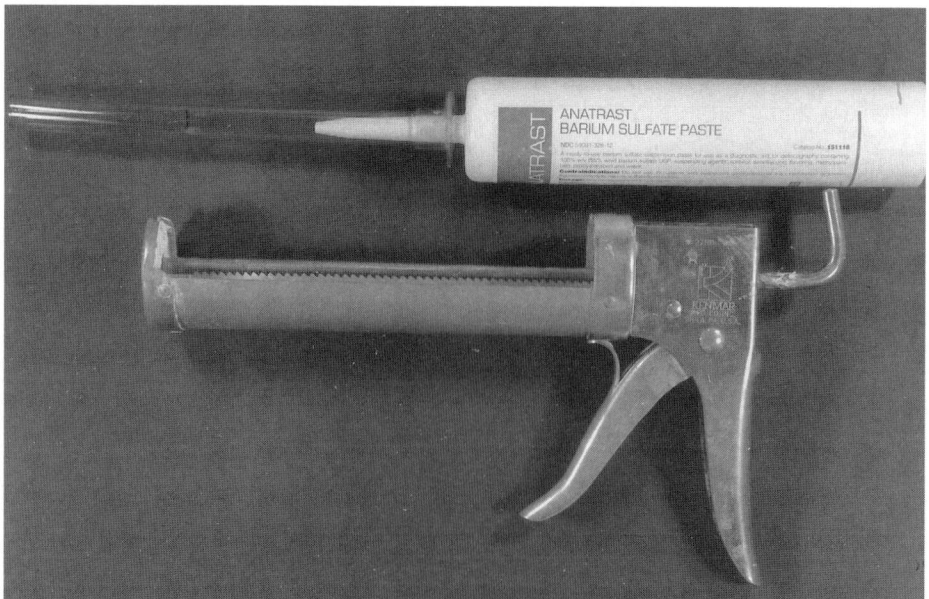

FIGURE 17-12. Thickened, barium paste (Anatrast) with a caulking gun to facilitate insertion.

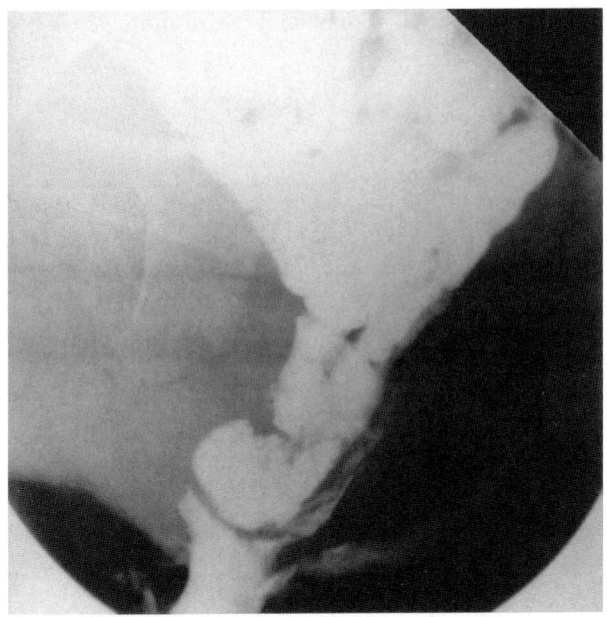

FIGURE 17-13. Defecogram with concomitant small bowel follow-through demonstrates a rectocele with a deep pouch of Douglas. An enterocele is also suspected and was consistent with the clinical observations.

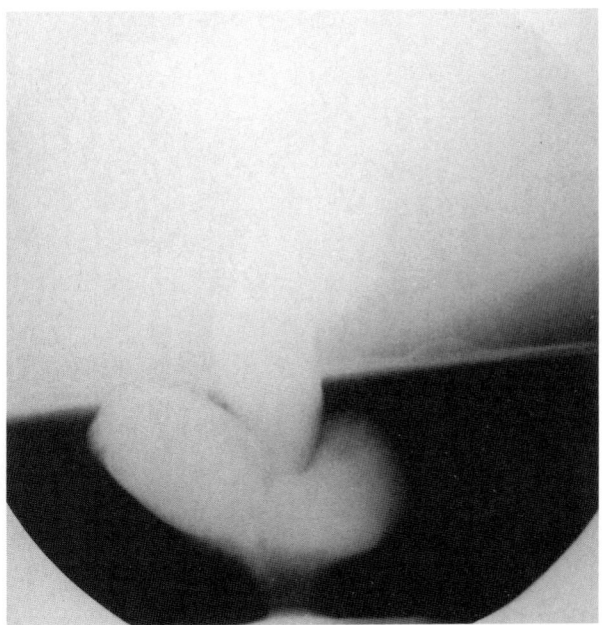

FIGURE 17-15. Defecogram. Colorectal intussusception (preprolapse).

leagues performed defecographic examination on 47 healthy volunteers in order to determine the range of normal findings.[215] They observed a broad spectrum of anorectal angle and pelvic floor descent changes that overlapped reported pathologic states. Others have also noted a wide range of measurements for anorectal angle in asymptomatic patients, as well as considerable variance from individual to individual for the position of the anorectal junction, perineal motility, and anal canal width.[73] Differences in observer interpretation further complicate the issue. However, most investigators remain convinced that defecography is the single most useful investigative tool for the evaluation of patients with presumed internal procidentia.[74] Still, in advising surgical intervention, there is no substitute for good clinical judgment.

Defecography has no place in the evaluation of individuals with *procidentia*, however. This is a clinical diagnosis that is merely reaffirmed by the radiologist if the

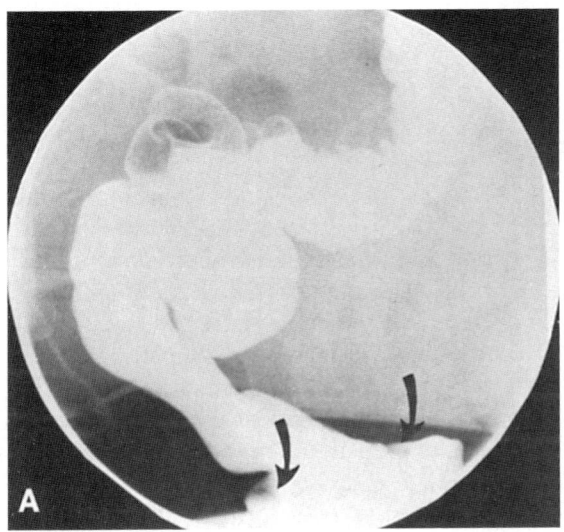

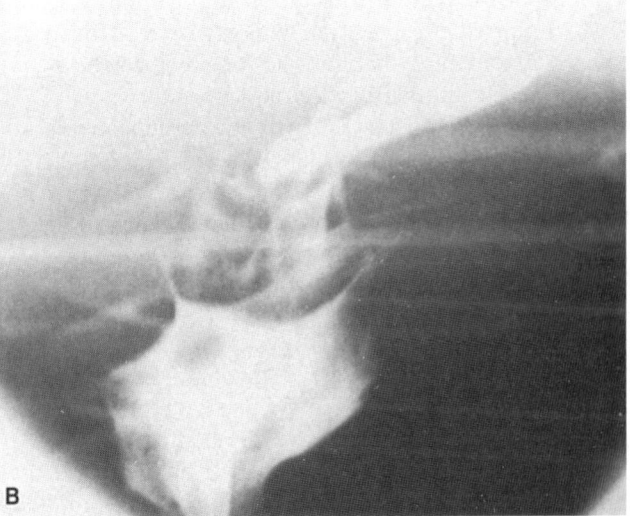

FIGURE 17-14. Defecogram of preprolapse. **(A)** A ring pocket *(arrows)* is demonstrated. **(B)** Intussusception is clearly evident.

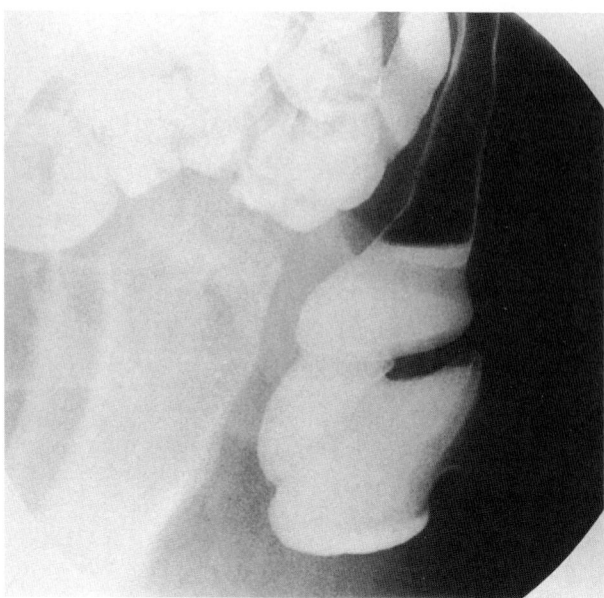

FIGURE 17-16. Complete rectal prolapse can be observed on this defecogram. One should not depend on the radiologist to make the diagnosis, however.

patient is submitted to this study (Figure 17-16). It is more than embarrassing to have the radiologist inform the surgeon that someone has a rectal prolapse.

Dynamic Magnetic Resonance Imaging Defecography

This procedure has been described for the assessment of pelvic floor disorders in proctologic patients. In a study by Rentsch and colleagues, patients were examined in the supine position and without a bowel preparation.[196] Images were taken during maximal straining after filling of the rectum with ultrasound gel enriched with gadolinium-diethylenetriamine pentaacetic acid. In a series of 20 patients, conditions such as rectocele, cystocele, enterocele, intussusception, and anismus were detected. Approximately one third of the patients were found to have additional abnormalities besides those that had been clinically suspected. Whether this new modality will prove to be as useful as defecography remains to be determined.

Colpocystodefecography

Hock and colleagues assessed through one single contrast study the complete female pelvis by means of colpocystodefecography (CCD).[96] This technique combines vaginal opacification, voiding cystography, and defecography. They performed 300 examinations and found CCD more useful than clinical evaluation for the diagnosis of preprolapse and enterocele. The authors concluded that CCD was useful in selecting the appropriate surgical

procedure for an individual with one or more pelvic floor anomalies.[96]

Treatment and Results

On the basis of the characteristic history and defecography evidence, Hoffman and colleagues performed retrorectal sacral fixation on eight patients with internal prolapse. All experienced relief of symptoms with no morbidity.[97] Berman and colleagues reported 65 patients with radiographic evidence of intussusception, and performed the Delorme procedure on 14 of them.[22] All had relief of pelvic symptoms and of severe constipation. A late follow-up (i.e., 3 years) revealed sustained symptomatic relief in greater than 70%.[21] Another alternative recommended by Berman and colleagues is reduction of rectal reservoir capacity by means of multiple rubber ring ligations or staple excision of the redundant mucosa.[20] McCue and Thomson performed polyvinyl alcohol sponge (i.e., Ivalon) abdominal rectopexy for internal prolapse in 12 individuals.[154] Although there was no suggestion of recurrence, the functional results were mixed. The authors caution that if obstructed defecation is part of the clinical presentation, this operation probably should not be offered. Christiansen and co-workers performed suspension operations in 24 patients with obstructed defecation resulting from preprolapse.[42] Defecographic abnormalities resolved following the procedure in 22, but none of the patients was completely relieved of his or her symptoms. They conclude that internal prolapse is probably a secondary phenomenon in patients with obstructed defecation and that a nonsurgical approach should be adopted.[42] Others assert that patients with fecal incontinence and intussusception do well with a surgical approach.[127] The surgical techniques are discussed later in the section on the operative management of rectal prolapse.

Opinion

There has been a dearth of publications on this subject since the late 1990s. I attribute this to a waning enthusiasm for operative intervention. Many surgeons' experiences suggest that at best the results are unimpressive. Clearly, one must be highly selective and circumspect. My own recommendation is to offer the patient an anterior resection if symptoms are classic and the defecogram is positive, the same philosophical approach and operation that I prefer to employ for procidentia (see later). The operation may also be considered for individuals with symptoms suggestive of obstructed defecation and in whom there is no objective evidence for this diagnosis. However, I make no promises as to the likelihood of alleviating symptoms.

SOLITARY RECTAL ULCER SYNDROME

Solitary ulcer of the rectum is an unusual condition that was initially described by Madigan and subsequently by Madigan and Morson; they collected a series of 68 cases.[145,146] Unfortunately, the term is rather confusing, because the syndrome does not necessarily have to be solitary, nor does it have to be confined to the rectum; in fact, it may be polypoid rather than ulcerating. The condition may be confused with nonspecific inflammatory bowel disease, villous adenoma, colitis cystica profunda, and other inflammatory and neoplastic diseases affecting the colon and rectum.

Etiology

The etiology of solitary rectal ulcer syndrome is uncertain, but chronic constipation and fecal impaction may play a role. Some believe that the victims are "unusual personalities, similar to that which is often ascribed to an individual with procidentia."[235] Patients who frequently resort to manual disimpaction may produce a local inflammatory reaction, with ulceration of the rectum and subsequent fibrosis. Because the anus and rectum are erogenous areas, autoeroticism has been thought to be involved with many of these individuals. Turnbull in fact suggested that the treatment of this condition should be bilateral long-arm casts (Turnbull, RB, personal communication).

The injudicious use of ergotamine suppositories has been reported to cause solitary rectal ulcer.[64] Another possible mechanism is the failure of inhibition of puborectalis muscle contraction. This may result in a repeated desire to defecate and cause the persistent need to strain to pass stool. However, most observers believe that the solitary ulcer syndrome is a distinct clinical inflammatory manifestation that is associated with rectal prolapse or, more specifically, the preprolapse condition (see earlier).[59,129,140,168,185] So disparate are the theories of causation and presentation that Sobin was inspired to pen a rather whimsical poem on the subject.[219] The following are the tenth to the thirteenth verses (out of 14):

> It is neither adenoma
> nor a type of carcinoid
> It's the sequel to a prolapse
> and mucosa that's destroyed.
> Called the solitary ulcer
> of the rectum this syndrome
> As the prolapse brings ischemia
> then mucosa's ulcer prone.
> Known as Cystica Profunda
> when there is a deep colitis
> And the submucosa's filled with
> Lakes of mucinous detritus.
> Pseudotumor on the surface
> is a lesion hyperplastic

> Called Cloacogenic Polyp
> it's enflamed but not dysplastic.[219]

Clinical Features

Solitary rectal ulcer syndrome is usually seen in women, especially those who harbor the bowel management problems previously described. However, in the St. Mark's Hospital (UK) experience of 119 patients, the condition occurred in men and women equally.[149] Symptoms usually consists of a variety of bowel complaints: constipation, diarrhea, passage of mucus, tenesmus, rectal bleeding, and proctalgia fugax. A classic history is one of blood and mucus per rectum associated with straining and a feeling of incomplete evacuation.[247]

Martin and co-workers reviewed 51 patients with the syndrome and noted that 98% presented with rectal bleeding, 96% with the passage of mucus, and 93% with tenesmus.[152] Approximately one half of the patients were constipated. Bleeding was severe enough to require transfusion in three individuals. In the experience at the Cleveland Clinic in Ohio, the principal symptoms were rectal bleeding (84%) and a disturbance of bowel function (56%).[239] Patients often present long after the onset of symptoms, sometimes more than 5 years.[247]

Examination

Classically, sigmoidoscopic examination usually reveals an ulcer with hyperemic edges and surrounding induration. Alternatively, exophytic lesions may be seen. In my own experience, a combination of ulcerating and polypoid lesions are often noted on the anterior rectal wall, usually at a level of 6 to 8 cm. Thomson and associates, in their report of six patients, found that the lesions were not necessarily solitary nor ulcerated.[234]

Histopathology

There are numerous characteristic features that permit the pathologist to distinguish solitary rectal ulcer from other lesions. Inflammatory changes may consist of replacement of the normal lamina propria by fibroblasts arranged at right angles to the muscularis mucosae (Figs. 17-17 and 17-18).[203,207] The microscopic appearance, however, is quite variable and can include loss of normal polarity of the glandular epithelial cells, shortening of the crypts, mucin depletion, mucosal thickening, and inflammatory reaction in the submucosa. Many of the manifestations are those that have been described in patients with inflammatory bowel disease. Electron microscopic changes have also been identified; these include dense collagen deposition within the lamina propria as well as numerous fibroblasts.[37]

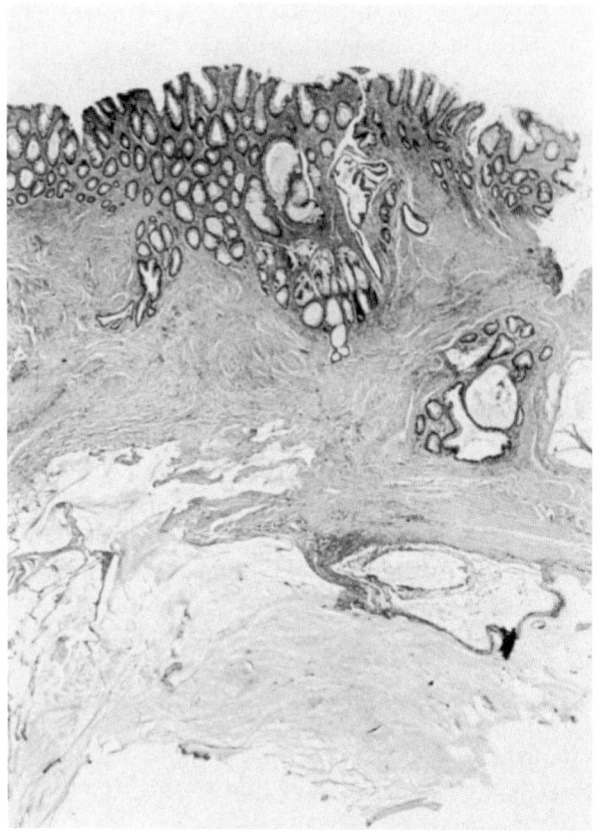

FIGURE 17-17. The submucosa of a solitary rectal ulcer contains a large mucous lake **(bottom)** and a group of glands in the submucosa between the lake and the overlying mucosa. (Original magnification ×20; courtesy of Rodger C. Haggitt, M.D.)

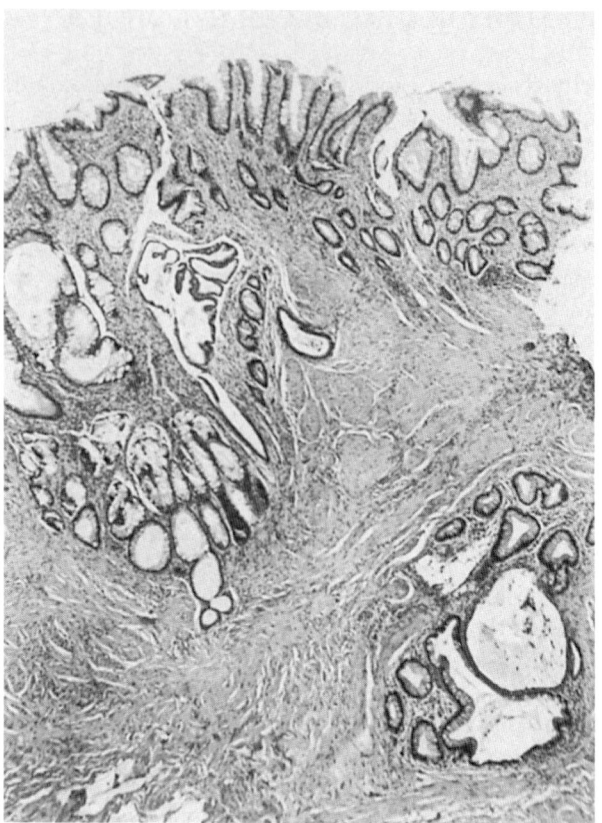

FIGURE 17-18. Solitary rectal ulcer. Markedly hyperplastic muscularis mucosa separates a group of glands in the submucosa **(lower right)** from the overlying mucosa. Fibers of muscularis mucosa extend into and obliterate the lamina propria between crypts. (Original magnification ×40; courtesy of Rodger C. Haggitt, M.D.)

Franzin and colleagues reported a follow-up study of 27 patients with solitary ulcer of the rectum.[70] The authors noted a striking change in the histologic pattern. Although the patient's symptoms may have improved, the histologic appearance seemed to suggest chronic ischemia and an evolution to a transitional mucosa.

Physiologic Evaluation and Contrast Studies

The diagnosis is made predominantly on the basis of symptoms, endoscopic appearance, and results of biopsy. Anorectal physiologic evaluation and radiologic studies of patients with solitary rectal ulcer has been reported but is of limited value.[247] Defecography has frequently revealed an occult rectal prolapse (see previous discussion). Other findings that have been noted include failure of the sphincter to relax on defecation, high intrarectal pressure, increased anorectal angle, perineal descent, and impaired sensation on balloon inflation of the rectum.[87,119,188,259,260] It has been suggested that a high evacuation pressure may cause mucosal ulceration by exposing the rectal wall to a high transmural pressure gradient.[261]

Goei and colleagues performed conventional barium enema studies on 15 individuals with histologically proven solitary rectal ulcer syndrome.[76] Findings included rectal stricture, granularity of the mucosa, and thickened rectal folds in 60%, but the remainder showed no abnormalities. Defecography demonstrated an intussusception in eight, and in four the puborectalis muscle failed to relax. There is general agreement on a high incidence and association of "rectoanal lack of coordination," perineal descent, and pudendal neuropathy in these individuals.[247]

Transrectal Ultrasound

Transrectal ultrasonography has been used in an attempt to understand the pathogenesis of solitary rectal ulcer syndrome. In a study by van Outryve and associates, involving 15 patients, a rigid linear endorectal probe was used.[250] All but two demonstrated a thickened rectal wall. Poor relaxation of the puborectalis muscle during straining was noted in 11 of the 15. The authors opined that thickening of the muscularis propria suggests a chronic mechanical load on the rectal wall, and that ulcerations are formed as a consequence of this phenomenon.[250] They concluded that nonrelaxation of the puborectalis muscle is an important element in the pathogenesis of this condition. The St. Mark's Hospital group performed *anal* endosonography on 20 patients with solitary rectal ulcer syndrome.[151] Thirteen were found to have an abnormally thick internal anal sphincter. The investigators observed that these individuals were significantly more likely to have defecographic evidence of internal prolapse and opine that this study (when positive) has a high predictive value for this association.

Management

Treatment of solitary rectal ulcer syndrome is rather problematic. I have been tempted on occasion to consider Turnbull's admonition; some of these patients are obviously psychologically disturbed. When the lesion is proximal to the rectum, every one of the patients in my experience subsequently proved to have inflammatory bowel disease, specifically Crohn's. Many individuals' symptoms may be ameliorated by a high-fiber diet and bowel management instructions.[249] With the characteristic rectal abnormality, the physician may consider a trial of hydrocortisone enemas, although I have not been impressed with any benefit. Others have observed marked improvement of symptoms through the use of sucralfate retention enemas; however, histologic changes persisted.[268] Fibrin sealant has also been suggested.[65] Rarely, a colostomy may be indicated for the treatment of symptoms and complications, such as massive rectal bleeding.

Biofeedback has been used both as the primary therapy and to supplement surgery, especially in individuals with obstructed defecation.[247] Transanal excision of localized lesions has been performed with mixed results—some recur, others do not. Because operations designed for the treatment of rectal prolapse have been reported to be of benefit in patients with the solitary ulcer syndrome (suspension, rectopexy and resection),[119,168,259] a high index of suspicion for the presence of sigmoidorectal intussusception (i.e., preprolapse) should be maintained if the examiner perceives the characteristic changes in the rectal mucosa. Anorectal physiologic evaluation, specifically defecography, is strongly encouraged under these circumstances.

Results

The St. Mark's group reported their results of behavioral treatment (biofeedback) in 13 patients with solitary ulcer syndrome.[147] Approximately one half improved, but there was significant deterioration over time (median follow-up, 36 months). In the experience of the Cleveland Clinic, intractable symptoms led to surgery in 60% of their patients, with symptomatic improvement noted in more

than two thirds.[239] They further observed that the optimal surgical procedure is still indeterminate, but rectopexy, local excision, and fecal diversion seem to achieve improvement in the majority of patients. The authors were rather circumspect with regard to recommendation of resective surgery for this condition. van Tets and Kuijpers performed rectopexy on 18 patients with solitary rectal ulcer syndrome.[251] All lesions healed, and patients became significantly less symptomatic. The authors believe that characteristic defecographic features and the presence of solitary rectal ulcer syndrome are indications for surgery, provided pelvic floor function during straining is normal—in other words, if there is no suggestion of obstructed defecation. In the experience of the St. Mark's Hospital group with 16 patients who remained symptomatic following rectopexy, they concluded that a prolonged preoperative evacuation time (obstructed defecation) may predict a poor surgical outcome.[87] A more recent publication from the same institution involved 81 patients who underwent surgery for this condition.[217] The ultimate stomal rate was 30%.

Surgery has a limited role in the treatment of solitary rectal ulcer. It should be reserved for those individuals with intractable symptoms, in whom behavioral therapy has failed, and/or who have incontrovertible evidence of internal prolapse.[247]

SYNDROME OF THE DESCENDING PERINEUM

When a healthy person increases intraabdominal pressure and relaxes the pelvic floor muscles, no significant change can be observed in the concavity of the perineum. However, in patients with chronic illness, malnutrition, and preprolapse, perineal descent may be observed, the normal concavity being obliterated when the patient strains.[185] In those with this syndrome, either the anal canal is situated several centimeters below a line drawn between the pubis and coccyx, or it descends 3 or 4 cm during straining.[185] The perineal area can even descend 5 or 6 cm in some persons (Figure 17-19). A "perineometer" has been described which can measure the amount of descent, but some authors question the accuracy of this instrument and advise standard defecographic techniques for this determination.[9,177,232] The Cleveland Clinic Florida group studied the reproducibility of measuring the anorectal angle and pelvic floor descent by two different methods.[40] The investigators concluded that both methods were consistently reliable.

A descending perineum is the result of injury to the pelvic floor muscles, especially the levators. Patients usually complain of tenesmus, difficulty evacuating, and incontinence. The problem with bowel control may be due to excessive straining with defecation, which stretches

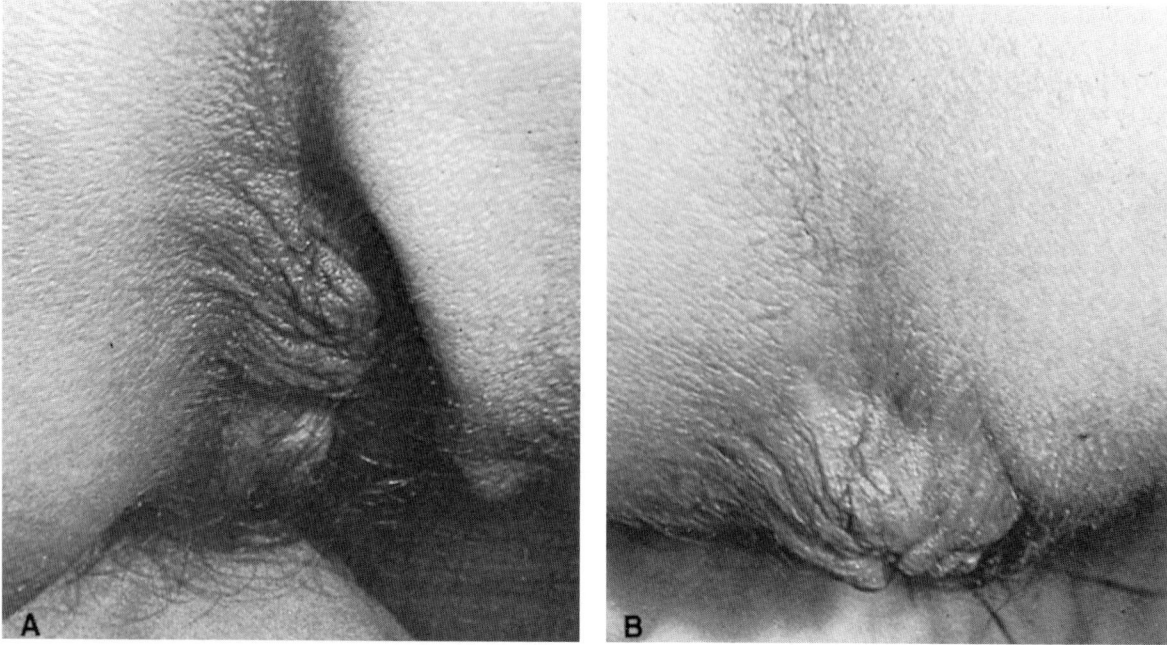

FIGURE 17-19. Descending perineum (perineal descensus). **(A)** At rest. **(B)** During straining. (From De los Rios Margrina E. *Color atlas of anorectal diseases.* Philadelphia: WB Saunders, 1980.)

the pudendal nerves and results in anorectal muscular atrophy. Jorge and co-workers at the Cleveland Clinic Florida performed a prospective study to assess the correlation between perineal descent and pudendal neuropathy in 213 consecutive patients.[113] There was no relationship found, leading the authors to conclude that these may represent independent findings despite being frequently observed in those with disordered defecation.

Treatment

Treatment is usually directed toward bowel management (e.g., diet, laxatives, suppositories) and to education (e.g., avoiding straining). When incontinence is the major complaint, restoration of the pelvic floor, with possible implantation of mesh, and resection or suspension of the rectum may be necessary. An alternative, suggested by Nichols, is to hitch the posterior wall of the rectum to the sacrum through a transcoccygeal (i.e., Kraske) approach (Figure 17-20).[169] The operation can be combined with plication of the levatores as well as an anterior perineorrhaphy. Unfortunately, almost irrespective of the various options that may be implemented, results are less than ideal. A possible exception to this is an innovation for the surgical treatment of pelvic floor laxity (including enterocele, rectocele, and cystocele) through the use of what Sullivan and Lee call a total pelvic Marlex mesh repair.[229] This is a most complicated operation that involves strip-

ping of the parietal and visceral peritoneum from the floor of the pelvis, separating the posterior vaginal wall from the rectum all the way down to the perineal body, and then implanting a trapezoid-shaped Marlex mesh with two additional strips—securing the mesh at the introitus, at the adjacent endopelvic fascia, and to the upper sacrum. In addition, the Marlex is secured to Cooper's ligament on each side as part of the anterior fixation.

The authors have reported their considerable experience (236 women) with this operation.[228] The median age was 64 years. The primary complaints were bladder protrusion, vaginal protrusion, or both (54%), but almost two thirds of these patients were found to have perineal descent. More than one third of patients required additional surgery for persistent or new complaints, but there have been no recurrences of rectal or vaginal prolapse. As one may appreciate, this is an esoteric operation indeed, the application of which thus far seems to be confined to the one center.

Collopy and colleagues reported a group of patients with rectal prolapse (see later) and posthysterectomy vaginal wall prolapse in whom they performed rectopexy, abdominal closure of the pelvic cul-de-sac, and a colpopexy (attaching forward extensions of the same mesh to the apex of the anatomically restored and reinforced vaginal vault; Figure 17-21).[45] Eighty-nine patients were provided considerable relief of symptoms without evident recurrent rectal or vaginal vault prolapse.

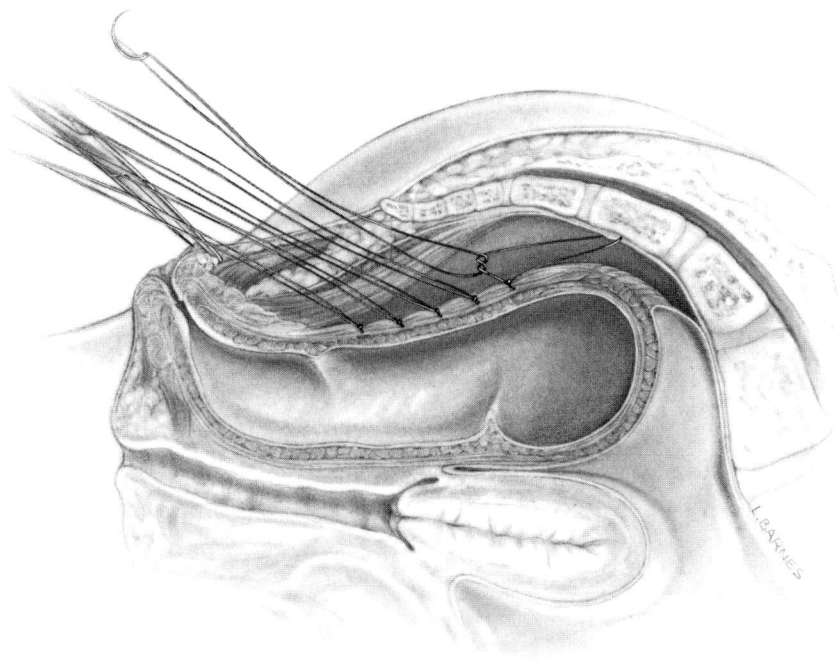

FIGURE 17-20. Series of plication sutures are placed 1 cm apart in the posterior wall of the rectum. Sutures are then sewn individually to the anterior periosteum of the sacrum. (Adapted from Nichols DH. Retrorectal levatorplasty for anal and perineal prolapse. *Surg Gynecol Obstet* 1982;154:251, with permission.)

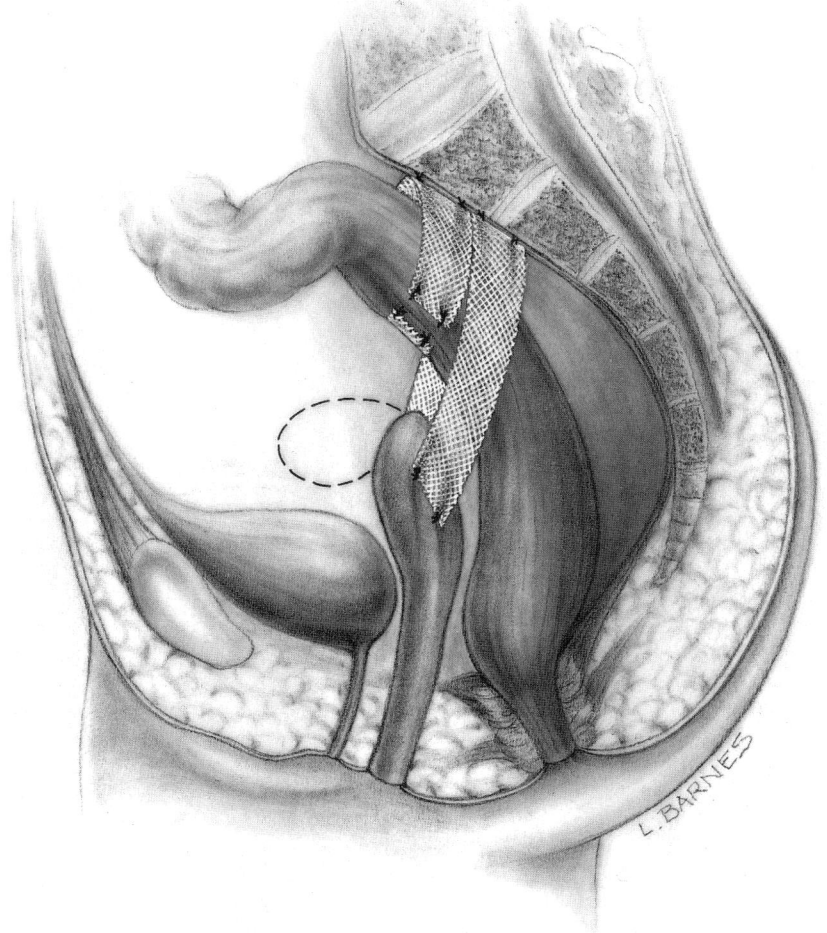

FIGURE 17-21. Abdominal colporectopexy with pelvic cul-de-sac closure. Lateral view of the completed procedure. Note that mesh is secured to the sacrum, to the rectum, and to the apex of the anatomically restored vagina. The *dotted line* indicates the obliterated cul-de-sac. (Redrawn from Collopy BT, Barham KA. *Dis Colon Rectum* 2002;45:523).

Comment

The management of perineal descent in an individual with disabling symptoms has been a frustratingly disappointing venture for me. Results following resection, suspension, and pelvic floor reconstruction with absorbable or nonabsorbable mesh has been less than uniformly successful. Furthermore, these patients are often elderly or infirm and are, therefore, not ideal candidates for a major reconstruction. Still, with a full understanding of the risks and potential benefits and with the failure of conservative measures, I am willing to offer an abdominal operation for this condition.

TREATMENT OF RECTAL PROLAPSE

In general, partial or incomplete (i.e., mucosal) prolapse should be treated by an anal operation. If only one quadrant is involved, simple excision, leaving the wound open, may be all that is required (see Figure 8-58). If the protruding area is circumferential, excision with an S-plasty may be considered (see Figs. 8-71 and 8-72). A more recent suggestion for the management of mucosal prolapse is the use of the circular stapler, especially the so-called PPH modification (stapled hemorrhoidopexy; see Chapter 8).[7]

With respect to the management of acute, incarcerated (i.e., irreducible) rectal prolapse (Figure 17-22), some have recommended a local anesthetic to paralyze the sphincters and to effect reduction (see Figure 8-32). Others suggest a spinal or general anesthetic. The placement of ordinary table sugar or powdered sugar on the bowel mucosa can result in decreased edema and sponta-

neous or easily induced reduction from the desiccating effect. This is a well-recognized technique in the veterinary literature.[163] Emergency resection is occasionally indicated, usually because of compromised viability.[193]

Nonoperative Treatment of Rectal Prolapse

If surgical treatment for incomplete or complete prolapse is contraindicated, or if the patient refuses an operation, numerous noninvasive approaches and limited office procedures may be employed, as follows:

Adhesive strapping of buttocks
Manual anal support during defecation
Correction of constipation
Establishment of workable time and method of defecation
Perineal strengthening exercises
Electronic stimulation (see Figure 13-13)
Injection of sclerosing agent
Rubber ring ligation
Infrared coagulation

Although instructing the patient on proper bowel management and perineal exercises may be salutary, and other methods may offer some degree of palliation of symptoms, these measures cannot be expected to produce a cure.

Modes of Surgical Therapy for Rectal Prolapse

More than 50 operations have been designed for the treatment of complete rectal prolapse. Most are variations of a few basic modes of therapy and depend on the surgeon's concept of the anatomic defect. The options for treatment include narrowing of the anal orifice, obliteration of the peritoneal pouch of Douglas, restoration of the pelvic floor, resection of the bowel (by an abdominal, perineal, or transsacral approach), and suspension or fixation of the rectum to the sacrum or to other structures. Additional operations are listed that combine one or more of these approaches.

Narrowing of the anal orifice
Obliteration of the peritoneal pouch of Douglas
Restoration of the pelvic floor
Resection of bowel
   Transabdominal
   Perineal
   Transsacral
Suspension or fixation of the rectum
   To sacrum
   To pubis
   To other structures
Combinations of two or more of the above[30]

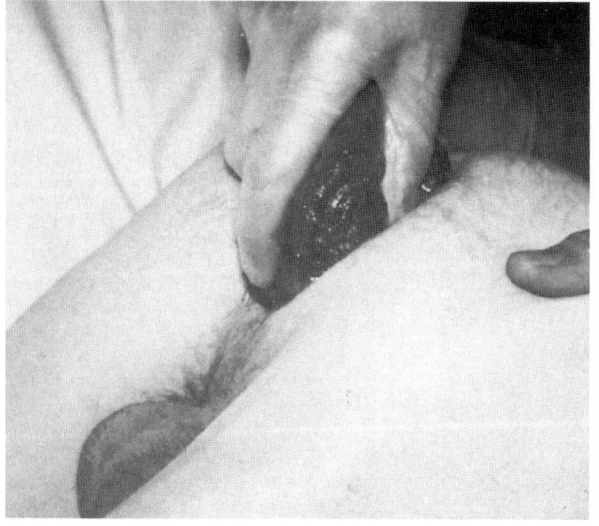

FIGURE 17-22. Manual replacement of incarcerated procidentia.

General Surgical Principles

All patients undergoing surgery for rectal prolapse should have a thorough mechanical cleansing of the bowel with an orally administered laxative. Colonic irrigation or small volume enemas may be unsuccessful with the often associated incontinence. Systemic, broad-spectrum antibiotics are advised during the perioperative period, especially if foreign material is to be implanted.

Postoperative care for abdominal operations is essentially the same as for any bowel resection (see Chapter 22). A progressive diet is instituted, and the patient is ideally discharged when the bowels have functioned. However, it is not unusual for there to be a longer period of ileus following rectal prolapse abdominal operations than when the same procedure is undertaken for other disease processes, such as cancer or diverticular disease.

Narrowing of the Anal Orifice

Thiersch Repair

In the older, poor-risk patient, some surgeons prefer to use the Thiersch operation.[77,92,121] This procedure can be performed with a local anesthetic, making it a satisfactory technique for these individuals. In the historic operation, silver wire was placed into the perianal space to encircle and narrow the anus. Today, surgeons have abandoned the use of wire because of the complications of breakage and ulceration. Other materials, such as nylon, Mersilene, Dacron, polypropylene mesh (i.e., Marlex), Teflon, fascia lata, silicone rubber, Silastic, and Dacron-impregnated Silastic mesh have been used for the same purpose.[63,89,101,103,121,132,142,174,189,191,204,231]

Operative Technique

The patient is placed in the lithotomy position on the operating table, and the perianal area is vigorously prepared with an antiseptic solution. A local anesthetic can be used to infiltrate the area. However, a general or spinal anesthetic may be more desirable. In the rare instance when I elect to employ this operation, I may use a double-armed 5-mm Mersilene suture (Figure 17-23). A small incision is made in the anterior and posterior positions, 1 cm outside the anal verge (Figure 17-24A). The

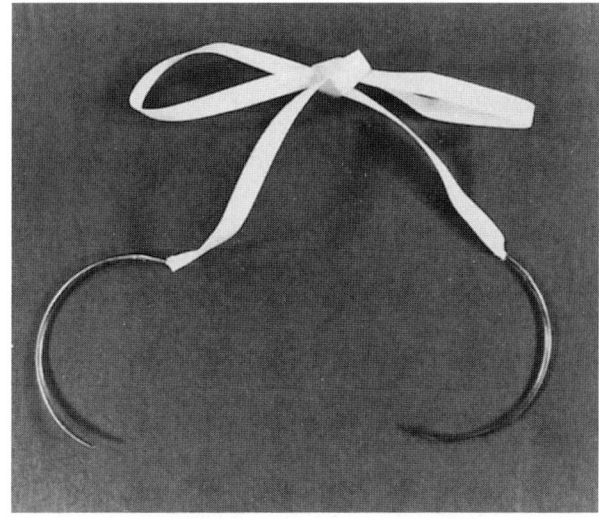

FIGURE 17-23. Double-armed, 5-mm Mersilene for Thiersch repair.

suture is passed from anterior to posterior on either side of the anus in the ischiorectal fossa (Figure 17-24B). The knot should be buried posteriorly. The recommendation that the diameter should equal the proximal interphalangeal joint of the operating surgeon is problematic (Figure 17-24C). The proximal interphalangeal joint is not a standard size; thus, one patient's anal canal orifice may be created relatively large and another is made relatively narrow. A No. 16 or 18 Hegar dilator (see Figure 23-117) is a better standard for determining luminal size. To avoid a bulky knot, suturing is required when using Mersilene tape. Alternatively, a stapling device may be used to secure the tape. I prefer the modification suggested by Thorlakson whereby an "eye" is cut near one end of the tape, and the other end brought through like a noose, doubled-back, and secured (Figure 17-24D).[237] The two wounds are primarily closed with absorbable sutures.

Postoperative Care

Frequent examinations are necessary to be certain that fecal impaction does not develop. Stool softeners, laxatives, suppositories, or enemas may be required. A topical antiseptic ointment, such as povidone-iodine (i.e.,

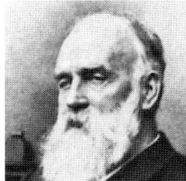

Carl Thiersch (1822–1895) Thiersch was born in Munich, Germany, to a very educated family. His father held the Professorship of Classics in the university and was president of the Academy of Science. Following his graduation from the gymnasium, the young Thiersch entered the study of medicine in his home university. Then, after a period of time at a number of European medical centers, he joined the Munich faculty. At the age of 32, he achieved professorial status. Shortly thereafter, he accepted a position as Professor of Surgery in Erlangen, and after 14 years, Leipzig. Like most of his contemporaries, he was expected to be a general surgeon, but his work with children and his head and neck surgery were particularly well recognized. The operation for which he was most famous was the preparation of thin skin grafts (i.e., Thiersch grafts), founded on his earlier microscopic investigations of granulation tissue. His name is also associated with the field of colon and rectal surgery for his suggestion of the management of procidentia by means of the circumanal placement of a silver wire.

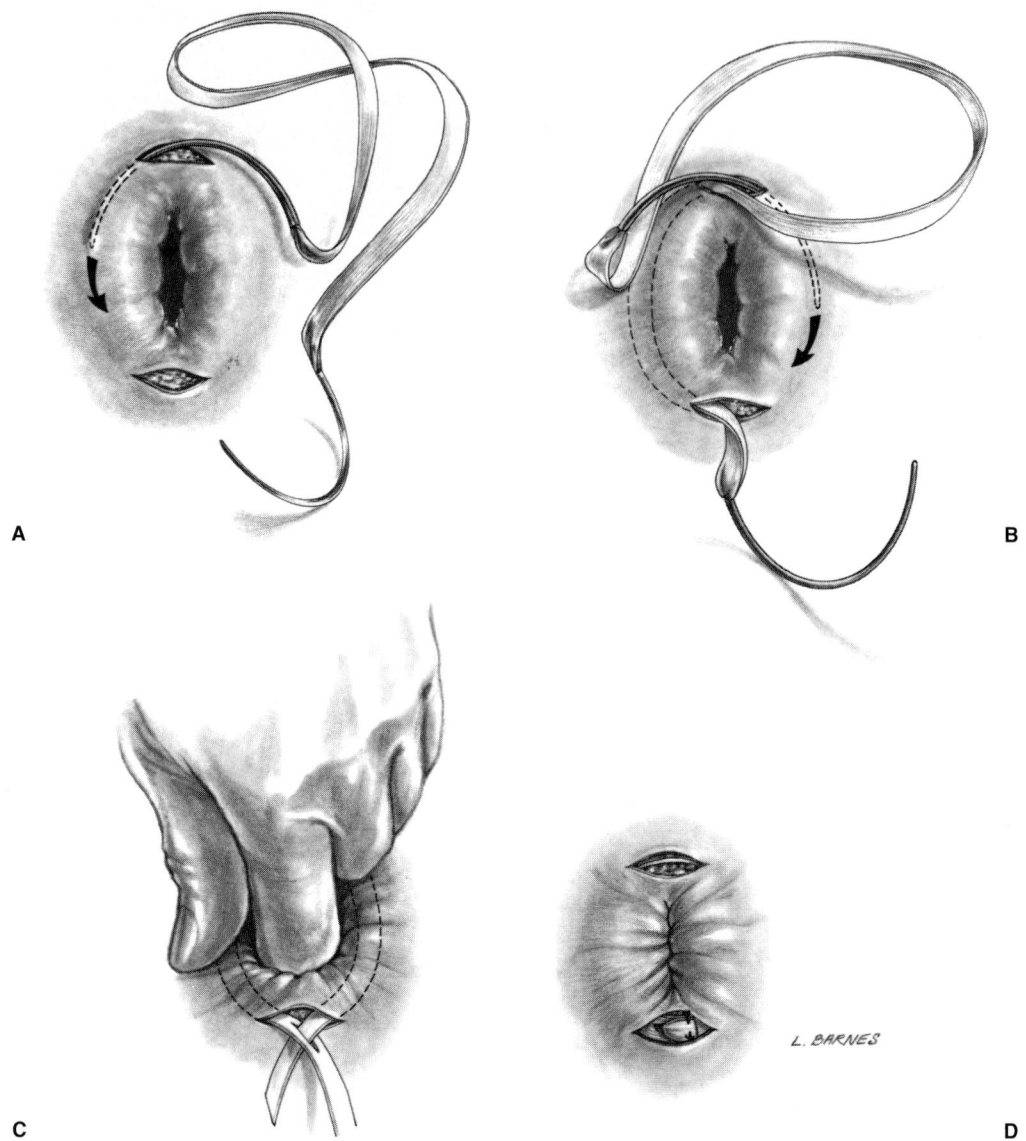

FIGURE 17-24. Thiersch repair with Mersilene tape. **(A,B)** Each needle arm is passed from anterior to posterior. **(C)** The tape is secured after tightening to the level of the proximal interphalangeal joint. A 18-French Hegar dilator is the preferred measuring device. **(D)** The tape is sutured to itself rather than knotted.

Betadine), is advised. In spite of the relative simplicity of the operation, the difficulty with postoperative management implies that the procedure ideally should be performed on an inpatient basis. The patient is discharged when bowel function has been established.

Complications

Complications are frequently seen with Thiersch and Thiersch-type repairs. Patients often complain of the sensation of "sitting on a lump." Tenesmus, a feeling of incomplete evacuation, and bowel management difficulties are the rule rather than the exception. The implant may profoundly narrow the anal opening to the extent that its removal becomes necessary. Fecal impaction often must

be managed in the operating room with an anesthetic. Wound infection is a common problem, the next most frequent reason for removal of the material. Finally, if the prolapse recurs, the rectum may become incarcerated and even strangulated. Recurrent prolapse following a Thiersch repair requires urgent evaluation and treatment. If erosion, sepsis, or obstruction supervenes, the material must be removed. The operation can be performed again once the wounds have healed.

Other Thiersch-Type Repairs

Other approaches have been advocated as alternatives to the Thiersch operation. Marlex mesh has been employed by Lomas and Cooperman.[142] Despite their wound infection rate of 33%, they believe this to be a rapid, safe procedure for use in the elderly patient who is not a candidate for a more extensive surgical operation.

Mersilene mesh, a woven polyester fiber, has been suggested as an alternative material for the Thiersch operation. Notaras used a ribbon of Mersilene (approximately 4 cm wide), passing it around the anus as has been described with the other material, except that a more extensive mobilization is required, and the mesh is placed more deeply.[174] The mesh is sutured together so that the opening permits the insertion of two fingers. Notaras reported an experience with 18 patients with no infection, breakage, or erosion.[174]

Sainio and colleagues reported 14 selected patients with prolapse who underwent anal encirclement with polypropylene mesh.[204] Although two had recurrences (15%), no breakage, erosion, or infection was observed. The authors caution that a history of fecal impaction implies that the surgeon should find another approach to the treatment of this condition.

Labow and associates described the use of an elastic fabric sling, a Dacron-impregnated Silastic sheet (see Figs. 13-58 and 13-59).[132] I have used this technique in the treatment of fecal incontinence in order to supplement the sphincter mechanism. The operation is similar to that of any Thiersch approach except that the authors recommend the prone jackknife position. A strip is cut to 1.5 cm wide, with care taken to prepare it in such a way that it is elastic along its longitudinal axis. An overlap of 1 cm is created, and a linear stapler is used to secure it in place. All wounds are primarily closed. The authors noted no problems with infection, erosion, or impaction in nine patients. The potential appeal of this material is that it theoretically can stretch, but stool is unlikely to open up this prosthesis. However, rectal examination reveals that it simulates a normal sphincter.

Hunt and colleagues treated 43 patients (mean age, 80 years) for full-thickness prolapse by implanting Silastic rods.[103] These are 4 mm in diameter and are inserted through two small stab incisions. The two ends are secured by a self-locking plastic clip, which fixes the overlapping ends of the rod and secures them into place by a cable gun.[103] The authors reported adequate control of the prolapse in 71% of patients, with no operative mortality.

Swerdlow addressed the issue of performing the operation through only one incision.[231] He describes a helical rod (the Encircler), a single loop having a diameter of 6 cm with an extension beyond 360 degrees, the end of which is adapted to accept varying tips (Figure 17-25). By rotating the handle, the tip can be passed circumferentially about the anus. The author recommends the use of Silastic tubing (Cooper Medical, Stamford, CT), but suggests that other material could be implanted as well with this device. Theoretically, this technique could reduce the incidence of septic complications.

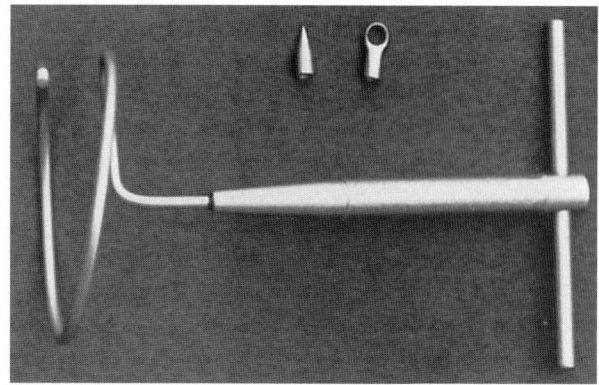

FIGURE 17-25. Encircler with a detachable mole and carrier tips. (Courtesy of Hyman Swerdlow, M.D.)

Khanduja and colleagues presented their experience with a compressible prosthesis composed of silicone elastomer surrounded by a silicone-coated Dacron tape.[121] Dacron mesh is embedded in the ends for reinforcement. Sixteen "extremely poor-risk" individuals were submitted to the procedure. Complications included breakage of the prosthesis in three, infection in one, and late sepsis in one individual. The device has never been marketed and is unavailable as of this writing.

Ladha and colleagues employed the Angelchik Anti-Reflux Prosthesis—a device that was introduced for the treatment of gastroesophageal reflux—for the repair of rectal prolapse in elderly patients.[133] The prosthesis is placed in a supralevator location around the rectum, a position which may help to restore the anorectal angle. The authors reported eight patients, with one death and one complication of wound sepsis.

Comment

It can be stated without equivocation that procidentia has stimulated more ingenious efforts at surgical treatment than virtually any other condition. Evaluation of the long-term results of the classical Thiersch procedure (i.e., using wire) is absent from contemporary writings, and even the newer materials are often described with little more than case report experience. The Thiersch-type operations, in my opinion, should rarely be employed; the complication rate is extremely high. Furthermore, the procedure does not cure the prolapse; it certainly would recur if the material were removed. Finally, the operation serves only to exacerbate bowel management problems.

However, there are certain limited situations in which the use of the Thiersch-type operation can be offered. For example, with a patient who "cannot tolerate a haircut," it is a simple and reasonably safe alternative. And for more convenient management of patients in nursing homes and psychiatric facilities, it is certainly appropriate to offer this suboptimal choice.

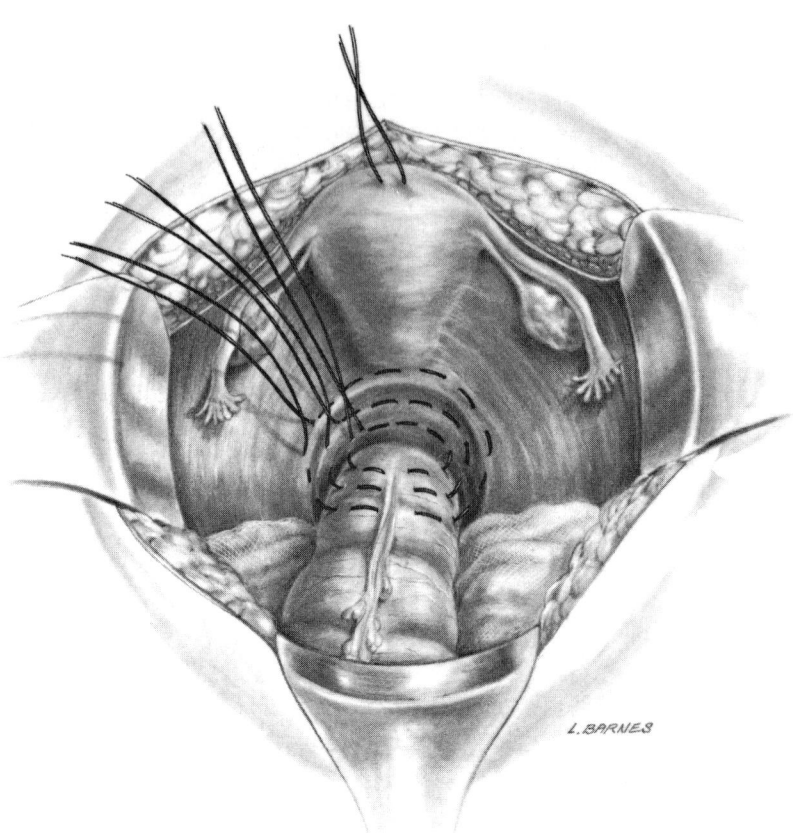

FIGURE 17-26. The Moschcowitz procedure involves the obliteration of the pouch of Douglas by serial purse-string sutures.

Obliteration of the Pouch of Douglas

The Moschcowitz procedure was designed with the theory that the cause of rectal prolapse is a sliding hernia.[132,161] The technique involves the placement of serial purse-string sutures into the floor of the pelvis to obliterate the pouch of Douglas (Figure 17-26). The recurrence rate, however, as reviewed by Theuerkauf and associates, was close to 50%.[233] Although I have had no experience with this technique, the lack of success of others and the theoretical premise on which it is based would seem to imply that the procedure should be abandoned.

Restoration of the Pelvic Floor

Restoration of the pelvic floor by means of plicating of the levators and obliteration of the pouch of Douglas was initially described by Graham in 1942.[83] In subsequent writings, other authors have advocated this operation, either alone or in combination with other modes of surgical therapy.[5,60,61,108,180] The procedure can be accomplished through the abdomen or the perineum (see also Chapter 13) or after removing the coccyx or lower sacrum.[108] Plicatinging the levators transabdominally can be performed anterior or posterior to the rectum, al-

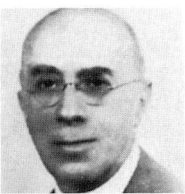

Alexis Victor Moschcowitz (1865–1937) Moschcowitz was born in Giralt, Hungary, and emigrated to the United States at the age of 15. He received a degree in pharmacy in 1885 and then entered the College of Physicians and Surgeons of Columbia University, graduating in 1891. He ultimately joined the staff of Mount Sinai Hospital in New York City and later became Professor of Clinical Surgery at his alma mater. During World War I, Moschcowitz was a consultant in the Surgeon General's Office in Washington, DC. His research as a member of the Empyema Commission resulted in a lowered mortality rate from this condition in soldiers. He contributed extensively to the surgical literature, reporting in 1907 an inguinal approach to femoral herniorrhaphy, a procedure that has come to be known as the Moschcowitz operation.

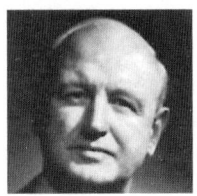

Roscoe Reid Graham (1890–1948) Graham was born in the village of Lobo, near London, Ontario, Canada, the son of a country physician. He received his medical degree at the University of Toronto, and after a year of internship went abroad to do postgraduate work in Great Britain and on the European Continent. He served with the Royal Canadian Medical Corps in England during World War I and returned to resume his practice at Toronto General Hospital, ultimately becoming Director of the Division of Surgery. He is credited with being the first to remove an islet cell tumor of the pancreas, and at the time was the youngest surgeon elected to the American Surgical Association.

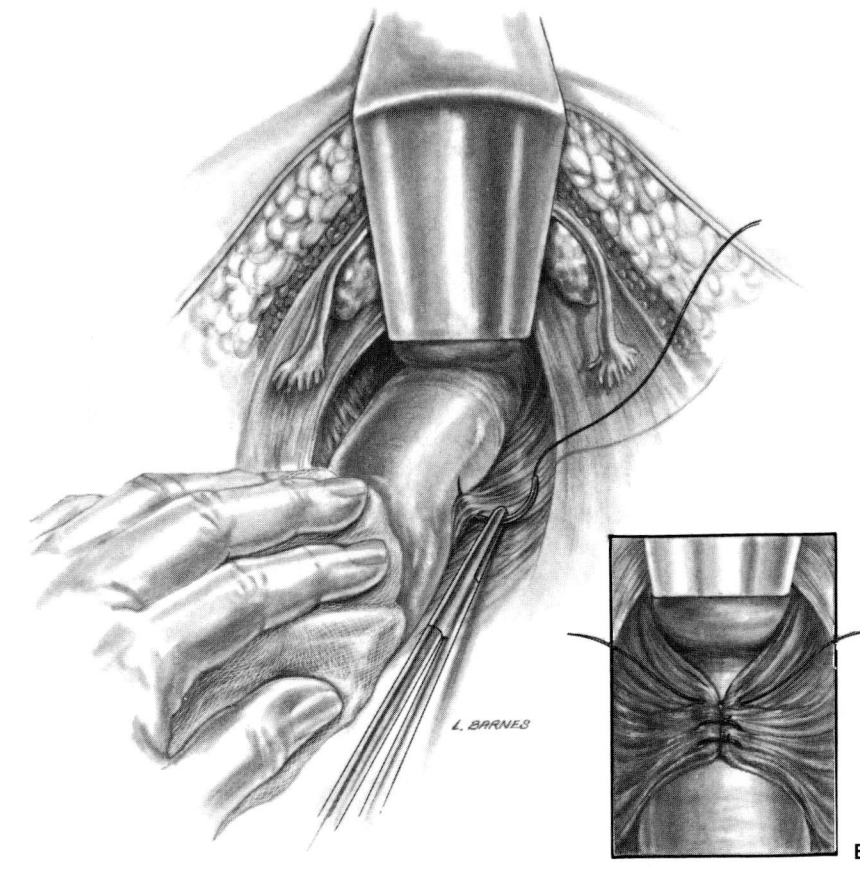

A

FIGURE 17-27. Roscoe Graham operation. **(A)** Reefing of the levator ani muscle is performed transabdominally. A suture is placed into the muscle adjacent to the right lateral aspect of the rectum. **(B)** Reefing or plication is accomplished anterior to the rectum.

B

though the latter may be technically difficult to accomplish (Figure 17-27). When it is employed with sacral fixation or resection, I believe that restoration of the pelvic floor is an unnecessary and often tedious maneuver that does not increase the likelihood of cure. If the physician were to use plication of the levatores as the sole method of treatment for rectal prolapse, the incidence of recurrence would be prohibitively high.

Resection of the Bowel

Anterior Resection

Anterior resection for the treatment of rectal prolapse has many advantages over other techniques, but it also has a number of potential concerns. One major advantage is the removal of the redundant sigmoid colon. This excess bowel can pose a problem with some patients who are to undergo suspension or fixation procedures (see Suspension or Fixation of the Rectum). A mobile sigmoid may predispose to torsion or to volvulus. Furthermore, those who undergo resection may have some bowel complaints ameliorated, especially constipation, if the redundant segment is removed. A sling operation may, however, worsen bowel symptoms, especially abdominal pain and constipation.

The major disadvantage of resection is the possibility of an anastomotic leak, but this risk should be minimal. The technique for performing anterior resection of the bowel is described in Chapter 22. The procedure has also been accomplished through a laparoscopically-assisted approach.[15] It is important to remember that when this operation is performed for prolapse, the rectum should be mobilized to the level of the lateral ligaments, but the anastomosis should be situated at or just below the sacral promontory (Figure 17-28). Mobilization of the rectum in these patients can be accomplished quite easily. The broad, deep pouch of Douglas, with lack of fixation of the rectum, expedites the dissection.

Results

Beahrs and colleagues reported on the treatment of rectal prolapse at the Mayo Clinic in Rochester, Minnesota.[17] Of 118 patients, 28 underwent anterior resection. One operative death occurred, and in one patient prolapse recurred. The cause of recurrence was thought to be a failure to free the rectum down to the level of the levator ani muscle. An updated report from the same institution included a total of 113 patients who underwent anterior resection.[209] This time a rather high recurrence rate was noted (9%), for which there was no ready explanation. A complication was experienced in 29%. Cirocco

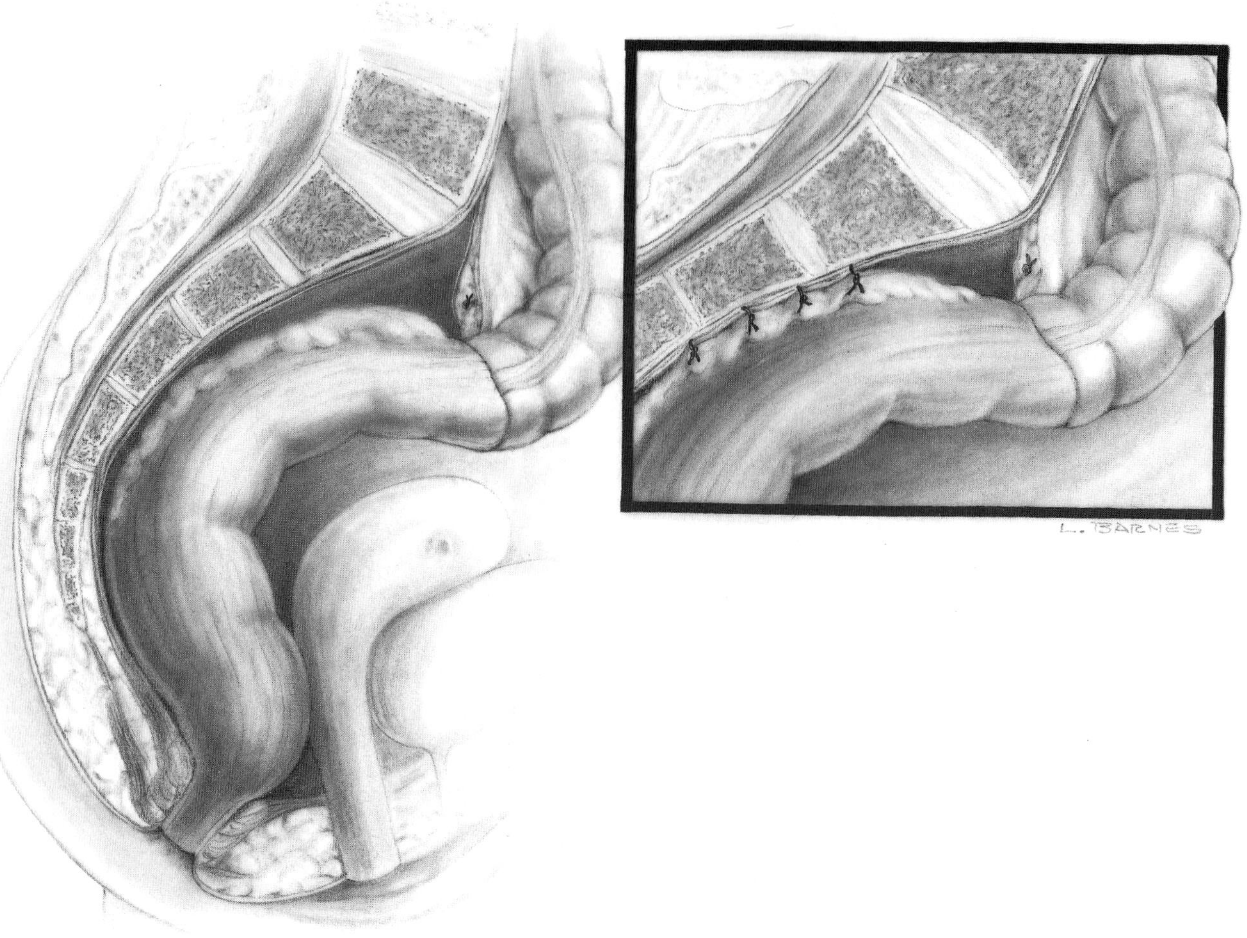

FIGURE 17-28. Anterior resection is performed with anastomosis at or just below the sacral promontory. Sacral fixation can be performed with or without concomitant resection. Sutures are placed directly into the muscularis of the rectum and through the periosteum of the sacrum.

and Brown performed anterior resection on 41 patients following full rectal mobilization down to the levator ani muscles.[44] There was no mortality. With a follow-up averaging 6 years, there was a 7% incidence of recurrence. A 15% morbidity was noted (three incisional hernias and two small bowel obstructions). None of the patients suffered an anastomotic leak.

Anterior Resection With Sacral Fixation

Despite the success of the foregoing operation, dependence on adhesions to fix the rectum posteriorly is unpredictable. Therefore, some authors advise rectal fixation concomitant with anterior resection. The posterior rectal wall or intact lateral ligaments are secured to the sacrum

Howard Martin Frykman (1917–1969) Howard Frykman was born on February 24, 1917 in North Dakota and received his undergraduate and medical school training at the University of Minnesota. He entered medical school but took time out to do research and to obtain a Masters Degree in neuroanatomy. After a 2-year stint in the United States Army, during which time he was wounded in the battle of Guadalcanal, he returned to Minnesota and received his M.D. degree in 1943. He completed his surgical residency at Minnesota and underwent additional training in proctology under the tutelage of Walter Fansler. He joined the University of Minnesota clinical faculty and ultimately achieved the rank of Clinical Professor of Surgery in the Division of Colon and Rectal Surgery. Early in his career he worked with Professor Clarence Dennis to study the role of vagotomy in the treatment of ulcerative colitis. In addition, he had an early interest in procidentia and popularized an intraabdominal repair combining several other previously described techniques. He also studied sepsis associated with bowel surgery and was an early advocate of an intraluminal bowel preparation prior to colonic surgery. He modified the Fansler technique of hemorrhoidectomy by completely closing all anorectal wounds following a submucosal hemorrhoidectomy. Frykman died on October 2, 1969, of a renal tumor. In 1970, the Division of Colon and Rectal Surgery at the University of Minnesota established the Annual Howard M. Frykman Memorial Lecture to honor this pioneer in the specialty. (With appreciation to David A. Rothenberger, M.D.)

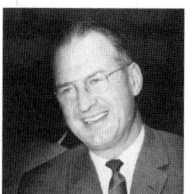

with three or four heavy, nonabsorbable sutures. The redundant sigmoid colon is then removed (Figure 17-28). Frykman and Goldberg described the addition of suture fixation of the anterior rectum to the endopelvic fascia as well as resection and posterior fixation (Figure 17-29).[72] I believe, however, that this is a meddlesome and an unnecessary addition to the technique. However, it is my understanding that the authors have abandoned it and limit the fixation to the sacrum only.

Results

Goldberg initially reported 125 cases using this technique with not a single recurrence.[195] A subsequent review from the same group of surgeons (University of Minnesota) included a follow-up of 102 patients in whom there were two recurrences.[255] When compared with other methods they had employed, the authors believed that not only was the operation eminently successful in curing the prolapse, but it also was much more likely to improve bowel control (see Rectal Prolapse and Fecal Incontinence). Sayfan and colleagues compared sutured posterior abdominal rectopexy and resection with Marlex rectopexy alone.[208] They found that the two procedures were comparable with respect to operative morbidity, curing the prolapse, and improving postoperative bowel control. However, because significantly fewer patients were constipated after the former operation, it seemed to them that this should be the preferred option.

Comment

Despite considerable experience with the Teflon sling repair (see Teflon or Marlex Sling Repair), I have since become much more enthusiastic about anterior resection. I have not found it necessary to suture the rectum or lateral ligaments to the sacrum and have experienced only two recurrences after operating on 117 patients. A particular concern when suturing the rectum to the presacral fascia is the possibility of causing hemorrage (see later). Because the results are so favorable without this

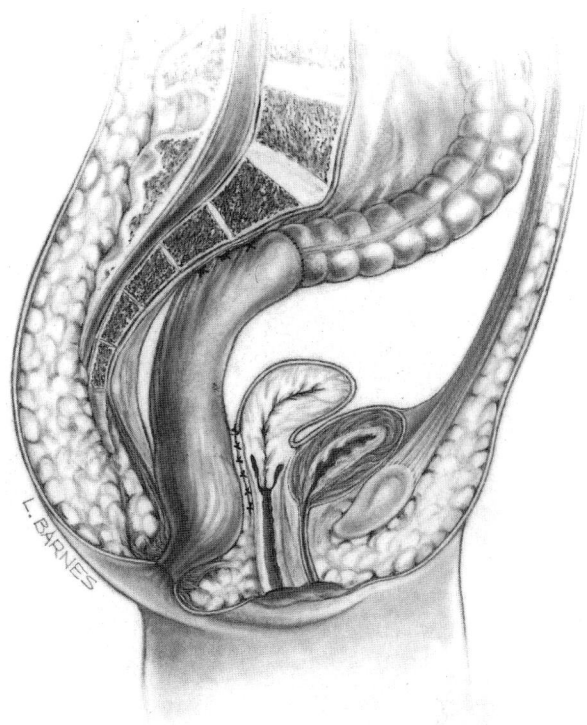

FIGURE 17-29. The rectum is mobilized and elevated, with suture of the lateral rectal stalks to the periosteum of the sacrum. The endopelvic fascia anterior to the rectum is also sutured, with obliteration of the cul-de-sac. The excess peritoneum is excised. (It is believed that the authors no longer apply an anterior fixation.—MLC) (Redrawn from Frykman HM, Goldberg SM. The surgical treatment of rectal procidentia. *Surg Gynecol Obstet* 1969;129:1225.)

added maneuver, it seems prudent to limit this risk. It is not surprising that, because most patients are constipated and are found to have a redundant sigmoid colon, anterior resection should yield optimal functional results.

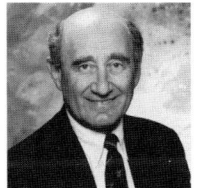

Stanley Morton Goldberg (1932–2003)   Stanley Goldberg was born May 20, 1932 in Minneapolis, Minnesota, the son of a physician. He was at the forefront of colon and rectal surgical education for nearly half a century. Goldberg attended the University of Minnesota for both his undergraduate and medical school education. After an internship at the Minneapolis General Hospital, he completed his general surgical residency training under Owen H. Wangensteen and his colon and rectal surgery training under William C. Bernstein. In 1962, he obtained an American Cancer Society grant in order to study colorectal surgery at St. Mark's Hospital in London. Upon his return to Minnesota, Goldberg joined the clinical faculty in the Division of Colon and Rectal Surgery at the University of Minnesota and in the private practice of Howard M. Frykman. Their partnership led to the publication of the 1969 classic article describing the "Frykman-Goldberg repair" for rectal procidentia. Following the retirement of Bernstein in 1972, Goldberg was appointed Chief of the Division of Colon and Rectal Surgery at the University of Minnesota. Under his leadership, the practice grew to become the largest colorectal specialty group in the world. He led the Division over the next 20 years as it evolved into a unique "town-gown" collaborative model for training of colorectal surgical residents, an environment combining a large, community-based surgical practice with a major teaching and research, university practice. International recognition for promoting the training of specialists in colon and rectal surgery was awarded to Stanley Goldberg by many surgical organizations from around the world, including Australia, Canada, Chile, England, France, Ireland, Mexico, the Philippines, and Scotland. In 2000, the University of Minnesota established the Stanley M. Goldberg Chair in Colon and Rectal Surgery in his honor. (With appreciation to David A. Rothenberger, M.D.)

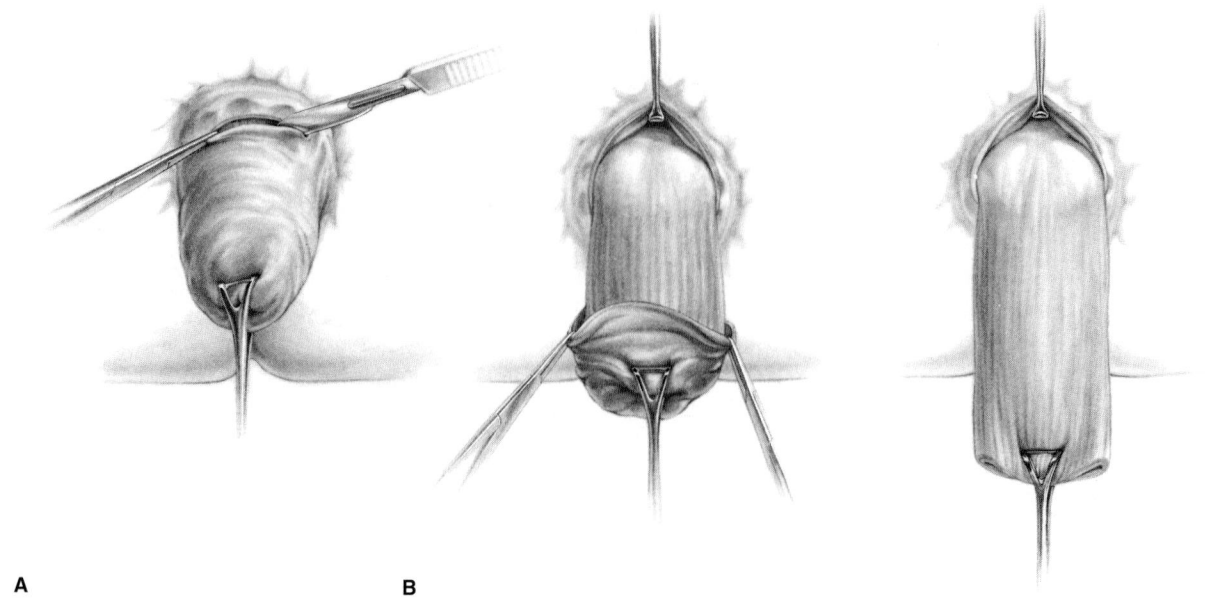

A   B   C

FIGURE 17-30. Altemeier procedure. **(A)** An incision is made circumferentially in the anal canal, just above the dentate line. **(B,C)** The rectum is mobilized and completely everted.

Perineal Procedures

Perineal resection of the prolapse, an operation that has been employed for more than 100 years, is a relatively simple means of addressing the problem. Unfortunately, the relatively high rate of recurrence (up to 25%) has dissuaded many surgeons from adopting this approach.[102] It may, however, be uniquely applicable in the rare instance of gangrene of the prolapsed bowel or even preferred when the patient is at an increased risk if a laparotomy is contemplated. The possibilities of anastomotic leak and stricture are still concerns, but with avoidance of tension on the suture line and attention to preservation of the blood supply, the risk should be minimal.

Altemeier Operation

Altemeier and Culbertson developed a modification of the perineal resection.[4,5] They advocated the operation with the patient placed in the lithotomy stirrups. Although this is the position that is illustrated in this text, my own preference is to place the patient in the prone jackknife position on the operating table. This permits one's assistants to be involved in the procedure and to offer the needed help. The prolapse is exteriorized, and its apex is grasped with clamps (Figure 17-30A). A circumferential incision is made through all layers of the outer bowel wall 1 cm proximal to the mucocutaneous junction (Figure 17-30A). When the circumferential incision is completed, clamps are reapplied to the distal edge of rectum (Figure 17-30B), and the prolapse is delivered as a single loop of exteriorized bowel (Figure 17-30C). With a deep pouch of Douglas, it is usually quite straightforward to enter the peritoneal cavity by incising the periteum anteriorly (Figure 17-31A). The redundant colon is delivered through the defect (Figure 17-31B). The peritoneum is ultimately repaired using a continuous suture to obliterate the sac, excising redundant peritoneum (if necessary), analogous to that of the technique employed for that of a sliding hernia (Figure 17-32).

A modification has been adopted for this procedure (in addition to the position of the patient) that involves plication of the levator ani muscle. This maneuver is thought by some to be associated with a lower incidence of recurrence and may have an ameliorative effect on

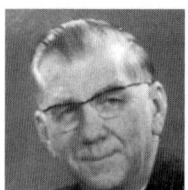

William Arthur Altemeier (1910–1983) Altemeier was born in Cincinnati, Ohio, the son of a railroad employee. He attended the University of Cincinnati, receiving a Bachelor of Science degree in 1930 and his doctorate in medicine 3 years later. After a surgical residency at Henry Ford Hospital in Detroit, Michigan and a period as an associate surgeon, he returned to Cincinnati General Hospital as an instructor. He rose to become Professor and Chairman of the Department of Surgery in 1952, positions he retained for 26 years. Altemeier was a member of at least 38 surgical societies, serving as president of ten of them, including the American College of Surgeons and the American Surgical Association. He developed a special interest in surgical infections and became one of the world authorities in this discipline. However, it is the management of procidentia with which his name is eponymously associated.

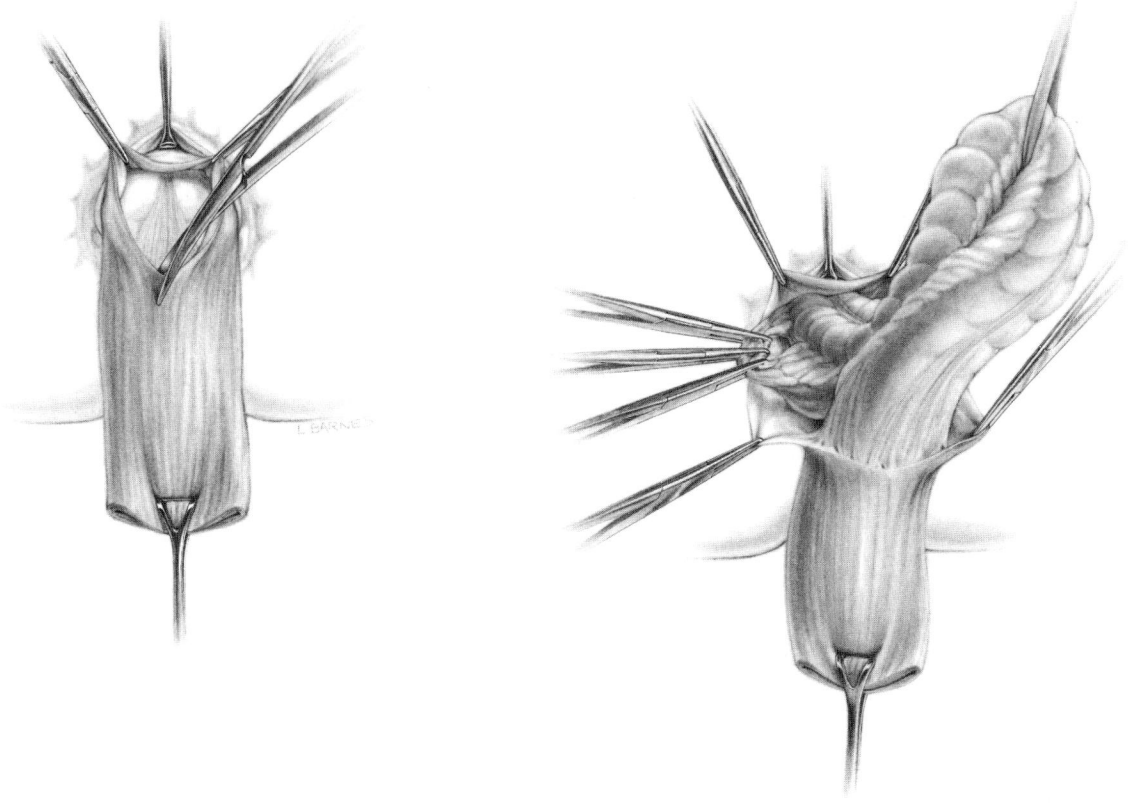

A

B

FIGURE 17-31. Altemeier procedure. **(A)** The peritoneal reflection is identified and opened. **(B)** Any redundant bowel is delivered through the peritoneal defect.

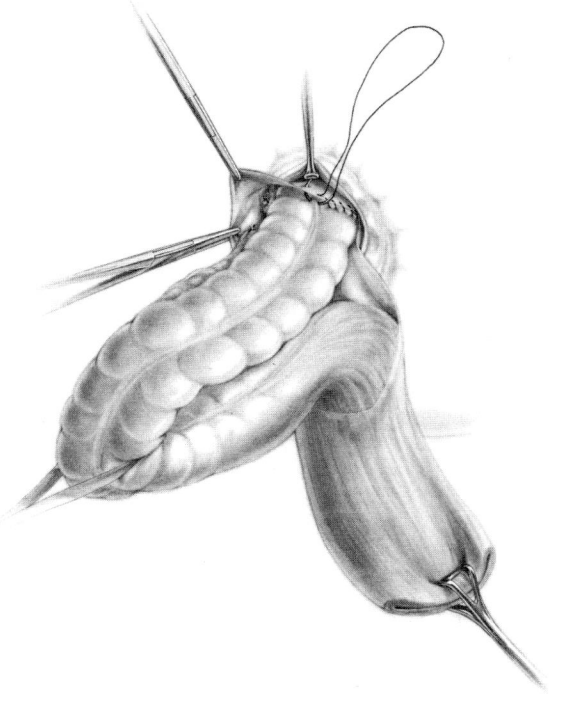

FIGURE 17-32. Altemeier procedure: the peritoneum is closed, and the sutures are anchored to the bowel wall as illustrated.

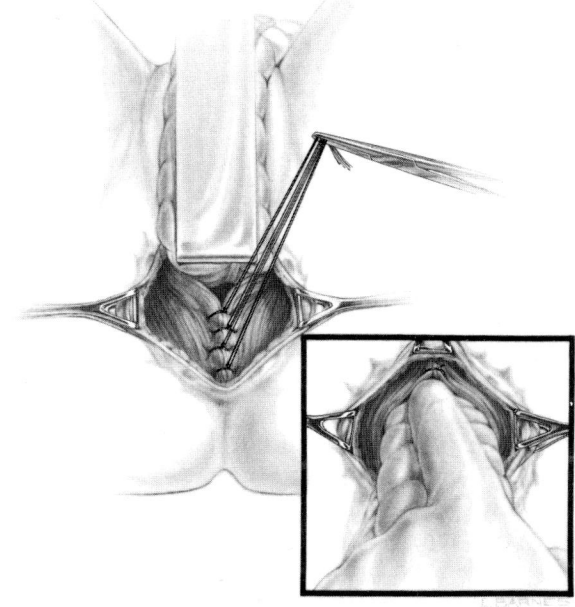

FIGURE 17-33. Altemeier procedure: the levator ani muscle is reefed anteriorly or, as illustrated, posteriorly, with long-term absorbable sutures. Care should be taken to avoid narrowing the rectum. A finger should be able to pass easily through the defect **(inset)**.

problems with bowel control.[43] The levator ani muscles are identified and plicated anterior or posterior to the bowel with interrupted long-term absorbable sutures (Figure 17-33). This eliminates the large defect in the pelvic diaphragm. The redundant intestine is then divided in half by anterior and posterior incisions carried to the point of the proposed resection (Figure 17-34). The intestine is transected obliquely and progressively, completing the anastomosis of the intestinal wall to the distal rectum/anal ring in each quadrant (Figure 17-34). The anastomosis is effected with an interrupted long-term absorbable suture technique; no drains are used. Others have successfully used the circular stapler for reestablishment of continuity.[18]

In principle, one ideally obliterates the pelvic pouch, plicates the levatores, and resects the redundant bowel. However, the rectum is not usually fixed to the sacrum.

Results Despite the successful experience of some authors, the relatively complex technique and the unfamiliar approach dissuade most surgeons from attempting this operation. Altemeier and colleagues reported on their results with 106 patients; three developed recurrences.[6] Gopal and colleagues noted only one failure with 18 elderly, debilitated individuals so treated.[80] Kimmins and co-workers performed the modified Altemeier procedure on 63 patients (mean age, 79 years), noting an overall recurrence rate of 6.4% (median follow-up, 20.8 months).[124] So benign is this operation for most patients that, in their experience, almost two thirds were discharged *the day of surgery*.

Others have described similarly favorable results with the addition of a posterior levator plication.[192] The Cleveland Clinic Florida group compared the outcomes of perineal rectosigmoidectomy with and without levatorplasty

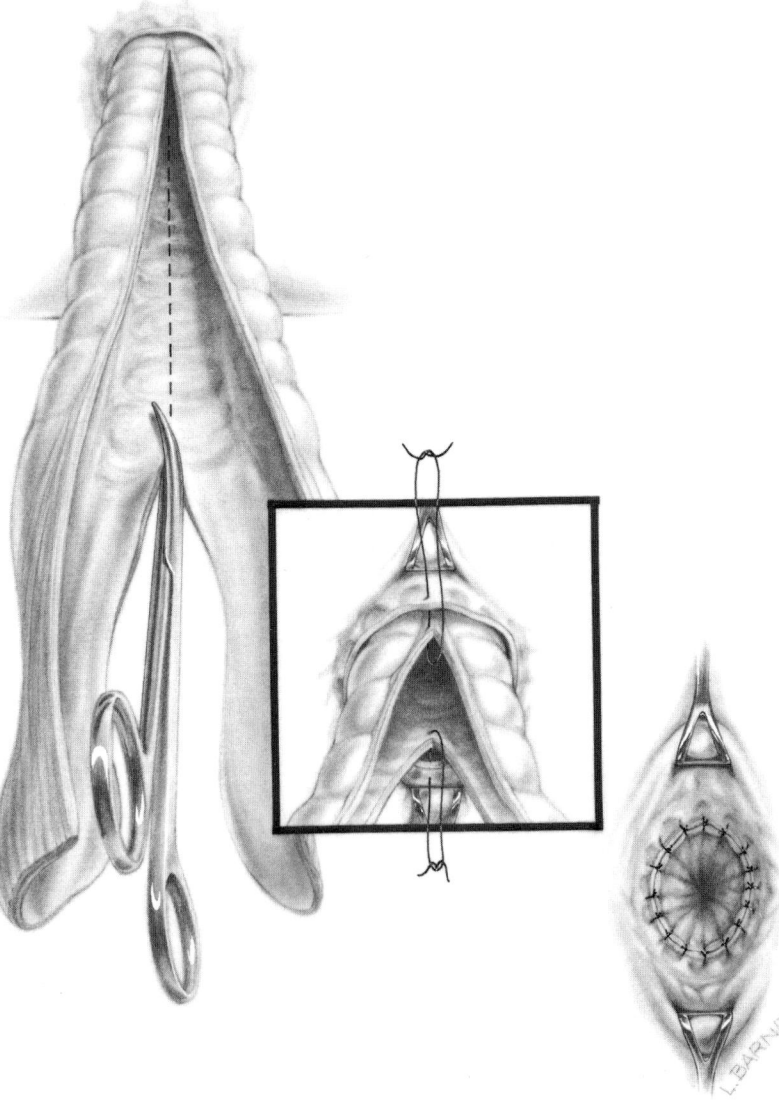

FIGURE 17-34. Altemeier procedure: the redundant bowel is incised longitudinally and sutured in the anterior and posterior midline to the residual cuff of the anal mucosa **(inset)**. After the redundant bowel is trimmed, interrupted sutures are placed between the anal canal and the underlying internal sphincter to the full thickness of the rectum.

in 109 patients.[43] Recurrence rates and mean time to recurrence were 20.6% and 13.3 months when rectosigmoidectomy alone was performed. When levatorplasty was added, the recurrence rate was 7.7%, and mean time to recurrence increased to 45.5 months.

However, Friedman and associates considered the Altemeier operation unsatisfactory.[71] In 27 patients, 50% experienced recurrence. When incontinence is discussed in publications, it seems that better functional results are achieved with concomitant levator plication than with proctosigmoidectomy alone.[1,194,257] The Cleveland Clinic Florida group noted that a prolonged PNTML was not shown to be an accurate predictor of postoperative incontinence nor was there a statistically significant difference in functional outcome, both groups having marked improvement in continence scores.[43,109] In the experience of the University of Minnesota group with 114 patients treated by perineal rectosigmoidectomy, a 10% incidence of recurrence was observed.[257] Ramanujam and co-workers performed this operation on 72 elderly, high-risk patients, nine of whom presented with acute, incarcerated rectal prolapse.[194] Their recurrence rate was 5.5%. In another report from the same group, eight elderly patients were treated for acute incarcerated prolapse, half of whom developed gangrene.[193] There were two anastomotic leaks (25%). There were, however, no deaths. Deen and colleagues performed a randomized trial, comparing anterior resection and rectopexy with perineal rectosigmoidectomy.[49] Pelvic floor repair was undertaken in both groups. There were no recurrences in the ten individuals who comprised the former group, but there was one after treatment by the latter method (10%). The abdominal operation was believed to be associated with better functional and physiologic results.

Vermeulen and associates reported another approach to perineal rectosigmoidectomy without levator plication by the use of the circular stapling device (Figure 17-35).[252] In nine women (mean age, 79 years), they noted no significant complications and no recurrences. They believed that this technique is the procedure of choice in the elderly, poor-risk patient.

Comment Perineal rectosigmoidectomy has become for me the standard operation in the elderly patient, especially someone who is at significant risk for a major abdominal operation. I fully recognize that the operation has a much higher incidence of recurrence (I quote 20% to my patients), but in this special group of individuals I believe that this is not an unreasonable compromise. If recurrence develops, the bowel may be resected again by the same approach. A real concern arises, however, if the surgeon plans an abdominal operation for recurrence following this operation. Resection is very dangerous indeed because of the risk of a devascularization injury to the distal bowel unless the surgeon performs a coloanal anastomosis. Therefore, a reasonable option if a laparotomy is undertaken with this history is to perform some type of suspension or fixation.

Delorme Procedure

The Delorme operation had not been commonly applied for many years since its original 1900 description but has reemerged as a good choice for the treatment of *mucosal prolapse* and as an alternative approach for managing full-thickness rectal prolapse.[51,240] The dissection may be facilitated by employing the suggestions of Sullivan and Garnjobst and Berman and colleagues.[21,226] With the patient in the lithotomy or the prone jackknife position, a circumferential incision is made 1 cm proximal to the dentate line, similar to that for the Altemeier procedure (Figure 17-36*A*). The bowel is not divided, however. This is a submucosal dissection with a mucosal stripping (Figure 17-36*B*). Using electrocautery, the mucosa is stripped to the apex of the protruding bowel. Dissection may be facilitated by infiltrating the submucosa with saline or a dilute epinephrine solution. Some have advocated the use of the Cavitron Ultrasonic Surgical Aspirator for the dissection (Extra-Corporeal Medical Specialties, King of Prussia, PA).[86] The redundant mucosa is excised, and the denuded muscularis propria is pleated longitudinally, collapsing the bowel like an accordion (Figure 17-37). The edges of the mucosa are then sutured. Alternatively, the mucosa-muscularis layers can be directly reapproximated in a circumferential fashion with multiple interrupted absorbable sutures.[86]

Complications from this operation are common and include hemorrhage, hematoma, suture line dehiscence, stricture, incontinence, and, of course, recurrence.

(text continues on page 30)

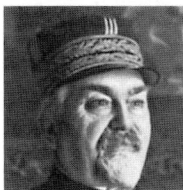

Edmond Delorme (1847–1929) Delorme was born in Lunéville, France, the son of a cabinetmaker. He demonstrated an interest in military sciences and enrolled in the medical military school at Strasbourg in 1866. He followed the army in its battles throughout Europe and North Africa, and in 1877 Delorme was named Professor of Operative Medicine at Val-de-Grace, and ultimately, Professor of Clinical Surgery. He was the director of a number of hospitals and introduced the concept of antisepsis into French military medicine. In 1903, he became head of all the health services of the French Army. A highly influential surgeon, he was elected successively President of the French Academy of Medicine, the Society of Surgery, and the Society of Military Medicine. He also held the title of Grand Officer of the Legion of Honor. His contributions to surgery were in the treatment of war injuries, fractures, lung decortication, and rectal surgery. In his publication of the operation for rectal prolapse that bears his name, Delorme reported three patients, one of whom died.

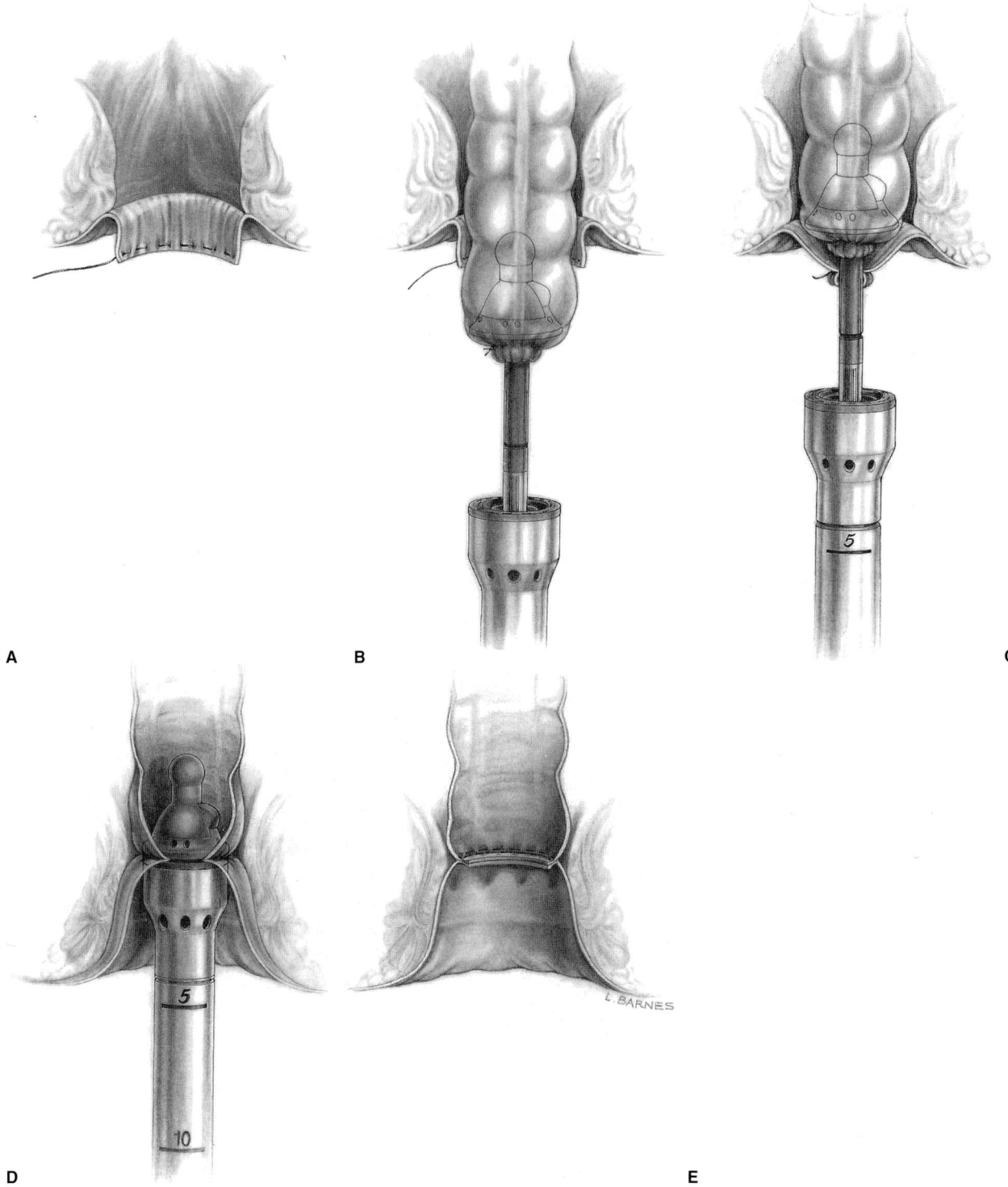

A   **B**   **C**

D   **E**

FIGURE 17-35. Perineal proctosigmoidectomy with circular stapler. **(A)** Purse-string sutures to the proximal and distal bowel after perineal resection. **(B)** The proximal segment is secured over the anvil. **(C)** The distal segment is secured. **(D)** The instrument is closed and fired. **(E)** Completed anastomosis. (Adapted from Vermeulen FD, Nivatvongs S, Fang DT, et al. A technique for perineal rectosigmoidectomy using autosuture devices. *Surg Gynecol Obstet* 1983;156:85, with permission.)

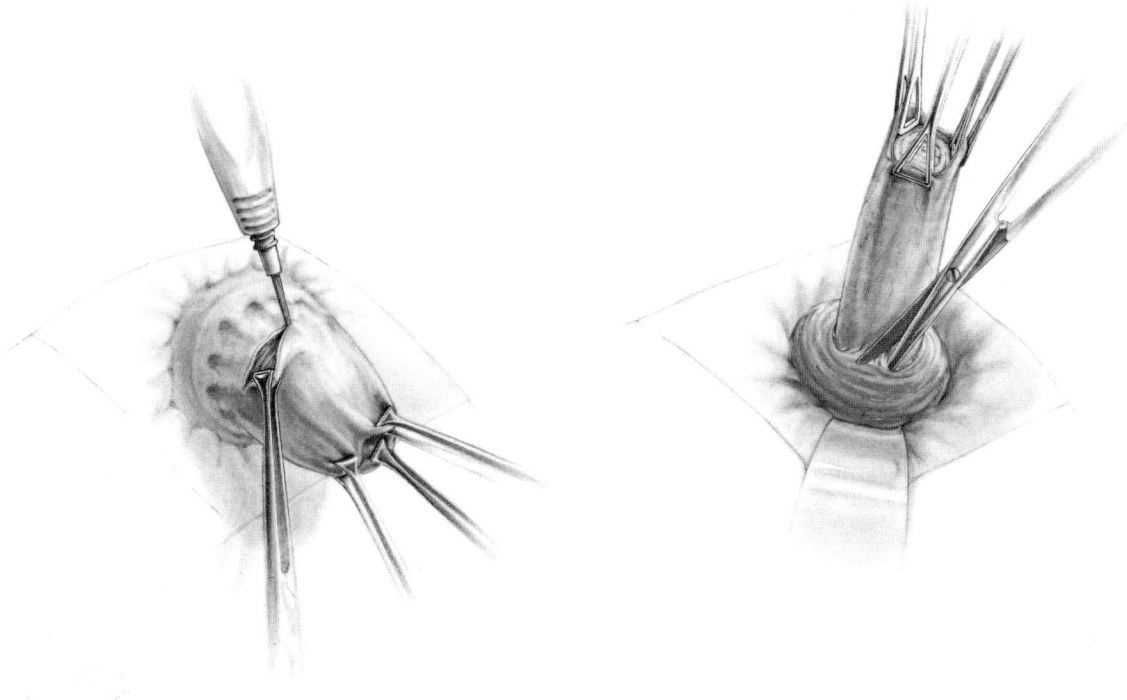

A   **B**

FIGURE 17-36. Delorme procedure. **(A)** The mucosa is circumferentially incised above the dentate line. **(B)** Submucosal stripping is carried out as far cephalad as is possible.

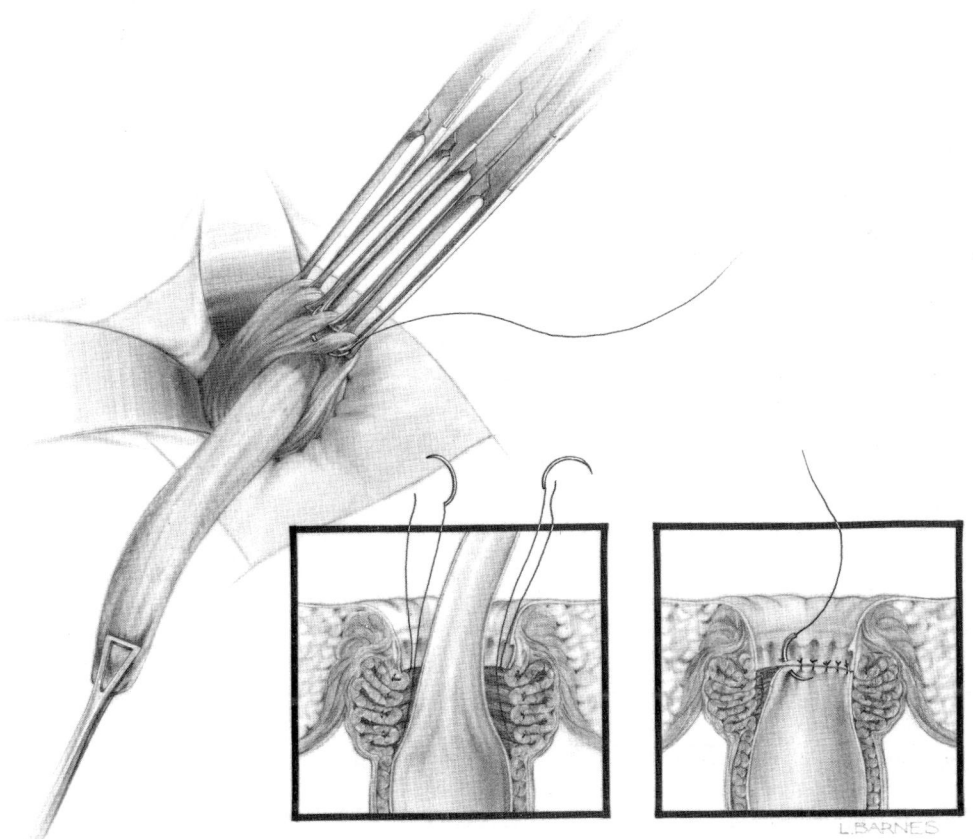

FIGURE 17-37. The circular muscle of the rectum is prepared for suturing by the placement of serial Allis clamps. Plication is carried out using 2–0 long-term absorbable sutures. The insets illustrate the completed "anastomosis" after the redundant mucosa has been amputated. (Adapted from Berman IR, Harris MS, Rabeler MB. Delorme's transrectal excision for internal prolapse: patient selection, technique, and three-year follow-up. *Dis Colon Rectum* 1990;33:573, with permission.)

The application of the stapler in performing mucosectomy for the treatment of hemorrhoids seems an ideal instrument for dealing with mucosal prolapse (see Chapter 8). Experience is just beginning to emerge with this alternative.

Results It is difficult to interpret the results of this operation, because those who have reported their experience often employ this option for the treatment of mucosal prolapse rather than true procidentia. In 30 patients treated by Nay and Blair, a 10% incidence of incontinence or recurrence was noted.[166] Uhlig and Sullivan have been quite enthusiastic about this technique, reporting only three failures in 44 patients—an incidence of less than 7%.[245] McCaffrey recommended this approach after a failed Ripstein operation.[153] He reported good results in three patients. Gundersen and colleagues noted "significant complications" in 17% of 18 patients so treated.[86]

The St. Mark's Hospital experience was published in 1994.[213] Only 32 operations were performed between 1978 and 1990. There was no mortality and one anastomotic dehiscence. With a mean follow-up of 24 months, there were four recurrences (12.5%). Approximately one half noted improved bowel control. The operation was recommended on so-called "unfit patients." Oliver and associates analyzed their experience of 41 patients who underwent this procedure.[178] This operation was selected when advanced age and/or poor health mitigated against an abdominal operation. The mean age was 82 years. They noted a 22% recurrence rate. One patient died, and minor complications were seen in 25%. The authors observed the importance of an adequate mucosectomy.[178] Others suggest also that elderly patients, those with failed prior prolapse procedures, and those with prior pelvic surgery or radiation should be considered for this procedure.[125,153]

Lechaux and co-workers reviewed their 85 patients who underwent this operation.[138] Their complication rate was 14%, with one death. The recurrence rate was 13.5% with approximately two thirds achieving improved bowel control. Plusa and colleagues evaluated physiologic changes following this procedure in 19 women.[190] There were no significant changes in anal sphincter pressures, but there was observed a decrease in the volume required for first rectal sensation as well as a decline in the maximum tolerated rectal volume. Furthermore, rectal compliance was reduced in addition to improved rectal sensation. Vachon and associates employed the procedure on 25 elderly patients with complex medical problems who were not candidates for a major abdominal operation.[246] All were undertaken with a local anesthetic supplemented by intravenous sedation. There were two recurrences (9.5%) and one operative death. Tsunoda and colleagues noted a 13% recurrence rate in their 31 patients (median follow up, 39 months).[244A] They also performed

physiologic assessment and found a statistically significant improvement in squeeze pressures, volume at first sensation, and maximum tolerable volume. The preoperative incontinence score improved from 11.5 to 6.0 (*p* < .0001). Watts and Thompson performed the Delorme procedure on 101 patients with "full-thickness rectal prolapse" and followed them for more than 1 year.[254] Thirty-eight had no recurrence, 33 died without recurrence and 30 developed a recurrence (30%).

Opinion Most surgeons are reluctant to consider this operation because of the cumbersome dissection and the high recurrence rate. Personally, I find the Delorme alternative tedious and, in my hands, floridly unsuccessful in those individuals with true procidentia. Even with surgeons who are the most experienced and the most enthusiastic, it is my opinion that the operation cannot possibly be as effective as the previously discussed Altemeier procedure for resecting a large (full-thickness) prolapse. These same respected surgeons could logically conclude that I do not know how to do the operation properly. I will not argue the point. I will affirm, however, that for mucosal prolapse I believe the operation to be a reasonable choice. In the poor-risk individual, this approach may be a quite acceptable alternative for some surgeons. There may even be a theoretical advantage in its contributing to improved bowel control through the creation of a "pseudosphincter" brought about by the plication of the muscularis. Still, I am not prepared to adopt this operation for a large prolapse.

Gant-Miwa Procedure

For an operative approach that is virtually unheard of in the West, it is interesting to note that the Gant-Miwa procedure is the most common surgical option employed for the treatment of rectal prolapse in Japan.[263] The concept is simply the placement of 20 to 40 absorbable sutures that incorporate the mucosa and submucosa, thereby creating tags or lumps from the apex of the prolapsed rectum to 1 cm from the dentate line.[263] The sutures should be placed at least 5 mm apart in order to avoid mucosal ulceration or necrosis. Gant introduced the procedure in Japan in the 1920s, but the recurrence rate was prohibitively high. Miwa suggested combining the operation with an anal encirclement to reduce the likelihood of recurrence. Still, even with the combined operation (i.e., the Gant-Miwa Procedure), recurrence rates in the range of approximately 15% are considered acceptable in Japan.[263]

Combined Abdominal and Perineal Operation

Dunphy reported a combined abdominal and perineal operation for rectal prolapse.[60] The perineal operation is essentially the same as that described by Altemeier and colleagues.[5,6] The abdominal operation, however, is accomplished several days later. Full mobilization of the rectum is carried out, and a plication of the ligamentous structures lateral to the rectum is performed. The pouch of Douglas is obliterated in the manner of Moschcowitz. Dunphy described this technique and results of treatment in four patients; no recurrence was noted.

Comment

This is an extensive operation requiring two major procedures. Although the belt-and-suspenders approach may be useful under some circumstances, there are simpler and equally reliable alternatives. The issue is undoubtedly moot because there have been no published reports in many years.

Transsacral Resection

The transsacral operation uses the approach to the rectum described by Kraske for resection of rectal cancer (see Chapter 23).[126] This procedure has been advocated by Davidian and Thomas and by Jenkins and Thomas.[48,108]

An incision is made overlying the sacrum and coccyx, and the latter is disarticulated and removed. The levator ani muscles are divided to expose the rectum. The peritoneum is incised anteriorly and the rectum fully mobilized. The redundant colon is liberated and delivered through the sacral wound (Figure 17-38A). The levator ani muscles are approximated anterior to the rectum (Figure 17-38B), the peritoneum is closed, and resection of the redundant bowel is carried out. After the anastomosis is completed, all wounds are primarily closed.

The theoretical advantages of this procedure are that the operation does not require a laparotomy and that the levator ani muscles are reconstituted, thus narrowing the defect in the pelvic floor. The pouch of Douglas is obliterated, and the rectum is secured posteriorly. The major disadvantage is that the patient has a painful sacrococcygeal wound that is subject to infection. The possibility of a fecal fistula, although not noted by Davidian and Thomas, is well recognized when this procedure has been undertaken for other indications. The authors reported 30 patients who underwent this operative approach; neither mortality nor recurrence occurred.[48]

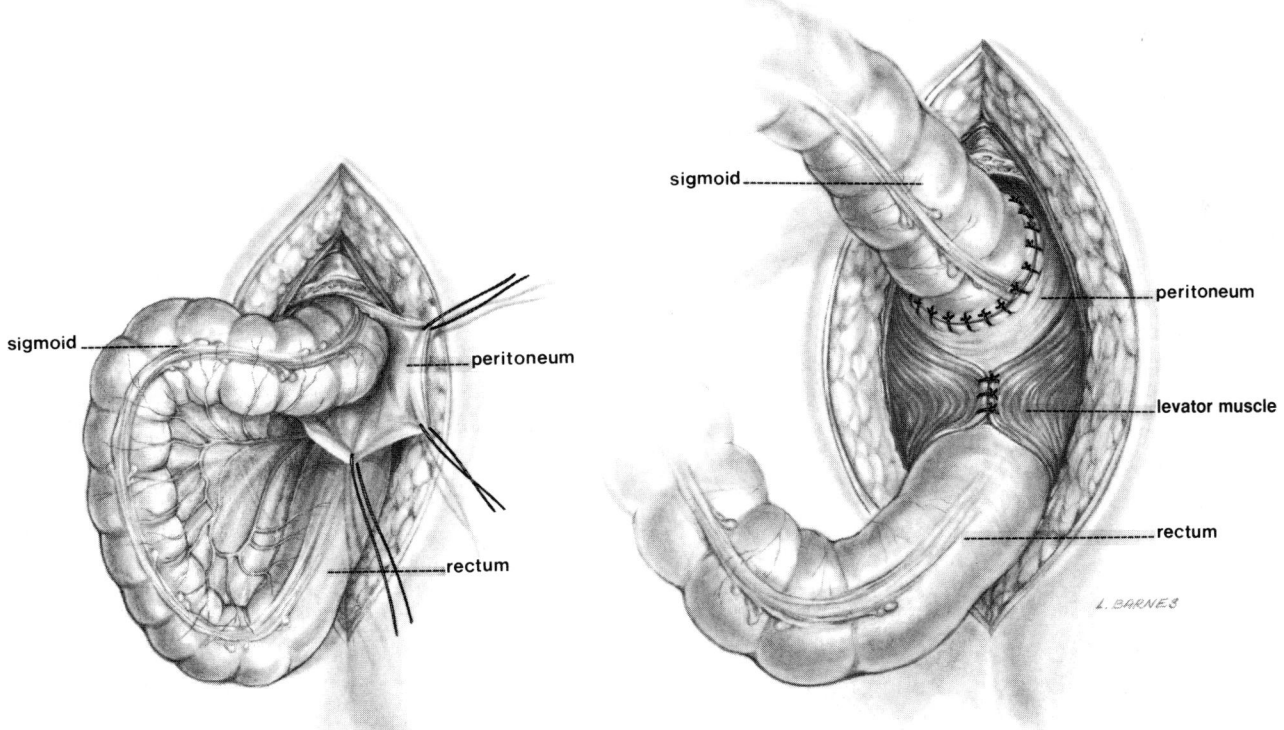

A   **B**

FIGURE 17-38. Thomas operation. **(A)** The hernial sac is identified anteriorly and opened, and the redundant sigmoid is delivered. **(B)** The hernial sac is excised and the floor of the pelvis reconstituted by suturing the seromuscular layer of the proximal bowel to the peritoneum. The levator ani muscle is plicated anterior to the rectum. The bowel is resected and an anastomosis is performed in the conventional way (not shown).

Comment

As with other procedures for the treatment of this condition, the esoteric, unfamiliar operation described earlier contraindicates its use for most surgeons, particularly in light of the simpler alternatives available for cure. Here also there have been no published reports of its use in a number of years.

Suspension or Fixation of the Rectum

Teflon or Marlex Sling Repair (Ripstein Operation)

Arguably the most common surgical approach for the treatment of rectal prolapse in the United States today is the sling repair, a procedure that was described initially by Ripstein in 1965, and is often called by his name.[198] The sling may be made out of Teflon, Marlex, or Gortex.

Technique

The patient is placed in the Trendelenburg position on the operating table, and a midline hypogastric incision is made. Exploration of the abdomen usually reveals the characteristic defect of redundant sigmoid colon, lack of fixation of the rectum to the sacrum, and a deep pouch of Douglas. The rectosigmoid is mobilized, usually without difficulty, with care taken to avoid injury to the ureters. The presacral space is entered, and the *inferior mesenteric vessels are carefully preserved*. Mobilization of the rectum to the level of the levator ani muscle can be accomplished easily. This is a particularly important maneuver that facilitates adhesion or passive fixation of the rectum to the sacrum. I suspect that if nothing more than mobilization were done, 50% to 60% of the patients would be cured by this maneuver alone.

Securing the Teflon mesh (or Marlex or Gore-Tex) to the sacrum can be accomplished in one of three ways. Sutures can be placed into the periosteum of the sacrum approximately 1 cm to the right of the midline by using a half circle Mayo trocar-point needle. Three or four nonabsorbable sutures are used (Figure 17-39A).

The mesh is trimmed to approximately 4 cm wide and secured in place along the right side of the sacrum (Fig-

ure 17-39B). At this point in the operation, it is important for the assistant to maintain proximal traction while the mesh is anchored to the muscularis propria of the rectum. If the rectum is not under cephalad tension and if redundant rectum is left below the mesh, a prolapse will recur. Nonabsorbable sutures are placed from the mesh into the rectal wall (Figure 17-39C). After the mesh has been laid around two thirds of the bowel, the redundant material is appropriately trimmed so that it can be secured without tension (Figure 17-39D). Sutures are then anchored in the sacrum on the left side and placed into the mesh. An approximately 1-cm defect is present posteriorly (Figure 17-39E). The remaining sutures on the left side are placed through the mesh and in the muscularis of the bowel (Figure 17-39F).

Another method of securing the mesh is to place a single row of sutures into the midline of the sacrum. The middle of the mesh is sutured into place and the material brought onto either side of the rectum (Figure 17-40). With proximal traction maintained on the rectum, the mesh is anchored, leaving a 1-cm defect anteriorly (Figure 17-40, *inset*). This is a simpler technique than the former, but it has the potential risk of leaving only a solitary row of sutures posteriorly with which to hold the rectum to the sacrum.

A simpler modification for attaching the mesh to the sacrum has been proposed by Nicosia and Bass.[170] A power fascial stapler was used successfully in 12 patients to accomplish fixation expeditiously and with essentially no risk of inducing hemorrhage (Figure 17-41).

Following suspension, it is not necessary to reperitonealize the floor of the pelvis, but it can be done at the surgeon's discretion. If hemostasis is secure, no pelvic drains are necessary, and with the foreign material the presence of a drain can pose a particular hazard for infection. However, when venous bleeding has been encountered, a closed suction drain may be placed into the pelvis and brought out through a stab wound in the left lower quadrant. This is usually maintained for 2 to 3 days.

Kuijpers and Mollen routinely perform a rectovaginoplasty in patients with complete prolapse, a procedure similar to that discussed earlier in this chapter (Figure

(text continues on page 534)

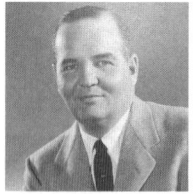

Charles Benjamin Ripstein (1913–2003) Charles Ripstein was born in Winnipeg, Manitoba, Canada, December 13, 1913, one of four children of a whiskey manufacturer. He wished to be an engineer but developed tuberculosis. He moved to Arizona to recuperate and while there attended the University of Tucson. Because of his own illness, he became interested in studying medicine. He then returned to Canada to enter medical school at McGill University, graduating first in his class. One of his classmates was Rupert Turnbull, his lifelong friend. Upon graduation in 1940, he enlisted in the Canadian Air Force as a flight surgeon and flew many bombing missions over Europe. Following the war, he returned to McGill for his surgical residency. His primary interest at that time was cardiothoracic surgery. He accepted a position as Professor of Thoracic Surgery at Downstate Medical Center (Brooklyn, New York) in 1949. During this time he developed an extensive cardiac surgery clinical, teaching, and research program. In 1955 he accepted the position as the first Professor of Surgery at the newly established Albert Einstein College of Medicine (New York) and Chief of General Thoracic Surgery, Brookside and Jacobi Hospitals. During the following decade, he developed a particular interest in colon and rectal surgery and ultimately became a Fellow of the American Society of Colon and Rectal Surgeons. In 1972 he moved to Miami, Florida, where he practiced colon and rectal surgery until he retired in his early eighties. (With appreciation to Linda Ripstein Dresnick, M.D. and Rene F. Hartmann, M.D.)

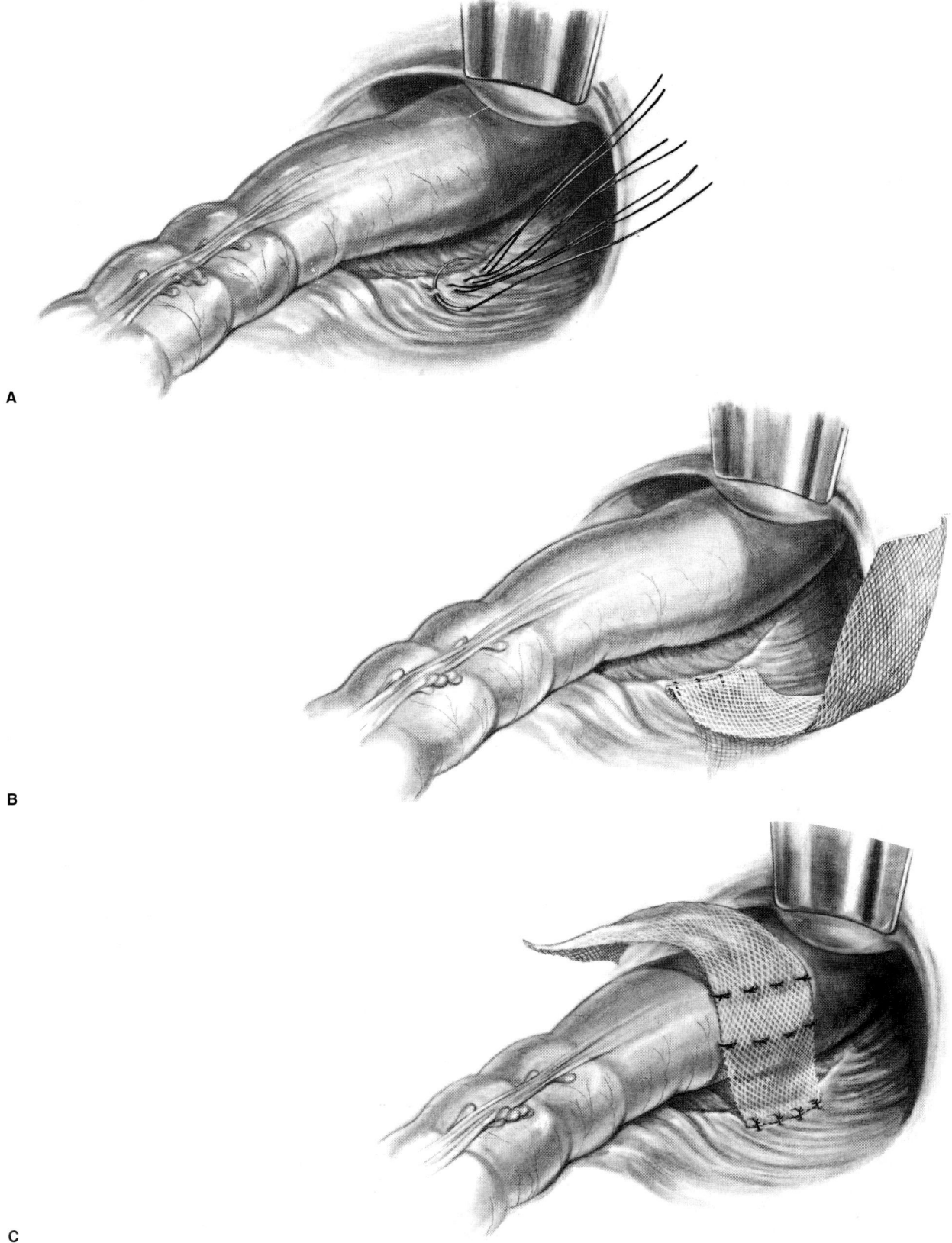

A

B

C

FIGURE 17-39. Teflon sling repair. **(A)** Sutures are placed into the periosteum on the right side of the sacrum. **(B)** The mesh is anchored into place after appropriate trimming. **(C)** With the rectum held under tension, the mesh is sutured to the muscularis of the bowel. **(D)** After the mesh has been placed approximately two thirds of the way around the rectum, it is trimmed so that it can be sutured without tension to the contralateral side of the sacrum. **(E)** The mesh is secured to the sacrum on the left side, leaving a defect of ~1 cm posteriorly. **(F)** A lateral view shows the position of the mesh as secured to the sacrum.

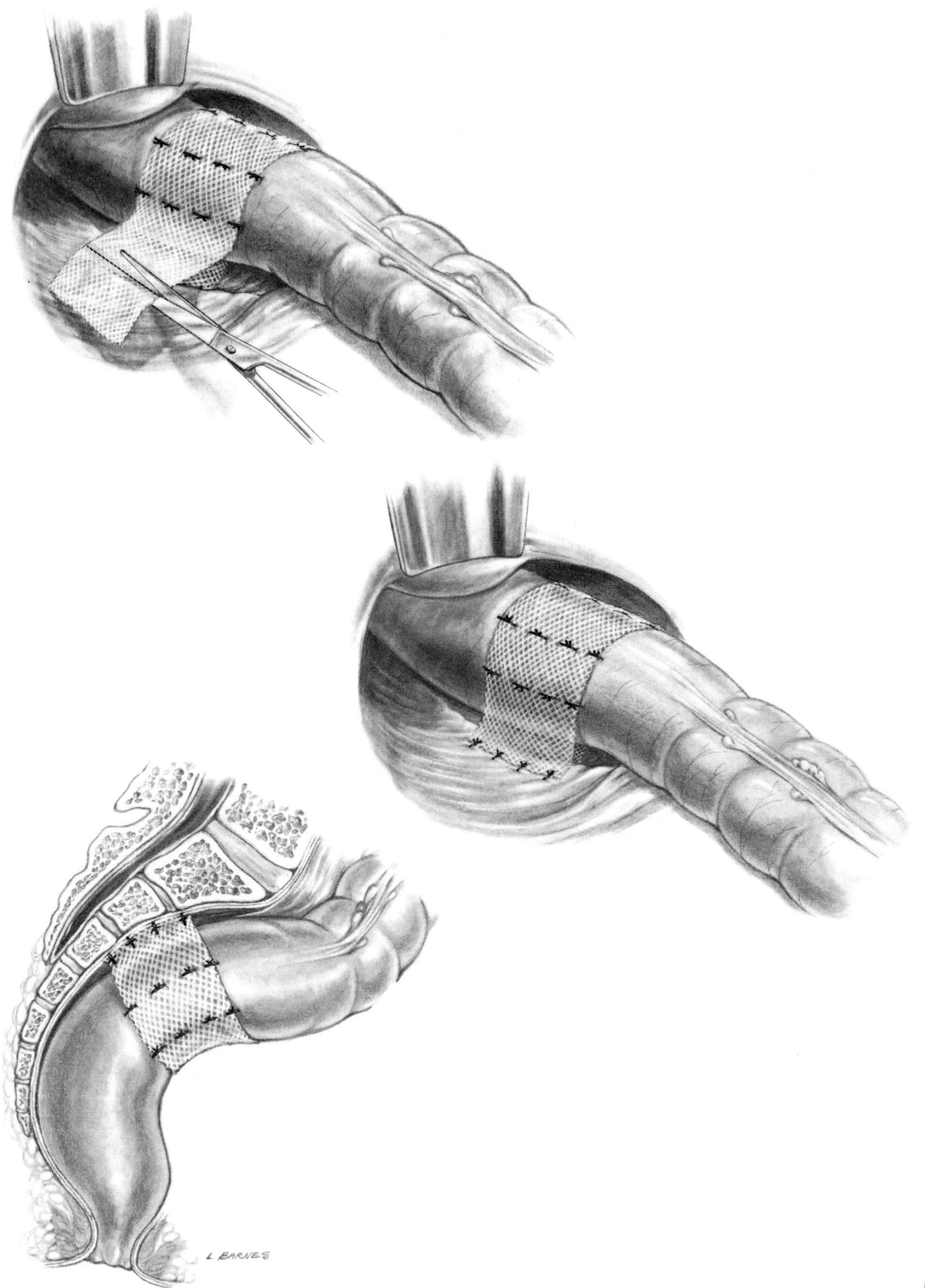

D

E

F

FIGURE 17-39. *(continued)*

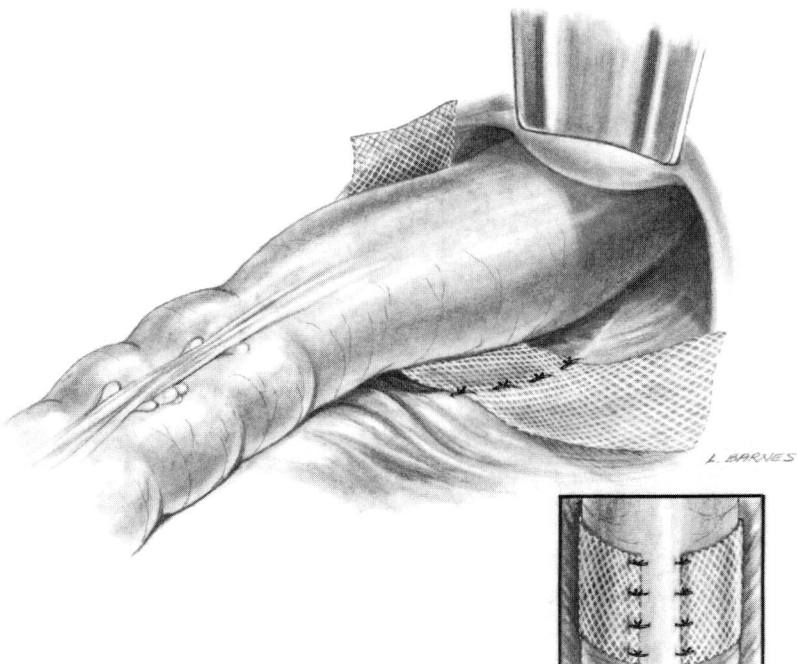

FIGURE 17-40. Alternative method of Teflon sling repair showing position of the mesh sutured in the midline. The mesh is brought around either side of the rectum and sutured to the anterior wall, leaving a defect of ~1 cm anteriorly **(inset)**.

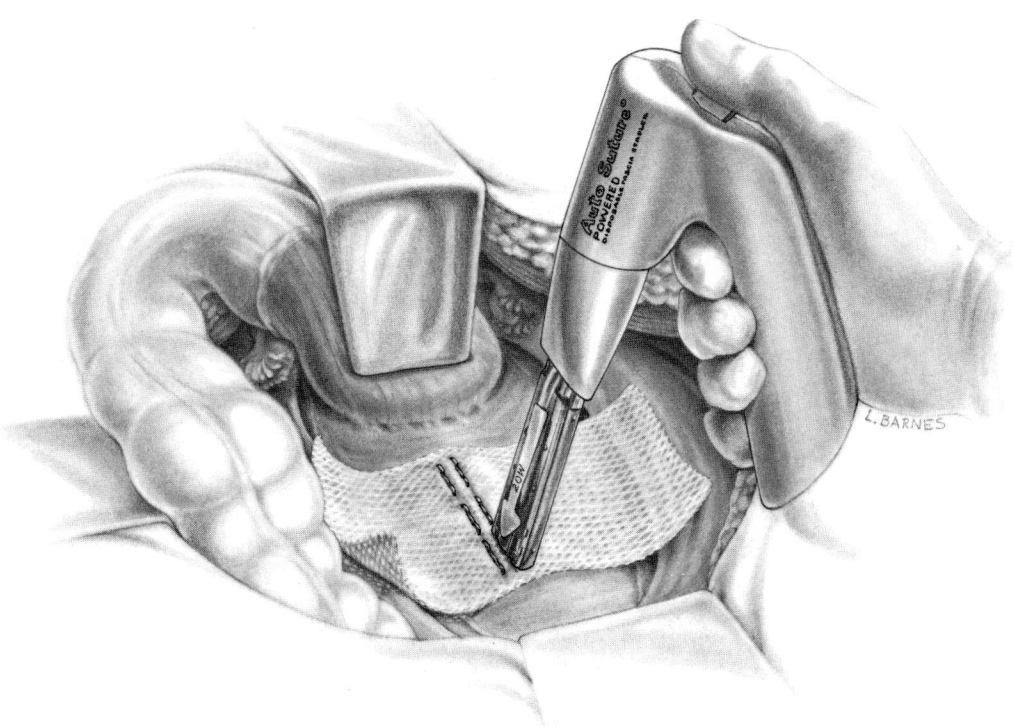

FIGURE 17-41. Securing Teflon mesh to sacrum with power fascial stapler. (Adapted from Nicosia JF, Bass NM. Use of the fascial stapler in proctopexy for rectal prolapse. *Dis Colon Rectum* 1987;30:900, with permission.)

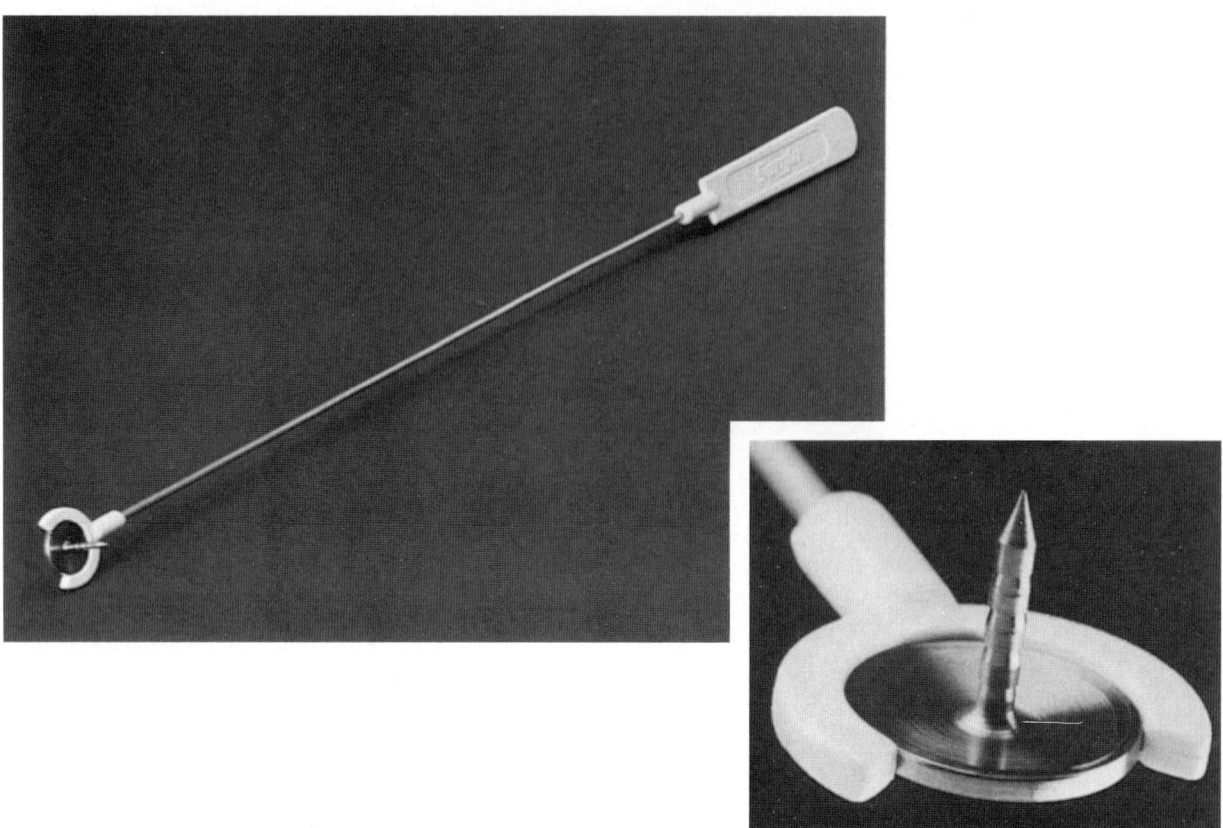

FIGURE 17-42. Titanium, preloaded, Hemorrhage Occluder Pin with applicator. Fingertip pressure is applied to the flat head of the pin until pin is flush with the bony cortex. (Courtesy of Surgin, Placentia, CA.)

17-21).[128] These surgeons believe that the incidence of concomitant genital prolapse is "at least 25%" or will surely develop later. They further emphasize that the pouch of Douglas should be obliterated.

Management of Presacral Hemorrhage

If a presacral vein is entered, the ligature can be tied. All too often, however, the basivertebral vein exits directly from the bone, and massive hemorrhage can ensue. Application of direct pressure to the area with an abdominal pad will usually stop the bleeding, especially if the surgeon leaves the operating room for 10 or 15 minutes while the assistant maintains compression. Dissecting the area in an attempt to visualize the bleeding point only adds to a potentially massive blood loss. Local measures to secure hemostasis include suturing, hemoclips, cauterization, packing, microfibillar collagen (Avitene), and absorbable gelatin sponges (Gelfoam).[31] Another alternative that has been suggested is to occlude the bleeding site with a titanium thumbtack inserted into the bone (Figure 17-42).[120,173] Other methods that have been described to deal with presacral bleeding include the use of the an endoscopic stapling device, a Silastic tissue expander for tamponade, a breast implant sizer, and pressure with a muscle fragment held into position over the bleeding area while indirect coagulation is performed through the muscle ("muscle-fragment welding").[31,47,89,94,262] This last technique involves harvesting a small piece of rectus abdominis muscle. The muscle is held in place over the bleeding site with a forceps while electrocautery at the highest setting is applied to the forceps.[88]

Comment Prevention of the bleeding, however, is obviously preferred. Direct visualization of the presacral space by sharp dissection is less likely to tear the fascia, rather than the blunt, manual maneuver that is all too often employed. Recognizing the welling up of venous blood and immediately applying direct pressure will forestall the needless loss of blood that inevitably occurs when one attempts to identify the bleeding site. With direct pressure, patience and sufficient time the bleeding should stop spontaneously. If it fails to do so, I am attracted to the "welding method," but thus far I have not had the opportunity of trying it.

Postoperative Management

Postoperative management of a sling repair is essentially the same as that for a bowel resection. An indwelling urinary catheter is recommended for several days. Patients are given intravenous fluids until a diet is tolerated. The patient is discharged when the bowel has functioned, usually by the sixth or seventh postoperative day. However, it is not unusual in elderly patients and with those who have concomitant slow intestinal transit to require a more prolonged hospital stay.

Results

Until I adopted the use of anterior resection, the Teflon sling repair had been my primary method for the treatment of rectal prolapse. One half of the patients in our reported experience had prior colorectal operations.[114] Most had undergone anorectal procedures; 20% had multiple operations. With an experience in excess of 100 such operations, the success rate was greater than 95%.[139] Four patients required reoperation, two because of recurrent rectal prolapse and two because of postoperative rectal stricture. One was a young woman in whom recurrent prolapse developed with the vaginal delivery of a child. Subsequent repair was performed without incident. The second person was 80 years old and quite active. The prolapse recurred within 6 weeks after the operation while the patient was building a stone wall and lifting an 80-pound bag of cement.

There were no operative deaths in our experience. On the basis of our initial report on 55 patients, 48 (87%) had an uneventful postoperative course.[114] The morbidity is summarized in Table 17-1.

Sepsis is an unusual complication of Teflon sling repair, but when it occurs, it is an extremely difficult problem to treat. Removal of the mesh inevitably becomes necessary, a technical *tour de force* that may eventuate in a bowel resection. It is primarily because of the risk of entering the bowel during some phase of the procedure that a mechanical preparation is strongly suggested. If the lumen is breached, the surgeon is advised to carry on with a resection rather than risk insertion of the foreign material in a contaminated field.

The mean follow-up period was 46 months in our series, with 35 patients available for evaluation more than 5 years later. Bowel management and incontinence remained persistent problems after the prolapse was corrected. Approximately one third complained of difficulty in regulating bowel function after the repair, and 11% reported incontinence or soiling. Of course, bowel function and incontinence problems are common complaints prior to surgical intervention. The habits of excessive straining to pass stool and dependence on laxatives are often long standing and not remedied by anatomic correction of the prolapse. It is for this reason that I have become much more enthusiastic about the resection option.

Gordon and Hoexter, in a study based on a questionnaire sent to members of the American Society of Colon and Rectal Surgeons, were able to gain information on 1,111 Teflon sling repairs performed by 129 surgeons.[81] The overall complication rate was 16.5%, with a recurrence rate of 2.3%. Fecal impaction was seen in 6.7%. It was the opinion of the authors that the complications seemed to be related primarily to applying the mesh too tightly around the rectum. The complication rate seems to diminish as the surgeon's experience increases.

Holmström and associates reported their initial experience with the Teflon sling repair in 59 patients.[98] The operative mortality was high (5%). However, in two of the three patients who died, the cause of death was coronary artery disease. The recurrence rate was 5.4%, with a mean observation period of 5 years. A later report from the same institution included 108 patients, 97 of whom were available for evaluation.[99] The recurrence rate in this study was 4.1%. The proportion of continent patients increased from 33% preoperatively to 72% postoperatively. However, problems with defecation were a major source of dissatisfaction; difficulties increased from 27% preoperatively to 43% postoperatively.

Biehl and colleagues reported on their experience at the Ochsner Clinic in New Orleans, Louisiana, and compared it with the Altemeier, sigmoidectomy, and Thiersch procedures that had been formerly used.[25] The Ripstein operation was associated with a lower recurrence rate and a lower morbidity rate.

Launer and colleagues reported the Cleveland Clinic experience with the Teflon sling repair.[137] Although there was no operative mortality in 57 patients, there was a rather high morbidity rate (26%). Seven (14%) developed recurrent mucosal prolapse, and six patients (12%) had a full-thickness recurrence. Despite the somewhat disappointing results, the authors believed that the Ripstein procedure remained the treatment of choice for rectal prolapse. A later report from the same institution in-

▶ **TABLE 17-1 Operative Morbidity**

Complication	Frequency	Percentage
None	48	87.3
Wound sepsis	4	7.3
Urinary tract infection	2	3.6
Wound separation	1	1.8
Pulmonary problems	1	1.8
Total	56*	

*One patient had both a urinary tract infection and wound sepsis.
From Jurgeleit HC, Corman ML, Coller JA, et al. Procidentia of the rectum: Teflon sling repair of rectal prolapse. Lahey Clinic experience. *Dis Colon Rectum* 1975; 18:464, with permission.

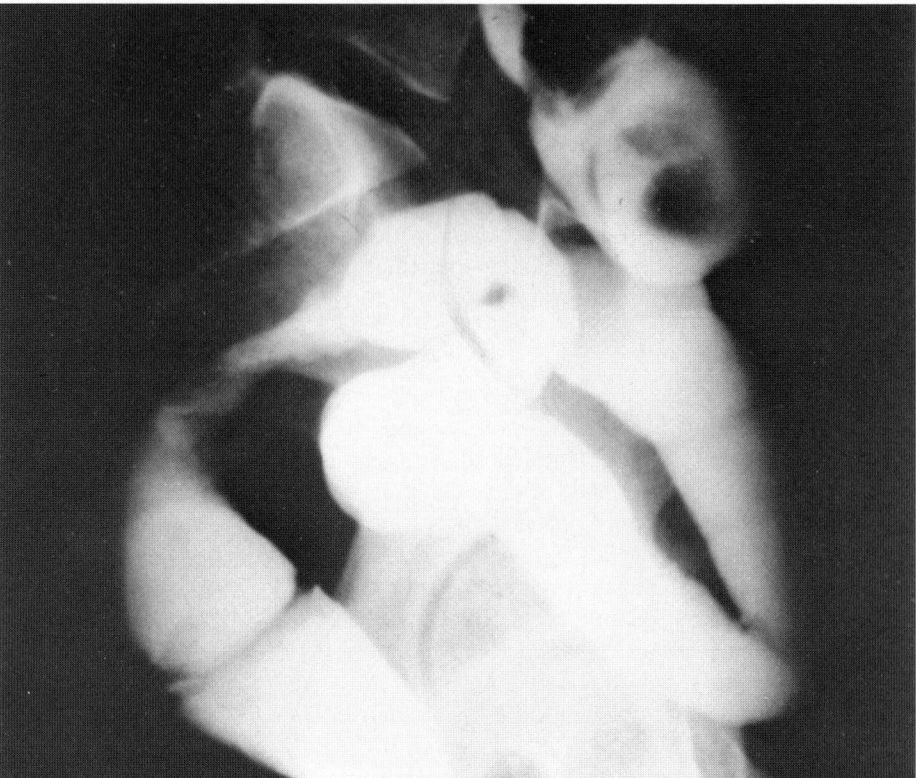

FIGURE 17-43. Barium enema study shows rectal stricture after Teflon sling repair. Note the redundant sigmoid colon. It is readily evident how this could predispose to volvulus. (From Lescher TJ, Corman ML, Coller JA, et al. Management of late complications of Teflon sling repair for rectal prolapse. *Dis Colon Rectum* 1979;22: 445, with permission.)

volved 142 patients.[238] The recurrence rate had now fallen to 8%. About one half of the patients experienced improvement in bowel control, but persistence or worsening of constipation was more common than after resection. Approximately one third remained dissatisfied with the functional results despite anatomic correction of the prolapse.

It has also been pointed out that enterocele is observed in about one third of patients with rectal prolapse.[159] Utilizing the Ripstein rectopexy, none had recurrent prolapse or enterocele in the experience of the group from the Department of Surgery at the Karolinska Institute of Stockholm.[159]

Late Complications

We have reported the late complications of Teflon sling repair, including our experience when the original procedure was performed elsewhere.[139] Rectal stricture developed in five patients. These individuals had in common a troublesome history of bowel management problems, specifically severe constipation that antedated insertion of the Teflon sling. Patients with rectal stricture also had a longer history of prolapse (79 months versus 37 months). Barium enema examination showed stenosis in all five of these individuals (Figs. 17-43 and 17-44), ranging from a diameter of 3 to 19 mm. The presence of narrowing was also identified by proctosigmoidoscopy.

McMahan and Ripstein confirmed that difficulties have arisen with Teflon as the suspension materialm.[156] They recommend Gore-Tex as being ideal because of its inert properties and its porous structure, which allows tissue incorporation. They also place the sling posteriorly, leaving the anterior rectal wall free to distend. No recurrences were seen in their series of 23 patients.[142]

Clearly constipation is not improved by the Teflon sling repair. On the contrary, abdominal pain, distension, and constipation may be exacerbated by the now-exaggerated redundancy of the sigmoid colon (Figs. 17-43 and 17-45).[33,264] Sigmoid volvulus has been reported to occur under these circumstances. In some individuals who present with obstructive symptoms relatively soon after the operation, faulty technique must be assumed. However, fibrotic reaction secondary to the mesh must also be considered as a possible contributing factor. In any patient with chronic constipation, particularly with a history of long-standing rectal prolapse, serious consideration should be given to performing an anterior resection initially. At the very least, these individuals should undergo careful preoperative investigation to identify those who have associated disturbances of function (e.g., slow-transit constipation, obstructed defecation).[56]

Recurrent rectal prolapse after Teflon sling repair usually is related to faulty surgical technique. The mesh may not be secured adequately to the presacral fascia or bone. In addition, as has been previously stated, when traction

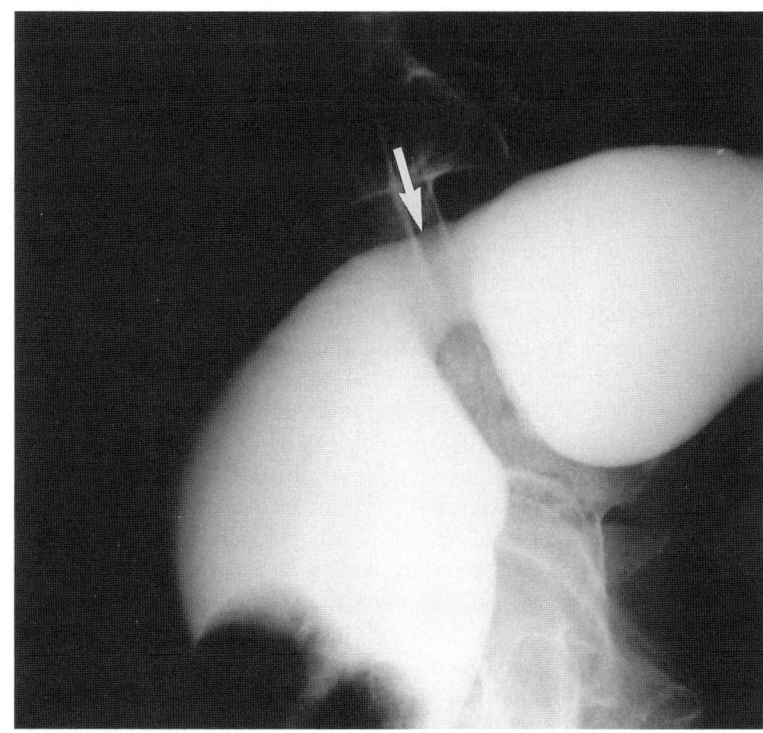

FIGURE 17-44. Profound rectal stricture *(arrow)* can be readily appreciated on this lateral film of the barium-filled rectum.

on the rectosigmoid is not maintained while the sling is inserted, the mesh will not be anchored sufficiently low on the rectum. The error is more likely to occur in a man whose pelvis is narrow and in whom mobilization and suture placement are more difficult. In our experience, a higher ratio of men to women is observed in the group of patients with this complication.

Comment

I believe that the sling repair should be abandoned in favor of anterior resection for all patients, but especially for men. An exception is the patient who develops a prolapse following an abdominal-anal pull-through operation or Altemeier procedure. Because there is a risk of devascularization of the lower rectal segment if resection is performed, a suspension operation is the better choice under these circumstances. Another exception is the patient who has severe diarrhea, especially if a subtotal colectomy had been previously performed. A suspension operation would be preferred to resection.

Laparoscopy

Another method of performing a suspension has become increasing popular in recent years, that of laparoscopic insertion and securing of the mesh.[14,19,82,91,131,220,221] Certainly, if any colon operation lends itself to the performance of minimally invasive surgery, it is this one (see also Chapter 27).

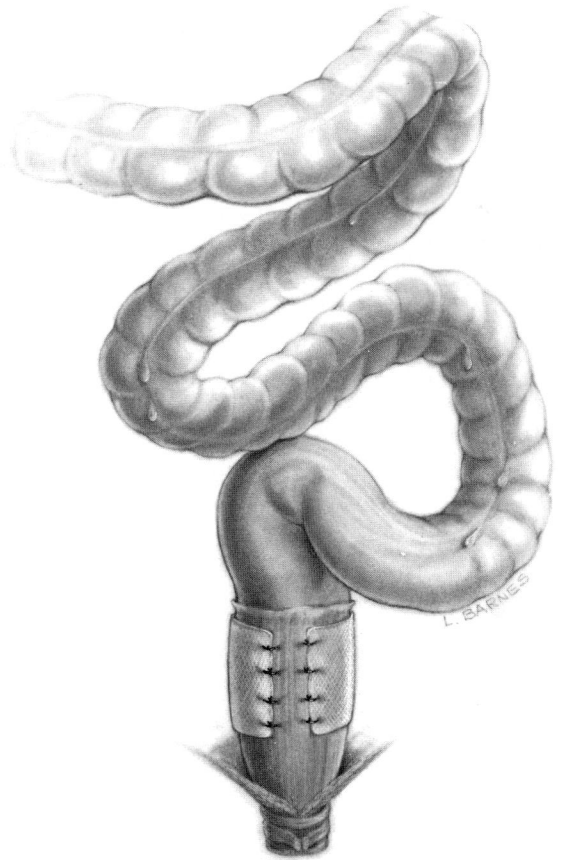

FIGURE 17-45. Rectal suspension procedures may exacerbate bowel management difficulties. Note the sigmoid redundancy that may result.

Solomon and co-workers randomized 40 patients to receive either open or laparoscopic rectopexy.[221] Their study was limited to in-hospital results as judged by their response to landmarks adopted through a clinical pathway regimen. The laparoscopic group was clearly superior in all areas (pain, diet advancement, bowel action) except for operative time. Kairaluoma and colleagues compared a consecutive series of patients who underwent an open operation with those who underwent laparoscopic repair. There were 53 patients in each group. Operating time was longer (210 versus 117 minutes), but median postoperative hospital stay was shorter (5 versus 7 days). There was no statistically significant difference in morbidity or mortality, rate of recurrence, and late complications.

Ivalon Sponge Implant or the Wells Operation

The use of Ivalon sponge as a wrapping about the rectum was initially described by Wells in 1959[256]; it has been enthusiastically advocated, primarily by the British and the Canadians.[3,13,29,30,36,150,155,160,187,202,225] However, because polyvinyl alcohol (i.e., Ivalon) has not been approved for this purpose in the United States, there is no American experience. The Ivalon sponge implant operation basically consists of the implantation of a synthetic polymer around the rectum. After full mobilization of the rectum, the appropriately tailored sponge is sutured to the sacrum in the posterior midline (Figs. 17–46A and B), not unlike the modified Teflon sling operation. It is then wrapped around the rectum, leaving a defect in the anterior midline (Figure 17-46C).

Results

Results of this procedure on 26 patients were reported by Boutsis and Ellis.[30] One operative death occurred, but no instance of pelvic sepsis or wound complication had developed. Follow-up study revealed nine mucosal recurrences—an incidence of 35%. Complete rectal prolapse developed in 11.5%. Stewart reported using this procedure in 41 patients; no operative deaths occurred, complete recurrence developed in three patients (7%), and a mucosal recurrence was noted in ten individuals (24%).[225] McCue and Thomson identified two recurrences in 53 patients (3.8%).[155] Boulos and associates reported 25 patients younger than 40 years of age who were followed for at least 5 years.[29] Twenty percent were found to have recurrences. Mann and Hoffman, however, noted no recurrences after 2 years in 44 patients.[150] A conscientious effort was made to fully mobilize the rectum, shorten the lateral ligaments, and excise the redundant peritoneum. Despite the absence of recurrence, constipation (47%) and incontinence (19%) caused difficult management problems. Rogers and Jeffery evaluated 24 indi-

viduals who were treated by concomitant Ivalon sponge rectopexy and postanal repair.[210] There was one recurrence (4%), with a maximum of 4 years of follow-up. Every patient was rendered continent in this uncontrolled study.

Allen-Mersh and colleagues noted a statistically significant increase in the prevalence of constipation following this operation.[3] One of the possible explanations that they suggest is the increased rectal wall thickness that occurs in some individuals. This may impede the passage of stool through the rectum and result in constipation.

Novell and co-workers performed a prospective, randomized trial of Ivalon sponge and sutured rectopexy (see later).[175] At a median follow-up of 47 months, prolapse had recurred in two patients (3%), one in each group; 22% suffered from incontinence, and 40% developed constipation. The authors concluded that the results of rectopexy by suture alone were equivalent to those obtained following the Ivalon sponge procedure. Therefore, they believed that the Ivalon rectopexy could now be abandoned.

Although septic problems are not common, removal of the sponge may be quite difficult, particularly when the physician attempts to identify foreign material within an abscess cavity.[134] Symptoms of this complication include sacral, coccygeal, or lower abdominal pain, pus per rectum, pus per vaginam, rectal discharge, and fever. No instance of recurrence was reported by the St. Mark's Hospital group (eight cases) after removal of the implant.[202] They recommend that removal of the implant be accomplished through the vagina or through the rectum if at all possible.

Comment

The apparent advantage of the Ivalon sponge implant operation is that fecal impaction has not been as great a problem.[160,187] However, because the incidence of recurrence is higher than that generally reported for the Teflon sling repair and for resection, I would not adopt the technique for my patients. Of course, the fact that it is not approved for use in the United States makes the matter academic.

Teflon Halter Operation

A unique approach to rectal suspension has been suggested by Nigro.[172] He believes the most effective way to correct prolapse is to use a method that most closely simulates the normal anatomic arrangement. It was his contention that the most important factor is the angulation and fixation provided by the pelvic floor musculature and that maximum support comes with contraction of the muscle as it lifts the lower rectum and tilts it forward toward the pubis.[171] Accordingly, he designed an intraabdominal sling approach that suspends the rectum from

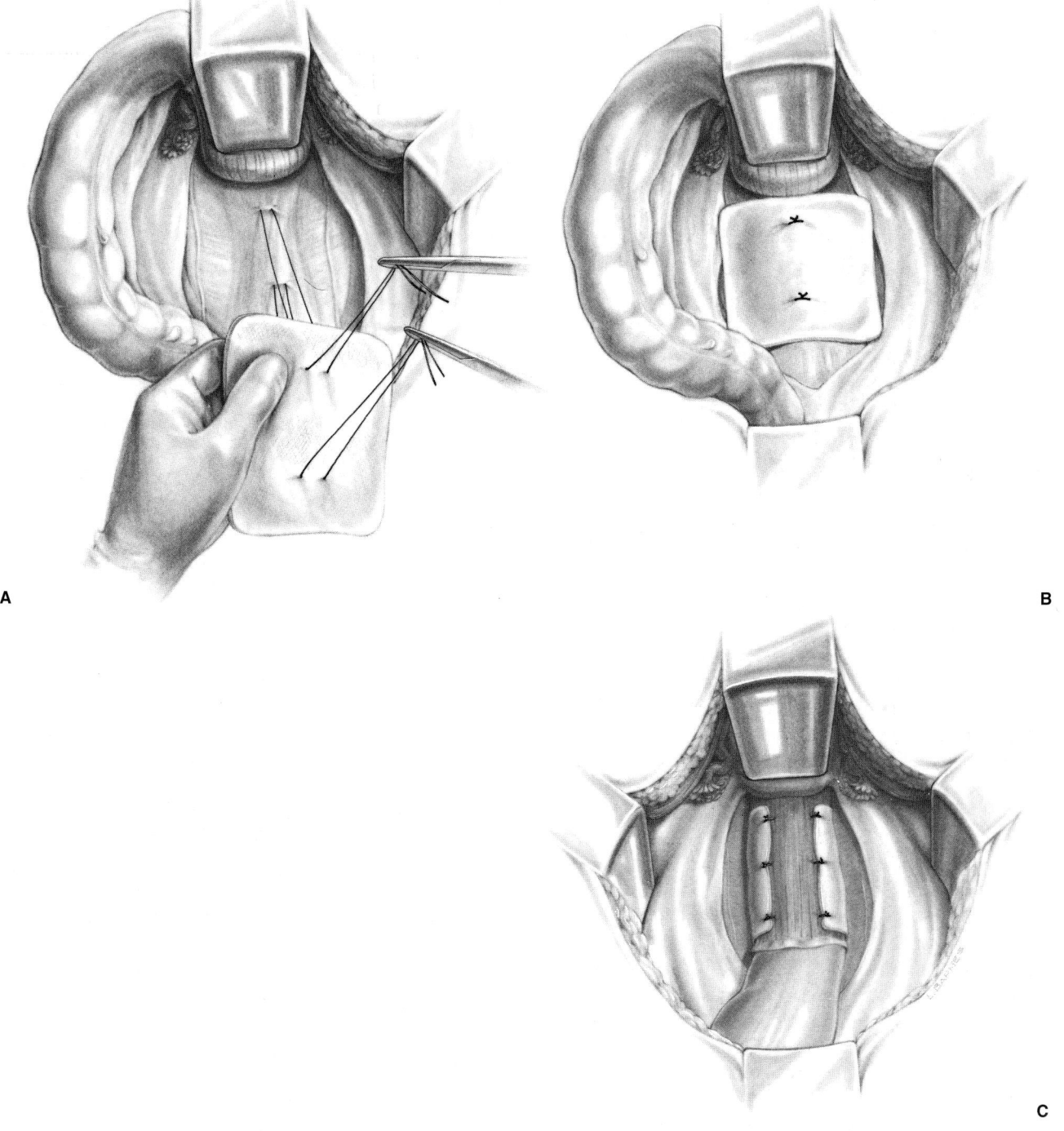

A

B

C

FIGURE 17-46. Technique of Ivalon sponge implant. **(A,B)** Suturing of sponge and anchoring to sacrum. **(C)** Suspension completed.

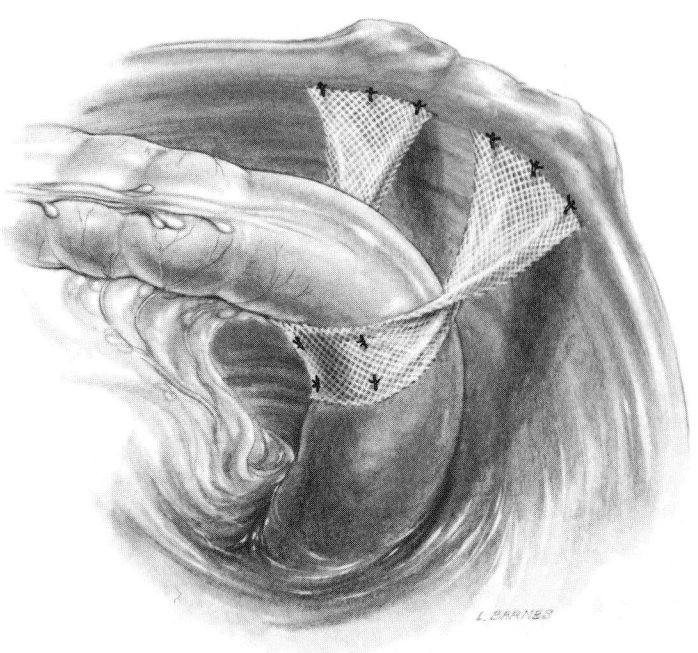

L. BARNES

FIGURE 17-47. Nigro procedure. The mesh is suspended from the pubis and brought around the posterior wall of the rectum as a halter.

the pubis. Successful results were experienced in all six patients.

The patient is placed in the Trendelenburg position on the operating table. A midline incision is made in the lower abdomen, and the rectum is mobilized in the same manner as that for a Ripstein or Wells repair. Care is taken to avoid injury to the inferior mesenteric vessels. The dissection is carried posteriorly down to the coccyx. The mesh is tailored to approximately 4 cm wide by 20 cm long. The central portion is secured to the rectum with interrupted nonabsorbable sutures. It is then sutured to the posterior and lateral walls of the rectum as low as possible.

The space of Retzius, in front of the bladder and close to the pubic rami, is opened. A long curved clamp is placed into this space and directed downward and posteriorly to the presacral space. The mesh is then grasped and pulled forward to lie on the pubic bone. The same is done on the contralateral side. Each end is then secured to the pubic ramus with interrupted nonabsorbable sutures. The length of graft is determined by holding it to the pubic bone with just enough tension to prevent slack (Figure 17-47). The presacral space is left open, and the abdomen is closed without drainage. Postoperative care is essentially the same as that for the conventional operation.

Results

Greene reported 15 patients who underwent this operation.[84] There was no mortality, no operative morbidity, and no recurrence with a minimum follow-up of 6 months. Severe incontinence was corrected in all but one patient, and this person was improved. There were no

problems with sexual function or urination. Greene believes that the particular advantage of this operation is its ameliorative effect on continence problems.

Comment

The utility of this operation is rather problematic. Dissection along the anterior pelvis places vital urinary and genital structures in jeopardy, and if carried out in a woman of childbearing age, a subsequent pregnancy will require a caesarean section. If the procedure is performed in a male patient, impotence is much more likely to be a complication than if the conventional alternative is used. Its theoretical advantage with respect to continence is probably overrated. Still, because I have had no experience with this technique, it is difficult to comment on its advisability. However, this point is probably irrelevant because there have been no publications in a number of years with this operation.

Fascia Lata Suspension (Orr)

In 1947, Orr described a suspension procedure by which the rectum is anchored to the sacrum with strips of fascia lata.[179] Loygue and co-workers and Orr modified the operation to include full rectal mobilization.[143,179] They reported their experience with 140 patients; two operative deaths were noted, and the incidence of recurrent prolapse was 3.6%. Christiansen and Kirkegaard reported two recurrences in 24 patients (8%) who underwent this procedure.[41] In 2003, Douard and associates assessed the functional results after the Orr-Loygue for complete rectal prolapse in 31 patients.[57] There were no recurrences, with a mean follow-up of 28 months. Continence improved in 24 of the 25 who were incontinent preoperatively. Evacuation difficulties increased significantly, however. A 10% increase in constipation rate was also observed.

Nylon Suspension

A modification that employs strips of nylon for the same purpose as that noted earlier has been described.[144] Loygue and colleagues reported 257 patients who underwent rectopexy by this technique.[144] There were two operative deaths. Recurrent rectal prolapse was observed in 4.3%, with a minimum follow-up of 5 years.

Suture Rectopexy

Perhaps the simplest abdominal approach to the treatment of rectal prolapse is suture rectopexy. The operation consists of mobilizing the rectum down to the levator ani muscle and securing the mesentery of the rectum and the muscularis to the sacral fascia or bone (Figure 17-48).

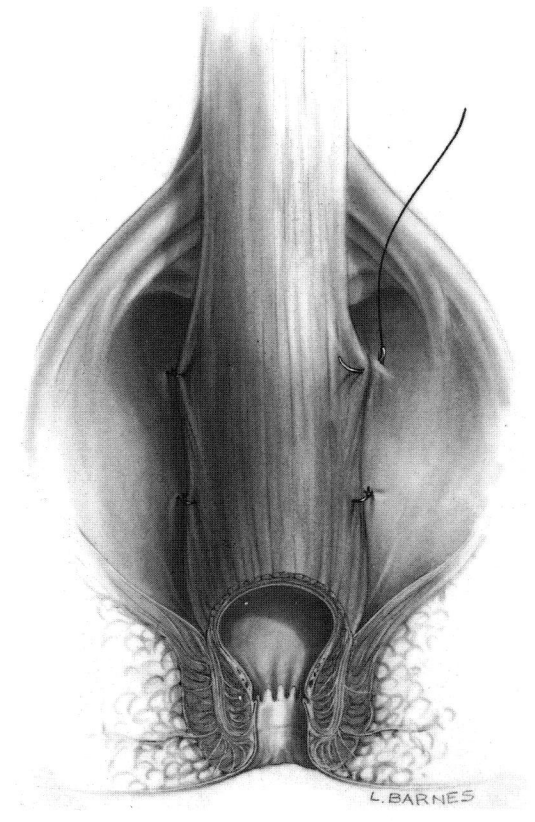

FIGURE 17-48. Suture rectopexy. The mobilized rectum is secured to the sacrum or presacral fascia with interrupted nonabsorbable sutures. (Redrawn from Blatchford GJ, Perry RE, Thorson AG, et al. Rectopexy without resection for rectal prolapse. *Am J Surg* 1989;158:574).

This can be performed through the use of interrupted nonabsorbable sutures.

Blatchford and colleagues undertook suture rectopexy on 43 patients.[27] Only one recurrence was noted (mean follow-up, 28 months). Others report two recurrences in 46 patients, a rate comparable to that of standard suspension procedures.[66]

Comment

It is evident that fixation of the rectum to the sacrum by whatever means has a high success rate with a low morbidity and mortality. Although I have had no experience with the foregoing techniques, their simplicity makes them quite appealing, although as with all suspension procedures there is an increased risk for evacuation disturbances, abdominal pain, constipation, and obstruction.

Rectal Prolapse and Fecal Incontinence

As implied from the aforementioned studies, the majority of patients will experience resolution of their incontinence difficulties once the prolapse has been adequately treated.[50,100] This is not surprising, because in addition to the prolapse no longer stretching and attenuating the sphincter, median perineal descent distance during attempted defecation usually decreases, and the anorectal angle becomes narrowed.[265] Farouk and co-workers performed ambulatory recordings utilizing a computerized anal EMG and anorectal manometry system on 32 patients with neurogenic fecal incontinence and rectal prolapse as well as on 33 controls.[68] They observed that recovery of continence occurs by abolition of high-pressure rectal waves. These waves produce maximal inhibition of sphincter activity before the operation. Others have shown that improvement in continence is not accompanied by changes in rectal sensation or reflexive functions of the internal sphincter.[205]

Keighley and Matheson reported 20 patients with prolapse and anal incontinence; rectopexy alone controlled the incontinence in all but four (20%).[117] Blatchford and colleagues noted that the proportion of continent patients increased from 36% preoperatively to 74% postoperatively following simple suture rectopexy.[27] In the experience of Yoshioka and co-workers, incontinence was observed in 58% before surgery, but in only 16% after Marlex mesh repair.[241]

There is, however, a small group of people for whom anal incontinence may be disabling despite correction of the rectal prolapse. Parks advocated postanal repair of the pelvic floor muscles for these individuals (see Chapter 13).[184] Although his overall failure rate for patients with incontinence was a respectable 17%, many did not have a prolapse initially. In fact, the results following this procedure were much less satisfactory when carried out after prolapse repair. Furthermore, the more severe the prolapse, the worse the result. Sainio and associates suggest that their preoperative and postoperative physiologic investigations lead them to the opinion that recovery of the resting and voluntary functions of the sphincter muscles is the cause of the improvement in continence.[205] Because anal manometry was unable to predict the outcome, they believe that supplementary procedures for restoration of continence are not advisable, and that rectopexy alone is as likely as rectopexy with the Parks operation to result in full restoration of bowel control. Williams and colleagues, however, have shown that patients who remained incontinent following surgery had a significantly lower preoperative resting anal pressure and lower maximum voluntary contraction pressure than those who improved.[258]

Shafik described an operative approach in the management of fecal incontinence by means of pudendal canal decompression (see also Chapter 13).[214] He performed the decompression by freeing the nerve on each side from the ischial spine through the pudendal canal. In an uncontrolled study involving 13 patients, seven improved with this operation. This is no better than one would expect without this decompression procedure.

Comment

I have rarely found it necessary to perform an operative procedure for fecal incontinence following repair of the prolapse. A Silastic-Dacron implant (Dow-Corning, Midland, MI) has been the surgical alternative I have used under these limited circumstances (see Chapter 13). The success of the operation from the surgeon's viewpoint, and, of course, from that of the patient, depends on many factors, not the least important of which is the ability to improve bowel habits. Perineal strengthening exercises, dietary measures, stool softeners, even periodic enemas or suppositories may be advisable. Although laxatives are usually discouraged, patients often return to their use. The physician cannot expect to remedy the bowel problems of a lifetime, but with appropriate counseling, one can anticipate that most patients will come to good terms with the condition.

Recommendations

The varied operative procedures available for rectal prolapse can be confusing. Some of the maneuvers are relatively esoteric and can be performed successfully only by the few surgeons who have developed the specialized techniques. It is recommended, therefore, that the surgeon who is less experienced with rectal prolapse adopt one of the standard operations. A rectopexy or suspension procedure without resection can be performed relatively safely with good results and with low morbidity and mortality rates. Anterior resection, with or without

sacral fixation, also offers an excellent cure rate and is a technique familiar to most surgeons.

The Thiersch-type approaches should probably be reserved for those individuals who cannot tolerate laparotomy. The material chosen should be one of the commercially available synthetic products. Wire should not be used. The Silastic-impregnated Dacron prosthesis for this operation has some potential benefit, especially for the incontinent patient. Results of further studies are awaited.

RECTAL PROLAPSE IN CHILDREN*

Rectal prolapse in children is an uncommon disease that occurs primarily in Western countries. It occurs most frequently in infants with cystic fibrosis. The condition can be associated with any illness that causes diarrhea (e.g., amebiasis, giardiasis, worms), constipation, frequent cough, especially whooping cough, or malnutrition; these associated conditions are described in more detail later[24,130,164,176,222,243]

Associated Conditions and Predisposing Factors for the Development of Rectal Prolapse in Children

Diarrhea (e.g., amebiasis, giardiasis, ulcerative colitis, trichuriasis)
Constipation
Straining to urinate (e.g., phimosis)
Vomiting
Cough (e.g., pertussis)
Malnutrition
Cystic fibrosis
Polyp or tumor[106,135]
Ehlers-Danlos syndrome[58]
Myelomeningocele
Spina bifida
Hirschsprung's disease[242]

Malnutrition is by far the most common predisposing factor for the development of rectal prolapse in infancy and childhood in developing countries. Most of the reports in the current literature emanate from Africa and Asia. The reasons for this geographic distribution are probably attributable to the diarrhea, in addition to the loss of ischiorectal fat and the lack of support for the rectum experienced by children in these regions. In 1914, Lockhart-Mummery stated that "rectal prolapse is a comparatively common affliction among children, especially in that class

---

*Reproduced in part from Corman ML. Rectal prolapse in children. *Dis Colon Rectum* 1985;28:535.

which attends hospitals".[141] The implication of this remark is that in the "better classes," children are better nourished and more quickly attended to if they become ill.

Soriano and colleagues reported ten cases of rectal prolapse associated with Trichuris trichiura as the only intestinal parasite (see Chapter 33).[222] Stern and co-workers noted that rectal prolapse occurred in 112 of 605 patients with cystic fibrosis (18.5%).[224] In one third of the prolapse patients, the prolapse preceded the diagnosis of cystic fibrosis. Kulczycki and Schwachman reported an incidence of almost 25% in 386 children afflicted with cystic fibrosis.[130]

Etiology

The etiology of rectal prolapse in infancy may be related to the loose attachment of the mucosa to the underlying muscularis. In this age group, the rectal mucosa may be normally rendundant.[206] Other anatomic factors in the child that tend to predispose to the development of prolapse are the vertical course of the rectum, flat sacrum and coccyx, low rectal position in relation to other pelvic organs, and lack of levator support. Rectal prolapse is most common in children younger than 3 years of age, with the most frequent incidence being in the first year of life. In this age group, it is the mucosa that tends to prolapse, not the full thickness of the bowel. Most studies report an approximately equal gender incidence.[24,62,164]

Symptoms and Findings

Symptoms may include protrusion, bleeding, passage of mucus, diarrhea, constipation, abdominal pain, and those complaints that may be referable to the associated or predisposing condition. Findings include the protrusion, lax sphincter tone and contractility, and, often, malnutrition (Figure 17-49). The most common differential

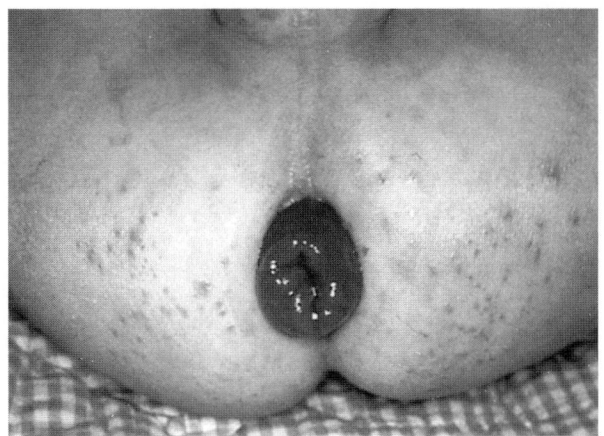

FIGURE 17-49. Rectal prolapse in an infant. (Courtesy of John Campbell, M.D. and Marvin W. Harrison, M.D.)

diagnostic condition is that of a juvenile polyp. Distinction between the two entities should not be difficult, however.

Treatment

Treatment usually consists of medical management, with normal growth of the child producing a cure in most patients. However, children with severe malnutrition and those without access to quality medical care and nutritional support are less likely to have spontaneous resolution of the prolapse condition.

Medical management consists of manual replacement, with sedation if necessary; the knee-chest position may be helpful. Supporting the perineum during defecation is also beneficial as well as to have the child defecate in the recumbent position. It may be necessary to tape the buttocks in order to prevent the prolapse from recurring spontaneously. Stool softeners are suggested for constipation and paregoric for diarrhea.

Surgical treatment has been advised for patients who are malnourished and for those who do not respond to medical management. Recommended procedures include the following:

- Excision of the mucosal prolapse[206]
- Anal encirclement with Silastic[55] or with catgut[164]
- Use of a sclerosing solution such as 30% saline[62,116] or 70% alcohol[148]
- Packing of the presacral space with gauze or Gelfoam[55,141,176]
- Linear cauterization of the anorectum[93]
- Transsacral rectopexy with obliteration of the pouch of Douglas and puborectalis plication[39]
- Transcoccygeal rectopexy and puborectalis plication[11]
- Perineal proctosigmoidectomy[165]
- Transanal rectopexy with delayed suture removal (Figs. 17-50 and 17-51)[90]

Results

Kay and Zachary employed a sclerosing solution of 30% saline in 51 children.[116] They noted 100% success with up to three treatments; however, two abscesses complicated the procedure. Dutta and Das used the same technique in 30 children.[62] They reported an 83% cure rate with one treatment and a 100% cure rate with three treatments. Malyshev and Gulin reported a series of 353 children from the former Soviet Union with rectal prolapse treated by perirectal 70% alcohol.[148] Ninety-six percent were cured. The authors advised, however, that no more than 35 mL should be employed, and that this treatment should be limited to those children who do not satisfactorily respond to medical measures.

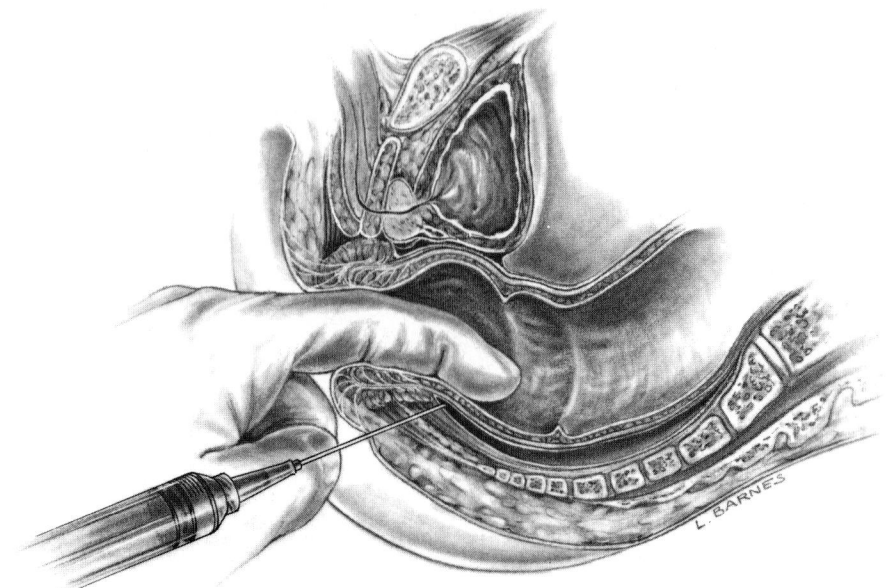

FIGURE 17-50. Injection technique. Sclerosing agent is infiltrated in the perirectal tissue posteriorly and laterally. The index finger is inserted into the rectum to confirm the position of the needle tip. (From Corman ML. Rectal prolapse in children. *Dis Colon Rectum* 1985;28:535, with permission.)

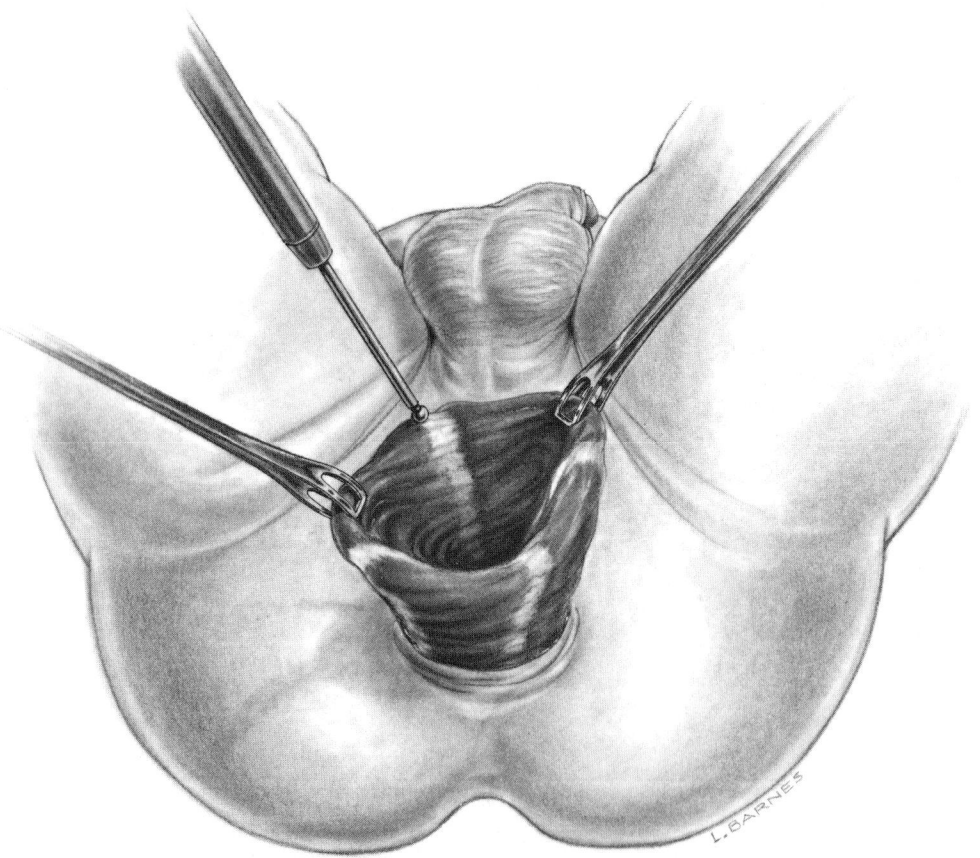

FIGURE 17-51. Linear cauterization. Four-quadrant electrocoagulation through the submucosa. (Adapted from Hight DW et al. Linear cauterization for pretreatment of rectal prolapse in infants and children. *Surg Gynecol Obstet* 1982;154:400; Corman ML. Rectal prolapse in children. *Dis Colon Rectum* 1985;28:535, with permission.)

Anal encirclement with Silastic is the approach that has been recommended in *Nelson's Textbook of Pediatrics*.[55] Narasanagi performed anal encirclement using No. 1 chromic catgut on 30 patients.[164] He reported one failure due to breakage of the suture. Subsequent treatment effectively cured the prolapse. Groff and Nagaraj advocate encirclement of the anus with a nonabsorbable suture (No. 0 or 1 Prolene) tightened over a Hegar dilator.[85] They observed that four patients required a repeat insertion and one required a third, but they believe that the safety and simplicity of the technique make it worthy of recommendation.

Packing the presacral space with gauze through a posterior approach, as well as excision of the prolapsed mucosa, have been recommended in the intractable case in Rudolph and Hoffman's textbook, *Pediatrics*.[206] Nwako packed the presacral space with Gelfoam in 100 patients and reported complete cure in every case.[176]

Hight and colleagues recommend a surgical approach for patients who do not respond to medical measures.[93] There were a total of 102 children in their series, 29 of whom responded adequately to medical measures. The remaining 73 underwent linear cauterization of the anorectum; all but two were successfully treated by this approach.

Heald, in a report of his experience with one child, was able to secure the rectum by means of transanal rectopexy, passing a suture through the full thickness of the rectum and skin overlying the coccyx.[90] The suture was removed at a later date.

Perineal proctosigmoidectomy has been used in intractable situations in children who had developed rectal prolapse as a consequence of spina bifida.[165] Chino and Thomas recommend transsacral rectopexy with obliteration of the pouch of Douglas and puborectalis plication, the technique that has been used for adults, except that resection is not recommended (Figure 17-38).[39] Successful repair was noted in four patients. Transcoccygeal rectopexy and puborectalis plication have been suggested by Ashcraft and colleagues, who treated and cured four children by this technique.[11]

Comment

My limited experience with this condition in children is such that I believe that medical measures are almost always successful. For the infant or child who fails to respond, it seems to me that a minimal surgical approach is appropriate: perirectal injection with a sclerosing agent, presacral packing, an anal encircling operation, or linear rectal cauterization. All have been reported in large series to have excellent results with minimal morbidity. Although more extensive adult-type operations are undoubtedly successful, I cannot justify their application in

children when I note the availability of simpler and safer, as well as effective, alternatives.

RECTOCELE

Rectocele is not a prolapse nor is it a descensus, but it does represent one of those conditions that occur as part of the pelvic laxity syndrome. In essence it is a hernial protrusion of part of the rectum into the vagina; it has also been referred to as a proctocele. The condition is often associated with anterior pelvic laxity, leading to cystocele and cystourethrocele. The literature concerning management of rectocele is found predominantly in gynecologic textbooks and journals catering to obstetricians and gynecologists. However, since the mid-1990s, some transanal approaches have been suggested, and these have been described in journals for colon and rectal and general surgeons. As of this writing, however, the two specialties appear to act independently and mutually exclusively with respect to their focus of management—that is, gynecologists address the transvaginal approach, whereas general and colon and rectal surgeons address the operation performed through the rectum or perineum. Figure 17-52 demonstrates the artist's conception of a typical rectocele.

Symptoms and Presentation

Repair is generally indicated when a rectocele is identified in a patient with the following symptoms:

- Constipation
- Rectal pain
- Need to insert a finger into the vagina to effect evacuation
- Stool pocketing
- Protrusion through the vagina
- Requirement for cystocele repair

Siproudhis and colleagues assessed symptomatic, anatomic, and physiologic features encountered in women with a clearly defined rectocele in order to determine the predisposing factors, symptoms, functional associations, and effects on quantified rectal emptying.[216] They compared clinical and manometric as well as anatomic features in 26 women with painful difficulty with elimination and a large rectocele with those patients complaining of similar symptoms *without* a rectocele. Those who harbored the rectocele had a statistically significant increased incidence of the requirement for endovaginal manipulation to effect defecation, more frequent symptoms of urinary incontinence, more frequent delayed rectal emptying, more frequent incomplete rectal emptying, and more frequently associated anismus. The

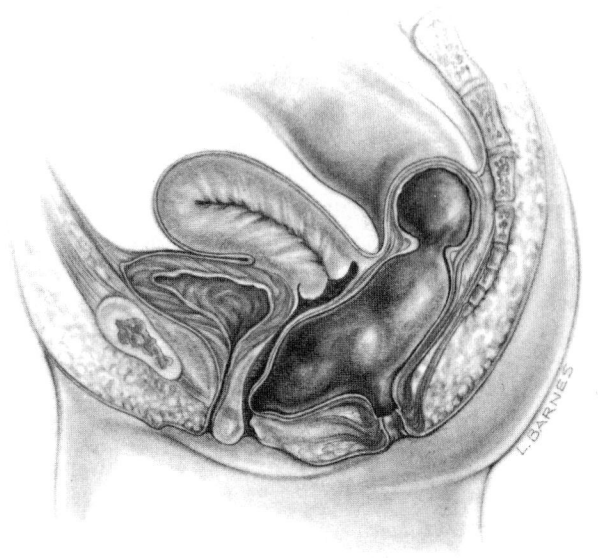

FIGURE 17-52. Sagittal view of a typical rectocele deformity.

observed.[111] Janssen and van Dijke demonstrated that anorectal manometry was useful in studying the beneficial physiologic effects of an endorectal repair.[107] For example, in those with no prior pelvic surgery, a large urge to defecate volume was found to be a predictor of a favorable clinical outcome.

Parenthetically, it is interesting to note that rectocele is not consistently associated with any physiologic change apart from an increased frequency of pelvic floor descent.[266] van Dam and colleagues noted that the main value of defecography was the objective demonstration of the rectocele and any other associated abnormalities.[248] The success of their transanal/transvaginal repair was not influenced by the concomitant presence of perineal descent, internal prolapse, radiologic signs of anismus or the size of the rectocele.

Rectocele in the Male

The existence of rectocele in the male seems a counterintuitive concept, especially if one defines the condition as that wherein there is a protrusion into the vagina. However, if one defines the condition as a bulge outside the line of the rectal wall that increases in size during straining or evacuation, it is possible to observe a rectocele in

authors recommend physiologic examination as part of the preoperative workup for any patient with a rectocele and dyschezia.[216] Others concur that careful preoperative investigations are important before surgically treating a rectocele because emptying difficulties are so frequently

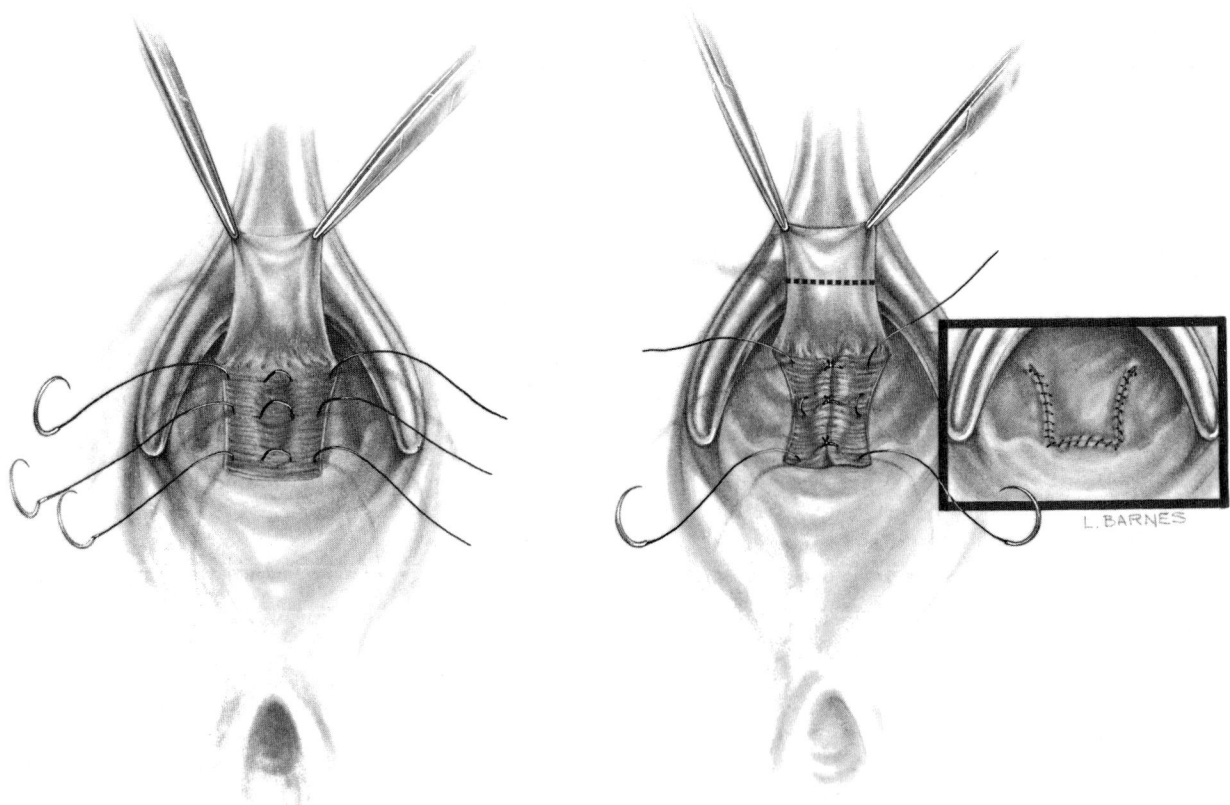

FIGURE 17-53. Transanal rectocele repair. Plication in layers of the lax rectovaginal septum.

men.[38] Chen and colleagues define a male rectocele as a bulging that fails to empty during defecography and is associated with obstructed defecation (anismus).[38] Forty patients (out of 234 male patients with evacuation disorders) in their series were found to have rectoceles by this definition. None was treated surgically because of this observation alone. The authors conclude that the clinical significance of this entity and the therapeutic strategy "remain unknown."

Techniques

Because of the multi-specialty clinic philosophy—rendering unto Caesar that which is Caesar's—I have often deferred to my colleagues in the gynecology department when I thought surgery advisable. Furthermore, because the operation is often performed concomitantly with cystocele repair, I felt even less comfortable in limiting my perspective to the rectum. However, this philosophy is changing, and some colon and rectal surgeons are now quite willing and able to perform a transanal or transperineal approach to the management of this condition, assuming that a concomitant anterior repair is not required. The initiative was seized by Sullivan and colleagues in 1968, when they advocated transrectal repair of rectocele concomitant with surgery for other anorectal conditions.[227]

One operation that has been suggested is basically a mucosal excision in the anterior quadrant with a plication of the deep external sphincter and levator ani muscle (Figure 17-53).[211] An obliterative, deep-suturing technique is advocated by Block as an expeditious (i.e., "6-minute") alternative to conventional rectocele repair (Figure 17-54).[28,123] Others advocate a combined transvaginal/transanal repair.[248] The combined procedure commences initially with a posterior colporrhaphy and then the repositioning the patient in the prone jackknife position. Any mucosal redundancy is excised from the anterior rectal wall through a transanal approach, followed by a transverse plication of the muscular layer of the rectal wall as is described in Figure 17-53. My preference, when a solitary posterior perineal weakness (rectocele) is present, is to perform a transperineal repair, an approach with which I am quite comfortable in that it is used frequently for repairing defects found following obstetric injuries (see Chapter 13). It is not within the province of this chapter to discuss the standard gynecologic operation for repair of rectocele.

Another approach to the surgical management of rectocele has been the use of the stapled hemorrhoidopexy instrument (see Chapter 8).[8] Altomare and co-workers employed a transperineal operation with the circular stapler, applying the device transanally but incorporating the rectal wall anteriorly.[8] Eight women were treated successfully by this technique as confirmed by defecography. Long-term results are awaited.

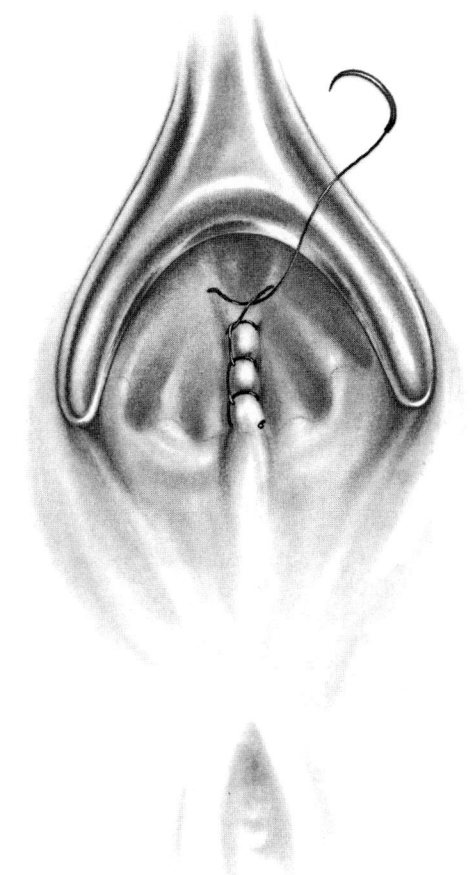

FIGURE 17-54. Transanal rectocele repair. Obliterative suture technique of Block.

Results

Some large series reveal excellent results of transanal operations, despite an infection rate in excess of 5% and the occurrence of quite a few postoperative rectovaginal fistulas.[58,132,215] Arnold and co-workers retrospectively compared 35 patients treated with a transanal approach with 29 who were treated by conventional transvaginal surgery.[10] When used for the treatment of constipation, more than one half were still symptomatic. The only apparent advantage of the anal operation was the fact that fewer individuals complained of pain. Watson and colleagues analyzed the results of a repair designed to deal with the cause (failure of the rectovaginal septum) rather than the effect (rectal and vaginal wall bulging).[253] Eight of the nine women achieved successful evacuation without the need for digital manipulation. Others report excellent functional results with improved evacuation by means of a transanal operation.[115,122,157,162]

Comment

I can remember with less than affection the long hours spent as a second assistant on the gynecology service when I was a medical student. Any alternative to the tedium of being a lithotomy position assistant must be regarded with favor. However, the procedures described earlier are not reasonable alternatives to conventional transvaginal surgery if the patient harbors a cystocele that requires repair. Still, application of a transanal or transperineal technique for those symptomatic patients who have an isolated rectocele or who are undergoing an anorectal operation for another problem seems prudent. I would wish to be certain preoperatively that the patient does not have a concomitant problem with obstructed defecation, and this concern should warrant appropriate testing.

REFERENCES

1. Agachan F, Pfeifer J, Joo JS, et al. Results of perineal procedures for the treatment of rectal prolapse. *Am Surg* 1997; 63:9.
2. Agachan F, Pfeifer J, Wexner SD. Defecography and proctography: results of 744 patients. *Dis Colon Rectum* 1996; 39:899.
3. Allen-Mersh TG, Turner MJ, Mann CV. Effect of abdominal Ivalon rectopexy on bowel habit and rectal wall. *Dis Colon Rectum* 1990;33:550.
4. Altemeier WA. One-stage perineal surgery for complete rectal prolapse. *Hosp Pract* 1972;7:102.
5. Altemeier WA, Culbertson WR. Technique for perineal repair of rectal prolapse. *Surgery* 1965;58:758.
6. Altemeier WA, Culbertson WR, Schowengerdt C, et al. Nineteen years' experience with the one-stage perineal repair of rectal prolapse. *Ann Surg* 1971;173:993.
7. Altomare DF, Rinaldi M, Chimarulo C, et al. Treatment of external anorectal mucosal prolapse with circular stapler: an easy and effective new surgical technique. *Dis Colon Rectum* 1999;42:1102.
8. Altomare DF, Rinaldi M, Veglia A, et al. Combined perineal and endorectal repair of rectocele by circular stapler: a novel surgical technique. *Dis Colon Rectum* 2002;45:1549.
9. Ambrose S, Keighley MRB. Outpatient measurement of perineal descent. *Ann R Coll Surg Engl* 1985;67:306.
10. Arnold MW, Stewart WRC, Aguilar PS. Rectocele repair: four years' experience. *Dis Colon Rectum* 1990;33:684.
11. Ashcraft KW, Amoury RA, Holder TM. Levator repair and posterior suspension for rectal prolapse. *J Pediatr Surg* 1977; 12:241.
12. Asman HB. Internal procidentia of the rectum. *South Med J* 1957;50:641.
13. Atkinson KG, Taylor DC. Wells procedure for complete rectal prolapse: a ten-year experience. *Dis Colon Rectum* 1984; 27:96.
14. Baker R, Senagore AJ, Luchtefeld MA. Laparoscopic-assisted vs. open resection: rectopexy offers excellent results. *Dis Colon Rectum* 1995;38:199.
15. Ballantyne GH. Laparoscopically assisted anterior resection for rectal prolapse. *Surg Laparosc Endosc* 1992;2:230.
16. Bartolo DCC, Roe AM, Virjee J, et al. Evacuation proctography in obstructed defaecation and rectal intussusception. *Br J Surg* 1985;72:111.
17. Beahrs OH, Theuerkauf FJ Jr, Hill JR. Procidentia: surgical treatment. *Dis Colon Rectum* 1972;15:337.
18. Bennett BH, Geelhoed GW. A stapler modification of the Altemeier procedure for rectal prolapse. *Am Surg* 1985; 51:116.
19. Berman IR. Sutureless laparoscopic rectopexy for procidentia: technique and implications. *Dis Colon Rectum* 1992;35:689.
20. Berman IR, Harris MS, Leggett IT. Rectal reservoir reduction procedures for internal rectal prolapse. *Dis Colon Rectum* 1987;30:765.
21. Berman IR, Harris MS, Rabeler MB. Delorme's transrectal excision for internal prolapse: patient selection, technique, and three-year follow-up. *Dis Colon Rectum* 1990;33:573.
22. Berman IR, Manning DH, Dudley-Wright K. Anatomic specificity in the diagnosis and treatment of internal rectal prolapse. *Dis Colon Rectum* 1985;28:816.
23. Berman IR, Manning DH, Harris MS. Streamlining the management of defecation disorders. *Dis Colon Rectum* 1990;33:778.
24. Bhandari B, Ameta DK. Etiology of prolapse rectum in children with special reference to amoebiasis. *Indian J Pediatr* 1977;14:635.
25. Biehl AG, Ray JE, Gathright JB Jr. Repair of rectal prolapse: experience with the Ripstein sling. *South Med J* 1978;71:923.
26. Birnbaum EH, Stamm L, Rafferty JF, et al. Pudendal nerve terminal motor latency influences surgical outcome in treatment of rectal prolapse. *Dis Colon Rectum* 1996;39: 1215.
27. Blatchford GJ, Perry RE, Thorson AG, et al. Rectopexy without resection for rectal prolapse. *Am J Surg* 1989;158: 574.
28. Block IR. Transrectal repair of rectocele using obliterative suture. *Dis Colon Rectum* 1986;29:707.
29. Boulos PB, Stryker SJ, Nicholls RJ. The long-term results of polyvinyl alcohol (Ivalon) sponge for rectal prolapse in young patients. *Br J Surg* 1984;71:213.
30. Boutsis C, Ellis H. The Ivalon-sponge-wrap operation for rectal prolapse: an experience with 26 patients. *Dis Colon Rectum* 1974;17:21.
31. B raley SC, Schneider PD, Bold RJ, et al. Controlled tamponade of severe presacral venous hemorrhage: use of a breast implant sizer. *Dis Colon Rectum* 2002;45:140.
32. Brodén B, Snellman B. Procidentia of the rectum studied with cineradiography: a contribution to the discussion of causative mechanism. *Dis Colon Rectum* 1968;11:330.
33. Brodén G, Dolk A, Holmström B. Evacuation difficulties and other characteristics of rectal function associated with procidentia and the Ripstein operation. *Dis Colon Rectum* 1988; 31:283.
34. Cali RL, Pitsch RM, Blatchford GJ, et al. Rare pelvic floor hernias: report of a case and review of the literature. *Dis Colon Rectum* 1992;35:604.
35. Capps WF Jr. Rectoplasty and perineoplasty for the symptomatic rectocele: a report of fifty cases. *Dis Colon Rectum* 1975;18:237.
36. Carter AE. Rectosacral suture fixation for complete rectal prolapse in the elderly, the frail and the demented. *Br J Surg* 1983;70:522.
37. Chanvitan A, Nopanitaya W. Solitary rectal ulcer: electron microscopy study of two cases. *Dis Colon Rectum* 1986;29: 421.
38. Chen HH, Iroatulam A, Alabaz O, et al. Associations of defecography and physiologic findings in male patients with rectocele. *Tech Coloproctol* 2001;5:157.
39. Chino ES, Thomas CG Jr. Transsacral approach to repair of rectal prolapse in children. *Am Surg* 1984;50:70.
40. Choi JS, Wexner SD, Nam YS, et al. Intraobserver and interobserver measurements of the anorectal angle and perineal descent in defecography. *Dis Colon Rectum* 2000;43: 1121.
41. Christiansen J, Kirkegaard P. Complete prolapse of the rectum treated by modified Orr operation. *Dis Colon Rectum* 1981;24:90.

42. Christiansen J, Zhu BW, Rasmussen O, Sørensen M. Internal rectal intussusception: results of surgical repair. *Dis Colon Rectum* 1992;35:1026.

43. Chun S, Pilarsky A, You S, et al. Perineal rectosigmoidectomy for rectal prolapse: role of levatorplasty. *Dis Colon Rectum* 2001;44:A5–A26.

44. Cirocco WC, Brown AC. Anterior resection for the treatment of rectal prolapse: a 20-year experience. *Am Surg* 1993;59:265.

45. Collopy BT, Barham KA. Abdominal colporectopexy with pelvic cul-de-sac closure. *Dis Colon Rectum* 2002;45:522.

46. Corman ML, Veidenheimer MC, Coller JA. Managing rectal prolapse. *Geriatrics* 1974;29:87.

47. Cosman BC, Lackides GA, Fisher DP, et al. Use of tissue expander for tamponade of presacral hemorrhage: report of a case. *Dis Colon Rectum* 1994;37:723.

48. Davidian VA, Thomas CG Jr. Trans-sacral repair of rectal prolapse: efficacy of treatment in thirty consecutive patients. *Am J Surg* 1972;123:231.

49. Deen KI, Grant E, Billingham C, et al. Abdominal resection rectopexy with pelvic floor repair versus perineal rectosigmoidectomy and pelvic floor repair for full-thickness rectal prolapse. *Br J Surg* 1994;81:302.

50. Delemarre JBVM, Gooszen HG, Kruyt RH, et al. The effect of posterior rectopexy on fecal continence: a prospective study. *Dis Colon Rectum* 1991;34:311.

51. Delorme E. Communication sur le traitement des prolapsus du rectum totaux par l'excision de la muqueuse rectale ou recto-colique. *Bull Soc Chir Paris* 1900;26:498. (Translated in *Dis Colon Rectum* 1985;28:544.)

52. Devadhar DS. A new operative treatment for complete prolapse of the rectum. *J Christ Med Assoc India* 1961;36:18.

53. Devadhar DS. New thoughts on the mechanism and treatment of rectal procidentia. *J Int Coll Surg* 1964;42:672.

54. Devadhar DS. A new concept of mechanism and treatment of rectal procidentia. *Dis Colon Rectum* 1965;8:75.

55. Doershuk CF, Boat TF. In: Behrman RE, Vaughan VC, eds. *Nelson's textbook of pediatrics*, 12th ed. Philadelphia: WB Saunders, 1983:1097.

56. Dolk A, Brodén G, Holmström B, et al. Slow transit of the colon associated with severe constipation after the Ripstein operation: a clinical and physiologic study. *Dis Colon Rectum* 1990;33:786.

57. Douard R, Frileux P, Brunel M, et al. Functional results after the Orr-Loygue transabdominal rectopexy for complete rectal prolapse. *Dis Colon Rectum* 2003;46:1089.

58. Douglas BS, Douglas HM. Rectal prolapse in the Ehlers-Danlos syndrome. *Aust Paediatr J* 1973;9:109.

59. Duff TH, Wright FF. Acute and chronic ulcers of the rectum. *Surg Gynecol Obstet* 1981;153:398.

60. Dunphy JE. A combined perineal and abdominal operation for the repair of rectal prolapse. *Surg Gynecol Obstet* 1948;86:493.

61. Dunphy JE, Botsford TW, Savlov E. Surgical treatment of procidentia of the rectum: an evaluation of combined abdominal and perineal repair. *Am J Surg* 1953;86:605.

62. Dutta BN, Das AK. Treatment of prolapse rectum in children with injections of sclerosing agents. *J Indian Med Assoc* 1977;69:275.

63. Earnshaw JJ, Hopkinson BR. Late results of silicone rubber perianal suture for rectal prolapse. *Dis Colon Rectum* 1987;30:86.

64. Eckardt VF, Kanzler G, Remmele W. Anorectal ergotism: another cause of solitary rectal ulcers. *Gastroenterology* 1986;91:1123.

65. Ederle A, Bulighin G, Orlandi PG, et al. Endoscopic application of human fibrin sealant in the treatment of solitary ulcer syndrome [Letter]. *Endoscopy* 1992;24:736.

66. Ejerblad S, Krause U. Repair of rectal prolapse by rectosacral suture fixation. *Acta Chir Scand* 1988;154:103.

67. Ekberg O, Nylander G, Fork F-T. Defecography. *Radiology* 1985;155:45.

68. Farouk R, Duthie GS, MacGregor AB, et al. Rectoanal inhibition and incontinence in patients with rectal prolapse. *Br J Surg* 1994;81:743.

69. Felt-Bersma RJF, Luth WJ, Janssen JJWM, et al. Defecography in patients with anorectal disorders: which findings are clinically relevant? *Dis Colon Rectum* 1990;33:277.

70. Franzin G, Dina R, Scarpa A, et al. The evolution of the solitary ulcer of the rectum: an endoscopic and histopathological study. *Endoscopy* 1982;14:131.

71. Friedman R, Muggia-Sulam M, Freund HR. Experience with the one-stage perineal repair of rectal prolapse. *Dis Colon Rectum* 1983;26:789.

72. Frykman HM, Goldberg SM. The surgical treatment of rectal procidentia. *Surg Gynecol Obstet* 1969;129:1225.

73. Goei R. Anorectal function in patients with defecation disorders and asymptomatic subjects: evaluation with defecography. *Radiology* 1990;174:121.

74. Goei R, Baeten C. Rectal intussusception and rectal prolapse: detection and postoperative evaluation with defecography. *Radiology* 1990;174:124.

75. Goei R, Baeten C, Arends JW. Solitary rectal ulcer syndrome: findings at barium enema study and defecography. *Radiology* 1988;168:303.

76. Goei R, Engelshoven Jv, Schouten H, et al. Anorectal function: defecographic measurement in asymptomatic subjects. *Radiology* 1989;173:137.

77. Goldman J. *Über Mastdarmvorfall mit besonderer berücksichtigung der Thiersch'schen operation (Concerning prolapse of the rectum with special emphasis on the operation by Thiersch).* Inaugural dissertation before the Faculty of Medicine at Kaiser-Wilhelms University, Strassburg. Strassburg: BC Goeller, 1892. (Translated in *Dis Colon Rectum* 1988;31:154.)

78. Goligher JC. *Surgery of the anus, rectum and colon*, 3rd ed. London: Baillière Tindall, 1975:293.

79. Gooley NA, Kuhnke M, Eusebio EB. Acute transanal ileal evisceration. *Dis Colon Rectum* 1987;30:479.

80. Gopal KA, Amshel AL, Shonberg IL, et al. Rectal procidentia in elderly and debilitated patients: experience with the Altemeier procedure. *Dis Colon Rectum* 1984;27:376.

81. Gordon PH, Hoexter B. Complications of the Ripstein procedure. *Dis Colon Rectum* 1978;21:277.

82. Graf W, Stefánsson T, Arvidsson D, et al. Laparoscopic suture rectopexy. *Dis Colon Rectum* 1995;38:211.

83. Graham RR. The operative repair of massive rectal prolapse. *Ann Surg* 1942;115:1007.

84. Greene FL. Repair of rectal prolapse using a puborectal sling procedure. *Arch Surg* 1983;118:398.

85. Groff DB, Nagaraj HS. Rectal prolapse in infants and children. *Am J Surg* 1990;160:531.

86. Gundersen AL, Cogbill TH, Landercasper J. Reappraisal of Delorme's procedure for rectal prolapse. *Dis Colon Rectum* 1985;28:721.

87. Halligan S, Nicholls RJ, Bartram CI. Proctographic changes after rectopexy for solitary rectal ulcer syndrome and preoperative predictive factors for a successful outcome. *Br J Surg* 1995;82:314.

88. Harrison JL, Hooks VH, Pearl RK, et al. Muscle fragment welding for control of massive presacral bleeding during rectal mobilization: a review of eight cases. *Dis Colon Rectum* 2003;46:1115.

89. Haskell B, Rovner H. A modified Thiersch operation for complete rectal prolapse using a Teflon prosthesis. *Dis Colon Rectum* 1963;6:192.

90. Heald CL. A simple, bloodless operation for anorectal prolapse in children. *Surg Gynecol Obstet* 1926;42:840.

91. Henry LG, Cattey RP. Rectal prolapse. *Surg Laparosc Endosc* 1994;4:357.

92. Henschen C. Ueber den Ersatz des Thierschschen Drahtringes bei der Operation des Mastdarmvorfalls durch geflochtene Seidenriemen, frei überpflanzte gefäss-sehnenperiost-oder Faszien stücke. *Munchen Med Wochenschr* 1912;59:128.

93. Hight DW, Hertzler JH, Philippart AI, et al. Linear cauterization for the treatment of rectal prolapse in infants and children. *Surg Gynecol Obstet* 1982;154:400.

94. Hill ADK, Menzies-Gow N, Darzi A. Methods of controlling presacral bleeding. *J Am Coll Surg* 1994;178:183.

95. Hiltunen K-M, Matikainen M, Auvinen O, et al. Clinical and manometric evaluation of anal sphincter function in patients with rectal prolapse. *Am J Surg* 1986;151:489.

96. Hock D, Lombard R, Jehaes C, et al. Colpocystodefecography. *Dis Colon Rectum* 1993;36:1015.

97. Hoffman MJ, Kodner IJ, Fry RD. Internal intussusception of the rectum: diagnosis and surgical management. *Dis Colon Rectum* 1984;27:435.

98. Holmström B, Ahlberg J, Bergstrand O, et al. Results of the treatment of rectal prolapse operated according to Ripstein. *Acta Chir Scand* 1978;482:51.

99. Holmström B, Brodén G, Dolk A. Results of the Ripstein operation in the treatment of rectal prolapse and internal rectal procidentia. *Dis Colon Rectum* 1986;29:845.

100. Holmström B, Brodén G, Dolk A, et al. Increased anal resting pressure following the Ripstein operation. *Dis Colon Rectum* 1986;29:485.

101. Hopkinson BR, Hardman J. Silicone rubber perianal suture for rectal prolapse. *Proc R Soc Med* 1973;66:1095.

102. Hughes ESR. Discussion on rectal prolapse of the rectum. *Proc R Soc Med* 1949;421:1007.

103. Hunt TM, Fraser IA, Maybury NK. Treatment of rectal prolapse by sphincteric support using silastic rods. *Br J Surg* 1985;72:491.

104. Ihre T. Internal procidentia of the rectum: treatment and results. *Scand J Gastroenterol* 1972;7:643.

105. Ihre T, Seligson U. Intussusception of the rectum—internal procidentia: treatment and results in 90 patients. *Dis Colon Rectum* 1975;18:391.

106. Impieri M, Zambarda E. Rectal prolapse in a child with Peutz-Jeghers syndrome. *Acta Gastroenterol Belg* 1982;45:429.

107. Janssen LWM, van Dijke CF. Selection criteria for anterior rectal wall repair in symptomatic rectocele and anterior rectal wall prolapse. *Dis Colon Rectum* 1994;37:1100.

108. Jenkins SG Jr, Thomas CG Jr. An operation for the repair of rectal prolapse. *Surg Gynecol Obstet* 1962;114:381.

109. Johansen OB, Wexner SD, Daniel N, et al. Perineal rectosigmoidectomy in the elderly. *Dis Colon Rectum* 1993;36:767.

110. Johansson C, Ihre T, Ahlbäck SO. Disturbances in the defecation mechanism with special reference to intussusception of the rectum (internal procidentia). *Dis Colon Rectum* 1985;28:920.

111. Johansson C, Nilsson BY, Holmström B, et al. Association between rectocele and paradoxical sphincter response. *Dis Colon Rectum* 1992;35:503.

112. Jorge JMN, Ger GC, Gonzalez L, et al. Patient position during cinedefecography. *Dis Colon Rectum* 1994;37:927.

113. Jorge JMN, Wexner SD, Ehrenpreis ED, et al. Does perineal descent correlate with pudendal neuropathy? *Dis Colon Rectum* 1993;36:475.

114. Jurgeleit HC, Corman ML, Coller JA, et al. Procidentia of the rectum: Teflon sling repair of rectal prolapse. Lahey Clinic experience. *Dis Colon Rectum* 1975;18:464.

115. Karlbom U, Graf W, Nilsson S, et al. Does surgical repair of a rectocele improve rectal emptying? *Dis Colon Rectum* 1996;39:1296.

116. Kay NR, Zachary RB. The treatment of rectal prolapse in children with injections of 30 percent saline solutions. *J Pediatr Surg* 1970;5:334.

117. Keighley MRB, Matheson DM. Results of treatment for rectal prolapse and fecal incontinence. *Dis Colon Rectum* 1981;24:449.

118. Keighley MRB, Shouler PJ. Abnormalities of colonic function in patients with rectal prolapse. *Br J Surg* 1984;71:892.

119. Keighley MRB, Shouler P. Clinical and manometric features of the solitary ulcer syndrome. *Dis Colon Rectum* 1984;27:507.

120. Khan FA, Fang DT, Nivatvongs S. Management of presacral bleeding during rectal resection. *Surg Gynecol Obstet* 1987;165:274.

121. Khanduja KS, Hardy TG Jr, Aguilar PS, et al. A new silicone prosthesis in the modified Thiersch operation. *Dis Colon Rectum* 1988;31:380.

122. Khubchandani IT, Clancy JP III, Rosen L, et al. Endorectal repair of rectocele revisited. *Br J Surg* 1997;84:89.

123. Khubchandani IT, Sheets JA, Stasik JJ, et al. Endorectal repair of rectocele. *Dis Colon Rectum* 1983;26:792.

124. Kimmins MH, Evetts BK, Isler J, et al. The Altemeier repair: outpatient treatment of rectal prolapse. *Dis Colon Rectum* 2001;44:565.

125. Kling KM, Rongione AJ, Evans B, et al. The Delorme procedure: a useful operation for complicated rectal prolapse in the elderly. *Am Surg* 1996;62:857.

126. Kraske P. Zur Exstirpation hochsitzender Mastdarmkrebse. *Verh Dtsch Ges Chir* 1885;14:464.

127. Kruyt RH, Delemarre JBVM, Gooszen HG, et al. Selection of patients with internal intussusception of the rectum for posterior rectopexy. *Br J Surg* 1990;77:1183.

128. Kuijpers HC, Mollen M. Invited commentary. *Dis Colon Rectum* 2002;45:526.

129. Kuijpers HC, Schreve RH, Hoedemakers HTC. Diagnosis of functional disorders of defecation causing the solitary ulcer syndrome. *Dis Colon Rectum* 1986;29:126.

130. Kulczycki LL, Schwachman H. Studies in cystic fibrosis of the pancreas: occurrence of rectal prolapse. *N Engl J Med* 1958;259.409.

131. Kwok SPY, Carey DP, Lau WY, et al. Laparoscopic rectopexy. *Dis Colon Rectum* 1994;37:947.

132. Labow S, Rubin RJ, Hoexter B, et al. Perineal repair of rectal procidentia with an elastic fabric sling. *Dis Colon Rectum* 1980;23:467.

133. Ladha A, Lee P, Berger P. Use of Angelchik Anti-Reflux Prosthesis for repair of total rectal prolapse in elderly patients. *Dis Colon Rectum* 1985;38:5.

134. Lake SP, Hancock BD, Lewis AAM. Management of pelvic sepsis after Ivalon rectopexy. *Dis Colon Rectum* 1984;27:589.

135. Lamesch AJ. An unusual hamartomatous malformation of the rectosigmoid presenting as an irreducible rectal prolapse and necessitating rectosigmoid resection in a 14-week-old infant. *Dis Colon Rectum* 1983;26:452.

136. Lane RH. Clinical application of anorectal physiology. *Proc R Soc Med* 1975;68:28.

137. Launer DP, Fazio VW, Weakley FL, et al. The Ripstein procedure: a 16-year experience. *Dis Colon Rectum* 1982;25:41.

138. Lechaux JP, Lechaux D, Perez M. Results of Delorme's procedure for rectal prolapse: advantages of a modified technique. *Dis Colon Rectum* 1995;38:301.

139. Lescher TJ, Corman ML, Coller JA, et al. Management of late complications of Teflon sling repair for rectal prolapse. *Dis Colon Rectum* 1979;22:445.

140. Levine DS. "Solitary" rectal ulcer syndrome: are "solitary" rectal ulcer syndrome and "localized" colitis cystica profunda analogous syndromes caused by rectal prolapse? *Gastroenterology* 1987;92:243.

141. Lockhart-Mummery P. *Diseases of the rectum and anus.* New York: William Wood, 1914.

142. Lomas MI, Cooperman H. Correction of rectal procidentia by use of polypropylene mesh (Marlex). *Dis Colon Rectum* 1972;15:416.

143. Loygue J, Huguier M, Malafosse M, et al. Complete prolapse of the rectum: a report on 140 cases treated by rectopexy. *Br J Surg* 1971;58:847.

144. Loygue J, Nordlinger B, Cunci O, et al. Rectopexy to the promontory for the treatment of rectal prolapse: report of 257 cases. *Dis Colon Rectum* 1984;27:356.

145. Madigan MR. Solitary ulcer of the rectum. *Proc R Soc Med* 1964;57:403

146. Madigan MR, Morson BC. Solitary ulcer of the rectum. *Gut* 1969;10:871.

147. Malouf AJ, Vaizey CJ, Kamm MA. Results of behavioral treatment (biofeedback) for solitary rectal ulcer syndrome. *Dis Colon Rectum* 2001;44:72.

148. Malyshev YI, Gulin VA. Our experience with the treatment of rectal prolapse in infants and children. *Am J Proctol* 1973;24:470.

149. Mann CV. Rectal prolapse. In: Morson BC, ed. *Diseases of the colon, rectum and anus.* New York: Appleton-Century-Crofts, 1969:238.

150. Mann CV, Hoffman C. Complete rectal prolapse: the anatomical and functional results of treatment by an extended abdominal rectopexy. *Br J Surg* 1988;75:34.

151. Marshall M, Halligan S, Fotheringham T, et al. Predictive value of internal anal sphincter thickness for diagnosis of rectal intussusception in patients with solitary rectal ulcer syndrome. *Br J Surg* 2002;89:1281.

152. Martin CJ, Parks TG, Biggart JD. Solitary rectal ulcer syndrome in Northern Ireland, 1971–1980. *Br J Surg* 1981;68:744.

153. McCaffrey JF. Delorme repair for prolapse of the rectum following "failed" Ripstein operation. *Am J Proctol Gastroenterol Colon Rectal Surg* 1983;34:5.

154. McCue JL, Thomson JPS. Rectopexy for internal rectal intussusception. *Br J Surg* 1990;77:632.

155. McCue JL, Thomson JPS. Clinical and functional results of abdominal rectopexy for complete rectal prolapse. *Br J Surg* 1991;78:921.

156. McMahan JD, Ripstein CB. Rectal prolapse: an update on the rectal sling procedure. *Am Surg* 1987;53:37.

157. Mellgren A, Anzén B, Nilsson B-Y, et al. Results of rectocele repair: a prospective study. *Dis Colon Rectum* 1995;38:7.

158. Mellgren A, Bremmer S, Johansson C, et al. Defecography: results of investigations in 2,816 patients. *Dis Colon Rectum* 1994;37:1133.

159. Mellgren A, Dolk A, Johansson C, et al. Enterocele is correctable using the Ripstein rectopexy. *Dis Colon Rectum* 1994;37:800.

160. Morgan CN, Porter NH, Klugman DJ. Ivalon (polyvinyl alcohol) sponge in the repair of complete rectal prolapse. *Br J Surg* 1972;59:841.

161. Moschcowitz AV. The pathogenesis, anatomy, and cure of prolapse of the rectum. *Surg Gynecol Obstet* 1912;15:7.

162. Murthy VK, Orkin BA, Smith LE, et al. Excellent outcome using selective criteria for rectocele repair. *Dis Colon Rectum* 1996;39:374.

163. Myers JO, Rothenberger DA. Sugar in the reduction of incarcerated prolapsed bowel: report of two cases. *Dis Colon Rectum* 1991;34:416.

164. Narasanagi SS. Rectal prolapse in children. *J Indian Med Assoc* 1973;62:378.

165. Nash DF. Bowel management in spina bifida patients. *Proc R Soc Med* 1972;65:70.

166. Nay HR, Blair CR. Perineal surgical repair of rectal prolapse. *Am J Surg* 1972;123:577.

167. Neill ME, Parks AG, Swash M. Physiological studies of the anal sphincter musculature in faecal incontinence and rectal prolapse. *Br J Surg* 1981;68:531.

168. Nicholls RJ, Simson JNL. Anteroposterior rectopexy in the treatment of solitary rectal ulcer syndrome without overt rectal prolapse. *Br J Surg* 1986;73:222.

169. Nichols DH. Retrorectal levatorplasty for anal and perineal prolapse. *Surg Gynecol Obstet* 1982;154:251.

170. Nicosia JF, Bass NM. Use of the fascial stapler in proctopexy for rectal prolapse. *Dis Colon Rectum* 1987;30:900.

171. Nigro ND. An evaluation of the cause and mechanism of complete rectal prolapse. *Dis Colon Rectum* 1966;9:391.

172. Nigro ND. A sling operation for rectal prolapse. *Proc R Soc Med* 1970;63:106.

173. Nivatvongs S, Fang DT. The use of thumbtacks to stop massive presacral hemorrhage. *Dis Colon Rectum* 1986;29:589.

174. Notaras MJ. The use of Mersilene mesh in rectal prolapse repair. *Proc R Soc Med* 1973;66:684.

175. Novell JR, Osborne MJ, Winslet MC, et al. Prospective randomized trial of Ivalon sponge versus sutured rectopexy for full-thickness rectal prolapse. *Br J Surg* 1994;81:904.

176. Nwako F. Rectal prolapse in Nigerian children. *Int Surg* 1975;60:284.

177. Oettle GJ, Roe AM, Bartolo DCC, et al. What is the best way of measuring perineal descent? A comparison of radiographic and clinical methods. *Br J Surg* 1985;72:999.

178. Oliver GC, Vachon D, Eisenstat TE, et al. Delorme's procedure for complete rectal prolapse in severely debilitated patients: an analysis of 41 cases. *Dis Colon Rectum* 1994;37:461.

179. Orr TG. A suspension operation for prolapse of the rectum. *Ann Surg* 1947;126:833.

180. Palmer JA. Prolapse of the rectum: treatment by the Moschcowitz-Graham operation. *Can J Surg* 1969;12:116.

181. Paramore RH. The supports-in-chief of the female pelvic viscera. *J Obstet Gynaecol* 1908;13:391.

182. Paramore RH. The pelvic floor aperture: with an appendix. *J Obstet Gynaecol* 1910;18.95.

183. Paramore RH. The Hunterian lecture on the intra-abdomino-pelvic pressure in man. *Lancet* 1911;2:1677.

184. Parks AG. Anorectal incontinence. *Proc R Soc Med* 1975;68:681.

185. Parks AG, Porter NH, Hardcastle J. The syndrome of the descending perineum. *Proc R Soc Med* 1966;59:477.

186. Parks AG, Swash M, Urich H. Sphincter denervation in anorectal incontinence and rectal prolapse. *Gut* 1977;18:656.

187. Penfold JC, Hawley PR. Experience of Ivalon-sponge implant for complete rectal prolapse at St. Mark's Hospital, 1960–1970. *Br J Surg* 1972;59:846.

188. Pescatori M, Maria G, Mattana C, et al. Clinical picture and pelvic floor physiology in the solitary rectal ulcer syndrome. *Dis Colon Rectum* 1985;28:862.

189. Plumley P. A modification to Thiersch's operation for rectal prolapse. *Br J Surg* 1966;53:624.

190. Plusa SM, Charig JA, Balaji V, et al. Physiological changes after Delorme's procedure for full-thickness rectal prolapse. *Br J Surg* 1995;82:1475.

191. Poole GV Jr, Pennell TC, Myers RT, et al. Modified Thiersch operation for rectal prolapse: technique and results. *Am Surg* 1985;51:226.

192. Prasad ML, Pearl RK, Abcarian H, et al. Perineal proctectomy, posterior rectopexy, and postanal levator repair for the treatment of rectal prolapse. *Dis Colon Rectum* 1986;29:547.

193. Ramanujam PS, Venkatesh KS. Management of acute incarcerated rectal prolapse. *Dis Colon Rectum* 1992;35:1154.

194. Ramanujam PS, Venkatesh KS, Fietz MJ. Perineal excision of rectal procidentia in elderly high-risk patients. *Dis Colon Rectum* 1994;37:1027.

195. Rectal prolapse [Symposium]. *Contemp Surg* 1980;17.54.

196. Rentsch M, Lenhart M, Feuerbach S, et al. Dynamic magnetic resonance imaging defecography: a diagnostic alternative in the assessment of pelvic floor disorders in proctology. *Dis Colon Rectum* 2001;44:999.

197. Ripstein CB. The repair of massive rectal prolapse. *Surg Proc* 1965;2:2.

198. Ripstein CB. Surgical care of massive rectal prolapse. *Dis Colon Rectum* 1965;8:34.

199. Ripstein CB. Procidentia of the rectum: internal intussusception of the rectum (stage I rectal prolapse). *Dis Colon Rectum* 1975;18:458.

200. Ripstein CB, Lanter B. Etiology and surgical therapy of massive prolapse of the rectum. *Ann Surg* 1963;157:259.

201. Rogers J, Jeffery PJ. Postanal repair and intersphincteric Ivalon sponge rectopexy for the treatment of rectal prolapse. *Br J Surg* 1987;74:384.

202. Ross AH McL, Thomson JPS. Management of infection after prosthetic abdominal rectopexy (Wells' procedure). *Br J Surg* 1989;76:610.

203. Rutter KRP, Riddell RH. The solitary ulcer syndrome of the rectum. *Clin Gastroenterol* 1975;4:505.

204. Sainio AP, Halme LE, Husa AI. Anal encirclement with polypropylene mesh for rectal prolapse and incontinence. *Dis Colon Rectum* 1991;34:905.

205. Sainio AP, Voutilainen PE, Husa AI. Recovery of anal sphincter function following transabdominal repair of rectal prolapse: cause of improved continence? *Dis Colon Rectum* 1991;34:816.

206. Santulli TV. Rectal prolapse. In: Rudolph AM, Hoffman JI, eds. *Pediatrics*, 17th ed. Norwalk, CT: Appleton-Century-Crofts, 1983:990.

207. Saul SH. Solitary rectal ulcer syndrome: its clinical and pathological underdiagnosis. *Am J Surg Pathol* 1985;9:411.

208. Sayfan J, Pinho M, Alexander-Williams J, et al. Sutured posterior abdominal rectopexy with sigmoidectomy compared with Marlex rectopexy for rectal prolapse. *Br J Surg* 1990;77:143.

209. Schlinkert RT, Beart RW Jr, Wolff BG, et al. Anterior resection for complete rectal prolapse. *Dis Colon Rectum* 1985; 28:409.

210. Schuster MM. The riddle of the sphincters. *Gastroenterology* 1975;69:249.

211. Sehapayak S. Transrectal repair of rectocele: an extended armamentarium of colorectal surgeons. A report of 355 cases. *Dis Colon Rectum* 1985;28:422.

212. Selvaggi F, Pesce G, Di Carlo ES, et al. Evaluation of normal subjects by defecographic technique. *Dis Colon Rectum* 1990;33:698.

213. Senapati A, Nicholls RJ, Chir M, et al. Results of Delorme's procedure for rectal prolapse. *Dis Colon Rectum* 1994;37:456.

214. Shafik A. Pudendal canal decompression for the treatment of fecal incontinence in complete rectal prolapse. *Am Surg* 1996;62:339.

215. Shorvon PJ, McHugh S, Diamant NE, et al. Defecography in normal volunteers: results and implications. *Gut* 1989; 30.1737.

216. Siproudhis L, Dautréme S, Ropert A, et al. Dyschezia and rectocele: a marriage of convenience? *Dis Colon Rectum* 1993;36:1030.

217. Sitzler PJ, Kamm MA, Nicholls RJ, et al. Long-term clinical outcome of surgery for solitary rectal ulcer syndrome. *Br J Surg* 1998;85:1246.

218. Snooks SJ, Henry MM, Swash M. Anorectal incontinence and rectal prolapse: differential assessment of the innervation to puborectalis and external anal sphincter muscles. *Gut* 1985;26:470.

219. Sobin LH. Tales of the ampulla of Vater: VIII. *Dis Colon Rectum* 1987;30:159.

220. Solomon MJ, Eyers AA. Laparoscopic rectopexy using mesh fixation with a spiked chromium staple. *Dis Colon Rectum* 1996;39:279.

221. Solomon MJ, Young CJ, Eyers AA, et al. Randomized clinical trial of laparoscopic versus open abdominal rectopexy for rectal prolapse. *Br J Surg* 2002;89:35.

222. Soriano LR, del Mundo F, Naguit-Sim L. Rectal prolapse in children with trichuriasis. *J Philippine Med Assoc* 1966;42:843.

223. Spencer RJ. Manometric studies in rectal prolapse. *Dis Colon Rectum* 1984;27:523.

224. Stern RC, Izant RJ Jr, Boat TF, et al. Treatment and prognosis of rectal prolapse in cystic fibrosis. *Gastroenterology* 1982;82:707.

225. Stewart R. Long-term results of Ivalon wrap operation for complete rectal prolapse. *Proc R Soc Med* 1972;65:777.

226. Sullivan ES, Garnjobst WM. Advantage of initial transanal mucosal stripping in ileo-anal pull-through procedures. *Dis Colon Rectum* 1982;25:170.

227. Sullivan ES, Leaverton GH, Hardwick CE. Transrectal perineal repair: an adjunct to improved function after anorectal surgery. *Dis Colon Rectum* 1968;11:106.

228. Sullivan ES, Longaker CJ, Lee PYH. Total pelvic mesh repair: a ten-year experience. *Dis Colon Rectum* 2001;44:857.

229. Sullivan ES, Stranburg CO, Sandoz IL, et al. Repair of total pelvic prolapse: an overview. *Perspect Colon Rectal Surg* 1990;3:119.

230. Sun WM, Read NW, Carmel T, et al. A common pathophysiology for full thickness rectal prolapse, anterior mucosal prolapse and solitary rectal ulcer. *Br J Surg* 1989;76:290.

231. Swerdlow H. The encircler: a new instrument for the performance of the Thiersch procedure for rectal procidentia. *Dis Colon Rectum* 1986;29:145.

232. Takano M, Hamada A. Evaluation of pelvic descent disorders by dynamic contrast roentgenography. *Dis Colon Rectum* 2000:43[Suppl]:S6.

233. Theuerkauf FJ Jr, Beahrs OH, Hill JR. Rectal prolapse: causation and surgical treatment. *Ann Surg* 1970;171:819.

234. Thomson G, Clark A, Handyside J, et al. Solitary ulcer of the rectum—or is it? A report of 6 cases. *Br J Surg* 1981; 68:21.

235. Thomson H, Hill D. Solitary rectal ulcer: always a self-induced condition? *Br J Surg* 1980;67:784.

236. Thomson JPS. Anal sphincter incompetence. In: Russell RCG, ed. *Recent advances in surgery*. London: Churchill-Livingston, 1986:155.

237. Thorlakson RH. A modification of the Thiersch procedure for rectal prolapse using polyester tape. *Dis Colon Rectum* 1982;25:57.

238. Tjandra JJ, Fazio VW, Church JM, et al. Ripstein procedure is an effective treatment for rectal prolapse without constipation. *Dis Colon Rectum* 1993;36:501.

239. Tjandra JJ, Fazio VW, Petras RE, et al. Clinical and pathologic factors associated with delayed diagnosis in solitary rectal ulcer syndrome. *Dis Colon Rectum* 1993;36:146.

240. Tobin SA, Scott IHK. Delorme operation for rectal prolapse. *Br J Surg* 1994;81:1681.

241. Todd IP. Etiological factors in the production of complete rectal prolapse. *Postgrad Med J* 1959;35:97.

242. Traisman E, Colon D, Sherman JO, et al. Rectal prolapse in two neonates with Hirschprung's disease. *Am J Dis Child* 1983;137:1126.

243. Traynor LA, Michener WM. Rectal procidentia—a rare complication of ulcerative colitis: report of two cases in children. *Cleve Clin Q* 1966;33:115.

244. Tsunoda, Yasuda N, Yokoyama N, et al. Delorme's procedure for rectal prolapse: clinical and physiological analysis. *Dis Colon Rectum* 2003;46:1260.

245. Uhlig BE, Sullivan ES. The modified Delorme operation: its place in surgical treatment for massive rectal prolapse. *Dis Colon Rectum* 1979;22:513.

246. Vachon DA, Oliver GC, Eisenstat TE, et al. The Delorme procedure for rectal prolapse in the poor risk surgical patient. Poster presentation at the 89th annual meeting of the American Society of Colon and Rectal Surgeons, St. Louis, MO, April 29 to May 4, 1990.

247. Vaizey CJ, van den Bogaerde JB, Emmanuel AV, et al. Solitary rectal ulcer syndrome. *Br J Surg* 1998;85:1617.

248. van Dam JH, Ginai AZ, Gosselink MJ, et al. Role of defecography in predicting clinical outcome of rectocele repair. *Dis Colon Rectum* 1997;40:201.

249. van den Brandt-Grädel V, Huibregtse K, Tytgat GNJ. Treatment of solitary rectal ulcer syndrome with highfiber diet and abstention of straining at defecation. *Dig Dis Sci* 1984;29:1005.

250. van Outryve MJ, Pelckmans PA, Fierens H, et al. Transrectal ultrasound study of the pathogenesis of solitary rectal ulcer syndrome. *Gut* 1993;34:1422.

251. van Tets WF, Kuijpers JHC. Internal rectal intussusception: fact or fancy? *Dis Colon Rectum* 1995;38:1080.

252. Vermeulen FD, Nivatvongs S, Fang DT, et al. A technique for perineal rectosigmoidectomy using autosuture devices. *Surg Gynecol Obstet* 1983;156:85.

253. Watson SJ, Loder PB, Halligan S, et al. Transperineal repair of symptomatic rectocele with Marlex mesh: a clinical, physiological and radiologic assessment of treatment. *J Am Coll Surg* 1996;183:257.

254. Watts AMI, Thompson MR. Evaluation of Delorme's procedure as a treatment for full-thickness rectal prolapse. *Br J Surg* 2000;87:218.

255. Watts JD, Rothenberger DA, Buls JG, et al. The management of procidentia: 30 years' experience. *Dis Colon Rectum* 1985;28:96.

256. Wells C. New operation for rectal prolapse. *Proc R Soc Med* 1959;52:602.

257. Williams JG, Rothenberger DA, Madoff RD, et al. Treatment of rectal prolapse in the elderly by perineal rectosigmoidectomy. *Dis Colon Rectum* 1992;35:830.

258. Williams JG, Wong WD, Jensen L, et al. Incontinence and rectal prolapse: a prospective manometric study. *Dis Colon Rectum* 1991;34:209.

259. Williams ND. Impact of new technology on anorectal disorders. *Br J Surg* 1987;74:236.

260. Womack NR, Williams NS, Holmfield JH, et al. Anorectal function in the solitary rectal ulcer syndrome. *Dis Colon Rectum* 1987;30:319.

261. Womack NR, Williams NS, Holmfield JH, et al. Pressure and prolapse: the cause of solitary rectal ulceration. *Gut* 1987;28:1228.

262. Xu J, Lin J. Control of presacral hemorrhage with electrocautery through a muscle fragment pressed on the bleeding vein. *J Am Coll Surg* 1994;179:351.

263. Yamana T, Iwadare J. Mucosal plication (Gant-Miwa procedure) with anal encircling for rectal prolapse: a review of the Japanese experience. *Dis Colon Rectum* 2003;46 [Suppl]:S94.

264. Yoshioka K, Heyen F, Keighley MRB. Functional results after posterior abdominal rectopexy for rectal prolapse. *Dis Colon Rectum* 1989;32:835.

265. Yoshioka K, Hyland G, Keighley MRB. Anorectal function after abdominal rectopexy: parameters of predictive value in identifying return of continence. *Br J Surg* 1989;76:64.

266. Yoshioka K, Matsui Y, Yamada O, et al. Physiologic and anatomic assessment of patients with rectocele. *Dis Colon Rectum* 1991;34:704.

267. Zainea GG, Szilagy EJ. Perineal repair of colorectoanal intussusception. *Dis Colon Rectum* 1996;39:1434.

268. Zargar SA, Khuroo MS, Mahajan R. Sucralfate retention enemas in solitary rectal ulcer. *Dis Colon Rectum* 1991; 34: 455.

Chapter 18

Pediatric Surgical Problems

Guest Contributors: Alberto Peña and Marc Levitt

I am delighted that Drs. Alberto Peña and Marc Levitt have consented to contribute to the fifth edition of this book. Dr. Peña's singular efforts with the second, third, and fourth editions have been well recognized by everyone who deals with surgery of the anus, rectum, and colon. Dr. Peña is considered one of the world's authorities on the management of congenital anomalies of the rectum and has devised unique approaches for dealing with imperforate anus and its myriad manifestations. This fifth edition now incorporates the thoughts of Dr. Marc Levitt, another well-recognized individual in the field of pediatric surgery. As one of his colleagues in the Department of Surgery, I have always valued his insight and his knowledge of colon and rectal problems in both the adult and the pediatric population.

MLC

> We can say with some assurance that,
> although children may be the victims
> of fate, they will not be the victims
> of our neglect.
>
> John F. Kennedy

In this chapter, the spectrum of three congenital anomalies that affect the anorectal area is discussed: aganglionosis, neuronal intestinal dysplasia (NID), and imperforate anus. In addition, a review of an acquired intestinal condition, necrotizing enterocolitis (NEC) is presented. Other diseases in the pediatric population are presented within the appropriate chapters.

CONGENITAL MEGACOLON OR HIRSCHSPRUNG'S DISEASE

Historical Review

In 1691, Fredrick Ruysch reported the autopsy findings of a child who died with what appeared to be a congenital megacolon.[81] The eponymous association for this disease, however, originated with Harold Hirschsprung, who, in 1886, at the Pediatric Congress in Berlin, described an infant with this condition.[62] The first reference relating the absence of ganglion cells to the underlying disturbance is that of Tittle in 1901.[154] In 1940, Tiffin and co-workers described the disturbed peristalsis of the aganglionic intestine.[153] Robertson and Kernohan in 1938, and Zuelzer and Wilson in 1948, were able to correlate the functional disturbances of the distal colon with aganglionosis.[124,164] Swenson and colleagues, in 1949, described the main principles for the radiologic diagnosis of this condition; these observations are still useful today.[150] The first rational surgical approach for the management of congenital megacolon was reported by Swenson and Bill in 1948.[149] Other modifications of this technique, such as the Duhamel approach[35] and the Soave operation,[139] were developed in order to avoid some of the complications seen with the

---

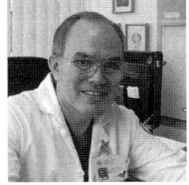 **Alberto Peña (1938–present)**   Alberto Peña was born August 16, 1938, in Mexico City, Mexico. He received his medical degree at the Military Medical School in Mexico City in 1962 and completed his general surgical training at the same institution in 1966. He then became interested in pediatric surgery and decided to do a Research Fellowship in Cardiovascular Surgery at Children's Hospital in Boston, Massachusetts. In pursuit of his pediatric surgery training, he continued at Children's Hospital for 2 additional years. Peña then returned to Mexico City to become the Surgeon-in-Chief and Professor of Pediatric Surgery at the National Institute of Pediatrics, a position he occupied until 1985. He then accepted the post of Chief of Pediatric Surgery and Professor of Surgery at the Schneider Children's Hospital in New Hyde Park, New York, a position he continues to hold. Peña has contributed to numerous areas in the field of pediatric surgery, including deformities of the chest wall, esophageal replacement, and pancreatectomy in the newborn. However, he is best known for his innovative approach to the management of congenital anorectal malformations. Peña has received numerous honors throughout the world, including recognition by the United Nations for his work with children in Africa, the Coe Medical from the Pacific Association of Pediatric Surgeons, and Honorary Fellowship of the Royal College of Surgeons of England. He continues to lecture and operate around the world and to teach pediatric surgeons his approach to the management of congenital anorectal malformations. (Courtesy of Avraham Belizon, M.D.)

Swenson method but were still based on the same principles of repair (see later).

More recently, babies with Hirschsprung's disease have undergone the surgery through a laparoscopic approach.[26,46,47,137] This is consistent with the contemporary trend to less invasive surgery for the treatment of children with congenital defects. Furthermore, a new and totally different technique has been applied for the treatment of this condition, the so-called *transanal approach* (see later).[28]

Pathophysiology and Embryology

Congenital megacolon is an anomaly characterized by partial or complete colonic obstruction associated with the absence of intramural ganglion cells.[63,92] The aganglionic portion of the colon is always located distally, but the length of the segment varies. This is the factor that determines the manifestations of the disease (Figure 18-1). The so-called "typical" and most frequent variation is the one in which the aganglionic segment includes the rectum and much of the sigmoid colon (Figure 18-1*B*). This type accounts for approximately two thirds of all patients. The long-segment variety represents approximately 10% of presentations (Figure 18-1*D*).[135] In this manifestation, the aganglionic portion may extend to any level between the hepatic flexure and the descending colon. Total colonic aganglionosis is a very serious condition in which the entire colon is aganglionic, frequently including a variable length of terminal ileum (Figure 18-1*C*). This type also represents approximately 10% of the entire group.[37] There is some debate

about the existence of so-called "ultrashort" aganglionosis or short-segment Hirschsprung's disease (see also Chapter 16). It is frequently misinterpreted as functional chronic constipation; its histologic confirmation is also a matter of some debate (see Figs. 16-4 and Figure 18-3).

Typically, the aganglionic portion of the colon appears narrow when compared with the distended, proximal part. Thus, the term "narrow segment" is somewhat misleading. The aganglionic portion demonstrates absence of intramural, submucosal, and intermuscular ganglion cells. Increased size and prominence of nerve fibers are also seen in this area. The proximal, normally innervated portion of the colon is usually distended, and its wall is thickened because of muscle hypertrophy. Mucosal ulcerations are also frequently seen. Between these two areas is the so-called "transition zone," a cone-shaped portion of colon that is often histologically described as hypoganglionic.

An increase in the enzyme acetylcholinesterase has been demonstrated in the aganglionic colon.[39,66,67] Acetylcholinesterase staining demonstrates a significant increase in the number of oversized nerve fibers located in the muscularis mucosa, the lamina propria, and the submucosa.

Congenital megacolon is believed to be a disease caused by the failure in the development of tissue derived from the neural crest. There appears to be an arrest in the craniocaudal migration of the neuroenteric ganglion cells from the neural crest into the upper gastrointestinal tract, down through the vagal fibers, and along the distal intestine.[101] As a consequence, ganglion cells are missing from Auerbach's myenteric plexus (located between the circular and longitudinal layers of bowel wall), Henle's plexus (located

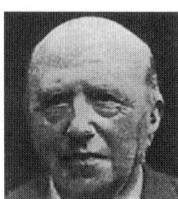

Harold Hirschsprung (1830–1916)   Hirschsprung was born in Copenhagen, Denmark. He passed his examinations in 1855 and was made a teacher in 1861. He was Professor of Pediatrics at the University of Copenhagen and Head Physician to the Queen Louise Children's Hospital. Hirschsprung is best known for his description of the disease that was named after him, perhaps because of his excellent account of the condition, given that his was not the original report. Parry actually described a case that is recorded in his collected papers in 1825. Levine of Chicago, in 1867, noted the first American case. In his paper, he does not identify the pathogenicity, nor does he offer a suggestion for treatment of aganglionic megacolon. Hirschsprung contributed extensively to the pediatric literature, publishing one of the first comprehensive reports on pyloric stenosis in 1888, and he was a pioneer in the use of hydrostatic pressure for the reduction of intussusception in 1905. Although theories abounded for 50 years, Lennander in 1900 was one of the first to suggest a neurogenic origin—there was so much confusion and there were so many differences of opinion that it was not until the 1940s that the absence of ganglion cells was believed to be the etiologic factor. (Hirschsprung H. Stuhltrúgheit neugeborener in folge von dilatation und hypertrophie des colon. *Jahrb Kinderheilkd* 1888;27:1.)

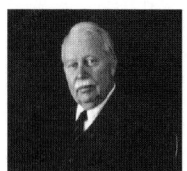

Orvar Swenson (1909–present)   Orvar Swenson was born in Halsingborg, Sweden, on February 7, 1909, the son of a Mormon missionary father. The family returned to the United States and settled in Independence, Missouri. Swenson attended William Jewell College in Liberty, Kansas, and received his Bachelor's degree in 1933. He then enrolled in Harvard Medical School, graduating in 1937. Following a year as an intern at Ohio State University Hospital, he returned to Boston and to the Peter Bent Brigham Hospital and the Boston Children's Hospital, where he completed training in general surgery and in pediatric surgery in 1945. Swenson remained on the staff of these two hospitals for 5 years, during which time he ascertained the etiology of and developed a surgical treatment for Hirschsprung's disease. In 1950, he took the position as Surgeon-in-Chief of the Boston Floating Hospital and Professor of Surgery at Tufts University School of Medicine. In 1960, he moved to Chicago to become Surgeon-in-Chief at Children's Memorial Hospital. In 1973, he moved on again, this time to the University of Miami, where he remained until his retirement in 1978. Swenson shared the second Mead Johnson Research Award in 1952 with Edward B. Neuhaser for their research on the elucidation, pathogenesis, and treatment of congenital megacolon. He later received the William Ladd Medal. (With appreciation to Avraham Belizon, M.D.; photograph, courtesy of Keith E. Georgeson, M.D.)

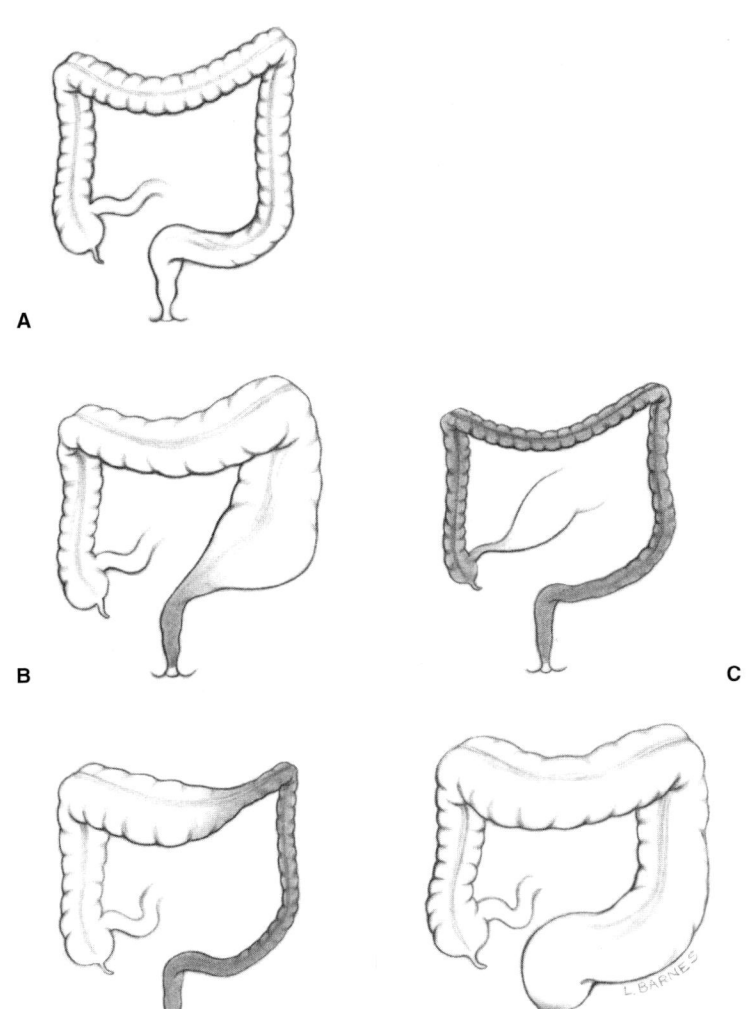

A

B

C

D

E

FIGURE 18-1. Different presentations of Hirschsprung's disease according to the length of the aganglionic segment. **(A)** Normal bowel. **(B)** Typical involvement. **(C)** Total colonic aganglionosis. **(D)** Long-segment disease. **(E)** Short-segment disease.

in the deep submucosa), and also Meissner's plexus in the superficial submucosa (Figs. 18-2 and 18-3; see also Figure 16-4). Under normal circumstances, the ganglia appear to act as a final common path for both sympathetic and parasympathetic influences. Their absence may perhaps produce the uncoordinated contractions of the affected bowel. Spasm, lack of propulsive peristalsis, and mass contraction of the aganglionic segment[61] have all been well documented, in addition to the lack of relaxation of the bowel and the spasm of the internal sphincter.[27,155] The clinical result of these pathophysiologic events is partial or total colonic obstruction with all of the usual sequelae. There is, however, a lack of correlation between the extent of the aganglionosis and the severity of the symptoms.

There has been a special interest in the role of nitric oxide as a neurotransmitter responsible for the inhibitory action elicited by the intrinsic enteric nerves. A lack of nitric oxide synthase (the enzyme required for nitric oxide production) has been demonstrated in the myenteric plexus of the aganglionic segment.[10,102] The significance of

this finding and the potential therapeutic implications are theoretically profound but have yet to be demonstrated.

Incidence and Associated Malformations

It is generally accepted that the incidence of Hirschsprung's disease is in the range of one in 5,000 births.[37] It also seems to be more common in whites. Although boys are much more frequently affected than girls, the long-segment manifestation is seen at least as often in female patients. Inheritance patterns seem to be multifactorial. The risk for a sibling sister of a male patient is 0.6%, whereas the risk for a brother of a female patient with long-segment disease is 18%.[1041]

Approximately 5% to 21% of all individuals affected with Hirschsprung's disease have an associated congenital anomaly.[64] Certainly, its association with anorectal malformations is well known. One may even suspect that Hirschsprung's disease could be erroneously overdiag-

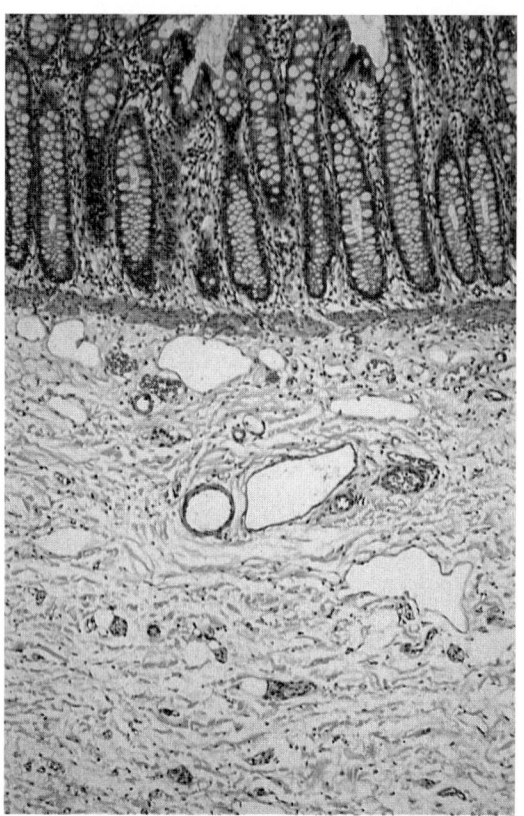

FIGURE 18-2. Histologic section including mucosa with submucosa of the rectum showing clusters of ganglion cells in the submucosal plexus. This excludes Hirschsprung's disease at this level. (See Color Fig. 18-2.) (Courtesy of Hector L. Monforte-Muñoz, M.D., Department of Pathology, Children's Hospital, Los Angeles, CA.)

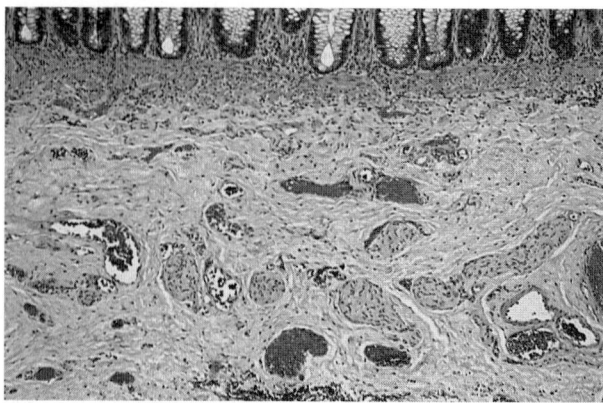

FIGURE 18-3. Histologic section including mucosa and submucosa of the rectum showing tortuous and hypertrophic nerve trunks of the submucosal plexus. There is no evidence of any ganglion cell present. This establishes the diagnosis of Hirschsprung's disease. (See Color Fig. 18-3.) (Courtesy of Hector L. Monforte-Muñoz, M.D., Department of Pathology, Children's Hospital, Los Angeles, CA.)

Clinical Manifestations and Differential Diagnosis

Infants suffering from Hirschsprung's disease usually become symptomatic during the first 24 to 48 hours of life. Occasionally, a child may have minimal or absent clinical manifestations during the first days or weeks and may exhibit moderate, intermittent bouts of symptoms at a later age (Fig.18-4; see also Chapter 16).

Abdominal distension, delayed passage of meconium, and vomiting represent the most frequent observations in

nosed because most patients who are born with anorectal malformations suffer some degree of constipation.[71] Another associated condition is Down's syndrome; this anomaly is found in 5% of these infants.[12,50]

There have been developments in determining the genetic defects associated with Hirschsprung's disease. A deletion in the long arm of chromosome 10 has been found.[90] More detailed evaluation indicates that the location of this mutation is between 10Q11.2 and Q21.2 2.[43,85] This deletion seems to overlap the region of the *RET* proto-oncogene. Patients with multiple endocrine neoplasia (MEN 2A) also have a deletion of this proto-oncogene. This genetic discovery is an important advance in the study of this complex disease. However, the identification of the gene and the exact sequence of the DNA code still elude us. Ultimately, it is hoped that this will provide information about the function of the gene and provide clues as to how and why the disease occurs. Molenaar opined that the contribution of mutations in the *RET* gene to the pathogenesis of Hirschsprung's disease and its associated anomalies will be clarified within the foreseeable future.[94] Certainly, new and exciting developments are occurring in the field of genetics in this condition.[4–8]

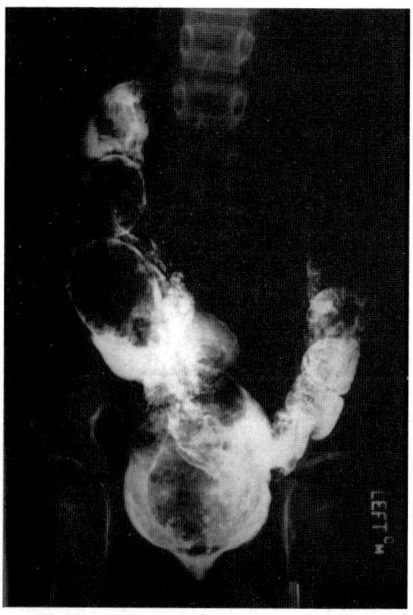

FIGURE 18-4. Barium enema study of young man with presumed short-segment Hirschsprung's disease with lifelong constipation. Note the dilated bowel and considerable fecal residue.

individuals with congenital megacolon. This triad of symptoms may be followed by a spontaneous or induced explosive, massively deflating passage of liquid bowel movement and gas, which dramatically improves the baby's condition. This is followed by a period of hours or days of relative absence of symptoms followed by recurrence of the same manifestations. Stools are frequently liquid and foul. When the abdomen is distended, the infant usually is very ill from sepsis, hypovolemia, and endotoxic shock. Ischemic enterocolitis with necrosis proximal to the aganglionic segment is the most serious complication. Other supervening problems are pneumatosis cystoides intestinalis, pericolic abscess, and cecal perforation.[141] There is a 25% to 30% mortality if the disease is unrecognized or untreated,[64] with some authors reporting a 50% mortality during the first year of life.[36]

Typically, rectal examination of an ill infant with Hirschsprung's disease produces an explosive bowel movement with immediate symptomatic improvement. The differential diagnosis includes any condition that causes intestinal obstruction in the newborn, probably the most frequent being the so-called *meconium-plug syndrome*. The expulsion of a plug of meconium with resolution of symptoms and the absence of other signs characteristic of Hirschsprung's disease help to establish this diagnosis. *Meconium ileus* is manifested by a clinical picture consistent with that of intestinal obstruction, with the child frequently exhibiting respiratory symptoms.[32] A family history of cystic fibrosis may be noted. The absence of air-fluid levels in an upright abdominal film and the "ground-glass" appearance of the lower abdomen are characteristic radiographic signs of this condition.

Another condition that may lead to confusion in differential diagnosis is the *small left colon syndrome*. Barium enema demonstrates a rather narrow left colon to the level of the splenic flexure. Symptoms usually improve following this study and resolve after several weeks. The mother is frequently diabetic.

Other, nonsurgical conditions that may be confused with Hirschsprung's disease include hypothyroidism, adrenal insufficiency, and cerebral injury.

Patients who survive despite inadequate treatment or who have relatively mild symptoms ultimately develop the classic clinical picture initially described for this condition. These children suffer severe constipation with an enormously distended abdomen. The proximal colon is huge and full of inspissated fecal material (Figure 18-4). At this stage, the diagnosis may be confused with chronic constipation (e.g., colon inertia or megarectum). In the latter condition, children usually become symptomatic after the sixth month of life; they neither vomit nor become seriously ill. A very important characteristic in this group of patients is overflow incontinence or encopresis, a constant, chronic soiling without evidence of neuromuscular disturbance (see Chapter 16). Rectal examination in these children reveals a severe fecal impaction just above the anal canal. Patients

with Hirschsprung's disease may have an empty rectum, or examination may disclose only a small amount of feces.

Diagnosis

Radiologic Studies

It is well known among pediatric surgeons, neonatologists, and pediatric radiologists that it is very difficult to differentiate a distended colon from a distended small bowel on the basis of a plain abdominal film of a neonate with intestinal obstruction. Therefore, one can only suspect the diagnosis of Hirschsprung's disease from this study. The presence of air-fluid levels is evidence of obstruction, but it is, of course, nonspecific. An enema examination performed with a rather dilute suspension of barium, or preferably with water-soluble contrast material, is the most valuable radiologic study for establishing the diagnosis.

No bowel preparation is required. The infant is placed in a lateral position, and a rectal tube is introduced to barely above the anal canal. Injection of contrast is optimally controlled by hand with a syringe. The introduction of a catheter beyond the limit of the anal canal will risk a misdiagnosis, because the tip may reach the distended colon and result in injection above the aganglionic portion. The dye is instilled until it reaches the distended portion of the intestine, at which point the study is terminated. Injection of excessive amounts of contrast material, especially barium, may produce further evacuation problems and impaction.

This study may reveal the presence of a very distended proximal colon, the transition zone, and a "contracted" distal rectosigmoid (Figure 18-5B). The older the patient, the more obvious the size difference between the normal ganglionic intestine and the abnormal aganglionic bowel will be. Therefore, sometimes the typical changes are not very obvious during the neonatal period (Figure 18-5A). A second barium enema performed a few days or weeks later may show a much more dramatic appearance than that seen previously (Figure 18-5B). Generally, however, the transition zone is indeed recognized in most newborns. Barium enema is less accurate in infants with very short aganglionosis or when the entire colon is involved.[130] In instances of total colonic aganglionosis, barium enema may reveal a rather short colon, with retraction of the hepatic and splenic flexures and straightening of the sigmoid.

Anorectal Manometry

Normally, when the rectum is distended with a balloon, pressure in the anal canal falls because of internal sphincter relaxation, the rectoanal inhibitory reflex. In infants with aganglionosis, this reflex is absent (see Chapter 6).[156] This abnormal response has been interpreted as diagnostic for this condition. However, this test has several limitations, the primary one being the technical difficulty

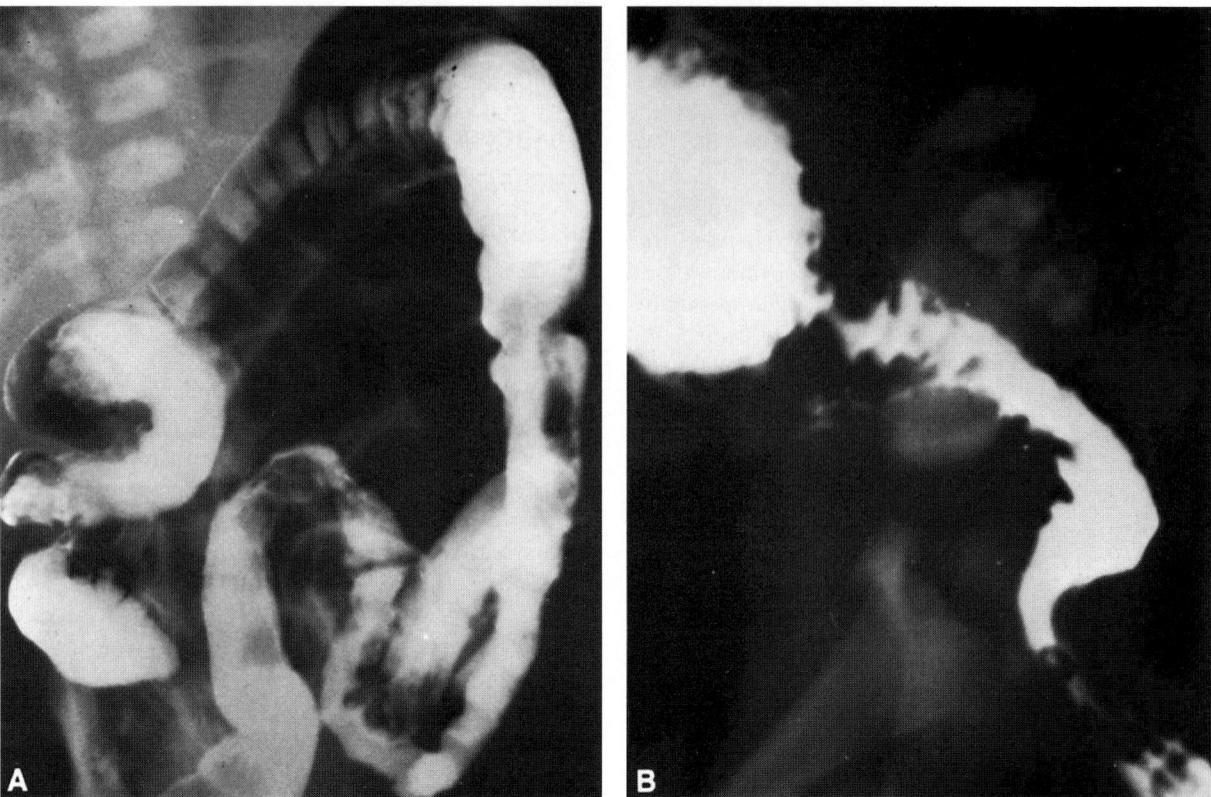

FIGURE 18-5. Hirschsprung's disease. **(A)** Barium enema performed in a newborn with Hirschsprung's disease. Often, classical changes are not obvious in the neonatal period. **(B)** A later barium enema demonstrates the typical megacolon, transition zone, and nondistended, aganglionic portion.

of evaluating the newborn. In our own experience, this test is useful primarily for older children (see Chapter 16).

Rectal Biopsy

The confirmation of the diagnosis is based on the absence of ganglion cells and the presence of an excess of non-myelinated nerves in an adequate rectal biopsy. The specimen must be taken at least 1.5 cm above the pectinate line. The traditional full-thickness rectal biopsy has obvious diagnostic value. However, the tissue is difficult to obtain in newborns because good rectal exposure requires a general anesthetic.[31,99] Suction biopsy (Model SBT-100 Medical Measurements, Inc., Hackensack, NJ), therefore, has gained wide acceptance because it is easily performed, is associated with virtually no risk of perforation, and does not require an anesthetic. The specimen usually measures 1 × 3 mm and should include mucosa and submucosa. Although interpretation requires expertise, this is the preferred study for establishing the diagnosis.

The presence of large amounts of acetylcholinesterase in the mucosa and submucosa has led to the use of this investigation as a diagnostic alternative.[39,66,67,91] The absence of nicotinamide adenine dinucleotide phospate diaphorase–containing neurons and an increase in the amount of acetylcholinesterase-containing nerve bundles are all characteristic.[95] Furthermore, nitric oxide synthase has gained increasing recognition as a candidate neurotransmitter responsible for relaxation of the internal anal sphincter. This observation is extremely important in the evaluation of individuals with short-segment Hirschsprung's disease.[95]

Opinion

There is considerable difference of opinion with respect to the reliability of the various diagnostic methods. It is our impression that the most important variable is the experience of the radiologist, physiologist, and pathologist. Barium enema, for us at least, has been the most valuable diagnostic test, with rectal suction biopsy a means for confirming the clinical and radiologic impression. Although biopsy may establish the diagnosis when the specimen is obtained through the rectum, it reveals nothing about the transition zone site. That valuable piece of information must be obtained radiologically, clinically, or by operative, full-thickness biopsy analysis.

Management

Medical Treatment

Bowel irrigation with saline solution is an extremely valuable procedure for the emergency management of distension and vomiting. By decompressing the bowel, the procedure may dramatically improve the condition of a very ill infant. However, continued treatment with enemas, as is used by some physicians, is extremely dangerous. Enterocolitis may rapidly develop, with fatal consequences. Therefore, bowel irrigation, although beneficial as an interim, emergency measure, should not be a substitute for surgical intervention.

It is extremely important to clarify the difference between an irrigation and an enema. To confuse these two terms may be dangerous for babies with Hirschsprung's disease. An enema is a procedure in which a determined amount of fluid is instilled into the rectum and colon. It is expected that this volume will be spontaneously expelled.

A rectal irrigation, conversely, is a procedure in which a large tube is introduced through the rectum, and small amounts of saline solution are instilled through the lumen of the tube in order to clear the bowel. The rectal and colonic content is expected to drain through the same lumen of the tube. The tube is then rotated in different directions and moved back and forth. The operator continues to instill small amounts of saline solution, allowing the evacuation of gas and liquid stool through the tube.

Patients with Hirschsprung's disease suffer from a very serious dysmotility disorder. This means that an enema, as defined here, may aggravate the condition of the patient rather than help him or her, because the patient does not have the capacity to expel the infused volume of fluid. With an irrigation, the patient benefits from the evacuation of the rectosigmoid contents through the lumen of the large tube.

Surgical Treatment

General Principles

The trend in the management of patients with Hirschsprung's disease is to perform a primary procedure during the neonatal period *without* a protective colostomy.[22,24,138] The advantage of this approach is to limit the number of operations (i.e., colostomy creation and closure) with the attendant morbidity. Some published reports have demonstrated that there is no difference in rate of complications associated with neonatal surgery when a protective colostomy is *not* employed.[8,21,138]

We believe that this trend is reasonable. However, consideration must be given to several important issues. The circumstances for performing the surgery are different from country to country, and there is often quite a variability in the experience of surgeons. In addition, the availability of fully trained, experienced clinical pathologists may be problematic. If one is to perform a primary neonatal pull-through procedure, the surgeon must rely on frozen-section analysis. For this, he or she must interact with an experienced pathologist, someone who is familiar with histologic diagnosis. Another concern is in the very ill, low-birth-weight newborn or one who suffers from associated defects or concomitant serious medical conditions. Such an individual may benefit from an initial fecal diversion. Finally, the long-term effects of a one-stage, primary repair in the newborn with Hirschsprung's disease, including the incidence of late constipation, enterocolitis, and fecal incontinence, remain to be seen. One must remember that a colostomy is still the optimal means for protecting the patient.

In addition to the issue of whether the performance of a colostomy is appropriate, there is a difference of opinion among surgeons as to the type and the location of the stoma. In our experience, if a colostomy is to be considered, a right transverse colon stoma is an effective and safe method for decompressing the bowel in the vast majority of infants with this condition. By using this location, the risk of falling victim to the tragic error of opening the colostomy in an aganglionic area is much reduced. It is a particularly useful option in the emergency situation, especially if the surgeon cannot rely on the radiologist, or if a pathologist capable of making the diagnosis on the basis of frozen-section analysis is unavailable. The primary disadvantage of this type of colostomy is that the individual may in actuality, harbor "long-segment" disease. Under these circumstances, when the definitive procedure is subsequently performed, the colostomy may interfere with the rectal pull-through because of the short length of bowel remaining between the stoma site and the transition zone.

Many surgeons advocate the creation of the colostomy immediately above the transition zone. This alternative obligates one to pull the colostomy down at the time of the definitive repair, thus depriving the patient of the protection of a proximal diversion unless a new one is created. Obviously, the advantage to this approach is that the child will require only a two-stage procedure, whereas a right transverse colostomy commits the surgeon to a three-stage operation.

Definitive Operations

Swenson's Procedure With the child in the lithotomy position, the abdomen is entered through a Pfannenstiel, hockey-stick incision.[149] Resection of the aganglionic portion of the colon is performed, including that of the

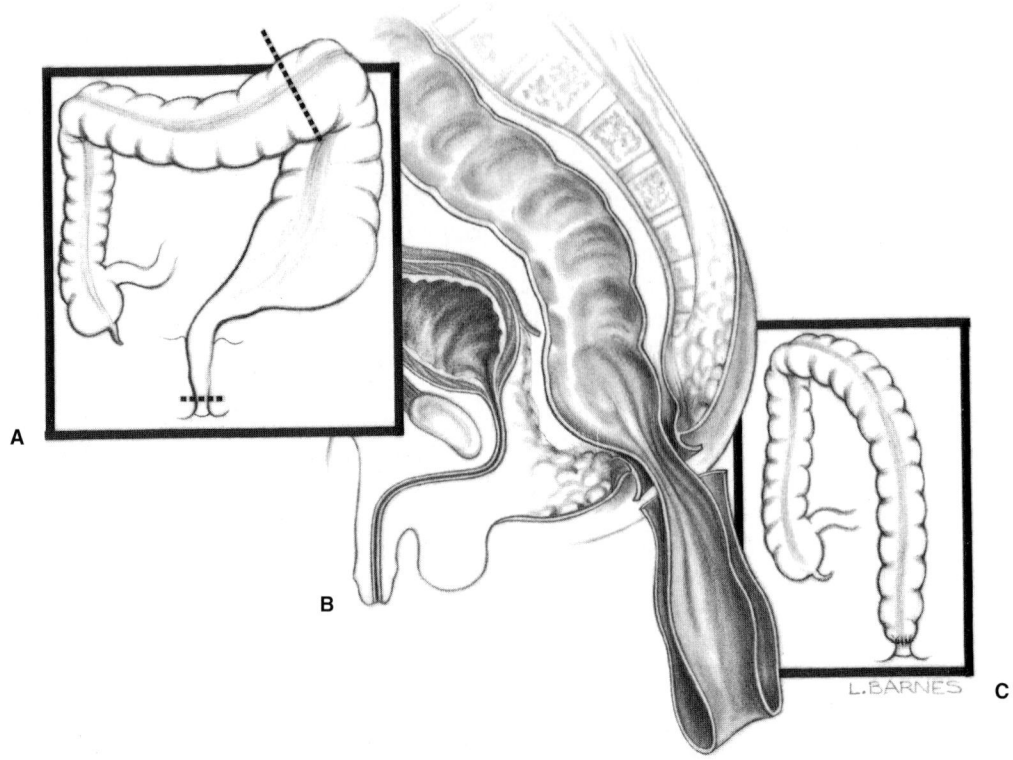

FIGURE 18-6. Swenson's procedure. **(A)** Bowel resection including aganglionic and distended bowel. **(B)** Pull-through of normally innervated colon. **(C)** Anastomosis completed.

most dilated portion of the bowel (Figure 18-6A). Typical Hirschsprung's disease may require only mobilization of the splenic flexure, but the long-segment type may necessitate mobilization of even the right colon in order to obtain sufficient length. Freeing of the aganglionic area below the peritoneal floor is carried out by precise dissection as close as possible to the rectal wall down to the level of the levator ani muscle. Dissection of the rectum includes ligation of the middle hemorrhoidal vessels and the use of diathermy to the perirectal vasculature (Figure 18-6B). Anastomosis is effected by a conventional, transanal, hand-sewn technique (Figure 18-6C). Because of the tedious pelvic dissection and the risk of anastomotic breakdown, most surgeons perform Swenson's operation only if the patient had previously undergone a protective colostomy.

Duhamel's Procedure Duhamel's procedure[35] was devised in order to avoid the extensive pelvic dissection required of Swenson's operation. This is accomplished by preserving the aganglionic rectum and dividing the bowel at the peritoneal reflection as distally as possible (Figure 18-7A). The rectal stump is then closed (Figure 18-7B). Normal (i.e., ganglionic) intestine, usually above the most dilated portion, is pulled through a presacral space that has been created by blunt dissection (Figure 18-7B and C). Attention is then turned to the perineal dissection. The posterior rectal wall is incised above the dentate line, entering the previously dissected retrorectal space (Figure 18-7D). The new, normally innervated colon is pulled through the rectal incision, and a gastrointestinal anastomosis or equivalent stapler or two large crushing clamps are used to effect anastomosis to the

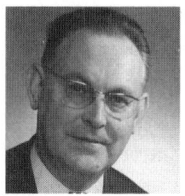

Bernard Georges Duhamel (1917–1996)   Bernard Duhamel was born in Paris, May 11, 1917. His father was a well-known author and a member of the Academie Française, and his mother was an artist. After completing his medical studies, he began his surgical training in 1939 in Paris. Following this, he undertook a Fellowship in Pediatric Surgery at the Sick Children's Hospital of Paris (Hôpital des Enfants Malades). In 1954, he was appointed Chairman of the Department of Pediatric Surgery at the Hôpital de Saint-Denis, and in 1955 he was elevated to Professor of Surgery. Duhamel made numerous contributions to neonatal surgery and wrote a number of books on surgical technique. He was elected President of the French Society of Pediatric Surgery in 1967 and was an influential member of the French Academy of Surgery. (With appreciation to Rolland F. Parc, M.D.)

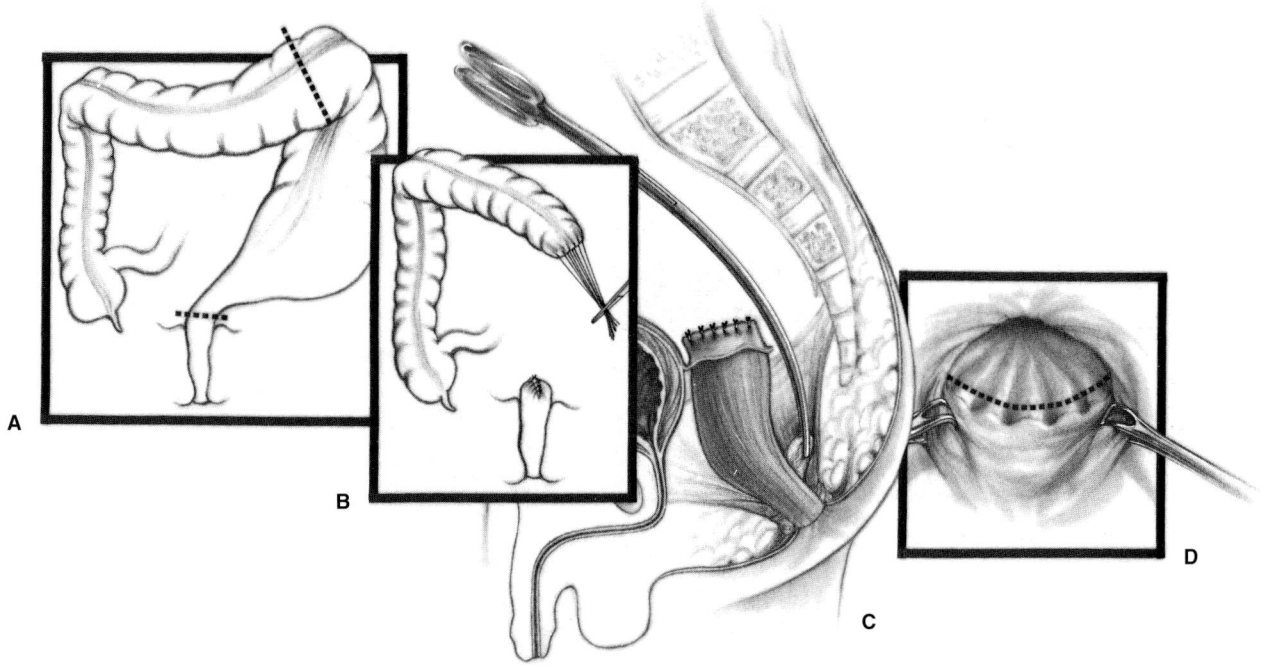

FIGURE 18-7. Duhamel's procedure. **(A)** Colon resection leaving the aganglionic portion in place. **(B)** Ganglionic bowel ready to be pulled down; the rectal stump has been closed. **(C)** Presacral dissection. **(D)** Posterior rectal wall incision.

aganglionic rectum (Figure 18-8*A* and *B*). The posterior wall of the colon is also sutured to the edge of the proctotomy (Figure 18-8*C*). The anastomosis between the colon and the aganglionic rectum must be created as wide as possible, and the rectal stump must be as small as possible in order to avoid fecal accumulation.

Soave's Procedure   Soave's procedure[139] is an ingenious and appealing operation because the aganglionic rectosigmoid is removed by an endorectal dissection, theoretically minimizing the risk of the pelvic injury associated with Swenson's procedure. The normally innervated colon is passed through a rectosigmoid muscular cuff. There is no aganglionic segment of rectum left, such as occurs with Duhamel's procedure. This operation was originally performed without a colostomy, leaving a portion of the pulled-through colon protruding well beyond the anal skin margin. This was then excised at a second operation 1 week later. This two-stage procedure was modified by Boley into a one-stage operation by effecting a primary anastomosis to the anal verge.[14] The endorectal dissection is initiated usually 1 or 2 cm above the peritoneal reflection (Figure 18-9). For some surgeons, this is a very tedious procedure requiring rather meticulous hemostasis. It is recommended that the endorectal dissection be carried down to approximately 1 or 2 cm above the dentate line in order to preserve the sensitive anal mucosa. The normal, ganglionic colon is anastomosed to the anorectal mucosa (Figure 18-10).

As previously mentioned, minimally invasive procedures are gaining more greater acceptance in pediatric surgery. A laparoscopically assisted approach in the treatment of Hirschsprung's disease has been advocated by a number of pediatric surgeons.[46,47,137]

In 1998, de la Torre and Ortega reported a transanal approach to the management of Hirschsprung's disease.[28] Others quickly adopted the concept and published large series with this operation.[78,79] The basic concept consisted of approaching the disease through the anus. A special retractor (Lone Star Medical Products, Inc., Houston, TX) is used (Figure 18-11). The circumferential traction exposes the anal canal, the pectinate line, and the rectal mucosa. Multiple fine sutures are placed in the rectal mucosa in a circumferential manner in order to exert uniform traction to facilitate the dissection of this part of the bowel. A circumferential incision distal to the multiple silk sutures is performed, and the dissection of the rectum commences (Figure 18-12).

Some surgeons prefer to perform this dissection submucosally (endorectally), but we prefer a full-thickness dissection as described in the original Swenson's procedure. A specific recommendation in both of these dissections is to stay as close as possible to the rectal wall in order to minimize risk of injury to important pelvic nerves. The peritoneal reflection is soon reached. As the dissection progresses, full-thickness biopsies are taken that are sent to the pathology department to look for

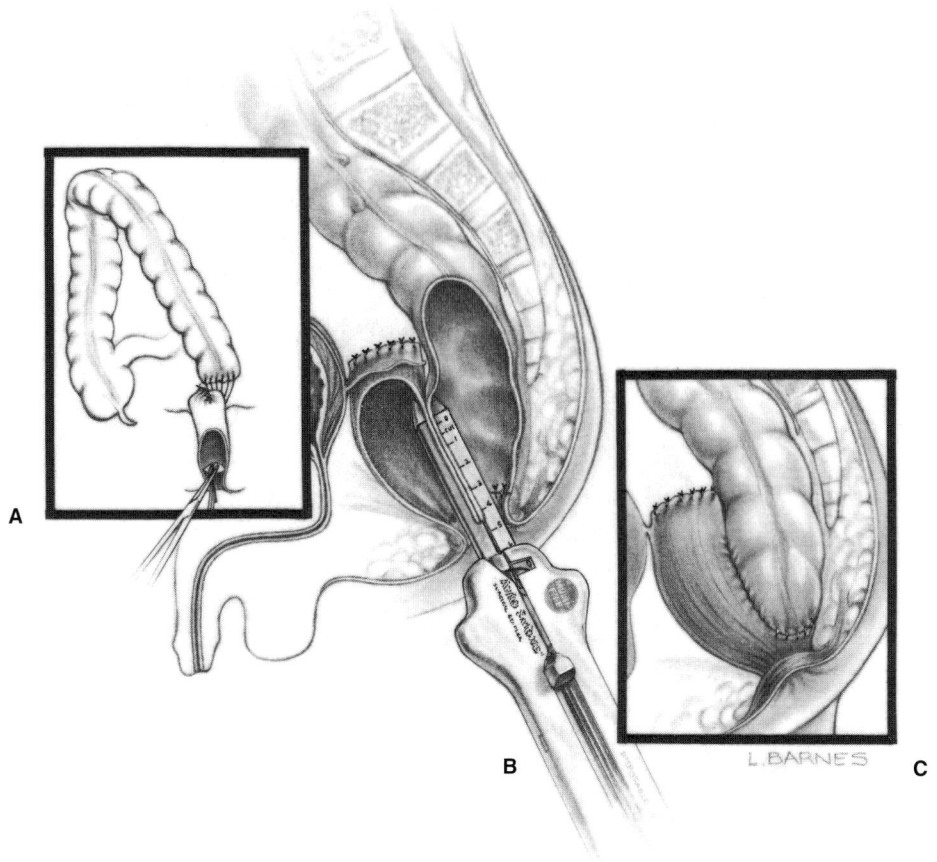

FIGURE 18-8. Duhamel's procedure. **(A)** Retrorectal pull-through. **(B)** Gastrointestinal anastomosis stapler used to join the colon to the aganglionic rectum. **(C)** Completed reconstruction.

ganglion cells. The transition zone sometimes shows an area of hypoganglionosis. It is recommended to continue the dissection until one reaches an area 4 cm above the transitional zone to be sure that normoganglionic bowel is pulled down. The normoganglionic bowel is transanally anastomosed to the anal canal 1 cm above the pectinate line (Figure 18-12C). Considering that most patients with Hirschsprung's disease have a transition zone in the sigmoid colon, it is possible to repair the entire defect using only the transanal approach without a laparotomy or laparoscopy. However, when the transition zone is located higher or the surgeon does not feel safe in conducting this dissection higher from below, then one must open the abdomen or perform a laparoscopic-assisted procedure in order to mobilize the colon. Some surgeons advocate commencing the procedure laparoscopically, performing a biopsy to identify the transition zone, mobilizing the sigmoid colon laparoscopically, and then dissecting transanally. It is important to keep in mind that the resection must include not only the aganglionic part but also the dilated part of the bowel. Pulling down a very dilated segment of colon will result in severe constipation later in life because dilated bowel tends to lose its peristaltic

ability. This approach is becoming increasing popular because it is straightforward in its concept, and the technique is generally reproducible.

Results

Swenson's operation as reported by Swenson and colleagues resulted in a mortality rate of 3.3%, a wound infection rate of 4.6%, an anastomotic leak rate of 5%, pelvic abscess in 2.9%, and rectal strictures in 6.2%.[151] Their patients had temporary soiling in 13% and suffered postoperative enterocolitis in 16% to 27%. In 1979, a survey revealed that only 23% of American surgeons preferred this approach.[74]

Advocates of Duhamel's procedure claim that this operation is a much simpler procedure and that postoperative enterocolitis is uncommon. Duhamel, himself, reported a 2.5% mortality and a 10% complication rate.[35] In the previously mentioned American survery, 30% of surgeons preferred the Duhamel option.[74]

Soave initially reported good results in 87% of patients and noted a 12% incidence of stricture.[139] A later experience with 339 children revealed an operative mortality of 3.5% and a complication rate of 3.4%.[140] The incidence of

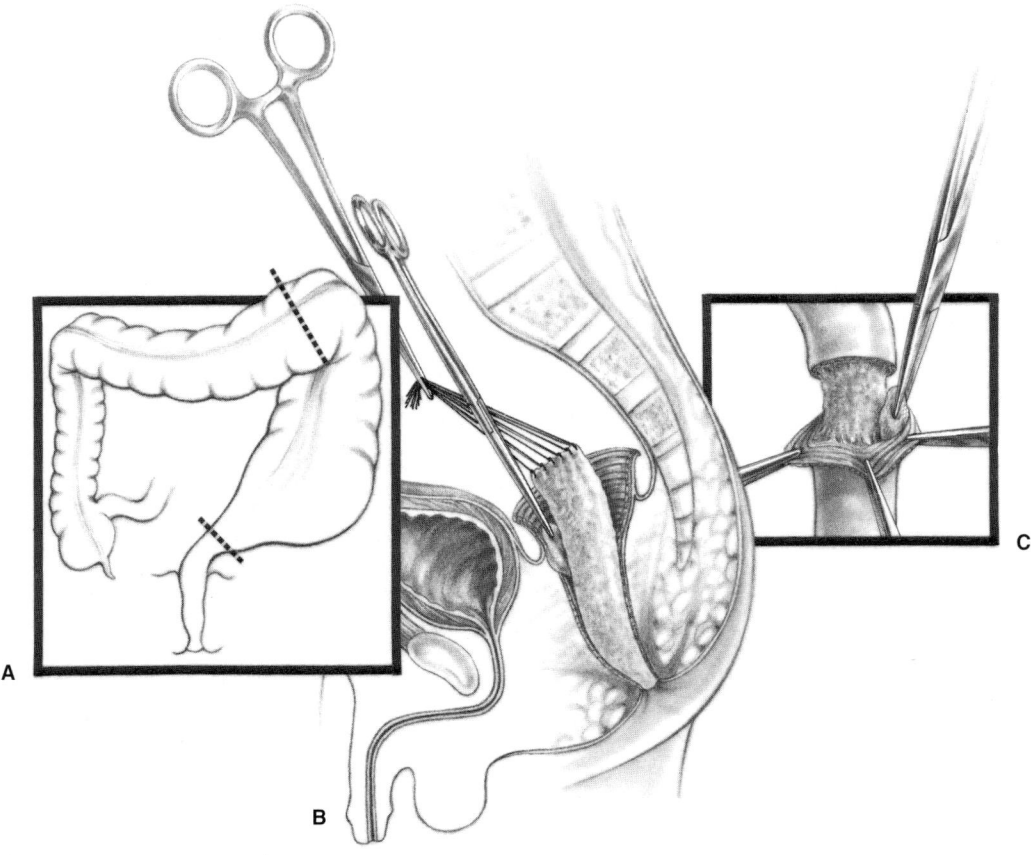

FIGURE 18-9. Soave's procedure. **(A)** Resection of most dilated portion of the bowel. **(B,C)** Endorectal dissection.

constipation was only 1.4%. Seventy-three children were followed for more than15 years. All had good rectal sensation, were able to defecate normally, and could discriminate among solid, liquid, and gas. Almost one half of the surgeons in the United States preferred this operation with the Boley modification.[135]

Fortuna and associates performed a retrospective view of 82 infants and children treated for Hirschsprung's disease during a 20-year period.[44] The most common operations (Soave's and Duhamel's) resulted in an uneventful recovery in only 60% and 67%, respectively. They further observed that both Soave's and Duhamel's pull-through operations have nearly identical reoperation rates (26% versus 29%), but complications after Soave's procedure often require multiple, more extensive procedures.[44] The authors cautioned that further refinement in operative technique and close follow-up are warranted because short-term continence rates for both procedures are less than 50%. However, all patients became continent at 15 years.

Rescorla and co-workers reported 260 children treated for Hirschsprung's disease.[119] Long-term follow-up was available in 103 patients who underwent Duhamel's procedure. Approximately two thirds had normal bowel

function, 27% used occasional enemas or stool softeners, and 8% had severe constipation or soiling. As with other investigators, the authors observed that bowel habits improved with time and were considered normal in 58% at 5 years and 88% at 15 years.

Opinion

At our institution, we are often referred patients who have undergone a procedure for Hirschsprung's disease only to suffer serious complications. The most common problem as a consequence of Duhamel's procedure is persistence of an aganglionic blind rectal pouch. This tends to grow with time and to produce chronic fecal impaction with multiple related symptoms.

Following Soave's procedure, we have seen patients suffering from perianal fistulas and abscesses related to the presence of islands of mucosal cells trapped in the pelvis. This is a consequence of a technical error that occurred during the endorectal dissection. These patients require an operation to excise these cells. We have actually found pieces of bowel that have been left trapped in the pelvis.

Complications and postoperative sequelae in patients with Hirschsprung's disease can be divided into two categories: preventable and nonpreventable. Preventable com-

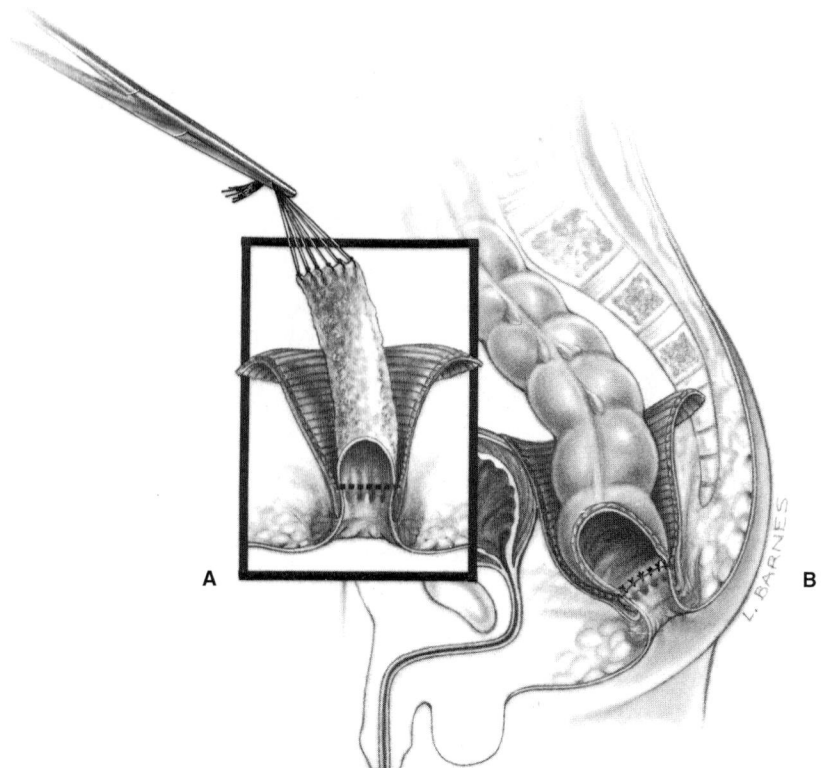

FIGURE 18-10. Soave's procedure. **(A)** Endorectal dissection completed above the dentate line. **(B)** Ganglionic bowel pulled through and anastomosis completed.

plications should truly not occur, because they are the result of technical errors. A feared and unfortunately frequent complication is fecal incontinence. This is most likely related to injury to the continence mechanism during one of these procedures. All operations for this condition are designed to prevent this from happening, provided the procedures are performed properly. Dehiscence, retraction, stricture, abscess, and fistula are all considered preventable because they are the result of technical errors.

A nonpreventable complication is enterocolitis. This problem is a true challenge for pediatric surgeons. Although the etiology is not known, it is believed that fecal stasis is a predisposing factor.

Constipation is, at least in part, a preventable consequence of surgery. One must anticipate the potential for its development and aggressively manage postoperative constipation in order to prevent subsequent difficulties. When a pull-through procedure includes a portion of very dilated colon, it is a self-fulfilling prophesy that these children will suffer from constipation. We have learned that a dilated colon is almost as severe a pathologic entity as an aganglionic segment. Therefore, it should be resected at the time of the pull-through. However, despite meticulous attention to surgical technique, constipation still occurs in approximately 15% of our cases.

Surgical Management
of Total Colonic Aganglionosis

In 1972, Martin described his technique for the treatment of total colonic aganglionosis, an unusual manifestation of the disease.[89] The procedure is based on the utilization of the aganglionic portion of the colon in order to take advantage of its resorptive capacity.

When the diagnosis is made, an ileostomy is required initially, and the definitive operation is performed after 1 year. At this time, the ileostomy is taken down and is sufficiently mobilized to reach the perineum. The ganglionic terminal ileum is pulled down through the retrorectal (i.e., presacral) space as described for Duhamel's procedure. The small bowel is drawn through the incised opening in the posterior rectal wall. The end of the ileum is then sutured to the opening in the posterior rectal wall. A stapler is used to remove a triangular segment of the common wall between rectum and small bowel. Up to this point, the procedure is no different from that of Duhamel's operation. The next step, however, consists of creating a long side-to-side anastomosis of the distal ileum and rectum, sigmoid, and descending colon up to the level of the splenic flexure. The proximal aganglionic intestine is excised. The primary complaint following this procedure is that of loose bowel movements, but after several months significant improvement should occur.

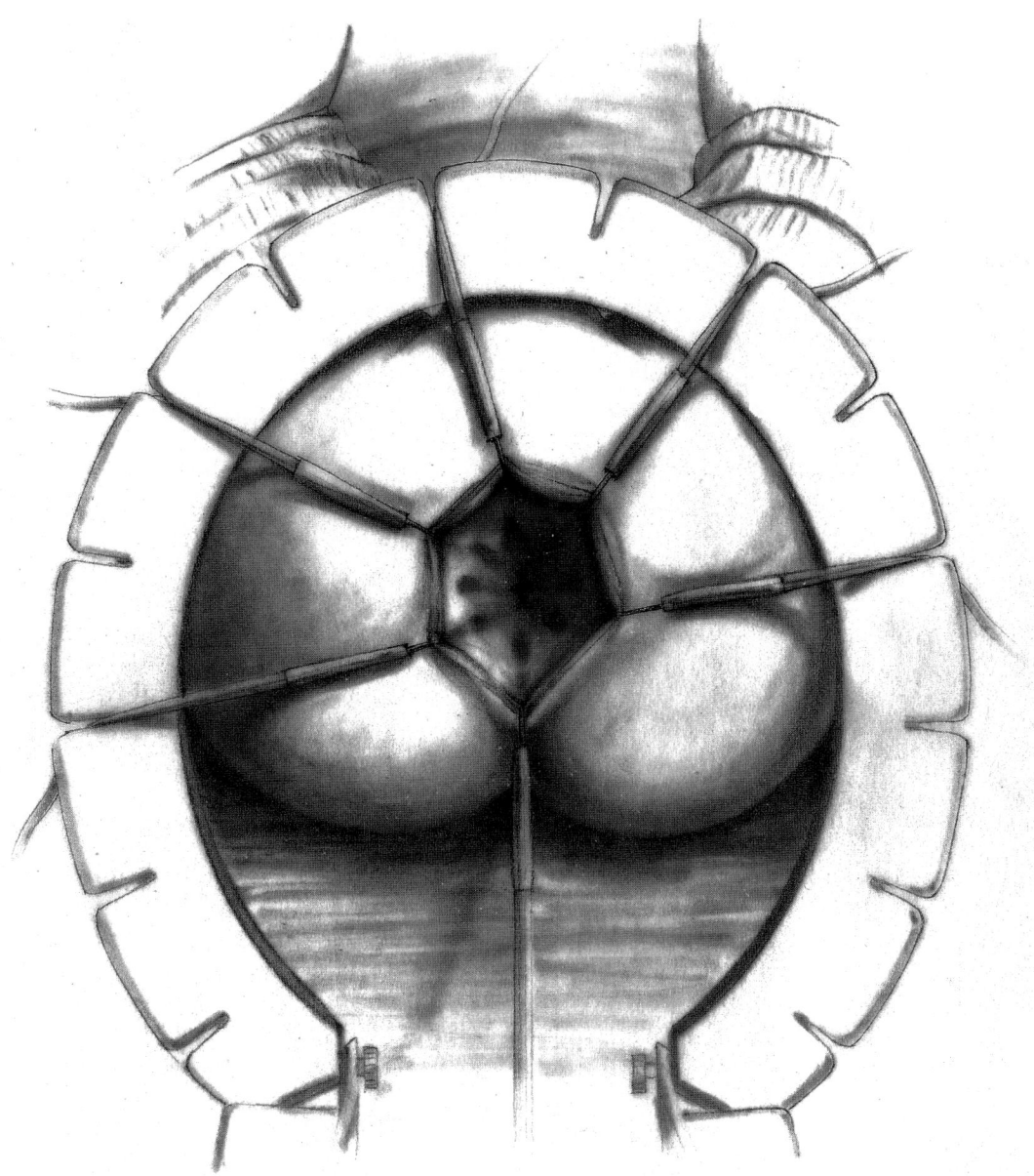

FIGURE 18-11. A Lone Star retractor in position with hooks in place to provide exposure for the dissection.

Kimura and colleagues advocate a staged approach, a modification of the foregoing technique that is ingenious as well as promising.[73] The first operation consists of an ileostomy. The second stage is a side-to-side ileum–ascending colon anastomosis. At the final stage, the terminal ileum, with the right colon as a free patch, is pulled down by employing any of the available techniques (i.e., Soave's, Duhamel's, or Swenson's).

Opinion The long-term follow up of patients with total colon aganglionosis convinced us that we have not yet found the ideal treatment for this very serious condition.

The concept of integrating a portion of aganglionic colon with a normal ganglionic bowel in order to create a pouch that will allow stasis of liquid stool, absorb fluid, decrease the number of bowel movements, and form solid stool, thereby improving the quality of life, has proven to be rather simplistic. Stasis of stool in the small bowel produces bacterial proliferation and an inflammatory process. Rather than absorbing water, very often the intestine secretes it into the lumen, producing what is essentially a secretory diarrhea. It is not uncommon that resection of the pouches becomes necessary in order to address the problems of malnutrition and fluid loss. We, as well as

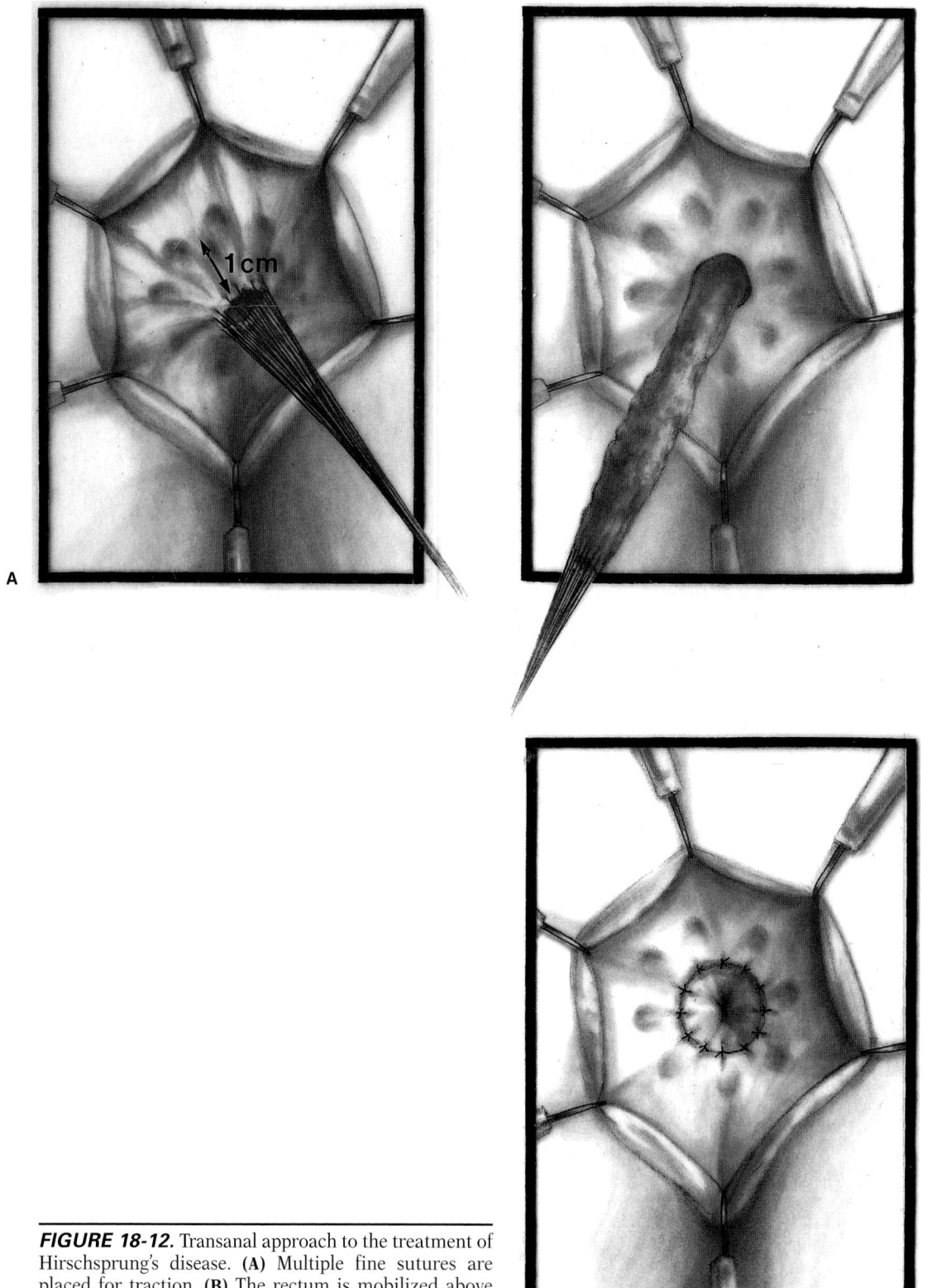

FIGURE 18-12. Transanal approach to the treatment of Hirschsprung's disease. **(A)** Multiple fine sutures are placed for traction. **(B)** The rectum is mobilized above the peritoneal reflection and above the aganglionic segment. **(C)** The anastomosis is completed.

others, believe that a straight ileorectal anastomosis is the preferred option because of the better long-term results.[152]

Total Intestinal Aganglionosis

Ziegler and co-workers, reporting from the Children's Hospital Medical Center at the University of Cincinnati in Ohio, described the management of the challenging problem of 16 neonates who presented with intestinal obstruction secondary to total (extending to the stomach) or near-total intestinal aganglionosis confirmed at one or more leveling operations.[163] Their operation included extending an antimesenteric myectomy-myotomy from the ganglionic-aganglionic transition zone for variable lengths, the operative design being to create sufficient small bowel length to support life (a minimum of 40 cm). Of ten survivors, two are totally gut nourished, six receive 20% to 80% of total calories enterally, and one receives minimal enteral feeding.[163]

Management of Short-Segment Aganglionosis

The management of the ultrashort or short-segment variant of aganglionosis is a source of considerable controversy (see Chapter 16). In 1975, Lynn reported his experience with anorectal myectomy for the treatment of this condition.[86] The procedure consisted basically of a posterior internal anal sphincterectomy, including excision of a strip of smooth muscle from the posterior wall of the rectum, 0.5 to 1 cm wide (see Figure 16-17). The strip is then oriented for histologic examination. If ganglion cells are absent at the lower end of the specimen but present at the upper end, significant clinical improvement may be anticipated. However, doubt has been raised concerning the validity of this criterion, and results have not been consistently satisfactory.

Neuronal Intestinal Dysplasia

There is evidence to suggest that the disorders of bowel innervation and ganglion distribution are represented by a spectrum of conditions, including an entity known as NID.[18,40,42,76,80,87,91,97,123,126,127,133,148] The implication of this observation is that the presence or absence of ganglion cells, such as in Hirschsprung's disease, may represent only a part of this spectrum. For example, the frequency of NID coexisting with Hirschsprung's disease has been reported to vary from 20% to 66%.[93,126] Other observations that have been described include hypertrophy of ganglion cells,[80] normal ganglion cells,[87] immature ganglia,[117] hypoganglionosis,[117] hyperplasia of the submucous and myenteric plexi with formation of giant ganglia, and hypoplasia or aplasia of sympathetic innervation of the myenteric plexus.[93] These histologic abnormalities may be localized or disseminated,[132] and they may or may not be associated with distal aganglionosis.[16,18,40,41,54,70,80,87,113,118,132] Although, as of this writing, a precise correlation between histology and clinical

manifestations is lacking, these observations may serve to explain why some individuals who have undergone a technically correct operation for Hirschsprung's disease, including the pull-through of a "normoganglionic" bowel, still suffer from symptoms of enterocolitis or of constipation.[41,70]

The histologic diagnosis of NID requires a high index of suspicion as well as the availability of special techniques and expertise.[45,84,91,117] Without these, the observer may have the false impression that the bowel is normally innervated. The staining methods used to establish the diagnosis include the acetylcholinesterase activity of the parasympathetic fibers. Suction rectal biopsies usually do not provide sufficient tissue to evaluate the sympathetic innervation of the muscularis propria. However, catecholamine staining by glyoxylic acid fluorescence, as described by Lindvall and Bjorklund, may help to detect aplastic or hypoplastic sympathetic innervation.[84]

The precise options for therapy have not been clearly established because of the lack of well-defined clinical, radiologic, and manometric findings.[25,76] It is to be hoped that, with the standardization of more sophisticated histologic methods, the surgeon will be able to resect areas with aganglionosis as well as areas with NID, thus limiting the likelihood of recurrent symptoms. For the present, it is suggested that bowel resection be undertaken in children with severe obstructive symptoms, and medical management be applied to those with lesser complaints. This is an important distinction, because clinical regression has been reported,[136] in addition to objective histologic improvement.[123]

Commentary

Hirschsprung's disease is a subject of active research and study. This has led to the production of a large number of publications causing one to hope that many of these patients will soon realize the benefits. For example, considerable effort has been made in transplanting ganglion cells.[129] Furthermore, advances in the field of genetics should ultimately allow us to predict which individuals are at risk for having babies with this condition. Additionally, genetic engineering may ultimately be used to prevent this condition, an exciting area of exploration indeed.

ANORECTAL MALFORMATIONS

Historical Review

Anorectal malformations have routinely been classified by the term, "imperforate anus." The condition has been recognized since antiquity (e.g., by Paulus Aegineta of Greece).[1] For many centuries, physicians understood that by creating an orifice in the perineum, many of the children with imperforate anus survived, some even with normal bowel function. Unfortunately, many developed an anal stricture. If the condition were uncorrected, intestinal obstruction and death frequently resulted. Ancient operations consisted of making an expeditious incision in the perineum deep enough both to open the rectal pouch and to obtain meconium. The surgeon packed the wound and changed the packing daily in an attempt to create a permanent perineal orifice. The primary concern was directed toward survival of the infant. Therefore, these operations took only a few minutes and were obviously undertaken without anesthesia, blood transfusion, or other adjunctive measures that are routinely used at the present time. In 1835, Amussat (see the biography in Chapter 23) was the first person not merely to open the rectal pouch, but also to suture it to the skin.[3] In retrospect, perhaps those who survived that operation were children who had "low malformations." Conversely, those for whom the operation was unsuccessful probably had a malformation now known as "high."

Chassaignac, in 1856, was the first person to perform a colostomy for the treatment of an anorectal malformation.[23] Hadra, in 1886, performed the first abdominoperineal procedure.[56] For the first part of the twentieth century, most surgeons used a preliminary colostomy and an abdominoperineal pull-through for the treatment of high malformations and a perineal approach without a colostomy for so-called "low malformations." In 1930, Wangensteen (see the biography in Chapter 22) and Rice described the invertogram, an x-ray film taken during the newborn period with the infant's head down, in order to measure the distance between the rectal pouch and the skin as a criterion for determining the height of the malformation.[161]

Although a perineal approach without a colostomy is still the preferred treatment for low defects, the method of approaching high malformations is still evolving. In 1948, Rhoads and colleagues reintroduced the neonatal one-stage abdominoperineal procedure.[120] In 1953, Stephens noted the importance of preservation of the puborectalis sling in maintaining fecal continence.[142] He proposed an initial sacral approach followed by an abdominoperineal operation, if necessary. Since 1980, I (A.P.) have suggested that these malformations be approached through a posterior sagittal incision, using an electrical stimulator to identify the striated muscle structures (see Figure 13-17).[30,105-107,110] This has been my preferred method of treatment, with the use of a protective colostomy in most cases. This technique has been instrumental in revealing a very important anatomic area that, until 1980, was a matter of speculation.

Incidence

Most authors report that one of every 5,000 newborns will have an anorectal malformation.[17,131,160] However, these numbers are quite variable. Male infants seem to suffer this condition more frequently than female infants. The most common type of malformation seen in boys is rectourethral fistula, and the most common type of anomaly in girls is vestibular fistula. There is an increased incidence of imperforate anus in children with Down's syndrome. In these patients, the anorectal malformation frequently consists of a low-lying rectal pouch without a genitourinary or perineal fistula.

Embryologic Considerations

These defects probably develop during gestational weeks 4 to 12.[143] The urinary, genital, and rectal tracts empty into a common channel, the cloaca. Ultimately, they will be segregated by the urorectal septum during its craniocaudal descent, separating the cloaca into an anterior urogenital sinus and a posterior intestinal canal. Two lateral folds of the cloaca also move simultaneously toward the midline. The perineal mound appears to be the caudal extension of the urorectal septum, which develops into the perineal body. In the male, the inner and outer genital ridges meet to form the urethra. In the female, these ridges do not coalesce but form the labia minora and majora. Various types of failures in this process have been postulated to explain each of the anorectal malformations. The resulting defects constitute a spectrum that ranges from the most severe examples (e.g., caudal regression and persistent cloaca) to the more easily managed concerns (e.g., perineal fistula, also known as low malformation).

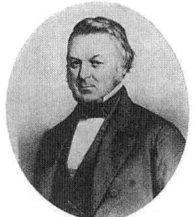

Edouard-Pierre-Marie Chassaignac (1804–1879) Edouard Chassaignac was born December 24, 1804, in Nantes, France. He received his medical school education at the University in Nantes and graduated in 1835. His great forte was the design of new instruments, and he was an ingenious experimenter. For example, he perfected the use of the then new product, rubber, for use as a fenestrated drain and developed the concept of the occlusive dressing for wounds. He became surgeon to the Lariboisiàre in 1852 and is recognized as the first surgeon to perform a colostomy for the management of an anorectal malformation. Other signal contributions included his classic dissertation on fractures of the femoral neck, his treatise on suppuration and surgical drainage, his classification of breast abscess, and his book (*The Subject of Surgical Anatomy and Pathology*), in which he relates his experiences in clinical surgery. He is also eponymously recognized for his description of the carotid (cervical) tubercle (Chassaignac's tubercle). In 1861, he was awarded the Legion of Honor, and in 1868 he was named a member of the Academy of Medicine. Chassaignac died in Versailles on August 26, 1879.

Classification

The classification of Ladd and Gross has been used for many years, particularly in the United States.[77] However, in 1970, an international classification was proposed in Melbourne, Australia.[145] Because this was considered rather complex and impractical, it was rarely used by pediatric surgeons. In 1984, Stephens and Smith pioneered another international reunion with the purpose of creating a more functional and practical classification.[146] This resulted in what has come to be known as the Wingspread classification. Some of the terminology of the Wingspread classification was taken from the Melbourne classification; it, therefore, has embryologic implications rather than therapeutic ones.

In our own experience, the posterior sagittal approach to these malformations has permitted the opportunity for directly exposing the anatomy of each of these defects. This has led to important therapeutic implications besides those of terminology and classification.

With imperforate anus, one is dealing with a spectrum of malformations. Thus, in attempting to separate these groups of defects into categories, one risks being arbitrary and artificial. The basic concept of a spectrum must always be kept in mind by the reader. With this cautionary note, the classification shown in Table 18-1 is considered practical for therapeutic purposes.

Anatomy

The posterior sagittal approach used for the repair of anorectal malformations, in addition to the management of tumors, rectal trauma, amebiasis, and rectal prolapse,

▶ **TABLE 18-1 Classification**

Male

Perineal fistula
Rectourethral fistula
    Bulbar
    Prostatic
Rectum–bladder neck fistula
Imperforate anus without fistula
Rectal atresia

Female

Perineal fistula
Vestibular fistula
Imperforate anus without fistula
Rectal atresia
Cloaca
Complex malformations

permitted me (A.P.) to conceptualize the anatomic details of a normal male (Figure 18-13) and a normal female (Figure 18-14). The external sphincter is represented by a group of parasagittal muscle fibers. The levator ani and external sphincter blend and become indistinguishable, forming a funnel-shaped continuum of muscle. The portion of muscle located between the parasagittal fibers of the external sphincter and the levator ani muscle is integrated mainly by vertical fibers that run parallel with the rectum, called the muscle complex. The levator ani, muscle complex, and external sphincter are indivisible structures working in concert. In the upper portion of the funnel, horizontal fibers predominate and push the rectum

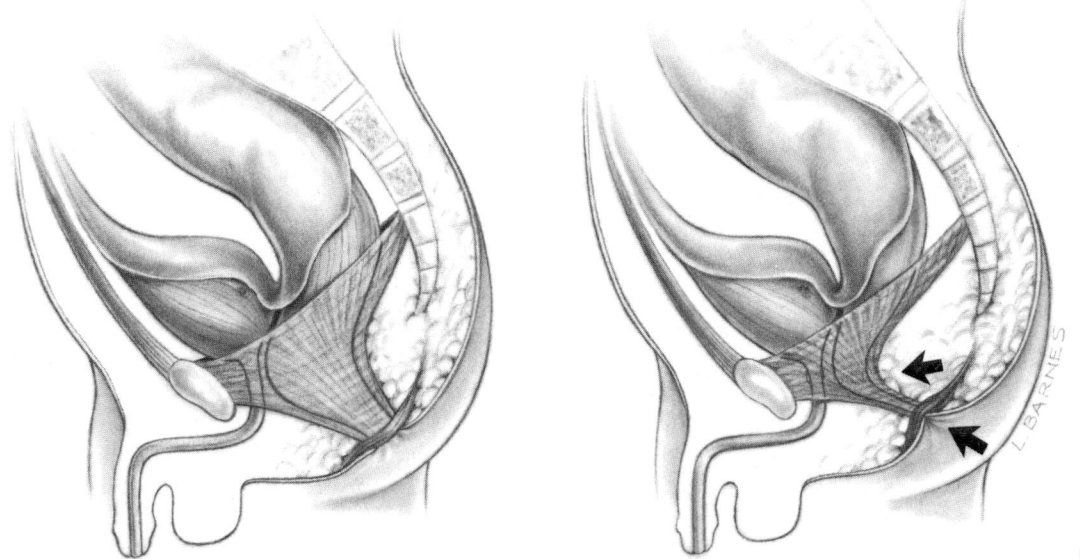

A   **B**

FIGURE 18-13. Normal male anatomy. **(A)** During defecation. **(B)** During sphincter contraction (i.e., retention).

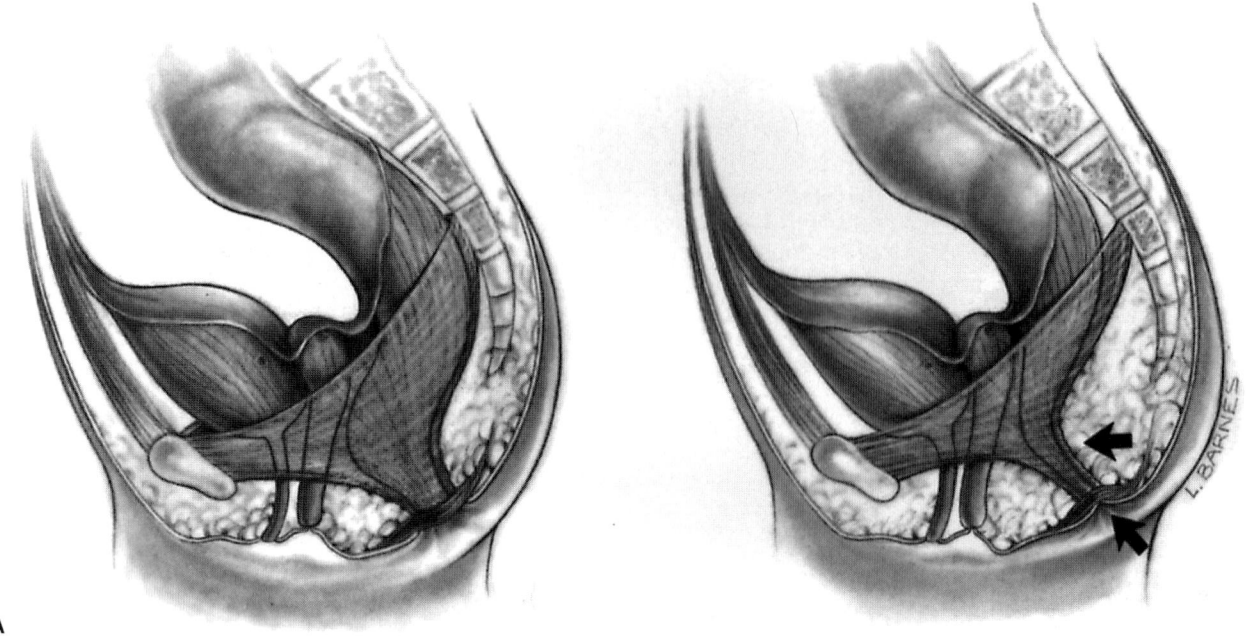

FIGURE 18-14. Normal female anatomy. **(A)** During defecation. **(B)** During sphincter contraction (i.e., retention).

forward. In the lower part of the funnel (i.e., muscle complex), vertical fibers predominate and elevate the anus. Because the parasagittal fibers meet together in front of the anus as well as posterior to it, contraction occludes the anus. This gives the fibers a circular appearance.

The problem of placing groups of malformations within specified categories and the use of the terms high, intermediate, and low confuse the issue of risk for fecal incontinence. When discussing results of surgical treatment, it is imperative to compare malformations that have a similar potential for bowel control. Thus, rather than comparing groups of malformations, one must examine the specific defects. The spectrum of such defects in the male patient is illustrated in Figure 18-15.

Description of Specific Defects in the Male Patient

Perineal Fistula

Perineal fistula consists of a very low malformation. The rectum has passed normally through much of the sphincter mechanism. However, the lowest part of the rectum is anteriorly deviated and ends as a perineal fistula anterior to the center of the external sphincter (Figure 18-15*A*). Frequently, the fistula tract lies immediately below a very thin layer of skin, with the external opening somewhere in the midline from the anus to the ventral portion of the penis. One often perceives beneath the midline skin, black, ribbonlike structure resulting from meconium (Figure 18-16). The infant does not require further inves-

tigation and can undergo surgery without a colostomy. Prognosis is excellent because the patient has all the necessary anatomic elements for maintaining bowel control.

In all anorectal malformations, the higher the defect, the less the likelihood will be of achieving bowel control. Conversely, the lower the malformation, the higher the incidence will be of constipation. Therefore, in treating an infant with a perineal fistula, the surgeon should anticipate the consequence of constipation and be prepared to treat it effectively.

Even when repair of a perineal fistula is accomplished by means of a relatively minor operation, the surgeon must be mindful of the fact that the anterior wall of the rectum is intimately attached to the posterior wall of the urethra. Meticulous dissection is, therefore, required in order to separate the two structures and to prevent a urethral injury. One must always perform the operation with a Foley catheter in place.

Anal Stenosis

Anal stenosis is another, rather benign defect that consists of a ring of fibrous tissue located at the anal verge. This causes a stricture that may result in varying degrees of functional abnormality, but the muscle structure is completely normal. From the external perspective, the anus also appears normal. One must introduce a Hegar dilator to detect the malformation, and digital rectal examination is impossible. The typical symptom is difficulty moving the bowels, with the parent describing a ribbonlike appearance to the feces. The patient can be

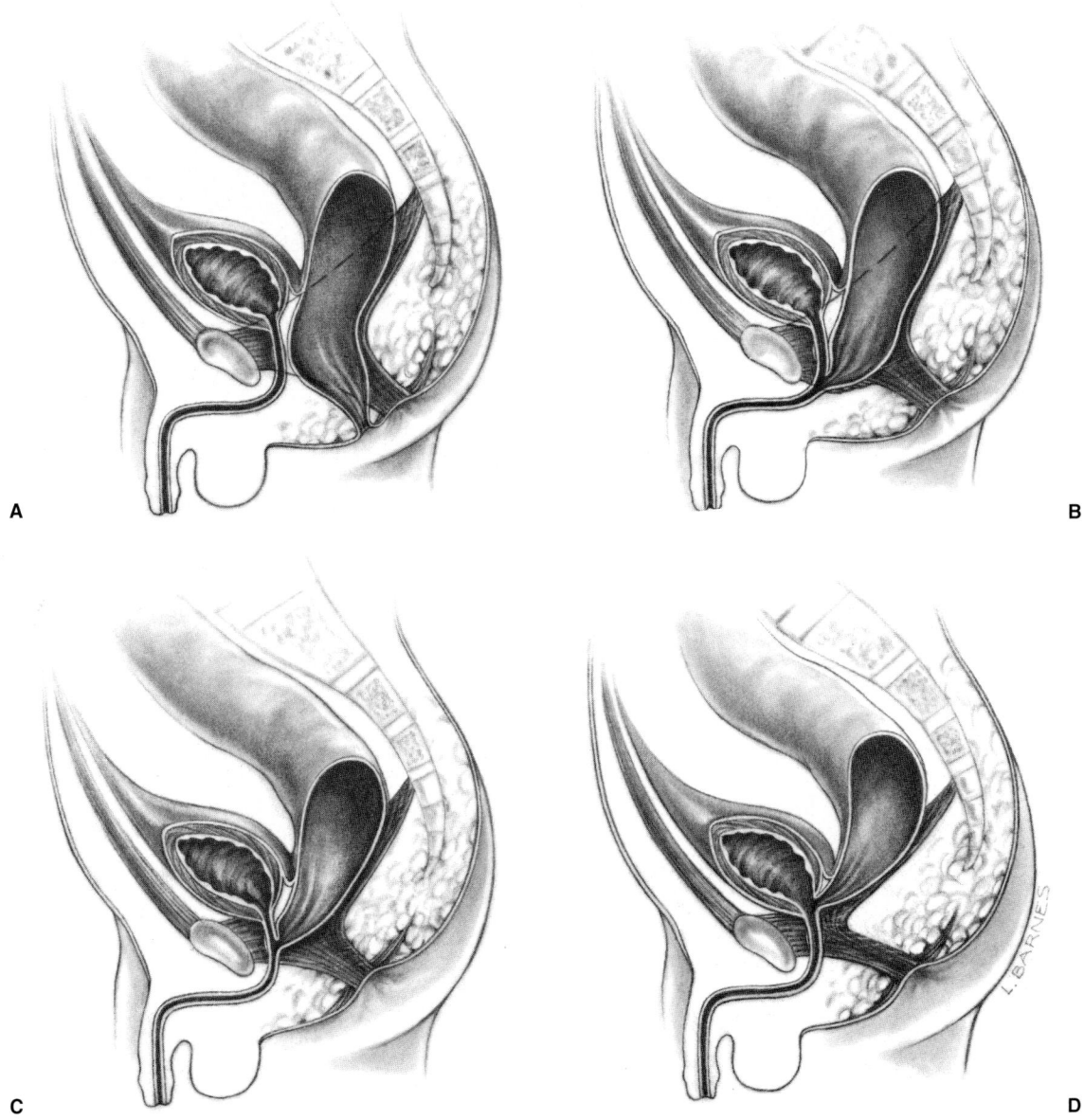

FIGURE 18-15. Spectrum of male defects. **(A)** Perineal fistula (low malformation). **(B)** Bulbar urethral fistula. **(C)** Prostatic urethral fistula. **(D)** Bladder neck fistula.

treated either by surgery or by dilatation; a colostomy is unnecessary.

Rectourethral Fistula

Rectourethral fistula is the most frequent malformation seen in the male patient. Congenitally, the rectum descends through a considerable portion of the funnel-shaped muscle structure, but at some point it deviates anteriorly and connects with the urethra. The most frequent site of the fistula is to the bulbar urethra (Figure 18-15B). However, significant numbers of urethral fistulas open at the prostatic urethra (Figure 18-15C). The rectum is usually very distended. Distal to the fistula site, the muscle structure becomes a solid mass, which is quite thin laterally and is situated very close to the posterior urethra. There is usually a considerable discrepancy between the size of the rectum and the available space through which the rectum must be pulled down. However, the quality of muscle in an infant with a rectourethral fistula is usually good. A patient with bulbar fistula usually has a better potential for continence because the rectum has already passed through much of the levator ani and muscle complex mechanism, the muscle quality is more satisfactory,

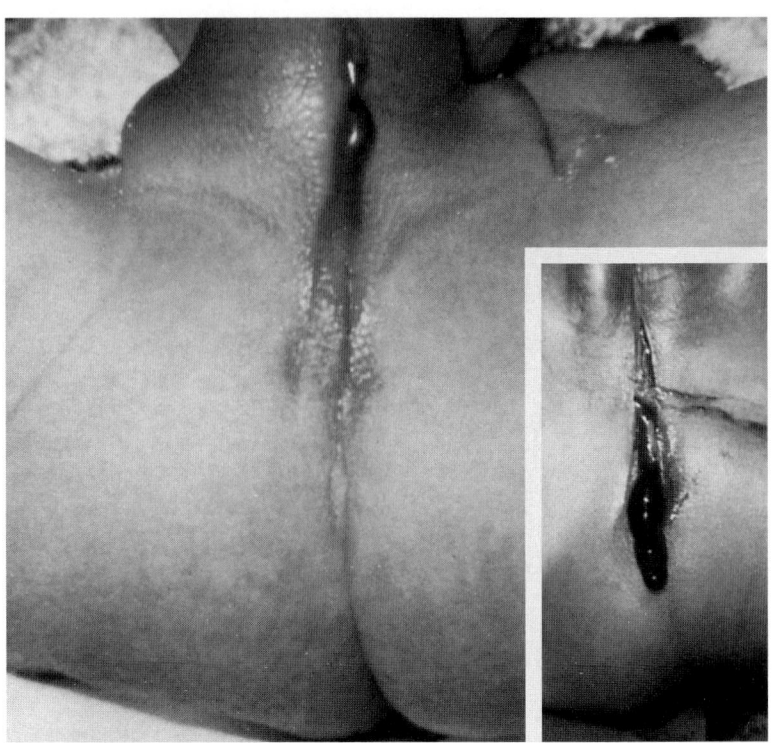

FIGURE 18-16. Perineal fistula (hooded anus). Note the ribbonlike structure containing meconium. The tract is unroofed **(inset)**.

and the sacrum is more normally developed. Higher malformations are more frequently associated with a poor sacrum and, consequently, poor innervation with a poor quality of muscle. The perineum in patients with rectourethral bulbar fistula usually exhibits a well-developed midline groove (natal cleft) and an easily recognized anal dimple or fossette (Figure 18-17). These signs are usually indicative of good muscle development.

Occasionally, however, a patient with a rectourethral fistula, usually *prostatic*, has a rather poor sacrum and a poor-looking perineum with a "flat" or "round bottom" consisting of an absent anal fossette and a very poor midline groove (Figure 18-18). All of these signs usually imply that the patient has poor striated muscle. Patients with rectoprostatic fistula frequently exhibit a bifid scrotum. Furthermore, the center of the sphincter mechanism is located very close to the scrotum. These findings do not occur as frequently in cases of rectourethral bulbar fistula. These infants require a posterior sagittal anorectoplasty (PSARP) preceded by a protective colostomy (see later).

Rectum–Bladder Neck Fistula

In the case of a rectovesical fistula, the rectum usually opens at the level of the bladder neck (Figure 18-15D). The levator ani muscle, muscle complex, and external sphincter are frequently underdeveloped. The available space between the posterior urethra and the levator ani muscle is very restricted and is often virtually absent.

The frequency of association with abnormal sacrum, "flat bottom," and poor-looking perineum—all signs of poor prognosis for fecal continence—is very high. Conversely, on occasion one may see a patient with a rectovesical fistula who has a good sacrum and fairly normal muscle structures. Often these patients have a rather narrow pelvis, especially in the anterior-posterior diameter. These infants must be treated with a colostomy followed by a PSARP and a laparotomy or laparoscopy. In our experience, this group represents approximately 10% of the series.

Ninety percent of infants with this anomaly have other defects. Unfortunately, the ultimate functional result is poor. These patients require a laparotomy or laparoscopy, in addition to the posterior sagittal approach, in order to reach a very high rectum.

Anorectal Agenesis without Fistula

Anorectal agenesis without fistula is a rather unusual anomaly, representing 5% of all children with anorectal malformations, half of whom suffer from Down's syndrome. More than 90% of the patients with Down's syndrome who have an anorectal malformation harbor this unusual specific defect. Even though these children have the trisomy 21 anomaly, 80% will have voluntary bowel control later in life.[158]

In our experience, the rectum usually ends blindly approximately 2 cm above the perineal skin. Even without a fistula, only a very thin membrane separates rectum from

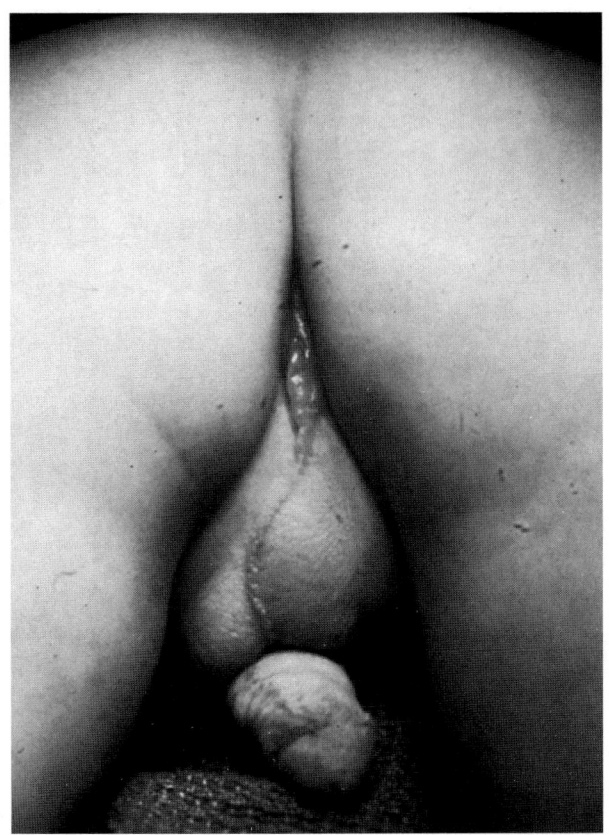

FIGURE 18-17. Perineum of a child with a rectourethral fistula. Note the prominent midline groove and a distinct anal dimple.

urethra. These infants usually have good muscle quality and a well-developed sacrum. We have not seen a blind pouch ending at the level of the bladder neck or close to the skin. The perineum in these infants usually exhibits signs implying a good prognosis. Treatment consists of a colostomy followed by a PSARP (see later).

Rectal Atresia

Rectal atresia is a rather unusual malformation that appears to be much more frequent in girls than in boys. It consists of a complete (i.e., atresia) or partial (i.e., stenosis) interruption of the rectal lumen between the anal canal and the rectum. The anal canal usually measures 1 to 2 cm in length and is rather narrow, whereas the rectum is usually quite distended. The distance between the rectal pouch and the anal canal in these patients is variable. One may see a very thin membrane separating both structures or a rather long fibrous space. These infants, in our experience, have all the necessary elements to achieve good fecal continence. Repair requires a PSARP with or without prior colostomy (see later). The results of treatment for this malformation are usually excellent.

Description of Specific Defects in the Female Patient

The characteristics of the striated muscle mechanism in female patients are very similar to those described earlier for male patients.

Perineal Fistula

Perineal fistula represents the most benign defect of the female spectrum. As with the male abnormality, the rectum traverses most of the sphincter mechanism, deviating in its most distal portion to communicate with the skin through a fistula located a few millimeters anterior to the center of the external sphincter (see Figure 18-23, *inset,* later). These infants have all the necessary elements for normal bowel control. The anterior rectal wall and the posterior vaginal wall are completely separated, as is seen during the surgical repair (see later). A simple anoplasty (i.e., minimal PSARP) is sufficient to treat this type of malformation without the need for a colostomy. It is well known that if patients do not undergo surgical treatment, they usually have normal bowel function and control. Treatment, therefore, is indicated primarily for cosmetic and psychological reasons.

Vestibular Fistula

Vestibular fistula is the malformation most frequently seen in female patients. The bowel is anteriorly deviated at a higher level, opening immediately behind the hymen into the vestibule (see Figure 18-25, *inset,* later). The rectum and the vagina are opposed, with only a very thin, common wall separating the two structures. The quality of muscle is similar to that seen in the male with a rectourethral bulbar fistula. Most patients have the potential for normal continence, a normal-appearing sacrum, adequate innervation, and a good-looking perineum. However, as with boys, there are exceptions in which one can find a vestibular fistula associated with rather inadequate muscle and a poor sacrum.

This malformation is frequently misdiagnosed as a *rectovaginal fistula.* A true vaginal fistula is extremely rare and is discussed in the following section. Meticulous examination of the genitalia of a newborn is required to localize the fistula site precisely.

Pediatric surgeons, worldwide, are operating on this specific defect during the newborn period or even later in life without a protective colostomy. In fact, at our institution, when an infant is born with this defect, has no associated defects, and is otherwise well, she is operated on within the first 48 hours without a colostomy. However, one must be mindful that a protective colostomy is still a very valuable adjunct under several circumstances. The most common one is the lack of experience in the

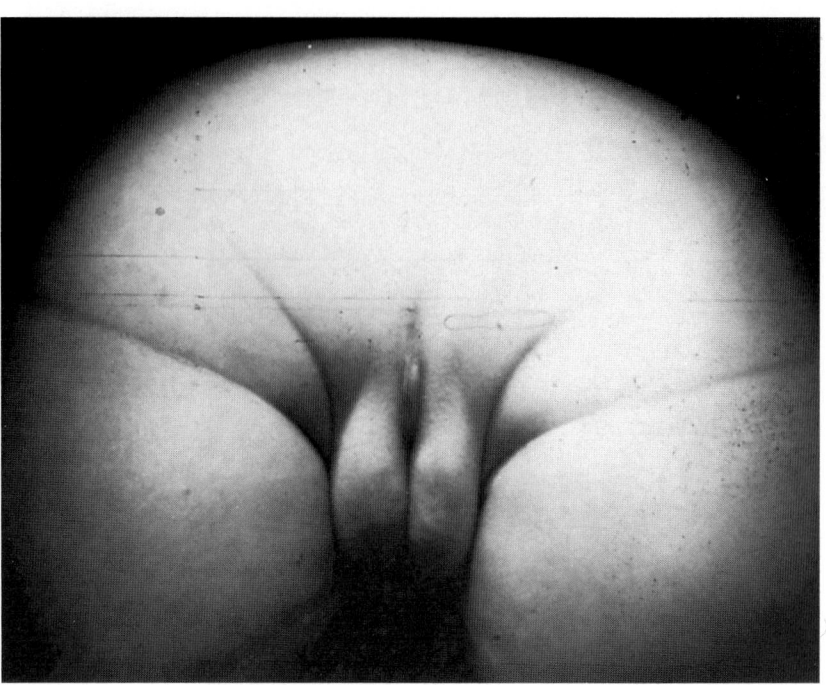

FIGURE 18-18. Perineum of a child with poor muscles (flat bottom).

performance of the definitive repair. In addition, a baby with an associated defect or in very poor clinical condition may be optimally managed with a colostomy.

This particular malformation is the one that we have seen most frequently managed incorrectly. Even when these children have an excellent potential for normal bowel control, a failed procedure will often jeopardize the success of a subsequent operation. A simple cut-back procedure, which does not include separating the vagina from the rectum, is still widely used as a surgical option. However, we are critical of this approach, because many of these children will ultimately require a secondary repair as a consequence of incontinence and of psychological problems that develop at the time of sexual awakening.

Vaginal Fistula

Vaginal fistula is a very unusual malformation in female patients. The rectum may open in the lower one half of the vagina or, as an even more uncommon manifestation, in the upper portion (see Figure 18-27A and B later). The higher the malformation is, the shorter the common wall between the rectum and vagina. A low vaginal fistula is usually associated with absence of the posterior rim of the hymen. One cannot see the fistula orifice by inspection, and the meconium seems to come from within the vagina. As with the male patient, the higher the fistula is, the greater the likelihood for an abnormal sacrum and a poor-looking perineum. There are exceptions to this dictum, however. The potential for normal continence in these infants is generally less than one would expect with vestibular fistula. Treatment consists of a diverting colostomy followed by a full PSARP.

Anorectal Agenesis without Fistula

Imperforate anus without fistula is also an uncommon malformation. The rectum is usually located more or less 2 cm above the skin. The rectovaginal septum is rather thin, there is a good sphincter muscle, a good-looking perineum, and a well-developed sacrum. Half of these babies, like the boys, suffer from Down's syndrome, and they have the same good prognosis for rectal function.[158] In these babies (when the condition is detected during the newborn period), one can see gas in the most distal part of the rectum below the coccyx on a cross-table lateral film with the patient in prone position.[98] The surgeon is justified in approaching the patient posterosagittally and without a colostomy in the patient during the newborn period, provided the surgeon has experience with this operation. The creation of a colostomy is still a reasonable alternative when the circumstances are not ideal.

Rectal Atresia

This condition is treated in the same manner in both the female and the male patient.

Persistent Cloaca

Persistent cloaca represents the extreme in the spectrum of complexity of female malformations. With this anomaly, the rectum, vagina, and urinary tract meet and fuse together into a single channel (see Figure 18-28, inset, later). Inspection of the perineum in these infants reveals rather small-looking external genitalia. Meticulous examination discloses a single orifice at the urethral site with no evidence of vagina or rectum.

Persistent cloaca, itself, is represented by a spectrum of defects. Many infants have a double or septated vagina, with different degrees of septation or division of the uterus. Frequently, the vaginal opening into the cloaca is obstructed, with a resultant severe hydrocolpos. The length of the common channel varies from 1 to 7 cm. This is considered a very important indicator of the potential difficulty that the surgeon will encounter when attempting to repair the defect. Lower, short cloacae, with good residual muscle and sacrum, are usually easier to repair. Longer cloacae are frequently associated with poor muscle and inadequate sacrum. These children, therefore, have an unlikely potential for continence.

In managing this malformation, one is committed to achieving normal bowel control, normal urinary continence, and normal sexual function, as well as childbearing potential. Success is more likely in children with a normal sacrum and an adequate vagina. As discussed, these malformations are frequently associated with severe obstructive uropathy. These patients require a colostomy and may often need some form of urinary diversion as well as vaginostomy for decompression of a hydrocolpos. At an appropriate interval, these procedures are followed by a posterior sagittal anorectovaginourethroplasty.

Associated Anomalies

Sacrum and Spine

The sacrum is frequently defective, with sacral vertebrae deformed or reduced in number. A hemisacrum is sometimes seen. A short sacrum, or a straight one without the normal anterior concavity, is frequently encountered. It is generally accepted that the more severe the sacral defect is, the less the potential for good bowel and urinary function. Usually, a patient with one or two vertebrae missing will have reasonably good potential for continence. However, an abnormal sacrum with a neurogenic bladder is considered a poor prognostic sign. Sacral anomalies are more frequently associated with a higher malformation. Other spinal defects include higher-level hemivertebrae with a consecutive scoliosis.

The advent of magnetic resonance imaging has permitted early detection and treatment of important associated defects, such as tethered cord, syrinx, and presacral masses (e.g., anterior meningocele, lipoma, dermoid, and teratoma).[103,116,128] This noninvasive study provides excellent imaging of the spine, cord, and pelvis. The limitation, however, is that an infant must be subjected to immobility and, therefore, adequate sedation for 30 to 45 minutes. Obviously, magnetic resonance imaging must be undertaken before repair of the major malformation. For example, in the situation of a tethered cord, release

must be accomplished by a separate neurosurgical procedure in order to avoid later nerve damage as a consequence of normal spinal growth. When a presacral mass has been identified, resection can be accomplished at the time of the PSARP. More recently, tethered cord has been detected by ultrasound by experienced pediatric radiologists, provided the study is performed when the baby is younger than 3 months of age (before the sacrum has ossified).[57]

Urogenital Defects

Genital and urinary abnormalities are often associated with anorectal malformations. The frequency of this association varies from 20% to 54% according to different authors.[11,144] This discrepancy is probably a reflection of the level of suspicion as well as the accuracy and thoroughness of the urologic workup in different institutions. Major urologic problems in children with imperforate anus are more common in those with high types of lesions.

In a review of our own series, we found that 48% of our patients (55% of girls; 44% of boys) had associated genital and urinary anomalies.[121] It is important to relate, however, that our patients tend to exhibit more complex malformations because of the referral nature of our institution. We were able to corroborate the concept that the higher the malformation is, the greater the association with urologic abnormalities. Additionally, we could determine the likelihood of an associated urologic malformation for every type of fistula. Thus, we observed that a patient with a persistent cloaca or rectovesical fistula has a 90% chance of an associated genital and urinary abnormality. Most of these are major, with the potential for significant morbidity if undiscovered and untreated. Conversely, children with a low fistula (i.e., perineal) exhibit less than a 10% incidence of associated malformations. In those infants with abnormal sacrum, the incidence of associated urologic malformations increased to 72%.

The most common genital and urinary anomaly encountered in our series and reported in the literature is renal agenesis. The incidence of renal agenesis (18%) and of vesicoureteral reflux (14%) were both found to correlate with the level of the fistula. Other important associated defects include cryptorchidism, ureteral duplication, hypospadias, rotated kidney, neurogenic bladder, renal dysplasia, renal ectopia, megaureter, hydronephrosis, and ureterovesical obstruction.[121]

Analysis of this data has helped us formulate guidelines for the urologic evaluation of infants with imperforate anus. We attempt to perform a renal and bladder ultrasound screening of all children born with imperforate anus before creation of a colostomy or performance of perineal surgery.[33] This precolostomy evaluation is considered a mandatory step, particularly in those with a persistent cloaca and a rectovesical fistula. If the study

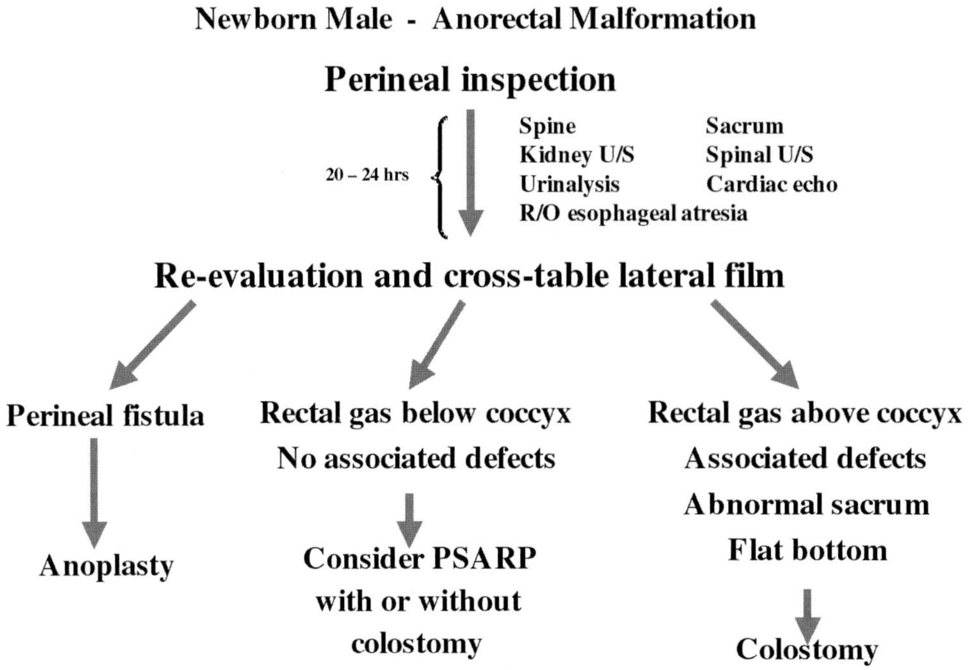

Newborn Male - Anorectal Malformation

Perineal inspection

20 – 24 hrs
{
Spine   Sacrum
Kidney U/S   Spinal U/S
Urinalysis   Cardiac echo
R/O esophageal atresia

Re-evaluation and cross-table lateral film

Perineal fistula

Rectal gas below coccyx
No associated defects

Rectal gas above coccyx
Associated defects
Abnormal sacrum
Flat bottom

Anoplasty

Consider PSARP
with or without
colostomy

Colostomy

FIGURE 18-19. Algorithm for the management of a newborn male child with an anorectal malformation.

discloses an abnormality, the surgeon should proceed with a more comprehensive urologic evaluation. Alternatively, male or female patients with perineal fistula may be subjected to ultrasound evaluation and urinalysis on an elective basis.

Algorithmic Approach to Decision Making

Figures 18-19 and 18-20 illustrate an algorithmic approach to decision making in the management of newborn infants (male and female) with anorectal malformations.

Male Patients

Mere inspection of the perineum and a urinalysis will permit one to determine whether the patient needs a colostomy 90% of the time. Usually, babies with anorectal malformations are not born with a distended abdomen. It takes at least 16 to 24 hours for the abdomen to develop this manifestation. The distal rectum (the blind portion, or the one connected to a fistula) is usually collapsed. Intraluminal pressure ultimately becomes sufficient to overcome the muscle tone of the sphincter mechanism, to allow the meconium or the gas to reach the most distal part of the bowel, and to be forced through a tiny fistula orifice. This explains why studies to determine the height of the malformation and the location of the fistula performed before 16 to 24 hours can lead to an

erroneous diagnosis, that of a "high" anorectal malformation. Diagnostic tests should, therefore, be performed after the baby is 24 hours old. However, during this first day, one should rule out potentially lethal conditions, such as cardiac, esophageal and urologic disorders. The baby receives intravenous fluids and antibiotics and remains fasting, and a nasogastric tube is inserted to avoid vomiting and the risk of bronchial aspiration.

The following studies are performed: abdominal ultrasound, x-ray study of the lumbar and sacral spine, and echocardiogram. The infant is observed for symptoms and signs of esophageal obstruction. After 24 hours of observation, the surgeon will obtain sufficient information to determine whether the baby requires a colostomy or whether a direct repair of the anorectal malformation may be performed. This is true in 90% of the cases. In the remaining 10%, that is, those in whom the surgeon does not obtain adequate information for a decision, a cross-table lateral film is taken with the baby in prone position. This will show the presence of gas in the distal rectum. The position of this bubble and its relationship to the coccyx are important for determining whether the surgeon can perform a reconstruction with or without a colostomy. Sometimes, the perineal fistula is a very obvious orifice that is located in the midline of the perineum between the genitalia and the anal dimple. One can see meconium coming out through it. Other times, the orifice is so tiny that it is not seen on first inspection. It requires a significant intraluminal bowel pressure to force

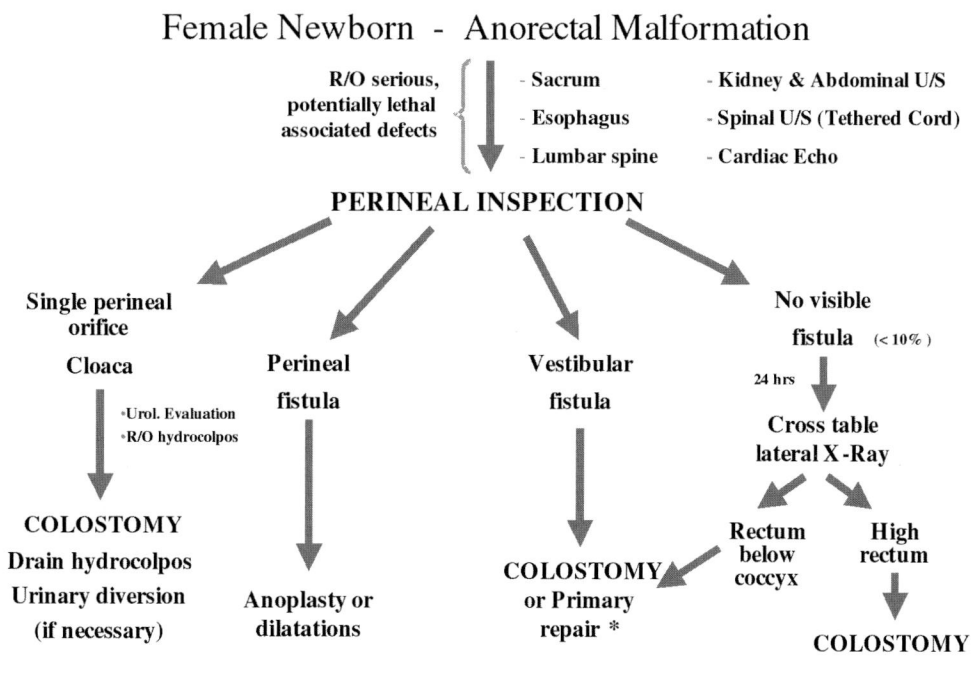

FIGURE 18-20. Algorithm for the management of a newborn female child with an anorectal malformation.

the meconium through it. Under these circumstances, it is not unusual, following 24 hours of observation, to see meconium appear to be coming through a tiny fistula orifice. The presence of a perineal fistula encourages the surgeon to perform an anoplasty without a protective colostomy within the infant's first 48 hours of life.

If the baby does not pass meconium in the urine, does not demonstrate a perineal fistula, and does not have a flat bottom, a cross-table lateral film is taken. If the rectal gas is located below the coccyx and the baby is in good condition, with no significant associated defects, the surgeon should consider the possibility of performing a primary posterior sagittal operation without a colostomy. This, as previously mentioned, will depend very much on the experience of the operator. Conversely, if the rectal gas is located well above the coccyx, the baby has significant associated defects, an abnormal sacrum, a flat bottom, and meconium in the urine, it is advisable to create a colostomy and avoid a primary approach to the perineum. Without evidence of the location of the rectum, this is a prudent policy in order to prevent injury to the urinary tract.

Female Patients

Determination of the need for a colostomy is an easier decision in female infants. The reason for this is that in 90% to 95%, the bowel opening is externally evident. The same rule applies for female babies—that is, decisions concerning colostomy or primary approach should not

be taken before 24 hours of life. The first day should be used, as mentioned for boys, to rule out the presence of potentially lethal conditions and to be certain that the baby does not have hydrocolpos, hydronephrosis, tethered cord, a cardiac malformation, esophageal atresia, or spinal defects. The presence of a perineal fistula (see Figure 18-23) is evidence of a very low malformation that can be treated with a minimal PSARP without a colostomy. As previously stated, the operation can be performed at any time. If these children are untreated, they will usually develop normal bowel control.

The presence of a vestibular fistula may be an indication for a colostomy or a primary reparative approach, depending on the circumstances. If the surgeon is experienced, and the baby is full term and has no significant associated malformations, the operation can be accomplished primarily within the first few days of life. Conversely, if the baby is very ill and has significant associated defects, or if the surgeon does not have the necessary experience, it is preferable to create a colostomy and to postpone the primary repair for a later date.

If the baby has a single perineal orifice, the diagnosis of a cloaca is immediately established. The surgeon should recognize that he or she is confronting a urologic problem. Therefore, this infant requires a complete urologic evaluation. The presence of hydrocolpos must be excluded. A colostomy is required, and it is mandatory to drain the hydrocolpos during the same operation. If the vagina is sufficiently capacious that it can reach the abdominal wall above the bladder, the patient can undergo a tubeless vaginostomy. Alternatively, if the vagina is dilated but does not reach above the bladder, a tube vaginostomy will be necessary.

Occasionally, an infant with a cloaca may have a virtual atresia of the urethra. Such an individual requires a temporary vesicostomy at the time of the colostomy. If the baby does not have a visible fistula (5% of the cases), a cross-table lateral x-ray film is indicated with the infant in the prone position. When the gas in the rectum is seen below the coccyx, depending on the surgeon's experience, the patient can be approached primarily posterosagittally. If the gas is located much higher than the coccyx, it is advisable to create a colostomy.

Surgical Technique

Colostomy

Diverting colostomy is considered a very important step in the management of anorectal malformations. Today, however, the pediatric surgical community is commonly utilizing a primary neonatal operation without a protective colostomy.[49,96] The advantages to this are that the patient will undergo fewer operations and will be able to avoid the potential morbidity associated with a colostomy.

At our institution, we are moving in the same direction. For example, we do not employ fecal diversion with babies who have perineal fistulas, vestibular fistulas, and imperforate anus without fistulas and rectourethral bulbar fistulas, provided the patients are in good condition and we have evidence that the rectum is located below the coccyx. We still advocate a colostomy for more complex defects.

The main limitation to the primary repair approach without colostomy is the lack of an accurate diagnostic test for delineating the precise anatomy of the malformation. The high-pressure distal colostogram is considered the most valuable diagnostic tool in these patients, because it allows one to see precisely the location of the rectum and the location of the fistula site (Figure 18-21).[53] A newborn infant should not be subjected to a procedure wherein the location of the rectum is unknown. This would lead essentially to a blind perineal exploration. We have seen many patients who were operated upon in this way only to suffer serious consequences. For example, the surgeon had been looking for a rectum that was located too high in the pelvis, and the search led to injury to urethra, vas deferens, seminal vesicles, prostate, and nerves affecting erection and bladder function.[65]

The ultimate result in these individuals depends largely upon preservation of whatever anatomic structures are present. A failed pull-through provokes severe scarring, fibrosis, and destruction of the original anatomy. A second repair, therefore, is less likely to succeed.

Thus, a diverting colostomy, specifically a left descending colostomy with separated stomas, still represents the safest method of treating these patients (Figure 18-22). A retracted or inadequately diverting loop colostomy may allow the passage of feces into the distal bowel and communication in most cases with the urinary tract through the fistula.

Repair of Specific Defects in the Female

Perineal Fistula

The most significant characteristic of this malformation is that the rectum and vagina are well separated without sharing a common wall. Therefore, the dissection between the two structures is relatively straightforward. Electrical stimulation will demonstrate that the fistula is not surrounded by muscle. Parasagittal fibers may be found on both sides of the fistula, but the anterior portion is usually devoid of muscle (Figure 18-23, *inset*).

The operation can be accomplished at any time, depending on the child's symptoms. Sometimes the fistula is efficient in emptying the rectum, and the treatment can be delayed. This is especially important if the infant has additional anomalies. Another limiting factor may be the surgeon's experience, but if one is familiar with the fine structures of a newborn, the operation can be accomplished during the first few days of life.

The infant is placed in the prone position with the pelvis elevated to expose the perineal area. The incision is of a "racket type" that encircles the fistula and extends posteriorly and midsagittally through the midportion of the external sphincter (Figure 18-23). Multiple 5–0 silk sutures are placed at the mucocutaneous junction of the fistula and are used for traction. A needle-tip electrocautery device is advised for performing this dissection because special emphasis is placed on meticulous hemostasis. The dissection is undertaken as close as is possible to the bowel wall in an attempt to preserve all the muscle lateral and posterior to the fistula. The dissection is also carried out as cephalad as is necessary in order to mobilize the rectum sufficiently so that satisfactory relation within the external sphincter, without tension on the suture line, is achieved (Figure 18-24).

After the mobilization has been completed, one is able to identify the vertical muscle fibers (i.e., muscle complex) that run parallel to the rectum and perpendicular to the parasagittal fibers (Figure 18-24A). The vertical fibers and the parasagittal fibers cross at two places, creating two corners that mark the limits of the new anus. The dissection does not reach the levator ani muscle. Tapering of the rectum is not required in these individuals. The rectum is then relocated within the limits of the muscle, and the perineal body is closed with 6–0 interrupted long-term absorbable sutures, bringing together the anterior limit of the muscle complex (Figure 18-24A).

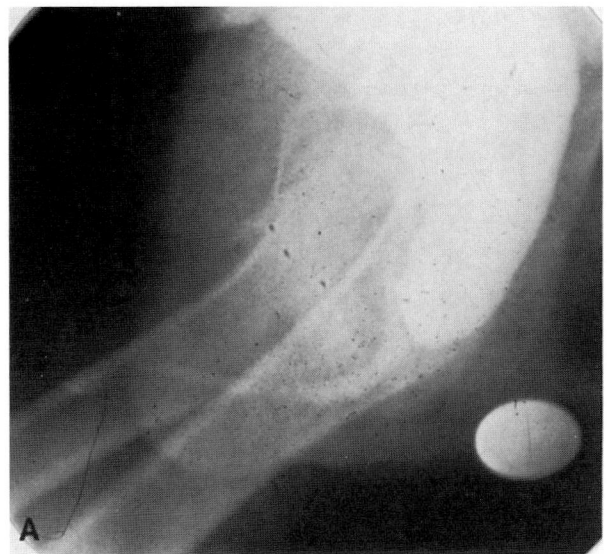

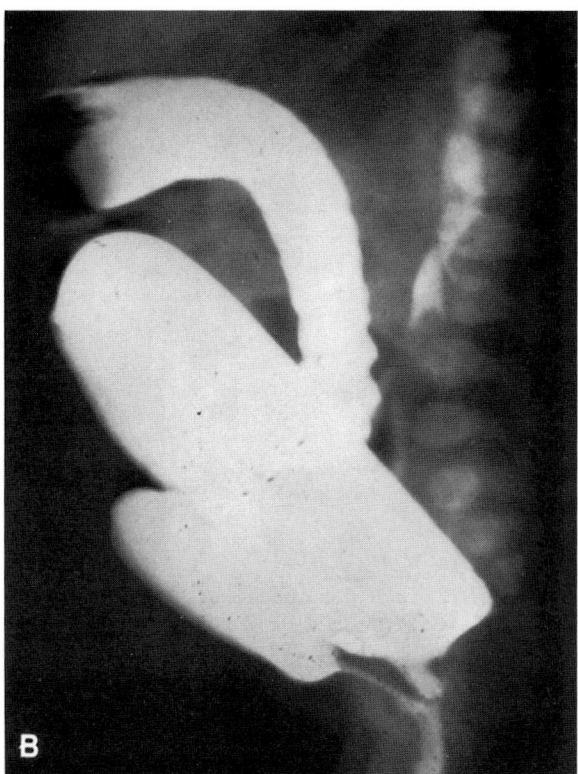

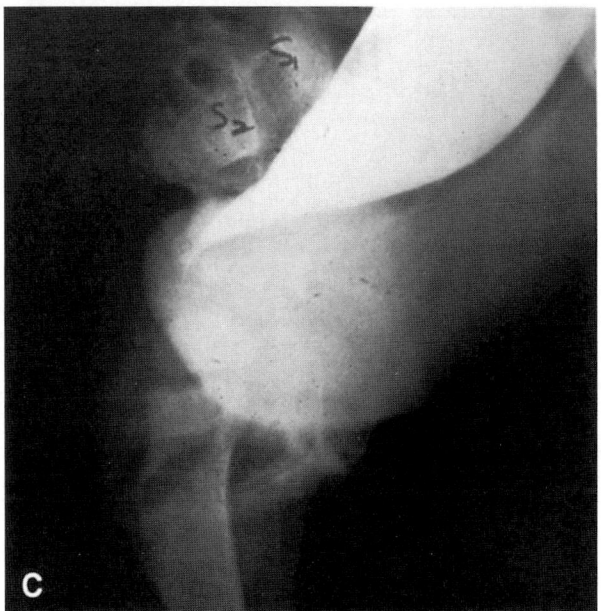

FIGURE 18-21. Distal colostograms. **(A)** Bulbar-urethral fistula. **(B)** Prostatic fistula. **(C)** Bladder fistula.

The posterior limit of the sphincter muscle is then sutured, incorporating part of the bowel wall to anchor the rectum and to prevent prolapse (Figure 18-24*A*). An anoplasty is accomplished by suturing the rectum to the skin after trimming, but as much tissue as possible is preserved (Figure 18-24*B*).

There is no requirement in the newborn for a bowel preparation, but prophylactic antibiotics (e.g., ampicillin, gentamicin) are administered for 2 days. The infant can usually eat the day following surgery and requires only local wound care (i.e., frequent washing with soap and water and an antibiotic ointment). Recovery is usually uneventful, and rectal dilatation is instituted 2 weeks following the procedure.

Vestibular Fistula

The primary characteristic with this defect is that the rectum and vagina share a common wall distally (Figure 18-25, *inset*). This must be kept in mind at the time of reconstruction, because it is imperative that complete separation of both structures be achieved in order to obtain a successful repair. The size of the fistula orifice is quite variable. As a consequence, these infants may manifest different degrees of obstruction, although normal bowel movement patterns may be evident during the newborn period.

Traditionally, surgical management of this malformation always required a completely diverting colostomy. However, if a surgeon feels comfortable with the

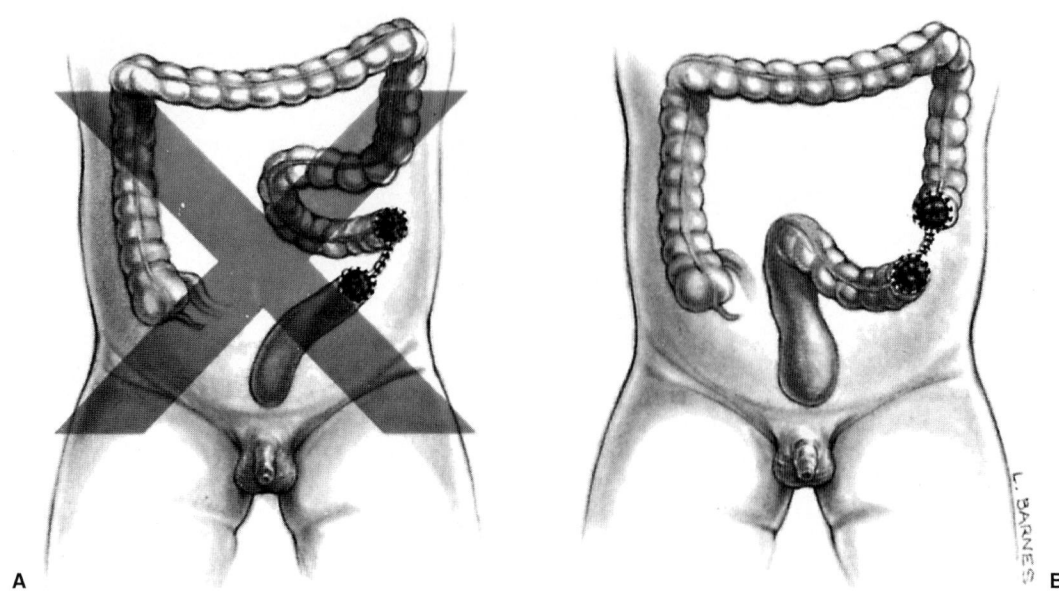

A
B

FIGURE 18-22. Possible colostomy alternatives. **(A)** Inadequate colostomy; short distal bowel interferes with the subsequent pull-through. **(B)** Recommended colostomy, located in the descending colon; redundant distal sigmoid permits subsequent pull-through. Note the separated stomas.

meticulous technique necessary for this reconstruction, a repair can be performed without diversion, either in the newborn period or delayed if the child has significant associated malformations. Not infrequently, the diagnosis of this defect is missed in the newborn period, and thus a surgeon may encounter it in an older child.

One may undertake a pull-through without diversion at that time.

At our institution, we adhere to a very strict preoperative bowel preparation. Furthermore, for 7 to 10 postoperative days, intravenous nutrition is maintained, and nothing is permitted by mouth. These precautions are employed in

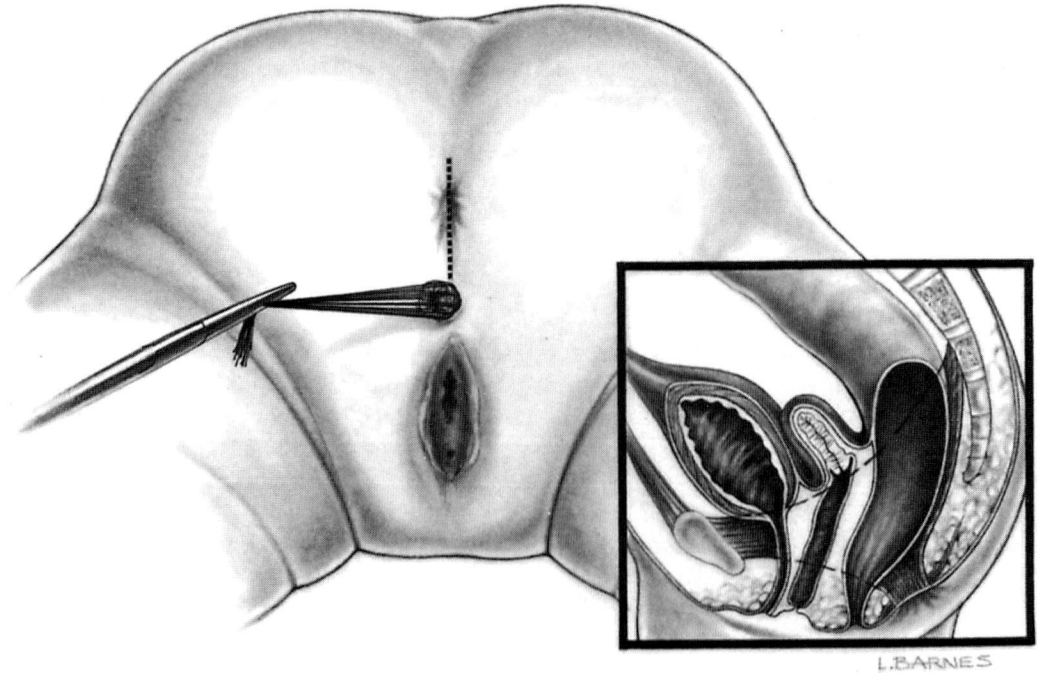

FIGURE 18-23. Perineal fistula. Surgical incision. Sagittal appearance of the perineal fistula **(inset).** Note the separation between the rectum and the vagina.

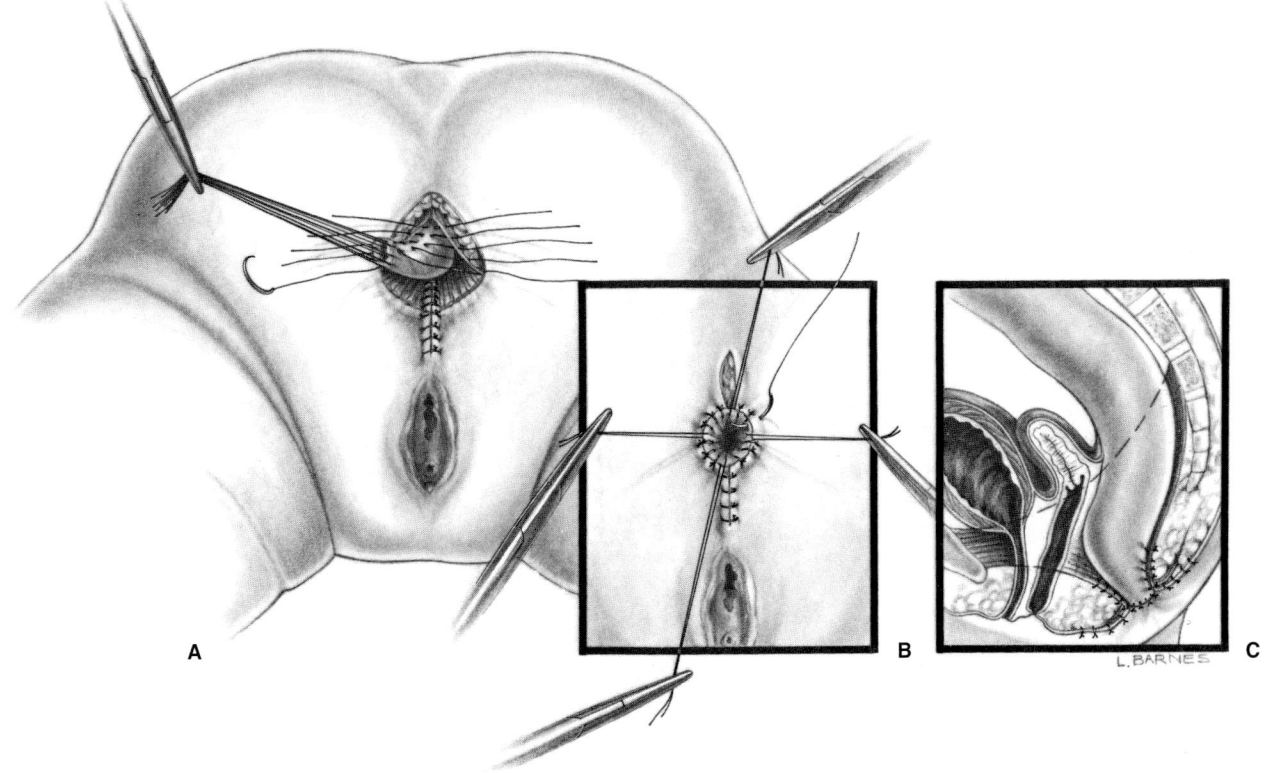

FIGURE 18-24. Repair of a perineal fistula. **(A)** The rectum has been dissected and the perineum reconstructed. Sutures are placed through the posterior edge of the muscle complex (behind the rectum) and include the bowel wall. **(B)** Anoplasty by means of interrupted mucocutaneous sutures. **(C)** Operation completed.

order to limit the likelihood of a perineal infection, a complication that can adversely affect prognosis.

The child is placed in the prone position with the pelvis elevated. Electrical stimulation demonstrates the contraction of the external sphincter muscle considerably posterior to the fistula site. The incision is longer than that which has been described for perineal fistula and is also of the racket type. Multiple 6–0 silk sutures are placed at the edge of the fistula and are used for traction. Because of the common wall, the most difficult part of the dissection consists of separating the rectum from the vagina. Often, it is helpful to inject epinephrine solution into this wall to facilitate the dissection. The use of a needle-tip electrocautery device also expedites the operation. Depending on the length of the common wall, the incision can be enlarged in order to obtain full separation of the rectum from the vagina. It must be made exactly in the midline so that the external sphincter is divided into two equal parts. The sagittal incision extends into the muscle complex and sometimes into the inferior portion of the levator ani. This procedure is called a limited PSARP because the dissection usually does not extend to the coccyx and levator ani muscle. With the application of an electrical stimulator, one can be certain that the dis-

section is in the midline. Mobilization of the rectum must be sufficiently adequate to permit relocation within the muscle complex and the external sphincter without tension. Tapering is usually not necessary with this malformation. The completed dissection reveals the intact vaginal wall, the anterior extent of the muscle complex, the perineal body with only subcutaneous fat, and the limits of the external sphincter, marked by the crossing of the vertical and parasagittal fibers (Figure 18-26A).

The anterior perineum is reconstructed with both anterior edges of the muscle complex approximated (Figure 18-26B). The posterior limit of the muscle complex is also sutured together, along with a portion of the posterior rectal wall (Figure 18-26C). This reduces the likelihood of a subsequent prolapse. An anoplasty is then created within the limits of the external sphincter in the same manner as that described for perineal fistula. The skin of the perineum is closed with interrupted 5–0 long-term absorbable sutures (Figs. 18-26D and E).

Postoperative Care The postoperative care requires perineal cleansing and the use of bacitracin ointment daily for 1 week. Dilatations are begun 2 weeks following the procedure. If a colostomy is in place, the child can usu-

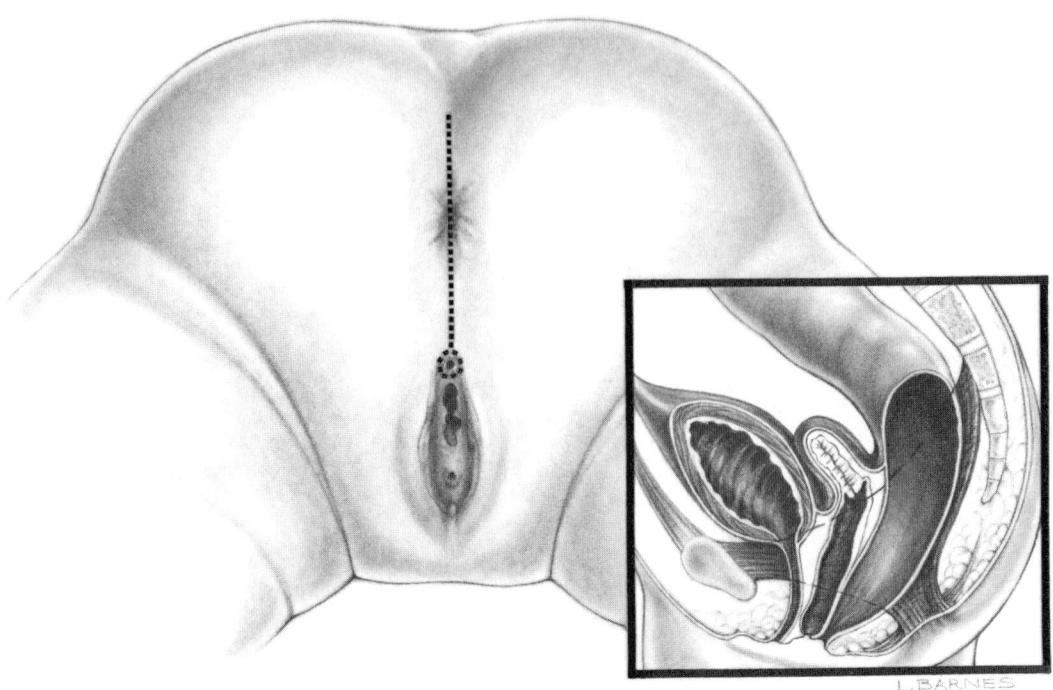

FIGURE 18-25. Surgical incision in a case of vestibular fistula. Sagittal appearance **(inset)**. Note the common, thin wall between rectum and vagina.

ally eat the day of the operation and is usually discharged the following day. Systemic antibiotics are administered as described with perineal fistula. With no colostomy is performed, we maintain the child on hyperalimentation with nothing by mouth for a period of 7 to 10 days in an attempt to avoid the passage of stool.

Vaginal Fistula

This is an extremely unusual defect, one that occurs in less than 1% of these anomalies. The perineum in these patients demonstrates no obvious anal orifice. It is not unusual to find that the posterior rim of the hymen is missing, an important clue for detecting a low vaginal fistula. The communication between rectum and vagina may be located in the lower part of the vagina (most frequent; Figure 18-27A) or in the upper portion (very unusual; Figure 18-27B). The lower the fistula is located, the longer the common wall will be. The sacrum may demonstrate different degrees of dysplasia, and the muscles may be deficient. Occasionally, however, a patient with a vaginal fistula may have excellent sphincter muscles. The external sphincter is found to be in its normal location.

These infants require a colostomy before repair. The operation can be performed on a child from 1 to 12 months of age, depending on the surgeon's experience. Management is similar to that described for the vestibular malformation. However, the incision is made from the

middle portion of the sacrum to the vaginal orifice. One must split the coccyx and divide the levator ani muscle throughout its length. This is a full PSARP. With this malformation, it is not unusual to find a considerable discrepancy between the size of the rectum and the space available between the levator ani muscle and the vagina. Commonly, therefore, one must taper the rectum (Figure 18-27C).

Once the levator ani has been divided in the midline, the rectum must be completely opened in order to expose the fistula directly. The rectum and vagina are separated by using multiple 5–0 silk traction sutures in the rectal mucosa. In the presence of a very high malformation, the rectum may not be found by this approach; a laparotomy is then required. When tapering is indicated, 20% to 70% of the rectal wall is resected, depending on the magnitude of the discrepancy between the rectum and the available space. The bowel is then closed in two layers with interrupted 5–0 long-term absorbable sutures. The posterior wall of the vagina should be repaired. The rectum must then be relocated in front of the levator ani muscle and behind the vagina. It is then directed 90 degrees posteriorly, following the direction of the muscle complex (Figure 18-27C). The new anus is created at the center of the external sphincter, and the parasagittal fibers are reapproximated with interrupted 5–0 long-term absorbable sutures. The coccyx is reconstituted with absorbable sutures, and the wound is closed with a subcuticular suture

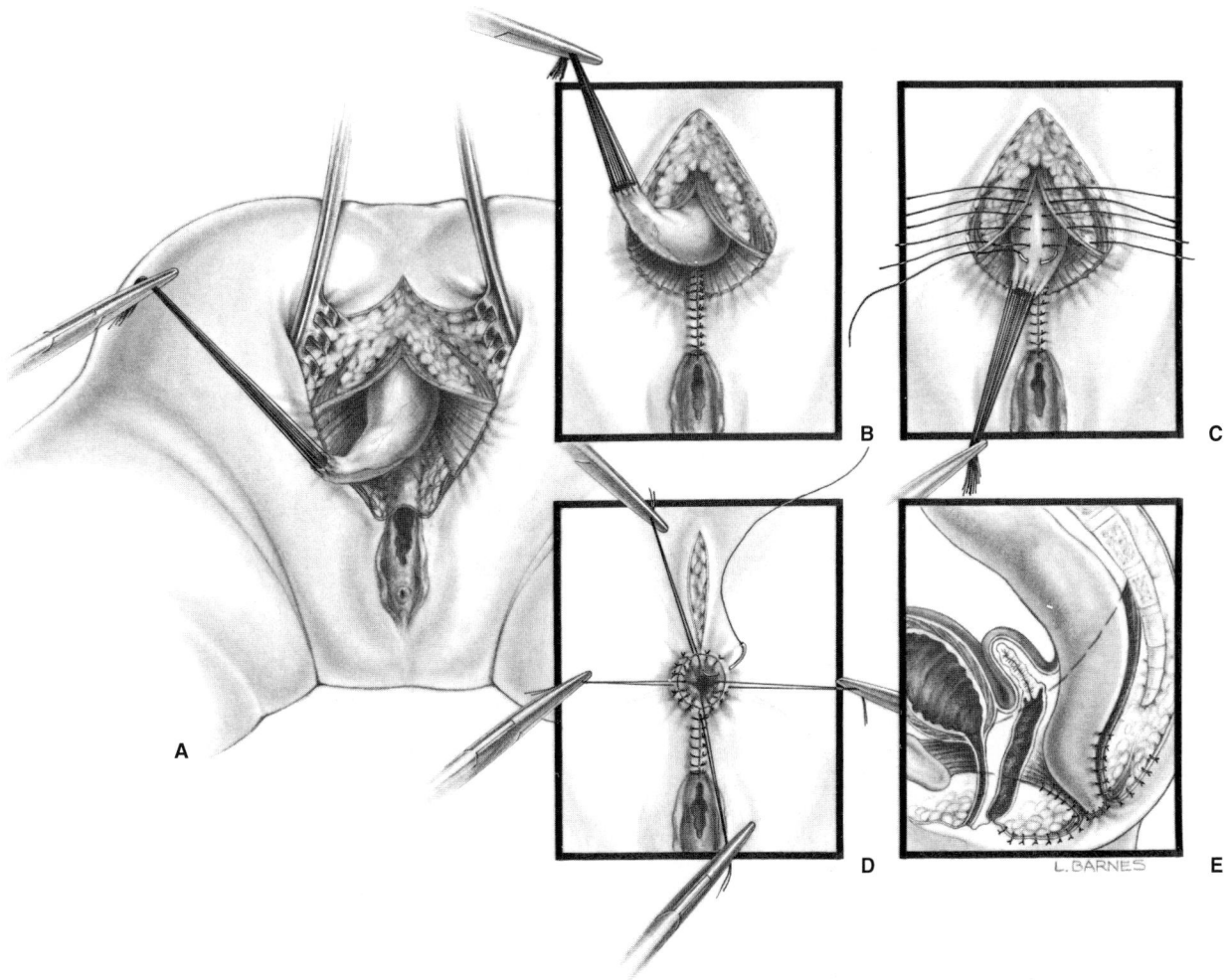

FIGURE 18-26. Repair of vestibular fistula. **(A)** The rectum has been dissected, including meticulous separation from the vagina. **(B)** The anterior perineum is reconstructed. The anterior edge of the muscle complex has been approximated anterior to the rectum. **(C)** Sutures are placed through the posterior edges of the muscle complex including the back of the rectal wall. **(D)** Anoplasty (mucocutaneous suture). **(E)** Completed operation.

of fine nylon. The perineal body, including the anterior edge of the muscle complex, is approximated as described for the vestibular fistula.

Perhaps because the operation is entirely accomplished through an incision in the midline raphe, it is relatively painless. A Foley catheter for urinary diversion is not used in any repair of perineal, vestibular or vaginal fistulas, because we do not believe that the presence of urine adversely affects suture lines. The patient can sit, walk, and be discharged the day after surgery.

Atresia and Stenosis of the Rectum

Although even today some surgeons still employ an abdominoperineal operation for atresia and stenosis of the rectum, we do not offer it, because these children have the necessary anatomic structures for continence.

PSARP offers a unique opportunity for repairing this malformation. This approach permits excellent exposure to the anomaly and makes the repair truly quite simple. The operation usually requires a full PSARP, with or without a diverting colostomy, depending on the baby's circumstances and the surgeon's experience. A midline incision is carried down to the levator ani and to the atretic rectum following the principles mentioned in the previous descriptions. Once the defect is exposed, the procedure consists of an end-to-end anastomosis of the proximal rectum to the distal anal canal. After this has been accomplished, the levator ani muscle, muscle complex, and parasagittal fibers are reapproximated with absorbable material. The skin is then closed with a subcuticular suture of 5–0 nylon. Even though the anus appears externally normal, anastomotic stricture

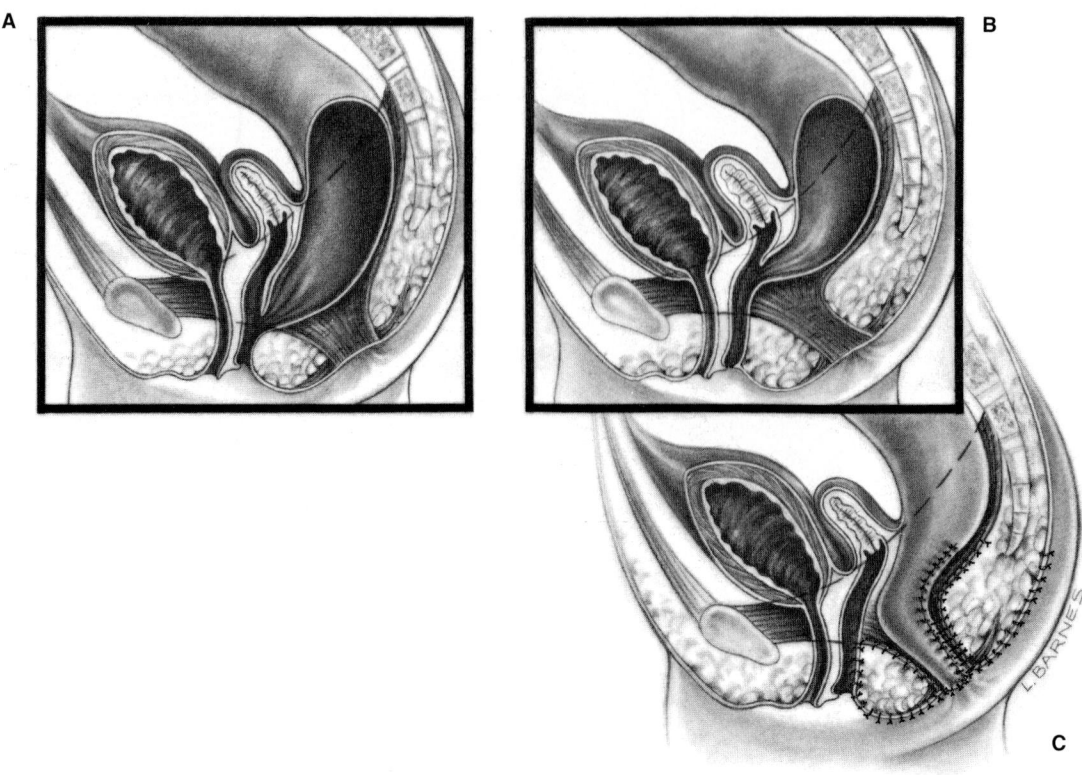

FIGURE 18-27. Vaginal fistula. **(A)** Low fistula. **(B)** High fistula. **(C)** Repaired malformation including tapering of the rectum.

may subsequently develop. These children, therefore, require dilatation.

Persistent Cloaca

Management of the complex malformation of persistent cloaca requires a number of surgical maneuvers. The procedure is called posterior sagittal anorectovaginourethroplasty.

The requisite incision is shown in Figure 18-28, extending from the middle portion of the sacrum. It passes through the center of the external sphincter and ends at the opening of the single channel or common cloaca. The external sphincter, muscle complex, and levator ani are divided in halves (Figure 18-29A). The rectum, including the common channel, is then opened exactly in the midline (Figure 18-29B). Once the entire visceral structure has been opened, one can identify the rectal, vaginal, and urethral orifices (Figure 18-29C). A Foley catheter is then inserted through the urinary opening. Attempts to pass the catheter before opening the cloaca are usually unsuccessful, because one cannot be certain which opening was entered.

Because the rectum and vagina share a common wall, there is no natural plane for separation. By placing multiple 5–0 or 6–0 silk sutures into the rectal mucosa for traction, the maneuver is expedited. The submucosal dissection continues cephalad to the point where the vagina and the rectum separate (Figure 18-30A). Then the maneuver

becomes simplified, because one is now dealing with the full thickness of the rectal wall. Until recently, once the rectum had been completely separated, the vagina was also separated from the urinary tract—an even more difficult procedure (Figure 18-30). A newer maneuver called "total urogenital mobilization" has been found to simplify the repair of the cloaca, to render better anatomic reconstruction, and to reduce the operative time.[109] After the rectum has been successfully separated from the vagina, no attempt is made to separate the vagina from the urinary tract. Rather, the entire urogenital sinus is dissected and mobilized. Multiple fine silk sutures are placed at the edge of the vagina and the common channel (Figure 18-31). Another series of 6–0 silk sutures is then placed across the common channel (urogenital sinus) and between 5 and 10 mm dorsal to the clitoris (Figure 18-31, *inset*). These sutures help to avoid tissue damage by distributing the tension on as many sutures as possible. The wall of the urogenital sinus is divided completely, ventral to the silk sutures. Anterior or ventral to the urogenital sinus, a well-defined space and plane separate this sinus from the pubis. The dissection must proceed lateral and ventral to the urogenital sinus to reach the retropubic space. Traction is exerted on the vaginal edges as the dissection continues in a circumferential manner, including vagina and urethra together (Figure 18-32). The urethra and vagina are held in the pelvis by avascular fibrous liga-

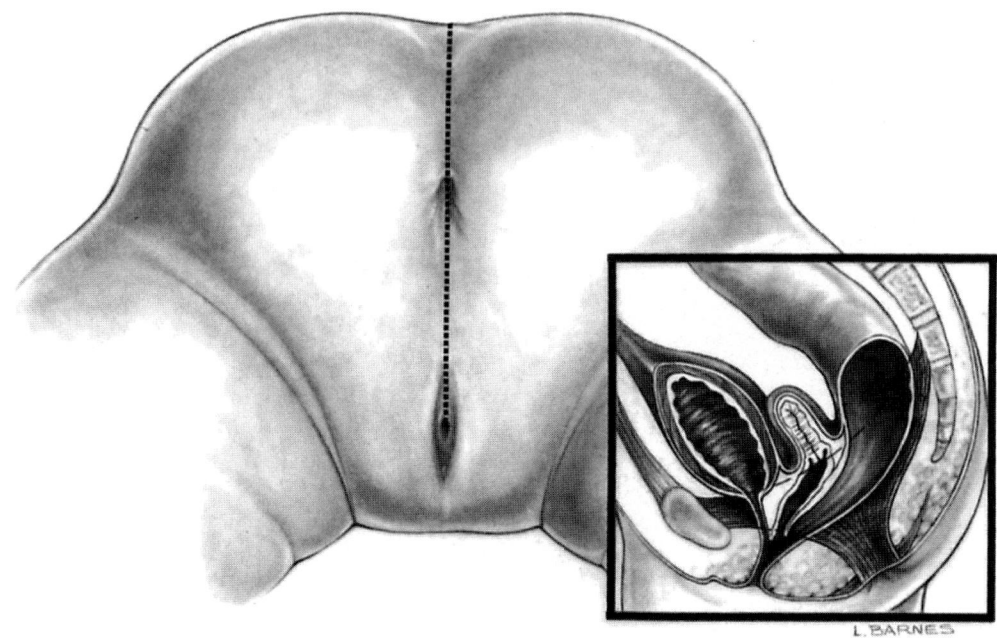

FIGURE 18-28. Persistent cloaca. Surgical incision; note the small-appearing vulva. Sagittal appearance **(inset)**; the rectum and vagina, as well as the vagina and urinary tract, share a common wall.

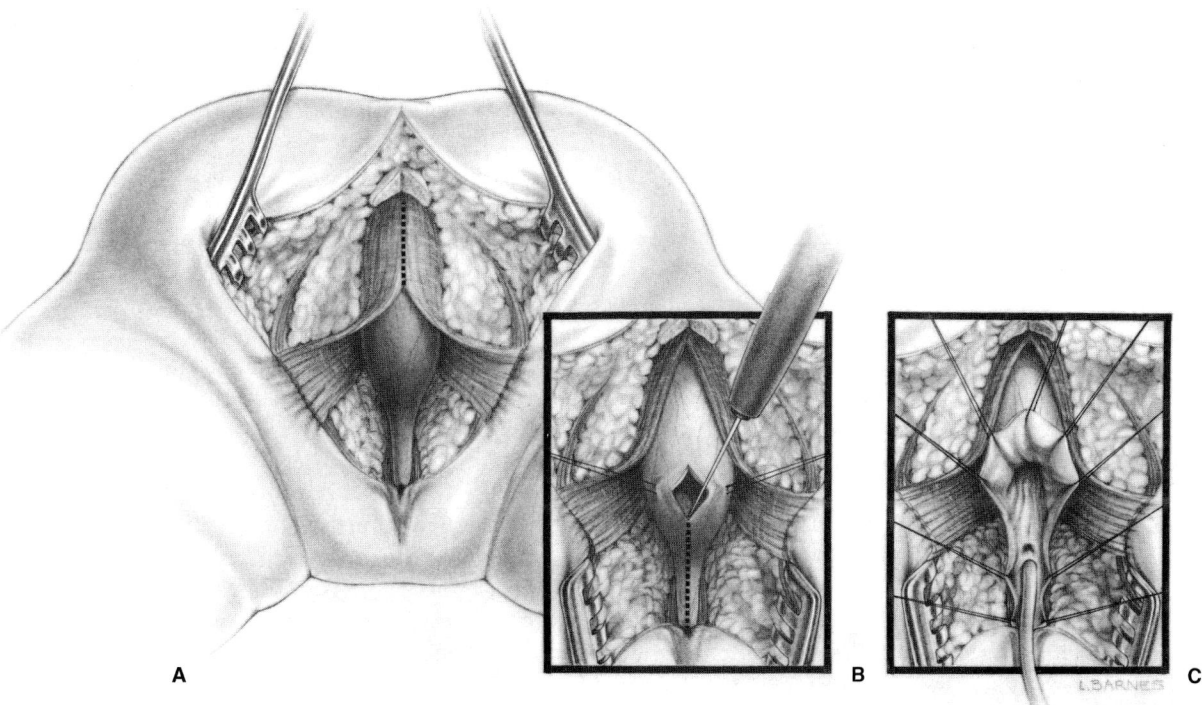

A   **B**   **C**

FIGURE 18-29. Repair of a persistent cloaca. **(A)** The external sphincter has been split in the middle. The levator ani muscle is divided to expose the persistent cloaca. **(B)** Opening the rectum. **(C)** The rectum and vagina are exposed; a catheter has been placed in the urethral orifice.

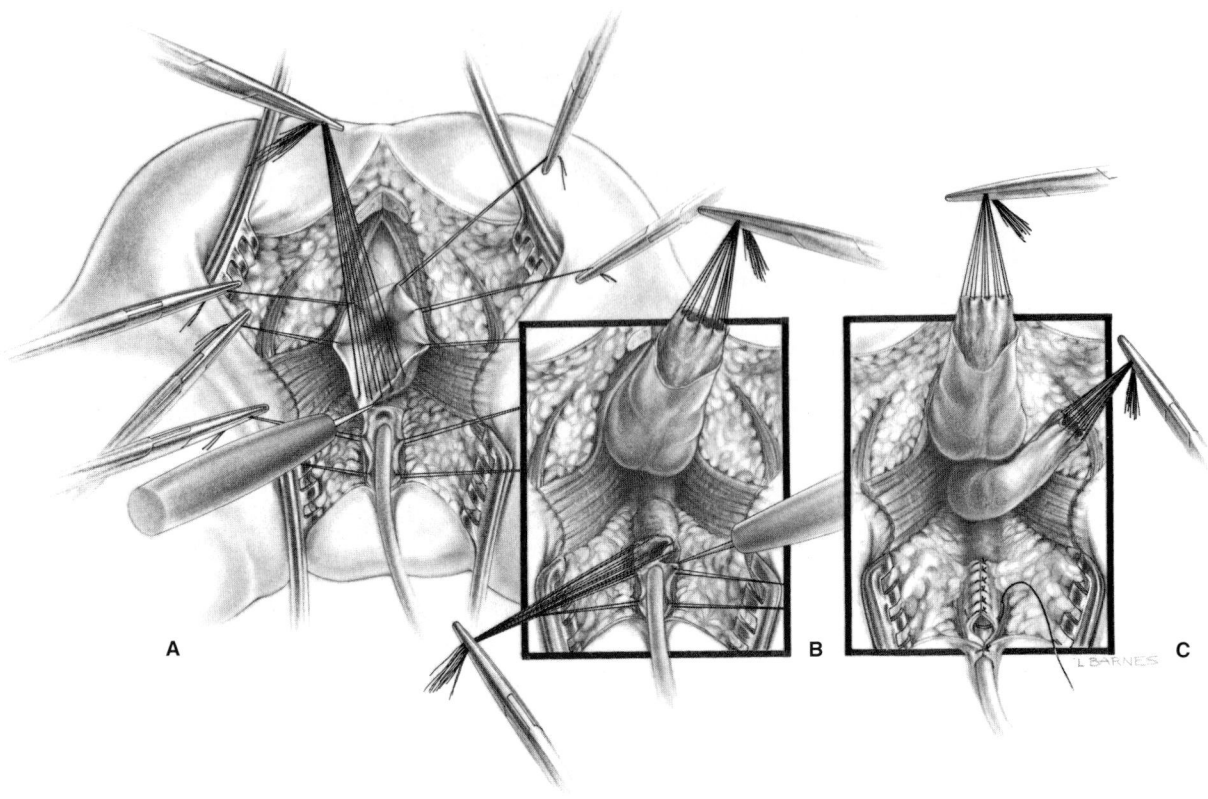

FIGURE 18-30. Former repair of persistent cloaca. **(A)** Rectum separated from vagina. **(B)** Separation of vagina from urinary tract. **(C)** Reconstruction of neourethra using the residual common channel of the cloaca.

ments attached to the pelvic rim. These ligaments must be divided to free the vagina, bladder, and urethra without the need for dividing the blood supply to these structures. The dissection continues circumferentially until enough length has been gained to connect the vaginal edges to the perineum (Figure 18-32, *inset*). Thus, a urethral and vaginal opening of a near-normal appearance is created (Figure 18-33). The vaginal edges are then sutured to the skin or the labia of the perineum with interrupted 5–0 long-term absorbable sutures. The urethral opening will then be located 5 to 8 mm from the clitoris.

This maneuver allows the reconstruction of urethra and vagina in greater than 50% of the patients with cloacas, namely, those who have a common channel of less than 3 cm. Additional maneuvers are required for the vaginal reconstruction in cases of a longer common channel.

One must remember that persistent cloaca represents a spectrum of malformations. A relatively simple repair is that of a short common channel associated with a rather large vagina and a low implanted rectum. Under these circumstances, rectum and vagina can be readily mobilized and reconstructed (Figure 18-34). At the other end of the spectrum, one may find a very high rectum that cannot even be recognized during posterior sagittal exploration. Under these circumstances, repair of this defect requires

a laparotomy. Another difficult problem arises when one must deal with a long (e.g., 7 cm) common channel and a very small vagina that cannot be mobilized to the perineum. In this particular situation, several options are possible. For example, one can interpose a segment of small or large bowel between the lower vaginal edge and the perineal skin or utilize the labia to fill the defect between vagina and perineum.[60,112] If the surgeon is confronted with a rather large vagina but a short common channel, it may be feasible to create a flap of the dome for interposition between the vagina and the perineum.

Occasionally, patients have two very large hemivaginas (bilateral hydrocolpos) and a long common channel, indicating that both hemivaginas are located far away from the perineum. The distance from one hemicervix to the other (transverse diameter of both hemivaginas together) is longer than the vertical length of both structures (Figure 18-35*A*). In this specific type of malformation, one can reconstruct the vagina doing a maneuver called a vaginal switch (Figure 18-35*B*). One hemiuterus is resected, including the fallopian tube, with special care taken to preserve the ovary. The vaginal dome in that specific site is switched down to the perineum and will be reanastomosed to the vulva. This maneuver has proved to be useful if the patient has this specific variant of malfor-

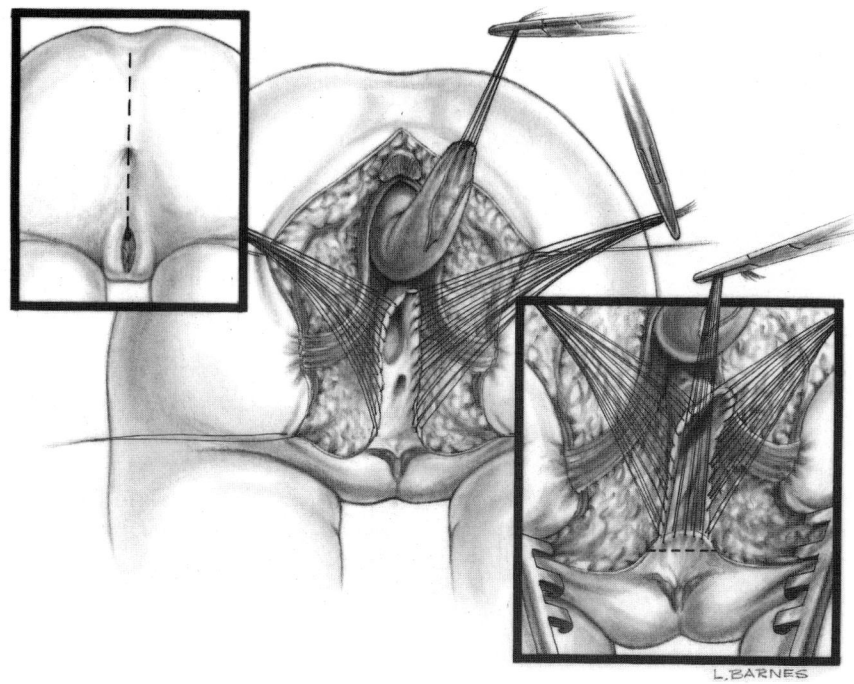

FIGURE 18-31. Management of a persistent cloaca. Total urogenital mobilization.

mation. After the urethra and vagina have been repaired, the rectum must be reconstructed.

With the aid of an electrical stimulator, the landmarks for the reconstruction, the center of the external sphincter, and the anterior limit of the muscle complex are determined. Fine, long-term absorbable sutures are placed to reapproximate the anterior edge of the muscle complex and the anterior portion of the external sphincter (Figure 18-34A). The rectum now is located within the muscle complex and the external sphincter. The posterior limit of the muscle complex is then reapproximated behind the rectum with 5–0 long-term absorbable sutures,

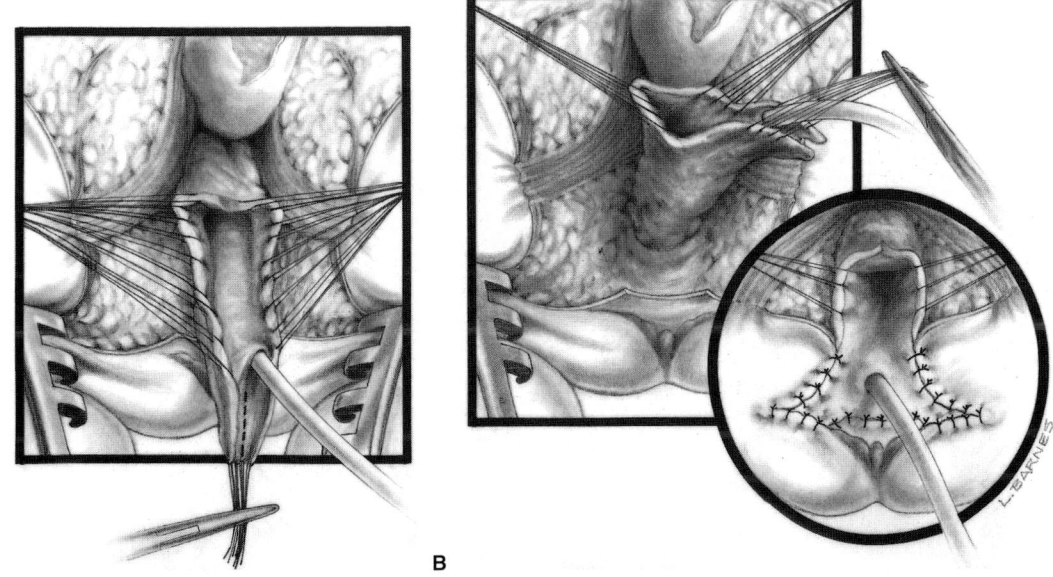

FIGURE 18-32. Management of a persistent cloaca. **(A)** Mobilized urogenital sinus. **(B)** Dissection of retropubic area. Reconstruction of the vulva **(inset)**.

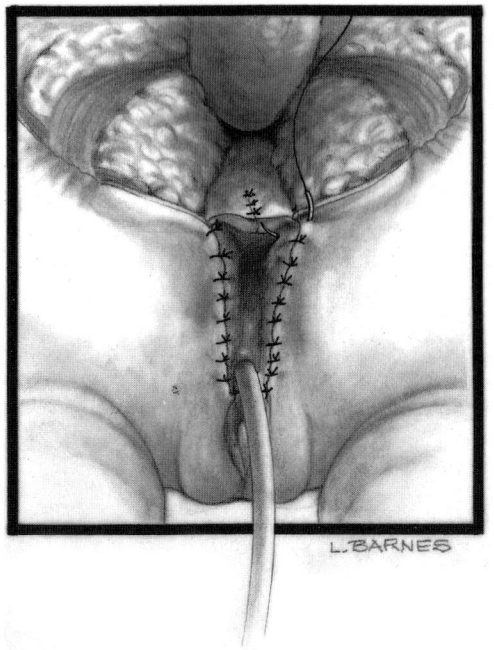

FIGURE 18-33. Management of a persistent cloaca. Total urogential mobilization is completed.

including the bowel wall (Figure 18-34*B*). An anoplasty is accomplished as described with the management of previous malformations, and the wound is closed in layers (Figure 18-34*C*).

A urinary catheter is usually left in place for approximately 10 days. Anal dilatations are started 2 weeks following the operation as is described for the other malformations.

Repair of these malformations represents the ultimate challenge in pediatric pelvic surgery and should be performed only by individuals who have considerable experience with this type of surgery.

Repair of Low Malformations in the Male Patient (Perineal Fistula), Previously Known as Cutaneous Fistula, Anal Stenosis, and Anal Membrane

Low malformations represent the most benign type of male anorectal defect. No colostomy is required with the reconstruction. The primary characteristic of patients with these anomalies is the location of the rectal fistula, immediately anterior to the center of the external sphincter (Figure 18-15*A*). The surgical technique used for the repair is very similar to that described for perineal fistula in female patients.

In male patients, the most common and feared intraoperative complication is a urethral injury. The surgeon

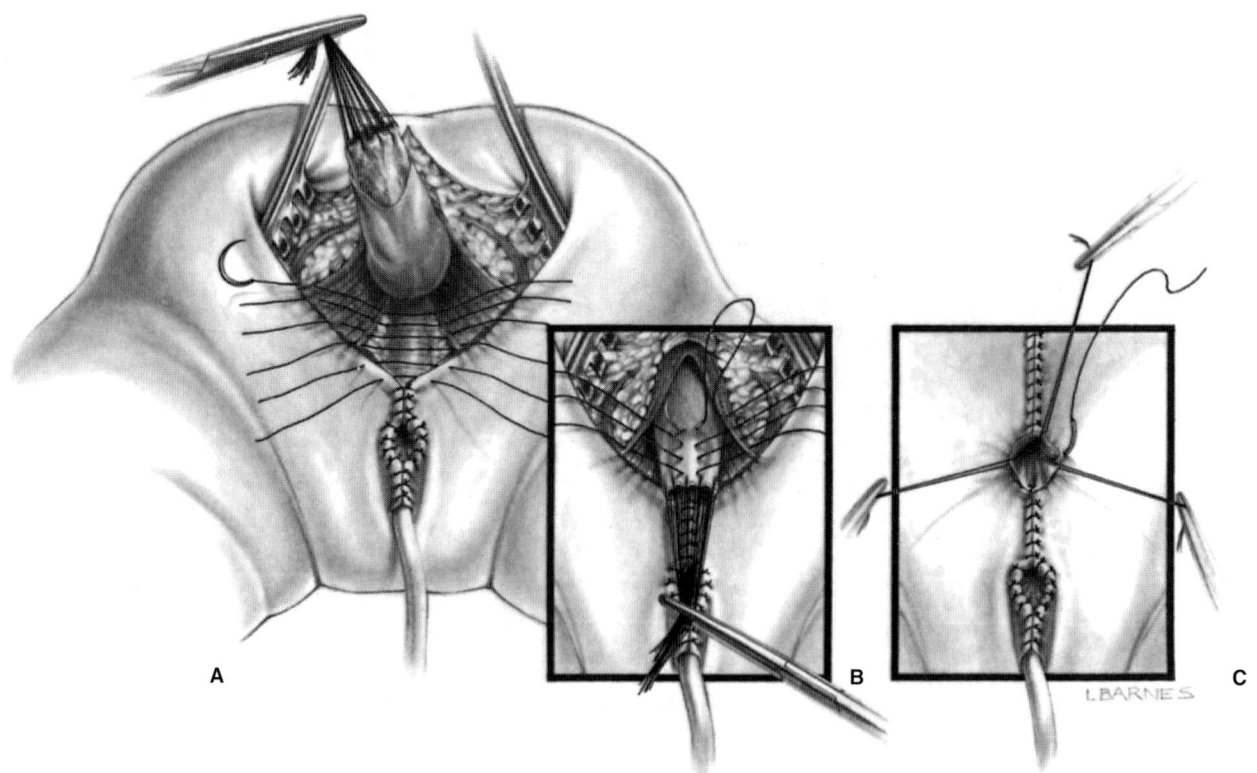

FIGURE 18-34. Repair of a persistent cloaca. **(A)** The urethra and the vagina have been reconstructed. Sutures are placed in the perineum. The anterior edge of the muscle complex is approximated anterior to the rectum. **(B)** The posterior edge of muscle complex is approximated behind the rectum. The sutures include the rectum. **(C)** Anoplasty.

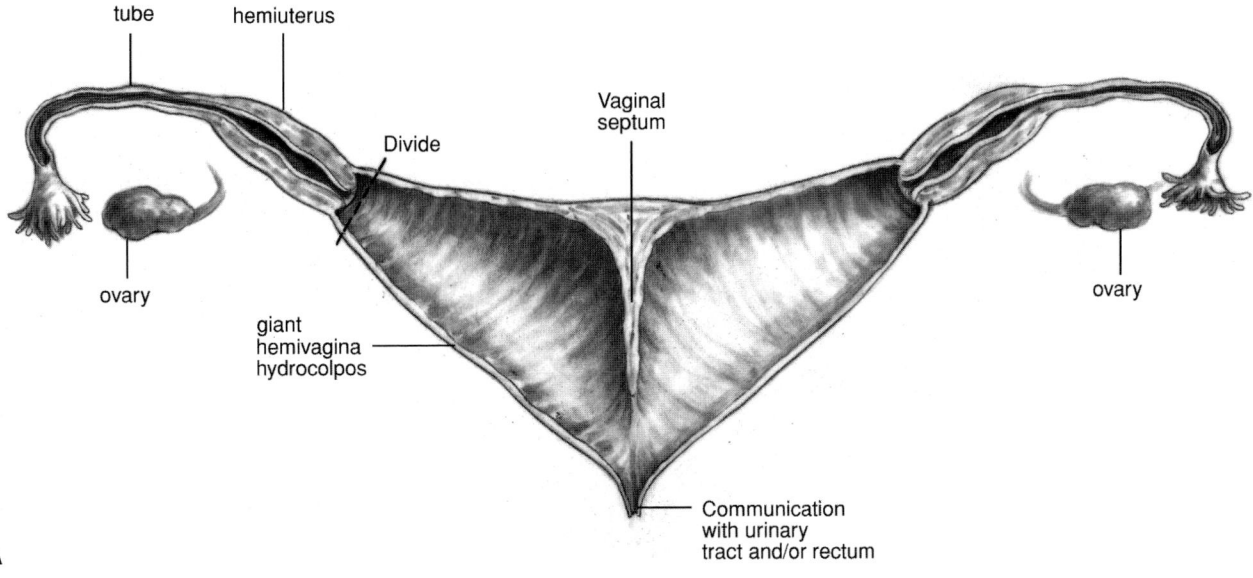

A

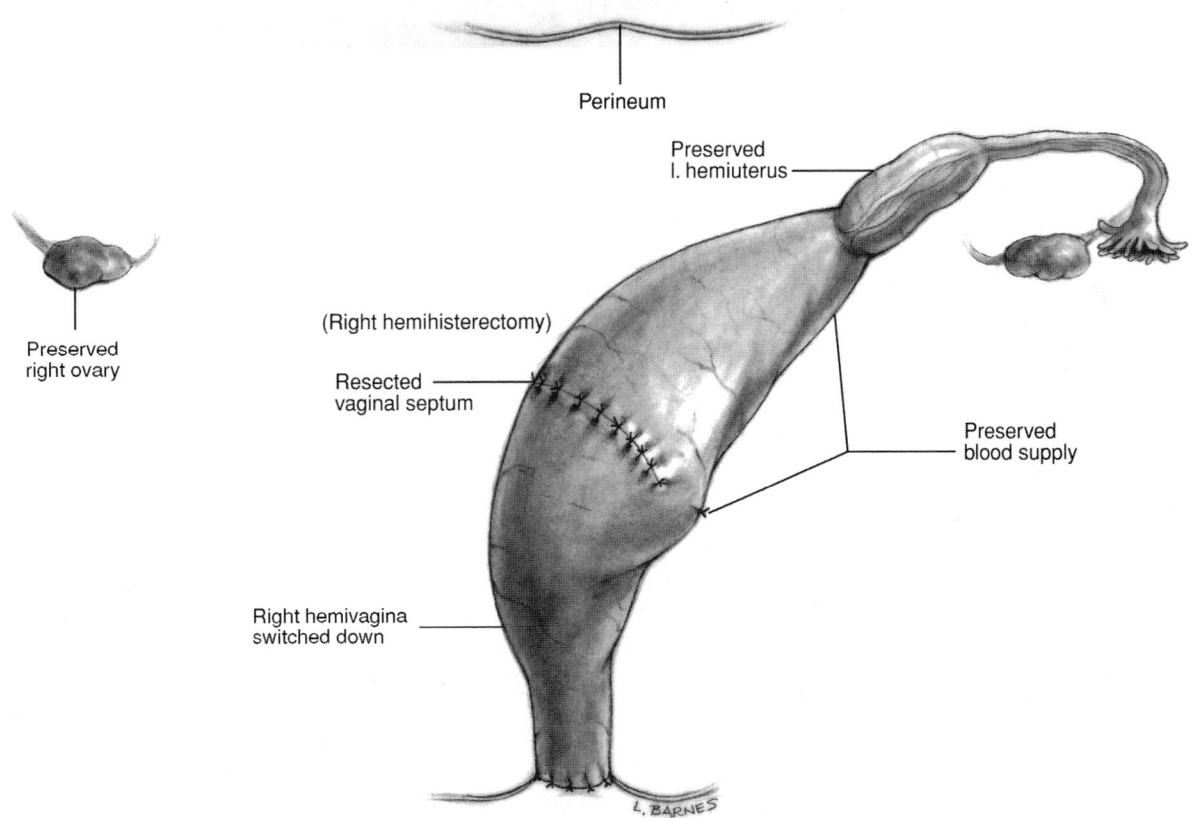

B

FIGURE 18-35. Persistent cloaca with hydrocolpos, hemivaginas, and hemiuterus. **(A)** Anatomic defect. **(B)** Vaginal reconstruction and switch maneuver.

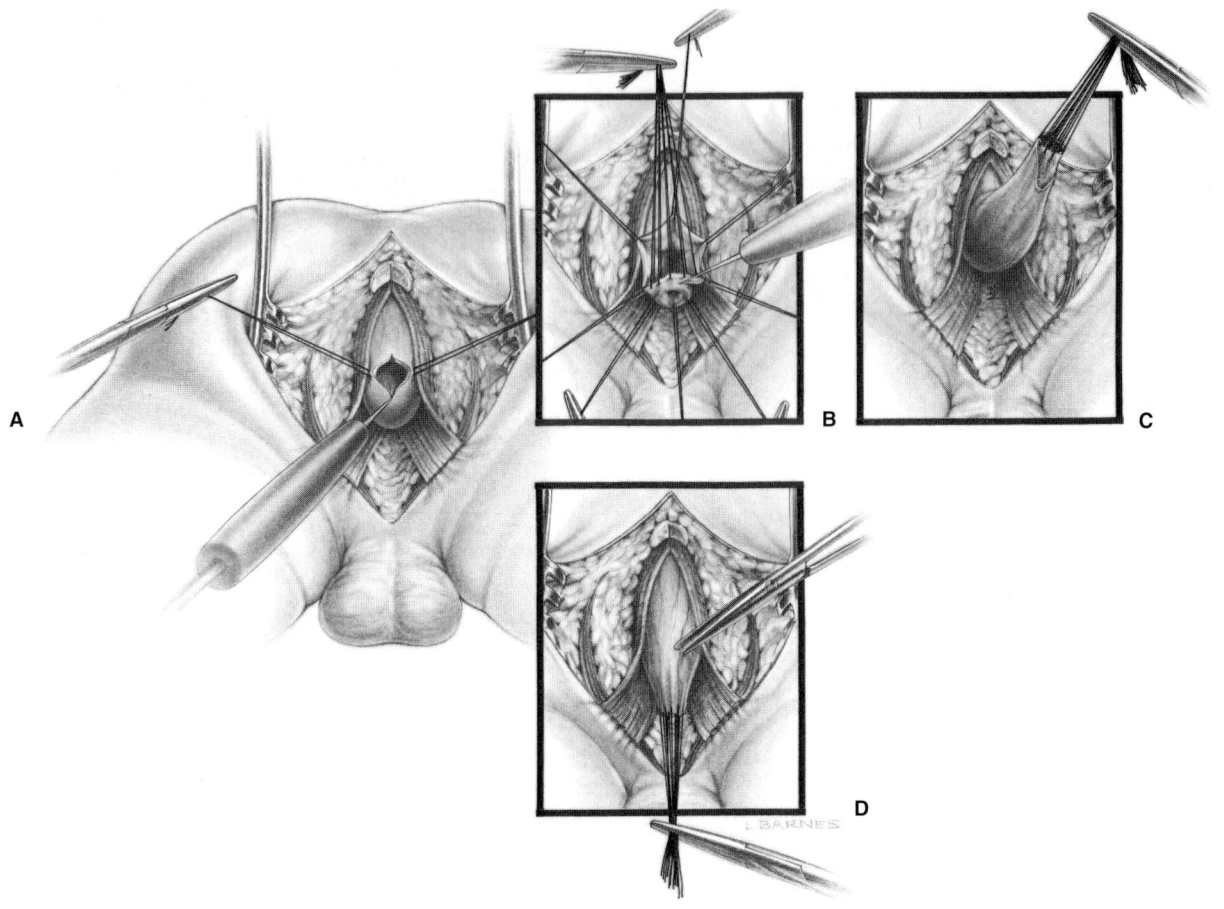

FIGURE 18-36. Repair of a rectourethral fistula. **(A)** The incision extends beyond the limits of the external sphincter. The levator ani muscle is divided, and the rectum is opened. **(B)** Separating the rectum from the urethra. **(C)** The rectum separated from urethra. **(D)** Dissection to gain rectal length.

must recognize that the anterior rectal wall is intimately attached to the posterior urethra. A Foley catheter must always be inserted before the operation.

Rectourethral Fistula

This is the rectal anomaly most commonly seen in male patients. The fistula may be located at the bulbar level (Figure 18-15*B*) or at the prostate (Figure 18-15*C*). Infants with a *prostatic fistula* require a colostomy before reconstruction (i.e., full PSARP). Some babies with *bulbar fistula* can be operated without a colostomy, provided that the surgeon has experience with this approach, the infant is healthy, and the surgeon is certain that the rectum is located below the coccyx as demonstrated by the presence of gas in a cross-table lateral x-ray film.

A Foley catheter is inserted, and a midsagittal incision is performed from the middle portion of the sacrum down to and through the center of the external sphincter. With rectoprostatic fistula, it may be possible to preserve the anterior limit of the external sphincter. However, in those patients with rectobulbar fistula, it is more conve-

nient to continue the incision slightly beyond the anterior limit of the external sphincter (Figure 18-36*A*). The parasagittal fibers of the external sphincter are separated, deepening the incision down to the levator ani and muscle complex. Once the muscle is incised, the rectum becomes evident, protruding through the defect in the levatores. The rectum is then secured with fine silk sutures and is opened in the midline with a needle-tip electrocautery device (Figure 18-36*A*). The fistula site in the lowest part of the rectum can now be identified. It is important to remember that rectum and urethra share a common wall immediately above the fistula site. The rectum is separated from the urethra by the use of rectal mucosal 6–0 silk traction sutures, in order to avoid injury to the prostate, seminal vesicles, and vas deferens. Approximately 2 cm above the fistula, both structures are complete, and the dissection can be expedited (Figure 18-36*B* and *C*). The urethral fistula is then closed with interrupted 5–0 long-term absorbable sutures. A careful rectal dissection is carried out, using traction on the silk sutures to gain rectal length for perineal reconstruction

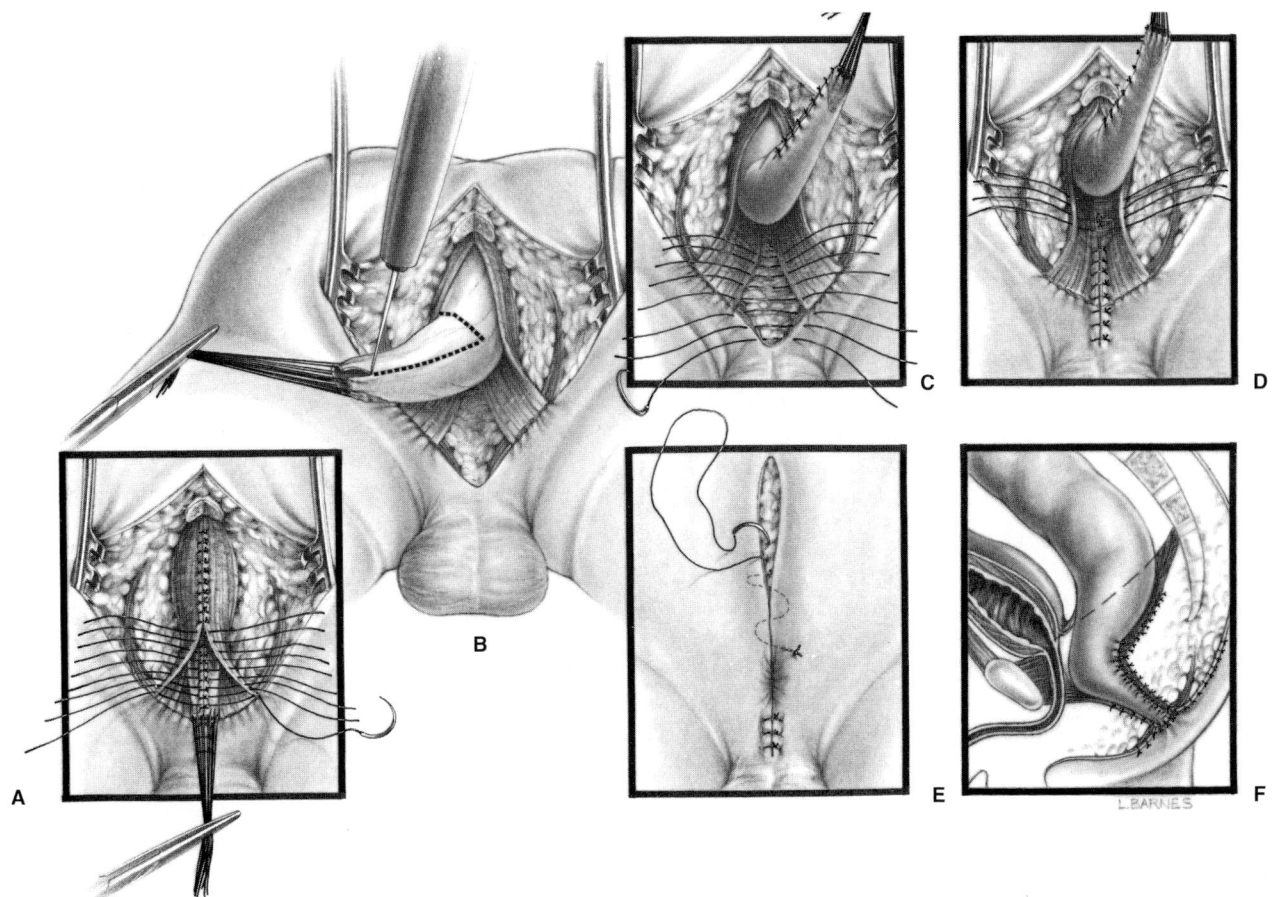

FIGURE 18-37. Repair of a rectourethral fistula. **(A)** Tapering of the rectum. **(B)** Repair of the perineal body. **(C)** Sutures placed at the levator ani edge. **(D)** Muscle complex sutures incorporating the rectal wall. **(E)** Closure of the wound. **(F)** Repaired malformation.

without tension (Figure 18-36*D*). Because the rectum is usually ectatic and distended, tailoring is often required to permit it to lie within the muscle structures (Figure 18-37*A*). The levator ani muscle must be constructed behind the rectum, with the distal bowel located within the confines of the muscle complex and external sphincter. The tapered rectum is reconstituted in two layers of interrupted 5–0 long-term absorbable sutures. The anterior extent of the muscle complex and external sphincter is reapproximated with like material (Figure 18-37*B*). Sutures are placed in both levator muscle edges (Figure 18-37*C*), and the rectum is then passed anteriorly. The remainder of the levator ani muscle is sutured together. The posterior edge of the muscle complex is then reapproximated behind the rectum with sutures that include the muscle complex and the rectal wall (Figure 18-37*D*). An anoplasty is performed as previously described, and the skin is closed with a subcuticular 5–0 nylon suture (Figure 18-37*E*). Figure 18-38*F* shows the completed repair with a tapered rectum. A urethral catheter is usually left in place for between 5 and 7 days.

Rectovesical Fistula

These malformations represent the extreme in the spectrum of male anorectal defects. The rectum usually opens at the level of the bladder neck (Figure 18-15*D*). The muscle complex and levator ani are frequently only rudimentary structures, and the space available between the urethra and the muscles is usually very narrow. Prognosis is not as satisfactory as that for rectourethral fistula. This malformation is often associated with varying degrees of sacral dysgenesis.

Because the rectum cannot be reached through a posterior sagittal approach, these children require a laparotomy or laparoscopy as well as a PSARP. The operation commences with a posterior sagittal incision, opening all layers down to the urethra. At this point, the presacral space is identified, following the path of the muscle complex.

The entire body from axilla to foot is prepared preoperatively, and the abdomen is entered either through a midline laparotomy or with a laparoscopic approach. The retroperitoneal space at the presacral location is identified, and the rectum is dissected below the peritoneal reflection to the level of the bladder fistula. This is usually located approximately 2 cm below the reflection. Because it is a very high malformation, there is no problem with a common wall between rectum and bladder. The dissection, therefore, is rather straightforward, but the surgeon must be careful to avoid injury to the vas deferens. This structure frequently courses very near the area. The fistula site is closed with interrupted absorbable sutures. The rectum is then mobilized so that it will reach the perineum. The rectum is then tapered if needed, taking as a reference the width of the presacral space. The tapered rectum is pulled to the perineum, bringing the rectum through the desired path. The operation is then completed with an anoplasty, and the abdomen is closed.[106,107]

Anorectal Agenesis Without Fistula

Surgical treatment for this defect in male and female patients is in accordance with the same principles. The rectum is usually found 2 cm deep to perineal skin. The technique is usually easier than that for patients with a fistula. Even in the absence of a communication between the rectum and vagina or urinary tract, one must be very cautious during the dissection of the anterior rectal wall in order to avoid injury to nearby structures. The approach is essentially the same as that previously described.

Rectal Atresia or Stenosis

The repair of these malformations in the male patient is the same as that for the female patient.

Secondary Operations for the Treatment of Fecal Incontinence

Infants who were born with an anorectal malformation and who had undergone a conventional procedure to repair the defect often continue to suffer from fecal incontinence (see Chapter 13). The posterior sagittal approach can be used to repair the muscle injured in prior operations as well as to relocate the rectum properly within the muscle structures.

The ideal candidate for this type of operation is an individual who has at least a favorable potential for continence: relatively normal sacrum and adequate residual muscle as evidenced by a good-looking perineum (e.g., midline raphe and anal dimple). Optimally, the patient should have clinical evidence of an inappropriately located rectum, with a well-preserved, intact external sphincter. The most common observations in these individuals are anteriorly or laterally mislocated anus and partial destruction of the lower portion of the levator ani muscle and anterior aspect of the muscle complex (Figure 18-38A). In those patients who had undergone an abdominoperineal procedure, considerable mesenteric fat may surround the rectum and interfere with muscle function. The anus, too, is usually surrounded by fat, because it lies in the anterior perineum. The rectum is usually identified very close to the posterior urethra, a finding reflecting the intention of the previous surgeon to preserve the puborectalis sling. The rectum can be seen to have been pulled in a straight manner, without following the normal curve of the muscle complex (Figure 18-38A).

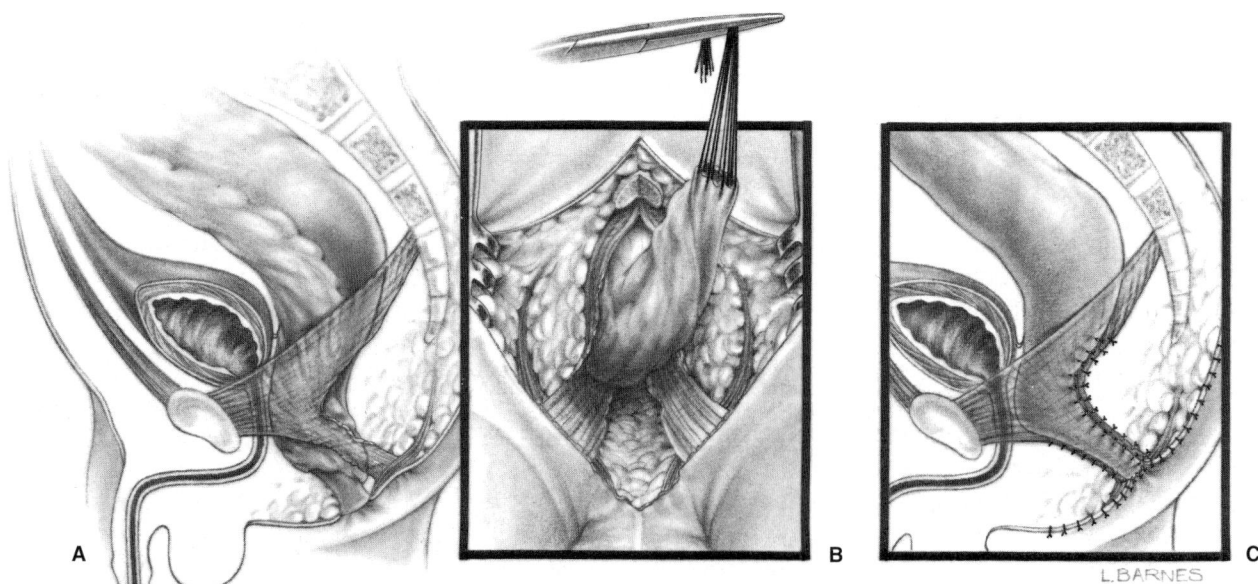

FIGURE 18-38. Secondary operation for the treatment of fecal incontinence. **(A)** Preoperative findings. The levator ani muscle and muscle complex are damaged. Mesenteric fat is surrounding the rectum. **(B)** Rectum dissected. **(C)** Operation completed. Mesenteric fat is removed, the rectum is relocated, and the muscle is reconstructed.

For several years, this reoperation had been preceded by a diverting colostomy, a procedure that seemed to limit the likelihood of postoperative septic problems. More recently, we have been performing this procedure without a protective stoma and have observed no infection in 50 consecutive children. The patients are admitted 2 days before the operation and are subjected to a strict program of total bowel irrigation with a balanced electrolyte solution (Golytely, 25 mL/kg of body weight/hour over 4 hours).[157] This regimen may be repeated up to three times, until one is certain that there has been adequate cleansing of the bowel. During the operation and for the following 2 days, the child receives intravenous triple antibiotics (i.e., ampicillin, gentamicin, clindamycin). In addition, no oral alimentation is permitted, but parenteral nutrition is maintained for 1 week.

The incision is carried out from the middle portion of the sacrum through the center of the external sphincter and around the anus. Multiple 5–0 silk sutures are placed at the mucocutaneous junction for traction. The incision is deepened, dividing the levator ani muscle and the muscle complex. Careful dissection is carried out as close as possible to the rectum, preserving all the striated muscle in the area. Figure 18-38*B* shows the rectum completely mobilized; the surrounding mesenteric fat can be easily appreciated. The repair consists of bringing together both anterior edges of the muscle complex and repairing the perineal body in a manner similar to that which has been previously described. The mesenteric fat is excised, with care taken to preserve adequate blood supply. Tapering of the rectum is rarely necessary, and the rectum is then relocated within the muscles. These are reconstructed as previously described (Figure 18-38*C*).

Because the urethra is not opened, a postoperative urinary catheter is not necessary. Anal dilatation is commenced 2 weeks following the operation.

Results of Treatment for Anorectal Malformations

It is not unexpected that results will vary depending on the potential for satisfactory repair that exists with each patient, because one is dealing with a spectrum of defects. For example, those individuals born with no sacrum or with more than three vertebrae missing will have very poor fecal and urinary continence. Infants with a normal sacrum and good muscle structures usually attain a degree of fecal and urinary control that allows them to enjoy a satisfactory quality of life. PSARP permits reconstruction of these defects by placing the rectum in the optimal position to achieve the best functional results. However, many patients continue to have bowel management problems, primarily because of sensory impairment and motility disturbance. These can contribute to varying degrees of soiling and of constipation.

Hassink and associates evaluated 58 *adult* patients who had undergone operative correction of high anorectal malformations.[59] Seven were found to have a permanent ileostomy or colostomy. Of the remaining 51, 61% were able to control defecation reasonably well without special aids, whereas 35% required enemas or bowel irrigations. Four percent were completely incontinent; 84% were satisfied with their level of cleanliness.

We have evaluated 1,500 patients on whom we have performed a primary reconstruction. Voluntary bowel movements were noted in 74.3% of the entire series. When separated by diagnosis, the percentages varied: 100% in patients with rectal atresia and perineal fistulas, 93% in those with vestibular fistula, 81% with rectourethral bulbar fistula, 71% with cloacas, 66% with rectourethral-prostatic fistula, and 16% in individuals with bladder neck fistula. Even though these patients had voluntary bowel movements, approximately 50% of them occasionally soiled their underwear. Of the entire series, 41% had voluntary bowel movements and never soiled their underwear, equivalent to the normal. Constipation was a problem in 43% of all children and was more frequently noted in those with simple defects. Urinary incontinence was present in 6% of male patients and 4% of female patients (excluding cloacal reconstructions). In those with cloacas, urinary incontinence was found in 19% of girls having a common channel shorter than 3 cm and in 69% of those who had longer common channels.[112] Sexual function and childbearing capacity have not been evaluated because these patients are still quite young.

Secondary operations for the treatment of fecal incontinence in patients with a normal sacrum revealed some improvement in approximately 80%. The same procedure, however, performed in individuals with an abnormal sacrum, was found to achieve significant improvement in only 20%, and at least 50% failed to benefit in this last group.

Complications

Wound infections were seen in four patients in whom the primary repair was accomplished without a protective colostomy or with a loop colostomy. Anorectal stricture was noted in three children who suffered devascularization injury in an attempt to gain rectal length. If anal dilatation is not performed properly, a ringlike stricture may develop at the mucocutaneous junction. It is, therefore, important to emphasize that anal dilatation be undertaken twice a day. The size of the dilator must be increased each week until normal caliber is achieved. At that point, the colostomy is closed, but dilatation must continue for 6 months, the required duration for complete healing. Once-weekly dilatation may cause recurrent laceration with resultant fibrosis.

When one performs the posterior sagittal approach in teenagers, with the patient in the prone position and the pelvis elevated, transient femoral nerve pressure palsy may result. This is an avoidable complication; padding of the vulnerable areas must be accomplished before the operation begins. Devascularization and retraction of the vagina during the repair of a persistent cloaca occurred in 3% of the patients; persistent urethrovaginal fistula has also been observed in 10% of the cases. The maneuver called "total urogenital mobilization" has eliminated these last two complications. Ectopic ureters opening into the posterior urethra or vas deferens may be injured during a posterior sagittal approach when one attempts to identify a very high rectum. A distal colostogram before performing the definitive repair will show the rectum opening at the bladder neck site. In this situation, a laparotomy is required, in addition to that of the posterior sagittal approach; the rectum should not be sought through the perineal incision.

Medical Management of Fecal Incontinence

Patients who suffer fecal incontinence as a consequence of either poor surgical technique or an inadequate sacrum and sphincter muscle can be improved by a number of medical regimens. Management must be individualized, because each patient may have a different problem. For example, some suffer primarily a bowel motility disturbance, as seen by severe constipation and overflow incontinence (i.e., encopresis). Judicious use of laxatives may be all that is required. However, sometimes the resultant loose stool may exacerbate incontinence difficulties. Under these circumstances, the use of a bisacodyl suppository is suggested, administered once daily after a main meal. In children younger than 8 years, the suppository should be divided in half. If abdominal pain or perianal irritation ensues, the medication must be discontinued. If these measures fail, a phosphate enema (Fleet) will usually keep the child clean for 24 hours, but it is important to be certain that the enema is instilled sufficiently high in the rectum to achieve adequate evacuation. A convenient method of obtaining this is to elevate the pelvis. Various methods of administering enemas are illustrated in Figure 18-39. Sometimes, the use of a rubber tube to give the enema achieves better rectosigmoid emptying.[111]

Some patients have a rather hyperactive colon or suffer from diarrhea and malabsorption. Others have lost part of their colon during prior operations. In such cases, a constipating diet and/or the use of loperamide, as well as the addition of phosphate enemas will usually keep them dry. Special dietary restrictions may include elimination of fried foods and dairy products, as well as limitation of the amount of fat consumed.[111]

The continued application of such bowel management programs for several months or even years may, through bowel regulation, occasionally permit the medication and enemas to be reduced or even eliminated (see Chapter 13). Some individuals, however, who receive enemas over a

long period of time express dissatisfaction with the logistical problem of administration. For these patients, one may consider offering a relatively new modality of management, creation of a continent appendicostomy (115 personal cases) or so-called Malone's procedure (see Chapter 13).[51,88] The appendix is exteriorized through the abdominal wall, and a one-way valve mechanism is created between the cecum and the appendix (a form of plication of the cecum around the appendix). The patient can then administer an enema through a narrow tube (no. 8 feeding tube) in an antegrade manner. Malone and colleagues proposed the sectioning of the appendix at its base and the subsequent reimplantation of it with an antireflux mechanism in the wall of the cecum.[88] In addition, the appendix is exteriorized through the abdominal wall in the right lower quadrant. We prefer to perform a plication of the cecum around the base of the appendix without sectioning it and to exteriorize the appendix through the umbilicus, thereby producing a more cosmetic result. Our patients are extremely satisfied with this procedure as an alternative to enema administration.[83]

NECROTIZING ENTEROCOLITIS

NEC is a serious intestinal disorder that affects predominantly premature infants.[2,55] There are approximately 24,000 cases per year in the United States, with a reported mortality varying between 10% and 50%.[68] Intestinal ischemia with or without necrosis seems to be the common denominator in all patients.

Progress in neonatal care since the mid-1970s years has created an increasing population of low-birth-weight neonatal survivors at risk for developing NEC. As many as 8% of preterm infants with birth weights of 750 to 1,500 g develop the condition, whereas fewer than 10% are full-term.[20,114] It has also been established that this condition occurs in episodic epidemics, usually after 10 days of life.[15,125]

Pathogenesis

The precise pathogenesis of this disease is unknown. However, the predisposing factors are well established and include prematurity, hyaline membrane disease, administration of synthetic hyperosmolar formulas, cardiac anomalies, hypovolemia, and sepsis.[75] Other less commonly associated factors are hypothermia, the use of umbilical catheters, and a history of maternal cocaine abuse.[34,159] Hyaline membrane disease, cardiac anomalies, hypovolemia, and hypotension are known to cause bowel ischemia. In addition, spasm of the mesenteric vessels, reminiscent of the defensive "diving reflex" seen in amphibious animals and associated with prematurity, has been postulated as a contributing factor for the development of bowel ischemia. Ischemic bowel allows enteric bacteria to invade

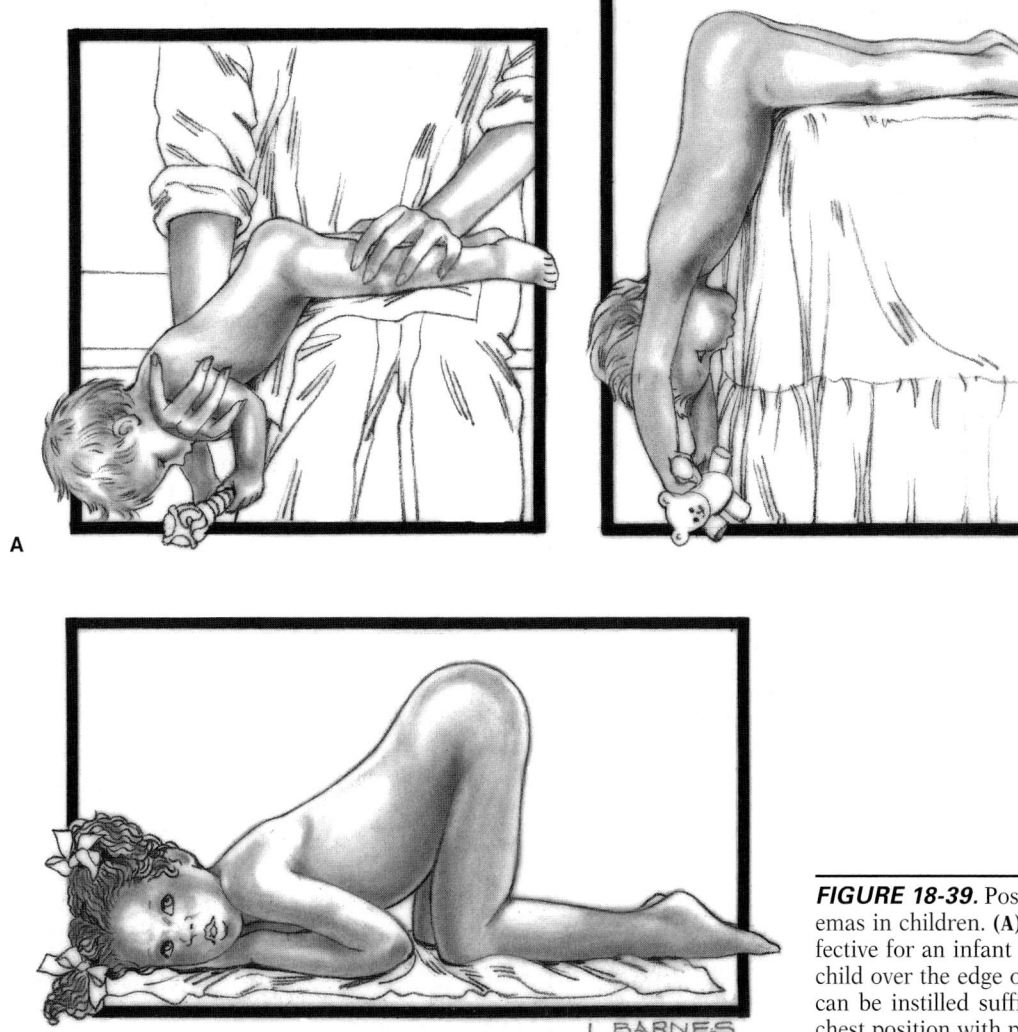

FIGURE 18-39. Positions for administrating enemas in children. **(A)** The lap position is very effective for an infant or small child. **(B)** With the child over the edge of a bed, the enema solution can be instilled sufficiently high. **(C)** The knee-chest position with pelvic tilt facilitates administration and adequate evacuation.

the wall and eventually to reach the portal circulation, a process known as bacterial translocation.[29]

Another factor is the failure to breast-feed. Lack of the mother's milk prevents the immature baby from creating an efficient gut barrier. Breast milk normally provides not only secretory immunoglobulin A, but also oligosaccharide, lactoferrin, lysozyme, epidermal growth factor, and immune cells.[48,100] The importance of breast milk is also supported by the fact that its administration frequently prevents NEC from developing.[9,29] Formula-fed babies suffer NEC six times more frequently than breast-fed newborns.[9,69]

Other etiologic agents are antibiotics. Broad-spectrum antibiotics, given to premature babies for a variety of indications, may alter the infant's gut flora, thereby contributing to colonization and overgrowth of potentially pathogenic organisms.[29] However, the specific offending bacterium remains elusive. Positive blood and stool cultures commonly grow *Klebsiella pneumonia, Escherichia coli, E. cloacae, Pseudomonas aeruginosa, Staphylococcus aureus* and *S. epidermidis,* and *Clostridium perfringens.*[162] Bacterial translocation most likely triggers an inflammatory cascade, with release of cellular mediators of injury that cause further bowel damage and severe systemic manifestations. In support of this scenario are the findings of an increased level of platelet-activating factor, tumor necrosis factor, and interleukin-6, in the serum of premature babies with NEC.[19,58]

There is no question that bacteria play a prominent role in the pathogenesis of this disease.[13] What remains controversial, however, is the sequence of events that eventually produces bowel necrosis, perforation, and generalized sepsis.

Ischemic and/or necrotic lesions most frequently occur in the terminal ileum, cecum, and ascending colon. Affected portions of bowel can be isolated, scattered, or generalized to the entire intestine (NEC totalis). Intraluminal bowel gas infiltrates the intestinal wall, appearing radiologically as intestinal pneumatosis. The gas frequently reaches the portal circulation, indicating a more serious and aggressive evolution.

Clinical Manifestations

Symptoms of NEC most frequently appear in relation to the onset of feeding. This commonly occurs after 10 days of life, generally after the baby has received an artificial formula. Initial, albeit subtle manifestations include increased gastric residual volumes, abdominal distension, and lethargy. More specific signs are blood-streaked stools and abdominal tenderness. The disease may then follow a variable clinical course depending on the efficiency of the initial medical management and other unknown factors. The baby may recover after effective treatment or may rapidly deteriorate. In the latter circumstance, the abdomen becomes markedly distended and may interfere with respiration. The abdominal wall is noted to be erythematous, and the presence of a palpable mass reflects the presence of inflamed and/or perforated matted loops of bowel. Manifestations of a systemic septic process become evident, including temperature instability, bradycardia, apnea, hypoglycemia, shock, and cyanosis.[115] The platelet and white blood cell counts are persistently low, and severe metabolic acidosis and hypoxia are the rule.

Radiologic Studies

Radiologic evaluation provides variable images, depending on the stage of the disease. Initial plain and decubitus films may show signs of a nonspecific ileus. Subsequently, intestinal and/or portal pneumatosis appears. Rapid changes in the radiologic images are not uncommonly observed as the disease evolves. Signs of bowel edema and increased peritoneal fluid, as evidenced by a separation of loops of bowel, frequently appear concomitant with the administration of intravenous fluids for resuscitative purposes. Free intraperitoneal gas is obviously a sign of bowel perforation (Figure 18-40). However, sometimes the bowel perforates, and there is no free air seen. Under such circumstances, more subtle radiologic findings may be appreciated: a persistently distended loop of bowel and bubbles of gas apparently outside of the intestinal lumen.

Treatment

NEC is basically a medical management condition. However, intervention by the surgeon is required if medical treatment fails. Nonoperative management must always be attempted in order to try to reverse the natural evolution of the disease or to stabilize and prepare the patient for surgery. The gastrointestinal tract is decompressed with a nasogastric tube. Reliable venous access is promptly established, and aggressive fluid resuscitation is started. Adequate oxygenation is mandatory, with endotracheal intubation and ventilatory assistance being fundamental. Broad-spectrum antibiotics are instituted initially, with change in antibiotic therapy guided by subsequent specific bacteriologic findings. The gastrointestinal tract must remain at rest, and, therefore, parenteral nutrition is mandatory. The response to medical treatment is clinically evaluated radiologically (every 4 to 8 hours) and with laboratory tests (platelet, white cell count, and arterial gases).

Ideally, surgical treatment should be initiated when the patient suffers full-thickness bowel necrosis that has not yet perforated. Bowel resection with anastomosis or diversion, accompanied by vigorous, supportive medical care inevitably will be associated with optimal operative results. Although the finding of perforated bowel means that the operation was indeed indicated, it may also reflect an unwarranted delay. Conversely, surgical exploration of a patient who suffers only from bowel dilatation or patches of ischemia without necrosis cannot be considered ameliorative. Unfortunately, specific symptoms and signs of bowel necrosis (without perforation) do not exist, and, therefore, it is not unusual for a surgeon to explore the abdomen and find no necrosis.

An absolute surgical indication is the presence of free intraperitoneal gas. A palpable mass with local tenderness and abdominal discoloration is also highly suggestive of bowel necrosis and sealed perforation (Figure 18-41). Clinical deterioration is a somewhat controversial indication for surgery because some patients rapidly fail and even die without necessarily suffering bowel necrosis. Therefore, if one observes that the patient is rapidly deteriorating, the surgeon is obligated to explore the ab-

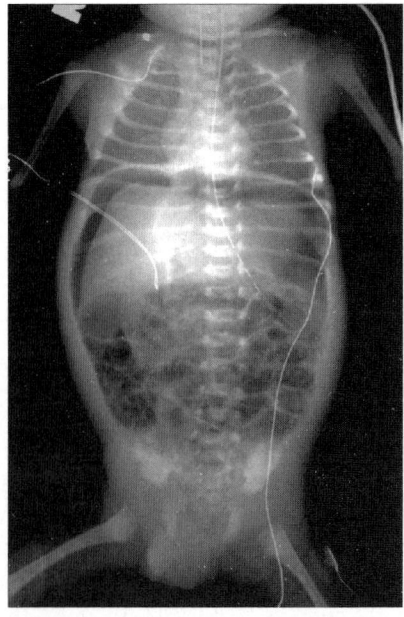

FIGURE 18-40. Free intraabdominal air in a baby with necrotizing enterocolitis and perforation.

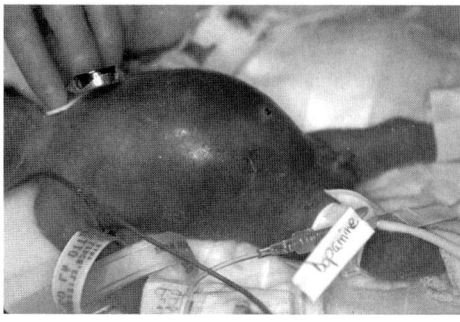

FIGURE 18-41. Abdominal wall discoloration in an infant with necrotizing enterocolitis as a consequence of perforation with bowel necrosis.

domen, because the consequences of not operating for bowel necrosis are far more serious than performing a laparotomy in an infant who does not have necrosis. A lack of clinical improvement and persistent radiologic signs of bowel distension during a 24-hour period are also considered indications for surgery.

Operative Treatment

The objectives of surgery are to resect obvious necrotic or perforated bowel and to preserve as much intestine as possible, including questionably necrotic areas. Several presentations of NEC are depicted in the operative photographs (Figure 18-42). Traditionally, most surgeons create one or more stomas after bowel resection. The reluc-

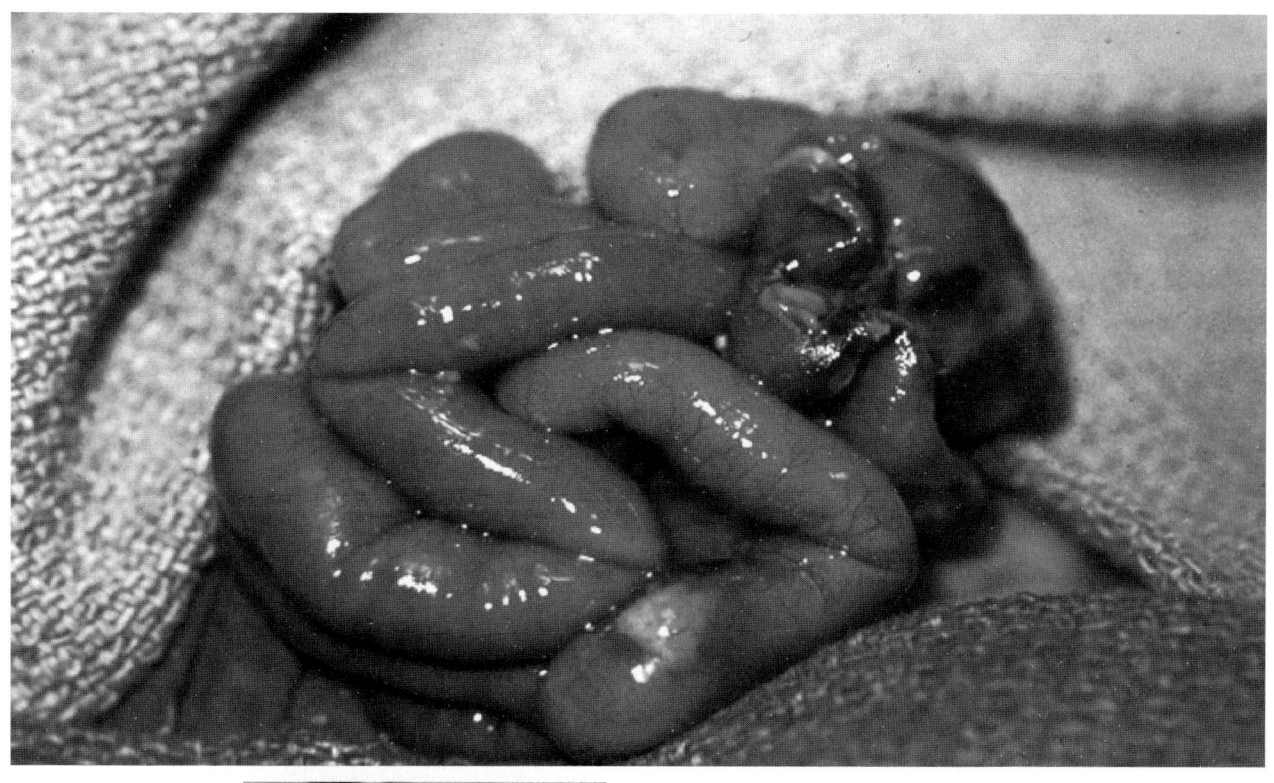

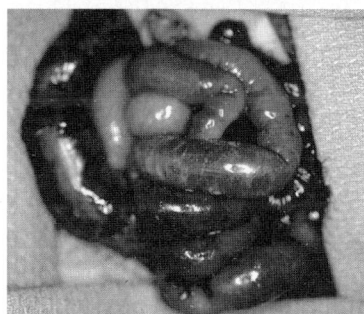
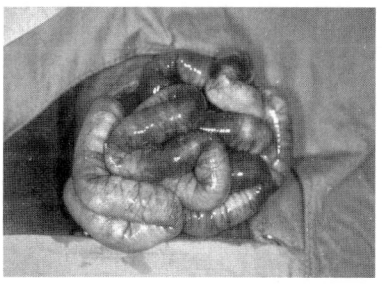

FIGURE 18-42. Operative presentations of necrotizing enterocolitis. **(A)** Mild patchy ischemic changes. **(B)** Severe ischemia with grossly gangrenous bowel and with some spared small intestine. **(C)** Total bowel necrosis.

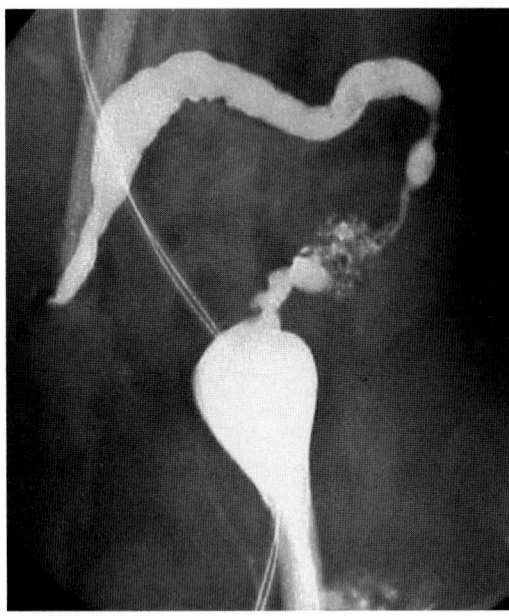

FIGURE 18-43. Colonic stricture following medical treatment for necrotizing enterocolitis.

tance to perform intestinal anastomoses is based on the fact that there is the potential for residual ischemic bowel. However, some advocate primary anastomosis, provided the remaining intestine exhibits good perfusion.[72,147] This avoids the morbidity related to creation of a stoma and the requirement for another operation. In such a difficult management situation, there is no substitute for good surgical judgment.

The finding of total bowel necrosis is tragic. In such instances, however, unexpectedly good results may be achieved by closing the abdomen, continuing medical management, and performing a "second-look" surgical exploration 48 hours later in the hope of finding some viable bowel. This may avoid a massive bowel resection with the ultimate result of a short bowel syndrome.

Bedside peritoneal drainage with local anesthesia has been advocated for the management of very small (micropremies, less than 1,000 g) and extremely ill infants who suffer from bowel perforation and severe abdominal distension that compromises ventilation.[38] Often, these babies are hemodynamically unstable and are poor candidates for a formal laparotomy. The abdominal cavity is decompressed with the insertion of a Penrose drain. This treatment improves ventilation and helps to stabilize the patient until such time as a formal laparotomy can be performed. Complete recovery without further surgery has been reported in up to 40% of these infants.[38]

Stomal closure can be performed several weeks later, provided the patient is stable and is growing. Injection of contrast material through the distal limb of the diversion is required before closure in order to rule out the presence of colonic strictures (Figure 18-43). These represent

scarring of intestine that suffered partial, usually circumferential necrosis without perforation. The incidence of stricture formation is approximately 10%.[134]

Survival in newborns suffering from NEC has been improving during recent years, with reports as high as 72.5% to 80%.[52,122]

REFERENCES

1. Aegineta P. On the imperforate anus. In: Adams F, trans. *The seven books*, book VI, section LXXXI. London: Syndenham Society, 1844:405.
2. Albanese CT, Rowe M. Necrotizing enterocolitis. *Semin Pediatr Surg* 1995;4:200–206.
3. Amussat JZ. Gustiure d'une operation d'anus artifical practiqué avec succàs par un nouveau procédé. *Gaz Med Paris* 1835;3:735.
4. Angrist M. Genomic structure of the gene for the SH2 and pleckstrin homology domain-containing protein GRB10 and evaluation of its role in Hirschsprung's disease. *Oncogene* 1998;17:3065.
5. Angrist M, Bolk S, Halushka M, et al. Germline mutations in glial cell line–derived neurotrophic factor (GDNF) and RET in a Hirschsprung disease patient. *Nat Genet* 1996; 14:341.
6. Angrist M, Bolk S, Thiel B, et al. Mutation analysis of the RET receptor tyrosine kinase in Hirschsprung disease. *Hum Mol Genet* 1995;4:821.
7. Angrist M, Jing S, Bolk S, et al. Human GFRAI: cloning, mapping, genomic structure, and evaluation as a candidate gene for Hirschsprung disease susceptibility. *Genomics* 1998;48:354.
8. Badner JA, Sieber WK, Garver KL, et al. A genetic study of Hirschsprung disease. *Am J Hum Genet* 1990;46:568.
9. Barlow B, Santulli TV, Heird WC, et al. An experimental study of neonatal enterocolitis: the importance of breast milk. *J Pediatr Surg* 1974;9:587–595.
10. Bealer JF,Natuzzi ES, Buscher C, et al. Nitric oxide synthase is deficient in the aganglionic colon of patients with Hirschsprung's disease. *Pediatrics* 1994;93:647–651.
11. Belman AB, King LR. Urinary tract abnormalities associated with imperforate anus. *J Urol* 1972;108:823.
12. Black CT, Sherman JO. The association of low imperforate anus and Down's syndrome. *J Pediatr Surg* 1989;24:92.
13. Blakely JL, Lubitz L, Campbell NT, et al. Enteric colonization in sporadic neonatal necrotizing enterocolitis. *J Pediatr Gastroenterol Nutr* 1985;4:591–595.
14. Boley SJ. A new modification of the surgical treatment of Hirschsprung's disease. *Surgery* 1964;56:1015.
15. Book LS, Overall JC, Herbst JJ, et al. Clustering of necrotizing enterocolitis: interruption by infection-control methods. *N Engl J Med* 1977;297:984–986.
16. Briner J, Oswald H, Hirsig J, et al. Neuronal intestinal dysplasia: clinical and histochemical findings and its association with Hirschsprung's disease. *Z Kinderschir* 1986;41: 282.
17. Brenner EC. Congenital defects of the anus and rectum. *Surg Gynecol Obstet* 1915;20:579.
18. Bussman H, Roth H, Nutzenadel W. Variabilitat Klinischer Symptome bei neuronaler intestinaler Dysplasie. *Monatschr Kinderheilk* 1990;138:284.
19. Caplan MS, Sun X-M, Hsueh W, et al. Role of platelet activating factor and tumor necrosis factor-alpha in neonatal necrotizing enterocolitis. *J Pediatr* 1990;116:960.
20. Caplan MS, Jilling T. New concepts in necrotizing enterocolitis. *Curr Opin Pediatr* 2001;13:111.
21. Carcassone M, Morisson LG, Letourneau JN. Primary corrective operation without decompression in infants less than three months of age with Hirschsprung's disease. *J Pediatr Surg* 1982;17:241.
22. Cass DT. Neonatal one-stage repair of Hirschsprung's disease. *Pediatr Surg Int* 1990;5:341.

23. Chassaignac M. Présentation de malades. *Bull Soc Chir* 1856;Feb. 20:410.
24. Cilley RE, Statter MB, Hirschl RB, et al. Definitive treatment of Hirschsprung's disease in the newborn with a one-stage procedure. *Surgery* 1994;115:551.
25. Csury L, Peña A. Intestinal neuronal dysplasia: myth or reality? *Pediatr Surg Int* 1995;10:441.
26. Curran TJ, Raffensperger JG. The feasibility of laparoscopic Swenson pull-through. *J Pediatr Surg* 1994;29:1273.
27. Davidson M. Alimentary canal. In: Code CF, Werner H, eds. *Handbook of physiology,* 5th ed. Baltimore: Williams & Wilkins, 1970:2783.
28. de la Torre L, Ortega J. Transanal endorectal pullthrough for Hirschsrpung's disease. *J Pediatr Surg* 1998;33:1283.
29. DeLemos, RA, Rogers JH, McLaughlin GW. Experimental production of necrotizing enterocolitis in newborn goats. *Pediatr Res* 1974;8:380.
30. deVries P, Peña A. Posterior sagittal anorectoplasty. *J Pediatr Surg* 1982;17:638.
31. Dobbins WO, Bill AH. Diagnosis of Hirschsprung's disease excluded by rectal suction biopsy. *N Engl J Med* 1965; 272:990.
32. Dochetry JG, Zaki A, Coutts JAP, et al. Meconium ileus: a review: 1972–1990. *Br J Surg* 1992;79:571.
33. Donaldson JS, Black CT, Reynolds M, et al. Ultrasound of the distal pouch in infants with imperforate anus. *J Pediatr Surg* 1989;24:465.
34. Downing GJ, Horner SR, Kilbride HW, et al. Characteristics of perinatal cocaine-exposed infants with necrotizing enterocolitis. *Am J Dis Child* 1991;145:26.
35. Duhamel B. Retrorectal and transanal pull-through procedure for the treatment of Hirschsprung's disease. *Dis Colon Rectum* 1964;7:455.
36. Eek S, Knutrud O. Megacolon congenitum Hirschsprung. *J Oslo City Hosp* 1962;12:245.
37. Ehrenpreis T. *Hirschsprung's disease: incidence.* Chicago: Year Book, 1970.
38. Ein SH, Shandling B, Wesson D, et al. A 13 year experience with peritoneal drainage under local anesthesia for necrotizing enterocolitis perforation. *J Pediatr Surg* 1990;25: 1034.
39. Elema JJ, deVries JA, Vos LJ. Intensity and proximal extension of acetylcholinesterase activity in the mucosa of the rectosigmoid in Hirschsprung's disease. *J Pediatr Surg* 1973;8:361.
40. Fadda B, Maier W, Meier-Ruge W, et al. Neuronal intestinal dysplasia: a critical 10 year analysis of clinical and biopsy results. *Z Kinderchir* 1983;38:305.
41. Fadda B, Pistor G, Meier-Ruge W, et al. Symptoms, diagnosis, and therapy of neuronal intestinal dysplasia masked by Hirschsprung's disease: report of 24 cases. *Pediatr Surg Int* 1987;2:76.
42. Fahr K, Nutzenadel W. Die neuronale Kolodysplasie. *Therapiewochenschr* 1979;29:8717.
43. Fewtrell MS, Tam PK, Thomson AH, et al. Hirschsprung's disease associated with a deletion of chromosome 10 (q11 2q21 2): a further link with the neurocristopathies? *J Med Genet* 1994;31:325.
44. Fortuna RS, Weber TR, Tracy TF Jr, et al. Critical analysis of the operative treatment of Hirschsprung's disease. *Arch Surg* 1996;131:520.
45. Fuxe K, Jonsson G. The histochemical fluorescence method for the demonstration of catecholamines: theory, practice and application. *J Histochem Cytochem* 1973;21: 293.
46. Georgeson KE, Cohen RD, Hebra A, et al. Primary laparoscopic assisted endorectal colon pullthrough for Hirschsprung's disease: a new gold standard. *Ann Surg* 1999;229:678.
47. Georgeson KE, Fuenfer MM, Hardin WD. Primary laparoscopic pullthrough for Hirschsprung's disease in infants and children. *J Pediatr Surg* 1995;30:1017.
48. Goldman AS, Thorpe LW, Goldblum RM, et al. Anti-inflammatory properties of human milk. *Acta Pediatr Scand* 1986;75:689.
49. Goon HK. Repair of anorectal anomalies in the neonatal period. *Pediatr Surg Int* 1990;5:246.
50. Gravier L, Sieber WK. Hirschsprung's disease and mongolism. *Surgery* 1966;60:458.
51. Griffith DM, Malone PS. The Malone antegrade continence enema (MACE). *J Pediatr Surg* 1995;30:68.
52. Grosfeld JL, Cheu H, Schlatter M, et al. Changing trends in necrotizing enterocolitis (NEC): experience with 302 cases in two decades. *Ann Surg* 1991;214:300.
53. Gross GW, Wolfson PJ, Peña A. Augmented-pressure colostogram in imperforate anus with fistula. *Radiology* 1991; 21:560.
54. Gulotta F, Straaten G. Hirschsprung's disease combined with aganglionosis and so-called neuronal colonic dysplasia (dysganglionosis colica). *Z Kinderchir* 1977;20:42.
55. Guthrie SO, Gordon PV, Thomas V, et al. Necrotizing enterocolitis among neonates in the United States. *J Perinatol* 2003;23:278.
56. Hadra. *Berlin Klin Wochenschr* 1886:7.
57. Levitt MA, Patel M, Rodriguez G, et al. The tethered spinal cord in patients with anorectal malformations. *J Pediatr Surg* 1997;32:462.
58. Harris HC, Costarino AT Jr, Sullivan JS, et al. Cytokine elevations in critically ill infants with sepsis and necrotizing enterocolitis. *J Pediatr* 1994;124:105.
59. Hassink EA, Rieu PN, Severijnen RS, et al. Are adults content or continent after repair for high anal atresia? A long-term follow-up study in patients 18 years of age and older. *Ann Surg* 1993;218:196.
60. Hendren WH. Repair of cloacal anomalies: current techniques. *J Pediatr Surg* 1986;21:1159.
61. Hiatt RB. A further description of the pathologic physiology of congenital megacolon and the results of surgical treatment. *Pediatrics* 1958;21:825.
62. Hirschsprung H. Stuhltrúgheit Neugeboreher in Folge von Dilatation und Hypertrophie des Colons. *Jahrb Kinderhkd* 1888;27:1.
63. Holschneider AM. Particular forms of Hirschsprung's disease. In: Holschneider A, ed. *Hirschsprung's disease.* Stuttgart: Hippokrates-Verlag, 1982:133.
64. Holschneider AM, ed. *Hirschsprung's disease.* Stuttgart: Hippokrates-Verlag, 1982.
65. Hong AR, Rosen N, Acuna MF, et al. Urologic injuries associated with the repair of anorectal malformations in male patients. *J Pediatr Surg* 2002;37:339.
66. Howard ER. Hirschsprung's disease: a review of the morphology and physiology. *Postgrad Med J* 1972;48:471.
67. Howard ER. Histochemistry in the diagnosis and investigation of congenital aganglionosis (Hirschsprung's disease). *Am Surg* 1973;39:602.
68. Jason JM. Infectious disease-related deaths of low birth weight infants, United States, 1968 to 1982. *Pediatrics* 1989; 84:296.
69. Jucas A, Cole TJ. Breast milk and neonatal necrotizing enterocolitis. *Lancet* 1990;336:1519.
70. Kessler S, Campbell J. Neuronal colonic dysplasia associated with short-segment Hirschsprung's disease. *Arch Pathol Lab Med* 1985;109:532.
71. Kiesewetter WB, Sukarochana K, Sieber WK. The frequency of aganglionosis. *Surgery* 1965;58:877.
72. Kiesewetter WB, Taghizadeh F, Bower RJ. Necrotizing enterocolitis: is there a place for resection and primary anastomosis? *J Pediatr Surg* 1979;14:360.
73. Kimura K, Nishij MAE, Muraji T, et al. A new surgical approach to extensive aganglionosis. *J Pediatr Surg* 1981; 16: 840.
74. Kleinhaus S, Boley SJ, Sheraw M, et al. Hirschsprung's disease: a survey of the members of the Surgical Section of the American Academy of Pediatrics. *J Pediatr Surg* 1979;14:588.
75. Kliegman RM. Neonatal necrotizing enterocolitis: implications for an infectious disease. *Pediatr Clin North Am* 1979;26:327.
76. Krebs C, Silva MC, Parra MA. Anorectal electromanometry in the diagnosis of neuronal intestinal dysplasia in childhood. *Eur J Pediatr Surg* 1991;1:40.

77. Ladd WE, Gross RE. Congenital malformations of anus and rectum: report of 162 cases. *Am J Surg* 1934;23:167.

78. Langer JC, Durrant AC, de la Torre L, et al. One-stage transanal Soave pullthrough for Hirschsprung's disease: a multicenter experience with 141 children. *Ann Surg* 2003;238:569.

79. Langer JC, Minkes RK, Mazziott MV, et al. Transanal one stage Soave procedure for infants with Hirschsprung's disease. *J Pediatr Surg* 1999;34:148.

80. Lassman G, Wurnig P. Local hypertrophy of the ganglion cells in the submucosa of the oral end of the aganglionic segment in Hirschsprung's disease. *Z Kinderchir* 1973;12:236.

81. Leenders E, Sieber WK. Congenital megacolon observation by Frederich Ruysch—1691. *J Pediatr Surg* 1970;5:1.

82. Levitt MA, Patel M, Rodriguez G, et al. The tethered spinal cord in patients with anorectal malformations. *J Pediatr Surg* 1997;32:462.

83. Levitt MA, Soffer SZ, Peña A. Continent appendicostomy in the bowel management of fecal incontinent children. *J Pediatr Surg* 1997;32:1630.

84. Lindvall O, Bjorklund A. The glyoxylic acid fluorescence histochemical method: a detailed account of the methodology of the visualization of central catecholamine neurons. *Histochemistry* 1974;39:97.

85. Luo Y, Ceccherini I, Pasini B, et al. Close linkage with the RET proto-oncogene and boundaries of deletion mutations in autosomal dominant Hirschsprung's disease. *Hum Mol Genet* 1993;2:1803.

86. Lynn HB. Rectal myectomy in Hirschsprung's disease: a decade of experience. *Arch Surg* 1975;110:991.

87. MacMahon RA, Moore CCM, Cussen LJ. Hirschsprung-like syndromes in patients with normal ganglion cells on suction rectal biopsy. *J Pediatr Surg* 1981;16:835.

88. Malone PS, Ransley PG, Kiely EM. Preliminary report: the antegrade continence enema. *Lancet* 1990;336:1217.

89. Martin LW. Surgical management of total colonic aganglionosis. *Ann Surg* 1972;176:343.

90. Martucciello G, Biocchi M, Dodero P, et al. Total colonic aganglionosis associated with interstitial deletion of the long arm of chromosome 10. *Pediatr Surg Int* 1992;7:308.

91. Meier-Rouge W. Hirschsprung's disease: its etiology, pathogenesis and differential diagnosis. *Curr Top Pathol* 1974;59:131.

92. Meier-Rouge W. Cause of colon disorder with symptoms of Hirschsprung's disease. *Verh Dtsch Ges Pathol* 1971;55:506.

93. Meier-Rouge W. Angeborene Dysganglionosen des Colon. *Kinderarzt* 1985;16:151.

94. Molenaar JC. Pathogenetic aspects of Hirschsprung's disease. *Br J Surg* 1995;82:145.

95. Moore BG, Singaram C, Eckhoff DE, et al. Immunohistochemical evaluations of ultrashort-segment Hirschsprung's disease. *Dis Colon Rectum* 1996;39:817.

96. Moore TC. Advantages of performing the sagittal anoplasty operation for imperforate anus at birth. *J Pediatr Surg* 1990;25:276.

97. Munakata K, Morita K, Okabe I, et al. Clinical and histologic studies of neuronal intestinal dysplasia. *J Pediatr Surg* 1985;20:231.

98. Narasimharao KL, Prasad GR, Katariya S. Prone crosstable lateral view: an alternative to the invertogram in imperforate anus. *AJR Am J Roentgenol* 1983;140:227.

99. Noblett HR. A rectal suction biopsy tube for use in the diagnosis of Hirschsprung's disease. *J Pediatr Surg* 1969;4:406.

100. Ogra SS, Weintraub D, Ogra PL. Immunologic aspects of human colostrum and milk. III. Fate and absorption of cellular and soluble components in the gastrointestinal tract of the newborn. *J Immunol* 1977;119:245.

101. Okamoto E, Veda T. Embryogenesis of intramural ganglia of the gut and its relation to Hirschsprung's disease. *J Pediatr Surg* 1967;2:437.

102. O'Kelly TJ, Davies JR, Tam PK, et al. Abnormalities of nitric oxide producing neurons in Hirschsprung's disease morphology and implications. *J Pediatr Surg* 1994;29:294.

103. Panuel M, Guys JM, Devred P, et al. Imagerie par résonance magnétique des malformations ano-rectales hautes. *Chir Pediatr* 1988;29:243.

104. Passarge E. Genetics of Hirschsprung's disease. *Clin Gastroenterol* 1973;2:507.

105. Peña A. Posterior sagittal anorectoplasty as a secondary operation for the treatment of fecal incontinence. *J Pediatr Surg* 1983;18:796.

106. Peña A. *Posterior sagittal approach for the correction of anorectal malformations*, vol. 19. Chicago: Year Book, 1985.

107. Peña A. Surgical treatment of high imperforate anus. *World J Surg* 1985;9:236.

108. Peña A. Anorectal malformations. *Semin Pediatr Surg* 1995;4:35.

109. Peña A. Total urogenital mobilization: an easier way to repair cloacas. *J Pediatr Surg* 1997;32:263.

110. Peña A, deVries P. Posterior sagittal anorectoplasty: important technical considerations and new applications. *J Pediatr Surg* 1982;17:796.

111. Peña A, Guardino K, Tovilla JM, et al. Bowel management for fecal incontinence in patients with anorectal malformations. *J Pediatr Surg* 1998;33:133.

112. Peña A, Levitt MA, Hong AR, Midulla PS. Surgical management of cloacal malformations: a review of 339 patients. *J Pediatr Surg* 2004;39–70.

113. Pistor G, Kapherr S, Grussner R, et al. Neuronal intestinal dysplasia: modern diagnosis and therapy—report of 23 patients. *Pediatr Surg Int* 1987;2:352.

114. Pokorny WJ, Garcia-Pratts JA, Barry YN. Necrotizing enterocolitis: incidence, operative care and outcome. *J Pediatr Surg* 1986;21:1149.

115. Polgin SE, Shlasko E, Levitt MA, et al. Alterations in respiratory status: early signs of severe necrotizing enterocolitis. *J Pediatr Surg* 1998;33:856.

116. Pomeranz AJ, Altman N, Sheldon JJ, et al. Magnetic resonance of congenital anorectal malformations. *Magn Reson Imaging* 1986;4:69.

117. Puri P, Fujimoto T. Diagnosis of allied functional bowel disorders using monoclonal antibodies and electron microscopy. *J Pediatr Surg* 1988;23:546.

118. Puri P, Lake BD, Nixon HH, et al. Neuronal colonic dysplasia: an unusual association of Hirschsprung's disease. *J Pediatr Surg* 1977;12:681.

119. Rescorla FJ, Morrison AM, Engles D, et al. Hirschsprung's disease: evaluation of mortality and long-term function in 260 cases. *Arch Surg* 1992;127:934.

120. Rhoads JE, Piper RL, Randall JP. A simultaneous abdominal and perineal approach in operations for imperforate anus with atresia of the rectum and rectosigmoid. *Ann Surg* 1948;127:552.

121. Rich MA, Brock WA, Peña A. Spectrum of genitourinary malformations in patients with imperforate anus. *Pediatr Surg Int* 1988;3:110.

122. Ricketts RR. Surgical therapy for necrotizing enterocolitis. *Ann Surg* 1984;200:653.

123. Rintala R, Rapola J, Louhimo I. Neuronal intestinal dysplasia. *Prog Pediatr Surg* 1989;24:186.

124. Robertson HE, Kernohan JW. The myenteric plexus in congenital megacolon. *Proc Staff Meet Mayo Clin* 1938;13:123.

125. Rothbart HA, Levin MJ. How contagious is necrotizing enterocolitis? *Pediatr J Infect Dis* 1983;2:406.

126. Sacher P, Briner J, Stauffer G. Clinical aspects of neuronal intestinal dysplasia. *Z Kinderchir* 1982;35:96.

127. Sacher P, Briner J, Stauffer UG. Unusual aspects of neuronal intestinal dysplasia. *Pediatr Surg Int* 1991;6:225.

128. Sachs TM, Applebaum, H, Touran T, et al. Use of MRI in evaluation of anorectal anomalies. *J Pediatr Surg* 1990;25:817.

129. Sandgren K, Ekblad E, Larsson LT. Survival of neurons and interstitial cells of Cajal after autotransplantation of myenteric ganglia from small intestine in the lethal spotted mouse. *Pediatr Surg Int* 2000;16:272.

130. Sane SM, Giardany BR. Total aganglionosis coli. *Radiology* 1973;107:397.

131. Santulli TV. Treatment of imperforate anus and associated fistulas. *Surg Gynecol Obstet* 1952;95:601.

132. Scharli F, Meier-Rouge W. Localized and disseminated forms of neuronal intestinal dysplasia mimicking Hirschsprung's disease. *J Pediatr Surg* 1981;16:164.

133. Schofield D, Yunis E. Intestinal neuronal dysplasia. *J Pediatr Gastroenterol Nutr* 1991;12:182.

134. Schwartz MZ, Hayden CK, Richardson CJ, et al. A prospective evaluation of intestinal stenosis following necrotizing enterocolitis. *J Pediatr Surg* 1982;17:764.

135. Sieber WK, Hirschsprung's disease. In: Welch KJ, Randolph JG, Ravitch MM, et al., eds. *Pediatric surgery*, vol. 2, 4th ed. Chicago: Year Book, 1986:995.

136. Simpser E, Kahn E, Kenigsberg K, et al. Neuronal intestinal dysplasia: quantitative diagnostic criteria and clinical management. *J Pediatr Gastroenterol Nutr* 1991;12:61.

137. Smith BM, Steiner RB, Lobe TE. Laparoscopic Duhamel pullthrough procedure for Hirschsprung's disease in childhood. *J Laparoendosc Surg* 1994;4:273.

138. So HB, Schwartz DL, Becker JM, et al. Endorectal "pullthrough" without preliminary colostomy in neonates with Hirschsprung's disease. *J Pediatr Surg* 1980;15:470.

139. Soave F. Hirschsprung's disease: a new surgical technique. *Arch Dis Child* 1964;39:116.

140. Soave F. Endorectal pull-through: 20 years experience. Address of the guest speaker, APSA, 1984. *J Pediatr Surg* 1985;20:568.

141. Soper RT, Ortiz JM. Neonatal pneumoperitoneum and Hirschsprung's disease. *Surgery* 1961;51:527.

142. Stephens FD. Imperforate rectum: a new surgical technique. *Med J Austr* 1953;1:202.

143. Stephens FD, Smith ED. *Ano-rectal malformations in children*, vol. 4. Chicago: Year Book, 1971.

144. Stephens FD, Smith ED. *Genito-urinary anomalies and their complications*, vol 4. Chicago: Year Book, 1971.

145. Stephens FD, Smith ED. *Proposed international classification*, vol. 4. Chicago: Year Book, 1971.

146. Stephens FD, Smith ED. Classification, identification and assessment of surgical treatment of anorectal anomalies. *Pediatr Surg Int* 1986;1:200.

147. Stevenson J, Oliver TK, Graham B, et al. Aggressive treatment of neonatal necrotizing enterocolitis: 38 patients with 25 survivors. *J Pediatr Surg* 1971;6:28.

148. Stoss F. Neuronal dysplasia: considerations for the pathogenesis and treatment of primary chronic constipation in adults. *Int J Colorect Dis* 1990;5:106.

149. Swenson O, Bill AH. Resection of rectum and rectosigmoid with preservation of the sphincter for benign spastic lesions producing megacolon: an experimental study. *Surgery* 1948;24:212.

150. Swenson O, Neuhauser EBD, Pickett LK. New concepts of etiology, diagnosis and treatment of congenital megacolon (Hirschsprung's disease). *Pediatrics* 1949;4:201.

151. Swenson O, Sherman JO, Fisher JH, et al. The treatment and postoperative complications of congenital megacolon: a 25 year follow-up. *Ann Surg* 1975;182:266.

152. Teitelbaum DH, Coran AG, Weitzman JJ, et al. Hirschsprung's disease and related neuromuscular disorders of the intestines. In: O'Neill JA Jr, Rowe MI, Grosfeld JL, et al, eds. *Pediatric surgery*. St. Louis: Mosby, 1998: 1381–1424.

153. Tiffin ME, Changler LR, Faber HK. Localized absence of ganglion cells of the myenteric plexus in congenital megacolon. *Am J Dis Child* 1940;59:1071.

154. Tittle K. Uber eine angeborene Missbildung des Dickdarmes. *Wien Klin Wochenschr* 1901;14:903.

155. Tobon F, Nigel CR, Ried W, et al. Non-surgical test for the diagnosis of Hirschsprung's disease. *N Engl J Med* 1968; 278:188.

156. Tobon F, Schuster M. Megacolon: special diagnostic (2nd) therapeutic features. *Johns Hopkins Med J* 1974;135:91.

157. Tolia V, Fleming S, Dubois RS. Use of Golytely in children and adolescents. *J Pediatr Gastroenterol Nutr* 1984;3:468.

158. Torres P, Levitt MA, Tovilla JM, et al. Anorectal malformations and Down's syndrome. *J Pediatr Surg* 1998;33:1.

159. Touloukian RJ. Etiologic role of the circulation. In: Brown EG, Sweet AY, eds. *Neonatal necrotizing enterocolitis*. New York: Grune and Stratton, 1980:41.

160. Trusler GA, Wilkinson RH. Imperforate anus: a review of 147 cases. *Can J Surg* 1962;5:169.

161. Wangensteen OH, Rice CO. Imperforate anus: a method of determining the surgical approach. *Ann Surg* 1930; 92:77.

162. Westra-Meijer CMM, Degener JE, Dzoljic-Danilovic G, et al. Quantitative study of the aerobic and anaerobic fecal flora in neonatal enterocolitis. *Arch Dis Child* 1983;58: 523.

163. Ziegler MM, Royal RE, Brandt J, et al. Extended myectomy-myotomy: a therapeutic alternative for total intestinal aganglionosis. *Ann Surg* 1993;218:504.

164. Zuelzer WW, Wilson JL. Functional intestinal obstruction on congenital neurogenic basis in infancy. *Am J Dis Child* 1948;75:40.

Chapter 19

Cutaneous Conditions

What's the matter, you dissentious rogues
That, rubbing the poor itch of your opinion,
Make yourselves scabs?
                    William Shakespeare: *Coriolanus* I, i, 168

Dermatologic anal problems are often trivialized by the surgeon, who may categorize them as complaints attributable to a psychoneurotic or anal-obsessive personality. The patient may be referred directly to a dermatologist or may be given any one of a number of proprietary creams or the ubiquitous topical steroid, without the benefit of a physical examination. Dermatologists are understandably more adept at establishing the diagnosis of skin problems and usually perform a biopsy for confirmation in questionable cases, but the dermatologist is loath to perform a rectal examination and rarely has endoscopic equipment available. In my opinion, therefore, patients with anal complaints, including perianal dermatologic problems, should be seen by a physician or surgeon who has the knowledge and the instruments necessary to perform a complete rectal evaluation. If the condition appears to be limited to the skin and of uncertain diagnosis, consultation with a dermatologist is certainly appropriate.

The purpose of this chapter is to describe the skin conditions that affect the perianal area, emphasizing the differential diagnosis, indications for biopsy, and treatment of the relevant diseases. Those conditions that may be found in the anal area that are only incidental to a systemic cutaneous process are mentioned *en passant* if recognition of the disease in the area is believed to be unique or of particular interest. This chapter is not meant to be a *précis* of a textbook of dermatology.

CLASSIFICATION

Dermatologic diseases may be categorized in a number of ways: on the basis of the type of lesion (e.g., flat, elevated, depressed), according to whether they are primary or secondary, histopathologically, or by the commonly employed classifications of inflammation, infection, and neoplasm. A modification using this last method is illustrated as follows:

Dermatologic Anal Conditions

Inflammatory Diseases

Pruritus ani
Psoriasis
Lichen planus
Lichen sclerosus et atrophicus
Atrophoderma
Contact (i.e., allergic) dermatitis
Seborrheic dermatitis
Atopic dermatitis
Radiodermatitis
Behçet's syndrome
Lupus erythematosus
Dermatomyositis
Scleroderma
Erythema multiforme
Familial benign chronic pemphigus (i.e., Hailey-Hailey)
Pemphigus vulgaris
Cicatricial pemphigoid

Infectious Diseases

Nonvenereal
    Pilonidal sinus
    Suppurative hidradenitis
    Anorectal abscess and anal fistula
    Crohn's disease
    Tuberculosis
    Actinomycosis
    Fournier's gangrene
    Ecthyma gangrenosum
    Herpes zoster
    Vaccinia
    Tinea cruris
    Candidiasis (i.e., moniliasis)
    "Deep" mycoses
    Amebiasis cutis
    Trichomoniasis
    Schistosomiasis cutis
    Bilharziasis
    Oxyuriasis (e.g., pinworm, enterobiasis)
    Creeping eruption (i.e., larva migrans)

Larva currens
Cimicosis (i.e., bedbug bites)
Pediculosis
Scabies
Venereal
Gonorrhea
Syphilis
Chancroid
Granuloma inguinale
Lymphogranuloma venereum (*Chlamydia* infection)
Molluscum contagiosum
Herpes genitalis
Condylomata acuminata

Premalignant and Malignant Diseases

Acanthosis nigricans
Leukoplakia
Mycosis fungoides
Leukemia cutis
Basal cell carcinoma
Squamous cell carcinoma
Malignant melanoma
Bowen's disease
Extramammary Paget's disease

In addition, a glossary of dermatologic terms (provided at the end of this chapter) may aid the reader in interpreting the description of the lesions.[80,108]

INFLAMMATORY CONDITIONS

Pruritus Ani

Itching in the perianal area, pruritus ani, is a frequently voiced complaint. In fact, it is a symptom that was well recognized in antiquity. In the earliest manuscript exclusively devoted to anorectal disorders, the Chester Beatty Medical Papyrus, ten of its 41 remedies were devoted to the management of anal itching and irritation.[19] By far the most common anorectal symptom presenting to the dermatologist is pruritus ani.[6] The rich nerve supply to the perianal area is thought to be the primary reason for the sensitivity to potential irritants.[178]

Symptoms

Itching is usually noted in the anal or occasionally the genital areas, but the condition is not generalized. Although the anus is frequently the site for autoeroticism, most individuals do not appear to fall into this category. The condition tends to be worse at night, awakening the patient from sleep. This leads to scratching, which exac-

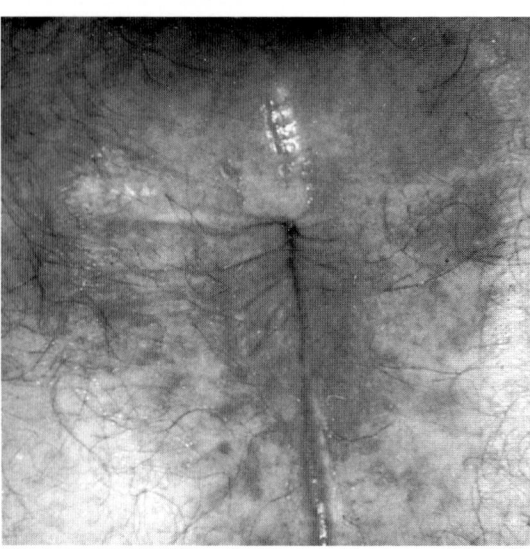

FIGURE 19-1. Perianal neurodermatitis is manifested with lichenification and fissuring. (See Color Fig. 19-1.) (Courtesy of William G. Robertson, M.D.)

erbates the complaint even further. Pruritus ani is more common in men.

Differential Diagnosis

Although the symptoms may be caused by a specific condition [e.g., hemorrhoids,[189], anal fissure, scarring from prior anal surgery] or an associated problem (e.g., constipation or diarrhea), most patients are not found to have significant anorectal pathology except for the obvious skin changes. Besides anorectal disease, allergic (i.e., contact) dermatitis, mycoses, seborrhea, diabetes, and oxyuriasis (pinworm) have all been implicated as causative factors. Other dermatologic problems, such as psoriasis (see later), should be considered. In addition, the possibility of harboring a systemic disease, such as diabetes, may necessitate further studies. Anal neurodermatitis may cause violent itching, which may lead to tearing of the perianal area (Figure 19-1). With chronicity, the skin can become atrophic or hypertrophic, with nodularity and scarring (Figure 19-2).

Special Studies

Physiologic studies have demonstrated that in patients with idiopathic pruritus ani, the anal sphincter relaxes in response to rectal distension more readily than in those with no anal disease.[102] Allan and colleagues showed that pruritic individuals without coexisting anal pathologic features had a significantly greater fall of anal pressure when a rectal balloon was inflated (57%) than did a control population (40%).[7] Others have observed that patients

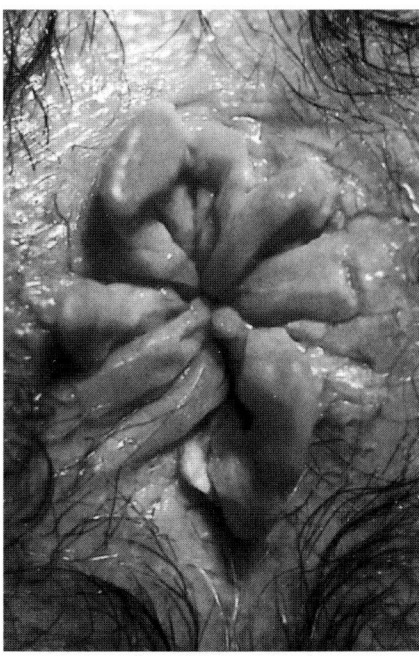

FIGURE 19-2. Marked edema with papillomatosis and nodularity resulting from chronic abrading is characteristic of pruritus ani. (See Color Fig. 19-2.) (Courtesy of William G. Robertson, M.D.)

with idiopathic pruritus ani have an abnormal rectoanal inhibitory reflex and a lower threshold for internal sphincter relaxation during such studies as the saline continence test.[104] It is, therefore, postulated that pruritus and soiling in some patients may occur as a result of a defect in anal sphincter function.

Evaluation

Physical examination should include anoscopy and proctosigmoidoscopy to look for a local cause of the symptoms. Daniel and colleagues reviewed 109 individuals with pruritus ani as the only presenting symptom and concluded that those with complaints of long duration should undergo evaluation for proximal colon and anorectal neoplasms.[72] Usually, however, the procedures are unrewarding. Examination with a magnifying lens may be helpful.[70] Evaluation with Wood's lamp may reveal fluorescence,[233] but this equipment is usually not readily available in the office practice of most physicians and surgeons. If suspicion warrants, skin scrapings of the perianal area should be examined using a potassium hydroxide slide preparation and should be cultured on Sabouraud's medium for yeast and fungi (see Fungal Infections). However, because there is no good evidence to suggest that abnormal fecal flora contributes to the symptoms, neither qualitative nor quantitative assessment of the stool is considered appropriate.[229]

Treatment

Pruritus ani has traditionally been considered a condition that eludes all attempts at cure. Numerous potions, nostrums, and lotions have been employed with varying success, as well as more aggressive treatment, such as injection of local anesthetics, phenol, and alcohol.[241,242] Excision and skin grafting have also been suggested. Eusebio and colleagues reported "long-term cure" with the use of up to 30 mL of 0.5% methylene blue (i.e., methylthionine chloride) injected intradermally and subcutaneously in 23 individuals with intractable pruritus ani.[101]

Psychological factors have been thought to play a role in contributing to symptoms. However, there has never been objective evidence to demonstrate a statistically significant deviation from a normal personality.[8] It is reasonable to assume that severe perianal itching, 24 hours a day, every day, is likely to make an individual rather irascible.

In recent years, attention has been drawn to the role of diet in the cause of the condition; therefore, an accurately obtained history will often dictate the appropriate treatment. Items that have been implicated include the following:

- Coffee (caffeine)
- Tea (caffeine)
- Carbonated beverages, especially caffeinated colas
- Milk products
- Alcohol, particularly wine and beer
- Tomatoes and tomato products, such as ketchup
- Cheese
- Chocolate
- Nuts[114,247]

Cigarette smoking is another factor. It is postulated that all these products induce mucous discharge, probably through a systemic route, or possibly in some instances by changing the pH of the stool.

Because most individuals indulge in one or more of the foregoing substances, it is probable that the physician will receive an affirmative response when inquiring about the dietary history. By recognizing the association of one of these agents with pruritus ani, a patient will become an ally of the surgeon. It is, therefore, important to solicit an individual's understanding and cooperation.[19] A patient may have been previously told that the problem is psychoneurotic, so that the physician's reassurance and sympathy are beneficial factors that contribute to a satisfactory resolution. Removing or changing the dietary factor may cause the symptoms to disappear. Additionally, promoting complete evacuation with increased fluids and bulking agents (e.g., bran, psyllium) may help avoid the irritation.[29] Rectal irrigation and a bowel management program also may be necessary for those individuals who experience incontinence or leakage of stool (see Chapter 13).

Despite the validity of the previous suggestions, the most important advice that can be given is usually directed toward the management of anal hygiene. Many individuals perceive their problem to be one of lack of cleanliness; the opposite is more likely. Vigorous scrubbing of the area with soap and water will cause the skin to be defatted, and contact dermatitis may supervene. Rarely have I identified a patient with pruritus who was not scrupulous with respect to anal cleanliness; the difficulty is to convince the person that the anal area need not be sterilized.

One should advise the patient to remove the soap from the area! The perineum should be cleansed with plain water, particularly when bathing or showering, and ideally even following defecation. Irrigating the rectum with warm water through a bulb syringe is often ameliorating. Some individuals may actually be allergic to toilet paper, so that in stubborn cases a moist cloth should be used for cleansing. Even in a public toilet, a moistened paper towel is preferable to the irritative effects of continued rubbing with toilet paper. For those with copious discharge, a cotton ball placed at the anal verge, changed as necessary, may be helpful.

A wealth of topical creams and ointments, obtained over the counter and by prescription, is available for the pruritus ani sufferer. The use of anesthetic ointments and creams [e.g., dibucaine (Nupercainal), pramoxine (Tronolane), benzocaine (Americaine), lidocaine (ELA-Max 5)] is not advised except on a highly limited basis. Symptoms are only temporarily masked, the underlying problem is not addressed, and allergic dermatitis can develop. Soothing creams and lotions are generally preferred to ointments; many are quite satisfactory [e.g., mineral oil and lanolin (Balneol), witch hazel and glycerin (Tucks), pramoxine (Prax)]. For more severe skin cracking, bath treatment with Aveeno Colloidal Oatmeal may be quite helpful. However, when the proprietary preparation fails, one must consider using a topical steroid; this almost inevitably will bring immediate relief. My own preference is to use Proctocort (1% hydrocortisone cream) or 2.5% Analpram-HC (hydrocortisone and pramoxine), because they are nicely packaged with a plastic applicator. The medication is applied at bedtime and once or twice more during the day, if necessary. It should be discontinued, however, as soon as symptoms resolve, to avoid skin atrophy (see Atrophoderma). Dasan and colleagues opine that patients with unresolved, long-standing pruritus ani, and with no other symptoms to suggest colorectal disease, should be referred to a dermatologist for assessment and patch testing (see Allergic Dermatitis).[74]

In the rare intractable case, sedatives and tranquilizers may be considered. In addition, biofeedback and self-hypnosis have been of demonstrable benefit with some

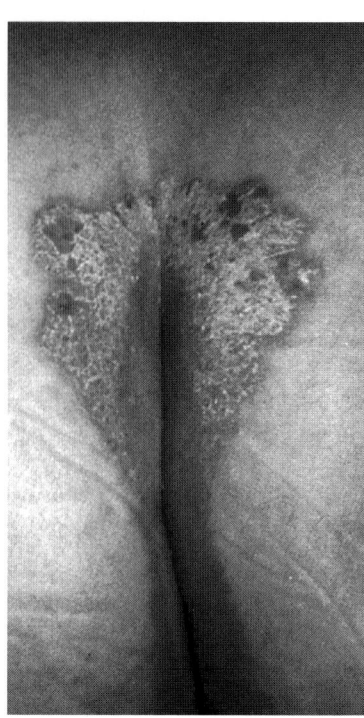

FIGURE 19-3. Well-marginated erythematosquamous plaque with characteristic silvery scales indicates psoriasis. (See Color Fig. 19-3.) (Courtesy of Arnold Medved, M.D.)

patients. Consultation with a professional familiar with these techniques may be advisable.

Psoriasis

Psoriasis is a common, chronic inflammatory disease of the skin, characterized by rounded, circumscribed, erythematous, dry, scaling patches covered by grayish white or silvery white scales. The lesions have a predilection for the scalp, nails, extensor surfaces of the limbs, elbows, knees, and the sacral region.[75] When the condition occurs in the anal area, it may cause severe pruritic symptoms. Perianal psoriasis is usually sharply marginated, with a characteristic butterfly distribution extending over the coccyx and sacrum (Figure 19-3). Psoriatic lesions are often present at other sites on the body.

Histologically, characteristic features include epidermal thickening (i.e., acanthosis), regular elongation of the rete ridges with broadening of the deeper aspect, and elongation with edema of the dermal papillae (Figure 19-4). There may be increased mitotic activity in the epidermis. Cells of the stratum corneum usually have retained nuclei (i.e., parakeratosis). Focal collections of neutrophils in the subcorneum are known as Munro's microabscesses.

Treatment may simply consist of moisturizers (emollients) and agents containing salicylic acid. Topical

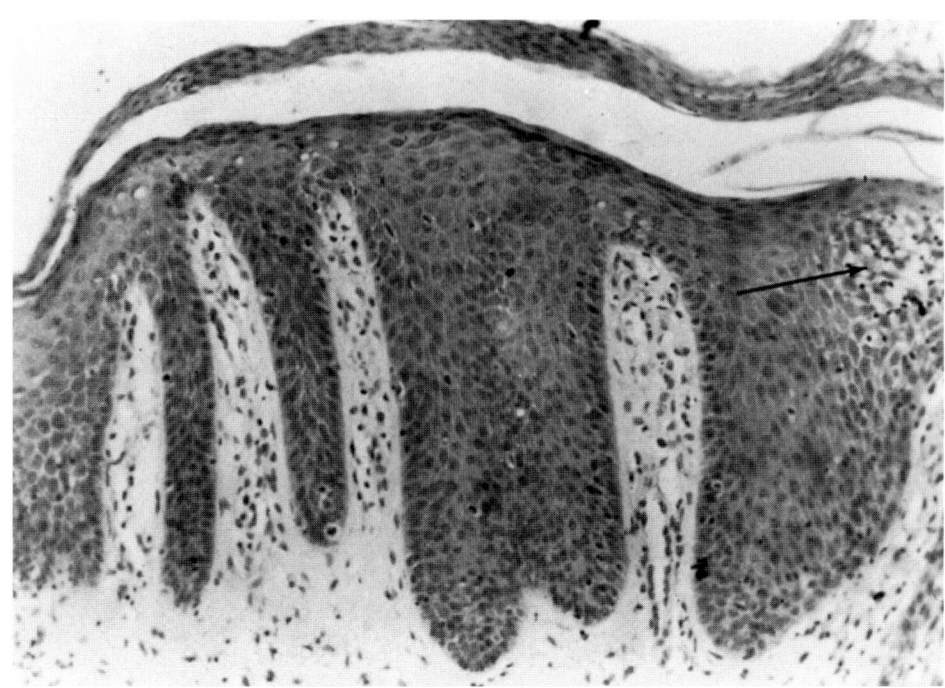

FIGURE 19-4. Psoriasis. Elongation of the rete ridges and edema of the dermal papillae are characteristic features of psoriasis. Note parakeratosis, Munro abscess *(arrow)*, and the absence of a granular cell layer. (Original magnification × 180; courtesy of Rudolf Garret, M.D.)

agents include corticosteroids, coal tar products, anthralin, retinoid (tazarotene), a vitamin D_3 derivative (calcipotriene), or a combination of these. In addition, the application of sunlight (not terribly practical for perianal disease) and the use of ultraviolet light B (UVB) have been found to be beneficial. More recently, the so-called PUVA treatment has been advocated. This consists of a combined systemic-external therapy, using a potent photoactive agent (i.e., psoralen) followed by administration of a special light system emitting long-wave UVA. Cancer chemotherapeutic drugs, such as methotrexate and cyclosporine, have also been advocated.

I am reluctant to treat psoriasis without dermatologic consultation unless the condition is localized to the perianal area and then only for a limited course.

Lichen Planus

Lichen planus is a skin condition that consists of an eruption of small, flat-topped papules with a distinct violaceous color and polypoid configuration. The lesion is characteristically found on the flexor surfaces, mucous membranes, genitalia (25%), and occasionally in the perianal area. There have rare reports of squamous cell carcinoma developing within lichen planus in the anal area.[116]

Histologically, the papule shows focal thickening of the granular layer, degeneration of the basement membrane and basal cells, and a bandlike lymphocytic infiltrate in the upper dermis (Figure 19-5). Biopsy of the skin establishes the diagnosis.

Treatment often has less than satisfactory results, with corticosteroids appearing to be the most helpful for this condition. Topical preparations with occlusive dressings are quite useful, and systemic administration and intralesional injections have also been employed. In mild cases, antipruritic lotions and antihistamines are suggested. Rest is also helpful.

Lichen Sclerosus et Atrophicus

Lichen sclerosus et atrophicus is an unusual condition of unknown cause. It occurs much more frequently in women than in men. The genital area appears to be the most commonly involved site.

Physical examination may reveal the characteristic "inverted keyhole" distribution. In this situation, the disease extends beyond the mucocutaneous border to involve the skin of the vulva, perineum, and perianal area. In the vulva, the condition affects the labia, vestibule, and introitus (Figure 19-6). Discomfort, pruritus, dysuria, and dyspareunia are common complaints.

The characteristic histologic changes in lichen sclerosus et atrophicus are edema and homogenization of the collagen below the epidermis (Figure 19-7). The epidermis also shows variable hyperkeratosis and follicular plugging. Lichen sclerosus et atrophicus may be associated with squamous cell carcinoma of the vulva. An association between the condition and squamous cell carcinoma of the perianal region has also been noted.[232]

Treatment is primarily directed to the relief of the pruritic complaints in the hope of lessening the risk for

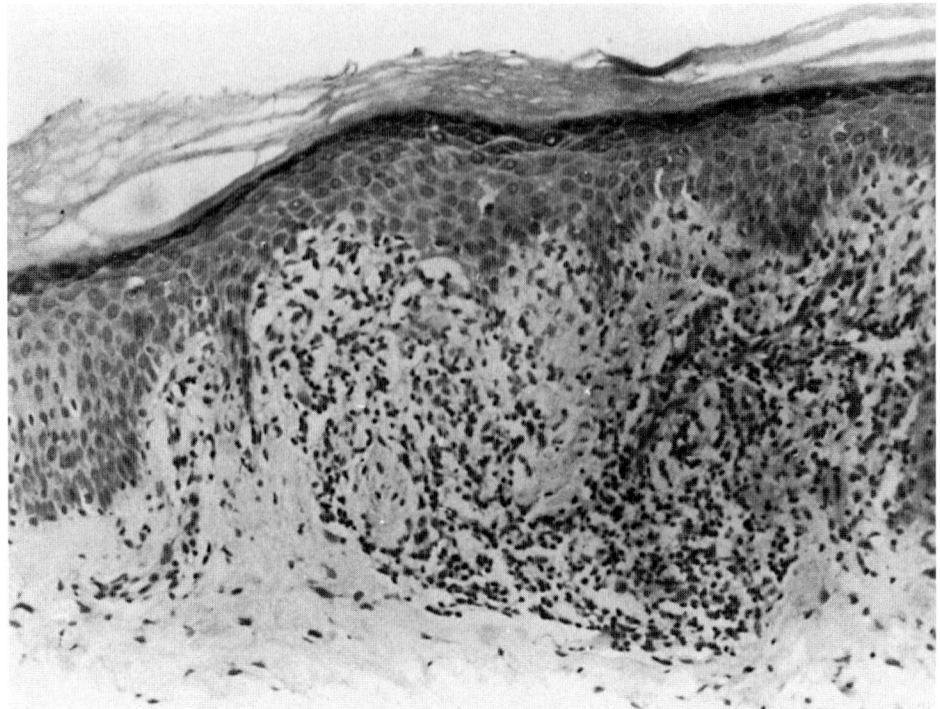

FIGURE 19-5. Characteristics of lichen planus include moderate hyperkeratosis, thickening of the stratum granulosum, sawtooth configuration of the rete ridges, and lymphocytic infiltration of the dermis and basal cell layer. Note the sharp demarcation of the lymphocytic infiltrate. (Original magnification × 120; courtesy of Rudolf Garret, M.D.)

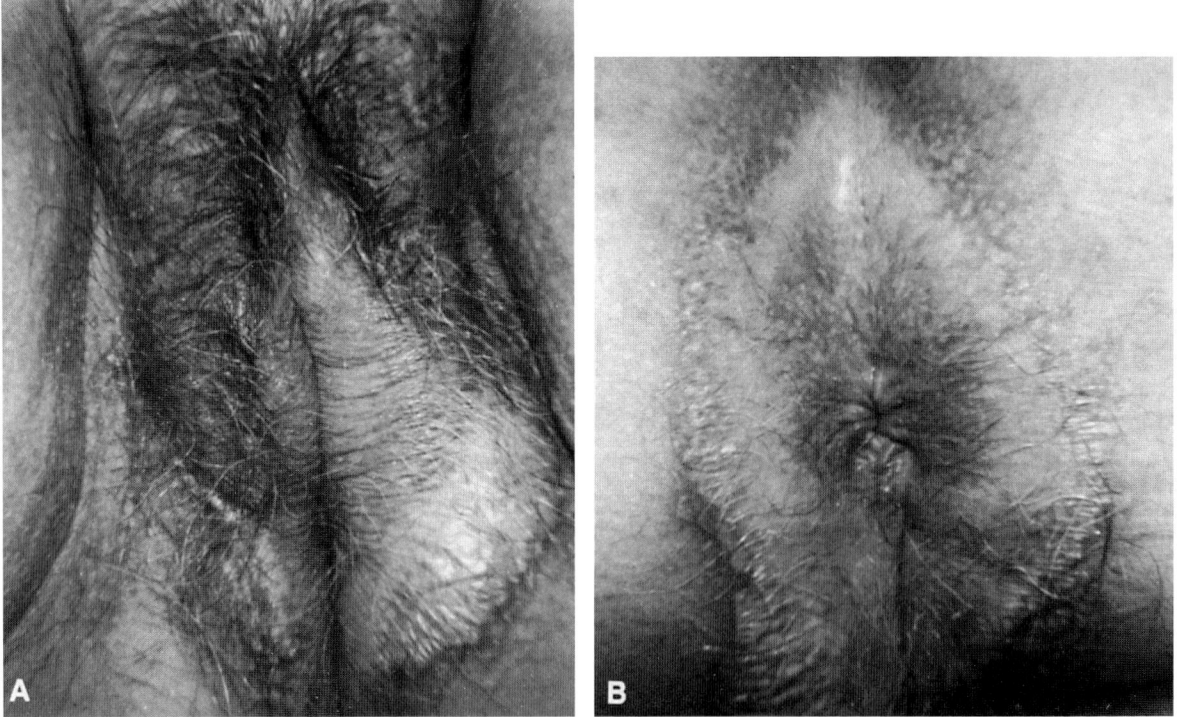

FIGURE 19-6. Characteristic of lichen sclerosus et atrophicus is a sharply defined dermatosis in the **(A)** vulvar area and **(B)** perianum with hypopigmentation centrally and hyperpigmentation peripherally. Note the lichenoid papules about the periphery. (Courtesy of John A. Clark, M.D.)

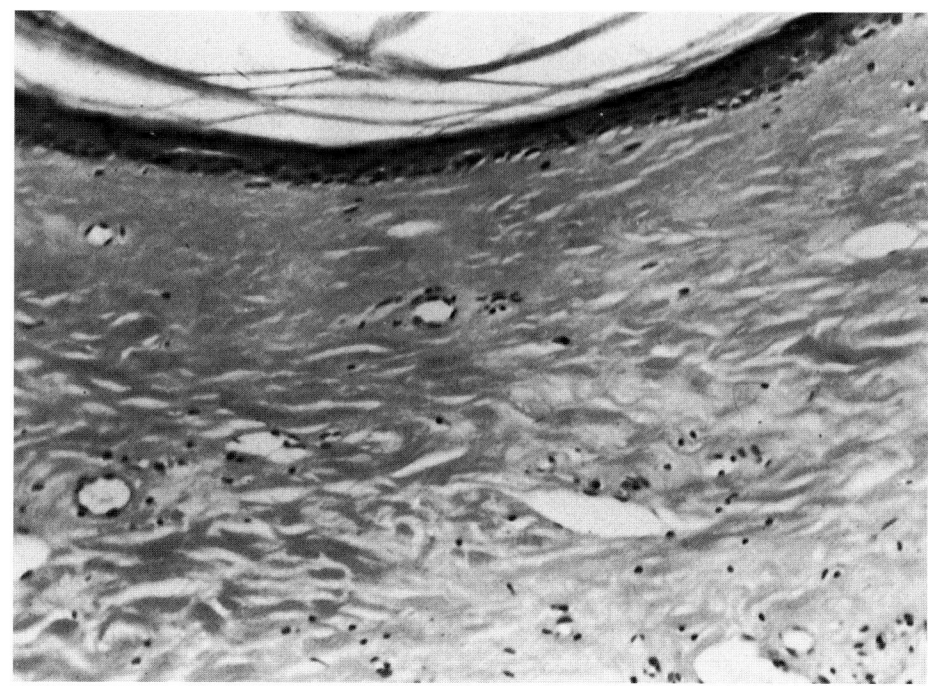

FIGURE 19-7. Atrophy of the epidermis and hyalinization of the dermis in lichen sclerosis et atrophicus. (Original magnification × 120; courtesy of Rudolf Garret, M.D.)

leukoplakia and carcinoma. A mild topical steroid sufficient to control the symptoms is advocated. Secondary infection should be treated with appropriate antibiotics.

Atrophoderma or Atrophy of the Skin

Atrophy of the skin is a reaction to the repeated and prolonged application of topical corticosteroids; it may also follow local injection of these products.[120] Telangiectasia occurs, indicating loss of dermal collagen, and the patient who initially complained of pruritus subsequently reports discomfort and burning.[234] The friction of walking rubs the already atrophic and thinned epidermis.

Patients usually report a history of self-application of topical corticosteroids for many years. Attempting to remove the medication is frequently unsuccessful. Biopsy may reveal atrophy and hyperkeratosis. Because of the risk for development of this condition, it is important to discontinue the use of cortisone treatment as soon as possible.

Irritant and Contact or Allergic Dermatitis

Two types of dermatitis are caused by substances coming into contact with the skin:

- Irritant dermatitis (caused by a nonallergic reaction following exposure to an irritating substance)
- Allergic (contact) dermatitis caused by allergic sensitization to a number of agents[82]

Irritants include alkalis, acids, metal salts, dusts, gases, and hydrocarbons. Allergic contact dermatitis results from

hypersensitivity of the delayed type, also known as cell-mediated hypersensitivity or immunity.[82] A person may be exposed to an allergen for many years before hypersensitivity develops. The allergens are numerous and varied, as follows:

- Dyes
- Oils
- Resins
- Chemicals used for fabrics, cosmetics, and insecticides
- Products or the substances of bacteria, fungi, and parasites[82]

The most common causes of contact dermatitis are as follows, in order of frequency:

1. Poison ivy, oak, and sumac
2. Paraphenylenediamine
3. Nickel
4. Common rubber compounds
5. Neomycin
6. Dichromates[107]

The patch test is used to detect hypersensitivity to a substance that is in contact with the skin (see Pruritus Ani). A nonirritating concentration of agents suspected to be the cause of the contact dermatitis is applied. The patches remain in place for 48 hours, less if burning or itching occurs. A positive reaction will produce severe pruritus and erythema or vesicles. It is wise to defer this test, however, until the rash has cleared, to limit the likelihood of a severe exacerbation.

Therapy obviously is directed toward removing the underlying cause of the skin problem or the allergen. Iodine and adhesive tape are common dermatitis-inducing products in patients who undergo anal surgery. Soothing compresses such as Aveeno Colloidal Oatmeal, in addition to corticosteroids and possibly antipruritics, may be advisable.

Seborrheic Dermatitis

Seborrheic dermatitis is a chronic, superficial, inflammatory disease of the skin, with a predilection for the scalp, eyebrows, nasolabial crease, ears, axillae, submammary folds, umbilicus, groin, and natal cleft. The disease is characterized by dry, moist, or greasy scales and by crusted, pink-yellow patches of diverse size and shape.[84] The condition is believed to be caused by hypersecretion of sebum and is apparently exacerbated by increased perspiration and emotional stress. A high fat intake is frequently noted.

Histologically, the picture is not dissimilar to that of psoriasis, but Munro's abscesses are not seen. According to one school of thought, the two conditions are so similar that there is some justification for thinking their origin may be the same. However, more recent evidence favors a role for yeast organisms in the etiology of the condition, with therapy being directed accordingly. Still, application of corticosteroids is the primary therapy.

Atopic Dermatitis or Atopic Eczema

The term *atopy* is derived from the Greek word meaning "out of place" or "strange." It is defined as the tendency for allergies to manifest themselves by systemic symptoms, such as asthma, hay fever, and eczema.[81] The condition is believed to be either a form of immunologic deficiency or possibly a blockade of β-adrenergic receptors in the skin.

Atopic dermatitis can occur as localized, erythematous, scaly, papular, or vesicular patches or in the form of pruritic, lichenified lesions.[84] The condition is often paroxysmal, with an emotional upset initiating some attacks. Other factors exacerbating the problem may be clothing, certain foods, and dryness of the skin. Superimposed infections such as intertrigo and dermatophytosis may produce further recurrences.

Histologically, hyperkeratosis and parakeratosis with acanthosis are noted (Figure 19-8). When lichenification is present, the acanthosis is increased, and there is papillomatosis, with long papillary bodies reaching to the stratum corneum. These changes may somewhat resemble those seen in psoriasis.

Treatment consists of avoiding emotional stress, if possible, avoiding extremes of cold and heat, limiting the use of stimulant beverages, and using oral antihistamines and topical corticosteroids. Prednisone, 30 to 40 mg orally for 4 to 6 weeks or possibly longer, is usually recommended. Alternatively, a parenteral preparation may be substituted.

Radiodermatitis

Radiodermatitis is a particular problem in the anal area, because current therapy for carcinoma of the rectum, anus, and prostate often involves ionizing radiation. In some individuals, unfortunately, the cancer treatment may be actually worse than the original disease (see Chapter 28).

Many changes are found in the cell as the result of radiation therapy. Mitoses are temporarily arrested, chro-

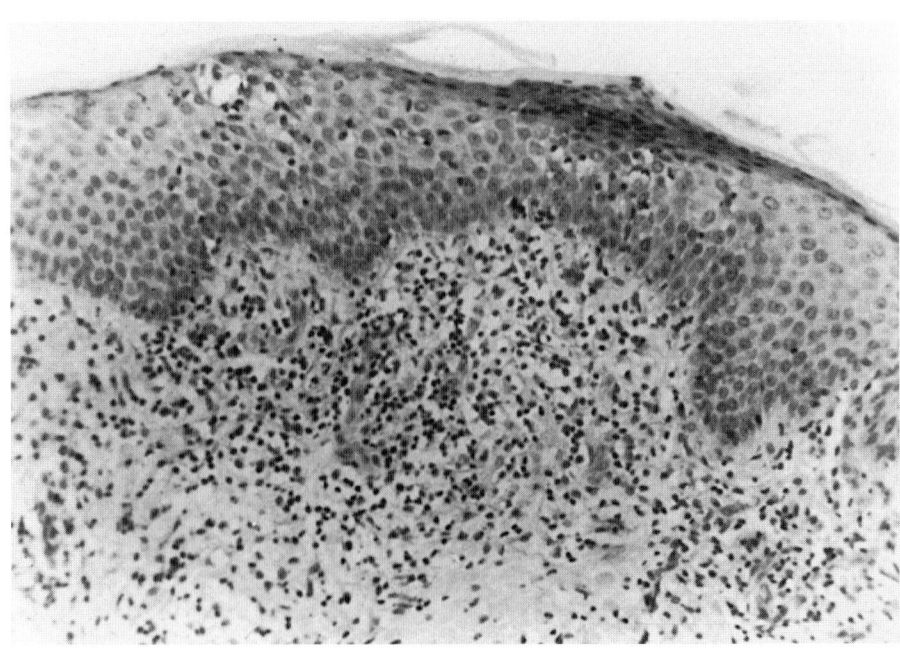

FIGURE 19-8. Histologic characteristics of atopic dermatitis include mild acanthosis, spongiosis, focal parakeratosis, and dermal mononuclear cell infiltrate. (Original magnification × 180; courtesy of Rudolf Garret, M.D.)

mosomal abnormalities occur, and there is at least a temporary halt in the normal cell cycle. The amount of skin change resulting from radiotherapy depends on the dose. Changes may be manifested as erythema, edema, and ulceration, and symptoms may include burning, itching, or severe pain. After a period of time, telangiectasia, atrophy, and freckling may appear. The skin becomes dry, thin, smooth, and shiny (Figure 19-9). Radiation injury may result in the subsequent development of malignancy, in most cases following a rather prolonged latent period. The manifestations of this complication increase with the passage of time.

Results of treatment are often less than satisfactory. However, symptomatic improvement has been reported with a regimen consisting of oral vitamin A, 8,000 IU, given twice daily.[167] Hyperbaric oxygen treatment has also been recommended. Cleansing the area with mild soap and water, in addition to the use of an emollient, a corticosteroid preparation, or both, may be of help. Biopsy specimens should be taken from any suspected lesions.

Behçet's Syndrome

Behçet's syndrome is characterized by four main symptoms: recurrent aphthous ulcers in the mouth, skin lesions, eye lesions, and genital ulcerations.[134] Genital ulcerations may be found in persons of both sexes on the genitocrural fold, on the anus, on the perineum, or in the rectum. Although the cause of the condition is unknown, there is some evidence to suggest that it is of viral origin or possibly represents an autoimmune disease. Histologically, the lesions usually show vasculitis.

The anal condition may be misdiagnosed as hemorrhoids, fissure, Crohn's disease, condylomata, or STI.[134] Surgery is contraindicated, and corticosteroid treatment, systemically or topically, is the preferred treatment (see also Chapter 28).

Lupus Erythematosus

Lupus erythematosus, like other connective tissue diseases, only rarely occurs in the anal area and still more rarely develops as an isolated finding in this location. The cutaneous manifestation is called discoid lupus erythematosus (DLE). It may begin with single or multiple lesions involving entire regions of the body, especially the head and neck, sternum, vulva, and perineum. The typical plaque is approximately 1 cm or more in diameter, with characteristic scales. Removal of the scales reveals patulous follicular orifices with dry, horny, keratinous plugs.[83] Occasionally, basal cell or squamous cell carcinoma may develop in long-standing DLE lesions.

In laboratory investigation, the LE cell test usually yields a negative result in DLE. Results of the direct immunofluorescence test are usually positive, however, as are antinuclear antibody test results.

Treatment consists of avoidance of strong sunlight, extremes in temperature, and localized trauma. Corticosteroid creams and ointments are particularly beneficial, with intralesional steroid therapy often helpful. Systemic therapy with antimalarials also has been advised.

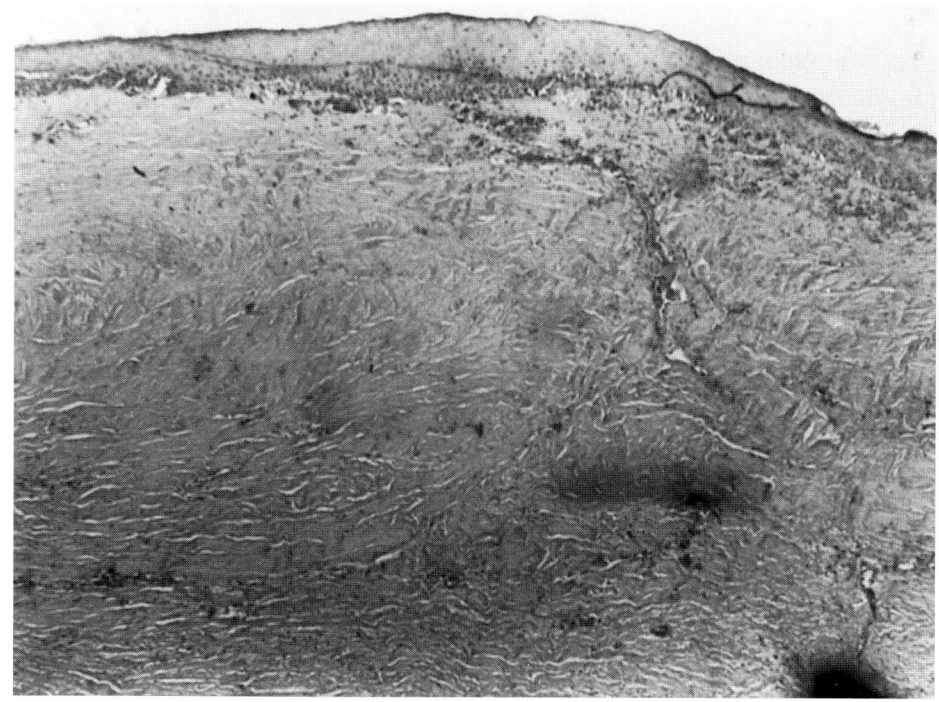

FIGURE 19-9. Histologic findings of radiodermatitis include fibrosis of the dermis with sclerosis, atrophy of the epidermis, and the absence of skin appendages. (Original magnification × 120; courtesy of Rudolf Garret, M.D.)

Dermatomyositis

Dermatomyositis (polymyositis) is an inflammatory condition that produces angiopathy in the skin, subcutaneous tissue, and muscles. The disease usually starts in the face and eyelids and may spread to other areas. It is associated with a number of other disturbances, including Raynaud's phenomenon, alopecia, urticaria, and erythema multiforme. Of particular interest to the surgeon is that in patients older than 40 years of age, visceral cancer is frequently associated with the condition. Histologic changes are similar to those of lupus erythematosus. Treatment consists of rest, salicylates, steroids, methotrexate, and azathioprine.

Scleroderma or Progressive Systemic Sclerosis

Scleroderma is characterized by the appearance of areas that are immobile and give the skin the appearance of being "hidebound."[83] The skin becomes smooth, yellowish, and firm, and it shrinks, so that the underlying structures are bound down. Although the condition frequently involves the face and hands, leading to an expressionless appearance on the former and a clawlike appearance of the latter, it can progress to involve most of the internal organs. Involvement of the small intestine may cause constipation, diarrhea, and abdominal distension. Although the colon is only rarely affected, it can produce the signs and symptoms of Ogilvie's syndrome (see Chapter 16). Treatment consists of supportive measures, baths, a high-protein diet, corticosteroids, and a number of other medications, including immunosuppressives.

Erythema Multiforme

Erythema multiforme is a clinically and histologically distinctive skin disease that is precipitated by the following conditions, among others:

- Viral infections
- Bacterial infections
- Radiotherapy
- Carcinomatosis
- Pregnancy
- Connective tissue diseases
- Drug reactions

The mechanism for this particular reaction is unknown. The lesions present as flat, dull-red maculopapules that may be rather small or may increase to 1 or 2 cm in 48 hours. The periphery may remain red, whereas the center is purpuric. The lesions look almost like targets. They commonly appear in the oral mucous membrane, but genital lesions are also frequent.

Histologically, the abnormality is confined to the upper dermis and lower epidermis. In more severe cases, there is necrosis of the whole epidermis. Bullae usually are subepidermal.

Treatment consists of symptomatic relief in mild cases, but in severe instances the use of corticosteroids has been suggested. Antibiotics are advised if secondary infection develops.

Familial Benign Chronic Pemphigus or Hailey-Hailey

Familial benign chronic pemphigus is a hereditary disease characterized by a recurrent bullous and vesicular dermatitis of the neck, axillae, flexors, and surfaces that appose. The condition has been found localized to the perianal area and may pose confusion in differential diagnosis (Figure 19-10).[266] The disease is transmitted as an autosomal dominant trait. The histologic pattern is unique, with prominent intraepidermal vesicles and bullae (Figure 19-11).

Treatment consists of local or systemic antibiotics and the use of topical corticosteroids. Additionally, low-dose radiation treatment has been recommended. Localized areas have been treated by excision and skin grafting.

Pemphigus Vulgaris

Pemphigus vulgaris is characterized by bullae appearing on apparently normal skin and mucous membranes.[87] The lesions usually begin first in the mouth

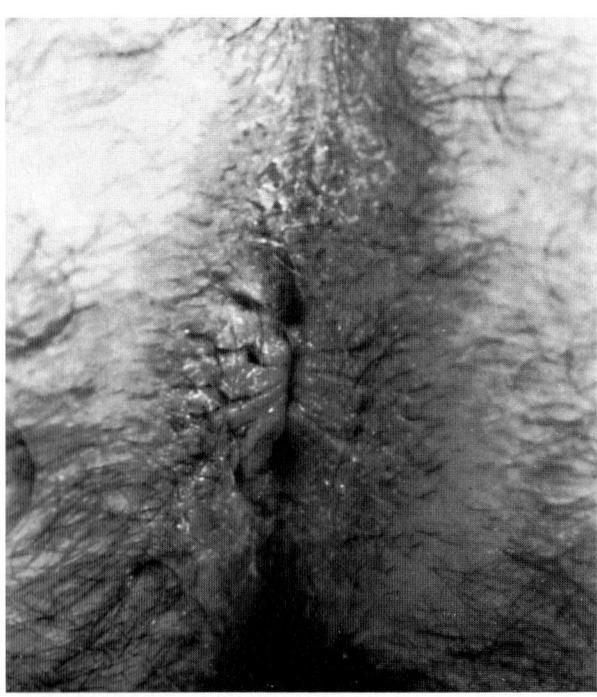

FIGURE 19-10. Hailey-Hailey. A macerated erythematous patch has well-defined borders. (Courtesy of Samuel L. Moschella, M.D.)

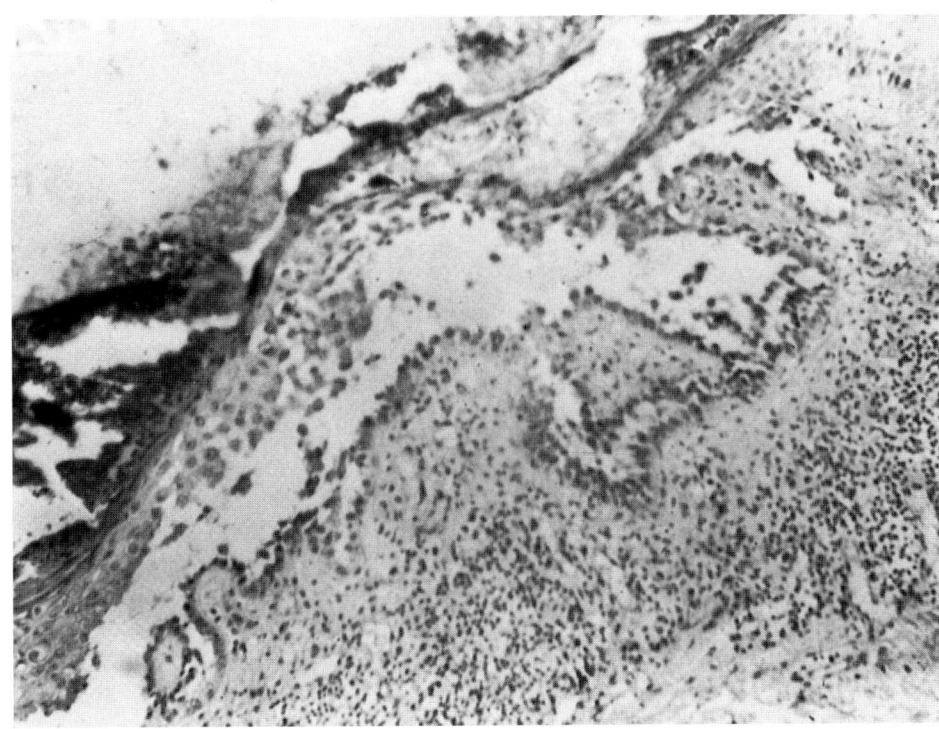

FIGURE 19-11. Benign familial chronic pemphigus (Hailey-Hailey) is characterized by suprabasal bullae, such as the one shown here, containing detached prickle cells and good preservation of acantholytic cells. Note the moderate inflammatory reaction in the underlying dermis. (Original magnification × 180; courtesy of Rudolf Garret, M.D.)

and next in the groin, scalp, face, neck, axillae, and genitals. It appears that an autoimmune mechanism is the cause. The condition occurs equally in both sexes, usually in adults in their fifth and sixth decades. Circulating intercellular antibodies may be demonstrated in these individuals.

The pathologic changes are acantholysis, cleft and blister formation in the intraepidermal areas just above the basal cell layer, and the formation of acantholytic cells (Figure 19-12).[87] Characteristic of the separation of keratinocytes is the presence of Tzanck's cell lining the bulla, as well as lying free in the cavity.

Because of the pain associated with advanced cases, prolonged daily baths with permanganate solution may be advised. Silver sulfadiazine (Silvadene) cream, which is effective in the treatment of burns, is also useful in this condition. High-dose corticosteroids (160 mg of prednisone daily) remain the primary therapy. Immunosuppressive agents, such as azathioprine, cyclophosphamide, cyclosporine, and methotrexate, are part of the multimodality approach, which may include antibiotics, antimalarials, gold, and plasmapheresis.

Cicatricial Pemphigoid or Benign Mucosal Pemphigoid

Cicatricial pemphigoid is characterized by the presence of transient vesicles that heal by scarring of mucous membranes. The condition most commonly occurs in the mouth and conjunctivae. Other areas of involvement include the pharynx, esophagus, genitalia, and anus. In rare cases, the lesion has been confined to the genital and anal areas.[143] Direct immunofluorescence of the lesion reveals the presence of antibodies at the basement membrane. The absence of acantholysis differentiates the condition from pemphigus vulgaris.

There is no effective medication for cicatricial pemphigoid. Obstructing areas in the larynx and esophagus may require tracheostomy or gastrostomy.

INFECTIOUS CONDITIONS

For the purposes of discussion, I have taken the liberty of classifying the infectious processes as those that are nonvenereal and those that are usually attributable to venereal causes.

Nonvenereal Infections

Pilonidal Sinus

Pilonidal sinus is a common infective process occurring in the natal cleft and sacrococcygeal region. It primarily affects young adults and teenagers. There is a 3:1 male predominance. In the military in particular, it has been a considerable source of concern with regard to personnel and economics. For example, more than 77,000 soldiers were admitted to army hospitals for symptoms from pilonidal sinus disease from 1942 through 1945, and they remained for an average of 44 days.[218] In 1973, more than 70,000 patients were admitted to nongovernmental hospitals in the

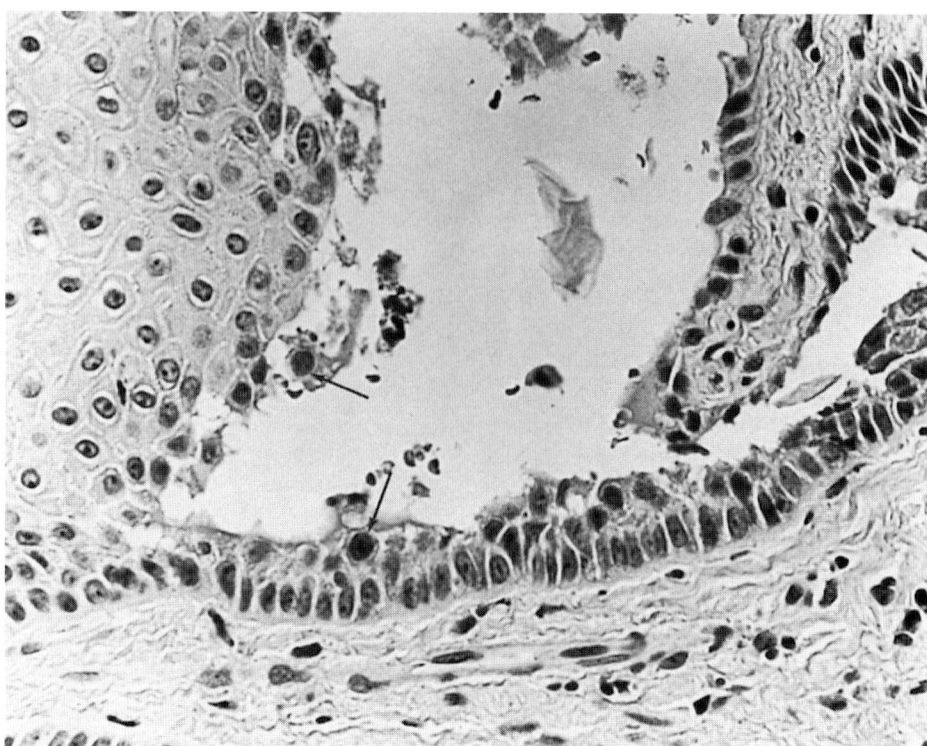

FIGURE 19-12. Intraepithelial vesicles such as this one are characteristic of pemphigus vulgaris. The *arrows* indicate cells with large hyperchromatic nuclei (Tzanck's cells). There is an absence of inflammatory reaction in the dermis. (Original magnification × 600.)

United States with the primary diagnosis of a pilonidal sinus.[174] As recently as 1980, more than 40,000 patients with pilonidal disease were hospitalized in the United States, averaging more than 5 days of in-hospital care.[21] Of course, this was before government and insurance company restrictions were applied concerning permissible days in the hospital for a given illness.

The condition was originally described by Anderson in a letter to the editor of the *Boston Medical Surgical Journal* of 1847 and was subsequently named "pilonidal sinus" by Hodges in 1880.[12,132] The term literally means "nest of hair"; this is because the epithelium-lined sinus usually is found to contain hair.

When the sinus becomes infected, commonly after puberty, it drains from an opening or openings overlying the coccyx and sacrum (Figure 19-13). The infected abscess may extend to the perianal area in a presentation that may be mistaken for anal fistula. The disease can also be confused with suppurative hidradenitis. Although the condition is by no means life-threatening, it does cause considerable disability for many individuals. Time lost from school or work can amount to months.

Abraham Wendell Anderson (1804–1876)   Anderson was born in Windham, Maine, the son of the first settlers in the town. He attended Gorham Academy and in 1829 graduated from Bowdoin Medical School. He established his practice in the town of Gray Corner, where he remained all his life. In 1868, he participated in the founding of the Cumberland County Medical Society and was elected its first president. In his letter, Anderson reports a 21-year-old man with what was thought to be a scrofulous sore on his back.[12] The author found "a fistula opening near the os coccygis," which he drained. Three weeks later, he drew out of the cavity "a hair, very finely matted, and about two inches in length." The discharge stopped, and the wound healed rapidly.

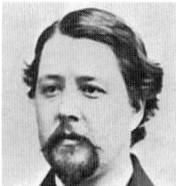

Richard Manning Hodges (1827–1896)   Hodges was born in Bridgewater, Massachusetts. He graduated from Harvard College in the class of 1847 and subsequently received his M.A. and M.D. at Harvard Medical School. He then joined the faculty there in the Department of Anatomy as a demonstrator, a position he held until 1861. He was befriended by the renowned Boston surgeon Henry Bigelow, who helped launch him toward a successful career in surgery. Hodges served on the Board of Overseers of Harvard College and as a visiting surgeon at the Massachusetts General Hospital and was a member of the American Academy of Arts and Sciences. Although many of his writings were on orthopedics and trauma, it is because of his article, read before the Boston Society for Medical Improvement, in which he names the condition "pilonidal sinus" that he is recognized today.

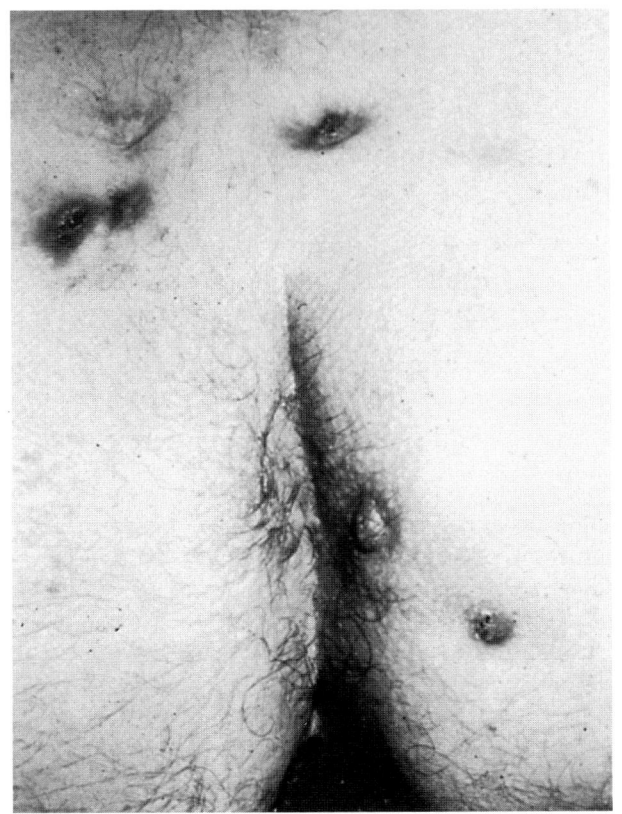

FIGURE 19-13. Pilonidal sinus. Note the multiple openings overlying the sacrum and buttocks.

Etiology

The etiology of the condition has been the subject of some controversy and discussion. One possible theory that has been espoused is the failure of fusion in the embryo, with resultant entrapment of hair follicles in the sacrococcygeal region. Proponents of this theory are quick to point out the frequent incidence of eyebrow hair that meets in the midline in such patients. Another theory attributes the problem to the result of trauma, with the introduction of hair shafts into the subdermal area.

Lord observed a number of interesting features of the condition.[172] He believed that there was a constant relationship between the lateral sinus openings and the midline pits; the openings were always cephalad to the pits. Lord further observed the presence of 23 hairs of exactly the same length, diameter, color, and orientation in a patient. He postulated that it would be impossible for this number of hairs to follow each other into a pilonidal sinus and be identical in every respect. Lord applied this observation by proposing that the treatment of pilonidal sinus could therefore be made quite simple. He suggested that all that is required is the removal of the offending hair follicle and the hairs that have been shed. These observations were subsequently confirmed by Bascom, a concept that led to his proposed surgical approach (see later).[21]

Symptoms and Findings

The patient usually presents with pain, swelling, and purulent drainage at and around the site of the pilonidal opening. A solitary midline opening or pit may be observed, or there may be numerous openings, with pus draining and hair protruding. The typical appearance of an abscess that can be found anywhere in the skin and subcutaneous tissue may be evident. Fever and leukocytosis may also accompany the symptoms.

Most individuals may merely observe periodic discharge or intermittent swelling and discomfort. The process may resolve spontaneously or progress to more obvious drainage, an abscess, and severe pain. Long-standing disease may be associated with the development of squamous cell carcinoma (see later). A critical symptom, *bleeding* in a sinus that has been present for many years, warrants special attention and surgical intervention.[268] An association with condylomata and human immunodeficiency virus (HIV) has also been described with squamous cell cancer.[34] Other reported complications of the condition are sacral osteomyelitis, necrotizing fasciitis, toxic shock syndrome, and meningitis.[258,268]

Treatment

As with other septic processes in the perianal area, antibiotics have little place in the therapy, except possibly as an adjunct to the surgical procedure in a septic or immunocompromised patient. For acute pilonidal abscess, incision and drainage should relieve the patient's symptoms. Regardless of the size of the septic process, this can usually be accomplished in a physician's office or in an ambulatory care facility. Whenever possible, it is advisable to drain the abscess and curette or excise the infected sinus simultaneously. The Standards Task Force of the American Society of Colon and Rectal Surgeons has established certain practice parameters for the performance of ambulatory surgery.[239] The following represents their complete statement:

> Localized pilonidal abscesses, either primary or recurrent, can usually be incised and drained under local anesthesia in an outpatient setting. For uncomplicated pilonidal sinuses, definitive surgical treatment, including but not limited to excision, curettage, and unroofing, can be accomplished as an outpatient procedure. More complicated surgical procedures, including but not limited to wide excision, creation of skin flaps, and grafting, may require inpatient stay for concern over skin viability or bleeding. Extensive cellulitis in association with pilonidal disease may require inpatient intravenous antibiotic therapy.[239]

Definitive elective treatment of pilonidal disease includes excision and primary closure, excision and grafting, excision leaving the wound open to close secondarily, incision and curettage, follicle excision, and cryosurgical destruction.

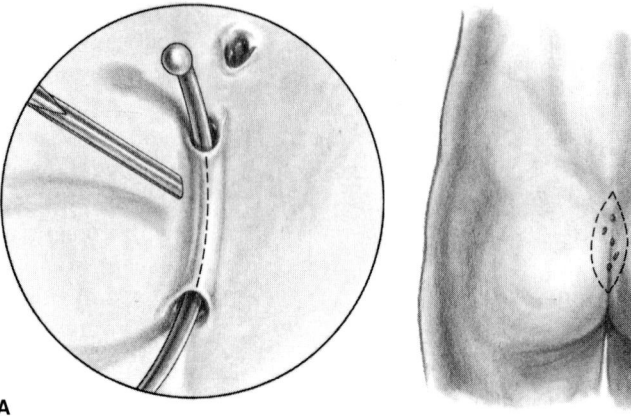

FIGURE 19-14. Excision and packing for the treatment of pilonidal sinus can be accomplished by **(A)** unroofing of the individual tract or by **(B)** an all-encompassing excision.

A

B

Drainage with or without Excision Incision or excision with drainage is rather simple to accomplish, requires minimal hospital stay, and in fact usually can be accomplished with a local anesthetic in the office. A probe is passed from opening to opening, and the sinus is unroofed (Figure 19-14A). Alternatively, the multiple openings can be excised *en bloc,* with further extensions or side tracts curetted out (Figure 19-14B). If the procedure is undertaken on an ambulatory basis, the patient is instructed to remove the packing the following morning, usually while taking a bath.

Shpitz and colleagues perform what they term a "controlled excision" by means of loop diathermy.[226] The procedure consists of incision and drainage of any pus, followed by excision of diseased tissue and lateral sinuses. With this approach, an expeditious surgical procedure and a shortened or eliminated hospital stay are, in essence, exchanged for a prolonged postoperative convalescence, especially if one is dealing with extensive or deep tissue involvement. All too often, these difficult wounds require frequent treatments, necessitating cauterization, shaving, cleansing, and packing. An approach to dealing with this problem has been suggested by Rosenberg.[219] He advocates taping the buttocks apart to flatten the intergluteal cleft during the healing process. However, there is little existing evidence to support the use of antimicrobial agents for chronic wound healing.[197]

It is not uncommon for pilonidal sinus wounds that extend toward the anal verge to take 6 months or longer to heal (Figure 19-15). Delayed healing may persist to the point where reexcision is advised; multiple operative procedures are frequent sequelae under these circumstances. It is for this reason that I am reluctant to advise this particular approach except for relatively small sinuses.

A more recent option for the management of a complex or large pilonidal sinus is *vacuum-assisted closure.*[181] This is a subatmospheric pressure dressing that consists of a foam pad cut to the internal shape of the wound and inserted with a plastic fenestrated tube applied to the center.[181] In theory, the vacuum device assists wound contraction by exerting a centripetal force and increases blood flow while reducing edema and tissue bacterial counts.[181] Disadvantages include the initial hospital charges, the relative immobility of the patient, and the cost associated with the use of the pump.

Marsupialization Excision with marsupialization is a compromise between a completely open wound and a completely closed one. This approach was initially described by Buie in 1937 and amplified later in his article on "jeep disease."[44] This operation permits a somewhat smaller opening than does the technique in which the wound is left totally open (Figure 19-16). If the catgut or long-term absorbable suture succeeds in holding the edges together, more rapid healing should occur. Unfortunately, the sutures frequently pull out, and the individual is left with as wide a wound as would have resulted had excision and packing been employed. Even without this complication, the wound still requires careful attention, including packing, shaving, and cleansing.

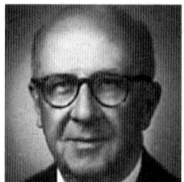

Louis A. Buie (1890–1975) Buie was born in Kingstree, South Carolina and received his bachelor's degree from the University of South Carolina in 1911. He graduated from the University of Maryland Medical School, and after internship in Maryland he entered the Mayo Clinic as a Fellow in Surgery. Following service in Italy during World War I, he returned to the Mayo Clinic and, at the request of William J. Mayo, established the Section of Proctology. A founder of the American Board of Proctology and twice president of the American Proctologic Society, he played a leading role in the development of proctology and, later, of colon and rectal surgery as a specialty in the United States. Other contributions included designs of a sigmoidoscope, proctoscopic table, and biopsy forceps. In addition, he authored or coauthored three texts on proctology and was a founder of the journal *Diseases of the Colon and Rectum,* serving as its editor-in-chief from 1957 to 1967. An international authority in the field, he was perhaps best known for his writings and treatment of pilonidal sinus.

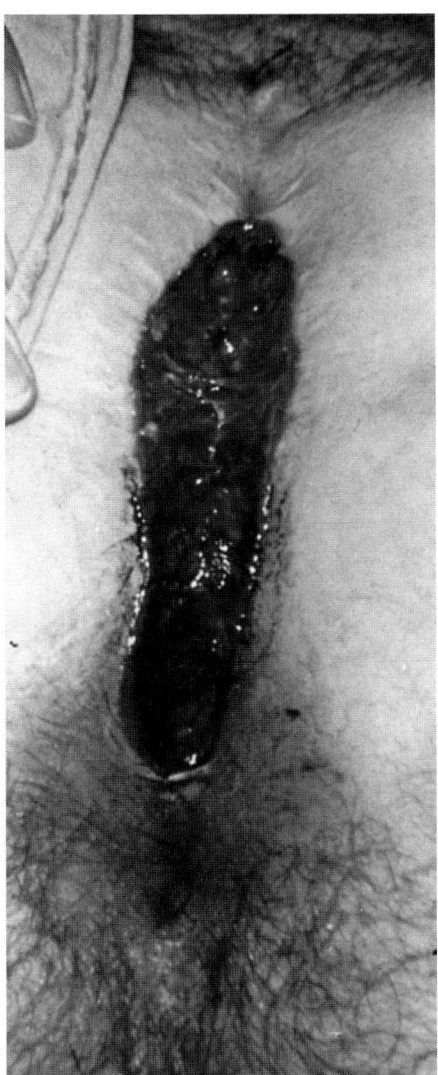

FIGURE 19-15. Indolent, granulating, nonhealing wound of a recurrent (persistent) pilonidal sinus.

complex pilonidal sinus problems, particularly when multiple procedures have been performed (Figure 19-15), the excision and primary closure technique may be very effective.

The pilonidal sinus is excised to the gluteal fascia (Figure 19-17A). The fascia is incised, and a periosteal elevator is used to lift the fascia off the sacrum (Figure 19-17B). This maneuver permits the placement of heavy retention sutures through all layers. These are laid into position, and the fascia is reapproximated with absorbable suture material (Figure 19-18A). The wound is copiously irrigated, and the skin is closed (Figure 19-18B). The retention sutures are secured over a stent dressing, and the dressing is left in place for approximately 10 days (Figure 19-18C). When the pilonidal sinus extends near the anal opening, it is better to confine the bowels for several days. This requires a clear liquid diet and the use of a bowel-confining regimen—deodorized tincture of opium, diphenoxylate hydrochloride, and codeine (see Chapter 13).

Excision with Grafting With considerable skin loss, as may occur following multiple operations, or as a primary procedure, it is sometimes useful to rotate skin flaps to cover the resultant wound defect.[126] This can be performed using the principles described in Chapter 8, advancement or rotation flaps (see Anoplasty for Severe Stenosis), or even, as has been suggested, by means of a gluteus maximus myocutaneous flap.[203] To eliminate the deep natal cleft and the conventional vertical wound, which tends to pull apart, some surgeons recommend a Z-plasty.[35,150,174,180,185–187,253] Others suggest excision in a rhomboid fashion, with coverage effected by means of a so-called Limberg buttock flap (Figure 19-19).[11,252,257] Another modification of the rhomboid flap design is the so-called Dufourmentel technique.[175] In the Z-plasty, the depth of the intergluteal fold with the associated pilonidal sinus disease is excised; skin flaps are then mobilized, rotated, and interdigitated (Figure 19-20).

Karydakis described a technique for limiting the likelihood of recurrence following excision of pilonidal sinus by means of a variation of excision with primary closure and grafting in more than 6,000 patients.[146] By this technique, each sinus is completely excised through a vertical, eccentric, elliptical incision. A thick flap is created by undermining the medial edge and advancing it across the midline so that the whole suture line is lateralized in order to reduce the risk for recurrence.[152]

Oncel and co-workers undertook a prospective, randomized study in which 40 consecutive patients with "limited, chronic pilonidal disease" were operated on with either excision or marsupialization.[198] Operation time, hospital stay, and time lost from work were all shorter in the former group. Furthermore, patient satisfaction was significantly greater in this group, primarily because the procedure was undertaken on an outpatient basis.

Excision with Primary Closure Excision with primary closure can be performed in an ambulatory surgical facility if the sinus is relatively small. However, for more extensive lesions, inpatient therapy is recommended. This approach has the disadvantage of a relatively prolonged hospital stay, but it provides the potential benefit of a healed wound within perhaps 10 to 14 days. For large,

Sinus Extraction The importance of avoiding the creation of a midline incision has been emphasized by Lord and Bascom.[21,22,172] This approach consists of lateral drainage of the abscess, removal of the hair, and excision

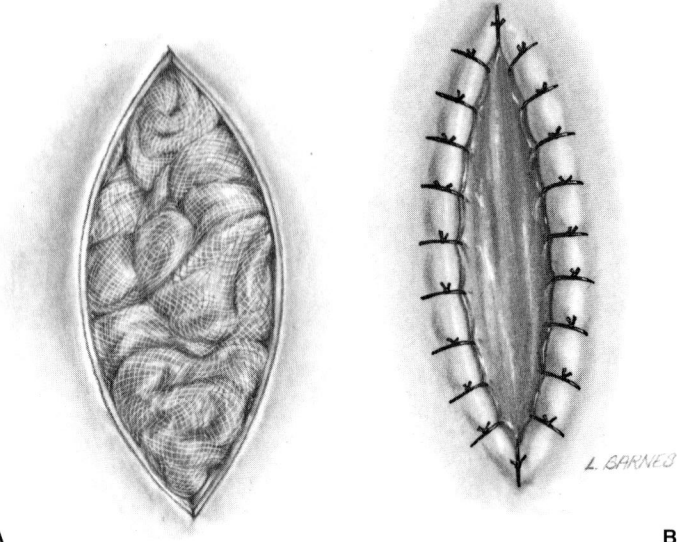

FIGURE 19-16. Appearance of the pilonidal sinus after two different surgical approaches: **(A)** open and packed, usually with iodoform gauze, and **(B)** marsupialized, suturing the full thickness of the skin to the underlying epithelialized tract or fascia.   **A**   **B**

of the hair follicle (if present). Minimal excision of a sinus tract may be performed. The cavity is cleansed through incisions adjacent to but not inside the pilonidal sinus. The cavity walls are not excised but are permitted to collapse. The procedure may be carried out in the office or at an ambulatory surgical facility. An alternative approach is to drain the acute abscess and allow the infection to subside before follicle removal is attempted.[22] According to Bascom, the enlarged follicles should be excised individually, leaving only small midline wounds, 2 to 4 mm in diameter (Figure 19-21).[22] Alternatively, these may be closed primarily to reduce healing time.

This technique may be analogous to that of the management of a "horseshoe" fistula, in which one endeavors

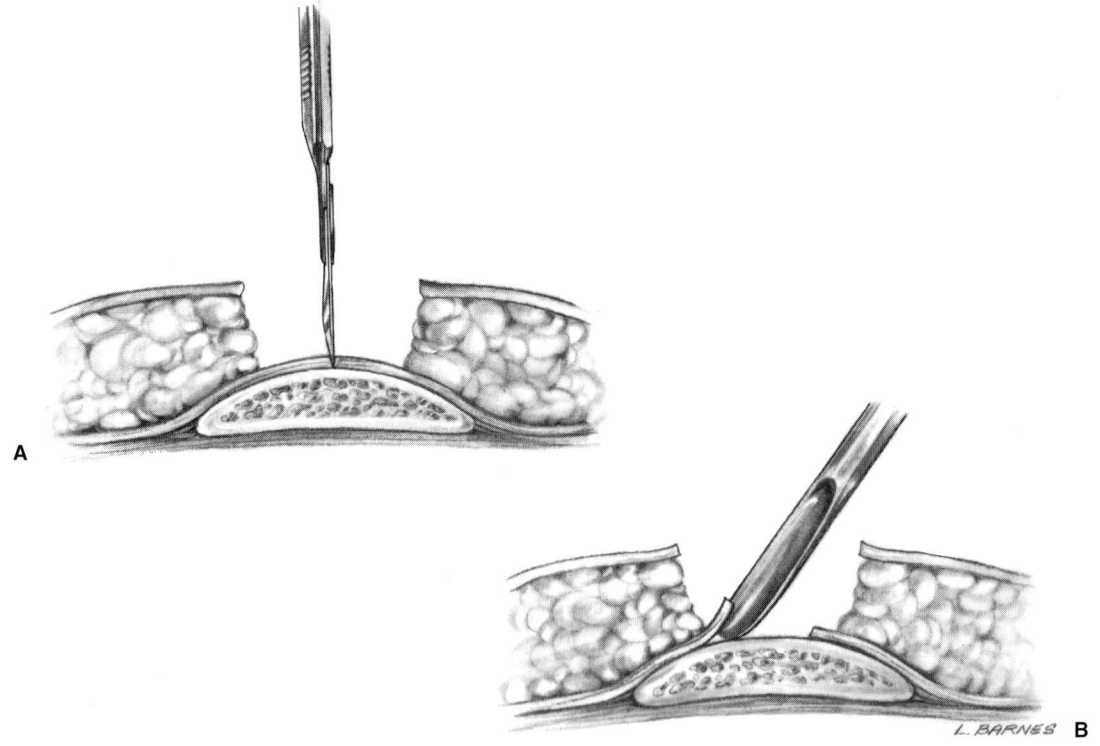

FIGURE 19-17. The first two steps in the primary closure technique for the treatment of pilonidal sinus infection. **(A)** The fascia is incised. **(B)** The fascia is elevated.

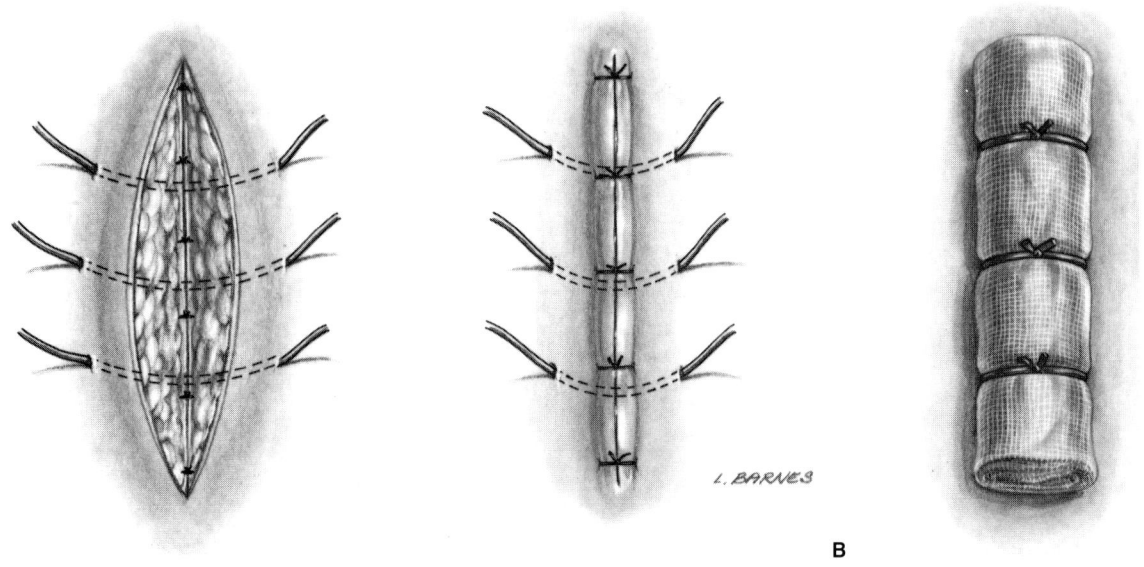

A   **B**   **C**

FIGURE 19-18. The last three steps in the primary closure technique for treating pilonidal sinus infection. **(A)** With retention sutures in place, the fascia is closed. **(B)** The skin is closed. **(C)** A stent dressing is secured.

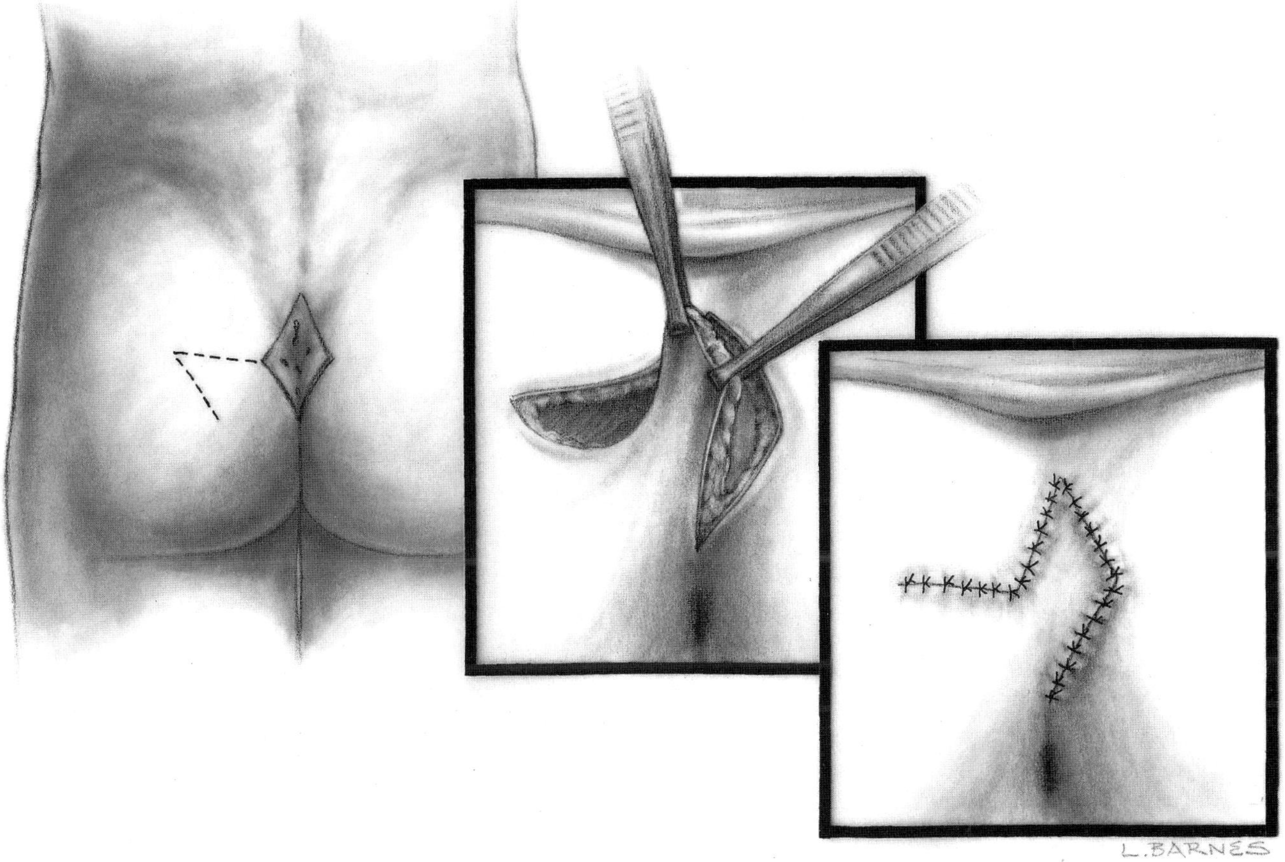

FIGURE 19-19. Pilonidal sinus treated by excision with a rhomboid design and a Limberg flap.

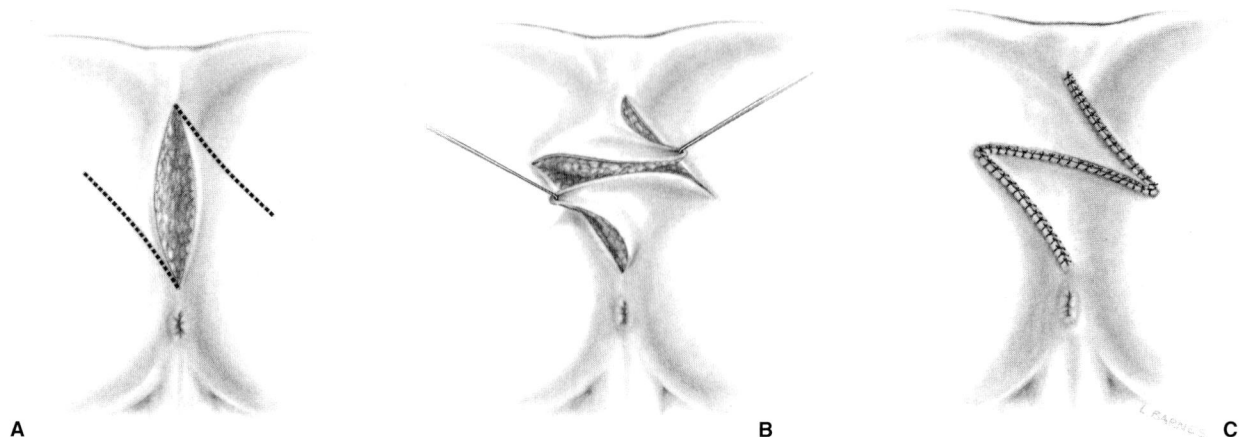

A   B   C

FIGURE 19-20. Treatment of pilonidal sinus by Z-plasty. **(A)** Incisions outlined. **(B)** Skin flaps rotated. **(C)** Primary closure obliterates the natal cleft defect.

merely to remove the crypt-bearing area and establish adequate drainage. Certainly, if one can accomplish this satisfactorily, healing will result with minimal deformity. The same "less is more" approach appears equally valid for selected instances of pilonidal sinus.

Sclerosing Injection Hegge and colleagues suggest a "conservative" approach to the treatment of pilonidal disease, injection of phenol (80%) into the sinus tract.[129] The procedure was carried out on 48 patients after they had undergone minimal drainage and hair removal. They were considered cured if there was no evidence of recurrent disease within 1 year of treatment. The authors reported a low recurrence rate—only 6.3%.

Cryosurgery The use of cryosurgical destruction has also been advocated in the surgical management of pilonidal sinus.[119,195] The technique consists of surgery (opening of the tracts and side branches), curettage, and electrocoagulation of bleeding points. The open wound is then sprayed with liquid nitrogen for approximately 5 minutes.

I have had no experience with this technique, but O'Connor has stated that there is less deformity and scarring than with a wider excision.[195] However, because it has been generally recognized that a wide excision is not a necessary part of the treatment, the comparison may be inappropriate.

Nonoperative Management As previously mentioned, the military has been quite concerned about the lost time associated with the surgical management of pilonidal sinus and its adverse consequences. Armstrong and Barcia examined the role of conservative, nonoperative treatment of pilonidal sinus disease at an army community hospital.[17] Complete healing over 83 occupied-bed days was observed in 101 consecutive cases managed through meticulous

hair control by natal cleft shaving, improved perineal hygiene, and limited lateral incision and drainage for abscess. This was compared with 4,760 occupied bed-days in 229 patients who had undergone 240 operative procedures during the previous 2 years. The prolonged hospitalization was explained by the army basic trainee population, who, by regulation, could not be discharged from the hospital until they were fit for duty. The authors further observed

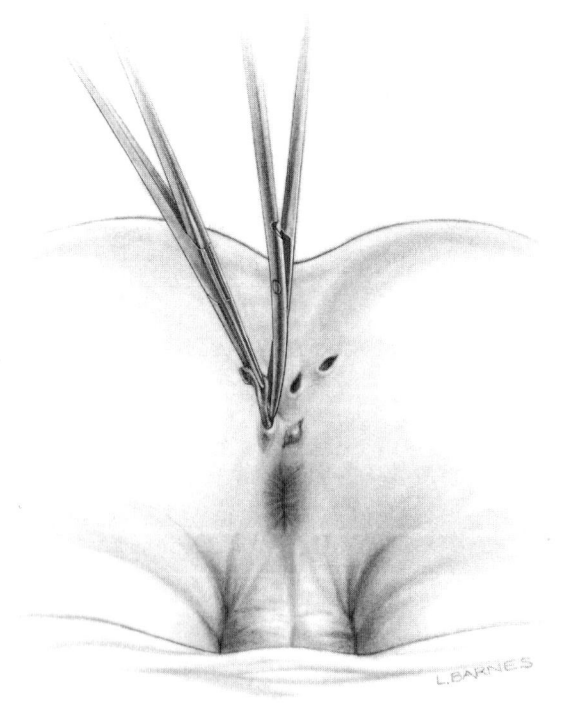

FIGURE 19-21. Pilonidal sinus excision by extraction technique (Bascom's). Each individual sinus opening is excised. The midline wounds are closed whenever possible, leaving the lateral wounds open to drain.

that with the application of conservative treatment over 17 years, only 23 excisional operations were performed.

Results of the Various Methods of Management

It is interesting to note that almost irrespective of the method of treatment applied, very few patients are troubled with symptoms of persistent pilonidal sinus disease beyond the age of 40 years. Perhaps one simply outgrows the condition. It is, therefore, important to understand that ultimate cure is an almost inevitable result when one compares the value of the various surgical alternatives. Another problem with analyzing the data is that there are very few so-called prospective, randomized, controlled studies that can survive critical review. One such report by Fùzun and colleagues randomly compared primary closure with excision in 110 consecutive patients.[117] Although primary closure was associated with hospital stays significantly longer than those in the open-treatment group, the patients returned to work significantly earlier. The primary closure group also had an increased risk for infection and a higher recurrence rate (4.1% versus 0%). The authors concluded that both treatments have their place. Therefore, the recommendation should be based on individual preference, especially employment status. Others concur in uncontrolled studies that the primary advantage of the closed techniques over open drainage is more rapid recovery, but this must be balanced against the risk of infection.[199,238]

Incision or Excision and Drainage Hanley has been an advocate of emergency surgery for acute pilonidal abscess by excision and open treatment.[127] With this technique, he reported uniform healing with no evidence of recurrence in a small group of patients. Jensen and Harling performed simple incision and drainage of 73 consecutive individuals who presented with an acute pilonidal abscess.[140] Healing *per primam* occurred in 42 (58%) within 10 weeks. The recurrence rate following initial primary healing was, however, 21%. The authors further observed that those with fewer pits and lateral tracts had a statistically significantly better chance of healing primarily. There is agreement in all current writings that wide excision of all tissue down to the sacrum, leaving the wound to heal by granulation, cannot be justified.[9]

Excision and Marsupialization This is still one of the most commonly employed options for the treatment of pilonidal sinus. Solla and Rothenberger reported that 125 of their 150 patients were so managed.[237] The average healing time was 4 weeks, with three individuals requiring up to 20 weeks for closure. The recurrence rate was 6%, all ultimately healing following remarsupialization.

Excision with Primary Closure Zimmerman reported outpatient excision and primary closure in 32 patients.[272]

Follow-up was for a mean of 24 months. In all cases, primary healing was obtained, a result that is not dissimilar to my own experience. In addition, Obeid noted primary healing in all 27 individuals managed by a modification of the primary closure technique illustrated in Figures 19-17 and 19-18.[194] Kronborg and colleagues reported the results of a randomized trial of treatment by one of three methods: excision, excision with suture, and excision with suture and antibiotic coverage with clinda-mycin.[157] Recurrence rates were, respectively, 13%, 25%, and 19%. As expected, healing was much quicker after primary suture than after excisional therapy alone (median, 14 days versus 64 days). Tritapepe and Di Padova reported 243 consecutive patients who underwent excision and primary closure with the use of a closed suction drain for 24 hours, followed by wound irrigation with an antiseptic solution.[254] With a follow-up of 5 to 15 years, there were no wound breakdowns and no recurrences.

Peterson and colleagues undertook a metaanalysis of data published over a period of 35 years with various primary closure techniques.[204] Seventy-four publications included a total of 10,090 patients. These investigators concluded that there appears to be a significant benefit with respect to healing when the asymmetric-oblique closure or the full-thickness flap technique is employed when compared with midline closure.[204]

Excision and Grafting Reports of the success of excision and grafting are somewhat difficult to interpret in light of the lack of a control in these studies.[126,174] In the report from the Cleveland Clinic in Ohio, 58 patients were reviewed who underwent extensive or recurrent pilonidal disease surgery with primary skin grafting.[126] More than 72% had recurrent disease when initially seen. The average hospital stay was 10 days, and the time lost from work averaged 28 days. The recurrence rate was 1.7%, and the failure rate was 3.4%. Using the Z-plasty technique, Mansoory and Dickson treated 120 patients.[174] There were two recurrences, a very favorable experience. Alver and colleagues reported 35 selected individuals with "small and moderate extent disease" treated by the fasciocutaneous Limberg flap method.[11] The rate of wound infection or dehiscence was 17%, with all individuals ultimately healing. Urhan and co-workers initially reported 110 Limberg flap procedures with five recurrences (4.9%),[257] with no further failures when 90 later patients were added.[252] Manterola and colleagues utilized the similar Dufourmentel technique in 25 patients and noted two instances of infection or dehiscence.[175] Kitchen reported 141 patients treated by the Karydakis operation and noted a recurrence rate of 4%.[152]

When skin is lost as a consequence of pilonidal sinus disease, particularly in the recurrent situation, mobilizing skin to cover the defect will more reliably lead to a satisfactory result. Bascom reported 30 patients with open midline wounds from recurrence.[23] All healed by closure of the natal cleft through the raising of skin flaps.

Sinus Extraction (Lord-Bascom Procedure) Bascom and Edwards reported their experiences with the Lord treatment: removal only of the follicles and hairs.[21,94] In an earlier report, 50 patients were treated in the office, and local anesthesia was used. Acute abscesses were treated by excision of the enlarged follicles from the midline skin. One to ten follicles were removed, individually if possible. Because incisions were kept smaller than 7 mm, the specimens weighed less than 1 g per patient. Follow-up averaged 24 months. The mean disability was 1 day, and the mean wound healing time was 3 weeks. Recurrences appeared in four patients (8%); all were healed 3 weeks following reoperation. There was no incident of a second recurrence. A later publication by Bascom of 161 patients so treated revealed comparable results.[22]

Edwards reported 102 patients treated by this technique.[94] The median number of days lost from work was 10, and the median number of days requiring healing was 39. Eighty-nine percent of these patients were free of recurrent disease provided they attended the follow-up clinic. Because some patients failed to attend, it is difficult to interpret the results of this study. It appears, however, that the author was not as successful as Bascom.

Senapati and associates performed 218 Bascom's operations as day cases.[225] Ten percent developed recurrences requiring reoperation. Theodoropoulos and colleagues opine, on the basis of their experience with this operation in a military hospital, that this operation is safe, with minimal morbidity, and can be reliably used as a second-line alternative for recurrent disease.[250]

Comment It is now generally agreed that minimal surgery should be applied to the treatment of pilonidal disease whenever possible. The concept of Lord and of Bascom in removing the hair follicles and the hairs themselves without extensive excision and debridement is an excellent one. Every attempt should be made to keep the patient out of the hospital and to limit the morbidity of the procedure. However, there are some individuals who will benefit from a more generous excision, particularly those who have undergone multiple procedures or have extensive disease. Under these circumstances, inpatient hospital treatment with excision and primary closure, with or without grafting, may offer a lower morbidity, shortened convalescence, and more rapid healing.

Pilonidal Sinus and Squamous Cell Carcinoma

Squamous cell carcinoma has been reported to arise in pilonidal sinus tracts, almost all inevitably involving long-standing active inflammation. Fasching and colleagues reviewed 36 cases that they identified in the literature.[105] As of 1996, there were 44 reported.[75] Treat-

ment consisted of wide excision and grafting. This is similar to the management of squamous cell carcinoma of the skin anywhere in the body that can lend itself to this approach. More recently, it has been suggested that because of the high recurrence rate of the malignancy, consideration should be given to adjuvant chemotherapy and radiation.[75,159]

Suppurative Hidradenitis or Hidradenitis Suppurativa

Suppurative hidradenitis is an uncommon, chronic, recurrent, indolent infection involving the skin and subcutaneous tissue arising in the apocrine glands (i.e., axillary, inguinal, genital, perineal, and mammary). The most frequent area of involvement is the axilla. The condition was originally described in 1839 by Velpeau.[259] The incidence is increased in women, with most cases occurring between the ages of 16 and 40 years, but most studies of operated cases affecting the perineum indicate a larger number of men.

Etiology

Suppurative hidradenitis does not occur before puberty because it is believed that the effect of sex hormones on the apocrine glands is the inciting factor. An androgen-based endocrine disorder has also been postulated. Harrison and colleagues demonstrated an androgen excess and a progesterone decrease through detailed hormonal profiles in 36 women and 14 controls.[128] Although the etiology is unknown, acne appears to be a predisposing factor, with stress, poor skin hygiene, obesity, excessive heat, hyperhidrosis, and chemical depilatories possibly playing a role.[61] There has been no documentation of an increased association with diabetes mellitus, but impaired glucose tolerance has been observed. There may be a genetic predisposition based on an increased familial incidence. Some observe an increased frequency in those with Crohn's disease, irritable bowel syndrome, herpes simplex, certain kinds of arthritis, and a number of other conditions.

Pathophysiology

Suppurative hidradenitis commences with obstruction of the apocrine gland duct, with resultant inspissated secretions. The gland may then rupture, which can lead to extension of the process into the dermis, with consequent secondary involvement of other glands and ducts. In rare instances, the process can extend through the fascia into the underlying muscle.

Differential Diagnosis

The condition may be confused with anal fistula, Crohn's disease, tuberculosis, pilonidal sinus, infected sebaceous cyst, furunculosis, granuloma inguinale, lymphogranuloma venereum, and other infections in the

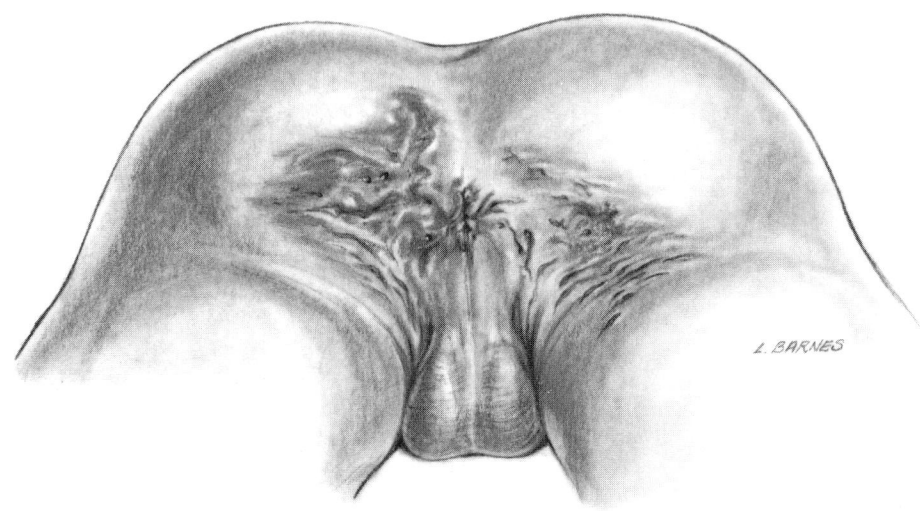

FIGURE 19-22. Artist's concept of suppurative hidradenitis with extensive involvement of perianal area and buttocks.

anal area. In cases in which the disease is of long standing, squamous cell carcinoma may develop.[42]

Physical Examination

Examination reveals painful, tender, erythematous, purulent lesions (Figure 19-22). These may be associated with adenopathy and systemic signs (i.e., fever, malaise, leukocytosis). The condition frequently produces burrowing sinuses that can extend for many inches around the anus, into the scrotum, buttocks, labia, medial thighs, and sacrum (Figure 19-23). Although the tracts are usually relatively superficial, they can actually invade deeply and extend to involve the area around the femoral ves-

sels. Urethral and rectal fistulas have been noted, but these are more likely caused by aggressive surgery rather than aggressive disease.

Histopathology

Microscopically, the earliest inflammatory changes are seen within and around the apocrine glands, the ducts of which may be distended with leukocytes (Figure 19-24). In the chronic stage, multiple abscesses, intercommunicating sinus tracts, and irregular hypertrophied scars form.[52] The scars, ulceration, and infection extend within the subcutaneous tissue to the fascia (Figure 19-25).

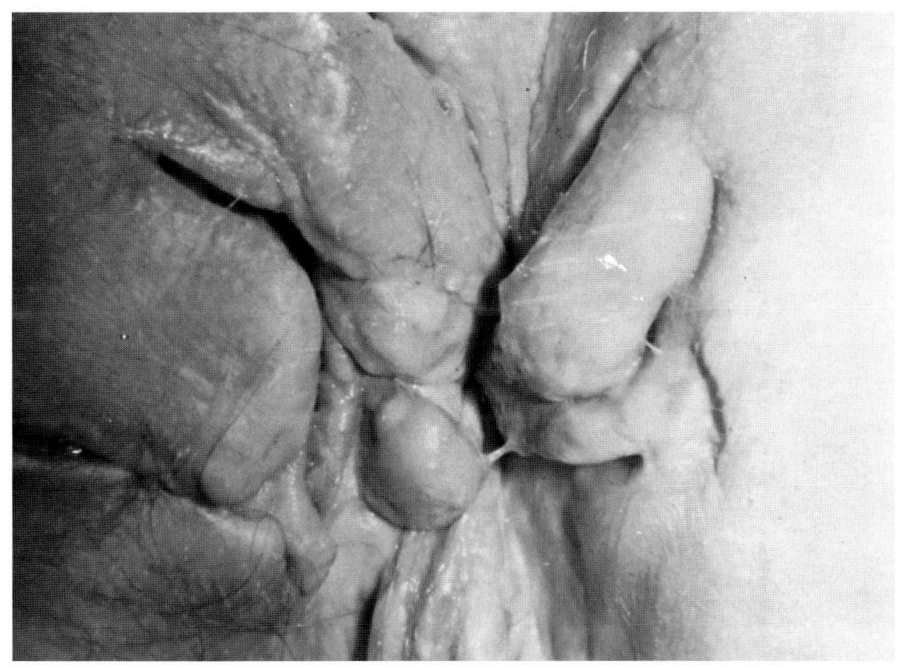

FIGURE 19-23. Suppurative hidradenitis with extensive perianal sinuses.

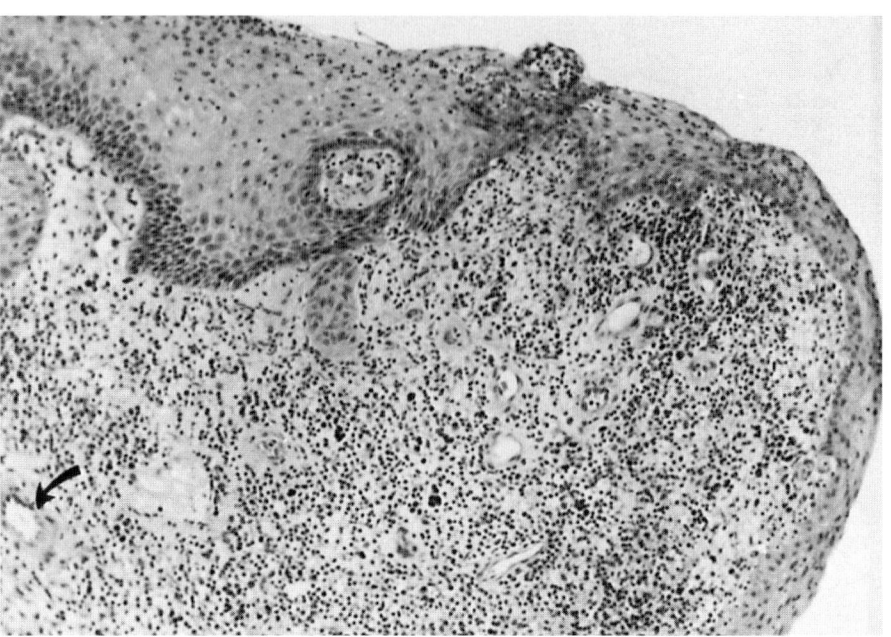

FIGURE 19-24. Suppurative hidradenitis. An apocrine gland *(arrow)* has surrounding inflammation. (Original magnification × 120.)

Treatment

It is generally believed that antibiotic therapy early in the course of the disease is of considerable value. Numerous bacteria have been isolated, including staphylococci, streptococci, *Escherichia coli*, and *Proteus* species. It is interesting to note, however, that in one study, a sample of the drained pus sent for culture and antibiotic sensitivity revealed no growth in approximately one half of the patients.[251] Still, local and systemic broad-spectrum antibiotics are advisable. These include penicillin, erythromycin, clindamycin, and tetracycline in those cases when acne is noted in other areas. The antibiotics should be used until resolution of the process is complete. Some patients require treatment for months or even years. Isotretinoin (Accutane) has been shown to benefit some patients. Unfortunately, there is a group of individuals who do not respond to any medical regimen, and disability is such that surgical intervention is required to treat the extensive sinus tracts and abscesses.

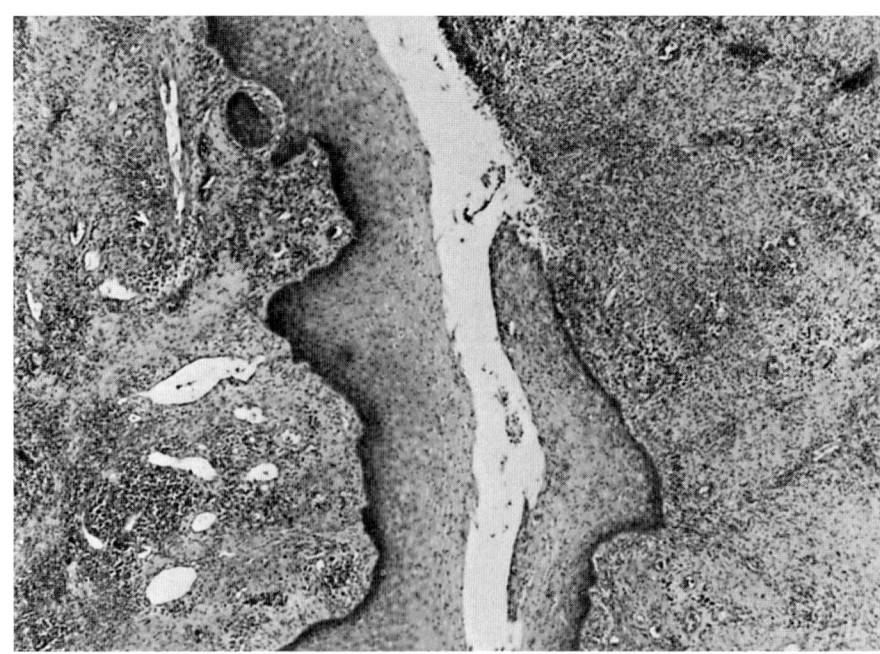

FIGURE 19-25. Suppurative hidradenitis. The sinus tract is lined by squamous epithelium with surrounding acute and chronic inflammation. (Original magnification × 120.)

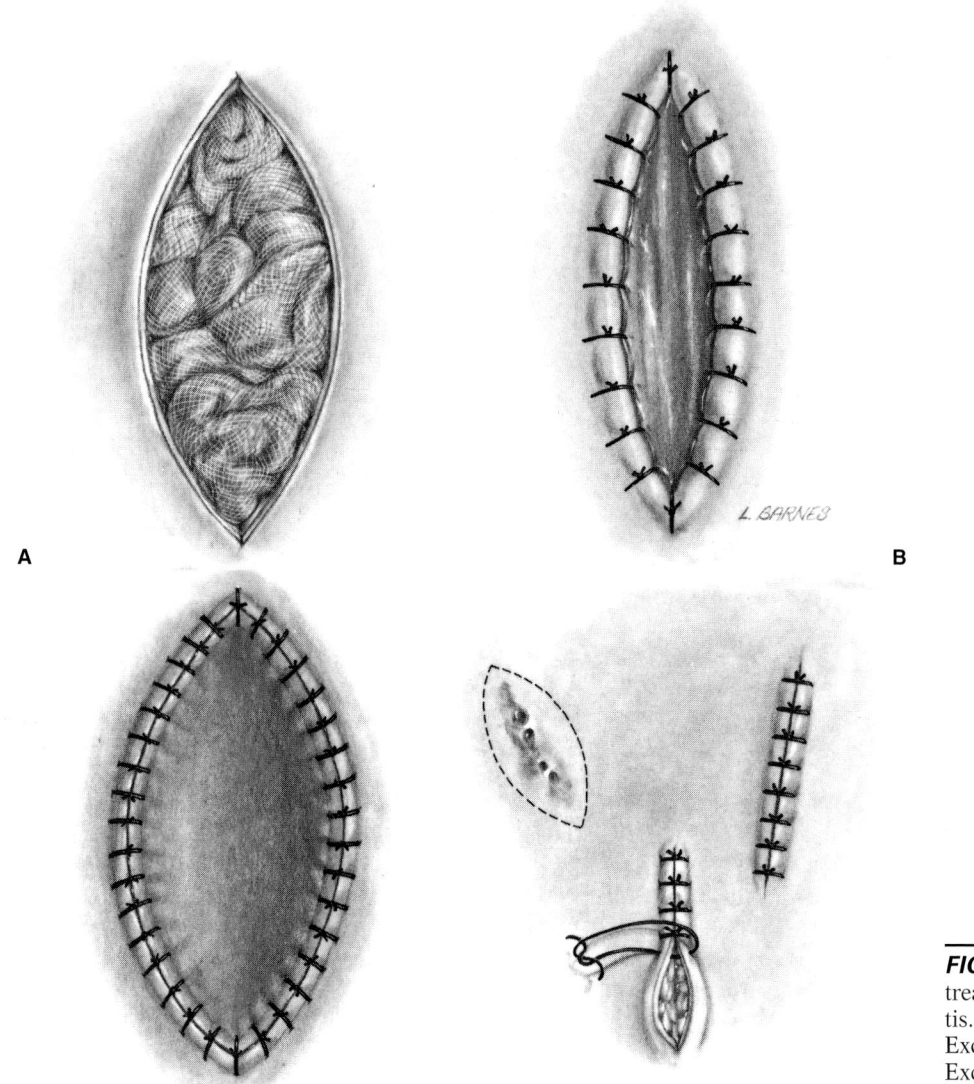

A

B

L. BARNES

C

D

FIGURE 19-26. Four methods of treatment for suppurative hidradenitis. **(A)** Excision with packing. **(B)** Excision with marsupialization. **(C)** Excision with grafting. **(D)** Excision and primary closure.

Operative Approaches With minimal involvement and inadequate palliation by medical means, incision and drainage of an abscess may result in cure. When the condition progresses to extensive sinus formation, excision is the only means by which the condition can be effectively ameliorated.

The four methods of surgical treatment are as follows (Figure 19-26):

1. Excision with primary closure
2. Excision with grafting
3. Excision with marsupialization
4. Excision with packing

All four methods can be applied usefully, even in the same patient. Primary closure usually requires a relatively narrow wound, but often by elevating the full thickness of skin on either side of the excision site, the wound may be approximated without tension. Wide excision, leaving the wound open to heal by second intention, is probably the most common method of surgical treatment. This has the obvious disadvantage of a prolonged healing time (Figure 19-27).

Methods to close the wound include the application of a split-thickness graft or some form of plastic procedure similar to that previously described for pilonidal sinus (e.g., Z-plasty or Limberg's flap).[212] It is certainly preferable to close the wound by some means if this is possible. Occasionally, it is necessary to perform a diverting colostomy if extensive surgery and grafting are required in the perianal area. Fortunately, the anal canal itself is usually spared. Involvement of the sphincter muscle is so unusual that this observation should encourage the surgeon to consider another diagnosis for the problem. Rarely does the disease progress to the point where there

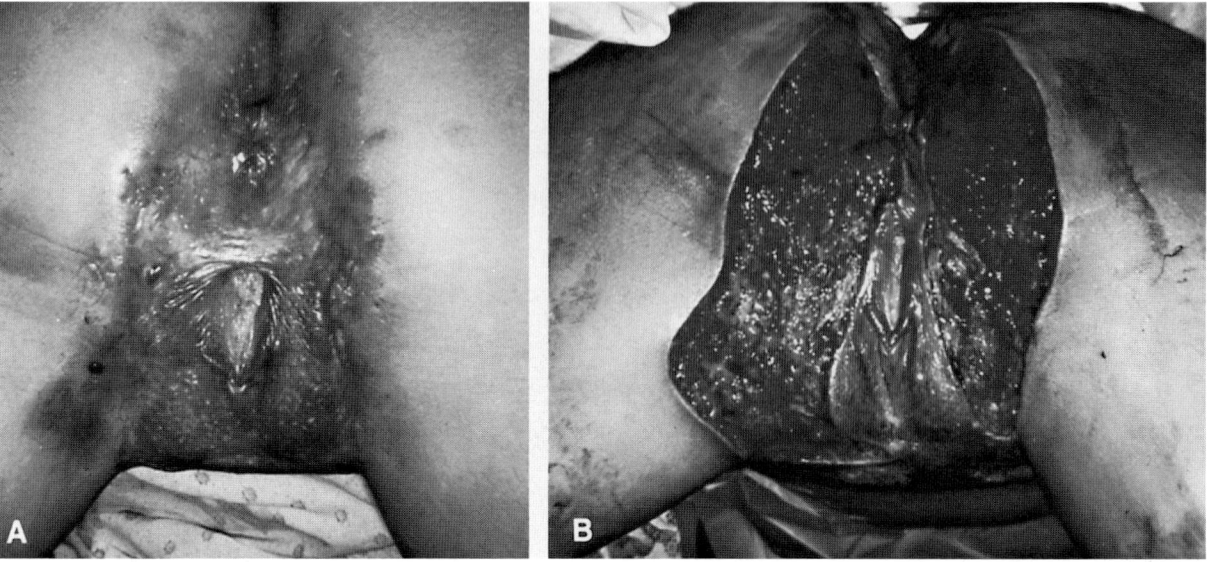

FIGURE 19-27. Suppurative hidradenitis. **(A)** Extensive perineal disease. **(B)** Treatment by wide excision.

is such significant deformity of the anal canal that a permanent colostomy becomes necessary. For those who harbor bilateral, circumferential, or anterior and posterior disease in the perineal area, it may be wise from the perspective of patient discomfort and disability to perform surgery on one side only and to treat the opposite side after healing has taken place.

Results

Culp reported the Mayo Clinic (Rochester, Minnesota) experience with 132 patients observed with anogenital hidradenitis suppurativa during a 6-year period.[69] Of the 30 individuals whose disease was limited to the anal canal and adjacent areas, two thirds were men. Most had undergone previous multiple attempts at surgical drainage or excision. The author commented that although excision with grafting had been used extensively in the past, such a program had not been necessary in recent years. Extensive excision was the method employed in 17 of the 30 patients; the wounds healed within 8 weeks in all cases. A diverting colostomy was not believed to be necessary. There was no recurrence in more than 1 year of follow-up.

Thornton and Abcarian reviewed 104 patients who underwent surgery for the condition at the Cook County Hospital in Chicago.[251] Approximately two thirds were men. The operative procedure for all patients consisted of wide excision down to normal fat or fascia using electrocautery. The wounds were then packed with iodoform gauze, and the patients were followed on a biweekly basis. The average hospital stay was approximately 1 week. However, those more than 40 years old had an av-

erage hospital stay of approximately 19 days. Healing times ranged from approximately 1 month for relatively small wounds to 2 months for larger ones. In four individuals, a recurrence developed.

Broadwater and colleagues reviewed their experience of 23 patients treated between 1967 and 1981.[40] Sixty-one percent were male, the average age was 30 years, and the mean duration of symptoms was in excess of 5 years. The authors' primary treatment included wide and deep excision with selective (i.e., individualized) closure. Although it is difficult to evaluate the reasons for selection of the procedure, the overall recurrence rate in those undergoing primary closure was 30%. Those who underwent excision with application of a split-thickness graft had a 13% incidence of recurrence. In one half of the patients treated by excision, with the wound left open to heal by secondary intention, recurrence developed. However, only four individuals were so treated.

Wiltz and colleagues reviewed the Lahey Clinic (Boston) experience involving 43 individuals.[269] Recurrence developed in two thirds after either wide excision with healing allowed by secondary intention or incision and drainage with or without limited local excision. Jemec reported a very limited cure rate with excision, only 21%.[138] However, patient satisfaction was quite high, implying that even temporary relief through surgical excision is preferable to the chronic draining illness. Others believe that wide excision is the preferred treatment and the one most likely to effect cure.[33]

Banerjee reviewed a number of publications reporting the results of surgical treatment of suppurative hidradenitis and concluded that no method satisfies all requirements for the ideal treatment.[18] Furthermore, good reports of the relative cure rates of the different surgical options are scarce, with controlled trials nonexistent. He considered that the preferred option in most instances is wide local excision, with healing taking place by secondary intention.[18]

Comment Suppurative hidradenitis is a complicated condition to treat, and the approach to each case must be individualized. My own preference, whenever possible, is to excise and to perform primary closure of relatively small areas of involvement. I am reluctant to embark on various plastic procedures because of my discomfort with opening up planes of dissection in the presence of known sepsis. For large lesions, I prefer to excise widely and marsupialize or leave the area to granulate. In some situations with extensive involvement, one may consider the application of a split-thickness graft 4 or 5 days after initial excision or a grafting maneuver to expedite the healing process. In my experience, the length of time for healing is considerable. Repeated operations may also be required for extension of the disease process that was inapparent at the time of the initial procedure.

Anorectal Abscess and Anal Fistula

Anorectal abscess and fistula (Figure 19-28) are perianal infective processes that may be confused with pilonidal sinus and suppurative hidradenitis. Chapters 10 and 11 are dedicated to the diagnosis and management of these conditions.

Crohn's Disease

Anal and perianal Crohn's disease presents a difficult management problem (see Figs. 11-43 and 11-48). This condition is discussed in Chapter 11, and the diagnosis and management of Crohn's disease are presented in Chapter 30.

Tuberculosis

Tuberculosis distal to the ileocecal valve is uncommon, and it is seldom even considered in the differential diagnosis when the disease process is located in the large intestine.[125] When it affects the perianal area, it can be confused with Crohn's disease, actinomycosis, anal fistula, colloid carcinoma, sarcoidosis, and other skin conditions. Anal fistula is the most frequent presentation of anorectal tuberculosis (80% to 90%), but there are no obvious distinguishing characteristics from that of cryptoglandular fistula.[248] Most reported cases occur in developing countries. The disease is seen most commonly in men, usually associated with pulmonary tuberculosis,

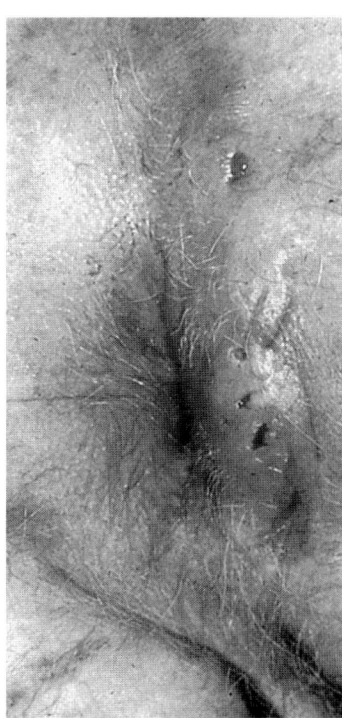

FIGURE 19-28. Multiple external openings are present in this patient with fistula-in-ano. (See Color Fig. 19-28.)

but there have been case reports of the process occurring in the absence of pulmonary infection.[155,265] Primary inoculation of the mycobacteria may result from trauma to the skin or mucosa.

The lesion may appear as a brownish red papule that can progress into an ulcerating plaque; this is known as a tuberculous chancre. The ulcers are usually painful and indolent, with blue, irregular edges. Regional lymphadenopathy is common. A high index of suspicion is necessary if one is to establish the diagnosis early and to initiate appropriate therapy. It has been suggested that an anal fissure in an unusual location that is slow to heal should be pathologically confirmed with appropriate staining and cultures to rule out the presence of the bacterium.[165]

The diagnosis can be established by the determination of acid-fast bacilli in the biopsy specimen (Ziehl-Nielsen stain), by positive guinea pig culture, and by the presence of caseating granulomas in the histologic examination of skin lesions. Because culture results take about 4 weeks, newer approaches may be more useful, such as the detection of the bacterial DNA by means of genomic amplification by polymerase chain reaction, a 48-hour test.[248] Chaudhary and Gupta and colleagues suggest that the biopsy be performed using an anesthetic, because considerable effort is required to obtain representative tissue from the depths of any fibrotic or strictured area.[50,125] Demonstration of active disease in the lungs and a positive tuberculin skin test result are helpful in confirming the true nature of the lesion (see Chapter 33).

In developed countries, tuberculosis is not likely to be considered in the differential diagnosis of a perianal ulcer.[4,142] In the absence of a pulmonary lesion, it would be very difficult for me *not* to work up and treat the patient, initially at least, for Crohn's disease. One should certainly consider performing a tuberculin skin test and obtaining cultures in individuals who harbor wounds that fail to heal, especially if the person comes from a developing country.

Obviously, antituberculous drugs are the treatment of choice. Therapy with isoniazid, rifampin, and ethambutol will usually resolve the anal condition in a matter of 2 or 3 weeks. However, treatment should be continued for many months following resolution of the local or systemic manifestations.

Actinomycosis

Actinomycosis is a chronic infectious disease involving the cervicofacial area, thorax, or abdomen. It is caused by an anaerobic, gram-positive bacterium, *Actinomyces israelii*. It produces a suppurative, fibrosing inflammation that forms sinus tracts, discharging granules (Figure 19-29). In the abdominal form, a mass is usually present, and a psoas abscess occasionally occurs (see Chapter 33).

The diagnosis is established by identification of the microorganism in cultures of tissue or the exudate of the lesion; the finding of sulfur granules leaves no doubt. In

the anal area, sinus tracts and fistulas may resemble Crohn's disease, anal fistula, suppurative hidradenitis, and tuberculosis.[10] The presence of the disease elsewhere, particularly in the abdomen, is helpful in alerting the surgeon to the nature of the problem. The possibility of perianal actinomycosis should be entertained in any individual who has extensive fistula tracts and in whom recurrence develops after what are considered adequate attempts at surgical treatment.

Management consists of surgical excision and drainage of the abscess as well as antibiotics, usually penicillin. A 4-week period of treatment is recommended.

Viral Infections

Virtually any viral infection that affects the skin can involve the perianal area. This may occur as part of a generalized cutaneous process or by autoinoculation from another site. When lesions are seen in an intertriginous zone, they may not resemble the typical appearance seen elsewhere. This may cause the physician to misdiagnose the condition as secondary syphilis.[147] Two common viral infections that are presumed to be nonvenereal in origin are mentioned briefly.

Herpes Zoster

Herpes zoster, caused by reactivation of varicella, may involve the anal area. The condition, also known as shingles, affects both sexes equally and may be particularly troublesome in patients who have been immunosuppressed by treatment for malignancy. The lesion is char-

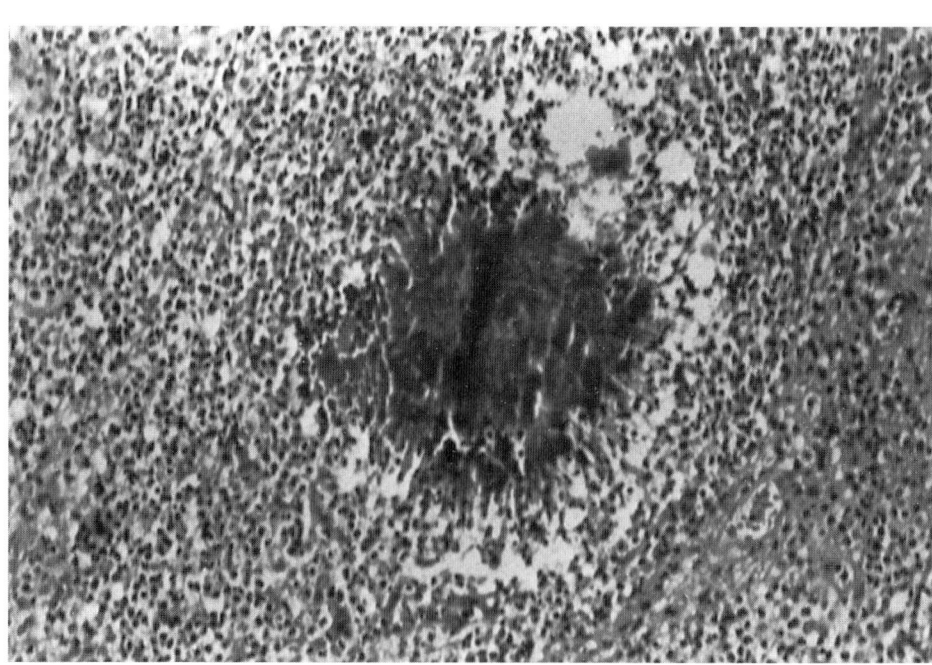

FIGURE 19-29. The basophilic "sulfur granule" of *Actinomyces* in actinomycosis. Note the homogeneous center and the club-shaped filaments at the periphery. (Original magnification × 120; courtesy of Rudolf Garret, M.D.)

Treatment consists of medical measures, including rest and the application of heat. Analgesics are advisable for acute neuralgia. Acyclovir (Zovirax), 800 mg orally four to five times per day for 7 to 10 days, is extremely helpful if initiated early in the course of the disease. For older patients with severe pain, systemic corticosteroid therapy may be considered.

Vaccinia

Vaccinia virus is an attenuated cowpox virus that has been propagated in laboratories for immunization against smallpox. Perianal vaccinia is a rare complication of vaccination and usually occurs in young children.[64] It has also been reported as a complication of diarrhea, with probable transmission to the excoriated area by the fingers.[67] In adults, the condition may be confused with syphilis or with herpes simplex infection. The history is helpful if the patient has undergone a recent vaccination or was exposed to someone who had done so.

Treatment is generally supportive, because complete recovery usually occurs spontaneously. However, vaccinia immune globulin has been recommended in severe cases or to expedite resolution of the process.

Bacterial Infections

Infective processes associated with bacterial organisms, such as pilonidal sinus and suppurative hidradenitis, have already been discussed. There is, however, a unique infective condition in the perianal area that is worthy of discussion, Fournier's gangrene.

Fournier's Gangrene or Necrotizing Perineal Infection

In 1883, Fournier described a necrotizing soft tissue infection of the perineum, groin, and genitalia that almost invariably ended fatally. Because of the prevalence of two or more species of bacteria in the infection, the term *synergistic gangrene* has been employed. *Necrotizing fasciitis* is another expression that has been used to describe the condition. It is important to distinguish this entity from clostridial myonecrosis, because the treatment is obviously different.[32]

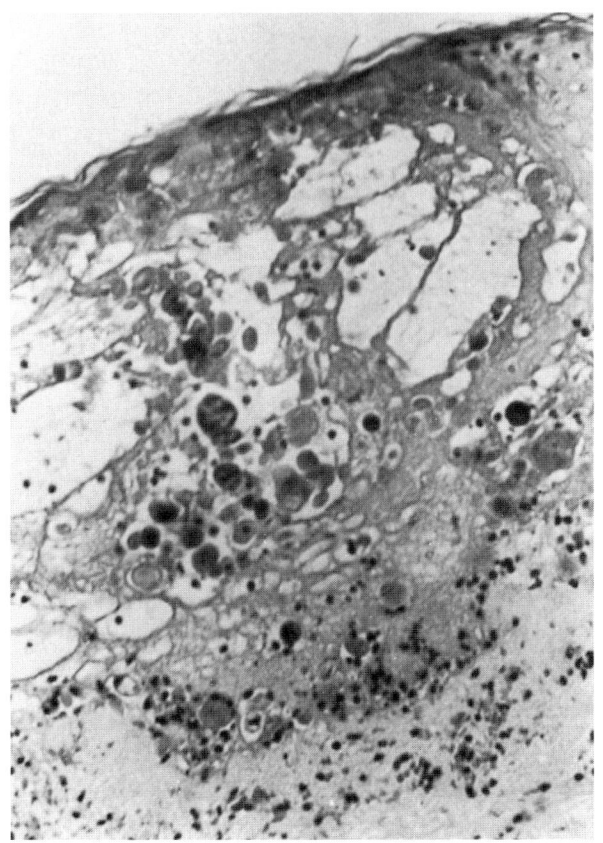

FIGURE 19-30. Ballooning degeneration of prickle cells with the formation of multilocular vesicles in herpes zoster. Note the cells with large inclusion bodies. (Original magnification × 240; courtesy of Rudolf Garret, M.D.)

acterized by groups of vesicles on an erythematous base along the distribution of a spinal nerve leading to a posterior ganglion. Itching, tenderness, and pain are characteristically located along the region supplied by the nerve. Jellinek and Tulloch described seven patients with retention, loss of sensation, or incontinence.[137]

Diagnosis can be established by means of tissue culture and by demonstration of antibodies in the serum by immunofluorescent techniques. Histologically, vesicles are seen to be intraepidermal; within these vesicles are found large, swollen cells called "balloon cells" (Figure 19-30).

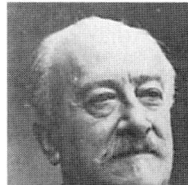

Jean-Alfred Fournier (1832–1914) Fournier was born in Paris. He became a pupil of Ricord, who exerted considerable influence over him and was responsible for stimulating Fournier to pursue investigations on STDs. In 1860, he graduated from the University of Paris Medical School, his thesis dealing with syphilitic contagion. Fournier is recognized as one of the pioneers in the diagnosis and management of STIs. In 1863, he became physician to the hospitals of Paris and Professeur Agrégé in the Faculty of Medicine. In 1868, he was appointed Chief of Service at the Lourcine Hospital, and in 1876, he was advanced to the Hôpital St. Louis, where he remained until retirement in 1902. The Academy of Medicine admitted Fournier to its ranks in 1879. His activities in writing and teaching brought him worldwide recognition and probably the largest clientele in the history of syphilology. Among the honors he received were the presidency of the French Society of Dermatology and Syphilology, Commander of the Legion of Honor, and the Order of Leopold of Belgium. In later years, his particular interest was the Society of Sanitary and Moral Prophylaxis, of which he was the founder and first president.

Why such a fulminant septic process develops in some patients with seemingly trivial septic problems in the rectum, perianal area, or urinary tract is not known. Delay in making the correct diagnosis and in initiating appropriate treatment of minor infections probably is the major contributing factor. The high mortality rate associated with these infections may in part be attributable to its occurrence in patients with debilitating illnesses, including diabetes.[20,153,163] Urinary tract infection, instrumentation, and surgery have all been implicated as contributing factors. Patients who undergo chemotherapy and those with acquired immunodeficiency syndrome (AIDS) are also more susceptible, implying that immunosuppression may play a role (see later and Chapters 20 and 33).[209] Some patients have a history of prior anorectal surgery or pelvic surgery for an infective process (e.g., perforated diverticulitis), but sometimes, especially when an anorectal procedure is performed, an underlying infection may not be recognized. Rubber ring ligation of hemorrhoids has been reported to be the precipitating event in a number of cases (see Chapter 8). Virtually all patients in published series have a demonstrable port of entry for the organism; specifically, perianal infection has become the most common cause.[77] Interestingly, the well-recognized entity in children of perianal cellulitis, caused by hemolytic streptococci, does not seem to predispose to the development of this complication.[214]

Stephens and colleagues reviewed the English language literature to determine whether there have been changes in demography, etiology, and outcome, compared with cases dating back to 1763.[240] They noted that in the decade 1979 to 1988, 449 cases were reported. The average age was 50 years, with 14% of cases occurring in female patients. The most common etiologic factors were colorectal (33%), idiopathic (26%), and genitourinary (21%).[240] The authors noted that the mortality associated with the disease as a consequence of colorectal disease was highest (one of three died). The overall mortality in the series was 22%.

Symptoms and Findings The usual presenting complaints are perineal pain and swelling. Frank suppuration or even gangrene of the overlying skin may be apparent in advanced cases (Figure 19-31). Fever and leukocytosis are invariably present.

Bacteriology There has been considerable disagreement about the specific bacteria involved in the infection. Numerous organisms have been identified, both aerobic and anaerobic, including *Clostridium welchii*.[131] More commonly, the gangrene is caused by such mixed bacterial flora as microaerophilic *Streptococcus*, *Staphylococcus aureus* and *S. albus*, *Bacteroides*, *Klebsiella*, *E. coli*,

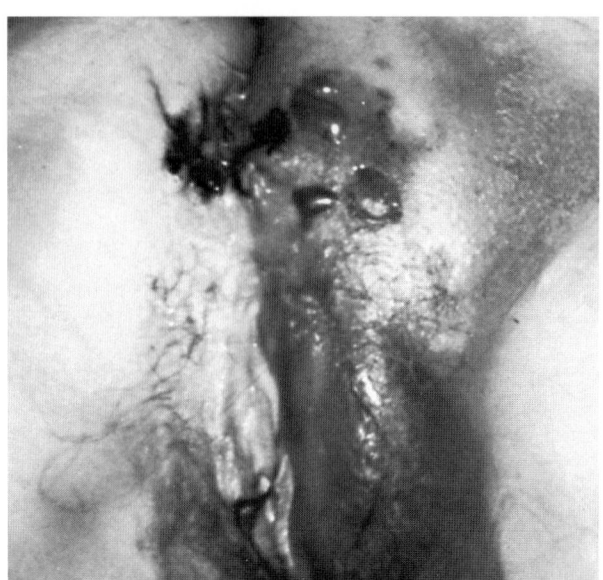

FIGURE 19-31. Fournier's gangrene. Note the necrotic areas of perianal skin, bullae, and introital edema. (Courtesy of Paul J. Kovalcik, M.D.)

Enterococcus, *Proteus*, and *Citrobacter*.[149] Gram stains and aerobic and anaerobic cultures should be obtained from the margins where infection is advancing.[149]

Treatment Broad-spectrum antibiotic therapy is, of course, recommended. Because most anaerobic isolates are reported to be sensitive to clindamycin and metronidazole, these have been suggested to be the first-line antibiotics of choice.[205] However, vigorous surgical excision and debridement of all nonviable tissue are imperative.[20,77,99,149,154,206] Treatment with hyperbaric oxygen is controversial and may be contraindicated unless the infection is caused by *C. welchii*.[77,99,149] A colostomy may be advisable to reduce fecal contamination of the area, but is mandatory if anorectal or colonic disease is the cause of the perineal sepsis. Debridement must be radical and should be continued until the skin and subcutaneous tissue cannot be readily separated from the fascia.[99] Histologic examination of the margins of excised tissue may be useful in determining the adequacy of debridement.[206] Because of the life-threatening nature of the illness, one should not be concerned about the need for subsequent skin coverage or reconstruction.[77,99] One exception to this dictum is the need to protect exposed testes from dessication. Because the scrotal skin has considerable elastic properties, this can often be used.[206] If this is not possible, the testicles can be implanted in thigh pouches.[211] The wounds are left open and packed, and the patient is returned to the operating room if further debridement is deemed advisable. Vigorous irrigation with antiseptic solution [e.g., peroxide, sodium hypochlorite (Dakin solution)] is recommended. Delayed primary closure, skin grafting, and other reconstructive procedures are often ultimately required.

An interesting approach to the management of Fournier's gangrene was proposed by Efem from the University Department of Surgery in Calabar, Nigeria.[95] He postulated that the organisms commonly associated with the condition are sensitive to the antimicrobial activity of unprocessed honey. In 20 consecutive cases, the author applied the honey topically along with systemic antibiotics. Utilizing historic controls, he observed that the response to treatment and the reduction of morbidity were better in the honey-treated group. It is theorized that its effectiveness is based on a combination of wound debridement, topical antibacterial activity, and local generation of oxygen.

Results Generally, the results of treatment for this condition, applying the principles outlined earlier, have improved considerably.[148] Eke identified 1,726 patients with Fournier's gangrene in the literature since the 1950s.[97] Enriquez and colleagues described 28 patients with necrotizing genital and perianal infections and noted an overall mortality of 25%.[99] Anorectal infections were more severe and carried a higher mortality than those from primary urologic causes. Di Falco and colleagues reported five patients, with one death.[77] Full-thickness skin grafts were required in three individuals. Barkel and Villalba reported eight cases, six of which were anorectal in origin.[20] One patient died following treatment by an abdominoperineal resection, and another expired of an unrelated cause. The interval from the onset of clinical symptoms to the initial surgical intervention is the most important factor that contributes to a successful outcome.[153]

Clayton and colleagues identified 57 men in whom necrotizing fasciitis of the male genitalia developed.[56] Forty-seven (82%) survived. Survival was associated with a younger age, a serum blood urea nitrogen level of less than 50 mg/dL at presentation, and fewer major compli-

cations after initial debridement. Interestingly, the authors found that the survival of those with a localized process was no better than that of individuals in whom extension into the abdominal wall or thigh developed. In the experience of Stephens and co-workers, the highest mortality was associated with a colorectal cause (33%).[240] Female mortality (49%) was not significantly greater than male mortality (17%) when obstetric origin was excluded. The overall mortality for the 11 reported cases was 22%.[240] The importance of combined aggressive surgical and medical management, utilizing a team comprising an infectious disease specialist, a surgeon, and, if necessary, a urologist, cannot be overestimated.

Ecthyma Gangrenosum

Ecythma gangrenosum is a skin condition found most commonly in immunocompromised children, such as those with leukemia.[115] It is usually caused by infection with the organism *Pseudomonas aeruginosa*. Most of the lesions are located in the anogenital area, axillae, and extremities. A report of the need for perineal reconstruction as a consequence of tissue destruction from this condition has been described.[115]

Fungal Infections

The primary site of involvement of recognized superficial fungal infections is the skin. This is presumably because fungi digest and live on keratin. These superficial fungi are called dermatophytes; they include *Microsporum*, *Trichophyton*, and *Epidermophyton*.[85]

Tinea Cruris (Jock Itch, Crotch Itch)

Tinea cruris, also known as ringworm of the groin, is caused by a species of *Trichophyton*. The condition occurs most commonly in the intertriginous areas and is exacerbated by heat and humidity (Figure 19-32). The differential diagnosis includes candidiasis, erythrasma, seborrheic dermatitis, psoriasis, and vegetative pemphigus. Demonstration of the fungus by potassium hydrox-

---

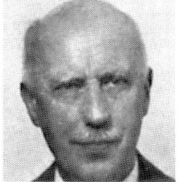

Henry Drysdale Dakin (1880–1952) Dakin was born in London, the son of a Leeds iron and steel merchant. In 1898, he entered Yorkshire College, now the University of Leeds, to study under the famous organic chemist Julius Cohen. Because of Dakin's particular interest in enzyme chemistry, Cohen gave him the nickname "Zyme," which became his mode of address by friends for the rest of his life. Indeed, he became one of the founding leaders in the emerging field of biochemistry. In 1902, Dakin was awarded a scholarship to study in other laboratories—the Jenner Institute in London and with Kossel in Heidelberg. While there, he shared in the discovery of arginase. When World War I broke out, he offered his services and was asked to cooperate with Alexis Carrel in a research effort in the treatment of injuries suffered by the French wounded at Compiègne. It was there that he developed the buffered hypochlorite solution that bears his name. Later, in the Dardenelles, the ship *Aquitania* was fitted with a special tank for the electrolysis of sea water, through which an unlimited supply of hypochlorite disinfectant solution was made available. On this converted hospital ship, an immediate reduction in the incidence of infection was noted. Among his other notable achievements were the synthesis of epinephrine, the discovery of glyoxalase, and the oxidation of fatty acids. The French government made him a Chevalier of the Legion of Honor.

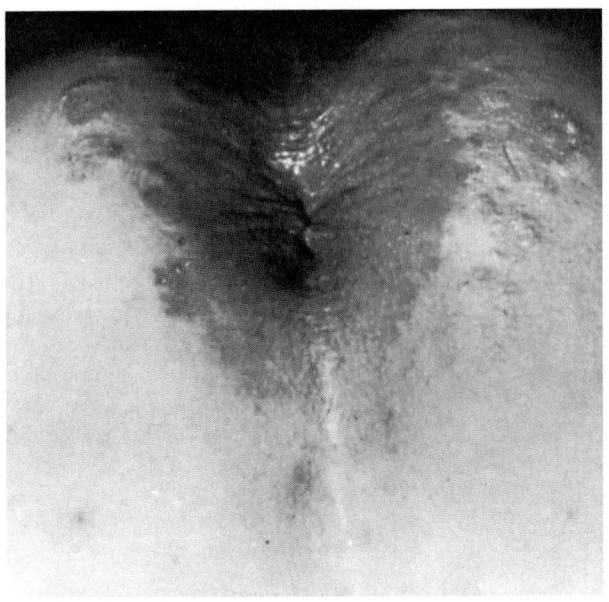

FIGURE 19-32. Dermatophytosis (tinea cruris), a superficial fungal infection. Note that patches have annular borders with scaling and a tendency toward central clearing. (Courtesy of Samuel L. Moschella, M.D.)

ide microscopic examination and culture confirms the diagnosis (Figure 19-33).

Treatment consists of reduction of perspiration and enhancement of evaporation from the crural area. Loose-fitting clothes are suggested. Griseofulvin has been considered the most effective drug in the treatment of all dermatophytes, but it is rarely needed.[262] Its action is believed to modify keratin so that the fungus will not invade. Treatment for 3 to 4 weeks is advised if topical fungicides such as tolnaftate, clotrimazole, miconazole, econazole, and ciclopirox are not helpful.[262]

Candidiasis or Moniliasis

Candidiasis is caused by the yeastlike fungus *Candida albicans*. The fungus is a frequent commensal in humans and is present in the alimentary tract and vagina of many healthy people.[262] Intertriginous areas are commonly affected, including the perianal and inguinal folds and the axillae.

The organism is usually found outside the epidermis and behaves primarily as an opportunistic infection, especially in patients who have impaired resistance (e.g., AIDS). The condition may be somewhat difficult to recognize. Pustules without surrounding inflammation may leave a "collarette" of scale, and satellite lesions can be often seen in adjacent skin. Some eruptions in the inguinal area may resemble tinea cruris, but usually there is less scaling and a greater tendency to fissure.[85] When the condition occurs in children, it is called diaper or napkin dermatitis.

The diagnosis of candidiasis is made by demonstrating the yeast, spores, or pseudomycelium under the microscope with potassium hydroxide. Culture on Sabouraud's glucose agar shows a growth of creamy, grayish, moist colonies in about 4 days.[85]

Treatment consists of topical nystatin, clotrimazole, or miconazole. For very severe cases, usually in those patients with an immunologic deficiency, oral ketoconazole (Nizoral), 200 mg, or intravenous amphotericin B can be administered.

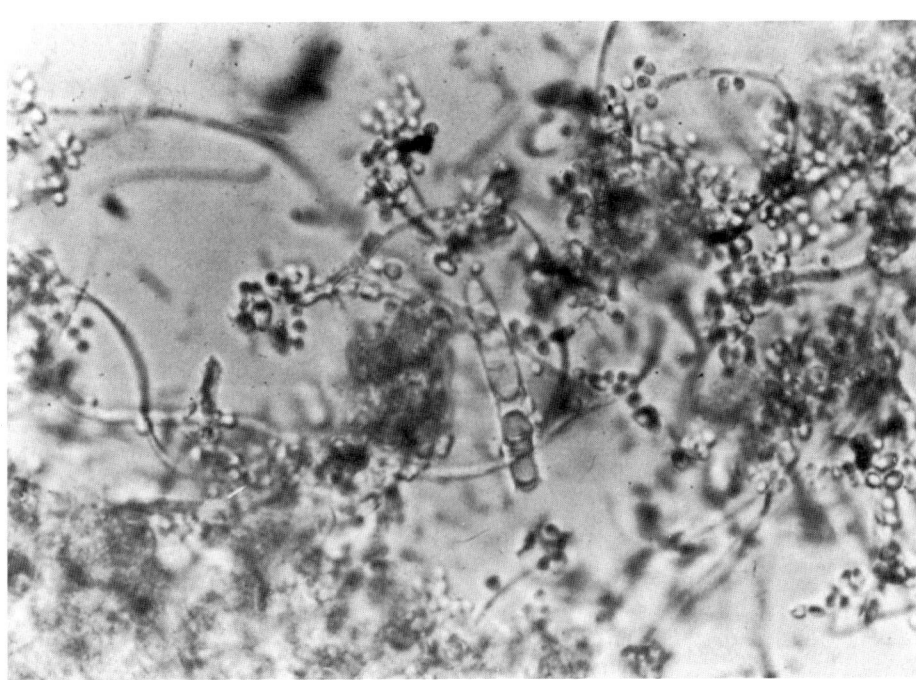

FIGURE 19-33. *Trichophyton mentagrophytes*, as seen in a potassium hydroxide preparation, a species of *Trichophyton* that can cause tinea cruris (ringworm) of the groin. (Original magnification × 600; courtesy of Rudolf Garret, M.D.)

Sporotrichosis, Coccidioidomycosis, Histoplasmosis, North American Blastomycosis, Chromomycosis, Cryptococcosis, Nocardiosis, and Mycetoma

These fungal infections are generally known as the "deep" mycoses. They usually come from inhalation of dust contaminated with the fungus, from droppings of animals infected by it, or from contamination from other sources.[85] All have associated skin lesions, which have a good prognosis in the case of primary cutaneous infections. However, when skin involvement is the result of dissemination from a visceral focus, the prognosis is usually much worse. Generally, skin biopsy will reveal the presence of the fungi.

Treatment varies with the type of fungus and with the extent of disease, either localized or systemic. The reader is referred to a textbook of medicine for the clinical features, diagnosis, and management of these conditions.

Parasitic Diseases

Numerous parasitic diseases exhibit cutaneous manifestations, and many of these also affect the alimentary tract. Included are infections caused by protozoa (i.e., single-cell organisms), nematodes (i.e., roundworms), arthropods, trematodes (i.e., flukes), cestodes (i.e., flatworms), annelids (i.e., leeches), and chordates. Some of these conditions are discussed in Chapter 33. The discussion that follows is limited to those cutaneous manifestations that may be of interest to the surgeon.

Amebiasis Cutis

Entamoeba histolytica is an organism that causes disease that is most common in the tropics. Cutaneous amebiasis occurs less frequently than the intestinal condition, except for cutaneous manifestations in the genitalia and perianal area. It is believed that the reason for its presentation in this location is direct extension from the involved bowel. Lesions begin as deep abscesses that rupture and form distinct ulcerations; there is usually an erythematous halo around the ulcer. Characteristically, skin lesions spread rapidly and may terminate fatally.

Histologically, there are areas of necrotic ulceration, with many lymphocytes, neutrophils, plasma cells, and eosinophils. The organism is frequently demonstrated in the fresh material from the base (see Chapter 33). Although abscesses may require surgical drainage, the cutaneous manifestation will usually respond to either metronidazole or emetine.

Trichomoniasis

Trichomonas vulvovaginitis causes vaginal pruritus, burning, and leukorrhea. The condition is caused by the protozoan *T. vaginalis*. Because of the discharge and pruritic symptoms, the anal area may be secondarily in-volved by the irritation. Eliciting a history of the vaginal discharge will alert the physician to the source of the problem. Treatment is metronidazole (Flagyl), 250 mg for 10 days.

Schistosomal Dermatitis (Schistosomiasis Cutis, Swimmer's Itch)

Schistosomal dermatitis is a severe pruritic, papular dermatitis caused by cercarial species of *Schistosoma*, a genus of trematodes. Exposure to the cercariae (see Figure 33-30) occurs by swimming or wading in water containing them. They attach by burrowing into the skin. Clinically, there is severe itching at the time of the exposure secondary to an urticarial reaction. The resultant papular, pruritic lesion spontaneously regresses after a few days, disappearing by 2 weeks. Antipruritic measures are used for treatment.

Visceral schistosomiasis (i.e., bilharziasis) may produce cutaneous manifestations as a result of deposition of eggs in the dermis. Fistulous tracts may develop in the perineum and buttocks, associated with hard masses, sinus tracts, and seropurulent discharge with a characteristic foul odor. In the severe vegetating form, malignant change in the granulomas has been noted. Treatment consists of trivalent antimony compounds [e.g., tartar emetic, stibophen, trivalent sodium antimonyl gluconate (Triostam), astiban].

Nematode Infections

Oxyuriasis (Pinworm, Threadworm, Enterobiasis) Enterobius (Oxyuris) vermicularis is the helminth that most commonly infects humans. Children are more frequently affected than adults, and the condition is more common in temperate climates than in the tropics. The worm lives in the proximal colon and is often found in the appendix (Figure 19-34), but the disease is not truly related to the bowel itself. The worms migrate to the rectum at night and emerge on the perianal skin to deposit thousands of ova (Figs. 19-35 and 19-36). The ova are returned to the mouth by the patient through scratching. The larvae then hatch in the duodenum and migrate to the small and large intestine. Fertilization occurs in the cecum, completing the life cycle.

The primary complaint is usually itching, especially interfering with the patient's sleep. Friction and maceration by tight-fitting clothes may lead to superficial or deep folliculitis of the buttocks and perineum.[110] Anal abscess complicating the condition has also been reported,[188] as has a perineal, subcutaneous nodule.[160]

The diagnosis is usually established by demonstration of the ova in smears taken from the anal area early in the morning. Applying cellophane tape against the perianal region, adding a drop of iodine, and examining the tape under a microscope slide may facilitate detection of the ova. Demonstration of the pinworm in the stool is rarely

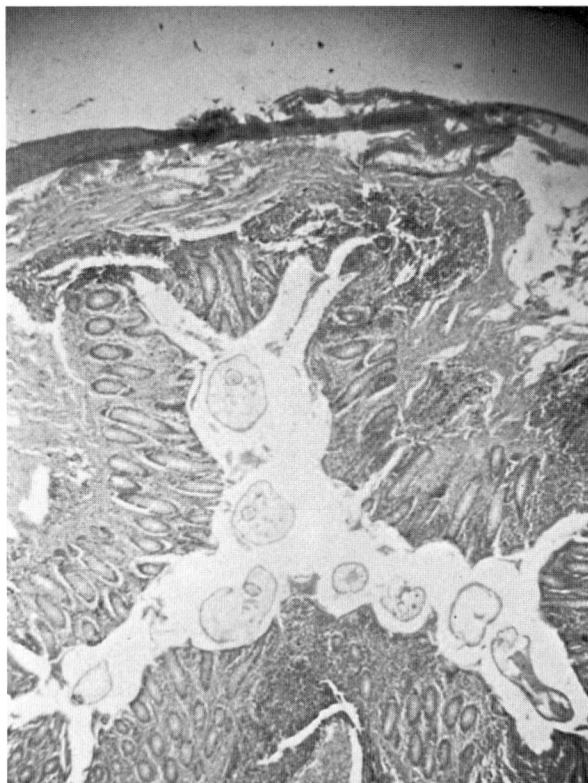

FIGURE 19-34. *Enterobius vermicularis* infection. Pinworms are in the appendix, in a cross-sectional view. (Original magnification × 80; courtesy of Rudolf Garret, M.D.)

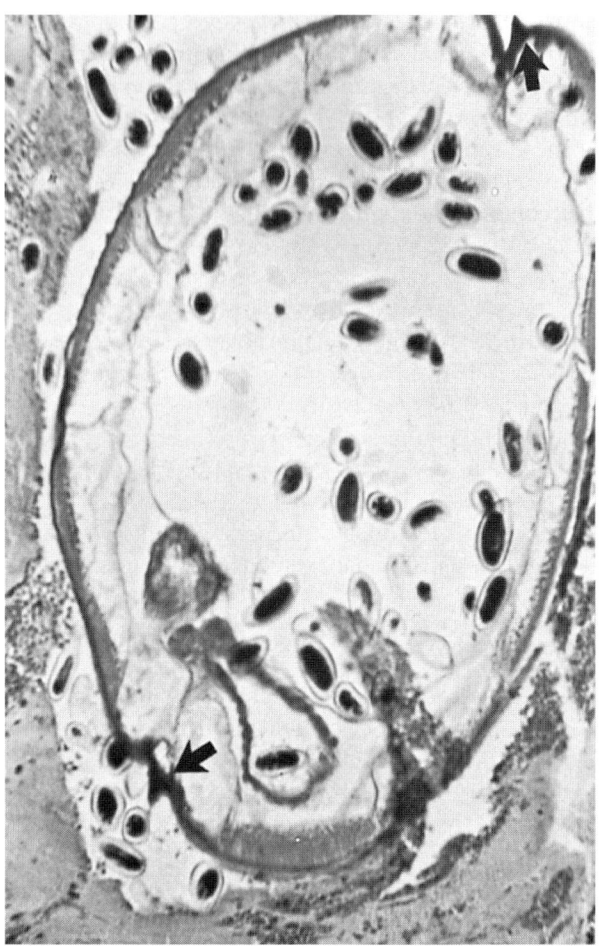

FIGURE 19-35. Adult pinworm *(Enterobius vermicularis)*. Note the prominent lateral alae *(arrows)*. Numerous ova are seen. (Original magnification × 170; courtesy of Rudolf Garret, M.D.)

successful, but occasionally the adult worms may be seen on the perianal skin. Because of the high likelihood of communication, it is appropriate to study members of the patient's family.

Current management of pinworm infestation is mebendazole (Vermox), 100 mg, as a chewable tablet, taken once. Other effective medications for the treatment of the condition are piperazine (Antepar) and pyrvinium pamoate (Povan). The former is given in single daily doses of 65 mg/kg (not to exceed 2,500 mg) taken 1 hour before breakfast for 8 consecutive days, and the latter is given in a single dose of 5 mg/kg; a second dose may be given 1 week after the first treatment.[86] Undergarments, towels, sheets, pajamas, and other clothing should be thoroughly laundered separately from those of other members of the family.

Creeping Eruption or Larva Migrans Larva migrans is a cutaneous eruption caused by larvae of several nematodes, most commonly the cat or dog hookworm, *Ancylostoma braziliense* or *A. caninum.* The ova of these hookworms are deposited in the soil and hatch into infectious larvae that penetrate the skin. People who go barefoot at the beach, children playing in sandboxes, carpenters and plumbers working under homes, and gardeners are the

most common victims.[86] The feet, buttocks, hands, and genitals are most frequently involved by the process. Raised, pruritic, thin, linear, tunnel-like lesions that contain serous fluid are noted.

The disease is usually self-limited, but freezing of the larvae with ethyl chloride or liquid nitrogen is effective. An alternative internal treatment is thiabendazole (Mintezol).

Larva Currens Larva currens is a form of cutaneous larva migrans caused by *Strongyloides stercoralis.* The condition is so called because of the speed of larval migration. It is caused in essence by an autoinfection, penetration of the perianal skin by larvae excreted in the feces. The eruption is usually associated with intestinal strongyloidiasis, beginning in the skin around the anus, and may involve the buttocks, thighs, and back. The itching is quite severe. As the larvae leave the skin to enter the bloodstream and settle in the intestinal mucosa, the

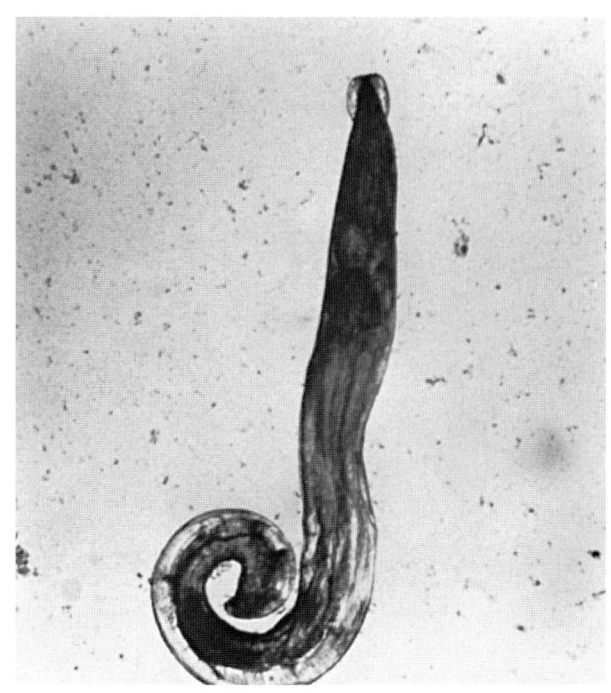

FIGURE 19-36. *Enterobius vermicularis,* the adult pinworm (female). (Courtesy of Rudolf Garret, M.D.)

rash disappears. The skin demonstrates a papular eruption with edema and urticaria. Treatment consists of thiabendazole, 25 to 50 mg/kg for 2 to 4 days.

Insect Diseases

Cimicosis or Bedbug Bites The bedbug (i.e., *Cimex lectularius*) hides in crevices during the daytime and feeds on human blood at night.[122] The bedbug usually produces a linear series of bites on the ankles and buttocks. Because the bites are painless, the patient may not be aware of what has happened until finding the bedclothes stained with blood. Some individuals may react with severe urticaria and pain. Treatment consists of soothing antipruritic lotions. The pests are eliminated by means of fumigation (e.g., with malathion).

Pediculosis Pubis (Phthiriasis) Several varieties of *Pediculus* affect humans, but the one that concerns us for the purpose of this discussion is *P. pubis* (*Phthirus pubis*), the pubic or crab louse. The condition is usually transmitted by sexual intercourse or acquired from contaminated bedding. The lice are found on the hair or skin and appear as yellowish brown or gray, glistening specks.[86] The so-called nits are attached to the hair shaft and are best seen under Wood's light. Symptoms include intense pruritus and the secondary effects of persistent excoriation. The condition frequently coexists with other sexually transmitted diseases. Treatment consists of 1% γ-benzene hexachloride cream or lotion to the pubic area, lindane (Kwell), or crotamiton (Eurax). Bed linen and clothing essentially require sterilization.

Arachnid Infection: Scabies

Scabies is a skin condition resulting from infestation by the mite *Sarcoptes scabiei.* The female burrows into the stratum corneum and there deposits her eggs. Patients complain primarily of itching that is worse at night. Areas commonly involved include the interdigital folds, flexor aspects of the wrist, nipples, navel, genitals, buttocks, and outer aspects of the feet. The lesion appears as a whitish burrow that is rather tortuous and threadlike. Papules and pustules are frequently seen. The condition is usually contracted by close contact with a person harboring the mite. The diagnosis is made by microscopic examination of scrapings or shave excision of suspected skin for eggs, larvae, adult mites, or feces (Figs. 19-37 and 19-38).[109] Treatment consists of permethrin (Elimite) cream, 10% crotamiton cream (Eurax), or thiabendazole, as well as decontamination of clothing.

Sexually Transmitted Diseases

> Two minutes with Venus,
> two years with mercury.
>
> J. Earle Moore: *Aphorism*

Sexually transmitted infections (STIs), once called STD, are among the most common infectious diseases in the United States today. More than 20 STIs have now been identified, and they affect more than 13 million men and women in the United States each year.[196] The annual comprehensive cost of STIs in the United States is estimated to be well in excess of $10 billion. STIs affect men and women of all backgrounds and economic levels but are most prevalent among teenagers and young adults. Nearly two thirds of all STIs occur in people younger than 25 years of age. The incidence of STIs is rising, in part because young people are sexually active earlier yet are marrying later. In addition, divorce is more common. The net result is that sexually active people today are more likely to have multiple sex partners during their lives. Sohn and Robilotti coined the phrase "gay bowel syndrome" to indicate a constellation of diseases and conditions to which male homosexuals fall victim.[236] Receptive anal intercourse is a particular risk factor, because of the greater fragility of the rectal mucosa in comparison with the squamous mucosa of the vagina.[200]

Most of the time, STIs cause no symptoms, particularly in women. When and if symptoms develop, they may be confused with those of other diseases not transmitted through sexual contact. Health problems caused

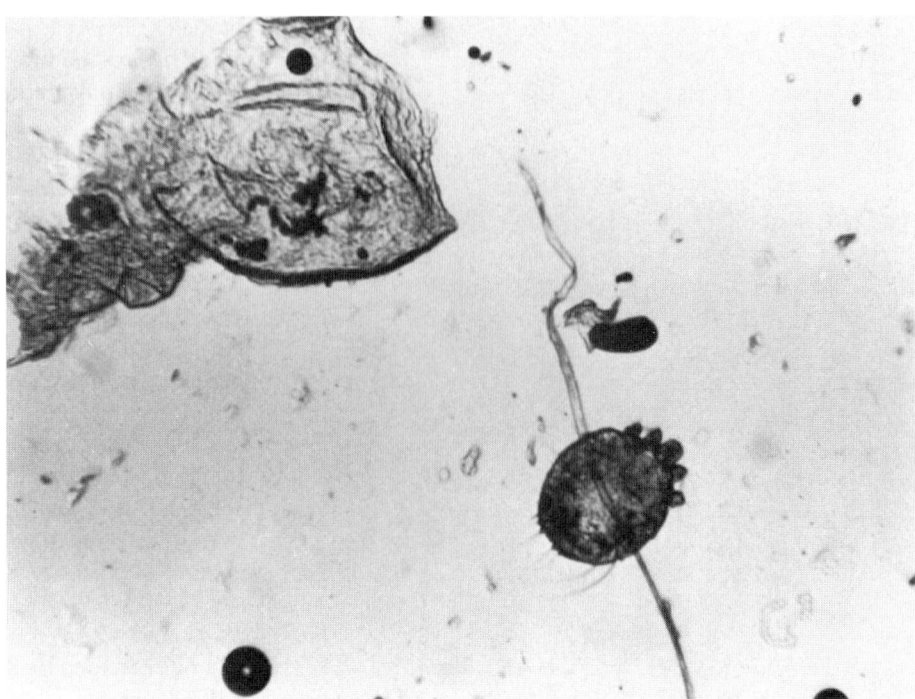

FIGURE 19-37. Scrapings from a scabies lesion showing the female mite. (Original magnification × 240; courtesy of Rudolf Garret, M.D.)

by STIs tend to be more severe and more frequent for women than for men, in part because the frequency of asymptomatic infection means that many women do not seek care until serious problems have developed. Some STIs can spread into the uterus and fallopian tubes to cause pelvic inflammatory disease, which, in turn, is a major cause of both infertility and ectopic pregnancy. STIs in women also may be associated with cervical cancer. One STI, human papillomavirus infection (HPV), causes genital warts and cervical and other genital cancers. The following is a list of STIs and the organisms responsible.

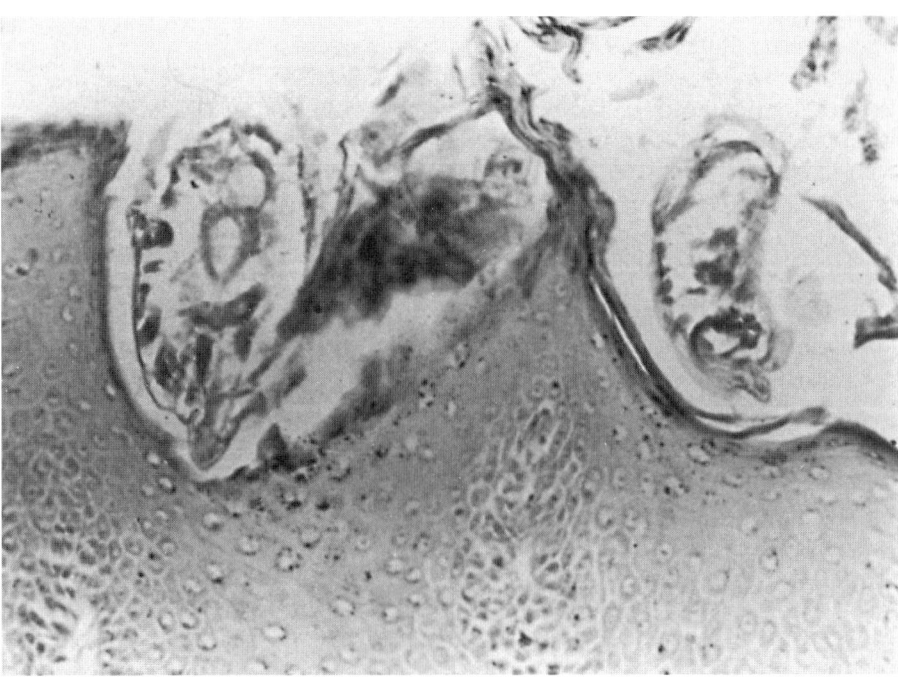

FIGURE 19-38. A biopsy specimen showing the female mite burrowing into the epidermis. (Original magnification × 280; courtesy of Rudolf Garret, M.D.)

Disease	Organism
AIDS HIV	
Bacterial vaginosis	*Bacteroides, Gardnerella vaginalis, Mobiluncus* sp., *Mycoplasma hominis, Ureaplasma urealyticum*
Chancroid	*Haemophilus ducreyi*
Chlamydial infections	*Chlamydia trachomatis*
Cytomegalovirus infections	Cytomegalovirus
Genital herpes	Herpes simplex virus
Genital (venereal) warts	HPV
Gonorrhea	*Neisseria gonorrhoeae*
Granuloma inguinale (donovanosis)	*Calymmatobacterium granulomatis*
Leukemia-lymphoma	Human T-cell lyphotrophic virus-I and II
Lymphogranuloma venereum	*Chlamydia trachomatis*
Molluscum contagiosum	Molluscum contagiosum virus
Pubic lice	*Pediculus pubis*
Scabies	*Sarcoptes scabiei*
Syphilis	*Treponema pallidum*
Trichomoniasis	*Trichomonas vaginalis*
Vaginal yeast infections	*Candida albicans*

The epidemic venereal conditions today are condylomata acuminata, anogenital herpes, and AIDS (see Chapter 20). With the changes in mores and attitudes toward sexual matters, it is incumbent upon the surgeon to be knowledgeable about the manifestations, differential diagnosis, and treatment of STIs.

Gonorrhea

Gonorrhea is a bacterial infection caused by *Neisseria gonorrhoeae*, a gram-negative diplococcus. Humans are the only known reservoir. The disease affects mucous membranes of the urethra, cervix, rectum, and oropharynx.

During the 1980s, the incidence of the disease declined markedly, but the condition is diagnosed at least ten times more often than syphilis. The incidence in the black population has been reported to be almost 40 times that of whites. The 1995 summary of reported cases by the United States Centers for Disease Control and Prevention (CDC) is 150 per 100,000 population.[49] Approximately 400,000 cases of gonorrhea are reported to the CDC each year.

The most common symptoms of gonorrhea are a discharge from the vagina or penis and painful or difficult urination. Gonococcal dermatitis is a rare infection that may develop in a wound that has come in contact with the bacterium, including wounds of the genital area. The most common and serious complications occur in women and, as with chlamydial infection, these complications include pelvic inflammatory disease, ectopic pregnancy, and infertility. The complication of gonorrheal proctitis is of particular interest to the surgeon. This is usually seen in the homosexual population as a result of infection from anal intercourse (see Chapter 20). In women, the condition is frequently caused by spread to the rectum from the genital tract. Historically, penicillin has been used to treat gonorrhea, but since the mid-1990s, antibiotic resistance has emerged. New antibiotics or combinations of drugs must be used to treat these resistant strains. The reader is referred to Chapter 33 for a discussion of gonococcal proctitis and its treatment.

Syphilis (Lues)

Know syphilis in all its manifestations
and relations, and all things clinical
will be added unto you.

William Osler: *Aequanimatas*

According to the United States Public Health Service, the incidence of primary and secondary syphilis in the United States is about 130,000 cases annually, with three cases in men reported for every one in a woman.[109] The disease is caused by the spirochete *Treponema pallidum*.

The organism enters the skin or mucous membrane, producing a chancre approximately 3 weeks following the infection. This is the primary stage of the disease. The lesion is usually single and is most commonly found as an open sore on the penis or vagina, but it can also be seen on the lips, tongue, tonsillar area, and in the anus. In women, it may be inapparent because of its location within the vagina or cervix. In the homosexual population, the chancre is usually situated at the anal margin or in the anal canal (Figure 19-39). The lesion is usually painless, but near the anal opening there may be severe discomfort, tenesmus, difficulty with defecation, and discharge. Unless there is a high index of suspicion, the condition may be confused with an anal fissure, but the presence of inguinal adenopathy should alert the examiner to this possibility. The aberrant location of the fissure (e.g., lateral) may create some suspicion, but this also could be a finding consistent with anal Crohn's disease.

Most writings on the subject state that the diagnosis can be established on the basis of identification of the organism by means of dark-field examination (Figure 19-40).

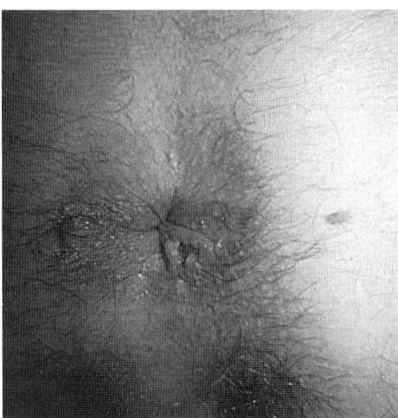

FIGURE 19-39. A noninflamed, punched out-appearing ulcerated chancre that was dark-field positive for *Treponema pallidum*. (See Color Fig. 19-39).

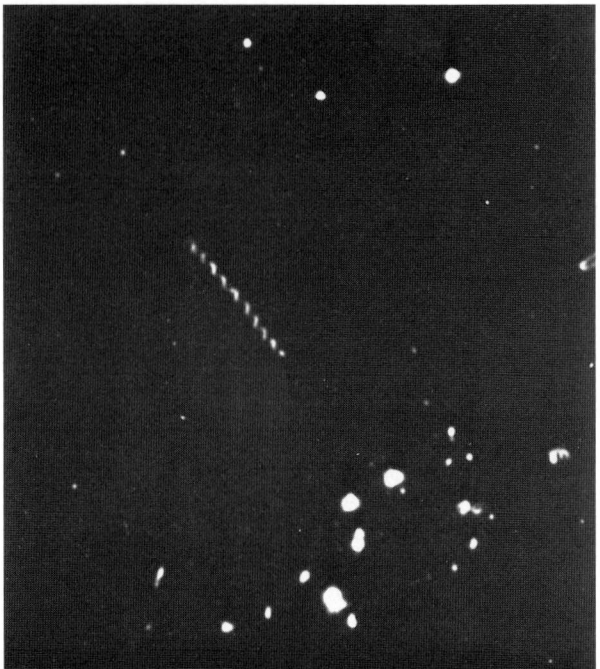

FIGURE 19-40. *Treponema pallidum*, the causative agent of syphilis, appears as a corkscrew-shaped organism on dark-field examination. (Original magnification × 600; courtesy of Rudolf Garret, M.D.)

Because the absence of a positive test result does not exclude the diagnosis, it is probably preferable to treat patients with suspected clinical lesions and await the results of serologic evaluation. It is important to remember, however, that serologic tests for syphilis do not yield positive results until the primary chancre has been present for several weeks.

Although excision of the lesion is not recommended, there are characteristic histopathologic changes (Figure 19-41).[90] There is dense infiltration by round cells, plasma cells, and fibroblasts. Proliferation of endothelial cells results in progressive arteritis.

Treatment

Benzathine penicillin is the treatment of choice in nonallergic patients, 2.4 million U intramuscularly, repeated 7 days later. For those who are allergic to penicillin, tetracycline, 500 mg orally four times daily for 15 days, is recommended.[90] Other tetracyclines can be used as well as erythromycin, 500 mg orally four times daily for 15 days (see Chapter 20).

Condylomata Lata

The other cutaneous manifestation of lues is the secondary stage of syphilis, condylomata lata. The signs and symptoms of secondary syphilis may develop 2 to 6 months after infection and usually 6 to 8 weeks after the appearance of the primary chancre. Both lesions may exist synchronously. A maculopapular rash develops, which gives rise to a proliferating, weeping mass containing the spirochetes. The lesions may appear rather flat, scaling, red, and indurated. In the anal area particularly, they may become papillomatous and vegetative with an associated foul odor (Figure 19-42). Although most literature suggests that the lesions are nonpruritic, some believe that this may be the primary complaint.[58]

The diagnosis may be established by demonstrating the organism using dark-field microscopic examination, but results of serologic tests are virtually always positive. The histopathology of secondary syphilis varies depending on the clinical presentation. The lesions of condylomata lata show acanthosis and edema in the epidermis with broadening of the rete ridges (Figure 19-43). Some lesions may demonstrate a nonspecific chronic inflammatory reaction with a large number of plasma cells (Figure 19-44).

Treatment with penicillin, erythromycin, or tetracycline is effective. An important part of the management of the patient includes the tracing of all sexual contacts, which, in the case of secondary syphilis, necessitates a 1-year retrospective review.

Chancroid

Chancroid is a rare sexually transmitted disease, but recent years have seen an increase in the incidence in the United States, presumably on the basis of individuals emigrating from the Caribbean, Mexico, and Southeast Asia.[109] The condition is most common in tropical and subtropical areas and in the poorer populations. The dis-

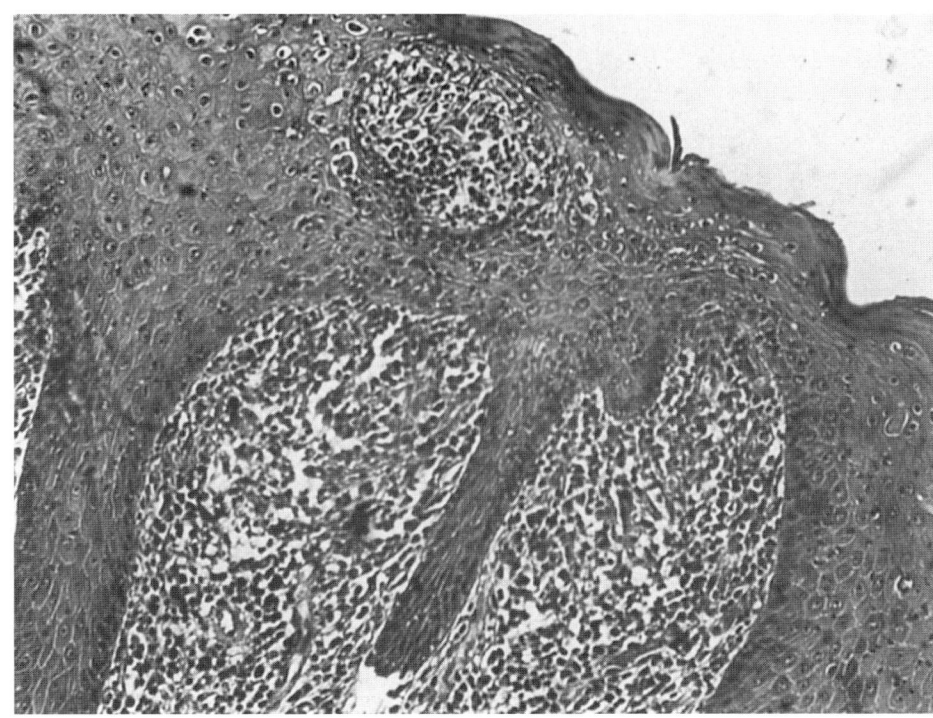

FIGURE 19-41. Syphilitic chancre demonstrating pseudoepitheliomatous hyperplasia and plasma cell infiltration of the dermis with dilated lymphatics. (Original magnification × 250; courtesy of Rudolf Garret, M.D.)

ease is caused by the gram-negative bacillus, *Haemophilus ducreyi.*

Chancroid begins on the genitals as an inflammatory macule or pustule; the latter ruptures, forming a punched-out ulcer with irregular edges. Within a few days to 2 weeks inguinal adenitis frequently develops, which may lead to perforation of the lymphatics. The inguinal node is called a *bubo.* Characteristic of chancroid is its tendency to autoinoculation. In addition to involvement of the anal area, extragenital lesions may be noted on the hands, eyelids, and elsewhere. The diagnosis is established by demonstrating the bacterium in smears from the ulcer grown on enhanced chocolate agar vancomycin.[109]

Because many cases are resistant to tetracycline, treatment usually consists of sulfonamides (i.e., double-strength trimethoprim-sulfamethoxazole), one tablet orally every 12 hours for 14 days. Third-generation cephalosporins are also effective.

Granuloma Inguinale (Granuloma Venereum, Donovanosis)

Granuloma inguinale is a chronic, granulomatous, ulcerative skin disease caused by *Calymmatobacterium granulomatis,* formerly known as *Donovania granulomatis.* In the United States, fewer than 100 cases are reported annually, almost exclusively in homosexual, African-American men.[109] There is some question whether it may be trans-

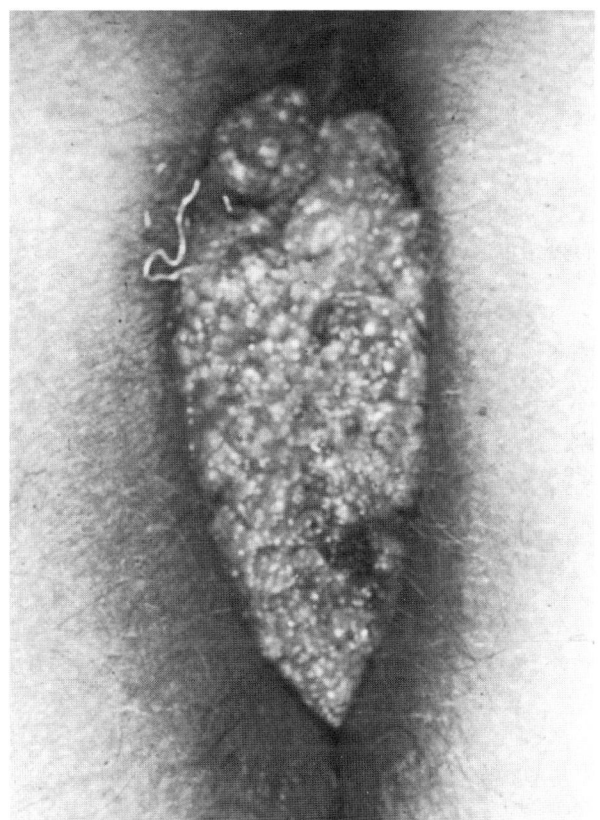

FIGURE 19-42. Condylomata lata. This large, perianal, mucoid, warty mass is composed of smooth-surfaced lobules. (Courtesy of Rudolf Garret, M.D.)

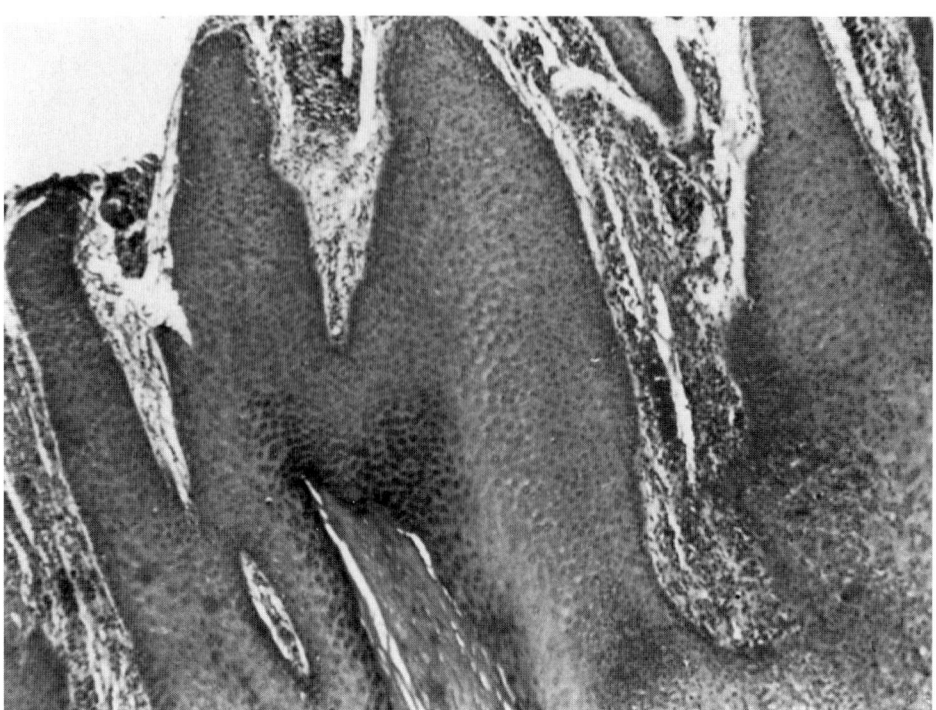

FIGURE 19-43. Condylomata lata demonstrating dilated lymphatics, proliferation of the prickle cell layer (acanthosis), and an inflammatory exudate. (Original magnification × 250; courtesy of Rudolf Garret, M.D.)

mitted nonvenereally as well as venereally. The lesions appear as cauliflower-like proliferations from which develop pustules and papules (Figure 19-45). Sinuses and scars are characteristic, with healed areas often devoid of pigment (Figure 19-46). The lesions may be quite uncomfortable. Adenopathy is not necessarily present, but secondary infection with abscess of inguinal nodes can occur. Squamous cell carcinoma may develop in long-standing, untreated lesions.

The diagnosis is usually established by the appearance, by the history, and by the staining of a punch biopsy specimen. Donovan bodies appear as deeply staining, bipolar, safety pin–shaped rods in the cytoplasm of macrophages (Figure 19-47). Biopsy usually reveals a massive, predominantly polymorphonuclear inflammatory reaction, thickening of the epidermis at the periphery, and pale-staining macrophages, usually in the upper parts of the granuloma (Figure 19-48).

Many antibiotics have been successful in the treatment; a 14-day course of tetracycline is preferred. If irreversible tissue destruction develops, resective surgery may be necessary.

Chlamydia Infection, Lymphogranuloma Venereum (Lymphogranuloma Inguinale, Lymphopathia Venereum)

Chlamydia infection is now the most common of all bacterial STIs in the United States, with an estimated 4 to 8 million new cases occurring each year. It is most frequently seen in the homosexual population, with a particularly high incidence among African-Americans. Lymphogranuloma venereum is a suppurative STI caused by *C. trachomatis*. It has been an uncommon disease in the United States, with fewer than 400 cases noted annually.[109,173] The infection is more common in Southeast Asia, Africa, Central and South America, and the Caribbean. However, the incidence is increasing as a complication in patients with AIDS patients (see Chapter 20).

Early symptoms are referable to the genitourinary tract, although 25% of men and 50% of women experience no initial symptoms. In both men and women, chlamydial infection may cause an abnormal genital discharge and burning with urination. In women, untreated chlamydial infection may lead to pelvic inflammatory disease, one of the most common causes of ectopic pregnancy and infertility in women. A case of the disease presenting as a rectovaginal fistula has been described.[173]

The lesion initially appears as a herpetiform vesicle on the genitalia or anal area. Complaints, when they occur, include dysuria, pyuria, and mucopurulent discharge. Lower abdominal pain may also be noted, especially in women. The diagnosis can be established by noting the clinical pattern of the genital lesion, followed 1 to 4 weeks later by marked unilateral lymphadenopathy and systemic symptoms. The nodes enlarge, form a large mass, become fluctuant, and drain.

Lymphogranuloma venereum may also start in the rectum as proctitis. Clinical symptoms under these circum-

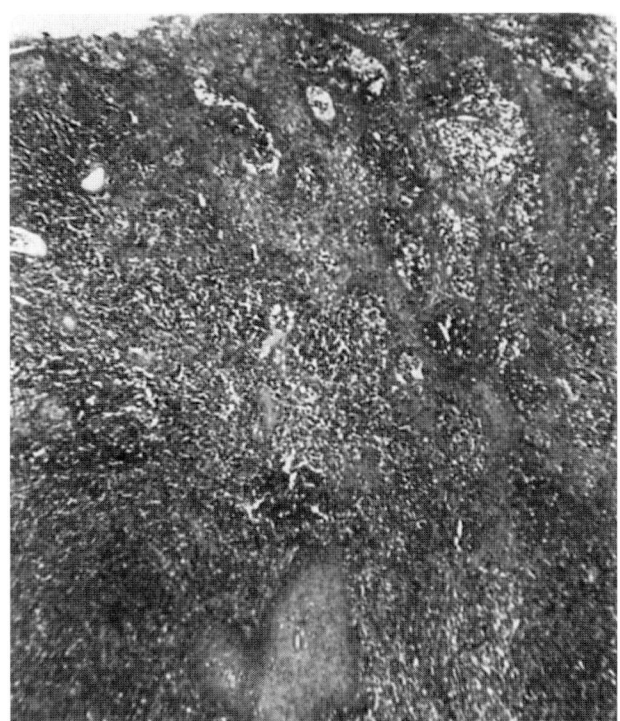

FIGURE 19-44. Condylomata lata showing pseudoepitheliomatous hyperplasia of the squamous epithelium. A heavy plasma cell infiltrate is evident in the dermis, with dilated lymphatics. (Original magnification × 250; courtesy of Rudolf Garret, M.D.)

stances are rectal discharge, bleeding, and tenesmus. An associated anal fissure is not uncommon. Perianal and rectovaginal fistulas may develop, and in late cases, progression to severe rectal stricture can occur. Approximately 2 weeks following the appearance of the primary lesion, inguinal lymphadenopathy is evident. Characteristically, in men the nodes fuse together in a large mass. If the primary lesion appears on the cervix or in the rectum, the perirectal and deep iliac nodes will enlarge.[109] Intestinal obstruction and elephantiasis of the genitals are late sequelae.

Histologically, the changes consist of an infectious granuloma with the formation of stellate abscesses (Figure 19-49). Laboratory studies reveal characteristic abnormalities, such as the frequently observed inversion of the albumin-globulin ratio. The so-called Frei test has been classically employed to establish the diagnosis of lymphogranuloma venereum; this is an intradermal test similar to the tuberculin test. However, the procedure has fallen into disrepute and in many places is no longer available. The lymphogranuloma venereum complement fixation test is considered positive at 1:80 or higher, but the microimmunofluorescent test is regarded as being more sensitive.[109] Elevated titers are noted approximately 1 month after the onset of the illness.

Recommended treatments include the following: tetracycline, 500 mg orally four times daily for 21 days; ery-

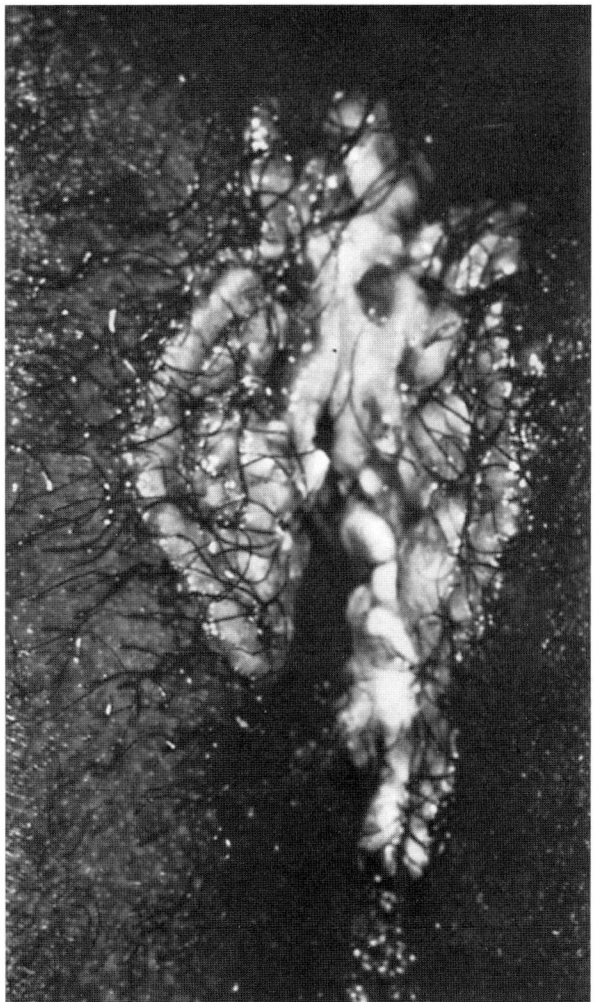

FIGURE 19-45. Cicatricial granulomatous nodule with a surrounding erythematous border, characteristic of granuloma inguinale. (Courtesy of Rudolf Garret, M.D.)

thromycin, 500 mg orally four times daily for 21 days; and double-strength trimethoprim-sulfamethoxazole, every 12 hours for 21 days.[71,109] Rectal stenosis may require a resective procedure or a diversion[63] (Figure 19-50).[63]

Molluscum Contagiosum

Molluscum contagiosum is a communicable skin disease caused by a poxvirus. It is seen principally in preschool and elementary school children. In adults, the condition can involve the skin of the abdomen, thighs, groin, genitalia, buttocks, and, in homosexual men, the perianal area. The lesions begin as papules, often develop central umbilication, and may be widely disseminated. They are often asymptomatic but may be pruritic.

Molluscum contagiosum has a characteristic histopathology. There is a downward proliferation of the rete

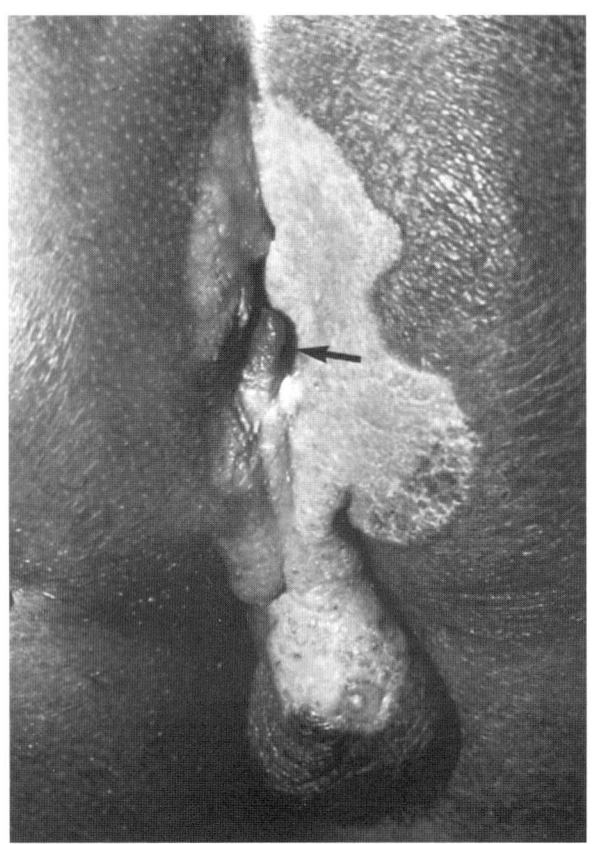

FIGURE 19-46. Granuloma inguinale. This is a chronic, irregularly shaped, enlarging ulceration of the perianal area *(arrow)*. Note the hypertrophic scarring devoid of pigment. (Courtesy of Samuel L. Moschella, M.D.)

ridges and envelopment by the connective tissue to form a deep crater. So-called molluscum bodies are found in the cytoplasm of the cells of the stratum malpighii (Figure 19-51).

Treatment may not be required, because the lesions usually heal without scarring unless secondarily infected. Curettage can be employed using ethyl chloride spray for freezing. Liquid nitrogen, electrocoagulation, 20% podophyllin, trichloracetic acid, carbon dioxide laser, and pulsed dye laser have also been effective.[271]

Herpes Genitalis, Genital Herpes, Herpes Simplex Infection, Herpes

Herpes simplex is a ubiquitous infection caused by a virus that has been associated with a number of acute, limited, vesicular eruptions near mucocutaneous junctions. Synonyms include fever blister, cold sore, herpes febrilis, herpes labialis, and genital herpes. According to the CDC, approximately 500,000 new cases occur annually, with 60 million Americans believed to be harboring the virus.[109]

Classically, herpes simplex virus type 1 (HSV-1) commonly appeared above the waistline and was not usually sexually acquired, whereas with the type 2 form (HSV-2), the opposite was often the case.[109] With the increased frequency of oral-genital sex, however, both types may be found in each location. The likelihood of reactivation of herpes simplex infection differs between HSV-1 and HSV-2 infections; the frequency of clinical recurrence with the genital form is six times that of the oral-labial type.[161]

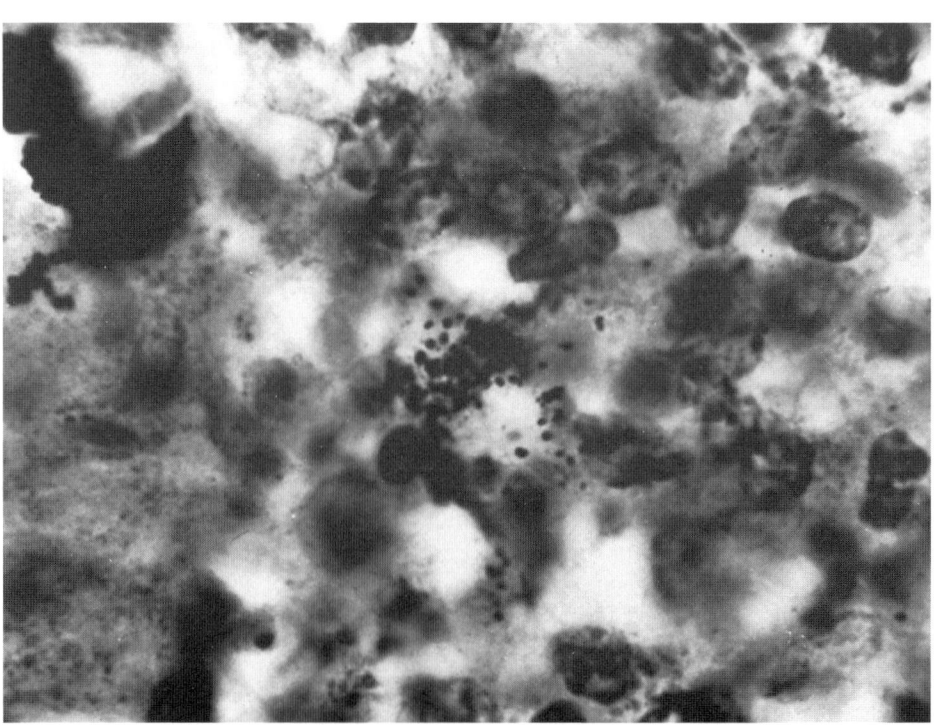

FIGURE 19-47. Granuloma inguinale. Donovan bodies in macrophages are demonstrated by Leishman's stain. (Original magnification × 600; courtesy of Rudolf Garret, M.D.)

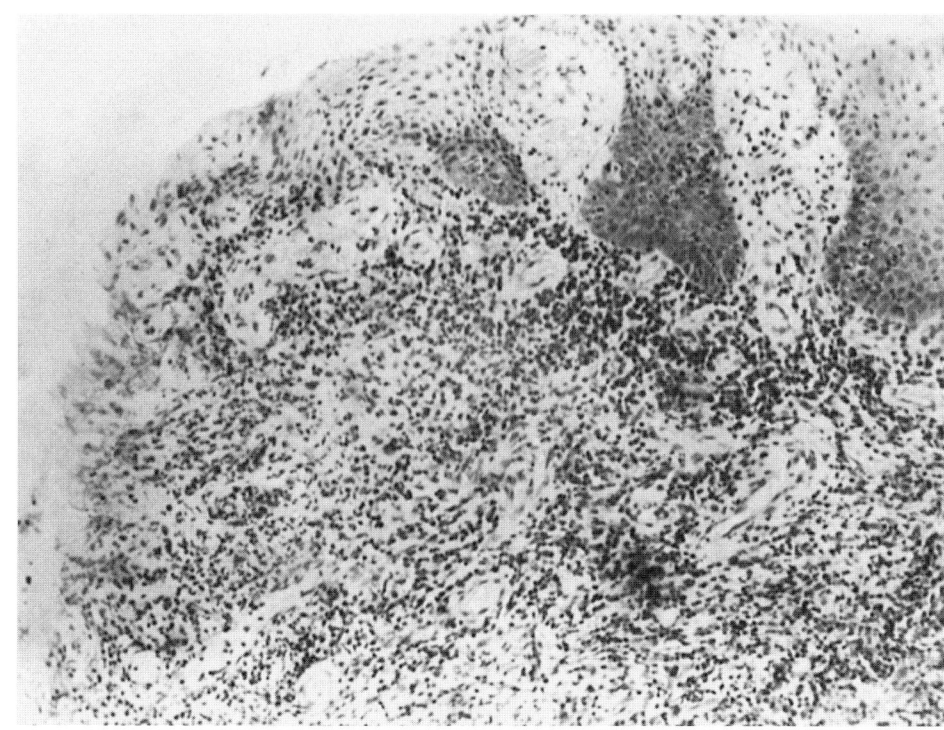

FIGURE 19-48. Granuloma inguinale. Mononuclear cell infiltrate in the dermis with an ulcer on the left is seen. (Original magnification × 120; courtesy of Rudolf Garret, M.D.)

The major symptoms of herpes infection are painful blisters or open sores in the genital area. These may be preceded by a tingling or burning sensation in the legs, buttocks, or genital region. The herpes sores usually disappear within 2 to 3 weeks, but the virus remains in the body for life, and the lesions may recur from time to time. Cutaneous lesions associated with herpes simplex infections are usually characteristic vesicles in small groups. However, patients are often not seen until the vesicles have ulcerated. In the genital area, painful lesions may appear on the prepuce, glans, shaft of the penis, labia, vulva, clitoris, and cervix. The inguinal nodes may be firm and tender. Healing is usually complete by 10 days.

The anal area and medial buttocks are also commonly involved, especially in homosexual men. Jacobs reported

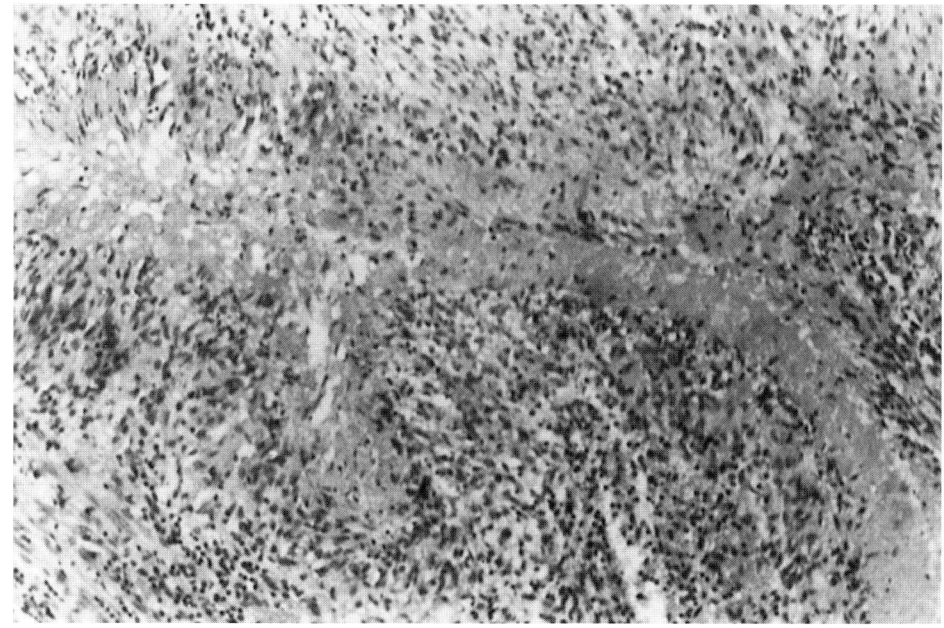

FIGURE 19-49. Lymphogranuloma venereum. Stellate granuloma in a lymph node is evident. (Original magnification × 280; courtesy of Rudolf Garret, M.D.)

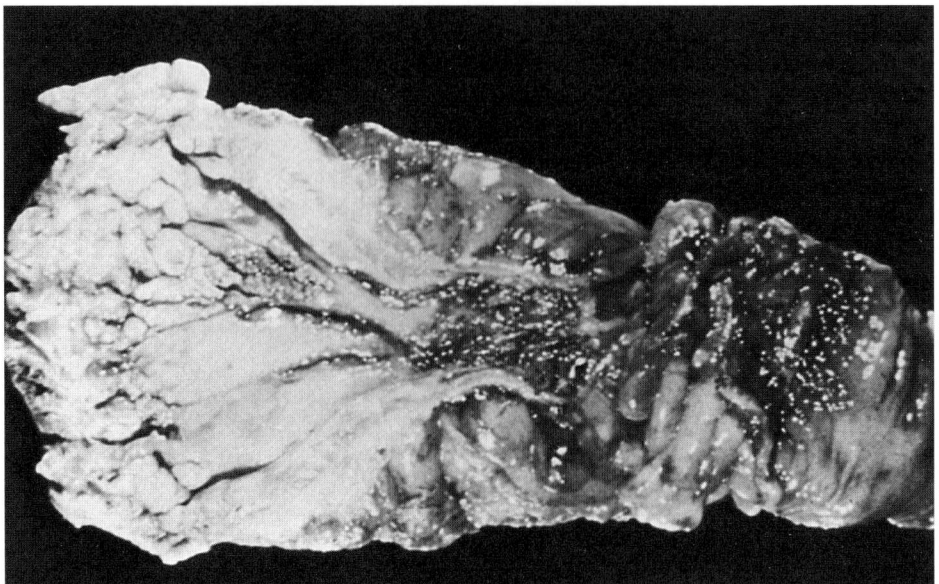

FIGURE 19-50. Severe rectal stricture caused by lymphogranuloma venereum necessitated proctectomy. If resection is necessary, reestablishment of intestinal continuity should be attempted if possible. (From Corman ML, Veidenheimer MC, Swinton NW. *Diseases of the anus, rectum and colon. Part I: neoplasms.* New York: Medcom, 1972, with permission.)

16 patients with herpes simplex infection of the perianal skin and anal canal over a 2-year period.[136] There were 14 men and two women; all were either homosexual or bisexual. Chronic perianal herpes is also more frequently seen in immunocompromised patients (see Chapter 20).[144]

Following infection, the virus travels by an afferent nerve to the associated ganglion (e.g., HSV-2 goes to the sacral ganglion) and remains in the body in a latent state. At this stage there are no clinical manifestations, but reactivation of the virus may occur, usually two or three

times a year, sometimes after a fever, emotional upset, trauma, or perhaps menstruation. Prodromal symptoms of exacerbation include itching, tingling, and radiating pain to the pelvis and legs. Recurrent episodes tend to be of shorter duration and intensity. Once infected, the patient is condemned to have herpes for life.

Concerns about herpes infections relate not only to the primary cutaneous process, but also to adverse psychological effects and to the risk for transmission from pregnant mothers to newborns. There may also be an in-

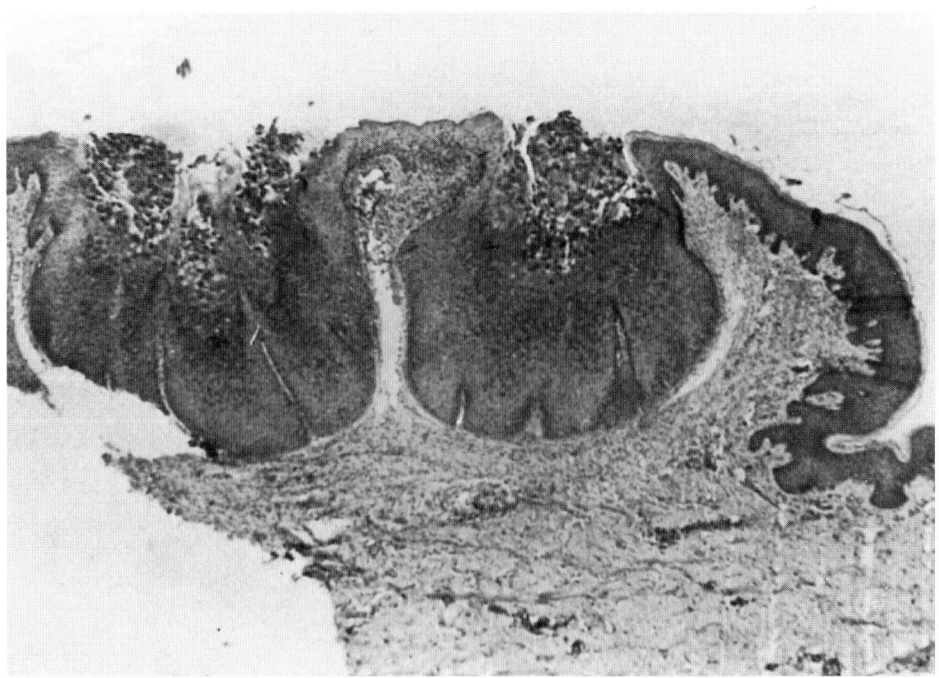

FIGURE 19-51. Proliferation of squamous cells with formation of pear-shaped lobules and molluscum bodies in the central, crater-like area, characteristic of molluscum contagiosum. (Original magnification × 120; courtesy of Rudolf Garret, M.D.)

creased frequency of cervical cancer. Untreated neonatal herpes is associated with a 50% mortality rate, but this risk can be reduced by cesarean delivery.

To determine the risk for sexual transmission of herpes simplex virus, Mertz and colleagues prospectively studied heterosexual couples in which one partner had symptomatic recurrent disease.[182] They concluded that transmission appeared to result from sexual contact during periods of asymptomatic viral shedding in 70% of individuals. Furthermore, they noted that the risk for acquisition of herpes simplex virus was higher in women than in men.

Diagnosis

A direct fluorescent antibody technique using the fluid from a vesicle is a rapid means for confirmation. Tzanck's preparation, in which scrapings are placed on a slide and stained, will reveal intranuclear inclusion bodies and giant cells. The most definitive method for the diagnosis of herpes simplex virus infection is viral culture, but this is a cumbersome, expensive study. The clinical picture of grouped vesicles on an erythematous base anywhere in the body suggests herpes infection, so that laboratory studies serve primarily for confirmation.

Treatment

Current therapy for the condition is the use of an antiviral preparation, acyclovir (Zovirax), but it does not cure the disease.[88,124,183,193,215,244] Acyclovir is a synthetic acyclic purine nucleoside analog that exhibits *in vitro* inhibitory activity against the virus. Treatment is directed to three areas: management of the initial episode, management of the recurrence, and maintenance between attacks. Primary herpes of less than 7 days' duration is treated by oral acyclovir, 200 mg five times daily for 10 days. Intermittent therapy, given at the first sign of recurrence, consists of 200 mg five times daily for 5 days. Long-term suppressive therapy for recurrent disease is 400 mg two times daily for up to 12 months. Patients who present after 1 week but who still have early vesicular lesions or constitutional symptoms may also benefit from therapy. However, acyclovir is not recommended for the management of crusted lesions and for patients who are asymptomatic.[124] Recurrent episodes must be treated within 48 hours if beneficial results are to be expected, but some clinicians believe that acyclovir has no measurable effect on the natural history of the disease.[124] Suppressive therapy is probably most effective in those patients who are subject to frequent exacerbations, but asymptomatic shedding of the virus implies that the individual is still infectious. Continuous or episodic oral acyclovir therapy has been demonstrated to be safe and reasonably effective, with annual rates of recurrence substantially reduced.[145,184] Some recommend interrupting any prolonged treatment to assess further need.[243]

Topical care should include frequent gentle cleansing of the area with alcohol. A cortisone-antibiotic ointment may be employed when the lesions are crusted but not vesicular. Acyclovir ointment applied to the affected area may also be of value during an attack.

Condylomata Acuminata (Venereal Warts)

Condylomata acuminata represent the most common STI in the practice of most surgeons. The condition is also among the most troublesome to eliminate. Health officials estimate that genital or anal warts develop in 1 million Americans annually, and two thirds of their sexual partners acquire the condition. The disease is caused by HPV, a DNA virus that is a member of the papovavirus group.[31] Evidence suggests that the virus is antigenically, biochemically, and immunologically distinct from the virus of the common wart, verruca vulgaris.[31] Although the condition may occur in heterosexual men and women, it is most commonly seen in male homosexuals. It may be found in association with other conditions, such as gonorrhea, lymphogranuloma venereum, and syphilis, especially in those who have had homosexual contact.[177] A retrospective review of 677 patients who tested positive for HIV revealed that 119 (19%) had anal condylomata.[27] The condition has also been reported in a child with HIV infection.[164] Because there is such a strong association, all patients who are observed to have anal condylomata should undergo appropriate blood testing for HIV (see Chapter 20).

Condylomata acuminata can also occur in infants and children. The increased incidence of anogenital warts in children is rising; sexual abuse has been implicated as a potential cause.[43] It is, therefore, important to be aware of this relationship and to report suspected cases of sexual abuse to the appropriate authorities, including child protection services.

Symptoms

Patients usually complain of a lump or lumps and often think that the problem is caused by hemorrhoids. Other symptoms include discharge, pruritus, difficulty with defecation, anal pain, tenesmus, foul odor, and rectal bleeding.

A characteristic scenario is one in which the patient reports having received some form of topical external therapy over many weeks or months. The fact that the treatment has failed precipitates the second opinion or referral. Clearly, treatment of the external component should not be undertaken unless the patient has undergone an adequate anoscopic examination. External application of various medicaments is doomed to failure if disease is present in the anal canal. However, I believe that I am probably preaching to the choir, because the initial treatment is often rendered by a nonsurgeon.

Examination

The appearance of the lesion usually makes the diagnosis quite obvious. The warts are usually small, discrete, elevated, pink to gray, vegetative excrescences in the anal canal, perianal skin, and urogenital region (Figure 19-52). They may be single or multiple or may coalesce to form polypoid masses. Lesions in the anal canal rarely extend into the rectum, but are confined to the squamous epithelium and transitional zones. The wart itself is histologically a hyperplastic epithelial growth with irregular acanthosis and marked hyperkeratosis (Figure 19-53).

Treatment

The previously mentioned Standards Task Force of the American Society of Colon and Rectal Surgeons has recommended certain practice parameters for ambulatory surgery of anal condylomata.[239] The statement reads as follows:

> When condylomata are limited to the perianal skin, treatment with topical medications, local destruction, or harvesting and immunotherapy can be administered in an outpatient setting. Patients with extensive perianal or anal canal condylomata or those patients with associated genital condylomata may require inpatient care.

Numerous methods of treating anal condylomata have been proposed, including the following:

- Podophyllin
- Bichloracetic acid and other caustic agents
- Immunotherapy
- Immunomodulation
- Chemotherapy
- Sublesional injection of interferon alfa
- Cryotherapy
- Electrocoagulation
- Laser therapy
- Surgical excision

Podophyllin Podophyllin is a chemical agent that is cytotoxic for the warts, but it has the disadvantage of being quite irritating to the skin. It is therefore important to apply the liquid with care, and then only to the warts. Podophyllum resin, derived from the plants *Podophyllum emodi* and *P. peltatum*, contains many biologically active lignin compounds, including podofilox, the most thoroughly characterized and the most active against genital warts.[30] The technique has the advantage of being simple and inexpensive, but its application is limited to external warts. As with all topical methods, no specimen is available for pathologic determination; this also is a theoretical disadvantage. Dysplasia has been reported with prolonged use, but whether this is from the warts or from the chemical itself has been a matter of some conjecture. Multiple treatments are often required.

Simmons performed a randomly allocated double-blind study of 10% and 25% podophyllin in 140 men with anogenital warts.[230] There was no significant difference in the effect of the two preparations; only 22% of the patients were free of warts following 3 months of therapy. Beutner and colleagues utilized a technique whereby patients applied the chemical to themselves without systemic adverse reactions and with satisfactory results.[30]

Bichloracetic Acid or Dichloracetic Acid Bichloracetic acid, an extremely powerful keratolytic and cauterant, has also been successfully employed in the management of condylomata. The chemical rapidly penetrates and cauterizes the skin, keratin, and other tissues. Like podophyllin, it is simple to apply and is inexpensive. Additionally, it has the advantage of being applicable to the anal canal. Multiple office visits are usually required, however, and there is the concern for skin irritation and discomfort.[264]

Swerdlow and Salvati treated 34 patients by bichloracetic acid only, in an uncontrolled study comparing patients who had undergone other forms of therapy.[249] The authors concluded that the recurrence rate was lower and discomfort was less.

Immunotherapy Abcarian and Sharon stimulated considerable interest in 1982 by employing another approach to the management of anal condylomata, that of immunotherapy.[2] A vaccine is created by excising and washing the condyloma tissue, and a 10% suspension is prepared in Medium 199 supplemented with antibiotics. Following homogenization and freezing, it is then centrifuged, and the supernatant is heated. The inactivated material is then centrifuged again, and the supernatant is collected and tested for bacterial sterility. The patient is vaccinated with six consecutive weekly injections of 0.5 mL, subcutaneously administered in the deltoid area, with the vaccine frozen between injections.[1–3]

Two hundred consecutive patients were studied during an 8-year period.[3] Excellent results were seen in 84%, and fair results in 11%; no improvement was noted in 5%. There were no adverse reactions or complications. The authors concluded that immunotherapy should be the recommended method of treatment for extensive, recurrent, or persistent anal condylomata.

Eftaiha and colleagues reported their own experience with immunotherapy and compared it with other more conventional forms of treatment.[96] Condylomata were successfully eradicated in approximately 94% of patients by this means. It was the authors' opinion, however, that this treatment modality should be reserved for recurrent and giant anal condylomata. Wiltz and co-workers compared surgical excision followed by vaccination using an autogenous condylomata acuminata vaccine for primary and recurrent perianal warts with other modalities.[270] They found this approach far superior to excision alone, bichloracetic

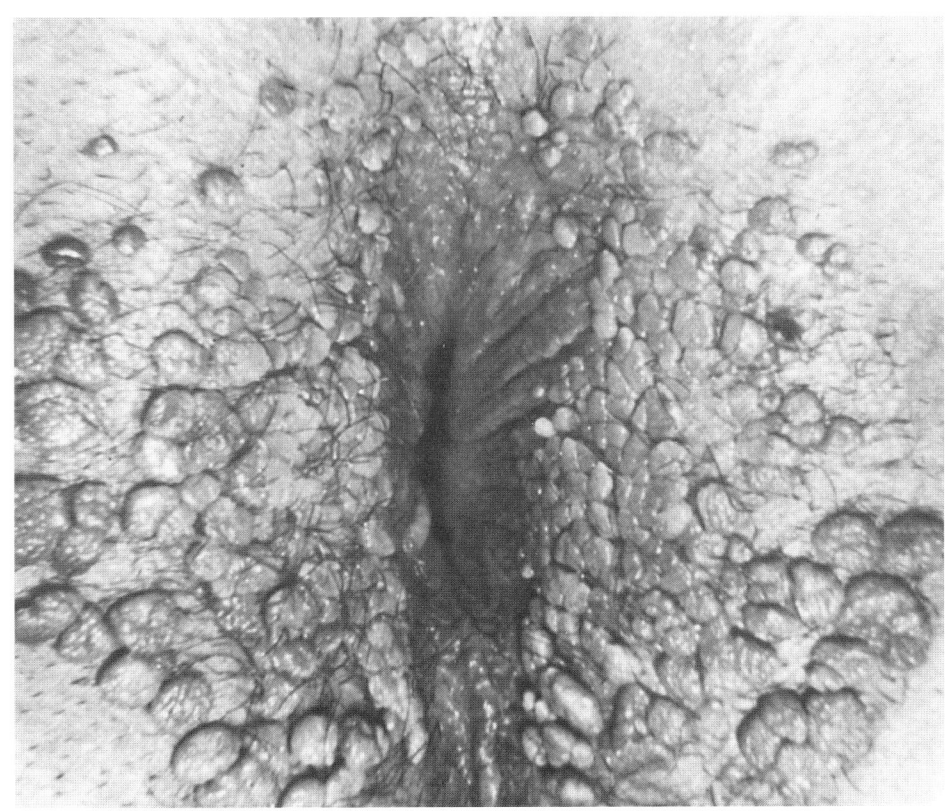

FIGURE 19-52. Condylomata acuminata. Multiple, closely grouped papillomas create a cauliflower-like appearance. (From Corman ML, Veidenheimer MC, Swinton NW. *Diseases of the anus, rectum and colon. Part I: neoplasms.* New York: Medcom, 1972, with permission.)

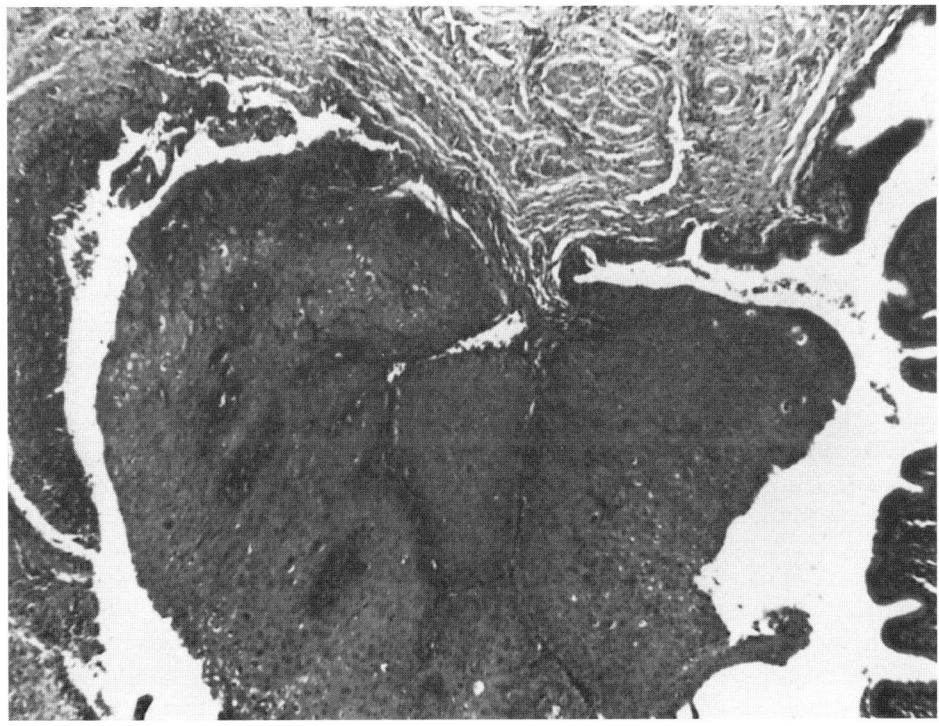

FIGURE 19-53. Condylomata acuminata in an anal duct. Note the proliferation of squamous cells, vacuolated squamous cells, and hyperchromatic nuclei, and the absence of a cornified layer. Note also the columnar epithelium lining the anal duct. (Original magnification × 120; courtesy of Rudolf Garret, M.D.)

acid, podophyllin, and interferon alfa. The recurrence rate with a mean follow-up of 13 months was only 4.6%.

Although the results of immunotherapy are really quite good, the application of this modality has become a moot issue, because convincing a laboratory to prepare it is virtually impossible. Because of the potential liability hazards and the considerable financial investment needed to perform the clinical and laboratory trials required by the United States Food and Drug Administration, no laboratory has been willing to assume the responsibility. However, if the physician is able to convince the appropriate personnel to become involved, the technique used for vaccine preparation is well within the capacity of a standard hospital laboratory.

Immunomodulators

IMIDAZOQUINOLINES. The imidazoquinolines are a new class of immune-response modifiers (immunomodulators) that have been introduced for the treatment of *external* genital and perianal warts. Imiquimod (Aldara) cream 5% (3M Pharmaceuticals) does not possess direct antiviral activity, nor does it cause direct, nonspecific cytolysis.[256] Although its mechanism of action is unknown, it is thought to play a role in the cytokine-induced activation of the immune system.

The product is self-applied three times per week at bedtime. The primary side effect is that of local skin reaction, especially erythema. Treatment is continued until the warts are eradicated or until 16 weeks have elapsed. Results of clinical studies have demonstrated early promise in the treatment of those affected with external condylomata.

CIDOFOVIR (HPMPC). Another immunomodulator has been reported from Belgium, cidofovir (Vistide Pharmacia, Brussels, Belgium).[62] This antiviral topical agent has been demonstrated to be effective in HPV infections. Coremans and colleagues found that this drug compared favorably with electrocoagulation in a noncontrolled study, but its primary value was to supplement conventional electrosurgery when recurrence developed.[62]

COMMENT. Further publications are awaited concerning the merits of both of these immunomodulators, but the fact that they are applicable only to the external component causes one to be quite circumspect as to the relative value for the practice of colon and rectal surgeons.

Topical Cytostatics Various chemotherapeutic agents have been advocated in the treatment of this condition, including 5-fluorouracil,[191] thiotepa,[51] and bleomycin.[106,207] Figueroa and Gennaro injected bleomycin intralesionally in ten patients at intervals of every 2 to 3 weeks.[106] An overall success rate of 70% was achieved. Three individuals experienced total resolution of the condylomata after the first treatment, but three patients failed to respond after

several sessions. With the exception of discomfort, there were no systemic effects following the treatment.

Interferon Human leukocyte interferon (Alferon N), because of its antiproliferative and antiviral properties, has been demonstrably effective in the treatment of condylomata acuminata.[100,113,133] Interferons are produced and secreted in response to viral infections and to a variety of other synthetic and biologic inducers. Alferon N is manufactured from pooled units of human leukocytes that have been induced by incomplete infection with an avian virus to produce interferon alfa-n3.

Eron and colleagues performed a randomized, controlled study involving 257 patients and injected the substance intralesionally into each wart.[100] There was a statistically significant reduction in wart area in the treated group. A later report revealed complete clearance of warts in 62% of patients.[113] Fleschner and Freilich performed a prospective, randomized controlled study in which one group of patients underwent surgical excision and fulguration immediately followed by an injection of 500,000 IU (0.1 mL) of interferon alfa-n3 into each quadrant of the anal canal.[111] The other group underwent surgical excision and fulguration but then received four injections of saline solution into each quadrant. After a mean follow-up of 3.8 months, condylomata recurred in 23%, but only 12% were noted to have recurrence in the interferon-treated group. A 39% recurrence rate was observed in the controls. The difference was statistically significant.

Individual warts may be readily treated by this technique, but patient intolerance would probably preclude its application for larger lesions. Under these circumstances, the recommendation of excision combined with interferon treatment has been demonstrated to have merit.[60]

The most commonly observed adverse effects are mild, transient, flulike symptoms. Cyclic therapy with low-dose interferon has also been believed to be very effective.[123] In asymptomatic individuals affected with HIV, the therapeutic response to intralesional treatment with interferon is considerably reduced.[89] The management of condylomata by this technique is also very expensive (see Chapter 20).

Current recommendation is to inject each wart with 0.05 mL (250,000 IU) twice weekly for up to 8 weeks. The maximum dose per session should not exceed 0.5 mL (2.5 million IU).

Cryotherapy Cryotherapy is an approach that is also advocated for the treatment of this condition.[190,223] Savin reported one failure in six patients.[223] It is certainly one of the most frequently utilized techniques by dermatologists for removal of conventional warts on the fingers and hands. Topical application of liquid nitrogen is simple to accomplish and requires the use of very little special equipment. This can be performed with a spray or with the use of a cotton-tipped applicator and can be applied with limited success within the anal canal. As with the foregoing methods, no pathologic specimen is obtained. Some patients report sufficient discomfort that either a local or regional anesthetic may be required.

Laser Therapy Some have recommended laser therapy in the treatment of condylomata, with early success noted in the range of 88% to 95%.[79,227] Contact lasers have been said to produce more predictable, sharply defined areas of thermal necrosis than electrosurgery, although noncontact neodymiun:yttrium-aluminum-garnet and carbon dioxide lasers have been successfully employed.[227] One of the concerns that has been expressed is the possibility of vaporizing the viral particles, with consequent risk to the surgeon and to the operating room team. Special mask precautions are, therefore, thought to be required. Other disadvantages are the absence of a pathologic specimen and the expensive equipment that is required.

Billingham and Lewis reported a controlled study of 38 patients.[31] Surgical therapy was performed on the left half of the anus (i.e., electrocoagulation), whereas the right half was treated with the carbon dioxide laser. The authors concluded that the laser was associated with at least as much pain as electrocoagulation. Furthermore, recurrences were seen more often on the laser side. These factors, along with the high cost of the equipment, implied no advantage to this form of treatment.

Another randomized trial also compared carbon dioxide laser therapy with conventional electrocoagulation.[92] There was no difference between the two groups with respect to number of recurrences, postoperative pain, healing time, and rate of scar formation. The authors believed that treat-

ment of recalcitrant condylomata acuminata with the laser did not offer any advantages over traditional surgery.

Electrocoagulation and Surgical Excision Electrocoagulation with excision of a portion of the specimen to submit for pathologic examination is the "gold standard" for the management of *anal canal* condylomata. The procedure can be undertaken in the office if there are only a few warts present. A local anesthetic injection is generally required because of the anticipated pain, however. For more extensive warts, a general anesthetic, field block, or spinal or epidural anesthetic is recommended.

The technique of electrocoagulation requires the creation of a first- or at most a second-degree burn. When the needle-tip electrode is used, the wart is virtually exploded, and the residual tissue is wiped away with a dry sponge (Figure 19-54). It is helpful to remove a sampling of the warts to submit for pathologic examination. This can be accomplished by simple scissors dissection. If the "burn" is not undertaken too deeply, pain is not very severe; it can usually be controlled with a nonnarcotic prescription. Creating a burn deep into the dermis or fat is wrong. Patients will likely complain bitterly of pain, and there is a risk for the subsequent development of an anal stricture if a large area is to be treated. The patient is advised to take sitz baths and is seen every 2 weeks for evaluation and possible office treatment.

Results Close follow-up examination is required to treat recurrent lesions as soon as they are evident, without, it is hoped, the need to return the patient to the operating room. Unfortunately, fewer than one half of my patients

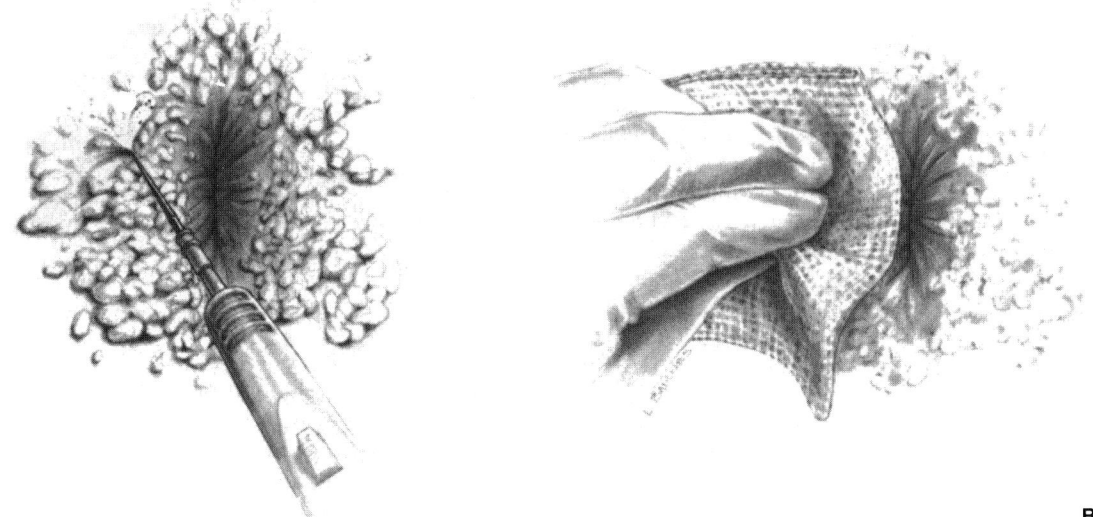

A   **B**

FIGURE 19-54. Technique of diathermy excision of anal condylomata. **(A)** With a needle-tip electrode, warts are individually electrocoagulated. **(B)** Wiping the debris with a dry sponge should leave behind intact skin, with evidence only of a first- or second-degree burn.

have resolution of the process after only one treatment. It is important, therefore, for the patient to understand that therapy may be rather prolonged. However, once the warts have been removed and the wounds have healed, the condition usually does not recur. Preoperative immune status has been shown to affect the likelihood of recurrence following surgical excision. de la Fuente and co-workers performed a retrospective review on 63 consecutive patients with anal condylomata who underwent excision.[76] Forty-five were immunocompromised (HIV-positive patients, patients with leukemia, transplant recipients), and 18 were immunocompetent. Recurrence developed with a statistically significantly increased frequency and within a shorter period of time in the immunocompromised group.

Khawaja prospectively compared podophyllin versus scissor excision in the treatment of condylomata acuminata.[151] With the former method, initial complete clearance was noted in 89% versus 79% with podophyllin. However, only one third were free of recurrence at 42 weeks with podophyllin, compared with 72% in the scissor excision group. A similar trial from another institution revealed comparable results.[139]

Anal Intraepithelial Neoplasia

Anal intraepithelial neoplasia (AIN) is a lesion that is thought to be a precursor of anal squamous cell carcinoma (see Chapter 24) and has been observed in those with HIV and AIDS (see Chapter 20). The incidence of subclinical AIN in patients with anal condylomata has been studied by the Cleveland Clinic Florida Group.[59] Thirty-one percent of 97 specimens were found to harbor unsuspected AIN. The incidence was higher in the HIV-positive group (51%) as compared with the HIV-negative patients (17%). The authors stress the importance of obtaining pathologic material.

Opinion

External condylomata without evidence of internal warts can usually be effectively treated by chemical means (e.g., podophyllin, bichloracetic acid, imiquimod). If the response is unsatisfactory, physical destruction by electrocoagulation is the preferred approach. If there are only a few warts, the use of a local anesthetic will permit adequate office treatment. For more extensive lesions, I prefer to use a general anesthetic, administered on an outpatient basis. Obtaining tissue for pathologic confirmation, especially with respect to premalignant or malignant change, is a prudent philosophy.

Giant Condyloma Acuminatum or Buschke-Löwenstein Tumor and Malignant Degeneration

The Buschke-Löwenstein tumor, also known as giant condyloma acuminatum, is a variant of anal condylomata that tends to behave in a locally malignant fashion, bur-

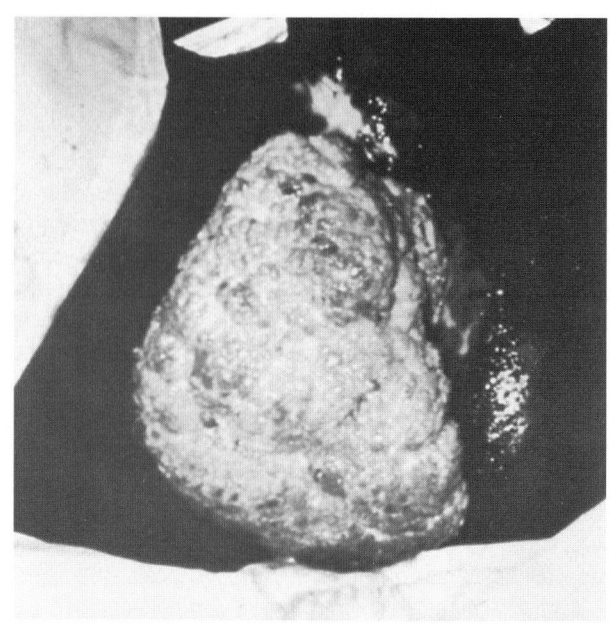

FIGURE 19-55. Verrucous squamous carcinoma, or tumor of Buschke-Löwenstein. (From Corman ML, Veidenheimer MC, Swinton NW. *Diseases of the anus, rectum and colon. Part I: neoplasms.* New York: Medcom, 1972, with permission.)

rowing deeply into adjacent structures (Figure 19-55).[5,98] According to Trombetta and Place, 52 cases were reported in the English literature from 1958 to 2000.[255]

Numerous articles have described the development of squamous cell carcinoma in these rare "giant" cases.[68,166,171,205] Creasman and colleagues hypothesize that this entity represents an intermediate lesion in a pathologic continuum from condyloma acuminatum to squamous cell carcinoma.[65] Chu and co-workers analyzed 42 cases in the English literature and reviewed the behavior and management of the lesion.[53] They observed the hallmark of the disease to be the high rate of recurrence (66%) and the high incidence of malignant transformation (56%). Recurrences developed in 50% of those who were initially treated with radical surgery.

Wide local excision, however, is the recommended initial surgical approach. If the margins are free of tumor, no further treatment is warranted. Occasionally, however, the lesion may be so extensive that it is deemed unresectable. Butler and colleagues reported a case successfully managed by intravenous 5-fluorouracil, mitomycin C, and extended-field radiation.[46] Adjuvant chemoradiation therapy has been found to be associated with an improved cure rate in comparison with surgery alone.[53] Others have report successful regression with radiation therapy.[235] Adjuvant therapy with lesions of this type should be considered in accordance with the protocol described in Chapter 24. In addition, malignant transformation in a virally caused illness, especially a condition that is common in the immunocompromised population, should alert the physician to the possibility of AIDS (see Chapter 20).

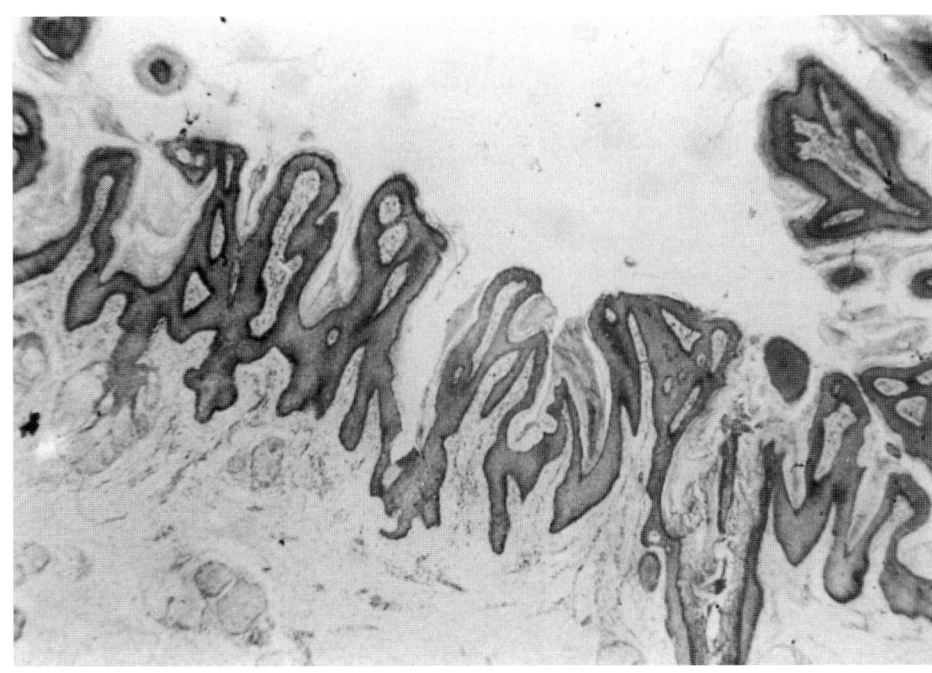

FIGURE 19-56. Acanthosis nigricans, epithelium in a papillary configuration with pigmented cells in the basal cell layer. (Original magnification × 260; courtesy of Rudolf Garret, M.D.)

Human Immunodeficiency Virus Infection and Acquired Immunodeficiency Syndrome

AIDS was first reported in the United States in 1981. It is caused by HIV, and an estimated 900,000 people in the United States are currently infected. Transmission of the virus primarily occurs during sexual activity and by sharing needles used to inject intravenous drugs. The colorectal manifestations are discussed in Chapter 20.

PREMALIGNANT AND MALIGNANT DERMATOSES

Malignant neoplasms of the anal margin and perianal skin include basal cell carcinoma, extramammary Paget's disease, Bowen's disease, malignant melanoma, and epidermoid carcinoma. The last two conditions are discussed in Chapter 24. Leukemic and lymphomatous infiltration also may involve the anal area. In addition to these, two other cutaneous lesions may be premalignant or associated with cancer elsewhere: acanthosis nigricans and leukoplakia.

Acanthosis Nigricans

Acanthosis nigricans is known chiefly to surgeons for its ominous association with abdominal cancer in adults.[38] Regions affected include the face, neck, axillae, external genitalia, groin, inner thighs, umbilicus, and anus. The condition appears usually as a grayish, velvety thickening or roughening of the skin. The pathologic changes are epidermal, with papillomatosis, hyperkeratosis, and hyperpigmentation (Figure 19-56). Pruritus is the most frequent symptom.

The malignant form of acanthosis nigricans may antedate, accompany, or follow the onset of the internal cancer. Most abdominal malignancies are adenocarcinomas, usually of gastric origin (60%). The tumor itself is usually advanced at the time of discovery and has a rapid progression. Treatment is directed to the primary malignant condition.

Leukoplakia

Leukoplakia is a whitish thickening of the mucous membrane epithelium occurring in patches of diverse size and shape. In the anal canal, it is seen mostly in

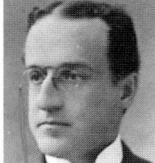

John Templeton Bowen (1857–1940) Bowen was born in Boston, Massachusetts, the son of a prominent family. He attended Boston Latin School, and graduated from Harvard College in 1879 and from Harvard Medical School in 1884. For most of the ensuing 3 years, he studied in Berlin, Munich, and Vienna. He must have developed an interest in dermatologic problems during this time, because in 1889 he was appointed assistant physician to outpatients with diseases of the skin at the Massachusetts General Hospital. In 1907, he became the first Wigglesworth Professor of Dermatology at Harvard Medical School, before which he was elected president of the American Dermatologic Association. Bowen is best remembered for his description of precancerous dermatoses. A man who loved quiet and solitude, he is recognized as one of the preeminent figures in the field of dermatology.

men and is occasionally associated with delayed wound healing (e.g., following excision of a fissure, hemorrhoids, and condylomata). Although the anal condition itself does *not* represent a malignancy, when it occurs in the gingival and buccal mucosa, there is a high risk for the development of epidermoid carcinoma. Bleeding, discharge, and pruritic symptoms are the most common complaints.

Microscopically, hyperkeratosis and squamous metaplasia are seen (Figure 19-57). Excision of the lesion has been unsuccessful in my experience; the condition simply recurs. However, the likelihood of recurrence may be reduced if an anoplasty is performed, covering the defect with new, full-thickness skin (see Chapter 8). Because of the theoretical potential for malignancy, annual proctosigmoidoscopy (anoscopy) with biopsy of any suspected area is advised.

Mycosis Fungoides

Mycosis fungoides is an uncommon, pruritic, usually fatal cutaneous malignant neoplasm of the lymphoreticular system, specifically the thymus-derived lymphocytes (T cells). Subsequent involvement of lymph nodes and internal organs develops as the disease progresses.

The cutaneous lesion can occur anywhere. The overlying skin may have only telangiectasia or be violaceous, often of varied vivid color (Figure 19-58). As the tumor advances, ulcerations occur (Figure 19-59), and pain is a predominant symptom. Microscopic changes include epi-

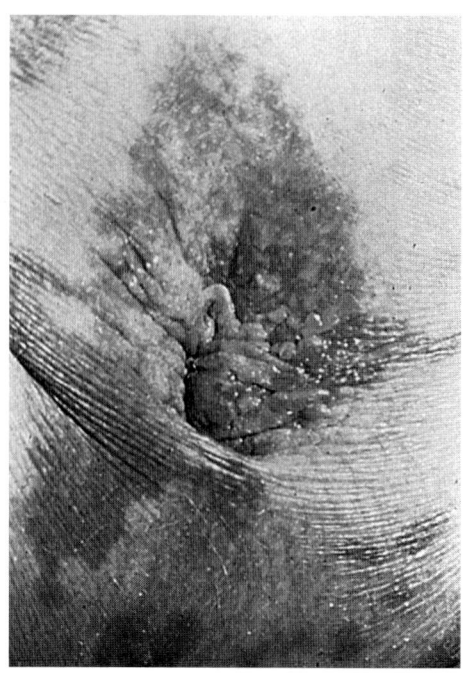

FIGURE 19-58. A violaceous tumor with adjacent reddish brown, irregularly shaped plaques is indicative of mycosis fungoides. (See Color Fig. 19-58.) (From Corman ML, Veidenheimer MC, Swinton NW. *Diseases of the anus, rectum and colon. Part I: neoplasms.* New York: Medcom, 1972, with permission.)

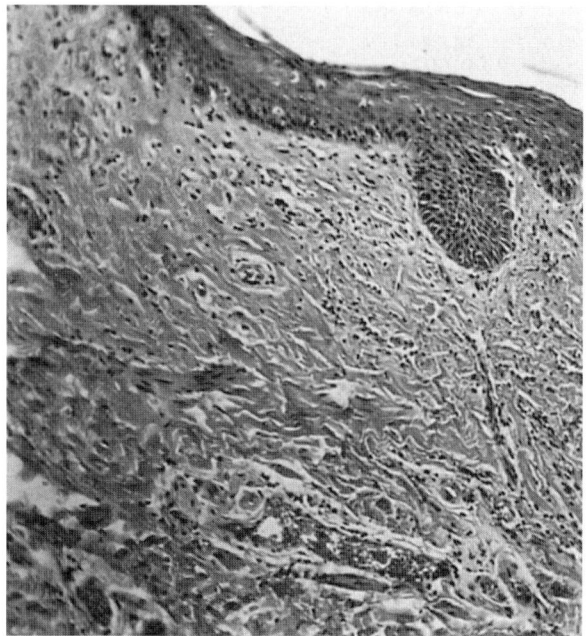

FIGURE 19-57. Leukoplakia. Parakeratosis with atrophy of the epidermis and fibrosis of the dermis is seen. Note the few cells with hyperchromatic nuclei close to the basal cell layer. (Original magnification × 240; courtesy of Rudolf Garret, M.D.)

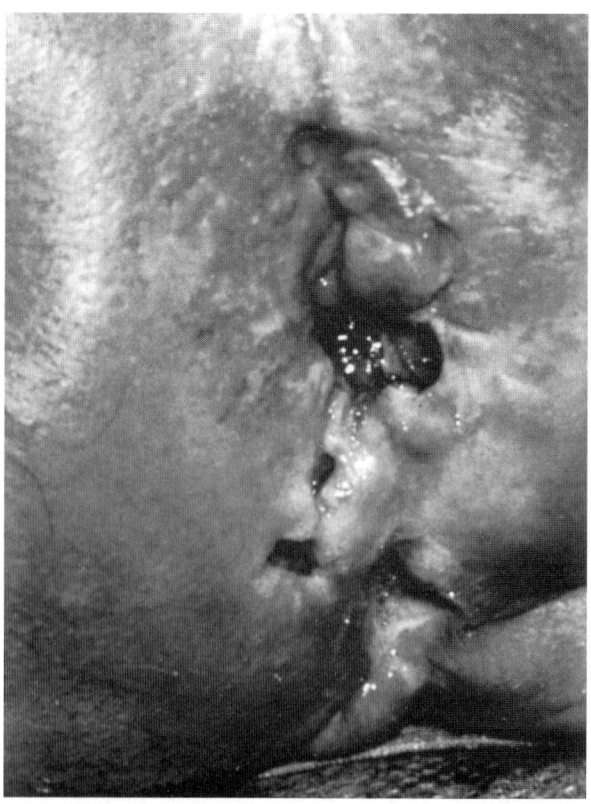

FIGURE 19-59. Perianal ulceration, nodules, and skin infiltration by biopsy-proven lymphomatous infiltrate. (Courtesy of Daniel Rosenthal, M.D.)

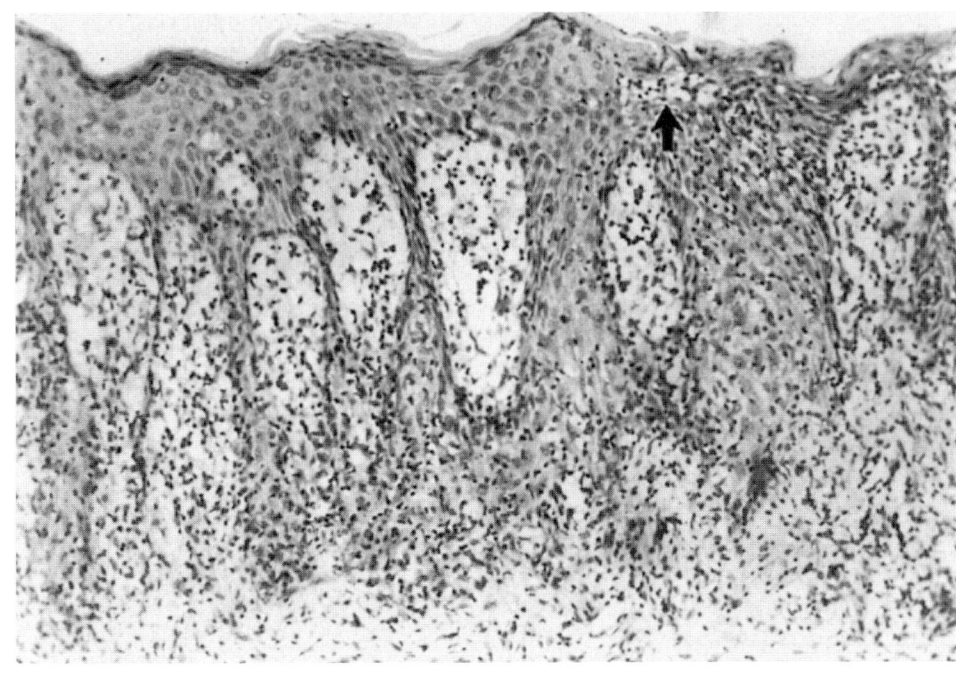

FIGURE 19-60. Mycosis fungoides, pleomorphic infiltrate of the dermis with characteristic Pautrier's abscess *(arrow)* within the epidermis. (Original magnification × 280; courtesy of Rudolf Garret, M.D.)

dermal invasion of small groups of abnormal-appearing lymphocytes and perivascular accumulation of lymphocytic cells. As the disease progresses, increased numbers of abnormal, malignant cells are demonstrated (Figure 19-60). Treatment is directed toward management of the systemic disease.

Leukemia Cutis

Infiltration of the perianal area by leukemic cells is quite uncommon.[66,68,91,231,261] Occasionally, this may be the first manifestation of the malignancy. Leukemia of the skin may consist of a diffuse infiltration, erythema, and ulceration (Figure 19-61). Lymphocytic leukemia characteristically may have a discrete nodular appearance (Figure 19-62). It may present as a fistula, an abscess, or a tender, erythematous area. Cellulitis may be quite marked.

Histologically, masses of cells may be seen in the upper dermis or as nodules in the dermis (Figure 19-63). The type of cells and immature forms are those of the systemic process. Mitoses are infrequently seen in the skin lesions.

Infections in the perianal area are relatively common in patients with myeloproliferative disorders. The incidence in those with acute leukemia is approximately 8% to 9%, with mortality rates as high as 55%.[47] Because the initial symptoms may be confined to the anal area, biopsy and appropriate hematologic studies may be the only means for establishing an early diagnosis.[48] In acute leukemia, the course of the neutrophil count is an important prognostic factor as well as a de-

terminant as to the appropriateness of operative intervention.[47] The reader is referred to Chapter 10 for a discussion of the management of perianal complications of leukemia.

Basal Cell Carcinoma

Basal cell carcinoma is the most common cutaneous malignancy, but in the anal area it is an extremely rare tumor. Only one case was reported in Gabriel's experi-

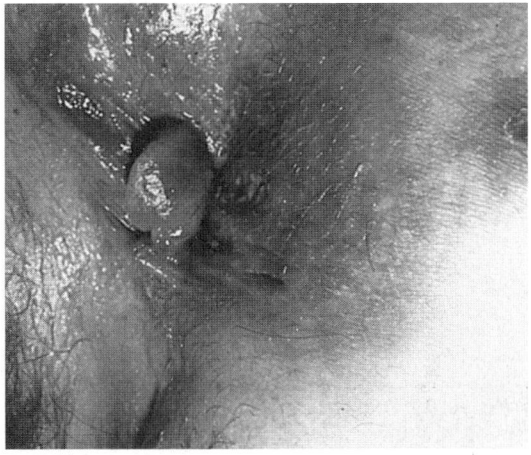

FIGURE 19-61. An ulcerating, violaceous nodule demonstrated leukemic cells on biopsy, indicating leukemia cutis. (See Color Fig. 19-61.) (From Corman ML, Veidenheimer MC, Swinton NW. *Diseases of the anus, rectum and colon. Part I: neoplasms.* New York: Medcom, 1972, with permission.)

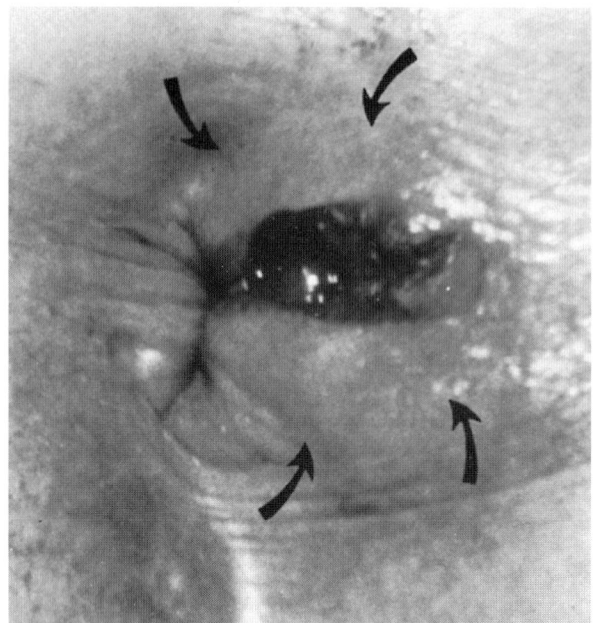

FIGURE 19-62. Leukemia cutis (lymphocytic leukemia). Diffuse swelling and infiltration *(arrows)* with ulceration are noted. (Courtesy of Daniel Rosenthal, M.D.)

ence of 1,700 malignant tumors of the anus and rectum.[118] Most published reports involve one or two patients.[15,45,156,220] Nielsen and Jensen reported the largest single series; 34 patients were treated over a 30-year period.[192] There was no gender predominance. Tumors were usually between 1 and 2 cm in size and localized to the anal margin. Symptoms include the sensation of a lump or of an ulcer in two thirds of patients. Bleeding,

pain, pruritus, and discharge were other observed complaints. Paterson and colleagues reported their experience with 21 patients, 17 of whom were treated by local excision, one by electrocautery, and one by Mohs' surgery.[202] No tumor recurred. One third of the individuals were found to have basal cell cancers at other sites, leading the reviewers to recommend careful assessment of the total skin surface rather than limiting oneself to the perhaps obvious primary complaint.

The characteristic appearance of the lesion is that of a chronic, indurated growth with rolled edges (i.e., pearly border) and a central depression or ulceration (Figure 19-64). Histologically, the tumor arises from the basal cells of the malpighian layer of the skin (Figure 19-65). Sheets of basophilic-staining cells are seen to contain large, blue-staining nuclei with minimal cytoplasm.

Local excision with adequate margins is the preferred treatment. Abdominoperineal resection is performed for neglected, extensive, or infiltrating tumors. There were no deaths caused by basal cell carcinoma in the series of Nielsen and Jensen.[192] Those tumors in other series that were reported to have metastasized were probably basaloid (i.e., cloacogenic) carcinomas with both squamous and basal cell histologic features (see Chapter 24).

Squamous Cell or Epidermoid Carcinoma

Squamous cell carcinoma of the perianal skin is manifested in the same way as lesions occurring in the skin elsewhere on the body. The tumor may appear superficial, discrete, and hard. With progression, it may ulcerate (Figure 19-66) or become papillomatous or cauliflower-

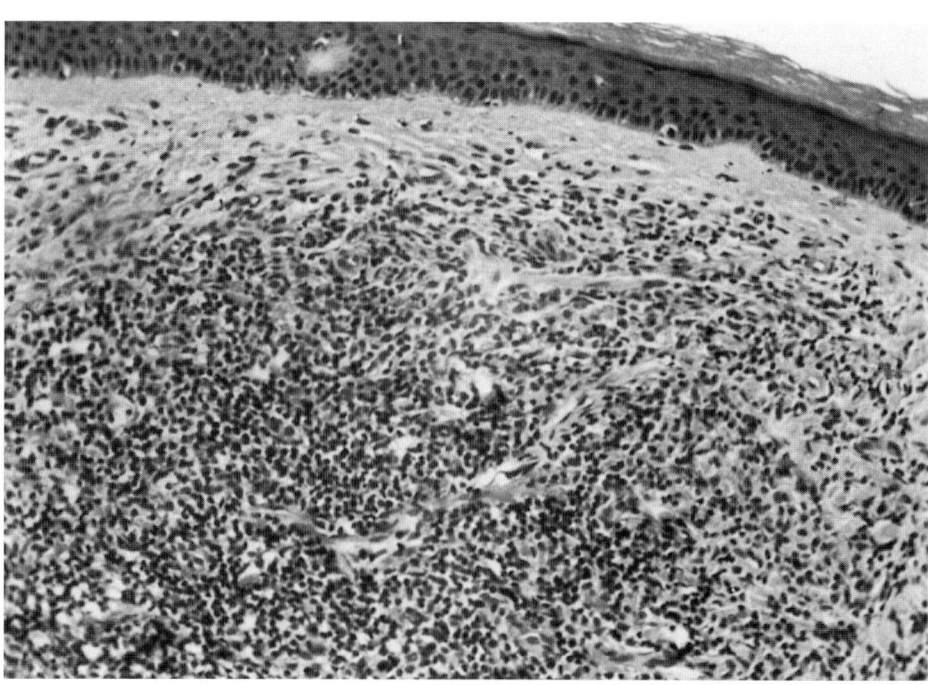

FIGURE 19-63. Leukemia cutis. Infiltration of the dermis by leukemic cells. Note the collagen bundle separating the mass of tumor cells from the underlying epidermis. (Original magnification × 240; courtesy of Rudolf Garret, M.D.)

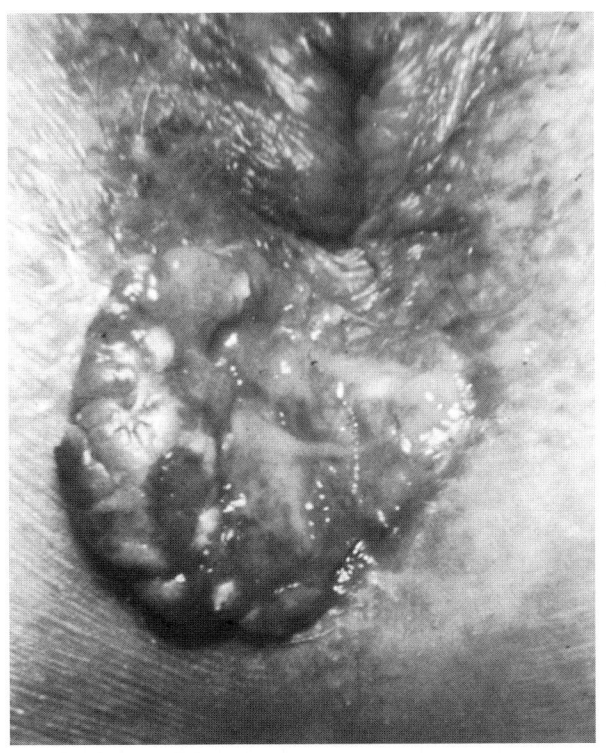

FIGURE 19-64. Basal cell carcinoma (rodent ulcer). This ulcerating tumor has a pearly border. (From Rosenthal D. Basal cell carcinoma of the anus: report of two cases. *Dis Colon Rectum* 1967;10:397, with permission.)

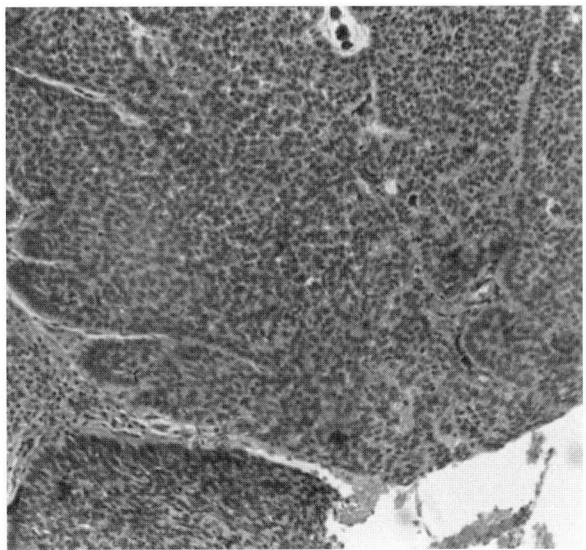

FIGURE 19-65. Basal cell carcinoma. Proliferating basal cells infiltrate the dermis. Note the peripheral palisading. (Original magnification × 240; courtesy of Rudolf Garret, M.D.)

like (Figure 19-67). Although this tumor is relatively slow growing, metastases to regional lymph nodes can occur. Wide local excision is the treatment of choice for most lesions (Figure 19-68).[78,208] If the anal canal or anal margin is involved, treatment in accordance with the protocol described in Chapter 24 is suggested.

Malignant Melanoma

Malignant melanoma is described in Chapter 24.

Bowen's Disease

Bowen's disease is an intraepidermal squamous cell carcinoma that tends to spread intraepidermally, but it may also invade. As with AIN, it is a precursor to squamous cell carcinoma of the anus, and it, too, is associated with HPV infection.[25,57,263] The condition is eponymously recognized through the author of the 1912 article.[36] It is more commonly seen on the trunk, but more than 100 cases involving the anus have been reported.[208] Graham and Helwig noted a relationship of this condition to malignant tumors elsewhere (e.g., thymoma, bronchogenic carcinoma, hypernephroma, gastrointestinal cancer).[121,122] Neoplasms developed in one third of their patients within 10 years of the original diagnosis. They suggested that

Bowen's disease could represent a cutaneous manifestation of a predisposition to the development of cancer. However, Reymann and colleagues, in a retrospective statistical study of 581 patients with Bowen's disease, failed to support the view that the condition is a marker for internal malignancy.[216] Others have also come to adopt this opinion, so the current consensus is that there is no such relationship.[39,54,55] Parenthetically, a case of Bowen's disease in association with Crohn's colitis has been described.[26]

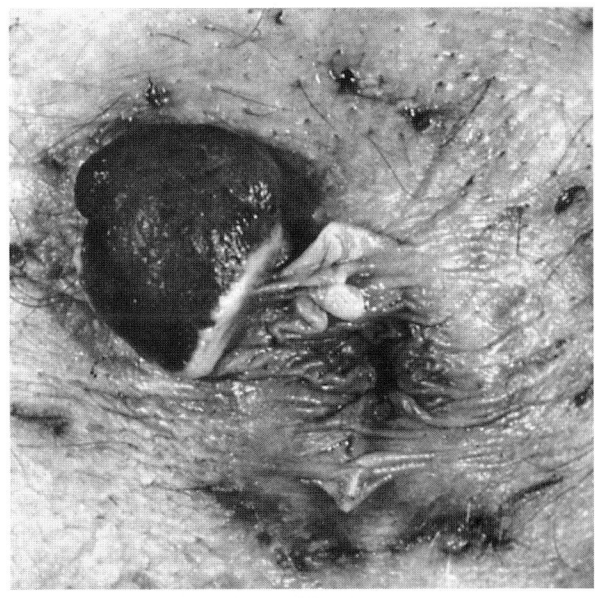

FIGURE 19-66. Squamous cell carcinoma. An ulcerating, friable tumor is noted. (Courtesy of Rudolf Garret, M.D.)

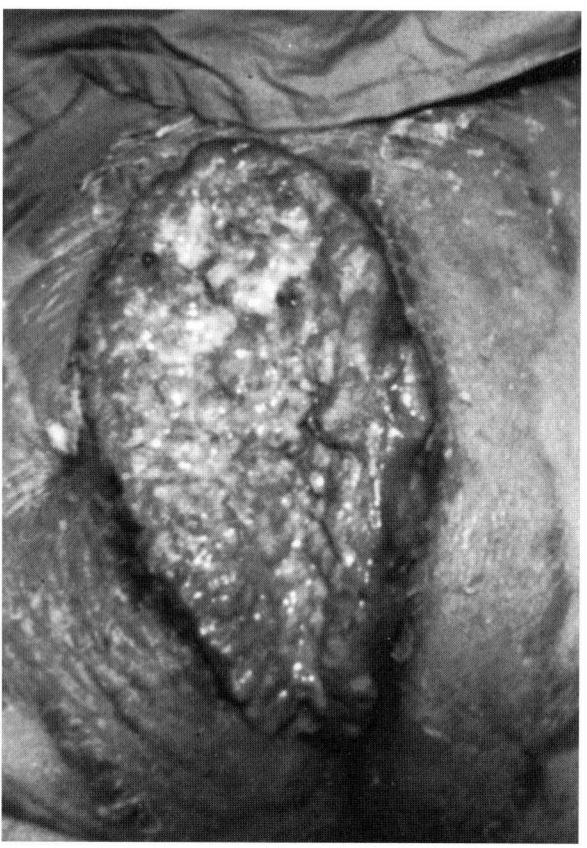

FIGURE 19-67. Squamous cell carcinoma. A fungating, cauliflower-like mass is present. (Courtesy of Daniel Rosenthal, M.D.)

Symptoms

The disease usually presents with itching and burning, although pain and bleeding may be noted.[224] Strauss and Fazio, in their report from the Cleveland Clinic of 12 patients, noted that the diagnosis was usually made as an incidental finding after anorectal surgery.[245] In a later publication from the same institution involving 33 patients with perianal Bowen's disease, 20 (61%) presented with symptoms, whereas 13 individuals (39%) were noted to harbor the condition upon pathologic evaluation of hemorrhoidectomy specimens.

Clinical Appearance and Histology

The lesion appears as an erythematous, slightly crusted, plaquelike area with well-defined margins (Figure 19-69). The condition may be confused with psoriasis and with Paget's disease. Topical staining with toluidine blue has been successfully applied as a screening technique for intraepithelial carcinoma of the cervix and vulva.[41] This approach may prove to have value in the diagnosis of Bowen's disease.

Microscopically, the epidermis is thickened by hyperkeratosis, and there may be parakeratosis and acanthosis (Figure 19-70). In contrast to what is noted in Paget's disease, a bowenoid cell does not pick up aldehyde-fuchsin stain (Figure 19-71).[208] Anal Bowen's disease and high-grade squamous intraepithelial lesions are histologically and immunochemically indistinguishable.[263]

Treatment

Treatment requires wide local excision with frozen-section examination to ensure adequate margins, although radical surgical extirpation has been used when this procedure fails.[93] The condition has also been reported to respond to topical dinitrochlorobenzene and 5-fluorouracil.[210] Photodynamic therapy has been described for the management of residual disease.[222]

Results

In the 12 individuals reviewed by the Cleveland Clinic group, there was no recurrence or metastasis when adequate excision with or without grafting was employed.[245] Seven of the patients previously had or subsequently developed a systemic or cutaneous cancer. In a later report involving 33 individuals, 27 were managed by wide local excision, three by simple excision, three by fulguration, and one by abdominoperineal resection.[25] During a follow-up period averaging 3.7 years, a new invasive skin cancer developed in one person, and a second was found to have recurrent Bowen's disease.

Of the 11 patients treated at the Memorial Sloan-Kettering Cancer Center in New York, five were free of dis-

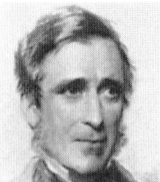

James Paget (1814–1899) Paget was born one of 17 children. He studied at St. Bartholomew's Hospital in London, where he made his first observation. Small, hard specks were often seen in muscle at that time, and he became quite curious as to their nature. Because St. Bartholomew's did not have a microscope, Paget traveled to the British Museum and discovered *Trichinella spiralis*. In 1842, he began to assist in the cataloging of the College of Surgeons' Museum. In the next year, he was given the lectureship in physiology at St. Bartholomew's and was appointed warden of the new residential college for medical students at that hospital. The Professorship of Anatomy and Surgery of the College of Surgeons came next. In 1849, the *Pathological Catalogue of the College of Surgeons Museum*, of which he was the greatest contributor, was completed; this volume formed an exact description of more than 3,500 specimens. Paget established himself as one of the most notable pathologists of all time, with 30 learned bodies conferring distinction on him. Although he did not describe the disease as it affects the anus, only the breast condition, Darier and Couillaud credit him with the identification of the peculiar cells that may be found in these locations. (Data from Graham H. *Surgeons all.* New York: Philosophical Library, 1957:370; and Power D. *British masters of medicine.* Baltimore: W. Wood, 1936:131.)

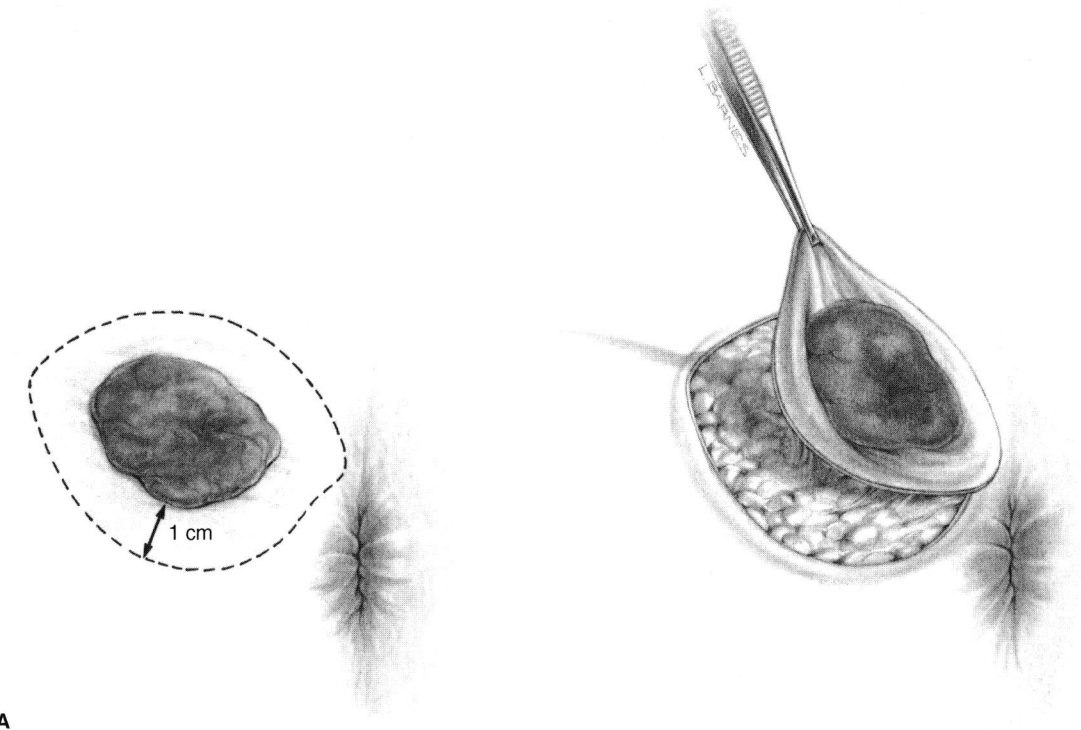

FIGURE 19-68. Technique for wide local excision of perianal skin cancer. **(A)** At least a 1-cm margin of normal skin should be excised with the lesion. **(B)** Full thickness of skin completes the excision. Margins should be checked by means of frozen section to ensure adequacy of removal. Depending on the size of the defect, various skin-grafting approaches may be used.

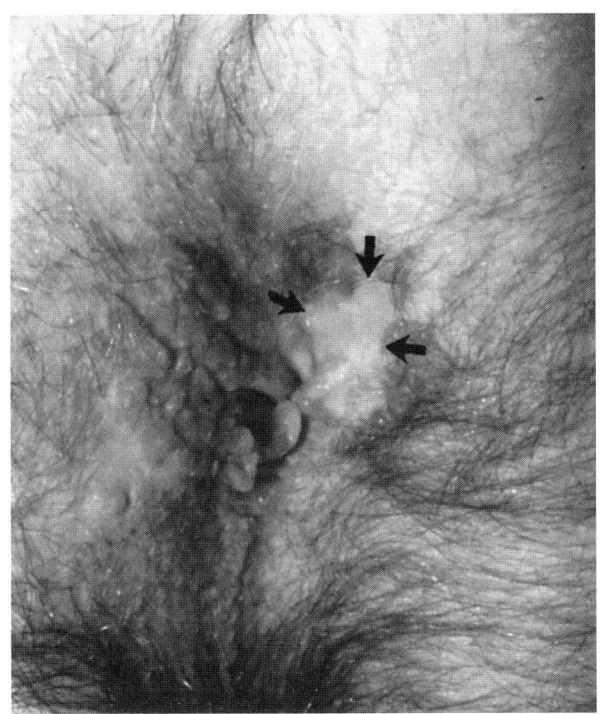

FIGURE 19-69. Bowen's disease. An indurated erythemato-squamous patch involves the perianal area *(arrows)*.

ease after 5 years and one died of colon cancer; the remainder had a limited follow-up.[208] Ramos and colleagues reported seven patients treated by local excision with "minimal margin of resection."[213] No recurrence was observed. Reynolds and colleagues noted one recurrence after total excision of the anal mucosa and grafting in six patients.[217] In the experience of the Cleveland Clinic Florida group, which involved 25 patients, no concomitant carcinomas were found by computed tomography and colonoscopy.[103] There were no recurrences in the 15 individuals without HPV or HIV infection, but five (50%) with this association developed recurrent disease. Although newer evidence suggests that a comprehensive search for malignancy in other organs is unwarranted, close follow-up evaluation for recurrence or invasive carcinoma is recommended.[176]

Bowenoid Papulosis

Bowenoid papulosis was described in 1979 by Wade and colleagues as a dermatosis affecting the genitalia, a condition that is quite similar to Bowen's disease.[260] The condition is often associated with anal condylomata or genital herpes. HPV is believed to be the causative agent. Immunocompromised individuals, especially those with

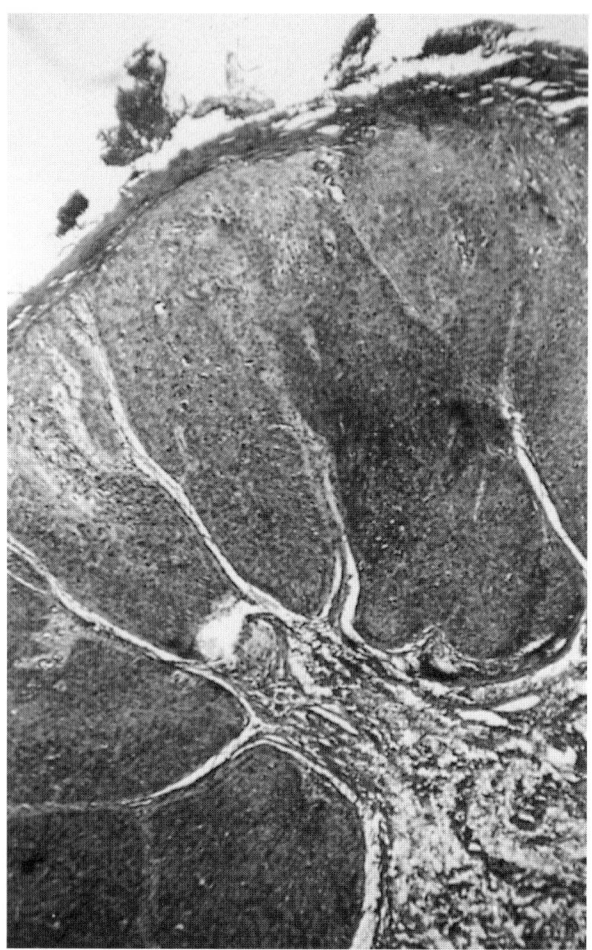

FIGURE 19-70. Bowen's disease. Disturbance of architecture of the squamous epithelium is noted. (Original magnification × 250; courtesy of Rudolf Garret, M.D.)

AIDS, may be at a higher risk for development of cancer on the basis of bowenoid papulosis.[221]

The lesions are described as multiple reddish brown or violaceous papules. Most individuals are asymptomatic or have pruritic complaints. Because the microscopic picture is essentially identical to that of Bowen's disease, the differential diagnosis between the two conditions is made on the basis of age (i.e., patients with bowenoid papulosis tend to be younger) and the fact that bowenoid lesions are small, papular, and multiple.[166] Local excision is the treatment of choice, but the prognosis following removal is unclear.

Extramammary Paget's Disease

In 1874, Sir James Paget described a cutaneous lesion of the breast that histologically demonstrated the presence of large, round, clear-staining cells with large nuclei.[201]

Darier and Couillaud subsequently described the condition in the perineal area, the lesions of extramammary Paget's disease being not unlike those seen in the breast.[73] This is a relatively rare condition, with only about 125 cases reported in the literature. The mean age of onset has been reported to be from 59 to 65 years.[28,130]

Presentation and Histopathology

Most patients complain of ulceration, discharge, pruritus, and occasionally bleeding and pain. They may be asymptomatic or have a florid type of eczema.[28]

Helwig and Graham reviewed material from the Armed Forces Institute of Pathology; 40 patients were identified with lesions in this area.[130] These investigators found that the dermatosis usually appeared erythematous to whitish-gray, elevated, crusty, scaly, eczematoid, and occasionally papillary (Figure 19-72).

Microscopically, hyperkeratosis, parakeratosis, acanthosis, and pale vacuolated cells are seen (pagetoid cells) within the epidermis (Figure 19-73). Sialomucin may be identified by periodic acid–Schiff stain (Figure 19-74). Conversely, Bowen's disease does not show this positive staining.

Association with Malignancy

Carcinoma in adjacent areas is found in a high percentage of patients, especially the anal canal and rectum (Figure 19-75). Thirteen of the 40 patients in the series of Helwig and Graham had an immediate underlying cutaneous carcinoma.[130] Another seven had primary internal or extracutaneous cancer. Lock and associates reported four patients, in three of whom carcinoma developed.[170] Others note a similar association—for example, with cloacogenic carcinoma and with villous adenoma of the rectum.[14,135,208,246,267] In addition, a familial occurrence has been described.[158] A special staining technique has been employed to assist in the distinction between Paget's disease and so-called pagetoid spread as a consequence of an anorectal malignancy.[16] Further studies are awaited.

Treatment

Treatment depends on the presence or absence of an underlying invasive carcinoma. The use of a retinoid, etretinate, taken orally may be beneficial in the treatment of the chronic or recurrent form when there is no concomitant invasive carcinoma.[169] It should be self-evident that all these individuals require a careful proctosigmoidoscopy and anoscopy. Linder and Myers suggest that a distinction be made between a carcinoma *in situ* and an infiltrating growth.[168] In the latter situation, abdomino-

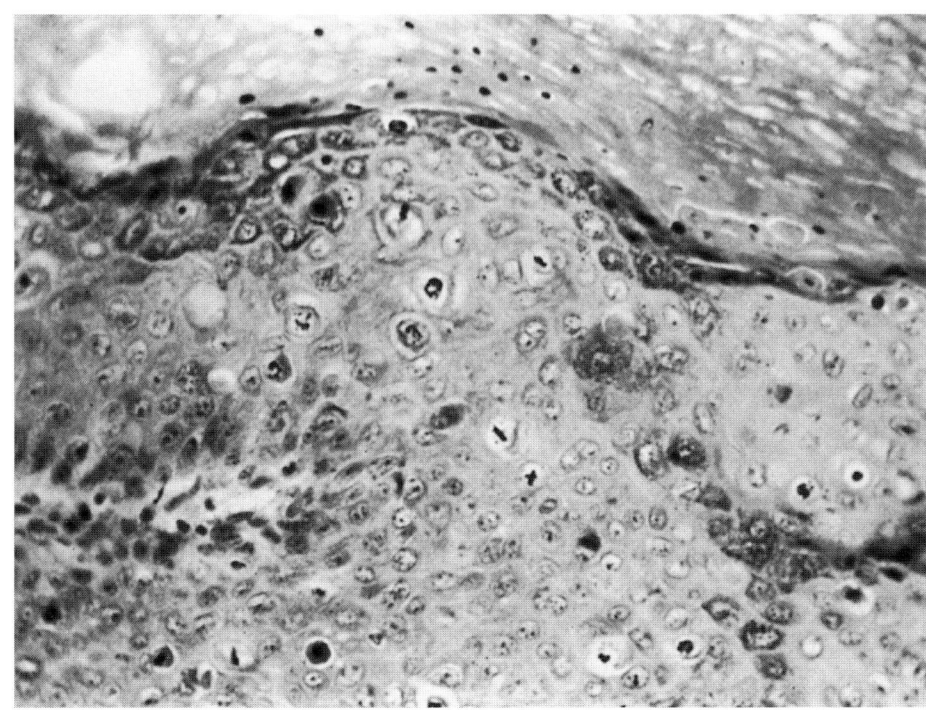

FIGURE 19-71. Bowen's disease. Note the cells with hyperchromatic nuclei (bowenoid cells) scattered throughout the epithelium. Many mitotic figures are seen. (Original magnification × 600; from Corman ML, Veidenheimer MC, Swinton NW. *Diseases of the anus, rectum colon. Part I: neoplasms.* New York: Medcom, 1972, from permission.)

perineal resection may be required, or consideration may be given to neoadjuvant therapy (see Chapter 24). Wide local excision with or without grafting should be adequate for noninvasive disease, however.[13,162,179] Usually, mapping biopsies with frozen section are utilized. Some have suggested that one can determine the extent of the disease by means of photodynamic diagnosis.[13] This is a noninvasive tool that uses a 20% 5-aminolevulinic acid (ALA) ointment applied around the lesion, which is then protected from light.[13] When pagetoid or cancer cells are exposed to ALA, they accumulate intrinsic protoporphyrin IX, which emits red fluorescence with ultraviolet light.[13]

Shutze and Gleysteen suggest a management classification based on the depth of invasion, a modification of which follows:[228]

Stage I. Localized perianal disease without carcinoma: wide local excision

Stage IIA. Localized disease with underlying malignancy: wide local excision

Stage IIB. Localized disease with associated anorectal carcinoma: abdominoperineal resection

Stage III. Associated carcinomatous spread to regional lymph nodes: abdominoperineal resection plus chemoradiation therapy; possible radical inguinal node dissection

Stage IV. Distant metastases: standard palliative cancer management

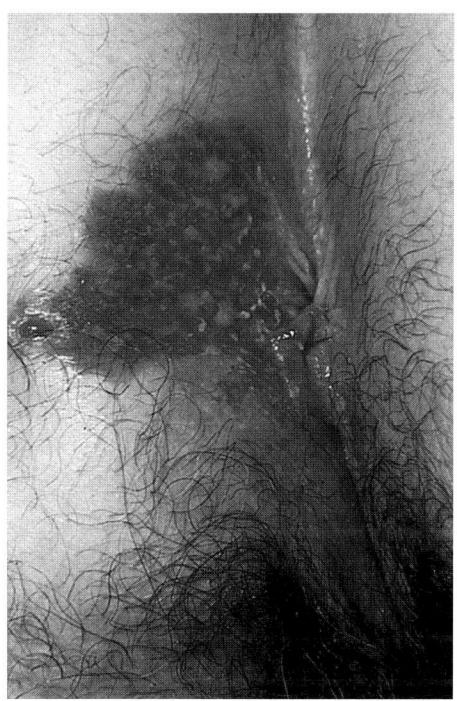

FIGURE 19-72. Extramammary Paget's disease has caused an irregular but well-marginated erythematous erosive patch with slightly indurated edges in this patient. (See Color Fig. 19-72.) (Courtesy of Arnold Medved, M.D.)

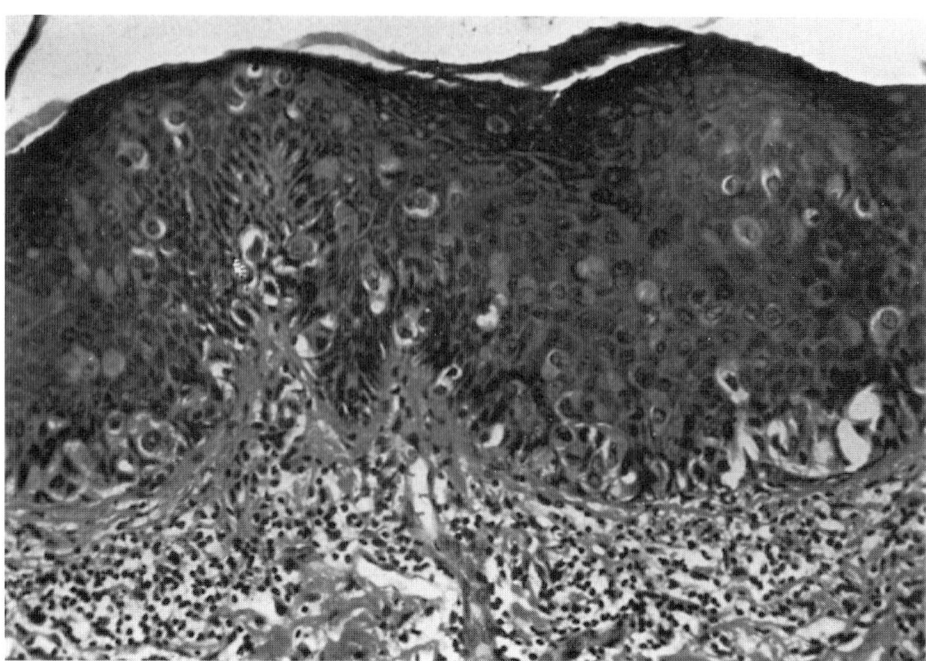

FIGURE 19-73. Extramammary Paget's disease. Note the large, pagetoid cells within the epithelium. These were mucicarmine-positive (Fig. 19-74), thus ruling out Bowen's disease. (Original magnification × 240; courtesy of Rudolf Garret, M.D.)

Results

In the experience of the Cleveland Clinic group (ten patients), most were free of disease when wide, local excision and skin grafting were performed.[24] The three patients in whom metastatic disease developed all presented with invasive carcinoma.

Jensen and colleagues evaluated 22 patients with Paget's disease of the anal margin.[141] Approximately three fourths suffered from persistent pruritus ani, and about one third had a malignancy. The 5- and 10-year crude sur vival rates of 54% and 45%, respectively, were significantly lower than what would be antici-

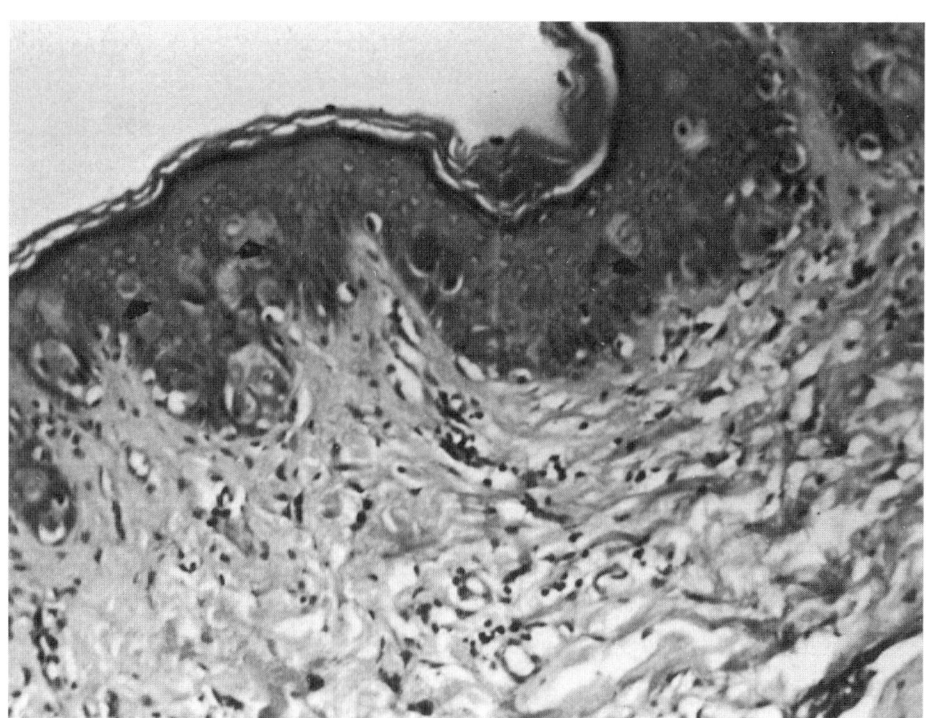

FIGURE 19-74. Extramammary Paget's disease. Mucicarmine-positive cells *(arrows)* are present within the epithelium. (Original magnification × 240; courtesy of Rudolf Garret, M.D.)

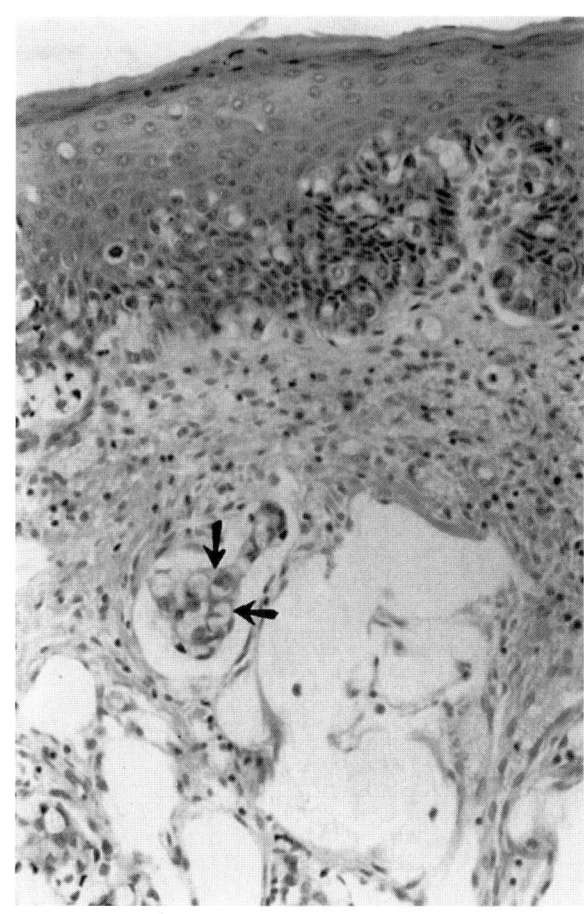

FIGURE 19-75. Perianal skin shows infiltration of lower portion of epidermis by Paget's cells. These are characterized by clear cytoplasm and nuclear pleomorphism. In the underlying dermis, a nest of mucin-secreting carcinoma is seen. The cells show a typical signet-ring appearance *(arrows)*. The spaces represent pools of mucin. On resection, the tumor was proved to arise from anal glands. (Original magnification × 240.)

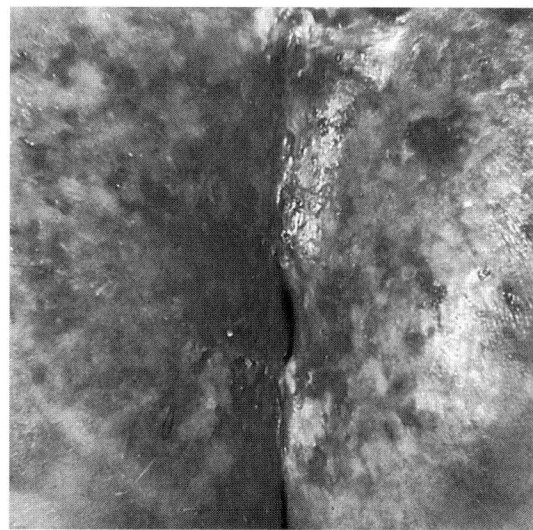

FIGURE 19-76. Extramammary Paget's disease that recurred after excision and skin grafting. (See Color Fig. 19-76). (Courtesy of William G. Robertson, M.D.)

pated in the normal population. The Memorial Sloan-Kettering Cancer Center experience was reported in 2003 and involved 27 patients who were identified between 1950 and 2000.[179] The median age was 63 years. Three fourths were treated with wide local excision, and the overall recurrence rate was 37%. Forty-four percent had an invasive component. The overall and disease-free survivals at 5 years was 59% and 64%, respectively, decreasing to 33% and 39%, respectively, at 10 years.[179]

Careful follow-up is considered essential, with recurrence probably dictating a wider excision, provided, of course, that there is no evidence of malignancy (Figure 19-76). Photodynamic therapy for recurrent disease has also been advocated.[222] Those managed by local excision should undergo frequent biopsy of any pruritic areas or skin lesions.[141]

REFERENCES

1. Abcarian H, Sharon N. The effectiveness of immunotherapy in the treatment of anal condylomata acuminatum. *J Surg Res* 1977;22:231.
2. Abcarian H, Sharon N. Long-term effectiveness of immunotherapy of anal condyloma acuminatum. *Dis Colon Rectum* 1982;25:648.
3. Abcarian H, Smith D, Sharon N. The immunotherapy of anal condyloma acuminatum. *Dis Colon Rectum* 1976;19:237.
4. Ahlberg J, Bergstrand O, Holmström B, et al. Anal tuberculosis: a report of two cases. *Acta Chir Scand* 1980;500 [Suppl]:45.
5. Alexander RM, Kaminsky DB. Giant condyloma acuminatum (Buschke-Löwenstein tumor) of the anus: case report and review of the literature. *Dis Colon Rectum* 1979;21:561.
6. Alexander S. Dermatological aspects of anorectal disease. *Clin Gastroenterol* 1975;4:651.
7. Allan A, Ambrose NS, Silverman S, et al. Physiological study of pruritus ani. *Br J Surg* 1987;74:576.
8. Allan A, Keighley MRB. Treatment for pruritus ani. *Surg Rounds* 1988;7:69.
9. Allen-Mersh TG. Pilonidal sinus: finding the right track for treatment. *Br J Surg* 1990;77:123.
10. Alvarado-Cerna R, Bracho-Riquelme R. Perianal actinomycosis a complication of a fistula-in-ano: report of a case. *Dis Colon Rectum* 1994;37:378.
11. Alver O, Kayabasi B, Ozcan M, et al. The complete rhombic excision of pilonidal sinus with primary closure by the use of fasciocutaneous Limberg flap. *Contemp Surg* 1988; 33:54.
12. Anderson AW. Hair extracted from an ulcer. *Boston Med Surg J* 1847;36:74.
13. Araki Y, Noake T, Hata H, et al. Perianal Paget's disease treated with a wide excision and gluteal fold flap reconstruction guided by photodynamic diagnosis: report of a case. *Dis Colon Rectum* 2003;46:1563.
14. Arminski TC, Pollard RJ. Paget's disease of the anus secondary to a malignant papillary adenoma of the rectum. *Dis Colon Rectum* 1973;16:46.

15. Armitage G, Smith I. Rodent ulcer of the anus. *Br J Surg* 1955;42:395.
16. Armitage NC, Jass JR, Richman PI, et al. Paget's disease of the anus: a clinicopathological study. *Br J Surg* 1989;76:60.
17. Armstrong JH, Barcia PJ. Pilonidal sinus disease. *Arch Surg* 1994;129:914.
18. Banerjee AK. Surgical treatment of hidradenitis suppurativa. *Br J Surg* 1992;79:863.
19. Banov L Jr. Pruritus ani and anal hygiene. *J SC Med Assoc* 1985;81:557.
20. Barkel DC, Villalba MR. A reappraisal of surgical management in necrotizing perineal infections. *Am Surg* 1986; 52:395.
21. Bascom J. Pilonidal disease: origin from follicles of hairs and results of follicle removal as treatment. *Surgery* 1980; 87:567.
22. Bascom J. Pilonidal disease: long-term results of follicle removal. *Dis Colon Rectum* 1983;26:800.
23. Bascom JU. Repeat pilonidal operations. *Am J Surg* 1987; 154:118.
24. Beck DE, Fazio VW. Perianal Paget's disease. *Dis Colon Rectum* 1987;30:263.
25. Beck DE, Fazio VW, Jagelman DG, et al. Perianal Bowen's disease. *Dis Colon Rectum* 1988;31:419.
26. Beck DE, Harford FJ, Roettger RH. Perianal Bowen's disease associated with Crohn's colitis: report of a case. *Dis Colon Rectum* 1989;32:252.
27. Beck DE, Jaso RG, Zajac RA. Surgical management of anal condylomata in the HIV-positive patient. *Dis Colon Rectum* 1990;33:180.
28. Berardi RS, Chen HP. Perianal extramammary Paget's disease. *Surg Gynecol Obstet* 1988;167:359.
29. Berman IR. Mechanisms, diagnosis, and management of anal irritation and itching. In: Schrock TR, ed. *Perspectives in colon and rectal surgery*, vol 3. St. Louis, MO: Quality Medical, 1990:82.
30. Beutner KR, Conant MA, Friedman-Kien AE, et al. Patient-applied podofilox for treatment of genital warts. *Lancet* 1989;1:831.
31. Billingham RP, Lewis FG. Laser versus electrical cautery in the treatment of condylomata acuminata of the anus. *Surg Gynecol Obstet* 1982;155:865.
32. Blanchard RJ. Fulminating nonclostridial gas-forming infection: a case of necrotizing fasciitis. *Can J Surg* 1975; 18:339.
33. Bocchini SF, Habr-Gama A, Kiss DR, et al. Gluteal and perianal hidradenitis suppurativa: surgical treatment by wide excision. *Dis Colon Rectum* 2003;46:944.
34. Borges VF, Keating JT, Nasser IA, et al. Clinicopathologic characterization of squamous-cell carcinoma arising from pilonidal disease in association with condylomata acuminatum in HIV-infected patients: report of two cases. *Dis Colon Rectum* 2001;44:1873.
35. Bose B, Candy J. Radical cure of pilonidal sinus by Z-plasty. *Am J Surg* 1970;120:783.
36. Bowen JT. Precancerous dermatoses: a study of two cases of chronic atypical epithelial proliferation. *J Cutan Dis* 1912;30:241.
37. Bozkurt MK, Tezel E. Management of pilonidal sinus with the Limberg flap. *Dis Colon Rectum* 1998;41:
38. Braverman IM. *Skin tags of systemic disease*. Philadelphia, WB Saunders, 1981:669.
39. Braverman IM. Bowen's disease and internal cancer. *JAMA* 1991;266:842.
40. Broadwater JR, Bryant RL, Petrino RA, et al. Advanced hidradenitis suppurativa: review of surgical treatment in 23 patients. *Am J Surg* 1982;144:668.
41. Broen EM, Ostergard DR. Toluidine blue and colposcopy for screening and delineating vulvar neoplasia. *Obstet Gynecol* 1971;38:775.
42. Brown SCW, Kazzazi N, Lord PH. Surgical treatment of perineal hidradenitis suppurativa with special reference to recognition of the perianal form. *Br J Surg* 1986;73:978.
43. Budayr M, Ankney RN, Moore RA. Condyloma acuminatum in infants and children: a survey of colon and rectal surgeons. *Dis Colon Rectum* 1996;39:1112.
44. Buie LA. Jeep disease (pilonidal disease of mechanized warfare). *South Med J* 1944;37:103.
45. Bunstock WH. Basal cell carcinoma of the anus. *Am J Surg* 1958;95:822.
46. Butler TW, Gefter J, Kletto D, et al. Squamous-cell carcinoma of the anus in condyloma acuminatum: successful treatment with preoperative chemotherapy and radiation. *Dis Colon Rectum* 1987;30:293.
47. Büyükasik Y, Özcebe OI, Sayinalp N, et al. Perianal infections in patients with leukemia: importance of the course of neutrophil count. *Dis Colon Rectum* 1998; 41:81.
48. Carle G. Anorectal involvement in leukaemia. *J R Coll Surg Edinb* 1982;27:118.
49. Centers for Disease Control (CDC). Summary of notifiable diseases. *MMWR Morb Mortal Wkly Rep* 1995;44:73.
50. Chaudhary A. Colorectal tuberculosis. *Dis Colon Rectum* 1986;29:738.
51. Cheng SF, Veenema RJ. Topical application of thiotepa to penile and urethral tumors. *J Urol* 1965;94:259.
52. Ching CC, Stahlgren LH. Clinical review of hidradenitis suppurativa: management of cases with severe perianal involvement. *Dis Colon Rectum* 1965;8:349.
53. Chu QD, Vezeridis MP, Libbey NP, Wanebo HJ. Giant condyloma acuminatum (Buschke-Löwenstein tumor) of the anorectal and perianal regions: analysis of 42 cases. *Dis Colon Rectum* 1994;37:950.
54. Chuang T-Y, Reizner GT. Bowen's disease and internal malignancy: a matched case-control study. *J Am Acad Dermatol* 1988;19:47.
55. Chute CG, Chuang T-Y, Bergstralh EJ, et al. The subsequent risk of internal cancer with Bowen's disease: a population-based study. *JAMA* 1991;266:816.
56. Clayton MD, Fowler JE Jr, Sharifi R, et al. Causes, presentation and survival of fifty-seven patients with necrotizing fasciitis of the male genitalia. *Surg Gynecol Obstet* 1990; 170:49.
57. Cleary RK, Schaldenbrand JD, Fowler JJ, et al. Perianal Bowen's disease and anal intraepithelial neoplasia: review of the literature. *Dis Colon Rectum* 1999;42:945.
58. Cole GW, Amon RB, Russell PS. Secondary syphilis presenting as a pruritic dermatosis. *Arch Dermatol* 1977;113:489.
59. Colquhoun P, Efron J, Eze G, et al. The incidence of subclinical anal intraepithelial neoplasia (AIN) in patients with anal condylomata. *Dis Colon Rectum* 2001;44:A5.
60. Congilosi SM, Madoff RD. Current therapy for recurrent and extensive anal warts. *Dis Colon Rectum* 1995;38:1101.
61. Conway H, Stark RB, Climo S, et al. The surgical treatment of chronic hidradenitis suppurativa. *Surg Gynecol Obstet* 1952;95:455.
62. Coremans G, Margaritis V, Snoeck R, et al. Topical cidofovir (HPMPC) is an effective adjuvant to surgical treatment of anogenital condylomata acuminate. *Dis Colon Rectum* 2003;46:1103.
63. Corman ML, Veidenheimer MC, Swinton NW. *Diseases of the anus, rectum, and colon. Part I: neoplasms*. New York: Medcom, 1972.
64. Crapp AR, Macbeth WAAG. Perianal vaccinia: a case report. *Aust NZ J Surg* 1976;46:83.
65. Creasman C, Haas PA, Fox TA Jr, et al. Malignant transformation of anorectal giant condyloma acuminatum (Buschke-Löwenstein tumor). *Dis Colon Rectum* 1989;32:481.
66. Cresson DH, Siegal GP. Chronic lymphocytic leukemia presenting as an anal mass. *J Clin Gastroenterol* 1985;7:83.
67. Crighton JL. Diarrhoea and perianal vaccinia. *BMJ* 1976;2:732.
68. Croxson T, Chabon AB, Rorat E, et al. Intraepithelial carcinoma of the anus in homosexual men. *Dis Colon Rectum* 1984;27:325.

69. Culp CE. Chronic hidradenitis suppurativa of the anal canal: a surgical skin disease. *Dis Colon Rectum* 1983;26:669.
70. Dailey TH. Pruritus ani. *Pract Gastroenterol* 1980;4:30.
71. Dan M, Rotmensch HH, Eylan E, et al. A case of lymphogranuloma venereum of 20 years' duration: isolation of *Chlamydia trachomatis* from perianal lesions. *Br J Vener Dis* 1980;56:344.
72. Daniel GL, Longo WE, Vernava AM III. Pruritus ani: causes and concerns. *Dis Colon Rectum* 1994;37:670.
73. Darier J, Couillaud P. Sur un cas de maladie de Paget de la région périnéo-anale et scrotale. *Soc Fr Dermatol Syphilogr* 1893;4:25.
74. Dasan S, Neill SM, Donaldson DR, et al. Treatment of persistent pruritus ani in a combined colorectal and dermatological clinic. *Br J Surg* 1999;86:1337.
75. Davis KA, Mock CN, Versaci A, et al. Malignant degeneration of pilonidal cysts. *Am Surg* 1994;60:200.
76. de la Fuente SG, Ludwig KA, Mantyh CR. Preoperative immune status determines anal condyloma recurrence after surgical excision. *Dis Colon Rectum* 2003;46:367.
77. Di Falco G, Guccione C, D'Annibale A, et al. Fournier's gangrene following a perianal abscess. *Dis Colon Rectum* 1986;29:582.
78. Dillard BM, Spratt JS Jr, Ackerman LV, et al. Epidermoid cancer of anal margin and canal. *Arch Surg* 1963;86:772.
79. Dixon JA, Gilbertson JJ. Cutaneous laser therapy. *West J Med* 1985;143:758.
80. Domonkos AN, Arnold HL Jr, Odom RB. Cutaneous symptoms, signs and diagnosis. In: Domonkos AN, Arnold HL, eds. *Andrew's diseases of the skin,* 7th ed. Philadelphia: WB Saunders, 1982:15.
81. Domonkos AN, Arnold HL Jr, Odom RB. Cutaneous symptoms, signs, and diagnosis. In: Domonkos AN, Arnold HL, eds. *Andrew's diseases of the skin,* 7th ed. Philadelphia: WB Saunders, 1982:75.
82. Domonkos AN, Arnold HL Jr, Odom RB. Cutaneous symptoms, signs, and diagnosis. In: Domonkos AN, Arnold HL, eds. *Andrew's diseases of the skin,* 7th ed. Philadelphia: WB Saunders, 1982:97.
83. Domonkos AN, Arnold HL Jr, Odom RB. Cutaneous symptoms, signs, and diagnosis. In: Domonkos AN, Arnold HL, eds. *Andrew's diseases of the skin,* 7th ed. Philadelphia: WB Saunders, 1982:175.
84. Domonkos AN, Arnold HL Jr, Odom RB. Cutaneous symptoms, signs, and diagnosis. In: Domonkos AN, Arnold HL, eds. *Andrew's diseases of the skin,* 7th ed. Philadelphia: WB Saunders, 1982:228
85. Domonkos AN, Arnold HL Jr, Odom RB. Cutaneous symptoms, signs, and diagnosis. In: Domonkos AN, Arnold HL, eds. *Andrew's diseases of the skin,* 7th ed. Philadelphia: WB Saunders, 1982:341.
86. Domonkos AN, Arnold HL Jr, Odom RB. Cutaneous symptoms, signs, and diagnosis. In: Domonkos AN, Arnold HL, eds. *Andrew's diseases of the skin,* 7th ed. Philadelphia: WB Saunders, 1982:526.
87. Domonkos AN, Arnold HL Jr, Odom RB. Cutaneous symptoms, signs, and diagnosis. In: Domonkos AN, Arnold HL, eds. *Andrew's diseases of the skin,* 7th ed. Philadelphia: WB Saunders, 1982:581.
88. Douglas JM, Critchlow C, Benedetti J, et al. A double-blind study of oral acyclovir for suppression of recurrences of genital herpes simplex virus infections. *N Engl J Med* 1984;310:1551.
89. Douglas JM Jr, Rogers M, Judson FN. The effect of asymptomatic infection with HTLV-III on the response of anogenital warts to intralesional treatment with recombinant 2 interferon. *J Infect Dis* 1986;154:331.
90. Drusin LM, Homan WP, Dineen P. The role of surgery in primary syphilis of the anus. *Ann Surg* 1976;184:65.
91. Dubois JD, Dilly SA, Gazet JC. Leukaemic infiltration of the anus. *Eur J Surg Oncol* 1985;11:365.
92. Duus BR, Philipsen T, Christensen JD, et al. Refractory condylomata acuminata: a controlled clinical trial of carbon dioxide laser versus conventional surgical treatment. *Genitourin Med* 1985;61:59.
93. Edwards M. Bowen's disease: a case report. *Dis Colon Rectum* 1965;8:297.
94. Edwards MH. Pilonidal sinus: a 5-year appraisal of the Millar-Lord treatment. *Br J Surg* 1977;64:867.
95. Efem SE. Recent advances in the management of Fournier's gangrene: preliminary observations. *Surgery* 1993;113:200.
96. Eftaiha MS, Amshel AL, Shonberg IL, et al. Giant and recurrent condyloma acuminatum: appraisal of immunotherapy. *Dis Colon Rectum* 1979;25:136.
97. Eke N. Fournier's gangrene: a review of 1726 cases. *Br J Surg* 2000;87:718.
98. Elliot MS, Werner ID, Immelman EJ, et al. Giant condyloma (Buschke-Loewenstein tumor) of the anorectum. *Dis Colon Rectum* 1979;22:497.
99. Enriquez JM, Moreno S, Devesa M, et al. Fournier's syndrome of urogenital and anorectal origin: a retrospective, comparative study. *Dis Colon Rectum* 1987;30:33.
100. Eron LJ, Judson F, Tucker S, et al. Interferon therapy for condylomata acuminata. *N Engl J Med* 1986;315:1059.
101. Eusebio EB, Graham J, Mody N. Treatment of pruritus ani. *Dis Colon Rectum* 1990;33:770.
102. Eyers AA, Thomson JPS. Pruritus ani: is anal sphincter dysfunction important in aetiology? *BMJ* 1979;2:1549.
103. Eze G, Park T, Efron J, et al. Perianal Bowen's disease: result of wide local excision and association with other carcinomas. *Dis Colon Rectum* 2001;44:A27-A59.
104. Farouk R, Duthie GS, Pryde A, et al. Abnormal transient internal sphincter relaxation in idiopathic pruritus ani: physiological evidence from ambulatory monitoring. *Br J Surg* 1994;81:603.
105. Fasching MC, Meland NB, Woods JE, et al. Recurrent squamous-cell carcinoma arising in pilonidal sinus tract: multiple flap reconstructions. Report of a case. *Dis Colon Rectum* 1989;32:153.
106. Figueroa S, Gennaro AR. Intralesional bleomycin injection in treatment of condyloma acuminatum. *Dis Colon Rectum* 1980;23:550.
107. Fisher AA. New advances in contact dermatitis. *Int J Dermatol* 1977;16:552.
108. Fitzpatrick TB. Fundamentals of dermatologic diagnosis. In: Fitzpatrick TB, Eisen AZ, Wolff K, et al, eds. *Dermatology in general medicine,* 2nd ed. St. Louis, MO: McGraw-Hill, 1979:10.
109. Fiumara NJ. *Pictorial guide to sexually transmitted diseases.* Secaucus, NJ: Hospital Publications, 1987.
110. Fiumara NJ, Tang S. Folliculitis of the buttocks and pinworms: a case report. *Sex Transm Dis* 1986;13:45.
111. Fleshner PR, Freilich MI. Adjuvant interferon for anal condyloma: a prospective, randomized trial. *Dis Colon Rectum* 1994;37:1255.
112. Fournier AJ. Gangrène foudroyante de la verge. *Semin Med* 1883;3:345.
113. Friedman-Kien AE, Eron LJ, Conant M, et al. Natural interferon alfa for treatment of condylomata acuminata. *JAMA* 1988;259:533.
114. Friend WG. The cause and treatment of idiopathic pruritus ani. *Dis Colon Rectum* 1977;20:42.
115. Freud E, Farkash U, Prieto F, et al. Perineal reconstruction for severe sequela of ecthyma gangrenosum: report of a case. *Dis Colon Rectum* 1999;42:961.
116. Fundarò S, Spallanzani A, Ricchi E, et al. Squamous-cell carcinoma developing within anal lichen planus: report of a case. *Dis Colon Rectum* 1998;41:111.
117. Fùzun M, Bakir H, Soylu M, et al. Which technique for treatment of pilonidal sinus: open or closed? *Dis Colon Rectum* 1994;37:1148.
118. Gabriel WB. *Principles and practice of rectal surgery,* 4th ed. London: HK Lewis, 1948:469.
119. Gage AA, Dutta P. Cryosurgery for pilonidal disease. *Am J Surg* 1977;133:249.

120. Goldman L, Kitzmiller KW. Perianal atrophoderma from topical corticosteroids. *Arch Dermatol* 1973;107:611.
121. Graham JH, Helwig EB. Bowen's disease and its relationship to systemic cancer. *Arch Dermatol* 1959;80:133.
122. Graham JH, Helwig EB. Bowen's disease and its relationship to systemic cancer. *Arch Dermatol* 1961;83:738.
123. Gross G. Interferon and genital warts. *JAMA* 1988;260:2066.
124. Guinan ME. Oral acyclovir for treatment and suppression of genital herpes simplex virus infection. *JAMA* 1986;255:1747.
125. Gupta AS, Sharma VP, Rathi GL. Anorectal tuberculosis simulating carcinoma. *Am J Proctol* 1976;27:33.
126. Guyuron B, Dinner MI, Dowden RV. Excision and grafting in treatment of recurrent pilonidal sinus disease. *Surg Gynecol Obstet* 1983;156:201.
127. Hanley PH. Acute pilonidal abscess. *Surg Gynecol Obstet* 1980;150:9.
128. Harrison BJ, Read GF, Hughes LE. Endocrine basis for the clinical presentation of hidradenitis suppurativa. *Br J Surg* 1988;75:972.
129. Hegge HGJ, Vos GA, Patka P, et al. Treatment of complicated or infected pilonidal sinus disease by local application of phenol. *Surgery* 1987;102:52.
130. Helwig EB, Graham JH. Anogenital (extramammary) Paget's disease. *Cancer* 1963;16:387.
131. Himal H, McLean AP, Duff JH. Gas gangrene of scrotum and perineum. *Surg Gynecol Obstet* 1974;139:176.
132. Hodges RM. Pilo-nidal sinus. *Boston Med Surg J* 1880;103:485.
133. Horowitz BJ. Interferon therapy for condylomatous vulvitis. *Obstet Gynecol* 1989;73:446.
134. Iwama T, Utzunomiya J. Anal complication in Behçet's syndrome. *Jpn J Surg* 1977;7:114.
135. Jackson BR. Extramammary Paget's disease and anaplastic basaloid small-cell carcinoma of the anus: report of a case. *Dis Colon Rectum* 1975;18:339.
136. Jacobs E. Anal infections caused by herpes simplex virus. *Dis Colon Rectum* 1976;19:151.
137. Jellinek EH, Tulloch WS. Herpes zoster with dysfunction of bladder and anus. *Lancet* 1976;2:1219.
138. Jemec GBE. Effect of localized surgical excisions in hidradenitis suppurativa. *J Am Acad Dermatol* 1988;18:1103.
139. Jensen SL. Comparison of podophyllin application with simple surgical excision in clearance and recurrence of perianal condylomata acuminata. *Lancet* 1985;2:1146.
140. Jensen SL, Harling H. Prognosis after simple incision and drainage for a first-episode acute pilonidal abscess. *Br J Surg* 1988;75:60.
141. Jensen SL, Sjolin KE, Shokouh-Amiri MH, et al. Paget's disease of the anal margin. *Br J Surg* 1988;75:1089.
142. Jones LM. Rectal tuberculosis. *Contemp Surg* 1985;26:41.
143. Joost TH v, Faber WR, Manuel HR. Drug-induced anogenital cicatricial pemphigoid. *Br J Dermatol* 1980;102:715.
144. Kalb RE, Grossman ME. Chronic perianal herpes simplex in immunocompromised hosts. *Am J Med* 1986;80:486.
145. Kaplowitz LG, Baker D, Gelb L, et al. Prolonged continuous acyclovir treatment of normal adults with frequently recurring genital herpes simplex virus infection. *JAMA* 1991;265:747.
146. Karydakis GE. Easy and successful treatment of pilonidal sinus after explanation of its causative processes. *Aust NZ J Surg* 1992;62:385.
147. Kennedy CTC, Lyell A. Perianal orf. *J Am Acad Dermatol* 1984;11:72.
148. Kent RB, Richards JJ. Fournier's perianal gangrene. *Surg Rounds* 1989;8:33.
149. Khan SA, Smith NL, Gonder M, et al. Gangrene of male external genitalia in a patient with colorectal disease. *Dis Colon Rectum* 1985;28:519.
150. Khatri VP, Espinosa MH, Amin AK. Management of recurrent pilonidal sinus by simple V-Y fasciocutaneous flap. *Dis Colon Rectum* 1994;37:1232.
151. Khawaja HT. Podophyllin versus scissor excision in the treatment of perianal condylomata acuminata: a prospective study. *Br J Surg* 1989;76:1067.
152. Kitchen PRB. Pilonidal sinus: experience with the Karydakis flap. *Br J Surg* 1996;83:1452.
153. Korkut M, İçöz G, Dayangaç M, et al. Outcome analysis in patients with Fournier's gangrene: report of 45 cases. *Dis Colon Rectum* 2003;46:649.
154. Kovalcik PJ, Jones J. Necrotizing perineal infections. *Am Surg* 1983;49:163.
155. Kraemer M, Gill SS, Seow-Cheon F. Tuberculous anal sepsis. *Dis Colon Rectum* 2000;43:1589.
156. Krause EW. Perianal basal cell carcinoma. *Arch Dermatol* 1978;114:460.
157. Kronborg O, Christensen K, Zimmermann-Nielsen C. Chronic pilonidal disease: a randomized trial with a complete 3-year follow-up. *Br J Surg* 1985;72:303.
158. Kuehn PG, Tennant R, Brenneman AR. Familial occurrence of extramammary Paget's disease. *Cancer* 1973;32:145.
159. Kulaylat MN, Gong M, Doerr RJ. Multimodality treatment of squamous cell carcinoma complicating pilonidal disease. *Am Surg* 1996;62:922.
160. Kumar N, Sharma P, Sachdeva R, et al. Perineal nodule due to enterobiasis: an aspiration cytologic diagnosis. *Diagn Cytopathol* 2003;28:58.
161. Lafferty WE, Coombs RW, Benedetti J, et al. Recurrences after oral and genital herpes simplex virus infection. *N Engl J Med* 1987;316:1444.
162. Lam DTY, Batista O, Weiss EG, et al. Staged excision and split-thickness skin graft for circumferential perianal Paget's disease. *Dis Colon Rectum* 2001;44:868.
163. Lamerton AJ. Fournier's gangrene: non-clostridial gas gangrene of the perineum and diabetes mellitus. *J R Soc Med* 1986;79:212.
164. Laraque D. Severe anogenital warts in a child with HIV infection. *N Engl J Med* 1989;320:1220.
165. LaVoo JW. Bowenoid papulosis. *Dis Colon Rectum* 1987;30:62.
166. Lee SH, McGregor DH, Kuziez MN. Malignant transformation of perianal condyloma acuminatum: a case report with review of the literature. *Dis Colon Rectum* 1981;24:462.
167. Levitsky J, Hong JJ, Jani AB, et al. Oral vitamin A therapy for a patient with a severely symptomatic postradiation anal ulceration: report of a case. *Dis Colon Rectum* 2003;46:679.
168. Linder JH, Myers RT. Perianal Paget's disease. *Am Surg* 1970;35:342.
169. Lingam MK, O'Dwyer PJ. Clinicopathological study of perineal Paget's disease. *Br J Surg* 1997;84:231.
170. Lock MR, Katz DR, Parks A, et al. Perianal Paget's disease. *Postgrad Med J* 1977;53:768.
171. Longo WE, Ballantyne GH, Gerald WL, et al. Squamous cell carcinoma in situ in condyloma acuminatum. *Dis Colon Rectum* 1986;29:503.
172. Lord PH. Etiology of pilonidal sinus. *Dis Colon Rectum* 1975;18:661.
173. Lynch CM, Felder TL, Schwandt RA, et al. Lymphogranuloma venereum presenting as a rectovaginal fistula. *Infect Dis Obstet Gynecol* 1999;7:199.
174. Mansoory A, Dickson D. Z-plasty for treatment of disease of the pilonidal sinus. *Surg Gynecol Obstet* 1982;155:409.
175. Manterola C, Barroso M, Araya JC, et al. Pilonidal disease: 25 cases treated by the Dufourmentel technique. *Dis Colon Rectum* 1991;34:649.
176. Marfing TE, Abel ME, Gallagher DM. Perianal Bowen's disease and associated malignancies: results of a survey. *Dis Colon Rectum* 1987;30:782.
177. Marino AWM Jr. Proctologic lesions observed in male homosexuals. *Dis Colon Rectum* 1964;7:121.
178. Marks MM. The influence of the intestinal pH on pruritus ani. *South Med J* 1968;61:1005.

179. McCarter MD, Quan SHQ, Busam K, et al. Long-term outcome of perianal Paget's disease. *Dis Colon Rectum* 2003;46:612.
180. McDermott FT. Pilonidal sinus treated by Z-plasty. *Aust NZ J Surg* 1967;37:64.
181. McGuinness JG, Winter DC, O'Connell PR. Vacuum-assisted closure of a complex pilonidal sinus. *Dis Colon Rectum* 2003;46:274.
182. Mertz GJ, Benedetti J, Ashley R, et al. Risk factors for the sexual transmission of genital herpes. *Ann Intern Med* 1991;116:197.
183. Mertz GJ, Critchlow CW, Benedetti J, et al. Double-blind placebo-controlled trial of oral acyclovir in first-episode genital herpes simple virus infection. *JAMA* 1984;252:1147.
184. Mertz GJ, Jones CC, Mills J, et al. Long-term acyclovir suppression of frequently recurring genital herpes simplex virus infection. A multicenter double-blind trial. *JAMA* 1988;260:201.
185. Middleton MD. Treatment of pilonidal sinus by Z-plasty. *Br J Surg* 1968;55:516.
186. Monro RS. A consideration of some factors in the causation of pilonidal sinus and its treatment by Z-plasty. *Am J Proctol* 1967;18:215.
187. Monro RS, McDermott T. The elimination of causal factors in pilonidal sinus treated by Z-plasty. *Br J Surg* 1965;52:177.
188. Mortensen NJ, Thomson JP. Perianal abscess due to *Enterobius vermicularis*. *Dis Colon Rectum* 1984;27:677.
189. Murie JA, Sim AJW, Mackenzie I. The importance of pain, pruritus and soiling as symptoms of haemorrhoids and their response to haemorrhoidectomy or rubber band ligation. *Br J Surg* 1981;68:247.
190. Nahra KS, Moschella SL, Swinton NW Sr. Condyloma acuminatum treated with liquid nitrogen: report of five cases. *Dis Colon Rectum* 1969;12:125.
191. Nel WS, Fourie ED. Immunotherapy and 5 percent topical 5-fluorouracil ointment in the treatment of condylomata acuminata. *S Afr Med J* 1973;47:45.
192. Nielsen OV, Jensen SL. Basal cell carcinoma of the anus: a clinical study of 34 cases. *Br J Surg* 1981;68:856.
193. Nilsen AE, Aasen T, Halsos AM, et al. Efficacy of oral acyclovir in the treatment of initial and recurrent genital herpes. *Lancet* 1982;2:571.
194. Obeid SAF. A new technique for treatment of pilonidal sinus. *Dis Colon Rectum* 1988;31:879.
195. O'Connor JJ. Surgery plus freezing as a technique for treating pilonidal disease. *Dis Colon Rectum* 1979;22:306.
196. Office of Communications and Public Liaison. National Institute of Allergy and Infectious Diseases. National Institutes of Health, Bethesda, MD 20892, 1999.
197. O'Meara SM, Cullum NA, Majid M, et al. Systematic review of antimicrobial agents used for chronic wounds. *Br J Surg* 2001;88:4.
198. Oncel M, Kurt N, Kement M, et al. Excision and marsupialization versus sinus excision for the treatment of limited chronic pilonidal disease: a prospective, randomized trial. *Tech Coloproctol* 2002;6:165.
199. Orland PJ, Rhei E, Brolin RE, et al. Comparison of open versus closed excision of chronic pilonidal sinus. *Contemp Surg* 1992;41:13.
200. Owen RJ. Role of biopsy in diagnosis of rectal infections. *Gastroenterology* 1986;91:770.
201. Paget J. On disease of the mammary areola preceding cancer of the mammary gland. *St Bartholomew Hosp Rep* 1874;10:87.
202. Paterson CA, Young-Fadok TM, Dozois RR. Basal cell carcinoma of the perianal region: 20-year experience. *Dis Colon Rectum* 1999;42:1200.
203. Perez-Gurri JA, Temple WJ, Ketcham AS. Gluteus maximus myocutaneous flap for the treatment of recalcitrant pilonidal disease. *Dis Colon Rectum* 1984;27:262.
204. Petersen S, Koch R, Stelzner S, et al. Primary closure techniques in chronic pilonidal sinus: a survey of the results of different surgical approaches. *Dis Colon Rectum* 2002;45:1458.
205. Prasad ML, Abcarian H. Malignant potential of perianal condyloma acuminatum. *Dis Colon Rectum* 1980;23:191.
206. Pruitt BA Jr. Invited commentary to Diettrich NA, Mason JH. Fournier's gangrene: a general surgery problem. *World J Surg* 1983;7:288.
207. Pyrhönen SO. Treatment of condyloma acuminatum and other warts. *Infect Surg* 1988;7:674.
208. Quan SHQ. Anal and para-anal tumors. *Surg Clin North Am* 1978;58:591.
209. Quinn TC. Gastrointestinal manifestations of AIDS. *Pract Gastroenterol* 1985;9:23.
210. Raaf JH, Krown SE, Pinsky CM, et al. Treatment of Bowen's disease with topical dinitrochlorobenzene and 5-fluorouracil. *Cancer* 1976;37:1633.
211. Ramanujam PS, Taylor LG, DeLaPava D, et al. Fournier's gangrene: importance of aggressive management. *Contemp Surg* 1989;35:21.
212. Ramasastry SS, Conklin WT, Granick MS, et al. Surgical management of massive perianal hidradenitis suppurativa. *Ann Plast Surg* 1985;15:218.
213. Ramos R, Salinas H, Tucker L. Conservative approach to the treatment of Bowen's disease of the anus. *Dis Colon Rectum* 1983;26:712.
214. Rehder PA, Eliezer ET, Lane AT. Perianal cellulitis: cutaneous group A streptococcal disease. *Arch Dermatol* 1988;124:702.
215. Reichman RC, Badger GJ, Mertz GJ, et al. Treatment of recurrent genital herpes simplex infections with oral acyclovir: a controlled trial. *JAMA* 1984;251:2103.
216. Reymann F, Ravnborg L, Schou G, et al. Bowen's disease and internal malignant disease. *Arch Dermatol* 1988;124:677.
217. Reynolds VH, Madden JJ, Franklin JD, et al. Preservation of anal function after total excision of the anal mucosa for Bowen's disease. *Ann Surg* 1984;199:563.
218. Rook A, Wilkinson DS. The principles of diagnosis. In: Rook A, Wilkinson DS, Ebling FJG, eds. *Textbook of dermatology,* 3rd ed. Oxford: Blackwell Scientific, 1979:57.
219. Rosenberg I. The dilemma of pilonidal disease: reverse bandaging for cure of the reluctant pilonidal wound. *Dis Colon Rectum* 1977;20:290.
220. Rosenthal D. Basal cell carcinoma of the anus: report of two cases. *Dis Colon Rectum* 1967;10:397.
221. Rüdlinger R, Buchmann P. HPV 16-positive bowenoid papulosis and squamous-cell carcinoma of the anus in an HIV-positive man. *Dis Colon Rectum* 1989;32:1042.
222. Runfola MA, Weber TK, Rodriguez-Bigas MA, et al. Photodynamic therapy for residual neoplasms of the perianal skin. *Dis Colon Rectum* 2000;43:499.
223. Savin S. The role of cryosurgery in management of anorectal disease: preliminary report on results. *Dis Colon Rectum* 1975;18:292.
224. Scoma JA, Levy EI. Bowen's disease of the anus. *Dis Colon Rectum* 1975;18:137.
225. Senepati A, Cripps NPJ, Thompson MR. Bascom's operation in the day-surgical management of symptomatic pilonidal sinus. *Br J Surg* 2000;87:1067.
226. Shpitz B, Kaufman Z, Kantarovsky A, et al. Definitive management of acute pilonidal abscess by loop diathermy excision. *Dis Colon Rectum* 1990;33:441.
227. Shumaker BP. Treatment of condylomata acuminata with the contact laser system. In: *Clinical procedures review,* vol 9. Surgical Laser Technologies, 1991.
228. Shutze WP, Gleysteen JJ. Perianal Paget's disease. Classification and review of management: report of two cases. *Dis Colon Rectum* 1990;33:502.
229. Silverman SH, Youngs DJ, Allan A, et al. The fecal microflora in pruritus ani. *Dis Colon Rectum* 1989;32:466.
230. Simmons PD. Podophyllin 10 percent and 25 percent in the treatment of ano-genital warts. *Br J Vener Dis* 1981;57:208.

231. Slater DN. Perianal abscess: "Have I excluded leukaemia?" *BMJ* 1984;289:1682.
232. Sloan PJM, Goepel J. Lichen sclerosus et atrophicus and perianal carcinoma: a case report. *Clin Exp Dermatol* 1981;6:399.
233. Smith LE, Henrichs D, McCullah RD. Prospective studies on the etiology and treatment of pruritus ani. *Dis Colon Rectum* 1982;25:358.
234. Sneddon IB. Atrophy of the skin: the clinical problems. *Br J Dermatol* 1976;94:121.
235. Sobrado CW, Mester M, Nadalin W, et al. Radiation-induced total regression of a highly recurrent giant perianal condyloma: report of a case. *Dis Colon Rectum* 2000;43:257.
236. Sohn N, Robilotti JG Jr. The gay bowel syndrome: a review of colonic and rectal conditions in 200 male homosexuals. *Am J Gastroenterol* 1977;67:478.
237. Solla JA, Rothenberger DA. Chronic pilonidal disease: an assessment of 150 cases. *Dis Colon Rectum* 1990;33:758.
238. Spivak H, Brooks VL, Nussbaum M, et al. Treatment of chronic pilonidal disease. *Dis Colon Rectum* 1996;39:1136.
239. Standards Task Force of the American Society of Colon and Rectal Surgeons. Practice parameters for ambulatory anorectal surgery. *Dis Colon Rectum* 1991;34:285.
240. Stephens BJ, Lathrop JC, Rice W, et al. Fournier's gangrene: historic (1764–1978) versus contemporary (1979–1988) differences in etiology and clinical importance. *Am Surg* 1993;59:149.
241. Stone HB. A treatment for pruritus ani. *Johns Hopkins Hosp Bull* 1916;27:242.
242. Stone HB. Pruritus ani: treatment by alcohol injection. *Surg Gynecol Obstet* 1926;42:565.
243. Straus SE, Croen KD, Sawyer MH, et al. Acyclovir suppression of frequently recurring genital herpes: efficacy and diminishing need during successive years of treatment. *JAMA* 1988;260:2227.
244. Straus SE, Takiff HE, Seidlin M, et al. Suppression of frequently recurring genital herpes: a placebo-controlled double-blind trial of oral acyclovir. *N Engl J Med* 1984;310:1545.
245. Strauss RJ, Fazio VW. Bowen's disease of the anal and perianal area: a report and analysis of twelve cases. *Am J Surg* 1979;137:231.
246. Subbuswamy SG, Ribeiro BF. Perianal Paget's disease associated with cloacogenic carcinoma: report of a case. *Dis Colon Rectum* 1981;24:535.
247. Sullivan ES, Garnjobst WM. Pruritus ani: a practical approach. *Surg Clin North Am* 1978;58:505.
248. Sultan S, Azria F, Bauer P, et al. Anoperineal tuberculosis: diagnostic and management considerations in seven cases. *Dis Colon Rectum* 2002;45:407.
249. Swerdlow DB, Salvati EP. Condyloma acuminatum. *Dis Colon Rectum* 1971;14:226.
250. Theodoropoulos GE, Vlahos K, Lazaris AC, et al. Modified Bascom's asymmetric midgluteal cleft closure technique for recurrent pilonidal disease: early experience in a military hospital. *Dis Colon Rectum* 2003;46:1286.
251. Thornton JP, Abcarian H. Surgical treatment of perianal and perineal hidradenitis suppurativa. *Dis Colon Rectum* 1978;21:573.
252. Topgül K, Özdemir E, Kiliç, et al. Long-term results of Limberg flap procedure for treatment of pilonidal sinus: a report of 200 cases. *Dis Colon Rectum* 2003;46:1545.
253. Toubanakis G. Treatment of pilonidal sinus disease with the Z-plasty procedure (modified). *Am Surg* 1986;52:611.
254. Tritapepe R, Di Padova C. Excision and primary closure of pilonidal sinus using a drain for antiseptic wound flushing. *Am J Surg* 2002;183:209.
255. Trombetta LJ, Place RJ. Giant condyloma acuminatum of the anorectum: trends in epidemiology and management. *Dis Colon Rectum* 2001;44:1878.
256. Tyring SK. Immune-response modifiers: a new paradigm in the treatment of human papillomavirus. *Curr Ther Res Clin Exp* 2000;61:584.
257. Urhan MK, Kücükel F, Topgül K, et al. Rhomboid excision and Limberg flap for managing pilonidal sinus: results of 102 cases. *Dis Colon Rectum* 2002;45:656.
258. Velitchkov N, Djedjev M, Kirov G, et al. Toxic shock syndrome and necrotizing fasciitis complicating neglected sacrococcygeal pilonidal sinus disease. *Dis Colon Rectum* 1997;40:1386.
259. Velpeau A. *Dictionnaire en 30 volumes.* Articles: Aiselle, II, p 91; Anus, III, p 304; Mamelles, XIX, 1839; Clinique chirurg, II, p 133. Quoted by Conway H, Stark RB, Climo S, et al. The surgical treatment of chronic hidradenitis suppurativa. *Surg Gynecol Obstet* 1952;95:455.
260. Wade TR, Kopf AW, Ackerman AB. Bowenoid papulosis of the genitalia. *Arch Dermatol* 1979;115:306.
261. Walsh G, Stickley CS. Acute leukemia with primary symptoms in the rectum: a rapid increase in the white cells and fatal outcome. *South Med J* 1934;96:684.
262. Warin RP. Antifungal agents. *Practitioner* 1974;213:494.
263. Welton M, Amerhauser A, Litle V, et al. Anal Bowen's disease and high-grade squamous intraepithelial lesions are histologically and immunohistochemically indistinguishable. *Dis Colon Rectum* 2001;44:A27.
264. Wexner SD. Managing common anorectal sexually transmitted diseases. *Infect Surg* 1990;9:9.
265. Whalen TV Jr, Kovalcik PJ, Old WL Jr. Tuberculous anal ulcer. *Dis Colon Rectum* 1980;23:54.
266. Wilkin JK. Chronic benign familial pemphigus: minimal involvement mimicking chronic perianal candidiasis. *Arch Dermatol* 1978;114:136.
267. Williams SL, Rogers LW, Quan SHQ. Perianal Paget's disease: report of seven cases. *Dis Colon Rectum* 1976;19:30.
268. Williamson JD, Silverman JF, Tafra L. Fine-needle aspiration cytology of metastatic squamous-cell carcinoma arising in a pilonidal sinus, with literature review. *Diagn Cytopathol* 1999;20:367.
269. Wiltz O, Schoetz DJ Jr, Murray JJ, et al. Perianal hidradenitis suppurativa: the Lahey Clinic experience. *Dis Colon Rectum* 1990;33:731.
270. Wiltz OH, Torregrosa M, Wiltz O. Autogenous vaccine: the best therapy for perianal condyloma acuminata? *Dis Colon Rectum* 1995;38:838.
271. Yoshinaga IG, Conrado LA, Schainberg SC, et al. Recalcitrant molluscum contagiosum in a patient with AIDS: combined treatment with CO_2 laser, trichloroacetic acid, and pulsed dye laser. *Lasers Surg Med* 2000;27:291.
272. Zimmerman CE. Outpatient excision and primary closure of pilonidal cysts and sinuses. *Am J Surg* 1978;136:640.

GLOSSARY OF DERMATOLOGIC TERMS

Elevated Lesions

Abscess localized collection of pus

Bulla (bullae) bleb; blisters containing serous or sero-purulent fluid

Crusts dried masses of serum, pus, or blood, with epithelial and bacterial debris

Cyst sac containing liquid or semisolid material

Desquamation scales; results from abnormal keratinization and exfoliation of cornified epithelial cells

Exfoliation scales; laminated masses of keratin; desquamated epidermis

Exudate crusts; dried blood or pus

Furuncle necrotizing form of folliculitis; many may coalesce to form a carbuncle

Hyperkeratosis increased thickening of the stratum corneum

Keratosis (keratotic) horny growth

Lichenification (lichenoid) thickened, leathery; exaggerated skin markings resembling a mosaic

Nodule (nodular) larger papule

Papule (papular, papilloma, papillomatosis) circumscribed solid elevations with no fluid

Plaque minimal height, relatively large surface area

Pustule "pimple"; elevation of the skin containing pus

Urticaria wheals

Vegetation (vegetative) luxuriant, funguslike growth

Vesicle blister; circumscribed epidermal elevation

Wheal evanescent, edematous, variably sized flat elevation

Flat Lesions

Macule (macular) circumscribed change in skin color

Sclerosis (sclerotic) induration or hardening

Telangiectasia condition caused by dilatation of capillary vessels and minute arteries

Depressed Lesions

Atrophy (atrophic) thin, almost transparent epidermis

Excoriation mechanical abrasion

Gangrene death and decay of body tissue characterized by both liquefactive and coagulative necrosis

Scar cicatrix secondary to injury or disease

Sinus tract from a suppurative cavity to skin surface

Ulcer excavation of variable depth involving loss of dermis as well as epidermis

Data from Domonkos AN, Arnold HL Jr, Odom RB. Cutaneous symptoms, signs and diagnosis. In *Andrew's diseases of the skin*, 7th ed. Philadelphia: WB Saunders, 1982:15; Fitzpatrick TB. Fundamentals of dermatologic diagnosis. In Fitzpatrick TB, Eisen AZ, Wolff K, et al, eds. *Dermatology in general medicine*, 2nd ed. St. Louis, MO: McGraw-Hill, 1979:10; and Rook A, Wilkinson DS. The principles of diagnosis. In Rook A, Wilkinson DS, Ebling FJG, eds. *Textbook of dermatology*, 3rd ed. Oxford: Blackwell Scientific, 1979:57.

Chapter 20

Colorectal Manifestations of Acquired Immunodeficiency Syndrome (HIV Infection)

Guest Contributors: Homayoon Akbari and Lester Gottesman

I have asked Drs. Lester Gottesman and Homayoon Akbari to contribute this chapter because of their considerable personal experience with this particular problem. Dr. Gottesman is a recognized national authority, and I respect very much his counsel in this regard. Dr. Gottesman is Associate Professor of Clinical Surgery, Columbia University College of Physicians and Surgeons, New York City. He is also Director of the Division of Colon and Rectal Surgery at St. Luke's–Roosevelt Hospital Center in New York. Dr. Akbari is Assistant Professor in the Department of Surgery at Thomas Jefferson University in Philadelphia and Attending Surgeon at Thomas Jefferson University Hospital. He is a former Resident in Colon and Rectal Surgery at St. Luke's–Roosevelt Hospital Center.

MLC

In human affairs the best stimulus for running is to have something we must run from.
Eric Hoffer: The Ordeal of Change (1964)

ACQUIRED IMMUNODEFICIENCY SYNDROME

Acquired immunodeficiency syndrome (AIDS) is caused by human immunodeficiency virus (HIV), a lentivirus, from the family of retroviruses, with an RNA genome. The disease was first recognized in the United States in 1981. HIV has since become the fourth leading cause of death worldwide, with an estimated 40 million men, women, and children infected according to 2001 figures.[170] In the United States, 41,113 new cases were diagnosed in 2000.[153] This suggests a decreased number of newly diagnosed cases compared with prior years, although more recent reports indicate the incidence to be again increasing.[152] Improved medical therapy with the development of highly active antiretroviral therapy (HAART) in the mid-1990s decreased the number of AIDS-related deaths, thus resulting in increased numbers of persons living with AIDS. In 2000, this number was estimated to be 337,731 in the United States.[153] Whereas AIDS was initially confined to the homosexual popula-

tion, intravenous drug users, and recipients of contaminated blood, there has been a noticeable increase in the incidence among the heterosexual population.

Mechanism of Viral Replication

HIV infects immune cells, thereby enabling replication of the virus. The HIV glycoprotein, gp 120, interacts with the cell surface CD4 molecule and either the CXCR4 chemokine receptor (expressed in CD4$^+$ T cells) or the CCR5 chemokine receptor (expressed in macrophages and primary T cells) to permit cellular entry of HIV. The viral RNA is reverse-transcribed into complementary (cDNA) by the enzyme reverse transcriptase (RT). The cDNA is then transported to the host cell nucleus and is integrated into the host cell DNA by the enzyme integrase, thereby permitting replication of the viral RNA and the synthesis of viral proteins. The enzyme, protease, sections the viral proteins into shorter pieces, which then encapsulate, allowing release of new virions.

HIV infection results in immune dysfunction, which, if untreated, leads to a progressive, profound immunocompromised state, with decreased cellular and humoral immunity, opportunistic infections, rare malignant tumors, and, ultimately, death.

Symptoms and Associated Conditions

HIV often causes a brief, flulike illness at the time of infection, but the virus may be harbored for many years without producing clinical manifestations. Because the acute infection generally produces mild, nonspecific symptoms, HIV infection is usually not diagnosed until several years after infection. Immunoglobulin M (IgM) antibodies to various HIV proteins are detectable within 2 weeks of infection by enzyme-linked immunoabsorbent assay and Western blot.[148] IgG antibody is generally detected by 6 weeks after the onset of acute infection, although Imagawa and colleagues demonstrated that HIV infection may actually occur 35 months before detection of antibodies.[118] However, this observation is generally thought to be the exception.

Acute HIV infection may manifest itself through fever, lymphadenopathy, pharyngitis, rash, weight loss, and fatigue.[46] Gastrointestinal symptoms such as abdominal pain, diarrhea, nausea, and anorexia have also been reported during the acute illness.[209,221] Immunologically, there is a precipitous drop in peripheral T-cell populations during the acute phase.[52] This is transient and is followed by a lymphocytosis 3 to 4 weeks later, although there is a decrease in CD4+ cells relative to CD8+ cells.[277]

Progression of HIV results in a gradual decline of CD4+ cells and an increase in the number of virions ("viral load"). CD4+ lymphocyte counts are used as an indicator of disease progression. Individuals with CD4+ cell counts lower than 200 are considered to have advanced immunodeficiency, and, by definition, AIDS, and those with CD4+ cell counts lower than 50 have end-stage disease. HIV continually destroys resident T cells at a fairly constant rate and, after initial infection, stabilizes the rate of viral replication (called the set point) in each individual. This continues until the capacity of the immune system to restore itself is exhausted. Because T4 cells are constantly being replenished and destroyed, measurement of plasma HIV-1 RNA now appears to be a better prognostic indicator of disease activity than the CD4 count.[82] Disease progression leads to increased opportunistic infections, AIDS-related malignancies, and, ultimately, death.

Colonic and anorectal problems in individuals who are HIV positive are mainly infectious in origin, as can be predicted from the immunodeficient status of the patients. Certain enteric infections have a high prevalence among homosexual men with and without AIDS, but especially if the latter condition supervenes. These include gonorrhea, syphilis, shigellosis, condylomata acuminata, campylobacteriosis, amebiasis, giardiasis, cryptosporidiosis, cytomegalovirus infection, isosporiasis, candidiasis, and infection with *Chlamydia trachomatis*, *Salmonella typhimurium*, and *Mycobacterium avium*.[191] Gastrointestinal tract hemorrhage is an uncommon manifestation.[37] Miles and colleagues noted that the most frequent reason for surgical referral was anorectal disease (5.9% of all HIV-positive patients), and warts comprised the single most common indication.[164]

Certain malignant tumors are seen more frequently in patients with AIDS. The most common are Kaposi's sarcoma and non-Hodgkin's lymphoma (NHL), both of which may have colonic involvement. The incidence of anal squamous carcinoma is also increased in patients with AIDS.[218]

Intestinal and Anorectal Immunology and Human Immunodeficiency Virus

The mucosal layer on the surface of the gut provides a barrier to the large number of bacteria within the intestinal tract. Nonspecific mucosal defenses are extrinsic to the mucosa and form a protective barrier. These include the mucous coat, resident microflora, which prevent overgrowth of pathogenic organisms, proteolytic secretions, and glycocalyx. Secretory IgA, the primary immunoglobulin in external secretions, is the main immunologic defense in the gastrointestinal tract, and it acts as a non–complement-binding antibody that captures pathogens before they can invade the mucosal surface. An antigen that succeeds in penetrating this defense is processed by specialized epithelial cells on the mucosal surface, microvillus (M) cells, and is presented to immunologically competent cells in the lamina propria. Gut-associated lymphoid tissue is found in Peyer's patches, solitary lymphoid follicles, and local, activated T cells within the lamina propria. Intraluminally, these lymphoid aggregates are covered with follicle-associated epithelium that contains M cells. M cells function to transport antigen to dendritic cells and tissue macrophages within the lymphoid aggregates, which, in turn, present antigen to CD4+ T cells and B cells.[185] Once activated, resident T cells initiate cellular immunity by release of cytokines and modulation of other cellular immune elements, and B cells produce antigen-specific antibody.

HIV can gain access to lymphoid tissue within the lamina propria either through a break in the mucosa or by M cell–mediated transport. Within the lamina propria and epithelium of the intestinal tract, HIV infects resident T-cell and macrophage populations in the lymphoid aggregates and diffuses activated memory T cells. As described earlier, this is mediated through the cell surface coreceptors CXCR4 and CCR5. Gut-associated lymphoid tissue contains more than 50% of total lymphocytes in the body and as such represents an important HIV reservoir. It is unique in the proportion of activated memory T cells it contains, which is higher than in peripheral blood and lymph nodes. It has been postulated to be an early site of HIV infection and replication, because the virus replicates more efficiently in activated memory T cells.[214,249,279] In a primate model using simian immunodeficiency virus (SIV), activated memory CD4 T cells were found to be rapidly depleted within days of SIV infection. The early, selective, rapid infection and depletion of intestinal lymphoid tissue led the authors to hypothesize that acute HIV and SIV infection is primarily a disease of the mucosal/intestinal immune system.[249] The early infection and apoptosis of intestinal mucosal CD4 T cells may explain the abdominal complaints common in early HIV infection described earlier. The depletion of CD4 T cells adversely affects immunoglobulin production and mucosal integrity, thereby promoting translocation of bacteria and subsequent bacterial invasion.[93] A similar phenomenon has been more recently described for vaginal mucosal CD4 T cells, which likewise serve as an early site of entry and replication of HIV.[248]

The squamous epithelium of the anal canal and anal verge also has immunologic function. Both CD4 and CD8 T lymphoctes and dendritic cells, which function as antigen-presenting cells, are present in the anal mucosa.[31,94] Dendritic cells, also known as Langerhans cells after migration to the epithelium, act as antigen-presenting cells to activate a cellular immune response.[243] In their capacity as antigen-presenting cells, epithelial and subepithelial dendritic cells of the anal canal may act to facilitate access of HIV to the mucosal lymphoid system. The capacity to migrate from initial points of entry, together with their capacity to activate the cellular immune response by recruiting and activating large numbers of T cells, led to some researchers to propose that these cells play an integral role in sexual transmission of HIV.[136]

The interaction of HIV, anal canal dendritic cells, and mucosal T cells may explain the effect of HIV on other viral infections of the anal canal in HIV-positive patients, including human papillomavirus (HPV). Persistent HPV infection in HIV-positive patients may be secondary to local immune dysfunction rather than to generalized immunosuppression.[58] Sobhani and co-workers have shown a decrease in the number of dendritic cells in the anal mucosa of HIV-positive patients with HPV infection compared with HIV-negative controls,[230] a finding that may explain the more aggressive nature of HPV infection in HIV-positive patients.

New antiviral therapies and mucosal vaccines are being investigated that would block the transmission of HIV to T cells by dendritic cells via the membrane protein, DC-SIGN, which binds the HIV-1 envelope.[25]

Antiretroviral Therapy

HAART has profoundly affected the progression of HIV disease. HAART reduces plasma viral load, increases CD4 T-cell counts, and reduces the incidence of opportunistic infections in HIV-infected patients.[80,184] HAART is a combination of three or more antiretroviral drugs from two or, sometimes, three different classes of drugs. Class-sparing regimens have been advocated to allow for second-line therapy in case of resistance.[1] The three classes of drugs used in HAART are the nucleoside RT inhibitors (NRTIs), the nonnucleoside RT inhibitors (NNRTIs), and the protease inhibitors (PIs). More recently, a fourth class, the fusion inhibitors, has been introduced and approved by the United States Food and Drug Administration (FDA). The NRTIs were the first class of antiretroviral drugs, introduced with zidovudine (formerly known as azidothymidine or AZT).[109] The NRTIs are dideoxynucleoside analogues that, once phosphorylated, can be incorporated into the cDNA, causing early chain termination and preventing HIV replication. The NNRTIs, like the NRTIs, prevent the transcription of the HIV RNA into cDNA. However, unlike the NRTIs, the NNRTIs do not act as substrates for the enzyme but rather bind to the active site of the enzyme, preventing viral DNA synthesis. PIs, introduced in 1995, inhibit the enzyme HIV protease, blocking the final cleavage of HIV proteins and preventing the assembly of new virions.[66] Combination antiviral therapy with a PI is more effective in reducing plasma HIV-1 RNA compared with regimens without a PI.[108] In March 2003, the FDA approved enfuvirtide (Fuzeon), the first fusion inhibitor to be approved for use in combination with other antiretroviral drugs. The fusion inhibitors, a novel class of drug, differ from previous HIV medications in that they do not disrupt the replication and release of HIV, but rather prevent the entry of HIV into the target cell.[122] Unlike other antiretrovirals, enfuvirtide lacks oral availability and is administered by subcutaneous injection twice daily.

The impact of HAART on the intestinal mucosal immune system has not yet been fully investigated. As mentioned earlier, the gut-associated lymphoid tissue represents a large reservoir for HIV infection and is affected by HIV early in the course of infection with a dramatic loss of lymphoid cells and, by extension, decrease in the immune function of the intestinal mucosa. Talal and coworkers examined the effects of HAART on gut-associated lymphoid tissue in a small, prospective study with eight patients. In all individuals, levels of HIV-1 RNA fell to less than detectable levels after 6 months of therapy in both gut-associated lymphoid tissue and plasma. Immune reconstitution, however, was less dramatic in intestinal lymphoid tissue compared with peripheral blood.[241] Other authors have documented a similar decrease in HIV-1 RNA but with a significant increase in CD4 T-cell counts in rectal biopsies.[140]

Although HAART has not yet been definitively shown to result in immune reconstitution of gut-associated lymphoid tissue, combination antiviral therapy has had a tremendously impact on intestinal manifestations of HIV. The incidence of AIDS-associated intestinal malignancies and opportunistic infections has decreased since the advent of HAART. The prevalence of opportunistic pathogens in endoscopic biopsy specimens in HIV-infected patients decreased from 69% to 13% following the introduction of HAART.[167] Similarly, the incidence of opportunistic infections causing chronic diarrhea in patients with AIDS decreased from 53% to 13% following the introduction of HAART.[31] However, the overall incidence of diarrhea remains high, a concern that may be secondary to PIs. Diarrhea is a common side effect of these inhibitors and is noted in up to 70% of patients. Treatment for opportunistic pathogens in HIV-infected patients with chronic diarrhea is more successful in patients receiving HAART. In a study of 282 individuals, those receiving PIs had a significantly higher response rate to the treatment for pathogen-identified diarrhea.[19] Immune reconstitution of gut-associated lymphoid tissue with an increase in CD4 T cells and recovery from cryptosporidiosis in an HIV-infected patient following initiation of HAART have been described.[211]

Surgery and Surgical Outcome

Surgical consultation is often sought in patients with HIV infection or AIDS for complaints of abdominal pain. Many of the opportunistic gastrointestinal diseases that are seen in patients with AIDS may present with severe abdominal pain that can mimic standard surgical conditions. The majority of these can safely be managed non-operatively. Generally, the goal in management of the acute abdomen in a patient with HIV is to *try to avoid surgery*.[74,81] Evaluating by means of computed tomography and endoscopy, understanding the natural history of the colonic manifestations, and knowing the expected responses from pharmacologic intervention will usually allow the surgeon to avoid an unnecessary and unhelpful laparotomy. However, intestinal perforation, gastrointestinal bleeding, and obstruction as a consequence of infection or malignancy may be seen in HIV-positive patients, and these manifestations often necessitate surgical intervention.

Numerous articles have been published on the results of surgery in individuals who harbor the AIDS virus and in those who have the full-blown picture of AIDS or AIDS-related complex.[63,103,215,267] Wolkomir and colleagues reported 474 patients who underwent abdominal and anorectal surgery with these conditions.[273] None required surgery for complications secondary to cytomegalovirus, visceral lymphoma, or visceral Kaposi's sarcoma. Although no deaths occurred within 30 days, the morbidity rate was 72%. The rate of wound healing was inversely related to the white blood cell count. Wilson and colleagues submitted their experience of 36 major abdominal operations performed on 35 patients with AIDS.[272] Cytomegalovirus was the most common pathogen. Mycobacterial infections presented as retroperitoneal adenopathy or splenic abscess, and NHL was the most common malignancy identified.[107] Elective mortality was 9% at 30 days and 46% when an emergency operation was necessary. In a study by Chambers and Lord, the outcome of laparotomy in patients with AIDS who were found to have AIDS-related pathology was compared with those with non–AIDS-related pathology.[39] Those in the former group were found at the time of laparotomy to have lower mean body weights, serum albumin levels, and CD4 T-cell counts. The most frequent postoperative AIDS-related pathology was B-cell NHL. The 30-mortal-

ity rate was 17%, and the complication rate was 70%, with no significant difference between patients with AIDS with AIDS-related pathology and those with non–AIDS-related pathology. More than 50% of postoperative complications were infectious in origin (pulmonary, wound, and systemic sepsis). This is in contrast to an earlier study in which a slightly higher mortality rate in patients with AIDS-related pathology at laparotomy was observed (47%) compared with patients with non–AIDS-related pathology.[20] Postoperative complications have been noted to occur with a higher frequency (61% versus 7%) in patients with AIDS than in asymptomatic HIV-infected patients. Again, most complications were infectious in origin.[275] In contrast to intraabdominal surgical procedures, perianal surgical procedures do not appear to carry a higher morbidity and mortality in HIV-infected patients.[35] Barrett and co-workers reported a 2% complication rate in 485 anorectal procedures, and there were no deaths.[9] This is consistent with our own experience.

Postoperative Complications and Wound Healing

Early reports about poor wound healing and fear of becoming infected through inadvertent exposure have contributed to the reluctance of many surgeons to operate on HIV-positive patients. Analysis of data suggests an inverse relationship between CD4 T-cell count and wound healing—that is, poor wound healing is associated with low CD4 T-cell counts in lesions not expected to heal, such as malignancies and ulcers.[50] More recently, a greater incidence of wound complications in HIV-positive patients has been reported.[65] CD4 T-cell counts do appear to be a prognostic factor in surgical outcome in patients with AIDS. Albaran and co-workers found that patients with CD4 T-cell counts lower than 200 cells/mm³ had increased morbidity and mortality rates following surgery.[2] An increased incidence of surgical infection, regardless of the type of operative procedure, has been noted in HIV-positive patients with CD4 T-cell counts lower than 200 cells/mm.[3,78] In experimental studies, abdominal wounds in thymectomized rats with depletion of CD4 lymphocytes have been found to have a significant decrease in strength, resilience, and toughness.[64]

Similar results of lower CD4 T-cell counts on wound healing and outcome following anorectal surgery have been reported. Viral load has also been studied as a prognostic indicator following surgery in HIV-positive patients,[266] although as noted earlier, more recent studies find no increased incidence of complications following anorectal surgery. Studies have demonstrated that viral load is the best single predictor of clinical outcome, followed by CD4 T-cell counts.[17,158] Unfortunately, no studies have examined the prognostic value of the extent of viremia on postoperative outcome.

Given the evidence available, increased wound and other infective complications should be expected following abdominal and, possibly, anorectal surgery.[120] The prognostic value of CD4 T-cell counts indicates that optimization of the patient with immune reconstitution through HAART should be beneficial before semielective and elective procedures. Obviously, this is not possible in the emergency situation.

COLONIC MANIFESTATIONS OF HUMAN IMMUNODEFICIENCY VIRUS INFECTION

Gastrointestinal disease is seen frequently in HIV-infected patients. Specifically, a variety of disease processes may affect the colon in an individual who harbors HIV. These may present in a number of ways. Diarrhea has been reported to affect up to 50% of patients with AIDS in North America and is a significant cause of morbidity and mortality among such persons.[229] Chronic diarrhea is seen more frequently in male homosexual HIV-infected patients and in those with severely depleted CD4 T-cell counts.[127,200] Gastrointestinal bleeding and perforation are most commonly seen in enteroinvasive infections, such as those caused by cytomegalovirus and *Clostridium difficile*, but they may be secondary to gastrointestinal involvement by HIV-associated malignancies. Obstruction may be seen with malignant disease, primarily Kaposi's sarcoma and NHLs. Finally, lymphadenopathy itself may cause severe abdominal pain and compression of viscera, primarily through a *Mycobacterium avium* complex (MAC) infection.

Diarrheal Conditions

Diarrhea is seen in approximately 50% of patients with AIDS.[229] Chronic diarrhea results in a decreased quality of life and contributes to the morbidity of HIV infection. The etiology is multifactorial. Certainly, the ability to identify an organism depends on how vigorously the cause is pursued.[24] Infection with HIV is thought to cause minor alterations in architecture of the villi, which may lead to mild malabsorption of carbohydrates;[128] this can cause diarrhea also. Furthermore, increased permeability resulting from cytokine activation by foreign antigens, as well as bacterial overgrowth in the small bowel, may also contribute to pathogen-negative diarrhea.[12] HIV has amino acid sequences similar to those of vasoactive intestinal peptide (VIP) and may induce diarrhea by upregulation of VIP receptors.[250] HIV infection of the intestinal tract may also affect the barrier function of the intestinal epithelium. Stockmann and co-workers have proposed a leak-flux mechanism for diarrhea in HIV-infected individuals, secondary to intestinal mucosal cytokine release with resultant disruption of the epithelial barrier.[238]

Patients who present with diarrhea and abdominal pain should be assessed with a detailed history and physical examination, routine laboratory studies, and stool studies. The patient's immune status should be assessed by CD4 T-cell count and viral load. Recent exposure history can be obtained by careful attention to sexual history, travel, diet (to rule out food intolerance), and medications (specifically, PIs and antibiotic use). The characteristics of the diarrhea should be assessed, including duration, severity, associated abdominal pain, hematochezia, weight loss, and fever. Frequent, small movements with associated tenesmus are more indicative of an anorectal cause, whereas bloody movements and fever suggest an enteroinvasive, colonic pathogen. Physical examination should include a careful abdominal examination with attention to organomegaly, tenderness, and distension, an anorectal examination to assess for perianal lesions that may highlight an infectious source (e.g., herpes simplex), and a general physical evaluation to determine temperature, the presence or absence of cachexia, and lymphadenopathy.[169]

The American Gastroenterological Society created guidelines for the evaluation and management of chronic diarrhea in HIV-infected patients.[270] Recommendations include stool samples for bacteria and parasites, as well as for *C. difficile* if there is a risk for antibiotic-associated diarrhea. In the febrile patient, blood cultures should be drawn for bacteria and, in severely immunocompromised patients with CD4 T-cell counts lower than 100 cells/mm³, for mycobacteria. For those in whom stool studies fail to identify an infectious cause, endoscopy and mucosal biopsy are recommended, particularly in patients whose symptoms indicate a rectal or colonic cause. Flexible sigmoidoscopy with mucosal biopsies for microscopic examination and for bacterial and mycobacterial culture should be performed. Total colonoscopy may be necessary in certain patients, particularly when cytomegalovirus infection is suspected, given the high incidence of isolated proximal colonic involvement. Finally, esophagogastroduodenoscopy should be performed with duodenal biopsies when other investigations have failed to reveal a source. This may aid in identifying *Giardia*, MAC, microsporidia, or *Isospora*. With a comprehensive investigation, an etiologic agent can be found in 90% of patients.[24] Among identified causes of diarrhea in patients with AIDS and chronic diarrhea, the most common opportunistic pathogens are cytomegalovirus, MAC, and the protozoans *Cryptosporidia* and *Microsporidia*.[270] Treatment of pathogen-negative diarrhea consists of rehydration and somatostatin analogues.[226]

Cytomegalovirus Infection

Cytomegalovirus is a double-stranded DNA virus from the herpesvirus family. It was first isolated in 1956 and has been found in urine, feces, semen, saliva, breast milk, blood, and cervical and vaginal secretions.[201] Although ubiquitous in humans, cytomegalovirus does not produce symptoms; it becomes an opportunistic infection as immune function deteriorates. Infection with cytomegalovirus is extremely common in patients with AIDS.[171] Disseminated cytomegalovirus has been identified in 90% of patients with AIDS at autopsy, with 94% of homosexual men testing positive at some venereal disease clinics.[267] Colonic cytomegalovirus is a common cause of diarrhea and abdominal pain in patients with AIDS, with resultant morbidity and mortality.[270]

Gastrointestinal manifestations of cytomegalovirus infection include ulcers, which may occur anywhere along the gastrointestinal tract, enteritis, colitis, ileocecal obstruction, perforation, and gastrointestinal hemorrhage. The colon is the main target in the gastrointestinal tract, and ileocolitis is the major colorectal manifestation.[71,197,263] In a study examining the colonoscopic findings of cytomegalovirus infection in patients with AIDS, ulcerations, colitis, and subendothelial hemorrhage were the most common findings. Disease limited to the right colon was seen in 13% of patients, again emphasizing the need for complete colonoscopy in those with suspected cytomegalovirus.[269] The diagnosis of cytomegalovirus colitis should always be considered in patients with AIDS who develop an acute abdomen, especially if a free perforation is diagnosed on radiographic study (see later).

Symptoms and Findings

The most common manifestation of colonic cytomegalovirus infection is watery diarrhea.[68,69,160] Bloody stools are common and may be seen in the absence of diarrhea. Abdominal pain may be severe, mimicking an acute surgical abdomen.[269] Up to 30% of patients may complain of fever and weight loss *without* diarrhea.[68] As the virally induced vasculitis progresses, thrombosis, occlusion, and ischemia of the affected area may occur. Toxic megacolon, hemorrhage, and perforation have been reported; this is of obvious interest to the surgeon.[97,257,267] Cytomegalovirus enterocolitis was the single most common reason for abdominal surgery in the AIDS population in the experience of Wilson and colleagues and is the most frequent life-threatening condition requiring emergency celiotomy in these individuals.[143,272] However, effective antiviral therapy has reduced the incidence of these severe complications.[257]

Diagnosis

The accurate diagnosis of cytomegalovirus colitis is sometimes quite difficult. Endoscopically, the mucosa in cytomegalovirus colitis is diffusely erythematous and friable with ulcerations. The ulcers themselves range from shallow, punctate lesions to deeply coalescing ulcers, the appearance of which may be difficult to distinguish from that of other colitides. Submucosal hemorrhage, sec-

ondary to cytomegalovirus-induced vasculitis, may be seen. Colonic involvement is patchy or limited to one region. As mentioned, patchy colitis localized to the right colon may be seen in 13% to 40% of patients, necessitating full colonoscopy rather than sigmoidoscopy.[68,143,269] However, in 25% of those with cytomegalovirus colitis, the mucosa appears endoscopically normal. For diagnosis, biopsy samples are taken randomly from the cecum, ascending colon, transverse colon, descending colon, and sigmoid colon. Cytomegalovirus may be demonstrated on histologic examination of grossly normal mucosa; therefore, samples of both inflamed and noninflamed areas should be taken.

Pathology

Biopsy usually reveals an inflammatory infiltrate, including lymphocytes and plasma cells with, in some areas, polymorphonuclear leukocytes and histiocytes.[70,203] Cellular changes seen under light microscopy are colonic mucosal cell enlargement with basophilic intranuclear inclusions, surrounded by a clear halo that gives the characteristic "owl's eye" appearance. (Figure 20-1).[114] The retrieval of cytomegalovirus inclusions appears to depend on the number of biopsy specimens, the skill of the pathologist, and whether the material was taken from an endoscopically abnormal colon.[99,160] Cultures for cytomegalovirus have been inconsistent in predicting the presence of active infection. *In situ* hybridization staining and polymerase chain reaction may increase the sensitivity of histologic analysis.[56,217] Polymerase chain reaction amplification of cytomegalovirus DNA offers the best method for both diagnosis and monitoring of the efficacy of therapy.[55]

Radiologic investigation, specifically computed tomography, usually reveals the nonspecific changes of colitis, with colonic thickening and diffuse ulcerations.

Management

Medical management includes ganciclovir (Cytovene, 5 mg/kg intravenously twice daily), an antiviral agent that has been demonstrated to be active against cytomegalovirus, and foscarnet, which usually improves both the histologic and macroscopic appearance within 3 weeks. Complete response to ganciclovir and/or foscarnet therapy can be expected in approximately 90%. If there is no improvement, foscarnet, at a dose of 60 to 90 mg/kg intravenously three times daily, should be used. However, because relapse is very common (50%), maintenance therapy should always be considered.[18,60] Patients receiving such treatment and those taking PIs have been demonstrated to have the lowest recurrence rates and an improved survival.[18]

Surgical intervention is reserved for perforation, massive bleeding, and toxic megacolon. However, a patient with mild peritoneal signs, without free air, and with the

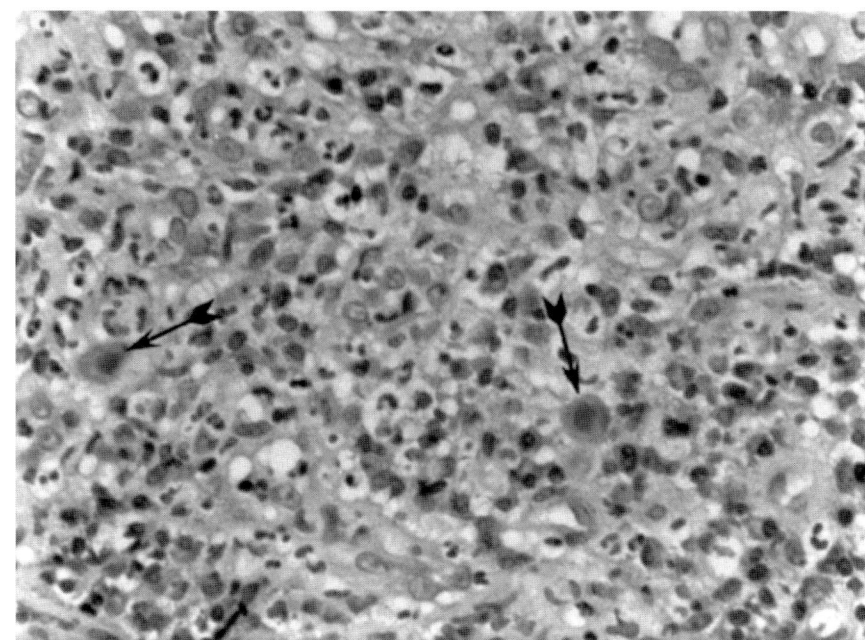

FIGURE 20-1. Cytomegalovirus entero-colitis. Acutely inflamed granulation tissue with cells positive for cytomegalo-virus demonstrating intranuclear inclusions *(arrows)*. (Original magnification × 400.)

presumptive diagnosis of cytomegalovirus colitis may be treated with both ganciclovir and appropriate antibiotics for aerobic and anaerobic organisms while he or she is observed carefully. Most individuals will respond without the need for surgical intervention. However, when emergency surgery is required, resection of the involved segment of colon is necessary. No anastomosis should be performed under these circumstances.

Results of Surgery

Approximately two thirds of patients with AIDS who underwent emergency bowel resection by Wexner and colleagues had cytomegalovirus ileocolitis.[267] The postoperative mortality was 28% at 1 day, 71% at 1 month, and 86% at 6 months. Death often is a consequence of sepsis and pneumonia caused by *Pneumocystis carinii*.[143] Elective resection of eight patients reported by Söderlund and co-workers resulted in one death.[234] Recurrent or persistent symptoms of cytomegalovirus enterocolitis occurred in four patients after a mean of 7 months.

Mycobacterium avium Complex Infection

MAC affects about 5% of severely immunocompromised HIV patients and is diagnosed in 50% of those with AIDS.[72] This is an environmental bacterium that enters through both the gastrointestinal and respiratory tracts.[145] Typically, patients with gastrointestinal MAC infection have low CD4 T-cell counts. In addition to severe diarrhea, patients may report abdominal pain, anorexia, and weight loss. Anemia may be identified upon laboratory evaluation. Abdominal pain may be secondary to intraabdominal lymphadenopathy. This is readily diagnosed by computed tomography and needle aspiration.[5] Colonic infection may result in obstruction, fistula formation, and perforation, although these are uncommon, and surgery is rarely indicated in the management of gastrointestinal MAC.[108]

Diagnosis is made on biopsy of either affected small intestine or colon. The endoscopic appearance of MAC is quite distinctive, with granular, small (4-mm), white nodules with surrounding erythema. Colonic mucosa may be edematous and, uncommonly, ulcerated. Biopsy cultures are used to confirm the diagnosis and permit sensitivity typing. Because MAC is a systemic disease, blood cultures may be taken to confirm the diagnosis and have been reported to be more helpful than either stool or respiratory specimens for establishing the diagnosis with certainty.[43]

Medical treatment of gastrointestinal MAC is with a combination of antituberculous drugs. Ethambutol (15 to 25 mg/kg daily), ciprofloxacin (500 to 750 mg twice daily), rifampin (600 mg daily), rifabutin (450 to 600 mg daily), amikacin (10 to 15 mg/kg daily), clofazimine (50 to 200 mg daily), and azithromycin (500 mg daily) may be used in three or four drug regimens for a 12-week treatment period.[14,33] Response to quadruple therapy is good, with more than one half of patients demonstrating complete response and resolution of symptoms.[130]

Protozoal Infections

Microsporidia Infection

Microsporidia, of which *Enterocytozoon bieneusi* accounts for the majority of cases in patients with AIDS, are obligate intracellular, spore-forming protozoa. Microsporidia have been identified in up to 60% of patients with AIDS with chronic diarrhea.[166,232] Microsporidiosis is usually seen in those with advanced AIDS with CD4 T-cell counts lower than 100 cells/mm³. Patients present with frequent, watery bowel movements (nonbloody), abdominal pain, and nausea.

Diagnosis Microsporidiosis most frequently affects the proximal jejunum. Upper endoscopy with a pediatric colonoscope is necessary to obtain biopsies. Histologically, characteristic small, round/oval plasmodia and spores within the infected enterocyte cytoplasm, typically supranuclear in the apical cytoplasm, are demonstrated.[176] Atrophy of intestinal villi and crypt hyperplasia are seen microscopically, and the resultant changes in absorption contribute to the diarrhea.[189]

Colonoscopy with terminal ileal biopsies may permit visualization of the organisms and should be performed when microsporidiosis is suspected. Although examination of biopsy specimens is the most sensitive method for detection, microscopic examination of stool samples, both with trichrome staining and indirect immunofluorescence, using polyclonal and monoclonal antibodies, may diagnose the condition.[259,280]

Treatment Treatment of microsporidiosis is difficult and generally does not result in eradication of the infection. The destruction of the resident T cells in the lamina propria of the gut is probably responsible for the persistence of these protozoal infections.[150] Albendazole, 400 mg twice daily, is the recommended drug. Clinically, a partial response of more than a 50% reduction in bowel movements was noted in one study, although repeat endoscopy revealed persistence of infection in all regardless of clinical response.[67] More recently, thalidomide has been investigated as a drug to treat the condition. Thalidomide, 100 mg daily for 30 days, was found to result in a complete clinical response in sevenof 28 patients.[220] Immune reconstitution with HAART has been noted to result in a complete clinical response in patients with microsporidiosis and cryptosporidiosis.[34]

Cryptosporidium Infection

Cryptosporidium is a protozoan parasite that primarily affects the small intestine and causes a profuse, watery diarrhea. *Cryptosporidium* oocysts are spread by person-to-person contact and by contaminated water transmission. It is a common source of diarrhea in immunocompetent individuals worldwide but is usually self-limiting in the nonimmunocompromised host. In HIV-positive patients, cryptosporidiosis is self-limited in up to one third of patients with CD4 T-cell counts higher than 200/µL. However, in patients with AIDS with lower CD4 T-cell counts, *Cryptosporidium* may result in a serious, chronic disease with abdominal pain, nausea, vomiting, and anorexia, in addition to diarrhea.[84] Infection can be fatal, with severe dehydration and electrolyte imbalances, and wasting.

Diagnosis Cryptosporidium affects primarily the jejunum and ileum, resulting in villous atrophy, malabsorption, and altered permeability.[100] Cryptosporidium may produce an enterotoxin that results in hypersecretion of fluid into the bowel and the large-volume diarrhea seen clinically.[106] Diagnosis is made by stool examination with modified acid-fast stain and light microscopy to detect oocysts. Alternatively, immunofluorescence antibody may be used with increased sensitivity.[92] Endoscopic biopsy demonstrates the intracellular protozoa, villous atrophy, and inflammation of the lamina propria.

Treatment Treatment of cryptosporidiosis is difficult, and there still remains no ideal regimen. As noted earlier, immune reconstitution with HAART may result in resolution of symptoms. A more recent study demonstrated that a combination of azithromycin and paromomycin may be promising, with almost complete eradication of oocyst excretion at 12 weeks.[228] Preventive measures include avoiding drinking water directly from lakes and waters, careful hand washing after contact with human and animal feces, and avoidance of oral-anal sexual practices.

Clostridium difficile *Infection*

C. difficile colitis is common among AIDS victims because many who are infected with HIV receive a variety of antimicrobial agents, either for prophylaxis or for treatment of bacterial illnesses. In addition, repeat hospital admissions predispose the patient to colonization with the organism. The typical presentation includes mucoid diarrhea, abdominal pain, and fever (see Chapter 33). The condition may progress to that of acute megacolon as well as to life-threatening diarrhea.[129]

Diagnosis is made by testing stool for toxin A or toxin B, both of which are produced by *C. difficile*. Endoscopy is usually not indicated and, in fact, should be discouraged in patients with severe disease without suspicion of necrosis. Endoscopically, the colonic mucosa appears inflamed, and ulcerations and pseudomembranes may be present. However, in the patient with AIDS, the colitis may lack characteristic pseudomembranes and may also involve a secondary pathogen, such as cytomegalovirus.[36]

Treatment is with either oral vancomycin (125 mg four times daily) or metronidazole (250 mg four times daily). In severe disease, a combination of intravenous metronidazole (Flagyl) and oral vancomycin is recommended. With profuse diarrhea, oral cholestyramine may be used to bind toxin and to reduce stool frequency. The reader is referred to Chapter 33 for a comprehensive discussion of antibiotic-associated colitis.

Histoplasmosis

Histoplasma capsulatum is a fungus that usually causes subclinical infection when its airborne spore is inhaled.[104] The risk of developing histoplasmosis and the severity of disease are dependent on the immune status of HIV-infected individuals. Disseminated histoplasmosis is usually seen in patients with CD4 T-cell counts lower than 200 cells/mm³.[268] Gastrointestinal involvement is common in disseminated histoplasmosis, although symptomatic gastrointestinal disease is only seen in a small percentage of patients.

Symptoms of gastrointestinal histoplasmosis are nonspecific and include abdominal pain, diarrhea, nausea, anorexia, and weight loss. Gastrointestinal histoplasmosis may also present with gastrointestinal bleeding, obstruction, or perforation.[86,112,131,237] Dissemination of the fungus may cause focal lesions affecting any segment of the gastrointestinal tract. However, the terminal ileum and ascending colon are the most frequently involved sites, probably because of the presence of considerable lymphoid tissue[10] The lesions may appear as polyps or may coalesce to form inflammatory masses that may mimic carcinoma.[8] An additional discussion concerning this fungal infection is found in Chapter 33.

Non-Hodgkin's Lymphoma

NHL is an AIDS-defining malignancy. HIV infection increases the risk of systemic NHL by 200-fold, with the greatest increase in high-grade NHL.[54] Extranodal NHL occurs in approximately 10% of HIV-infected individuals, and it had become the most common malignant disease associated with AIDS in certain areas until the mid-1990s.[105] However, after a steady increase in the number of NHL cases up until 1995, there has since been a decline.[62] Unlike Kaposi's sarcoma (see later), there is little variation in the incidence of NHL between different HIV exposure groups. It tends to occur in advanced disease in those individuals with a CD4-cell count of less than 50/mm³.[195]

Pathogenesis

The biology and presentation of NHL in HIV-positive individuals are different from those of the general population in that high-grade lymphomas are more frequent with HIV infection. The biology of these lymphomas varies in relationship to morphologic type, anatomic site, and overall state of immunodeficiency.[138] Large cell immunoblastic lymphomas are the most common (see Figure 25-21).[15] Many AIDS-associated large cell lymphomas represent polyclonal proliferation suggestive of lymphokine-induced expansion of a B-cell population.[216] In addition, most patients with HIV infection and NHL

present with advanced disease; 90% have extranodal disease at presentation, and more than 50% present with stage IV disease.[126,135] Age greater than 35 years, advanced stage at diagnosis, and a CD4 count of less than 100 cells/mm³ are adverse prognostic factors. HAART is associated with a decreased incidence of NHL and an improved prognosis.[154] The gastrointestinal tract is the most common site of extranodal NHL, and in approximately 25% of the time, the gastrointestinal tract is the only site of disease.[119] More than 90% of these lymphomas are B-cell lymphomas, and Epstein-Barr virus expression is seen in the majority.[137,223]

It has been postulated that HIV infection results in immune dysfunction and altered cytokine release that, when combined with chronic antigenic exposure to other viral pathogens, namely, the Epstein-Barr virus or human herpesvirus-8, result in proliferation of B-cell clones that subsequently undergo malignant transformation secondary to genetic instability.[139] More recently, it has been hypothesized that integration of the HIV genome into the genome of infected macrophages results in overexpression of stimulatory cytokines that enhances B-cell proliferation and potentiates malignant transformation.[156]

Diagnosis

NHL may present as a rectal or colonic mass causing abdominal pain, bleeding or obstruction.[32] Radiographically, a nodule or nodules that may be ulcerated can be seen on a computed tomography scan. These may be quite large and show evidence of central necrosis. Endoscopically, submucosal masses may be noted, and these should undergo biopsy for tissue diagnosis. If tumors cannot be safely accessed or sampled for biopsy by means of endoscopy, percutaneous biopsy or surgery may be necessary in order to obtain a tissue diagnosis.

Treatment and Results

Chemotherapy is generally an effective treatment, with surgery reserved for bleeding, perforation, or obstruction.[121] One of the complications of chemotherapy, however, is perforation; fortunately, this is quite rare. Resection should be reserved for localized disease, and then only after an extensive search has been made for a disseminated process. A primary anastomosis may be safely performed in the absence of concomitant severe colitis.

In the past, survival was quite limited once the diagnosis of NHL was made, but with improvement in the treatment of HIV, especially with the introduction of HAART, as well as improvement in life expectancy in those with AIDS, patients with NHL are being treated more aggressively.[235,246] Results of the survival benefits of these regimens is awaited.

Kaposi's Sarcoma

Kaposi's sarcoma is usually an indolent cutaneous disorder in older men of central European origin, but the neoplasm is more aggressive in immunocompromised patients and resembles the more aggressive "endemic" form of Kaposi's sarcoma seen in sub-Saharan Africa.[49] The increased incidence of Kaposi's sarcoma early in the AIDS epidemic resulted in its becoming a specific diagnostic criterion for this condition in HIV-positive individuals. The recognition of an increased incidence of Kaposi's sarcoma in the homosexual population was made in the early 1980s.[90] This was identified as a much more aggressive form, with frequent metastatic spread to lymph nodes and the gastrointestinal tract.

Epidemiology, Etiology, and Pathogenesis

The incidence of Kaposi's sarcoma peaked at approximately 32 per 100,000 white men in the early 1990s, but since the advent of HAART, much like NHL, it has steadily declined to approximately 2.8 per 100,000 white men in 1998.[76] In fact, it has been noted that triple-antiretroviral therapy may decrease the incidence of Kaposi's sarcoma by 50% in HIV-infected homosexual men.[123] Kaposi's sarcoma is predominantly a disease of homosexual men with AIDS and is not commonly seen among other HIV exposure groups. This prompted the search for an infective cofactor as the etiologic agent. Initially, cytomegalovirus was implicated but could not be consistently identified by *in situ* hybridization probes.[4,71] Eventually, a herpes-like virus was identified as the cause of Kaposi's sarcoma,[41] and it has since been named Kaposi's sarcoma–associated herpes virus or human herpesvirus-8. The mode of transmission of human herpesvirus-8 is still not clear. However, a sexual mode of transmission has been hypothesized, because the incidence of Kaposi's sarcoma is related to the number of sexual partners in men who have sex with men.[22,174] Interestingly, heterosexual transmission is not common; in the endemic form of the disease in Africa, transmission via saliva is hypothesized.[194]

It is postulated that Kaposi's sarcoma lesions are fed by the massive cytokine levels that circulate in the HIV-infected patient.[77] Kaposi's sarcoma is more common in HIV-1 infection than in HIV-2 infection in patients with similar herpesvirus-8 infection rates, a finding raising the possibility that HIV-1 may have an etiologic role in Kaposi's sarcoma.[6] In an experimental animal model, Vogel and co-workers have demonstrated a role for HIV tat, which is an angiogenesis factor and induces secretion of inflammatory cytokines, in the development of Kaposi's sarcoma–like lesions in mice.[252] In addition, it appears that female sex hormones are inhibitory for Kaposi's sarcoma and may be used in treatment.[110]

Clinical Presentation

Kaposi's sarcoma lesions vary in their clinical presentations. The lesions range in color from light pink to purple and may appear as papules, plaques, and nodules. Although skin lesions are the most common, up to 50% of patients with AIDS with cutaneous lesions also have oral and gastrointestinal manifestations.[196,208] The gastrointestinal tract appears to be uniquely susceptible to dissemination by this tumor, and occasionally gastrointestinal lesions antedate skin changes.[258] The stomach, duodenum, small bowel, and colon may be affected simultaneously, or the tumor may be localized to one site.[112] Rectal involvement is quite common.[79]

Symptoms

Symptoms may include diarrhea, mucous discharge, bleeding, rectal pain, and incontinence, but patients are more often troubled with systemic problems related to opportunistic infections. The presence of characteristic raised, purple, nontender skin lesions, especially on the feet, should alert the physician to the diagnosis.

In view of the increased incidence in AIDS, a diagnosis of Kaposi's sarcoma should be considered in homosexual men presenting with persistent diarrhea for which no infectious cause can be ascertained.[258] Advanced gastrointestinal disease may present with both upper and lower gastrointestinal bleeding. Large lesions may result in acute obstruction, either directly or through intussusception of the affected bowel. Rectal lesions may be mistaken for thrombosed external hemorrhoids, given their purple, nodular appearance.

Endoscopy

The lesions appear submucosal, purple, spongy, and irregularly shaped.[233] When viewed endoscopically, they may vary in size from a few millimeters up to 2 cm.[49] There may be a resemblance to angiodysplasia, characterized by maculopapular tumors with a stellate vascular pattern.[264] In larger lesions, a central umbilication may develop in the ulcerated area.[198] Biopsy specimens can be taken if clinical management may be altered by the results. A deep biopsy is usually needed because of the location of the lesions. Because of the tendency to hemorrhage following rectal biopsy, Sohn recommends performing a rubber band ligation of the site and then sampling the more superficial portion.[233] However, attempts at biopsy confirmation may be frustrating because of the submucosal nature of the lesions and the sometimes firm consistency.[49,75] False-negative biopsy results are common, and rates of up to 77% have been reported.[89] Oral cavity and skin lesions are more accessible and are therefore preferred for biopsy.

Histopathology

When the biopsy is successful in obtaining histologic material, spindle-like cells with hemorrhage are frequently demonstrated (Figure 20-2).[198] Kaposi's sarcoma cells are thought to arise from the mesenchymal cells and are characterized by intense neovascularization with spindle cells.[165,262] Three features make up the histologic appearance of Kaposi's sarcoma: proliferation of vascular spaces, a background of spindle cells, and extravasation of red cells. Cytochemical and phenotypic marker studies have demonstrated Kaposi's sarcoma cells to have features of vascular channel and endothelial cell lineage.

Radiologic Studies

Contrast study may reveal changes in the stomach and duodenum suggestive of diffuse nodularity, multiple polypoid lesions, or the presence of an infiltrative mass. In the small bowel, thickening and irregularity of the folds may be noted. In the limited number of articles published to date, barium enema investigation sometimes reveals any one or more of the changes seen in the upper gastrointestinal tract.[88,255]

Computed tomography of the rectum reveals a high incidence of rectal and perirectal abnormalities, but the changes are nonspecific because many of these patients harbor other inflammatory conditions of the rectum.[3]

Identification of the site of massive bleeding by means of angiography has been demonstrated in a patient with ileal Kaposi's sarcoma.[172]

Treatment

"Aggressive" attempts at surgical management are not indicated except for the rare case of bleeding or obstruction.[149,151] Medically, antiretroviral therapy in the HAART era with immune reconstitution is essential to the management of Kaposi's sarcoma. Immune reconstitution may not only decrease active human herpesvirus-8 infection but may also decrease HIV viral load. Controlling HIV replication would decrease levels of the HIV tat protein and decrease the cytokine driven proliferation of the sarcoma. In addition, certain PIs have direct antineoplastic effects in Kaposi's sarcoma.[188,219]

Local therapies include intralesional injection with vinblastine or 3% sodium tetradecyl sulfate, interferon-alfa, and cryotherapy.[202,260] Cutaneous lesions have been irradiated successfully.[49] Gastrointestinal lesions, if symptomatic, necessitate systemic therapy. Chemotherapy includes recombinant human interferon-alfa, the vinca alkaloids, etoposide, and doxorubicin.[49,125,147,258] Interferon-alfa as a single agent has been found to have a 20% response rate.[253] High-dose interferon-alfa (8 million units daily, subcutaneously) plus the antiretroviral, zidovudine, resulted in a 31% response rate.[144] Systemic chemotherapy may be used for symptomatic gastrointestinal disease and rapidly progressive disease. It may have an indolent course or progress aggressively with significant mortality and morbidity. The single agents ap-

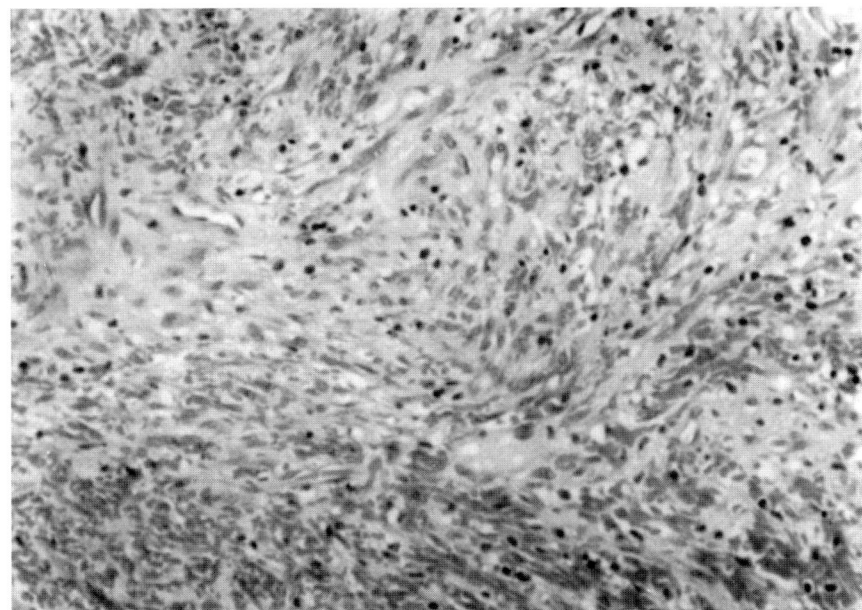

FIGURE 20-2. Kaposi's sarcoma. Spindle cell proliferation with slitlike vascular spaces. There are a few inflammatory cells, and endothelial cellular atypia is noted. Few extravasated red cells are seen. (Original magnification × 400.)

proved for use in Kaposi's sarcoma by the FDA are liposomal doxorubicin, liposomal daunorubicin, and paclitaxel.[254]

ANORECTAL DISEASE IN THE HIV-INFECTED PATIENT

A host of coexisting factors can make evaluation of the anorectum in the HIV-infected patient perplexing. The anorectum in the practicing homosexual is infected by a variety of pathogens, some living comfortably and clandestinely and some wreaking havoc. To this must be added the effects of HIV infection on the integrity of the mucosal cells (making them extremely friable), of anoreceptive intercourse on sphincter function, and of intermittent, indolent infections (herpes simplex) and routine anorectal diseases (fissures, fistulas). It is hoped that the following contribution will help the clinician to understand these varied, unusual processes.

Examination and Diagnosis: General Principles

Despite increased reliance on expensive laboratory evaluation, much can be ascertained by clinical examination in the HIV-positive patient. Visual inspection of the perineum may reveal condylomata, the blisters of herpes simplex, the linear lesions of a sacral root herpes zoster, the erythema of an ischiorectal abscess, or the excoriated anus of a patient with intractable diarrhea and a lax sphincter. Before performing a digital examination, it is important to manipulate the perianal tissue, to look for the discharge of pus or air bubbles that would suggest a deep infection. Spreading the buttocks gently can identify an anal fissure. Palpation of the anus and low rectum may demonstrate a mass or an ulcer. Careful attention should be paid to the prostate, because a patient with a prostatic abscess may present with vague, deep-seated rectal pain and fever, and the condition can be mistaken for an ischiorectal abscess. Rigid sigmoidoscopy will assess the rectal mucosa for evidence of proctitis. In any patient in whom evaluation is too painful, it is wise to proceed to an examination under anesthesia.

An examination under anesthesia should be performed before any definitive therapy is entertained, including sphincterotomy. A few caveats are helpful as well as cost-effective. Any exudate associated with a fistula or ulcer should be sent for acid-fast stain and culture. Rarely is useful information obtained from routine aerobic and anaerobic culture. Furthermore, *any exudate found in the anus or distal rectum without a demonstrable fistula should be cultured and stained for Neisseria gonorrhoeae, Chlamydia, amoebae, acid-*

fast bacilli, and herpes simplex virus (HSV). For inflammation extending proximal to 15 cm from the anal verge, cultures for all enteric pathogens, ova and parasites, and *C. difficile* should be requested and colonoscopy performed if preliminary results are nondiagnostic. Tissue from all ulcerative lesions that are shallow and not suggestive of an idiopathic AIDS-related ulcer should be sent for cytomegalovirus and HSV culture as well as for histopathology. A noncutting seton should be placed in all identified fistula tracts (Figure 20-3). Biopsy should be performed on any mass. Frozen-section examination generally does not alter immediate therapy and should, therefore, be used judiciously. One should not risk complications such as bleeding by obtaining large biopsy specimens for tissue typing in patients with NHL. It is safer to oversew biopsy sites in a patient with a friable mucosa with 2–0 long-term absorbable sutures. Thinner material may cut through with resultant bleeding. This adds to everyone's concerns, because postoperative hemor-

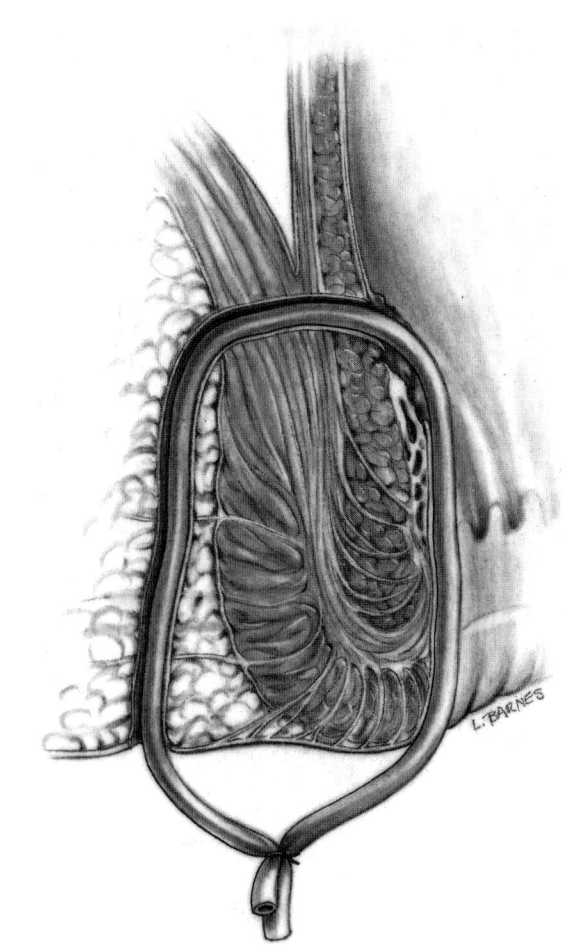

FIGURE 20-3. Noncutting seton placed for a high anal fistula in HIV-positive patients.

rhage poses a hazard for both patient and health care providers.

Nonsexually Transmitted Anal Disease

The anus of the HIV-infected patient may be affected by a number of conditions not necessarily related to HIV. This is important to note, because in addition to the reluctance of many physicians to treat HIV-positive patients, there is the natural tendency to ascribe all diseases in this population to specifically HIV-related problems.

Anal Fissure

The differentiation of an anal fissure from an idiopathic AIDS-related ulcer is critical to proper management. This is discussed later and also in Chapter 9. Anal fissures present with pain and bleeding, the same as in the general population. Chronic diarrhea and anoreceptive intercourse may contribute to the development of anal fissures and may delay their healing. Benign anal fissure should be initially managed conservatively with sitz baths and fiber supplements. Sources of chronic diarrhea are sought and appropriately treated. If conservative management fails, topical therapy with 0.2% nitroglycerin cream, 2% diltiazem, or botulinum toxin injection may be tried before surgical therapy (see Chapter 9).

Uncontrolled diarrhea is a relative contraindication to a definitive procedure, such as lateral internal anal sphincterotomy. Generally, however, the results of internal anal sphincterotomy are satisfactory.[206] However, if there is heightened concern about the possibility of impairment for bowel control, anorectal manometry can be performed to assess the anal canal pressure preoperatively and to determine whether the procedure can be undertaken with minimal morbidity.

Perianal Suppuration

Perianal abscess in the HIV-positive patient is analogous to the problem observed in an individual with Crohn's disease. One must distinguish between the standard cryptoglandular infection and that caused by erosion from ulcer or malignancy. Studies have shown that incision and drainage of abscesses can be successful, with salutary results.[261] Therefore, there is no place for nonoperative management in the presence of perianal suppuration.

A generous incision should be made, but the wound should not be packed. If a fistula is found, a noncutting seton should be placed (Figure 20-3). Any purulent material should be sent for acid-fast stain and for culture. Untreated perianal sepsis may progress to necrotizing gangrene (see Chapter 19) or can lead to disseminated abscesses.[51]

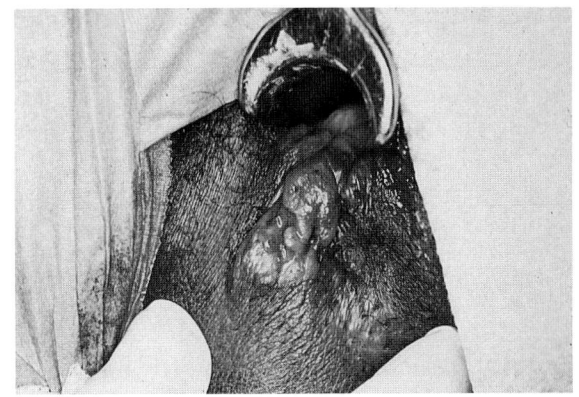

FIGURE 20-4. Fistula caused by *Mycobacterium avium* complex that spontaneously healed. (See Color Fig. 20-4.)

Fistula-in-Ano

Generally, any anal fistula should be treated conservatively, without performing a definitive operation. As previously mentioned, diarrhea can lead to disabling incontinence in many of the patients with attenuated sphincters. A fistulotomy may be considered only when the tract is superficial. High fistulas can be managed with seton drainage, changed or removed if necessary (see also Chapter 11). Spontaneous healing can occur, but this is unpredictable and may be related to the response to treatment of an underlying specific infection (Figure 20-4).

Hemorrhoids

The frequency of hemorrhoidal symptoms does not appear to be increased in HIV-infected patients. In fact, the physician needs to be aware that many so-called exacerbations of hemorrhoidal disease are in reality acute HSV infections.

External thrombosed hemorrhoids may be safely excised, with similar indications for surgery as in the HIV-negative patient. Rubber band ligation of symptomatic hemorrhoids has been reported to result in a higher complication rate.[212] However, we have not found this to be true in our practice and offer it to appropriate patients as a therapeutic option. Although hemorrhoidectomy has been reported to be safe in HIV-positive individuals,[113] only one third actually underwent a full hemorrhoidectomy. It is our practice to offer surgical hemorrhoidectomy to the patient with symptomatic grade III hemorrhoids if the HIV disease is early in its course. However, it is extremely difficult to treat grades III and IV hemorrhoids in advanced AIDS. The accompanying diarrhea aggravates hemorrhoidal prolapse and is a significant source of morbidity.

Pruritus Ani

Severe pruritus occurs secondary to leakage of pus, fecal incontinence, and fungal overgrowth. This is readily treated by antifungal powders and the avoidance of sensitizing over-the-counter preparations (see Chapter 19). If possible, the source of the excessive moisture should be eliminated. Persistence of pruritus despite therapy should lead one to consider biopsy to rule out Bowen's disease and other specific perianal conditions (see Chapter 19).

Sexually Transmitted Disease in the HIV-Infected Population

Gonorrhea

Gonorrhea is caused by *Neisseria gonorrhoea* and is considered to be the most common sexually transmitted disease in homosexual men. Historically, carrier rates have been reported in up to 55% of homosexual men.[124] Although the incidence of gonorrhea initially declined with the advent of safe-sex practices, more recently the incidence has been reported to be increasing (see also Chapter 19).[222,247] The gonorrheal organism is thought to be a cofactor in the transmission of HIV.[57]

Presentation and Diagnosis

The classic clinical presentation of rectal gonorrhea is that of a thick, yellow mucopurulent discharge, with or without proctitis, occurring 5 days after inoculation. In addition to mucoid rectal discharge, patients may present with tenesmus, pruritus, or rectal bleeding. Evaluation of the anorectum reveals friable, erythematous rectal mucosa with mucopurulent exudates. Mucopurulent discharge may be noted from the anal crypts or may be elicited by gentle external pressure. Diagnosis is confirmed by the presence of gram-negative intracellular diplococci on culture of rectal swabs on Thayer-Martin medium. At the time of diagnosis, patients should also be screened for syphilis.

Treatment

Rectal gonorrhea has been reported to be more resistant to therapy because of the antibiotic inactivation attributed to the microflora of the rectum.[85] Empiric treatment is initiated with a single dose of ceftriaxone, 125 mg intramuscularly, while awaiting culture results. Alternative regimens are ciprofloxacin, 500 mg orally, or levofloxacin, 500 mg orally, in a single dose. Because of the high coinfection rate with *Chlamydia trachomatis*, current recommendations are to treat with a regimen effective against uncomplicated chlamydial infection.[274]

If left untreated, gonorrhea may progress to disseminated gonococcal infection. Disseminated infection results in petechial skin lesions, septic arthritis, and tenosynovitis. Less commonly, it may manifest as fulminant perihepatitis, meningitis, or endocarditis. Hospitalization with intravenous antibiotics is recommended for disseminated gonococcal infection. Endocarditis requires 4 weeks of therapy. The reader is referred to Chapters 19 and 33 for a more comprehensive discussion of this infection.

Chlamydia Infection and Lymphogranuloma Venereum

C. trachomatis is the most common sexually transmitted infectious pathogen in the United States. Anal chlamydial infection is transmitted by anal receptive intercourse and oral-anal intercourse. After a 10-day incubation period, symptomatic chlamydial infection may occur, although the large number of asymptomatic infections explains the high prevalence among sexually active individuals. Depending on the serotype, the infection may present as mild proctitis or may progress to lymphogranuloma venereum. Ten days after inoculation, non–lymphogranuloma venereum proctitis presents with pain, tenesmus, fever, and nonulcerative proctitis, with a bloody or mucoid discharge. Upon proctoscopy, the rectal mucosa appears erythematous, friable, and granular. When lymphogranuloma venereum develops, ulceration, abscesses, and strictures mimicking Crohn's disease occur. However, whereas lymphadenopathy is present in lymphogranuloma venereum, it is absent with Crohn's disease. Once a stricture develops, fecal diversion is the preferred option.

Diagnosis is most reliably made with culture of a rectal biopsy. Unfortunately, the biopsy needs to be transported on ice for tissue culture, thus making it expensive and time-consuming. Antichlamydial antibodies can be assayed with a complement fixation test. A titer of 1:80 or greater is confirmatory of chlamydial infection. Elevated titers are not seen, however, less than 1 month after infection. A newly developed urinary polymerase chain reaction test for chlamydia may allow for more rapid confirmation.[155]

Chlamydial infection is treated with a single dose of azithromycin, 1 g orally, or doxycycline, 100 mg orally, twice a day for 7 days. As mentioned in the section on gonorrhea, treatment for concurrent gonorrhea infection is recommended. Further details concerning epidemiology, symptoms, and treatment are found in Chapter 19.

Syphilis

Anal syphilis, caused by *Treponema pallidum*, is a condition that develops 2 to 6 weeks following inoculation. The primary lesion of syphilis is the chancre, a rounded ulcer with well-defined margins that may be mistaken for an anal fissure. Although typically painless at other sites, anal chancres may result in severe anal pain. The ulcerative lesions may be single (most common) or multiple. When multiple and situated opposite one another, the pathognomic "kissing" ulcers may be observed. Additionally, one may find mild proctitis. Even without treatment, the primary chancre of syphilis heals within 3 to 6 weeks.

The disease progresses in approximately one third of patients, and in one third it remains latent. When it progresses, the second stage usually is recognized 2 months following resolution of the chancre. The presentation at this time is that of verrucous, flat lesions (condylomata lata) that are associated with pruritus and discharge, a maculopapular rash on the soles of the feet and the palms of the hand, fever, and malaise.

Diagnosis is made by dark-field immunofluorescent microscopy and nontreponemal serology testing, that is, the Venereal Disease Research Laboratory (VDRL) assay. Although the classic treatment consists of intramuscular benzathine penicillin, complicating factors in the HIV-positive population include the high incidence of neurosyphilis and the lack of a predictable serologic response to treatment.[26,276] This translates into either doing a spinal tap at the time of diagnosis or empirically treating all patients for neurosyphilis. Following treatment, patients should undergo quantitative serologic testing at 3-month intervals for 1 year in order to document falling titers and to aid in identifying treatment failures. The reader is referred to Chapter 19 for an additional discussion.

Herpes Simplex

HSV is a large DNA virus transmitted by anal intercourse (HSV type II, accounting for 90% of anal herpes) and oral-anal contact (HSV type I, accounting for 10% of anal herpes).[53,265] HSV infection is important not only because of its high incidence, but also because the associated break in the epithelial integrity of the skin probably facilitates the transmission of HIV.[102,224] The incubation period for HSV type II infections is 4 to 21 days. Initially, small vesicles with associated perivesicular erythema develop that may then coalesce to form larger ulcers within the anal canal and distal rectum and on the perianal skin. The disease is usually self-limiting, and ulcers heal after 2 weeks. In severely immunocompromised individuals, the disease may persist. Persistence of herpetic vesicles and ulcers beyond 1 month is an AIDS-defining condition (Figure 20-5).

Clinically, patients typically complain of exquisite anorectal pain, which is exacerbated by defecation and anoreceptive intercourse, pruritus, and tenesmus. The initial infection may be accompanied by systemic signs, including fever, general malaise, and inguinal lymphadenopathy.[96] Following resolution of the initial infection, the virus remains latent in the sacral root ganglia with frequent reactivations. Upon reactivation, in addition to anorectal ulcerations, it can cause root symptoms along the affected dermatomes, leading to urinary dysfunction, paresthesias, constipation, and impotence.

Both tissue culture and biopsy specimens for histopathology are recommended, rather than the use of simple swabs. Biopsies of ulcer beds reveal the typical multinucleated giant cells or intranuclear inclusions bodies as seen in Figure 20-6. Tissue should be sent for cell culture to isolate

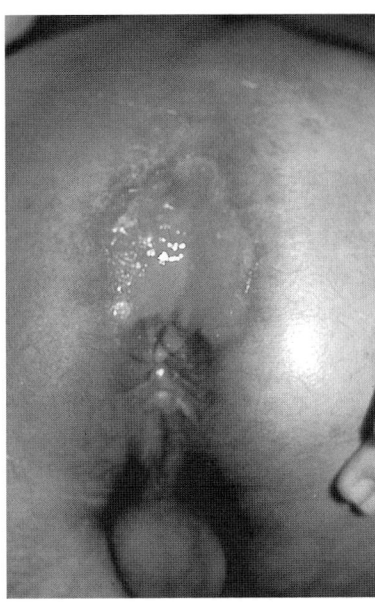

FIGURE 20-5. Severe erosive perianal herpes simplex. (See Color Fig. 20-5.)

HSV. However, sensitivity declines after healing of lesions starts. Therefore, empiric treatment with antiviral therapy should be undertaken before results of biopsy are obtained. Acyclovir promotes healing of lesions and decreases the duration of anorectal pain.[205] The dosage of acylclovir used for herpetic proctitis (400 to 800 mg five times per day for 7 days) is higher than the recommended regimen for genital herpes. However, no studies have documented a clear advantage to the higher dosage. Alternative drugs for the acute treatment of herpes are valacyclovir (1000 mg twice/day) and famciclovir (500 mg twice/day). Both have been shown to have comparable efficacy to acyclovir in the treatment of anogenital herpes in HIV-infected patients.[48,204] The twice-daily dosing regimens of valacyclovir and famciclovir offer the added advantage of a reduced medication burden. Supportive care, including sitz baths and topical anesthetic agents, help to minimize pain during the active infection. Those who are acyclovir resistant (thymidine kinase–deficient HSV-2 mutants) usually respond well to foscarnet (Foscavir).[7,207] Suppressive therapy with antivirals reduces the frequency of herpetic recurrences with no cumulative toxicity. They should be considered in patients with frequent recurrence or in severely immunocompromised patients because the severity and frequency of recurrences vary inversely with the CD4 count.[7,42,161] The daily suppressive dose of acyclovir is 400 mg twice daily. Topical acyclovir, however, has little utility in the HIV-positive patient. Valacyclovir, at a dose of 500 mg, twice a day, has been shown to have comparable efficacy to that of acyclovir as suppressive therapy in patients with CD4 T-cell counts greater than 200 cells/mm^3.[48] Patients with severe disease or with evidence of disseminated disease (i.e., pneumonitis, meningitis, or hepatitis) should

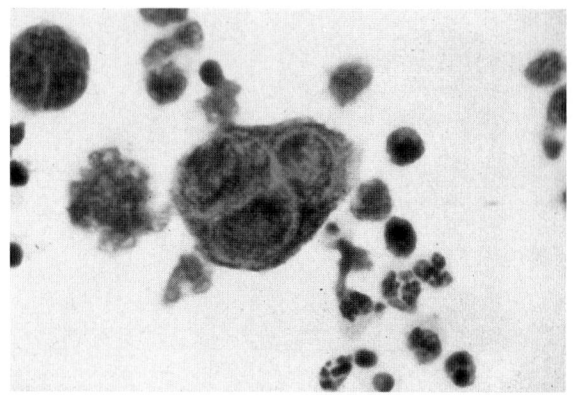

FIGURE 20-6. Characteristic multinucleated giant cell of herpes simplex virus infection. (See Color Fig. 20-6.)

be hospitalized and treated with intravenous acyclovir therapy at a dose 5 to –10 mg/kg body weight, every 8 hours, until clinical improvement is noted.[274]

Herpes genitalis is also discussed in Chapter 19, and herpes simplex proctitis is discussed in Chapter 33.

Cytomegalovirus Infection

Cytomegalovirus has been implicated in causing anorectal ulceration.[117] Because cytomegalovirus is ubiquitous in the AIDS population, it may actually be a nonpathogenic bystander or secondary pathogen rather than a primary cause of disease. In addition, it has a predilection for endothelial cells found in the granulation tissue of many inflammatory anal conditions.

It has been suggested that a diagnosis of cytomegalovirus infection can be made by an "erosive or ulcerative process in the wall of the gut in which the presence of cytomegalovirus is shown by routine histological examination, culture, or antigen or DNA staining, and in a person in whom other explanations for the lesion(s) have been excluded."[98]

Opinion

Our skepticism in implicating cytomegalovirus in anal disease arises from the lack of ability to retrieve cytomegalovirus from anal lesions and the lack of predictable response to therapy from lesions in which cytomegalovirus has been identified. It is our opinion that cytomegalovirus plays very little role in anal disease in HIV-infected patients.

Anal Condylomata Acuminata

Etiology and Pathogenesis

Condylomata are caused by HPV, a sexually transmitted virus. HPV is a double-stranded DNA virus. More than 80 subtypes have been identified, with subtypes 6 and 11

responsible for most anal condylomata acuminata.[240] Certain subtypes, notably 16, 18, and perhaps 31, 33, 45, and 46, have a greater oncogenic potential. HPV typically causes infection by direct inoculation, infecting basal keratinocytes, but anoreceptive intercourse is not required for anal infection. Viral replication occurs in basal keratinocytes, and the viral genome is carried to upper layers of the epithelium. As the virus propagates upward through the layers of the epithelium, the characteristic lesions are seen.

Anogenital HPV infection is more common in HIV-infected patients, and among HIV-positive men, it is more common in the homosexual population.[28,134] In one study, the prevalence of anal HPV infection in HIV-positive homosexual men was found to be 85%, compared with 46% in HIV-positive heterosexual men with no history of anal receptive sex.[192] The prevalence of this virus is probably a confounding factor in a variety of pathologic conditions affecting the anorectum in the HIV-positive patient.[16] Shedding of HPV, extent of disease, and recurrence of anal condylomata all increase as CD4 T-cell counts decrease.[45,181]

Malignant transformation is believed to be secondary to integration of the HPV DNA into the host genome. The integration of the viral DNA results in loss of the regulatory viral genes *E1* and *E2* and leads to overexpression of the *E6* and *E7* viral genes. The *E6* gene binds to the tumor suppressor protein p53, resulting in its degradation. *E7* binds to pRB, a cellular protein that normally inhibits transcriptional activity. Together, the result is increased DNA synthesis and decreased DNA repair of the host cell producing in malignant transformation.[73,210,242,265] HIV may be a cofactor in *E6* and *E7* gene expression.[30]

Presentation

Clinically, patients with anal warts may present with only a complaint of perianal lesions, or they may complain of perianal discomfort, itching, bleeding, or discharge. On examination, anal warts are easily identified by their white or pigmented, exophytic, hyperkeratotic appearance (see Chapter 19). Acetic acid may be used to help illuminate the warts in order to aid in their identification, particularly small warts or the less common flat warts. Microscopic changes show characteristic orderly papillomatosis, poikilocytosis, and hyperkeratosis (Figure 20-7).

Anal Intraepithelial Neoplasia

As previously noted, HPV infection is more common in HIV-infected individuals. Infection with multiple subtypes of HPV and more extensive disease are seen in HIV-positive patients. The incidence of anal cancer is higher in HIV-infected individuals, with a relative risk of 6.8 in women and 37.9 in men.[91] Sobhani and co-workers examined the prevalence of anal dysplasia and anal cancer with respect to HIV status, CD4 T-cell counts, and HPV. They found HIV positivity, HIV viral loads (but not CD4 counts), and condyloma relapse to be risk factors for high-grade dysplasia and

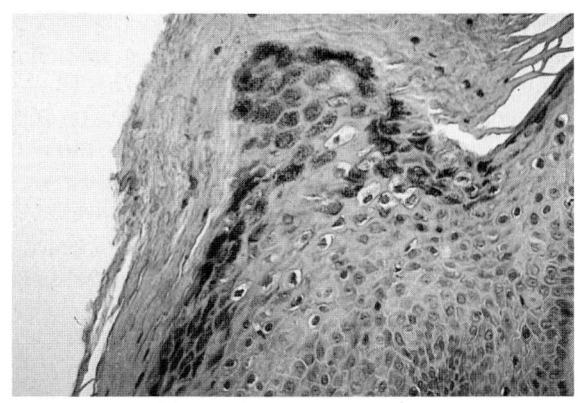

FIGURE 20-7. Histopathology of anal condyloma acuminatum, showing orderly papillomatosis, poikilocytosis, and hyperkeratinization. (See Color Fig. 20-7.)

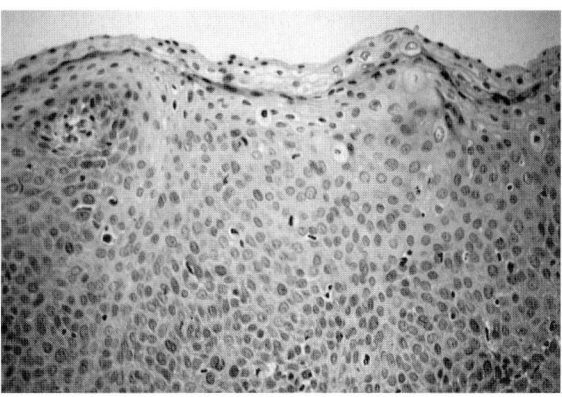

FIGURE 20-8. Histopathology of a flat lesion showing anal intraepithelial neoplasia (AIN III) with severe dysplasia. (See Color Fig. 20-8.)

invasive carcinoma. Of note, the same study found decreased local immunity, as measured by Langerhans' cells in the anal mucosa, and increased prevalence of oncogenic HPV subtypes in HIV-positive patients.[231] A prospective study examining HPV as a risk factor for anal and perianal skin cancer found an increased risk in patients seropositive for IgG antibodies to HPV-16 and HPV-18.[21] It should be noted that anal HPV infection and anal intraepithelial neoplasia (AIN) can be observed in HIV-positive patients in the absence of prior anal intercourse.[192]

The association among HPV infection, HIV-positivity, AIN and the possible progression of these dysplastic lesions to invasive anal carcinoma have stimulated a great deal of debate on screening and management in the HIV-positive patient. Initially, a similarity was found between AIN and cervical intraepithelial neoplasia, a precursor to cervical cancer (Figure 20-8).[11] The finding of AIN in routine scrapings from the anus of HIV-positive male patients, in addition to an increase in both prevalence and progression of cytologic changes, engendered fear of a potential epidemic of anal cancer.[182,183] It appears that in HIV-infected men, HPV infection may occur with clinically normal but histologically abnormal epithelium.[239] Progression to AIN appears to be directly related to the level of immunosuppression rather than to the specific subtype of HPV retrieved, although more recent reports examining the effect of HAART on the severity of AIN have not shown any benefit.[59,162,256] In a study examining the natural history of AIN following initiation of HAART in 200 patients, rates of progression or regression of AIN remained unchanged in the first 6 months after HAART use was started, even though there was an increase in the CD4 T-cell counts of treated patients.[179] Because the benefits of HAART do not appear to extend to AIN and do not affect progression of low-grade lesions to high-grade lesions, the question of screening and treatment of subclinical lesions in the HIV-infected patient has been raised.

Presumably, as life expectancy of these patients is improved, rates of progression to invasive squamous carcinoma will increase. Adding further to the confusion is the observation of infection with multiple concurrent subtypes, variability of retrieval of HPV by different methods utilized, and overall higher retrieval rate of oncogenic HPV subtypes in the immunosuppressed patient.[29,225,227]

Palefsky and co-workers have proposed an AIN screening protocol in which anal cytologic examination is performed in a fashion similar to the Papanicolaou's smear for cervical cytology with a water-moistened Dacron swab of the anal canal. In their protocol, all patients with abnormal cytology are then referred for high-resolution anoscopy, which may be added by acetic acid illumination of abnormal tissue and biopsy of all visualized lesions.[180] Although no studies have clearly documented progression to anal invasive squamous cell carcinoma, and, in fact, two small reports failed to demonstrate progression of AIN to squamous cell cancer, ablative therapy for treatment of AIN has been proposed.[44,83,87,173] Chin-Hong and Palefsky recommend treating lesions smaller than 1 cm² with local topical therapy and treating larger lesions with surgery, although for very large and/or circumferential disease, they recommend no treatment, because of the high morbidity of the extensive surgical procedure involved.[44] Given that progression rates to invasive cancer remain unknown as well as the high rates of persistent or recurrent AIN following surgical treatment (23 of 29 patients in one study), one may be legitimately concerned that vigorous screening for subclinical lesions will lead to unnecessarily debilitating surgery.[40]

Principles of Management

Anal warts should be destroyed, with follow-up every 2 months. Topical treatments that are available include podophyllin, bichloroacetic acid, and imiquimod. Podophyllin is cytotoxic to warts provided it is applied directly to the external component. However, its use is limited by its local toxicity. The success rate with podophyllin is problematic. In a study comparing surgical therapy versus podophyllin, the recurrence rate at 42 weeks was 68% for podophyllin versus 28% in the surgery group.[132] Bichloroacetic acid, a caustic agent, is similarly limited in its utility because of the poor response and high recurrence rate. Imiquimod is a newer agent that was approved for use in 1997. Application of imiquimod results in a local release of cytokines, including interferon.[244] Although it does have efficacy against anal warts, it does not appear to be effective as monotherapy in our experience.[101] However, in our practice, we have found imiquimod effective as adjunctive therapy in select patients following cytodestruction.

Because of the poor response and high recurrence rates following topical therapy, our preferred alternative is cytodestruction (electrocautery) after acetic acid staining (Figure 20-9). In patients with aggressive disease, topical imiquimod as an adjunct is used. This technique combines the antiproliferative and antiviral properties of imiquimod with cytodestruction to maximize eradication of both clinical and subclinical disease. It is our belief that aggressive treatment of clinical lesions should be performed in all patients with good performance status. Larger flat lesions should be excised. Noninvasive flat lesions that are determined to be carcinoma-*in-situ* with negative margins do not require additional therapy.[168] *HPV subtyping* should be reserved for research protocols only, because it is expensive and really does not affect treatment. We also believe that *anal cytology* has no value other than in research protocols. Furthermore, ablative prophylactic therapy for AIN is not indicated. These patients should be observed at 3-month intervals. Biopsy specimens can safely be taken from any suspected lesions, which can be treated as they become apparent.

Although various methods have been described for treating anal condyloma acuminata, high recurrence rates remain a problem. However, decreased relapse rates in HIV-positive patients with improved management of their underlying HIV infection with HAART have been reported.[177]

Research has focused on the development of both prophylactic and therapeutic HPV vaccines. Prophylactic vaccines are based on the viral capsid protein L1. Preliminary results at 17 months from a controlled trial of a prophylactic vaccine against HPV-16 virus–like particles created from self-assembly of the HPV-16 capsid protein have been favorable.[142] Women in the study were randomly assigned to receive three doses of either HPV-16 virus–like particle vaccine or placebo at day 0, month 2, and month 6. Genital samples for HPV-16 DNA were obtained at enrollment, 1 month after the last vaccination, and at 6-month intervals. The primary end point was defined as persistent HPV infection. Forty-one cases of persistent HPV-16 infection occurred in the placebo group and none in the vaccinated group. Of these women, nine had HPV-16–associated cervical intraepithelial neoplasia. An additional 33 were transiently positive for HPV-16 DNA at a

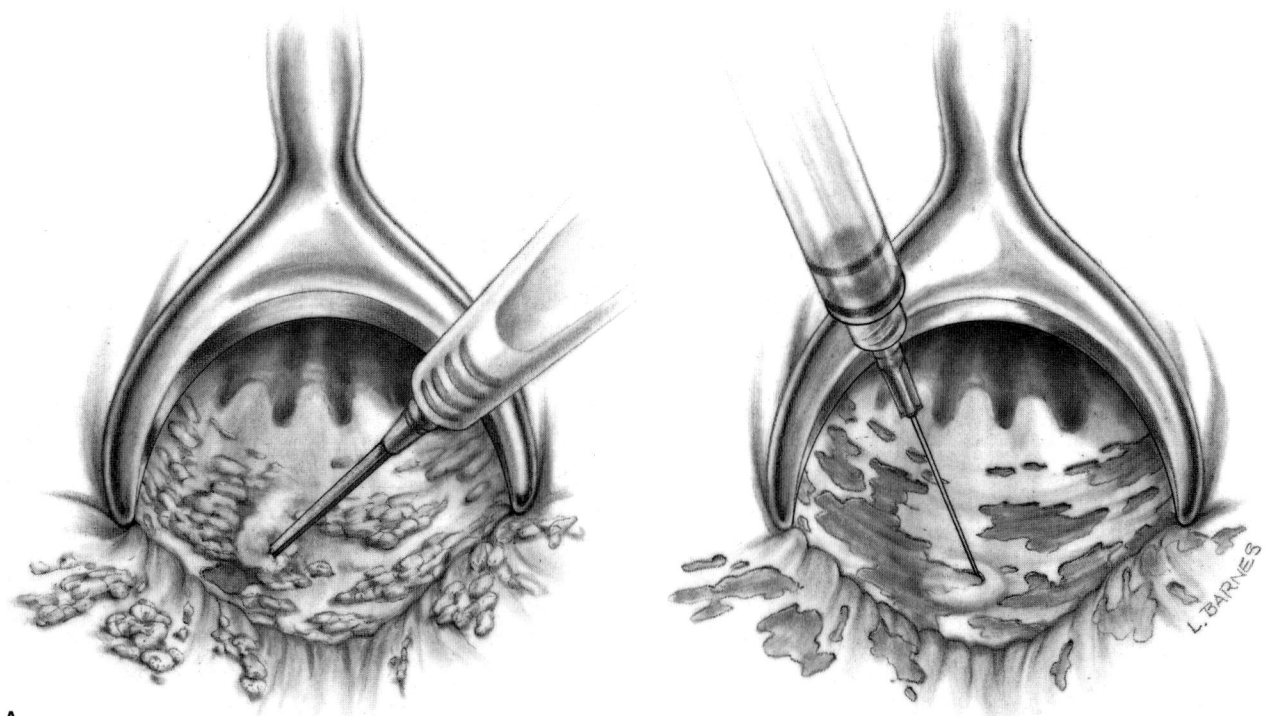

A

B

FIGURE 20-9. Fulguration after acetic acid staining of anal condyloma acuminatum.

single visit, six of whom were vaccine recipients. These preliminary results support the contention that the vaccine may prevent persistent infection by reducing viral load rather than by providing a sterilizing immunity. Clinically, a longer follow-up is necessary before the efficacy of a prophylactic vaccine can be evaluated. Furthermore, multivalent vaccines with efficacy against a range of HPV subtypes will need to be developed.

Therapeutic vaccines to eradicate infected cells are being investigated as potential treatments for HPV intraepithelial neoplasia and invasive cancer. As mentioned earlier, the HPV proteins, E6 and E7, are overexpressed in cells undergoing malignant transformation. Therefore, therapeutic vaccines have largely been based on these oncoproteins and the establishment of a cytotoxic T-cell response to cells expressing the E6 and E7 proteins. A vaccine developed from fusing the HPV-16 E7 protein to the bacille Calmette-Guérin heat-shock protein 65 was tested in patients with persistent high-grade squamous intraepithelial lesions in an open-label trial. Goldstone and co-workers reported complete resolution of warts in three of 14 patients at baseline, at week 24 following vaccination, and a 70% to 95% reduction in warts in ten of the 14 patients.[95] At 15 months, 95% of men with high-grade anal dysplasia showed at least a reduction in pathologic staging to low-grade anal dyspla-

sia, and 44% demonstrated a complete pathologic response.[178] Other therapeutic vaccines, including a HPV6 L2/E7 fusion protein, have shown similar effects in reducing or eradicating warts and are being tested for their efficacy in the treatment of high-grade dysplasia.[146] Although still in trials, the development of prophylactic and therapeutic vaccines will, we hope, allow for the gradual eradication of anogenital warts (see also Chapter 19).

AIDS-Specific Disease

The most debilitating lesions seen in the anorectum of patients with AIDS are idiopathic AIDS-related ulcers. These occur in advanced disease, usually when the CD4 T-cell counts fall to less than 200 cells/μL. Although no study has examined the effect of immune reconstitution on the natural history of idiopathic AIDS-related ulcers, the incidence of these anal ulcers in the era of HAART has predictably decreased. Their characteristic appearance is one of an extremely erosive and ulcerative process that occurs more proximally than do benign anal fissures, undermines what appears to be normal mucosa, and traverses normal tissue planes (Figs. 20-10 through 20-13).[251] Whereas benign fissures are associated with hypertonia, idiopathic HIV-associated anal ulcers typi-

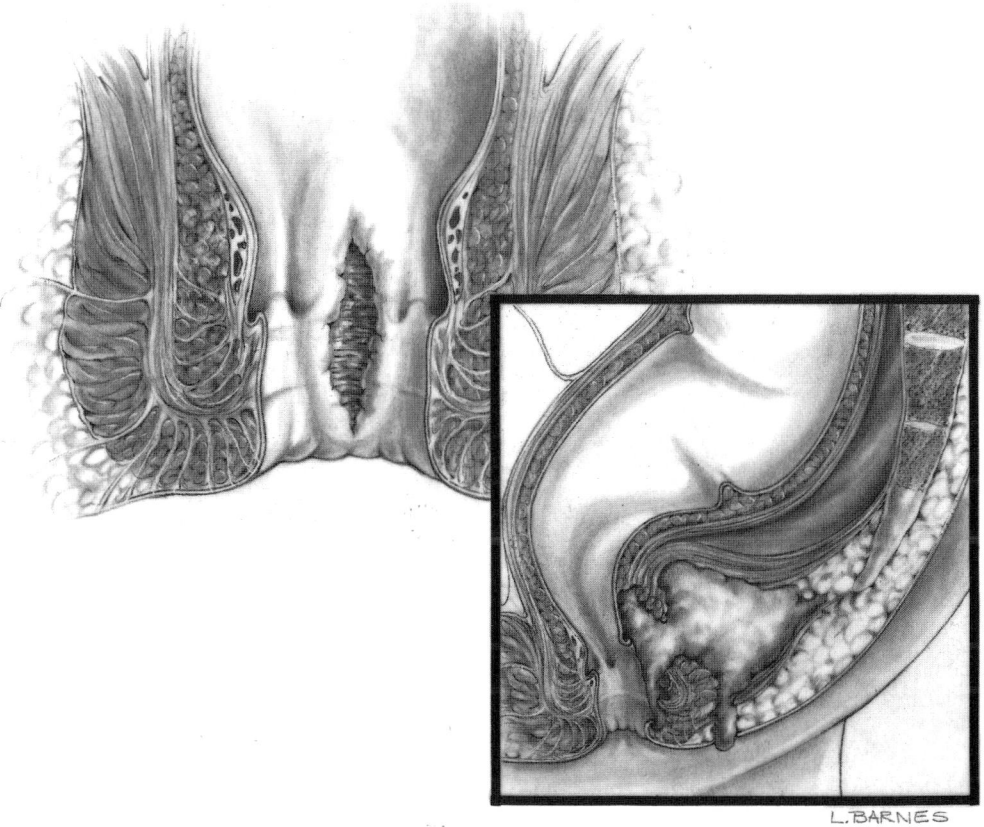

FIGURE 20-10. AIDS-related ulcer showing erosion in submucosal planes with destruction of the intersphincteric plane and formation of a deep postanal space collection *(inset)*. The "bottleneck" causes a sensation of pressure.

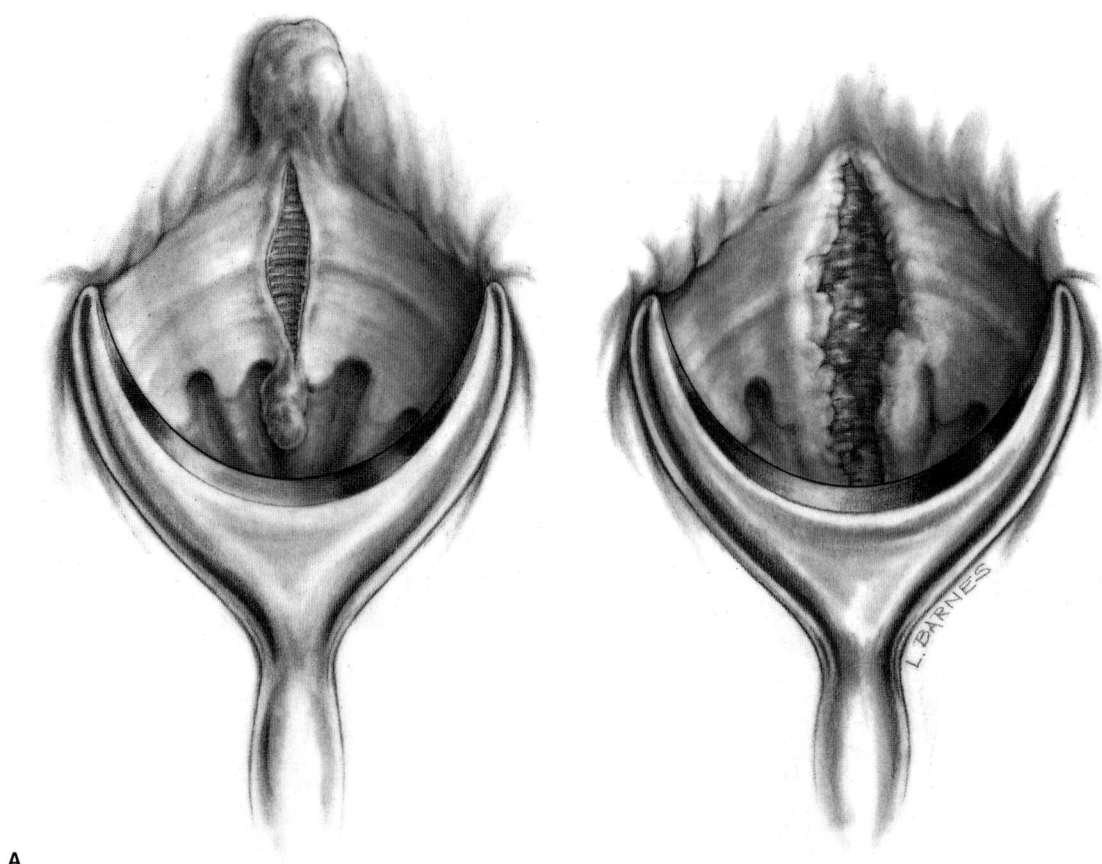

A   B

FIGURE 20-11. Anal ulcers. Artist's conception of the clinical appearances differentiating between a so-called benign lesion (**A**) and an idiopathic AIDS-related ulcer (**B**).

cally are associated with hypotonia of the anal sphincter. Symptoms include a sensation of pressure caused by pocketing of stool, pus, and vegetable matter and severe pain that is worse on defecation.

An aggressive workup for the cause of idiopathic AIDS-related ulcers is usually a fruitless exercise except,

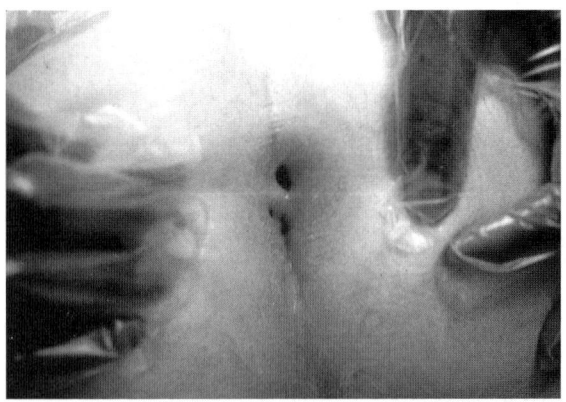

FIGURE 20-12. Erosion of an idiopathic AIDS-related ulcer into the deep postanal space, exiting into the perianal skin. (See Color Fig. 20-12.)

of course, for an underlying malignancy.[151,213] Neither HSV nor cytomegalovirus is considered a causative agent, so therapy against retrieved pathogens is futile. In our experience, one half of these patients harbor oncogenic HPV in adjacent mucosa.[186] This may be purely coincidental or may suggest HPV-induced initiation of a cytodestructive cytokine cascade.[159]

Treatment consists of operative debridement to eliminate the pocketing effect and injection of a depot steroid preparation into the base and sides of the ulcers (Figs. 20-14 and 20-15). As we have reported, this protocol has produced uniformly satisfying results.[251] It is thought that the steroids may downregulate cytokine reduction in aphthous ulceration in the same way as a model seen in the esophagus.[141] Another agent, thalidomide, has been used anecdotally in both anal and oral aphthous ulceration.[187] Its presumed mechanism of action is also downregulation of cytokine production. Some authors have advocated operative debridement and a rectal mucosal advancement flap and have reported favorable results.[50] In patients with severe pain in whom anal procedures have failed, fecal diversion may be considered. Laparoscopic stoma creation has been reported to have the benefit of improved postoperative recovery and decreased

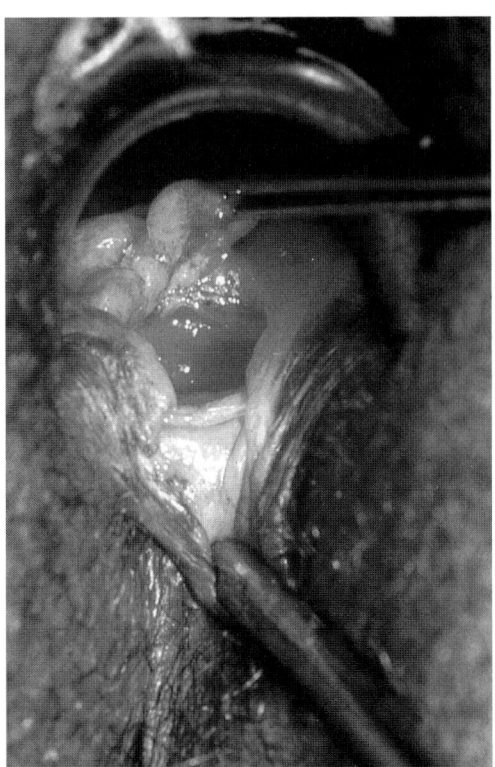

FIGURE 20-13. Idiopathic AIDS-related ulcer showing dissection in the submucosal and intersphincteric plane. (See Color Fig. 20-13.)

compromise of immune function when compared with laparotomy.[175]

Anorectal Malignancy

As stated previously, the anorectum may be the initiating site for NHL (Figure 20-16). It may present as either a mass or a fissure; biopsy is diagnostic. Because chemotherapy is so effective, a diverting stoma is now rarely utilized in the management of NHL. With respect to Kaposi's sarcoma, this is usually an incidental finding and rarely causes significant anorectal symptoms.[151]

The greatest controversy in the AIDS-infected individual concerns the management of squamous cell carcinoma (Figure 20-17). The incidence of this tumor in the homosexual population has been rising, and with the onset of HIV, incidence rates have further increased.[157,271] Combined-modality therapy replaced abdominoperineal resection in the 1980s and remains the standard of care (see Chapter 24).[61] Combined-modality therapy is often difficult for the patient and is associated with a high morbidity. Acutely, adverse effects of radiation therapy include desquamation of the perineal region, diarrhea, and severe anal pain. Anal stenosis and ulcers are late manifestations of radiation toxicity. Toxic effects of chemo-

therapy include exacerbation of chronic diarrhea, weight loss (in an already nutritionally challenged patient), and bone marrow suppression. Several small series, including our unpublished experience, have documented the inability of patients with advanced HIV disease or coincidental diarrhea to complete the protocol without intolerable consequences.[27,38,111,116] More recently, two studies examining toxicity of combined-modality therapy in HIV-positive patients found very high rates of toxicity. Hoffman and co-workers reported an 82% incidence of grade 3 or 4 toxicity in HIV-positive patients, with 50% requiring a colostomy for control of symptoms in those with CD4 T-cell counts lower than 200.[115] Kim and co-workers similarly found higher rates of acute toxicity in HIV-positive patients when compared with HIV-negative patients (80% versus 30%). Late toxic effects of combined-modality therapy were likewise increased (38% versus 15%).[133] In an attempt to limit the toxicity of therapy, the dose of radiation therapy was lowered to 30 Gy in one small study, with no impact on local control.[190] The impact of HAART on the toxicity profile of combined-modality therapy has not been studied in large studies. However, a report on 12 patients, nine of whom were receiving HAART, indicates no significant difference in the toxicity rates.[47]

The outcome of combined-modality therapy in anal squamous cell cancers in HIV-positive patients has also been examined. In a retrospective study, poor local control and persistent disease were noted in more than 50% of patients with invasive cancer.[193] In the study by Kim and co-workers, only 62% of HIV-positive patients had a complete response to combined-modality therapy as compared with 85% of HIV-negative patients.[133] In our own unpublished experience, we have noted a similar increase in the toxicity profile of combined-modality therapy, necessitating more treatment breaks, and a decrease in local control in HIV-positive patients, particularly in patients with advanced disease. Larger, multicenter trials are needed to assess the impact of HAART and CD4 T-cell counts on the treatment of invasive anal squamous cell carcinoma by combined-modality therapy and the role of surgical resection in patients with advanced AIDS.

PROTECTION OF THE SURGEON

Seroconversion to an HIV-positive state following percutaneous exposure with a hypodermic needle (0.3%) and mucous membrane exposure (0.09%) has been documented. However, there have been no reported seroconversions after being stuck with a suture needle.[245] This is thought to be a consequence of the fact that the needle is solid. Furthermore, there have been no seroconversions following exposure when the skin is intact. The quantifi-

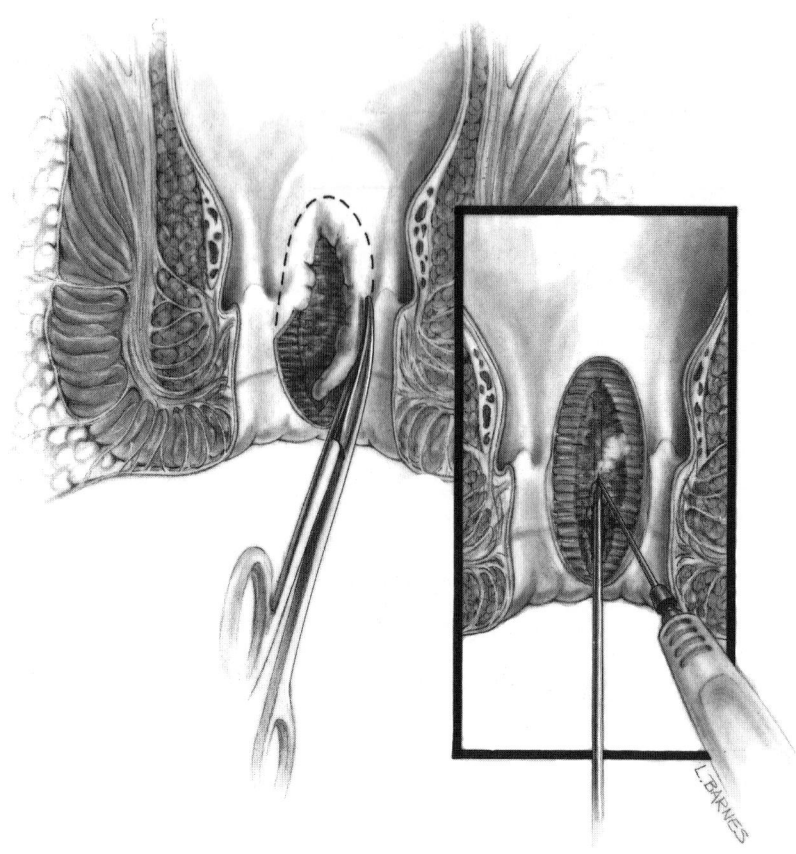

FIGURE 20-14. Treatment of an AIDS-related ulcer by debridement of the mucosal overhanging edges and incision of the internal anal sphincter to allow better drainage **(inset)**.

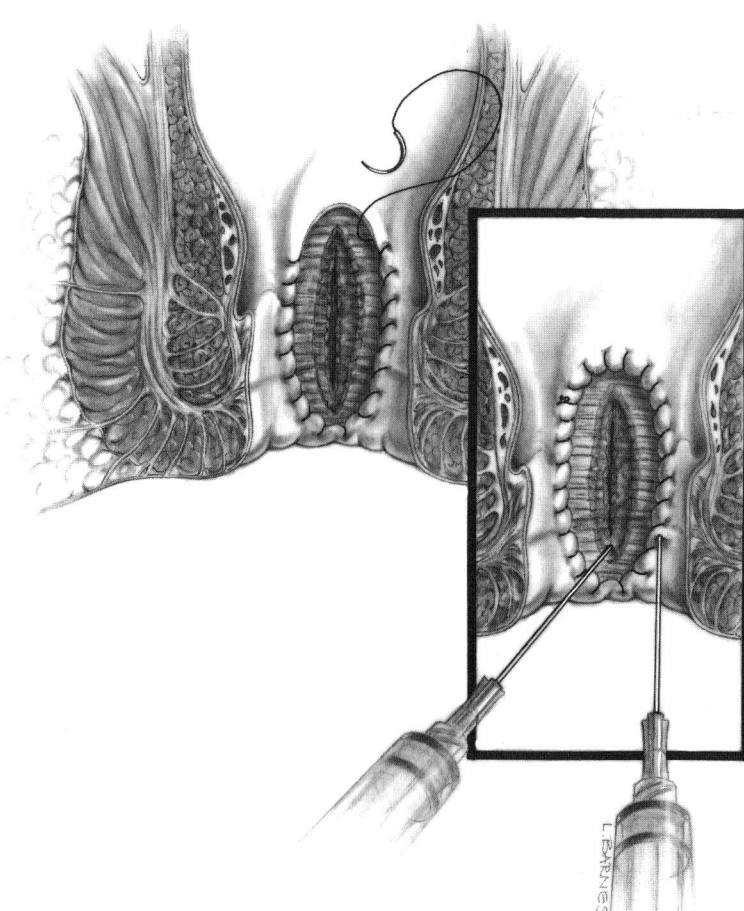

FIGURE 20-15. Treatment of an AIDS-related ulcer by marsupialization of the mucosal edges with heavy absorbable suture and injection of methylprednisolone (Depo-Medrol) into the submucosal and deep tissues **(inset)**.

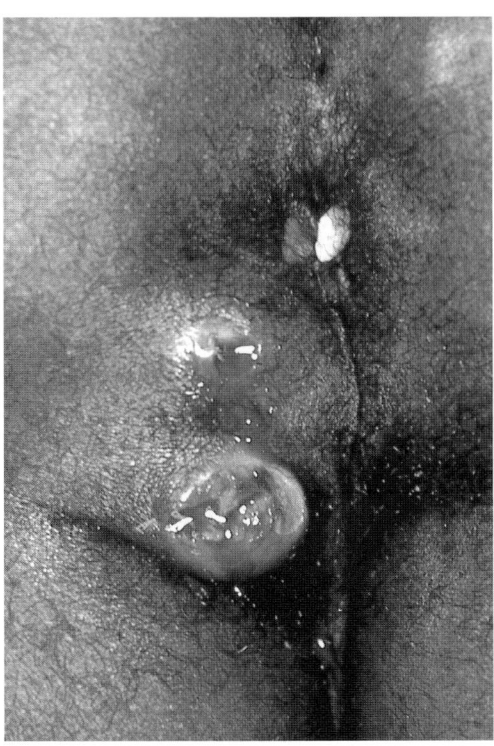

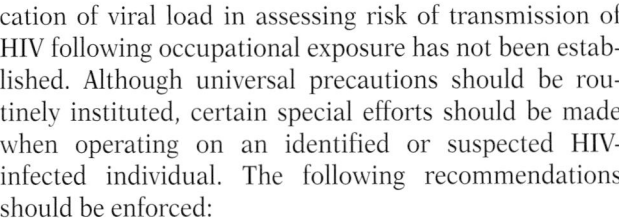

FIGURE 20-16. Large non-Hodgkin's rectal lymphoma eroding through the perianal skin. (See Color Fig. 20-16.)

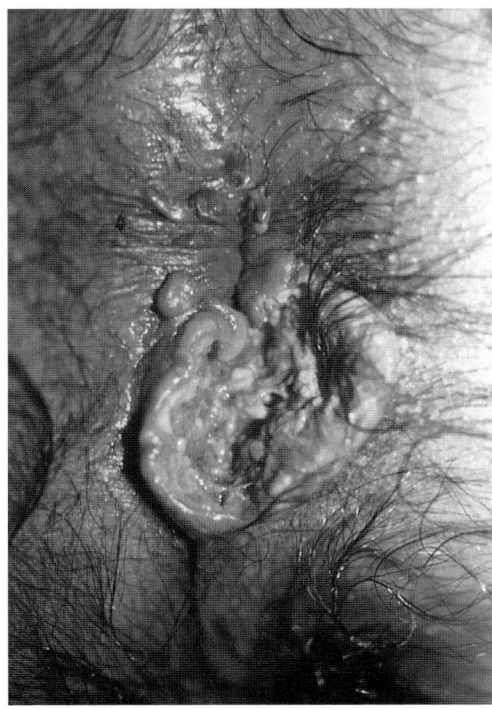

FIGURE 20-17. Squamous cell carcinoma of the anus in a patient with AIDS. (See Color Fig. 20-17.)

cation of viral load in assessing risk of transmission of HIV following occupational exposure has not been established. Although universal precautions should be routinely instituted, certain special efforts should be made when operating on an identified or suspected HIV-infected individual. The following recommendations should be enforced:

- Eyeglasses should be worn, in addition to water-resistant foot covering.
- Double gloves with a disposable sleeve insert should be used to prevent blood from reaching the wrists of the surgeon.
- Scalpels should be disposed of once skin incisions have been made.
- A choreographed procedure is dictated by the senior surgeon when suturing is being performed.[257]
- Triple therapy is recommended if a serious exposure occurs.

CONCLUSIONS

The introduction of HAART has radically changed the clinical course of HIV infection and AIDS. Although not curative, HAART does lead to significant and sustained elevations in CD4 T-cell counts and immune function as well as decreased serum viral levels to almost undetectable levels. This has resulted in a reduction in the

number of opportunistic infections and malignancies associated with AIDS and an improved survival and life expectancy.

In this chapter, we attempt to discuss the major colonic and anorectal problems encountered in the HIV-positive patient. Controversies in the management of several disorders, including AIN and invasive squamous cell carcinoma of the anal canal will, we hope, be resolved by the next edition because large multicenter studies are being currently conducted. Lest we be lulled into a false sense of security, it should be remembered that the incidence of HIV is once again rising, and the compliance of HIV-positive patients, particularly younger people with HAART regimens, is dropping. Sadly, although HAART improves life expectancy through inhibition of viral replication and immune reconstitution, 90% of the world's HIV-infected individuals do not have access to these drugs.

REFERENCES

1. *Aidsinfo.nih.gov.* Accessed 08/03.
2. Albaran RG, Webber J, Steffes CP. CD4 cell counts as prognostic factor of major abdominal surgery in patients infected with the human immunodeficiency virus. *Arch Surg* 1998;133:626.
3. Albin J, Lewis E, Eftekhari F, et al. Computed tomography of rectal and perirectal disease in AIDS patients. *Gastrointest Radiol* 1987;12:67.
4. Andersen CB, Karkov J, Bjerregaard B, et al. Cytomegalovirus infection in classic endemic and epidemic Kaposi's

sarcoma analyzed by in situ hybridization. *APMIS* 1991;99:
893.
5. Angelici A, Palumbo P, Piermattei A, et al. Exploratory laparotomy for diagnosis of abdominal painful syndromes in
HIV-positive patients. *Int Conf AIDS* 1993;9:447.
6. Ariyoshi K, Schim van der Loeff M, Cook P, et al. Kaposi's
sarcoma in the Gambia, West Africa is less frequent in
human immunodeficiency virus type 2 than in human immunodeficiency type 1 infection despite a high prevalence
of human herpesvirus 8. *J Hum Virol* 1998;1:193.
7. Bagdades EK, Pillay D, Squire SB, et al. Relationship between herpes simplex virus ulceration and CD4+ cell counts
in patients with HIV infection. *AIDS* 1992;6:1317.
8. Balthazar EJ, Megibow AJ, Barry M, et al. Histoplasmosis
of the colon in patients with AIDS: imaging findings in four
cases. *AJR Am J Roentgenol* 1993;161:585.
9. Barrett WL, Callahan TD, Orkin BA. Perianal manifestations of human immunodeficiency virus infection: experience with 260 patients. *Dis Colon Rectum* 1998;41:606.
10. Becherer PR, Sokol-Anderson M, Joist JH, et al. Gastrointestinal histoplasmosis presenting as hematochezia in
human immunodeficiency virus–infected hemophiliac patients. *Am J Hematol* 1994;47:229.
11. Beck DE, Jaso RG, Zajac RA. Surgical management of anal
condylomata in the HIV+ patient. *Dis Colon Rectum* 1990;
33:180.
12. Belistos PC, Greenson JK, Yarley JH, et al. Association of
gastric hypoacidity with opportunistic enteric infections in
patients with AIDS. *J Infect Dis* 1992;166:277.
13. Benhamou G, Potet F. Quantitative analysis of the immune cells in the anal mucosa. *Pathol Res Pract* 1995;191:
1067.
14. Benson CA. Treatment of disseminated disease due to the
Mycobacterium avium complex in patients with AIDS. *Clin
Infect Dis* 1994;18:S237.
15. Beral V, Peterman T, Berkelman R, et al. AIDS-associated
non-Hodgkin lymphoma. *Lancet* 1991;337:805.
16. Bernard C, Mougin C, Madoz L, et al. Viral co-infections in
human papillomavirus–associated anogenital lesions according to the serostatus for the human immunodeficiency
virus. *Int J Cancer* 1992;52:731.
17. Binderow SR, Cavallo RJ, Freed J. Laboratory parameters
as predictors of operative outcome after major abdominal
surgery in AIDS and HIV-infected patients. *Am Surg*
1993;59:754.
18. Bini EJ, Gorelick SM, Weinshel EH. Outcome of AIDS-associated cytomegalovirus colitis in the era of potent antiretroviral therapy. *J Clin Gastroenterol* 2000;30:414.
19. Bini EJ, Cohen J. Impact of protease inhibitors on the
outcome of human immunodeficiency virus–infected patients with chronic diarrhea. *Am J Gastroenterol* 1999;94:
3553.
20. Bizer LS, Pettorino R, Ashikari A. Emergency abdominal
operations in the patient with acquired immunodeficiency
syndrome. *J Am Coll Surg* 1995;180:205.
21. Bjorge T, Engeland A, Luostarinen T, et al. Human papillomavirus as a risk factor for anal and perinal skin cancer in
a prospective study. *Br J Cancer* 2002;87:61.
22. Blackbourn DJ, Osmond D, Levy JA, et al. Increased
human herpesvirus 8 seroprevalence in young homosexual
men who have multiple sex contacts with different partners. *J Infect Dis* 1999;179:237.
23. Blanshard C, Gazzard BG. An algorithm for the investigation of diarrhoea in HIV infection. *Gut* 1991;32:A1225.
24. Blanshard C, Gazzard BG. Natural history and prognosis
of diarrhoea of unknown cause in patients with acquired
immunodeficiency syndrome (AIDS). *Gut* 1995;36:283.
25. Blauvelt A, Piguet V. Essential roles for dendritic cells in
the pathogenesis and potential treatment of HIV disease. *J
Invest Dermatol* 2002;119:365.
26. Bordon J, Martinez-Vasquez C, Alvarez M, et al. Neurosyphilis in HIV–infected patients. *Eur J Clin Microbiol
Infect Dis* 1995;14:864.
27. Bottomley D, Gershuny A, Govindaraju S, et al. Epidermoid anal cancer in HIV–infected patients. *Br J Cancer*
1994;70[Suppl 22]:17.
28. Breese PL, Judson FN, Penley KA, et al. Anal human papillomavirus infection among homosexual and bisexual
men: prevalence of type-specific infection and association
with human immunodeficiency virus. *Sex Transm Dis* 1995;
22:7.
29. Brown DR, Bryan JT, Harven C, et al. Detection of multiple
human papilloma virus types in condylomata acuminata
from immunosuppressed patients. *J Infect Dis* 1994;170:
759.
30. Buonaguro FM, Tornesello ML, Buonaguro L, et al. Role of
HIV as cofactor in HPV oncogenesis: in vitro evidence of
virus interactions. *Antibiot Chemother* 1994;46:102.
31. Call SA, Heudebert G, Saag M, et al. The changing etiology
of chronic diarrhea in HIV-infected patients with CD4 cell
counts less than 200 cells/mm^3. *Am J Gastroenterol* 2000;
95:3142.
32. Cappell MS, Botros N. Predominantly gastrointestinal
symptoms and signs in 11 consecutive AIDS patients with
gastrointestinal lymphoma: a multicenter, multiyear study
including 763 HIV-seropositive patients. *Am J Gastroenterol* 1994;89:545.
33. Cappell MS, Mandell W, Grimes MM, et al. Immunophe-
notypic and molecular analysis of acquired immune deficiency syndrome-related and Epstein-Barr virus-associ-
ated lymphomas: a comparative study. *Dig Dis Sci* 1988;
33:353.
34. Carr A, Marriott D, Field A, et al. Treatment of HIV-1 associated microsporidiosis and cryptosporidiosis with combination antiretroviral therapy. *Lancet* 1998;351:256.
35. Carr ND, Mercey D, Slack WW. Non-condylomatous perianal disease in homosexual men. *Br J Surg* 1989;76:1064.
36. Case records of the Massachusetts General Hospital. *N
Engl J Med* 1996;334:1461.
37. Cello JP, Wilcox CM. Evaluation and treatment of gastrointestinal tract hemorrhage in patients with AIDS. *Gastroenterol Clin North Am* 1988;17:639.
38. Chadha M, Rosenblatt EA, Malamud S, et al. Squamous
cell carcinoma of the anus in HIV-positive patients. *Dis
Colon Rectum* 1994;37:861.
39. Chambers AJ, Lord RSA. Incidence of acquired immune
deficiency syndrome (AIDS)-related disorders at laparotomy in patients with AIDS. *Br J Surg* 2001;88:294.
40. Chang G, Berry J, Jay N, et al. Surgical treatment of high-
grade anal squamous intraepithelial lesions: a prospective
study. *Dis Colon Rectum* 2002;45:453–458.
41. Chang Y, Cesarman E, Pessin MS, et al. Identification of
herpes virus–like DNA sequences in AIDS-associated Kaposi's sarcoma. *Science* 1994;266:1865.
42. Change E, Absar N, Beall G. Prevention of recurrent herpes
simplex virus infections in HIV-infected persons. *AIDS Patient Care* 1995;9:252.
43. Chin DP, Hopewell PC, Yajko DM, et al. *Mycobacterium
avium* complex in the respiratory or gastrointestinal tract
and the risk of *M. avium* complex. *J Infect Dis* 1994;169
:289.
44. Chin-Hong PV, Palefsky JM. Natural history and clinical
management of anal human papillomavirus disease in men
and women infected with human immunodeficiency virus.
Clin Infect Dis 2002;35:1127.
45. Chopra KF, Tyring SK. The impact of the human immunodeficiency virus on the human papillomavirus epidemic.
Arch Dermatol 1997;133:629.
46. Clark SJ, Saag MS, Decker WD, et al. High titers of cytopathic virus in plasma of patients with symptomatic primary HIV-1 infection. *N Engl J Med* 1991;324:954.
47. Cleator S, Fife K, Nelson M, et al. Treatment of HIV-associated invasive anal cancer with combined chemoradiation.
Eur J Cancer 2000;36:754.
48. Conant MA, Shacker TW, Murphy RL, et al. Valaciclovir
versus acyclovir for herpes simplex virus infection in HIV-

infected individuals: two randomized trials. *Int J STD AIDS* 2002;13:12.

49. Cone LA, Woodard DR, Potts BE, et al. An update on the acquired immunodeficiency syndrome (AIDS): associated disorders of the alimentary tract. *Dis Colon Rectum* 1986; 29:60.

50. Consten ECJ, Slors FJ, Noten HJ, et al. Anorectal surgery in human immunodeficiency virus-infected patients. *Dis Colon Rectum* 1995;38:1169.

51. Consten EC, Slors JF, Danner SA, et al. Severe complications of perianal sepsis in patients with human immunodeficiency virus. *Br J Surg* 1996;83:778.

52. Cooper DA, Tindall B, Wilson EJ, et al. Characterization of T lymphocyte responses during primary HIV infection. *J Infect Dis* 1987;155:1113.

53. Corey L, Nahmias AJ, Guinan ME, et al. A trial of topical acyclovir in genital herpes simplex virus infections. *N Engl J Med* 1982;306:1313.

54. Cote TR, Bigger R, Rosenberg PS, et al. Non-Hodgkin's lymphoma among people with AIDS: incidence, presentation and public health burden. *Int J Cancer* 1997;73:645.

55. Cotte L, Drout E, Bailly F, et al. Cytomegalovirus DNA level on biopsy specimens during treatment of cytomegalovirus gastrointestinal disease. *Gastroenterology* 1996;111:439.

56. Cotte L, Drouet E, Bissuel F, et al. Diagnostic value of cytomegalovirus-DNA amplification from gastrointestinal biopsies in HIV-infected patients. *Int Conf AIDS* 1993; 9:1(abst).

57. Craib KJ, Meddings DR, Strathdee SA, et al. Rectal gonorrhea as an independent risk factor for HIV infection in a cohort of homosexual men. *Genitourin Med* 1995;71:150.

58. Critchlow CW, Hawes SE, Kuypers JM, et al. Effect of HIV infection on the natural history of anal human papillomavirus infection. *AIDS* 1998;12:1177.

59. Critchlow CW, Surawicz CM, Holmes KK, et al. Prospective study of high-grade anal squamous intraepithelial neoplasia in a cohort of homosexual men: influence of HIV infection, immunosuppression and human papillomavirus infection. *AIDS* 1995;9:1255.

60. Crumpacker CS. Ganciclovir. *N Engl J Med* 1996;335:721.

61. Cummings BJ. Concomitant radiotherapy and chemotherapy for anal cancer. *Semin Oncol* 1992;19:102.

62. Dal Maso L, Franceschi S. Epidemiology of non-Hodgkin lymphoma and other haemolymphopoietic neoplasms in people with AIDS. *Lancet Oncol* 2003;4:110.

63. Davidson T, Allen-Mersh TG, Miles AJG, et al. Emergency laparotomy in patients with AIDS. *Br J Surg* 1991;78:924.

64. Davis PA, Corless DJ, Aspinall R, et al. Effect of CD4+ and CD8+ cell depletion on wound healing. *Br J Surg* 2001; 88:298.

65. Davis PA, Corless DJ, Gazzard BG, et al. Increased risk of wound complications and poor healing following laparotomy in HIV-seropositive and AIDS patients. *Dig Surg* 1999;16:60.

66. Deeks SG, Volberding PA. HIV-1 protease inhibitors. *AIDS Clin Rev* 1997–98;145.

67. Dieterich DT, Lew EA, Kotler DP, et al. Treatment with albendazole for intestinal disease due to *Enterocytozoon bieneusi* in patients with AIDS. *J Infect Dis* 1994;169:178.

68. Dieterich DT, Rahmin M. Cytomegalovirus colitis in AIDS: presentation in 44 patients and a review of the literature. *J Acquir Immune Defic Syndr* 1991;4:S29.

69. Drew WL. Cytomegalovirus infection in patients with AIDS. *J Infect Dis* 1988;158:449.

70. Drew WL, Buhles W, Erlich KS. Herpesvirus infections (cytomegalovirus, herpes simplex virus, varicella-zoster virus): how to use ganciclovir (DHPG) and acyclovir. *Infect Dis Clin North Am* 1988;2:495.

71. Drew WL, Mills J, Hauer LB, et al. Declining prevalence of Kaposi's sarcoma in homosexual AIDS patients paralleled by fall in cytomegalovirus transmission. *Lancet* 1988;1:66.

72. Dryden MS, Shanson DC. The microbial cause of diarrhea in patients infected with the human immunodeficiency virus. *J Infect* 1988;17:107.

73. Dyson N, Howley PM, Munger K, Harlow E, et al. The human papillomavirus-16 E7 oncoprotein is able to bind the retinoblastoma gene produce. *Science* 1989;243:934.

74. Science and Technology. Hope. *Economist* 1996;Jun 29: 82–84.

75. Ell CH, Matek W, Gramatzki M, et al. Endoscopic findings in a case of Kaposi's sarcoma with involvement of the large and small bowel. *Endoscopy* 1985;17:161.

76. Eltom MA, Hemal A, Mbulaiteye SM, et al. Trends in Kaposi's sarcoma and non-Hodgkin's lymphoma incidence in the United States from 1973 through 1998. *J Natl Cancer Inst* 2002;94:1204.

77. Emmanoulides C, Miles SA, Mitsuyasu RT. Pathogenesis of AIDS-related Kaposi's sarcoma. *Oncology* 1996;10:335.

78. Emparan C, Iturburu IM, Ortiz J, et al. Infective complications after abdominal surgery in patients infected with human immunodeficiency virus: role of CD4+ lymphocytes in prognosis. *World J Surg* 1998;22:778.

79. Endean ED, Ross CW, Strodel WE. Kaposi's sarcoma appearing as a rectal ulcer. *Surgery* 1987;101:767.

80. Eron JJ, Benoit SL, Jemesk J et al. Treatment with lamivudine, zidovudine, or both in HIV-positive patients with 200 to 500 CD4+ cells per cubic millimeter. *N Engl J Med* 1995;333:1662.

81. Fauci AS. AIDS in 1996: much accomplished, much to do. *JAMA* 1996;276:155.

82. Feinberg M. Changing the natural history of HIV disease. *Lancet* 1996;348:239.

83. Fenger C, Nielson V. Precancerous changes in the anal canal epithelium in resection specimens. *Acta Pathol Microbiol Immunol Scand* 1986;94:63.

84. Flanigan T, Wahlen C, Turner J, et al. *Cryptosporidium* infection and CD4 counts. *Ann Intern Med* 1992;116:840.

85. Fluker JL, Deherogoda P, Platt DJ, et al. Rectal gonorrhoea in male homosexuals: presentation and therapy. *Br J Vener Dis* 1980;56:397.

86. Forsmark CE, Wilcox CM, Darragh TM, et al. Disseminated histoplasmosis in AIDS: an unusual case of esophageal involvement and gastrointestinal bleeding. *Gastrointest Endosc* 1990;36:604.

87. Foust RL, Dean PJ, Stoler MH, et al. Intraepithelial neoplasia of the anal canal in hemorrhoidal tissue: a study of 19 cases. *Hum Pathol* 1991;22:528.

88. Frager DH, Frager JD, Brandt LJ, et al. Gastrointestinal complications of AIDS: radiologic features. *Radiology* 1986; 158:597.

89. Friedman SL, Wright TL, Altman DF. Gastrointestinal Kaposi's sarcoma in patients with AIDS. *Gastroenterology* 1985; 89:102.

90. Friedman-Kein A, Laubenstein L, Marmor M, et al. Kaposi's sarcoma and *Pneumocystis* pneumonia among homosexual men. *MMWR Morb Mortal Wkly Rep* 1981;30:305.

91. Frisch M, Biggar RJ, Engels EA, et al. Association of cancer with AIDS-related immunosuppression in adults. *JAMA* 2001;285:1736.

92. Garcia LS, Brewer TC, Bruckner DA. Fluorescence detection of *Cryptosporidium* oocysts in human fecal specimens by using monoclonal antibodies. *J Clin Microbiol* 1987; 31:1468.

93. Gautreaux MD, Gelder FB, Deitch EA, et al. Adoptive transfer of T lymphocytes to T-cell-depleted mice inhibits *Escherichia coli* translocation from the gastrointestinal tract. *Infect Immun* 1995;63:3827.

94. Gervaz E., Dauge-Geffroy MD, Sobhani I, et al. Quantitative analysis of the immune cells in the anal mucosa. *Pathol Res Pract* 1995;191:1067.

95. Goldstone S, Palefsky J, Winnett M. Activity of HspE7, a novel immunotherapy in patients with anogenital warts. *Dis Colon Rectum* 2002;45:502.

96. Goodell SE, Quinn TC, Mkrtichian E, et al. Herpes simplex virus proctitis in homosexual men: clinical, sigmoidoscopic, and histopathological features. *N Engl J Med* 1983; 308:868.

97. Goodgame MD, Porter DD. Cytomegalovirus vasculitis with fatal colonic hemorrhage. *Arch Pathol* 1973;96:281.

98. Goodgame RW. Gastrointestinal cytomegalovirus disease. *Ann Intern Med* 1993;119:924.

99. Goodgame RW, Genta RM, Estrada R, et al. Frequency of positive tests for cytomegalovirus in AIDS patients: endoscopic lesions compared with normal mucosa. *Am J Gastroenterol* 1993;88:338.

100. Goodgame, RW, Kimball K, Ou CN, et al. Intestinal function and injury in acquired immunodeficiency syndrome-related cryptosporidiosis. *Gastroenterology* 1995;108: 1075.

101. Gottesman L. Adjuvant operative bed alfa-interferon 2b in the treatment of persistent and recalcitrant anal condylomata acuminata. American Society of Colon and Rectal Surgery, Seattle, 1996 (abst).

102. Gottesman L. Ulcerative disease of the anorectum in AIDS. *Int J STD AIDS* 1995;6:4.

103. Gottesman LG, Miles AJG, Milsom JW, et al. The management of anorectal disease in HIV-positive patients. *Int J Colorectal Dis* 1990;5:61.

104. Graybill JR. AIDS commentary. Histoplasmosis and AIDS. *J Infect Dis* 1988;158:623.

105. Grulich AE, Li Y, McDonald AM, et al. Decreasing rates of Kaposi's sarcoma and non-Hodgkin's lymphoma in the era of potent combination anti-retroviral therapy. *AIDS* 2001; 15:629.

106. Guarino A, Canani P, Pozio E, et al. Enterotoxic effect of stool supernatant of cryptosporidosis-infected calves on human jejunum. *Gastroenterology* 1994;106:28.

107. Haddad FS, Ghossain A, Sawaya E, et al. Abdominal tuberculosis. *Dis Colon Rectum* 1987;30: 724.

108. Gulick RM, Mellors JW, Havlir D, et al. Treatment with indinavir, zidovudine, and lamivudine in adults with human immunodeficiency virus infection and prior antiretroviral therapy. *N Engl J Med* 1997;337:734.

109. Hamilton JD, Hartigan PM, Simberkoff MS, et al. A controlled trial of early versus late treatment with zidovudine in symptomatic human immunodeficiency virus infection: results of the Veterans Affairs Cooperative Study. *N Engl J Med* 1992;326:437.

110. Harris PJ. Treatment of Kaposi's sarcoma and other manifestations of AIDS with human chorionic gonadotropin. *Lancet* 1995;346:118.

111. Harrison M, Tomlinson D, Steward S. Squamous cell carcinoma of the anus in patients with AIDS. *Clin Oncol* 1995;7:50.

112. Heneghan SJ, Li J, Petrossian E, et al. Intestinal perforation from gastrointestinal histoplasmosis in acquired immunodeficiency syndrome: case report and review of the literature. *Arch Surg* 1993;128:464.

113. Hewitt WT, Sokol RP, Fleshner PR. Should HIV status alter indications for hemorrhoidectomy? *Dis Colon Rectum* 1996;39:615.

114. Hinant KL, Rotterdam HZ, Bell ET, et al. Cytomegalovirus infection of the alimentary tract: a clinicopathological correlation. *Am J Gastroenterol* 1986;81:944.

115. Hoffman R, Welton ML, Klencke B, et al. The significance of pretreatment CD4 count on the outcome and treatment tolerance of HIV-positive patients with anal cancer. *Int J Radiat Oncol Biol Phys* 1999;44:127.

116. Holland JM, Swift PS. Tolerance of patients with human immunodeficiency virus and anal carcinoma to treatment with combined chemotherapy and radiation therapy. *Radiology* 1994;193:251.

117. Horn RD, Hood AF. Cytomegalovirus is predictably present in perineal ulcers from immunosuppressed patient. *Arch Dermatol* 1990;26:646.

118. Imagawa DT, Lee MH, Wolinsky SM, et al. Human immunodeficiency virus type I infection in homosexual men who remain seronegative for prolonged periods. *N Engl J Med* 1989;320:1458.

119. Imrie K, Sawka C, Kutas G, et al. HIV-associated lymphoma of the gastrointestinal tract. *Proc Ann Meeting Am Soc Clin Oncol* 1993;12:A1(abst).

120. Irizarry E, Gottesman L. Rectal sexual trauma including foreign bodies. *Int J STD AIDS* 1996;7:166.

121. Jarrin G, Kemeny M, Lee M. Abdominal surgery in patients with AIDS-related lymphomas: bacteremia in patients with human immunodeficiency virus infection. *J Infect Dis* 1994;169:289; *Proc Ann Meeting Am Soc Clin Oncol* 1992; 11:A17(abst).

122. Jiang S, Zhao Q, Debnath AK. Peptide and non-peptide HIV fusion inhibitors. *Curr Pharm Des* 2002;8:563.

123. Jones JL, Hanson DL, Dworkin MS, et al. Incidence and trends in Kaposi's sarcoma in the era of effective antiretroviral therapy. *J Acquir Immune Defic Syndr Hum Retrovirol* 2000;24:270.

124. Judson FN, Penley KA, Robinson ME, et al. Prevalence and site pathogen studies of *Neisseria meningitidis* and *Neisseria gonorrhoeae* in homosexual men. *Am J Epidemiol* 1980; 112:836.

125. Kaplan LD, Wofsy CB, Volberding PA. Treatment of patients with acquired immunodeficiency syndrome and associated manifestations. *JAMA* 1987;257:1367.

126. Kaplan, LD, Abrams D, Feigal E, et al. AIDS-associated non-Hodgkin's lymphomas in San Francisco. *JAMA* 1989; 261:719.

127. Kaslow RA, Phair JP, Friedman HB, et al. Infection with the human immunodeficiency virus: clinical manifestations and their relationship to immunodeficiency. A report from the Multicenter AIDS Cohort Study. *Ann Intern Med* 1987;107:474.

128. Keating J, Bjarnason I, Somasundaram S, et al. Intestinal absorptive capacity, intestinal permeability and jejunal histology in HIV and their relationship to diarrhoea. *Gut* 1995;37:623.

129. Kelly CP, Pothoulakis C, LaMont JT. *Clostridium difficile* colitis. *N Engl J Med* 1994;330:257.

130. Kemper CA, Meng TC, Nussbaum J, et al. Treatment of *Mycobacterium avium* complex bacteremia in AIDS with a four drug oral regimen. *Ann Intern Med* 1992;116:466.

131. Kerr A, Dix J, Quinnonez C. A case of fatal hemorrhage caused by intestinal histoplasmosis. *Am J Gastroenterol* 1991;86:910.

132. Khawaja Ht. Podophyllin versus scissor excision in the treatment of perianal condylomata: a prospective study. *Br J Surg* 1989;76:1067.

133. Kim JH, Sarani B, Orkin BA, et al. HIV-positive patients with anal carcinoma have poorer treatment tolerance and outcome than HIV-negative patients. *Dis Colon Rectum* 2001;44:506.

134. Kiveat N, Rompalo A, Bowden R, et al. Anal human papillomavirus among human immunodeficiency virus–seropositive and seronegative men. *J Infect Dis* 1990;162:358.

135. Klencke B, Kaplan L. Advances and future challenges in non-Hodgkin's lymphoma. *Curr Opin Oncol* 1998;10:422.

136. Knight SC, Patterson S. Bone marrow–derived dendritic cells, infection with human immunodeficiency virus, and immunopathology. *Annu Rev Immunol* 1997;15:593.

137. Knowles DM, Chadburn A. AIDS-associated lymphoid proliferations. In Knowles DM, ed. *Neoplastic hematopathology.* Baltimore: Williams & Wilkins;1992.

138. Knowles DM. Biologic aspects of AIDS-associated non-Hodgkin's lymphoma. *Curr Opin Oncol* 1993;5:845.

139. Knowles D. Etiology and pathogenesis of AIDS-related non-Hodgkin's lymphoma. *Hematol Oncol Clin North Am* 1996;10:1081.

140. Kotler DP, Shimda T, Snow G, et al. Effect of combination anti-retroviral therapy upon rectal mucosal HIV RNA burden and mononuclear cell apoptosis. *AIDS* 1998; 12:597.

141. Kotler DP, Reka S, Orenstein JM, et al. Chronic idiopathic esophageal ulceration in the acquired immunodeficiency syndrome: characterization and treatment with corticosteroids. *J Clin Gastroenterol* 1992;15:284.

142. Koutsky LA, Ault KA, Wheeler CM, et al. A controlled trial of a human papillomavirus type 16 vaccine. *N Engl J Med* 2002;347:1645.

143. Kram HB, Shoemaker WC. Intestinal perforation due to cytomegalovirus infection in patients with AIDS. *Dis Colon Rectum* 1990;33:1037.

144. Krown SE, Gold JWM, Niedzwiecki D, et al. Interferon-alpha with zidovudine: safety, tolerance, and clinical and virologic effects in patients with Kaposi's sarcoma associated with the acquired immunodeficiency syndrome (AIDS). *Ann Intern Med* 1990;112:812.

145. Kuzell Institute for Arthritis and Infectious Disease, San Francisco. Immunobiology of *Mycobacterium avium* infection. *Eur J Clin Microbiol Infect Dis* 1994;11:1000.

146. Lacey CJ, Thompson HS, Monteiro EF, et al. Phase IIa safety and immunogenicity of a therapeutic vaccine, TA-GW, in persons with genital warts. *Dis Colon Rectum* 2002; 45:502.

147. Laine L, Amerian J, Rarick M, et al. The response of symptomatic gastrointestinal Kaposi's sarcoma to chemotherapy: a prospective evaluation using an endoscopic method of disease quantification. *Am J Gastroenterol* 1990; 85:959.

148. Lange JMA, Parry JV, de Wolf F, et al. Diagnostic value of specific IgM antibodies in primary HIV infection. *BMJ* 1986;293:1459.

149. Lew EA, Dieterich DT. Severe hemorrhage caused by gastrointestinal Kaposi's sarcoma in patients with the acquired immunodeficiency syndrome: treatment with endoscopic injection sclerotherapy. *Am J Gastroenterol* 1992;87: 1471.

150. Lim SG, Condez A, Lee CA, et al. Loss of mucosal CD4 lymphocytes is an early feature of HIV infection. *Clin Exp Immunol* 1993;92:448.

151. Lorenz HP, Wilson W, Leigh B, et al. Kaposi's sarcoma of the rectum in patients with the acquired immunodeficiency syndrome. *Am J Surg* 1990;160:681.

152. MMWR. Advancing HIV prevention: new strategies for a changing epidemic. United States 2003. *MMWR Morb Mortal Wkly Rep* 2003;52:329.

153. MMWR. Diagnosis and reporting of HIV and AIDS in states with HIV/AIDS surveillance. United States, 1994–2000. *MMWR Morb Mortal Wkly Rep* 2002;51:595.

154. Matthews G, Bower M, Mandalia S, et al. Changes in acquired immunodeficiency syndrome–related lymphoma since the introduction of highly active antiretroviral therapy. *Blood* 2000;96:2730.

155. Marrazzo JM, Whittington WL, Celum CL, et al. Urine-based screening for *Chlamydia trachomatis* in men attending sexually transmitted disease clinics. *Sex Transm Dis* 2001;28:219.

156. McGrath MS, Herndier B. Clonal HIV in the pathogenesis of AIDS-related lymphoma: sequential pathogenesis. In: Goedert JJ, ed. *Infectious causes of cancer: targets for intervention.* Totowa, NJ: Humana Press, 2000.

157. Melbye M, Cote TR, Kessler L, et al. High incidence of anal cancer among AIDS patients: the AIDS/Cancer Working Group. *Lancet* 1994;343:636.

158. Mellors JW, Rinaldo CR Jr, Grupta P, et al. Prognosis in HIV-1 infection predicted by the quantity of virus in plasma. *Science* 1996;272:1167.

159. Memar OM, Arany I, Trying SK. Skin-associated lymphoid lesions in human immunodeficiency virus, HPV, and herpes simplex virus infection. *J Invest Dermatol* 1995;105 [Suppl 1]:99s.

160. Mentec H, Leport C, Leport J, et al. Cytomegalovirus colitis in HIV-1 infected patients: a prospective research in 55 patients. *AIDS* 1994;8:461.

161. Mertz GJ, Jones CC, Mills J, et al. Long-term acyclovir suppression of frequently recurring genital herpes simplex virus infection: a multicenter double-blind trial. *JAMA* 1988;260:201.

162. Metcalf AM, Dean T. Risk of dysplasia in anal condyloma. *Surgery* 1995;118:724.

163. Miles AJG, Allen-Mersh TG, Wastell C. Effect of anoreceptive intercourse on anal function. *J R Soc Med* 1993; 86:144.

164. Miles AJG, Mellor CH, Gazzard B, et al. Surgical management of anorectal disease in HIV-positive homosexuals. *Br J Surg* 1990;77:869.

165. Mitsuyasu RT. Kaposi's sarcoma in the acquired immunodeficiency syndrome. *Infect Dis Clin North Am* 1989;2: 511.

166. Molina JM, Sarfati C, Beauvais B, et al. Intestinal microsporidiosis in human immunodeficiency virus–infected patients with chronic unexplained diarrhea: prevalence and clinical and biological features. *J Infect Dis* 1993; 167:217.

167. Monkemuller KE, Call SA, Lazenby AJ, et al. Declining prevalence of opportunistic gastrointestinal disease in the era of combination antiretroviral therapy. *Am J Gastroenterol* 2000;95:457.

168. Morgan AR, Miles AJ, Wastell C. Anal condyloma acuminatum and squamous carcinoma-in-situ of the anal canal. *J R Soc Med* 1994;87:15.

169. Mortensen NJ, Thomson JP. Perianal abscess due to *Enterobius vermicularis*. *Dis Colon Rectum* 1984;27:677.

170. Moylett EH, Shearer WT. HIV: clinical manifestations. *J Allergy Clin Immunol* 2002;110:3.

171. Murray JG, Evans SJ, Jeffrey PB, et al. Cytomegalovirus colitis in AIDS: CT features. *AJR Am J Roentgenol* 1995; 165:67.

172. Neff R, Kremer S, Voutsinas L, et al. Primary Kaposi's sarcoma of the ileum presenting as massive rectal bleeding. *Am J Gastroenterol* 1987;82:276.

173. Northfelt DW. Anal neoplasia in persons with HIV infection. *AIDS Clin Care* 1996;8:63.

174. O'Brien TR, Kedes D, Ganem D, et al. Evidence for concurrent epidemics of human herpesvirus 8 and human immunodeficiency virus type 1 in US homosexual men: rates, risk factors, and relationship to Kaposi's sarcoma. *J Infect Dis* 1999;180:600.

175. Oliveira L, Wexner SD. Laparoscopically assisted sigmoid colectomy in human immunodeficiency virus (HIV) patients: a good indication for laparoscopic surgery. *Surg Laparosc Endosc* 1996;6:414.

176. Orenstein, JM, Tenner M, Kotler DP. Localization of infection by the microsporidian *Enteroctyozoon bieneusi* in the gastrointestinal tract of AIDS patients with diarrhea. *AIDS* 1992;6:195.

177. Orlando G, Fasolo MM, Signori R, et al. Impact of highly active antiretroviral therapy on clinical evolution of genital warts in HIV-1–infected patients. *AIDS* 1999;13:291.

178. Palefsky JM, Goldstone SE, Winnett M, et al. HspE7 treatment of anal dysplasia: results of an open label trial of HspE7 and comparison with a prior controlled trial of low dose HspE7. 41st Interscience Conference on Antimicrobial Agents and Chemotherapy, Chicago, 2001 (abst).

179. Palefsky JM, Holly EA, Ralston ML, et al. Effect of highly active antiretroviral therapy on the natural history of anal squamous intraepithelial lesions and human papillomavirus infection. *J Acquir Immune Defic Syndr Hum Retrovirol* 2001;28:422.

180. Palefsky JM, Holly E, Hogeboom CJ, et al. Anal cytology as a screening tool for anal squamous intraepithelial lesions. *J Acquir Immune Defic Syndr Hum Retrovirol* 1997;14:415.

181. Palefsky JM. Cutaneous and genital HPV-associated lesions in HIV-infected patients. *Clin Dermatol* 1997;15:439.

182. Palefsky J, Gonzales J, Greenblatt R, et al. High prevalence of anal intraepithelial neoplasia and anal papillomavirus infection among males with group IV HIV disease. *JAMA* 1990;263:2911.

183. Palefsky J, Gonzales J, Greenblatt R, et al. Natural history of anal cytologic abnormalities and papillomavirus infection among homosexual men with group IV HIV disease. *J Acquir Immune Defic Syndr Hum Retrovirol* 1992; 5:1258.

184. Palella FJ Jr, Delaney KM, Moorman AC, et al. Declining morbidity and mortality among patients with advanced human immunodeficiency virus infection: HIV Outpatient Study investigators. *N Engl J Med* 1998;338:853.

185. Panja A, Mayer L. Diversity and function of antigen-presenting cells in mucosal tissue. In: Ogra PL, Lamm ME,

McGhee JR, eds. *Handbook of mucosal immunology.* San Diego: Academic Press, 1994:177.

186. Pare A, Gottesman L. Oncogenic human papillomavirus in idiopathic AIDS ulcers: cause or bystander? *Presentation, NY Soc Colon Rect Surg* 1995.

187. Paterson DL, Georghiou PR, Allworth AM, et al. Thalidomide as treatment of refractory aphthous ulceration related to human immunodeficiency virus infection. *Clin Infect Dis* 1995;20:250.

188. Pati S, Pelser CB, Dufraine J, et al. Antitumorigenic effects of HIV protease inhibitor ritonavir: inhibition of Kaposi's sarcoma. *Blood* 2002;99:3771.

189. Peacock CS, Blanchard C, Tovey DG, et al. Histological diagnosis of intestinal microsporidiosis in patients with AIDS. *J Clin Pathol* 1991;44 :558.

190. Peddada AV, Smith DE, Rao AR, et al. Chemotherapy and low-dose radiotherapy in the treatment of HIV-infected patients with cancer of the anal canal. *Int J Radiat Oncol Biol Phys* 1997;37:1101.

191. Peppercorn MA. Enteric infections in homosexual men and without AIDS. *Contemp Gastroenterol* 1989;2:23.

192. Piketty C, Darragh TM, Da Costa M, et al. High prevalence of anal human papillomavirus infection and anal cancer precursors among HIV-infected persons in the absence of anal intercourse. *Ann Intern Med* 2003;138:453.

193. Place RJ, Gregorcyk SG, Huber PJ, et al. Outcome analysis of HIV-positive patients with anal squamous cell carcinoma. *Dis Colon Rectum* 2001;44:506.

194. Plancoulaine S, Abel L, van Beveren M, et al. Human herpesvirus 8 transmission from mother to child and between siblings in an endemic population. *Lancet* 2000; 356:1062.

195. Pluda JM, Venson DJ, Tosato G, et al. Parameters affecting the development of non-Hodgkin's lymphoma in patients with severe human immunodeficiency virus infection receiving antiretroviral therapy. *J Clin Oncol* 1993;11: 1099.

196. Port JH, Traube J, Winans CS. The visceral manifestations of Kaposi's sarcoma. *Gastrointest Endosc* 1982;28:179.

197. Puy-Montbrun T, Ganansia R, Lemarchand N, et al. Anal ulcerations due to cytomegalovirus in patients with AIDS: report of six cases. *Dis Colon Rectum* 1990;33:1041.

198. Neff R, Kremer S, Voutsinas L, et al. Primary Kaposi's sarcoma of the ileum presenting as massive rectal bleeding. *Am J Gastroenterol* 1987;82:276.

199. Quinn TC. Global burden of the HIV pandemic. *Lancet* 1996;348:99.

200. Rabeneck L, Crane MM, Risser JMH, et al. Effect of HIV transmission category and CD4 count on the occurrence of diarrhea in HIV-infected patients. *Am J Gastroenterol* 1993;88:1720.

201. Rabinowitz M, Bassan I, Robinson MJ. Sexually transmitted cytomegalovirus proctitis in a woman. *Am J Gastroenterol* 1988;83:885.

202. Ramirez-Amador V, Esquivel-Pedraza L, Lozada-Nur F, et al. Intralesional vinblastine vs 3% sodium tetradecyl sulfate for the treatment of oral Kaposi's sarcoma: a double-blind, randomized clinical trial. *Oral Oncol* 2002;38:460.

203. Rene E, Marche C, Chevalier T, et al. Cytomegalovirus colitis in patients with acquired immunodeficiency syndrome. *Dig Dis Sci* 1988;33:741.

204. Romanowski B, Aoki FY, Martel AY, et al. Efficacy and safety of famciclovir for treating mucocutaneous herpes simplex infection in HIV-infected individuals. *AIDS* 2000; 14:1211.

205. Rompalo AM, Mertz GJ, Davis LG, et al. Oral acyclovir for treatment of first-episode herpes simplex virus proctitis. *JAMA* 1988;259:2879–2881.

206. Safavi A, Gottesman L, Dailey TH. Anorectal surgery in the HIV+ patient: update. *Dis Colon Rectum* 1991;34:299.

207. Safrin S. Treatment of acyclovir-resistant herpes simplex virus infection in patients with AIDS. *J Acquir Immune Defic Syndr Hum Retrovirol* 1992;5[Suppl 1]:S29.

208. Saltz RK, Kurtz RC, Lightdale CJ et al. Kaposi's sarcoma: gastrointestinal involvement correlation with skin findings and immunologic function. *Dig Dis Sci* 1984;29:817.

209. Schacker T, Collier AC, Hughes J, et al. Clinical and epidemiological features of primary HIV infection. *Ann Intern Med* 1996;125:257.

210. Scheffner M, Whitaker NJ. Human papillomavirus-induced carcinogenesis and the ubiquitin-proteasome system. *Semin Cancer Biol* 2003;13:59.

211. Schmidt W, Wahnschaffe U, Schafer M, et al. Rapid increase in mucosal CD4 T cells followed by clearance of intestinal cryptosporidiosis in an AIDS patient receiving highly active antiretroviral therapy. *Gastroenterology* 2001; 120:984.

212. Schmitt SL, Wexner SD. Treatment of anorectal manifestations of AIDS: past and present. *Int J STD AIDS* 1994;8:8.

213. Schmitt SL, Wexner SD, Nogueras JJ, et al. Is aggressive treatment of perianal ulcers in homosexual HIV-seropositive men justified? *Dis Colon Rectum* 1993;36:240.

214. Schnittman SM, Lane HC, Greenhouse J, et al. Preferential infection of CD4+ memory T cells by human immunodeficiency virus type 1: evidence for a role in the selective T-cell functional defects observed in infected individuals. *Proc Natl Acad Sci USA* 1990;87:6058.

215. Scholefield JH, Northover JMA, Carr ND. Male homosexuality, HIV infection and colorectal surgery. *Br J Surg* 1990;77:493.

216. Schulz TF, Boshoff CH, Weiss RA. HIV infection and neoplasia. *Lancet* 1996;348:587.

217. Schwartz DA, Wilcox CM. Atypical cytomegalovirus inclusions in gastrointestinal biopsy specimens from patients with the acquired immunodeficiency syndrome: diagnostic role of in situ nucleic acid hybridization. *Hum Pathol* 1992;23:1019.

218. Selik RM, Rabkin CS. Cancer death rates associated with human immunodeficiency virus infection in the United States. *J Natl Cancer Inst* 1998;90:1300.

219. Sgadari C, Barillari G, Toschi E, et al. HIV protease inhibitors are potent anti-angiogenic molecules and promote regression of Kaposi's sarcoma. *Nat Med* 2002;8:225.

220. Sharpstone D, Rowbottom A, Francis N, et al. Thalidomide: a novel therapy for microsporidiosis. *Gastroenterology* 1997;112:1823.

221. Sharpstone D, Gazzard B. Gastrointestinal manifestations of HIV infection. *Lancet* 1996;348:379.

222. Sherrard J, Forsyth JR. Homosexually acquired gonorrhoea in Victoria, 1983–1991. *Med J Aust* 1993;158:450.

223. Shiramizu BS, Herndier B, McGrath MS. Identification of a common clonal HIV integration site in HIV-associated lymphomas. *Cancer Res* 1994;54:2069.

224. Siegel FP, Lopez C, Hammer GS, et al. Severe acquired immunodeficiency in male homosexuals manifested by chronic perianal ulcerative herpes simplex lesions. *N Engl J Med* 1981;305:1439.

225. Sillman FH, Sedlis A. Anogenital papillomavirus infection and neoplasia in immunodeficient women. *Obstet Gynecol Clin North Am* 1987;14:537.

226. Simon DM, Cello JP, Valenzuela J. Multicenter trial of octreotide in patients with refractory acquired immunodeficiency syndrome-associated diarrhea. *Gastroenterology* 1995; 109:1024.

227. Skyldberg B, Hagmer B, Johannson B, et al. HPV detection in cytological cases with condylomatous or dysplastic changes: a study with PCR and in situ hybridization on cytological material. *Diagn Cytopathol* 1995;13:8.

228. Smith NH, Cron S, Valdez LM, et al. Combination drug therapy for cryptosporidiosis in AIDS. *J Infect Dis* 1998 178:900.

229. Smith PD, Quinn TC, Strober W, et al. NIH conference: gastrointestinal infections in AIDS. *Ann Intern Med* 1992; 116:63.

230. Sobhani I, Walker F, Aparicio T, et al. Effect of anal epidermoid cancer–related viruses on the dendritic (Langerhans')

cells of the human anal mucosa. *Clin Cancer Res* 2002;8:2862.

231. Sobhani I, Vuagnat A, Walker F, et al. Prevalence of high-grade dysplasia and cancer in the anal canal in human papillomavirus–infected individuals. *Gastroenterology* 2001;120:857.

232. Sobottka I, Schwartz DA, Schottelius J, et al. Prevalence and clinical significance of intestinal microsporidiosis in human immunodeficiency virus–infected patients with and without diarrhea in Germany: a prospective coprodiagnostic study. *Clin Infect Dis* 1998;26:475.

233. Sohn N. Surgical conditions of the anus and rectum in male homosexuals. *Pract Gastroenterol* 1985;9:46.

234. Söderlund C, Bratt GA, Engstrom L, et al. Surgical treatment of cytomegalovirus enterocolitis in severe immunodeficiency virus infection: report of eight cases. *Dis Colon Rectum* 1994;37:63.

235. Sparano JA. Clinical aspects and management of AIDS-related lymphoma. *Eur J Cancer* 2001;37:1296.

236. Spetz A, Strominger J, Groh-Spies V. T-cell subsets in normal human epidermis. *Am J Pathol* 1996;149:665.

237. Spivak H, Schlasinger MH, Tabanda-Lichauco R, et al. Small bowel obstruction from gastrointestinal histoplasmosis in acquired immune deficiency syndrome. *Am Surg* 1996;62:369.

238. Stockmann M, Schmitz H, Fromm M, et al. Mechanisms of epithelial barrier impairment in HIV infection. *Ann NY Acad Sci* 2000;915:293.

239. Surawicz CM, Critchlow C, Sayer J, et al. High-grade anal dysplasia in visually normal mucosa in homosexual men: seven cases. *Am J Gastroenterol* 1995;90:1776.

240. Sykes NL Jr. Condyloma accuminatum. *Int J Dermatol* 1995;34:297.

241. Talal AH, Monard S, Vesanen M, et al. Virologic and immunologic effect of antiretroviral therapy on HIV-1 in gut-associated lymphoid tissue. *J Acquir Immune Defic Syndr Hum Retrovirol* 2001;26:1.

242. Thomas M, Massimi P, Jenkins J, et al. HPV-18 E6 mediated inhibition of p53 DNA binding activity is independent of E6 induced degradation. *Oncogene* 1995;10:261.

243. Teunissen MB. Dynamic nature and function of epidermal Langerhans cells in vivo and in vitro: a review, with emphasis on human Langerhans cells. *Histochem J* 1992;24:697.

244. Tyring S. Imiquimod applied topically: a novel immune response modifier. *Skin Ther Lett* 2001;6:1.

245. United States Public Health Service. Updated U.S. Public Health Service guidelines for the management of occupational exposures to HBV, HCV, and HIV and recommendations for post-exposure prophylaxis. *MMWR Recommen Rep* 2001;50:1–52.

246. Vaccher E, Spina M, Tirelli U. Clinical aspects and management of Hodgkin's disease and other tumours in HIV-infected individuals. *Eur J Cancer* 2001;37:1306.

247. Van den Hoek JAR, van Griensven GJP, Coutinho RA. Increase in unsafe homosexual behavior. *Lancet* 1990;336:179.

248. Veazy RS, Marx PA, Lackner AA. Vaginal CD4+ T cells express high levels of CCR5 and are rapidly depleted in simian immunodeficiency virus infection. *J Infect Dis* 2003;187:769.

249. Veazy RS, DeMaria M, Chalifoux LV, et al. Gastrointestinal tract as a major site of CD4+ T cell depletion and viral replication in SIV infection. *Science* 1998;280:427.

250. Veljkovic V, Metlas R, Raspopovic J, et al. Spectral and sequence similarity between vasoactive intestinal peptide and the second conserved region of human immunodeficiency virus type 1 envelope glycoprotein (gp120): possible consequences on prevention and therapy of AIDS. *Biochem Biophys Res Commun* 1992;189:705.

251. Viamonte M, Dailey TH, Gottesman L. Ulcerative disease of the anorectum in the HIV+ patient. *Dis Colon Rectum* 1993;6:801.

252. Vogel J, Hinrichs SH, Reynolds RK, et al. The HIV tat gene induces dermal lesions resembling Kaposi's sarcoma in transgenic mice. *Nature* 1998;335:606.

253. Volberding PA, Mitsuyasu RT, Golando JP, et al. Treatment of Kaposi's sarcoma with interferon alpha-2b (Intron A). *Cancer* 1987;59:620.

254. Von Roenn JH, Clinical presentations and standard therapy of AIDS-associated Kaposi's sarcoma. *Hematol Oncol Clin North Am* 2003;17:747.

255. Wall SD, Friedman SL, Margulis AR. Gastrointestinal Kaposi's sarcoma in AIDS: radiographic manifestations. *J Clin Gastroenterol* 1984;6:165.

256. Wallace M, Bower M, Allen-Mersh T. The severity of anal intraepithelial neoplasia is not affected by antiretroviral therapy in HIV positive men. *Dis Colon Rectum* 2002;45:A30.

257. Wastell C, Corless D, Keeling N. Surgery and human immunodeficiency virus-1 infection. *Am J Surg* 1996;172:89.

258. Weber JN, Carmichael DJ, Boylston A, et al. Kaposi's sarcoma of the bowel presenting as apparent ulcerative colitis. *Gut* 1985;26:295.

259. Weber R, Bryan RT, Owen RL, et al. Improved light-microscopical detection of microsporidia spores in stool and duodenal aspirates. *N Engl J Med* 1992;326:161.

260. Webster GF. Local therapy for mucocutaneous Kaposi's sarcoma in patient's with acquired immunodeficiency syndrome. *Dermatol Surg* 1995;21:205.

261. Weiss EG, Wexner SD. Surgery for anal lesions in the HIV-infected patients. *Ann Med* 1995;27:467.

262. Welch HA, Salahuddin SZ, Gill P, et al. AIDS-associated Kaposi's sarcoma–derived cells in long-term culture express and synthesize smooth-muscle alpha-actin. *Am J Pathol* 1991;139:1251.

263. Weller IVD. The gay bowel. *Gut* 1985;26:869.

264. Weprin L, Zollinger R, Clausen K, et al. Kaposi's sarcoma: endoscopic observations of gastric and colon involvement. *J Clin Gastroenterol* 1982;4:357.

265. Wexner SD. Sexually transmitted diseases of the colon, rectum, and anus: the challenge of the nineties. *Dis Colon Rectum* 1990;33:1048.

266. Wexner SD, Smithy WB, Milsom JW, et al. The surgical management of anorectal diseases in AIDS and pre-AIDS patients. *Dis Colon Rectum* 1986;29:719.

267. Wexner SD, Smithy WB, Trillo C, et al. Emergency colectomy for cytomegalovirus ileocolitis in patients with the acquired immune deficiency syndrome. *Dis Colon Rectum* 1988;31:755.

268. Wheat J. Endemic mycosis in AIDS: a clinical review. *Clin Microbiol Rev* 1995;8:146–159.

269. Wilcox CM, Chalasani N, Lazenby A, et al. Cytomegalovirus colitis in acquired immunodeficiency syndrome: a clinical and endoscopic study. *Gastrointest Endosc* 1998;48:39.

270. Wilcox CM, Rabeneck L, Friedman S. AGA Technical review: malnutrition and cachexia, chronic diarrhea, and hepatobiliary disease in patients with human immunodeficiency virus infection. *Gastroenterology* 1996;111:1724.

271. Williams GR, Talbott IC. Anal carcinoma: a histological review. *Histopathology* 1994;25:507.

272. Wilson SE, Robinson G, Williams RA, et al. Acquired immune deficiency syndrome (AIDS): indications for abdominal surgery, pathology, and outcome. *Ann Surg* 1989;210:428.

273. Wolkomir AF, Barone JE, Hardy HW III, et al. Abdominal and anorectal surgery and the acquired immune deficiency syndrome in heterosexual intravenous drug users. *Dis Colon Rectum* 1990;33:267.

274. Workowski KA, Levine WC. Selected topics from the Centers for Disease Control and Prevention sexually transmitted diseases treatment guidelines 2002. *HIV Clin Trials* 2002;3:421.

275. Yii MK, Saunder A, Scott DF. Abdominal surgery in HIV/AIDS patients: indications, operative management, pathology and outcome. *Aust NZ J Surg* 1995;65:320.

276. Yinnon AM, Coury-Donger P, Polito R, et al. Serologic response to treatment of syphilis in patients with HIV infection. *Arch Intern Med* 1996;156:321.

277. Zaunders J, Carr A, McNally L, et al. Effects of primary HIV-1 infection on subsets of CD4+ and CD8+ T lymphocytes. *AIDS* 1995;9:561.

278. Zeitz M, Ullrich R, Schneider T, et al. Cell differentiation and proliferation in the gastrointestinal tract with respect to the local immune system. *Ann NY Acad Sci* 1994;733:75.

279. Zeitz M, Greene WC, Peffer NJ, et al. Lymphocytes isolated from the intestinal lamina propria of normal nonhuman primates have increased expression og genes associated with T-cell activation. *Gastroenterology* 1988;94:647.

280. Zierdt CH, Gill VJ, Zierdt WS. Detection of microsporidian spores in clinical samples by indirect fluorescent-antibody assay using whole-cell antisera to *Encephalitozoon cuniculi* and *Encephalitozoon hellem*. *J Clin Microbiol* 1993;31:3071.

Chapter 21

Polypoid Diseases

If people are falling over the edge of a cliff and sustaining injuries, the problem could be dealt with by stationing ambulances at the bottom or erecting a fence at the top. Unfortunately, we put far too much effort into the provision of ambulances and far too little into the simple approach of erecting fences.

Denis Burkitt

This chapter consists of a discussion of benign polypoid conditions that are commonly observed in the practice of general and colon and rectal surgeons. A *polyp* is a well-circumscribed projection above the surface epithelium. It may be pedunculated or sessile. It can vary in size from 1 or 2 mm to more than 10 cm. It is not a histologic diagnosis, however. Polyp is merely a descriptive term. Three types of polyps are discussed in this chapter: hyperplastic (metaplastic), hamartomatous, and adenomatous.

HYPERPLASTIC OR METAPLASTIC POLYP

In 1934, Westhues described a nonneoplastic mucosal lesion that has come to be known in the United States as a hyperplastic polyp.[441] In England, the tumor is called metaplastic; this term was introduced by Morson in his 1962 article.[270] He preferred the latter terminology because the former has a connotation suggestive of neoplasm. In truth, the lesion is associated with cancer in the resected specimen as frequently as 50% of the time (see Figure 22-25). Still, it had been believed that this type of growth bears no relationship to benign or malignant neoplastic lesions of the colon and rectum in that it does not serve as a marker for the concomitant presence of either. Some have challenged this opinion with the belief that there is an association (see later). Hayashi and colleagues suggest that the cells forming the hyperplastic polyp grow more slowly and have a longer life span than adjacent normal mucosal cells.[171] The retained epithelium fails to detach, becoming "hypermature."[171]

Clinical Appearance

Hyperplastic polyps are usually found in the rectum and sigmoid colon, often at the summit of mucosal folds and on the apex of the valves of Houston (Figure 21-1). They are nearly always multiple and can present in such large numbers that on both endoscopic examination and barium enema they may simulate familial (multiple) polyposis.[146] Their usual size is 2 to 5 mm. They appear approximately the same color as the rectal mucosa or slightly paler. Often they are overlooked.

Histology

Microscopically, crypts are seen to be lined by a hyperplastic epithelium that gives the crypt lumen a scalloped appearance (Figure 21-2). The structure is quite different

---

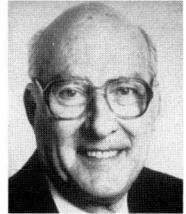

Basil Morson (1921–present) Basil Morson was born November 13, 1921. He enrolled in Oxford University in 1939 with the intent of studying medicine. However, in 1943 he deferred his degree and joined the British Royal Navy as an Ordinary Seaman. Within 6 months, he was promoted to Sublieutenant. Upon demobilization, Morson returned to Oxford and qualified as a physician in 1949 before gaining his Doctorate in 1955 with his thesis on intestinal metaplasia of the gastric mucosa. He ultimately succeeded Cuthbert Dukes as Consultant Histopathologist at St Mark's Hospital, London, and served in that position for 30 years, 1956 to 1986. Among his notable academic achievements are a detailed description of the adenoma-carcinoma sequence (with Tetsuichiro Muto), the first description of large bowel Crohn's disease (with Sir Hugh Lockhart-Mummery), and the standard book of British gastrointestinal pathology, known colloquially as Morson and Dawson, now in its fourth edition. He is recognized throughout the world as the father of the specialty of gastrointestinal pathology. A prolific writer, he has been honored by both colleges and medical societies. He was made a Fellow both of the Royal College of Surgeons of England and the Royal College of Physicians. He was awarded the John Hunter Medal of the Royal College of Surgeons in 1987 and served as President of the Proctology Section of the Royal Society of Medicine, President of the British Society of Gastroenterology (the first pathologist so to be so honored), and both Vice-President and Honorary Treasurer of the Royal College of Pathologists. He was made CBE (Commander of the British Empire) just after his retirement in 1987 and currently lives in Sussex. (Courtesy of Robin K.S. Phillips.)

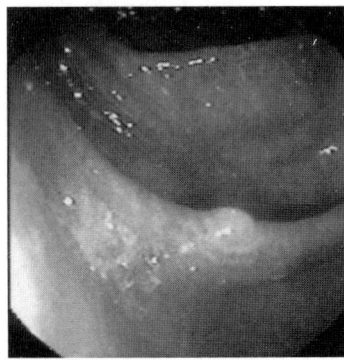

FIGURE 21-1. A hyperplastic polyp can be seen on the surface of one of the valves of Houston. Note the co-existing melanosis coli, which serves to demarcate clearly the nonpigmented lesion. (See Color Fig. 21-1.)

from that of an adenomatous polyp. The lining epithelium loses its regular columnar and goblet cell pattern and appears serrated because of flattening of the cells (Figure 21-3).[270] Goblet cells are diminished, and the lamina propria may demonstrate increased inflammatory reaction: plasma cells, and lymphocytes (Figure 21-4).

Evaluation and Management

Because it has been generally accepted that hyperplastic polyps are not neoplasms and do not, in themselves, connote increased risk for the development of neoplasms, either benign or malignant, the question of how to treat them demands a decision. The fact that a patient harbors

hyperplastic polyps would seem of little clinical significance; hence, therapy may be deemed unnecessary. The problem arises, however, in establishing with certainty the nature of the tumor. This can be accomplished only by submitting the lesion for pathologic confirmation. This is an important consideration, because if it is discovered that the tumor is actually a neoplasm (e.g., a polypoid adenoma), the need for total colonic evaluation and follow-up is theoretically different.

Waye and Bilotta suggested a technique to help differentiate between adenomas and hyperplastic polyps.[433] It is their contention that some diminutive hyperplastic polyps, especially those in the rectum, will flatten and lose their configuration during maximal air insufflation and will blend into the surrounding mucosa. With the application of suction, the lesion reappears. Such a phenomenon is not seen with true neoplasms, hence the distinction. They concluded that when such "disappearing" polyps are observed, neither biopsy nor polypectomy need be performed.

Church and colleagues, reporting from the Cleveland Clinic, found that small *colonic* polyps are usually neoplastic, but even if hyperplastic, they are associated with adenomas elsewhere in 75% of cases.[60] Small rectal polyps are usually hyperplastic but still were associated with neoplasms elsewhere in 63% of the patients in their report.[60] The authors, therefore, recommended total colonoscopy for even proved hyperplastic polyps. Ansher and associates found that almost one third of their patients in whom an isolated hyperplastic polyp was found in the left colon harbored a proximal adenomatous polyp.[5] They opined that hyperplastic colonic polyps *do* serve as a

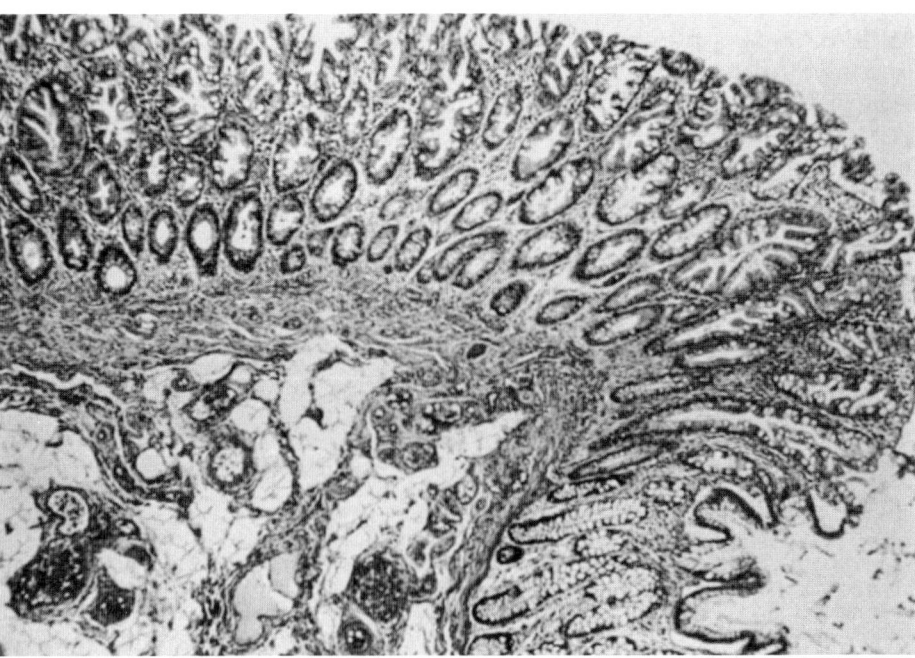

FIGURE 21-2. Hyperplastic (metaplastic) polyp. Note the hyperplastic changes in the mucosa and the serrated glands near the surface with papillary projections. (Original magnification × 240; from Corman ML, Veidenheimer MC, Swinton NW. *Diseases of the anus, rectum, and colon. Part I: neoplasms.* New York: Medcom, 1972, with permission.)

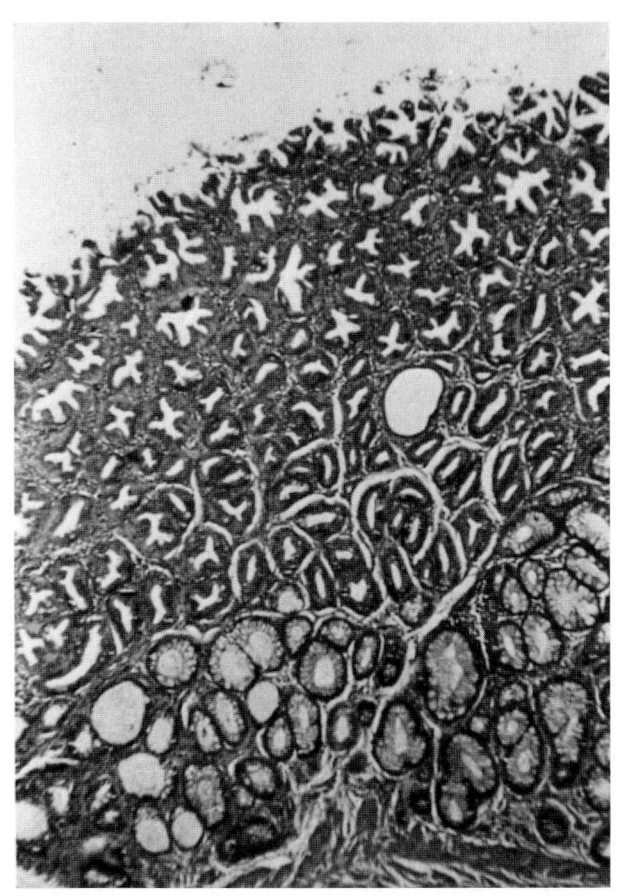

FIGURE 21-3. Hyperplastic (metaplastic) polyp. A lesion has serrated glands, some of which are cystically dilated. (Original magnification × 280; courtesy of Rudolf Garret, M.D.)

marker for adenomatous colonic neoplasms. Conversely, Provenzale and colleagues reviewed the records of 1,836 consecutive colonoscopic examinations.[332] Following statistical analysis, these investigators concluded that distal hyperplastic polyps were *not* strong predictors of the risk for concomitant proximal benign or malignant neoplasms. They did advocate biopsy, however, to confirm the true nature of the lesion. Others also have concluded that small adenomatous and hyperplastic polyps cannot reliably be distinguished by their endoscopic appearance.[294] Tonooka and co-workers reported a case of carcinoma in a 12-mm hyperplastic polyp in the cecum diagnosed by a magnifying colonoscope.[413] When the lesion was seen in the magnified view, an irregularly-shaped pit was evident in the center. Biopsy confirmed malignant change at that location.

Waye and colleagues noted that 73% of all polyps in the right colon were neoplastic, but 65% of the polyps in the rectum were nonneoplastic.[435] Azimuddin and associates believe that hyperplastic polyps that are "large" and right sided have an uncertain clinical significance and should be excised, with the patient placed on a surveillance program.[9] Jass opined that subsets of hyperplastic polyps may have malignant potential.[208] These include multiple, large, and proximal location. Cappell and Forde demonstrated that hyperplastic polyps show spatial clustering with neoplastic polyps and suggested that regions with prior polyps merit close surveillance.[50]

Hyperplastic Polyposis

Numerous cases of so-called hyperplastic polyposis have appeared in the literature. As would be anticipated from the foregoing opinions, this particular entity seems to

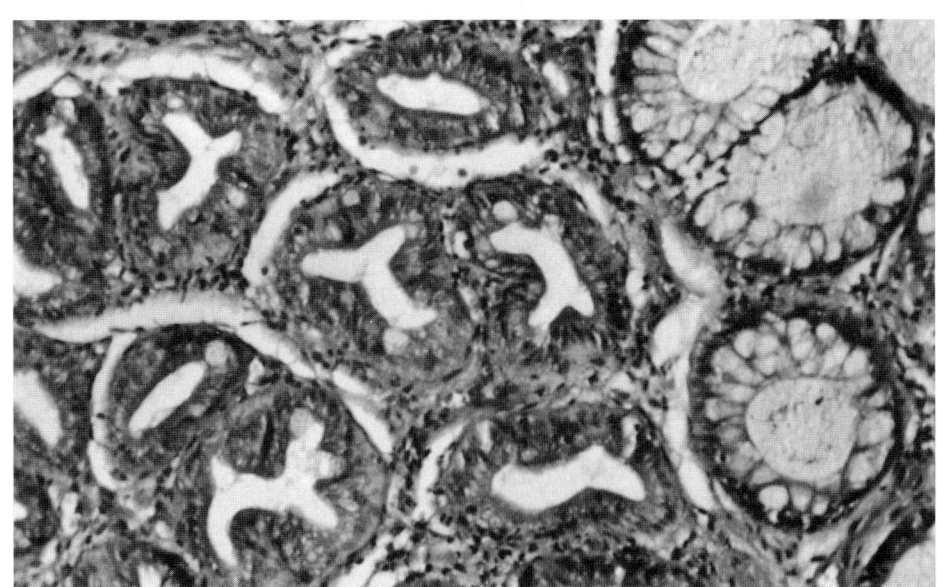

FIGURE 21-4. Hyperplastic (metaplastic) polyp. Compare the normal glands on the **right** with the serrated glands on the **left**. (Original magnification × 600; courtesy of Rudolf Garret, M.D.)

have an increased association with colorectal cancer. Interestingly, disappearance of the hyperplastic polyps has been reported following resection.[235]

Opinion

My own philosophy is to effect a compromise between an aggressive "search and destroy" attitude with every identifiable mucosal excrescence and a laissez-faire approach. The following protocol is recommended.

Excise the lesion initially to confirm the diagnosis. No follow-up other than the routine colorectal cancer screening appropriate for any patient free of a prior history of neoplasm is suggested, if the polyp is nonneoplastic. If an individual is found on subsequent routine endoscopic examination to harbor additional lesions, no treatment is advised, except possibly fulguration or cold biopsy of the relatively larger ones. There are four reasons why I suggest continuing to ignore them. First, they tend to disappear spontaneously and recur elsewhere (I agree with the observation of Waye and Bilotta); some patients simply are hyperplastic polyp creators. Second, I am reluctant to create further anxiety by reinforcing the phobia most people have about cancer. Third, there are complications associated with excision of lesions; bleeding and perforation are encountered more frequently when small lesions are removed than when large tumors are sampled for biopsy. This occurs because sometimes normal bowel must be injured in order to extirpate the growth completely. If the surgeon performs procedures through the endoscope frequently enough, inevitably a complication will result. Finally, it adds considerably to the cost of medical care.

Despite my impression that I am usually able to determine on clinical inspection alone the likelihood that lesion is hyperplastic, there are times when I am certainly mistaken. Neale and co-workers reported an accuracy rate of 80% in this regard.[286] In their study, the diagnostic sensitivity of detecting adenomas was 69%, whereas specificity (the accurate diagnosis of hyperplastic polyps) was 86%. There were also a number of false-negative and false-positive diagnoses. I concur with the authors that there is probably a relationship between physician experience and accuracy. The surgeon must establish his or her own criteria and philosophical approach to removal, fulguration, or nonintervention of presumed hyperplastic polyps.

HAMARTOMAS

A hamartoma is defined as a nonneoplastic growth that is composed of an abnormal mixture of normal tissue. In the colon, this includes juvenile and Peutz-Jeghers polyps.[438]

Juvenile Polyps

The juvenile polyp (congenital polyp, retention polyp, juvenile adenoma) is usually found in children less than 10 years of age, but it is also seen in older children and in adults at any age.[270] It is an uncommon condition, occurring in approximately 1% of asymptomatic children.[141] The age distribution has been reported to have a bimodal pattern.[349] According to Roth and Helwig, the childhood group has a modal age of 4 years whereas the adult group has a modal age of 18 years.[349] The incidence is twice as frequent in boys, and there is a 13:1 ratio of men to women in adults.[349]

Although juvenile polyps are the most common colorectal tumors in children, benign and malignant neoplasms can present at virtually any age.[22,228] Billingham and colleagues observed that solitary adenomas accounted for 7.4% of all polyps found in patients less than 20 years of age.[28]

Symptoms and Signs

The most common presenting complaint is rectal bleeding, followed by prolapse or protrusion of the mass, passing of tissue, and abdominal pain.[129,186,261,349] Autoamputation is noted in up to 10% of patients. Diarrhea, mucus, proctalgia, tenesmus, and rectal prolapse are also identifiable complaints.[45]

Distribution

Mazier and associates reported 258 patients with juvenile polyps.[261] Sixty percent of the polyps were located within 10 cm of the anal verge. Only 10% were located farther away than 20 cm, but these were scattered throughout the colon. Approximately three fourths were greater than 1 cm in diameter. Jalihal and colleagues found that 80% of the more than 100 colonoscopy polypectomies performed for juvenile polyps were found in the rectosigmoid region.[204]

Appearance

Macroscopically, the lesions are usually round or oval, with a smooth, continuous surface, in contrast to the papillary surface that characterizes the adenomatous polyp.[225] They usually have a short stalk. The cut surface demonstrates numerous cystic spaces filled with mucus (Figure 21-5).

Histology

Microscopic examination reveals that juvenile polyps are composed of an epithelial and a connective tissue element, with the latter contributing the bulk of the tumor

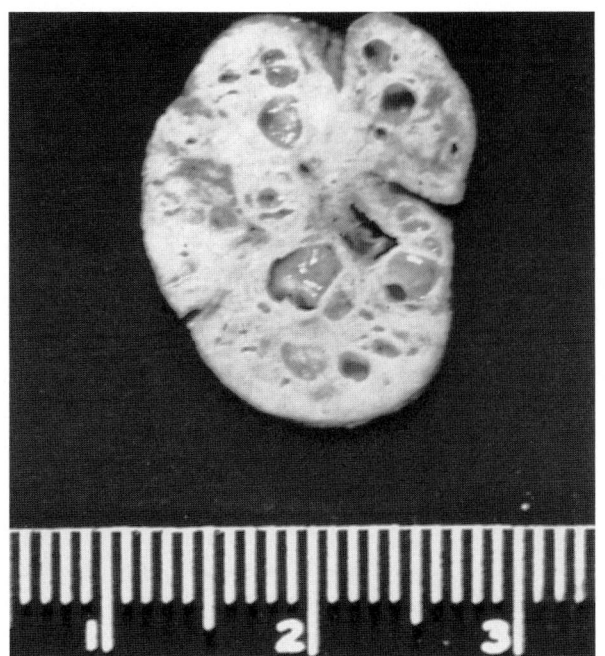

FIGURE 21-5. Juvenile polyp. Note the characteristic cystic spaces in cross section. (Courtesy of Rudolf Garret, M.D.)

mass (Figure 21-6).[216] Acute and chronic inflammatory cells are frequently seen.

Etiology

Alexander and colleagues noted that a frequent microscopic finding is infiltration by eosinophils.[2] They postulated that because eosinophils usually connote an allergic response, the polyps are the result of allergy. In support of this theory is the observation that there was a statistically significant increased incidence of allergy in children with polyps and in the families of those children.

Despite the suggestion by some that juvenile polyps may be neoplastic, most pathologists today agree with Morson that the lesion is a hamartoma.[270] Morson based his conclusion on the observations that there is an abnormality of the mucosal connective tissue or lamina propria and that this connective tissue stroma bears a resemblance to primitive mesenchyme. This concept lends support to the contention that the lesion is a malformation rather than a neoplasm. One theory holds that the polyp is a form of retention cyst that takes on a polypoid form from traction as a result of peristalsis. Juvenile polyps also have been reported at the site of a ureterosigmoidoscopy.[423]

Diagnosis and Management

The diagnosis is usually confirmed by means of proctosigmoidoscopy, and the lesion is removed transanally. In those polyps beyond the reach of the instrument, barium enema has succeeded in identifying the lesion. In the past, before the advent of colonoscopy, many of these patients were observed, because the alternative meant colostomy and polypectomy. With the availability of colonoscopy, there is no reason to adopt such an approach. In many centers, colonoscopy is the initial means employed for investigating children with undiagnosed rectal bleeding.[103,204,386]

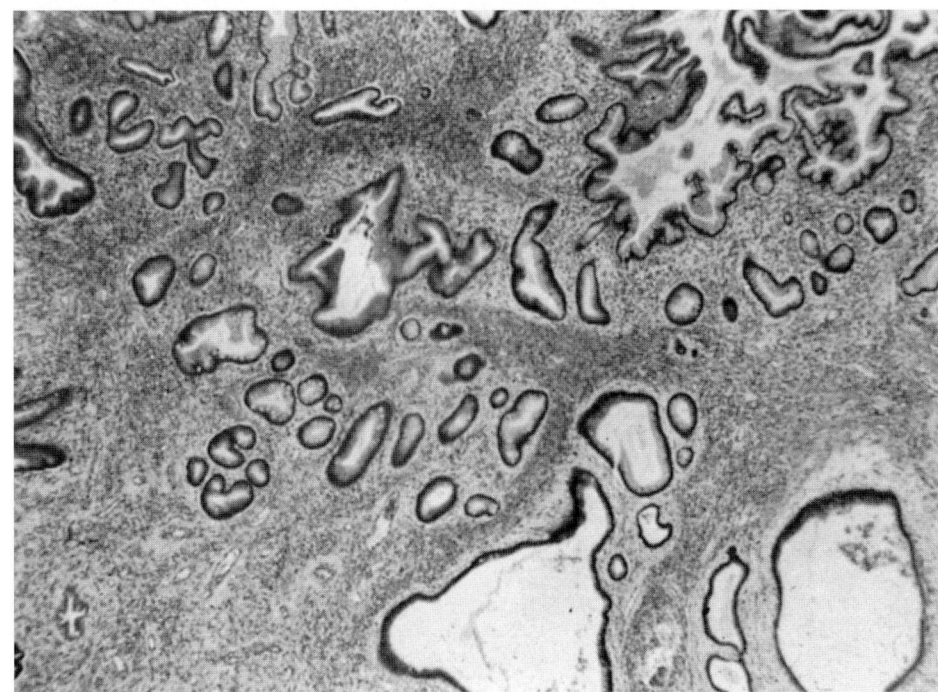

FIGURE 21-6. Juvenile polyp. Note the cystically dilated glands lined by normal-appearing epithelium. (Original magnification × 170; courtesy of Rudolf Garret, M.D.)

Despite the likelihood that a lesion proximal to a juvenile polyp in the rectum is most probably another juvenile polyp, an aggressive attitude should be taken to confirm its true histologic nature. It is, however, generally agreed that a juvenile polyp, itself, is neither a neoplasm nor a premalignant condition. Once the polyp is removed, no further follow-up is required.

Juvenile Polyposis

Juvenile polyposis is an uncommon condition characterized by the development of multiple juvenile polyps primarily in the colon, but also in the remainder of the intestinal tract.[97] The condition initially was described by McColl and associates in a number of children.[263] Many of these individuals have a family history of adenomatous polyposis and of carcinoma of the colon.[163,206,381] A family history is found in 20% to 50% of patients, with an apparent autosomal dominant hereditary pattern. The gene has not, as of this writing, been identified. There is a strong association with benign and malignant neoplasms of the colon as well as with gastroduodenal polyps. The condition usually presents in childhood, with only 15% being identified in the adult population.

Juvenile polyposis should be distinguished from multiple juvenile polyps (Figure 21-7).[344] As suggested, in addition to the colon, the polyps can occasionally be found in the small intestine and stomach.[339] Reed and Vose reported simultaneous diffuse juvenile polyposis and adenomatous polyps in a 17-year-old girl.[340] The authors theorized that the two histologically different lesions may represent phases in a spectrum of diffuse colonic polyposis that may be initiated or exacerbated by a yet undetermined stimulus. The recurrence rate for solitary juvenile polyps is less than 20%, whereas the rate approaches 90% in familial cases.[163]

Patients with juvenile polyposis have a much different clinical course when compared with those who have solitary juvenile polyps. Hematochezia, iron-deficiency anemia, hypoproteinemia, hypokalemia, anergy, finger clubbing, and a failure to thrive are much more likely to occur in the former condition.[159] Other extracolonic congenital and acquired manifestations in this condition include macrocephaly, alopecia, bony swellings, cleft lip, cleft palate, abnormalities of the vitellointestinal duct, double renal pelvis and ureter, acute glomerulonephritis, undescended testicle, and bifid uterus and vagina.[97] Of course, some of the associations may be purely coincidental. The quite rare and often fatal form, juvenile polyposis of infancy, is associated with profuse diarrhea, protein-losing enteropathy, bleeding, and rectal prolapse.[97]

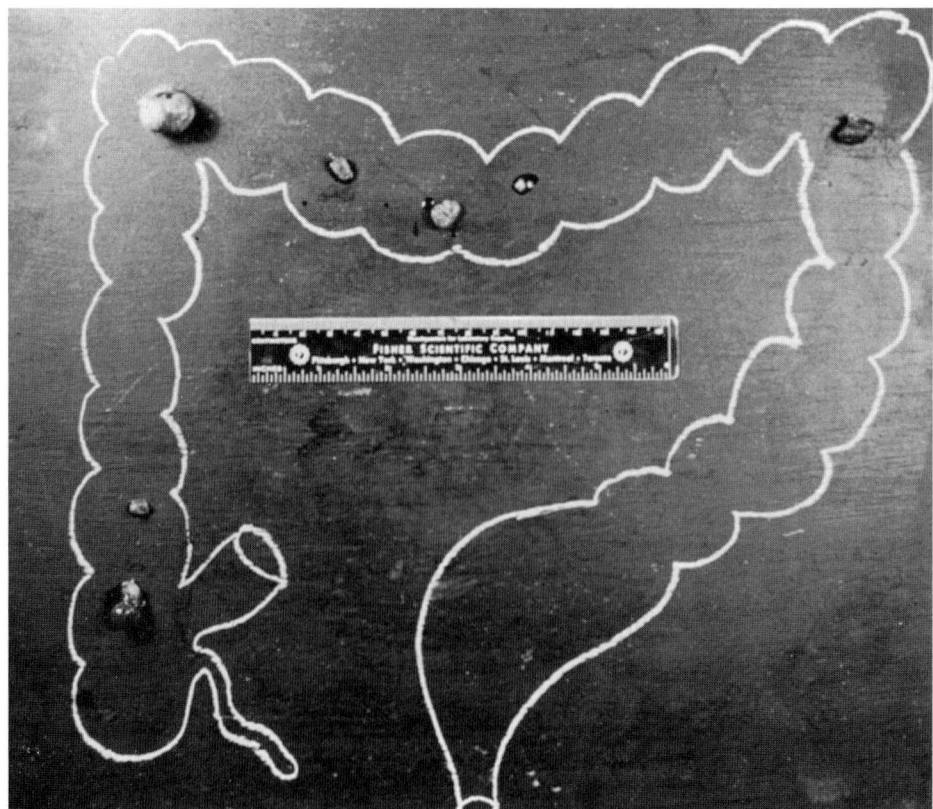

FIGURE 21-7. Multiple juvenile polyps removed from one patient. (Courtesy of Rudolf Garret, M.D.)

Management

Because juvenile polyposis should be considered a potentially premalignant condition, an aggressive approach to management is indicated.[245,338] Unless one is truly satisfied that the colon has been "cleared" (usually by means of colonoscopy and polypectomies), total colectomy is the recommended procedure.[159] Consideration should be given to ileoanal anastomosis with intervening pouch if the rectum is densely involved (see later and Chapter 29).[370] Neoplasms within the ileal reservoir following this operation have been reported.[394] Periodic endoscopic surveillance of the ileal pouch as well as upper gastrointestinal endoscopy should be considered following restorative proctocolectomy. Proctocolectomy and ileostomy may be required in some cases. Finally, family members should undergo colorectal evaluation.

Cronkhite-Canada Syndrome

In 1955, Cronkhite and Canada described a syndrome of gastrointestinal polyposis, hyperpigmentation, alopecia, and nail dystrophy.[85] Other cases have since been reported.[148,212] The syndrome is believed to be a variant of juvenile polyposis with ectodermal changes and without evidence of genetic transmission.[337] Some have suggested that the disease is the result of an abnormality of ectodermal and endodermal proliferation.[130] The polyps may be seen in association with neoplasms of the colon and are considered by some authors to represent a premalignant condition.[253,337]

Symptoms and Signs

Diarrhea and malabsorption produce severe vitamin deficiency, hypoproteinemia, and fluid and electrolyte abnormalities. Anemia and rectal bleeding are commonly reported.[89] Other symptoms include weight loss, abdominal pain, weakness, nausea and vomiting, hypogeusia (loss of taste), and a variety of neurologic complaints.[89] Hair loss and nail and skin changes may be evident before the gastrointestinal symptoms become manifest.[131]

Polyps involve the stomach and large bowel in virtually every case, but the small intestine probably contains the tumors as frequently; it is simply that the small bowel is more difficult to evaluate. As with juvenile polyposis, pathologic study confirms their hamartomatous nature. Malhotra and Sheffield recommend that Cronkhite-Canada syndrome be included with other gastrointestinal syndromes that have a malignant potential.[253] The observation of dysplasia in a biopsy specimen should encourage the endoscopist to pursue an aggressive surveillance program.

Management

Most patients have been treated symptomatically by means of nutritional support, including home parenteral nutrition.[121] Resection is indicated when involvement is limited to a segment amenable to excision, whether it be stomach, small bowel, or colon.[79] This has been applied to an individual with protein-losing enteropathy as a consequence of localized right colon involvement.[169] The causes of death in those who have expired are attributable to the disease and its complications (e.g., cachexia, malnutrition, septicemia, and shock).[89]

Peutz-Jeghers Polyps

In 1921, Peutz reported a familial syndrome of polyps of the gastrointestinal tract with pigmentation of the mouth and other parts of the body.[321] Later, Jeghers and his col-

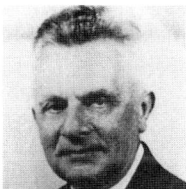

Johannes Laurentius Augustinus Peutz (1886–1957) Johannes Peutz was born in Holland and educated at Rolduc, where he began the study of medicine in 1905. After qualification in 1914, Peutz trained in internal medicine at the Coolsingel Hospital in Rotterdam, as well as at clinics in Germany, Italy, and Belgium. In 1917, he became Principal Physician to the Hospital of St. Joannes de Deo, a Roman Catholic Hospital at The Hague, where he remained for 34 years until his retirement in 1951. He is credited with the establishment of an independent department of internal medicine and a laboratory with electrocardiographic facilities built to his specifications. Peutz was a dedicated clinician and a keen observer, with broad scientific and humanitarian interests. In 1921, he was conferred the degree of Doctor of Medicine for his thesis involving the diagnosis and treatment of disorders of the pancreas. In recognition of his many contributions, Peutz was awarded the Pro Ecclesia et Pontifice Medal, the Order of St. Gregorius the Great, and the Order of Oranje-Nassau. (Courtesy of Faisal Aziz. Photograph courtesy of Udo Rudloff, M.D.)

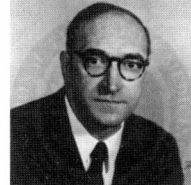

Harold Joseph Jeghers (1904–1990) Harold Jeghers was born September 26, 1904. He received his Bachelor of Science degree in 1928 from the Rensselaer Polytechnic Institute in Troy, New York and then attended the Case Western Reserve University Medical School in Cleveland, Ohio, graduating in 1932. There followed training in internal medicine at the Evans Memorial Institute for Clinical Research in Boston and at the Boston City Hospital. He then became consultant physician to the Boston City Hospital, where he held a teaching post from 1937 to 1946. In 1946, he was appointed Professor of Medicine and Physician-in-Chief at Georgetown University School of Medicine in Washington, DC while also serving as consultant to the Walter Reed Army Medical Center and the National Naval Hospital. Jeghers returned to Boston as Professor of Medicine at Tufts University Medical School in 1966 and retired in 1974. Jeghers was active as a visiting lecturer at a large number of American institutions and English universities. In 1935, Jeghers began building a medical library based on his own method of indexing, which today is known as the Jeghers Medical Index System. (With appreciation to Faisal Aziz.)

leagues established the syndrome by describing a number of cases.[210,211] The disease appears to be transmitted in an autosomal dominant fashion, but *de novo* cases have been reported without any suggestive family history.

The polyps are found most frequently in the small bowel, particularly the jejunum, but they also can occur in the stomach, colon, and rectum.[270] Several hundred patients with the syndrome have been described.

Signs, Symptoms, and Diagnosis

Cutaneous pigmentation usually is noted at birth or in infancy, but the skin changes may actually disappear after puberty.[439] They consist of clusters of black or dark brown spots resembling freckles, 1 to 2 mm in diameter, on and around the lips and buccal mucosa, fingers, and toes.[43] The most common symptom and the one most difficult to manage is abdominal pain, often caused by intestinal obstruction. The obstruction is usually the result of a polyp or of an intussusception. The other frequent complaint is rectal bleeding. Additional signs and symptoms include prolapse of the polyp, passage of the polyp, hematemesis, and anemia. Diagnosis of the syndrome can usually be made on the basis of family history, skin pigmentation, and gastrointestinal symptoms. Contrast studies in addition to endoscopy confirm the extent of the polypoid disease.

Pathology

Macroscopically, the polyps vary in size. They may be as large as several centimeters in diameter, and with increasing size, they tend to become pedunculated. In visual appearance, they look very much like adenomatous polyps (see Polypoid Adenoma, Adenomatous Polyp, and Tubular Adenoma).

Microscopically, the polyps seem to originate from intestinal glandular epithelium along with a muscular branching framework that arises from the muscularis mucosa (Figure 21-8).[146] The tubules of epithelium rest on the branching bands of smooth muscle in a relationship similar to that of the glandular epithelium with the muscularis mucosa of the normal bowel.[270] Because there is no evidence of hyperplasia, cytologic variation, or loss of differentiation, Morson suggested that the lesion represents a hamartomatous process or malformation, rather than a neoplasm.[270]

Treatment

The major problem with this condition lies with the treatment, particularly for the most frequent manifestation, small bowel involvement. Many of these young individuals undergo multiple abdominal operations because of

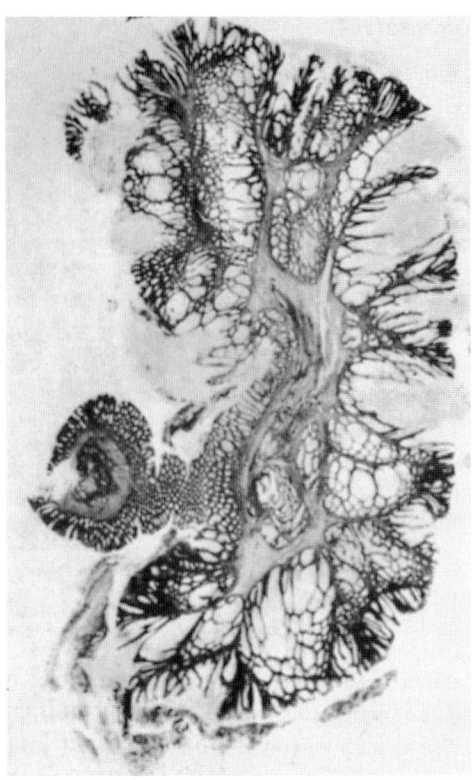

FIGURE 21-8. Peutz-Jeghers polyp of the large intestine. Note the treelike muscular framework. (From Morson BC. Some peculiarities in the histology of intestinal polyps. *Dis Colon Rectum* 1962;5:337, with permission.)

small bowel obstruction and bleeding.[16] Under these circumstances, multiple polyps can be removed by enterotomy and invagination, not resection, or by endoscopic polypectomies through enterotomy. Alternatively, an orally introduced endoscope has been successfully employed at the time of laparotomy by telescoping the small bowel over the instrument.[390,422] Panos and colleagues have used a small-diameter endotracheal tube. They further emphasized the need to lyse all adhesions, to reduce the small bowel intussusception whenever necessary, to "Kocherize" the duodenum, and to use the 170-cm colonoscope.[305] Another approach is to perform operative endoscopy by means of an enterotomy (intraoperative enteroscopy). Edwards and colleagues used this method on 25 patients and identified 350 polyps not detectable by palpation or transillumination.[107] No patient required operative polypectomy within 4 years of clearance by this method. Holt reported the use of small bowel plication, on a prophylactic basis, in a patient who had undergone multiple prior bowel resections because of complications of the disease.[187] Massive small bowel resection should rarely be necessary, thus avoiding the consequences of a short bowel syndrome.

Williams and associates, of St. Mark's Hospital in the United Kingdom, reported the management of ten patients with Peutz-Jeghers syndrome by means of upper and lower gastrointestinal endoscopy.[447] As many as 17 polypectomies were performed in one patient. These investigators recommended upper and lower gastrointestinal endoscopy every other year, the same evaluation if the patient develops symptoms, and laparotomy for any small bowel polyp 1.5 cm in diameter or greater. There is evidence to suggest that an aggressive follow-up approach is justified because the frequency of recurrent tumors increases as the patient becomes older.

Relationship to Cancer

Another concern that has been expressed is the suggestion that there may be an association between Peutz-Jeghers syndrome and the development of gastrointestinal benign and malignant tumors.[67,191,227,259,341,378,388,389] In a review by Konishi and colleagues, 117 neoplasms were found in 103 patients.[227] There were 50 carcinomas of the gastrointestinal tract, the colon and rectum being the most common site. It was established that some of these tumors arose within a Peutz-Jegher polyp, but many probably originated in otherwise normal mucosa. Giardiello and colleagues investigated 31 patients with this syndrome and found that 48% developed a malignancy; this rate was 18 times greater than would be expected.[145] The increased frequency was noted for cancers of both gastrointestinal and nongastrointestinal origin. Spigelman and associates reviewed 72 individuals and found malignant tumors to have developed in 16 (22%), with only one survival.[389] These investigators calculated the chance of dying of cancer by the age of 57 years was 48%. They concluded that there is evidence to suggest a hamartoma-carcinoma sequence in this syndrome and suggested that the gene locus may be relevant to the development of malignancy in general.[389] Hizawa and coworkers investigated 75 gastrointestinal polyps resected surgically or endoscopically from seven patients with this syndrome.[182] Nine were accompanied by an adenomatous component, two of which demonstrated malignant transformation with pedicle invasion. The authors opined that neoplastic transformation was not a rare event and that their results suggested a hamartoma-adenoma-carcinoma sequence in Peutz-Jeghers polyposis.[182]

Linos and colleagues, conversely, reported the considerable Mayo Clinic (Rochester, MN) experience (48 patients) and failed to document one definite instance of cancer; the median follow-up period was 33 years.[242] The authors, furthermore, found that survival was similar to that of the population at large. They recommended that every effort should be made to conserve intestine in the management of this condition. Another reason to be concerned about an aggressive surgical approach is the possibility of misinterpretation of the histologic appearance.

Dippolito and colleagues suggested that careful evaluation may reveal most of these lesions to be, in reality, enteritis cystica profunda (see Chapter 25).[101]

As of this writing, the question of surveillance for malignancy is an unresolved issue. With the probability of an increased incidence of breast, ovarian, and pancreatic cancers, annual mammography and ultrasound studies may be useful.[377]

Of course, it is of paramount importance to distinguish and identify those lesions that represent true (adenomatous) polyps from the hamartomatous tumors. The malignant potential of the former is not a subject for debate.

ADENOMAS

Polyps in the large bowel keep bad company.
Rupert B. Turnbull

Whereas a hyperplastic polyp is the most common "tumor" of the colon and rectum, the adenoma is by far the most frequently observed neoplasm. Adenomas are classified into three categories: polypoid, villous, and mixed. The lesions are by definition benign, but their relationship to the subsequent development of cancer is important (see Polyp-Cancer Sequence).

Polypoid Adenoma, Adenomatous Polyp, and Tubular Adenoma

Probably the seminal if not the most comprehensive study of polyps was published in 1975 by Muto, Bussey, and Morson.[278] More than 3,000 patients were evaluated at St. Mark's Hospital during a period of almost 12 years. Approximately 4,500 benign and malignant neoplasms were interpreted pathologically in these individuals. Seventy-five percent of the benign tumors were classified as adenomatous polyps and 10% as villous adenomas.

The lesions may be as small as 1 mm or greater than 5 cm. They may be pedunculated (Figure 21-9) or sessile (Figure 21-10), with a relatively smooth surface broken by clefts into multiple nodules. The smaller tumors are more likely to have a regular outline and the larger adenomas a lobulated pattern.[177]

Histology

Microscopically, polypoid adenomas consist of closely packed epithelial tubules separated by normal lamina propria, which grow and branch horizontally to the muscularis mucosae.[91] There is, however, no consistent appearance of the tubules; they may be quite regular or

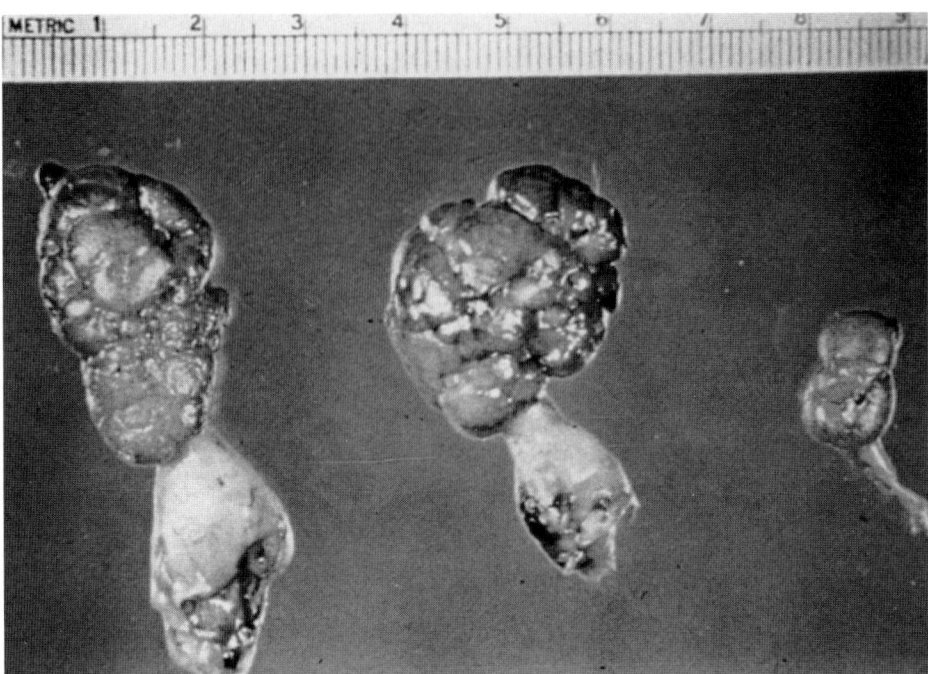

FIGURE 21-9. Adenomatous polyps. These three pedunculated tumors were removed from the same patient. (From Corman ML, Veidenheimer MC, Swinton NW. *Diseases of the anus, rectum, and colon. Part I: neoplasms.* New York: Medcom, 1972, with permission.)

irregular, with or without inflammatory reaction (Figure 21-11). The epithelial cells may become distorted, the nuclei may be hyperchromic (stain more deeply) with increased number, and mucus is reduced (Figure 21-12). Mitoses can be quite frequently observed, but there is no invasion of the muscularis mucosae. Whereas some authors describe certain changes as representative of carcinoma-*in-situ*, others may call the same phenomenon "atypia" or "dysplasia." I prefer not to use the expression carcinoma-*in-situ*, because the term is confusing. If there is no invasion of the muscularis mucosae, the lesion, as far as I am concerned, is benign (Figs. 21-13 and 21-14).

Minute adenomas can actually be detected microscopically as single-gland structures. Oohara and colleagues studied their histogenesis and concluded that they originate from basal cells of the deep layer of mucosa, with those on the lymphoid follicles most likely to undergo neoplastic change.[300] The glands then grow by branching.

The frequency of aneuploidy (see Tumor DNA Content, Chapter 22) and the proliferative activity of adenomatous polyps was investigated by Matthews and colleagues.[258] Twenty percent of the adenomas contained aneuploid cells compared with 63% of adenocarcinomas, and this correlated with increasing degrees of dysplasia. There was a positive correlation between the size of the diploid adenomas and proliferative activity.

Rate of Growth

Normal surface epithelial cells of the colonic mucosa are replaced every 4 to 8 days.[91] Exfoliation of the cells is balanced by cell division and migration. Elias and associates, using stereologic methods, determined that epithelial surfaces were increased up to 226 times in adenomatous polyps when compared with the normal mucosa.[111] These investigators demonstrated, furthermore, that the

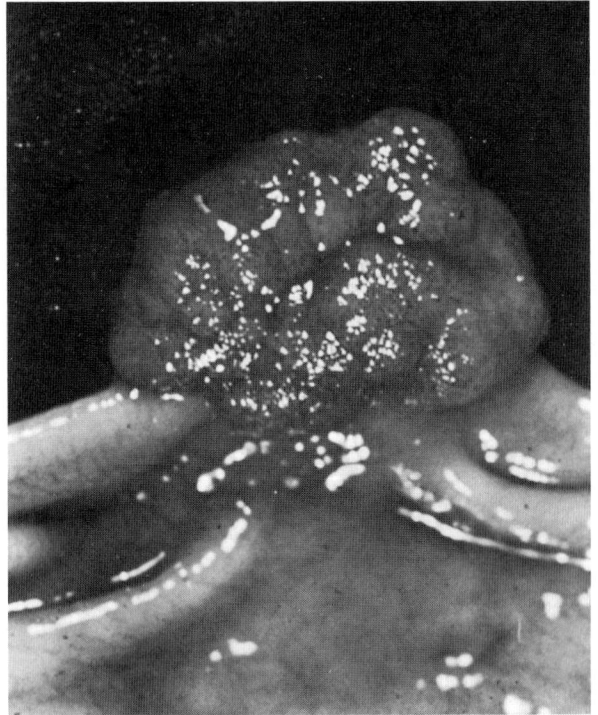

FIGURE 21-10. Sessile adenomatous polyp. (Courtesy of Rudolf Garret, M.D.)

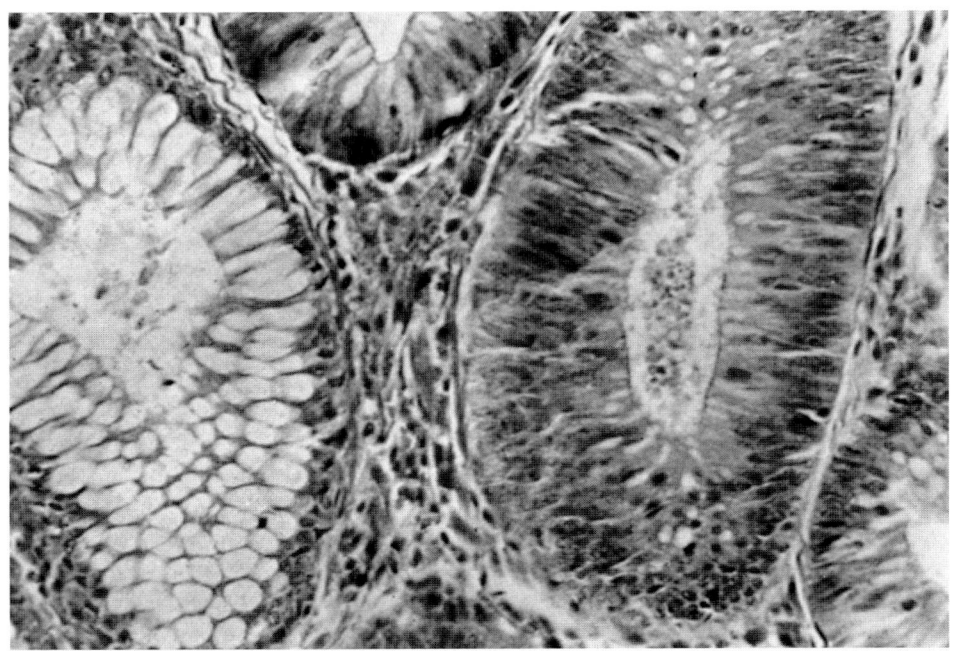

FIGURE 21-11. This section from the edge of a polypoid adenoma illustrates a neoplastic and a normal gland, side by side. Note the crowding of cells, piling up of nuclei, and the loss of ability to produce mucus in the neoplastic gland **(right)**. (From Corman ML, Veidenheimer MC, Swinton NW. *Diseases of the anus, rectum, and colon. Part I: neoplasms.* New York: Medcom, 1972, with permission.)

number of cells was increased up to 370 times. The authors concluded that the increased number was not primarily dependent on mitotic activity but upon amitotic nuclear fragmentation.

Pseudocarcinomatous Invasion

Benign-appearing glandular tissue has been described deep to the muscularis mucosae. This condition has been termed pseudocarcinomatous invasion.[278] It is believed to be associated with larger tumors, those with a long pedicle, and lesions of the sigmoid colon.[91] Day and Morson suggested that the histologic appearance is the result of trauma, possibly secondary to repeated twisting of the stalk.[91] Histologic examination reveals glandlike or cystlike structures in the submucosa that show a cytologic appearance similar to that of the overlying benign tumor (Figure 21-15).

Differentiation of pseudocarcinomatous invasion from invasive cancer is important. In the St. Mark's Hospital series of 56 patients, no one developed a recurrence or metastasis following local excision.[75]

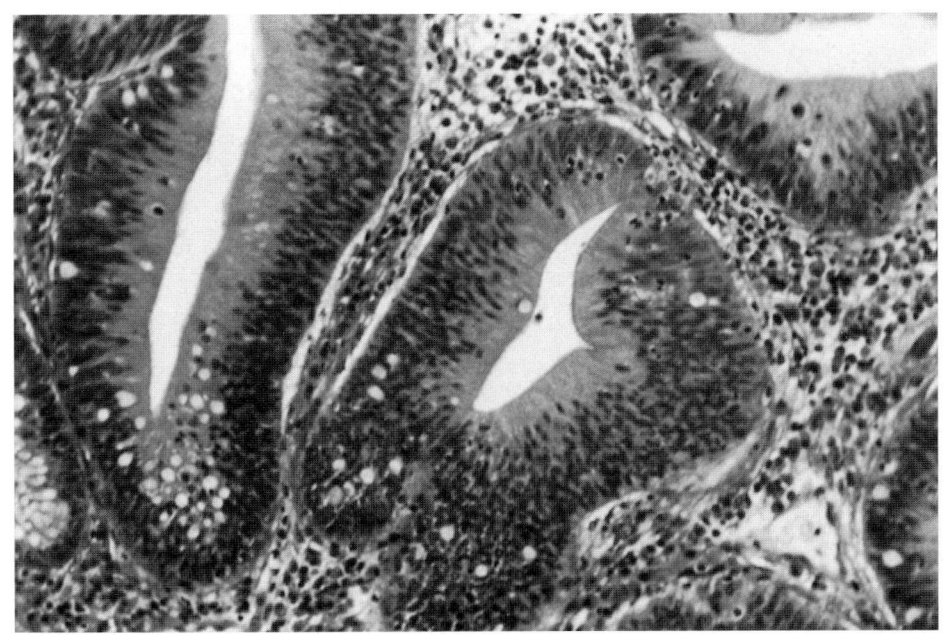

FIGURE 21-12. Adenomatous polyp. Note the dysplasia characterized by loss of polarity with some mitotic figures. (Original magnification × 600; courtesy of Rudolf Garret, M.D.)

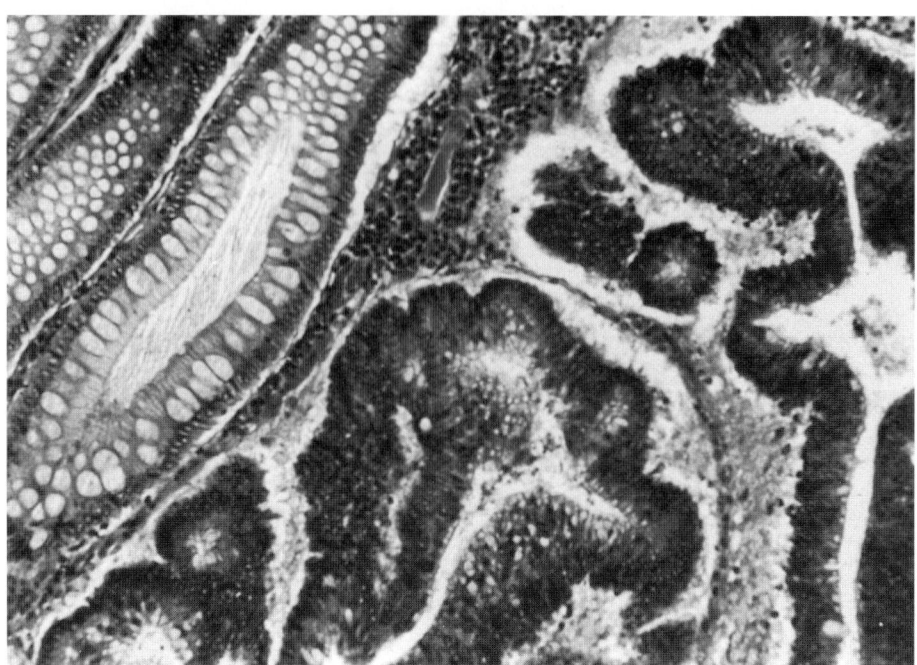

FIGURE 21-13. Adenomatous polyp with severe dysplasia **(right)**; normal glands **(left)**. (Original magnification × 600; courtesy of Rudolf Garret, M.D.)

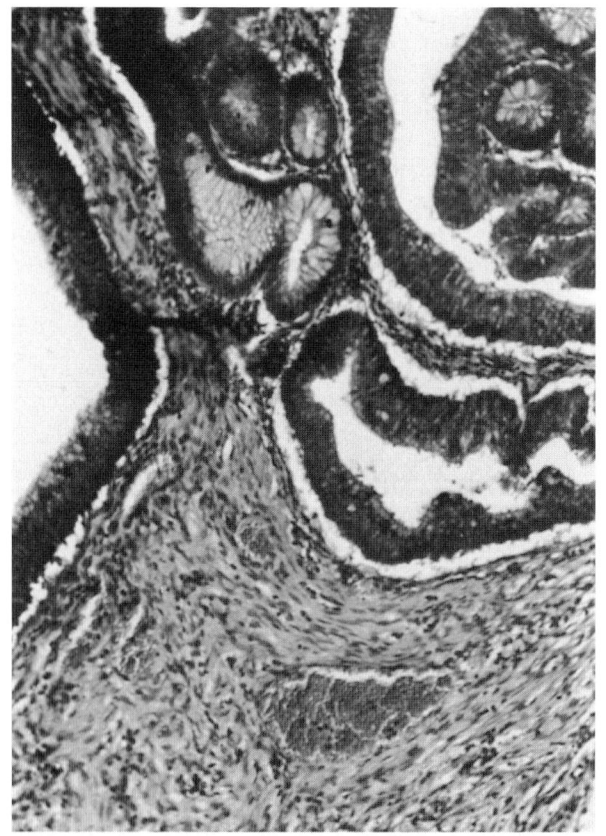

FIGURE 21-14. Adenomatous polyp with severe dysplasia; the whole thickness of the glandular epithelium shows total loss of polarity. (Original magnification × 600; courtesy of Rudolf Garret, M.D.)

Villous Adenoma or Villous Papilloma

The villous adenoma generally appears larger than a polypoid adenoma and is more frequently sessile (Figure 21-16). The margins are usually less well defined than with adenomatous polyps. Despite its size, however, its velvety soft texture may cause it to be missed on digital examination of the rectum (Figure 21-17*A*). However, sigmoidoscopy will readily demonstrate the presence of a lesion. Large tumors can prolapse through the anal canal (Figure 21-18).

Chiu and Spencer reported the Mayo Clinic experience with villous lesions of the colon.[55] During the decade 1964 through 1973, 331 such patients without an associated carcinoma were identified. The median age was 64 years (range, 36 to 82 years); one third of these patients were asymptomatic. Whereas other investigators have noted a more distal location for the lesions, in the Mayo Clinic experience the lesions were evenly distributed throughout the colon. Seven percent of the lesions were smaller than 1 cm, and 61% were smaller than 3 cm.

Symptoms

Although rectal bleeding is the most frequent presenting complaint for both adenomatous conditions, change in bowel habits and mucous discharge are much more frequent concerns in a patient with a large villous adenoma. In fact, there is a unique symptom complex asso-

have been published.[90,152,203,333,352] Jeanneret-Grosjean and Thompson noted that sodium loss is as frequently seen and may actually be the dominant feature of this syndrome in some cases.[209]

Histology

Microscopically, the villous adenoma consists of finger-like processes, each made up of a core of lamina propria covered by epithelial cells growing vertically toward the bowel lumen (Figure 21-20).[91] The epithelium sits on the muscularis mucosae, and in the benign lesion there is no evidence of invasion (Figure 21-21). Whereas there is decreased mucus in polypoid adenomas, some villous adenomas may actually demonstrate an increase (Figure 21-22). Atypia or dysplasia is commonly observed (Figs. 21-23 and 21-24).

Tubulovillous Adenoma, Villoglandular Adenoma, Papillary Adenoma, Villoglandular Polyp, Mixed Adenoma, and Polypoid-Villous Adenoma

The combination of polypoid and villous elements is frequently seen in benign neoplasms of the colon and rectum (Figure 21-25). Histologically, the changes are intermediate between a villous and a polypoid adenoma (Figure 21-26). The distinction, however, between this presentation and that of a "pure" polypoid adenoma is academic. The patient's symptoms, the methods of diagnosis, and the therapy for the benign lesion are identical.

Evaluation and Diagnosis

Adenomas are commonly observed in countries where there is a high incidence of colorectal cancer; their frequency increases with the age of the patient.[92] Depending on the mean age in the various reported series, benign neoplasms of the colon and rectum have been observed in 12% to 60%. Published studies based on radiographic findings generally identify fewer polyps than do postmortem examination results.[92,108,134,344] There are four methods for diagnosing polypoid disease: proctosigmoi-

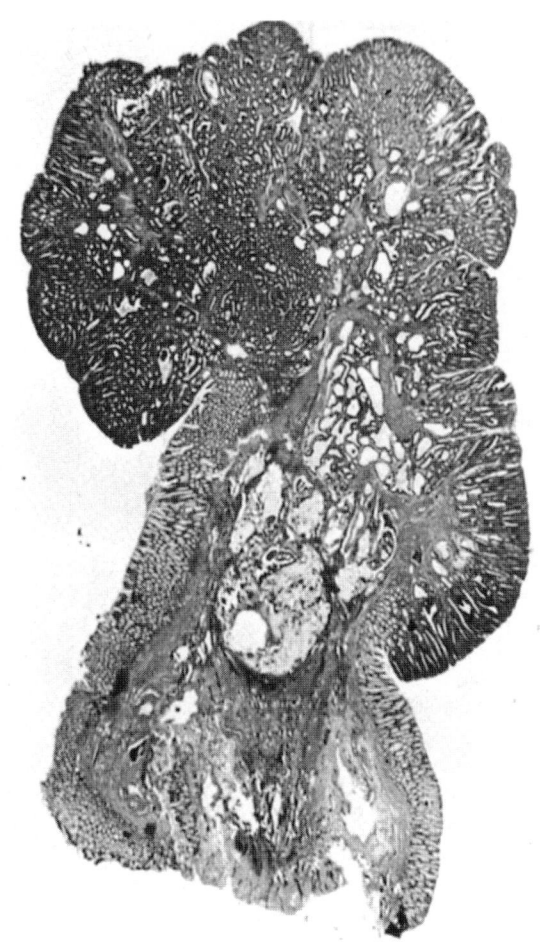

FIGURE 21-15. Adenomatous polyp with pseudoinvasion of the pedicle. The glands are cystically dilated and look identical to those in the polyp. The glands in the stalk are lined by normal-appearing epithelium. (Original magnification × 80; from Corman ML, Veidenheimer MC, Swinton NW. *Diseases of the anus, rectum, and colon. Part I: neoplasms.* New York: Medcom, 1972, with permission.)

ciated with villous adenoma that today has become quite rare: hypokalemia and dehydration. The syndrome was originally reported by McKittrick and Wheelock in 1954 and is attributed to the loss of copious fluid and electrolytes from the mucus-secreting tumor (Figure 21-19).[265] Since this original article, many other reports

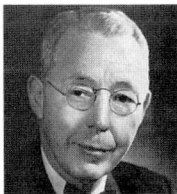

Leland Sterling McKittrick (1893–1978) Leland McKittrick was born in Thorp, Wisconsin, the son of a town physician. He attended the University of Wisconsin and graduated from Harvard Medical School in 1918. McKittrick began his surgical experience at the University of Minnesota but then transferred to the Massachusetts General Hospital in Boston. Following the completion of his training, he joined the surgical practice of a preeminent Boston surgeon, Daniel Fiske Jones. McKittrick was a thoughtful and innovative clinician. He introduced synchronous resection with ileostomy for ulcerative colitis, rather than employ the multistaged approach that was in vogue, and he was also an advocate of side-to-end anastomoses in the bowel. In addition to his technical mastery, he was an authority on gastrointestinal pathophysiology. He was the first to recognize the electrolyte imbalance and fluid loss associated with villous adenomas of the large bowel. McKittrick took on a leadership role in surgery, not only in New England, but also nationally. He was elected President of the American Surgical Association in 1965. He retired from surgical practice at the age of 78 but pursued an active life until his death at age 85. (Reproduced in part from Drazan KE. Leland Sterling McKittrick. *Dis Colon Rectum* 1997;40:1494. Photograph courtesy of John McKittrick, M.D.)

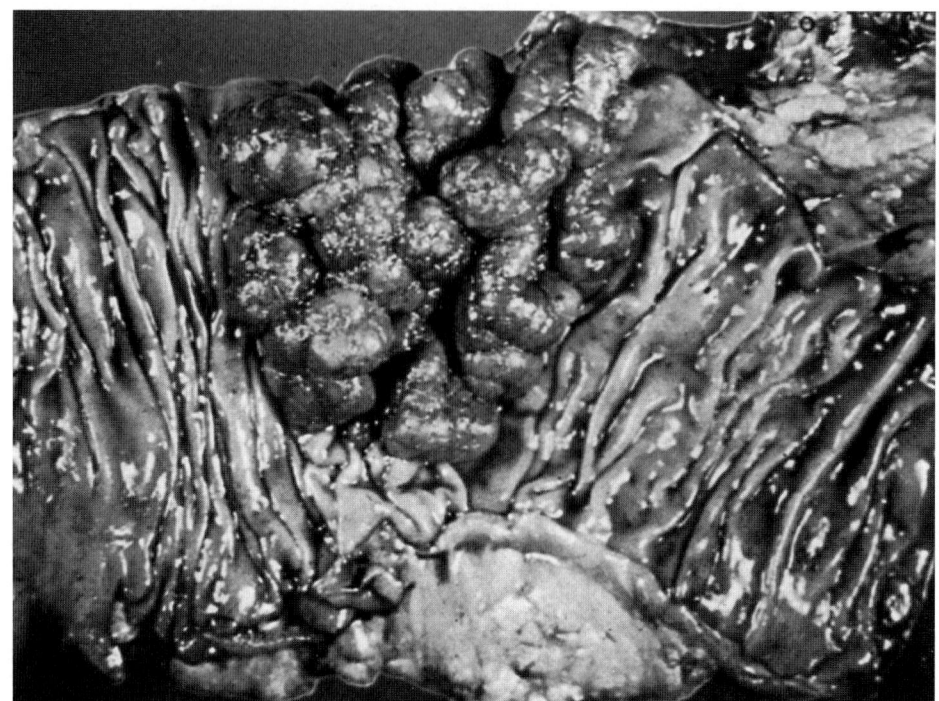

FIGURE 21-16. A villous adenoma in a resected specimen demonstrates the soft, velvety appearance of this lesion. (From Corman ML, Veidenheimer MC, Swinton NW. *Diseases of the anus, rectum, and colon. Part I: neoplasms.* New York: Medcom, 1972, with permission.)

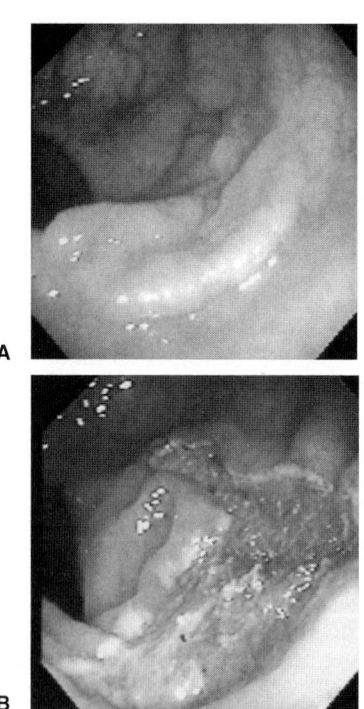

FIGURE 21-17. **(A)** The velvety appearance of sessile villous adenoma can be seen with the colonoscope. **(B)** Snare electrocoagulation reveals an extensive open wound that encompasses approximately one half of the bowel circumference. (See Color Fig. 21-17.)

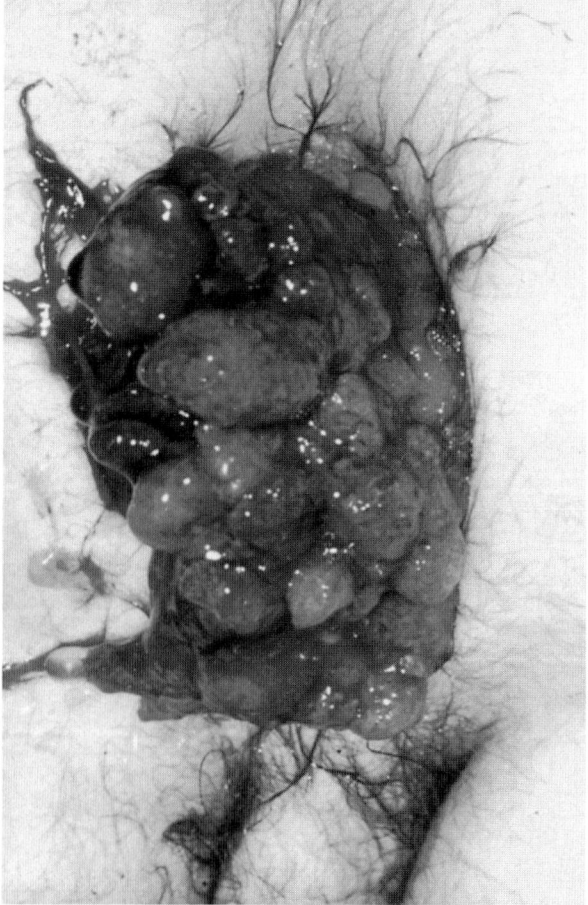

FIGURE 21-18. Villous adenoma presenting outside the anus. (Courtesy of Rudolf Garret, M.D.)

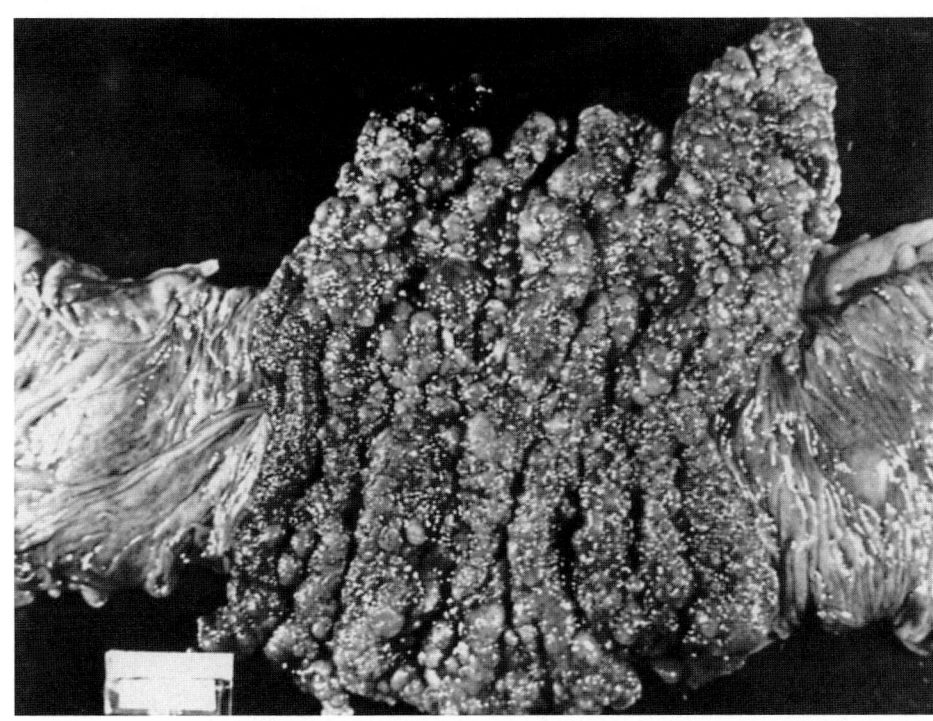

FIGURE 21-19. A large villous adenoma. This huge lesion produced electrolyte depletion. (From Corman ML, Veidenheimer MC, Swinton NW. *Diseases of the anus, rectum, and colon. Part I: neoplasms.* New York: Medcom, 1972, with permission.)

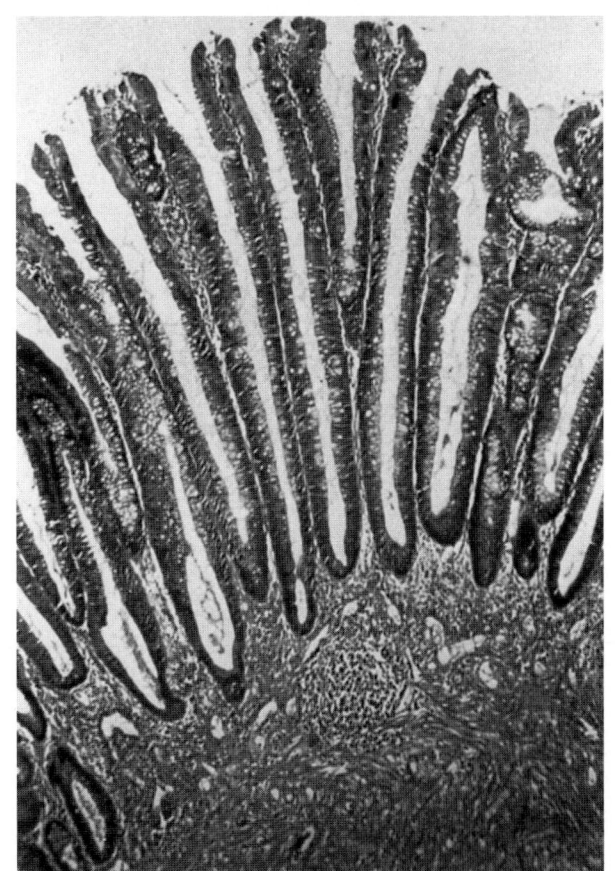

FIGURE 21-20. Villous adenoma. Papillary fronds extend from the mucosa. (Original magnification × 280; from Corman ML, Veidenheimer MC, Swinton NW. *Diseases of the anus, rectum, and colon. Part I: neoplasms.* New York: Medcom, 1972, with permission.)

doscopy (flexible sigmoidoscopy), endoscopic colonoscopy, virtual (radiologic) colonoscopy, and barium enema (with or without air).[329] The relative merits of these approaches and the techniques, themselves, are discussed in Chapters 4 and 5. It is perhaps worth mentioning again, however, some of the more obvious limitations and advantages.

Sigmoidoscopy

We reported results of rigid proctosigmoidoscopy as peformed on an asymptomatic population.74 Three fourths were men (mean age, 51 years), and one fourth were women (mean age, 55 years). The mean depth of insertion of the instrument was 20 cm. Benign lesions were found in 220 patients (9%).

Radiologic Evaluation

Depending on the barium enema technique employed, polyps of the colon can be identified in 1% to 13% of patients; the double-contrast (air-contrast) approach gives a higher yield (see Chapter 4).[4,24,232,303] The air-contrast enema is considered the preferred option by many radiologists for evaluating the colon, but especially when the patient has a prior history of polyps or carcinoma. Lesions as small as 2 or 3 mm may be identified by this technique. We determined, in 200 asymptomatic patients who were found to have one or more rectal polyps, that a barium enema demonstrated a synchronous, proximal neoplasm in 2.5%.[76]

(text continues on page 718)

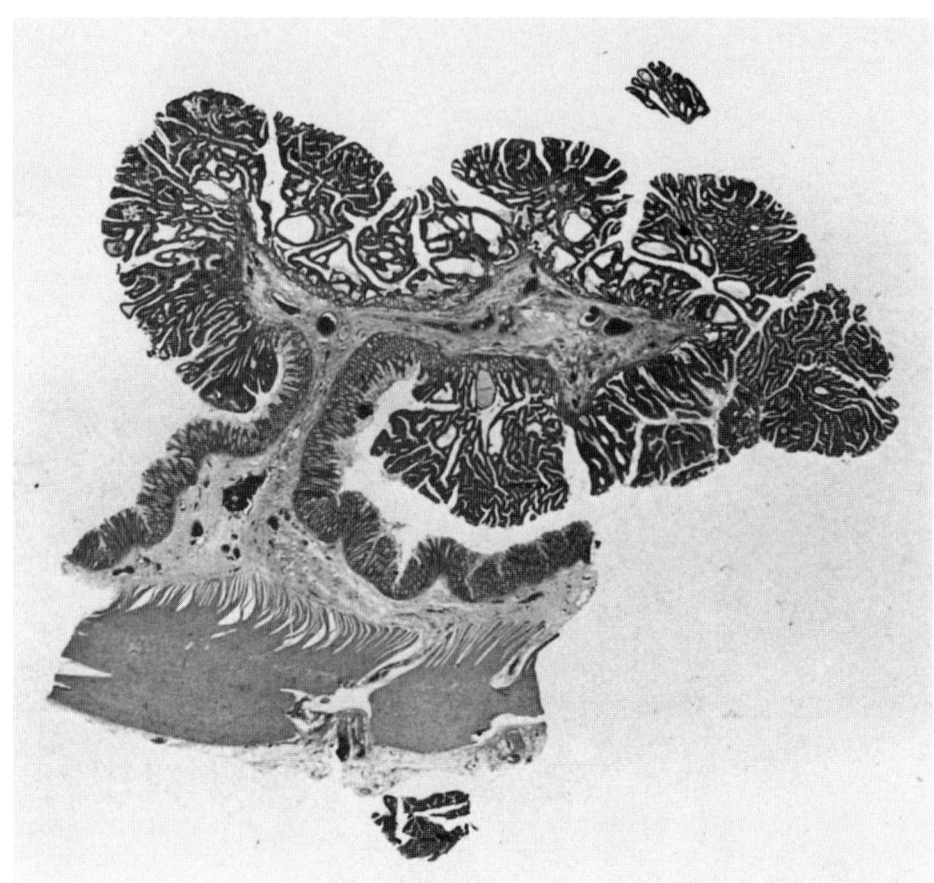

FIGURE 21-21. Villous adenoma (whole mount specimen). Note the papillary projections with transition between the normal large bowel mucosa and the polyp. (Courtesy of Rudolf Garret, M.D.)

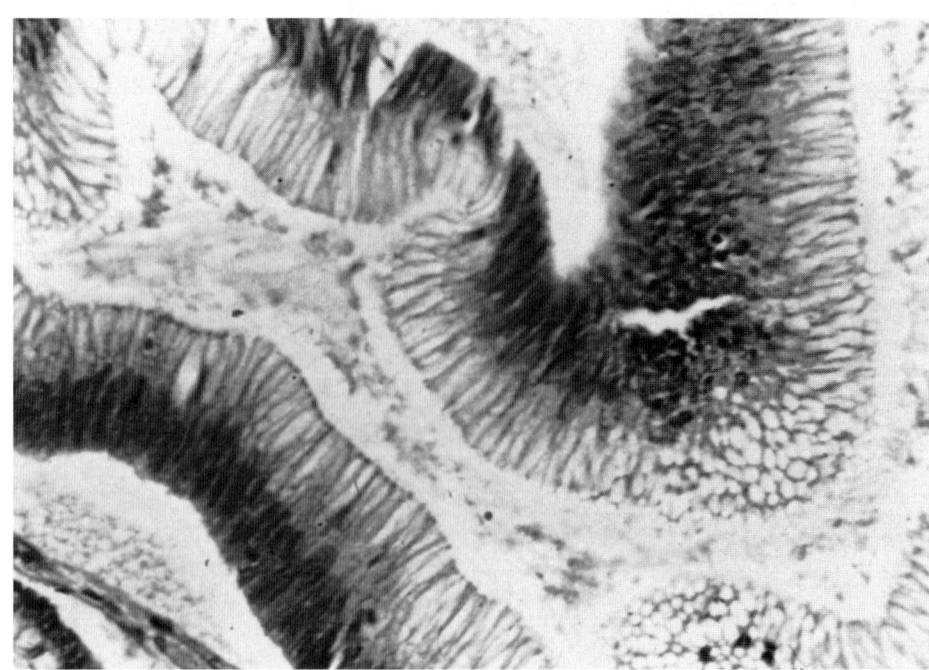

FIGURE 21-22. Villous adenoma. The neoplastic gland is lined by cells that have retained their capacity for the production of mucus. Rich in electrolytes, this mucus accounts for the occasionally observed abnormalities that occur in patients with large lesions. (Original magnification × 600; from Corman ML, Veidenheimer MC, Swinton NW. *Diseases of the anus, rectum, and colon. Part I: neoplasms.* New York: Medcom, 1972, with permission.)

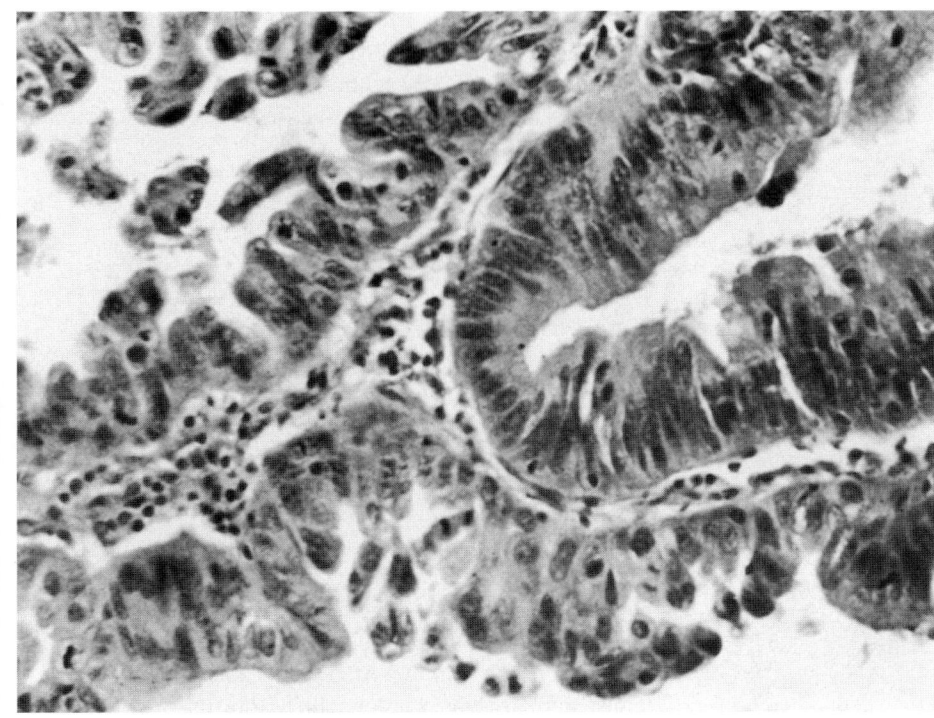

FIGURE 21-23. Villous adenoma. Foci of atypical epithelial hyperplasia. (Original magnification × 600; from Corman ML, Veidenheimer MC, Swinton NW. *Diseases of the anus, rectum, and colon. Part I: neoplasms.* New York: Medcom, 1972, with permission.)

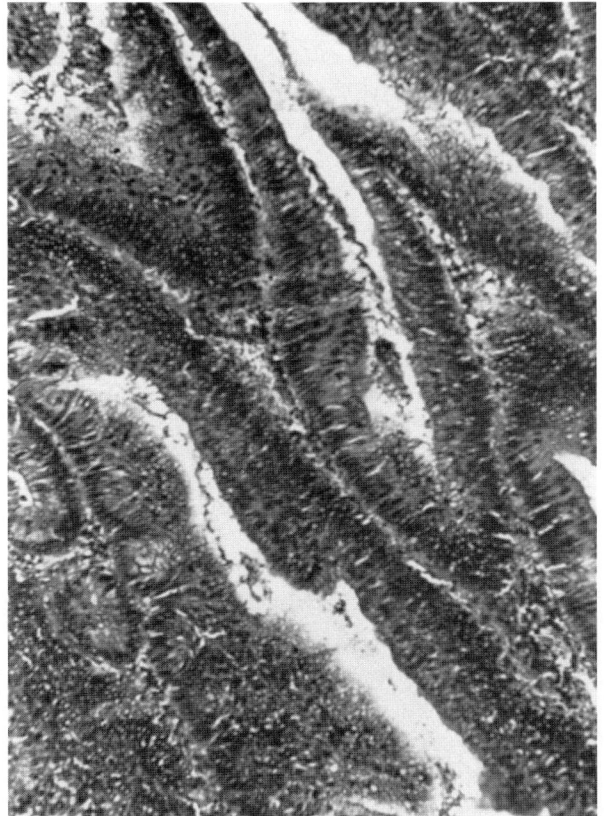

FIGURE 21-24. Villous adenoma. The lining cells of the glandular epithelium show a loss of polarity; this represents a mild dysplastic change. (Original magnification × 600; courtesy of Rudolf Garret, M.D.)

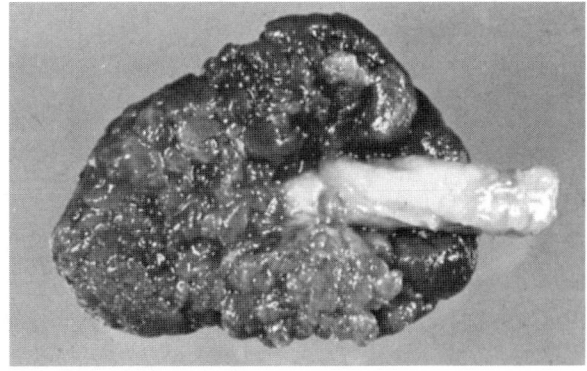

FIGURE 21-25. Villoglandular polyp. This pedunculated lesion has areas of varied coloration that, on microscopic examination, showed both villous and adenomatous changes. (From Corman ML, Veidenheimer MC, Swinton NW. *Diseases of the anus, rectum, and colon. Part I: neoplasms.* New York: Medcom, 1972, with permission.)

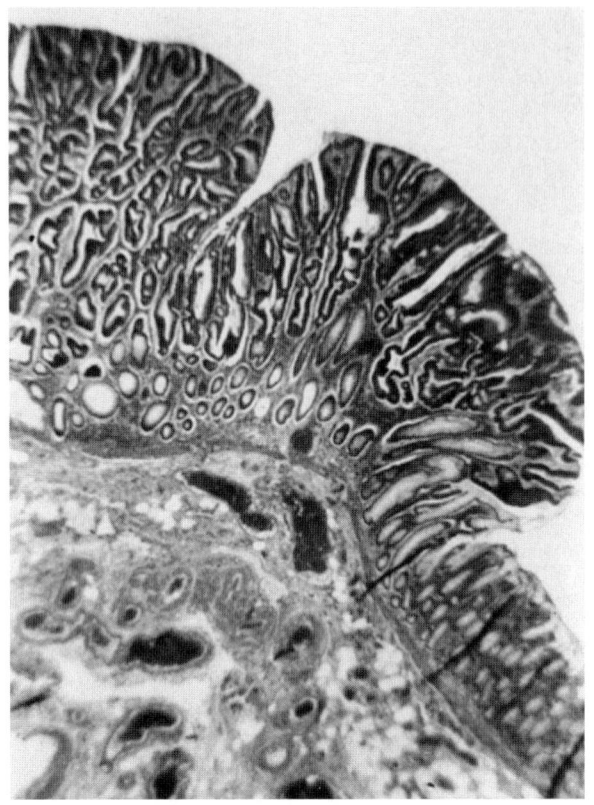

FIGURE 21-26. Villoglandular polyp. (Original magnification × 280; courtesy of Rudolf Garret, M.D.)

The radiologist cannot ascertain the histologic nature of a polyp, although certain characteristic features may be identified. Of particular importance is to note the presence or absence of a pedicle or stalk (Figs. 21-27 through 21-29). Although a pedicle does not connote benignity, it implies that one should at least attempt to remove the lesion by means of the colonoscope, and that an adequate margin will probably be obtained (see Figure 5-18). Sessile lesions are more likely to be malignant and are more difficult to remove by means of colonoscopy (Figure 21-30; see Figure 5-33). Again, the radiologist should not be the arbiter of the pathologic diagnosis.

Villous adenomas often have a characteristic radiologic appearance. They have an irregular surface because of the frondlike growths; barium in the interstices of the tumor surface produces striated or lacelike radiographic features (Figure 21-31).[28]

Colonoscopy

Colonoscopy and colonoscopy-polypectomy are the diagnostic and therapeutic modalities that have been responsible for the quantum advance in our knowledge of polypoid disease over the past 25 years. The indications, equipment, technique, and complications are discussed in Chapter 5. Although the procedure of polypectomy required hospitalization in the past, outpatient management is now considered safe if the patient is without serious illness, is reliable, and is near adequate medical facilities should the need for care arise.[293] The following is a summary of opinions and results in a number of selected studies, although again the reader is referred to Chapter 5.

Knutson and Max reported their experience of 662 patients;[226] 421 polypoid lesions, three fourths of which were benign, were seen in 281 patients. In this report, the comparative overall inaccuracy rate for air-contrast barium enema (false-positive and false-negative) was 30%. The major morbidity was the "lost polyp." Cowen and associates reported 741 polyps removed during 300 examinations.[81] Thirty-six were excised in one patient, and a 7-cm villous adenoma was removed in another. Forty percent were not identified by barium enema. Other investigators, in a comparison of two techniques, demonstrated 90% accuracy of air-contrast enema and 91% accuracy of colonoscopy.[127]

A colonoscopic survey of adenomas was reported from St. Mark's Hospital.[149] More than 1,000 polyps were removed, three fourths of which were left sided. With increasing polyp size there was a greater tendency to villous involvement; this was associated with a higher incidence of malignant change. Shinya and Wolff, in an analysis of 7,000 polyps endoscopically removed, found that polyp size was related to malignant change, but they noted that invasive cancer was found in polyps less than 1 cm in diameter.[378]

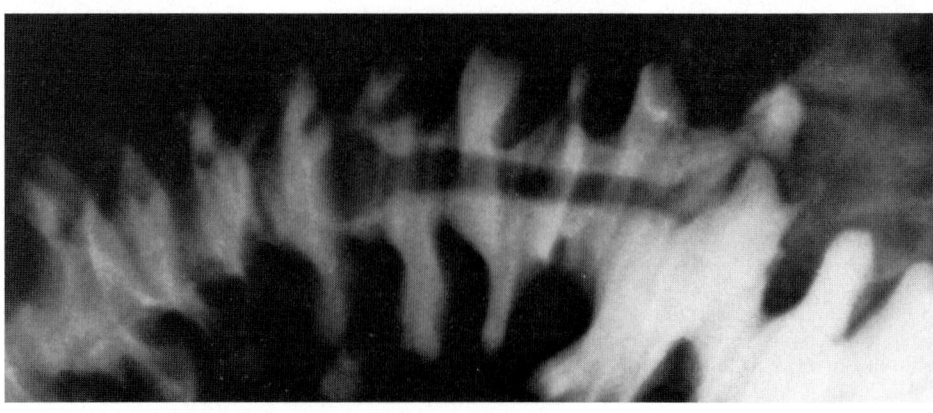

FIGURE 21-27. Adenomatous polyp. Barium enema demonstrates a 1.5-cm lesion on a very long pedicle.

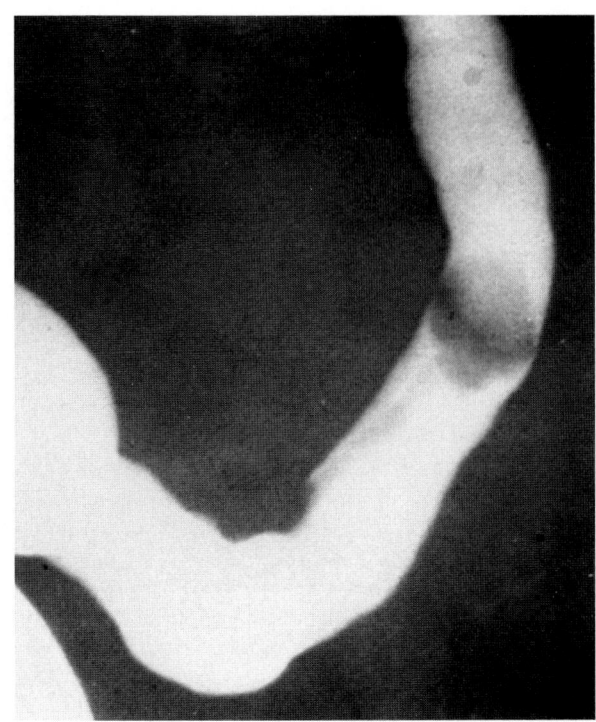

FIGURE 21-28. Villoglandular polyp. Note the slightly lobulated filling defect on a long pedicle demonstrated by barium enema. (From Corman ML, Veidenheimer MC, Swinton NW. *Diseases of the anus, rectum, and colon. Part I: neoplasms.* New York: Medcom, 1972, with permission.)

Visual determination of the neoplastic or nonneoplastic, benign or malignant natures of polyps is often an unsuccessful exercise, as has been mentioned. Despite generalizations concerning size, color, and the presence or absence of a pedicle, the only definitive means for establishing the diagnosis is histologic confirmation. Webb and Dyess offered five criteria suggestive of malignant change: friability, ulceration, firmness, lobulation, and asymmetry.[436] To this, they also added the "dunce cap" appearance (a broad base tapering to a narrow tip) as indicative of invasive carcinoma.[436]

Tedesco and co-workers, in a study of small polyps (less than 5 mm), reported that approximately one half were neoplastic and one half were metaplastic (hyperplastic).[406] Nishizawa and colleagues used the magnifying fiberoptic colonoscope and dissecting microscope.[291] They could detect a characteristic "pit pattern" of abnormality in apparently normal colonic mucosa (as small as 1 mm) with the frequent presence of an "incipient" adenoma. Chapuis and associates, using the flexible sigmoidoscope, attempted to diagnose the nature of the lesion by inspection; the diagnosis was correct in 82% of the cases.[51] Although the size of the polyp prejudiced the examiner, this was not a reliable indicator of the diagnosis.

One question that must be asked is whether endoscopic measurements of colonic polyps are truly reliable. Fennerty and co-workers conducted a study using artificial polyps in an endoscopy teaching model, utilizing the services of eight experienced endoscopists.[119] The sizes of 13 polyps were estimated at two separate sessions 2 weeks

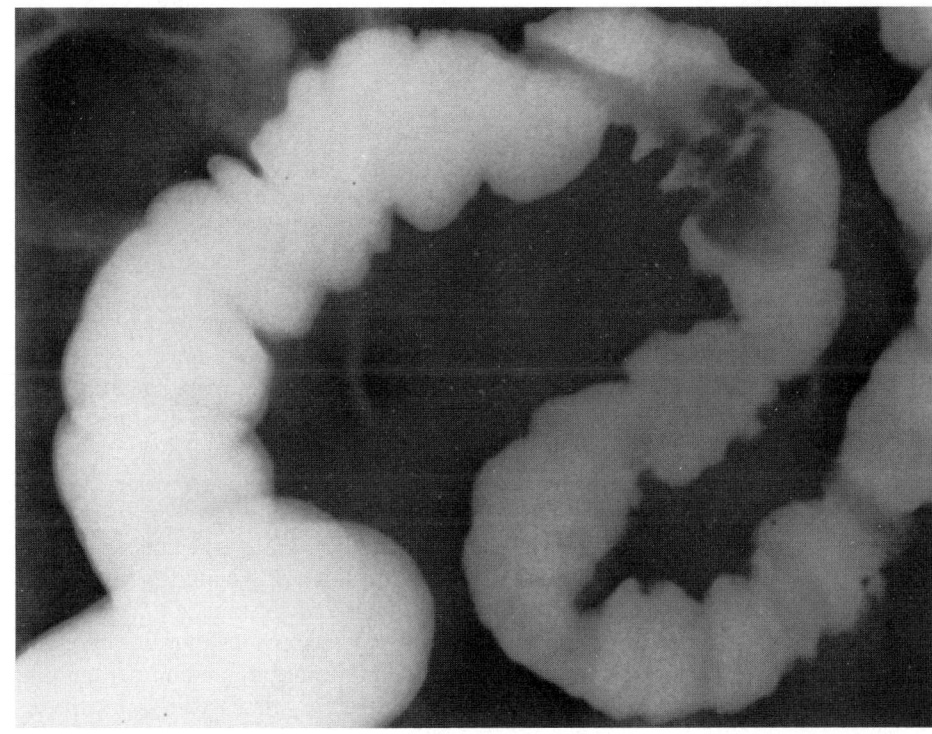

FIGURE 21-29. Villous adenoma. This large lesion (3.5 cm) is on a long pedicle. Barium enema demonstrates irregularity of the surface resulting from a frondlike growth.

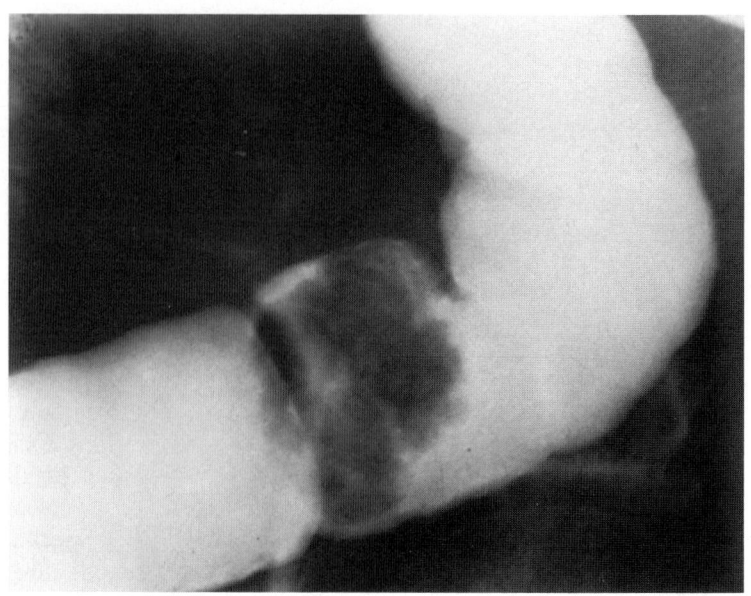

FIGURE 21-30. Villoglandular polyp. This sessile 3-cm lesion was found to be benign; it was removed by colonoscopy-polypectomy.

apart. The investigators observed that estimates of polyp size tended to be significantly lower than the true polyp size for all lesions and by all endoscopists at both sessions. They also found a statistically significant difference in the magnitude of the underestimation between the first and the second session.[119]

Total colonoscopy is a requisite for patients found to harbor a neoplasm of the colon. We reported colonoscopic examination of the entire colon performed on 146 patients for radiographically suspected benign polypoid disease.[73] Of 36 who did not have a neoplastic lesion at the suspected site, seven (19%) had unsuspected small, benign polypoid adenomas elsewhere in the colon. Sixty-two of 110 individuals (56%) who were found to have a

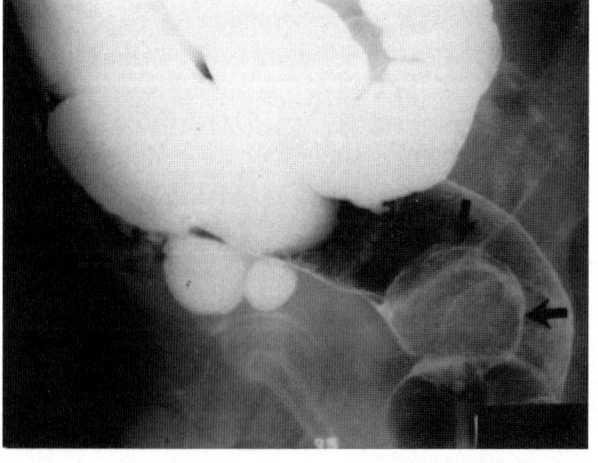

FIGURE 21-31. Villous adenoma of the rectum. Barium enema shows a slightly lobulated, broad-based filling defect on the anterior wall *(arrows)*. The frondlike appearance is suggestive of a villous adenoma.

lesion at the radiographically demonstrated location harbored a total of 128 additional, unsuspected polyps. Whereas the radiographically demonstrated polyps were predominantly on the left side, two thirds of the unsuspected neoplasms were found proximal to the splenic flexure, resulting in a more uniform distribution of neoplastic colonic polypoid disease (Figure 21-32).[73]

Read and co-workers prospectively analyzed the importance of so-called diminutive polyps (less than or equal to 5 mm in diameter) detected by sigmoidoscopy with respect to the identification of a proximal colon tumor.[339] They found that 29% of patients with small polyps and 57% with large polyps had one or more proximal neoplasms in the colon. The authors concluded that the substantial prevalence of proximal colonic neoplasms, including advanced lesions, warranted total colonoscopy in individuals, even with rectosigmoid adenomas 5 mm in diameter or smaller.[339] Pennazio and associates reached a similar conclusion in their study of 733 small colorectal neoplasms.[320] They recommended total colonoscopy in all patients with distal polyps, regardless of their size and, furthermore, regardless of histology. Others have also recommended that any patient with polyps seen during screening sigmoidoscopy, regardless of histopathology, should undergo colonoscopy.[302]

There has been a change in the distribution of colon and rectal cancer to a more proximal location, an observation originally reported by Cady and colleagues (see Chapter 22).[46] Others, in analyzing benign polypoid disease, have shown a similar left-to-right shift.[156]

What of screening colonoscopy in the asymptomatic patient? At this time, the procedure should certainly be performed on individuals at an increased risk for the development of neoplasms, but it is reasonable to consider

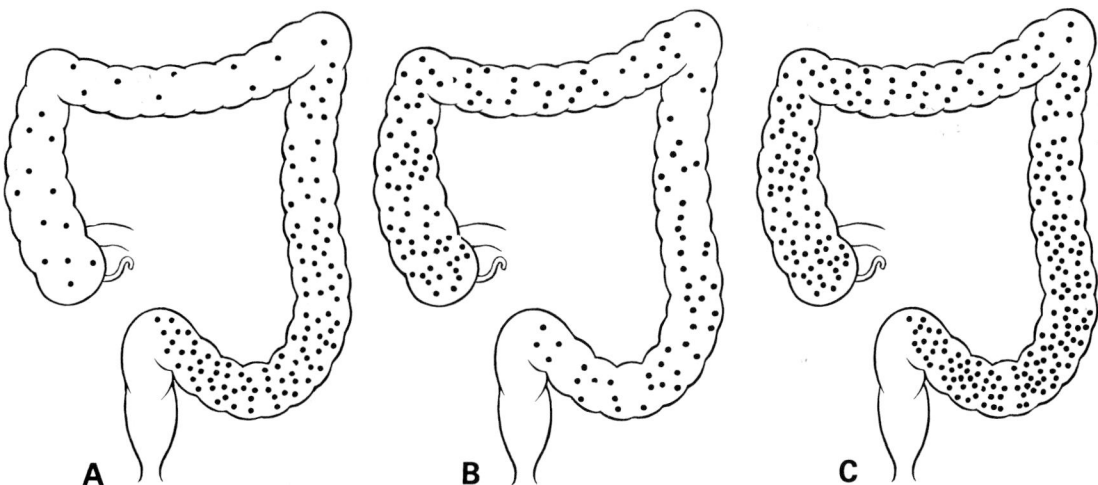

FIGURE 21-32. Distribution of colonic polyps. **(A)** Radiologically suspected. **(B)** Unsuspected. **(C)** Total distribution. (Illustration by FE Steckel; based on data from Coller JA, Corman ML, Veidenheimer MC. Colonic polypoid disease: need for total colonoscopy. *Am J Surg* 1976;131:490.)

this evaluation every 5 to 10 years for all asymptomatic adults.[287] Surveillance in patients with a history of adenomas requires colonoscopy at 4- or 5-year intervals when the colon has been found to be clear on an interim study.[31]

Polyp-Cancer Sequence

The significance of neoplastic polyps would be merely of academic interest were it not for the relationship between these lesions and the subsequent development of carcinoma.[411,428] This relationship has already been alluded to, but it is important to discuss the evidence for this conclusion. Some documentation is indeed circumstantial, but it is not without validity. It may seem that this observation has been well known and established for more than 100 years, but it has been only about 40 years since the validity of the polyp-cancer sequence has been generally accepted. In was in 1939 that Swinton and Warren published their seminal article on the subject, and then it was roundly criticized.[400] At the time, most physicians believed cancers of the colon arose *de novo*, in otherwise normal bowel.

Synchronous Cancer

Morson and Dawson demonstrated that about one third of resected specimens for colon and rectal cancer harbor one or more adenomas.[273] Greene reported an incidence of 13%.[156] In a postmortem study, Helwig was able to

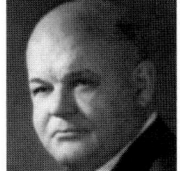

Neil Williams Swinton (1907–1980)   Swinton was born in Ontonagon, Michigan and spent his early years in Marquette. He attended Lehigh University and the University of Michigan, and he obtained his medical degree from the latter institution in 1929. Following postgraduate training in the Department of Surgery at the university, he became a fellow in surgery at the Lahey Clinic in Boston. He volunteered for duty at the start of World War II and served with distinction as Commanding Officer in a portable surgical hospital in the Southwest Pacific Theatre. Following the war, he returned to the Lahey Clinic as a staff surgeon and ultimately became one of the leaders in the field of proctology in the United States. Swinton wrote or coauthored 144 scientific papers, including the paper quoted earlier that he wrote with his colleague, Shields Warren, Chairman of the Department of Pathology at the New England Deaconess Hospital. Swinton was recognized by his colleagues through serving as President of the American Proctologic Society, now the American Society of Colon and Rectal Surgeons. He was an Honorary Fellow of the Section of Proctology of the Royal Society of Medicine. After 40 years as a surgeon at the clinic, he retired to Arizona, where he died.

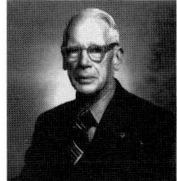

Shields Warren (1898–1980)   Shields Warren was born in Cambridge, Massachusetts on February 26, 1898, the grandson of the first president of Boston University. He received a classical Greek and Latin education and entered Boston University, from which he graduated in 1918. Following a period of ill health and travel, he was admitted to Harvard Medical School, where he developed a lifelong interest in pathology. He received an appointment to the then world-reknowned Pathology Department at Boston City Hospital. In 1927, he went to the New England Deaconess Hospital in Boston and established their Department of Pathology, remaining as Chairman until 1963. Warren was recognized by his clinical peers as the "pathologist to the living" because of their reliance on his expertise in the decision-making process for the care of their patients. In 1948, he was appointed Professor at Harvard Medical School. His interest in radiation and radiation injuries resulted in his involvement in the shipment of uranium ore during the Second World War. From 1947 until 1952, he assumed the post of Head of the Division of Biology and Medicine at the Atomic Energy Commision. He died, on July 1, 1980 on Cape Cod, Massachusetts. (Abstracted from Corman ML. Landmark Articles of the 20th Century. *Semin Colon Rectal Surg* 1999;10:209.)

show adenomas in one half the patients found to have a large bowel carcinoma (Figure 21-33).[177] In ten other patients who were found to have "an adenoma with carcinomatous transition," eight harbored additional adenomas.[177] In those patients found to have two or more synchronous carcinomas, Heald and Bussey found that 75% had an associated adenoma.[173] Numerous colonoscopy studies have confirmed this frequent association.

Metachronous Cancer

Gilbertsen's studies from the University of Minnesota Medical Center have demonstrated a marked reduction in the incidence of large bowel cancers by a program of follow-up proctosigmoidoscopy after polypectomy.[147] Only 15% of the statistically anticipated carcinomas developed, and each of these was an early lesion. Prager and associates traced approximately 300 patients 15 years following sigmoidoscopy-polypectomy for a benign neoplasm.[329] Twelve were found to have developed a carcinoma in the interval. The number of malignancies was twice that which would be expected, and the distribution of these lesions was more proximal in location. The authors concluded as follows: first, patients with colorectal polyps have a greater tendency to develop colorectal cancer than do unaffected persons; second, carcinomas develop in areas not previously the site of polyps; third, proctosigmoidoscopy is inadequate as the only modality of surveillance; and finally, without the prior polypec-

tomy, the incidence of cancer would in all probability have been higher. Winawer and colleagues also have concluded that colonoscopy-polypectomy prevents the development of future colorectal cancers.[452] In their study of more than 1,000 patients who underwent complete colonoscopy and removal of all benign polyps, with a follow-up of 8,401 person-years, five asymptomatic early-stage colorectal cancers were detected. This is much fewer than would be expected over this period of time, and the results are highly statistically significant.[452]

It has long been known that patients who have undergone colon resection for carcinoma are at an increased risk for the subsequent development of a malignancy.[44] Morson reported that the metachronous cancer rate at St. Mark's Hospital was approximately 4%.[271] The average time interval was about 10 years, implying that the polyp-cancer development period, specifically, is that length of time. The frequency of identifying benign neoplasms in such patients is also high. In a later study from the same institution, Morson and Bussey reported that 50% of patients who had single adenomas initially developed a metachronous adenoma within 15 years, but the risk for cancer was much less (one in 15 patients).[272] The magnitude of risk increased considerably, however, when the individual presented with more than one adenoma.

Henry and colleagues reported 154 patients who had previously undergone polypectomy and were followed for a mean of 7 years.[178] Thirty percent developed recurrent polyps; the rate was 16 times that expected in a popula-

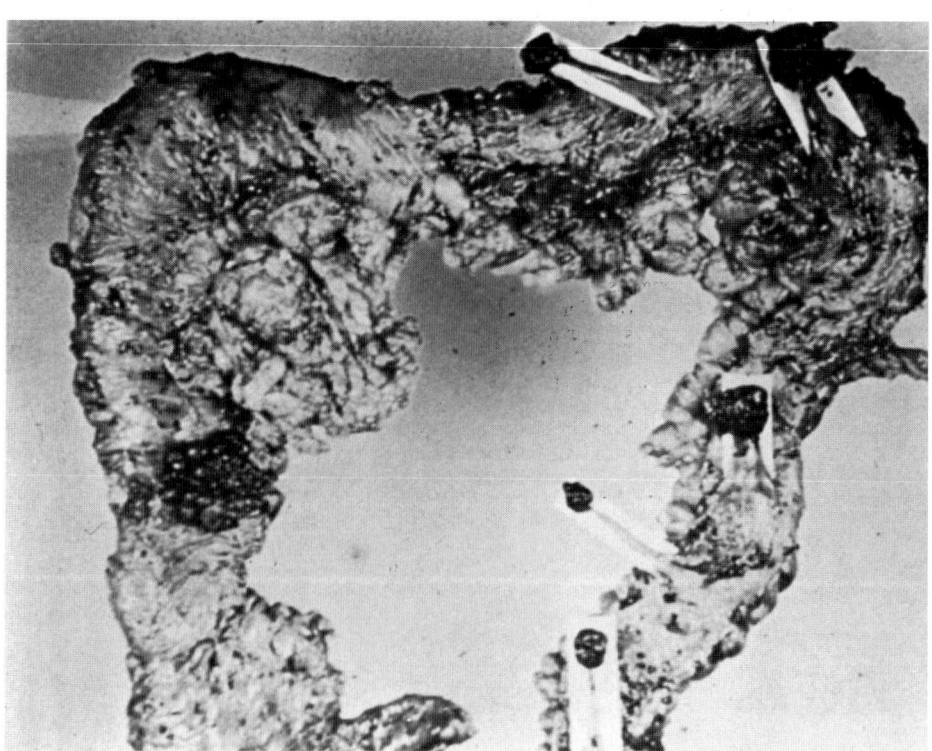

FIGURE 21-33. Carcinoma with multiple polyps. There are five pedunculated, adenomatous polyps in the left and transverse colon and a carcinoma in the ascending colon. (From Corman ML, Veidenheimer MC, Swinton NW. *Diseases of the anus, rectum, and colon. Part I: neoplasms.* New York: Medcom, 1972, with permission.)

tion of similar age and gender during the first year. Furthermore, in those who developed a recurrent polyp, one third developed another recurrence.

Geographic Distribution

Carcinoma of the colon and rectum is primarily a disease of Western civilization. Adenomatous polyps parallel the geographic distribution, with a high incidence in Europe and in the United States, in other countries with high meat consumption, and in urban populations. The epidemiology of carcinoma is discussed in Chapter 22.

Anatomic Distribution

The distribution of benign tumors of the colon is similar to that of cancers: more frequent in the distal bowel, with a relatively high incidence in the cecum. Ekelund, in an autopsy study, found more than one half of patients to have adenomas of the rectum and sigmoid colon, slightly fewer than those who were found to have a carcinoma.[110] Nineteen percent of the benign lesions were in the right colon, virtually the same as the distribution for cancer. In Helwig's series, the sigmoid colon was the most common site of adenomas, adenomas with malignant transformation, and carcinomas.[177] Other sites were correspondingly involved. Additional studies have demonstrated a more uniform distribution for adenomas than for carcinomas; this observation may be anticipating a further trend to more proximal cancers. Greene noted that a left-to-right shift was apparent in the decade from 1971 to 1980 in comparison with the prior 10-year period.[156] Thirty-two percent of adenomas were found in the rectum in the former decade and 13% in the latter.

Age

It should be expected that adenomatous polyps antedate cancer by several years, but until recently this could not be well documented. The probable reason for this is that patients with cancer are usually symptomatic, and the date of onset can be quite accurately reported. Polyps, especially when small, may be asymptomatic for a considerable period of time. Morson estimates that evolution of the polyp-cancer sequence is approximately 10 years.[271] In my own experience, the mean age of patients who underwent colonoscopy-polypectomy was 55, compared with patients with colorectal cancer, whose mean age was 62.

Gender

Men and women have an approximately equal frequency of colorectal cancer; the same observation is true for adenomas. Women have a slightly greater number of right-sided lesions (both benign and malignant).

Miscellaneous Factors

The high incidence of polyps parallels that of colorectal cancer in every population-based study. Whether this is related to diet or to other environmental factors, one cannot deny the validity of the observation. Kikendall and colleagues observed that cigarette smoking and beer consumption are independent risk factors for the development of colonic adenomas.[221] In a Japanese study, cigarette smoking was found to be a risk factor for the development of colorectal adenoma.[280] Naveau and colleagues reported that cirrhosis is an independent risk factor for colorectal adenomatous polyps and confirmed that alcoholism increases this risk.[2284] Immunodeficiency has also been suggested to play a possible role in the pathogenesis,[1] but Parikshak and co-workers noted that transplant recipients are not more likely to develop metachronous polyps than the general population.[306]

Family History

The adenoma-carcinoma sequence suggests an increased risk of colorectal cancer in the families of patients who harbor adenomatous polyps. Winawer and colleagues interviewed a random sample of participants in the National Polyp Study who had newly diagnosed adenomatous polyps with respect to the history of colorectal cancer in parents and siblings.[451] There were 1,031 patients found with adenomas, 1,865 parents and 2,381 siblings. The authors concluded that siblings and parents of patients with adenomatous polyps are at an increased risk for the development of colorectal cancer, particularly if the adenoma were diagnosed before the age of 60 years, or in the case of siblings, when a parent has had a colorectal cancer.[451]

Evolution

There are three situations in which the life history of the adenoma-carcinoma sequence can be demonstrated: first, in the unusual opportunity in which a patient with a benign polyp refuses removal of the lesion and subsequently develops a carcinoma at the same site; second, in familial polyposis, a condition that always results in a bowel cancer if the colon is not resected (see later); and third, in hereditary nonpolyposis colorectal cancer (see Lynch Syndromes, Chapter 22). Because the histologic nature of the polyps in the familial polyposis condition is no different from that seen in the common, solitary adenoma, one must infer that there is a cause and effect relationship. The huge number of polyps present in the bowel implies that the risk is multiplied many times.

Lanspa and colleagues reviewed 44 individuals with asymptomatic Lynch syndrome by means of a colonoscopy screening program.[238] Thirty percent were found to have at least one adenoma; in 20% the lesions were multiple. The prevalence was greater than an unselected reference group, a finding supporting the hypothesis that adenomatous change is the premalignant lesion in the Lynch syndrome.

Muto and co-workers reported four patients who had untreated adenomatous polyps.[278] In one, cancer was diagnosed at the same site after 5 years; in the second, cancer was found after 6 years. The third patient had cancer of the rectum that develop 13 years after the original observation of a benign polyp. In the fourth case, after 11 years the tumor was still benign. The authors concluded that the life history of the cancer sequence is probably at least 5 years and may in some cases be more than 10 years.

A retrospective review of Mayo Clinic records from a 6-year period before the development of colonoscopy revealed 226 patients with colonic polyps at least 1 cm in diameter for whom periodic radiographic examination was elected rather than colostomy and polypectomy.[395] Actuarial analysis revealed that the cumulative risk of diagnosis of cancer at the polyp site at 5, 10, and 20 years was 2.5%, 8%, and 24%, respectively.

Patients with large, sessile, villous adenomas represent a special situation, because the lesions are frequently removed locally by a transanal approach and have a tendency to recur. Muto and associates observed the long-term follow-up in ten such patients (5 to 30 years).[278] All had periodic evaluation and further treatment as necessary for recurrence. Two patients subsequently developed cancers—one after 10 years and one at 28 years.

In individuals with familial polyposis, the onset of the cancer is on average approximately 15 years following establishment of the initial diagnosis. In the St. Mark's series, the mean age at diagnosis of polyposis without cancer was 27 years, and polyposis with cancer, 39 years, a 12-year time interval.[278]

Histologic Change

The most direct evidence for the polyp-cancer sequence is the demonstration of all stages in the development of malignancy within the same specimen: normal epithelium, adenomatous tissue, atypia, and frank invasion (Figure 21-34). Occasionally, from macroscopic examination alone, an otherwise benign lesion may appear to have undergone malignant change (Figure 21-35). In large series of colonoscopy polypectomies, 4% to 5% of polyps demonstrate some element of invasive carcinoma.[112,149,456]

Generally, the larger the lesion the greater the likelihood of malignant degeneration. Polypoid adenomas smaller than 1 cm have been shown to have a 1% incidence of malignant change; those from 1 to 2 cm have a 10% incidence, and those larger than 2 cm, a 35% incidence.[278]

In patients with *villous adenomas*, the incidence of malignant change has been reported as follows: less than 1 cm, 10%; 1 to 2 cm, 10%; and greater than 2 cm, 53%.[278] Stulc and colleagues, reporting from the Roswell Park Memorial Institute (Buffalo, NY), identified 65 villous and tubovillous adenomas ≥ 4 cm.[396] They noted that 85% contained invasive adenocarcinoma.

Flat Adenoma

Muto and colleagues collected 33 small *flat adenomas*, not more than 1 mm in diameter, and described their histologic characteristics.[279] They are easily missed at endoscopy, presenting as small reddish spots with or without a central depression.[47] The grade of atypia seemed to increase with the size of the polyp, emphasizing the importance of recognizing and removing even small lesions. Although the natural history of these small, early lesions is not definitively understood, most investigators believe that they have important implications for screening and for the polyp-cancer sequence. Because of their difficulty in detection, special magnification instruments, as well as chromoscopic colonoscopy, have been suggested.[193]

De Novo *Carcinoma Versus the Polyp-Cancer Sequence*

If carcinomas of the large bowel arose *de novo* from normal mucosa, without passing through the stage of benignity, it would not be uncommon to observe a cancer 0.5 cm in diameter.[92] Because this is not the case, one must assume that the most colorectal cancers arise from benign polyps. It has been said that if one seeks vigorously enough and performs sufficient serial sections of the pathologic specimen, an element of benign polyp can virtually always be found in a cancer, particularly if the tumor is relatively small. There is, however, compelling evidence to suggest that some malignant tumors of the rectum and colon arise from the mucosa without passing through a benign stage. Kuramoto and colleagues identified a number of flat, early cancers and concluded that a "flat route of cancer can occur *de novo*" in a polyp-free large intestine.[234] They found four such cancers with a mean size of 11 mm. Jass emphasized that infiltrating carcinoma can arise within small, flat foci of severely dysplastic epithelium (indistinguishable from carcinoma-*in-situ*).[208] The implications of this observation are applied to the follow-up evaluation of individuals with long-standing ulcerative colitis (see Relationship to Malignancy, Chapter 29).

Molecular Genetic Evidence for the Colorectal Adenoma-Carcinoma Sequence

The most recent and largest body of data relates to molecular genetic events and their cellular effects.[241] The value of these observations has not been clearly defined. It is,

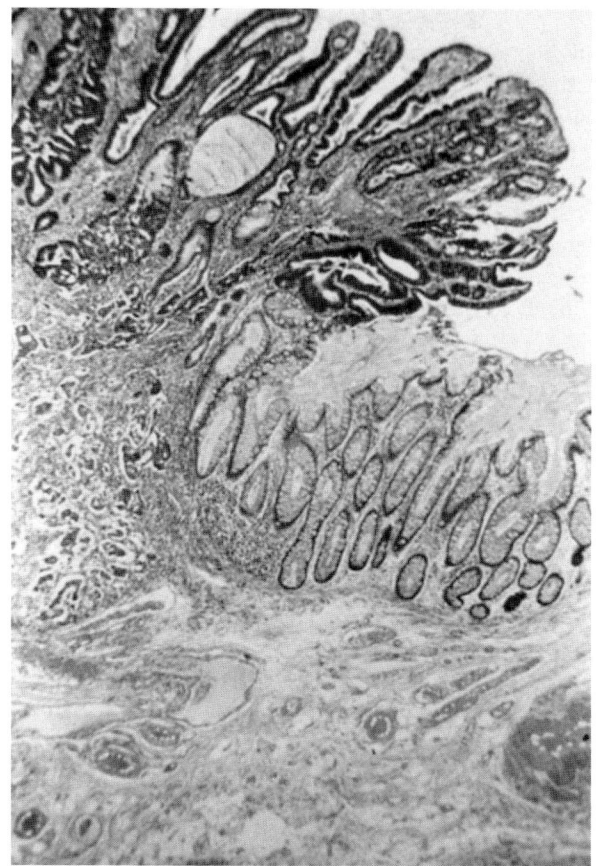

FIGURE 21-34. Villous adenoma. Note the marked dysplasia of the lining cells on the **left**, with infiltrating well-differentiated adenocarcinoma penetrating the muscularis mucosae. (Original magnification × 260; courtesy of Rudolf Garret, M.D.)

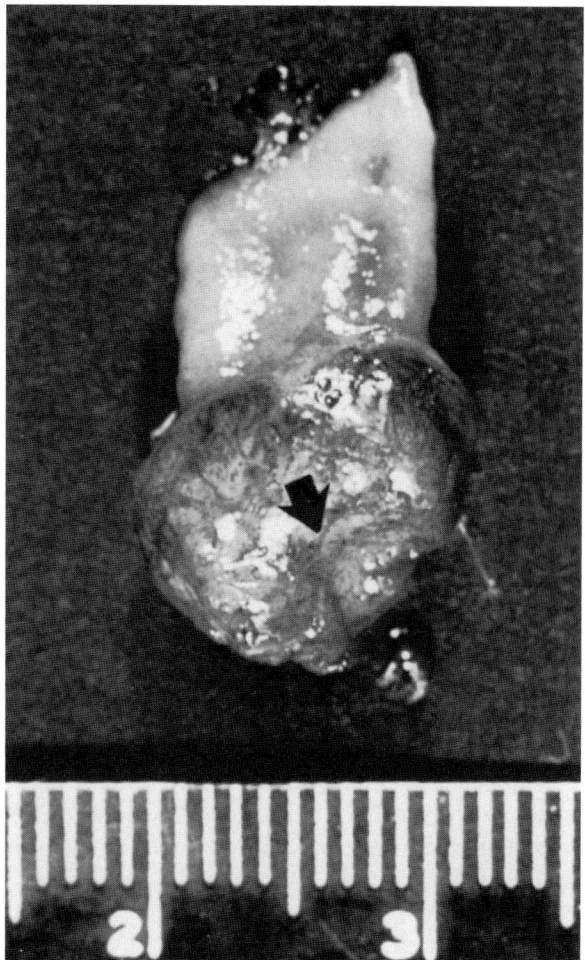

FIGURE 21-35. A polypoid adenoma with carcinoma at the tip. An ulcer is indicated *(arrow)*. (Courtesy of Rudolf Garret, M.D.)

however, worth making the effort at this point to discuss the fundamentals of the molecular and genetic evidence that clinicians should be aware of in this rapidly evolving field.

Genetics

This section on genetics has been contributed by Dr. Anthony A. Goodman. Dr. Goodman's teaching skills are well demonstrated by this contribution. His clarity of writing on a highly complex subject, especially for an audience of surgeons who, in many cases, are light years away from their basic science studies, makes his presentation truly invaluable. Dr. Goodman is retired from the practice of general and colorectal surgery. He lives in Montana, where he holds two teaching posts at Montana State University: Adjunct Professor of Medicine in the W.W.A.M.I. Medical Sciences Program and Adjunct Professor of Microbiology—MLC.

Carcinogenesis has been well established as a multistep process involving the accumulation of mutations in the genome of somatic cells and, less commonly, germ cells. In the case of colorectal cancers, the progression from normal cells to benign adenomas and finally to carcinomas has been among the best studied. Because of ready access through colonoscopic assessment of the mucosa, as well as the ease of biopsy of colonic lesions, it has been possible to document many of the steps in the process of tumorogenesis and to correlate the gross and microscopic pathologic changes with alterations in the molecular biology of the precursor and tumor cells. It is now well established that virtually all colorectal carcinomas derive from preexisting benign adenomas. The following discussion focuses on the mutational events that are the basis of the phenotypic changes seen in both adenomas and carcinomas of the colon and rectum. Although sporadic colorectal cancers are far more common than the familial forms, the genetic changes seen in the latter have provided a great deal of information about the carcinogenesis of both types of cancer.

Cancer and Natural Selection

Microevolution It has become increasingly clear that the development of all forms of cancer is based upon the accumulation of mutations that favor accelerated growth in the cellular DNA and the subsequent effects of natural selection on these mutated clones of cells. This is true micromolecular or molecular evolution. The mutations can give rise to a single abnormal cell, thereby providing a significant growth advantage to that cell. Its progeny will predominate over its neighbors. Mutations that do not result in a growth advantage will either drop out of the population (if the mutations are deleterious) or remain neutral. This can be viewed as a microevolutionary process in which the rules of survival of the fittest cell (or the fittest DNA) will predominate.

Multistep Carcinogenesis

Steps of Carcinogenesis: Initiation, Promotion, Conversion, and Progression The process of carcinogenesis can be seen to occur in four basic steps. This multistep process has been well worked out in the cases of chemical environmental carcinogens, but it also applies to other kinds of carcinogens, including those of viral and physical agents.

Each step or phase of the multistep process is driven by random genetic damage primarily to somatic cells, as well as germ line cells in familial syndromes. The DNA is exposed to some form of carcinogen (chemical, viral, physical), which permanently alters the structure of the DNA.[53] This confers a selective growth advantage upon the cell by increasing the cell's responsiveness to intracellular and intercellular growth signals, while ignoring signals that restrain growth.

The mutations involved in the genesis of cancer must occur in stem cells or determined cells, rather than fully differentiated cells. The theory of the "histogenic assumption" popular in the mid-1900s assumed that mutations occurred in fully differentiated cells, which then underwent a "loss of differentiation." We now know that this is not correct. The mutations must occur in cells which are still undergoing differentiation and will never reach the state of full differentiation because of the changes in the DNA caused by the carcinogens. So the real process is that of "failure to differentiate" rather than "loss of differentiation." Fully differentiated cells replicate only rarely, so that opportunities for mutation are also rare. This suggests that tissues that have the most rapid turnover, and therefore the most active stem cells, should have higher rates of cancer formation. Indeed, this is the case. Nearly 90% of cancers are carcinomas, originating in epithelial and endothelial cells in which turnover rate is high and in which the tissues are exposed to environmental carcinogens. More indolent tissues in, for example, mesothelial structures, form far fewer cancers.

In the case of colorectal cancers, the mucosal stem cells are exposed to many carcinogens contained in the fecal mass. Because of the rapid turnover rate of the mutated, emerging stem cells, these changes will lead to selective clonal expansion and natural selection, which ultimately increase the overall turnover rate, leading to still more DNA damage. The speeding up of cell replication interferes with the processes that allow for discovery and repair of DNA errors. Finally, after accumulation of sufficient mutations, usually over decades, the mutated cell will express the malignant phenotype, emerging with the clinical characteristics that define cancer:

- Failure to differentiate
- The potential to invade normal tissue
- The potential to metastasize
- This process may ultimately lead to lethality as a consequence of invasion and metastases to vital organ systems

Initiation The first step in this multistep process is called *initiation*. This involves modification of cellular DNA by the carcinogen to produce irreversible genetic damage. Usually, the carcinogen (especially in the case of chemicals and viruses) forms an adduct with the host DNA. Radiation and physical agents, conversely, tend to disrupt chemical bonds in the cellular DNA. At the molecular level, what usually take place during initiation are the activation of an oncogene (more specifically, the conversion of a proto-oncogene to an oncogene) and the inactivation of a tumor suppressor gene. Proto-oncogenes are cellular genes that are present in the genome of a normal cell and are generally involved with the regulation of the rate of growth and replication. The proto-oncogenes are the "wild-type" or normal form of the oncogene. These proto-oncogenes may be inappropriately activated to cause the dysregulation of cell growth and differentiation. The resulting oncogenes may cause growth abnormalities by one or more of several mechanisms:

- Overexpression of a gene product, which leads to an increase in concentration of an active protein (dosage hypothesis)
- Expression of a gene at an inappropriate time in the cell cycle, bypassing resting phases (G_0) and increasing rate of replication (unscheduled gene expression)
- Expression of a gene product in an inappropriate cell type
- Structural alteration of a gene protein or product to make the same amount of product more potent

Oncogenes, therefore, are the mutated form of normal cellular genes whose "overexpressed" gene products expand the cellular population of the mutated cell at an inappropriately rapid rate.

In general, oncogenes behave as if they were dominant genes, as described in mendelian inheritance. Because the mutation of a single gene in the allele pair is sufficient to turn on rapid replication, only one mutation may be necessary. As will be seen, another form of gene, the tumor suppressor gene, generally behaves as if it were a recessive mendelian gene. However, in the case of colorectal cancers, as with other cancers, there are exceptions to these rules of dominant and recessive gene function (see later, mutated p53 and the dominant negative effect). Finally, the mutations that occur during initiation will ultimately confer upon the mutated cell a growth and survival advantage, in addition to the ability to invade later and to mutate further. In general, because mutations are random events, it is the accumulation of the mutations over time, and not the order of their occurrence in the stages of tumorogenesis, that is important in the development of cancers of all kinds. However, in the case of colorectal cancer, it appears that the order, as well as the accumulation of mutations, may also have some importance.[117,427] It is of some interest that mutations converting proto-oncogenes to oncogenes have been seen only in somatic cells and not in the germ line cells of familial colon cancer syndromes. Tumor suppressor gene mutations have been documented in both.

Promotion The second phase of carcinogenesis is called promotion. During this phase, the predominant events involve expansion of the initiated clone of cells. It is at this stage that more errors are made because the rate of accumulation of mutations (replication errors) parallels the rate of cell division. This explains why the majority of human cancers are carcinomas, because the most rapidly proliferating cells are, in general, epithelial or endothelial. The immediate effect of environmental promoters (chemical, viral and physical) is to stimulate division in cells that would not ordinarily be dividing. Tumor promoters are not generally mutagenic after initiation is complete. Although initiators and promoters tend to be separate classes of carcinogens, there are some chemicals that can both initiate and promote. These are called "complete carcinogens" and include such substances as benzo-α-biphenyl and 4-aminobiphenyl. Common promoters include dioxin, saccharin, cigarette smoke condensates, ultraviolet–B light, cyclamates, estrogens, chronic inflammation, and aflatoxins produced by *Aspergillus flavus*. The promoters can act by either directly promoting genetic damage (tobacco smoke, aflatoxin) or by enlarging the tumor cell populations. These can then undergo further genetic damage through more mutations (similar to estrogen, which influences the rate of cell growth in breast tissue). The promoters can also induce tumor formation in conjunction with doses of initiators that would have been too low for carcinogenesis.

Cells that have undergone initiation and promotion, although containing permanent genetic damage, are still in a reversible stage. Until these cells express a malignant phenotype, the process can generally be reversed. After the next step (malignant conversion), the process becomes irreversible. At this point, clinical cancer is present, although not necessarily able to be diagnosed.

Malignant Conversion The change from the stages of promotion to *malignant conversion* requires that more genetic alteration occurs in the DNA. The important steps here include multiple frequent doses of tumor promoters over time, rather than a single large dose. If that critical point (conversion) does not occur, the process may be reversed, as, for example, in smokers whose risk returns to that of a nonsmoker after about 10 to 15 years following the discontinuance of tobacco use. Malignant conversion is often mediated by the activation of more oncogenes and the loss of more tumor suppressor genes. p53 is particularly important at this stage.

Tumor Progression The final stage in multistep carcinogenesis is called *tumor progression*. This stage represents the clinical expression of the malignant phenotype. It is here that the physician or surgeon deals with the clinical aspects of invasion and metastases in the individual with clinically evident cancer. The process of natural selection continues, with the most aggressive and resistant tumor cell clones dominating the clinical picture. The time course for these changes is often measured in decades. One of the shortest documented latency periods between initiation and clinical diagnosis is that of the survivors of the nuclear detonations at Hiroshima and Nagasaki. These patients developed leukemias as early as 7 years following exposure to the massive, nonlethal doses of radiation.

Molecular Mechanisms of Carcinogenesis

General release of growth constraints derives mainly from mutations that result in either activation of proto-oncogenes to oncogenes or inactivation of tumor suppressor genes. The role of the oncogene as it relates to the stimulation of inappropriate growth of cells has been discussed. Many authors have likened this to the car with its accelerator stuck on the floor. Tumor suppressor genes can be thought of as failure of the brakes. This combination, whether in cells or on the highway, sets up conditions that can lead inexorably to accidents, often fatal.

Again, oncogenes function as "dominant" genes, in that a mutation in only one of the alleles is necessary to initiate tumorogenesis. It is actually the abnormal proteins made by the mutant allele that are sufficient for carcinogenesis. The tumor suppressor gene, conversely, behaves in most instances as if it were a "recessive" gene, requiring both alleles to be mutated or inactivated before it fails to act as a "brake" on abnormal replication. This is because the single wild-type tumor suppressor gene can still function as the cell's brake even when the other allele is inactivated or absent. There is an important exception to this last concept, called the "dominant negative." It seems that, in certain situations, the protein of the mutated tumor suppressor gene can overwhelm the wild-type protein in a number of ways and can still destroy the brake function of the remaining allele. Such may be the case with the p53 protein.

p53 is a gene whose function it is to detect errors in the replication of DNA and is thought to be central to the development of a high proportion of human tumors.[392] Its protein checks for errors in DNA replication. When such errors are detected, p53 can halt the cell cycle while repairs are made. However, if the damage is too serious to repair, p53 can trigger apoptosis, programmed cell death, thereby eliminating the damaged cell from the population. More recent information suggests that p53 works by activating another nearby gene, called WAF1 (identical to p21). WAF1/p21 is a powerful suppressor of tumor growth; it acts by inhibiting cell cycle-controlling kinase systems. At this time, there is a known cascade of genes that act in sequence following activation by p53.

The mutated form of p53 not only fails to do its job as a brake on replication, but in the worst-case mutations, it can actually stimulate even faster replication. p53 protein, acting as a dimmer or higher-order polymer, can bind to and inactivate wild-type p53, creating the dominant negative effect. Thus, whereas most tumor suppressor genes act in a recessive fashion, mutated p53 can neutralize otherwise functioning p53, in essence resembling dominant gene action.

Furthermore, loss of p53 can confer resistance upon the tumor cell to therapies such as radiation and chemotherapy. In reality, therapeutic radiation does not "fry" tumor cells, but rather acts by doing sufficient damage to the DNA that p53 then can take over and trigger apoptosis. A similar event occurs with some chemotherapy protocols. If the p53 is inactivated, then the damage done by the radiation or chemotherapy will fail to trigger apoptosis, and cell death may not occur.

Finally, there is a group of genes that function neither as oncogenes nor as tumor suppressor genes. These are what have been called "mutator genes."[419] This class of genes does not control the intrinsic pathways for regulation of growth and replication, but rather controls the rate at which other genes may mutate. Because these mutations also occur in proto-oncogenes and tumor suppressor genes, aberrant mutator genes increase the probability of tumorogenesis.

Molecular Changes Leading to Colorectal Cancers

There are at least five alterations common to the cellular biology of most colorectal cancers. These occur in both the sporadic as well as the hereditary forms of the disease. As discussed previously, virtually all colorectal cancers arise from preexisting benign adenomas. The sequential steps from the first changes in these adenomas appear to be quite consistent as they progress from small adenomas to large adenomas, and thence through stages of hyperplasia, dysplasia, and finally to invasive cancer.[282]

There are several features that should be kept in mind as the steps in colorectal carcinogenesis are analyzed. First, both the activation of proto-oncogenes to oncogenes and the inactivation of tumor suppressor genes are vital to the early initiation and promotion of these tumors. Second, it is now generally agreed that the total accumulation of the genetic changes is a critical factor in tumorogenesis, as well as the actual temporal sequence of the changes.

Specific Genetic Alterations in the Development of Colorectal Cancers

One of the most commonly mutated genes in the evolution of colon polyps to cancer is the adenomatous polyposis coli (APC) gene. This gene is altered in the germ line of families with familial adenomatous polyposis (FAP) as well as in sporadic polyps and cancers. It is located at 5q21 (on the "q" or long arm of chromosome 5).[222,311,387] This is a tumor suppressor gene, and the loss of heterozygosity at this location is found in more than 70% of colorectal cancers and small adenomatous polyps. The wild-type APC gene functions in cell-to-cell adhesion and intercellular communication.[86] Mutations or inactivation of the APC gene produces a pattern of hyperplasia, often without dysplastic changes. The resultant cell pattern is seen in early adenomas. Also located on chromosome 5q is a tumor suppressor gene named "mutated in colon carcinoma" (MCC). This gene is present in invasive colon carcinomas and is often classified as a tumor initiator.[315] Another epigenetic event that appears to occur early in the genesis of colon cancer is the hypomethylation of DNA.[29,117,366] This loss of methyl groups has been postulated to inhibit the condensation of chromosome material and lead to nondisjunction. The affected chromosomes would then be at risk for possible allelic losses.

Of the several genes involved in the evolution of colorectal cancers, perhaps the most important is the *ras* oncogene.[116] This is located on chromosome 12p (chromosome 12, on the small "p" or "petite" arm) and is named for its discovery in rat *sarcoma*. The gene is found mutated in approximately 50% of adenomas greater than or equal to 1 cm in diameter and in fewer than 10% of adenomas less than 1 cm.[34,428] The wild-type K-*ras* gene (other family members include H-*ras* and N-*ras*) produces a protein whose function in normal cells is to stimulate cell division and differentiation when signaled to do so by extracellular growth factors. It is involved, therefore, in what is called intracellular signal transduction, as a mitogenic signaling pathway from cell surface receptors. The mutated version (*ras* oncogene) continues to promote cell division even in the absence of any signals to do so. The result is continued replication in an inappropriate setting, as well as failure to enter terminal differentiation. This mutation tends to enter the carcinogenesis progression in the conversion from an early small adenoma to the larger and more dysplastic intermediate adenoma. Cells affected by K-*ras* mutations show abnormal histologic patterns of differentiation and are seen in dysplastic polyps.[117]

The next important mutation or allelic loss involves a tumor suppressor gene that is rare in polyps but very common in colon carcinomas (70%) and in late adenomas (50%).[117] This gene is called "deleted in colon carcinoma" (DCC) and is located on chromosome 18q21. The gene product of the wild type is a 190-kDa protein, which appears to function in cell-cell and cell–extracellular matrix adhesion processes. It also appears to function in cell differentiation. The degree of mutation of this gene has been found to correlate with prognosis in Dukes' B colorectal cancer. The tumors in patients with allelic loss of DCC behave more like those of Dukes' C cancer, whereas those with intact DCC behave more like those of Dukes' A cancer.[376]

DCC is not, however, found in hereditary nonpolyposis colon cancer syndromes (HNPCC; see Chapter 22). There is a locus on chromosome 2p22–21 that has been found in HNPCC (Lynch syndrome), called *MSH2* (the human homologue of the bacterial gene, *mutS*).[124] The gene at this location has been shown to be responsible for mismatch repairs. These were found in both somatic and germ line cells in patients with this disease. Other genes that are commonly mutated in HNPCC include *MLH1, PMS1,* and *PMS2*. Each of these *(MSH2, MLH1, PMS1, PMS2)* encodes substances involved in the detection and correction of mismatch repairs of DNA.[66] As would be expected, patients with HNPCC tend to have large numbers of cells with errors in their DNA replication. Carcinogenesis and the natural selection that takes place among the aberrant cells seem to be the consequence of these accumulated errors.

The clinical differences between the familial cancer syndromes (FAP and HNPCC) can be correlated with differences in the molecular biology of the two diseases. In FAP, patients develop thousands of benign polyps that have a relatively low rate of further mutation to cancer. Only one or a few will go on to develop a carcinoma. In HNPCC, there are only small numbers of benign tumors, but with a high propensity for conversion to the malignant phenotype. Both diseases become clinically evident decades before sporadic colon cancers arise. Therefore, if one looks to the general theory of carcinogenesis, FAP seems to be a defect in tumor initiation (APC gene leading to multiple benign adenomas), whereas HNPCC is a disease characterized by the changes that take place in tumor promotion and conversion.

The latest event in the chronology and accumulation of genetic mutations or losses in colon cancer involves p53. This tumor suppressor gene is mutated in more than 50% of all cancers worldwide and in the majority of colon cancers. Its mutated form is uncommon in adenomas. The wild-type p53 protein functions as the last brake on cell replication in the presence of DNA errors. The "guardian of the genome," as it has been called, checks the DNA for errors. If errors are found, it will generally halt the cell cycle until repairs can be made. If the damage is too extensive, it will initiate cellular apoptosis or cell suicide. The mutated form of p53 is doubly dangerous in the genesis of cancers. In many cases, it will not only fail to stop the cell cycle and fail to trigger apoptosis, but it may actually increase the rate of replication of the abnormal cells. p53 can also act in the pathway of tumor angiogenesis.[88] p53, in its wild type, acts to stimulate the release of thrombospondin-1, a potent angiogenesis inhibitor. The mutated form of p53 loses this function, and, therefore, the inhibition of angiogenesis is lost as well. Tumor angiogenesis is critical to the development of tumors from microscopic to larger masses, as well as for permitting and encouraging blood-borne metastases.

The loss of p53 in the final stages of colon carcinogenesis not only allows the cells to divide at an unrestrained rate, but also further promotes the development of even more cellular genetic mutations because the cell cycle is not interrupted when errors are detected.

The complex sequences of oncogene activation and tumor suppressor gene inactivation fit well into the classic concepts of tumorogenesis (Figure 21-36). However, it should be remembered that APC, *ras*, and p53 mutations or deletions do not occur in all colorectal cancers. The remainder of the colon cancers have other aberrations in their genome, aberrations that may develop from another, different set of errors. However, the action of promoters to enhance rapid replication and perpetuate genetic errors will not occur if the initiating event has not taken place. For example, mutant p53 may not have as ominous an effect in a normally replicating cell if its rate has not been stepped up by the loss of an APC brake.

Other genes have been identified in the genesis of colorectal cancers as well as other malignancies. A metastasis suppressor gene called nm23-h1 has been implicated with high tumor metastasis potential and a poor prognosis in colon and breast cancers.[353,402] This gene appears to be involved in signal transduction through transforming growth factor-α.[190] Its mutated expression has been used as a predictor for staging colorectal cancers. Decrease in motility and responsiveness to motility signals may account for the mode of action of normal nm23. Similarly, a protective effect by normal nm23 has also been noted in the outcome of colorectal cancers.[353]

Microsatellite Instability Another category of genomic change has been identified in many malignancies, but has become of special interest in HNPCC. This has to do with what is called *microsatellite instability*. Microsatel-

Model of colorectal carcinogenesis

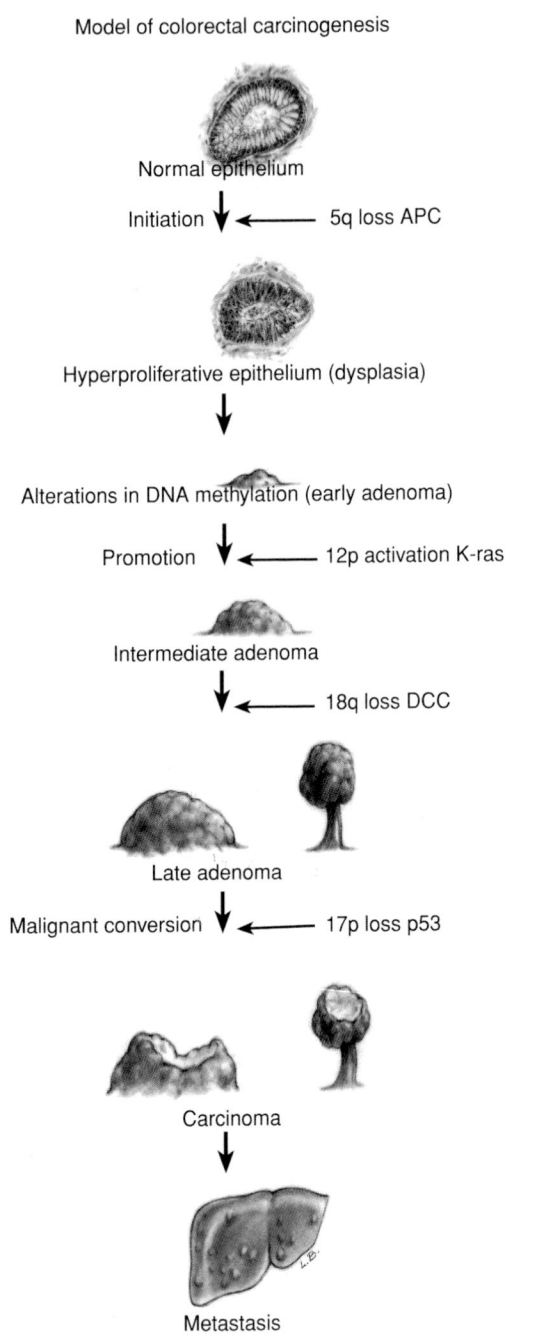

FIGURE 21-36. Model of colorectal carcinogenesis. (Redrawn from Fearon ER, Vogelstein B. A genetic model of colorectal cancer tumorigenesis *Cell* 1990;61:759.)

lites are short repeat segments of DNA in which certain sequences of nucleotides are repeated in varying lengths. These are noncoding segments of DNA and play no significant role in functional protein production. The human genome contains hundreds of thousands of sets of such repeats. During replication some of these repeats

may be shortened or lengthened because of errors or misalignments in the sequences. Normal cells generally try to repair these units using mismatch repair genes. However, in tumors in which there are abnormal mismatch repair genes, the defects go unchanged, and the "instability" in the satellites persists. In virtually all patients with HNPCC, these satellites can serve as markers, leading to areas where there are mutations in functioning genes.[250,314] It has been established that HNPCC results from a germ line defect in mismatch repair genes. Thus, microsatellite instability may be used as a marker for HNPCC.

Summary and Conclusions

The molecular and genetic changes in colorectal cancers are among the best studied and delineated in the field of human oncology. The progress to date has included the elucidation of certain genetic defects that appear to be common to the majority of colorectal lesions, adenomas, or carcinomas. Although the normal function of many of these genes is not fully understood, progress has been made that ultimately should benefit the patient with colorectal cancer. Understanding the expression and overexpression of several of these molecules can now enable the physician to select patients who may be at a higher or lower risk for future recurrence. The status of expression of the DCC gene or the nm23 gene, for example, may influence the decision concerning the advisability of adjuvant or neoadjuvant therapy in certain individuals. Some patients may be considered to be at less risk when evaluated by conventional means, such as histologic grade and lymph node status. Furthermore, recent studies on the specific molecular mutations formed in HNPCC patients are being used to determine the most efficient and effective forms of surveillance and therapy.[249,424,425] The era of gene therapy, utilizing genetic manipulations to correct defects in the genome, is now upon us. Although a practical method for the introduction of genes into human tumor cells is as yet an unachieved ideal, promising methods are now in the early stages of investigation. It may be within the lifetime of this reader that one will be able to alter and to correct cellular genetic defects in the treatment of most, if not all, human cancers.

Treatment and Results

The presence of a polypoid lesion virtually dictates endoscopic evaluation and, in most cases, polypectomy.[302,320,339,451] There is no justification for observation to determine the lesion's change in appearance or size with the passage of time, except in the rare situation when the risk of endoscopy is too great.

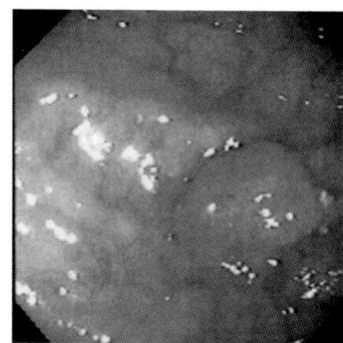
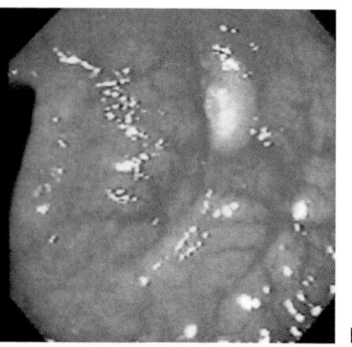

FIGURE 21-37. (A) A 1-cm polyp on short stalk can be easily snare excised by colonoscopy-polypectomy. (B) A whitish area of coagulated mucosa remains at the excision site. (See Color Fig. 21-37.)

Colonoscopy-Polypectomy

The technique of colonoscopy-polypectomy is discussed in Chapter 5, and the protocol for follow-up evaluation is presented in the following section. Pedunculated polyps can usually be snare excised (Figure 21-37) as can small sessile lesions (Figure 21-38). Tappero and colleagues recommended cold snare excision of small colorectal polyps.[403] In a series of 210 consecutive patients, no case of perforation, significant bleeding, or mortality was observed. Their data lend further support to the concept that all visible polypoid lesions should be removed. Even relatively large, flat villous lesions can be reasonably extirpated by means of colonoscopy, provided the tumor is benign (Figure 21-17).

The problem of the management of the sessile lesion has been the subject of debate.[87] Most examiners today, however, depending on the "aggressiveness" and experience of the endoscopist, would recommend at least an attempt at colonoscopic removal of a benign-appearing lesion.[95] Christie reported the removal of 47 sessile tumors, from 2 to 6 cm in size.[56] There was one incident of complication requiring operative intervention. The author recommended that the appearance at endoscopy determines the advisability of resection by this approach. Smooth, soft, lobulated, nonulcerated tumors were considered excisable, provided one has good instrument tip control at the level of the lesion.[56] For those patients considered poor candidates for anesthesia and laparotomy,

the endoscopist should attempt removal of even very large tumors.[19,88]

Doniec and co-workers published their experience with endoscopic removal of 186 polyps greater than 3 cm in diameter.[102] The incidence of bleeding was 2%. Perforation occurred in one patient (0.5%). None of the patients with invasive carcinoma who subsequently underwent resection (ten) had evidence of tumor in the resected specimen. With a mean follow-up of 40 months, 3% developed a benign recurrence.[102] Church reported the Cleveland Clinic Ohio experience with 58 patients who had *colonic* polyps who were referred for surgery.[57] Endoscopic resection was successfully performed in all but 15 (74%). The author encouraged a second opinion before surgery is undertaken for a presumably benign lesion.

Comment

There is a reflexive tendency on the part of the surgeon to perform whatever operative procedure the referring physician or gastroenterologist wishes. As discussed in Chapter 5, a surgeon undertaking colonoscopy is much more likely to attempt removal of a large or sessile polyp than a nonsurgeon. Clearly, this is because a surgeon can deal with the complications, whereas the gastroenterologist must ask for help, an issue not merely of one's ego, but also that of a potentially litigious concern. The surgeon understandably is reluctant to submit a referred patient to a second colonoscopy. When one makes such a suggestion,

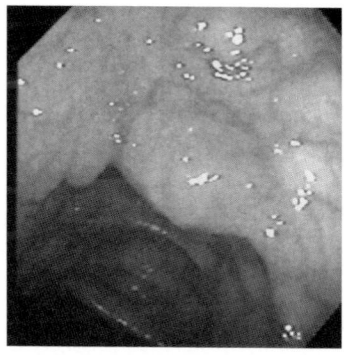
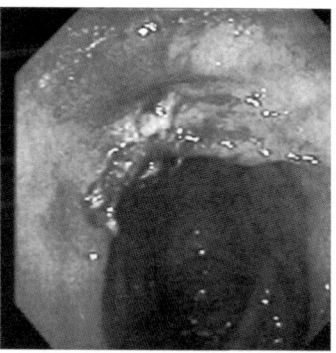

FIGURE 21-38. (A) A benign-appearing 1.5-mm sessile polyp can be removed by snare excision. (B) This creates a rather broad ulcer. Whether additional treatment is appropriate will depend on the histologic interpretation of the biopsy. (See Color Fig. 21-38.)

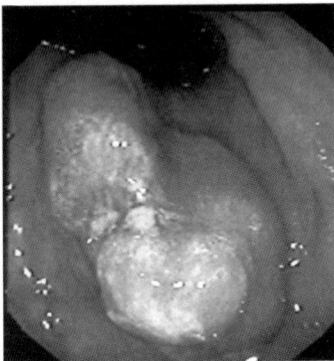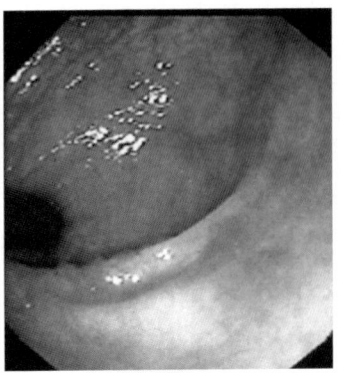

A **B**

FIGURE 21-39. **(A)** A large adenomatous polyp was found to contain invasive carcinoma. **(B)** The postpolypectomy site appeared relatively benign. Resection revealed lymph node involvement with adenocarcinoma. (See Color Fig. 21-39.)

the the implication is that there may be a question about the gastroenterolgist's judgment or capability. This becomes a special problem for the surgeon who relies on the gastroenterologist for patient referrals. How can one reconcile this potential conflict of interest? One method is to obtain the photographs of the lesion. The macroscopic appearance may help to resolve any doubt as to the appropriateness of operative resection. However, if there is reason to question the need for a major operation, the surgeon must communicate this to the referring doctor. In these circumstances, one should be able to afford what cannot be considered a luxury, that of integrity.

Management of Malignant Polyp

The most controversial management issue is the problem of what to do if invasive carcinoma is found in the polypectomy specimen (Figure 21-39).[20,23,80,274,343,365,373,379,455] Some advise resection selectively (e.g., in individuals with poorly differentiated lesions or simply in young patients). Wolff

and Shinya recommend resection if the cancer is close to the plane of resection, if there is tumor in the lymphatics, or if the lesion is poorly differentiated.[455] Interestingly, however, in five patients with small polypoid cancers (no benign element present), no residual cancer was identified by the authors. However, Colacchio and associates, in analyzing size, depth of invasion of the pedicle, degree of differentiation, and involvement of lymphatics within the stalk, could not accurately predict the likelihood of tumor spread to regional lymph nodes.[71] They recommended conventional colonic resection in all patients who harbor polyps with invasive carcinoma.

Haggitt and colleagues determined the prognostic significance of invasion at different levels in 129 colorectal carcinomas arising in adenomas.[162] The level of invasion was defined according to the following criteria:

Level 1: carcinoma invading through the muscularis mucosae into the submucosa but limited to the head of the polyp

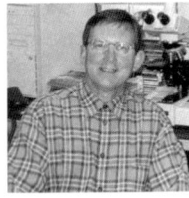

Rodger C. Haggitt (1942–2000) Rodger Haggitt was born in Detroit, Michigan on August 28, 1942. At the age of 11, he and his family moved to Tennessee. At age 16, he was introduced to what would become a lifelong passion while assisting a local pathologist with an autopsy. By the time he entered medical school, literally hundreds of autopsies later, he took pride in his finely honed autopsy skills and knack for making visual observations. He began his formal pathology training at the Baptist Memorial Hospital in Memphis and completed it at the New England Deaconess Hospital in Boston with Shields Warren (see the biography earlier in this chapter), William Meissner, and Merle Lagg. After fulfilling his military obligation at Tripler Army Medical Center in Honolulu, he returned to Boston and the Deaconess Hospital as one of pathology's rising stars. In 1977, Haggitt returned to the University of Tennessee and the Baptist Memorial Hospital, where he directed the Division of Surgical Pathology. In 1984, he moved to the University of Washington in Seattle as Director of the Division of Gastrointestinal Pathology. Haggitt's interest in this specialty developed when the era of colonoscopy and of gastrointestinal endoscopic biopsy began. Because of his desire to combine clinical relevance with pathologic interpretation, he enjoyed a close interaction with his gastrointestinal medical and surgical colleagues. His study of prognostic factors for adenocarcinoma arising in endoscopically resected colonic adenomas has come to be known as the Haggitt Classification. His collaboration with the late Warren Nugent, Chief of Gastroenterology at the Lahey Clinic in Boston, resulted in the publication of one of the first long-term, prospective, follow-up studies of neoplastic progression in ulcerative colitis. They showed that endoscopic surveillance reduced mortality from colorectal cancer. At Tripler in Hawaii, while fulfilling his military obligation, Haggitt worked with Larry Johnson and Tom DeMeester to establish esophageal 24-hour pH monitoring as the gold standard for investigating gastroesophageal reflux disease. In 1978, he and his colleagues at the Deaconess Hospital published a landmark study documenting that dysplasia was the precursor of adenocarcinoma in Barrett's esophagus and suggested that its detection by endoscopic biopsy could lead to earlier surgical intervention in order to prevent cancer in these patients. Haggitt also made important contributions to hepatic pathology, including the first American description of nonalcoholic steatohepatitis and, with James Williams at the University of Tennessee, the initial implementation of hepatic allograft biopsies. These protocol biopsies are now standard practice in many transplant centers. Dr. Haggitt was a dedicated and generous mentor to a generation of pathology residents and fellows. Through his activities with the American Society of Clinical Pathologists, he taught more practicing pathologists and had more influence on the practice of gastrointestinal pathology than any other person working with that organization. Haggitt was an active member of the national society, the Gastrointestinal Pathology Club. In 2001, after his tragic and untimely death on June 28, 2000, at the hands of a disturbed pathology resident, the name of the society was officially changed to the Rodger C. Haggitt Gastrointestinal Pathology Society. (With special appreciation to the Departments of Pathology and Gastroenterology, University of Washington, Seattle.)

Level 2: carcinoma invading to the level of the junction between adenoma and stalk

Level 3: carcinoma invading any part of the stalk

Level 4: carcinoma invading into the submucosa of the bowel wall but above the muscularis propria (Figure 21-40)[162]

Level 0 lesions are not defined as carcinomas because the muscularis mucosae is not breached. Level 4 invasion and rectal location were the only statistically significant adverse prognostic factors.

Morson and colleagues reviewed 60 patients with malignant polyps who were followed up for a minimum of 5 years.[274] There was no recurrence in the 46 individuals judged to have complete excision of the lesion. Two of the remaining 14 patients who underwent resection had residual tumor at the site of the polypectomy; regional lymph nodes were not involved. One patient with a poorly differentiated lesion developed metastatic disease despite the operative specimen's being free of tumor.

Nivatvongs and colleagues reported the Mayo Clinic experience with 151 patients who underwent bowel resection after removal of polyps containing invasive carcinoma.[292] In those patients with sessile polyps, the incidence of lymph node metastasis was 10%. Eighty percent of these had lymphovascular invasion. For pedunculated polyps, the incidence of lymph node metastasis was 6%, but it was zero when the depth of invasion was limited to levels 1, 2, or 3 (see earlier).

The St. Mark's group strongly believes that with the application of proper histopathologic evaluation, malignant polyps can be successfully treated by polypectomy alone. DeCosse agreed with the foregoing conclusions in his editorial comments.[93] He and others affirmed that the patient can be treated for pedunculated lesions by endoscopic polypectomy alone if the following criteria are applied:[69,83,93,132,277,292,343,398,457]

Visual confidence of complete excision

Proper preparation and examination of the removed malignant polyp

Absence of a poorly differentiated tumor

Absence of lymphatic or vascular invasion

Absence of invasion at the margin

Preparation of the specimen by using an elastic tissue, van Gieson's stain, is very helpful for identifying venous invasion (see Figure 22-32).

Russell and colleagues identified four factors that had prognostic value for increased risk of residual cancer: size of tumor greater than 1.5 cm, sessile as opposed to pedunculated form, cancer in at least 50% of the specimen by volume, and the presence of an invasive carcinoma.[355] Virtually everyone agrees that surgery is recommended for all patients with sessile polyps with invasive cancer and for those with level 4 lesions.[323,325]

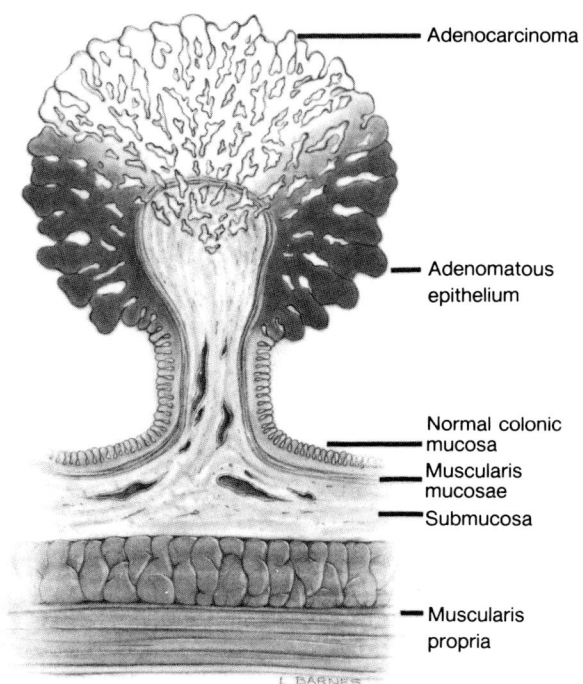

FIGURE 21-40. A pedunculated adenoma has various structures that determine the significance of invasion at different levels. (Adapted from Haggitt RC, Glotzbach RE, Soffer EE, et al. Prognostic factors in colorectal carcinomas arising in adenomas: implications for lesions removed by endoscopic polypectomy. *Gastroenterology* 1985;89:328, with permission.)

The key to proper management, therefore, is competent interpretation of the microscopic findings. This is particularly difficult when so many terms are used by different pathologists: severe dysplasia, adenoma with atypia, carcinoma-*in-situ*, superficial carcinoma, focal carcinoma, and intramucosal carcinoma.[345] The surgeon is well advised to look at the slides personally, so that with the pathologist he or she can make a reasoned judgment about the validity of pursuing a more aggressive approach. It must be remembered that the polyp must be totally removed; biopsy alone is inadequate in the decision-making process.

Opinion and Recommendations

With respect to pedunculated tumors, if the cancer invades the pedicle, it is theoretically possible for the tumor to metastasize. The likelihood, however, is remote if the margin is free. In this situation, my preference is to inform the patient that in all probability cure has been achieved, but there is the possibility (perhaps 1% or 2%) that residual tumor may still be present. The determination for or against resection is left to the individual on that basis. This is usually a highly personal decision, based on age, risk of surgery, anxiety level, and a host of subjective concerns. However, if the margin is not clear, resection is strongly encouraged.

If laparotomy is performed, it is important for the surgeon to know exactly where the lesion originally was located. If the specimen is opened, it is usually possible to recognize the site of the polypectomy, even up to 5 weeks later.[165] One alternative to facilitate identification of the polypectomy site and to avoid blind colon resection is preoperatively to tattoo the area endoscopically with a dye, such as India ink, indocyanine green, or methylene blue.[33,120,166,328,461] The color can be easily perceived on the serosal aspect. Another option is to perform intraoperative colonoscopy (see later).[68]

Colotomy-Polypectomy

Colotomy-polypectomy for pedunculated lesions is a procedure that has been relegated almost completely to the realm of historical interest (Figure 21-41). If the technique of colonoscopy is unavailable, if the lesion is believed to be beyond the limit of the endoscopist's ability, if the instrument cannot be passed to the level of the lesion, or if adequate control cannot be obtained during an attempt at polypectomy, abdominal operation may be justified. Even with one of these criteria fulfilled, however, a second opinion from another endoscopist would be the prudent alternative (see prior Comment). Figure 21-42 illustrates the classic technique of colotomy-polypectomy for a pedunculated lesion.

The major concerns for laparotomy as the method for removing the lesion are, of course, the operative morbidity and mortality, hospital costs, and time lost from work. Before the advent of colonoscopy, the generally quoted operative mortality was 1% to 2%. There may be some rationale for deferring surgery in the high-risk patient who harbors a relatively small lesion, because there is little risk of cancer (less than 1% for a tumor of less than 1 cm). Unfortunately, this information is not terribly helpful in management, because lesions of this diameter can usually be removed by means of the colonoscope. Those that cannot are larger, and hence the likelihood of the presence of a cancer is that much greater. Whether laparoscopic-assisted colon surgery will reestablish the validity of colotomy and polypectomy is a matter of conjecture at this time (see Chapter 27).[17,109,331] It will be interesting to see whether the indications for this operation will ultimately include this once commonly employed technique.

Comment

When laparotomy is required for pedunculated polyps, colotomy-polypectomy is, indeed, an adequate operation. However, the preferred treatment of sessile lesions for which laparotomy is required is resection. Frozen-section examination should be performed when sessile tumors are removed (if resection is not performed) and for pedunculated tumors with a short pedicle or in which there is some indication of possible cancerous change. It is more than embarrassing to return for a second laparotomy because the histologic appearance mandated a more extensive resection. The techniques of bowel resection are described in Chapter 22.

Operative Colonoscopy

An alternative to colotomy and polypectomy when colonoscopy has been unsuccessfully employed is the procedure of operative colonoscopy: laparotomy and transanal polypectomy. Wilson and associates describe the technique as follows:[449]

The patient is placed in the perineolithotomy position as if for combined abdominoperineal resection (see Figure 23-12). Following laparotomy, the colonoscope is inserted into the rectum; a noncrushing clamp is placed proximal to the tumor to avoid air insufflation beyond the area for polyp excision. With the guidance of the abdominal surgeon, the endoscope is expeditiously passed, and the polyp is removed by the endoscopist.

Others have been pleased with the technique in the infrequent circumstance when it has been advised.[255] In addition to cases of unsuccessful colonoscopy, the procedure can be usefully employed in combination with laparotomy for other conditions (e.g., cholelithiasis), in order to avoid opening the colon and for localization of nonpalpable but known colonic lesions. Although the advantages of the approach are limited, consideration should be given to its application in the occasional difficult polypectomy problem. Without the ability to palpate, this alternative needs to be available to any surgeon who performs laparoscopic colon procedures (see Chapter 27).

Management of Benign Rectal Tumors

Large benign neoplasms of the rectum, those that do not lend themselves readily to endoscopic excision, are tumor management problems that present a challenge to all surgeons. Villous adenomas, in particular, have an increased likelihood of malignant degeneration when compared with polypoid adenomas. This may in part be the result of the usually larger size of villous lesions. However, even when comparing the two histologic types size for size, an increased frequency of cancerous change is noted.

Biopsy results of a large, grossly benign polyp are notoriously inaccurate, but with villous adenoma this dictum is especially true. The tumor should be inspected

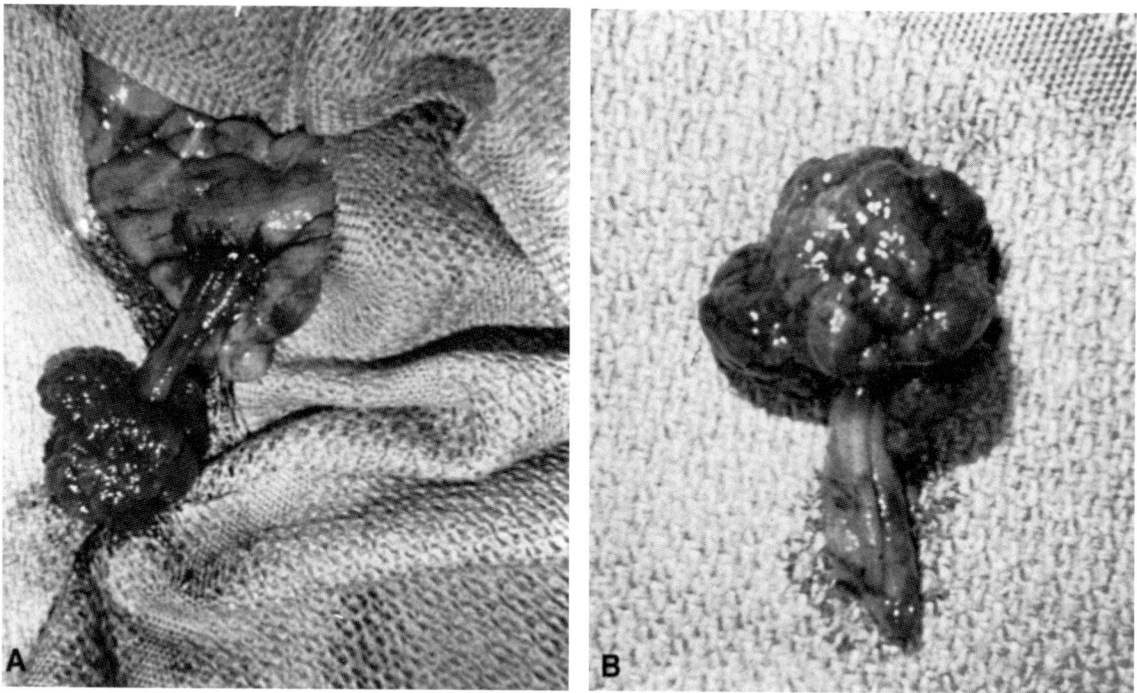

FIGURE 21-41. Pedunculated adenomatous polyp. **(A)** Delivered through colotomy. **(B)** Polypectomy performed.

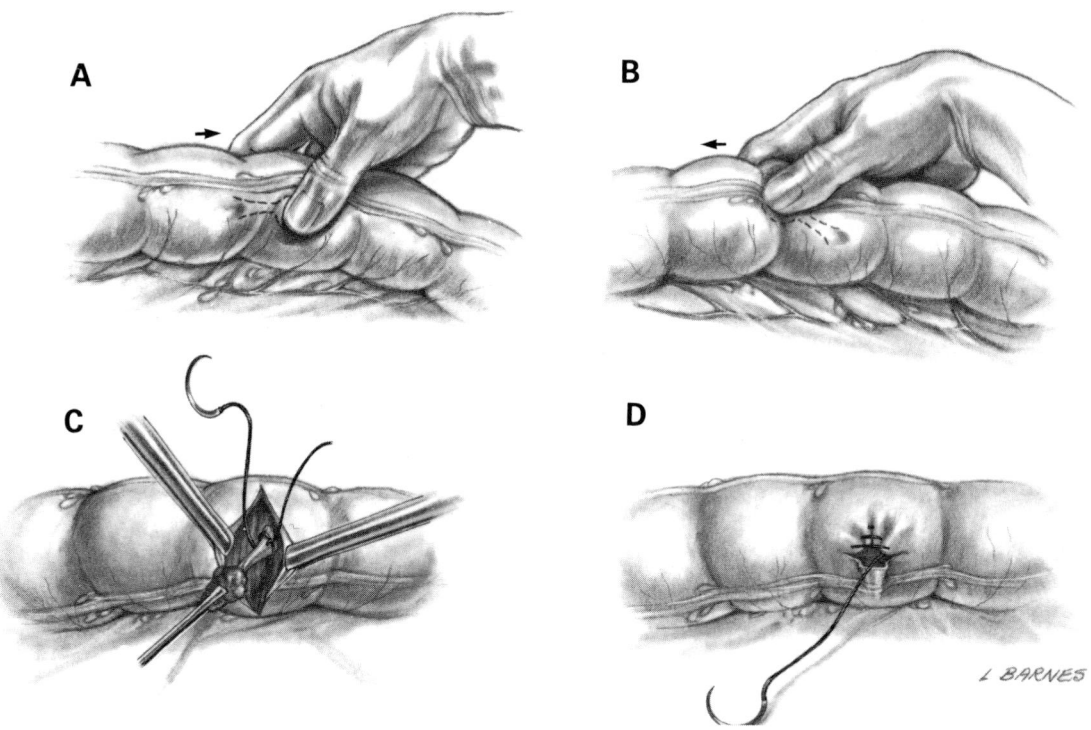

FIGURE 21-42. Colotomy and polypectomy. The base of the pedicle is determined by traction to create dimpling **(A)**, or the polyp is moved in both directions **(B)**, with the site **(C)** for colotomy determined by splitting the difference. Transverse colotomy is preferred, and the base is suture ligated. Longitudinal enterotomy **(D)** with transverse closure to avoid luminal narrowing is also acceptable.

carefully, and pale or white areas that may be suggestive of malignant change should be noted. These are the sites that should be examined by biopsy. Palpation is often very helpful in identifying firm or hard areas for biopsy. Certainly, the presence of ulcer implies cancerous change.

Taylor and colleagues reported their experience with preoperative assessment of villous adenomas.[405] Forty-four percent of the biopsy reports were misleading when compared with the interpretation when the specimen was completely excised. Most disturbing was a 10% false-positive incidence. Therefore, the most important criterion for determining the type of operative approach in my opinion is the clinical impression gained by palpation and inspection. Transrectal ultrasound (see Chapters 4 and 23) may be helpful when the surgeon knows that he or she is dealing with a malignant growth, but for the purpose of this discussion, the procedure should merely confirm that which is, in all probability, self-evident. If one is convinced that the lesion harbors no invasive cancer, every effort should be made to perform a sphincter-saving approach.

Techniques

There are basically five methods of removing rectal tumors: transanal excision, transcoccygeal excision (Kraske's), transsphincteric excision (Mason's), transperineal excision, and rectal resection with or without restoration of intestinal continuity. These methods are discussed in Chapter 23, but transanal excision and the transcoccygeal and transperineal approaches are reviewed here.

Transanal Excision Transanal excision is the preferred operation for benign neoplasms, especially if resection precludes restoration of continuity. The procedure can be performed by snare electrocoagulation, by laser therapy, by conventional excision with some type of retractor, or by means of transanal endoscopic microsurgery (TEM). Generally, I prefer to use the first approach for larger lesions and transanal excision for the smaller ones. The reason for this apparent contradiction is that it is helpful to have the specimen removed intact and submitted for pathologic evaluation. With a small lesion, this can usually be achieved by excision; however, excision of large or circumferential tumors requires a tedious, often bloody dissection. A compromise is suggested, wherein a wire-loop snare is used to remove the bulk of the mass, and the base is electrocoagulated. Grice suggested a method for maintaining hemostasis by means of suturing with a hemostatic clip (Poly Surgiclip) applied to the end of the ligature.[157] This permits bleeding areas to be secured without the problem of having to attempt knot tying in a confined space. A second clip is used to maintain firm positioning.

SNARE-ELECTROCOAGULATION With snare-electrocoagulation of a large tumor, inpatient management may be necessary. A mechanical bowel preparation as if for colectomy is advisable. However, only a small-volume enema is given for relatively small tumors; this type of problem can usually be dealt with on an outpatient basis. The patient is placed in the prone jackknife position if the lesion is situated anteriorly and in the lithotomy position if the tumor is primarily posterior. A moderate sphincter stretch is undertaken and, depending on the level of the lesion, an operating anoscope (see Figure 23-139) or any one of a number of anal retractors is inserted. The tumor is pared down with the wire loop until there remains only a minimal residual or it has been completely extirpated (Figure 21-43A). Using the needle-tip electrode, the base is coagulated along with any residual tumor; one needs to make certain that an adequate margin has been created (Figure 21-43B). It may be helpful to inject saline solution submucosally to facilitate excision and to minimize bleeding.[217] Some surgeons prefer to use a dilute epinephrine solution, but most believe that this is unnecessary.

EXCISION One can perform complete excision of the tumor by means of electrocautery without paring down the tumor. The lesion is outlined by the needle tip in order to be certain that the excision margins will be adequate, and then the tumor is completely excised (Figure 21-44).

Another option is "cold" knife or scissors dissection. The tumor is visualized, and an anchoring suture is placed distally (Figure 21-45). As mentioned, it is often helpful to infiltrate the submucosa with saline solution or possibly dilute epinephrine to facilitate dissection and to limit blood loss. If necessary, the full thickness of the bowel may be excised in order to obtain an adequate margin around the tumor. The rectum may be reapproximated as the dissection proceeds. Each suture is held for traction. It is important to place the suture distally initially. An error is made when the surgeon attempts to place the suture proximally and then carry the dissection in a distal manner. Traction can also be effected by elevating a flap of mucosa somewhat distal to the tumor (Figure 21-46).[313] Grice suggested a method for maintaining hemostasis by means of suturing with a hemostatic clip (Poly-Surgiclip) applied to the end of the ligature.[157] This permits bleeding areas to be secured without the problem of having to attempt knot tying in a confined space. A second clip is used to maintain firm positioning. These techniques have the advantage of obtaining a complete, undistorted pathologic specimen.

Another approach has been described in which a pseudostalk composed of normal mucosa and submucosa is created by traction on the tumor with Allis or Babcock forceps, and a stapling device is applied across the base

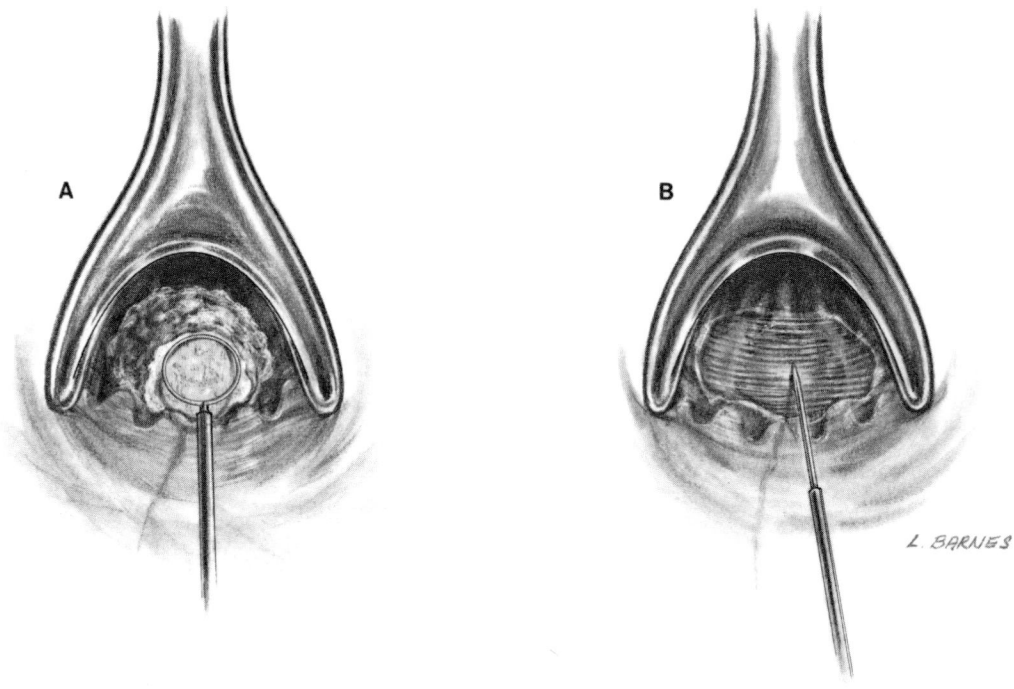

FIGURE 21-43. Transanal snare electrocoagulation. **(A)** A wire loop snare is used to pare down the tumor mass. **(B)** A needle electrode is employed for electrocoagulation of residual tumor.

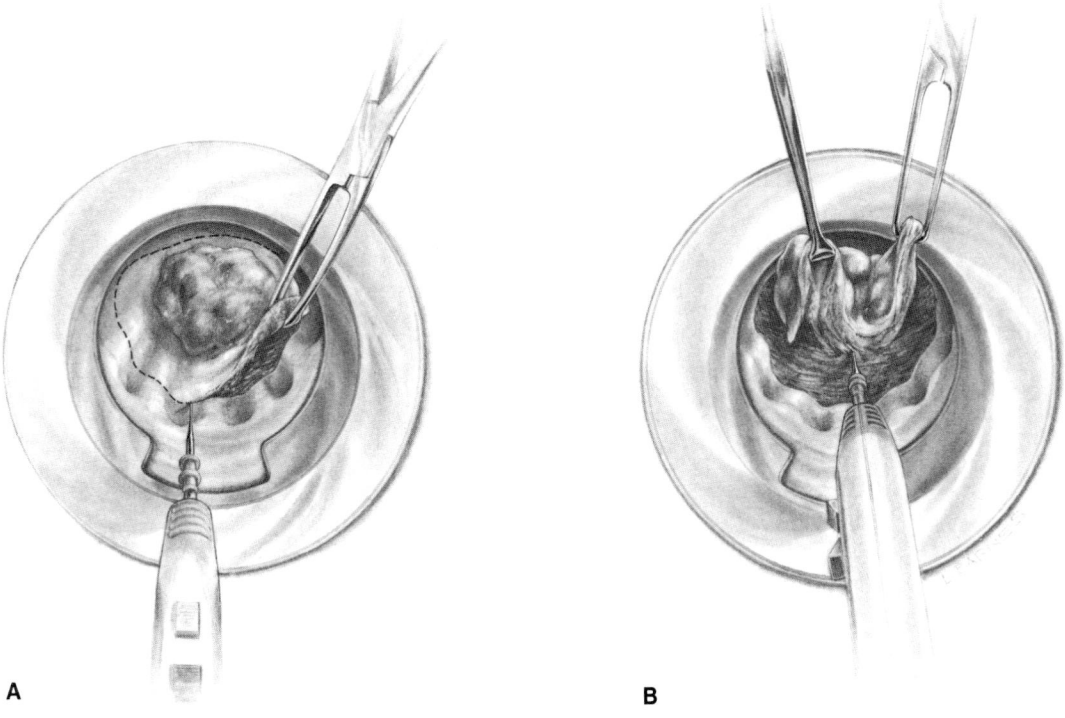

FIGURE 21-44. Transanal excision of rectal tumor by means of electrocautery. **(A)** The tumor is outlined with the needle-tip electrode with an adequate margin. **(B)** Complete excision of lesion with good hemostatic control.

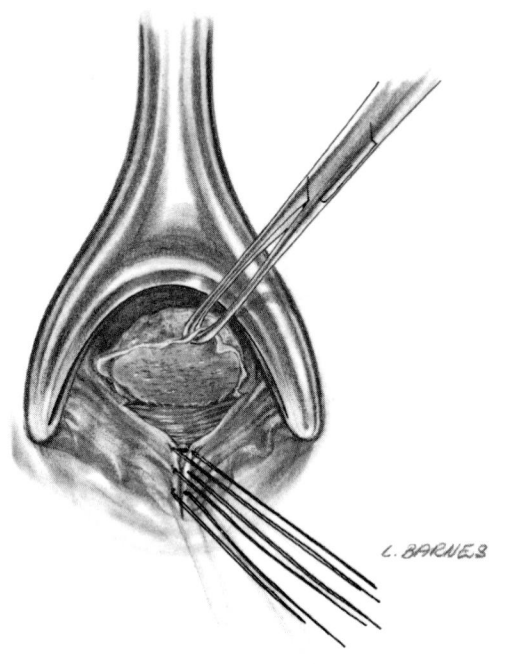

FIGURE 21-45. Transanal excision. An anchoring suture is placed distal to the tumor; the lesion is excised in a stepwise fashion; and the bowel is reapproximated as the polypectomy proceeds.

(Figure 21-47).[269] Another option is to utilize a laparoscopic stapler to excise the lesion and to maintain hemostasis (Figure 21-48).[94,334] The tumor is then removed. Even if the muscularis is incorporated by the staple line, bowel closure should still be secure. Another alternative is to utilize an endoscopic clipping apparatus as one ex-

cises the polyp in order to maintain hemostasis.[195] The concept of rectal mucosectomy, as adapted from restorative proctocolectomy, has been used to manage large benign tumors of the rectum. Keck and colleagues utilized this approach in 12 patients with lesions, on average, 8.5 cm in diameter.[218] After a mean follow-up of 47 months, the incidence of tumor persistence was 17% in this group with a high recurrence rate. This approach is recommended for large or circumferential benign lesions and is illustrated in Figure 21-49.

PHOTOABLATION With respect to photoablation, there is no question that the laser is an effective tool for vaporizing and destroying rectal tumors with minimal risk of bleeding. Numerous investigators have successfully used either the noncontact neodymium:yttrium-aluminum-garnet (Nd:YAG) laser or the contact endoprobe with coaxial water to destroy both benign and malignant lesions.[247,256,362] The major problem, however, is that because the target site is destroyed, it is not available for complete histologic study.[36] The equipment is expensive, the technique is time-consuming, and operating room safety is always a concern. I have not found it useful to apply this technique in my practice.

TRANSANAL ENDOSCOPIC MICROSURGERY TEM is a procedure that has been available primarily through its German inventors since 1983.[260,359] It is an endoluminal, minimally invasive technique that permits transanal excision of rectal lesions up to a level of about 20 cm without the requirement for a major abdominal operation. The procedure has been recommended primarily for benign

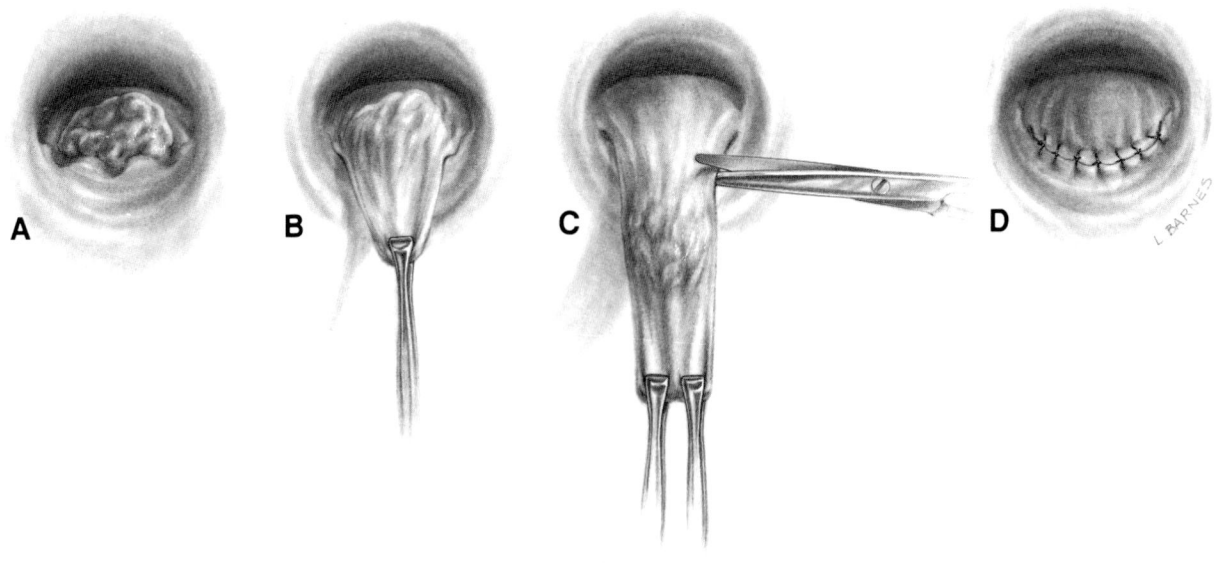

FIGURE 21-46. Transanal excision of tumor using mucosa for traction. **(A)** Lesion identified. **(B)** Flap mobilization with tumor. **(C)** Excision. **(D)** Closure. (Adapted from Pello MJ. Transanal excision of large sessile villous adenomas using an endorectal traction flap. *Surg Gynecol Obstet* 1987;164:281, with permission.)

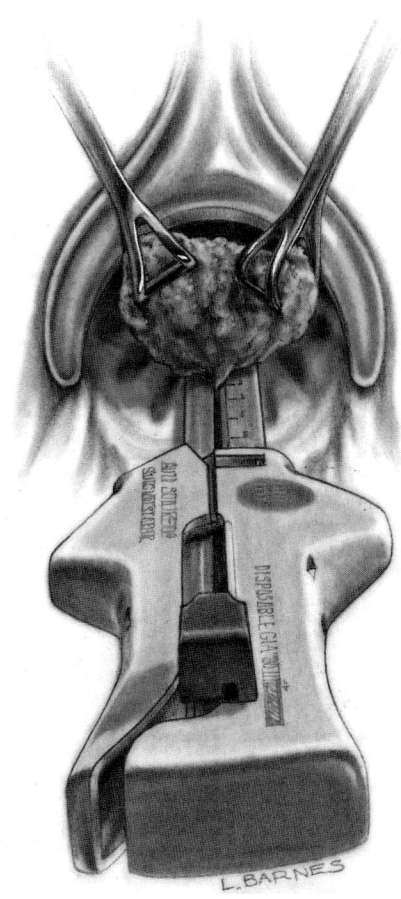

FIGURE 21-47. Transanal excision of rectal tumor. A gastrointestinal anastomosis stapling device is applied to the base of the tumor. The normal mucosa is incorporated and, when applicable, is an effective method for excision while maintaining hemostasis. (Redrawn from Miskowiak J, Lindenberg S. Excision of rectal villous adenoma using a TA or GIA stapler. *Br J Surg* 1986;73:630.)

tumors at a higher level, especially those that would require an abdominal operation to extirpate.

The instrument is a modified operating rectoscope, 4 cm in diameter. It holds a stereoscopic optical visual attachment with four gas-tight ports to allow simultaneous use of four instruments. Carbon dioxide is constantly infused, and various instruments such as tissue graspers, a high-frequency knife, suction devices, and needle holders, are inserted through the face-piece.[359] Adenomas that are even circumferential as well as selected carcinomas can be removed with TEM instrumentation. Wetherall and colleagues utilized a urologic resectoscope to perform 61 endoscopic resections.[443] The complication rate was minimal.

The two major disadvantages are that there is a limited space within the lumen to undertake suturing, and the equipment is quite expensive, especially because it cannot be readily applied to other uses.[207] Nakagoe and co-workers described their experience with a modifica-

tion of TEM, that of gasless video endoscopic excision that incorporates a standard laparoscopic video camera and requires no carbon dioxide insufflation system.[281] One hundred five rectal tumors were so managed.

OPINION I have had no personal experience with TEM. However, its prohibitively high cost for most individuals and most medical centers would obviously limit the ability of most surgeons to gain experience. Furthermore, there are more readily available, simpler, virtually equally effective options.

ENDOSCOPIC EXCISION WITH UROLOGIC RESECTOSCOPE This alternative, local approach for removing rectal tumors has been employed for palliation in the treatment of rectal cancers as well as for removing benign lesions. The procedure consists of inserting a 24-French 30-degree urologic resectoscope, 1.5% glycine solution as an irrigant, and the use of a loop-cutting electrode.[399] Sutton an colleagues reported 104 patients who underwent this procedure during a 10-year period.[399] The median distance from the anal verge was 10 cm, and the median operative time was 25 minutes. Lesions up to 16 cm from the anal verge were removed by this technique.

Transcoccygeal Excision or Resection Transcoccygeal excision is a very satisfactory alternative approach to the removal of benign midrectal lesions that do not permit resection and reestablishment of intestinal continuity by a more conventional means. It can also be employed for excision of a more distal lesion when the surgeon wishes to accomplish partial rectal resection rather than simply tumor excision. However, the operation should not be performed for malignant lesions because there is no removal of the associated lymph-bearing area. The so-called Kraske[229] approach is discussed elsewherewithin this text as applied to several conditions (e.g., rectal prolapse, rectourethral fistula, rectal cancer, and rectal stricture). The reader is advised to consult the respective sections for the particular application. A historical review, including that of Kraske, is presented in Chapter 23.

TECHNIQUE A bowel preparation is recommended as with any conventional colon operation. The patient is placed in the prone (jackknife) position with the buttocks taped apart. Through a midline incision from just outside the anal verge to just above the coccyx, the coccyx is exposed (Figure 21-50). The dissection can be facilitated by removal of the coccyx and even the lower sacral segments, if necessary. The levatores are incised, in addition to the deep portion of the external sphincter. The entire sphincter can be divided and repaired if this is required for complete excision of the tumor (see Transsphincteric Excision, Chapter 23). The posterior wall of the rectum is then exposed (Figure 21-50, *inset*). Guide sutures may be placed on the cut edge of the levatores and external

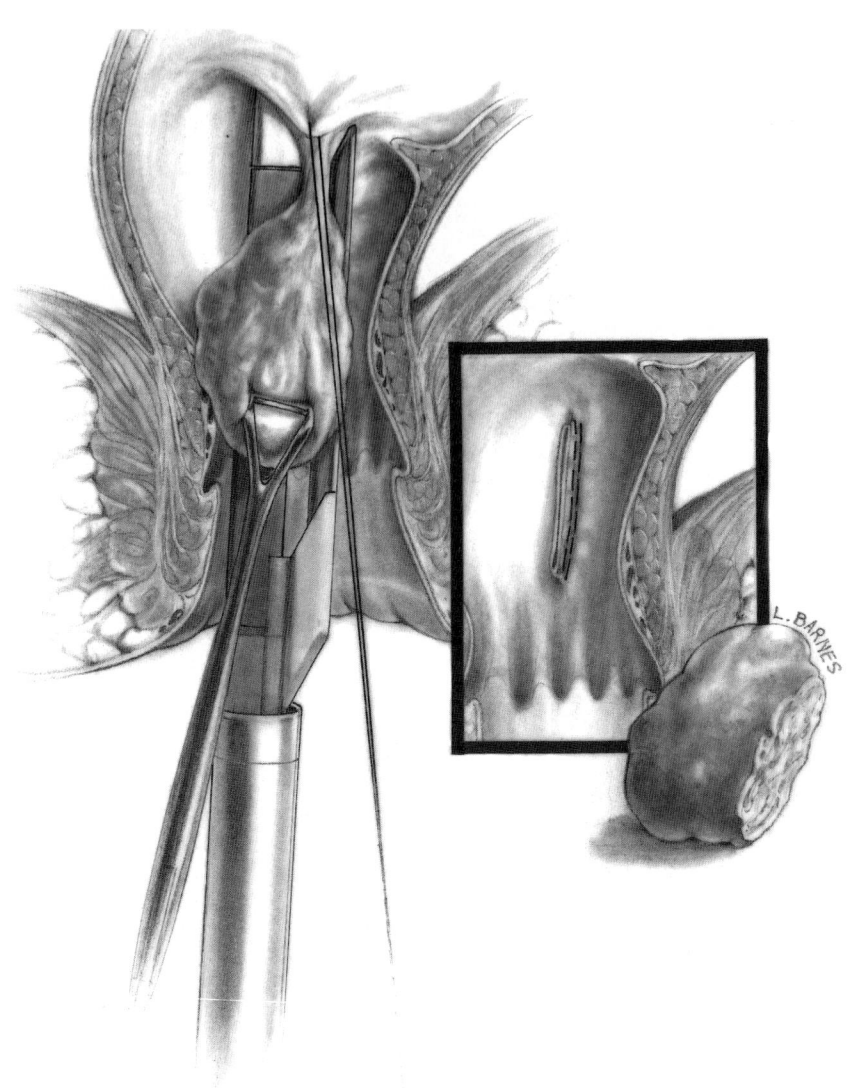

FIGURE 21-48. Transanal excision of rectal tumor utilizing a principle similar to that outlined in Figure 21-47. A laparoscopic stapling device is employed. (Redrawn from De Gennaro VA, Lescher TC. Transanal excision of rectal tumors using a laparoscopic stapler. *Dis Colon Rectum* 1995; 38:327.)

sphincter to facilitate subsequent identification at the time of closure and sphincter repair. Allis forceps are placed on the posterior rectal wall, and a transverse proctotomy is performed. This usually poses no problem when the tumor is located anteriorly; a partial wall excision is then performed (Figure 21-51). The rectal incisions can then be closed individually (Figure 21-51A) and the sphincter repair accomplished with interrupted No. 1 long-term, absorbable sutures (Figure 21-51B). The defect created as a consequence of removal of the coccyx cannot be closed. It is often advisable to place a small, closed-suction drain into this area through a stab wound in the buttock. The skin wound is reapproximated with a continuous subcuticular closure of fine absorbable suture.

If it is necessary to resect the bowel or to perform an excision of a tumor on the posterior wall, it is especially important to make the proctotomy incision at the correct level (not through the tumor!). Partial wall excision or proctectomy can be performed and an anastomosis ef-

fected by either a hand-sewn or stapling technique (Figure 21-52; see Figure 23-136). One can usually safely resect only 5 or 6 cm without opening the peritoneal cavity to obtain sufficient bowel for performing an anastomosis. If necessary, this can be accomplished by opening the anterior peritoneum and delivering the sigmoid colon through the pelvic pouch of Douglas (see Figure 17-37).

Intersphincteric Excision Selvaggi and colleagues suggested an unusual approach for the treatment of benign tumors of the rectum, that of anterior intersphincteric access.[369] This apparently offers a good view of the posterior rectal wall and enables the surgeon to perform excision of the neoplasm. The operation is, in essence, the reverse of transcoccygeal excision.

A transverse, curvilinear, transperineal, anterior incision is made outside the anal verge. Through the intersphincteric plane, the supralevator area is exposed. An anterior proctotomy is created, and the tumor on the posterior rec-

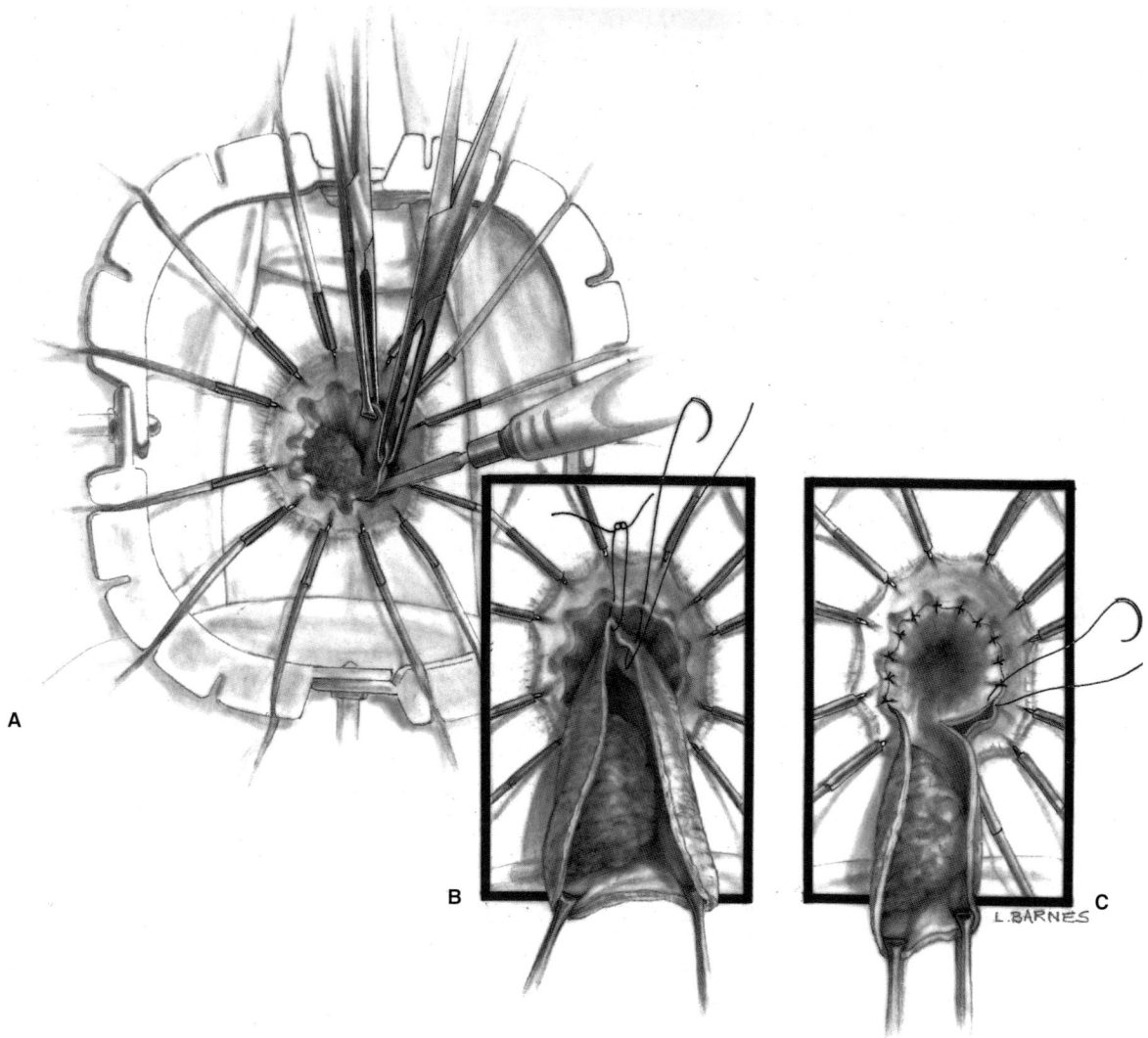

FIGURE 21-49. Excision of a large rectal tumor. **(A)** A Lone Star self-retaining retractor provides exposure of the anal canal and lower rectum. A circumferential incision is made distal to the tumor, just above the dentate line. **(B)** Following dissection and freeing of the rectal mucosa circumferentially, including the tumor, the rectal mucosal sleeve is incised. Sutures are placed between the proximal rectal mucosa and the dentate line to prevent retraction. **(C)** The rectal mucosa above the tumor is progressively divided, and the anastomosis is completed with interrupted sutures as the tumor is being excised. (Redrawn from Keck JO, Schoetz DJ Jr, Roberts PL, et al. Rectal mucosectomy in the treatment of giant rectal villous tumors. *Dis Colon Rectum* 1995;38:233.)

tal wall is directly visualized and excised. Repair follows the general principles of standard layered closure.

OPINION I have had no personal experience with this operation, but I see no advantage over the transcoccygeal alternative. Generally, the lithotomy position should be avoided for any major operation, except under very special circumstances. As stated many times throughout this book, the prone jackknife position is technically easier and more comfortable for the surgeon, and uses the assistant or assistants more effectively.

Transsphincteric Excision See Chapter 23.

Medical Treatment

As mentioned previously and as discussed in Chapter 22, a diet high in vegetables and fruits is associated with a lower risk of cancer of the colon. There has been a particular interest in supplementary antioxidant vitamins to prevent colorectal cancer, because these vitamins are present in these food groups. A clinical trial of such antioxidant vitamins (β-carotene, vitamin C, and vitamin E) was undertaken to determine their efficacy in prevention of colorectal adenomas. In the experience of Greenburg and his associates in the Polyp Prevention Study Group, in which 751 patients completed a 4-year clinical trial,

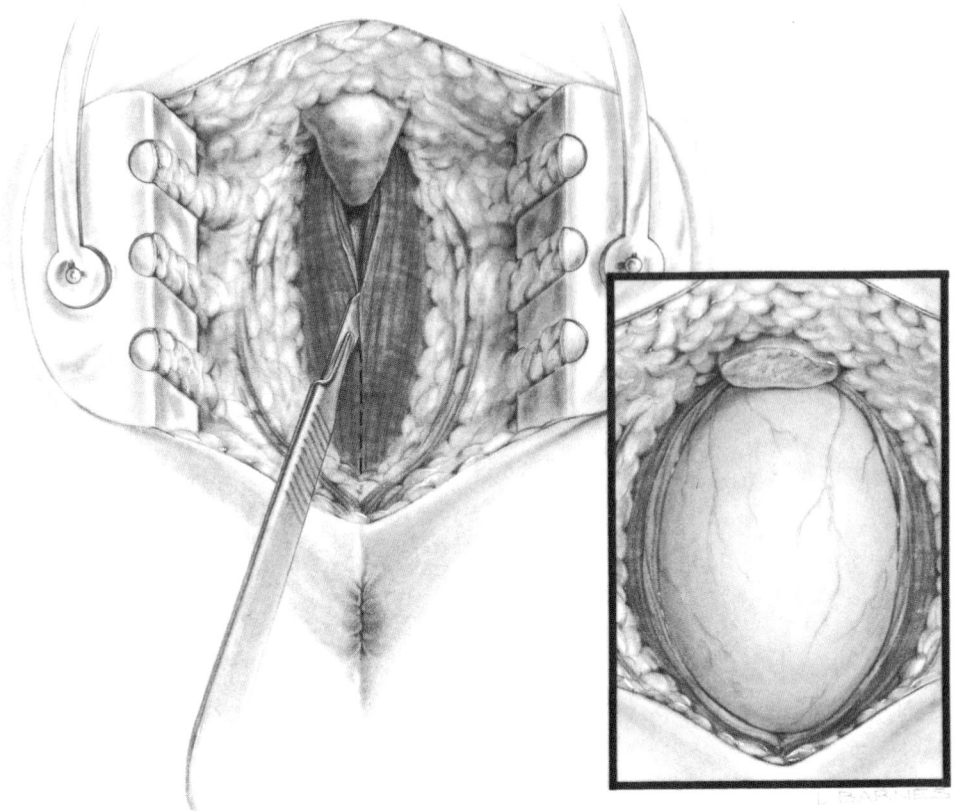

FIGURE 21-50. Transcoccygeal approach to removal of rectal tumors. A midline incision is made, and the levator ani muscle is divided. The coccyx is excised, and the posterior wall of the rectum is exposed **(inset)**.

there was no demonstrable benefit with the use of supplemental β-carotene and vitamins C and E.[155] However, in a publication by Whelan and colleagues, the use of multivitamins, vitamin E, and calcium supplements was found to be associated with a lower incidence of *recurrent* adenomas.[444] There is one case report demonstrating that the nonsteroidal antiinflammatory drug, piroxicam, was effective in causing tumor regression in a patient with a villous adenoma who refused surgical excision.[125]

Results

There are no meaningful (i.e., prospective, randomized, controlled) studies of the results of surgical treatment of benign rectal tumors by means of transanal excision, snare excision, electrocoagulation, or any other method. This is perhaps because there is the perception that the results are satisfactory, the complications minimal, and the rate of recurrence low, irrespective of the method of treatment.

Laser Excision

There seems to have been be a particular interest in publishing the results of laser treatment for this condition, although much less information has appeared since

the late 1990s.[35,246,247,256] A cynic could observe that this is an attempt to justify an expensive technique. I believe that laser excision of rectal tumors is another example of technology's seeking an application. However, I believe that the indications for its use as expressed by Low and colleagues are quite reasonable:[247]

- A broad-base istologically benign colonic polyp that cannot be removed by snare resection
- Malignant polyp in an individual who is not a candidate for or refuses radical resection
- Recurrent benign or malignant tumor that cannot optimally be approached by another method

One can add a fourth potential indication: failure of a prior approach to establish tumor control or elimination.

Mathus-Vliegen and Tytgat performed Nd:YAG laser photocoagulation on 100 individuals with colorectal adenomata and rectal polyps following colectomy and ileorectal anastomosis for FAP.[256] With tumors greater than 4 cm, 69% recurred. Those with tumors between 1 and 4 cm experienced a 55% recurrence rate. Brunetaud and colleagues performed endoscopic laser treatment of 264 patients with benign rectosigmoid villous adenomas and noted a 13% rate of recurrence.[35] These investigators

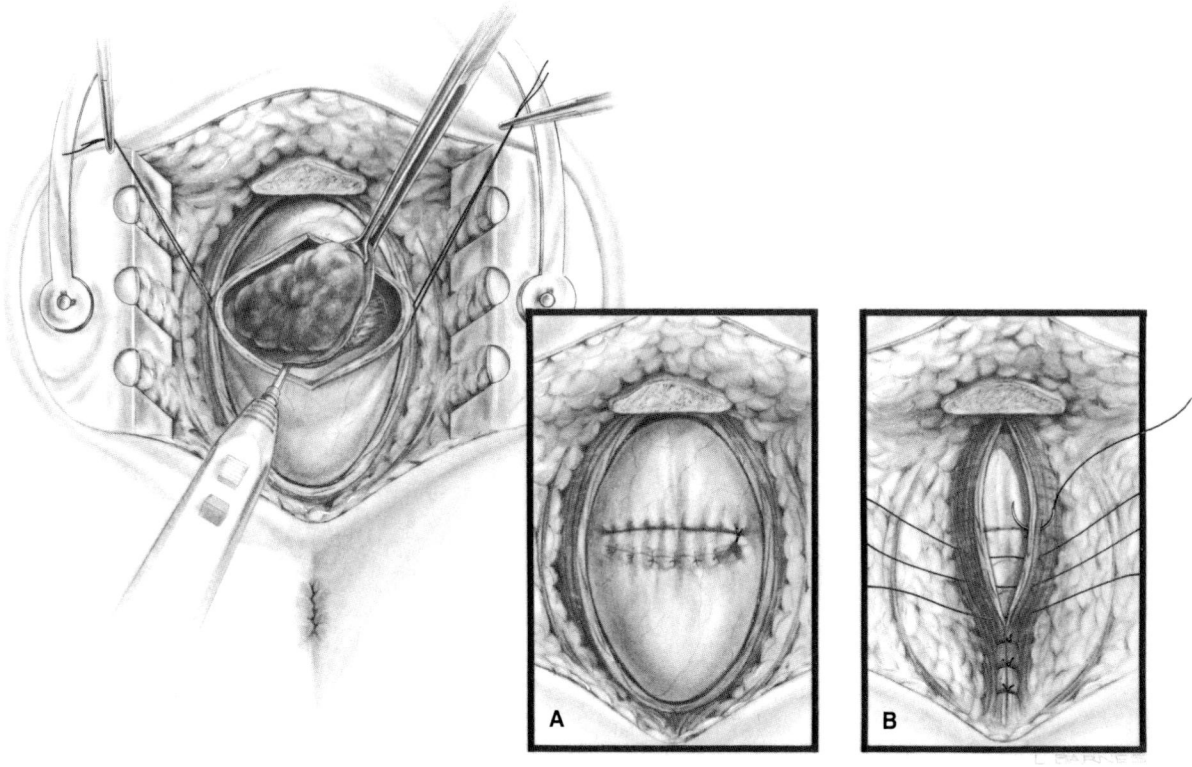

FIGURE 21-51. Transcoccygeal approach to removal of rectal tumors. A posterior proctotomy reveals a tumor on the anterior wall. This is excised by means of electrocautery. Tumor excision alone or full-thickness excision of the bowel wall can be accomplished. **(A)** The enterotomy wounds can be closed separately. **(B)** Repair of the sphincter muscles is accomplished in a layered fashion.

concluded that because this approach is time-consuming and technically difficult to accomplish, laser photocoagulation of extensive lesions should be limited to those individuals who are not candidates for surgical resection.

Other Results

Chiu and Spencer reported the Mayo Clinic experience of 331 villous adenomas treated over a 10-year period.[55] Excluded were patients with synchronous carcinomas. Numerous methods were employed, depending on the location and size of the tumors. Only three individuals underwent abdominoperineal resection. Sixty-nine electrocoagulations were associated with four recurrences, whereas 26 transanal excisions yielded seven patients who developed recurrences. The authors reiterated the importance of nonradical resection for lesions without invasive carcinoma.

Sakamoto and colleagues reviewed the experience from the Ferguson Clinic (Grand Rapids, MI), involving 118 individuals with villous adenoma treated by transanal excision.[361] With a mean follow-up period of 55 months, 30% developed recurrences. Important compli-

cations included ten instances of hemorrhage and two of perforation (complication rate, 10%).

In the Memorial Hospital (New York) experience, 72 patients underwent local excision, and nine developed recurrences.[333] The authors advocated local excision by means of cautery snare for all benign-appearing villous adenomas. Because of the 12% recurrence rate, frequent follow-up examination is recommended. The recurrence rate in 24 patients who underwent transanal excision as reported by Jahadi and Bailey was also 12%.[203] Other investigators confirmed general satisfaction with the standard approaches used for complete removal of benign rectal tumors.[100,360,462]

Westbrook and colleagues reported 19 patients who underwent transsacral (transcoccygeal) or transsphincteric operations; nine patients had villous adenomas.[440] Despite four fecal fistulas, two wound dehiscences, one rectal stricture, and one sacrococcygeal hernia, the authors stated that "the posterior approach to the rectum is safe and effective. . . ." I cannot agree; the procedure may be effective (there were no recurrences), but in the authors' experience, as well as in my own and that of oth-

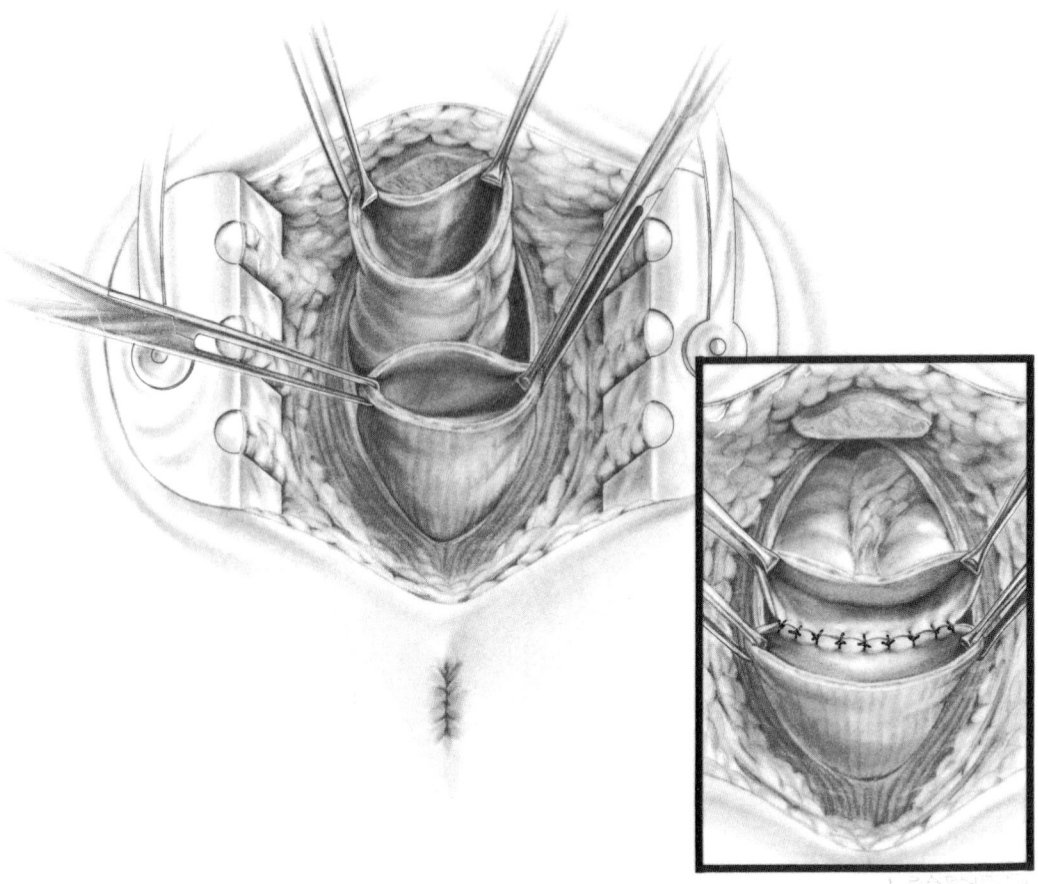

FIGURE 21-52. Transcoccygeal approach to removal of rectal tumors. Sleeve resection can be performed, if necessary, but additional length may be required through the floor of the pelvis. Anastomosis is shown by means of an interrupted suture technique **(inset)**.

ers,[54] the morbidity rate is appreciable. Transanal snare electrocoagulation and transanal excision are, with rare exception, the approaches on which one should rely in the treatment of benign tumors of the rectum.

Polyp Follow-Up

How to follow up patients who have undergone colonoscopy-polypectomy is a subject of some controversy. As mentioned, if the patient has had only a polypectomy and a limited examination, complete endoscopic evaluation of the entire colon should be accomplished as soon as feasable. Unfortunately, however, there has been little objective evidence upon which to recommend the correct intervals for follow-up examination.[445]

According to Nava and colleagues, individuals who harbored a single adenomatous polyp were diagnosed with new ones after a mean time of 23 months compared with 13.5 months in patients with two or more initial lesions.[283] Williams and colleagues reported a prospective study from St. Mark's Hospital.[448] Recall of 300 patients

who had previously undergone colonoscopic polypectomy was conducted using multiple diagnostic tests (occult blood testing, proctosigmoidoscopy, double-contrast barium enema, fiberoptic sigmoidoscopy, and total colonoscopy). The mean follow-up interval since the polypectomy was 3.6 years. Because double-contrast barium enema examination missed 71% of adenomas, the authors suggested that colonoscopy is the preferred method for follow-up.

Waye and Braunfeld reported more than 200 patients with a "cleared" colon who underwent a repeat colonoscopy within 1 year of endoscopic polypectomy.[434] Further adenomas were found in 56%. Those with single adenomas had as much likelihood of having further lesions as did those with multiple tumors. Of the remaining patients in whom no adenomas were found at 1 year, 35% developed new growths within 4 years; those with a single tumor initially had one half the rate of a subsequent neoplasm when compared with patients who had multiple adenomas. The authors recommended colonoscopy every 2 years if more than one adenoma was removed and every 3 years in patients with only one index lesion. Most reports seem to agree that the presence of multiple polyps on initial examination is a significant consideration in predicting the likelihood of the subsequent development of tumors.[8,188,288,460]

Ransohoff and colleagues submitted a study design to determine whether colonoscopic surveillance after polypectomy is cost-effective.[336] They found that a program of colonoscopy every 3 years would incur cumulatively a 1.4% risk of colonic perforation, a 0.11% risk for a perforation-related death, and direct physician costs in excess of $2,000 per examination (1991 statistics). They estimated that one death from cancer could be prevented per 283 examinations. The authors concluded that colonoscopic surveillance can be justified financially only in the individual at high risk (e.g., with multiple polyps).

Kronbörg and colleagues reported the results of 629 colonoscopies and 130 double-contrast examinations performed during the first 2 years of a prospective program.[232] Three months following polypectomy, 13 patients required an additional polypectomy. The yield was highest with patients who had sessile villous adenomas, those with dysplasia, and those with carcinoma. In a later study, Kronbörg reported several prospective colonoscopic follow-up programs.[231] The author recommended increasing the interval length of reexamination from 6 to 24 months. Although the chance of missing an earlier lesion was obviously more likely, he believed this position could be reconciled by the morbidity and mortality of the examination. There was no demonstrable difference in survival rates between the group with more frequent examinations and the other group.

Hofstead and co-workers, in a prospective evaluation of individuals with colorectal polyps, identified an apparent falling off of new polyp formation in patients more than 60 years of age.[185] These investigators concluded that these individuals are at a reduced risk once their colons have been cleared. Therefore, a policy of discharge from surveillance following removal of small adenomous polyps, provided the lesions are solitary, is worthy of consideration.[185,401]

Winawer and associates sought to determine whether follow-up colonoscopy at 3 years would detect important colonic lesions following initial excision of one or more adenomas.[453] Patients were randomly assigned to have follow-up colonoscopy at 1 and 3 years or at 3 years only. The authors concluded that colonoscopy performed at 3 years following colonoscopic removal of adenomatous polyps detects important colonic lesions as effectively as follow-up at 1 and 3 years. It was believed that this recommendation should reduce the cost of postpolypectomy surveillance and screening.

Epidemiologic studies have demonstrated that relatives of patients with colorectal cancer are at an increased risk for the development of malignancy.[450] Rozen

and colleagues also confirmed this observation, not only in families of patients with cancer, but also in families in which relatives harbored adenomatous polyps (excluding the polyposis syndromes).[354] Therefore, these individuals also should be subjected to a screening and follow-up protocol (see also Chapter 22).

Opinion

One must assume that the risk of the presence of a synchronous adenoma in a patient with a known neoplasm is at least 25%. There is, therefore, no debate about the merits of "clearing the colon." Even after such a procedure, however, published studies of colonoscopic examinations performed 1 year later usually find that 25% or more of the patients have additional neoplasms.[69,289,358,437,446] How important are these benign tumors? Because they are invariably small, the fact that they are merely present is not a threat to survival. Therefore, if one is to carry out a vigorous, effective, polyp-cancer surveillance program for an individual who had undergone prior polypectomy for neoplastic disease (benign or malignant), I advocate no radiologic investigation and limit the procedure to colonoscopy every 3 years. In order to help ensure maximum patient commitment to follow-up, a flexible sigmoidoscopy is advised at a yearly visit.

Exceptions to this regimen include individuals believed to be at an increased risk. This group includes those who have had multiple adenomas removed, those who initially harbored a large neoplasm, especially if there is an increased risk for local recurrence, those who had a sessile tumor, or those who had evidence of invasive carcinoma. These people may require more frequent examinations.

With respect to villous adenomas, local recurrence is not uncommon, especially when large, sessile lesions of the rectum are removed by snare electrocoagulation or by local excision. Although there is a higher incidence of malignant degeneration, when it occurs the tumors are usually well differentiated and relatively slow growing.[135] Frequent follow-up examination is mandatory. Examination every 3 months is recommended until recurrence is no longer observed. Usually, if the patient is free of recurrence after 1 year, I am willing to pursue an annual follow-up program. Even when confronted with tumor at each visit, I am willing to continue to perform local treatment, as long as the biopsy results are benign, if the alternative is an abdominoperineal resection.

Familial Adenomatous Polyposis

FAP is an inheritable (autosomally dominant) disease with close to 100% penetrance (i.e., the risk of colorectal cancer approximates 100%), occurring in one of every

7,000 to 10,000 births and in which the colon is involved with innumerable adenomatous polyps. The most reliable figures are those derived from registers. The Danish Register is considered the most complete, reporting an incidence of one in 7,000.[49] Campbell and colleagues believed that the probable incidence ranges from one in 7,000 to one in 16,000 live births, with a prevalence of approximately one in 25,000.[49] Despite the well-recognized inheritance pattern, approximately 20% of patients have no family history. Presumably, these cases represent spontaneous genetic mutations. A retrospective review of the FAP registry at the Cleveland Clinic revealed an incidence of spontaneous mutation of 22%.[356]

Some individual case reports of patients with multiple polyps were described in the eighteenth and nineteenth centuries, but Cripps is generally credited with being the first to note the condition in two members of the same family (see Chapter 23).[52,77,84] Handford described the association of cancer in 1890.[168] The establishment of the St. Mark's Hospital register was the result of the initial observations of Lockhart-Mummery (see Chapter 9); this was succeeded by other reports from the same institution.[104,105,244] Following these publications, some families were identified by other authors as harboring this genetic defect.[38] Gardner and co-workers, although not the first to identify extracolonic manifestations, accumulated sufficient data to isolate a group of patients who were subsequently determined to have Gardner's syndrome (see later).[137,139,140]

The largest experience with FAP was published by Bussey in a monograph based upon more than 300 families contained in the St. Mark's Hospital Polyposis Register.[42] Bussey stressed that distinction should be made between FAP and the condition of multiple adenomas. In the former, colon polyps number as many as several thousand (Figure 21-53), whereas in the latter it is usually fewer than 100. The author suggests that the number, 100, be the cutting-off point to distinguish between the two conditions.[42] The severity of the manifestation, that is, the number of polyps, varies in accordance with the age at presentation.

FAP becomes apparent during youth, and if colectomy is not performed it is associated with a high incidence of colorectal cancer, usually by the age of 40 years. Cancer occurs rarely in those younger than 20 years, and only one case has been reported in someone younger than 15 years.[63] The condition is believed to be responsible for 0.5% to 1% of colorectal cancers.

Attenuated Familial Adenomatous Polyposis

The attenuated form of FAP (AFAP) is characterized by fewer polyps and later onset of colorectal cancer. The diagnosis of polyps and cancer in AFAP is usually made a decade or more later than in FAP. In a report by Church and associates, polyps were diagnosed at a mean of 44 years, with cancer diagnosed at a mean of 56 years.[62] AFAP may be part of a spectrum that includes FAP but is caused by different mutations within the adenomatous polyposis coli (APC) gene.[62]

Gene Identification

Studies have demonstrated that a gene on chromosome 5q21 is responsible for the inheritance of FAP (the *APC* gene) and, therefore, is important for the development of colorectal carcinoma (see the earlier discussion of genetics in this chapter).[222,311] Mutations in in the *APC* gene result in FAP.[335] Additionally, two genes that are tightly linked to FAP have been found to be somatically altered in tumors from patients with sporadic colorectal cancer.[290] The identification and characterization of the FAP gene have been accomplished by demonstrating mutations that were essentially base substitutions or deletions.[158,216] Park and co-workers performed linkage studies using two polymorphic systems close to or at the *APC* locus from which they could determine the haplotypes of individuals in order to make the diagnosis a FAP.[307] These investigators found that their method, utilizing RSA1 site polymorphism and cytosine-adenine repeat length polymorphism, as well as the polymerase chain reaction–based sequencing method, provided accurate and efficient tools for presymptomatic diagnosis of FAP in families of those with known disease. Identification of these genes should permit a better understanding of the pathogenesis of colorectal neoplasms and, therefore, in the counseling of individuals with a possible predisposition to these tumors.

Genetic Testing and Counseling

Genetic testing and counseling are complex and problematic issues with respect to both FAP and hereditary nonpolyposis cancer (see Chapter 22). The interpretation of genetic tests is not as straightforward as that of obtaining a blood glucose concentration, and there are implications that transcend the purely clinical (e.g., the potential of discrimination for insurance and in employment).[458] Theoretical candidates for testing include first-degree relatives of patients with FAP and AFAP as well as relatives of an individual with a confirmed *APC* germ line mutation. One must recognize that genetic testing is regulated by governments and by governmental agencies, and in the United States, Institutional Review Board approval is also required.[335] However, there are potential benefits if not to the patient, then to our knowledge. For example, Groden and colleagues were able to show that DNA from parents of one of their patients had a deletion that represented a new mutation; this was then transmitted to two of the children.[158]

FAP DNA testing for patients, family members, and by prenatal investigation (amniocentesis) is commercially available (Myriad Genetic Laboratories, Salt Lake City,

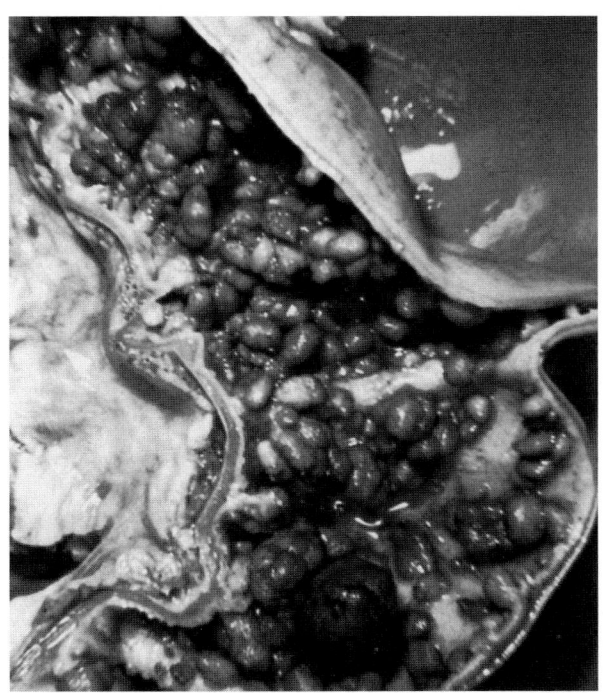

FIGURE 21-53. Familial adenomatous polyposis. This portion of a sigmoid colon demonstrates numerous, variable-sized polypoid excrescences throughout the bowel. (From Corman ML, Veidenheimer MC, Swinton NW. *Diseases of the anus, rectum, and colon. Part I: neoplasms.* New York: Medcom, 1972, with permission.)

UT). Giardiello and associates utilized the commercial test for the *APC* gene in a nationwide sample of 177 patients from 125 families.[142] Eighty-three percent had clinical features of FAP or were at risk for the disease. The authors emphasized the importance of adequate genetic counseling not only if the test is positive, but even if the test is ordered. If a mutation in APC is identified in the patient's germ line DNA, the immediate family and other branches of the family can be encouraged to come forward for genetic counseling and to learn their risk status if they wish.[335] Importantly, if no mutation is detected, genetic testing for APC mutations in the family is *not* indicated.

As mentioned, gene therapy of somatic cells may in the future provide a nonsurgical means for dealing with this condition. In the prenatal situation, if somatic gene therapy could be successfully applied to fetuses with FAP, it could possibly obviate the decision to terminate pregnancies.[387] This issue raises important ethical and legal questions concerning altering the human gene pool, with its unknown effect on future generations.[387]

Signs, Symptoms, and Manifestations

Polyps may be present for a number of years before the onset of symptoms. That is why family members of patients with known polyposis should be routinely screened for the presence of such polyps. The mean age of the appearance of polyps in the St. Mark's Hospital series was 22 years. Bussey theorized that polyps exist for at least a decade before causing symptoms of sufficient import to stimulate the patient to seek medical attention.[42] With the formation of polyposis registries, however, there has been a significant decrease in the percentage of patients who have cancer at the time of colon resection.[36,176]

Bleeding is the most common complaint (80%), followed by diarrhea (70%), abdominal pain, and mucous discharge. Weight loss, anemia, and intestinal obstruction are ominous signs, implying the presence of cancer. In the experience from the Mt. Sinai Medical Center in New York, 27% of the 115 patients who were reviewed had colorectal cancer at the time of presentation.[205]

In addition to the complaints and findings indicative of intestinal polyloid disease, patients may develop symptoms resulting from extracolonic manifestations.

Gardner's Syndrome

Gardner's syndrome is characterized by the presence of multiple osteomas (usually skull and mandible), cysts, and soft tissue tumors. Other conditions associated with the syndrome include the following: desmoid tumors of the abdominal wall, mesentery, and retroperitoneum; dental abnormalities; thyroid carcinoma; periampullary carcinoma; and gastrointestinal adenomatosis and carcinoma. It is now understood that all these features may be seen, with variable expression, in many patients with FAP, and Gardner's syndrome should not be considered a genetically distinct variant.[237] With careful scrutiny of individuals with FAP, the presence of extracolonic manifestations probably represents the rule rather than the exception.[371]

Osteomas Osteomas were originally described in the skull and mandible but more recently have been shown to involve other areas; they may be the only extracolonic manifestations.[421,431] The bony tumors may be present for many years before the onset of intestinal symptoms.[42] Because of the potential for use as a marker for Gardner's syndrome, some clinicians have suggested screening x-ray studies of the skull and mandible. Woods and colleagues had the x-ray films of 51 individuals independently reviewed from the Cleveland Clinic Registry by a dental surgeon and by a neuroradiologist.[459] Only 14% of patients were found to have a significant lesion, each of whom harbored other extracolonic manifestations. The authors believed that such screening was, therefore, not useful.

Epidermoid Cysts (Oldfield's Syndrome) The association of epidermoid (sebaceous) cysts with FAP has been termed Oldfield's syndrome.[298] Because of the common occurrence in the general population of these cutaneous lesions, little thought is usually given to the possibility of the cysts' being associated with the condition. However, in young patients with FAP, the distribution is different—face, scalp, and extremities rather than the back.[237] Furthermore, because they are uncommon before the age of puberty, the presence of epidermoid cysts in this age group should alert the physician to pursue colorectal investigation.[42,240]

Desmoid Tumors Desmoid tumors are usually benign fibromas that tend to infiltrate locally into adjacent tissue. They are reported to arise in 3.5% to 5.7% of patients who have Gardner's syndrome.[42,382] Although the lesion appears occasionally to emulate fibrosarcoma, metastasis does not occur. Local recurrence is the rule rather than the exception. The mass tends to develop in abdominal incisions, in the abdominal cavity (particularly the

small bowel mesentery), and the retroperitoneum (Figure 21-54).[153,262] The condition may antedate the appearance of the polyposis by developing in an abdominal incision performed for another purpose (e.g., appendectomy). Usually, however, desmoid tumors become manifest from 1 to 3 years following surgery for polyposis.[42] Studies have shown that the absolute risk of desmoids in patients with FAP is 2.56/1,000 person-years, with the comparative risk 852 times that of the general population.[21] Desmoids can, however, occur in the absence of Gardner's syndrome.[128] Clark and Phillips and others confirmed that intraabdominal desmoids behave unpredictably but are an important source of mortality in those with FAP.[65] The authors also observed that signal inten-

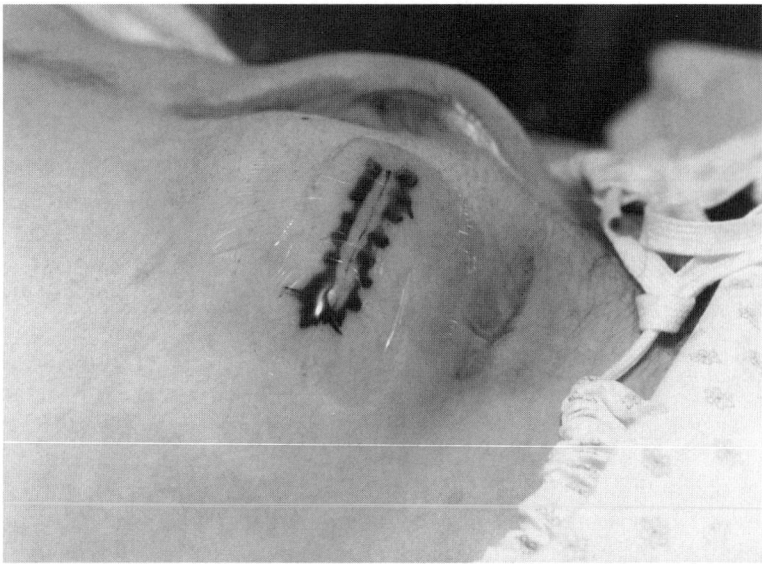

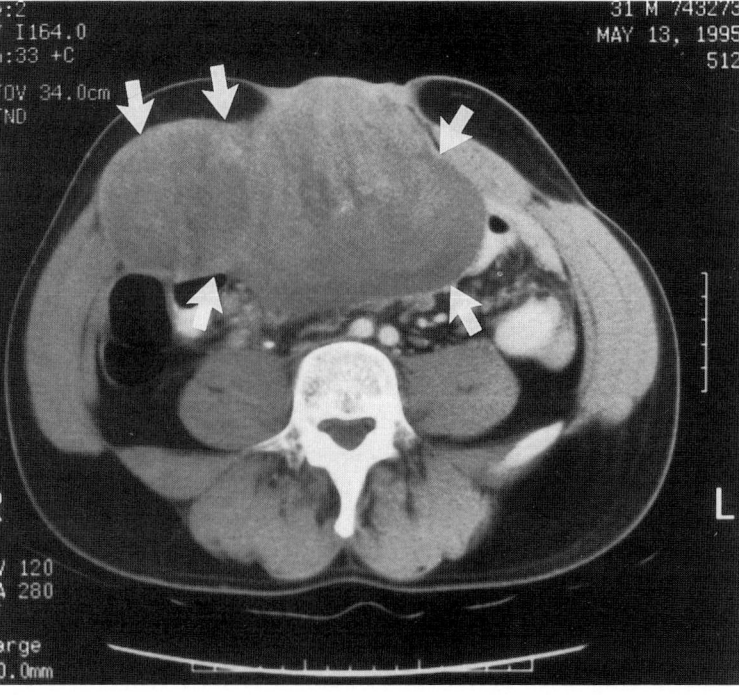

FIGURE 21-54. Desmoid tumor of the abdomen in a young man who had previously undergone total colectomy for familial adenomatous polyposis. **(A)** Massive tumor can be appreciated in the midabdomen. Note the broad scar from the prior surgical procedure. An excisional biopsy was performed in the left side of the abdomen to confirm the diagnosis. (Note the adhesive dressing.) **(B)** Computed tomography demonstrates huge mass involving the abdominal wall *(arrows)*.

sity on magnetic resonance imaging reflects tumor cellularity, which may, in part, determine progression; this may aid in management of these individuals.[65]

Dental Anomalies Dental abnormalities have been recognized as part of the syndrome complex, including impacted supernumerary teeth, unerupted teeth, early cavities, edentulousness, dentigerous cysts, and abnormal mandibular bone structure.[42,138]

Thyroid Disease Thyroid carcinoma has been reported to be associated with Gardner's syndrome.[48,82,144,219,239,324,383,384] Unique about this observation is that the proliferative abnormalities of the syndrome as listed earlier are of mesenchymal origin, whereas thyroid tumors are not; this suggests a broader potential for the genetic defect.[48] Review of the St. Mark's Hospital Polyposis Registry revealed that young women (less than 35 years old) are at a particular risk for developing thyroid cancer, mainly of the papillary type.[324] This group especially warrants periodic thyroid

evaluation. An association with thyroiditis has also been observed.[180]

Upper Gastrointestinal Tumors Periampullary carcinoma is a well-recognized disease that is associated with Gardner's syndrome.[397] Twelve percent of patients in the St. Mark's Hospital series who survived for 5 years after colectomy developed carcinoma of the duodenum, ampulla of Vater, or pancreas.[42] Sugihara and associates reviewed the literature and identified 29 such patients, with a mean age of 45 years.[397] Eleven patients developed colorectal cancer, all of them having presented with symptoms before the periampullary malignancy. Many studies have been published that confirm this association.[41,70,144,210,371,393]

Gastrointestinal polyps and cancer have been frequently reported with this syndrome (Figs. 21-55 through 21-57).[39,40,363,371] Invasive upper gastrointestinal adenocarcinoma was found in 4.5% of patients with FAP as recorded in ten polyposis registries.[202] de Vos tot

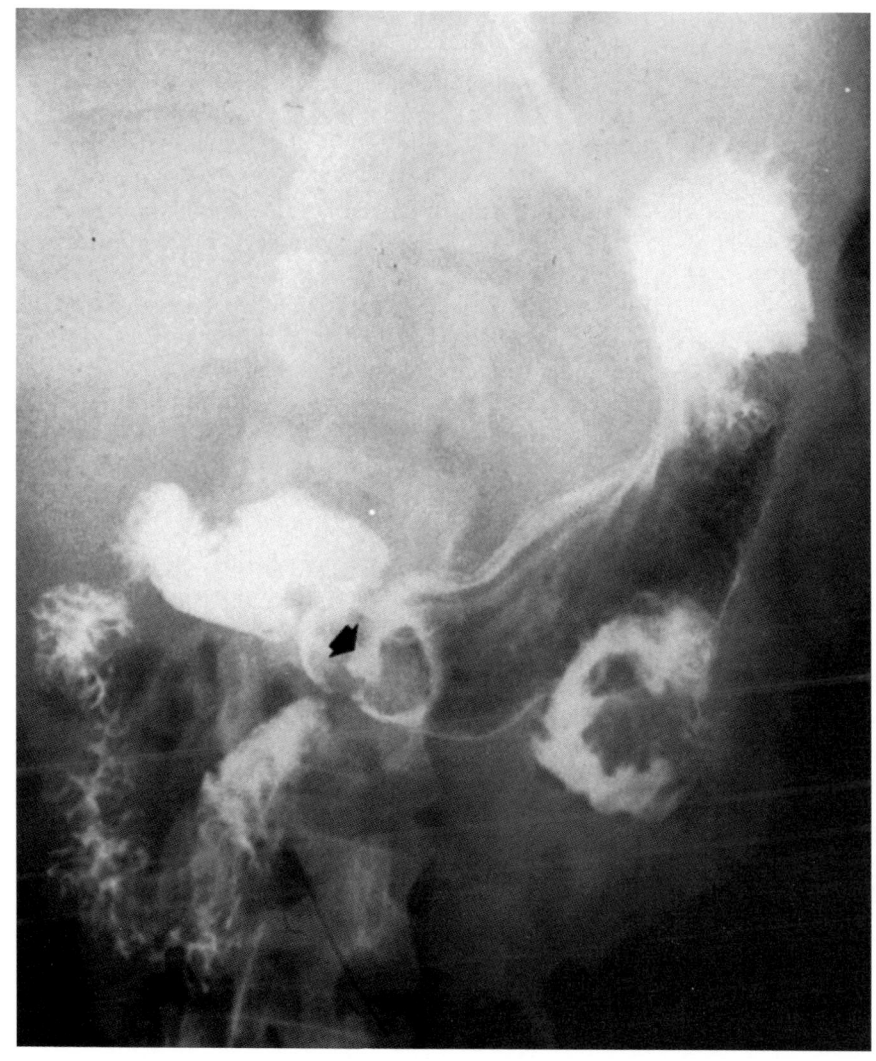

FIGURE 21-55. Antral polypoid lesion with central ulceration *(arrow)* on an upper gastrointestinal series in a patient with familial adenomatous polyposis.

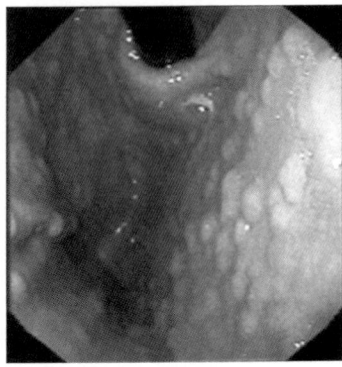

FIGURE 21-56. Upper gastrointestinal endoscopy in a patient with familial adenomatous polyposis reveals a gastric fundus showing a sheet of polyps. (See Color Fig. 21-56.)

Nederveen Cappel and associates calculated that the lifetime risk of developing duodenal cancer in FAP is 5%.[98] The most frequent sites for upper gastrointestinal tumors are duodenum, followed by pancreatic ampulla and then stomach. Japanese studies reveal the incidence of gastric polyps to be as high as 70% with Gardner's syndrome, whereas the incidence of duodenal polyps approaches 100%.[397,430] In Korea, where carcinoma of the stomach is the most common neoplasm, one survey identified 72 patients with FAP, three of whom (4.2%) were found to harbor gastric cancer.[308] This is a much higher risk than would be anticipated from the general population in that country.

Numerous case reports indicate the association of gastroduodenal polyps (including villous adenoma), as well as an association with small bowel carcinoma.[32,41,164,184,219,257,322,348] In a study from the Cleveland Clinic of 100 patients with FAP, one third were found to have duodenal adenomas on upper gastrointestinal endoscopy.[363] Periodic upper gastrointestinal radiologic investigation (optimally with double-contrast technique),

or preferably endoscopy at intervals in all patients found to have FAP is recommended in order to diagnose and treat lesions at an earlier stage, before invasive carcinoma supervenes.[18,96,170,196,363] This should be accomplished every 6 months to 4 years, depending on the polyp load.[4430] Their kindred should also be studied.

Pancreatitis Acute pancreatitis has been reported to be associated with FAP.[41,70,371,393] The pancreatitis may be secondary to the duodenal tumor or possibly the result of trauma when one attempts to sample the lesion for biopsy. However, there have been suggestions of pancreatitis developing before recognition of the periampullary tumor.

Hepatobiliary Tumors Cholangiocarcinoma, pancreatic adenocarcinoma, and hepatoblastoma have all been reported in association with FAP.[237] Hepatoblastoma is a rare childhood tumor affecting one in 100,000 children less than 15 years old. Twenty-seven cases of patients with a history of FAP had been identified in the literature as of 1992.[26] The condition may precede the development of FAP by many years.

Congenital Hypertrophy of the Retinal Pigment Epithelium Pigmented ocular fundus lesions—such as congenital hypertrophy of the retinal pigment epithelium (CHRPE)—have been noted in patients with Gardner's syndrome and in some family members.[10,25,181,415] When such lesions are identified in both retinas, they suggest inheritance of the gene for polyposis. Absence of this ophthalmologic finding, however, does not guarantee that an individual is protected. Iwama and colleagues performed eye examinations on patients with FAP and noted that the prevalence of CHRPE was higher in those with exostosis or desmoid tumors.[200] Other investigators have confirmed the association with extracolonic manifestations.[25] The Cleveland Clinic group has shown that the existence of four or more CHRPE lesions in both eyes is a congenital marker for FAP in about two thirds of families.[181] Morton and colleagues undertook an evaluation of this manifestation as a disease marker in a defined population with FAP.[275] Indirect ophthalmoscopy was performed on 75 individuals from 25 known families with FAP. Using a combined set of diagnostic criteria, CHRPE identified affected patients with a specificity of at least 94% and a sensitivity of 84%. The authors suggested that a combined screening program utilizing DNA analysis and indirect ophthamologic examination should be included with bowel evaluation.[275]

Miscellaneous Associations Other conditions that are believed to represent manifestations of this syndrome include carcinoid of the small bowel, adrenal cancer, adrenal adenoma, pheochromcytoma, skin pigmentation, and lymphoid polyposis.[172,213,254,304,409,426,442] There is, however,

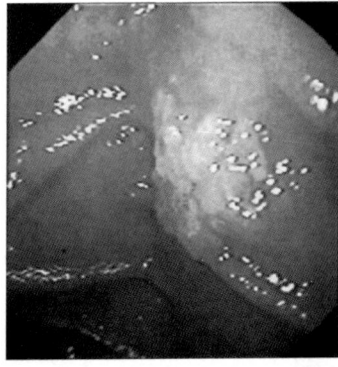

FIGURE 21-57. Duodenoscopy reveals a sessile villous tumor of the duodenum in a patient with familial adenomatous polyposis. (See Color Fig. 21-57.)

the possibility that the observations may merely be coincidental. A single case report of a duodenal lymphoma (mucosa-associated lymphoid tissue) called into question the possibility of an association, because there are other reports of lymphoma in patients with FAP.[133]

By considering Gardner's syndrome in terms of a family unit rather than for a specific, affected individual, the physician will be alerted to the increased risk for the development of colorectal tumors as well as the possibility of extracolonic manifestations.[70]

Turcot's Syndrome

Turcot's syndrome is the eponym given to FAP in association with malignant tumors of the central nervous system, that is, tumors of neuroepithelial origin. The condition was originally described by Turcot and colleagues in 1959.[418] Other reports have been published confirming the relationship between the two diseases.[13,48,78,197,230,233,368,414] Rothman and associates noted the development of a medulloblastoma before the colonic condition was recognized.[351]

Itoh and Ohsato suggested that there are three areas of difference with respect to the colon pathology in patients with Turcot's syndrome and with FAP.[197] These investigators believed that there are fewer polyps present (20 to 100), there is a higher frequency of larger polyps (greater than 3 cm), and there is an earlier development of colon cancer (70% to 100% during the second or third decade).[197] The authors suggested that if a patient with polyposis fits into this pattern, intracranial investigations be undertaken in the hope of identifying a brain tumor at an earlier stage. However, the Cleveland Clinic group does not believe it is appropriate to screen all at-risk children with FAP for brain tumors.[233]

Turcot's syndrome is thought to be distinct from Gardner's syndrome because of the pattern of inheritance, in that a generation is frequently missed. Some have attributed this observation to variable gene penetrance.[78,384] Others suggest that the disease is transmitted as an autosomal recessive trait.[113,198]

Turcot's syndome can be classified into two different manifestations: type 1 and type 2. The former type includes those with central nervous system tumors (especially gliomas that occur before the age of 20 years), colorectal adenomas without FAP, and the occasional presence of skin lesions (e.g., *café-au-lait* spots).[237] Type 2 is less common and includes those with medulloblastoma and characteritic FAP. Skin lesions are less frequently observed.[237]

Evaluation

Historically, proctosigmoidoscopy has been the procedure employed for identification of FAP in relatives of a family member known to harbor the condition. The rectum, however, may be relatively or even totally spared, and patients may be given false reassurance.[996]

In addition to considering the means of evaluation, the age at which screening should begin must be addressed. Naylor and Lebenthal reported three children (all asymptomatic) with evidence of polyps who were related to an individual with Gardner's syndrome.[285] They were 18 months, 6 years, and 9 years of age. Because barium enema was not always diagnostic of polyps, the authors recommend colonoscopy and biopsy in at-risk children. In their opinion, by deferring colonic examination until adolescence, the opportunity to diagnose polyposis and possibly prevent cancer may be jeopardized.

Pavlides and colleagues assessed colonoscopy, barium enema, and occult blood determination in families of patients with hereditary polyposis.[312] Colonoscopy was demonstrated to be superior to barium enema. Results of occult blood determination were positive in 30% of those with polyposis, more than five times as frequently as in those without polyposis. Although barium enema or double-contrast study will demonstrate the disease in most patients (Figure 21-58), small lesions, such as those illustrated in Figure 21-59, may be missed. There is little controversy today in that one should utilize colonoscopy as the screening tool for the at-risk family member. In children especially, one must be sensitive to radiation exposure.

The following surveillance recommendations have been established by the American Medical Association:

- FAP: Flexible sigmoidoscopy annually beginning at age 10 years
- AFAP: Colonoscopy/esophagogastroduodenoscopy; baseline at genetic testing or by age 15 years; if no polyps, repeated at age 20, then annually

Morton and co-workers emphasized the importance of the development of a polyposis registry.[276] They found that since establishing the registry, the median age of diagnosis of the affected patients was reduced from 32 to 23 years, and the incidence of colorectal cancer fell from 35% to 14%. These differences were statistically significant. These investigators and others recommended the establishment of a regional registry as an essential component of screening for this disease.[267,276]

Treatment

There are four resective operations that may be considered for the treatment of FAP:

- Proctocolectomy and ileostomy
- Total colectomy with ileorectal anastomosis (periodically fulgurating or excising residual or recurrent rectal polyps)
- Total proctocolectomy and ileoanal anastomosis
- Proctocolectomy with ileoanal reservoir (restorative proctocoloectomy)

The technical aspects of total colectomy and ileorectal anastomosis are discussed in Chapter 22; the other procedures are detailed in Chapter 29. Total colectomy with ileorectal anastomosis for this condition has also been undertaken laparoscopically.[268] Performing restorative proctocolectomy for FAP is somewhat different from that of ulcerative colitis. It is important that all rectal mucosa be removed in order to limit the risk for the development of a neoplasm. In my opinion, the double-stapling technique, the maneuver that facilitates the operation for ulcerative colitis, should not be used unless one is certain that the linear stapler has been placed sufficiently low—that is, the dentate line, unless one wishes to make a compromise. Consideration should certainly be given to stripping the mucosa whenever this cannot be accomplished. Of course, if one elects to leave behind viable rectal mucosa, close follow-up is required. One other possibility is to strip the mucosa at a later operation, perhaps concomitant with closure of the ileostomy. Still, there is always the tradeoff between neoplasia control and functional results.[317]

Results

All patients with FAP will develop colorectal carcinoma if untreated. The Cleveland Clinic group recommended *total colectomy and ileorectal anastomosis* for this condition, especially if the rectum is relatively spared.[150,151] Their protocol includes early surgical intervention (before age 20), with anastomosis at approximately 12 cm from the dentate line, and with close follow-up (every 6 months).[150] In a 1996 publication, the same group reiterated their conclusion that colectomy and ileorectal anastomosis is a relatively safe operation that results in minimal disturbance of bowel function.[61] This review included a total of 51 patients. It is certainly agreed that the choice of operation should be based upon the perceived risk of cancer's developing in the residual rectum.[372] In a later publication from the Cleveland Clinic group (2001), the value and reliability of the preoperative rectal polyp count were discussed.[58] The authors concluded that the finding of fewer than five rectal adenomas at presentation almost always predicts mild disease; these patients do well with an ileorectal anastomosis. Finding 20 or more adenomas implies severe disease. The investigators concluded that proctoscopy is a useful test for triage of patients with FAP according to disease severity to the preferred operation.[58] Another article from the Cleveland Clinic group compared the risk for the development of rectal cancer in patients treated by ileorectostomy (IR) before and after 1983, the year when ileo-pouch–anal anastomosis (IPAA) became a generally available alternative.[59] Sixty-two such operations were performed in the prepouch era (median follow-up, 212 months), and 135 in the

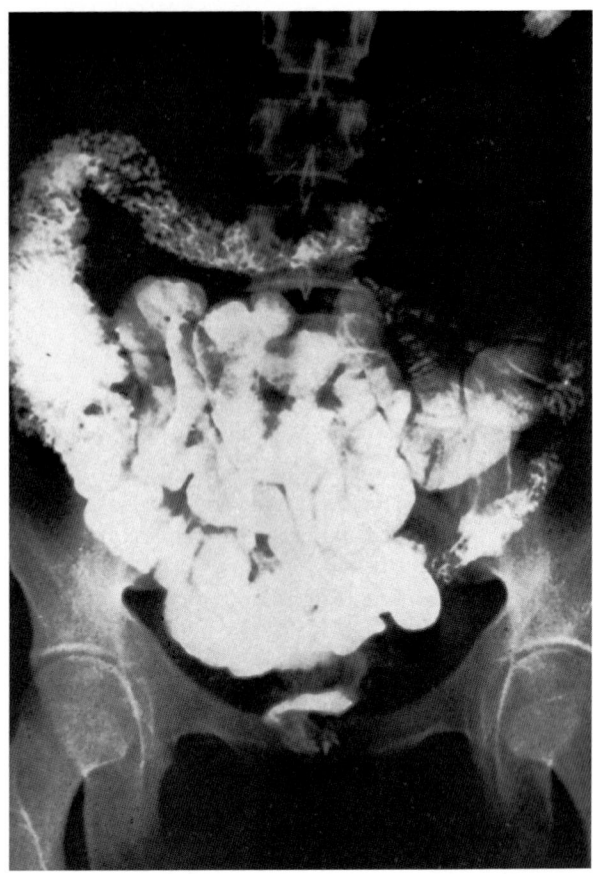

FIGURE 21-58. Barium enema reveals multiple filling defects throughout the colon and rectum. The air-contrast technique is preferred. (From Corman ML, Veidenheimer MC, Swinton NW. *Diseases of the anus, rectum, and colon. Part I: neoplasms.* New York: Medcom, 1972, with permission.)

pouch era (median follow-up, 60 months). Despite the shorter follow-up, almost one third of the earlier patients had to undergo subsequent proctectomy compared with only 2% since 1983. The authors concluded that the improved results probably are based in part on the ability to select patients appropriately for IR and to offer IPAA only to those with severe polyposis.

The Cleveland Clinic Ohio group also reported 119 patients who were submitted to IPAA for FAP, 42 mucosectomies and 77 stapled anastomoses.[342] These investigators concluded that patients with *stapled* IPAA had better functional results than patients who underwent *mucosectomy*, they may avoid a temporary ileostomy, but IPAA was associated with a 28% incidence of adenomas in the anal transition zone. All patients were managed with a local procedure. One was found to have cancer in the residual rectum. Fourteen percent of those who underwent mucosectomy developed adenomas. A later report from this center involved 146 patients who underwent IPAA for FAP.[301] None whom they actually operated upon developed an anal transitional zone can-

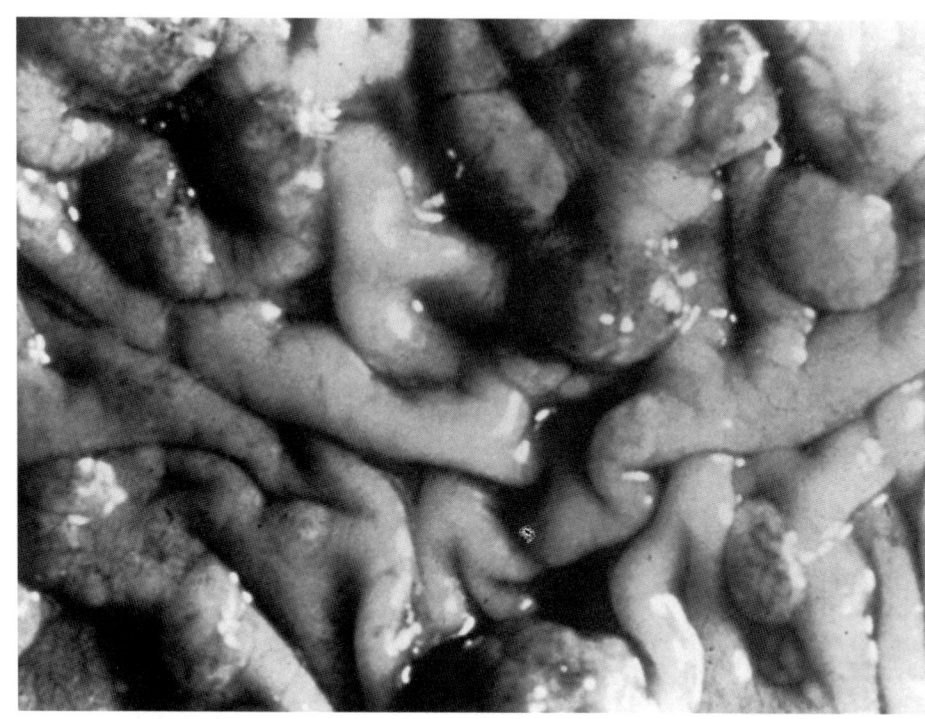

FIGURE 21-59. Familial adenomatous polyposis. These multiple small mucosal excrescences may be inapparent upon barium enema study. (From Corman ML, Veidenheimer MC, Swinton NW. *Diseases of the anus, rectum, and colon. Part I: neoplasms.* New York: Medcom, 1972, with permission.)

cer, but two patients whom they were following and who were operated elsewhere developed this complication (one after a double-stapled anastomosis and one after mucosectomy).

Beart commented on the Mayo Clinic experience with total colectomy and ileorectal anastomosis.[14] More than 100 patients were admitted for fulguration of recurrent or persistent adenomas. The only major complication was bleeding (2.8%). He believed at the time (1985 publication) that until the IPAA operations could be as demonstrably satisfactory, total colectomy and ileorectal anastomosis should be the primary modality of surgical therapy. A 1992 publication from the Mayo Clinic seemed to imply that the time had arrived.[3] A comparison was made between 21 individuals who underwent IR and 94 with IPAA. There was no statistically significant difference between the groups with respect to age and gender and no difference in postoperative morbidity. Sixty-one percent of the patients who underwent IR needed fulguration of rectal polyps, and 7% of the patients who underwent IPAA developed pouchitis (see Chapter 29). There was no difference in average stool frequency, but nighttime soiling was noted in 4% of those who underwent IPAA, a significant increase. The authors now recommend IPAA for most patients with polyposis, except for those who do not wish to risk impairment of sexual function.[3,22,179] Parenthetically, other investigators have also observed pouchitis to develop following reservoir construction for FAP.[224] Obviously, this complication is not limited to patients who undergo the procedure for inflammatory bowel disease.

Pouch polyposis following this procedure has also been observed. In fact, proctocolectomy and IPAA do not truly cure FAP. One must be aware that adenomatous polyps develop commonly in the reservoir itself.[27,64] In the experience of Thompson-Fawcett and colleagues, 60% of their patients developed adenomas or "microadenomas."[410] The importance of regular endoscopic surveillance, therefore, applies not only to the anastomotic area, but also to the reservoir itself. With this operation or one of the modifications, it is important for the patients to undergo lifelong proctoscopic surveillance.[183]

In addition to the concern for neoplasms developing in the rectal remnant of patients who have undergone IR, in the reservoir after IPAA, and in the anal transitional zone, *ileal adenomas* have been observed following colectomy. Iida and colleagues performed endoscopy and biopsy of the terminal ileum in 18 patients with FAP who had previously undergone total colectomy and IR.[194] All these patients were found to harbor numerous polypoid lesions; 83% had adenomas. The authors cautioned that endoscopic examination of the terminal ileum is necessary, not merely rectal evaluation following IR. Carcinoma of an ileostomy in an individual who had undergone proctocolectomy many years previously has also been described.[330]

The Mayo Clinic group opined that IPAA should be considered in favorable cancers complicating FAP, although reservations are expressed if the rectal cancer is advanced or even is an advanced proximal bowel malignancy.[404] Penna and colleagues studied the results of ileal J-pouch-anal anastomosis in 6 patients with rectal carcinoma.[316] There was a statistically significant increased frequency of defecation during the day as well as nocturnal defecation when compared with those who did not harbor a rectal cancer. The authors concluded that the relatively poor functional outcome was related to mesorectal excision.

Total colectomy with ileorectal anastomosis had been for many years the procedure of choice at St. Mark's Hospital. Regression of the polyps seemed to take place in the first decade after surgery, but this trend was reversed in the second decade. Of the 89 patients surviving surgery, two subsequently developed carcinoma of the rectum. Because these patients had been followed closely, at the time of subsequent proctectomy all were found to have Dukes' A lesions. Only one other required proctectomy. This individual originally had more than 5,000 polyps; the numerous recurrences finally made further surgery necessary. Bussey computed the cumulative risk of the development of cancer in the retained rectum at 3.6%.[42] The Cleveland Clinic group reported ten of 133 patients to have developed cancer in the rectal remnant.[364] Others reported a similar relatively favorable experience.[199,296,380] Another report from St. Mark's Hospital compared morbidity and bowel function after IR and IPAA, but these investigators arrived at the opposite conclusion from that at the Mayo Clinic.[252] There was a statistically significant increase in morbidity with the latter procedure. As with the Mayo experience, the bowel frequency was not appreciably different, but nighttime soiling was indeed a problem in 43% of patients who had undergone IPAA. The authors concluded that the greater morbidity of IPAA should limit its application to those at higher risk for developing rectal cancer, those who refuse or cannot undergo close follow-up, those with large or confluent rectal polyps, and those with curable colon cancer at the initial operation.[252]

Soave reported the functional results of endorectal ileal pull-through performed on eight patients with FAP.[385] Modest soiling was observed with occasional nighttime incontinence. Three years following the procedure, the average stool frequency ranged between three and five times per day. Reports with the same operation from other institutions revealed stool frequency to be up to ten times per day.[189]

Parks and associates initially reported four patients with FAP who underwent proctocolectomy with an ileal reservoir and ileoanal anastomosis.[310] There was no disturbance of urinary or sexual function. Everyone was continent during the day; one patient was incontinent at night. The average frequency of evacuation was approximately four times in 24 hours. The authors believed that this operation was a reasonable alternative to proctocolectomy and ileostomy. Others agree that the pelvic reservoir procedure is a desirable option.[37,125,126,167,175,214,318,350,407] Utsunomiya and colleagues reported the use of multiple operative variations to

effect ileoanal anastomosis in 11 patients with polyposis.[420] The side-to-end ileoanal anastomosis with J-loop reservoir provided the best functional results in their experience. Irrespective of the method of pouch construction, reports from every series indicate that patients with polyposis have better bowel control and fewer evacuations than those who undergo the operation for ulcerative colitis.

Olsen and associates studied 230 women from the Danish, Finnish, Swedish, and Norwegian polyposis registers with respect to *fecundity*, the biologic ability to conceive.[299] The results were compared with the general population and those who had ulcerative colitis. Although patients who underwent IR had fecundity comparable to that of the general population and to those individuals with FAP before surgery, there was a significant reduction in the ability to conceive after IPAA. The authors cautioned that this concern should be a matter of discussion with women when operative choices are being discussed.[299]

Even after conventional total colectomy with ileorectal anastomosis, IPAA can still be performed secondarily.[316] Björk and colleagues presented the Swedish experience of IPAA in FAP (120 patients) and compared this operation with IR and with IPAA as a secondary procedure after an initial IR.[30] Complications occurred in 40% of the patients who underwent IPAA initially and in 56% who underwent IPAA as a secondary procedure. When the IR procedure was added to the subsequent IPAA, the total complication rate for the two operations was 67%. Two patients with IR developed rectal cancer. Functional outcome did not differ between an initial IPAA and IPAA as a secondary procedure. However, as with other studies studies, IR gave the best functional results with respect to stool frequency, soiling, and continence.[30]

Nugent and co-workers reviewed the St. Mark's Hospital experience between 1948 and 1990 with respect to life expectancy.[297] In their 222 patients, comparing them with age and sex-matched controls, the relative risk of dying was calculated to be 3.35 times as great. The three main causes of death were upper gastrointestinal malignancy, desmoid disease, and perioperative complications.[28] Others confirmed that in recent years, a greater percentage of deaths in patients with FAP appears to be attributable to extracolonic manifestations of the disease.[21]

Regression of Rectal Polyps

Numerous authors have pointed out that polyps may spontaneously regress following total colectomy.[72,122,154,192,243,374] A lowered pH of the stool has been stated to be a possible factor. The administration of antioxidant vitamins and lactulose has also been believed to increase the tendency to regression.[432] Although the regression may be only temporary, the avoidance of a high-morbidity operation or an ileostomy in an individual who is likely to comply with the follow-up regimen makes colectomy with ileorectal anastomosis a very appealing surgical option for many patients. As discussed, when the rectum is relatively free of polyps, total colectomy with ileorectal anastomosis is the preferred alternative. It is important to reemphasize that initial polyp regression does not prevent the subsequent development of rectal cancer. The Cleveland Clinic group cautioned that although spontaneous regression occurred in 64% of patients following ileorectal anastomosis, continuous follow-up is necessary in order to fulgurate recurrent tumors and to screen for the development of cancer.[118]

The drug, sulindac, a nonsteroidal anti-inflammatory agent (a long-acting analogue of indomethacin), 150 or 200 mg twice a day in adults, has been demonstrated to produce regression of rectal polyps following total colectomy.[114,143,236,295,412,429,454] This drug has been applied orally and even rectally. In the experience of Winde and colleagues, a low-dose rectal sulindac maintenance therapy achieved complete adenoma remission without relapse in 87% of patients after a 33-month follow-up.[454] Long-term treatment is, of course, mandated. In a study by Guldenschuh and co-workers, 17 patients with FAP were treated with 300 mg of oral sulindac for 4 months followed by a "washout phase" of 6 months.[160] Ten of the patients still had intact colons. There was a statistically significant decrease in the number of adenomas, with a more pronounced affect in the proximal colon. After cessation of treatment, the number of adenomas increased but remained significantly lower than at baseline. Furthermore, even in spite of continuous treatment with sulindac, malignant degeneration of residual retained polyps has been observed.[412]

Oral calcium has been shown to inhibit rectal epithelial proliferation in patients with FAP.[115,408] The mechanism of action is believed to be the ability of calcium to reduce colorectal cell turnover.

Extracolonic Manifestations

Desmoid Tumors

A desmoid tumor is by far the most troublesome, indeed disabling, consequence of Gardner's syndrome.[161] Complete extirpation in some individuals may not be possible, but resection certainly represents the best possibility for cure. Involvement of retroperitoneal structures may cause urinary obstruction, which, in turn, may require a diversionary procedure. Because of the variation in the way desmoid tumors present, there is no one specific method of management. Even after aggressive surgical excision, recurrence is likely. In the experience of the Cleveland Clinic group, 90% of individuals with desmoids had intraabdominal involvement.[215] Twenty-one percent died of the desmoid itself. In fact, in another report from the same institution, the major causes of death in FAP individuals were as follows:[7]

- Metastatic colorectal carcinoma, 58%
- Desmoid tumors, 11%
- Periampullary carcinoma, 8%
- Brain tumors, 7%
- Adrenal carcinoma, 1%

If the tumor is incorporated within the small bowel mesentery and excision is to be attempted, meticulous dissection of the mesenteric vessels must be carried out in order to preserve the blood supply to the bowel.[220] A bypass procedure is often the wiser alternative. Abdominal wall tumors can usually be treated by wide excision, with abdominal wall reconstruction if necessary.[375] A case of successful excision of a pelvic desmoid tumor arising from the reservoir in a woman who had undergone IPAA for FAP has been reported.[123] The mass interfered with defecation and voiding and interfered with growth and development of a fetus.

For unresectable lesions, radiotherapy and chemotherapy have been employed with limited success. Bataini and colleagues reported 26 patients with desmoid tumors treated at the Institut Curie in Paris with megavoltage irradiation, one fourth of whom had intraabdominal tumors.[12] Clinical regression after treatment was slow, with complete disappearance taking up to 2 years. Postoperative radiotherapy with doses of at least 5,000 to 6,000 rads (50 to 60 Gy) was effective in achieving local control of inoperable or incompletely resected tumors. In the experience of others, however, intraabdominal desmoids do not respond to radiation therapy.[264] The complication of radiation enterocolitis has also been reported.[416] The Paris group further emphasized the importance of computed tomography in assessment of tumor extension in the preoperative and preradiation evaluation process (Figure 21-54*B*). In fact, a computed tomography scoring system has been proposed that can be used to compare phenotypic progression of patients with FAP who have desmoid precursor lesions.[266] Posner and colleagues identified five factors by means of univariate analysis that were predictive of local failure:[327]

Age between 18 and 30 years
Presentation with recurrent disease
Partial or limited margin excision
Tumor at or near microscopic margin of resection
Radiation therapy not administered for gross residual disease

Inhibition of prostaglandin synthesis has been attempted in order to enhance the immune response. If the tumor is not resectable, the nonsteroidal antiinflammatory drug, sulindac (Clinoril), 100 mg, twice daily, has been reported to diminish the size of the tumor.[22,215] Another possible alternative, the antiestrogen and prostaglandin inhibitor, tamoxifen (Nolvadex), has also been suggested. Tsukada and colleagues employed sulindac (with and without tamoxifen), indomethacin, tamoxifen alone, progesterone (Depo-Provera), and testolactone in a total of 16 patients.[417] Therapy was continued for at least 6 months and resulted in three complete remissions and seven partial remissions. There were marked benefits in the treatment group when compared with controls.

A combined chemotherapy program with vincristine, azathioprine, cyclophosphamide, and prednisone has also been suggested.[223] Others avow that chemotherapy should be reserved for those individuals who do not respond to a trial of noncytotoxic drug therapy.[416] Some investigators have found a substantial response to treatment through a cytotoxic chemotherapeutic regimen of doxorubicin and dacarbazine.[326,367] Others have also experienced success in a limited number of patients who have failed to respond to other agents.[248] Although many pharmacologic approaches have been advocated, it is difficult to evaluate the results, because the experience is often anecdotal.[106] Penna and colleagues found that none of the aforementioned medical therapies was effective in their patients.[319] A newer chemotherapeutic approach has been suggested by Heidemann and colleagues, that of the use of drugs to block angiogenesis.[174] These investigators noted a substantial response in two patients who were treated with toremifene and interferon-alfa-2b.

Anthony and co-workers recommend the following protocol for treatment of patients with desmoid tumors.[6] In patients with abdominal wall and extraabdominal involvement, sulindac or tamoxifen should used. If the mass enlarges, consideration is given to wide local excision. If the bowel mesentery is involved or if the process is in an intraabdominal location, the authors recommended sulindac or tamoxifen if the individual is asymptomatic. However, if symptoms are present, palliative resection is advised, with the addition of supplementary chemotherapy if the tumor is growing rapidly. It is self-evident, however, that these tumors are essentially locally malignant soft tissue neoplasms that require aggressive therapy.[327]

Baliski and associates recommended a different protocol for potentially resectable lesions on the basis of their experience with 13 patients.[11] This consists of doxorubicin and radiotherapy (10 × 300 cGy) with resection 4 to 6 weeks later.

Gastroduodenal Tumors

Lynch and Lynch recognized that polyps of the duodenum present a special challenge.[251] However, they opined that only a minority will require more than surveillance, because the natural history is quite indolent.[251] Tumors of the stomach and duodenum may be treated by endoscopic removal. Gastric resection is necessary for malignant lesions, and pancreaticoduodenectomy (Whipple's operation) is required for periampullary carcinomas. Villous tumors of the duodenum present a particular management problem, because even when biopsies are performed, malignant change is often missed. Ryan and colleagues, reporting from the Massachusetts General Hospital in Boston, observed a 56% false-negative rate.[3357] Complete excision either by endoscopy or duodenotomy is necessary if one is to advise the patient accurately.[201] The authors recommended that pancreaticoduodenectomy be performed if the patient can tolerate the operation, in order to effect better local control of both extensive benign and nonmetastasizing malignant lesions.[357]

As previously mentioned, some reports have demonstrated regression or disappearance of colonic polyps with sulindac therapy. Interestingly, a case of such a disappearance with duodenal polyps has been reported.[309] Others now believe that it is useful to consider this drug as an adjunctive measure following duodenal clearance.[295]

It is important to appreciate the survival rates following removal of duodenal villous tumors from patients who do not have polyposis. This should be a valid comparison because the histologic nature of the lesions is identical. The records of 32 patients with villous and tubulovillous adenomas of the duodenum treated at the Cleveland Clinic were reviewed.[136] The incidence of malignancy was 47%. A 28% recurrence rate was observed, all following segmental resection, local excision, or endoscopic excision. The 2- and 5-year survival rates for those found to harbor invasive cancer were 22% and zero, respectively.

Practice Parameters

In 2003, the Standards Task Force of the American Society of Colon and Rectal Surgeons published practice parameters for the treatment of FAP.[391] The following are the salient recommendations:

- Treatment must be preceded by thorough counseling about the nature of the syndrome, its history, its extracolonic manifestations, and the need for compliance, with recommendations for management and surveillance.
- Prophylactic colectomy or proctocolectomy is required. The timing and type of surgery depend on the severity of the polyposis phenotype and to a lesser extent on the genotype, age, and clinical and social circumstances of the patient.
- Lifetime follow-up of the rectum (after IR), pouch (after IPAA), and ileostomy (after total proctocolectomy) is required. Increasing neoplasia on the rectum is an indication for proctectomy.
- The use of chemoprevention as primary therapy for colorectal polyps is neither proven nor recommended.
- Treatment of duodenal adenomas depends on adenoma size and the presence of severe dysplasia. Small

tubular adenomas with mild dysplasia may be managed by surveillance, but adenomas with severe dysplasia must be removed.

- Duodenectomy or pancreaticoduodenectomy is recommended for patients with persistent or recurrent severe dysplasia in the papilla or duodenal adenoma.
- Surgery for intraabdominal desmoid tumors should be reserved for small, well-defined lesions with the expectation of a clear margin. Abdominal wall desmoids should be excised whenever possible.
- Intraabdominal desmoid tumors involving the small bowel mesentery are treated according to their rate of growth and their presentation. Clinically inert tumors should be treated with sulindac or not treated at all. Slowly growing or mildly symptomatic tumors may be treated with less toxic regimens, such as sulindac and tamoxifen or vinblastine and methotrexate. Rapidly growing tumors require aggressive therapy with either very high-dose tamoxifen or anti-sarcoma-type chemotherapy. Radiotherapy may also be considered.

Comment

Conventional proctocolectomy and ileostomy achieve complete extirpation of the polyp-bearing intestine but at the expense of the loss of intestinal continuity. The fear of having a permanent stoma may dissuade some patients from having needed surgery or members of families with polyposis from undergoing screening evaluation. If one is to consider retaining the rectum, however, a considerable burden of responsibility falls upon the surgeon and the patient. The confidence of being relatively asymptomatic lulls patients into a false sense of security. Rationalization and denial are frequently employed defense mechanisms. Under such circumstances, when rectal bleeding or a change in bowel habits develops, the cancer is often far advanced. Of the four patients upon whom I operated for rectal cancer who did not undergo periodic evaluation and who became symptomatic following total colectomy, all had metastatic disease.

The patient must be informed of the risk and be willing to undergo sigmoidoscopy every 6 months for the reminder of his or her life. It is easier to justify this position if the rectum is relatively spared. If rectal polyposis cannot be adequately treated by local means, an IPAA or complete proctectomy must be performed. Although IPAA is generally preferred to conventional ileostomy, the procedure is associated with a high morbidity, and the functional results are certainly less than perfect.

In summary, total colectomy with ileorectal anastomosis is my recommended approach to the treatment of FAP if the rectum is relatively spared. IPAA is considered if there are extensive rectal polyps, if cancer is present any-

where in the colon, or if the patient is unwilling to submit to close follow-up. Proctocolectomy is advised for those with invasive rectal cancer and for those who wish the best operation for minimizing future contact with the surgical profession. This also includes patients unwilling to undergo surveillance. The operation is also suggested for those who are not candidates for IPAA (e.g., incontinence, sphincter injury).

REFERENCES

1. Adachi Y, Mori M, Kido A, et al. Multiple colorectal neoplasms in a young adult. *Dis Colon Rectum* 1992;35:197.
2. Alexander RH, Beckwith JB, Morgan A, et al. Juvenile polyps of the colon and their relation to allergy. *Am J Surg* 1970;120:222.
3. Ambroze WL Jr Dozois RR, Pemberton JH, et al. Familial adenomatous polyposis: results following ileal pouch-anal anastomosis and ileorectostomy. *Dis Colon Rectum* 1992; 35:12.
4. Andren L, Frieberg S, Welin S. Roentgen diagnosis of small polyps in colon and rectum. *Acta Radiol (Stockh)* 1955; 43:201.
5. Ansher AF, Lewis JH, Fleischer DE, et al. Hyperplastic colonic polyps as a marker for adenomatous colonic polyps. *Am J Gastroenterol* 1989;84:113.
6. Anthony T, Rodríguez-Bigas MA, Weber TK, et al. Desmoid tumors. *J Am Coll Surg* 1996;182:369.
7. Arvanitis ML, Jagelman DG, Fazio VW, et al. Mortality with familial adenomatous polyposis. *Dis Colon Rectum* 1990; 33:639.
8. Atkin WS, Morson BC, Cuzick J. Long-term risk of colorectal cancer after excision of rectosigmoid adenomas. *N Engl J Med* 1992;326:658.
9. Azimuddin K, Statsik JJ, Khubchandani IT, et al. Hyperplastic polyps: "more than meets the eye"? Report of sixteen cases. *Dis Colon Rectum* 2000;43:1309.
10. Baba S, Tsuchiya M, Watanabe I, et al. Importance of retinal pigmentation as a subclinical marker in familial adenomatous polyposis. *Dis Colon Rectum* 1990;33:660.
11. Baliski CR, Temple WJ, Arthur K, et al. Desmoid tumors: a novel approach for local control. *J Surg Oncol* 2002; 80:96.
12. Bataini JP, Belloir C, Mazabraud A, et al. Desmoid tumors in adults: the role of radiotherapy in their management. *Am J Surg* 1988;155:754.
13. Baughman FA Jr, List CF, Williams JR, et al. The glioma-polyposis syndrome. *N Engl J Med* 1969;281:1345.
14. Beart RW Jr. Familial polyposis. *Br J Surg* 1985;72:29.
15. Beart RW Jr, Dozois RR, Kelly KA. Ileoanal anastomosis in the adult. *Surg Gynecol Obstet* 1982;154:826.
16. Beck AR, Jewett TC Jr. Surgical implications of the Peutz-Jeghers syndrome. *Ann Surg* 1967;165:299.
17. Beck DE, Karulf RE. Laparoscopic-assisted full-thickness endoscopic polypectomy. *Dis Colon Rectum* 1993;36: 693.
18. Beckwith FS, van Heerden JA, Dozois RR. Prognosis of symptomatic duodenal adenomas in familial adenomatous polyposis. *Arch Surg* 1991;126:825.
19. Bedogni G, Bertoni G, Ricci E, et al. Colonoscopic excision of large and giant colorectal polyps: technical implications and results over eight years. *Dis Colon Rectum* 1986;29:831.
20. Behringer GE. Polypoid lesions of the colon: which should be removed? *Surg Clin North Am* 1974;54:699.
21. Belchetz LA, Berk T, Bapat BV, et al. Changing causes of mortality in patients with familial adenomatous polyposis. *Dis Colon Rectum* 1996;39:384.
22. Belliveau P, Graham AM. Mesenteric desmoid tumor in Gardner's syndrome treated by sulindac. *Dis Colon Rectum* 1984;27:53.

23. Berci G, Panish J, Morgenstern L. Diagnostic colonoscopy and colonoscopic polypectomy. *Arch Surg* 1973;106:818.
24. Berk RN. Polypoid lesions of the colon. In: Greenbaum EI, ed. *Radiographic atlas of colon disease*. Chicago: Year Book, 1980:401.
25. Berk T, Cohen Z, McLeod RS, et al. Congenital hypertrophy of the retinal pigment epithelium as a marker for familial adenomatous polyposis. *Dis Colon Rectum* 1988; 31:253.
26. Bernstein IT, Bülow S, Mauritzen K. Hepatoblastoma in two cousins in a family with adenomatous polyposis: report of two cases. *Dis Colon Rectum* 1992;35:373.
27. Beveridge IG, Swain DJW, Groves CJ, et al. Large villous adenomas arising in ileal pouches in familial adenomatous polyposis: report of two cases. *Dis Colon Rectum* 2004;47: 123.
28. Billingham RP, Bowman HE, MacKeigan JM. Solitary adenomas in juvenile patients. *Dis Colon Rectum* 1980;23:26.
29. Bishop JM, Weinberg RA. Molecular oncology. In: *Introduction to molecular medicine*. Scientific American, 1996: 187.
30. Björk J, Åkerbrant H, Iselius L, et al. Outcome of primary and secondary ileal pouch-anal anastomosis and ileorectal anastomosis in patients with familial adenomatous polyposis. *Dis Colon Rectum* 2001;44:984.
31. Blumberg D, Opelka FG, Hicks TC, et al. Significance of a normal surveillance colonoscopy in patients with a history of adenomatous polyps. *Dis Colon Rectum* 2000;43: 1984.
32. Boley SJ, McKinnon WM, Marzulli VF. The management of familial gastrointestinal polyposis involving stomach and colon. *Surgery* 1961;50:691.
33. Botoman VA, Pietro M, Thirlby RC. Localization of colonic lesions with endoscopic tattoo. *Dis Colon Rectum* 1994;37: 775.
34. Bos JL, Fearon ER, Hamilton SR, et al. Prevalence of ras gene mutations in colorectal cancers. *Nature* 1987;327:293.
35. Brunetaud JM, Maunoury V, Cochelard D, et al. Endoscopic laser treatment for rectosigmoid villous adenoma: factors affecting the results. *Gastroenterology* 1989;97: 272.
36. Brunetaud JM, Mosquet L, Houcke M, et al. Villous adenomas of the rectum: results of endoscopic treatment with argon and Nd:YAG lasers. *Gastroenterology* 1985;89: 832.
37. Bubrick MP, Jacobs DM, Levy M. Experience with the endorectal pull-through and S pouch for ulcerative colitis and familial polyposis in adults. *Surgery* 1985;98:689.
38. Bülow S. Clinical features in familial polyposis coli: results of the Danish polyposis register. *Dis Colon Rectum* 1986;29: 102.
39. Bülow S, Lauritsen KB, Johansen A, et al. Gastroduodenal polyps in familial polyposis coli. *Dis Colon Rectum* 1985; 28:90.
40. Burt RW, Berenson MM, Lee RG, et al. Upper gastrointestinal polyps in Gardner's syndrome. *Gastroenterology* 1984; 86:295.
41. Burt RW, Rikkers LF, Gardner EJ, et al. Villous adenoma of the duodenal papilla presenting as necrotizing pancreatitis in a patient with Gardner's syndrome. *Gastroenterology* 1987;92:532.
42. Bussey HJR. *Familial polyposis coli*. Baltimore: Johns Hopkins University Press, 1975.
43. Bussey HJR. Polyposis syndromes. In: Morson BC, ed. *The pathogenesis of colorectal cancer*. Philadelphia: WB Saunders, 1978:81.
44. Bussey HJR, Wallace MH, Morson BC. Metachronous carcinoma of the large intestine and intestinal polyps. *Proc R Soc Med* 1967;60:208.
45. Cabrera A, Lega J. Polyps of the colon and rectum in children. *Am J Surg* 1960;110:551.
46. Cady B, Persson AV, Monson DO, et al. Changing patterns of colorectal carcinoma. *Cancer* 1974;33:422.
47. Cairns S, Quirke P. Flat adenomas. *Br J Surg* 1999;86:1489.
48. Camiel MR, Mulé JE, Alexander LL, et al. Association of thyroid carcinoma with Gardner's syndrome in siblings. *N Engl J Med* 1968;278:1056.
49. Campbell WJ, Spence RAJ, Parks TG. Familial adenomatous polyposis. *Br J Surg* 1994;81:1722.
50. Cappell MS, Forde KA. Spatial clustering of multiple hyperplastic, adenomatous, and malignant colonic polyps in individual patients. *Dis Colon Rectum* 1989;32:641.
51. Chapuis PH, Dent OF, Goulston KJ. Clinical accuracy in the diagnosis of small polyps using the flexible fiberoptic sigmoidoscope. *Dis Colon Rectum* 1982;25:669.
52. Chargelaigue A. *Des polypes du rectum*. Paris: Thesis, 1859.
53. Cheng J-Y, Sheu L-F, Lin J-C, et al. Detection of human papillomavirus DNA in colorectal adenomas. *Arch Surg* 1995; 10:73.
54. Christiansen J. Excision of mid-rectal lesions by the Kraske sacral approach. *Br J Surg* 1980;67:651.
55. Chiu YS, Spencer RJ. Villous lesions of the colon. *Dis Colon Rectum* 1978;21:493.
56. Christie JP. Colonoscopic excision of large sessile polyps. *Am J Gastroenterol* 1977;67:430.
57. Church JM. Avoiding surgery in patients with colorectal polyps. *Dis Colon Rectum* 2003;46:1513.
58. Church J, Burke C, McGannon E, et al. Predicting polyposis severity by proctoscopy: how reliable is it? *Dis Colon Rectum* 2001;44:1249.
59. Church J, Burke C, McGannon E, et al. Risk of rectal cancer in patients after colectomy and ileorectal anastomosis for familial adenomatous polyposis: a function of available surgical options. *Dis Colon Rectum* 2003;46:1175.
60. Church JM, Fazio VW, Jones IT. Small colorectal polyps: are they worth treating? *Dis Colon Rectum* 1988;31:50.
61. Church JM, Fazio VW, Lavery IC, et al. Quality of life after prophylactic colectomy and ileorectal anastomosis in patients with familial adenomatous polyposis. *Dis Colon Rectum* 1996;39:1404.
62. Church JM, Hernegger GS, Moore HG, et al. Attenuated familial adenomatous polyposis: an evolving and poorly understood entity. *Dis Colon Rectum* 2002;45:127.
63. Church JM, McGannon E, Burke C, et al. Teenagers with familial adenomatous polyposis: what is their risk for colorectal cancer? *Dis Colon Rectum* 2002;45:887.
64. Church JM, Oakley JR, Wu JS. Pouch polyposis after ileal pouch-anal anastomosis for familial adenomatous polyposis: report of a case. *Dis Colon Rectum* 1996;39:584.
65. Clark SK, Phillips RKS. Desmoids in familial adenomatous polyposis. *Br J Surg* 1996;83:1494.
66. Cleaver JE. It was a very good year for DNA repair. *Cell* 1994;76:1.
67. Cochet B, Carrel J, Desbaillets L, et al. Peutz-Jeghers syndrome associated with gastrointestinal carcinoma: report of two cases in a family. *Gut* 1979;20:169.
68. Cohen JL, Forde KA. Intraoperative colonoscopy. *Ann Surg* 1988;207:231.
69. Cohen LB, Waye JD. Treatment of colonic polyps-practical considerations. *Clin Gastroenterol* 1986;15:359.
70. Cohen SB. Familial polyposis coli and its extracolonic manifestations. *J Med Genet* 1982;19:193.
71. Colacchio TA, Forde KA, Scantlebury VP. Endoscopic polypectomy: inadequate treatment for invasive colorectal carcinoma. *Ann Surg* 1981;194:704.
72. Cole JW, Holden WD. Postcolectomy regression of adenomatous polyps of the rectum. *Arch Surg* 1959;79:385.
73. Coller JA, Corman ML, Veidenheimer MC. Colonic polypoid disease: need for total colonoscopy. *Am J Surg* 1976; 131:490.
74. Corman ML, Coller JA, Veidenheimer MC. Proctosigmoidoscopy-age criteria for examination in the asymptomatic patient. *CA Cancer J Clin* 1975;25:286.
75. Corman ML, Veidenheimer MC, Swinton NW. *Diseases of the anus, rectum, and colon. Part I: Neoplasms*. New York: Medcom, 1972.

76. Corman ML, Veidenheimer MC, Coller JA. Barium enema study findings in asymptomatic patients with rectal polyps. *Dis Colon Rectum* 1974;17:325.

77. Corvisart L. Hypertrophie partielle de la muqueuse intestinale. *Bull Soc Anat* 1847;22:400.

78. Costa OL, Silva DM, Colnago FA, et al. Turcot syndrome: autosomal dominant or recessive transmission? *Dis Colon Rectum* 1987;30:391.

79. Cotterill JA, Day JL, Hughes JP, et al. The Cronkhite-Canada syndrome. *Postgrad Med J* 1973;49:268.

80. Coutsoftides T, Sivak MV Jr, Benjamin SP, et al. Colonoscopy and the management of polyps containing invasive carcinoma. *Ann Surg* 1978;188:638.

81. Cowen AE, Stitz RW, Ward M. Colonoscopic polypectomy. *Med J Aust* 1981;1:627.

82. Crail HW. Multiple primary malignancies arising in the rectum, brain and the thyroid. *US Nav Med Bull* 1949;49:123.

83. Cranley JP, Petras RE, Carey WD, et al. When is endoscopic polypectomy adequate therapy for colonic polyps containing invasive carcinoma? *Gastroenterology* 1986;91:419.

84. Cripps WH. Two cases of disseminated polypus of the rectum. *Trans Pathol Soc Lond* 1882;33:165.

85. Cronkhite LW, Canada WJ. Generalized gastrointestinal polyposis: unusual syndrome of polyposis, pigmentation, alopecia and onychotrophia. *N Engl J Med* 1955;252:1011.

86. Cunningham C, Dunlop MG. Molecular basis of colorectal cancer susceptibility. *Br J Surg* 1996;83:321.

87. Dagradi AE, Riff DS, Ford EA. Colonoscopic polypectomy excision of a huge villous adenoma. *Am J Gastroenterol* 1976;66:464.

88. Damerson KM, Volpert OV, Tainsky MA, et al. Control of angiogenesis by p53 regulation of thrombospondin-1. *Science* 1994;265:1582.

89. Daniel ES, Ludwig SL, Lewin KJ, et al. The Cronkhite-Canada syndrome. *Medicine (Baltimore)* 1982;61:293.

90. Davis JE, Seavey PW, Sessions JT Jr. Villous adenomas of the rectum and sigmoid colon with severe fluid and electrolyte depletion. *Ann Surg* 1962;155:806.

91. Day DW, Morson BC. Pathology of adenomas. In: Morson BC, ed. *The pathogenesis of colorectal cancer.* Philadelphia: WB Saunders, 1978:43.

92. Day DW, Morson BC. The polyp problem. In: Hunt RH, Waye JD, eds. *Colonoscopy: techniques, clinical practice and colour atlas.* London: Chapman & Hall, 1981:301.

93. Decosse JJ. Malignant colorectal polyp. *Gut* 1984;25:433.

94. De Gennaro VA, Lescher TC. Transanal excision of rectal tumors using a laparoscopic stapler. *Dis Colon Rectum* 1995;38:327.

95. Dell'Abate P, Iosca A, Galimberti A, et al. Endoscopic treatment of colorectal benign-appearing lesions 3 cm or larger: techniques and outcome. *Dis Colon Rectum* 2001;44:112.

96. Denzler TB, Harned PK, Pergam CJ. Gastric polyps in familial polyposis coli. *Radiology* 1979;130:63.

97. Desai DC, Neale KF, Talbot IC, et al. Juvenile polyposis. *Br J Surg* 1995;82:14.

98. de Vos tot Nederveen Cappel WH, Järvinen HJ, Björk J, et al. Worldwide survey among polyposis registries of surgical management of severe duodenal adenomatosis in familial adenomatous polyposis. *Br J Surg* 2003;90:705.

99. Dick JA, Owen WJ, McColl I. Rectal sparing in familial polyposis coli. *Br J Surg* 1984;71:664.

100. Dickinson AJ, Savage AP, Mortensen NJMC, et al. Long-term survival after endoscopic transanal resection of rectal tumors. *Br J Surg* 1993;80:1401.

101. Dippolito AD, Aburano A, Bezouska CA, et al. Enteritis cystica profunda in Peutz-Jeghers syndrome: report of a case and review of the literature. *Dis Colon Rectum* 1987;30:192.

102. Doniec JM, Löhnert MS, Schniewind B, et al. Endoscopic removal of large colorectal polyps: prevention of unnecessary surgery? *Dis Colon Rectum* 2003;46:340.

103. Douglas JR, Campbell CA, Salisbury DM, et al. Colonoscopic polypectomy in children. *BMJ* 1980;281:1386.

104. Dukes CE. The hereditary factor in polyposis intestine or multiple adenomata. *Cancer Rev* 1930;5:241.

105. Dukes CE. Familial intestinal polyposis. *Ann Eugen Lond* 1952;17:1.

106. Easter DW, Halasz NA. Recent trends in the management of desmoid tumors: summary of 19 cases and review of the literature. *Ann Surg* 1989;210:765.

107. Edwards DP, Khosraviani K, Staggerton R, et al. Long-term results of polyp clearance by intraoperative enteroscopy in the Peutz-Jeghers syndrome. *Dis Colon Rectum* 2003;46:48.

108. Eide TJ, Stalsberg H. Polyps of the large intestine in northern Norway. *Cancer* 1978;42:2839.

109. Eijsbouts QAJ, Heuff G, Sietses C, et al. Laparoscopic surgery in the treatment of colonic polyps. *Br J Surg* 1999;86:505.

110. Ekelund G. On cancer and polyps of colon and rectum. *Acta Pathol Microbiol Scand* 1963;59:165.

111. Elias H, Hyde DM, Mullens RS, et al. Colonic adenomas: stereology and growth mechanisms. *Dis Colon Rectum* 1981;24:331.

112. Enterline HT, Evans GW, Mercado-Lugo R, et al. Malignant potential of adenomas of colon and rectum. *JAMA* 1962;179:322.

113. Erbe RW. Inherited gastrointestinal polyposis syndromes. *N Engl J Med* 1976;294:1101.

114. Esaki M, Matsumoto T, Mizuno M, et al. Effect of sulindac treatment for attenuated familial adenomatous polyposis with a new germline APC mutation at codon 161: report of a case. *Dis Colon Rectum* 2002;45:1397.

115. Farmer KCR, Phillips RKS. Colectomy with ileorectal anastomosis lowers rectal mucosal cell proliferation in familial adenomatous polyposis. *Dis Colon Rectum* 1993;36:167.

116. Farr CJ, Marshall CJ, Easly DJ, et al. A study of ras mutation in colorectal adenomas from familial polyposis coli patients. *Oncogene* 1988;3:673.

117. Fearon ER, Vogelstein B. A genetic model of colorectal cancer tumorigenesis. *Cell* 1990;61:759.

118. Feinberg SM, Jagelman DG, Sarre RG, et al. Spontaneous resolution of rectal polyps in patients with familial polyposis following abdominal colectomy and ileorectal anastomosis. *Dis Colon Rectum* 1988;31:169.

119. Fennerty MB, Davidson J, Emerson SS, et al. Are endoscopic measurements of colonic polyps reliable? *Am J Gastroenterol* 1993;88:496.

120. Fennerty MB, Sampliner RE, Hixson LJ, et al. Effectiveness of India ink as a long-term mucosal marker. *Am J Gastroenterol* 1992;87:79.

121. Ferney DM, DeSchryver-Kecskemeti K, Clouse RE. Treatment of Cronkhite-Canada syndrome with home total parenteral nutrition. *Ann Intern Med* 1986;104:588.

122. Feinberg SM, Jagelman DG, Sarre RG, et al. Spontaneous resolution of rectal polyps in patients with familial polyposis following abdominal colectomy and ileorectal anastomosis. *Dis Colon Rectum* 1988;31:169.

123. Firoozmand E, Prager E. Pelvic desmoid tumor: threat to mother and fetus. *Am Surg* 2001;67:1213.

124. Fishel R, Lescoe MK, Rao MRS, et al. The human mutator gene homolog MHS2 and its association with hereditary nonpolyposis colon cancer. *Cell* 1993;75:1027.

125. Fonkalsrud EW. Endorectal ileal pullthrough with ileal reservoir for ulcerative colitis and polyposis. *Am J Surg* 1982;144:81.

126. Fonkalsrud EW. Endorectal ileal pullthrough with isoperistaltic ileal reservoir for colitis and polyposis. *Ann Surg* 1985;202:145.

127. Fork F-T. Double contrast enema and colonoscopy in polyp detection. *Gut* 1981;22:971.

128. Forte MD, Brant WE. Spontaneous isolated mesenteric fibromatosis: report of a case. *Dis Colon Rectum* 1988;31:315.

129. Franklin R, McSwain B. Juvenile polyps of the colon and rectum. *Ann Surg* 1972;175:887.

130. Freeman K, Anthony PP, Miller DS, et al. Cronkhite-Canada syndrome: a new hypothesis. *Gut* 1985;26:531.

131. Freeman K, Anthony PP, Miller DS, et al. Cronkhite-Canada syndrome. *J R Soc Med* 1984;77:4.

132. Fried GM, Hreno A, Duguid WP, et al. Rational management of malignant colon polyps based on long-term follow-up. *Surgery* 1984;96:815.

133. Frizelle FA, Hemmings CT, Whitehead MR, et al. Familial adenomatous polyposis and duodenal lymphoma: report of a case. *Dis Colon Rectum* 2003;46:1698.

134. Gabrielsson N, Granqvist S, Ohlsén H, et al. Malignancy of colonic polyps: diagnosis and management. *Acta Radiol Diagn* 1978;19:479.

135. Galandiuk S, Fazio VW, Jagelman DG, et al. Villous and tubulovillous adenomas of the colon and rectum. *Am J Surg* 1987;153:41.

136. Galandiuk S, Hermann RE, Jagelman DG, et al. Villous tumors of the duodenum. *Ann Surg* 1988;207:234.

137. Gardner EJ. A genetic and clinical study of intestinal polyposis, a predisposing factor for carcinoma of the colon and rectum. *Am J Hum Genet* 1951;3:167.

138. Gardner EJ. Gardner's syndrome re-evaluated after twenty years. *Proc Utah Acad* 1969;46:1.

139. Gardner EJ, Plenk HP. Hereditary pattern for multiple osteomas in a family group. *Am J Hum Genet* 1952;4:31.

140. Gardner EJ, Richards RC. Multiple cutaneous and subcutaneous lesions occurring simultaneously with hereditary polyposis and osteomatosis. *Am J Hum Genet* 1953;5:139.

141. Gelb AM, Minkowitz S, Tresser M. Rectal and colonic polyps occurring in young people. *NY State J Med* 1962:513.

142. Giardiello FM, Brensinger JD, Petersen GM, et al. The use and interpretation of commercial APC gene testing for familial adenomatous polyposis. *N Engl J Med* 1997;336:823.

143. Giardiello FM, Hamilton SR, Krush AJ, et al. Treatment of colonic and rectal adenomas with sulindac in familial adenomatous polyposis. *N Engl J Med* 1993;328:1313.

144. Giardiello FM, Offerhaus GJA, Lee DH, et al. Increased risk of thyroid and pancreatic carcinoma in familial adenomatous polyposis. *Gut* 1993;34:1394.

145. Giardiello FM, Welsh SB, Hamilton SR, et al. Increased risk of cancer in the Peutz-Jeghers syndrome. *N Engl J Med* 1987;316:1511.

146. Gibbs NM, Katz D. Hyperplastic polyps. In: Morson BC, ed. *The pathogenesis of colorectal cancer.* Philadelphia: WB Saunders, 1978:13.

147. Gilbertsen VA. Proctosigmoidoscopy and polypectomy in reducing the incidence of rectal cancer. *Cancer* 1974;34:936.

148. Gill W, Wilkin BJ. Diffuse gastrointestinal polyposis associated with hypoproteinaemia. *J R Coll Surg Edinb* 1967;12:149.

149. Gillespie PE, Chambers TJ, Chan KW, et al. Colonic adenomas: a colonoscopy survey. *Gut* 1979;20:240.

150. Gingold BS, Jagelman DG. Sparing the rectum in familial polyposis: causes for failure. *Surgery* 1981;89:314.

151. Gingold BS, Jagelman DG, Turnbull RB Jr. Surgical management of familial polyposis and Gardner's syndrome. *Am J Surg* 1979;137:54.

152. Gjöres JE, Örndahl B. Villous adenoma with severe fluid imbalance. *Acta Chir Scand* 1974;140:82.

153. Gorlin RJ, Chaudhry AP. Multiple osteomatosis, fibromas, lipomas and fibrosarcomas of the skin and mesentery, epidermoid inclusion cysts of the skin, leiomyomas and multiple intestinal polyposis. *N Engl J Med* 1960;263:1151.

154. Gowen GF. Complete regression of villous adenomas of the colon using piroxicam, a nonsteroidal anti-inflammatory drug. *Dis Colon Rectum* 1996;39:101.

155. Greenberg ER, Baron JA, Tosteson TD, et al. A clinical trial of antioxidant vitamins to prevent colorectal adenoma. *N Engl J Med* 1994;331:141.

156. Greene FL. Distribution of colorectal neoplasms: a left to right shift of polyps and cancer. *Am Surg* 1983;49:62.

157. Grice OD. A technique for suturing soft viscera using compression sutures. *Surg Gynecol Obstet* 1988;167:523.

158. Groden J, Thliveris A, Samowitz W, et al. Identification and characterization of the familial adenomatous polyposis coli gene. *Cell* 1991;66:589.

159. Grosfield JL, West KW. Generalized juvenile polyposis coli. *Arch Surg* 1986;121:530.

160. Guldenschuh I, Hurlimann R, Muller A, et al. Relationship between APC genotype, polyp distribution, and oral sulindac treatment in the colon and rectum of patients with familial adenomatous polyposis. *Dis Colon Rectum* 2001;44:1090.

161. Gurbuz AK, Giardiello FM, Petersen GM, et al. Desmoid tumours in familial adenomatous polyposis. *Gut* 1994;35:377.

162. Haggitt RC, Glotzbach RE, Soffer EE, et al. Prognostic factors in colorectal carcinomas arising in adenomas: implications for lesions removed by endoscopic polypectomy. *Gastroenterology* 1985;89:328.

163. Haggitt RC, Pitcock JA. Familial juvenile polyposis of the colon. *Cancer* 1970;26:1232.

164. Halstead JA, Harris E, Bartlett MK. Involvement of the stomach in familial polyposis of the gastro-intestinal tract: report of a family. *Gastroenterology* 1950;15:763.

165. Hambrick E. Fiberoptic colonoscopy: the fate of colonoscopic polypectomy sites. *Dis Colon Rectum* 1976;19:400.

166. Hammond DC, Lane FR, Mackeigan JM, et al. Endoscopic tattooing of the colon: clinical experience. *Am Surg* 1993;59:205.

167. Handelsman JC, Fishbein RH, Hoover HC Jr, et al. Endorectal pull-through operation in adults after colectomy and excision of rectal mucosa. *Surgery* 1983;93:247.

168. Handford H. Disseminated polypi of the large intestine becoming malignant. *Trans Pathol Soc Lond* 1890;41:133.

169. Hanzawa M, Yoshikawa N, Tezuka T, et al. Surgical treatment of Cronkhite-Canada syndrome associated with protein-losing enteropathy. *Dis Colon Rectum* 1998;41:932.

170. Harned RK, Williams SM. Familial polyposis coli and periampullary malignancy. *Dis Colon Rectum* 1982;25:227.

171. Hayashi T, Yatani R, Apoltol J, et al. Pathogenesis of hyperplastic polyps of the colon: a hypothesis based on ultrastructure and in vitro kinetics. *Gastroenterology* 1974;66:347.

172. Heald RJ. Gardner's syndrome in association with two tumours in the ileum. *Proc R Soc Med* 1967;60:914.

173. Heald RJ, Bussey HJR. Clinical experiences at St. Mark's Hospital with multiple synchronous cancers of the colon and rectum. *Dis Colon Rectum* 1975;18:6.

174. Heidemann J, Ogawa H, Otterson MF, et al. Antiangiogenic treatment of mesenteric desmoid tumors with toremifene and interferon alfa-2b: report of two cases. *Dis Colon Rectum* 2004;47:118.

175. Heimann TM, Gelernt I, Salky B, et al. Familial polyposis coli: results of mucosal proctectomy with ileoanal anastomosis. *Dis Colon Rectum* 1987;30:424.

176. Heimann TM, Greenstein AJ, Bolnick K, et al. Colorectal cancer in familial polyposis coli and ulcerative colitis. *Dis Colon Rectum* 1985;28:658.

177. Helwig EB. Adenomas and the pathogenesis of cancer of the colon and rectum. *Dis Colon Rectum* 1959;2:5.

178. Henry LG, Condon RE, Schulte WJ, et al. Risk of recurrence of colon polyps. *Ann Surg* 1975;182:511.

179. Heppell J, Kelly KA, Phillips SF, et al. Physiologic aspects of continence after colectomy, mucosal proctectomy, and endorectal ileo-anal anastomosis. *Ann Surg* 1982;195:435.

180. Herrera L, Carrel A, Rao U, et al. Familial adenomatous polyposis in association with thyroiditis. *Dis Colon Rectum* 1989;32:893.

181. Heyen F, Jagelman DG, Romania A, et al. Predictive value of congenital hypertrophy of the retinal pigment epithelium as a clinical marker for familial adenomatous polyposis. *Dis Colon Rectum* 1990;33:1003.

182. Hizawa K, Iida M, Matsumoto T, et al. Neoplastic transformation arising in Peutz-Jeghers polyposis. *Dis Colon Rectum* 1993;36:953.

183. Hoehner JC, Metcalf AM. Development of invasive adenocarcinoma following colectomy with ileoanal anastomosis for familial polyposis coli: report of a case. *Dis Colon Rectum* 1994;37:824.
184. Hoffmann DC, Goligher JC. Polyposis of the stomach and small intestine in association with familial polyposis coli. *Br J Surg* 1971;58:126.
185. Hofstad B, Vatn MH, Andersen SN, et al. Growth of colorectal polyps: redetection and evaluation of unresected polyps for a period of three years. *Gut* 1996;39:449.
186. Holgersen LO, Miller RE, Zintel HA. Juvenile polyps of the colon. Surgery 1971;69:288.
187. Holt RW. Prevention of intussusception in Peutz-Jeghers syndrome. *Dis Colon Rectum* 1979;22:274.
188. Holtzman R, Poulard J-B, Bank S, et al. Repeat colonoscopy after endoscopic polypectomy. *Dis Colon Rectum* 1987;30:185.
189. Hrabovsky EE, Watne AL, Carrier JM. Changing management in familial polyposis. *Am J Surg* 1984;147:130.
190. Hsu S, Huang F, Ossowski L, et al. Colon carcinoma cells with inactive nm23 show increased motility and response to motility factors. *Carcinogenesis* 1995;16:2259.
191. Hsu S-D, Zaharopoulos P, May JT, et al. Peutz-Jeghers syndrome with intestinal carcinoma: report of the association in one family. *Cancer* 1979;44:1527.
192. Hubbard TB Jr. Familial polyposis of the colon: the fate of the retained rectum after colectomy in children. *Am Surg* 1957;23:577.
193. Hurlstone DP, Fujii T, Lobo AJ. Early detection of colorectal cancer using high-magnification chromoscopic colonoscopy. *Br J Surg* 2002;89:272.
194. Iida M, Matsui T, Mibu R, et al. Ileal adenomas in postcolectomy patients with familial adenomatosis coli/Gardner's syndrome: incidence and endoscopic appearance. *Dis Colon Rectum* 1989;32:1034.
195. Iida Y, Miura S, Munemoto Y, et al. Endoscopic resection of large colorectal polyps using a clipping method. *Dis Colon Rectum* 1994;37:179.
196. Iida M, Yao T, Itoh H, et al. Natural history of gastric adenomas in patients with familial adenomatosis coli/Gardner's syndrome. *Cancer* 1988;61:605.
197. Itoh H, Ohsato K. Turcot syndrome and its characteristic colonic manifestations. *Dis Colon Rectum* 1985;28:399.
198. Itoh H, Ohsato K, Yao T, et al. Turcot's syndrome and its mode of inheritance. *Gut* 1979;20:414.
199. Iwama T, Mishima Y. Factors affecting the risk of rectal cancer following rectum-preserving surgery in patients with familial adenomatous polyposis. *Dis Colon Rectum* 1994;37:1024.
200. Iwama T, Mishima Y, Okamoto N, et al. Association of congenital hypertrophy of the retinal pigment epithelium with familial adenomatous polyposis. *Br J Surg* 1990;77:273.
201. Iwama T, Tomita H, Kawachi Y, et al. Indications for local excision of ampullary lesions associated with familial adenomatous polyposis. *J Am Coll Surg* 1994;179:462.
202. Jagelman DG, DeCosse JJ, Bussey HJR. Upper gastrointestinal cancer in familial adenomatous polyposis. *Lancet* 1988;1:1149.
203. Jahadi MR, Bailey W. Papillary adenomas of the colon and rectum: a twelve year review. *Dis Colon Rectum* 1975;18:249.
204. Jalihal A, Misra SP, Arvind AS, et al. Colonoscopic polypectomy in children. *J Pediatr Surg* 1992;27:1220.
205. Jang Y-S, Steinhagen RM, Heimann TM. Colorectal cancer in familial adenomatous polyposis. *Dis Colon Rectum* 1997;40:312.
206. Järvinen H, Franssila KO. Familial juvenile polyposis coli: increased risk of colorectal cancer. *Gut* 1984;25:792.
207. Jass JR. Do all colorectal carcinomas arise in preexisting adenomas? *World J Surg* 1989;13:45.
208. Jass JR. Hyperplastic polyps of the colorectum: innocent or guilty? *Dis Colon Rectum* 2001;44:163.
209. Jeanneret-Grosjean AJ, Thompson WG. Villous adenoma with hyponatremia and syncope: report of a case. *Dis Colon Rectum* 1978;21:118.
210. Jeghers H. Pigmentation of skin. *N Engl J Med* 1944;231:88.
211. Jeghers H, McKusick VA, Katz KH. Generalized intestinal polyposis and melanin spots of the oral mucosa, lips and digits: a syndrome of diagnostic significance. *N Engl J Med* 1949;241:993.
212. Johnson MM, Vosburgh JW, Wiens AT, et al. Gastrointestinal polyposis associated with alopecia, pigmentation, and atrophy of the fingernails and toenails. *Ann Intern Med* 1962;56:935.
213. Johnson Smith TGP, Clark SK, Katz DE, et al. Adrenal masses are associated with familial adenomatous polyposis. *Dis Colon Rectum* 2000;43:1739.
214. Johnston D, Williams NS, Neal DE, et al. The value of preserving the anal sphincter in operations for ulcerative colitis and polyposis: a review of 22 mucosal proctectomies. *Br J Surg* 1981;68:874.
215. Jones I, Fazio VW, Weakley FL, et al. Desmoid tumors in familial polyposis coli. *Ann Surg* 1986;204:94.
216. Joslyn G, Carlson M, Thliveris A, et al. Identification of deletion mutations and three new genes at the familial polyposis locus. *Cell* 1991;66:601.
217. Kanamori T, Itoh M, Yokoyama Y, et al. Injection-incision-assisted snare resection of large sessile colorectal polyps. *Gastrointest Endosc* 1996;43:189.
218. Keck JO, Schoetz DJ Jr, Roberts PL, et al. Rectal mucosectomy in the treatment of giant rectal villous tumors. *Dis Colon Rectum* 1995;38:233.
219. Keshgegian AA, Enterline HT. Gardner's syndrome with duodenal adenomas, gastric adenomyoma and thyroid papillary-follicular adenoma. *Dis Colon Rectum* 1978;21:255.
220. Khorsand J, Karakousis CP. Desmoid tumors and their management. *Am J Surg* 1985;149:215.
221. Kikendall JW, Bowen PE, Burgess MB, et al. Cigarettes and alcohol as independent risk factors for colonic adenomas. *Gastroenterology* 1989;97:660.
222. Kinzler KW, Nilbert MC, Su L-K, et al. Identification of FAP locus genes from chromosome 5q21. *Science* 1991;253:661.
223. Kitamura A, Kanagawa T, Yamada S, et al. Effective chemotherapy for abdominal desmoid tumor in a patient with Gardner's syndrome: report of a case. *Dis Colon Rectum* 1991;34:822.
224. Kmiot WA, Williams MR, Keighley MRB. Pouchitis following colectomy and ileal reservoir construction for familial adenomatous polyposis. *Br J Surg* 1990;77:1283.
225. Knox WG, Miller RE, Begg CF, et al. Juvenile polyps of the colon: a clinicopathologic analysis of 75 polyps in 43 patients. *Surgery* 1960;48:201.
226. Knutson CO, Max MH. Diagnostic and therapeutic colonoscopy. *Arch Surg* 1979;114:430.
227. Konishi F, Wyse NE, Muto T, et al. Peutz-Jeghers polyposis associated with carcinoma of the digestive organs: report of three cases and review of the literature. *Dis Colon Rectum* 1987;30:790.
228. Kottmeir PK, Clatworthy HW Jr. Intestinal polyps and associated carcinoma in childhood. *Am J Surg* 1965;110:709.
229. Kraske P. Zur exstirpation hochsitzender Mastdarmkrebse. *Arch Klin Berl* 1886;33:563. [Extirpation of high carcinomas of the bowel. *Dis Colon Rectum* 1984;27:499].
230. Krokowicz P. The Turcot syndrome. *Acta Chir Scand* 1979;145:113.
231. Kronborg O. Follow-up after removal of colorectal adenomas and radical surgery for colorectal carcinomas. *Br J Surg* 1985;72:26.
232. Kronborg O, Hage E, Deichgraeber E. The clean colon: a prospective, partly randomized study of the effectiveness of repeated examinations of the colon after polypectomy and radical surgery for cancer. *Scand J Gastroenterol* 1981;16:879.

233. Kropilak M, Jagelman DG, Lavery IL, et al. Brain tumors in familial adenomatous polyposis. *Dis Colon Rectum* 1989; 32:778.

234. Kuramoto S, Mimura T, Yamasaki K, et al. Flat cancers do develop in the polyp-free large intestine. *Dis Colon Rectum* 1997;40:534.

235. Kusunoki M, Fujita S, Sakanoue Y, et al. Disappearance of hyperplastic polyposis after resection of rectal cancer. *Dis Colon Rectum* 1991;34:829.

236. Labayle D, Discher D, Vielh P, et al. Sulindac causes regression of rectal polyps in familial adenomatous polyposis. *Gastroenterology* 1991;101:635.

237. Lal G, Gallinger S. Familial adenomatous polyposis. *Semin Surg Oncol* 2000;18:314.

238. Lanspa SJ, Lynch HT, Smyrk TC, et al. Colorectal adenomas in the Lynch syndromes: results of a colonoscopy screening program. *Gastroenterology* 1990;98:1117.

239. Lee FI, MacKinnon MD. Papillary thyroid carcinoma associated with polyposis coli. *Am J Gastroenterol* 1981;76:138.

240. Leppard B. Epidermoid cysts and polyposis coli. *Proc R Soc Med* 1974;67:1036.

241. Leslie A, Carey FA, Pratt NR, et al. The colorectal adenoma-carcinoma sequence. *Br J Surg* 2002;89:845.

242. Linos DA, Dozois RR, Dahlin DC, et al. Does Peutz-Jeghers syndrome predispose to gastrointestinal malignancy? *Arch Surg* 1981;116:1182.

243. Localio SA. Spontaneous disappearance of rectal polyps following subtotal colectomy and ileoproctostomy for polyposis of the colon. *Am J Surg* 1962;103:81.

244. Lockhart-Mummery JP. Cancer and heredity. *Lancet* 1925; 1:427.

245. Longo WE, Touloukian RJ, West AB, et al. Malignant potential of juvenile polyposis coli: report of a case and review of the literature. *Dis Colon Rectum* 1990;33:980.

246. Low DE, Kozarek RA, Ball TJ, et al. Colorectal neodymium-YAG photoablative therapy: comparing applications and complications on both sides of the peritoneal reflection. *Arch Surg* 1989;124:684.

247. Low DE, Kozarek RA, Ball TJ, et al. Nd-YAG laser photoablation of sessile villous and tubular adenomas of the colorectum. *Ann Surg* 1988;208:725.

248. Lynch HT, Fitzgibbons R Jr, Chong S, et al. Use of doxorubicin and dacarbazine for the management of unresectable intra-abdominal desmoid tumors in Gardner's syndrome. *Dis Colon Rectum* 1994;37:260.

249. Lynch HT, de la Chapelle A. Genetic susceptibility to non-polyposis colorectal cancer. *J Med Genet* 1999; 36:801–818.

250. Lynch HT, de la Chapelle A. Hereditary colorectal cancer. *N Engl J Med* 2003;348:919–932.

251. Lynch HT, Lynch PM. Invited commentary. *Dis Colon Rectum* 2002;45:1402.

252. Madden MV, Neale KF, Nicholls RJ, et al. Comparison of morbidity and function after colectomy with ileorectal anastomosis or restorative proctocolectomy for familial adenomatous polyposis. *Br J Surg* 1991;78:789.

253. Malhotra R, Sheffield A. Cronkhite-Canada syndrome associated with colon carcinoma and adenomatous changes in C-C polyps. *Am J Gastroenterol* 1988;83:772.

254. Marshall WH, Martin FIR, Mackay IR. Gardner's syndrome with adrenal carcinoma. *Aust Ann Med* 1967;16:242.

255. Martin PJ, Forde KA. Intraoperative colonoscopy: preliminary report. *Dis Colon Rectum* 1979;22:234.

256. Mathus-Vliegen EMH, Tytgat GNJ. Nd:YAG laser photocoagulation in colorectal adenoma: evaluation of its safety, usefulness and efficacy. *Gastroenterology* 1986;90:1865.

257. Matsumoto T, Iida M, Kobori Y, et al. Progressive duodenal adenomatosis in a familial adenomatous polyposis pedigree with APC mutation at codon 1556. *Dis Colon Rectum* 2002;45:229.

258. Matthews J, Sousha S, Parkins RA, et al. Proliferation patterns and aneuploidy in adenomatous polyps of the colon. *Br J Surg* 1988;75:906.

259. Matuchansky C, Babin P, Coutrot S, et al. Peutz-Jeghers syndrome with metastasizing carcinoma arising from a jejunal hamartoma. *Gastroenterology* 1979;77:1311.

260. Mayer J, Mortensen NJMC. Transanal endoscopic microsurgery: a forgotten minimally invasive operation. *Br J Surg* 1995;82:435.

261. Mazier WP, MacKeigan JM, Billingham RP, et al. Juvenile polyps of the colon and rectum. *Surg Gynecol Obstet* 1982; 154:829.

262. McAdam WAF, Goligher JC. The occurrence of desmoids in patients with familial polyposis coli. *Br J Surg* 1970;57:618.

263. McColl I, Bussey HJ, Veale AMO, et al. Juvenile polyposis coli. *Proc R Soc Med* 1964;57:896.

264. McKinnon JG, Neifield JP, Kay S, et al. Management of desmoid tumors. *Surg Gynecol Obstet* 1989;169:104.

265. McKittrick LS, Wheelock FC Jr. *Carcinoma of the colon.* Springfield, IL: Charles C Thomas, 1954:61.

266. Middleton SB, Clark SK, Matravers P, et al. Stepwise progression of familial adenomatous polyposis-associated desmoid precursor lesions demonstrated by a novel CT scoring system. *Dis Colon Rectum* 2003;46:481.

267. Mills SJ, Chapman PD, Burn J, et al. Endoscopic screening and surgery for familial adenomatous polyposis: dangerous delays. *Br J Surg* 1997;84:74.

268. Milsom JW, Ludwig KA, Church JM, et al. Laparoscopic total abdominal colectomy with ileorectal anastomosis for familial adenomatous polyposis. *Dis Colon Rectum* 1997; 40:675.

269. Miskowiak J, Lindenberg S. Excision of rectal villous adenoma using a TA or GIA stapler. *Br J Surg* 1986;73:630.

270. Morson BC. Some peculiarities in the histology of intestinal polyps. *Dis Colon Rectum* 1962;5:337.

271. Morson BC. Evolution of cancer of the colon and rectum. *Cancer* 1974;34:845.

272. Morson BC, Bussey HJR. Magnitude of risk for cancer in patients with colorectal adenomas. *Br J Surg* 1985;72:23.

273. Morson BC, Dawson IMP. *Gastrointestinal pathology.* Oxford: Blackwell Scientific, 1972.

274. Morson BC, Whiteway JE, Jones EA, et al. Histopathology and prognosis of malignant colorectal polyps treated by endoscopic polypectomy. *Gut* 1984;25:437.

275. Morton DG, Gibson J, Macdonald F, et al. Role of congenital hypertrophy of the retinal pigment epithelium in the predictive diagnosis of familial adenomatous polyposis. *Br J Surg* 1992;79:689.

276. Morton DG, Macdonald F, Haydon J, et al. Screening practice for familial adenomatous polyposis: the potential for regional registers. *Br J Surg* 1993;80:255.

277. Muller S, Chesner IM, Egan MJ, et al. Significance of venous and lymphatic invasion in malignant polyps of the colon and rectum. *Gut* 1989;30:1385.

278. Muto T, Bussey HJR, Morson BC. The evolution of cancer of the colon and rectum. *Cancer* 1975;36:2251.

279. Muto T, Kamiya J, Sawada T, et al. Small "flat adenoma" of the large bowel with special reference to its clinicopathologic features. *Dis Colon Rectum* 1985;28:847.

280. Nagata C, Shimizu H, Kametani M, et al. Cigarette smoking, alcohol use, and colorectal adenoma in Japanese men and women. *Dis Colon Rectum* 1999;42:337.

281. Nakagoe T, Ishikawa H, Sawai T, et al. Surgical technique and outcome of gasless video endoscopic transanal rectal tumor excision. *Br J Surg* 2002;89:769.

282. Nakamura Y, While R, Smits AMM, et al. Genetic alterations during colorectal tumor development. *N Engl J Med* 1988;319:525.

283. Nava H, Carlsson G, Petrelli NJ, et al. Follow-up colonoscopy in patients with colorectal adenomatous polyps. *Dis Colon Rectum* 1987;30:465.

284. Naveau S, Chaput JC, Bedossa P, et al. Cirrhosis as an independent risk factor for colonic adenomas. *Gut* 1992;33: 535.

285. Naylor WE, Lebenthal E. Early detection of adenomatous polyposis coli in Gardner's syndrome. *Pediatrics* 1979;63: 222.

286. Neale AV, Demers RY, Budev H, et al. Physician accuracy in diagnosing colorectal polyps. *Dis Colon Rectum* 1987; 30:247.

287. Neugut AI, Forde KA. Screening colonoscopy: has the time come? *Am J Gastroenterol* 1988;83:295.

288. Neugut AI, Jacobson JS, Ahsan H, et al. Incidence and recurrence rates of colorectal adenomas: a prospective study. *Gastroenterology* 1995;108:402.

289. Neugut AI, Johnsen CM, Forde KA, et al. Recurrence rates for colorectal polyps. *Cancer* 1985;55:1586.

290. Nishisho I, Nakamura Y, Miyoshi Y, et al. Mutations of chromosome 5q21 genes in FAP and colorectal cancer patients. *Science* 1991;253:665.

291. Nishizawa M, Okada T, Sato F, et al. A clinicopathological study of minute polypoid lesions of the colon based on magnifying fiber-colonoscopy and dissecting microscopy. *Endoscopy* 1980;12:124.

292. Nivatvongs S, Rojanasakul A, Reiman HM, et al. The risk of lymph node metastasis in colorectal polyps with invasive adenocarcinoma. *Dis Colon Rectum* 1991;34:323.

293. Norfleet RG. Colonoscopy and polypectomy in nonhospitalized patients. *Gastrointest Endosc* 1982;28:15.

294. Norfleet RG, Ryan ME, Wyman JB. Adenomatous and hyperplastic polyps cannot be reliably distinguished by their appearance through the fiberoptic sigmoidoscope. *Dig Dis Sci* 1988;33:1175.

295. Nugent KP, Farmer KCR, Spigelman AD, et al. Randomized controlled trial of the effect of sulindac on duodenal and rectal polyposis and cell proliferation in patients with familial adenomatous polyposis. *Br J Surg* 1993;80: 1618.

296. Nugent KP, Phillips RKS. Rectal cancer risk in older patients with familial adenomatous polyposis and an ileorectal anastomosis: a cause for concern. *Br J Surg* 1992; 79:1204.

297. Nugent KP, Spigelman AD, Phillips RKS. Life expectancy after colectomy and ileorectal anastomosis for familial adenomatous polyposis. *Dis Colon Rectum* 1993;36:1059.

298. Oldfield MC. The association of familial polyposis of the colon with multiple sebaceous cysts. *Br J Surg* 1954;41: 534.

299. Olsen K<asO>, Juul S, Bülow S, et al. Female fecundity before and after operation for familial adenomatous polyposis. *Br J Surg* 2003;90:227.

300. Oohara T, Ogino A, Tohma H. Histogenesis of microscopic adenoma and hyperplastic (metaplastic) gland in nonpolyposis coli. *Dis Colon Rectum* 1981;24:375.

301. Ooi BS, Remzi FH, Gramlich T, et al. Anal transitional zone cancer after restorative proctocolectomy and ileoanal anastomosis in familial adenomatous polyposis: report of two cases. *Dis Colon Rectum* 2003;46:1418.

302. Opelka FG, Timmcke AE, Gathright JB Jr, et al. Diminutive colonic polyps: an indication for colonoscopy. *Dis Colon Rectum* 1992;35:178.

303. Ott DJ, Gelfand DW. Colorectal tumors: pathology and detection. *AJR Am J Roentgenol* 1978;131:691.

304. Painter TA, Jagelman DG. Adrenal adenomas and adrenal carcinomas in association with hereditary adenomatosis of the colon and rectum. *Cancer* 1985;55:2001.

305. Panos RG, Opelka FG, Nogueras JJ. Peutz-Jeghers syndrome: a call for intraoperative enteroscopy. *Am Surg* 1990;56:331.

306. Parikshak M, Pawlak SE, Eggenberger JC, et al. The role of endoscopic colon surveillance in the transplant population. *Dis Colon Rectum* 2002;45:1655.

307. Park J-G, Han H-J, Kang M-S, et al. Presymptomatic diagnosis of familial adenomatous polyposis coli. *Dis Colon Rectum* 1994;37:700.

308. Park J-G, Park KJ, Ahn Y-O, et al. Risk of gastric cancer among Korean familial adenomatous polyposis patients. *Dis Colon Rectum* 1992;35:996.

309. Parker AL, Kadakia SC, Maccini DM, et al. Disappearance of duodenal polyps in Gardner's syndrome with sulindac therapy. *Am J Gastroenterol* 1993;88:93.

310. Parks AG, Nicholls RJ, Belliveau P. Proctocolectomy with ileal reservoir and anal anastomosis. *Br J Surg* 1980;67:533.

311. Paul P, Jagelman DG, Fazio VW, et al. Evaluation of polymorphic genetic markers for linkage to the familial adenomatous polyposis locus on chromosome 5. *Dis Colon Rectum* 1990;33:740.

312. Pavlides GP, Milligan FD, Clarke DN, et al. Hereditary polyposis coli I: the diagnostic value of colonoscopy, barium enema, and fecal occult blood. *Cancer* 1977;40:2632.

313. Pello MJ. Transanal excision of large sessile villous adenomas using an endorectal traction flap. *Surg Gynecol Obstet* 1987;164:281.

314. Peltomaki P, Lothe RA, Aaltonen LA, et al. Microsatellite instability is associated with tumors that characterize the hereditary non-polyposis colorectal cancer syndrome. *Cancer Res* 1993; 53:5853–5855.

315. Pendanna N, Mendis R, Holt S, et al. Genetics of colorectal cancer. *Int J Oncol* 1996;9:327.

316. Penna C, Kartheuser A, Parc R, et al. Secondary proctectomy and ileal pouch-anal anastomosis after ileorectal anastomosis for familial adenomatous polyposis. *Br J Surg* 1993;80:1621.

317. Penna C, Tiret E, Daude F, et al. Results of ileal J-pouch-anal anastomosis in familial adenomatous polyposis complicated by rectal carcinoma. *Dis Colon Rectum* 1994;37: 157.

318. Penna C, Tiret E, Kartheuser A, et al. Function of ileal J pouch-anal anastomosis in patients with familial adenomatous polyposis. *Br J Surg* 1993;80:765.

319. Penna C, Tiret E, Parc R, et al. Operation and abdominal desmoid tumors in familial adenomatous polyposis. *Surg Gynecol Obstet* 1993;177:263.

320. Pennazio M, Arrigoni A, Risio M, et al. Small rectosigmoid polyps as markers of proximal neoplasms. *Dis Colon Rectum* 1993;36:1121.

321. Peutz JLA. Very remarkable case of familial polyposis of mucous membrane of intestinal tract and nasopharynx accompanied by peculiar pigmentations of skin and mucous membrane. *Ned Maandschr Geneeskd* 1921;10:134.

322. Phillips LG Jr. Polyposis and carcinoma of the small bowel and familial colonic polyposis. *Dis Colon Rectum* 1981;24: 478.

323. Pines A, Bat L, Shemesh E, et al. Invasive colorectal adenomas: surgery versus colonoscopic polypectomy. *J Surg Oncol* 1990;43:53.

324. Plail RO, Bussey HJR, Glazer G, et al. Adenomatous polyposis: an association with carcinoma of the thyroid. *Br J Surg* 1987;74:377.

325. Pollard CW, Nivatvongs S, Rojanasakul A, et al. The fate of patients following polypectomy alone for polyps containing invasive carcinoma. *Dis Colon Rectum* 1992;35: 933.

326. Poritz LS, Blackstein M, Berk T, et al. Extended follow-up of patients treated with cytotoxic chemotherapy for intra-abdominal desmoid tumors. *Dis Colon Rectum* 2001;44: 1268.

327. Posner MC, Shiu MH, Newsome JL, et al. The desmoid tumor: not a benign disease. *Arch Surg* 1989;124:191.

328. Poulard JB, Shatz B, Kodner I. Preoperative tattooing of polypectomy site. *Endoscopy* 1985;17:84.

329. Prager ED, Swinton NW, Young JL, et al. Follow-up study of patients with benign mucosal polyps discovered by proctosigmoidoscopy. *Dis Colon Rectum* 1974;17:322.

330. Primrose JN, Quirke P, Johnston D. Carcinoma of the ileostomy in a patient with familial adenomatous polyposis. *Br J Surg* 1988;75:384.

331. Prohm P, Weber J, Bönner C. Laparoscopic-assisted coloscopic polypectomy. *Dis Colon Rectum* 2001;44:746.

332. Provenzale D, Garrett JW, Condon SE, et al. Risk for colon adenomas in patients with rectosigmoid hyperplastic polyps. *Ann Intern Med* 1990;113:760.

333. Quan SHQ, Castro EB. Papillary adenomas (villous tumors): a review of 215 cases. *Dis Colon Rectum* 1971;14: 267.

334. Qureshi MA, Monson JRT, Lee PWR. Transanal MULTI-FIRE ENDO GIA technique for rectal polypectomy. *Dis Colon Rectum* 1997;40:116.

335. Rabelo R, Foulkes W, Gordon PH, et al. Role of molecular diagnostic testing in familial adenomatous polyposis and hereditary nonpolyposis colorectal cancer families. *Dis Colon Rectum* 2001;44:437.

336. Ransohoff DF, Lang CA, Kuo HS. Colonoscopic surveillance with polypectomy: considerations of cost effectiveness. *Ann Intern Med* 1991;114:177.

337. Rappaport LB, Sperling, HV, Stavrides A. Colon cancer in the Cronkhite-Canada syndrome. *J Clin Gastroenterol* 1986;8:199.

338. Ramaswamy G, Elhosseiny AA, Tchertkoff V. Juvenile polyposis of the colon with atypical adenomatous changes and carcinoma in situ: report of a case and review of the literature. *Dis Colon Rectum* 1984;27:393.

339. Read TE, Read JD, Butterly LF. Importance of adenomas 5 mm or less in diameter that are detected by sigmoidoscopy. *N Engl J Med* 1997;336:8.

340. Reed K, Vose PC. Diffuse juvenile polyposis of the colon: a premalignant condition. *Dis Colon Rectum* 1981;24:205.

341. Reid JD. Intestinal carcinoma in the Peutz-Jeghers syndrome. *JAMA* 1974;229:833.

342. Remzi FH, Church JM, Bast J, et al. Mucosectomy vs. stapled ileal pouch-anal anastomosis in patients with familial adenomatosis polyposis: functional outcome and neoplasia control. *Dis Colon Rectum* 2001;44:1590.

343. Richards WO, Webb WA, Morris SJ, et al. Patient management after endoscopic removal of the cancerous colon adenoma. *Ann Surg* 1986;205:665.

344. Rickert RR, Auerbach O, Garfinkel L, et al. Adenomatous lesions of the large bowel: an autopsy study. *Cancer* 1979;43:1847.

345. Riddell RH. Hands off "cancerous" large bowel polyps. *Gastroenterology* 1985;89:432.

346. Rolles CJ. Juvenile intestinal polyps-are they always benign? *BMJ* 1987;294:529.

347. Roncucci L, Di Donato P, Carati L, et al. Antioxidant vitamins or lactulose for the prevention of the recurrence of colorectal adenomas. *Dis Colon Rectum* 1993;36:227.

348. Ross JE, Mara JE. Small bowel polyps and carcinoma in multiple intestinal polyposis. *Arch Surg* 1974;108:736.

349. Roth SI, Helwig EB. Juvenile polyps of the colon and rectum. *Cancer* 1963;16:468.

350. Rothenberger DA, Vermeulen FD, Christenson CE, et al. Restorative proctocolectomy with ileal reservoir and ileoanal anastomosis. *Am J Surg* 1983;145:82.

351. Rothman D, Su CP, Kendall AB. Dilemma in a case of Turcot's (glioma-polyposis) syndrome: report of a case. *Dis Colon Rectum* 1975;18:514.

352. Roy AD, Ellis H. Potassium-secreting tumours of the large intestine. *Lancet* 1959;1:759.

353. Royds JA, Cross SS, Silcocks PB, et al. Nm23 "antimetastatic" gene product expression in colorectal carcinoma. *J Pathol* 1994;172:261.

354. Rozen P, Fireman Z, Figer A, et al. Family history of colorectal cancer as a marker of potential malignancy within a screening program. *Cancer* 1987;60:248.

355. Russell JB, Russell MP, Chan CH, et al. When is polypectomy sufficient treatment for colorectal cancer in a polyp? *Am J Surg* 1990;160:665.

356. Rustin RB, Jagelman DG, McGannon E, et al. Spontaneous mutation in familial adenomatous polyposis. *Dis Colon Rectum* 1990;33:52.

357. Ryan DP, Schapiro RH, Warshaw AL. Villous tumors of the duodenum. *Ann Surg* 1986;203:301.

358. Ryo UY, Roh SK, Balkin RB, et al. Extensive metastases in Peutz-Jeghers syndrome. *JAMA* 1978;239:2268.

359. Saclarides TJ, Smith L, Ko S-T, et al. Transanal endoscopic microsurgery. *Dis Colon Rectum* 1992;35:1183.

360. Said S, Huber P, Pichlmaier H. Technique and clinical results of endorectal surgery. *Surgery* 1993;113:65.

361. Sakamoto GD, MacKeigan JM, Senagore AJ. Transanal excision of large, rectal villous adenomas. *Dis Colon Rectum* 1991;34:880.

362. Sankar MY, Joffe SN. Laser surgery in colonic and anorectal lesions. *Surg Clin North Am* 1988;68:1447.

363. Sarre RG, Frost AG, Jagelman DG, et al. Gastric and duodenal polyps in familial adenomatous polyposis: a prospective study of the nature and prevalence of upper gastrointestinal polyps. *Gut* 1987;28:306.

364. Sarre RG, Jagelman DG, Beck GJ, et al. Colectomy with ileorectal anastomosis for familial adenomatous polyposis: the risk of rectal cancer. *Surgery* 1987;101:20.

365. Schapiro M. What to do with the adenoma-carcinoma intermezzo. *Gastroenterology* 1986;91:256.

366. Schmid M, Haaf T, Grunert D. 5-Azacytidine-induced undercondensations in human chromosomes. *Hum Genet* 1984;67:257.

367. Schnitzler M, Cohen Z, Blackstein M, et al. Chemotherapy for desmoid tumors in association with familial adenomatous polyposis. *Dis Colon Rectum* 1997;40:798.

368. Schröder S, Moehrs D, von Weltzien J, et al. The Turcot syndrome: report of an additional case and review of the literature. *Dis Colon Rectum* 1983;26:533.

369. Selvaggi F, di Carlo ES, Maffettone V, et al. Intersphincteric surgical access to the rectum for the treatment of villous adenomas. *Dis Colon Rectum* 1992;35:92.

370. Sene A, Thomas PE, Gautam V, et al. Juvenile polyp in an ileoanal J pouch following restorative proctocolectomy for juvenile polyposis coli. *Br J Surg* 1989;76:801.

371. Sener SF, Miller HH, DeCosse JJ. The spectrum of polyposis. *Surg Gynecol Obstet* 1984;159:525.

372. Setti-Carraro P, Nicholls RJ. Choice of prophylactic surgery for the large bowel component of familial adenomatous polyposis. *Br J Surg* 1996;83:885.

373. Shatney CH, Lober PH, Gilbertsen VA, et al. The treatment of pedunculated adenomatous colorectal polyps with focal cancer. *Surg Gynecol Obstet* 1974;139:845.

374. Shepard JA. Familial polyposis of the colon with special reference to regression of rectal polyposis after subtotal colectomy. *Br J Surg* 1971;58:85.

375. Sheridan R, D'Avis J, Seyfer AE, et al. Massive abdominal wall desmoid tumor. Treatment by resection and abdominal wall reconstruction. *Dis Colon Rectum* 1986;29:518.

376. Shibata D, Reale MA, Lavin P, et al. DCC protein and progress in colorectal cancer. *N Engl J Med* 1996;335:1727.

377. Shields HM. Peutz-Jeghers syndrome: perhaps not so benign [Editorial]. *Gastroenterology* 1987;93:1135.

378. Shinya H, Wolff WI. Morphology, anatomic distribution and cancer potential of colonic polyps: an analysis of 7,000 polyps endoscopically removed. *Ann Surg* 1979;190:679.

379. Silverberg SG. Focally malignant adenomatous polyps of the colon and rectum. *Surg Gynecol Obstet* 1970;131:103.

380. Skinner MA, Tyler D, Branum GD, et al. Subtotal colectomy for familial polyposis. *Arch Surg* 1990;125:621.

381. Smilow PC, Pryor CA, Swinton NW. Juvenile polyposis coli: a report of three patients in three generations of one family. *Dis Colon Rectum* 1966;9:248.

382. Smith WG. Desmoid tumors in familial multiple polyposis. *Mayo Clin Proc* 1959;34:31.

383. Smith WG. Familial multiple polyposis: research tool for investigating the etiology of carcinoma of the colon? *Colon Rectum* 1968;11:17.

384. Smith WG, Kern BB. The nature of the mutation in familial multiple polyposis: papillary carcinoma of the thyroid, brain tumors, and familial multiple polyposis. *Dis Colon Rectum* 1973;16:264.

385. Soave F. Endorectal ileal pull-through for ulcerative colitis and polyposis in children. *Dis Colon Rectum* 1985;28:76.

386. Sokhi GS, Hashemi K. Colonoscopic polypectomy in children. *BMJ* 1981;282:145.

387. Spigelman AD. Familial adenomatous polyposis: recent genetic advances. *Br J Surg* 1994;81:321.

388. Spigelman AD, Arese P, Phillips RKS. Polyposis: the Peutz-Jeghers syndrome. *Br J Surg* 1995;82:1311.
389. Spigelman AD, Murdey V, Phillips RKS. Cancer and the Peutz-Jeghers syndrome. *Gut* 1989;30:1588.
390. Spigelman AD, Thomson JPS, Phillips RKS. Towards decreasing the relaparotomy rate in the Peutz-Jeghers syndrome: the role of preoperative small bowel endoscopy. *Br J Surg* 1990;77:301.
391. Standards Task Force of the American Society of Colon and Rectal Surgeons. Practice parameters for treatment of patients with dominantly inherited colorectal cancer (familial adenomatous polyposis and hereditary nonpolyposis colorectal cancer). *Dis Colon Rectum* 2003;46:1001.
392. Steele RJC, Thompson AM, Hall PA, et al. The *p53* tumour suppressor gene. *Br J Surg* 1998;85:1460.
393. Stevenson JK, Reid BJ. Unfamiliar aspects of familial polyposis coli. *Am J Surg* 1986;152:81.
394. Stoltenberg RL, Madsen JA, Schlack SC, et al. Neoplasia in ileal pouch mucosa after total proctocolectomy for juvenile polyposis: report of a case. *Dis Colon Rectum* 1997; 40:726.
395. Stryker SJ, Wolff BG, Culp CE, et al. Natural history of untreated colonic polyps. *Gastroenterology* 1987;93:1009.
396. Stulc JP, Petrelli NJ, Herrera L, et al. Colorectal villous and tubulovillous adenomas equal to or greater than four centimeters. *Ann Surg* 1988;207:65.
397. Sugihara K, Tetsuichiro M, Kamiya J, et al. Gardner's syndrome associated with periampullary carcinoma, duodenal and gastric adenomatosis: report of a case. *Dis Colon Rectum* 1982;25:766.
398. Sugihara K, Muto T, Morioka Y. Management of patients with invasive carcinoma removed by colonoscopic polypectomy. *Dis Colon Rectum* 1989;32:829.
399. Sutton CD, Marshall L-J, White SA, et al. Ten-year experience of endoscopic transanal resection. *Ann Surg* 2002;235: 355.
400. Swinton NW, Warren S. Polyps of the colon and rectum and their relation to malignancy. *JAMA* 1939;113:1927.
401. Talbot IC. Redetection and growth of colorectal polyps. *Gut* 1996;39:492.
402. Tannapfel A, Köckerling F, Katalini A, et al. Expression of nm23-H-1 predicts lymph node involvement in colorectal carcinoma. *Dis Colon Rectum* 1995;38:651.
403. Tappero G, Gaia E, De Giuli P, et al. Cold snare excision of small colorectal polyps. *Gastrointest Endosc* 1992;38: 310.
404. Taylor BA, Wolff BG, Dozois RR, et al. Ileal pouch-anal anastomosis for chronic ulcerative colitis and familial polyposis coli complicated by adenocarcinoma. *Dis Colon Rectum* 1988;31:358.
405. Taylor EW, Thompson H, Oates GD, et al. Limitations of biopsy in preoperative assessment of villous papilloma. *Dis Colon Rectum* 1981;24:259.
406. Tedesco FJ, Hendrix JC, Pickens CA, et al. Diminutive polyps: histopathology, spatial distribution, and clinical significance. *Gastrointest Endosc* 1982;28:1.
407. Telander RL, Perrault J. Colectomy with rectal mucosectomy and ileoanal anastomosis in young patients: its use for ulcerative colitis and familial polyposis. *Arch Surg* 1981;116:623.
408. Thomas MG, Thomson JPS, Williamson RCN. Oral calcium inhibits rectal epithelial proliferation in familial adenomatous polyposis. *Br J Surg* 1993;80:499.
409. Thomford NR, Greenberger NJ. Lymphoid polyps of the ileum associated with Gardner's syndrome. *Arch Surg* 1968;96:289.
410. Thompson-Fawcett MW, Marcus VA, Redston M, et al. Adenomatous polyps develop commonly in the ileal pouch of patients with familial adenomatous polyposis. *Dis Colon Rectum* 2001;44:347.
411. Tierney RP, Ballantyne GH, Modlin IM. The adenoma to carcinoma sequence. *Surg Gynecol Obstet* 1990;171:81.
412. Tonelli F, Valanzano R, Messerini L, et al. Long-term treatment with sulindac in familial adenomatous polyposis: is there an actual efficacy in prevention of rectal cancer? *J Surg Oncol* 2000;74:15.
413. Tonooka T, Sano Y, Fujii T, et al. Adenocarcinoma in solitary large hyperplastic polyp diagnosed by magnifying colonoscope: report of a case. *Dis Colon Rectum* 2002;45: 1407.
414. Torres CF, Korones DN, Pilcher W. Multiple ependymomas in a patient with Turcot's syndrome. *Med Pediatr Oncol* 1997;28:59.
415. Traboulsi EI, Krush AJ, Gardner EJ, et al. Prevalence and importance of pigmented ocular fundus lesions in Gardner's syndrome. *N Engl J Med* 1987;316:661.
416. Tsukada K, Church JM, Jagelman DG, et al. Systemic cytotoxic chemotherapy and radiation therapy for desmoid in familial adenomatous polyposis. *Dis Colon Rectum* 1991; 34:1090.
417. Tsukada K, Church JM, Jagelman DG, et al. Noncytotoxic drug therapy for intra-abdominal desmoid tumor in patients with familial adenomatous polyposis. *Dis Colon Rectum* 1992;35:29.
418. Turcot J, Despres JP, St. Pierre F. Malignant tumors of the central nervous system associated with familial polyposis of the colon. *Dis Colon Rectum* 1959;2:465.
419. Umar A, Kunkel TA. DNA replication fidelity, mismatch repair and genome instability in cancer cells. *Eur J Biochem* 1996;238:297.
420. Utsunomiya J, Iwama T, Imajo M, et al. Total colectomy, mucosal proctectomy and ileoanal anastomosis. *Dis Colon Rectum* 1980;23:459.
421. Utsunomiya J, Nakamura T. The occult osteomatous changes in the mandible in patients with familial polyposis coli. *Br J Surg* 1975;62:45.
422. van Coevorden F, Mathus-Vliegen EMH, Brummelkamp WH. Combined endoscopic and surgical treatment in Peutz-Jeghers syndrome. *Surg Gynecol Obstet* 1986;162: 426.
423. van Driel MF, Ziers W, Grond J, et al. Juvenile polyps at the site of a ureterosigmoidostomy: report of five cases. *Dis Colon Rectum* 1988;31:553.
424. Vasen HFA, Wijnen JT, Menko FH, et al. Cancer risk in families with hereditary nonpolyposis colorectal cancer diagnosed by mutational analysis. *Gastroenterology* 1996;110: 1020.
425. Vasen HFA, Wijnen JT. Clinical implications of genetic testing of hereditary nonpolyposis colorectal cancer. *Cytogenet Cell Genet* 1999; 86: 136.
426. Venkitachalam PS, Hirsch E, Elguezabal A, et al. Multiple lymphoid polyposis and familial polyposis of the colon: a genetic relationship. *Dis Colon Rectum* 1978;21:336.
427. Vogelstein B, Fearon ER, Hamilton S, et al: Genetic alterations during colorectal-tumor development. *N Engl J Med* 319:525, 1988.
428. Vogelstein B, Fearon ER, Hamilton SR, et al. The adenoma to carcinoma sequence. *Surg Gynecol Obstet* 1990;171:81.
429. Waddell WR, Ganser GF, Cerise EJ, et al. Sulindac for polyposis of the colon. *Am J Surg* 1989;157:175.
430. Wallace MH, Phillips RKS. Upper gastrointestinal disease in patients with familial adenomatous polyposis. *Br J Surg* 1998;85:742.
431. Watne AL, Core SK, Carrier JM. Gardner's syndrome. *Surg Gynecol Obstet* 1975;141:53.
432. Watne AL, Lai HY, Carrier J, et al. The diagnosis and surgical treatment of patients with Gardner's syndrome. *Surgery* 1977;82:327.
433. Waye JD, Bilotta JJ. Rectal hyperplastic polyps: now you see them, now you don't—a differential point. *Am J Gastroenterol* 1990;85:1557.
434. Waye JD, Braunfeld S. Surveillance intervals after colonoscopic polypectomy. *Endoscopy* 1982;14:79.
435. Waye JD, Lewis BS, Frankel A, et al. Small colon polyps. *Am J Gastroenterol* 1988;83:120.
436. Webb WA, Dyess L. Endoscopic criteria for malignancy in colon adenoma. *Dis Colon Rectum* 1986;29:896.
437. Wegener M, Börsch G, Schmidt G. Colorectal adenomas: distribution, incidence of malignant transformation, and rate of recurrence. *Dis Colon Rectum* 1986;29:383.

438. Welch CE, Hedberg SE. *Polypoid lesions of the gastrointestinal tract*, 2nd ed. Philadelphia: WB Saunders, 1975:131.

439. Welch CE, Hedberg SE. *Polypoid lesions of the gastrointestinal tract*, 2nd ed. Philadelphia: WB Saunders, 1975: 186.

440. Westbrook KC, Lang NP, Broadwater JR, et al. Posterior surgical approaches to the rectum. *Ann Surg* 1982;195: 677.

441. Westhues M. *Die pathologisch-anatomischen Grundlagen der Chirurgie des Rektumkarzinoms*. Leipzig: Georg Thieme Verlag, 1934.

442. Weston SD, Weiner M. Familial polyposis associated with a new type of soft-tissue lesion (skin pigmentation): report of three cases and a review of the literature. *Dis Colon Rectum* 1967;10:311.

443. Wetherall AP, Williams NMA, Kelly MJ. Endoscopic transanal resection in the management of patients with sessile rectal adenomas, anastomotic stricture and rectal cancer. *Br J Surg* 1993;80:788.

444. Whelan RL, Horvath KD, Gleason NR, et al. Vitamin and calcium supplement use is associated with decreased adenoma recurrence in patients with a previous history of neoplasia. *Dis Colon Rectum* 1999;42:212.

445. Williams CB. Follow-up after polypectomy [Editorial]. *Endoscopy* 1982;14:73.

446. Williams CB. Polyp follow-up: how, who for and how often? *Br J Surg* 1985;72:25.

447. Williams CB, Goldblatt M, Delaney PV. "Top and tail endoscopy" and follow-up in Peutz-Jeghers syndrome. *Endoscopy* 1982;14:82.

448. Williams CB, Macrae FA, Bartram CI. A prospective study of diagnostic methods in adenoma follow-up. *Endoscopy* 1982;14:74.

449. Wilson SM, Poisson J, Gamache A, et al. Intraoperative fiberoptic colonoscopy: "the difficult polypectomy." *Dis Colon Rectum* 1976;19:136.

450. Winawer SJ, O'Brien MJ, Waye JD, et al. Risk surveillance of individuals with colorectal polyps. *WHO Bull* 1990;68: 789.

451. Winawer SJ, Zauber AG, Gerdes H, et al. Risk of colorectal cancer in the families of patients with adenomatous polyps. *N Engl J Med* 1996;334:82.

452. Winawer SJ, Zauber AG, Ho MN, et al. Prevention of colorectal cancer by colonoscopic polypectomy. *N Engl J Med* 1993;329:1977.

453. Winawer SJ, Zauber AG, O'Brien MJ, et al. Randomized comparison of surveillance intervals after colonoscopic removal of newly diagnosed adenomatous polyps. *N Engl J Med* 1993;328:901.

454. Winde G, Schmid KW, Schlegel W, et al. Complete reversion and prevention of rectal adenomas in colectomized patients with familial adenomatous polyposis by rectal low-dose sulindac maintenance treatment: advantages of a low-dose nonsteroidal anti-inflammatory drug regimen in reversing adenomas exceeding 33 months. *Dis Colon Rectum* 1995;38:813.

455. Wolff WI, Shinya H. Definitive treatment of "malignant" polyps of the colon. *Ann Surg* 1975;182:516.

456. Wolff WI, Shinya H. Endoscopic polypectomy: therapeutic and clinicopathologic aspects. *Cancer* 1975;36:683.

457. Wolff WL, Shinya H, Cwern M, et al. Cancerous colonic polyps: "hands on" or "hands off." *Am Surg* 1990;56:148.

458. Wong N, Lasko D, Rabelo R, et al. Genetic counseling and interpretation of genetic tests in familial adenomatous polyposis and hereditary nonpolyposis colorectal cancer. *Dis Colon Rectum* 2001;44:271.

459. Woods RJ, Sarre RG, Ctercteko GC, et al. Occult radiologic changes in the skull and jaw in familial adenomatous polyposis coli. *Dis Colon Rectum* 1989;32:304.

460. Woolfson IK, Eckholdt GJ, Wetzel CR. Usefulness of performing colonoscopy one year after endoscopic polypectomy. *Dis Colon Rectum* 1990;33:389.

461. Yeh T-M, Boonswang P, Smith DH. Endoscopic tattooing prior to colon resection. *Contemp Surg* 1988;33:73.

462. Yokota T, Sugihara K, Yoshida S. Endoscopic mucosal resection for colorectal neoplastic lesions. *Dis Colon Rectum* 1994;37:1108.

Chapter 22

Carcinoma of the Colon

There is a tremendous literature on cancer, but what we know for sure about it can be printed on a calling card.

August Bier

Excluding cancer of the skin, colorectal carcinoma is the second most common malignancy found in most Western countries. In women, lung and breast cancers are more common, whereas in men, lung and prostate cancers are more frequently observed. In 2004, the American Cancer Society estimated that 146,940 new cases would be diagnosed in the United States, and 56,730 deaths would occur.[451] The chance of colorectal carcinoma developing during the life of an infant born in the United States today is 5%.

The incidence of colorectal cancer had been relatively stable for the 40 years before the last decade, even as death rates were falling. However, the incidence appears to be decreasing. This suggests that the fall in colorectal cancer incidence, especially among whites, may be attributable to more effective preventive measures. The trends in cancer incidence, mortality, and patient survival in the United States are derived from the SEER Program (Survey of Epidemiology and End Results) of the National Cancer Institute.[678]

ETIOLOGY AND EPIDEMIOLOGY

The epidemiology of large bowel cancer has become a major area of investigative interest. Interpopulation and nationality differences were the inspiration for Burkitt's hypothesis on the contributory role of a low-residue, high-carbohydrate diet in causing colorectal cancer.[118,121] His observations generated additional reports about the incidence and mortality of large bowel cancer, and other hypotheses have been suggested.[81,361,363,367,408,687]

Distribution and Nationality

The mortality rates for colorectal cancer in Western European countries are generally high.[237,781] Scotland is the leader in the world, with rates much higher than even those of England.[842] Spain and Portugal, conversely, have relatively low rates, more consistent with those of Eastern Europe.[237] The two populations with risks similar to those of Western Europe are the people of Israel and the Chinese in Singapore. In Israel, a considerable difference has existed between Israelis born in Europe and those born in North Africa or Asia. The incidence in the former is 2.5 times that of the latter. With the exception of Singapore, Asia has a low incidence. African countries generally have

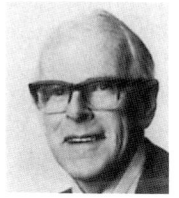

Denis Parsons Burkitt (1911–1993)   Denis Burkitt was born February 28, 1911, in Enniskillen, Northern Ireland, the son of an engineer. Without any particular interest in medicine, he followed in his father's footsteps to engineering school at Dublin University. An indifferent student, he learned of a letter the don had written to his father in which he expressed doubt as to Denis' ability to obtain a university degree and warned about the risk of forfeiting the £10 enrollment fee. It is therefore ironic that many years later he received the university's highest award, an honorary fellowship of Trinity College, Dublin. Interestingly, in light of Burkitt's subsequent career, the British Colonial Office rejected his offer for service in Africa because he had lost an eye in an accident at the age of 11. He abandoned the course he had initiated, instead seeking and obtaining admission to medical school, an act he attributed to a commitment to the highest ideals and principles of his Christian faith. Burkitt completed medical school at Dublin in 1936, received his Fellowship in the Royal College of Surgeons in Edinburgh in 1938, and his doctorate in 1946. Through the Second World War, he served with the Royal Army Medical Corps, and in 1946 he joined His Majesty's Colonial Service in Uganda as a government surgeon and lecturer at the Makerere University College Medical School. He became committed to serving less privileged people than himself. The rest is medical history. In 1957, he treated a child with swellings in both maxillae and mandibles, a condition that ultimately came to be known as Burkitt's lymphoma. This led to the discovery of the cause and to the subsequent identification of the Epstein-Barr virus. His keen sense of observation and knowledge of epidemiology helped him to recognize that the most common diseases of Western civilization were virtually unknown in rural populations of developing countries. Modestly, he stated that were it not for the reputation of his eponymous association with a lymphoma, no one would have listened to his thoughts concerning the epidemiology of colon cancer. Numerous honors came to Burkitt, including the Harrison Prize of the Royal Society of Medicine, the Stuart Prize of the British Medical Association, and the Walker Prize of the Royal College of Surgeons. Honorary degrees and fellowships were awarded to him by numerous universities and organizations throughout the world. The author of six books and more than 300 scientific publications, he actively wrote from his home in Gloucester, England, until the end of his life. When autographing a book, he always penned these thoughts: "Attitudes are more important than abilities; motives are more important than methods; character is more important than cleverness; and stick-to-it-iveness is more important than the starting place."

a very low frequency of colorectal cancer; in Latin American countries, the incidence rates vary.[181,409,995]

In addition to the differences in the incidence of colorectal cancer from one population to another, observations have been made concerning the variations in the distribution within the colon and rectum. It has been postulated that low-risk populations have a relatively increased incidence of right-sided cancers, whereas relatively high-risk communities have an increased risk of left-sided malignancies.[96,118,121,364]

A difference in the incidence of cancer has been observed from country to country when urban populations are compared with rural populations.[80,162,225,530,675,890,937] The nature of the urban-rural gradient with respect to risk has been extensively investigated in the United States. By comparing metropolitan and nonmetropolitan counties, Haenszel and Dawson showed that in the United States, increased risk for large bowel cancer is found in urban populations in each major region of the country.[366]

With respect to immigrants, colorectal cancer is less common among Japanese Americans than among white Americans.[871] However, the rates for Japanese Americans are higher than those for Japanese living in Japan. The children of these immigrants have an incidence approximating that of native white Americans.[367] A similar phenomenon has been seen in other populations.[889]

Race

Very little difference is found in the incidence of colorectal cancer between African-Americans and whites within each community and region of the country.[192,1053] However, the risk for large bowel cancer in American Indians is less than one half that in whites.[183,872] There is a higher death rate among African-American men and women, presumably because they are less likely to be diagnosed at a localized stage. Survival rates are actually lower for each stage of diagnosis, suggesting the possible influences of differences in receipt of care and the presence of comorbid conditions.[451]

SOCIOECONOMIC STATUS AND OCCUPATION

Some studies have shown a higher death rate for colorectal cancer in more affluent people.[163,697] Colombia, a country with a low incidence, reported a higher rate in this group.[365]

Occupation has been investigated as a possible causative factor.[632,697] The relative affluence associated with some occupations appears to be the reason why certain professionals have a higher incidence of colorectal cancer.

RELIGION

In studies of the religion of patients, Jews have a higher incidence than people of other religions.[361,362,682,843] Members of the Church of Jesus Christ of Latter-Day Saints (Mormons) have a low incidence.[115,251,564] Their religion prohibits the use of tobacco, alcohol, tea, and coffee. Seventh-Day Adventists have a significantly lower rate of colorectal cancer; their church proscribes tobacco and alcohol.[526,527,733]

ALCOHOL AND TOBACCO

A prospective study of Japanese men in Hawaii reveals an association between the consumption of alcohol and rectal cancer, attributable to a monthly consumption of beer of 500 oz (15 L) or more.[743]

Some studies have been published evaluating the association of tobacco and cancer.[142,224,375,407,462,835] In these studies, there appears to be no causative relationship between smoking and malignancy of the colon and rectum. A report from Quebec, Canada evaluated the effects of smoking on the risk of colorectal cancer according to anatomic subsite.[853] A positive association with cigar smoking and rectal cancer was observed. There was no statistically significant association with cigarette smoking, but these was a "positive association" with proximal colon cancer.

Diet

Diet is the epidemiologic area that has received the most attention since the mid-1980s 20 years, especially since Burkitt's observations.[117-121] He and Painter postulated that a high content of fiber was the primary factor responsible for the low incidence of colorectal cancer in African natives.[719] In essence, their theory states that whatever carcinogen is ingested or produced should be present in a relatively diluted form, and when the transit time is decreased, it is excreted rapidly. Fleiszer and colleagues and Chen and co-workers found that parenteral administration of dimethylhydrazine, a known colon carcinogen, conferred great protection on rats, provided their dietary fiber was increased.[151,271]

Other studies have demonstrated correlations between colorectal cancer and additional dietary factors. For example, Nigro (see Biography, Chapter 24) and colleagues demonstrated that cancer in the animal model can be inhibited by an increased fiber intake only when the fat content is relatively low.[687-689] They presented a program for possible prevention of colorectal cancer: a 10% reduction in fat consumption, the addition of 25 g of dietary fiber per day, and plant steroids.[687] These substances have been shown to inhibit the cancer that can be induced by carcinogens. One theory holds that inositol hexaphosphate (phytic acid), an abundant plant seed component present in many fiber-rich diets, is one of the specific agents responsible for suppression of colon carcinogenesis.[328]

The mechanism by which increased dietary fiber achieves protection from the development of large bowel cancer remains speculative. One of the theories is that because fiber is heterogeneous, its mechanism of action within the gut may vary. McIntyre and colleagues studied the effects of three types of dietary fiber in fermentative production of butyrate in the distal colon to ascertain the influence on tumor mass in a rat model of bowel cancer.[611] They observed that the fiber associated with high butyrate concentrations in the distal large bowel is protective against large bowel cancer, whereas soluble fibers that do not raise distal butyrate concentrations are not protective.

Sengupta and co-workers conducted a literature search on the effect of dietary fiber on tumor incidence through the use of the Medline database of all case-control, longitudinal, and randomized, controlled studies published in English between 1988 and 2000, as well as animal model studies in the period, 1986 to 2000.[847] Thirteen of 24 case-control studies demonstrated a protective effect of dietary fiber against colorectal neoplasms; conversely, only three of 13 longitudinal studies in various cohorts demonstrated a protective effect of fiber. The animal studies were more impressive; 15 of 19 demonstrated protection against tumor induction when compared with controls.

Fecal Bile Acids

Fecal bile acid concentration is increased by dietary fat and decreased by dietary cereal fiber. Others have shown an unambiguous connection between the fecal bile acid level and the incidence of dimethylhydrazine-induced colon cancer.[663] Hill and associates determined that the feces of people in Western countries exhibit a high concentration of bile acids when compared with the feces of residents of African and Eastern countries.[410]

Cholesterol

Some investigators have demonstrated a strong correlation between colorectal cancer and a high intake of animal fat and protein.[27,421,422] Others opine that the consumption of red meat, or total or saturated fat, has only a weak association with the development of colorectal cancer.[945] Populations with a high consumption of beef generally have the highest incidence of bowel cancer.[223,225] The

epidemiologic evidence is conflicting, but there seems to be an inconsistent relationship of colorectal cancer with respect to fat and sugar consumption, serum cholesterol, and serum β-lipoprotein.[105,584,681,952,1016] Winawer and colleagues performed a time-trend, case-control study in which serum cholesterol was determined at several intervals before the diagnosis of colon cancer.[1025] They concluded that although individuals in whom colorectal cancer developed had the same levels of serum cholesterol as the general population initially, during the 10 years before the diagnosis of cancer was established, they demonstrated a decline in cholesterol values. This took place in a population of "control" individuals whose serum cholesterol levels tended to increase with age.

Bacteria

Bacteria are thought to play a role in the causation of colorectal cancer; presumably, their action on ingested fat or metabolites is a critical factor. Hill and associates demonstrated that people in the United States and Great Britain have a higher colony count of anaerobic flora and a lower count of aerobic bacteria.[410] Others have confirmed this observation.[24] The similarity between the chemical structure of bile salts and the carcinogen, methylcholanthrene, has been observed. It is not unreasonable to hypothesize that the action of bacteria on bile salts may produce a substance capable of inducing malignant degeneration. Burkitt, in fact, postulated that one of the reasons for the preponderance of carcinoma in the distal bowel is the higher concentration of bacteria in this location.[118]

Cholecystectomy

Because of the clinical evidence for an increased quantity of secondary bile acids in the feces of patients with bowel cancer, and experimental studies demonstrating that secondary bile acids promote chemical carcinogenesis, cholecystectomy has been implicated as a possible precipitating factor.[961,979] This operation increases secondary bile acids in the enterohepatic circulation.[961] Other reports have failed to confirm a relationship between gallbladder removal and the subsequent development of colorectal cancer.[2,6,83,463] There is, however, some opposing evidence to suggest that more than 10 years following cholecystectomy, older women may have an increased risk, especially for right-sided lesions.[585,653] Johansen and co-workers evaluated 40,000 patients with gallstones identified in the Danish Hospital Discharge Register.[455] A borderline significant association was seen between gallstones and cancer of the colon. Jorgensen and Rafaelsen believe that cholecystectomy *per se* is not responsible for the apparent association, but rather that gallstone disease itself accounts for the relationship.[460]

Jejunoileal Bypass

With respect to jejunoileal bypass, an operation that in animals promotes the development of chemically induced bowel cancers, there has been no evidence to date to suggest an increased risk in humans,[610] despite profound alterations in transit time, bile salt metabolism, and fecal flora. In a long-term follow-up study (up to 17 years), Sylvan and associates examined these patients postoperatively by means of colonoscopy and biopsy as well as by flow cytometric DNA analysis.[918] These investigators were not able to verify any colorectal malignant transformation.

Ulcer Surgery

An association has been reported between colorectal cancer and prior peptic ulcer surgery, specifically truncal vagotomy.[664] Mullan and colleagues observed increased proportions of chenodeoxycholic acid and lithocholic acid as well as decreased proportions of cholic acid in the duodenal bile of these individuals.[664] They proposed that abnormalities in bile acid metabolism as a consequence of vagotomy could explain the increased risk for the development of colorectal cancer.

ASPIRIN

There is considerable evidence to suggest that regular use of aspirin and other nonsteroidal anti-inflammatory agents reduces the risk for the development of colorectal cancer.[925,945,946] Giovannucci and colleagues determined the rates of colorectal cancer among women in the Nurses' Health Study who reported regular aspirin use, comparing the rates in this group with those of women who stated that they did not use aspirin.[305] They concluded that the risk for colorectal cancer is reduced only after 10 or more years of aspirin use. Thun and co-workers found that dietary consumption of vegetables and grains and regular use of aspirin were the only factors having an independent and statistically significant association with prevention of colon cancer.[945]

Estrogen

Studies suggest that the use of estrogen reduces the risk of colorectal cancer. In a report by Paganini-Hill of 7,701 women who were initially free of cancer and used estro-

gen replacement therapy, there was a statistically significant reduction in the incidence of colorectal cancer and colorectal cancer deaths compared with those individuals who did not take this replacement medication.[718]

Inflammatory Bowel Disease

Patients with inflammatory bowel disease, especially ulcerative colitis, are at increased risk for the development of a malignancy; this risk is as high as 60% with 30 years of active, total-bowel disease (see Chapter 29).[565,630] With respect to Crohn's disease, some reports have been published implicating an association between regional enteritis and small bowel carcinoma.[533,659,808,857] The relationship between granulomatous colitis and large bowel cancer is less well documented but appears to be real (see Chapter 30).[1057]

Radiation

There have been considerable differences of opinion about the risk for development of colorectal cancer following pelvic irradiation. One report demonstrated an increased risk for women who were irradiated for gynecologic cancer.[819] Additional studies are required for an accurate assessment of any relationship, especially in light of the increased application of neoadjuvant therapy, but as of this writing there appears to be no clear evidence.

Immmunosuppression

Immunosuppressive therapy, especially following organ transplantation, is associated with an increased risk for the development of malignant tumors, including that of the colon and rectum. A surveillance colonoscopy program for these individuals is recommended.

Appendectomy

McVay reported an appreciably increased incidence of colorectal carcinoma in patients who had undergone appendectomy.[616] He suggested that the relationship could be explained by immunologic factors. Others have failed to substantiate this relationship.[347,423,431] However, a prior history of appendectomy has been found to be an independent risk factor for decreased survival, worsening the prognosis for those in whom carcinoma of the cecum subsequently developed.[26]

Ureterosigmoidostomy

Numerous authors have recognized the relationship between ureterosigmoidostomy and carcinoma of the colon at the site of the ureteral implant into the colon.[359,377,501,567,629,888,908,966,1006] The frequency of this complication may be several hundred times greater than that expected in the general population. The origin of this complication is not clearly understood. It may be related to bathing of the colonic mucosa by urine, the presence of a carcinogen in the urine, or the effects of the ureter itself implanted into the colon. It is suggested that this type of diversion of the urinary tract be abandoned, especially in young patients with benign disease.[852] Periodic endoscopic evaluation of the bowel is required. Consideration should be given to resecting that area of the colon, with conversion to another diversionary procedure.[252,491,888]

Congenital Urinary Tract Anomalies

Atwell and co-workers believed they had recognized an association between a family history of congenital anomalies of the urinary tract and the development of colorectal cancer.[36] Their observations should be taken with caution, because the numbers reported were small.

Extracolonic Tumors

With respect to the incidence and risk for the development of a metachronous colorectal cancer following an extracolonic primary tumor, one study demonstrates that a patient with breast cancer has the same risk for a colorectal malignancy as for a second primary tumor in the opposite breast.[11]

An association between sebaceous gland tumors and internal malignancies has been called the *Muir-Torre syndrome*. Approximately 120 cases have been reported. The incidence of colorectal malignancies is estimated to be almost 50%.[982] It is important to screen all individuals with sebaceous gland tumors for underlying gastrointestinal as well as genitourinary and breast malignancies.

Genetic Predisposition

Genetic influences have been known for some time to be an independent risk factor for the development of colorectal cancer. There was always the possibility, however, that this observation was a consequence of common environmental exposures, primary genetic factors, the interaction of environment and heredity, or simply of chance.[558] However, in a prospective study, Rozen and colleagues confirmed the relationship of the family history, even when one member harbors a large bowel neoplasm.[800] As a consequence, they and others have advocated a screening program for such family members.[673] Conversely, there is no evidence to suggest a greater frequency of bowel tumors in spouses of colorectal cancer victims. Fuchs and co-workers conducted a prospective

study of almost 120,000 patients who had not been previously examined by colonoscopy or sigmoidoscopy and who provided data on first-degree relatives with colorectal cancer.[285] The relative risk of cancer in persons with affected first-degree relatives, compared with persons without a family history, was 1.72 for one relation and 2.75 for two or more. This increased risk for disease was especially evident among younger individuals (5.37).

Rapid advances in the identification of genetic events that are important in colonic carcinogenesis have been made in the past few years.[13] Specifically inherited abnormalities, such as that for familial adenomatous polyposis, have been discussed in Chapter 21. Both acquired and genetic anomalies (*ras* gene point mutations; c-*myc* gene amplification; allelic deletion at specific sites on chromosomes 5, 17, and 18) seem to be capable of mediating steps in the progression from normal to malignant colonic mucosa (see Figure 21-36 and Chapter 21).[13] Chromosomal studies have succeeded in identifying a gene on chromosome 18q that is altered in colorectal cancers.[259] Allelic deletions have been found to occur in more than 70% of such tumors. These are thought to signal the existence of a tumor suppressor gene in the affected region.[259] Specifically, an abnormality of the *p53* tumor suppressor gene, the most commonly mutated gene in human cancer, is thought to be critical to the development of the majority of human tumors.[893] In essence, the presence of the gene through its product (the p53 protein) acts to induce cell-cycle arrest or apoptosis in response to DNA damage.[893]

Lynch Syndromes

Excluding the polyposis syndromes, carcinoma of the colon has been reported in cancer families, the so-called cancer family syndrome or hereditary nonpolyposis colorectal cancer (HNPCC).[546,553,555,556,744] This hereditary predisposition has been reported to account for 5% to 10% of all cases of colorectal cancer.[974] However, Kee and Collins suggest that the frequency is much less—1% to 2%.[469] In a prospective multicenter study from Finland, Mecklin and co-workers investigated family history and other risk factors during a 1-year period for all new patients in whom colorectal cancer was diagnosed.[621] Lynch and colleagues estimate that the risk for development of colorectal cancer is three times greater than that of the general population if one has a first-degree relative with this condition.[558] Familial colorectal cancer, however, requires the presence of the disease in two or more first-degree relatives. Itoh and colleagues noted a sevenfold increased risk for colon cancer.[438] Unfortunately, it has been shown that although family cancer history is commonly obtained during the initial surgical consultation of patients with colorectal cancer, there is a tendency to underestimate the extent and its implications.[804]

On the basis of early observations by Warthin,[992] Lynch and colleagues have defined two clinical variants: Lynch syndrome I or HNPCC and Lynch syndrome II or hereditary site-specific nonpolyposis colonic cancer HSSCC.[552]

Lynch syndrome I is characterized by the following features:

- Autosomal dominance
- Early age at onset
- Predominance of proximal bowel involvement
- Multiple primary colon tumors

Lynch syndrome II is characterized by the same features, but additionally shows an excess of other adenocarcinomas, particularly involving the endometrium and the ovary.[556,558,563] Others have added stomach, small bowel, and urinary tract cancers to the spectrum.[554,562,975] Itoh and co-workers noted that the risk for breast cancer was increased fivefold, and the lifetime risk was estimated at 1 in 3.7 for first-degree relatives of persons with Lynch syndrome II.[438] Even carcinoma of the larynx has been suggested to be associated.[557]

It is useful at this point to define three terms that have entered the literature in this field: Amsterdam Criteria, Bethesda Guidelines, and Microsatellite Instability.

Amsterdam Criteria

In 1991, the following clinical criteria (*Amsterdam Criteria*) were established to facilitate consistency in research and are often applied in diagnosing HNPCC:[975]

- Three or more cases of colorectal cancer in a minimum of two generations
- One affected individual a first-degree relative of the others with colorectal cancer
- One case of colorectal cancer diagnosed before age 50 years

- Exclusion of a diagnosis of familial adenomatous polyposis

The criteria have since been modified as follows:

- Two cases of colorectal cancer when families are small (one less than 55 years old)
- Two cases of colorectal cancer and one of endometrial cancer, or other early-onset cancer

Bethesda Guidelines

The Bethesda Guidelines were developed in 1997 from the results of a National Cancer Institute workshop on HNPCC.[788] These guidelines include all of the criteria described in Amsterdam I and Amsterdam II. Because it was believed that the Amsterdam criteria alone led to an underestimation of the true incidence of HNPCC, additional criteria were added. These include histopathologic (signet ring cell, poorly differentiated), morphologic (right-sided), and less selective clinical criteria. Additionally, the guidelines were proposed to assist in the selection of patients whose tumors should be analyzed for microsatellite instability.[1047]

Microsatellite Instability

Colorectal cancers demonstrate increased rates of intragenic mutation, characterized by generalized instability of short, tandemly repeated DNA sequences known as microsatellites.[349] A high frequency of microsatellite instability (defined as 40% or more of the microsatellite loci) has been found in most patients with HNPCC. This is because of the inactivation of mismatch repair function by the subsequent loss of the second allele that results in length variations of short sequences in HNPCC colorectal cancers.[1047] This alteration of dinucleotide repeats in microsatellite sequences, MSI or replication error, is used as a diagnostic criterion of mismatch repair deficiency.[700] Early-age-at-onset colorectal cancer has been demonstrated to be correlated with high-frequency microsatellite instability tumor status.[751] It

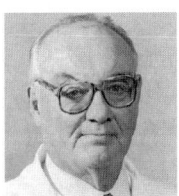

has also been shown to be a marker for predicting development of metachronous colorectal carcinoma after surgery.[865]

Specific findings of the patients in accordance with Lynch and co-workers were as follows: mean age at the initial colon cancer diagnosis was 44.6 years; of first colon cancers, 72.3% were located in the right side of the colon and only 25% were in the sigmoid and rectum; 18.1% of the patients had synchronous colon cancer, with a risk for metachronous lesions at 10 years of 40%.[558] Studies have shown the existence of a genetic defect with a population frequency of 19%, that is transmitted in a mendelian, dominant mode.[238] This defect may predispose the bowel epithelium to the effects of fecal carcinogens.

What clinical clues should lead a physician to suspect the diagnosis of HNPCC? The following have been determined:

- Early onset of carcinoma of the colon, especially in the proximal bowel (in the absence of multiple colonic polyps)
- Presence of multiple primary cancers (e.g., of the colon, endometrium, ovary)
- Having a first-degree relative with early-onset cancers integral to Lynch syndrome II[561]

It must be remembered, however, that in the experience of Mecklin and Järvinen, only 40% of patients had a positive family history at the time the tumor was diagnosed.[619] Some have suggested that the flat adenoma, a slightly raised lesion with adenomatous tubules concentrated near the luminal surface, or even a small, flat carcinoma, may represent markers for the syndrome (see Chapter 21).[92,429,507] When cancers do develop, the incidence of the mucinous type is high.[3,558,622] Svendsen and colleagues suggest that young individuals with metachronous colorectal cancer developing after a previous diagnosis of colorectal carcinoma could in fact have HNPCC.[915] The possibility of HNPCC should certainly be considered in adolescents in whom colorectal cancer is diagnosed.[575] Such consideration would inevitably lead the surgeon to make a recommendation concerning the nature of the operation. For example, some have suggested that because there is a high risk for the development of a metachronous colorectal cancer following a limited resection, a total colectomy may be indicated.[970] Others concur that close relatives of early-onset cases warrant more intensive colonoscopic screening at an earlier age than do relatives of patients in whom disease is diagnosed at an older age.[370,371]

Screening

The American Society of Colon and Rectal Surgeons established a Task Force that led to the publication of *Practice Parameters* for the identification and testing of patients at risk for dominantly inherited colorectal cancer. The following are the conclusions of that collaborate group:[884,885]

- Take a family history.
- Document a suspicious pedigree. Request medical records to confirm the diagnosis.
- Identify criteria for genetic testing (Amsterdam, Bethesda, microsatellite instability in tumors).
- Offer surveillance to families not meeting the above criteria for genetic testing.
- Adhere to all protocols for genetic testing, including Institutional Review Board, informed consent, and counseling.

Surveillance

Because the lifetime risk for the development of colorectal cancer approaches 80% in HNPCC, a surveillance program is recommended. In Lynch syndrome I, the surveillance approach is directed to the bowel exclusively. However, with Lynch syndrome II, one must also be aware of the increased risk for the development of extracolonic tumors. Annual colonoscopy is generally believed to be the preferred screening modality for bowel cancer in these individuals, although some believe that this is too frequent; evaluation of the stool for occult blood is unsatisfactory for this purpose.[419,506,558] Because of the increased risk for harboring benign and malignant tumors, colonoscopy is recommended for screening asymptomatic individuals with first-degree relatives having colon cancer, even in the absence of one of the Lynch syndromes.[353,905] Indeed, colonoscopy has superceded prophylactic surgery in those with the an inherited mutation.[515] Lynch and associates point out the potential for adverse medicolegal consequences because of failure to diagnose colorectal cancer.[560]

Green and colleagues performed colonoscopic screening on 61 asymptomatic individuals with an affected first-degree relative who had HNPCC.[336] Neoplasms were found in 15% and malignancies in 3%. Because of the high incidence of multiple lesions, consideration should be given to the performance of subtotal or total colectomy if surgery becomes necessary for colon cancer.[136] A regular, annual endoscopic follow-up of the residual rectum is still necessary, of course.[620] The risk for development of rectal cancer has been estimated to be 3% every 3 years after abdominal colectomy for the first 12 years.[789] There is no doubt that the familial cancer risk associated with early-onset disease outside of the recognized cancer predisposition syndromes is markedly increased.[456]

With respect to Lynch syndrome II patients, annual pelvic examinations are recommended beginning at age 25, including endometrial aspiration biopsy and ovarian ultrasonography.[558] Prophylactic hysterectomy with bilateral salpingo-oophorectomy should be considered in postmenopausal women and in those who have completed childbearing.[558]

Lynch and Lynch have made a plea for the establishment of computerized registries, such as have been developed for familial adenomatous polyposis, to transmit information about the diagnosis, surveillance, and management of hereditary colon cancer syndromes.[551,559] Recognizing high-risk families and individuals who would benefit from surveillance should help reduce the incidence of this common malignancy.[99]

In the Netherlands, families with HNPCC are monitored in an intensive surveillance program. Of the 35 cancers detected while patients were on the program, all but two were reported as identified at a local stage.[214]

Genetic Testing and Counseling

It is known that HNPCC is caused by germ-line mutations in one of four DNA mismatch repair (MMR) genes, *hMSH2*, *hMLH1*, *hPMS1*, or *hPMS2* (see also Chapter 21). It is estimated that defects in two of the known MMR genes, *hMSH2* and *hMLH1*, account for 90% of mutations found in HNPCC families.[62,753] Although many mutations in these genes have been found in HNPCC kindreds, thereby complying with the so-called Amsterdam criteria, little is known about the involvement of these genes in families not satisfying these criteria but showing clear-cut familial clustering of colorectal cancer and other cancers.[1011] Wijnen and colleagues found *hMSH2* and *hMLH1* mutations in 49% of the kindreds that fully complied with the Amsterdam criteria, whereas a disease-causing mutation could be identified in only 8% of the families in which the criteria were not satisfied fully.[1011] These results imply that there are significant consequences to genetic testing and counseling in the management of colorectal cancer families.

Once the diagnosis has been established, the importance of genetic counseling has been strongly emphasized by Lynch and colleagues and by others.[562,901] It is recommended that all families with suggestive pedigrees should be referred to a geneticist for genetic testing. If the test result is negative for carrying the gene, the family member's cancer risk drops to that of the general population.[625] Conversely, the lifetime cancer risk for a gene carrier is approximately 90%. However, individuals need to know the implications and consequences of genetic test results before acquiescing to the testing.[1042]

Commercial testing is available in the United States through OncorMed.* The company has produced a protocol for testing. People who meet the following inclusion criteria should be tested:

- A person with colorectal cancer who has three relatives with colorectal cancer (at least one being a first-degree relative to the other two)
- A person with colorectal cancer who has two or more first- or second-degree blood relatives with colorectal cancer
- A person with colorectal cancer with onset before 30 years of age
- A person with colorectal cancer with onset between 30 and 50 years who has at least one other first- or second-degree relative with colorectal cancer
- A person with colorectal cancer with multiple colon primary tumors
- A person with colorectal cancer and another related primary cancer
- A relative of an individual with a documented *MSH2* or *MLH1* mutation

The following people should not be tested:

- A person less than 18 years old
- A person with a known diagnosis of ulcerative colitis for 7 or more years, familial adenomatous polyposis/Gardner's syndrome, hereditary flat adenoma syndrome, Peutz-Jeghers syndrome, familial juvenile polyposis syndrome, or hereditary discrete polyp-carcinoma syndrome
- A cognitively impaired person or one unable to provide informed consent
- Someone who has a psychological condition precluding testing

Treatment

The Standards Task Force of the American Society of Colon and Rectal Surgeons established Practice Parameters for the treatment of patients with dominantly inherited colorectal cancer (HNPCC).[886] The following guidelines have been published:

- Treatment must be preceded by thorough counseling about the nature of the syndrome, its natural history, its extracolonic manifestations, and the need for compliance with all recommendations for management and surveillance.
- When patients with HNPCC as defined by genotype or compliance with Amsterdam I criteria are diagnosed with more than one advanced adenoma or a colon cancer, they should be offered the options of prophylactic total colectomy and ileorectal anastomosis or hemicolectomy plus yearly colonoscopy.

---

*OncorMed, 205 Perry Parkway, Gaithersburg, MD 208777; 301–208–1888.

- Patients with HNPCC who have *rectal cancer* should be offered the options of total proctocolectomy and ileo-pouch–anal anastomosis or anterior proctosigmoidectomy, assuming that the sphincters can be saved.
- Female patients with HNPCC and uterine cancer in their families may be offered prophylactic hysterectomy once childbearing is complete or when they undergo surgery for other intraabdominal conditions.

AGE AND GENDER

The incidence of carcinoma of the colon and rectum increases with age, but the progression also varies by anatomic site, population, and sex. In our experience, the mean age at diagnosis for men was 63 years, and for women, 62 years.[178] Cook and associates computed the slopes of the logarithm of the incidence against the logarithm of the age from a number of cancer registries and demonstrated that the slopes of the curves for colon and rectal cancer for men were consistently higher than the slopes of curves for women in almost every population.[171] They noted, furthermore, that this variation in male-female difference was greater for colon than for rectal carcinoma.

In women, colorectal cancer ranks third in the United States in number of cancer deaths, 10%. Lung (25%) and breast (17%) are first and second, respectively. The 2003 estimated cancer incidence is third, after breast and lung (30%, 13%, and 11%, respectively).

In men, colorectal cancer (9%) ranks third, after lung (32%) and prostate (14%), for deaths. Prostate cancer is now the single most common cancer (43%); lung is second (13%), and colorectal, third (8%). Men have a preponderance of rectal cancer and a slight excess of cancer of the descending and transverse colon. The incidence of cancer of the ascending colon and cecum is essentially the same for both sexes according to one report,[141] but according to another, women were found to have more right-sided tumors.[907]

SYMPTOMS AND SIGNS

Change in Bowel Habits

Change in bowel habits is the most frequent complaint of patients with colorectal cancer. The change may be as insignificant as that from a bowel movement every other day to one daily. All too often, people place little emphasis on this observation until a profound alteration occurs. Generally, a more distal lesion creates more obvious symptoms than a proximal one. The reasons for this are threefold: first, it is more "difficult" for formed stool in the distal colon to pass through an area of narrowing than for the relatively liquid stool present in the proximal bowel; second, the lumen of the bowel itself is larger proximally than distally; and third, because of the presence of other symptoms (bleeding, pain, discharge), the patient is more likely to pay attention when a distal tumor produces a change in bowel habits.

Bleeding

Bleeding is the second most common symptom of colorectal cancer. It may be overt or occult. The blood may be bright red, purple, mahogany, black, or inapparent. The more distal the location of the lesion, the less altered the blood will be, and the redder it will appear. Although bleeding can represent a relatively early sign of cancer of the bowel, it is often a neglected symptom. Helfand and colleagues performed a prospective cohort study of 201 individuals who mentioned rectal bleeding as part of their review of systems evaluation and then determined whether such a complaint merits investigation for significant pathology.[399] They identified 24% with "serious disease," including benign and malignant neoplasms and inflammatory bowel disease. The authors concluded that physicians should ask all adults about visible rectal bleeding and should visualize the entire colon in those who manifest such symptoms. Individuals frequently attribute bleeding to hemorrhoids, particularly if they have had prior difficulty with hemorrhoids. For this reason, it is important to treat bleeding hemorrhoids, so that the presence of this symptom succeeds in alerting the patient to seek medical attention.

Conversely, the physician may mistakenly attribute the bleeding to hemorrhoids. Nothing is more tragic than the misdiagnosis of a potentially curable cancer because of inadequate examination or investigation. Too often, patients are managed with suppositories, creams, and laxatives, and only when symptoms become severe enough is proper investigation undertaken.

Mucus

The presence of mucus, either as a discharge (implying a distal lesion) or mixed with the stool, is another symptom; it often accompanies bleeding. The presence of mucus and bleeding should be considered a highly suggestive combination that necessitates bowel investigation.

Pain

Rectal pain is an unlikely presenting symptom of cancer. The most common reasons for anorectal pain are thrombosed hemorrhoids, anal fissure, abscess, and proctalgia fugax. When rectal cancer produces pain, the lesion usually is very distal or very large. Pain may result from infiltration of the sensitive anal canal or from sphincteric invasion. Such invasion may produce tenesmus, a painful urgency to defecate.

Abdominal pain resulting from tumor implies an obstructing or partially obstructing lesion. This pain is usually colicky in nature and may be associated with abdominal distension, nausea, or vomiting. Intestinal obstruction is a presenting complaint in 5% to 15% of individuals with colorectal cancer. Back pain from retroperitoneal extension of a tumor of the ascending or descending colon is an unusual and late sign.

Mass

A palpable or visible abdominal mass in the absence of other signs and symptoms implies a slow-growing, infiltrative process that may be much more amenable to surgical extirpation than might otherwise be anticipated. Such tumors often metastasize quite late in the course of disease.

Weight Loss

Weight loss, in the absence of other symptoms, is a poor prognostic sign. Inanition and loss of strength and appetite suggest metastatic disease, most commonly to the liver. Presentation with symptoms of metastatic disease occurs in approximately 5% of patients with colorectal cancer. Hepatomegaly is a frequent observation, but pulmonary, cerebral, and osseous metastases as isolated findings may reveal an occult colorectal primary on investigation.

Peritonitis

Perforation with peritonitis is an unusual presentation today (except in certain hospitals that serve an indigent population). Differentiating carcinoma from perforated diverticulitis, particularly with a sigmoid lesion, may be extremely difficult (see Surgical Treatment).

"Appendicitis"

Rarely, carcinoma of the cecum can obstruct the lumen of the appendix and cause signs and symptoms of acute appendicitis.[690] An even more uncommon phenomenon is perforation of the appendix from obstructing carcinoma of the more distal bowel.[914] The development of a fecal fistula after appendectomy should lead the physician to suspect an underlying malignancy. Although such presentations are uncommon, any individual more than 50 years old with a presentation of acute appendicitis

should be evaluated carefully at the time of surgery for underlying carcinoma.

Inguinal Hernia

It has been thought that inguinal hernia in older men is associated with colorectal carcinoma, especially if the hernia is of relatively short duration.[198,601,750,938] Because of this observation, some have advised routine barium enema examination for all patients before herniorrhaphy. However, Brendel and Kirsh reported no such association.[101] I have not been impressed with the yield of such screening studies and do not advocate routine barium enema examination or colonoscopy in patients before performing inguinal herniorrhaphy. The high incidence of colorectal neoplasms in the general population suggests that the theoretical relationship is more likely to be coincidental. That said, it is known that carcinoma of the colon can present, albeit rarely, as an incarcerated hernia.[417] It is therefore prudent to perform colonoscopic examination before hernia repair in patients experiencing a change in bowel habits or other symptoms suggestive of underlying bowel pathology.

Septicemia

Septicemia from *Streptococcus bovis* is associated with gastrointestinal neoplasms, especially colonic neoplasms.[68] Kline and colleagues prospectively studied individuals with sepsis caused by this organism.[486] Eight of 15 who completed gastrointestinal evaluation, including colonoscopy, were found to harbor colon carcinoma. The differential diagnosis of a fever of unknown origin includes colorectal cancer and demands appropriate evaluation.[613] Additionally, fevers of undetermined origin in individuals with known colorectal carcinoma should lead one to investigate the possibility of bacterial endocarditis.[795] Secondary infections of hepatic metastases in an individual with a known primary tumor of the colon are well recognized. However, it is much less appreciated that colonic cancer can be an underlying cause of pyogenic liver abscesses in the absence of metastases. After the usual causes have been excluded, an asymptomatic colon cancer should be considered in the differential diagnosis.[931] The presence of an organism normally found in the colon should heighten the clinician's suspicion.

Cutaneous Manifestations

Nonmetastatic cutaneous presentations of colorectal cancer have been reviewed by Rosato and associates.[793] They noted a number of conditions associated with gastrointestinal malignancy, including acanthosis nigricans, dermatomyositis, pemphigoid, and others (see Chapter 19). Such manifestations are rare, but any disseminated skin condition that is unresponsive to conventional therapy should encourage the physician to consider gastrointestinal investigation.

Cutaneous metastases from colorectal carcinoma are extremely unusual except, of course, in the incision or port site (see later). Even rarer is the individual who presents with skin lesions as the initial complaint.[197] Certainly, the incidence must be less than 1%. Biopsy will usually clarify any confusion as to the diagnosis.

Intussusception

Intussusception in the adult is always a condition that requires surgical treatment. This is in contradistinction to children, for whom medical management (e.g., reduction by barium enema) may result in cure. Patients usually present with signs and symptoms of intestinal obstruction.

Nagorney and associates reviewed the Mayo Clinic experience with 144 cases of adult intussusception treated at that institution since 1910.[670] Almost 9 in 10 were associated with a definitive pathologic process: malignant neoplasm, benign tumor, metastatic lesion, or Meckel's diverticulum (see Figs. 22-84 and 22-87 later). Two thirds of the colonic intussusceptions were associated with primary carcinoma of the colon, whereas only one third of the intussusceptions of the small intestine were associated with an underlying cancer; most of those malignancies were metastatic. Others have also recognized the association between colonic intussusception and the presence of underlying tumors in the adult.[103,261,679,818,1003] The importance of resection without reduction is discussed later.

Duration of Symptoms

Unfortunately, one continues to be impressed by the long history of symptoms reported by many patients who come to surgery for colorectal cancer. Symptoms were present for longer than 6 months in one third of our patients. Some had sought help earlier, but lack of suspicion of carcinoma or inadequate examination at the time of evaluation delayed operative intervention. However, those with a short history of symptoms do not have a better prognosis. Individuals with symptoms of less than 5 months' duration have a higher incidence of resection for cure, but the actual long-term survival has not been shown to be improved.[435,827]

Delay in Diagnosis: Legal Implication

A question asked by attorneys in medicolegal actions is when an earlier diagnosis will make a difference with respect to prognosis (see Chapter 34). Clearly, the issue of tumor doubling time does not provide the answer. In an unofficial poll of the Chicago Society of Colon and Rectal Surgeons (1997), all but two of the more than 50 surgeons who were in attendance responded, "6 months." I believe that this is an appropriate time frame for one honestly to be able to accept.

EVALUATION

Practice Parameters for the Detection of Colorectal Neoplasms

Colorectal cancer screening is relatively inexpensive compared with screening for breast and cervical cancer, with cost estimates suggesting that the amount necessary to prevent one cancer is essentially equivalent to that required to treat a symptomatic patient.[390] Although the most cost-effective approach has yet to be identified, screening can decrease mortality by making possible the identification of tumors at an earlier stage and the removal of benign lesions before they become malignant, thus preventing the subsequent development of cancer.[951] Several protocols have been established by a number of organizations for the detection of colorectal neoplasms at the earliest possible stage.

Clinical guidelines and a rationale for colorectal screening have been endorsed by the American Cancer Society, the American College of Gastroenterology, the American Gastroenterological Association, the American Society of Colon and Rectal Surgeons, the American Society for Gastrointestinal Endoscopy, the Crohn's and Colitis Foundation of America, the Oncology Nursing Society, and the Society of American Gastrointestinal Endoscopic Surgeons (SAGES). These have been published in a 1997 report that appeared in the journal *Gastroenterology*.[1026] The following general guidelines have been proposed:

- People with symptoms that suggest the presence of colorectal cancer or polyps should have appropriate diagnostic evaluation; they are not candidates for screening.
- Personal and familial risk factors need to be evaluated when screening is being considered.
- Screening for colorectal cancer and adenomatous polyps should be offered to all men and women without risk factors beginning at age 50.
- Physicians should recommend a diagnostic evaluation of the colon to follow up a positive result of a screening test.
- Follow-up surveillance should be considered after treatment of colorectal cancer or removal of adenomatous polyps or in the presence of underlying premalignant conditions such as inflammatory bowel disease.

- Health care providers who perform the tests should have appropriate proficiency, and the tests should be performed correctly.
- Screening should be accompanied by efforts to optimize the participation of both patients and health care providers in screening tests and appropriate diagnostic follow-up.
- People who are candidates for screening should be given adequate information on the risks and benefits of the various screening procedures.

In 1992, the American Society of Colon and Rectal Surgeons published guidelines for the detection of colorectal neoplasms.[882,883] These guidelines are reproduced in Table 22-1.

Determination of Occult Blood

The stool guaiac or orthotoluidine test has been the subject of a number of reports (see Chapter 4). Gregor studied patients with known asymptomatic colorectal cancers and found the presence of blood in at least one of three stool specimens.[335] Because of the relatively high false-positive rate, he recommended a special diet that succeeded in reducing this rate to approximately 1%. The diet is free of meat, fish, and chicken and is relatively high in roughage (fiber) to stimulate bleeding from an existing lesion. Norfleet's study, however, failed to demonstrate any benefit with respect to sensitivity or specificity from this diet.[692] Ostrow and associates studied healthy volunteers and found that the test slide preparation gave consistently positive results after the administration of 25 mL of blood and usually gave positive results with only 10 mL.[712]

A study from the United Kingdom by Tate and colleagues compared three fecal occult tests—Hemoccult, Fecatwin, and E-Z Detect—to determine which is best suited for use in asymptomatic patients.[929] The test most sensitive for blood was Fecatwin; it found 93% of cancers and 69% of other mucosal diseases, but the incidence of false-positive results was three times that of Hemoccult. Home testing methods have thus far demonstrated no advantage through increased compliance to outweigh the lower sensitivity.[752]

In Gilbertsen's study, guaiac testing revealed that cancer was responsible for positive test results in 5.1% of patients, and benign tumors in 24%, with no evidence of gastrointestinal neoplasms in 68%.[302] A later report from this center evaluated 48,000 asymptomatic patients during a period of approximately 4 years.[691] Invasive carcinoma was found in 113; more than one half of the tumors had not breached the seromuscular surface of the bowel wall. Hardcastle and Pye believe that the predictive value of a positive test result for invasive cancer is 11% to 17%,

and for adenomas, 36% to 41%.[379] In another report, from the Minnesota Colon Cancer Control study, annual fecal occult blood testing with rehydration of the samples decreased the 13-year cumulative mortality from colorectal cancer by 33%.[583]

In a prospective randomized trial, Kewenter and coworkers investigated a number of new colorectal neoplasms that developed during the first 7 years after the end of a rescreening program by means of occult blood determination.[476] One hundred one carcinomas were diagnosed in the screened group and 128 in the control group during the follow-up period. The results indicated that screening and rescreening of a population had little influence on the stage of the cancers in the test group compared with controls during this 7-year period.

Robinson and colleagues reported the use of an immunologic fecal occult blood test called Hemeselect, comparing this with standard guaiac testing in almost 1,500 patients who completed both evaluations.[784] Hemeselect had a much higher positive predictive value for cancer and adenomas than did Hemoccult.

Evaluation of a patient with a positive occult blood determination can be expensive, but other pathologic entities that may be of significance are worth identifying.[244] Although the cost versus the benefit of a massive screening program is debatable, no one doubts the value of early diagnosis, especially before a malignancy supervenes.[18,302,477,574,582,1023,1028] Scudamore showed that when a patient has no gastrointestinal symptoms, a 100% possibility of curative resection can be expected, with an 88% 5-year survival.[839] Mapp and co-workers found that screening by means of occult blood determination improved survival in a randomized, controlled study.[586] Others challenge the concept of unsupervised mass screening from the point of view of cost-effectiveness, but because of voluntary services and supplies, such projects are probably useful in educating the public about colon and rectal cancer and the value of early detection.[144,479] Lieberman suggests that screening with fecal occult blood testing and sigmoidoscopy, as recommended by the American Cancer Society, may not be as cost-effective as screening with colonoscopy.[531] The guidelines previously mentioned, as published under the auspices of multiple societies, recommend fecal occult blood test screening on an annual basis.[1026] Testing of two samples from each of three consecutive stools for the presence of occult blood, followed by colonoscopy, has been demonstrated to reduce the risk of death from colorectal cancer. Average-risk people with an abnormal screening test result by fecal occult blood testing (i.e., a trace-positive or positive test result from any sample) require an accurate examination of the entire colon and rectum, ideally by colonoscopy.[1026] The other option would be to perform a double-contrast barium enema, preferably with flexible sigmoidoscopy (see later

▶ **TABLE 22-1 Screening Guidelines***

Risk	*Procedure*	*Onset*	*Frequency*
I. Asymptomatic low risk	Digital and fecal occult blood Sigmoidoscopy	Age 40 Age 50	Yearly 3–5 years
II. Asymptomatic high risk	Fecal occult blood Colonoscopy or barium enema and sigmoidoscopy	Age 35 Age 40	Yearly 3–5 years
III. Familial adenomatous polyposis	Sigmoidoscopy	Age 10	Yearly until age 40; then follow asymptomatic high-risk guidelines
IV. A. Ulcerative colitis (pancolitis)	Colonoscopy	Disease years 7 and 8	Every 2 years until 20 years of disease; then annually
B. Ulcerative left-sided colitis (or Crohn's colitis)	Colonoscopy	Disease year 15	Every 2 years
V. Symptomatic patient	Barium enema or colonoscopy (preferred if bleeding, occult blood, or melena)	—	—
VI. A. Polyp surveillance (adenoma)	Colonoscopy	—	Yearly until colon cleared; then every 3–5 years
B. Hyperplasia	Colonoscopy	—	Repeat colonoscopy in 1 year; then revert to asymptomatic low-risk guidelines if colon cleared
VII. Colon cancer surveillance after resection A. If colonoscopy or barium enema cleared colon preoperatively	Colonoscopy or barium enema	—	One year postoperatively; then every 3 years until colon is cleared
B. If colon not cleared preoperatively by barium enema or colonoscopy	Colonoscopy or barium enema	—	Within 6 months; then every 3 years if colon cleared

*Refer to Practice Parameters for the Detection of Colorectal Neoplasms—Supporting Documentation (*Dis Colon Rectum* 1992;35:391–393).

and Chapter 4). Newer approaches to screening and additional data are also discussed in Chapter 4.

Digital Rectal Examination

William J. Mayo remarked, "The physician often hesitates to make the necessary examination because it involves soiling the finger."[603] Or, simply stated, if you do not put your finger in, you'll put your foot in. The index finger has also been termed "God's bioprobe." However, the efficacy of digital examination today for identifying cancer of the rectum is less compelling than previously thought. Only 10% of colorectal cancers are potentially within reach of the examiner's finger. Even when the cancer is palpable, the physician may not be sufficiently cautious and diligent to permit discovery of a lesion. The risks of the examination, however, are nonexistent, and no one can argue the cost versus the benefit.

Digital examination will identify the location of the tumor, anterior or posterior, and whether it occupies part or the whole of the circumference. The tumor may be fixed or movable, ulcerated or scirrhous, exophytic or invasive. Careful palpation of the presacral space may reveal hard lymph nodes suggestive of tumor metastases; this may be a valuable prognostic sign. The fact that the tumor is palpable will often suggest the type of operation possible or whether the lesion is indeed resectable. Fixity may indicate a need for supplemental treatment, such as neoadjuvant therapy. Therefore, despite the numerous, often esoteric studies available to evaluate today's patient, digital examination of the rectum is still a very important adjunct.

Proctosigmoidoscopy

The rigid sigmoidoscope is one of the most valuable diagnostic tools used (see also Chapter 4). Examination with this instrument may reveal mucosal excrescences, polyps, polypoid lesions, cancer, inflammatory changes, strictures, vascular malformation, and anatomic distortion from extraluminal masses. It may also detect numerous anal conditions, such as fistulas, hemorrhoids, fissures, and abscesses. When the instrument is passed to its full length of 25 cm, almost two thirds of all cancers of the colon and rectum may be identified. Unfortunately, with the rigid instrument, insertion to its full length is possible in only about 50% of patients, the average penetration being approximately 20 cm.

Many investigators have advocated routine proctosigmoidoscopy for early diagnosis,[132,160,301,406,454,746,851,916] but others have questioned the need for this procedure on an annual basis.[230,231,648] The American Cancer Society encourages physicians to search for colorectal cancer before the onset of symptoms. Optimally, an annual proctosigmoidoscopic examination for all patients 40 years of age and older would be recommended. However, with more than 90 million such persons in the United States, this is indeed an awesome task. It was estimated in 1980 that annual sigmoidoscopic examination on all people more han 40 years old in the United States would cost approximately $2.75 billion.[244] We studied 2,500 consecutive asymptomatic patients with the rigid sigmoidoscope as part of a general examination. Excluded from the study were symptomatic patients and those with a prior history of colorectal disorders. The proctoscope was inserted to a mean length of 20 cm. Adenocarcinoma was found in eight patients, and in two of these, carcinoma developed in polypoid adenomas. A total of 432 benign polypoid lesions were found in 228 patients (9.1%).[173]

In this study, all lesions found in patients less than 50 years old were benign; no cancers were detected before the sixth decade of life. This is not surprising, because only 5% of colorectal cancers occur in patients less than 45 years old.[40] Although bowel cancer can develop in a person at any age, because of the limitations of time, space, and personnel, we suggested that routine proctosigmoidoscopic examination be performed in those age groups most likely to benefit from the procedure: patients 50 years old and older. If this criterion were met, 30% fewer examinations would need to be performed.

Selby and colleagues provided the strongest possible evidence of the value of screening rigid sigmoidoscopy.[845] In a case-control study, they determined that individuals who had undergone one or more screening sigmoidoscopic examinations in the preceding 10 years had a 60% to 70% reduction in the risk of death from rectal or distal colon cancer in comparison with those who had not undergone such an examination. Furthermore, their finding that the risk for death from these cancers was markedly reduced for 10 years *following* a single examination is of considerable interest.[529] The authors concluded that screening once every 10 years may be nearly as efficacious as more frequent examinations.[845]

The flexible sigmoidoscope has, in recent years, virtually replaced the rigid instrument for screening purposes (see later and Chapter 5). Although no one can argue against the value of screening a greater colonic surface, it is a sad commentary that many surgical residents coming out of training programs today do not know how to use the rigid instrument. There is no question that the rigid instrument is far superior to the flexible one for determining the level of the lesion when a cancer is identified in the rectum or rectosigmoid. It is also generally superior for evaluating the state of the anastomosis as part of a follow-up protocol or when the patient experiences symptoms following resective surgery.

Biopsy

Obviously when a patient has symptoms, a proctosigmoidoscopic examination, at least, is mandatory. When a tumor is identified, a biopsy of the lesion should be performed. This is usually a simple office procedure requiring no anesthetic and the very minimum of special tools. For polypoid, exophytic lesions, appreciable bleeding is rarely a concern after a biopsy. If electrocoagulation equipment is not readily available and bleeding is encountered, pressure with a long, cotton-tip applicator soaked in a topical solution of adrenaline will usually suffice.

The sample for biopsy should be taken from the edge of the lesion at the junction of the tumor and the normal-appearing bowel, and placed in a fixative solution. Notation should be made of the distance from the anal verge to the lower level of the lesion. The size, macroscopic appearance (ulcerated or polypoid), and location should also be recorded.

Flexible Sigmoidoscopy, Video-endoscopy, and Colonoscopy

The flexible sigmoidoscope has been recommended as the preferred initial screening tool for colorectal cancer (see also Chapter 5).[976,951,1029] Its primary advantage is that it allows more proximal evaluation of the bowel. It remains to be seen whether the relatively high cost of the instrument and the time spent in examination are justified by the increased yield. It must be remembered, however, that the rectum is evaluated better by the rigid sigmoidoscope than by the flexible instrument.

The examiner must be wary of performing such procedures as biopsy-cautery and snare excision with the flexible instrument in an inadequately prepared colon. With the limited cleansing regimen commonly employed for this instrument examination, there is a serious risk for explosion when electrical equipment is used for tumor biopsy or removal.

The place of colonoscopy as a screening tool in the asymptomatic, low-risk population has been somewhat controversial. Lieberman and co-workers reported the Veterans Cooperative Study Group experience with 3,197 patients who had been enrolled.[532] In this group of almost exclusively men, colonoscopic examination demonstrated one or more neoplasms in 37.5% of the patients. As a consequence of this and other studies, the United States government insurance program, Medicare, will pay for colonoscopy as a screening test every decade beginning at age 50. Furthermore, colonoscopic screening for neoplasms in asymptomatic first-degree relatives of patients with colon cancer is strongly recommended.[352,617,716] The aforementioned multiorganizational cancer screening guideline protocol recommends that close relatives (e.g., siblings, parents, and children) of a person who has had colorectal cancer or an adenomatous polyp should be offered the same options as average-risk people, but beginning at the age of 40 years.[1026] If colorectal cancer has been diagnosed in the close relative before the age of 55 years, or an adenomatous polyp before the age of 60, special effort should be made to ensure that screening takes place. Interestingly, transplant patients have the same risk for the development of colorectal neoplasms as the general population.[722] In the absence of risk factors, consideration should be given to offering a colonoscopy every 10 years.

Colonoscopy has been of demonstrable value for the patient with a known neoplasm by identifying a synchronous tumor (Figure 22-1). Barium enema, of course, serves the same purpose, although usually not as effec-

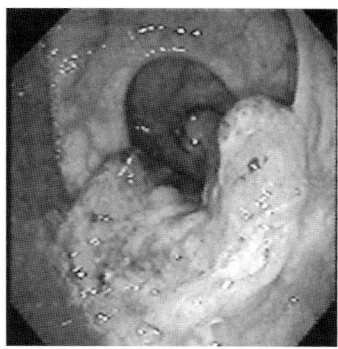

FIGURE 22-1. Colonscopic examination reveals an ulcerating tumor of the sigmoid colon. The tumor encompasses approximately one third of the bowel circumference. There is a small polyp proximal to the tumor that should emphasize the importance of total colonoscopic evaluation. (See Color Fig. 22-1.)

tively. Herbst and associates, in a retrospective study of 55 patients, found that nine (16%) harbored another lesion.[402] This discovery caused the operation to be modified. In the report of Reilly and associates, 7.6% of 92 patients had a synchronous cancer.[775] All were missed on barium enema examination, and none was more invasive than the index lesion. Other studies have demonstrated that 2% to 8% of patients will have a synchronous carcinoma elsewhere in the colon.[437,504,714,717,775,944,998] When polyps are present, the risk is even higher. Conversely, perhaps as many as 50% of patients with colon cancer harbor one or more colon polyps.[714]

Because many symptomatic patients undergo proctosigmoidoscopy and barium enema sequentially, Winawer suggests that the colonoscope be used if small to moderate tumors are present, because the instrument can usually slip past the lesion.[1024] He believes that the procedure is more valuable in evaluating patients with known right-sided tumors of the colon. The yield is higher, and the distal bowel can be more easily examined. These studies confirm what has long been suspected: often, the metachronous tumor actually represents the missed synchronous one.

Gilbertsen and co-workers believe that barium enema examination is not sufficiently reliable in evaluating patients for suspected colorectal cancer and have abandoned the routine use of this modality in favor of colonoscopy for patients in whom a colorectal lesion is suspected.[303] They hold that barium enema examination often need not be performed if colonoscopy is diagnostic. Others have recommended the technique as a valuable screening tool for those who are at an increased risk for development of colon cancer (e.g., with a positive family history).[350,545] Most concur, however, that the detection rate of colon cancer is about the same with both studies, provided that they are competently performed and bowel preparation is adequate. Colonoscopy, though, is believed to be superior to barium enema in detecting rectal carcinoma.[772] One must remember that even colonoscopy is imperfect. Byrd and colleagues noted a 97% correlation with the resected specimen, but in 3%, lesions were missed.[126] Blind areas in the colon plus misjudgment that the instrument had been inserted to the perceived level were responsible for the majority of colonoscopic errors. Recognizing the limits of this procedure, colonoscopy should be the initial examination that is performed on anyone who presents with signs and symptoms suggestive of a large bowel problem.[870]

Complete visualization of the colon must be accomplished within a reasonable time following identification of a bowel neoplasm. Optimally, this should be performed preoperatively, because it may alter the type of operation.[420] Many patients are submitted to this investigation the day before or the day of colon resection in order to obviate the need for a second bowel preparation. Preoperative barium enema is utilized only when the size of the lesion precludes passage of the instrument. If total colonoscopy is not undertaken before surgery, it should be carried out by the sixth postoperative week.

Comment and Opinion

From the economic and manpower perspective frequent *colonoscopy* as a screening test cannot be justified in an asymptomatic individual who is not in a high-risk group. The procedure often requires sedation and is not without complication (e.g., a perforation rate of 0.1% to 0.5%). In any event, the reality is that there are insufficient resources for performing total colonoscopy on everyone more than 50 years old, even if this were accomplished every 5 years. The real question is how much is a human life worth, or putting it in another way, how much "good medicine" can one afford! Of course, the bureaucratic low-dull-normals who regulate the health care industry in the United States and make these decisions for us all are often the same cretinous flotsam who implement such critically important reconstruction such as earthquake retrofitting of bridges without regard to cost and to benefit (see later, equally opinionated comments on follow-up evaluation).

Cytology

Establishing the diagnosis of carcinoma of the colon by means of cytologic evaluation, washing out the colon with saline solution, has been advocated by some authors (see Chapter 4).[152,757] Winawer and colleagues performed brush cytology and lavage on selected patients with colonic neoplasms.[1027] They and others believe that brush cytology improves the yield of tissue diagnosis when combined with biopsy, but lavage cytology alone does not

seem to be as useful.[661,1027] Chen suggests that cell brushings may be of particular value when colonic stricture and obstruction prevent the colonoscope from reaching the lesion for biopsy.[152]

Although I have had only limited experience with this technique, the addition of brushing or lavage appears relatively academic. If the nature of the lesion can be identified with an accuracy rate of only 90%, exploratory laparotomy and segmental resection are advisable. I believe this technique should be relegated to that of a historical curiosity.

Stool DNA

Because of the utility of identification of mutations in oncogenes and tumor-suppressor genes, it has been suggested that this observation may have a demonstrable advantage over such indirect studies of the stool, such as occult blood determination.[12,528,956] Some studies have been reported which utilize purified DNA from stool samples in individuals known to harbor colorectal cancer and have detected these mutations.[496,956] Additional work is needed to determine the specificity of these genetic tests in asymptomatic patients and to define more precisely the prevalence of the mutations and the sensitivity of the assay.[228] A commercially available, stool-based, DNA colorectal cancer screening test, Pre-Gen, can be obtained in the United States through EXACT Sciences (*www.exactsciences.com*).

Barium Enema: Air-Contrast Enema Examination

There are no studies evaluating whether screening double-contrast (air-contrast) barium enema alone reduces the incidence or mortality of colorectal cancer in individuals who are at average risk for development of the disease.[1026] The previously mentioned cooperative recommendation on colorectal cancer screening suggests that an individual be offered this radiologic study every 5 to 10 years.

The barium enema has traditionally been the most commonly employed investigative study for evaluation of carcinoma of the large bowel, but for screening and preoperative assessment it has essentially been replaced by colonoscopy. Most people believe that despite meticulous double-contrast technique, the examination cannot be performed with the accuracy of colonoscopy (see Chapter 4). Even the most careful and competent of radiologists can overlook a colon carcinoma through failure to observe such subtle points as missing haustral folds, disharmony of interhaustral fold patterns, small, radiolucent filling defects, local contractions, and residue-like masses.[274] Obviously, the absence of any therapeutic potential relegates this examination to a second choice for most physicians.

When barium enema is performed in the presence of a known rectal carcinoma, it should be accomplished with great care (Figure 22-2). After the procedure, the rectum must be cleansed vigorously by multiple enemas to avoid the possibility of obstruction from inspissated barium.

Figure 22-3 demonstrates a typical apple-core lesion at the rectosigmoid juncture. This segment is fairly long; the normal mucosal pattern is lost in the involved bowel, and characteristically the mucosa overhangs the lesion. Another frequent appearance of carcinoma of the sigmoid is shown in Figure 22-4.

The presence of a pedicle (Figure 22-5) does not rule out the diagnosis of carcinoma. In fact, the illustration shows a polypoid carcinoma on a stalk measuring more than 2 cm in length. However, the radiologist is not in a position to comment whether a polyp is benign or malignant.[180]

Barium enema study (Figure 22-6) reveals complete retrograde obstruction to the flow of barium at the level of the mid-sigmoid colon. Retrograde obstruction, although an impressive radiologic finding, is not necessarily indicative of antegrade obstruction. Occasionally, patients will report minimal change in bowel habits, even with this radiologic picture. The resected specimen is shown in Figure 22-7.

The barium enema study shown in Figure 22-8 demonstrates carcinoma of the sigmoid colon with associated diverticular disease. Differentiating between these two conditions is often difficult. It is sometimes said that the presence of diverticula, as seen in this patient, excludes the diagnosis of carcinoma. This is certainly not true. The most important radiologic distinction is that the mucosal pattern usually is maintained in diverticular disease, whereas in carcinoma the mucosa is destroyed or the pattern is lost. In some patients, however, it is impossible to distinguish between the two conditions, and without further information a resection must be performed.

Carcinoma of the sigmoid colon with perforation is shown in Figure 22-9. Under such circumstances, differentiation between carcinoma and diverticular disease is virtually impossible. Another complication of colon cancer is fistulization. Figure 22-10 demonstrates reflux of barium into the upper intestinal tract from a carcinoma near the hepatic flexure.

Figure 22-11 demonstrates carcinoma involving one wall of the cecum in a patient who presented with anemia. Careful bowel preparation is necessary for evaluation of cecal tumors, because fecal matter frequently obscures this area.

It is important to remember that not all tumors of the colon originate within the bowel. Metastases of cancers

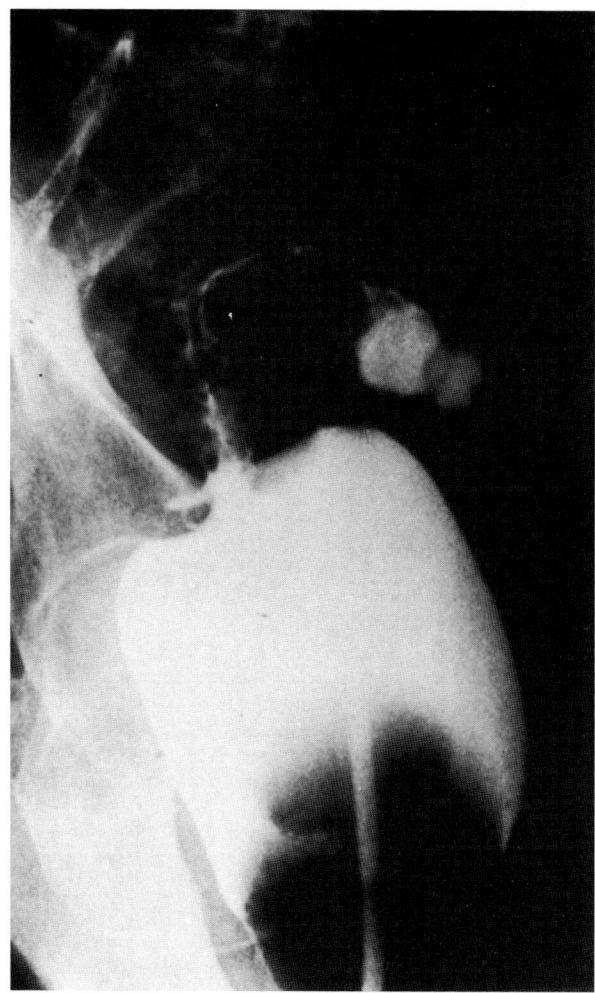

FIGURE 22-2. Barium enema study of a patient with known rectal carcinoma invites the hazard of inspissated barium precipitating colonic obstruction. The physician must weigh the value of screening the proximal bowel against this risk. (From Corman ML, Veidenheimer MC, Swinton NW. *Diseases of the anus, rectum, and colon. Part I: neoplasms.* New York: Medcom, 1972, with permission.)

from an ovary, breast, or other sites, as well as direct extension from adjacent organs, can produce a radiologic picture virtually identical to that of an intrinsic lesion. For example, the transverse colon is involved in 8% of pancreatic malignancies (Figure 22-12).[247] This is another area in which colonoscopy with biopsy has a particular advantage. Despite the plethora of illustrative radiologic material shown, colonoscopy has indeed become the standard for evaluation and interpretation of colonic tumors. In fact, a barium enema for neoplastic disease is almost a historical curiosity, so effectively has colonoscopy replaced this examination. There is so little interest in gastrointestinal radiology on the part of radiologists today that it is virtually impossible to recruit such an individual with this expertise to any radiology

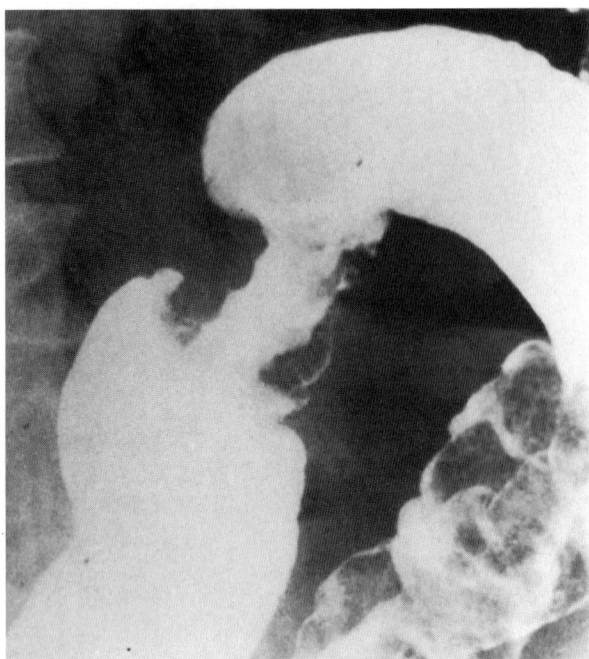

FIGURE 22-3. Apple-core carcinoma at the rectosigmoid juncture. (From Corman ML, Veidenheimer MC, Swinton NW. *Diseases of the anus, rectum, and colon. Part I: neoplasms.* New York: Medcom, 1972, with permission.)

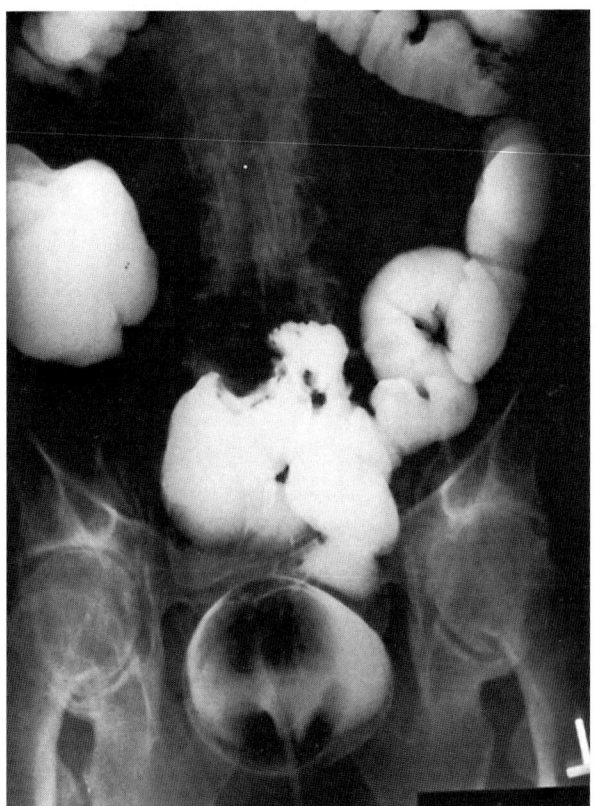

FIGURE 22-4. Carcinoma of the sigmoid. An irregularly marginated mass projecting into the lumen of the colon shows the characteristic shoulders of a malignancy.

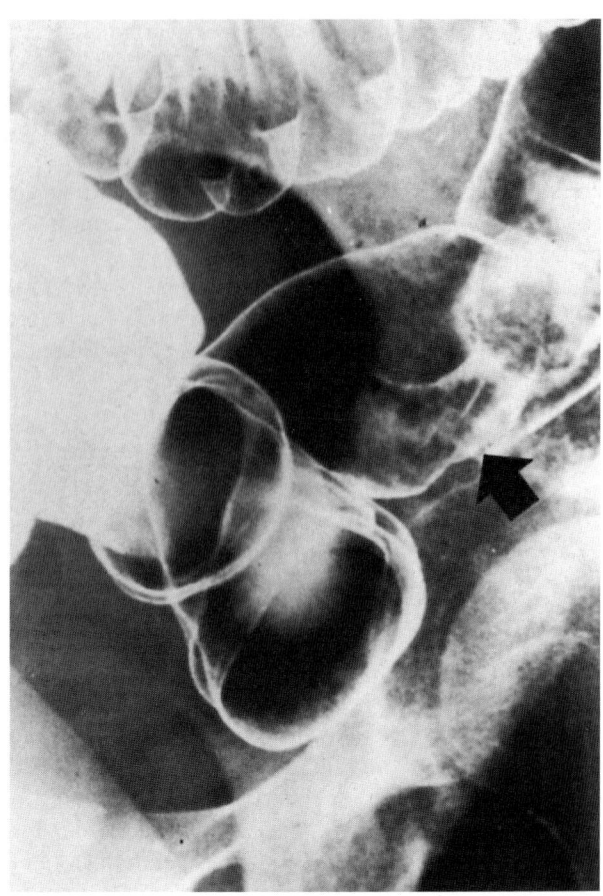

FIGURE 22-5. The presence of a pedicle *(arrow)* does not exclude carcinoma. This lesion was entirely malignant. (From Corman ML, Veidenheimer MC, Swinton NW. *Diseases of the anus, rectum, and colon. Part I: neoplasms.* New York: Medcom, 1972, with permission.)

department. Although there is no denying that colonoscopy is a superior study for the evaluation of mucosal disease, barium enema is much preferred for understanding colonic anatomy, extrinsic compression, and identification of intramural lesions. Even in this area, however, barium enema has been relegated to a secondary role because of the advent of computed tomography (CT).

Urologic Evaluation

For many surgeons in the past, an integral part of the preoperative evaluation of a patient about to undergo bowel surgery was intravenous pyelography (IVP).[980] One cannot help but be impressed by the unexpected findings identified through its routine use (see Tables 4-1 and 4-2). In our experience, ureteral duplication was seen in 2.2% of patients, in addition to a number of other congenital anomalies and serendipitous find-

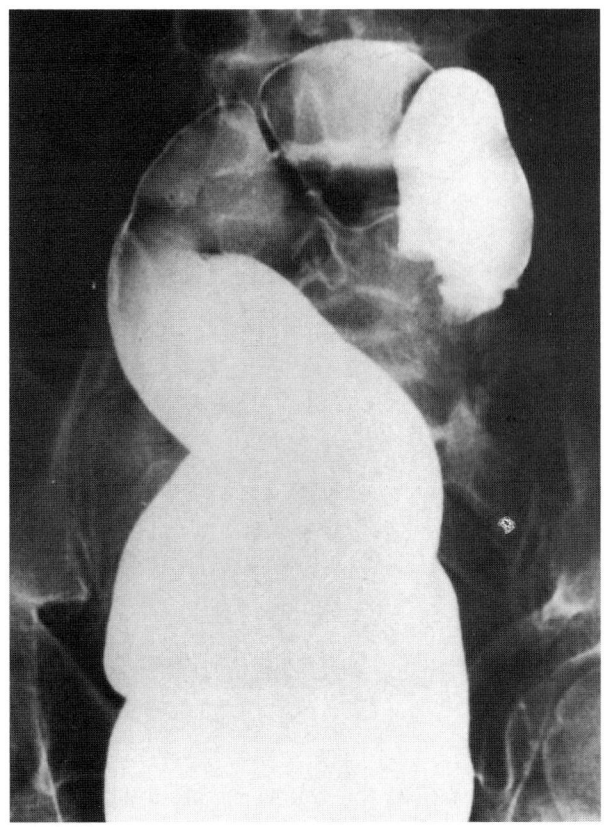

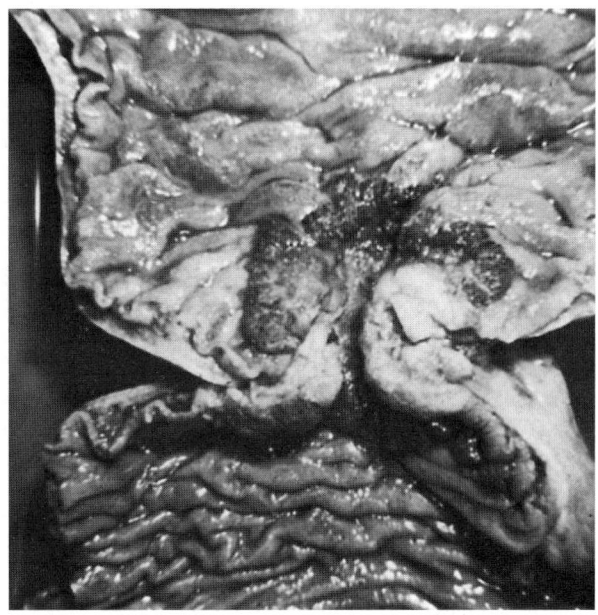

FIGURE 22-7. String stricture. Resected specimen of the carcinoma causing obstruction shown in Figure 22-6. (From Corman ML, Veidenheimer MC, Swinton NW. *Diseases of the anus, rectum, and colon. Part I: neoplasms.* New York: Medcom, 1972, with permission.)

FIGURE 22-6. Retrograde obstruction to the flow of barium from a carcinoma may or may not be associated with significant obstructive symptoms clinically. (From Corman ML, Veidenheimer MC, Swinton NW. *Diseases of the anus, rectum, and colon. Part I: neoplasms.* New York: Medcom, 1972, with permission.)

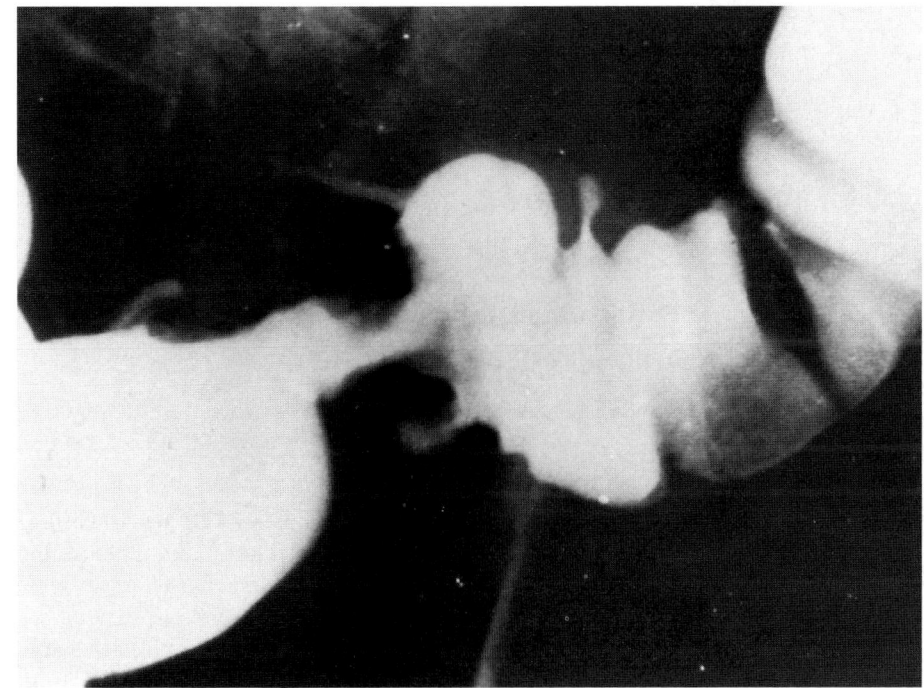

FIGURE 22-8. Carcinoma of the sigmoid with diverticular disease. Because of the relative frequency of both conditions, this is not an uncommon picture. (From Corman ML, Veidenheimer MC, Swinton NW. *Diseases of the anus, rectum, and colon. Part I: neoplasms.* New York: Medcom, 1972, with permission.)

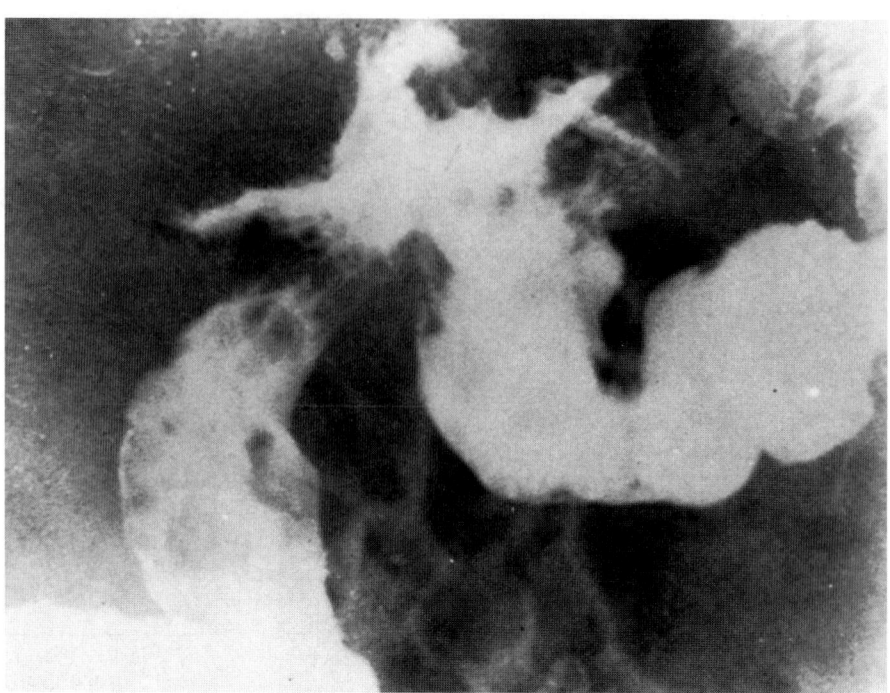

FIGURE 22-9. Perforated carcinoma may be indistinguishable from diverticulitis. (From Corman ML, Veidenheimer MC, Swinton NW. *Diseases of the anus, rectum, and colon. Part I: neoplasms.* New York: Medcom, 1972, with permission.)

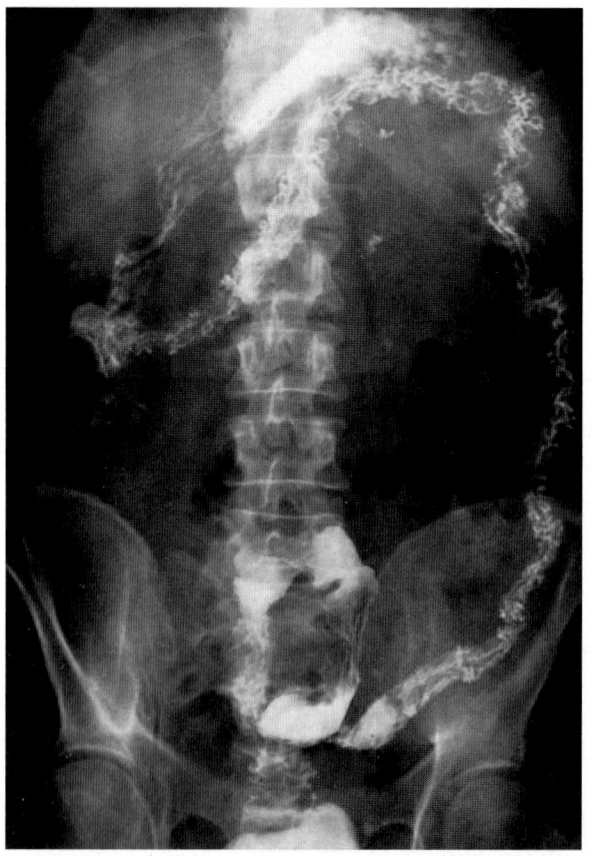

FIGURE 22-10. Carcinoma with fistula. Note the reflux of barium into the duodenum and stomach through a fistula from a hepatic flexure lesion.

ings.[748] In addition, the course of the ureters and the presence of ureteral obstruction can be ascertained, and the postvoiding residual may be estimated. However, in a retrospective study of more than 500 patients, the incidence of complications was the same in patients with normal and abnormal IVP results as well as in patients who did not undergo IVP.[927] Because most injuries occur after low anterior resection or abdominoperineal resection, it seems reasonable to apply the technique to the preoperative evaluation of those whose surgical procedure predisposes them to an increased risk. However, with the ubiquitous application of CT with intravenous contrast in the preoperative assessment of individuals with colorectal cancer, IVP is unnecessary. The urinary tract is generally well visualized by means of this investigation.

Virtual Colonoscopy

See Chapters 4 and 5.

Computed Tomography

Sophisticated radiologic studies may be worthwhile if they can help in therapeutic decision-making before the operation. However, it has been said that CT is not useful in this respect, because the presence of metastases does not, in and of itself, contraindicate palliative surgery.[711] I am not certain that this is a valid objection.

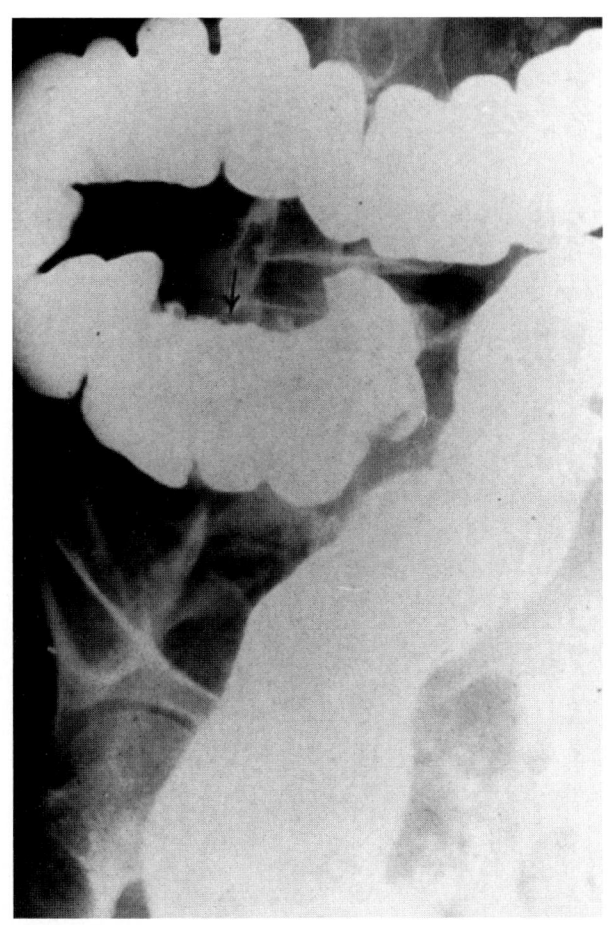

FIGURE 22-11. Carcinoma of the cecum occupying one wall of the bowel *(arrow)*. (From Corman ML, Veidenheimer MC, Swinton NW. *Diseases of the anus, rectum, and colon. Part I: neoplasms.* New York: Medcom, 1972, with permission.)

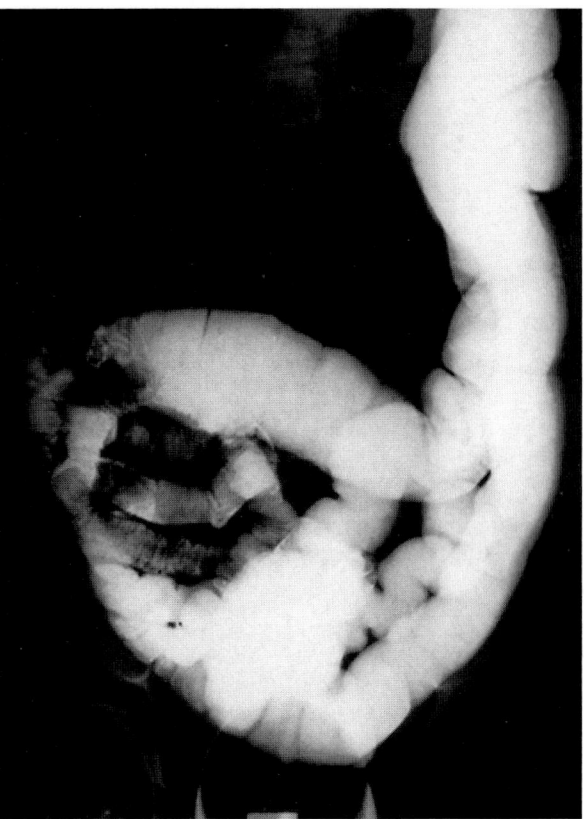

FIGURE 22-12. Partial obstruction to flow of barium at hepatic flexure. The lesion was caused by an invasive carcinoma of the head of the pancreas.

Still, although useful information may be obtained, it rarely causes the proposed colon surgery to be altered (Figs. 22-13 and 22-14). Kerner and colleagues studied 158 consecutive patients who underwent CT as part of the preoperative evaluation for primary colorectal carcinoma.[475] Fifty-six percent had unsuspected findings, of which 35% were considered clinically important. These observations caused the surgeon to alter the proposed operative procedure, or they added additional technical information that was meaningful in the preoperative assessment. Still, the single most common finding was liver metastasis, with abdominal wall or contiguous organ invasion as the second most common finding.

The issue of performing closed liver biopsy with the potential risk of dissemination of tumor was addressed by Rodgers and colleagues.[786] The investigators undertook a multicenter, retrospective review which involved 43 individuals who underwent preoperative biopsy. The authors concluded that there is a significant risk of local dissemination of the tumor, but there was no demonstrated effect on resectability or survival.[786] Liver surgeons uniformly recommend against percutaneous biopsy if surgery is contemplated.

The accuracy of CT scan for liver evaluation has improved considerably with the incorporation of methods that can assess volume—that is, injection of contrast medium in order to permit visualization of the parenchyma in the arterial, portal, and delayed phases.[23]

CT has also been used to assess the stage of the *primary tumor*, but studies have failed to demonstrate that the technique is sufficiently accurate (Figure 22-15).[283] Hypodense contrast media (air or 1,000 to 1,200 mL of water) by retrograde administration (CT enteroclysis) immediately before scanning allow the entire large bowel to be visualized for such lesions.[23] The density of the tumor with respect to the adjacent wall markedly increases following injection of the contrast.

The main advantage of preoperative CT is that it provides a means for comparison should the patient require subsequent evaluation for the possibility of recurrent tumor.[309] Depending on the timing of planned surgery, I

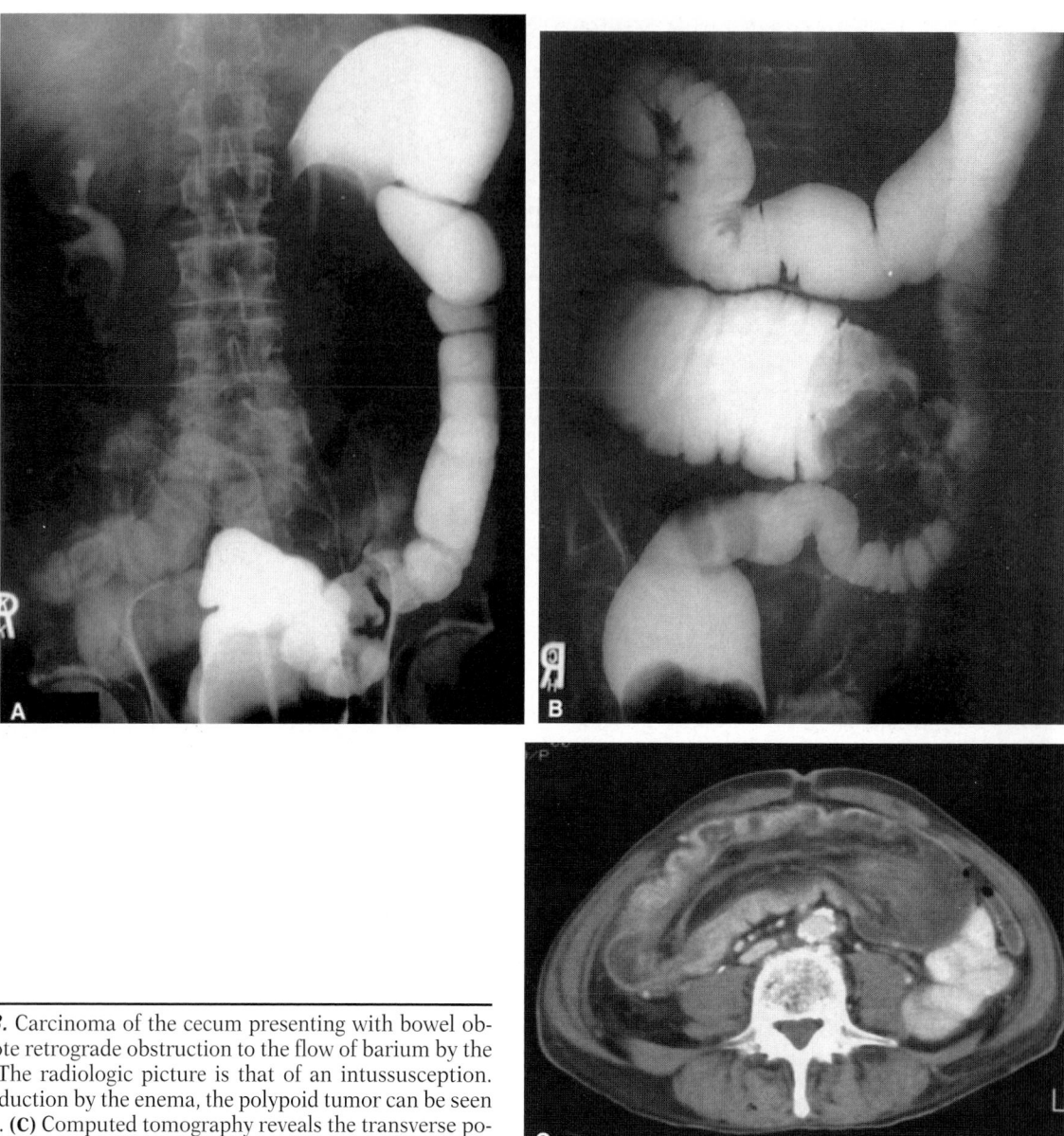

FIGURE 22-13. Carcinoma of the cecum presenting with bowel obstruction. **(A)** Note retrograde obstruction to the flow of barium by the rounded mass. The radiologic picture is that of an intussusception. **(B)** Following reduction by the enema, the polypoid tumor can be seen to fill the cecum. **(C)** Computed tomography reveals the transverse position of the right colon, with a soft tissue mass in the cecum.

always try to obtain a preoperative CT scan. This study is a requisite, however, if one plans to remove the bowel by a laparoscopic technique (Figure 22-16; see Chapter 27). The place of CT and ultrasonographic evaluation of an individual with known or suspected metastatic disease is discussed later in this chapter.

Ultrasonography

Ultrasonographic examination has become well established for the evaluation of a host of conditions within the abdominal cavity—most commonly, assessment of gallstones or gallbladder disease. With the use of sonography alone, however, it has been considered impossi-

ble to detect lesions of the colon with any reliability. Figure 22-17 illustrates a classic ultrasonographic finding in a patient with carcinoma of the colon, the "pseudokidney," or "target" sign. Limberg studied this modality and compared it with hydrocolonic sonography in the diagnosis and staging of colonic tumors.[534] The latter method consisted of instillation of up to 1,500 mL of water into the colon following the injection of a bowel relaxant. Continuous transabdominal sonographic examination of the large intestine was then carried out beginning at the time of water instillation. In every case, colonoscopy was performed following the examination. With the instillation of water into the colon, it was possible to display the bowel sonographically from the rec-

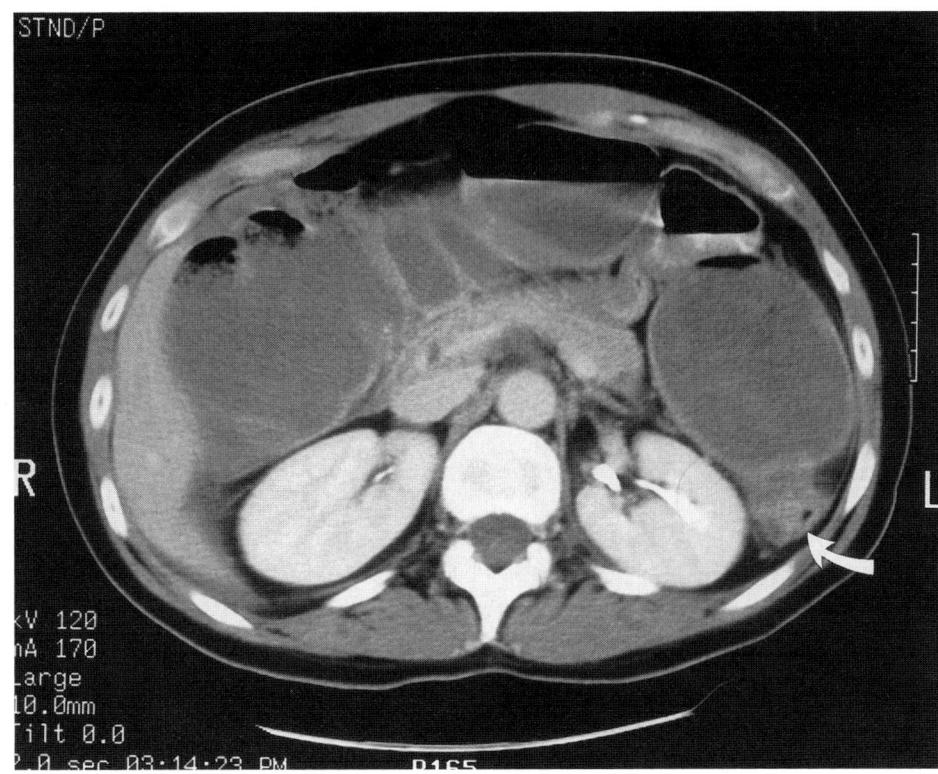

FIGURE 22-14. Computed tomography demonstrates profound colonic dilatation secondary to an obstructing carcinoma of the descending colon *(arrow)*.

tosigmoid to the cecum in 97% of the patients examined.[534] A further advantage was the fact that the layers of the colonic wall could be seen in detail so that the depth of invasion by tumor could be determined. The authors confirmed the lack of value of conventional abdominal sonography. Hydrocolonic sonography is certainly an interesting diagnostic procedure that merits further evaluation.

Transcolorectal endosonography has been suggested to offer an important advantage. The application of this modality for assessing rectal cancers is well established and is discussed in Chapters 4, 6, and 23. Tio and colleagues performed echoendoscopy, in some cases with newer instruments that were prototypes being developed.[949] The accuracy of staging rectal and colonic carcinomas was 81% and 93%, respectively. Although the po-

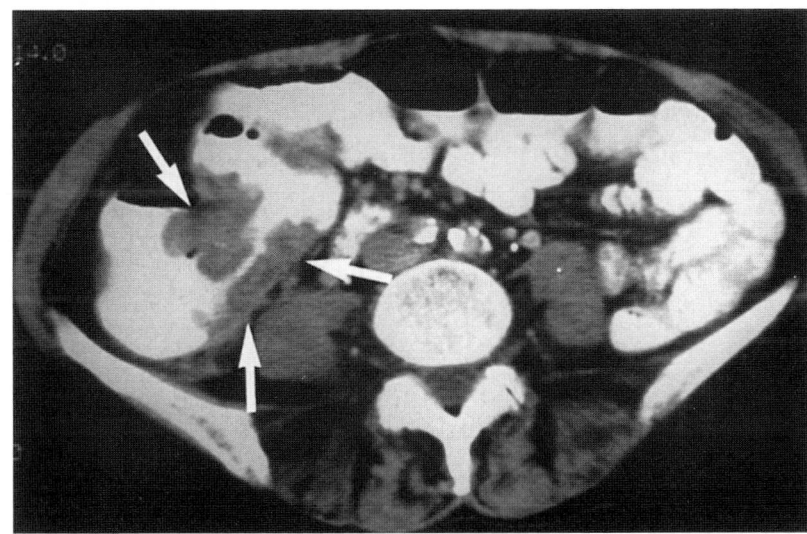

FIGURE 22-15. Computed tomography demonstrates polypoid mass filling part of the ascending colon, consistent with the subsequently demonstrated apple-core lesion observed on barium enema study *(arrows)*.

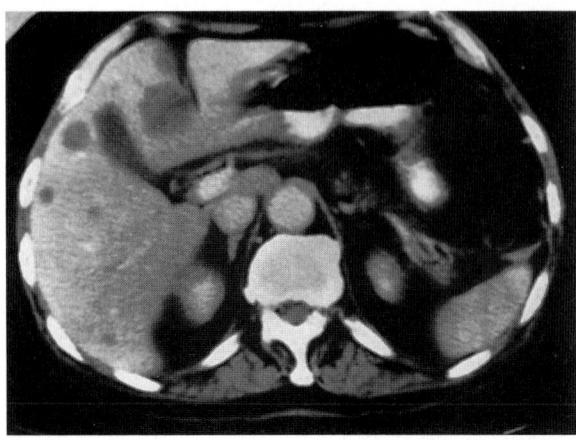

FIGURE 22-16. Computed tomography demonstrates multiple defects in the liver parenchyma, consistent with metastases.

tential for benefit in managing patients with rectal cancer is genuine (there may be other surgical options besides resection), the alternatives to colon resection constitute a less valid proposition.

Carcinoembryonic Antigen

Attention to the immunologic aspects of bowel cancer has been stimulated by the findings of Gold and Freedman, who identified an antigen in extracts from colon cancer tissue.[311,312] This antigen is a glycoprotein absent from normal adult intestinal mucosa but present in primitive endoderm. It was, therefore, called carcinoembryonic antigen (CEA). Thomson and associates described a radioimmunoassay for CEA in the serum and reported

positive results in 97% of patients with colon cancer.[940] However, the high accuracy of CEA as a diagnostic test for bowel cancer reported in earlier articles apparently resulted from the fact that most of the patients studied had advanced disease with extensive metastases. In such individuals, CEA is not only frequently detected but also is present at very high levels in the blood, especially when the liver is involved. In cancer localized to the mucosa and submucosa, without invasion into the muscularis propria, the percentage of patients with an elevated test result falls to between 30% and 40%. Even when recurrence is confined to the bowel wall, the results of the test are usually negative. Therefore, the use of CEA as a screening technique for the asymptomatic population cannot be justified.[310,401,779]

Despite this admonition, levels of CEA can be applied usefully in assessing the prognosis of individuals with colorectal cancer. If the tumor has been completely excised, any elevated level preoperatively should return to normal within a few days. A limited fall to an intermediate, albeit elevated, level is indicative of incomplete excision. Subsequent elevation after return to normal implies recurrence of tumor (see later). There have been many articles attesting to the fact that preoperative and postoperative assessment of the serum CEA level is extremely helpful in determining whether tumor has been left behind after operation. This is true not only after resection of the primary cancer but also after resection for recurrent tumor.[414] Specifically, by determining preoperative and postoperative CEA levels, one can identify patients in a poorer prognostic group who may benefit from early introduction of adjuvant therapy.[155]

The preoperative CEA level in and of itself also has some prognostic significance. Patients with localized disease (as evaluated by clinical methods) have a higher re-

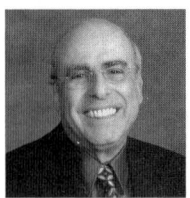

Phil Gold (1936–present) Phil Gold was born in Montreal, Canada and attended McGill University in that city, where he obtained four degrees. He received a Bachelor of Science in Physiology in 1957 and his Doctorate in Medicine as well as Master of Science in 1961. Medical graduation was accompanied by the Wood Gold Medal, the J. Francis Williams Scholarship in Medicine and Clinical Medicine, the Women's Pavilion Prize in Obstetrics and Gynecology, and the Prize of the College of Physicians and Surgeons of the Province of Quebec in Pathology and Medicine. After a year of rotating internship and another of residency in internal medicine, the next 2 years were spent in the laboratories of the Montreal General Hospital Research Institute; he obtained a Ph.D. for his thesis *Carcinoembryonic Antigens of the Human Digestive System*. Gold's discovery of the carcinoembryonic antigen (CEA), along with the description of α-fetoprotein at about the same time, ushered in the modern era of human tumor marker research. The radioimmunoassay for circulating serum CEA has become the most frequently used marker for human cancer. During training at the Public Health Research Institute of New York City in 1967 and 1968 as a Centennial Fellow of the Medical Research Council of Canada, Gold acquired the concepts and technology for electromicroscopy, tissue culture, virology, and cell biology. He then returned to the Montreal General Hospital, its Research Institute, and McGill University as an Assistant Professor of Medicine and a Medical Research Council Career Investigator. In 1972, he was appointed Professor of Medicine. In 1977, he became Director of the Division of Clinical Immunology and Allergy at the Montreal General Hospital, and the following year he assumed the position as the first Director of the McGill Cancer Centre, now the Department of Oncology of McGill's Faculty of Medicine. In 1980, Gold returned to the Montreal General Hospital as Physician-in-Chief and served as the Chairman of the Department of Medicine at McGill University for the statutory 5-year period between 1985 and 1990. In 1995, he became Executive Director of the Clinical Research Centre of the Research Institute of the McGill University Health Centre. The other positions he currently holds include Douglas G. Cameron Professor of Medicine and Professor, Departments of Physiology and Oncology, McGill University. In recognition of the scientific contributions made by Phil Gold, he has been the recipient of numerous international awards and honors and has been elected to a wide variety of scientific organizations. These include Companion of the Order of Canada, Officer of the L'Ordre Nationale du Québec, and recipient of the Gold Medal Award of Merit of the Graduate Society of McGill University. (Courtesy of Faisal Aziz.)

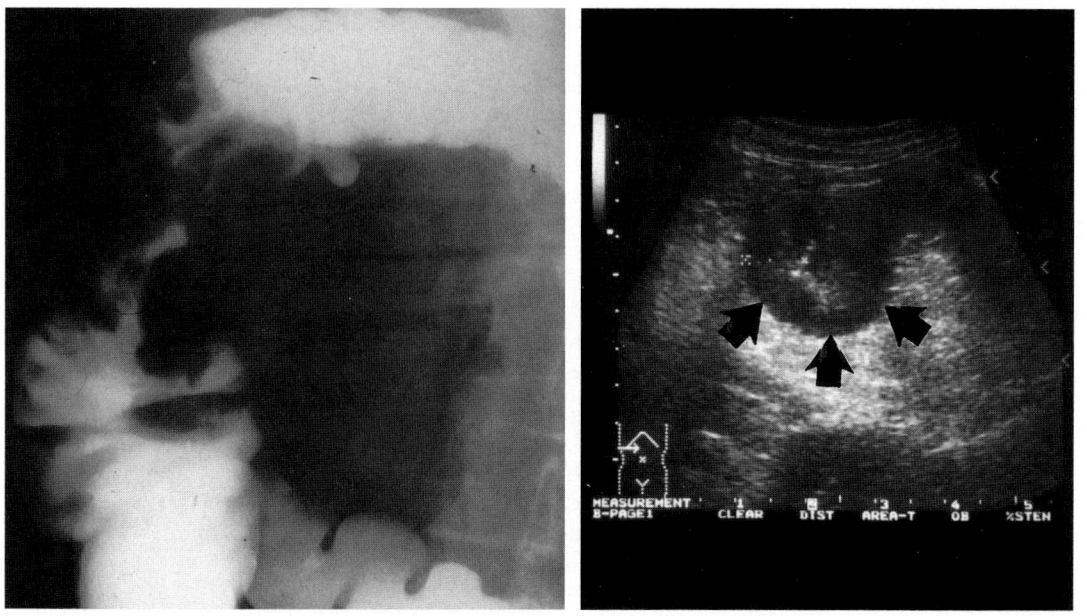

FIGURE 22-17. Carcinoma of the colon. **(A)** Barium enema study reveals classic napkin ring tumor with destruction of the mucosa. **(B)** Ultrasonography demonstrates so-called "pseudokidney" or "target sign." A hypoechoic mass can be seen *(arrows)* with an echogenic center. The echogenic portion represents the "bull's-eye" of the target. This is the narrowed lumen. The thickened bowel wall, a consequence of tumor, can be clearly seen. (Courtesy of Cynthia Withers, M.D.)

currence rate when a high preoperative CEA level is noted than when the preoperative level is low. Such an elevation may be suggestive of inapparent spread of the tumor. Wiratkapun and co-workers noted that CEA levels about 15 ng/mL predicted an increased risk of metastatic recurrence in potentially curative colonic cancer.[1032] This suggests undetected disseminated disease. Ashton and colleagues demonstrated a statistically significant association between survival and a high preoperative CEA level.[33] Others have demonstrated a relationship between the preoperative CEA level and the depth of invasion according to Dukes' classification (see later).[1039] Tumor fixation has also been correlated with the level of CEA elevation.[240] Sener and colleagues showed, through the use of a cancer registry system in a retrospective analysis, that the preoperative serum CEA level can be an indicator of survival that is independent of the stage of disease at diagnosis.[846]

CEA is of limited value in the search for a primary site if metastatic carcinoma is noted. The antigen is detected in about 50% of tumors of the breast, stomach, lung, and in other solid tumors. Levels higher than normal have also been found in heavy smokers and in persons with cirrhosis, pancreatitis, uremia, peptic ulcer, intestinal metaplasia of the stomach, as well as ulcerative colitis. The antigen has been reported in tissue of intestinal polyps, colonic inflammatory mucosa, and normal intestinal mucosa of children. CEA has also

been found in cancerous tissue from the breast, liver, and lung, as well as in body fluids exposed to cancer. In colonic washings, high levels of CEA have been found in patients with colon cancer and colon polyps, intermediate levels in those with ulcerative colitis, and lower levels in normal subjects.[1022] Yeatman and colleagues demonstrated an elevated CEA in gallbladder bile in some individuals who showed no evidence of hepatic metastasis at the time of surgery for the primary tumor.[1051] They suggested that those with slight increases should be followed closely for the possible subsequent appearance of such lesions.

Nuclear Medicine Studies

Liver Scan

The liver scan has been virtually abandoned for the evaluation of this organ in patients with colorectal cancer, either preoperatively or postoperatively. The study has been supplanted by CT.

Pelvic Lymphoscintigraphy

Pelvic lymphoscintigraphy has been used to try to discriminate between normal and diseased large bowel and to determine the extent of nodal uptake, but it has no demonstrable value in the diagnosis or staging of colorectal cancer.[767] Angiography of the mesenteric arteries likewise has not been proved useful in the preoperative evaluation of colon carcinoma.[468]

Radiolabeled Antibody Imaging

Anti-Carcinoembryonic Antigen

A modification of the CEA assay involves the use of radiolabeled antibodies to the antigen followed by an external photoscan.[314–316] Goldenberg and co-workers evaluated 50 patients by injecting antibody against CEA labeled with iodine-131 and performing total-body scans.[315] In this study, 83% of the preoperative group and approximately 90% of the postoperative group were found to have the tumors correctly localized. The authors conclude that among other potential benefits, this technique can help to stage the tumor preoperatively and complement other methods used to assess tumor response to therapy.

Beatty and colleagues studied 100 patients with known or suspected colorectal cancer by radioimmunoscintigraphy, using murine monoclonal anti-CEA antigen labeled with indium.[55] Sensitivity was 76% for primary tumors, 44% for hepatic metastases, 38% for extrahepatic abdominal metastases, and 78% for extraabdominal metastases.

Lechner and co-workers submitted 47 patients to radioimmunoscintigraphic investigations for primary or recurrent colorectal cancer by means of technetium-99m (^{99m}Tc)-fab' fragment (Immu 4).[518] The advantage of this particular commercially available product is that it has a short half-life with high photon abundance. It can be administered at high doses and permits early imaging with a gamma camera. The overall accuracy of this study was 93.75% in primary and 91.6% in recurrent colorectal cancer. The investigators concluded that immunoscintigraphy had a decisive influence on treatment planning in one third of patients with primary colorectal cancer and was superior to CT in the detection of early recurrences (see the later discussion under follow-up evaluation).[518]

Gastrointestinal Cancer Antigen

Gastrointestinal cancer antigen (CA 19–9) is a monoclonal antibody produced against human colorectal carcinoma cell line SW1116.[439,760] However, this antigen is not specific for cancer and has been found in certain normal tissues, most notably pancreas, gallbladder, and gastric mucosa.[439] As of this writing, there is no evidence to suggest that CA 19–9 is superior to CEA in predicting recurrence, although there may be some advantage in screening high-risk patients for colorectal cancer.[760]

Other Antibody Imaging Options

Yiu and colleagues used the same concept through the application of monoclonal antibodies that react with epithelial membrane antigen.[1052] Indium-111 (^{111}In)-M8 detected 13 of 16 tumor sites, whereas In[111]–77–1 detected ten of 15 tumor sites. The implication again is that these monoclonal antibodies may have a role in the preoperative immunolocalization of colorectal cancers. Additionally, others have shown unsuspected tumor sites using a similar technique, a method that directly affected treatment in 18% of patients.[220]

Yamaguchi and colleagues used another tumor marker, NCC-ST 439, in the preoperative and postoperative evaluation of individuals with colorectal cancer.[1049] This is a monoclonal antibody obtained using ST-4, a cell line derived from poorly differentiated stomach cancer. The authors demonstrated results comparable with those obtained with the other markers, especially when it was used in combination with CEA.

Shibata and co-workers studied circulating anti-p53 antibodies in patients with known colorectal carcinoma to evaluate the clinical application of this technique.[861] Circulating anti-p53 antibodies were detected in 68% of their patients.[861] The authors concluded that this particular analysis may become an important diagnostic indicator of colorectal malignancies (see earlier discussion).

Carpelan-Holmström and associates investigated whether there are differences in serum levels of CA 242, a tumor marker demonstrated to have a high preoperative sensitivity for colorectal cancer and CEA.[138] The authors concluded that the two studies supplement each other, in that the two markers together show a higher sensitivity than either one alone.

Van Kamp and co-workers assessed CA M43, a serum marker for colorectal cancer, to determine its clinical utility.[972] This monoclonal antibody study identifies tumor-associated mucin. The investigators concluded that this marker shows a positivity rate equivalent to that of CEA, and as was demonstrated with CA 242, it appears to complement CEA. Together, they reached 87% positivity in the presence of metastatic disease.[972]

Vasoactive Intestinal Peptide Receptor Imaging

Vasoactive intestinal peptide (VIP) is a major regulator of water and electrolyte secretion in the gut. Various endocrine tumors, as well as intestinal adenocarcinomas, express large numbers of high-affinity receptors for VIP. Virgolini and associates evaluated the usefulness of scanning with VIP-labeled iodine-123 to localize gastrointestinal tumors.[984] Among those with colorectal cancer, primary recurring tumors were visualized in all ten patients, liver metastases were seen in 15 of 18, and lung metastases were detected in two of three. All four patients with lymph node metastases were identified with this technique. It appears that scanning with radiolabeled VIP permits visualization of intestinal tumors and metastases, provided, of course, that they express receptors for VIP.

Comment

The advent of monoclonal antibody technology has permitted the development of a number of radiolabeled tumor-reactive probes. These can be used in conjunction with gamma camera imaging equipment to identify the anatomic distribution of colorectal cancer within an individual. The reader is referred to the discussion on the postoperative application of these techniques in the section on follow-up evaluation. The real excitement will occur when it will be possible to attach a therapeutic agent to the monoclonal antibody to treat the primary or metastatic cancer.

Serum Gastrin

Kameyama and colleagues evaluated the relationship between serum gastrin levels and liver metastases in colorectal cancer to determine whether serum gastrin can be used as a predictor of liver metastases, independent of other prognostic variables.[464] In a series of 140 patients who underwent surgery for colorectal cancer, the fasting serum gastrin level was determined preoperatively. The incidence of liver metastases was statistically significantly higher in those patients with a serum gastrin level of 150 pg/mL or greater than in those with a serum gastrin level less than this number.[464] These results suggest that serum gastrin serves as a useful predictor of liver metastases that correlates well with the pathologic determination of venous invasion.

Leukocyte Adherence Inhibition

The leukocyte adherence inhibition assay is an *in vitro* test based on the observation that, following incubation with tumor extracts from the same organ, leukocytes from cancer patients lose their ability to adhere to glass surfaces.[41] Reports have demonstrated relatively consistent identification of malignant processes.[348,928,941] Theoretically, it may be possible to utilize this phenomenon to improve the detection rate of colorectal cancer.[536] However, the lack of specificity for localization of the growth and inconsistencies in the performance of the technique

relegate the procedure at this time to the status of a research tool.

PATHOLOGY

By far the most common malignant lesion affecting the colon and rectum is adenocarcinoma. The tumor arises from the glandular epithelium, and it can invade microscopic blood vessels as well as metastasize to distant organs, most commonly the liver. It can spread by way of the lymphatics to regional lymph nodes and ultimately pass into the systemic circulation. The tumor may also extend locally into adjacent organs (e.g., posterior vaginal wall, uterus, bladder, small bowel, stomach, and retroperitoneal structures).

Microscopic Appearance

Histologically, the cancer may appear well differentiated (Figure 22-18), moderately differentiated (Figure 22-19), or poorly differentiated (Figure 22-20). The tumor may produce so much mucin that the nucleus is pushed to one side of the cell, creating a signet ring appearance (Figure 22-21). This last type has been the subject of some debate with respect to its prognostic implications. Minsky has observed that the incidence of this manifestation in patients with colorectal cancer is approxi-

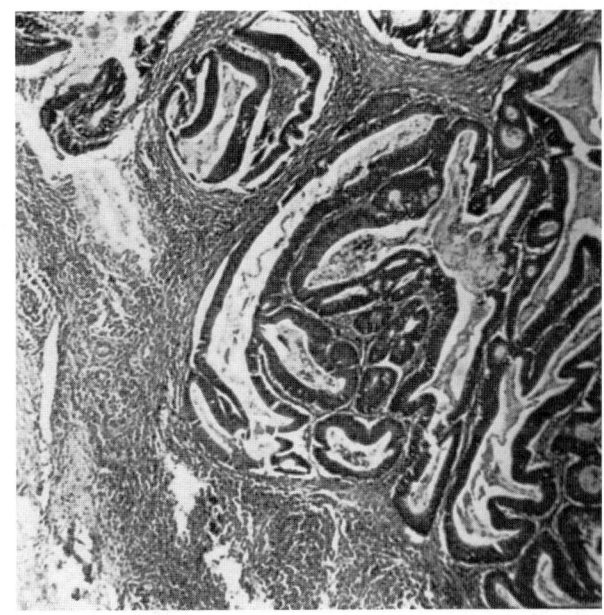

FIGURE 22-18. Well-differentiated adenocarcinoma. The neoplastic glands display somewhat oriented epithelium and resemble crypts in their overall architecture. (Original magnification × 250; courtesy of Rudolf Garret, M.D.)

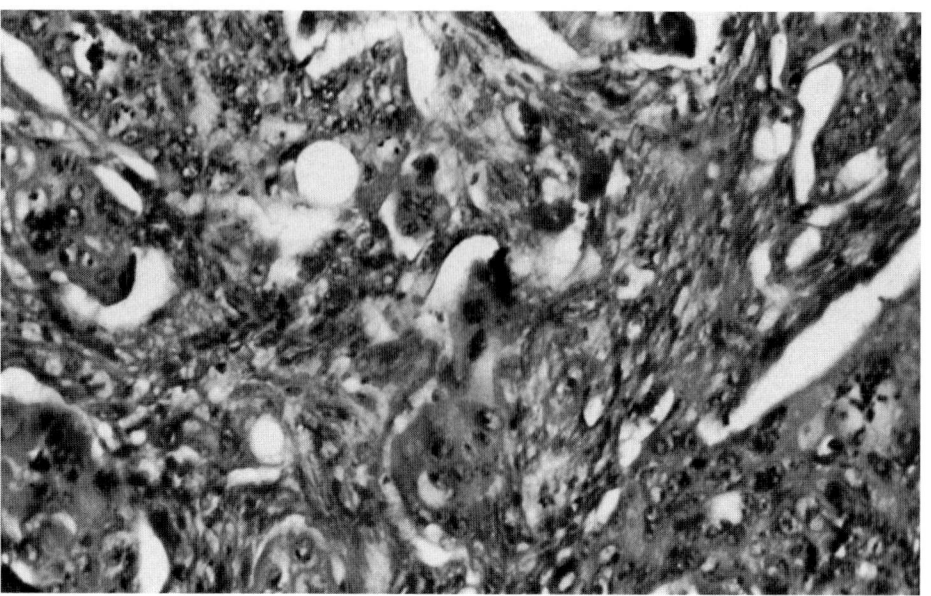

FIGURE 22-19. Moderately differentiated adenocarcinoma. The glands are more irregular and exhibit less orientation of the epithelium. (Original magnification × 250; courtesy of Rudolf Garret, M.D.)

mately 17%.[634] He found that colloid carcinoma was not an independent prognostic factor for survival, but believed that it should be reported separately from other histologic patterns in order to achieve a better understanding of its natural history. Generally, the more poorly differentiated tumors are more invasive at the time of diagnosis, and the more invasive the tumor, the poorer the prognosis.

Macroscopic Appearance

In addition to degree of differentiation, tumor morphology—whether polypoid, infiltrative, or ulcerated—has been found to be an important prognostic variable. It,

too, should be reported as part of a comprehensive pathologic evaluation of the patient.[898] Macroscopically, the tumor can display a number of forms (Figs. 22-22 through 22-30).

Factors Affecting Rates of Growth and Spread of Tumor

Carcinomas of the colon and rectum are relatively slow-growing tumors. Symptoms usually appear early in the development of the disease, and metastases occur relatively late. Tumor growth and spread display considerable variation, depending partly on histologic grade (based on cellular arrangement and differentiation), in-

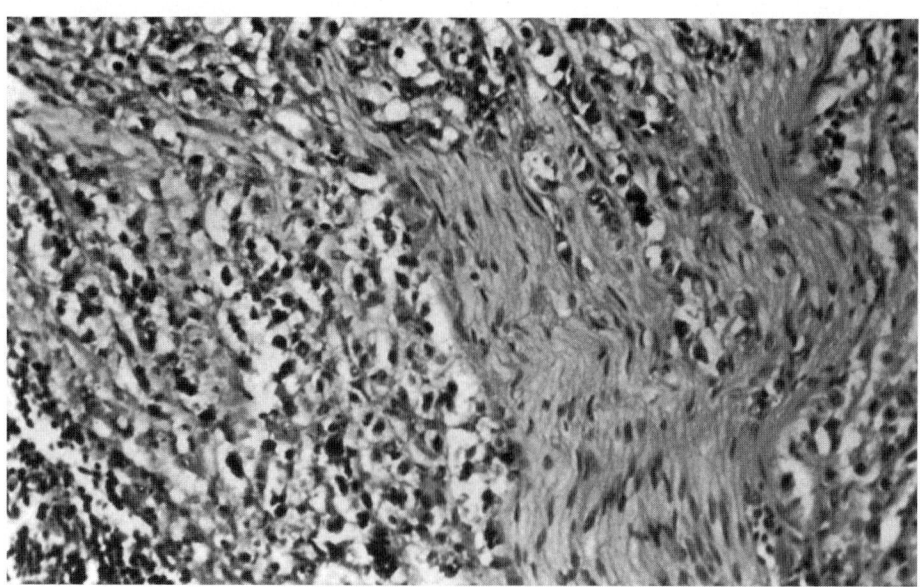

FIGURE 22-20. Poorly differentiated (undifferentiated) adenocarcinoma. There is no definite formation of glands. (Original magnification × 250; courtesy of Rudolf Garret, M.D.)

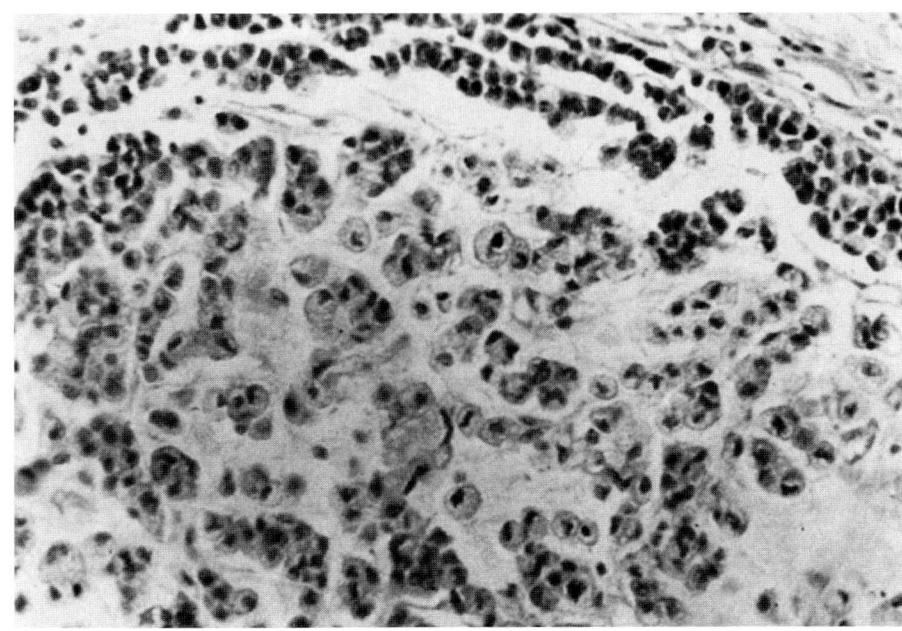

FIGURE 22-21. Signet ring carcinoma. In this malignant variant, mucin displaces the nucleus to one side. This is occasionally seen in lesions of the right side and when carcinoma arises in ulcerative colitis. (Original magnification × 600; from Corman ML, Veidenheimer MC, Swinton NW. *Diseases of the anus, rectum, and colon. Part I: neoplasms.* New York: Medcom, 1972, with permission.)

creased ameboid action of some cancer cells, enzymes such as hyaluronidase, decreased adhesiveness of the tumor cells, size of the lesion at the primary site, and length of time the tumor has been present.[343,917] Daneker and colleagues showed the interaction of the tumor with the basement membrane to be an important factor in predicting spread.[194] They noted that in general, more poorly differentiated cancers tend to adhere and there-

fore to invade much more readily. Additional variables include location of the tumor, indeterminate host factors, manipulation at surgery, and the age and sex of the person.[38,166,242,405,820]

Histochemical studies assess those factors that contribute to tumor growth and spread. These include changes in sialomucin in the distal resection margin and the presence of human chorionic gonadotropin.[201,866] For

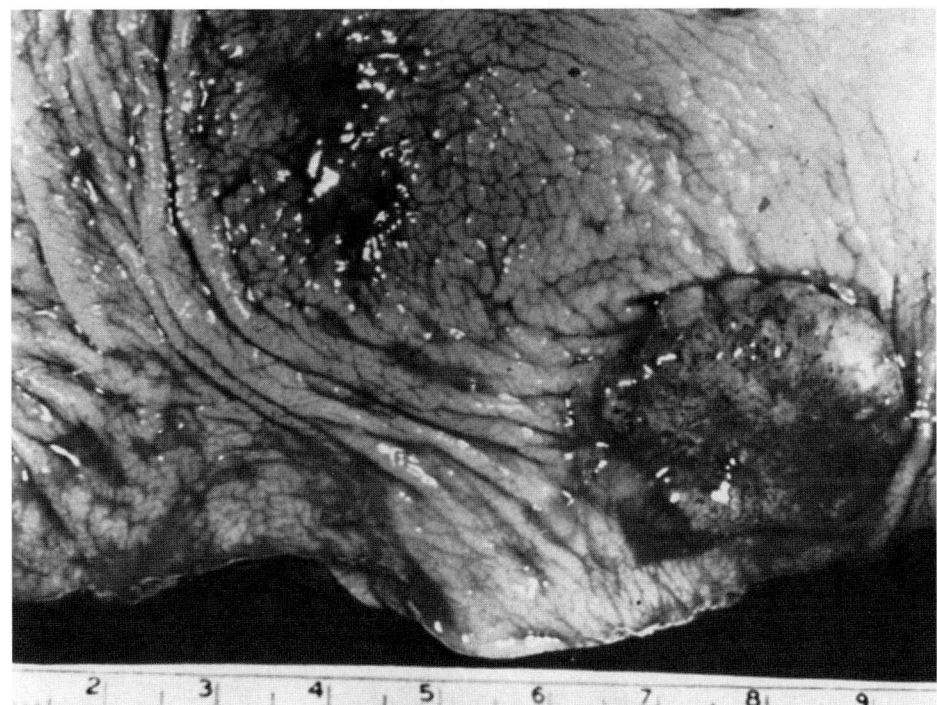

FIGURE 22-22. Relatively small polypoid carcinoma. (From Corman ML, Veidenheimer MC, Swinton NW. *Diseases of the anus, rectum, and colon. Part I: neoplasms.* New York: Medcom, 1972, with permission.)

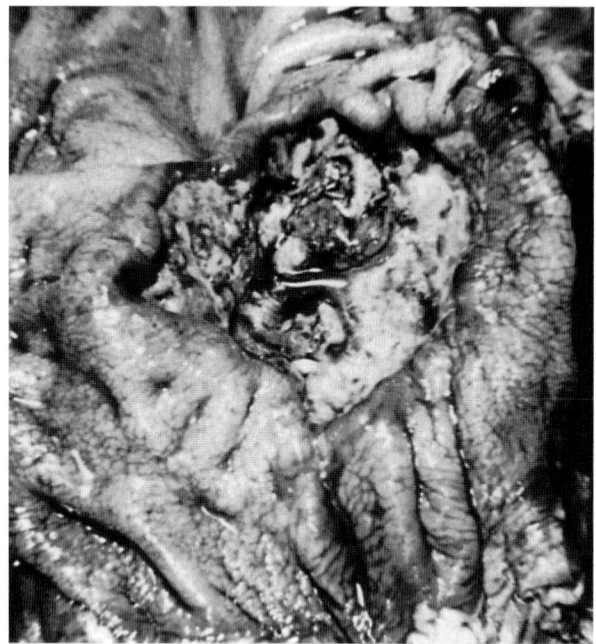

FIGURE 22-23. Ulcerating carcinoma. (From Corman ML, Veidenheimer MC, Swinton NW. *Diseases of the anus, rectum, and colon. Part I: neoplasms.* New York: Medcom, 1972, with permission.)

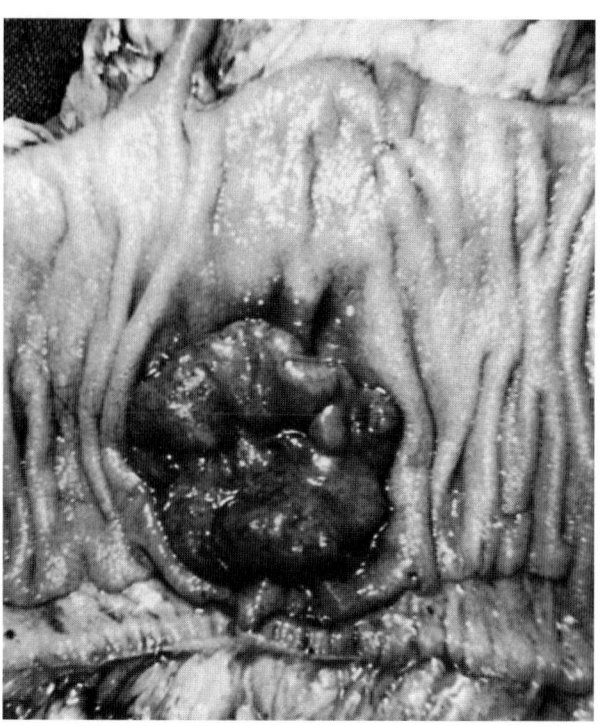

FIGURE 22-24. Polypoid carcinoma with ulceration. (From Corman ML, Veidenheimer MC, Swinton NW. *Diseases of the anus, rectum, and colon. Part I: neoplasms.* New York: Medcom, 1972, with permission.)

FIGURE 22-25. Polypoid carcinoma with mucosal hyperplasia *(arrow).* This association is commonly seen (see Chapter 10). (From Corman ML, Veidenheimer MC, Swinton NW. *Diseases of the anus, rectum, and colon. Part I: neoplasms.* New York: Medcom, 1972, with permission.)

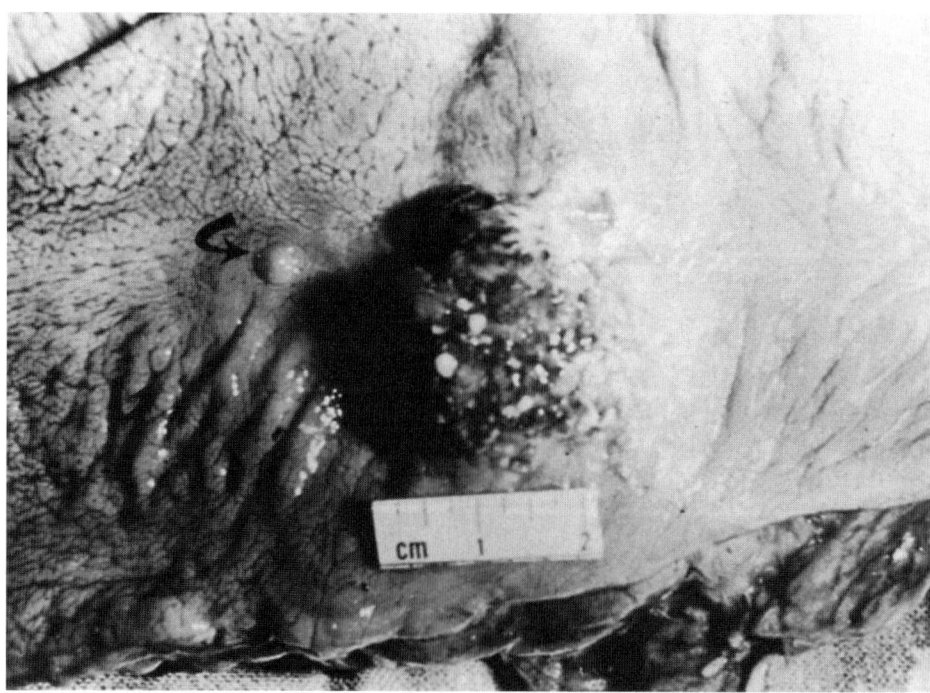

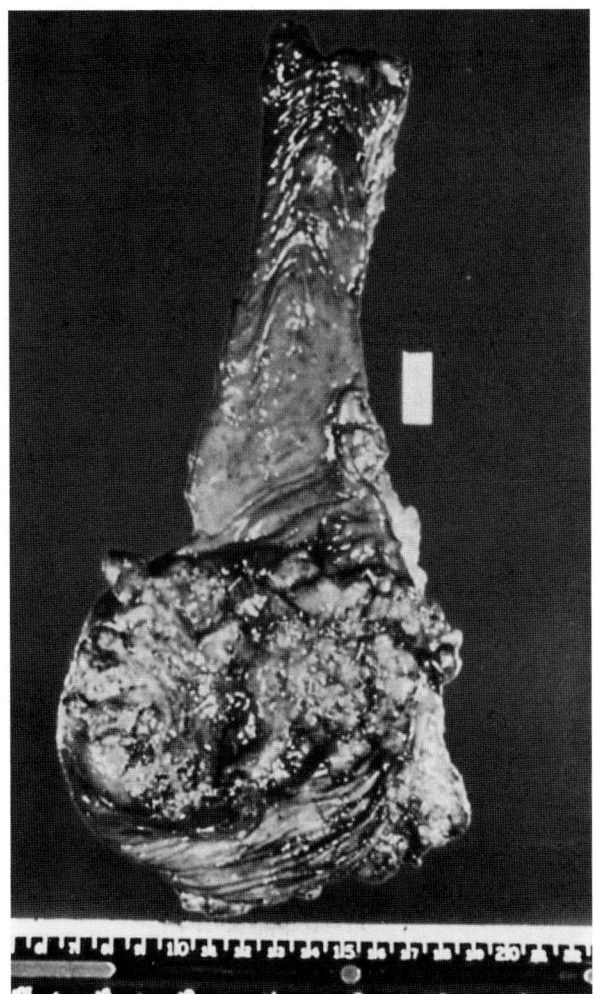

FIGURE 22-26. Large polypoid carcinoma. Despite its size, the prognosis is better with this tumor than with a smaller, invasive lesion. (From Corman ML, Veidenheimer MC, Swinton NW. *Diseases of the anus, rectum, and colon. Part I: neoplasms.* New York: Medcom, 1972, with permission.)

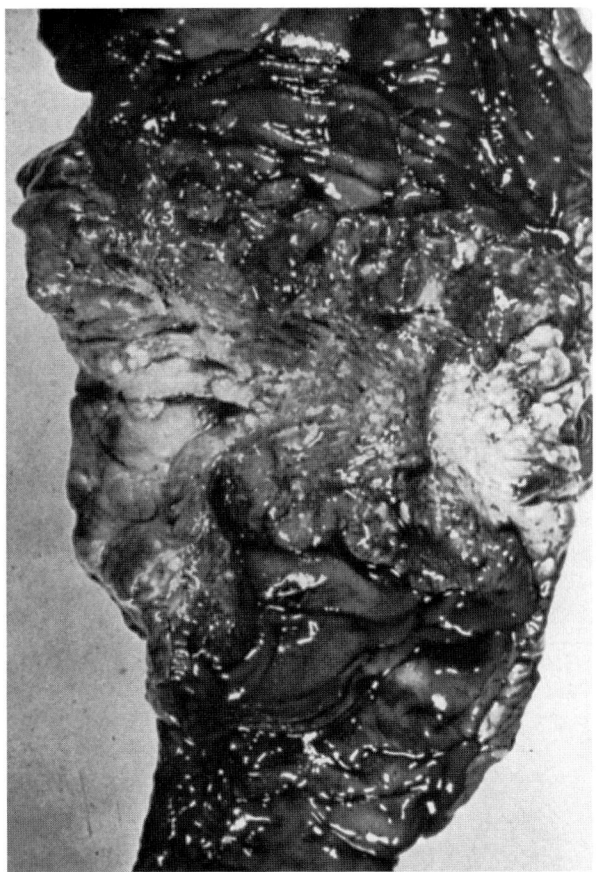

FIGURE 22-27. Scirrhous or infiltrating carcinoma is associated with a poorer prognosis. (From Corman ML, Veidenheimer MC, Swinton NW. *Diseases of the anus, rectum, and colon. Part I: neoplasms.* New York: Medcom, 1972, with permission.)

example, Dawson and colleagues showed that sialomucin adjacent to a primary colorectal cancer provides a crude assessment of tumor invasiveness, and therefore the risk for local recurrence.[200] Ideally, as more information is developed about prognostic factors, more meaningful recommendations with respect to supplementary therapy will be made.

The first opportunity to measure the growth of colonic cancer at its site of origin was reported in 1961 by Spratt and Ackerman.[880] In this study, nine air-contrast enemas were performed during a period of 7.5 years.[879] Radiographic measurements of the tumor were taken, and by appropriate plotting on a graph, the growth curve was shown to conform to an exponential increase in volume. The tumor was calculated to have a doubling time of 636.5 days. When desquamation from the sur-

face was taken into account, it was postulated that a net increase of only one cell per 1,000 cells per day was adequate to account for the observed rate of growth. Another study demonstrated the mean doubling time of tumor volume to be only 130 days.[91] The authors believed that this high rate of growth could be attributed to the large size of the tumors, and therefore their greater likelihood of being malignant at the initial examination.

Doubling time of pulmonary metastases from colon and rectal carcinomas has been calculated radiographically and found to be 109 days.[878] Metastatic tumors increase their cellular complement six times faster than primary cancers.[879] It is theorized that the absence of desquamation in the metastatic site accounts for this observed difference.

Finlay and colleagues studied the growth rate of hepatic metastases by means of serial CT.[267] They discovered that the mean doubling time for obvious metastases

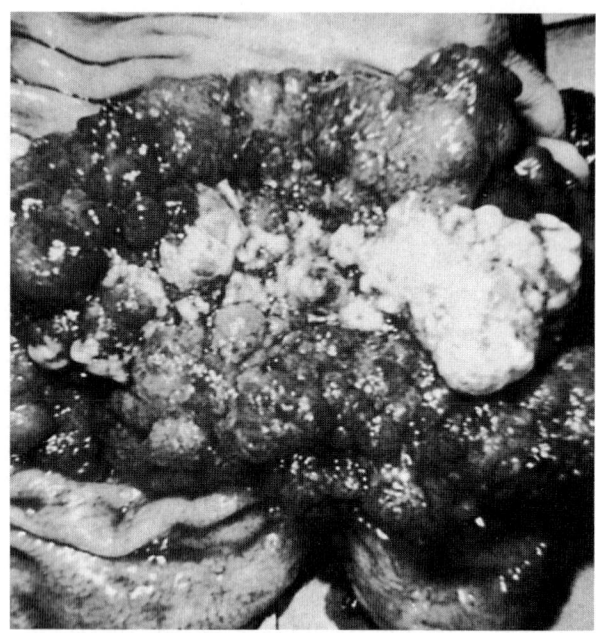

FIGURE 22-28. Colloid carcinoma. Prognosis has generally been believed to be poorer with this variant of carcinoma. Note the gelatinous appearance. (From Corman ML, Veidenheimer MC, Swinton NW. *Diseases of the anus, rectum, and colon. Part I: neoplasms.* New York: Medcom, 1972, with permission.)

(those discovered at the time of laparotomy) was 155 days, compared with 86 days for occult metastases. By means of extrapolation, the authors concluded that the mean age of the former lesions was 3.7 years, and the latter was 2.3 years.

The metastatic behavior of neoplasms varies. According to Spratt, examination of the cancer-host interface is helpful in determining the behavioral pattern of the tumor.[878] One that is less likely to metastasize exhibits a well-circumscribed, intact margin. The tumor that is more likely to metastasize to lymph nodes has a loose or infiltrating margin with little inflammatory reaction. Sacchi and co-workers looked at the border between normal tissue and tumor in colorectal cancer and opined that it is the mast cell, probably influenced by the inflammatory infiltrate and/or colorectal cancer cells themselves, which destroy lymphatic vessels, thereby preventing spread into the lymphatic system.[807]

Some investigators have suggested that the concentration of circulating C-reactive protein may play a role in predicting recurrence and survival in colorectal cancer. McMillan and colleagues studied the presence of a systemic inflammatory response as measured by circulating C-reactive protein in 174 patients who were believed to have undergone a curative resection.[614] C-reactive protein concentration was found to be an independent predictor for survival—that is, the presence of elevated concentrations predicts a poor outcome.

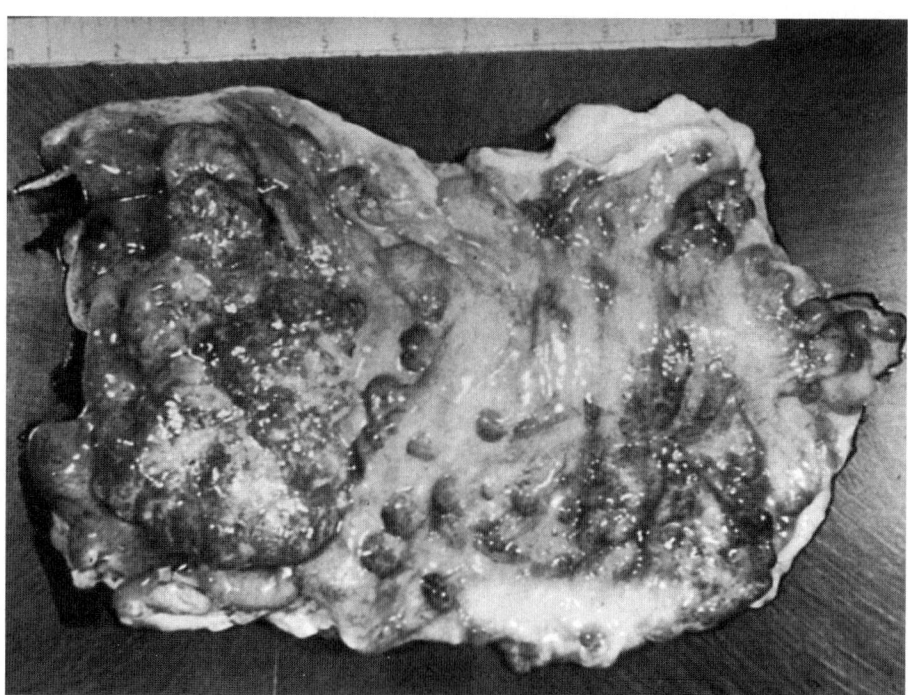

FIGURE 22-29. Carcinoma **(light area, center)** arising in villous adenoma. (From Corman ML, Veidenheimer MC, Swinton NW. *Diseases of the anus, rectum, and colon. Part I: neoplasms.* New York: Medcom, 1972, with permission.)

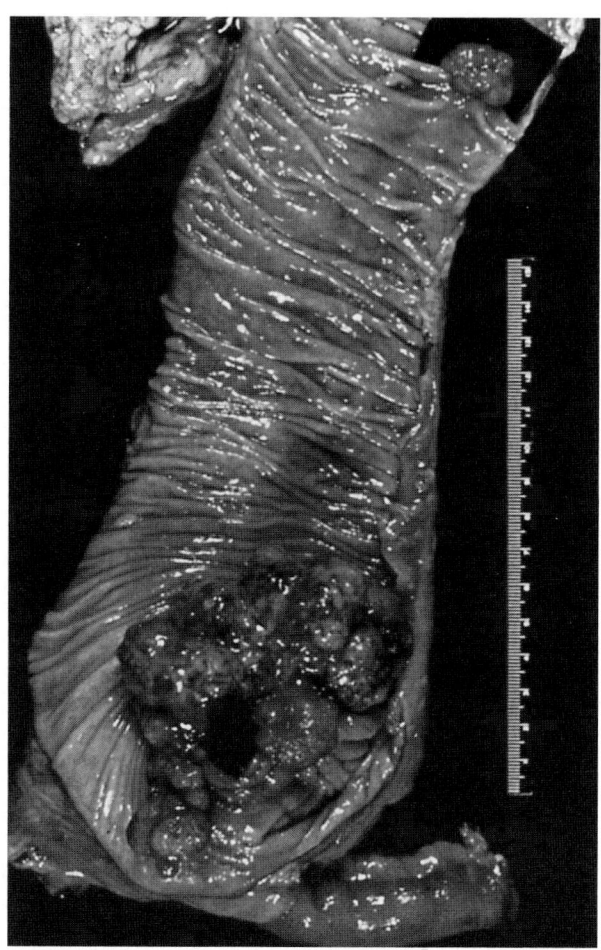

FIGURE 22-30. Perforated cecal carcinoma.

Comment

The one article by Spratt and Ackerman has been responsible for more confusion, misinterpretation, and misrepresentation in the sphere of medical litigation with respect to the accusation of delay in diagnosis than all other variables combined. For the record, the concept of cancer doubling time is without merit in considering the likelihood of survival and its applicability to earlier diagnosis and prognosis in the individual patient.

Staging and Prognosis

Classifications

The importance of tumor invasion and its prognostic implications was postulated by Dukes in 1930 and was subsequently revised by him in 1932.[233,234] This has come to be known as Dukes' classification (not Duke's). The classification was originally directed toward rectal cancer (Table 22-2). After performing numerous meticulous dissections of resected specimens to identify metastases to lymph nodes, Dukes further modified his classification in 1944.[235] Those tumors with lymph node involvement but with a negative node at the ligation of the inferior mesenteric artery he called C1. Lesions classified as C2 had metastases to the node at the level of the ligature (Table 22-3). The addition of the D category has been generally accepted as representative of tumor spread beyond the reach of potential surgical cure but was not included in his classification (Table 22-4).

Others have introduced their own classifications, expanding and subdividing Dukes' system and broadening it to include colon cancer and disseminated metastases, degree of differentiation, tumor morphology, and histogram pattern, among others.[34,263,482,726,960,1056] Jass and colleagues suggested a classification based on prognosis:[446]

I. Excellent prognosis
II. Good
III. Fair
IV. Poor

A scoring system was developed based on several factors that appear to influence survival—number of lymph nodes with metastatic tumor, character of the invasive margin, presence of peritumoral lymphocytic infiltration, and local spread. Most observers believe that the classification of Dukes is of greater prognostic value and more reproducible than that of Jass.[205]

Figure 22-31 illustrates the more popular staging systems. Obviously, the more one "substages," the greater the refinement potential to predict tumor behavior, and therefore to gain more information about the possible outcome.[683] There is even a Japanese Classification (Kikuchi) which subdivides vertical invasion of the submucosa into

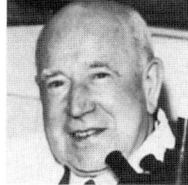

Cuthbert Esquire Dukes (1890–1977) Cuthbert Dukes was born in Bridgwater, Somerset, England and graduated in medicine from Edinburgh University in 1914. He served in World War I in the Royal Army Medical Corps, receiving the Order of the British Empire. After the war, he became a demonstrator in bacteriology at University College, London and joined the staff of St. Mark's Hospital in 1922 as its first pathologist. It was there that he produced his classification of cancer of the rectum that became so valuable as a guide to prognosis. His many writings include the pioneering work on familial polyposis (and the Polyposis Registry at St. Mark's Hospital) and several books. He became successively president of the Royal Society of Medicine (1944), the section of urology (1957), and the section of the history of medicine (1959), and was elected to honorary fellowship in the Royal College of Surgeons and the American Society of Colon and Rectal Surgeons.

▶ **TABLE 22-2 Dukes' Classification of Rectal Cancer (1932)**

Stage	Classification
A	Carcinoma limited to wall of rectum
B	Carcinoma spread by direct continuity to extrarectal tissues; no lymph node metastases
C	Metastases present in regional lymph nodes

Sm1 (upper third of the submucosa), Sm2 (middle third), and Sm3 (invasion near the "inner surface of the muscularis propria"). The question, however, is whether this is really important, especially in the absence of adjuvant therapy specific to disease-invasion subsets. The TNM system has become the most popular classification in use in the United States and indeed in the world (*Tumor-Node-Metastasis*; Table 22-5). Additionally, the TNM system utilizes a staging method on the basis of the characteristics as follows:

TNM Stage	Characteristics
0	T_{is}, N_0, M_0
I	T_1, N_0, M_0 T_2, N_0, M_0
II	T_3, N_0, M_0 T_4, N_0, M_0
III	Any T, N_1, M_0 Any T, N_2, M_0
IV	Any T, Any N, M_1

Fisher and colleagues compared the relative prognostic value of the Dukes, Astler-Coller, and TNM staging systems in 745 pathologically evaluable individuals with rectal cancer.[269] They concluded that the Dukes method was the simplest and most consistent algorithm related to prognosis. They observed, however, that the Astler-Coller C1 and C2 designations were a uniquely valuable contribution to prognostic discrimination.

▶ **TABLE 22-3 Dukes' Classification of Rectal Cancer (1944)**

Stage	Classification
A	Carcinoma confined to wall of rectum
B	Carcinoma spread by direct continuity to perirectal tissue; no lymph node metastasis
C_1	Metastasis present in nodes but not to ligature
C_2	Metastasis present in nodes to level of ligature

▶ **TABLE 22-4 Modified Dukes' Clinicopathologic Classification of Colorectal Cancer**

Stage	Classification
A	Carcinoma confined to wall of bowel
B	Carcinoma spread by direct continuity to perirectal or pericolonic tissue; no lymph node metastasis
C	Metastasis present in regional lymph node
D	Omental implant; peritoneal seeding; metastasis beyond the confines of surgical resection

Opinion

I agree with Goligher that the various classifications proposed can create only confusion and mislead the reader interpreting the surgical results from one institution to another. He observed:

> It is the unalienable right of every pathologist and surgeon to evolve his own system for categorizing the extent of spread of cancers of the colon and rectum . . . [but] I suggest that it would be more useful to restrain his urge to classify and accept Dukes' categorization exactly as it was defined by him.[318]

Despite this suggestion, the Council of the American Society of Colon and Rectal Surgeons (1991) endorsed the TNM staging classification. More's the pity, for I believe that the clinicopathologic classification of Dukes fulfills all reasonable criteria for prognostication. Other studies comparing the various staging classifications concur with this conclusion.[146,205,268,269,535,674] Sadly, the plea for romance and historical precedent has inevitably fallen on deaf ears—the TNM classification has become the benchmark that we all must accept and adopt.

Lymphatic Invasion

The importance of lymph node involvement by tumor has been well established in providing important prognostic information.[299,304,333,346] It seems reasonable, therefore, that if one were to use special clearing techniques, a greater number of lymph nodes will be identified, thereby improving the ability to prognosticate.[346,432,735] Koren and colleagues proposed the use of a new lymph node–revealing solution composed of various traditional fixatives and fatty solvents to clear the mesentery and identify more lymph nodes.[493] In 30 problematic cases, in which an unsatisfactory number of lymph nodes were found by the traditional method, this approach resulted in upstaging a number of tumors from Dukes' B to C. The number of positive nodes has been shown in one study to be a more accurate predictor of survival than depth of tumor penetration.[1038] I have not routinely employed a clearing technique, but I believe that if

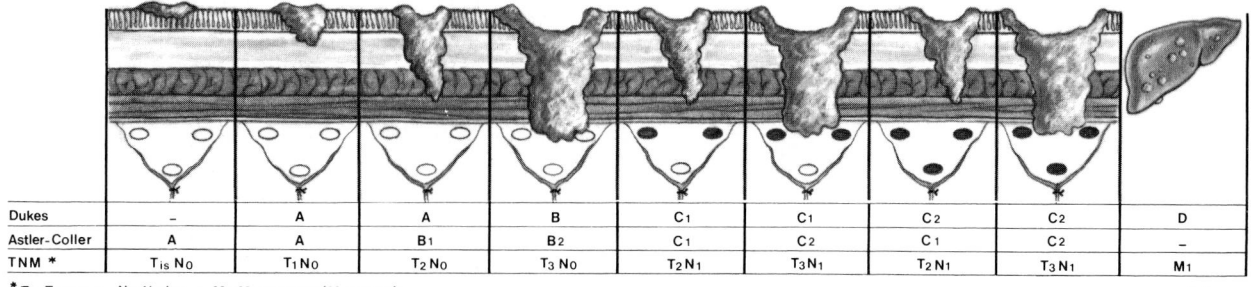

FIGURE 22-31. Comparison of staging classifications for colorectal carcinoma.

Dukes	–	A	A	B	C₁	C₁	C₂	C₂	D
Astler-Coller	A	A	B₁	B₂	C₁	C₂	C₁	C₂	–
TNM *	Tis N0	T₁N0	T₂N0	T₃N0	T₂N₁	T₃N₁	T₂N₁	T₃N₁	M₁

* T = Tumor · N = Nodes · M = Metastases (M₀= none)

all laboratories vigorously pursued lymph node identification, a greater consistency in reporting the results of treatment would be achieved.

Tsakraklides and colleagues evaluated the histologic morphology of lymph nodes in an attempt to improve prognostic ability.[959] They found a higher rate of survival (which was not statistically significant) in patients whose nodes showed germinal center predominance compared with those whose nodes showed lymphocyte predominance, the "unstimulated pattern."

Cutait and colleagues demonstrated that by using immunoperoxidase staining of CEA and cytokeratins of lymph nodes previously considered free of disease, restaging of 22 nodes became necessary.[189] However, follow-up at 5 years failed to show any statistically significant difference in survival.

TABLE 22-5 Tumor Staging with Tumor-Node-Metastasis (TNM) System

Stage	Description
T_x	Primary tumor cannot be assessed
T_0	No evidence of primary tumor
T_{is}	Carcinoma-*in-situ*
T_1	Tumor invades submucosa
T_2	Tumor invades muscularis propria
T_3	Tumor invades through muscularis propria into the subserosa or into the nonperitonealized pericolic or perirectal tissue
T_4	Tumor directly invades other organs or structures and/or perforates the visceral peritoneum
N_x	Regional lymph nodes cannot be evaluated
N_0	No invasion of regional lymph nodes
N_1	Invasion of one to three lymph nodes
N_2	Invasion of four or more regional lymph nodes
M_x	Distant metastases cannot be determined
M_0	No distant metastases or residual tumor
M_1	Distant metastases or residual tumor present

Blood Vessel Invasion

Compared with lymph node involvement, the importance of blood vessel invasion (Figure 22-32) has been emphasized to a much lesser extent.[102,107,270] However, the prognostic implication of blood vessel invasion has been well established,[177,864] a fact that has stimulated different approaches to the technique of surgical removal of the tumor (see later).[48,270,815,960] It should be axiomatic that the pathologist seek to identify and report invasion of blood vessels with the same concern applied to identifying involvement of lymph nodes.

Neural Invasion

Like blood vessel invasion, neural invasion has prognostic import—that is, the presence of perineural invasion implies a more ominous prognosis than if such invasion were not present.

DNA Content or DNA Ploidy

Some studies have suggested that tumor DNA content, as determined by flow cytometry, can provide valuable information about the biologic behavior of neoplastic cells and is therefore an important prognostic factor in determining survival.[25,46,489,838,1017] Aneuploid (nondiploid) tumors contain a population of cells that exhibit a DNA content distinctly different from the DNA noted in "normal" (diploid) malignant cells. For example, Scott and colleagues reported that DNA nondiploid rectal carcinomas were associated with a statistically significant increased incidence of vascular invasion, tumor fibrosis, and advanced Dukes' stage.[837] In another study from the same unit, these cancers also were associated with a significantly poorer prognosis in patients with unresectable disease.[838] Kokal and colleagues demonstrated that in comparison with diploid tumors, tumors with abnormal DNA content tended to be less well differentiated, to invade the serosa or extend beyond, and to have lymph node metastases.[490] It should be remembered, however, that tumor cell DNA content, although it can be an independent prognostic factor, is not as

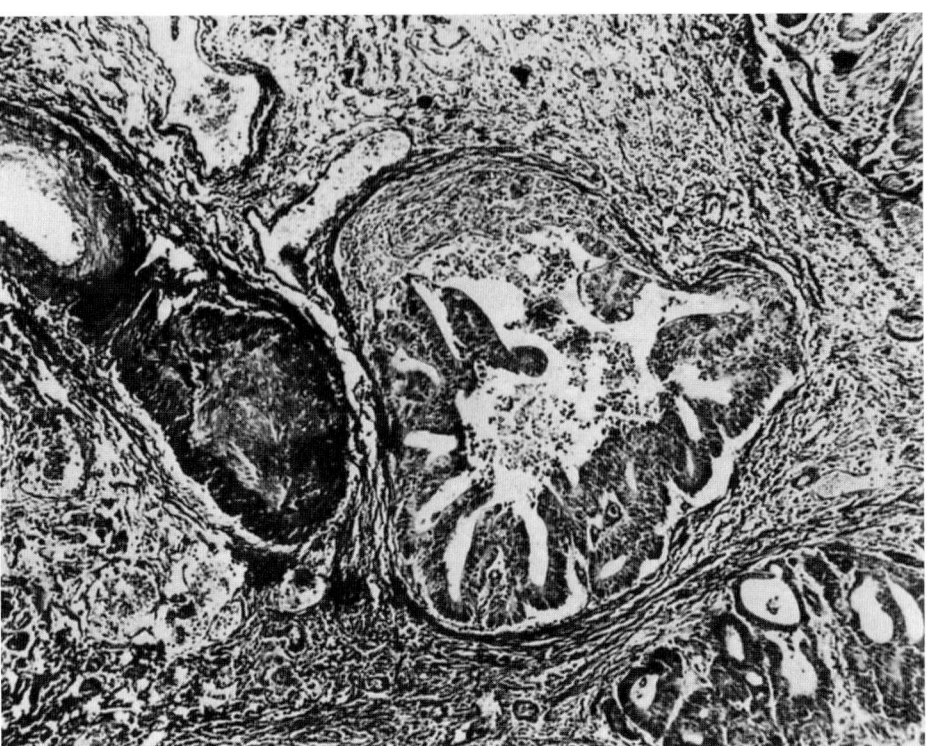

FIGURE 22-32. Blood vessel invasion by colonic adenocarcinoma. Note the extensive growth of tumor inside the vein that has thin, black elastica in its wall and fibrous thickening of the intima in the artery **(left)**. (Original magnification × 80; from Corman ML, Swinton NW Sr, O'Keefe DD, et al. Colorectal carcinoma at the Lahey Clinic, 1962–1966. *Am J Surg* 1973; 125:424.)

accurate as Dukes' classification in this respect.[95,398,832] Deans and associates performed flow cytometry on 312 patients with adenocarcinoma of the colon and rectum and found by univariate survival analysis that no flow cytometric variable was statistically significantly related to survival.[206] They concluded that Dukes' stage, patient age, and tumor differentiation are the variables most closely related to survival, and that conventional histologic variables remain the best predictors of prognosis for this condition.[206] Others believe, however, that tumor DNA content is the single most important prognostic factor among all the clinical and pathologic variables available.[204,490,491] Although there may be some controversy in this respect, there is no disagreement that nondiploid lesions are generally associated with a greater level of invasion and therefore a more advanced Dukes' stage.

Oncogene Analysis

Rowley and colleagues compared DNA ploidy and nuclear-expressed p62 c-*myc* oncogene in the prognosis of colorectal cancer.[797] As discussed earlier, oncogenes exist in the normal human genome as proto-oncogenes but may be activated by various means in tumors, including overexpression and mutation (see also Chapter 21).[797] The authors could not suggest a replacement for Dukes' staging system for prognostication, but observed that the combination of ploidy status and oncogene expression predicted survival better than ploidy alone.

Nucleolar Organizer Regions

Nucleolar organizer regions are loops of ribosomal DNA in nuclei that direct ribosome and protein formation.[655] Moran and colleagues studied the prognostic implication of these regions, as well as ploidy, in individuals with advanced colorectal cancer.[655] They concluded that nucleolar organizer regions are the most important individual variable for predicting survival, whereas ploidy values are equivalent to histologic differentiation.

Nuclear Morphology

Mitmaker and colleagues studied nuclear shape as a possible factor in determining prognosis.[639] The nuclear shape factor was defined as the degree of circularity of the nucleus, with a perfect circle recorded as 1.0. A shape value greater than 0.84 was associated with a poor outcome, and indeed was the most significant predictor of survival even when corrections were made for sex, age, histologic grade, and Dukes' classification.

Doppler Perfusion Index

Leen and co-workers assessed the relative value of Dukes' staging and the Doppler perfusion index (DPI) as prognostic indices in individuals who underwent apparently curative surgery for colorectal cancer.[520] This index, the ratio of hepatic arterial to total liver blood flow, was measured before resection by means of duplex/color Doppler sonography. The authors observed that the DPI identified two groups of individuals—78% of those with an abnormally elevated DPI value had recurrent disease or died, whereas 97% of those with a normal DPI value survived. The implications concerning the suitability for adjuvant therapy following apparent curative resection are clear.

Tumor Budding

Tumor "budding" refers to the presence of microscopic clusters of undifferentiated cancer cells ahead of the invasive front of the lesion. This has been believed to have prognostic significance with respect to cure rates following resection for colon and rectal cancer. Hase and colleagues analyzed all surgical specimens for this phenomenon in 663 patients who underwent curative resection.[392] The presence of severe budding was associated with a poorer prognosis and paralleled a more invasive Dukes' classification.

Miscellaneous

Lindmark and co-workers, in an attempt to identify better prognostic predictors than Dukes' classification, studied 212 patients by means of clinical, histopathologic, cellular, and serologic tumor characteristics.[535] Dukes' stage was the most powerful variable. Others found significant survival associations with erythrocyte sedimentation rate, leukocyte blood count, alkaline phosphatase level, aspartate aminotransferase level, number of small blood vessels, age of the patient, and six different serum tumor markers.

Proliferating Cell Nuclear Antigen Expression

Cellular proliferative activity has been shown to be a useful indicator of biologic aggressiveness in colorectal carcinoma. Choi and associates investigated the correlation between proliferative activity and malignancy potential in colorectal cancers to determine whether the proliferative index of cancer cells has prognostic significance.[153] Utilizing immunohistochemical methods involving a monoclonal antibody to proliferating cell nuclear antigen (PCNA), they obtained 86 pathologic sections and compared PCNA with conventional clinicopathologic factors as well as other prognostic parameters. The authors determined that PCNA at the invasive tumor margin was a valuable predictor for determining those individuals with a higher potential for metastasis or recurrence.[153]

Anatomic Distribution

Numerous reports have demonstrated a change in the distribution of colorectal carcinoma.[1,130,184,323,338,657,869] It had long been thought that 75% of colorectal cancers were within the range of the rigid proctosigmoidoscope.

More recent data suggest that the figure should be closer to 60%.

Whether the trend to more proximal location of tumors will continue is impossible to say. Figure 22-33 illustrates the distribution of tumors based on our decade report of the 1970s.[178] In the beginning and at the end of the decade, we noted no change in the location of cancers. Rectal and sigmoid lesions together encompassed 67% in the previous 5-year study and 68% in the most recent report. Ascending colonic lesions were present in 18% of the patients in each group.

Cady and associates reviewed almost 6,000 resected specimens of the large bowel that had been removed during a 40-year period (1928 to 1967).[130] During this time, the incidence of cancer of the right side of the colon increased from 7% to 22%, and the incidence of rectosigmoid, sigmoid, and rectal carcinomas fell from 80% to 62%. These changes represented statistically significant differences. A trend to smaller tumors was also evident, with less frequent lymph node involvement of the distal lesions, possibly reflecting an improvement in early detection. Beart and colleagues reviewed the Mayo Clinic experience by studying the new cases diagnosed among residents of Rochester, Minnesota, between 1940 and 1979.[53]

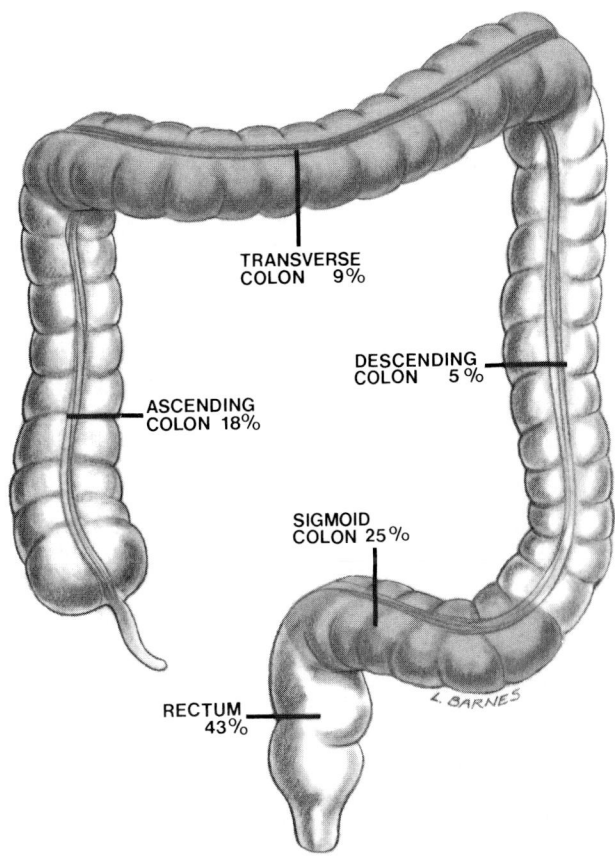

FIGURE 22-33. Distribution of colon and rectal cancer.

They found an increase in the incidence of proximal lesions (from 15.1/100,000 person-years in 1940 to 1959 to 17.3/100,000 in 1960 to 1979). This coincided with a fall in distal lesions (from 35.5/100,000 person-years to 28.2/100,000 person-years). In a 2002 report from the Netherlands, the incidence of colorectal cancer has almost doubled from 1981 to 1996 while the proportion of proximal cancers increased from 25% to 37%.[626] Gonzalez and colleagues found that increased age, female gender, black non-Hispanic race, and the presence of comorbid illnesses were factors associated with a greater likelihood of developing colorectal cancer in a proximal location.[323] In a Veterans Administration study, black race was likewise shown to be associated with a higher incidence of right-sided tumors than that of whites.[184]

A possible explanation for the observed increase in the proportion of more proximal colon cancers is the "search and destroy" concept for the management of colorectal polyps. This is particularly true when the polyp is within range of the shorter instrument. By clearing the rectum through electrocoagulation, biopsy excision, and snare excision, one essentially prevents the subsequent development of a distal malignancy. Another obvious implication is the limitation of proctoscopy or flexible sigmoidoscopy as a screening tool.

SURGICAL TREATMENT

Historical Perspective

Resection of the bowel with intestinal anastomosis is a relatively recent operation. In 1818, Zang declared that "every intestinal suture is a mighty procedure in a highly vulnerable organ, and therefore a dangerous, yes, a very dangerous undertaking."[281] Exteriorization was the method of treatment for intestinal disease and injury, a technique that had remained essentially unchanged for more than two millennia.

Reybard of Lyons in 1833 was the first to perform a successful resection of the sigmoid colon; for this he was criticized by the Paris Academy of Medicine.[14,778] Colostomy was advocated as a palliative procedure as early as 1839. Before this time, an occasional obstructing carcinoma of the colon was relieved by the spontaneous formation of a fecal fistula, when it was relieved at all. Before 1889, the mortality rate for colonic resection was 60%, but this figure had been reduced to 37% by 1900.[656] Because of the high mortality for intraabdominal resection and anastomosis, the staged extraperitoneal operations of Paul,[725] von Mikulicz,[631] and Bloch[86] (exteriorization-resection) were usually employed.

Jean-François Reybard (1790–1863) Reybard was born in Cloisia (Jura) in France near the Swiss border. His parents were farmers. His father was also the mayor of the community and was therefore able to send his son to college at Nantes and then to Lyons for the completion of his studies. Reybard developed an interest in medicine while at the university and became an assistant at the Hôtel-Dieu in 1813 when he was 18 years old. While at the Charity Hospital, he had the opportunity of seeing the horrible consequences of war injuries, the result of Napoleon's campaigns. When the city of Lyons was occupied by the Austrians, Reybard treated the wounds of both sides. In 1816, he was appointed to the Faculty of Medicine at Lyons. In 1827, he reported the results of his experiments on intestinal suturing. In May, 1833, he successfully performed a resection of the sigmoid colon with a primary anastomosis on a 28-year-old man, although the tumor recurred 6 months later. Because of skepticism from the Academy, he offered to repeat the procedure on dogs, but all seven died. While performing an operation for anal fistula, he stuck himself, developed septicemia, and succumbed 5 days later.

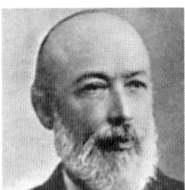

Frank Thomas Paul (1851–1941) Paul was born at Pentney, Norfolk, England and was educated at the Yarmouth grammar school. In 1869, he entered Guy's Hospital and qualified as a Member of the Royal College of Surgeons in 1873. After a year as resident house surgeon, he left London for Liverpool, where he practiced for the rest of his professional life. In 1875, he was made the first resident medical officer at the Liverpool Royal Infirmary. He became successively pathologist, lecturer in dental surgery, professor of medical jurisprudence, and surgeon to the Royal Infirmary. His 1891 article on exteriorization-resection, using "Paul's tube," antedated the modification described by von Mikulicz by a dozen years. Although he wrote little else, he was considered a masterful technician. Lord Moynihan of Leeds often visited his theater, observing that Paul was "the neatest operator he had ever seen." Another visitor stated, "Paul, operating in the heyday of his manual efficiency, always made me think that he did with his hands what Pavlova did with her feet, only Paul's work was much more useful." He retired to grow orchids and died in his ninetieth year. (Photo from *Br J Surg* 1951;39:195, with permission.)

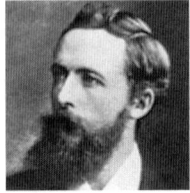

Johann von Mikulicz-Radecki (1850–1905) Mikulicz was born in Cernowicz in the Balkan Peninsula, then a part of the Austro-Hungarian Empire. He was educated at Hermannstadt and earned his way through the university by giving piano lessons and playing the organ. He achieved the M.D. degree in Vienna in 1875 and became an assistant to Billroth. At the age of 32, he was appointed director and professor of surgery at Krakow, Poland. While there, he performed the first esophageal resection and introduced lateral pharyngotomy for excision of malignant tumors of the tonsillar region. In 1887, Mikulicz became director of the clinic and professor of surgery at Konigsburg. At the age of 40 (1890), he moved to Breslau as Professor of Surgery, a position he held until his death. One of the great innovative minds of nineteenth-century surgery, Mikulicz's name has been used eponymously for varied conditions and procedures, including Mikulicz's cells, disease, drain, line, mask, ointment, and at least ten operations (e.g., exteriorization-resection of the colon).

The initial attempts to coapt ends of intestine involved insertion of various objects into the lumina of the cut ends of the bowel, with or without the addition of sutures. These procedures involved the use of a reed pipe, goose trachea, cardboard smeared with sweet oil, a cylinder of fish glue, a wax ring, and a silver ring, to name a few.[281,503] Balfour suggested the use of a tube stent.[44] Probably the most famous internal stent was the Murphy "button" (Figure 22-34).[667] Introduced in 1892, it quickly became the primary method of anastomosing bowel.

Until the nineteenth century, most surgeons regarded wounds of the intestine as a *noli me tangere* (do not touch), believing that nature would be more successful in the healing process than any artificial attempt to effect closure.[848] Travers (1812) is believed to be the pioneer in the use of sutures to perform intestinal anastomoses.[955] Lembert (1826) is eponymously associated with a type of intestinal suturing that produced a serosa-to-serosa apposition.[525] As he was with so many other operative innovations, Billroth was also

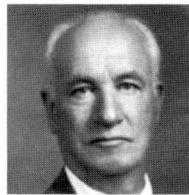

Donald Church Balfour (1882–1963)   Donald Balfour was born in Toronto, Canada and obtained his undergraduate education at the Hamilton Collegiate Institute. He was graduated from the University of Toronto Medical School in 1906. In 1907, Balfour became an assistant in pathology at the Mayo Clinic in Rochester, Minnesota and became, successively, a junior surgeon and, in 1912, Head of a Section of General Surgery. In 1937, he became Director of the Department of Surgery. In 1910, he married Carrie Mayo, daughter of William J. Mayo. Balfour wrote on varied subjects, including tonsillectomy and thyroid and biliary procedures, but he gradually focused his research and writings on gastrointestinal surgery. He devised a number of instruments—an abdominal retractor, an operating table, and an operating room mirror. Among his many offices and honorary fellowships, he was one of the founders of the World Medical Organization and a charter member of the World Health Organization.

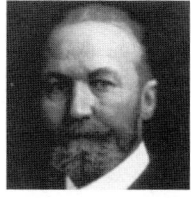

John B. Murphy (1857–1916)   John Murphy was born in Appleton, Wisconsin, the son of Irish immigrant pioneers. He entered the Rush Medical College in Chicago and graduated in 1879, winning the "first place" position as intern at the Cook County Hospital. In 1882, following 2 years of medical practice, he traveled for 18 months throughout Europe and came under the direction of Billroth in Vienna. On his return to practice in Chicago, he became known as a bold, brilliant surgeon and teacher, an indefatigable worker, and an innovator. Although he was often the subject of controversy ("the stormy petrel of surgery"), he was always greatly respected. In succession, he became Chief Surgeon at Chicago's Mercy Hospital, Professor of Surgery at the Northwestern University Medical School, Chief of the Editorial Staff of the journal *Surgery, Gynecology and Obstetrics*, and President of the American Medical Association. He was a founder and regent of the American College of Surgeons and a recipient of numerous honorary titles. His writings were diverse and numerous and included treatises on the following: gunshot wounds of the abdomen; appendicitis; ileus; and vascular, pulmonary, neurologic, and orthopedic surgery. His interests in experimental surgery inspired the anastomotic button. Although controversial even in his day, it is still appreciated and indeed imitated as an ingenious method of circumventing some of the risks of conventional suture technique.

Antoine Lembert (1802–1851)   Lembert was born April 19, 1802 in Nancy, France. Very little biographic information is available concerning his life, and no rendering of his likeness has been found. He studied under Guillaume Dupuytren in Paris, where he was epidemiologist to the Seine-Départment. In 1828, he won a 5,000-franc prize from the Académie des Sciences for his essay, *la Méthode Endermique*. He is particularly remembered for his intestinal suture, an inverting technique used in circular enterorrhaphy which was published in 1826 *(Mémoire sur l'entéroraphie avec la description d'un procédé nouveau pour pratiquer cette opération chirurgicale)*. What has come to be known as Lembert's approach ensures serosa-to-serosal apposition, the cornerstone of contemporary gastric and intestinal suturing. Johann Dieffenbach is credited with being the first person to employ his method successfully. Lembert died of stomach cancer at the age of 49.

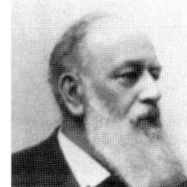

Christian Albert Theodor Billroth (1829–1894)   Billroth was born in Bergen, on the Baltic Sea island of Rgen. When he was 5 years old, his father, an impoverished preacher, died, leaving a young widow with five sons, the youngest being Theodor. Billroth was considered a poor student, possibly, by today's terminology, dyslexic. He wished to pursue a musical career; however, his mother and physician uncle encouraged him to enter medical school at the University of Greifswald in 1848. Although he was an indifferent student at that institution, he became inspired when he followed Professor Baum to the University of Göttingen. After 3 years of physiologic and pathologic investigations in a number of areas, he completed his studies in Berlin under von Langenbeck. After a year and a half of military service, travel, and failure to establish a general practice, Billroth fortunately obtained a position as assistant in the Langenbeck Clinic, his entree into surgery. In 1859, he was appointed Professor of Surgery in Zurich. It was there that he wrote his famous textbook, *General Surgical Pathology and Therapy*, which ran through 11 editions. He also wrote a number of musical pieces. In 1867, Billroth accepted a professorship of surgery in Vienna. He was the first surgeon to resect the stomach for cancer, the first to resect the esophagus, and the first to perform a laryngectomy. Billroth declined many offers of other positions, including the chair in Berlin, preferring to remain in his adopted Austrian homeland with his close musical companions, Johannes Brahms and Johann Strauss. Billroth's classic paper on intestinal anastomosis is printed in translation (Concerning enterorrhaphy. *Dis Colon Rectum* 1986;29:284–287 [Über enteroraphie. *Wien Med Wochenschr* 1879;1:1–6]).

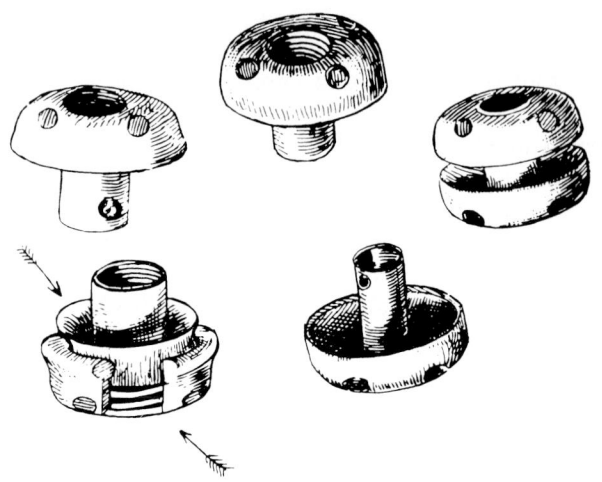

FIGURE 22-34. Murphy button, with and without spring cup attachment. (From Murphy JB. Cholecysto-intestinal, gastro-intestinal and entero-intestinal anastomosis, and approximation without sutures. *Med Rec N Y* 1892;42:665.)

one of the leaders of intestinal anastomotic surgery. In 1887, Halsted reported an experimental study demonstrating the submucosa to be the primary layer responsible for a safe and secure anastomosis and emphasized the importance of inversion of the intestinal suture line.[372] This was confirmed in a subsequent report.[373] Later, Connell described his continuous inverting suture.[170] Allis simplified the technique of suturing intestine when he introduced his tenaculum forceps in 1901.[17] For an excellent, comprehensive review of the history and evolution of the diverse anastomotic techniques developed before the twentieth century, one should read Senn's classic article on the subject.[848] A wonderful, contemporary perspective can be gleaned from the article by Steichen and Ravitch.[894]

In the twentieth century, resection of the colon and primary anastomosis did not become generally used until the antibiotic era. In fact, in many centers, resection of the sigmoid colon was not attempted without a diversionary colostomy until the 1950s. Dixon, among others, is regarded as one of the advocates of primary anastomosis

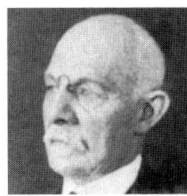

William Stewart Halsted (1852–1922)   William Halsted was born in New York City to a prominent, affluent family. He attended Phillips Academy in Andover, Massachusetts and received his A.B. degree from Yale University in 1874. He entered medical school at the Columbia University College of Physicians and Surgeons in New York and graduated first in his class in 1877. After a time at Bellevue Hospital in New York, he became the first house physician at New York Hospital. In 1878, he went to Europe to study at the great institutions of the day. It was through his association with the German, Austrian, and Swiss masters that he developed his passionate interest in clinical and laboratory investigation. Returning to New York in the fall of 1880, he began his practice of surgery. Within a period of 6 years, he held appointments, including chief surgeon, in at least eight hospitals. His clinical duties were awesome, but he still managed to be actively involved in teaching and research. When an infected finger became complicated by painful neuritis, Halsted sought relief by the use of cocaine and became habituated. As an invalid unable to carry on his practice, he came to Baltimore in 1887, having been attracted to the university under the leadership of William Welch. It was there that his genius for investigation flourished. In 1899, Halsted was elected Surgeon-in-Chief of the Johns Hopkins Hospital, subsequently leading that department for 33 years. He laid the foundation for a model training school for surgeons and introduced numerous instruments and techniques: rubber gloves, hemostat, "mosquito" forceps, and "cigarette" drain, to mention only a few. He was an advocate of fine silk sutures, as opposed to catgut. His study of a comparison of suture techniques to effect intestinal anastomosis is generally regarded as the best example of the importance of laboratory investigation to the clinical setting. Halsted can with justification be called the father of American surgery.

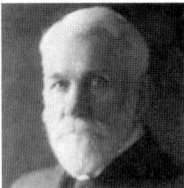

Oscar Huntington Allis (1836–1921)   Oscar Allis was born in Holley, New York, a direct descendant of a Puritan settler of the first colony at Salem, Massachusetts. He attended Lafayette College, receiving an M.A. degree in 1864, and graduated from Jefferson Medical College in 1866. Following an internship at the Philadelphia General Hospital, he ultimately became one of the original surgeons at the Presbyterian Hospital of Philadelphia. Allis acquired a special interest in orthopedic surgery and was recognized as an authority on fractures and dislocations. Relaxation of the fascia between the iliac crest and the greater trochanter, a sign of fracture of the neck of the femur, is Allis' sign. Among his many valuable contributions to surgery were his dissector, his ether inhaler, and his splint—all called by his name. Today, Allis forceps continue to be one of the standard instruments in any general kit.

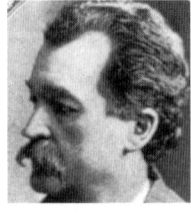

Nicholas Senn (1844–1908)   Nicholas Senn was born in the canton of St. Gall in Switzerland. In 1852, he came with his parents to the United States and settled in the frontier town of Ashford, Wisconsin. Following 2 years at a local country school, he attended Northwestern University. In 1865, he entered the Chicago Medical College, and on completing the course of study there, he won the competitive examination for residency at the Cook County Hospital. He practiced for 5 years in the small town of Elmore, Wisconsin, and in 1877 he traveled to Munich, where he spent a year studying bacteriology. Returning to Milwaukee, he was called to the Chair in Surgery at the College of Physicians and Surgeons in Chicago. In 1888, he became Professor of Surgical Pathology at the Rush Medical College. Senn was a prolific writer, his manuscripts comprising 160 volumes. His personal library was believed to be the best private medical collection in America. Senn was one of the first surgeons in the Western hemisphere to recognize the importance of the animal laboratory as a resource for improving and modifying surgical technique. In association with Connell, it was said that he "constructed the arch and placed the keystone in the structure of intestinal anastomosis."

without colostomy.[217] Numerous articles have been written that address the means to avoid fecal contamination with bowel resection (closed anastomosis with noncrushing clamps; rubber-shod clamps) and to avoid inverting too much tissue (e.g., the Gambee suture).[290] To complicate the issue further, Getzen and associates advocated the use of eversion, concluding that it produces a more secure anastomosis than inversion.[297] Although this contention was supported by some studies,[134,374,396,540] other reports refuted the observation.[322,806] The hand-sewn eversion technique is in disfavor and should not be used.

De Petz was not the first person to describe a stapling device, but he is generally credited with having produced the initial practical instrument, employing it for gastrectomy.[213] Stapling techniques, however, were developed as early as 1908 by Hültl and Fischer.[895] However, the real credit must be given to the Russians for producing the contemporary stapling instruments.[281] They, as well as others, performed stapled anastomoses that were sometimes everting and sometimes inverting.[22,761,762] Ultimately, the Russian SPTU gun was described. It produced an inverting end-to-end anastomosis by means of a circular row of staples placed within the lumen of the bowel. The United States Surgical Corporation (Norwalk, CT) was the initial developer of stapling instruments in this country, and other American companies produced further modifications. Reports of their successful application are myriad.[319,321,394,763,773] The latest major innovations involve the application to laparoscopic bowel surgery (see Chapter 27).

Preoperative Preparation

For elective colon resection in the United States, patients are usually admitted to the hospital the day of surgery, depending on the likelihood of achieving an adequate bowel cleansing if the preparation is undertaken on an outpatient basis. A more prolonged hospitalization to prepare the bowel or to perform preoperative testing is generally not believed to be necessary and, in the era of cost containment, can rarely be justified to insurance carriers, even when the indications are reasonable.

Several studies have been published comparing inpatient and outpatient preparation for elective colorectal surgery.[282,376,519,731] Results of both approaches are certainly comparable with respect to surgical complications.

However, individuals with medical problems may not tolerate extensive fluid shifts and may require intravenous supplementation and monitoring.[519] Certainly, if the preoperative preparation cannot be performed with safety because of medical conditions (cardiac, renal, hepatic) or because of certain logistic concerns, the procedure should be undertaken in a hospital setting.

Mechanical Preparation

A bowel preparation regimen consists of appropriate dietary restriction and mechanical cleansing. The use of nonabsorbable antibiotics the day before surgery is still considered an option, but more and more surgeons have accepted the comparably favorable results reported in many studies and utilize perioperative systemic antibiotics on the day of surgery. Generally, the patient is placed on a clear liquid diet 24 hours before the operation. Ideally, the mechanical preparation begins at noon the day before surgery. A vigorous cathartic is administered at this time so that its effect will have dissipated in time for the patient to have a reasonable night of sleep. The choice of laxative is a matter of the surgeon's personal experience or prejudice, because when adjusted for dosage, most laxatives have a comparable effect. However, patients may prefer the taste of one to another or perceive that one produces less discomfort than another. Castor oil (2 oz), magnesium citrate (10 oz), and X-Prep liquid (2.5 oz) are relatively equivalent in producing the desired results. Some surgeons prefer "whole-gut" irrigation with or without a nasogastric tube; others adopt an oral colonic lavage with a 10% mannitol solution (see Chapter 5).[59,60,232,272,386,441] In a survey of 269 members of the American Society of Colon and Rectal Surgeons published in 1990, 51% used cathartics and enemas as the primary method of bowel cleansing, whereas 43% used a polyethylene glycol (PEG) lavage.[58] My own preference is a well-tolerated and effective regimen, oral Fleet phosphosoda ACCU-PREP (60 to 90 mL). Another option that has achieved some converts is the use of Visicol tablets (sodium phosphate monobasic monohydrate, USP, sodium phosphate dibasic anhydrous, USP). This has the advantage of the patient consuming virtually tasteless tablets with comparable cleansing efficacy in clinical trials. At least of equal or perhaps greater importance than the administration of the cathartic itself, according to many surgeons, is the use of enemas until the returns are clear on the morning of the

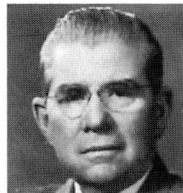

Claude F. Dixon (1893–1968) Claude Dixon was born in Piedmont, Kansas and received his Doctor of Science degree from the University of Kansas in 1919 and his medical degree from the same institution in 1921. Following an internship at the University of Kansas Hospital, he entered the Mayo Graduate School in Rochester, Minnesota as a resident in surgery. In 1928, he became a member of the Mayo Clinic staff and Head of the Section of General Surgery, a post he held until he retired in 1957. With a special interest in abdominal surgery, particularly surgery of the colon, Dixon became one of the leaders in the development of anterior resection. He was also a recognized authority in surgery of the head and neck and contributed more than 300 articles to the surgical literature.

operation. The fact is that most surgeons base their protocol in this area on their subjective experience and habit.[1059]

Wolters and colleagues undertook a prospective, randomized study of preoperative bowel cleansing utilizing three different methods—gut irrigation with Ringer's lactate, Prepacol (a combined preparation comprising bisacodyl tablets and sodium phosphate solution), and PEG.[1040] All were equally effective in cleansing the bowel. However, the postoperative complication rate was significantly increased in the Prepacol group despite its being tolerated better. Overall, the authors observed that PEG is the recommended bowel preparation for individuals undergoing elective colorectal surgery. Oliveira and colleagues also performed a randomized, controlled study in which sodium phosphate and PEG-based oral lavage solutions were compared.[706] Although the two were equally effective and safe, patient tolerance was much greater with the sodium phosphate.

The question has been posed as to whether mechanical bowel preparation is truly necessary. This seems counterintuitive, suggesting that one turn back the clock to those bad-old-days of a high incidence of septic complications following elective colon surgery. Still, all surgeons agree that it is preferable to deal with formed stool in the bowel rather than to have watery feces spilling into the peritoneal cavity as a consequence of an incomplete preparation.

van Geldere and colleagues prospectively analyzed 250 consecutive operations without a mechanical bowel preparation, with no deleterious consequences observed.[971] Burke and co-workers also reported whether a mechanical bowel preparation for elective colorectal surgery was indeed required.[116] Patients were randomized to receive a standard mechanical preparation or none. The overall morbidity rate (18%) was similar in the two groups. The two deaths that occurred were both in individuals who had received bowel preparations. The authors concluded that bowel preparation does not affect the outcome after elective colorectal surgery.[116] Zmora and associates randomized patients undergoing elective colon surgery into two groups: ethylene glycol bowel preparation and no mechanical preparation.[1058] Almost 200 patients were allocated to each group. There were no statistically significant differences between the two with respect to overall septic complications (10.2 versus 8.8%), wound infection (6.4 versus 5.7%), anastomotic leak (3.7 versus 2.1%), and abdominal abscess (1.1 versus 1%). In a metaanalysis of randomized trials, Wille-Jørgensen and colleagues found no evidence in the literature for any beneficial effects from the use of bowel cleansing.[1015]

Antibiotics

The nonabsorbable antibiotic regimen advocated by Nichols and co-workers has been believed to reduce the incidence of infectious complications.[684] This consists of neomycin (1 g) and an erythromycin base (1 g) at 1 PM, 2 PM, and 11 PM the day before surgery. The use of a broad-spectrum systemic antibiotic immediately preoperatively, intraoperatively, and for one or two doses postoperatively has been suggested in numerous experimental regimens to reduce the incidence of infection following elective colon resection.[210,255,326,609,624,997,1019] In a survey of 352 colon and rectal surgeons, all favored some antibiotic preparation.[874] Eighty-eight percent preferred a combined regimen with oral and systemic antibiotics. Condon and associates, as well as others, have demonstrated no discernible benefit from adding parenteral antibiotic prophylaxis in elective colon surgery if mechanical cleansing and neomycin and erythromycin are employed.[169,900] However, other investigators have found that the addition of perioperative parenteral cefoxitin, in comparison with oral antimicrobial agents alone, greatly reduces the incidence of wound infections in patients undergoing elective colorectal surgery.[510] We showed that single preoperative doses of cefuroxime and metronidazole are as effective in the prevention of postoperative infections associated with colorectal surgery as standard therapy with four doses of cefoxitin, but single doses of either cefuroxime or cefoxitin were less effective than the combination regimen.[176] Others reached a similar conclusion with the use of a single 2-g dose of cefotetan, given preoperatively and 12 hours postoperatively.[442,662] Favorable results were reported with a single intravenous dose of Timentin (ticarcillin-clavulanic acid),[82,191,965] metronidazole-netilmicin,[82] ceftizoxime,[1030] and mezlocillin.[965] Still others have found that oral ciprofloxacin offers advantages in efficacy and ease of administration and is as effective as other parenteral antibiotics.[605] Jensen and colleagues concluded, on the basis of their prospective, randomized trial, that a single dose of an appropriate antibiotic in acute or elective colorectal surgery is as protective for infection as a triple-dose regimen.[453]

Song and Glenny utilized several databases and found 147 relevant trials in order to assess the relative efficacy of antimicrobial prophylaxis for the prevention of postoperative wound infection in patients undergoing elective colorectal surgery.[875] Although they confirmed that antibiotic prophylaxis is indeed effective, they could not demonstrate statistically significant benefit with one or another regimen. Still, they were able to show that certain regimens are *inadequate*. These include metronidazole alone, doxycycline alone, piperacillin alone, and *oral neomycin and erythromycin the day before surgery* (note the earlier discussion). Furthermore, they concluded that a single dose administered immediately (or within 1 hour) before the operation is as effective as long-term postoperative antimicrobial prophylaxis.[875]

Opinion and Recommendations

It is clear that systematic antibiotic prophylaxis is indicated for elective colon surgery. Furthermore, there is no good evidence to suggest that the oral preparations administered the day before add any benefit. Therefore, the so-called Nichols/Condon preparation should be abandoned. All studies which determine effective blood levels with systemically administered antibiotics indicate that the drug should be circulating within 1 hour before making the incision, ideally less. The likely pathogens when performing colorectal surgery are enteric gram-negative bacilli, anaerobes, and enterococci. Therefore, the most beneficial and cost-effective drugs for elective, uncomplicated colorectal surgery are cefotetan, cefmetazole, or cefoxitin. Another alternative is cefazolin plus metronidazole. In the individual who is allergic to penicillin, flouroquinolone plus clindamycin is preferred (Medicare Quality Improvement Preoject, 2002). When there has been gross fecal contamination, in the presence of obstruction, perforation, abscess, when there has been a prolonged operative time or excessive blood loss, I believe that antibiotics should be continued beyond the recommended one or two postoperative doses. A patient with valvular heart disease and immunocompromised individuals require special consideration with respect to antibiotics (see Chapter 4).

Urinary Catheter

An indwelling urinary catheter should be placed for all bowel operations in my opinion. It may be removed the day after surgery if there has been no pelvic dissection. For an abdominoperineal resection or low pelvic operation, the urinary catheter should remain in place for 5 to 7 days in order to minimize the likelihood of subsequent urinary retention.

Ureteral Catheters

The routine placement of ureteral catheters before colonic surgery has been advised by some surgeons. However, I limit their use selectively, especially for those individuals who are to have reoperative pelvic surgery. One must remember, however, that although they may aid in identifying the ureters (by palpation), care must be taken not to rely too much on them. The precaution of seeking and carefully dissecting the ureters away from the area of the surgical dissection should be taken, regardless of the ease or difficulty of the operation or the presence or absence of ureteral catheters. Fiberoptic catheters, of course, permit easier visualization without the need to palpate, but they are quite expensive. Darkening the operating room to facilitate identification by these means is for me, at least, a nuisance. Ureteral catheters are not harmless—ureteral edema, oliguria, and anuria, as well as ureteral injury itself, are potential consequences.[856] However, one unquestioned benefit is that there is no doubt as to the location or nature of the injury when the catheter is divided. It is suggested that the reader peruse an excellent article on ureteral stents by Saltzman.[817] The approaches to the management of ureteral injuries are discussed in the Chapter 23.

It is wise to remove one catheter at a time. Generally, the first may be taken out at the end of the operation. The second can usually be removed the following day. Still, prudence suggests that one utilize the services of the urologist in determining the timing of withdrawal—after all, he or she is the individual responsible for inserting the catheter in the first place and should be given the opportunity to provide an opinion.

Hydration

Overnight intravenous hydration before operation is advisable for any patient who may be prone to adverse cardiac or renal consequences of excessive fluid loss. Oral hydration during catharsis is also helpful and is one of the reasons why a PEG preparation may be the better mechanical cleansing for high-risk individuals.

Hyperalimentation and Nutritional Assessment

Hyperalimentation has been advocated before operation for the nutritionally depleted patient in order to prepare for the assault on the patient's metabolic processes. Many individuals with colorectal cancer have lost weight, are anemic and hypoalbuminemic, or have a variety of fluid and electrolyte problems. With the exception of weight loss, however, laboratory abnormalities can usually be corrected by 2 or 3 days of appropriate therapy. Delaying surgical intervention for a week or more to administer hyperalimentation is an expensive, time-consuming extravagance that has in itself an associated morbidity.

Nutritional assessment has also been advised because of its potential in anticipating postoperative morbidity and mortality. In the experience of Thompson and colleagues, subnormal findings for triceps skin-fold thickness and percentage of ideal body weight were associated with a higher complication rate, but these occurred so infrequently that the routine use of such tests was not recommended.[939] Ondrula and co-workers identified a number of preoperative factors that increased the risk of colon resection: emergency operation, age greater than 75 years, congestive heart failure, prior abdominal or pelvic radiation therapy, corticosteroid use, serum albumin less than 2.7 g/dL, chronic obstructive pulmonary disease, previous myocardial infarction, diabetes, cirrhosis, and renal insufficiency.[708]

Opinion

I am impressed by the salutary effects of surgery, and the consequent improvement in the nutritional status after the expeditious removal of colonic pathology. The patient can usually commence a regular diet by the fifth postoperative day. Therefore, I am not an advocate of the use of hyperalimentation in the preoperative management of patients who need surgery for malignant disease.

Nasogastric Intubation

The routine use of a nasogastric tube is discouraged for colon resections. It does not protect the anastomosis and merely causes patient discomfort. In a prospective study by Colvin and colleagues comparing the preoperative use of a long intestinal tube (Cantor), a nasogastric tube, and no tube, there were no significant differences in the lengths of hospital stay, duration of postoperative ileus, adequacy of intraoperative intestinal decompression, gastric dilatation, and postoperative complications.[168] Wolff and colleagues counsel that even though there is an increase in the rate of minor symptoms of nausea, vomiting, and abdominal distension when nasogastric decompression is not employed, nasogastric intubation still is not warranted prophylactically.[1035] My only caveat with respect to advocating the prophylactic use of a nasogastric tube is in the patient who is obtunded or who is at serious risk for aspiration. Obviously, on a therapeutic basis (intestinal obstruction, postoperative vomiting), gastric drainage is indicated.

Thrombophlebitis Prophylaxis

There has been a tendency for many surgeons to eschew deep vein thrombosis prophylaxis because of the fear of bleeding and to a lesser extent because of the misconception that their patients are not at risk for this complication. The likelihood of bleeding is small, about 1%, while the risk of a hematoma is approximately 3%. The fact is that the highest risk patients are the ones that are being discussed in this chapter—major surgery, older than 40 years, and cancer—each is an independent variable for increased thromboembolism risk. The use of antiembolism stockings has been of proven value in the prevention of postoperative thrombophlebitis and pulmonary embolism. It has been suggested that these be worn before surgery, ideally placed on the night before (an impossible criterion if the patient is admitted the day of surgery). Both the use of low-dose heparin and low-molecular-weight heparin have been shown to significantly reduce the incidence of deep vein thrombosis and pulmonary embolism in the moderate and high risk patient. An excellent, contemporary review and consensus on thromboembolic prophylaxis appears in the journal *Chest* (2001; 119:132S–175S).

Operative Technique

> Surgeons must be careful when they take their knife,
> Underneath their fine incisions stirs the culprit—life!
>   Emily Dickinson

General Principles

Incision

Generally, most surgeons prefer to perform colon operations through a midline incision. This permits ready access to both sides of the abdomen and allows rapid entry into the peritoneal cavity. Furthermore, it leaves both sides of the abdomen free should a colostomy or ileostomy be required. The wound heals strongly and is easily closed in a single layer. Some surgeons utilize a right-sided oblique incision for right colon resections. These wounds heal well and are perhaps associated with less discomfort, but one may compromise on the exposure.

Older surgeons have been trained through the adage, "a big surgeon means a big incision." However, the advent of minimally invasive surgery has resulted in earlier return of bowel function, the ability to feed patients sooner, less discomfort, and a shortened hospital stay (see Chapter 27). This has stimulated some surgeons to perform open colon resections through a much smaller incision, the so-called minilaparotomy. Minilaparotomy has been defined as complete resection performed through a skin incision less than 7 cm long. Nakagoe and co-workers in Japan reported that this exposure could be successfully accomplished for colonic cancer in 72 out of 84 patients.[671] Using historical controls they found statistically significant shorter hospitalizations and lower analgesia requirements. However, some surgeons may argue that the body habitus of the average Japanese patient is more conducive to minilaparotomy than that of the frequently large and obese Western patient.

A Pfannenstiel incision can be used for its cosmetic benefit, but exposure may be limited. The rectus muscles, however, can be divided in order to permit better visualization (Maylard incision; Figure 22-35), an operative approach that has merit especially in pelvic surgery (e.g., low anterior resection). Furthermore, this incision may be easily extended, if necessary, to facilitate taking down the splenic flexure. A self-retaining (e.g., Balfour, Bookwalter) retractor is often inserted for retraction of the abdominal wall. My own preference, especially because I have converted to performing a limited incision as often

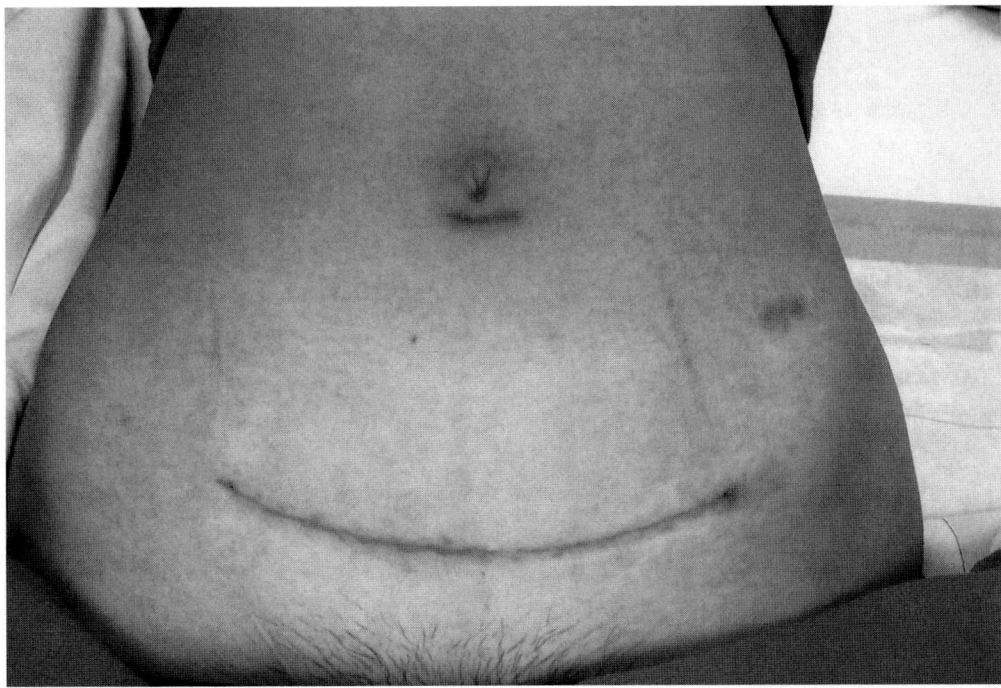

FIGURE 22-35. Maylard incision for a total colectomy. Note the small infraumbilical incision from prior port site for a laparoscopic cholecystectomy.

as feasible, is to use a disposable, self-retaining retractor, the Protractor (Figure 22-36).

Exploration

The abdominal contents are examined carefully for the presence of metastatic disease and any other incidental lesion. The cancer itself is examined last. It is important to determine whether the tumor is freely movable or fixed, whether sepsis or perforation is present, whether the mesentery is invaded by tumor, and whether seeding of the peritoneal cavity has occurred. It is often difficult to determine by inspection alone whether lymph nodes contain tumor or are uninvolved. Large, firm nodes may prove to be inflamed when examined under the microscope.

Tumoricidal agents

The use of topical tumoricidal agents has been suggested to minimize the risk for implantation metastases, especially with respect to resection of the rectum (see Chapter 23). Long and Edwards instilled dilute formalin (as a cancericidal agent) into the lumen of the bowel in 40 patients before opening it.[544] A statistically significant difference in actuarial survival was observed in comparison with

historical controls. I remain unconvinced as to the merits of this technique and do not use it.

Drains

In the absence of pus, no drains are employed. Some studies have demonstrated that the prophylactic use of drains is at best ineffective and poses a potential hazard for further complications, especially an anastomotic leak.[413]

Wound Closure

For wound closure, I prefer a single layer of interrupted long-term absorbable sutures placed through all layers except the skin. In our controlled trial of three different suture materials for abdominal wound closure (a nonabsorbable monofilament suture, a nonabsorbable multifilament suture, and a long-term absorbable suture), no statistically significant difference was seen in the incidence of wound infection, wound dehiscence, and incisional hernia.[179] It was believed that closure of the abdominal wall with long-term absorbable suture is the preferred method. A another alternative is to use a continuous suturing technique, such as looped No. 1 polydioxanone suture (PDS). Carlson and Condon performed a prospective, randomized comparison of nylon versus polyglyconate (Maxon), utilizing a looped suture in a running mass

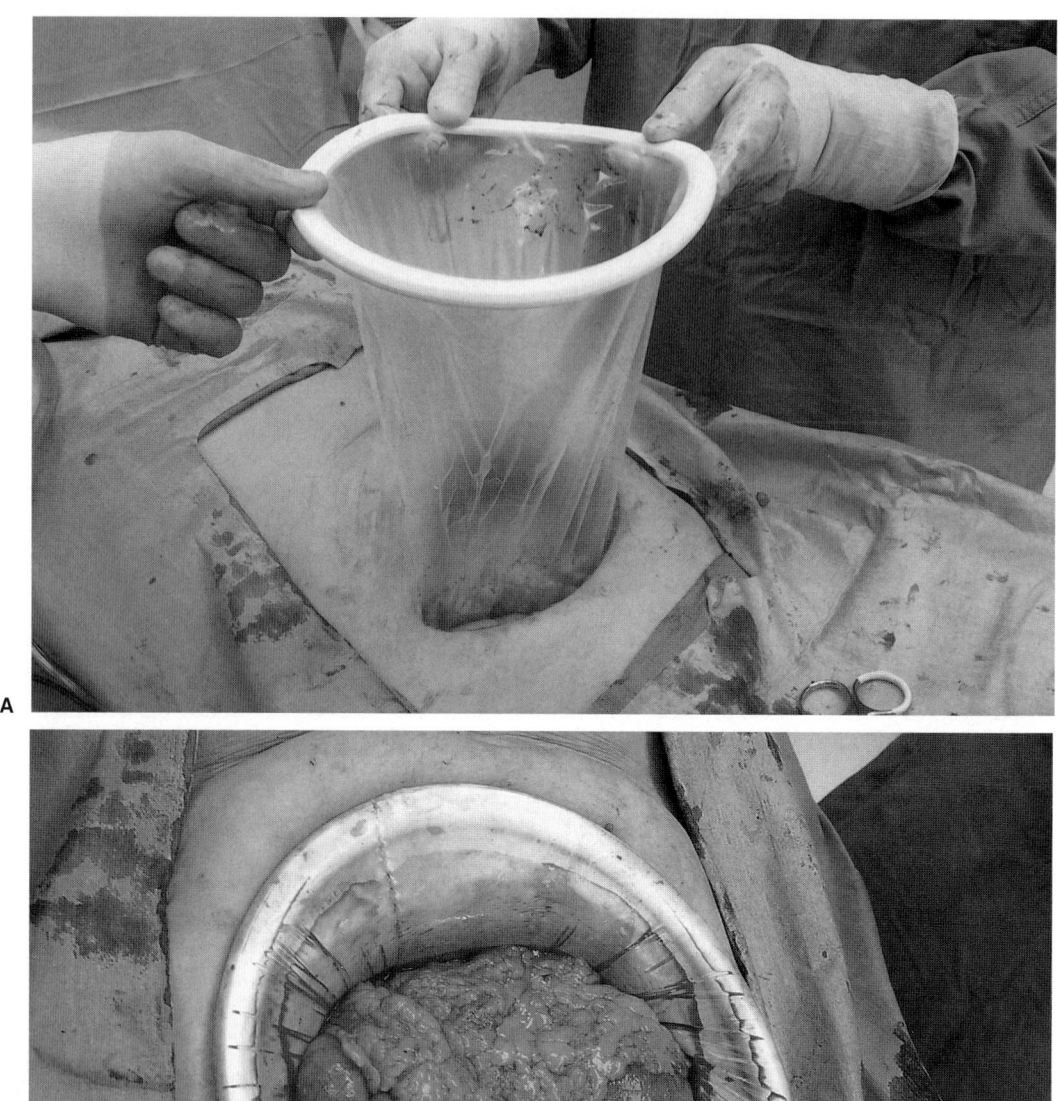

FIGURE 22-36. Protractor disposable wound retractor through Maylard incision. **(A)** Protractor inserted; gasket will be folded down. **(B)** Final position of Protractor in place.

closure of midline abdominal incisions in 225 patients.[137] There was no significant difference in the overall rate of ventral hernia and dehiscence between the two groups with a 2-year follow up. Needless to say, other surgeons involved in many varied trials conclude that different materials and methods are preferred.[256,320,596,781]

The general or trauma surgeon may be faced with a situation wherein abdominal wound closure may not be possible without tension. Numerous methods are available, including the use of polyglycolic acid (Vicryl) mesh, Marlex, Gore-Tex, "Bogota bag", and sandwich-vacuum pack, just to name a few.[677] Fortunately, it is unusual that one cannot close the abdomen in colon and rectal surgery, but the occasion may arise, especially in the presence of bowel obstruction, perforation, an anastomotic leak, with intraabdominal packing, following abdominal radiation, with the abdominal compartment syndrome, or when tumor invades the abdominal wall (see also Chapter 14).

Operations

As with all operations for malignancy, the objective of surgical treatment for carcinoma of the colon is to remove the growth with an adequate margin through performing a wide excision of the tumor-bearing area and associated lymphatics, with attention to the blood supply to that segment (see Figure 1-15) and the creation of an anastomosis without tension. What the actual distance is between the tumor margin and the cut edge of bowel may be somewhat problematic. Depending on when it is measured, a margin of 5 cm unstretched *in situ* has been noted to shrink to under 2 cm.[1000]

The operations that are generally employed for cancer above the rectum include right colectomy, transverse colectomy, left colectomy, sigmoid colectomy, high anterior resection, subtotal colectomy, and total colectomy. Other, more limited resections are occasionally performed for palliation, but these generally should be condemned because of the potential for inadequate blood supply, insufficient mesenteric removal, and tension on the anastomosis.

Right Hemicolectomy

Lesions of the cecum, ascending colon, and hepatic flexure usually are treated by right hemicolectomy, because the blood supply to this area comes from the ileocolic and right colic arteries. The dissection may be expedited if the surgeon stands on the patient's left side, although this is a matter of personal preference. Resectability of the tumor is evaluated with a minimum of manipulation. The small bowel is retracted into the left half of the abdominal cavity, and the root of the

mesentery and the base of the transverse mesocolon are exposed. Many surgeons ligate the right colic and right branch of the middle colic arteries and veins as the initial maneuver (Figure 22-37). This procedure is not difficult unless the patient is obese, in which case preliminary ligation of the blood vessels may be neither convenient nor safe. The small incision in the root of the mesentery required for this preliminary main trunk ligation is now extended to the point on the transverse colon and ileum where division of the bowel is to take place. The vessels in the mesentery and mesocolon are ligated, and the entire blood supply to the tumor is divided. An alternative to ligating the mesenteric blood supply is to employ a vessel sealing device, the LigaSure vessel-sealing system (Figure 22-38). This unique approach can be used in place of clips, sutures, and other energy-based ligation methods. In essence, it produces within a few seconds a consistent seal of vessels up to 7 mm in diameter without dissection or isolation.

Although I am not an advocate of the no-touch technique (see later), it certainly makes sense not to manipulate the bowel or handle the tumor unnecessarily. However, I believe that one may still adhere to this principle and yet expedite the operation by initially mobilizing the colon. The terminal ileum and right colon are elevated

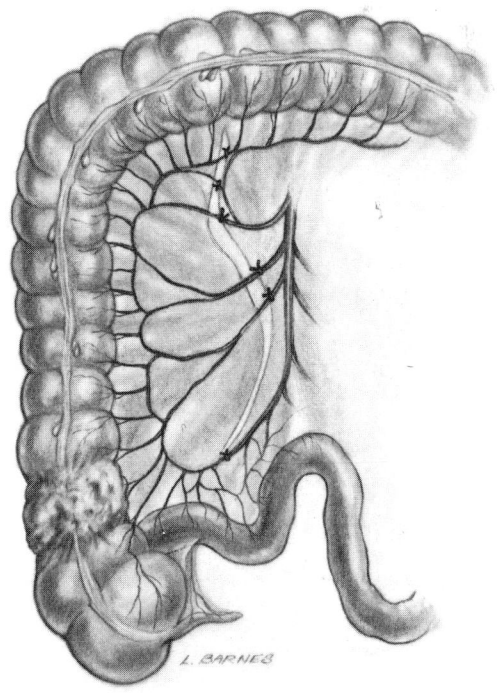

FIGURE 22-37. Right hemicolectomy. Early ligation of the vascular supply to the right colon is illustrated.

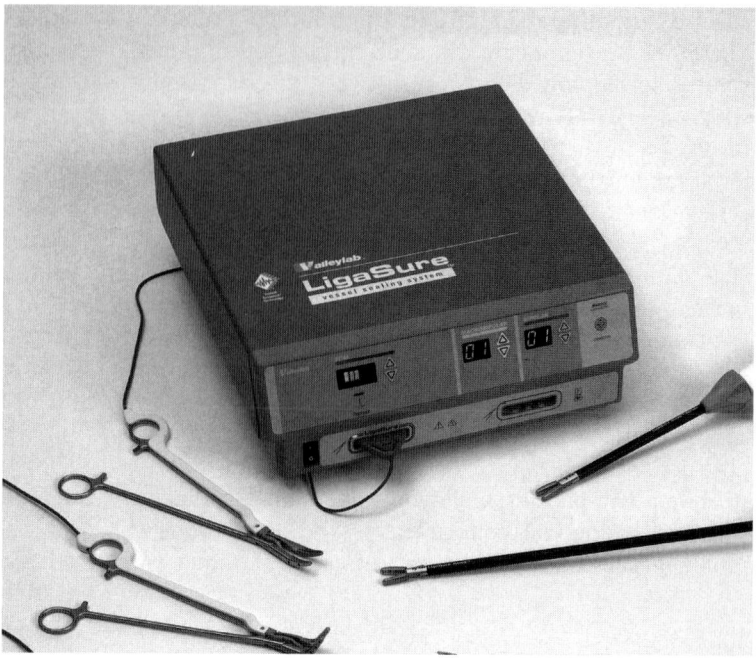

FIGURE 22-38. The LigaSure system offers nine instruments for open and laparoscopic procedures. (Courtesy of Valleylab, a Division of Tyco Healthcare, Boulder, CO; *www.valleylab.com*.)

from the retroperitoneal structures by dividing the peritoneum along the lateral gutter, at the so-called "white line of Toldt" (Figure 22-39). Included in the resected specimen is any lateral peritoneum involved by serosal tumor. Care must be taken to avoid injury to the ureter, spermatic or ovarian vessels, and inferior vena cava. The terminal ileum is prepared by incising the antimesenteric fold of Treves.

The next structure of concern is the second portion of the duodenum. This must be displaced carefully as the colon is freed from its retroperitoneal attachments. The developmental adhesions from the gallbladder and liver

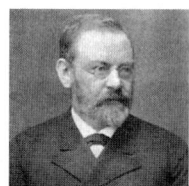

Carl Florian Toldt (1840–1920)   Carl Toldt was born May 3, 1840 in Bruneck, Austria, the second of ten children. As a young man, he spent much of his free time learning to assemble and repair clocks with a local clockmaker. He believed that this experience was beneficial to both his analytical skills and to his manual dexterity. Toldt attended medical school at Joseph's University in Vienna, from which he received his doctorate in 1864. His expertise encompassed a number of areas in medicine, but he held a special interest for anatomy. He was first appointed Professor of Anatomy at the University of Vienna in 1875, then went on to become Professor of Anatomy at the German University in Prague. In 1884, he returned to Vienna where he created the Anatomy Institute of Vienna together with his colleague, Langer. Toldt was responsible for many publications on histology, tissue growth, forensic medicine, and anatomy. His best-known work is his anatomic atlas, *Anatom Atlas fur Studierende und Aerzte*, which was translated into English and last published in New York in 1926. In addition to his writing, Toldt showed his creative nature by inventing an electrical lighting system for dissecting rooms. Toldt died of pneumonia in Vienna on November 13, 1920. (With appreciation to Brian de Rubertis.)

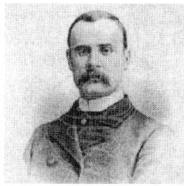

Frederick Treves (1853–1923)   Frederick Treves was born in Dorchester, Dorset, England on February 15, 1853. He received his medical education at the London School of Medicine, and in 1879 he became Surgical Registrar and Assistant Surgeon at the London Hospital. For a time he worked as a lecturer of practical anatomy and demonstrator in anatomy at that hospital and become, in 1883, surgeon as well as Head of the Department of Anatomy. Later in this year, he met Joseph Merrick, known as the "Elephant Man." Treves rescued Merrick from destitution and created a home for him in the attic of the London Hospital until Merrick died in 1890. Treves was a prolific author as well as a brilliant investigator and observer. In 1883, the Royal College of Surgeons awarded him the Jacksonian Prize for his dissertation, *Pathology, Diagnosis and Treatment of Obstruction of the Intestine*. His best recognized works are his Hunterian lectures, delivered to the Royal College of Surgeons, on *The Anatomy of the Intestinal Canal and Peritoneum* (1885). In 1884, Treves, at the age of 31, became Full Surgeon to the London Hospital. He was one of the first to devote special attention to diseases of the appendix. He concluded that the disease, then known as perityphlitis, involved the appendix and not the cecum. His consulting rooms at 6 Wimpole Street became among the best known in England. In 1899, upon the outbreak of the Boer War, he was called to serve as consulting surgeon to the field forces. The following year, he published an account of his experiences in charge of No. 4 Field Hospital and being present at the relief of Ladysmith, in his *Tale of a Field Hospital*. Treves was a brilliant lecturer and a very able surgeon who made original contributions to surgical anatomy, peritonitis, intestinal obstruction, and appendicitis. He was knighted by King Edward VII, on whom he performed an appendectomy in June 1902. Later that year, Treves retired from medical practice to become an author, moving in 1918 to Lake Geneva, Switzerland because of poor health. Treves had by this time become quite a successful travel writer, by publishing a series of books based on his experiences. His last book was devoted to recollections of his medical experiences and was entitled *The Elephant Man and Other Reminiscences* (1923). He died of peritonitis on December 7, 1923 in Lausanne, Switzerland. His lifelong friend, the author and poet, Thomas Hardy, arranged for and spoke at the funeral in Dorset. (Photograph courtesy of the Wellcome Library, London.)

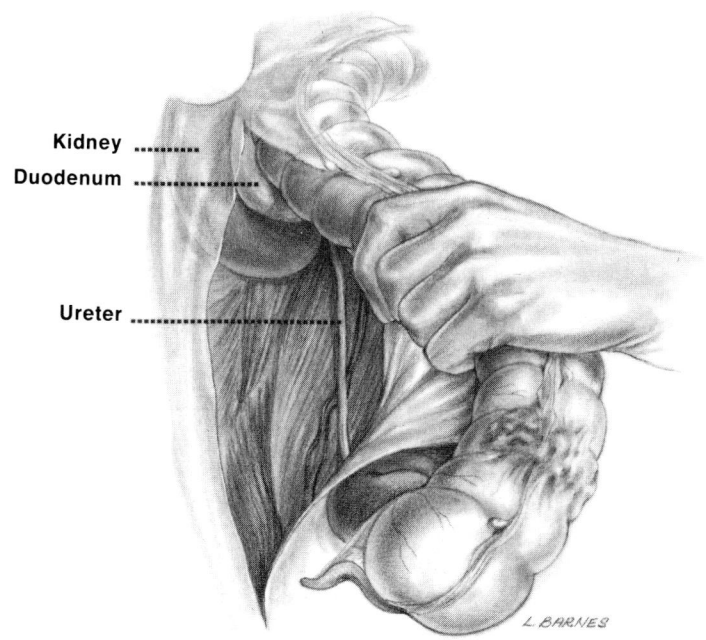

Kidney ....
Duodenum ....
Ureter ....

L. BARNES

FIGURE 22-39. Right hemicolectomy. The dissection proceeds along the right paracolic gutter, and the retroperitoneal structures are identified and preserved.

to the hepatic flexure are incised. When the head of the pancreas is in view (Figure 22-40), the duodenum is sufficiently clear from the dissection so that clamping of the blood supply can be accomplished with safety. This can be performed by passing a hand around the vessels through the avascular plane (Figure 22-41).

It is often advisable to enter the lesser sac, dividing the gastrocolic omentum as far to the left as possible. This maneuver expedites entrance into the sac and permits the posterior wall of the stomach to be retracted out of harm's way. The remainder of the gastrocolic omentum is then divided until the hepatic flexure is no longer tethered. The omentum is incised to the point where the anastomosis will be performed. With all the blood supply divided to the segment, the bowel is resected (Figure 22-42).

Bokey and co-workers emphasize as in rectal surgery that mobilization of the colon along anatomic planes is an important principle and an independent prognostic factor that influences outcome.[89] Curley and

colleagues comment that fixation may occur to the duodenum or pancreas, albeit rarely.[187] They reported *en bloc* pancreaticoduodenectomy or lateral duodenectomy in 12 individuals. Others have found that locally advanced right-sided cancer can be safely treated with *en bloc* pancreaticoduodenectomy.[71] Cure can still be achieved by such in-continuity resections (see later).

Suturing Principles: Personal Perspective

In this era of stapling, I find that many residents have little or no experience with hand-sewn techniques. Although I recognize the ease and rapidity of performing a side-to-side stapled ileocolic anastomosis, residents often wish to gain more experience with sewing. Not uncommonly, a discrepancy exists between the luminal sizes of the ileum and the transverse colon, the latter being considerably larger. Under such circumstances, it is usually advisable to make a Cheatle cut into the antimesen-

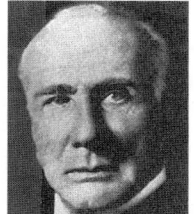

George Lenthal Cheatle (1865–1951)   George Cheatle was born in Belvedere, Kent, England on June 13, 1865. He was educated at King's College, London. Following graduation and while awaiting his house appointment at King's College Hospital, he acted as Assistant Demonstrator of Anatomy. He was the last to serve as Lord Lister's Assistant in Surgery. In 1900, he became full surgeon to King's while also teaching surgical pathology. In the South African War (Boer War), he served as consulting surgeon, and in the First World War he held the rank of Surgeon Rear Admiral in the Royal Navy, receiving the honor of Knight Commander of the Bath for his services. In his obituary in *The Lancet* (1951;1:115) the following statement was made about him: "The accumulation of a large, consulting practice was inevitable to a man of such distinction, but he remained a keen and conscientious teacher and a rabid research-worker." In 1931, he was awarded the Walker Prize for his work on cancer. Among his many recognitions were Honorary Fellow of the American College of Surgeons, Chevalier of the French Legion of Honor, and Officer of the Grand Cross of Italy. He was so esteemed that in order to lecture at Hines Hospital, Chicago, a privilege accorded to none but American nationals, he was granted American citizenship for 1 week. Sir Lenthal died at his home in London on January 3, 1951, at the age of 85. (Photograph from journal, *Cancer* 1951;4:220, with permission.)

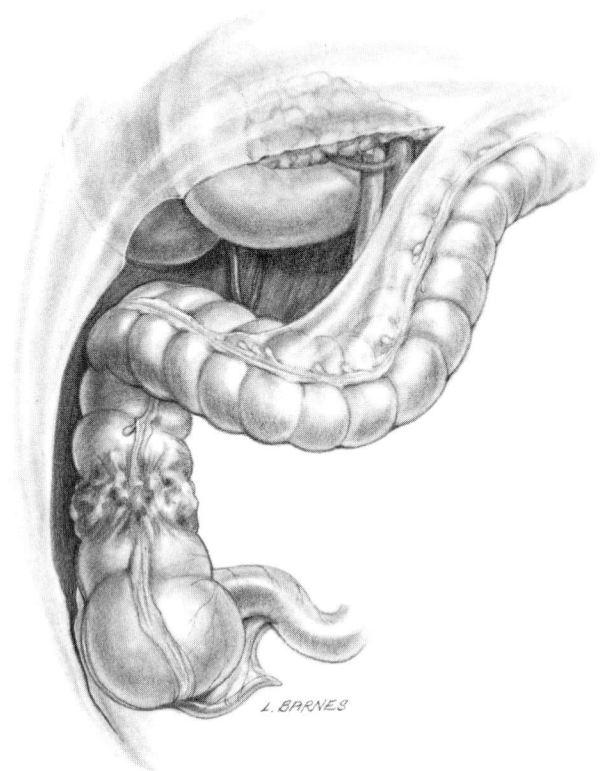

L. BARNES

FIGURE 22-40. Right hemicolectomy. The hepatic flexure is mobilized, exposing the duodenum and the head of the pancreas.

teric portion of the ileum when performing a hand-sewn anastomosis (Figure 22-43A). I do not like nor do I perform a hand-sewn ileocolic side-to-end or end-to-side anastomosis.

My own preference when sewing is to undertake all colonic anastomoses by an interrupted, single-layer, inverting technique through the application of long-term absorbable sutures (Figure 22-43). Small bites of mucosa are taken, with a relatively deeper passage through the seromuscular layer. Although the submucosal layer is the most important, there is little consequence of incorporating a small amount of mucosa. The use of a second row of seromuscular sutures is not necessary. It adds nothing to the security of the anastomosis, inverts more tissue, and further narrows the lumen. I recognize, however, that we are talking about a subject that is pervaded by prejudice and dogma and is always a reflection of an individual's training, experience, and personal preference. I will defend to your death your right to utilize whatever technique with which you are comfortable. Every suture material has been used, and everything works reasonably well. Logically, one cannot blame the suture material if an anastomosis fails, but this excuse is still postulated. Prolene and wire work but they

are tedious to tie, and braided, nonabsorbable material creates more tissue reaction, which, theoretically, can serve as a nidus for sepsis. Catgut is acceptable, but objectively it has no advantage over a long-term absorbable suture. Reasonable people have differences of opinion with respect to choice of suture material and technique (whether a single or a double layer is preferable, interrupted or continuous), but there is little disagreement that an inverting approach is the proper one for all colonic anastomoses when a conventional hand-sewn technique is used.

After a satisfactory anastomosis has been achieved, the mesenteric defect may be closed with either an interrupted or a continuous technique. Theoretically, this may prevent herniation of small bowel through the defect in the mesentery, but there is no evidence to support this claim. Many surgeons always leave the defect open, but it is probably prudent to close a small opening. It is also useful to place omentum around all colonic anastomoses to protect further against the possibility of leakage (see later).

Suture Technique: Study Results

Max and colleagues prefer a single-layer continuous technique, using polypropylene (Figure 22-44); they reported a successful experience with 1,000 intestinal anastomoses.[600] Carty and co-workers advocate a single-layer extramucosal approach.[139] Thomson and Robinson also prefer a one-layer continuously sutured anastomosis, using a double-ended absorbable monofilament suture placed in an extramucosal fashion.[943] Clark and co-workers performed a randomized trial of polyglycolic acid sutures and catgut in colonic anastomoses, but with a double-layer approach.[159] Interrupted silk was used as a seromuscular suture, and a continuous inverting mucosal suture was employed with either of the two materials. Although clinical evidence of anastomotic breakdown occurred with equal frequency in the two groups studied, radiologic evidence of anastomotic leak was twice as common with the catgut.[159]

Some investigators are of the opinion that the type of suture material may have an effect on the risk for anastomotic recurrence. In an experimental study, Hubens and colleagues found that persisting suture material at a colonic anastomosis affected the distribution of tumor formation when a chemical carcinogen was administered.[424] They opined that the actual elimination process of such material may influence the crypt cell proliferation rate. In view of these observations, the authors suggest that either inert suture material be used or sutureless anastomotic techniques be applied.[424]

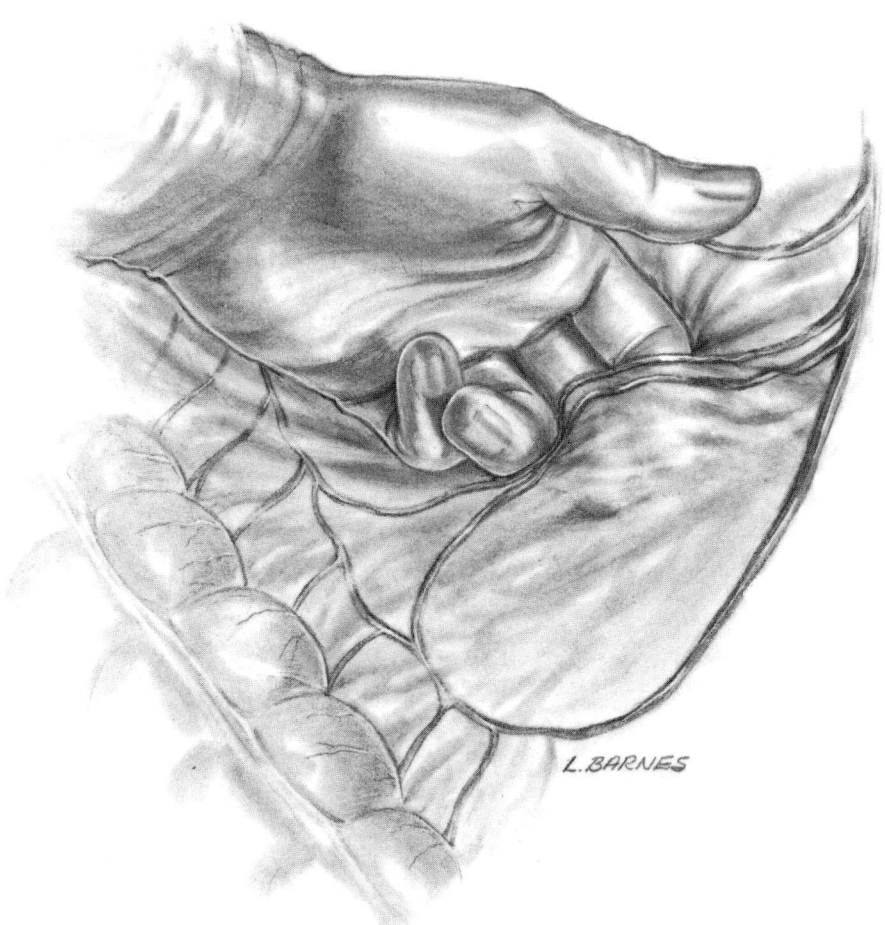

FIGURE 22-41. Right hemicolectomy. Technique of identification and manual isolation of major blood supply to the right colon.

Surgery for Carcinoma of the Transverse Colon

Carcinoma of the transverse colon often presents a challenge in the choice of operative procedure. The blood supply to this area is derived from the middle colic artery as well as from the right and left colic vessels. Anastomosis in the region of the splenic flexure poses some risk for compromise of the blood supply to the bowel, because with the middle colic artery divided, the blood supply must come from the inferior mesenteric artery. In the region of the hepatic flexure, however, blood supply is not usually a problem, because of the contribution from the ileocolic and right colic vessels.

In addition to the concerns about blood supply with an anastomosis in the transverse colon, another problem is the lymph-bearing area. Carcinoma in this location can spread to regional lymphatics through the middle colic, right colic, and left colic branches. Because of this risk, subtotal colectomy has been advocated as the optimal approach to the treatment of carci-

noma of the transverse colon. My own philosophy for removing such tumors depends on the location in the transverse colon. For proximal lesions, right hemicolectomy is advised. For distal transverse colon lesions, left partial or left hemicolectomy is reasonable (Figure 22-45) with anastomosis of the transverse colon to the sigmoid colon (Figure 22-46). However, for lesions of the mid-transverse colon, limited transverse colectomy may be considered for palliation or as a compromise for other indications. As mentioned, however, as a cancer operation it may be inadequate. If tension or other technical difficulty prevents a safe anastomosis between the proximal and distal transverse colon (Figure 22-47), subtotal or total colectomy and ileosigmoid or ileorectal anastomosis is strongly recommended. The result of tension on a transverse colon anastomosis is illustrated in Figure 22-48.

Mobilization of the splenic flexure is facilitated by, first, division of the gastrocolic omentum to within a few centimeters of the flexure and, second, incision of the lateral peritoneal attachments along the descending and

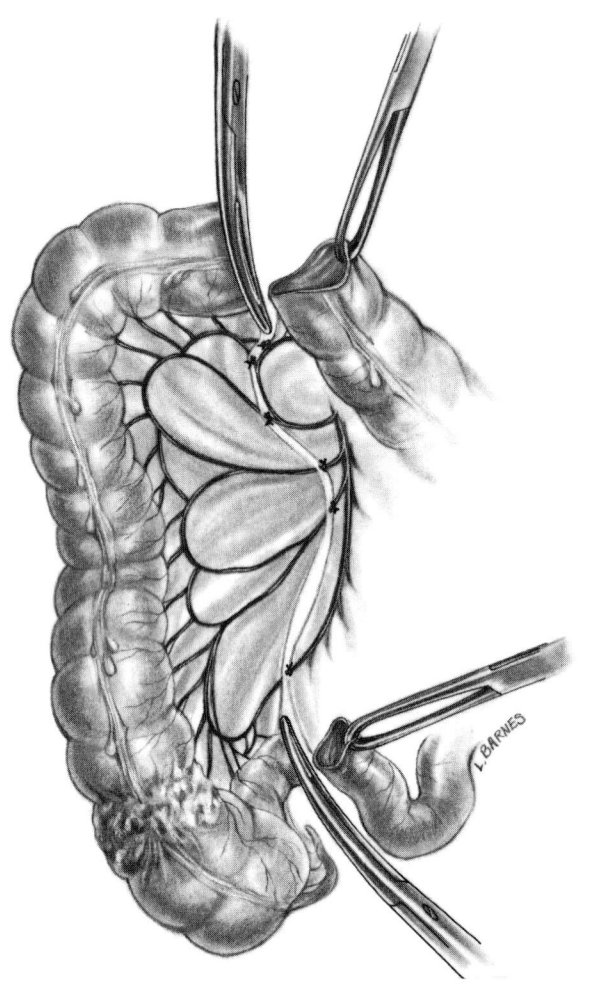

FIGURE 22-42. Right hemicolectomy. After ligation of the vascular supply and mobilization of the bowel, crushing clamps are applied to the ileum and transverse colon, and the bowel is divided with a scalpel, leaving the ends open for anastomosis.

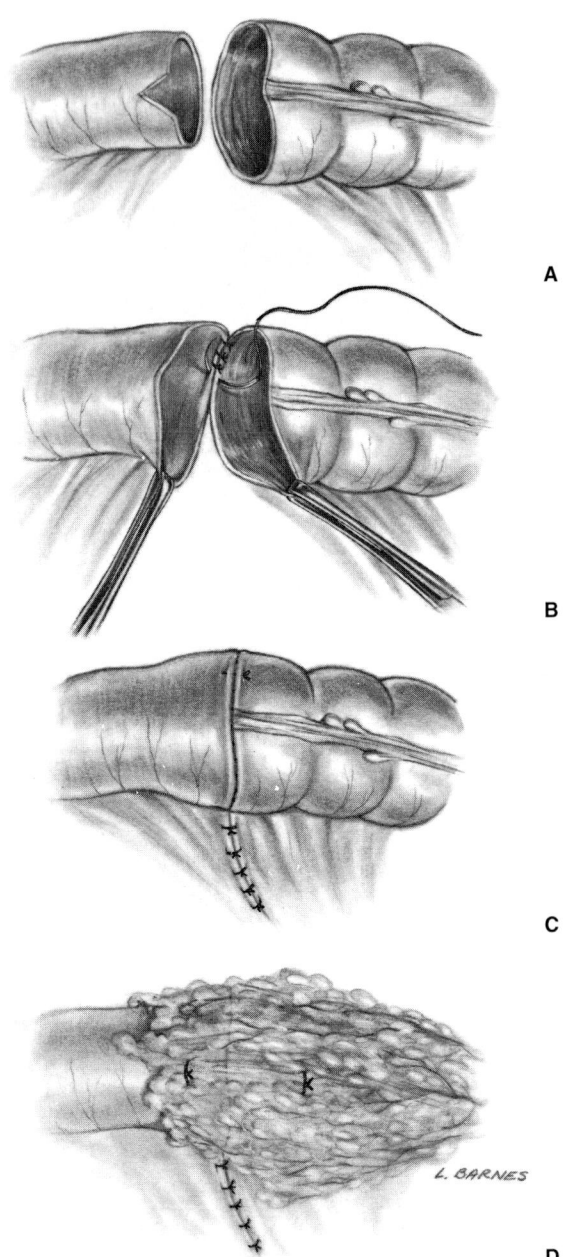

FIGURE 22-43. Right hemicolectomy. **(A)** Any disparity between the luminal ends can be corrected by dividing the smaller segment of bowel along its antimesenteric border. **(B)** The anastomosis is accomplished using a single layer of interrupted sutures. **(C)** Note the single mattress suture used to effect final closure. The rent in the mesentery is closed. **(D)** Omentum is placed around the anastomosis.

sigmoid colon (Figure 22-49). As the splenic flexure is approached, the spleen is seen, and the lienocolic and phrenocolic ligaments are divided (Figure 22-50). Only one clamp should be used to avoid tearing the splenic capsule. The splenic flexure is delivered into the wound, and any back-bleeding can be clamped at this point without concern about injury to the spleen (Figure 22-51). The technique of anastomosis does not differ from that already described.

Splenectomy

Locally invasive tumors of the splenic flexure usually are not amenable to wide excision unless the spleen and tail of the pancreas are also removed. Removal of the spleen, whether intentional or inadvertent in conjunction with a colonic resection, is associated with a high morbidity and an increased mortality rate (Figure 22-52).[158,195,485,505,798] Langevin and colleagues reviewed 993 consecutive colon and rectal operations and found that the spleen was injured in eight.[505] Splenectomy was required in three. Therefore, the incidence of splenectomy during splenic flexure mobilization is approximately 1%. Varty and colleagues reviewed the experience of splenectomy con-

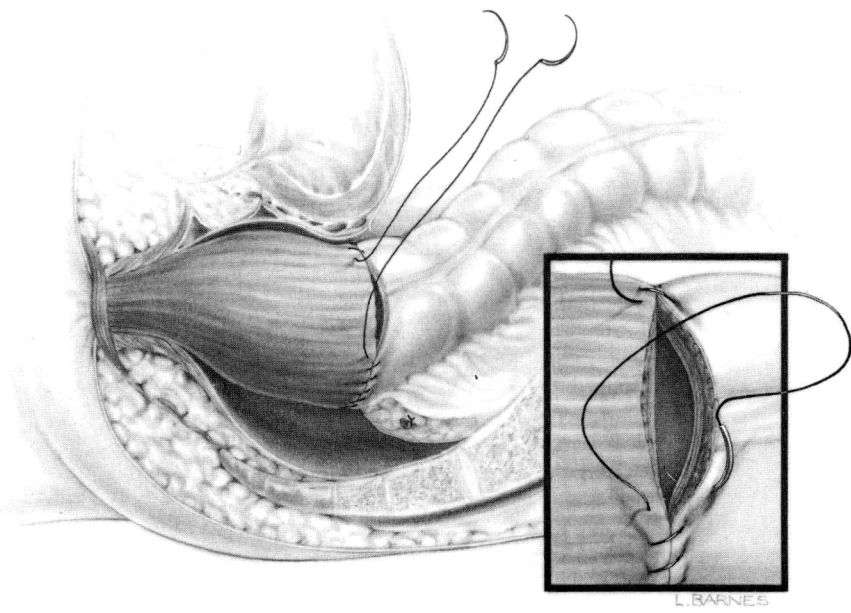

FIGURE 22-44. Colorectal anastomosis by continuous suturing, incorporating minimal mucosa. The method illustrated uses a no. 4–0, double-armed polypropylene suture, as advocated by Max and colleagues.[600]

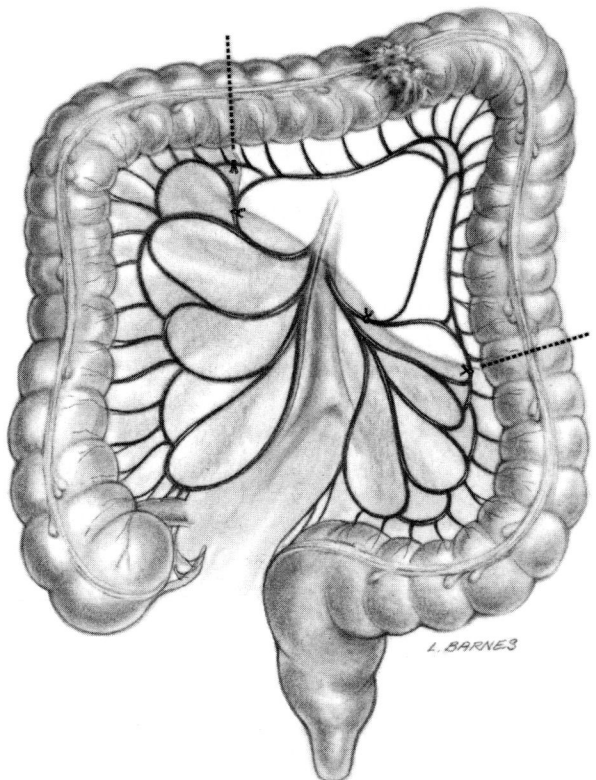

FIGURE 22-45. Left partial colectomy. With tumors of the left portion of the transverse colon, resection of the descending colon is required to obtain a safe anastomosis while removing lymphatic drainage areas.

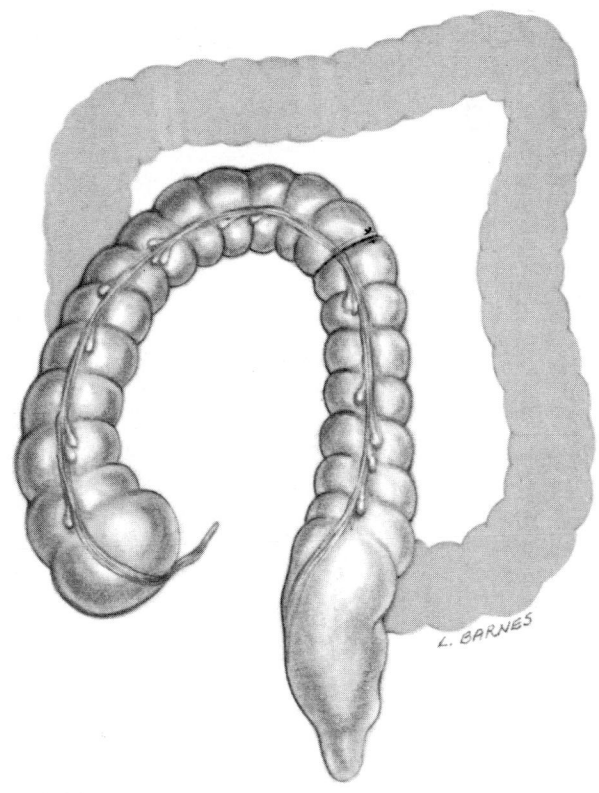

FIGURE 22-46. Left partial colectomy. Anastomosis between the midtransverse colon and the upper sigmoid is usually possible without difficulty, except in very obese patients.

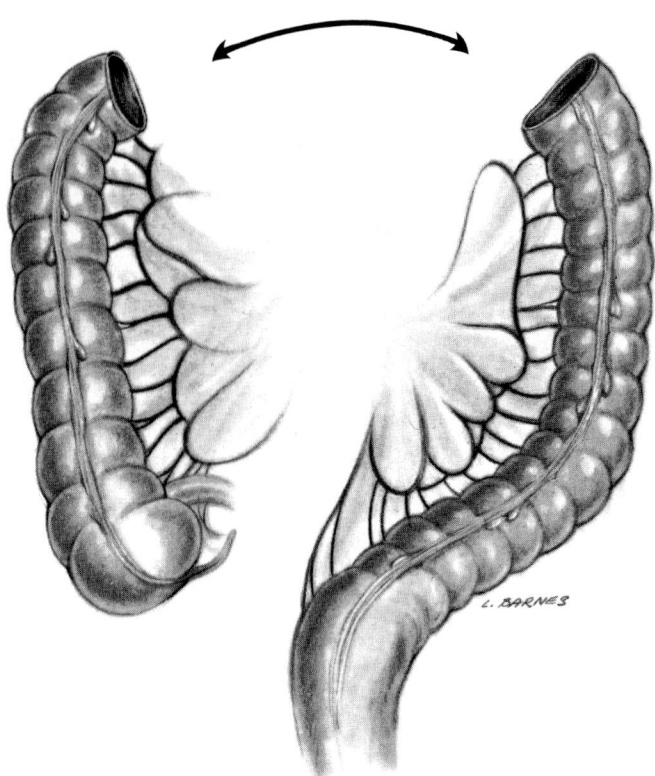

FIGURE 22-47. Transverse colon resection. Anastomosis may not be feasible because of tension.

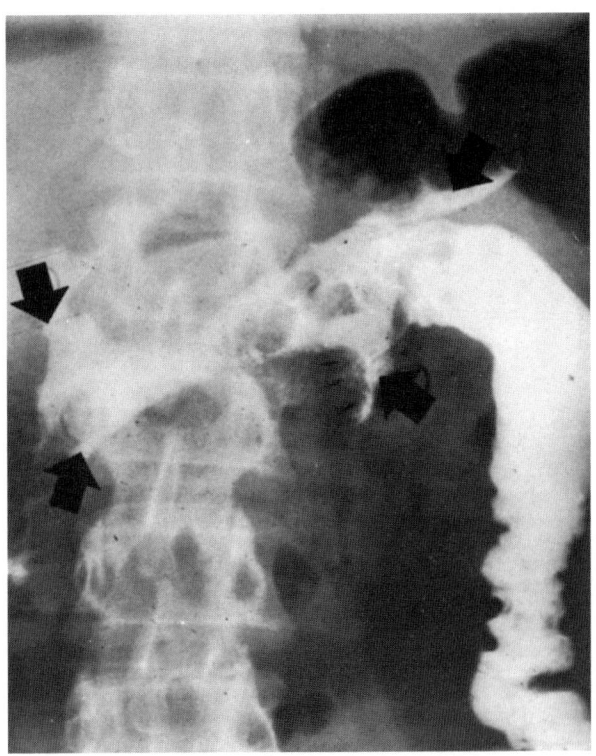

FIGURE 22-48. Anastomotic leak *(arrows)* demonstrated on a postoperative barium enema study 2 weeks after transverse colectomy for carcinoma. At the second operation, the ends of the bowel were found to have separated completely.

comitant with resections for colon and rectal cancer at University College, London, comparing the patients with individually matched controls.[973] There was no influence on long-term survival, although there was an increased incidence of postoperative sepsis.

Because most injuries to the spleen are capsular tears caused by inadequate exposure and too vigorous traction, every effort should be made to conserve the organ. Topical hemostatic agents such as Avitene, Surgicel, Helistat, and Gelfoam have been recommended as well as primary suture repair and even partial splenectomy. If removal is required, the incidence of septic complications is increased. Drains should not be used except in the presence of sepsis or gross contamination. Under such circumstances, closed drainage with sump suction is preferred. Appropriate counseling concerning the implications of the loss of the spleen is advised, and the administration of polyvalent pneumococcal vaccine (Pneumovax) is a requisite.

Left Partial Colectomy or Hemicolectomy

Left partial colectomy is the preferred operation for tumors involving the distal transverse colon, splenic flexure, and descending colon. The right branch of the middle colic artery should be kept intact proximally, and the left colic artery is ligated, care being taken to preserve the origin of

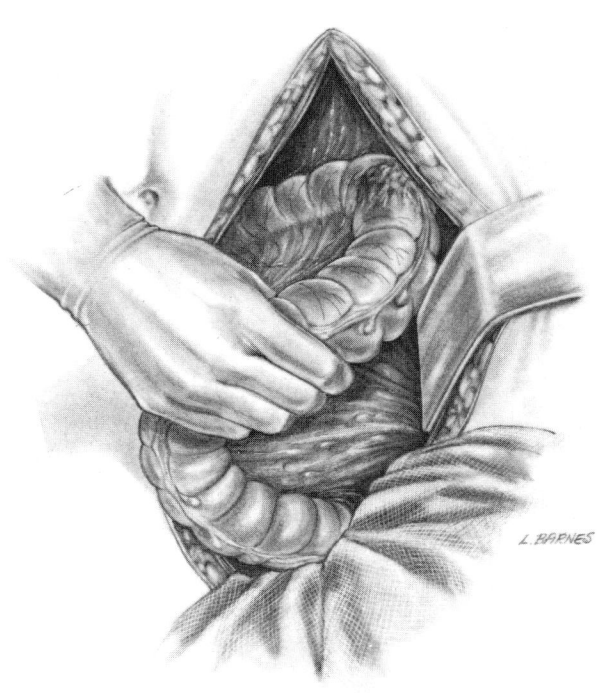

FIGURE 22-49. Mobilization of the splenic flexure is facilitated by freeing the descending colon.

the inferior mesenteric artery (Figure 22-53). The anastomosis is effected between the midtransverse colon and the upper sigmoid. In most instances, sufficient redundancy of the sigmoid colon is present to permit an anastomosis without tension. Occasionally, with an obese patient or with someone who has undergone a prior resection, such an anastomosis is not possible. Under these circumstances, total or subtotal colectomy is a reasonable alternative. Whereas one can virtually always close the defect in the mesentery following a right hemicolectomy, it is often not possible to accomplish such a closure on the left. One prefers to leave a large opening rather than to attempt suturing and have it partially disrupt. As I mentioned earlier, the risk for entrapment of small bowel is theoretically greater when a small defect is present. I never attempt to close the mesentery after a left colon resection.

Sigmoid Colectomy and High Anterior Resection (Anastomosis into the Upper Rectum)

Removal of the sigmoid colon for carcinoma is the standard operation for tumors in this location. With respect to blood supply, the operation preserves the left colic artery, dividing only the sigmoid branches of the inferior mesenteric artery. Viability of the distal bowel should present no problem, because of the usually excellent

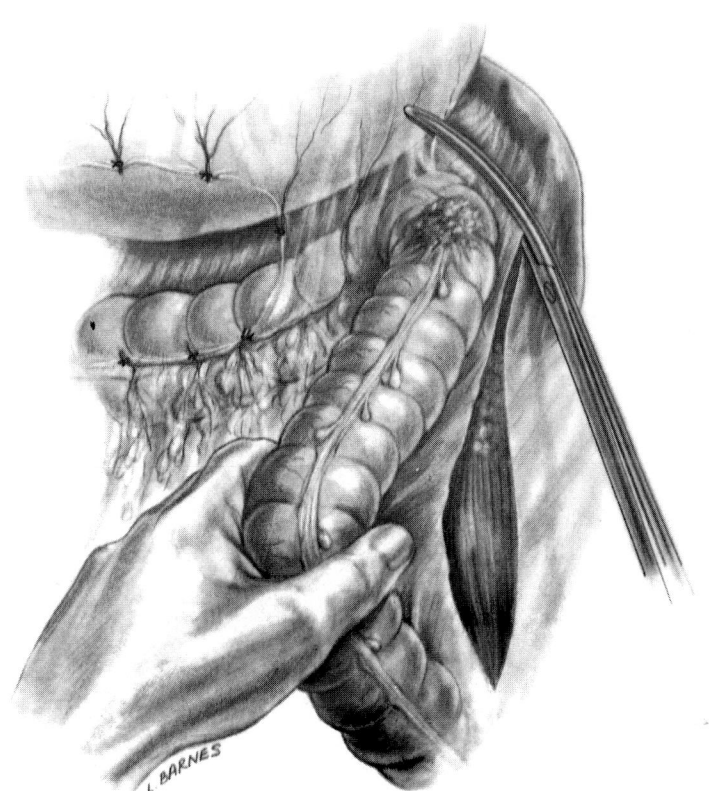

FIGURE 22-50. The lienocolic ligament is divided. Back-bleeding can be dealt with as the splenic flexure is brought into the wound.

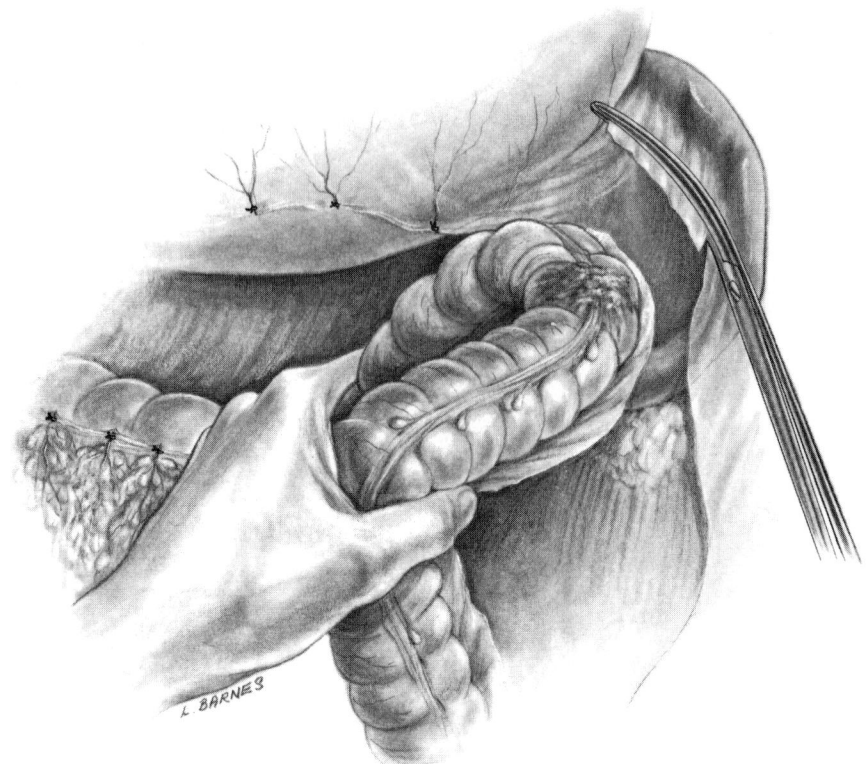

FIGURE 22-51. With traction on the transverse colon and descending colon, the splenic flexure is delivered from its retroperitoneal attachments.

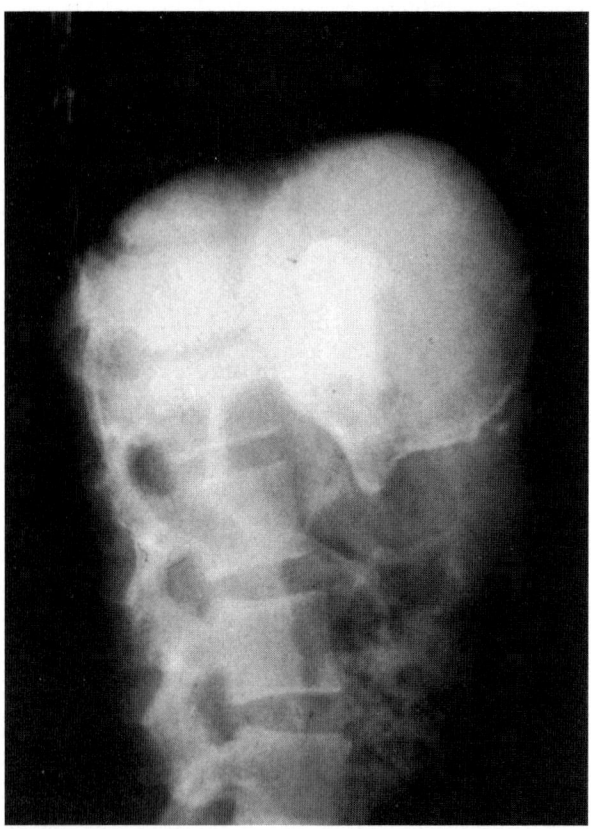

FIGURE 22-52. Subphrenic abscess that developed following colectomy and splenectomy.

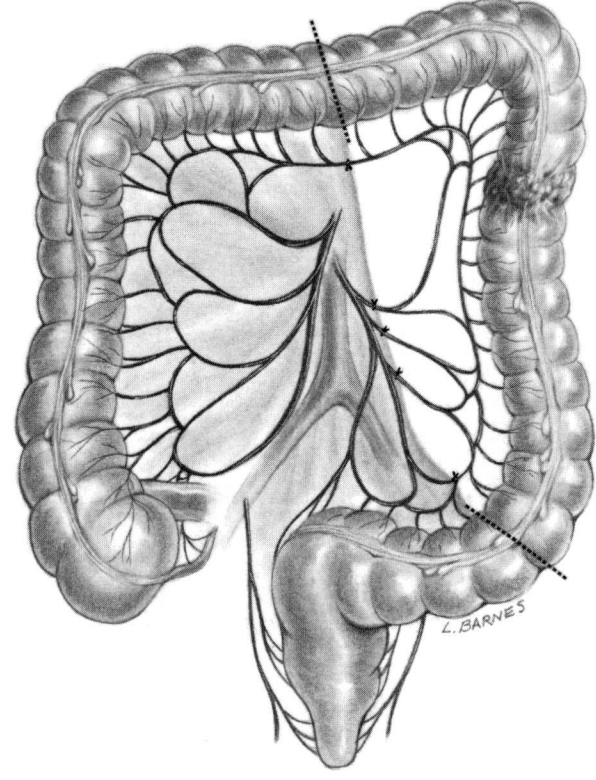

FIGURE 22-53. Left partial colectomy. Area of resection for lesion of descending colon, with preservation of sigmoid and rectal vessels.

blood supply from the middle hemorrhoidal arteries and the upper sigmoid vessels. The proximal blood supply is usually adequate through the left colic artery. Some surgeons stress the importance of high ligation of the inferior mesenteric artery (on the aorta).[345] However, if a node at this level harbors cancer, the chance for cure is very remote indeed. At least three studies have demonstrated that there is no survival advantage of high ligation of the inferior mesenteric artery.[488]

In mobilization of the sigmoid colon, a major concern is to avoid traumatizing the left ureter. Most injuries to this structure take place at the level of the iliac vessels. The left ureter should be retracted laterally and displaced from the area of resection (Figure 22-54). The surgeon's left hand is passed beneath the inferior mesenteric vessels, and the peritoneum is incised on the right side (Figure 22-55). The left hand is then withdrawn and passed around the vessels and through the defect between the left colic artery and the sigmoid vessels (Figure 22-56). The inferior mesenteric vessels are cross-clamped, divided, and ligated, and the arcade vessels to the upper sigmoid are divided. Rather than perform an anastomosis between the upper sigmoid and lower

sigmoid (because of a potential problem with distal blood supply), I prefer to do a high anterior resection, anastomosing the bowel to the upper rectum at or just below the peritoneal reflection. For distal sigmoid lesions, it may be necessary to mobilize the rectum slightly and preserve a portion of proximal sigmoid to effect a safe anastomosis without tension. Conversely, for proximal sigmoid lesions, I prefer to preserve the distal sigmoid and perform an anastomosis between the lower descending colon and the distal sigmoid colon rather than to mobilize the splenic flexure. This allows adequate length without tension. This is different from the principle of resection described for sigmoid diverticulitis, in which the anastomosis is always placed into the non-tenia-bearing rectum (see Chapter 26).

The technique that many surgeons use for dividing the mesorectum is often unnecessarily nitpicking. A right-angle clamp is placed into the mesorectum; by vigorous exertion of proximal traction, the mesentery is divided (Figure 22-57). This maneuver effectively strips the bowel in preparation for the anastomosis. Alternatively, a finger or a large clamp can be passed along the posterior rectal wall, separating the mesentery of the rectum. The mesorectum is

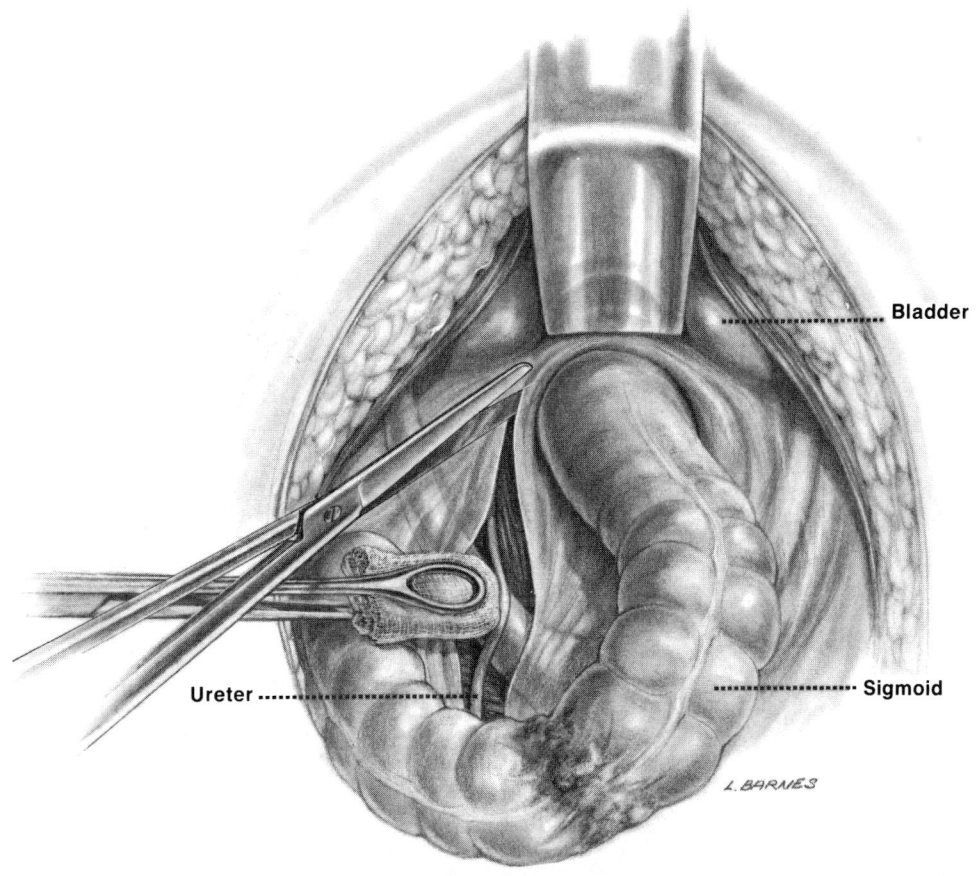

FIGURE 22-54. High anterior resection. The sigmoid colon is mobilized, with care taken to avoid injury to the ureter.

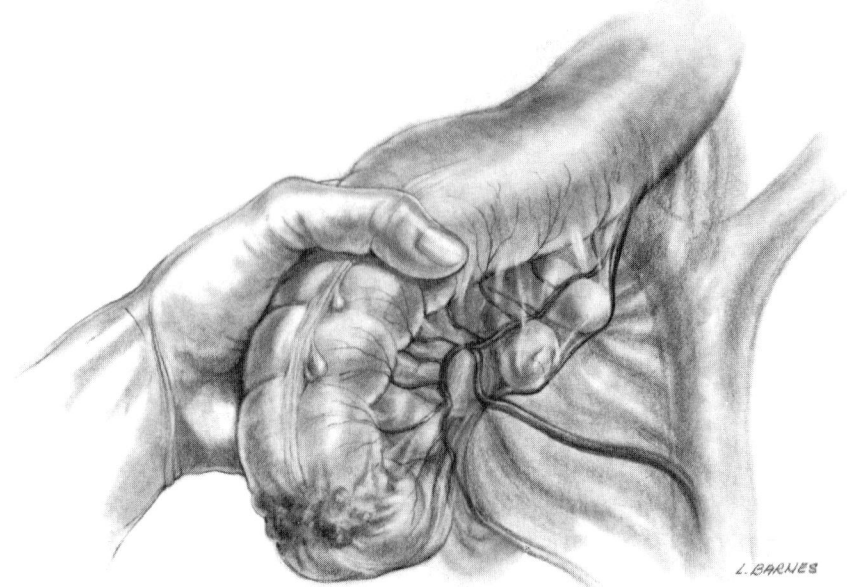

FIGURE 22-55. High anterior resection. The left hand is passed behind the bowel and beneath the vessels.

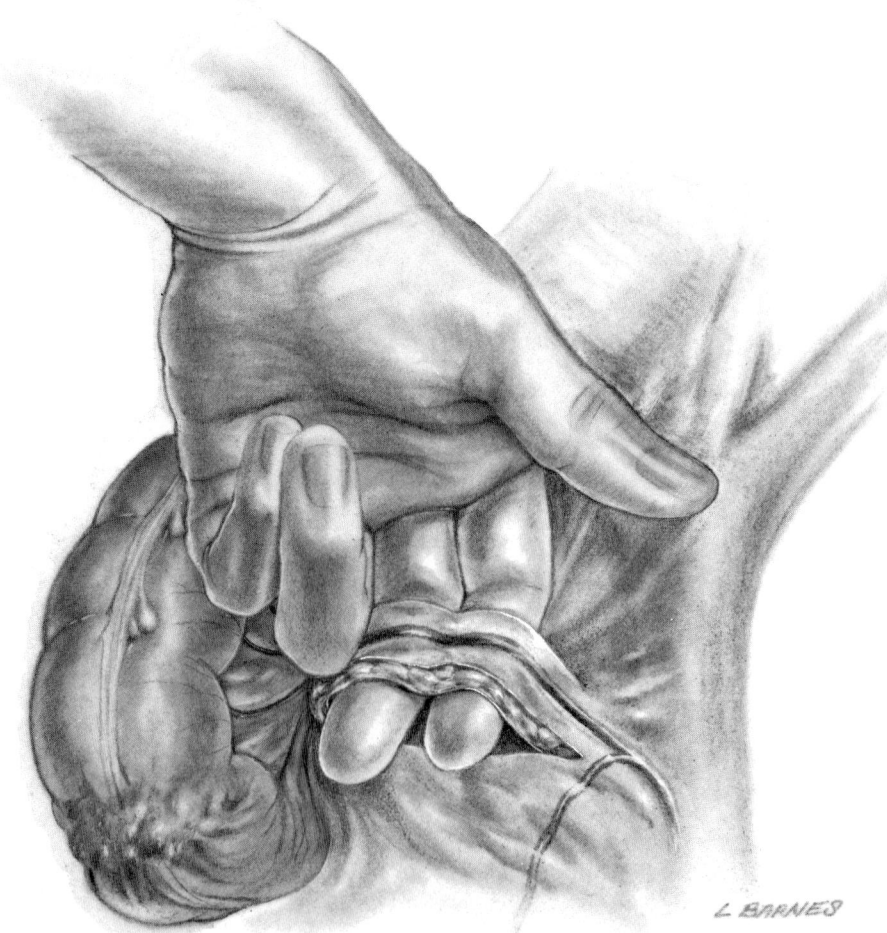

FIGURE 22-56. High anterior resection. The left hand is repositioned to pass around the mesenteric vessels. The vascular pedicle is clamped as it is held by the left hand.

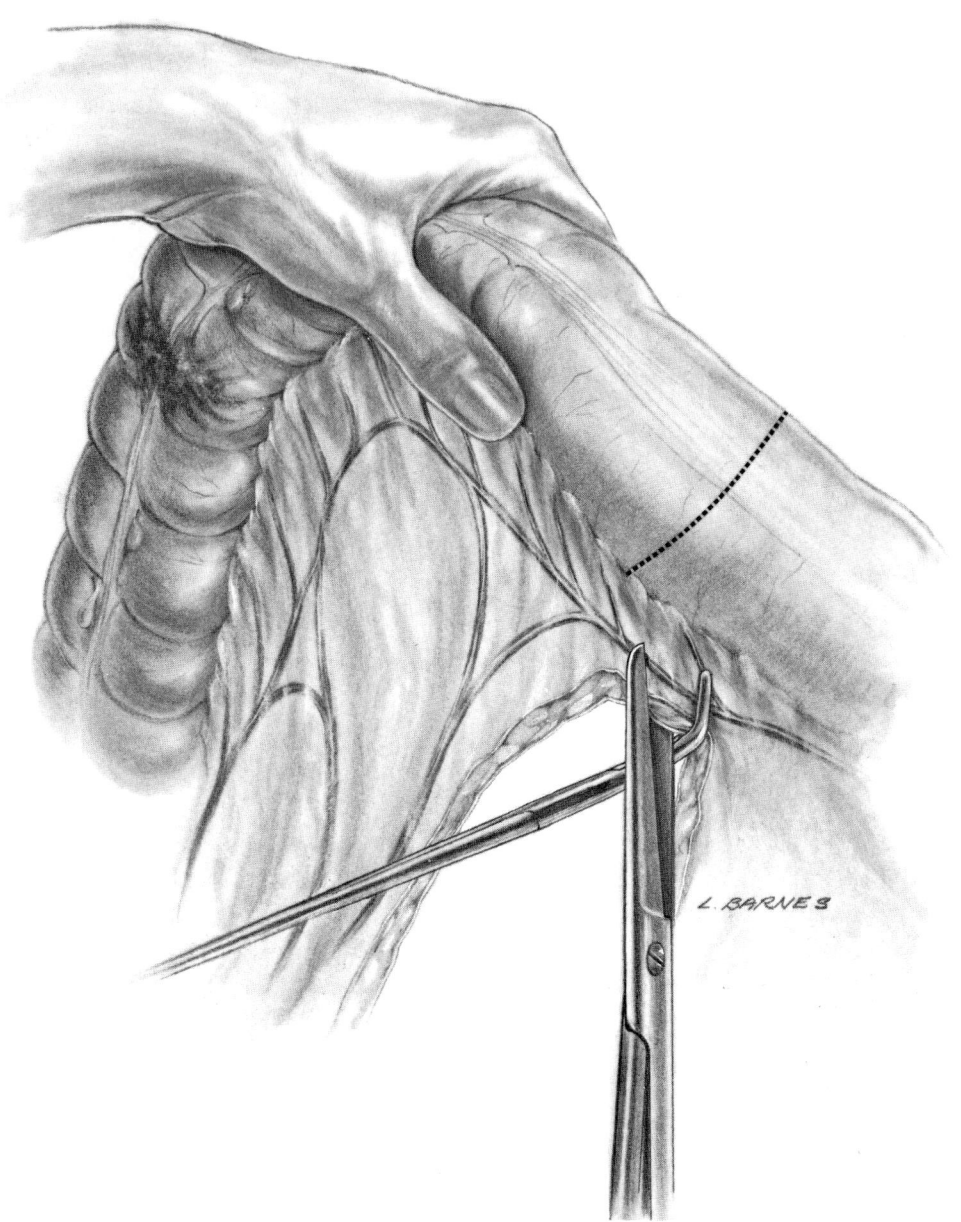

FIGURE 22-57. High anterior resection. The mesentery is clamped with vigorous cephalad traction as the mesocolon is divided.

then clamped with the large instrument, and the rectum is "stripped" of its mesentery in one maneuver.

Left Hemicolectomy

Left hemicolectomy should rarely be necessary for sigmoid colon lesions. Despite the potential advantage of radical removal of the lymphatics, the additional dissection required, the prolongation of the operative time, the possibility of injury to the spleen, and the technical difficulty associated with a transverse colorectal anastomosis all militate against this approach. Le and Gathright recognized the difficulty in reestablishing rectal continuity following a left hemicolectomy and developed an anastomotic ap-

proach to facilitate this maneuver.[516] The procedure involves bringing the proximal ascending colon or transverse colon through a distal ileal mesenteric defect in order to reach the rectum without tension (Figure 22-58).

Use of Drains

The application of intraabdominal drains following elective colon resection has traditionally been a stimulating subject for debate at surgical meetings. Johnson and colleagues reported a prospective study of 49 patients who were randomized to a group that had a corrugated Silastic drain placed next to the anastomosis or

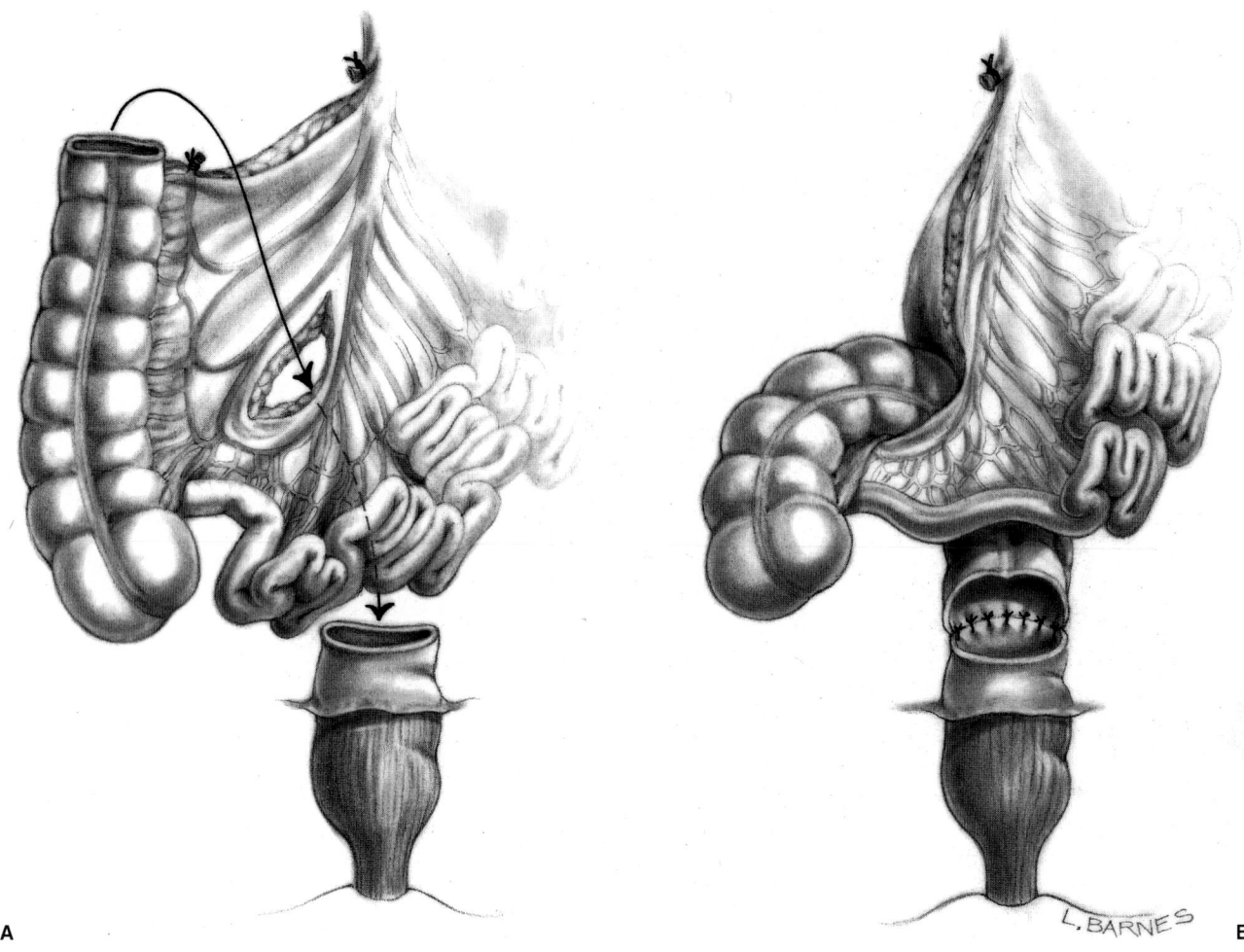

A   **B**

FIGURE 22-58. Reconstitution of intestinal continuity following extended left colectomy. **(A)** A mesenteric defect is created following resection. **(B)** The proximal ascending or transverse colon stump is brought through the ileal mesenteric defect to reach the rectum without tension. (Adapted from Le TH, Gathright JB Jr. Reconstitution of intestinal continuity after extended left colectomy. *Dis Colon Rectum* 1993;36:197.)

to a control group without drainage.[457] There was absolutely no difference in outcome between the groups. There has never been a study to my knowledge that provides evidence in support of drains under the circumstances mentioned. Therefore, I do not use them unless I am draining something (pus or anticipating transient bleeding). Parenthetically, if an abdominal drain is used, it should ideally be a closed-suction system. If the drain is placed prophylactically, it should be removed by 48 hours, assuming that the drainage is minimal (less than 75 mL in 24 hours).

Subtotal or Total Colectomy

Removal of all or most of the colon and anastomosing the bowel to the upper rectum or sigmoid colon comprises a more extensive operation but permits a techni-
cally straightforward anastomosis. It also has the advantage of maximal removal of lymph-bearing tissue. The procedure is indicated or should be considered when tumors are found synchronously on the left and right sides of the colon (Figure 22-59), when multiple tumors (benign or malignant or both) are present, in those individuals with familial adenomatous polyposis or HNPCC, when a resection has been performed previously, when the distal colon is obstructed (see the discussion of management of obstruction), or when technical factors preclude a limited bowel resection.[102,307,344,425,868] I recognize that synchronous resections of two bowel segments with two intestinal anastomoses can be relatively safely performed without a diversionary procedure if the bowel preparation is satisfactory, with minimal fecal soilage and with lack of tension on the suture lines,[1005] I rarely employ this alternative.

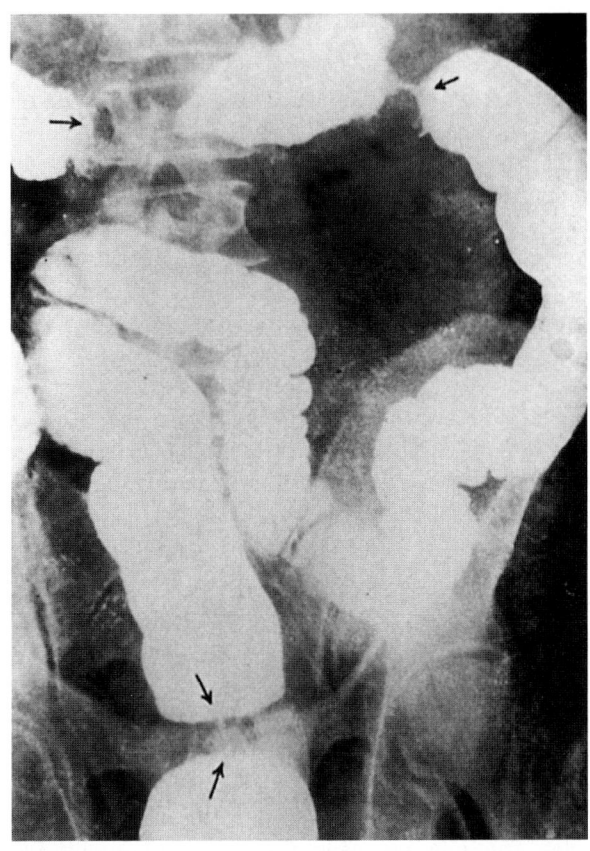

FIGURE 22-59. Three synchronous, stricturing carcinomas of the colon *(arrows):* midtransverse, at the splenic flexure, and at the rectum. (From Corman ML, Veidenheimer MC, Swinton NW. *Diseases of the anus, rectum, and colon. Part I: neoplasms.* New York: Medcom, 1972, with permission.)

Usually, an end-to-end anastomosis between the ileum and the rectum or sigmoid colon can be accomplished easily, but occasionally, because of discrepancy between the bowel lumina or because of the angulation of the mesentery when the ileum is turned down onto the rectum, a side-to-end anastomosis may be usefully applied (Figure 22-60).

Some of the expressed concerns of subtotal or total colectomy, as opposed to the so-called "lesser alternatives," are the morbidity and mortality rates, and the patient's quality of life. Walsh and colleagues reviewed 107 consecutive total abdominal colectomies performed for a number of indications.[987] There were two anastomotic leaks leading to deaths (1.8%). These were attributable to a failure to divert the fecal stream. In other words, no anastomosis should have been performed. Morbidity was 10.3%, with only 5% complaining of debilitating diarrhea. Beckwith and colleagues reported the experience with this operation in 32 patients more than 60 years of age at the Mayo Clinic.[64] The average increase in number of bowel movements immediately following surgery was 3.6 per day, and this gradually decreased over time. After 5 years, the average number was only 1.5 times the preoperative number. One should, however, be circumspect before contemplating the procedure on a prophylactic basis for the potential development of a metachronous cancer.[102] With proper surveillance by means of colonoscopy, I limit the procedure to the indications previously mentioned, unless the person is in the younger age group.

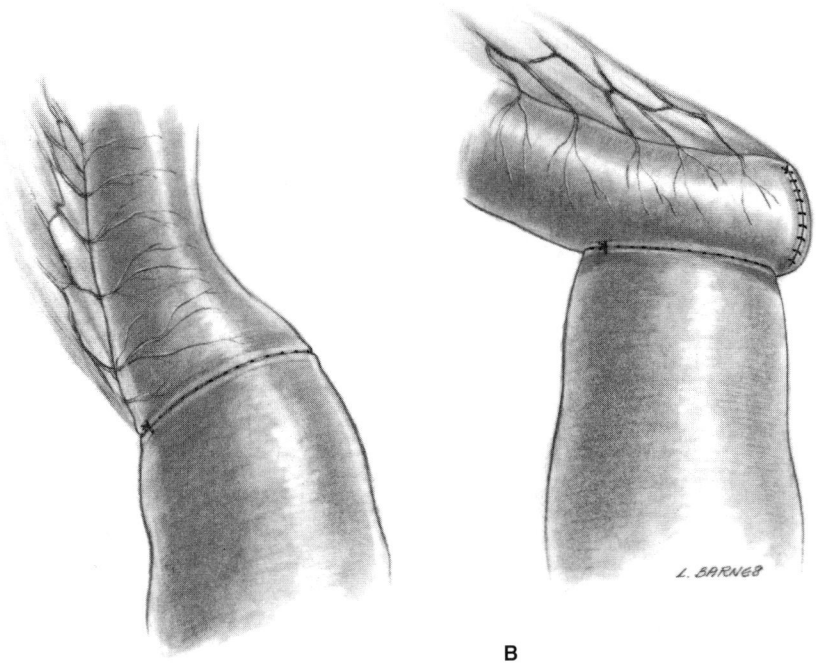

A   B

FIGURE 22-60. Ileorectal anastomosis can usually be accomplished end-to-end **(A)**, with or without a Cheatle cut of the ileum, or as a side-to-end anastomosis **(B)**.

No-Touch Technique

In 1954, the studies of Cole and associates with respect to circulating cancer cells and others prompted Turnbull and colleagues to ligate the vascular pedicle before mobilizing the colon and to develop the method known as the no-touch technique.[167,270,448,960] In Turnbull's operation, the cancer-bearing segment is mobilized last. I have already alluded to this principle in the removal of lesions of the right side of the colon.

Although the theoretical value of early ligation of the vascular pedicle seems reasonable, it is difficult to understand how the excellent cure rates reported by the Cleveland Clinic (Ohio) group are achieved solely by this maneuver. Many patients already harbor inapparent tumor above the ligature. They obviously would not be cured by this technique. One possible explanation for Turnbull's results is that a somewhat different classification was used for staging cancers of the colon. However, in a prospective, randomized trial of 236 patients operated on for colon cancer, Jeekel reported that liver metastases appeared later, particularly where there was evidence of blood vessel invasion in the resected specimen.[449,1010] Fielding comments that modest gains in prognosis for colon cancer can be expected in some individuals if this method is used.[264] García-Olmo and associates studied whether "conventional" surgery could provoke the circulation of tumor cells as detected by genetic technology.[291] They used the reverse transcriptase-polymerase chain reaction to analyze tumor biopsy specimens and blood samples obtained from the antecubital vein before and after surgery, as well as from the main drainage vein of the tumor when the tumor had been removed. The investigators concluded that there was no evidence to suggest detachment of cells from the tumor at surgery.[291] Bessa and colleagues found that neither intraoperative nor postoperative detection of blood circulating tumor cells had prognostic significance in patients with colorectal cancer operated on for cure.[73] Others have concluded that there is no statistically significant advantage in the no-touch technique.[488] In my opinion, the value of the no-touch technique has been greatly overstated, and I never use it.

Radical Lymphadenectomy

As has been mentioned previously, the concepts of high ligation of the inferior mesenteric artery and of radical lymphadenectomy have failed to show any survival benefit. With respect to radical lymphadenectomy, the complications for me, at least, far outweigh the theoretical advantages.[488] That stated, if there are only a small number of lymph nodes identified in the resected specimen, there is the real possibility that the patient's tumor extent will be understaged.[749] This may have implications for adjuvant therapy (see the following discussion on sentinel lymph node mapping).

Sentinel Lymph Node Mapping and "Ultrastaging"

If one were to ask the question, "what is the single most important variable for determining prognosis in colorectal cancer?" most surgeons and oncologists would state, "the presence or absence of lymph node involvement." An improved understanding of the likelihood of harboring such metastases would, therefore, seem to have merit. The first possible sites of metastasis along the route of lymphatic drainage from the primary lesion are known as sentinel nodes.[483] These are, therefore, the lymph nodes that are most likely to harbor metastases. Beside sentinel node evaluation, the concept of "ultrastaging" by serial sectioning, combined with immunohistochemical techniques, improves one's ability to detect lymph node micrometastases (smaller than 2 mm).[472,665]

Technique

"Mapping" may be performed *in vivo* at the time of laparotomy or following removal of the specimen. Typically, lymphatic mapping is performed intraoperatively through the subserosal injection of blue dye. Regional nodes take up the dye in about 5 minutes. Another technique is to employ colloidal antimony sulfide in blue dye or other agents, with detection by the use of a gamma probe. This may be accomplished by endoscopic injection or by injection directly around the tumor. One may then perform a standard lymphadenectomy or remove additional mesentery containing lymphatics and nodes when there appears to be atypical drainage.

Ex vivo mapping involves the injection of blue dye around the tumor and then massaging the mesentery to propel the dye through the lymphatics and into the nodes. Such identified nodes are then harvested for microscopic sectioning.

Results

Kitagawa and colleagues enrolled 56 patients with curatively resectable colorectal carcinoma in order to test the feasibility of performing the technique and the accuracy of radioactivity-guided mapping of the first lymph nodes found in draining the primary tumor site.[483] They used a technique that involved preoperative endoscopic injection of ^{99m}Tc–labeled tin colloid. Diagnostic accuracy according to sentinel node status was determined to be 92%.[483] As expected, the incidence of metastasis in the sentinel node (22%) was significantly higher than that in the nonsentinel nodes (3%). Joosten and associates injected blue dye around the tumor in 50 patients.[459] Routine pathologic assessment was made of all nodes, with the blue-stained ones additionally tested immunohistochemically. A false-negative of 60% was observed, leading the authors to conclude that the concept of lymph node mapping and sentinel node identification is not valid for colorectal cancer.[459] Esser and colleagues injected 31 colorectal cancers with lymphazurin blue dye, reporting a sensitivity of 67%, a specificity and positive predictive value of 100%, and a negative predictive value of 94%.[253] Trocha and associates emphasize that dual-agent lymphatic mapping (radiotracer plus blue dye) more accurately identifies sentinel node metastases than blue dye alone and allows a more focused histopathologic examination.[958] Mulsow and co-workers in 2003 reviewed the literature as it applies to mapping of colorectal cancer and noted a false-negative rate of approximately 10%.[665] They and others conclude that further follow-up studies are necessary in order truly to assess the prognostic significance of micrometastases and staging benefits with respect to therapeutic implications.[472,1044]

Radioimmunoguided Surgery

Radioimmunoguided surgery (RIGS) utilizes a hand-held gamma-detecting probe to identify radioactivity following injection of one of a number of radiolabeled monoclonal antibodies. This approach is discussed later in this chapter, especially as it applies to second-look operations. Some, however, have explored the use of RIGS in the management of colorectal cancer at the time of the initial procedure. Through this technique, it has been shown that RIGS enables surgeons to define lymphatic metastases with a higher degree of sensitivity and specificity than can be determined by clinical assessment alone (see later discussion).[351]

As with the discussion on sentinel node mapping, the critical issue is whether these applications improve cure rates. That is unlikely. However, such techniques are potentially useful in improving the staging of colorectal cancer.

Peritoneal Cytology

Intraoperative peritoneal washings have been performed in order to examine whether the presence or absence of positive cytology has prognostic implications. Kanellos and colleagues undertook 110 such examinations by placing 100 mL of saline over the tumor site and then aspirating the fluid for cytologic assessment.[465] Patients with positive cytology were found to have a significantly higher rate of recurrence, but the survival rate did not correlate with the findings.

Intraoperative Colonoscopy

The importance of complete evaluation of the colon before undertaking a colectomy for cancer cannot be overestimated. However, there are instances when such an evaluation may not be feasible. Under such circumstances, one may consider utilizing intraoperative colonoscopy. Various clinical settings have been suggested—assessment of a new anastomosis to determine whether any air leakage is present or to identify any suture line defects, identification of a prior polypectomy site, inability to do a complete or adequate preoperative colonoscopy, detection of a source of intestinal bleeding, and detection of a colon lesion that cannot be palpated.[812] With respect to resection of colon tumors, however, the primary indications are identification of a nonpalpable lesion and an incomplete or inadequate preoperative colonoscopy.

Although the procedure may be somewhat awkward and generally requires a skilled endoscopist as well as the operating surgeon, it can be performed safely as the instrument is guided through the bowel by the surgeon, but not necessarily easily or expeditiously. Clamping the region of the distal ileum is important to avoid reflux of air back into the small bowel; this can result in dilatation. When an obstructing tumor is present, the procedure can be undertaken in an antegrade fashion through a cecotomy or in a retrograde fashion after resection of the tumor-bearing segment. Obviously, the patient must be placed in the perineolithotomy position on the operating table to provide appropriate exposure. Still, this is not necessarily a straightforward procedure.

Stapling Techniques

The use of staplers in colonic operations has been proven to be at least as safe as conventional suturing and in some circumstances offers distinct advantages. Three types of stapling devices are available to perform intestinal anastomoses: linear staplers [United States Surgical TA series—30, 45, 60, and 90 mm; Ethicon (Somerville, NJ) Proximate RL series—30, 60, and 90 mm], which apply two rows of staggered staples (Figure 22-61); the gastrointestinal anastomosis (GIA) stapler (United States Surgical—60 and 80 mm) and Proximate linear cutter (Ethicon—55, 75, and 100 mm), which apply two staggered rows of staples and divide the tissue by means of a contained knife (Figure 22-62); and the circular, end-to-end (EEA, CEEA) anastomosis stapler (United States Surgical) and ILS, DHC (Ethicon) see Figs. 23-71 through 23-73, which secure two rows of staples from within the lumen of the bowel to produce an inverting anastomosis in a circular fashion. The 3M Company (St. Paul, MN) also produces internal stapling devices, such as the Precise ILA-50 and 100-mm and the Flexistapler circular stapling instruments.

Stapling of the bowel requires stripping the mesentery and fat from the ends of the intestine. This should be carried out for a distance of approximately 5 mm, but the critical issue is to remove any fat and blood vessels at the

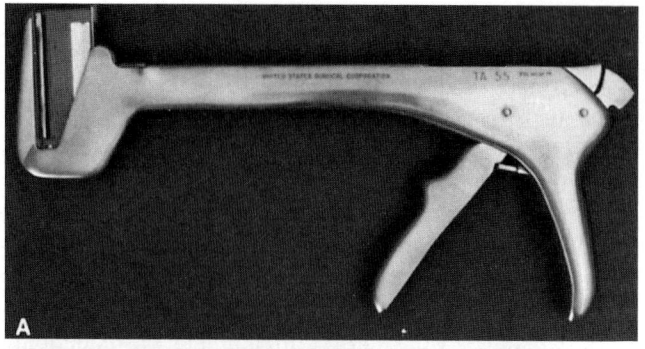

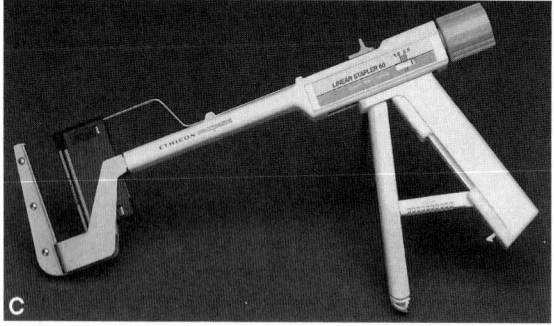

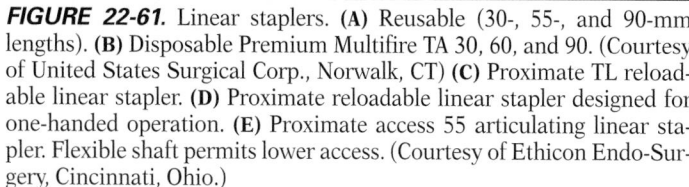

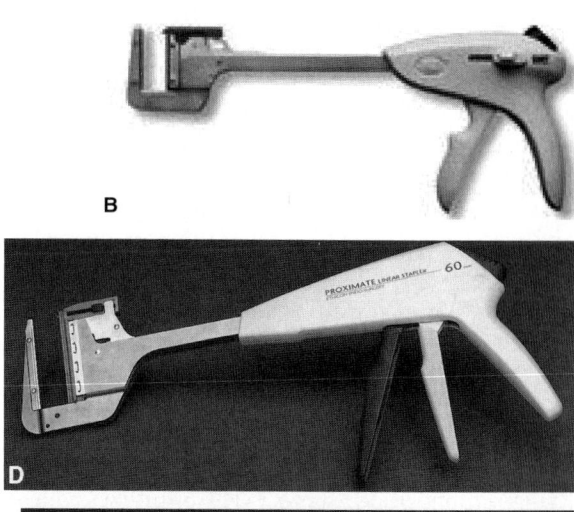

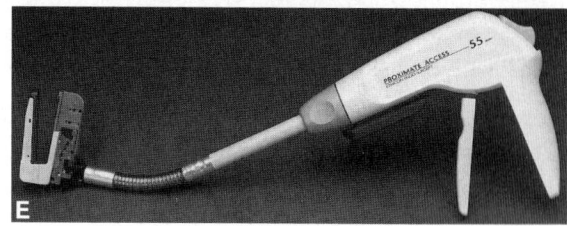

FIGURE 22-61. Linear staplers. **(A)** Reusable (30-, 55-, and 90-mm lengths). **(B)** Disposable Premium Multifire TA 30, 60, and 90. (Courtesy of United States Surgical Corp., Norwalk, CT) **(C)** Proximate TL reloadable linear stapler. **(D)** Proximate reloadable linear stapler designed for one-handed operation. **(E)** Proximate access 55 articulating linear stapler. Flexible shaft permits lower access. (Courtesy of Ethicon Endo-Surgery, Cincinnati, Ohio.)

level where the instrument closes.[773] Attention to that detail minimizes the risk of bleeding.

Anastomosis of the bowel can be accomplished by a number of methods. Figure 22-63 demonstrates the application of the linear stapler by a triangulation technique. The staple lines should cross each other. This produces an everting anastomosis that, although contraindicated when used with conventional suturing, does not seem to be a problem with the stapling device. An alternative approach is to invert the posterior row, everting the two anterior limbs (Figure 22-64). Venkatesh and colleagues utilized the triangulation stapling technique to perform colorectal anastomoses in 259 patients.[977] The incidence of anastomotic leak was certainly comparable with that of the circular stapled anastomoses performed for this purpose (1.1%). Still, this method is rarely employed, having been replaced by the following.

The GIA or linear cutter stapler creates a side-to-side anastomosis, but the tissue is divided, producing a functional end-to-end anastomosis. Figure 22-65 illustrates the closed technique and subsequent closure of the enterotomies (Figure 22-66). Alternatively, an open method can be employed (Figs. 22-67 and 22-68). Other variations include division of the bowel with a linear stapler

(Figure 22-69) or with the GIA stapler (Figure 22-70). A final modification to effect right hemicolectomy has been suggested by Meagher and Wolff by use of the GIA stapler or linear cutter (Figure 22-71).[618]

The circular stapling devices can also be used to effect colonic anastomoses. Figure 22-72 demonstrates this procedure. Additionally, an ileocolic anastomosis can be accomplished with the circular stapler (Figure 22-73). Other methods of application are illustrated in Chapter 23.

A new concept on circular stapling is called the Surg-ASSIST (Power Medical Interventions, New Hope, PA; www.pmi2.com). This is a long, flexible power source that is passed through the anus and guided by the surgeon to effect a circular stapled anastomosis higher up in the colon than may be achieved by the conventional circular stapling instruments. The device consists of a computer-mediated closure and is available in diameters of 21, 25, 29, and 33 mm. The loading unit is disposable. The company also makes a linear cutter. All instrument movements with both devices are automated and executed via push-button remote control. With the linear cutter, two double-rows of staples are deployed with the incorporated cutting blade. It remains to be seen whether this advanced concept has sufficient practicality for one to justify its purchase.

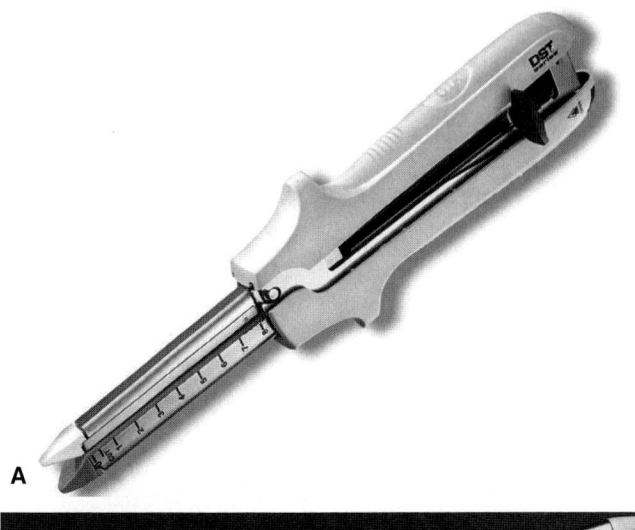

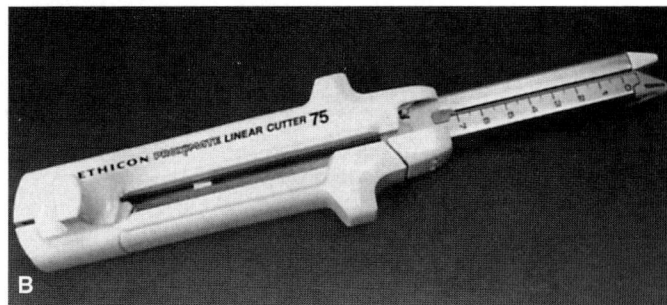

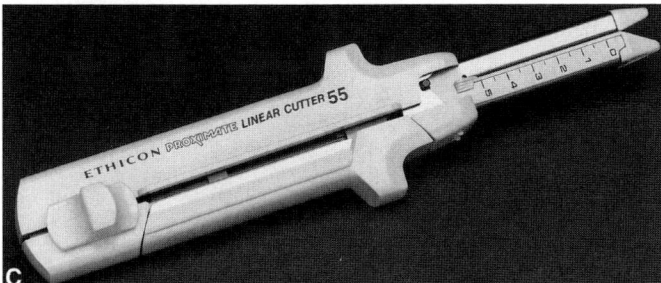

FIGURE 22-62. Intestinal anastomosis staplers. **(A)** Disposable Multifire DST-GIA, available in 60 mm and 80 mm lengths. (Courtesy of Tyco/United States Surgical Corp., Norwalk, CT) **(B)** Disposable, reloadable Proximate linear cutter (TLC75). This is also available in 50- and 100-mm lengths. **(C)** Ethicon TVC55 linear cutter for mesenteric division. This is a vascular stapler. (Courtesy of Ethicon Endo-Surgery, Cincinnati, Ohio.)

Complications and Results of Anastomoses

Disruption of the suture or staple line is clinically apparent in approximately 5% of all colonic anastomoses, but the true incidence of this complication is probably much higher.[834] The rate of anastomotic disruption low in the rectum, when studied thoroughly, may be as high as 69% (see Chapter 23).[834] Factors that contribute to anastomotic leakage are discussed in Chapter 23 (see Table 23-1). Irrespective of the technique employed to reapproximate the bowel, the rates of complications (fecal fistula, hemorrhage, stricture) are about the same.[149,219, 254,478,774,993,996] However, Dunn and colleagues, in a study on dogs, believed that the one-layer, hand-sewn anastomosis was superior.[239] Reiling and associates, in a controlled trial, reported that operating time, nasogastric intubation, and total length of hospitalization were about the same for both techniques.[774] This implies that the variables responsible for complications have less to do with the method of anastomosis than with other factors, such as tension, blood supply, presence of sepsis, and nutritional state of the patient. Friend and colleagues, in a randomized trial of 250 patients who underwent elective surgery involving an anastomosis in the left colon, observed no differences in the clinical or radiologic leakage rate.[284] However, when the results were analyzed according to surgeon, it became evident that those in training did less well with suturing. Perhaps the relatively standardized approach to stapling was able to account for the observed difference. Alternatively, it may have represented a lack of experience by surgical residents with the suturing technique. In the area of experience, it has been shown that not only surgeon procedure volume but also hospital procedure volume is an important predictor of outcome with respect to morbidity, mortality, and cure rates following colon cancer resection.[833]

A problem that appears to be more specific with stapled intestinal anastomoses is bleeding. Many surgeons make a conscientious effort to visualize the staple line before final closure in a functional end-to-end anastomosis. Any bleeding point can be managed with a simple suture ligature. Atabek and colleagues have successfully employed vasopressin to control bleeding from a stapled intestinal anastomosis in the postoperative period.[35] This method of treatment is frightening to me because of the risk of causing ischemia.

Comment

Stapling instruments have replaced conventional suture techniques for many surgeons today. In fact, as mentioned, in some teaching centers residents have only

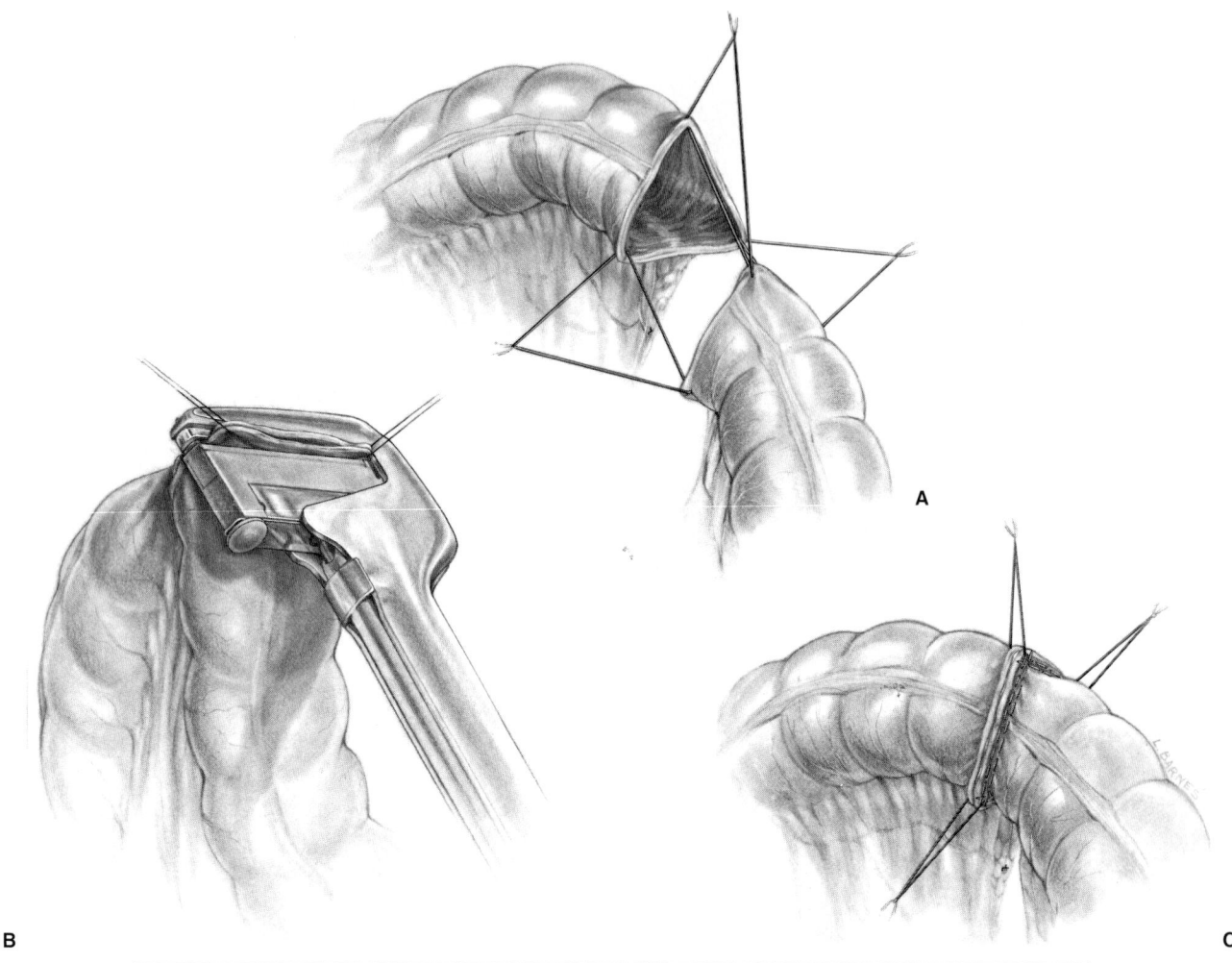

FIGURE 22-63. Anastomosis by triangulation using the linear stapler. **(A)** Everting anastomosis using three stay sutures. **(B)** The TA stapler. **(C)** Eversion of all three applications.

minimal exposure to the traditional approach. It is true that as one gains experience an anastomosis may be constructed more quickly with a stapling instrument. It is difficult to believe, however, that operative time can, as has been claimed, be reduced by 25% and even 50%. The fact is that the performance of the anastomosis, itself, represents only a part of the time invested in the whole operation. Opening and exploring the abdomen, dissecting out the bowel, resecting the specimen, and closing the abdomen represent efforts that may require a considerable expenditure of time. Intestinal stapling, obviously, fails to expedite these. Except for avoidance of the risk for needle injury and some slight savings in time, I believe that the stapling devices offer no great advantages over conventional suture technique for standard colon anastomoses other than low pelvic procedures (see Chapter 23). However, I recognize that a large coterie of respected, competent surgeons believes otherwise. I stated in the second edition of this text,

"Perhaps it is simply intransigence that causes me to persist in using conventional suturing, but if truth be told I must confess that I enjoy sewing." I still enjoy sewing, but because of the risk for injury to operating room personnel, I find that I am eschewing suturing much more frequently today in favor of the application of a stapling alternative.

Other Anastomotic Devices

Biofragmentable Ring (Valtrac)

In 1985, Hardy and colleagues described a biofragmentable ring for sutureless intestinal anastomosis.[383] The ring is composed of two segments containing polyglycolic acid (Dexon) and 12% barium sulfate. The major advantage when compared with the classic Murphy button (Figure 22-34) is that it does not produce necrosis but fragments during the third week following implantation. The procedure is probably somewhat more rapid than

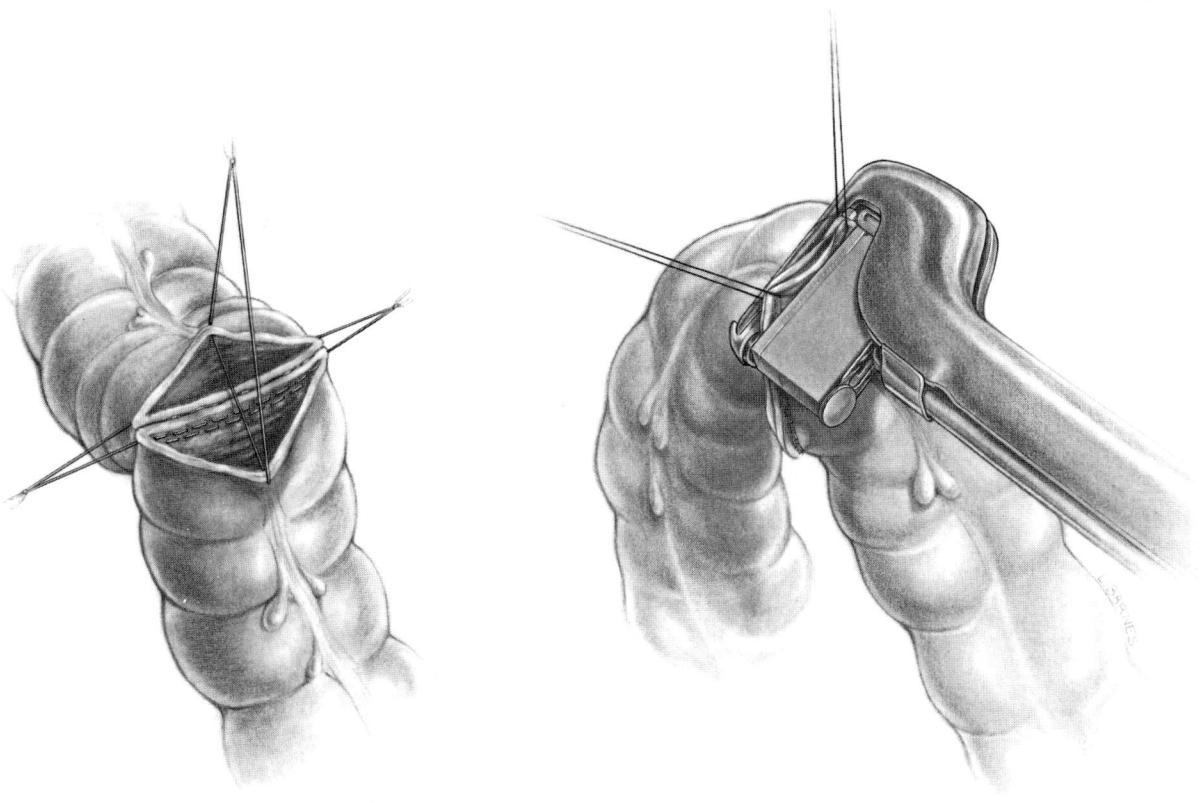

A   **B**

FIGURE 22-64. Triangulation anastomosis by inversion of the posterior (mesenteric) wall **(A)** and eversion of the anterior walls **(B)**.

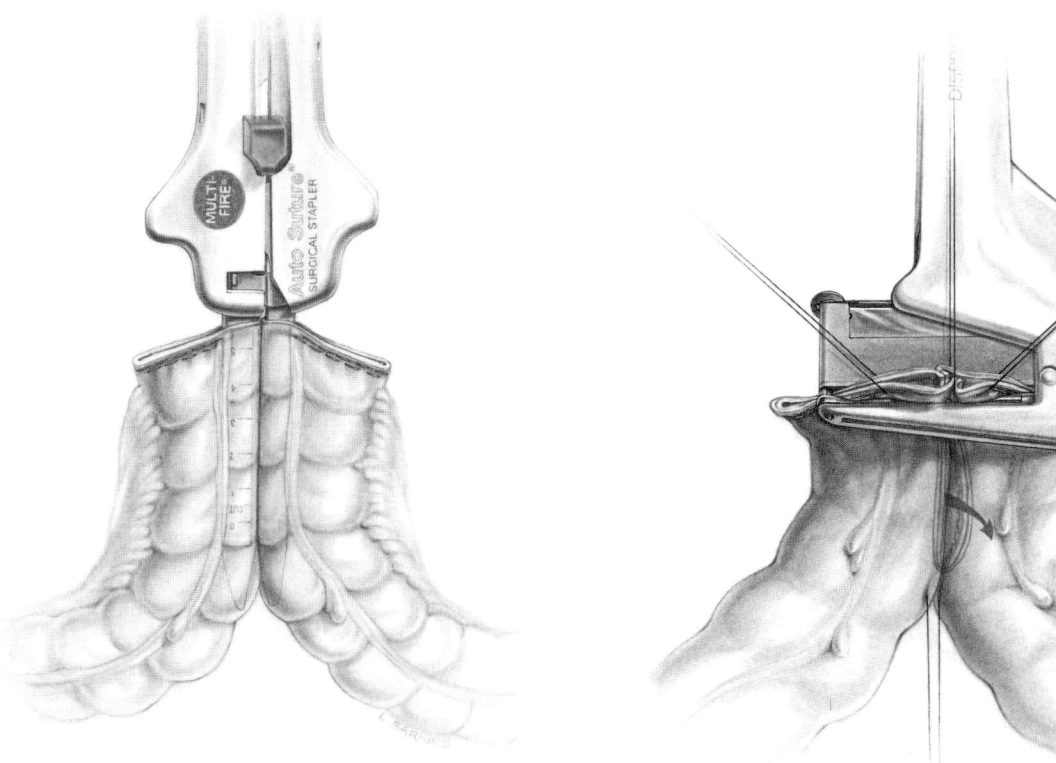

FIGURE 22-65. Functional end-to-end anastomosis by the closed technique after creation of two enterotomies for insertion of the separate limbs of the gastrointestinal anastomosis stapler.

FIGURE 22-66. Closure of the enterotomies using the TA stapler.

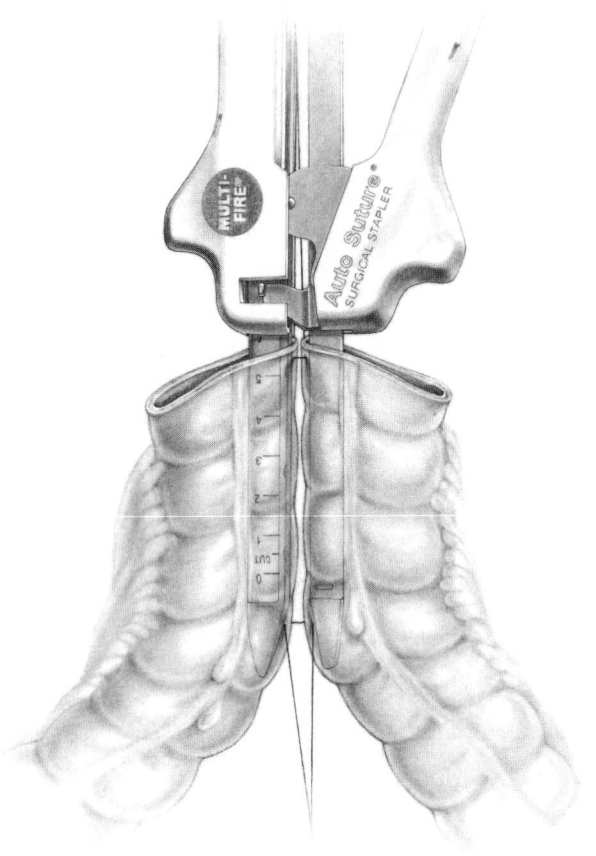

FIGURE 22-67. Functional end-to-end anastomosis by the open technique with the gastrointestinal anastomosis stapler.

conventional suturing and has the advantage of applicability to all parts of the intestine. However, it is quite limiting with respect to low rectal anastomoses, especially when compared with the circular stapling device, although an adapter for transanal placement has been reported from Taiwan.[150] However, it is at least as safe as other anastomotic alternatives. The rings are available in six sizes represented by the outside diameter, inside diameter, and closed position gap. The outside diameters are 28, 31, and 34 mm, and the gap width varies between 1.5 and 2.5 mm.

Technique Figure 22-74 illustrates the bowel anastomosis ring in the open position with the holder in place. The method of performing the anastomosis is as follows: After the bowel has been mobilized, a purse-string suture is placed (Figs. 22-75 and 22-76). As with the placement of a purse-string for the circular stapling instrument, a monofilament suture, preferably absorbable, is recommended. Three Allis clamps are triangulated on the proximal limb if a colorectal anastomosis is contemplated. A sizing device is available to determine which diameter ring is applicable (Figure 22-77). It is important to place the device into the proximal end first, because it is easier to pull the rectum onto the ring

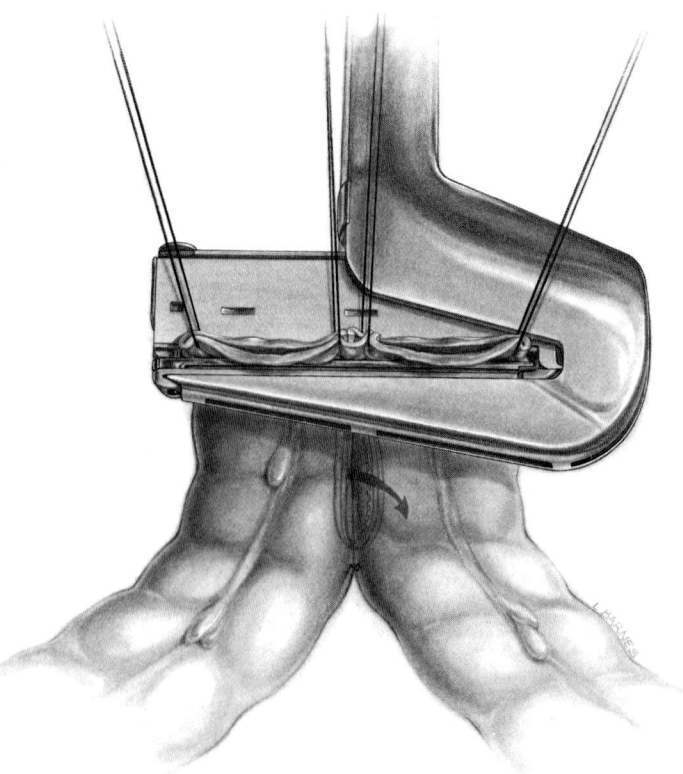

FIGURE 22-68. Closure of the bowel ends with the TA stapler and open functional end-to-end anastomosis.

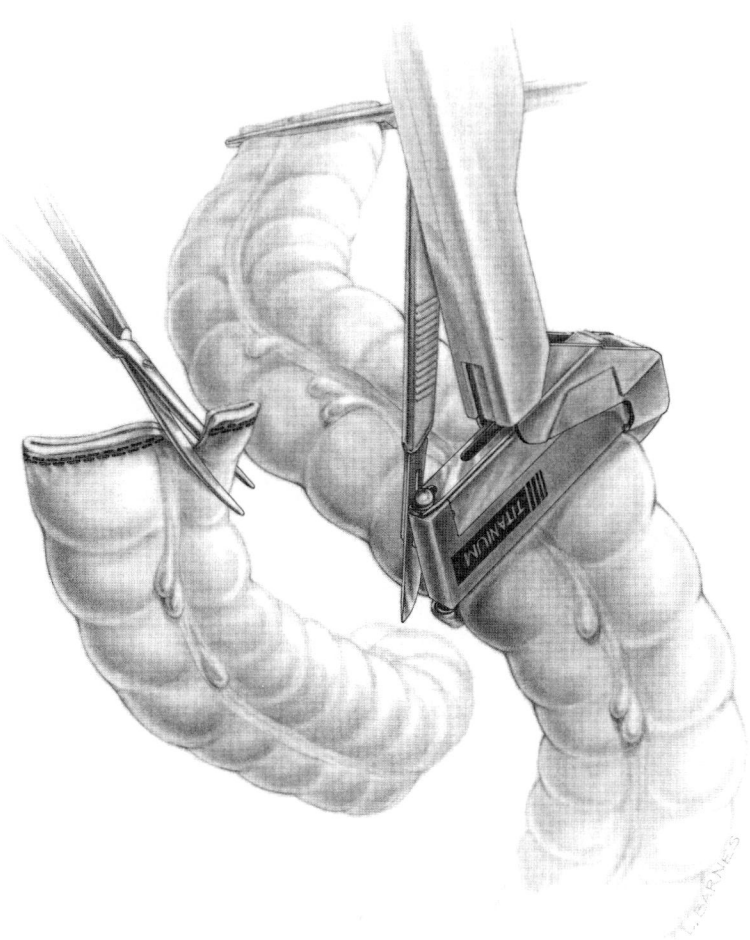

FIGURE 22-69. One option for resection and division of the bowel in preparation for the anastomosis is to use the linear stapler.

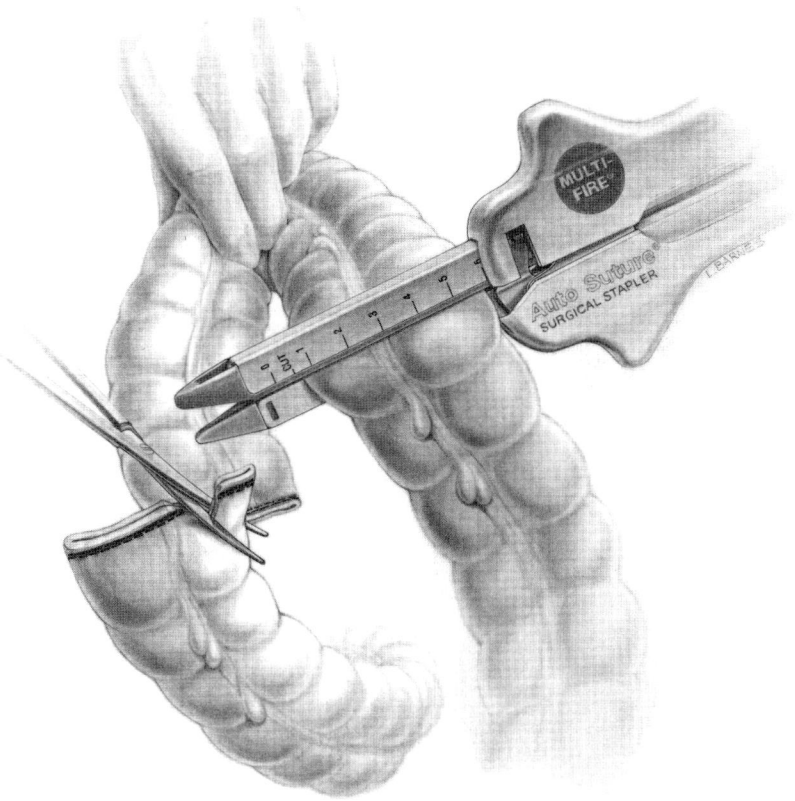

FIGURE 22-70. Most common method of creating a stapled anastomosis involves division of the bowel with the gastrointestinal anastomosis stapler and anastomosis through several firings of the instrument. Linear closure of the created defect is then accomplished.

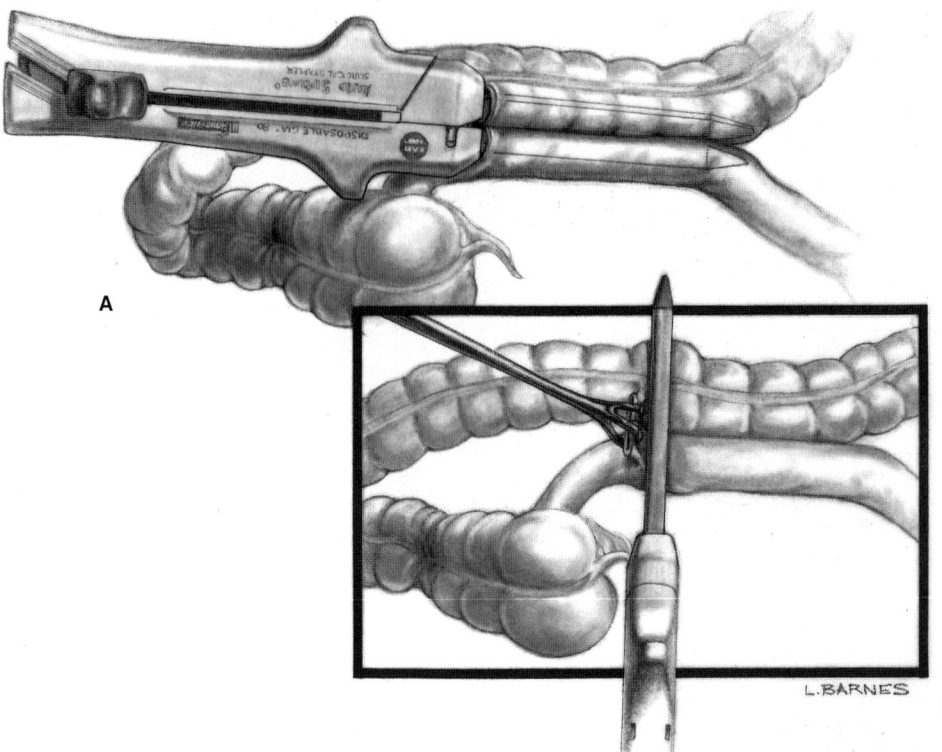

FIGURE 22-71. Colon anastomosis is facilitated following mobilization of the right colon by use of the gastrointestinal anastomosis stapling device to create a functional end-to-end anastomosis **(A)** and simultaneous firing of the instrument across both the ileum and colon **(B)**. (Adapted from Meagher AP, Wolff BG. Right hemicolectomy with a linear cutting stapler. *Dis Colon Rectum* 1994; 37:1043.)

L.BARNES

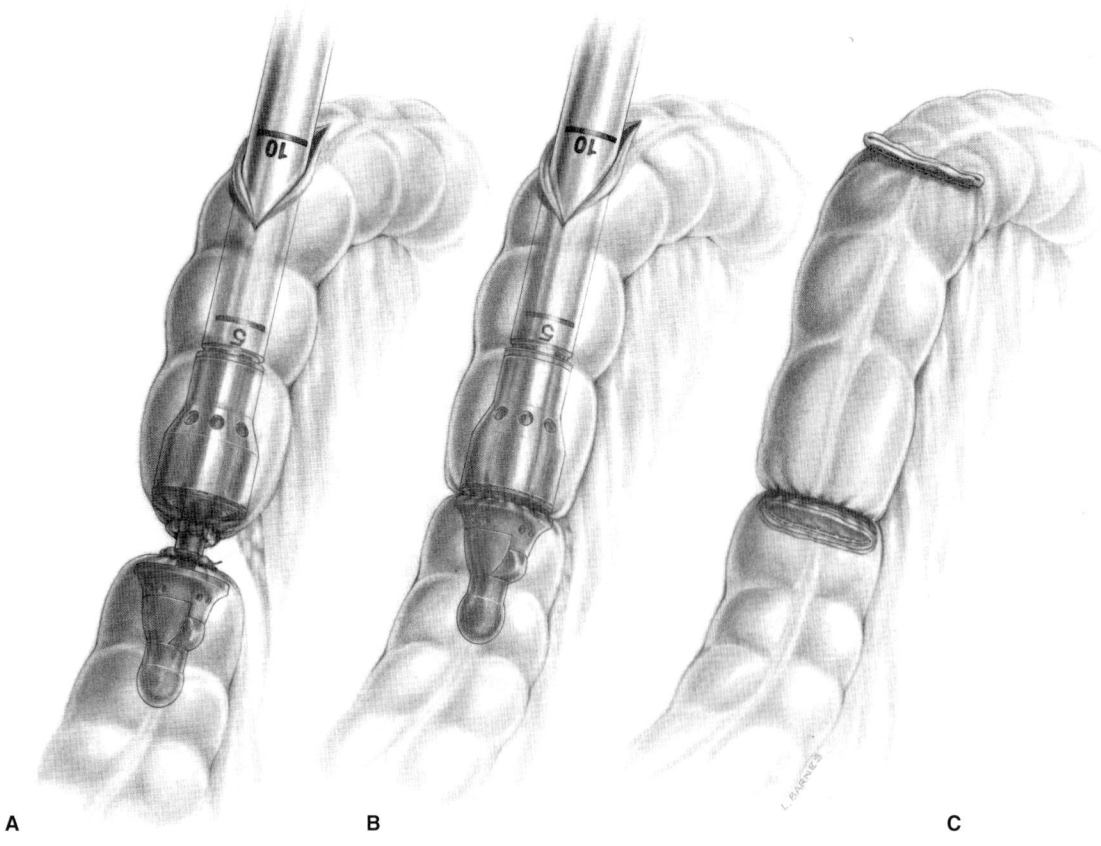

A B C

FIGURE 22-72. (A,B) Steps of circular end-to-end anastomosis stapler used in colonic anastomosis through a proximal colotomy. **(C)** Note the stapled closure of the colotomy converting the longitudinal incision to a transverse closure.

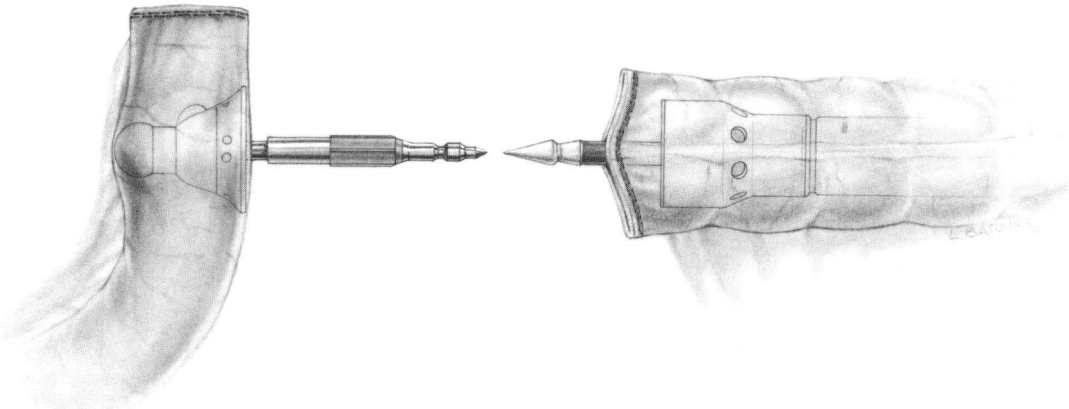

FIGURE 22-73. Anastomosis of the distal ileum to the transverse colon by means of the circular stapler. The proximal anvil can be placed either in the end of the ileum or in the side (as illustrated). The stapling device is placed through an enterotomy in the colon with anastomosis shown by a double-stapling technique (note the trocar). A purse-string suture is another option. There are several possible variations on this theme.

rather than to push the proximal bowel down (Figure 22-78). It does not matter whether the proximal or distal end is secured initially if the anastomosis is well out of the pelvis. The purse-string suture is then secured (Figure 22-79). With the use of a triangulation technique, the ring is inserted into the distal bowel (Figure 22-80). A "holding" device is available that may make this maneuver easier to accomplish (Figure 22-81). The second purse-string suture is then tied (Figure 22-82). The ring is then snapped shut with an audible and tactile click, and an inverted serosa-to-serosa anastomosis is created (Figure 22-83). The security of the closure needs to be checked by the application of gentle pressure between the two anvils, to make certain that they cannot be separated (Figure 22-84).[143]

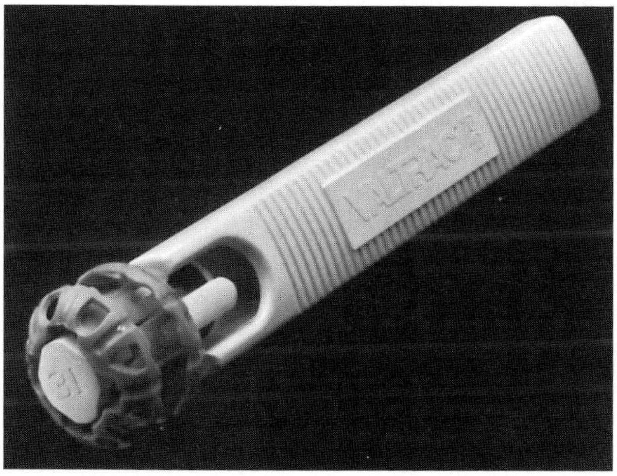

Results Because the ring is impregnated with barium, it is radiopaque and can be seen on a plain abdominal x-ray film (Figure 22-85). Fragmentation usually takes place between 17 and 21 days (Figure 22-86). The material at this time is soft and is rarely noted by the patient when it is passed during defecation.

Since the original publication of the experimental reports, hundreds of patients have undergone resection and anastomosis by this method.[257,273,381,385] In randomized, multicenter, prospective clinical trials that compared the biofragmentable ring with suture technique and with stapling, there was no significant difference in morbidity, mortality, or clinical course of the patients.[111,354] The safety and efficacy of this device were confirmed in several other trials.[135,175,1043] Gullichsen and colleagues studied the late results after colonic anastomosis performed with the biofragmentable ring in 30 patients at a mean of 2 years.[355] One had undergone reoperation because of a stricture. Endoscopic and radiology examination could not identify the anastomotic site in approximately half of the patients.

Comment The Valtrac device is indeed still available, but no one seems motivated to write about it. There are apparently only a very few surgeons who continue to employ it, however. Along these same lines, there has also been a virtual absence of publications in the last few years on the whole subject of stapling and suturing. Perhaps everything has been said, taught, and learned with

(text continues on page 840)

FIGURE 22-74. Valtrac biofragmentable ring. (Courtesy of United States Surgical Corporation, Norwalk, CT.)

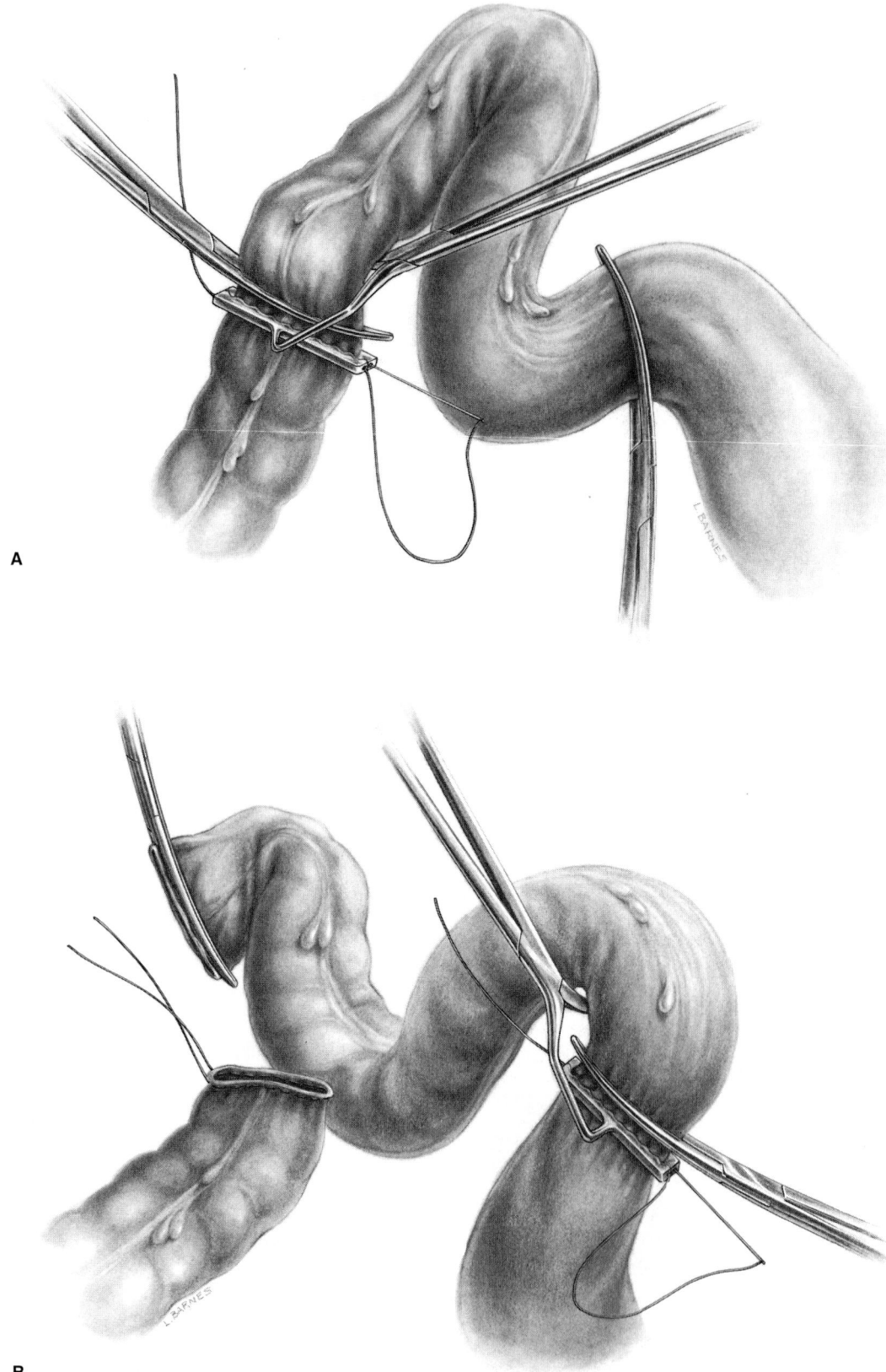

FIGURE 22-75. (A,B) Anastomosis by biofragmentable ring. Purse-string technique with an applicator.

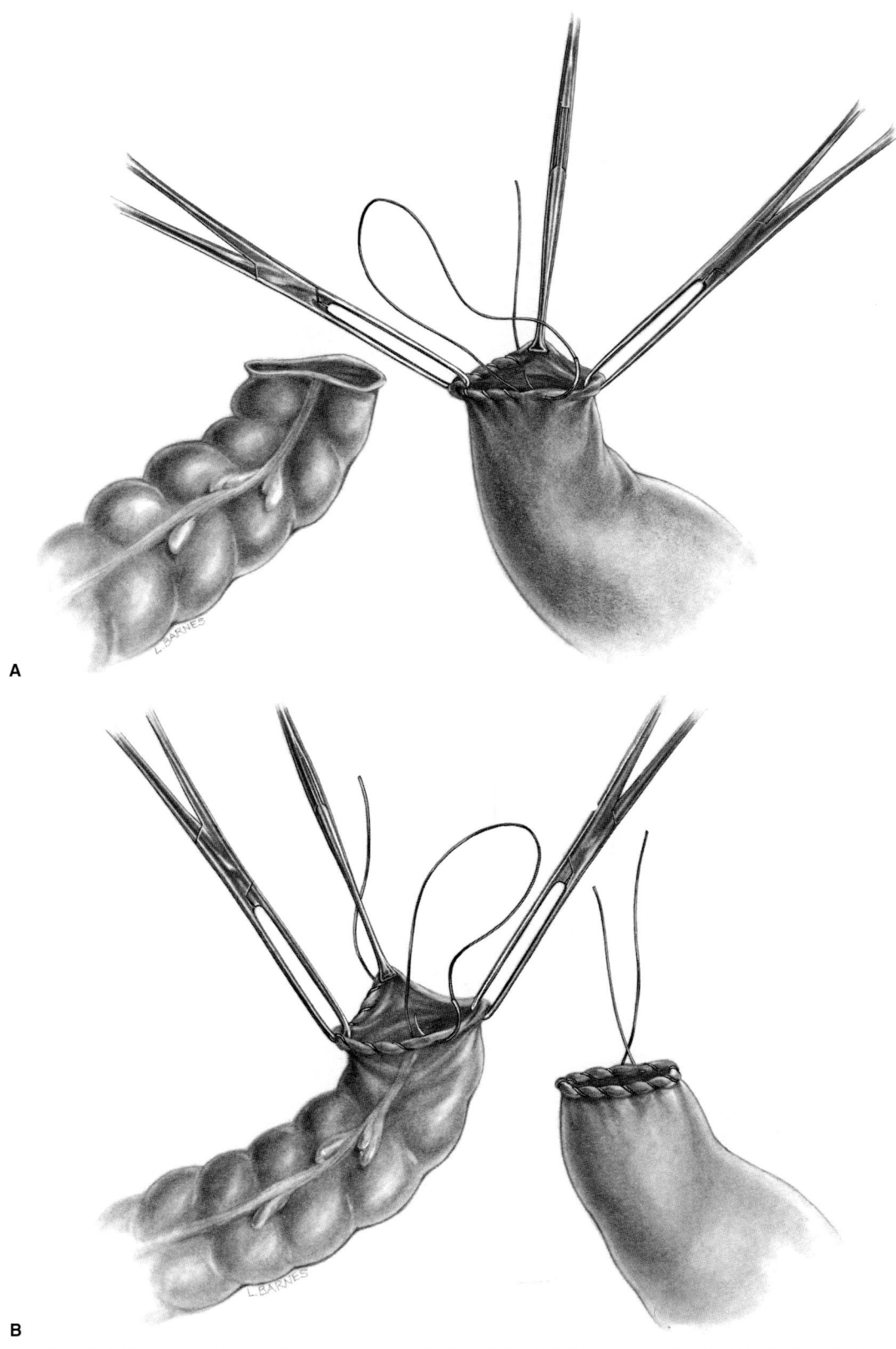

FIGURE 22-76. (**A,B**) Anastomosis by biofragmentable ring. Hand-sewn purse string.

A

B

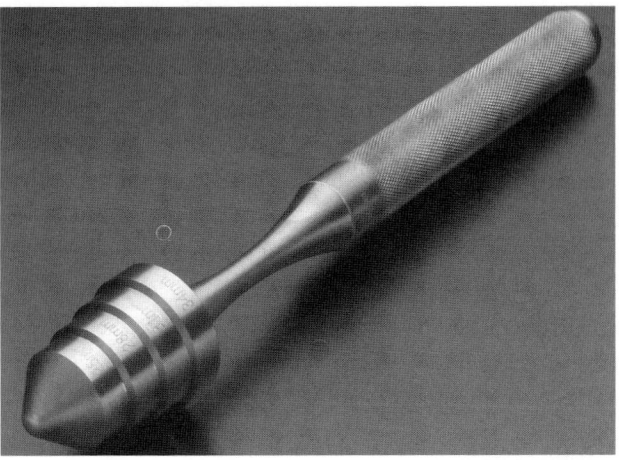

FIGURE 22-77. Sizing device for determining which diameter Valtrac ring is appropriate. (Courtesy of United States Surgical Corporation, Norwalk, CT.)

regard to the technical aspects of reestablishing intestinal continuity—I hope not.

Circular Compression Device

In 1988, Rosati and colleagues described a mechanical device for creating a circular anastomosis through compression.[791] This is much more like the Murphy button, in that both innovations effect an anastomosis by means of compression. The apparatus consists of three molded polypropylene rings carried by a gun that introduces them into the bowel. For a colorectal anastomosis, transanal insertion is undertaken in the same way that the conventional circular stapling instruments are employed (see Chapter 23). Firing of the gun causes simultaneous assemblage of the rings, expulsion of the entire anastomotic apparatus, and disengagement of the gun, with the creation of two tissue rings.[791] The rings are evacuated

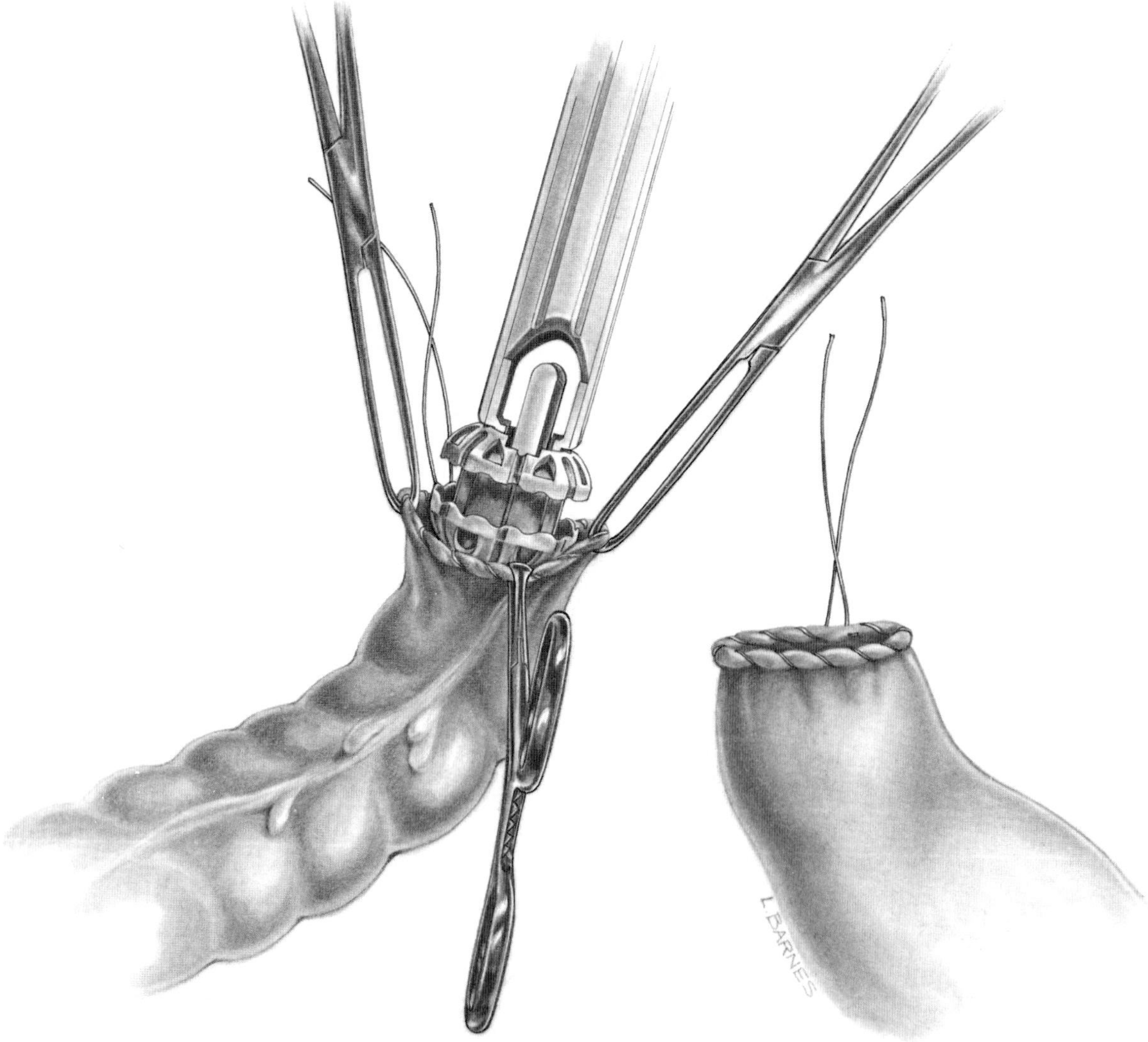

FIGURE 22-78. Anastomosis by biofragmentable ring. Insertion of Valtrac ring into proximal limb of bowel.

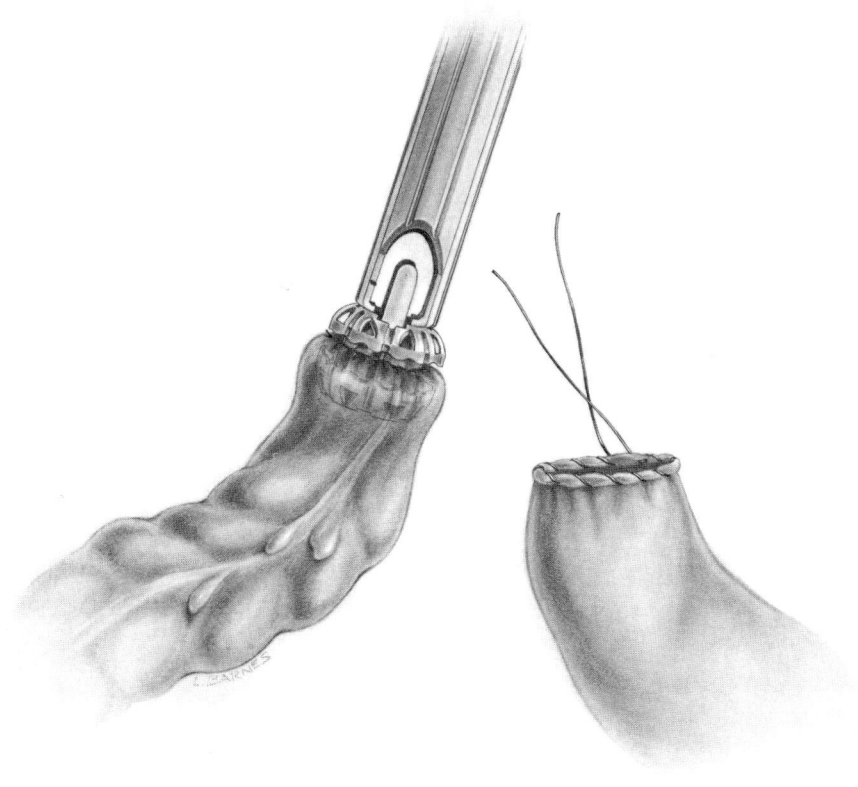

FIGURE 22-79. Anastomosis by biofragmentable ring. A purse-string suture is secured around the device.

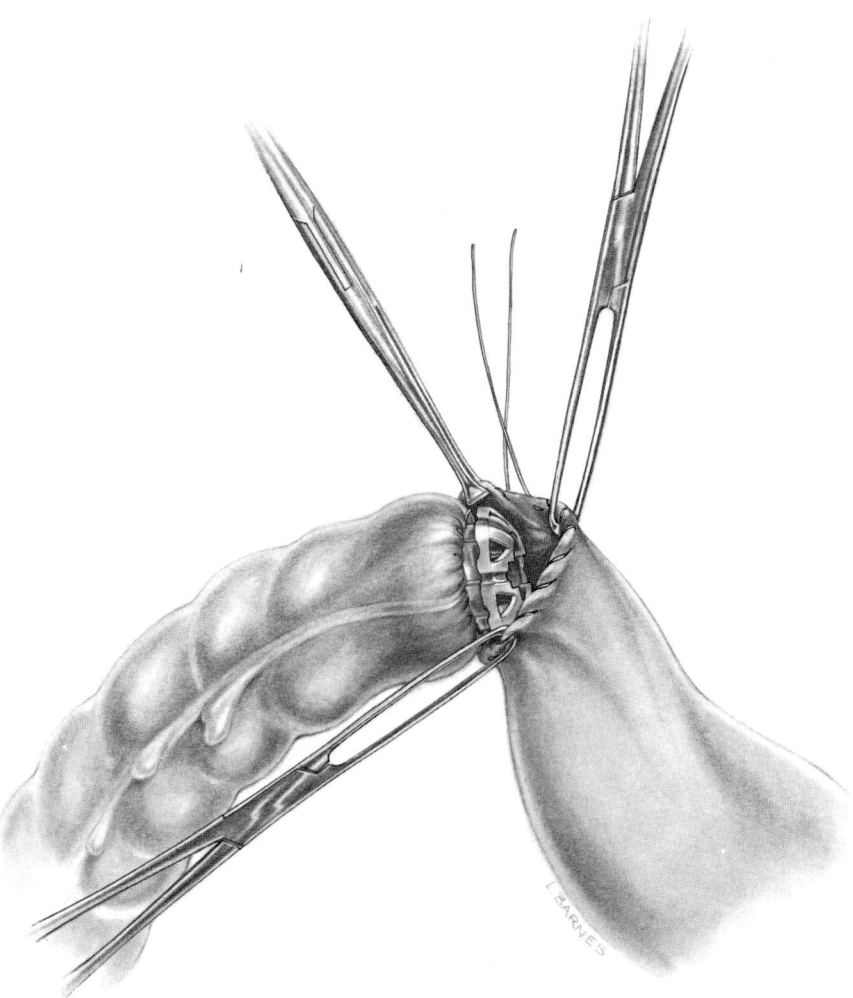

FIGURE 22-80. Anastomosis by biofragmentable ring. The ring is inserted into the distal bowel.

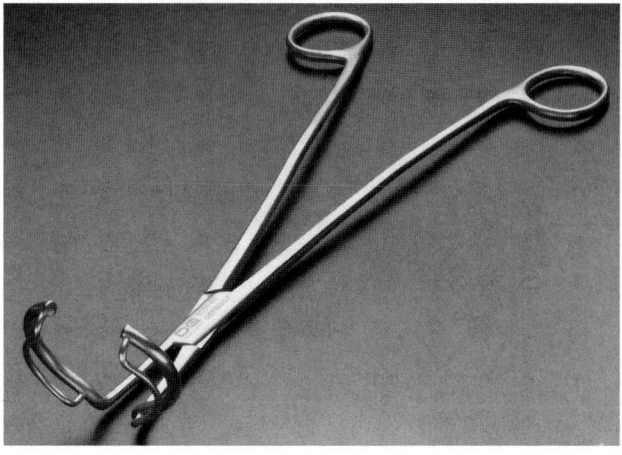

FIGURE 22-81. Device for holding the biofragmentable ring while the distal bowel is pulled upward. (Courtesy of United States Surgical Corporation, Norwalk, CT.)

between the ninth and thirteenth postoperative days. In contrast to the circular stapler, it leaves no staples or foreign material within the bowel.

Results Malthaner and colleagues employed the device experimentally in dogs and compared it with the circular stapler.[580] They noted that the button was easier to use, caused less ulceration, fibrosis, and inflammation, and was associated with better reepithelialization at the anastomotic site. Rebuffat and colleagues used the technique for 56 patients in diverse colon operations.[768] There was one operative death (myocardial infarction) and one anastomotic leak.

As of this writing, I have had no experience with this device and have been able to identify no recent literature on the subject.

Magnetic Ring Anastomosis

A modification of the Murphy button has been described by Jansen and colleagues.[445] An anastomotic apparatus consisting of two magnetic rings embedded in polyester progressively compresses and causes necro-

sis in the intervening bowel through increasing magnetic force while healing takes place. After 7 to 12 days, the magnets cut through and are eliminated through the stool.

I have had no experience with this method. Furthermore, since the publication of the third edition of this text, there have been no further contributions to the literature.

Specific Management Situations

Obstruction

Proximal Colon Obstruction

The management of intestinal obstruction was an area of particular interest for one of the singular individuals in American surgery in the twentieth century, Claude E. Welch.[1004] Obstructing carcinoma of the proximal colon usually can be treated by resection and primary anastomosis without a diversionary procedure (Figure 22-87). Technically, the resection can be relatively easily performed and an anastomosis effected between the ileum and the distal bowel.

When the ileocecal valve is intact, the distal ileum is usually of normal caliber. Even when the small bowel is dilated, an anastomosis can usually be accomplished with relative safety. Whenever carcinoma of the right and transverse colon presents with obstruction, the resected bowel proximal to the lesion should always include the colon to the level of the distal ileum. If the surgeon believes that diversion of a proximal colonic obstruction is necessary at the first stage, or if a protective stoma after ileocolonic anastomosis is indicated, loop ileostomy is the preferred option (see Figs. 31-67 through 31-69).

Left Colon Obstruction

Ninety percent of colonic obstructions occur distal to the splenic flexure. When carcinoma precipitates a left-sided obstruction, the surgeon faces a more difficult decision. Should primary resection be undertaken? Should an

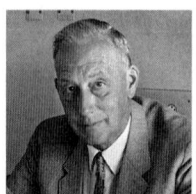

Claude E. Welch (1907–1996)   Claude Welch was born in Stanton, Nebraska, February 25, 1907. He attended Doane College in Crete, Nebraska and graduated in 1927. He then obtained a Master's Degree in Chemistry from the University of Missouri. He entered medical school at Harvard and graduated in 1932. There followed a Residency in Pathology at Boston City Hospital and a Residency in Surgery at Pondville Hospital in suburban Boston and at the Massachusetts General Hospital. He joined the faculty at Harvard in 1937 and remained there for the rest of his life. His role model was Arthur Allen, Chief of the East Service at the General. In 1942, Welch joined the Harvard medical group in North Africa and then in Italy, returning in 1945. That same year, he performed the first vein graft at Massachusetts General Hospital. He became recognized as a brilliant technical surgeon and clinical investigator. His principal contributions were the introduction of catheter duodenostomy, the management of intestinal obstruction, and the treatment of respiratory failure concomitant with peritonitis. In 1981, he was called to Rome to assist in the care of Pope John Paul II following his gunshot wound to the abdomen. Welch won numerous awards, including the Bigelow Medal of the Boston Surgical Society and the Nathan Smith Award of the New England Surgical Society. In 1992, on the occasion of the sixtieth anniversary of his graduation from Harvard Medical School, the University established an endowed Chair of Surgery in his honor. He died on March 9, 1996, of a cerebrovascular accident. (With appreciation to Harvard Medical School. Photograph, Courtesy of Dr. Welch.)

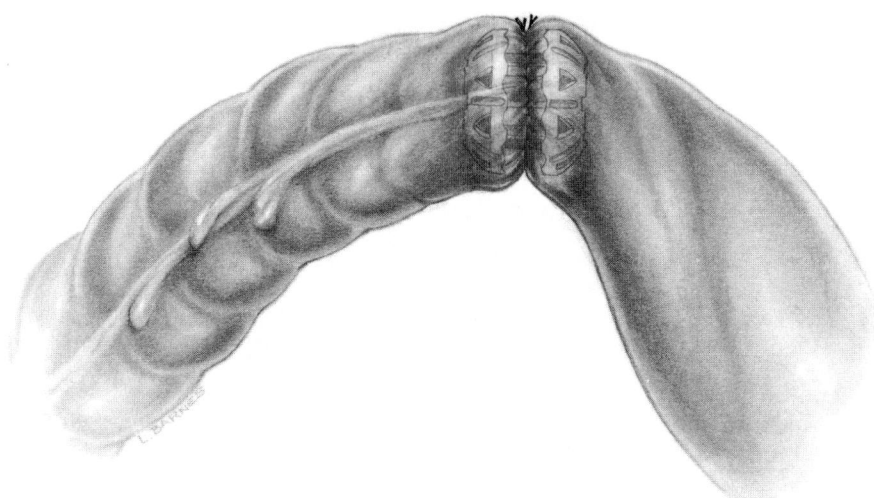

FIGURE 22-82. Anastomosis by bio-fragmentable ring. The distal purse-string suture is now tied.

anastomosis be performed? Should a diversion be created? It is difficult to answer these questions dogmatically, because nuances in the presentation or in the findings may lead the surgeon to take an alternative course of action. One of the important considerations is to note whether the obstruction is complete or partial (Figs. 22-88 and 22-89). If the patient continues to have bowel movements or to pass flatus or is seen to have gas distal to the site of obstruction on a plain film of the abdomen, the obstruction is incomplete. Conversely, if the patient has not passed flatus or defecated for many hours or even days and no gas is visible distally, the obstruction is probably complete. At exploratory laparotomy, the degree of dilatation of the proximal bowel can be assessed and the choice of operation determined. Obstruction as a result of a malignancy does not necessarily mandate an exploratory operation. For example, when carcinomatosis is known to be present, it may be prudent to observe the patient and to treat the condition

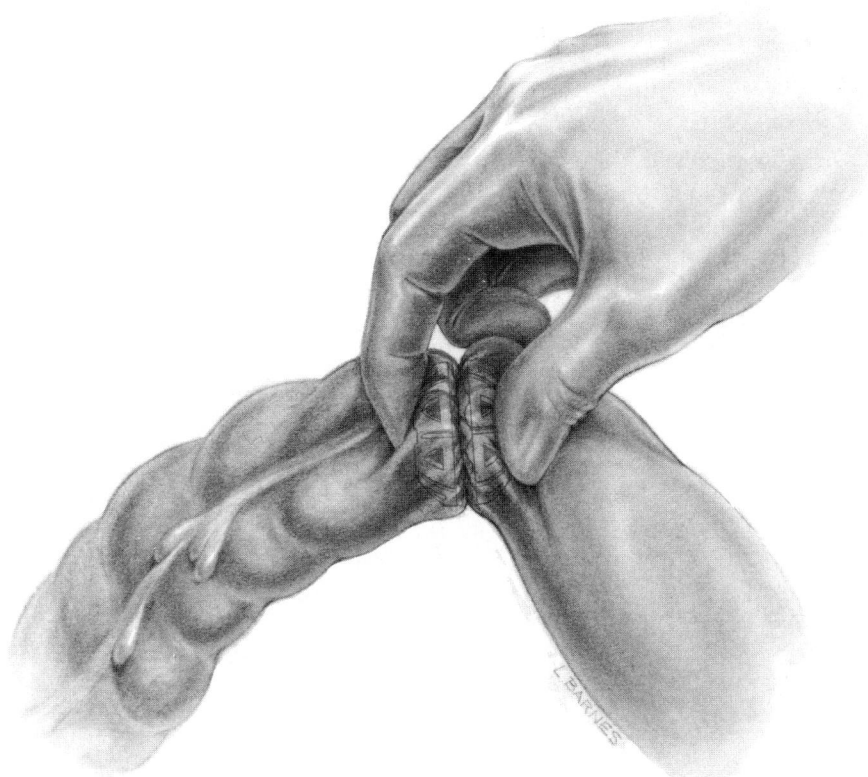

FIGURE 22-83. Anastomosis by bio-fragmentable ring. The ring is closed.

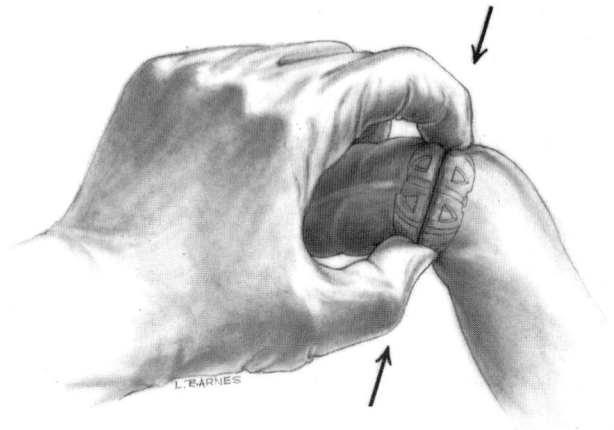

FIGURE 22-84. Testing the security of the Valtrac biofragmentable anastomotic ring by attempted distraction of the anvils through gentle pressure. (Adapted from Celoria G, Falco E, Nardini A, et al. Intraoperative testing of the Valtrac biofragmentable anastomotic ring. *Br J Surg* 1993;80:618.)

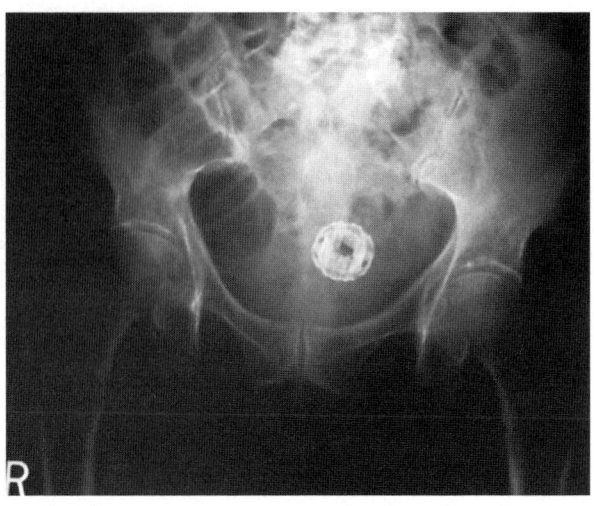

FIGURE 22-85. Plain abdominal roentgenogram reveals radiopaque ring at the site of rectal anastomosis.

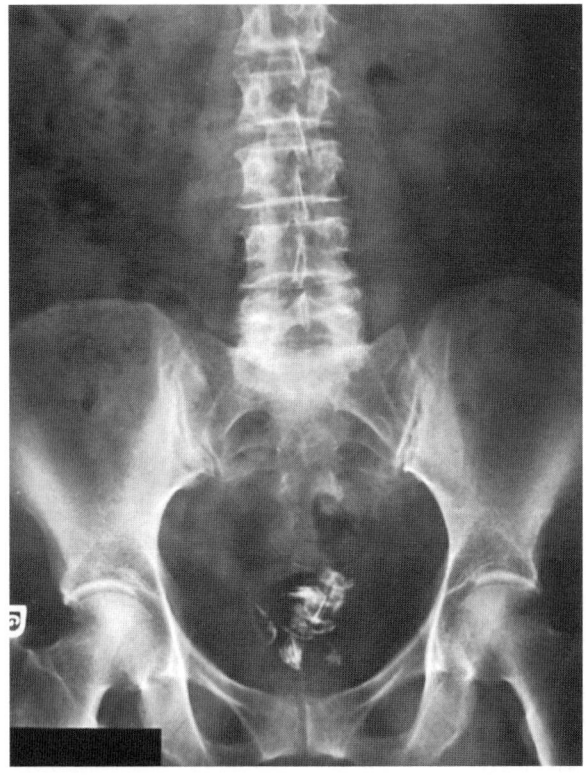

FIGURE 22-86. Fragmented ring apparent on a plain abdominal x-ray film just before its passing.

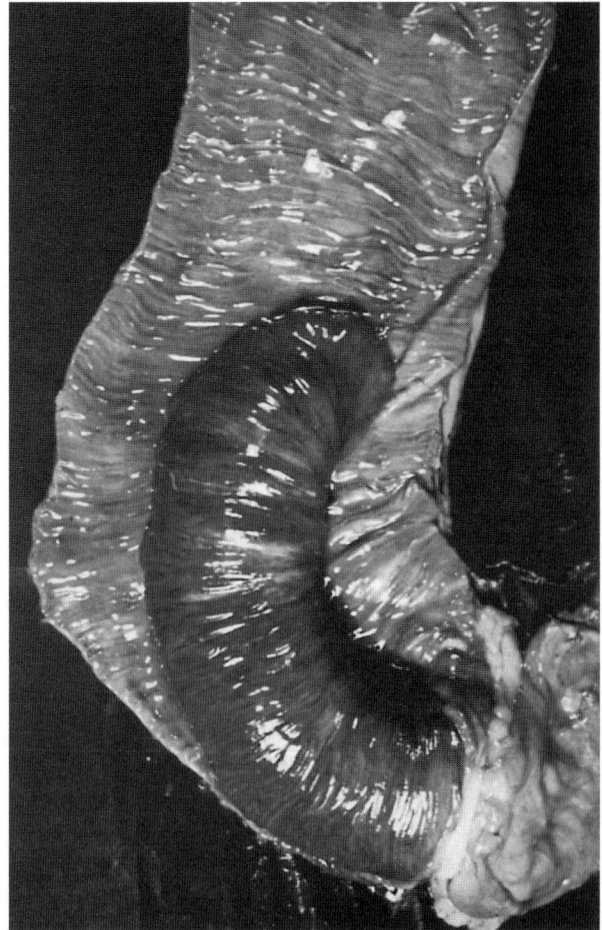

FIGURE 22-87. Ileocecal intussusception from cecal carcinoma producing intestinal obstruction. (Courtesy of Rudolf Garret, M.D.)

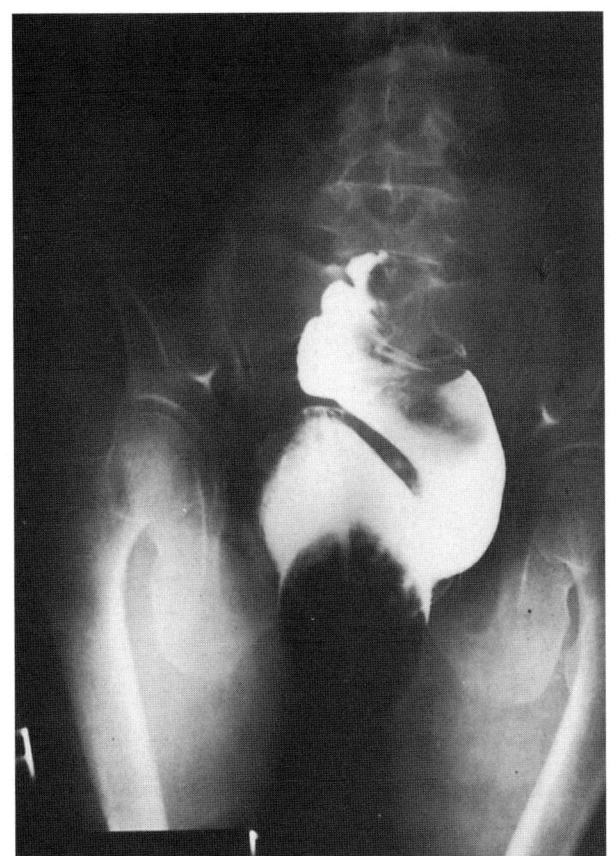

FIGURE 22-88. Partial colonic obstruction secondary to carcinoma of the sigmoid with intussusception. Note the characteristic coiled-spring appearance of the intussusceptum.

nonoperatively in the hope that the obstruction may resolve. In any event, it is reasonable to at least consider this alternative under these circumstances.

For a primary tumor, if the dilatation is minimal or moderate and removal can be accomplished without an extensive dissection (as for a sigmoid lesion), resection is advisable. It is always preferred to extirpate a mass initially and obtain a definitive pathology report. An anastomosis may then be considered. If a limited distal colon resection is accomplished, however, a proximal diversion should be performed. Not to do so in a situation in which the bowel is unprepared and the colon is dilated invites disaster. In the experience of Phillips and co-workers, immediate anastomosis in the obstructed left colon was associated with a high rate of clinical leakage (18%).[732] Another report demonstrated an operative mortality of 12% and a wound infection rate of 40%.[19] Emergency surgery for colon carcinoma has been shown to have a strong negative influence on immediate surgical morbidity and mortality.[873] Setti Coraro and colleagues reported 528 patients who underwent colonic resection over a 10-year period (1980 to 1989) wherein 179 presented with obstructing tumors.[850] There was a statistically significant increased risk of the development of metastases and death in the obstructed group.

Fecal Diversion The surgeon may elect to decline an anastomosis in favor of, for example, a colostomy or ileostomy (see Chapter 31)—a safe, acceptable alternative. It should be remembered, however, that a dilated stoma (especially sigmoid colostomy) tends to retract. An extra length should be delivered to avoid this complication. Ten days to 2 weeks later, elective resection can be undertaken, or the stoma may be allowed to remain. The stoma may or may not be closed or resected at the same time. However, there is an increased risk when two anastomoses are closed synchronously.

My own preference is to create a loop ileostomy if resection cannot be performed. It is always easier to make an ileal stoma than a colostomy. It is also easier to manage the appliance (see Chapter 31). With respect to end versus loop ostomy, one must be circumspect with regard to a distal obstruction. There is the theoretical possibility that an end stoma will result in a blown stump in the distal bowel, thus exposing the patient to the risk of fecal contamination and peritonitis. One can avoid this problem by creating an end-loop colostomy (see Figure 31-35) or a loop ileostomy (see Figs. 31-67 through 31-69). I am unalterably opposed to a separate opening for a mucus fistula. Often this will lead to intolerable drainage that may even require an appliance. Furthermore, it may be more difficult to manage than the functioning stoma, itself.

de Almeida and colleagues compared two methods of dealing with a left colon acutely obstructed by cancer in a retrospective fashion.[202] Colostomy alone was associated with 10% mortality and 30% morbidity. Subtotal colectomy (see later) was associated with 9% mortality but only 18% morbidity.

Cecostomy Tube cecostomy has been recommended by some as a conservative option for the patient believed to be at a prohibitively high risk for a more major procedure.[318,412] This operation, however, although it may succeed in venting the bowel, truly does not divert the fecal stream. If the obstruction can be relieved by enemas or by endoscopic decompression, thereby permitting the surgeon sufficient time to prepare the bowel, this may be optimal.[524]

Salim performed percutaneous decompression and irrigation through a small cecostomy tube in 28 individuals, in preparation for elective operation.[813] This is not the same technique as colonoscopically assisted cecostomy, performed for the treatment of Ogilvie's syndrome (see Chapter 16). This procedure cannot be undertaken with the use of a colonoscope because of the distal obstruction. I believe this is a risky concept indeed, with the possible consequences of precipitating a perforation in addition to the obstruction.

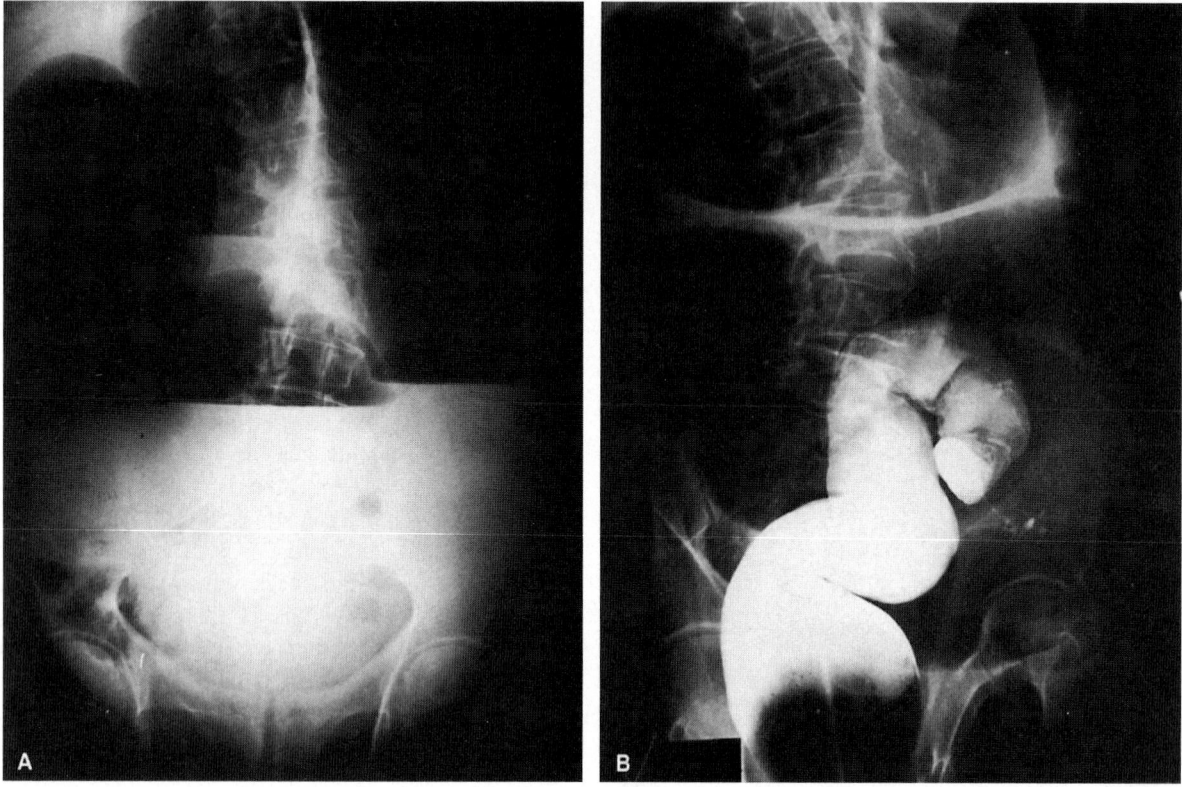

FIGURE 22-89. Complete colonic obstruction. **(A)** Huge gas- and fluid-filled loops of colon are characteristic of mechanical obstruction. **(B)** Barium enema demonstrates sigmoid obstruction.

There are, however, several other options that permit resection and ultimate reestablishment of intestinal continuity in the first instance for malignant left-sided colonic obstruction.

Colonic Stenting Nonoperative alternatives to relieve colonic obstruction have been attempted with indifferent results. These include balloon dilation, placement of a plastic nonexpandable rectal tube, cryosurgical destruction, electrocoagulation, and laser ablation. Most apply to the palliative management of rectal cancer (see Chapter 23). The concept of using a self-expandable metal stent to relieve obstruction in an occluded lumen was first introduced in 1985, when Wright and co-workers successfully placed stents in the canine jugular vein and abdominal aorta.[196] Dohmoto was the first to describe this application in the colon.[222] The procedure may be performed as a bridge to elective surgery, for palliation, and it may be successfully maintained through neoadjuvant therapy until resection is undertaken.[7]

The endoluminal Wallstent enteral endoprosthesis (Boston Scientific/Microvasive, Natick, MA; *www.bsci.com*) is a metal self-expanding stent with an internal diameter of 20 mm and a column length of 80 mm (Figure 22-90). It is placed endoscopically, usually under fluoroscopic guidance, to palliate colon obstruction (Figs. 22-90 and 22-91). Figure 22-92 demonstrates the stent in place in the sigmoid colon on a plain film of the abdomen, and Figure 22-93 is an artist's concept of the stent in position. The resected specimen, incorporating the stent, is illustrated in Figure 22-94. A technical precaution that should be mentioned is the attention necessary for performing the resection without unnecessarily handling the area of the stent placement. There is a real possibility that the sharp metal ends may have penetrated the bowel sufficiently to cause a laceration if one is not careful.

Numerous articles have been published on the use of this device.[576,577,777,932,933] One of the largest experiences has been reported from Spain by Tejero and colleagues.[9326] Thirty-eight patients underwent insertion of the stent for malignant obstruction of the left colon. The obstruction was relieved in 35 (92%), and in 13 individuals the stent constituted definitive palliative treatment. In approximately two thirds, definitive elective surgery was successfully concluded. We reported our experience with 26 patients.[196] In 14, the stents were placed for palliation, whereas in 12, they were placed as a bridge to ultimate resection. In 22 individuals (85%), stent placement was successful initially, and in one, subsequently.

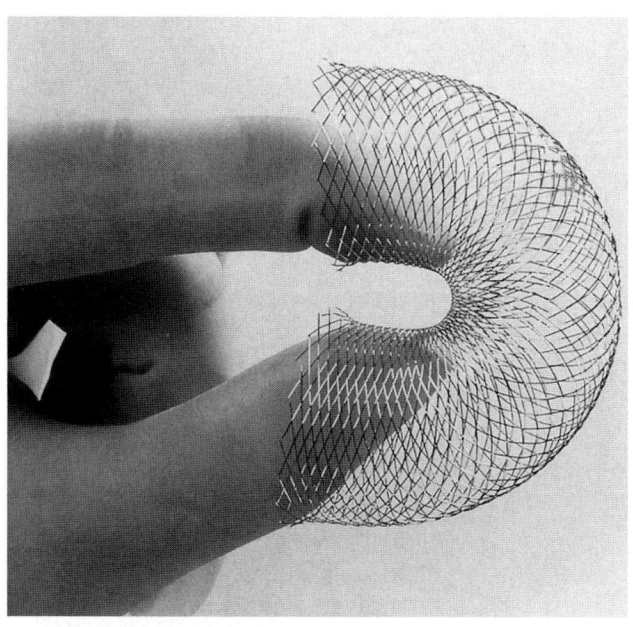

FIGURE 22-90. Wallstent metallic enteral endoprosthesis. (Courtesy of Schneider, Inc., Plymouth, MN.)

The remaining four required emergency surgery. Nine of the 12 patients (75%) in the bridge-to-surgery group underwent elective colon resection. In the palliative group, four (29%) developed recurrent obstruction, and in one (9%), the stent migrated. In the remaining nine (64%), the stent was patent until the patient expired or until the end of the follow-up (median, 156 days).[196] Martinez-Santos and co-workers assigned patients to either preoperative stenting followed by elective resection or palliative stenting versus emergency surgery.[595] Obstruction was relieved in 41 of 43 patients after stent placement (95%). Eight-five percent ultimately underwent resection and primary anastomosis without a stoma. Only 41% avoided a stoma when emergency resection was performed. Others report comparable success.[513,51,811,921] Endoscopic transanal decompression with a drainage tube has also been described for acute colonic obstruction.[924]

On-Table Lavage The literature abounds, especially from the United Kingdom, with various approaches that attempt to prepare the bowel for primary anastomosis.[227,279,380,384,495,500,666,742,754,863,868,942] The technique is particularly applicable to obstructing rectal cancers, but it has been recommended as an alternative for left-sided colon lesions as well. The irrigation can be accomplished in an antegrade or retrograde fashion, either before or after the tumor has been removed, through the open bowel, a cecotomy, or an appendicostomy (Figure 22-95).[97,1021] Some authors report relatively good results (a clinical anastomotic leak rate of 5% to 7%),[331,495,754,906,942]

but others note a clinical and radiologic leak rate of 10% to 14% and a mortality rate of up to 17%.[742] The SCOTIA Study Group, reporting from Aberdeen, Scotland, developed a prospective, randomized trial comparing subtotal colectomy with segmental resection and primary anastomosis and the use of intraoperative irrigation for malignant left-sided colonic obstruction.[836] Hospital mortality and complication rates did not differ significantly, but 4 months after operation, increased bowel frequency was significantly more common in the subtotal colectomy group. Because of this complaint, the authors concluded that segmental resection following intraoperative irrigation is the preferred alternative for uncomplicated left-sided bowel obstruction. Tan and colleagues noted an operative mortality of 13% and a wound infection rate of 30%.[922] Nonetheless, all who describe their experiences are quite enthusiastic.

OPINION I am rather surprised that this procedure has been welcomed with such enthusiasm. Despite modifications designed to simplify the method, it involves insertion of a catheter into the cecum (thus necessitating at least an additional enterotomy), the instillation of several liters of saline solution, and the evacuation of the contents through a large-bore tube (into a collecting bag, it is hoped, rather than onto the floor of the operating room). The other problem I have is the definition of "large bowel obstruction." One finds in articles and in verbal presentations examples of large bowel obstruction that to me often represent mild dilatation. In many cases, these individuals could in all probability have undergone bowel preparation and elective surgery. Still, I must respect the opinions of well-recognized surgeons. For myself, however, I continue to employ subtotal or total colectomy for this indication (see later).

Intracolonic or Intraluminal Bypass In 1985, Ravo and Ger described a unique approach to effecting reestablishment of intestinal continuity in situations in which one would hesitate to undertake such a procedure, the intracolonic bypass.[764] The procedure, which involves only a limited resection, is applicable to obstruction and to perforation.[792] The technique and results are described in Chapter 26, but the product is not available in the United States.

Subtotal or Total Colectomy From my perspective and that of others, the optimal way of dealing with an obstructed colon is to perform subtotal or total colectomy and ileosigmoid or ileorectal anastomosis.[102,113,307,369] This operation has the additional merit of removing any synchronous lesions, especially if unsuspected.[51] The procedure is obviously technically somewhat more difficult, but results indicate that the morbidity and mortality do not exceed, and in most series are con-

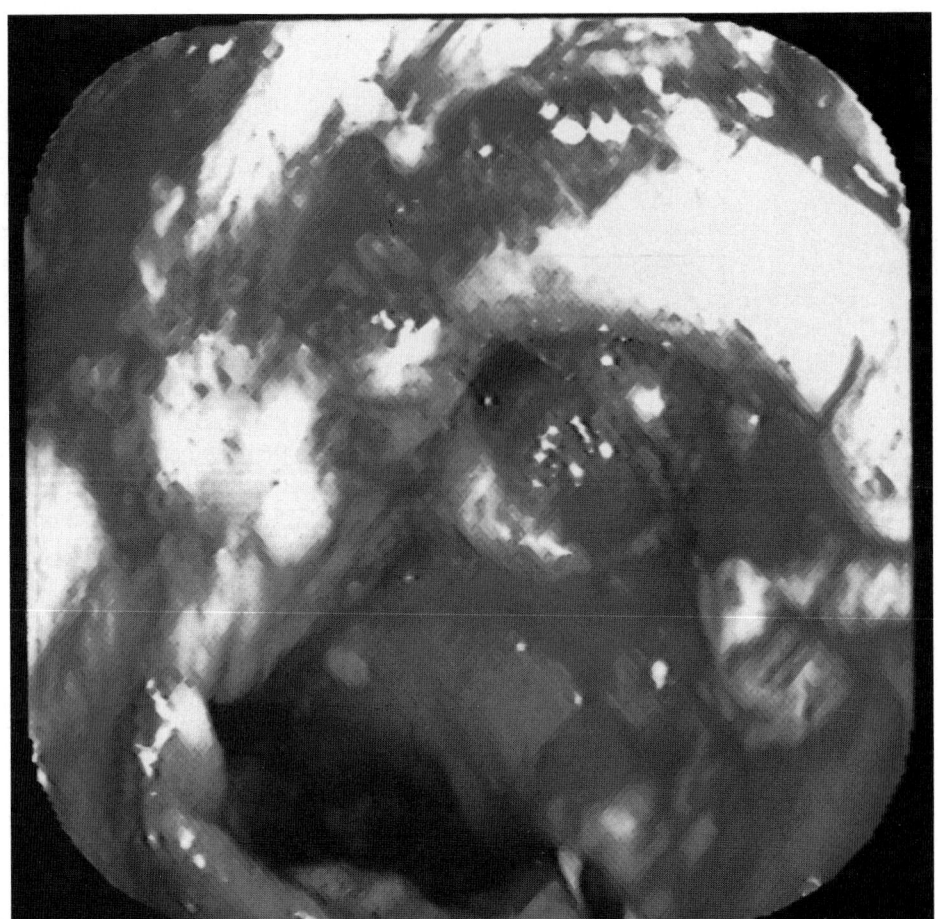

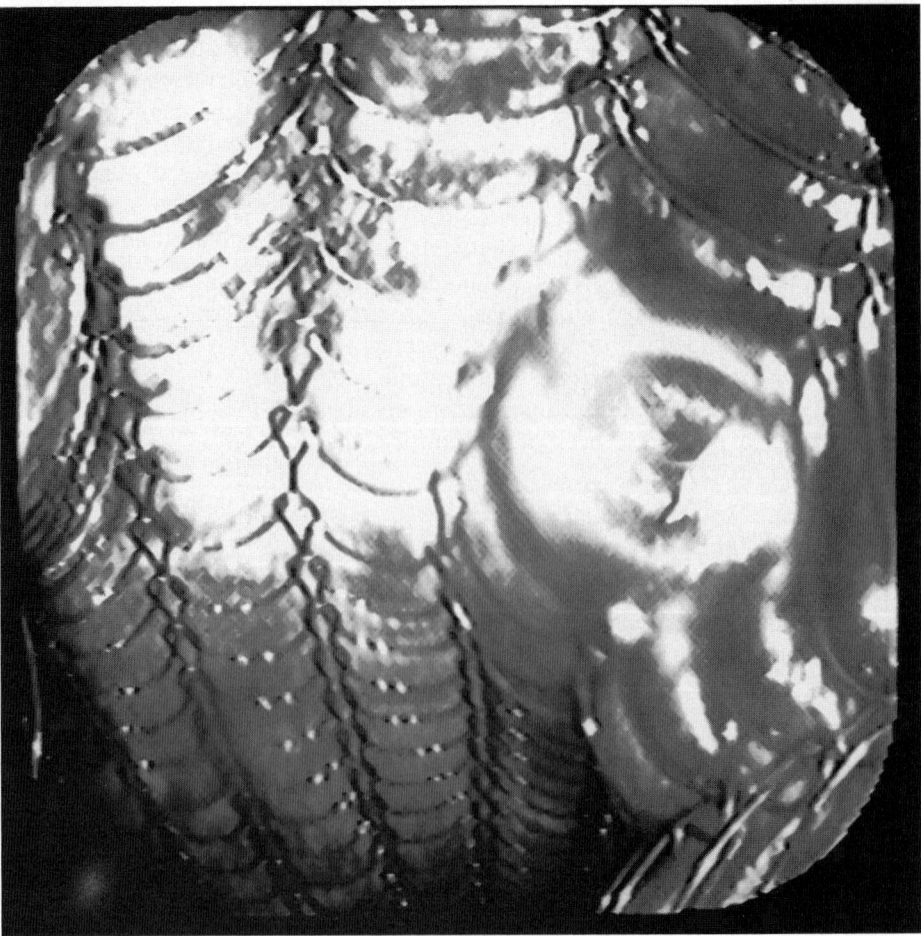

FIGURE 22-91. Obstructing sigmoid colon cancer. **(A)** Stricture seen through the colonoscope. **(B)** Endoscopic view of the stent's having been deployed.

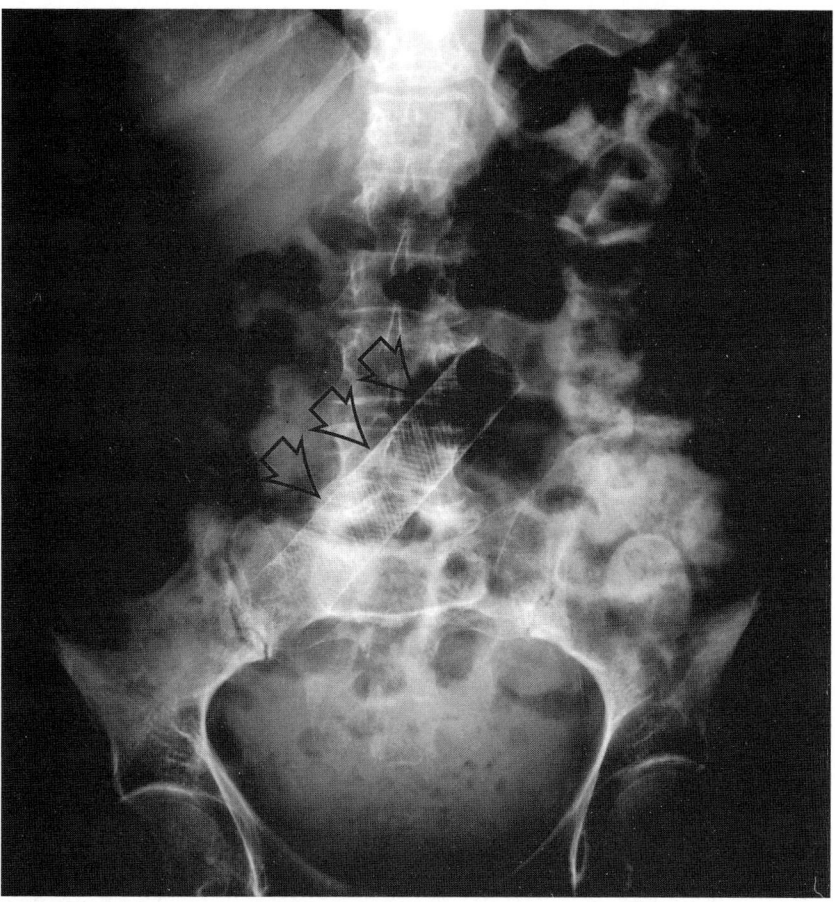

FIGURE 22-92. Plain film of the abdomen demonstrates the stent in place *(arrows)* in the patient shown in Figure 22-91.

siderably better, than those of staged operations.[265,426,484,902,1007] All patients can tolerate a virtually normal diet, and those with an ileorectal anastomosis stabilize at about two or three bowel movements per day.[369] Occasionally, an individual may have to resort to one of the "slowing" medications. This procedure is also preferred for the management of perforation, in which situation it is of paramount importance to remove the bowel in the first instance (see later). The functional results following total (subtotal) colectomy are reviewed in Chapter 16.

Colitis Proximal to a Partially Obstructing Carcinoma of the Colon

A nonspecific type of ulcerative colitis proximal to a partially obstructing carcinoma is an uncommon condition. It is a clinical and pathologic entity that must be distinguished from idiopathic ulcerative colitis, from which a carcinoma may subsequently develop.[260,809,948,1008,1036] The location of the colitis is in-variably proximal to the tumor, with the bowel distal to the tumor normal. In almost all reported cases, a short segment of normal mucosa separates the area of colitis from the tumor. The pathologic description of the colitis varies from involvement of the entire bowel wall with hemorrhagic necrosis to superficial mucosal ulcerations only.

The colitis is frequently unsuspected and discovered only at the time of surgery for the colonic tumor. Although often apparent from the macroscopic appearance of the proximal intestine and mesentery, the extent of the inflammatory process may not be fully appreciated until the bowel is opened. The limits of resection will be dictated not only by the requirement of an adequate cancer operation but also by the length of the inflamed bowel.

Bypass

As mentioned earlier, resection of right-sided obstructing lesions can generally be performed with reestablish-

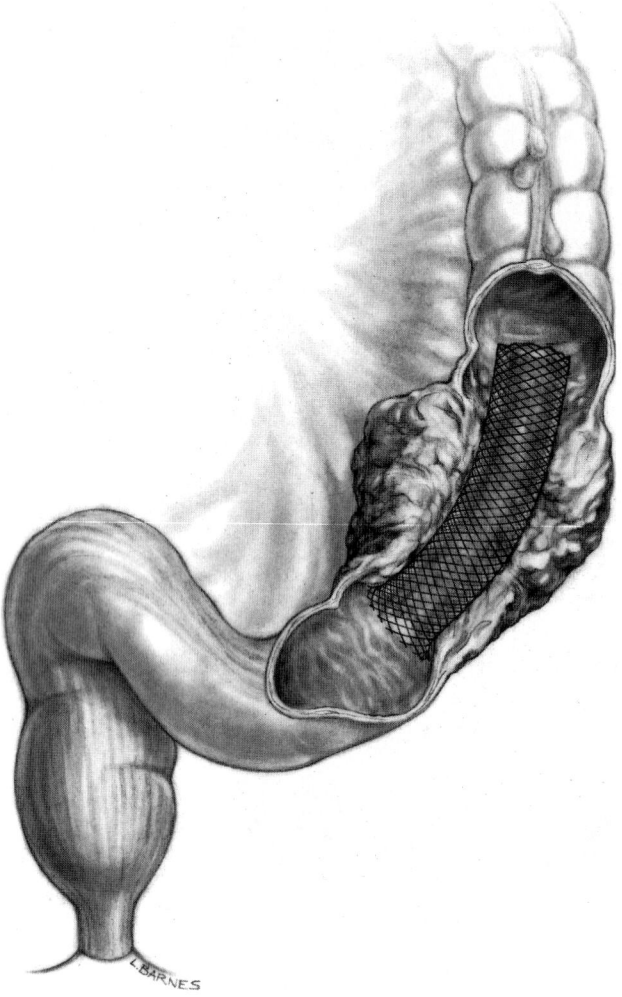

FIGURE 22-93. Artist's concept of a Wallstent in place through an obstructing carcinoma of the sigmoid colon.

ment of intestinal continuity, even with unprepared bowel and small bowel dilatation. Obviously, clinical judgment remains the primary criterion. The alternative is resection and ileostomy.

Enteroenterostomy is a reasonably safe alternative for patients with obstructing tumors and for those unresectable cancers that are likely to obstruct (Figure 22-96). To effect a safe bypass, the enterostomy should ideally be at least 20 cm from the lesion proximally and distally, and the anastomosis should be free of areas of tumor implantation if this is possible. A colocolostomy is the preferred approach whenever it can be accomplished, in order to save as much useful bowel as possible and to decrease the likelihood of diarrhea (Figure 22-96B). For right-sided lesions, an ileocolostomy is usually very effective (Figure 22-96A), but if the entire colon is in jeopardy for recur-

rent tumor, ileorectal or ileosigmoid bypass is suggested (Figure 22-96C).

Perforation

Carcinoma of the colon with perforation is another challenging surgical problem. All too often, the pathologic diagnosis is not clearly established preoperatively or even intraoperatively. The patient often presents with a rigid abdomen, generalized peritonitis, and a pneumoperitoneum. Surgery often is required without benefit of gastrointestinal investigation or even a meaningful history from the patient. Even though extravasation is demonstrated on a limited water-soluble enema, the differential diagnosis (especially for a sigmoid lesion) always includes diverticulitis. Colonoscopy will usually fail to define the nature of the lesion because of inadequate bowel preparation, the general condition of the patient, and the inflammatory reaction in the area.[203] Failure to demonstrate a carcinoma by means of colonoscopy at or near the site of a known perforation does not exclude cancer. Realistically, if one makes an attempt to perform a colonoscopy in the presence of free gas within the peritoneal cavity, it is not merely an exercise in futility, but it is likely to increase the amount of contamination and certainly to expand the pneumoperitoneum. Performing a flexible instrument examination under the circumstances is, in my opinion, poor judgment.

The establishment of the diagnosis can usually be confirmed with certainty only by an exploratory laparotomy and resection of the involved segment of bowel. It should be emphasized repeatedly to all surgical trainees that limited exploration and blind diversionary procedures for suspected colonic perforation are to be condemned. Passing the hand into the pelvis to attempt diagnosis in the presence of inflammatory reaction, adhesions, pus, or feces is a gesture in futility. A transverse colostomy for a perforated cecal carcinoma is a totally preventable tragedy. The lesion should be clearly demonstrable before definitive treatment is undertaken. Parenthetically, it is important to evaluate the rectum before an incision is made. It is more than embarrassing to perform a resection and leave behind a synchronous carcinoma of the rectum. It is impossible to evaluate the extraperitoneal rectum through an exploratory laparotomy. By simply passing a rigid sigmoidoscope with the patient on the operating table, the surgeon should be able to confirm adequately that the rectum is spared of disease.

Treatment

The surgical options in the treatment of perforation are somewhat more limited than those for obstruction.

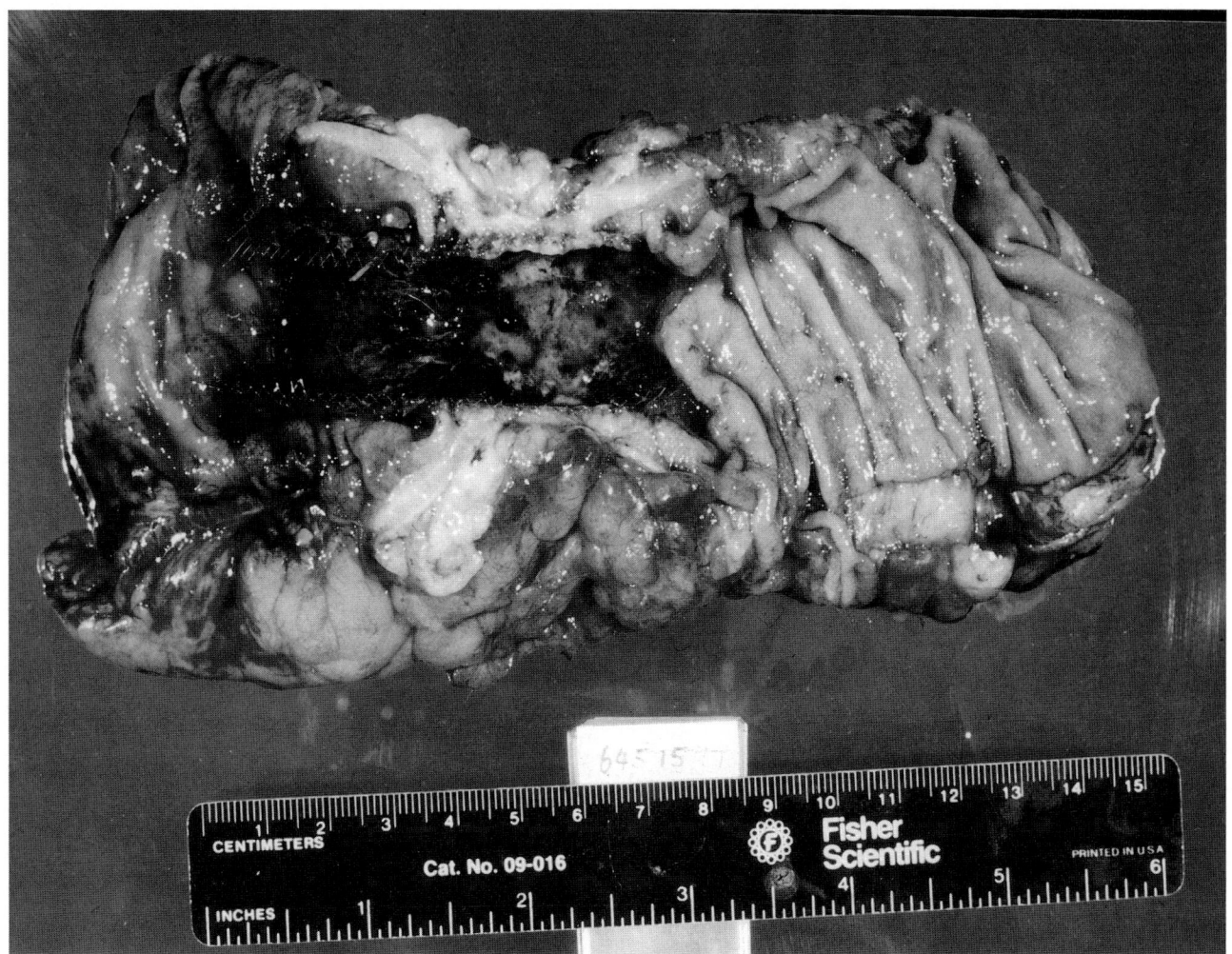

FIGURE 22-94. Resected, opened sigmoid colon specimen showing an incised stent in place with transmural invasion by cancer. Note that there is very little difference in luminal size between the proximal and distal bowel.

The goal should be to remove the diseased segment. As mentioned, if a colostomy and drainage procedure is performed for a sigmoid lesion, the actual histology may not be defined for several weeks. However, if a carcinoma is diagnosed but not removed, resection should be undertaken in 10 to 14 days unless neoadjuvant therapy is planned. If diverticular disease is the cause, resection theoretically may be deferred for 6 weeks to many months (see Chapter 26).

Another reason for initially resecting the lesion is to remove the septic process. Even with drainage and proximal diversion, the contamination will continue, because a foot or more of stool-filled bowel may be situated between the stoma and the perforation. In addition, desquamated cells from the tumor itself may continue to seed the abdomen and further worsen the already grim prognosis.

Surgical alternatives for removal of a perforated bowel include resection of the disease-bearing segment, anastomosis if appropriate, *always* a protective colostomy or ileostomy, and drainage of the area of contamination. With a right-sided perforation, the surgeon may elect to perform end ileostomy and adjacent mucous fistula of the colon (at the same site), ileocolic anastomosis with protective loop ileostomy, or end ileostomy with closure of the colonic stump. With more distal lesions, the surgeon can attempt an anastomosis with protective loop colostomy or loop ileostomy, end stoma with adjacent mucous fistula, or end stoma with closure of the distal stump.

Subtotal or total colectomy with ileosigmoid or ileorectal anastomosis is another alternative for the treatment of perforation. It fulfills the criterion of removing the disease, and it permits a relatively safe anastomosis for left-

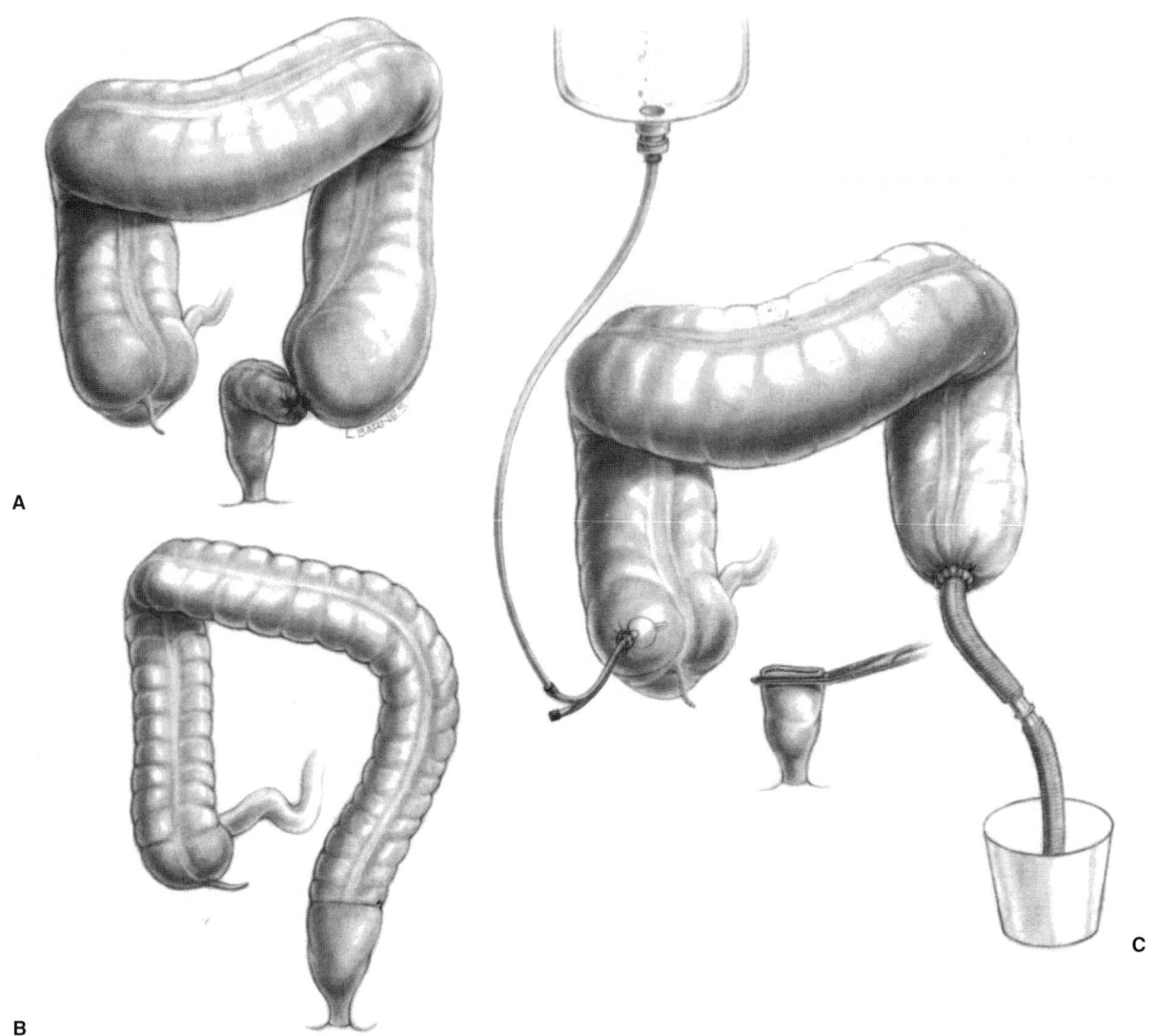

FIGURE 22-95. Technique of on-table lavage for bowel obstruction. **(A)** Profound large bowel obstruction from cancer is conceptually illustrated. **(B)** Lavage is performed by insertion of a large-bore catheter into the cecum, with drainage from the distal end effected by means of corrugated anesthetic-gas tubing. **(C)** Anastomosis is completed by the usual means, without a diversionary procedure and without removing the entire colon.

sided perforations. It also treats synchronous lesions that could otherwise be overlooked. However, dissection in the upper part of the abdomen in the presence of a hypogastric perforation increases the risk for spreading the septic process under the diaphragms and below the liver. Even with a technically secure anastomosis, loop ileostomy should be considered when contamination has occurred. Although possibly applicable to a number of situations, concomitant loop ileostomy is the procedure of choice in one circumstance—when obstructing carcinoma of the left colon produces perforation of the right colon. Under these circumstances, subtotal or total colectomy is preferred despite the more extensive dissection required.

When an emergency resection is performed, blunt dissection should be employed as often as possible. Unless invasion by the tumor has caused fixation of the bowel, sharp dissection invites injury to the ureter and other retroperitoneal structures. If unusual difficulty is encountered, the area should be drained, with proximal diversion of the fecal stream. Although this is not the optimal course of action, it is an acceptable alternative under these circumstances. In addition, because of the poor prognosis of perforating carcinomas of the colon and the high risk for local recurrence, clips should be applied to serve as markers for subsequent radiotherapy. I believe that adjuvant postoperative radiotherapy should be initi-

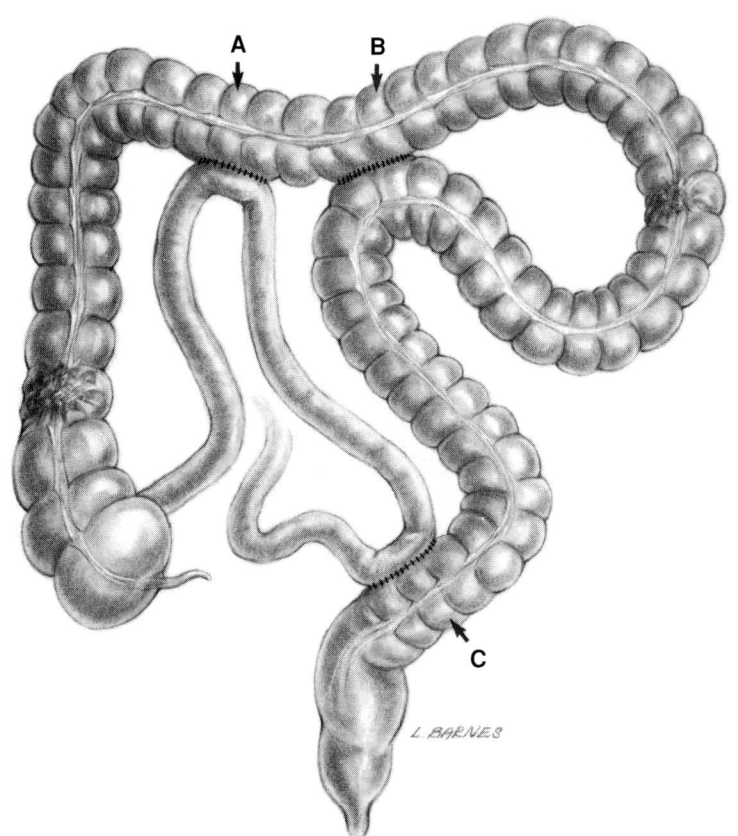

FIGURE 22-96. Bypass procedures. **(A)** Ileotransverse colostomy. **(B)** Colocolostomy. **(C)** Ileosigmoidostomy.

ated for the perforated tumor (see later). Metallic clips (e.g., stainless steel), although readily visible on plain radiographs, often distort and interfere with the interpretation of CT sans. Plastic clips cannot be seen on the plain film, but because they produce much less artifact than steel, titanium clips are preferred.[1001]

Finally, vigorous irrigation of the peritoneal cavity should be performed with many liters of saline solution.[39,452,612,633] Continuous postoperative lavage may also be helpful for up to 72 hours. Placement of antibiotics or povidone-iodine in the irrigating solution is not advised. This opinion is based on the absence of literature to support its application, although many surgeons like to use this method.

Prevention of Adhesions

In recent years, there has been a renewed concern and therapeutic effort regarding the prevention of intestinal adhesions. The magnitude of the problem is not insignificant. In a prospective analysis of 210 patients undergoing a laparotomy, Menzies and Ellis found that 93% had intraabdominal adhesions that were the result of prior surgery.[628] This compared with 115 first-time laparotomies in which only 10.4% were found to have adhesions. The authors noted that approximately 1% of adult general surgical admissions to the hospital were for intestinal obstruction. Furthermore, 3.3% of laparotomies were for adhesive obstruction.[628] The majority of the surgical procedures that produced intestinal obstruction principally involved the colon. It is obvious that the economic consequences of such a formidable incidence are considerable. Ray and colleagues noted, in an article published in 1993, that hospitalizations in which adhesiolysis was performed in the United States in 1988 were responsible for expenditures of more than $1 billion.[765] Cox and co-workers performed a retrospective analysis of all patients admitted with a diagnosis of acute adhesive small bowel obstruction during a 9-year period in Victoria, Australia.[182] The following was the breakdown of the prior operations: appendectomy, 23.3%; colorectal resection, 20.8%; gynecologic surgery, 11.7%; upper gastrointestinal and biliary surgery, 90.2%; small bowel surgery, 8.3%; and more than one prior abdominal operation, 23.6%.[182]

Ellis and associates used data from the Scottish National Health Service from patients who underwent abdominal or pelvic surgery in 1986 and followed them for up to 10 years.[249] Overall, 34.6% of the 29,790 patients who underwent surgery were readmitted a mean of 2.1 times over 10 years for adhesions or for abdominal surgery that could be complicated by adhesions.[249] Beck and colleagues, in the United States, used Health Care Financing Administration data to evaluate a random 5% sample of all Medicare patients who underwent open colorectal and general surgery in 1993.[61] *Within 2 years* of the surgery for incision, excision, and anastomosis of intestine [International Classification of Diseases (ICD-9) code 45], 14.3% developed intestinal obstruction, 2.6% required adhesiolysis, and 12.9% underwent additional colorectal or general surgery. Furthermore, of those with ICD-9 code 46 (other operations on the intestine), 17% developed obstruction (3.1 having to undergo adhesiolysis), and 20.2% underwent additional colorectal or general surgery. Numerous other articles have been published attesting to the enormity of the problem.[627,651,710]

Physical barriers have been developed to prevent adhesion formation by limiting tissue apposition during the early stages of mesothelial repair.[218] Although certain agents have been proposed, including solutions and physical barriers, none has been demonstrated to be consistently effective. However, hyaluronic acid has indeed been shown to protect tissue from injury and to prevent adhesion development. A bioresorbable membrane has been developed to provide a mechanical barrier for this purpose.[122] The product, Seprafilm, is composed of a sodium salt of hyaluronic acid, sodium hyaluronate, combined with another polyanionic polysaccharide, carboxymethyl cellulose. This membrane is produced by Genzyme Corp. (Cambridge, MA; *www.genzyme.com*). Other available products that have been demonstrated to reduce adhesion formation are Interceed (Johnson & Johnson Medical Co., Arlington, TX) and Gore-Tex Surgical Membrane (W. L. Gore, Flagstaff, AZ).[218]

Results and Recommendations

Seprafilm has been shown to decrease adhesion formation and has been recommended as a potentially safe adjuvant for preventing postoperative abdominal adhesions through both clinical and animal studies.[56,623] A randomized, controlled, blinded, prospective multicenter study was performed involving 183 patients who underwent restorative proctocolectomy and ileal J-pouch anastomosis with diverting ileostomy.[56] All patients would subsequently require closure of the ileostomy, so that the patients were ideal candidates for reassessment of the magnitude of the adhesion formation with and without the bioresorbable membrane. It was found that Seprafilm decreased the rate of adhesion formation by nearly 50%.[56] Fifty-one percent of recipients were adhesion free compared with only 6% of untreated patients. There were no adverse reactions that could be attributed to the product. A similar multicenter study was reported by Becker and co-workers.[63] Eleven centers enrolled 183 patients with ulcerative colitis or familial polyposis who were scheduled for colectomy and ileal pouch-anal anastomosis with loop ileostomy. Only 6% of control patients were found to be without adhesions, whereas 51% with Sepra-

film were free of adhesions. There was no increased incidence of complications attributable to the use of the bioresorbable membrane.

A large, prospective, randomized, multicenter, controlled study was published on the safety of Seprafilm (Adhesion Study Group Steering Committee) and involved 1,791 patients.[57] Just before closure, patients were randomized to receive Seprafilm or no treatment. Complications within the first month were evaluated. This report concluded that there were no increased risks related to abdominal abscess, pelvic abscess, and pulmonary embolism. However, the authors commented that wrapping the suture or staple line of a new bowel anastomosis with Seprafilm is unwise, because the data suggested that it may increase the risk of an anastomotic leak. Another study by Oikonomakis and associates showed that Seprafilm did not adversely affect the short-term recurrence rate after curative resection of colorectal cancer.[705]

Technique

Depending on the amount of surface that one would hope to treat prophylactically will determine how many sheets of Seprafilm to apply. Generally, the full length of the incision, the floor of the pelvis, and the stoma, itself, are the most critical areas. The raw retroperitoneal surfaces where the bowel has been mobilized as well as any sites that required excessive handing are recommended for application. It is easier and preferable to wrap the stoma before it is brought through the abdominal wall. Furthermore, it is important to keep the sheet dry, applying it to the areas to be treated by means of a dry sponge-stick rather than the surgeon's fingers.

Opinion

I have been extremely impressed, both as a participant in a randomized, clinical trial, and as a treating surgeon who has utilized Seprafilm off protocol, with the remarkable reduction in the amount and the severity of adhesions whenever I have had to reoperate on the patient. As a consequence, I always use this product in all of my abdominal surgeries. Whether its application will inevitably prevent the development of subsequent intestinal obstruction is now part of a prospective, randomized, long-term, follow-up evaluation.

Liver Metastases

What to do with metastatic liver disease at the time of colon resection is a problem that often confronts the surgeon. CT will usually provide adequate evaluation of the liver to determine the presence or absence of metastases. However, as mentioned previously, this rarely changes the approach to the management of the primary tumor.

Color Plates

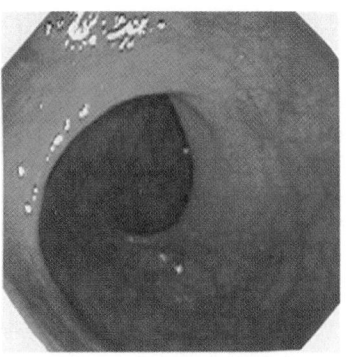

COLOR FIGURE 4-12. The middle and upper rectal valves of Houston. (See Fig. 4-12.)

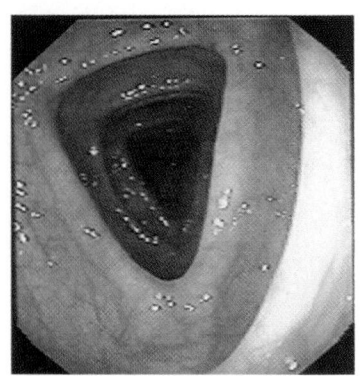

COLOR FIGURE 5-18. Normal transverse colon. (See Fig. 5-18.)

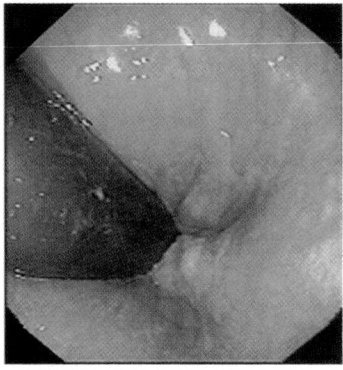

COLOR FIGURE 5-8. Retroflexion of the flexible sigmoidoscope. (See Fig. 5-8.)

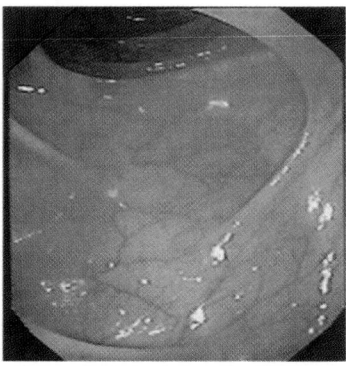

COLOR FIGURE 5-20. Hepatic flexure. (See Fig. 5-20.)

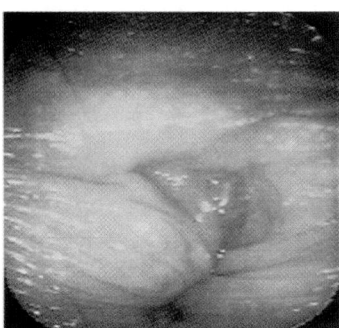

COLOR FIGURE 5-9. Anal fissure can be seen with the flexible sigmoidoscope. However, this is not the optimal way for making the diagnosis. (See Fig. 5-9.)

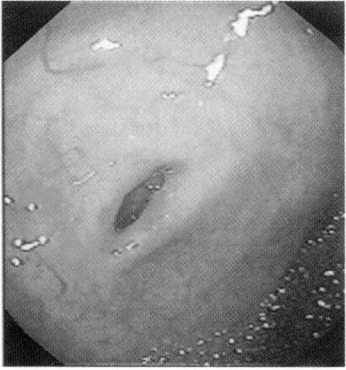

COLOR FIGURE 5-21. The appendiceal orifice. (See Fig. 5-21.)

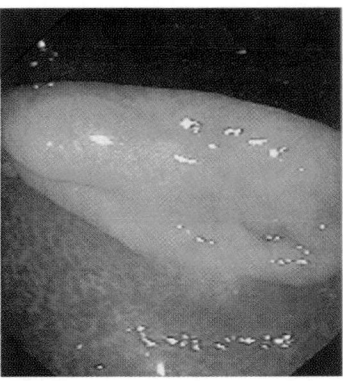

COLOR FIGURE 5-22. The ileocecal valve seen from a retroflexed instrument position. (See Fig. 5-22.)

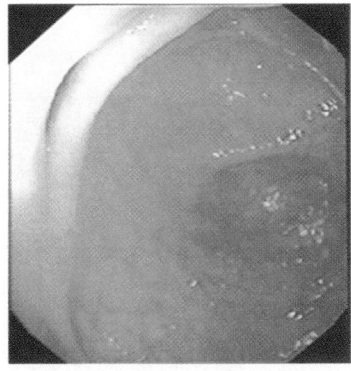

COLOR FIGURE 5-23. The ileocecal valve as is appears entering the cecum. (See Fig. 5-23.)

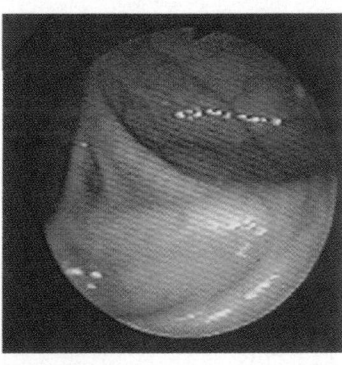

COLOR FIGURE 5-24. Normal cecal base with triangulation of the tinea. (See Fig. 5-24.)

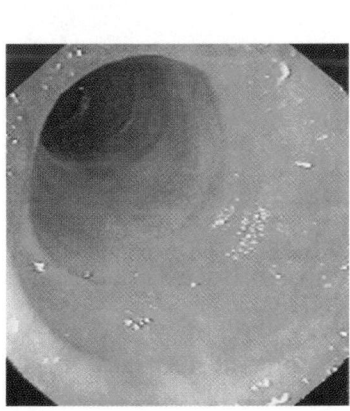

COLOR FIGURE 5-25. Normal terminal ileum. (See Fig. 5-25.)

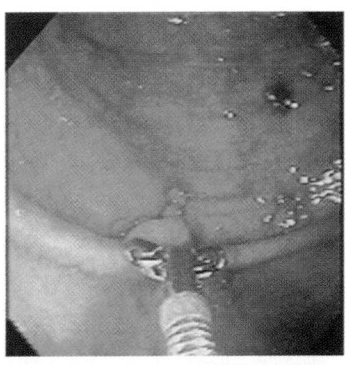

COLOR FIGURE 5-28. A small polyp is removed with biopsy forceps. (See Color Figure 5-28.)

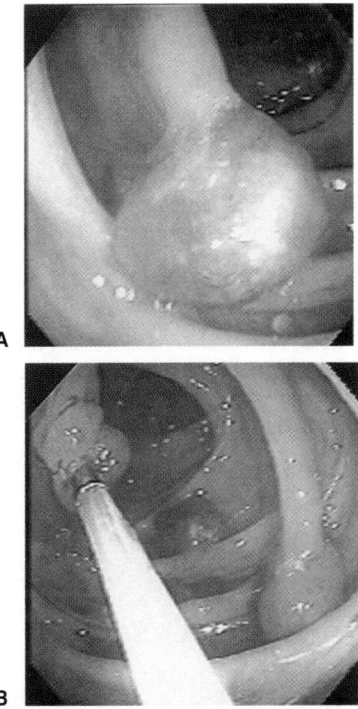

COLOR FIGURE 5-29. Technique of snare polypectomy. **(A)** A polyp on a stalk is seen in the midsigmoid colon. **(B)** The snare encompasses the head of the polyp; an adjacent pedunculated polyp can be seen. (See Fig. 5-29.)

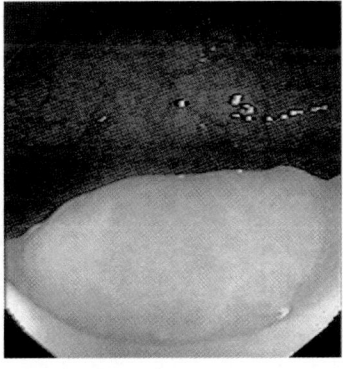

COLOR FIGURE 5-30. Sessile polypoid tumor of the rectosigmoid. (See Fig. 5-30.)

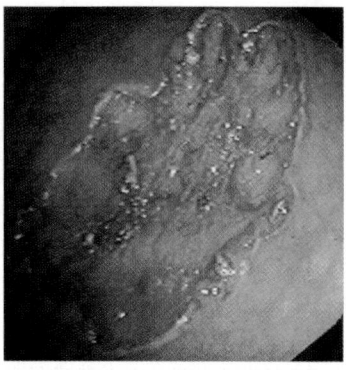

COLOR FIGURE 5-31. Removal of a tumor has been effected with snare cautery. (See Fig. 5-31.)

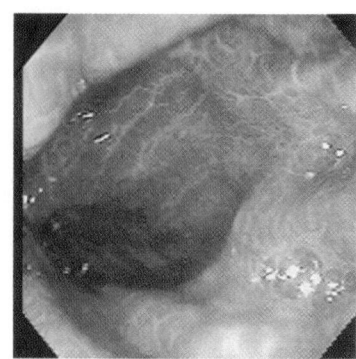

COLOR FIGURE 16-10. Colonoscopy demonstrates the typical cobblestone pattern of melanosis coli. (See Fig. 16-10.)

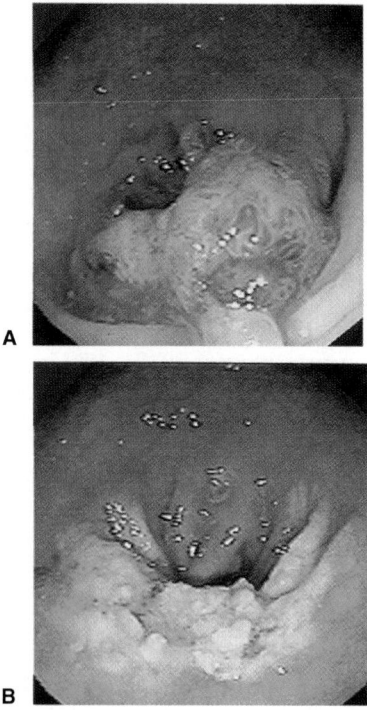

COLOR FIGURE 5-32. Snare excision of large polyp. **(A)** Snare is passed around polypoid lesion. **(B)** Coagulum appears at the site of polyp removal. (See Fig. 5-32.)

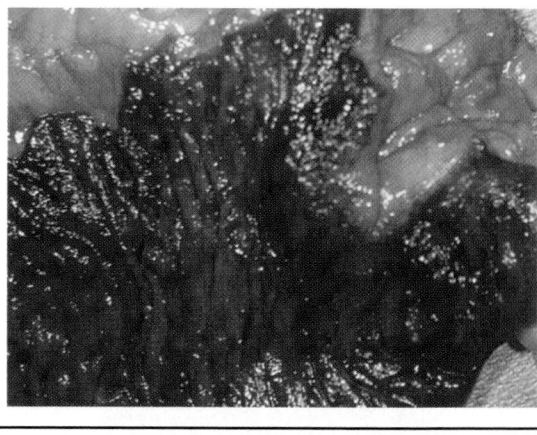

COLOR FIGURE 16-11. Note the dark black pigment characteristic of melanosis coli in a resected specimen. (See Fig. 16-12.)

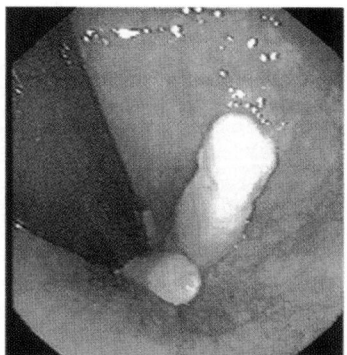

COLOR FIGURE 9-3. Hypertrophied anal papillae are seen through a retroflexed video-endoscope in a patient with a chronic anal fissure. (See Fig. 9-3.)

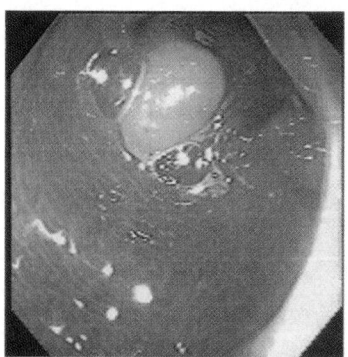

COLOR FIGURE 16-13. A polypoid lesion is clearly evident against the background of the darkly pigmented normal mucosa. (See Fig. 16-13.)

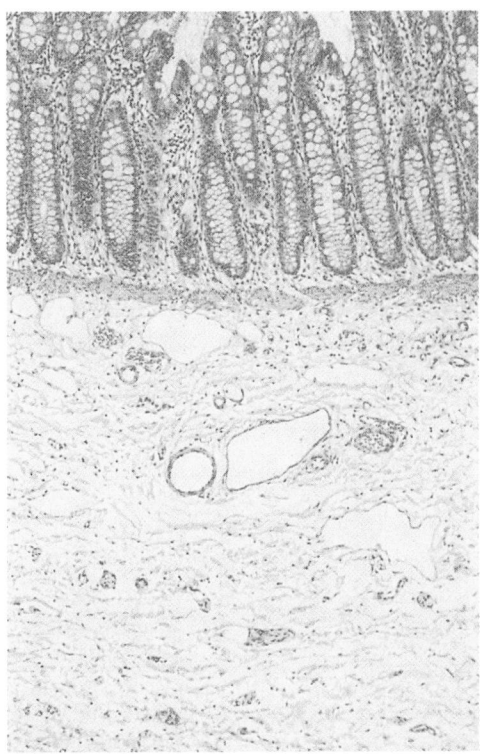

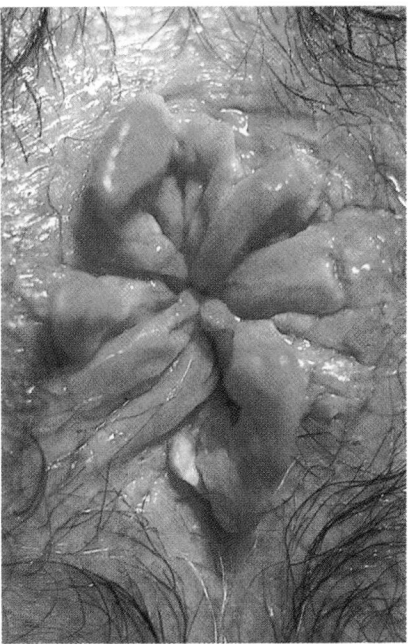

COLOR FIGURE 19-2. Marked edema with papillomatosis and nodularity resulting from chronic abrading is characteristic of pruritus ani. (Courtesy of William G. Robertson, M.D.) (See Fig. 19-2.)

COLOR FIGURE 18-2. Histologic section including mucosa with submucosa of the rectum showing clusters of ganglion cells in the submucosal plexus. This excludes Hirschsprung's disease at this level. (Courtesy of Hector L. Monforte-Muñoz, M.D., Department of Pathology, Children's Hospital, Los Angeles, CA.) (See Fig. 18-2.)

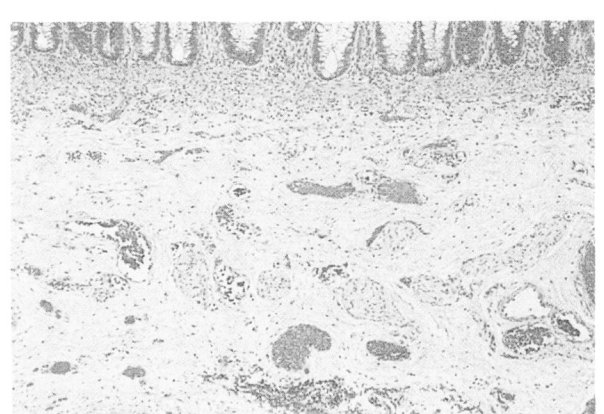

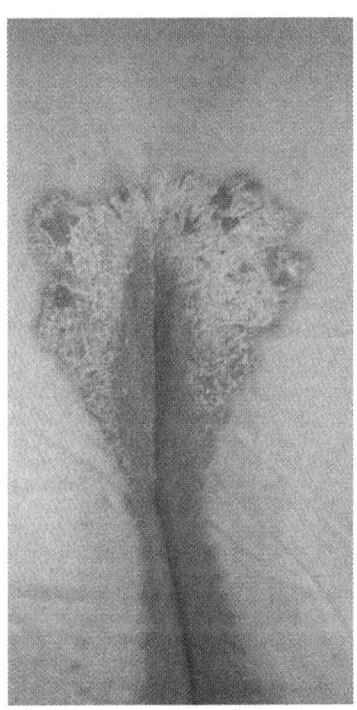

COLOR FIGURE 18-3. Histologic section including mucosa and submucosa of the rectum showing tortuous and hypertrophic nerve trunks of the submucosal plexus. There is no evidence of any ganglion cell present. This establishes the diagnosis of Hirschsprung's disease. (Courtesy of Hector L. Monforte-Muñoz, M.D., Department of Pathology, Children's Hospital, Los Angeles, CA.) (See Fig. 18-3.)

COLOR FIGURE 19-3. Well-marginated erythematosquamous plaque with characteristic silvery scales indicates psoriasis. (Courtesy of Arnold Medved, M.D.) (See Fig. 19-3.)

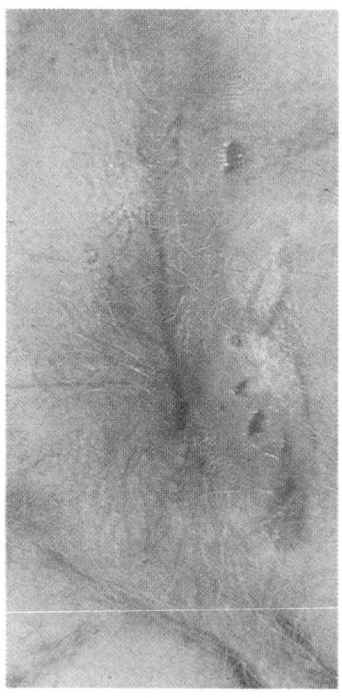

COLOR FIGURE 19-28. Multiple external openings are present in this patient with fistula-in-ano. (See Fig. 19-28.)

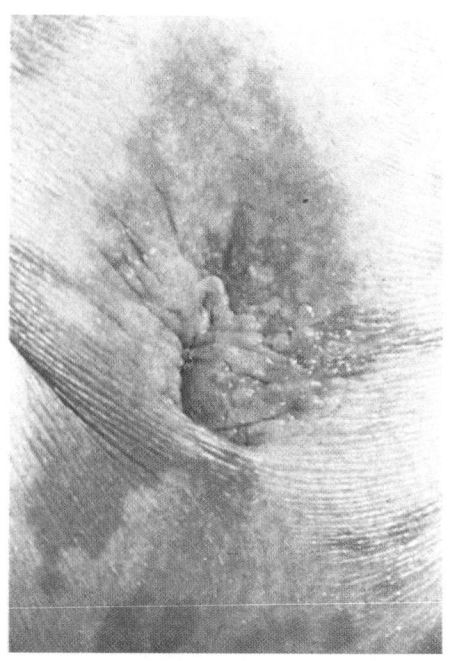

COLOR FIGURE 19-58. A violaceous tumor with adjacent reddish brown, irregularly shaped plaques is indicative of mycosis fungoides. (From Corman ML, Veidenheimer MC, Swinton NW. *Diseases of the anus, rectum and colon. Part I: neoplasms.* New York: Medcom, 1972, with permission.) (See Fig. 19-58.)

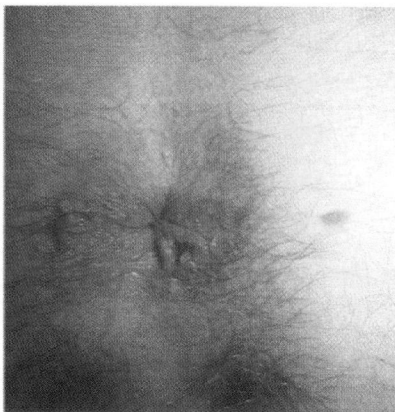

COLOR FIGURE 19-39. A noninflamed, punched out-appearing ulcerated chancre that was dark-field positive for *Treponema pallidum*. (See Fig. 19-39.)

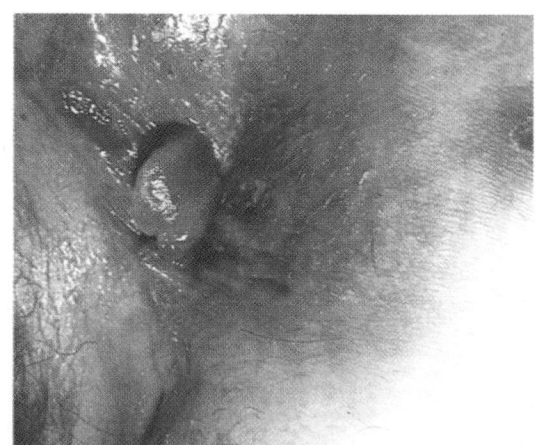

COLOR FIGURE 19-61. An ulcerating, violaceous nodule demonstrated leukemic cells on biopsy, indicating leukemia cutis. (From Corman ML, Veidenheimer MC, Swinton NW. *Diseases of the anus, rectum and colon. Part I: neoplasms.* New York: Medcom, 1972, with permission.) (See Fig. 19-61.)

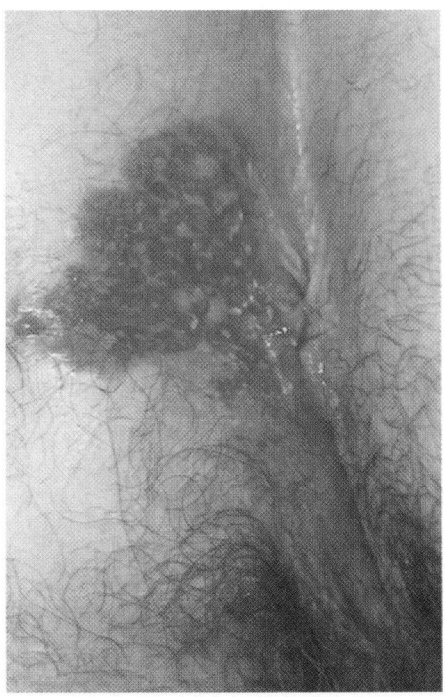

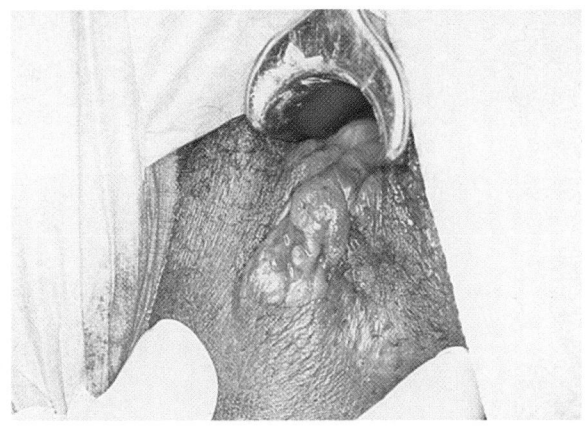

COLOR FIGURE 20-4. Fistula caused by *Mycobacterium avium* complex that spontaneously healed. (See Fig. 20-4.)

COLOR FIGURE 19-72. Extramammary Paget's disease has caused an irregular but well-marginated erythematous erosive patch with slightly indurated edges in this patient. (Courtesy of Arnold Medved, M.D.) (See Fig. 19-72.)

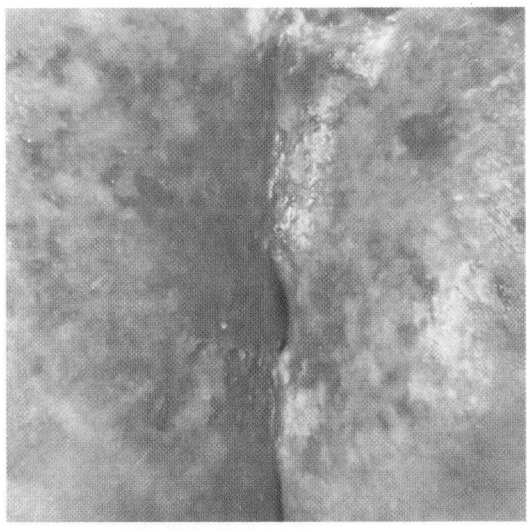

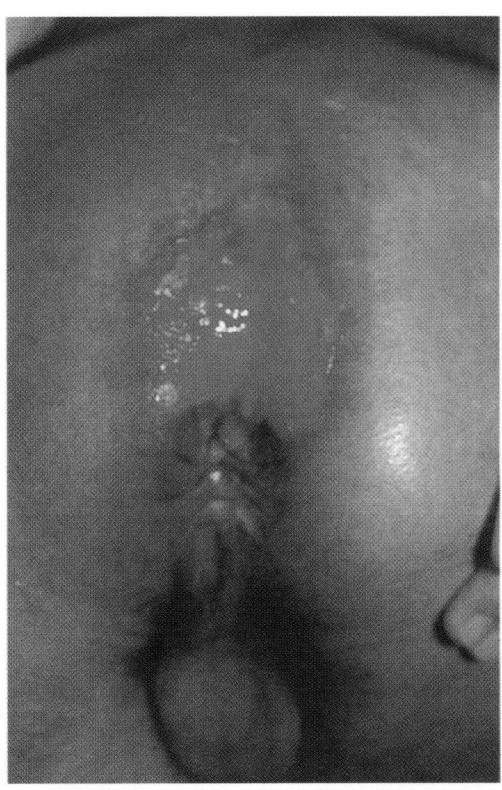

COLOR FIGURE 19-76. Extramammary Paget's disease that recurred after excision and skin grafting. (Courtesy of William G. Robertson, M.D.) (See Fig. 19-76.)

COLOR FIGURE 20-5. Severe erosive perianal herpes simplex. (See Fig. 20-5.)

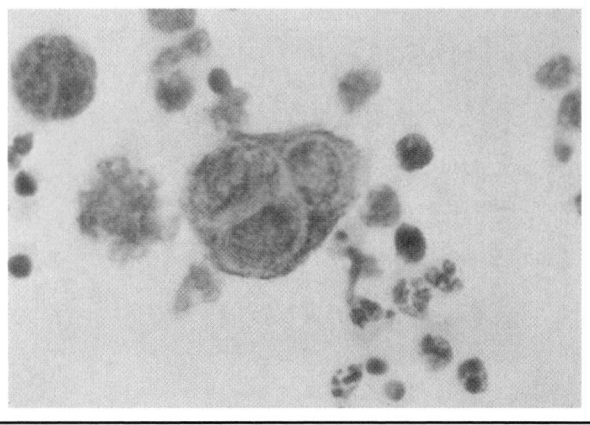

COLOR FIGURE 20-6. Characteristic multinucleated giant cell of herpes simplex virus infection. (See Fig. 20-6.)

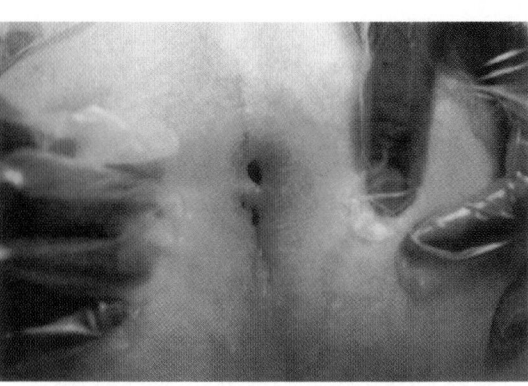

COLOR FIGURE 20-12. Erosion of an idiopathic AIDS-related ulcer into the deep postanal space, exiting into the perianal skin. (See Fig. 20-12.)

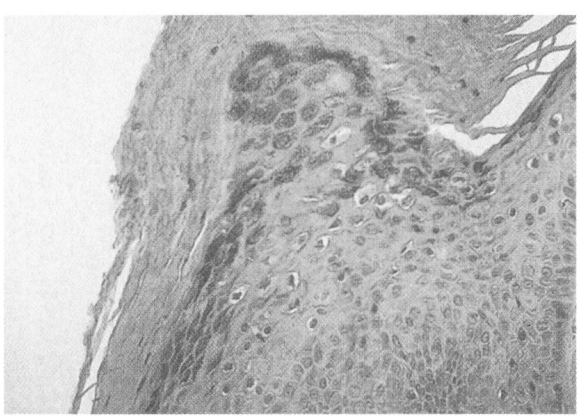

COLOR FIGURE 20-7. Histopathology of anal condyloma acuminatum, showing orderly papillomatosis, poikilocytosis, and hyperkeratinization. (See Fig. 20-7.)

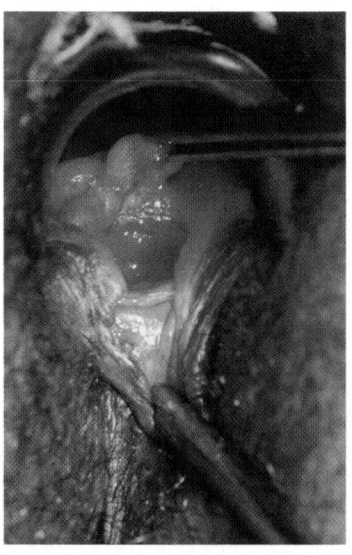

COLOR FIGURE 20-13. Idiopathic AIDS-related ulcer showing dissection in the submucosal and intersphincteric plane. (See Fig. 20-13.)

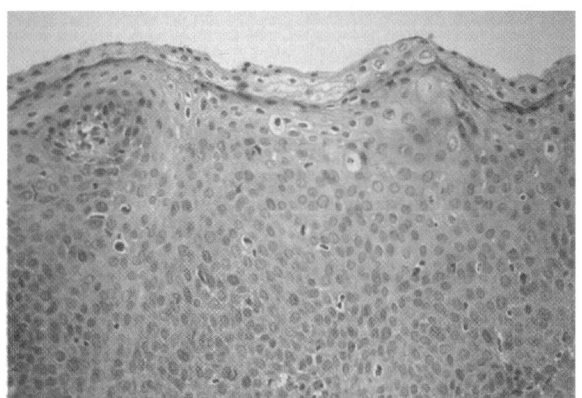

COLOR FIGURE 20-8. Histopathology of a flat lesion showing anal intraepithelial neoplasia (AIN III) with severe dysplasia. (See Fig. 20-8.)

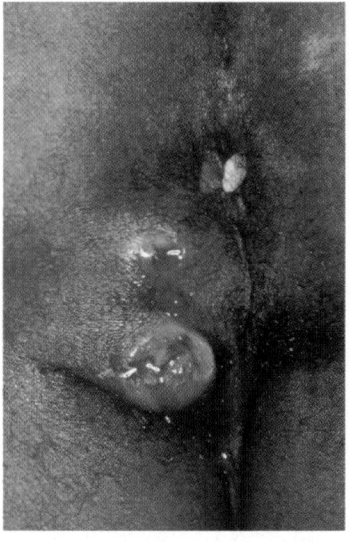

COLOR FIGURE 20-16. Large non-Hodgkin's rectal lymphoma eroding through the perianal skin. (See Fig. 20-16.)

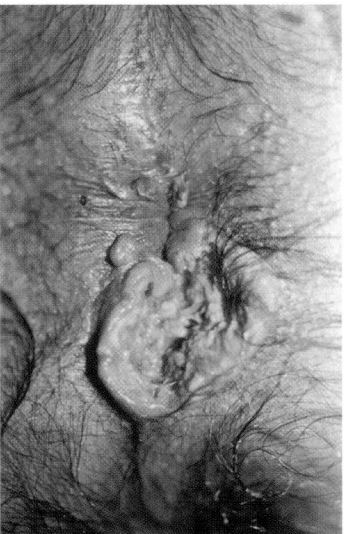

COLOR FIGURE 20-17. Squamous cell carcinoma of the anus in a patient with AIDS. (See Fig. 20-17.)

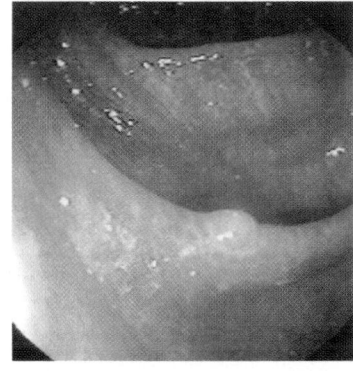

COLOR FIGURE 21-1. A hyperplastic polyp can be seen on the surface of one of the valves of Houston. Note the co-existing melanosis coli, which serves to demarcate clearly the nonpigmented lesion. (See Fig. 21-1.)

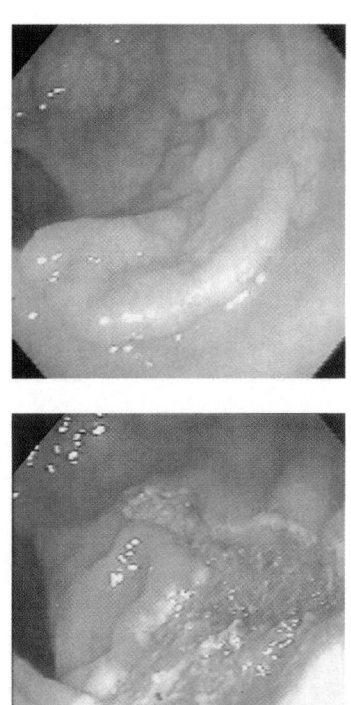

COLOR FIGURE 21-17. (A) The velvety appearance of sessile villous adenoma can be seen with the colonoscope. (B) Snare electrocoagulation reveals an extensive open wound that encompasses approximately one half of the bowel circumference. (See Fig. 21-17.)

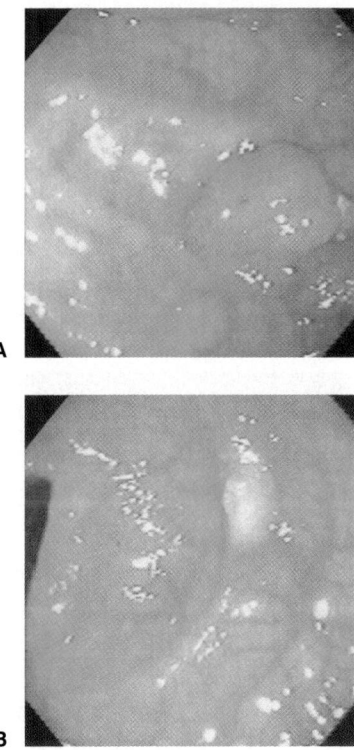

COLOR FIGURE 21-37. (A) A 1-cm polyp on short stalk can be easily snare excised by colonoscopy-polypectomy. (B) A whitish area of coagulated mucosa remains at the excision site. (See Fig. 21-37.)

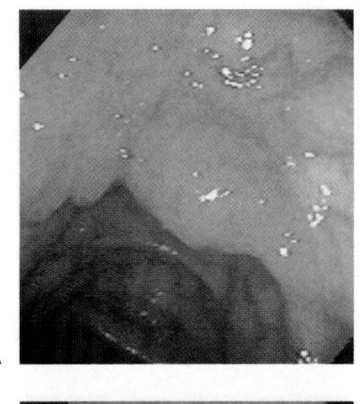

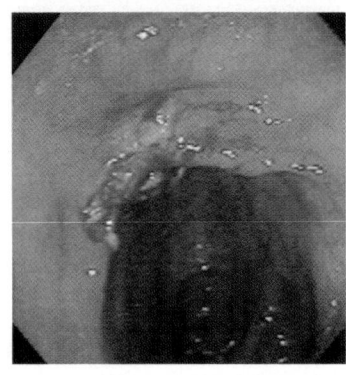

COLOR FIGURE 21-38. (A) A benign-appearing 1.5-mm sessile polyp can be removed by snare excision. (B) This creates a rather broad ulcer. Whether additional treatment is appropriate will depend on the histologic interpretation of the biopsy. (See Fig. 21-38.)

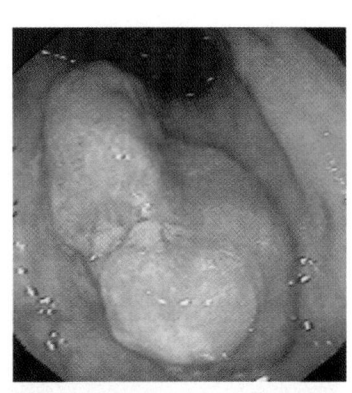

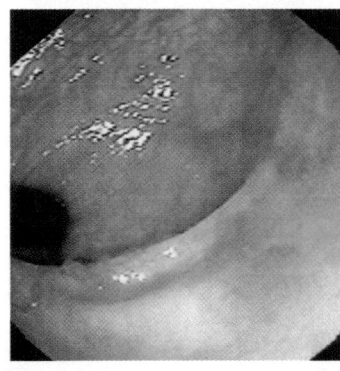

COLOR FIGURE 21-39. (A) A large adenomatous polyp was found to contain invasive carcinoma. (B) The postpolypectomy site appeared relatively benign. Resection revealed lymph node involvement with adenocarcinoma. (See Fig. 21-39.)

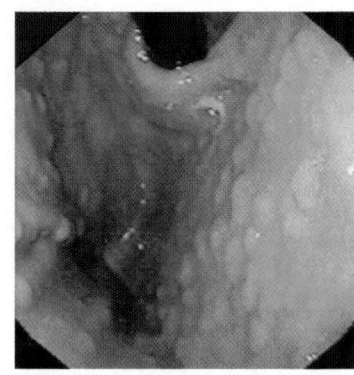

COLOR FIGURE 21-56. Upper gastrointestinal endoscopy in a patient with familial adenomatous polyposis reveals a gastric fundus showing a sheet of polyps. (See Fig. 21-56.)

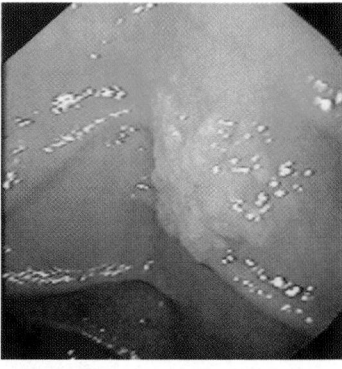

COLOR FIGURE 21-57. Duodenoscopy reveals a sessile villous tumor of the duodenum in a patient with familial adenomatous polyposis. (See Fig. 21-57.)

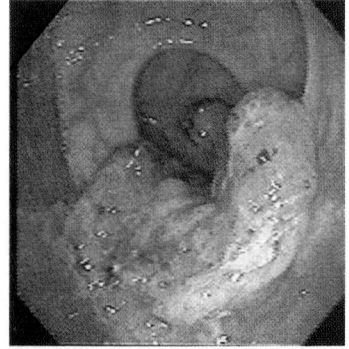

COLOR FIGURE 22-1. Colonscopic examination reveals an ulcerating tumor of the sigmoid colon. The tumor encompasses approximately one third of the bowel circumference. There is a small polyp proximal to the tumor that should emphasize the importance of total colonoscopic evaluation. (See Fig. 22-1.)

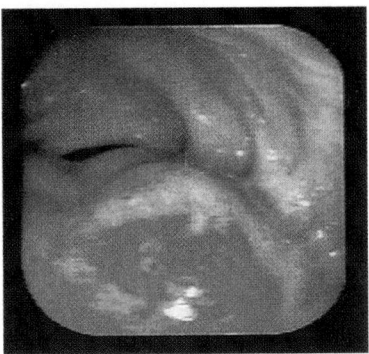

COLOR FIGURE 23-5. Proctoscopy demonstrates an exophytic, polypoid lesion, which on palpation was found to be freely movable. This tumor, theoretically, may be removed by local excision. (See Fig. 23-5.)

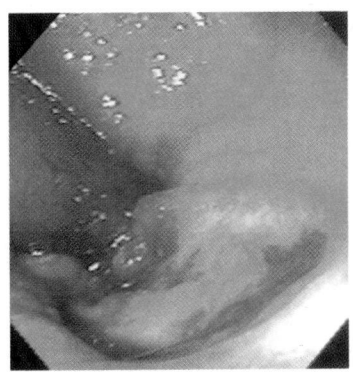

COLOR FIGURE 24-11. Retroflexion with the endoscope in the rectum reveals an ulcerating lesion in the transitional zone at the top of the anal canal and lower rectum. Biopsy confirmed the presence of a cloacogenic carcinoma. (See Fig. 24-11.)

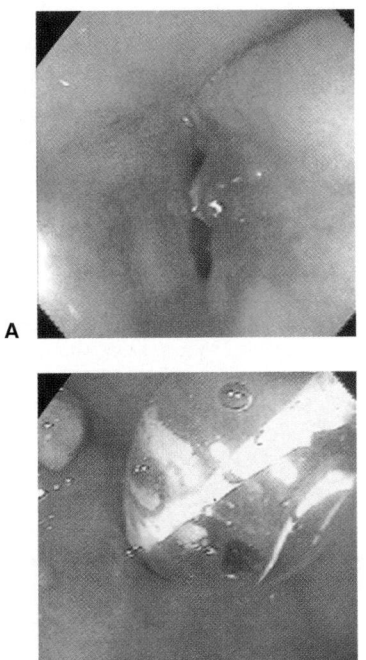

COLOR FIGURE 23-118. A benign rectal stricture is discovered following high anterior resection. **(A)** Marked narrowing can be seen through the flexible endoscope. **(B)** The stricture is dilated by the insertion of an endoscopic balloon. (See Fig. 23-118.)

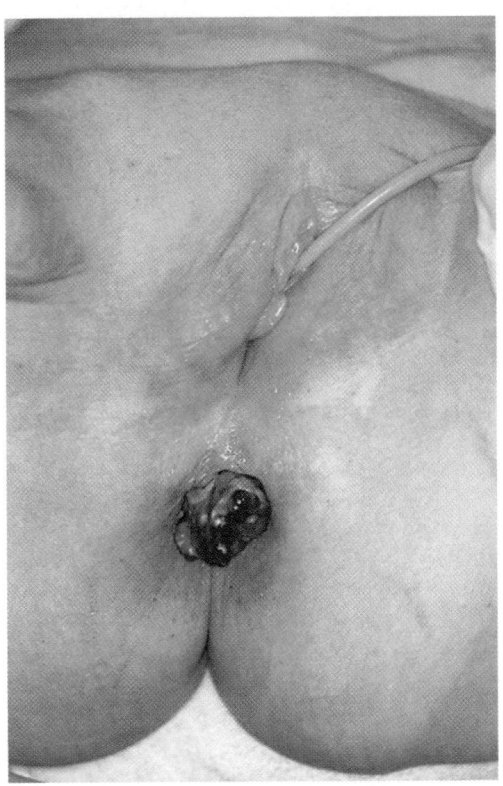

COLOR FIGURE 24-17. Malignant melanoma of the anus. A pigmented polypoid mass can be seen outside the anal verge. (See Fig. 24-17.)

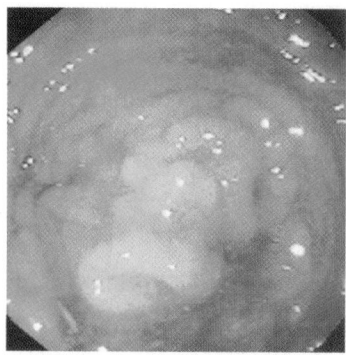

COLOR FIGURE 25-13. Colonoscopy reveals numerous confluent, sessile, mucosal nodules. Biopsy was consistent with nodular lymphoid hyperplasia. (See Fig. 25-13.)

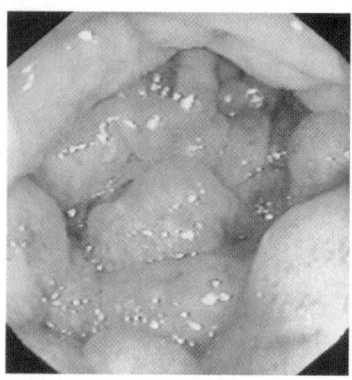

COLOR FIGURE 25-60. Submucosal cystic nodules were proven on biopsy to be lymphatic cysts. (See Fig. 25–60.)

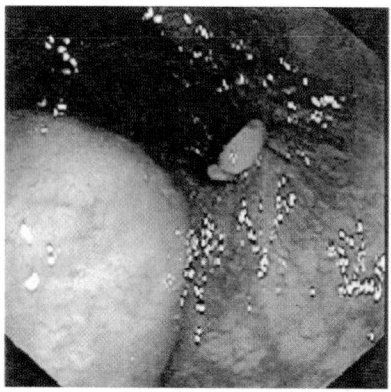

COLOR FIGURE 25-27. Malignant gastrointestinal stromal tumor (GIST). Extrarectal mass *(arrows)* seen on retroflexion of colonoscope demonstrating mucosal preservation. (See Fig. 25-27A.)

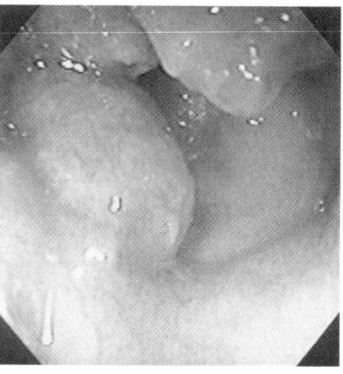

COLOR FIGURE 25-94. Pneumatosis cystoides intestinalis. Colonoscopy demonstrates cystic masses that pose a potential problem in differential diagnosis. Biopsy, however, revealed the histologic picture consistent with this condition. (See Fig. 25-94.)

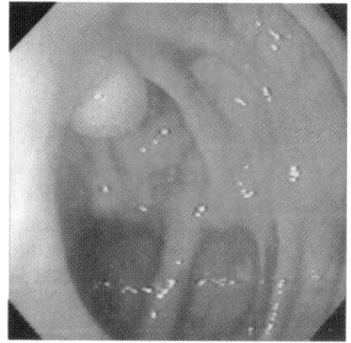

COLOR FIGURE 25-44. Lipoma of the ileocecal valve can be seen through the colonoscope. (See Fig. 25-44.)

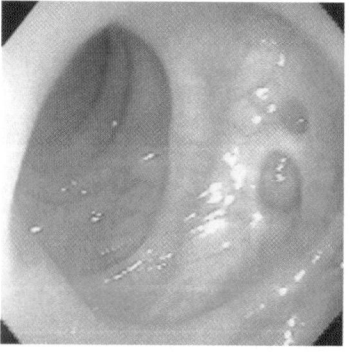

COLOR FIGURE 26-2. Colonoscopy reveals two diverticular openings in the region of the lower sigmoid colon. (See Fig. 26-2.)

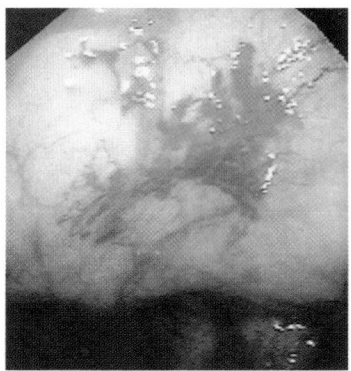

COLOR FIGURE 28-3. An angiodysplastic lesion, seen on colonoscopy, is characteristically a focal, submucosal, vasular ectasia. (See Fig. 28-3.)

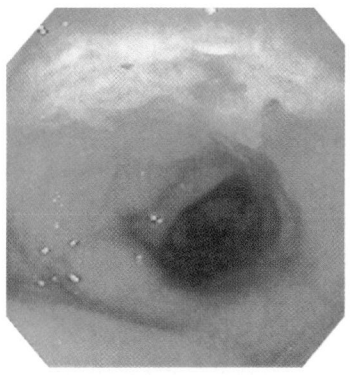

COLOR FIGURE 28-34. Endoscopy reveals a whitish area of scar surrounded by erythematous mucosa with evident stenosis characteristic of radiation proctitis. (See Fig. 28-34.)

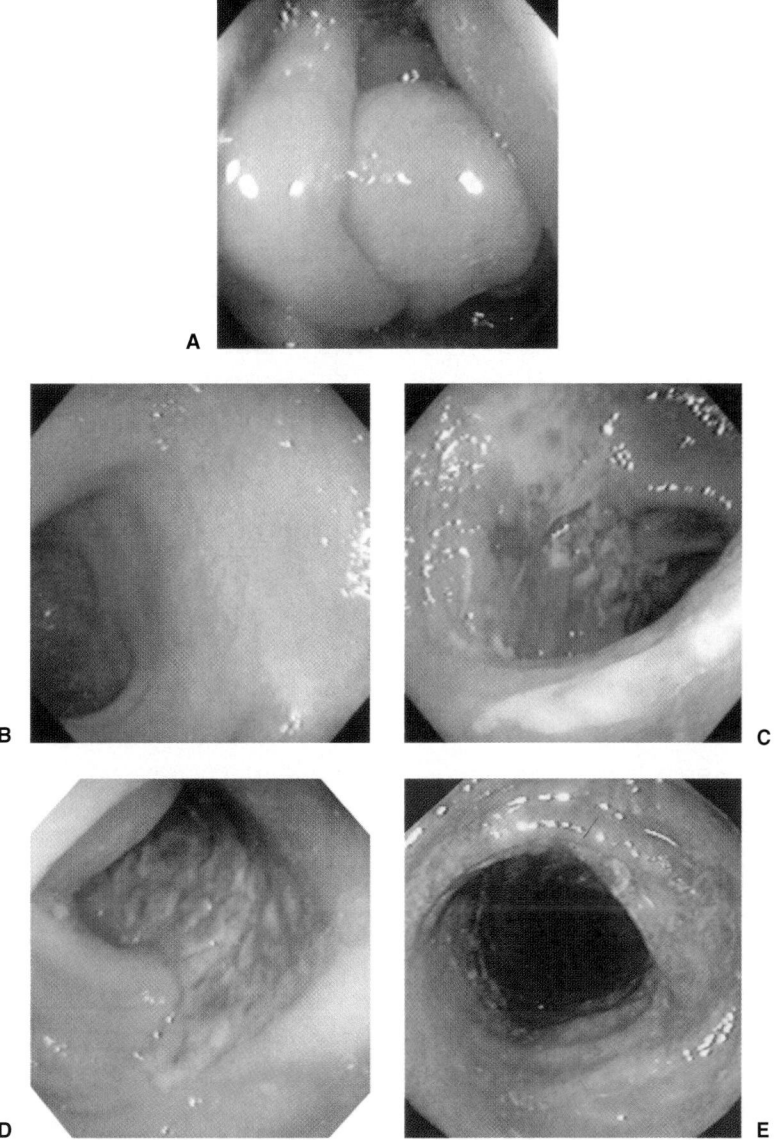

COLOR FIGURE 28-26. Colonoscopy reveals all of the characteristic changes of ischemic colitis in the region of the sigmoid colon of the same patient. **(A)** Edema. **(B)** Hyperemia. **(C)** Contact bleeding. **(D)** Mucosal pallor and necrosis. **(E)** Hemorrhagic, ulcerated mucosa. The condition is difficult to differentiate from inflammatory bowel disease. (See Fig. 28-26.)

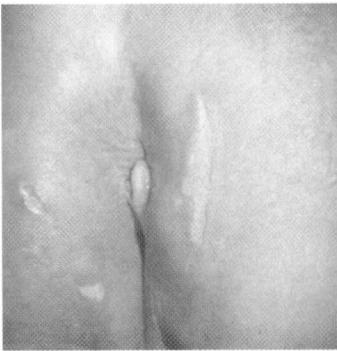

COLOR FIGURE 28-35. Erythema and linear ulcerations of the buttocks are evident in this patient who is undergoing radiation therapy for a carcinoma of the anal canal. Part of the lesion is apparent protuding from the anal verge. (See Fig. 28-35.)

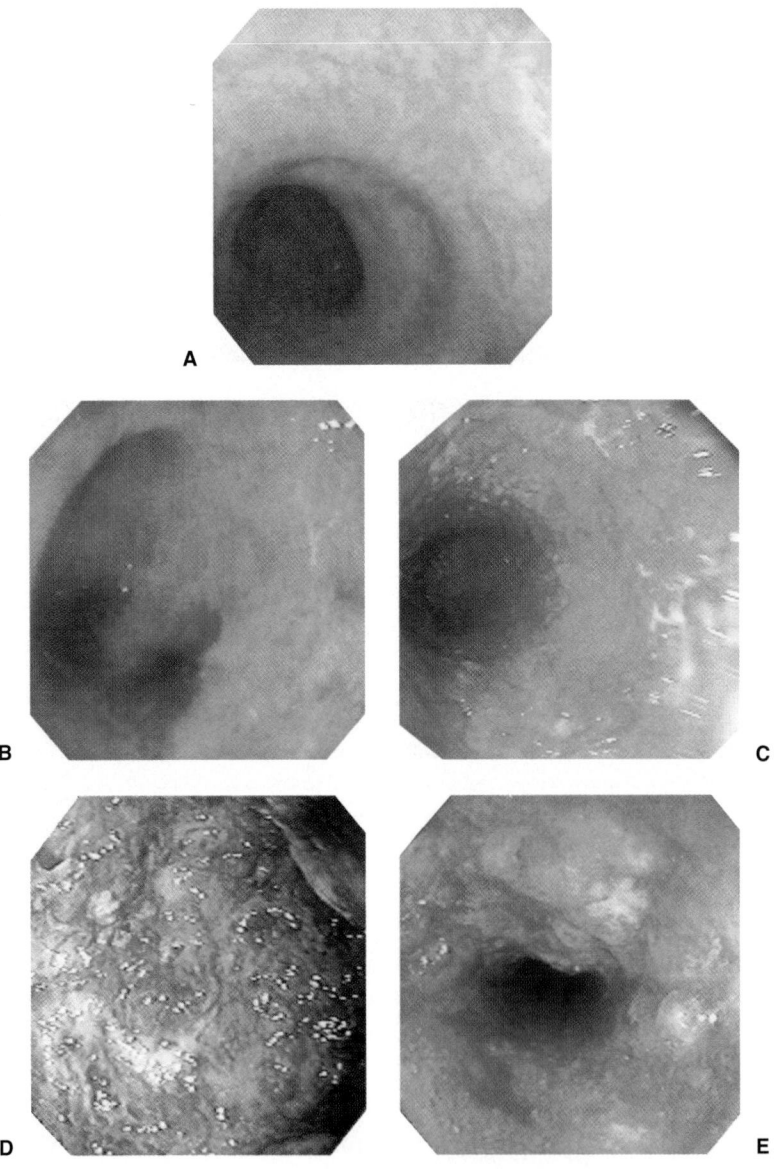

COLOR FIGURE 29-1. Colonoscopic changes in ulcerative colitis. **(A)** Loss of the normal vessel pattern is the earliest endoscopic change. **(B)** Contact bleeding. The friability of the mucosa is demonstrated by contact with the instrument. **(C)** Granularity appears in ulcerative colitis of longer duration. **(D)** Florid changes in an ulcerated mucosa. **(E)** A colonic stricture in a patient with ulcerative colitis proved on biopsy to be malignant. (See Fig. 29-1.)

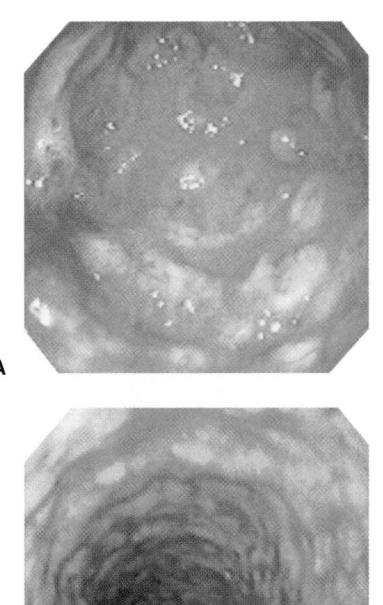

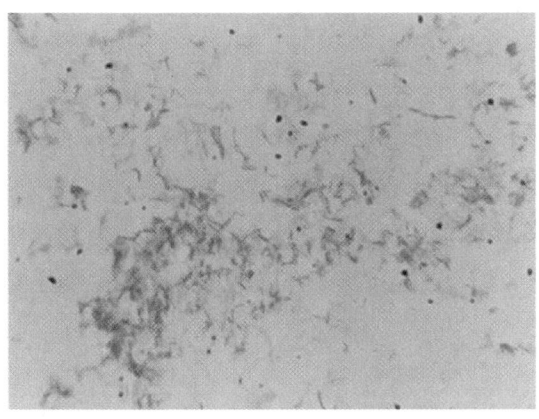

COLOR FIGURE 33-8. (**A, B**) Colonoscopy clearly demonstrates the patterns of yellow and yellow white adherent plaques in pseudomembranous colitis. (See Fig. 33-8.)

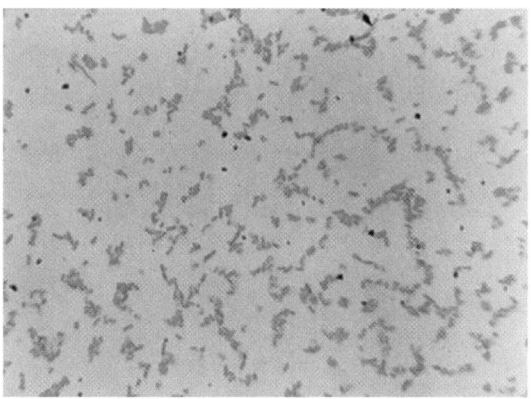

COLOR FIGURE 33-19. Shigella. Gram-negative bacillae, which, on biochemical and serological testing, reveal *Shigella*. (Original magnification ×1,060.) (See Fig. 33-19.)

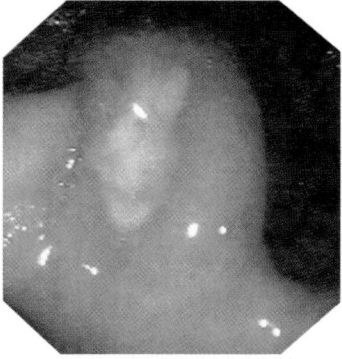

COLOR FIGURE 33-25. Colonoscopy demonstrates an exudative amebic ulcer that appears flask-shaped, even in this projection. Overhanging mucosa and undermining margins are present. Microscopic examination of the stool was positive for the trophozoites. (See Fig. 33-25.)

COLOR FIGURE 33-14. Pleiomorphic red-staining bacilli that are acid-fast because they retain carbol fuchsin and resist decolorization with acid alcohol. (Original magnification ×1,060). (See Fig. 33-14.)

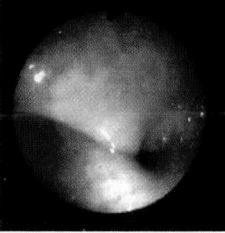

COLOR FIGURE 33-33. Proctosigmoidoscopic appearance of classic narrowing as a consequence of a sigmoid volvulus in a patient with Chagas disease. (Courtesy of T. Cristina Sardinha, M.D.) (See Fig. 33-33.)

There are a number of options for treatment when a known or unsuspected hepatic metastatic tumor is identified preoperatively or intraoperatively (see later). What is actually accomplished, however, may depend on the availability of specialized equipment.

Intraoperative Ultrasonography

Numerous articles have been published attesting to the value of intraoperative ultrasonography for identifying tumor in the liver that may not be apparent by means of palpation alone (Figure 22-97).[161,570,707,758,957] Often, the equipment employed is an ordinary real-time, linear-array, B-mode scanner not specifically designed for operative use.[957] A smaller probe is preferred, however, if available. The sterile probe is placed directly on the liver surface by the surgeon who performs the examination. A technician or radiologist may facilitate interpretation of the visual picture. A complete examination consists of identifying the vascular landmarks (three hepatic veins and inferior vena cava) and assessing the liver parenchyma segment by segment.

Olsen performed intraoperative ultrasonography on 213 patients with carcinoma of the colon and rectum and compared preoperative ultrasonography and inspection of the liver during surgery with this technique.[707] Intraoperative ultrasonography detected 116 previously unrecognized metastatic lesions. The authors concluded that the procedure is safe and more accurate than either standard exploratory methods or preoperative imaging.

Intraoperative ultrasonography is particularly applicable for assessment of the liver when a resection of metastatic tumor is planned, and it is an excellent substitute for manual palpation in someone who is undergoing laparoscopically assisted colectomy for cancer (see later and Chapter 27).

General Principles of Management

Surgical resection is the only potentially curative treatment for colorectal liver metastases, but only 20% to –25% of such lesions are considered resectable.[294] If a small focus of disease is present on the margin of the liver and no other lesion can be palpated or identified by means of operative ultrasonography, it is reasonable to remove it. For any other situation, resection is not advised. The location and size of the residual tumor or tumors are determined, and the patient is reevaluated following the operation. A CT scan (Figure 22-16) is obtained during the postoperative convalescence. If multiple or bilobar tumors are confirmed, no attempt is made to perform a resection. If solitary or unilobar disease is seen on the first scan, the study is repeated in 3 weeks. If only localized disease persists, the patient is admitted to the hospital for selective hepatic angiography. If there is still no evidence of extension, exploratory laparotomy and resection are recommended in accordance with the protocol discussed in Liver Metastases in the section Treatment of Recurrence.

Weber and colleagues, however, emphasize that the surgical strategy for treatment of synchronous colorectal liver metastases is still controversial.[999] They were able to simultaneously resect 36% of 97 patients from 1987 to 2000, and the remainder underwent delayed resection. The morbidity with the synchronous resection did not differ from that of the delayed resection, nor did the extent of liver resection. The overall survival rate was 94%, 45%, and 21% at 1, 3, and 5 years, respectively, after simultaneous resection, and 92%, 45%, and 22% after delayed resection.[999] Geoghegan and Scheele, following an extensive MEDLINE literature search, concluded that patients with colorectal liver metastases should be assessed in units that can offer all of the specialized techniques necessary in order to deliver optimal care.[294] I concur.

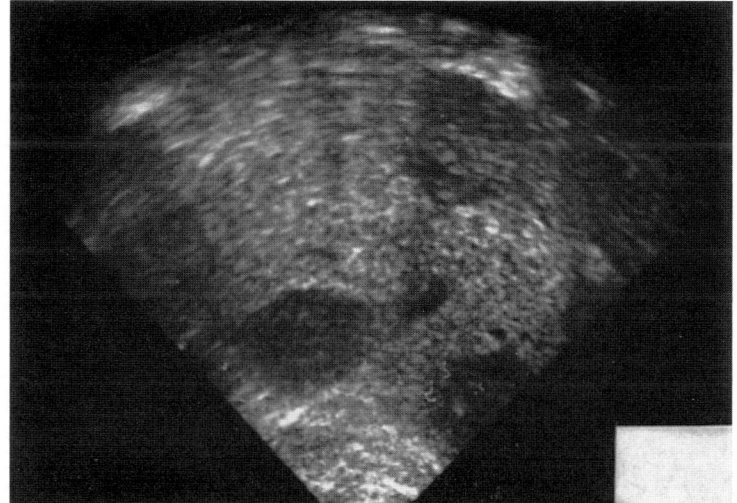

FIGURE 22-97. Intraabdominal ultrasonography demonstrates multiple filling defects in the liver, consistent with metastatic disease.

Resection of Other Organs

Excision in Continuity

Resection of adjacent small or large intestine, bladder wall, uterus, tubes and ovaries, stomach, spleen, tail of pancreas, duodenum, kidney, and portions of the abdominal wall may be performed for cure or to offer better palliation.[502] Because of the differences in the biologic nature of neoplasms, occasionally a tumor will invade locally and not metastasize until late in the course of the disease. If this locally invasive tumor is not removed, the patient may experience many months or years of pain. Intestinal obstruction or a visible protrusion of the tumor may develop—all situations that may be preventable by a more aggressive attempt at extirpation at the time of the initial operation. In the experience of Gall and Altendorf, operative mortality following multivisceral resections was 12%, as compared with a 6% mortality with bowel resection alone.[289] *En bloc* resection, removal in continuity with adjacent organs, is preferable to individual organ resection, with the recognition that adhesions may be inflammatory rather than neoplastic. However, the risk of seeding viable tumor cells justifies this approach. Eisenberg and colleagues have shown that survival in locally advanced colorectal carcinoma depends more on lymph node status than on the extent of local invasion.[245] Others have confirmed that the most important predictors of survival are lymph node status and involvement of the resection margins by tumor.[548,740] Therefore, the importance of obtaining tumor-free margins, even if radical resection is required for locally advanced colorectal cancer, should be emphasized. However, major resections of the abdominal wall, alloplasty, hemicorporectomy, and total pelvic exenteration, in the hope of improving the likelihood of cure for colorectal cancer, should be discouraged except in highly selected instances. The morbidity and mortality rates associated with these operations are so high that they almost preclude the possibility of a meaningful lifestyle.

Oophorectomy

There is no doubt that therapeutic removal of ovaries containing metastatic tumor is an appropriate and necessary treatment. The incidence of such involvement, usually found in younger, premenopausal women, often concomitantly with diffuse intraabdominal metastases, is approximately 6%.[45,78,660] The incidence of carcinoma of the ovary in women with carcinoma of the colon and rectum is approximately five times that of a primary ovarian malignant neoplasm.[696] The ovarian tumor may produce symptoms in advance of the colon cancer.[403,597] In the past, women were not uncommonly submitted to panhysterectomy for an ovarian tumor only to discover subsequently that the histologic nature of the lesion was consistent with a colonic primary tumor. A cure is only rarely obtained even when all the obvious visual disease is removed. Even so, unremoved ovarian tumors may grow to such an enormous size that symptoms may dictate an additional operation.

The question of the role of prophylactic oophorectomy has been a matter of some controversy. Blamey and colleagues noted that only 1.4% of 882 women who underwent resection for colorectal cancer subsequently required an operation for ovarian recurrence.[83] The low incidence of clinical recurrence indicated to these authors that prophylactic oophorectomy could not be supported. Young-Fadok and co-workers undertook a prospective, randomized trial to evaluate the influence of oophorectomy on recurrence and survival in patients with Dukes' B and C cancers.[1054] No patient had evidence of gross or microscopic metastatic disease among the 77 individuals randomized to oophorectomy. Others, however, have reported the occasional cure of a patient found to have micrometastases and strongly recommend prophylactic oophorectomy.[329,573] Still others believe that these successes are merely anecdotal, but they continue to recommend prophylactic oophorectomy in postmenopausal women if for no other reason than to prevent primary ovarian cancer.[78,190]

Rozario and colleagues found, depending on the age of the patient, that prophylactic oophorectomy results in a 4% to 11% reduction in the incidence of ovarian carcinoma, a rate that increases to 16.6% to 26.9% if general surgery procedures in which access could be more difficult are considered.[799] The additional procedure adds minimal risk and increases operative time only slightly. However, in the premenopausal patient, replacement estrogen therapy is required, and the operation will obviously precipitate early menopause.[78] To date, therefore, there are no objective, compelling data to support prophylactic oophorectomy in the premenopausal woman. However, the need for closer follow-up by means of pelvic ultrasonography or CT has been suggested for these individuals.[243]

Incidental Cholecystectomy

The risk of additional intraabdominal procedures at the time of colectomy was reviewed by Biggers and colleagues.[75] In a series of 242 patients from the Mayo Clinic in whom an adequate bowel preparation had been performed, the risk was minimal. Cholecystectomy represented the most frequently applied incidental operation (81 patients; 33%). There were two deaths and one complication in this group. The morbidity and mortality did not differ significantly from those previously reported following colon resections without cholecystectomy. Others have confirmed the relative merit of incidental, simultaneous cholecystectomy.[859] It is my policy always to perform a cholecystectomy during elective colon resection when cholelithiasis is present, unless the operative time would be inappropriately prolonged or the incision would need to be extended for an unreasonable length.

Appendectomy

It has been advocated in the past that appendectomy should be performed concomitantly with cholecystectomy, gynecologic procedures, and bowel resections. However, the incidence of acute appendicitis in the older population—that is, the patient population most likely to require surgery for colon cancer—is extremely small. It has been estimated that to prevent a single lifetime case of acute appendicitis in someone 60 years of age, 166 incidental appendectomies would be required.[1034] On the basis of a number of actuarial studies, it has been concluded that appendectomy as a preventive measure in individuals more than 40 years old is not cost effective. Furthermore, although the morbidity associated with the appendectomy itself is extremely low, the differential diagnostic concerns may be increased when an intraabdominal septic problem develops in a patient following colectomy. Therefore, I do not recommend incidental appendectomy and do not perform it.

Meckel's Diverticulectomy

Meckel's diverticulum is the most common congenital abnormality of the small intestine. When symptomatic, it may lead to rectal bleeding, intussusception, and Meckel's diverticulitis. Abdominal pain and lower gastrointestinal hemorrhage are the usual presentations (see Chapter 28). Children most often present with bowel obstruction and/or bleeding, whereas in adults intestinal obstruction is more likely to develop. After a thorough review of the literature, Wolff concluded that, as with appendectomy, Meckel's diverticulum in the older patient should be left alone.[1034] I agree.

Incidental Abdominal Aortic Aneurysmectomy

The incidence of colonic cancer coexisting with an aneurysm of the abdominal aorta is approximately 2%.[539] As a general surgeon specializing in colon and rectal surgery, I have never given much consideration to the potential dilemma of being confronted with an unsuspected abdominal aortic aneurysm. My preoperative plan would not waiver; the aneurysm would be duly noted and dealt with by a vascular surgeon at the appropriate interval.

Lobbato and colleagues reported the opinions of 46 professors of general and vascular surgery.[539] Whenever the preoperative diagnosis was clearly established, approximately one third favored excision of the carcinoma first, one third stated that priority should be given to the aneurysm, and the remaining one third stated that they would make a decision at the time of the laparotomy. Only two individuals believed that simultaneous operations should be attempted. Because of risk for sepsis in the graft and the potentially catastrophic consequences

of such a complication, I believe that this last position is without justification.

Minu and colleagues reported the clinical courses of three patients who concomitantly underwent resection for colorectal cancer and wrapping of the aneurysm with a Dacron or Teflon mesh.[638] With a follow-up in excess of 2 years, no complications relative to the procedures or to the subsequent development of symptoms referable to the aneurysm were encountered. The authors concluded that in the absence of an impending rupture of the aneurysm, the tumor can be resected and an interim aneurysmal wrapping performed. Baxter and co-workers retrospectively reviewed the Mayo Clinic experience with colorectal cancer and concomitant abdominal aortic aneurysm.[52] Eighty-three such patients were identified between the years 1986 and 2000. In 64 of these, the colorectal cancer was treated initially (44 with aneurysms less than 5 cm in diameter). No complication referable to the aneurysm was encountered in the postoperative period. Twenty patients had an aneurysm 5 cm or greater in diameter and underwent solely colorectal cancer resection. In two, the aneurysms ruptured in the postoperative period. Twelve patients underwent treatment of both conditions concomitantly without graft complication (median follow-up, 3.2 years). Seven patients underwent graft repair before colon resection. There was a highly significant delay in resection of the colon cancer (median, 122 days) when compared with the other groups. The authors conclude that patients requiring aneurysm surgery for smaller lesions, less than 5 cm, should undergo colon resection first. Larger aneurysms present a risk of rupture and, therefore, can be reasonably treated concomitantly with the cancer. Treating the aneurysm without resecting the colon leads to an unacceptable delay in cancer therapy for many patients. However, the newer modality of endovascular repair may be considered, followed by colon resection shortly thereafter.[52]

POSTOPERATIVE CARE

The relative merits of postoperative antibiotics and the use of an indwelling urinary catheter have been previously discussed. The relative lack of benefit of a nasogastric tube has also been addressed.

Pain Control

One of the most important concerns to the patient and to the surgeon is the ability to control pain. The use of an epidural catheter and a patient-controlled intravenous analgesic regimen are my personal preferences.[790] However, Petros and colleagues found that patient-controlled analgesia after uncomplicated colectomy increases the risk for postoperative ileus.[730] This has not been my observation, however, in those patients in whom meperidine (Demerol) is the agent employed for pain control by this method.

The use of continuous epidural analgesia is discussed in Chapter 7. Lehman and Wiseman studied the effect of epidural analgesia and the return of peristalsis and length of stay following elective colorectal surgery.[522] No statistically significant difference was found between this modality and traditional analgesia with respect to either variable. Furthermore, there was no increased complication rate and, specifically, no increased incidence of anastomotic leaks. Certainly, any individual who poses a risk because of pulmonary difficulties will benefit from epidural analgesia.[100] Despite the foregoing conclusions and the fact that I do like to use it, I have not found continuous epidural analgesia to be the panacea that many people believe. Reasons for problems in management include inconsistent dosing, catheter migration, and inability to adjust the medication or to supply additional medications without the advice and consent of the anesthesiology department. Clearly, success with this technique is very much dependent on the skill of the individual performing the procedure.

Diet

It has been generally believed that patients who undergo colon resection should be given only minimal oral alimentation until flatus has passed, at which time a progressive diet is instituted. Since the advent of laparoscopic surgery, the concept of early feeding has been explored. Based on the experience of early postoperative feeding in patients who have undergone laparoscopically-assisted surgery, the principles have been applied to open colon resection. Numerous articles have confirmed that early feeding, if tolerated, decreases the length of hospital stay and may not be uniquely applicable to laparoscopy.[76,114,154,391,450,776]

Some have observed in a prospective, randomized, controlled study that gum chewing aids in the early recovery from abdominal surgery by limiting ileus, and it is an inexpensive means for stimulating the return of intestinal activity.[32] In an experience from the Kaiser Permanente Medical Center, when a protocol consisting of a clear liquid diet on the second postoperative day and a regular diet on the third was utilized, two thirds of patients who underwent colon resection were able to be discharged home by the fourth postoperative day.[154] Such reports have led me to introduce oral alimentation sooner, with progression more quickly advanced in those individuals who seem to tolerate it.

Holte and Kehlet pointed out that the pathogenesis of ileus involves inhibitory neural reflexes and inflammatory mediators released from the site of injury.[416] They strongly encouraged a multimodal rehabilitation strategy in order to minimize this problem. This may include epidural analgesia, avoidance of nasogastric tubes, immediate enforced oral nutrition, early mobilization, protein drinks, laxatives, and planned early discharge.[49,50,211,471]

Without doubt, the use of opioids contributes to the prolongation of ileus. In 1972, opioid receptors were discovered in the gut, on presynaptic nerve terminals in the myenteric plexus.[470] These receptors are believed to send signals that decrease propulsive contractions when bound with opioids. There are currently studies on the use of pharmacologic agents to block the peripheral or so-called *mu* (μ) receptors in the bowel wall and yet simultaneously allow the central analgesic effects.[470,1018] Alvimopam (Adolor Corporation, Exton, PA) is such a proposed agent which, as of this writing, is in the process of clinical trials.[828]

COMPLICATIONS

The complications of colon and rectal surgery, especially as applied to cancer, are discussed in Chapter 23.

MORTALITY AND RECURRENCE AFTER RESECTION

Considerable difficulty is encountered in analyzing the survival results after resection for colorectal carcinoma from various institutions. Many reports use actuarial methods, correcting the data for the age of the patient, thereby theoretically giving more accurate survival statistics. However, confusion may still arise. For example, only a few patients who are more than 90 years old and whose disease is cured survive 5 years. If a patient in this age group dies of carcinoma of the colon 4 years after resection, this is still considered a cure. Another method commonly employed to analyze results divides patients who have undergone surgery into two categories: those who have had resection and in whom the surgeon believes the disease is potentially curable and those whose disease is considered incurable and for whom the operation is palliative.

A third method of analysis is to determine the "crude" survival rate. This is calculated on the basis of the number of patients alive 5 years after treatment. Obviously, this may not be a true estimate of the number of deaths from cancer, because the patient may have died of another cause during the interim. Determinate survivors are those individuals who die within 5 years with no evidence of recurrent disease. Some institutions employ this means for reporting data. The obvious implication is that the survival figures are improved if patients are considered cured even if they die, albeit free of disease, before 5 years have elapsed. A need exists for uniformity in reporting the results of treatment for colorectal cancer and for the use of consistently comparable classifications of staging. What is more, there seems to be less interest in reporting overall survival statistics, at least for colon cancer. Moreover, what data exist, including our own earlier reports, often combine colon and rectal cancer mortalities when there is a recognized difference in survival between the two areas, especially in light of the fact that the confines of the pelvis tend to limit the ability for one to widely resect the tumor. In the literature, there is much greater attention to survival with rectal cancer, especially with respect to, for example, neoadjuvant therapy, total mesorectal excision, and palliative treatment. Therefore, one must presume that surgery has accomplished all it can for colon cancer stage for stage.

In order better to evaluate and compare the morbidity and mortality rates associated with major surgery, a scoring system has been developed. The *Physiologic* and *Operative Severity Score* for the en*U*meration of *Mortality* and morbidity (POSSUM) and *Portsmouth* (P-POSSUM) equations were derived from a heterogeneous general surgical population to provide this information.[70,934] Tekkis and colleagues evaluated these scoring systems in patients undergoing colorectal surgery and found that both systems overpredicted mortality in young patients and underpredicted mortality in the elderly.[934] Emergency surgical deaths were also underpredicted.

Mitry and co-workers studied specifically operative mortality after colorectal cancer surgery over a 20-year period (1976 to 1995).[640] Overall mortality decreased from 17.7% to 8.1%, whereas rates after curative resection fell from 12.6% to 6.2%. These still seem very high mortality numbers, the consequence of which was the dramatic improvement in overall survival based on this criterion alone. In 1979, we reported 1,008 patients who underwent treatment for carcinoma of the colon and rectum.[178] Of these, 15 (1.5%) did not undergo operation. Thirty-nine operative deaths occurred, a mortality rate of 3.9%. Operative mortality in patients operated on for cure, however, was 1.8%. These data are summarized as follows:

As discussed earlier in the chapter, the prognostic implication of Dukes' classification has been well established. When the lesion is confined to the bowel wall, the chance of cure is great. In our experience, the uncorrected survival rate for a patient with a Dukes' A lesion is 81%.[178] For Dukes' B lesions, the uncorrected rate is 62%, and for Dukes' C lesions, 35%. Actuarially corrected rates were 95%, 90%, and 55%, respectively (Table 22-6). Table 22-7 compares our results with those of others.

Survival rates generally correlate with the extent of lymph node involvement. Table 22-8 illustrates the survival rate in comparison with the number of positive lymph nodes. If more than three nodes were positive, the overall survival rate was only 18%. These results lend further support to the contention that ultraradical resection for colorectal carcinoma is not justifiable. The number of positive nodes in the specimen appears to be as important as the level of nodes involved by tumor. Others have also concluded that the location, rather than the number, of nodal metastases has a greater impact on prognosis in colorectal cancer patients.[862] This is not to say that involvement of an apical lymph node is not an important criterion for survival (see earlier discussion on the sentinel lymph node). Wong and associates conducted a study on 345 patients with M_0 disease to determine whether increasing the number of *negative* nodes recovered would better stage the patient and more accurately predict disease-free survival.[1041] When compared with a national registry (OncoPool), they observed a significantly greater number of lymph nodes sampled in their study population and a statistically significantly improved survival between their patients and the National Cancer Registry population.[1041] Komuta and co-workers noted that the identification of extracapsular invasion of metastatic lymph nodes has a negative effect on survival when compared with lymph node invasion that does not extend outside the capsule.[492]

Malassagne and colleagues explored the relationships between a host of pathologic parameters, including the

Results of Operation for Colorectal Carcinoma (1962 to 1971)

Number of patients: 1,008
  Men: 548
  Women: 460
Mean age: 63 years
  Men: 63 years
  Women: 62 years
Not operated: 15
Operated: 993
Not resected: 51
Resectability: 95%
Operative mortality: 39 (3.9%)[178]

▶ **TABLE 22-6** **Survival Rate by Dukes' Classification (1962–1971)**

Uncorrected	Number of Cases	Percentage	Corrected* (%)
A	225	81	95
B	332	62	90
C	204	35	55
D	<u>247</u>	0	1
	1008		

*Data from United States National Center for Health Statistics. *Table of expectation of life and mortality rates from vital statistics for the United States (1974)*, vol 2, sect 5, life tables. Washington, DC: United States Government Printing Office, 1976.

▶ **TABLE 22-7 Five-Year Survival**

	Source	*Study Years*	*Number of Patients*	*Uncorrected 5-Year Survival (%)*
Dukes' Classification A	Gilbertsen[300]	1940–1959	359	67
	Dukes and Bussey[236]	1928–1952	308	81
	Corman et al.[178]	1962–1971	225	81
Dukes' Classification B	Dukes and Bussey[236]	1928–1952	692	64
	Corman et al.[178]	1962–1971	332	62
	Gilbertsen[300]	1940–1959	174	51
Dukes' Classification C	Dukes and Bussey[236]	1928–1952	1,037	32
	Grinnell[343]	1936–1945	221	36
	Corman et al.[178]	1962–1971	204	35
	Gilbertsen[300]	1940–1950	173	33
	Botsford et al.[94]	1960–1965	146	44

location and number of lymph nodes involved, blood vessel invasion, depth of tumor penetration, and metastases.[579] The 5-year survival rates were 45% and 17% for patients without and with apical lymph node involvement, respectively, and 44% and 6% with four or fewer nodes involved and more than four involved, respectively. These differences were statistically significant.

In addition to lymph node involvement, we have been particularly interested in the presence or absence of blood vessel invasion (Figure 22-32). Table 22-9 shows the uncorrected survival rate in patients with Dukes' C lesions with and without blood vessel invasion. The survival rate of patients with blood vessel invasion was 31%, compared with 43% in those without blood vessel invasion. These differences are not statistically significant, but they do suggest that the combination of blood vessel invasion and lymph node involvement is associated with a poorer prognosis for survival than lymph node involvement alone. The importance of blood vessel invasion is evident in Table 22-10. With Dukes' B lesions, 5-year survival was 70% in those without blood vessel invasion but only 55% in those with such invasion. This difference is statistically significant ($p < .05$). The mean ages of patients with and without blood vessel invasion, alive or dead, were identical. Oh-e and associates opine that intratumor microvessel count at the site of deepest penetration of the cancer is a predictor for the presence of lymph node metastasis.[703]

Gervaz and co-workers studied Dukes' B colorectal cancers with respect to p53 protein expression and determined that it is an independent factor for survival.[296] Furthermore, this also correlated with tumor location; 86% of p53-positive tumors were located in the distal colon and rectum.

Galandiuk and colleagues reviewed the patterns of recurrence after curative resection for carcinoma of the colon and rectum.[288] As expected, colon cancer had a better prognosis than rectal cancer (52% versus 40%). The most frequent sites for recurrence were hepatic (33%),

▶ **TABLE 22-8 Survival Versus Number of Lymph Nodes Involved (1962–1971)**

Number of Positive Lymph Nodes	*Total*	*Deaths*	*5-Year Survival*	
			Number	*Percent*
1	71	39	32	45
2	47	33	14	30
3	30	15	15	50
4	20	16	4	20
5	11	9	2	18
6	8	6	2	25
7	7	6	1	14
8 or more	9	8	1	11
Total	**203**	**132**	**71**	**35**

From Corman ML, Veidenheimer MC, Coller JA. Colorectal carcinoma: a decade of experience at the Lahey Clinic. *Dis Colon Rectum* 1979;22:477, with permission.

▶ **TABLE 22-9 Uncorrected Survival Rates, Dukes' Classification C Colorectal Carcinoma (1962–1966)**

Blood Vessel Invasion	*5-Year Survival*	*Deaths*	*Living*	
			Total	*Percent*
Present	19	43	62	31
Absent	24	32	56	43

From Corman ML, Veidenheimer MC, Coller JA. Colorectal carcinoma: a decade of experience at the Lahey Clinic. *Dis Colon Rectum* 1979;22:477, with permission.

▶ **TABLE 22-10** Uncorrected Survival Rates, Dukes' Classification B Colorectal Carcinoma (1962–1966)

Blood Vessel Invasion	Living	Deaths	Total	Living (%)
Present	32	26	58	55
Absent	82	35	117	70
Total	**114**	**61**	**175**	**65**

From Corman ML, Swinton NW Sr, O'Keefe DD, et al. Colorectal carcinoma at the Lahey Clinic, 1962–1966. *Am J Surg* 1973;125:424, with permission.

pulmonary (22%), local or regional (21%), intraabdominal (18%), retroperitoneal (10%), and peripheral lymph nodes (4%). There was a much higher incidence of local recurrence in rectal sites than in colonic, a fact that is attributable to the difficulties with the technique of wide excision within the confines of the pelvis. This has been confirmed in a number of reports.[695]

Mzabi and colleagues undertook a retrospective study to determine the factors associated with mortality and survival after resection for colonic cancer.[668] As could be expected, patients who presented for operation with no symptoms had a significantly better rate of survival than those who presented with symptoms. Furthermore, these investigators and others demonstrated that rectal bleeding as a symptom was a better prognostic sign than the other presenting complaints of colonic cancer.[668,897] Other variables, ranked according to their relative importance independent of stage according to one study, were as follows: histologic grade, level of direct spread, presence of venous invasion, age and sex of the patient, and presence of obstruction.[145] The Cleveland Clinic surgeons reported their observations on the factors affecting local recurrence in colon cancer and concluded that the location of the tumor is not relevant.[387] In their experience, fixity to another viscus, perforation or fistulization, advanced stage of disease, and dedifferentiation of tumor increase the risk of recurrence following curative resections.[387] In the Mayo Clinic experience, whereas the grade of anaplasia and ploidy had a strong influence on the rate of recurrence, these factors did not influence the timing or the pattern.[288] Goodman and Irvin studied the effect of a delay of diagnosis on prognosis following resection of carcinoma of the right side of the colon.[324] The authors observed that a delayed presentation was not associated with a different rate of survival than an early presentation.

Significance of Gender

Some reports suggest that survival after colorectal cancer surgery is better in women when controlled for tumor stage. The previously alluded to anatomic differences be-

tween the male and female pelvis may play an important factor with respect to rectal cancer resection from the technical perspective, but that does not account for improved survival with colon cancer. McArdle and colleagues noted in their 3,200 patients that overall survival at 5 years was higher in women, better in women with colonic tumors, in those who underwent elective surgery, and in those who underwent apparently curative resection.[604] It has been suggested that immunologic factors may play a role.[1009]

Significance of Blood Transfusion

Perioperative blood transfusion, possibly because of the potential for immunosuppression, may be associated with an increased risk for recurrence according to some studies, even when this variable is controlled for age, sex, Dukes' stage, and histologic differentiation.[74,723,925] Wobbes and colleagues noted a statistically significant worsening of disease-free survival when more than 6 units of blood were administered in comparison with a lesser amount.[1033] Marsh and colleagues found that the risk for recurrence in patients who received a transfusion of plasma was twice that in patients who did not receive any.[589] These investigators were not able to show a harmful effect of transfusion with packed cells. These data suggest that the plasma protein rather than the cellular component of whole blood mediates the accelerated tumor recurrence.[589] However, others have found no relationship between transfusion status and tumor recurrence, tumor behavior, or patient survival.[156,280,867,1002] Conversely, Houblers and colleagues found that their patients had a lower 3-year survival than those who were not transfused, but this poor survival was not related to recurrent cancer.[418] Busch and co-workers opine that the association between blood transfusions and prognosis in colorectal cancer is a result of circumstances that necessitate the transfusions in the first place.[124] Furthermore, the association may be greater with the development of local recurrence than with distant metastases.[124]

Obstructing and Perforating Carcinoma

Patients who present with obstruction or perforation have a poorer prognosis than other individuals with colorectal carcinoma.[898] The operative morbidity and mortality are also much higher.[803] Often, patients have evidence of metastatic disease at the time of presentation.[963,981] As previously mentioned, perforated carcinoma should be treated by primary resection whenever possible. In addition, primary resection should be carried out for proximal obstructing lesions. The concept of intraoperative colonic lavage with primary anastomosis in the presence of perforation (even peritonitis in certain instances) and obstruction has been advocated by a number of investigators (see earlier discussion).[77]

Some studies suggest that operative mortality and even prognosis are better when primary resection with anastomosis is performed rather than a staged approach. Umpleby and Williamson reported a 48% 5-year survival in curative resections with anastomosis, compared with an 18% survival rate with a staged resection.[963] Gennaro and Tyson noted an overall operative mortality of 14% for obstructing carcinoma.[293] The uncorrected survival rate at 5 years was approximately 9%, whereas only 18% of patients who underwent curative resection survived 5 years. Glenn and McSherry reported an operative mortality of 13% in patients with obstruction and a 5-year survival rate of approximately 20%.[308] Their experience with perforated carcinoma revealed an equally poor prognosis. The operative mortality was 15%, and the 5-year survival rate, 28%.[308] Serpell and colleagues reviewed 148 patients with colonic obstruction and found a significantly higher incidence of recurrence after curative resection and a lower survival rate.[849] Kriwanek and co-workers commented on the recognized high postoperative mortality for malignant perforation, concluding that it is the cumulative effect of the malignancy and sepsis that is responsible.[497]

Carcinoma in Younger Patients

Colorectal carcinoma has been believed to be associated with a poor prognosis when it develops in young patients. Only a small percentage of these individuals will have a predisposing factor, such as familial adenomatous polyposis. Although the incidence is much lower in the younger group, it is imperative for the physician at least to consider investigating anyone who presents with symptoms suggestive of a bowel tumor (vague abdominal pain, nausea and vomiting, weight loss, rectal bleeding, or change in bowel habits). Determination of occult blood in the stool may be helpful. Because of the symptoms at presentation and the difficulty in interpreting their significance, delay in diagnosis and treatment is one of the major factors responsible for the poor survival rates. In the experience of Palmer and colleagues, no Dukes' A or B lesions were seen in individuals less than 20 years of age, and only 11% were observed in those in their 20s.[720]

Even for the same stage of lesion, however, younger persons have been believed to do less well when compared with older individuals. This may be because younger patients have a higher incidence of mucinous and poorly differentiated tumors.[8,466,739] Recalde and associates reported a 13% 5-year survival rate in 40 patients 35 years of age or younger.[769] Furthermore, they noted that no 5-year survivors were found among individuals who had lymph node metastases, visceral metastases, or tumors larger than 5 cm in diameter. Sanfelippo and Beahrs reported on 118 patients less than 40 years of age who underwent resection for colorectal carcinoma.[821] Their overall 5-year survival rate was 39%. Patients with Dukes' C lesions had a 5-year survival rate of 21%.

Carcinoma of the colon is extremely uncommon in children. In contrast to the presentation in adults, the most frequent symptom is abdominal pain, often with vomiting. The diagnosis was delayed for more than 1 year in more than one half of the adolescents reviewed by Steinberg and co-workers.[896] Pemberton reported on the cure of a 9-year-old child and stated that no other report was found in the literature of a survivor in whom the disease developed at such an early age.[727] He further observed that in children, the colon is affected more frequently by cancer than any other part of the digestive system.

Fundamentally, three factors contribute to the increased mortality in these individuals: delay in diagnosis, advanced stage of disease, and poorly differentiated histology.[109,188] Mitry and colleagues emphasized that inadequate screening and treatment of young people with familial adenomatous polyposis or a family history of early age-at-onset colorectal cancer are the primary factors contributing to poorer prognosis rather than young age, itself.[641]

Carcinoma in the Elderly

Simply stated, there is no justification for avoiding needed surgery simply on the basis of a patient's age. Generally, there are no differences with respect to presentation, location, Dukes' classification, and prognosis in comparison with younger individuals. All studies confirm that there are no statistically significant differences in age-corrected survival curves.[434] However, emergency operations are associated with a higher morbidity and mortality in this age group.[69]

Carcinoma in Pregnancy

Colorectal carcinoma in pregnancy is extremely unusual. Nesbitt and colleagues reported their experience with five patients and reviewed the literature.[680] As with carcinoma in young patients, and for essentially the same reasons, prognosis is poor. Management is determined by the gestational age of the fetus at the time of diagnosis, as well as by religious and ethical considerations. The question of concomitant oophorectomy is problematic, especially during the first trimester, because of the risk for spontaneous abortion.[680]

Palliative Resection

Because carcinoma of the colon is a relatively slow-growing tumor, palliative resection should be performed whenever possible, subject to a few relative contraindications. Even with extensive metastatic disease, patients may live a relatively long time and be free of the often miserable sequelae associated with an untreated primary lesion.

Cady and co-workers reported that during the years from 1941 to 1960, patients with liver metastases diagnosed at operation survived a mean of 13 months.[128] Factors that adversely influenced survival included weight loss, intestinal symptoms, ascites, peritoneal seeding, extension of the primary cancer to other viscera, histologic involvement of lymph nodes or blood vessels, and extent of surgical treatment.[128] Takaki and associates noted a mean survival time of approximately 12 months in 59 patients who underwent palliative resection.[920] Goslin and colleagues reported a similar median survival.[325] With the newer adjuvant approaches to the treatment of metastatic cancer (see later), patients now live longer, especially with liver metastases. Those whose tumors are poorly differentiated or who have weight loss of greater than 10% at presentation (with metastases) survive a median of only 6 months.[325]

Contraindications to performing palliative resection include the presence of ascites, massive peritoneal seeding, jaundice, or severe debilitation. Jayne and colleagues found that the median survival with peritoneal carcinomatosis from colorectal cancer for synchronous disease was 7 months.[447] Liu and co-workers found that palliative resection of primary colon cancers is associated with a relatively high postoperative mortality but that it should be performed as long as hepatic metastases occupy less than 50% of liver volume.[537] Obviously, the decision to carry out such a procedure is a matter of surgical judgment.

The decision to perform a palliative resection in someone with bleeding, a profound anemia, perforation, or obstruction is usually not difficult. However, when a relatively asymptomatic colorectal cancer is found in someone with metastastic disease, one must consider whether the primary tumor should be removed. Sarela and colleagues identified 24 such patients and managed them with systemic chemotherapy without surgery.[823] Four patients developed bowel obstructions requiring operative management in two and stents in two. Additionally, three subsequently underwent right hemicolectomy for abdominal pain with poor relief. One other patient was downstaged and underwent a curative resection. The overall median survival was 10.3 months. The problem clearly is that some patients live longer than one anticipates. Ruo and co-workers reported the experience of the Memorial-Sloan Kettering Cancer Center in New York with patients with asymptomatic stage IV disease who underwent *elective* resection (127 individuals) and compared the results with 103 patients with stage IV disease who did not undergo resection.[805] Resected patients had longer median (16 versus 9 months) and 2-year survivals (25% versus 6%). The investigators concluded that patients with stage IV disease who were selected for elective palliative resection of asymptomatic primary colorectal cancers had a substantial postoperative survival that was significantly better than those not submitted to resection.[805]

FOLLOW-UP EVALUATION

How to follow patients who have undergone resection for carcinoma of the colon is a subject worthy of some discussion. Methods of evaluation include physical examination, fecal occult blood testing, proctosigmoidoscopy, colonoscopy, barium enema examination, chest radiography, determination of CEA levels, liver function studies, liver scan, ultrasonographic evaluation, CT, and exploratory laparotomy at an interval after operation, among others.[258,978]

Besides the variety of examinations, tests, and procedures that are available to follow the patient with cancer postoperatively, the frequency with which such evaluation should be undertaken is also the subject of some debate. One school of thought postulates that the patient should be discharged after recovery from surgery and report only if symptoms develop, so nihilistic is the attitude of many physicians and surgeons that earlier diagnosis and treatment of recurrent disease fail to result in a sufficiently improved survival rate to justify the cost and the effort.

Moertel and colleagues contributed an article in 1993 that stimulated considerable debate about the value of monitoring patients following resection of colon cancer.[645] The authors concluded that cancer cures attributable to monitoring of CEA are, at best, infrequent. Therefore, they question whether this small gain justifies the substantial cost and physical and emotional stress that this intervention usually causes patients. Obviously, cost is a major issue today, with no indication that higher-cost strategies increase the survival or quality of life.[983] Clearly, an intensive follow-up program is associated with, at best, only a minimally increased survival rate, but for those individuals fortunate enough to have recurrent tumors that are amenable to curative reresection, it would seem very important.[88,246,547,578,715,794,810,831,954] Bruinvels and colleagues found that patients with an intensive follow-up regimen noted a 9% better 5-year survival than those with minimal or no follow-up.[110] The fact is that few patients are salvaged in whom a recurrence of cancer develops. However, there is a group of individuals for whom a cure can still be achieved, or at least for whom lifestyle can be improved and long-term survival possible, if recurrent tumor is recognized early. These include those with a longer disease-free interval between initial resection and recurrence, with negative margins of resection, and smaller recurrent tumor size.[860]

In one area, at least, there appears to be no controversy: there is an increased risk for the development of a metachronous lesion. The calculated annual incidence for metachronous tumors was determined by Cali and colleagues to be 0.35%.[133] The cumulative incidence of 18 years was 6.3%. If for no other reason than this observation, the patient should never be discharged from follow-up study but should be evaluated periodically for the development of a second primary tumor in the bowel.

Heald and Lockhart-Mummery showed that the chance of cure was much improved in those patients who attended a follow-up clinic at the time of the occurrence of a second growth.[395] It has also been shown that metachronous cancers are diagnosed at earlier stages than the index cancers.[133] Ovaska and colleagues compared the results of 368 individuals who underwent regular follow-up evaluation with 139 who did not.[714] The cancer-related 5-year survival rate was 72% in the former group and 62% in the latter. Curative reoperations were performed in 21% of the former, but in only 7% of the latter. These investigators concluded that regular follow-up detects more recurrent tumors, enabling radical reoperations to be performed significantly more often than when this is not undertaken.

Physical Examination

Physical examination is quite unrewarding in my opinion for identifying an early recurrence. By the time palpation of the abdomen reveals a tumor in the liver or a recurrent lesion in the peritoneal cavity, the cancer is always nonresectable. Therefore, palpation of the abdomen, pelvic examination, and evaluation of supraclavicular and inguinal nodes serve primarily to reassure the patient and the physician. The primary value of such examinations and findings is to follow the response to adjuvant treatment once an obvious tumor has been identified.

Occult Blood Determination

The importance of examination of the stool for occult blood has been emphasized earlier in this chapter and in Chapter 4. As with the early identification of a primary tumor, the main purpose of performing this test is to look for a second (metachronous) lesion. It has been suggested that a lifelong follow-up regimen following resection of colorectal carcinoma for cure should include an annual occult blood determination.[87]

Proctosigmoidoscopy and Flexible Sigmoidoscopy

On an annual basis, or even more frequently, proctosigmoidoscopy is of particular value if the anastomosis can be seen with the instrument. Recurrence at the suture line, which most often results from inward growth of the tumor from the pelvis and not from residual cancer within the bowel wall or mucosa, can be identified, so that reresection for possible cure may be performed. Flexible sigmoidoscopy serves the same purpose if the anastomosis can be seen within range of this instrument. If the anastomosis is above this level, the only purpose of either examination is to identify a metachronous lesion within the limitations of the instrument.

Colonoscopy

Colonoscopy should be employed to evaluate the residual colon following resection if the procedure was not performed preoperatively or if visualization of the entire bowel was not accomplished. Many studies have demonstrated the high incidence of benign and malignant lesions harbored in the residual colon, presumably missed at the time of resection.[287,480,498,509,512,676,964] Harris and colleagues described the colonoscopic features of anastomoses in 117 postoperative patients.[388] The following were identified:

- Neovascularity (89.7%)
- White anastomotic edge (54.7%)
- Disruption of haustral pattern (54.7%)
- Radial suture tracks (38.0%)
- Exposed suture (11.9% of those sutured)
- Exposed staples (24% of those stapled)
- Scar tissue adjacent to anastomotic line (6.8%)
- Nondistensibility (4.3%)
- Blind colonic pouch (8.5%)

The site of seven anastomoses (5.5%) could not be identified.[388]

Reilly and associates performed perioperative colonoscopy on 92 patients.[775] Synchronous cancers were found in almost 8%. Approximately 3 or more years following treatment of the index cancer, a metachronous malignancy was demonstrated in an additional 8%.

The procedure is also of value in identifying recurrent disease at the anastomosis. Colonoscopy is advised by some authors every 3 years once the bowel has been demonstrated to be completely free of neoplasm,[87] but others believe that an annual evaluation with this instrument for the first 4 years after curative resection is preferable.[509,714] Leggett and co-workers performed colonoscopy within 6 months of surgery and then at intervals of 3 years thereafter on 433 individuals.[521] They calculated the rate of development of metachronous cancer at 0.61% annually. Juhl and colleagues performed annual colonoscopy in their surveillance program of 174 individuals.[461] The combined findings of anastomotic recurrences, metachronous colon cancers, and polyps represented an interval yield of 3% to 5% annually. Based on these results, they suggest an annual colonoscopy for at least the initial 6 years after resection.

My own preference is to perform an annual colonoscopic examination until the bowel is clear; then colonoscopy is performed every 3 years. It must be remembered that endoscopy is a poor tool for evaluating extramucosal, locally recurrent disease. Any follow-up program must, therefore, address this concern through alternative studies.[47]

Barium Enema Examination

The barium enema examination is of limited benefit in the follow-up evaluation of the patient with colorectal cancer. It is unlikely that recurrent disease at the suture line will be identified more readily by this technique than by colonoscopy. A possible exception to this dictum, however, is that extrinsic compression might be perceived more readily with a barium enema study than by means of colonoscopy. As suggested, in the follow-up evaluation of the bowel of patients who have undergone resection for colorectal cancer, colonoscopy appears to be the preferred technique, certainly for identifying a mucosal lesion.

Chest Radiography

Chest radiography should be performed annually to identify patients with possible pulmonary metastases; some of these individuals may still be operated on for cure (see Pulmonary Metastases in the section Treatment of Recurrence).

Liver Function Studies

Liver function studies have traditionally been considered useful in the follow-up evaluation of patients with colorectal cancer. In my experience, the alkaline phosphatase determination has been about as effective in diagnosing liver metastases as has the CEA determination, but the most sensitive overall test for detecting occult metastases has been CEA. One study has demonstrated that if patients with elevated serum alkaline phosphatase values are not found to have metastases to the liver at the time of laparotomy, then these individuals are at no greater risk for the development of liver tumors than those with normal serum levels.[926] Rocklin and colleagues believe that liver function tests should be deleted from follow-up of cancer patients, because the CEA heralds the onset of liver metastases much more frequently.[785]

Liver Scan

Postoperatively, in a patient with known liver metastases, the liver scan is useful to confirm the location and presence of the lesion or lesions. However, in the absence of a positive CEA determination or elevated level of alkaline phosphatase, this study has no place in postoperative screening. CT has replaced this study in the evaluation of colorectal cancer patients.

Computed Tomography

CT offers a simple, noninvasive method for the evaluation of metastatic colon tumor by enabling visualization of the liver, pelvis, retroperitoneum, and adrenal glands (Figs. 22-16 and 22-98). Some clinicians and investigators suggest that it be employed as a baseline study after surgery and then used at intervals to detect local recurrence.[248] It has also proved valuable in the evaluation of patients for supplemental therapy. Most studies confirm that both postoperative baseline CEA values and CT of the abdomen have the highest positive predictive rate when metastases or persistent disease is suspected.[298] In addition, the CT-guided aspiration technique is useful for obtaining cytologic confirmation of malignancy.

Glover and colleagues prospectively assessed the accuracy of a number of imaging techniques in 100 patients who were considered free of liver metastases after colorectal cancer resections.[309] These included CT, magnetic resonance imaging (MRI), ultrasound, isotope assessment, and serum CEA. The most sensitive technique was CT. CT and MRI (but not ultrasound) were completely accurate in differentiating liver metastases from other hepatic lesions, but only two thirds of affected patients were identified.

Magnetic Resonance Imaging

MRI is a promising modality that has certain advantages in comparison with CT, even replacing it as the diagnostic study of choice for lesions of the central nervous system. However, this advantage does not translate as well to the evaluation of tumor in other organs. As of this writing, CT is still the preferred alternative for the detection and follow-up of metastatic liver tumors.

Tumor Markers

The primary role of tumor markers today is in the postoperative surveillance of individuals who, theoretically, underwent surgery for cure and therefore are at risk for recurrence.[1046] The most frequently employed such marker is serum CEA. In addition, monoclonal antibodies labeled

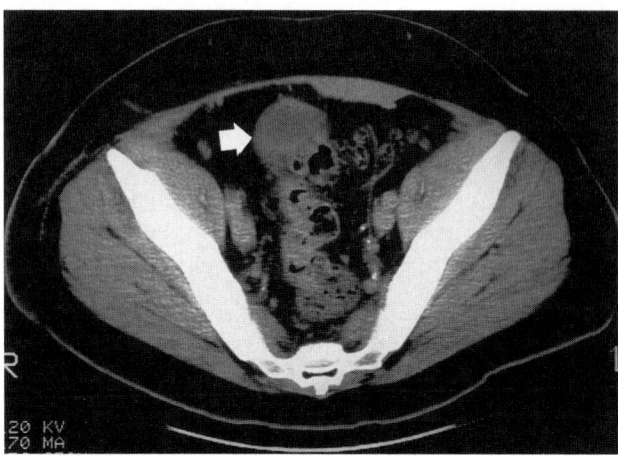

FIGURE 22-98. Computed tomography of the abdomen reveals tumor mass adjacent to the colon *(arrow)*. The radiologic study was pursued because of an elevation in the carcinoembryonic antigen determination. Because no other site of spread was identified, the patient underwent reexploration with resection of this solitary recurrence.

with radioisotopes are being used to identify possible sites of recurrent disease.

Carcinoembryonic Antigen

Although the studies of Gold and Freedman demonstrated that elevated titers of CEA preceded clinical signs of disease by 2 weeks to 10 months, Moertel and co-workers opined that the CEA test is grossly insensitive in the diagnosis of recurrent colorectal carcinoma.[311,312,649] They tested 36 patients with histologically demonstrable recurrent or residual malignant disease after resection but with no clinical evidence of distant metastases. Only nine patients (25%) had abnormal CEA levels even though most of them had had symptoms of recurrence for several months. Sugarbaker and colleagues studied the serial monthly CEA determinations of 33 individuals after resection for large bowel cancer.[912] Confirmed recurrent malignant disease subsequently developed in 12 of these patients. A rising titer was the first evidence of recurrence in only four of these 12, and all four had distant metastases.

Despite objections about the lack of specificity of CEA and the question whether it is a sufficiently early diagnostic marker of recurrent disease to make cure possible, most researchers generally agree that increasing levels are found with more advanced disease, a failure of elevated levels of CEA to return to normal after resection is associated with a poor prognosis, and elevated levels usually appear before any clinical evidence of recurrence.[28,332,538,542,547,591–593,685,692,693,702,876,1014,1055] Chu and colleagues further showed that the preoperative and postop-

erative levels were predictive of recurrence and survival independently of tumor stage.[155] Many asymptomatic patients suspected of having recurrent colorectal cancer based on an elevated CEA will be spared unnecessary surgery if strict attention is paid to the preoperative assessment.[702] McCall and co-workers found that CEA was the first indicator of recurrent disease in 58% of their patients and in 80% of those with liver metastases.[606]

Carcinoembryonic Antigen Concentration Gradient

Another possible application of the CEA determination has been reported by Patt and co-workers.[724] By means of selective angiographic techniques, a CEA concentration gradient can be determined by sampling from appropriate vessels. Identification of the site of recurrence may be possible with this method.

CA 19–9

CA 19–9 has been a widely used tumor marker for colorectal cancer, especially in Japan. Morita and co-workers undertook a retrospective investigation of 118 patients who underwent curative colorectal cancer surgery, analyzing and comparing CEA with CA 19–9 as indicators of prognosis for recurrent disease.[658] This study failed to demonstrate evidence to support the use of CA 19–9 to predict prognosis or to detect recurrence of colorectal cancer.

CA 242

CA 242 is a mucin tumor marker of interest in colorectal cancer. In a prospective study comparing it with CEA, Engarås found that CEA is preferred for postoperative surveillance.[250]

Messenger RNA of a Tumor-Specific Antigen (L6)

Schiedeck and colleagues compared CEA levels with the detection of messenger RNA (mRNA) coding for the tumor-associated antigen L6 in patients with colorectal cancer.[825] These investigators concluded that L6 is more sensitive and precise than CEA in diagnosing and monitoring colorectal cancer.

Acute-Phase Response

It has been postulated that measurement of acute-phase proteins in serum may serve as a useful marker for tumor recurrence. McMillan and co-workers examined this phenomenon in 36 patients with colorectal cancer who had undergone an apparently curative resection.[615] The authors found a significantly higher recurrence rate in individuals with an acute-phase response (11 of 15) than in those with no such response (two of 21). The place of this particular study in the postoperative assessment of persons who have undergone resection for colorectal cancer needs further exploration.

Radiolabeled Imaging

The advent of monoclonal antibody technology has permitted the development of radiolabeled tumor reactive probes, which can be used in conjunction with gamma camera imaging equipment to identify the presence of a malignancy within a patient.[650] Some studies have been published concerning the value of radioimmunolocalization with radiolabeled antibody to CEA in individuals with no physical signs of local recurrence but with elevated CEA levels.[67] Generally, these tests can distinguish between localized and disseminated disease and often are more accurate than conventional radiologic studies, including CT. For example, an antibody fragment (Fab') specific to CEA and labeled with ^{99m}Tc (CEA-Scan, Arcitumomab, Immunomedics, Morris Plains, NJ) is a nuclear imaging test for clinical use. Although this nuclear medicine study depends on the presence of the same antigen as the serum CEA test, it is apparently more sensitive than the serum evaluation.

Other monoclonal antibodies have been developed.[919] One such agent, monoclonal antibody B72.3 (Oncoscint CR/OV, Cytogen Corp., Princeton, NJ), has been the focus of study because of its pattern of extensive reactivity with a wide variety of mucin-producing adenocarcinomas. Because of its well-documented selectivity in binding to such tumors, it has been a useful target for patients with colorectal carcinoma. Monoclonal antibody B72.3 is a murine monoclonal antibody of the immunoglobulin G1 subclass that detects a glycoprotein, TAG-72, associated with high-molecular-weight tumors. This glycoprotein is expressed on certain human colon and breast carcinoma cell lines. To serve as a useful diagnostic agent, however, it must be coupled or conjugated to a radionuclide for imaging purposes. We have reported the use of this monoclonal antibody conjugate, termed CYT-103, labeled with ^{111}In for diagnostic imaging of colorectal carcinoma in 103 patients.[174] Enrollment was restricted to cases in which standard diagnostic modalities did not provide sufficient information for patient management decisions. Forty-nine of these individuals had rising CEA levels with no evidence of a site for recurrence. The antibody imaging study detected occult (inapparent) disease in 70%, a finding responsible for altering or canceling the planned procedure (Figure 22-99). A total of 83% of the patients was found to have benefited from the study. Others have demonstrated that mono-

clonal antibody labeled with ^{111}In is safe and can be helpful in the detection of extrahepatic abdominal and pelvic tumors.[221,226,584,728,734,1031] Because this is a physiologic study, it has proved to be more sensitive than CT in the detection of disease in the pelvis and extrahepatic abdomen.[588] Confusion with radiation changes or postoperative scarring may be resolved in many instances through the use of radioimaging techniques.

Numerous factors influence the success of imaging, including the experience of the individual interpreting the scan as well as the level of tissue antigen expression.[935] Problems may arise with certain studies, such as the use of monoclonal antibody B72.3, in that murine antibodies may produce human antimouse antibody (HAMA) response, which can lead to allergic reactions and difficulty in interpreting findings of subsequent studies, including CEA determination. Of course, there is the concern for false-positive and false-negative imaging.

Comment

Radiolabeled imaging techniques that have been applied to the follow-up management of patients who have undergone resection for colorectal cancer certainly have added much to our knowledge of the pathologic processes. Questions remain, however, as to the sensitivity

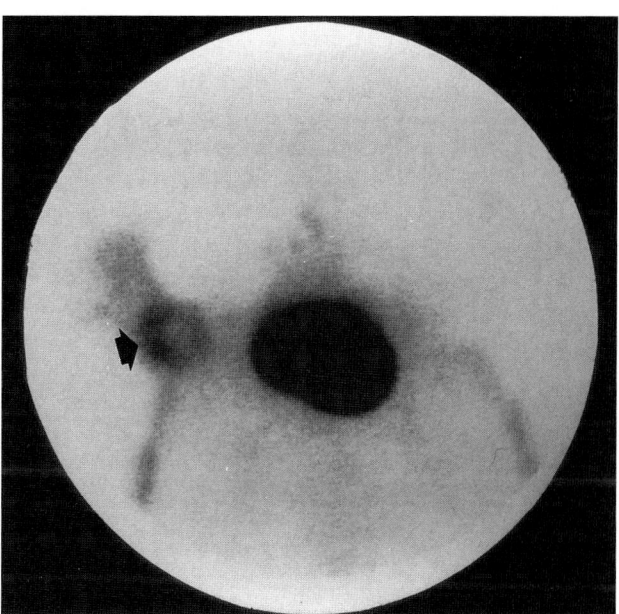

FIGURE 22-99. Oncoscint scan demonstrating uptake in the right hip, which on subsequent biopsy proved to be metastatic adenocarcinoma consistent with a colon primary tumor *(arrow)*. The patient had been asymptomatic. Results of all other studies were negative, except for a rising carcinoembryonic antigen value.

and whether there is a tangible survival benefit. For the present, I believe these modalities are of value in only two scenarios—that of an individual who will be submitted to reexploration for a presumed isolated recurrence and that of someone with a rising CEA in whom other evaluations fail to identify the site of recurrence. Before embarking on a second-look procedure (see later), I believe that radiolabeled imaging should be considered. In some instances, the tumor will be localized, and in others, one may be able to identify cancer beyond the limits of surgical cure. In both instances, the operative procedure would be changed. As the technology improves, it is hoped that the sensitivity and specificity will be high enough so that the surgeon can make an appropriate recommendation to the patient concerning the advisability of reexploration.

Other Markers

Other markers that have been employed in an attempt to increase the sensitivity of monitoring for tumor recurrence include serum protein hexose, transferrin, and ceruloplasmin.[332] More work must be done, however, before the true value of all these newer techniques can be accurately assessed.

Positron Emission Tomography

Initially developed for brain evaluation in the 1970s and unlike conventional nuclear medicine technology, positron emission tomography (PET) uses unique radiopharmaceuticals or "tracers" labeled with isotopes that are the basic elements of biologic substrates. These isotopes mimic natural substrates such as sugars, water, proteins, and oxygen. The technique uses CT imaging equipment and rings of detectors surrounding the patient to record gamma radiation produced when positrons (positively charged particles) emitted by the tracer collide with electrons. As a result, PET will often reveal more about the cellular-level metabolic status of a disease than other types of imaging modalities. Furthermore, PET images can be acquired quantitatively to reflect the actual amounts of tracer in the regions of interest. Therefore, recurrent disease may be diagnosed before structural changes become detectable by anatomic imaging techniques, such as CT.

As with radiolabeled imaging, PET may be helpful for localizing tumor recurrence following resection of colorectal cancer. Beets and colleagues performed a prospective study to evaluate the clinical impact of this whole-body imaging technique utilizing fluoride-18fluorodeoxyglucose.[66] The investigators found that whole-body PET affected management in 14 of their 35 patients who were studied. Johnson and co-workers correlated CT and PET scan with operative findings in 41 patients with metastatic colorectal cancer.[458] PET scanning was found to be more sensitive for the liver, for the extrahepatic region, and within the abdomen, but results were comparable in the pelvis.

The main disadvantages of PET are the cost and the limited availability. As with radiolabeled imaging, the indications for the use of this modality are limited: an equivocal evaluation or a presumed isolated recurrence. PET may be of particular usefulness in the evaluation of the resectability of a presacral mass of equivocal nature on CT or MRI.[66]

Second-Look Operation (Reexploration of the Abdomen)

When recurrence of tumor is discovered, surgical resection offers the best possible chance for cure in those patients who have localized disease. Wangensteen first proposed the second-look procedure in the management of colorectal cancer in 1949 in an attempt to increase the cure rate for patients with nodal disease at the time of resection.[990] Patients were subjected to an exploratory laparotomy 6 months to 1 year after operation. Obviously, this meant that some patients underwent exploration who had no evidence of recurrent disease underwent exploration. Only 15% of Wangensteen's patients actually had recurrence at the time of exploratory laparotomy. For this reason, the second-look concept was abandoned until the advent of the CEA determination. Since the mid-1950s, we have sought less invasive and more sensitive ways of detecting early recurrence.

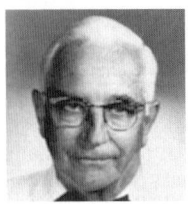

Owen H. Wangensteen (1899–1981) Owen Wangensteen was born on a farm in Lake Park, Minnesota and received all his degrees (A.B., M.B., M.D., and Ph.D.) from the University of Minnesota. In addition, he pursued virtually his entire surgical training there and became Chairman of the Department of Surgery, a post he held for 37 years. His surgical "progeny" included more than 60 professors of surgery or heads of departments. Wangensteen was a great believer in the importance of the laboratory in the training of surgeons. He stated, "The laboratory trains the surgeon's hand while it schools him in the disciplines of observation, thinking and reasoning." Among his many recognitions were the American Medical Association's Distinguished Service Award, the American Cancer Society's Award, and the Samuel D. Gross Award of the Philadelphia Academy of Surgery. His many writings and books cover the spectrum of surgery, including gastric freezing, open heart surgery, the "conservative" management of bowel obstruction, and the "second-look" operation. He was made an honorary fellow of the Royal College of Surgeons of Edinburgh, and served as president of the American Surgical Association and president of the American College of Surgeons.

Minton and associates reoperated 36 patients on the basis of progressive elevation of the CEA determination and found recurrent tumor in 30 of them.[637] The last 11 patients were able to have the tumor removed. They attributed their later improved results to a decrease in the time delay between identification of an appreciable rise in CEA and reoperation. They recommended serial CEA determination every 2 months, but whether these patients have been cured is another matter. Many studies fail to report 5-year follow-up evaluations after reresection.

Steele and associates reported on 75 patients with Dukes' B and C lesions followed for a median of 24 months.[892] Of 15 individuals found to have a tumor at a second-look operation (based on successive increased elevations of the CEA value), four underwent resection. Tong and colleagues performed a laparotomy on 64 patients with known recurrent disease.[950] Seventeen percent underwent attempted curative resection; "prolonged" survival was achieved in three. Some reports suggest that second-look surgical procedures appear to be beneficial in selected patients.[212,989]

Gamma-Guided Surgery; Radioimmunoguided Surgery

It is axiomatic that accurate assessment of the extent and location of tumor within the abdomen is necessary if one is to perform a truly useful exercise by reoperation. Standard methods of visual examination and palpation at the time of surgery are, of course, supplemented by the information gleaned through the preoperative methods previously discussed. It has been suggested that radioimmunolocalization using labeled monoclonal an-

tibodies potentially may complement the traditional approaches.[29,31,165,199,411,499,590,594,686,822,899,947]

Technique

One of the monoclonal antibody tumor markers previously discussed, such as anti-CEA labeled with ^{111}In (^{111}In-MoAb), is injected preoperatively. At the time of laparotomy, a hand-held gamma-detecting probe is used to locate foci of malignancy (e.g., Neoprobe Corp., Dublin, OH) (Figure 22-100). Depending on the location of the tumor or tumors, an *en bloc* excision or "tumorectomy" is performed. If one is dealing with lymph nodes that are producing the uptake seen on the imager, the operation may become little more than "cherry picking."

Results

The results of studies with the various gamma-guided alternatives are still preliminary. Whether there will truly be long-term benefits, represented by a decreased incidence of recurrence and a higher cure rate, remains to be determined with longer follow-up. Martin and colleagues used labeled monoclonal antibody B72.3 in 66 individuals with tissue-proven tumor.[594] Positive probe counts were detected in 83% with primary colon cancer and in 79% with recurrent tumor. The technique failed to identify known tumor in 20%. The authors suggest that improvements in specificity and sensitivity will depend on the availability of higher-affinity, newer-generation antibodies, alternate routes of antibody administration, other radionuclides, and more sophisticated, bioengineered antibodies and antibody combinations.[594]

Using the same antibody, Cohen and co-workers noted an overall sensitivity of 77% and a predictive value of a positive detection of 78%.[165] They concluded that the an-

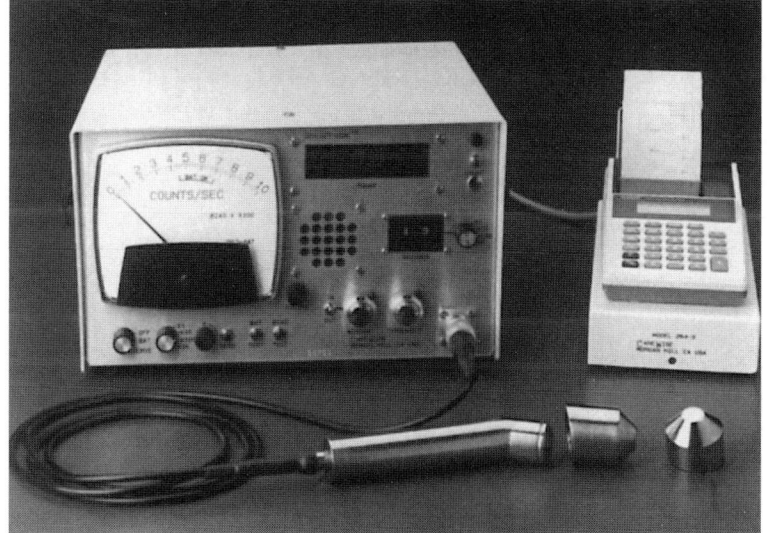

FIGURE 22-100. A C-Trak system with probe for gamma detection of recurrent tumor at the time of laparotomy. (Courtesy of Care Wise Medical Products Corp., Morgan Hill, CA)

tibody study provided unique data that contraindicated resection in ten individuals (9.6%), and in another eight (7.7%) it extended the potentially curative procedure. Others have also found that the gamma-guided system is more dependable in localizing clinically inapparent metastases than are other methods.[822] It is stated by the advocates of this technique that RIGS system has the advantage of providing immediate staging information that may affect therapeutic decision making and upstaging of tumors, even in the initial management of a primary colorectal cancer.[30,581]

Lunniss and associates used RIGS in 40 patients with recurrent colorectal cancer and noted that 25% were "benefited."[550] For the majority of their patients, however, accurate detection of recurrent disease was not associated with the possibility of cure. The authors believed that there is a need for a prospective, randomized trial to confirm the utility of this technique.

In the opinion of all investigators, RIGS is of particular value in the accurate selection of patients with disease deemed potentially resectable at second-look surgery for recurrent colorectal cancer.[29,199,411,481,499,590,686] It has also been successfully applied to patients with recurrent tumor or suspected recurrent tumor who have negative results on intraabdominal exploration and by all other radiographic criteria for identification of "micrometastases."[215] Finally, in patients who are to be submitted to exploration and resection of liver metastases, the use of the RIGS system may be a valuable adjunct for the detection of periportal lymph node metastases.[830]

Opinion

The problem that I have with RIGS is that therapeutic efforts to remove lymph nodes by identification through radiolocalization are not consistent with the concepts of cancer operative technique. In other words, "cherry picking" lymph nodes adds nothing to the survival benefit for an individual with metastatic disease at that focus. This has been discussed previously with respect to apical nodes in the resected specimen. Still, there is value in the technique, particularly with respect to upstaging. The pathologist can identify tumor only within the specimens submitted for examination. The surgeon, conversely, may be able to identify tumor beyond the reach of surgical excision. This obviously would have an influence on subsequent management decisions (e.g., adjuvant therapy). One must weigh the theoretical benefit of changing the classification of the patient's tumor against the additional cost, in terms of both equipment and increased operative time.

The philosophical issue of the relative merits of an aggressive follow-up regimen must focus on the unanswerable question, "How much is a human life worth?" A pragmatic, if rhetorical question in response would be, "How much *good medicine* can one afford?" I do not pretend to know the answer to either of these questions. Ob-

viously, cost effectiveness is inversely correlated with the frequency of screening. As mentioned previously, Moertel and colleagues opined that CEA assay could not be justified in colorectal cancer follow-up.[645] Their rationalization was that the cost of evaluation (including other studies when the CEA was elevated) turned out to be $1,415 per patient, wherease the cost per patient saved was $62,500 and change. Frankly, I think that is cheap, but we can be even more perspicacious in our testing, and, therefore, we can reduce costs even further.

One can calculate approximately how much it costs to perform annual occult blood determinations to save one life—the Minnesota Group computed it to be $24,660. The same is true for sigmoidoscopy and colonoscopy. Annual sigmoidoscopy starting at age 60 costs about $4,800 per life-year saved (1998 dollars). In a Norwegian follow-up program involving CEA, ultrasound, chest radiography, and colonoscopy, the cost of the program was $3,200 per patient, and the cost per life saved was $26,720.[694] For many years, no one seemed to question the value and cost of annual Papanicolaou testing for cervical cancer; in 1999, Brown and Garber determined that the cost per life saved was $166,000.[108]

It is useful to put the costs of screening for colorectal cancer in proper perspective. To do so requires that one examine the costs and the benefits of other governmental screening and safety programs. There is little question about the value of a mass media antismoking campaign for adolescents. The cost per student exposed has been determined to be $41, the cost per student smoker averted is $754, the cost per life saved is $969, and the cost per year of cigarettes at one pack per day is $1,460 (1997 dollars).[841] One is able to compute the cost per life saved with the use of motorcycle helmets, automobile shoulder harnesses, and air bags. Driver's-side air bags cost $24,000 per life saved, and passenger-side air bags cost $61,000 per life saved (1997 dollars).[330,508] The cost of head injury avoided with the use of bicycle helmets has been determined to be $144,500, and the cost per life saved in primary school children is $100,000, secondary school children, $750,000, and adults, $900,000 (1995 dollars).[378,393] Would anyone not advocate bicycle helmets for children? And what of the cost per human life saved of earthquake retrofitting—who knows?

Some suggest that potentially curative recurrences are detected primarily by liver imaging and colonoscopy.[85] The inference is the yields of CEA measurements, chest radiography, and physical examination are so low that they should not be part of a routine program. Clearly there must be some rationale or an algorithm that one must apply to a follow-up protocol for individuals who underwent curative colorectal cancer surgery. I have already addressed the issue of the metachronous lesion and the requirement for all patients to undergo follow-up on that basis alone. However, there is no point in pursuing further investigations if the physician will do nothing in response to an abnormal test. Therefore, it is only a patient in whom one would perform additional surgery or adjuvant treatment that testing should be performed.

The following regimen is suggested:

■ For Dukes' A (Stage I) tumors, no testing for recurrent disease is necessary.
■ For Dukes' B and C (Stage II and III) tumors, CEA determination should be done every 3 months for 2 years. If the test is elevated, repeat the CEA study; if it is still elevated, complete the full workup, including chest x-ray, colonoscopy, CT scan, PET scan (or antibody scan). If localized (resectable) disease is identified, one should perform a complete medical and preoperative workup and attempt surgical extirpation, having available intraoperative ultrasound for the liver and consider the application of RIGS.

The burden of proof that there is no recurrence once the CEA level remains persistently elevated must rest with the surgeon. Some studies have demonstrated prolonged survival after reresection with and without objective preoperative evidence of localized or definitive disease.[593,881] However, there appears to be a relative consistency with respect to the salvage rates in those who are identified as having recurrent disease, and that is about 2%.[246,715,794,810,954] Most cures are in patients with isolated liver metastases. In a study from Sweden in which patients who underwent curative resection for colorectal cancer were randomized either to no follow-up or *intense* follow-up, one third developed recurrent disease in each group.[704] Three patients in the "no-follow-up group" were submitted to reresection, but none was cured. Conversely, five individuals in the "intense follow-up group" underwent reresection, and two were cured. Despite the small numbers, these differences were statistically significant.[704] Even more impressive results were described in a study from the University of Parma, Italy.[737] In a randomized trial involving 207 patients who were submitted to either conventional or intensive follow-up, curative reresection was possible in only 10% of those conventionally followed, but was 65% in those who underwent intensive follow-up. The survival rates were 2.5% and 12.2%, respectively (p = .0004). Whether the morbidity, mortality, and cost of a second-look procedure are justified remains unanswered.[693]

TREATMENT OF RECURRENCE

Anastomotic Recurrence

Anastomotic recurrence following resection for colon carcinoma is much less commonly seen than after resection for rectal cancer. It is usually much more feasible to per-

form an adequate, wide excision of the cancer-bearing segment than when limitations are imposed by the confines of the pelvis. Symptoms of recurrence include abdominal pain, anorexia, nausea, vomiting, weight loss, change in bowel habits, and rectal bleeding. If a tumor is identified in the bowel, an aggressive surgical attitude should be adopted because the so-called recurrence may, in reality, be a missed synchronous lesion. Excluding this possibility, in contrast to recurrence following rectal resection, in which an inadequate lateral or distal margin is often the precipitating factor, anastomotic recurrence that develops after a more proximal bowel resection is usually a result of initial retroperitoneal fixation by that tumor. In one series, the median survival following "curative" reresection was 23 months.[909] A few patients are actually cured, but this is quite unusual.[826,906,990] However, surgical alternatives, such as reresection, bypass, and diversion, are recommended for palliation whenever possible.

The specific problems of anastomotic recurrence and local recurrence following rectal excision are discussed in Chapter 23.

Pulmonary Metastases

Solitary lung metastases from colorectal cancer have been resected for cure more often than metastases to all other sites combined.[802] Cahan and co-workers reported that in a patient with a history of colorectal carcinoma, a solitary lung lesion will be metastatic from that primary one half of the time.[131] It still should be remembered, however, that primary lung cancer is the most common visceral malignancy when both sexes are combined. An isolated pulmonary metastasis should not contraindicate radical surgical removal of the bowel tumor. In fact, the chance of a cure is better for resection of a solitary lung lesion that has metastasized from a primary colon carcinoma than when the lesion is a primary bronchogenic carcinoma.

Bronchoscopy, mediastinoscopy, and sputum cytology are useful in identifying the histologic nature of the neoplasm. Lung tomograms are essential to rule out the presence of additional nodules.

In the experience of McCormack and Attiyeh, the 5-year survival rate following excision was 22% and was significantly improved when the primary colonic cancer was a Dukes' A or B lesion.[607] Wilking and colleagues reported a 14% 5-year survival for patients with solitary lesions.[1013] Brister and associates found a 5-year survival of 21%.[104] McCormack and colleagues found that the overall 5- and 10-year survival rates in 144 patients who underwent resection for pulmonary metastases at the Memorial Sloan-Kettering Cancer Center were 40% and 30%, respectively.[608] Watanabe and co-workers noted a 5-year survival rate of 56% in their 49 patients.[994] Pihl and co-workers noted that lung recurrence is significantly more common after potentially curative resection of rectal than of colonic carcinoma.[738] Scheele and associates, however, noted no difference between colon and rectal primaries in this respect.[824] Several studies have found that the only factor that appears to be significant is the disease-free interval—the longer the interval, the better the survival rate.[104,433,858]

Yano and colleagues investigated whether *multiple pulmonary metastases* from colorectal cancer preclude surgical resection.[1050] The rate of disease-free survival at 5 years was 62% for solitary lesions, 35% for two metastases, and 0% for four or more. Additionally, the incidence of local recurrence at the primary site increased with the number of lesions identified in the lung. The authors concluded that one should search for the presence of a local recurrence at the primary site when multiple pulmonary metastases are identified.[1050]

Comment

I believe a vigorous approach to the surgical treatment of solitary pulmonary metastases when there are no signs of other metastatic lesions is appropriate. Wedge resection, preserving as much lung tissue as possible, is usually performed, although resection of the lobe is sometimes necessary to remove the lesion completely.

Ovarian Metastases

The ovary may be the only site of macroscopic spread of disease; it is the site of metastases in 3% to 5% of patients. Bilateral oophorectomy has been recommended on a prophylactic basis in all postmenopausal women who have colorectal cancer because of the risk for harboring a metastatic focus as well as for the prevention of primary ovarian carcinoma (see earlier discussion). There is no question as to the advisability of therapeutic oophorectomy when macroscopic tumor is evident in the adnexa. The likelihood of cure in such circumstances, however, is virtually nil.

Liver Metastases

As has been discussed earlier, the overall mean survival of patients with untreated metastatic colorectal cancer to the liver is approximately 16 months.[721] However, with contemporary adjuvant therapy protocols (see later), this may be too low a figure. Stangl and colleagues prospectively analyzed 566 patients with unresectable hepatic metastases from colorectal cancer who received no treatment.[887] They were able to identify six independent determinants of survival in the following order: percentage of liver volume replaced by tumor, grade of malignancy of the primary tumor, presence of extrahepatic disease, mesenteric lymph node involvement, serum CEA deter-

mination, and age. They believed able to provide a prognostic tree that displayed median survival times for a number of subgroups of these variables.[887]

The poor prognosis has stimulated a number of approaches that have yielded successful results, including neoadjuvant chemotherapy before resection.[10,37,125,127, 277,278,428,440,494,541,729,755,923] Fortner and associates estimated that 15% to 25% of individuals with metastatic disease are candidates for these procedures.[276] Before embarking on such an effort, however, it is imperative to determine the extent of disease and the surgical anatomy. This can be accomplished by several preoperative and intraoperative methods. Radiolabeled imaging, CT, and the gamma-guided approach have already been discussed. It has been estimated that standard CT will detect approximately two thirds of all tumors (12% of lesions smaller than 1 cm).[985] The characterization of liver metastases by CT is the single most important independent prognostic factor in patients undergoing curative hepatic resection.[669]

Computed Tomography with Arterial Portography

Although CT is important in the preliminary assessment of an individual who is being evaluated for a rising CEA, particularly with respect to identification of liver metastases, it is not as sensitive as one would wish. It is now well established that CT undertaken during arterial portography (CTAP) is the most sensitive preoperative imaging technique for the detection of hepatic metastases from colorectal cancer.[877] Knowledge of the extent of the metastases is important not only in intraoperative decision making, but also in determining which patients are not candidates for a resective approach. Karl and colleagues compared CTAP with conventional CT in 109 consecutive patients who had evidence of hepatic tumors.[467] They, too, observed that CTAP is the most sensitive test for assessing the distribution of intrahepatic disease. Soyer and associates undertook a prospective study to compare the sensitivities of intraoperative ultrasonography (see later) and CTAP.[877] Fifty-one of the 56 metastases were preoperatively identified by means of CTAP (91%), whereas intraoperative ultrasonography identified 54 of the 56 metastases (96%). It is clear, therefore, that the two studies are complementary. Vogel and coworkers attempted to predict the surgical resectability of hepatic colorectal metastases by comparing conventional CT, CTAP, and hepatic artery perfusion scintigraphy.[985] As previously mentioned, 64% of all lesions greater than 1 cm were identified by standard CT. These investigators found that of the 40 patients who had resection for possible cure, CTAP and hepatic artery scintigraphy falsely predicted *unresectability* in 15% and 25% of patients, respectively. The positive predictive value for unresectability of the two studies was 73% and 60%, respectively. The authors concluded that false-positive results by the two evaluations may limit the ability to predict accurately unresectibility before surgery and may actually deny patients the chance for surgical resection and cure.[985]

Matsui and colleagues compared the total detection rate (sensitivity) of liver metastases with a number of modalities and discovered the following: ultrasonography (58% success), CT (63%), selective celiac arteriography (27%), infusion hepatic angiography (50%), and CTAP (84%).[598] Others have also found that CTAP is the most accurate technique for identifying hepatic neoplasms and suggest that it be employed preoperatively for all individuals who are being considered for liver resection.[397,1048]

Hepatic Angiography

Liver angiography has been believed to be a useful guide in the preoperative assessment of known hepatic metastatic tumor as well as in the evaluation of vascular anatomy, particularly if a major hepatic resection is contemplated. Lundstedt and co-workers, however, showed that based on the findings at laparotomy, angiography adequately demonstrated tumor growth in the right lobe of the liver but repeatedly failed to do so in the left.[549] CT was believed to be more accurate.

The primary roles of angiography are in the accurate assessment of the sources of blood supply to the liver and of vascular anomalies and as a method of visualizing the conduit for intraarterial chemotherapy.

Hepatic Resection

The precise steps in the performance of the various hepatic resection maneuvers are not within the purview of this text. Options include right hepatic lobectomy, right trisegmentectomy, left hepatectomy, left lateral segmentectomy, wedge resection, extended left hepatectomy (left trisegmentectomy), and segmental resections.

Results

Many studies confirm that hepatic resection for colorectal metastatic disease can be undertaken in a number of individuals for cure.[340,400,427,636,770,913] The Mayo Clinic group was among the early advocates of resection and reported 60 patients with hepatic metastases from colorectal cancer.[9,1020] Two thirds of the lesions were solitary. The results were "unexpectedly favorable." Forty-two percent of the individuals with apparent solitary lesions survived 5 years, although a later report revealed that the overall 5-year survival rate was 25%.[10] Contrary to the earlier observations, this later study justified removal of some multiple hepatic metastases. A later report from the Mayo Clinic, involving 280 consecutive individuals who under-

went hepatic resection for colorectal cancer metastases, revealed an overall 5-year survival of 27%.[444] Rees and associates found that 37% of their patients survived 5 years.[771] Wanebo and co-workers advise that resection of bilobar disease should generally be avoided, especially in medically compromised patients.[988] Steele and Ravikumar have concluded that major liver resection can be performed safely, with less than a 5% operative mortality, and a cure rate between 20% and 25%.[891]

An early Dukes' stage initially, absence of extrahepatic metastases, and female sex are relatively favorable prognostic findings.[10] In reports from the National Cancer Institute in Bethesda, Maryland, and from other institutions, however, the Dukes' stage of the primary lesion was not predictive of survival after resection.[37,729] Other factors reported to improve the outcome include resection margins of at least 1 cm and fewer than four metastatic nodules.[98,127,341,428,440] Rodgers and McCall note that there are few 5-year survivors after liver resection, with or without lymph node dissection, for colorectal hepatic metastases involving the hepatic lymph nodes.[787] The biologic behavior of the tumor is probably the vital criterion that determines survival, not the timing of the resection or perhaps even the vigor and frequency with which one pursues the CEA level.[37,127] Geoghegan and Scheele undertook a literature review based on a Medline search from 1970 to 1998 on the treatment of colorectal liver metastases.[294] They concluded that with the use of multimodality regimens, 5-year survival rates of patients with lesions that were even *unresectable* are being reported.

Fortner observed a median survival time of 31 months after complete removal of a *second hepatic recurrence*, considerably greater than the median of 14 months when excision was not possible.[275] Others confirm that repeat hepatic resection for isolated metastases can result in long-term survival in selected patients.[5,79,342,967]

Intraoperative Ultrasonography

The area of occult hepatic metastases has been emphasized earlier with respect to the application of intraoperative ultrasonography (see Figure 22-97).[90,141,266,327,569,758] Many centers are recommending its routine use during surgery for colorectal cancer. Charnley and colleagues found that more metastases were diagnosed by intraoperative ultrasonography than by palpation, abdominal ultrasonography, or CT.[148]

Operative ultrasonography has certain advantages that are of particular importance in hepatic surgery: (1) because no energy is lost in passage through the abdominal wall, greater resolution is possible and smaller lesions can be detected; (2) landmarks on the liver parenchyma can be easily correlated with the position of the probe; and (3) ultrasonographic guidance can facilitate biopsy as well as other hepatobiliary procedures.[141] The technique can be used to confirm the presence of tumor in the liver that was suspected on the basis of preoperative evaluation. It can prevent the surgeon from embarking on an ill-advised resection when cure is unattainable (e.g., when multiple lesions are involved). Finally, it can establish the relationship between tumor and intrahepatic vessels, thus possibly preventing vascular injury and perhaps making radical hepatic resection safer.[327]

Rifkin and colleagues evaluated 49 patients with suspected liver disease by means of intraoperative ultrasonography.[783] In 19% new information was gathered that changed the operative approach. Finlay and McArdle demonstrated unsuspected hepatic metastases in 17 of 24 patients (24%) by this technique.[266] It was their contention that the presence or absence of occult metastases predicts the majority of deaths from disseminated cancer following apparently curative resections. Other articles attest to the better accuracy of intraoperative ultrasonography in diagnosing liver metastases in comparison with other screening methods.[161,570]

Cryosurgery

Intraoperative ultrasonography has been employed not only to identify the location of hepatic metastases, but also to direct the application of treatment, specifically cryotherapy. *In situ* destruction of tumors by means of freezing has been applied to the management of skin, rectal, prostatic, gynecologic, and head and neck cancers, so it is not surprising that some centers have begun to utilize this approach in the treatment of primary and metastatic lesions of the liver.[758] The cryoprobe, which utilizes circulating liquid nitrogen and produces a spherical ball of ice around each treated metastatic site, is controlled by the imaging technique.[147] A method has also been described that utilizes cryosurgery in combination with hepatic resection, in essence excising the ice ball.[741]

Cryodestruction can accomplish a number of possibilities:

■ Treat multiple areas of involvement focally.
■ Preserve a maximal amount of normal liver tissue.
■ Destroy tumors deep in the liver parenchyma without the need for major resection.
■ Avoid large vessels or vital structures.
■ Minimize blood loss.
■ Cause lower morbidity and mortality than resection.
■ Combine with other modalities—for example, resection of one lobe and cryosurgical destruction in other areas.[708]

Ravikumar and colleagues utilized this approach in the treatment of multiple unresectable hepatic metastases from colorectal carcinoma.[758] There were no significant complications. One patient subsequently underwent repeated laparotomy and resection of the frozen lesions; there was no residual tumor. A later report from the same group involved 32 patients, 28% of whom remained disease-free after a follow-up period of 5 to 60 months.[759] Onik and co-workers treated 18 patients with unresectable tumors, 14 of whom had bilobar disease.[709] Mean survival of the 14 cases with recurrence was 21.4 months, with two individuals still living. Adam and colleagues reported their experience with 25 patients who had nonresectable metastases from colorectal cancer.[4] At a mean follow-up of 16 months, the local recurrence rate was 44%. The survival rate was 52% at that time, with 20% free of disease.

Osseous Metastases

Osseous metastases from colonic and rectal cancer are relatively uncommon, occurring in up to 9% of reported series.[112] The usual locations correspond to the areas where there is active hematopoiesis, but involvement of the phalanges has also been described.[112] In the experience of the Memorial Sloan-Kettering Cancer Center, 6.9% of patients with disseminated colorectal carcinoma had osseous metastases.[48,72] Most of these tumors had spread to bone in association with widespread metastases elsewhere. In a study from the Roswell Park Memorial Institute, 19 of 47 patients (40%) had osseous metastases only.[93] The median survival time from establishment of the diagnosis was 7 months.

Bone scanning is believed to be more sensitive for diagnosing metastases than is radiography.[93] Palliative treatment by means of radiation therapy for the bone pain is usually quite effective.

Cerebral Metastases

Metastatic carcinoma to the brain is uncommon and is usually associated with metastatic disease elsewhere, especially in the lung. Rarely will a metastatic focus be present in the brain with no other evidence of disease. Ko and colleagues found that brain metastases are more common with rectal cancer.[487] Craniotomy is indicated to remove the metastatic lesion, with the expectation that good palliation of neurologic signs and symptoms can be accomplished. Nakajima and associates reported on a patient who had removal of a metastatic lesion of the brain; at postmortem examination 2 years later no evidence of intracranial metastases was found.[672]

Occasionally, a patient will present with neurologic signs and symptoms as the initial manifestation of colorectal cancer. Subsequent gastrointestinal investigation may be stimulated by the histologic interpretation after the intracranial tumor has been removed.

Penile Metastases

Metastatic tumors to the penis are uncommon. More than 80% of them originate in the bladder, prostate, rectum, sigmoid colon, and kidney.[747] Direct invasion, retrograde venous extension, retrograde lymphatic extension, perineural spread, and arterial embolism are proposed mechanisms for the spread.[360,747]

Extent of involvement of the urethra may be determined by urethrography, but cavernosography may be able to give a more precise definition of the size and extent of the nodule or nodules.[360] Surgical excision with or without chemoradiation therapy is the primary treatment. Prognosis for long-term survival is poor.

Chemotherapy

In light of the extraordinarily rapid changes in the chemotherapeutic approaches to the management of colorectal cancer I have asked Herbert M. Dean, a board-certified hematologist and medical oncologist, Assistant Professor of Medicine at the University of Massachusetts Medical School, and Medical Director of Verax Biomedical, to provide this completely rewritten and contemporary perspective. MLC

This section reviews advances in the treatment of metastatic colorectal cancer and then discusses the current status and recommendations for adjuvant chemotherapy. Since the last edition, major advances in the treatment of colorectal cancer have occurred through the application of three chemotherapeutic agents: irinotecan, oxaliplatin, and capecitabine. In addition, promising new agents called biologic response modifiers are being used, which unlike conventional chemotherapeutic agents that act as cellular poisons and effect DNA synthesis and growth of cancer cells, have different mechanisms of action. These include interference with membrane receptors, alteration of signal pathways necessary for tumor growth, and inhibition of tumor-supported angiogenesis to promote cancer cell death (apoptosis). Two have demonstrated efficacy in phase III trials, cetuximab and bevacizumab (BV).[65,186,430,801,968]

When response to the standard chemotherapeutic agents, 5-fluorouracil (FU) or leucovorin (LV),[164,193,216,286,292,368,436,903,911,930] becomes resistant or refractory, newer agents must be considered. Such newer candidate drugs that were found to be effective in the setting of advanced or metastatic disease have been entered into phase I and II trials. Those agents that appear promising by virtue of their activity in these trials have been entered into phase III clinical studies, comparing them to the established standard FU/LV as the control arm. Studies have identified effectiveness of the drugs mentioned earlier, resulting the incorporation of these newer agents in combination with FU/LV (so-called, triplets). This has given rise to a new nomenclature—IFL, FOLFOX (FU/LV and oxaliplatin), and FOLFIRI, which have become the standard for treating patients with metastatic disease. Furthermore, these new agents in a variety of combinations are being evaluated in the adjuvant and neoadjuvant settings (with radiation) for colorectal cancers that present with advanced local stage (large tumors, those adherent to adjacent structures) in order to shrink and downstage the malignancy and, therefore, to increase the likelihood of surgical resection.[21,229,816]

Since the 1950s, intravenous FU, biomodulated with LV, has been the most effective of all the chemotherapeutic regimens employed in treating colon cancer, both in the metastatic or advanced disease setting and as adjuvant chemotherapy.[602,644] In an attempt to improve the results, the FU/LV regimen has been administered in various dose schedules, including the Mayo Clinic regimen developed by Moertel and colleagues.[745] This involves the intravenous administration of FU/LV daily for 5 days as a bolus at 425 mg/m^2 along with LV at 20 mg/m^2 for 5 days each 4-week cycle; or on a weekly schedule at doses of between 600 and 750 mg/m^2 along with LV at doses between 20 mg/m^2 (low dose) up to using 500 mg/m^2 (high dose) weekly for six cycles every 8 weeks; or as infusional FU, usually at 300 mg/m^2 per 24-hour period for several days up to 20 days depending on toxicity.[123,543,652,745] The use of intraperitoneal chemotherapy has not been shown to prolong survival and is considered investigational.[587]

Bolus FU has been more commonly used for simplicity and the avoidance of a catheter, usually a requisite in infusional FU schedules. Comparable median survival data are reported with infusional FU, although there are generally higher response rates. Different toxicities are seen with the bolus programs, including bone marrow suppression with neutropenia and thrombocytopenia, along with mucositis, nausea, vomiting, and diarrhea. The hand-foot syndrome is the main side effect seen with prolonged infusional treatment.

In stage III colon cancer, FU/LV administered as adjuvant chemotherapy (after surgery) has demonstrated improved disease-free and overall survival, but in the metastatic setting results have generally been disappointing—that is, only slight improvement in survival when compared with optimal supportive care.[511,572,652] A meta-analysis of 18 randomized studies of metastatic colon cancer, using the combination of FU/LV versus FU alone, demonstrated a doubling of the response rate from 11% to 23% with the "doublet" but no difference in the median survival (11.5 versus 11 months).[736] A small, statistically significant increase in the 1-year survival of 48% versus 43% was noted. A European study compared the

Mayo Clinic schedule with that which is commonly referred to as the de Gramont schedule.[208] This latter protocol consisted of bimonthly intravenous LV, 200 mg/m^2, as a 2-hour infusion, followed by bolus FU, 400 mg/m^2; then a 22-hour infusion of FU at 600 mg/m^2 was given for 2 consecutive days every 2 weeks until disease progression demonstrated a statistically significant improvement in response rate. The de Gramont schedule, combining infusional and bolus FU, had a response rate of 33% versus only a 14% response with the bolus arm alone. A progression-free interval of 28 versus 22 weeks was noted, but there was no significant survival benefit (62 versus 57 weeks).[208]

Irinotecan

Based on the results of a randomized, multicenter, three-arm trial, IFL, consisting of irinotecan and FU/LV (Saltz regimen), was approved as first-line treatment for metastatic colon cancer in March, 2000. Six hundred eighty-three patients were randomized to irinotecan, 125 mg/m^2 weekly for 4 weeks every 6 weeks, FU/LV administered by the Mayo schedule (control arm), or irinotecan as administered as a single agent combined with weekly FU, 500 mg/m^2 for 4 weeks every 6 weeks. The control arm (FU/LV) showed a response rate, time to progression, and overall survival of 21%, 4.2 months, and 12 months, respectively, essentially the same as that of the single agent, irinotecan. With IFL, the response rate was 39%, the time to progression was 7 months, and the overall survival was 14.4 months.[816] A European study of 387 patients compared FU/LV with IFL, employing the de Gramont schedule of FU/LV and irinotecan, either 80 mg/m^2 for 6 weeks every 7 weeks or 180 mg/m^2 day 1 every 2 weeks. This showed similar results to the Saltz study, with a response rate, time to progression, and median survival in the FU/LV arm of 23%, 4.4 months, and 14 months, respectively, with 59% alive at 1 year. The IFL arm demonstrated a 41% response rate, a time to progression of 6.7 months, and a median survival of 16.8 months, with 69% alive at 1 year.[229]

Toxicity with irinotecan includes both an acute and delayed diarrhea that can cause significant fluid loss. This is associated with an increased 60-day mortality rate, a fact that led to a manufacturer's alert and increased efforts to control the diarrhea with anticholingeric drugs during and after the administration of the agent. Close monitoring of fluids and electrolytes is a requisite.[796]

Oxaliplatin

Unlike other platinum compounds, oxaliplatin demonstrates activity in human tumor xenografts and in cisplatinum and carboplatin-resistant colon cancer cell lines.[766]

de Gramont compared FU/LV, the control arm using the de Gramont schedule, versus the addition of oxaliplatin, 85 mg/m^2, given 1 day every 2 weeks (FOLFOX). The response rate was 49% compared with 22% for the control arm. Progression-free survival was 8.9 versus 5.9 months, and median survival was 15.9 months compared with 14.7 months.[209]

An Intergroup study was undertaken that ultimately became a three-arm trial: IFL, FOLFOX, and irinotecan combined with oxaliplatin (IROX). The following were the results of that effort[313,1012] (Table 22-11).

The interpretation of the results is impacted by the crossover design that led to 60% of patients who were on the FOLFOX arm to subsequently receive irinotecan because of disease progression. However, only 24% of patients who received IFL received oxaliplatin because that agent had not yet been approved for second-line treatment in the United States. Although FOLFOX appears to be a superior regimen to IFL and IROX for first-line treatment of metastatic disease and is less toxic, except for peripheral neuropathy, differences with respect to those who received second-line treatment in the IFL arm with the crossover drug create difficulty in the interpretation of the results.

Oxaliplatin is associated with neurosensory side effects, including acute dysesthesia that occurs in up to 80% of patients, with numbness and tingling of the distal extremities. This is usually mild and brief and aggravated by cold, including chilled beverages. Oral and perioral pharangolaryngeal tingling occurs in fewer than 2% of patients, but this can be quite distressing. Chronic sensory neuropathy that is dose related can cause grade III toxicity when doses greater than 850 mg/m^2 are administered (less than 10% to 15% of patients). This generally improves over several months with discontinuance of the drug.[313,1012]

Capecitabine

FU given in various schedules often requires the placement of an indwelling, long-term, intravenous access catheter, with frequent office visits for treatment and for catheter care as well as complications related to the device.[43,157,382,756,904,1045] Oral fluropyrimidine, capecitabine (Xeloda), undergoes a three-step conversion to FU and can achieve blood levels and efficacy comparable to that obtained with infusional chemotherapy while offering greater patient convenience and a more acceptable side effect profile.[523] The main toxicity is the hand-foot syndrome, the same as seen with infusional FU. However, the frequency of this side effect has greatly diminished since the initial recommended dose of 2,500 mg/m^2 in two divided daily doses has been reduced to 2,000 mg/m^2.

A trial of combined capecitabine, 1000 mg/m^2 twice daily for 14 days, followed by 7 days off, combined with

▶ **TABLE 22-11 Results of Intergroup N9741 Trial of First-Line IFL versus FOLFOX versus IROX**

	IFL	IROX	FOLFOX
Response rates	31%	34%	45%
Medium time to progression (mo)	6.9	6.5	8.7
Overall survival (mo)	14.8	17.4	19.5
Grade III Toxicity (%)			
	IFL	IROX	FOLFOX
Neutropenia	40	36	50
Febrile neutropenia	15	11	4
Nausea	16	19	6
Vomiting	14	22	3
Diarrhea	28	24	12
Paresthesia	3	7	18

FOLFOX, 5-fluorouracil, leucovorin, and oxaliplatin; IFL, irinotecan, 5-fluorouracil, and leucovorin; IROX, irinotecan and oxaliplatin.

oxaliplatin, 130 mg/m^2, as a 2-hour infusion on day 1 at 3-week intervals, achieved in a trial of 96 patients a response rate of 45%, progression-free survival of 7.6 months, and an overall survival of 19.5 months.[969] Grade III toxicities included neutropenia in 7%, nausea and vomiting in 13%, diarrhea in 16%, and neuropathy in 16%.

Novel Agents

Since the pioneering work of Judah Folkman, which demonstrated that tumor growth requires the cancer to induce the host to provide new blood vessels (angiogenesis) by means of chemical mediators secreted by the tumor, efforts to develop antiangiogenesis agents have been sought to inhibit new blood vessel formation and tumor growth.[262,443] Tumor angiogenesis can be assessed noninvasively by measuring angiogenic cytokine concentrations in peripheral circulation and by dynamic contrast-enhanced MRI.[295] BV (Avastin) is a humanized monoclonal antibody developed against vascular endothelial growth factor.[334] A trial involving 815 patients comparing IFL/Placebo with IFL/ BV as first line therapy demonstrated in the BV arm a response rate of 45% versus a 35% response in the IFL, progression free survival of 10.6 months versus 6.3 months, and a median survival of 20.3 months versus 15.6 months.[430] Grade III hypertension was noted in 10.9% of those in the BV arm versus 2.3% in the IFL arm.

Cetuximab (Erbitux) is a chimeric monoclonal antibody to the epidermal growth factor receptor (EGFR). By attaching to the receptor on the cancer cell, this drug inhibits the binding and signal activity of epidermal growth factor and transforming growth factor-α and is synergistic with chemotherapy and radiation.[701] A trial in irinotecan-refractory, EGFR-positive patients with metastatic colorectal disease compared cetuximab alone versus cetuximab combined with irinotecan.[185] Cetuximab was given at an initial dose of 400 mg/m^2, intravenously, followed by 250 mg/m^2 weekly, and combined with irinotecan at the same dose the patient was on while the disease had progressed. A partial response was seen in 11% on cetuximab alone, and 23% in the combined arm. Time to progression was noted to be 1.5 and 4.1 months, respectively, and overall survival was 6.9 versus 9.4 months.

Epidemiologic studies have suggested that aspirin and cyclooxygenase-2 (COX-2) inhibitors reduce the risk of polyps, colon cancer, and mortality, and COX-2 inhibitors and aspirin have demonstrated activity in reducing polyp formation in patients with familial adenomatous polyps.[337,910] A study of 47,900 male health care professionals showed that those taking at least two aspirin tablets per week over 20 years reduced their risk of cancer by 50%.[306]

COX-2 expression demonstrated by immunochemistry has been shown to be present in colorectal carcinomas, with greater staining noted in larger tumors and in those with advanced stage (e.g., nodal involvement).[854] This observation supports a possible therapeutic role for COX-2 inhibitors. Trials are currently underway that incorporate COX-2 inhibitors and the previously described agents as well as combinations in both the metastatic and adjuvant settings.[654,840]

Further attempts to improve the results with chemotherapy and biologic response modifiers have led to additional trials using various combinations of agents. These include sequencing the two major combinations, FOLFOX and irinotecan, FU/LV (FOLFIRI, Saltz), and additional trials that combine cetuximab, BV, and COX-2 inhibitors with the various doublets and triplets as well as capecitabine.[20,334,953,962,969] Other agents in clinical testing include premetrexed, gefinitib (Iressa), bortezomib (Velcade), erlotinib (Tarceva), panitumumab (ABX-EGF), and tezacitabine.

Adjuvant Chemotherapy

The TNM classification system for colon cancer has replaced the Dukes' classification and its modification, Astler-Coller, for oncologists, especially. Published series have reported a range of survival in Dukes' C patients from 35% to 50%, and in Dukes' B, 60% to 80%. Dukes' classification fails to distinguish the differences in prognosis and risk for metastatic disease stratified according to the number of involved nodes, nor does it take into account the size of the primary tumor. The TNM classification improves one's ability to predict the course and survival more accurately, because it stratifies stage by tumor penetration and size as well as the number of involved nodes.

The latest revision of the sixth edition of the American Joint Committee on Cancer's staging manual includes several modifications. Stage II is now subdivided into IIA if the primary tumor is T3 and into IIB for T4 lesions. Stage III is split into IIIA for T1, T2, N_1, M_0 tumors, IIIB for T3, T4, N1, M0 lesions, and IIIC for any T, N2, M0. The surgeon is asked to define the completeness of his resection as follows: RO for complete resection and negative margins, R1 for incomplete resection because of a positive microscopic margin, or R2 with nonresected gross residual tumor.[339]

Adjuvant chemotherapy has been shown to be effective in 929 stage III colon cancer patients who had undergone curative surgery by a randomized trial with levamisole alone, levamisole plus FU, or observation alone. The treatment was continued for 1 year with the levamisole given every 2 weeks or for 48 weeks on the combined arm. At a median follow-up of 6.5 years, the combination of FU/levamisole reduced the recurrence rate by greater than 40% and the death rate by 33% compared with observation alone.[643,646,647,699] No survival benefit was seen in stage II patients using this adjuvant chemotherapy.

The International Multicenter Pooled Analysis of stage II cancers (Astler-Coller B2), comprising more than 1,000 patients randomized to FU/levamisole or observation alone, demonstrated event-free survival of 76% in the treated arm versus 73% in the observation alone arm.[647] Certain lesions, including T4 tumors or obstructing tumors now classified as stage IIB, III, or IV lesions, and evidence of lymphovascular invasion, are believed to warrant adjuvant chemotherapy.

Another trial evaluated FU/LV versus FU/levamisole. This showed that the FU/LV arm given on the Mayo Clinic schedule was as effective as FU/levamisole, and that 12 months of treatment offered no significant advantage over 6 months of treatment. A 6-month regimen of FU has become the standard adjuvant program for stage III colorectal cancers against which the new doublet and triplet combinations are being evaluated.[652,698,699]

Radiation treatment, preoperatively or after surgery, should be considered along with chemotherapy for lesions adherent to adjacent structures, in those with perforation, and especially in T3 and T4 lesions of the rectum and lower sigmoid (see Chapter 23).[635,936]

Several adjuvant trials for colorectal cancer incorporating the newer agents have commenced. The Mosaic trial, an international adjuvant study of 2,248 patients, 40% stage II and 60% stage III, were randomized to the de Gramont schedule of FU/LV versus FOLFOX. At 3 years, FOLFOX showed an overall risk reduction, 23% com-

pared with FU/LV, 24% in stage III, and 18% in stage II.[207] Ongoing studies by various collaborative groups employing the newer chemotherapeutic combinations in the adjuvant setting, together with one of the novel agents that interfere with receptor sites, signal pathways, and angiogenesis, are in clinical trials.

Summary and Conclusions

Chemotherapy in both the metastatic setting and as adjuvant treatment has shown modest improvement in response rates, time to progression, and overall survival with FU/LV. The addition of either irinotecan or oxaliplatin and the ability to administer an oral fluropyrimidine, capecitabine, that achieves infusional concentrations of the drug, thereby providing a more convenient outpatient program for patients, have led to at least a 50% increase in response rates, time to progression, and improvement in overall survival. Oxaliplatin combinations (FOLFOX) may have a better side effect profile than IFL, except for that of temporary and mild acute and cumulative sensory neuropathy. This concern generally is reversible with discontinuance of the drug in the long-term setting. Several newer agents with different mechanisms of action are being employed, together with the foregoing agents, for their potentially enhanced effectiveness in the treatment of colorectal cancer.

Author's Comment

It is self-evident that despite the high rate of resectability and the improvement in the surgical management of patients with colorectal cancer, almost one half die of recurrent disease. Colorectal cancer has proved extremely resistant to chemotherapeutic agents, and chemotherapy has been completely ineffectual in the treatment of peritoneal seeding.[106]

In addition to long-term survival or even cure, tumor response, defined as clinical or radiologic tumor shrinkage, is the primary objective of chemotherapy. Allen-Mersh and colleagues assessed whether a fall in the serum CEA concentration after chemotherapy is a predictor of prolonged survival, and compared it with "tumor response."[16] They observed that monitoring the serum CEA, especially during the first 2 months of treatment, appears to provide a sensitive and economical means for identifying those individuals whose survival is likely to be prolonged by the treatment.[16] Others have shown that FU-based adjuvant chemotherapy benefited patients with stage II or stage III colon cancers with microsatellite-stable tumors or tumors exhibiting low-frequency microsatellite instability, but not those with tumors exhibiting high-frequency microsatellite instability.[780]

One must remember that chemotherapy is not innocuous. The potential complications are myriad, a partial list of which includes bone marrow depression, alopecia, sepsis, renal and hepatic toxicity, gastrointestinal hemorrhage, mutagenesis, typhlitis, and bowel wall necrosis.[473] Obviously, the toxicity and expense of chemotherapy must be weighed against the potential benefits. Drug resistance is the principal reason why chemotherapy often fails. However, as one may appreciate from Dean's contribution, patients today no longer have limited treatment options. Furthermore, one even has the possibility of identifying drug resistance through an *in vitro* test, the tumor stem cell assay (clonogenic chemosensitivity test—Oncotech, Tustin, California—*www.oncotech.com*).[814,844] Although surgery has been and continues to be the mainstay in the treatment of colorectal cancer, it is exciting to contemplate the day when this cancer and all cancers may be either prevented or completely eliminated without the need for operation.

Hepatic Artery Infusion, Ligation, Dearterialization; Portal Vein Infusion

Hepatic artery infusion is sometimes recommended for the treatment of metastatic disease to the liver that is unresectable. In the opinion of some authors, it produces higher regression rates and slightly longer remissions than other techniques.[129,474] However, these advantages are at the cost of increased morbidity, time in the hospital, and technical difficulties, which may make this route less than desirable. Because of the risk for inducing chemical cholecystitis by this approach, some authors recommend elective cholecystectomy at the time of the placement of the arterial catheter.[713]

Usually, hepatic artery infusion is applied to those individuals who have failed to show improvement with more conventional systemic techniques. Miyanari and colleagues assessed the value of hepatic arterial infusion chemotherapy, noting that it was possible to perform resection of metastatic liver disease in those who responded.[642] The survival rate for all patients was about two thirds after 1 year and 10% after 5 years. Of the 25% who responded (16 of 64 patients), however, 35.1% were alive after 5 years.

Hepatic artery ligation and hepatic dearterialization also have been employed, but similarly have not been shown to produce worthwhile benefit either in terms of palliation or survival.[930] Portal vein infusion with has also been performed, with mixed results.[54] Allen-Mersh and colleagues employed continuous hepatic artery infusion with floxuridine in a randomized study of 100 patients, who were compared with patients receiving conventional pallia-

tion only.[15] A significant prolongation of survival was noted in the former group, as well as a qualitative and quantitative improvement in a host of other variables.

Immunotherapy

Chemotherapeutic agents, especially FU, have been used in combination with other modalities of treatment, such as surgery, radiation, and immunotherapy. The value of chemoimmunotherapy has been studied, and in reports from the M.D. Anderson Hospital and the Southwest Oncology Group, FU plus bacille Calmette-Guérin (BCG) has been shown to produce a longer disease-free period with increased survival in some patients.[42,358] These studies have not yet been confirmed by randomized, controlled trials from other institutions.

Immunotherapy with BCG is most effective when the tumor mass is reduced to a minimum, when it is administered directly into or close to the tumor, when the patient is able to respond to BCG, and when a large enough dose is given. Routes of administration include direct insertion into the tumor; administration may also be intradermal (by skin scarification), intracavitary, or oral.[404,566]

Although the number of patients with reported colorectal cancer for whom BCG immunotherapy has been used is still small, this regimen has occasionally produced increased survival, most striking in those individuals with liver metastases. Mavligit and co-workers reported on 83 patients with Dukes' C colorectal carcinoma who received postoperative BCG alone or in combination with orally administered FU.[599] The BCG was administered by the scarification method at weekly intervals. Patients were followed for as long as 30 months, with an appreciable prolongation of both disease-free interval and overall survival. The conclusion of these observers is that adjuvant immunotherapy without chemotherapy improves the prognosis of patients with surgically treated Dukes' C colorectal carcinoma. Wolmark and colleagues compared patients who received postoperative BCG with controls and with patients given chemotherapy (FU, semustine, and vincristine) in a randomized trial involving individuals with Dukes' B and C colon cancer.[1037] The authors found no significant difference in survival advantage with the use of BCG.

Another study employed adjuvant immunochemotherapy with PSKR, an immunomodulator comprising a protein-bound polysaccharide extracted from mycelia of *Coriorus versicolor*.[172] The PSKR group received this agent orally over 3 years, in addition to mitomycin C and FU. The median follow-up time was four years. When the PSKR patients were compared with the control group (chemotherapy alone), a statistically significant improvement was noted in the disease-free survival curve.

Immunotherapy with agents such as interferon-alfa-2a, monoclonal antibody 17–1, and autologous tumor vaccines is also under investigation, and preliminary results suggest improved survival.[140] The German Cancer Aid 17–1A study group designed a protocol in which a monoclonal antibody (17–1A) was used to target minimal residual disease (i.e., Dukes' C patients).[782] Patients were randomly assigned to an observation regimen or to postoperative treatment with this antibody, infused each month. Antibody treatment reduced the overall death rate by 30% and decreased the recurrence rate by 27%.[782]

Gene Therapy

Note: the following information is abstracted from the United States Office of Biological and Environmental Research, Human Genome Program. MLC

Gene therapy is a research technique for correcting defective genes responsible for causing diseases. Investigators may use several approaches for accomplishing this:

- A normal gene may be inserted into a nonspecific location within the genome to replace a nonfunctional gene.
- An abnormal gene may be swapped for a normal gene through homologous recombination.
- The abnormal gene may be repaired through selective reverse mutation, which returns the gene to its normal function.
- The regulation (the degree to which a gene is turned on or off) of a particular gene may be altered.

In most gene therapy studies, a "normal" gene is inserted into the genome to replace an "abnormal," disease-causing gene. A carrier molecule called a vector must be used to deliver the therapeutic gene to the patient's target cells. Currently, the most common vector is a virus that has been genetically altered to carry normal human DNA. Viruses have evolved a method of encapsulating and delivering their genes to human cells in a pathogenic manner. Target cells, such as the patient's liver, are infected with the viral vector. The vector then unloads its genetic material containing the therapeutic human gene into the target cell. The generation of a functional protein product from the therapeutic gene restores the target cell to a normal state. Some of the different types of viruses used as gene therapy vectors are:

- Retroviruses: A class of viruses that can create double-stranded DNA copies of their RNA genomes. These copies of its genome can be integrated into the chromosomes of host cells. Human immunodeficiency virus is a retrovirus.
- Adenoviruses: A class of viruses with double-stranded DNA genomes that cause respiratory, intestinal, and eye infections in humans. The virus that causes the common cold is an adenovirus.
- Adenoassociated viruses: A class of small, single-stranded DNA viruses that can insert their genetic material at a specific site on chromosome 19.
- Herpes simplex viruses: A class of double-stranded DNA viruses that infect neurons.

Besides virus-mediated gene-delivery systems, there are several nonviral options for gene delivery. The simplest method is the direct introduction of therapeutic DNA into target cells. This approach is limited in its application because it can be used only with certain tissues and requires large amounts of DNA. Another nonviral approach involves the creation of an artificial lipid sphere with an aqueous core. This liposome, which carries the therapeutic DNA, is capable of passing the DNA through the target cell's membrane.

Therapeutic DNA also can get inside target cells by chemically linking the DNA to a molecule that will bind to special cell receptors. Once bound to these receptors, the therapeutic DNA constructs are engulfed by the cell membrane and passed into the interior of the target cell. This delivery system tends to be less effective than other options.

Sheen and co-workers applied gene therapy principles through the use of patient-derived T lymphocytes to target and eradicate hepatic metastases.[855] The T lymphocytes that had been isolated preoperatively were modified genetically with recombinant retroviruses and tested for functional activity against freshly isolated harvested autologous tumor cells. The potential for this approach to therapy was believed to be encouraging.

Radiotherapy

Radiotherapy has been applied primarily in the treatment of rectal cancer (see Chapter 23). However, conventional external radiation therapy should still be considered when macroscopic tumor remains or when fixity of the lesion precludes complete excision. Usually, 45 to 60 Gy (4,500 to 6,000 rads) is administered over a period of 5 to 6 weeks. There is evidence to suggest that this reduces the likelihood of local recurrence and improves survival rates.[241]

Gunderson and associates reported a unique method of administering radiation therapy for colon carcinoma, intraoperative radiation.[356] For treatment of inoperable, residual, or recurrent cancer, doses in excess of 60 Gy (6,000 rads) were given by means of an intraoperative technique at the time of laparotomy. This required transporting the patient, while anesthetized and with the abdomen open, to a different area of the hospital for radiation therapy. The authors postulated that if this technique proved feasible, it could be possible to ablate the tumor by radiation therapy, a result that could not be expected with a lower-dose, externally applied method. Other institutions are employing this technique and have designed operating room suites to accommodate the requisite radiation therapy equipment.[389] Results of further experience are awaited.

When FU is combined with radiation therapy, a modest improvement takes place in length of remission and survival compared with survival after radiation therapy alone in patients with local, inoperable, or recurrent disease.

Holt and colleagues have used intraoperative interstitial radiation therapy in the treatment of hepatic metastases from colorectal carcinomas.[415] It is premature to assess the results of this concept.

Comment

In reviewing the experience with colorectal carcinoma since the 1950s, it is evident that no significant improvements in operative mortality and cure rate have taken place. It appears, then, that surgery has accomplished all it possibly can for this condition. Any further improvement in survival rates will depend on bringing patients to operation earlier and on the effectiveness of other modalities of therapy.

REFERENCES

1. Abrams JS. Elective resection for colorectal cancer in Vermont: 1971–1975. *Am J Surg* 1980;139:78.
2. Abrams JS, Anton JR, Dreyfuss DC. The absence of a relationship between cholecystectomy and the subsequent occurrence of cancer of the proximal colon. *Dis Colon Rectum* 1983;26:141.
3. Abusamra H, Maximova S, Bar-Meir S, et al. Cancer family syndrome of Lynch. *Am J Med* 1987;83:981.
4. Adam R, Akpinar E, Johann M, et al. Place of cryosurgery in the treatment of malignant liver tumors. *Ann Surg* 1997; 225:39.
5. Adam R, Bismuth H, Castaing D, et al. Repeat hepatectomy for colorectal liver metastases. *Ann Surg* 1997;225:51.
6. Adami H-O, Krusemo UB, Meirik O. Unaltered risk of colorectal cancer within 14–17 years of cholecystecomy: updating of a population-based cohort study. *Br J Surg* 1987; 74:675.
7. Adler DG, Young-Fadok TM, Smyrk T, et al. Preoperative chemoradiation therapy after placement of a self-expanding metal stent in a patient with an obstructing rectal cancer: clinical and pathologic findings. *Gastrointest Endosc* 2002;55:435.
8. Adloff M, Arnaud J-P, Schloegel M, et al. Colorectal cancer in patients under 40 years of age. *Dis Colon Rectum* 1986; 29:322.
9. Adson MA, van Heerden JA. Major hepatic resections for metastatic colorectal cancer. *Ann Surg* 1980;191:576.
10. Adson MA, van Heerden JA, Adson MH, et al. Resection of hepatic metastases from colorectal cancer. *Arch Surg* 1984; 119:647.
11. Agarwal N, Cayten CG, Ulahannan MJ, et al. Increased risk of colorectal cancer following breast cancer. *Ann Surg* 1986;203:307.
12. Ahlquist DA, Skoletsky JE, Boynton KA, et al. Colorectal cancer screening by detection of altered human DNA in stool: feasibility of a multitarget assay panel. *Gastroenterology* 2000;119:1219.
13. Ahnen DJ. Genetics of colon cancer. *West J Med* 1991; 154: 700.
14. d'Allaines F, Morgan CN, Lloyd-Davies OV. Discussion on conservative resection in carcinoma. *Proc R Soc Med* 1950; 43:697.
15. Allen-Mersh TG, Earlam S, Fordy C, et al. Quality of life and survival with continuous hepatic-artery floxuridine infusion for colorectal liver metastases. *Lancet* 1994;344: 1255.
16. Allen-Mersh TG, Kemeny N, Niedzwiecki D, et al. Significance of a fall in serum CEA concentration in patients treated with cytotoxic chemotherapy for disseminated colorectal cancer. *Gut* 1987;28:1625.
17. Allis OH. Intestinal anastomosis with suturing of the entire thickness of the intestinal wall. *Am J Obstet* 1902;60.
18. Allison JE, Feldman R. Cost benefits of hemoccult screening for colorectal carcinoma. *Dig Dis Sci* 1985;30:860.
19. Amsterdam E, Krispin M. Primary resection with colocolostomy for obstructive carcinoma of the left side of the colon. *Am J Surg* 1985;150:558.
20. Andre T, Figer A, Cervantes A, et al. FOLFOX7 compared to FOLFOX4, Preliminary results of the randomized optimox study. *Proc ASCO* 2003;22(abst 1016).
21. Andre T, Louvet C, Raymond E, et al. Bimonthly high-dose leucovorin, 5-fluorouracil 48 hour infusion and oxaliplatin (FOLFOX) for metastatic colorectal cancer resistant to the same LV-5FU regimen. *Ann Oncol* 1998;9:1251.
22. Androsov PI. Experience in the application of instrumental suture in surgery of the stomach and rectum. *Acta Chir Scand* 1970;136:57.
23. Angelelli G, Stabile Ianora AA, Scardapane A, et al. Role of computerized tomography in the staging of gastrointestinal neoplasm's. *Semin Surg Oncol* 2001;20:109.
24. Aries V, Crowther JS, Drasar BS, et al. Bacteria and the aetiology of cancer of the large bowel. *Gut* 1969;10:334.
25. Armitage NC, Robins RA, Evans DF, et al. The influence of tumour cell DNA abnormalities on survival in colorectal cancer. *Br J Surg* 1985;72:828.
26. Armstrong CP, Ahsan Z, Hinchley G, et al. Appendicectomy and carcinoma of the caecum. *Br J Surg* 1989;76:1049.
27. Armstrong B, Doll R. Environmental factors and cancer incidence and mortality in different countries, with special reference to dietary practices. *Int J Cancer* 1975;15:617.
28. Arnaud JP, Koehl C, Adloff M. Carcinoembryonic antigen (CEA) in diagnosis and prognosis of colorectal carcinoma. *Dis Colon Rectum* 1980;23:141.
29. Arnold MW, Schneebaum S, Berens A, et al. Intraoperative detection of colorectal cancer with radioimmunoguided surgery and CC49, a second-generation monoclonal antibody. *Ann Surg* 1992;216:627.
30. Arnold MW, Schneebaum S, Berens A, et al. Radioimmunoguided surgery challenges traditional decision making in patients with primary colorectal cancer. *Surgery* 1992;112:624.
31. Arnold MW, Young DC, Hitchcock CL, et al. Radioimmunoguided surgery in primary colorectal carcinoma: an intraoperative prognostic tool and adjuvant to traditional staging. *Am J Surg* 1995;170:315.
32. Asao T, Kuwano H, Nakamura J-I, et al. Gum chewing enhances early recovery from postoperative ileus after laparoscopic colectomy. *J Am Coll Surg* 2002;195:30.
33. Ashton WS, Sariego J, Byrd M, et al. A multivariate analysis of colon cancer, preoperative carcinoembryonic antigen levels, and patient survival. *Contemp Surg* 1993;43:11.
34. Astler VB, Coller FA. Prognostic significance of direct extension of carcinoma of colon and rectum. *Ann Surg* 1954; 139:846.
35. Atabek U, Pello MJ, Spence RK, et al. Arterial vasopressin for control of bleeding from a stapled intestinal anastomosis: report of two cases. *Dis Colon Rectum* 1992;35:1180.

36. Atwell JD, Taylor I, Cruddas M. Increased risk of colorectal cancer associated with congenital anomalies of the urinary tract. *Br J Surg* 1993;80:785.

37. August DA, Sugarbaker PH, Ottow RT, et al. Hepatic resection of colorectal metastases. Influence of clinical factors and adjuvant intraperitoneal 5-fluorouracil via Tenckhoff catheter on survival. *Ann Surg* 1985;201:210.

38. Ault GW. Carcinoma of rectum: factors responsible for recurrent or residual disease. *Am Surg* 1953;19:1035.

39. Aune S, Norman E. Diffuse peritonitis treated with continuous peritoneal lavage. *Acta Chir Scand* 1970;136:401.

40. Axtell LM, Cutler SJ, Myers MH, eds. *End results in cancer.* Report No 4. Publication No. (NIH) 73–272. Bethesda, MD: US Department of Health, Education, and Welfare, 1972: 217.

41. Ayeni AO, Thomson DMP, MacFarlane JK. A comparison of tube leukocyte adherence inhibition assay and standard physical methods for diagnosing colorectal cancer. *Cancer* 1981;48:1855.

42. Baker LH, Matter R, Talley R, et al. 5-FU vs. 5-FU and Me CCNU in gastrointestinal cancers: a phase III study of the South West Oncology Group. *Proc Am Assoc Cancer Res* 1975;16:229(abst).

43. Balch CM, Urist MM, McGregor ML. Continuous regional chemotherapy for metastatic colorectal cancer using a totally implantable infusion pump: a feasibility study in 50 patients. *Am J Surg* 1983;145:285.

44. Balfour DC. A method of anastomosis between sigmoid and rectum. *Ann Surg* 1910;51:239.

45. Ballantyne GH, Reigel MM, Wolff BG, et al. Oophorectomy and colon cancer. *Ann Surg* 1985;202:209.

46. Banner BF, Tomas de la Vega JE, Roseman DL, et al. Should flow cytometric DNA analysis precede definitive surgery for colon carcinoma? *Ann Surg* 1985;202:740.

47. Barkin JS, Cohen ME, Flaxman M, et al. Value of a routine follow-up endoscopy program for the detection of recurrent colorectal carcinoma. *Am J Gastroenterol* 1988;88:1355.

48. Barringer PL, Dockerty MB, Waugh JM, et al. Carcinoma of the large intestine: a new approach to the study of venous spread. *Surg Gynecol Obstet* 1954;98:62.

49. Basse L, Billesbølle P, Kehlet H. Early recovery after abdominal rectopexy with multimodal rehabilitation. *Dis Colon Rectum* 2002;45:195.

50. Basse L, Jacobsen DH, Billesbølle P, et al. Colostomy closure after Hartmann's procedure with fast-track rehabilitation. *Dis Colon Rectum* 2002;45:1661.

51. Bat L, Neumann G, Shemesh E. The association of synchronous neoplasms with occluding cancer. *Dis Colon Rectum* 1985;28:149.

52. Baxter NN, Noel AA, Cherry K, et al. Management of patients with colorectal cancer and concomitant abdominal aortic aneurysm. *Dis Colon Rectum* 2002;45:165.

53. Beart RW, Melton JL III, Maruta M, et al. Trends in right- and left-sided colon cancer. *Dis Colon Rectum* 1983;26:393.

54. Beart RW Jr, Moertel CG, Wieand HS, et al. Adjuvant therapy for resectable colorectal carcinoma with fluorouracil administered by portal vein infusion: a study of the Mayo Clinic and the North Central Cancer Treatment Group. *Arch Surg* 1990;125:897.

55. Beatty JD, Hyams DM, Morton BA, et al. Impact of radiolabeled antibody imaging on management of colon cancer. *Am J Surg* 1989;157:13.

56. Beck DE. The role of Seprafilm bioresorbable membrane in adhesion prevention. *Eur J Surg* 1997;577:49.

57. Beck DE, Cohen Z, Fleshman JW, et al. A prospective, randomized multicenter, controlled study of the safety of Seprafilm adhesion barrier in abdominopelvic surgery of the intestine. *Dis Colon Rectum* 2003;46:1310.

58. Beck DE, Fazio VW. Current preoperative bowel cleansing methods: results of a survey. *Dis Colon Rectum* 1990;33:12.

59. Beck DE, Fazio VW, Jagelman DG. Comparison of oral lavage methods for preoperative colonic cleansing. *Dis Colon Rectum* 1986;29:699.

60. Beck DE, Harford FJ, DiPalma JA, et al. Bowel cleansing with polyethylene glycol electrolyte lavage solution. *South Med J* 1985;78:1414.

61. Beck DE, Opelka FG, Bailey HR, et al. Incidence of small-bowel obstruction and adhesiolysis after open colorectal and general surgery. *Dis Colon Rectum* 1999;42:241.

62. Beck NE, Tomlinson IPM, Homfray T, et al. Genetic testing is important in families with a history suggestive of hereditary non-polyposis colorectal cancer even if the Amsterdam criteria are not fulfilled. *Br J Surg* 1997;84:233.

63. Becker JM, Dayton MT, Fazio VW, et al. Prevention of postoperative abdominal adhesions by a sodium hyaluronate-based bioresorbable membrane: a prospective, randomized, double-blind multicenter study. *J Am Coll Surg* 1996; 183:297.

64. Beckwith PS, Wolff BG, Frazee RC. Ileorectostomy in the older patient. *Dis Colon Rectum* 1992;35:301.

65. Becouam Y, Ychou M, Ducreux M, et al. Oxaliplatin as first line chemotherapy in metastatic colorectal patients. *J Clin Oncol* 1998;8:2739.

66. Beets G, Penninckx F, Schiepers C, et al. Clinical value of whole-body positron emission tomography with [^{18}F]fluorodeoxyglucose in recurrent colorectal cancer. *Br J Surg* 1994;81:1666.

67. Begent RHJ, Keep PA, Searle F, et al. Radioimmunolocalization and selection for surgery in recurrent colorectal cancer. *Br J Surg* 1986;73:64.

68. Belinkie SA, Narayanan NC, Russell JC, et al. Splenic abscess associated with *Streptococcus bovis* septicemia and neoplastic lesions of the colon. *Dis Colon Rectum* 1983; 26:823.

69. Bender JS, Magnuson TH, Zenilman ME, et al. Outcome following colon surgery in the octagenerian. *Am Surg* 1996;62:276.

70. Bennett-Guerrero E, Hyam JA, Shaefi S, et al. Comparison of P-POSSUM risk-adjusted mortality rates after surgery between patients in the USA and the UK. *Br J Surg* 2003; 90:1593.

71. Berrospi F, Celis J, Ruiz E, et al. En bloc pancreaticoduodenectomy for right colon cancer invading adjacent organs. *J Surg Oncol* 2002;79:194.

72. Besbeas S, Stearns MW Jr. Osseous metastases from carcinomas of the colon and rectum. *Dis Colon Rectum* 1978; 21:266.

73. 57A. Bessa X, Piñol V, Castellví-Bel S, et al. Prognostic value of postoperative detection of blood circulating tumor cells in patients with colorectal cancer operated on for cure. *Ann Surg* 2003;237:368.

74. Beynon J, Davies PW, Billings PJ, et al. Perioperative blood transfusion increases the risk of recurrence in colorectal cancer. *Dis Colon Rectum* 1989;29:975.

75. Biggers OR, Ready RL, Beart RW Jr. Risk of additional intra-abdominal procedures at the time of colectomy. *Dis Colon Rectum* 1982;15:185.

76. Binderow SR, Cohen SM, Wexner SD, et al. Must early postoperative oral intake be limited to laparoscopy? *Dis Colon Rectum* 1994;37:584.

77. Biondo S, Jaurrieta E, Jorba R, et al. Intraoperative colonic lavage and primary anastomosis in peritonitis and obstruction. *Br J Surg* 1997;84:222.

78. Birnkrant A, Sampson J, Sugarbaker PH. Ovarian metastasis from colorectal cancer. *Dis Colon Rectum* 1986;29:767.

79. Bismuth H, Adam R, Lévi F, et al. Resection of nonresectable liver metastases from colorectal cancer after neoadjuvant chemotherapy. *Ann Surg* 1996;224:509.

80. Bjelke E. *Epidemiologic studies of cancer of the stomach, colon, and rectum: with special emphasis on the role of diet: abstracts and literature review.* Oslo: Universitets Forlaget, 1974.

81. Bjelke E. Epidemiologic studies of cancer of the stomach, colon, and rectum: with special emphasis on the role of diet. *Scand J Gastroenterol Suppl* 1974;9:1.

82. Blair JE, McLeod RS, Cohen Z, et al. Ticarcillin/clavulanic acid (Timentin) compared to metronidazole/ netilmicin in preventing postoperative infection after elective colorectal surgery. *Can J Surg* 1987;30:120.

83. Blamey SL, McDermott FT, Pihl E, et al. Resected ovarian recurrence from colorectal adenocarcinoma: a study of 13 cases. *Dis Colon Rectum* 1981;24:272.

84. Blanco D, Ross RK, Paganini-Hill A, et al. Cholecystectomy and colonic cancer. *Dis Colon Rectum* 1984;27:290.

85. Bleeker WA, Mulder NH, Hermans J, et al. Value and cost of follow-up after adjuvant treatment of patients with Dukes' C colonic cancer. *Br J Surg* 2001;88:101.

86. Bloch OT. Om extra-abdominal behandlung af cancer intestinalis (rectum derfra undtaget) med en frem stilling af de for denne sygdom foretagne operationer og deres resultater. *Nord Med Ark* 1892;24:1.

87. Bülow S, Svendsen LB, Mellemgaard A. Metachronous colorectal carcinoma. *Br J Surg* 1990;77:502.

88. Böhm B, Schwenk W, Hucke HP, et al. Does methodic long-term follow-up affect survival after curative resection of colorectal carcinoma? *Dis Colon Rectum* 1993;36:280.

89. Bokey EL, Chapuis PH, Dent OF, et al. Surgical technique and survival in patients having a curative resection for colon cancer. *Dis Colon Rectum* 2003;46:860.

90. Boldrini G, de Gaetano AM, Giovannini I, et al. The systematic use of operative ultrasound for detection of liver metastases during colorectal surgery. *World J Surg* 1987;11:622.

91. Bolin S, Nilsson E, Sjdahl R. Carcinoma of the colon and rectum: growth rate. *Ann Surg* 1984;198:151.

92. Boman B, Fitzgibbons RJ, Lanspa SJ, et al. Hereditary nonpolyposis colon cancer (Lynch syndrome I and II): a challenge for the clinician. *Nebr Med J* 1989;74:2.

93. Bonnheim DC, Petrelli NJ, Herrera L, et al. Osseous metastases from colorectal carcinoma. *Am J Surg* 1986;151:457.

94. Botsford TW, Aliapoulios MR, Fogelson FS. Results of treatment of colorectal cancer at the Peter Bent Brigham Hospital from 1960 to 1965. *Am J Surg* 1971;121:398.

95. Böttger TC, Gabbert HE, Stöckle M, et al. DNA image cytometry: a prognostic tool in rectal cancer? *Dis Colon Rectum* 1992;35:436.

96. Boyd JT, Langman M, Doll R. The epidemiology of gastrointestinal cancer with special reference to causation. *Gut* 1964;5:196.

97. Bradnock B. Speeding up colonic lavage. *Br J Surg* 1987;74:464.

98. Bradpiece HA, Benjamin IS, Halevy A, et al. Major hepatic resection for colorectal metastases. *Br J Surg* 1987;74:324.

99. Bralow SP, Green S. Forewarned is forearmed: some colorectal cancer is hereditary. *Contemp Gastroenterol* 1990; 3:57.

100. Bredtmann RD, Herden HN, Teichmann W, et al. Epidural analgesia in colonic surgery: results of a randomized prospective study. *Br J Surg* 1990;77:638.

101. Brendel TH, Kirsh IE. Lack of association between inguinal hernia and carcinoma of the colon. *N Engl J Med* 1971;284:369.

102. Brief DK, Brener BJ, Goldenkranz R. An argument for increased use of subtotal colectomy in the management of carcinoma of the colon. *Am Surg* 1983;49:66.

103. Brisson PA, Morere D. Colorectal intussusception. *Contemp Surg* 1990;36:30.

104. Brister SJ, de Varennes B, Gordon PH, et al. Contemporary operative management of pulmonary metastases of colorectal origin. *Dis Colon Rectum* 1988;31:786.

105. Bristol JB, Emmett PM, Heaton KW, et al. Sugar, fat, and the risk of colorectal cancer. *BMJ* 1985;291:1467.

106. Brodsky JT, Cohen AM. Peritoneal seeding following potentially curative resection of colonic carcinoma: implications for adjuvant therapy. *Dis Colon Rectum* 1991;34:723.

107. Brown CE, Warren S. Visceral metastasis from rectal carcinoma. *Surg Gynecol Obstet* 1938;66:611.

108. Brown AD, Garber AM. Cost-effectiveness of three methods to enhance the sensitivity of Papanicolaou testing. *JAMA* 1999;281:347.

109. Brown RA, Rode H, Millar AJW, et al. Colorectal carcinoma in children. *J Pediatr Surg* 1992;27:919.

110. Bruinvels DJ, Stiggelbout AM, Kievit J, et al. Follow-up of patients with colorectal cancer: a meta-analysis. *Ann Surg* 1994;219:174.

111. Bubrick MP, Corman ML, Cahill CJ, et al. Prospective, randomized trial of the biofragmentable anastomosis ring. *Am J Surg* 1991;161:136.

112. Buckley N, Brown DAP. Metastatic tumors in the hand from adenocarcinoma of the colon. *Dis Colon Rectum* 1987;30:141.

113. Buechter KJ, Boustany C, Caillouette R, et al. Surgical management of the acutely obstructed colon. A review of 127 cases. *Am J Surg* 1988;156:163.

114. Bufo AJ, Feldman S, Daniels GA, et al. Early postoperative feeding. *Dis Colon Rectum* 1994;37:1260.

115. Burbank F. Patterns in cancer mortality in the United States: 1950–1967. *Natl Cancer Inst Monogr* 1971;33:1.

116. Burke P, Mealy K, Gillen P, et al. Requirement for bowel preparation in colorectal surgery. *Br J Surg* 1994;81:907.

117. Burkitt DP. Relationship as a clue to causation. *Lancet* 1970;2:1237.

118. Burkitt DP. Epidemiology of cancer of the colon and rectum. *Cancer* 1971;28:3.

119. Burkitt DP. Some neglected leads to cancer causation. *J Natl Cancer Inst* 1971;47:913.

120. Burkitt D. An approach to the reduction of the most common Western cancers: the failure of therapy to reduce disease. *Arch Surg* 1991;126:345.

121. Burkitt DP, Walker AR, Painter NS. Effect of dietary fibre on stools and the transit times, and its role in the causation of disease. *Lancet* 1972;2:1408.

122. Burns JW, Skinner K, Colt J, et al. Prevention of tissue injury and postsurgical adhesions by precoating tissues with hyaluronic acid solutions. *J Surg Res* 1995;59:644.

123. Buroker TR, O'Connell MJ, Wieand HS, et al. Randomized comparison of two schedules of fluorouracil and leucovorin in the treatment of advanced colorectal cancer. *J Clin Oncol* 1994;12:14.

124. Busch ORC, Hop WCJ, Marquet RL, et al. Blood transfusions and local tumor recurrence in colorectal cancer: evidence of a noncausal relationship. *Ann Surg* 1994;220:791.

125. Butler J, Attiyeh FF, Daly JM. Hepatic resection for metastases of the colon and rectum. *Surg Gynecol Obstet* 1986; 162:109.

126. Byrd RL, Boggs HW Jr, Slagle GW, et al. Reliability of colonoscopy. *Dis Colon Rectum* 1989;32:1023.

127. Cady B, McDermott WV. Major hepatic resection for metachronous metastases from colon cancer. *Ann Surg* 1985;201:204.

128. Cady B, Monson DO, Swinton NW Sr. Survival of patients after colonic resection for carcinoma with simultaneous liver metastases. *Surg Gynecol Obstet* 1970;131:697.

129. Cady B, Oberfield RA. Regional infusion chemotherapy of hepatic metastases from carcinoma of the colon. *Am J Surg* 1974;127:220.

130. Cady B, Persson AV, Monson DO, et al. Changing patterns of colorectal carcinoma. *Cancer* 1974;33:422.

131. Cahan WG, Castro El B, Hajdu SI. The significance of a solitary lung shadow in patients with colon carcinoma. *Cancer* 1974;33:414.

132. Cahill CJ, Betzler M, Gruwez J, et al. Sutureless large-bowel anastomosis: European experience with the biofragmentable anastomosis ring. *Br J Surg* 1989;76:344.

133. Cali RL, Pitsch RM, Thorson AG, et al. Cumulative incidence of metachronous colorectal cancer. *Dis Colon Rectum* 1993;36:388.

134. Cameron BH, William G, Fitzgerald N, et al. Hereditary site-specific colon cancer in a Canadian kindred. *Can Med Assoc J* 1989;140:41.

135. Camp TF Jr, Connolly JM. Colorectal polypoid lesions. *Arch Surg* 1966;93:625.

136. Canalis F, Ravitch MM. Study of healing of inverting and everting intestinal anastomoses. *Surg Gynecol Obstet* 1968; 126:109.

137. Carlson MA, Condon RE. Polyglyconate (Maxon) versus nylon suture in midline abdominal incision closure: a prospective randomized trial. *Am Surg* 1995;61:980.

138. Carpelan-Holmström MA, Haglund CH, Roberts PJ. Differences in serum tumor markers between colon and rectal cancer: comparison of CA 242 and carcinoembryonic antigen. *Dis Colon Rectum* 1996;39:799.

139. Carty NJ, Keating J, Campbell J, et al. Prospective audit of an extramucosal technique for intestinal anastomosis. *Br J Surg* 1991;78:1439.

140. Casillas S, Pelley RJ, Milsom JW. Adjuvant therapy for colorectal cancer: present and future perspectives. *Dis Colon Rectum* 1997;40:977.

141. Castaing D, Emond J, Bismuth H, et al. Utility of operative ultrasound in the surgical management of liver tumors. *Ann Surg* 1986;204:600.

142. Cederlf R, Friberg L, Hrubec Z, et al. *The relationship of smoking and some social covariables to mortality and cancer morbidity: a ten-year follow-up in a probability sample of 55,000 Swedish subjects ages 18 to 69.* Stockholm: Karolinska Mediko-Kirurgiska Institutet, 1975.

143. Celoria G, Falco E, Nardini A, et al. Intraoperative testing of the Valtrac biofragmentable anastomotic ring. *Br J Surg* 1993;80:618.

144. Chang FC, Jackson TM, Jackson CR. Hemoccult screening for colorectal cancer. *Am J Surg* 1988;156:457.

145. Chapuis PH, Dent OF, Fisher R, et al. A multivariate analysis of clinical and pathological variables in prognosis after resection of large-bowel cancer. *Br J Surg* 1985; 72:698.

146. Chapuis PH, Dent OF, Newland RC, et al. An evaluation of the American Joint Committee (pTMN) staging method for cancer of the colon and rectum. *Dis Colon Rectum* 1986; 29:6.

147. Charnley RM, Doran J, Morris DL. Cryotherapy for liver metastases: a new approach. *Br J Surg* 1989;76:1040.

148. Charnley RM, Morris DL, Dennison AR, et al. Detection of colorectal liver metastases using intraoperative ultrasonography. *Br J Surg* 1991;78:45.

149. Chassin JL, Rifkind KM, Sussman B, et al. The stapled gastrointestinal tract anastomosis: incidence of postoperative complications compared with the sutured anastomosis. *Ann Surg* 1978;188:689.

150. Chen T-C, Ding K-C, Yang M-J, et al. New device for biofragmentable anastomotic ring in low anterior resection. *Dis Colon Rectum* 1994;37:834.

151. Chen W-F, Patchefsky AS, Goldsmith HS. Colonic protection from dimethylhydrazine by a high-fiber diet. *Surg Gynecol Obstet* 1978;147:503.

152. Chen YL. The diagnosis of colorectal cancer with cytologic brushings under direct vision at fiberoptic colonoscopy: a report of 59 cases. *Dis Colon Rectum* 1987;30:342.

153. Choi HJ, Jung IK, Kim SS, et al. Proliferating cell nuclear antigen expression and its relationship to malignancy potential in invasive colorectal carcinomas. *Dis Colon Rectum* 1997;40:51.

154. Choi J, O'Connell TX. Safe and effective early postoperative feeding and hospital discharge after open colon resection. *Am Surg* 1996;62:853.

155. Chu DZJ, Erickson CA, Russell MP, et al. Prognostic significance of carcinoembryonic antigen in colorectal carcinoma. *Arch Surg* 1991;126:314.

156. Chung M, Steinmetz OK, Gordon PH. Perioperative blood transfusion and outcome after resection for colorectal carcinoma. *Br J Surg* 1993;80:427.

157. Cioffiro W, Schein CJ, Gliedman ML. Splenic injury during abdominal surgery. *Arch Surg* 1976;11:167.

158. Clark CG. Implantable vascular access devices in the treatment of colorectal liver metastases. *Br J Surg* 1986;73:419.

159. Clark CG, Harris J, Elmasri S, et al. Polyglycolic acid sutures and catgut in colonic anastomoses: a controlled clinical trial. *Lancet* 1972;2:1006.

160. Clark TW, Schor SS, Elsom KE, et al. The periodic health examination: evaluation of routine tests and procedures. *Ann Intern Med* 1961;54:1209.

161. Clarke MP, Kane RA, Steele GS Jr, et al. Prospective comparison of preoperative imaging and intraoperative ultrasonography in the detection of liver tumors. *Surgery* 1989;106:849.

162. Clemmesen J. Statistical studies in the aetiology of malignant neoplasms. *Acta Pathol Microbiol Scand Suppl* 1974; 247:1.

163. Clemmesen J, Nielsen A. Social distribution of cancer in Copenhagen, 1943 to 1947. *Br J Cancer* 1951;5:159.

164. Cohen AM, Kaufman SD, Wood WC. Treatment of colorectal cancer hepatic metastases by hepatic artery chemotherapy. *Dis Colon Rectum* 1985;28:389.

165. Cohen AM, Martin EW Jr, Lavery I, et al. Radioimmunoguided surgery using iodine 125 B72.3 in patients with colorectal cancer. *Arch Surg* 1991;126:349.

166. Cohn I Jr. Implantation in cancer of the colon. *Surg Gynecol Obstet* 1967;124:501.

167. Cole WH, Packard D, Southwick HW. Carcinoma of the colon with special reference to prevention of recurrence. *JAMA* 1954;155:1549.

168. Colvin DB, Lee W, Eisenstat TE, et al. The role of nasointestinal intubation in elective colonic surgery. *Dis Colon Rectum* 1986;29:295.

169. Condon RE, Bartlett JG, Greenlee H, et al. Efficacy of oral and systemic antibiotic prophylaxis in colorectal operations. *Arch Surg* 1983;118:496.

170. Connell ME. Intestinal anastomosis—by a new method, without plates and with but two knots—either silk or catgut sutures may be used. *JAMA* 1893;21:150.

171. Cook PJ, Doll R, Fellingham SA. A mathematical model for the age distribution of cancer in man. *Int J Cancer* 1969;4:93.

172. The Cooperative Study Group of Surgical Adjuvant Immunochemotherapy for Cancer of Colon and Rectum (Kanagawa). Mitomi T, Tsuchiya S, Ijima N, et al. Randomized controlled study on adjuvant immunochemotherapy with PSKR in curatively resected colorectal cancer. *Dis Colon Rectum* 1992;35:123.

173. Corman ML, Coller JA, Veidenheimer MC. Proctosigmoidoscopy: age criteria for examination in the asymptomatic patient. *CA Cancer J Clin* 1975;24:286.

174. Corman ML, Galandiuk S, Block GE, et al. Immunoscintigraphy with ^{111}In-Satumomab pendetide in patients with colorectal adenocarcinoma: performance and impact on clinical management. *Dis Colon Rectum* 1994;37: 129.

175. Corman ML, Prager ED, Hardy TG Jr, et al. Comparison of the Valtrac biofragmentable anastomosis ring with conventional suture and stapled anastomosis in colon surgery: results of a prospective, randomized clinical trial. *Dis Colon Rectum* 1989;32:183.

176. Corman ML, Robertson WG, Lewis TH, et al. A controlled clinical trial: cefuroxime, metronidazole, and cefoxitin as prophylactic therapy for colorectal surgery. *Contemp Surg* 1993;12:36.

177. Corman ML, Swinton NW Sr, O'Keefe DD, et al. Colorectal carcinoma at the Lahey Clinic, 1962–1966. *Am J Surg* 1973; 125:424.

178. Corman ML, Veidenheimer MC, Coller JA. Colorectal carcinoma: a decade of experience at the Lahey Clinic. *Dis Colon Rectum* 1979;22:477.

179. Corman ML, Veidenheimer MC, Coller JA. Controlled clinical trial of three suture materials for abdominal closure after bowel resections. *Am J Surg* 1981;141:510.

180. Corman ML, Veidenheimer MC, Swinton NW. *Diseases of the anus, rectum, and colon. Part I: neoplasms.* New York: Medcom, 1972.

181. Correa P, Llanos G. Morbidity and mortality from cancer in Cali, Colombia. *J Natl Cancer Inst* 1966;36:717.

182. Cox MR, Gunn IF, Eastman MC, et al. The operative aetiology and types of adhesions causing small-bowel obstruction. *Aust N Z J Surg* 1993;63:848.

183. Creagan ET, Fraumeni JF Jr. Cancer mortality among American Indians. *J Natl Cancer Inst* 1972;49:959.

184. Cucino C, Buchner AM, Sonnenberg A. Continued rightward shift of colorectal cancer. *Dis Colon Rectum* 2002;45:1035.

185. Cunningham D, Humblet Y, Siena S, et al. Cetuximab (C225) alone or in combination with irinotecan (CPT-11) in patients with epidermal growth factor receptor (EGFR)-positive, irinotecan-refractory metastatic colorectal cancer (MCRC). *Proc ASCO* 2003;22(abst 1012).

186. Cunningham D, Purhonen S, James RD, et al. Randomized trial of irinotecan plus supportive care versus supportive care alone after fluorouracil failure for patients with metastatic colorectal cancer. *Lancet* 1998;352:1413.

187. Curley SA, Evans DB, Ames FC. Resection for cure of carcinoma of the colon directly invading the duodenum or pancreatic head. *J Am Coll Surg* 1994;179:587.

188. Cusack JC, Giacco GG, Cleary K, et al. Survival factors in 186 patients younger than 40 years old with colorectal adenocarcinoma. *J Am Coll Surg* 1996;183:105.

189. Cutait R, Alves VAF, Lopes LC, et al. Restaging of colorectal cancer based on the identification of lymph node micrometastases through immunoperoxidase staining of CEA and cytokeratins. *Dis Colon Rectum* 1991;34:917.

190. Cutait R, Less ML, Enker WE. Prophylactic oophorectomy in surgery for large-bowel cancer. *Dis Colon Rectum* 1983; 16:6.

191. Cuthbertson AM, McLeish AR, Penfold CB, et al. A comparison between single- and double-dose intravenous Timentin for the prophylaxis of wound infection in elective colorectal surgery. *Dis Colon Rectum* 1991;34:151.

192. Cutler SJ, Young JL Jr, eds. The third national cancer survey: incidence data: cancer morbidity. *Natl Cancer Inst Monogr* 1975;41:1.

193. Daly JM, Butler J, Kemeny N, et al. Predicting tumor response in patients with colorectal hepatic metastases. *Ann Surg* 1985;202:384.

194. Daneker GW Jr, Piazza AJ, Steele GD Jr, et al. Interactions of human colorectal carcinoma cells with basement membranes: analysis and correlation with differentiation. *Arch Surg* 1989;124:183.

195. Danforth DN Jr, Thorbjarnarson B. Incidental splenectomy: a review of the literature and the New York Hospital experience. *Ann Surg* 1976;183:124.

196. Dauphine CE, Tan P, Beart RB Jr, et al. Placement of self-expanding metal stents for acute malignant large-bowel obstruction: a collective review. *Ann Surg Oncol* 2002;9: 574.

197. Davis TP, Knollmann-Ritschel B, DeNobile JW. An unusual cutaneous presentation of metastatic colon cancer. *Dis Colon Rectum* 1995;38:670.

198. Davis WC, Jackson FC. Inguinal hernia and colon carcinoma. *CA Cancer J Clin* 1968;18:143.

199. Dawson PM, Blair SD, Begent RHJ, et al. The value of radioimmunoguided surgery in first- and second-look laparotomy for colorectal cancer. *Dis Colon Rectum* 1991;34: 217.

200. Dawson P, Habib NA, Fane S, et al. Association between extent of colonic mucosal sialomucin change and subsequent local recurrence after curative excision of primary colorectal cancer. *Br J Surg* 1990;77:1279.

201. Dawson PM, Habib NA, Rees HC, et al. Mucosal field change in colorectal cancer. *Am J Surg* 1987;153:281.

202. de Almeida ACM, Gracias CW, dos Santos NM, et al. One-stage colectomy in the management of acutely obstructed left colon cancer. *Dig Surg* 1992;9:155.

203. Dean ACB, Newell JP. Colonoscopy in the differential diagnosis of carcinoma from diverticulitis of the sigmoid colon. *Br J Surg* 1973;60:633.

204. Dean PA, Vernava AM III. Flow cytometric analysis of DNA content in colorectal carcinoma. *Dis Colon Rectum* 1992; 35:95.

205. Deans GT, Heatley M, Anderson N, et al. Jass' classification revisited. *J Am Coll Surg* 1994;179:11.

206. Deans GT, Williamson K, Heatley M, et al. The role of flow cytometry in carcinoma of the colon and rectum. *Surg Gynecol Obstet* 1993;177:377.

207. de Gramont A, Banzi M, Navarro M, et al. Oxaliplatin/5FU/LV in adjuvant colon cancer: Results of the international randomized Mosaic trial. *Proc ASCO* 2003;22(abst 1015).

208. de Gramont A, Bosset JF, Milan C, et al. Randomized trial comparing monthly low-dose leucovorin and fluorouracil bolus with bimonthly high-dose leucovorin and fluorouracil bolus plus continuous infusion for advanced colorectal cancer: a French intergroup study. *J Clin Oncol* 1997;15:808.

209. de Gramont A, Figer A, Seymour M, et al. Leucovorin and fluorouracil with or without oxaliplatin as first line treatment in advanced colorectal cancer. *J Clin Oncol* 2000; 18:2938.

210. de la Hunt MN, Karran SJ. Sulbactam/ampicillin compared with cefoxitin for chemoprophylaxis in elective colorectal surgery. *Dis Colon Rectum* 1986;29:157.

211. Delaney CP, Zutshi M, Senagore AJ, et al. Prospective, randomized, controlled trial between a pathway of controlled rehabilitation with early ambulation and diet and traditional postoperative care after laparotomy and intestinal resection. *Dis Colon Rectum* 2003;46:851.

212. Delpero JR, Pol B, Le Treut YP, et al. Surgical resection of locally recurrent colorectal adenocarcinoma. *Br J Surg* 1998;85:372.

213. de Petz A. Aseptic technic of stomach resections. *Ann Surg* 1927;83:388.

214. de Vos tot Nederveen Cappel WH, Nagengast FM, Griffioen G, et al. Surveillance for hereditary nonpolyposis colorectal cancer: a long-term study on 114 families. *Dis Colon Rectum* 2002;45:1588.

215. Di Carlo V, Badellino F, Stella M, et al. Role of B72.3 iodine in 125-labeled monoclonal antibody in colorectal cancer detection by radioimmunoguided surgery. *Surgery* 1994; 115:190.

216. Didolkar MS, Elias EG, Whitley NO, et al. Unresectable hepatic metastases from carcinoma of the colon and rectum. *Surg Gynecol Obstet* 1985;160:429.

217. Dixon CF. Anterior resection for malignant lesions of the upper part of the rectum and lower part of the sigmoid. *Ann Surg* 1948;128:425.

218. diZerega GS. Contemporary adhesion prevention. *Fertil Steril* 1994;61:219.

219. Docherty JG, McGregor JR, Akyol AM, et al. Comparison of manually constructed and stapled anastomoses in colorectal surgery. *Ann Surg* 1995;221:176.

220. Doerr RJ, Abdel-Nabi H, Baker JM, et al. Detection of primary colorectal cancer with indium 111 monoclonal antibody B72.3. *Arch Surg* 1990;125:1601.

221. Doerr RJ, Kulaylat MN, Bumpers H, et al. The role of immunoscintigraphy in the staging and management of colorectal cancer. *Am Surg* 1996;62:956.

222. Dohmoto M. New method: endoscopic implantation of rectal stent in palliative treatment of malignant stenosis. *Endosc Digest* 1991;3:1507.

223. Doll R. The geographical distribution of cancer. *Br J Cancer* 1969;23:1.

224. Doll R, Hill AB. Mortality in relation to smoking: ten years' observations of British doctors. *BMJ* 1964;1:1399.

225. Doll R, Muir C, Waterhouse J, eds. *Cancer incidence in five continents: technical reports of the International Union Against Cancer.* New York: Springer-Verlag, 1970.

226. Dominguez JM, Wolff BG, Nelson H, et al. ^{111}In-CYT-103 scanning in recurrent colorectal cancer: does it affect standard management? *Dis Colon Rectum* 1996;39:514.

227. Donaldson DR, Hughes LE. Notes on "on table" lavage. *Br J Surg* 1987;74:465.

228. Dong SM, Traverso G, Johnson C, et al. Detecting colorectal cancer in stool with the use of multiple genetic targets. *J Natl Cancer Inst* 2001;93:858.

229. Douillard JY, Cunningham D, Roth AD, et al. Irinotecan combined with fluorouracil compared with fluorouracil alone as first line treatment for metastatic colorectal cancer: a multicenter randomized trial. *Lancet* 2000;355:1041.

230. Drexler J. Asymptomatic polyps of the colon and rectum. 3. Proximal and distal polyp relationships. *Arch Intern Med* 1971;127:466.

231. Drexler J. Proctosigmoidoscopy: when and why? *N Engl J Med* 1972;286:668.

232. Dueholm S, Rubinstein E, Reipurth G. Preparation for elective colorectal surgery: a randomized blinded comparison between oral colonic lavage and whole-gut irrigation. *Dis Colon Rectum* 1987;30:360.

233. Dukes CE. The spread of cancer of the rectum. *Br J Surg* 1930;17:643.

234. Dukes CE. The classification of cancer of the rectum. *J Pathol Bacteriol* 1932;35:323.

235. Dukes CE. The surgical pathology of rectal cancer. (President's address.) *Proc R Soc Med* 1944;37:131.

236. Dukes CE, Bussey HJ. The spread of rectal cancer and its effect on prognosis. *Br J Cancer* 1958;12:309.

237. Dunham LJ, Bailar JC III. World maps of cancer mortality rates and frequency ratios. *J Natl Cancer Inst* 1968;41:155.

238. Dunlop MG. Inheritance of colorectal cancer susceptibility. *Br J Surg* 1990;77:245.

239. Dunn DH, Robbins P, Decanini C, et al. A comparison of stapled and hand-sewn anastomoses. *Dis Colon Rectum* 1978;21:636.

240. Durdey P, Williams NS, Brown DA. Serum carcinoembryonic antigen and acute-phase reactant proteins in the preoperative detection of fixation of colorectal tumours. *Br J Surg* 1984;71:881.

241. Duttenhaver JR, Hoskins RB, Gunderson LL, et al. Adjuvant postoperative radiation therapy in the management of adenocarcinoma of the colon. *Cancer* 1986;57:955.

242. Dwight RW, Higgins GA, Keehn RJ. Factors influencing survival after resection in cancer of the colon and rectum. *Am J Surg* 1969;117:512.

243. Dwyer WA Jr. The role of the ovary in colon cancer management. *Contemp Surg* 1991;38:15.

244. Eddy D. Cancer of the colon and rectum. *CA Cancer J Clin* 1980;30:208.

245. Eisenberg SB, Kraybill WG, Lopez MJ. Long-term results of surgical resection of locally advanced colorectal carcinoma. *Surgery* 1990;108:779.

246. Ekman C-A, Gustavson J, Henning A. Value of a follow-up study of recurrent carcinoma of the colon and rectum. *Surg Gynecol Obstet* 1977;145:895.

247. Eldar S, Meguid MM. Pancreatic cancer presenting as colonic obstruction. *Contemp Surg* 1984;25:36.

248. Ellert J, Kreel L. The value of CT in malignant colonic tumors. *CT* 1980;4:225.

249. Ellis H, Moran BJ, Thompson JN, et al. Adhesion-related hospital readmissions after abdominal and pelvic surgery: a retrospective cohort study. *Lancet* 1999;353:1476.

250. Engarås B. Individual cutoff levels of carcinoembryonic antigen and CA 242 indicate recurrence of colorectal cancer with high sensitivity. *Dis Colon Rectum* 2003;46:313.

251. Enstrom JE. Cancer mortality among Mormons. *Cancer* 1975;36:825.

252. Eraklis AJ, Folkman MJ. Adenocarcinoma at the site of ureterosigmoidostomies for exstrophy of the bladder. *J Pediatr Surg* 1978;13:730.

253. Esser S, Reilly WT, Riley LB, et al. The role of sentinel lymph node mapping in staging of colon and rectal cancer. *Dis Colon Rectum* 2001;44:850.

254. Everett WG, Friend PJ, Forty J. Comparison of stapling and hand-suture for left-sided large bowel anastomosis. *Br J Surg* 1986;73:345.

255. Fabian TC, Mangiante EC, Boldreghini SJ. Prophylactic antibiotics for elective colorectal surgery or operation for obstruction of the small bowel: a comparison of cefonicid and cefoxitin. *Rev Infect Dis* 1984;6:896.

256. Fagniez P-L, Hay JM, Lacine F, et al. Abdominal midline incision closure: a multicentric randomized prospective trial of 3,135 patients, comparing continuous versus interrupted polyglycolic acid sutures. *Arch Surg* 1985;120:1351.

257. Fansler RF, Mero K, Steinberg SM, et al. Utility of the biogfragmentable anastomotic ring in traumatic small-bowel injury. *Am Surg* 1994;60:379.

258. Fantani GA, De Cosse JJ. Surveillance strategies after resection of carcinoma of the colon and rectum. *Surg Gynecol Obstet* 1990;171:267.

259. Fearon ER, Cho KR, Nigro JM, et al. Identification of a chromosome 18q gene that is altered in colorectal cancers. *Science* 1990;247:49.

260. Feldman PS. Ulcerative disease of the colon proximal to partially obstructive lesions: report of two cases and review of the literature. *Dis Colon Rectum* 1975;8:601.

261. Felix EL, Cohen MH, Bernstein AD, et al. Adult intussusception: case report of recurrent intussusception and review of the literature. *Am J Surg* 1976;131:758.

262. Fernando N, Hurwitz H. Inhibition of vascular endothelial growth factor in the treatment of colorectal cancer. *Semin Oncol* 2003;30[Suppl 6]:39.

263. Fielding LP. Clinical-pathologic staging of large-bowel cancer: a report of the ASCRS Committee. *Dis Colon Rectum* 1988;31:204.

264. Fielding LP. The portal vein and colorectal cancer. *Br J Surg* 1988;75:402.

265. Fielding LP, Stewart-Brown S, Blesovsky L. Large-bowel obstruction caused by cancer: a prospective study. *BMJ* 1979;2:515.

266. Finlay IG, McArdle CS. Occult hepatic metastases in colorectal carcinoma. *Br J Surg* 1986;73:732.

267. Finlay IG, Meek D, Brunton F, et al. Growth rate of hepatic metastases in colorectal carcinoma. *Br J Surg* 1988;75:641.

268. Fisher ER, Robinsky B, Sass R, et al. Relative prognostic value of the Dukes and the Jass systems in rectal cancer: findings from the National Surgical Adjuvant Breast and Bowel Projects (Protocol R-01). *Dis Colon Rectum* 1989;32:944.

269. Fisher ER, Sass R, Palekar A, et al. Dukes' classification revisited: findings from the National Surgical Adjuvant Breast and Bowel Projects (Protocol R-01). *Cancer* 1989;64:2354.

270. Fisher ER, Turnbull RB Jr. The cytologic demonstration and significance of tumor cells in the mesenteric venous blood in patients with colorectal carcinoma. *Surg Gynecol Obstet* 1955;100:102.

271. Fleiszer D, MacFarlane J, Murray D, et al. Protective effect of dietary fibre against chemically induced bowel tumours in rats. *Lancet* 1978;2:552.

272. Fleites RA, Marshall JB, Eckhauser ML, et al. The efficacy of polyethylene glycol-electrolyte lavage solution versus traditional mechanical bowel preparation for elective colonic surgery: a randomized, prospective, blinded clinical trial. *Surgery* 1985;98:708.

273. Forde KA, McLarty A, Tsai J, et al. Murphy's button revisited: clinical experience with the biofragmentable anastomotic ring. *Ann Surg* 1993;217:78.

274. Fork F-T. Radiographic findings in overlooked colon carcinomas. *Acta Radiol* 1988;29:331.

275. Fortner JG. Recurrence of colorectal cancer after hepatic resection. *Am J Surg* 1988;155:378.

276. Fortner JG, Kim DK, Barrett MK, et al. Eight years' experience with surgical management of 321 patients with liver tumors. In: Fox BW, ed. *Advances in medical oncology research and education: Basis for cancer therapy I*, vol 5. Oxford: Pergamon Press, 1979:257.

277. Foster JH. Survival after liver resection for secondary tumors. *Am J Surg* 1978;135:389.

278. Foster JH, Berman M. *Solid liver tumors.* Philadelphia: WB Saunders, 1977.

279. Foster ME, Johnson CD, Billings PJ, et al. Intraoperative antegrade lavage and anastomotic healing in acute colonic obstruction. *Dis Colon Rectum* 1986;29:255.

280. Fowler DL, White SA. Laparoscopy-assisted sigmoid resection. *Surg Laparosc Endosc* 1991;1:183.

281. Fraser I. An historical perspective on mechanical aids in intestinal anastomosis. *Surg Gynecol Obstet* 1982;155:566.

282. Frazee RC, Roberts J, Symmonds R, et al. Prospective, randomized trial of inpatient versus outpatient bowel preparation for elective colorectal surgery. *Dis Colon Rectum* 1992; 35:223.

283. Freeny PC, Marks WM, Ryan JA, et al. Colorectal carcinoma evaluation with CT: preoperative staging and detection of postoperative recurrence. *Radiology* 1986;158:347.

284. Friend PJ, Scott R, Everett WG, et al. Stapling or suturing for anastomoses of the left side of the large intestine. *Surg Gynecol Obstet* 1990;171:373.

285. Fuchs CS, Giovannucci EL, Colditz GA, et al. A prospective study of family history and the risk of colorectal cancer. *N Engl J Med* 1994;331:1669.

286. Fujimoto S, Miyazaki M, Kitsukawa Y, et al. Long-term survivors of colorectal cancer with unresectable hepatic metastases. *Dis Colon Rectum* 1985;28:588.

287. Gabrielsson N, Grangvist S, Ohlsn H. Recurrent carcinoma of the colon in the anastomosis diagnosed by roentgen examination and colonoscopy. *Endoscopy* 1976;8:47.

288. Galandiuk S, Wieand HS, Moertel CG. Patterns of recurrence after curative resection of carcinoma of the colon and rectum. *Surg Gynecol Obstet* 1992;174:27.

289. Gall FP, Altendorf JT. Multivisceral resections in colorectal cancer. *Dis Colon Rectum* 1987;30:337.

290. Gambee LP. Single-layer open intestinal anastomosis applicable to small as well as large intestine. *West J Surg* 1951;59:1.

291. García-Olmo D, Ontañón J, García-Olmo DC, et al. Experimental evidence does not support use of the "no-touch" isolation technique in colorectal cancer. *Dis Colon Rectum* 1999;42:1449.

292. Gastrointestinal Tumor Study Group. Adjuvant therapy of colon cancer: results of a prospectively randomized trial. *N Engl J Med* 1984;310:737.

293. Gennaro AR, Tyson RR. Obstructive colonic cancer. *Dis Colon Rectum* 1978;21:346.

294. Geoghegan JG, Scheele J. Treatment of colorectal liver metastases. *Br J Surg* 1999;86:158.

295. George ML, Dzik-Jurasz ASK, Padhani AR, et al. Non-invasive methods of assessing angiogenesis and their value in predicting response to treatment in colorectal cancer. *Br J Surg* 2001;88:1628.

296. Gervaz P, Bouzourene H, Cerottini J-P, et al. Dukes B Colorectal cancer: distinct genetic categories and clinical outcome based on proximal or distal tumor location. *Dis Colon Rectum* 2001;44:364.

297. Getzen LC, Roe RD, Holloway CI. Comparative study of intestinal anastomotic healing in inverted and everted closures. *Surg Gynecol Obstet* 1966;123:1219.

298. Gianola FJ, Dwyer A, Jones AE, et al. Prospective studies of laboratory and radiologic tests in the management of colon and rectal cancer patients: I. Selection of useful preoperative tests through an analysis of surgically occult metastases. *Dis Colon Rectum* 1984;27:811.

299. Gilbertsen VA. Improving the prognosis for patients with intestinal cancer. *Surg Gynecol Obstet* 1967;124:1253.

300. Gilbertsen VA. The earlier diagnosis of adenocarcinoma of the large intestine: a report of 1,884 cases, including 5-year follow-up survival data, results of surgery for the disease, and effect on survival prognosis of treatment earlier in the development of the disease. *Cancer* 1971;27:143.

301. Gilbertsen VA. Proctosigmoidoscopy and polypectomy in reducing the incidence of rectal cancer. *Cancer* 1974;34 [Suppl]:936.

302. Gilbertsen VA. The detection of colorectal cancers. Paper presented at the International Symposium on Colorectal Cancer, New York, March 1979.

303. Gilbertsen VA, Williams SE, Schuman L, et al. Colonoscopy in the detection of carcinoma of the intestine. *Surg Gynecol Obstet* 1979;149:877.

304. Gilchrist RK, David VC. A consideration of pathological factors influencing 5 year survival in radical resection of the large bowel and rectum for carcinoma. *Ann Surg* 1947;126:421.

305. Giovannucci E, Egan KM, Hunter DJ, et al. Aspirin and the risk of colorectal cancer in women. *N Engl J Med* 1995;333:609.

306. Giovannucci E, Rimm E, Stampfer M, et al. Aspirin use and the risks for colorectal cancer and adenoma in male health professionals. *Ann Intern Med* 1994; 121:241.

307. Glass RL, Smith LE, Cochran RC. Subtotal colectomy for obstructing carcinoma of the left colon. *Am J Surg* 1983; 145:335.

308. Glenn F, McSherry CK. Obstruction and perforation in colorectal cancer. *Ann Surg* 1971;173:983.

309. Glover C, Douse P, Kane P, et al. Accuracy of investigations for asymptomatic colorectal liver metastases. *Dis Colon Rectum* 2002;45:476.

310. Go VLW. Carcinoembryonic antigen: clinical application. *Cancer* 1976;37:562.

311. Gold P, Freedman SO. Demonstration of tumor-specific antigens in human colonic carcinomata by immunological tolerance and absorption techniques. *J Exp Med* 1965; 121:439.

312. Gold P, Freedman SO. Specific carcinoembryonic antigens of the human digestive system. *J Exp Med* 1965;122:467.

313. Goldberg RN, Sargent DJ, Morton RF, et al. A randomized controlled trial of fluorouracil plus leucovorin, irinotecan, and oxaliplatin combinations in patients with previously untreated metastatic colorectal cancer. *J Clin Oncol* 2004; 22: 23.

314. Goldenberg DM, DeLand FH, Kim E, et al. Use of radiolabeled antibodies to carcinoembryonic antigen for the detection and localization of diverse cancers by external photoscanning. *N Engl J Med* 1978;298:1384.

315. Goldenberg DM, Kim EE, Bennett SJ, et al. Carcinoembryonic antigen radioimmunodetection in the evaluation of colorectal cancer and in the detection of occult neoplasms. *Gastroenterology* 1983;84:524.

316. Goldenberg DM, Kim EE, DeLand FH, et al. Radioimmunodetection of cancer with radioactive antibodies to carcinoembryonic antigen. *Cancer Res* 1980;40:2984.

317. Goldstein SD, Salvati EP, Rubin RJ, et al. Tube cecostomy with cecal extraperitonealization in the management of obstructing left-sided carcinoma of the large intestine. *Surg Gynecol Obstet* 1986;162:379.

318. Goligher JC. The Dukes' A, B and C categorization of the extent of spread of carcinomas of the rectum. *Surg Gynecol Obstet* 1976;143:793.

319. Goligher JC. Use of circular stapling gun with peranal insertion of anorectal purse-string suture for construction of very low colorectal or coloanal anastomoses. *Br J Surg* 1979;66:501.

320. Goligher JC, Irvin TT, Johnston ID, et al. A controlled clinical trial of three methods of closure of laparotomy wound. *Br J Surg* 1975;62:823.

321. Goligher JC, Lee PWR, Macfie J, et al. Experience with the Russian Model 249 suture gun for anastomosis of the rectum. *Surg Gynecol Obstet* 1979;148:517.

322. Goligher JC, Morris C, McAdam WAF, et al. A controlled trial of inverting versus everting intestinal suture in clinical large-bowel surgery. *Br J Surg* 1970;57:817.

323. Gonzalez EC, Roetzheim RG, Ferrante JM, et al. Predictors of proximal vs. distal colorectal cancer. *Dis Colon Rectum* 2001;44:251.

324. Goodman D, Irvin TT. Delay in the diagnosis and prognosis of carcinoma of the right colon. *Br J Surg* 1993;80:1327.

325. Goslin R, Steele G, Zamcheck N, et al. Factors influencing survival in patients with hepatic metastases from adenocarcinoma of the colon or rectum. *Dis Colon Rectum* 1982;25:749.

326. Gottrup F, Diederich P, Sorensen K, et al. Prophylaxis with whole-gut irrigation and antimicrobials in colorectal surgery. *Am J Surg* 1985;149:317.

327. Gozzetti G, Mazziotti A, Bolundi L, et al. Intraoperative ultrasonography in surgery for liver tumors. *Surgery* 1986; 99:523.

328. Graf E, Easton JW. Dietary suppression of colonic cancer: fiber or phytate? *Cancer* 1985;56:717.

329. Graffner HOL, Alm POA, Oscarson JEA. Prophylactic oophorectomy in colorectal carcinoma. *Am J Surg* 1983; 146:233.

330. Graham JD, Thompson KM, Goldie DJ, et al. The cost-effectiveness of air bags by seating position. *JAMA* 1997; 278:1148.

331. Gramegna A, Saccomani G. On-table colonic irrigation in the treatment of left-sided large-bowel emergencies. *Dis Colon Rectum* 1989;32:585.

332. Gray BN, Walker C. Monitoring of patients with carcinoma of the large intestine by use of acute-phase proteins and carcinoembryonic antigen. *Surg Gynecol Obstet* 1983;156:777.

333. Gray JH. The relation of lymphatic vessels to the spread of cancer. *Br J Surg* 1939;26:462.

334. Gray R, Giantonio BJ, O'Dwyer PJ, et al. The safety of adding angiogenesis inhibition into treatment for colorectal, breast, and lung cancer: the Eastern Cooperative Oncology Group's (ECOG) experience with bevacizumab (anti-VEGF). *Proc ASCO* 2003;22(abst 825).

335. Greegor DH. Occult blood testing for detection of asymptomatic colon cancer. *Cancer* 1971;28:131.

336. Green SE, Chapman PD, Burn J, et al. Clinical impact of colonoscopic screening in first-degree relatives of patients with hereditary non-polyposis colorectal cancer. *Br J Surg* 1995;82:1338.

337. Greenberg E, Baron J, Freeman D, et al. Reduced risks of large bowel adenomas among aspirin users: the Polyp Prevention Study Group. *J Natl Cancer Inst* 1993;85:912.

338. Greene FL. Distribution of colorectal neoplasms. *Am Surg* 1983;49:62.

339. Greene F, Page D, Fleming T, et al. *AJCC cancer staging manual*, 6th ed. New York: Springer-Verlag, 2002.

340. Greenwald P, Korns RF, Nasca PC, et al. Cancer in United States Jews. *Cancer Res* 1975;35:3507.

341. Greenway B. Hepatic metastases from colorectal cancer: resection or not. *Br J Surg* 1988;75:513.

342. Griffith KD, Sugarbaker PH, Change AE. Repeat hepatic resections for colorectal metastases. *Surgery* 1990;107:101.

343. Grinnell RS. The spread of carcinoma of the colon and rectum. *Cancer* 1950;3:641.

344. Grinnell RS. The rationale of subtotal and total colectomy in the treatment of cancer and multiple polyps of the colon. *Surg Gynecol Obstet* 1958;106:288.

345. Grinnell RS. Results of ligation of inferior mesenteric artery at the aorta in resections of carcinoma of the descending and sigmoid colon and rectum. *Surg Gynecol Obstet* 1965;120:1031.

346. Grinnell RS. Lymphatic block with atypical and retrograde lymphatic metastasis and spread in carcinoma of the colon and rectum. *Ann Surg* 1966;163:272.

347. Gross L. Incidence of appendectomies and tonsillectomies in cancer patients. *Cancer* 1966;19:849.

348. Grosser N, Thomson DMP. Cell-mediated anti-tumor immunity in breast cancer patients evaluated by antigen-induced leukocyte adherence inhibition in test tubes. *Cancer Res* 1975;35:2571.

349. Gryfe R, Kim H, Hsieh ETK, et al. Tumor microsatellite instability and clinical outcome in young patients with colorectal cancer. *N Engl J Med* 2000;342:69.

350. Gryska PvR, Cohen AM. Screening asymptomatic patients at high risk for colon cancer with full colonoscopy. *Dis Colon Rectum* 1987;30:18.

351. Gu J, Zhao J, Li Z, et al. Clinical application of radioimmunoguided surgery in colorectal cancer using ^{125}I-labeled carcinoembryonic antigen-specific monoclonal antibody submucosally. *Dis Colon Rectum* 2003;46:1659.

352. Guillem JG, Forde KA, Treat MR, et al. Colonoscopic screening for neoplasms in asymptomatic first-degree relatives of colon cancer patients: a controlled, prospective study. *Dis Colon Rectum* 1992;35:523.

353. Guillem JG, Neugut AI, Forde KA, et al. Colonic neoplasms in asymptomatic first-degree relatives of colon cancer patients. *Am J Gastroenterol* 1988;83:271.

354. Gullichsen R, Havia T, Ovaska J, et al. Colonic anastomosis using the biofragmentable anastomotic ring and manual suture: a prospective, randomized study. *Br J Surg* 1992;79:578.

355. Gullichsen R, Ovaska J, Havia T, et al. What happens to the Valtrac anastomosis of the colon? A follow-up study. *Dis Colon Rectum* 1993;36:362.

356. Gunderson LL, Cohen AM, Welch CE. Interaction of surgery and radiotherapy. *Am J Surg* 1980;139:518.

357. Gunderson LL, Sosin H. Areas of failure found at reoperation (second or symptomatic look) following "curative surgery" for adenocarcinoma of the rectum: clinicopathologic correlation and implications for adjuvant therapy. *Cancer* 1974;34:1278.

358. Gutherman JU, Mavligit GM, Blumenshein G, et al. Immunotherapy of human solid tumors with Bacillus Calmette-Guérin: prolongation of disease-free interval and survival in malignant melanoma, breast and colorectal cancer. *Ann N Y Acad Sci* 1976;277:135.

359. Guy RJ, Handa A, Traill Z, et al. Rectosigmoid carcinoma at previous uterosigmoidostomy in a renal transplant patient. *Dis Colon Rectum* 2001;44:1534.

360. Haddad FS, Manne RK. Involvement of the penis by rectocolic adenocarcinoma: report of a case and review of the literature. *Dis Colon Rectum* 1987;30:123.

361. Haenszel W. Cancer mortality among the foreign-born in the United States. *J Natl Cancer Inst* 1961;26:37.

362. Haenszel W. Cancer mortality among U.S. Jews. *Isr J Med Sci* 1971;7:1437.

363. Haenszel W, Berg JW, Segi M, et al. Large-bowel cancer in Hawaiian Japanese. *J Natl Cancer Inst* 1973;51:1765.

364. Haenszel W, Correa P. Cancer of the colon and rectum and adenomatous polyps: a review of epidemiological findings. *Cancer* 1971;28:14.

365. Haenszel W, Correa P, Cuello C. Social class in differences among patients with large-bowel cancer in Cali, Colombia. *J Natl Cancer Inst* 1975;54:1031.

366. Haenszel W, Dawson EA. A note on the mortality from cancer of the colon and rectum in the United States. *Cancer* 1965;18:265.

367. Haenszel W, Kurihara M. Studies of Japanese migrants. I. Mortality from cancer and other diseases among Japanese in the United States. *J Natl Cancer Inst* 1968;40:43.

368. Hafstrm L, Rudenstam C-M, Domellf, et al. A randomized trial of oral 5-fluorouracil versus placebo as adjuvant therapy in colorectal cancer Dukes' B and C: results after 5 years' observation time. *Br J Surg* 1985;72:138.

369. Halevy A, Levi J, Orda R. Emergency subtotal colectomy: a new trend for treatment of obstructing carcinoma of the left colon. *Ann Surg* 1989;210:220.

370. Hall NR, Bishop DT, Stephenson BM, et al. Hereditary susceptibility to colorectal cancer: relatives of early-onset

cases are particularly at risk. *Dis Colon Rectum* 1996;39: 739.

371. Hall NR, Finan PJ, Ward B, et al. Genetic susceptibility to colorectal cancer in patients under 45 years of age. *Br J Surg* 1994;81:1485.

372. Halsted WS. Circular suture of the intestine: an experimental study. *Am J Med Sci* 1887;94:436.

373. Halsted WS. Intestinal anastomosis. *Bull Johns Hopkins Hosp* 1891;2:1.

374. Hamilton JE. Reappraisal of open intestinal anastomoses. *Ann Surg* 1967;165:917.

375. Hammond EC. Smoking in relation to the death rates of one million men and women. *Natl Cancer Inst Monogr* 1966;19:127.

376. Handelsman JC, Zeiler S, Coleman J, et al. Experience with ambulatory preoperative bowel preparation at the Johns Hopkins Hospital. *Arch Surg* 1993;128:441.

377. Haney MJ, McGarity WC. Ureterosigmoidostomy and neoplasms of the colon: report of a case and review of the literature. *Arch Surg* 1971;103:69.

378. Hansen P, Scuffham PA. Cost-effectiveness of compulsory bicycle helmets in New Zealand. *Aust J Pub Health* 1995; 19:450.

379. Hardcastle JD, Pye G. Screening for colorectal cancer: a critical review. *World J Surg* 1989;13:38.

380. Hardy TG Jr, Aguilar PS, Stewart WRC. Complete obstruction of the sigmoid colon treated by primary resection and anastomosis: an improved technique (preliminary report): report of three cases. *Dis Colon Rectum* 1989;32:528.

381. Hardy TG Jr, Aguilar PS, Stewart WRC, et al. Initial experience with a biofragmentable ring for sutureless bowel anastomosis. *Dis Colon Rectum* 1987;30:55.

382. Hardy TG Jr, Hartmann RF, Samson RB, et al. Percutaneous intrahepatic chemotherapy via indwelling portal vein catheter and subcutaneous injection reservoir. *Dis Colon Rectum* 1982;25:292.

383. Hardy TG Jr, Pace WG, Maney JW, et al. A biofragmentable ring for sutureless bowel anastomosis. *Dis Colon Rectum* 1985;28:484.

384. Hardy TG Jr, Stewart WRC, Aguilar PS. Prevention of colostomy in partial colonic obstruction by intraoperative rectal tube irrigation. *Dis Colon Rectum* 1985;28:122.

385. Hardy TG Jr, Stewart WRC, Aguilar PS, et al. Biofragmentable ring for sutureless bowel anastomosis: early clinical experience. *Contemp Surg* 1987;31:39.

386. Hares MM, Alexander-Williams J. The effect of bowel preparation on colonic surgery. *World J Surg* 1982;6:175.

387. Harris CGJ, Church JM, Senagore AJ, et al. Factors affecting local recurrence of colonic adenocarcinoma. *Dis Colon Rectum* 2002;45:1029.

388. Harris MT, Laudito A, Waye JD. Colonoscopic features of colonic anastomoses. *Gastrointest Endosc* 1994;40:554.

389. Harrison LB, Enker WE, Anderson LL. High-dose-rate intraoperative radiation therapy for colorectal cancer. *Oncology* 1995;9:679.

390. Hart AR, Wicks ACB, Mayberry JF. Colorectal cancer screening in asymptomatic populations. *Gut* 1995;36:590.

391. Hartsell PA, Frazee RC, Harrison JB, et al. Early postoperative feeding after elective colorectal surgery. *Arch Surg* 1997;132:518.

392. Hase K, Shatney C, Johnson D, et al. Prognostic value of tumor "budding" in patients with colorectal cancer. *Dis Colon Rectum* 1993;36:627.

393. Hatziandreu EJ, Sacks JJ, Brown R, et al. The cost-effectiveness of three programs to increase use of bicycle helmets among children. *Public Health Rep* 1995;110:251.

394. Heald RJ, Leicester RJ. The low stapled anastomosis. *Br J Surg* 1981;68:333.

395. Heald RJ, Lockhart-Mummery HE. The lesion of the second cancer of the large bowel. *Br J Surg* 1972;59:16.

396. Healey JE Jr, McBride CM, Gallagher HS. Bowel anastomosis by inverting and everting techniques. *J Surg Res* 1967;7:299.

397. Heiken JP, Weyman PJ, Lee JKT, et al. Detection of focal hepatic masses: prospective evaluation with CT, delayed CT, CT during arterial portography, and MR imaging. *Radiology* 1989;171:47.

398. Heimann TM, Martinelli G, Szporn A, et al. Prognostic significance of DNA content abnormalities in young patients with colorectal cancer. *Ann Surg* 1989;210:792.

399. Helfand M, Marton KI, Zimmer-Gembeck MJ, et al. History of visible rectal bleeding in a primary care population: initial assessment and 10-year follow-up. *JAMA* 1997; 277:44.

400. Hemming AW, Scudamore CH, Davidson A, et al. Evaluation of 50 consecutive segmental hepatic resections. *Am J Surg* 1993;165:621.

401. Herberman RB. Immunologic approaches to the diagnosis of cancer. *Cancer* 1976;37:549.

402. Herbst CA Jr, Sessions JT, Lapis JL. Fiberoptic colonoscopic examination in surgical patients with colorectal cancer. *South Med J* 1980;73:548.

403. Herrera-Ornelas L, Natarajan N, Tsukada Y, et al. Adenocarcinoma of the colon masquerading as primary ovarian neoplasia: an analysis of ten cases. *Dis Colon Rectum* 1983;26:377.

404. Hersh EM, Gutterman JU, Mavligit GM, et al. BCG vaccine and its derivatives: potential, practical considerations, and precautions in human cancer immunotherapy. *JAMA* 1976; 235:246.

405. Herter FP, Slanetz CE Jr. Preoperative intestinal preparation in relation to the subsequent development of cancer at the suture line. *Surg Gynecol Obstet* 1968;127:49.

406. Hertz RE, Deddish MR, Day E. Value of periodic examinations in detecting cancer of the rectum and colon. *Postgrad Med* 1960;27:290.

407. Higginson J. Etiological factors in gastrointestinal cancer in man. *J Natl Cancer Inst* 1966;37:527.

408. Higginson J. Etiology of gastrointestinal cancer in man. *Natl Cancer Inst Monogr* 1967;25:191.

409. Higginson J, Oettle AG. Cancer incidence in the Bantu and "Cape Colored" races of South Africa: report of a cancer survey for the Transvaal (1953–1955). *J Natl Cancer Inst* 1960;24:589.

410. Hill MJ, Drasar BS, Aries V, et al. Bacteria and aetiology of cancer of large bowel. *Lancet* 1971;1:95.

411. Hitchcock CL. Radioimmunoguided surgery and the staging of colorectal carcinoma. *Semin Colon Rectal Surg* 1995; 6:207.

412. Hoffmann J, Jensen H-E. Tube cecostomy and staged resection for obstructing carcinoma of the left colon. *Dis Colon Rectum* 1984;27:24.

413. Hoffmann J, Shokouh-Amiri M, Damm P, et al. A prospective, controlled study of prophylactic drainage after colonic anastomoses. *Dis Colon Rectum* 1987;30: 449.

414. Hohenberger P, Schlag PM, Gerneth T, et al. Pre- and postoperative carcinoembryonic antigen determinations in hepatic resection for colorectal metastases: predictive value and implications for adjuvant treatment based on multivariate analysis. *Ann Surg* 1994;219:135.

415. Holt RW, Nauta RJ, Lee TC, et al. Intraoperative interstitial therapy for hepatic metastases from colorectal carcinomas. *Am Surg* 1988;54:231.

416. Holte K, Kehlet H. Postoperative ileus: a preventable event. *Br J Surg* 2000;87:1480.

417. Horowitz J, Tessier J, Rodriguez-Bigas M, et al. Sigmoid carcinoma presenting in an inguinal hernia sac. *Contemp Surg* 1995;47:78.

418. Houblers JGA, Brand A, van de Watering LMG, et al. Randomised controlled trial comparing transfusion of leucocyte-depleted or buffy-coat-depleted blood in surgery for colorectal cancer. *Lancet* 1994;344:573.

419. Houlston RS, Murdey V, Harocopos C, et al. Screening and genetic counselling for relatives of patients with colorectal cancer in a family cancer clinic. *BMJ* 1990;301:366.

420. Howard ML, Greene FL. The effect of preoperative endoscopy on recurrence and survival following surgery for colorectal carcinoma. *Am Surg* 1990;56:124.

421. Howell MA. Factor analysis of international cancer mortality data and per capita food consumption. *Br J Cancer* 1974;29:328.

422. Howell MA. Diet as an etiological factor in the development of cancer of the colon and rectum. *J Chronic Dis* 1975;28:67.

423. Howie JGR, Timperley WR. Cancer and appendectomy. *Cancer* 1966;19:1138.

424. Hubens G, Totté E, Verhulst A, et al. The influence of the interaction of sutures with the mucosa on tumour formation at colonic anastomoses in rats. *Eur Surg Res* 1993; 25:213.

425. Hughes ESR, Cuthbertson AM. Subtotal colectomy for obstructing carcinoma of the upper left colon. *Dis Colon Rectum* 1965;8:411.

426. Hughes ESR, McDermott FT, Polglase AL, et al. Total and subtotal colectomy for colonic obstruction. *Dis Colon Rectum* 1985;28:162.

427. Hughes KS, Rosenstein RB, Songhorabodi S, et al. Resection of the liver for colorectal carcinoma metastases: a multi-institutional study of long-term survivors. *Dis Colon Rectum* 1988;31:1.

428. Hughes KS, Simon R, Songhorabodi S, et al. Resection of the liver for colorectal carcinoma metastases: a multi-institutional study of patterns of recurrence. *Surgery* 1986; 100:278.

429. Hunt DR, Cherian M. Endoscopic diagnosis of small flat carcinoma of the colon: report of three cases. *Dis Colon Rectum* 1990;33:143.

430. Hurwitz H, Fehrenbacher L, Cartwright T, et al. Bevacizumab (a monoclonal antibody to vascular endothelial growth factor) prolongs survival in first-line colorectal cancer (CRC): results of a phase III trial of bevacizumab in combination with bolus IRL (irinotecan, 5-fluorouracil, leucovorin) as first line therapy in subjects with metastatic CRC. *Proc ASCO* 2003;23(abst 3646).

431. Hyams L, Wynder EL. Appendectomy and cancer risk: an epidemiological evaluation. *J Chronic Dis* 1968;21:391.

432. Hyder JW, Talbott TM, Maycroft TC. A critical review of chemical lymph node clearance and staging of colon and rectal cancer at Ferguson Hospital, 1977 to 1982. *Dis Colon Rectum* 1990;33:923.

433. Ike H, Shimada H, Ohki S, et al. Results of aggressive resection of lung metasases from colorectal carcinoma detected by intensive follow-up. *Dis Colon Rectum* 2002;45: 468.

434. Irvin TT. Prognosis of colorectal cancer in the elderly. *Br J Surg* 1988;75:419.

435. Irvin TT, Greaney MG. Duration of symptoms and prognosis of carcinoma of the colon and rectum. *Surg Gynecol Obstet* 1977;144:883.

436. Irvin T, Vowles KDJ, Golby MG. Fluorouracil in chemoprophylaxis of colorectal cancer: results of a controlled clinical trial. *Dis Colon Rectum* 1986;29:704.

437. Isler JT, Brown PC, Lewis FG, et al. The role of preoperative colonoscopy in colorectal cancer. *Dis Colon Rectum* 1987;30:435.

438. Itoh H, Houlston RS, Harocopos C, et al. Risk of cancer death in first-degree relatives of patients with hereditary non-polyposis cancer syndrome (Lynch type II): a study of 130 kindreds in the United Kingdom. *Br J Surg* 1990; 77:1367.

439. Itzkowitz SH, Kim YS. New carbohydrate tumor markers [Editorial]. *Gastroenterology* 1986;92:491.

440. Iwatsuki S, Esquivel CO, Gordon RD, et al. Liver resection for metastatic colorectal cancer. *Surgery* 1986;100:804.

441. Jacobs, Verdeja JC, Goldstein HS. Minimally invasive colon resection (laparoscopic colectomy). *Surg Laparosc Endosc* 1991;1:144.

442. Jagelman DG, Fazio VW, Lavery IC, et al. A prospective, randomized, double-blind study of 10 percent mannitol mechanical bowel preparation, combined with oral neomycin and short-term, perioperative, intravenous Flagyl as prophylaxis in elective colorectal operations. *Surgery* 1985; 98:861.

443. Jain RK. Tumor angiogenesis and accessibility: role of vascular endothelial growth factor. *Semin Oncol* 2002;29 [Suppl 16]:3.

444. Jamison RL, Donohue JH, Nagorney DM, et al. Hepatic resection for metastatic colorectal cancer results in cure for some patients. *Arch Surg* 1997;132:505.

445. Jansen A, Brummelkamp WH, Davies GAG, et al. Clinical applications of magnetic rings in colorectal anastomosis. *Surg Gynecol Obstet* 1981;153:537.

446. Jass JR, Love SB, Northover JMA. A new prognostic classification of rectal cancer. *Lancet* 1987;1:1303.

447. Jayne DG, Fook S, Loi C, et al. Peritoneal carcinomatosis from colorectal cancer. *Br J Surg* 2002;89:1545.

448. Jeekel J. Curative resection of primary colorectal cancer. *Br J Surg* 1986;73:687.

449. Jeekel J. Can radical surgery improve survival in colorectal cancer? *World J Surg* 1987;11:412.

450. Jeffery KM, Harkins B, Cresci GA, et al. The clear liquid diet is no longer a necessity in the routine postoperative management of surgical patients. *Am Surg* 1996;62:167.

451. Jemal A, Tiwari RC, Murray T, et al. Cancer statistics, 2004. *CA Cancer J Clin* 2004;54:8.

452. Jennings WC, Wood CD, Guernsey JM. Continuous postoperative lavage in the treatment of peritoneal sepsis. *Dis Colon Rectum* 1982;25:641.

453. Jensen LS, Andersen A, Fristrup SC, et al. Comparison of one dose versus three doses of prophylactic antibiotics, and the influence of blood transfusion, on infectious complications in acute and elective colorectal surgery. *Br J Surg* 1990;77:513.

454. Jenson CB, Shahon DB, Wangensteen OH. Evaluation of annual examinations in the detection of cancer: special reference to cancer of the gastrointestinal tract, prostate, breast, and female generative tract. *JAMA* 1960;174: 1783.

455. Johansen C, Chow W-H, Jörgensen T, et al. Risk of colorectal cancer and other cancers in patients with gall stones. *Gut* 1996;39:439.

456. Johns LE, Kee F, Collins BJ, et al. Colorectal cancer mortality in first-degree relatives of early-onset colorectal cancer cases. *Dis Colon Rectum* 2002;45:681.

457. Johnson CD, Lamont PM, Orr N, et al. Is a drain necessary after colonic anastomoses? *J R Soc Med* 1989;82:661.

458. Johnson K, Bakhsh A, Young D, et al. Correlating computed tomography and positron emission tomography scan with operative findings in metastatic colorectal cancer. *Dis Colon Rectum* 2001;44:354.

459. Joosten JJA, Strobbe LJA, Wauters CAP, et al. Intraoperative lymphatic mapping and the sentinel node concept in colorectal carcinoma. *Br J Surg* 1999;86:482.

460. Jorgensen T, Rafaelsen S. Gallstones and colorectal cancer: there is a relationship, but it is hardly due to cholecystectomy. *Dis Colon Rectum* 1992;35:24.

461. Juhl G, Larson GM, Mullins R, et al. Six-year results of annual colonoscopy after resection of colorectal cancer. *World J Surg* 1990;14:255.

462. Kahn HA. The Dorn study of smoking and mortality among U.S. veterans: report on eight and one-half years of observation. *Natl Cancer Inst Monogr* 1966;19:1.

463. Kaibara N, Wakatsuki T, Mizusawa K, et al. Negative correlation between cholecystectomy and the subsequent development of large-bowel carcinoma in a low-risk Japanese population. *Dis Colon Rectum* 1986;29:644.

464. Kameyama M, Fukuda I, Imaoka S, et al. Level of serum gastrin as a predictor of liver metastasis from colorectal cancer. *Dis Colon Rectum* 1993;36:497.

465. Kanellos I, Demetriades H, Zintzaras E, et al. Incidence and prognostic value of positive peritoneal cytology in colorectal cancer. *Dis Colon Rectum* 2003;46:535.

466. Kanemitsu Y, Kato T, Hirai T, et al. Survival after curative resection for mucinous adenocarcinoma of the colorectum. *Dis Colon Rectum* 2003;46:160.

467. Karl RC, Morse SS, Halpert RD, et al. Preoperative evaluation of patients for liver resection: appropriate CT imaging. *Ann Surg* 1993;217:226.

468. Karlsson S, Jonsson K, Rosengren J-E, et al. Angiography in colonic carcinoma. *Dis Colon Rectum* 1984;27:648.

469. Kee F, Collins BJ. How prevalent is cancer family syndrome? *Gut* 1991;32:509.

470. Kehlet H, Holte K. Review of postoperative ileus. *Am J Surg* 2001;182(Suppl Nov):3S.

471. Kehlet H, Mogensen T. Hospital stay of 2 days after open sigmoidectomy with a multimodal rehabilitation programme. *Br J Surg* 1999;86:227.

472. Kell MR, Winter DC, O'Sullivan GC, et al. Biological behaviour and clinical implications of micrometastases. *Br J Surg* 2000;87:1629.

473. Keidan RD, Fanning J, Gatenby RA, et al. Recurrent typhlitis: a disease resulting from aggressive chemotherapy. *Dis Colon Rectum* 1989;32:206.

474. Kemeny N, Daly J, Reichman B, et al. Intrahepatic or systemic infusion of fluorodeoxyuridine in patients with liver metastases from colorectal carcinoma: a randomized trial. *Ann Intern Med* 1987;107:459.

475. Kerner BA, Oliver GC, Eisenstat TE, et al. Is preoperative computerized tomography useful in assessing patients with colorectal carcinoma? *Dis Colon Rectum* 1993;36:1050.

476. Kewenter J, Brevinge H, Engarås B, et al. Follow-up after screening for colorectal neoplasms with fecal occult blood testing in a controlled trial. *Dis Colon Rectum* 1994;37:115.

477. Kewenter J, Engars B, Haglind E, et al. Value of retesting subjects with a positive hemoccult in screening for colorectal cancer. *Br J Surg* 1990;77:1349.

478. Khoury GA, Waxman BP. Large-bowel anastomoses. I. The healing process and sutured anastomoses: a review. *Br J Surg* 1983;70:61.

479. Khubchandani IT, Karamchandani MC, Kleckner FS, et al. Mass screening for colorectal cancer. *Dis Colon Rectum* 1989;32:754.

480. Kiefer PJ, Thorson AG, Christensen MA. Metachronous colorectal cancer: time interval to presentation of a metachronous cancer. *Dis Colon Rectum* 1986;29:378.

481. Kim JA, Triozzi PL, Martin EW Jr. Radioimmunoguided surgery for colorectal cancer. *Oncology* 1993;7:55.

482. Kirklin JW, Dockerty MB, Waugh JM. Role of peritoneal reflection in prognosis of carcinoma of rectum and sigmoid colon. *Surg Gynecol Obstet* 1949;88:326.

483. Kitagawa Y, Watanabe M, Hasegawa H, et al. Sentinel node mapping for colorectal cancer with radioactive tracer. *Dis Colon Rectum* 2002;45:1476.

484. Klatt GR, Martin WH, Gillespie JT. Subtotal colectomy with primary anastomosis without diversion in the treatment of obstructing carcinoma of the left colon. *Am J Surg* 1981;141:577.

485. Klaue P, Eckert P, Kern E. Incidental splenectomy: early and late postoperative complications. *Am J Surg* 1979;138:296.

486. Kline RS, Catalano MT, Edberg SC, et al. *Streptococcus bovis* septicemia and carcinoma of the colon. *Ann Intern Med* 1979;91:560.

487. Ko F-C, Liu JM, Chen W-S, et al. Risk and patterns of brain metastases in colorectal cancer: 27-year experience. *Dis Colon Rectum* 1999;42:1467.

488. Köhler L, Eypasch E, Paul A, Troidl H. Myths in management of colorectal malignancy. *Br J Surg* 1997;84:248.

489. Kokal WA, Duda RB, Azumi N, et al. Tumor DNA content in primary and metastatic colorectal carcinoma. *Arch Surg* 1986;121:1434.

490. Kokal WA, Gardine RL, Sheibani K, et al. Tumor DNA content in resectable, primary colorectal carcinoma. *Ann Surg* 1989;209:188.

491. Kokal W, Sheibani K, Terz J, Harada JR. Tumor DNA content in the prognosis of colorectal carcinoma. *JAMA* 1986;255:3123.

492. Komuta K, Okudaira S, Haraguchi M, et al. Identification of extracapsular invasion of the metastatic lymph nodes as a useful prognostic sign in patients with resectable colorectal cancer. *Dis Colon Rectum* 2001;44:1838

493. Koren R, Siegal A, Klein B, et al. Lymph node-revealing solution: simple new method for detecting minute lymph nodes in colon carcinoma. *Dis Colon Rectum* 1997;40:407.

494. Kortz WJ, Meyers WC, Hanks JB, et al. Hepatic resection for metastatic cancer. *Ann Surg* 1984;199:182.

495. Koruth NM, Krukowski ZH, Youngson GG, et al. Intraoperative colonic irrigation in the management of left-sided large-bowel emergencies. *Br J Surg* 1985;72:708.

496. Koshiji M, Yonekura Y, Saito T, et al. Microsatellite analysis of fecal DNA for colorectal cancer detection. *J Surg Oncol* 2002;80:34.

497. Kriwanek S, Armbruster C, Dittrich K, et al. Perforated colorectal cancer. *Dis Colon Rectum* 1996;39:1409.

498. Kronborg O, Hage F, Deichgraeber E. The remaining colon after radical surgery for colorectal cancer: the first three years of a prospective study. *Dis Colon Rectum* 1983;26:172.

499. Kuhn JA, Corbisiero RM, Buras RR, et al. Intraoperative gamma detection probe with presurgical antibody imaging in colon cancer. *Arch Surg* 1991;126:1398.

500. Kwok SPY, Varma JS, Li AKC. Quicker intraoperative colonic irrigation. *Br J Surg* 1989;76:604.

501. Labow SB, Hoexter B, Walrath DC. Colonic adenocarcinomas in patients with ureterosigmoidostomies. *Dis Colon Rectum* 1979;22:157.

502. Landercasper J, Stolee RT, Steenlage E, et al. Treatment and outcome of right colon cancers adherent to adjacent organs or the abdominal wall. *Arch Surg* 1992;127:841.

503. Lanfranco of Milan. *Science of chirurgerie*. Fleischhaker R, trans. London: Early English Text Society, Kegan Paul, Trench, Trubner and Co, 1894.

504. Langevin JM, Nivatvongs S. The true incidence of synchronous cancer of the large bowel. *Am J Surg* 1984;147:330.

505. Langevin JM, Rothenberger DA, Goldberg SM. Accidental splenic injury during surgical treatment of the colon and rectum. *Surg Gynecol Obstet* 1984;159:139.

506. Lanspa SJ, Lynch HT, Smyrk TC, et al. Colorectal adenomas in the Lynch syndrome. *Gastroenterology* 1990;98:1117.

507. Lanspa SJ, Smyrk TC, Lynch HT. The colonoscopist and the Lynch syndromes. *Gastrointest Endosc* 1990;36:156.

508. Larkin GL, Weber JE. Cost-effectiveness of air bags in motor vehicles. *JAMA* 1998;279:506.

509. Larson GM, Bond SJ, Shallcross C, et al. Colonoscopy after curative resection of colorectal cancer. *Arch Surg* 1986;121:535.

510. Lau WY, Chu KW, Poon GP, et al. Prophylactic antibiotics in elective colorectal surgery. *Br J Surg* 1988;75:782.

511. Laurie JA, Moertel CG, Fleming TR, et al. Surgical adjuvant therapy of large-bowel carcinoma: an evaluation of levamisole and the combination of levamisole and fluorouracil. *J Clin Oncol* 1989;7:1447.

512. Lautenbach E, Forde KA, Neugut AI. Benefits of colonoscopic surveillance after curative resection of colorectal cancer. *Ann Surg* 1994;220:206.

513. Law WL, Choi HK, Chu KW. Comparison of stenting with emergency surgery as palliative treatment for obstructing primary left-sided colorectal cancer. *Br J Surg* 2001;90:1429.

514. Law WL, Choi HK, Lee YM, et al. Palliation for advanced malignant colorectal obstruction by self-expanding metallic stents: prospective evaluation of outcomes. *Dis Colon Rectum* 2004;47:31.

515. Lawes DA, SenGupta SB, Boulos PB. Pathogenesis and clinical management of hereditary non-polyposis colorectal cancer. *Br J Surg* 2002;89:1357.

516. Le TH, Gathright JB Jr. Reconstitution of intestinal continuity after extended left colectomy. *Dis Colon Rectum* 1993;36:197.

517. Leadbetter GW Jr, Zickerman P, Pierce E. Uretero-sigmoidoscopy and carcinoma of the colon. *J Urol* 1979;121:732.

518. Lechner P, Lind P, Binter G, et al. Anticarcinoembryonic antigen immunoscintigraphy with a ^{99m}Tc-Fab′ fragment (Immu 4) in primary and recurrent colorectal cancer. *Dis Colon Rectum* 1993;36:930.

519. Lee EC, Roberts PL, Taranto R, et al. Inpatient versus outpatient bowel preparation for elective colorectal surgery. *Dis Colon Rectum* 1996;39:369.

520. Leen E, Angerson WG, Cooke TG, et al. Prognostic power of Doppler perfusion index in colorectal cancer: correlation with survival. *Ann Surg* 1996;223:199.

521. Leggett BA, Cornwell M, Thomas LR, et al. Characteristics of metachronous colorectal carcinoma occurring despite colonoscopic surveillance. *Dis Colon Rectum* 1997;40:603.

522. Lehman JF, Wiseman JS. The effect of epidural analgesia on the return of peristalsis and the length of stay after elective colonic surgery. *Am Surg* 1995;61:1009.

523. Leichman C, Lyman G, Remedios P, et al. Molecular biologic correlates with continuous infusion 5-FU (CIFU) or capecitabine(C) in disseminated colorectal cancer (CRC). *Proc ASCO* 2002;(abst 1720).

524. Lelcuk S, Klausner JM, Merhav A, et al. Endoscopic decompression of acute colonic obstruction: avoiding staged surgery. *Ann Surg* 1986;203:292.

525. Lembert A. Mémoire sur l'enterorrhaphie avec la description d'un procédé nouveau pour pratiquer cette operation chirurgicale. *Rep Gen Anat Physiol Pathol* 1826;2:100.

526. Lemon FR, Walden RT. Death from respiratory system disease among Seventh-Day Adventist men. *JAMA* 1966;198:117.

527. Lemon FR, Walden RT, Woods RW. Cancer of the lung and mouth in Seventh-Day Adventists: preliminary report on a population study. *Cancer* 1964;17:486.

528. Lev Z, Kislitsin D, Rennert G, et al. Utilization of *k*-ras mutations identified in stool DNA for the early detection of colorectal cancer. *J Cell Biochem Suppl* 2000;34:35.

529. Levin B. Screening sigmoidoscopy for colorectal cancer. *N Engl J Med* 1992;326:700.

530. Levin ML, Haenszel W, Carroll BE, et al. Cancer incidence in urban and rural areas of New York State. *J Natl Cancer Inst* 1960;24:1243.

531. Lieberman D. Cost-effectiveness of colon cancer screening. *Am J Gastroenterol* 1991;86:1789.

532. Lieberman DA, Weiss DG, Bond JH, et al. Use of colonoscopy to screen asymptomatic adults for colorectal cancer. *N Engl J Med* 2000;343:162.

533. Lightdale CJ, Sternberg SS, Posner G, et al. Carcinoma complicating Crohn's disease: report of seven cases and review of the literature. *Am J Med* 1975;59:262.

534. Limberg B. Diagnosis and staging of colonic tumors by conventional abdominal sonography as compared with hydrocolonic sonography. *N Engl J Med* 1992;327:65.

535. Lindmark G, Gerdin B, Påhlman L, et al. Prognostic predictors in colorectal cancer. *Dis Colon Rectum* 1994;37:1219.

536. Liu H-P, Yan Z-S, Zhang S-S. The application of leukocyte adherence inhibition assay to patients with colorectal cancer: comparison with serum level of carcinoembryonic antigen and sialic acid. *Dis Colon Rectum* 1989;32:210.

537. Liu SKM, Church JM, Lavery IC, et al. Operation in patients with incurable colon cancer: is it worthwhile? *Dis Colon Rectum* 1997;40:11.

538. Livingstone AS, Hampson LG, Shuster J, et al. Carcinoembryonic antigen in the diagnosis and management of colorectal carcinoma: current status. *Arch Surg* 1974;109:259.

539. Lobbato VJ, Rothenberg RE, LaRaja RD, et al. Coexistence of abdominal aortic aneurysm and carcinoma of the colon: a dilemma. *J Vasc Surg* 1985;2:724.

540. Loeb MJ. Comparative strength of inverted, everted and end-on-intestinal anastomoses. *Surg Gynecol Obstet* 1967;125:301.

541. Logan SE, Meier SJ, Ramming KP. Hepatic resection of metastatic colorectal carcinoma. *Arch Surg* 1982;117:25.

542. Lo Gerfo P, Herter FP. Carcinoembryonic antigen and prognosis in patients with colon cancer. *Ann Surg* 1975;181:81.

543. Lokich J, Ahlgren J, Gullo J, et al. A prospective randomized comparison of continuous infusion fluorouracil with a conventional bolus schedule in metastatic colorectal cancer: a Mid-Atlantic Oncology Program Study. *J Clin Oncol* 1989;7:425.

544. Long RTL, Edwards RH. Implantation metastasis as a cause of local recurrence of colorectal carcinoma. *Am J Surg* 1989;157:194.

545. Love RR, Morrissey JF. Colonoscopy in asymptomatic individuals with a family history of colorectal cancer. *Arch Intern Med* 1984;144:2209.

546. Lovett E. Family studies in cancer of the colon and rectum. *Br J Surg* 1976;63:13.

547. Lucha PA Jr, Rosen L, Olenwine JA, et al. Value of carcinoembryonic antigen monitoring in curative surgery for recurrent colorectal carcinoma. *Dis Colon Rectum* 1997;40:145.

548. Luna-Pérez P, Rodríguez-Ramírez SE, Gutiérez de la Barrera M, et al. Multivisceral resection for colon cancer. *J Surg Oncol* 2002;80:100.

549. Lundstedt C, Ekberg H, Halldorsdottir A, et al. Angiography as diagnostic, prognostic and therapeutic tool in liver metastases from a colorectal primary tumor. *Acta Radiol Diagn* 1985;4:373.

550. Lunniss PJ, Skinner S, Britton KE. Effect of radioimmunoscintigraphy on the management of recurrent colorectal cancer. *Br J Surg* 1998;86:244.

551. Lynch HT. Frequency of hereditary nonpolyposis colorectal carcinoma (Lynch syndromes I and II). *Gastroenterology* 1986;90:486.

552. Lynch HT. The surgeon and colorectal cancer genetics: case identification, surveillance, and management strategies. *Arch Surg* 1990;125:698.

553. Lynch HT, Bronson EK, Strayhorn PC, et al. Genetic diagnosis of Lynch syndrome II in an extended colorectal cancer-prone family. *Cancer* 1990;66:2233.

554. Lynch HT, Ens JA, Lynch JF. The Lynch syndrome II and urological malignancies. *J Urol* 1990;143:24.

555. Lynch HT, Guirgis H, Swartz M, et al. Genetics and colon cancer. *Arch Surg* 1973;106:669.

556. Lynch HT, Kimberling W, Albano WA, et al. Hereditary nonpolyposis colorectal cancer (Lynch syndromes I and II). I. Clinical description of recurrence. *Cancer* 1985;56:934.

557. Lynch HT, Kriegler M, Christiansen TA, et al. Laryngeal carcinoma in a Lynch syndrome II kindred. *Cancer* 1988;62:1007.

558. Lynch HT, Lanspa SJ, Boman BM, et al. Hereditary nonpolyposis colorectal cancer: Lynch syndromes I and II. *Gastroenterol Clin North Am* 1988;17:679.

559. Lynch HT, Lynch J. Genetic predictability and minimal cancer clues in Lynch syndrome II. *Dis Colon Rectum* 1987;30:243.

560. Lynch HT, Paulson J, Severin M, et al. Failure to diagnose hereditary colorectal cancer and its medicolegal implications. *Dis Colon Rectum* 1999;42:31.

561. Lynch HT, Smyrk TC, Lynch PM, et al. Adenocarcinoma of the small bowel in Lynch syndrome II. *Cancer* 1989;64:2178.

562. Lynch HT, Watson P, Lanspa SJ, et al. Natural history of colorectal cancer in hereditary nonpolyposis colorectal cancer (Lynch syndromes I and II). *Dis Colon Rectum* 1988;31:439.

563. Lynch PM, Lynch HT, Harris RE. Hereditary proximal colonic cancer. *Dis Colon Rectum* 1977;20:662.

564. Lyons JL, Klauber MR, Gardner JW, et al. Cancer incidence in Mormons and non-Mormons in Utah, 1966–1970. *N Engl J Med* 1976;294:129.

565. MacDougall IPM. The cancer risk in ulcerative colitis. *Lancet* 1964;2:655.

566. MacGregor AB, Falk RE. Immunotherapy of malignant disease: part 2. *J R Coll Surg Edinb* 1976;21:43.

567. MacGregor AMC. Mucus-secreting adenomatous polyp at the site of ureterosigmoidostomy: a case report and review of the literature. *Br J Surg* 1968;55:591.

568. Mach J-P, Jaeger P, Bertholoet M-M, et al. Detection of recurrence of large-bowel carcinoma by radioimmunoassay of circulating carcinoembryonic antigen (CEA). *Lancet* 1974;2:535.

569. Machi J, Isomoto H, Kurohiji T, et al. Detection of unrecognized liver metastases from colorectal cancers by routine use of operative ultrasonography. *Dis Colon Rectum* 1986; 29:405.

570. Machi J, Isomoto H, Kurohiji T, et al. Accuracy of intraoperative ultrasonography in diagnosing liver metastasis from colorectal cancer: evaluation with postoperative follow-up results. *World J Surg* 1991;15:551.

571. Machi J, Isomoto H, Yamashita Y, et al. Intraoperative ultrasonography in screening for liver metastases from colorectal cancer: comparative accuracy with traditional procedures. *Surgery* 1987;101:678.

572. Machover D, Diaz-Rubio E, de Gramont A, et al. Modulation of fluorouracil by LV in patients with advanced colorectal cancer: evidence in terms of response rate: Advanced Colorectal Cancer Meta-Analysis Project. *J Clin Oncol* 1992;10:896.

573. MacKeigan JM, Ferguson JA. Prophylactic oophorectomy and colorectal cancer in premenopausal patients. *Dis Colon Rectum* 1979;22:401.

574. Macrae F, St John DJB. Hemoccult tests. *Dig Dis Sci* 1987; 32:947.

575. Madlensky L, Bapat B, Redston M, et al. Using genetic information to make surgical decisions: report of a case of a 13-year-old boy with colon cancer. *Dis Colon Rectum* 1997; 40:240.

576. Mainar A, de Gregorio Ariza MA, Tejero E, et al. Acute colorectal obstruction: treatment with self-expandable metal stents before scheduled surgery: results of a multicenter study. *Radiology* 1999;210:65.

577. Mainar A, Tejero E, Maynar M, et al. Colorectal obstruction: treatment with metallic stents. *Radiology* 1996;198: 761.

578. Mäkelä JT, Laitinen SO, Kairaluoma MI. Five-year follow-up after radical surgery for colorectal cancer: results of a prospective randomized trial. *Arch Surg* 1995;130:1062.

579. Malassagne B, Valleur P, Serra J, et al. Relationship of apical lymph node involvement to survival in resected colon carcinoma. *Dis Colon Rectum* 1993;36:645.

580. Malthaner RA, Hakki FZ, Saini N, et al. Anastomotic compression button: a new mechanical device for sutureless bowel anastomosis. *Dis Colon Rectum* 1990;33:291.

581. Manayan RC, Hart MJ, Friend WG. Radioimmunoguided surgery for colorectal cancer. *Am J Surg* 1997;173:386.

582. Mandel JS, Bond JH, Bradley M. Sensitivity, specificity, and positive predictivity of the Hemoccult test in screening for colorectal cancers. *Gastroenterology* 1989;97:597.

583. Mandel JS, Bond JH, Church TR, et al. Reducing mortality from colorectal cancer by screening for fecal occult blood. *N Engl J Med* 1993;328:1365.

584. Mannes GA, Maier A, Thieme C, et al. Relation between the frequency of colorectal adenoma and the serum cholesterol level. *N Engl J Med* 1986;315:1634.

585. Mannes AG, Weinzierl M, Stellaard F, et al. Adenomas of the large intestine after cholecystectomy. *Gut* 1984;25:863.

586. Mapp TJ, Hardcastle JD, Moss SM, et al. Survival of patients with colorectal cancer diagnosed in a randomized controlled trial of faecal occult blood screening. *Br J Surg* 1999;86:1286.

587. Markman M. Intraperitoneal chemotherapy in the management of colon cancer. *Semin Oncol* 1999;26:536.

588. Markowitz A, Saleemi K, Freeman LM. Role of In-111-labeled CYT-103 immunoscintigraphy in the evaluation of patients with recurrent colorectal carcinoma. *Clin Nucl Med* 1993;18:685.

589. Marsh J, Donnan PT, Hamer-Hodges DW. Association between transfusion with plasma and the recurrence of colorectal carcinoma. *Br J Surg* 1990;77:623.

590. Martin EW Jr, Carey LC. Second-look surgery for colorectal cancer: the second time around. *Ann Surg* 1991; 214:321.

591. Martin EW Jr, James KK, Hurtubise PE, et al. The use of CEA as an early indicator for gastrointestinal tumor recurrence and second-look procedures. *Cancer* 1977;39:440.

592. Martin EW Jr, Kibbey WE, DiVecchia L, et al. Carcinoembryonic antigen: clinical and historical aspects. *Cancer* 1976;37:62.

593. Martin EW Jr, Minton JP, Carey LC. CEA-directed second-look surgery in the asymptomatic patient after primary resection of colorectal carcinoma. *Ann Surg* 1985;202:310.

594. Martin EW Jr, Mojzisik CM, Hinkle GH Jr, et al. Radioimmunoguided surgery using monoclonal antibody. *Am J Surg* 1988;156:386.

595. Martinez-Santos C, Lobato RF, Fradejas JM, et al. Self-expandable stent before elective surgery *vs.* emergency surgery for the treatment of malignant colorectal obstructions: comparison of primary anastomosis and morbidity rates. *Dis Colon Rectum* 2002;45:401.

596. Martyak SN, Curtis LW. Abdominal incision and closure, a systems approach. *Am J Surg* 1976;131:476.

597. Mason MH III, Kovalcik PJ. Ovarian metastases from colon carcinoma. *J Surg Oncol* 1981;17:33.

598. Matsui O, Takashima T, Kadoya M, et al. Liver metastases from colorectal cancers: detection with CT during arterial portography. *Radiology* 1987;165:65.

599. Mavligit GM, Burgess MA, Seibert GB, et al. Prolongation of postoperative disease-free interval and survival in human colorectal cancer by B.C.G. or B.C.G plus 5-fluorouracil. *Lancet* 1976;1:171.

600. Max E, Sweeney WB, Bailey HR, et al. Results of 1,000 single-layer continuous polypropylene intestinal anastomoses. *Am J Surg* 1991;162:461.

601. Maxwell JW Jr, Davis WC, Jackson FC. Colon carcinoma and inguinal hernia. *Surg Clin North Am* 1965;45:1165.

602. Mayer, RJ. Moving beyond fluorouracil for colorectal cancer. *N Engl J Med* 2000;343:963.

603. Mayo WJ. The cancer problem. *Lancet* 1915;35:339.

604. McArdle CS, McMillan DC, Hole DJ. Male gender adversely effects survival following surgery for colorectal cancer. *Br J Surg* 2003;90:711.

605. McArdle CS, Morran CG, Pettit L, et al. Value of oral antibiotic prophylaxis in colorectal surgery. *Br J Surg* 1995; 82:1046.

606. McCall JL, Black RB, Rich CA, et al. The value of serum carcinoembryonic antigen in predicting recurrent disease following curative resection of colorectal cancer. *Dis Colon Rectum* 1994;37:875.

607. McCormack PM, Attiyeh FF. Resected pulmonary metastases from colorectal cancer. *Dis Colon Rectum* 1979;22: 553.

608. McCormack PM, Burt ME, Bains MS, et al. Lung resection for colorectal metastases: 10-year results. *Arch Surg* 1992; 127:1403.

609. McCulloch PG, Blamey SL, Finlay IG, et al. A prospective comparison of gentamicin and metronidazole and moxalactam in the prevention of septic complications associated with elective operations of the colon and rectum. *Surg Gynecol Obstet* 1986;162:521.

610. McFarland RJ, Talbot RW, Woolf N, et al. Dysplasia of the colon after jejuno-ileal bypass. *Br J Surg* 1987;74:21.

611. McIntyre A, Gibson PR, Young GP. Butyrate production from dietary fibre and protection against large-bowel cancer in a rat model. *Gut* 1993;34:386.

612. McKenna JP, Currie DJ, MacDonald JA. The use of continuous postoperative peritoneal lavage in the management of diffuse peritonitis. *Surg Gynecol Obstet* 1970;130: 254.

613. McMahon AJ, Auld CD, Dale BAS, et al. *Streptococcus bovis* septicaemia associated with uncomplicated colonic carcinoma. *Br J Surg* 1991;78:883.

614. McMillan DC, Canna K, McArdle CS. Systemic inflammatory response predicts survival following curative resection of colorectal cancer. *Br J Surg* 2003;90:215.

615. McMillan DC, Wotherspoon HA, Fearon KCH, et al. A prospective study of tumor recurrence and acute-phase response after apparently curative colorectal cancer surgery. *Am J Surg* 1995;170:319.

616. McVay JR Jr. The appendix in relation to neoplastic disease. *Cancer* 1964;17:929.

617. Meagher AP, Stuart M. Colonoscopy in patients with a family history of colorectal cancer. *Dis Colon Rectum* 1992; 35:315.

618. Meagher AP, Wolff BG. Right hemicolectomy with a linear cutting stapler. *Dis Colon Rectum* 1994;37:1043.

619. Mecklin J-P, Järvinen HJ. Clinical features of colorectal carcinoma in cancer family syndrome. *Dis Colon Rectum* 1986;29:160.

620. Mecklin J-P, Järvinen H. Treatment and follow-up strategies in hereditary nonpolyposis colorectal carcinoma. *Dis Colon Rectum* 1993;36:927.

621. Mecklin J-P, Järvinen HJ, Hakkiluoto A, et al. Frequency of hereditary nonpolyposis colorectal cancer: a prospective multicenter study in Finland. *Dis Colon Rectum* 1995; 38:588.

622. Mecklin J-P, Sipponen P, Järvinen HJ. Histopathology of colorectal carcinomas and adenomas in cancer family syndrome. *Dis Colon Rectum* 1986;29:849.

623. Medina M, Paddock HN, Connolly RJ, et al. Novel antiadhesion barrier does not prevent anastomotic healing in a rabbit model. *J Invest Surg* 1995;8:179.

624. Menaker GJ. The use of antibiotics in surgical treatment of the colon. *Surg Gynecol Obstet* 1987;164:581.

625. Menko FH, Wijnen JT, Vasen HFA, et al. Genetic counseling in hereditary nonpolyposis colorectal cancer. *Oncology* 1996;10:71.

626. Mensink PBF, Kolkman JJ, van Baarlen J, et al. Change in anatomic distribution and incidence of colorectal carcinoma over a period of 15 years: clinical considerations. *Dis Colon Rectum* 2002;45:1393.

627. Menzies D. Peritoneal adhesions: incidence, cause, and prevention. *Surg Ann* 1992;24:27.

628. Menzies D, Ellis H. Intestinal obstruction from adhesions: how big is the problem? *Ann R Coll Surg Engl* 1990;72:60.

629. Metzger PP. Adenocarcinoma developing in a rectosigmoid conduit used for urinary diversion: report of a case. *Dis Colon Rectum* 1989;32:247.

630. Michener WM, Gage RP, Sauer WG, et al. The prognosis of chronic ulcerative colitis in children. *N Engl J Med* 1961;265:1075.

631. Mikulicz J von. Chirurgische erjahrun ber das Darmcarcinom [Surgical experience with intestinal carcinoma]. *Arch Klin Chir Berl* 1903;69:28. (Translated in *Med Classics* 1937–1938;2:210 and reproduced in *Dis Colon Rectum* 1980;23:513.)

632. Milham S Jr. *Occupational mortality in Washington State, 1950–1971*, vols 2 and 3. Cincinnati, OH: United States Dept of Health, Education and Welfare, Public Health Service; Centers for Disease Control; and National Institute for Occupational Safety and Health, Division of Surveillance, Hazard Evaluation, and Field Studies, 1976.

633. Minervini A, Bentley S, Young D. Prophylactic saline peritoneal lavage in elective colorectal operations. *Dis Colon Rectum* 1980;23:392.

634. Minsky BD. Clinicopathologic impact of colloid in colorectal carcinoma. *Dis Colon Rectum* 1990;33:714.

635. Minsky BD. Adjuvant therapy of rectal cancer. *Semin Oncol* 1999;26:540.

636. Minton JP, Hamilton WB, Sardi A, et al. Results of surgical excision of one to 13 hepatic metastases in 98 consecutive patients. *Arch Surg* 1989;124:46.

637. Minton JP, James KK, Hurtubise PE, et al. The use of serial carcinoembryonic antigen determinations to predict recurrence of carcinoma of the colon and the time for a second-look operation. *Surg Gynecol Obstet* 1978;147:208.

638. Minu AR, Takemura K, Iwai T, et al. Role of wrapping in concomitant intra-abdominal aneurysm and colorectal carcinoma: report of three cases. *Dis Colon Rectum* 1992; 35:991.

639. Mitmaker B, Begin LR, Gordon PH. Nuclear shape as a prognostic discriminant in colorectal carcinoma. *Dis Colon Rectum* 1991;34:249.

640. Mitry E, Bouvier A-M, Esteve J, et al. Benefit of operative mortality reduction on colorectal cancer survival. *Br J Surg* 2002;89:1557.

641. Mitry E, Benhamiche A-M, Jouve J-L, et al. Colorectal adenocarcinoma in patients under 45 years of age: comparison with older patients in a well-defined French population. *Dis Colon Rectum* 2001;44:380.

642. Miyanari N, Mori T, Takahashi K, et al. Evaluation of aggressively treated patients with unresectable multiple liver metastases from colorectal cancer. *Dis Colon Rectum* 2002; 45:1503.

643. Moertel CG. Chemotherapy for colorectal cancer. *N Engl J Med* 1994;330:1136.

644. Moertel CG, Fleming TR, MacDonald JS, et al. Levamisole and fluorouracil for adjuvant therapy of resected colon carcinoma. *N Engl J Med* 1990;322:352.

645. Moertel CG, Fleming TR, MacDonald JS, et al. An evaluation of the carcinoembryonic antigen (CEA) for monitoring patients with resected colon cancer. *JAMA* 1993;270:943.

646. Moertel CG, Fleming TR, MacDonald JS, et al. Fluorouracil plus levamisole as effective adjuvant therapy after resection of stage III colon carcinoma: a final report. *Ann Intern Med* 1995;122:321.

647. Moertel CG, Fleming TR, MacDonald JS, et al. Intergroup study of fluorouracil plus levamisole adjuvant therapy for stage III Dukes' B2 colon cancer. *J Clin Oncol* 1995;13:2936.

648. Moertel CG, Hill JR, Dockerty MB. The routine proctoscopic examination: a second look. *Mayo Clin Proc* 1966; 41:368.

649. Moertel CG, Schutt AJ, Go VLW. Carcinoembryonic antigen test for recurrent colorectal carcinoma. *JAMA* 1978; 239:1065.

650. Moffat FL Jr, Pinsky CM, Hammershaimb L, et al. Clinical utility of external immunoscintigraphy with IMMU-4 technetium-99m Fab' antibody fragment in patients undergoing surgery for carcinoma of the colon and rectum: results of a pivotal, phase III trial. *J Clin Oncol* 1996;14:2295.

651. Monk BJ, Berman ML, Montz FJ. Adhesions after extensive gynecologic surgery: clinical significance, etiology, and prevention. *Am J Obstet Gynecol* 1994;170:1396.

652. Moore HC, Haller DG. Adjuvant therapy of colon cancer. *Semin Oncol* 1999;59:545.

653. Moorehead RJ, Kernohan RM, Patterson CC, et al. Does cholecystectomy predispose to colorectal cancer? A case-control study. *Dis Colon Rectum* 1986;29:36.

654. Morabito A, Gattuso D, Sarmiento R, et al. Rofecoxib associated with an antiangiogenic schedule of weekly irinotecan and infusional 5-fluorouracil as second line treatment of patients with metastatic colorectal cancer: results of a dose-finding study. *Proc ASCO* 2003;22(abst 1311).

655. Moran K, Cooke T, Forster G, et al. Prognostic value of nucleolar organizer regions and ploidy values in advanced colorectal cancer. *Br J Surg* 1989;76:1152.

656. Morgan CN. The management of carcinoma of the colon. *Ann R Coll Surg Engl* 1952;10:305.

657. Morgenstern L, Lee SE. Spatial distribution of colonic carcinoma. *Arch Surg* 1978;113:1142.

658. Morita S, Nomura T, Fukushima Y, et al. Does serum CA 19–9 play a practical role in the management of patients with colorectal cancer? *Dis Colon Rectum* 2004;47:227.

659. Morowitz DA, Block GE, Kirshner JB. Adenocarcinoma of the ileum complicating chronic regional enteritis. *Gastroenterology* 1968;55:397.

660. Morrow M, Enker WE. Late ovarian metastases in carcinoma of the colon and rectum. *Arch Surg* 1984;119:1385.

661. Mortensen NJMcC, Eltringham WK, Mountford RA, et al. Direct vision brush cytology with colonoscopy: an aid to

the accurate diagnosis of colonic strictures. *Br J Surg* 1984;71:930.

662. Morton AL, Taylor EW, Lindsay G, et al. A multicenter study to compare cefotetan alone with cefotetan and metronidazole as prophylaxis against infection in elective colorectal operations. *Surg Gynecol Obstet* 1989;169:41.

663. Morvay K, Szentlleki K, Trk G, et al. Effect of change of fecal bile acid excretion achieved by operative procedures on 1,2-dimethylhydrazine-induced colon cancer in rats. *Dis Colon Rectum* 1989;32:860.

664. Mullan FJ, Wilson HK, Majury CW, et al. Bile acids and the increased risk of colorectal tumours after truncal vagotomy. *Br J Surg* 1990;77:1085.

665. Mulsow J, Winter DC, O'Keane JC, et al. Sentinel lymph node mapping in colorectal cancer. *Br J Surg* 2003;90:659.

666. Munro A, Steele RJC, Logie JRC. Technique for intra-operative colonic irrigation. *Br J Surg* 1987;74:1039.

667. Murphy JB. Cholecysto-intestinal, gastro-intestinal and entero-intestinal anastomosis, and approximation without sutures. *Med Rec N Y* 1892;42:665.

668. Mzabi R, Himal HS, Demers R, et al. A multiparametric computer analysis of carcinoma of the colon. *Surg Gynecol Obstet* 1976;143:959.

669. Nagakura S, Shirai Y, Hatakeyama K. Computed tomographic features of colorectal carcinoma liver metastases predict posthepatectomy patient survival. *Dis Colon Rectum* 2001;44:1148.

670. Nagorney DM, Sarr MG, McIlrath DC. Surgical management of intussusception in the adult. *Ann Surg* 1981;193:230.

671. Nakagoe T, Sawai T, Tsuji T, Ayabe H. Use of minilaparotomy in the treatment of colonic cancer. *Br J Surg* 2001;88:831.

672. Nakajima N, Ramadan H, Lapi N, et al. Rectal carcinoma with solitary cerebral metastasis: report of a case and review of the literature. *Dis Colon Rectum* 1979;22:252.

673. Narod SA, Ginsburg O, Jothy S. Family history and colorectal cancer. *N Engl J Med* 1995;332:1578.

674. Nathanson SD, Schultz L, Tilley B, et al. Carcinomas of the colon and rectum: a comparison of staging classifications. *Am Surg* 1986;52:428.

675. National Board of Health and Welfare. *Cancer incidence in Sweden, 1959–1965.* Stockholm: Swedish Cancer Registry, 1971.

676. Nava HR, Pagana TJ. Postoperative surveillance of colorectal carcinoma. *Cancer* 1982;49:1043.

677. Navsaria PH, Bunting M, Omoshoro-Jones J, et al. Temporary closure of open abdominal wounds by the modified sandwich-vacuum pack technique. *Br J Surg* 2003;90:718.

678. Nelson RL, Persky V. The rise and fall of colorectal cancer. *Dis Colon Rectum* 1994;37:1163.

679. Nesbakken A, Haffner J. Colo-recto-anal intussusception: case report. *Acta Chir Scand* 1989;155:201.

680. Nesbitt JC, Moise KJ, Sawyers JL. Colorectal carcinoma in pregnancy. *Arch Surg* 1985;120:636.

681. Neugut AI, Johnsen CM, Finl DJ. Serum cholesterol levels in adenomatous polyps and cancer of the colon: a case-control study. *JAMA* 1986;255.365.

682. Newill VA. Distribution of cancer mortality among ethnic subgroups of the white population of New York City, 1953–1958. *J Natl Cancer Inst* 1961;26:405.

683. Newland RC, Chapuis PH, Smyth EJ. The prognostic value of substaging colorectal carcinoma: a prospective study of 1117 cases with standardized pathology. *Cancer* 1987;60: 852.

684. Nichols RL, Broido P, Condon RE, et al. Effect of preoperative neomycin-erythromycin intestinal preparation on the incidence of infectious complications following colon surgery. *Ann Surg* 1973;178:453.

685. Nicholson JR, Aust JC. Rising carcinoembryonic antigen titers in colorectal carcinoma: an indication for the second-look procedure. *Dis Colon Rectum* 1978;21:163.

686. Nieroda CA, Mojzisik C, Sardi A, et al. The impact of radio-immunoguided surgery (RIGS) on surgical decision making in colorectal cancer. *Dis Colon Rectum* 1989;32:927.

687. Nigro ND. A strategy for prevention of cancer of the large bowel. *Dis Colon Rectum* 1982;25:755.

688. Nigro ND, Bull AW. Experimental intestinal carcinogenesis. *Br J Surg* 1985(Sept);72(Suppl):S36.

689. Nigro ND, Bull AW, Klopfer BA, et al. Effect of dietary fiber on azoxymethane-induced intestinal carcinogenesis in the rat. *J Natl Cancer Inst* 1979;62:1097.

690. Nitschke J, Richter H, Herguth D, et al. Acute appendicitis and postoperative fecal fistula: symptoms of an unrecognized carcinoma of the colon. *Dis Colon Rectum* 1976; 19:605.

691. Nivatvongs S, Gilbertsen VA, Goldberg SM, et al. Distribution of large-bowel cancers detected by occult blood test in asymptomatic patients. *Dis Colon Rectum* 1982; 25:420.

692. Norfleet RG. Effect of diet on fecal occult blood testing in patients with colorectal polyps. *Dig Dis Sci* 1986;31:498.

693. Northover J. Carcinoembryonic antigen and recurrent colorectal cancer. *Gut* 1986;27:117.

694. Norum J, Olsen JA. Cost-effectiveness approach to the Norwegian follow-up programme in colorectal cancer. *Ann Oncol* 1997;8:1081.

695. Obrand DI, Gordon PH. Incidence and patterns of recurrence following curative resection for colorectal carcinoma. *Dis Colon Rectum* 1997;40:15.

696. O'Brien PH, Newton BB, Metcalf JS, et al. Oophorectomy in women with carcinoma of the colon and rectum. *Surg Gynecol Obstet* 1981;153:827.

697. *Occupational mortality. Decennial Supplement England and Wales. Population Censuses and Surveys Office, 1970–1972.* London: HM Stationery Office, 1978.

698. O'Connell M, Laurie J, Kahn M, et al. Prospective randomized trial of postoperative adjuvant therapy in patients with high risk colon cancer. *J Clin Oncol* 1998;16:295.

699. O'Connell M, Malliard J, MacDonald J, et al. An Intergroup trial of intensive 5-FU and low dose leucovorin as surgical adjuvant for high-risk colon cancer. *Proc ASCO* 1993;12 (abst 190).

700. Oda S, Oki E, Maehara Y, et al. Precise assessment of microsatellite instability using high resolution fluorescent microsatellite analysis. *Nucl Acids Res* 1997;25:3415.

701. O'Dwyer PJ, Benson A. Epidermal growth factor receptor targeted therapy in colorectal cancer. *Semin Oncol* 2002; 29 [Suppl 14]:10.

702. O'Dwyer PJ, Mojzisik C, McCabe DP, et al. Reoperation directed by carcinoembryonic antigen level: the importance of a thorough preoperative evaluation. *Am J Surg* 1988; 155:227.

703. Oh-e H, Tanaka S, Kitadai Y, et al. Angiogenesis at the site of deepest penetration predicts lymph node metastasis of submucosal colorectal cancer. *Dis Colon Rectum* 2001;44: 1129.

704. Ohlsson B, Breland U, Ekberg H, et al. Follow-up after curative surgery for colorectal carcinoma: randomized comparison with no follow-up. *Dis Colon Rectum* 1995;38:619.

705. Oikonomakis I, Wexner SD, Gervaz P, et al. Seprafilm: a retrospective preliminary evaluation of the impact on short-term oncologic outcome in colorectal cancer. *Dis Colon Rectum* 2002;45:1376.

706. Oliveira L, Wexner SD, Daniel N, et al. Mechanical bowel preparation for elective colorectal surgery: a prospective, randomized, surgeon-blinded trial comparing sodium phosphate and polyethylene glycol-based oral lavage solutions. *Dis Colon Rectum* 1997;40:585.

707. Olsen AK. Intraoperative ultrasonography and the detection of liver metastases in patients with colorectal cancer. *Br J Surg* 1990;77:998.

708. Ondrula DP, Nelson RL, Prasad ML, et al. Multifactorial index of preoperative risk factors in colon resections. *Dis Colon Rectum* 1992;35:117.

709. Onik G, Rubinsky B, Zemel R, et al. Ultrasound-guided hepatic cryosurgery in the treatment of metastatic colon carcinoma: preliminary results. *Cancer* 1991;67:901.

710. Operative Laparoscopy Study Group. Postoperative adhesion development after operative laparoscopy: evaluation at early second-look procedures. *Fertil Steril* 1991; 55:700.

711. Oren JW, Folse R, Kraudel KL, et al. The preoperative liver scan and surgical decision making in patients with colorectal cancer. *Am J Surg* 1986;151:452.

712. Ostrow JD, Mulvaney CA, Hansell JR, et al. Sensitivity and reproducibility of chemical tests for fecal occult blood with an emphasis on false-positive reactions. *Am J Dig Dis* 1973; 18:930.

713. Ottery FD, Scupham RK, Weese JL. Chemical cholecystitis after intrahepatic chemotherapy. The case for prophylactic cholecystectomy during pump replacement. *Dis Colon Rectum* 1986;29:187.

714. Ovaska J, Järvinen H, Kujari H, et al. Follow-up of patients operated on for colorectal carcinoma. *Am J Surg* 1990;159:593.

715. Ovaska J, Järvinen HJ, Mecklin JP. The value of a follow-up programme after radical surgery for colorectal carcinoma. *Scand J Gastroenterol* 1989;24:416.

716. Overholt BF. Colonoscopy and colon cancer: current clinical practice. *CA Cancer J Clin* 1982;32:180.

717. Pagana TJ, Ledesma EJ, Mittelman A, et al. The use of colonoscopy in the study of synchronous colorectal neoplasms. *Cancer* 1984;53:356.

718. Paganini-Hill A. Estrogen replacement therapy and colorectal cancer risk in elderly women. *Dis Colon Rectum* 1999;42:1300.

719. Painter NS, Burkitt DP. Diverticular disease of the colon: a deficiency disease of Western civilization. *BMJ* 1971; 2:450.

720. Palmer ML, Herrera L, Petrelli NJ. Colorectal adenocarcinoma in patients less than 40 years of age. *Dis Colon Rectum* 1991;34:343.

721. Palmer M, Petrelli NJ, Herrera L. No treatment option for liver metastases from colorectal adenocarcinoma. *Dis Colon Rectum* 1989;32:698.

722. Parikshak M, Pawlak SE, Eggenberger JC, et al. The role of endoscopic colon surveillance in the transplant population. *Dis Colon Rectum* 2002;45:1655.

723. Parrott NR, Lennard TWJ, Taylor RMR, et al. Effect of perioperative blood transfusion on recurrence of colorectal cancer. *Br J Surg* 1986;73:970.

724. Patt YZ, Mavligit G, Chuang VP, et al. Arteriovenous carcinoembryonic antigen gradient: determination by selective angiography for localization of metastatic colorectal cancer. *Arch Surg* 1980;115:1122.

725. Paul FT. Colectomy. *BMJ* 1895;1:1136.

726. Payne JE. International colorectal carcinoma staging and grading. *Dis Colon Rectum* 1989;32:282.

727. Pemberton M. Carcinoma of the large intestine with survival in a child of nine and in his father: a study of carcinoma of the colon with particular reference to children. *Br J Surg* 1970;57:841.

728. Petersen BM Jr, Bass BL, Bates HR, et al. Use of radiolabeled murine monoclonal antibody, ^{111}In-CYT-103, in the management of colon cancer. *Am J Surg* 1993;165:137.

729. Petrelli NJ, Nambisan RN, Herrera L, et al. Hepatic resection for isolated metastasis from colorectal carcinoma. *Am J Surg* 1985;149:205.

730. Petros JG, Realica R, Ahmad S, et al. Patient-controlled analgesia and prolonged ileus after uncomplicated colectomy. *Am J Surg* 1995;170:371.

731. Philip RS. Efficacy of preoperative bowel preparation at home. *Am Surg* 1995;61:368.

732. Phillips RKS, Hittinger R, Fry JS, et al. Malignant large-bowel obstruction. *Br J Surg* 1985;72:296.

733. Phillips RL. Role of life-style and dietary habits in risk of cancer among Seventh-Day Adventists. *Cancer Res* 1975; 35[Suppl II]:3513.

734. Philpott GW, Siegel BA, Schwarz SW, et al. Immuno-scintigraphy with a new indium-111-labeled monoclonal antibody (Mab 1A3) in patients with colorectal cancer. *Dis Colon Rectum* 1994;37:782.

735. Pickren JW. Nodal clearance and detection. *JAMA* 1975; 231:969.

736. Piedbois P, Michiels S. Survival benefit of 5FU/LV over 5FU bolus in patients with advanced colorectal cancer: an updated meta-analysis based on 2,751 patients. *Proc ASCO* 2003;22(abst 1180).

737. Pietra N, Sarli L, Costi R, et al. Role of follow-up in management of local recurrences of colorectal cancer: a prospective, randomized study. *Dis Colon Rectum* 1998;41:1 127.

738. Pihl E, Hughes ESR, McDermott FT, et al. Lung recurrence after curative surgery for colorectal cancer. *Dis Colon Rectum* 1987;30:417.

739. Pitluk H, Poticha SM. Carcinoma of the colon and rectum in patients less than 40 years of age. *Surg Gynecol Obstet* 1983;157:335.

740. Poeze M, Houbiers JGA, van de Velde CJH, et al. Radical resection of locally advanced colorectal cancer. *Br J Surg* 1995;82:1386.

741. Polk W, Fong Y, Karpeh M, et al. A technique for the use of cryosurgery to assist hepatic resection. *J Am Coll Surg* 1995;180:171.

742. Pollack AV, Playforth MJ, Evans M. Peroperative lavage of the obstructed left colon to allow safe primary anastomosis. *Dis Colon Rectum* 1987;30:171.

743. Pollack ES, Nomura AMY, Heilbrun LK, et al. Prospective study of alcohol consumption and cancer. *N Engl J Med* 1984;310:617.

744. Ponz de Leon M, Sassatelli R, Sacchetti C, et al. Familial aggregation of tumors in the three-year experience of a population-based colorectal cancer registry. *Cancer Res* 1989;49:4344.

745. Poon M, O'Connell M, Moertel C, et al. Biochemical modulation of fluorouracil: evidence of significant improvement of survival and quality of life in patients with advanced colorectal cancer. *J Clin Oncol* 1989;7: 1407.

746. Portes C, Majarakis JD. Proctosigmoidoscopy: incidence of polyps in 50,000 examinations. *JAMA* 1957;163:411.

747. Powell BL, Craig JB, Muss HB. Secondary malignancies of the penis and epididymis: a case report and review of the literature. *J Clin Oncol* 1985;3:110.

748. Prager E, Swinton NW, Corman ML, et al. Intravenous pyelography in colorectal surgery. *Dis Colon Rectum* 1973; 16:479.

749. Prandi M, Lionetto R, Bini A, et al. Prognostic evaluation of stage B colon cancer patients is improved by an adequate lymphadenectomy: results of a secondary analysis of a large scale adjuvant trial. *Ann Surg* 2002;235: 458.

750. Pratt SM, Weaver FA, Potts JR III. Preoperative evaluation of patients with inguinal hernia for colorectal disease. *Surg Gynecol Obstet* 1987;165:53.

751. Pucciarelli S, Agostini M, Viel A, et al. Early-age-at-onset colorectal cancer and microsatellite instability as markers of hereditary nonpolyposis colorectal cancer. *Dis Colon Rectum* 2003;46:305.

752. Pye G, Jackson J, Thomas WM, et al. Comparison of Colo-screen Self-Test and haemoccult faecal occult blood tests in the detection of colorectal cancer in asymptomatic patients. *Br J Surg* 1990;77:630.

753. Rabelo R, Foulkes W, Gordon PH, et al. Role of molecular diagnostic testing in familial adenomatous polyposis and hereditary nonpolyposis colorectal cancer families. *Dis Colon Rectum* 2001;44:437.

754. Radcliffe AG, Dudley HAF. Intraoperative antegrade irrigation of the large intestine. *Surg Gynecol Obstet* 1983; 156:721.

755. Rajpal S, Dasmahapatra KS, Ledesma EJ, et al. Extensive resections of isolated metastasis from carcinoma of the colon and rectum. *Surg Gynecol Obstet* 1982;155:813.

756. Ramming KP, O'Toole K. The use of the implantable chemoinfusion pump in the treatment of hepatic metastases of colorectal cancer. *Arch Surg* 1986;121:1440.

757. Raskin HF, Pleticka S. The cytologic diagnosis of cancer of the colon. *Acta Cytol (Baltimore)* 1964;8:131.

758. Ravikumar TS, Kane R, Cady B, et al. Hepatic cryosurgery with intraoperative ultrasound monitoring for metastatic colon carcinoma. *Arch Surg* 1987;122:403.

759. Ravikumar TS, Kane R, Cady B, et al. A 5-year study of cryosurgery in the treatment of liver tumors. *Arch Surg* 1991;126:1520.

760. Ravikumar TS, Steele G Jr. Conventional and new tumor markers in the diagnosis and therapy of colorectal cancer. *Surg Rounds* 1987;10:30.

761. Ravitch MM, Lane R, Cornell WP, et al. Closure of duodenal, gastric and intestinal stumps with wire staples: experimental and clinical studies. *Ann Surg* 1966;163: 573.

762. Ravitch MM, Steichen FM. Technics of staple suturing in the gastrointestinal tract. *Ann Surg* 1972;175:815.

763. Ravitch MM, Steichen FM. A stapling instrument for end-to-end inverting anastomoses in the gastrointestinal tract. *Ann Surg* 1979;189:791.

764. Ravo B, Ger R. Temporary colostomy: an outmoded procedure? A report on the intracolonic bypass. *Dis Colon Rectum* 1985;28:904.

765. Ray NF, Larsen JW Jr, Stillman RJ, et al. Economic impact of hospitalizations for lower abdominal adhesiolysis in the United States in 1988. *Surg Gynecol Obstet* 1993;176:271.

766. Raymond E, Faivre S, Waynarowski, et al. Oxaliplatin: Mechanisms of action and anti-neoplastic activity. *Semin Oncol* 1998;25(Suppl 5):4.

767. Reasbeck PG, Manktelow A, McArthur AM, et al. An evaluation of pelvic lypmphoscintigraphy in the staging of colorectal carcinoma. *Br J Surg* 1984;71:936.

768. Rebuffat C, Rosati R, Montorsi M, et al. Clinical application of a new compression anastomotic device for colorectal surgery. *Am J Surg* 1990;159:330.

769. Recalde M, Holyoke ED, Elias EG. Carcinoma of the colon, rectum, and anal canal in young patients. *Surg Gynecol Obstet* 1974;139:909.

770. Redwine DB, Sharpe DR. Laparoscopic segmental resection of the sigmoid colon for endometriosis. *J Laparoendosc Surg* 1991;1:217.

771. Rees M, Plant G, Bygrave S. Late results justify resection for multiple hepatic metastases from colorectal cancer. *Br J Surg* 1997;84:1136.

772. Registry of Hepatic Metastases. Resection of the liver for colorectal carcinoma metastases: a multi-institutional study of indications for resection. *Surgery* 1988;103:278.

773. Reiling RB. Staplers in gastrointestinal surgery. *Surg Clin North Am* 1980;60:381.

774. Reiling RB, Reiling WA Jr, Bernie WA, et al. Prospective controlled study of gastrointestinal stapled anastomoses. *Am J Surg* 1980;139:147.

775. Reilly JC, Rusin LC, Theuerkauf FJ Jr. Colonoscopy: its role in cancer of the colon and rectum. *Dis Colon Rectum* 1982; 25:532.

776. Reissman P, Teoh T-A, Cohen SM, et al. Is early oral feeding safe after elective colorectal surgery? A prospective randomized trial. *Ann Surg* 1995;222:73.

777. Rey J-F, Romanczyk T, Greff M. Metal stents for palliation of rectal carcinoma: a preliminary report on 12 patients. *Endoscopy* 1995;27:501.

778. Reybard JF. Mémoire sur une tumeur cancéreuse affectant l'iliaque du colon: ablation de la tumeur et de l'intestin. *Bull R Med* 18833;296.

779. Reynoso G, Chu TM, Holyoke D, et al. Carcinoembryonic antigen in patients with different cancers. *JAMA* 1972;220: 361.

780. Ribic CM, Sargent DJ, Moore MJ, et al. Tumor microsatellite-instability status as a predictor of benefit from fluorouracil-based adjuvant chemotherapy for colon cancer. *N Engl J Med* 2003;349:247.

781. Richards PC, Balch CM, Aldrete JS. Abdominal wound closure: a prospective study of 571 patients comparing continuous versus interrupted suture techniques. *Ann Surg* 1983;197:238.

782. Riethmüller G, Schneider-Gädicke E, Schlimok G, et al. Randomised trial of monoclonal antibody for adjuvant therapy of resected Dukes' C colorectal carcinoma. *Lancet* 1994;343:1177.

783. Rifkin MD, Rosato FE, Branch HM, et al. Intraoperative ultrasound of the liver: an important adjunctive tool for decision making in the operating room. *Ann Surg* 1987; 205:466.

784. Robinson MHE, Marks CG, Farrands PA, et al. Population screening for colorectal cancer: comparison between guaiac and immunological faecal occult blood tests. *Br J Surg* 1994;81:448.

785. Rocklin MS, Senagore AJ, Talbott TM. Role of carcinoembryonic antigen and liver function tests in the detection of recurrent colorectal carcinoma. *Dis Colon Rectum* 1991; 34:794.

786. Rodgers MS, Collinson R, Desai S, et al. Risk of dissemination with biopsy of colorectal liver metastases. *Dis Colon Rectum* 2003;46:454.

787. Rodgers MS, McCall JL. Surgery for colorectal liver metastases with hepatic lymph node involvement: a systematic review. *Br J Surg* 2000;87:1142.

788. Rodríguez-Bigas MA, Boland CR, Hamilton SR, et al. A National Cancer Institute workshop on hereditary nonpolyposis colorectal cancer syndrome: meeting highlights and Bethesda guidelines. *J Natl Cancer Inst* 1997;89:1758.

789. Rodríguez-Bigas MA, Vasen HFA, Pekka-Mecklin J, et al. Rectal cancer risk in hereditary nonpolyposis colorectal cancer after abdominal colectomy. *Ann Surg* 1997;225: 202.

790. Rogers DA, Dingus D, Stanfield J, et al. A prospective study of patient-controlled analgesia: impact on overall hospital course. *Am Surg* 1990;56:86.

791. Rosati R, Rebuffat C, Pezzuoli G. A new mechanical device for circular compression anastomosis. *Ann Surg* 1988; 207:245.

792. Rosati R, Smith L, Deitel M, et al. Primary colorectal anastomosis with the intracolonic bypass tube. *Surgery* 1992; 112: 618.

793. Rosato FE, Shelley WB, Fitts WT Jr, et al. Non-metastatic cutaneous manifestations of cancer of the colon. *Am J Surg* 1969;117:277.

794. Rosen M, Chan L, Beart RW Jr, et al. Follow-up of colorectal cancer: a meta-analysis. *Dis Colon Rectum* 1998; 41:1116.

795. Roses DF, Richman H, Localio SA. Bacterial endocarditis associated with colorectal carcinoma. *Ann Surg* 1973;179: 190.

796. Rothenberg M, Meropol N, Poplin E, et al. Mortality associated with irinotecan plus bolus fluorouracil/leucovrin: summary findings of an independent panel. *J Clin Oncol* 2001;19:3801.

797. Rowley S, Newbold KM, Gearty J, et al. Comparison of deoxyribonucleic acid ploidy and nuclear expressed p62 c-*myc* oncogene in the prognosis of colorectal cancer. *World J Surg* 1990;14:545.

798. Roy M, Geller JS. Increased morbidity of iatrogenic splenectomy. *Surg Gynecol Obstet* 1974;139:392.

799. Rozario D, Brown I, Fung MFK, et al. Is incidental prophylactic oophorectomy an acceptable means to reduce the incidence of ovarian cancer? *Am J Surg* 1997;173:495.

800. Rozen P, Fireman Z, Figer A, et al. Family history of colorectal cancer as a marker of potential malignancy within a screening program. *Cancer* 1987;60:248.

801. Rubin MS, Shin DM, Pasmantier M, et al. Monoclonal antibody (MoAb) IMC-C225. An epidermal growth factor receptor (EGFr) for patients with EGFr positive tumors refractory to or in relapse from previous therapeutic regimens. *Proc ASCO* 2000;19(abst 1860).

802. Rubin P, Green J. *Solitary metastases*. Springfield, IL: Charles C Thomas, 1968.

803. Runkel NS, Schlag P, Schwarz V, et al. Outcome after emergency surgery for cancer of the large intestine. *Br J Surg* 1991;78:183.

804. Ruo L, Cellini C, La-Calle JPJr, et al. Limitations of family cancer history assessment at initial surgical consultation. *Dis Colon Rectum* 2001;44:98.

805. Ruo L, Gougoutas C, Paty PB, et al. Elective bowel resection for incurable stage IV colorectal cancer: prognostic variables for asymptomatic patients. *J Am Coll Surg* 2003; 196:722.

806. Rusca JA, Bornside GH, Cohn I. Everting versus inverting gastrointestinal anastomoses: bacterial leakage and anastomotic disruption. *Ann Surg* 1969;169:727.

807. Sacchi G, Weber E, Aglianó M, et al. Lymphatic vessels in colorectal cancer and their relation with inflammatory infiltrate. *Dis Colon Rectum* 2003;46:40.

808. Saeed W, Kim S, Burch BH, et al. Development of carcinoma in regional enteritis. *Arch Surg* 1974;108:376.

809. Saegesser F, Sandblom P. Ischemic lesions of the distended colon. *Am J Surg* 1975;129:309.

810. Safi F, Link KH, Beger HG. Is follow-up of colorectal cancer patients worthwhile? *Dis Colon Rectum* 1993;36: 636.

811. Saida Y, Sumiyama Y, Nagao J, Uramatsu M. Long-term prognosis of preoperative "bridge to surgery" expandable metallic stent insertion for obstructive colorectal cancer: comparison with emergency operation. *Dis Colon Rectum* 2003;46[Suppl]:S44.

812. Sakanoue Y, Nakao K, Shoji Y, et al. Intraoperative colonoscopy. *Surg Endosc* 1993;7:84.

813. Salim AS. Percutaneous decompression and irrigation for large-bowel obstruction. New approach. *Dis Colon Rectum* 1991;34:973.

814. Salmon SE, Hamburger AW, Soehnlen B, et al. Quantitation of differential sensitivity of human tumor stem cells to anticancer drugs. *N Engl J Med* 1978;298:1321.

815. Salsbury AJ, McKinna JA, Griffiths JD, et al. Circulating cancer cells during excision of carcinomas of the rectum and colon with high ligation of the inferior mesenteric vein. *Surg Gynecol Obstet* 1965;120:1266.

816. Saltz LB, Cox JV, Blanke C, et al. Irinotecan Study Group. Irinotecan plus fluorouracil and leucovorin for metastatic colorectal cancer. *N Engl J Med* 2000;343: 905.

817. Saltzman B. Ureteral stents; indications, variations and complications. *Urol Clin North Am* 1988;15:481.

818. Sanders GB, Hagan WH, Kinnaird DW. Adult intussusception and carcinoma of the colon. *Ann Surg* 1958;147:796.

819. Sandler RS, Sandler DP. Radiation-induced cancers of the colon and rectum: assessing the risk. *Gastroenterology* 1983; 84:51.

820. Sanfelippo PM, Beahrs OH. Factors in the prognosis of adenocarcinoma of the colon and rectum. *Arch Surg* 1972;104:401.

821. Sanfelippo PM, Beahrs OH. Carcinoma of the colon in patients under forty years of age. *Surg Gynecol Obstet* 1974; 138:169.

822. Sardi A, Workman M, Mojzisik C, et al. Intra-abdominal recurrence of colorectal cancer detected by radioimmunoguided surgery (RIGS system). *Arch Surg* 1989;124:55.

823. Sarela AI, Guthrie JA, Seymour MT, et al. Non-operative management of the primary tumour in patients with incurable stage IV colorectal cancer. *Br J Surg* 2001;88:1352.

824. Scheele J, Altendorf-Hofmann A, Stangl R, et al. Pulmonary resection for metastatic colon and upper rectum cancer: is it useful? *Dis Colon Rectum* 1990;33:745.

825. Schiedeck THK, Wellm C, Roblick UJ, et al. Diagnosis and monitoring of colorectal cancer by L6 blood serum polymerase chain reaction is superior to carcinoembryonic antigen-enzyme-linked immunosorbent assay. *Dis Colon Rectum* 2003;46:818.

826. Schiessel R, Wunderlich M, Herbst F. Local recurrence of colorectal cancer: effect of early detection and aggressive surgery. *Br J Surg* 1986;73:342.

827. Schillaci A, Cavallaro A, Nicolanti V, et al. The importance of symptom duration in relation to prognosis of carcinoma of the large intestine. *Surg Gynecol Obstet* 1984;158:423.

828. Schlinkert RT. Laparoscopic-assisted right hemicolectomy. *Dis Colon Rectum* 1991;34:1030.

829. Schmidt WK. Alvimopan (ADL 8–2698) is a novel peripheral opioid antagonist. *Am J Surg* 2001;182[Suppl]:27S.

830. Schneebaum S, Arnold MW, Houchens DP, et al. The significance of intraoperative periportal lymph node metastasis identification in patients with colorectal carcinoma. *Cancer* 1995;75:2809.

831. Schneebaum S, Arnold MW, Young D, et al. Role of carcinoembryonic antigen in predicting resectability of recurrent colorectal cancer. *Dis Colon Rectum* 1993;36:810.

832. Schoetz DJ Jr, Roberts RL, Murray JJ, et al. Addition of parenteral cefoxitin to regimen of oral antibiotics for elective colorectal operations: a randomized prospective study. *Ann Surg* 1990;212:209.

833. Schrag D, Panageas KS, Riedel E, et al. Surgeon volume compared to hospital volume as a predictor of outcome following primary colon cancer resection. *J Surg Oncol* 2003; 83:68.

834. Schrock TR, Deveney CW, Dunphy JE. Factors contributing to leakage of colonic anastomoses. *Ann Surg* 1973; 177:513.

835. Schwartz D, Flamant R, Lellouch J, et al. Results of a French survey on the role of tobacco, particularly inhalation, in different cancer sites. *J Natl Cancer Inst* 1961;26: 1085.

836. SCOTIA Study Group. Single-stage treatment for malignant left-sided colonic obstruction: a prospective randomized clinical trial comparing subtotal colectomy with segmental resection following intraoperative irrigation. *Br J Surg* 1995;82:1622.

837. Scott NA, Rainwater LM, Weiand HS, et al. The relative prognostic value of flow cytometric DNA analysis and conventional clinicopathologic criteria in patients with operable rectal carcinoma. *Dis Colon Rectum* 1987;30: 513.

838. Scott NA, Weiand HS, Moertel CG, et al. Colorectal cancer: Dukes' stage, tumor site, preoperative plasma CEA pattern. *Arch Surg* 1987;122:1375.

839. Scudamore HH. Cancer of the colon and rectum—general aspects, diagnosis, treatment, and prognosis: a review. *Dis Colon Rectum* 1969;12:105.

840. Searle/Pharmacia Corporation. Data on File.

841. Secker-Walter RH, Worden JK, Holland RR, et al. A mass media programme to prevent smoking among adolescents: costs and cost effectiveness. *Tobacco Control* 1997; 6:207.

842. Segi M. *Cancer mortality for selected sites in 24 countries: 1950–1957.* Sendai, Japan: Department of Public Health, Tohoku University School of Medicine, 1960.

843. Seidman H. Cancer death rates by site and sex for religious and socioeconomic groups in New York City. *Environ Res* 1970;3:234.

844. Selby P, Buick RN, Tannock I. A critical appraisal of the human tumor stem-cell assay. *N Engl J Med* 1983;308:129.

845. Selby JV, Friedman GD, Quesenberry CP Jr, et al. A case-control study of screening sigmoidoscopy and mortality from colorectal cancer. *N Engl J Med* 1992;326:653.

846. Sener SF, Imperato JP, Chmiel J, et al. The use of cancer registry data to study preoperative carcinoembryonic antigen level as an indicator of survival in colorectal cancer. *CA Cancer J Clin* 1989;39:50.

847. Sengupta S, Tjandra JJ, Gibson PR. Dietary fiber and colorectal neoplasia. *Dis Colon Rectum* 2001;44:1016.

848. Senn N. Enterorrhaphy: its history, technique and present status. *JAMA* 1893;21:215.

849. Serpell JW, McDermott FT, Katrivessis H, et al. Obstructing carcinomas of the colon. *Br J Surg* 1989;76:965.

850. Setti Carraro PG, Segala M, Cesana BM, et al. Obstructing colonic cancer: failure and survival patterns over a

ten-year follow-up after a one-stage curative surgery. *Dis Colon Rectum* 2001;44:243.

851. Shahon DB, Wangensteen OH. Early diagnosis of cancer of the gastrointestinal tract. *Postgrad Med* 1960;27:306.

852. Shapiro A, Berlatsky Y, Lijovetsky G, et al. Carcinoma of colon after ureteric anastomosis. *Urology* 1979;13:617.

853. Sharpe CR, Siemiatycki JA, Rachet BP. The effects of smoking on the risk of colorectal cancer. *Dis Colon Rectum* 2002;45:1041.

854. Sheehan KM, Sheahan K, O'Donoghue D, et al. The relationship between cyclooxygenase-2 expression and colorectal cancer. *JAMA* 1999; 282:1254.

855. Sheen AJ, Irlam J, Kirillova N, et al. Gene therapy of patient-derived T lymphocytes to target and eradicate colorectal hepatic metastases. *Dis Colon Rectum* 2003;46: 793.

856. Sheikh FA, Khubchandani IT. Prophylactic ureteric catheters in colon surgery: how safe are they? *Dis Colon Rectum* 1990;33:508.

857. Sheil F O'M, Clark CG, Goligher JC. Adenocarcinoma associated with Crohn's disease. *Br J Surg* 1968;55:53.

858. Sheiner NM, Brister SJ, Gordon PH. Management of pulmonary metastases of colorectal origin. *Surg Rounds* 1988; 11:29.

859. Shennib H, Fried GM, Hampson LG. Does simultaneous cholecystectomy increase the risk of colonic surgery? *Am J Surg* 1986;151:266.

860. Shibata D, Paty PB, Guillem JG, et al. Surgical management of isolated retroperitoneal recurrences of colorectal carcinoma. *Dis Colon Rectum* 2002;45:795.

861. Shibata Y, Kotanagi H, Andoh H, et al. Detection of circulating anti-p53 antibodies in patients with colorectal carcinoma and the antibody's relation to clinical factors. *Dis Colon Rectum* 1996;39:1269.

862. Shida H, Ban K, Matsumoto M, et al. Prognostic significance of location of lymph node metastases in colorectal cancer. *Dis Colon Rectum* 1992;35:1046.

863. Shimotsuma M, Takahashi T, Yamane T, et al. Intraoperative cleansing of the impacted colon using an endotracheal tube. *Dis Colon Rectum* 1990;33:241.

864. Shirouzu K, Isomoto H, Kakegawa T. A prospective clinicopathologic study of venous invasion in colorectal cancer. *Am J Surg* 1991;162:216.

865. Shitoh K, Konishi F, Miyakura Y, et al. Microsatellite instability as a marker in predicting metachronous multiple colorectal carcinomas after surgery: a cohort-like study. *Dis Colon Rectum* 2002;45:328.

866. Shousha A, Chappell R, Matthews J, et al. Human chorionic gonadotrophin expression in colorectal adenocarcinoma. *Dis Colon Rectum* 1986;29:558.

867. Sibbering DM, Locker AP, Hardcastle JD, et al. Blood transfusion and survival in colorectal cancer. *Dis Colon Rectum* 1994;37:358.

868. Slater G, Aufses AH Jr, Szporn A. Synchronous carcinoma of the colon and rectum. *Surg Gynecol Obstet* 1990;171: 283.

869. Slater GI, Haber RH, Aufses AH Jr. Changing distribution of carcinoma of the colon and rectum. *Surg Gynecol Obstet* 1984;158:216.

870. Smith GA, Oien KA, O'Dwyer PJ. Frequency of early colorectal cancer in patients undergoing colonoscopy. *Br J Surg* 1999;86:1328.

871. Smith RL. Recorded and expected mortality among the Japanese of the United States and Hawaii, with special reference to cancer. *J Natl Cancer Inst* 1956;17:459.

872. Smith RL. Recorded and expected mortality among the Indians of the United States with special reference to cancer. *J Natl Cancer Inst* 1957;18:385.

873. Smothers L, Hynan L, Fleming J, et al. Emergency surgery for colon carcinoma. *Dis Colon Rectum* 2003;46:24.

874. Solla JA, Rothenberger DA. Preoperative bowel preparation: a survey of colon and rectal surgeons. *Dis Colon Rectum* 1990;33:154.

875. Song F, Glenny A-M. Antimicrobial prophylaxis in colorectal surgery: a systematic review of randomized controlled trials. *Br J Surg* 1998;85:1232.

876. Sorokin JJ, Sugarbaker PH, Zamcheck N, et al. Serial carcinoembryonic antigen assays: use in detection of cancer recurrence. *JAMA* 1974;228:49.

877. Soyer P, Levesque M, Elias D, et al. Detection of liver metastases from colorectal cancer: comparison of intraoperative US and CT during arterial portography. *Radiology* 1992;183:541.

878. Spratt JS Jr. The rates and patterns of growth of neoplasms of the large intestine and rectum. *Surg Clin North Am* 1965;45:1103.

879. Spratt JS Jr. Gross rates of growth of colonic neoplasms and other variables affecting medical decisions and prognosis. In: Burdette WJ, ed. *Carcinoma of the colon and antecedent epithelium.* Springfield, IL: Charles C Thomas, 1970:66.

880. Spratt JS Jr, Ackerman LV. The growth of a colonic adenocarcinoma. *Am Surg* 1961;27:23.

881. Staab HJ, Anderer FA, Stumpf E, et al. Eighty-four potential second-look operations based on sequential carcinoembryonic antigen determinations and clinical investigations in patients with recurrent gastrointestinal cancer. *Am J Surg* 1985;149:198.

882. Standards Task Force, American Society of Colon and Rectal Surgeons. Practice parameters for the detection of colorectal neoplasms. *Dis Colon Rectum* 1992;35:389.

883. Standards Task Force, American Society of Colon and Rectal Surgeons. Practice parameters for the detection of colorectal neoplasms: supporting documentation. *Dis Colon Rectum* 1992;35:391.

884. Standards Task Force of the American Society of Colon and Rectal Surgeons. Practice parameters for the identification and testing of patients at risk for dominantly inherited colorectal cancer. *Dis Colon Rectum* 2001;44: 1403.

885. Standards Task Force of the American Society of Colon and Rectal Surgeons. Practice parameters for the identification and testing of patients at risk for dominantly inherited colorectal cancer: supporting documentation. *Dis Colon Rectum* 2001;44:1404

886. Standards Task Force of the American Society of Colon and Rectal Surgeons. Practice parameters for the treatment of patients with dominantly inherited colorectal cancer (familial adenomatous polyposis and hereditary nonpolyposis cancer). *Dis Colon Rectum* 2003;46:1001.

887. Stangl R, Altendorf-Hofmann A, Charnley RM, et al. Factors influencing the natural history of colorectal liver metastases. *Lancet* 1994;343:1405.

888. Starling JR, Uehling DT, Gilchrist KW. Value of colonoscopy after ureterosigmoidoscopy. *Surgery* 1984;96: 784.

889. Staszewski J, McCall MG, Stenhouse NS. Cancer mortality in 1962–66 among Polish migrants to Australia. *Br J Cancer* 1971;25:599.

890. *Statistical Review of England and Wales. Supplement on cancer, 1968–1970.* London: HM Stationery Office, 1975.

891. Steele G Jr, Ravikumar TS. Resection of hepatic metastases from colorectal cancer. *Ann Surg* 1989;210:127.

892. Steele G Jr, Zamcheck N, Wilson R, et al. Results of CEA-initiated second-look surgery for recurrent colorectal cancer. *Am J Surg* 1980;139:544.

893. Steele RJC, Thompson AM, Hall PA, et al. The p53 tumour suppressor gene. *Br J Surg* 1998;85:1460.

894. Steichen FM, Ravitch MM. History of mechanical devices and instruments for suturing. *Curr Probl Surg* 1982;19:1.

895. Steichen FM, Ravitch MM. Contemporary stapling instruments and basic mechanical suture techniques. *Surg Clin North Am* 1984;64:425.

896. Steinberg JB, Tuggle DW, Postier RG. Adenocarcinoma of the colon in adolescents. *Am J Surg* 1988;156:460.

897. Steinberg SM, Barkin JS, Kaplan RS, et al. Prognostic indicators of colon tumors: the Gastrointestinal Tumor Study Group experience. *Cancer* 1986;57:1866.

898. Steinberg SM, Barwick KW, Stablein DM. Importance of tumor pathology and morphology in patients with surgically resected colon cancer: findings from the Gastrointestinal Tumor Study Group. *Cancer* 1986;58:1340.

899. Stella M, De Nardi P, Paganelli G, et al. Avidin-biotin system in radioimmunoguided surgery for colorectal cancer: advantages and limits. *Dis Colon Rectum* 1994;37:335.

900. Stellato TA, Danziger LH, Gordon N, et al. Antibiotics in elective colon surgery: a randomized trial of oral, systemic, and oral/systemic antibiotics for prophylaxis. *Am Surg* 1990;56:251.

901. Stephenson BM, Finan PJ, Gascoyne J, et al. Frequency of familial colorectal cancer. *Br J Surg* 1991;78:1162.

902. Stephenson BM, Shandall AA, Farouk R, et al. Malignant left-sided large bowel obstruction managed by subtotal/total colectomy. *Br J Surg* 1990;77:1098.

903. Sterchi JM. Hepatic artery infusion for metastatic disease. *Surg Gynecol Obstet* 1985;160:477.

904. Sterchi JM, Fulks D, Cruz J, et al. Operative technique for insertion of a totally implantable system for venous access. *Surg Gynecol Obstet* 1986;163:381.

905. Stevenson GW, Hernandez C. Single-visit screening and treatment of first-degree relatives: colon cancer pilot study. *Dis Colon Rectum* 1991;34:1120.

906. Stewart J, Diament RH, Brennan TG. Management of obstructing lesions of the left colon by resection, on-table lavage, and primary anastomosis. *Surgery* 1993;114:502.

907. Stewart RJ, Stewart AW, Turnbull PRG, et al. Sex differences in subsite incidence of large bowel cancer. *Dis Colon Rectum* 1983;26:658.

908. Strachan JR, Woodhouse CRJ. Malignancy following ureterosigmoidoscopy in patients with exstrophy. *Br J Surg* 1991;178:1216.

909. Stule JP, Petrelli NJ, Herrera L, et al. Anastomotic recurrence of adenocarcinoma of the colon. *Arch Surg* 1986;121:1077.

910. Sub O, Mettlin C, Petrelli N. Aspirin use, cancer, and polyps of the large bowel. *Cancer* 1993;72:1171.

911. Sugarbaker PH, Gianola FJ, Speyer JC, et al. Prospective, randomized trial of intravenous versus intraperitoneal 5-fluorouracil in patients with advanced primary colon or rectal cancer. *Surgery* 1985;98:414.

912. Sugarbaker PH, Zamcheck N, Moore FD. Assessment of serial carcinoembryonic antigen (CEA) assays in postoperative detection of recurrent colorectal cancer. *Cancer* 1976;38:2310.

913. Sugihara K, Hojo K, Moriya Y, et al. Pattern of recurrence after hepatic resection for colorectal metastases. *Br J Surg* 1993;80:1032.

914. Sumpio BE, Ballantyne GH, Zdon MJ, et al. Perforated appendicitis and obstructing colonic carcinoma in the elderly. *Dis Colon Rectum* 1986;29:668.

915. Svenden LB, Blow S, Mellemgaard A. Metachronous colorectal cancer in young patients: expression of the hereditary nonpolyposis colorectal cancer syndrome? *Dis Colon Rectum* 1991;34:790.

916. Swinton NW Sr, Nahra KS, Khazei AM, et al. The evolution of colorectal cancer. *Dis Colon Rectum* 1968;11:413.

917. Swinton NW Sr, Scherer WP. The value of proctosigmoidoscopic examinations. *CA Cancer J Clin* 1968;18:88.

918. Sylvan A, Sjölund B, Janunger KG, et al. Colorectal cancer risk after jejunoileal bypass: dysplasia and DNA content in longtime follow-up of patients operated on for morbid obesity. *Dis Colon Rectum* 1992;35:245.

919. Takahashi H, Carlson R, Ozturk M, et al. Radioimmunolocation of hepatic and pulmonary metastasis of human colon adenocarcinoma. *Gastroenterology* 1989;96:1317.

920. Takaki HS, Ujiki GT, Shields TS. Palliative resections in the treatment of primary colorectal cancer. *Am J Surg* 1977;133:548.

921. Tamin WZ, Ghellai A, Counihan TC, et al. Experience with endoluminal colonic wall stents for the management of large bowel obstruction for benign and malignant disease. *Arch Surg* 2000;135:434.

922. Tan SG, Nambiar R, Rauff A, et al. Primary resection and anastomosis in obstructed descending colon due to cancer. *Arch Surg* 1991;126:748.

923. Tanaka K, Adam R, Shimada H, et al. Role of neoadjuvant chemotherapy in the treatment of multiple colorectal metastases to the liver. *Br J Surg* 2003;90:963.

924. Tanaka T, Furukawa A, Murata K, et al. Endoscopic transanal decompression with a drainage tube for acute colonic obstruction. *Dis Colon Rectum* 2001;44:418.

925. Tartter PI. The association of perioperative blood transfusion with colorectal cancer recurrence. *Ann Surg* 1992;216:633.

926. Tartter PI, Slater G, Papatestas AE, et al. The prognostic significance of elevated serum alkaline phosphatase levels preoperatively in patients with carcinoma of the colon and rectum. *Surg Gynecol Obstet* 1984;158:569.

927. Tartter PI, Steinberg BM. The role of preoperative intravenous pyelogram in operations performed for carcinoma of the colon and rectum. *Surg Gynecol Obstet* 1986;163:65.

928. Tataryn DN, MacFarlane JK, Murray D, et al. Tube leukocyte adherence inhibition (LAI) assay in gastrointestinal (GIT) cancer. *Cancer* 1979;43:898.

929. Tate JJT, Northway J, Royle GT, et al. Faecal occult blood testing in symptomatic patients: comparison of three tests. *Br J Surg* 1990;77:523.

930. Taylor I. Colorectal liver metastases: to treat or not to treat? *Br J Surg* 1985;72:511.

931. Teitz S, Guidetti-Sharon A, Manor H, et al. Pyogenic liver abscess: warning indicator of silent colonic cancer: report of a case and review of the literature. *Dis Colon Rectum* 1995;38:1220.

932. Tejero E, Fernández-Lobato R, Mainar A, et al. Initial results of a new procedure for treatment of malignant obstruction of the left colon. *Dis Colon Rectum* 1997;40:432.

933. Tejero E, Mainar A, Fernández L, et al. New procedure for the treatment of colorectal neoplastic obstructions. *Dis Colon Rectum* 1994;37:1158.

934. Tekkis PP, Kessaris N, Kocher HM, et al. Evaluation of POSSUM and P-POSSUM scoring systems in patients undergoing colorectal surgery. *Br J Surg* 2003;90:340.

935. Tempero M. Pitfalls in antibody imaging in colorectal cancer. *Cancer* 1993;71:4248.

936. Tepper JE, O'Connell M, Niedzwiecki D, et al. Adjuvant therapy in rectal cancer: analysis of stage, sex and local control-Final Report of Intergroup 0114. *J Clin Oncol* 2002;20:1744.

937. Teppo L, Hakamd M, Hakulinen T, et al. *Cancer in Finland, 1953–1970: incidence, mortality, prevalence.* Copenhagen: Munksgaard, 1975.

938. Terezis NL, Davis WC, Jackson FC. Carcinoma of the colon associated with inguinal hernia. *N Engl J Med* 1963;268:774.

939. Thompson JS, Beart RW Jr, Anderson CF. Limitations of nutritional assessment in predicting the outcome of colorectal operations. *Dis Colon Rectum* 1986;29:488.

940. Thomson DMP, Krupey J, Freedman SO, et al. The radioimmunoassay of circulating carcinoembryonic antigen of the human digestive system. *Proc Natl Acad Sci USA* 1969;64:161.

941. Thomson DMP, Tataryn DN, Lopez M, et al. Human tumor-specific immunity assayed by a computerized tube leukocyte adherence inhibition. *Cancer Res* 1979;39:638.

942. Thomson WHF, Carter SStC. On-table lavage to achieve safe restorative rectal and emergency colonic resection without covering colostomy. *Br J Surg* 1986;73:61.

943. Thomson WHF, Robinson MHE. One-layer continuously sutured colonic anastomosis. *Br J Surg* 1993;80:1450.

944. Thorsen AG, Christensen MA, Davis SJ. The role of colonoscopy in the assessment of patients with colorectal cancer. *Dis Colon Rectum* 1986;29:306.

945. Thun MJ, Calle EE, Namboodiri MM, et al. Risk factors for fatal colon cancer in a large prospective study. *J Natl Cancer Inst* 1992;84:1491.

946. Thun MJ, Namboodiri MM, Health CW Jr. Aspirin use and reduced risk of fatal colon cancer. *N Engl J Med* 1991; 325:1593.

947. Thurston MO, Kaehr JW, Martin EW III, Martin EW Jr. Radionuclide of choice for use with an intraoperative probe.

948. Tietjen GW, Markowitz AM. Colitis proximal to obstructing colonic carcinoma. *Arch Surg* 1975;110:1133.

949. Tio TL, Coene PPLO, van Delden OM, et al. Colorectal carcinoma: preoperative TNM classification with endosonography. *Radiology* 1991;179:165.

950. Tong D, Russell AH, Dawson LE, et al. Second laparotomy for proximal colon cancer: sites of recurrence and implications for adjuvant therapy. *Am J Surg* 1983;145:382.

951. Toribara NW, Sleisenger MH. Screening for colorectal cancer. *N Engl J Med* 1995;332:861.

952. Törnberg SA, Holm L-E, Cartensen JM, et al. Risks of cancer of the colon and rectum in relation to serum cholesterol and beta-lipoprotein. *N Engl J Med* 1986;315:1629.

953. Tournigand C, Louvet C, Quinaux E, et al. FOLFIRI followed by FOLFOX versus FOLFOX followed by FOLFIRI in metastatic colorectal cancer (MCRC): Final results of a phase III study. *Proc ASCO* 2001;20(abst 494).

954. Tornqvist A, Ekelund G, Leandoer L. The value of intensive follow-up after curative resection for colorectal carcinoma. *Br J Surg* 1982;69:725.

955. Travers B. *An inquiry into the process of nature in repairing injuries of the intestine.* London: Longmans, Green and Co, 1812.

956. Traverso G, Shuber A, Levin B, et al. Detection of *APC* mutations in fecal DNA from patients with colorectal tumors. *N Engl J Med* 2002;346:311.

957. Traynor O, Castaing D, Bismuth H. Peroperative ultrasonography in the surgery of hepatic tumours. *Br J Surg* 1988;75:197.

958. Trocha SD, Nora DT, Saha SS, et al. Combination probe and dye-directed lymphatic mapping detects micrometastases in early colorectal cancer. *J Gastrointest Surg* 2003; 7:340.

959. Tsakraklides V, Wanebo HJ, Sternberg SS, et al. Prognostic evaluation of regional lymph node morphology in colorectal cancer. *Am J Surg* 1975;129:174.

960. Turnbull RB Jr, Kyle K, Watson FR, et al. Cancer of the colon: the influence of the no-touch isolation technic on survival rates. *Ann Surg* 1967;166:420.

961. Turunen MJ, Kivilaakso EO. Increased risk of colorectal cancer after cholecystectomy. *Ann Surg* 1981;194:639.

962. Twelves C, Wong A, Nowacki MP, et al. Improved safety results of a phase III trial of capecitabine vs. bolus 5-FU/leucovorin (LV) as adjuvant therapy for colon cancer (the X-ACT Study). *Proc ASCO* 2003;22(abst 1182).

963. Umpleby HC, Williamson RCN. Survival in acute obstructing colorectal carcinoma. *Dis Colon Rectum* 1984; 27:299.

964. Unger SW, Wanebo HJ. Colonoscopy: an essential monitoring technique after resection of colorectal cancer. *Am J Surg* 1983;145:71.

965. University of Melbourne Colorectal Group. A comparison of single-dose systemic Timentin with mezlocillin for prophylaxis of wound infection in elective colorectal surgery. *Dis Colon Rectum* 1989;32:940.

966. Urdaneta LF, Duffell D, Creevy CD, et al. Late development of primary carcinoma of the colon following ureterosigmoidostomy: report of three cases and literature review. *Ann Surg* 1966;164:503.

967. Valliant J-C, Balladur P, Nordlinger B, et al. Repeat liver resection for recurrent colorectal metastases. *Br J Surg* 1993;80:340.

968. Van Custem E, Twelves C, Cassidy J, et al. Oral capecitabine compared with intravenous fluorouracil plus leucovorin in patients with metastatic colorectal cancers: results of a large phase III study. *J Clin Oncol* 2001;19:4097.

969. Van Cutsem E, Twelves C, Taberno J, et al. XELOX: Mature results of a multinational, phase 11 trial of capecitabine plus oxaliplatin, an effective 1st line option for patients (pts) with metastatic colorectal cancer (MCRC). *Proc ASCO* 2003;22(abst 1023).

970. van Dalen R, Church J, McGannon E, et al. Patterns of surgery in patients belonging to Amsterdam-positive families. *Dis Colon Rectum* 2003;46:617.

971. van Geldere D, Fa-Si-Oen P, Noach LA, et al. Complications after colorectal surgery without mechanical bowel resection. *J Am Coll Surg* 2002;194:40.

972. van Kamp GJ, von Mensdorff-Pouilly S, Kenemans P, et al. Evaluation of colorectal cancer-associated mucin CA M43 assay in serum. *Clin Chem* 1993;39:1029.

973. Varty PP, Linehan IP, Boulos PB. Does concurrent splenectomy at colorectal cancer resection influence survival? *Dis Colon Rectum* 1993;36:602.

974. Vasen HFA, Johan G, Offerhaus A, et al. The tumour spectrum in hereditary non-polyposis colorectal cancer: a study of 24 kindreds in the Netherlands. *Int J Cancer* 1990;46:31.

975. Vasen HFA, Mecklin J-P, Khan PM, et al. Hereditary non-polyposis colorectal cancer. *Lancet* 1991;338:877.

976. Vellacott KD, Smith JHF, Mortensen NJMcC. Rising detection rate of symptomatic Dukes' A colorectal cancers. *Br J Surg* 1987;74:18.

977. Venkatesh KS, Morrison N, Larson DM, et al. Triangulating stapling technique: an alternative approach to colorectal anastomosis. *Dis Colon Rectum* 1993;36:73.

978. Verne JECW, Northover JMA. Screening strategies for the secondary prevention of colorectal cancer. *Gastroenterology J Club* 1990;2:6.

979. Vernick LJ, Kuller LH, Lohsoonthorn P, et al. Relationship between cholecystectomy and ascending colon cancer. *Cancer* 1980;45:392.

980. Vezeridis MP, Petrelli NJ, Mittelman A. The value of routine preoperative urologic evaluation in patients with colorectal carcinoma. *Dis Colon Rectum* 1987;30:758.

981. Vigder L, Tzur N, Huber M, et al. Management of obstructive carcinoma of the left colon: comparative study of staged and primary resection. *Arch Surg* 1985;120:825.

982. Vigo FC, Pardo R, Saenz D, et al. Muir-Torre syndrome with multiple neoplasia. *Br J Surg* 1992;79:1161.

983. Virgo KS, Vernava AM, Longo WE, et al. Cost of patient follow-up after potentially curative colorectal cancer treatment. *JAMA* 1995;273:1837.

984. Virgolini I, Raderer M, Kurtaran A, et al. Vasoactive intestinal peptide-receptor imaging for the localization of intestinal adenocarcinoms and endocrine tumors. *N Engl J Med* 1994;331:1116.

985. Vogel SB, Drane WE, Ros PR, et al. Prediction of surgical resectability in patients with hepatic colorectal metastases. *Ann Surg* 1994;219:508.

986. Walsh HPJ, Schofield PF. Is laparotomy for small-bowel obstruction justified in patients with previously treated malignancy? *Br J Surg* 1984;71:933.

987. Walsh RM, Aranha GV, Freeark RJ. Mortality and quality of life after total abdominal colectomy. *Arch Surg* 1990;125: 1564.

988. Wanebo HJ, Chu QD, Vezeridis MP, Soderberg C. Patient selection for hepatic resection of colorectal metastases. *Arch Surg* 1996;131:322.

989. Wanebo HJ, Llaneras M, Martin T, et al. Prospective monitoring trial for carcinoma of colon and rectum after surgical resection. *Surg Gynecol Obstet* 1989;169:479.

990. Wangensteen OH. Cancer of the colon and rectum: with special reference to (1) earlier recognition of alimentary tract malignancy; (2) secondary delayed re-entry of the

abdomen in patients exhibiting lymph node involvement; (3) subtotal primary excision of the colon; (4) operation in obstruction. *Wis Med J* 1949;48:591.

991. Warden MJ, Petrelli NJ, Herrera L, et al. The role of colonoscopy and flexible sigmoidoscopy in screening for colorectal carcinoma. *Dis Colon Rectum* 1986;30:52.

992. Warthin AS. Heredity with reference to carcinoma. *Arch Intern Med* 1913;12:546.

993. Wassner JD, Yohai E, Heimlich HJ. Complications associated with the use of gastrointestinal stapling devices. *Surgery* 1977;82:395.

994. Watanabe I, Arai T, Ono M, et al. Prognostic factors in resection of pulmonary metastasis from colorectal cancer. *Br J Surg* 2003;90:1436.

995. Waterhouse J, Muir C, Correa P, et al, eds. *Cancer incidence in five continents*, vol 3. New York: Springer-Verlag, 1976.

996. Waxman BP. Large-bowel anastomoses. II. The circular staplers. *Br J Surg* 1983;70:64.

997. Weaver M, Burdon DW, Youngs DJ, et al. Oral neomycin and erythromycin compared with single-dose systemic metronidazole and ceftriaxone prophylaxis in elective colorectal surgery. *Am J Surg* 1986;151:437.

998. Weber CA, Deveney KE, Pellegrini CA, et al. Routine colonoscopy in the management of colorectal carcinoma. *Am J Surg* 1986;152:87.

999. Weber JC, Bachellier P, Oussoultzoglou E, et al. Simultaneous resection of colorectal primary tumour and synchronous liver metastases. *Br J Surg* 2003;90:956.

1000. Weese JL, O'Grady MG, Ottery FD. How long is the five-centimeter margin? *Surg Gynecol Obstet* 1986;163:101.

1001. Weese JL, Rosenthal MS, Gould H. Avoidance of artifacts on computerized tomograms by selection of appropriate surgical clips. *Am J Surg* 1984;147:684.

1002. Weiden PL, Bean MA, Schultz P. Perioperative blood transfusion does not increase the risk of colorectal cancer recurrence. *Cancer* 1987;60:870.

1003. Weilbaecher D, Bolin JA, Hearn D, et al. Intussusception in adults: review of 160 cases. *Am J Surg* 1971;121:531.

1004. Welch CE. The treatment of combined intestinal obstruction and peritonitis by refunctionalization of the intestine. *Ann Surg* 1955;142:739.

1005. Whelan RL, Wong WD, Goldberg SM, et al. Synchronous bowel anastomoses. *Dis Colon Rectum* 1989;32:365.

1006. Whitaker RH, Pugh RC, Dowe D. Colonic tumours following uretero-sigmoidostomy. *Br J Urol* 1971;43:562.

1007. White CM, Macfie J. Immediate colectomy and primary anastomosis for acute obstruction due to carcinoma of the left colon and rectum. *Dis Colon Rectum* 1985;28:155.

1008. Whitehouse GH, Watt J. Ischemic colitis associated with carcinoma of the colon. Gastrointest Radiol 1977;2:31.

1009. Wichmann MW, Müller C, Hornung HM, et al. Gender differences in long-term survival of patients with colorectal cancer. *Br J Surg* 2001;88:1092.

1010. Wiggers T, Jeekel J, Arends JW, et al. No-touch isolation technique in colon cancer: a controlled prospective trial. *Br J Surg* 1988;75:409.

1011. Wijnen J, Khan PM, Vasen H, et al. Hereditary nonpolyposis colorectal cancer families not complying with the Amsterdam criteria show extremely low frequency of mismatch-repair-gene mutations. *Am J Hum Genet* 1997;61:329.

1012. Wilkes G. Oxaliplatinin: third-generation platinum analog. *Clin J Oncol Nurs* 2003;7:353.

1013. Wilking N, Petrelli NJ, Herrera L, et al. Surgical resection of pulmonary metastases from colorectal adenocarcinoma. *Dis Colon Rectum* 1985;28:562.

1014. Wilking N, Petrelli NJ, Herrera L, et al. Abdominal exploration for suspected recurrent carcinoma of the colon and rectum based upon elevated carcinoembryonic antigen alone or in combination with other diagnostic methods. *Surg Gynecol Obstet* 1986;162:465.

1015. Wille-Jørgensen P, Guenaga KF, Castro AA, et al. Clinical value of preoperative mechanical bowel cleansing in elective colorectal surgery: a systematic review. *Dis Colon Rectum* 2003;46:1013.

1016. Willett WC, MacMahon B. Diet and cancer: an overview (second of two parts). *N Engl J Med* 1984;310:697.

1017. Williams NN, Daly JM. Flow cytometry and prognostic implications in patients with solid tumors. *Surg Gynecol Obstet* 1990;171:257.

1018. Wilmore DW. Can we minimize the effects of opioids on the bowel and still achieve adequate pain control? *Am J Surg* 2001;182[Suppl]:1S.

1019. Wilson SE, Sokol T. Antimicrobials in elective colon surgery. *Infect Surg* 1985;4:609.

1020. Wilson SM, Adson MA. Surgical treatment of hepatic metastases from colorectal cancers. *Arch Surg* 1976;111:330.

1021. Wimpson AHRW, Thomson WHF. Technical modifications making on-table washout easier. *Br J Surg* 1987;74:464.

1022. Winawer SJ. The role of CEA in the diagnosis of colonic cancer and other lesions. *Natl Large-Bowel Cancer Project Newslett* 1975;3:7.

1023. Winawer SJ. Screening for colorectal cancer. Presented at the International Symposium on Colorectal Cancer, New York, March 1979.

1024. Winawer SJ. Colon cancer. In: Hunt RH, Waye JD, eds. *Colonoscopy: techniques, clinical practice and colour atlas.* London: Chapman & Hall, 1981:327.

1025. Winawer SJ, Flehinger BJ, Buchalter J, et al. Declining serum cholesterol levels prior to diagnosis of colon cancer: a time-trend case-control study. *JAMA* 1990;263:2083.

1026. Winawer SJ, Fletcher RH, Miller L, et al. Colorectal cancer screening: clinical guidelines and rationale. *Gastroenterology* 1997;112:594.

1027. Winawer SJ, Leidner SD, Hajdu SI, et al. Colonoscopic biopsy and cytology in the diagnosis of colon cancer. *Cancer* 1978;42:2849.

1028. Winawer SJ, Leidner SD, Miller DG, et al. Results of a screening program for the detection of early colon cancer and polyps using fecal occult blood testing. *Gastroenterology* 1977;72:1150(abst A127).

1029. Winawer SJ, Miller C, Lightdale C, et al. Patient response to sigmoidoscopy: a randomized, controlled trial of rigid and flexible sigmoidoscopy. *Cancer* 1987;60:1905.

1030. Winslet MC, Youngs D, Burdon DW, et al. Short-term chemoprophylaxis with ceftizoxime versus five-day aminoglycoside with metronidazole in "contaminated" lower gastrointestinal surgery. *Dis Colon Rectum* 1990;33:878.

1031. Winzelberg GG, Grossman SJ, Rizk S, et al. Indium-111 monoclonal antibody B72.3 scintigraphy in colorectal cancer: correlation with computed tomography, surgery, histopathology, immunohistology, and human immune response. *Cancer* 1992;69:1656.

1032. Wiratkapun S, Kraemer M, Seow-Choen F, et al. High preoperative serum carcinoembryonic antigen predicts metastatic recurrence in potentially curative colonic cancer: results of a five-year study. *Dis Colon Rectum* 2001;44:231.

1033. Wobbes T, Joosen KHG, Kuypers HHC, et al. The effect of packed cells and whole-blood transfusions on survival after curative resection for colorectal carcinoma. *Dis Colon Rectum* 1989;32:743.

1034. Wolff BG. Current status of incidental surgery. *Dis Colon Rectum* 1995;38:435.

1035. Wolff BG, Pemberton JH, van Heerden JA, et al. Elective colon and rectal surgery without nasogastric decompression. *Ann Surg* 1989;209:670.

1036. Wolloch Y, Zer M, Lurie M, et al. Ischemic colitis proximal to obstructing carcinoma of the colon. *Am J Proctol* 1979;30:17.

1037. Wolmark N, Fisher B, Rockette H, et al. Postoperative adjuvant chemotherapy or BCG for colon cancer: results from NSABP protocol C-01. *J Natl Cancer Inst* 1988; 80:30.

1038. Wolmark N, Fisher B, Weiand HS. The prognostic value of the modifications of the Dukes' C class of colorectal cancer: an analysis of the NSABP clinical trials. *Ann Surg* 1986;203:115.

1039. Wolmark N, Fisher B, Wieand S, et al. The prognostic significance of preoperative carcinoembryonic antigen levels in colorectal cancer. *Ann Surg* 1984;199:375.

1040. Wolters U, Keller HW, Sorgatz S, et al. Prospective randomized study of preoperative bowel cleansing for patients undergoing colorectal surgery. *Br J Surg* 1994;81: 598.

1041. Wong JH, Bowles BJ, Bueno R, et al. Impact of the number of negative nodes on disease-free survival in colorectal cancer patients. *Dis Colon Rectum* 2002;45:1341.

1042. Wong N, Lasko D, Rabelo R, et al. Genetic counseling and interpretation of genetic tests in familial adenomatous polyposis and hereditary nonpolyposis colorectal cancer. *Dis Colon Rectum* 2001;44:271.

1043. Wood JS, Frost DB. Results using the biofragmentable anastomotic ring for colon anastomosis. *Am Surg* 1993; 59:642.

1044. Wood TF, Nora DT, Morton DL, et al. One hundred consecutive cases of sentinel lymph node mapping in early colorectal carcinoma: detection of missed micrometastases. *J Gastrointest Surg* 2002;6:322.

1045. Wool NL, Straus AK, Roseman DL. Hickman catheter placement simplified. *Am J Surg* 1983;145:283.

1046. Woolfson K. Tumor markers in cancer of the colon and rectum. *Dis Colon Rectum* 1991;34:506.

1047. Wüllenweber H-P, Sutter C, Autschbach F, et al. Evaluation of Bethesda guidelines in relation to microsatellite instability. *Dis Colon Rectum* 2001;44:1281.

1048. Yamaguchi A, Ishida T, Nishimura G, et al. Detection by CT during arterial portography of colorectal cancer metastases to liver. *Dis Colon Rectum* 1991;34:37.

1049. Yamaguchi A, Kurosaka Y, Ishida T, et al. Clinical significance of tumor markers NCC-ST 439 in large bowel cancers. *Dis Colon Rectum* 1991;34:921.

1050. Yano T, Fukuyama Y, Yokoyama H, et al. Failure in resection of multiple pulmonary metastases from colorectal cancer. *J Am Coll Surg* 1997;185:120.

1051. Yeatman TJ, Bland KI, Copeland EM III, et al. Relationship between colorectal liver metastases and CEA levels in gallbladder bile. *Ann Surg* 1989;210:505.

1052. Yiu CY, Baker LA, Boulos PB. Anti-epithelial membrane antigen monoclonal antibodies and radioimmunolocalization of colorectal cancer. *Br J Surg* 1991;78:1212.

1053. Young JL Jr, Devesa SS, Cutler SJ. Incidence of cancer in United States blacks. *Cancer Res* 1975;35:3523.

1054. Young-Fadok TM, Wolff BG, Nivatvongs S, et al. Prophylactic oophorectomy in colorectal carcinoma: preliminary results of a randomized prospective trial. *Dis Colon Rectum* 1998;41:277.

1055. Zamcheck N, Moore TL, Dhar P, et al. Immunologic diagnosis and prognosis of human digestive-tract cancer: carcinoembryonic antigens. *N Engl J Med* 1972;286:83.

1056. Zinkin LD. A critical review of the classifications and staging of colorectal cancer. *Dis Colon Rectum* 1983;26: 37.

1057. Zinkin LD, Brandwein C. Adenocarcinoma in Crohn's colitis. *Dis Colon Rectum* 1980;23:115

1058. Zmora O, Mahajna A, Bar-Zakai B, et al. Colon and rectal surgery without mechanical bowel preparation: a randomized prospective trial. *Ann Surg* 2003;237:363.

1059. Zmora O, Pikarsky AJ, Wexner SD. Bowel preparation for colorectal surgery. *Dis Colon Rectum* 2001;44:1537.

Chapter 23

Carcinoma of the Rectum

To preserve and to renew is almost as noble as to create.
Voltaire: *A Philosophical Dictionary*

Any fool can cut off a leg—it takes a surgeon to save one.
George G. Ross

Chapter 22 addresses the diagnosis and treatment of cancer of the colon. In this chapter, the presentation, evaluation, management, and results of treatment of cancer of the rectum are presented.

SIGNS, SYMPTOMS, AND DIAGNOSIS

The signs and symptoms of cancer of the rectum are discussed in Chapter 22. Bleeding is the most common complaint (35% to 40%), followed by diarrhea, change in bowel habits, and abdominal pain. Rectal pain, however, as a presenting symptom is quite uncommon and implies a more distal lesion, one that invades deeply, or one that impinges or extends into the anal canal.

Carcinoma of the Prostate

Potential confusion may occasionally exist in the differential diagnosis. One must be wary of the rectal mass that results from invasion by carcinoma of the prostate. A tumor of the prostate may actually lead to rectal ulceration. The lesion may become so large that the rec-

tum is completely encircled and obstructive symptoms are produced (Figure 23-1). In a review by Fry and colleagues of 13 such patients, six had rectal bleeding, and all had constipation.[227] In ten cases, the lesion was annular.

Biopsy may show adenocarcinoma, but if it is poorly differentiated, special staining may be required to establish the tumor to be of prostatic origin (acid phosphatase; prostate-specific antigen).[638] Because of the frequency of both conditions, the two tumors may occasionally occur synchronously (Figure 23-2). If computed tomography (CT) is performed, a consistent finding is the presence of ureteral dilatation.[227]

The significance of an incorrect diagnosis cannot be overestimated because the treatment of the two conditions is obviously so different.

HISTORICAL NOTES

Colostomy as a diverting procedure has its origins in antiquity. Praxagoras (*circa* 400 BC) was alleged to have employed some form of decompression maneuver for ileus. Alexis Littre (1710) is usually credited with the concept of ultimately performing a colostomy when he performed a postmortem examination on an infant who died with an imperforate anus. He is quoted as stating: " . . . it would be necessary to make an incision into the belly, open the two ends of the closed bowel, . . . bring the bowel to the surface of the body wall where it would never close, but perform the function of an anus."[479] Colostomy, however, did not

---

Alexis Littre (1658–1726) Alexis Littre's name is often confused with that of another eminent French anatomist, Emile Littré, who lived about a century later (note the accent over the "e"). Littre was born on July 21, 1658, at Cordes, Tarn-et-Garonne, France. He studied in Montpellier and in Paris. In 1690, he became licensed in medicine and received a doctorate in 1691. As an anatomist and surgeon, Littre lectured extensively and is credited with numerous advances in surgical techniques. He was the first to suggest that a deliberate colostomy could be successfully performed when he examined the body of a 6-day-old infant born with an imperforate anus. His concept was extraordinarily prescient. His many papers were published in *L'Histoire de l'Académie des Sciences*. Littre's name is associated with the mucus glands of the male urethra and the diverticular hernia. He died on February 3, 1726.

achieve an important role until Amussat (1839),[12] a French surgeon, urged that it be the routine procedure for obstructing rectal cancer.[513] For most of the nineteenth and into the twentieth century, the stoma was placed in the inguinal or iliac region. This avoided entering the peritoneal cavity. Luke,[500] however, was an exception, and was the first to bring the bowel out in the area of the rectus muscle, whereas Deaver[158] was an advocate of lumbar colostomy.

The treatment of carcinoma of the rectum by some form of excisional or amputative procedure dates back more than 250 years, but it was not until 1826 that Lisfranc successfully excised the rectum for this condition.[478] His was a transanal approach and, as such, was of necessity used only for low-lying rectal lesions. This procedure and merely supportive care were the only available options. Modifications were introduced by

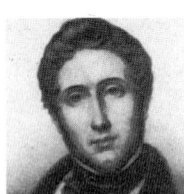

Jean Zulema Amussat (1796–1855) Amussat was born at St. Maixent in the Poitou, France. He was the son of a physician, and he received his basic tutelage at the hands of his father and from another surgeon in the town. At the age of 17, Amussat joined the army in a position equivalent to today's medic and performed many battlefield operations during the Napoleonic Wars. He became quite knowledgeable in anatomy through his wartime experiences and by dissecting the corpses of Russian soldiers. Following the war, he went to Paris to complete his medical studies. While there, he developed an interest in neurologic disease and is credited with having invented the rachitome. In 1822, he described a technique for removing foreign bodies from the bladder and for dilating urethral strictures. In 1826, he described the different kinds of groin hernias as they related to the inferior epigastric artery. In 1835, he published an experimental technique of intestinal anastomosis. He also presented classic works on experimental air embolism in animals, surgery for uterine fibroids, surgery for strabismus, and hemorrhoidectomy. He is believed to be the first person to perform a colostomy for an obstructing carcinoma of the rectum and was considered one of the most ingenious and innovative surgeons of his time. He was recognized by his colleagues through his elevation to membership in the Imperial Academy of Medicine and was a Chevalier of the French Legion of Honor.

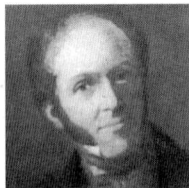

James Luke (1799–1881) Luke was born at Exeter, England, the son of a merchant and banker. At the age of 17, and upon the death of his father, he became attached to John Andrews of the London Hospital. He attended the lectures and, 3 years later, was appointed Demonstrator of Anatomy. In 1827, he was elected Assistant Surgeon and ultimately achieved the position of Consulting Surgeon in 1861. At the Royal College of Surgeons, Luke was a member of the Council for 20 years and was President in 1853 and again in 1862. He was a Hunterian Orator in 1852. Luke was a tall man who was said to harbor an irascible temper. A rapid surgeon, he once amputated a leg at the hip and removed the limb in 27 seconds. He was particularly interested in the treatment of cleft palate and of fractures and in the repair of groin hernias. He is believed to have been the first surgeon to perform a pararectus incision for bowel obstruction, bringing the proximal colon out in this location. He recommended this approach in preference to Amussat's suggestion, particularly when the site of the obstruction had not been clearly delineated preoperatively. Luke retired to Buckinghamshire, where he lived as a country gentleman, employing himself in woodcarving until his death.

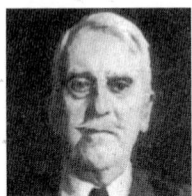

John Blair Deaver (1855–1931) Deaver was born in Lancaster County, Pennsylvania, the son of a country physician. He attended Nottingham Academy near his home and matriculated in America's first medical school, the University of Pennsylvania in Philadelphia, graduating in 1878. Following internship at the German Hospital and Children's Hospital of Philadelphia, he embarked in clinical practice. In 1886, he joined the staff of the German Hospital and developed an enormous personal practice in surgery. His Saturday afternoon operative clinics were attended by surgeons throughout the world while he performed as many as 25 operations in an afternoon. It was, in fact, at the German Hospital that he achieved his greatest recognition, although he was called to the post of Professor of the Practice of Surgery at the University of Pennsylvania in 1911 and assumed the Chair 7 years later. Deaver was considered an aggressive and radical surgeon—a great "slasher." He was among the early advocates of immediate appendectomy for acute appendicitis. He often stated, "An inch and a half, a minute and a half, a week and a half," to mean respectively the length of the incision, the time it took to perform the operation, and the duration of the hospital stay. "Cut well, get well, stay well," was another of his favorite aphorisms. He was also responsible for using the word "pathology" to mean pathologic finding or lesion rather than the study (e.g., "what is the pathology?"). Deaver's name is well-recognized by every medical student and surgical house officer who has had the displeasure of holding "his" retractor. He, in fact, never permitted his assistants to perform any aspect of the operation. He insisted that all be done by his own hand. Although he was accorded many honors, including that of President of the American College of Surgeons, the practice of surgery was his total commitment—this, and the writing of five books and almost 250 articles.

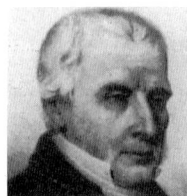

Jacques Lisfranc (1790–1847) Lisfranc was born in Saint-Paul-Jarrest (Loire), France, the son of a physician. He accomplished his preliminary studies at the Lyceum in Lyons and then went to Paris to continue his medical training at the Hôtel-Dieu. It was there that he came under the tutelage of Dupuytren. Later, however, the two became rivals and developed a vigorous animosity toward each other. Lisfranc received his doctorate in medicine in 1812 at a time when France was involved in the Napoleonic Wars. He was commissioned as a surgeon and distinguished himself in campaigns in Saxony and in France. Following the wars, he established his practice in Paris. Fortuitously, one day Lisfranc rescued a magistrate who fell from a horse, and through this serendipitous meeting he was invited to join the Faculty of Medicine at the Hospital of Pity. He rose rapidly to become Chief of Surgery. For more than 20 years, he was affiliated with this institution and wrote numerous articles on such diverse subjects as shoulder disarticulation, the application of the stethoscope in the diagnosis of fractures, and diseases of the uterus. It has been generally attributed that Lisfranc was the first person to remove a cancerous tumor from the rectum, essentially by means of a transanal operation. A man of formidable reputation, Lisfranc was a founding member and ultimately President of the French Academy of Medicine and a Chevalier of the Legion of Honor.

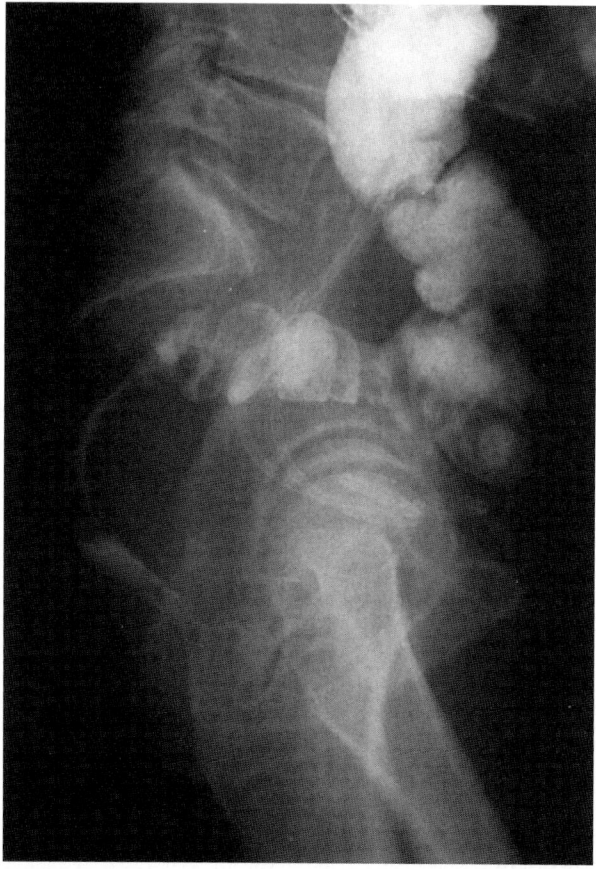

FIGURE 23-1. Barium enema study demonstrates profound rectal stricture, which on subsequent evaluation was proved to result from a circumferential narrowing as a consequence of invasive prostatic cancer.

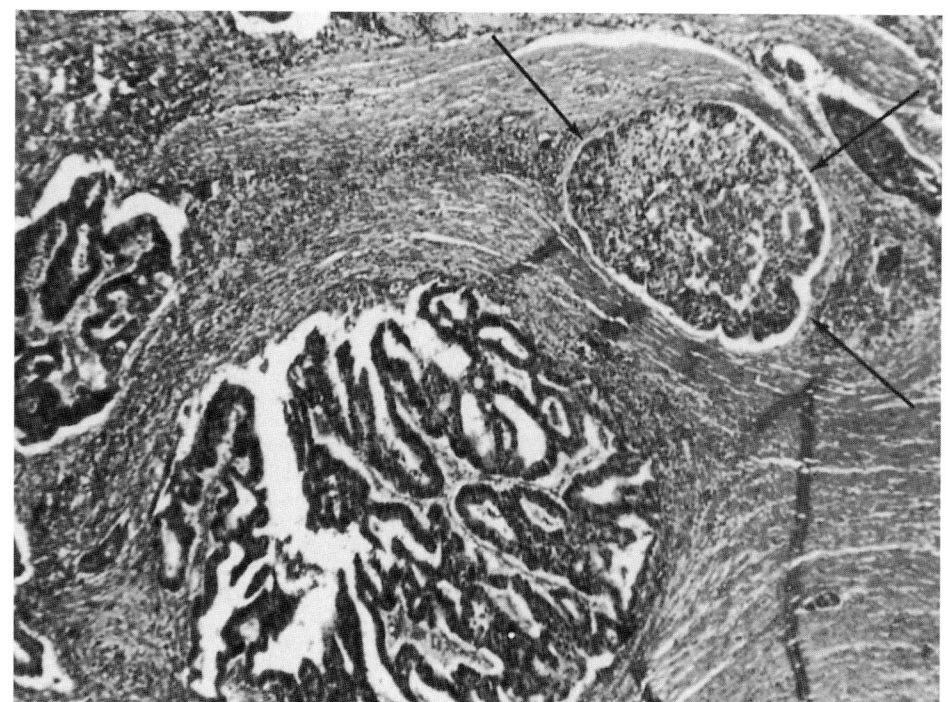

FIGURE 23-2. Prostatic carcinoma *(arrows)* invading the rectal wall with an associated primary rectal cancer. This is known as a collision tumor. (Original magnification × 250; courtesy of Rudolf Garret, M.D.)

von Volkmann,[849] Cripps,[138] and others, but the results of the perineal operation were poor. There was frequent incontinence, a high recurrence rate, and a high mortality rate.[671]

In 1885, Kraske removed the coccyx and part of the sacrum (a maneuver that had been accomplished many times as an extension of the perineal proctectomy), but he preserved the anus and sphincters to effect an anastomosis.[436,437] Often, however, continuity of the bowel could not be restored, either because of too much tension on the upper segment, impairment of the blood supply, or both, and the procedure was often completed by the establishment of a sacral anus. The operation was quite popular for a time but ultimately fell into disrepute because of the complications of sepsis, anastomotic leak, and recurrent disease.

In 1894, Czerny was unable to remove a rectal cancer and combined the extirpation with an abdominal opera-

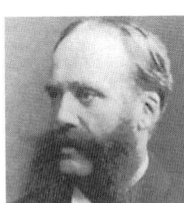

Richard von Volkmann (1830–1889) von Volkmann was born at Leipzig, Germany, the son of the Professor of Anatomy and Physiology at the University of Halle. All of his life he was associated with the university at which his father taught. In 1856, he was appointed Deputy to the Surgical Clinic of Professor Blasius, and in 1867, von Volkmann achieved the Chair in Surgery. After a time in military service during the Franco-Prussian War, he returned to his own hospital to confront the ravages of sepsis, having become familiar with Lister's work. He was so successful in applying listerian principles that it was to Volkmann's unit rather than to Britain that surgeons came from throughout the world to learn these methods. A visitor to the clinic he designed would be impressed with the terrazzo paving, constructed in such a manner as to permit efficient drainage. This was extremely important, because flushing the wounds with carbolic solution from gardening pots was always employed during a procedure, given that sepsis was such a pervasive problem. Volkmann's primary interests were orthopedics and general surgery. He emphasized the importance of open drainage and widening of wounds and made other contributions to the management of hydatid cyst of the liver, intraabdominal abscess, ulcer disease, tuberculous arthritis, joint dislocation, and compound fractures. His "improved" operation for excision of the rectum is less familiar than that of his pupil, Kraske. In fact, his name is recognized today primarily because of his description of the pathophysiology of ischemic muscle contracture. Besides being a master surgeon with an enormous private practice, von Volkmann was a superb orator. He could lecture fluently in several languages, including Latin. He was also well recognized and extremely popular throughout Germany as a published author of poems and fairy tales for children.

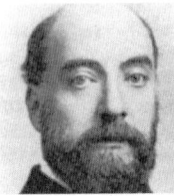

William Harrison Cripps (1850–1923) Cripps was born in Gloucestershire, England, of a prominent family. He received his medical education at St. Bartholomew's Hospital, obtaining his membership in the Royal College of Surgeons in 1872. He was attached to St. Bartholomew's for the remainder of his professional life. In 1876, he was awarded the Jacksonian Prize by the Royal College of Surgeons for his monograph, *Carcinoma of the Rectum*. Cripps was not a particular enthusiast for listerian methods. For example, he did not operate under the carbolic spray, which was then in vogue. He was, however, the only surgeon at the hospital at that time who would make a complete change of clothes before surgery. Cripps was one of the early British advocates of inguinal colostomy, often employing the procedure both for palliation and before perineal and transsacral excision for rectal cancer.

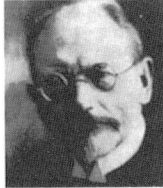

Paul Kraske (1851–1930) Kraske was born in Berg, near Muskau, Germany, and obtained his surgical training in Halle under the tutelage of Richard von Volkmann, whom he assisted from 1876 through 1883. For several years, Kraske demonstrated a particular interest in colorectal cancer and produced a number of papers on the subject. It was this, the foundation for his fame, that caused him to be selected as Director of the Surgical Clinic in Freiburg at the age of 32 years. In 1885, he presented a lecture at the Fourteenth Congress of the German Society of Surgery on the subject of the transsacral approach to the removal of rectal cancer. His experience was based on cadaver dissections and the treatment of two patients. Kraske was also considered a great patriot, having volunteered as a soldier in the Franco-Prussian War of 1870 to 1871 and as a medical officer in the beginning of the First World War. His particular interest in his later years was in the value of early laparotomy for abdominal wounds. Kraske remained faithful to the University of Freiburg until his death and led the clinic for 36 years until he retired in 1919.

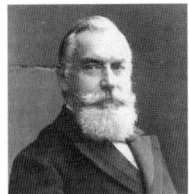

Vincenz Czerny (1842–1916) Vincenz Czerny was born in Trautenau, Bohemia, on November 19, 1842, the son of a pharmacist. Having become fascinated with the microscope, he became quite interested in the study of botany and zoology. He entered the University of Prague in 1860 to study medicine. He continued his education at the University of Vienna and achieved his medical degree, *summa cum laude*, in 1866. In 1868, he was appointed assistant to the great Theodor Billroth. He soon developed an abiding commitment to general surgery, especially the performance of pioneering work in gastric and esophageal surgery. In addition, he was the first to remove the larynx. In 1870 and 1871, he served with the German army in France and upon his return was appointed Professor of Surgery at the University of Freiburg, at the remarkable age of 29. At this time, his writings were numerous and diverse, including those on tuberculosis, intestinal suturing, embolism, and tumor transplantation, to name only a few. In 1877, Czerny was appointed Professor of Surgery at Heidelberg, where he served for 25 years. It was there that he performed the first vaginal hysterectomy and, in 1884, the first abdominoperineal resection. In 1906, he established the Institute for Cancer Research in Heidelberg following an international tour, which included a visit to the New York State Institute for the Study of Malignant Disease in Buffalo. Czerny was recognized with numerous honors and awards, including Honorary Fellowship in the American Surgical Association (1885) and Presidency of the International Association for Cancer Research.

tion, thus becoming the first person to perform an abdominoperineal resection (APR).[151] In 1908, Miles described his modification of Czerny's operation, placing emphasis on meticulous dissection and removing the zone of upward spread of the cancer (Figure 23-3).[568] He concluded as follows:

(1) that an abdominal anus is a necessity; (2) that the whole of the pelvic colon, with the exception of the part from which the colostomy is made, must be removed because its blood-supply is contained in the zone of upward spread; (3) that the whole of the pelvic mesocolon below the point where it crosses the common iliac artery, together with a strip of peritoneum at least one-inch wide on either side of it, must be cleared away; (4) that the group of lymph nodes situated over the bifurcation of the common iliac artery are in all instances to be removed; and lastly (5) that the perineal portion of the operation should be carried out as widely as possible so that the lateral and downward zones of spread may be effectively extirpated.

Although initially presenting 12 patients, with an operative mortality of 42%, Miles believed that with improved technique and further experience the operation could be performed relatively safely. Later, as performed by him, it was a most impressive display of operative technique—one of the noted sites of London surgery in the 1920s and 1930s.[271] The abdominal phase, carried out with the patient lying flat on the table and in a steep Trendelenburg tilt, seldom took more than 35 to 40 minutes. Miles was quite prescient: the Miles resection has become the standard operation for the treatment of cancers of the low rectum. A presumably less radical but perhaps safer procedure was the attitude taken by Miles'

rival, Percy Lockhart-Mummery (see Biography, Chapter 9), who favored a perineal excision, preceded 2 or 3 weeks earlier by a minilaparotomy to determine that the growth was resectable.[271] When this was the case, a loop-iliac colostomy was established.

An alternative operation for treatment of cancer of the middle to upper rectum or of the rectosigmoid was proposed by Hartmann in 1923.[318] This procedure succeeded in removing the tumor following establishment of a colostomy, but avoided the perineal dissection. However, the operation was useful for higher lesions only and, of course, was not designed for eventual reestablishment of intestinal continuity, although the Hartmann resection is frequently applied today in the initial surgical management of complicated sigmoid diverticulitis. The original article probably is worth reproducing in translation. It must represent a record for the briefest article to produce eponymous immortality for the author, because Hartmann's fame is based on only two paragraphs of narrative:

It is the rule that, in order to remove cancers of the distal pelvic colon, it is necessary to perform a very serious operation when removing the rectum by means of an abdominoperineal excision. In two patients who underwent colostomy for intestinal obstruction, at the second operation I limited resection to the intermediate portion of the colon between the artificial anus and the rectum, including the corresponding area of innervation. Following this, I closed the upper end of the rectum and reperitonealized it, without reconstructing the perineal floor.

Following the operation both cases were as uneventful as an operation for a cold appendix. The conservation of a small *cul-de-sac* of the rectum above the

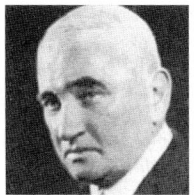

W. Ernest Miles (1869–1947) The name Miles is probably the best-recognized eponym in surgery of the colon and rectum. Miles was born in Trinidad, British West Indies, and trained at St. Bartholomew's Hospital, but the area of rectal surgery attracted him, and he became house surgeon to St. Mark's Hospital in London. Within a few years, he was appointed to the Gordon Hospital for Diseases of the Rectum and attained the senior honorary staff at the Royal Cancer Hospital in 1903. Much of his early training he owed to David Goodsall, to whose memory he dedicated his own book, *Rectal Surgery*, in 1939, and with whom he collaborated 40 years earlier on a two-volume work entitled *Diseases of the Rectum and Anus*. Miles did much to clarify the pathologic anatomy of hemorrhoids and their operative treatment; he classified and had unique success in the treatment of anal fistula, but his pecten band failed to endure. It is, however, in connection with the operation of abdominoperineal resection of the rectum that posterity will forever honor him. It was an operation that, as he planned it in 1906, required unswerving conviction and remarkable courage. A master surgeon, a brilliant and dexterous craftsman, he eventually was able to perform the entire operation in less than 30 minutes. He was the recipient of numerous honors, not only from his own country, but also from Ireland, the United States, France, and Greece. (Adapted from Burghard FF. In memoriam: W. Ernest Miles. *Br J Surg* 1947;35:320.)

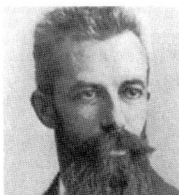

Henri Albert Hartmann (1860–1952) Hartmann was born in Paris. He apparently developed an early interest in pursuing a medical career, becoming a prosector in anatomy in 1884 at the University of Paris. Following graduation from the Medical School in 1887, he continued on the staff of the Hôtel Dieu and ultimately became Professor and Chairman of the Department of Surgery in 1909. Hartmann developed a huge clinical practice, performing in excess of 1,000 operations each year for 20 years. He took meticulous notes of each procedure and of the postoperative course. Most of his writings were in the areas of breast, gastric, and biliary surgery, but he also wrote books on gynecology, war injuries, and cancer. Hartmann achieved international recognition, and his clinic at the Hôtel Dieu became a mecca for surgeons from all over the world. He was accorded tributes in many countries, including honorary fellowship in the American Surgical Association and the Royal College of Surgeons of England and of Ireland. In his own country, he was a Grand Officer of the Legion of Honor. He died in Paris, January 2, 1952, at the age of 91.

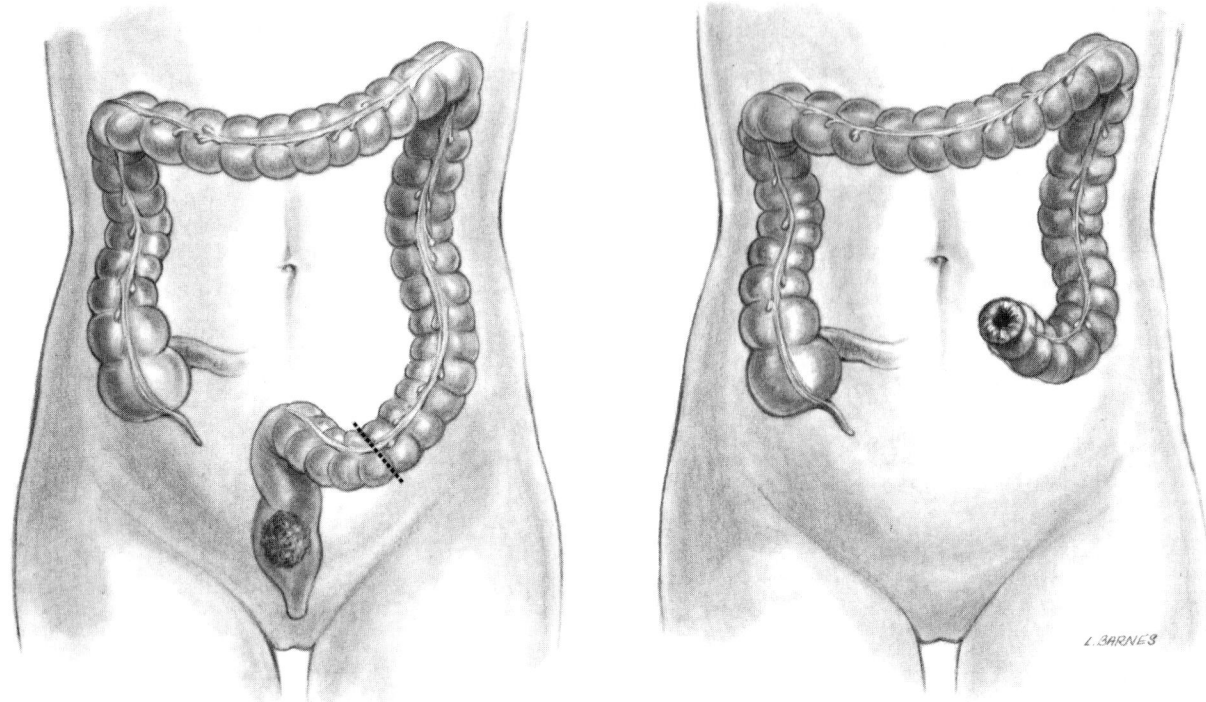

A

B

FIGURE 23-3. Carcinoma of the rectum. **(A)** Extent of removal in classic abdominoperineal resection. **(B)** The sigmoid colostomy is created in the left iliac fossa.

sphincters did not present a particular problem, and follow-up 9 and 10 months later revealed the patients to be quite well.[318]

The first documented attempt at abdominal resection with restoration of continuity is generally attributed to Reybard of Lyons (see Biography, Chapter 22).[681] He performed a partial sigmoid resection; the patient survived approximately 10 months. The fear of sepsis and anastomotic leak inspired Murphy, in 1892, to create his "button" (see Biography, Chapter 22; see Figure 22-34).[599] The same year, Maunsell[543] reported a technique using an anastomotic method employed by Hochenegg[353] in what has come to be called the "pull-through" procedure. A more practical modification of this approach was suggested by Weir[864] in 1901.

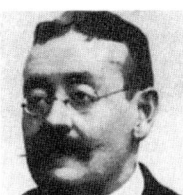

Henry Widenham Maunsell (1847–1895)   Maunsell was born in Dublin in 1847 and obtained his degree from the College of Surgeons in 1867. He moved to Melbourne, Australia, the following year and became Resident Medical Officer at the Melbourne Hospital. Following this appointment, he took a similar post in Hokitika, New Zealand. After achieving his M.D. degree from the College of Surgeons in Dublin, he returned to New Zealand and settled in Dunedin. In 1892, he reemigrated to the South Kensington section of London and devoted his efforts to writing, lecturing, and illustrating. He was quite well known as a fine artist who supplemented his surgical tutorials with his own beautiful drawings. The Maunsell method, the abdominoanal pull-through procedure, became for many surgeons the sphincter-saving operation of choice for the treatment of carcinoma of the rectum. He was an innovative surgeon and is credited with original concepts in the technique of intraabdominal hysterectomy. He was elected to the fellowship of the British Gynecological Society in 1889 and was appointed a Councillor in 1893. Maunsell died of bronchitis following a bout of influenza.

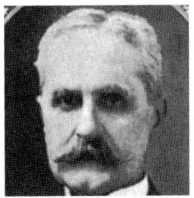

Robert Fulton Weir (1838–1927)   Weir was born in New York City, the son of a prominent pharmacist. His early education was in public school, and in 1854 he graduated, the youngest in his class, from the College of the City of New York, then known as the Free Academy. In 1857, he earned the degree of Master of Arts from the same institution. By clerking for his father and through contacts with local physicians, he developed an interest in surgery. In 1859, he received his degree in medicine from the New York College of Physicians and Surgeons and became a pupil and assistant to Gurdon Buck (who originated Buck's extension). In 1861, Weir entered the army and for most of the Civil War was in charge of the general hospital at Frederick, Maryland. Following the war, he practiced in New York City, ultimately becoming Chief of the Surgical Service at Roosevelt Hospital and Professor of Surgery at Women's Medical College and at the College of Physicians and Surgeons. Weir was one of the first in the United States to adopt Lister's technique of antisepsis; he was among the early workers in surgery of the brain and was one of the first persons to recognize duodenal ulcer as a distinct pathologic entity. Weir went on to become President of the American Surgical Association, the New York Surgical Society, and the New York Academy of Medicine. He was made an honorary Fellow of the Royal College of Surgeons of England and was one of five surgeons honored by the American College of Surgeons at its initial convocation.

During the first half of the twentieth century, restoration of continuity by means by primary anastomosis evolved through abdominosacral resection and the familiar operation of anterior resection. The introduction of newer suture materials, the advocacy by some of interrupted suture technique, and the application of the stapling devices all indicate that the operation can nevertheless be improved and that the risk of complications can still be diminished.

FACTORS INFLUENCING THE CHOICE OF OPERATION

To save or not to save the sphincter is a perennial question. Is there a level below which an anastomosis should not be attempted? When is an APR inappropriate or an anterior resection the operation of choice? Unfortunately, there is no reliable answer to these questions. Some may even advise with the simple adage, "If you can feel the lesion you should not perform a sphincter-saving operation"—the rule of the index finger. However, this is much too simplistic an approach and may prejudice the surgeon to embark upon an inappropriate proctectomy.

Conversely, surgeons, in a zealous effort to avoid a colostomy and to reestablish intestinal continuity, may compromise on the margins of resection. The consequences can be tragic: recurrent disease, anastomotic obstruction, unremitting pelvic pain, and the requirement for subsequent surgery, including a colostomy. Obviously, an APR is no panacea, but it is an operation that can be accomplished with relative safety and is at least as effective as any other modality of treatment for the cure of carcinoma of the rectum.

There are a number of available procedures that can, under particular circumstances, be the preferred approach for a given patient:

- APR
- Low anterior resection (with colorectal or coloanal anastomosis; with or without J colonic pouch)
- Colostomy or ileostomy
- Hartmann's resection
- Abdominoanal pull-through
- Abdominosacral (coccygeal) resection
- Transsacral resection (Kraske's)
- Transsphincteric excision
- Transanal (local) excision
- Electrocoagulation
- Laser coagulation
- Cryosurgical destruction
- Interstitial or intracavitary radiation (obviously not an operation, but it can be the sole modality of treatment in some instances)

The alternatives to APR are, therefore, numerous and are discussed individually. However, if another resective procedure is contemplated, it should rarely be other than an anterior resection. If one embarks upon what may be called an esoteric sphincter-saving operation (e.g., abdominoanal pull-through, abdominosacral resection, electrocoagulation, transanal excision, transcoccygeal excision), one must be able to justify it as the optimal or at least a reasonable a option under the given circumstances.

Many surgeons utilize a more scientific approach to determining the proper surgical alternative. Sophisticated staging techniques have been suggested, including not only standard examination with biopsy and hematologic and radiologic studies, but also tumor DNA content, acute-phase reactive proteins, and endoluminal ultrasonography.[54,878] Factors that are helpful in determining the choice of operation for cancer in the rectum are summarized as follows:

- Level
- Macroscopic appearance (ulcerated, polypoid)
- Extent of circumferential involvement
- Fixity
- Degree of differentiation (histologic appearance)
- Tumor cell DNA content
- Endorectal ultrasound determination
- Magnetic resonance imaging (MRI) assessment
- CT
- Presacral adenopathy
- Body habitus
- Gender
- Age
- Metastatic disease
- Other systemic disease
- Other conditions that may affect one's ability to manage a colostomy (e.g., blindness, severe arthritis, mental incapacity)

The reader is referred to a publication by the American Society of Colon and Rectal Surgeons. This organization has established practice parameters for the preoperative evaluation and treatment of rectal cancer.[817]

Level of the Lesion

The distance of the lower edge of the tumor from the anal verge is probably the single most important variable that aids the surgeon in the choice of operation. This distance should be carefully measured using the rigid proctosigmoidoscope, and the result should be recorded (Figure 23-4). The flexible sigmoidoscope is not as accurate for this determination. When measuring, care must be taken to spread the buttocks, so that the instrument can be seen emerging from the anus, not from the buttocks fat.

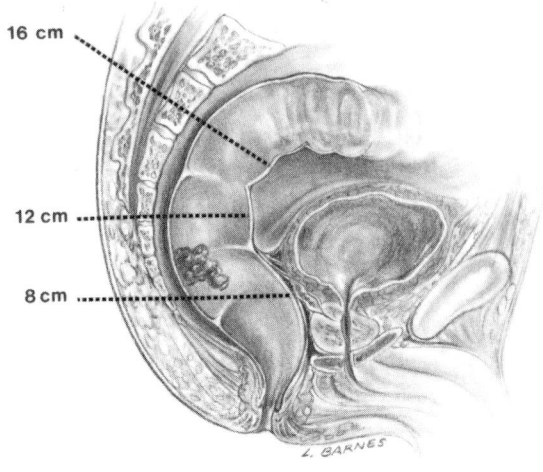

FIGURE 23-4. Rectal cancer. Tumors of the upper one third (23 to 16 cm) are amenable to anterior resection. Tumors of the lower one third (0 to 8 cm) usually require an abdominoperineal resection. It is the tumor in the middle one third that most often represents the management problem.

The preconceived notion that a tumor 7 cm from the anal verge requires APR but the one at 8 cm can be treated by anterior resection is erroneous. Other factors may prove the opposite to be true in both cases (e.g., fixity, size, degree of differentiation, pelvic anatomy).

Macroscopic Appearance

Generally, the distal margin of resection should be approximately 2 cm below the tumor, but for infiltrative carcinomas, one may not be "safe" from the risk of anastomotic recurrence even with a margin of 7 cm. The length of distal intramural spread of tumor in resected specimens is extremely variable, with three fourths of the rectal tumors in one study demonstrated to have no intramural spread.[876] A small, exophytic, well-differentiated lesion may be adequately removed with a 1-cm cuff of normal distal bowel. Ascertaining the appearance of the lesion, whether ulcerated, scirrhous (infiltrative), or polypoid, is very helpful in aiding the surgeon in the choice of operation (Figure 23-5).

Extent of Circumferential Involvement

Usually, more highly aggressive tumors tend to involve a greater circumference of the bowel wall when they present. Under these circumstances, a greater margin of resection is required. An anterior resection may be a poor choice even though resection and anastomosis can be technically effected.

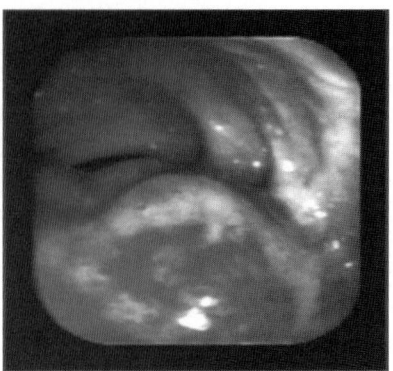

FIGURE 23-5. Proctoscopy demonstrates an exophytic, polypoid lesion, which on palpation was found to be freely movable. This tumor, theoretically, may be removed by local excision. (See Color Fig. 23-5.)

Fixity

Fixity of the tumor in the pelvis implies a poor prognosis. There is greater likelihood of residual tumor following resection, and anastomotic recurrence is a frequent sequela. An APR, although no guarantee of obviating the problem of recurrent disease, would probably offer better palliation, because the need for subsequent reoperation would be less likely. The presence of a fixed tumor should encourage the surgeon to consider neoadjuvant therapy (see later).

Histologic Appearance

A biopsy is, of course, mandatory and is done routinely, usually at the time of initial discovery of the lesion. Ideally, the material obtained should be from the edge of the lesion, because much useful information can be obtained. For example, an "expanding" margin implies that the area of invasion is pushing or reasonably well circumscribed, whereas an "infiltrating" margin suggests diffuse or widespread penetration of normal tissue.[388] All too often, however, the surgeon pays scant attention to the details of the report, except for noting whether the tumor is indeed malignant. However, it is important to be aware of the specific histologic appearance of a malignant tumor. Is it poorly differentiated, moderately well differentiated, or well differentiated (see Figs. 22-18 through 22-21)? Generally, tumors regarded as poorly differentiated have highly irregular glands or no glandular differentiation.[388] The more anaplastic, the more aggressive is the lesion; and the more aggressive, the greater is the resection margin that would be required. The chance of local recurrence is much higher with a poorly differentiated cancer than with one that is well differentiated. It is axiomatic that one must choose the most favorable cancers for performing less than a radical resection (see later). Therefore, one cannot overestimate the importance of degree of differentiation (Broder's classification), depth of penetration, and the presence or absence of venous or perineural invasion (PNI) in making the appropriate choice.

Shirouzu and colleagues evaluated whether PNI is an independent prognostic factor in individuals who underwent curative surgery.[754] There was a significant difference in local recurrence rates between those individuals with stage III lesions who were found to have PNI and those without PNI. In addition, the investigators found that patients with PNI and stage III lesions had a significantly lower survival rate.

Gagliardi and colleagues studied the effect of microacinar growth patterns on survival following radical surgery for rectal cancer in 138 consecutive patients.[236] They found that acinar size (whether microacinar or macroacinar) had independent prognostic value. Patients with microacinar tumors had a significantly reduced 5-year survival rate compared with those with macroacinar lesions. Saclarides and colleagues attempted to determine which features were predictors of nodal metastases.[710] They utilized nine histologic and morphologic features of 62 radically excised rectal cancers to determine which were associated with nodal disease. Statistically significant variables were worsening differentiation, increasing depth of penetration, microtubular configuration of 20% or more, the presence of venous invasion or PNI, and, of course, lymphatic invasion. Exophytic tumor morphology, mitotic count, and tumor size were not significant predictors.[710] In an analysis of all the variables or combination of factors, Broder's classification was the strongest predictor of nodal disease.

A particularly useful microscopic variable to identify is the extent of lymphocytic infiltration at the border of the tumor.[387] Jass and colleagues regarded this observation as "conspicuous" when there is a distinctive and delicate connective tissue mantle or cap at the invasive margin of the growth.[388] Patients who harbor tumors that demonstrate pronounced lymphocytic infiltration have a better prognosis than those who do not. If the pathologist fails to supply this information, he or she should be asked to review the slides and to amend the report. Optimally, the surgeon should view the histologic evidence himself or herself, in order to make the most reasoned recommendation to the patient.

Tumor Cell DNA Content

As with other solid cancers, malignant tumors of the bowel may demonstrate abnormalities in their chromosomal composition (see Chapter 22).[832] Reports of DNA measurements in human cancers suggest that flow cytometry assays of DNA ploidy have prognostic value.[106,395,558,832,884] Even with small rectal cancers, it appears that DNA content seems to provide useful prognostic information.[335] Hence, this may affect the choice of operation. A DNA histogram of normal colonic epithelium reveals that more than 90% of the cells have a single diploid peak. Carcinomas that are near diploid have a better prognosis than those that are aneuploid. Aggressive tumor behavior appears to correlate especially closely with aneuploidy in locally treated rectal cancers.[106] Although, the available data have not been subjected to long-term follow-up evaluation, analysis of DNA distribution may ultimately prove to be a more accurate predictor of extent of involvement and, therefore, prognosis, than is degree of differentiation. However, as of this writing, it appears that DNA ploidy parallels histologic differentiation, and it is therefore unlikely that this particular innovation will add more than microscopy.

Presacral Adenopathy

By careful palpation of the rectum, feeling for masses outside the wall, the surgeon can occasionally identify a hard lesion, a lymph node with metastasis. Such a finding can suggest (although by no means prove) that the tumor has spread beyond the bowel wall and that recurrence is, therefore, more likely, especially if a local procedure is performed. This is the type of situation in which neoadjuvant therapy may be of benefit. Of course, endorectal ultrasound is much more useful for identifying lymph nodes in this area (see later).

Computed Tomography

Numerous imaging modalities exist today for local staging, including three-dimensional reconstruction. These include endorectal ultrasonography, MRI with a phased-array coil, and multidetector CT with continuous scanning.[873] Since its introduction, CT had been thought to be a reasonably effective means for determining the depth of invasion of rectal cancer preoperatively.[95,117,430,750,843] Unfortunately, this has not proved to be the case. One thing is certain, however; CT is of great value in identifying metastatic disease, especially in the liver (see Figure 22-16) and elsewhere within the abdomen (Figs. 23-6 and 23-7).

Magnetic Resonance Imaging

MRI has also been used for preoperative assessment, but it has not been of particular advantage when compared with CT.[300,355] McNicholas and colleagues evaluated MRI

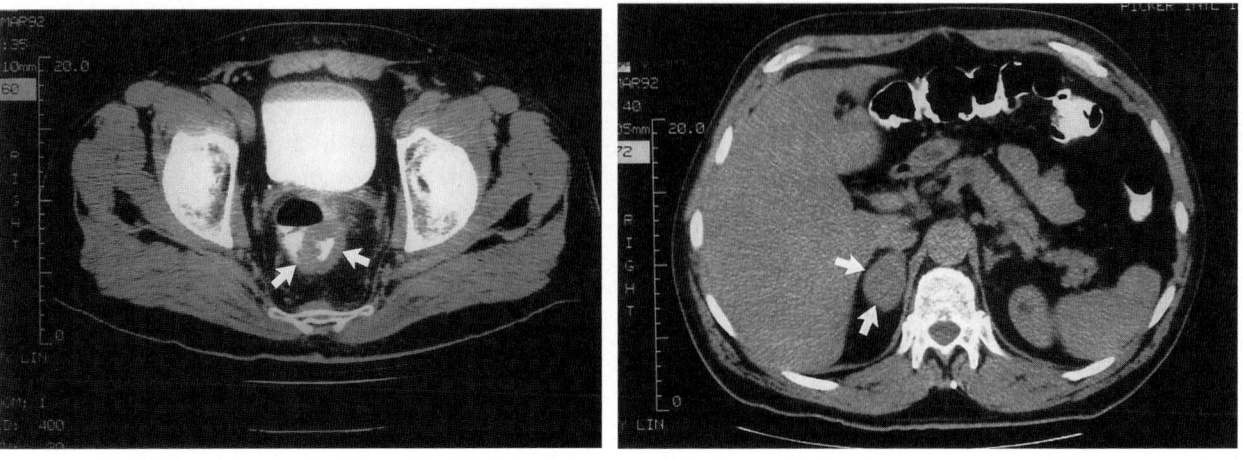

FIGURE 23-6. (**A**) Computed tomography demonstrates a tumor in the wall of the rectum *(arrows)*. (**B**) Metastatic tumor to the adrenal gland in this same patient can be appreciated *(arrows)*.

in 20 consecutive patient with rectal cancer who were to undergo curative surgery.[555] MRI staging concurred with histologic staging in 18 of 20 patients when Dukes' classification was used, but in only 14 when the Astler-Coller model was employed. The technique was effective in all but one patient with microscopic muscle wall invasion. The overall accuracy was 95%. Brown and co-workers used high-resolution MRI and compared their stagings with the pathologic specimens.[84] There was a 94% weighted agreement between MRI and pathology assessment of T stage.

Visualization of the endopelvic fascia and its relationship to the primary tumor is of critical importance with respect to staging and prognosis.[873] Both CT and MRI are believed by most radiologists to be comparable investigations for this purpose. Gagliardi and associates concluded, on the basis of their study of 28 patients, that MRI with *external* phase-array coils was more costly and not as accurate as endorectal ultrasound.[234] Others believe that MRI may be useful in the selection of patients for neoadjuvant chemoradiation therapy.[533]

Magnetic Resonance Imaging with Endorectal Coil

An improvement in MRI technique is the use of surface MRI coils to allow a higher definition of obtainable image with a smaller field of view.[304] By allowing identification of all the layers of the bowel wall, more accurate local staging is possible when compared with conventional MRI. As with endoluminal ultrasound, the technology is available for the office evaluation of patients (Medrad, Inc., Pittsburgh, PA). Initial reports implicated that this modality was promising for local staging of rectal cancer,[105] but some opine that the use of a pelvic phased-array coil does not improve the staging accuracy of MRI to a clinically useful level.[180,304]

Gualdi and colleagues staged 26 patients with rectal cancer by both endorectal coil MRI and transrectal ultrasound (TRUS), comparing their interpretations with the pathologically determined resected specimens.[297] Similar results were obtained. When there were staging errors, both modalities were more likely to overstage than to understage. The authors remind us of the fact that ultra-

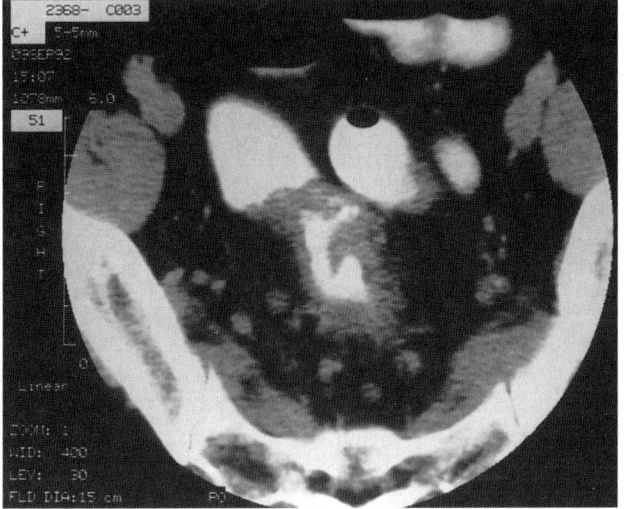

FIGURE 23-7. Computed tomography scan demonstrates a rectal tumor that obviously traverses the full thickness of the bowel wall. Lymph nodes are evident, but it cannot be determined with certainty whether these represent inflammatory perirectal nodes or tumor.

sound is more operator dependent, whereas MRI with endorectal coil is much more expensive.

Endorectal or Transrectal Ultrasound Examination

Endorectal ultrasound (Brüel & Kjaer Instruments, Inc., North Billerica, MA) has developed into an extremely useful tool for the preoperative assessment of patients with rectal cancer (see Figure 6-20).[13,53,77,124,262,347,407,432, 435,574,684,718] After a small enema is administered, the probe (Figure 23-8) is introduced into the rectum beyond the tumor. A balloon is filled with approximately 50 mL of water, and an acoustic contact is produced between the rotating part of the transducer and the rectal wall.[348] During withdrawal, the monitor is observed and the findings recorded.

Each of the layers of the rectum can be sonographically visualized, with a tumor usually appearing as a hypoechoic disruption of the rectal wall. The procedure may also reveal whether underlying lymph nodes are affected. Detection of invasive carcinoma within an otherwise villous lesion can be achieved with this technique.[6,450] In the experience of Hildebrandt and colleagues, lymph node metastases can be predicted with an accuracy of 72% and inflammatory lymph nodes with a specificity of 83%.[349] Many investigators, however, have expressed concern about the lack of specificity in distinguishing benign from malignant nodes.[392,704] The Memorial Sloan-Kettering Cancer Center (New York) group observed that the overall risk of undetected and untreated (if a local procedure is embarked upon) is 15%.[70]

Accurate preoperative staging with endorectal ultrasound implies the patients may be selected for a less than radical operation (see Local Procedures).[261] There is uniformity of agreement that optimal results can only be obtained if there is consistency in technique and in interpretation. Certainly, accuracy improves considerably with experience.[626] Mackay and colleagues emphasized that one needs to undertake 50 or more ultrasound procedures before optimal accuracy is achieved.[505] It is, therefore, preferable for the surgeon to be the individual responsible for performing and evaluating the study. Some investigators have commented that tumors of the lower rectum are incorrectly staged much more frequently than those of the middle and upper rectum.[342]

Technique

Wong (Memorial Sloan-Kettering Cancer Center) is regarded as an international authority on TRUS and in its interpretation. He has kind been kind enough to provide me a narrative of his technique, and I thought it useful to reproduce it here.

> The patient is instructed to take a Fleet enema 1 hour prior to the examination. The procedure is carefully explained to the patient and pertinent questions answered. The assistant enters the demographic data in the ultrasound computer as well as the frequency of the ultrasound probe and its focal range. The patient is placed in the left lateral position on the examining table. The study is preceded by a digital rectal examination to evaluate the size,

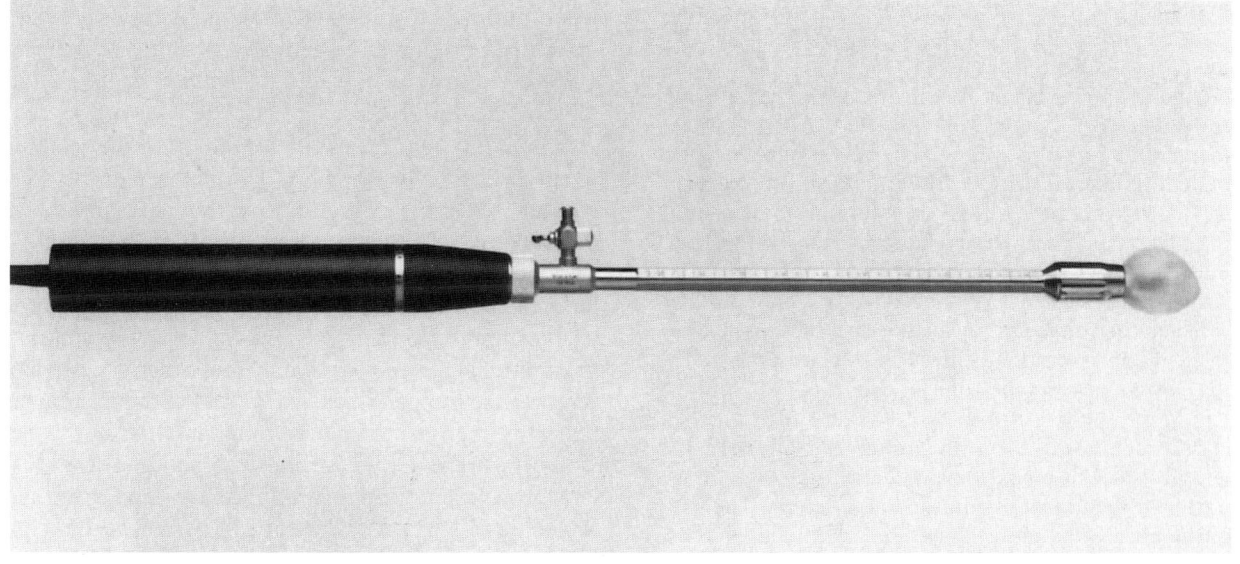

FIGURE 23-8. Ultrasound probe. (Courtesy of Brüel & Kjaer Instruments, Inc., North Billerica, MA.)

fixation, location, and morphology of the rectal lesion. In most instances the use of a large-bore proctoscope serves several purposes. It allows visual examination of the rectal tumor with exact determination of its location both with respect to circumferential involvement of the rectal wall and the distance from the anal verge. Second, it allows suctioning of any residual stool or enema fluid that might interfere with the acoustic pathways of the ultrasound waves that may distort the image. Most important, however, it allows easy passage of the probe above the tumor to ensure that the transducer is advanced above the rectal lesion to allow complete imaging. This is significant since the lower border of a rectal cancer can differ in the depth of invasion than the center or upper portions of the cancer, and lymph nodes in the perirectal region are often seen just above the level of the tumor. They will be missed if complete imaging is not obtained. Small distal lesions can be adequately imaged with the ultrasound inserted blindly and advanced above the lesion, but for most midrectal, bulky tumors the use of a proctoscope will facilitate the passage of the transducer.

The probe is prepared by placing a condom over the transducer head followed by a metal ring or rubber band that secures the base of the balloon. The assistant holds the probe with the balloon in the most dependent position and fills the balloon with about 50 mL of water via the connector at the base of the metal shaft. Any air in the system is aspirated through the syringe and expelled. A water-soluble lubricant is liberally applied to the outside of the balloon. The probe is now ready for insertion. The proctoscope is then advanced above the rectal lesion, and water-soluble lubricant is inserted into the lumen of the proctoscope to facilitate passage of the probe. The probe is then gently introduced through the proctoscope and advanced such that the transducer is sited above the rectal cancer. Once the 20 cm mark on the shaft of the probe is at the proximal end of the proctoscope, the proctoscope is then pulled back on the probe as far as possible, thus exposing the transducer for 7 cm beyond the end of the instrument, thus positioned about the rectal cancer. The balloon is then instilled with 30 to 60 mL of water; this is the volume required to obtain optimal imaging. The transducer is activated by depressing the button on the proximal end of the probe, and the image on the screen is visualized.

When the connector for introducing the water into the balloon is pointing upwards (towards the ceiling), by convention the anterior aspect of the rectum will be on the superior part of the screen, the right lateral rectum will be on the examiner's left, the left lateral wall will be on the examiner's right, and the posterior rectum will be in the lower screen. The tip of the ultrasound probe should be maintained in the center of the rectal lumen in order to achieve optimal imaging of the rectal wall and perirectal structures.

Some adjustments may have to be made on the *gain* of the ultrasound unit in order to provide better imaging. Occasionally, it is possible to perfectly depict all five layers of the rectum circumferentially, but usually only a portion of the rectal wall at a time will be optimally imaged. Minor adjustments will have to be made in the location of the probe relative to the rectal wall at various locations to optimally image all five layers clearly. Once optimal imaging of the rectal wall and surrounding structures has been achieved, the ultrasound probe is gradually withdrawn while carefully observing the screen and the images obtained. Several hard-copy images should be obtained for future reference through the use of a Polaroid image recorder. These images can be obtained by stopping the rotation of the transducer by depressing the activation/deactivation button and holding it longer, thus activating the recorder.

When a critical area of the tumor needs to be visualized at a higher magnification, the window can be activated which gives a large image of the area being examined. The entire length of the rectal tumor is evaluated. It is not uncommon for one to perform several passes along the full length of the tumor in order to acquire all the relevant information.

Attention must also be focused on the perirectal tissues in order to search for potentially involved lymph nodes. In general, normal lymph nodes are not visualized with the ultrasound, and, therefore, any hypoechoic structure in the surrounding perirectal tissue should be suspected of harboring metastatic disease. Lymph nodes often exhibit hypoechoic echogeneicity comparable to that of the primary tumor, are more often round than oval, and are frequently irregular in appearance. Lymph nodes can be distinguished from blood vessels which are also circular hypoechoic areas, but when followed distally and proximally they seem to extend further and may be seen to elongate and to branch. Once the study is completed the balloon is deflated, and the probe is removed.

Figure 23-9 illustrates the five layers of the rectal wall seen schematically and in the TRUS image of the normal rectum. The inner white line represents the interface of the balloon with the mucosal surface of the rectal wall. The inner black line represents the mucosa and muscularis mucosa, whereas the middle white line corresponds to the submucosa. It is this middle white line that is the most crucial layer to visualize in order to determine whether the tumor is invasive.[391] The outer black line corresponds to the muscularis propria whereas the outer white line represents the interface between the muscularis propria and the perirectal fat. Once it has been ascertained that the middle white line is broken, then the presence of an invasive tumor has been confirmed. It is then a matter of determining the depth of invasion. Figure 23-10

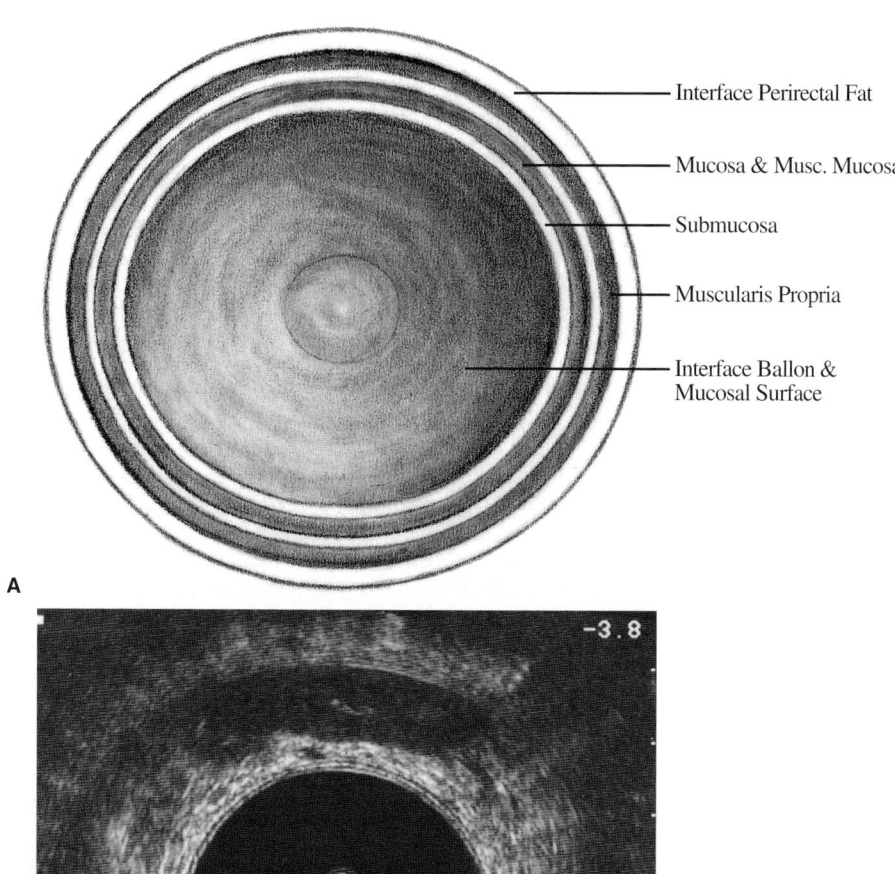

A

B

FIGURE 23-9. Endorectal ultrasound. **(A)** Schematic diagram of normal rectal wall anatomic layers. **(B)** Endorectal ultraound imaging of normal rectum.

demonstrates an ultrasound of a minimally invasive cancer with the corresponding resected, microscopic area. Figure 23-11 shows transmural involvement by tumor.

The TNM (tumor, node, metastasis) classification is used with a *u* modifier to describe depth of invasion and the presence or absence of metastatic lymph nodes as described by Beynon and co-workers:[53,56]

T Stage	Ultrasound Characteristics
uT_0	Noninvasive lesion. Hyperechoic submucosal interface is intact.
uT_1	Invasion of submucosa only. Hyperechoic middle white line is stippled and irregular but not disrupted.
uT_2	Breaching of hyperechoic middle white line indicates invasion of hypo choic muscularis propria (Figure 23-12). Outer white line is intact. Deep uT_2 lesions have a scalloped appearance.
uT_3	Invasion through muscularis propria into perirectal fat (Fig. 23-11). Outer (hyperechoic) white line (junction of muscularis propria with perirectal fat) is disrupted.
uT_4	Extension into adjacent organ or structure (e.g., vagina, prostate, bladder, cervix, seminal vesicles). Plane between any of these structures and the rectum is obliterated.

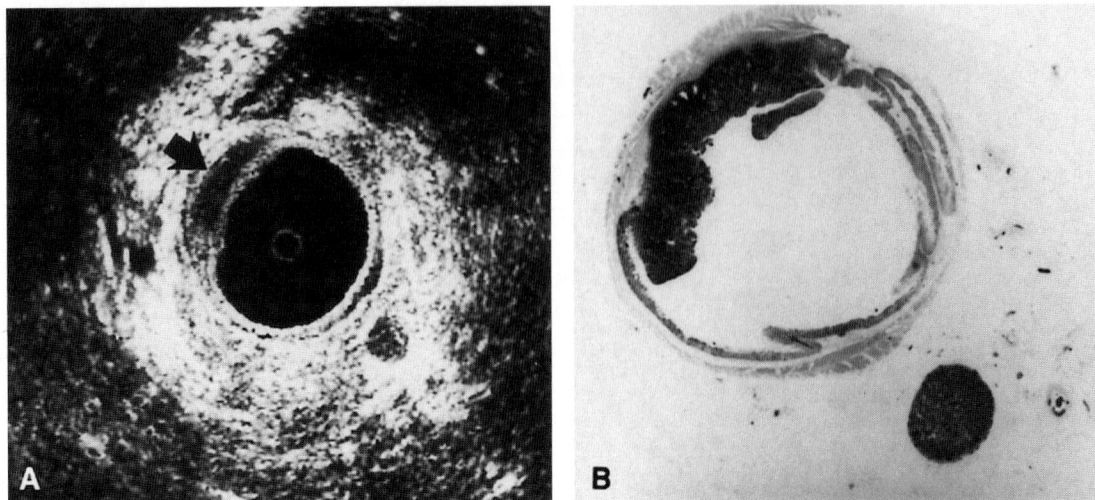

FIGURE 23-10. Endorectal ultrasound. **(A)** Sonogram of a rectal cancer confined to wall of the bowel *(arrow)*. The *black cavity* is the water-filled balloon with the *white circle in the center* corresponding to the transducer. A hyperechoic lymph node can be seen in the **lower right**. **(B)** Corresponding photomicrograph of the excised specimen confirms the depth of invasion by tumor. The lymph node in the lower right was free of tumor. (Courtesy of Ulrich Hildebrandt, M.D.)

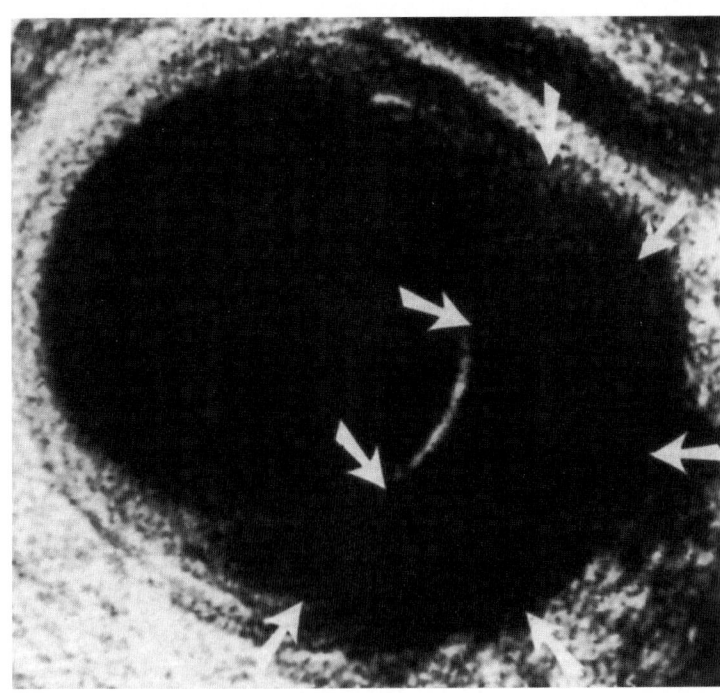

FIGURE 23-11. Endorectal ultrasound. Sonogram of a rectal cancer that penetrates into perirectal fat. Note the hypoechoic area *(arrows)*. The outermost layer of the bowel wall has been interrupted. (Courtesy of Ulrich Hildebrandt, M.D.)

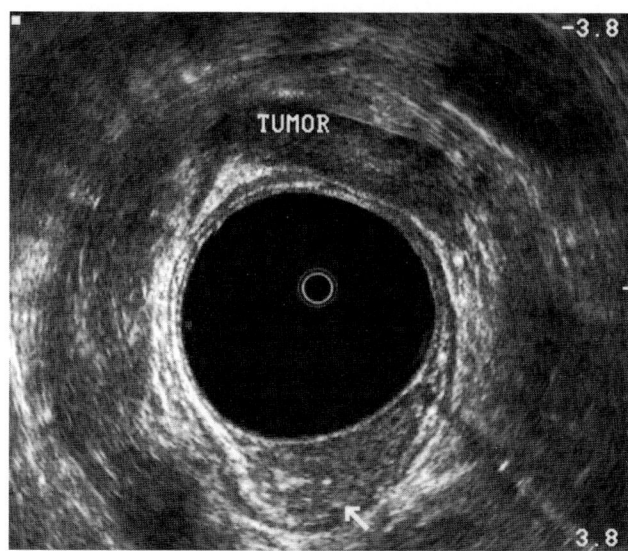

FIGURE 23-12. Endorectal ultrasound scan of a uT_2 tumor. Note disruption of the *middle white line* with the intact *outer white line*.

In the foregoing, uN_0 represents evidence of lymph nodes, uN_1 represents lymph nodes positive for tumor, M_X indicates metastatic tumor status unknown, M_0 represents no evidence of metastatic tumor, and M_1 means that metastatic tumor is present.

In addition to the foregoing indications, this technique offers the opportunity for clear visualization of the full thickness of an anastomotic area in those patients who have undergone restoration of rectal continuity, especially with respect to the possibility of early detection of recurrent cancer and for assessing the effects of preoperative radiotherapy.[55,109,396,536,602,689] Further information can be obtained by means of ultrasonographically guided biopsy and histologic determination of lymph node status.[749,895]

Published Experience and Comparative Results

The Creighton University group in Omaha, Nebraska, performed preoperative ultrasound staging on 107 patients with rectal cancer.[4] TRUS identified 18 of 19 patients with uT_3 tumors and 44 of 51 individuals with less invasion than uT_3 (86.3%). Garcia-Aguilar and colleagues reported the University of Minnesota group's experience of 1,184 patients with rectal adenocarcinoma or villous adenoma who underwent TRUS, comparing their assessment with pathologic specimens obtained by either resection or transanal excision without neoadjuvant treatment.[244] Somewhat disappointingly, overall accuracy in assessing the degree of rectal wall invasion was only 69%, with 18% overstaged and 13% understaged. Overall accuracy in assessing nodal involvement in those who underwent radical surgery (238 patients) was 64%, with 25% overstaged and 11% understaged. The primary benefits appear to have been in determining which tumors were benign and those that either went completely through the rectal wall and those that did not.[244]

Numerous studies have been published comparing TRUS, MRI, and CT. Roubein and colleagues showed that CT agreed with histopathology in 33% of cases, whereas TRUS agreed in 78%.[704] Some opine that TRUS is not sufficiently reliable for the evaluation of neoplasms because of interobserver differences.[775] However, this is a minority viewpoint. Goldman and colleagues found that TRUS had an accuracy of 81%, a sensitivity of 90%, and a specificity of 67%, whereas the corresponding figures for CT were 52%, 67%, and 27%, respectively.[266] Milsom and co-workers found that endoluminal ultrasound accurately predicted wall and lymph node status with 95% confidence intervals of 0.88 to 0.99 and 0.87 to 0.99, respectively, in 81 patients.[575] Thaler and colleagues compared the utility of endoluminal ultrasound with MRI in the preoperative staging of rectal cancer.[829] There was no statistically significant difference between the two methods in identifying T staging. Nodal staging was correct in 80% by ultrasound but only in 60% by MRI. A comprehensive preoperative staging, that is nodal and tumor extent, was correctly made in 68% with the use of endoluminal ultrasound, but in only 48% with the use of MRI. However, these differences were not statistically significant.

Kim and associates compared TRUS with pelvic CT, with MRI, and with endorectal coil in 89 patients.[416] Both TRUS and MRI with endorectal coil exhibited similar accuracies and were superior to conventional CT. Others affirm the better reliability of TRUS when compared with CT and conventional MRI in preoperative assessment,[54,300,313,338] but when recurrent disease is being sought, MRI and CT are at least as accurate as TRUS, if not more so.[690,851] It has also been shown that preoperative radiation therapy makes TRUS and CT less effective for staging, but the absence of lymph nodes before and after radiation can be considered reliable.[216,358,400,747,881]

A newer modality has been introduced—that of three-dimensional endoluminal ultrasound.[374,381] Although it has many of the limitations associated with conventional TRUS, it seems to provide significantly greater information for spatial relationships. This is particularly useful if one is to consider biopsy of extrarectal lymph nodes, for example.[573] Whether this modality will ultimately result in improved staging of rectal cancer awaits further investigations.

Rectal Endoscopic Lymphoscintigraphy

Arnaud and colleagues performed preoperative evaluation of patients with known rectal cancer in order to identify evidence of lymphatic spread.[19] The procedure involved the endoscopic injection of 0.1 mL of radiocolloid (rhenium sulfur marked with technetium-99m) into the submucosa of the extraperitoneal rectum bilaterally. The diffusion of the tracer along the lymphatics was registered by means of a computerized gamma camera. In ten control subjects and in a series of 85 patients with rectal cancer, the technique was found to have a sensitivity rate of 85%, a specificity of 68%, an overall accuracy of 76%, a positive predictive value of 71%, and a negative predictive value of 71%. The authors concluded that rectal endoscopic lymphoscintigraphy represented the only currently available method for evaluating lymphatic spread in rectal cancer.[19]

Other Factors

The previously discussed studies concern the tumor itself. The following variables that may influence the choice of operation are patient related.

Body Habitus

A rectal resection carried out on an asthenic patient usually permits a technically lower anastomosis than does an operation for the same level of lesion in an obese individual. In preoperative evaluation and counseling, therefore, the factor of body habitus may lead the surgeon to present an optimistic or pessimistic view of the likelihood of reestablishing intestinal continuity.

Gender

An anastomotic procedure is more likely to be possible in women than in men. A broad pelvis, furthermore, usually permits a wider resection, whereas a narrow pelvis tends to impede dissection, potentially limiting the adequacy of tumor margins and the use of conventional anastomotic techniques. This is especially true when one performs a low anterior resection.

Age

A resection involving an anastomosis is in some ways a higher-risk procedure than an APR. It has been facetiously remarked that an anastomosis that isn't made doesn't leak. Furthermore, the possibility of a second operation (i.e., closure of a colostomy) adds incrementally to the risk. Obviously radical resection is not contraindicated in patients solely because of age. Still, some elderly patients may be ideal candidates for a local approach to treatment.

Metastatic Disease

Palliative anastomotic procedures may be mistakenly embarked upon in order to avoid a colostomy during the terminal phase of the patient's illness. Unfortunately, even if the procedure is initially successful, the patient may return to undergo a colostomy because of symptoms related to pelvic recurrence. Operative mortality, furthermore, is much higher for palliative resections, including APR. Colostomy or Hartmann's resection may be adequate, or a local procedure may be the best choice if symptoms can be controlled by one of these means.

Systemic Disease

Any patient, regardless of age, is at an increased risk if systemic disease (e.g., cardiovascular, pulmonary, renal) is present. Such individuals are more safely treated by a procedure that does not involve an anastomosis. The surgeon must balance the risks with the advantage of avoiding a colostomy.

Ondrula and colleagues analyzed the predictive value of a number of preoperative risk factors on operative outcomes in 825 patients.[621] Those factors that were found to be statistically significant in predicting a greater risk were emergency operation, age of greater than or equal to 75 years, congestive heart failure, prior abdominal or pelvic radiation therapy, corticosteroid use, serum albumin less than 2.7 g/dL, chronic obstructive pulmonary disease, prior myocardial infarction, diabetes, cirrhosis, and renal insufficiency. The authors assigned a "risk score" for each category in order to determine a strategy for management based on the sum total of the risks.

Other Conditions

Avoiding a colostomy in a patient who cannot cope with an appliance or a stoma is an unusual, albeit legitimate, reason for choosing an alternative procedure. The quality of life may be poor, indeed, if a patient must be relegated to a nursing home or terminal care facility because the person cannot manage a stoma at home. This can happen if the individual is blind, has severe impairment in the use of hands (e.g., arthritis), or cannot be taught. Obviously, alternatives exist to support the patient, such as care by a family member, a visiting nurse, or a home helper. Of course, there may be no choice except to create a stoma to cure the disease or to palliate the condition effectively.

Comment

In the choice of operation, the surgeon must consider all of the foregoing factors and make a recommendation based upon what is the appropriate procedure for each individual. A tumor may require quite different treatment for one patient than the same lesion in the same location in another.

Each operation for carcinoma of the rectum is discussed in the following pages on its own merits.

ABDOMINOPERINEAL RESECTION

As previously observed, the description in 1908 by W. Ernest Miles of the abdominoperineal approach to tumors of the rectum was a landmark in the history of large bowel surgery.[568] This operation, as originally advocated, in-

volved an abdominal dissection and mobilization of the rectum. The rectum was then buried beneath the reconstituted pelvic floor. It was then excised through the perineal route, classically in the left lateral position. Since the original publication, only minor modifications in the surgical technique have been introduced. For example, J. P. Lockhart-Mummery of St. Mark's Hospital in the United Kingdom (see Biography, Chapter 9) introduced an extended perineal excision with preliminary colostomy and reported an improved mortality rate.[487] This method, however, did not remove the inferior mesenteric lymph nodes, nor was the technique applicable for higher rectal growths. However, it was used for more than 80% of the excisions of the rectum at that institution from 1928 to 1932, with Miles' operation being applied for the remainder.

Another option was proposed by Gabriel, an assistant to Lockhart-Mummery for many years.[2331] Gabriel started out as a perineal excisionist, but after careful study of the lymphatic spread of rectal cancer, he switched to his version of proctectomy, the perineoabdominal excision.

In 1939, Lloyd-Davies[480] reaffirmed the value of the synchronous-combined (two-team) APR that had been originally proposed by Mayo as early as 1904.[546] Mayo

---

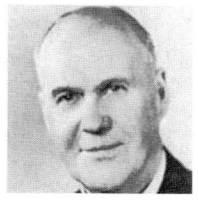

William Bashall Gabriel (1893–1975)   Gabriel was born in Oulton Broad, Suffolk, England, the son of an engineer. He attended Epsom College and distinguished himself as a very capable athlete. In 1912, he entered the Middlesex Hospital Medical School in London as the Freer Lucas Scholar. He was an outstanding student, winning a medal and scholarship for proficiency in surgery and another medal for theoretical and practical medicine. Following graduation, he served in World War I on a destroyer in the Mediterranean. In 1919, he became House Surgeon at St. Mark's Hospital in London, subsequently joining Sir Charles Gordon-Watson, J. P. Lockhart-Mummery, and Lionel Norbury. One of his most outstanding achievements was the establishment of a cancer follow-up department, the first of its kind in Great Britain. From this evolved the cumulative data of survival statistics for cancer treatment at St. Mark's. Gabriel was best known for his advocacy of the so-called perineoabdominal excision, a procedure that he performed more than 1,000 times. He was also renowned as the author of a major textbook that went through five editions, *Principles and Practice of Rectal Surgery*.

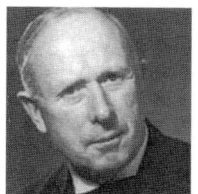

Oswald Vaughan Lloyd-Davies (1905–1987)   Lloyd-Davies was born the son of a Welsh clergyman and was educated at Caterham School. He received his medical education at the Middlesex Hospital in London. In 1935, at the age of 30, he was appointed to the staff of St. Mark's Hospital. Lloyd-Davies was regarded as a slow and meticulous surgeon. He was also an original thinker and designer of instruments for colon and rectal surgery. Among these was a small-bore sigmoidoscope with a proximal light source that he produced to permit outpatient and bedside evaluation of the lower bowel. His best-recognized contribution, however, was the development of specially designed leg supports as a means for providing access to the abdomen and to the perineum in the abdominoperineal resection. As a consequence, the lithotomy-Trendelenburg position has come to be associated with the his name. Lloyd-Davies was a modest and self-effacing man. In spite of his international reputation, few surgeons outside the United Kingdom knew him personally. He was, however, recognized as President by the Section of Proctology of the Royal Society of Medicine and was an Honorary Fellow of the American Society of Colon and Rectal Surgeons. (Adapted from Obituary. *BMJ* 1987;295:676; Obituary. *Lancet* 1987;1:465.)

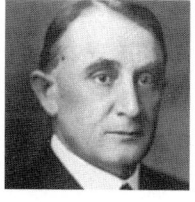

Charles Horace Mayo (1865–1939)   Mayo was born in Rochester, Minnesota, the son of William Worrall Mayo, a native of England and a general practitioner of medicine who had settled in the Territory of Minnesota in 1855. The young boy accompanied his father and elder brother, William J. Mayo, on numerous trips throughout the area as the father ministered to his patients. Charles Mayo studied in the public schools of Rochester and took the degree of Doctor of Medicine from Northwestern University in 1888. He returned to Rochester and joined his father and brother in their practice. In about 1903, what has come to be known as the Mayo Clinic had acquired sufficient form to warrant the use of that term by persons who sought the services of the brothers and their associates. Charles Mayo was considered, at least by his brother, to be the better surgeon. He could master a difficult situation with exceptional speed, and he had a facility for performing a variety of challenging operations (e.g., excision of a knee joint, sectioning the gasserian ganglion). Honors of every description were conferred upon Charles Mayo, as they were upon his brother. He was elected president of numerous medical organizations, including the Western Surgical Association, the Society of Clinical Surgery, the American Medical Association, the American College of Surgeons, and the American Surgical Association.

suggested that the synchronous combined approach be considered "if the surgeon has a good assistant." By 1963, the Lloyd-Davies technique was the most commonly employed alternative at the St. Mark's Hospital, and the operative mortality had been reduced to less than 3%.[589]

The procedure ideally involves two teams of surgeons operating synchronously once the resectability of the tumor has been ascertained. This method permits easier access to the pelvis and allows an attack on the area from two directions. It is particularly helpful when one is confronted with a bulky or fixed tumor or a patient with a narrow pelvis. With all appropriate deference to Miles and to his statement that the operation takes no more than 1 hour and that his patients suffer "no more shock than after an ordinary perineal excision,"[568] blood loss can be reduced and operative time decreased by using a two-team method. Interestingly, Miles' resection as performed by Richard Cattell of the Lahey Clinic in Boston (see Biography, Chapter 31) was called by his assistants "the *hour* of charm."

Others (e.g., Lahey) believed that if the operation were divided into two stages, it could be better tolerated by the patient.[453] The first stage consisted of making a median incision, dividing the sigmoid colon, and creating a left iliac colostomy with a mucous fistula of the distal segment delivered through the lower part of the abdominal incision. Care was taken to preserve the superior hemorrhoidal artery to the distal bowel. In the second stage, the proctectomy was carried out.

Although the two-stage procedure was successful in reducing morbidity and mortality before the availability of blood transfusion and in the preantibiotic era, it was gradually abandoned because of the improved safety of the one-stage approach.

Indications

Classically, it had been held that when tumors are less than 8 cm from the anal verge, the standard treatment is APR. Higher lesions generally permit restoration of intestinal continuity, usually by means of a conventional low anterior resection. Today, however, lower lesions can be satisfactorily managed by low anterior resection with restoration of continuity by any number of methods (see later). In fact, the only absolute contraindications for performing an anastomosis are invasion of the anal canal and invasion of the sphincter mechanism (i.e., levatores). As a palliative procedure (even in the presence of metastatic disease), if the patient's life expectancy may be several months or more, greater patient comfort can often be achieved with resection than by a diversionary procedure alone. This is particularly true when the tumor invades the sphincter mechanism to produce tenesmus, when it extends to the perineum, or when bleeding is a major concern. APR is the most consistently successful operation for carcinoma, and it is the procedure against which alternative sphincter-saving operations must be compared.

Preoperative Preparation

The routine preoperative screening studies are discussed in Chapter 22. Evaluation of the proximal bowel by means of colonoscopy or barium enema (to look for synchronous lesions) should be undertaken except when the rectal tumor appears to be virtually obstructing. A CT scan is strongly recommended, not only to ascertain whether there is evidence of metastatic disease, but also to evaluate tumor extent and whether there is any compression, dilatation, or deviation of the ureters. The bowel preparation consists of laxatives and enemas, as well as systemic perioperative antibiotics (see Chapter 22).

The importance of preoperative stomal site marking cannot be overestimated. One should determine the optimal location before surgery through any of a number of means. These are discussed in Chapters 29, 31, and 32.

Intraoperative Preparation and Anesthesia

A general, endotracheal anesthetic is advised for this procedure, but a spinal anesthetic can also be used. A Foley catheter with a 30-mL balloon is inserted into the bladder

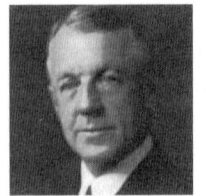

Frank Howard Lahey (1880–1953)   Lahey was born in Haverhill, Massachusetts, the only child of a bridge-building contractor. An outstanding athlete, Lahey attended Harvard University both as an undergraduate and as a medical student. Following graduate training at Boston City Hospital, he joined the staffs of Harvard and Tufts Medical Schools, when World War I interrupted his career. He became a Major in the Medical Corps and went to France to be the Chief of Surgery at an evacuation hospital. Following the war, he opened an office and shortly thereafter was joined by a surgeon and then an anesthesiologist. It was at this time that he conceived the idea of developing a multiple-specialty clinic, a practice that had been successful in the Midwest, but not in New England. The concept of staged operations was vigorously applied at the Lahey Clinic for many conditions—thyrotoxicosis, esophageal diverticulum, subphrenic and subhepatic abscess, pancreatic cancer, and diverticular disease. By staging the operation, Lahey and others were able to reduce the operative mortality considerably. The two-stage operation for cancer of the rectum was the procedure employed by surgeons on the staff of the Lahey Clinic until the early 1940s, more than 30 years after Miles' original publication. Lahey was a master surgeon; he was consistent and thorough. He often cautioned, "Be not the first to adopt a new technique nor the last to discard an old one." His most cherished award, the Bigelow Medal of the Boston Surgical Society, stated in part, ". . . superlative surgeon, doctor who teaches doctors, redoubtable administrator, advisor of Presidents in war and peace and, above all, a man who has the courage to be honest with himself. . . ."

when the patient is in the operating room. A Silastic catheter is preferred because there is less tissue reactivity, and it is less likely to cause a urethral stricture. Some surgeons prefer suprapubic bladder drainage, because it permits voluntary micturition.[78,423] Use of a nasogastric tube is not advised.

The issue of whether to place ureteral catheters prophylactically in operations involving the rectum is somewhat controversial, at least at the initial procedure. However, in reoperative pelvic surgery, when tumor extends into the area of the urinary tract, when there is evidence of ureteral obstruction, or when pelvic radiation had been performed, placement of ureteral stents is strongly recommended. The risk of ureteral injury as a direct result of catheter insertion is small (1.1%).[74] Although the presence of such catheters does not ensure the prevention of ureteral injuries, immediate recognition of the injury is evident. In a retrospective study by Bothwell and colleagues, 16.4% of experienced surgeons requested prophylactic ureteral catheter placement before sigmoid and rectosigmoid colon resections.[74] In a retrospective study by Kyzer and Gordon, ureteral catheterization was deemed necessary in 27.5% of cases.[451] Complications of stenting included renal colic, oligura, and anuria, but these were infrequently observed.

Technique

The two-team approach is the method I prefer for removal of the rectum, but with restoration of continuity being so frequently performed, and APR relatively uncommonly accomplished, I find that residents are not sufficiently familiar with the perineal dissection to permit independent responsibility for that part of the dissection. Hence, I usually place the patient in the perineolithotomy position, but I perform the operation as if we are one team. The leg supports may be similar to those described by Lloyd-Davies (Crown Brothers, Decatur, GA),[480] but they should not be the type that are usually employed for gynecologic procedures (i.e., "candy-canes"), although obstetric or urologic stirrups (with knee and foot crutch) may be substituted. My own preference is to use the Allen universal stirrups (Allen Medical Systems, Inc., Mayfield Heights, OH; *www.allenmedical.com;* Figure 23-13). It is relatively simple to position the patient, and there is no pressure on the popliteal fossa. The knees can be flexed, but the hips should be relatively extended and the thighs abducted in order to allow simultaneous, unlimited access to the abdomen and to the perineum. Too much hip flexion can interfere with the abdominal operator's maneuverability. Furthermore, if the patient is not properly positioned and the abdominal part of the operation requires a second assistant, adequate access may not be possible. A moderate degree of Trendelenburg (head-down) tilt aids in the dissection.

One of the concerns of placing the patient in the perineolithotomy position is its association with the development of a compartment syndrome. This occurs when elevated pressure in an osteofascial compartment compromises local perfusion.[740] This can result in neurovascular damage and permanent disability. Some authors emphasize the importance of prevention and early diagnosis.[220,738,740] The use of intermittent sequential compression of the lower limbs is strongly encouraged to prevent venous stasis.[738]

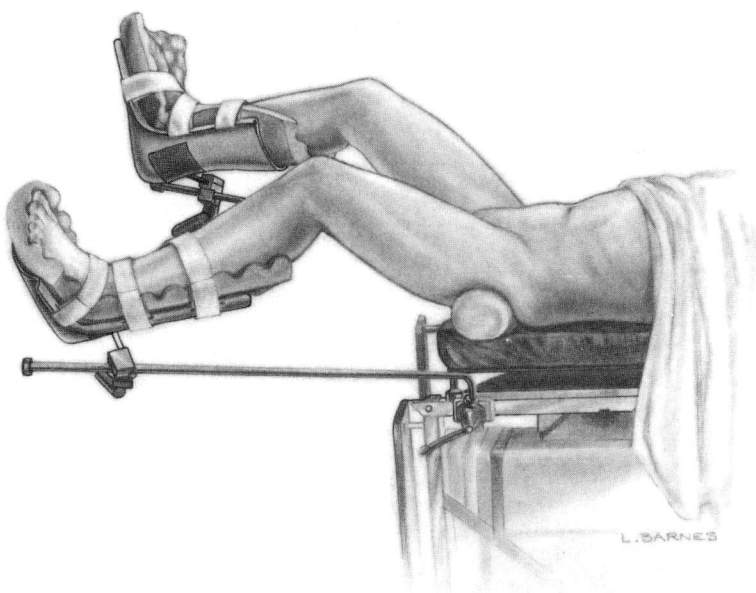

FIGURE 23-13. Perineolithotomy position with Allen's universal stirrups. The thighs are abducted and extended.

The Mayo stand should be placed over the patient's head, as low as the anesthesiologist will permit. No ether screen is employed; sterility on the upper end of the operative field is achieved with intravenous poles.

A purse-string suture is placed around the anus using a nonabsorbable retention suture (Figure 23-14). The abdomen and perineum are then cleansed with an antiseptic solution. Draping can be expedited by using a split sheet on the abdomen, with the open end down, in order to limit the amount of bulky covering over the perineum. Mayo-stand covers placed over the legs also simplify the draping.

Arthur H. Keeney has said, "Pray before surgery, but remember that God will not alter a faulty incision." The location of the incision is extremely important, not only for the obvious reason of access to the abdomen, but also to avoid interference with the subsequent placement of the stoma. A midline hypogastric incision is usually advised, extending through the umbilicus if necessary. However, as discussed in Chapter 22, I find Maylar's incision to be quite useful for both low anterior resection and APR. Ideally, the colostomy should be sited over the rectus muscle and brought out through the split thickness of the muscle. Paracolostomy herniation is less likely to occur if the stoma is brought through the muscle rather than in a pararectus location. Without question, it should never be brought out through the incision. A left paramedian incision, therefore, is contraindicated. Furthermore, ideally the stoma should be situated below the beltline at a distance from bony promontories and from the umbilicus (Figure 23-15). The consequences and management of poorly placed stomas are discussed in Chapters 31 and 32.

After the insertion of a self-retaining retractor (e.g., Balfour, Bookwalter, Protractor), the abdomen is explored for evidence of metastatic disease, the presence of synchronous colon lesions, or other pathologic features. The small intestine is packed into the upper abdomen using three moist pads: one over the cecum, one along the descending colon, and the third from side to side across the abdomen. Rarely should it be necessary to exteriorize the bowel. By keeping the viscera warm and moist and within the abdomen, there is less likelihood of postoperative ileus, and a nasogastric tube may be avoided. This can be more easily accomplished if the incision can be kept below the umbilicus.

Mobilization of the sigmoid colon and rectum commences along the left colic gutter, lysing the developmental adhesions in order to obtain sufficient mobility to deliver the bowel to the abdominal wall at the level of the proposed colostomy.

The peritoneum on the left lateral aspect is incised, and the left ureter is identified and retracted laterally (see Figure 22-51). Injury to the ureter most commonly occurs during this phase of the procedure, at the level of the iliac artery; therefore, it should always be visualized and protected. Incision of the peritoneum is continued anteriorly to the base of the bladder.

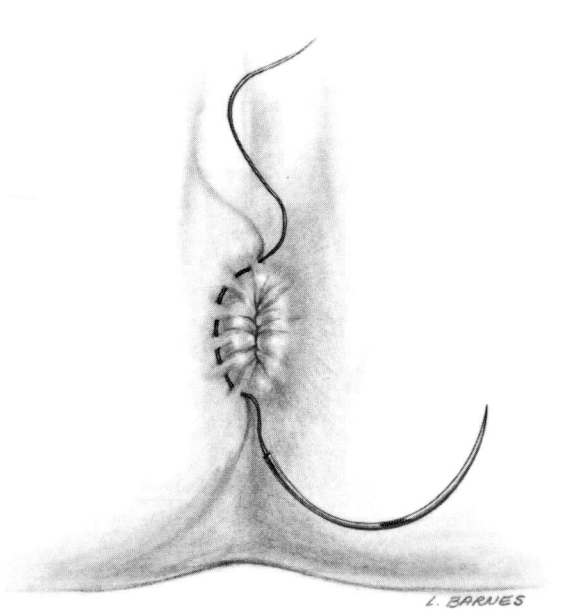

FIGURE 23-14. Abdominoperineal resection. A purse-string suture is secured, closing the anus.

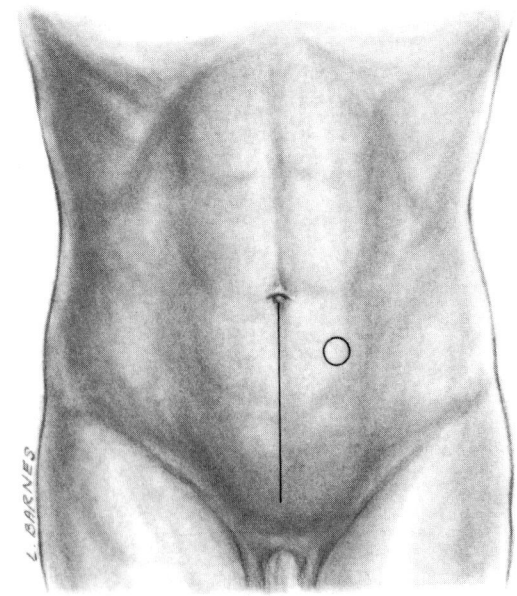

FIGURE 23-15. The proper position of the sigmoid colostomy site for abdominoperineal resection is away from bony promontories, the umbilicus, scars, and skin folds and within the rectus muscle.

The technique of APR requires identification and control of the inferior mesenteric vessels, the middle hemorrhoidal arteries (which pass adjacent to the lateral ligaments of the rectum), and the inferior hemorrhoidal vessels (Figure 23-16).

The left hand is then passed beneath the inferior mesenteric vessels, and a peritoneal incision is performed in a similar fashion on the right side (see Figure 22-52). The mesenteric vascular pedicle is ligated between clamps. One should always check to be certain that the left ureter has not been incorporated (see Figure 22-53). It is less important to visualize the right ureter because it should not be involved in this aspect of the dissection. Exceptions to this dictum include a congenital anomaly or a history of prior surgery that may have caused medial deviation of this structure. Injury to the right ureter is usually caused at the time of pelvic floor reconstruction by mobilization and suture of the peritoneum on that side.

Ligation of the inferior mesenteric artery at its origin is unnecessary because, in my experience and that of others, nodal involvement at that level is found only in patients with incurable cancer, and survival rates are not improved.[657] This may be useful information, however, for staging purposes and for prognosis (see Chapter 22). In a study of more than 4,000 patients who underwent surgery for rectal carcinoma at St. Mark's Hospital, no improved survival was seen when the inferior mesenteric artery was ligated above the origin of the left colic artery.[804] Ligation distal to the first branch of the inferior mesenteric artery ensures a viable blood supply to the bowel from which the stoma will be created. Pelvic peritoneal incisions are then joined across the base of the bladder (or at the vaginal apex in women).

Attention is then turned to the retrorectal space. Often, surgeons commence blunt dissection at the level of the sacral promontory, but when doing so the plane may be improperly entered, and the presacral vessels can be torn. This can result in rather profuse bleeding. Hemorrhage, in fact, is often the result of bleeding from basivertebral veins through the sacral foramina and not of injury to the presacral venous plexus.[664] When such vessels are encountered, attempt at ligation may be unsuccessful, especially if the bleeding emanates directly from bone. Rather than attempt to electrocoagulate and accept additional blood loss, direct pressure with a large pad for a few minutes is suggested. Failure to achieve hemostasis may necessitate the use of packing,[567,896] or even the application of a hemorrhage occluder pin (thumbtack) placed into the sacrum (see Figure 17-41).[792] I believe that the risk of bleeding can be mini-

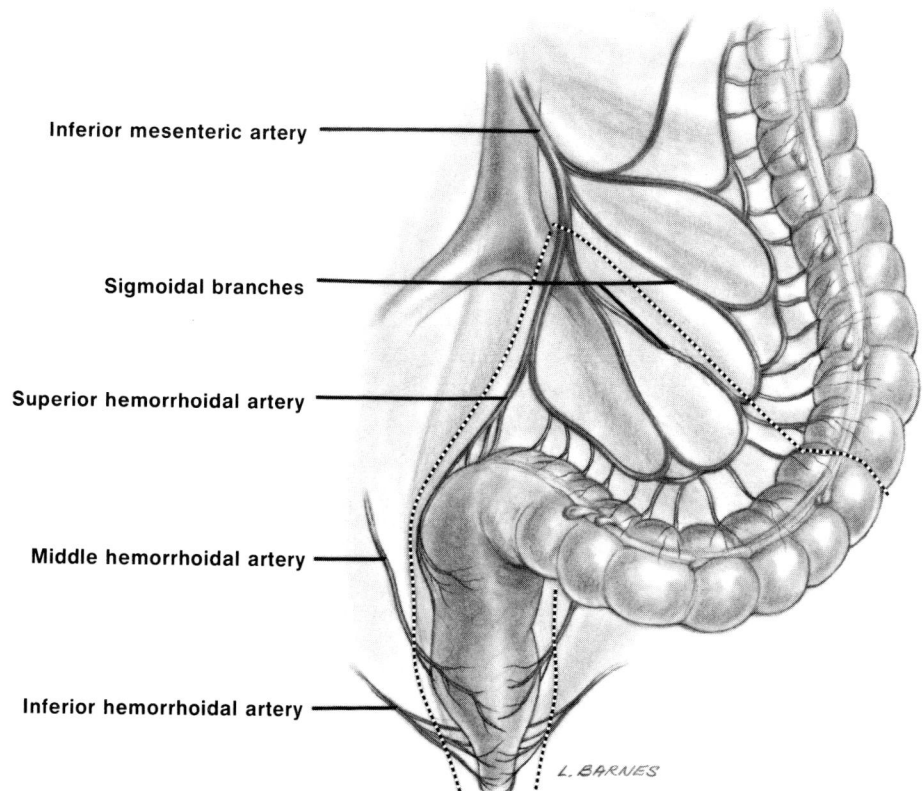

FIGURE 23-16. Blood supply to the rectum and sigmoid colon.

mized if the dissection is performed, as much as possible, under direct visualization and by sharp dissection (Figure 23-17).

Another important consideration besides the risk of bleeding in the presacral space is the possibility of breaching the visceral endopelvic fascia, the investing fascia of the mesentery. This may lead to confusion as to the anatomy and cause the surgeon to operate in the improper plane, leaving behind mesentery with its lymphatics (see Total Mesorectal Excision). Gentle anterior traction is placed on the rectosigmoid, and the scissors are inserted anterior to the sacral promontory. The presacral space is relatively avascular and usually readily entered. The loose areolar tissue is identified and incised. The presacral (sympathetic) nerves can usually be seen quite clearly and can, therefore, be displaced out of harm's way.

Once the presacral space has been opened as far as convenient by retraction and under direct visualization, the right hand can be inserted and the dissection carried out bluntly (Figure 23-18). It is often helpful to drape a gauze sponge over the fingers to facilitate this maneuver. However, it is still preferable to perform as much of the dissection under direct visualization, cutting with the scissors as distally as possible. The rectum is freed to the tip of the coccyx in a plane anterior to the sacral fascia, thereby avoiding injury to the presacral veins (Figure 23-19).

In the synchronous-combined operation, if posterior mobilization of the rectum is impeded by tumor extension, the abdominal operator should wait for the perineal surgeon to develop a plane, rather than to proceed blindly. If a synchronous-combined procedure is not being performed or if no plane can be developed from either direction, the surgeon must dissect wherever he or she presumes the plane to have been, fully recognizing that the possibility for cure may be compromised. If one is performing a synchronous approach, it is at this point in the operation that the abdominal operator meets the perineal surgeon (in the posterior midline), when the rectococcygeus ligament has been divided. Of course, depending on the anatomic knowledge and dexterity of the perineal surgeon, much more can be accomplished from "below". For example, John Goligher was able to accomplish the entire proctectomy through the perineal route except for a high tie on the inferior mesenteric artery.

Attention is then turned to the anterior part of the dissection. The posterior wall of the bladder and the seminal vesicles (or uterus and posterior vaginal wall in a woman) are visually demonstrated. This can be accomplished by using a 7-inch St. Mark's pattern retractor with turned-back lip (Thackray Instruments, Inc., Woburn, MA) and by a combination of sharp and blunt dissection (Figure 23-20). Denonvilliers' fascia must be incised in order to separate the rectum completely from the prostate and the

FIGURE 23-17. Abdominoperineal resection. The presacral space is entered by sharp dissection.

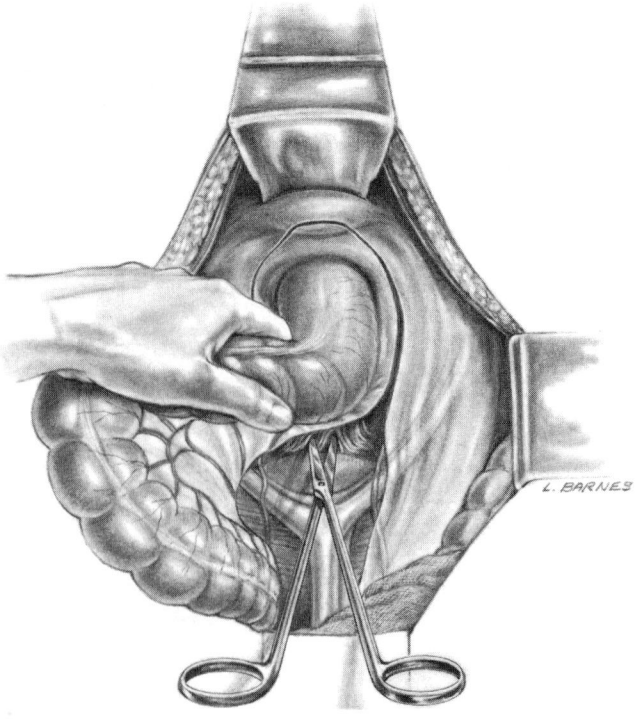

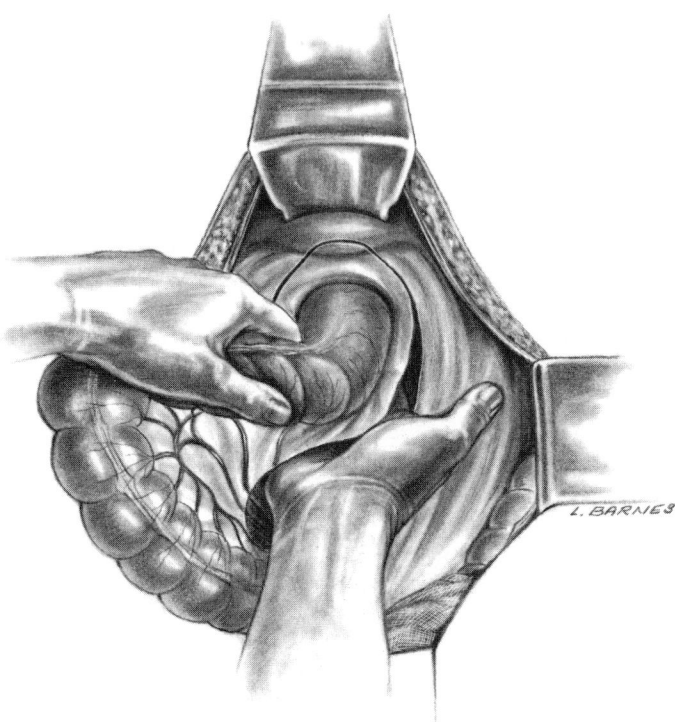

FIGURE 23-18. Abdominoperineal resection. The rectum is mobilized from the lower pelvic adhesions by blunt dissection; this produces a characteristic "sucking" sound.

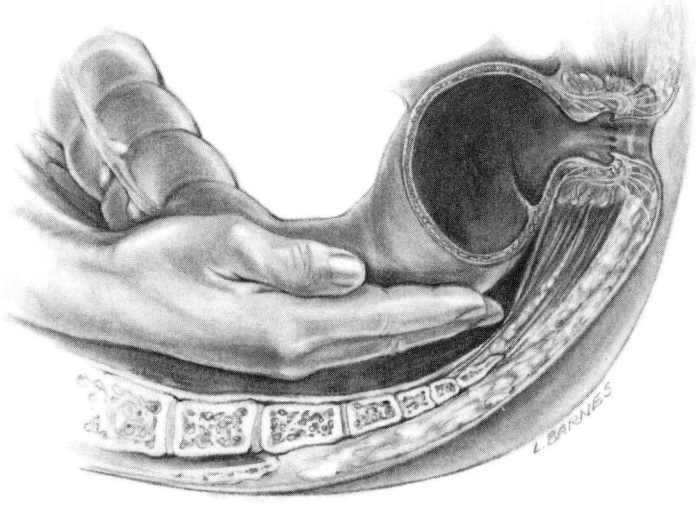

FIGURE 23-19. Abdominoperineal resection. The lateral view illustrates that, ideally, the sacral fascia is not breached when the rectum is bluntly dissected.

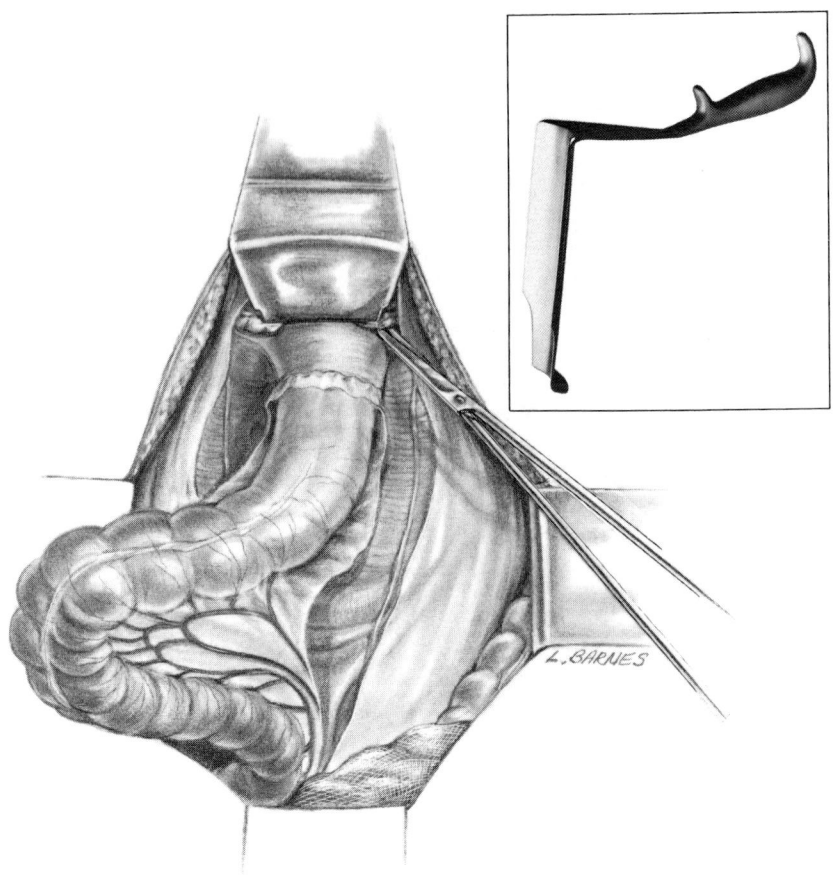

FIGURE 23-20. Abdominoperineal resection. The anterior peritoneal dissection in the male patient reveals the seminal vesicles and prostate. The mobilization is facilitated by use of the St. Mark's pattern retractor **(inset)**.

seminal vesicles. By means of retraction of the bladder and prostatic area and countertraction on the rectum, the dissection is carried distally until the inferior margin of the prostate and the urethra with its contained catheter can be palpated. In women, the posterior vaginal wall is swept anteriorly to the point where it is to be incised or removed (Figure 23-21). Dissection is facilitated by placing the left hand as distally as possible and compressing the anterior rectal wall.

Attention is then turned to the lateral ligaments and to the middle hemorrhoidal vessels. The space distal to the lateral ligaments is entered using a long scissors, and the scissors are spread in the anterior-posterior plane. The index finger of the left hand is then passed beneath the ligament and the adjacent vessels on the right side. There is often a firm fascial band that must be traversed bluntly. The ligament is then straddled with the index and long fingers of the left hand and retracted medially (Figure 23-22). A single crushing clamp is used, and the lateral ligament and the middle hemorrhoidal vessel transected medial to the clamp. Back-bleeding from the artery rarely occurs but can easily and safely be controlled by rotating the rectum and directly visualizing the bleeding point. When the lateral

ligament has been divided, the rectum on that side is readily mobilized.

The left lateral ligament is divided in a similar way, but the maneuver is slightly more difficult to perform. The left index and long fingers again straddle the structures, but the rectum is pushed toward the right side, and the clamp is applied adjacent to the dorsum of the hand (Figure 23-23).

Takahashi and colleagues emphasized that the lateral ligaments are not true ligamentous structures, but rather that they contain branches of the middle rectal (hemorrhoidal) artery, branches of the autonomic nerves to the pelvis, variable amounts of fat, and overlying fascia derived from the junction of the parietal and visceral layers of the endopelvic and pelvic fasciae.[812] The ligaments are, therefore, believed to be critical both with respect to defining the adequacy of cancer resection and the preservation of sexual function. This is the location where parasyzmpathetic nerves responsible for potency are most likely to be injured. Upon completion of this last step, the rectum is completely isolated anteriorly, laterally, and posteriorly. A few fibrous strands may require division, but no important vascular structures need to be controlled in order to complete the pelvic dissection.

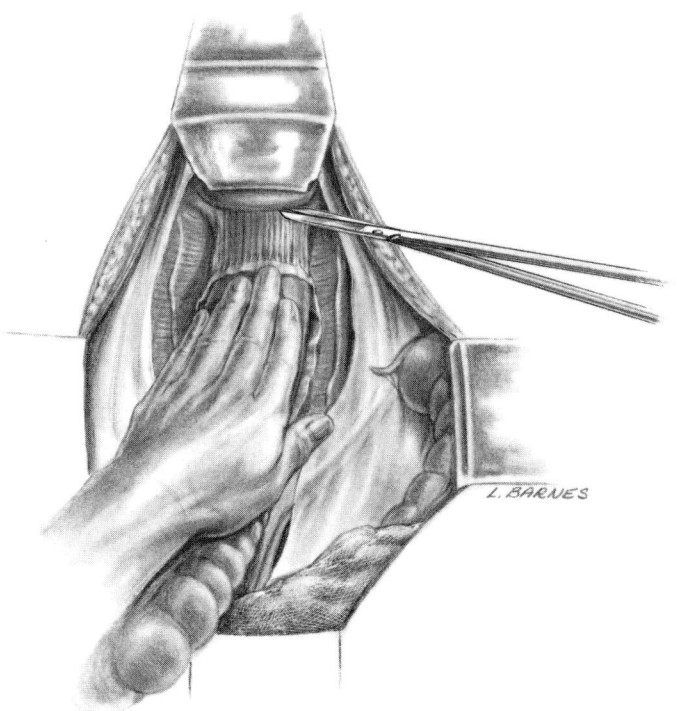

FIGURE 23-21. Abdominoperineal resection. The posterior vaginal wall is exposed below the retractor. By using the St. Mark's pattern retractor with the turned-back lip, the dissection between the rectum and vagina is facilitated.

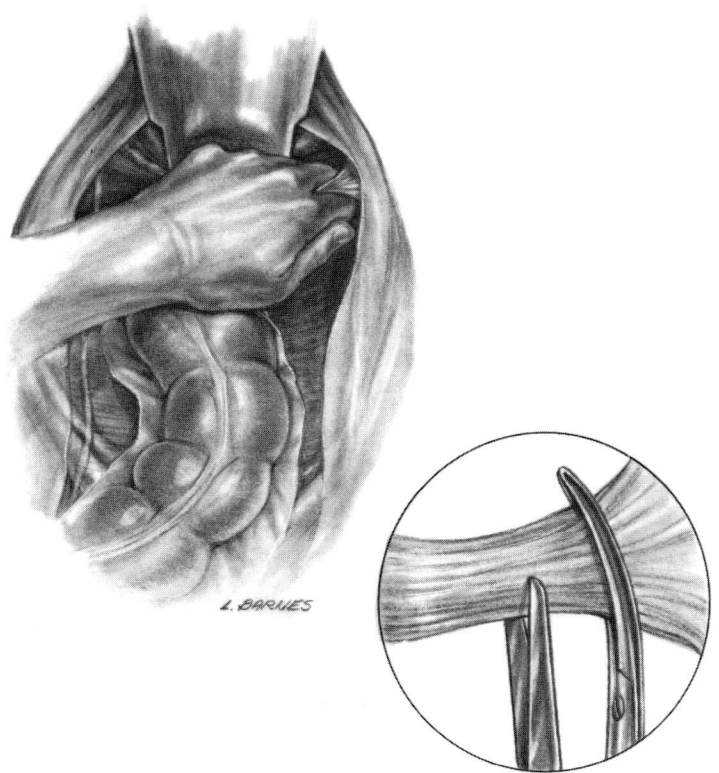

FIGURE 23-22. Abdominoperineal resection. The right lateral ligament is isolated between the index and long fingers of the left hand. The ligament and middle hemorrhoidal artery are clamped laterally and are divided on the rectal side **(inset)**.

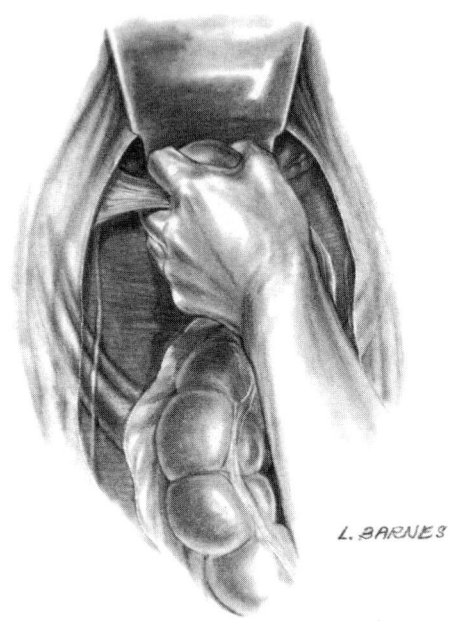

L. BARNES

FIGURE 23-23. Abdominoperineal resection. The left lateral ligament is isolated with the left hand, and the rectum is pushed toward the right side. A single clamp is then placed laterally.

The sigmoid colon is then held up to the abdominal wound, and a point (usually at the apex) is selected for creation of the colostomy. If the abdominal wall is thick, a slightly more distal point is selected. If the sigmoid colon is redundant, a more cephalad site is chosen. The arcade vessel is then divided.

The site of the colostomy is now prepared by grasping the skin with a Kocher clamp and by excising a disk of skin, the diamet er of which should approximate the diameter of the sigmoid colon to be used for the stoma (Figure 23-24A). The subcutaneous, fatty tissue is bluntly retracted (not excised), and the anterior sheath of the rectus muscle is incised in a cruciate fashion (Figure 23-24B,C). The rectus muscle fibers are then split in a longitudinal direction, and the peritoneal cavity is entered with scissors or an electrocautery device (Figure 23-24D). The colostomy aperture in the peritoneum, muscle, and skin should permit the insertion of two fingers.

The surgeon should now inspect the abdominal wall for possible injury to the inferior epigastric vessels. Frequently, an attempt is made to control bleeding from the colostomy site by exploring the wound through the skin opening. Because the vascular structures lie just above the peritoneum, this is a cumbersome and often futile exercise. By placing a sponge through the opening and out the abdominal incision and by applying traction, exposure of the epigastric artery and vein is facilitated (Figure 23-25). Hemostasis then can be easily established.

A crushing clamp is passed through the colostomy wound into the abdominal cavity to grasp the prepared colon at the site of the proposed stoma (Figure 23-26). The distal rectosigmoid is also clamped, and the bowel is divided between the two clamps. The proximal bowel is drawn through the abdominal wall to lie without tension on the anterior abdominal surface. Mavroidis and Koltun suggested the use of a Penrose drain to ensheathe the distal bowel to protect it and to facilitate delivery through the abdominal wall.[544]

The divided distal bowel is sealed from contamination by grasping it with a doubly gloved hand and tying the removed outer glove over the stump of the rectosigmoid as the clamp is released (Figure 23-27). Doubled no. 2 silk or catgut is used. The rectum is then delivered through the perineal opening (in a synchronous-combined operation) or buried in the pelvic cavity (with the classic Miles approach).

When it is certain that hemostasis has been established, Kocher clamps are placed on the cut edge of the peritoneum. By gentle finger dissection and judicious use of the scissors, the peritoneum is mobilized to a degree that will permit closure without tension; a continuous absorbable suture is suggested (Figure 23-28). Closure of the lateral, paracolostomy opening (gutter) is not recommended. Too often, a narrow opening results if a suture cuts through or breaks, and a large defect is preferred to a narrow one.

Following abdominal wound closure, the redundant bowel is excised and the colostomy primarily "matured" by using approximately eight sutures of no. 3–0 or 4–0 chromic catgut through the full thickness of the bowel and the skin (Figure 23-29). Another approach that has been described is to mature the stoma by means of the circular stapler, but I see no merit in the application of this technique.

Perineal Dissection

In the synchronous-combined excision, the perineal dissection is commenced as soon as the abdominal operator determines that the lesion is resectable. If two teams are not available, the perineal portion of the operation is performed after the entire abdominal operation has been completed, and the pelvic peritoneum has been closed above the stump of the rectosigmoid. Under no circumstances should the perineal operation be undertaken initially, that is, not until resectability has been determined. If the perineal proctectomy is accomplished with the patient in the left lateral position (the classic Miles' approach), the surgeon is usually more comfortable when

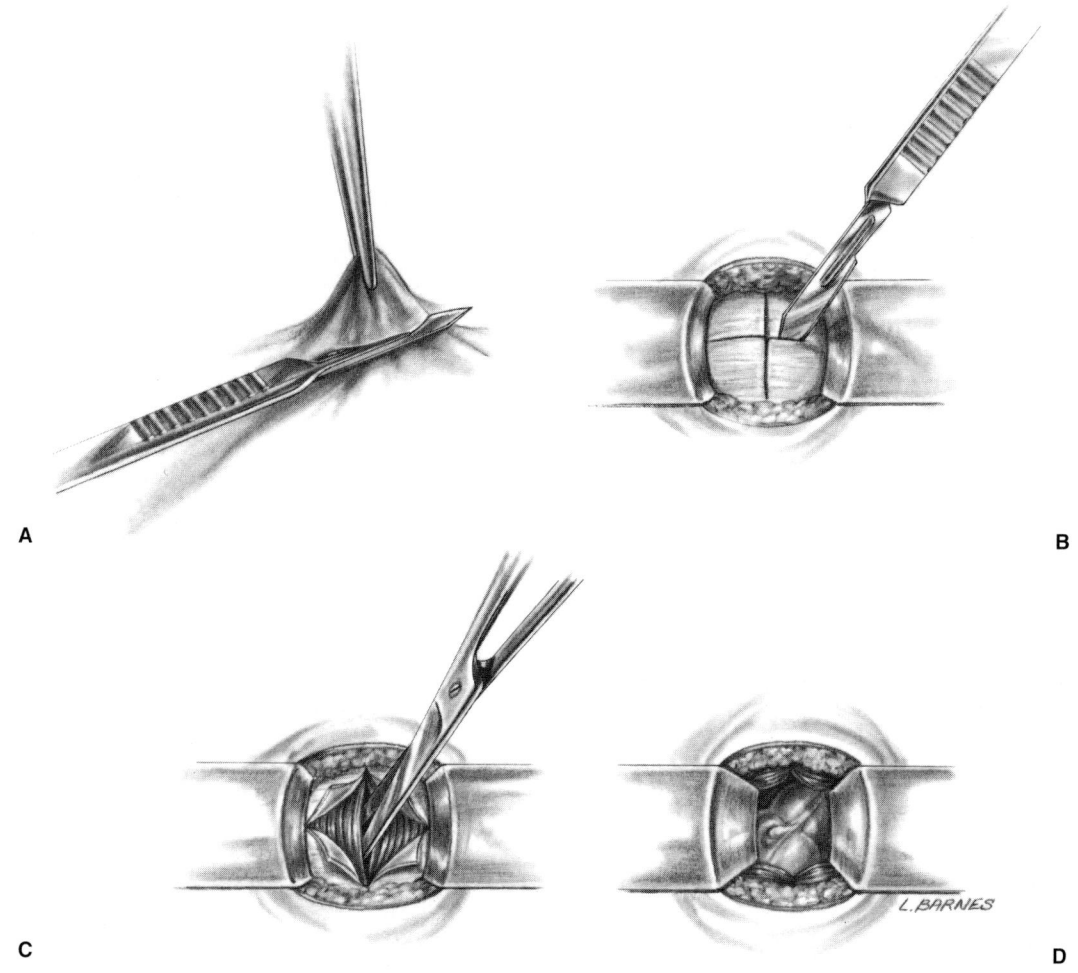

FIGURE 23-24. Abdominoperineal resection. Creating the abdominal wall opening for the colostomy. **(A)** A disk of skin is excised. **(B)** A cruciate incision is made in the anterior rectus fascia. **(C)** The rectus muscle is split longitudinally. **(D)** The completed abdominal wall opening.

seated. The light is directed from the foot, and the first assistant stands on a platform on the opposite side (Figure 23-30). The following illustrations, however, demonstrate the procedure in the perineolithotomy position, although the principles are the same.

An elliptical incision is made outside of the sphincter muscle, including a generous margin of perianal skin (Figure 23-31). The skin edges are grasped on each side with Kocher clamps. The dissection is carried out at least initially with electrocautery, and the assistant clamps any bleeding vessel with a curved hemostat. By touching the tip of the electrocautery device to the hemostat, one can continue dissecting without the need for frequent scraping of debris off the coagulating tip. Usually, two vascular bundles are encountered lying anteriorly and posteriorly on either side in the ischiorectal fat. These are the inferior hemorrhoidal vessels (Figure 23-32).

Once the ischiorectal fossa has been entered, a self-retaining (Lace) retractor (Crown Brothers, Decatur, GA) facilitates the exposure. The anterior dissection proceeds by incising the deep transverse perineal muscle (Figure 23-33).

The presacral space is now entered by dividing the rectococcygeus muscle, commencing at the level of the tip of the coccyx (Figure 23-34). The coccyx is not removed unless the tumor proves to be so large that it cannot be delivered through the perineal opening. To remove the coccyx, a scalpel is inserted into the joint by flexing the bone with the thumb (Figure 23-34, *inset*). It is then separated and removed by means of a knife or heavy scissors. Care should be taken to dissect sufficiently anterior to the sacrum All too often, the perineal procedure is carried out too far posteriorly, stripping the presacral fascia and causing considerable bleeding. Conversely, one must be

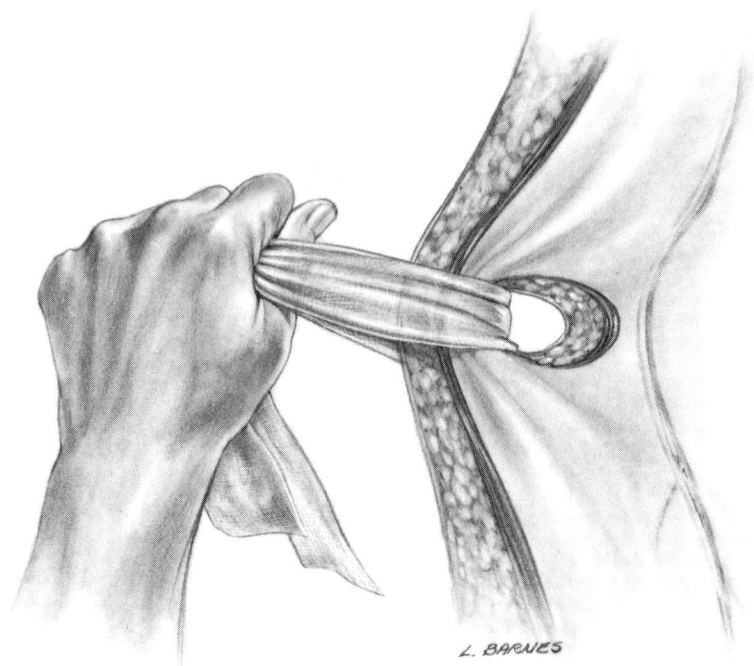

FIGURE 23-25. Abdominoperineal resection. Exposure of the epigastric vessels by sponge retraction.

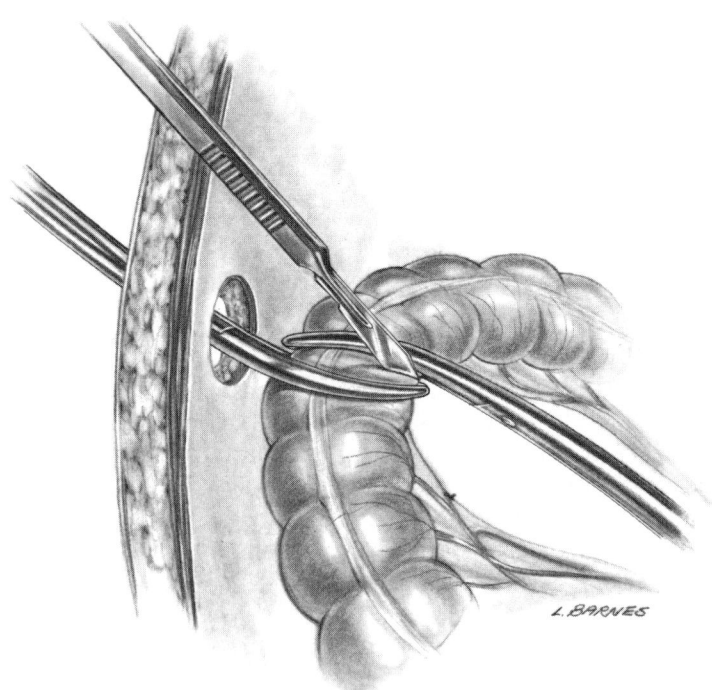

FIGURE 23-26. Abdominoperineal resection. A clamp is passed through the abdominal wall opening to grasp the bowel at the site for the creation of the colostomy. This maneuver eliminates one step and reduces the risk of fecal spillage when both clamps are placed within the abdomen.

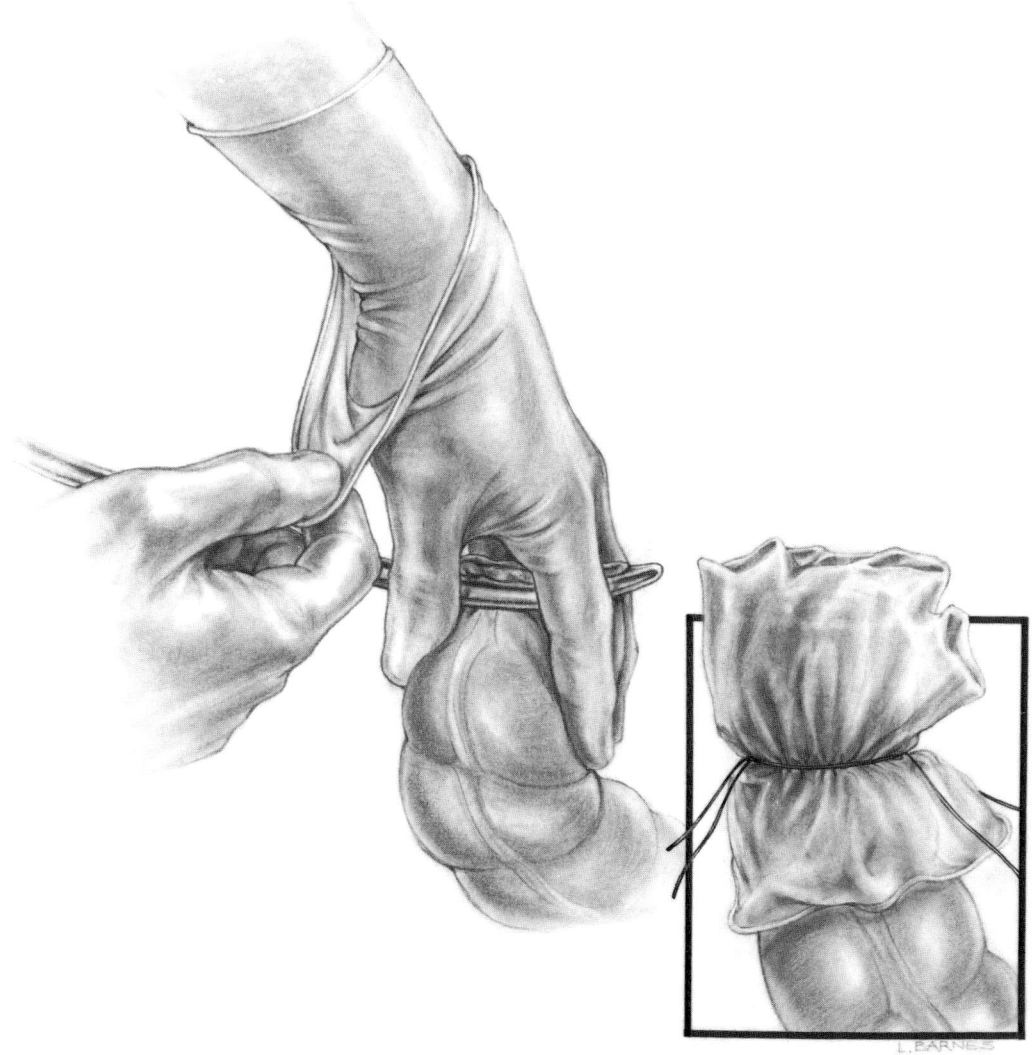

FIGURE 23-27. Abdominoperineal resection. The distal colonic stump is encompassed by a rubber glove. It is then everted and secured with heavy ligatures **(inset)**.

careful not to dissect too far anteriorly because of the risk of entering the rectum. This is particularly likely to occur if the tumor is relatively fixed posteriorly. With the synchronous-combined operation, the abdominal operator can direct the perineal surgeon into the proper plane. The rectum and anus should now be free in the midline posteriorly.

After the presacral space is entered, a finger is swept across the superior aspect of the levator muscles on the left and right sides of the pelvis. The levatores are then divided near the pelvic wall attachments with scissors or electrocautery. This is a relatively avascular dissection (Figure 23-35).

Sometimes one or both lateral ligaments are divided from below. The perineal operator must take care to

avoid injury to the ureters by this maneuver. The distal ureter is cut more frequently by the perineal operator during combined APR than by the abdominal surgeon.

The proximal rectum may now be delivered out of the pelvis. By vigorous traction, the remaining attachments of the rectourethralis muscle and fascia in the region of the urethra are sharply divided. There is no plane through which this can be undertaken bluntly (Figure 23-36). By palpating the catheter, the surgeon should be able to determine the location of the urethra and avoid it.

If the perineal surgeon moves along expeditiously, or if the abdominal surgeon is delayed in mobilizing the rectum, the anterior perineal dissection should be continued. One must recognize, however, that this is a more difficult maneuver and should not be left to an uninitiated

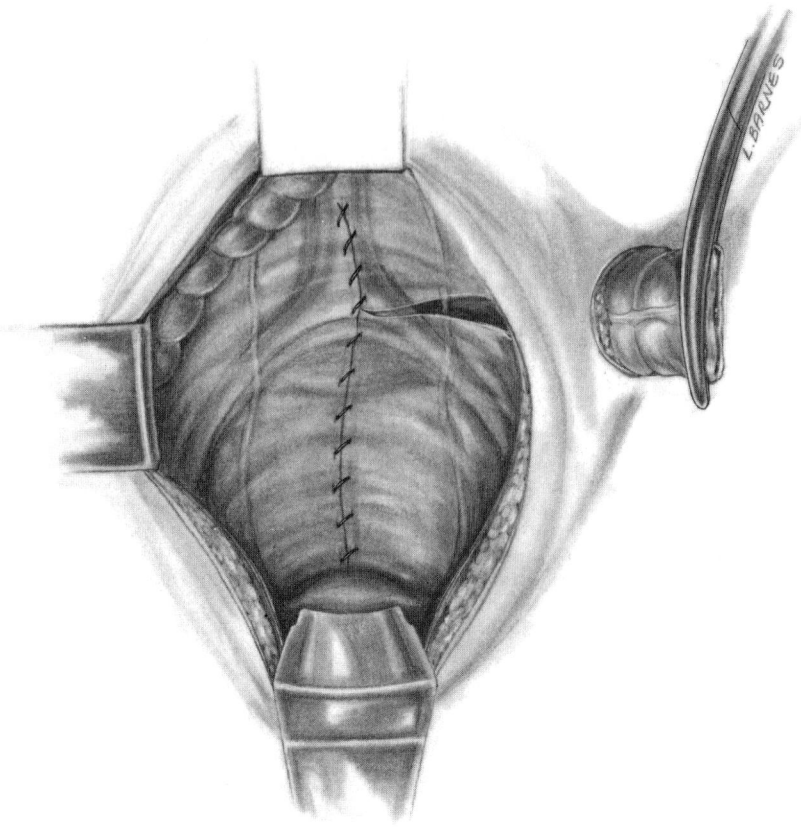

FIGURE 23-28. Abdominoperineal resection. The floor of the pelvis is reconstituted.

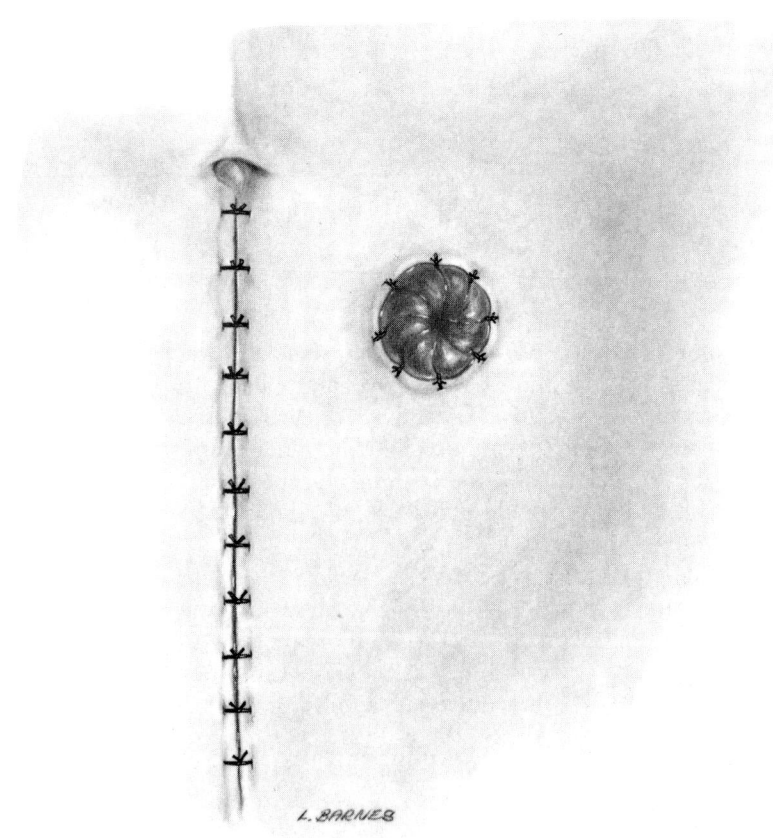

FIGURE 23-29. Abdominoperineal resection. The wound is closed and the colostomy matured.

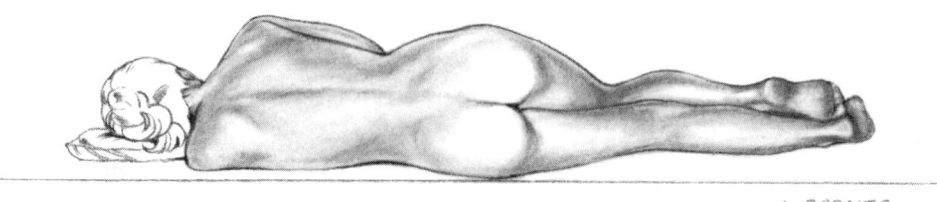

FIGURE 32-30. Perineal dissection is carried out with the patient in the left lateral position in the classical Miles' operation. The surgeon can be seated.

assistant. By posterior retraction on the rectum, the muscles are further divided with scissors (Figure 23-37). In men, it is dangerous to employ electrocautery because of the risk of injuring the urethra. Even when using scissor dissection, there is still a risk of injury to the urethra and to the prostate. Dissecting too far posteriorly, of course, may cause the rectum to be entered and compromise the cancer resection. APR is much more likely to be associated with rectal injury than low anterior resection, especially by the perineal operator. The high local recurrence rate and reduced survival following such injury should alert every surgeon to avoid this complication.[196]

If one can draw an imaginary line to the promontory of the sacrum and dissect in that direction, dividing the transverse perineal and rectourethralis muscles anteriorly, the posterior aspect of the prostate gland will be clearly identified. It is hoped that by keeping close to the rectum, one can avoid damage to the neural plexus supplying the external sphincter urethrae and the membranous urethra, although bladder dysfunction itself may

not be attributable to the perineal dissection (see later discussion).[716] With the division of the fascia of Denonvilliers, the peritoneal cavity is entered.

Posteriorly, the proximal dissection may be in some instances carried to the level of the sacral promontory if necessary, and the lateral ligaments can be clamped and divided by the perineal operator. Again, care must be taken to avoid injury to the ureter. After the bowel has been removed, the perineal wound is copiously irrigated with saline solution and the skin closed. I am personally not an advocate of continuous irrigation or of irrigating with antibiotics.[237] No attempt is made to reapproximate the levatores in a cancer operation, a different approach from when proctectomy is performed for inflammatory bowel disease (see Chapter 29). A closed suction drain (e.g., Jackson-Pratt) is placed into the pelvic cavity and brought out either through the incision, itself, or preferably through a stab wound in the buttock (Figure 23-38). Alternatively, some surgeons prefer to use a system of drainage through the abdominal wall, but the principle is the same.[632] In either case, the perineal wound is closed primarily.

As mentioned previously, diffuse bleeding from pelvic veins may persist. This may result from difficulty encountered because of tumor extension, prior pelvic surgery, or dissection in the improper plane. Under these circumstances, packing the pelvis with gauze, Kling, or Kerlex will usually control the source of the bleeding. If this is necessary, the packing is left in place for 3 to 4 days and then removed at the patient's bedside with the aid of a narcotic analgesic.

Palliative Abdominoperineal Resection

Palliative APR has been advocated by a number of authors.[29,73,485] Others have suggested that alternative forms of therapy should be considered because of the high surgical morbidity and mortality rates.[409,587,670] Individuals who have extensive liver metastases, lung metastases, or disseminated disease (e.g., bone, brain) are poor candidates. Those with ascites or multiple peritoneal implants are also extremely high operative risks. However, because the mean survival time in patients with Dukes' D lesions approximates 1 year, there

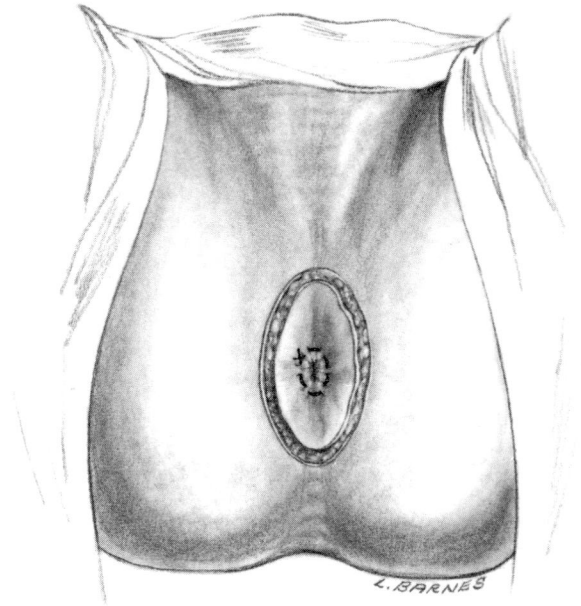

FIGURE 23-31. Perineal dissection. An elliptical incision is made outside the anus.

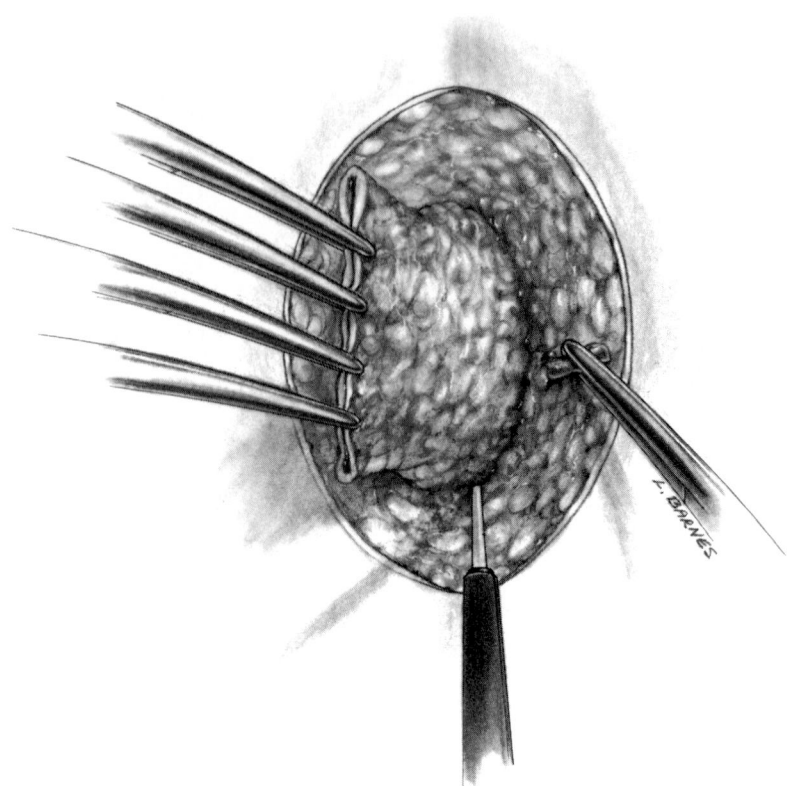

FIGURE 23-32. Perineal dissection. Serial Kocher clamps are applied to the perianal skin, and the incision is deepened. The inferior hemorrhoidal vessels are clamped and divided.

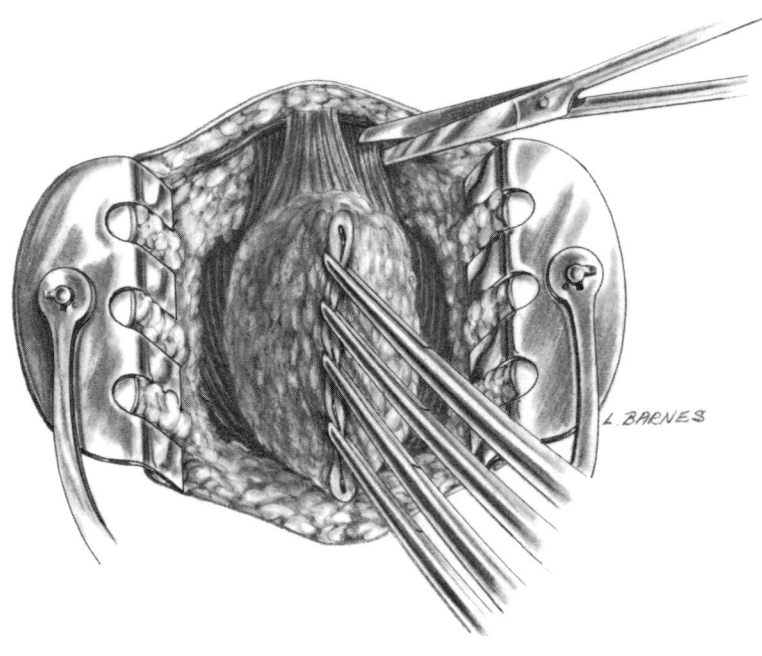

FIGURE 23-33. Perineal dissection. A Lace retractor is inserted, which facilitates the dissection by giving optimal exposure. The rectum is freed anteriorly by dividing the transverse perineal muscle.

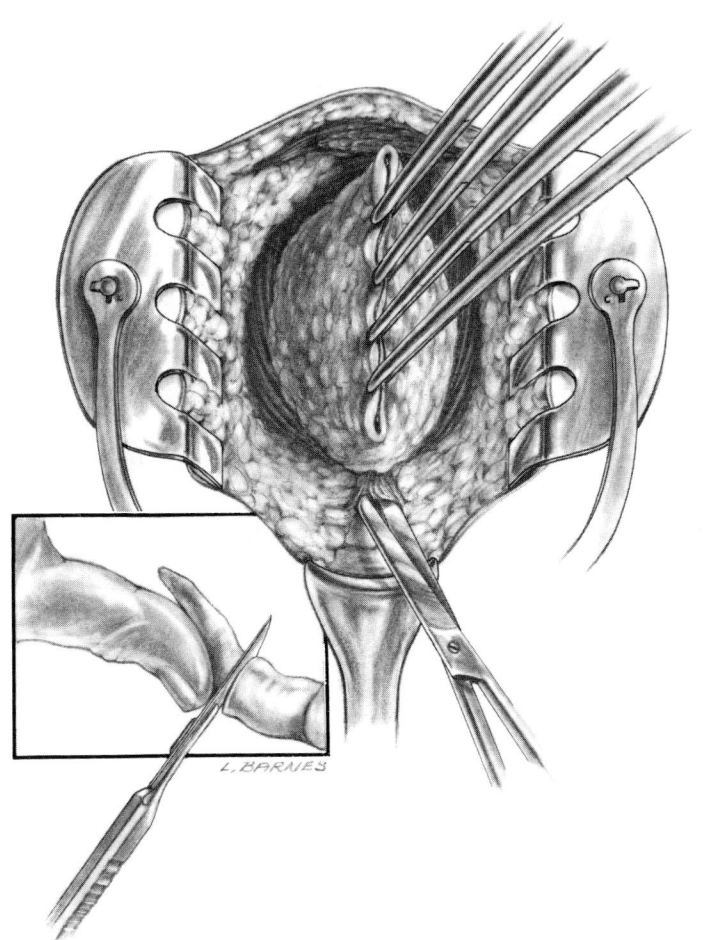

L. BARNES

FIGURE 23-34. Perineal dissection. The presacral space is entered, usually at the level of the tip of the coccyx. If necessary, the coccyx can be disarticulated **(inset)**.

is a group who should be considered for a palliative resection; these include patients with perineal pain, tenesmus, or hemorrhage. If the tumor can be extirpated, a better quality of life may be anticipated. In the experience of Moran and colleagues with 125 patients who underwent palliative surgical treatment, the median survival was 6.4 months for those treated by diverting colostomy, 14.8 months for abdominal resection, and 14.7 months for transanal excision.[587]

The fact that there are long-term survivors when so-called palliative procedures are performed implies that some individuals may still be well managed surgically, even though they have locally advanced disease. Extended resection in these patients, if feasible, has the potential of providing excellent palliation and even, occasionally, a cure.[465,652]

Pelvic Lymphadenectomy

Lateral pelvic lymph node dissection has been believed, especially by the Japanese, to be a requisite for proper rectal resection, especially of advanced cancer. Yamakoshi and co-workers found metastases to lymph nodes or lymphatic permeation in the tissue around the autonomic nerves in 14.3% of lower rectal cancers.[889] They, therefore, cautioned about the use of nerve-sparing techniques that fail to remove these nodes (see the following section). Fujita and colleagues noted that individuals with lymph node metastases had an overall 5-year disease-free survival rate of 73.3% for those who underwent lateral pelvic lymph node dissection compared with a 35.3% survival rate for those who did not (p = .013).[229] The authors caution, however, that what is needed is a randomized clinical trial. Moriya and colleagues reported a 5-year survival rate of 69% in their patients who did not undergo extended lymphadectomy, as compared with a rate of 76% for those who did.[593]

I am not an advocate of so-called *en bloc* pelvic lymphadenectomy, although I recognize that some institutions, through their retrospective studies, believe that survival rates are increased.[192] Others have demonstrated that patients with Dukes' A tumors do not benefit from lateral lymph node dissection and that local recurrence rates in those with Dukes' B and C lesions are not significantly decreased.[588]

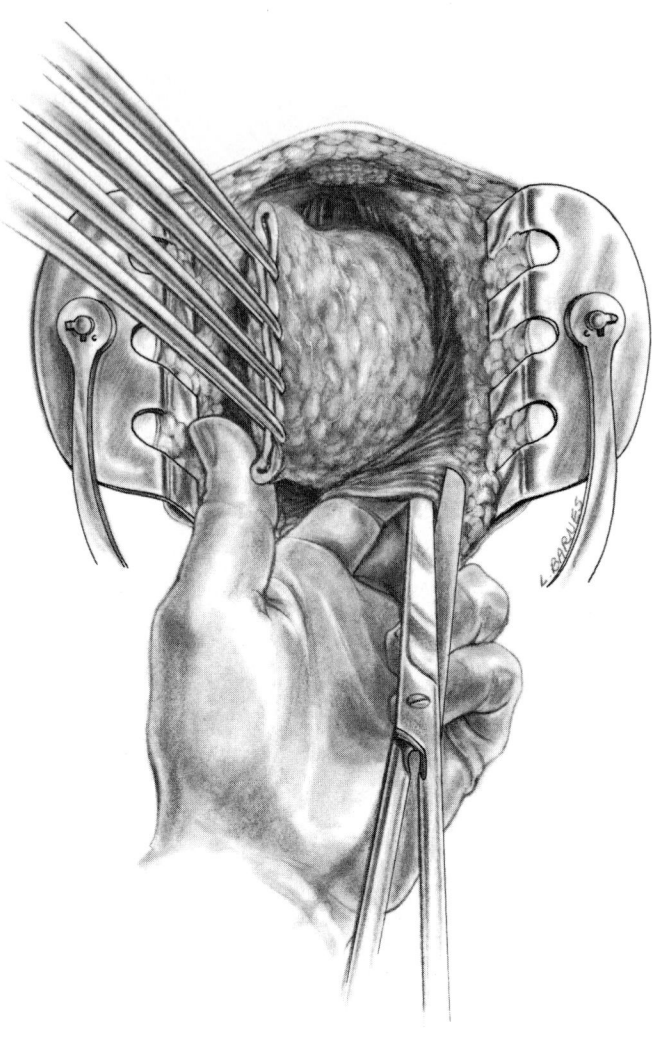

FIGURE 23-35. Perineal dissection. The levatores are divided from posterior to anterior on each side.

Inguinal Node Metastases

Inguinal node metastases with *rectal cancer* are an ominous prognostic finding. Graham and Hohn found no 5-year survivors irrespective of the method of management.[289] They still recommend therapeutic node dissection for purposes of local control and "possible cure." However, these unfortunate individuals indeed have surgically incurable disease. Therefore, one should endeavor to employ adjuvant measures, such as chemotherapy and radiotherapy, rather than to attempt a major resection. Depending on the findings and symptoms associated with the primary tumor, it may not be possible to achieve adequate palliation other than by operation. In 21 patients so observed by Tocchi and associates, the mean survival was 14.8 months (range, 2 to 42).[825]

Nerve-Preserving Operation

Urinary dysfunction and sexual dysfunction are common sequelae of APR (see later). Impotence is directly related to the extent of lateral pelvic dissection, hence my reluc-

tance to perform so-called radical lymphadenectomy as a routine in the treatment of rectal cancer. Injury to the parasympathetic nerves, especially in relation to the lateral ligaments where their course may be quite variable, is a clear risk (see Figure 1-19).[191,477] In recent years, there have been a number of publications that addressed the issue of autonomic nerve-preserving pelvic wall dissection, which theoretically combines the benefits of *en bloc* parietal pelvic dissection with nerve preservation.[191] In fact, there is an intraoperative tool that has been designed for locating the parasympathetic nerves, the CaverMap Surgical Aid (UroMed Corporation, Norwood, MA; *www.uromed.com*). Urologists have used this technique for many years when performing nerve-sparing radical prostatic surgery. A tumescence sensor is placed around the base of the penis. In preliminary studies, stimulation of the nerves resulted in a positive response in 40 patients (UroMed Publication).

It is relatively straightforward to preserve the paired hypogastric nerves beginning anterior to the sacral promontory (see Technique). Following identification of these

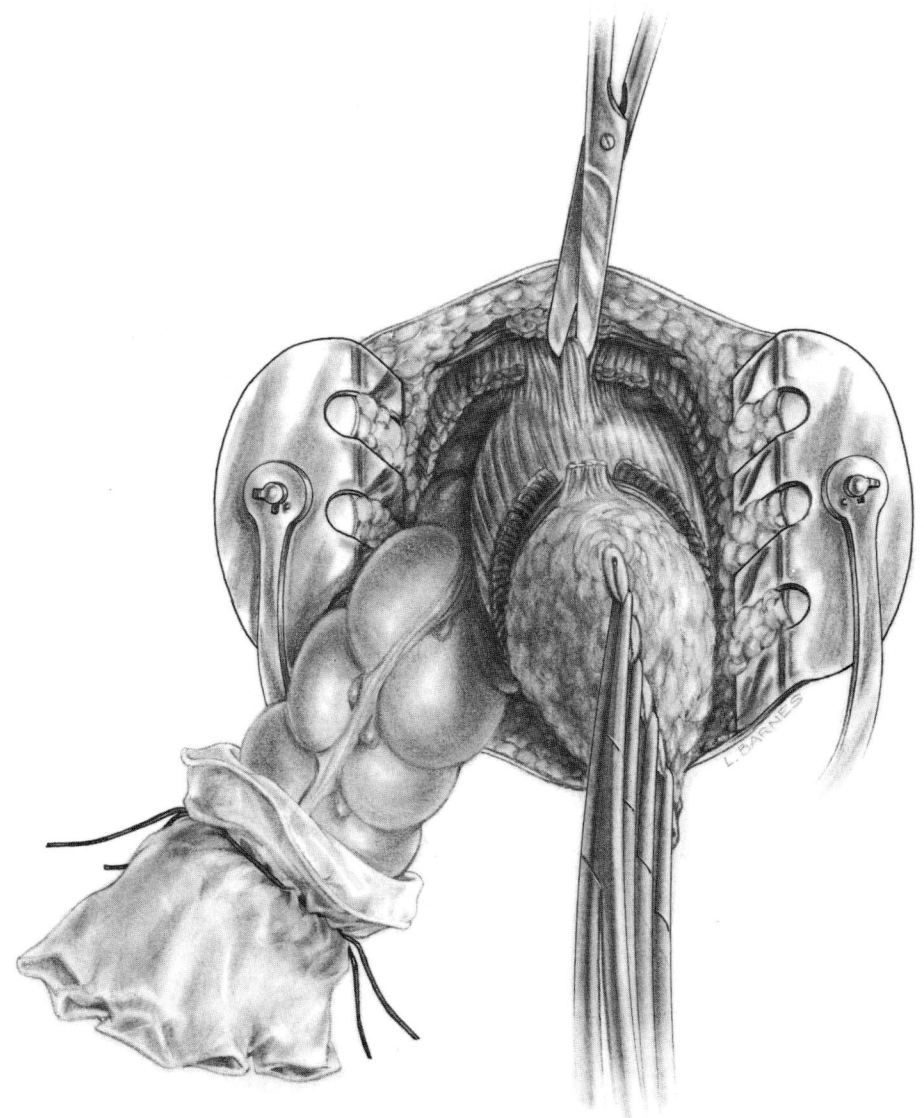

FIGURE 23-36. Perineal dissection. The proximal colon has been delivered through the pelvic defect. The rectourethralis muscle and the visceral fascia are the only structures remaining to be divided.

nerves, one can merely sweep them aside. The technique involves identification, dissection, and preservation of the hypogastric (sympathetic) nerves from above the aortic bifurcation to the lateral ligaments of the rectum.[191] Preservation of the sympathetic nerves can be readily achieved because they can be clearly visualized if one makes and effort to do so. Identification of the parasympathetic nerves is another matter. When one reads of the description of visualization and preservation of the nerves adjacent to the lateral ligaments, I, personally, am confounded. Even observation of video presentations on this subject fails to impress me as to the validity of the technical aspects of the dissection. In other words, I see no difference with the methods described from that which has previously been presented. Frankly, as is discussed later, the preoperative libido seems to be the most important issue with respect to

postoperative potency, not the nature of the dissection, except, of course if an ultraradical operation is undertaken.

Enker applied autonomic nerve-preserving pelvic wall dissection in 42 men undergoing sphincter-saving operations for the treatment of rectal cancer—not APR.[191] The incidence of potency was 86.7%, with 87.8% having normal ejaculation. Others report equally favorable results with this approach.[399,501,540,889]

Perineal Dissection in Women

Unless the tumor is quite small and exophytic, or localized only to the posterior wall of the rectum, a posterior vaginectomy should always be performed coincident with an APR. One must remember that the distance between the rectum and vagina is, in some areas, less

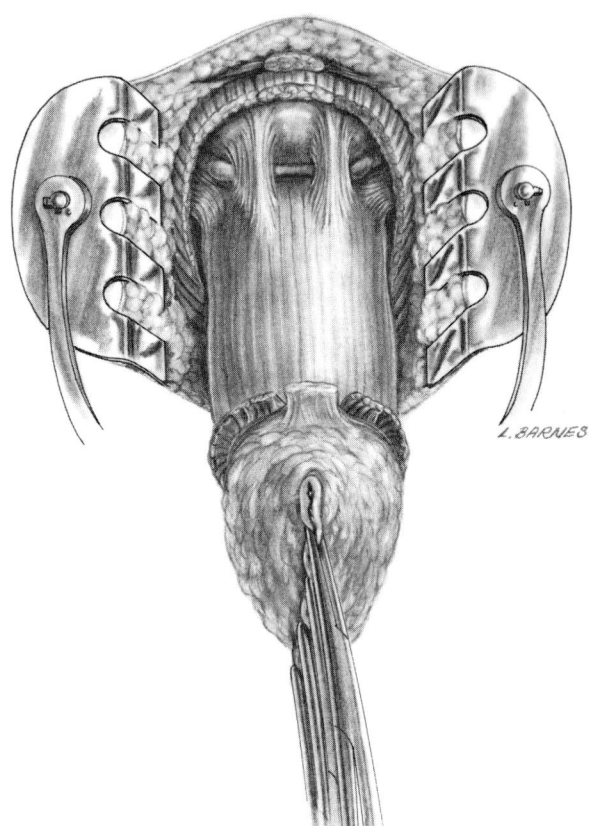

FIGURE 23-37. Perineal dissection. The rectourethralis muscle has been divided, exposing the prostate. With the division of the fascia of Denonvilliers, the peritoneal cavity can be entered anteriorly.

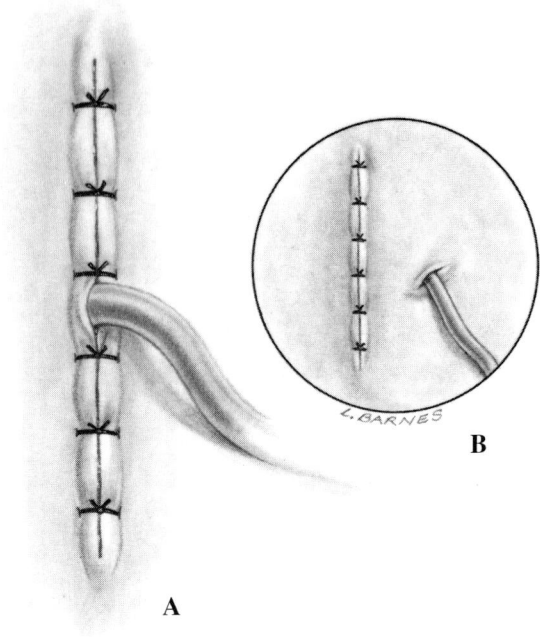

FIGURE 23-38. Perineal dissection. The wound is closed primarily and the pelvis is drained, either through the incision (**A**) or through a stab wound (**B**).

than 1 mm. For distal lesions, excision of the lower one third or the lower portion of the posterior vaginal wall may be all that is required, but for more extensive or more proximal tumors, the vagina should be excised to the level of the posterior *cul-de-sac* (Figure 23-39). Alternatively, a transverse incision can be made at the cephalad limit of the dissection in the vagina and the two lateral incisions connected.

Following posterior vaginectomy, the perineal skin closure is carried out until the forchette has been reconstituted. The posterior vaginal defect is left open, but the cut edges are sutured with an absorbable material for hemostasis. A drain is brought out through the defect in the vaginal wall rather than through the perineum (Figure 23-40). The vagina will eventually heal with minimal or no narrowing, depending on the extent of the vaginectomy. Obviously, if much of the vagina is removed, stenosis will result.

Concomitant Hysterectomy

Hysterectomy concomitant with APR should not be employed routinely, unless the presence of the uterus precludes visualization of the area of dissection. However, if the tumor breaches the muscular wall with invasion of the cervix, lower uterine segment, or body of the uterus, an in-continuity hysterectomy must be performed in order to extirpate the tumor adequately.

The incision of the peritoneum in the floor of the pelvis must be wider than that for APR (Figure 23-41). Both ureters are in greater danger of injury when this operation is performed. They should, therefore, be clearly identified virtually throughout their lengths. The peritoneum is swept off the uterus, and the bladder is bluntly pushed away from the cervix and vaginal wall. The infundibulopelvic and round ligaments are cross-clamped, divided, and ligated (Figure 23-42). The broad ligament is dissected away from the pelvic wall, exposing the uterine artery. By retraction of the uterus to the contralateral side, the uterine artery is cross-clamped, divided, and ligated. Division of the cardinal ligament poses the greatest threat to the ureter. If the tumor approaches this area, the cardinal ligament should be clamped close to the pelvic wall; thus the ureter must be clearly visualized (Figure 23-43). I prefer to use a single curved Kocher clamp, dividing the tissue on the medial aspect, a maneuver analogous to the technique employed for division of the lateral ligaments. The clamp is replaced more distally after each suture ligature is tied.

When the dissection has been completed on both sides, the anterior vaginal wall is incised and the posterior vaginal wall removed with the proctectomy specimen. The vagina may be closed or left open in order to fa-

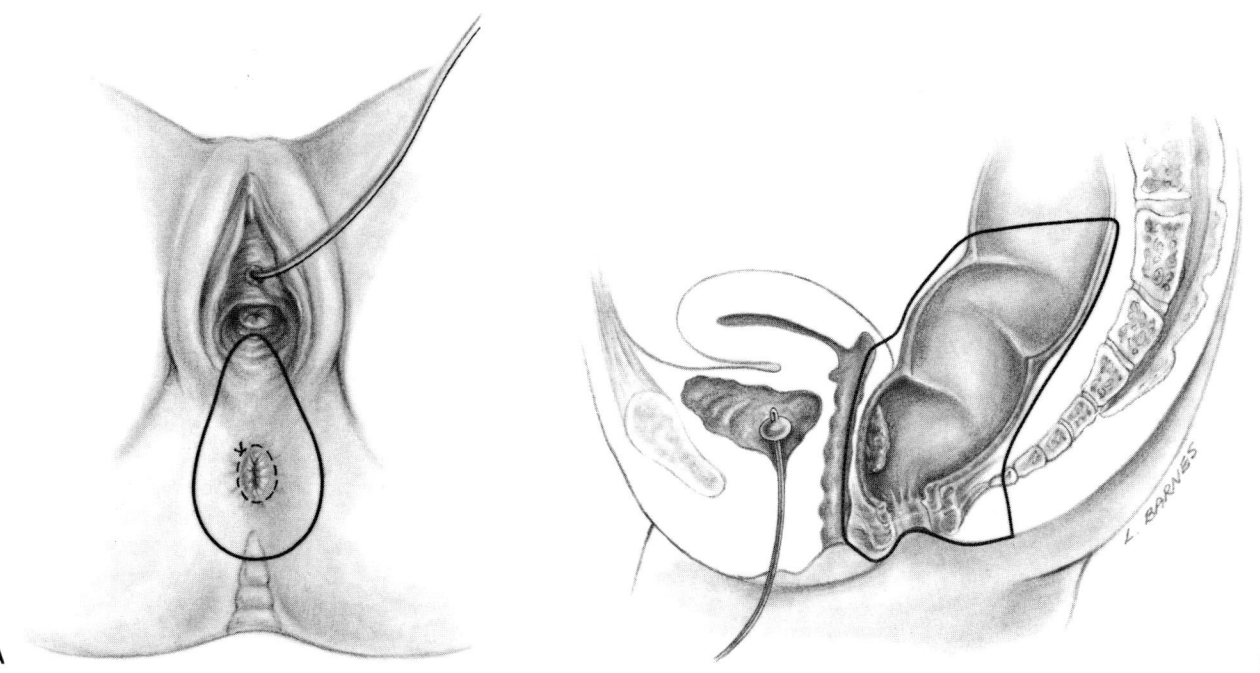

FIGURE 23-39. Perineal dissection in women. **(A)** Outline of the incision for excising the posterior vaginal wall. **(B)** Lateral view showing the extent of removal.

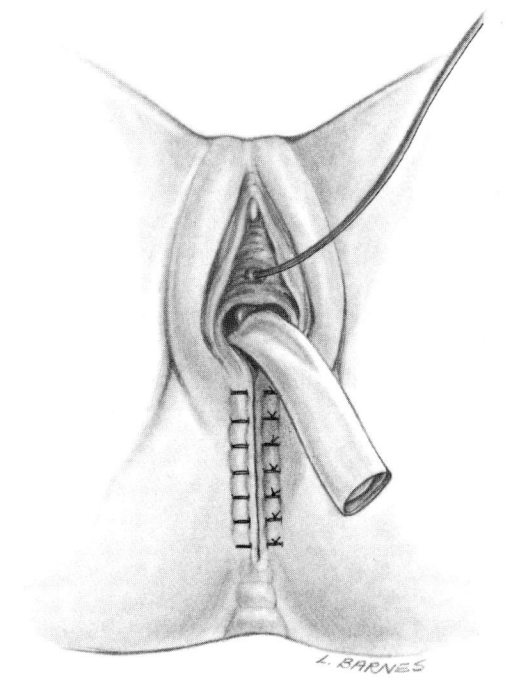

FIGURE 23-40. Perineal dissection in women. The skin wound is completely closed, and the perineal body is reconstructed. The drain is placed in the pelvis and brought out through the defect in the posterior vaginal wall.

cilitate drainage, depending on how much of the posterior vaginal wall has been excised.

Oophorectomy

Metastatic disease apparent at the time of surgery is an indication for therapeutic oophorectomy, but the value of prophylactic oophorectomy has been the subject of debate.[15,66,67,425,506] This controversy is discussed in Chapter 22, but it appears that the prevention of primary ovarian cancer is probably the main benefit.[149] With the low incidence of microscopic metastatic involvement, it is difficult to justify prophylactic oophorectomy in the premenopausal age group, but removal of the ovaries in the postmenopausal patient appears to me to be a reasonable course. Parenthetically, oophorectomy is as appropriate for cecal carcinoma as it is for a rectal or sigmoid lesion.

Reconstruction of the Pelvic Floor

One of the concerns expressed in the application of postoperative as well as preoperative radiotherapy (see later) is the possibility of injury to the small bowel. The likelihood of such a complication is considerably reduced if doses do not exceed 50 Gy. However, there is evidence to suggest that if higher dosages are applied, recurrence rates may diminish. Certain techniques have been suggested to minimize radiation to this relatively vulnerable

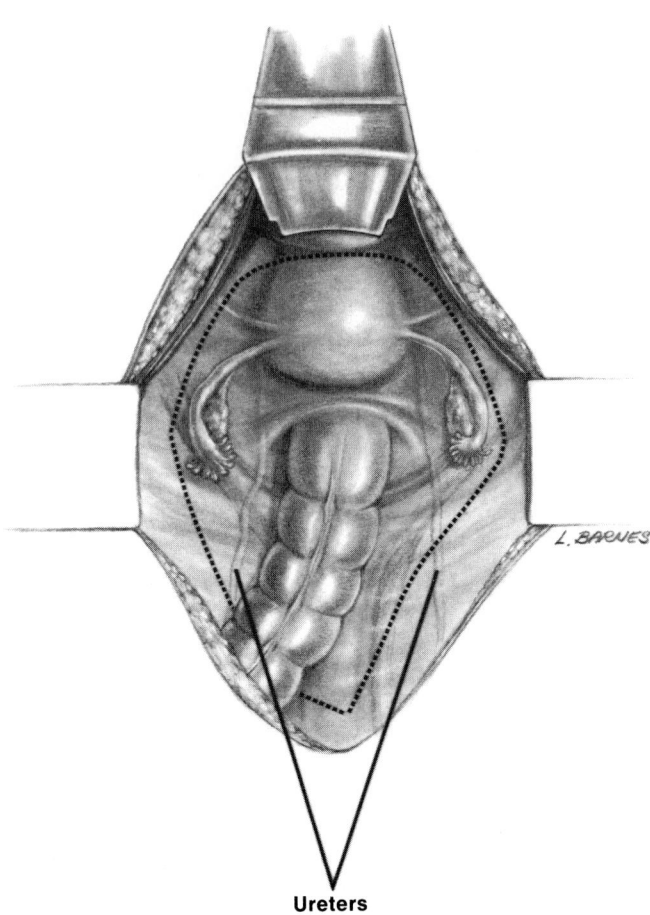

Ureters

FIGURE 23-41. Hysterectomy concomitant with abdominoperineal resection. Peritoneal incision *(dotted line)* must be quite wide to incorporate the uterus and rectum for removal in continuity.

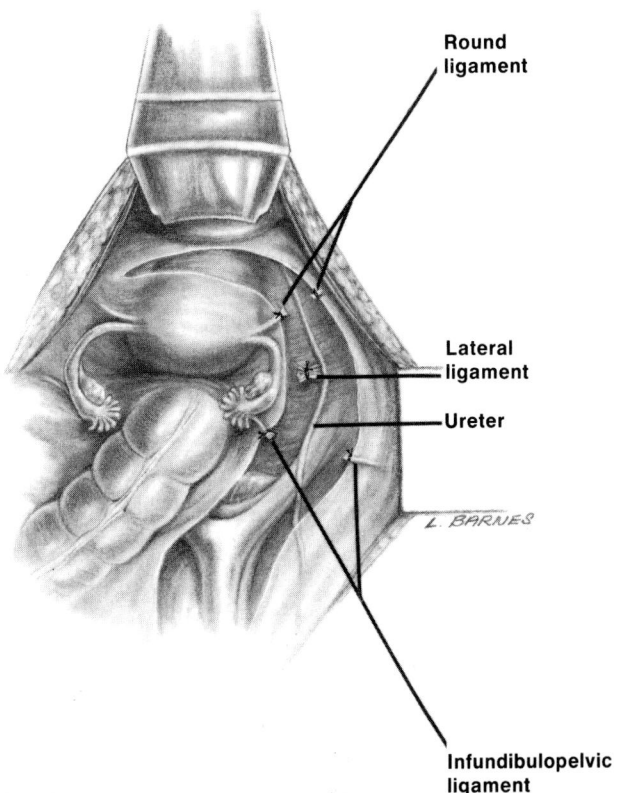

Round ligament

Lateral ligament

Ureter

Infundibulopelvic ligament

FIGURE 23-42. Concomitant hysterectomy. The uterus and rectum are mobilized on the right side by division of the round, infundibulopelvic, and lateral ligaments.

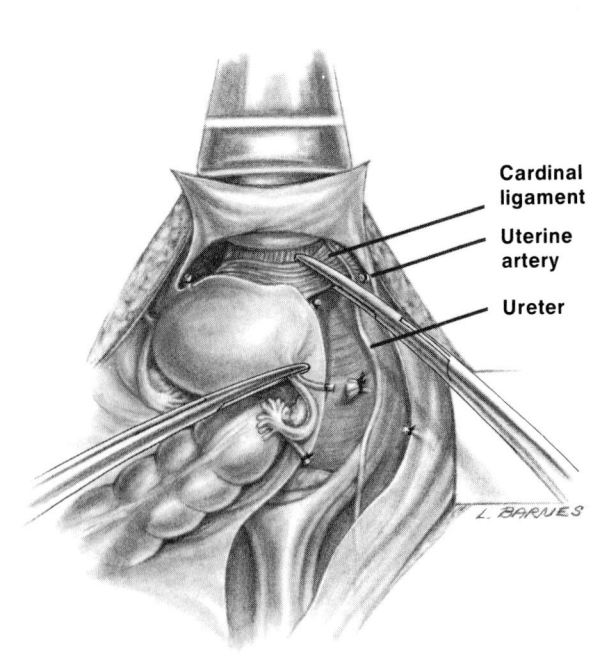

Cardinal ligament

Uterine artery

Ureter

FIGURE 23-43. Concomitant hysterectomy. The uterine artery has been divided, and the cardinal ligament is clamped. The ureter is extremely vulnerable to injury at this point.

organ by excluding the small bowel from the pelvis. These include suturing the terminal ileum and its mesentery around the linea terminalis,[850] construction of an omental envelope, the use of the rectus abdominis muscle, and placement of a synthetic absorbable or nonabsorbable mesh sling, a breast prosthesis, and a synthetic polymer mold.[86,168,171–173,185,199,291,301,433,464,745,802] The possibility of infection with nonabsorbable material is, of course, a concern, as well as the inconvenience if one must remove it.

Technique

My own preference is to use polyglycolic acid mesh (either Dexon or Vicryl mesh) for this procedure, a technique that is recommended whenever postoperative radiation, following either APR or even anterior resection, is being considered. Because the mesh that is provided is not usually of sufficient size to create the sling, two are used and sutured together. Commencing at the level of the sacral promontory, the mesh is anchored (Figure 23-44). Using a continuous, locking suture technique, one anchors the mesh laterally on each side to the peritoneum (Figure 23-45). The mesh is then brought to the anterior abdominal wall and secured in place, creating a halter or sling that keeps the small bowel out of the pelvis (Figure 23-46).

Results

Devereux and colleagues reported 19 patients who underwent resection with simultaneous use of the sling procedure.[173] Postoperatively, all received contrast-simulation studies that documented the small bowel above the sacral promontory. Fractional tumoricidal doses ranging from 5,200 to 5,800 cGy were administered. No patient demonstrated obstruction, infection, nausea, vomiting, cramps, diarrhea, or acute radiation-associated small bowel injury.[173] When three individuals subsequently came to surgery, all mesh had been resorbed, there were no adhesions, and there was no suggestion of recurrent tumor. Dasmahapatra and Swaminathan used this technique in 45 patients without an early mesh-related complication (two individuals later developed small bowel obstruction, not resulting from the mesh).[156] However, Sener and colleagues experienced three perioperative complications in their eight patients who underwent reconstruction of the pelvic floor with polyglactin mesh—a pelvic abscess, a wound dehiscence, and a herniation of the small bowel between the mesh and the pelvic sidewall.[745]

Lechner and Cesnik employed omentopexy in 43 patients to create an artificial diaphragm between the abdominal cavity and the pelvis.[464] With subsequent adjuvant radiotherapy, no complication related to the small bowel was recognized. Voros and colleagues utilized the ileum and mesentery to reconstruct the pelvic floor.[850] Imaging studies on postoperative day 10 confirmed the position of the bowel out of the pelvis.

Incidental Appendectomy

Incidental appendectomy is not recommended at the time of proctectomy or with any bowel resection. It is sufficiently difficult to evaluate postoperative lower abdominal signs and symptoms, fever, and leukocytosis, without adding an unnecessary variable.

Bladder Resection

The urinary bladder is not uncommonly directly invaded by rectal cancer. As such, one should always attempt resection in-continuity with the bladder whenever the surgeon is confronted with this problem. One errs if he or she assumes that the adherence is inflammatory, rather than neoplastic. Clearly, wide excision with adequate margins is much preferred to that of leaving behind gross or microscopic tumor. The surgeon cannot depend on postoperative radiation treatment to "sterilize" the field. Carne and colleagues analyzed 53 patients who underwent *en bloc* bladder resection for colorectal cancer in New Zealand.[97] Forty-five had a partial cystectomy. All who did not have *en bloc* resection developed local recurrence. The authors noted that the decision whether to perform partial or total cystectomy depends on the site of the bladder invasion.

Sacrectomy and Pelvic Exenteration

Total pelvic exenteration is defined as the removal of the distal colon and rectum, along with the lower ureters, bladder, internal reproductive organs, perineum, draining lymph nodes, and pelvic peritoneum.[494] In a highly selected series from the Ellis Fischel State Cancer Center, Columbia, Missouri involving 24 patients over a 30-year period, Lopez and colleagues reported an operative mortality of about 20% (9% during the last decade).[494] The overall survival rate was a remarkable 42%. A review by Williams and colleagues, summarizing the results of several series, concluded that the procedure can be carried out with a mortality rate of less than 10%.[875]

Sugarbaker has advocated *en bloc* excision of rectal cancer with sacrectomy for lesions that are fixed posteriorly.[801] In reporting his experience with six patients, he noted that four survived more than 3 years. Pearlman and colleagues carried out 12 pelvic and seven sacropelvic exenterations.[651] Of the 15 patients without extrapelvic disease, there was one operative death, two

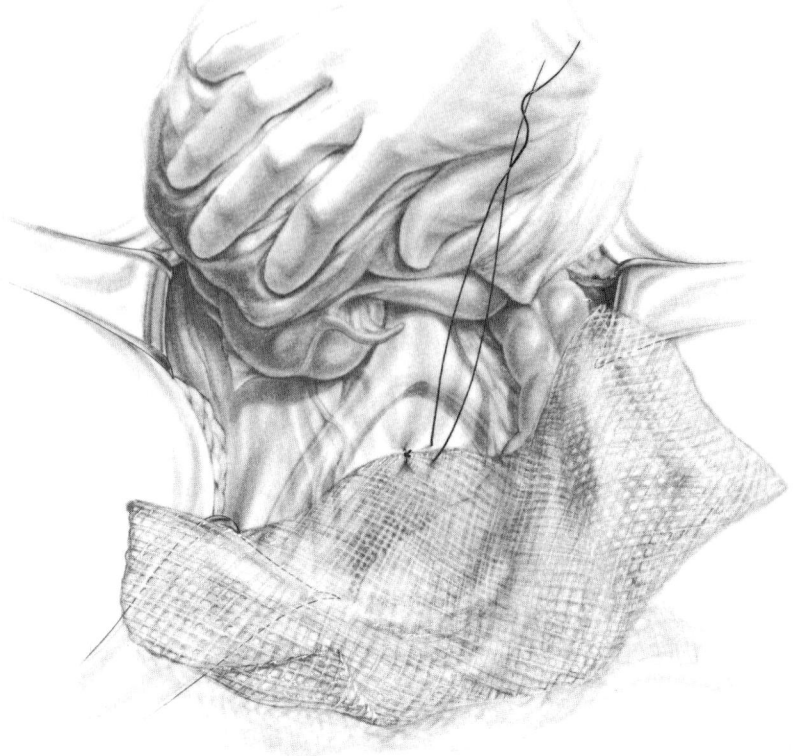

FIGURE 23-44. Implantation of mesh for postoperative radiation. The mesh is anchored to the sacral promontory.

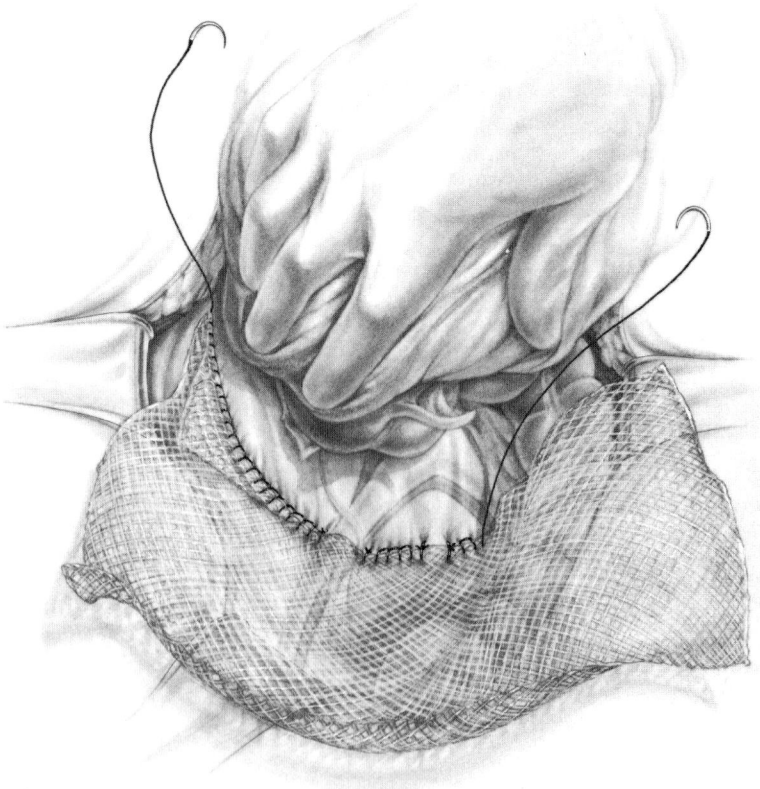

FIGURE 23-45. Implantation of mesh for postoperative radiation. Using a continuous, interlocking suture technique, the mesh is anchored to the posterior and lateral peritoneal surfaces. Two pieces of mesh may be required to effect this maneuver.

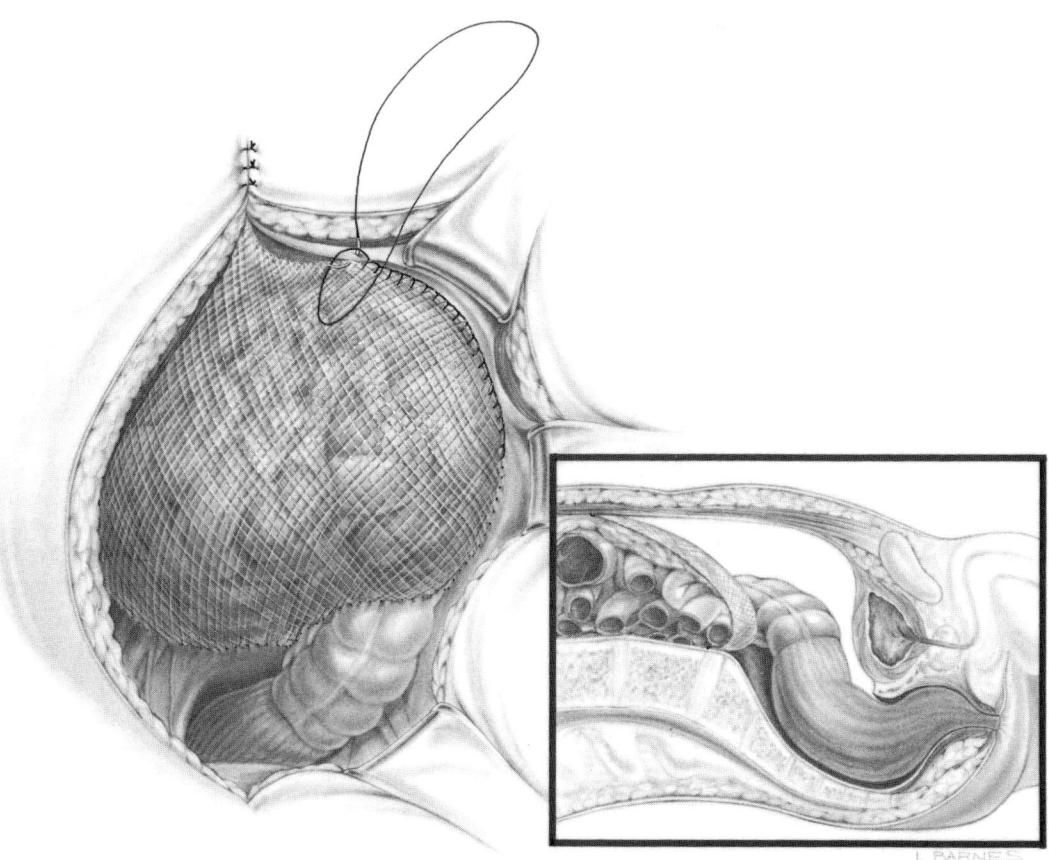

FIGURE 23-46. Implantation of mesh for postoperative radiation. The completed suspension requires the mesh to be anchored to the anterior abdominal wall. Care must be taken not to impede the exit of the bowel for the stoma. The abdominal wound should be closed without incorporating the mesh, but anterior fixation can be achieved to the peritoneum. Final position of the fixation in an individual who has undergone an anterior resection **(inset)**.

died free of disease, three died of cancer, one was alive with recurrence, and the remainder were free of disease (none had achieved 5 years). Shirouzu and colleagues performed total pelvic exenteration on 26 patients for locally advanced colorectal cancer.[755] The operative mortality was 8%. In those with stage II primary disease, the recurrence rate after curative surgery was three of seven, but the mean survival time was 58 months, with a 5-year survival of 71%. Those with stage IV disease had a mean survival time of only 5 months. Others have demonstrated that pelvic exenteration (APR and cystectomy) in selected patients may produce a 25% to 50% 5-year survival.[139,378,421]

Jiminez and colleagues reported the Memorial Sloan-Kettering Cancer Center experience with total pelvic exenteration in the treatment of rectal cancer.[390] Fifty-five patients were identified—71% with recurrent disease and 29% for the primary tumor. At the time of the procedure 49% received intraoperative radiation treatment, and 20% required sacrectomy. The perioperative mortality was 5.5%. Median disease-specific survival was 48.9 months. Univariate analysis identified five factors associated with decreased survival: male gender, recurrent disease, prior APR, positive surgical margins, and the administration of intraoperative radiation.[390] Koda and co-workers commented that total pelvic exenteration for locally advanced cancers can be selectively performed with reestablishment of both bowel and urinary continuity when the tumor invades neither the anal canal nor the urogenital diaphragm.[427]

Comment

It is often difficult to interpret the results of this procedure from the literature because the indications are variable and may include a large percentage of individuals with carcinoma of the uterine cervix.[434] Furthermore, a major problem with most published studies is that, in order to report more than an anecdotal experience, authors tend to supplement their reports with patients who have limited follow-up. It is well advised that optimal care is facilitated by specialist urologic consultation.[554] It certainly seems appropriate that evaluation of potential candidates for this operation and the procedure, itself (if indicated), should be undertaken by individuals who have a particular interest and experience with this operation.

Reconstruction with a Neosphincter

Mercati and colleagues initially described a technique whereby an APR was carried out, but a gracilis muscle transposition was employed to create a new sphincter mechanism around the pulled down proximal colon (see Chapter 13).[566] Restoration was simultaneously effected in four individuals, with three sphincter reconstructions performed at a later time. Williams and colleagues described a similar operation in which a neorectum and neoanal sphincter are constructed by means of the gracilis muscle and by using low-frequency stimulation to alter the muscles characteristics (fast-twitch to slow-twitch; see Chapter 13).[879] The patient was continent with the stimulator on and was able to evacuate when the stimulator was turned off. Others have employed a seromuscular graft for this purpose.[830]

Since these initial contributions, numerous articles have been published concerning reconstruction with reestablishment of intestinal continuity following APR. Cavina has the world's largest experience and in 1996 published a 10-year follow-up report with 81 patients.[102] Thirty-seven surviving patients who underwent APR with gracileplasty were followed for a mean of 78.6 months. The overall complication rate was 37%, with a 5-year survival rate of 58%. Fecal continence was obtained in 90% of patients, with apparently no pejorative effect on survival. Others, too, confirm that total anorectal reconstruction is possible in selected patients without adverse consequences for survival.[2] Geerdes and colleagues utilized double dynamic gracileplasty with and without an intervening reservoir.[248] The authors caution that further modifications in the technique will be required before the procedure can be undertaken with minimal morbidity. Of the 15 patients evaluable, 53% were continent, but five underwent conversion to an abdominal stoma (33%). In the experience of Santoro and colleagues, of the 11 patients available for long-term evaluation, eight demonstrated adequate stool control.[723] The authors concluded that the sphincter is really an elastic stenosis. Abercombie and colleagues measured anorectal sensory function following APR and total anal reconstruction in six individuals.[1] No patient appreciated neorectal distension, a desire to

defecate, or a feeling of passage of flatus. The authors concluded that the loss of rectal sensation suggests that the prime sensors of rectal feeling probably lie within the rectum itself.[1]

Romano and co-workers performed anorectal reconstruction with the artificial bowel sphincter (Acticon; see Chapter 13).[691] Eight underwent reconstruction—five with a synchronous operation and three as a delayed procedure. All but one achieved a good incontinence score (Cleveland Clinic Score). Sato and colleagues have explored the possibility of a perineal colostomy with pudendal nerve anastomosis to a reconstructed gluteus muscle as a staged procedure.[725,726]

Comment

Because one must be concerned about the risk of recurrent tumor, I question whether the synchronous application for malignant disease is an appropriate choice, except in highly selected patients. Furthermore, the need for subsequent radiotherapy in some individuals could adversely affect the reconstruction. Still, the concept is exciting and merits consideration and further study. One awaits the results of longer follow-up and greater experience.

Postoperative Care

An indwelling catheter should be left in place for 5 to 7 days, longer if the patient has had a history of difficulty in voiding or has prostatic hypertrophy. In fact, in those individuals whose prostatic enlargement has seriously interfered with urinary function preoperatively, transurethral resection of the prostate may ultimately be necessary. I prefer to defer such a procedure for some weeks, even if it is necessary for the patient to be discharged with a catheter, in order to avoid further urinary tract complications (see later). Generally, women have fewer problems with micturition following APR than men.

A nasogastric tube is not routinely employed. With reasonably expeditious surgery and no intraoperative complications or extenuating circumstances, most patients tolerate the absence of a tube quite well (see Chapter 22). Occasionally, a patient complains of nausea, but antiemetic medication usually suffices. If vomiting ensues, a nasogastric tube should be placed until gas is passed or gastric output is minimal.

In the past, ice chips or only small amounts of clear liquids had been permitted by mouth until flatus had been passed through the colostomy. However, as discussed in the previous chapter, there has arisen a concerted effort to institute oral feedings sooner and progress the patient's diet more rapidly. Certainly, as long as an individual can tolerate this kind of regimen, it is reasonable to encourage it. However, because it usually takes 48 to 96 hours for flatus to pass, this dietary approach may not always be possible. Generally, a progressive diet is instituted, advancing through full liquids and then to a selected diet. This usually encompasses 2 to 3 days.

At one time it was believed that patients should be kept at bed rest following APR because of the fear that the intestines would fall out of the perineum. This is an extraordinarily unusual complication, however. Early ambulation is, therefore, advised. Patients may be asked to sit or stand the evening of surgery and encouraged to walk on the first postoperative day. The use of a foam rubber donut will ameliorate the patient's discomfort.

The perineal drain is removed on the third postoperative day, if the drainage is less than 75 mL in 24 hours. Otherwise, it is left in place until the drainage reaches this level. If the wound has been left open, it is vigorously irrigated with saline, three times daily. If the drainage appears foul, one-half strength Dakin's solution or povidone-iodine (Betadine) is used. Sitz baths are also useful for comfort and are advised immediately following the irrigation. Sitz baths alone, however, are inadequate for cleansing the pelvic cavity. Hematoma, pus, and debris are effectively removed only by irrigation.

If the perineal wound required packing, the pack is removed at 3 or 4 days. This is done at the bedside and usually requires a parenteral narcotic. Rarely is it necessary to return the patient to the operating room for the purpose of having the pack removed.

During the patient's hospital convalescence, the colostomy is managed by means of a disposable transparent bag (see Chapters 31 and 32). By the fourth day, the patient is involved in stomal care and appliance change. The relative merits of spontaneous evacuation versus irrigation are always a subject for debate, but I believe that patients should be permitted the opportunity of choosing. Accordingly, instructions are given for both management options if the individual is willing to learn, but this is usually deferred until the patient has left the hospital because patients are discharged earlier than previously (see Chapter 32). Therefore, the responsibility for providing this information will usually rest with a visiting nurse.

Complications

Complications following APR are extremely common, with reported incidences in the range of 60%.[661]

Intraoperative Complications

Injury to small bowel usually is easily dealt with by standard reparative techniques, as long as the problem is recognized at the time of surgery. Likewise, slippage of ligatures on vessels or injury to vessels can be readily addressed by conventional hemostatic maneuvers.

By far the greatest fear that confronts the surgeon performing an APR is that of injury to the ureter. However, the operator can take some solace in the fact that, in most cases, recognition of the injury at that time will usually lead to a good functional result through the application of proper principles of repair. The degree of difficulty in effecting a delayed repair is much greater, and the results of such maneuvers are not as successful when compared with early recognition. The same techniques are applicable in the situation when part of the ureter is intentionally excised as a consequence of invasion by tumor.

Ureteral Injury

In spite of advances in the surgical treatment of patients, ureteral injuries still occur relatively frequently during the performance of pelvic operations, especially hysterectomy, low anterior resection, and APR. It is because of this risk that it is often helpful to have the benefit of CT, so that the surgeon can embark on repair knowing the status of urinary tract anatomy. It is also useful to know that the patient had two functioning kidneys before the operation. Factors predisposing to ureteral injury that are not related to tumor include congenital anomalies, such as duplication, megaureter, and ectopic ureter or kidney.[687]

Injury to the ureter occurs usually at one of three points during the procedure of removal of the rectum. First, during the ligation of the inferior mesenteric vessels, the left ureter can be incorporated in the ligature or divided when the vessels themselves are divided. Care must be taken to displace the left ureter laterally, away from the vascular pedicle. In addition, when dividing the inferior mesenteric vessels, one should always look a second time to be certain that the left ureter is out of harm's way.

The second area of injury occurs deep in the pelvis and is produced usually coincident with the division of the lateral ligaments. The ureter is particularly exposed to danger if a synchronous hysterectomy is carried out. In fact, hysterectomy is the commonest cause of ureteral injury even without rectal resection.[687] The risk of injury can obviously be reduced by retracting both ureters laterally and visualizing them throughout their lengths. However, this is often cumbersome and unnecessary if the growth is not adherent to the pelvic wall or if there has not been prior surgery to cause displacement. A practical means for avoiding ureteral injury during the course of division of the lateral ligaments is to employ only one clamp. Minimal dissection is required, so there is less likelihood of incorporating the ureter in the laterally placed hemostat. Back-bleeding is rarely evident, but it can be easily controlled by separate applications of a clamp with the rectum freed and the vascular area rotated anteriorly (see earlier, Technique).

The use of ureteral stents does not necessarily protect the ureter from harm (see earlier and Chapter 22). However, when the surgeon has a high index of suspicion of direct involvement of the bladder or ureters, when the operation is undertaken following radiation treatment, when the procedure represents repeat pelvic surgery, or when a difficult dissection is expected (especially for tumor extension), preoperative placement of ureteral catheters may aid the surgeon in identifying the structures. Moreover, if the ureter containing the catheter is divided, the injury is usually self-evident.

Injury to the lower ureter is more likely to occur during synchronous-combined APR than if the single-team approach is used.[287] This is because a more extensive perineal operation is performed by the perineal surgeon. If the lateral ligaments are divided from below or blind scissor dissection is employed, the ureter can be unknowingly injured. Great care must be taken by the perineal surgeon when dividing the ligaments or when dissecting in the supralevator area.

The third area of vulnerability is a consequence of mobilization of the peritoneum and the closure of the pelvic peritoneal floor. One or both ureters may be divided as the peritoneum is elevated, or they may be incorporated in the suture during the closure. It is imperative that the ureters be clearly visualized during the reperitonealization maneuver and that they be displaced laterally.

Unfortunately, only 20% to 30% of ureteral injuries are recognized at the time of operation.[900] If one is concerned about the possibility of ureteral injury during a difficult pelvic dissection, identification of the injury site may be revealed by injecting 12.5 g of mannitol intravenously followed by the intravenous administration of 5 mL of indigo carmine dye. The presence of a blue stain in the operative field is diagnostic of injury. If the distal ureter cannot be identified, a cystotomy should be made and a ureteral catheter placed through the ureteral orifice until it presents in the operative field. If ligation without penetration is suspected, a proximal linear ureterotomy permits antegrade insertion of a ureteral catheter to test the patency.[900]

As mentioned, most ureteral injuries go unrecognized and, indeed, may forever be unrecognized if a single ureter has been ligated. Flank pain, fever, leukocytosis, and tenderness are the most often presenting signs and symptoms of ureteral ligation during the early postoperative period. Urinary fistula can be suspected if there is copious serous or serosanguineous perineal wound drainage in the early postoperative period. A blue stain appearing on the perineal or abdominal wound dressing after intravenous administration of indigo carmine confirms the diagnosis. When there is no perineal wound, such as after low anterior resection, it often takes a number of days before the presence of urine within the abdominal cavity is appreciated.

Late urinary fistula can occur because of ureteral necrosis from devascularization injury, from the membranous urethra or from the base of the bladder.

Treatment With crush injury from a hemostat or with partial ligation, removing the ligature and performing a limited repair or tube decompression require careful patient selection in order to avoid postoperative difficulties. Occasionally, if the patient's poor general condition precludes prolonging the operation by the performance of a definitive reconstruction, a temporary feeding-tube proximal diversion can be employed.[900] Proximal ureteral ligation with the expectation of renal death in the poor-risk patient who has a limited life expectancy is generally to be condemned because of the risks of sepsis and fistula formation.[900] One also must be concerned about the function of the contralateral kidney.

INJURY TO THE LOWER URETER *Ureteroneocystotomy* is the preferred procedure for injuries of the pelvic ureter. Injuries within 5 cm of the bladder and often at greater distances are suitable for this approach. The technique has been described by Politano and Leadbetter, and by others.[473,474,660] The procedure achieves an anti-refluxing ureteral anastomosis. The following operations have been advocated by Libertino, Rote, and Zinman.[473,474]

A midline cystotomy is made, and 3 mL of saline solution is injected through a 23-gauge needle, raising a small bleb of mucosa (Figure 23-47). An ellipse of mucosa is excised, and a 3-cm submucosal tunnel is created with a right-angle clamp (Figure 23-48). The clamp is then rotated to point through the bladder wall, and the detrusor muscle is pierced. The distal ureter is pulled through the tunnel with the aid of traction sutures and spatulated for approximately 1 cm.[474] A no. 6 or 8 French catheter is inserted to make certain that the ureter pursues a direct course. The ureter is then sutured to the bladder with interrupted 5–0 chromic catgut sutures. Deep bites of detrusor must be included in the two distal sutures at the five and seven o'clock positions to help restore normal ureterovesical function.[473] A no. 5 feeding tube is used as a ureteral stent and is brought out alongside a suprapubic cystotomy catheter. This is removed on the seventh day.

Ureteral reimplantation into the bladder is the best method for restoring continuity following ureteral injury. Therefore, every effort should be made to accomplish this. If the ureter cannot be brought down without tension, a Boari bladder flap tube technique can be employed, or preferably a so-called psoas bladder hitch maneuver can be used.[49,61,837] These techniques are best

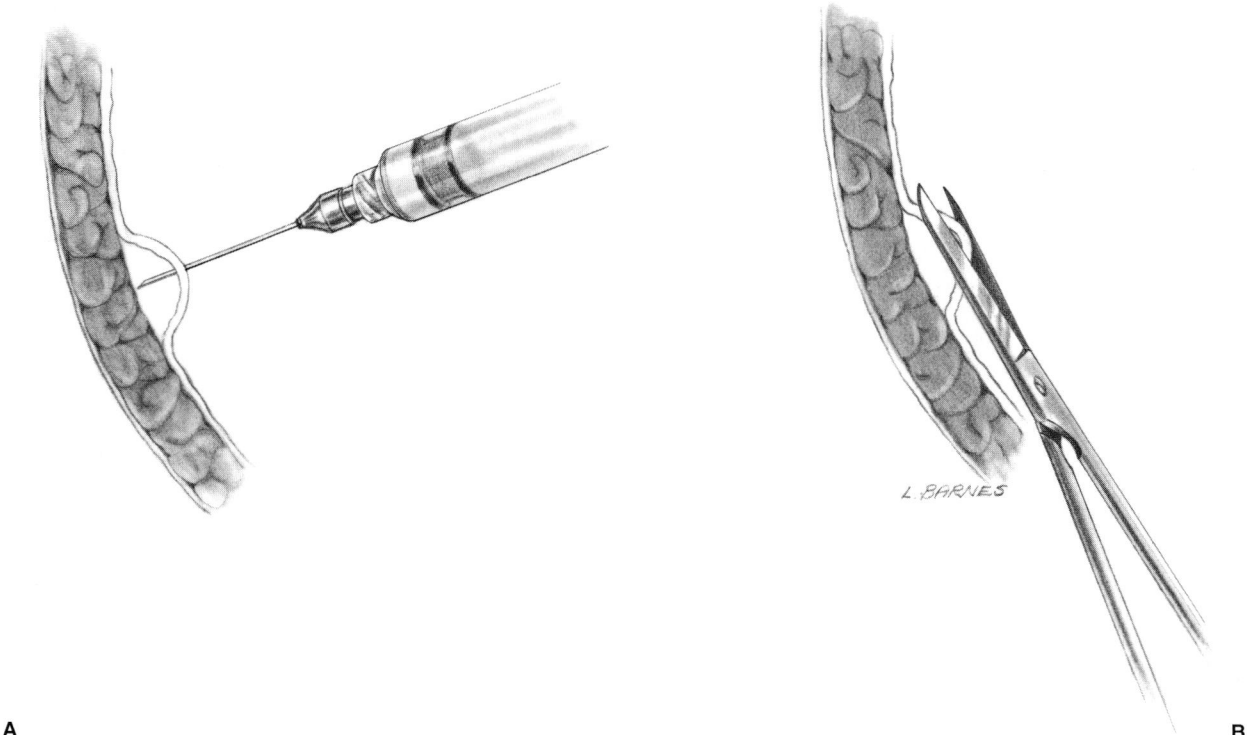

A

B

FIGURE 23-47. Ureteroneocystotomy. **(A)** Submucosal injection of saline. **(B)** A small ellipse of bladder mucosa is excised to allow creation of a submucosal tunnel. (Adapted from Libertino JA, Zinman L. Technique for uretero-neocystotomy in renal transplantation and reflux. *Surg Clin North Am* 1973;53:459, with permission.)

accomplished by a urologist who is familiar with the specialized approaches to ureterovesical surgery. It is always wise to take advantage of the availability of urologic consultation when injury to the urinary tract has occurred.

INJURY TO THE MIDDLE AND UPPER URETER Injuries to the proximal ureter are the most difficult and least satisfactory to treat. Fortunately, this is a rare complication of bowel surgery. Because of the distance, reimplantation into the bladder is not possible, and the blood supply is less adequate. Direct repair by *end-to-end ureteroureterostomy* is the treatment of choice. With loss of ureteral length from excision or necrosis, defects of up to 8 cm can be traversed by this method if one uses a renal-lowering technique.[474] If direct repair is impossible, one can consider the highly specialized techniques of *ileal interposition* and *autotransplantation*. Benson and colleagues reported success with ureteral reconstruction in 17 of their 18 patients by the selective application of ileal interposition, autotransplanation, psoas hitch, or Boari bladder tube.[49] *Nephrectomy* may be used if the surgeon is satisfied that contralateral kidney function is adequate and calculous disease or other conditions that may affect the kidney are not present.

Transureteroureterostomy is another alternative that may be employed for the injured ureter. Hodges and colleagues reported a large, successful experience with this technique,[354] but because of the possibility of injury to the recipient ureter, it should be used only sparingly and then limited to injuries of the upper pelvic ureter when re-implantation cannot be accomplished.[474] The technique is shown in Figure 23-49. The injured ureter should be resected at a point of certain viability, with care being taken to preserve the adventitia and blood supply. The recipient ureter should not be mobilized from its bed.

Whenever a direct repair of a ureteral injury is performed, proximal diversion is advised. Zinman and colleagues recommend a no. 7 French polyurethane double pigtail ureteral stent (Figure 23-50A).[900] The cut edges of the ureter are debrided and spatulated, and the kidney, ureter, or both, is adequately mobilized.[474] The ureter is spatulated on opposing sides of each end to prevent stricture (Figure 23-50B). Anastomosis is effected with interrupted 5–0 chromic catgut or long-term absorbable sutures placed full thickness, with the knots on the outside, inverting the mucosa (Figure 23-50C). Noncrushing vascular forceps can be used to grasp the tissue whereas the

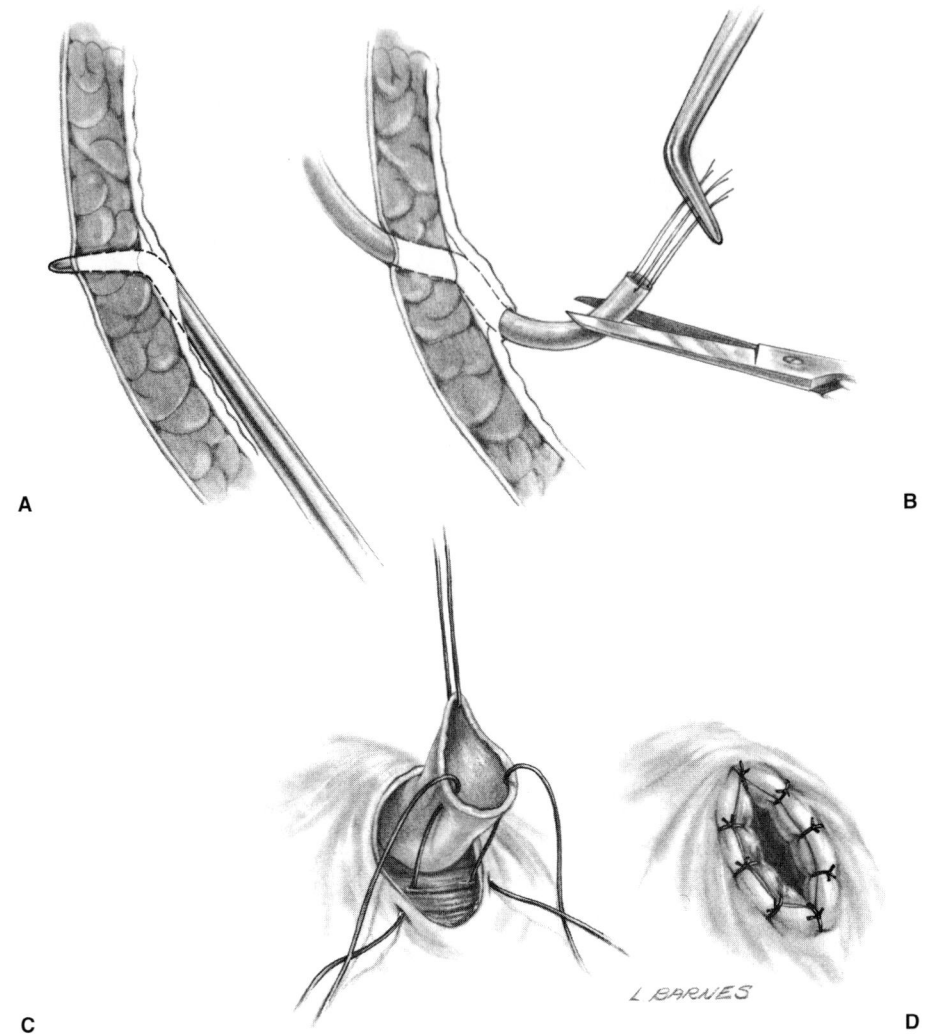

A

B

C

D

L BARNES

FIGURE 23-48. Ureteroneocystotomy. **(A)** A right-angle clamp pierces the detrusor muscle. **(B)** The ureter is pulled through the submucosal tunnel; the distal ureter is cut at a 45-degree angle, creating a new ureteral meatus. **(C)** The ureter is anchored to the bladder detrusor muscle. **(D)** Completion of the anastomosis to the bladder mucosa. (Adapted from Libertino JA, Zinman L. Technique for uretero-neocystotomy in renal transplantation and reflux. *Surg Clin North Am* 1973;53:459, with permission.)

presence of a catheter within the lumen facilitates the procedure. A continuous suture should never be employed. The ureter can be wrapped in omentum if the anastomosis is believed to be precarious. A soft rubber drain (Penrose) is placed at the site of the ureteroureterostomy and brought out through a stab wound. The stent is usually removed on postoperative day 10, followed by the drain 48 hours later (if no urine drainage is present).

Before discharge, CT with intravenous contrast should be performed for all patients who undergo ureteral repair, in order to determine the adequacy of the reconstruction.

Bladder Injury

Bladder injury that is recognized at the time of surgery can usually be repaired by means of a layered closure of 2–0 chromic catgut or long-term absorbable suture. When injury to the bladder neck or trigone has occurred, great care must be taken to avoid incorporating the distal ureters in the suture. A cystotomy with insertion of small catheters in a retrograde fashion through the ureteral orifices is useful to prevent this complication. Drainage of the area is advised. Suprapubic cystotomy is prudent when the injury is to the bladder neck or trigone.

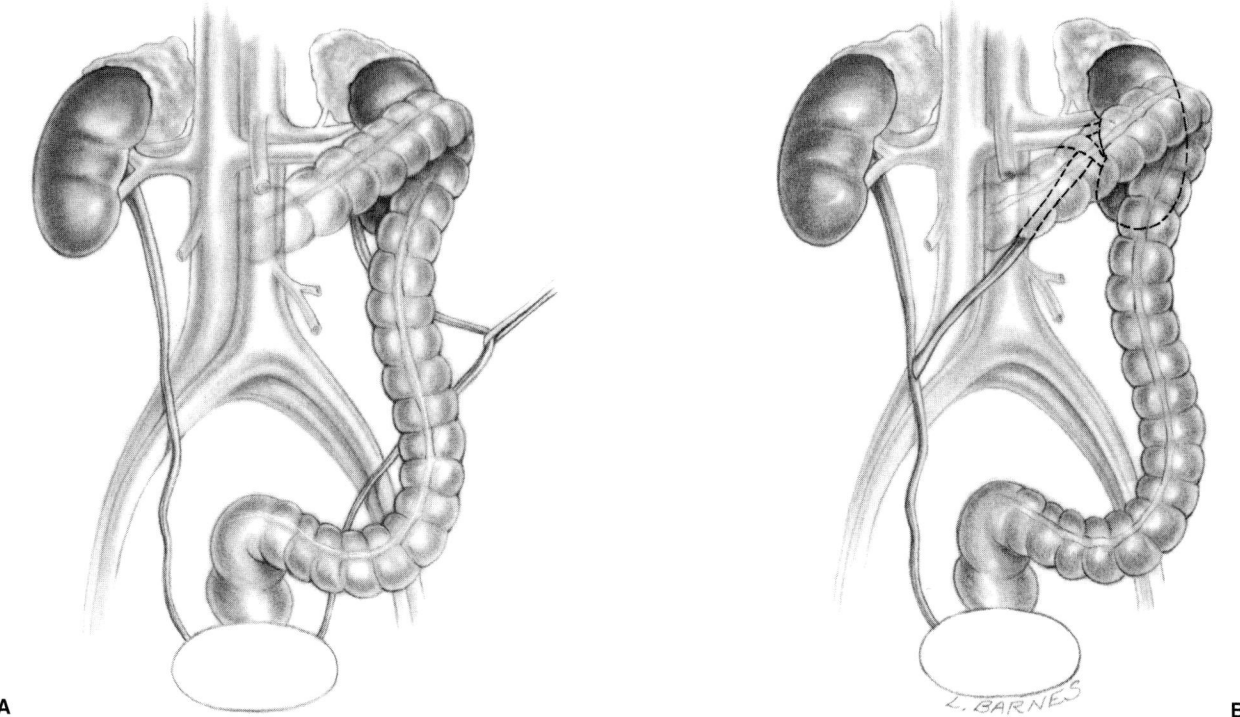

FIGURE 23-49. Transureteroureterostomy. (**A**) A tunnel is developed by retroperitoneal dissection after exposure of the upper ureter lateral to the colon. (**B**) The ureter is brought across the retroperitoneal space and is anastomosed. (Adapted from Libertino JA, Zinman L. Technique for ureteroneocystotomy in renal transplantation and reflux. *Surg Clin North Am* 1973;53:459, with permission.)

Urethral Injury

Injury to the urethra occurs most often as a result of too vigorous electrocoagulation in the prostatic area. In addition, tumor may invade the prostate, and, in an attempt to perform a curative resection, the prostatic urethra may be entered. External trauma can cause a delayed urethral stricture, which may require catheterization or subsequent reconstruction. If injury to this area is recognized at the time of proctectomy, direct repair or urethroplasty may be indicated. A urologist should be consulted if the surgeon is not experienced with reparative approaches.

Urethral stricture may require dilatation, internal urethrotomy, or reconstructive urethroplasty.[899] Here again, one should seek the advice of someone who has expertise in the management of such a complication.

Seminal Vesicle Injury

Injury to the seminal vesicles probably occurs much more frequently than is generally suspected. This may be responsible for some problems related to fertility, but should otherwise be of no consequence. However, a case of seminal vesicle–rectal fistula has been reported.[265] Moreover, a fistula to the perineum following an APR has been seen.[431] Treatment in this case included percuta-

neous drainage of the abscess, antibiotics, and oral administration of finasteride (Proscar).

Postoperative Complications

Perineal Hemorrhage

Bleeding from the perineal wound in the recovery room has a characteristic scenario. It usually begins with the surgeon's noting "moderate pelvic oozing" in the operating room. After some effort at clamping vessels in the sacral area, under the raised peritoneal flap, in the prostatic bed, from the lateral ligaments, levatores, and subcutaneous tissue, it is decided to close and drain the area. The bleeding is often noticed by the circulating nurse while the patient is still in the operating room. Unfortunately, however, the surgeon may direct that the patient be removed to the recovery area in the expectation that the bleeding will cease.

Returning the patient to the operating room is certainly a defeat for the surgeon and a risk to the patient. Happily, perineal hemorrhage can usually be controlled by opening the perineal wound and finding the bleeding vessel or by packing. Occasionally, however, laparotomy must be undertaken again.

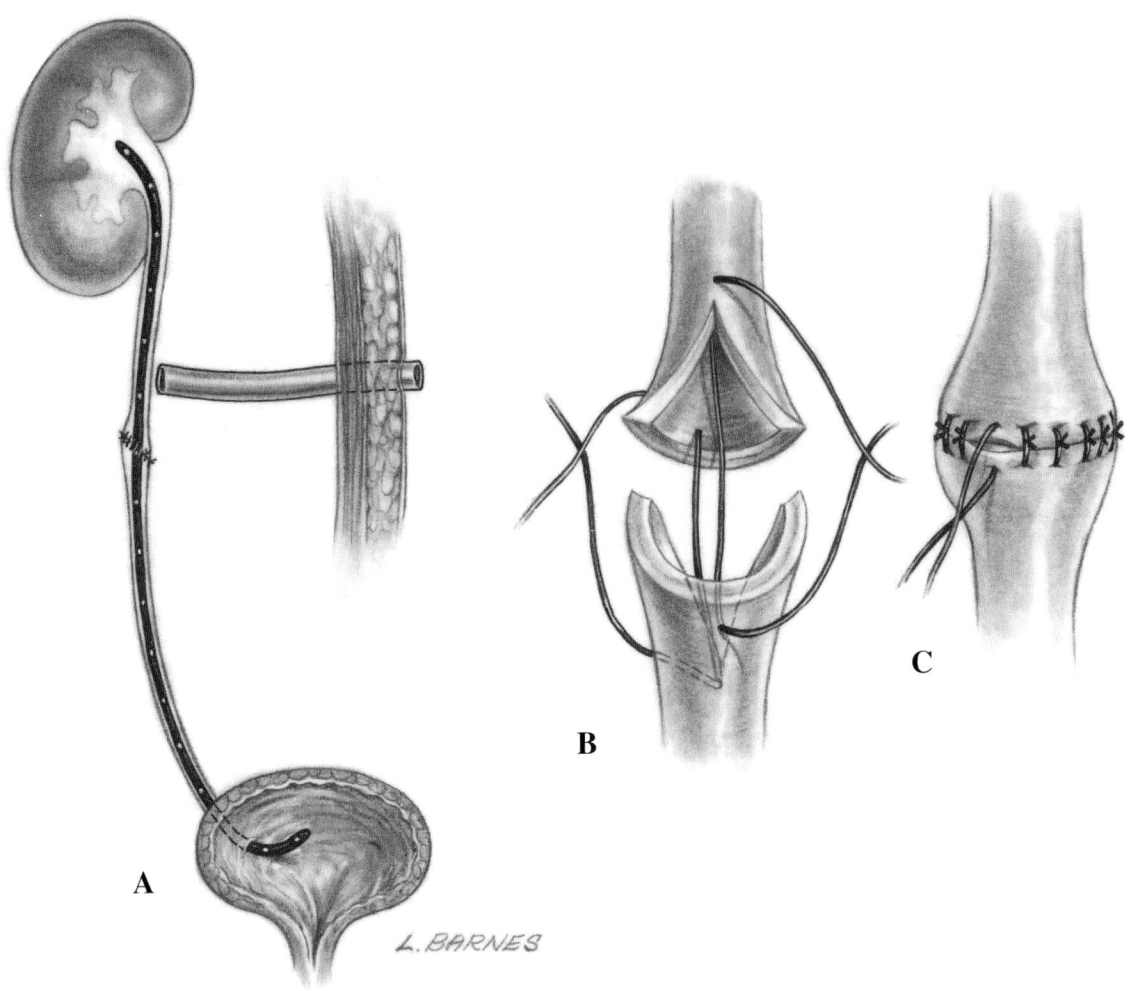

FIGURE 23-50. Ureteroureterostomy. (**A**) Midureteroureterosotomy is diverted by a Silastic double-J stent. (**B**) The ureters are spatulated on opposing sides of each end to achieve oblique anastomosis. (**C**) The edges are approximated with interrupted fine catgut sutures placed through the full thickness of the ureteral wall, thus inverting the mucosa. (Adapted from Libertino JA, Zinman L. Technique for ureteroneocystotomy in renal transplantation and reflux. *Surg Clin North Am* 1973;53:459, with permission.)

This complication is usually preventable. Perineal wound hemostasis should be adequate before the patient is permitted to leave the operating room. If the bleeding is so diffuse that a specific vessel cannot be identified, packing with or without a supplementary hemostatic agent may be necessary.

Necrotic Colostomy

I have mentioned that I do not advocate a high ligation of the inferior mesenteric artery because it does not increase the likelihood of cure. Furthermore, by preserving the first branch of the artery, blood supply to the descending colon and residual sigmoid colon is less likely to be impaired. In spite of this precaution, division of the inferior mesenteric artery or one of its major branches may result in necrosis or frank gangrene of the bowel.[405,751] This may occur when the colon receives much or all of its vascular supply from the inferior mesenteric artery. Goligher demonstrated that approximately 25% of patients who underwent high ligation of the inferior mesenteric artery during rectal excision developed gangrene or sloughing.[270] Some have suggested the use of Doppler ultrasound to determine the adequacy of the blood supply to the intestine at the time of surgery.[132–134,382,888] Others recommend endoscopic examination of the distal bowel through the stoma or the intravenous injection of 5 mL of fluorescein dye, followed by the use of a long-wave ultraviolet lamp.[772] Strong fluorescence of the mucosa assures viability. In my opinion, such relatively esoteric studies are unnecessary, because bowel ischemia can usually be assessed adequately by clinical inspection alone.

In spite of careful attention to the viability of the intestine, the colostomy at the time of abdominal wound closure may appear ischemic. This is usually noted when the surgeon has difficulty obtaining adequate length in creating the stoma, either because of the patient's obesity or because of tension on the bowel or blood supply itself. By making certain that there is sufficient bowel available to create the stoma without tension and by preparing a large enough opening in the abdominal wall, this difficulty can be avoided. All too often, however, the surgeon does not place sufficient importance on the creation of the stoma. One must remember, however, that to the patient it is the most important part of the operation.

If the bowel looks ischemic, it probably is ischemic. If the mucosa looks blue, it probably is blue. The optimal time to redo the stoma is at the time of the laparotomy, not 2 or 3 days later, when it has retracted into the peritoneal cavity or has become gangrenous. The treatment of stomal problems is addressed in Chapter 31.

Intestinal Obstruction

Small bowel obstruction is not uncommon following APR. Some element of ileus is normally present for a few days following surgery, but if flatus fails to pass by the sixth or seventh postoperative day, one must entertain the possibility that obstruction is present. Goligher and colleagues reported an incidence of obstruction of approximately 3% in 1,302 patients who underwent this operation.[277]

Obstruction is most commonly caused by adhesions between loops of bowel, a complication that can occur after laparotomy for any purpose, but there are two specific situations that are directly related to APR: herniation below the pelvic floor and herniation through the lateral colostomy gutter. The former usually occurs when the suture breaks or pulls out of the peritoneum, leaving a hole through which a loop of small intestine descends and becomes entrapped. Repair requires liberation of the bowel and closure of the defect. Rarely, the loop of bowel descends to the perineal skin or actually through the wound. Gangrene can also occur, but this is also unusual. Small bowel resection under such circumstances would obviously be required.

Harshaw and colleagues advocated leaving the peritoneum open and closing the skin primarily, thereby avoiding this complication.[317] However, it is preferable to close the pelvic floor if for no other reason than to keep the small bowel out of the pelvis should postoperative radiotherapy be deemed advisable (see earlier discussion and Postoperative Radiotherapy).

Herniation of the small bowel through the defect in the lateral gutter can produce a small bowel obstruction (Figure 23-51). Although some recommend a purse-string, interrupted, or continuous suture to close the space, and others prefer an extraperitoneal approach, I like to leave the defect widely patent on the theory that entrapment is less likely to take place if the opening is sufficiently large. In my experience, most patients who subsequently developed obstruction had undergone closure of the lateral space. At the time of reoperation, the suture was found to have either broken or pulled out.

If surgery is required, the bowel is reduced and the opening enlarged. If the gutter had been left open and herniation with obstruction did occur, it is probably wiser to attempt closure of the defect, but this is advice based on theory, not experience.

Urinary Retention and Infection or Bladder Dysfunction

Urinary tract infection and urinary retention are the most common complications following abdominoperineal or low anterior resection. Marks and Ritchie reported an incidence of 34%.[527] Janu and colleagues noted that 25% of their patients developed a urinary tract infection, whereas bladder dysfunction occurred in 22%.[386] In the experience of Cunsolo and colleagues, urinary retention occurred in 41% of men and 35% of women.[146] Wide iliopelvic lymphadenectomy increases the risk of voiding difficulties.[91,357] Urinary retention may the result of injury to the sympathetic or parasympathetic nerves to the bladder, postoperative distension, local trauma, prostatic hypertrophy, or prolapse of the bladder into the pelvis.

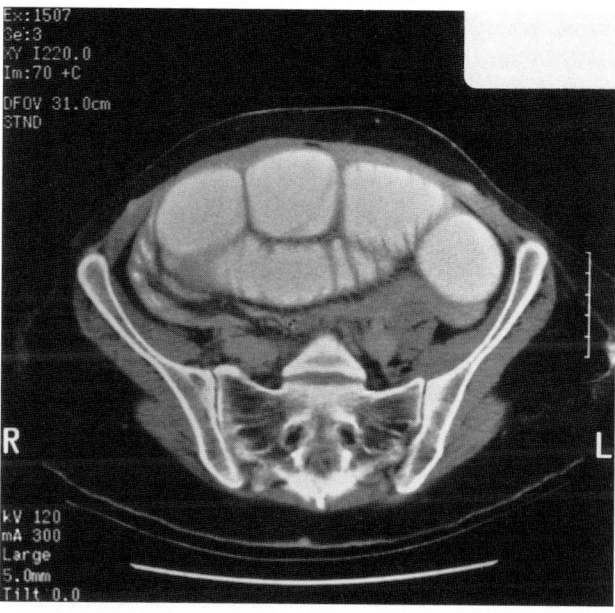

FIGURE 23-51. Computed tomography demonstrates small bowel obstruction. This was secondary to herniation through a defect in the pelvic floor. Note the decompressed small bowel.

The most important preventive maneuver that one may employ is to retain a Foley catheter in place for 5 to 7 days. The effects of direct trauma to the bladder necessitate a period of recovery. The catheter is removed at 6:00 AM and the voiding pattern carefully observed. If the patient is unable to void or urinates frequently in small amounts, a residual urine determination should be made. If it is more than 300 mL, the catheter should be reinserted and left for an additional 2 or 3 days. During this interval, it is reasonable to place the patient on bethanechol chloride (Urecholine), 25 to 50 mg, four times daily. This is suggested in an effort to improve detrusor tone. Urodynamic studies are advised if the patient is unable to void after removal of the catheter.

A cystometrogram usually will demonstrate a flaccid type of bladder, but the urethral pressure profile will probably be normal. What is important is to determine the external sphincter electromyogram (EMG). Very often after an APR, the internal pudendal nerve is compromised, and the patient loses the innervation of the external sphincter. Continence, therefore, is maintained by the internal sphincter or bladder neck mechanism only. The cystometrogram, urethral pressure profile, and external sphincter EMG should be correlated with the anatomic findings of cystourethroscopy. If the patient has an obstructed prostate and a normal sphincter EMG, then it is reasonable to carry out a transurethral resection. It is safer, however, to defer prostatectomy for 6 weeks in a patient who has recently undergone APR, in order to minimize the risk of a urinary-perineal fistula. If the external sphincter EMG shows a flaccid external sphincter, one would be loath to carry out a transurethral resection of the prostate or any form of prostatectomy for fear of making the patient incontinent. Under these circumstances, it is advisable to leave the catheter in place for a period of 6 weeks to 2 months or to instruct the patient in the use of intermittent catheterization. Hopefully, this respite will allow the bladder residual urine to be of small enough volume to avoid overdistension of the bladder and decompensation of the detrusor musculature. Intermittent catheterization is preferable to the patient's incontinence. Current urologic practice discourages clamping and unclamping the catheter in an attempt to restore detrusor tone. If the goal of keeping the bladder empty is achieved, the detrusor tone will ultimately return.

By evaluating preoperatively the urologic situation in a systematic way, Leadbetter and Leadbetter believed that they could selectively perform prostatectomy at the time of the APR and decrease the incidence of postoperative urinary retention.[462] From a limited experience with this approach, I believe that such a combined operation should be condemned. There is an associated high incidence of urinary tract infection, pelvic sepsis, and urinary-perineal fistula (Figure 23-52).

In women, the procedure should be essentially the same as that described earlier. If the woman has difficulty voiding after an additional period of catheter drainage and treatment with bethanechol, she should be taught the technique of intermittent self-catheterization until the bladder tone returns and normal voiding occurs. Self-catheterization is an option in men also.

Perineal Wound Sepsis

Perineal sepsis is not uncommon following APR. It may be caused by contamination at the time of proctectomy from injury to the rectal wall, fecal spillage, the presence of a perforated carcinoma, an infected hematoma, or the presence of perineal disease (e.g., fistula or abscess). A prolonged operative time may also predispose to the subsequent development of sepsis. Patients with perineal infection after APR have an increased incidence of local recurrence.[442]

Characteristically, the patient develops a low-grade fever on the third or fourth postoperative day, which progresses to a higher spiking fever elevation. In the absence of another obvious source for pyrexia, the perineal wound should be carefully explored with a gloved finger. Loculations should be broken and, if necessary, the wound reopened. Irrigating with one half strength Dakin's solution (using a rubber catheter) is important to remove clot and debris. A sitz bath, even with the wound wide open, is inadequate for treating or preventing perineal sepsis.

There is a means for avoiding this complication, and that is to leave the perineal wound widely open to heal by second intention. The disadvantage of a prolonged healing time (not infrequently for more than 4 months) makes this alternative inadvisable. Conversely, primary closure without drainage is contraindicated because of the high likelihood of sepsis.

A satisfactory compromise is to close the skin and to bring a drain through the wound or through a separate incision (Figure 23-38). A suction catheter drains more effectively and probably reduces the likelihood of pelvic sepsis.

Abdominal Wound Infection and Intraabdominal Sepsis

Although wound infection alone is rarely fatal, it adds considerably to morbidity and prolongs the patient's hospital stay. The incidence of wound infection following APR is the same as that for any colon resection. We reported an incidence of 8.6%, a rate that at the time compared favorably with that of others for colonic operations.[50,140,141,163,735,758,793,816,865] However, with the current protocol for preoperative preparation and wound management, I believe that a rate today in the range of 5% is more appropriate.

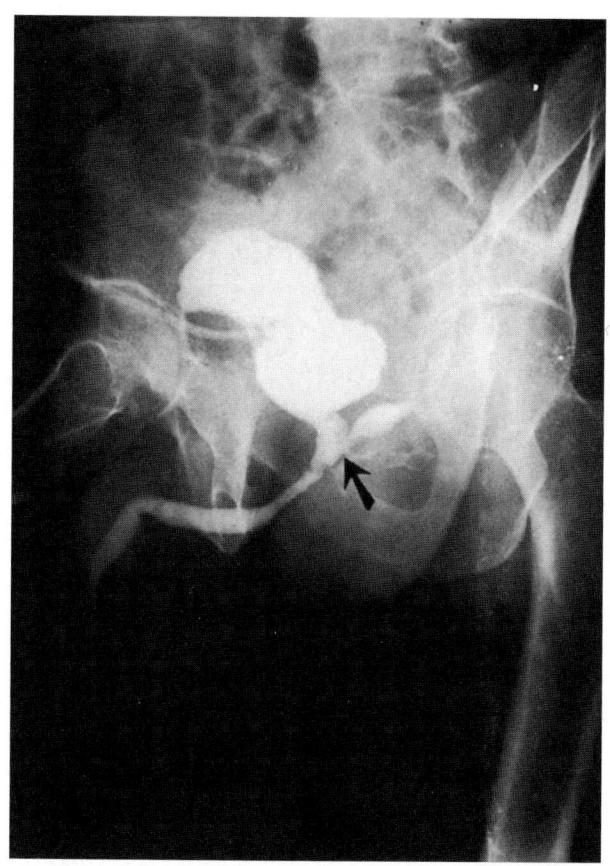

FIGURE 23-52. Urethroperineal fistula *(arrow)* is a serious consequence of an ill-advised concomitant proctectomy and prostatectomy.

The necessary ingredients of wound infection are contamination with pathogenic organisms and a susceptible host. Because of the nature of colonic and rectal surgery, some contamination is present in all patients, but certain factors are known to predispose to this complication (Table 23-1). Splenic trauma and the requirement for splenectomy concomitant with any colon operation increase the risk of infection in the early postoperative period. Combined spleen-colon trauma should be an indication rather than a contraindication for splenic salvage.[65]

Many methods have been devised to decrease the incidence of wound infection in contaminated incisions, including the use of subcutaneous drains.[258] Numerous bowel preparations and antibiotics have also been advocated (see Chapter 22).[130,131] In the past, the lowest incidence of wound infection occurred among patients who were administered the combination of oral erythromycin and neomycin, as popularized by Nichols and colleagues.[611] More recent evidence suggests that oral antibiotics are unnecessary, and the use of perioperative, systemic, broad-spectrum antibiotics is preferable for limiting the incidence of wound infections.[89,339,408,610,722,828,861]

TABLE 23-1 Predisposing Factors for the Development of Wound Infections after Colonic Surgery

Factor	Percentage of Infections	Statistical Significance
Preoperative irradiation	22.2	$p < .04$
Serum albumin < 2.9 g/dL	20.1	$p < .02$
Preoparative stoma	19.1	$p < .001$
Blood loss > 2 units	17.4	$p < .03$
Crohn's disease	14.3	$p < .002$
Bowel preparation		
Other than mechanical preparation plus nonabsorbable antiobiotic	14.1	$p < .001$
Antibiotic other than erythromycin base and neomycin	7.7	$p < .001$
Operative time > 2 hr	11.7	$p < 0.06$

(Adapted from DeGennaro V, Corman ML, Coller JA, et al. Wound infections after colectomy. *Dis Colon Rectum* 1978;21:567, with permission.)

The wound infection rate for elective colon surgery in the absence of radiation, pus, or gross contamination should be no greater than 5%. This incidence can be reduced still further by leaving the wound open and performing a delayed primary closure. In contrast to my previous thinking and to the opinion expressed in the first edition of this text, I no longer recommend the use of drains in the subcutaneous tissue. With adequate hemostasis, debridement of devitalized tissue, copious saline irrigation, careful tissue handling, and reduction of the operative time, wound infection should be an infrequent complication.

Neurologic and Vascular Complications

The perineolithotomy position has been associated with a number of intraoperative and postoperative complications, especially as related to the compartment syndrome. It is for this reason that special care needs to be taken in positioning the patient to minimize the risk of vascular injury. Another complication that has been noted has been related to the self-retaining retractor, that of femoral neuropathy. This complication has been reported to be a consequence of a number of operations, most commonly inguinal hernia repair. However, three instances have been associated with the use of the self-retaining Bookwalter retractor.[79] In a slender patient, the same phenomenon can occur if the Balfour retractor is used or if the O'Connor-O'Sullivan instrument is employed. Brasch and colleagues attribute risk factors to be as follows: a transverse incision, anticoagulation, uremia, diabetes, and those patients of thin, short stature or those who have poorly developed rectus muscles.[79] With careful attention to the location of the retractor blades, this complication should be preventable.

Acute arterial occlusion is a rare complication of low pelvic surgery. Underlying perpheral vascular disease may contribute to the development of this complication, but the use of the perineolithotomy position, the common hypercoagulable state of many patients with cancer, and the prolonged use of sequential compression devices all may be factors.[99]

Impotence, Infertility, and Dyspareunia

Impotence following proctectomy for carcinoma of the rectum is the rule rather than the exception, especially in the older age group, and particularly when a wide iliopelvic lymphadenectomy is applied.[32,357,418,454,863] This complication is such an important concern, especially for younger patients, that it becomes critical to discuss the possibility of this eventuality with the patient. A man may choose to "bank" his sperm prior to undergoing this operation, or he may elect alternative therapy (e.g., local excision). Cunsolo and colleagues reported that 59% of the preoperatively sexually active men who underwent APR became impotent.[146] The resection requires extensive pelvic dissection, which may result in injury to the parasympathetic nerves (nervi erigentes). Additionally, the patient's preoperative sexual function may have been less than adequate, and even minimal trauma may be sufficient to precipitate impotence. This may be an important explanation for why young people who undergo proctectomy for inflammatory bowel disease rarely have such difficulty when compared with older patients with cancer. In other words, preoperative libido may be the critical issue with respect to postoperative sexual function.

Women seem less likely to experience problems with orgasms, although most reports include a high number of widowed, elderly women who have no sexual partners. Retained menstrual blood, colpitis, chronic discharge from the vagina, and dyspareunia are not uncommon symptoms after proctectomy.[765] In one study, the incidence of dyspareunia was 50%.[146] Sjödahl and colleagues recommend an operation for this complaint that they attribute to dorsocaudal dislocation of the posterior vaginal wall (the horizontal vagina syndrome).[765] This involves coccygectomy, separation of the posterior fornix from the lower part of the sacrum, and interposition of muscle flaps from the right and left gluteus maximus muscle.

In men, infertility can result even if tumescence is not impaired, because of injury to the sympathetic nerves and the consequence of retrograde ejaculation. Injury to the vas or seminal vesicles has also been reported and may be associated with infertility.[469]

In the past, organic impotence was reported to be rather unsuccessfully treated with drugs, but in order that the patient may satisfy a sexual partner and gain an element of self-satisfaction, penile prosthetic implants have been used.[44,209,247,488,653,654] However, Lindsey and colleagues found that sildenafil (Viagra) improved erectile dysfunction in 79% of their patients.[476] They further observed that nocturnal penile tumescence, although diminished, is not always ablated by surgical dissection, suggesting that some of the cavernous nerves that govern inflow to the corpora cavernosa are intact, and that the nerve injury responsible for erectile dysfunction is partial.[4475] This helps to explain the response to sildenafil. Penile implantation should not be performed for at least 1 year after APR because of the possibility of return of this function.

Unhealed Perineal Wound and Persistent Perineal Sinus

The problem of delayed healing following proctectomy for cancer is quite unusual. This is in contradistinction to the frequency of the complication in individuals who undergo proctectomy for inflammatory bowel disease (see Chapter 29). However, with the use of preoperative and postoperative radiation therapy, the incidence of perineal wound breakdown and delayed healing is significantly increased. This is a particular concern if the radiation dose approaches 60 Gy. Techniques have been employed to ameliorate the condition and to effect healing, including reoperation and curettage, excision and grafting, muscle transposition,[14,31,443] and the use of fibrin adhesive fibrinogen concentrate and thrombin.[350] Radice and co-workers found that immediate myocutaneous flap closure in patients who underwent extended resection for locally advanced malignancy (including chemoradiation) achieved complete healing with reduced re–quirement for readmission and re-operation than those who underwent primary skin closure.[666] Numerous articles have been published concerning recommendations for managing sacral and perineal defects following APR, often with the use of muscle flaps.[489]

Perineal Hernia

Symptomatic perineal hernia is a rare, late complication of APR (Figure 23-53). Only a handful of cases have been reported.[42,83,103,293] The condition is much more common in women. Symptoms may include perineal pressure, fullness, pain, or feeling as if sitting on a lump. The hernia may produce skin breakdown or may be associated with an evisceration. Two patients who were reported from the Cleveland Clinic had symptoms of partial small bowel obstruction.[42]

So and colleagues identified 13 patients who underwent APR and developed a perineal hernia postopera-

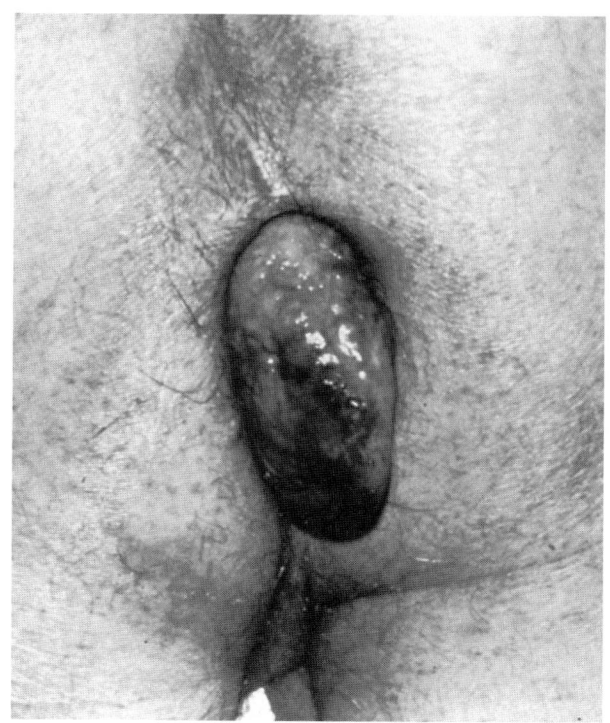

FIGURE 23-53. Perineal hernia developing 6 months following abdominoperineal resection. Treatment requires laparotomy and reconstruction of the pelvic floor.

tively, an incidence of 0.62%.[773] No definitive predisposing factors could be clearly identified. The authors emphasized the importance of the standard surgical principles for repairing a hernia in any other location—mobilization of the sac, reduction of its contents, excision of the sac, and repair of the defect—usually with mesh.

Treatment should be directed to an abdominal or a combined abdominal and perineal approach. Attempting repair from the perineum alone is unlikely to be successful. In principle, the bowel must be delivered out of the pelvis and the pelvic floor reconstituted, usually with mesh such as Marlex.[42,724] The pelvis should be drained and if necessary the redundant skin excised. Brotschi and colleagues reported a successful result after two operations using the gracilis muscle following a failed Marlex mesh repair.[83]

Phantom Sensations

Phantom sensations are quite common after amputation of extremities, so it is not surprising that patients may experience feelings of an urge to defecate or to pass flatus after excision of the rectum. In a review by Lubbers of 40 patients who underwent proctectomy, 65% reported the presence of these sensations.[498] Theoretically, such feelings are a normal response to removal of the rectum, because innervation is still represented at the level of the cerebral cortex. Reassurance and the passage of time usually alleviate patient anxiety.

Perineal Pain

Intractable pain in the perineum in an individual who has undergone proctectomy for carcinoma of the rectum is the result of recurrent tumor until proved otherwise. However, patients may occasionally complain bitterly of severe, deep-seated pain that is truly analogous to that of levator spasm (proctalgia fugax; see Chapter 16). This is a most difficult problem to treat. Inevitably, one resorts to sitz baths and analgesic medications with indifferent success. Perineal strengthening exercises and the use of muscle relaxants are more likely to be ameliorative. In a woman, one may use the vaginal stimulating attachment of the electrogalvanic stimulator (see Figure 16-19), but this is obviously not a possible recourse for a man. Injection with steroids is uniformly unsuccessful and worrisome if one is dealing with a postoperative patient with cancer. Likewise, the injection of sclerosing agents is fraught with hazard. In spite of every available study's being negative, persistent pain, unresponsive to any of the foregoing measures, will ultimately prove to be recurrent carcinoma in most instances.

Entrapped Ovary Syndrome

Matthews and colleagues reported retroperitoneal cysts with entrapped ovaries in the retroperitoneal pelvis of six patients who had undergone proctectomies.[542] Patients may present with abdominal pain, a mass, or distension. If the ovary is to be preserved, excision of the cyst and oophoropexy is advised.[542] Care should be taken at the time of the initial operation to be certain that the ovary remains as an intraperitoneal structure when the pelvic floor is closed, but because oophorectomy is recommended in all postmenopausal women, this should be a rare complication.

Stomal Problems

Colostomy retraction, stenosis, prolapse, and hernia, as well as peristomal dermatitis and appliance management problems, are discussed in Chapters 31 and 32.

Results

Morbidity and Operative Mortality

The operative mortality rate following APR has essentially remained unchanged since the mid-1960s. My associates and I reported in-hospital mortality to be 1% to 2%.[697] Others have noted a mortality rate of between 2% and 6.5% (Table 23-2).

▶ **TABLE 23-2** Operative Mortality following Abdominoperineal Resection

Author, Year	Percentage (%)
Lockhart-Mummery et al., 1976[486]	2.1
Localio et al., 1978[483]	2.3
Deddish and Stearns, 1961[161]	2.0
Bordos et al., 1974[73]	2.9
Williams et al., 1966[880]	4.3
Palumbo and Sharpe, 1968[636]	4.4
Glenn and McSherry, 1966[263]	4.7
Walz et al., 1977[853]	3.2
MacLennan et al., 1976[507]	3.2
Stearns, 1974[781]	3.5
Strauss et al., 1978[800]	3.5
Slanetz et al., 1972[766]	5.4
Enker et al., 1979[193]	6.4
Zollinger and Sheppard, 1971[901]	6.5

(From Rosen L, Veidenheimer MC, Coller JA, et al. Mortality, morbidity, and patterns of recurrence after abdominoperineal resection for cancer of the rectum. *Dis Colon Rectum* 1982;25:202, with permission.)

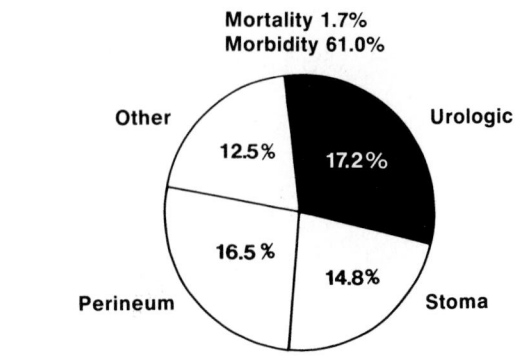

FIGURE 23-54. Morbidity and mortality following abdominoperineal resection in 230 patients. (From Rosen L, Veidenheimer MC, Coller JA, et al. Mortality, morbidity, and patterns of recurrence after abdominoperineal resection for cancer of the rectum. *Dis Colon Rectum* 1982;25:202, with permission.)

Most institutions report a high complication rate following this operation.[213,766] In our experience, 61% were found to have complications (Figure 23-54).[697] Urologic problems were most frequently observed (Table 23-3). Lapides noted a 15% incidence of poor micturition following this procedure.[457] Gerstenberg and associates in fact went so far as to recommend the routine application of urinary flow measurements and cystometry for all postoperative patients who undergo APR in order to detect potential problems before they become manifest (see discussion on urinary complications).[250]

Long-Term Results

The uncorrected 5-year survival for APR in our experience between the years 1963 and 1976 is shown in Table 23-4 according to Dukes' classification (see Figure 22-31). The mean age of patients was 62 years. The uncorrected 5-year survival rate approaches 90% for patients with Dukes' A lesions. This fell to 65% for Dukes' B and 23% for Dukes' C tumors. This is essentially the same as the uncorrected survival rate for colon resections during the same period. The uncorrected survival rate for all patients who underwent APR was 54%. The 10-year survival rate is illustrated in Figure 23-55. It can be appreciated that there is no significant falloff in survival after 5 years. This implies that it is a rare patient indeed who dies of recurrent cancer of the rectum following this length of time. A comparative survival rate from other investigators is shown in Table 23-5.

We analyzed retrospectively the patterns of recurrence in 180 of our patients who underwent an APR in anticipation of a cure.[697] Seventy-eight (43%) developed recurrent cancer (Figure 23-56). In 18 of these patients (23%) the first recurrence was local, whereas in 60 (77%) the initial manifestation of the recurrence was in a distant location. No one who initially had a Dukes' A lesion developed a local recurrence (Table 23-6). Penetration through the bowel wall with presumed residual tumor in the pelvis is the most important factor that contributes to recurrent pelvic and perineal disease.

Local recurrence appears much earlier in patients with Dukes' C lesions than in those who initially harbored a Dukes' B tumor. However, once recurrence develops, there is no statistically significant difference in median survival time between the two groups of individuals. Furthermore, there is no statistically significant difference in survival time irrespective of whether the initial recurrence was local or distant.

In the experience of Hojo and colleagues, statistically significant differences in survival rates and the incidence of local recurrence were observed when wide iliopelvic lymphadenectomy was compared with conventional lymphadenectomy.[357] This was accomplished, however, with the problems of a much higher incidence of bladder and potency difficulties. The Mayo Clinic group reported a 5-year survival rate of 52% in those individuals who underwent extended resection for locally advanced primary tumors.[625] Hafner and colleagues reviewed their 68 patients who underwent pelvic exenteration for rectal carcinoma and noted recurrences in 44%.[305] The overall survival was 43% when the procedure was performed for primary disease and 20% for recurrence.

Some reports emphasize the value of neoadjuvant chemoradiation therapy for reducing tumor size and limiting the incidence of local recurrence (see Radiotherapy) and that pelvic wall involvement carries with it a grim prognosis.[164,290,613,892] The incidence of recurrence increases

▶ **TABLE 23-3** Complications following Abdominoperineal Resection

Complication	Number of Patients	Percentage (%)*
Urologic		
Benign prostatic hypertrophy requiring TURP	13	8.1
Urinary tract infection	13	5.6
Neurogenic bladder	8	3.5
Orchitis	2	1.2
Urethral stricture	1	0.4
Fistula		
Vesicovaginal	1	—
Vesicoperineal	1	0.4
Ureteroperineal	1	0.4
Perineal		
Abscess	26	11.3
Hemorrhage	10	4.3
Hernia	2	0.9
Stomal Operation		
Stenosis, retraction, or prolapse	25	10.9
Hernia	7	3.0
Abscess	2	0.9
Miscellaneous		
Abdominal wound infection	6	2.6
Wound evisceration	7	3.0
Small bowel obstruction	10	4.3
Myocardial infarction	1	2.6
Atrial fibrillation	1	2.6
Hepatitis	1	2.6
Pulmonary embolism	1	2.6
Iliac vein injury	1	2.6
Pelvic abscess	1	2.6

TURP, transurethral resection.
Percentages are calculated according to the number of men (160) and the number of women (70) in the series, when applicable.
(From Rosen L, Veidenheimer MC, Coller JA, et al. Mortality, morbidity, and patterns of recurrence after abdominoperineal resection for cancer of the rectum. *Dis Colon Rectum* 1982;25:202, with permission.)

▶ **TABLE 23-4** Survival following Abdominoperineal Resection

Dukes' Classification	Number of Patients	Uncorrected 5-Year Survival (%)
A	45	86
B	75	65
C	60	33
D	20	0
Total	200	54

(From Rosen L, Veindenheimer MC, Coller JA, et al. Mortality, morbidity, and patterns of recurrence after abdominoperineal resection for cancer of the rectum. *Dis Colon Rectum* 1982;25:202, with permission.)

in the last few years. Both in the lay press and in medical journals, a heightened awareness of the differences with respect to the indications for surgery and the variability in the recommendations of operations, the potential risks, the obvious concern for mortality, and the attention to outcomes are all subjects of intense scrutiny. Wexner and Rotholtz emphasized that "surgeons should be cognizant of their own practice patterns, volume, capabilities . . . and results."[866] Furthermore, and equally important, they encourage all of us to submit to frequent auditing and willingly to share the information with our patients.

Read and co-workers reviewed the records of 384 consecutive patients with rectal cancer treated by colorectal

with the length of the follow-up period. Completeness, longer follow-up, and an intensive search for recurrence, including a high autopsy rate, are some of the factors that will inevitably yield higher recurrence rates.[96]

Surgeon Variables

Although not in a limited way applicable to APR or even to colon cancer surgery specifically, the issue of surgeon variability has been a subject of great interest

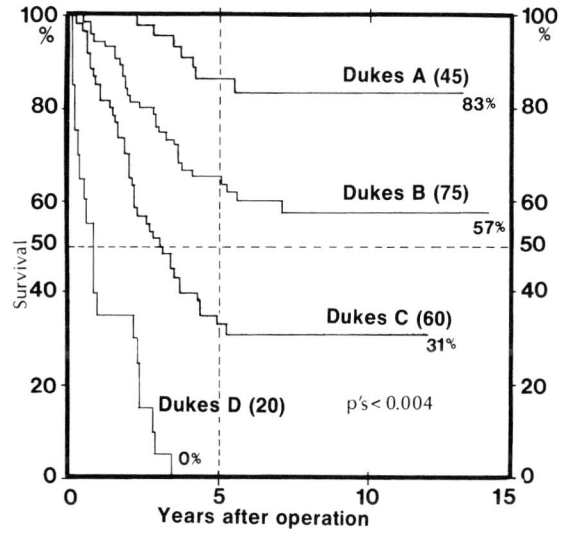

FIGURE 23-55. Survival after abdominoperineal resection. (From Rosen L, Veidenheimer MC, Coller JA, et al. Mortality, morbidity, and patterns of recurrence after abdominoperineal resection for cancer of the rectum. *Dis Colon Rectum* 1982; 25:202, with permission.)

▶ **TABLE 23-5** Abdominoperineal Resection: 5-Year Survival Rate

Author, Year	Dukes' Lesion:		
	A	B	C
Dukes, 1940[181]	93	65	23
Gilbertsen, 1960[254]	80	50	23
Slanetz et al., 1972[766]	81	52	33
MacLennan et al., 1976[507]	91	59	25
Strauss et al., 1978[800]	82	40	15
Walz et al., 1977[853]	78	45	22

(From Rosen L, Veindenheimer MC, Coller JA, et al. Mortality, morbidity, and patterns of recurrence after abdominoperineal resection for cancer of the rectum. *Dis Colon Rectum* 1982;25:202, with permission.)

surgeons (n = 251) and noncolorectal surgeons (n = 133) and concluded with the following statistically significant differences in results:[676]

Variable	Colorectal Surgeons	Noncolorectal Surgeons
Disease-free survival	77%	68%
Local control rates	93%	84%
Sphincter preservation	52%	30%

Smedh and colleagues in Sweden noted that establishment of a centralized colorectal unit was instrumental in reducing postoperative mortality from 8% to 1% and total complication rate from 57% to 24%.[768] From Germany, Marusch and co-workers reported the impact of hospital caseload on the short-term postoperative out- come of patients with rectal carcinoma.[535] In the 75 hospitals that formed the basis for this study, the authors concluded that a large caseload in rectal cancer surgery results in a significant reduction in the requirement for a permanent stoma and a significant decrease in postoperative morbidity. Others noted similar findings.[734] Birbeck and associates (University of Leeds, England) analyzed the variability in rates of circumferential resection margin involvement between different surgeons as a predictor of outcome after rectal cancer surgery.[58] They opined that circumferential resection margin may be employed as an indicator of the quality of the surgery. Hool and colleagues distributed a questionnaire to all colorectal surgeons in North America and observed that there is a considerable variation in the management of low rectal cancer, with divided opinion about which operation is optimal for each histologic and pathologic stage.[364]

Fleshman expressed his viewpoint on this subject in a 2002 editorial in the journal *Annals of Surgery*, as follows:[214]

> What more can we do? Academic surgeons can commit to training residents and community surgeons to perform the appropriate *en bloc* cancer resection based on anatomic planes, primary vascular ligation, and clear radial margins. We can be relentless in our requests for adequate staging of colon and rectal cancer by our pathologists. It is time to face issues such as centers of excellence or specialty practice for the treatment of cancer regardless of the site. Our goal of *excellence* must be turned to action rather than empty words in order to fulfill our promise to provide outstanding care for our patients.

Follow-up Regimen

The appropriateness and timing of the follow-up regimen after resection for rectal cancer are discussed in Chapter 22. As previously stated, the potential benefit for

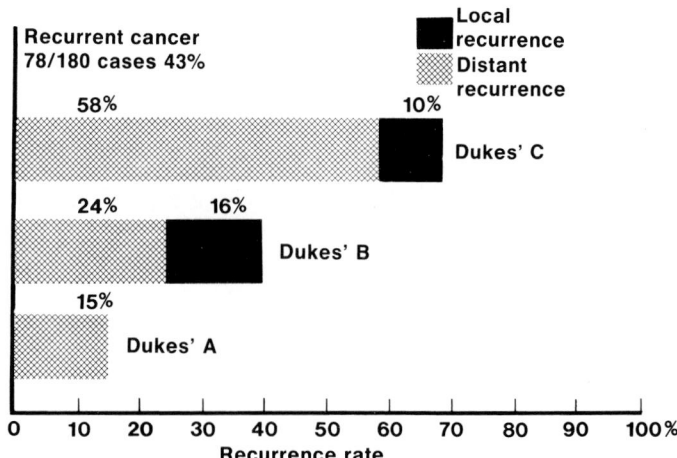

FIGURE 23-56. Rate of recurrence according to Dukes' classification. (From Rosen L, Veidenheimer MC, Coller JA, et al. Mortality, morbidity, and patterns of recurrence after abdominoperineal resection for cancer of the rectum. *Dis Colon Rectum* 1982;25:202, with permission.)

▶ **TABLE 23-6** Survival According to the Initial Site of Recurrence

Site	Dukes' Stage	Number of Patients	Median Time from Operation to Recurrrence (mo)	Median Time from Recurrence to Death (mo)	Overall Median Survival
Local (23%)	A	0	—	—	—
	B	12	21.5	17	38.5
	C	6	6	10.5	16.5
Distant (77%)	A	7	20	18	44
	B	18	12	11.5	22.5
	C	35	12	9	24

(From Rosen L, Veindenheimer MC, Coller JA, et al. Mortality, morbidity, and patterns of recurrence after abdominoperineal resection for cancer of the rectum. *Dis Colon Rectum* 1982;25:202, with permission.)

individuals from intensive evaluations following curative surgery has not been proved. In a study by Kjeldsen and colleagues involving almost 600 patients treated by radical surgery for colorectal cancer, the survival results suggest that individuals subjected to intense follow-up have recurrence diagnosed earlier and have more operations for recurrence, but survival rates are not significantly improved.[422] However, Barillari and colleagues opined that a follow-up program based on carcinoembryonic antigen (CEA) tissue plasminogen activator and CA 19–9 assays is associated with an earlier diagnosis, with a good resectability rate for both metastatic disease and local recurrence.[37]

Numerous factors suggest an increased risk for the development of recurrence, such as stage of the tumor, degree of differentiation, the presence of lymphatic invasion, and increased vascularity—all of which have been discussed previously.[549,711] The relevance, at least for rectal cancer, is that individuals may be selected for preoperative or postoperative radiotherapy based on a number of these characteristics or variables (see later).

Moran and colleagues studied DNA ploidy in 188 patients operated on for rectal cancer in order to define different risk groups for the development of recurrence.[586] Three variables had prognostic implications: more than three lymph nodes positive, macroscopic local tumor invasion, and DNA ploidy.

Treatment of Local Recurrence

The treatment of metastatic disease following resection of colorectal carcinoma is presented in Chapter 22. The discussion that follows is limited to the specific problem of recurrence following APR.

Symptoms and Diagnosis

One of the concerns that has been expressed with laparoscopically assisted colon resection for cancer is the possible increased incidence of trocar site recurrence

(see Chapter 27). However, one must remember that wound recurrence *does* develop following conventional surgical treatment of colorectal cancer, albeit uncommonly. Reilly and colleagues identified 11 patients (0.6%) with documented incisional recurrences (nine abdominal, one perineal, and one stomal) in their retrospective study of patients who underwent resection for colorectal carcinoma.[678] As with perineal recurrence in general, its presence usually implies more extensive disease.

With perineal recurrence, patients may complain of a painful mass (Figure 23-57). This may be the result of implantation in the skin, but more commonly it is a consequence of downward extend of pelvic tumor. Biopsy usually confirms the diagnosis. With pelvic recurrence, an individual may be asymptomatic, but usually the patient will report perineal, pelvic, or low abdominal pain. There may be the feeling as if sitting on a lump. The pain may radiate to the back, to the buttock, or have a sciatic distribution. If the tumor involves the bladder, prostate, or urethra, urinary symptoms (including hematuria) may develop. Urethral obstruction can supervene, but the most troubling, indeed disabling, complaint is the pain.

The diagnosis can be made without special studies and without positive biopsy evidence of recurrence, so characteristic is the syndrome. Knowledge of a previously "unfavorable" pathology report is helpful. A mass may be felt in the perineum or in the vagina. CT and MRI have been used successfully to delineate both the presence of a tumor mass and the extent of pelvic spread, as well as evidence of ureteral obstruction (Figure 23-58 and 23-59).[376] These studies have also been suggested as potentially valuable adjuncts for follow-up evaluation in order to anticipate recurrence before symptoms appear. CT-guided percutaneous biopsy has been demonstrated to be a particularly useful tool for establishing the histologic diagnosis of recurrent carcinoma in the pelvis.[93,466,612,897] Still, one should not need histologic confirmation in order to implement therapy. Elevation of the CEA level is certainly suggestive of recurrent disease, but all too often this laboratory study is

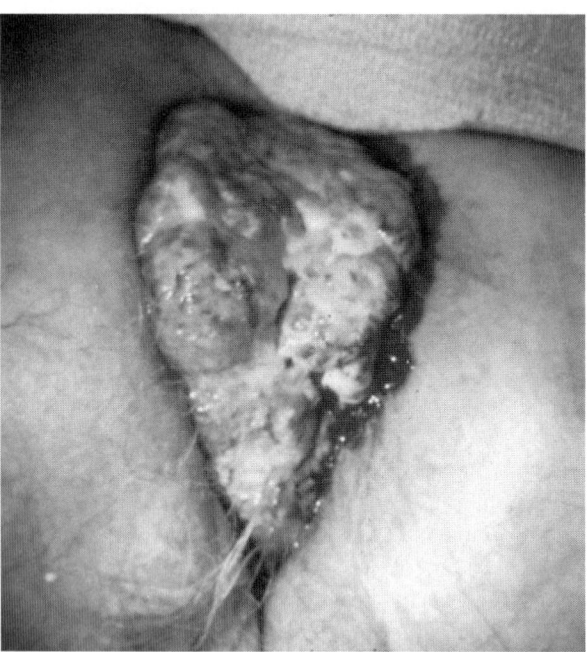

FIGURE 23-57. Fungating recurrent carcinoma of the perineum following abdominoperineal resection.

within the normal range if the recurrence is confined to the pelvis. This is in contradistinction to those patients who have involvement of the liver or another organ (see Chapter 22). An intravenous pyelogram may be performed, especially if there is concern for impingement on the ureters on the basis of the CT study (Figure 23-60). An elevated serum creatinine is obviously an ominous finding. Treatment, at least initially, requires decompression by means of an internal stent.

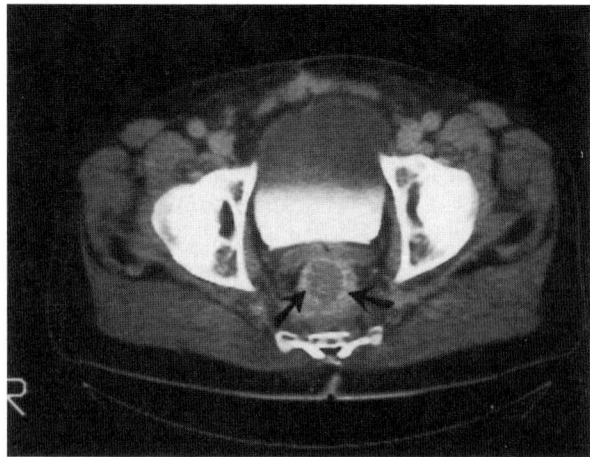

FIGURE 23-58. Computed tomography scan of pelvis. Recurrent pelvic carcinoma following abdominoperineal resection. Note the tumor mass with central necrosis *(arrows)*. The seminal vesicles can be clearly seen.

Surgical Treatment

Fazio has described a number of technical tips for reoperative abdominal and pelvic surgery for cancer.[207] Extensive preoperative investigation is mandatory, including CT. T_1- and T_2-weighted imaging is important to exclude bony erosion or pelvic side wall involvement. The presence of such tumor extension implies nonresectability and contraindication to adventuresome surgery.[207] It is wise to begin this type of surgery first thing in the morning and to not schedule any other difficult operations during that day. One should anticipate the need for specialty help, such as urology, orthopedics, and neurosurgery. A list of recommendations according to Fazio (which I totally support) follows:[207]

- Conduct a colon study for local and remote metastases.
- Provide ureteral stents.
- Schedule the case early in the day.
- Anticipate the need for other specialists.
- Ensure the availability of experienced assistance.
- Plan the incision carefully.
- Allow for a steep Trendelenburg position.
- Position the patient's arms at the sides.
- Utilize lighted instruments and/or head lights.
- Anticipate excessive blood loss.

The foregoing list is only a means for preoperatively reminding the surgeon of the magnitude of reoperative cancer surgery. It is by no means exhaustive.

The value of monoclonal antibody scans is discussed Chapter 22. As stated, ureteral stents are strongly encouraged in any reoperative surgical procedure within the pelvis.

Results Unfortunately, there is no truly satisfactory treatment for perineal or pelvic recurrence. There is, however, the rare instance when *perineal* (the equivalent of suture line) *recurrence* develops secondary to implantation or to an inadequate skin excision. It still may be possible to cure the condition by reexcising the perineal wound. With recurrent *pelvic malignancy*, rarely can resection be successfully effected. Stearns, in a 1980 report of the experience from the Memorial Sloan-Kettering Cancer Center stated, "Pelvic recurrence, in our experience, has not been curable by surgical excision or by any other modality of treatment."[782] Others concur that a surgical procedure can offer more effective palliation than other options and may prolong life in selected instances, but even the most radical resection rarely cures this disease.[314,514,571,618,715]

In the experience of Cunningham and colleagues, the only patients who had a survival benefit from reoperative pelvic surgery for rectal cancer were those whose disease could be completely resected (an uncommon situation).[145] Gagliardi and colleagues showed that recur-

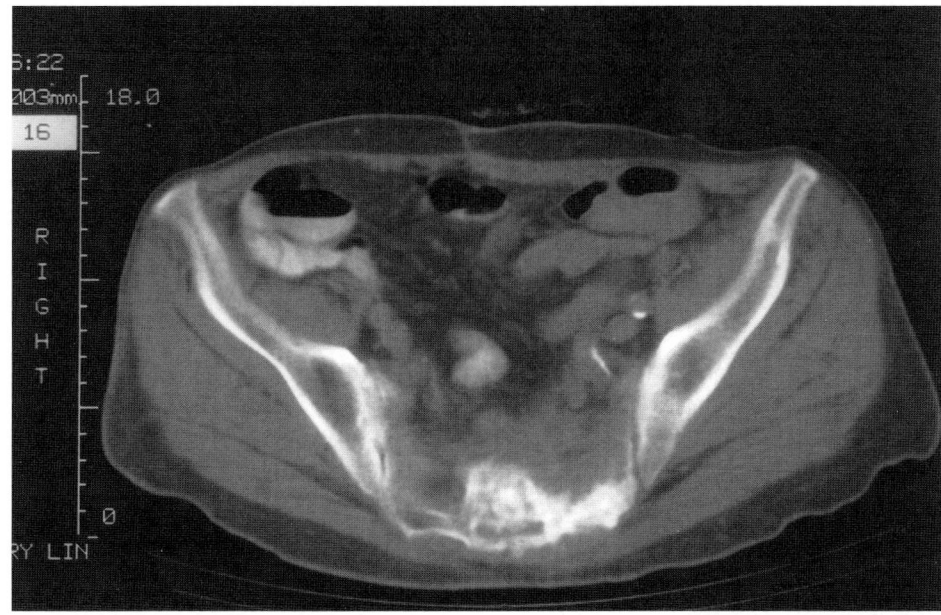

FIGURE 23-59. Computed tomography demonstrates erosion of the sacral bone from recurrent rectal cancer.

rent tumor diameter was the only prognostic variable, in that a diameter of less than 5 cm in the resected specimen achieved local control in 47% of their patients.[235] Others have shown that independent variables for resectability include younger age at diagnosis, earlier stage of the primary tumor, and initial treatment by a sphincter-saving approach.[242] In a report from the Mayo Clinic published in 1996, 224 patients with a preoperative diagnosis of recurrent rectal cancer underwent additional surgery.[805] Of these, 65 underwent surgery with the hope of cure. Three-year, 5-year, and median survival were 57, 34, and 44.7 months, respectively. Survival tended to be greater in women and those without pain. Cumulative probability of local treatment failure was 24%, 41%, and 47% at 1, 3, and 5 years, respectively. The authors concluded that complete excision of locally recurrent rectal cancer can provide meaningful survival benefits.[805] Wanebo and colleagues, reporting from Brown University in Rhode Island, observed that pelvic recurrence can be safely resected with expectation of long-term survival in approximately one third.[856] Salvage surgery for properly selected patients based on known risk factors is recommended and may lead to long-term palliation and the improving the length of disease-free survival.[495] There is little disagreement, however, that unilateral or bilateral hydronephrosis appears to be a contraindication for potentially curative surgical resection for recurrent rectal carcinoma.[688]

Radiotherapy

Surgical extirpation for pelvic recurrence has been used for palliation.[854,857] However, radiation therapy has been and continues to be the most effective treatment for palliating symptoms of locally recurrent disease (see later, Radiotherapy). Wang and Schulz, for example, reported a palliative benefit lasting from several months up to 10 years.[858] This may imply an increased survival rate, but our patients survived a median of only 15 months following radiotherapy for pelvic recurrence, the same as the median survival rate of those reported by Moossa and colleagues, with no radiotherapy.[585,670] There is, however, little controversy concerning improvement of symptoms. Radiation therapy is effective in the treatment of pain for approximately three fourths of patients. It may also decrease the size of a mass, and for an ulcerating lesion, the amount of perineal or vaginal drainage.

Radiotherapy can be administered to a total of 60 Gy (depending on whether the patient received preoperative treatment; see later). The Memorial Sloan-Kettering group recommend short treatments of 20 Gy when symptoms develop rather than a large-dose course.[782,787] In the experience of Villalon and Green with 85 patients who developed pelvic recurrence following APR, 92% with pain and 80% with a mass responded to 45 to 50 Gy.[847] Symptomatic relief was achieved in 80% of 143 patients reported by Pacini and colleagues.[629] They noted no significant difference in response to the three dose levels: 40, 50, and 60 Gy. Others reported comparable results.[175] Patients who are severely debilitated may be treated by so-called hypofractionation—the delivery of a single large dose (10 Gy) once a month for 3 months.[760]

One of the burdens that the patient and the surgeon may be forced to deal with is the radionecrosis that develops after high-dose radiation therapy for extensive primary or recurrent rectal cancer. Managing this type

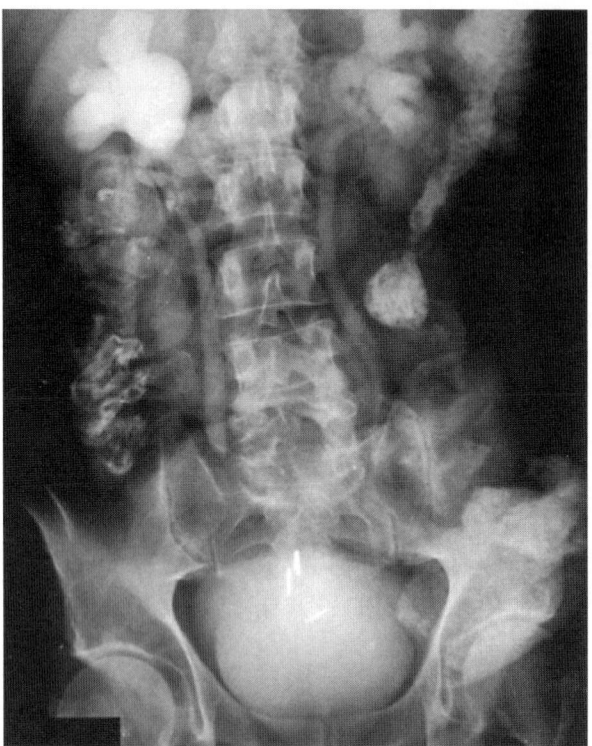

FIGURE 23-60. Intravenous pyelogram demonstrates hydroureters with marked dilatation of the renal pelvises and calyces, a consequence of recurrent rectal cancer.

of problem often presents extraordinary challenges for the surgeon. Associated complications, such as enterocutaneous fistula, urinary fistula, pelvic abscess, osteomyelitis, and persistent sinuses, further complicate the picture. Treating the foul-smelling discharge, alleviating the pain, and addressing the need for frequent dressing changes are of paramount concern.

Intraoperative Radiotherapy Intraoperative radiotherapy (IORT) is a technique by which a fundamentally resectable lesion is removed and the remaining cancer cells "sterilized" at the time of the operation, with the patient's abdomen open.[759] The procedure may be of value for those who are found to have fixed, unresectable rectal or rectosigmoid primary or recurrent tumors.[302,759,820] According to Sischy, in 1986 there were approximately 40 institutions in the United States employing this modality.[759] He suggested that the following criteria be used to identify patients who may be suitable for IORT:

- Tumor must be localized.
- Tumor must be accessible to treatment applicator and in an area from which normal tissue may be displaced.
- The condition must be potentially curable, yet the tumor is unable to be controlled by surgery alone.

Usually, the patient receives external beam radiation of 45 to 50 Gy. Four to 6 weeks following completion of this treatment, and after CT evaluation is performed to ascertain that there is no evidence of disseminated disease, the patient undergoes re-exploration and resection. If there is microscopic residual tumor as determined by frozen-section examination or if it is believed that cure is unlikely, an appropriate-sized Lucite "radiation applicator" is selected.[820] Few institutions have dedicated IORT operating suites, so it may be necessary to transport the patient to the radiation therapy unit for "booster therapy." A dose of 15 to 20 Gy is then delivered as a single treatment.

It is difficult to offer firm conclusions about the relative merits of this approach. According to Sischy, 3- to 5-year results from a number of centers for marginally resectable disease are approximately 50% and, for recurrent disease, approximately 40%.[759] Farouk and colleagues reviewed the evidence to support aggressive preoperative chemoradiation followed by surgical resection and IORT.[204] An overall 5-year survival of 42% was reported, even in those with locally unresectable primary rectal cancer. Some reports indicate that better local control and palliation of individuals with locally recurrent disease is achieved with IORT in combination with multi-modality treatment.[445,521] Hashiguchi and coworkers concluded that those with nonresectable distant metastasis, those with pain, elevated preoperative CA19–9, fixed tumors, or gross residual tumor after surgical resection are not suitable candidates for IORT.[320] The Memorial Sloan-Kettering Cancer Center group performed IORT with curative intent for recurrent rectal cancer in 111 patients.[757] Median disease-free survival was 31.2 months for complete resection compared with 7.9 months when the patient had microscopic or grossly positive margins. The presence of vascular invasion was also an independent variable for a poorer outcome. Numerous articles have been published that support the concept of combined sacropelvic resection with intraoperative radiation therapy to effect palliation and possible cure in selected patients with locally advanced or recurrent disease.[316,321,497,515,774]

Sadahiro and co-workers utilized IORT in 78 individuals for "curatively resected" rectal cancer.[712] The electron beam was administered as uniformly as possible to the entire dissected surface of the pelvis. Using historical controls, these investigators found that survival, disease-free survival, and local recurrence-free survival in the IORT group were all significantly more favorable than in the non-IORT group.

Radiofrequency Ablation A limited approach, that of CT-guided, percutaneous radiofrequency ablation has been described for nonresectable recurrence.[619]

Chemotherapy

Other treatment modalities for recurrence include radium implantation and chemotherapy (see also Chapter 22). Systemic chemotherapy as conventionally administered has not proved beneficial. However, there has been some palliation achieved by pelvic intraarterial perfusion of 5-fluorouracil (5-FU).[306,647] In one study, the percutaneous placement of catheters in the internal iliac arteries, the administration of 5-FU and mitomycin-C, and the application of whole-body hyperthermia were reported to offer better pain relief than that of perfusion/chemotherapy alone.[198] The use of radiosensitizers (5-FU and mitomycin-C) also have been suggested to improve the response to radiotherapy (see later).

Pain Management

For pain that cannot be effectively treated by radiotherapy and that is no longer responsive to narcotic analgesics, neurosurgical consultation is advised. Placement of epidural, intrathecal, and intraventricular catheters for narcotic drug delivery as well as the use of intrathecal alcohol or chordotomy may be appropriate alternatives in an intractable situation.[217]

HARTMANN'S RESECTION

Occasionally, a patient with metastatic disease can be adequately treated by the so-called Hartmann's resection (Figure 23-61; see Biography).[318] ReMine and Dozois reported 107 such procedures, approximately one half of which were considered palliative.[679] However, they were able to perform a subsequent colorectal anastomosis on only 10% of their patients.

The procedure certainly has the potential advantage of removing the symptomatic tumor mass, an important objective in a palliative resection. Unfortunately, when the operation is undertaken in an attempt to cure the condition, the colostomy is often permanent. In spite of numerous techniques devised to reestablish intestinal continuity, a major procedure is still required.[136,512,669] It is for this reason that I do not recommend Hartmann's resection for patients whose disease is potentially curable. Still, as a palliative procedure in those with advanced or metastatic rectal cancer, Hartmann's operation has the potential for offering excellent relief of rectal symptoms if the tumor can be completely extirpated by this means, especially because the patient will not have to contend with the consequences of a perineal wound.[327] However, the application today is primarily applied to those undergoing emergency surgery for diverticulitis (see Chapter 26).

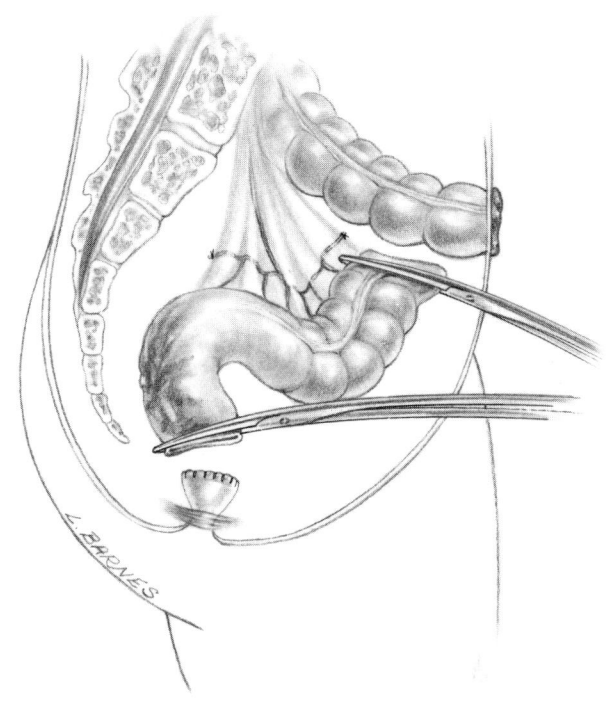

FIGURE 23-61. Hartmann's resection. The rectal stump is inverted by conventional suture technique or is closed with a linear stapler distal to the tumor. A sigmoid colostomy is created.

COLOSTOMY OR ILEOSTOMY

The use of a diversionary procedure without resection for cancer of the rectum is applied most frequently when the patient presents with obstruction or an impending obstruction. However, the difficult question is whether to perform a rectal excision at that time. The answer will depend on a number of factors: the degree of bowel dilatation, whether there is an opportunity to "prepare" the colon, whether an anastomosis can be effected, whether the tumor is resectable, whether supplementary radiotherapy is contemplated, and, of course, the condition of the patient. In general, when the surgeon is confronted with an obstruction, it is probably wiser to perform a colostomy and to return another day. An alternative approach may be to consider the methods of antegrade irrigation discussed in Chapter 22 and to resect (with or without an anastomosis). Further options are the use of a Wallstent (see Figs. 22-85 and 22-86), other prostheses,[380] and endoscopic, palliative approaches (see later). The techniques of stomal construction are discussed in Chapter 31.

If the patient's primary complaint is bleeding, colostomy is notoriously ineffective. Despite diversion, the bleeding often persists. Palliative APR is one option, and electrocoagulation and laser photocoagulation therapy are others (see later). Radiotherapy has not been of proved benefit in this situation. Another possibility for establishment of hemostasis is the application of a gauze soaked in 1% solution of alum (aluminum ammonium sulfate/aluminum potassium sulfate) as a styptic agent.[630]

LOW ANTERIOR RESECTION

The first resection of the sigmoid colon was performed in 1833 by Reybard of Lyons,[681] but for the next 100 years practically all operative approaches to the treatment of carcinoma either involved extirpation of the rectum or another sphincter-saving procedure, such as the various modifications of the pull-through operation. Murphy introduced his button in 1892 to perform a rapid and safe anastomosis,[599] but it was not until the 1940s, and even the 1950s in some centers, that conventional anastomotic techniques were believed safe enough to be employed for most cases of carcinoma of the rectum when intestinal continuity may be reestablished. Generally, it was the work of Dixon and of Wangensteen that contributed much to the ultimate success of this operation.[174,419,860]

Indications

The most important factor that determines the likelihood of performing an anastomosis is the level of the lesion, although if one is strongly motivated to reestablishing intestinal continuity, it can virtually always be accomplished—the obvious question is not so much, can you put the bowel together, but should you. Table 23-7 summarizes the various procedures and the method of reconstruction.

Favorable indices such as good differentiation, diploid histogram, limited bowel wall penetration with endorectal ultrasound, small size, and polypoid configuration may safely reduce the distal margin of resection to 1 or 2 cm. As mentioned previously, the only absolute contraindications to performing a low colorectal or coloanal anastomosis are invasion into the anal canal and invasion of the sphincter mechanism. When compared with other resective sphincter-saving operations, the low anterior resection is the one that is preferred. To embark upon an esoteric approach, one must believe rather strongly that an APR is inappropriate and a low anterior resection with conventional sutured or stapled techniques is impossible to accomplish.

Technique

There is often confusion about what constitutes a low anterior resection. This operation requires complete mobi-

TABLE 23-7 Options for Low-Lying Rectal Cancer

Exposure of distal rectum
  Abdominal
  Abdominotransanal
  Abdominosacral
  Abdominotranssphincteric
Resection
  Ultralow anterior resection
  Intersphincteric resection
  Transanal endoscopic microsurgery
  Abdominoperineal resection and neosphincter
Reconstruction
  Straight (end-to-end, side-to-end, end-to side)
  J-Pouch
  Coloplasty
Level of anastomosis
  Distal rectum
  Pelvic floor (anorectal ring)
  Anal canal
Type of anastomosis
  Hand-sewn
    Peranal
    Eversion of stump
  Stapled
    Single
    Double
    Triple

(Adapted from Tytherleigh MG, Mortensen NJ McC. Options for sphincter preservation in surgery for low rectal cancer. *Br J Surg* 2003;90:922.)

lization of the rectum from the hollow of the sacrum and division of the lateral ligaments with the middle hemorrhoidal arteries. Anastomosis is effected in the extraperitoneal rectum, that is, distal to the visceral peritoneum. Unless these criteria are met, the procedure is not by definition a low anterior resection.

The patient may be positioned in the perineolithotomy (Lloyd-Davies) position or supine on the operating table. When the surgeon feels confident that an anterior abdominal approach will permit anastomosis by a conventional suture method, the supine position is preferred. However, if there is some doubt whether an anastomosis can be effected readily from above or if a transanal stapling technique is contemplated (see later), the perineolithotomy position should be adopted. By using this position, alternative anastomotic techniques can be employed, if necessary (see Other Anastomotic Techniques), or an APR can be synchronously performed should an anastomotic procedure be considered unwise or technically impossible to accomplish. I do not believe that irrigating the rectum before resection is essential. Hence, this is not in itself an indication for using this position in my opinion. Of course, it makes sense to cleanse the rectum of residual stool if the patient has been inadequately prepared.

An exploratory laparotomy is performed and a determination made of the possibility and advisability of performing a resection. This is based on the presence or absence of metastatic disease and the fixity of the tumor in the pelvis. It may not be possible, however, to determine resectability until the rectum has been fully mobilized.

On occasion, the surgeon may elect to perform a resection on a patient who had previously undergone a polypectomy and in whom an invasive carcinoma was found. At laparotomy, it is sometimes impossible to identify the site of the lesion. This may then necessitate a "blind" or even inadequate resection. To avoid this potential dilemma, the area that had been excised can be infiltrated with India ink a day or more before the operation (Figure 23-62). This produces a black pigment in the lymphatics and permits ready identification of the tumor area from within the pelvis.

The initial steps of the procedure are identical to those described for APR. I prefer to mobilize the splenic flexure selectively (as needed), not routinely. I also do not believe in performing a high tie of the inferior mesenteric artery. Corder and colleagues studied 143 consecutive patients but failed to show any association between the method of vascular ligation and the risk of tumor recurrence and death.[135] Furthermore, anastomotic leak rates were not related to the method of vascular ligation.

Having been satisfied that an anastomosis can be performed, the surgeon's next task is to divide the mesorectum. Large clamps are placed posteriorly and the

mesentery divided above the clamps. Tension on the proximal bowel permits separation of the mesentery from the posterior rectal wall (Figure 23-63). With a very low anastomosis, there is usually little or no mesentery to divide.

Total Mesorectal Excision

Although tumor at the margin of resection and a second primary lesion are potential sources of recurrent disease, these are quite uncommon causes of recurrence. It is generally believed that most suture-line recurrences are the result of residual tumor left in the pelvis (the so-called tangential, circumferential or lateral margin) that subsequently grows into the lumen through the anastomosis.

Some reports have emphasized the importance of mesorectal spread of the tumor in determining risk of recurrence and survival.[104,346,404] Ono and co-workers in Tokyo examined the frequency, mode, and extent of *discontinuous spread* of rectal cancer in the mesorectum and also determined the optimal distal clearance margin.[622] Seventeen of 40 patients (43%) were found to have discontinuous cancer spread in the mesentery. The maximum extent of distal microscopic spread in this series was calculated to have been 24 mm *in situ*.

Heald and his colleagues in Basingstoke, England, have been in the forefront of emphasizing the importance of removing the "tongue" of mesorectum to reduce the incidence of recurrence—that is, total mesorectal excision (TME).[404,502] They have reported no local

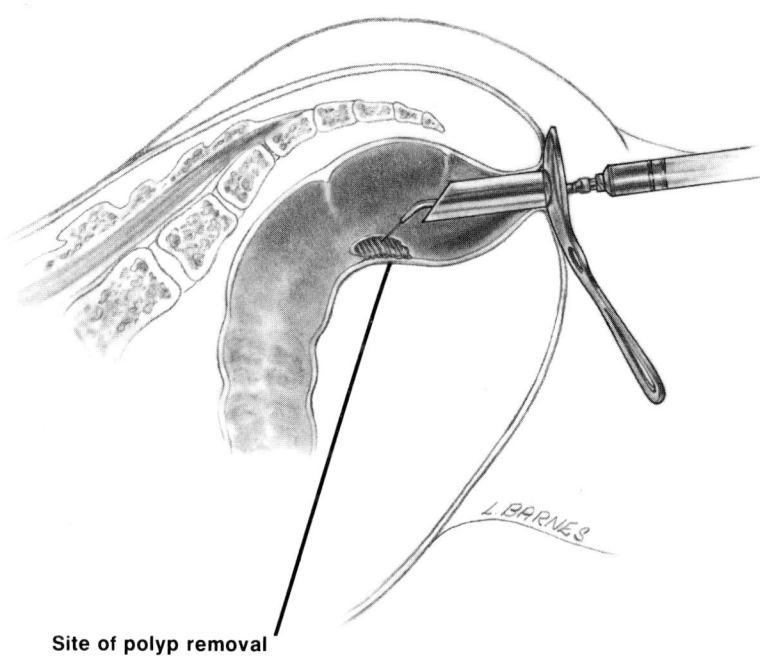

Site of polyp removal

L. BARNES

FIGURE 23-62. Technique of India ink injection of a previously removed tumor area.

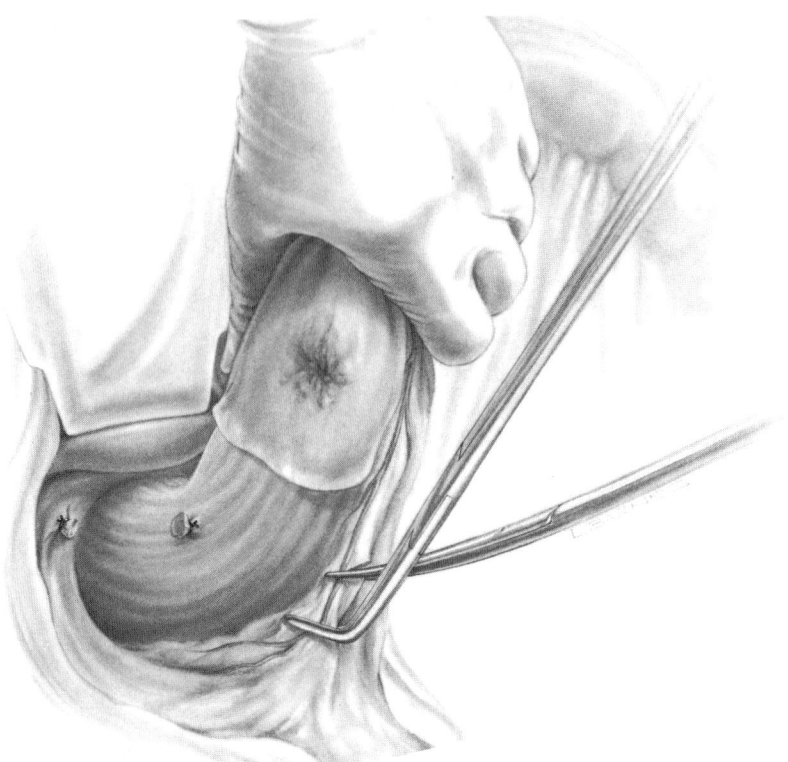

FIGURE 23-63. Anterior resection. Division of the mesorectum is expedited by application of right-angle clamps and vigorous cephalad tension as the mesentery is cut.

recurrences with a resection margin of greater than 1 cm and only a 3.6% incidence of recurrence if the margin is less. In theory, failure to excise the mesorectum completely has the potential to leave gross or microscopic residual disease, and this may predispose to local treatment failure.[682] Heald and colleagues went so far as to state that TME appears to be an oncologically superior operation than abdominoperineal excision.[330] The primary basis for this statement is that in their opinion and experience, three fourths of patients with cancer of the lower one third of the rectum can be offered sphincter-sparing surgery. Heald further suggested that optimal TME surgery can be widely implemented with the expectation that outcome improvement could be four times as great as that achievable by adjuvant therapy.[329] In Norway and Sweden, rectal cancer surgery has essentially been removed from general surgical training programs, and surgery is now exclusively performed by TME surgeons.[329,870]

One of the concerns that has been expressed is the increased morbidity associated with removing the mesentery to the rectum distal to the anastomosis. Devascularization may be a consequence, with an increased incidence of anastomotic leak. Hainsworth and colleagues suggested that the operation is not appropriate for the treatment of tumors in the upper third of the rectum for that reason.[309] Arbman and colleagues compared the results of resection by means of TME with an earlier period

of cases performed without that modification.[18] Actuarial analysis demonstrated a significant reduction in local recurrence rate as well as an increase in survival with TME. The problem with the study, however, is that the second group of patients underwent surgery by a limited number of surgeons familiar with TME. Others expressed enthusiasm for the technique, with some commenting that the procedure is compatible with autonomic nerve preservation as well as sphincter preservation.[90,195,323] Inevitably however, the "controls," such as they may be considered, are historical. Moreover, the authors compared TME with prior unacceptably high local recurrence rates, at least by my standards.

The problem with accepting without question often remarkable results is that when an APR is performed (removing all of the mesorectum), the risk of recurrence in the pelvis is significantly higher than that reported by Heald and colleagues as well as other investigators. How is this possible? For me, this is a conundrum that defies explanation. The fact is, local recurrence has been demonstrated to be closely related to tumor at the lateral or circumferential rectal margins.[5,607,665] In the experience of Ng and colleagues, 53% of patients with lateral resection margin involvement developed recurrent tumor.[607] In the experience of Adam and associates, tumor involvement of the circumferential margin was seen in 25% of 144 specimens for which the surgeon thought the resection was potentially curative.[5] Seventy-eight percent developed local recurrence under these circumstances. Wibe and co-workers, reporting from Norway, identified 686 patients *who underwent TME* with tumor found at the circumferential margin.[871] With a limited follow-up, 22% developed local recurrence and 40% were found to have distant metastases. This was even though many patients had been submitted to adjuvant therapy. Inarguably, TME adds nothing to the conventional operation when a surgeon is confronted with lateral tumor spread.

Opinion

It is difficult for me to understand what the excitement is about when reading reports of so-called TME. No one would argue that mobilization of the rectum consistent with a complete understanding of the anatomy is critical.[62,107] People do feel strongly about what the implications are, however. Chapuis and colleagues in Australia stated that the use of the word "mesorectum" is anatomically inaccurate, and the implication that total excision of all the perirectal fat contained within the perirectal fascia *en bloc* in all patients with rectal cancer will minimize local recurrence remains contentious.[107]

The operation, as described by Heald, is essentially the same procedure that most surgeons who are experienced in removing the rectum for cancer have employed for many years. The only difference, perhaps, is the removal of the "tongue" of mesorectum distal to the site of a low rectal tumor. However, this is a dangerous exercise for middle and upper rectal tumors. Actually, there is no "tongue" when a low rectal cancer is resected. The mesentery does not even exist at this level.

TME is a subject that tends to cause great ire whenever the issue arises among experienced surgeons. In his letter to the editor of the journal *Diseases of the Colon and Rectum,* van Langenberg wrote: "Any colorectal surgeon worth his salt in performing an abdominoperineal or low anterior resection would have been doing this operation long before it was christened 'TME.' Who in his right mind would plow through the mesorectum when it is well known that a plane exists between it and the sacrum that is almost bloodless, making it possible to remove the mesorectum (or whatever you choose to call it) *en bloc* with the rectum?"[842]

I, myself, do not understand why this operation is such a success in individuals with circumferential tumor involvement or where the tumor spreads laterally. The only conclusions I can reach for such remarkable achievements are as follows:

- My patients' cancers are different from their patients' cancers.
- I don't know what I'm doing.

- I don't understanding what they are doing.
- They preselect and determine which patients they consider "curable" and do not count them as recurrence failures.

Clearly, the results of TME defy logic. What is more, I am most concerned about devascularizing the rectum for any distance below my anastomosis.

Heald and others do deserve credit, however, for reminding us of the importance of the proper plane of dissection and the need to divide the mesentery (if present) below the tumor. One's attention to precise, sharp dissection in the areolar tissue between the visceral and parietal layers of the pelvic fascia, performed under direct vision,[600] such as I have earlier described, is the method that I have been taught and is the technique I have uniformly applied for 35 years. This is indeed worth reiterating. Furthermore, I concur with the comments of Gordon when he stated: "The key would seem to be careful not to cone down through the mesentery, but rather to proceed in the areolar plane outside the investing fascia of the rectum. When the appropriate distal margin is obtained, a sharp incision is made *perpendicular* [italics mine] to the bowel, thus including in the mesorectum any potential extramural retrograde spread."[279]

Conventional Suturing

A crushing clamp is applied, usually 4 cm below the distal margin of the tumor. An angled or curved clamp placed in the anteroposterior plane is preferred (Figure 23-64). Only one is used. Anchoring sutures are placed, and the bowel is divided distal to the clamp. Long Allis clamps may be used to identify the cut edge of the rectum (Figure 23-65). With the proximal bowel divided and the specimen removed, an open end-to-end anastomosis (EEA) is performed. Interrupted 3–0 or no. 4–0 long-term absorbable sutures are recommended, but the type of suture material is of less importance than is the meticulous approach to the technique employed. Simple, interrupted sutures are placed as a single layer, taking deeper bites in the muscularis and minimal mucosa (the rectum has no serosa at this level). With a low anastomosis, it is easier to place all of the sutures into the posterior row initially, before tying (Figure 23-66). It is usually more convenient to place the initial suture through the sigmoid on the ventral aspect of the mesenteric side and then through the right anterolateral part of the rectum. The knots are then secured and the anterior row completed. The last suture is usually a horizontal mattress suture in order to invert the mucosa (Figure 23-67). A single layer is considered adequate, although the surgeon may prefer to pull the anterior peritoneum over the anastomosis with Lembert sutures. A continuous suture technique, such as has been

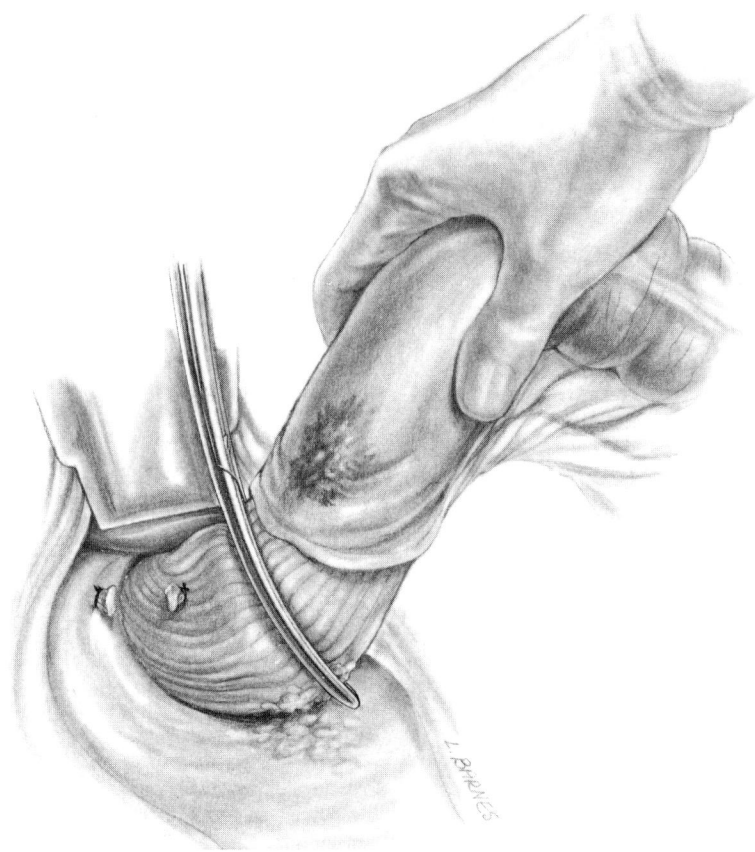

FIGURE 23-64. Anterior resection. An angled or curved clamp is applied at an adequate distance below the tumor.

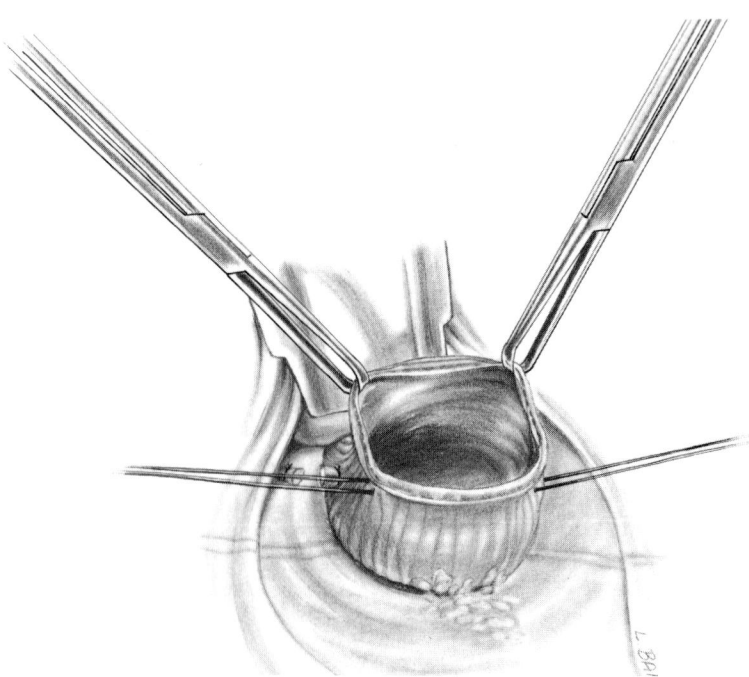

FIGURE 23-65. Anterior resection. The open distal rectum is prepared for anastomosis. Allis clamps and guide sutures are helpful.

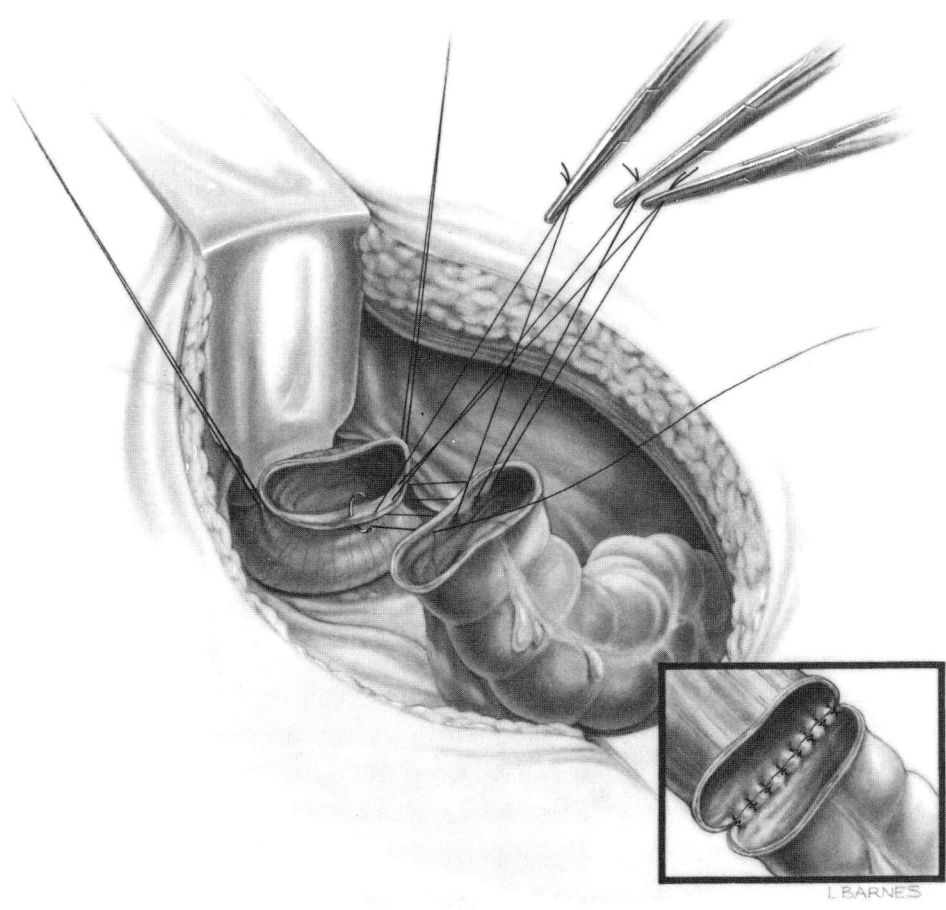

FIGURE 23-66. Anterior resection. Sutures are initially placed in the posterior row but not secured. The **inset** demonstrates the posterior row completed.

described in Figure 22-41, is also perfectly satisfactory. Deen advises the use of a Foley catheter to prevent bowel contamination and to facilitate placement of the sutures (Figure 23-68).[162] The floor of the pelvis is not reconstituted but is vigorously irrigated with saline.

Omental Wrapping

The placement of omentum around the anastomosis has been advocated by a number of investigators.[267,268,456,552] The procedure can be accomplished by freeing the omentum from the transverse colon with care to avoid injury to the blood supply (Figure 23-69). The appropriately tailored omentum is then brought down the lateral gutter into the pelvis, and an anchoring suture is placed below and posterior to the anastomosis (Figure 23-70).

Tocchi and colleagues performed a prospective, randomized study to evaluate the incidence of complications with and without omental wrapping in 112 patients.[826] Although there was no statistically significant difference in the incidence of anastomotic leaks, the authors believed that omentoplasty was responsible for better containment. My concern is that the use of omentoplasty may actually mask an otherwise significant anastomotic

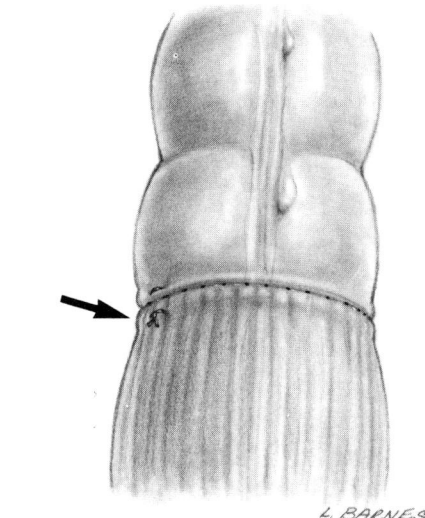

FIGURE 23-67. Anterior resection. Anastomosis completed. Note the final inverting mattress suture *(arrow)*.

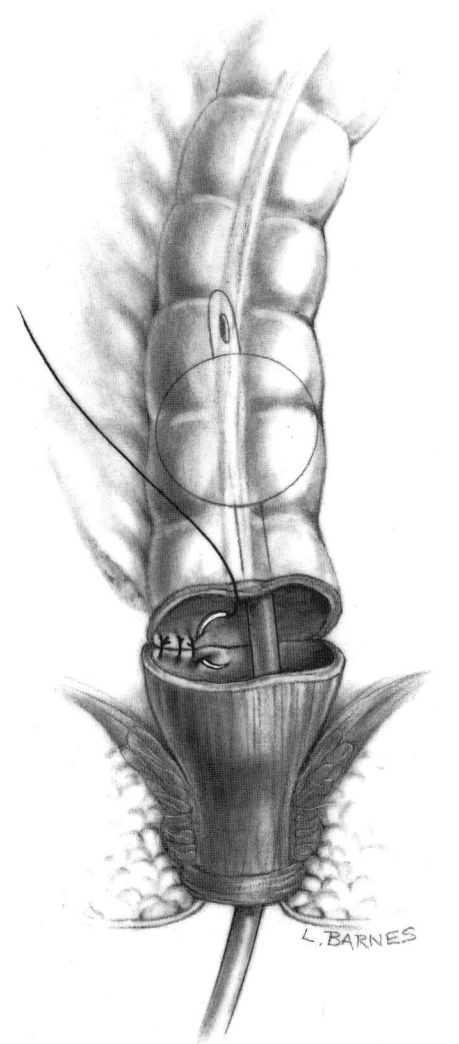

FIGURE 23-68. Foley catheter–assisted sutured colorectal anastomosis. (Adapted from Deen KI. Foley catheter–assisted sutured colorectal anastomosis. *Br J Surg* 1995;82:324.)

disruption, thereby delaying implementation of needed surgical treatment.

Rectal Irrigation

Rectal washout before performing the anastomosis in the hope that this will minimize local recurrence brought about by implantation of viable tumor cells is advocated by many surgeons. The application of cytocidal agents in the irrigant has been recommended, but it is more likely that the mechanical cleansing eliminates any exfoliated cells.[253] Agaba was unable to demonstrate any benefit in the use of cytocidal agents in reducing the incidence of local recurrence.[7] In a study by Sayfan and colleagues, 14 patients underwent rectal washout after the rectal stump was closed before performing a stapled anastomosis.[728]

Eleven individuals were found to have malignant cells after the first washing, and the fifth washing was still positive in seven. However, there are no randomized trials demonstrating that there is an improvement in local control with rectal stump irrigation, nor does it mean to suggest that one can compromise on the distal margin of resection through the application of this maneuver. I don't believe in it, and I don't use it—full stop!

Use of Drains

The routine use of drains for pelvic anastomoses is not advised. In a number of studies, the presence of a drain did not influence the postoperative morbidity or mortality. Furthermore, if the anastomosis leaked, the presence of a drain did not prevent the need for reoperation, nor does pus or feces emerge from the drain in those individuals in whom a leak occurs.[713,714,739] That said, if a significant amount of drainage is anticipated, such as following an unusually bloody pelvic dissection, it would seem prudent to leave a closed suction drain in the pelvis for 1 or 2 days, or at least until the serosanguineous drainage is minimal.

Stapled Anastomosis

The application of stapling instruments to effect colonic anastomoses is discussed in Chapter 22, but the creation of a low rectal anastomosis is usually not possible with the conventional instruments and maneuvers described in that chapter.

In 1978, the United States Surgical Corporation (Norwalk, CT) introduced a circular stapling device (similar to the Russian stapler, PKS) that was uniquely advantageous for effecting low colorectal anastomoses. The EEA (reusable) and CEEA (disposable) staplers (Figure 23-71) and the intraluminal stapler (ILS; Figure 23-72) create an inverted, circular anastomosis with two staggered rows of staples (Figure 23-73) and remove tissue "doughnuts" (rings) of bowel from each end to create an adequate lumen (Figure 23-74). Cartridges are available in several diameters: 25, 28, and 31 mm with the CEEA and 21, 25, 29, and 33 mm with the ILS.

Technique

Various stapling techniques have been suggested for performing an anastomosis in the rectum.[672] The most commonly employed is the EEA using the circular stapling instrument passed through the anal canal. The patient is placed in the perineolithotomy position in order to facilitate access to the anus and to the abdomen. After the bowel has been mobilized above and below the tumor and the blood supply has been divided, the proximal site for the anastomosis is prepared. In contrast to conven-

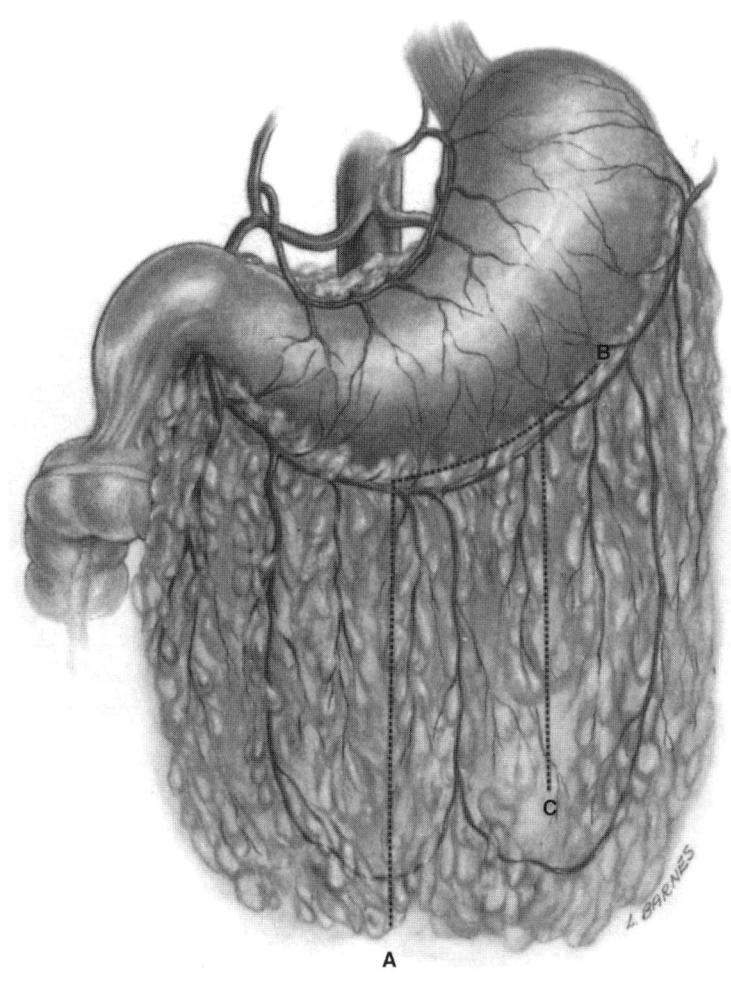

FIGURE 23-69. Tailoring of the omentum. Adequate length can usually be achieved if the apron is divided along lines *A* and *B*. If still more length is required, another incision *C* will usually suffice.

tional suturing technique, the bowel must be meticulously debrided of all fat for 1.5 to 2 cm. A crushing clamp is placed distally, and a purse-string monofilament suture (e.g., 2–0 Prolene) is placed proximally. If the purse-string instrument is used (Figure 23-75), a straight Keith needle of 2–0 Prolene is passed through both channels (Figure 23-76). A monofilament, nonabsorbable suture is required in order to prevent dragging when the purse-string suture is secured. The bowel is then divided between the clamps. Another option is to use the Purstring instrument, which actually applies the purse-string by means of a series of staples to the muscularis of the colon or rectal wall (Figure 23-77). Regrettably, I have found neither device to be satisfactory. Too often, the suture fails to incorporate the bowel wall properly, and the purse-string must be manually redone.

In like manner, the distal bowel below the tumor is freed and the mesentery debrided. Ideally, the purse-string clamp is placed an adequate distance below the tumor (Figure 23-78). Unfortunately, the applicator often cannot be usefully employed for anastomoses low in the pelvis. In this situation, the purse-string must be applied manually, although the Purstring device may accomplish this (Figure 23-79). Alternatively, a double-stapling technique may be used (see later).

A crushing clamp is placed on the bowel distal to the tumor. It is helpful to apply a noncrushing intestinal clamp or vascular clamp on the distal rectal stump to use as a handle or to place several guide sutures to elevate the rectum. The bowel is then divided, and the specimen is removed. A monofilament, nonabsorbable, purse-string suture is then inserted in an "over-and-over" fashion (Figure 23-80), although the more tedious "weaving" technique may be used (Figure 23-81A). Moseson and associates facilitate the application of the suture by elevation of the rectal cuff with traction on a Foley catheter.[597] Other articles have been published that address the issue of the inadequate or difficult purse-string and how to overcome the problem.[446,458,667,771,827] For example, pressure on the perineum with the fist will often elevate the rectal remnant sufficiently to permit placement of the purse-string (Figure 23-82). Thorlakson described specially designed occlusive clamps that facilitate the placement of either a hand-sewn purse-string or sutured anas-

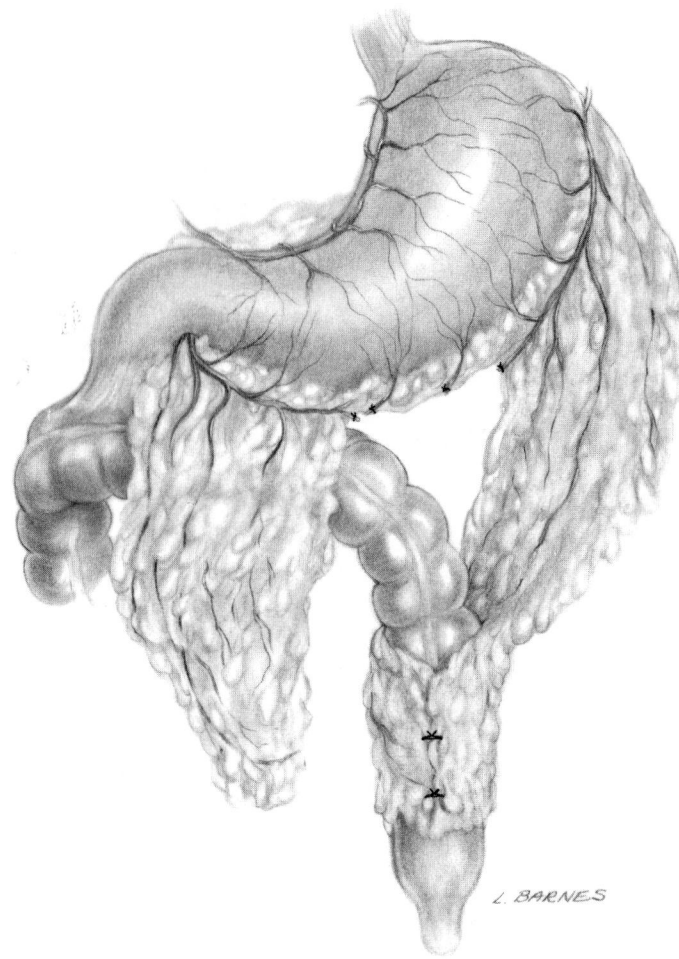

FIGURE 23-70. Tailoring of the omentum. The omentum is brought down the lateral gutter posterior to the anastomosis. It is then wrapped anteriorly and is fixed to the rectum and pelvic floor.

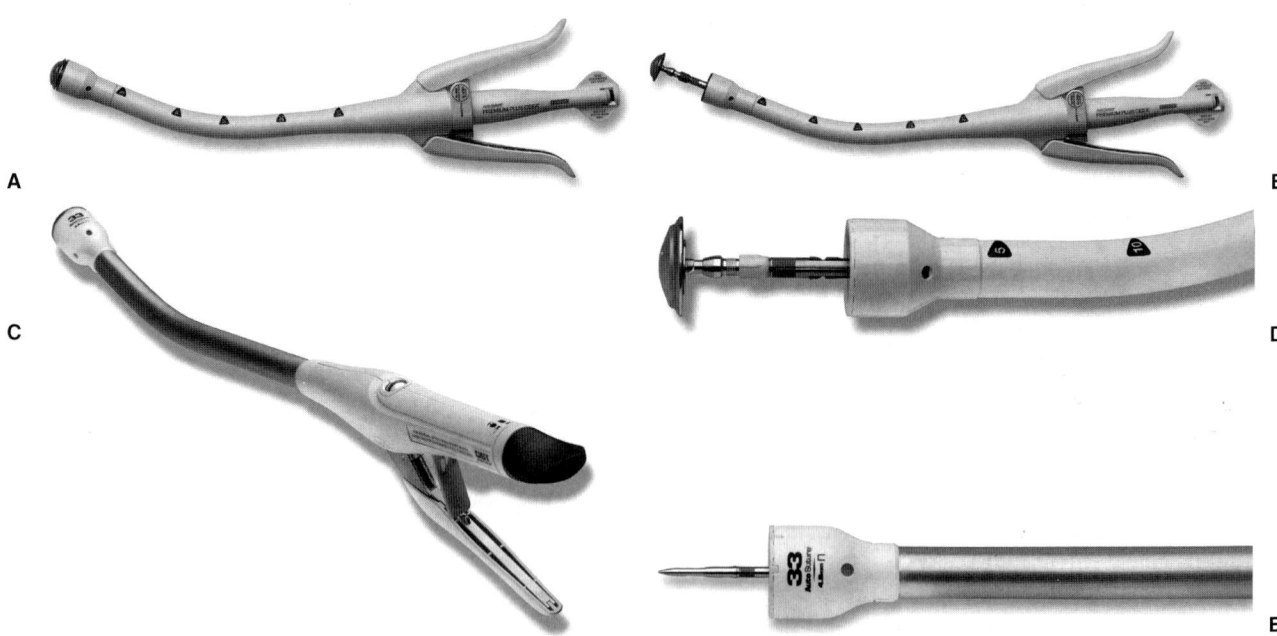

A

B

C

D

E

FIGURE 23-71. Multiple options are available in the circular instruments. Disposable curved CEEA (end-to-end circular stapler) with integrated flip-top anvil. This permits a low profile for ease of insertion and removal. **(A)** Closed instrument. **(B)** Opened instrument. **(C)** End-to-end anastomosis (EEA) Open/XL—available in two shaft lengths, ergonomic handle and knob, and one-handed firing. **(D)** Close-up view of open instrument. **(E)** Distal anvil removed. (Courtesy of the United States Surgical Corp, Norwalk, CT.)

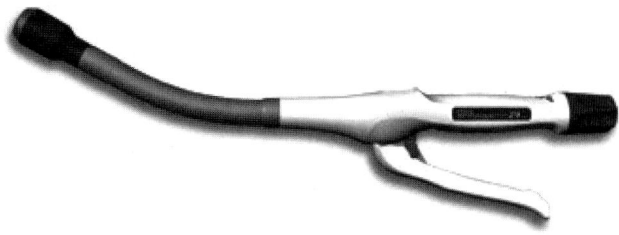

FIGURE 23-72. Proximate ILS curved intraluminal stapler with detachable head and with low-profile anvil. This is available in sizes 21, 25, 29, and 33 mm. (Courtesy of Ethicon Endo-Surgery, Inc., Cincinnati, Ohio.)

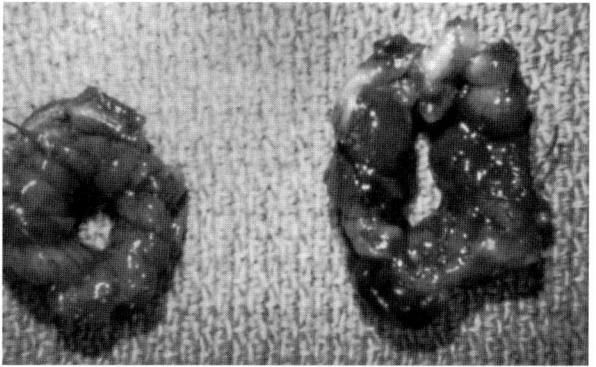

FIGURE 23-74. Intact "doughnuts" from the two bowel ends.

tomosis.[823] Kumashiro and colleagues facilitated the placement of the purse-string suture by securing a 2–0 Prolene suture on the edge of the distal stump by means of a disposable skin stapler (Figure 23-83).[447] Gingold and colleagues utilized a gasket that fixes the rectum to the center-rod, a technique analogous to rubber ring ligation of a hemorrhoid.[259]

An alternative technique involves inverting the rectal stump with the aid of guide sutures and passing the stump to the perineal operator.[675,767] If the rectum is of sufficient length, it is sometimes possible to apply the purse-string device outside the anal verge (Figure 23-81*B*). Realistically, however, if there is sufficient rectum remaining to permit this maneuver, it should be possible to apply the instrument through the abdomen, although there is the occasional situation in which this alternative can be a useful technique. After the suture has been placed, the rectum is returned to the pelvis.

Attention is then turned to the cartridge. With experience, the surgeon should be able to select the appropriate

size, but the largest should be used whenever possible. The sigmoid colon usually has the smaller lumen, but with the aid of a sizer, the luminal discrepancy may be somewhat obviated (Figs. 23-84 and 23-85). When bowel spasm presents a problem, the intravenous administration of 2 mg of glucagon has been recommended, as has the use of a Foley catheter balloon.[312,576] Shlasko and colleagues suggested the topical placement of 1% lidocaine to the cut edges of the mucosa.[756] After a few minutes, "relaxation" of the spasm may be observed. Oblique application of a purse-string clamp on the proximal bowel has also been proposed as a means for widening the lumen.[818]

The current generation of circular stapling instruments permits two important characteristics for effecting a low intestinal anastomosis: a detachable head and a trocar-tip (Figs. 23-86 to 23-89). The trocar is used for penetrating the closed bowel end (see later, Technique).

The perineal surgeon gently dilates the anus, and the well-lubricated instrument is inserted into the rectum.

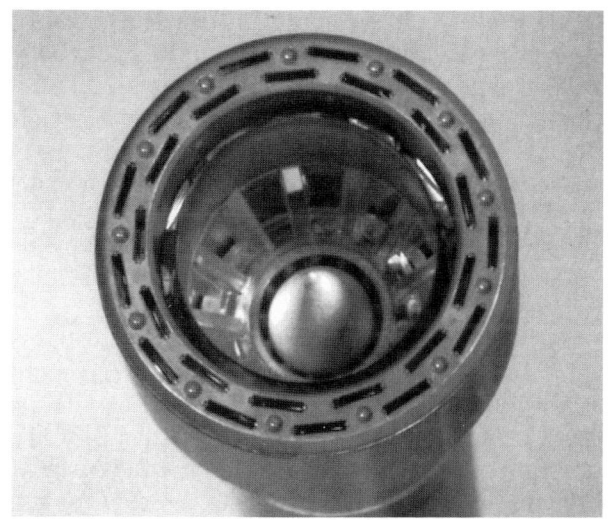

FIGURE 23-73. Cartridge containing two staggered rows of staples. (Courtesy of United States Surgical Corp, Norwalk, CT.)

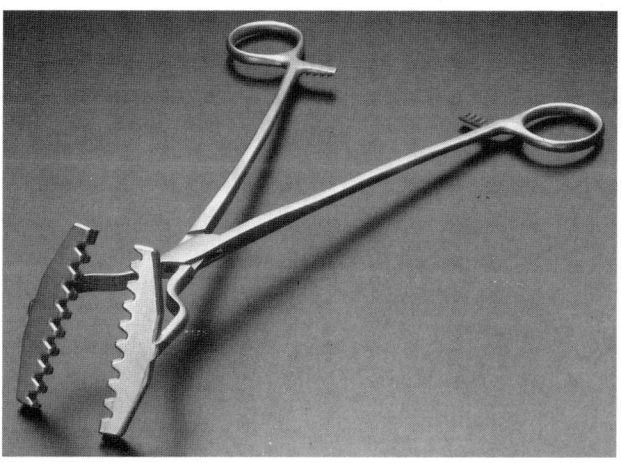

FIGURE 23-75. Purse-string instrument. (Courtesy of Sherwood—Davis and Geck, Inc., Danbury, CT.)

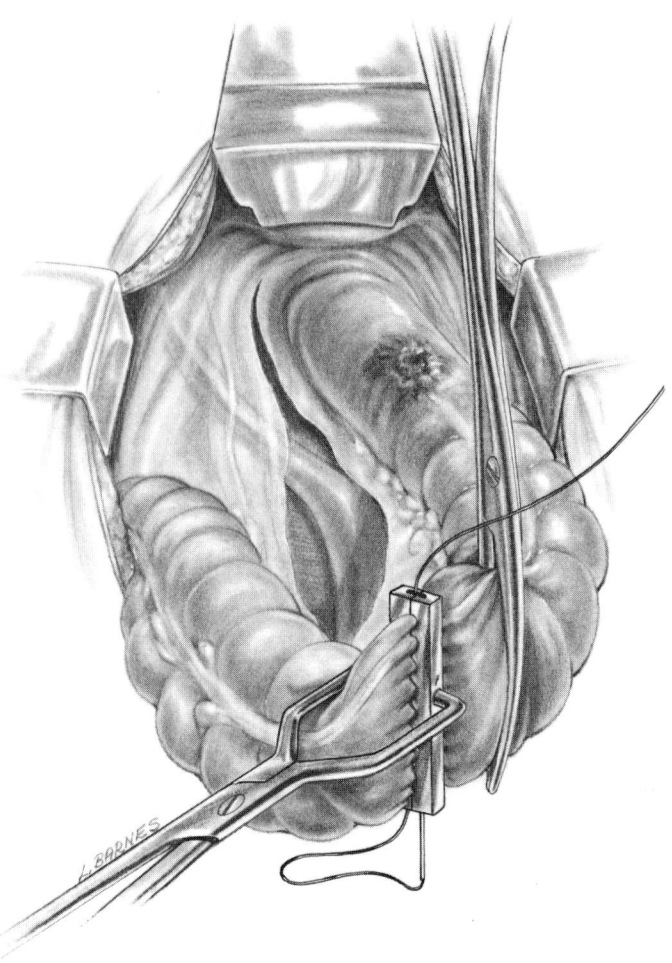

FIGURE 23-76. Circular stapled anastomosis. Application of purse-string instrument to proximal bowel.

The abdominal surgeon should guide the device anteriorly, because there is a tendency for the perineal operator to direct the instrument into the sacrum. The adjusting knob is turned counterclockwise, and the anvil is advanced from the cartridge into the pelvis (Figure 23-90). The distal purse-string suture is then tied over the shaft (Figure 23-91).

Then, by using one's hand or Allis or Babcock forceps, the proximal bowel is eased over the anvil and the proximal purse-string suture secured (Figure 23-92). Both sutures are then cut. Most of the time, the surgeon will first secure the distal purse-string. Occasionally, however, this maneuver will lead to great difficulty when attempting to tie the proximal one, particularly if the pelvis is deep and narrow. Under these circumstances, one should consider tying the colon purse-string first.[120] The surgeon is cautioned that this approach should be used only selectively, however, because the proximal bowel may interfere with tying of the distal purse-string. The judgment that must be made is which end is the more difficult to secure, and that is the end that should be tied initially. The concern about this issue

is truly academic with the availability of the CEEA and Proximate ILS instruments and the use of the double-stapling technique (see next section).

The perineal surgeon then tightens the adjusting knob, and the bowel ends are approximated. The abdominal surgeon makes certain that no tissue comes between the anvil and the cartridge. The posterior vaginal wall is especially vulnerable to incorporation by the stapler. The safety catch is released, and the handle grip is tightened to fire the staples and to cut the redundant bowel (Figure 23-93). The anvil is advanced, and by using a gentle rotational movement, the instrument is withdrawn with careful guidance by the abdominal operator.

Finally, the excised tissue rings, which are the cut edges of both ends of the anastomosis (with the purse-string sutures), are examined for completeness (Figure 23-74). If the rings are not intact, the anastomosis will require careful evaluation and perhaps need to be redone or reinforced with sutures.

One of the concerns that is frequently expressed is the difficulty in passing the instrument through the anal

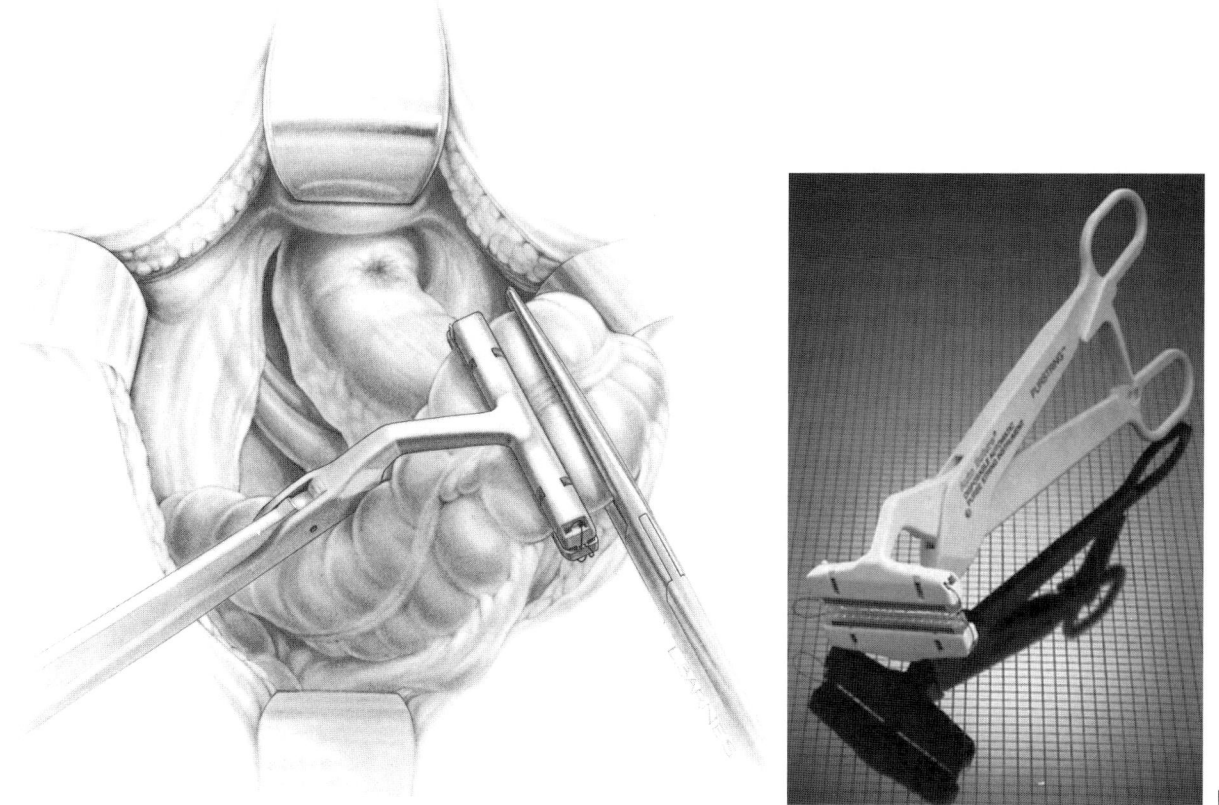

A

B

FIGURE 23-77. Purstring applicator (**inset**; Courtesy of United States Surgical Corp, Norwalk, CT) used to create a purse-string suture that is stapled to the muscularis of the bowel wall.

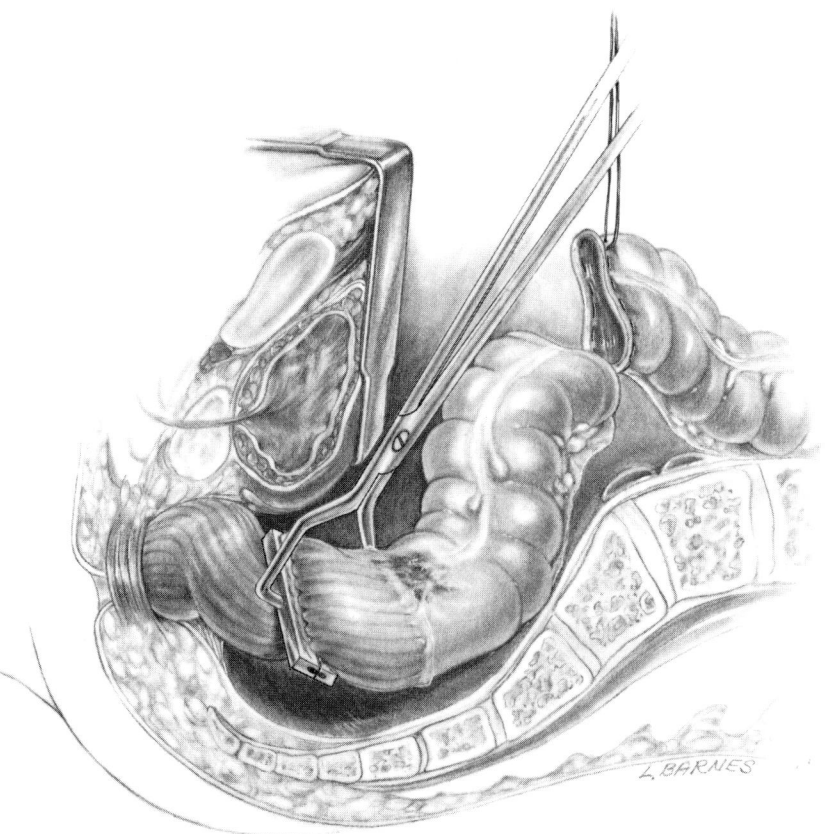

FIGURE 23-78. Circular stapled anastomosis. Application of a purse-string instrument distal to the tumor. The proximal suture is in place. Clamps are omitted for ease of illustration.

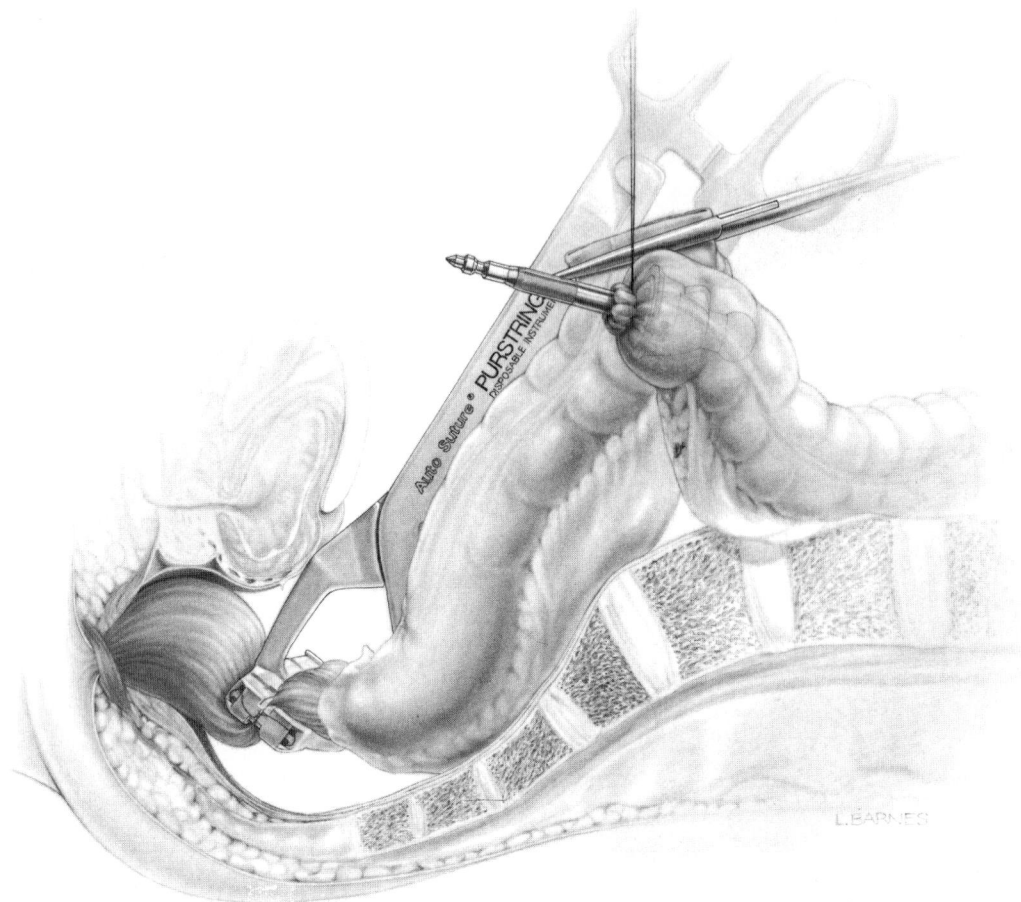

FIGURE 23-79. Resection of the bowel with reanastomosis by the transanal insertion of a circular stapler. Application of the Purstring instrument distally with insertion of the separated, proximal anvil.

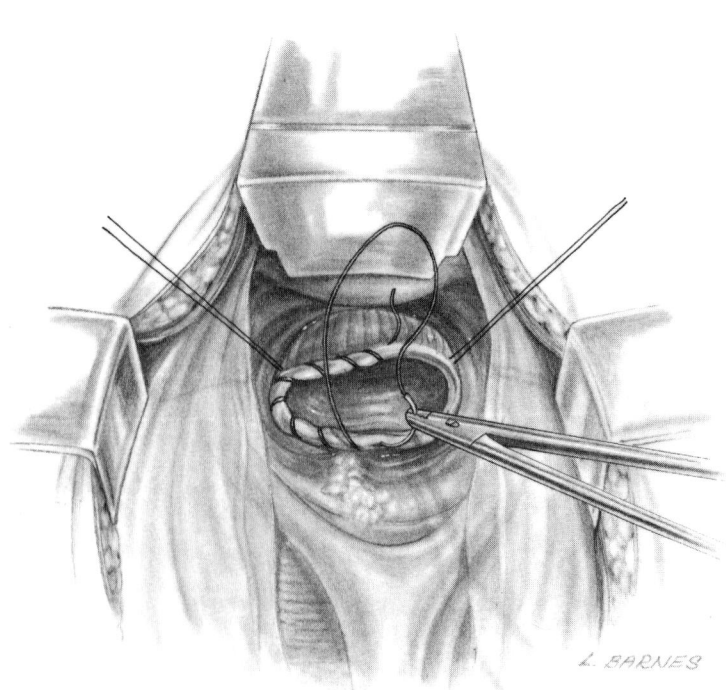

FIGURE 23-80. Circular stapled anastomosis. A hand-sewn purse-string suture is placed in the rectal stump.

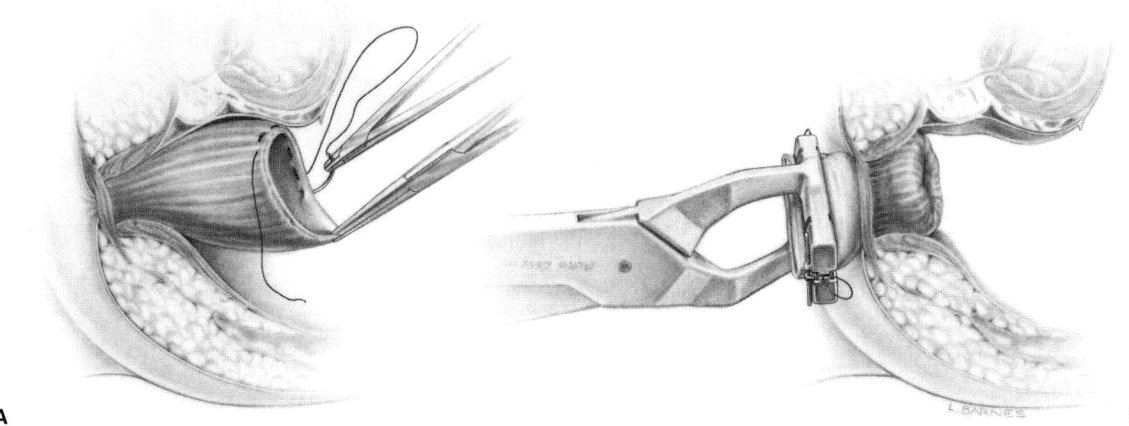

FIGURE 23-81. Circular stapled anastomosis. **(A)** Hand-sewn purse-string suture placed using "weaving" technique. **(B)** Purstring applicator employed on an inverted rectal stump.

canal without causing trauma. Numerous suggestions have been made, including incorporating the anvil within a Penrose drain to permit smooth passage. Additionally, various anal retractors have been developed that allow passage into the proximal bowel.[513] The Faensler operating anoscope (Figure 23-94) certainly helps to reduce the risk of injury and perhaps the incidence of stretch consequences that may ultimately lead to impairment for bowel control following low anterior resection (see later discussion).[412]

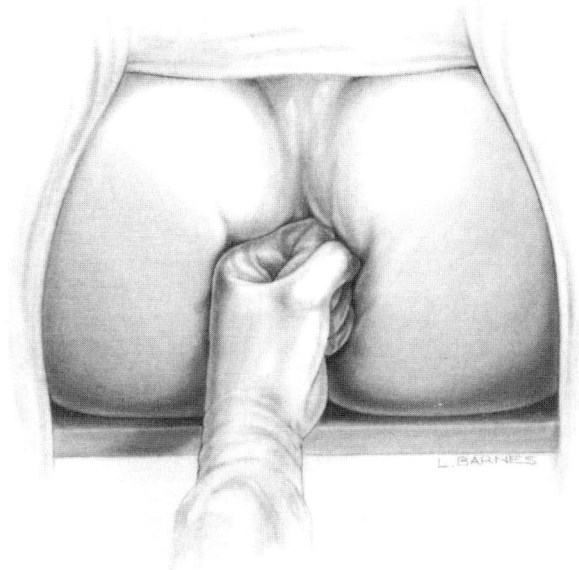

FIGURE 23-82. Pressure on the perineum by the fist or some other blunt object facilitates the placement of sutures into the rectal remnant.

Testing the Anastomosis

The anastomosis may be tested by placing saline solution in the pelvis and looking for bubbles when air is insufflated into the rectum via a proctoscope and with the proximal bowel occluded with fingers or a noncrushing clamp (Figure 23-95). Proctosigmoidoscopic visualization of the adequacy of the lumen may also be helpful. If the technique has been properly performed and there is no evidence of leak, no reinforcing sutures are necessary.

Beard and colleagues randomized 145 consecutive patients who underwent colorectal anastomoses to a test or to no test.[39] Any demonstrable leaks following testing were repaired. The two groups were well matched for age, sex, diagnosis, and operative details. Contrast studies were performed on postoperative day 10. There was a statistically significant increased frequency of clinical and radiologic leaks demonstrated in the no test group. The authors concluded that intraoperative air testing and repair significantly reduces the risk of postoperative clinical and radiologic leak.[39]

Double-Stapling Technique

An alternative to the placement of the distal purse-string is to close the rectal stump by means of a linear stapler and to perform an EEA using the so-called double-stapling technique.[125,294,397,424,608] This method affords a relatively safe way to perform a low colorectal anastomosis, an option that may not otherwise be technically possible. The only downside is the added cost associated with the use of a second stapler application. The technique may also be limited when the stapler needs to be applied low in the pelvis.

In this approach, the distal rectum is closed with a linear stapling instrument (Figs. 23-96 and 23-97). Eisenstat

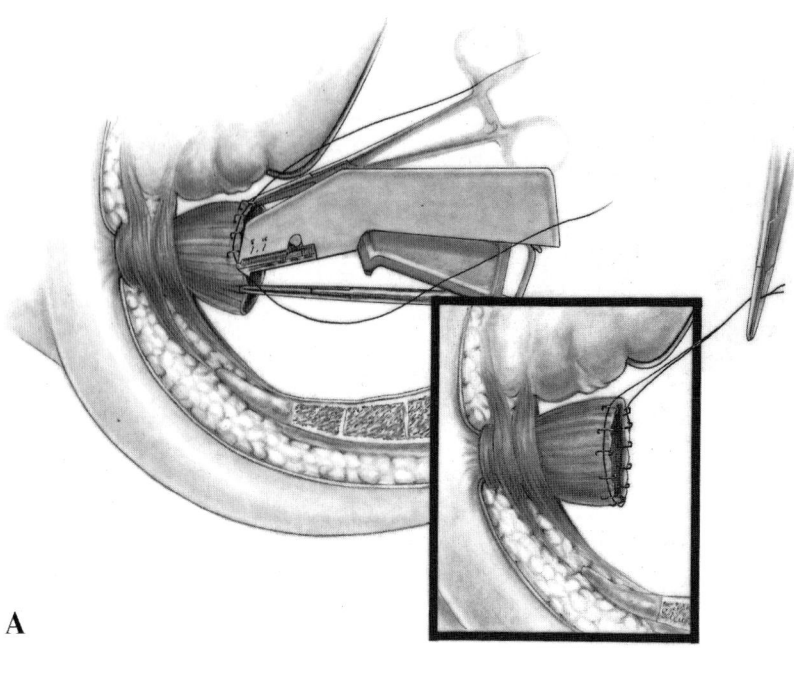

A

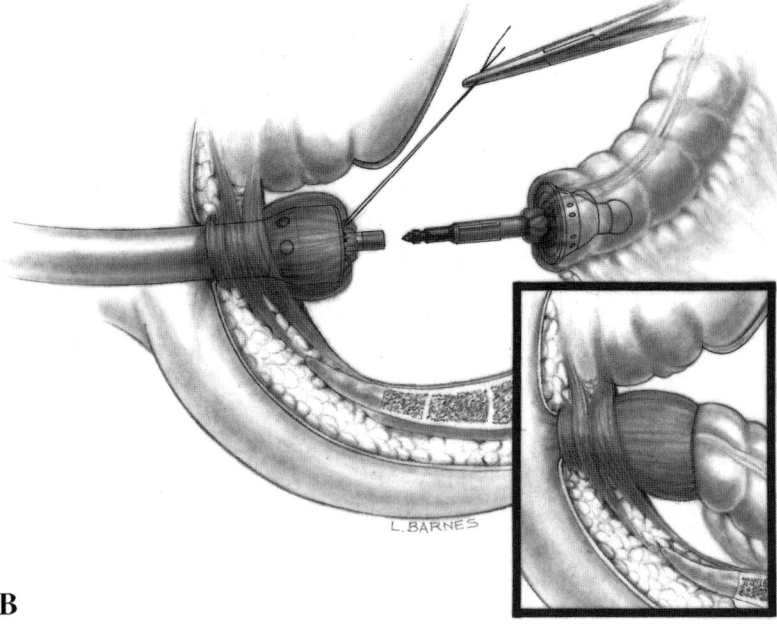

L. BARNES

B

FIGURE 23-83. (A) Application of distal purse-string suture utilizing a Prolene suture with a skin stapling device. The **inset** demonstrates the position before transanal placement. **(B)** The completed anastomosis. (Adapted from Kumashiro R, Sano C, Ugaeri H, et al. A new improved technique for placement of a purse-string suture on the edge of the distal part of the rectal stump using a skin stapler for low anterior resection. *J Am Coll Surg* 1994;178:405.)

and colleagues suggested, however, that closure may be effected more easily by means of the GIA90 instrument in certain individuals whose body habitus precludes the application of a linear stapler (Figure 23-98).[189] Ganchrow and Facelle suggested the use of double Roticulator placement so that a more distal closure of the rectal stump can be achieved.[241] As implied from the foregoing, I find it sufficiently difficult to apply one Roticulator, much less two.

My personal preference is to use the 30-mm instrument for low rectal double-stapled anastomoses. At this level, the rectal diameter is usually relatively narrow, and

there is minimal or no mesentery to deal with. This permits the lowest application that I can achieve with a stapling device. However, if the bowel is too large to permit the single application of the 30-mm instrument, another possibility is to apply the same stapler twice. One passes the pin through the rectal wall before firing and then reapplies the instrument with care to be certain that the staple lines *overlap* (Figure 23-99).

Hazama and colleagues modified the double-stapling approach to incorporate each corner of the staple line by a suture in order to obliterate remnants of the staple line

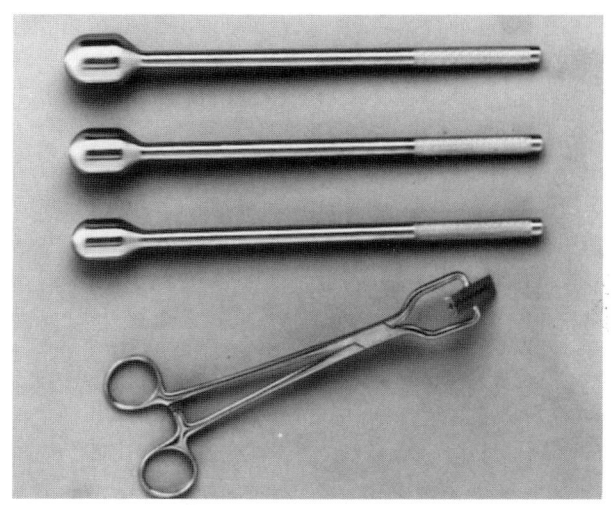

FIGURE 23-84. Sizers and purse-string instrument. (Courtesy of United States Surgical Corp, Norwalk, CT.)

that have not been removed by the circular device.[326] The theoretical objection of having the "dog ears" is not a real concern from my point of view. What is important is to make certain that the circular and linear staple lines overlap in order to avoid devascularizing the area between the staple lines. However, Asao and co-workers believed that removing these so-called dog ears may be useful in preventing local recurrence through total excision of the distal rectal staple line.[22] Falco and colleagues recommended an eversion technique (Figure 23-100A)[202], whereas Scotté and colleagues incorporated a drain in the staple line to pull the bowel through (Figure 23-100B,C).[741]

As discussed previously, after mild dilation of the anus has been performed, the well-lubricated circular stapling device is inserted into the rectum and the trocar-tipped center rod advanced (Figure 23-101). As mentioned earlier, Thorlakson and others have suggested the use of operating proctoscopes to facilitate insertion of the blunt-ended instrument.[822,824] Another option is to create an opening from above and to pass a catheter down through the rectum, so that by placing the catheter onto the rod, the anvil can be guided to its desired position (see Figure 26-40).

The center rod is passed through the closed rectum adjacent to or through the staple line, so that when the anastomosis is complete the linear row of staples will be partially excised (Figure 23-102). The hand is used to help direct the trocar tip to the proper location for penetration, to reinforce the linear staple line to keep it from tearing, and to keep adjacent structures, such as the posterior vaginal wall, out of harm's way. Theoretically, if there is intact bowel wall between the circular and linear rows of staples, the tissue may become ischemic, and necrosis could result. This is of less concern, however, if the operation is performed at a later date, such as when Hartmann's pouch is reconnected to the colon (see Figure 26-40). The stab wound in the rectum may be reinforced with a suture around the center rod if the surgeon is concerned about the possibility of an incomplete tissue ring. This may not be technically possible to accomplish, however. A singular advantage of the detachable anvil and shaft is the ability of the surgeon to facilitate securing the proximal purse-string (Figure 23-103). A simple alternative for placing this purse-string is to ligate the bowel around the center rod. Debridement of the mesentery can then be undertaken rather expeditiously (Figure 23-104). The extension is then reattached to the instrument shaft (Figure 23-105), and the knob is turned in a clockwise fashion until the marking site appears on the handle, indicating adequate approximation of the two ends (Figure 23-106). The stapler is closed and fired in the manner previously described (Figure 23-107). The roentgenographic appearance of the staple lines can be appreciated in Figure 23-108 as well as the findings on CT (Figure 23-109).

The anastomosis is secure because the tissue and staple lines are held firmly in place before the staple-cutting stage.[673] The intersecting staples may be transferred to the removed doughnut, but the knife will bend the intersecting staple rather than cut it.[673]

Side-to-End and Side-to-Side Anastomoses

Baker advocated side-to-end anastomosis of the colon to the rectum in order to deal with the disparity between the two lumina.[30] Others have also found this to be a useful technique.[414] In my opinion, anastomosis can be more readily accomplished in an end-to-end fashion, with the

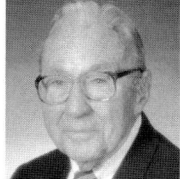

Joel W. Baker (1905–1999) Joel Baker was born in Shenandoah, Virginia. Thanks to the influence of his uncle, the town physician, Baker always wanted to pursue medicine. Baker graduated from the University of Virginia Medical School in 1928 and went to Seattle, Washington for his internship, having been recruited by the founder of the Virginia Mason Hospital, James Mason. He continued his training under Mason and remained as a member of the medical staff. Concomitantly, he went on to train at the Mayo Clinic in Rochester, Minnesota, and at the Lahey Clinic in Boston. Returning to Seattle, he became Chief of Surgery at the Virginia Mason Clinic, a position he held for 34 years. He was a champion of medical education and research and founded the department's general surgery residency program. He published 136 papers, including landmark articles on techniques and new instruments that carry his name (e.g., Baker tube and anastomosis). He served as President of the American College of Surgeons and was awarded honorary fellowship in the Royal College of Surgeons of England and Scotland. In his capacity as Inspector General of the United States Army, Navy, and Air Force, he was awarded the Outstanding Civilian Service Medal by the United States Army. Baker died on July 4, 1999. (With appreciation to Richard C. Thirlby, M.D. and to John Baker; photograph courtesy of Virginia Mason Medical Center, Seattle, WA.)

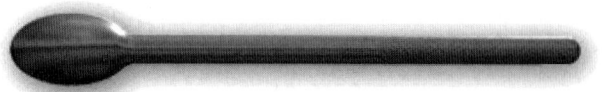

FIGURE 23-85. Ethicon sizer, available in three diameters. (Courtesy of Ethicon Endo-Surgery, Inc., Cincinnati, Ohio.)

addition of a Cheatle cut if necessary to deal with the luminal discrepancies (see Figure 22-56) or the circular stapling device can be employed.

One modification, however, is worth describing, that of restoring intestinal continuity by means of a double-stapling technique to create a side-to-end anastomosis (Figure 23-110). The detachable anvil is inserted in the open proximal bowel, and the end is closed. Anastomosis is effected in the manner just described.[398]

Another method of accomplishing an anastomosis is to close the rectal stump and to perform what is essentially a low side-to-side anastomosis with the gastrointestinal anastomosis or PLC instrument (Figure 23-111).

I have had no experience with this modification and can see no particular advantage in employing it.

Comment

There is little doubt that the various stapling techniques can permit a secure anastomosis. The savings in time, albeit limited, as well as the reduced risk of injury from needles in this AIDS-conscious environment, will inevitably lead to almost complete replacement of conventional suturing for the great majority of surgeons performing low pelvic surgery. Fazio has outlined what are the important principles for minimizing complications related to the use of staplers.[206] I believe it is worth restating them here:

- Use the largest-caliber instrument that the anastomosis will accommodate.
- Place the purse-strings so that excessive bulk of tissue does not appear around the shaft.
- Ensure that the purse-string can be tightened close to the shaft.

(text continues on page 84)

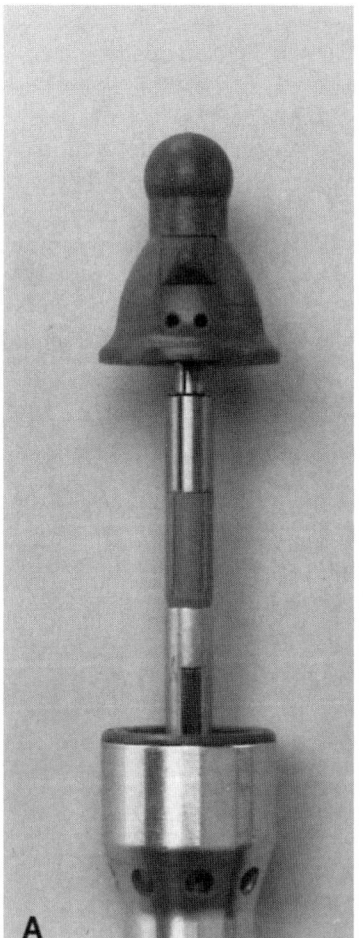
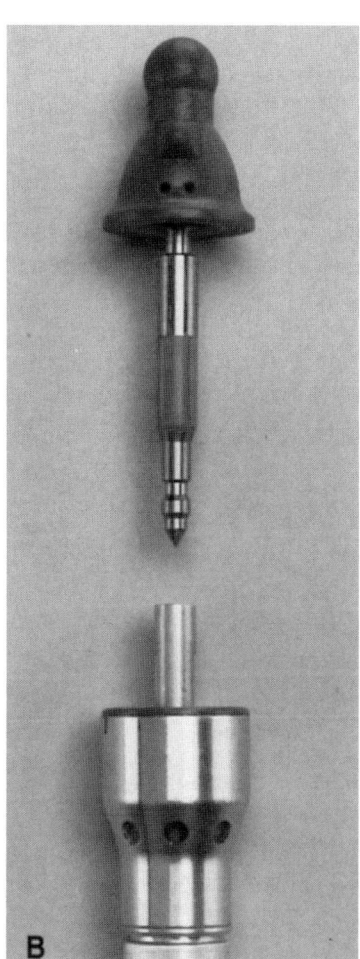
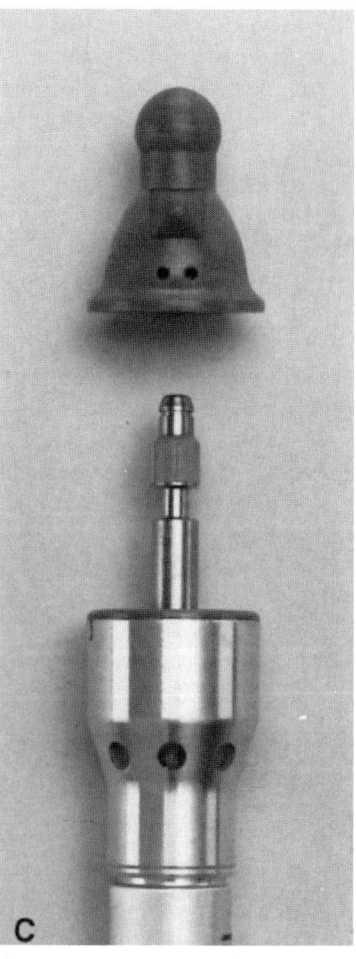

FIGURE 23-86. CEEA instrument. **(A)** Center rod advanced. **(B)** Anvil attached to the separated extension rod. **(C)** Anvil completely detached. (Courtesy of United States Surgical Corp, Norwalk, CT.)

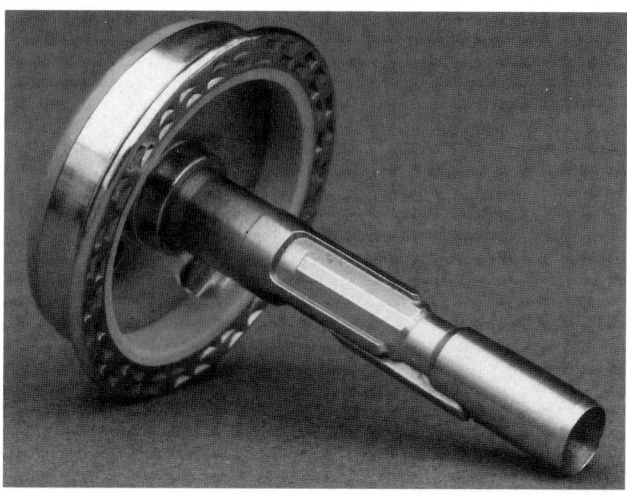

FIGURE 23-87. Low-profile anvil of the Proximate ILS curved intraluminal stapler detachable head. (Courtesy of Ethicon Endo-Surgery, Inc., Cincinnati, Ohio.)

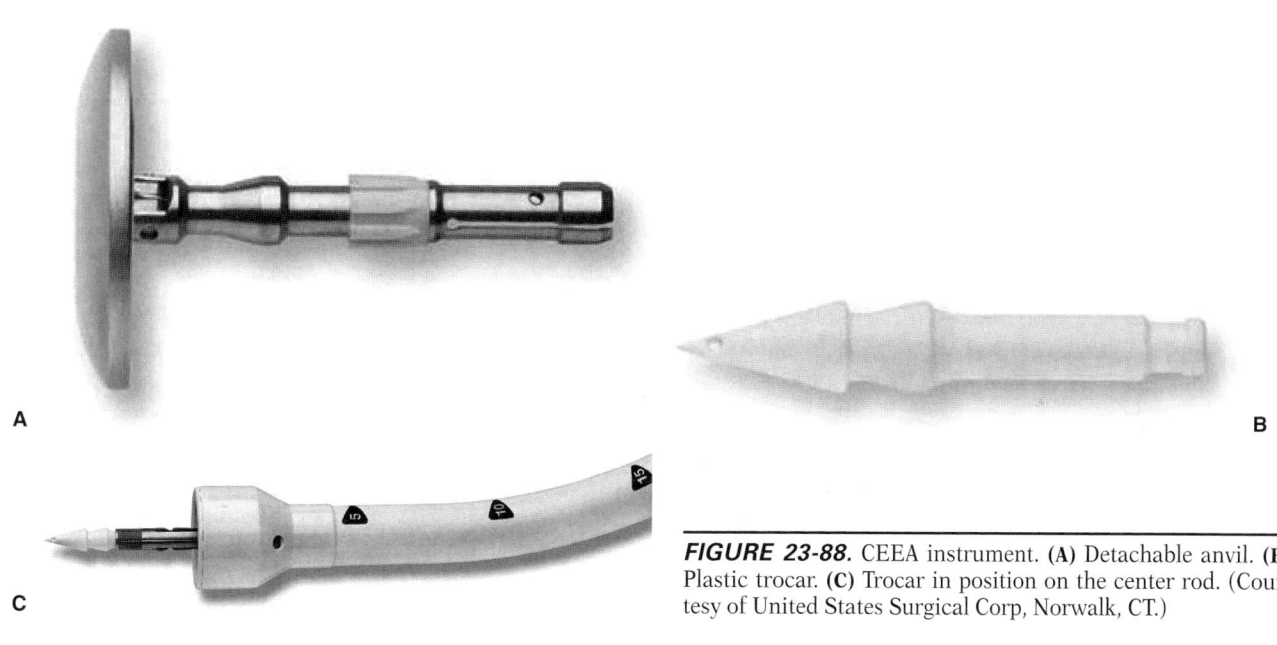

A

B

C

FIGURE 23-88. CEEA instrument. **(A)** Detachable anvil. **(B)** Plastic trocar. **(C)** Trocar in position on the center rod. (Courtesy of United States Surgical Corp, Norwalk, CT.)

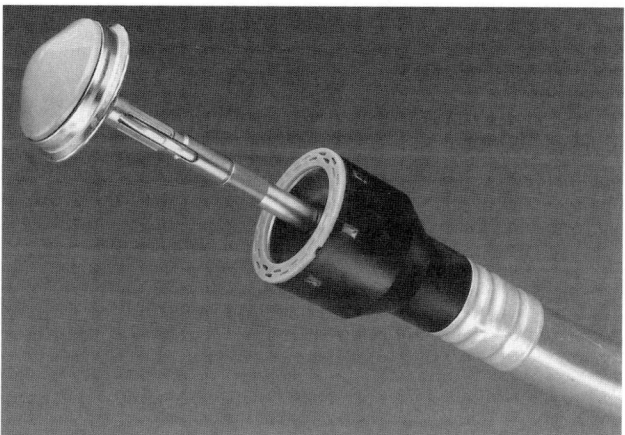

FIGURE 23-89. Proximate ILS curved intraluminal stapler with detachable head and low-profile anvil. (Courtesy of Ethicon, Inc., Cincinnati, Ohio.)

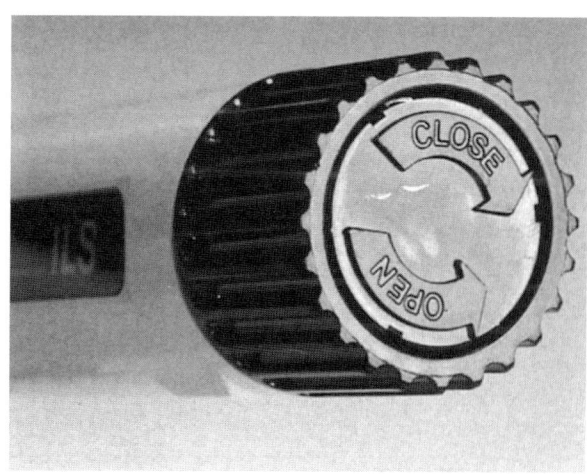

FIGURE 23-90. Close-up view of adjusting knob of the Proximate ILS stapler. (Courtesy of Ethicon, Inc., Cincinnati, Ohio.)

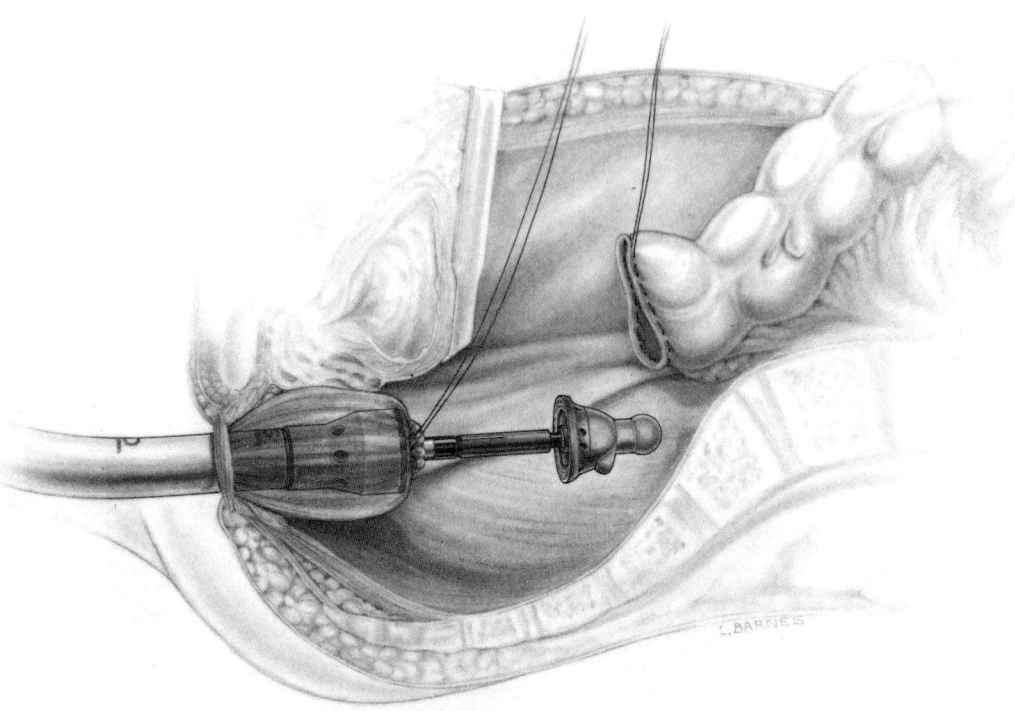

FIGURE 23-91. Circular stapled anastomosis instrument is inserted through the anus, and the distal purse-string is secured.

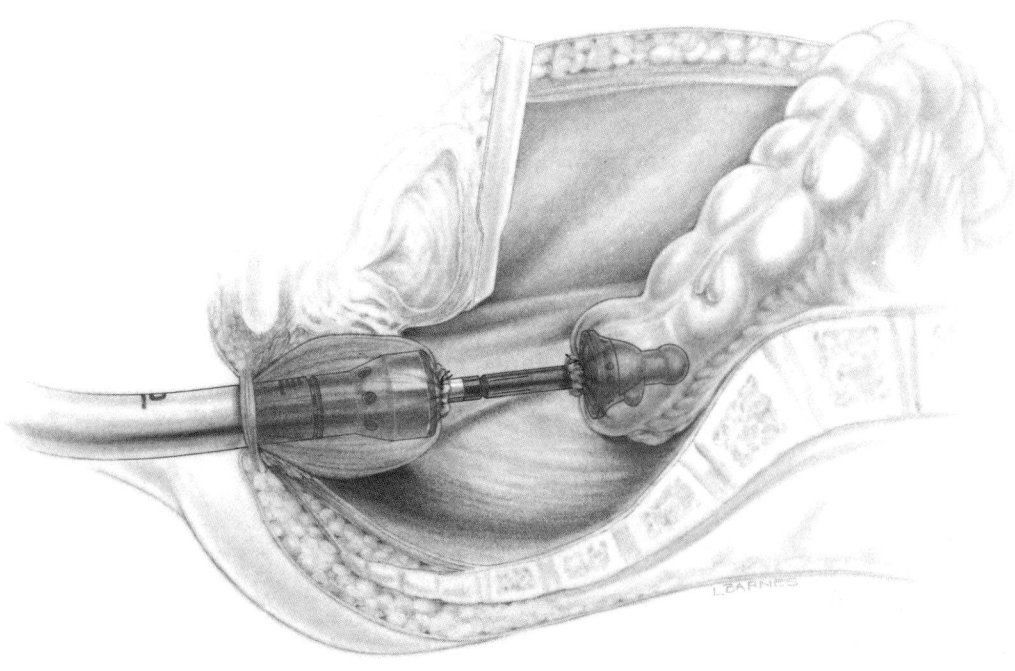

FIGURE 23-92. Circular stapled anastomosis. Proximal and distal purse-string sutures are secured.

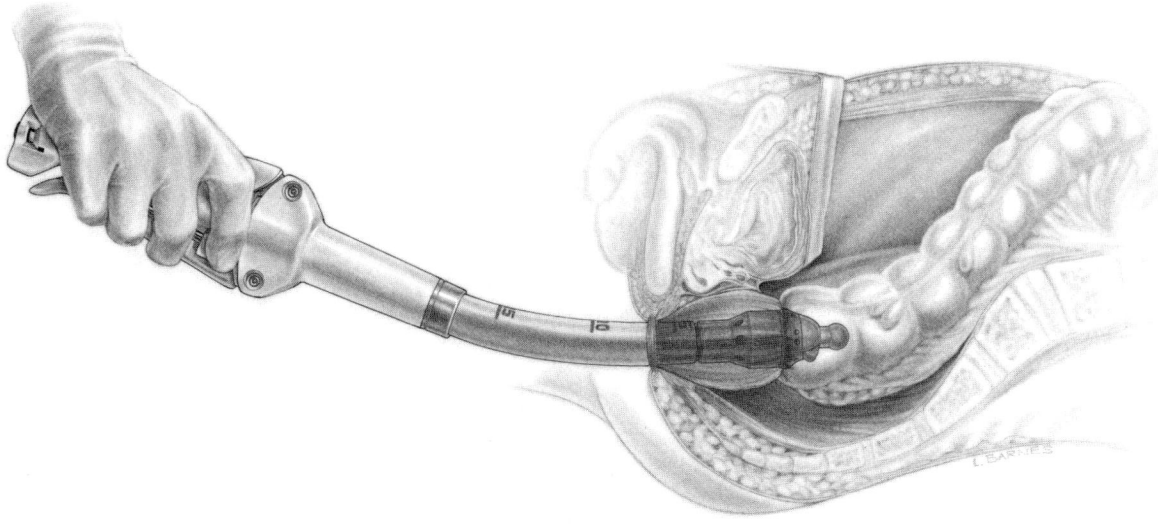

FIGURE 23-93. Circular stapled anastomosis. The instrument is fired after the ends of the bowel have been approximated.

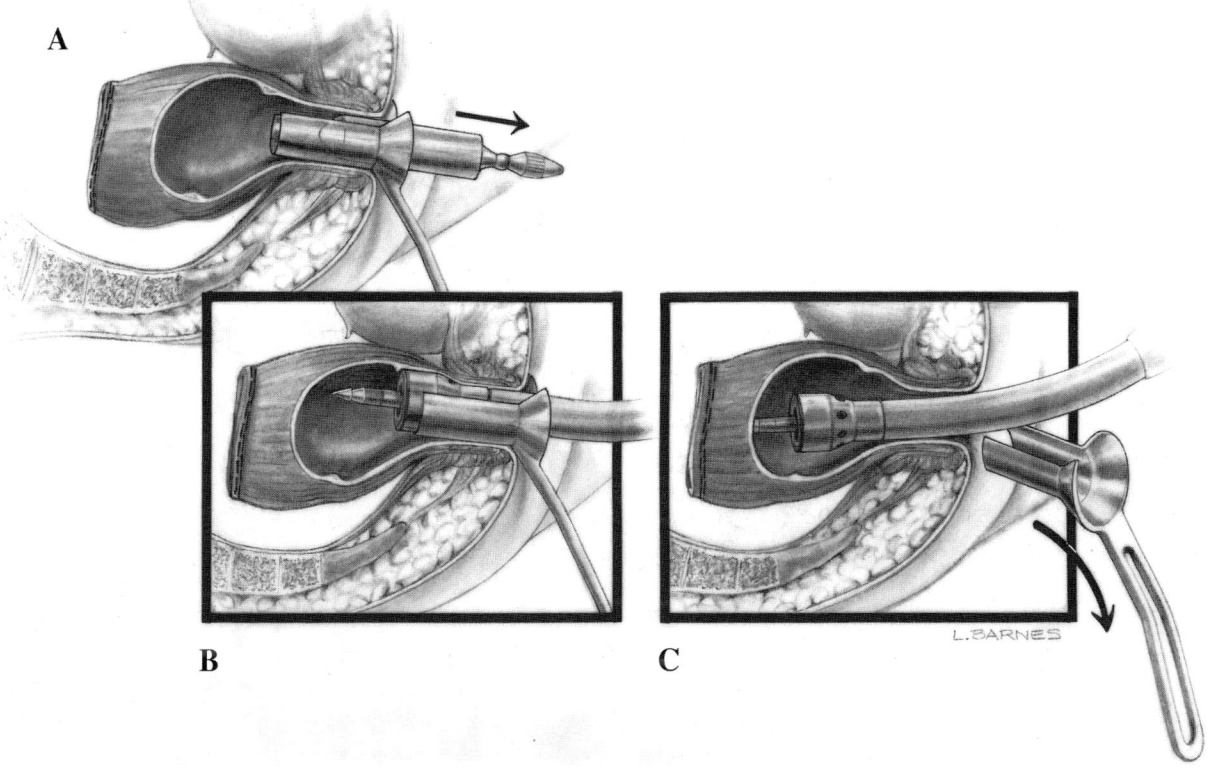

FIGURE 23-94. **(A)** Placement of the Faensler anoscope. **(B)** This facilitates insertion of the circular stapling instrument. **(C)** The instrument is then withdrawn before anastomosis. This is illustrated with the double-stapling anastomosis, but it can be used to equal advantage with other stapling approaches. (Adapted from Khoury DA, Opelka FG. Anoscopic-assisted insertion of end-to-end anastomosing staplers. *Dis Colon Rectum* 1995;38:553.)

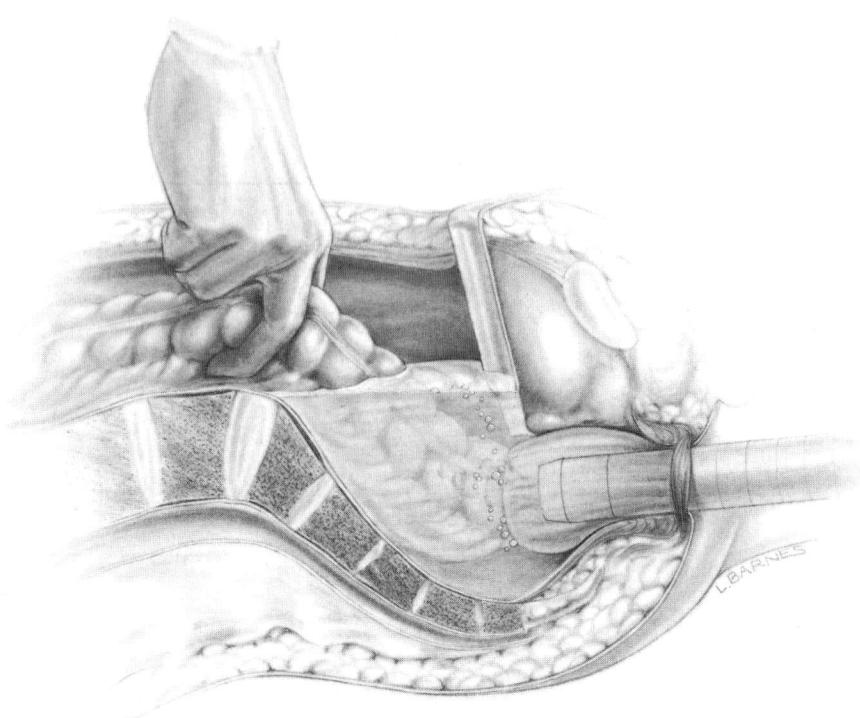

FIGURE 23-95. Method of testing for integrity of low rectal anastomosis. Inspection can be achieved by means of the rigid sigmoidoscope. By compression of the proximal bowel with the fingers or a noncrushing clamp, and by the insufflation of air with saline in the pelvis, bubbles may be seen to escape from a leak. The site can than be identified and possibly repaired.

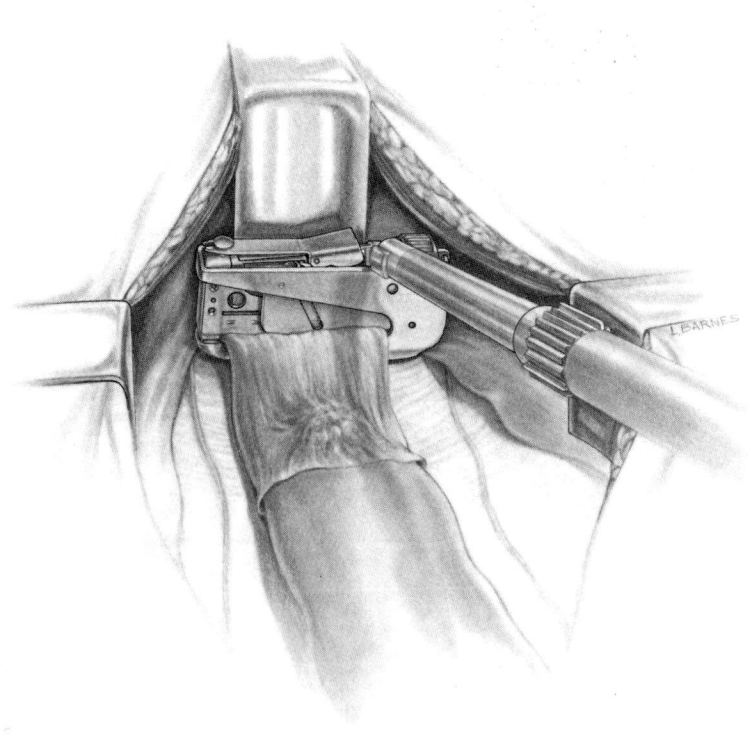

FIGURE 23-96. Double-stapling anastomosis. Closure of the distal rectum with linear stapler (Roticulator United States Surgical Corporation. Norwalk, CT). This instrument can be rotated in all three planes to permit accessibility to the low pelvis.

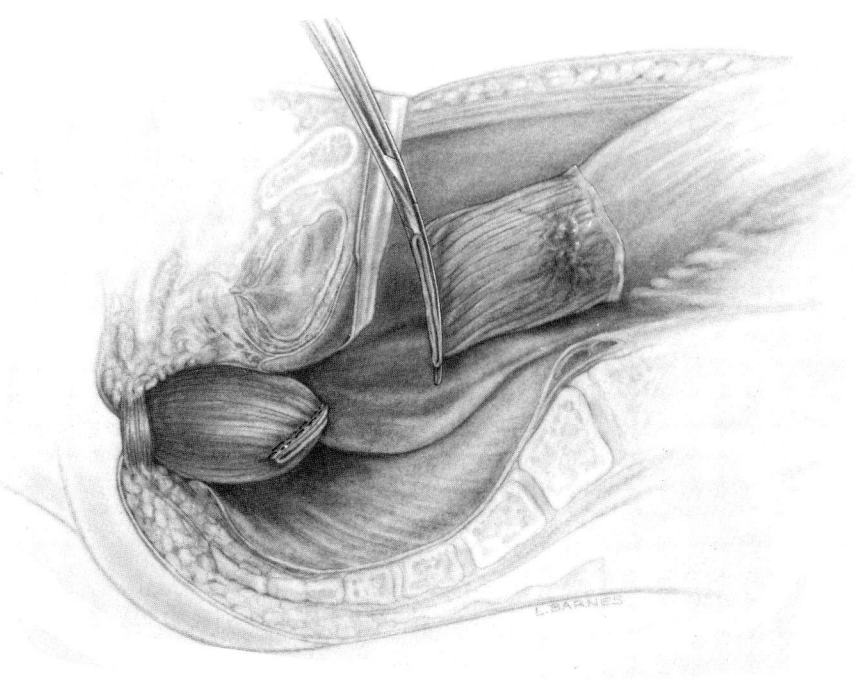

FIGURE 23-97. Double-stapling anastomosis. Rectal stump is closed.

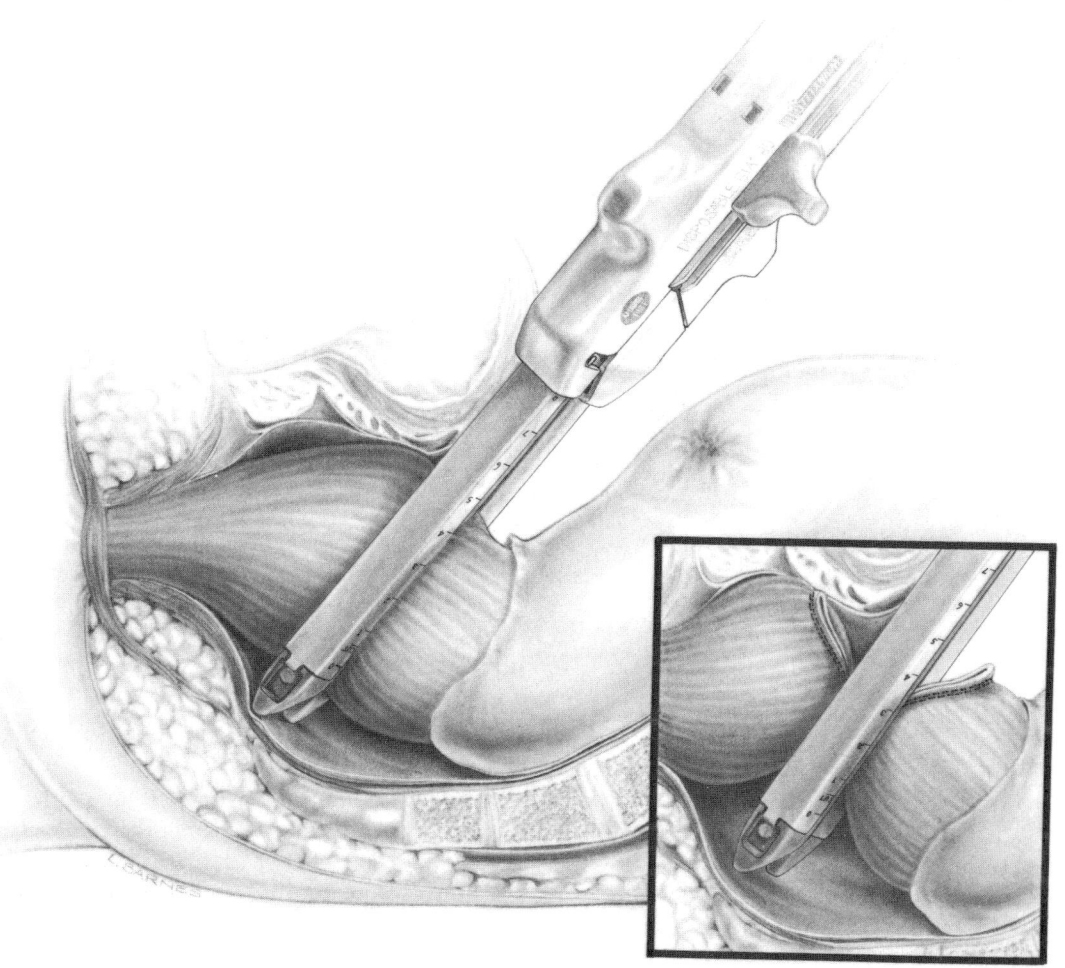

FIGURE 23-98. Closure of a rectal stump by means of the GIA90 instrument. This is optimally accomplished by placing the instrument in an anteroposterior direction. (Adapted from Eisenstat TE, Rubin RJ, Salisti EP, et al. New method for low transection of the rectum. *Dis Colon Rectum* 1990;33:346, with permission.)

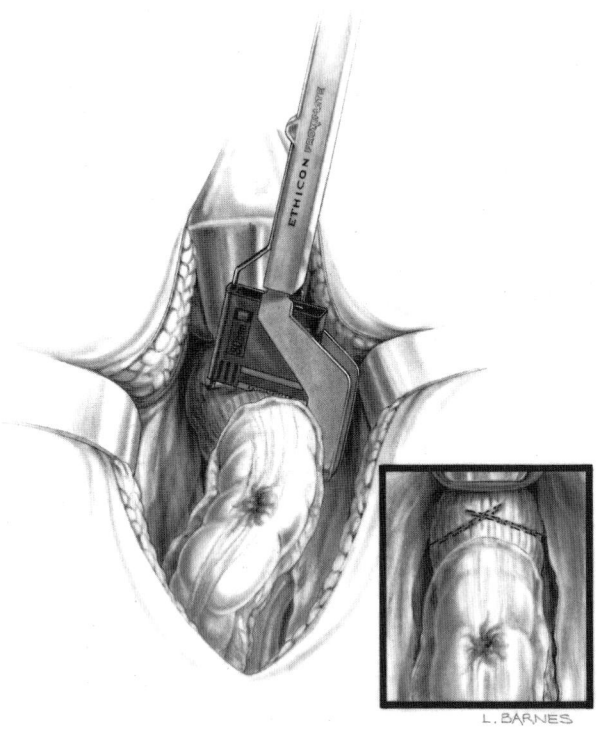

FIGURE 23-99. Application of a 30-mm linear stapler to the distal rectum in preparation for a double-stapled anastomosis. The staple lines are overlapped. This can be accomplished by application from either side **(inset)**, or the bowel may be divided partway before the second application.

- Reinforce the purse-string if one is concerned about the possibility of a gap.
- Use the detachable anvil shaft, especially if faced with a "formidable" pelvis.
- Repair any identified defect.
- Failure to effect a satisfactory repair mandates a diverting colostomy.[206]

I will add one personal caveat—if the surgeon is unhappy with the status of the anastomosis, take it down and do it over!

Concomitant Stoma (Colostomy or Ileostomy)

The decision whether to perform a protective colostomy or ileostomy at the time of low anterior resection is often not a matter of objective analysis but one of emotion. "The operation was technically difficult to perform, there was considerable blood loss, the tumor was stuck in the pelvis, the patient had multiple medical problems, metastases were present, metastases weren't present, the anastomosis looked tenuous, there was some tension on the suture line, I didn't feel good about it, I'll be able to sleep better tonight"—all are reasons expressed for protecting the anastomosis with a transverse colostomy or loop ileostomy. Karanjia and colleagues believe that diversion of the fecal stream should be routinely applied for any individual who undergoes an anastomosis at 6 cm or lower.[403] Others suggest that selective defunctioning of low rectal anastomoses can produce lower rates of anastomotic breakdown while limiting the morbidity associated with a temporary stoma.[285]

Probably the most common reason for subsequent anastomotic complications is tension on the suture line. This may compromise healing, not only because of distraction of the anastomosis itself, but also because of vascular insufficiency (Figure 23-112). Although mobilizing the splenic flexure is, in my opinion, usually unnecessary in the performance of a low anterior resection, every effort must be made to free the proximal bowel so that there is no tension. Placing the omentum around the anastomosis also helps to minimize the risk of leak (see earlier discussion).

If the foregoing precautions are taken, proximal diversion is usually unnecessary. Pelvic sepsis, excessive blood loss, immunocompromised status (e.g., high-dose steroids), radiated field, other systemic disease and poor nutritional status, however, are relative indications for protecting the anastomosis. If the patient is believed to have limited survival, however, APR or Hartmann's resection may be preferable to exposing the patient to the risk of an anastomotic complication. By creating a sigmoid colostomy rather than a more difficult-to-manage transverse colostomy or even ileostomy, better palliation may be achieved.

It is generally believed that a temporary stoma is avoided more often if a stapled anastomosis is created than if a hand-sewn technique is used.[789] This may reflect a greater confidence in the uniform technique offered by a mechanical device when compared with the variability associated with the manual placement of each suture. Fielding and colleagues reported a prospective multicenter study of the management of more than 2,000 patients who had elective colorectal anastomoses.[211] Of these, approximately 16% underwent a synchronous protective colostomy. Although the anastomotic leak rate was high in patients with a stoma, no overall differences were observed in mortality between those patients who had a stoma and those who did not.[211] The problem, of course, with this type of analysis is that there is considerable variation with respect to one surgeon's judgment and technical proficiency and another's. The routine use of proximal colostomy with low anterior resection has been shown through a number of reports to reduce mortality of anastomotic septic and fistula complications.[275,503,534,735] Clearly, even though the incidence of anastomotic leak with and without fecal diversion is identical, the significance of the leak carries a different valence if fecal diversion has been accomplished. Obviously, whenever a sur-

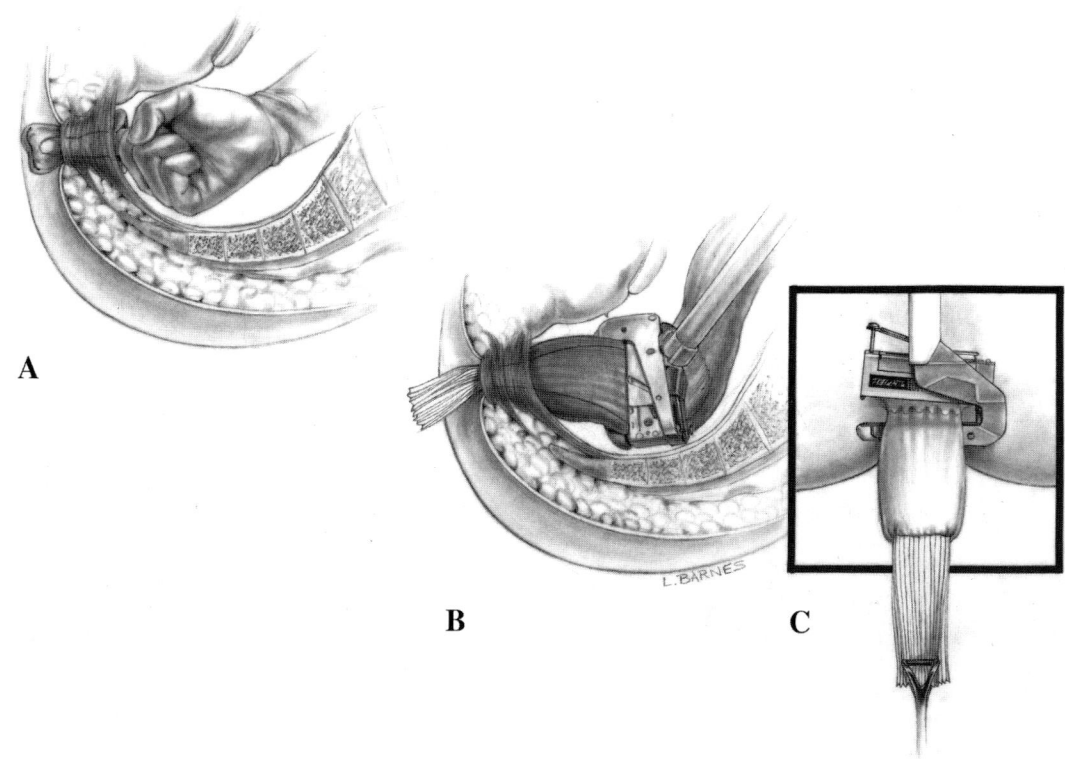

FIGURE 23-100. Eversion technique to facilitate anastomosis utilizing the double-stapling approach. **(A)** Manual eversion. **(B)** Eversion after insertion of a corrugated rubber drain. **(C)** Application of a linear stapler distal to the initial stapling to permit resection and very low anastomosis. (Adapted from Scotté M, Ténière P, Planet M, et al. Eversion of the rectum: a simplified technical approach to ileoanal anastomosis. *Dis Colon Rectum* 1995;38:96.)

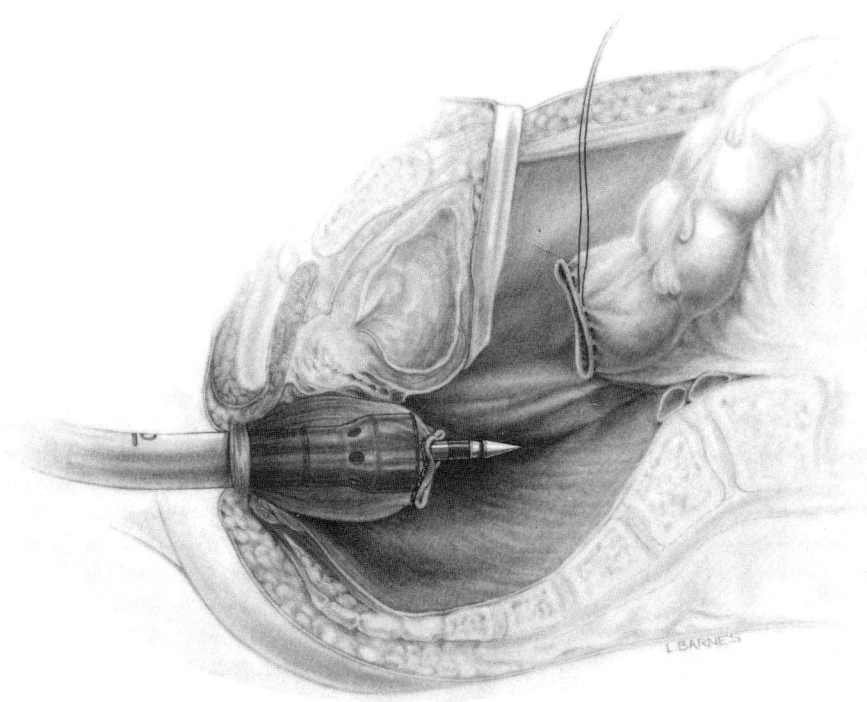

FIGURE 23-101. Double-stapling anastomosis. CEEA with a trocar tip penetrates the closed rectum at or adjacent to the linear staple line.

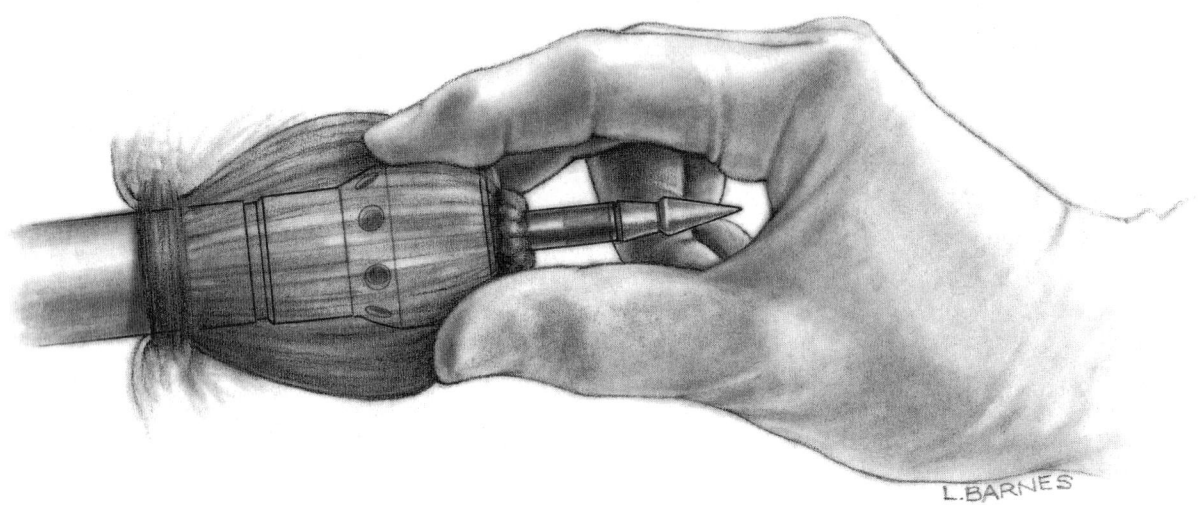

FIGURE 23-102. The surgeon's hand helps to direct the site where the trocar penetrates the rectal stump. This buttresses the bowel, thereby limiting the likelihood of tearing.

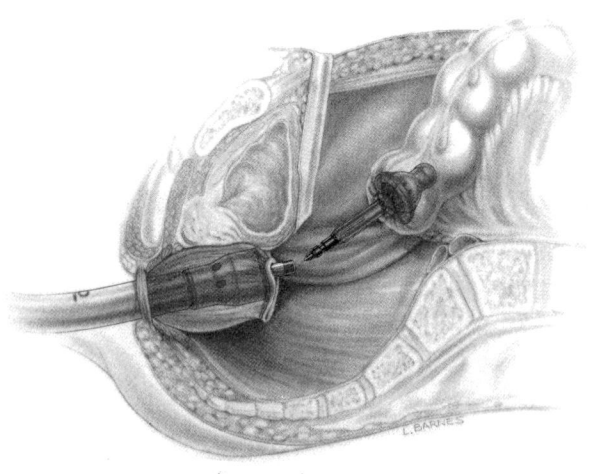

FIGURE 23-103. Double-stapling anastomosis. Detachable shaft and anvil secured into proximal colon.

geon must reoperate on the patient with an anastomotic leak, it is axiomatic that he or she wishes that fecal diversion had been performed initially (see later discussion on anastomotic leak).

Whether preferentially to employ diversion with a transverse colostomy or an ileostomy is a subject that has undergone quite a transition since the mid-1980s. Loop transverse colostomy had been the routine operation for proximal diversion because left-sided anastomoses have been undertaken, but today most colon and rectal surgeons prefer a loop ileostomy. The reasons for this choice are many. First, surgeons now know how to do a proper loop ileostomy, and they have discovered that it is indeed fully diverting. Second, transverse colostomies are more offensive—located in the epigastrium, foul-smelling, more likely to lead to parastomal hernia, and tending to prolapse. Third, experienced surgeons have found that creation of an ileostomy is technically easier to accomplish than a loop colostomy, especially in the obese patient. One can always perform a loop ileostomy; the same is not always true of a loop colostomy. Finally, with the excellent appliances currently available, loop ileostomy, being placed in the hypogastrium, being much less odorous, and being straightforward to close, make this operation

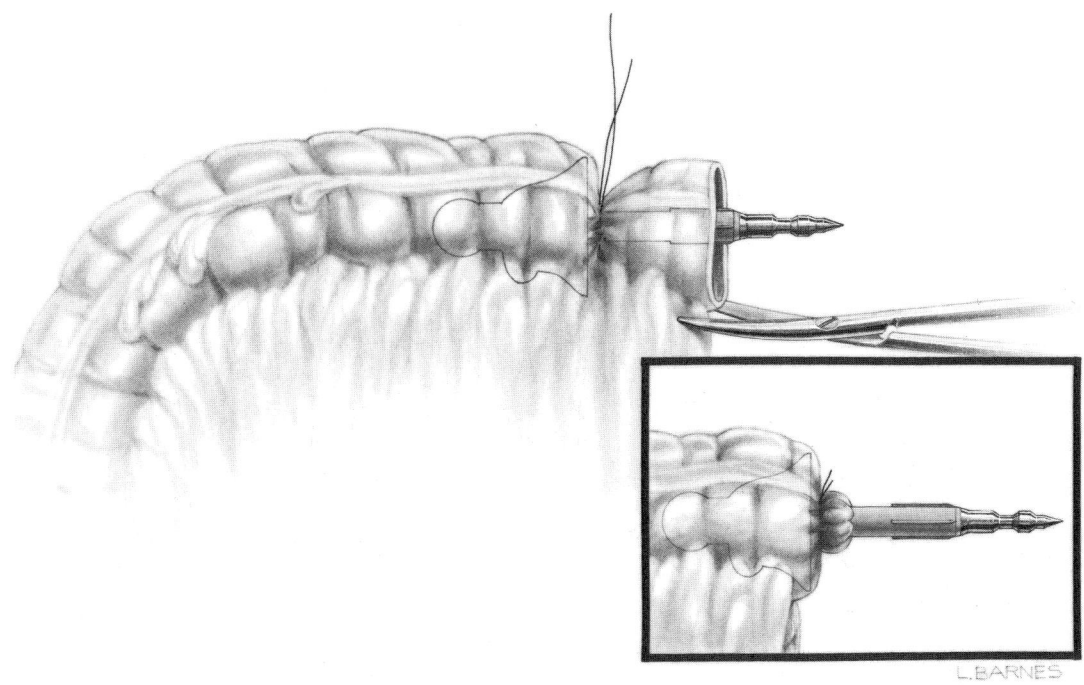

FIGURE 23-104. Expeditious method for securing the proximal anvil with ligation of the bowel around the anvil, followed by debridement of the excess mesentery.

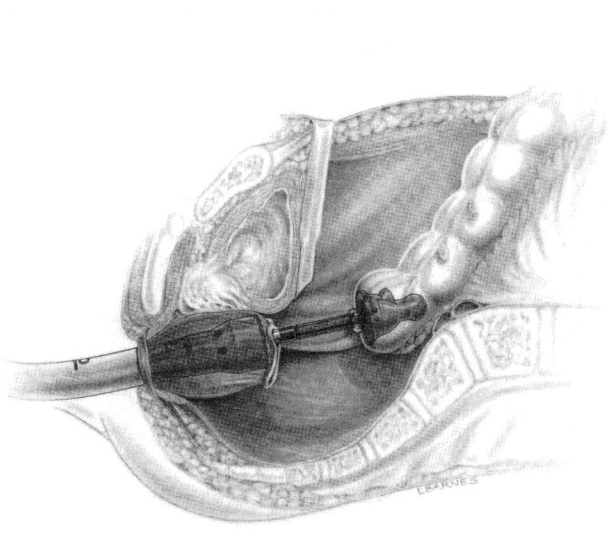

FIGURE 23-105. Double-stapling anastomosis. Anvil shaft reattached to the center rod in preparation for closure.

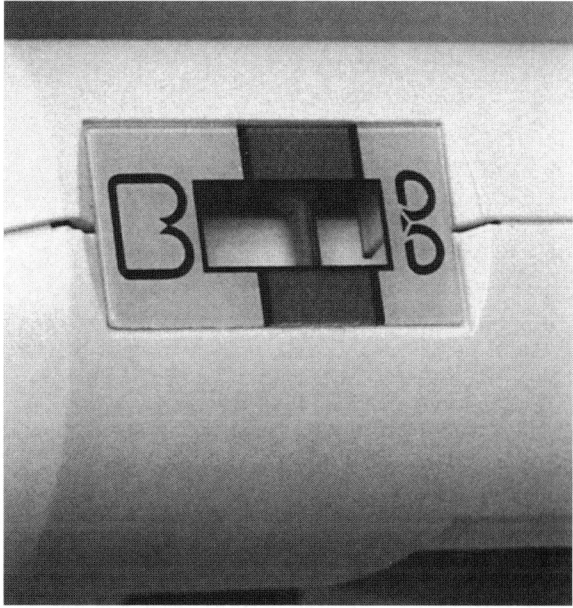

FIGURE 23-106. Close-up view of gap-setting scale, which indicates the proper position of the ends of the bowel prior to firing the instrument. (Courtesy of Ethicon, Inc., Endo-Surgery, Inc., Cincinnati, Ohio.)

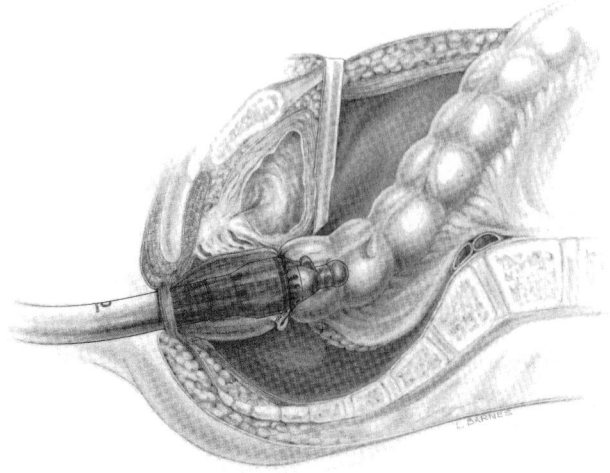

FIGURE 23-107. Completion of double-stapling anastomosis.

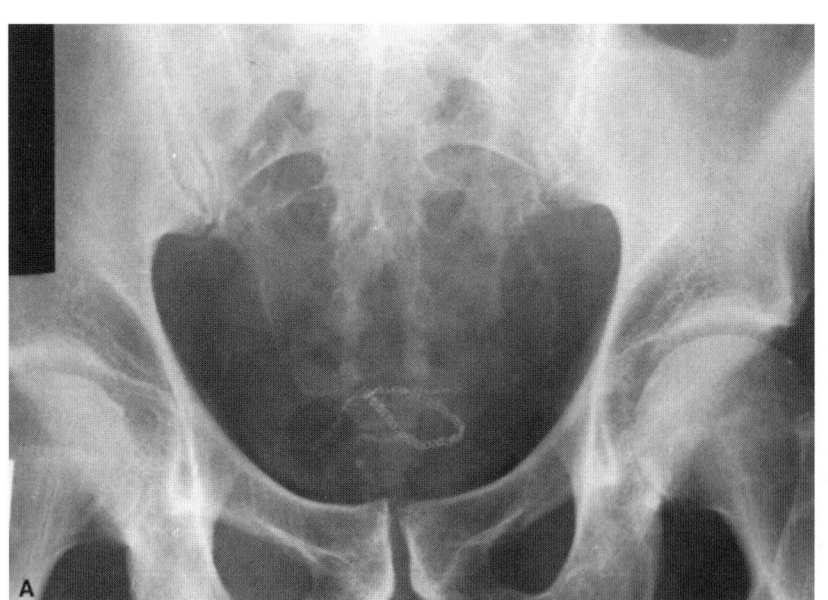
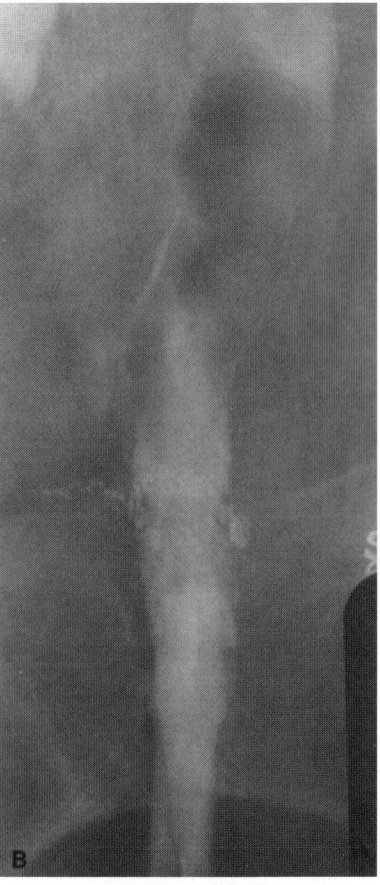

FIGURE 23-108. Double-stapling technique. **(A)** Intersecting staple lines can be seen on plain abdominal film. **(B)** Barium enema study of another patient with anastomosis by this technique reveals neither narrowing nor extravasation.

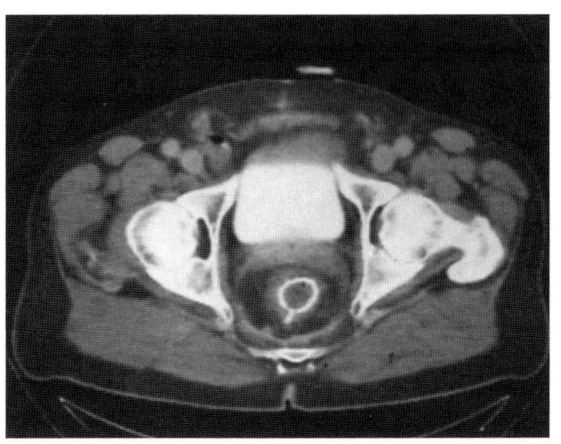

FIGURE 23-109. Computed tomography of the pelvis reveals linear and circular staples.

determination of the factors preoperatively that contribute to the subsequent development of anastomotic leakage will facilitate the intraoperative decision (Table 23-9). The techniques for creating and closing a transverse colostomy and loop ileostomy are discussed in Chapter 31.

Postoperative Care

Postoperative care following low anterior resection is essentially the same as that for any operation on the colon and the same. Prophylactic use of a nasogastric tube is not advised. An indwelling urinary catheter, however, is suggested for approximately 6 or 7 days. The amount of

(text continues on page 92)

more satisfactory (see further discussion in Chapters 31 and 32).

Ravo and Ger and others have tried to avoid a colostomy by performing an intracolonic bypass using a specially prepared soft tube (see Chapter 26).[674,694,706,893] This option, however, is not available in the United States.

There has been some evidence to suggest that fecal diversion is accompanied by depression of collagen turnover in the wall of the excluded colon.[68] It is, therefore, possible that the presence of a stoma proximal to an anastomosis may actually contribute to or cause breakdown. However, in controlled animal studies with and without a proximal colostomy, Senagore and colleagues demonstrated no significant difference in anastomotic blood flow, inflammatory scores, incidence of leak or stenosis, and bursting pressure.[744] They concluded that neither the presence of a proximal colostomy nor the choice of technique contributed any adverse effects to anastomotic healing. There is no question, however, that prolonged defunctioning of the rectum does result in mucosal hypoplasia and a transient, reversible, diversion colitis (see Chapter 33).[17]

Overall morbidity rates in our experience were 21% for colostomy construction and 49% for colostomy closure.[581] Although the morbidity of colostomy closure has decreased, it is still an important concern (see Chapter 31). Closure of the colostomy without resection produces the lowest incidence of complications when compared with other types of closure. If a colostomy is created, the interval between creation and closure should be at least 6 weeks. The longer the subsequent closure is deferred, the safer the procedure will be (Table 23-8).

Obstructed or perforated tumors are associated with a high incidence of anastomotic breakdown. Therefore, the advisability of performing a proximal stoma or delaying the anastomosis for a later time should be considered. The

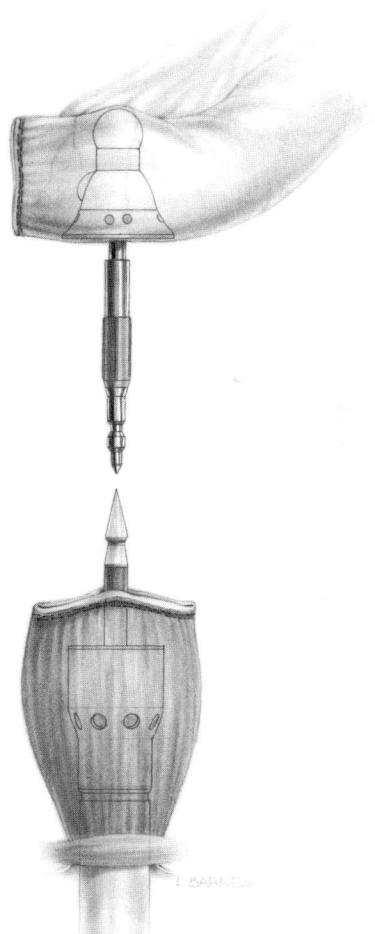

FIGURE 23-110. Side-to-end ileorectal anastomosis by the double-stapling method. Proximal anvil is inserted in open ileum and passed through the antimesenteric wall. The distal ileum is closed, and the stapling completed in the usual manner. The same principle can be applied to the colon, but this is rarely necessary.

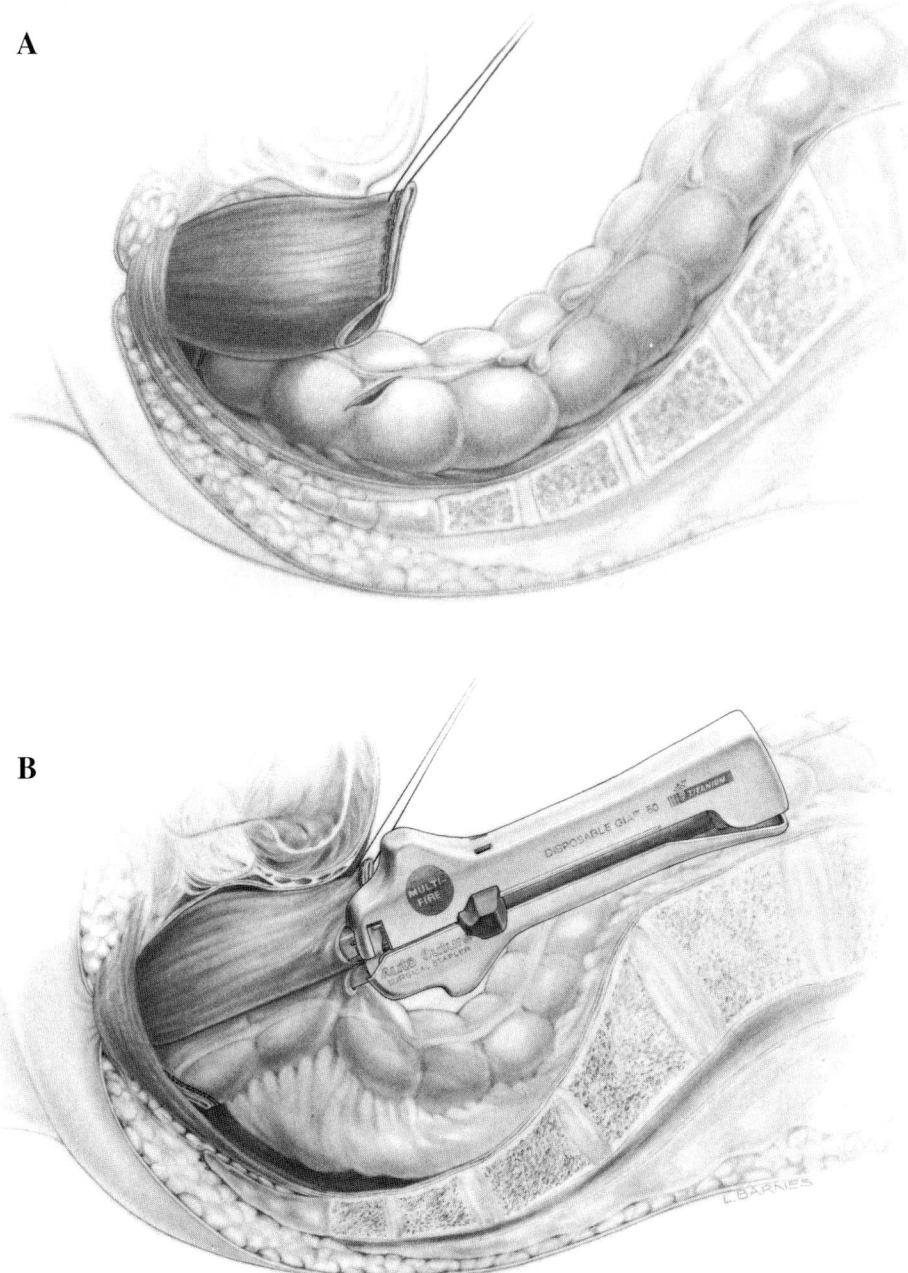

FIGURE 23-111. "Bayonet" anastomosis. **(A)** The proximal bowel is delivered low in the pelvis following closure of the rectal stump. Two small enterotomies are created. **(B)** Each limb of the gastrointestinal anastomosis instrument is inserted, and the instrument is fired. **(C)** The defect is closed by hand sewing. (Adapted from Ravitch MM, Steichen FM. Staples and staplers. *Adv Surg* 1983;17:241, with permission.) *(CONTINUED)*

C

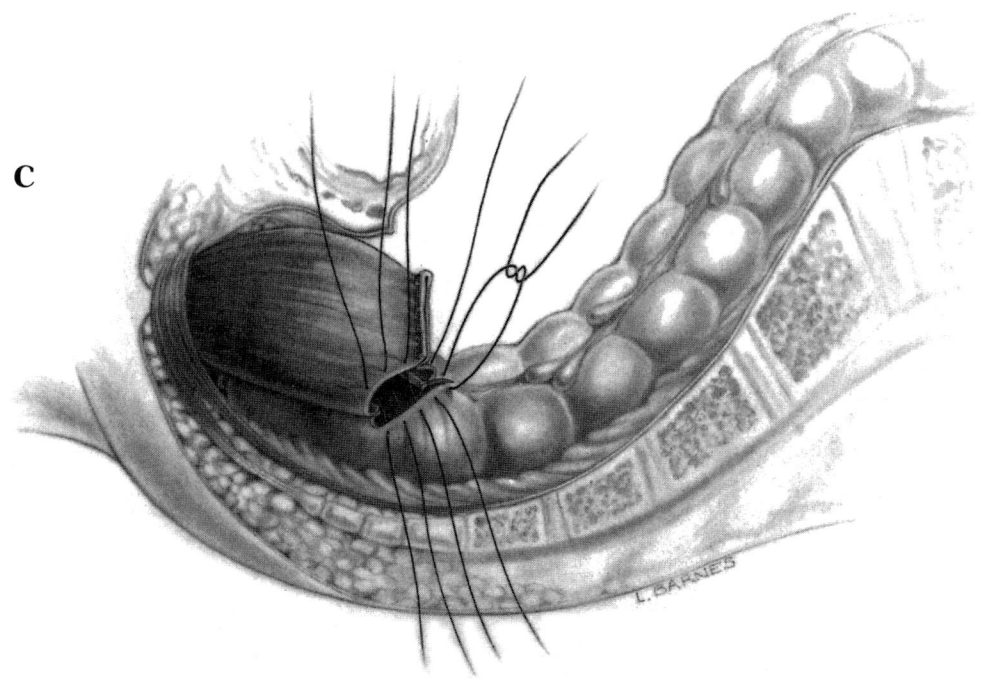

FIGURE 23-111. *(CONTINUED)*

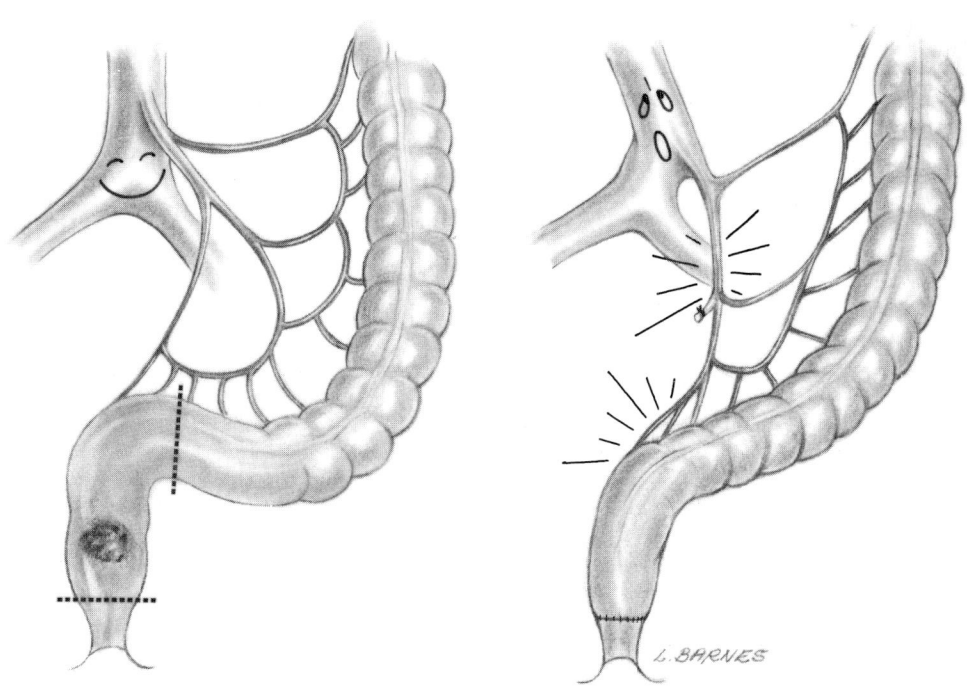

FIGURE 23-112. The etiology of anastomotic leaks: tension on the suture line with vascular compromise. (Suggested by John A. Coller, M.D.)

▶ **TABLE 23-8** Interval between Colostomy and Closure and Its Relation to Complications

Interval (mo)	Number of Patients	Number with Complications	Percentage with Complications (%)
0–3	41	21	51.2
4–6	35	12	34.2
7–12	26	9	34.6
>12	16	3	18.8
Total	118	45	—

(From Mirelman D, Corman ML, Veidenheimer MC, et al. Colostomies—indications and contraindications: Lahey Clinic experience, 1973–1974. *Dis Colon Rectum* 1978;21:172, with permission.)

pelvic dissection necessary to excise the rectum and to effect a low anastomosis is equivalent to that required for an APR. A progressive diet is instituted after the patient has passed flatus, or sooner, at the surgeon's discretion. Discharge follows toleration of the diet, and after bowel and bladder functions have been established. This usually requires approximately 6 or 7 days, but with economic concerns being the overriding issue, this is not always possible. Furthermore, with a regimented program of early ambulation, with special attention to pain management and early feeding, discharge from the hospital can be expedited (see Chapter 22).

▶ **TABLE 23-9** Significance of Related Factors in Anastomotic Complications (i.e., Obstruction, Sepsis, and Fistula) in 152 Patients

Factor*	Significance
Atherosclerotic disease	$p < .001$
Anemia	$p < .001$
Anastomosis below the peritoneal reflection	$p < .001$
Obstruction and perforation	$p < .001$
Anastomosis below the closed peritoneum	$p < .005$
Use of drains, anastomosis below the peritoneal reflection	$p < .01$
Diabetes	$p < .019$
Increased age	$p < .02$
Use of drains, entire series	$p < .05$

*The following factors were not significant for anastomotic complications: operative transfusions, $p < .1$; abnormal serum albumin levels, $p < .2$; cancer in the margin of resection, $p < .3$; other organ involvement, $p < .3$; all other abnormal liver function tests, $p < .5$; other colonic disease (diverticulitis, diverticulosis) in specimen, $p < .5$; extent of disease (Dukes), $p < .5$; operative blood loss, $p < .5$; anesthesia time, $p < .5$; gender, $p < .5$; abnormal prothrombin time, $p < .6$. Sample size for history of previous radiation therapy, for use of steroids, and for other debilitating diseases was too small for accurate calculations.

(From Manson PN, Corman ML, Coller JA, et al. Anterior resection for adenocarcinoma: Lahey Clinic experience from 1963 through 1969. *Am J Surg* 1976;131:434, with permission.)

Complications

Intraoperative Complications

With the exceptions of the problems resulting from the creation of a stoma and the perineal wound, the intraoperative complications encountered with a low anterior resection by conventional suture technique are identical to those of APR. Specific intraoperative difficulties related to the use of the stapler include serosal tears, incomplete tissue rings, instrument failure, and difficulty extracting the the instrument.[280,467] The anastomosis may require reconstruction if the problem cannot be addressed by simpler means.

Postoperative Complications

Neurologic and Vascular Complications

Peripheral neuropathy and peripheral vascular occlusion are discussed earlier in this chapter as presumed consequences of the perineolithotomy position as well as other contributing factors. A case of aortic thrombosis following low anterior resection for rectal cancer has been reported.[99]

Anastomotic Bleeding Hemorrhage from the anastomosis is seen in approximately 1% of patients.[523] This may be the result of inadequate hemostasis at the suture line itself or rupture of a hematoma in the pelvis through the posterior wall of the anastomosis. The former situation usually presents within the first 48 hours, whereas the latter may not become apparent for 7 days or more. The problem may be managed expectantly, although one must be concerned about an anastomotic dehiscence. Endoscopic electrocoagulation may be used effectively in the early postoperative period to control anastomotic bleeding.[115] Hemorrhage was at one time thought to be a problem with the single row of staples associated with the early Russian instrument. However, with the double row of interlocking staples, bleeding is an unusual complication.[331]

Cirocco and Golub reviewed the literature and identified 17 patients with postoperative hemorrhage from a combined total of 775 (1.8%) after stapled colorectal anastomoses that required blood transfusion and/or emergency surgery.[115] Nonoperative therapy was successful in 82%. The frequency of this complication is probably more common than is evident from the literature, but the fact that most spontaneously cease and do not go on to anastomotic leak implies that this is a relatively minor concern.

Postoperative Hemorrhage The complication of postoperative intraabdominal hemorrhage as specifically applied to colon surgery is important to consider. Clearly, the decision whether to reoperate rests with the good judgment of the surgeon. Whether this is based upon a fall in the hematocrit, a drop in the blood pressure, or the development of tachycardia, the surgeon should have a low threshold for reexploration, especially in the patient who has undergone colectomy. Waiting for abdominal distension to convince the surgeon as to the appropriateness of operative intervention is a poor idea. Considerable blood must be lost before this becomes evident.

The combination of blood and enteric organisms is an invitation to subsequent intraabdominal sepsis, pelvic abscess, and possible anastomotic leak. However, there is no evidence to suggest that evacuation of a hematoma and irrigation of the abdominal cavity predisposes to the development of a leak. It is better to perform a negative laparotomy (truly, it is never negative) rather than to leave 2 or 3 L of blood within the abdomen.

Prolonged Ileus

See Chapter 22.

Obstruction at the Anastomosis

Obstruction at the anastomosis without evidence of sepsis is not commonly seen, but when colonic ileus is associated with an "intact" ileocecal valve, perforation can result (Figure 23-113). Usually, conservative treatment (nasogastric tube) will suffice; rarely is it necessary to perform a laparotomy. Digital rectal examination may be helpful, but the use of a rectal tube is relatively contraindicated because of the danger of perforating the anastomosis. If unrelieved, this may be one of the rare indications for cecostomy (see Figs. 28-45 and 31-44).

Anastomotic Leak

Anastomotic leak is the greatest fear of every surgeon who performs low anterior resections and is the primary cause of surgically related mortality (Figure 23-114). Numerous factors have been associated including disease of the bowel itself (inflammation), inadequate blood supply, tension on the suture line, inaccurate suture placement, trauma, high-dose steroids, radiated field, and failure to

obtain a watertight seal.[159,325,735] The amount of transfused blood has been determined to be an independent risk factor for postoperative infectious complications.[811] Our results in a study of 152 patients indicate that diseases that affect local blood flow and response to infection (anemia, atherosclerotic disease, and diabetes) are important risk factors (Table 23-9).[523] Others have demonstrated that factors predictive of anastomotic leak include chronic obstructive pulmonary disease, peritonitis, bowel obstruction, malnutrition, use of corticosteroids, and perioperative blood transfusion.[278] Mäkelä and coworkers identified 44 of their patients with left-sided colonic anastomotic leaks and found the following variables to be associated with an increased risk for this complication: malnutrition, weight loss, hypoalbuminemia, cardiovascular disease, two or more underlying diseases, and the use of alcohol.[517] Moreover, they found surgery-related factors to be American Society of Anesthesiologists physical status, operating time greater than 2 hours,

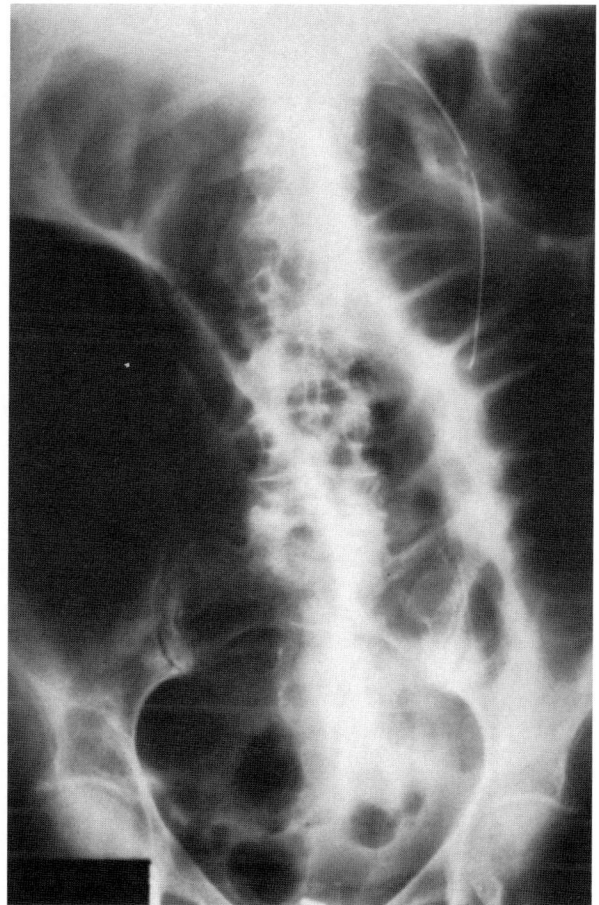

FIGURE 23-113. Colonic ileus. A massively dilated colon (especially the cecum) in a patient who underwent a low anterior resection. With an "intact" ileocecal valve, there is danger of perforation.

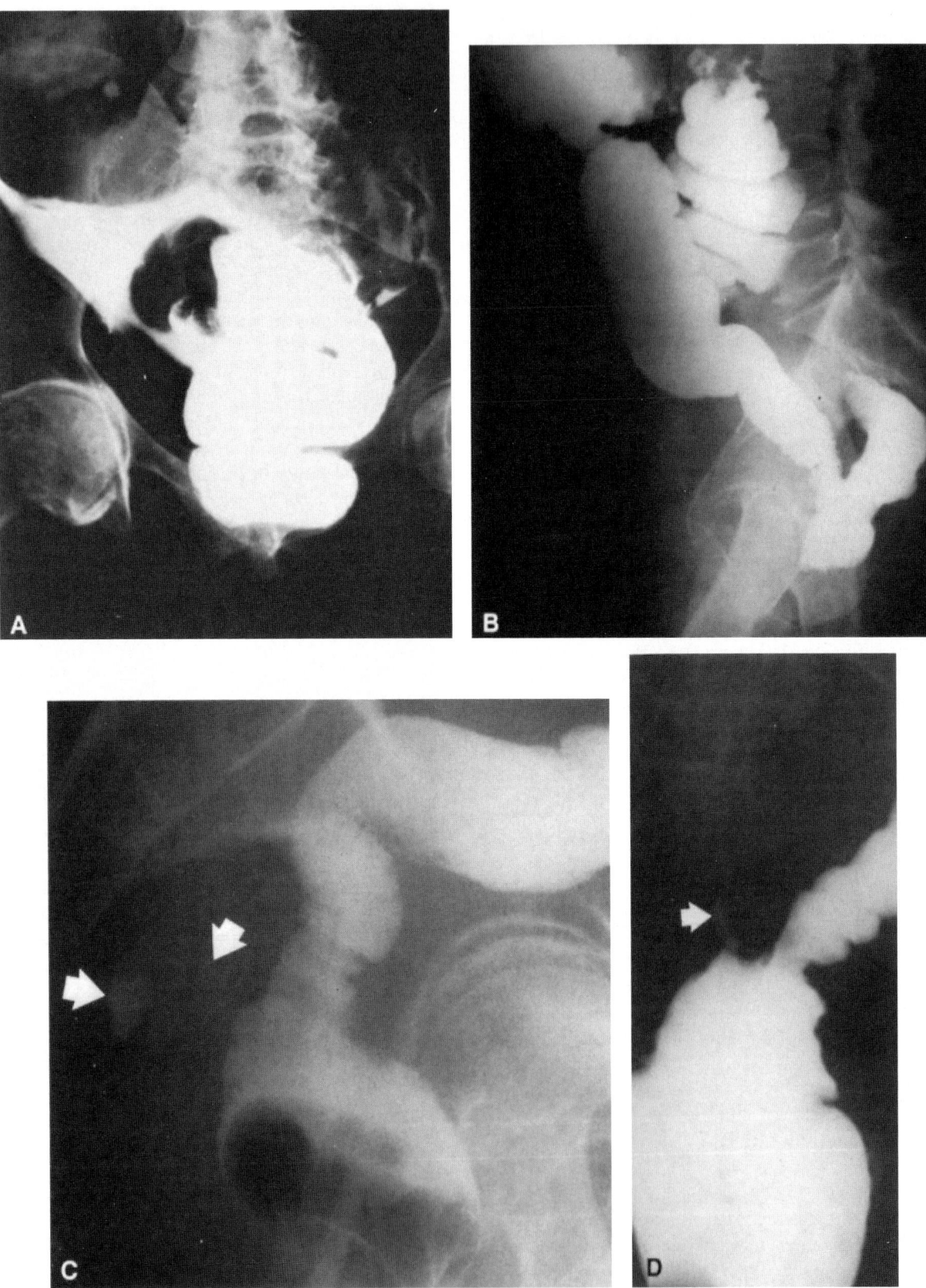

FIGURE 23-114. Anastomotic leaks. **(A)** Gastrografin enema demonstrates extravasation into the pelvis 1 week following anterior resection. **(B)** Large, abscess cavity in presacral space. **(C)** Fistula tract with abscess *(arrows)*. **(D)** Short anastomotic sinus tract *(arrow)*.

multiple blood transfusions, and intraoperative contamination of the operative field.[517] Sørensen and associates noted that smoking and alcohol abuse are major risk factors.[776] Others opined that male sex and level of the anastomosis are the only independent risk factors for the development of anastomotic leakage.[706] It has also been shown that leakage following a colorectal anastomosis, after potentially curative resection, is an independent predictor for local recurrence.[45]

When a leak occurs, it is usually located on the posterior aspect of the anastomosis. Foster and colleagues demonstrated a midline paucity of vessels both anteriorly and posteriorly by means of angiography of cadaver specimens.[219] They suggested that one of the reasons why wrapping the omentum is protective is that neovascularization may be stimulated.

Management Classically, a patient will develop signs of peritoneal irritation, a fever, and leukocytosis on the fourth, fifth, or sixth postoperative day, but the timing and presentation can be quite variable. There is an understandable reluctance on the part of most surgeons to face the possibility that their patient has developed this complication. Denial and rationalization are frequently employed defense mechanisms. Because there is often a coexisting respiratory problem, one may delay needed surgical intervention while the patient is submitted to vigorous pulmonary resuscitative measures. When metabolic acidosis supervenes, however, this is ominous. The fact is if one suspects the possibility of a leak, investigation at the minimum is mandatory.[570]

The preferred study is a water-soluble contrast enema, such as with Gastrografin (the use of barium is contraindicated). This may demonstrate a leak into the abdomen (Figure 23-114*A*) or into the presacral (retrorectal) space (Figure 23-114*D*). However, one does not need to perform such investigations if there is clinical suspicion. Reexploration requires no justification except concern for the possibility of a leak. At the time of reoperation, care should be taken to make certain that drainage of the affected area is adequate, but the anastomosis, itself, should not be taken down. Unless it is completely or at least halfway disrupted, one has a right to assume that eventual healing will take place. A breakdown of 25% of the circumference is most likely to result in uneventful healing. A breakdown of 25% to 50% likely will heal with stricture formation. Greater than 50% breakdown will not heal, however. Attempt at suture repair is usually an exercise in futility, but even if "successful," a proximal colostomy or ileostomy should *always* be performed.

There is the theoretical concern about leaving a stool-filled proximal bowel above a leaking anastomosis. Some think that the patient would, therefore, be better served with conversion to an end-sigmoid colostomy and closure of the rectal stump. However, there is no evidence

to support this contention. What is known, however, is that restoration of continuity following the equivalent of Hartmann's resection is associated with a much higher morbidity and indeed mortality than is closure of a loop ileostomy.

Occasionally, a patient will have an anastomotic leak but will fail to develop abdominal signs and symptoms suggestive of this complication. It is usually evident to the surgeon, however, that the patient is not having an uneventful postoperative course. Fever and leukocytosis should certainly arouse suspicion. Diarrhea, rectal pain, tenesmus, low back pain, and sciatic symptoms may result from an abscess in the presacral space, a consequence of an anastomotic leak. Rectal examination may demonstrate an anastomotic defect, and cautious proctoscopy may confirm the breakdown or the presence of purulent material. CT may demonstrate an abscess and air outside the bowel. If the process is localized, CT-guided drainage by means of a transgluteal, transabdominal, or transvaginal catheter may be employed in the hope that laparotomy and fecal diversion can be avoided (Figure 23-115). In my experience, however, this technique is of value only for those individuals who present at least 10 days after the operation. Almost inevitably, a diversionary procedure will be necessary if the patient develops an abscess during the postoperative period.

Stomal Closure The question of when to close the stoma often arises, especially if there remains evidence of a small leak (Figure 23-114*D*). My own philosophy is to close the ileostomy or colostomy if the tract as demonstrated on the water-soluble enema is relatively short and at least 2 months have elapsed since the original procedure. One cannot argue with the concept of delaying closure for another 4 to 6 weeks and repeating the study, but it is inappropriate to compel the patient to tolerate a stoma for a longer time. Should one wait 6 months or 1 year? Radiologic extravasation may persist indefinitely, but the stoma still can be taken down. If the tract is long or if it continues up into the abdominal cavity, and if such a radiologic appearance fails to improve, repeat resection is advised. The technical details of closing the stoma are discussed in Chapter 31.

Pelvic Abscess In any patient who develops a pelvic abscess after low anterior resection, consideration must be given to the possibility of an anastomotic leak as the proximate cause. This can be determined by CT-guided drainage (Figure 23-115). If feculent material appears at the time or subsequently, anastomotic breakdown must be assumed. This can be confirmed by means of a water-soluble contrast enema. In the absence of systemic signs and symptoms, reoperation may be deferred as long as the drainage can be managed by the patient. If surgical

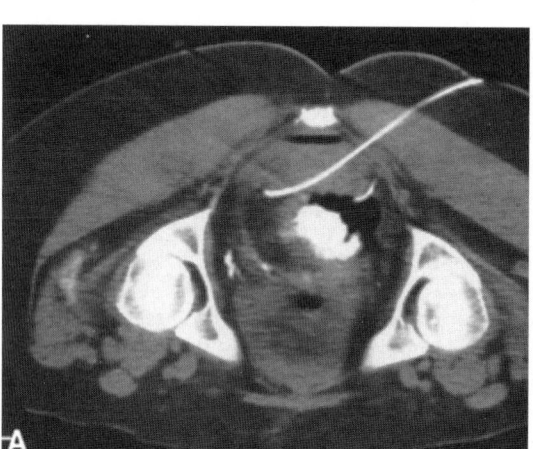
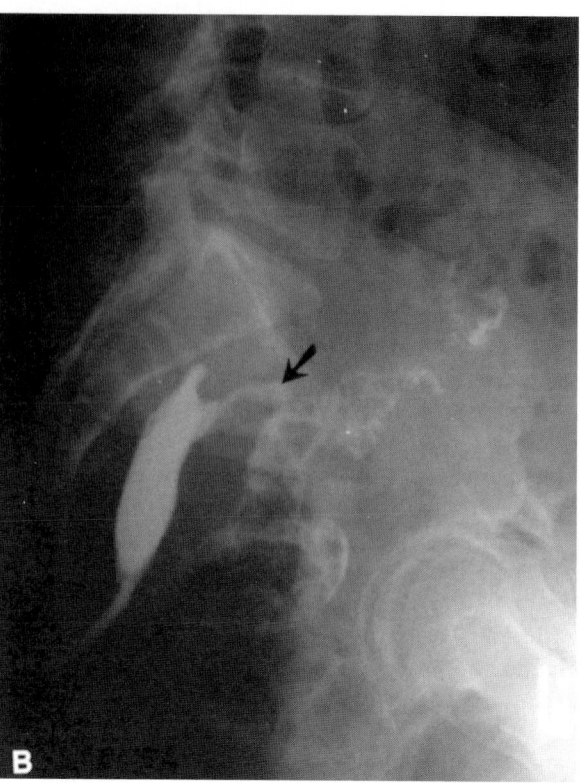

FIGURE 23-115. Anastomotic leak. **(A)** Computed tomography–guided transgluteal drainage. **(B)** Lateral view demonstrates contrast material in the presacral cavity and communication with rectum *(arrow)*.

drainage is required, it is usually accomplished from below (see Figs. 10-14 through 10-16). If signs of peritonitis are present, laparotomy is required for drainage. Concomitant fecal diversion should always be performed under these circumstances irrespective of one's ability to identify a leak.

Fecal Fistula Fecal fistula may develop in the postoperative period as a consequence of an anastomotic leak (see earlier discussion). Usually, this complication requires abdominal drainage and a diversionary procedure. However, if the fistula arises at a later time, perhaps following drainage of an intraabdominal or pelvic abscess, it can often be treated expectantly if there is absence of sepsis and the patient continues to have bowel movements. Without distal obstruction or persistent tumor, the fistula will usually close within a matter of a few weeks. If drainage is excessive, a stomal appliance may be used (see Chapters 31 and 32).

There is no need to limit dietary intake for a colonic fistula. This will not expedite the healing process, and, moreover, outputs generally are not excessive. Total parenteral nutrition and an elemental diet are both costly and unhelpful for patients with a fistula in this location.

If the patient *does* experience quite a bit of drainage, one must be certain of the location of the fistula and that small bowel is not involved. A fistulogram may be helpful. One can limit the amount of drainage through the use of a "slowing" regimen, including codeine, deodorized tincture of opium, and diphenoxylate with atropine (Lomotil) or loperamide (Immodium).

Failure to heal suggests the formation of an epithelialized tract or recurrent tumor. The presence of foreign material is another possibility, and an obstructed anastomosis must be ruled out. When is surgical repair indicated in the absence of sepsis or high output management issues? The answer is when the patient and the surgeon are discomforted by the failure to heal. Personally, I would allow 3 to 6 months for spontaneous healing to occur.

Rectovaginal Fistula Rectovaginal fistula following low anterior resection may result from pelvic sepsis and an anastomotic leak, with spontaneous drainage through the vagina. Transvaginal drainage of a pelvic collection may ultimately yield feculent material. In the absence of sepsis, there is usually no urgency to reoperate on these women, unless the amount of drainage cannot be tolerated. Recurrent urinary tract infections may develop, however (see Chapter 12). Unfortunately, rectovaginal fistulas will spontaneously heal only rarely. This is especially true if the vagina has been incorporated into the staple line (see Fig. 12-XXX).[803] Even with fecal diversion, direct repair or resection of the communication will almost inevitably be necessary. This usually requires repeat resection of the anastomosis.

Anastomotic Leak: Results There is an extensive and somewhat confusing literature on anastomotic leaks. This confusion is based on the difficulty in interpreting one surgeon's experience or one institution's experience with that of another. For example, it is not always clear if the study comingles anastomotic leak results from resections of different parts of the colon and/or rectum. This is critically important when one compares rectal anastomotic data, especially the issue of the level of the anastomosis. Furthermore, when a concomitant stoma is created, this will inevitably obfuscate the results, at least with respect to the incidence of clinically significant leaks. In the past, the complication rate of anastomotic leak following anterior resection was variously reported to be 17% to 77%.[116,159,183,275,325,379,523,591,735,743] More recently, however, studies seem to indicate lower rates (less than 10% to 22%).[94,98,110,334,375,545,706] This change may reflect the more frequent use of the transanal circular stapling technique, in addition to the implementation of intraoperative air testing and direct visualization by means of the sigmoidoscope. This was clearly demonstrated in the prospective trial performed by Beard and colleagues from the Leicester Royal Infirmary in the United Kingdom.[39] There were three clinical leaks (4%) in the "test group", and ten were noted (14%) in the "no test" group. These differences, both for clinical and for radiologic leaks, were statistically significant. For anastomoses below the peritoneal reflection, protection is afforded, as mentioned earlier, if the floor of the pelvis is left open and omental wrapping is employed.

The presence of drains is associated with an increased incidence of anastomotic complications, although when one analyzes published data, it is possible that only less secure anastomoses are drained. However, there is certainly support for the concept that drains adversely affect anastomotic healing.[269,525]

The incidence of anastomotic breakdown following stapled anastomoses has been reported by Heald and Leicester.[331] They noted 13 clinical leaks in 100 stapled anastomoses. They attributed their high breakdown rate primarily to the low level of the anastomosis (all occurred below 7 cm). They caution that blood supply is more adequate if the left colon is fully mobilized and used for the anastomosis rather than the sigmoid colon (conserving the inferior mesenteric artery). In an experience from the same unit with leakage from stapled low anastomoses

after TME, major anastomotic leaks associated with peritonitis or a pelvic collection were identified in 11.0% of patients.[402] An additional 6.4% of patients were found to have minor, asymptomatic leaks that were detected by radiologic study.

The Mayo Clinic group reported a controlled randomized trial.[41] Sixty percent of the hand-sewn anastomoses were considered difficult, whereas only 36% of the stapled anastomoses fell into this category. The time for anastomosis was significantly different for hand-sewn (19 minutes) and stapled (11 minutes; $p = .01$). The authors believed that approximately12% of their patients had the rectum preserved by stapling. Conversely, in a controlled trial of 118 patients reported by McGinn and colleagues, the incidence of clinical leaks with sutured anastomoses was 3% (radiologic, 7%), whereas the rate with the stapled technique was 12% (radiologic, 24%).[550] Other randomized trials comparing the two techniques have failed to demonstrate any statistically significant difference in leakage rate.[40,200,862]

The Cleveland Clinic group reported the results of 125 intestinal anastomoses using the Proximate ILS circular stapler.[208] Radiologic evaluation of 79 patients with Gastrografin demonstrated a leak in three (3.8%). There was only one clinically apparent leak in the series. A more recent report from the same institution comprised more than 1,000 patients who underwent stapled anastomoses.[846] Clinically apparent anastomotic leaks developed in 2.9%, with inapparent anastomotic dehiscence occurring in 7.7%. However, the incidence of anastomotic leaks above the level of 7 cm from the anal verge was only 1%. The authors further concluded that diabetes mellitus, the use of pelvic drains, and the duration of surgery were significantly related to the occurrence of anastomotic leaks.

Docherty and colleagues compared the morbidity associated with manually constructed and stapled anastomoses.[176] In a series of 732 patients, there was a significant increase in radiologic leakage in the sutured group (14.4% versus 5.2%), but there was no difference in clinical anastomotic leak rates, morbidity, or postoperative mortality. Marti and associates reported three clinical and seven radiologic leaks in 79 patients anastomosed with the EEA stapler, and others noted 11 complications in 19 low anterior resections performed with this technique.[532,729] Lack of experience is the suggested reason for the poor results. Eleven anastomotic leaks in 100 patients were reported by Detry and Kestens.[170]

Kennedy and associates experienced a 20% incidence of stapler-related complications in 265 patients.[410] There was a 3% incidence of clinical anastomotic leaks. Antonsen and Kronborg, in a prospective trial of low anterior resection using the EEA instrument with 178 patients, noted a clinical anastomotic leak rate of 15%.[16] Bokey and colleagues noted a clinically significant anastomotic leak rate following anterior resection of 2.9%.[71] Nesbakken and co-workers reported an 18% leak rate following low anterior resection in their 92 patients.[604] Stoma closure was not possible in five of the 17. Issues of concern when compared with those who had not developed this complication were a reduced neorectal capacity (p = .04), more evacuation problems (p = .02), increased fecal urgency (p = .09), and fecal incontinence (p = .06).

Feinberg and colleagues reported the results of 79 patients who underwent low anterior resection by the double-stapling technique.[210] The mean level of the cancer from the dentate line was 9 cm, and the clinical anastomotic leak rate was 8%. Griffen and colleagues observed an anastomotic leak rate of 2.7% with a double-stapling approach applied to 75 patients.[295]

If there is one inarguable conclusion one can make from the plethora of data, it is that the lower the anastomosis, the greater the risk of leak. One must weigh the relative merit of fecal diversion against the encumbrance of a stoma, the morbidity associated with an operation for ostomy closure, and the morbidity and mortality of reoperation for an anastomotic leak. This decision inevitably will be formulated on the basis of an individual surgeon's personal experience and judgment.

Late Complications

Rectal Stricture

Rectal stricture has been defined by members of the American Society of Colon and Rectal Surgeons by one's inability to pass a 12-mm diameter sigmoidoscope through the narrowed area.[499] Symptoms are quite variable, however, and do not necessarily parallel the degree of narrowing. These may include constipation, tenesmus, fecal soiling, urgency, diarrhea, and signs and symptoms of large bowel obstruction. Much depends on stool consistency and the level of the anastomosis, not only the degree narrowing. Benign stricture following anterior resection is usually a consequence of an anastomotic breakdown with subsequent fibrosis (Figure 23-116). As mentioned earlier, if there is a dehiscence of 25% to 50% of the circumference, healing will usually result in stricture formation. Stricture has been shown to develop more frequently following a fecal diversion, even in the absence of a leak, if a stapled anastomosis has been performed.[286] A stapled anastomosis may "need" the effect of dilatation by the passage of stool. However, conventional suture technique appears to be associated with stenosis less commonly if a proximal stoma has been performed. In a survey of members of the American Society of Colon and Rectal Surgeons, preoperative risk factors for development of this complication were obesity and abscess.[499] Anastomotic leak, incomplete tissue ring, postoperative

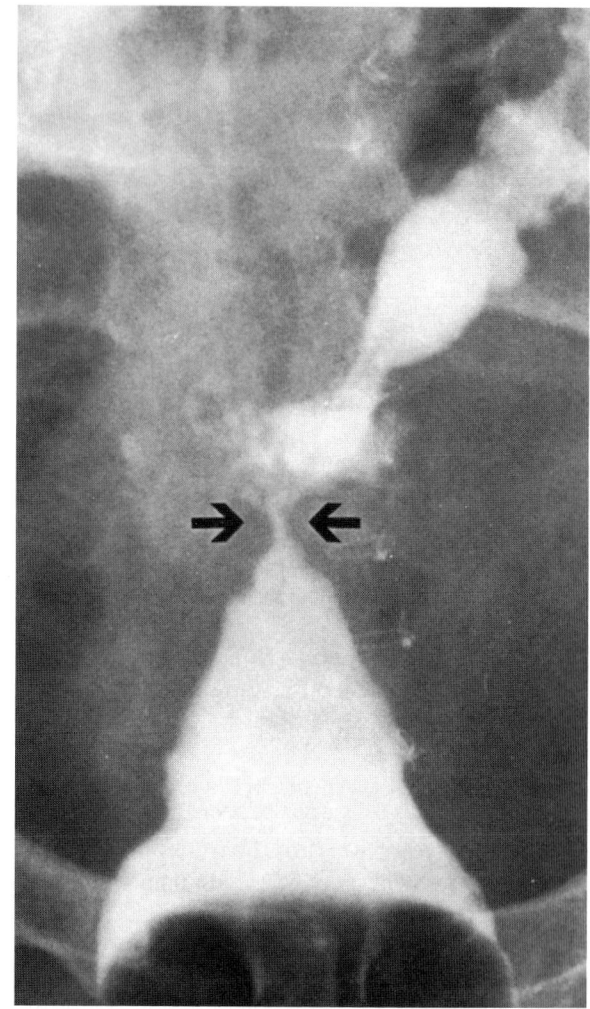

FIGURE 23-116. Barium enema reveals rectal stricture *(arrows)* following anastomotic leak. This proved to be benign.

radiation, and pelvic infection are also believed to be contributing factors.

Management Nonsurgical treatment of an anastomotic stricture consists of the use of stool softeners, enemas, or suppositories. Dilatation can be performed manually if it is within reach of the finger. For higher strictures (i.e., at a level of 8 to 12 cm) a double-ended Hegar's dilator (17 to 18 mm) or a flexible bougie may be used (Figure 23-117). Another alternative is to pass a narrow (1.1 cm) sigmoidoscope with its obturator through the stricture, gradually dilating the opening with serial passage of instruments of increasing diameter. For higher level strictures, Hood and Lewis recommend a curved metal dilator, modeled after the Lister urethral dilator, because the curvature of the sacrum and the angulation of the bowel may make passage impossible.[363] The application of the

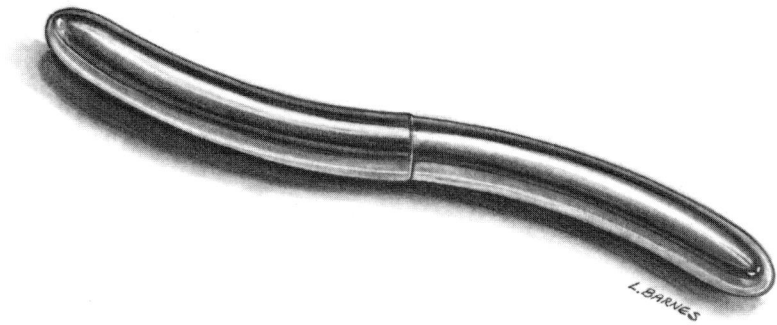

FIGURE 23-117. The double-ended Hegar's dilator is a useful tool in the treatment of strictures in the middle and upper rectum.

technique of endoscopic balloon dilatation, with or without the use of a guide wire, has also been reported (Figure 23-118).[23,36,43,553,605,628] Most patients require two to four dilatations, repeated at 3-month intervals.[417] There is a risk, of course, of perforating the bowel, a particular concern if the stricture is above the level of the peritoneal reflection. One must weigh the morbidity of the procedure itself against the alternative of a major abdominal operation.

If a symptomatic stricture persists, transanal lysis with sharp knife or electrocautery in the posterior midline may ameliorate the condition (Figure 23-119A). The use of the optical urethrotome knife has also been described,[113] as well as a device called a "staple cutter" (a variation of a bone cutter).[753] Another option is the use of an endostapler (Figure 23-120).[111,631] The application of the technique used for endoscopic papillotomy has also been suggested for the treatment of stricture,[3] as has the Eder Puestow dilatation over a guide wire, the technique employed for the management of esophageal strictures.[887]

Following the procedure, frequent office visits with dilatation as necessary is recommended for a number of weeks. This requirement may be obviated if it is possible to perform a proctoplasty, closing a proctotomy in a transverse fashion (Figure 23-119B). Analogous to the Heinecke-Mikulicz pyloroplasty as applied to the rectum, it is hoped that the diameter can be maintained without recurrent stenosis. The Wallstent prosthesis has also been advocated for relieving obstruction, not only for malignant tumors, but also for benign stricture (see Chapter 22 and Figs. 22-85 and 22-86).[719]

If all such treatments are of no avail, repeat resection may be indicated. An alternative to a standard resection is to pass the circular stapling instrument transanally without the anvil, with the center rod traversing the stricture. An enterotomy is created proximal to the strictured anastomosis, and the rod is visualized (Figure 23-121). The anvil is replaced and the instrument closed and fired (Figure 23-121, *inset*). A *single* tissue ring is created, which is the actual stricture (Figure 23-122). The enterotomy is then closed. Ovnat and colleagues describe the same method, using multiple applications of the circular stapler to create a larger lumen.[627]

One must always keep in mind that the cause of the stricture may be recurrent tumor. Evaluation by means of CT scan may be helpful, but biopsy or cytologic study is mandatory for establishing the diagnosis.[874] Obviously, the use of dilatation as a palliative measure has some merit,[794,831] but most successful reports employ cutting and ablating tools, such as the laser and electrocoagulator, for malignant disease (see later).[628]

Virtually all of the reports concerning the management of rectal strictures are essentially individual case studies. The long-term effectiveness of the various modalities has not been subjected to critical analysis. One exception is the publication of Johansson in a prospective study of 18 patients with rectal stricture.[393] Through

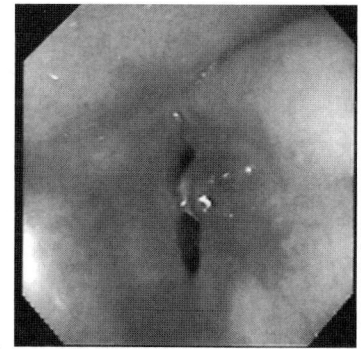

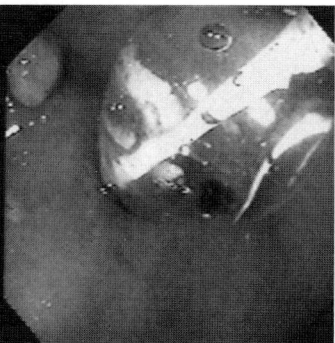

FIGURE 23-118. A benign rectal stricture is discovered following high anterior resection. **(A)** Marked narrowing can be seen through the flexible endoscope. **(B)** The stricture is dilated by the insertion of an endoscopic balloon. (See Color Fig. 23-118.)

A   B

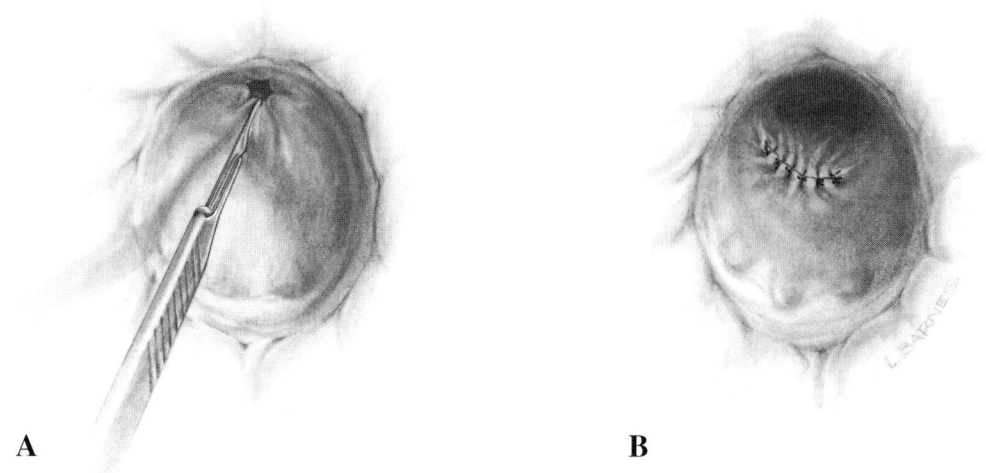

A   B

FIGURE 23-119. Rectal stricture at the site of a low colorectal anastomosis. **(A)** Lysis is performed posteriorly. **(B)** Ideally, a proctoplasty is accomplished by means of transverse closure of the longitudinal proctotomy.

the use of endoscopic balloon dilation, two-thirds had complete relief of their obstructive symptoms. Two of the patients considered the results to be poor, and four were not subjected to follow-up evaluation. One perforation developed as a consequence of the procedure. Schlegel and colleagues in Paris identified 13 patients who had been referred for surgical treatment of rectal anastomotic strictures whose original procedure was for rectal cancer.[733] Repeat resection was performed using various techniques for reestablishment of anal continuity without recurrence and with satisfactory functional results.

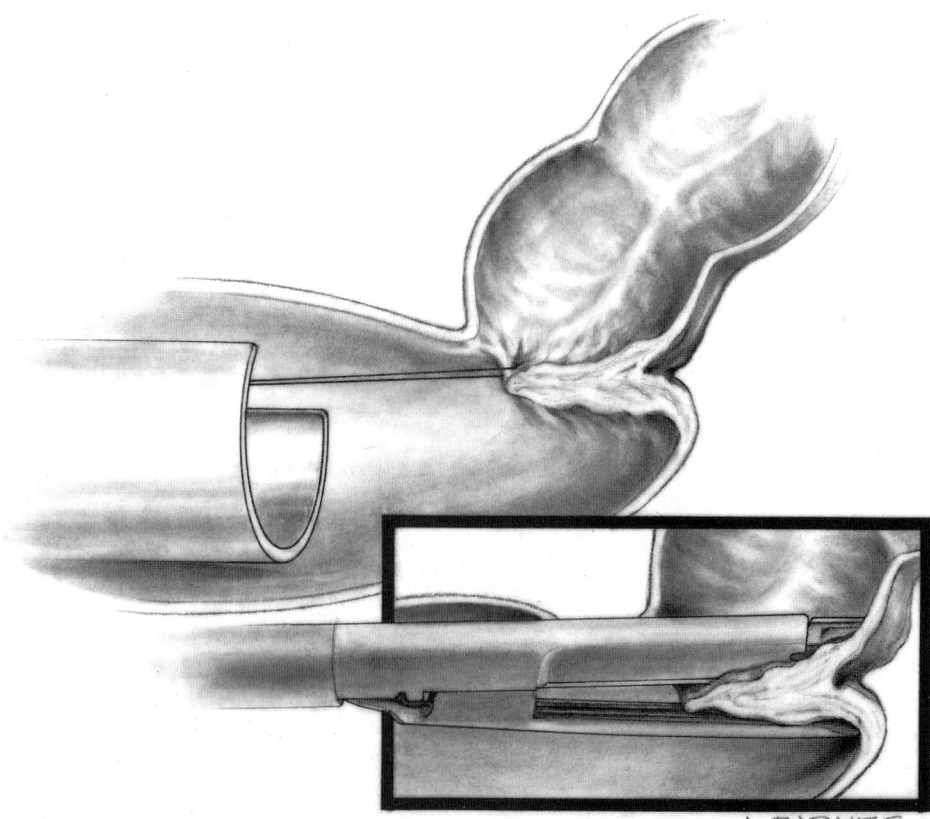

FIGURE 23-120. Technique of division of anastomotic stricture as performed through a Faensler rectoscope utilizing the endoGIA stapler. (Adapted from Pagni S, McLaughlin CM. Simple technique for the treatment of strictured colorectal anastomosis. *Dis Colon Rectum* 1995;38:433.)

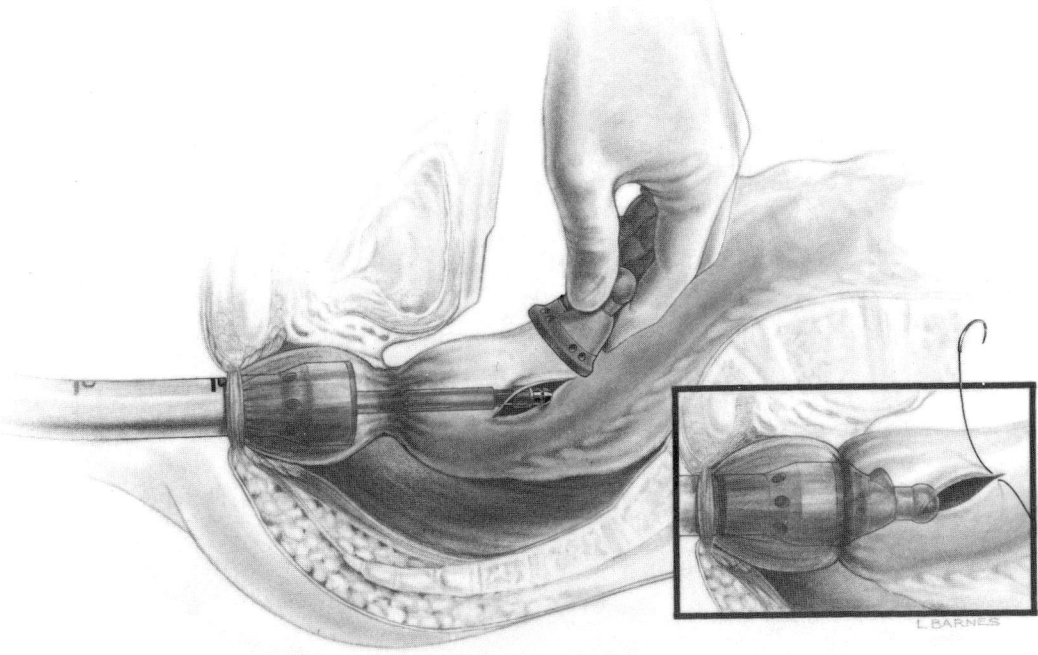

FIGURE 23-121. Excision of strictured anastomosis with CEEA. Enterotomy in proximal bowel permits replacement of anvil. The enterotomy is then closed **(inset).**

Incontinence and Irregular Bowel Function

Low anterior resection, irrespective of anastomotic technique, may be associated with control problems and other bowel management difficulties.[272,276] One concern about the stapling technique is that sphincter disruption can occur from dilatation associated with the passage of the instrument. The issue of stretching the internal and external sphincters is addressed in the chapter on anal fissure (see Chapter 3). Injury to the sphincters during transanal instrumentation has been demonstrated by a number of techniques, including endorectal ultrasound, and has been found to be associated with reduced resting and squeeze pressures when compared with patients who underwent hand-sewn anastomoses.[203,351,583] Long-term functional impairment may also be a consequence of anastomotic leakage (see earlier).[311]

Studies by Pedersen and colleagues of anorectal function following low anterior resection revealed that most patients demonstrate an abnormal rectoanal inhibitory reflex.[655] Rectal compliance was also lower 3 months after operation but had returned to normal in every individual by 12 months. Nakahara and colleagues found that all of their patients who underwent low anterior resection with anastomosis by the circular stapling device suffered from frequent bowel actions and soiling.[601] These symptoms improved to a virtually normal state by 6 months, as did rectal sensation and reservoir capacity. However, abnormal rectoanal inhibitory reflex, anal canal resting pressure, and maximum squeeze pressure per-

sisted. O'Riordain and colleagues found that in the majority of patients who underwent low anterior resection, the rectoanal inhibitory reflex was abolished and remained absent throughout the first year.[624] However, in their experience, this reflex had recovered by the end of the second postoperative year in all patients. Lewis and associates opined that continence after anterior resection is related to the sampling response that the anal sphincter develops to activity within the neorectum.[471,472] The length of the residual rectum is believed to be of critical importance in maintaining effective function. Yamana and co-workers performed preoperative and postoperative physiologic studies on patients who underwent low anterior resection.[891] They found that a longer preoperative high pressure zone, a larger preoperative maximum tolerable volume, and a lower sensory threshold were associated with better postoperative defecatory function. Older age has been thought by some to be an independent prognostic factor for increased incontinence risk. When patients older than 75 years were asked at 1 year following some form of restorative proctectomy, Phillips and colleagues found that 78 of their 92 patients (85%) denied "significant problems."[658]

Inflammatory reaction, narrowing at the anastomosis, sensory impairment, and bowel denervation all may contribute to impairment of control and irregular bowel habits. However, as long as the anal canal and sphincter muscles have been preserved and there is no anatomic abnormality, the symptoms usually resolve in a matter of

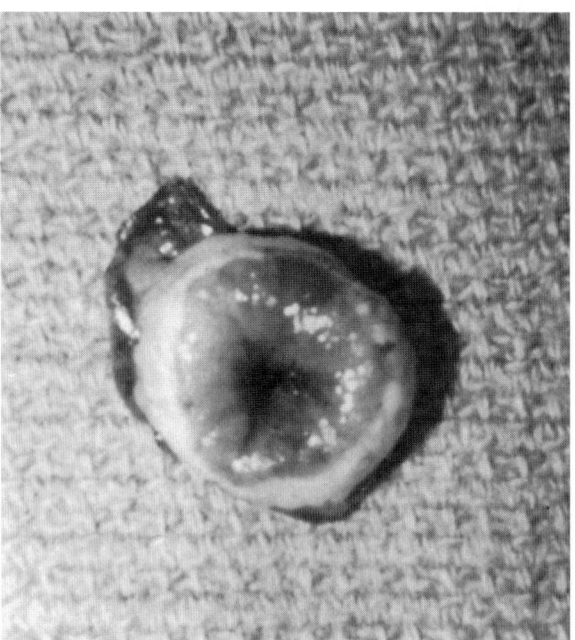

FIGURE 23-122. Single "doughnut" demonstrates marked luminal narrowing following staple resection of a stricture.

a few months. Most patients are able to regulate themselves by paying more attention to their diet than had been their custom. Eventually, for most patients, dietary restrictions become unnecessary.

Recurrence and Survival Results Following Anterior Resection

We reported our experience with anterior resection in 152 patients.[523] The mean age for both men and women was 62 years. There were two in-hospital deaths, a mortality rate of 1.3%. Survival data according to Dukes' classification are shown in Table 23-10. There was no statistically significant difference in survival rates between APR and anterior resection in those with Dukes' A and Dukes' B lesions. However, patients with Dukes' C tumors who underwent APR had a

significantly poorer survival rate than those who had a lesion sufficiently proximal to permit an anterior resection.

The most difficult problem following anterior resection is the management of locally recurrent disease (Figure 23-123). There is a dramatic decrease in the frequency of recurrence when the lesion is greater than 13 cm from the anal verge.[522] Furthermore, it has been shown that most recurrences involve tumors that initially penetrated the rectal wall and extended into the surrounding tissue.[901] In our experience, 88% of recurrent malignant lesions in so-called curative cases followed resections for this type of tumor.[522]

In order to minimize the risk of recurrence, it is crucial to identify preoperatively such individuals and offer them neoadjuvant therapy (see earlier discussion). Table 23-11 lists those variables that are statistically significant in their association with an increased risk of anastomotic recurrence. Table 23-12 shows the incidence of recurrence versus the histology. Table 23-13 compares the recurrence rate with Dukes' classification, and Table 23-14, the recurrence rate versus the distal margin of resection.

In summary, the incidence of anastomotic recurrence in our experience is as follows:

- It increases with more distal lesions.
- It increases with resection margins less than 6 cm.
- It is higher with ulcerating tumors.
- It is low with exophytic lesions.
- It is prohibitively high with poorly differentiated growths.
- It is low with well-differentiated tumors.
- It is low when the tumor does not penetrate the bowel.
- It is high with Dukes' B and C lesions.
- It is high in the presence of metastatic disease.

If the tumor is low lying (less than 8 cm from the anal verge), but especially if it is poorly differentiated, fixed, infiltrative, or ulcerating, then a sphincter-saving operation may be relatively contraindicated. Still, controversy concerning the ideal distal margin for anterior resection is unresolved. Vernava and colleagues prospectively studied 243 patients and found that there was no significant

▶ **TABLE 23-10 Rates of 5-Year Survival for Anterior Resection According to Dukes' Classification**

Dukes' Stage	Number of Patients	Percentage of Series	Number of 5-Year Survivors	Uncorrected 5-Year Survival (%)	Actuarially Corrected 5-Year Survival (%)
A	49	2.2	37	75.5	86.1
B	45	29.6	31	68.8	78.8
C	39	25.7	20	51.3	57.0
D	19	12.5	0	0.0	0.0
A, B, C	133	87.5	88	66.2	71.7
All stages	152	100.0	88	57.9	72.8

(From Manson PN, Corman ML, Coller JA, et al. Anterior resection for adenocarcinoma: Lahey Clinic experience from 1963 through 1969. *Am J Surg* 1976;131:434, with permission.)

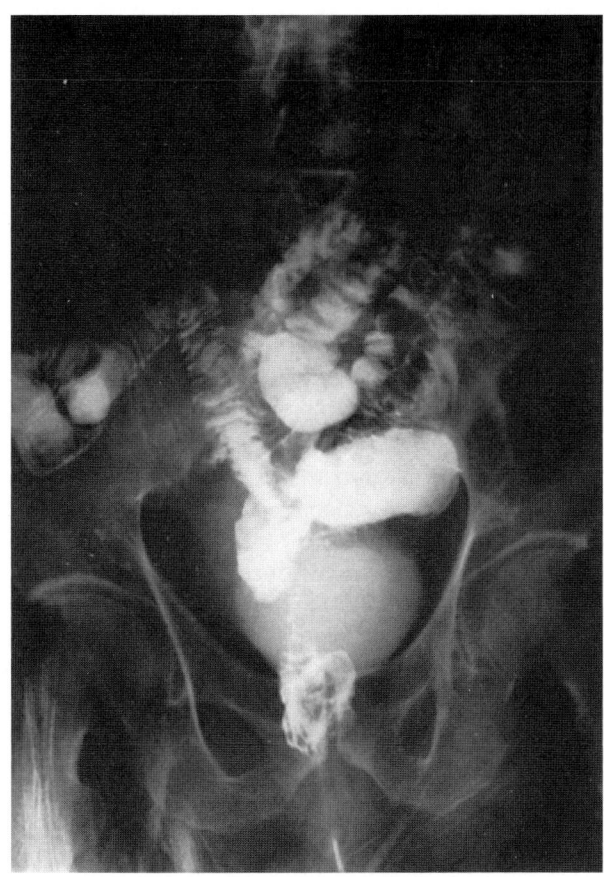

FIGURE 23-123. Rectal stenosis resulting from anastomotic recurrence. Note also reflux of barium into the small intestine because of an ileal fistula at the site of the colorectal anastomosis. In addition, a cystogram has been performed.

TABLE 23-11 Anastomotic Recurrence After Anterior Resection: Related Factors

Factor*	Significance
Penetration of coats of bowel by cancer	$p < .003$
Increased dedifferentiation	$p < .005$
Ulcerating cancer	$p < .005$
Tumor below peritoneal reflection	$p < .01$
Distal margin of resection	$p < .01$
Distal margin of resection of <6 cm	$p < .05$

*The following factors were not significant for anastomotic recurrence: lymph node involvement, $p < .07$; size of lesion, $p < .3$; proximal margin of resection, $p < .3$; previous colonic cancer, $p < .5$; polyps in specimen, $p < .5$; extent of disease (Dukes), $p < .5$; other organ involvement, $p < .5$; blood vessel invasion, $p < .5$; age, $p < .5$; gender, $p < .6$.

(From Manson PN, Corman ML, Coller JA, et al. Anastomotic recurrence after anterior resection for carcinoma: Lahey Clinic experience. *Dis Colon Rectum* 1976;19:219, with permission.)

In the experience of Horn and colleagues, neural invasion had the strongest association with local recurrence, whereas venous invasion was found to be the third most significant independent factor for subsequent metastases (following lymph node status and extent of tumor infiltration).[365]

Recurrence has been attributed to unresected tumor (in the pelvis or the bowel wall itself),[161,184,193,255–257,481,490,547,569,766,779,781] to a zone of potentially malignant mucosa,[490] to a new primary tumor,[273,490,493] to spillage of viable malignant cells,[126–129,490,551,777,841,848] and to implantation by suture material.[221] It has been also demonstrated that recurrence rates are higher for the same stage of lesion in men when compared with women.[88] This is presumably because the pelvic anatomy is such that the operation can be undertaken with a greater distal and circumferential margins in women than can be accomplished in most men.

Numerous measures have been propounded that have been reported to reduce recurrence rates,[340,452,590,662,701,777,833,835] but in these nonrandomized studies one wonders whether the alleged improved results are a consequence of

difference in local or distant recurrence or survival when each centimeter interval was studied down to 1 cm.[844] However, those with a distal margin of less than 0.8 cm had a statistically significantly increased incidence of anastomotic recurrence when compared with those of a greater distal margin. The concept of a 5-cm rule would, therefore, be antiquated.

TABLE 23-12 Anterior Resection for Carcinoma: Anastomotic Recurrence versus Histology

Type	Number of Patients	Number with Recurrences	Percentage of Recurrences (%)
Well differentiated	107	5	4.7
Moderately differentiated	33	6	18.2
Poorly differentiated	5	4	80.0
Villous	7	3 (2 benign)	42.9
Total	152	18	11.8

(From Manson PN, Corman ML, Coller JA, et al. Anastomotic recurrence after anterior resection for carcinoma: Lahey Clinic experience. *Dis Colon Rectum* 1976;19:219, with permission.)

▶ **TABLE 23-13** Anterior Resection for Carcinoma: 5-Year Survival (Uncorrected)

Dukes' Stage	Number of Patients	Number Survived	Percentage Survived (%)
A	49	38	77.6
B	45	30	66.6
C	39	19	48.7
D	19	1	5.3
All stages	152	88	57.9

(From Manson PN, Corman ML, Coller JA, et al. Anastomotic recurrence after anterior resection for carcinoma: Lahey Clinic experience. *Dis Colon Rectum* 1976;19:219, with permission.)

patient selection or of attention to other details, such as a wide resection. For myself, I do not believe the type of suture material is important. I do not utilize the no-touch technique, and I do not perform rectal irrigation with cytotoxic agents (or with anything for that matter). My opinion on TME I believe should be clear to the reader.

Results With Stapled Anastomoses

Because it is possible for surgeons to effect reestablishment of intestinal continuity for relatively low-lying lesions, concern has been expressed about the risk of tumor recurrence following stapled anastomosis. There has been a case report of tumor implantation in the anal canal, possibly as a consequence of trauma from the insertion of the circular stapler.[614] Malignant cells have also been demonstrated in up to 90% of tissue rings.[251] However, the real question is whether surgeons are compromising on the adequacy of the distal margin, and the corollary question is whether it is truly important. A few studies suggest that there may be a higher rate of recurrence with the circular stapling device, but most investigators believe that this may be attributable to factors other than the length of the distal margin of resection (e.g., anatomic considerations, anastomotic leak).[550,606, 695,727] Most reports reveal no increase in local recurrence when the stapler is used, and some believe the incidence is actually reduced (when compared with the suture technique), because one may possibly obtain a greater distal margin.[468,518,617,886] Akyol and colleagues suggested that the use of stapling instruments could be associated with a reduction in the incidence of local recurrence and cancer-specific mortality by as much as 50%.[8] Others have shown that tumor recurrence and cancer-specific mortality were higher in sutured patients and in those who sustained anastomotic leaks.[176] Some studies have demonstrated that there is no statistically significant correlation between the incidence of recurrence and the length of distal margin when one controls for the other variables, unless the margin is minimal (less than 2 cm).[332,336,356,371,459,511,659] In a pathologic study of 42 colorectal cancers reported by Hughes and colleagues, only two demonstrated intramural spread, the maximum length being 2 cm.[371] Others have observed that all potentially curable carcinomas would have been ad-

▶ **TABLE 23-14** Anterior Resection for Carcinoma: Anastomotic Recurrence versus Distal Margin of Resection

Distal Margin (cm)	Number of Patients	Number of Recurrences	Percentage of Recurrences (%)
0	2	0	0.0
1	10	1	10.0
2	17	3	17.6
3	23	2	8.7
4	24	3	12.5
5	31	6	19.4
6	16	2	12.5
7	14	1	7.1
>7	15	0	0.0

(From Manson PN, Corman ML, Coller JA, et al. Anastomotic recurrence after anterior resection for carcinoma: Lahey Clinic experience. *Dis Colon Rectum* 1976;19:219, with permission.)

equately resected with a distal margin of only 1.5 cm.[511] Some have suggested that aggressive pelvic dissection to achieve resection margins greater than 3.5 cm may actually contribute to tumor dissemination and subsequent distant metastases.[685] In general, local recurrence rates following low anterior resection are essentially the same as the rates for APR when comparing the same degree of differentiation and stage of tumor.[877,885]

Significance of Mucus Production

Habib and colleagues investigated the histochemical characteristics of mucus overlying tumor areas and evaluated the proximal and distal margins of resected cancers in patients proved to have local tumor recurrence.[303] They noted a differential pattern of mucus production in the patients who developed recurrence when compared with those who remained tumor free. Mucus from tumors and the adjacent area is composed mainly of sialomucins, whereas normal mucus is composed predominantly of sulfated mucins.[303] Dawson and colleagues, in a multicenter prospective trial of 358 patients followed for 18 months who underwent curative surgery for colorectal cancer, observed that the presence of sialomucin was the optimal prognostic variable for anticipating local recurrence.[157] It was not quite as accurate in its predictive ability for subsequent death or other recurrences; Dukes' classification was better for those patients. These studies may lead one to anticipate individuals who are at an increased risk for the development of local recurrence. Clearly, the most effective method to limit the likelihood of local recurrence is to select those patients who are at an increased risk and either perform an APR or implement neoadjuvant therapy (see later).

Management of Recurrence Following Anterior Resection

When anastomotic recurrence develops, it usually presents within 2 years following resection. The patient may be without symptoms, but a suspicious mass may be noted either by palpation (digital examination) or by proctosigmoidoscopy as part of the cancer follow-up regimen. Unfortunately, anastomotic recurrence usually implies incurable disease because the presentation is virtually always a consequence of pelvic recurrence. Many patients who present with recurrent cancer in the pelvis do not have disseminated disease, and under these circumstances the CEA is often not elevated. When symptoms develop, they may include bleeding, change in the caliber of the stool, and pelvic, abdominal, or sacral pain. Biopsy or scrapings for cytologic examination usually will confirm the diagnosis, but MRI and CT also may be helpful (Figure 23-124). Positron emission tomography has been used to follow-up individuals with colorectal malignancy to differentiate between recurrent tumor and scar (see Chapter 22).[21] The method employs the injection of fluorine-18–labeled deoxyglucose (FDG) to assess tumor metabolism. In the experience of Schlag and Strauss and their colleagues, nonmalignant lesions had a low FDG accumulation as compared with the high levels seen with recurrent cancer.[732,799] Based on subsequent histologic confirmation, the test was 100% accurate in

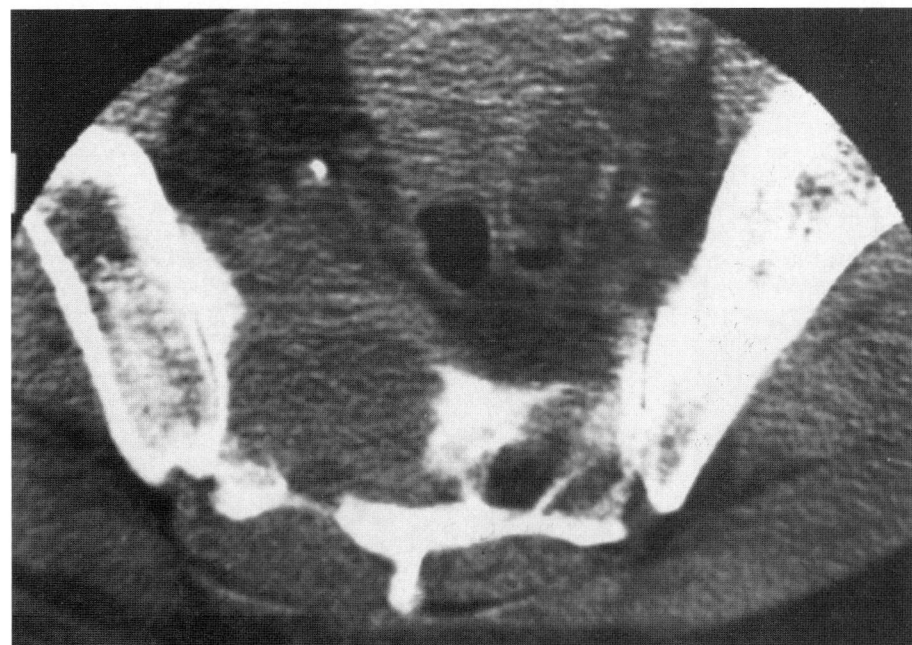

FIGURE 23-124. Recurrent rectal cancer. Computed tomography scan shows marked bony erosion.

their hands. The application of monoclonal antibody scanning is discussed in Chapter 22.

The only hope for cure is repeat resection. This usually involves an APR (Figure 23-125). Before undertaking reoperation, however, it is imperative to determine whether the patient has evidence of disseminated disease. Because of the possibility of retroperitoneal extension of the tumor and the likelihood of urinary tract involvement (ureteral obstruction is common; Figure 23-126), a CT scan or intravenous pyelogram is mandatory.

Principles of Surgery for Recurrent Disease

See the earlier discussion on treatment of recurrence.

Results of Reoperation

Studies of APR following anastomotic recurrence have limited numbers of patients and are difficult to interpret.[742] Overall cure rates are certainly less than 25% in those considered resectable for cure. Wanebo and colleagues reported limited success with a combined ab-dominosacrectomy, with more than one half of the patients requiring a bladder resection.[855] The operative mortality was 12%.

It is my feeling that cure is rarely achieved except when a second primary lesion is found rather than recurrent disease or when the pathologist reports that the recurrence is confined to, but does not breach, the bowel wall. This may be the rare circumstance when mucosal seeding produces the recurrence rather than inward growth of residual pelvic disease. The results of the treatment of pelvic recurrence are discussed earlier in this chapter.

OTHER ANASTOMOTIC TECHNIQUES

> Be not the first by whom the first is tried, nor yet the last to lay the old aside.
>
> Alexander Pope

Transanal or Coloanal Anastomosis

An alternative technique for reestablishing intestinal continuity is the transanal or coloanal anastomosis, described initially by Parks in 1972.[645] A hand-sewn technique may be employed. A Parks self-retaining, three-bladed anal retractor (see Figure 29-84), paired Gelpi retractors place at right

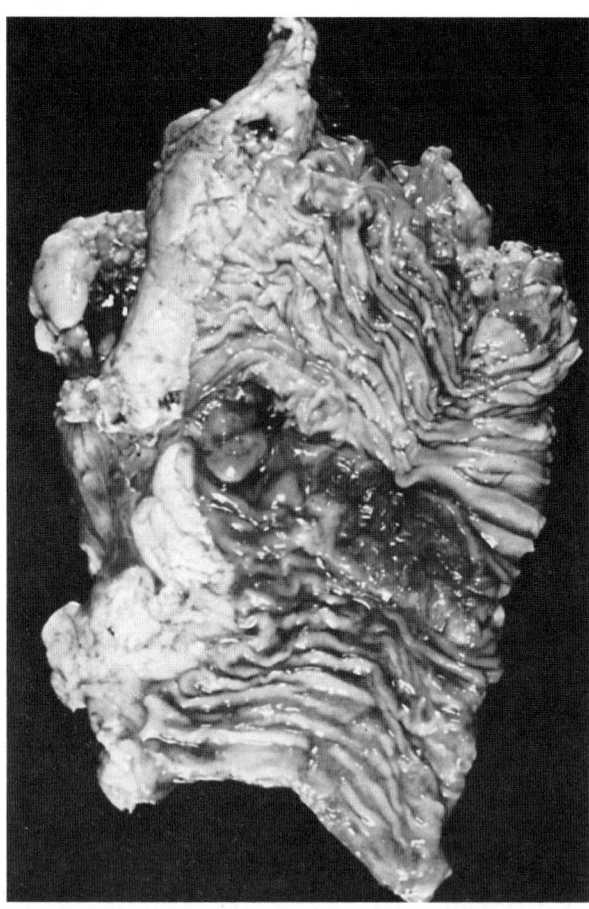

FIGURE 23-125. A portion of resected specimen showing suture line recurrence of tumor.

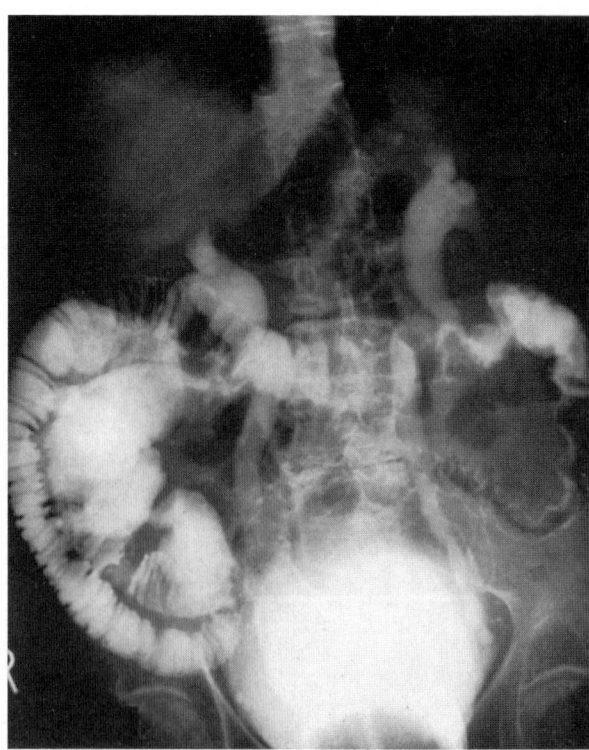

FIGURE 23-126. Recurrent rectal cancer with ureteral obstruction.

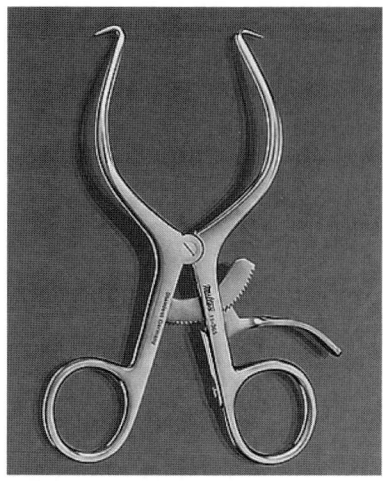

FIGURE 23-127. Gelpi Retractor. (Courtesy of Milltex Instruments, York, PA; *www.Milltex.com*.)

angles to each other (Figure 23-127), a Lone Star Retractor (see Figure 29-85), or a Bookwalter rectal kit (Codman, Randolph, MA), can facilitate exposure for a hand-sewn transanal anastomosis (Figure 23-128). A ⅝-circle needle is particularly helpful for placing the sutures—for example, a round-bodied modification of a Turner-Warwick urethro-plasty needle or a long-term absorbable suture. This is the technique employed for reestablishing continuity after colectomy, proctectomy, and ileal pouch for inflammatory bowel disease (see Chapter 29). The sutures incorporate the full thickness of the colon with the anal canal and the underlying internal sphincter. An alternative approach is to use a double-stapling technique.

Results

Parks reported 76 patients who underwent rectal excision for carcinoma with restoration of bowel continuity by coloanal anastomosis.[646] Ten developed pelvic sepsis, two with anastomotic breakdown. Sixty-nine of 70 patients reviewed had a good functional result. Although not all were followed for 5 years, Parks believed that the preliminary survival data were comparable to that for patients treated by APR.

Enker and colleagues reported their experience with 41 individuals treated by this anastomotic technique.[194] The mean distance of the tumor from the anal verge was 6.7 cm. At the time of their publication, the median follow-up period was only 31 months, with 73% free of disease. The authors recommend that every patient undergo a temporary diverting colostomy and that the left colon

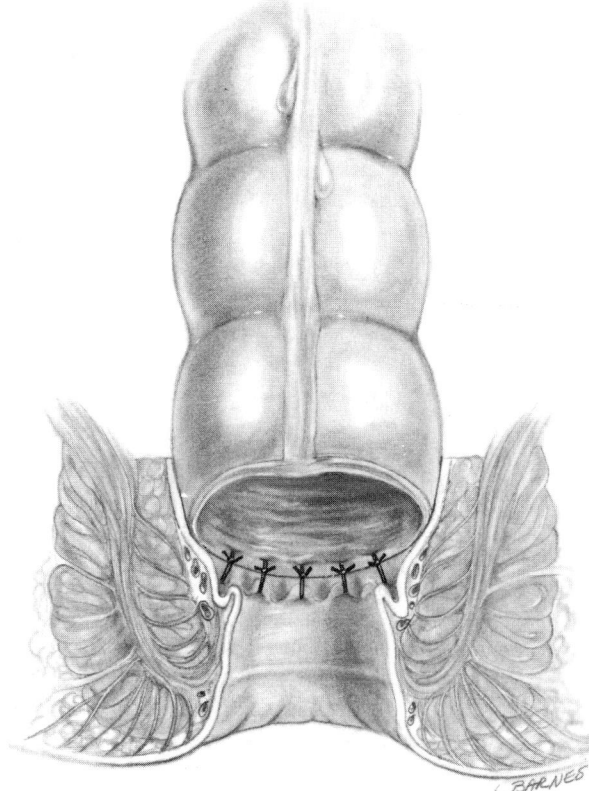

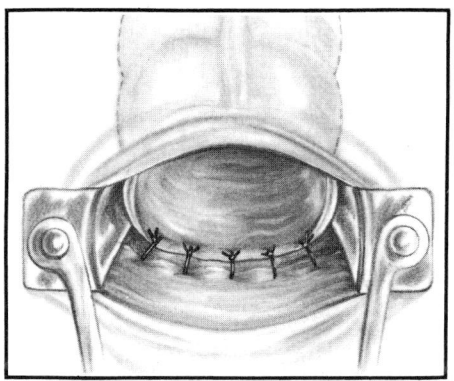

FIGURE 23-128. A Parks retractor facilitates the insertion of sutures (**inset**) coloanal anastomosis.

be completely mobilized to avoid tension on the anastomosis. A more recent report from the same institution (Memorial Sloan-Kettering Cancer Center) involved 134 patients.[648] Actuarially corrected 5-year survival for all patients was 73%. Mesenteric implants, positive microscopic resection margin, T_3 tumor, positive nodal involvement, blood vessel invasion, and high tumor grade were associated with increased risk for pelvic recurrence. Gamagami and co-workers performed coloanal anastomoses on 174 patients.[240] Mean follow-up was 66 months. The mean anastomotic height was 2.3 cm, and the overall recurrence rate was 7.9%. The 5-year survival was comparable to that of APR. Others report at least as satisfactory results in terms of both bowel function and recurrent disease.[100,121,194,322,705,809,845]

In the experience of the Memorial Sloan-Kettering Cancer Center, the median stool frequency was two per day, with 22% of patients reporting four or more stools in 24 hours.[649] Stool frequency tended to decrease with time, with the use of postoperative adjuvant radiotherapy influencing the frequency and difficulty with evacuation. Poor sphincter function has been found to be significantly more common in women than in men.[572] All agree that the surgical morbidity is significantly higher than that of low anterior resection.

Comment

I previously opined that the issue is not whether one can reestablish intestinal continuity, but whether one should. The technical ability to accomplish this must be weighed against the risk of recurrent disease. The only absolute contraindications for performing a coloanal anastomosis are invasion of the sphincter mechanism and invasion of the anal canal. However, some believe that the latter instance is not an absolute, and that through excision of the internal anal sphincter satisfactory cure can still be achieved, even with tumors that invade the anal canal (see later). With regard to fecal diversion, it is my belief that coloanal anastomosis should *always* be accompanied by a proximal colostomy or ileostomy.

Transanal or Coloanal Anastomosis With Colonic Reservoir

In 1986, Lazorthes and colleagues and Parc and associates developed the concept of restoration of continuity by means of a colonic reservoir in order to address the functional concerns associated with a straight coloanal anastomosis.[461,644] However, this "problem" would appear to be a nonissue if one reviews the references in the earlier section.[372] The technique is essentially the same as that for a J-pouch ileal reservoir (see Chapter 29), except that the colon is used (Figure 23-129). Banerjee and Parc attempted to develop a model for appropriate pouch size.[35] According to the authors, ideal pouch dimensions should be 6 to 7 cm of nondistended bowel circumference, with limb lengths of 8 to 10 cm. Others suggest that a shorter limb is satisfactory, and that there is no justification for creating a limb of 10 or more cm. Ho and co-workers, in fact, demonstrated in a randomized, controlled trial by means of scintigraphy, that a small colonic J-pouch improves retention of liquid stool.[352] All investigators emphasized the importance of mobilizing the splenic flexure and preserving the first branch of the inferior mesenteric artery.

A theoretical advantage of the J-reservoir when compared with a straight coloanal anastomosis is that the blood supply may be superior, and that better healing may be anticipated with less chance of an anastomotic leak. A potential problem is that a narrow, male pelvis may preclude the possibility of creating a reservoir. Likewise, a thickened, fatty mesentery may cause the operation to be technically nonfeasible. Finally, some surgeons selectively recommend the use of the descending colon rather than to create a reservoir with a thickened sigmoid colon, but others have found that pouches made from sigmoid or descending colon provide similar bowel function.[328] The same principle of fecal diversion applies to the colonic J-pouch as it does to the straight coloanal anastomosis—namely, diversion, in my opinion, is a requisite. In the experience of Dehni and colleagues, there was a clinical anastomotic leak rate of 17% in those without a defunctioning stoma.[167]

Results

Drake and colleagues reported the Mayo Clinic experience with 29 individuals suffering from either benign or malignant disease.[179] Anastomotic stricture was found in 28%, and a 3.4% leak rate was noted. Fourteen percent could not have their colostomy or ileostomy closed. A later report incorporating the experience from both Mayo and Cleveland Clinics, involving 117 patients most of whom had undergone a straight coloanal anastomosis, satisfactory fecal continence was achieved in 78%.[101] No J-pouch recipient had frequent incontinence. Five-year survival was 69%, but 62% had complications (anastomotic leak, 18%). Some institutions have found that stool frequencies are fewer with this method, especially during the first year,[48,166,169,344, 345,470,596,668,748,859] than with patients who undergo reconstruction procedures without a reservoir, but others note that approximately 25% of individuals must evacuate with a small enema.[461,644,656] This is the primary reason for limiting the size of the reservoir, and, furthermore, to use this option only for anastomoses at the level of the anal canal. Evacuation problems are more likely to occur with an intact lower rectum.

Sailer and associates in Würzburg, Germany, performed a prospective trial in which 64 patients were randomized to either a straight (n = 32) or coloanal J pouch (n = 32).[717] These investigators found that patients who

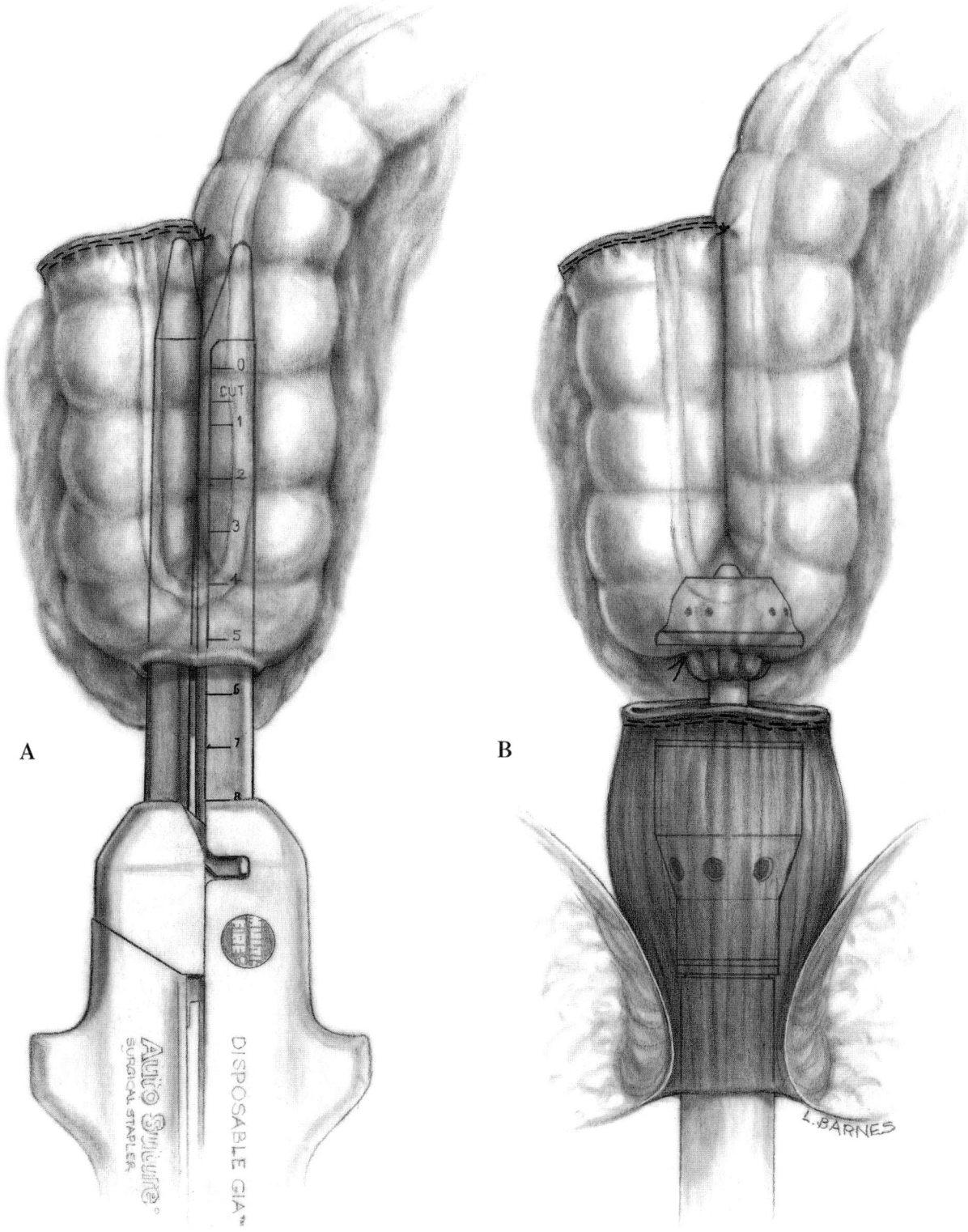

FIGURE 23-129. Coloanal anastomosis utilizing intervening J-pouch. **(A)** The pouch is constructed either by a hand-sewn technique or by using a stapler (as shown). **(B)** The double-stapled anastomosis is being completed.

underwent pouch reconstruction had better functional results as well as an improved quality of life in the early months. Nicholls and colleagues compared the St. Mark's Hospital experience with the colonic reservoir and straight coloanal anastomoses.[609] They found no significant difference in balloon expulsion testing, defecation proctography, or methylcellulose evacuation in the two groups. Frequency of defecation and daytime soiling were inversely correlated with the maximal tolerable volume.[449] Hallböök and colleagues perfomed a randomized comparison of straight and J-pouch anastomoses in 100 consecutive patients with rectal cancer in whom a sphincter-saving procedure was considered appropriate.[310] The incidence of symptomatic anastomotic leakage was lower in the pouch group (2% versus 15%). At 1 year, the patients who had undergone the pouch procedure had significantly fewer bowel movements in 24 hours and less nocturnal evacuation, urgency, and incontinence.[310] Those familiar with the technique report no increase in morbidity or mortality attributable to the reservoir itself. Machado and co-workers in Stockholm showed that either a colonic J-pouch or a side-to-end anastomosis performed in the descending colon, in a prospective randomized trial, can be utilized with the expectation of similar functional and surgical results.[504]

The Cleveland Clinic group identified seven reasons why the J-pouch could not be constructed and stipulated that coloplasty has reduced the frequency of these problems (see the following section).[315] They were as follows:

- Narrow pelvis
- Bulky sphincters or mucosectomy
- Diverticulosis
- Insufficient colon length
- Pregnancy
- Complex surgery
- Distant metastases

One of the concerns for any operation that restores continuity in the patient with rectal cancer is the impact of adjuvant or neoadjuvant chemoradiotherapy. The Cleveland Clinic group assessed individuals who underwent either preoperative or postoperative treatment and concluded that chemoradiation therapy adversely affects continence and evacuation in those who underwent colonic J-pouches.[252] The authors expressed concern over long-term functional results with radiation of the anal canal, sphincter mechanism, and neorectum (in the adjuvant patient) and offered the suggestion that consideration should be given to excluding the anal canal from the field of irradiation in those with stage II and III rectal cancer whenever a sphincter-preserving operation is contemplated.[252] Others have found that preoperative radiotherapy significantly increases the frequency of nocturnal defecation and diarrhea when compared with nonirradiated patients.[165]

Coloanal Anastomosis with Coloplasty

Following a series of experimental studies, Z'graggen and co-workers in Bern, Switzerland, conceptually explored whether a coloplasty, equivalent to a very small pouch, could decrease stool frequency without the technical and functional problems associated with the J-pouch.[898] Forty-three patients were so treated, all with a proximal stoma. The early results were comparable to those of the J-pouch reservoir procedure.

Technique

Z'graggen's group used a segment of descending colon for the coloplasty. The procedure is analygous to that of the Heineke-Mikulicz pyloroplasty as applied to the colon—that is, a linear colotomy with a transverse closure. After the anvil is secured in the colon, an 8-cm incision is made longitudinally between the tenia, 2 cm proximal to the rim of the anvil (Figure 23-130). Lateral traction by stay sutures develops the appearance of the reservoir. The colostomy is closed in two layers (their preference) with the stapled anastomosis performed in the usual manner. The procedure can also be accomplished with a hand-sewn coloanal anastomosis. All patients require fecal diversion.

Results

Besides Z'graggen and colleagues, other surgeons have expressed satsfaction with this procedure. Fürst and co-workers randomized 40 consecutive patients to either a J-pouch or coloplasty.[230] The construction of a coloplasty pouch was possible in every instance, but four of 20 (20%) in the J-pouch group could not undergo the procedure because of a fatty mesentery. At 6 months, there was no significant difference in stool frequency and no significant difference in resting and squeeze pressures, as well as neorectal volume. However, there was an increased neorectal sensitivity in the coloplasty group. The authors concluded the coloplasty is a particularly attractive alternative because of its simplicity and one's ability to apply it for all patients. The Cleveland Clinic group members were of like opinion, based on their report of 20 patients.[524]

Coloanal Anastomosis with Intersphincteric Resection

In an effort to restore intestinal continuity in those patients who have even invasion of the anal canal, some have suggested restoration by incorporating intersphincteric resection. By these means, the anal canal and internal sphincter are removed with preservation of the external sphincter mechanism. In other words, if the tumor has a low rectal transmural infiltration without invasion of the levator ani or external sphincter, this operation may be undertaken.[707,840] Others opined that tumors close to the anal canal, not infiltrating the external sphincter,

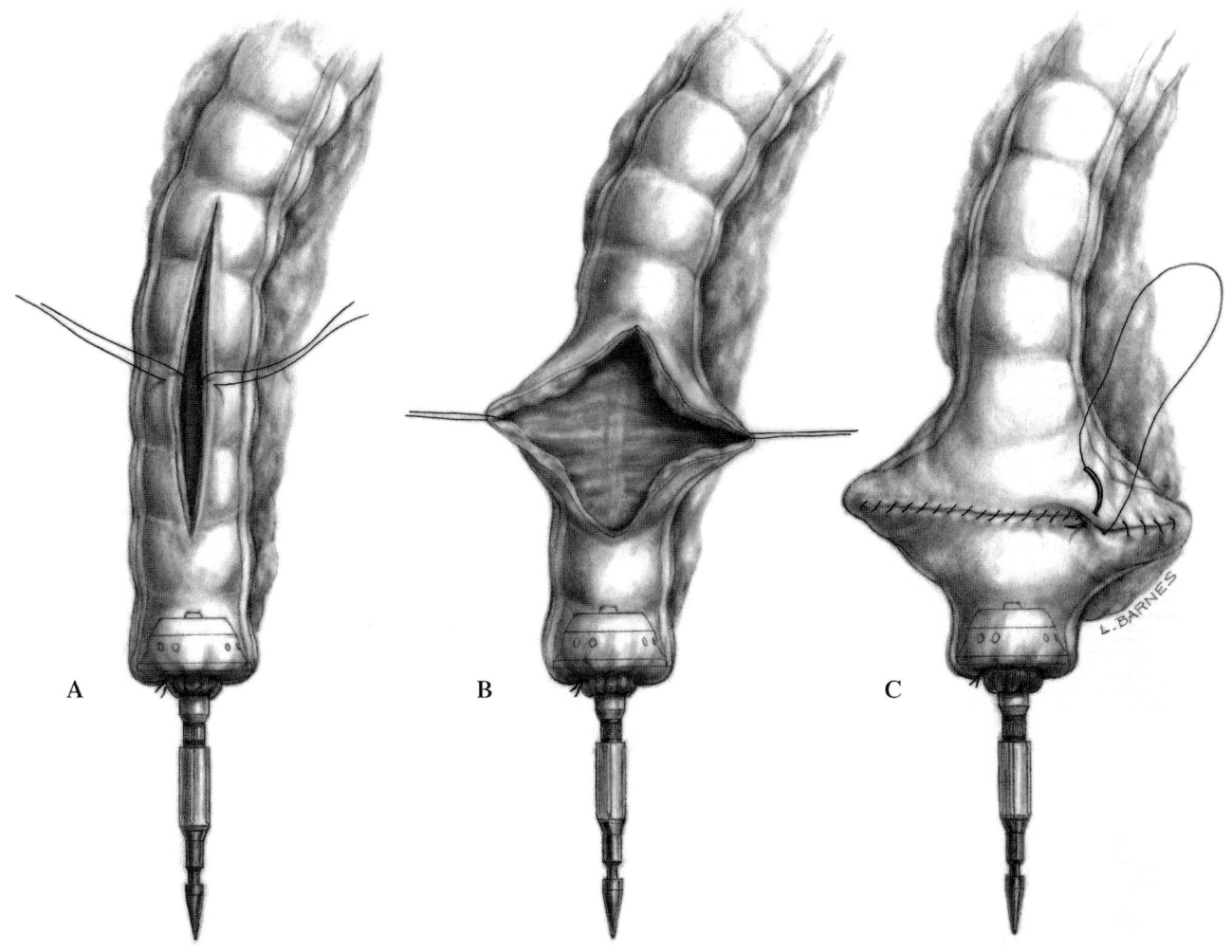

FIGURE 23-130. Coloplasty. **(A)** Linear incision is made between the taeniae. **(B)** Guide sutures are placed in preparation for transverse closure. **(C)** Pouch is completed.

and with good to moderate differentiation may be removed by intersphincteric resection and coloanal reconstruction.[680] This removes, at least theoretically in the minds of some individuals, one of the absolute contraindications to restoration of bowel continuity, namely, invasion of the anal canal. Figure 23-131 illustrates the concept of the extent of resection.

Rullier and colleagues in Bordeaux, France, prospectively studied 16 patients with infiltrating T_2 and T_3 rectal tumors located between 2.5 and 4.5 cm from the anal verge.[707] Six underwent partial resection of the internal sphincter and ten complete resection. A colonic J-pouch was performed in one half of their patients. Twelve had undergone neoadjuvant radiation therapy. There were no deaths. No local recurrence developed (median, 44 months). Two required proctectomy for complications, and two died of metastatic disease. Continence was normal in one half of the patients.

Clearly, the concept of sphincter sparing by this new approach will require a larger series before accepting the premise that this procedure can be performed without compromising the possibility for cure.

Alternatives to Fecal Diversion

Intraluminal Bypass

The indications and method for performing the so-called intraluminal bypass[674,709] for effecting a colorectal anastomosis are discussed in Chapter 15. However, this method is no longer available in the United States.

Transanal Stent

Amin and colleagues report the use of a transanal stent to perform "distal decompression."[11] Although the results are preliminary, the authors suggest that such a device may obviate the need for fecal diversion with coloanal anastomoses.

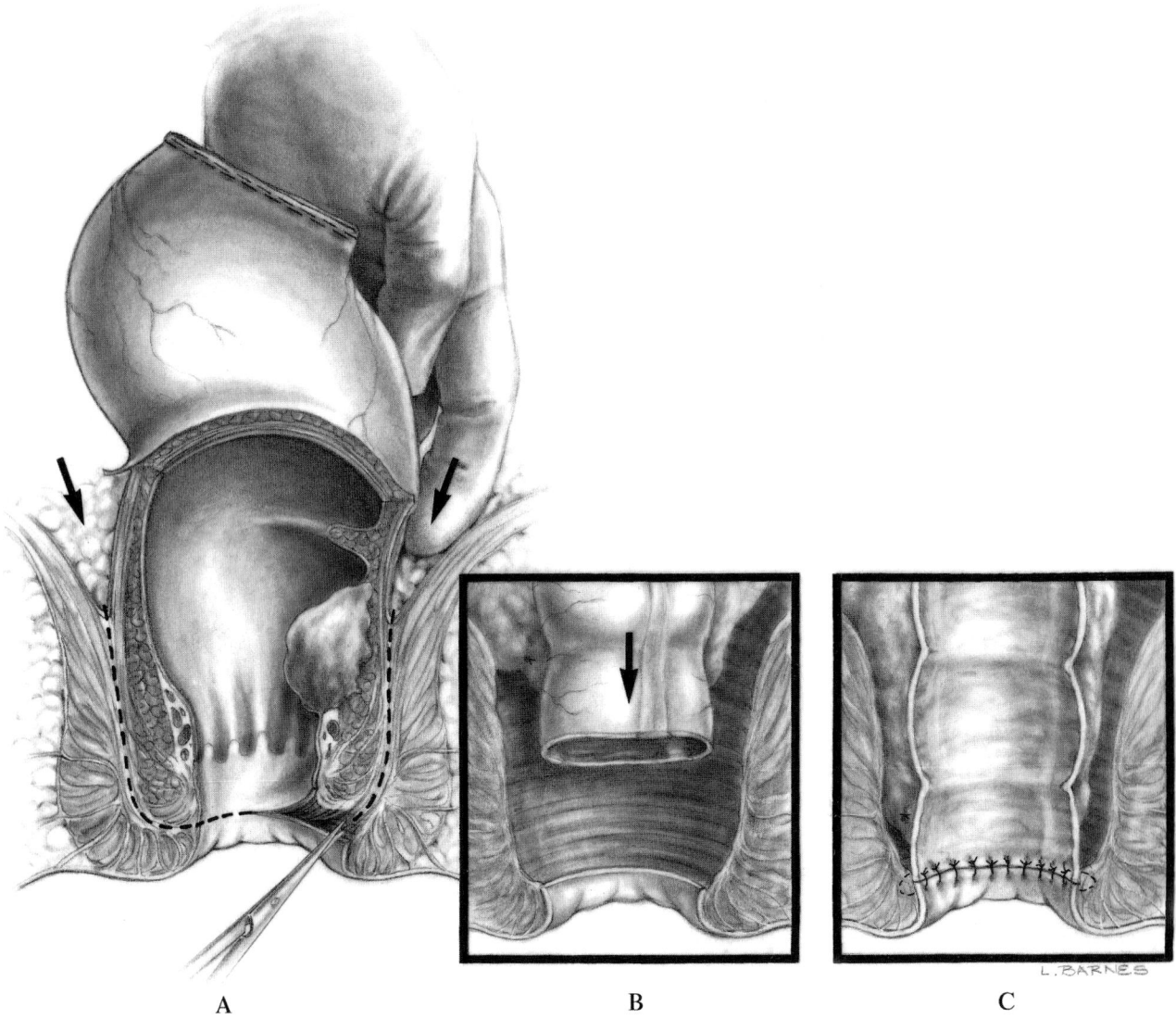

A   B   C

FIGURE 23-131. Intersphincteric resection. **(A)** The *dashed line* indicates the extent of resection in the intersphincteric plane. Note the artist's conception of a small tumor invading the internal sphincter at the top of the anal canal. **(B)** The external sphincter is intact, and the proximal colon is pulled through. **(C)** Completed anastomosis.

Abdominoanal Pull-Through Procedures

An alternative method for reestablishing intestinal continuity following rectal resection is the pull-through procedure. The operation was initially described by Maunsell in 1892 and was supported by Weir in 1901 (see Biographies).[543,864] It was developed primarily as an alternative to the transsacral excision of Kraske (see Transsacral Resection) and the Murphy anastomotic button (see Chapter 22).[437,599] Pull-through procedures are generally applied for anastomoses below 7 cm, but they are relatively infrequently employed today because of the preference for other techniques (i.e., double-stapling, coloanal, and abdominosacral anastomoses) and other treatment modal-

ities (e.g., local excision). As with other esoteric sphincter-saving alternatives, the surgeon should be wary of using the pull-through procedure for malignant disease unless the operation fully meets the principles of oncologic resection. There are several methods for accomplishing anal anastomosis by the pull-through approach.

Eversion Techniques

The patient is placed in the perineolithotomy position, and the operation proceeds as if for a low anterior resection. However, when a pull-through operation is undertaken, greater length of proximal colon needs to be liberated. In virtually every instance, the splenic flexure requires mobilization. The bowel is divided as low as is possible and the specimen resected.

The safest anastomosis and the one that offers the best functional result is accomplished with Weir's procedure. The rectal stump is everted, the proximal bowel is "pulled-through," and the anastomosis is performed by the perineal operator with interrupted 3–0 long-term absorbable sutures (Figure 23-132). The anastomotic area returns to the pelvis spontaneously. The pelvic peritoneal floor is left open, and a proximal colostomy is usually advised.

A modification of Weir's technique has been described by Turnbull (see Biography) and Cuthbertson and by Cutait and Figliolini.[148,834] The rectal stump is everted, but the bowel is pulled through and left to project on the perineum for 7 or 8 cm. The cut edge of the rectum is sutured to the seromuscular surface of the intussuscepting colon, but not penetrating the lumen (Figure 23-133). A catheter is secured into the protruding bowel. After 10 days to 2 weeks, the redundant colon is amputated and the anastomosis accomplished with full-thickness sutures secured via the perineum. The rectum then immediately retracts into the pelvis. Fecal diversion is not required.

Delayed Union: Amputation Techniques

A more distal pull-through anastomosis can be effected using the Babcock, Bacon, or Black technique.[25,26,28,64] Babcock described his method of one-stage abdominoperineal proctosigmoidectomy with perineal anus in 1939.[25] After a generous posterior sphincterotomy has been performed, the bowel is amputated at the top of the anal canal and pulled through. This allegedly reduces the risk of necrosis of the exteriorized colon. Healing takes place between the cut edge of the anorectum and the serosa of the colon. Amputation of the stump is performed 2 weeks later. In the Black modification, no sphincterotomy is undertaken.[64]

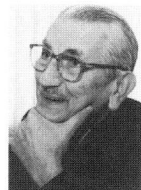

Daher Elias Cutait (1913–2001) Daher Cutait was born in São Paulo, Brazil, where he attended the University of São Paulo Medical School, graduating in 1939. From 1941 to 1943, as the recipient of a scholarship provided by the Institute of International Education of New York and later by the Kellogg Foundation (Michigan), he came to the United States to the Presbyterian Hospital of Columbia University. From there, he went to the University of Michigan Hospital, where Frederick Coller trained him in colorectal surgery. Upon his return to Brazil, Cutait initiated an active career at the University of São Paulo Hospital das Clinicas. In 1947, he was appointed Head of Colo-Proctology, a position he held until his retirement in 1983. During his tenure of service, he became one of the most prestigious colorectal surgeons, not only in Brazil, but throughout Latin America, having trained hundreds of surgeons. He published more than 120 papers and three books. His unique technical abilities were applied to a host of colorectal conditions, but he is eponymously remembered for his pull-through procedure, an operation that was designed for the treatment of chagasic megacolon (see Chapter 33). Cutait received numerous international awards and recognitions. He was President of the Brazilian Society of Colo-Proctology, the Brazilian College of Surgeons, and the Brazilian Chapter of the American College of Surgeons, a member of the American Society of Colon and Rectal Surgeons, and honorary member of the Royal College of Surgeons of England and Ireland and the French Society of Medicine, to name only a few. In the early 1960s, he established the Hospital Sirion Libanes, a referral center for surgery in São Paulo. He directed this hospital until his last days. Daher Cutait died on June 6, 2001. (With appreciation to his son, Raul Cutait, M.D.)

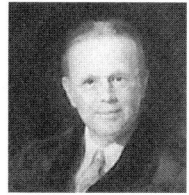

William Wayne Babcock (1872–1963) Babcock was born in East Worcester, New York. After 2 years as a preceptee, when he studied medicine and the classics, he enrolled in the College of Physicians and Surgeons in Baltimore, graduating with honors in 1895. After 1 year as a resident physician in Salt Lake City, Utah, he matriculated for an additional year of medical training at the University of Pennsylvania in Philadelphia, receiving his second M.D. degree in 1895. During the ensuing 7 years, Babcock held a number of positions, including surgeon and pathologist. When he completed his training in gynecology, he was offered the Chair in this specialty at Temple Medical College of Philadelphia. However, he elected to accept the Chair of Surgery at the same school when he was only 31 years of age. He served as Professor and Head of the Department for 40 years and was one of America's most renowned surgeons. His textbook, *Principles of Surgery*, was highly regarded through several revisions. His list of accomplishments was extraordinary. He was the first person in the United States to employ a spinal anesthetic. He is eponymously associated with an operation for stripping varicose veins and for inguinal herniorraphy. He was the inventor of the acorn-shaped vein stripper; he introduced the use of alloy steel wire sutures, wire mesh in hernia repairs, and, of course, his bowel clamp. With respect to his pull-through procedure, he was often criticized for applying it inappropriately or too often. Certainly, with Babcock and with Bacon, Temple University became the center for this particular procedure. (Photograph courtesy of the Department of Surgery, Temple University School of Medicine, Philadelphia.)

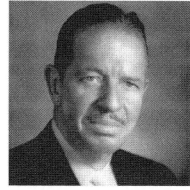

Harry Ellicott Bacon (1900–1981) Harry Bacon was born in Philadelphia on August 25, 1900, the son of a Professor of Surgery at Temple University Medical School. He received his Bachelor of Science degree from Villanova University and his Doctorate in Medicine from Temple University in 1925. Following an internship in surgery at the Philadelphia General Hospital, he became interested in proctology. He pursued further training at the Graduate Hospital in that city, St. Mark's Hospital in London, St. Antoine in Paris, and the Algemeine Krankenhuis in Vienna. Returning to Philadelphia, he became Associate Professor of Proctology at the University of Pennsylvania and subsequently Professor of Surgery and Chairman of the Department of Colon and Rectal Surgery at Temple University, a position he held until 1972, when he achieved emeritus status. Bacon was a prolific writer, with six books plus numerous scientific articles to his credit. Additionally, he published three volumes of poetry as well as musical arrangements for the piano and organ. He played a principal role in the establishment of the journal *Diseases of the Colon and Rectum* and served in an editorial capacity from its inception until his death. He received numerous awards and recognitions throughout his life, including a silver medallion from Pope Pius XII and a gold medallion from Pope John XXIII. He was the founder of the Pennsylvania Society of Colon and Rectal Surgery, a founding member of the International Society of University Colon and Rectal Surgeons, and President of the American Proctologic Society (he was instrumental in changing the name to the American Society of Colon and Rectal Surgeons), and he received honorary degrees from eight universities and honorary fellowships from 18 international surgical organizations. Bacon died on May 12, 1981. (With appreciation to Indru T. Khubchandani, M.D.)

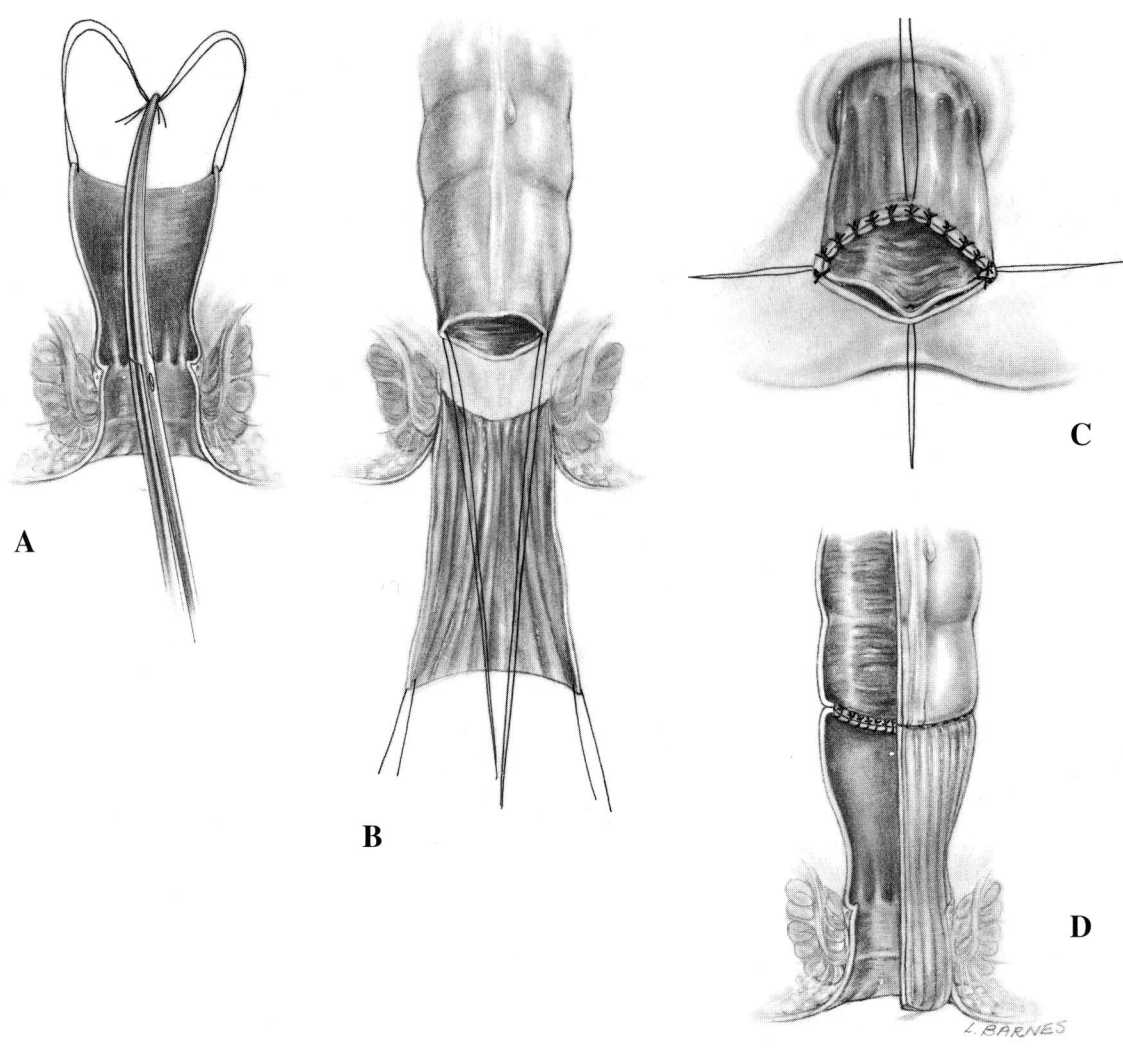

FIGURE 23-132. Weir pull-through technique. **(A)** Guide sutures evert the rectal stump. **(B)** The proximal bowel is delivered through the everted rectal stump with guide sutures. **(C)** The anastomosis is performed in one layer by the perineal surgeon. **(D)** The bowel returns to the pelvis.

Bacon first described his alternative in 1945.[28] He removed the anal canal by way of the perineal route, dividing the bowel at or above the levatores. This permits a wider surface area to come in contact with the pulled-through bowel, a theoretical advantage in that healing may be more effective. As with the other procedures, the redundant bowel is amputated approximately 2 weeks later.

Results

Cutait and colleagues have considerable experience with the various pull-through operations; in 1985, they reported a total of 728 patients treated by several methods.[147] Only 57 individuals, however, underwent the operation for rectal cancer. These investigators noted that the incidence of leakage was 31.9% in immediate anastomoses and only 2.2% in delayed anastomoses. Likewise, the incidence of septic complications was much less when the delayed technique was used (6.8% versus 27.9%). Operative mortality was also less with the delayed method (2.2% versus 6.1%).

Rosen and colleagues and Khubchandani and coworkers reported the results of 28 patients with respect to defecation, to continence, and to survival after the Bacon-type of pull-through operation had been performed.[413,696] Although these patients all were continent, 83% failed to defecate spontaneously and required an enema. Rather than abstract the results of the moderately extensive earlier literature on the subject, I have appended a list of references.[27,46,47,63,274,420,438,439,455,780,834] All studies are uncontrolled or, at best, relate only to historical controls. Morbidity is generally higher than with APR, as is the length of hospitalization. Mortality rates generally are also higher with the pull-through procedures. Cure rates and problems with pelvic recurrence are comparable, however.

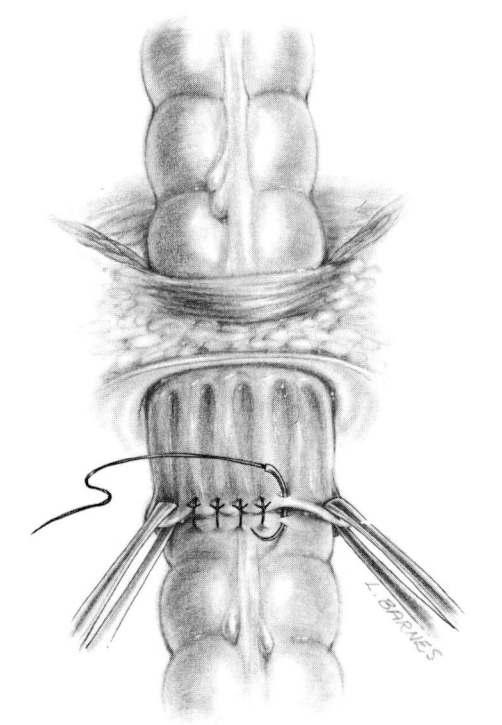

FIGURE 23-133. Pull-through by eversion and seromuscular suture (first stage).

Comment

The delayed union–amputative techniques permit a lower anastomosis than can be achieved through eversion. Hence, one can effect an anastomosis in situations when an anterior abdominal approach with any suture technique, other than coloanal, is impossible. However, the anastomosis may be less secure, and subsequent continence may not be as satisfactory as with the former methods. With the temporary, perineal "colostomy," a proximal diversion, however, should be unnecessary.

One problem in my experience has been that of the wet anus (see Figure 17-3). The mucosal ectropion associated with nonanastomotic pull-through procedures can be a source of considerable discharge and discomfort.

The advantage of Weir's (Maunsell's) procedure is that it is tidier, because an anastomosis is performed *per primam*. The staging method, however, creates an uncomfortable, often frightening, foul-smelling, necrotic, perineal protrusion, but it can accomplish an anastomosis safely, without the need for a diversionary procedure. Hence, it has this advantage. The fact of the matter is that both procedures are rarely useful alternatives to low anterior resection. In order to create an eversion of sufficient length to deliver the rectum to the perineum, a minimum of 6 cm of residual rectum is required. With less rectum available, eversion is virtually impossible; the tethering of the levatores tends to draw the bowel back into the pelvis. Most patients are able to have continuity reestablished by more conventional means (if reestablishment is considered advisable).

One is tempted to be skeptical of the frequent application of an esoteric operation when most other surgeons use another, standard approach. Although I hesitate to accuse surgeons who favor these operations of provincialism or of unwarranted enthusiasm, I have difficulty in placing great credence on the objectivity of their reports. It is useful to note that since the publication of the second edition of this text (1989), no new references on the pull-through procedure have been added. I do not believe this is because I have failed to pursue the literature with sufficient vigor.

In my opinion, these operations should be performed rarely, having been replaced by coloanal anastomosis. Essentially, it should be relegated to the realm of historical curiosity, resurrected only when a surgeon wishes to apply it as an alternative to one of the esoteric sphincter-saving procedures and when no other resective or local operation is appropriate, an extraordinarily unusual situation indeed.

Transsacral or Transcoccygeal Resection

Sacral excision had been performed by Theodor Kocher as early as 1875.[426] However, it has been associated with the name of Kraske ever since he described the

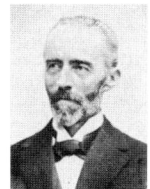
Emil Theodor Kocher (1841–1917)   Emil Kocher was born in Switzerland on August 25, 1841 and graduated from medical school *summa cum laude* from the University of Bern. He visited distinguished professors such as Billroth, Lister, Pasteur, and Nelaton and settled in Bern in 1866. He was awarded the Chair of Surgery at this University in 1875 and held the position for the next 45 years. He was the first to excise the thyroid for goiter (1876) and ultimately performed more than 5,000 thyroid operations. In 1909, Kocher won the Nobel Prize for Physiology or Medicine for his work on the physiology, pathology, and surgery of the thyroid gland. He has been described as a calm and imperturbable operator, while also maintaining total asepsis in an era of frequent infections. His name is eponymously associated with numerous techniques and instruments—an incomplete list includes his incisions (abdominal and thyroid), his maneuver, his methods (uterine fixation, inguinal herniorraphy, shoulder dislocation), his reflex, his sign, his syndrome (for thyrotoxicosis), his forceps, his clamp, his drain, and his probe. He even has a verb named after him—every surgeon knows what it means to kocherize the duodenum. Kocher contributed extensively to the literature in general surgery, endocrine surgery, urology, gynecology, neurosurgery, and war-related injuries. His lifelong efforts were compiled in his textbook, *Operative Surgery (Chirurgische Operationslehre,* 1892), a monumental tome that was published in a number of editions and translations. He was named the first President of the International Surgical Society. In 1909, the Kocher Institute in Bern was established as a permanent memorial to him. He retired as Professor of Surgery in 1911 and died on July 25, 1917. (Photograph courtesy of Archiv fur Kunst und Geschichte, Berlin.)

technique in detail to the Fourteenth Congress of the German Association of Surgeons in 1884 (see Historical Notes).[436] Interestingly, in the classic description of the procedure, the bowel was brought out by establishing a sacral anus at the posterior end of the wound, amputating the entire distal rectum. This, in essence, was a sacral colostomy. Others, such as Turner, modified the operation by performing an EEA to the residual anorectum.[836]

Technique

Routine bowel preparation is carried out as if for an anterior resection. The operation is performed with the patient in the prone position and with the buttocks taped. Some surgeons prefer the lateral position, but the prone jackknife position is easier (Figure 23-134). An incision is made in the midline from just above the anal verge to the lower sacrum and carried through the subcutaneous tissue to expose the levator ani muscle and coccyx (see Figs. 21-50 to 21-52). The levator ani muscle is then divided, exposing the posterior wall of the rectum. The coccyx is then freed from its muscular attachments, disarticulated, and removed. If it is apparent that sufficient exposure has been achieved, then no part of the sacrum is removed. However, if further exposure is necessary, the lower portion (two sacral segments) are excised using a Gigli saw. It is imperative when dividing the sacrum that the third sacral nerve on one side be preserved in order to avoid problems with incontinence.

The rectum is then completely mobilized. Care must be taken to avoid injuring the anterior rectum where it is adherent to the vagina or to the prostate. A Penrose drain is placed around the rectum for traction and the dissection is completed. The peritoneum may be opened on the anterior rectal surface. The bowel is then drawn downward as far as is possible and the superior hemorrhoidal vessels divided (Figure 23-135). The bowel is divided at the desired level and an anastomosis is effected with interrupted 3–0 long-term absorbable sutures as a single layer. The circular stapling technique has also been recommended (Figure 23-136).[384] A Silastic drain is placed through a stab wound of the buttock into the presacral space and connected to suction. It is usually left in place for 48 to 72 hours or until drainage ceases.

Postoperatively, management is essentially the same as that for a low anterior resection. When flatus is passed, a progressive diet is instituted. During the time of convalescence, the patient is instructed on perineal strengthening exercises (see Chapter 13). A degree of incontinence occurs for several days to a few weeks, but in all cases virtually normal control will be restored eventually, assuming that there has been preservation of the nerve supply.

Results of this operation in contemporary writings are essentially anecdotal. However, Sweeney and Deshmukh performed the procedure on 11 patients, but in only one was primary rectal carcinoma the diagnosis.[811] These investigators reported no morbidity or mortality. McCready and colleagues used this approach combined with radiotherapy as a means for effecting a local excision of selected patients with rectal cancer (see later).[548] Wound infection or a fistula was noted in 29%. Although no recurrences were identified, follow-up was only 13 months.

Comment

Sacral excision rapidly had become the most popular modality of treatment for carcinoma of the rectum by the end of the nineteenth century, but the problems of anastomotic breakdown, fecal fistula, wound sepsis, and tumor recurrence have since caused the procedure to fall into disrepute. The Kraske operation usually permits resection of 8 to 10 cm of rectum without difficulty. However, by contemporary standards, the operation must be regarded as inadequate for the management of rectal cancer because it fails to remove the "zone of upward spread."

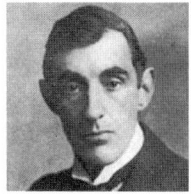

George Grey Turner (1877–1951) Turner was born in Tynemouth, the county of Northumberland, England. He was educated at a private school and graduated from the Newcastle Medical School of Durham University with first-class honors in 1898. He obtained his M.S. in 1901 and his F.R.C.S. in 1903. After holding resident surgical posts at Newcastle, Turner went to London and continued his postgraduate studies at King's College Hospital. After visiting a number of surgical clinics on the continent, he returned to Newcastle and to the staff of the Royal Victoria Infirmary. Because of his dexterity, daring, and extraordinary capacity for work, his operating theater became a center for visitors comparable to that of the great Lord Moynihan. In 1927, he was named Professor of Surgery at the University of Durham, and in the following year was made President of the Association of Surgeons of Great Britain and Ireland. Grey Turner was more of a "generalist" and was considered one of the boldest individuals, because of his aggressive treatment of malignant disease. His point of view with respect to the anal sphincter was perhaps somewhat less radical, however. Preservation of the "wonderful sphincteric apparatus" did appear to be a priority concern. Grey Turner was recognized through numerous awards and honors. He was Hunterian Professor on two occasions and Honorary Fellow of the American and Royal Australasian Colleges of Surgeons. He was elected President of the Proctologic and General Surgical Sections of the Royal Society of Medicine. He delivered the John B. Murphy Oration in Philadelphia and received the Bigelow Medal in Boston for the advancement of surgery. His name is eponymously associated with the sign that produces local discoloration of the skin of the flank in acute pancreatitis. (Photograph courtesy of the Royal College of Surgeons of England.)

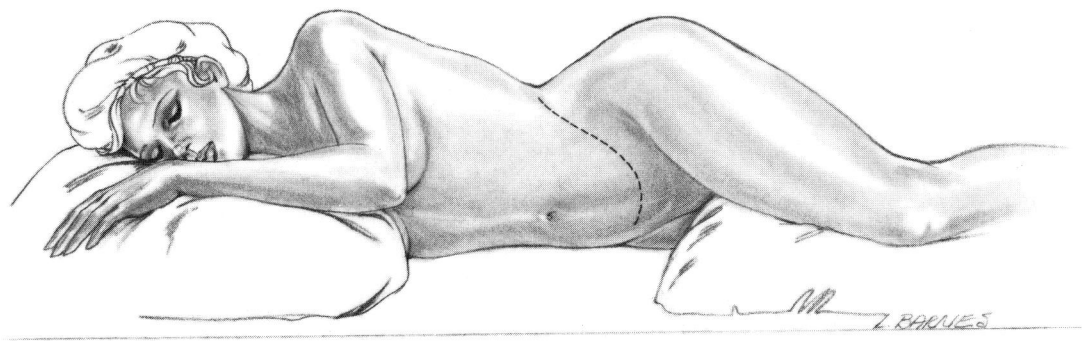

FIGURE 23-134. Position of the patient for synchronous abdominosacral resection and anastomosis (not recommended).

Some surgeons, however, still recommend this alternative for small malignant tumors, but I believe that better local procedures are available for such conditions (see later). The operation does, however, have application in carefully selected patients for benign disease: villous adenoma, benign rectal stricture, rectovaginal fistula, and rectoprostatic fistula (see Chapters 12 and 21).

Abdominosacral Resection

Kraske was the first to suggest a combined abdominosacral resection to overcome the disadvantage of failure to remove the lymphatics of the rectum and rectosigmoid. In the early 1930s, Goetz[264] and Pannett[637] resected the rectum and were able to reestablish intestinal continuity by the sacral approach. In the United States, Donaldson and colleagues, Localio and Stahl, and Marks and associates revived interest in this operation for the treatment of rectal cancer.[177,484,528]

Technique

In the modification described by Localio and Stahl, access to the abdomen and the sacrum is achieved simultaneously by placing the patient in the right lateral position (Figure 23-134).[484] Two teams can then operate

independently on the abdomen and over the sacrum. I have found this approach cumbersome, however, and much prefer the patient to be placed in the perineolithotomy position. The abdominal phase is completed as if for a low anterior resection. The lateral stalks are divided, and the surgeon then decides on the advisability of reestablishing continuity and the choice of operation to accomplish this. If the sacral approach is elected, the abdomen is closed. It is important fully to mobilize the entire left colon and splenic flexure so that the bowel can be easily delivered and so that there is no tension on the subsequent anastomosis. The bowel is not divided during the abdominal phase of the procedure. A transverse colostomy or, preferably, a loop ileostomy is routinely performed.

The patient is then placed in the prone jackknife position, and Kraske's approach is used (see Figs. 21-50 through 21-52). With the rectum already fully mobilized, the bowel containing the tumor can be delivered through the incision and resected (Figure 23-135). Anastomosis is accomplished with an interrupted single-layer technique or alternatively by the circular stapling instrument (Figure 23-136). The muscles are repaired with heavy long-term absorbable sutures, and a Silastic drain is placed into the hollow of the sacrum and brought out through a stab wound in the buttock.

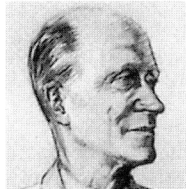

Charles Aubrey Pannett (1884–1969) Pannett was born in the Shepherd's Bush area of London, the only surviving son of an ironmonger. Coming from a poor family, he was discouraged from attempting a career in medicine; however, having gained entrance to St. Mary's Hospital, he obtained a scholarship. Alexander Fleming was also a scholarship recipient in the same class. The two were rivals, sharing between them all the medical school prizes. Pannett obtained his degree of Doctor of Medicine in 1907 with a gold medal and his fellowship in the Royal College of Surgeons in 1910. Shortly thereafter, he contracted tuberculosis and was forced to spend most of the ensuing 4 years in a sanitorium, performing light work as a house surgeon. In 1914, he became registrar at St. Mary's. During World War I, Pannett served as a surgeon on a hospital ship and in the Middle East. Following the war, he returned to St. Mary's and ultimately achieved the Professorship of Surgery in the University of London. He was best known for his skill in performing a partial gastrectomy at a time when gastrojejunostomy was the preferred and safer procedure for ulcer disease. In 1929, he reported 100 consecutive operations without a death, a remarkable achievement for that or any time. He was the first British surgeon to perform the sphincter-saving operation by means of the abdominosacral approach. Later, he abandoned the operation in favor of anterior resection. A master surgeon, his motto was "cut well, see well, and your patients will get well."

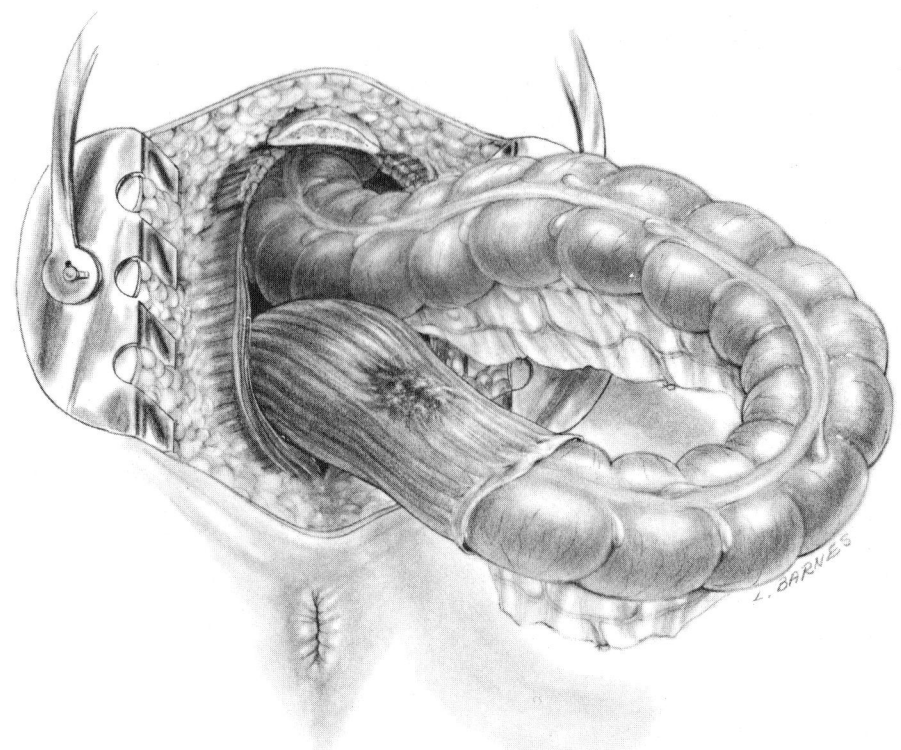

FIGURE 23-135. Abdominosacral resection. The colon is delivered through the sacral defect and is resected. Anastomosis is readily performed through the sacral wound.

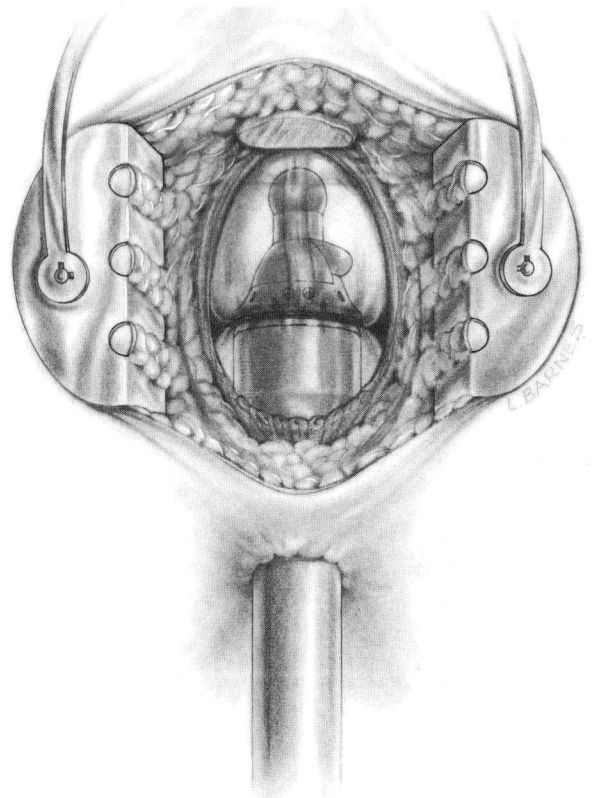

FIGURE 23-136. Circular-stapled anastomosis by transcoccygeal approach. Note the coccyx has been removed.

Results

Localio and colleagues had probably the largest experience with this operation, reporting the results of 427 patients with carcinoma of the rectum.[482,483] Preoperative assessment was made to determine the type of operation that the patient would require: APR, anterior resection, or abdominosacral resection. A total of 100 abdominosacral resections was performed. Although recurrence rates and mortality rates were comparable for the three procedures, the morbidity of abdominosacral resection was much higher. Twelve percent of the patients developed either a fecal fistula or peritonitis (Figure 23-137). Because of these complications, the authors advised that a colostomy should always be performed.

Marks and colleagues reported the results of this operation as performed following radiotherapy.[528] Only those presumed to have locally unfavorable disease were selected. The tumors were located from 3 to 7 cm from the anal verge. Twenty-four patients were followed from 20 to 84 months with no evidence of pelvic or perineal recurrence.[528] This is probably attributable to the use of preoperative radiation (see later), rather than to the choice of operation. In fact, the radiotherapy was undoubtedly responsible for "downgrading" of the depth of invasion as determined by the subsequent pathology report (see later). However, the authors succeeded in demonstrating that preoperative radiation

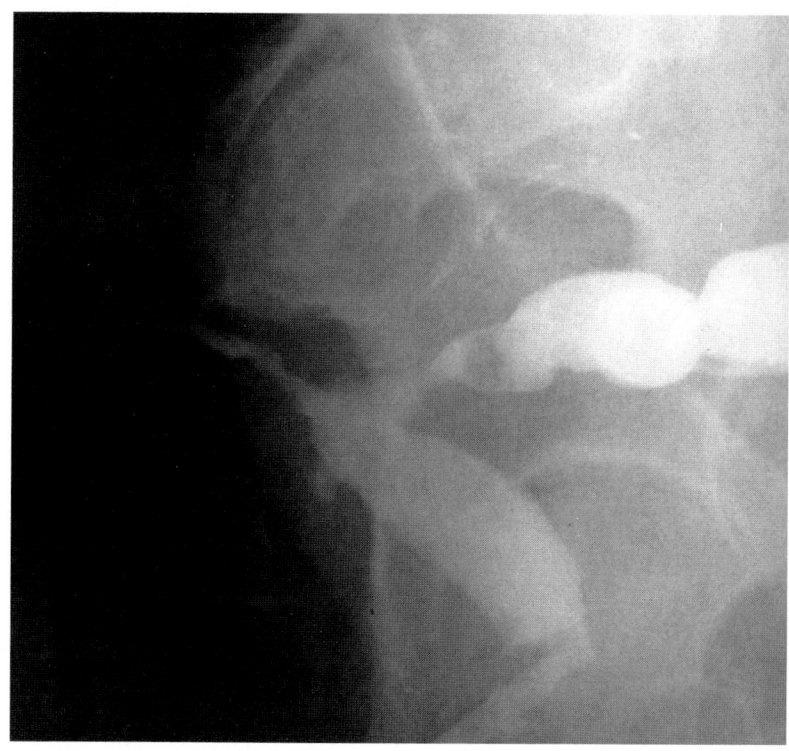

FIGURE 23-137. Anastomotic fistula following an abdominosacral procedure. Note the absence of the coccyx and lower sacrum, which have been resected.

therapy (40 to 50 Gy) permitted the safe application of this anastomotic alternative.

Comment

Although I have had only a limited experience with this operation, and that primarily for benign conditions, I am not enthusiastic about its value in the treatment of rectal cancer. It is true that the procedure effectively removes the cancer-bearing segment and lymphatics and that a low anastomosis can satisfactorily be achieved, but a candidate for its application is infrequent indeed. The fact that the patient must contend with a sacral wound as well as an abdominal incision causes me to look for an al-

ternative operation for preserving the anal sphincter when such an approach is desirable.

TRANSSPHINCTERIC EXCISION

Interest was stimulated in transsphincteric excision as a method for removal of selected, low-lying cancers of the rectum by Mason in 1970.[537] The procedure, however, is not new, having been advocated by Bevan in 1917 for "small carcinomas of the rectum without any radial involvement."[52] Interestingly, however, the author did not seem to repair the sphincter, simply stating, "I do not hope to attain anything like complete continence," nor did he comment about the risk of the development of a fistula.

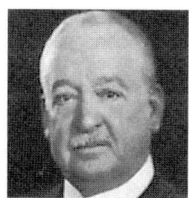

Arthur Dean Bevan (1861–1943) Bevan was born in Chicago, the son of a physician. He graduated from the Sheffield Scientific School of Yale University in 1879 and Rush Medical College in 1883. Bevan began his medical career at the United States Marine Hospital in Portland and as a Professor of Anatomy at Oregon State University. In 1888, he returned to Chicago as Professor of Anatomy at Rush Medical College, holding the Chair until 1902, when he assumed the position of Professor of Surgery. Seven years later, he was appointed Head of the Department, succeeding Nicholas Senn. As Chairman of the Council of Medical Education of the American Medical Association for one quarter of a century, he was instrumental in establishing minimum requirements for admission to medical school and for virtually eliminating the so-called homeopathic and eclectic schools in the United States. Bevan was the first to perform an operation using ethylene anesthesia. His lateral rectus approach for gallbladder surgery is known as the Bevan incision. He devised operations for undescended testis and for the repair of ventral hernia. During World War I, Bevan became Director of the Surgical Division of the Office of the Surgeon General of the United States Army. He took an active part in organizing physicians for the war effort, for which he received the French Legion of Honor. In 1932, he served as president of the American Surgical Association.

Technique

With the patient in the prone jackknife position, the levator ani and external sphincter muscles are completely divided in the posterior midline. The bowel is opened, offering excellent exposure of the low and middle rectum (Figure 23-138). Although tumors on the anterior wall are the easiest to demonstrate, those on the posterior or lateral walls can be brought into view by fully mobilizing the rectum.

In an experience with 14 patients, Mason reported a recurrence rate of 13%.[538] Allgöwer and colleagues reported 36 patients with rectal cancers treated by a sphincter-splitting approach.[9,10] There were no operative deaths, but there were nine recurrences. The authors recommend frozen-section examination of the surgical margins and depth of penetration by the tumor. The results of the experience with 116 patients from the same unit are rather difficult to interpret.[368] The authors reported this application for many indications, approximately one half of which were for malignancy.

Comment

Although I have had no experience with this technique, the obvious criticism of failure to remove the associated lymphatics would relegate this procedure to one of palliation in the poor-risk patient. Yet I cannot see why one would have to divide the sphincter muscles to accomplish this. I have no reservations, however, about dividing the sphincter muscles, because good functional results can be expected with direct repair. One may consider this option as an alternative to local excision (transanal excision; see later). It may be useful to include the procedure in one's "repertoire of operations on the rectum," as some have suggested,[324] but it is doubtful that the treatment of cancer should be one of the indications.

ABDOMINOTRANSSPHINCTERIC RESECTION

Mason also reported the foregoing technique an alternative means for effecting an anastomosis following an abdominoanal pull-through.[539] By dividing the sphincter muscles as described in the preceding section, an anastomosis can be performed quite readily at the anal verge.

Lazorthes and colleagues undertook this operation in 65 patients.[460] More than one half received preoperative radiotherapy. In 57 cases, a diverting colostomy was performed. There were no operative deaths, but six patients (9%) developed pelvic sepsis or an anastomotic leak. Of those surviving 1 year, 91% reported normal control for feces.

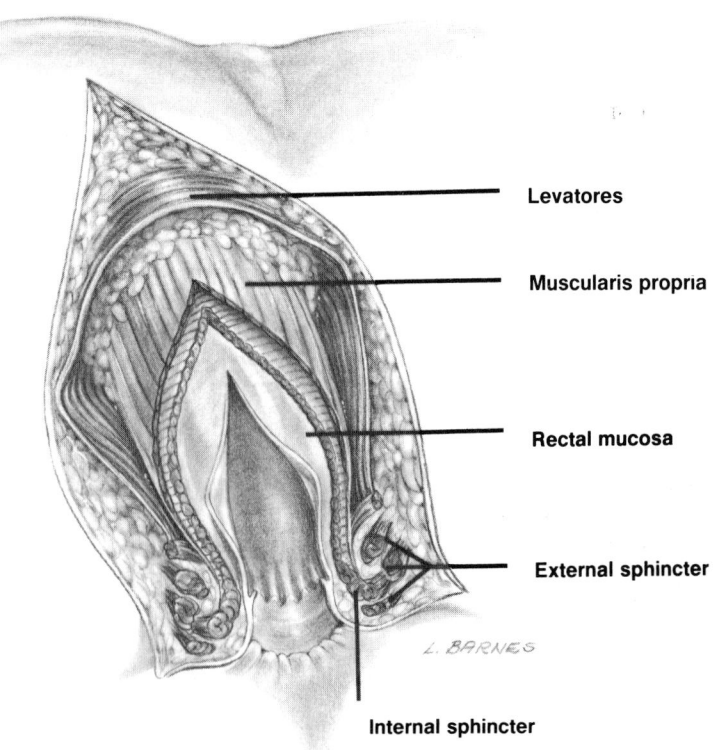

FIGURE 23-138. Transsphincteric excision. The rectum is opened like a book, posteriorly.

Levatores

Muscularis propria

Rectal mucosa

External sphincter

Internal sphincter

Comment

As with other esoteric sphincter-saving approaches, it is not difficult for me to control my enthusiasm.

LOCAL PROCEDURES

In addition to transsacral (transcoccygeal) excision and transsphincteric excision, there are a number of local procedures that can be used both for palliation and as curative approaches for the management of carcinoma of the rectum. With respect to cure, extensive preoperative evaluation should be obtained to be certain that a curative approach can be reasonably achieved through some form of local treatment. This includes clinical assessment, biopsy, degree of differentiation, CT or MRI, endorectal ultrasound, and a number of other possible studies—all of which are addressed earlier in this chapter and in Chapter 22. Individuals who are poor candidates for curative attempt at local incision include those with transmural involvement (T_3 lesions), poorly differentiated tumors, those with evident lymph node metastases, those in whom a sphincter-saving operation can be carried out by conventional means, and those that can tolerate a major operation. Hase and colleagues identified five histopathologic characteristics as risk factors for lymph node metastases:[319]

- Small clusters of undifferentiated cancer cells ahead of the invasive front of the lesion ("tumor budding")
- A poorly demarcated invasive front
- Moderately or poorly differentiated cancer cells in the invasive front
- Extension of the tumor to the middle or deep submucosal layer
- Cancer cells in the lymphatics

The investigators concluded that those individuals with three or fewer risk factors had no nodal spread, whereas the rate of lymph node involvement with four or more risk factors was 33% and 67%, respectively.[319] Such a classification may be useful in determining those individuals who

may be preferred candidates for local excision. Others suggest that the incidence of lymph node metastases is higher for lesions greater than 1 cm in diameter, for those showing "massive" submucosal invasion, and for moderately differentiated adenocarcinomas.[813]

It has been noted that lymph node–clearing techniques may demonstrate tumor in lymph nodes as small as 1 mm, suggesting that even the best methods for preoperative assessment may miss tumors that are theoretically beyond surgical curability through local excision.[341] The implication of this observation is that one should consider supplementary radiotherapy, either preoperatively or postoperatively, whenever a local procedure is recommended or performed. In a study by Huddy and colleagues, involving 109 rectal excision specimens in which the tumors were locally confined to the bowel wall, 20% had metastases to local lymph nodes.[369] Although less well-differentiated tumors were more likely to have metastasized, there was no statistically significant difference in the size of tumors or in the depth of invasion between patients with or without lymph node metastases. The reality is that patients who undergo local procedures do so without complete assurance that the operation is as effective in curing cancer as is the conventional, radical approach.

Electrocoagulation

Destruction of tumors by electric current has been reported virtually since electricity was harnessed. In 1913, Strauss advocated electrocoagulation for palliation in poor-risk patients with carcinoma of the rectum and in those individuals with extensive lesions.[795–798] His indications were gradually broadened to include almost all stages of carcinoma of the rectum. Subsequent reports advocating electrosurgical destruction have dotted the literature, but their authors emphasized that the primary value of the procedure was in those patients who had incurable carcinoma or in those who refused colostomy.[383,411,699] Despite Strauss' results, which were reported to be at least as satisfactory as those for surgically resected carcinomas, the value of this technique failed to have any significant impact on surgical thinking until Madden and Kandalaft

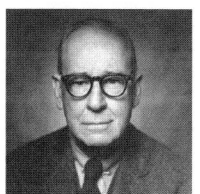

John Leo Madden (1912–1999) John Madden was born in Washington, DC, and received his medical degree from the George Washington University in 1937. He completed his surgical residency training at the Long Island College Hospital-Kings County Hospital in New York. During World War II, Madden served in the Army Medical Corps in the Pacific theater. Upon returning to New York City, he joined the staff of St. Clare's hospital and in 1948 was appointed Director of Surgery, a position he held until 1975. He was also on the staff of New York Hospital/Cornell University Medical Center as well as Clinical Professor of Surgery at Cornell. Madden was a prolific author and innovative thinker. His contributions were varied and numerous. In 1952, he received the Ludwig Hektoen gold medal from the American Medical Association for his work illustrating blood vessels. Madden was a true pioneer in the emerging field of vascular surgery. He also has been credited with singular approaches to the treatment of breast and colorectal disease, especially that of diverticulitis and rectal cancer. He was also an innovator in video teaching. The American College of Surgeons video library contains almost 50 of his procedures. Madden received numerous recognitions and awards during his long and fruitful career, including President of the New York Academy of Medicine, Chairman of the Section on Surgery of the American Medical Association, President of the International Cardiovascular Society, and membership in the French Academy of Surgery. He died on March 25, 1999. (With appreciation to Keith P. Meslin, M.D.; photograph courtesy of the New York Academy of Medicine.)

reported their series in 1967.[508] They believed electrocoagulation to be the preferred treatment for carcinoma of the rectum. Subsequently, they updated their study in 1971, and Crile and Turnbull reported a series with favorable results in 1972.[137,509] As a consequence, others have been encouraged to selectively apply this technique.[440,720,882] Because of these reports, many surgeons had begun to use this treatment not only for palliation, but also for the potentially curable lesion.

The decision of attempting to avoid APR, a surgical procedure that has been reasonably successful in the primary treatment of carcinoma of the rectum for a century, requires careful consideration. It would be helpful if there were a prospective, randomized, controlled clinical study comparing APR with electrocoagulation or other local procedure for that matter. However, it is unlikely that we shall ever see one, although even in the absence of a controlled study, sufficient evidence has accumulated to warrant adoption of a policy of advising a local procedure for selected patients with carcinoma of the rectum.

Indications

Electrocoagulation may be considered when the tumor encompasses less than 50% of the circumference of the bowel wall, when the lesion is exophytic and well differentiated (or of a low-grade malignancy), when the tumor is confined to the bowel wall, when the patient with known metastases can have symptoms effectively palliated by this means, when debilitating disease is present, or when the patient refuses or cannot manage a colostomy. Relative contraindications include a circumferential lesion, a poorly differentiated or anaplastic tumor, a deeply ulcerating growth, an anterior lesion in a woman, or a tumor that extends above the peritoneal reflection. Certainly, if the growth is high enough to be removed by anterior resection, this is the treatment of choice.

Informed Consent

Before operation, the surgeon should explain the alternative forms of therapy available and the pros and cons of each procedure. If electrocoagulation is contemplated, the importance of close follow-up examination and the possibility of readmission to the hospital must be stressed. This places a considerable emotional burden on both the patient and the surgeon, and this clearly must be recognized at the outset. It is much easier for a surgeon to perform an abdominoperineal excision knowing that there is little more to offer the patient from the surgical point of view if the tumor recurs. However, if tumor recurs following electrocoagulation, it is extremely difficult to judge when this approach should be abandoned and when abdominoperineal excision should be undertaken. Even after unsuccessful electrocoagulation, the patient may be cured by radical surgery many months after the initial therapy.

Technique

All individuals are treated in the hospital, not as outpatients, unless one is dealing with a very small lesion. Regional or general anesthesia is required. The technique has been described by Madden and Kandalaft.[508] The patient is placed in the prone position if the tumor is primarily anterior and in the lithotomy position if the tumor is essentially posterior. Following sphincter stretch, a plastic operating anal retractor (Ferguson Clinic, Grand Rapids, MI) of appropriate diameter and length is inserted (Figure 23-139). These instruments were initially advocated by Schultz and Muldoon and by Muldoon and

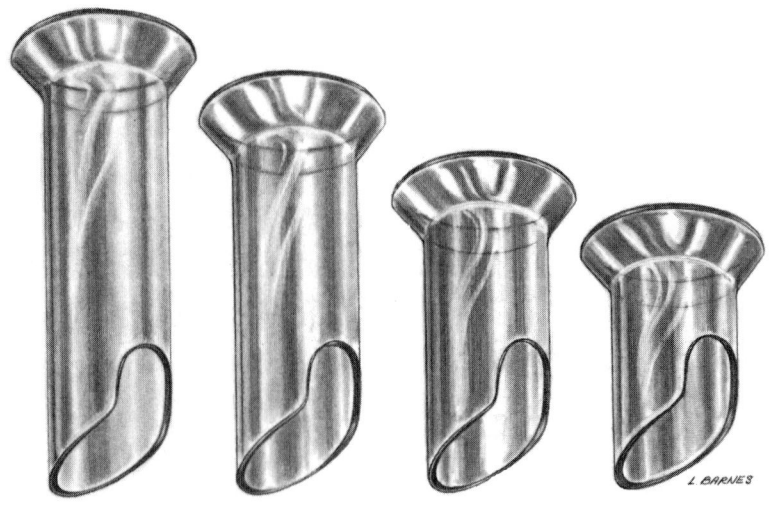

FIGURE 23-139. Plastic retractors of varied lengths and diameters permit excellent visualization for electrocoagulation.

Capehart for use in excision of polyps of the colon and rectum.[598,736] However, I have found them ideal for exposing the tumor preparatory to electrocoagulation or local excision. Other retractors may, of course, be used. Salvati and Rubin suggested the use of local infiltration with bupivacaine and epinephrine to improve anal relaxation and to limit the depth of anesthesia required.[720]

The goal of electrocoagulation is to destroy by coagulating current the entire tumor and a margin of normal tissue both deep to and around it. A standard electrocautery unit is used with the needle-tip adapter, and only coagulating current is employed. The area for electrocoagulation is outlined by means of the needle (Figure 23-140A). The tip is then plunged into the tumor while the current is applied, and the process is repeated until the entire area has been treated[46] (Figure 23-140B). Necrotic tissue is removed by scraping with the aid of an electrified wire-loop or endometrial curette (Figure 23-140C). When normal tissue is encountered (muscular wall or perirectal adipose tissue), the procedure is terminated. It is helpful to have available special lighting. This may include a headlamp, fiberoptic light source, or lighted retractor. A Frazier-tip suction is helpful for smoke as well as bleeding because it is quite small and is not as likely to impede the already limited view. Frequent irrigation with a bulb syringe is also a requisite. Operative time varies according to the size of the lesion and the degree of penetration; it may be as long as 2 hours (Figure 23-141). By no means should this procedure be considered a minor undertaking. For larger tumors, more than one session may be required, each necessitating hospitalization and an anesthetic.

After a large tumor has been ablated, the patient, ideally, is confined in the hospital for several days, at which time further biopsies are taken, and a repeat coagulation is performed if necessary. Unfortunately, in the United States today, ideal management is often not possible because of economic constraints. As a consequence, one must be willing to assume the risk of sepsis and delayed hemorrhage with the individual's having been discharged. The patient is seen at monthly intervals for the first 6 months and is readmitted to the hospital (if possible) for biopsy and electrocoagulation if a recurrent tumor is suspected. After 6 months without evidence of tumor, the intervals between office visits are gradually lengthened to approximately four times a year.

Complications

The most common postoperative complication is a pyrexia. An oral temperature of 103°F (39.4°C) on the evening after surgery is not uncommon. It is because of this problem that broad-spectrum antibiotic treatment is recommended preoperatively and postoperatively for 24

at least 24 hours. Pelvic peritonitis may occur without rectal perforation, but abdominal exploration, drainage, and colostomy are rarely indicated.

Hemorrhage at the time of surgery may necessitate multiple blood transfusions. All patients should have blood available when electrocoagulation is performed for large lesions. This can be a time-consuming operation, a procedure during which blood loss may appear to be minimal, but it can be persistent and ultimately not inconsequential. Late hemorrhage can occur up to several weeks after the procedure, probably secondary to sloughing of the eschar. This often requires readmission to the hospital and transfusion, and it has been reported to occur in as many as 22% of patients who undergo electrocoagulation.[509] I think, however, this is too high a figure. Five of 48 patients (10%) had hemorrhage sufficiently severe to require transfusion in our early experience.[370]

Rectal stricture may result from electrocoagulation if more than 50% of the bowel wall is involved by tumor. Repeated procedures increase the risk of this complication. Furthermore, the development of a stricture may impede the ability of the surgeon to visualize the area for possible recurrence. Benign stricture may be treated by lysis and the frequent insertion by the patient of Hegar's dilator (Figure 23-117; see Complications of Anterior Resection). Strictures occurred in 8% of our patients.[370]

In women, rectovaginal fistula may result from vigorous burning of an anterior lesion. Electrocoagulation, therefore, should be performed only for small, exophytic lesions when they occur in this location.

Results

Madden and Kandalaft updated their experience in 1983 to include a total of 204 patients treated by electrocoagulation.[510] Their 5-year survival rates even with ulcerating tumors were very impressive (57% with lesions larger than 3 cm and 63% if smaller than 3 cm). Patients with polypoid tumors had a 70% 5-year survival rate for the smaller tumors and a 64% rate for the larger ones.

In our experience, 39 patients were operated upon for cure.[370] Twenty-one were men, and 18 were women. The median age was 70 years (range, 48 to 89 years), as compared with a median age of 62 years for the group of individuals who underwent APR. Ten were 80 years old or older. The approximate sizes of the lesions were up to 2 cm in 14 patients, 3 cm in 13 patients, 4 cm in eight patients, and 6 cm or larger in four patients. Twenty-four individuals had exophytic tumors, and 15 had ulcerative lesions. Only three of the exophytic tumors were greater than 3 cm, whereas nine of the ulcerating tumors were greater than 3 cm. Thirty-seven patients had well-differentiated or moderately well-differentiated tumors. The remaining two patients had poorly differentiated lesions. Ten patients re-

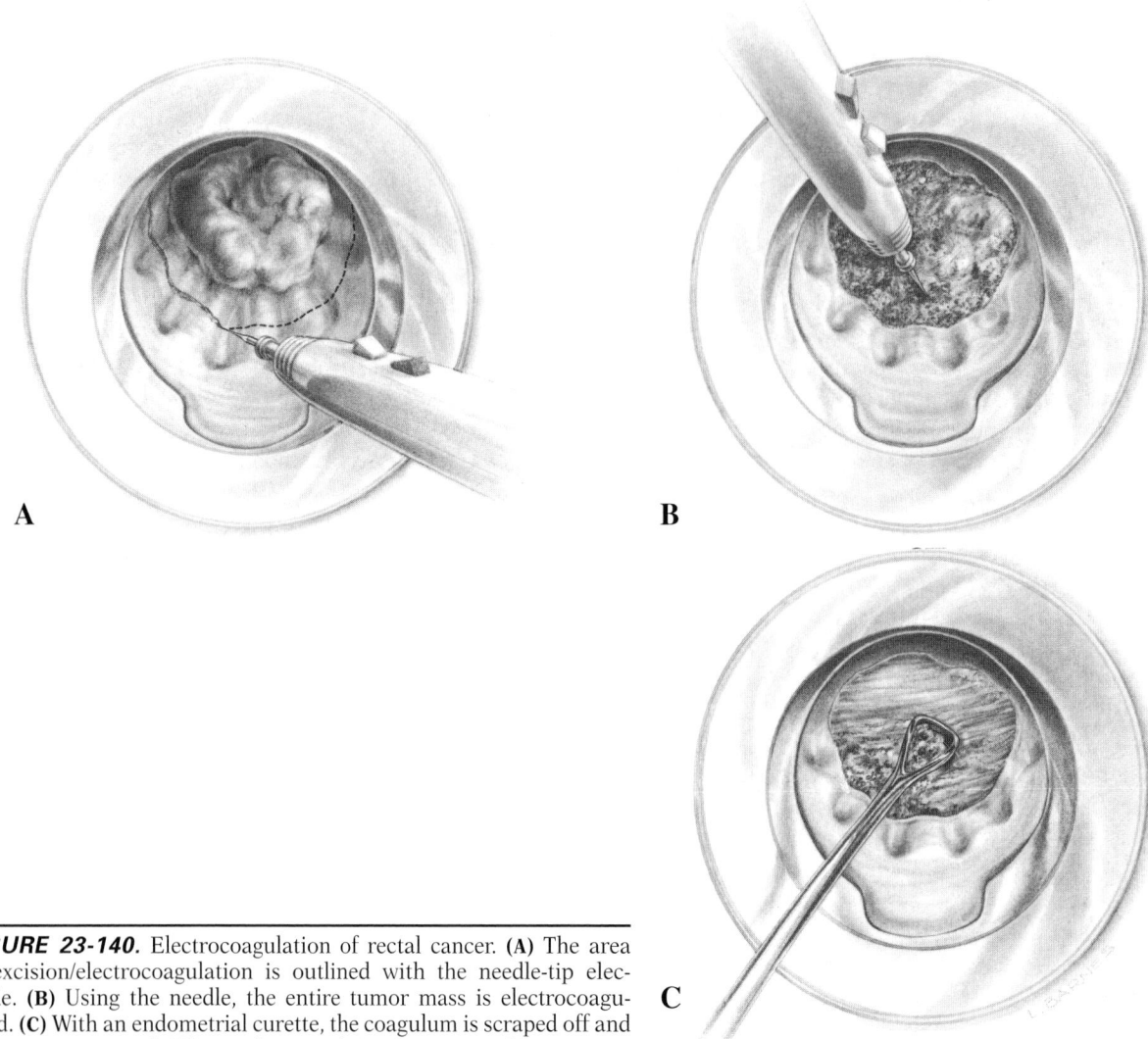

FIGURE 23-140. Electrocoagulation of rectal cancer. **(A)** The area of excision/electrocoagulation is outlined with the needle-tip electrode. **(B)** Using the needle, the entire tumor mass is electrocoagulated. **(C)** With an endometrial curette, the coagulum is scraped off and the process repeated. When only normal tissue remains, the operation is complete.

quired only a single session for treatment. Nine underwent two sessions, four underwent four sessions, and four patients underwent six or more sessions. There were two operative deaths related to cardiac problems, which should remind the surgeon that this is not a benign procedure.

In 27 of the 39 patients (69%), no evidence of disease was apparent at the end of the follow-up period. Twenty patients were alive, and seven had died of causes unrelated to the rectal cancer. Of the 24 patients with exophytic tumors, 22 (92%) had no evidence of the disease. However, only five of the 15 patients with ulcerative tumors (33%) had no evidence of disease (Table 23-15). Forty percent of patients who initially had ulcerative lesions could not have their local disease controlled by electrocoagulation; 27% required APR.

Salvati and colleagues reported 81 patients who underwent electrocoagulation for cure and in whom at least a 5-year follow-up was available.[721] The criteria for selection

were essentially the same as those previously discussed. The overall 5-year survival rate was 47%, but 38% required conversion to an APR. This last group had a 29% 5-year survival. The morbidity rate for electrocoagulation was 21%. Others have also become advocates of the judicious application of this technique.[868] The subsequent colostomy rate, however, has been reported to be as high as 25%.[34]

Palliation by Electrocoagulation

Christiansen and Kirkegaard employed electrocoagulation after recurrence developed following low anterior resection in an attempt to avoid colostomy.[114] Of 15 patients so treated, nine were alive without colostomy 8 to 16 months after the first treatment, and three had died without a stoma. There was one death, a consequence of the procedure. Kurz and colleagues reported the use of the urologic resectoscope for palliating symptoms from obstructing and

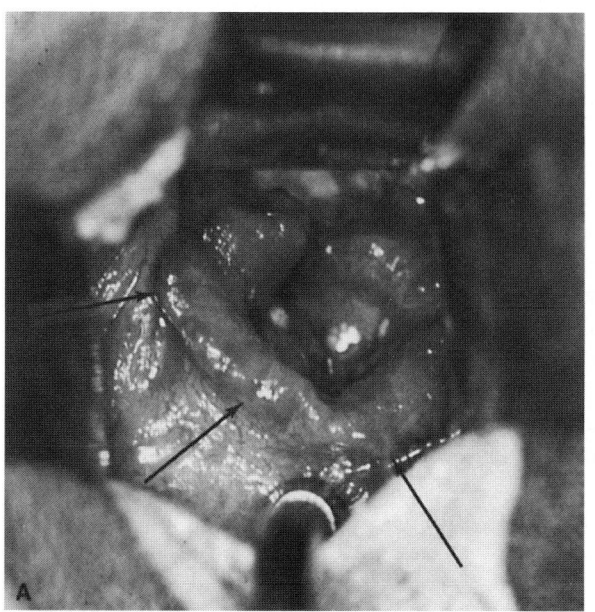

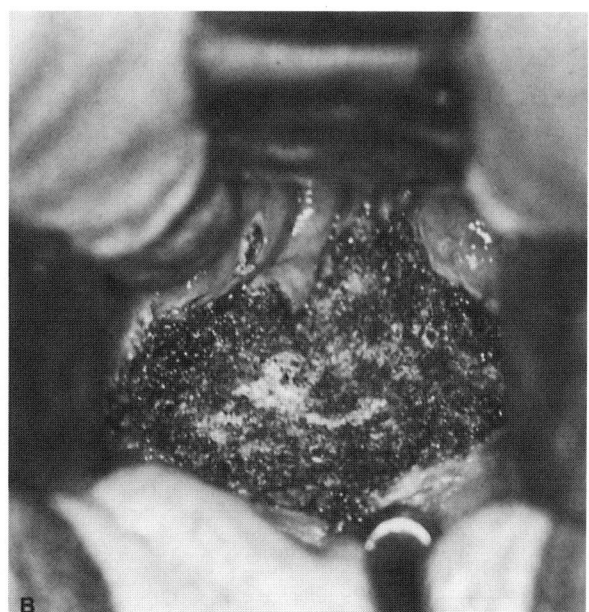

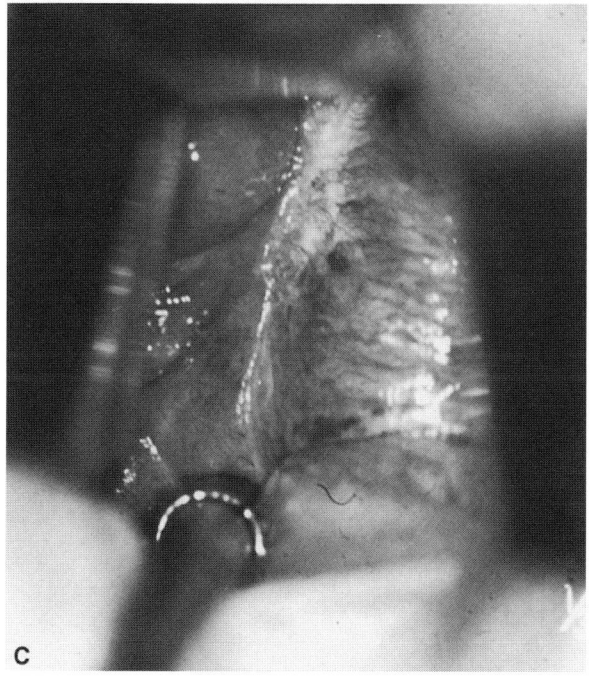

FIGURE 23-141. Electrocoagulation. **(A)** Rectal cancer is exposed *(arrows)*. **(B)** The tumor has been completely electrocoagulated. **(C)** Only the scar remains 2 months following treatment. (Courtesy of John L. Madden, M.D.)

bleeding lesions.[448] They emphasize the unique benefit of cutting current with continuous fluid irrigation to provide excellent visibility. Berry and colleagues used the same technique both for benign and malignant lesions.[51] Salvati and Rubin reported that colostomy was avoided in all but three of the 19 patients they treated for palliation.[720]

Opinion

I remain unconvinced that electrocoagulation is an effective modality of therapy for the patient with incurable disease. In seven such individuals whom we treated, four required a colostomy.[370] The median number of operative sessions was three, hardly an encouraging experience.

Sequential Treatment (Electrocoagulation Followed by Resection)

Eisenberg combined electrocoagulation with subsequent resection in the treatment of 250 patients.[188] The author preferred to perform low anterior resection, which calls into question the issue of performing this sphincter-saving alternative in the first instance. The survival results were exceptionally good: 85% following low anterior resection

▶ **TABLE 23-15 Results of Electrocoagulation on Morphologic Appearance of the Lesion**

Results	Exophytic	Ulcerative
Median age	68 y	73 y
Size		
<3 cm	21	6
>3 cm	3	9
Median treatments	—	4
No evidence of disease	92%	33%
Disease not controlled	4%	40%
Subsequent abdominoperineal resection	4%	27%

(From Hughes EP, Veidenheimer MC, Corman ML, Coller JA. Electrocoagulation of rectal cancer. *Dis Colon Rectum* 1982;25:215, with permission.)

and 61% after APR. Despite these favorable results, no one else has been motivated to report their experience.

Comment

In order for electrocoagulation to be successfully employed, careful preoperative assessment must be made, including endorectal ultrasound. Tumors should be mobile, exophytic, and well differentiated or moderately well differentiated. Flow cytometric evaluation has been thought to be helpful, but probably not more so that degree of differenetiation. The chance of lymph node metastases is considerably reduced if this protocol is followed.[137,260,292]

Probably the most important criticism of this method is the failure to obtain a complete pathologic specimen. One must depend on clinical assessment, personal experience, and biopsy and frozen section to determine the adequacy of tumor removal, and evidence obviously may be incomplete or inaccurate.

An additional concern is what to do if the tumor recurs. When should one abandon this modality of treatment? The answer, in my experience, lies in the quality of the doctor-patient relationship. The patient who accepts electrocoagulation in the first instance will often help to guide the surgeon in making future operative decisions. Finally, it is important to recognize that 5-year survival figures of 50%, 60%, 70%, or even 80% may not be laudatory, especially if the patients who are being selected for this treatment harbor the most favorable tumors (i.e., Dukes' A lesions—T_1 or T_2).

Transanal Excision

Transanal excision has been advocated by a number of surgeons for the definitive treatment of small (less than 3 cm), exophytic, movable, well-differentiated lesions.[57,150, 160,415,520,595,786,869] As with electrocoagulation, the preoperative evaluation should include, among all of the other criteria, histopathologic confirmation, especially the degree of differentiation, as well endorectal ultrasound (see prior discussion). The policy of less than resection is based on the knowledge that there is only a 10% risk of synchronous metastasis to regional lymph nodes when the cancer is confined to the rectal wall.[594] Conversely, the Mayo Clinic group observed that the risk of harboring lymph nodes metastases with T_1 low rectal cancers that have lymphovascular invasion on biopsy or invasion into the lower third of the submucosa was sufficiently high as to mandate either radical resection or adjuvant therapy.[603]

The singular advantage of local excision over that of electrocoagulation is that it offers the opportunity for histologically evaluating a "total biopsy." Theoretically, if local excision is judged by the pathologist to be "complete" and the tumor is well or moderately well differentiated, then one may reasonably recommend that no additional surgical treatment is required.[594] The essential variables, therefore, are the capability and the interest of the pathologist. It is also extremely important to orient the specimen for histologic examination accurately. Sweeney suggests that one use 25-gauge needles to pin the specimen onto a cautery cleansing pad for this purpose.[810] Whether one is truly satisfied with the margins of the excision and whether there is evidence of lymphatic or blood vessel invasion may create additional concerns about the wisdom of performing a limited procedure. Guillem and colleagues at Memorial Sloan-Kettering suggested using the following criteria in order to determine which tumors are theoretically suitable for transanal excision:[298]

- Size less than 4 cm
- Tumor confined to less than one quadrant
- Site less than 9 cm from anal verge
- Mobility
- Well-differentiated appearance
- Absence of lymphovascular invasion
- Absence of nodal involvement
- Ultrasonographic T_1, T_2, N_0 lesion
- On CT scan, no metastases

Unfortunately, there are no statistically meaningful studies available concerning the risk of harboring additional tumor, and there have been no prospective randomized clinical trials.

Technique

The procedure can be performed through an operating proctoscope (depending on the location and the size of the lesion), but more commonly it is accomplished by dilating the anus and inserting retractors. The technique is essentially the same as that illustrated in Figures 21-44 and 21-45 for benign lesions. As with electrocoagulation, proper positioning is crucial. Anterior lesions are best managed with the patient in the prone, jackknife position, and posterior lesions are optimally treated with the patient in the lithotomy position. Ideally, one attempts to achieve a 1-cm margin, but lesser margins may be as satisfactory. The tumor is outlined with an adequate margin by means of the needle-tip electrocautery. Some individuals prefer injection of saline with or without epinephrine to facilitate hemostasis and to aid in the dissection. Generally, it is easier to begin the dissection from below the tumor utilizing a clamp to hold the specimen as the dissection proceeds cephalad. A full-thickness rectal wall excision is performed; one should not attempt to preserve part of the bowel wall.

Results

Hager and associates reported 95 patients treated by local excision.[307] The 5-year survival rate for tumors confined to the mucosa and submucosa was 90%, and 78% when the cancer invaded the muscularis propria. Biggers and colleagues reported the Mayo Clinic experience of 234 patients.[57] Of these, 180 never developed a recurrence, five developed metastases, and 49 had local recurrences. Although it may seem that the overall failure rate is excessive (23%), many patients who had undergone this treatment would today not fulfill the previously mentioned criteria for selection. For example, if one limits the indications for this treatment to those tumors that have a pedicle or pseudopedicle, Grigg and colleagues reported that 100% of their 16 patients survived for 5 years.[296]

Graham and colleagues identify three pathologic features that correlate with a high risk of recurrence and a poor outcome: positive surgical margins, poorly differentiated histology, and increasing depth of bowel wall invasion.[288] Coco and associates employed local excision in 36 patients, adding postoperative radiation therapy if the tumor unexpectedly had breached the rectal wall.[119] The complication rate was 9.3%. The results were not sufficiently long term to give meaningful cure or recurrence rates. Close follow-up examination is emphasized. Bleday and colleagues noted an 8% recurrence rate with local excision and concluded that either a positive margin or lymphatic invasion were believed to be indications for resection.[69] Faivre and colleagues noted a 28% incidence of recurrence in their 126 patients.[201] Vascular invasion and a mucinous component were believed to be poor prognostic factors. Rouanet and associates opined that local control should improve if postoperative radiotherapy is given for more invasive tumors and those greater than 3 cm in diameter.[703] Others reported a reasonably satisfactory experience in a highly selected group of patients.[222,238,367]

Mellgren and colleagues reported the University of Minnesota experience.[560] One hundred eight patients with T_1 and T_2 rectal cancers treated by local excision were compared with 153 individuals with T_1N_0 and T_2N_0 rectal cancers managed by radical resection. Mean follow-up was greater than 4 years in each group. The estimated 5-year recurrence rate was 18% for T_1 and 47% for T_2 tumors. The rate following radical resection was 9% for T_1 and 16% for T_2 cancers. The authors concluded that local excision carries with it a much greater risk of recurrence than radical resection, and despite salvage surgery (see the following), local excision for T_2 tumors especially may compromise overall survival.[560]

Löhnert and co-workers, as part of their follow-up routine, evaluated by means of endorectal ultrasound all of their 116 patients who had undergone local excision, in addition to the usual clinical and laboratory investigations.[491] Evidence of local recurrence suggested by endorectal ultrasound was confirmed by ultrasound-guided needle biopsy. All 25 patients who were found to have *occult* rectal cancer recurrences were alive at the end of the study period (four with recurrences). Because endoluminal ultrasound can apparently detect local recurrence at an earlier and subclinical stage, the authors encouraged the routine application of this modality as part of the follow-up regimen.

Local Excision and Radiotherapy

Downstaging with neoadjuvant therapy followed by local excision is another controversial issue. Schell and co-workers found that some of their patients with T_3 lesions experienced significant downstaging and submitted 11 to local excision.[731] There were no local recurrences in these individuals (median follow-up, 47.9 months). Marks and colleagues reported their experience of 20 patients with preoperative radiation (45 Gy) followed by full-thickness local excision 4 to 6 weeks later.[530] They found a recurrence rate of 21%. As a consequence, they believed that this approach is of value only for the individual who cannot tolerate a standard resection.

Ellis and colleagues performed local excision of favorable rectal cancers followed by radiotherapy (45 Gy).[190] They found no evidence of disease in their eight patients, with a mean of 67 months of follow-up. The obvious question, however, is whether the patients would have been equally served without the radiation. A less successful experience was noted by others.[579]

Salvage Resection

The decision about what to do when recurrence develops or tumor persists is discussed in the section on electrocoagulation. Baron and colleagues retrospectively reviewed 155 patients who were submitted to initial curative treatment by a local procedure.[38] A total of 21 patients underwent radical resection because of an unfavorable pathology report, either APR or low anterior resection immediately following the local treatment. An additional 21 patients underwent a so-called salvage resection for local recurrence. The disease-free survival for those who had undergone immediate resection was 94.1% as compared with the delayed group survival rate of 55.5%. The authors recommended that when adverse pathologic features are present in the excision specimen, immediate resection should be performed.[38] The 5-year survival rate as reported by Rouanet and colleagues was 30% for those individuals subjected to resection for recurrent disease.[703]

The aforementioned University of Minnesota group identified 24 of 27 patients with recurrence after local excision who underwent salvage surgery.[560] The estimated 5-year survival rate was 72% for T_1 tumors and 65% after salvage surgery for what was initially T_2 lesions. Another report from the same institution revealed that the stage of recurrent tumor was more advanced than that of the primary in 93%.[225] The authors emphasized the importance of appropriate selection for those offered local excision. In still another publication from the Memorial Sloan-Kettering Cancer Center involving 125 patients, the investigators concluded that two thirds of the patients who developed recurrence have local treatment failure, implicating inadequate excision.[650] Furthermore, neither adjuvant radiotherapy nor salvage surgery was believed to be reliable in controlling or preventing local recurrence.

Recommendations and Comment

The advantage of having a pathologic specimen has stimulated me to utilize excision as the primary technique for those who are to undergo a local procedure. I employ electrocoagulation primarily for palliation in those individuals who have larger lesions and who are not candidates for or refuse to have APR. As discussed in the section on electrocoagulation, the primary conundrums are what to do with an unfavorable pathology report and how to treat recurrence.

Until relatively recently, I had recommended chemoradiation therapy for lesions that were subsequently found to be transmural and/or in the presence of lymphatic or vascular invasion. However, I now believe that adjuvant therapy should be offered to those who have been found to harbor T_2 tumors as well. Following completion of the treatment, the patient is reevaluated and a decision made as to whether a radical operation is appropriate. Unfortunately, there are no meaningful statistics to determine whether additional surgery is necessary. However, there is certainly ample evidence to suggest that chemoradiation therapy can control local disease and downstage tumors (see later). I agree with the comments made by the Melbourne, Australia group, that there is a need for a randomized, controlled trial for T_2 lesions in which local excision with adjuvant chemoradiation therapy is compared with radical resec-

tion.[746] Whether we shall ever see it, however, is problematic.

If resection is recommended, it should be performed not sooner than 3 weeks following completion of the chemoradiation therapy, in my opinion. I do not recommend proceeding immediately to resection with an unfavorable pathology report before adjuvant therapy has been undertaken. It is technically impossible to remove the rectum without entering a contaminated field, thereby increasing the risk of infection, and perhaps even jeopardizing the potential for cure through implantation of malignant cells. This concern may be theoretical, but there is a certain logic to it.

Transanal Endoscopic Microsurgery

Because of the technical problems associated with attempts at local excision of lesions at higher distances from the anal verge, Buess and colleagues developed a minimally invasive technique by means of a resectoscope.[87] The procedure permits a stereoscopic, magnified view of a gas-dilated rectum, a feature that allows precise surgery to be performed in a difficult-to-reach area. The rectoscope has a diameter of 40 mm, with lengths available in either 12 or 20 cm (Figure 23-142). All instruments are designed for endoscopic work and include scissors, angled forceps, needle holder, suction device, and clip applicator.

Results

Buess and colleagues utilized this techniques initially in 74 patients.[87] Their results are comparable to those of other local procedures that have been discussed. A later experience from the same unit in Tübingen, Germany, involved 113 patients.[564] There were no operative deaths. In a limited follow-up, only two patients developed a local recurrence. The complication rate resulting from perforation was 7%. One must remember, however, that the technique is often employed for higher-level lesions than one would or could attempt by conventional transanal excision or electrocoagulation. Others strongly advocate this procedure because of the excellent visualization obtained with this instrument.[883]

Winde and colleagues reported a 5-year survival rate of 96% in their 50 patients.[883] Only 4.2% developed a local recurrence. Others reported comparable success with this technique.[441,565,791] All concluded that the results are superior to alternative local approaches in the middle and upper rectum.[770]

One particular concern that has been expressed is the adverse effect of prolonged anal dilatation with this 4-cm–diameter instrument. Hemingway and colleagues performed anorectal manometry on six patients and discovered that no individual reported incontinence at a mean of 16 weeks of follow-up.[337]

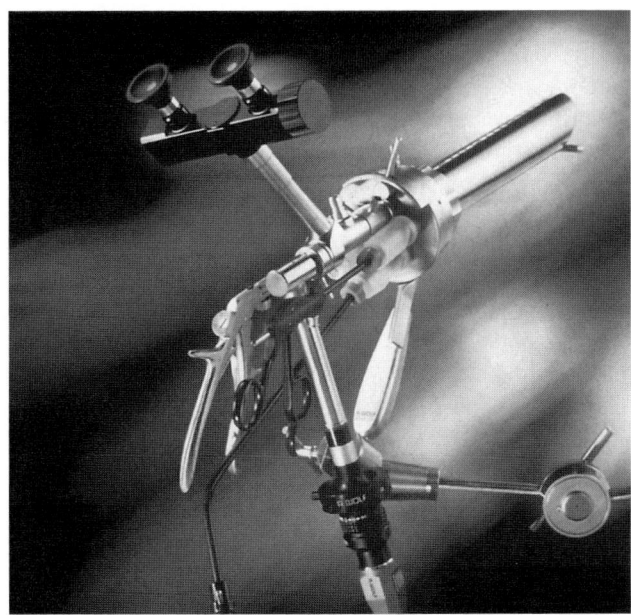

FIGURE 23-142. Transanal endoscopic microsurgery system. The stereoscopic system permits excellent visualization. Up to four surgical instruments can be inserted at the same time. The assistant can follow the procedure through the use of a fiberoptic channel or through a video monitor. (Courtesy of Richard Wolf Medical Instruments, Inc. Vernon Hills, IL.)

Comment

Transanal endoscopic microsurgery can obviously accomplish what amounts to alocal excision. However, there are two major disadvantages or concerns as I see it. First, the cost is considerable. Because of the limited applicability of this technique, it is doubtful whether very many surgeons or institutions can justify the expense associated with this particular investment. Certainly, for distal rectal lesions, there is no advantage of the technology when one has the option of merely using an anorectal retractor. The second concern that I have is the problematic application of this method for higher lesions, because these can usually be resected by conventional means, with reestablishment of intestinal continuity. Therefore, although the instrument is indeed impressive and offers beautiful visualization, I do not see its entering the mainstream for most specialty surgeons in the management of carcinoma of the rectum.

Laser Photocoagulation

There are at least three ablative methods for palliative endoscopic treatment of malignant strictures of the rectum: laser photocoagulation, electrocoagulation, and cryosurgical destruction. These are discussed previously in this chapter and in Chapter 22. The neodymium:yttrium-aluminum-garnet (Nd:YAG) laser (see Chapter 1) has been applied by many groups for the palliative treatment of rectal cancer.[76,85,112,492,496,519,541,737] No one, however, is advocating this approach for the management of curable cancers of the rectum. However, for the unresectable tumor, or when bleeding is a problem, the laser can restore luminal patency and achieve at least temporary hemostasis.[541] When compared with other local procedures, laser therapy is unique in that it is of equal applicability to tumors above the peritoneal reflection as it is to those below. Eckhauser and colleagues employed the Nd:YAG laser as a preresective treatment for obstructing rectal carcinoma.[187] They found that recanalization by this method permitted primary resection and anastomosis to be accomplished.

The procedure may be performed selectively on an outpatient basis, but it usually requires hospitalization. Standard bowel preparation is employed; sedation alone may be adequate. Concern has been expressed that the energy delivered by the laser can be quite misleading. The actual tissue effect is as much related to the technique of application as it is to the laser power settings.[496] Although laser endoscopy permits change of these settings to enhance a hemostatic or vaporizing effect, this must be recognized if one is to avoid excessive cavitation.[496]

Initial relief of symptoms has been reported to be approximately 90% in several published series, but after a few months individuals may require an additional treatment.[76,85,112,492,541,616,852] The primary aim is to avoid a colostomy, and this is usually successful because patients are not expected to survive for very long. Perirectal abscess and bowel perforation are reportedly infrequent complications. Mandava and co-workers experienced a 15% complication rate in their 27 patients.[519]

Escudero-Fabre and Sack have proposed what seems to me to be reasonable indications for this technique:[197]

- For palliation of malignant neoplasms in individuals with extensive local disease, disseminated disease, high operative risk, or refusal to undergo surgery
- As a temporizing measure to improve preoperative status in those individuals with lesions complicated by obstruction or bleeding
- As an alternative approach for the management of benign lesions

Farouk and colleagues reported that laser treatment offered adequate palliation for 78% of their 41 patients.[205] They further observed that those who survived more than 2 years were more likely to require surgical intervention.

Bright and associates had a less favorable experience with this approach in their report of 38 patients.[81] Two thirds of those with large tumors required an alternative surgical approach. Furthermore, the overall mortality rate within 1 month of treatment was 21%. The authors concluded that tumors that are circumferential or those involving the anal sphincters are better managed by approaches other than laser therapy.[81]

Laser photocoagulation may be used in combination with either implantation of a plastic prosthesis or a self-expanding metal stent (see Chapter 22).[708] The advantage of stent placement is to maintain luminal patency to prevent the need for repetitive laser treatments. Rupp successfully utilized self-expanding metal stents in combination with palliative laser therapy.[708] Serious complications or signs of reobstruction were not observed until the patient's death, with survival time up to 25 months.

Comment

The application of the laser to the treatment of benign and malignant neoplasms of the colon and rectum is a relatively recent phenomenon. I stated before the second edition of this text, "It is probable that by the time this book is published, there will be a number of papers describing this technique for the primary treatment of favorable rectal cancers that might otherwise be managed by electrocoagulation or by local excision." Not only did this prove to be untrue, but it still remains untrue as writing for the fifth edition proceeds. However, with the increased use of endorectal ultrasound and other staging techniques, it is not unreasonable to expect that, at some point, patients with potentially curable cancers will be offered this alternative. This option, however, *does* require special expertise, and the equipment is quite expensive. Whether one is justified in becoming proficient at this time is a matter of conjecture. Regardless, it is doubtful that laser photocoagulation will prove to be more advantageous than the other methods available for nonresectional treatment.

Cryosurgery

Gage reported the use of cryotherapy for palliation of symptoms in seven patients with inoperable rectal cancer and one with perineal recurrence after APR.[232] Bleeding was controlled, obstruction was relieved, and colostomy was not required. These benefits were believed to be related to the reduction of tumor bulk. Gage believed that cryotherapy can compete successfully with radiation and electrocoagulation in the management of selected cases of inoperable rectal cancer.[233]

Fritsch and colleagues treated 219 patients with this technique but only for palliation.[226] At 6 months to 7 years following treatment, local tumor was eradicated in 30% and reduced in size sufficiently to relieve symptoms in 24%. Fourteen percent of patients experienced hemorrhage, and 26% developed stenoses. Other major complications (e.g., peritonitis) were seen in 8%. Disadvantages included frequent discharge of necrotic tissue and malodorous secretions, as well as rather costly equipment. Heberer and colleagues utilized cryosurgery for palliation in 268 patients.[333] A colostomy was avoided in 80% (mean observation time, 2.3 years). The experience of others suggests that the cryosurgical technique provides therapeutic benefits for selected patients with advanced rectal cancer and for those who cannot tolerate a major operation.[890]

Comment

I have had no experience with this technique. Cautious consideration may be given to its application for patients who harbor symptomatic rectal cancers too proximal to electrocoagulate or as an alternative to laser therapy and in whom metastatic disease is present. Interestingly, there have been no reports of the use of this technique that I have been able to locate since the publication of the third edition of this text.

Endocavitary Irradiation

The use of radium needles and radiation therapy has been employed in the palliative treatment of incurable or recurrent rectal cancer for more than 50 years. In fact, Sir Charles Gordon-Watson presented a paper on the use

---

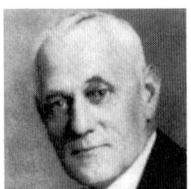

Sir Charles Gordon-Watson (1874–1949) Gordon-Watson was born one of 12 children who survived into adulthood, the fifth son of a Buckinghamshire (England) vicar. His youthful ambition was to become a soldier, but because life in the army during those days was impossible for a man without means, he endeavored to establish himself in country life by becoming apprenticed to a land agent. When a position failed to materialize, with no science background and upon a whim, he applied and was accepted to St. Bartholomew's Medical College and Hospital in London. Following his qualification in 1898 and a period as house surgeon, he volunteered to serve as a Civil Surgeon in the Boer War. After 2 years, he returned to England and became a Fellow of the Royal College of Surgeons. In 1908, he joined the staff of St. Mark's Hospital in London, and in 1910 he was elected Assistant Surgeon to St. Bartholomew's. When World War I broke out, he joined the expeditionary forces in France, and while there he received many tributes for field military service. He was the first person to describe the syndrome of trench foot. In 1919, he had conferred upon him a Knighthood of the Order of the British Empire. In 1931, he was made an Honorary Fellow of the American College of Surgeons. He is remembered for his numerous contributions to coloproctology through his association with St. Mark's Hospital.

of radium in the treatment of rectal cancer as early as 1927.[281] Although he recognized in several publications in the 1930s that in most cases the results were somewhat less than gratifying, he believed that there was indeed a place for this method, especially in the nonresectable situation.[282-284] However, it was not until Papillon reported his experience in 1973 that radiation was applied as an alternative to surgery for a potentially curable lesion.[639]

Technique

The procedure requires a special device that can be inserted through a large-diameter proctoscope. The contact unit, manufactured by Phillips (Eindhoven, the Netherlands; Figure 23-143), develops a high-radiation output (10 to 20 Gy/minute) with low-voltage (50-kV) x-rays. The effective area is approximately 3 cm in diameter, with absorption of the x-rays essentially limited to a depth of 2 cm. Papillon recommended 25 to 40 Gy at each treatment, administered within 3 minutes.[641] The procedure is repeated from 1 to 3 weeks later, for a total dose of between 80 and 150 Gy over a period of 4 to 10 weeks. Most patients can be managed outside of a hospital setting, and no anesthesia is usually required.

In a later publication, Papillon suggested that in patients younger than 60 years old, a perirectal lymphadenectomy be considered.[642] He also added a combination of external-beam radiation (30 Gy in 12 days), followed by iridium-192 implant 2 months later, to extend the field of radiation in the poor-risk patient in whom one wishes to use a "conservative" treatment.[642]

Patient Selection

According to Papillon, certain criteria must be met if a patient is to be considered for this treatment:[640]

- Accessibility of the entire lesion
- Small size (<4.5 cm)
- Noninfiltrating status
- Histologically well-differentiated status
- Palpability
- Mobility
- Absence of palpable mesorectal nodes

Results

Papillon reported initially 106 patients, 70% of whom were alive and free of disease after 5 years.[640] Local recurrence developed in 14 individuals (13%). Sixteen patients (15%) died of malignant disease. A later report from his center included 245 patients followed for more than 5 years.[642] A local failure rate of 5.3% was noted. The death rate from cancer was 8.9%, and the 5-year survival rate, 76%.

Sischy and Remington reported 23 of 25 patients to have responded to treatment and to be free of disease, but the follow-up period was considerably shorter.[762,763] Fleshman and colleagues noted one failure in treating eight patients (13%).[215] From the Cleveland Clinic came a report of 199 patients treated by means of endocavitary radiation, 126 of whom were managed with curative intent.[373] Twenty-nine percent developed a recurrence. With additional treatment, 11% were rendered free of disease. With more than 5 years of follow-up, 91% had no evidence of disease with additional treatment, but only 68% were cured on the basis of endocavitary irradiation alone.

Birnbaum and colleagues reported the Washington University (St. Louis, MO) experience with combined external and endocavitary radiation in order to identify factors predictive for recurrence of rectal cancer.[60] Seventy-two patients underwent pretreatment assessment by means of endorectal ultrasound staging. After a median follow-up of 31 months, there were no recurrences in the uT_1 group, a 22% recurrence rate in the uT_2 individuals, and a 51% recurrence for uT_3 lesions.

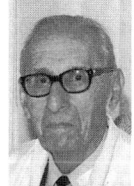

Jean Papillon (1914–1993) Jean Papillon was born in Lyons, France, September 18, 1914, the city in which he resided for his entire life. He graduated from the Medical School in 1936 and entered the Internship Program at Lyons Hospital. He completed his training in radiology at the University of Lyons in 1944 with his thesis *Radiological Studies of Bronchial Obstruction.* In 1946, he became radiologist physician to the Hôpitaux de Lyons. In 1943, he also worked at the Centre Léon Bérard, a well-recognized institution devoted to oncology. Through these auspices, he contributed more than 500 articles and lectures on a variety of tumor problems, such as Hodgkin's disease, head and neck malignancies, and thoracic, gynecologic, and osseous tumors. In 1950, he became interested in the management of cancer of the anus and rectum. Utilizing the concepts initially advocated by Lamarque in Montpellier, Papillon developed the techniques of intrarectal contact x-ray therapy and anal cancer curietherapy. As a consequence of his initial observations, he formulated the protocol of treatment utilizing radiation therapy alone or in combination with surgery for the management of anal and rectal cancers in order to effect sphincteric preservation. Papillon was appointed Head of Radiotherapy at the Centre Léon Bérard in 1951 and in 1955 became Professor of Radiotherapy at Lyons University. Author of a text dedicated to Rupert Turnbull, *Conservative Treatment by Irradiation—An Alternative to Radical Surgery,* he received international recognition for his contributions through honorary fellowship in the Royal College of Radiologists, the Canadian College of Radiologists, and the American College of Radiologists.

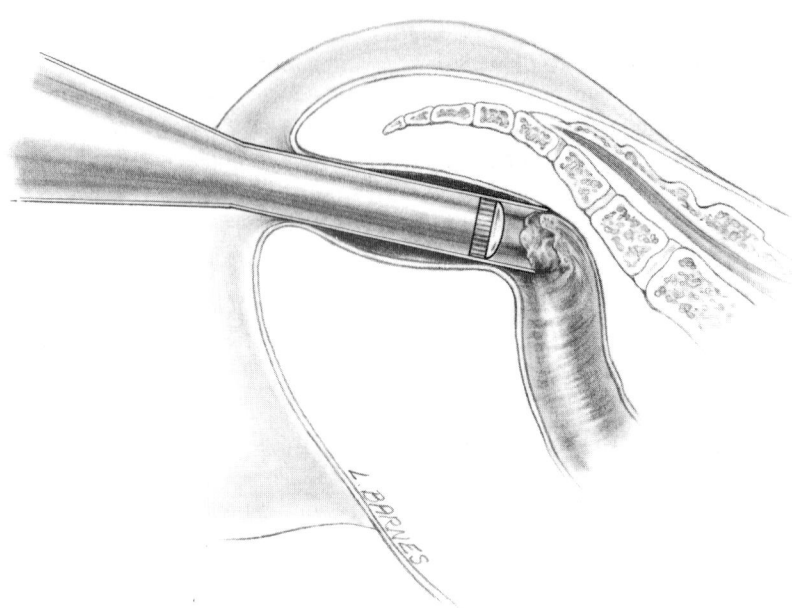

FIGURE 23-143. Endocavitary irradiation. The unit is introduced by means of a rectoscope.

Complications

Very few complications are attributable to the treatment. Jelden reported mild proctitis of short duration and occasional bleeding.[389] Rectovaginal fistula has also been seen. Deaths directly related to the therapy have not been reported.

Comment

As with all local procedures, it is difficult to assess the results of endocavitary radiation by comparison with standard resective treatment. Only those who have the most favorable prognoses are selected. A patient who undergoes APR for a Dukes' A lesion has a chance of cure that approaches 90%, so that claiming a cure rate less than this figure does not represent a great breakthrough in the treatment of cancer of the rectum. Furthermore, as with any local treatment, one wonders whether some patients are being deprived of the only possibility for cure if they harbor lymph node metastases. As previously discussed, even with careful patient selection, the decision whether to employ any local procedure requires a dedication to preoperative counseling and to close follow-up.

RADIOTHERAPY

The use of external-beam radiotherapy in the management of rectal cancer has received considerable attention in recent years as an adjunctive treatment to surgery, either preoperatively or postoperatively. In theory, preoperative treatment may decrease the size and the extent of tumor invasion and permit complete removal as well as minimize the risk of local recurrence. Preoperative treatment may also limit the likelihood of dissemination of viable tumor cells during surgical manipulation.

Postoperative therapy offers the distinct advantage of one having the availability of a pathology report. Thus, the known extent of disease determines the field of treatment. In the postoperative patient who is known to have a less favorable lesion (Dukes' B or C), radiotherapy may reduce the risk of pelvic recurrence. The downside of postoperative radiotherapy is the likelihood of adverse functional consequences because one will inevitably be radiating the rectum if continuity has been reestablished.

Preoperative Radiotherapy (Neoadjuvant Radiation Therapy)

Background and Indications

The rationale for neoadjuvant radiation therapy in the management of rectal cancer is to alter the viability of cancer cells so that they are no longer capable of local implantation.[760] When the concept was first proposed, however, there was concern that delay in initiating surgical treatment could increase the risk of tumor spread, but there is no evidence today to suggest that this is in fact the case. The primary issue is identifying those patients in advance who would most likely benefit from neoadjuvant radiotherapy. How can one make this determination? Clinical assessment is probably the gold standard, but endorectal ultrasound, CT, and MRI may also be quite helpful. Staging laparotomy has been suggested in order to determine mobility, resectability, staging, and the possibility of constructing a diversionary stoma before embarking upon radiotherapy.[89] Some authors believe that every rectal cancer should be treated by preoperative radiation, but most surgeons are selective in their approach. The following variables are generally considered appropriate indications for performing preoperative radiation:

- Fixed tumor
- Evidence of ureteral obstruction
- Invasion of adjacent structures (e.g., bladder, seminal vesicles, vagina)
- Presacral adenopathy
- Anal canal invasion
- Ultrasound uT_3 or uT_4 lesion
- Poorly differentiated histology

The impetus for the application of preoperative radiotherapy can be attributed to the reports by Quan and Stearns and their colleagues that emanated from the Memorial Sloan-Kettering Cancer Center in New York.[463,778,783–785] Although their initial studies indicated improved survival, a prospective evaluation demonstrated that the overall survival rate was not better, but that the incidence of failure because of local recurrence was reduced.[785] At that institution, Stearns and colleagues used external radiation through opposing anterior and posterior portals, 2.5 Gy daily to 20 Gy. The resection was carried out 2 days to 6 weeks following treatment.

The classic article that evaluated preoperative radiation was reported by Dwight and Higgins and their col-

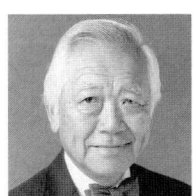

Stuart H.Q. Quan (1920–present)   Stuart Quan was born in Oakland, California on July 4, 1920, the youngest of ten children and the son of a physician from China who practiced Chinese medicine in San Francisco. Although Quan was only 3 years old when his father passed away, he knew as early as 6 years old that we wished to become a doctor. He completed his undergraduate education at Stanford University and graduated from Harvard Medical School in Boston in 1945. There followed 3 years of residency in Boston before his initial visit to New York. In 1949, his interest in oncologic surgery took him to the Memorial Hospital for Cancer and Allied Diseases as an Assistant Resident in Surgery. Except for 2 years serving with the United States Air Force as a flight surgeon in France and Libya, he has been continuously on the Surgical Staff at the Memorial Sloan-Kettering Cancer Center in New York to this day. Quan has contributed extensively to his chosen field, that of colorectal cancer surgery. As such, he has been recognized through numerous awards and honors, including Presidency of the American Society of Colon and Rectal Surgeons and an endowed Chair in his honor at Memorial-Sloan Kettering. He and his colleagues were pioneers in promoting preoperative irradiation for cancer of the rectum. After 51 years of caring for a huge number of patients, he retired from the practice of surgery, but not from his academic pursuits.

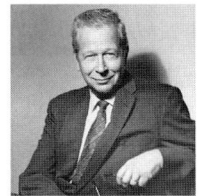

Maus W. Stearns, Jr. (1914–present)   Maus Stearns was born in Schenectady, New York. He accomplished his premedical studies at Union College in that city and graduated from the Albany Medical College in 1939. Following his internship in Port Chester, New York, he began his long association with the Memorial Hospital from resident surgeon to Chief of the Rectal and Colon Service. In 1942, his training was interrupted by World War II. Stearns served 3 years in the China-Burma-India theater, and he helped to operate on 25,000 Chinese patients and cared for such legendary soldiers as Merrill's Marauders and others under the command of General Stillwell. Following his demobilization, he received a National Cancer Institute Fellowship through the Memorial Hospital for 3 years. Stearns then joined the Colon and Rectal Service, which had been organized by George Binkley, a man who had been recruited by James Ewing to treat rectal cancer with radium. This experience led to the comprehensive evaluation of radiation by Stearns and his colleagues at that institution. Many important publications were the result of his leadership of the department, with Stearns being the prime motivator for accumulating and publishing the Memorial Hospital's experience. In response to Turnbull's description of the "no-touch" technique, Stearns opined that the time-honored tenet of sound surgical technique to encompass radical *en bloc* excision of the primary tumor with the lymphatics was the critical issue and that it is the radical treatment and completeness of the resection responsible for optimal results—not the so-called "no-touch" approach. Stearns received many honors and recognitions, including Presidency of the Society of Surgical Oncology (now the James Ewing Society) and Presidency of the American Society of Colon and Rectal Surgeons. He lives in retirement in California. (Photograph courtesy of Blackstone-Shelburne, New York.)

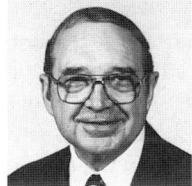

George Alfred Higgins, Jr. (1917–1994)   George Higgins was born in Towanda, Kansas, but grew up in Mountainair, New Mexico, where he attended the University of New Mexico. Following graduation, he entered Harvard Medical School in Boston in 1942 and then pursued a residency in surgery at the Boston City Hospital. His training was interrupted by World War II. Following his service as a battalion surgeon at Fort Hood, Texas and at the Walter Reed Hospital in Washington, DC, he completed his surgical training at the Veterans Administration (VA) Hospital in Washington, DC. Following appointments as Chief of Surgery at the Wichita, Kansas and Kansas City, Missouri VA Hospitals, he accepted the position as Chief of Surgery at the Washington, DC VA. Certified in general and thoracic surgery, he achieved the rank of Professor of Surgery at both Georgetown University and the George Washington University Medical Schools. At the age of 65, he retired from the VA and embarked on a new career—that of Director of Surgical Education at the Santa Barbara Cottage Hospital in California. He remained in that position until his death. Higgins was the quintessential academician, holding numerous research grants and writing or stimulating the writing of hundreds of peer-reviewed papers and three books. However, his greatest love and commitments were to the training surgical residents. Higgins assumed the position of Chairman of the VA Surgical Adjuvant Chemotherapy Study Group and provided the leadership and inspiration for the 34 clinical research protocols that were developed for the neoadjuvant and adjuvant treatments of cancer of the lung, stomach, colon, rectum, and pancreas. Among his many honors and recognitions were the Gold Medal Paper Award of the Southeastern Surgical Congress, the Arthur Shipley Award of the Southern Surgical Association, and the Lucy Wortham James Clinical Research Award of the Society of Surgical Oncology. He died on September 3, 1994. (With appreciation to Elliot D. Prager, M.D. and to the American Surgical Association.)

leagues from the Veterans Administration (VA).[186] This study randomly allocated 700 men either to surgery or to preoperative radiotherapy plus surgery. These investigators found a statistically significant decreased incidence of positive nodes in the irradiated group and a lower incidence of recurrent disease in those who died. Roswit and associates used 20 Gy over 2 weeks, with a booster dose of 5 Gy if the tumor was less than 9 cm from the anal verge.[702]

Since these initial reports, there have been numerous papers that attest to the success of radiotherapy in reducing the size of the tumor, downstaging the degree of invasion, and decreasing the risk of local recurrence.[75,80,92, 108,142–144,152,178,212,218,239,243,245,246,299,343,377,385,406,429,531,557,559–5 63,578,633,643,692,698,700,761,764,769,821,839] Some have stated that survival rates are better.[224,808] Kandioler and co-workers observe that a tumor with a normal p53 genotype is predictive for response to preoperative short-term radiotherapy and increased patient survival.[401] However, there remains disagreement as to whether preoperative radiation therapy has any effect on survival.[249]

Methods

Minsky commented about the weaknesses of the prospective, randomized trials.[577] He stated that none utilizes standard dosages of radiation therapy. Second, he opined that the interval between the completion of radiation and surgery is generally considered to be inadequate. The Memorial Sloan-Kettering Cancer Center group demonstrated a trend toward an increased pathologic response rate and downstaging when an interval between completing the radiotherapy and surgery is at least 44 days.[584] Most recommend 4 to 6 weeks following completion of the treatment in order to achieve maximum downstaging and tissue recovery. Moreover, he affirmed that utilizing anterior-posterior/ posterior-anterior portals, rather than multiple-field techniques, predisposes to increased morbidity associated with the radiation.[577] Others confirmed that the morbidity and mortality of both preoperative and postoperative radiotherapy are higher when two-portal rather than three-portal or four-portal radiation technique is employed.[623] This is especially true for elderly patients who may have an increased risk of impairment for blood supply. Stein and colleagues concluded in the analysis of their patients that a longer time interval (beyond 8 weeks) between completion of neoadjuvant chemoradiation and surgical resection did not increase the tumor response rate or reduce the morbidity associated with the surgery.[788]

There is considerable controversy as to what the optimal dose for preoperative radiation treatment should be. Some have recommended a short course of high-dose therapy, whereas most centers in the United States suggest 40 to 45 Gy, delivered in 4 to 6 weeks. Surgery is recommended approximately 4 to 6 weeks after the completion of the treatment because tumoricidal benefits may continue for some time. Data show no increased morbidity or mortality associated with supplementary treatment.[182,663]

Results

The largest prospective, randomized trials come from Sweden—actually a combination of two Swedish protocols (the Stockholm Rectal Cancer Study Group and the Swedish Rectal Cancer Trial).[228,359–362,806–808] In the Stockholm trial, the most recent publication analyzed postoperative morbidity, mortality, local recurrence, and death from rectal cancer in 1,399 patients who were prospectively randomized to preoperative radiotherapy or no radiotherapy.[360] Those allocated to preoperative radiotherapy received a total dose of 35 Gy in five fractions over 1 week, with surgery performed within 1 week thereafter. Interestingly, patients operated on by surgeons who were certified specialists for at least 10 years had a lower risk of local recurrence and death from rectal cancer.[360] A significantly reduced risk of local recurrence was observed, but there was no clear improvement in survival. However, the investigators also found that the postoperative mortality rate may be increased in the radiotherapy group.[362]

In the Swedish Rectal Cancer Trial involving 1,168 patients (as of the most recent date), preoperative radiation was accomplished through 25 Gy and five fractions in 1 week, also followed by operation within 1 week.[807] In this randomized, prospective study, the local recurrence rate during a period of 2 years was reduced by approximately 65%. Furthermore, this short-term regimen of high-dose preoperative radiotherapy was found to improve survival.[808] The overall 5-year survival rate was 58% in the radiotherapy plus surgery group and 48% in the surgery-alone group ($p = .004$). This appears to be truly the first clear demonstration of improved survival by means of preoperative radiotherapy. In another report from the Uppsala, Sweden, group involving patients who underwent preoperative radiotherapy followed by low anterior resection, using historical controls, there was strong evidence for improved long-term survival.[154] In still another prospective, randomized trial that was undertaken by the Medical Research Council Rectal Cancer Working Party in Birmingham, England, investigators utilized 40 Gy given in 20 fractions of 2 Gy over 4 weeks in those individuals randomized to preoperative radiotherapy.[556] At 5-year follow-up, those who were randomized to radiation therapy had a statistically significantly lower incidence of local recurrence as well as fewer distant metastases. However, survival results were equivocal.

There is an inherent problem concerning a well-controlled, randomized trial with this group of patients. Stratification by the usual criterion, namely depth of invasion (e.g., Dukes' classification) cannot be applied. One must utilize other, less well-defined criteria such as clinical judgment. Endorectal ultrasound is of help for staging the depth of penetration,[602,730] and DNA ploidy seems to be an independent factor for predicting response to radiotherapy,[335] but for the present time one must await the results of the studies currently in progress.

Complications and Functional Results

Wichmann and associates concluded, on the basis of their evaluation of 30 patients who underwent preoperative chemoradiotherapy, that this treatment results in significant immune dysfunction as indicated by depression of lymphocyte subpopulations, monocytes, granulocytes, and proinflammatory cytokine release.[872] They believed that these observations are important in contributing to the increased perioperative morbidity that is seen as a consequence of neoadjuvant therapy. Experienced surgeons are well aware of the problem of delayed healing of the perineal wound after proctectomy when preoperative radiation is performed.[677] The safety of performing anastomosis in the rectum following radiation therapy has been a matter of some conjecture. Some studies, however, have demonstrated that colorectal anastomoses can be performed without concern for an increased risk of complications if the radiation dose does not exceed 45 Gy.[121,122,223,366,529,580,582,686,867] Still, preoperative radiotherapy may have an adverse effect on long-term anorectal function.[867] For example, the Cleveland Clinic group reviewed anal canal specimens following pelvic radiation and noted damage to the myenteric plexus of the internal anal sphincter.[155] A tendency to increased collagen deposition was also observed. Birnbaum and colleagues prospectively evaluated the acute effect of preoperative radiation (45 Gy) on anal function in 20 individuals.[59] These investigators concluded that preoperative radiation therapy has minimal immediate effect on the anal sphincter and is not a major contributing factor to postoperative incontinence after sphincter-saving operations for rectal cancer. However, preoperative radiotherapy alters endosonographic staging and interferes with the endosonographic interpretation of the anastomotic area.[602] Others have observed that preoperative radiothereapy may have a pejorative effect on male sexual and urinary function.[72]

Dahlberg and co-workers ascertained the long-term effects on bowel function by means of a questionnaire of 171 patients who could be evaluated and who were included in the Swedish Rectal Cancer Trial.[153] Mean bowel frequency per week, incontinence for loose stool, urgency, and emptying difficulties were statistically significantly more common following preoperative radiation when compared with those operated upon without radiation. This serves to emphasize the importance of patient selection in order to limit the consequences of nonbeneficial neoadjuvant therapy.

Comment

I believe that unless one is to participate in a controlled, randomized clinical trial, preoperative radiotherapy should be limited to those patients in whom the surgeon believes a chance for cure by resection is problematic or when transmural invasion is likely. If radiotherapy is to be considered under these circumstances, it should be carried to approximately 45 to 50 Gy over 5 or 6 weeks, with resection performed (with or without anastomosis) 6 to 8 weeks later.

Postoperative Radiotherapy (Adjuvant Therapy)

In 1991, Krook and colleagues demonstrated encouraging results with postoperative chemoradiation therapy.[444] A total of 204 patients with rectal carcinoma that was either deeply invasive or metastatic to lymph nodes was randomly assigned to postoperative radiation alone (45 to 50 Gy) or to radiation plus 5-FU, which was both preceded and followed by a cycle of systemic therapy with 5-FU plus semustine (methyl-CCNU).[444] After a median follow-up of more than 7 years, the combined regimen reduced the recurrence rate by 34%. Initial local recurrence was reduced by 46% and distant metastasis by 37%. Additionally, the combined treatment reduced the rate of cancer-related deaths by 36% and the overall death rate by 29%.

O'Connell and colleagues, reporting from the Mayo Clinic, administered 5-FU by protracted infusion throughout the duration of radiation therapy in 660 patients with Dukes' B and C tumors.[615] With a median follow-up of 46 months among surviving patients, those who received the infusion had a significantly increased time before relapse as well as an improved survival. Others confirmed that 5 FU combined with irradiation appears to maximize control of both local and distant metastatic disease.[683] A 1-month protocol reported on behalf of the Norwegian Adjuvant Rectal Cancer Project Group, utilizing 5-FU, revealed a reduced local recurrence rate and increased recurrence-free survival and overall survival, without serious side effects when compared with those who did not undergo such treatment.[838] More recent studies of adjuvant protocols incorporate the newer chemotherapeutic agents discussed in the prior chapter.

As previously stated, the primary advantage of postoperative radiotherapy is that selected patients may be submitted to this additional treatment based on their "unfavorable" pathology reports. Conversely, disadvantages of this alternative include the risk that cells may be seeded outside the treatment area, wound healing may be delayed, and the physiology of residual tumor may be altered by reduction in the vascular supply.[760] Furthermore, there is the concern for the possibility of prolonged delay in initiating the therapy when postoperative complications arise, such as wound infection, the need for reoperation, medical problems, and other issues.

Romsdahl and Withers delivered a total of 55 Gy following APR to patients who were found to have Dukes' B and C lesions.[693] The local recurrence rate was 8%, as compared with a 27% rate in historical controls. According to Brizel and Tepperman, among 51 patients who received at least 45 Gy of pelvic irradiation, only five tumors recurred (10%) when there was no gross residual disease at the time of resection.[82] Arnaud and colleagues undertook a prospective, randomized trial involving 172 patients who had previously undergone resection for either a Dukes' B or C rectal cancer.[20] Patients received 46 Gy for 5 days/week within a 30- to 38-day period. This trial failed to demonstrate any improvement in overall survival or local control when postoperative radiation was given compared with those who did not receive radiation therapy. Tang and associates, utilizing historic controls, also treated patients with Dukes' B and C rectal cancer and likewise found no improvement in survival or local recurrence.[814] Others believe that prophylactic postoperative adjuvant radiotherapy is not justified because the incidence of local recurrence in the absence of disseminated disease is relatively low.[24] In two studies, that figure was approximately 10%.[33,635] Several prospective randomized trials are currently in progress, but as of this writing, 5-year follow-up conclusions are not available.[633,700]

Problems

Generally, there is the perception that postoperative radiotherapy is not as well tolerated as preoperative treatment.[635,752] Anastomotic strictures have been reported to occur as a consequence of this regimen.[634] In the long term, small bowel complications are of most concern (see Chapter 28).[526] Ooi and colleagues, in their MEDLINE and literature search, noted that with postoperative radiotherapy, small bowel obstruction occurs in 5% to 10%, delay in commencing radiotherapy because of wound healing problems, 6%, postoperative fatigue, 14%, and toxicities precluding completion of adjuvant therapy, 49% to 97%.[623] Other symptoms and complications include abscess and fistula formation, mucus discharge, urgency, tenesmus, and bleeding.[394]

Comment

Until the results of controlled studies are available, my attitude is to advise supplementary radiotherapy for patients who are at a high risk of tumor recurrence: those with poorly differentiated tumors and those with Dukes' B or C lesions. In my opinion, the treatment should begin not sooner than 1 month following the operation (in order to avoid problems with wound healing) or later than 2 months (in order to limit the likelihood of spread). The dosage to the tumor bed should be approximately 60 Gy.

Radiotherapy is not without significant complication: urinary tract infection, diarrhea, small bowel injury, and skin and wound breakdown. Therefore, before embarking on such treatment one must consider other factors, such as the age of the patient and the anticipated quality of life.

Palliative Radiotherapy

Radiotherapy can be uniquely beneficial in the treatment of patients with recurrent disease who have pelvic pain. This is discussed earlier in this chapter. It has also been suggested for use in those patients with locally advanced lesions, in combination with chemotherapy and/or surgery.[123,819] Kodner and colleagues definitively treated by means of external radiation 84 patients with invasive rectal carcinoma.[428] The use of external radiation before endocavitary radiation achieved local control in 93% of patients with favorable lesions. However, the investigators found that there was little place for nonresective management of aggressive rectal cancers, even for palliation, unless an individual's life expectancy was less than 6 months. Still, Zacherl and co-workers opined that partial sacral resection as a means for achieving palliation of perineosacral pain is justified even though cure can very rarely be achieved.[894] Others have demonstrated that many patients with locally recurrence rectal cancer can benefit from multimodality therapy.[308]

The implications of these studies are such that any individual with pathologic confirmation of a Dukes' B or C (T_3, T_4, or N_1) lesion should be considered for a postoperative protocol.

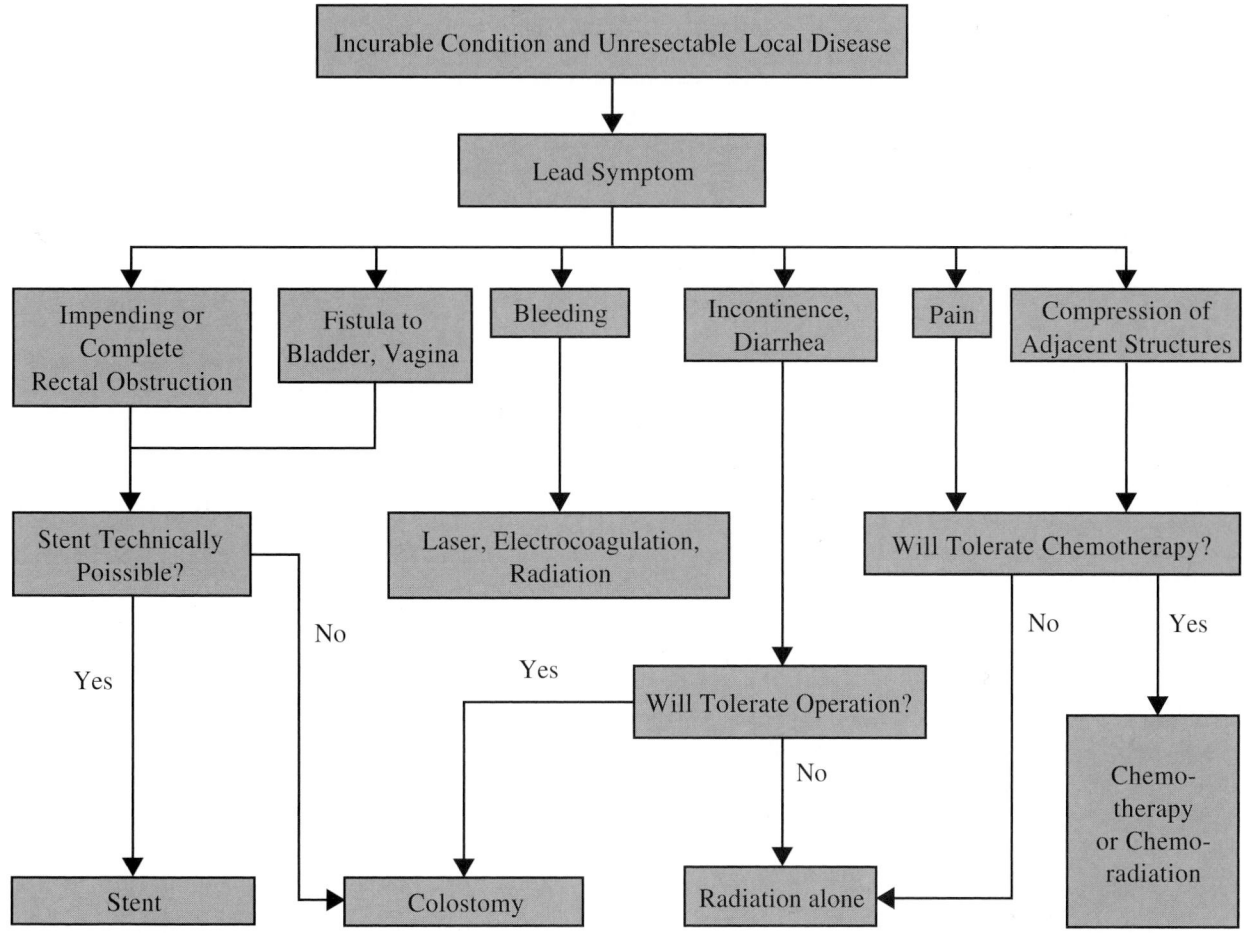

FIGURE 23-144. Algorithm for palliative care of patients with locally unresectable rectal cancer. (From Stelzner M. Palliative therapy of rectal cancer: summary statement. *J Gastrointest Surg* 2004;8:253, with permission.)

Intraoperative Radiotherapy

See the earlier discussion.

CHEMOTHERAPY

The role of chemotherapy in colorectal cancer is discussed in Chapter 22.

Hyperthermochemoradiotherapy

Mori and colleagues have reported the application of a multimodality approach in the management of patients with rectal cancer, that of hyperthermochemoradiotherapy.[592] This consists of a preoperative combination of hyperthermia at 42 to 45°C for 40 minutes (twice per week for 2 weeks), 5-FU intravenously, and a total of 30 Gy irradiation. Reduction in tumor size was evident in their

11 patients with either no or only a few viable cancer cells present in the resected specimen. A later report from the same institution involving 36 patients revealed that 5-year survival rates were 91% compared with historical controls of 74% in those not receiving hyperthermochemoradiotherapy.[620] Whether this approach will prove to have merit in the management of patients with rectal cancer remains to be determined.

Palliative Therapy: An Algorithmic Approach

At the 2003 Annual Meeting of the Society for Surgery of the Alimentary Tract, Stelzner suggested an algorithmic approach to the palliative management of nonresectable and resectable rectal cancer.[790] I personally am attracted to this for providing a useful perspective on all of the management alternatives discussed within this chapter (Figs. 23-144 and 23-145).

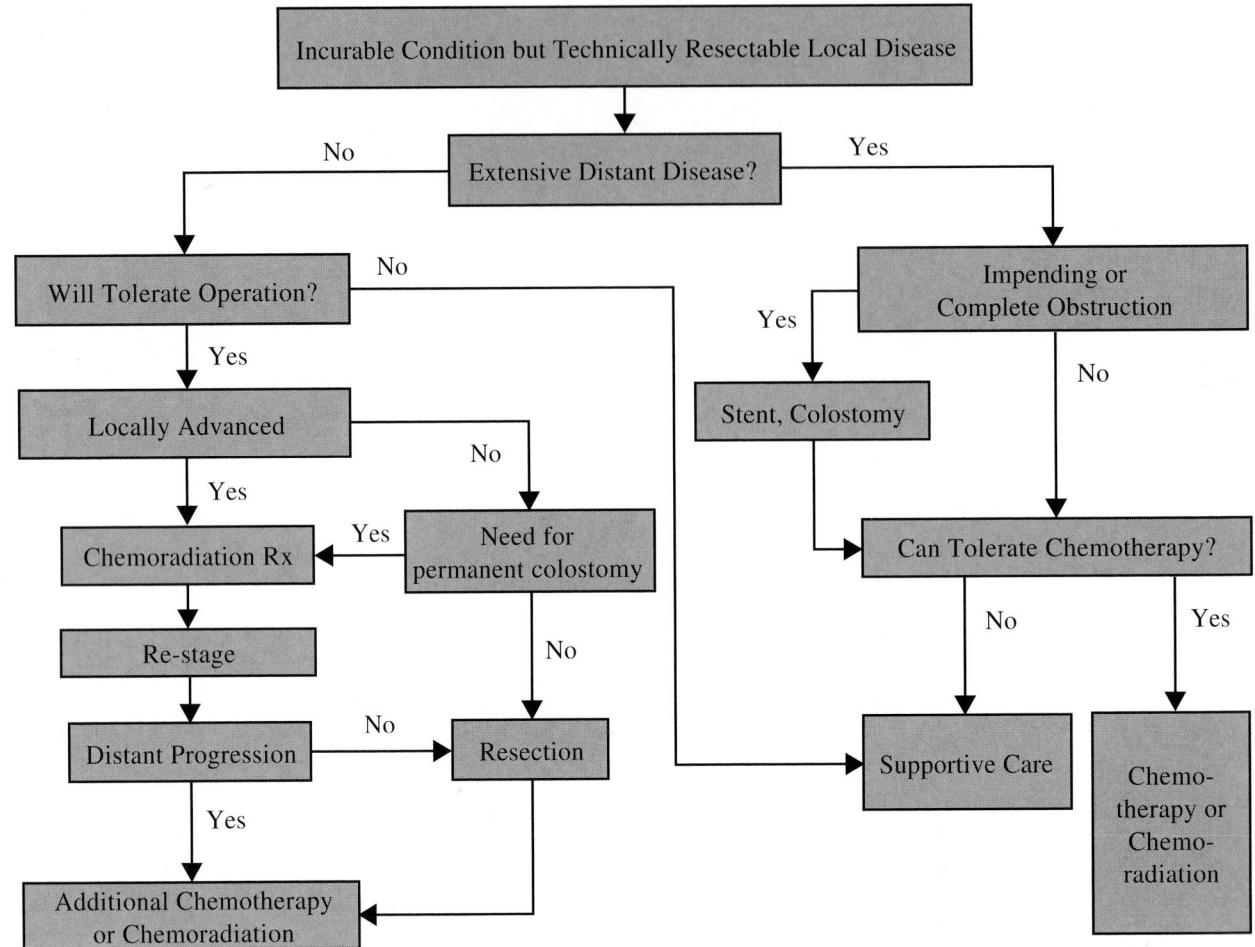

FIGURE 23-145. Algorithm for palliative care of patients with locally resectable rectal cancer. (From Stelzner M. Palliative therapy of rectal cancer: summary statement. *J Gastrointest Surg* 2004;8:253, with permission.)

REFERENCES

1. Abercrombie JF, Rogers J, Williams NS. Total anorectal reconstruction results in complete anorectal sensory loss. *Br J Surg* 1996;83:57.
2. Abercrombie JE, Williams NS. Total anorectal reconstruction. *Br J Surg* 1995;82:438.
3. Accordi F, Sogno O, Carniato S, et al. Endoscopic treatment of stenosis following stapler anastomosis. *Dis Colon Rectum* 1987;30:647.
4. Adams DR, Blatchford GJ, Lin KM, et al. Use of preoperative ultrasound staging for treatment of rectal cancer. *Dis Colon Rectum* 1999;42:159.
5. Adam IJ, Mohamdee MO, Martin IG, et al. Role of circumferential margin involvement in the local recurrence of rectal cancer. *Lancet* 1994;344:707.
6. Adams WJ, Wong WD. Endorectal ultrasonic detection of malignancy within rectal villous lesions. *Dis Colon Rectum* 1995;38:1093.
7. Agaba EA. Does rectal washout during anterior resection prevent local tumor recurrence? *Dis Colon Rectum* 2004; 47:291.
8. Akyol AM, McGregor JR, Galloway DJ, et al. Recurrence of colorectal cancer after sutured and stapled large bowel anastomoses. *Br J Surg* 1991;78:1297.
9. Allgöwer M. Sphincter-splitting approach to the rectum. *Am J Surg* 1983;145:5.
10. Allgöwer M, Dürig M, Hochstetter AV, et al. The parasacral sphincter-splitting approach to the rectum. *World J Surg* 1982;6:539.
11. Amin AI, Ramalingam T, Sexton R, et al. Comparison of transanal stent with defunctioning stoma in low anterior resection for rectal cancer. *Br J Surg* 2003;90:581.
12. Amussat J-Z. *Mémoire sur la possibilité d'établir un anus artificiel dans la région lombaire sans pénétrer dans le péritoine*. [Notes on the possible establishment of an artificial anus in the lumbar region without entering the peritoneal cavity.] Paris: Germer-Bailliére, 1839. Translated in *Dis Colon Rectum* 1983;26:483.
13. Anderson BO, Hann LE, Enker WE, et al. Transrectal ultrasonography and operative selection for early carcinoma of the rectum. *J Am Coll Surg* 1994;179:513.
14. Anthony JP, Mathes SJ. The recalcitrant perineal wound after rectal extirpation: applications of muscle flap closure. *Arch Surg* 1990;125:1371.
15. Antoniades K, Spector HB, Heckscher RH Jr. Prophylactic oophorectomy in conjunction with large-bowel resection for cancer: report of two cases. *Dis Colon Rectum* 1977; 20:506.
16. Antonsen HK, Kronborg O. Early complications after low anterior resection for rectal cancer using the EEA;Lt sta-

pling device: a prospective trial. *Dis Colon Rectum* 1987; 30:579.

17. Appleton GVN, Williamson RCN. Hypoplasia of defunctioned rectum. *Br J Surg* 1989;76:787.
18. Arbman G, Nilsson E, Hallböök O, et al. Local recurrence following total mesorectal excision for rectal cancer. *Br J Surg* 1996;83:375.
19. Arnaud JP, Bergamaschi R, Schloegel M, et al. Progress in the assessment of lymphatic spread in rectal cancer: rectal endoscopic lymphoscintigraphy. *Dis Colon Rectum* 1990; 33:398.
20. Arnaud JP, Nordlinger B, Bosset JF, et al. Radical surgery and postoperative radiotherapy as combined treatment in rectal cancer: final results of a phase III study of the European Organization for Research and Treatment of Cancer. *Br J Surg* 1997;84:352.
21. Arulampalam THA, Costa DC, Loizidou M, et al. Positron emission tomography and colorectal cancer. *Br J Surg* 2001;88:176.
22. Asao T, Kuwano H, Nakamura J-I, et al. Use of a mattress suture to eliminate dog ears in double-stapled and triple-stapled anastomoses. *Dis Colon Rectum* 2002;45:137.
23. Aston NO, Owen WJ, Irving JD. Endoscopic balloon dilatation of colonic anastomotic strictures. *Br J Surg* 1989; 76:780.
24. Auld RM, Chapman S, Kuster GGR, et al. Local recurrence of adenocarcinoma of the rectosigmoid: is postoperative adjuvant radiotherapy justified? *Dis Colon Rectum* 1986; 29:326.
25. Babcock WW. Experiences with resection of the colon and the elimination of colostomy. *Am J Surg* 1939;4:186.
26. Babcock WW. Radical single-stage extirpation for cancer of the large bowel, with retained functional anus. *Surg Gynecol Obstet* 1947;85:1.
27. Bacon HE. Abdominoperineal proctosigmoidectomy with sphincter preservation: five-year and ten-year survival after "pull-through" operation for cancer of rectum. *JAMA* 1956; 160:628.
28. Bacon HE. Evaluation of sphincter muscle preservation and re-establishment of continuity in the operative treatment of rectal and sigmoidal cancer. *Surg Gynecol Obstet* 1945;81:113.
29. Bacon HE, Martin PV. The rationale of palliative resection for primary cancer of the colon and rectum complicated by liver and lung metastasis. *Dis Colon Rectum* 1964;7:211.
30. Baker JW. Low end to side rectosigmoidal anastomosis: description of technique. *Arch Surg* 1950;61:143.
31. Baird WL, Hester TR, Nahai F, et al. Management of perineal wounds following abdominoperineal resection with inferior gluteal flaps. *Arch Surg* 1990;125:1486.
32. Balslev I, Harling H. Sexual dysfunction following operation for carcinoma of the rectum. *Dis Colon Rectum* 1983;26:785.
33. Balslev I, Pedersen M, Teglbjaerg PS, et al. Postoperative radiotherapy in rectosigmoid cancer Dukes' B and C: interim report from a randomized multicentre study. *Br J Cancer* 1982;46:551.
34. Banerjee AK, Jehle EC, Shorthouse AJ, et al. Local excision of rectal tumours. *Br J Surg* 1995;82:1165.
35. Banerjee AK, Parc R. Prediction of optimum dimensions of colonic pouch reservoir. *Dis Colon Rectum* 1996;39:1293.
36. Banerjee AK, Walters TK, Wilkins R, et al. Wire-guided balloon coloplasty: a new treatment for colorectal strictures. *J R Soc Med* 1991;84:136.
37. Barillari P, Bolognese A, Chirletti P, et al. Role of CEA, TPA, and Ca 19–9 in the early detection of localized and diffuse recurrent rectal cancer. *Dis Colon Rectum* 1992;35:471.
38. Baron PL, Enker WE, Zakowski MF, et al. Immediate vs. salvage resection after local treatment for early rectal cancer. *Dis Colon Rectum* 1995;38:177.
39. Beard JD, Nicholson ML, Sayers RD, et al. Intraoperative air testing of colorectal anastomoses: a prospective, randomized trial. *Br J Surg* 1990;77:1095.
40. Beart RW Jr, Kelly KA. Randomized prospective evaluation of the EEA stapler for colorectal anastomoses. *Am J Surg* 1981;141:143.
41. Beart RW Jr, Wolff BG. The use of staplers for anterior anastomoses. *World J Surg* 1982;6:525.
42. Beck DE, Fazio VW, Jagelman DG, et al. Postoperative perineal hernia. *Dis Colon Rectum* 1987;30:21.
43. Bedogni G, Ricci E, Pedrazzoli C, et al. Endoscopic dilation of anastomotic colonic stenosis by different techniques: an alternative to surgery? *Gastrointest Endosc* 1987;33:21.
44. Beheri GE. Surgical treatment of impotence. *Plast Reconstr Surg* 1966;38:92.
45. Bell SW, Walker KG, Rickard MJFX, et al. Anastomotic leakage after curative anterior resection results in a higher prevalence of local recurrence. *Br J Surg* 2003;90:1261.
46. Bennett RC. The place of pull-through operations in treatment of carcinoma of the rectum. *Dis Colon Rectum* 1976;19:420.
47. Bennett RC, Hughes ES, Cuthbertson AM. Long-term review of function following pull-through operations of the rectum. *Br J Surg* 1972;59:723.
48. Benoist S, Panis Y, Boleslawski E, et al. Functional outcome after coloanal versus low colorectal anstomosis for rectal carcinoma. *J Am Coll Surg* 1997;185:114.
49. Benson MC, Ring KS, Olsson CA. Ureteral reconstruction and bypass: experience with ileal interposition, the Boari flap-psoas hitch and renal autotransplantation. *J Urol* 1990;143:20.
50. Bernard HR, Cole WR. The prophylaxis of surgical infection: the effect of prophylactic antimicrobial drugs on the incidence of infection following potentially contaminated operations. *Surgery* 1964;56:151.
51. Berry AR, Souter RG, Campbell WB, et al. Endoscopic transanal resection of rectal tumours-a preliminary report of its use. *Br J Surg* 1990;77:134.
52. Bevan AD. Carcinoma of the rectum: treatment by local excision. *Surg Clin Chicago* 1917;1:1233.
53. Beynon J, Foy DMA, Roe AM, et al. Endoluminal ultrasound in the assessment of local invasion in rectal cancer. *Br J Surg* 1986;73:474.
54. Beynon J, Mortensen NJMC, Foy DMA, et al. Pre-operative assessment of local invasion in rectal cancer: digital examination, endoluminal sonography or computed tomography? *Br J Surg* 1986;73:1015.
55. Beynon J, Mortensen NJMC, Foy DMA, et al. The detection and evaluation of locally recurrent rectal cancer with rectal endosonography. *Dis Colon Rectum* 1989;32:509.
56. Beynon J, Mortensen NJMC, Foy DMA, et al. Preoperative assessment of mesorectal lymph node involvement in rectal cancer. *Br J Surg* 1989;76:276.
57. Biggers OR, Beart RW Jr, Ilstrup DM. Local excision of rectal cancer. *Dis Colon Rectum* 1986;29:374.
58. Birbeck KF, Macklin CP, Tiffin NJ, et al. Rates of circumferential resection margin involvement vary between surgeons and predict outcomes in rectal cancer surgery. *Ann Surg* 2002;235:449.
59. Birnbaum EH, Dreznik Z, Myerson RJ, et al. Early effect of external beam radiation therapy on the anal sphincter: a study using anal manometry and transrectal ultrasound. *Dis Colon Rectum* 1992;35:757.
60. Birnbaum EH, Ogunbiyi OA, Gagliardi G, et al. Selection criteria for treatment of rectal cancer with combined external and endocavitary radiation. *Dis Colon Rectum* 1999; 42:727.
61. Bischoff PF. Boari-plasty and vesicorenal reflux. In: Whitehead ED, ed. *Current operative urology*. New York: Harper & Row, 1975:708.
62. Bissett IP, Hill GL. Extrafascial excision of the rectum for cancer: a technique for the avoidance of the complications of rectal mobilization. *Semin Surg Oncol* 2000;18:207.
63. Black BM, Botham RJ. Combined abdominoendorectal resection: a critical reappraisal based on 91 cases. *Surg Clin North Am* 1957;37:989.

64. Black BM, Kelly AH. Recurrent carcinoma of the rectum and rectosigmoid: results of treatment after continence preserving procedures. *Arch Surg* 1955;72:538.

65. Blackwood JM, Hurd T, Machiedo GW. Intra-abdominal infection following combined spleen-colon trauma. *Am Surg* 1988;54:212.

66. Blamey SL, McDermott FT, Pihl E, et al. Resected ovarian recurrence from colorectal adenocarcinoma. *Dis Colon Rectum* 1981;24:272.

67. Blamey S, McDermott F, Pihl E, et al. Ovarian involvement in adenocarcinoma of the colon and rectum. *Surg Gynecol Obstet* 1981;153:42.

68. Blomquist P, Jiborn H, Zederfeldt B. Effect of diverting colostomy on collagen metabolism in the colonic wall. *Am J Surg* 1985;149:330.

69. Bleday R, Breen E, Jessup JM, et al. Prospective evaluation of local excision for small rectal cancers. *Dis Colon Rectum* 1997;40:388.

70. Blumberg D, Paty PB, Guillem JG, et al. All patients with small intramural rectal cancers are at risk for lymph node metastasis. *Dis Colon Rectum* 1999;42:881.

71. Bokey EL, Chapuis PH, Fung C, et al. Postoperative morbidity and mortality following resection of the colon and rectum for cancer. *Dis Colon Rectum* 1995;38:480.

72. Bonnel C, Parc YR, Pocard M, et al. Effects of preoperative radiotherapy for primary resectable rectal adenocarcinoma on male sexual and urinary function. *Dis Colon Rectum* 2002;45:934.

73. Bordos DC, Baker RR, Cameron JL. An evaluation of palliative abdominoperineal resection for carcinoma of the rectum. *Surg Gynecol Obstet* 1974;139:731.

74. Bothwell WN, Bleicher RJ, Dent TL. Prophylactic ureteral catheterization in colon surgery. *Dis Colon Rectum* 1994;37:330.

75. Botti C, Cosimelli M, Ambesi Impiombato F, et al. Improved local control and survival with the sandwich technique of pelvic radiotherapy for resectable rectal cancer: a retrospective, multivariate analysis. *Dis Colon Rectum* 1994;37:S6.

76. Bown SG, Barr H, Matthewson K, et al. Endoscopic treatment of inoperable colorectal cancers with the Nd YAG laser. *Br J Surg* 1986;73:949.

77. Boyce GA, Sivak MV Jr, Lavery IC, et al. Endoscopic ultrasound in the pre-operative staging of rectal carcinoma. *Gastrointest Endosc* 1992;38:468.

78. Branagan GW, Moran BJ. Published evidence favors the use of suprapubic catheters in pelvic colorectal surgery. *Dis Colon Rectum* 2002;45:1104.

79. Brasch RC, Bufo AJ, Kreienberg PF, et al. Femoral neuropathy secondary to the use of a self-retaining retractor: report of three cases and review of the literature. *Dis Colon Rectum* 1995;38:1115.

80. Brierley JD, Cummings BJ, Wong CS, et al. Adenocarcinoma of the rectum treated by radical external radiation therapy. *Int J Radiat Oncol* 1995;31:255.

81. Bright N, Hale P, Mason R. Poor palliation of colorectal malignancy with the neodymium yttrium-aluminium-garnet laser. *Br J Surg* 1992;79:308.

82. Brizel HE, Tepperman BS. Postoperative adjuvant irradiation for adenocarcinoma of the rectum and sigmoid. *Am J Clin Oncol* 1984;7:679.

83. Brotschi E, Noe JM, Silen W. Perineal hernias after proctectomy. *Am J Surg* 1985;149:301.

84. Brown G, Radcliffe AG, Newcombe RG, et al. Preoperative assessment of prognostic factors in rectal cancer using high-resolution magnetic resonance imaging. *Br J Surg* 2003;90:355.

85. Brunetaud JM, Maunoury V, Ducrotte P, et al. Palliative treatment of rectosigmoid carcinoma by laser endoscopic photoablation. *Gastroenterology* 1987;92:663.

86. Buchsbaum HJ, Christopherson W, Lifshitz S, et al. Vicryl mesh in pelvic floor reconstruction. *Arch Surg* 1985;120:1389.

87. Buess G, Mentges B, Manncke K, et al. Technique and results of transanal endoscopic microsurgery in early rectal cancer. *Am J Surg* 1992;163:63.

88. Buhre LMD, Mulder NH, DeRuiter AJ, et al. Effect of extent of anterior resection and sex on disease-free survival and local recurrence in patients with rectal cancer. *Br J Surg* 1994;81:1227.

89. Buhre LM, Verschueren RCJ, Mehta DM, et al. Staging laparotomy for inoperable or borderline operable cancer of the rectum. *Dis Colon Rectum* 1987;30:352.

90. Bülow S, Christensen IJ, Harling H, et al. Recurrence and survival after mesorectal excision for rectal cancer. *Br J Surg* 2003;90:974.

91. Burgos FJ, Romero J, Fernandez E, et al. Risk factors for developing voiding dysfunction after abdominoperineal resection for adenocarcinoma of the rectum. *Dis Colon Rectum* 1988;31:682.

92. Buroker T, Nigro N, Correa J, et al. Combination preoperative radiation and chemotherapy in adenocarcinoma of the rectum: a preliminary report. *Dis Colon Rectum* 1976;19:660.

93. Butch RJ, Wittenberg J, Mueller PR, et al. Presacral masses after abdominoperineal resection for colorectal carcinoma: the need for needle biopsy. *AJR Am J Roentgenol* 1985;144:309.

94. Cade D, Gallagher P, Schofield PF, et al. Complications of anterior resection of the rectum using the EEA stapling device. *Br J Surg* 1981;68:339.

95. Cance WG, Cohen AM, Enker WE, et al. Predictive value of a negative computed tomographic scan in 100 patients with rectal carcinoma. *Dis Colon Rectum* 1991;34:748.

96. Carlsson U, Lasson A, Ekelund G. Recurrence rates after curative surgery for rectal carcinoma with special reference to their accuracy. *Dis Colon Rectum* 1987;30:431.

97. Carne PWG, Frye JNR, Kennedy-Smith A, et al. Local invasion of the bladder with colorectal cancers: surgical management and patterns of local recurrence. *Dis Colon Rectum* 2004;47:44.

98. Carty NJ, Keating J, Campbell J, et al. Prospective audit of an extramucosal technique for intestinal anastomosis. *Br J Surg* 1991;78:1439.

99. Casillas S, Nicholson JD. Aortic thrombosis after low anterior resection for rectal cancer: report of a case. *Dis Colon Rectum* 2002;45:829.

100. Castrini G, Toccaceli S. Cancer of the rectum sphincter-saving operation: a new technique of coloanal anastomosis. *Surg Clin North Am* 1988;68:1383.

101. Cavaliere F, Pemberton JH, Cosimelli M, et al. Coloanal anastomosis for rectal cancer: long-term results at the Mayo and Cleveland Clinics. *Dis Colon Rectum* 1995;38:807.

102. Cavina E. Outcome of restorative perineal graciloplasty with simultaneous excision of the anus and rectum for cancer: a ten-year experience with 81 patients. *Dis Colon Rectum* 1996;39:182.

103. Cawkwell I. Perineal hernia complicating abdominoperineal resection of the rectum. *Br J Surg* 1963;50:431.

104. Cawthorn SJ, Parums DV, Gibbs NM, et al. Extent of mesorectal spread and involvement of lateral resection margin as prognostic factors after surgery for rectal cancer. *Lancet* 1990;335:1055.

105. Chan TW, Kressel HY, Milestone B, et al. Rectal carcinoma: staging at MR imaging with endorectal surface coil: work in progress. *Radiology* 1991;181:461.

106. Chang K-J, Enker WE, Melamed M. Influence of tumor cell DNA ploidy on the natural history of rectal cancer. *Am J Surg* 1987;153:184.

107. Chapuis P, Bokey L, Fahrer M, et al. Mobilization of the rectum: anatomic concepts and the bookshelf revisited. *Dis Colon Rectum* 2002;45:1.

108. Chari RS, Tyler DS, Anscher MS, et al. Preoperative radiation and chemotherapy in the treatment of adenocarcinoma of the rectum. *Ann Surg* 1995;221:778.

109. Charnley RM, Pyf G, Amar SS, et al. The early diagnosis of recurrent rectal carcinoma by rectal endosonography. *Br J Surg* 1988;75:1232.

110. Chassin JL, Rifkind KM, Sussman B, et al. The stapled gastrointestinal tract anastomosis: incidence of postoperative complications compared with the sutured anastomosis. *Ann Surg* 1978;188:689.

111. Chew SSB, King DW. Use of endoscopic titanium stapler in rectal anastomotic stricture. *Dis Colon Rectum* 2002;45: 283.

112. Chia YW, Ngoi SS, Goh PMY. Endoscopic Nd:YAG laser in the palliative treatment of advanced low rectal carcinoma in Singapore. *Dis Colon Rectum* 1991;34:1093.

113. Chia YW, Ngoi SS, Tung KH. Use of the optical urethrotome knife in the treatment of a benign low rectal anastomotic stricture. *Dis Colon Rectum* 1991;34:717.

114. Christiansen J, Kirkegaard P. Treatment of recurrent rectal cancer by electroresection/coagulation after low anterior resection. *Dis Colon Rectum* 1983;26:656.

115. Cirocco WC, Golub RW. Endoscopic treatment of postoperative hemorrhage from a stapled colorectal anastomosis. *Am Surg* 1995;61:460.

116. Clark CG, Harris J, Elmasri S, et al. Polyglycolic acid sutures and catgut in colonic anastomosis: a controlled clinical trial. *Lancet* 1972;2:1006.

117. Clark J, Bankoff M, Carter B, et al. The use of computerized tomography scan in the staging and follow-up study of carcinoma of the rectum. *Surg Gynecol Obstet* 1984; 159:335.

118. Clarke JS, Condon RE, Bartlett JG, et al. Preoperative oral antibiotics reduce septic complications of colon operations: results of prospective, randomized, double-blind clinical study. *Ann Surg* 1977;185:251.

119. Coco C, Magistrelli P, Granone P, et al. Conservative surgery for early cancer of the distal rectum. *Dis Colon Rectum* 1992;35:131.

120. Cohen AM. Purse-string placement for transanal intraluminal circular stapling. *Dis Colon Rectum* 1986;29:532.

121. Cohen AM, Enker WE, Minsky BD. Proctectomy and coloanal reconstruction for rectal cancer. *Dis Colon Rectum* 1990;33:40.

122. Cohen AM, Minsky BD. A phase I trial of preoperative radiation, proctectomy, and endoanal reconstruction. *Arch Surg* 1990;125:247.

123. Cohen AM, Minsky BD. Aggressive surgical management of locally advanced primary and recurrent rectal cancer. *Dis Colon Rectum* 1990;33:432.

124. Cohen JL, Grotz RL, Welch JP, et al. Intrarectal sonography: a new technique for the assessment of rectal tumors. *Am Surg* 1991;57:459.

125. Cohen Z, Myers E, Langer B, et al. Double stapling technique for low anterior resection. *Dis Colon Rectum* 1983; 26:231.

126. Cohn I. Implantation in cancer of the colon. *Surg Gynecol Obstet* 1967;124:501.

127. Cohn I. Cause and prevention of recurrence following surgery for colon cancer. *Cancer* 1971;28:183.

128. Cole WH. Recurrence in carcinoma of colon and proximal rectum following resection for carcinoma. *Arch Surg* 1952; 65:264.

129. Cole WH, Packard D, Southwick W. Carcinoma of the colon with special reference to prevention of recurrence. *JAMA* 1954;155:1549.

130. Condon RE. Antibiotic preparation of the colon or rectum for elective resection. *Infect Surg* 1982;1:15.

131. Condon RE, Bartlett JG, Greenlee H, et al. Efficacy of oral and systemic antibiotic prophylaxis in colorectal operations. *Arch Surg* 1983;118:496.

132. Cooperman M, Martin EW Jr, Evans WE, et al. Assessment of anastomotic blood supply in operations upon the colon by Doppler ultrasound. *Surg Gynecol Obstet* 1979;149:15.

133. Cooperman M, Martin EW Jr, Keith LM, et al. Use of Doppler ultrasound in intestinal surgery. *Am J Surg* 1979;138: 856.

134. Cooperman M, Pace WG, Martin EW Jr, et al. Determination of viability of ischemic intestine by Doppler ultrasound. *Surgery* 1978;83:705.

135. Corder AP, Karanjia ND, Williams JD, et al. Flush aortic tie versus selective preservation of the ascending left colic artery in low anterior resection for rectal carcinoma. *Br J Surg* 1992;79:680.

136. Criado FJ, Wilson TH Jr. Technique for reestablishing continuity after the Hartmann operation. *Am Surg* 1981;47: 366.

137. Crile G Jr, Turnbull RB Jr. The role of electrocoagulation in the treatment of carcinoma of the rectum. *Surg Gynecol Obstet* 1972;135:391.

138. Cripps WH. *Cancer of the rectum: its pathology, diagnosis and treatment (including a portion of the Jacksonian Prize Essay for 1876)*. London: Churchill, 1880.

139. Crowe PJ, Temple WJ, Lopez MJ, et al. Pelvic exenteration for advanced pelvic malignancy. *Semin Surg Oncol* 1999; 17:152.

140. Cruse PJ. Incidence of wound infection on the surgical services. *Surg Clin North Am* 1975;55:1269.

141. Cruse PJ, Foord R. A five-year prospective study of 23,649 surgical wounds. *Arch Surg* 1973;107:206.

142. Cummings BJ. Adjuvant radiation therapy for rectal adenocarcinomas. *Dis Colon Rectum* 1984;27:826.

143. Cummings BJ. A critical review of adjuvant preoperative radiation therapy for adenocarcinoma of the rectum. *Br J Surg* 1986;73:332.

144. Cummings BJ, Rider WD, Harwood AR, et al. Radical external beam radiation therapy for adenocarcinoma of the rectum. *Dis Colon Rectum* 1983;26:30.

145. Cunningham JD, Enker W, Cohen A. Salvage therapy for pelvic recurrence following curative rectal cancer resection. *Dis Colon Rectum* 1997;40:393.

146. Cunsolo A, Bragaglia RB, Manara G, et al. Urogenital dysfunction after abdominoperineal resection for carcinoma of the rectum. *Dis Colon Rectum* 1990;33:918.

147. Cutait DE, Cutait R, Ioshimoto M, et al. Abdominoperineal endoanal pull-through resection. *Dis Colon Rectum* 1985; 28:294.

148. Cutait DE, Figliolini FJ. A new method of colorectal anastomosis in abdominoperineal resection. *Dis Colon Rectum* 1961;4:335.

149. Cutait R, Enker WE. Prophylactic oophorectomy in surgery for large-bowel cancer. *Dis Colon Rectum* 1983;26:6.

150. Cuthbertson AM, Kaye AH. Local excision of carcinomas of the rectum, anus and anal canal. *Aust N Z J Surg* 1978; 48:412.

151. Czerny V. Casuistische Mittheilungen aus der Chirurg. Klin zu Heidelberg. *Munch Med Wochenschr* 1894:11.

152. Dahl O, Horn A, Morild I, et al. Low-dose preoperative radiation postpones recurrences in operable rectal cancer: results of a randomized multicenter trial in western Norway. *Cancer* 1990;66:2286.

153. Dahlberg M, Glimelius B, Graf W, et al. Preoperative irradiation affects functional results after surgery for rectal cancer: results from a randomized study. *Dis Colon Rectum* 1998;41:543.

154. Dahlberg M, Påhlman L. Bergström R, et al. Improved survival in patients with rectal cancer: a population-based register study. *Br J Surg* 1998;85:515.

155. da Silva GM, Berho M, Wexner SD, et al. Histologic analysis of the irradiated anal sphincter. *Dis Colon Rectum* 2003; 46:1492.

156. Dasmahapatra KS, Swaminathan AP. The use of a biodegradable mesh to prevent radiation-associated small-bowel injury. *Arch Surg* 1991;126:366.

157. Dawson PM, Habib NA, Rees HC, et al. Influence of sialomucin at the resection margin on local tumour recurrence and survival of patients with colorectal cancer: a multivariate analysis. *Br J Surg* 1987;74:366.

158. Deaver JB. Lumbar versus iliac colotomy. *J Phila County Med Soc* 1891;12:97.

159. Debas HT, Thomson FB. A critical review of colectomy with anastomosis. *Surg Gynecol Obstet* 1972;135:747.

160. Deddish MR. Local excision. *Surg Clin North Am* 1974; 54:877.

161. Deddish MR, Stearns MW Jr. Anterior resection for carcinoma of the rectum and rectosigmoid area. *Ann Surg* 1961;154:961.

162. Deen KI. Foley catheter-assisted sutured colorectal anastomosis. *Br J Surg* 1995;82:324.

163. DeGennaro V, Corman ML, Coller JA, Veidenheimer MC. Wound infections after colectomy. *Dis Colon Rectum* 1978; 21:567.

164. Dehni N, McFadden N, McNamara DA, et al. Oncologic results following abdominoperineal resection for adenocarcinoma of the low rectum. *Dis Colon Rectum* 2003;46:867.

165. Dehni N, McNamara DA, Schlegel RD, et al. Clinical effects of preoperative radiation therapy on anorectal function after proctectomy and colonic J-pouch-anal anastomosis. *Dis Colon Rectum* 2002;45:1635.

166. Dehni N, Parc R. Colonic J-pouch-anal anastomosis for rectal cancer. *Dis Colon Rectum* 2003;46:667.

167. Dehni N, Schlegel RD, Cunningham C, et al. Influence of a defunctioning stoma on leakage rates after low colorectal anastomosis and colonic J pouch-anal anastomosis. *Br J Surg* 1998;85:1114.

168. DeLuca FR, Ragins H. Construction of an omental envelope as a method of excluding the small intestine from the field of postoperative irradiation to the pelvis. *Surg Gynecol Obstet* 1985;160:365.

169. Dennett ER, Parry BR. Misconceptions about the colonic J-pouch: what the accumulating data show. *Dis Colon Rectum* 1999;42:804.

170. Detry RJ, Kestens PJ. Colorectal anastomoses with the EEA stapler. *World J Surg* 1981;5:739.

171. Deutsch AA, Stern HS. Technique of insertion of pelvic Vicryl mesh sling to avoid postradiation enteritis. *Dis Colon Rectum* 1989;32:628.

172. Devereux DF, Chandler JJ, Eisenstat T, et al. Efficacy of an absorbable mesh in keeping the small bowel out of the human pelvis following surgery. *Dis Colon Rectum* 1988; 31:17.

173. Devereux DF, Eisenstat T, Zinkin L. The safe and effective use of postoperative radiation therapy in modified Astler Coller stage C3 rectal cancer. *Cancer* 1989;63:2393.

174. Dixon CF. Anterior resection for malignant lesions of the upper part of the rectum and lower part of the sigmoid. *Ann Surg* 1948;128:425.

175. Dobrowsky W, Schmid AP. Radiotherapy of presacral recurrence following radical surgery for rectal carcinoma. *Dis Colon Rectum* 1985;28:917.

176. Docherty JG, McGregor JR, Akyol AM, et al. Comparison of manually constructed and stapled anastomoses in colorectal surgery. *Ann Surg* 1995;221:176.

177. Donaldson GA, Rodkey GV, Behringer GE. Resection of the rectum with anal preservation. *Surg Gynecol Obstet* 1966; 123:571.

178. Dosoretz DE, Gunderson LL, Hedberg S, et al. Preoperative irradiation for unresectable rectal and rectosigmoid carcinomas. *Cancer* 1983;52:814.

179. Drake DB, Pemberton JH, Beart RW Jr, et al. Coloanal anastomosis in the management of benign and malignant rectal disease. *Ann Surg* 1987;206:600.

180. Drew PJ, Farouk R, Turnbull LW, et al. Preoperative magnetic resonance staging of rectal cancer with an endorectal coil and dynamic gadolinium enhancement. *Br J Surg* 1999; 86:250.

181. Dukes CE. Cancer of the rectum: an analysis of 1000 cases. *J Pathol Bacteriol* 1940;50:527.

182. Duncan W. Adjuvant radiotherapy in rectal cancer: the MRC trials. *Br J Surg* 1985;72:59.

183. Dunphy JE. The cut gut. Presidential address. *Am J Surg* 1970;119:1.

184. Durdey P, Williams NS. The effect of malignant and inflammatory fixation of rectal carcinoma on prognosis after rectal excision. *Br J Surg* 1984;71:787.

185. Dürig M, Steenblock U, Herberer M, et al. Prevention of radiation injuries to the small intestine. *Surg Gynecol Obstet* 1984;159:162.

186. Dwight RW, Higgins GA, Roswit B, et al. Preoperative radiation and surgery for cancer of the sigmoid colon and rectum. *Am J Surg* 1972;123:93.

187. Eckhauser ML, Imbembo AL, Mansour EG. The role of pre-resectional laser recanalization for obstructing carcinomas of the colon and rectum. *Surgery* 1989;106:710.

188. Eisenberg HW. Sequential electrocoagulation and resection for carcinoma of the rectum. *Surg Gynecol Obstet* 1984;159:471.

189. Eisenstat TE, Rubin RJ, Salvati EP, et al. New method for low transection of the rectum. *Dis Colon Rectum* 1990; 33:346.

190. Ellis LM, Mendenhall WM, Bland KI, et al. Local excision and radiation therapy for early rectal cancer. *Am Surg* 1988;54:217.

191. Enker WE. Potency, cure, and local control in the operative treatment of rectal cancer. *Arch Surg* 1992;127:1396.

192. Enker WE, Heilweil ML, Hertz RL, et al. En bloc pelvic lymphadenectomy and sphincter preservation in the surgical management of rectal cancer. *Ann Surg* 1986;203:426.

193. Enker WE, Laffer UT, Block GE. Enhanced survival of patients with colon and rectal cancer is based upon wide anatomic resection. *Ann Surg* 1979;190:350.

194. Enker WE, Stearns MW Jr, Janov AJ. Perianal coloanal anastomosis following low anterior resection for rectal carcinoma. *Dis Colon Rectum* 1985;28:576.

195. Enker WE, Thaler HT, Cranor ML, et al. Total mesorectal excision of the operative treatment of carcinoma of the rectum. *J Am Coll Surg* 1995;181:335.

196. Eriksen MT, Wibe A, Syse A, et al. Inadvertent perforation during rectal cancer resection in Norway. *Br J Surg* 2004; 91:210.

197. Escudero-Fabre A, Sack J. Endoscopic laser therapy for neoplastic lesions of the colorectum. *Am J Surg* 1992; 163:260.

198. Estes NC, Morphis JG, Hornback NB, et al. Intraarterial chemotherapy and hyperthermia for pain control in patients with recurrent rectal cancer. *Am J Surg* 1986;152: 597.

199. Evans DB, Shumate CR, Ames FC, et al. Use of Dexon mesh for abdominal partitioning above the peritoneal reflection. *Dis Colon Rectum* 1991;34:833.

200. Everett WG, Friend PJ, Forty J. Comparison of stapling and hand-suture for left-sided large bowel anastomosis. *Br J Surg* 1986;73:345.

201. Faivre J, Chaume J-C, Pigot F, et al. Transanal electroresection of small rectal cancer: a sole treatment? *Dis Colon Rectum* 1996;39:270.

202. Falco E, Celoria G, Nardini A. Simple method for very low colorectal anastomosis with the double staple technique. *Br J Surg* 1995;82:1049.

203. Farouk R, Drew PJ, Duthie GS, et al. Disruption of the internal anal sphincter can occur after transanal stapling. *Br J Surg* 1996;83:1400.

204. Farouk R, Nelson H, Gunderson LL. Aggressive multimodality treatment for locally advanced irresectable rectal cancer. *Br J Surg* 1997;84:741.

205. Farouk R, Ratnaval CD, Monson JRT, et al. Staged delivery of Nd:YAG laser therapy for palliation of advanced rectal carcinoma. *Dis Colon Rectum* 1997;40:156.

206. Fazio VW. Cancer of the rectum-sphincter-saving operations. *Surg Clin North Am* 1988;68:1367.

207. Fazio VW. Technical tips for re-operative abdomino/pelvic surgery. Personal communication.

208. Fazio VW, Jagelman DG, Lavery IC, et al. Evaluation of the proximate-ILS circular stapler: a prospective study. *Ann Surg* 1985;210:108.

209. Fein RL, Needell MH, Winton L. An orderly approach to the impotent male and the dorsal approach for insertion of the Jonas penile prosthesis. *Contemp Surg* 1983;23:93.

210. Feinberg SM, Parker F, Cohen Z, et al. The double stapling technique for low anterior resection of rectal carcinoma. *Dis Colon Rectum* 1986;29:885.

211. Fielding LP, Stewart-Brown S, Hittinger R, et al. Covering stoma for elective anterior resection of the rectum: an outmoded operation? *Am J Surg* 1984;147:524.

212. Fisher B, Wolmark N, Rockette H, et al. Postoperative adjuvant chemotherapy or radiation therapy for rectal cancer: results from NSABP Protocol R-01. *J Natl Cancer Inst* 1988; 80:21.

213. Fitzgibbons RJ Jr, Harkrider WW, Cohn I Jr. Review of abdominoperineal resections for cancer. *Am J Surg* 1977;134: 624.

214. Fleshman JW. The effect of the surgeon and the pathologist on patient survival after resection of colon and rectal cancer. *Ann Surg* 2002;235:464.

215. Fleshman JW, Kodner IJ, Fry RD, et al. Adenocarcinoma of the rectum: results of radiotherapy and resection, endocavitary irradiation, local excision, and preoperative clinical staging. *Dis Colon Rectum* 1985;28:810.

216. Fleshman JW, Myerson RJ, Fry RD, et al. Accuracy of transrectal ultrasound in predicting pathologic stage of rectal cancer before and after preoperative radiation therapy. *Dis Colon Rectum* 1992;35:823.

217. Foley KM. The treatment of cancer pain. *N Engl J Med* 1985;313:84.

218. Fortier GA, Constable WC. Preoperative radiation therapy for rectal cancer. *Arch Surg* 1986;121:1380.

219. Foster ME, Lancaster JB, Leaper DJ. Leakage of low rectal anastomosis: an anatomic explanation? *Dis Colon Rectum* 1984;27:157.

220. Fowl RJ, Akers DL, Kempczinski RF. Neurovascular lower extremity complications of the lithotomy position. *Ann Vasc Surg* 1992;6:357.

221. Franklin R, McSwain B. Carcinoma of the colon, rectum, and anus. *Ann Surg* 1970;171:811.

222. Frazee RC, Patel R, Belew M, et al. Transanal excision of rectal carcinoma. *Am Surg* 1995;61:714.

223. Friedmann P, Garb JL, McCabe DP, et al. Intestinal anastomosis after preoperative radiation therapy for carcinoma of the rectum. *Surg Gynecol Obstet* 1987;164:257.

224. Friedmann P, Garb JL, Park WC, et al. Survival following moderate-dose preoperative radiation therapy for carcinoma of the rectum. *Cancer* 1985;55:967.

225. Friel CM, Cromwell JW, Marra C, et al. Salvage radical surgery after failed local excision for early rectal cancer. *Dis Colon Rectum* 2002;45:875.

226. Fritsch A, Seidl W, Walzel C, et al. Palliative and adjunctive measures in rectal cancer. *World J Surg* 1982;6:569.

227. Fry DE, Amin M, Harbrecht PJ. Rectal obstruction secondary to carcinoma of the prostate. *Ann Surg* 1979;189: 488.

228. Frykholm GJ, Glimelius B, Påhlman L. Preoperative or postoperative irradiation in adenocarcinoma of the rectum: final treatment results of a randomized trial and an evaluation of late secondary effects. *Dis Colon Rectum* 1993;36:564.

229. Fujita S, Yamamoto S, Akasu T, et al. Lateral pelvic lymph node dissection for advanced lower rectal cancer. *Br J Surg* 2003;90:1580.

230. Fürst A, Suttner S, Agha A, et al. Colonic J-pouch vs. coloplasty following resection of distal rectal cancer: early results of a prospective, randomized, pilot study. *Dis Colon Rectum* 2003;46:1161.

231. Gabriel WB. Perineal-abdominal excision of the rectum in one stage. *Lancet* 1934;2:69.

232. Gage AA. Cryotherapy for inoperable rectal cancer. *Dis Colon Rectum* 1968;11:36.

233. Gage AA. Cryosurgery in the treatment of cancer. *Surg Gynecol Obstet* 1992;174:73.

234. Gagliardi G, Bayar S, Smith R, et al. Preoperative staging of rectal cancer using magnetic resonance imaging with external phase-arrayed coils. *Arch Surg* 2002;137:447.

235. Gagliardi G, Hawley PR, Hershman MJ, et al. Prognostic factors in surgery for local recurrence of rectal cancer. *Br J Surg* 1995;82:1401.

236. Gagliardi G, Stepniewska KA, Hershman MJ, et al. New grade-related prognostic variable for rectal cancer. *Br J Surg* 1995;82:599.

237. Galandiuk S, Fazio VW. Postoperative irrigation-suction drainage after pelvic colonic surgery. A prospective randomized trial. *Dis Colon Rectum* 1991;34:223.

238. Gall FP, Hermanek P. Cancer of the rectum-local excision. *Surg Clin North Am* 1988;68:1353.

239. Galloway DJ, Cohen AM, Shank B, et al. Adjuvant multimodality treatment of rectal cancer. *Br J Surg* 1989;76:440.

240. Gamagami RA, Liagre A, Chiotasso P, et al. Coloanal anastomosis for distal third rectal cancer: prospective study of oncologic results. *Dis Colon Rectum* 1999;42:1272.

241. Ganchrow MI, Facelle TL. Double Roticulator stapling technique for low-lying rectal tumors. *Am J Surg* 1993; 166:54.

242. Garcia-Aguilar J, Cromwell JW, Marra C, et al. Treatment of locally recurrent rectal cancer. *Dis Colon Rectum* 2001; 44:1743.

243. Garcia-Aguilar J, Hernandez de Anda E, Sirivongs P, et al. A pathologic complete response to preoperative chemoradiation is associated with lower local recurrence and improved survival in rectal cancer patients treated by mesorectal excision. *Dis Colon Rectum* 2003;46:298.

244. Garcia-Aguiler J, Pollack J, Lee S-H, et al. Accuracy of endorectal ultrasonography in preoperative staging of rectal tumors. *Dis Colon Rectum* 2002;45:10.

245. Gastrointestinal Tumor Study Group. Prolongation of the disease-free interval in surgically treated rectal carcinoma. *N Engl J Med* 1985;312:1465.

246. Gastrointestinal Tumor Study Group. Survival after postoperative combination treatment of rectal cancer. *N Engl J Med* 1986;315:1294.

247. Gee WF, McRoberts JW, Ansell JS. Penile prosthetic implant for the treatment of organic impotence. *Am J Surg* 1973;126:698.

248. Geerdes BP, Zoetmulder FAN, Heineman E, et al. Total anorectal reconstruction with a double dynamic graciloplasty after abdominoperineal reconstruction for low rectal cancer. *Dis Colon Rectum* 1997;40:698.

249. Gérard A, Buyse M, Nordlinger B, et al. Preoperative radiotherapy as adjuvant treatment in rectal cancer: final results of a randomized study of the European Organization for Research and Treatment of Cancer (EORTC). *Ann Surg* 1988;208:606.

250. Gerstenberg TC, Nielsen ML, Clausen S, et al. Bladder function after abdominoperineal resection of the rectum for anorectal cancer: urodynamic investigations before and after operation in a consecutive series. *Ann Surg* 1980; 191:81.

251. Gertsch P, Baer HU, Kraft R, et al. Malignant cells are collected on circular staplers. *Dis Colon Rectum* 1992;35:238.

252. Gervas P, Rotholtz N, Wexner SD, et al. Colonic J-pouch function in rectal cancer patients: impact of adjuvant chemoradiotherapy. *Dis Colon Rectum* 2001;44:1667.

253. Gibbs P, Chao MW, Tjandra JJ. Optimizing the outcome for patients with rectal cancer. *Dis Colon Rectum* 2003;46:389.

254. Gilbertsen VA. Adenocarcinoma of the rectum: incidence and locations of recurrent tumor following present-day operations performed for cure. *Ann Surg* 1960;151:340.

255. Gilbertsen VA. The results of surgical treatment of cancer of the rectum. *Surg Gynecol Obstet* 1962;114:313.

256. Gilchrist RK, David VC. Consideration of pathological factors influencing five year survival in radical resection of large bowel and rectum for carcinoma. *Ann Surg* 1947;126: 421.

257. Gilchrist RK, David VC. Prognosis in carcinoma of bowel. *Surg Gynecol Obstet* 1948;86:359.

258. Gingold BS, Berardis J, Knight P. Reducing the risk of wound infection in operations upon the colon. *Surg Gynecol Obstet* 1984;158:9.

259. Gingold BS, Cooper MI, Wallack MK. Ligation device assisting low anterior anastomosis. *Dis Colon Rectum* 1995; 38:1322.

260. Gingold BS, Mitty WF Jr, Tadros M. Importance of patient selection in local treatment of carcinoma of the rectum. *Am J Surg* 1983;145:293.

261. Glaser F, Kuntz C, Schlag P, et al. Endorectal ultrasound for control of preoperative radiotherapy of rectal cancer. *Ann Surg* 1993;217:64.

262. Glaser F, Schlag P, Herfarth CH. Endorectal ultrasonography for the assessment of invasion of rectal tumours and lymph node involvement. *Br J Surg* 1990;77:883.

263. Glenn F, McSherry CK. Carcinoma of the distal large bowel: 32-year review of 1,026 cases. *Ann Surg* 1966;163: 838.

264. Goetz O. Das Rektumkarzinom als Exstirpationsobjekt; Vorschläge zur sakralen und abdominosakralen Operation. *Zentralbl Chir* 1931;58:1746.

265. Goldman HS, Sapkin SL, Foote RF, et al. Seminal vesicle-rectal fistula: report of a case. *Dis Colon Rectum* 1989;32: 67.

266. Goldman S, Arvidsson H, Norming U, et al. Transrectal ultrasound and computed tomography in preoperative staging of lower rectal adenocarcinoma. *Gastrointest Radiol* 1991;16:259.

267. Goldsmith HS. Protection of low rectal anastomosis with intact omentum. *Surg Gynecol Obstet* 1977;144:584.

268. Goldsmith HS. Use of the omentum in the presacral space. *Dis Colon Rectum* 1978;21:405.

269. Goldstein M, Duff JH. Reconsideration of colostomy in elective left colon resection. *Surg Gynecol Obstet* 1972; 134:593.

270. Goligher JC. The adequacy of the marginal blood-supply to the left colon after high ligation of the inferior mesenteric artery during excision of the rectum. *Br J Surg* 1954;41: 351.

271. Goligher JC. Ernest Miles: the rise and fall of abdomino-perineal excision in the treatment or carcinoma of the rectum. *J Pelv Surg* 1996;2:53.

272. Goligher JC. Further reflections on preservation of the anal sphincters in the radical treatment of rectal cancer. *Proc R Soc Med* 1962;55:341.

273. Goligher JC, Dukes CE, Bussey HJR. Local recurrences after sphincter-saving excisions of carcinoma of rectum and rectosigmoid. *Br J Surg* 1951;39:199.

274. Goligher JC, Duthie HL, DeDombal FT, et al. Abdomino-anal pull-through excision for tumors of the mid-third of the rectum: a comparison with low anterior resection. *Br J Surg* 1965;52:323.

275. Goligher JC, Graham NG, DeDombal FT. Anastomotic dehiscence after anterior resection of rectum and sigmoid. *Br J Surg* 1970;57:109.

276. Goligher JC, Hughes ESR. Sensibility of the rectum and colon: its role in the mechanism of anal continence. *Lancet* 1951;1:543.

277. Goligher JC, Lloyd-Davies OV, Robertson CT. Small-gut obstructions following combined excision of rectum, with special reference to strangulation around the colostomy. *Br J Surg* 1951;38:467.

278. Golub R, Golub RW, Cantu R Jr, et al. A multivariate analysis of factors contributing to leakage of intestinal anastomoses. *J Am Coll Surg* 1997;184:364.

279. Gordon PH. Is total mesorectal excision really important? *J Surg Oncol* 2000;74:177.

280. Gordon PH, Vasilevsky C. Experience with stapling in rectal surgery. *Surg Clin North Am* 1984;64:555.

281. Gordon-Watson C. Treatment of cancer of the rectum with radium by open operation. *Proc R Soc Med* 1927;21:309.

282. Gordon-Watson C. The treatment of carcinoma of the rectum with radium. *Br J Surg* 1930;17:649.

283. Gordon-Watson C. How far can radium replace radical surgery for cancer of the rectum? *Ann Surg* 1931;93:467.

284. Gordon-Watson C. Discussion on the radium treatment of malignant disease of the rectum and anus. *Proc R Soc Med* 1935;28:1251.

285. Grabham JA, Moran BJ, Lane RHS. Defunctioning colostomy for low anterior resection: a selective approach. *Br J Surg* 1995;82:1331.

286. Graffner H, Fredlund P, Olsson S-A, et al. Protective colostomy in low anterior resection of the rectum using the EEA stapling instrument-a randomized study. *Dis Colon Rectum* 1983;26:87.

287. Graham JW, Goligher JC. The management of accidental injuries and deliberate resections of the ureter during excision of the rectum. *Br J Surg* 1954;42:151.

288. Graham RA, Garnsey L, Jessup JM. Local excision of rectal carcinoma. *Am J Surg* 1990;160:306.

289. Graham RA, Hohn DC. Management of inguinal lymph node metastases from adenocarcinoma of the rectum. *Dis Colon Rectum* 1990;33:212.

290. Grann A, Minsky BD, Cohen AM, et al. Preliminary results of preoperative 5-fluorouracil, low-dose leucovorin and concurrent radiation therapy for clinically resectable T3 rectal cancer. *Dis Colon Rectum* 1997;40:515.

291. Granai CO, Gajewski W, Madoc-Jones H, et al. Use of the omental J flap for better delivery of radiotherapy to the pelvis. *Surg Gynecol Obstet* 1990;171:71.

292. Greaney MG, Irvin TT. Criteria for the selection of rectal cancers for local treatment; a clinicopathologic study of low rectal tumors. *Dis Colon Rectum* 1977;20:463.

293. Gregory JS, Muldoon JP. Perineal herniation-a late complication of abdominoperineal resection of the rectum: report of a case. *Dis Colon Rectum* 1969;12:33.

294. Griffen FD, Knight CD. Stapling technique for primary and secondary rectal anastomoses. *Surg Clin North Am* 1984; 64:579.

295. Griffen FD, Knight CD Sr, Whitaker JM, et al. The double stapling technique for low anterior resection. Results, modifications, and observations. *Ann Surg* 1990;211:745.

296. Grigg M, McDermott FT, Pihl EA, et al. Curative local excision in the treatment of carcinoma of the rectum. *Dis Colon Rectum* 1984;27:81.

297. Gualdi GF, Casciani E, Gaudalaxara A, et al. Local staging of rectal cancer with transrectal ultrasound and endorectal magnetic resonance imaging: comparison with histologic findings. *Dis Colon Rectum* 2000;43:338.

298. Guillem JG, Paty PB, Cohen AM. Surgical treatment of colorectal cancer. *CA Cancer J Clin* 1997;47:113.

299. Guillem JG, Puig-La Calle JJr, Akhurst T, et al. Prospective assessment of primary rectal cancer response to preoperative radiation and chemotherapy using 18-fluorodeoxyglucose positron emission tomography. *Dis Colon Rectum* 2000; 43:18.

300. Guinet C, Buy J-N, Ghossain MA, et al. Comparison of magnetic resonance imaging and computed tomography in the preoperative staging of rectal cancer. *Arch Surg* 1990; 125:385.

301. Gunderson LL, Cohen AM, Welch CE. Residual, inoperable or recurrent colorectal cancer: interaction of surgery and radiotherapy. *Am J Surg* 1980;139:518.

302. Gunderson LL, Martin JK, Beart RW, et al. Intraoperative and external beam irradiation for locally advanced colorectal cancer. *Ann Surg* 1988;207:52.

303. Habib N, Salem R, Luck RJ, et al. A histochemical method that predicts local recurrence after curative resection in carcinoma of the colon and rectum. *Surg Gynecol Obstet* 1984;159:436.

304. Hadfield MB, Nicholson AA, MacDonald AW, et al. Preoperative staging of rectal carcinoma by magnetic resonance imaging with a pelvic phased-array coil. *Br J Surg* 1997; 84:529.

305. Hafner GH, Herrera L, Petrelli NJ. Patterns of recurrence after pelvic exenteration for colorectal adenocarcinoma. *Arch Surg* 1991;126:1510.

306. Hafström L, Jönsson P-E, Landberg T, et al. Intraarterial infusion chemotherapy (5-FU) in patients with inextirpable or locally recurrent rectal cancer. *Am J Surg* 1979;137:757.

307. Hager TH, Gall FP, Hermanek P. Local excision of cancer of the rectum. *Dis Colon Rectum* 1983;26:149.

308. Hahnlosser D, Nelson H, Gunderson LL, et al. Curative potential of multimodality therapy for locally recurrent rectal cancer. *Ann Surg* 2003;237:502.

309. Hainsworth PJ, Egan MJ, Cunliffe WJ. Evaluation of a policy of total mesorectal excision for rectal and rectosigmoid cancers. *Br J Surg* 1997;84:652.

310. Hallböök O, Påhlman L, Krog M, et al. Randomized comparison of straight and colonic J pouch anastomosis after low anterior resection. *Ann Surg* 1996;224:58.

311. Hallböök O, Sjödahl R. Anastomotic leakage and functional outcome after anterior resection of the rectum. *Br J Surg* 1996;83:60.

312. Harford FJ. Use of glucagon in conjunction with the end-to-end anastomosis (EEA) stapling device for low anterior anastomoses. *Dis Colon Rectum* 1979;22:452.

313. Harnsberger JR, Charvat P, Longo WE, et al. The role of intrarectal ultrasound (IRUS) in staging of rectal cancer and detection of extrarectal pathology. *Am Surg* 1994;60:571.

314. Harris GJC, Church JM, Senagore AJ, et al. Factors affecting local recurrence of colonic adenocarcinoma. *Dis Colon Rectum* 2002;45:1029.

315. Harris GJC, Lavery IJ, Fazio VW. Reasons for failure to construct the colonic J-pouch. what can be done to improve the size of the neorectal reservoir should it occur? *Dis Colon Rectum* 2002;45:1304.

316. Harrison LB, Enker WE, Anderson LL. High-dose-rate intraoperative radiation therapy for colorectal cancer. *Oncology* 1995;9:737.

317. Harshaw DH, Gardner B, Vives A, et al. The effect of technical factors upon complications from abdominal perineal resections. *Surg Gynecol Obstet* 1974;139:756.

318. Hartmann H. Nouveau procédé d'ablation des cancers de la partie terminale du colon pelvien. In: *Trentiéme Congrès de Chirurgie.* Strasbourg, France, 1923:411.

319. Hase K, Shatney CH, Mochizuki H, et al. Long-term results of curative resection of minimally invasive colorectal cancer. *Dis Colon Rectum* 1995;38:19.

320. Hashiguchi Y, Sekine T, Kato S, et al. Indicators for surgical resection and intraoperative radiation therapy for pelvic recurrence of colorectal cancer. *Dis Colon Rectum* 2003;46:31.

321. Hashiguchi Y, Sekine T, Sakamoto H, et al. Intraoperative irradiation after surgery for locally recurrent rectal cancer. *Dis Colon Rectum* 1999;42:886.

322. Hautefeuille P, Valleur P, Perniceni T, et al. Functional and oncologic results after coloanal anastomosis for low rectal carcinoma. *Ann Surg* 1988;207:61.

323. Havenga K, Enker WE, McDermott K, et al. Male and female sexual and urinary function after total mesorectal excision with autonomic nerve preservation for carcinoma of the rectum. *J Am Coll Surg* 1996;182:495.

324. Hawkins FE Jr, Marks C. The parasacral approach to the rectum. *Am Surg* 1984;50:623.

325. Hawley PR. Infection-the cause of anastomotic breakdown: an experimental study. *Proc R Soc Med* 1970;63:752.

326. Hazama S, Oka M, Suzuki T. Modified technique for double stapling of colorectal anastomosis following low anterior resection. *Br J Surg* 1996;83:1110.

327. Heah SM, Eu KW, Ho YH, et al. Hartmann's procedure *vs.* abdominoperineal resection for palliation of advanced low rectal cancer. *Dis Colon Rectum* 1997;40:1313.

328. Heah SM, Seow-Choen F, Eu KW, et al. Prospective, randomized trial comparing sigmoid vs. descending colonic J-pouch after total rectal excision. *Dis Colon Rectum* 2002;45:322.

329. Heald RJ. Total mesorectal excision is optimal surgery for rectal cancer: a Scandinavian consensus. *Br J Surg* 1995;82:1297.

330. Heald RJ, Smedh RK, Kald A, et al. Abdominoperineal excision of the rectum: an endangered operation. *Dis Colon Rectum* 1997;40:747.

331. Heald RJ, Leicester RJ. The low stapled anastomosis. *Dis Colon Rectum* 1981;24:437.

332. Heald RJ, Ryall RDH. Recurrence and survival after total mesorectal excision for rectal cancer. *Lancet* 1986;1:1479.

333. Heberer G, Denecke H, Demmel N, et al. Local procedures in the management of rectal cancer. *World J Surg* 1987; 11:499.

334. Heberer G, Denecke H, Pratschke E, et al. Anterior and low anterior resection. *World J Surg* 1982;6:517.

335. Heimann TM, Miller F, Martinelli G, et al. Significance of DNA content abnormalities in small rectal cancers. *Am J Surg* 1990;159:199.

336. Heimann TM, Szporn A, Bolnick K, et al. Local recurrence following surgical treatment of rectal cancer: comparison of anterior and abdominoperineal resection. *Dis Colon Rectum* 1986;29:862.

337. Hemingway D, Flett M, McKee RF, et al. Sphincter function after transanal endoscopic microsurgical excision of rectal tumours. *Br J Surg* 1996;83:51.

338. Heriot AG, Grundy A, Kumar D. Preoperative staging of rectal carcinoma. *Br J Surg* 1999;86:17.

339. Herter FP, Colacchio TA. The influence of antibiotics on infection and anastomotic recurrence after colon resection for cancer. *World J Surg* 1982;6:188.

340. Herter FP, Slanetz CA Jr. Preoperative intestinal preparation in relation to the subsequent development of cancer at the suture line. *Surg Gynecol Obstet* 1968;127:49.

341. Herrera L, Villarreal JR. Incidence of metastases from rectal adenocarcinoma in small lymph nodes detected by a clearing technique. *Dis Colon Rectum* 1992;35:783.

342. Herzog U, von Flüe M, Tondelli P, et al. How accurate is endorectal ultrasound in the preoperative staging of rectal cancer? *Dis Colon Rectum* 1993;36:127.

343. Hickey RC, Romsdahl MM, Johnson DE, et al. Recurrent cancer and metastases. *World J Surg* 1982;6:585.

344. Hida J-I, Yasutomi M, Maruyama T, et al. Indications for colonic J-pouch reconstruction after anterior resection for rectal cancer: determining the optimum level of anastomosis. *Dis Colon Rectum* 1998;41:558.

345. Hida J-I, Yasutomi M, Fujimoto K, et al. Functional outcome after low anterior resection with low anastomosis for rectal cancer using the colonic J-pouch. *Dis Colon Rectum* 1996;39:986.

346. Hida J-I, Yasumoti M, Maruyama T, et al. Lymph node metastases detected in the mesorectum distal to carcinoma of the rectum by the clearing method: justification of total mesorectal excision. *J Am Coll Surg* 1997;184:584.

347. Hildebrandt U, Feifel G. Preoperative staging of rectal cancer by intrarectal ultrasound. *Dis Colon Rectum* 1985; 28:42.

348. Hildebrandt U, Feifel G, Scherr O. Endorectal ultrasound: instrumentation and clinical aspects. *Int J Colorect Dis* 1986;1:203.

349. Hildebrandt U, Klein T, Feifel G, et al. Endosonography of pararectal lymph nodes. In vitro and in vivo evaluation. *Dis Colon Rectum* 1990;33:863.

350. Hjortrup A, Moesgaard F, Kjaergård J. Fibrin adhesive in the treatment of perineal fistulas. *Dis Colon Rectum* 1991; 34:752.

351. Ho Y-H, Tsang C, Tang CL, et al. Anal sphincter injuries from stapling instruments introduced transanally: randomized, controlled study with endoanal ultrasound and anorectal manometry. *Dis Colon Rectum* 2000;43:169.

352. Ho Y-H, Yu S, Ang E-S, et al. Small colonic J-pouch improves colonic retention of liquids: randomized, controlled trial with scintigraphy. *Dis Colon Rectum* 2002;45:76.

353. Hochenegg J. Die Sakrale Methode der Exstirpation von Mastdarmkrebsen nach Prof. Kraske. *Wien Klin Wochenschr* 1888;1:254.

354. Hodges CV, Moore RJ, Lehman TH, et al. Clinical experiences with transureteroureterostomy. *J Urol* 1963;90:552.

355. Hodgman CG, MacCarty RL, Wolff BG, et al. Preoperative staging of rectal carcinoma by computed tomography and 0.15T magnetic resonance imaging. *Dis Colon Rectum* 1986;29:446.

356. Hojo K. Anastomotic recurrence after sphincter-saving resection for rectal cancer. *Dis Colon Rectum* 1986;29:11.

357. Hojo K, Sawada T, Moriya Y. An analysis of survival and voiding, sexual function after wide iliopelvic lymphadenectomy in patients with carcinoma of the rectum, compared with conventional lymphadenectomy. *Dis Colon Rectum* 1989;32:128.

358. Holdsworth PJ, Johnston D, Chalmers AG, et al. Endoluminal ultrasound and computed tomography in the staging of rectal cancer. *Br J Surg* 1988;75:1019.

359. Holm T, Cedermark B, Rutqvist L-E. Local recurrence of rectal adenocarcinoma after curative surgery with and without preoperative radiotherapy. *Br J Surg* 1994;81:452.

360. Holm T, Johansson H, Cedermark B, et al. Influence of hospital- and surgeon-related factors on outcome after treatment of rectal cancer with or without preoperative radiotherapy. *Br J Surg* 1997;84:657.

361. Holm T, Rutqvist L-E, Johansson H, et al. Abdominoperineal resection and anterior resection in the treatment of rectal cancer: results in relation to adjuvant preoperative radiotherapy. *Br J Surg* 1995;82:1213.

362. Holm T, Rutqvist L-E, Johansson H, et al. Postoperative mortality in rectal cancer treated with or without preoperative radiotherapy: causes and risk factors. *Br J Surg* 1996; 83:964.

363. Hood K, Lewis A. Dilator for high rectal strictures. *Br J Surg* 1986;73:633.

364. Hool GR, Church JM, Fazio VW. Decision-making in rectal cancer surgery: survey of North American colorectal residency programs. *Dis Colon Rectum* 1998;41:147.

365. Horn A, Dahl O, Morild I. Venous and neural invasion as predictors of recurrence in rectal adenocarcinoma. *Dis Colon Rectum* 1991;34:798.

366. Horn A, Halvorsen JF, Dahl O. Preoperative radiotherapy in operable rectal cancer. *Dis Colon Rectum* 1990;33:823.

367. Horn A, Halvorsen JF, Morild I. Transanal extirpation of early rectal cancer. *Dis Colon Rectum* 1989;32:769.

368. Huber A, von Hockstetter A, Allgöwer M. Anatomy of the pelvic floor for translevatoric-transsphincteric operations. *Am Surg* 1987;53:247.

369. Huddy SPJ, Husband EM, Cook MG, et al. Lymph node metastases in early rectal cancer. *Br J Surg* 1993;80:1457.

370. Hughes EP, Veidenheimer MC, Corman ML, et al. Electrocoagulation of rectal cancer. *Dis Colon Rectum* 1982;25:215.

371. Hughes TG, Jenevein EP, Poulos E. Intramural spread of colon carcinoma. *Am J Surg* 1983;146:697.

372. Huguet C, Harb J, Bona S. Coloanal anastomosis after resection of low rectal cancer in the elderly. *World J Surg* 1990;14:619.

373. Hull TL, Lavry IC, Saxton JP. Endocavitary irradiation: an option in select patients with rectal cancer. *Dis Colon Rectum* 1994;37:1266.

374. Hünerbein M, Schlag PM. Three-dimensional endosonography for staging of rectal cancer. *Ann Surg* 1997;225:432.

375. Hunt TK. Anastomotic failure. In: Simmons RL, ed. *Topics in intraabdominal surgical infection.* Norwalk, CT: Appleton-Century-Crofts, 1982:101.

376. Husband JE, Hodson NJ, Parsons CA. The use of computed tomography in recurrent rectal tumors. *Radiology* 1980; 134:677.

377. Hyams DM, Mamounas EP, Petrelli N, et al. A clinical trial to evaluate the worth of preoperative multimodality therapy in patients with operable carcinoma of the rectum: a progress report of national surgical adjuvant breast and bowel project protocol R-03. *Dis Colon Rectum* 1997;40: 131.

378. Ike H, Shimada H, Yamaguchi S, et al. Outcome of total pelvic exenteration for primary rectal cancer. *Dis Colon Rectum* 2003;46:474.

379. Irvin TT, Goligher JC. Aetiology of disruption of intestinal anastomoses. *Br J Surg* 1973;60:461.

380. Itabashi M, Hamano K, Kameoka S, et al. Self-expanding stainless steel stent application in rectosigmoid stricture. *Dis Colon Rectum* 1993;36:508.

381. Ivanov KD, Diacov CD. Three-dimensional endoluminal ultrasound: new staging techniques in patients with rectal cancer. *Dis Colon Rectum* 1997;40:47.

382. Iwai H, Sato S, Sakurazawa K, et al. Use of transanal intubation in Doppler ultrasonic assessment of blood flow of the rectal wall. *Surg Gynecol Obstet* 1989;169:263.

383. Jackman RJ. Conservative management of selected patients with carcinoma of the rectum. *Dis Colon Rectum* 1961;4:429.

384. Jacobson YG. Posterior rectal resection using EEA stapler. *Dis Colon Rectum* 1985;28:681.

385. James RD, Schofield PF. Resection of "inoperable" rectal cancer following radiotherapy. *Br J Surg* 1985;72:279.

386. Janu NC, Bokey EL, Chapuis PH, et al. Bladder dysfunction following anterior resection for carcinoma of the rectum. *Dis Colon Rectum* 1986;29:182.

387. Jass JR. Lymphocytic infiltration and survival in rectal cancer. *J Clin Pathol* 1986;39:585.

388. Jass JR, Love SB, Northover JMA. A new prognostic classification of rectal cancer. *Lancet* 1987;1:1303.

389. Jelden GL. Presentation to American Society of Therapeutic Radiologists, Miami Beach (as reported in *Medical News*). *JAMA* 1981;246:2419.

390. Jiminez RE, Shoup M, Cohen AM, et al. Contemporary outcomes of total pelvic exenteration in the treatment of colorectal cancer. *Dis Colon Rectum* 2003;46:1619.

391. Jin Kim H, Wong WD. Role of endorectal ultrasound in the conservative management of rectal cancers. *Semin Surg Oncol* 2000;19:358.

392. Jochem RJ, Reading CC, Dozois RR, et al. Endorectal ultrasonographic staging of rectal carcinoma. *Mayo Clin Proc* 1990;65:1571.

393. Johansson C. Endoscopic dilation of rectal strictures: a prospective study of 18 cases. *Dis Colon Rectum* 1996;39: 423.

394. Johnston MJ, Robertson GM, Frizelle FA. Management of late complications of pelvic radiation in the rectum and anus: a review. *Dis Colon Rectum* 2003;46:247.

395. Jones DJ, Moore M, Schofield PF. Prognostic significance of DNA ploidy in colorectal cancer: a prospective flow cytometric study. *Br J Surg* 1988;75:28.

396. Jones DJ, Zaloudik J, James RD, et al. Predicting local recurrence of carcinoma of the rectum after preoperative radiotherapy and surgery. *Br J Surg* 1989;76:1172.

397. Julian TB, Ravitch MM. Evaluation of the safety of end-to-end (EEA) stapling anastomoses across linear stapled closures. *Surg Clin North Am* 1984;64:567.

398. Julian TB, Wolmark N. Stapled Baker type anastomosis for low anterior resections. *Surg Gynecol Obstet* 1990;171:169.

399. Junginger T, Kneist W, Heintz A. Influence of identification and preservation of pelvic autonomic nerves in rectal cancer surgery on bladder dysfunction after total mesorectal excision. *Dis Colon Rectum* 2003;46:621.

400. Kahn H, Alexander A, Rakinic J, et al. Preoperative staging of irradiated rectal cancers using digital rectal examination, computed tomography, endorectal ultrasound, and magnetic resonance imaging does not accurately predict T0, N0 pathology. *Dis Colon Rectum* 1997;40:140.

401. Kandioler D, Zwrtek R, Ludwig C, et al. TP53 genotype but not p53 immunohistochemical result predicts response to preoperative short-term radiotherapy in rectal cancer. *Ann Surg* 2002;235:493.

402. Karanjia ND, Corder AP, Bearn P, et al. Leakage from stapled low anastomosis after total mesorectal excision for carcinoma of the rectum. *Br J Surg* 1994;81:1224.

403. Karanjia ND, Corder AP, Holdsworth PJ, et al. Risk of peritonitis and fatal septicaemia and the need to defunction the low anastomosis. *Br J Surg* 1991;78:196.

404. Karanjia ND, Schache DJ, North WRS, et al. "Close shave" in anterior resection. *Br J Surg* 1990;77:510.

405. Karmody AM, Jordan FR, Zaman DYS. Left colon gangrene after acute inferior mesenteric artery occlusion. *Arch Surg* 1976;111:972.

406. Katin MJ, Dosoretz DE, Gunderson L. The role of radiation therapy in the treatment of unresectable, residual, or recurrent colorectal carcinoma. *Contemp Surg* 1984;24:25.

407. Katsura Y, Yamada K, Ishizawa T, et al. Endorectal ultrasonography for the assessment of wall invasion and lymph node metastasis in rectal cancer. *Dis Colon Rectum* 1992; 35:362.

408. Keighley MRB, Crapp AR, Burdon DW, et al. Prophylaxis against anaerobic sepsis in bowel surgery. *Br J Surg* 1976; 63:538.

409. Kelly SR, Nugent KP. Formalin instillation for control of rectal hemorrhage in advanced pelvic malignancy: report of two cases. *Dis Colon Rectum* 2002;45:121.

410. Kennedy HL, Rothenberger DA, Goldberg SM, et al. Colocolostomy and coloproctostomy utilizing the circular intraluminal stapling devices. *Dis Colon Rectum* 1983;26:145.

411. Kergin FG. Diathermy fulgurization in treatment of certain cases of rectal carcinoma. *Can Med Assoc J* 1953;69:14.

412. Khoury DA, Opelka FG. Anoscopic-assisted insertion of end-to-end anastomosing staplers. *Dis Colon Rectum* 1995; 38:553.

413. Khubchandani IT, Karamchandani MC, Sheets JA, et al. The Bacon pull-through procedure. *Dis Colon Rectum* 1987;30:540.

414. Khubchandani IT, Trimpi HD, Sheets JA. Low end-to-side rectoenteric anastomosis with single-layer wire. *Dis Colon Rectum* 1975;18:308.

415. Killingback MJ. Indications for local excision of rectal cancer. *Br J Surg* 1985;72:54.

416. Kim NK, Kim MJ, Yun SH, et al. Comparative study of transrectal ultrasonography, pelvic computerized tomography, and magnetic resonance imaging in preoperative staging of rectal cancer. *Dis Colon Rectum* 1999;42:770.

417. Kingsley AN. Colonic strictures: management by endoscopic balloon dilation. *Contemp Surg* 1991;38:50.

418. Kinn A-C, Öhman U. Bladder and sexual function after surgery for rectal cancer. *Dis Colon Rectum* 1986;29:43.

419. Kirwan WO, O'Riordain MG, Waldron R. Declining indications for abdominoperineal resection. *Br J Surg* 1989;76:1061.

420. Kirwan WO, Turnbull RB Jr, Fazio VW, et al. Pull-through operation with delayed anastomosis for rectal cancer. *Br J Surg* 1978;65:695.

421. Kiselow M, Butcher HR Jr, Bricker EM. Results of the radical surgical treatment of advanced pelvic cancer: a fifteen-year study. *Ann Surg* 1967;166:428.

422. Kjeldsen BJ, Kronborg O, Fenger C, et al. A prospective randomized study of follow-up after radical surgery for colorectal cancer. *Br J Surg* 1997;84:666.

423. Klaaborg K-E, Kronborg O. Suprapublic bladder drainage in elective colorectal surgery. *Dis Colon Rectum* 1986;29: 260.

424. Knight CD, Griffen FD. An improved technique for low anterior resection of the rectum using the EEA stapler. *Surgery* 1980;88:710.

425. Knoepp LF, Ray JE, Overby I. Ovarian metastases from colorectal carcinoma. *Dis Colon Rectum* 1973;16:305.

426. Kocher T. Quoted in Rankin FW, Bargen JA, Buie LA, eds. *The colon, rectum and anus.* Philadelphia: WB Saunders, 1932.

427. Koda K, Tobe T, Takiguchi N, et al. Pelvic exenteration for advanced colorectal cancer with reconstruction of urinary and sphincter functions. *Br J Surg* 2002;89:1286.

428. Kodner IJ, Gilley MT, Shemesh EI, et al. Radiation therapy as definitive treatment for selected invasive rectal cancer. *Surgery* 1993;114:850.

429. Kodner IJ, Shemesh EI, Fry RD, et al. Preoperative irradiation for rectal cancer: improved local control and long-term survival. *Ann Surg* 1989;209:194.

430. Koehler PR, Feldberg MAM, van Waes PFGM. Preoperative staging of rectal cancer with computerized tomography. *Cancer* 1984;54:512.

431. Kollmorgen TA, Kollmorgen CF, Lieber MM, et al. Seminal vesicle fistula following abdominoperineal resection for recurrent adenocarcinoma of the rectum. *Dis Colon Rectum* 1994;37:1325.

432. Konishi F, Muto T, Takahashi H, et al. Transrectal ultrasonography for the assessment of invasion of rectal carcinoma. *Dis Colon Rectum* 1985;28:889.

433. Kouraklis G. Reconstruction of the pelvic floor using the rectus abdominis muscles after radical pelvic surgery. *Dis Colon Rectum* 2002;45:836.

434. Kraybill WG, Lopez MJ, Bricker EM. Total pelvic exenteration as a therapeutic option in advanced malignant disease of the pelvis. *Surg Gynecol Obstet* 1988;166:259.

435. Kramann B, Hildebrandt U. Computed tomography versus endosonography in the staging of rectal carcinoma: a comparative study. *Int J Colorect Dis* 1986;1:216.

436. Kraske P. Ueber die Entstehung sek undarer Krebsqeschwüre durch Impfung. *Zentralbl Chir* 1884;11:801.

437. Kraske P. Zur exstirpation hochsitzender Mastdarmkrebse. [Extirpation of high carcinomas of the large bowel.] *Arch Klin Chir (Berl)* 1886;33:563. Translated in *Dis Colon Rectum* 1984;27:499.

438. Kratzer GL. The pull-through operation. *Dis Colon Rectum* 1967;10:112.

439. Kratzer GL. Modification of the pull-through operation. *Dis Colon Rectum* 1972;15:288.

440. Kratzer GL, Onsanit T. Fulguration of selected cancers of the rectum. *Dis Colon Rectum* 1972;15:431.

441. Kreis ME, Jehle EC, Haug V, et al. Functional results after transanal endoscopic microsurgery. *Dis Colon Rectum* 1996; 39:1116.

442. Kressner U, Graf W, Mahteme H, et al. Septic complications and prognosis after surgery for rectal cancer. *Dis Colon Rectum* 2002;45:316.

443. Kroll SS, Pollock R, Jessup JM, et al. Transpelvic rectus abdominis flap reconstruction of defects following abdomino-perineal resection. *Am Surg* 1989;55:632.

444. Krook JE, Moertel CG, Gunderson LL, et al. Effective surgical adjuvant therapy for high-risk rectal carcinoma. *N Engl J Med* 1991;324:709.

445. Kuehne H, Kleisli T, Biernacki P, et al. Use of high-dose-rate brachytherapy in the management of locally recurrent rectal cancer. *Dis Colon Rectum* 2003;46:895.

446. Kumashiro R, Sano C, Inutsuka S. An adapter for stapling a colorectal anastomosis. *Dis Colon Rectum* 1990;33:243.

447. Kumashiro R, Sano C, Ugaeri H, et al. A new improved technique for placement of a pursestring suture on the edge of the distal part of the rectal stump using a skin stapler for low anterior resection. *J Am Coll Surg* 1994;178 :405.

448. Kurz KR, Pitts WR, Speer D, et al. Palliation of carcinoma of the rectum and pararectum using the urologic resectoscope. *Surg Gynecol Obstet* 1988;166:60.

449. Kusunoki M, Shoji Y, Yanagi H, et al. Function after anoabdominal rectal resection and colonic J pouch-anal anastomosis. *Br J Surg* 1991;78:1434.

450. Kusunoki M, Yanagi H, Gondoh N, et al. Use of transrectal ultrasonography to select type of surgery for villous tumors in the lower two thirds of the rectum. *Arch Surg* 1996; 131:714.

451. Kyzer S, Gordon PH. The prophylactic use of ureteral catheters during colorectal operations. *Am Surg* 1994;60:212.

452. Labow SB, Salvati EP, Rubin RJ. Suture-line recurrences in carcinoma of the colon and rectum. *Dis Colon Rectum* 1975;18:123.

453. Lahey FH. Two-stage abdominoperineal removal of cancer of the rectum. *Surg Gynecol Obstet* 1930;51:622.

454. La Monica G, Audisio RA, Tamburini M, et al. Incidence of sexual dysfunction in male patients treated surgically for rectal malignancy. *Dis Colon Rectum* 1985;28:937.

455. Lane RHS, Parks AG. Function of the anal sphincters following colo-anal anastomosis. *Br J Surg* 1977;64:596.

456. Lanter B, Mason RA. Use of omental pedicle graft to protect low anterior colonic anastomosis. *Dis Colon Rectum* 1979;22:448.

457. Lapides J. Urologic complications of abdominoperineal surgery. *Contemp Surg* 1974;5:81.

458. Last MD, Fazio VW. The rational use of the purse-string device in constructing anastomoses with the circular stapler. *Dis Colon Rectum* 1985;28:979.

459. Laxamana A, Solomon MJ, Cohen Z, et al. Long-term results of anterior resection using the double-stapling technique. *Dis Colon Rectum* 1995;38:1246.

460. Lazorthes F, Fages P, Chiotasso P, et al. Synchronous abdominotranssphincteric resection of low rectal cancer: new technique for direct colo-anal anastomosis. *Br J Surg* 1986;73:573.

461. Lazorthes F, Fages P, Chiotasso P, et al. Resection of the rectum with construction of a colonic reservoir and colo-anal anastomosis for carcinoma of the rectum. *Br J Surg* 1986;73:136.

462. Leadbetter GW, Leadbetter WF. A new approach to the problem of urinary retention following abdominoperineal resection for carcinoma of the rectum. *Surg Gynecol Obstet* 1958;107:333.

463. Leaming RH, Stearns MW, Deddish MR. Preoperative irradiation in rectal carcinoma. *Radiology* 1961;77:257.

464. Lechner P, Cesnik H. Abdominopelvic omentopexy: preparatory procedure for radiotherapy in rectal cancer. *Dis Colon Rectum* 1992;35:1157.

465. Lee PH, Khauli RB, Baker S, et al. Prognostic and therapeutic observations of manifestations in the genitourinary tract of adenocarcinoma of the colon and rectum. *Surg Gynecol Obstet* 1989;169:511.

466. Leer JWH, Scholten RE, Heslinga T, et al. Role of computed tomography in the diagnosis and radiotherapy planning of recurrent rectal carcinoma. *Diagn Imaging* 1980;49:208.

467. Leff EI, Hoexter B, Labow SB, et al. The EEA stapler in low colorectal anastomoses: initial experience. *Dis Colon Rectum* 1982;25:704.

468. Leff EI, Hoexter B, Labow S, et al. Anastomotic recurrences after low anterior resection: stapled vs. hand-sewn. *Dis Colon Rectum* 1985;28:164.

469. Lelcuk S, Yavez H, Klausner JM, et al. "Spermatocele" following abdominoperineal resection and radiotherapy. *Dis Colon Rectum* 1986;29:355.

470. Leo E, Belli F, Baldini MT, et al. New perspective in the treatment of low rectal cancer: total rectal resection and coloendoanal anastomosis. *Dis Colon Rectum* 1994;37:S62.

471. Lewis WG, Holdsworth PJ, Stephenson BM, et al. Role of the rectum in the physiological and clinical results of coloanal and colorectal anastomosis after anterior resection for rectal carcinoma. *Br J Surg* 1992;79:1082.

472. Lewis WG, Martin IG, Williamson MER, et al. Why do some patients experience poor functional results after anterior resection of the rectum for carcinoma? *Dis Colon Rectum* 1995;38:259.

473. Libertino JA, Rote AR, Zinman L. Ureteral reconstruction in renal transplantation. *Urology* 1978;12:641.

474. Libertino JA, Zinman L. Technique for uretero-neocystotomy in renal transplantation and reflux. *Surg Clin North Am* 1973;53:459.

475. Lindsey I, Cunningham C, George BD, et al. Nocturnal penile tumescence is diminished but not ablated in postproctectomy impotence. *Dis Colon Rectum* 2003;46:14.

476. Lindsey I, George B, Kettlewell M, et al. Randomized, double-blind, placebo-controlled trial of sildenafil (Viagra) for erectile dysfunction after rectal excision for cancer and inflammatory bowel disease. *Dis Colon Rectum* 2002;45:727.

477. Lindsey I, Mortensen NJ McC. Iatrogenic impotence and rectal dissection. *Br J Surg* 2002;89:1493.

478. Lisfranc J. Mémoire sur l'excision de la partie inférieure du rectum devenue carcinomateuse. [Observation on a cancerous condition of the rectum treated by excision.] *Rev Med Franc* 1826;2:380. Translated in *Dis Colon Rectum* 1983;26:694.

479. Littre A. *Mémoire de l'academie des sciences*. 1710;10:36.

480. Lloyd-Davies OV. Lithotomy-Trendelenburg position for resection of rectum and lower pelvic colon. *Lancet* 1939;2:74.

481. Localio SA. Curative surgery of midrectal cancer with preservation of the sphincters. *Surg Ann* 1974;6:213.

482. Localio SA, Baron B. Abdomino-transsacral resection and anastomosis for mid-rectal cancer. *Ann Surg* 1973;178:540.

483. Localio SA, Eng K, Gouge TH, et al. Abdominosacral resection for carcinoma of the mid-rectum: ten years experience. *Ann Surg* 1978;188:475.

484. Localio SA, Stahl WH. Simultaneous abdomino-transsacral resection and anastomosis for mid-rectal cancer. *Am J Surg* 1969;117:282.

485. Lockhart-Mummery HE. Surgery in patients with advanced carcinoma of the colon and rectum. *Dis Colon Rectum* 1959;2:36.

486. Lockhart-Mummery HE, Ritchie JK, Hawley PR. The results of surgical treatment for carcinoma of the rectum at St. Mark's Hospital from 1948 to 1972. *Br J Surg* 1976;63:673.

487. Lockhart-Mummery JP. Two hundred cases of cancer of the rectum treated by perineal excision. *Br J Surg* 1926;14:110.

488. Loeffler RA, Sayegh ES. Perforated acrylic implants in the management of organic impotence. *J Urol* 1960;84:559.

489. Loessin SJ, Meland NB, Devine RM, et al. Management of sacral and perineal defects following abdominoperineal resection and radiation with transpelvic muscle flaps. *Dis Colon Rectum* 1995;38:940.

490. Lofgren EP, Waugh JM, Dockerty MB. Local recurrence of carcinoma after anterior resection of the rectum and the sigmoid: relationship with the length of normal mucosa excised distal to the lesion. *Arch Surg* 1957;74:825.

491. Löhnert MSS, Doniec JM, Henne-Bruns D. Effectiveness of endoluminal sonography in the identification of occult local rectal cancer recurrences. *Dis Colon Rectum* 2000;43:483.

492. Loizou LA, Grigg D, Boulos PB, et al. Endoscopic Nd:YAG laser treatment of rectosigmoid cancer. *Gut* 1990;31:812.

493. Long JW, Mayo CW, Dockerty MB, et al. Recurrent versus new and independent carcinomas of the colon and rectum. *Mayo Clin Proc* 1950;25:169.

494. Lopez MJ, Kraybill WG, Downey RS, et al. Exenterative surgery for locally advanced rectosigmoid cancers: is it worthwhile? *Surgery* 1987;102:644.

495. Lopez-Kostner F, Fazio VW, Vignali A, et al. Locally recurrent cancer predictors and success of salvage surgery. *Dis Colon Rectum* 2001;44:173.

496. Low DE, Kozarek RA, Ball TJ, et al. Colorectal neodymium-YAG photoablative therapy. *Arch Surg* 1989;124:684.

497. Lowy AM, Rich TA, Skibber JM, et al. Preoperative infusional chemoradiation, selective intraoperative radiation, and resection for locally advanced pelvic recurrence of colorectal adenocarcinoma. *Ann Surg* 1996;223:177.

498. Lubbers E-JC. Phantom sensations after excision of the rectum. *Dis Colon Rectum* 1984;27:777.

499. Luchtefeld MA, Milsom JW, Senagore A, et al. Colorectal anastomotic stenosis: results of a survey of the ASCRS membership. *Dis Colon Rectum* 1989;32:733.

500. Luke J. A case of obstruction of the colon relieved by an operation performed at the groin. *Med Chir Trans* 1850;34: 263.

501. Maas CP, Moriya Y, Steup WH, et al. Radical and nerve-preserving surgery for rectal cancer in the Netherlands: a prospective study on morbidity and functional outcome. *Br J Surg* 1998;85:92.

502. MacFarlane JK, Ryall RDH, Heald RJ. Mesorectal excision for rectal cancer. *Lancet* 1993;341:457.

503. Machado M, Hallböök O, Goldman S, et al. Defunctioning stoma in low anterior resection with colonic pouch for rectal cancer: a comparison between two hospitals with a different policy. *Dis Colon Rectum* 2002;45:940.

504. Machado M, Nygren J, Goldman S, et al. Similar outcome after colonic pouch and side-to-end anastomosis in low anterior resection for rectal cancer: a prospective randomized trial. *Ann Surg* 2003;238:214.

505. MacKay SG, Pager CK, Joseph D, et al.. Assessment of the accuracy of transrectal ultrasonography in anorectal neoplasia. *Br J Surg* 2003;90:346.

506. MacKeigan JM, Ferguson JA. Prophylactic oophorectomy and colorectal cancer in premenopausal patients. *Dis Colon Rectum* 1979;22:401.

507. MacLennan G, Stogryn RD, Voitk AJ. Abdominoperineal resection: treatment of choice for carcinoma of the rectum. *Cancer* 1976;38:953.

508. Madden JL, Kandalaft S. Electrocoagulation: a primary and preferred method of treatment for cancer of the rectum. *Ann Surg* 1967;166:413.

509. Madden JL, Kandalaft S. Clinical evaluation of electrocoagulation in the treatment of cancer of the rectum. *Am J Surg* 1971;122:347.

510. Madden JL, Kandalaft SI. Electrocoagulation as a primary curative method in the treatment of carcinoma of the rectum. *Surg Gynecol Obstet* 1983;157:164.

511. Madsen PM, Christiansen J. Distal intramural spread of rectal carcinomas. *Dis Colon Rectum* 1986;29:279.

512. Madura JA, Fiore AC. Reanastomosis of a Hartmann rectal pouch: a simplified procedure. *Am J Surg* 1983;145:279.

513. Maeda K, Hashimoto M, Katai H, et al. Peranal introduction of the stapler in colorectal anastomosis with a double-stapling technique. *Br J Surg* 1994;81:1057.

514. Maetani S, Nishikawa T, Iijima Y, et al. Extensive en bloc resection of regionally recurrent carcinoma of the rectum. *Cancer* 1992;69:2876.

515. Magrini S, Nelson H, Gunderson LL, et al. Sacropelvic resection and intraoperative electron irradiation in the management of recurrent anorectal cancer. *Dis Colon Rectum* 1996;39:1.

516. Mahteme H, Påhlman L, Glimelius B, et al. Prognosis after surgery in patients with incurable rectal cancer: a population-based study. *Br J Surg* 1996;83:1116.

517. Mäkelä JT, Kiviniemi H, Laitinen S. Risk factors for anastomotic leakage after left-sided colorectal resection with rectal anastomosis. *Dis Colon Rectum* 2003;46:653.

518. Malmberg M, Graffner H, Ling L, et al. Recurrence and survival after anterior resection of the rectum using the end to end anastomotic stapler. *Surg Gynecol Obstet* 1986;163:231.

519. Mandava N, Petrelli N, Herrera L, et al. Laser palliation for colorectal carcinoma. *Am J Surg* 1991;162:212.

520. Mann CV. Techniques of local surgical excision for rectal carcinoma. *Br J Surg* 1985;72:57.

521. Mannaerts GHH, Rutten HJT, Martijn H, et al. Comparison of intraoperative radiation therapy-containing multimodality treatment with historical treatment modalities for locally recurrent rectal cancer. *Dis Colon Rectum* 2001;44:1749.

522. Manson PN, Corman ML, Coller JA, et al. Anastomotic recurrence after anterior resection for carcinoma: Lahey clinic experience. *Dis Colon Rectum* 1976;19:219.

523. Manson PN, Corman ML, Coller JA, et al. Anterior resection for adenocarcinoma: Lahey clinic experience from 1963 through 1969. *Am J Surg* 1976;131:434.

524. Mantyh CR, Hull TL, Fazio VW. Coloplasty in low colorectal anastomosis: manometric and functional comparison with straight and colonic J-pouch anastomosis. *Dis Colon Rectum* 2001;44:37.

525. Manz CW, LaTendresse C, Sako Y. The detrimental effects of drains on colonic anastomosis: an experimental study. *Dis Colon Rectum* 1970;13:17.

526. Marijnen CAM, van de Velde CJH. Preoperative radiotherapy for rectal cancer. *Br J Surg* 2001;88:1556.

527. Marks CG, Ritchie JK. The complications of synchronous combined excision for adenocarcinoma of the rectum at St. Mark's Hospital. *Br J Surg* 1975;62:901.

528. Marks G, Mohiuddin M, Borenstein BD. Preoperative radiation therapy and sphincter preservation by the combined abdominotranssacral technique for selected rectal cancers. *Dis Colon Rectum* 1985;28:565.

529. Marks G, Mohiuddin M, Eitan A, et al. High-dose preoperative radiation and radical sphincter-preserving surgery for rectal cancer. *Arch Surg* 1991;126:1534.

530. Marks G, Mohiuddin M, Masoni L, et al. High-dose preoperative radiation and full-thickness local excision: a new option for patients with select cancers of the rectum. *Dis Colon Rectum* 1990;33:735.

531. Marsh PJ, James RD, Schofield PF. Adjuvant preoperative radiotherapy for locally advanced rectal carcinoma: results of a prospective, randomized trial. *Dis Colon Rectum* 1994;37:1205.

532. Marti MC, Fiala JM, Rohner A. EEA stapler in large bowel surgery. *World J Surg* 1981;5:735.

533. Martling A, Holm T, Bremmer S. Prognostic value of preoperative magnetic resonance imaging of the pelvis in rectal cancer. *Br J Surg* 2003;90:1422.

534. Marusch F, Koch A, Schmidt U, et al. Value of a protective stoma in low anterior resections for rectal cancer. *Dis Colon Rectum* 2002;45:1164.

535. Marusch F, Koch A, Schmidt U, et al. Hospital caseload and the results achieved in patients with rectal cancer. *Br J Surg* 2001;88:1397.

536. Mascagni D, Corbellini L, Urciuoli P, et al. Endoluminal ultrasound for early detection of local recurrence of rectal cancer. *Br J Surg* 1989;76:1176.

537. Mason AY. Surgical access to the rectum-a transsphincteric exposure. *Proc R Soc Med* 1970;63:91.

538. Mason AY. The place of local resection in the treatment of rectal carcinoma. *Proc R Soc Med* 1970;63:1259.

539. Mason AY. Trans-sphincteric exposure for low rectal anastomosis. *Proc R Soc Med* 1972;65:974.

540. Masui H, Ike H, Yamaguchi S, et al. Male sexual function after autonomic nerve-preserving operation for rectal cancer. *Dis Colon Rectum* 1996;39:1140.

541. Mathus-Vliegen EMH, Tytgat GNJ. Laser photocoagulation in the palliation of colorectal malignancies. *Cancer* 1986;57:2212.

542. Matthews JM, Kodner IJ, Fry RD, et al. Entrapped ovary syndrome. *Dis Colon Rectum* 1986;29:341.

543. Maunsell HW. A new method of excising the two upper portions of the rectum and the lower segment of the sigmoid flexure of the colon. *Lancet* 1892;2:473.

544. Mavroidis D, Koltun WA. Technique for atraumatic delivery of intestine through the abdominal wall during stoma formation. *Dis Colon Rectum* 1996;39:461.

545. Max E, Sweeney WB, Bailey HR, et al. Results of 1,000 single-layer continuous polypropylene intestinal anastomoses. *Am J Surg* 1991;162:461.

546. Mayo CH. Cancer of the large bowel. *Med Sent* 1904;12:37.

547. Mayo CW, Schlicke CP. Carcinoma of the colon and rectum: a study of metastasis and recurrences. *Surg Gynecol Obstet* 1942;74:83.

548. McCready DR, Ota DM, Rich TA, et al. Prospective phase I trial of conservative management of low rectal lesions. *Arch Surg* 1989;124:67.

549. McDermott FT, Hughes ESR, Pihl E, et al. Local recurrence after potentially curative resection for rectal cancer in a series of 1008 patients. *Br J Surg* 1985;72:34.

550. McGinn FP, Gartell PC, Clifford PC, et al. Staples or sutures for low colorectal anastomoses: a prospective randomized trial. *Br J Surg* 1985;72:603.

551. McGrew EA, Laws JF, Cole WH. Free malignant cells in relation to recurrence of carcinoma of colon. *JAMA* 1954;154:1251.

552. McLachlin AD. Anastomotic leakage below the peritoneal reflection, a study in the dog. *Dis Colon Rectum* 1978;21:400.

553. McLean GK, Cooper GS, Hartz WH, et al. Radiologically guided balloon dilation of gastrointestinal strictures. Part I. Technique and factors influencing procedural success. *Radiology* 1987;165:35.

554. McNamara DA, Fitzpatrick JM, O'Connell PR. Urinary tract involvement by colorectal cancer. *Dis Colon Rectum* 2003;46:1266.

555. McNicholas MMJ, Joyce WP, Dolan J, et al. Magnetic resonance imaging of rectal carcinoma: a prospective study. *Br J Surg* 1994;81:911.

556. Medical Research Council Rectal Cancer Working Party. Randomised trial of surgery alone versus radiotherapy followed by surgery for potentially operable locally advanced rectal cancer. *Lancet* 1996;348:1605.

557. Medich D, McGinty J, Parda D, et al. Preoperative chemoradiotherapy and radical surgery for locally advanced distal rectal adenocarcinoma: pathoogic findings and clinical implications. *Dis Colon Rectum* 2001;44:1123.

558. Melamed MR, Enker WE, Banner P, et al. Flow cytometry of colorectal carcinoma with three-year follow-up. *Dis Colon Rectum* 1986;29:184.

559. Mella O, Dahl O, Horn A, et al. Radiotherapy and resection for apparently inoperable rectal adenocarcinoma. *Dis Colon Rectum* 1984;27:663.

560. Mellgren A, Sirivongs P, Rothenberger DA, et al. Is local excision adequate therapy for early rectal cancer? *Dis Colon Rectum* 2000;43:1064.

561. Mendenhall WM, Bland KI, Copeland EM III, et al. Does preoperative radiation therapy enhance the probability of local control and survival in high-risk distal rectal cancer? *Ann Surg* 1992;215:696.

562. Mendenhall WM, Bland KI, Pfaff WW, et al. Initially unresectable rectal adenocarcinoma treated with preoperative irradiation and surgery. *Ann Surg* 1987;205:41.

563. Mendenhall WM, Million RR, Bland KI, et al. Preoperative radiation therapy for clinically resectable adenocarcinoma of the rectum. *Ann Surg* 1985;202:215.

564. Mentges B, Buess G, Effinger G, et al. Indications and results of local treatment of rectal cancer. *Br J Surg* 1997;84:348.

565. Mentges B, Buess G, Schäfer D, et al. Local therapy of rectal tumors. *Dis Colon Rectum* 1996;39:886.

566. Mercati U, Trancanelli V, Castagnoli GP, et al. Use of the gracilis muscle for sphincteric construction after abdominoperineal resection: technique and preliminary results. *Dis Colon Rectum* 1991;34:1085.

567. Metzger PP. Modified packing technique for control of presacral pelvic bleeding. *Dis Colon Rectum* 1988;31:981.

568. Miles WE. A method of performing abdomino-perineal excision for carcinoma of the rectum and the terminal portion of the pelvic colon. *Lancet* 1908;2:1812.

569. Miles WE. Cancer of the rectum. *Trans Med Soc Lond* 1923;46:127.

570. Mileski WJ, Joehl RJ, Rege RV, et al. Treatment of anastomotic leakage following low anterior colon resection. *Arch Surg* 1988;123:968.

571. Miller AR, Cantor SB, Peoples GE, et al. Quality of life and cost effectiveness analysis of therapy for locally recurrent rectal cancer. *Dis Colon Rectum* 2000;43:1695.

572. Miller AS, Lewis WG, Williamson MER, et al. Factors that influence functional outcome after coloanal anastomosis for carcinoma of the rectum. *Br J Surg* 1995;82:1327.

573. Milsom JW, Czyrko C, Hull TL, et al. Preoperative biopsy of pararectal lymph nodes in rectal cancer using endoluminal ultrasonography. *Dis Colon Rectum* 1994;37:364.

574. Milsom JW, Graffner H. Intrarectal ultrasonography in rectal cancer staging and in the evaluation of pelvic disease. *Ann Surg* 1990;212:602.

575. Milsom JW, Lavery IC, Stolfi VM, et al. The expanding utility of endoluminal ultrasonography in the management of rectal cancer. *Surgery* 1992;112:832.

576. Minichan DP Jr. Enlarging the bowel lumen for the EEA stapler. *Dis Colon Rectum* 1982;25:61.

577. Minsky BD. Preoperative combined modality treatment for rectal cancer. *Oncology* 1994;8:53.

578. Minsky B, Cohen A, Enker W, et al. Preoperative 5-fluorouracil, low-dose leucovorin, and concurrent radiation therapy for rectal cancer. *Cancer* 1994;73:273.

579. Minsky BD, Cohen AM, Enker WE, et al. Sphincter preservation in rectal cancer by local excision and postoperative radiation therapy. *Cancer* 1991;67:908.

580. Minsky BD, Cohen AM, Enker WE, et al. Sphincter preservation with preoperative radiation therapy and coloanal anastomosis. *Int J Radiat Oncol* 1995;31:553.

581. Mirelman D, Corman ML, Veidenheimer MC, et al. Colostomies-indications and contraindications: Lahey clinic experience, 1973–1974. *Dis Colon Rectum* 1978;21:172.

582. Mohiuddin M, Marks G. Patterns of recurrence following high-dose preoperative radiation and sphincter-preserving surgery for cancer of the rectum. *Dis Colon Rectum* 1993;36:117.

583. Molloy RG, Moran KT, Coulter J, et al. Mechanism of sphincter impairment following low anterior resection. *Dis Colon Rectum* 1992;35:462.

584. Moore HG, Gittleman AE, Minsky BD, et al. Rate of pathologic complete response with increased interval between preoperative combined modality therapy and rectal cancer resection. *Dis Colon Rectum* 2004;47:279.

585. Moossa AR, Ree PC, Marks JE, et al. Factors influencing local recurrence after abdominoperineal resection for cancer of the rectum and rectosigmoid. *Br J Surg* 1975;62:727.

586. Moran MR, Rothenberger DA, Gallo RA, et al. Multifactorial analysis of local recurrences in rectal cancer, including DNA ploidy studies: a predictive model. *World J Surg* 1993;17:801.

587. Moran MR, Rothenberger DA, Lahr CJ, et al. Palliation for rectal cancer. Resection? Anastomosis? *Arch Surg* 1987;122:640.

588. Moreira LF, Hizuta A, Iwagaki H, et al. Lateral lymph node dissection for rectal carcinoma below the peritoneal reflection. *Br J Surg* 1994;81:293.

589. Morgan CN. Carcinoma of the rectum. *Ann R Coll Surg Engl* 1965;36:73.

590. Morgan CN, Lloyd-Davies OV. Discussion on conservative resection in carcinoma of the rectum. *Proc R Soc Med* 1950;43:701.

591. Morgenstern L, Yamakawa T, Ben-Shashkan M, et al. Anastomotic leakage after low colonic anastomosis: clinical and experimental aspects. *Am J Surg* 1972;123:104.

592. Mori M, Sugimachi K, Matsuda H, et al. Preoperative hyperthermochemoradiotherapy for patients with rectal cancer. *Dis Colon Rectum* 1989;32:316.

593. Moriya Y, Hojo K, Sawada T, et al. Significance of lateral node dissection for advanced rectal carcinoma at or below the peritoneal reflection. *Dis Colon Rectum* 1989;32:307.

594. Morson BC. Histological criteria for local excision. *Br J Surg* 1985;72:53.

595. Morson BC, Bussey HJ, Samoorian S. Policy of local excision for early cancer of the colorectum. *Gut* 1977;18:1045.

596. Mortensen NJM, Ramirez JM, Takeuchi N, et al. Colonic J pouch-anal anastomosis after rectal excision for carcinoma: functional outcome. *Br J Surg* 1995;82:611.

597. Moseson MD, Salvati EP, Rubin RJ, et al. Technique for placement of distal pursestring. *Dis Colon Rectum* 1982;25:59.

598. Muldoon JP, Capehart RJ. Two scope technique for the transrectal removal of lesions high in the rectum and sigmoid colon. *Surg Gynecol Obstet* 1973;137:1019.

599. Murphy JB. Cholecysto-intestinal, gastro-intestinal, entero-intestinal anastomosis, and approximation without sutures. *Med Rec* 1892;42:665.

600. Murty M, Enker WE, Martz J. Current status of total mesorectal excision and autonomic nerve presentation in rectal cancer. *Semin Surg Oncol* 2000;19:321.

601. Nakahara S, Itoh H, Mibu R, et al. Clinical and manometric evaluation of anorectal function following low anterior

resection with low anastomotic line using an EEATM stapler for rectal cancer. *Dis Colon Rectum* 1988;31:762.

602. Napoleon B, Pujol B, Berger F, et al. Accuracy of endosonography in the staging of rectal cancer treated by radiotherapy. *Br J Surg* 1991;78:785.

603. Nascimbeni R, Burgart LJ, Nivatvongs S, et al. Risk of lymph node metastasis in T1 carcinoma of the colon and rectum. *Dis Colon Rectum* 2002;45:200.

604. Nesbakken A, Nygaard K, Lunde OC. Outcome and late functional results after anastomotic leakage following mesorectal excision for rectal cancer. *Br J Surg* 2001;88: 400.

605. Neufeld DM, Shemesh EI, Kodner IJ, et al. Endoscopic management of anastomotic colon strictures with electrocautery and balloon dilation. *Gastrointest Endosc* 1987;33: 24.

606. Neville R, Fielding LP, Amendola C. Local tumor recurrence after curative resection for rectal cancer: a ten-hospital review. *Dis Colon Rectum* 1987;30:12.

607. Ng IOL, Luk ISC, Yuen ST, et al. Surgical lateral clearance in resected rectal carcinomas: a multivariate analysis of clinicopathologic features. *Cancer* 1993;71:1972.

608. Nicholls RJ, Hall C. Treatment of non-disseminated cancer of the lower rectum. *Br J Surg* 1996;83:15.

609. Nicholls RJ, Lubowski DZ, Donaldson DR. Comparison of colonic reservoir and straight colo-anal reconstruction after rectal excision. *Br J Surg* 1988;75:318.

610. Nichols RL. Postoperative wound infection. *N Engl J Med* 1982;307:1701.

611. Nichols RL, Broido P, Condon RE, et al. Effect of preoperative neomycin-erythromycin intestinal preparation on the incidence of infectious complications following colon surgery. *Ann Surg* 1973;178:453.

612. Nielsen MB, Pedersen JF, Hald J, et al. Recurrent extraluminal rectal carcinoma: transrectal biopsy under sonographic guidance. *AJR Am J Roentgenol* 1992;158:1025.

613. Nissan A, Guillem JG, Paty PB, et al. Abdominoperineal resection for rectal cancer at a specialty center. *Dis Colon Rectum* 2001;44:27.

614. Norgren J, Svensson JO. Anal implantation metastasis from carcinoma of the sigmoid colon and rectum-a risk when performing anterior resection with the EEA stapler? *Br J Surg* 1985;72:602.

615. O'Connell MJ, Martenson JA, Wieand HS, et al. Improving adjuvant therapy for rectal cancer by combining protracted-infusion fluorouracil with radiation therapy after curative surgery. *N Engl J Med* 1994;331:502.

616. O'Connor JJ. Endoscopic palliative management of rectal cancer. *South Med J* 1991;84:472.

617. Odou MW, O'Connell TX. Changes in the treatment of rectal carcinoma and effects on local recurrence. *Arch Surg* 1986;121:1114.

618. Ogunbiyi OA, McKenna K, Birnbaum EH, et al. Aggressive surgical management of recurrent rectal cancer: is it worthwhile? *Dis Colon Rectum* 1997;40:150.

619. Ohhigashi S, Nishio T, Watanabe F, et al. Experience with radiofrequency ablation in the treatment of pelvic recurrence in rectal cancer: report of two cases. *Dis Colon Rectum* 2001;44:741.

620. Ohno S, Tomoda M, Tomisaki S, et al. Improved surgical results after combining preoperative hyperthermia with chemotherapy and radiotherapy for patients with carcinoma of the rectum. *Dis Colon Rectum* 1997;40:401.

621. Ondrula DP, Nelson RL, Prasad ML, et al. Multifactorial index of preoperative risk factors in colon resections. *Dis Colon Rectum* 1992;35:117.

622. Ono C, Yoshinaga K, Enomoto M, et al. Discontinuous rectal cancer spread in the mesorectum and the optimal distal clearance margin *in situ*. *Dis Colon Rectum* 2002; 45:744.

623. Ooi BS, Tjandra JJ, Green MD. Morbidities of adjuvant chemotherapy and radiotherapy for resectable rectal cancer: an overview. *Dis Colon Rectum* 1999;42:403.

624. O'Riordain MG, Molloy RG, Gillen P, et al. Rectoanal inhibitory reflex following low stapled anterior resection of the rectum. *Dis Colon Rectum* 1992;35:874.

625. Orkin BA, Dozois RR, Beart RW Jr, et al. Extended resection for locally advanced primary adenocarcinoma of the rectum. *Dis Colon Rectum* 1989;32:286.

626. Orrom WJ, Wong WD, Rothenberger DA, et al. Endorectal ultrasound in the preoperative staging of rectal tumors. *Dis Colon Rectum* 1990;33:654.

627. Ovnat A, Peiser J, Avinoah E, et al. A new approach to rectal anastomotic stricture. *Dis Colon Rectum* 1989;32:351.

628. Oz MC, Forde KA. Endoscopic alternatives in the management of colonic strictures. *Surgery* 1990;108:513.

629. Pacini P, Cionini L, Pirtoli L, et al. Symptomatic recurrences of carcinoma of the rectum and sigmoid: the influence of radiotherapy on the quality of life. *Dis Colon Rectum* 1986;29:865.

630. Paes TRF, Marsh GDJ, Morecroft JA, et al. Alum solution in the control of intractable haemorrhage from advanced rectal carcinoma. *Br J Surg* 1986;73:192.

631. Pagni S, McLaughlin CM. Simple technique for the treatment of strictured colorectal anastomosis. *Dis Colon Rectum* 1995;38:433.

632. Pahlman L, Enblad P, Stahle E. Abdominal vs. perineal drainage in rectal surgery. *Dis Colon Rectum* 1987;30:372.

633. Påhlman L, Glimelius B. Pre- or postoperative therapy in rectal and rectosigmoid carcinoma: report from a randomized multicenter trial. *Ann Surg* 1990;211:187.

634. Påhlman L, Glimelius B, Frykholm G. Ischaemic strictures in patients treated with a low anterior resection and perioperative radiotherapy for rectal carcinoma. *Br J Surg* 1989;76:605.

635. Påhlman L, Glimelius B, Graffman S. Pre- versus postoperative radiotherapy in rectal carcinoma: an interim report from a randomized multicentre trial. *Br J Surg* 1985;72: 961.

636. Palumbo LT, Sharpe WS. Anterior versus abdominoperineal resection: resection for rectal and rectosigmoid carcinoma. *Am J Surg* 1968;115:657.

637. Pannett CA. Resection of the rectum with restoration of continuity. *Lancet* 1935;2:423.

638. Papa MZ, Koller M, Klein E, et al. Prostatic cancer presenting as a rectal mass: a surgical pitfall. *Br J Surg* 1997;84:69.

639. Papillon J. Endocavitary irradiation of early rectal cancers for cure: a series of 123 cases. *Proc R Soc Med* 1973;66: 1179.

640. Papillon J. Endocavitary irradiation in the curative treatment of early cancers. *Dis Colon Rectum* 1974;17:172.

641. Papillon J. Intracavitary irradiation of early rectal cancer for cure: a series of 186 cases. *Cancer* 1975;36:696.

642. Papillon J. New prospects in the conservative treatment of rectal cancer. *Dis Colon Rectum* 1984;27:695.

643. Papillon J. The future of external beam irradiation as initial treatment of rectal cancer. *Br J Surg* 1987;74:449.

644. Parc R, Tiret E, Frileux P, et al. Resection and colo-anal anastomosis with colonic reservoir for rectal carcinoma. *Br J Surg* 1986;73:139.

645. Parks AG. Transanal technique in low rectal anastomosis. *Proc R Soc Med* 1972;65:975.

646. Parks AG. Per-anal anastomosis. *World J Surg* 1982;6:531.

647. Patt YZ, Peters RE, Chuang VP, et al. Palliation of pelvic recurrence of colorectal cancer with intra-arterial 5-fluorouracil and mitomycin. *Cancer* 1985;56:2175.

648. Paty PB, Enker WE, Cohen AM, et al. Treatment of rectal cancer by low anterior resection with coloanal anastomosis. *Ann Surg* 1994;219:365.

649. Paty PB, Enker WE, Cohen AM, et al. Long-term functional results of coloanal anastomosis for rectal cancer. *Am J Surg* 1994;167:90.

650. Paty PB, Nash GM, Baron P, et al. Long-term results of local excision for rectal cancer. *Ann Surg* 2002;236:522.

651. Pearlman NW, Donohue RE, Steigmann GV, et al. Pelvic and sacropelvic exenteration for locally advanced or recurrent anorectal cancer. *Arch Surg* 1987;122:537.

652. Pearlman NW, Stiegmann GV, Donohue RE. Extended resection of fixed rectal cancer. *Cancer* 1989;63:2438.

653. Pearman RO. Treatment of organic impotence by implantation of a penile prosthesis. *J Urol* 1967;97:716.

654. Pearman RO. Insertion of a Silastic penile prosthesis for the treatment of organic sexual impotence. *J Urol* 1972; 107:802.

655. Pedersen IK, Hint K, Olsen J, et al. Anorectal function after low anterior resection for carcinoma. *Ann Surg* 1986;204: 133.

656. Pélissier EP, Blum D, Bachour A, et al. Functional results of coloanal anastomosis with reservoir. *Dis Colon Rectum* 1992;35:843.

657. Pezim ME, Nicholls RJ. Survival after high or low ligation of the inferior mesenteric artery during curative surgery for rectal cancer. *Ann Surg* 1984;200:729.

658. Phillips PS, Farquharson SM, Sexton R, et al. Rectal cancer in the elderly: patients' perception of bowel control after restorative surgery. *Dis Colon Rectum* 2004;47:287.

659. Phillips RKS, Hittinger R, Blesovsky L, et al. Local recurrence following "curative" surgery for large bowel cancer. II. The rectum and rectosigmoid. *Br J Surg* 1984;71:17.

660. Politano VA, Leadbetter WF. An operative technique for the correction of vesicoureteral reflux. *J Urol* 1958;79:932.

661. Pollard CW, Nivatvongs S, Rojanasakul A, et al. Carcinoma of the rectum: profiles of intraoperative and early portoperative complications. *Dis Colon Rectum* 1994;37: 866.

662. Pollett WG, Nicholls RJ. The relationship between the extent of distal clearance and survival and local recurrence rates after curative anterior resection for carcinoma of the rectum. *Ann Surg* 1983;198:159.

663. Porter NH, Nicholls RJ. Pre-operative radiotherapy in operable rectal cancer: interim report of a trial carried out by the Rectal Cancer Group. *Br J Surg* 1985;72:62.

664. Qinyao W, Weijin S, Youren Z, et al. New concepts in severe presacral hemorrhage during proctectomy. *Arch Surg* 1985; 120:1013.

665. Quirke P, Dixon MF, Durdey P, et al. Local recurrence of rectal adenocarcinoma due to inadequate surgical resection: histopathological study of lateral tumour spread and surgical excision. *Lancet* 1986;2:996.

666. Radice E, Nelson H, Mercill S, et al. Primary myocutaneous flap closure following resection of locally advanced pelvic malignancies. *Br J Surg* 1999;86:349.

667. Ramanujam P, Prasad ML, Abcarian H. Modification of rectal pursestring suture for end-to-end anastomotic stapler use. *Surg Gynecol Obstet* 1983;157:79.

668. Ramirez JM, Mortensen NJM, Takeuchi N, et al. Colonic J-pouch rectal reconstruction is it really a neorectum? *Dis Colon Rectum* 1996;39:1286.

669. Ramirez OM, Hernandez-Pombo J, Marupudi SR. New technique for anastomosis of the intestine after the Hartmann's procedure with the end-to-end anastomosis stapler. *Surg Gynecol Obstet* 1983;156:367.

670. Ramsey WH. Treatment of inoperable cancer of the rectum by fulguration. *Dis Colon Rectum* 1963;6:114.

671. Rankin FW, Graham AS. *Cancer of the colon and rectum.* Springfield, IL: Charles C Thomas, 1939.

672. Ravitch MM. Varieties of stapled anastomoses in rectal resection. *Surg Clin North Am* 1984;64:543.

673. Ravitch MM. Intersecting staple lines in intestinal anastomoses. *Surgery* 1985;97:8.

674. Ravo B, Ger R. Temporary colostomy-an outmoded procedure? A report on the intracolonic bypass. *Dis Colon Rectum* 1985;28:904.

675. Ravo B, Ger R. A modified technique for perineal colorectal, coloanal or ileoanal anastomosis with the EEA stapler. *Surg Gynecol Obstet* 1987;164:83.

676. Read TE, Myerson RJ, Fleshman JW, et al. Surgeon specialty is associated with outcome in rectal cancer treatment. *Dis Colon Rectum* 2002;45:904.

677. Reed WP, Garb JL, Park WC, et al. Long-term results and complications of preoperative radiation in the treatment of rectal cancer. *Surgery* 1988;103:161.

678. Reilly WT, Nelson H, Schroeder G, et al. Wound recurrence following conventional treatment of colorectal cancer: a rare but perhaps underestimated problem. *Dis Colon Rectum* 1996;39:200.

679. ReMine SG, Dozois RR. Hartmann's procedure: its use with complicated carcinomas of sigmoid colon and rectum. *Arch Surg* 1981;116:630.

680. Renner K, Rosen HR, Novi G, et al. Quality of life after surgery for rectal cancer: do we still need a permanent colostomy? *Dis Colon Rectum* 1999;42:1160.

681. Reybard JF. Mémoire sur une tumeur cancéreuse affectant l'iliaque du colon; ablation de la tumeur et de l'intestin: réunion directe et immédiate des deux bouts de cet organe. *Bull Acad Med Paris* 1843–44;9:1031.

682. Reynolds JV, Joyce WP, Dolan J, et al. Pathological evidence in support of total mesorectal excision in the management of rectal cancer. *Br J Surg* 1996;83:1112.

683. Rich TA. Infusional chemoradiation for operable rectal cancer: post-, pre-, or nonoperative management? *Oncology* 1997;11:295.

684. Rifkin MD, Marks GJ. Transrectal US as an adjunct in the diagnosis of rectal and extrarectal tumors. *Radiology* 1985; 157:499.

685. Rinnert-Gongora S, Tartter PI. Multivariate analysis of recurrence after anterior resection for colorectal carcinoma. *Am J Surg* 1989;157:573.

686. Roberson SH, Heron HC, Kerman HD, et al. Is anterior resection of the rectosigmoid safe after preoperative radiation? *Dis Colon Rectum* 1985;28:254.

687. Rodriguez L, Payne CK. Management of urinary fistulas. In: Taneja SS, Smith RB, Ehrlich RM. *Complications of urologic surgery,* 3rd ed. Philadelphia: WB Saunders, 2001: 186.

688. Rodriguez-Bigas MA, Herrera L, Petrelli NJ. Surgery for recurrent rectal adenocarcinoma in the presence of hydronephrosis. *Am J Surg* 1992;164:18.

689. Romano G, de Rosa P, Vallone G, et al. Intrarectal ultrasound and computed tomography in the pre- and postoperative assessment of patients with rectal cancer. *Br J Surg* 1985;72:117.

690. Romano G, Esercizio L, Santangelo M, et al. Impact of computed tomography vs. intrarectal ultrasound on the prognosis of locally recurrent rectal cancer. *Dis Colon Rectum* 1993;36:261.

691. Romano G, La Torre F, Cutini G, et al. Total anorectal reconstruction with the artificial bowel sphincter: report of eight cases. A quality-of-life assessment. *Dis Colon Rectum* 2003;46:730.

692. Rominger CJ, Gelber RD, Gunderson LL, et al. Radiation therapy alone or in combination with chemotherapy in the treatment of residual or inoperable carcinoma of the rectum and rectosigmoid or pelvic recurrence following colorectal surgery. *Am J Clin Oncol* 1985;8:118.

693. Romsdahl M, Withers H. Radiotherapy combined with curative surgery: its use as therapy for carcinoma of the sigmoid colon and rectum. *Arch Surg* 1978;113:446.

694. Rosati C, Smith L, Deitel M, et al. Primary colorectal anastomosis with the intracolonic bypass tube. *Surgery* 1992; 112:618.

695. Rosen CB, Beart RW Jr, Ilstrup DM. Local recurrence of rectal carcinoma after hand-sewn and stapled anastomoses. *Dis Colon Rectum* 1985;28:305.

696. Rosen L, Khubchandani IT, Sheets JA, et al. Clinical and manometric evaluation of continence after the Bacon two-stage pull-through procedure. *Dis Colon Rectum* 1985;28: 232.

697. Rosen L, Veidenheimer MC, Coller JA, et al. Mortality, morbidity, and patterns of recurrence after abdominoperineal resection for cancer of the rectum. *Dis Colon Rectum* 1982; 25:202.

698. Rosenberg SA. Combined-modality therapy of cancer: what is it and when does it work? *N Engl J Med* 1985; 312:1512.

699. Rosenthal II, Turell R. Surgical diathermy (electrothermia) of cancer of the rectum. *JAMA* 1958;167:1602.

700. Rosenthal SA, Trock BJ, Coia LR. Randomized trial of adjuvant radiation therapy for rectal carcinoma: a review. *Dis Colon Rectum* 1990;33:335.

701. Rosi PA, Cahill WJ, Carey J. A ten year study of hemicolectomy in the treatment of carcinoma of the left half of the colon. *Surg Gynecol Obstet* 1962;114:15.

702. Roswit B, Higgins G, Keehn R. Preoperative irradiation for carcinoma of the rectum and rectosigmoid colon: report of a National Veterans Administration randomized study. *Cancer* 1975;35:1597.

703. Rouanet P, Saint Aubert B, Fabre JM, et al. Conservative treatment for low rectal carcinoma by local excision with or without radiotherapy. *Br J Surg* 1993;80:1452.

704. Roubein LD, David C, DuBrow R, et al. Endoscopic ultrasonography in staging rectal cancer. *Am J Gastroenterol* 1990;85:1391.

705. Rudd WWH. The transanal anastomosis: a sphincter-saving operation with improved continence. *Dis Colon Rectum* 1979;22:102.

706. Rullier E, Laurent C, Garrelon JL, et al. Risk factors for anastomotic leakage after resection of rectal cancer. *Br J Surg* 1998;85:355.

707. Rullier E, Zerbib F, Laurent C, et al. Intersphincteric resection with excision of internal anal sphincter for conservative treatment of very low rectal cancer. *Dis Colon Rectum* 1999, 42:1168.

708. Rupp KD, Dohmoto M, Meffert R, et al. Cancer of the rectum palliative endoscopic treatment. *Eur J Surg Oncol* 1995;21:644.

709. Sackier JM, Wood CB. Low anterior resection and the intraluminal bypass tube. *Br J Surg* 1988;75:1232.

710. Saclarides TJ, Bhattacharyya AK, Britton-Kuzel C, et al. Predicting lymph node metastases in rectal cancer. *Dis Colon Rectum* 1994;37:52.

711. Saclarides TJ, Speziale NJ, Drab E, et al. Tumor angiogenesis and rectal carcinoma. *Dis Colon Rectum* 1994;37:921.

712. Sadahiro S, Suzuki T, Ishikawa K, et al. Intraoperative radiation therapy for curatively resected rectal cancer. *Dis Colon Rectum* 2001;44:1689.

713. Sagar PM, Couse N, Kerin M, et al. Randomized trial of drainage of colorectal anastomosis. *Br J Surg* 1993;80:769.

714. Sagar PM, Hartley MN, Macfie J, et al. Randomized trial of pelvic drainage after rectal resection. *Dis Colon Rectum* 1995;38:254.

715. Sagar PM, Pemberton JH. Surgical management of locally recurrent rectal cancer. *Br J Surg* 1996;83:293.

716. Saha SK. A critical evaluation of dissection of the perineum in synchronous combined abdominoperineal excision of the rectum. *Surg Gynecol Obstet* 1984;158:33.

717. Sailer M, Fuches K-H, Fein M, et al. Randomized clinical trial comparing quality of life after straight and pouch coloanal reconstruction. *Br J Surg* 2002;89:1108.

718. Saitoh N, Okui K, Sarashina H, et al. Evaluation of echographic diagnosis of rectal cancer using intra-rectal ultrasonic examination. *Dis Colon Rectum* 1986;29:234.

719. Salinas JC, Quintana J, De Gregorio MA, et al. Management of benign rectal stricture by implantation of a self-expanding prosthesis. *Br J Surg* 1997;84:674.

720. Salvati EP, Rubin RJ. Electrocoagulation as primary therapy for rectal carcinoma. *Am J Surg* 1976;132:583.

721. Salvati EP, Rubin RJ, Eisenstat TE, et al. Electrocoagulation of selected carcinoma of the rectum. *Surg Gynecol Obstet* 1988;166:393.

722. Sandusky WR. Use of prophylactic antibiotics in surgical patients. *Surg Clin North Am* 1980;60:83.

723. Santoro E, Tirelli C, Scutari F, et al. Continent perineal colostomy by transposition of gracilis muscles: technical

724. Sarr MG, Stewart JR, Cameron JC. Combined abdominoperineal approach to repair of postoperative hernia. *Dis Colon Rectum* 1982;25:597.

725. Sato T, Konishi F, Kanazawa K. Anal sphincter reconstruction with a pudendal nerve anastomosis following abdominoperineal resection: report of a case. *Dis Colon Rectum* 1997;40:1497.

726. Sato T, Konishi F, Kanazawa K. Functional perineal colostomy with pudendal nerve anastomosis following anorectal resection: a cadaver operation study on a new procedure. *Surgery* 1997;121:569.

727. Sauven P, Playforth MJ, Evans M, et al. Early infective complications and late recurrent cancer in stapled anastomoses. *Dis Colon Rectum* 1989;32:33.

728. Sayfan J, Averbuch F, Koltun L, et al. Effect of rectal stump washout on the presence of free malignant cells in the rectum during anterior resection for rectal cancer. *Dis Colon Rectum* 2000;43:1710.

729. Schaeffer CJ, Giordano JM. Complications associated with EEA stapler in performance of low anterior resections. *Am Surg* 1981;47:426.

730. Schaldenbrand JD, Siders DB, Zainea GG, et al. Preoperative radiation therapy for locally advanced carcinoma of the rectum: clinicopathologic correlative review. *Dis Colon Rectum* 1992;35:16.

731. Schell SR, Zlotecki RA, Mendenhall WM, et al. Transanal excision of locally advanced rectal cancers downstaged using neoadjuvant chemoradiotherapy. *J Am Coll Surg* 2002;194:584.

732. Schlag P, Lehner B, Strauss LG, et al. Scar or recurrent rectal cancer: positron emission tomography is more helpful for diagnosis than immunoscintigraphy. *Arch Surg* 1989; 124:197.

733. Schlegel RD, Dehni N, Parc R, et al. Results of reoperations in colorectal anastomotic strictures. *Dis Colon Rectum* 2001;44:1464.

734. Schrag D, Panageas KS, Riedel E, et al. Surgeon volume compared to hospital volume as a predictor of outcome following primary colon cancer resection. *J Surg Oncol* 2003;83:68.

735. Schrock TR, Deveney CW, Dunphy JE. Factors contributing to leakage of colonic anastomoses. *Ann Surg* 1973;177: 513.

736. Schultz PE, Muldoon JP. A transrectal approach to the high-lying lesion in the rectosigmoid. *Dis Colon Rectum* 1969;12:417.

737. Schulze S, Lyng K-M. Palliation of rectosigmoid neoplasms with Nd:YAG laser treatment. *Dis Colon Rectum* 1994; 37:882.

738. Schwenk W, Böhm B, Junghans T, et al. Intermittent sequential compression of the lower limb prevents venous stasis in laparoscopic and conventional colorectal surgery. *Dis Colon Rectum* 1997;40:1056.

739. Scott H, Brown AC. Is routine drainage of pelvic anastomosis necessary? *Am Surg* 1996;62:452.

740. Scott JR, Daneker G, Lumsden AB. Prevention of compartment syndrome associated with the dorsal lithotomy position. *Am Surg* 1997;63:801.

741. Scotté M, Téniére P, Planet M, et al. Eversion of the rectum: a simplified technical approach to ileoanal anastomosis. *Dis Colon Rectum* 1995;38:96.

742. Segall MM, Nivatvongs S, Balcos E, et al. Abdominoperineal resection for recurrent cancer following anterior resection. *Dis Colon Rectum* 1981;24:80.

743. Sehapayak S, McNatt M, Carter HG, et al. Continuous sump-suction drainage of the pelvis after low anterior resection: a reappraisal. *Dis Colon Rectum* 1973;16:485.

744. Senagore A, Milsom JW, Walshaw RK, et al. Does a proximal colostomy affect colorectal anastomotic healing? *Dis Colon Rectum* 1992;35:182.

remarks and results in 14 cases. *Dis Colon Rectum* 1994; 37:S73.

745. Sener SF, Imperato JP, Blum MD, et al. Technique and complications of reconstruction of the pelvic floor with polyglactin mesh. *Surg Gynecol Obstet* 1989;168:475.

746. Sengupta S, Tjandra JJ. Local excision of rectal cancer: what is the evidence? *Dis Colon Rectum* 2001;44:1345.

747. Sentovich SM, Blatchford GJ, Falk PM, et al. Transrectal ultrasound of rectal tumors. *Am J Surg* 1993;166:638.

748. Seow-Choen F. Colonic pouches in the treatment of low rectal cancer. *Br J Surg* 1996;83:881.

749. Shami VM, Parmar KS, Waxman I. Clinical impact of endoscopic ultrasound and endoscopic ultrasound-guided fine-needle aspiration in the management of rectal carcinoma. *Dis Colon Rectum* 2004;47:59.

750. Shank B, Dershaw DD, Caravelli J, et al. A prospective study of the accuracy of preoperative computed tomographic staging of patients with biopsy-proven rectal carcinoma. *Dis Colon Rectum* 1990;33:285.

751. Shaw RS, Green TH. Massive mesenteric infarction following inferior mesenteric-artery ligation in resection of the colon for carcinoma. *N Engl J Med* 1953;248:890.

752. Shehata WM, Meyer RL, Jazy FK, et al. Total abdominopelvic irradiation and a boost for cancer of the colon: a pilot study. *Appl Radiol* 1989;March:26.

753. Shimada S, Matsuda M, Uno K, et al. A new device for the treatment of coloproctostomic stricture after double stapling anastomoses. *Ann Surg* 1996;224:603.

754. Shirouzu K, Isomoto H, Kakegawa T. Prognostic evaluation of perineural invasion in rectal cancer. *Am J Surg* 1993;165:233.

755. Shirouzu K, Isomoto H, Kakegawa T. Total pelvic exenteration for locally advanced colorectal carcinoma. *Br J Surg* 1996;83:32.

756. Shlasko E, Gorfine SR, Gelernt IM. Using lidocaine to ease the insertion of the circular stapler. *Surg Gynecol Obstet* 1992;174:70.

757. Shoup M, Guillem JG, Alektiar KM, et al. Predictors of survival in recurrent rectal cancer after resection and intraoperative radiotherapy. *Dis Colon Rectum* 2002;45:585.

758. Simchen E, Shapiro M, Sacks TG, et al. Determinants of wound infection after colon surgery. *Ann Surg* 1984;199:260.

759. Sischy B. Intraoperative electron beam radiation therapy with particular reference to the treatment of rectal carcinomas-primary and recurrent. *Dis Colon Rectum* 1986;29:714.

760. Sischy B. The role of radiation therapy in the management of carcinoma of the rectum. *Contemp Surg* 1987;30:13.

761. Sischy B, Graney MJ, Hinson EJ, et al. Preoperative radiation therapy with sensitizers in the management of carcinoma of the rectum. *Dis Colon Rectum* 1985;28:56.

762. Sischy B, Remington JH. Treatment of carcinoma of the rectum by intracavitary irradiation. *Surg Gynecol Obstet* 1975;141:562.

763. Sischy B, Remington JH, Sobel SH. Treatment of rectal carcinomas by means of endocavity irradiation. *Cancer* 1978;42:1073.

764. Sischy B, Remington JH, Sobel SH, et al. Treatment of carcinoma of the rectum and squamous carcinoma of the anus by combination chemotherapy, radiotherapy and operation. *Surg Gynecol Obstet* 1980;151:369.

765. Sjödahl R, Nyström P-O, Olaison G. Surgical treatment of dorsocaudal dislocation of the vagina after excision of the rectum: the Kylberg operation. *Dis Colon Rectum* 1990;33:762.

766. Slanetz CA Jr, Herter FP, Grinnell RS. Anterior resection versus abdominoperineal resection for cancer of the rectum and rectosigmoid: an analysis of 524 cases. *Am J Surg* 1972;123:110.

767. Slutzki S, Bogokowsky H, Negri M, et al. The everted rectal stump technique for the application of the distal pursestring suture in the construction of stapled anastomoses. *Surg Gynecol Obstet* 1985;161:287.

768. Smedh K, Olsson L, Johansson H, et al. Reduction of postoperative morbidity and mortality in patients with rectal cancer following the introduction of a colorectal unit. *Br J Surg* 2001;88:273.

769. Smith DE, Muff NS, Shetabi H. Combined preoperative neoadjuvant radiotherapy and chemotherapy for anal and rectal cancer. *Am J Surg* 1986;151:577.

770. Smith LE, Ko ST, Saclarides T, et al. Transanal endoscopic microsurgery: initial registry results. *Dis Colon Rectum* 1996;39:S79.

771. Snook CW. An alternate technique to apply a low rectal purse-string when using the EEA stapler for low pelvic anastomosis. *Dis Colon Rectum* 1986;29:69.

772. Snyder CL, Kauffman DB. A simple technique for assessing the viability of stomas of the intestines. *Surg Gynecol Obstet* 1991;172:399.

773. So JB, Palmer MT, Shellito PC. Postoperative perineal hernia. *Dis Colon Rectum* 1997;40:954.

774. Sofo Luigi, Ratto C, Doglietto GB, et al. Intraoperative radiation therapy in integrated treatment of rectal cancers: results of phase II study. *Dis Colon Rectum* 1996;39:1396.

775. Solomon MJ, McLeod RS, Cohen EK, et al. Reliability and validity studies of endoluminal ultrasonography for anorectal disorders. *Dis Colon Rectum* 1994;37:546.

776. Sørensen LT, Jørgensen T, Kirkeby LT, et al. Smoking and alcohol abuse are major risk factors for anastomotic leakage in colorectal surgery. *Br J Surg* 1999;86:927.

777. Southwick HW, Harridge WH, Cole WH. Recurrence at the suture line following resection for carcinoma of the colon: incidence following preventive measures. *Am J Surg* 1962;103:86.

778. Stearns MW Jr. Preoperative radiation in carcinoma of the rectum. *Proc Natl Cancer Conf* 1964;5:489.

779. Stearns MW Jr. Surgical management of colo-rectal cancer. *Proc Natl Cancer Conf* 1973;7:481.

780. Stearns MW Jr. The choice among anterior resection, the pull-through, and abdominoperineal resection of the rectum. *Cancer* 1974;34:969.

781. Stearns MW Jr. Carcinoma of the rectum: results of abdominoperineal resection (symposium). *Dis Colon Rectum* 1974;17:586.

782. Stearns MW Jr. Diagnosis and management of recurrent pelvic malignancy following combined abdominoperineal resection. *Dis Colon Rectum* 1980;23:359.

783. Stearns MW Jr, Bert JW, Deddish MR. Preoperative irradiation of cancer of the rectum. *Dis Colon Rectum* 1961;4:403.

784. Stearns MW Jr, Deddish MR, Quan SHQ. Preoperative roentgen therapy for cancer of the rectum. *Surg Gynecol Obstet* 1959;109:225.

785. Stearns MW Jr, Deddish MR, Quan SHQ, et al. Preoperative roentgen therapy for cancer of the rectum and rectosigmoid. *Surg Gynecol Obstet* 1974;138:584.

786. Stearns MW Jr, Sternberg SS, DeCosse JJ. Treatment alternatives: localized rectal cancer. *Cancer* 1984;54:2691.

787. Stearns MW Jr, Whiteley HW Jr, Leaming RH, et al. Palliative radiation therapy in patients with localized cancer of the colon and rectum. *Dis Colon Rectum* 1970;13:112.

788. Stein DE, Mahmoud NN, Anné PR, et al. Longer time interval between completion of neoadjuvant chemoradiation and surgical resection does not improve downstaging of rectal carcinoma, *Dis Colon Rectum* 2003;46:448.

789. Steinhagen RM, Weakley FL. Anastomosis to the rectum: operative experience. *Dis Colon Rectum* 1985;28:105.

790. Stelzner M. Palliative therapy of rectal cancer: summary statement. *J Gastrointest Surg* 2004;8:253.

791. Stipa S, Chiavellati L, Nicolanti V, et al. Microscopic endoluminal tumorectomy. *Dis Colon Rectum* 1994;37:S81.

792. Stolfi VM, Milsom JW, Lavery IC, et al. Newly designed occluder pin for presacral hemorrhage. *Dis Colon Rectum* 1992;35:166.

793. Stone HH, Hooper CA, Kolb LD, et al. Antibiotic prophylaxis in gastric, biliary and colonic surgery. *Ann Surg* 1976;184:443.

794. Stone JM, Bloom RJ. Transendoscopic balloon dilatation of complete colonic obstruction: an adjunct in the treat-

ment of colorectal cancer: report of three cases. *Dis Colon Rectum* 1989;32:429.

795. Strauss AA. *Immunologic resistance to carcinoma produced by electrocoagulation: based on fifty-seven years of experimental and clinical results.* Springfield, IL: Charles C Thomas, 1969.

796. Strauss AA, Appel M, Saphir O, et al. Immunologic resistance to carcinoma produced by electrocoagulation. *Surg Gynecol Obstet* 1965;121:989.

797. Strauss AA, Strauss SF, Crawford RA, et al. Surgical diathermy of carcinoma of rectum: its clinical end results. *JAMA* 1935;104:1480.

798. Strauss AA, Strauss SF, Strauss HA. New method and end results in treatment of carcinoma of stomach and rectum by surgical diathermy (electrical coagulation). *South Surg* 1936;5:348.

799. Strauss LG, Clorius JH, Schlag P, et al. Recurrence of colorectal tumor: PET evaluation. *Radiology* 1989;170:329.

800. Strauss RJ, Friedman M, Platt N, et al. Surgical treatment of rectal carcinoma: results of anterior resection vs abdominoperineal resection at a community hospital. *Dis Colon Rectum* 1978;21:269.

801. Sugarbaker PH. Partial sacrectomy for en bloc excision of rectal cancer with posterior fixation. *Dis Colon Rectum* 1982;25:708.

802. Sugarbaker PH. Intrapelvic prosthesis to prevent injury of the small intestine with high dosage pelvic irradiation. *Surg Gynecol Obstet* 1983;157:269.

803. Sugarbaker PH. Rectovaginal fistula following low circular stapled anastomosis in women with rectal cancer. *J Surg Oncol* 1996;61:155.

804. Surtees P, Ritchie JK, Phillips RKS. High versus low ligation of the inferior mesenteric artery in rectal cancer. *Br J Surg* 1990;77:618.

805. Suzuki K, Dozois RR, Devine RM, et al. Curative reoperations for locally recurrent rectal cancer. *Dis Colon Rectum* 1996;39:730.

806. Swedish Rectal Cancer Trial. Initial report from a Swedish multicentre study examining the role of preoperative irradiation in the treatment of patients with resectable rectal carcinoma. *Br J Surg* 1993;80:1333.

807. Swedish Rectal Cancer Trial. Local recurrence rate in a randomised multicentre trial of preoperative radiotherapy compared with operation alone in resectable rectal carcinoma. *Eur J Surg* 1996;162:397.

808. Swedish Rectal Cancer Trial. Improved survival with preoperative radiotherapy in resectable rectal cancer. *N Engl J Med* 1997;336:980.

809. Sweeney JL, Ritchie JK, Hawley PR. Resection and sutured peranal anastomosis for carcinoma of the rectum. *Dis Colon Rectum* 1989;32:103.

810. Sweeney WB. Local excision of rectal tumors: specimen orientation. *Dis Colon Rectum* 1992;35:204.

811. Sweeney WB, Deshmukh N. Modified Kraske approach for disease of the mid-rectum. *Am J Gastroenterol* 1991;86:75.

812. Takahashi T, Ueno M, Azekura K, et al. Lateral ligament: its anatomy and clinical importance. *Semin Surg Oncol* 2000;19:386.

813. Tanaka S, Yokota T, Saito D, et al. Clinicopathologic features of early rectal carcinoma and indications for endoscopic treatment. *Dis Colon Rectum* 1995;38:959.

814. Tang R, Wang J-Y, Chen J-S, et al. Postoperative adjuvant radiotherapy in Astler-Coller stages B2 and C rectal cancer. *Dis Colon Rectum* 1992;35:1057.

815. Tartter PI. Blood transfusion and infectious complications following colorectal cancer surgery. *Br J Surg* 1989; 75:789.

816. Tartter PI, Quintero S, Barron DM. Perioperative blood transfusion associated with infectious complications after colorectal cancer operations. *Am J Surg* 1986;152:479.

817. Task Force. American Society of Colon and Rectal Surgeons. Practice parameters for the treatment of rectal carcinoma. *Dis Colon Rectum* 1993;36:989.

818. Tchervenkov CI, Gordon PH. Simple techniques of enlarging the diameter of the bowel lumen for the performance of end-to-end anastomoses using the EEA stapler. *Dis Colon Rectum* 1984;27:630.

819. Temple WJ, Ketcham AS. Surgical palliation for recurrent rectal cancers ulcerating in the perineum. *Cancer* 1990;65: 1111.

820. Tepper JE, Cohen AM, Wood WC, et al. Intraoperative electron beam radiotherapy in the treatment of unresectable rectal cancer. *Arch Surg* 1986;121:421.

821. Theodoropoulos G, Wise WE, Padmanabhan A, et al. T-level downstaging and complete pathologic response after preoperative chemoradiation for advanced rectal cancer result in decreased recurrence and improved disease-free survival. *Dis Colon Rectum* 2002;45:895.

822. Thorlakson RH. Operating proctoscopes designed for use in rectal anastomosis by stapling techniques. *Dis Colon Rectum* 1986;29:214.

823. Thorlakson RH. New upper and lower clamps for use in anterior resection of the rectum by hand suture, or stapling techniques. *Surg Gynecol Obstet* 1986;103:569.

824. Thorlakson RH. A new operating proctoscope designed for use in rectal anastomosis by stapling techniques. *Surg Gynecol Obstet* 1988;166:367.

825. Tocchi A, Lepre L, Costa G, et al. Rectal cancer and inguinal metastases: prognostic role and therapeutic indications. *Dis Colon Rectum* 1999;42:1464.

826. Tocchi A, Mazzoni G, Lepre L, et al. Prospective evaluation of omentoplasty in preventing leakage of colorectal anastomosis. *Dis Colon Rectum* 2000;43:951.

827. Tolls RM, Herrera-Ornelas L, Petrelli N, et al. An aid in the construction of a stapled anterior rectal anastomosis. *Surg Gynecol Obstet* 1986;163:177.

828. Törnquist A, Ekelund G, Forsgren A, et al. Single dose doxycycline prophylaxis and preoperative bacteriological culture in elective colorectal surgery. *Br J Surg* 1981;68: 565.

829. Thaler W, Watzka S, Martin F, et al. Preoperative staging of rectal cancer by endoluminal ultrasound vs. magnetic resonance imaging. *Dis Colon Rectum* 1994;37:1189.

830. Torres RA, González MA. Perineal continent colostomy: report of a case. *Dis Colon Rectum* 1988;31:957.

831. Triadafilopoulos G, Sarkisian M. Dilatation of radiation-induced sigmoid stricture using sequential Savary-Guilliard dilators: a combined radiologic-endoscopic approach. *Dis Colon Rectum* 1990;33:1065.

832. Tribukait B, Hammarberg C, Rubio C. Ploidy and proliferation patterns in colorectal adenocarcinomas relating to Dukes' classification and to histopathological differentiation. *Acta Pathol Microbiol Immunol Scand (A)* 1983;91:89.

833. Turnbull RB Jr. Cancer of the colon: the five- and ten-year survival rates following resection utilizing the isolation technique. *Ann R Coll Surg Engl* 1970;46:243.

834. Turnbull RB Jr, Cuthbertson A. Abdominorectal pull-through resection for cancer and for Hirschsprung's disease: delayed posterior colorectal anastomosis. *Cleve Clin Q* 1961;28:109.

835. Turnbull RB Jr, Kyle K, Watson FR, et al. Cancer of the colon: the influence of the no-touch isolation technic on survival rates. *Ann Surg* 1967;166:420.

836. Turner GG. Conservative resection of the rectum by the lower route: the after results in seventeen cases. *Acta Chir Scand* 1932;72:519.

837. Turner-Warwick R, Worth PH. The psoas bladder-hitch procedure for the replacement of the lower third of the ureter. *Br J Urol* 1969;41:701.

838. Tveit KM, Guldvog I, Hagen S, et al. Randomized controlled trial of postoperative radiotherapy and short-term time-scheduled 5-fluorouracil against surgery alone in the treatment of Dukes B and C rectal cancer. *Br J Surg* 1997;84:1130.

839. Twomey P, Burchell M, Strawn D, et al. Local control in rectal cancer: a clinical review and meta-analysis. *Arch Surg* 1989;124:1174.

840. Tytherleigh MG, Mortensen NJ McC. Options for sphincter preservation in surgery for low rectal cancer. *Br J Surg* 2003;90:922.

841. Umpleby HC, Fermor B, Symes MO, et al. Viability of exfoliated colorectal carcinoma cells. *Br J Surg* 1984;71:659.

842. van Langenberg A. Total mesorectal excision is not a "new" operation. *Dis Colon Rectum* 2002;45:1120.

843. van Waes PFGM, Koehler PR, Feldberg MAM. Management of rectal carcinoma: impact of computed tomography. *AJR Am J Roentgenol* 1983;140:1137.

844. Vernava AM III, Moran M, Rothenberger DA, et al. A prospective evaluation of distal margins in carcinoma of the rectum. *Surg Gynecol Obstet* 1992;175:333.

845. Vernava AM III, Robbins PL, Brabbee GW. Restorative resection: coloanal anastomosis for benign and malignant disease. *Dis Colon Rectum* 1989;32:690.

846. Vignali A, Fazio VW, Lavery IC, et al. Factors associated with the occurrence of leaks in stapled rectal anastomoses: a review of 1,014 patients. *J Am Coll Surg* 1997;185:105.

847. Villalon AH, Green D. The use of radiotherapy for pelvic recurrence following abdominoperineal resection for carcinoma of the rectum: a 10-year experience. *Aust N Z J Surg* 1981;51:149.

848. Vink M. Local recurrence of cancer in large bowel: role of implantation metastases and bowel disinfection. *Br J Surg* 1954;41:431.

849. von Volkmann R. *Ueber den Mastdarmkrebs und die Exstirpatio recti.* [Concerning rectal cancer and the removal of the rectum.] *Sammlung klinischer vorträge in verbindung mit deutschen klinikern.* [Collection of clinical lectures in cooperation with German clinicians.] Nos. 29–53. Leipzig: Breitkopf and Hartel. Translated in *Dis Colon Rectum* 1986; 29:679.

850. Voros D, Fragoulidis G, Theodosopoulos T, et al. Pelvic floor reconstruction after major cancer surgery. *Dis Colon Rectum* 1996;39:1232.

851. Waizer A, Powsner E, Russo I, et al. Prospective comparative study of magnetic resonance imaging versus transrectal ultrasound for preoperative staging and follow-up of rectal cancer: preliminary report. *Dis Colon Rectum* 1991; 34:1068.

852. Walfisch S, Stern H, Ball S. Use of Nd-Yag laser ablation in colorectal obstruction and palliation in high-risk patients. *Dis Colon Rectum* 1989;32:1060.

853. Walz BJ, Lindstrom ER, Butcher HR Jr, et al. Natural history of patients after abdominal perineal resection: implications for radiation therapy. *Cancer* 1977;39:2437.

854. Wanebo HJ. Resection of pelvic recurrence of rectal cancer. *Contemp Surg* 1982;21:21.

855. Wanebo HJ, Gaker DL, Whitehill R, et al. Pelvic recurrence of rectal cancer: options for curative resection. *Ann Surg* 1987;205:482.

856. Wanebo HJ, Koness RJ, Vezeridis MP, et al. Pelvic resection of recurrent rectal cancer. *Ann Surg* 1994;220:586.

857. Wanebo HJ, Marcove RC. Abdominal sacral resection of locally recurrent rectal cancer. *Ann Surg* 1981;194:458.

858. Wang CC, Schulz MO. The role of radiation therapy in the management of carcinoma of the sigmoid, rectosigmoid, and rectum. *Radiology* 1962;79:1.

859. Wang J-Y, You Y-T, Chen H-H, et al. Stapled colonic J-pouch-anal anastomosis without a diverting colostomy for rectal carcinoma. *Dis Colon Rectum* 1997;40:30.

860. Wangensteen OH. Primary resection (closed anastomosis) of rectal ampulla for malignancy with preservation of sphincteric function together with further account on primary resection of colon and rectosigmoid and note on excision of hepatic metastases. *Surg Gynecol Obstet* 1945;81:1.

861. Washington JA, Dearing WH, Judd ES, et al. Effect of preoperative antibiotic regimen on development of infection after intestinal surgery: prospective, randomized, double-blind study. *Ann Surg* 1974;180:567.

862. Waxman BP. Large bowel anastomoses. II. The circular staplers. *Br J Surg* 1983;70:64.

863. Weinstein M, Roberts M. Sexual potency following surgery for rectal carcinoma. *Ann Surg* 1977;185:295.

864. Weir RF. An improved method of treating high-seated cancers of the rectum. *JAMA* 1901;37:801.

865. Welch CE, Hedberg SE. Complications in surgery of the colon and rectum. In: Artz CP, Hardy JD, eds. *Management of surgical complications,* 3rd ed. Philadelphia: WB Saunders, 1975:600.

866. Wexner SD, Rotholtz NA. Surgeon influenced variables in resectional rectal cancer surgery. *Dis Colon Rectum* 2000;43:1606.

867. Wheeler JMD, Warren BF, Jones AC, et al. Preoperative radiotherapy for rectal cancer: implications for surgeons, pathologists and radiologists. *Br J Surg* 1999;86:1108.

868. Whelan CS, Deckers PJ. Electrocoagulation: its value in treating skin, internal, and rectal cancers. *Contemp Surg* 1988;33:35.

869. Whiteway J, Nicholls RJ, Morson BC. The role of surgical local excision in the treatment of rectal cancer. *Br J Surg* 1985;72:694.

870. Wibe A, Møller B, Norstein J, et al. A national strategic change in treatment policy for rectal cancer-implementation of total mesorectal excision as routine treatment in Norway. a national audit. *Dis Colon Rectum* 2002;45:857.

871. Wibe A, Rendedal PR, Svensson E, et al. Prognostic significance of the circumferential resection margin following total mesorectal excision for rectal cancer. *Br J Surg* 2002; 89:327.

872. Wichmann MW, Meyer G, Adam M, et al. Detrimental immunologic effects of preoperative chemoradiotherapy in advanced rectal cancer. *Dis Colon Rectum* 2003;46:875.

873. Wiggers T. Staging of rectal cancer. *Br J Surg* 2003;90:895.

874. Williams JG, Williams LA. Colonoscopy and brush cytology in the diagnosis of colonic strictures. *J R Coll Surg Edinb* 1988;33:119.

875. Williams LF Jr, Huddleston CB, Sawyers JL, et al. Is total pelvic exenteration reasonable primary treatment for rectal carcinoma? *Ann Surg* 1988;207:670.

876. Williams NS, Dixon MF, Johnston D. Reappraisal of the 5 centimetre rule of distal excision for carcinoma of the rectum: a study of distal intramural spread and of patients' survival. *Br J Surg* 1983;70:150.

877. Williams NS, Durdey P, Johnston D. The outcome following sphincter-saving resection and abdomino-perineal resection for low rectal cancer. *Br J Surg* 1985;72:595.

878. Williams NS, Durdey P, Quirke P, et al. Pre-operative staging of rectal neoplasm and its impact on clinical management. *Br J Surg* 1985;72:868.

879. Williams NS, Hallan RI, Koeze TH, et al. Restoration of gastrointestinal continuity and continence after abdominoperineal excision of the rectum using an electrically stimulated neoanal sphincter. *Dis Colon Rectum* 1990; 33:561.

880. Williams RD, Yurko AA, Kerr G, et al. Comparison of anterior and abdominoperineal resections for low pelvic colon and rectal carcinoma. *Am J Surg* 1966;111:114.

881. Williamson PR, Hellinger MD, Larach SW, et al. Endorectal ultrasound of T3 and T4 rectal cancers after preoperative chemoradiation. *Dis Colon Rectum* 1996;39:45.

882. Wilson E. Local treatment of cancer of the rectum. *Dis Colon Rectum* 1973;16:194.

883. Winde G, Nottberg H, Keller R, et al. Surgical cure for early rectal carcinomas (T1). *Dis Colon Rectum* 1996;39:969.

884. Wolley RC, Schreiber K, Koss LG, et al. DNA distribution in human colon carcinomas and its relationship to clinical behavior. *J Natl Cancer Inst* 1982;69:15.

885. Wolmark N, Fisher B. An analysis of survival and treatment failure following abdominoperineal and sphincter-saving resection in Dukes' B and C rectal carcinoma. *Ann Surg* 1986;204:480.

886. Wolmark N, Gordon PH, Fisher B, et al. A comparison of stapled and handsewn anastomoses in patients undergoing resection for Dukes' B and C colorectal cancer. *Dis Colon Rectum* 1986;29:344.

887. Woodward A, Tydeman G, Lewis MH. Eder Puestow dilatation of benign rectal stricture following anterior resection. *Dis Colon Rectum* 1990;33:79.

888. Wright CB, Hobson RW. Prediction of intestinal viability using Doppler ultrasound technics. *Am J Surg* 1975;129: 642.

889. Yamakoshi H, Ike H, Oki S, et al. Metastasis of rectal cancer to lymph nodes and tissues around the autonomic nerves spared for urinary and sexual function. *Dis Colon Rectum* 1997;40:1079.

890. Yamamoto Y, Sano K, Kimoto M. Cryosurgical treatment for anorectal cancer: a method of palliative or adjunctive management. *Am Surg* 1989;55:252.

891. Yamana T, Oya M, Komatsu J, et al. Preoperative anal sphincter high pressure zone, maximum tolerable volume, and anal mucosal electrosensitivity predict early postoperative defecatory function after low anterior resection for rectal cancer. *Dis Colon Rectum* 1999;42:1145.

892. Yiu R, Wong SK, Cromwell J, et al. Pelvic wall involvement denotes a poor prognosis in T4 rectal cancer. *Dis Colon Rectum* 2001;44:1676

893. Yoon W-H, Song I-S, Chang E-S. Intraluminal bypass technique using a condom for protection of coloanal anastomosis. *Dis Colon Rectum* 1994;37:1046.

894. Zacherl J, Scheissel R, Windhager R, et al. Abdominosacral resection of recurrent rectal cancer in the sacrum. *Dis Colon Rectum* 1999;42:1035.

895. Zainea GG, Lee F, McLeary RD, et al. Transrectal ultrasonography in the evaluation of rectal and extrarectal disease. *Surg Gynecol Obstet* 1989;169:153.

896. Zama N, Fazio VW, Jagelman DG, et al. Efficacy of pelvic packing in maintaining hemostasis after rectal excision for cancer. *Dis Colon Rectum* 1988;31:923.

897. Zelas P, Haaga JR, Fazio VW. The diagnosis by percutaneous biopsy with computed tomography of a recurrence of carcinoma of the rectum in the pelvis. *Surg Gynecol Obstet* 1980;151:525.

898. Z'graggen K, Maurer CA, Birrer S, et al. A new surgical concept for rectal replacement after low anterior resection: the transverse coloplasty pouch. *Ann Surg* 2001;234:780.

899. Zinman LM, Libertino JA. Surgical management of urethral strictures. *Surg Clin North Am* 1973;53:465.

900. Zinman LM, Libertino JA, Roth RA. Management of operative ureteral injury. *Urology* 1978;12:290.

901. Zollinger RM, Sheppard MH. Carcinoma of the rectum and the rectosigmoid: a review of 729 cases. *Arch Surg* 1971; 102:335.

Malignant Tumors of the Anal Canal

While there are several chronic diseases more destructive to life than cancer, none is more feared.

Charles H. Mayo

Carcinomas of the anal canal and perianal skin are uncommon clinical entities, accounting for only 2% or fewer of all colorectal carcinomas. At the Memorial Sloan-Kettering Cancer Center in New York, between 1929 and 1974 approximately 400 uncommon neoplasms were found in this area, as compared with almost 10,000 adenocarcinomas of the rectum.[111] This is an incidence of 4% in a specialized referral center.

Anal canal cancer is almost three times more common than carcinoma of the anal margin.[87] If the dentate line is taken as the distal limit of the anal canal, approximately 70% of all anal tumors will occur in the anal canal.[31] However, if the anal canal is assumed to extend from the anorectal ring to the anal verge (the junction of modified squamous epithelium with the hair-bearing, keratinized perianal skin), 85% of anal tumors will arise in the anal canal.[31] Anal canal tumors are more frequently seen in women (3:2), whereas carcinoma of the anal margin is more common in men (4:1). Morson and Pang noted the same median age for both genders at presentation (57 years).[87]

ANATOMY AND HISTOLOGY

There is some controversy about the anatomic limits of the anal canal, although it is generally agreed that the proximal extent corresponds to the anorectal ring.[52] The distal end has been variously proposed to be the dentate line, Hilton's line, and the anal verge.[50,52] My interpretation of the anal canal is that portion of the distal segment of the intestinal tract that lies between the termination of the rectal mucosa above and the beginning of the perianal skin below (i.e., the mucocutaneous junction; Figure 24-1). It is divided into a proximal transitional zone encompassing the columns and sinuses of Morgagni and a distal zone lined by squamous epithelium (Figure 24-2). The transitional zone is derived from the embryonic cloaca and separates the rectal mucosa from the squamous epithelium of the distal anal canal. The anal glands and ducts arise from this area and are lined by stratified columnar epithelium (Figure 24-3). The median number of anal glands is six, with 80% extending to the submucosa, 8% to the circular internal sphincter, 8% to the longitudinal internal sphincter, 2% to the intersphincteric space, and only 1% penetrating the external anal sphincter.[121] The implications of the depth of penetration of the anal glands concerning the etiology of fistula-in-ano are discussed in Chapter 11. The anal glands have definite secretory activity and are presumed to be responsible for lubricating the anal canal.

The transitional zone contains epithelium resembling that found in the urethra, but much variability exists in the region. Patches of squamous epithelium are frequently present, especially over the crests of the columns of Morgagni. The junction between the transitional zone and squamous mucosa lies at the inferior limit of the columns of Morgagni and has been referred to as the dentate or pectinate line. However, some authors place the dentate line at the proximal limit of the anal canal, at the junction between the rectal mucosa and transitional zone.[54,68] The more distal zone of the anal canal is lined by stratified squamous epithelium and can be differentiated histologically from perianal skin by the absence of the epidermal appendages found in the skin. Thus, a finger examining the anal canal first passes the perianal skin, the squamous epithelium of the distal anal canal, the transitional zone, and finally reaches the rectal mucosa. Separating tumors that arise in the anal canal from those of the perianal skin is important because their biologic behavior and, consequently, the treatments are distinctly different.

CARCINOMA OF THE PERIANAL SKIN AND ANAL MARGIN

Neoplasms of the anal margin and perianal skin include squamous cell carcinoma, Bowen's disease, Paget's disease, and basal cell carcinoma. It is generally accepted that wide surgical excision is adequate treatment for

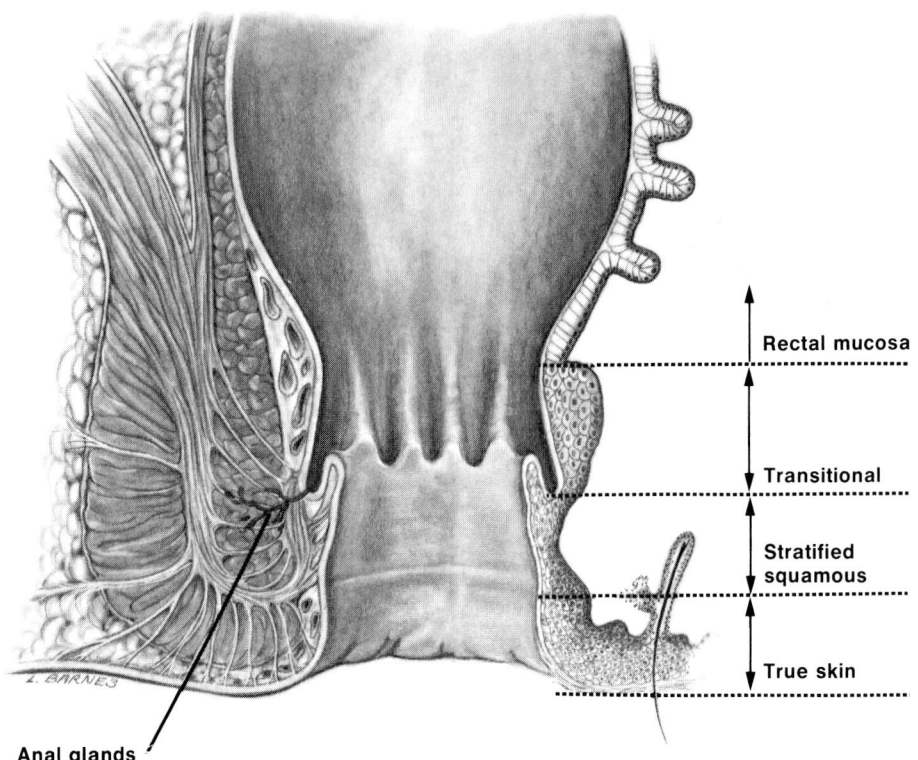

FIGURE 24-1. Anatomy of the anus with histologic pattern schematically illustrated.

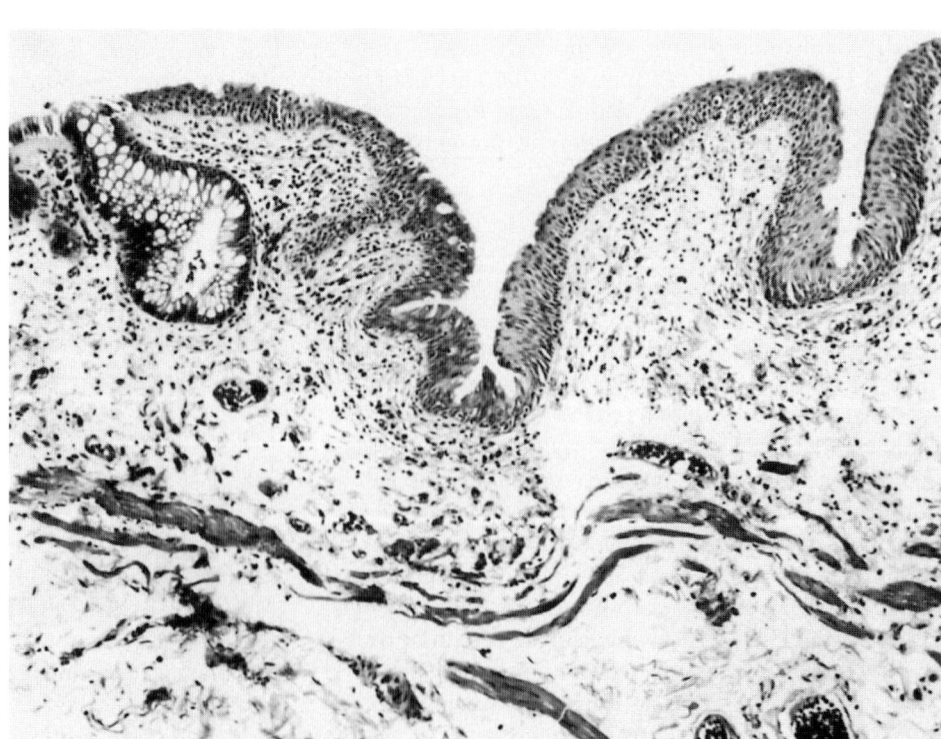

FIGURE 24-2. Normal anal canal at the junction between the glands of the rectal mucosa and the transitional zone **(left)**. The epithelium of the transitional zone **(center, right)** resembles the transitional epithelium of the lower genitourinary tract. (Original magnification × 100.)

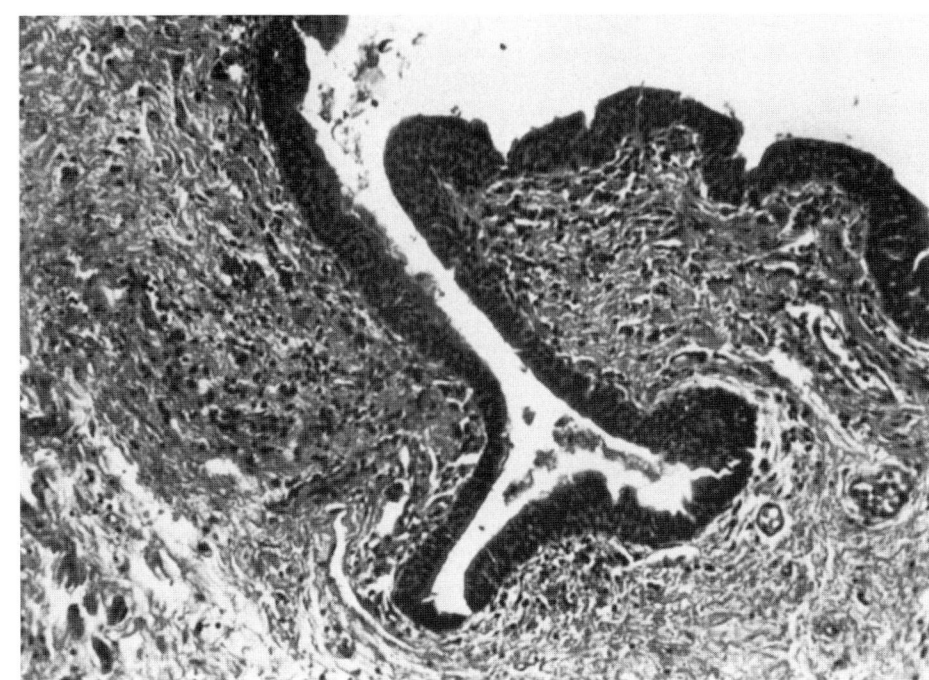

FIGURE 24-3. Cross-section of a normal anal duct. (Original magnification × 250; courtesy of Rudolf Garret, M.D.)

lesions of the perianal skin (Figure 24-4).[105] Management of these conditions is discussed in Chapter 19. Carcinomas of the anal margin have a better prognosis than that of tumors of the anal canal. Mendenhall and colleagues reviewed the experience at the University of Florida, Gainesville, of squamous cell carcinoma of the anal margin.[86] They concluded that superficial, well- to moderately differentiated T1 cancers of the anal margin may be successfully treated with radiotherapy alone or by local excision. However, because stage T2 lesions have an increased risk for lymph node metastases to the groin, they recommended radiotherapy to the primary tumor in conjunction with elective inguinal lymph node radiation. Furthermore, abdominoperineal resection (APR) is reserved for those who have complications secondary to the radiation therapy or locally recurrent disease.[86] Greenall and colleagues reported the results of treatment of 48 patients with anal margin lesions.[51] Local excision was associated with a corrected 5-year survival rate of 88%, but 46% of these individuals developed a local or regional recurrence. Additional treatment contributed to the satisfactory results, but APR did not improve survival.

Recommendation

It is self-evident that any suspicious lesion around the anus should be examined by biopsy. If the lesion is confirmed to be a malignant neoplasm, the usual treatment is to perform wide local excision, because these lesions

tend not to metastasize (see Figure 19-67). The defect created by excision can be left to granulate, covered by a split-thickness skin graft, or, in some instances, may be closed by rotating a flap of adjacent skin, such as described in Chapter 8.

CLASSIFICATION OF ANAL CANAL TUMORS

Several histologic types of tumors are identified in the anal canal: epidermoid (squamous cell) and mucoepidermoid carcinoma, transitional-cloacogenic carcinoma, adenocarcinoma, and malignant melanoma. Some physicians regard transitional-cloacogenic carcinoma as a manifestation of epidermoid carcinoma,[96,100] whereas others believe it is a separate entity that arises from the transitional zone of the anal canal with different morphologic and clinical features.[41,68] Although it is true that transitional-cloacogenic carcinomas are generally recognizable as a distinct group of tumors, there is some overlap with standard epidermoid carcinomas. They, therefore, form one part of a spectrum that ranges from pure transitional-cloacogenic tumors through lesions with mixtures of squamous elements to those with purely squamous differentiation. The Memorial Sloan-Kettering Cancer group recommends that tumors be classified as squamous or basaloid (transitional-cloacogenic), according to the predominant cell type, although the authors recognize that this may be quite subjective and depen-

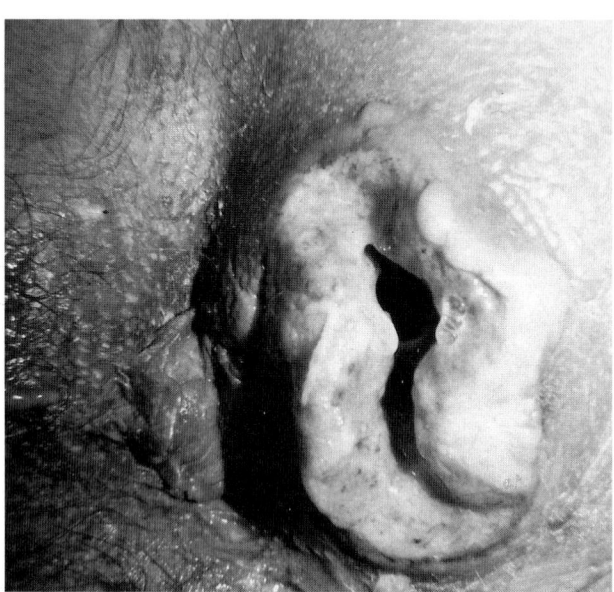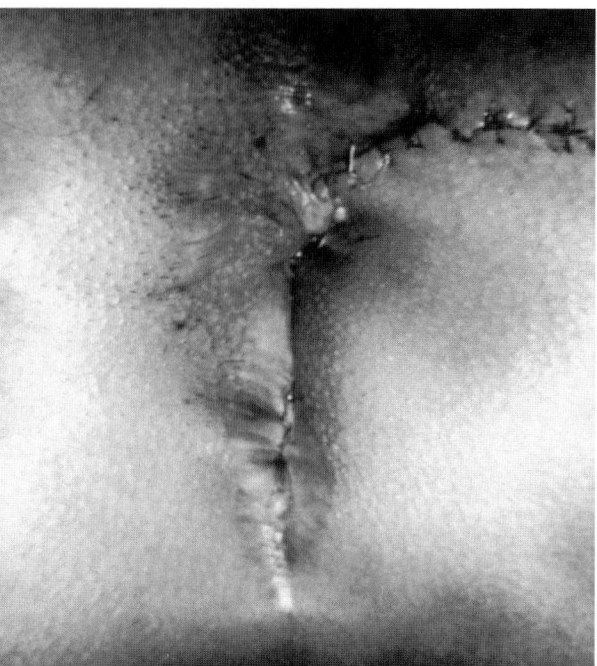

A   **B**

FIGURE 24-4. Ulcerating squamous cell carcinoma of the buttock. **(A)** The lesion has been excised. **(B)** A rotation flap of full-thickness skin covers the defect.

dent upon tissue sampling.[50] With the exception of melanoma, the clinical behavior of carcinoma of the anal canal appears to be relatively independent of the morphologic subtype when compared stage for stage and grade for grade.

Epidermoid (squamous cell) carcinoma accounted for the majority of the tumors of the anal canal in our series (almost two thirds), transitional-cloacogenic carcinomas comprised approximately one fourth, and melanomas made up the remainder (14%).[22]

EPIDERMOID OR SQUAMOUS CELL CARCINOMA OF THE ANUS

Incidence

As mentioned, epidermoid carcinoma of the anus is a rare condition. It can be multifocal in the anal canal as well as in the perianal skin, perineum, and vulvar areas. Most published articles describe each institution's rather limited experience. Failes and Morgan reported 59 patients over a 20-year period; Sawyers and colleagues reported 42 patients over a period of 35 years (2.4% of cancers of the colon, rectum, and anus); and Cattell and Williams reported a 1.7% incidence of epidermoid carcinoma in 600 rectal and anal neoplasms.[16,35,118] Grinnell noted a 1.8% incidence of epidermoid carcinoma in colorectal cancers.[53] Golden and Horsley reported on 26 patients, an incidence of 1.8% of all colorectal cancers.[43] Beahrs and Wilson at the Mayo Clinic in Rochester, Minnesota, reported on 113 patients with epidermoid carcinoma, an incidence of approximately 1% of all colorectal carcinomas seen during the 20-year review.[6] Stearns and Quan (see biographies in Chapter 23) identified 234 epidermoid carcinomas, which represented approximately 3.9% of all malignant tumors detected in the terminal 18 cm of the alimentary tract.[129] The annual incidence of anal cancer among men in the United States is 0.7 per 100,000, but in homosexual men the incidence has been estimated to be as high as 37 in 100,000.[108]

Maggard and co-workers undertook a study in 2003 to obtain an updated population-based perspective on anal canal cancer incidence rates, demographics, and outcomes through the use of a national database from 1973 to 1998 (United States Surveillance Epidemiology and End Results Cancer Registry).[81] The study included a total of 4,841 patients. Female patients were significantly older than male patients (65 versus 58 years), there was a yearly increase in incidence, and blacks were less likely to have localized disease. The disease prevalence by stage at diagnosis was as follows:

- Localized (53%)
- Regional (38%)
- Distant (9%)

Age and Gender

Epidermoid carcinoma can occur at almost any age, but absent human immunodeficiency virus (HIV)–positivity, the condition is usually found in the sixth and seventh decades. As mentioned previously, most studies have shown a preponderance of carcinoma of the anal canal in women. However, in our non-HIV experience, the gender incidence was approximately the same (15 women and 14 men).[22] The mean age of the 29 patients was 59 years, with a range of 39 to 84 years. In Sweden, the annual age-adjusted incidence per 100,000 population for squamous cell carcinoma is 1.40 for women and 0.68 for men. However, where there are centers with a large patient population of men at high risk, the female-to-male ratio may approach unity.[31]

Predisposing Conditions and Etiology

An increased incidence of anal cancer is seen with a number of anorectal inflammatory conditions, such as chronic anal fistula (see Chapter 11) and anal condylomata, as well as in those with HIV infection (see Chapters 19 and 20). This includes patients with Crohn's disease (see Chapter 30). An association with smoking, anoreceptive intercourse, and immunosuppression has also been described. A relationship with human papillomavirus (HPV) types that are known to be associated with cervical and other genital cancers has been suggested. Individuals who engage in anal intercourse and who are infected with HPV type 16 have a relative risk of developing anal canal cancer as high as 33% over the general population.[67] Palmer and colleagues affirmed that both HPV types 16 and 18 are involved in the development of anal and genital squamous cell carcinoma.[95] Youk and associates identified HPV type 16 in all 21 of their patients with anal cancer.[142] Holmes and associates found associations between positive herpes simplex virus 2 titer, cigarette smoking, a prior positive or questionable cervical Papanicolaou smear, and an increasing number of sexual partners with the development of anal cancer.[59] An increased incidence of cancers in the anogenital region has also been observed in patients who have undergone renal transplantation, presumably as a consequence of immunosuppression.[103] Anal cancers have occurred following radiation therapy for pruritus.[31]

Several reports have suggested a significantly higher incidence in patients with Crohn's disease.[126] Although it is unlikely that a patient with an anal fistula or condylomata would be treated with expectant observation, individuals with Crohn's disease are often managed in this way. Therefore, it is important to perform a biopsy of any unusual lesion. It may even be good counsel to suggest random anal biopsies at intervals for patients with this condition.

Frisch and colleagues examined the risk of anal cancer developing in individuals who harbored benign anal lesions, including fissures, fistulas, perianal or perirectal abscesses, and hemorrhoids.[40] Whereas these investigators concluded that there was a strong temporal association between the diagnosis of benign anal lesions and the diagnosis of anal cancer, their data did not support the view that there was an association for these diagnoses.

Melbye and co-workers compared the numbers of observed cases and expected cases of anal cancer among patients with acquired immunodeficiency syndrome (AIDS) by utilizing registries in seven health departments in the United States.[85] These investigators found that there was a strikingly increased risk of the development of this malignancy in individuals with AIDS. Lorenz and co-workers retrospectively reviewed six patients with squamous cell carcinoma treated between 1985 and 1988.[79] All six were homosexual men; five had AIDS, and one was HIV positive. Because of the increased incidence of venereal disease in the homosexual population, there is increasing evidence to suggest that homosexual men are at a particular risk for the development of anal cancer.[73] Even in the absence of AIDS, anal canal carcinoma, Kaposi's sarcoma, and anorectal lymphoma are seen in younger patients and much more frequently than would be expected.[29,32,62,70,90] Daling and colleagues demonstrated that two correlates of homosexual behavior, unmarried status and positive serologic test result for syphilis, are related to an increased incidence of anal cancer.[28,29] Because having had syphilis and being single are associated with the practice of anal intercourse in men, but not in women, the authors suggest that this act is an independent risk factor for the development of anal cancer. Goldstone and associates recommend that all men who have sex with men with presumed benign anorectal disease undergo high-resolution anoscopy and multiple biopsies of all abnormal areas in order to look for high-grade, squamous intraepithelial lesions that represent precursors of invasive carcinoma (see Chapter 20).[49] Place and co-workers opined that anal squamous cell carcinoma in an HIV-positive patient should be considered an AIDS-defining illness.[108]

It can be appreciated, therefore, that certain predisposing conditions are associated with the development of malignant anal canal tumors. This implies that the etiology probably represents an interaction between genetic and environmental factors.[31] The genetic aspect may be related to changes in chromosome 11 (11q22) or the short arm of chromosome 3 (3p22).[89]

In summary, the following variables are related to the development of anogenital carcinoma:

- Prior radiotherapy
- Chronic anal fistula
- Crohn's disease

- Smoking
- Positive Papanicolaou smear
- Cervical carcinoma
- HPV infection
- Hodgkin's disease
- Renal transplantation
- Promiscuity
- Positive herpes simplex virus 2 titer
- HIV infection
- Male homosexuality
- Anoreceptive intercourse
- Immunosuppression
- Positive serologic test for syphilis
- Anal condylomata

Current evidence indicates that the etiology of anal cancer is a multifactorial interaction among environmental factors, HPV infection, immune status, and suppressor genes.[31]

Signs and Symptoms

Symptoms of anal canal carcinoma include rectal bleeding, anal pain, pruritus, mucous discharge, tenesmus, the sensation of a lump in the anus, and a change in bowel habits (Figure 24-5). Rectal bleeding occurs in more than one half of individuals. The duration of symptoms is of little prognostic significance.[50] Complaints such as discharge, incontinence, change in bowel habits, pelvic pain, or the passage of stool or gas through the vagina suggest an advanced lesion.[31] Tenesmus, the painful urgency to defecate, implies invasion of the sphincter mechanism. Presentation is often late, with the mean size of tumor at diagnosis between 3 and 4 cm.[31] Occasionally, a patient may present with a mass in the groin, a manifestation of a metastasis before the primary tumor causes significant symptoms. The condition may also be identified incidentally upon review of the histology of a hemorrhoidectomy specimen (see later).

Examination and Biopsy

Rectal examination may reveal an ulcerating, hard, tender, bleeding mass in the anal canal or lower rectum. Examination of an advanced lesion may be excruciatingly tender and may require evaluation using an anesthetic to identify the extent truly and to perform a biopsy of the lesion. The lesion may fungate through the anal canal and appear on the perianal skin or present through a chronic draining anal fistula (Figure 24-6).

Proctosigmoidoscopic examination usually shows that the tumor is confined to the anal canal. However, in far-advanced cases, the lesion may extend upward to involve the rectum. Conversely, a carcinoma that seems to arise within the anal canal may occasionally be a rectal cancer that has spread downward (Figure 24-7). Another possi-

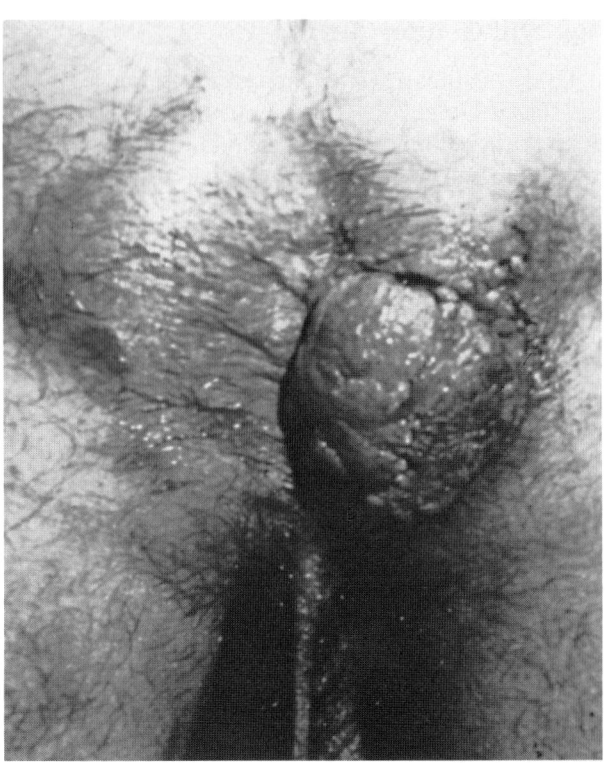

FIGURE 24-5. Squamous cell carcinoma. The patient complained of a lump. (From Corman ML, Veidenheimer MC, Swinton NW. *Diseases of the anus, rectum and colon. Part I: neoplasms.* New York: Medcom, 1972, with permission.)[23]

bility is implantation from a colon tumor, a particular concern if hemorrhoidectomy is performed at the time of a colectomy for cancer. Scott and colleagues demonstrated by flow cytometric DNA analysis that an anal malignancy was actually the result of a "dropped" metastasis from a sigmoid colon carcinoma.[120] Biopsy of the lesion will establish its histologic nature.

Pathology

Epidermoid Carcinoma

Epidermoid carcinoma originates from the stratified squamous epithelium of the distal anal mucosa and therefore morphologically resembles carcinoma arising from the buccal mucosa, esophagus, uterine cervix, and so forth. The tumor is composed of squamous epithelial cells that resemble normal anal mucosa to a varying extent, depending on the degree of differentiation (Figure 24-8). The more differentiated tumors have readily apparent keratin formation, either as pearls or as individual cell keratinization. The lesions can be graded on the basis of the degree of keratinization and the nuclear morphology, and this grade correlates with the behavior of the tumor: that is, well-differentiated tumors tend to be less deeply invasive and are less likely to metastasize. More

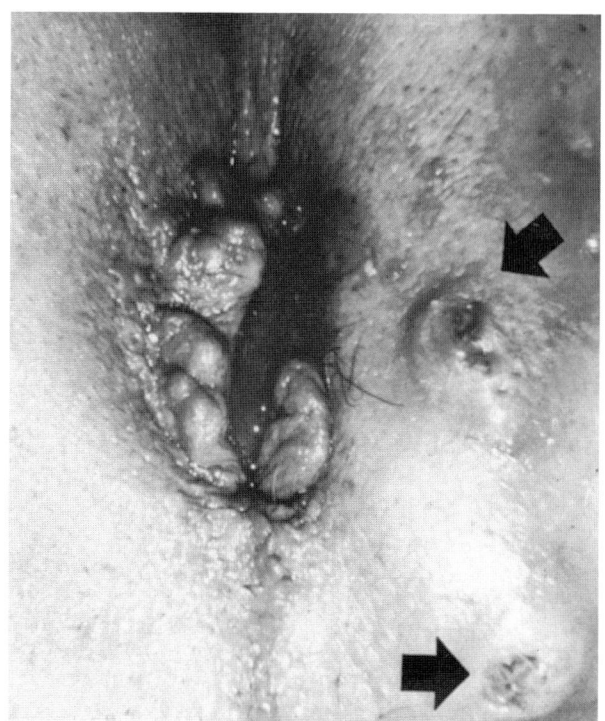

FIGURE 24-6. Two fistulous openings *(arrows)* from anal canal carcinoma. Biopsy of the tracts confirmed the presence of tumor. (From Corman ML, Veidenheimer MC, Swinton NW. *Diseases of the anus, rectum and colon. Part I: neoplasms.* New York: Medcom, 1972, with permission.)

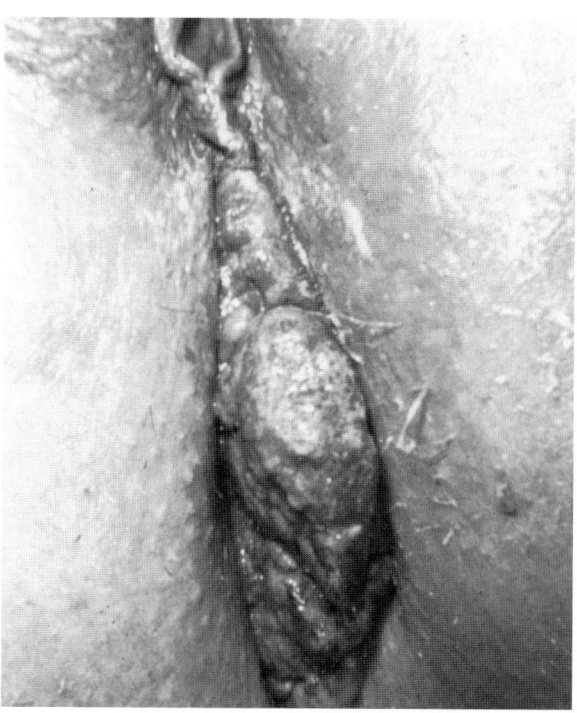

FIGURE 24-7. Adenocarcinoma of the rectum fungating through the anal canal. (From Corman ML, Veidenheimer MC, Swinton NW. *Diseases of the anus, rectum and colon. Part I: neoplasms.* New York: Medcom, 1972, with permission.)

than 50% of anal canal tumors are nonkeratinizing, whereas 80% are poorly differentiated.[31] This is in contrast to anal margin tumors, with 80% demonstrating keratinization and 85% being well differentiated.[31]

Goldman and colleagues examined 15 patients with anal carcinoma by means of percutaneous and transanorectal fine needle aspiration cytology, confirming the diagnosis by this means.[48] Interestingly, despite the predominance in women, neither estrogen receptors nor progesterone receptors could be detected. Surawicz and coworkers utilized anal cytology and biopsy to determine the presence of anal dysplasia (anal intraepithelial neoplasia) in 90 homosexual men with abnormalities of the anal canal.[131] Eighty-six percent had HPV-associated abnormalities, including condylomata. Dysplasia was detected by cytology in 36% and by biopsy in 92% (27% high grade).[131] The authors concluded that further studies are indicated to determine the clinical significance of the dysplastic phenomenon and its rate of progression to cancer (see also Chapter 20). Obviously, this has implications with respect to screening and to treatment.

A careful search using mucin stains may disclose a focus of mucin-producing cells in as many as 10% to 15% of patients.[88] Such tumors have been classified separately as mucoepidermoid carcinomas, but little evidence exists that differences in the behavior of this subgroup warrant

its separation. A spindle cell carcinoma (pseudosarcoma) has been reported to be another variant.[65]

Squamous cell carcinoma tumor-associated antigen (SCC antigen) has been shown to be a tumor marker that seems to be related to the histologic characteristics of differentiated epidermoid tumors rather than to tumor site.[106] Fontana and colleagues measured SCC antigen in epidermoid carcinoma of the anal canal in 66 patients at diagnosis, before treatment, and during follow-up.[38] There did not appear to be a correlation with the primary tumor, itself, except with respect to nodal involvement. These investigators concluded that there was no prognostic value of this study at the time of diagnosis, but that the level of SCC antigen correlated well with the development of recurrence.

Transitional-Cloacogenic Carcinoma

In 1956, Grinvalsky and Helwig published a study of the anatomy of the anal canal in which they detailed the features of the transitional or "cloacogenic" zone and suggested that tumors which arise in this area differ from the usual epidermoid carcinomas originating in the squamous epithelium of the distal anal canal.[54] They proposed the term transitional-cloacogenic for these lesions. Subsequent studies have confirmed the morphologic difference from that of the usual squamous carcinomas.[68,96]

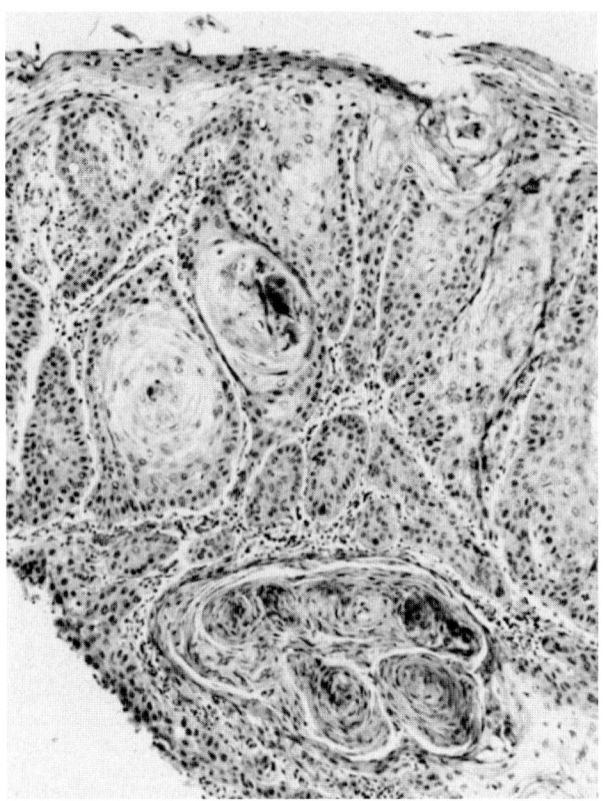

FIGURE 24-8. This well-differentiated squamous cell carcinoma resembles normal squamous epithelium and is producing keratin pearls **(bottom)**. Less well-differentiated lesions lose their resemblance to squamous epithelium, lack keratin pearls, and behave more aggressively. (Original magnification × 100.)

Transitional-cloacogenic carcinomas may resemble carcinomas of urothelium to a certain extent, or they may have patterns similar to those of basal cell carcinoma of skin—hence the term basaloid, because the cells at the periphery are arranged in an orderly, palisade fashion (Figure 24-9). However, this variation in cell pattern must not be confused with basal cell carcinoma. The former is a malignant tumor that frequently metastasizes, whereas the latter is relatively benign (see Chapter 19).

Those tumors resembling urothelial carcinomas are composed of islands or nests of cells that have indistinct borders and oval nuclei (Figure 24-10). A focus of keratinization is often present. As stated previously, varying amounts of squamous elements produce a spectrum of lesions ranging from purely transitional through mixed varieties to purely squamous tumors. Some examples of transitional-cloacogenic carcinoma appear to arise in the lower part of the rectum above the transitional zone, whereas others may not even involve the mucosa. The probable explanation for these phenomena is that such tumors may originate from the transitional epithelium that lines the anal ducts deep to

the mucosa or in proximal ramifications of the ducts beneath rectal mucosa.

As stated before, transitional-cloacogenic tumors form a histologically recognizable subgroup of anal canal carcinomas, but on the basis of grade and stage of the lesions, their behavior appears to be comparable to that of epidermoid carcinomas of similar grade and stage (Figure 24-11). There are fewer published studies of transitional-cloacogenic tumors than that of epidermoid carcinoma, but evidence suggests that there is sufficient overlap in the epidemiology (e.g., an increased incidence in anal-receptive homosexual men),[20] the clinical presentation, and the results of treatment that, for the purposes of management, one should consider the two entities identical.

Melanoma

The histopathology of malignant melanoma is discussed later in this chapter.

Adenocarcinoma

Adenocarcinoma of the anus is usually seen as a downward extension of a primary rectal tumor. However, glandular epithelium may be found on biopsy from ectopic glands of the anal wall, from sebaceous glands of the perineum, from anal fistulas, or from tumors arising in anal glands or ducts (Figure 24-12). Hobbs and colleagues found that a useful and discriminating definition of anal gland carcinoma is an anal tumor composed of "haphazardly dispersed, small glands with scant mucin production invading the wall of the anorectal area without an intraluminal component" (see later).[58] As discussed in Chapter 19, the association with an underlying mucinous adenocarcinoma and Paget's disease has been well documented.

Staging

No satisfactory method for staging anal canal tumors has been developed. Dukes' classification is not applicable because invasion to groin nodes may occur when lymph node involvement is not evident in the resected specimen. The TNM system has been criticized because it is difficult to distinguish tumor invasion limited to the internal sphincter from that involving the external sphincter and because extension into the rectum or perianal skin does not necessarily imply a poorer prognosis.[50,52]

Goldman and colleagues examined specimens from 47 cases of squamous cell carcinoma of the anus with respect to clinical stage, histologic grade, and DNA content

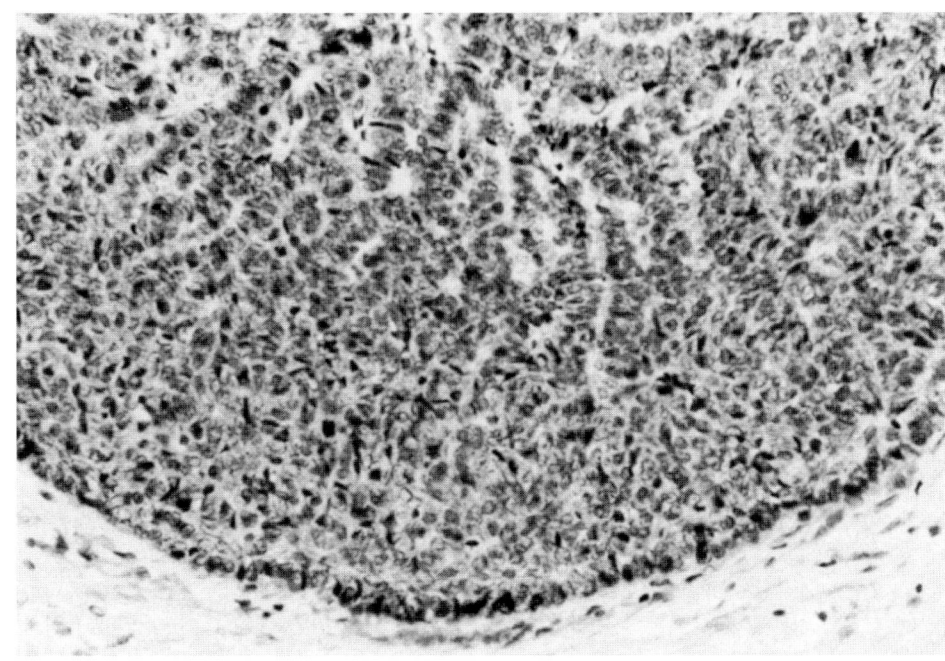

FIGURE 24-9. Transitional-cloacogenic carcinoma. In this tumor, the cells at the periphery tend to arrange themselves in a palisade, thus resembling basal cell carcinoma of the skin. This variant of transitional-cloacogenic carcinoma is sometimes called basaloid carcinoma. (Original magnification × 80.)

of the tumor cells.[44] Because most tumors were aneuploid, no statistically significant difference could be demonstrated with respect to DNA content and survival. The authors affirmed that histologic grade and clinical stage seem to be the best predictors of patient outcome.

Treatment

Until the middle to late 1970s, APR was believed by most surgeons to be the only curative approach to the management of anal canal carcinoma.[115] Before the advent of neoadjuvant therapy, selective application of local excision could also be considered.[45] The choice of treatment depended on the stage of the tumor as determined by depth of invasion.

Local Excision

For carcinoma confined to the mucosa and submucosa or carcinoma-*in-situ* (Figure 24-10), wide local excision with or without anoplasty will usually be curative (see Chapter 8). For more deeply invading tumors, such as those that invade the internal sphincter, local excision, including the internal sphincter, may also achieve cure. However, for tumors that invade more deeply than the internal sphincter, APR has, historically, been the preferred alternative. These differences in therapy based on the stage of the tumor require precise preoperative evaluation, including careful digital examination to assess the depth of invasion and endoanal ultrasound. Tarantino

and Bernstein evaluated 13 consecutive patients with biopsy-proven squamous cell carcinoma of the anal canal by means of endoanal ultrasound.[132] These investigators proposed the following staging system:

uT_1 = Tumor confines to the submucosa
uT_{2a} = Tumor invaded internal sphincter
uT_{2b} = Tumor invades external sphincter
uT_3 = Tumor invades through sphincter complex into perianal tissues
uT_4 = Tumor invades adjacent structures

The authors concluded that endoanal ultrasound can accurately determine the depth of penetration and can also be used to determine the efficacy of neoadjuvant therapy.[132]

Scholefield and colleagues reported the management of 70 patients with anal intraepithelial neoplasia.[119] In concert with the foregoing recommendations, the authors performed local excision and in some cases skin grafting to those larger lesions that were more invasive. Chang and co-workers performed excision and cauterization directed by high-resolution anoscopy in HIV-negative and HIV-positive patients with high-grade intraepithelial lesions.[17] No HIV-negative patient developed recurrence (mean follow-up, 32 months), but 23 of 29 individuals who were HIV positive had persistent or recurrent lesions.

Other options in the management of small, superficial, or minimally invasive anal canal cancers include cryosurgery, laser vaporization, and possibly the use of chemical or immunoablational topical agents (especially for

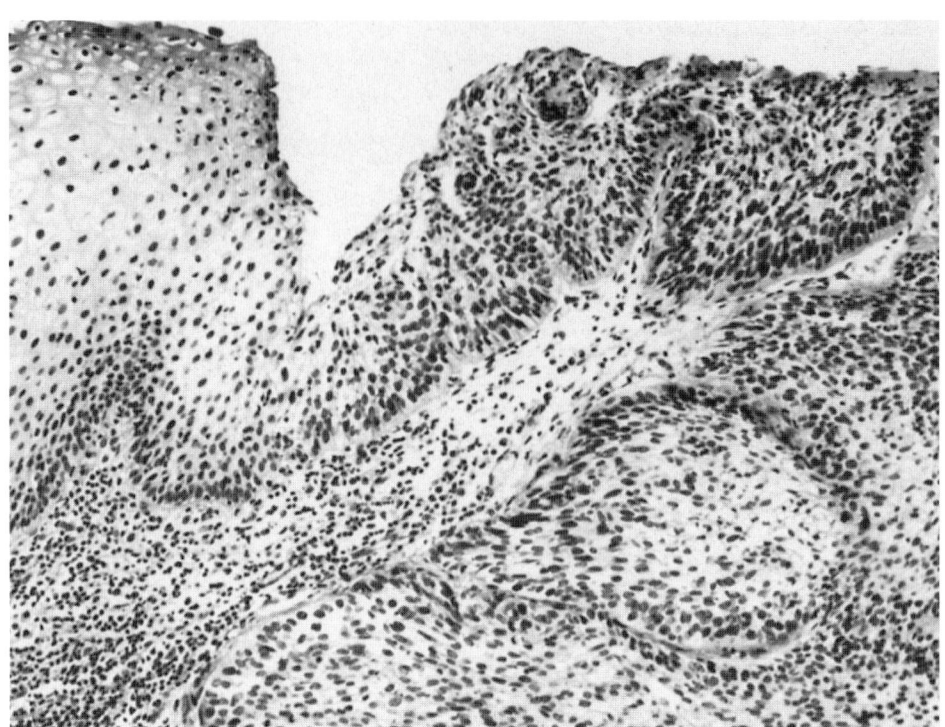

FIGURE 24-10. Transitional-cloacogenic carcinoma. The tumor has an *in situ* component **(upper right)** resembling a transitional cell carcinoma of the urinary bladder, hence its name. (Original magnification × 125.)

intraepithelial neoplasia).[119] Hamdan and co-workers reported the use of photodynamic therapy for the treatment of this condition.[57] This consists of a two-step process that involves the topical or systemic application of a photosensitizer followed by illumination of the treatment area with a non-thermal laser or nonlaser light of a specific wavelength.[57] The effect is to create a local cytotoxic action.

Abdominoperineal Resection

The technique of APR is described in Chapter 23. An important principle to remember is that when the anal margin is involved by tumor, a wider excision of perianal skin

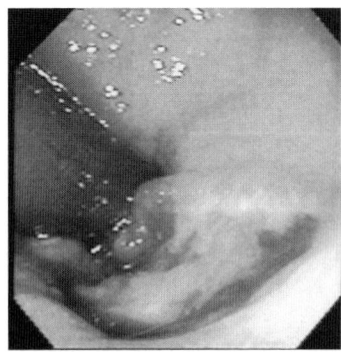

FIGURE 24-11. Retroflexion with the endoscope in the rectum reveals an ulcerating lesion in the transitional zone at the top of the anal canal and lower rectum. Biopsy confirmed the presence of a cloacogenic carcinoma. (See Color Fig. 24-11.)

is required than is customary for adenocarcinoma of the rectum (Figs. 24-13 and 24-14).

Results of Conventional, Non-neoadjuvant Abdominoperineal Resection and Local Excision ("Historical" Data)

Five-year survival after APR has been reported to be between 20% and 70% and depends on tumor size, histologic grading, and depth of invasion.[47,50,52,110] Pelvic or perineal recurrence accounts for 50% to 70% of failures, with only 10% of patients dying of disseminated disease.[50] Welch and Malt noted a 30% recurrence rate in the perineum of 37 patients who underwent APR.[139] Carcinoma was present in 20% of the resection margins. The authors, therefore, caution the surgeon to perform posterior vaginectomy in women as well as wide excision of the perianal skin. Madden and colleagues reported a 21% survival rate in 29 patients after 5 years.[80]

Singh and associates reported 65 patients from Roswell Park Memorial Institute in Buffalo, New York, two thirds of whom had epidermoid carcinoma of the anal canal.[124] The remainder harbored cloacogenic cancers. The overall survival rate depended on the depth of invasion, but it was approximately 50% in both groups. Wide local excision for tumors that invaded through the submucosa was accompanied by a recurrence rate of 100%. Of all surgical approaches, APR with posterior exenteration had the lowest recurrence rate.

The Memorial Sloan-Kettering Cancer group observed that they had treated very few patients with epi-

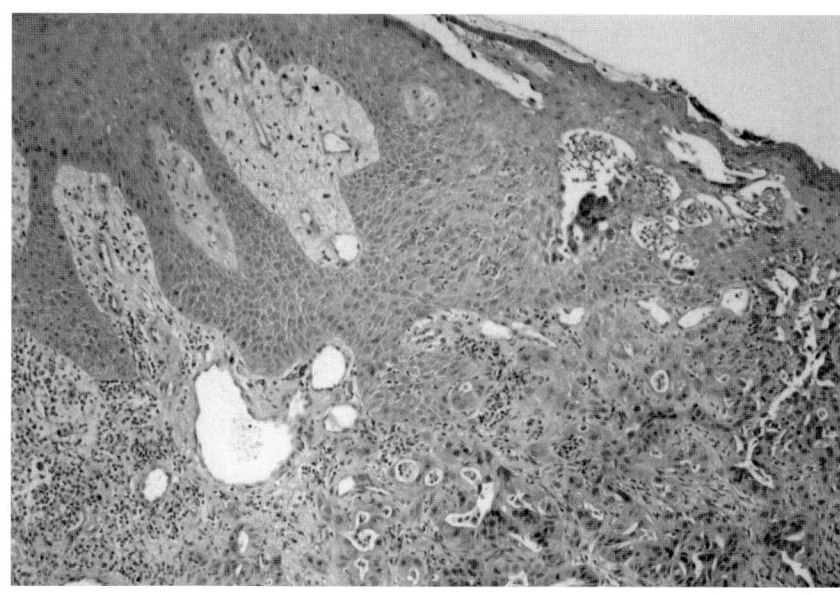

FIGURE 24-12. Adenocarcinoma arising from an anal gland. Note the abutting squamous epithelium. (Original magnification × 200.)

dermoid cancer of the anal canal by local excision, and interpretation of the results may be somewhat confusing because these individuals may be combined with those who had tumors of the anal margin.[50] The fact is that fewer than 10% of tumors were suitable for local excision, and more than 60% of these patients developed recurrence.[50]

In our experience, all patients who had disease confined to the mucosa or submucosa were cured by local excision or by APR. Likewise, all patients who had APR were cured (without supplemental therapy) when the disease was confined to muscle.[22]

With lymph node involvement or invasion into the perirectal or perianal fat, the prognosis is much less optimistic. With lymph node involvement, we observed a 29% 5-year survival rate.[22] It is generally agreed that the depth of invasion and the presence or absence of lymph node involvement are the major criteria for determining length of survival. The prognosis after resection for transitional-cloacogenic carcinoma is essentially the same as that for

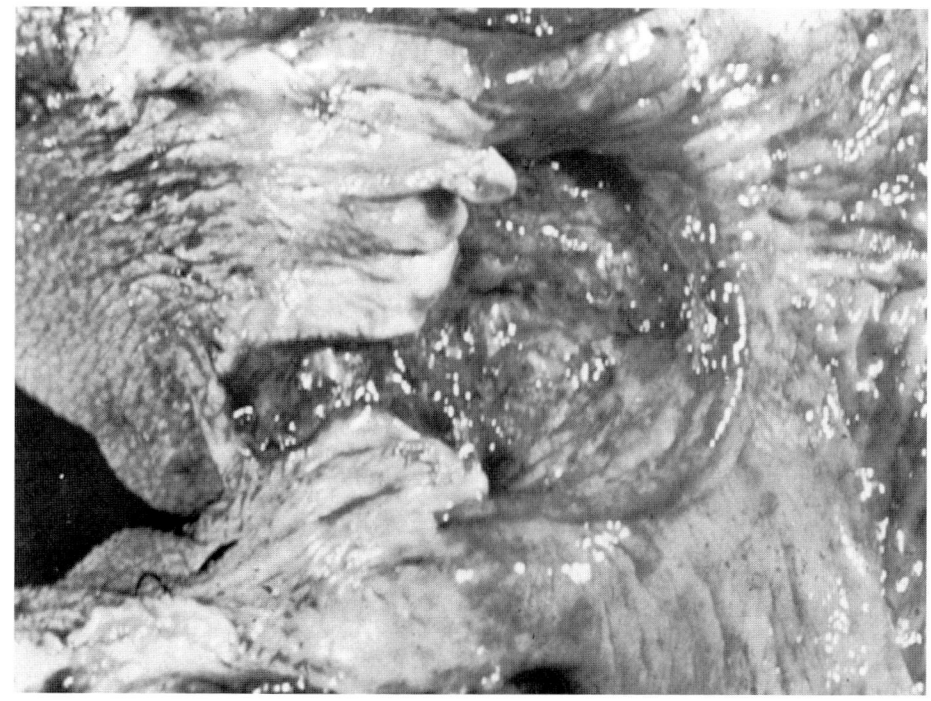

FIGURE 24-13. Proctectomy specimen of squamous cell carcinoma of the anus infiltrating the pectinate line. (Courtesy of Rudolf Garret, M.D.)

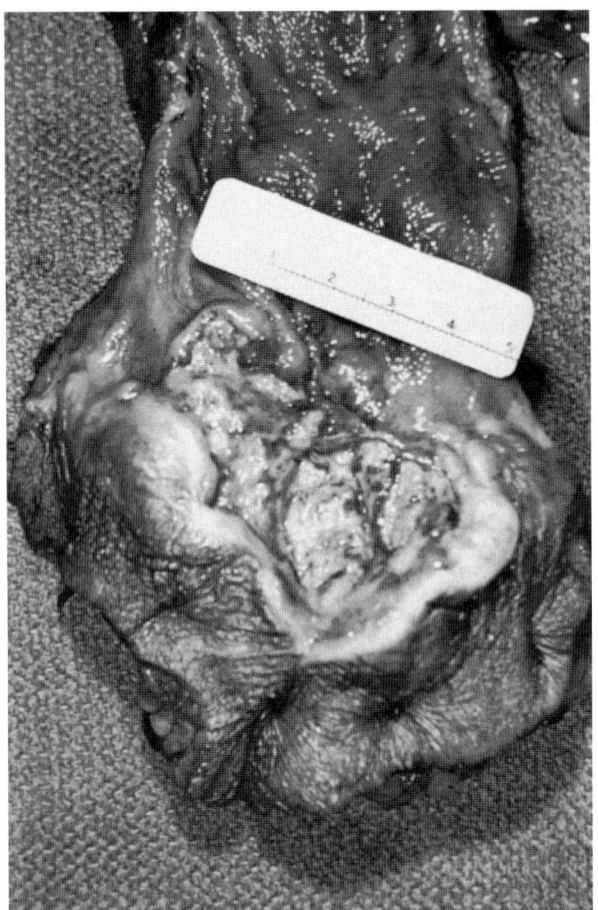

FIGURE 24-14. Cloacogenic carcinoma. Resected specimen of an ulcerated tumor impinging on the pectinate line. (Courtesy of Rudolf Garret, M.D.)

epidermoid carcinoma for the same depth of invasion. In analyzing survival with respect to cell differentiation, no relationship is apparent except that the more poorly differentiated lesions tend to present at a more advanced stage.

To all intents and purposes, the foregoing results are of historical interest only. Today it is not within the standard of care to go directly to APR for carcinoma of the anal canal. This is because of the advances made with the application of neoadjuvant therapy.

Groin Dissection

Radical groin dissection was advocated in the past as a valuable adjunctive procedure in the primary treatment of carcinoma of the anal canal because of the possibility of spread to inguinal nodes. Later reports have been highly critical of this approach, however.[6,22,129,130] Because of its high morbidity and because it is an unnecessary operation in most patients, radical groin dissection

as a therapeutic modality should be employed only when adenopathy is subsequently discovered.[117] For diagnostic and staging purposes, it seems reasonable to excise a large inguinal mass. Even though the cure rate is still low, some authors believe that this procedure reduces the risk of groin complications from tumor growth.[117] It is unlikely that radical inguinal node dissection will lead to the cure of a patient with groin node involvement by tumor. However, one should consider chemotherapy and radiotherapy for these individuals in light of the responsiveness of this tumor to such an approach (see later).

Sentinel Node Biopsy

Damin and colleagues, in 2003, undertook a study to assess the feasibility of inguinal sentinel node biopsy and staging in 14 patients with anal canal cancer and with no evident inguinal node involvement.[30] The procedure consisted of a combination of preoperative lymphoscintigraphy with technetium-99m dextran 500 injected around the tumor and intraoperative detection of the sentinel node with a gamma probe. Patent blue V dye was also injected to permit identification of the blue-stained node. The investigators were able to detect and remove sentinel nodes in all patients and found one individual with a metastatic node. The authors opined that the results of a sentinel lymph node procedure may have a role in directing a different approach to management. Perera and co-workers used injections of antimony sulfide around the tumor with gamma scanning of the inguinal area in order to identify sentinel nodes in 12 patients.[104] The sentinel node was found in eight (67%). In two individuals, metastases were histologically confirmed.

Pelvic Lymphadenectomy

Pelvic lymphadenectomy in conjunction with APR may be performed relatively easily in some patients. The value of obtaining lymph nodes to determine the prognosis and the advisability of adding other treatment may justify this approach, but it should not be performed if the dissection is difficult (see Chapter 23). Wade and colleagues accomplished a retrospective study of 29 patients who underwent potentially curative APR and whose surgical specimens were treated by a clearing technique of the lymph nodes.[136] These investigators found a lack of association between the size of the primary tumor and the lymph nodes and noted that metastasis to small nodes (less than 5 mm) was a common occurrence. This, perhaps, is an explanation for understaging of some patients.

Neoadjuvant (Combined Modality) Therapy (Nigro Protocol)

In 1974, Nigro and associates reported dramatic results in the treatment of epidermoid carcinoma of the anus by means of preoperative radiation therapy and chemotherapy.[94] Subsequent reports from Nigro's unit at Wayne State University School of Medicine in Detroit revealed continued enthusiasm.[12,13,71,91,92] Its remarkable success in the management of even locally extensive tumors or in individuals with regional node metastases has revolutionized the approach to the management of this condition.

The protocol initially consisted of preoperative radiation (a total of 30 Gy) to the tumor and to the pelvic and inguinal nodal areas in 15 treatments over a 3-week period (2 Gy per day, 5 days a week). The first day that radiotherapy is commenced, the patient is administered 5-fluorouracil in 5% glucose, 1,000 mg/m^2 per day, for 4 days as a continuous 24-hour infusion, and again from days 29 through 32. In addition, the patient is given mitomycin-C, 15 mg/m^2, as a single bolus on the first day. This protocol is usually associated with only a mild degree of thrombocytopenia and leukopenia. The most frequent side effects are low-grade stomatitis and moderate diarrhea.[71] There are now numerous variations on this radiation-chemotherapy scheme in terms of both drugs used and radiation dosage and frequency. For example, Löhnert and colleagues in Kiel, Germany, utilize a three-dimensional, endosonographic-based radiation target simulation method, using an afterloading needle application.[77] The anal cancer is restaged following external beam radiation with 45 Gy. The Memorial Sloan-Kettering group suggested that in patients who are selected to undergo an initial excisional biopsy followed by combined modality therapy, 30 Gy may be an adequate radiation dose.[61]

Results

Analysis of 45 patients treated at Wayne State University School of Medicine revealed that 38 of 45 patients (84%) were rendered free of cancer.[71] Although the follow-up period of many patients was less than 5 years, 34 (89%) were alive and free of disease. All patients with residual tumor, even after APR had been performed, died of disseminated disease. The initial median size of those with persistent tumor was 5 cm, as compared with 3.5 cm for those lesions with no residual tumor.

Others have reported favorable experience.[8,19,26,34,36,55,107,112,125,128] Enker and colleagues noted that 59% of their patients had no residual tumor at the time of proctectomy.[34] Seventy-seven percent were free of disease at follow-up. Sischy and co-workers reported 15 patients who received chemotherapy and radiotherapy with a complete response, thereby avoiding APR.[125] Cummings and associates achieved tumor control in all six patients by the protocol, and Wanebo and colleagues had good results even in patients with recurrent and locally advanced disease.[26,137]

Cummings and co-workers compared the results of treatment by radical external beam radiation alone with the combined modality approach.[25] Although the uncorrected 5-year survival rate for the two groups was approximately 70%, control of the primary tumor was much better with combination treatment (93%) than with radiation therapy alone (60%). Almost one half of the patients who underwent chemoradiation therapy developed hematologic toxicity, and in one third the course was complicated by enterocolitis that did not respond to antidiarrheal agents. This is a higher complication rate than that reported by the Nigro group and caused the authors to recommend interrupting the course of therapy for 1 week. None of the patients who underwent combination therapy required a colostomy for uncontrolled tumor, but four of 30 had treatment complications that necessitated a stoma.

The United Kingdom Coordinating Committee on Cancer Research trial compared the results of treatment, randomizing radiation therapy alone versus radiotherapy and chemotherapy (5-fluorouracil and mitomycin).[135] A total of 585 individuals participated in the protocol. Clinical responses were assessed 6 weeks following initial treatment. Good responders were recommended for boost radiotherapy, whereas poor responders were submitted to "salvage surgery." After a median follow-up of

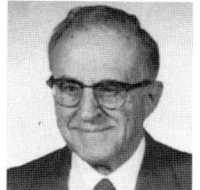

Norman D. Nigro (1912–present) Norman Nigro was born in Syracuse, New York, but moved to Detroit for his early education. He returned to attend Syracuse University, graduating Phi Beta Kappa with a liberal arts degree in 1934 and a doctorate in medicine in 1937. Following internship at Syracuse, he became a preceptee in surgery in Detroit under the tutelage of L. J. Hirshmann. In World War II, he was assigned to the Seventeenth Army General Hospital with the Fifth Army in Italy. At the conclusion of the war, he returned to Wayne State University in Detroit, where he remained for his entire distinguished career. His experiences with Hirshmann led him to develop an interest in colon and rectal surgery, and eventually he achieved the position of secretary to the American Proctologic Society. In 1965, Nigro was elected president of this organization, now known as the American Society of Colon and Rectal Surgeons. He also served as secretary to the American Board of Colon and Rectal Surgery from 1972 to 1986. As a consequence of his work on the combined therapy for anal canal cancer, numerous honors have been bestowed on him, including an honorary lectureship in his name at the annual convention of the American Society of Colon and Rectal Surgeons. His papers have been among the most requested and quoted from the National Library of Medicine. In more recent years, he has made notable contributions to the understanding of the role of nutrition in the etiology of cancer of the large bowel. Nigro retired from active practice in 1989.

42 months, patients receiving radiation therapy alone had a local treatment failure rate of 59%, whereas those receiving combined modality therapy had a local failure rate of only 36%. These differences were highly statistically significant. The only downside was that early morbidity was significantly more frequent with the combined treatment, but late morbidity was about the same. The working party concluded that standard treatment should be a combined approach. They further recommended that surgery should be reserved for patients in whom this regimen fails.[135]

Doci and colleagues treated 56 consecutive patients with a modified protocol, emphasizing that because of variable toxicity it may be necessary to suspend or alter treatment for certain individuals.[33] A complete response was noted in 87%, eight of whom had evidence of positive nodes. The actuarially corrected 5-year survival was 81%.

Flam and associates reported that 26 of 30 patients were rendered free of disease as a result of initial combined modality treatment.[36] The four patients with demonstrable residual tumor were subjected to additional treatment with radiation and chemotherapy. None underwent an operation and none had evidence of recurrence, although follow-up for many was relatively short. The authors counsel that a salvage regimen, such as 5-fluorouracil infusion and cisplatin or sequential methotrexate–5-fluorouracil–leukovorin with radiotherapy, should be instituted before consideration of radical resective measures.[36]

It has been thought that HIV-positive patients do less well with anal cancer than HIV-negative individuals. Kim and co-workers tested this hypothesis by analyzing 98 patients in accordance with their HIV status.[67] The HIV-positive and HIV-negative groups differed by age (42 versus 62 years), gender (92% versus 42% males), and homosexuality (46% versus 15%). Acute treatment toxicities also differed significantly (positive, 80% versus negative, 30%). Finally, only 62% of HIV-positive patients were disease free after initial therapy as compared with 85% of HIV-negative persons. Median time to cancer-related death was also statistically significantly shorter in HIV-positive patients (1.4 as compared with 5.3 years).[67]

In the previously mentioned population-based study that utilized data from the Surveillance Epidemiology and End Results Cancer Registry, the overall 5-year survival for the entire cohort (4,841 patients) was 53%, and cancer-specific survival was 84%.[81]

Treatment and Results of Cloacogenic Carcinoma

As with all invasive anal canal cancers, classical treatment had been APR (Figure 24-14). Results following resection (without chemoradiation) have been essentially the same as that reported for epidermoid carcinoma, the 5-year survival rate being approximately 50%.[24,60,66,122] However, the applicability of the combined-modality approach is as valid for this histologic type as it is for epidermoid carcinoma, and this should be the approach to management. As has been implied by a number of authors, survival rates should be the same.

Post-therapy Evaluation and Treatment

The question of how to address the posttherapy evaluation is still a matter of some debate. Biopsy or local excision of the scar site may be performed 6 weeks after completion of the regimen. If no tumor is found, the patient is observed at intervals, perhaps every 2 to 3 months. Any suspicious area is subsequently examined by biopsy. Some surgeons prefer observation without biopsy if no suspicious area is evident. Most clinicians believe that recurrent or persistent tumor following chemoradiation therapy mandates radical resection. Others assert that an additional course of chemoradiation therapy may be warranted.[36]

It is not unusual to develop radiation-induced injury after combined-modality treatment. Problems such as stricture, fistula, and ulceration may supervene. Oral vitamin A therapy has been anecdotally suggested for those with symptomatic postradiation anal ulceration (see Chapter 28).[72]

Petrelli and colleagues reported the application of SCC antigen as a tumor marker for the follow-up of patients with carcinoma of the anal canal.[105] The procedure was initially developed and used primarily for women with carcinoma of the uterus, but its applicability for epidermoid carcinoma of the anal canal has been proposed. In the report from the Roswell Park Cancer Institute, 33 patients with histologic documentation of squamous cell carcinoma of the anal canal underwent serial collection for radioimmunoassay of SCC antigen.[105] In the 33 individuals analyzed, the sensitivity of this antigen was 76%, specificity 86%, and positive predictive value 62%. The implication of this is that with longer follow-up and greater accumulation of patients, SCC antigen may prove to be a valuable tumor marker in the long-term follow-up of individuals with squamous cell carcinoma of the anal canal.

Salvage Surgery

There are now numerous articles reporting the results of so-called "salvage" surgery following chemoradiation therapy—that is, APR. In the experience of Longo and colleagues, 53% of those who underwent APR for persistent tumor were alive.[78] Not all achieved a 5-year follow-up, however. Zelnick and co-workers analyzed 30 patients who underwent APR for treatment failures.[143] The mean follow-up was 35 months. In their experience and that of others, the mortality rate within 3 years was 71%.

Pocard and associates in Paris identified 21 patients with residual or recurrent anal canal carcinoma following radiotherapy on whom an APR had been performed.[109] Of these, 11 had residual disease following treatment, and ten subsequently developed recurrence. With a mean follow-up of 40 months, the overall survival was 58%. However, 60% of those with residual disease were alive at 5 years, whereas there were no survivors in the group that developed recurrences.[109] Clearly there is a need for adjuvant treatment in addition to APR for those who develop recurrence.

Nilsson and colleagues in Stockholm analyzed 35 individuals from the Stockholm Health Care Region who had locoregional failure after multimodality treatment and who underwent APR.[93] There were no postoperative deaths. However, there was considerable morbidity associated with healing of the perineal wound. The crude 5-year survival was 52% (median follow up, 33 months). The issue of management of the perineal wound is discussed in Chapter 23. Tei and co-workers advocated the use of a transpelvic rectus abdominis musculocutaneous flap concomitant with APR that is undertaken following radiation therapy for anal cancer.[133] Primary healing occurred in all 14 patients so managed.

Overview Opinion

The following protocol is recommended for management of carcinoma of the anal canal:

Local excision may be an adequate operation for patients with invasion into the submucosa or the internal sphincter only. Endoanal ultrasound may be useful in staging the tumor. Close follow-up evaluation should be pursued, and biopsies of suspicious areas should be undertaken. Chemoradiation therapy should be considered for recurrent tumor, with APR reserved for those in whom this therapy fails.

Those with *suspected invasion into the muscle, perirectal, or perianal soft tissue* should undergo preoperative combined-modality therapy in accordance with the Nigro protocol.

Persistent tumor following chemoradiation therapy should be managed by APR and with the possible addition of chemoradiation therapy. *Recurrent tumor* that develops during follow-up after combined-modality treatment requires APR with adjuvant therapy to the level of tolerance.

If *metastatic inguinal nodes* persist or subsequently develop following chemoradiation therapy, interval radical groin dissection should be considered.

The Nigro protocol has clearly become the standard for the treatment of anal canal cancer against which all other options must be compared. However, the optimal dosage for radiation and the timing and choices of chemotherapeutic regimens are evolving. Still, because there are now sufficient numbers of patients from many centers who have undergone combined-modality treatment for this condition, one is justified in making a dogmatic statement. Results are so impressive that unless otherwise contraindicated, contemporary medical treatment mandates that this approach be used initially for all patients with invasive anal canal cancer.

Radiation Therapy Alone

As previously discussed, squamous cell carcinoma is a radiosensitive tumor. The application of external beam radiation therapy as the sole method for the treatment of carcinoma of the anal canal, without chemotherapy, therefore, still has relevance. In a retrospective review of 51 patients who were treated with radiation therapy alone, with surgery reserved for those with residual carcinoma, Cummings and associates noted a survival rate of 59%.[27] More than one half of the patients' tumors were controlled by this approach. Twenty-three of 30 long-term survivors did not require a colostomy.

Following treatment with 45 to 50 Gy, 183 patients at the Curie Institute in Paris were examined by both the radiotherapist and the surgeon.[96] When there was evidence to suggest a lack of response, the patient underwent excisional surgery. Otherwise, the radiation treatment was carried to 60 or 65 Gy. An operation was performed only for persistent tumor or for recurrence. One hundred fifty-eight patients received curative radiotherapy, 115 of whom did not undergo operation. Eighty were alive with no evidence of disease with a minimum of 3 years of follow-up. Five-year survival was 56% for squamous cancers and 62% for cloacogenic cancers.[116]

Experience from the Mayo Clinic utilizing external radiation therapy without chemotherapy revealed that the overall 5-year survival rate was in excess of 90%.[83] However, most of these patients had very favorable initial lesions, some of which were completely excised before radiation. Still, in this group of individuals, especially, a radiation therapeutic approach without chemotherapy would seem reasonable. Touboul and colleagues advocated a treatment protocol that differentiates the approach according to tumor stage and tumor size.[134] They recommended radiation therapy alone for those individuals who harbor a tumor of 4 cm or smaller and limit chemoradiation therapy to those with larger tumors or those that are fixed. One thing is clear: chemotherapy when combined with radiation reduces the amount of radiation required. Hence, fewer late complications may be anticipated.

As with chemoradiation therapy, the options following recurrence with radiation therapy alone are essentially the same—additional nonsurgical treatment, radical resection, and local excision. Zoetmulder and Baris performed local excision with reconstitution of the anal canal by means of myocutaneous flaps.[144] The advantage of this approach is that it theoretically brings nonirradiated tissue into the field, thereby increasing the likelihood of effecting primary healing.

Interstitial Curie Therapy

In 1973, Papillon (see Chapter 23) reported 98 epidermoid carcinomas treated by interstitial Curie therapy over a 20-year period.[97] This was usually accomplished with the patient under general anesthesia and by using radium needles inserted either through the skin or the anal mucosa. The dose was less than 40 Gy in 2 or 3 days. A second implant was usually performed for residual tumor 2 months after the first implant, and external irradiation could also be given coincident with the implantation. Sixty-four patients were followed for more than 5 years, 44 of whom were alive and free of disease (68%).

James and colleagues reported their experience from Manchester, England, with 74 patients who underwent this treatment.[63] Thirty-five developed recurrences (47%), of whom 26 underwent surgery (28 with curative intent). The local control rate for patients with tumors smaller than 5 cm and with negative inguinal nodes was significantly better than that for patients with more advanced disease.

Papillon cautioned that treatment must be planned carefully to avoid radionecrosis. Later, he and Montbarbon suggested a split course of irradiation with cobalt-60 and iridium-192, and they have been adding chemotherapy during the first few days.[99]

Although selective in the choice of patients for this procedure, including only those with the most favorable prognosis, the results are encouraging and imply that this approach is worthy of further study. In a still later report from Papillon's center in Lyon, France, the following conclusion was reached: "The treatment of carcinoma of the anal margin is not as simple as it may seem to be at first sight. It should be conceived as a team effort by surgeons, radiotherapists, and medical oncologists to define the most appropriate treatment strategy."[98]

Carcinoma in a Hemorrhoidectomy Specimen

The problem of what to do when the pathologist reports a focus of carcinoma in a hemorrhoidectomy specimen is one of the quandaries that occasionally confronts the surgeon (Figs. 24-15 and 24-16). Some have criticized the technique of rubber ring ligation for hemorrhoids, because it fails to obtain a specimen that could harbor an occult neoplasm. However, the surgeon often wishes that

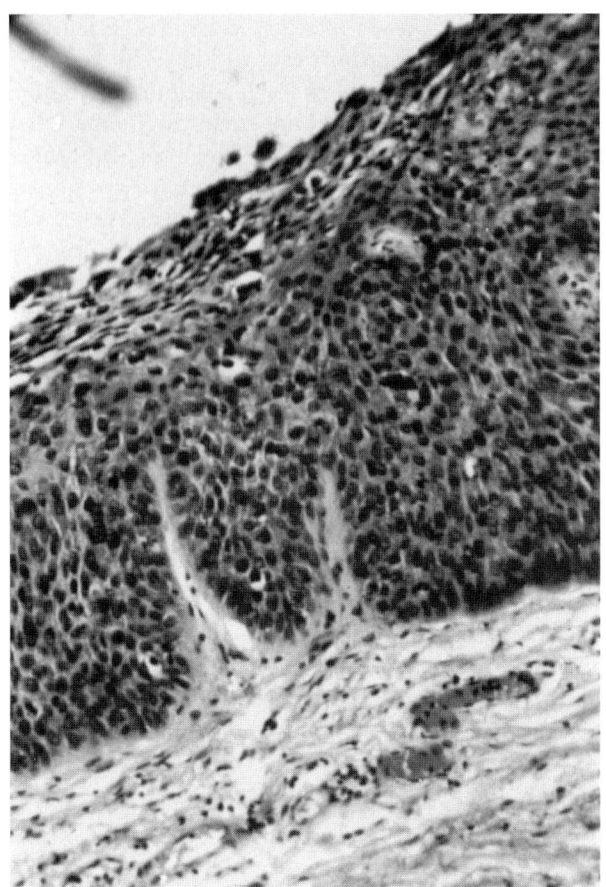

FIGURE 24-15. Squamous cell carcinoma-*in-situ*. Note the complete destruction of the architecture of the squamous epithelium with absence of maturation and preserved basement membrane. (Original magnification × 250; courtesy of Rudolf Garret, M.D.)

he or she were not aware of the focus of carcinoma, because it carries with it the burden of having to make some sort of recommendation. Some have suggested that the hemorrhoid tissue not be submitted for pathologic evaluation in order to avoid any confusion, so rare is malignant change observed and so favorable the prognosis with no treatment (see Chapter 8). However, if one is unfortunate enough to obtain a pathology report that describes the presence of *invasive* carcinoma, the microscopic appearance should at least be confirmed and the depth of invasion ascertained. It is usually not helpful to examine the patient again until the wounds are healed. Parenthetically, the presence of carcinoma-*in-situ* does not require further evaluation or treatment. The following protocol is recommended for invasive cancer:

Reexamine the patient under anesthesia in 4 to 6 weeks when the wounds are healed, and perform multiple biopsies, mapping the source in the anus from which the biopsy specimens were taken. It is always impossi-

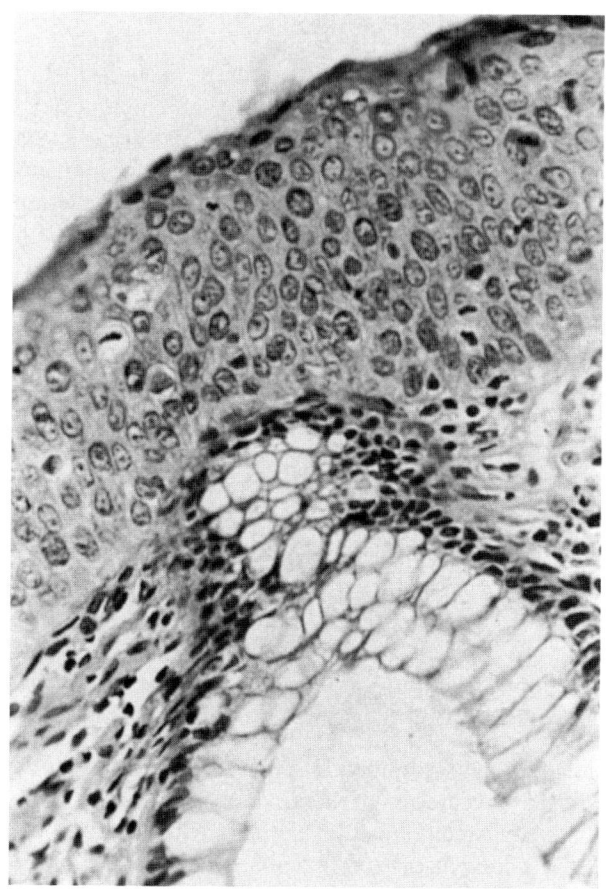

FIGURE 24-16. Squamous cell carcinoma-*in-situ* discovered in a hemorrhoidectomy specimen. Note the atypical squamous cells occupying the full thickness of the epithelium. Normally, surface mucosa consists of columnar cells, as in the gland seen here. (Original magnification × 250; from Corman ML, Viedenheimer MC, Swinton NW. *Diseases of the anus, rectum and colon. Part I: neoplasms.* New York: Medcom, 1972, with permission.)

ble to know from which site the hemorrhoid tissue harboring the tumor was obtained.

If results of the biopsies are negative, follow the patient's status at 3-month intervals for 1 year, and perform a biopsy of any suspicious areas.

If no recurrence develops by 1 year, the patient is considered cured. If a recurrence is identified, the patient may be considered for local excision or the standard therapy protocol for anal canal carcinoma.

MALIGNANT MELANOMA

Although the anal canal represents the most common site for the development of malignant melanoma in the alimentary tract, it is an extremely rare condition, accounting for only 0.2% of all melanomas and 0.5% of tumors of the anorectum.[10] The tumor is presumed to arise from melanocytes present in the squamous mucosa of the lower anal canal. Mason and Helwig reviewed 17 cases seen at the Armed Forces Institute of Pathology in Washington, DC, and concluded that all the evidence argued against any melanoma arising from the rectal mucosa.[84] Other authors, however, have claimed that melanoma may be primary in the lower rectum as well as in the anal canal.[2] Cooper and associates analyzed 255 cases and added 12 of their own, but fewer than 500 cases had been reported as of 1982.[21] The largest series from one institution is from the Memorial Sloan-Kettering Cancer Center.[3,113] The most recent paper, presented in 1994 and published in 1995, reviewed their experience from 1929 to 1993.[10] A total of 85 patients was identified: 46 female and 39 male. Others have shown a higher incidence of female predominance (2.4:1).[127] Goldman and colleagues analyzed the total Swedish population between 1970 and 1984 and found 49 people with this disease.[46]

Cagir and associates of Jefferson Medical College in Philadelphia utilized the National Cancer Institute Surveillance, Epidemiology, and End Results database covering the period 1973 through 1992.[15] They identified 117 patients. This represents 0.048% of all colorectal malignancies. The male-to-female ratio was 1:1.72, and the mean age at diagnosis was 66 years, but men tended to be younger. There is a suggestion from this study that there is an increased predisposition to the development of malignant melanoma perhaps in a less virulent form in the HIV-positive population, but these observations require more data.

Symptoms

Rectal bleeding is the commonest complaint, 54% in the Memorial Sloan-Kettering Cancer Center series.[3,10] Anorectal pain and change in bowel habits are also frequently reported. Many patients note a feeling of a lump or a "hemorrhoid," with its attendant discomfort. A mass in the groin may also be the initial complaint. In the experience of the Memorial Sloan-Kettering Cancer Center, 8% had the melanoma discovered upon pathologic review of hemorrhoidectomy specimens.[10]

Physical Findings

Findings on physical examination vary from a small, hemorrhoidlike, pigmented lesion to a deeply ulcerating or polypoid mass at or near the anorectal junction (Figure 24-17). Pigment may be readily apparent, but Quan and associates reported that 29% of these lesions were histologically amelanotic, an incidence similar to that noted by Cooper and colleagues.[10,21,113] In the Sloan-Kettering experience, an indication of the advanced stage of the disease and, therefore, the poor prognosis was reflected by the fact that 75% of individuals harbored tumors

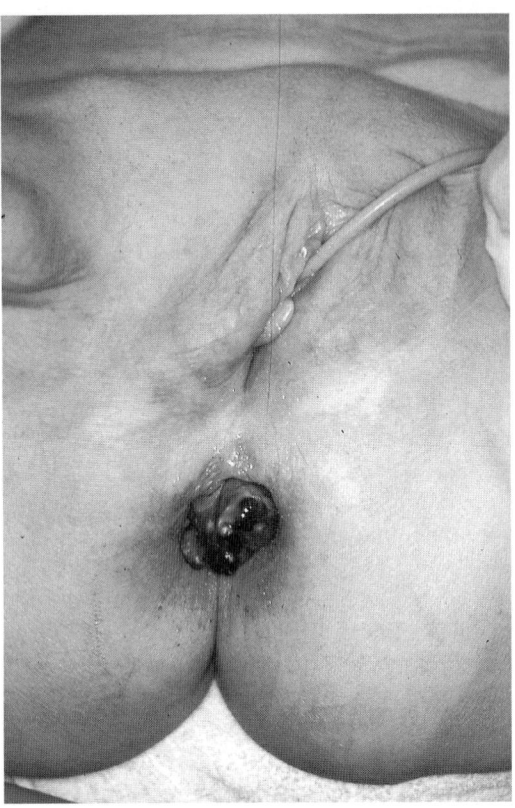

FIGURE 24-17. Malignant melanoma of the anus. A pigmented polypoid mass can be seen outside the anal verge. (See Color Fig. 24-17.)

greater than 1 cm in diameter (average, 4 cm). A later report revealed the median tumor size in individuals undergoing APR to be 3.0 cm.[10] This compared with a median tumor size of 3.3 cm in individuals undergoing local procedures.[3]

Histology

Cells comprising the lesion usually assume either a polygonal or a spindle shape (Figs. 24-18 through 24-21) and are often arranged in nests to produce an alveolar pattern. If the mucosa overlying the lesion is not ulcerated, evidence of a junctional component, such as nests of melanoma cells within the squamous epithelium, may be found. This finding confirms the squamous mucosa of the anal canal as the primary site of origin. Identification of melanin within the tumor cells permits diagnosis of the lesion as a melanoma rather than as a poorly differentiated carcinoma. Melanin pigmentation was readily apparent in 11 of the 17 tumors reported by Mason and Helwig and was demonstrable by special staining techniques in four additional lesions.[84] Electron microscopy can be of value in identifying apparently amelanotic melanomas by demonstrating melanosomes within the tumor cells.

Treatment and Results

Because anorectal melanoma is more likely to metastasize to mesenteric lymph nodes than squamous cell carcinoma of the anus, APR (Figure 24-21) has been the standard of treatment. This and radical groin lymph node dissection had been the mainstays of surgical therapies for this condition. However, because the prognosis has been so grim, a case has been made for either no treatment at all or simply local excision.[114] Several reports have noted no statistically significant difference in survival rate of patients treated for cure by local excision versus APR.[11,21,127] As a consequence wide local excision for a tumor that can be removed by this method is frequently suggested.[11,82] The major benefit of radical resection may be for controlling local and regional disease.[46,127] Quan and associates reported one survivor (5%),[113] and most other series report either none or only the occasional cure at 5 years.[5,9,18,22,39,114,123,127,138] Bullard and Tuttle in Minneapolis, Minnesota, noted that two patients out of seven (29%) were alive at 5 years.[11] Based on the Memorial Sloan-Kettering experience, two conclusions were set forth:[10]

Most patients with anorectal melanoma will die of their disease regardless of therapy.
There is a small subset of patients with localized, relatively early disease or favorable tumor biology in whom a surgical cure can be achieved.

The Memorial Sloan-Kettering group, therefore, opined that APR with pelvic lymphadenectomy is a reasonable alternative for those individuals without locally advanced tumors or evidence of regional lymph node involvement. In these patients, they emphasized the importance of pelvic lymphadenectomy. One pertinent observation was that all of their long-term survivors were women. It appears that female sex was a favorable prognostic factor in individuals with cutaneous melanoma as well. Women with operable melanoma of the anus according to the criteria set forth by the Memorial Sloan-Kettering Cancer group have a 29% survival following APR. However, the previously mentioned report by Cagir and co-workers, based upon 117 patients in the National Cancer Institute Registry, found that male patients (especially young and positive for HIV) do better than female patients, but it appears that age rather than sex is the more important variable.[15] The overall survival rate in both sexes was less than 20% at 5 years.

Supplementary treatment with radiotherapy has been of no consistent benefit, nor have the various chemotherapeutic agents uniformly helped. Immunotherapy, usually with bacille Calmette-Guérin vaccine, has been employed for malignant melanoma in other sites, but recommendations concerning its value with malignant melanoma of the anal canal have been anecdotal and dis-

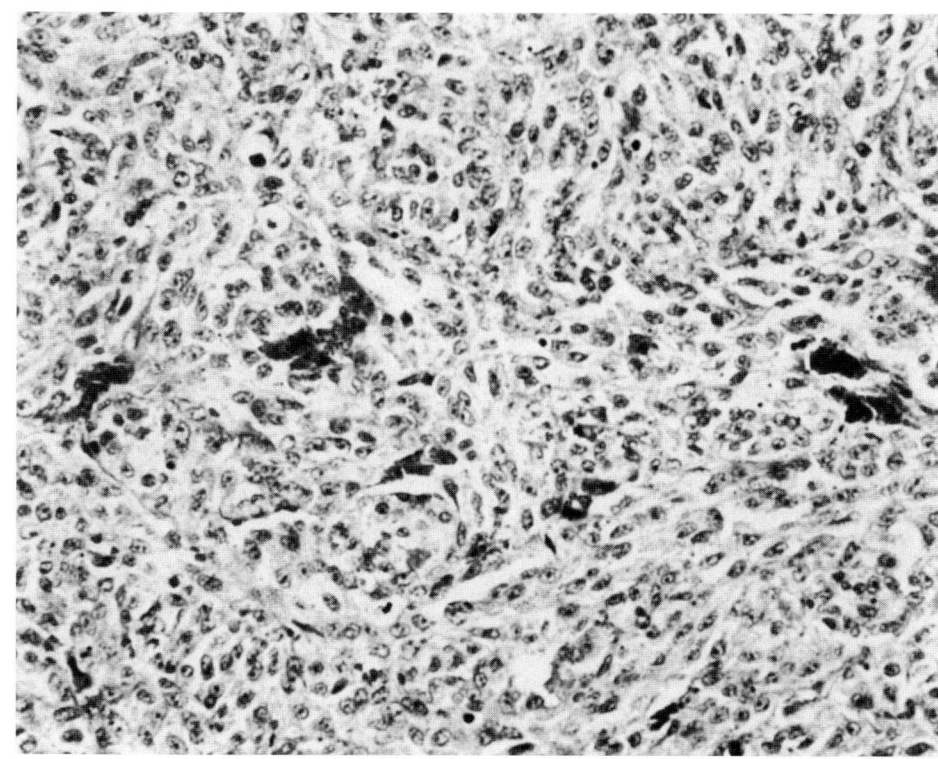

FIGURE 24-18. Melanoma of the anus. This very poorly differentiated tumor is recognizable as a melanoma only because of the black pigment being produced. (Original magnification × 250.)

couraging. Most investigators, however, recommend an aggressive multimodality approach, but there has been no consistency in the patient selection, pathologic extent, or treatment employed with the relatively few long-term survivors reported.

MISCELLANEOUS ANAL CONDITIONS

Verrucous Squamous Carcinoma

A very rare tumor, verrucous squamous carcinoma, has come to be known as the tumor of Buschke and Löwenstein because of their description of it in 1925.[14] The lesion is frequently confused with benign anal conditions, especially condyloma (see Chapter 19). It may appear as a pale, pink, cauliflowerlike mass on the perianal skin or in the anal canal (see Figure 19-54).

Histologically, the tumor is so well differentiated that it closely resembles benign proliferative lesions of squamous epithelium, and it may not be recognizable as a carcinoma until invasion of underlying structures can be identified. For this reason, superficial biopsies of verrucous squamous cell carcinomas are frequently not diagnosed as carcinoma. Biopsies should be taken from the base of the lesion to demonstrate invasion.

Classical treatment consists of wide local excision or APR for invasive tumors.[42,76,130] However, the value of combined-modality therapy needs to be explored (for additional discussion, see Chapter 19).

Keratoacanthoma

Keratoacanthoma is an exophytic, benign skin tumor, usually with a central crater, 0.5 to 2.0 cm in diameter, that is most often associated with exposure to the sun.[64] Only three cases involving the perianal skin and one in the anal canal have been reported.[64] Local excision or electrocoagulation should be curative, although the histologic appearance may mimic that of squamous cell carcinoma.

Pseudosarcomatous Carcinoma

Pseudosarcoma has been described in the esophagus, larynx, oral cavity, and other areas, but Kuwano and associates reported the first and only case of such a tumor in the anal canal.[69] The patient presented with a pedunculated 4-cm mass. Microscopic examination of the locally excised specimen revealed epithelial elements in sarcomalike areas. No recurrence was noted after a 25-month follow-up.

Carcinoma of the Anal Glands and Ducts

Colloid or mucinous adenocarcinoma of anal glandular or ductal origin is a rare entity.[56,140,141] Parks stated, however, that although the condition is extremely uncommon, it may not be as infrequent as the literature suggests.[101] This, he postulated, is explained by the fact that the site of origin is destroyed early by the malignant

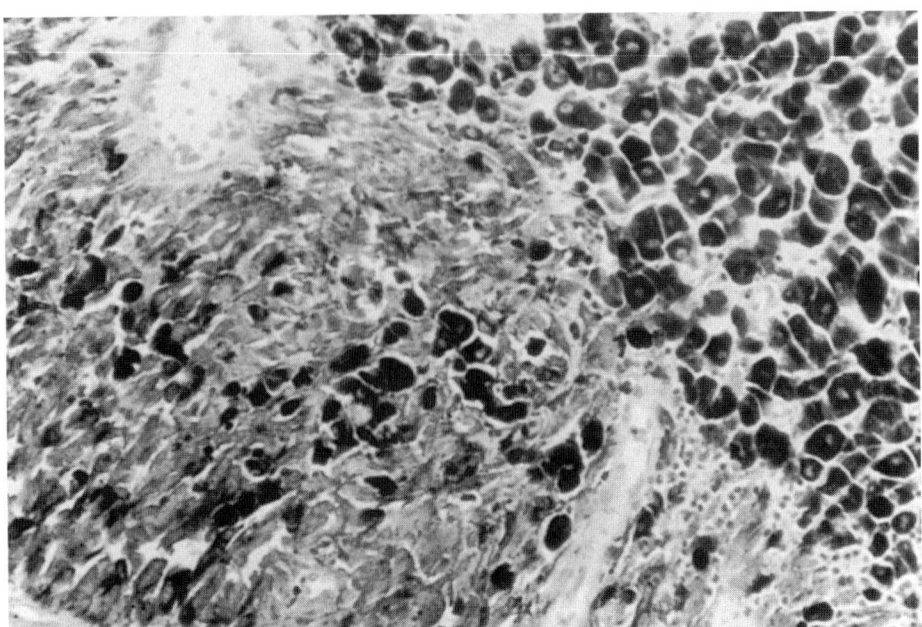

FIGURE 24-19. Melanoma of the anal canal. Another variant displaying an epithelioid pattern with extensive melanin pigment present. (Original magnification × 360.)

growth. Lindkaer Jensen and colleagues identified 21 individuals treated from Denmark from 1943 to 1982.[74] Nine lesions were found in a perianal location, seven within the anal canal, and five in anal fistulas. Three were found serendipitously in hemorrhoidectomy specimens. The presence of Paget's disease may be a consequence of an underlying carcinoma, such as can arise from the anal ducts (see Chapter 19).

Abel and colleagues surveyed the members of the American Society and Colon and Rectal Surgeons and identified 52 cases for analysis.[1] Symptoms of anal pain were found in 58% and rectal bleeding in 40%. Thirty-seven percent perceived a mass, whereas more than half presented with a fistula.

Treatment

Because this is a highly malignant variant, APR is usually recommended. Local excision, however, may be considered for early lesions, but radical resection is generally required to control disease.[1] The place of chemoradiation therapy is probably similar to that of conventional ade-

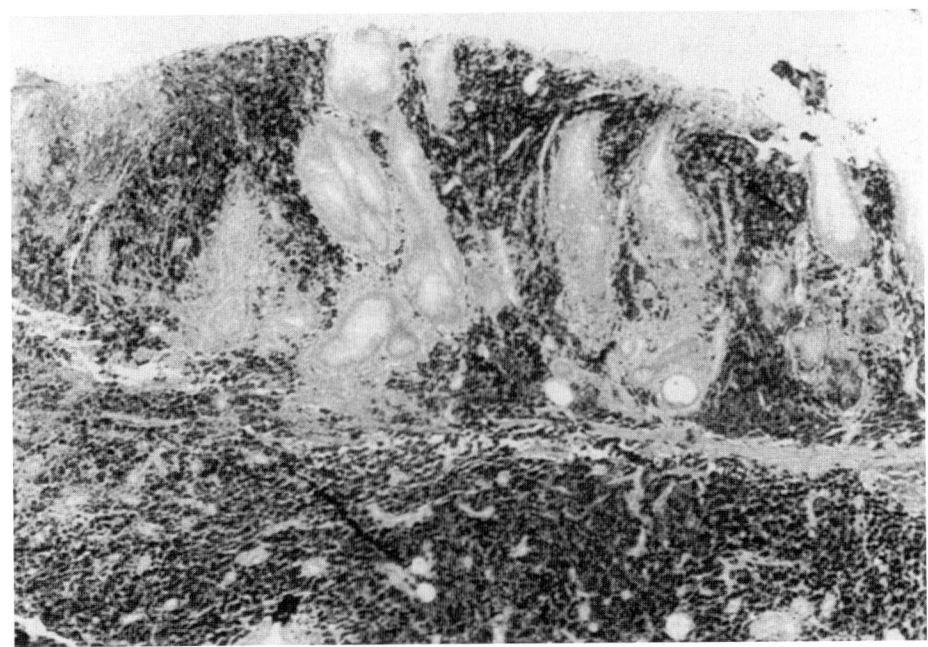

FIGURE 24-20. Malignant melanoma of the anus reveals sheets of melanin-pigmented cells infiltrating the mucosa and submucosa of the lower rectum. Foci of residual glands may still be seen. (Original magnification × 250.)

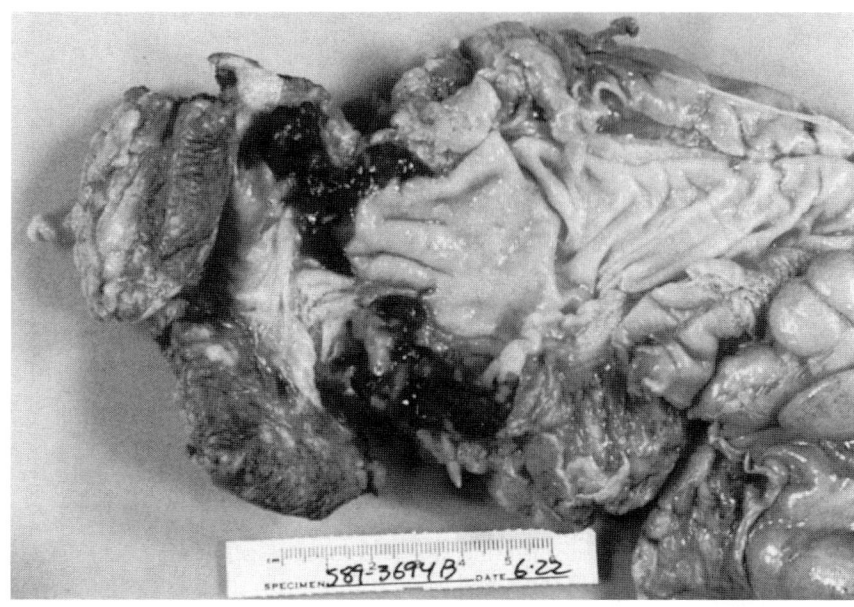

FIGURE 24-21. Proctectomy specimen reveals densely melanotic pigmentation of a practically circumferential lesion of the anal canal.

nocarcinoma of the rectum, but this has not been clearly defined. The Memorial Sloan-Kettering Cancer Center group in 2003 treated 13 patients with primary adencarcinoma of the anal canal with three operative and chemoradiation therapy alternatives.[7] In a relatively short-term follow-up and with a small number of patients with this unusual tumor, the authors concluded that a combined-therapy approach is reasonable.

Results

Basik and co-workers reviewed the prognosis of anal adenocarcinoma from the Roswell Park Cancer Institute.[4] Eight patients underwent radical resection and two local excision. Median survival was 29 months, with seven patients developing recurrence. It is evident that anal adenocarcinoma is associated with a poor prognosis despite radical surgery.

Adenosquamous Carcinoma

This rare tumor of the large bowel can even more rarely affect the anal canal. The condition is discussed in Chapter 25.

Merkel Cell (Neuroendocrine) Carcinoma

Merkel cell tumors are rare neuroendocrine, small cell malignancies usually found on the skin, most commonly on exposed surfaces. These tumors behave aggressively when found in less typical areas.[102] A single example of this condition affecting the anal canal has been re-

ported.[102] In this one instance that was treated by local excision, the patient died 13 months later of metastatic disease. Neuroendocrine tumors affecting the colon and rectum are discussed in Chapter 25.

Malignant Fibrous Histiocytoma

Malignant fibrous histiocytoma is a pleiomorphic sarcoma that classically arises in the extremities and metastasizes to the lungs and regional lymph nodes, but it also can occur rarely in the gastrointestinal tract.[37] Flood and colleagues identified the first and only case involving the anal canal.[37] This was managed by APR and radiotherapy.

Inflammatory Cloacogenic Polyp

Inflammatory cloacogenic polyp is a nonneoplastic anal tumor that may be analogous to a prolapse in the area of the transitional zone. Lobert and Appelman identified eight such cases and noted that the primary complaint is usually rectal bleeding.[75] The polyp in their experience was found primarily on the anterior wall of the anal canal, not unlike the distribution seen in solitary rectal ulcer (see Chapter 17). However, in the eight cases identified by Lobert and Appelman, instead of the usual female predominance, there were five men.[75] The etiology of the condition is uncertain, but theories include ischemia, trauma (manual, stercoral), congenital, and early prolapse. Histologically, the lesion is characterized by a tubulovillous pattern of growth, superficial ulceration, displaced crypts, and extension of chronically inflamed fibromuscular stroma into the lamina propria (Figure 24-22).[75] Treatment consists simply of local excision.

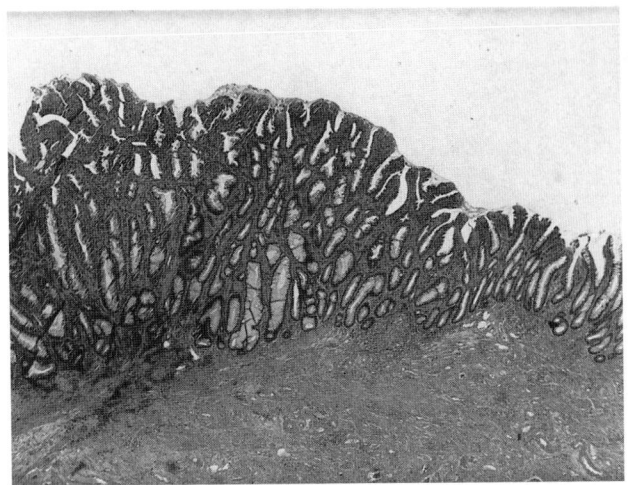
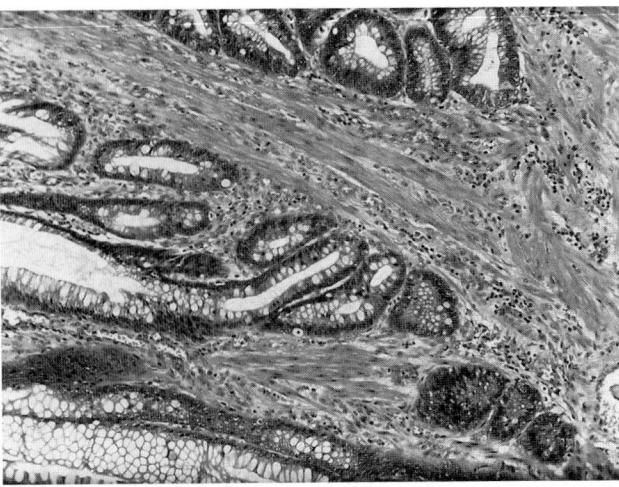

FIGURE 24-22. Inflammatory cloacogenic polyp. **(A)** Nonulcerated surface showing glandular hyperplasia with a thickened submucosa. (Original magnification × 20.) **(B)** Higher power demonstrates colonic glands and inflammatory cells with muscle bundles extending between the glands into the submucosa. (Original magnification × 100.)

Basal Cell Carcinoma, Bowen's Disease, and Paget's Disease

See Chapter 19.

REFERENCES

1. Abel ME, Chiu YSY, Russell TR, et al. Adenocarcinoma of the anal glands: results of a survey. *Dis Colon Rectum* 1993; 36: 383.
2. Alexander RM, Cone LA. Malignant melanoma of the rectal ampulla: report of a case and review of the literature. *Dis Colon Rectum* 1977;20:53.
3. Banner WP, Quan SHQ, Woodruff JM. Malignant melanoma of the anorectum. *Surg Rounds* 1990;13:28.
4. Basik M, Rodriguez-Bigas MA, Penetrante R, et al. Prognosis and recurrence patterns of anal adenocarcinoma. *Am J Surg* 1995;169:233.
5. Baskies AM, Sugarbaker EV, Chretien PB, et al. Anorectal melanoma: the role of posterior pelvic exenteration. *Dis Colon Rectum* 1982;25:772.
6. Beahrs OH, Wilson SM. Carcinoma of the anus. *Ann Surg* 1976;184:422.
7. Beal KP, Wong D, Guillem JG, et al. Primary adenocarcinoma of the anus treated with combined modality therapy. *Dis Colon Rectum* 2003;46:1320.
8. Beck DE, Karulf RE. Combination therapy for epidermoid carcinoma of the anal canal. *Dis Colon Rectum* 1994;37: 1118.
9. Braastad FW, Dockerty MB, Dixon CF. Melano-epithelioma of anus and rectum: report of cases and review of literature. *Surgery* 1949;25:82.
10. Brady MS, Kavolius JP, Quan SHQ. Anorectal melanoma: a 64-year experience at Memorial Sloan-Kettering Cancer Center. *Dis Colon Rectum* 1995;38:146.
11. Bullard KM, Tuttle TM, Rothenberger DA, et al. Surgical therapy for anorectal melanoma. *J Am Coll Surg* 2003;196: 206.
12. Buroker TR, Nigro N, Bradley G, et al. Combined therapy for cancer of the anal canal: a follow-up report. *Dis Colon Rectum* 1977;20:677.
13. Buroker T, Nigro N, Correa J, et al. Combination preoperative radiation and chemotherapy in adenocarcinoma of the rectum: preliminary report. *Dis Colon Rectum* 1976; 19:660.
14. Buschke A, Loewenstein L. Condylomata acuminata simulating cancer on penis. *Klin Wochenschr* 1925;4:1726.
15. Cagir B, Whiteford MH, Topham A, et al. Changing epidemiology of anorectal melanoma. *Dis Colon Rectum* 1999; 42:1203.
16. Cattell RB, Williams AC. Epidermoid carcinoma of the anus and rectum. *Arch Surg* 1943;46:336.
17. Chang GJ, Berry JM, Jay N, et al. Surgical treatment of high-grade anal squamous intraepithelial lesions: a prospective study. *Dis Colon Rectum* 2002;45:453.
18. Chiu YS, Unni KK, Beart RW Jr. Malignant melanoma of the anorectum. *Dis Colon Rectum* 1980;23:122.
19. Cho CC, Taylor CW III, Padmanabhan A, et al. Squamous-cell carcinoma of the anal canal: management with combined chemo-radiation therapy. *Dis Colon Rectum* 1991;34: 675.
20. Cooper HS, Patchefsky AS, Marks G. Cloacogenic carcinoma of the anorectum in homosexual men: an observation of four cases. *Dis Colon Rectum* 1979;22:557.
21. Cooper PH, Mills SE, Allen MS Jr. Malignant melanoma of the anus; report of 12 patients and analysis of 255 additional cases. *Dis Colon Rectum* 1982;25:693.
22. Corman ML, Haggitt RC. Carcinoma of the anal canal. *Surg Gynecol Obstet* 1977;145:674.
23. Corman ML, Veidenheimer MC, Swinton NW. *Diseases of the anus, rectum and colon. Part I: neoplasms.* New York: Medcom, 1972.
24. Cullen PK Jr, Pontius EE, Sanders RJ. Cloacogenic anorectal carcinoma. *Dis Colon Rectum* 1966;9:1.
25. Cummings B, Keane T, Thomas G, et al. Results and toxicity of the treatment of anal canal carcinoma by radiation therapy or radiation therapy and chemotherapy. *Cancer* 1984;54:2062.
26. Cummings BJ, Harwood AR, Keane TJ, et al. Combined treatment of squamous cell carcinoma of the anal canal: radical radiation therapy with 5-fluorouracil and mitomycin-C, a preliminary report. *Dis Colon Rectum* 1980;23: 389.
27. Cummings BJ, Thomas GM, Keane TJ, et al. Primary radiation therapy in the treatment of anal canal carcinoma. *Dis Colon Rectum* 1982;25:778.
28. Daling JR, Weiss NS, Hislop TG, et al. Sexual practices, sexually transmitted diseases, and the incidence of anal cancer. *N Engl J Med* 1987;217:973.
29. Daling JR, Weiss NS, Klopfenstein LL, et al. Correlates of homosexual behavior and the incidence of anal cancer. *JAMA* 1982;247:1988.

30. Damin DC, Rosito MA, Gus P, et al. Sentinel lymph node procedure in patients with epidermoid carcinoma of the anal canal: early experience. *Dis Colon Rectum* 2003;46: 1032.
31. Deans GT, McAleer JJA, Spence RAJ. Malignant anal tumors. *Br J Surg* 1994;81:500.
32. DeGennaro VA, Grossi C, Nealon T Jr. Anorectal malignancy in male homosexuals. *Surg Rounds* 1986;9:82.
33. Doci R, Zucali R, Bombelli L, et al. Combined chemoradiation therapy for anal cancer: a report of 56 cases. *Ann Surg* 1992;215:150.
34. Enker WE, Heilwell M, Janov AJ, et al. Improved survival in epidermoid carcinoma of the anus in association with preoperative multidisciplinary therapy. *Arch Surg* 1986; 121:1386.
35. Failes D, Morgan BP. Squamous-cell carcinoma of the anus. *Dis Colon Rectum* 1973;16:397.
36. Flam MS, John MJ, Lovalvo LJ, et al. Definitive combined modality therapy of carcinoma of the anus: a report of 30 cases including results of salvage therapy in patients with residual disease. *Dis Colon Rectum* 1987;30:495.
37. Flood HD, Salman AA. Malignant fibrous histiocytoma of the anal canal: report of a case and review of the literature. *Dis Colon Rectum* 1989;32:256.
38. Fontana X, Lagrange JL, Francois E, et al. Assessment of "squamous cell carcinoma antigen" (SCC) as a marker of epidermoid carcinoma of the anal canal. *Dis Colon Rectum* 1991;34:126.
39. Freedman LS. Malignant melanoma of the anorectal region: two cases of prolonged survival. *Br J Surg* 1984;71: 164.
40. Frisch M, Olsen JH, Bautz A, et al. Benign anal lesions and the risk of anal cancer. *N Engl J Med* 1994;331:300.
41. Gillespie JJ, MacKay B. Histogenesis of cloacogenic carcinoma: fine structure of anal transitional epithelium and cloacogenic carcinoma. *Hum Pathol* 1978;9:579.
42. Gingrass PJ, Bubrick MP, Hitchcock CR, et al. Anorectal verrucose squamous carcinoma: report of two cases. *Dis Colon Rectum* 1978;21:120.
43. Golden GT, Horsley JS III. Surgical management of epidermoid carcinoma of the anus. *Am J Surg* 1976;131:275.
44. Goldman S, Auer G, Erhardt K, et al. Prognostic significance of clinical stage, histologic grade, and nuclear DNA content in squamous-cell carcinoma of the anus. *Dis Colon Rectum* 1987;30:444.
45. Goldman S, Glimelius B, Glas U, et al. Management of anal epidermoid carcinoma: an evaluation of treatment results in two population-based series. *Int J Colorectal Dis* 1989; 4:234.
46. Goldman S, Glimelius B, Påhlman L. Anorectal malignant melanoma in Sweden: report of 49 patients. *Dis Colon Rectum* 1990;33:874.
47. Goldman S, Ihre TH, Seligson U. Squamous-cell carcinoma of the anus: a follow-up study of 65 patients. *Dis Colon Rectum* 1985;28:143.
48. Goldman S, Skoog L, Wilking N. Immunocytochemical analysis of receptors for estrogen and progesterone in fine needle aspirates from anal epidermoid carcinoma. *Dis Colon Rectum* 1992;35:163.
49. Goldstone SE, Winkler B, Ufford LJ, et al. High prevalence of anal squamous intraepithelial lesions and squamous-cell carcinoma in men who have sex with men as seen in a surgical practice. *Dis Colon Rectum* 2001;44:690.
50. Greenall MJ, Quan SHQ, DeCosse JJ. Epidermoid cancer of the anus. *Br J Surg* 1985;72:97.
51. Greenall MJ, Quan SHQ, Stearns MW, et al. Epidermoid cancer of the anal margin. *Am J Surg* 1985;149:95.
52. Greenall MJ, Quan SHQ, Urmacher C, et al. Treatment of epidermoid carcinoma of the anal canal. *Surg Gynecol Obstet* 1985;161:509.
53. Grinnell RS. An analysis of 49 cases of squamous cell carcinoma of the anus. *Surg Gynecol Obstet* 1954;98:29.
54. Grinvalsky HT, Helwig EB. Carcinoma of the anorectal junction: histological considerations. *Cancer* 1956;9:480.
55. Habr-Gama A, da Silva e Sousa AH Jr, Nadalin W, et al. Epidermoid carcinoma of the anal canal: results of treatment by combined chemotherapy and radiation therapy. *Dis Colon Rectum* 1989;32:773.
56. Hagihara P, Vazquez MT, Parker JC, et al. Carcinoma of anal duct origin: report of a case. *Dis Colon Rectum* 1976;19:694.
57. Hamdan KA, Tait IS, Nadeau V, et al. Treatment of Grade III anal intraepithelial neoplasia with photodynamic therapy. *Dis Colon Rectum* 2003;46:1555.
58. Hobbes CM, Lowry MA, Owen D, et al. Anal gland carcinoma. *Cancer* 2001;92:2045.
59. Holmes F, Borek D, Owen-Kummer M, et al. Anal cancer in women. *Gastroenterology* 1988;95:107.
60. Hsu Y-H, Guzman LG. Cloacogenic carcinoma of the anal canal-Experience in eight cases and review of the literature. *Am J Proctol Gastroenterol Colon Rectal Surg* 1984; 35:5.
61. Hu K, Minsky BD, Cohen AM, et al. 30 Gy may be an adequate dose in patients with anal cancer treated with excisional biopsy followed by combined-modality therapy. *J Surg Oncol* 1999;70:71.
62. Ioachim HL, Weinstein MA, Robbins RD, et al. Primary anorectal lymphoma: a new manifestation of the acquired immune deficiency syndrome (AIDS). *Cancer* 1987;60: 1449.
63. James RD, Pointon RS, Martin S. Local radiotherapy in the management of squamous carcinoma of the anus. *Br J Surg* 1985;72:282.
64. Jensen SL, Sjolin K-E. Keratoacanthoma of the anus: report of three cases. *Dis Colon Rectum* 1985;28:743.
65. Kalogeropoulos NK, Antonakopoulos GN, Agapitos MB, et al. Spindle cell carcinoma (pseudosarcoma) of the anus: a light, electron microscopic and immunocytochemical study of a case. *Histopathology* 1985;9:987.
66. Kheir S, Hickey RC, Martin RG. Cloacogenic carcinoma of the anal canal. *Arch Surg* 1972;104:407.
67. Kim JH, Sarani B, Orkin BA, et al. HIV-positive patients with anal carcinoma have poorer treatment tolerance and outcome than HIV-negative patients. *Dis Colon Rectum* 2001;44:1496.
68. Klotz RG Jr, Pamukcoglu T, Souilliard DH. Transitional cloacogenic carcinoma of the anal canal: clinicopathologic study of three hundred seventy three cases. *Cancer* 1967; 20:1727.
69. Kuwano H, Iwashita A, Enjoji M. Pseudosarcomatous carcinoma of the anal canal. *Dis Colon Rectum* 1983;26:123.
70. Lee MH, Waxman M, Gillooley JF. Primary malignant lymphoma of the anorectum in homosexual men. *Dis Colon Rectum* 1986;29:413.
71. Leichman L, Nigro N, Vaitkevicius VK, et al. Cancer of the anal canal: model for preoperative adjuvant combined modality therapy. *Am J Med* 1985;78:211.
72. Levitsky J, Hong JJ, Jani AB, et al. Oral vitamin A therapy for a patient with a severely symptomatic postradiation anal ulceration: report of a case. *Dis Colon Rectum* 2003; 46:679.
73. Li FP, Osborn D, Cronin CM. Anorectal squamous carcinoma in two homosexual men. *Lancet* 1982;2:391.
74. Lindkaer Jensen S, Shokouh-Amiri MH, Hagen K, et al. Adenocarcinoma of the anal ducts: a series of 21 cases. *Dis Colon Rectum* 1988;31:268.
75. Lobert PF, Appelman HD. Inflammatory cloacogenic polyp: a unique inflammatory lesion of the anal transitional zone. *Am J Surg* Pathol 1981;5:761.
76. Lock MR, Katz DR, Samoorian S, et al. Giant condyloma of the rectum: report of a case. *Dis Colon Rectum* 1977; 20:154.
77. Löhnert M, Doniec JM, Kovács G, et al. New method of radiotherapy for anal cancer with three-dimensional tumor reconstruction based on endoanal ultrasound and ultrasound-guided afterloading therapy. *Dis Colon Rectum* 1998;41:169.
78. Longo WE, Vernava AM III, Wade TP, et al. Recurrent squamous cell carcinoma of the anal canal: predictors of initial treatment failure and results of salvage therapy. *Ann Surg* 1994;220:40.

79. Lorenz HP, Wilson W, Leigh B, et al. Squamous cell carcinoma of the anus and HIV infection. *Dis Colon Rectum* 1991;34:336.

80. Madden MV, Elliot MS, Botha JBC, et al. The management of anal carcinoma. *Br J Surg* 1981;68:287.

81. Maggard MA, Beanes SR, Ko CY. Anal canal cancer: a population-based reappraisal. *Dis Colon Rectum* 2003;46:1517.

82. Malik A, Hull TL, Milsom J. Long-term survivor of anorectal melanoma: report of a case. *Dis Colon Rectum* 2002;45:1412.

83. Martenson JA, Gunderson LL. External radiation therapy without chemotherapy in the management of anal cancer. *Cancer* 1993;71:1736.

84. Mason JK, Helwig EB. Ano-rectal melanoma. *Cancer* 1966;19:39.

85. Melbye M, Coté TR, Kessler L, et al. High incidence of anal cancer among AIDS patients. *Lancet* 1994;343:636.

86. Mendenhall WM, Zlotecki RA, Vauthey J-N, et al. Squamous cell carcinoma of the anal margin. *Oncology* 1996;10:1843.

87. Morson BC, Pang LSC. Pathology of anal cancer. *Proc R Soc Med* 1968;61:623.

88. Morson BC, Volkstadt H. Muco-epidermoid tumours of the anal canal. *J Clin Pathol* 1963;16:200.

89. Muleris M, Salmon RJ, Giordet J, et al. Recurrent deletions of chromosome 11q and 3p in anal canal carcinoma. *Int J Cancer* 1987;39:595.

90. Nash G, Allen W, Nash S. Atypical lesions of the anal mucosa in homosexual men. *JAMA* 1986;256:873.

91. Nigro ND. An evaluation of combined therapy for squamous cell cancer of the anal canal. *Dis Colon Rectum* 1984;27:763.

92. Nigro ND, Vaitkevicius VK, Buroker T, et al. Combined therapy for cancer of anal canal. *Dis Colon Rectum* 1981;24:73.

93. Nilsson PJ, Svensson C, Goldman S, et al. Salvage abdominoperineal resection in anal epidermoid cancer. *Br J Surg* 2002;89:1425.

94. Nigro ND, Vaitkevicius VK, Considine B Jr. Combined therapy for cancer of the anal canal: a preliminary report. *Dis Colon Rectum* 1974;17:354.

95. Palmer JG, Scholefield JH, Coates PJ, et al. Anal cancer and human papillomaviruses. *Dis Colon Rectum* 1989;32:1016.

96. Pang LS, Morson BC. Basaloid carcinoma of the anal canal. *J Clin Pathol* 1967;20:128.

97. Papillon J. Radiation therapy in the management of epidermoid carcinoma of the anal region. *Dis Colon Rectum* 1974;17:181.

98. Papillon J, Chassard JL. Respective roles of radiotherapy and surgery in the management of epidermoid carcinoma of the anal margin: series of 57 patients. *Dis Colon Rectum* 1992;35:422.

99. Papillon J, Montbarbon JF. Epidermoid carcinoma of the anal canal: a series of 276 cases. *Dis Colon Rectum* 1987;30:324.

100. Paradis P, Douglass HO Jr, Holyoke ED. The clinical implications of a staging system for carcinoma of the anus. *Surg Gynecol Obstet* 1975;141:411.

101. Parks TG. Mucus-secreting adenocarcinoma of anal gland origin. *Br J Surg* 1970;57:434.

102. Paterson C, Musselman L, Chorneyko K, et al. Merkel cell (neuroendocrine) carcinoma of the anal canal: report of a case. *Dis Colon Rectum* 2003;46:676.

103. Penn I. Cancers of the anogenital region in renal transplant recipients. *Cancer* 1986;58:611.

104. Perera D, Pathma-Nathan N, Rabbit P, et al. Sentinel node biopsy for squamous-cell carcinoma of the anus and anal margin. *Dis Colon Rectum* 2003;46:1027.

105. Petrelli NJ, Cebollero JA, Rodriguez-Bigas M, et al. Photodynamic therapy in the management of neoplasms of the perianal skin. *Arch Surg* 1992;127:1436.

106. Petrelli NJ, Palmer M, Herrera L, et al. The utility of squamous cell carcinoma antigen for the follow-up of patients with squamous cell carcinoma of the anal canal. *Cancer* 1992;70:35.

107. Pinna Pintor M, Northover JMA, Nicholls RJ. Squamous cell carcinoma of the anus at one hospital from 1948 to 1984. *Br J Surg* 1989;76:806.

108. Place RJ, Gregorcyk SG, Huber PJ, et al. Outcome analysis of HIV-positive patients with anal squamous cell carcinoma. *Dis Colon Rectum* 2001;44:506.

109. Pocard M, Tiret E, Nugent K, et al. Results of salvage abdominoperineal resection for anal cancer after radiotherapy. *Dis Colon Rectum* 1998;41:1488.

110. Pyper PC, Parks TG. The results of surgery for epidermoid carcinoma of the anus. *Br J Surg* 1985;72:712.

111. Quan SHQ. Anal and para-anal tumors. *Surg Clin North Am* 1978;58:591.

112. Quan SHQ, Magill GB, Leaming RH, et al. Multidisciplinary preoperative approach to the management of epidermoid carcinoma of the anus and anorectum. *Dis Colon Rectum* 1978;21:89.

113. Quan SHQ, White JE, Deddish MR. Malignant melanoma of the anorectum. *Dis Colon Rectum* 1959;2:275.

114. Ross M, Pezzi C, Pezz T, et al. Patterns of failure in anorectal melanoma; a guide to surgical therapy. *Arch Surg* 1990;125:313.

115. Salmon RJ, Fenton J, Asselain B, et al. Treatment of epidermoid anal canal cancer. *Am J Surg* 1984;147:43.

116. Salmon RJ, Zafrani B, Labib A, et al. Prognosis of cloacogenic and squamous cancers of the anal canal. *Dis Colon Rectum* 1986;29:336.

117. Sawyers JL. Current management of carcinoma of the anus and perianus. *Am J Surg* 1977;43:424.

118. Sawyers JL, Herrington JL Jr, Main FB. Surgical considerations in the treatment of epidermoid carcinoma of the anus. *Ann Surg* 1963;157:817.

119. Scholefield JH, Ogunbiyi OA, Smith JHF, et al. Treatment of anal intraepithelial neoplasia. *Br J Surg* 1994;81:1238.

120. Scott NA, Taylor BA, Wolff BG, et al. Perianal metastasis from a sigmoid carcinoma-objective evidence of a clonal origin: report of a case. *Dis Colon Rectum* 1988;31:68.

121. Seow-Choen F, Ho JMS. Histoanatomy of anal glands. *Dis Colon Rectum* 1994;37:1215.

122. Shindo K, Bacon HE. Transitional-cell cloacogenic carcinoma of the perianal region, anal canal, and rectum: report of seven cases. *Dis Colon Rectum* 1971;14:222.

123. Sinclair DM, Hannah G, McLaughlin IS, et al. Malignant melanoma of the anal canal. *Br J Surg* 1970;57:808.

124. Singh R, Nime F, Mittleman A. Malignant epithelial tumors of the anal canal. *Cancer* 1981;48:411.

125. Sischy B, Remington JH, Hinson EJ, et al. Definitive treatment of anal-canal carcinoma by means of radiation therapy and chemotherapy. *Dis Colon Rectum* 1982;25:685.

126. Slater G, Greenstein A, Aufses AH Jr. Anal carcinoma in patients with Crohn's disease. *Ann Surg* 1984;199:348.

127. Slingluff CL Jr, Vollmer RT, Seigler HF. Anorectal melanoma: clinical characteristics and results of surgical management in twenty-four patients. *Surgery* 1990;107:1.

128. Smith DE, Muff NS, Shetabi H. Combined preoperative neoadjuvant radiotherapy and chemotherapy for anal and rectal cancer. *Am J Surg* 1986;151:577.

129. Stearns MW Jr, Quan SH. Epidermoid carcinoma of the anorectum. *Surg Gynecol Obstet* 1970;131:953.

130. Sturm JT, Christenson CE, Uecker JH, et al. Squamous-cell carcinoma of the anus arising in a giant condyloma acuminatum: report of a case. *Dis Colon Rectum* 1975;18:147.

131. Surawicz CM, Kirby P, Critchlow C, et al. Anal dysplasia in homosexual men: role of anoscopy and biopsy. *Gastroenterology* 1993;105:658.

132. Tarantino D, Bernstein MA. Endoanal ultrasound in the staging and management of squamous-cell carcinoma of the anal canal. *Dis Colon Rectum* 2002;45:16.

133. Tei TM, Stolzenburg T, Buntzen S, et al. Use of transpelvic rectus abdominis musculocutaneous flap for anal cancer salvage surgery. *Br J Surg* 2003;90:575.

134. Touboul E, Schlienger M, Buffat L, et al. Epidermoid carcinoma of the anal canal. *Cancer* 1994;73:1569.

135. UKCCCR Anal Cancer Trial Working Party. Epidermoid anal cancer: results from the UKCCCR randomised trial of radiotherapy alone versus radiotherapy, 5-fluorouracil, and mitomycin. *Lancet* 1996;348:1049.

136. Wade DS, Herrera L, Castillo NB, et al. Metastases to the lymph nodes in epidermoid carcinoma of the anal canal studied by a clearing technique. *Surg Gynecol Obstet* 1989; 169:238.

137. Wanebo HJ, Futrell W, Constable W. Multimodality approach to surgical management of locally advanced epidermoid carcinoma of the anorectum. *Cancer* 1981;47: 2817.

138. Wanebo HJ, Woodruff JM, Farr GH, et al. Anorectal melanoma. *Cancer* 1981;47:1891.

139. Welch JP, Malt RA. Appraisal of the treatment of carcinoma of the anus and anal canal. *Surg Gynecol Obstet* 1977;145:837.

140. Wellman KF. Adenocarcinoma of anal duct origin. *Can J Surg* 1962;5:311.

141. Winkleman J, Grosfeld J, Bigelow B. Colloid carcinoma of anal-gland origin: report of a case and review of the literature. *Am J Clin Pathol* 1964;42:395.

142. Youk E-G, Ku J-L, Park J-G. Detection and typing of human papillomavirus in anal epidermoid carcinomas: sequence variation in the E7 gene of human papillomavirus Type 16. *Dis Colon Rectum* 2001;44:236.

143. Zelnick RS, Haas PA, Ajlouni M, et al. Results of abdominoperineal resections for failures after combination chemotherapy and radiation therapy for anal canal cancers. *Dis Colon Rectum* 1992;35:574.

144. Zoetmulder FAN, Baris G. Wide resection and reconstruction preserving fecal continence in recurrent anal cancer: report of three cases. *Dis Colon Rectum* 1995; 38:80.

Less Common Tumors and Tumorlike Lesions of the Colon, Rectum, and Anus

To pathology we owe the realization that the contrast between health and disease is not to be sought in a fundamental difference of two kinds of life, nor in an alteration of essence, but only in an alteration of conditions.

Rudolf Virchow: Disease, Life, and Man

Although adenoma and adenocarcinoma constitute the most commonly seen neoplasms of the colon, rectum, and anus, many other tumors and tumorlike conditions in this anatomic region have been described.[499] Of these, some represent extraordinarily rare lesions and may thus be the source of difficult decisions in the therapeutic approach to the patient. Others are important because they represent benign conditions that may be mistaken for malignant processes. Many lesions present a similar clinical picture despite their diverse pathologic natures. Understanding the biology of each is vital to sound therapeutic intervention. The importance of adequate pathologic examination, therefore, cannot be overstressed.

The following classification scheme organizes diseases essentially by their tissue of origin.

CLASSIFICATION OF UNUSUAL TUMORS AND TUMORLIKE CONDITIONS

Tumors of Epithelial Origin

Neuroendocrine (NE) carcinoma
Carcinoid tumor
Bowen's disease
Perianal Paget's disease
Basal cell carcinoma
Cloacogenic carcinoma
Malignant melanoma
Squamous cell carcinoma
Adenosquamous carcinoma (adenoacanthoma)
Stem cell carcinoma

Tumors of Lymphoid Origin

Lymphoid hyperplasia (benign lymphoma, lymphoid polyp)
Malignant lymphoma
Extramedullary plasmacytoma

Mesenchymal Tumors

Fibrous tissue origin
  Fibroma
  Inflammatory fibroid polyp (eosinophilic granuloma)
  Fibrosarcoma
  Malignant fibrous histiocytoma
Gastrointestinal stromal tumor (GIST)
Smooth muscle origin
  Leiomyoma
  Leiomyosarcoma
  Rhabdomyosarcoma
Adipose tissue origin
  Lipoma
  Liposarcoma

Tumors of Neural Origin

Neurofibroma
Ganglioneuromatosis
Neurilemoma (schwannoma)
Granular cell tumor

Vascular Lesions

Hemangioma
Lymphangioma
Hemangiopericytoma
Malignant vascular tumors (angiosarcoma, Kaposi's sarcoma)

Heterotopias and Hamartomas

Endometriosis
Hamartoma
Dermoid cyst and teratoma
Colitis cystica profunda (enterogenous cysts)
Ectopic tissue

Exogenous, Extrinsic, and Miscellaneous Conditions

Extraskeletal osteosarcoma
Choriocarcinoma
Metastatic tumor
Barium granuloma
Oleoma
Sarcoidosis
Wegener's granulomatosis
Amyloidosis
Malacoplakia
Sacrococcygeal chordoma
Ependymoma
Extramedullary (extraadrenal) myelolipoma
Anterior sacral meningocele
Extramedullary hematopoiesis
Pneumatosis cystoides intestinalis (pneumatosis coli)
Duplication

TUMORS OF EPITHELIAL ORIGIN

Neuroendocrine Carcinoma

A type of NE malignancy usually found in the lung (oat cell carcinoma, small cell carcinoma) has on occasion been reported in extrapulmonary sites, including the colon and rectum.[92,407,448] The so-called NE system includes endocrine cells distributed throughout the GI tract, pancreas, lung, thyroid, adrenal gland, skin, and elsewhere, with intestinal NE cells being the largest component. Staren and colleagues defined NE carcinoma as a malignant epithelial neoplasm of predominantly NE differentiation and reserved the term carcinoid for their benign or very low-grade malignant counterparts (see the following section).[463] Neoplastic proliferation of these cells occurs primarily in the appendix, ileum, and rectum, although tumors occur at other sites as well.[419] A case of presacral NE carcinoma arising in a tailgut cyst has been reported.[348] Another NE tumor, the very rare Merkel cell carcinoma, has been described in the anal canal.[377]

Associated Concerns

It is important to remember that there are certain colorectal manifestations of endocrine diseases that are not primary to the GI tract. Symptoms such as constipation are frequently observed in diabetic patients. Unexplained diarrhea should alert the clinician to the possibility of a pancreatic endocrine tumor.[439] Furthermore, thyroid disorders may be associated with refractory constipation, diarrhea, or steatorrhea, and hyperparathyroidsm often presents with constipation.[439] In short, endocrine diseases can and often do present or are associated with intestinal symptoms.

Diagnosis

NE tumors may be identified by immunohistochemical stains with application of a limited battery of available antibodies. Robidoux and colleagues suggested that electron microscopic examination is essential for diagnosis of the poorly differentiated tumor.[407] Many of the so-called poorly differentiated GI malignancies are probably NE tumors, but through the application of appropriate markers the true incidence and distribution may become apparent.[463] Saclarides and co-workers found that NE differentiation occurred in at least 3.9% of colon and rectal cancers.[419] Many were initially diagnosed as carcinoids, but the diagnosis was altered to NE carcinoma after appropriate immunohistochemical staining. In the experience of New York's Memorial Sloan-Kettering Cancer Center involving 38 patients, 22 were categorized as small cell carcinomas and 16 large cell.[53] Eighty percent of these tumors stained positive by means of immunohistochemistry, including chromogranin, synaptophysin, and/or neuron-specific enolase. These cancers must be differentiated from other small cell cancers, such as lymphoma.

Slooter and co-workers opined that somatostatin-receptor scintigraphic imaging with indium-111 octreotide is essential in the diagnostic evaluation.[454] Moreover, they believed that such expression *in vivo* predicts the outcome with somatostatin analogue treatment.

Results

Generally, these tumors are extremely aggressive and are associated with a very poor prognosis. Extensive preoperative workup is suggested, because there is a high rate of concomitant metastases, with the bone marrow frequently involved. In spite of the aggressive clinical behavior that is characteristic of the tumor in the lung, the Mayo Clinic of Rochester, Minnesota, reported that more than one half of the patients whose records were available survived 5 years.[92] In the Memorial Sloan-Kettering Cancer Center experience, metastatic disease was detected at the time of diagnosis in more than two thirds of their patients.[53] There was no significant difference in survival found among pathologic subtypes. Chemotherapy is often the same as that used for oat cell carcinoma of the lung.[76,407]

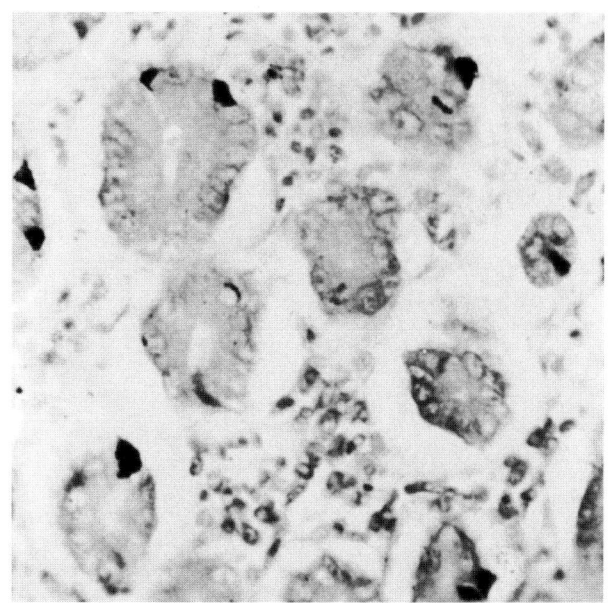

FIGURE 25-1. Normal bowel showing dark-staining argy-rophilic granules (in Kulchitsky cells) from which carcinoid tumors arise. (Original magnification × 600; courtesy of Rudolf Garret, M.D.)

Carcinoid Tumor

Carcinoids are slow-growing tumors of neuroectodermal origin that belong to the amine precursor uptake and decarboxylation system (APUD). They are the most common of the NE neoplasms of the GI tract. Lubarsch, in 1888, was the first to describe a clinical case of carcinoid disease.[301] The term *Karzinoid*, meaning carinomalike, was introduced by Oberndorfer in 1907.[361] It was believed that the tumor was similar to carcinoma because metastases could develop, but the clinical course often tended to be relatively benign. Although carcinoids occur most commonly as primary tumors of the GI tract, they can also be found in such diverse locations as the bronchus, ovary, and kidney.

Carcinoids arise from Kulchitsky's or basogranular enterochromaffin cells located in the crypts of Lieberkühn (Figure 25-1). A report of a patient with multiple carcinoid tumors of the rectum demonstrated numerous proliferations of extraglandular endocrine cells with no increase in intraglandular cell production.[317] In the past few decades, numerous investigators have suggested that the histochemical, chemical, and clinical characteristics vary depending on the site of origin.[57,370,524]

Classification and Diagnosis

The current classification relates to both the anatomic site of the tumor and the reactivity to silver incorporation by cytoplasmic granules.[61] A positive argentaffin reaction (argentaffinity) involves the reduction of silver salts to metallic silver by strong endogenous reducing substances.[484] Argentaffinity usually implies that the argyrophil reaction will be positive, but the mechanism for the latter reaction is unknown.[484] A positive argyrophil reaction occurs when metallic silver added in solution is precipitated on the cytoplasmic granules of the carcinoid cells. Two distinctive types of neurosecretory granules have been observed by electron microscopy.[539] A relatively small granule appears to be associated with argyrophil carcinoids and a larger one with argentaffin (Figure 25-2).

Midgut carcinoids (midduodenum to midtransverse colon) are usually both argyrophil and argentaffin positive, are frequently multicentric in origin, and often are associated with the carcinoid syndrome. The syndrome is characterized by a complex of symptoms thought to be related to overproduction of serotonin (5-hydroxytryptamine), but less than 10% of all patients with carcinoid tumors exhibit this manifestation. Hindgut carcinoids have been reported to be rarely argyrophil or argentaffin positive, are usually unicentric, and are not associated with the carcinoid syndrome.[370] Saegesser and Gross, however, reported the carcinoid syndrome in an individual with carcinoid of the rectum, and Taxy and associates noted, in 23 patients, that most rectal carcinoids are argyrophillic if the more sensitive Grimelius method is employed.[420,484] In this same group of patients, only three were argentaffin positive. The authors concluded that the Grimelius argyrophil stain is the most accurate light-microscopic means for confirming the diagnosis of a rectal carcinoid.

Determination of urine 5-hydroxyindoleacetic acid (5-HIAA) excretion is not helpful in defining metastatic disease in rectal tumors, because hindgut lesions are generally argentaffin negative and do not produce a detectable

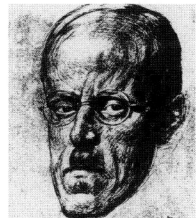
Siegfried Oberndorfer (1876–1944) Siegfried Oberndorfer was born in Munich, Germany, on June 24, 1876. He attended medical school in Munich and finished his studies in 1900. After an internship in pathology with Hellers, he entered a residency at the Pathological Institute of the University of Munich. Subsequently, he joined the faculty and accomplished his thesis in 1906, focusing on appendicitis. In 1910, he became Professor of Pathology at the University of Munich. In World War I, he worked as a military pathologist, but after the rise of the Third Reich, he was dismissed from his position because he was a Jew. He emigrated to Turkey and soon became Chair of the Department of Pathology at the University of Istanbul. Oberndorfer's first publication (1900) concerned the gastrointestinal manifestations of congenital syphilis. He was the first to describe carcinoid tumor of small bowel in 1907 in a presentation before the German Congress of Pathology (*Karzinoide Tumoren des Dünndarms*). He also precisely described the pathology of the male genital tract in his textbook, *Prostata, Hoden, Geschwülste* (1931). He also wrote a handbook of pathology in the Turkish language and published a German textbook on cancer, *Allgemeine Geschwülstlehre*. Oberndorfer died March 1, 1944, in Istanbul, at the age of 68. (With appreciation to Oliver Pfaar and Udo Rudloff for the biographic sketch and to Udo Rudloff for the drawing.)

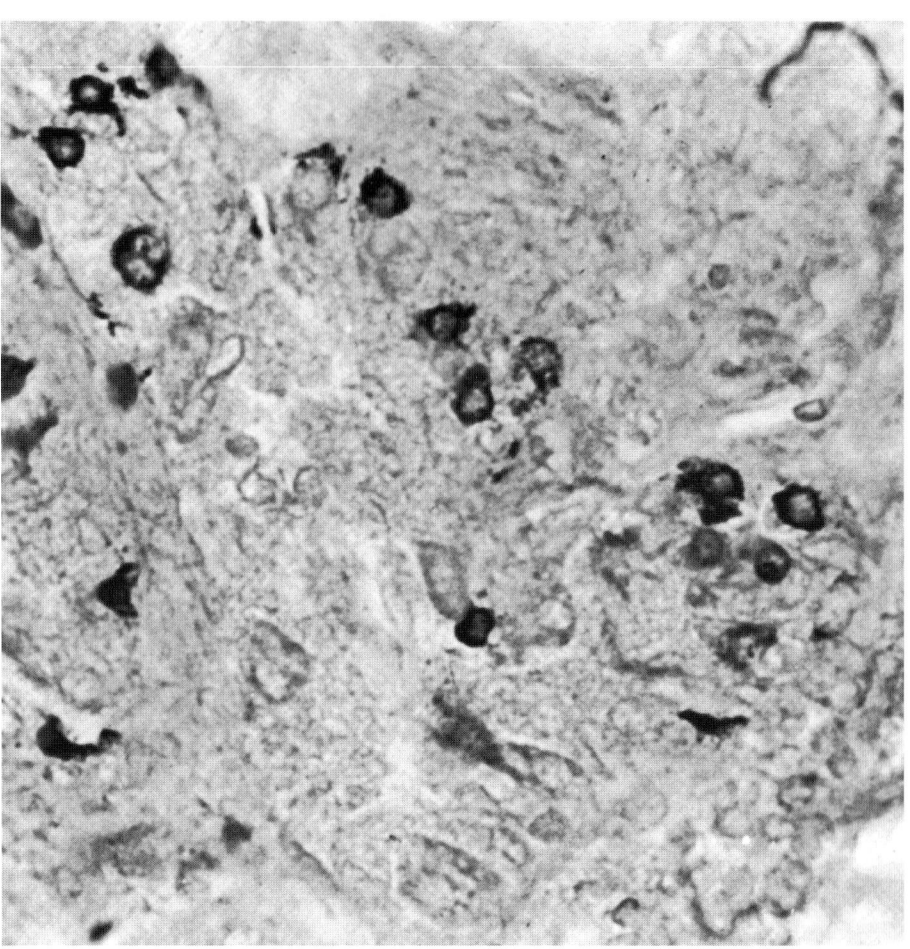

FIGURE 25-2. Carcinoid tumor showing argyrophilic granules in the cytoplasm. (Fontana stain; original magnification × 600; courtesy of Rudolf Garret, M.D.)

increase in tryptophan metabolites.[57] Table 25-1 summarizes the classic differences between carcinoids based on gut location.

Incidence, Distribution, and Associated Conditions

The incidence of GI carcinoid tumors increases from duodenum to ileum, with more than 80% located in the distal small bowel. They arise most commonly in the appendix and are found in 0.26% of appendectomy specimens.[82] The next most common location is the small intestine, followed by the rectum and stomach. Colonic involvement is infrequent, comprising 2.5% of GI carcinoids.[82] Orloff collected 3,000 cases of such carcinoids from the literature and noted 38 patients with rectal tumors.[370] Morson reported only 21 cases of rectal carcinoids seen at St. Mark's Hospital in London in 25 years.[347]

In a collective review, Neary and colleagues analyzed the results of a number of studies.[353] For example, in the United Kingdom, an incidence of 0.7 per 100,000 population was found. This is consistent with other reports from both the United States and Spain.

Modlin and associates evaluated 10,878 carcinoid tumors that were identified by the Surveillance, Epidemiology, and End Results (SEER) Program of the National Cancer Institute from 1973 to 1999 in addition to 2,837 carcinoid tumors that were registered previously by two earlier NCI programs.[338] Two thirds were found in the GI tract and about 25% in the bronchopulmonary system. The following was the distribution within the GI tract:

- Small intestine (41.8%)
- Gastric (20.5%)
- Colonic (20.0%)
- Appendiceal (18.2%)

Carcinoid tumors, irrespective of their site of origin, are associated with an increased incidence of other malignant tumors, especially those of the GI tract. Moreover, an increased incidence of breast and uterine malignancies, as well as cancer of the hematopoetic system, has been described. The reported rates of the development of a second primary malignancy with GI carcinoid tumors is as high as 55%.[193] This includes an increased risk for synchronous colorectal, small bowel, gastric and esophageal cancers as well as metachronous lung, prostate, and urinary tract neoplasms.[492] Because of the possible asso-

▶ **TABLE 25-1 Classic Differences Among Foregut, Midgut, and Hindgut Carcinoids**

	Foregut	*Midgut*	*Hindgut*
Location	Lungs, stomach, first part of duodenum	Duodenum through right colon, appendix	Transverse or left colon, rectum
Staining	Nonargentaffin but argyrophilic	Argentaffin + argyrophilic	Nonargentaffin but argyrophilic
Bioactivity	5-Hydroxytryptophan, ACTH, tachykinins, neurotensin, HCG; gastrin; low 5-HT content; high MAO activity without DAO activity	5-HT, tachykinins, rarely ACTH or 5-hydroxytryptophan; lower MAO activity than foregut carcinoids but higher DAO activity	Low 5-HT or ACTH content; may secrete somatostatin, tachykinins, glicentin, PYY, 5-hydroxytryptophan, neurotensin, pancreatic polypeptide, dopamine
Metastasis	25%, particularly to bone; metastases not required for systemic symptoms	60% to 80% (proportional to tumor size) to liver; rarely to bone	5% to 40% to bone
Presentation	Pulmonary obstruction, atypical neurohumoral symptoms	Bowel obstruction, classic carcinoid syndrome (diarrhea and flushing) if metastatic	Usually discovered by chance; rarely cause humoral symptoms

ACTH, adrenocorticotropic hormone; DAO, diamine oxidase; HCG, human chorionic gonadotropin; 5-HT = serotonin; MAO, monoamine oxidase; PYY, peptide YY.

From Basson MD, Ahlman H, Wangberg B, et al. Biology and management of the midgut carcinoid. *Am J Surg* 1993;165:288, with permission.

ciation with myelofibrosis, evaluation of the bowel in an individual with hematologic disease may be a useful exercise.[355] An association between ulcerative colitis and rectal carcinoid tumors has also been postulated.[431] The reason for the predisposition to develop other cancers may be due to the tumorigenic properties of the peptides secreted by NE cells, such as secretin, gastrin, bombesin, cholecystokinin, and vasoactive intestinal peptide.[193]

Age, Gender, and Race

The condition occurs most commonly in individuals in their sixth and seventh decades.[353] The mean age in Orloff's series was 55,[370] and the previously mentioned SEER study showed the mean age to be 61.4 years.[338] Appendiceal tumors had been seen most frequently in women at a 2:1 ratio,[413] but this has decreased to 57% in current reports. The male-to-female ratio is 0.93 for colonic carcinoids and 1.0 to 1.11 for rectal carcinoids.[338] For all sites, age-adjusted incidence rates are highest in black male patients.[338]

Signs, Symptoms, and Diagnosis

Appendix

The presentation is usually that of an individual with right lower quadrant abdominal pain and signs and symptoms of appendicitis. The identification of the tumor, itself, usually awaits pathologic confirmation. This often is a fortuitous finding that presents somewhat of a controversy in subsequent management (see later). The prevalence of carcinoids has been estimated to be 0.32%, based on a series of more than 34,000 appendec-

tomies.[342] Most are present at the tip (67%), with the body comprising 21%, and only 7% seen at the base.[342]

Small Bowel

Carcinoid tumors in the small bowel are frequently asymptomatic.[46] In those who are symptomatic, change in bowel habits, weight loss, and abdominal pain are the most frequent complaints. Moertel and colleagues advised that the presence of an abdominal mass on the right side and a long history of weight loss and diarrhea should raise suspicion of a carcinoid in the small intestine.[341] The frequency of metastases at diagnosis depends on the clinical presentation and ranges from 33% to 64%. In asymptomatic individuals, 93% who are diagnosed with small bowel carcinoids harbor metastases.[341]

The ileum is second only to the appendix as the site of origin of foregut carcinoid tumors.[63] Quantification of 5-hydroxytryptamine and its metabolites, especially 24-hour urinary 5-HIAA have been found to detect up to 84% of carcinoid tumors.[63] Unfortunately, small bowel carcinoids commonly present late because of the nonspecific signs and symptoms that occur. This leads to failure to pursue investigative studies that could identify the lesion at an earlier stage. The single most common presenting complaint is that of small bowel obstruction, but most patients have nonspecific GI symptoms.

The most rewarding diagnostic study for the evaluation of a suspected small bowel carcinoid is enteroclysis (see Chapter 4). However, a routine small bowel series is usually sufficient (Figure 25-3). It is important to remember that small carcinoids are frequently multiple. The use of computed tomography (CT) scan to evaluate the small bowel has also been recommended, but knowledge

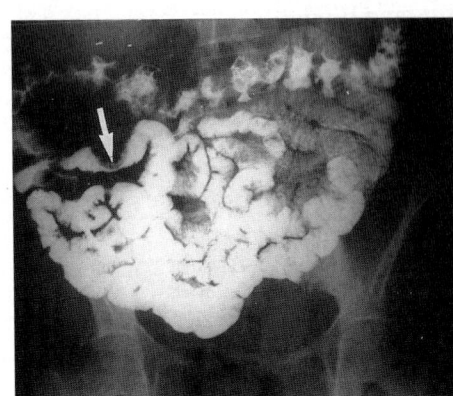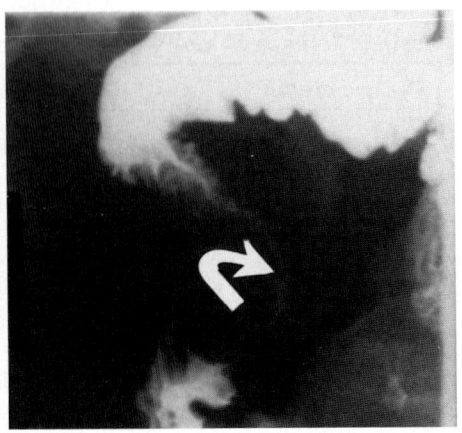

FIGURE 25-3. Carcinoid of the small bowel. Small bowel series. A right upper quadrant mass can be seen infiltrating the mesentery of the small bowel and proximal colon. **(A)** Note the filling defect *(arrow)*. **(B)** Spot film of the same patient reveals another lesion producing a profound stricture *(arrow)*.

gleaned is often *ex post facto*, the diagnosis of metastatic disease having already been established. Magnetic resonance imaging (MRI) has also been used for evaluation of GI carcinoid tumors. In the experience of Bader and co-workers, the primary tumor could be identified in eight of 12 of their patients.[32] The appearance was that of a nodular mass or bowel wall thickening with moderate enhancement on postgadolinium imaging. Liver metastases are commonly hypervascular and may be demonstrable only on immediate postgadolinium images.[32]

Colon

Colonic carcinoids usually grow to a large size before they become symptomatic. Even then, they are less likely to cause obstruction or rectal bleeding than adenocarcinoma of the colon. Thirty-two percent of Orloff's patients were asymptomatic, and an additional 21% had symptoms that were the result of another condition.[370] When the lesion does produce symptoms, they are indistinguishable from those caused by adenocarcinoma (e.g., bleeding, change in bowel habits, abdominal pain). Colonic carcinoids have a similar 5-year survival to that of adenocarcinoma.

Radiologic evaluation of colonic carcinoids reflects the appearance of the clinically seen lesion (Figure 25-4). For larger tumors, it is virtually impossible to distinguish the pathology from that of an adenocarcinoma. This is true even on colonoscopy or direct visualization. In the experience of Ballantyne and colleagues, 48% of the colon carcinoids were located in the cecum, 16% in the ascending colon, 6% in the transverse colon, 11% in the descending colon, and 13% in the sigmoid.[36] The remainder were not assigned. As previously mentioned, patients with carcinoid tumors have an increased incidence of GI adenocarcinoma.[36,47,70,393] Thorough evaluation of the entire GI tract is, therefore, essential.

Rectum

In the rectum, a carcinoid tumor usually is observed as a small, circumscribed, yellowish, submucosal nodule, 1 cm or less in diameter. It is often found incidentally, either at the time of pathologic examination of an excised rectum for another condition or in the course of clinical assessment for other complaints (Figs. 25-5 and 25-6). In the Ochsner Clinic experience in New Orleans, one half of rectal carcinoids were discovered at the time of anorectal examination of asymptomatic individuals.[235] The remainder were found primarily by evaluation of patients whose symptoms were the result of other, benign conditions. In a review by Mani and co-workers, the most common finding at the time of presentation was described as "nonspecific."[311] The most common complaint was that of anorectal discomfort, with rectal bleeding being the second most common. Other complaints included constipation, weight loss, change in bowel habits, rectal obstruction, "hemorrhoids," diarrhea, and the presence of an abdominal mass.[311] Endoscopic ultrasonography has been found to be applicable for determining depth of invasion, a useful consideration if one were to consider performing a local excision.

Presacral Lesion

The presentation of presacral lesions is discussed later in this chapter. It is of interest to note here, however, that an unusual presentation of carcinoid has been described within the presacral space.[127] In the absence of a demonstrable primary mucosal lesion, the authors concluded that the tumor arose from an enterochromaffin cell or teratoma within the presacral space or possibly a metastatic lymph node from an unknown primary.

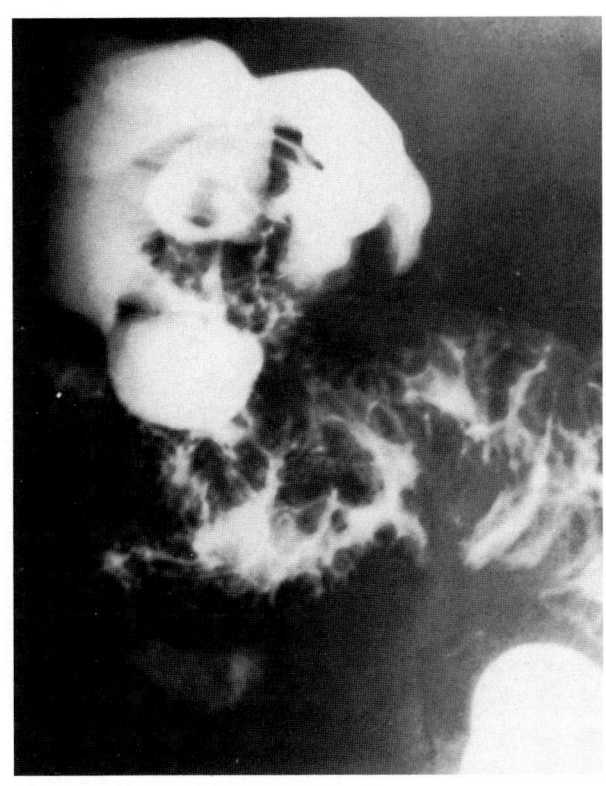

FIGURE 25-4. Carcinoid tumor of the hepatic flexure. Spot film on barium enema reveals distension of the colon with thickened folds. This appearance is caused by intense fibrosis and desmoplastic response produced by the carcinoid tumor.

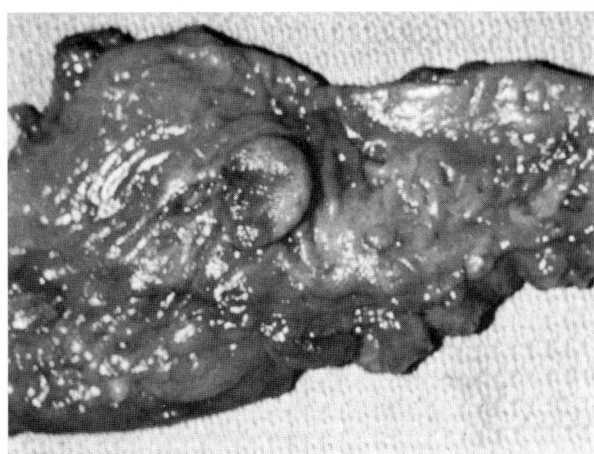

FIGURE 25-5. Carcinoid tumor. An ulcerated nodule protruding from the rectum in a resected specimen. (Courtesy of Rudolf Garret, M.D.)

Histopathology and DNA Ploidy

Microscopically, it is very difficult to differentiate between benign and malignant carcinoid. The usual criteria of malignancy, such as mitotic activity or pyknotic nuclei, are often lacking. The incidence of malignancy varies from 8% to 40%, with the evidence based on the presence of local extension or metastasis.[520] The tumor is composed of uniform, small, round or polygonal cells with prominent, round nuclei and eosinophilic cytoplasmic granules (Figs. 25-7 through 25-9). Johnson and colleagues suggest that there are five generally accepted carcinoid histologic growth patterns: insular, trabecular, glandular, undifferentiated, and mixed.[239] They further observed differences in median survival times in 138 patients based on these patterns and recommend the use of such stratification in future studies.

Tsioulas and co-workers studied the nuclear DNA pattern of 22 rectal carcinoids, finding that the three with metachronous or synchronous metastatic disease had an aneuploid pattern.[498] Conversely, all of the 19 tumors with no metastases exhibited a diploid pattern. The authors concluded that DNA ploidy is an important, independent prognostic indicator. Others have confirmed the association of aneuploidy with stage, size, and invasion by tumor, but in one study the data suggested that a near-hypertriploid pattern was the most precise and reliable parameter for predicting the prognosis of colorectal carcinoid tumors.[84]

Management

Appendix

Moertel and associates recommended appendectomy, alone, as adequate treatment for appendiceal carcinoids of less than 2 cm in diameter, even if lymphatic invasion is noted on subsequent histologic examination.[340] These investigators found no recurrence in a group of more than 100 patients who had microscopic evidence of lymphatic invasion who were so treated. A later report involving 150 patients revealed no other recurrences with the same criterion.[340] The authors further suggest that if the individual is elderly or at high operative risk, appendectomy alone is appropriate for even larger lesions.

A right colectomy is suggested for larger lesions in young patients and for those tumors identified to have vascular involvement or to have invasion of the mesoappendix.[340] Gouzi and co-workers opined that a further indication for secondary right hemicolectomy is the presence of mucinous-producing cells.[179]

Small Bowel

As suggested earlier, the major difficulty in managing patients with small bowel carcinoid is the fact that these individuals present quite late. There is a concern to which one must be sensitive, that of limiting the resection when the root of the mesentery is involved in order to minimize the risk of causing short-bowel problems. It is extremely important to examine the entire small bowel, looking for the presence of synchronous lesions. If at all possible, resection of obvious nodal involvement is encouraged, including removal of superficial hepatic metastases as well as performing a cholecystectomy. This

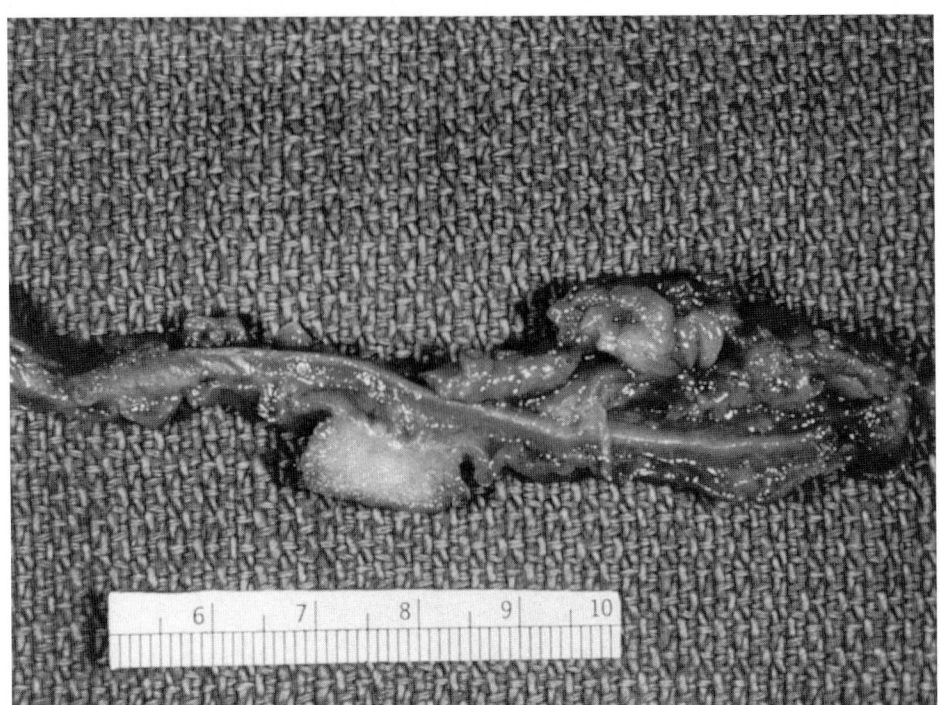

FIGURE 25-6. Longitudinal section of the specimen shown in Figure 25-5. Note the absence of infiltration of muscularis. (Courtesy of Rudolf Garret, M.D.)

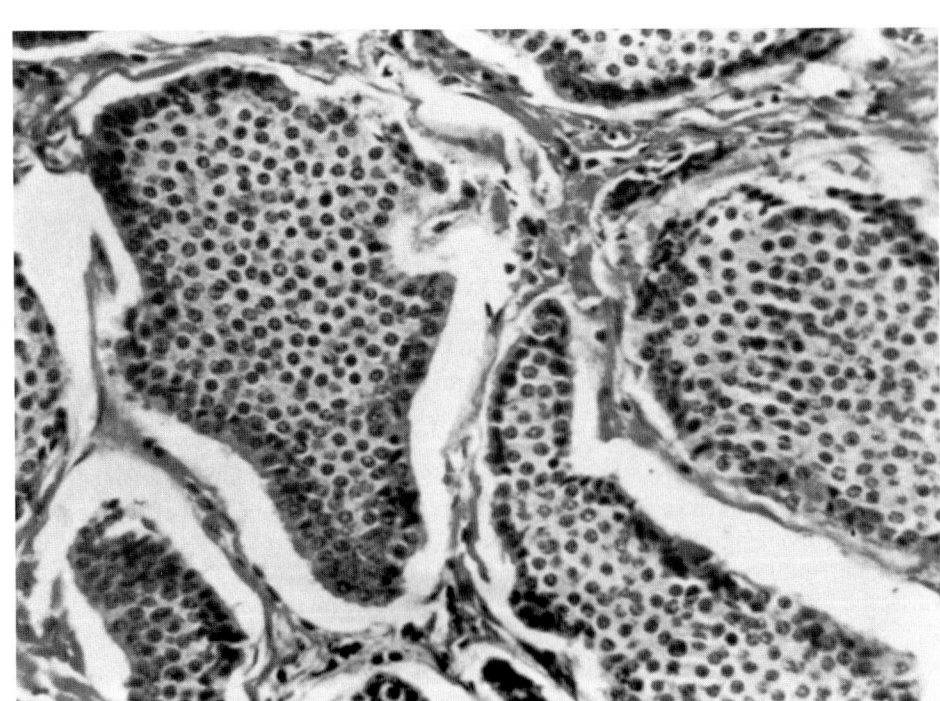

FIGURE 25-7. Carcinoid. Uniform cells with minimal variation of cell nuclei in clusters within the lymphatic spaces. (Original magnification × 280; from Corman ML, Veidenheimer MC, Swinton NW. *Diseases of the anus, rectum and colon. Part I: neoplasms.* New York: Medcom, 1972.)

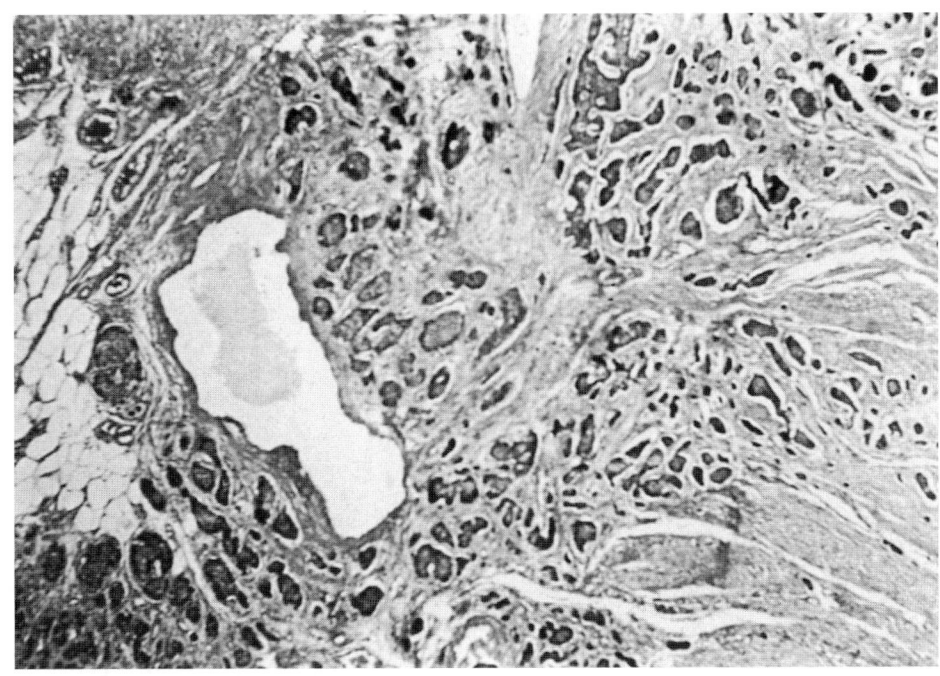

FIGURE 25-8. Malignant carcinoid infiltrating the whole wall of the rectum and invading adipose tissue. Note the cluster of tumor cells in tissue spaces and lymphatics. (Original magnification × 80; courtesy of Rudolf Garret, M.D.)

last procedure is advised if prolonged somatostatin analogue therapy is anticipated.[63]

Colon

Treatment for colonic carcinoid is resection. Because these tumors are relatively slow growing, metastatic disease is not a contraindication to resection of the primary lesion. Metastases occur more frequently with carcinoids of the large bowel than with carcinoids of the small intestine. Perhaps this can be explained by the fact that carcinoid tumors may attain a considerable size in the colon before they become symptomatic.

Rectum

In the rectum, the size of the carcinoid is the distinguishing feature that determines treatment. Most tumors of less than 2 cm in diameter require only local,

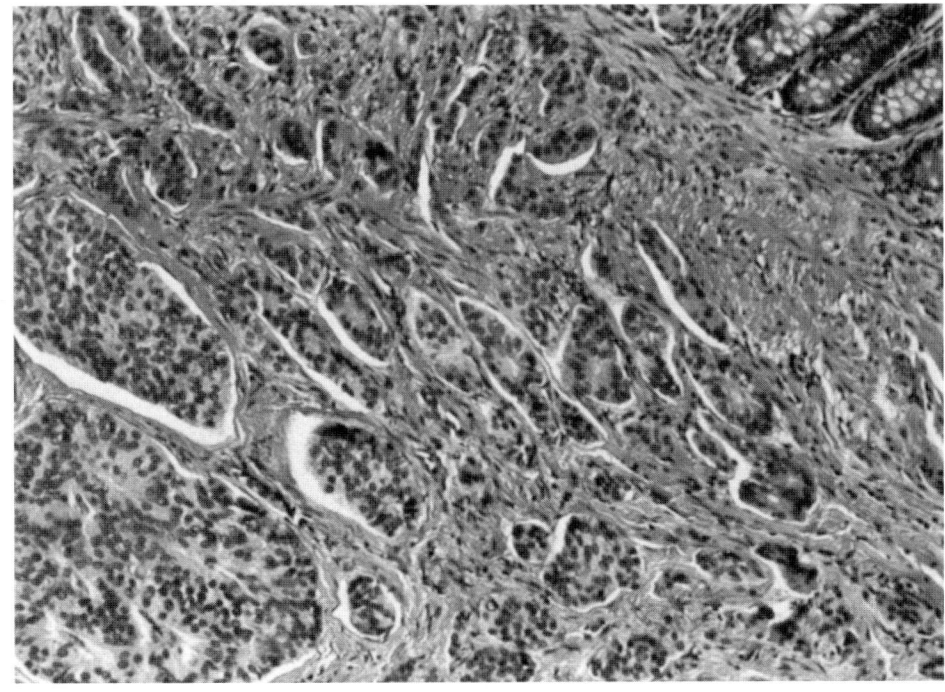

FIGURE 25-9. Malignant carcinoid. Uniform cells in tissue spaces, some forming abortive glandular structures. (Original magnification × 280; courtesy of Rudolf Garret, M.D.)

transanal excision. In the experience of Shirouzu and associates, rectal carcinoids of less than 2 cm in diameter had neither muscle invasion nor lymph node metastasis.[443] Other investigators confirmed the appropriateness of transanal excision for smaller lesions.[235] However, those lesions that are demonstrably invasive or are 2 cm in diameter or greater should probably be treated by a cancer type of resection.[311] Laparoscopic excision of a proximal rectal carcinoid has also been described.[286]

Carcinoid Syndrome

With the exception of tumors that originate outside of the intestinal tract, carcinoid syndrome develops only in those individuals whose cancers have spread to the liver. The classic symptoms and signs are those of skin flushing, diarrhea, and a heart murmur (most commonly, tricuspid insufficiency). The flushing may involve only the face or the entire body and may last anywhere from a few minutes to several hours. There may be excessive tearing, salivation, and facial edema, and the condition may be associated with respiratory symptoms, such as wheezing. With increased involvement of the liver the symptoms often become disabling. The likelihood of developing the syndrome is dependent on the site of the cancer. Up to 60% of those with metastatic small bowel carcinoids will develop symptoms, whereas only about 1% of those with appendiceal primary disease will develop the syndrome. With the exception of the rare "case report," virtually no one with a rectal carcinoid will ultimately develop the symptoms of carcinoid syndrome.

Because of the secretion of serotonin, the diagnosis is made through its byproduct, 5-HIAA, which is excreted in the urine. Some individuals with carcinoid syndrome may have normal urinary 5-HIAA levels. In such instances, the serum serotonin level must be measured in order to establish the diagnosis.

Treatment of symptoms of diarrhea include loperamide, diphenoxylate/atropine, cyproheptadine, and methysergide. For flushing, management includes antihistamines (e.g., diphenhydramine) and antiulcer medications, such as ranitidine. Phenoxybenzamine has also been recommended for the flushing.

In addition to chemotherapy, which is often offered but usually unhelpful, a somatostatin [octreotide (Sandostatin)] is advised, because it inhibits the severe diarrhea and flushing episodes associated with the disease. The suggested daily program during the first 2 weeks of therapy ranges from 100 to 600 µg/day, in two to four divided, subcutaneously injected doses. Along these lines, the resected specimen should be tested for somatostatin receptors. Somatostatin analogues, such as octreotide, lanreotide, and somatuline, have shown variable inhibition of tumor growth and therapeutic tolerance.[63] Lanreotide requires injection every 10 days compared with twice-daily injections of octreotide—therefore, the former may

be preferred.[371] An antiproliferative effect of octreotide on metastatic carcinoid, with regression of the tumors, has been reported to occasionally occur.[288] The addition of interferon-α has also been successfully employed for controlling symptoms and possibly retarding tumor growth.[266] Adjuvant chemotherapeutic and biomodulating therapies are under clinical investigation.[63]

The most efficacious program for the treatment of the carcinoid syndrome is surgically to remove (debulk) as much of the primary and secondary tumors as is possible in order to limit production of the polypeptides. Other options include hepatic artery embolization, radiation therapy, and selective hepatic artery infusion chemotherapy.

Adjuvant Therapy

Radiotherapy and chemotherapy have not proved to be effective in the treatment of carcinoid tumors of the colon and rectum. Adequate surgical excision remains the quintessential treatment. With respect to metastatic disease to the liver, drug combinations of 5-fluorouracil and strepozotocin have achieved high, albeit brief, response rates, whereas hepatic dearterialization and embolization are also useful palliative approaches.[28,490]

Results

Appendix

Anderson and Bergdahl reported results of treatment of carcinoid of the appendix in 25 children under the age of 15 years.[14] All underwent appendectomy, but one patient was subjected to right hemicolectomy because of tumor in the margin of the resected appendix. Despite serosal extension in nine children and lymph node metastases in one, no signs of recurrence were seen with a mean follow-up period of 12 years.

Gouzi and collegues reviewed the records of 181 patients with carcinoid tumor of the appendix seen during a 10-year period ending in 1987.[179] Appendectomy was the sole treatment in 146 individuals, with right hemicolectomy performed on the remainder. None of those treated by appendectomy alone developed recurrent tumor. However, there were five instances of residual tumor upon reexploration, with one death at 2 years and one patient alive with metastatic disease.

Small Bowel

Cure following resection of carcinoid of the small bowel is quite unusual because of the frequent late stage at presentation. In the unusual circumstance of disease confined to the bowel itself, without lymph node involvement or metastatic disease, the likelihood of cure is excellent.[63] For tumors of 1 to 2 cm in diameter, 18% to 44% have been found to be metastatic to the liver, with spread to the lymph nodes in up to 85% of cases reported by Box and colleagues.[63] Size appears to be the variable that correlates most well with survival.

Colon

According to Berardi, the average length of survival after resection of colonic carcinoids is 26 months.[50] Welch and Donaldson stated that the 5-year survival rate for patients with colonic carcinoids is similar to that of those with carcinoma of the colon and rectum.[521] When a distinction is made between cecal and other colonic sites, the former is found to be associated with a 71% incidence of metastasis, whereas the latter has a 33% incidence.[427] Ballantyne and co-workers noted a 5-year survival rate of 37% in their 54 patients.[36] Tumors larger than 2 cm had metastasized in approximately three-quarters of their patients, whereas only one in six less than 2 cm metastasized. Spread and colleagues noted that survival for carcinoids of the colon was significantly lower when compared with carcinoids of the rectum or appendix or with colonic adenocarcinomas.[462] They, however, believed that size and tumor invasion were not the major prognostic factors. Rather, tumor stage, histologic pattern, tumor differentiation, nuclear grade, and mitotic rate were found to influence the survival rate significantly.[462]

Rectum

Orloff applied his therapeutic principle to the management of rectal carcinoids.[370] All 23 of his patients with lesions less than 2 cm survived 5 years. The survival rate of the 15 patients with lesions measuring 2 cm or greater in diameter was 40%. However, the report from St. Mark's Hospital was less encouraging.[67] All with malignant tumors died irrespective of radical surgical treatment, but there were only four such individuals. Sauven and colleagues observed that rectal carcinoid tumors were cured only when they were discovered before the T3 stage, measured less than 2 cm in diameter, and when lymph nodes were not involved.[431] These investigators concluded that if local excision permits complete removal, radical resection provides little benefit. Others opined that extensive surgery offers no survival advantage over local excision.[270] Additional studies confirm that the two criteria, tumor size and depth of invasion, complement each other as prognostic indicators.[311]

Bowen's Disease, Perianal Paget's Disease, and Basal Cell Carcinoma

See Chapter 19.

Cloacogenic Carcinoma and Primary Malignant Melanoma

See Chapter 24.

Squamous Cell Carcinoma

Primary squamous cell carcinoma of the colon and rectum is an extremely rare tumor; approximately 75 cases have been reported.[66,96,164,289,505,525] The incidence of this tumor is believed to be 1 per 3,000 malignant tumors of the bowel.[96,505] These lesions tend to be distributed uniformly throughout the colon.[330]

Numerous theories have been postulated about the etiology and pathogenicity. These include metaplasia of glandular epithelium, embryonal rests, squamous metaplasia of existing adenoma or adenocarcinoma, damaged epithelium from toxic substances, and basal cell anaplasia.[51,96,304,505] Balfour believed that this entity is either a metastatic lesion or degeneration of a poorly differentiated adenocarcinoma.[37] Others suggest that this condition may represent an adenoacanthoma with primarily squamous elements (see later). Specific predisposing factors that have been associated are ulcerative colitis, radiotherapy, colonic duplication, and schistosomiasis.

Gelas and co-workers identified certain criteria that must be satisfied before one can definitively establish the diagnosis of primary squamous cell carcinoma of the *rectum*.[164] They are as follows:

- Metastases from another site must be excluded.
- A squamous-lined fistula tract must *not* involve the affected bowel.
- Squamous cell carcinoma of the anus with proximal extension must be excluded.

Symptoms are the same as those of adenocarcinoma, especially bleeding and change in bowel habits. Evaluation of the patient should proceed in the manner outlined in Chapters 22 and 23. Total colonoscopy is suggested because of the not uncommon association of synchronous benign and malignant tumors.

Histologic examination may demonstrate squamous metaplasia of the colonic mucosa as well as the carcinoma (Figure 25-10).

In the absence of metastases, the lesion should be treated in the same manner as that of adenocarcinoma. However, consideration should be given to implementing the multimodality approach described in Chapter 24, especially if abdominoperineal resection appears to be the surgical alternative.[282] A case report of squamous cell carcinoma of the sigmoid colon with metastatic disease to the liver is described that responded well to systemic chemotherapy.[244]

Adenosquamous Carcinoma or Adenoacanthoma

Adenosquamous carcinoma of the colon is an extremely rare tumor. In 1987, Chevinsky and colleagues identified 35 cases in the literature and also noted 25 re-

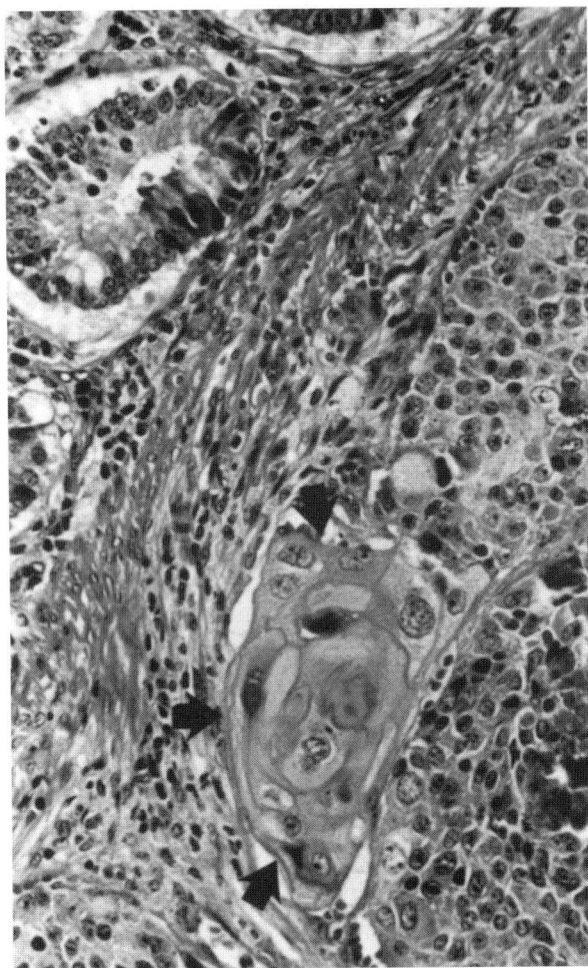

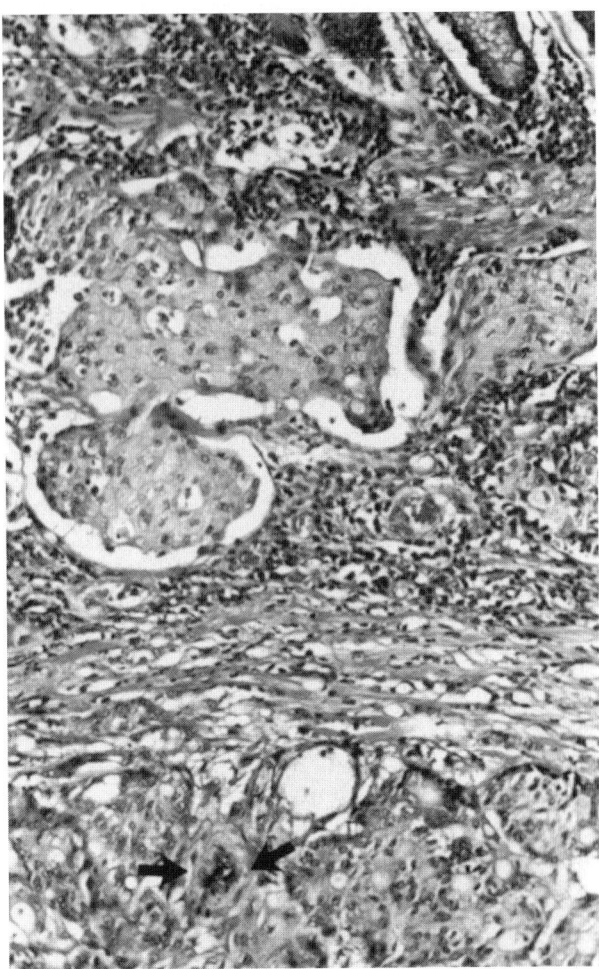

FIGURE 25-10. Squamous cell carcinoma of the cecum. Note the island of malignant squamous cells *(arrows)* near benign colonic glandular mucosa. (Original magnification × 50; courtesy of Rodger C. Haggitt, M.D.)

FIGURE 25-11. Adenoacanthoma of the colon. Islets of malignant squamous epithelium immediately underneath the mucosa and gland-forming tumor below that *(arrows)*. (Original magnification × 40; courtesy of Rodger C. Haggitt, M.D.)

ports of squamous carcinoma primary to the colon.[85] However, some authors believe that if careful review of the histologic pattern of tumors thought to be squamous carcinomas are undertaken, some of the lesions would prove to be adenosquamous cancers (adenoacanthomas), a mixture of both glandular and squamous features (Figure 25-11).[91] Petrelli and colleagues retrospectively reviewed the experience at the Roswell Park Cancer Institute in Buffalo, New York, between the years 1971 and 1994.[382] Seven patients were identified, representing 0.18% of the adenocarcinomas at that institution. Cagir and associates identified 145 patients with adenosquamous carcinoma of the colon, rectum, and anus in the National Cancer Institute's SEER database for the years 1973 through 1992.[69] The mean age was 67 years. Twenty-eight percent of the lesions were in the right colon.

Theoretical causes of this histologic manifestation include embryonal rests, indeterminate basal cells, squa-

mous metaplasia, and a germ or pluripotential stem cell.[85] An increased association with ulcerative colitis has been suggested.[331]

Adenosquamous cancers in general are very aggressive tumors and are associated with a less favorable prognosis than is adenocarcinoma.[77] Because the squamous component may have a greater potential for metastasizing and can do so as an undifferentiated carcinoma, Cerezo and colleagues as well as others suggested that all such lesions be carefully evaluated by means of immunoperoxidase stains and/or electron microscopy in order to identify squamous features.[77,268] This would also imply that evidence of metastatic squamous cell carcinoma does not preclude the possibility of the source being the colon. In the Roswell Park experience, all patients had stage III or IV disease upon presentation.[342] Median survival was only 23 months. In three individuals, the tumor was associated with ulcerative colitis. All died of their disease.

An assessment of the Mayo Clinic experience revealed a total of 31 patients with adenosquamous cancers of the colon and rectum and 11 pure squamous cell carcinomas.[157] They did not separate the two groups but reported an overall 5-year survival of 34% with a 65% survival for stage I to stage III disease. When there was nodal involvement, the survival rate was 23%, whereas without nodal involvement it was 85%. In Cagir and associates' SEER report, the overall adjusted 5-year survival rate was 30.7%.[69] The survival rate for tumors that did not demonstrate nodal involvement was comparable to that of adenocarcinoma, but more advanced lesions were associated with a poorer survival rate than adenocarcinoma stage for stage.

Stem Cell Carcinoma

Another highly aggressive tumor of the colon and rectum may be a variant of adenoacanthoma, the so-called *stem cell carcinoma*. In theory, there may be a pluripotential stem cell in the mucosa of the GI tract capable of differentiation in several directions.[373] Only a few cases have been reported. Palvio and colleagues reviewed tumors with adenosquamous and carcinoid elements in one patient and exocrine, NE, and squamous differentiation in another.[373]

TUMORS OF LYMPHOID ORIGIN

Lymphoid Hyperplasia, Benign Lymphoma, Lymphoid Polyp

Lymphoid hyperplasia is a benign, focal, or diffuse condition that occurs typically where clusters of lymphoid follicles are present (terminal ileum, rectum).[103,104,124,206] Although the etiology is unknown, the possibility of an inflammatory reaction as well as a hereditary predisposition has been suggested. In children, an infectious process is thought to precipitate the acute form of the disease.[242]

One of the earliest reports of benign lymphoid hyperplasia was by Cohnheim, who, in 1865, introduced the term *gastrointestinal pseudoleukemia*.[89] He described a hyperplasia of the lymphoid follicles of the GI tract with polyp formation but without the blood picture of lymphatic leukemia. In 1940, Ewing stated that "the gastrointestinal tract is the seat of a remarkable form of primary lymphoid hyperplasia which lacks the destructive character of lymphosarcoma and fails to give lymphocytosis in the blood."[138] He pointed out that lesions of the GI tract may be limited or diffuse and sometimes are associated with widespread lymphoid hyperplasia but never with leukemia. Symmers confirmed these findings in 1948.[480] Since that time, isolated cases have been reported sporadically, all of which confirm the benign nature of the disease.[68,95,105,228,242]

In 1961, Cornes and colleagues reviewed 100 such patients.[104] The tumors were described as usually single and most frequently found in the lower one third of the rectum. They may be seen in an individual at any age, but in adults they are most commonly noted during the third and fourth decades.[68,104,391] In children, the peak incidence is between 1 and 3 years and is twice as common in boys as in girls.[12,242]

Gruenwald suggested that the lesions are congenital malformations or hamartomas, a hypothesis that is supported by their occasional familial occurrence.[189] Granet reported solitary benign lymphomas in identical twins.[180] Keeling and Beatty noted the lesions in three siblings, ages 6, 7, and 9 years.[254] Others have observed an association with familial polyposis.[186,504]

Lymphoid hyperplasia is characterized radiographically by small, uniform, localized or generalized polypoid lesions (Figure 25-12). A fleck of barium may be seen in the center of the polyp on contrast study, representing umbilication at the apex of the lymphoid nodule. A central dimple in the nodule is considered good evidence for making the diagnosis.[240] Endoscopic examination with biopsy confirms the nature of the lesion. The nodules are usually small, firm, and sessile but occasionally may be large and can become pedunculated (Figure 25-13). When removed and sectioned, the tumors are found to be composed of well-differentiated lymphoid tissue with follicles separated by white fibrous bands and covered by a rather thin mucous membrane. The macroscopic and microscopic appearance may resemble malignant lymphoma or Hodgkin's disease. In fact, the condition has been regarded by some as a form of malignant lymphoma and has even been designated as pseudolymphoma.[480] However, the lesion lacks the infiltrating and destructive characteristics of malignant lymphoma and does not become disseminated. In the benign lymphoid polyp, a follicular pattern with a clearly defined germinal center is seen (Figure 25-14), whereas malignant lymphoma shows a poorly defined and irregular pattern with no germinal centers.[391] The condition also can resemble leukemic infiltration of the bowel, but in leukemia the lesion tends to have a segmental distribution (Figure 25-15). In addition, evidence of the disease is usually apparent in the peripheral blood smear.

Symptoms

Although it may produce no symptoms if located in the rectum, a lymphoid polyp may cause considerable pain when it occurs in the anal canal. Colonic lesions may cause bleeding, abdominal pain, change in bowel habits, and symptoms related to intussusception, the last especially in children.[12,242] Anemia and weight loss may be seen in the chronic form. Collins and associates have reported a case in which the clinical presentation was identical to that of neurofibromatosis with neurovisceral involvement.[95] How-

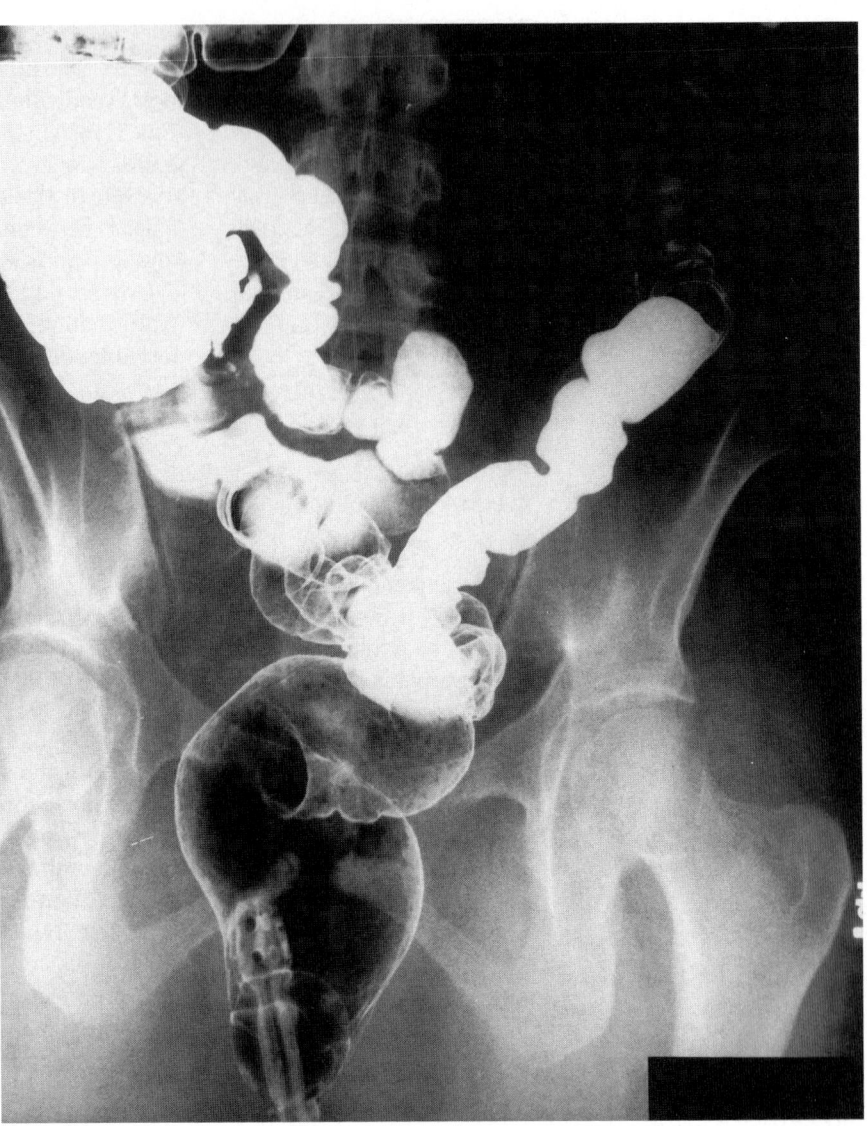

FIGURE 25-12. Lymphoid hyperplasia. Numerous small filling defects are evident in the rectum on this air-contrast barium enema study.

ever, no similarity exists between the bowel lesions of lymphoid hyperplasia and neurofibromatosis.

Treatment

Local excision is indicated and is adequate for isolated or scattered lesions.[104,202,219] Removal is important in order to differentiate the condition from other neoplasms. In 100 patients so treated by Cornes and associates, only five developed recurrences, even though some polyps were incompletely removed.[104]

When the condition mimics acute appendicitis, a common presentation in children, appendectomy is performed. With chronic symptoms and extensive involvement of the terminal ileum, an ileocecal resection may be advisable.[242] Adults with lymphoid polyposis have been treated by colectomy with and without ileorectal anastomosis.[95,105] In other instances, less extensive bowel resections have been performed in those with lymphoid hyper-

plasia who were misdiagnosed preoperatively.[155,476] It is crucial that one is aware of this entity and differentiates it from multiple polyposis.

Because radiotherapy and cytotoxic agents are often beneficial in the treatment of malignant lymphomas of the GI tract, similar treatment has been proposed for benign lymphoid polyposis.[103] Symmers stated that radiation is the accepted method of treatment.[480] Cosens claimed that the lesions may respond well to roentgen therapy, although no response occurred in his own case.[105] In my opinion, in the absence of symptoms, management should be expectant because spontaneous regression may occur without treatment.

Malignant Lymphoma

Malignant lymphoma, as a primary lesion or as part of a generalized malignant process, may involve the GI tract. This is the most common site for extranodal non-Hodgkin's

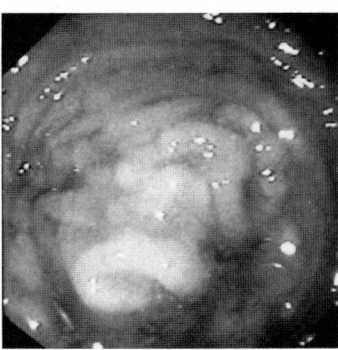

FIGURE 25-13. Colonoscopy reveals numerous confluent, sessile, mucosal nodules. Biopsy was consistent with nodular lymphoid hyperplasia. (See Color Fig. 25-13.)

lymphomas.[423] As a primary tumor, lymphoma comprises between 1% and 4% of all GI malignancies but only 0.5% of colonic and 0.1% of rectal cancers.[323,440] Gastric involvement is more common than that of small or large intestinal lymphoma and carries a better prognosis.[99] Colonic lymphoma preferentially involves the cecum and the rectum. However, concurrent tumors elsewhere in the large bowel, the small bowel, and the stomach have been reported.

Malignant lymphoma of the colon has been reported in association with a variety of other entities, especially those of altered immune status [e.g., acquired immune deficiency syndrome (AIDS); see Chapter 20].[8,117,139,226, 248,258,287,290,356,366,380,475,511] A high-grade B-cell lymphoma in an individual infected with human immunodefi-

ciency virus (HIV) is considered an AIDS-defining condition.[421] Most intestinal lymphomas in the AIDS population are of the non-Hodgkin's type. GI non-Hodgkin's lymphoma represents 17% of those with extranodal involvement.[421]

Waldenström pointed out considerable overlap among macroglobulinemia, lymphoma, and lymphocytic leukemia.[511] This was exemplified by a case reported by Levy and co-workers, in which cecal lymphoma developed in an 81-year-old individual while the patient was receiving immunosuppressive therapy for macroglobulinemia.[290] Associations with chronic ulcerative colitis, Crohn's disease, and celiac disease have also been observed.[292] With the concern for possible concomitant leukemia, total and differential white blood cell counts are mandated as part of an evaluation.[528]

In most series, the incidence is greater in men than in women by a ratio of almost two to one.[533] Most patients are more than 50 years of age at diagnosis, but the condition can occur at any age.

Signs and Symptoms

Many individuals complain of abdominal pain that is usually cramping and localized to the area of the tumor. Other prominent symptoms include weight loss, change in bowel habits, diarrhea, weakness, nausea, vomiting, anorexia, bleeding, and fever. Discrete intraabdominal masses are generally not appreciated until late in the course of the disease. The breakdown of signs and symp-

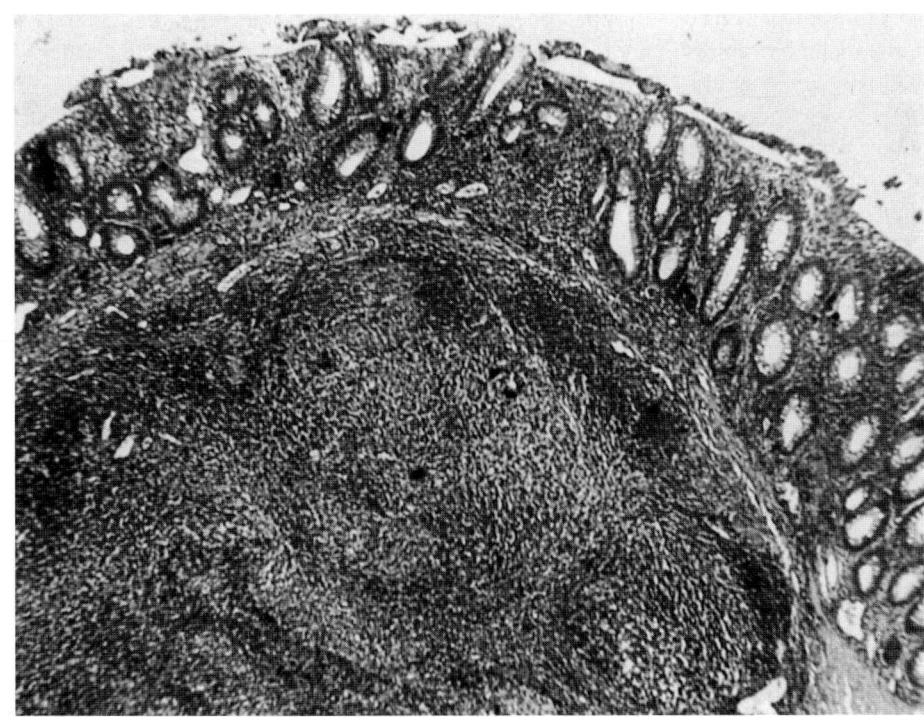

FIGURE 25-14. Lymphoid polyp of the rectum. Lymphocytic infiltration with irregular germinal centers in the submucosa. (Original magnification × 250; courtesy of Rudolf Garret, M.D.)

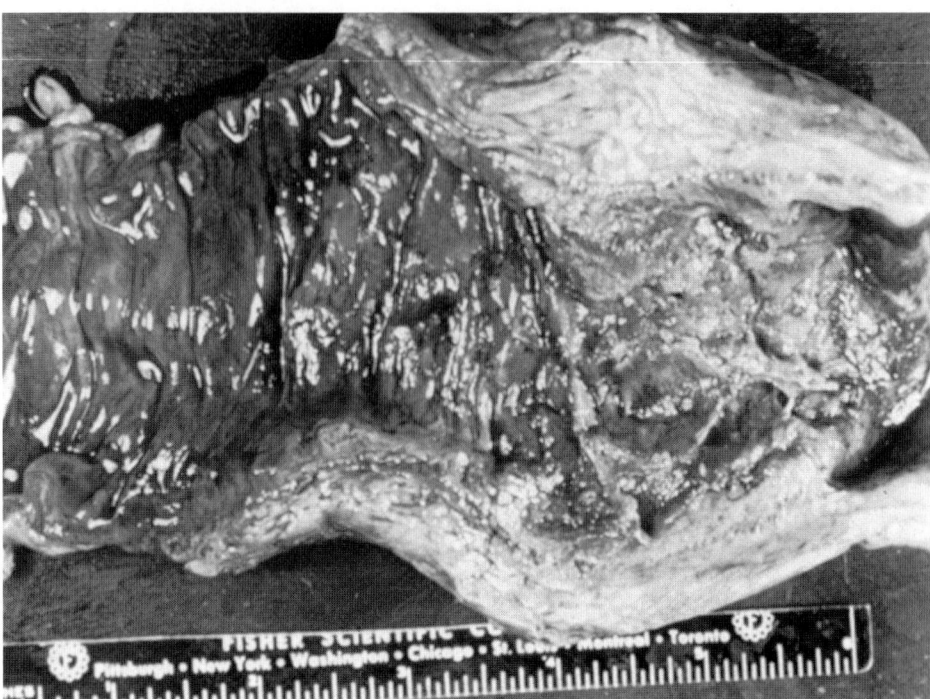

FIGURE 25-15. Autopsy specimen showing leukemic infiltration of the bowel wall simulating scirrhous carcinoma. (Courtesy of Rudolf Garret, M.D.)

toms according to Fan and co-workers (37 patients) is as follows:[140]

- Abdominal pain (65%)
- Abdominal mass (54%)
- Weight loss (43%)

The symptoms produced by *rectal involvement* are variable and largely depend on whether the growth has become ulcerated. In early stages, with an intact mucosa, symptoms consist of a bearing-down sensation or a feeling of fullness in the rectum, with some rectal irritability and low backache. When ulceration of the overlying mucosa has developed, bleeding and mucous discharge may be noticed. Later, pain and soreness are described if the growth begins to encroach on the anal canal. A high index of suspicion must be maintained in homosexual patients, and obviously if AIDS is known or suspected. Obstructive symptoms are unlikely to occur because the primary growth often remains fairly localized to one quadrant and does not usually extend in an annular fashion as is seen with carcinoma.

Pathogenesis

It is thought that malignant lymphoma starts in the submucosal lymphoid tissue, which in places extends into the mucosa. It is not known whether it begins multicentrically or arises from a single area and later spreads by direct extension or through lymphatic channels. At presentation, a large segment of colon may be involved in a uniform and continuous fashion. Submucosal infiltra-

tion often extends beyond the area of obvious involvement, and additional lesions may be found apart from that region. Marked involvement is most common in the ileocecal or the rectosigmoid area, where tumors sometimes become confluent and form a large conglomerate mass. This may cause intussusception and intestinal obstruction. In the ileocecal region, the process usually extends into the appendix and into the ileum for a variable distance. When the rectum is the site of the tumor, inguinal nodes may be enlarged and palpable. Extensive serosal or retroperitoneal involvement is not characteristic of diffuse lymphoma.

Endoscopy and Radiology

Clinical and radiographic diagnosis of colonic and rectal lymphoma may be obscured by the variety of appearances it may assume. Usher reported ten patients with rectal lymphoma from the Mayo Clinic and observed that in all cases the lesion was visualized on proctoscopic examination.[502] In no instance could a definite diagnosis of lymphoma be made by the appearance of the lesion. Usually, it was described as a polypoid tumor, diffuse proctitis, a submucosal nodule, or carcinoma (Figure 25-16). The endoscopic appearance may resemble that of Crohn's disease, such as has been described for the extremely rarely reported cases of granulocytic sarcoma and malignant histiocytosis.[75,422]

From the radiologic point of view, diffuse lymphoma of the colon must be differentiated from familial polyposis, ulcerative colitis with pseudopolyposis, granulomatous

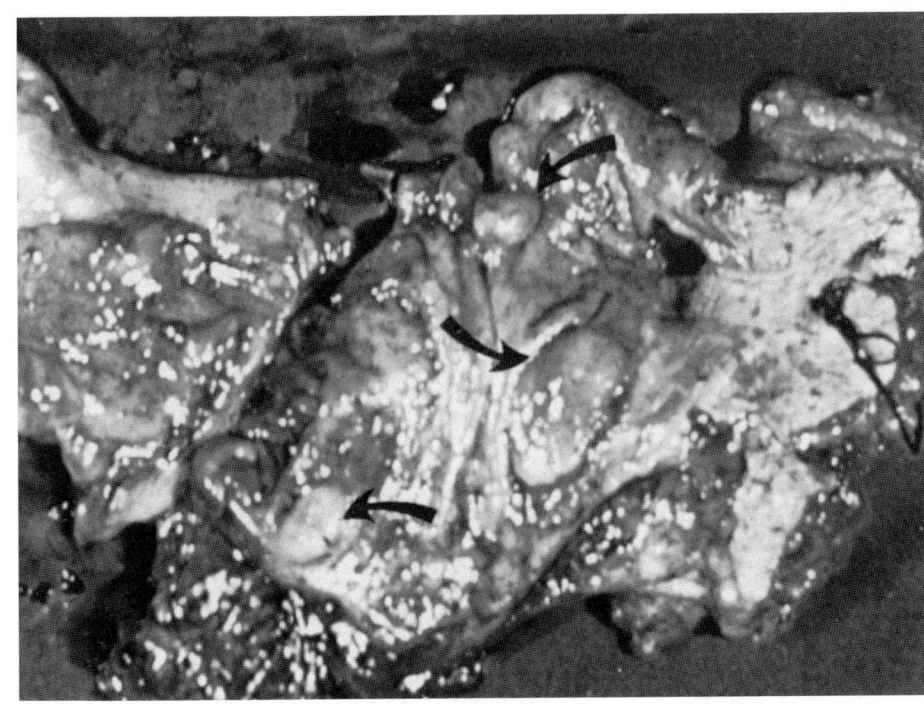

FIGURE 25-16. Lymphomatous infiltration of the rectum treated by abdominoperineal resection. Multiple lesions *(arrows)* are noted. (Courtesy of Rudolf Garret, M.D.)

colitis, nodular lymphoid hyperplasia, and schistosomiasis. Although radiologic differentiation from carcinoma may be impossible, Halls pointed out that certain presentations strongly suggest lymphoma: presence of a bulky extra-colonic component, concentric dilatation of the lumen, and a polypoid filling defect of the terminal ileum and ileocecal valve (Figs. 25-17 and 25-18).[196]

Histopathology

Macroscopic examination of the tumor reveals a polypoid or ulcerated mass resembling carcinoma or a diffuse process extending over a large segment of colon, sometimes with numerous polypoid intraluminal excrescences. The bowel wall is thickened and rubbery in consistency, and its cut surface demonstrates a greatly thickened mucosa, often with prominent convoluted folds resembling the surface of brain and reaching a thickness of 1 or 2 cm (Figure 25-19). The submucosa is markedly thickened as a result of infiltration by closely packed tumor cells. In contrast to disease in the small bowel, deep ulceration and perforation are uncommon. However, superficial ulceration and necrosis may be seen.

The presence of a nonulcerated, submucous tumor in the rectal wall requires differentiation from benign lesions, such as lipoma, myoma, and nodular lymphoid hyperplasia, and also from an inflammatory condition, such as an intramuscular abscess. Thus, biopsy and histologic examination are crucial to the evaluation of such lesions (Figs. 25-20 and 25-21). Microscopic examination usually readily distinguishes lymphoma from other malignancies.[212] How-

ever, a nonspecific lymphoid infiltrate in the mucosa and submucosa may present a problem with differential diagnosis. Under these circumstances, some investigators have recommended immunocytochemical studies as well as gene rearrangement analysis with DNA probes to elucidate the precise nature of the process.[365]

Regional lymph nodes are involved in approximately one half of the patients at the time of laparotomy. The presence of enlarged nodes may, however, represent reactive lymphoid hyperplasia and must be carefully examined histologically to document the presence of tumor. Because involvement beyond a single segment of bowel and its regional nodes excludes the diagnosis of primary lymphoma, a careful search for additional diseased nodes is necessary.

Classification

Malignant lymphoma is classified on the basis of its cellular morphology and immunologic surface markers. Included are the following histologic types: lymphocytic lymphoma, lymphosarcoma, reticulum cell sarcoma, giant follicular lymphoma, and Hodgkin's disease. Hodgkin's disease of the colon or rectum is the rarest.

Tumors are also classified on the basis of extent of involvement:

Class I: confined to bowel wall
Class II: regional node involvement within the drainage area of the bowel primary tumor
Class III: paraaortic node involvement; direct extension to adjacent viscera

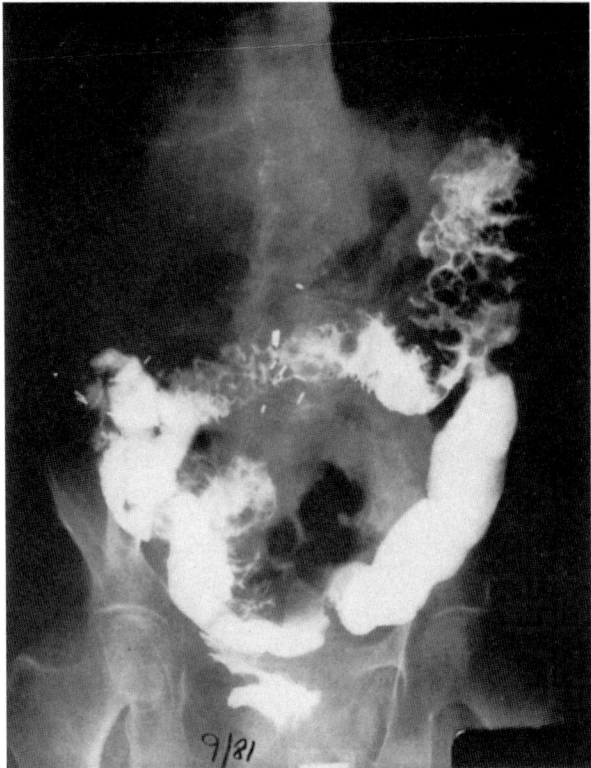

FIGURE 25-17. Malignant lymphoma. Postevacuation barium enema demonstrates multiple polypoid filling defects of varying size with areas of ulceration.

As pointed out by Wychulis and associates and by others, the prognosis of primary extranodal lymphoma in the colon or rectum is not clearly related to cell type but is affected by stage.[140,292,424,533]

Treatment

Most agree that resection is preferred whenever malignant lymphoma is confined to the bowel (including regional nodes).[25] The Mayo Clinic group recommended that if lymphoma is confined to the rectum and the tumor is resectable, surgical excision should be followed by radiation therapy.[115] In those tumors considered unresectable, radiation therapy is of definite benefit. A combined program with chemotherapy is recommended for systemic disease. Adjuvant therapy may include cyclophosphamide, doxorubicin (or epirubicine), vincristine, prednisone, and bleomycin.[25] Another approach utilizes mitoxantrone, chlorambucil, and prednisone.[423]

Results

Contreary and colleagues reported a 50% 5-year survival in those patients operated upon for cure.[99] When the tumor was confined to the bowel or involved only local

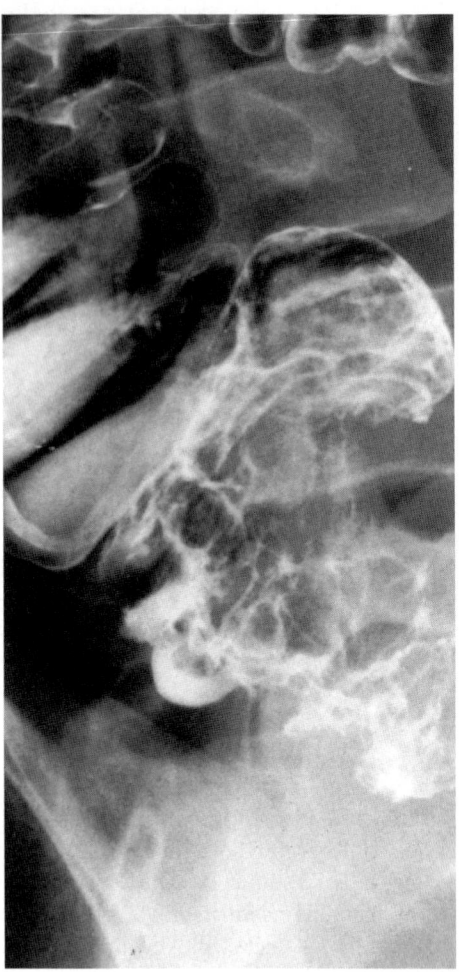

FIGURE 25-18. Malignant lymphoma of the cecum. Note the large, lobulated mass.

nodes, the survival rate in both situations was also 50%. When regional nodes were involved, 5-year survival fell to 12%. Although this was not a controlled study, the difference in survival rates between those patients operated upon for cure with supplementary radiotherapy and without it was 83% versus 16%. Moertel reported an overall 5-year survival rate of 55%.[339]

The treatment of non-Hodgkin's lymphoma in the setting of HIV infection has been much less effective than in individuals without immunodeficiency (see Chapter 20). The use of cytotoxic agents exacerbates the already existing immune impairment and leaves the person with prolonged neutropenia and at further risk for opportunistic infection.[421] Survival times are generally less than 1 year.

Extramedullary Plasmacytoma

Primary plasmacytoma is a localized plasma cell tumor that is most commonly found in the nasopharynx, although it has been described in many other parts of the

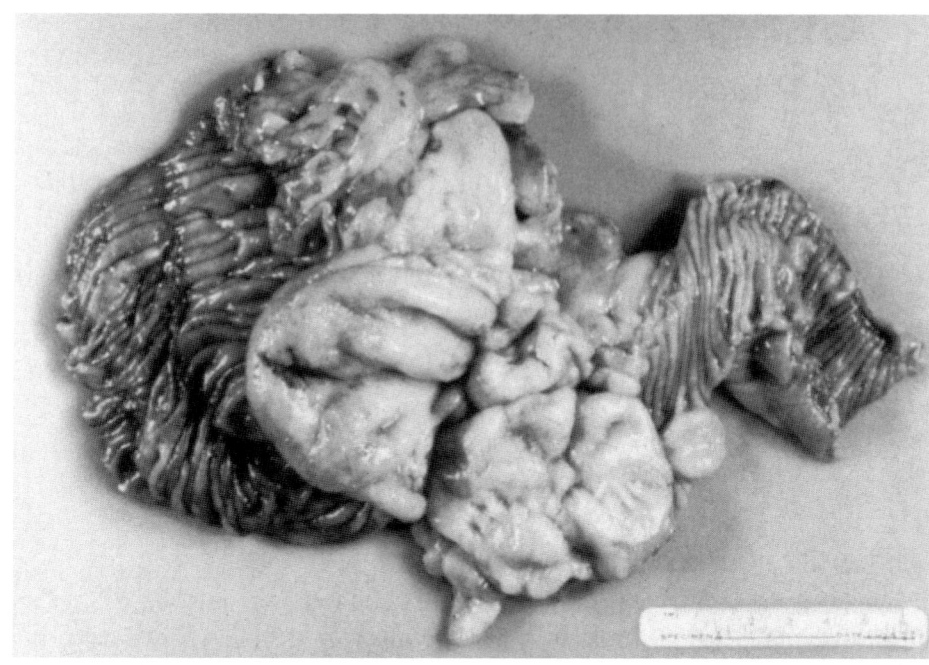

FIGURE 25-19. Lymphoma of the cecum. Note the convoluted folds.

body. Plasma cell neoplasms are classified in five categories: multiple myeloma, solitary myeloma, extramedullary plasmacytoma (with multiple myeloma), plasma cell leukemia, and primary plasmacytoma.[445]

The condition involves the colon extremely rarely with fewer than ten cases having been reported as a primary disease. Some have involved the bowel secondarily. Primary tumors elsewhere in the GI tract have also been noted.[176,199,205] Disseminated multiple myeloma is often diagnosed in patients who have a localized plasmacytoma if these patients are followed for a sufficiently long period. Therefore, a bone marrow examination should be performed at some point once an extramedullary plasmacytoma has been diagnosed. Primary and secondary colorectal plasmacytoma is commoner in men than in women by a ratio of 3:2.

Presenting symptoms include abdominal pain, bleeding, anorexia, nausea, vomiting, and weight loss. The tumor can be single or multiple and may consist of diffuse cellular infiltrates or of polypoid or nodular protrusions. Microscopic examination demonstrates the characteristic population of plasma cells (Figure 25-22). Identification by means of immunoperoxidase staining has also been advised.[172]

Treatment ideally consists of total excision when possible. If, for example, a GI lesion has been excised for purposes of diagnosis and the entire tumor was removed, no additional treatment would in all probability be indicated. Of the cases reviewed by Sidani and associates, none metastasized to any organ other than lymph nodes.[445] Plasmacytomas that are not readily resectable may be responsive to radiotherapy. The use of chemotherapy is restricted to disseminated disease.

MESENCHYMAL TUMORS

Fibrous Tissue Origin

Fibroma

Fibroma of the colon is a very rare tumor that belongs to the uncommon spindle cell group of benign tumors that also includes leiomyomas.[464] Its incidence is only one tenth that of leiomyoma, however.[64]

Although many authors use the terms fibroma, leiomyoma, and fibromyoma interchangeably, Rose emphasized that differential histologic tissue staining techniques distinguish the true fibroma from other spindle cell tumors.[411] According to Aird, the tumor may originate in any layer of the bowel wall but arises most frequently in the submucosa.[6] Fibromas have been reported in the appendicular stump and near the mesentery.[145,496] Reports of fibroma of the colon are few.[23,141,368,411] Abdominal pain and distension may be noted, and resection is the treatment of choice.

Fibroma of the anorectal region is very rare. It may arise from an hypertrophied papilla or by fibrous infiltration of a large prolapsing internal hemorrhoid, generally as a result of repeated attacks of thrombosis and strangulation without sloughing. It is encapsulated, firm, slightly movable, ovoid, of small to moderate size, and has little tendency to ulcerate. It is usually situated in the wall. In

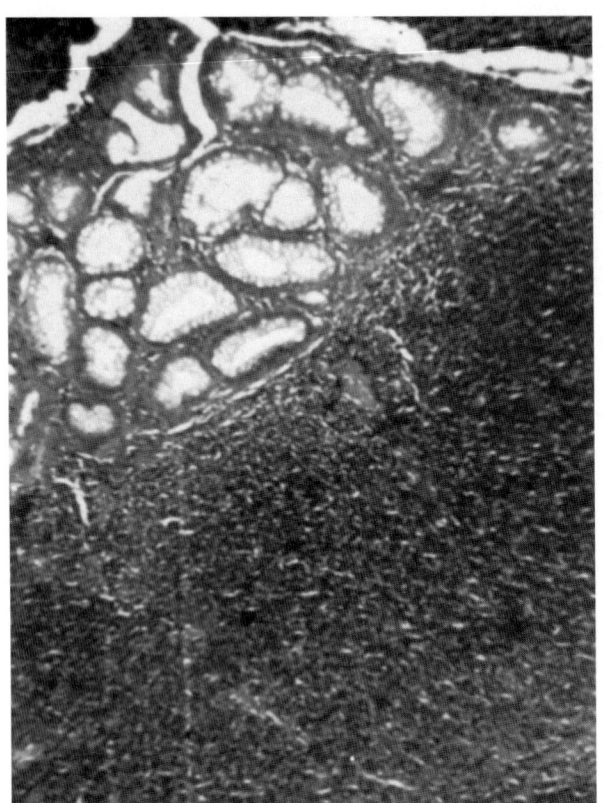

FIGURE 25-20. Lymphoma of the sigmoid colon. Note the heavy infiltrate of lymphocytic tumor cells involving the mucosa and submucosa. (Original magnification × 80; courtesy of Rudolf Garret, M.D.)

time, the covering of columnar epithelium becomes converted into squamous epithelium. A smooth, pale fibrous polyp results. The tumor may remain in the wall of the rectum or become polypoid and extend into the lumen. In general, it is single and of slow growth. However, fibrous polyps may be multiple, so a careful proctoscopy is essential.

Symptoms include tenesmus and a sense of heaviness in the rectum. If ulceration has occurred (an exception), bleeding may be noted. The diagnosis is seldom made without microscopic examination. Transanal excision is the appropriate treatment.

Inflammatory Fibroid Polyp or Eosinophilic Granuloma

Inflammatory fibroid polyp is a rare, focal lesion occurring in the submucosa of the GI tract, least commonly in the colon.[241,293,386] Only a few cases have been reported.[322,326,374,507] Another term for the condition is eosinophilic granuloma. Although the etiology is uncertain, the observation of the proliferation of submucosal mesenchymal fibrous tissue as well as variable eosinophilic infiltration suggests the effect of an inflammatory stimulus (Figure 25-23).[293]

Rectal bleeding, tenesmus, change in bowel habits, and diarrhea are the most common symptoms. Obstruction resulting from intussusception has also been reported.[293] Radiographically, the impression may be that of a carcinoma.[326] Because malignant degeneration has not been

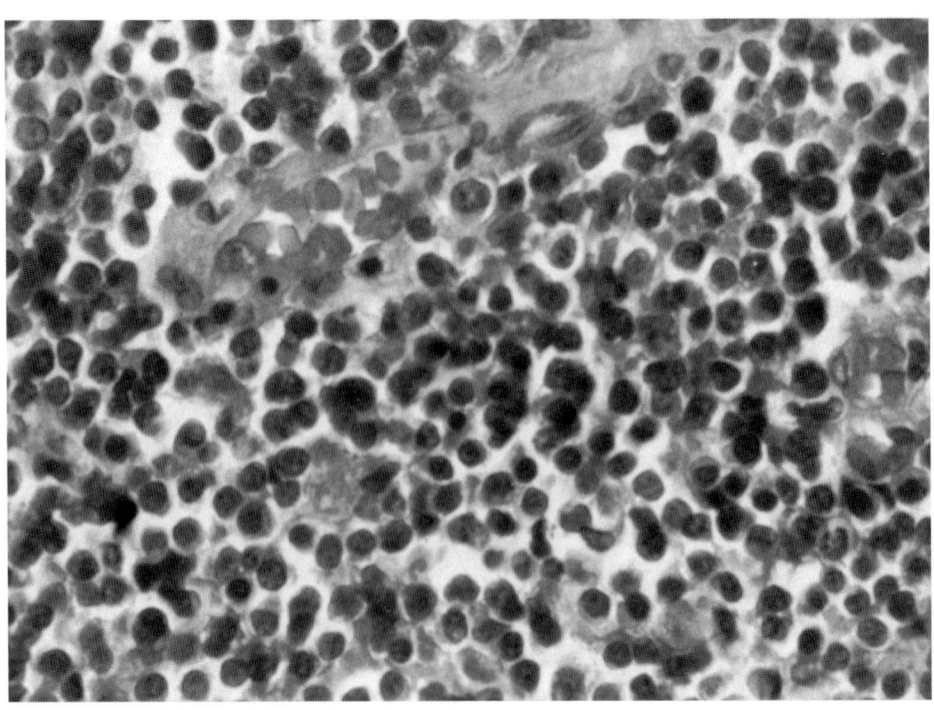

FIGURE 25-21. Lymphoma of the cecum. Note the lymphoblasts in the wall of the bowel. (Original magnification × 600; courtesy of Rudolf Garret, M.D.)

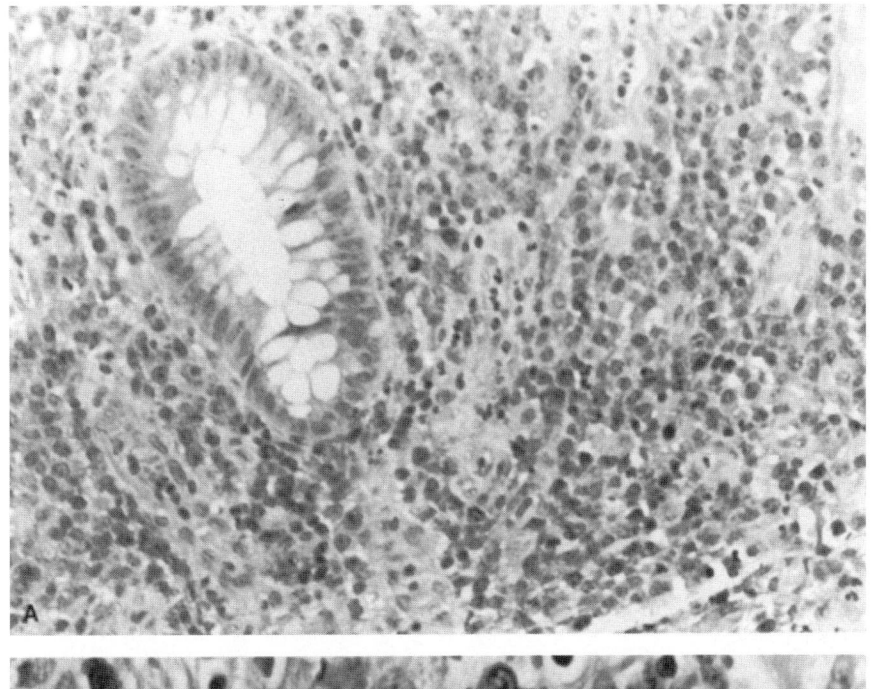

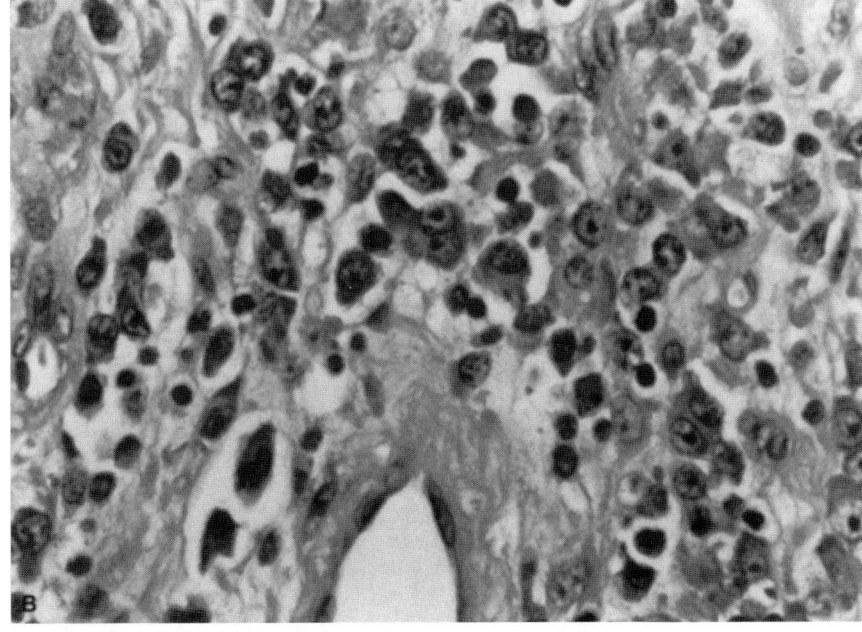

FIGURE 25-22. Extramedullary plasmacytoma. **(A)** Colonic gland surrounded by atypical, infiltrative plasma cells. (Original magnification × 100.) **(B)** Many plasma cells, some of which demonstrate hyperchromatic and eccentric nuclei. Note the apophyllic cytoplasm, a characteristic feature of plasma cells. There are also binucleate forms with discernible nucleoli. (Original magnification × 400.)

noted, however, endoscopic removal is suggested. A concern is that lesions may be sessile and submucosal and have a tendency to bleed readily. If colonoscopic resection is unsuccessful or inadvisable, colectomy or colotomy and polypectomy should be performed.

Fibrosarcoma

Of the sarcomas involving the GI tract, fibrosarcoma is one of the rarest. Stoller and Weinstein reported 21 cases of fibrosarcoma of the rectum in the literature from 1927 until 1954 and added two cases of their own.[468] The mean age of the patients in this series was 51 years. All tumors were situated in the rectum within 10 cm of the dentate line. Only two cases of fibrosarcoma of the colon have been reported.[45,216] Espinosa and Quan identified the only case of anal fibrosarcoma.[136] The lesion apparently arose at the site of a previous fistulectomy incision.

The most common presenting symptom of fibrosarcoma of the rectum is difficulty with defecation. Pain is the second most common symptom, and bleeding, third.[468] Proctosigmoidoscopic examination may reveal

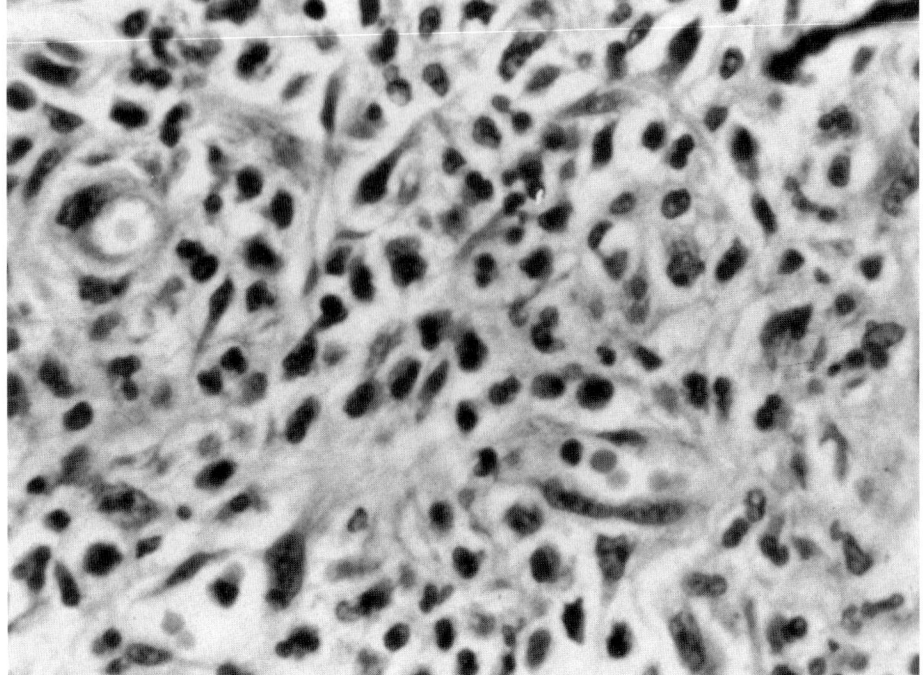

FIGURE 25-23. Inflammatory fibroid polyp. The bowel wall is infiltrated by many eosinophils. Note some fibroblasts and small blood vessels lined by prominent endothelial cells. (Original magnification × 280; courtesy of Rudolf Garret, M.D.)

the tumor to be consistent with an adenocarcinoma, and only histologic determination can establish the definitive diagnosis.

Microscopically, the tumor is characterized by strands of fibrous tissue that infiltrate the adjacent structures of the bowel wall but tend to spare the mucosa until late in the disease (Figs. 25-24 and 25-25).[468] The presence of mitoses is helpful in confirming the malignant nature of the lesion.

Treatment is essentially the same as that for adenocarcinoma: radical resection of the involved bowel with or without a sphincter-saving approach. Neither radiotherapy nor chemotherapy has been helpful in the management of this rare condition.

Malignant Fibrous Histiocytoma

Malignant fibrous histiocytoma is an extremely rare fibrosarcoma variant in which histiocyte-like cells are present.[39,438,514] The term was originally proposed by O'Brien and Stout to describe tumors composed of both fibroblasts and histiocytes (Figure 25-26).[363] The lesion is usually found in the lower extremity.

It is difficult to present a meaningful evaluation of the signs, symptoms, diagnosis, therapy, and prognosis with such an uncommon condition. Tumors tend to be large, present with obstructive symptoms, and are thought clinically to be adenocarcinomas. Treatment is radical resection, but prognosis is presumably poor. A partial response has been reported with chemotherapy.[197]

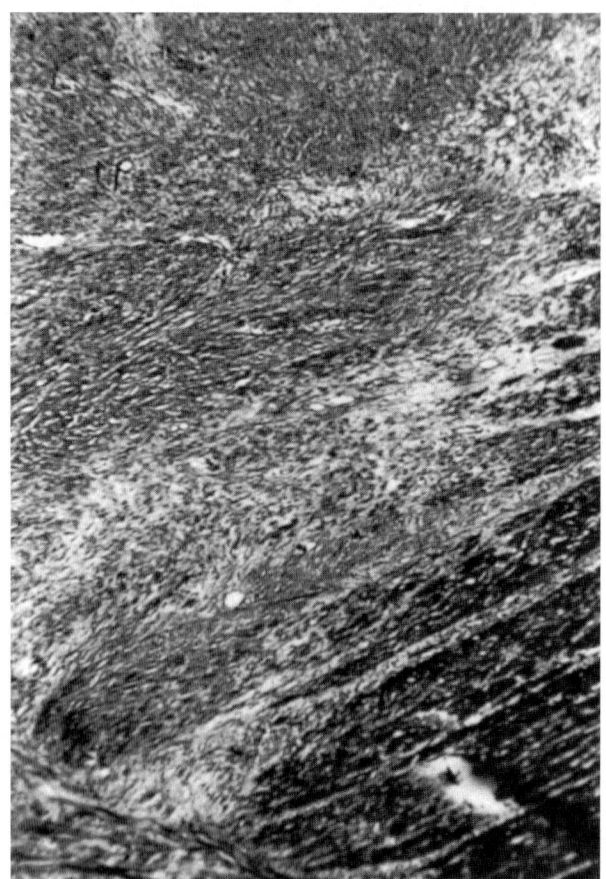

FIGURE 25-24. Fibrosarcoma. A well-differentiated tumor infiltrating the wall of the bowel. (Trichrome stain; original magnification × 80; courtesy of Rudolf Garret, M.D.)

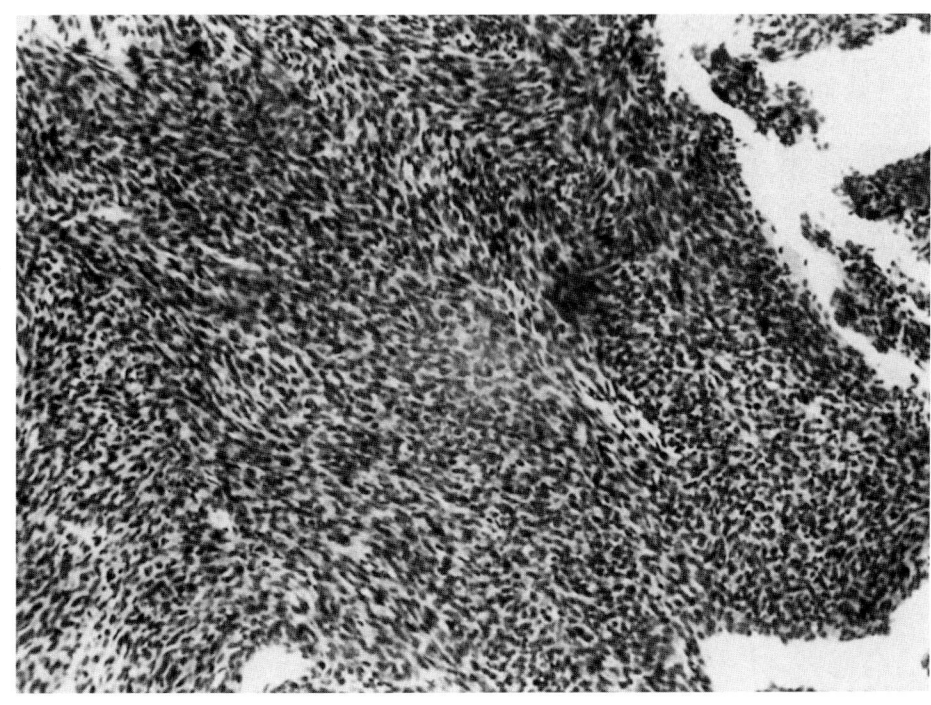

FIGURE 25-25. Cellular fibrosarcoma. Tumor consisting of bundles of undifferentiated fibroblasts. (Original magnification × 280; courtesy of Rudolf Garret, M.D.)

Stromal Origin

Gastrointestinal Stromal Tumors

GISTs are sarcomas arising from mesenchymal tissue. They are believed to represent the most common nonepithelial sarcoma of the GI tract, comprising approximately 0.1% to 3% of all GI cancers and approximately 5% of soft tissue sarcomas. This observation has been arrived at after a long period of presumed inaccurate diagnosis as having arisen from smooth muscle cells. GISTs are related to the muscle-like nerve cells, the interstitial cells of Cajal, which coordinate the autonomic movements of the GI tract. They may occur anywhere along the length of the digestive tract from the esophagus to the anus. Although the exact incidence is still somewhat unclear, it is now estimated that between 5,000 and 10,000

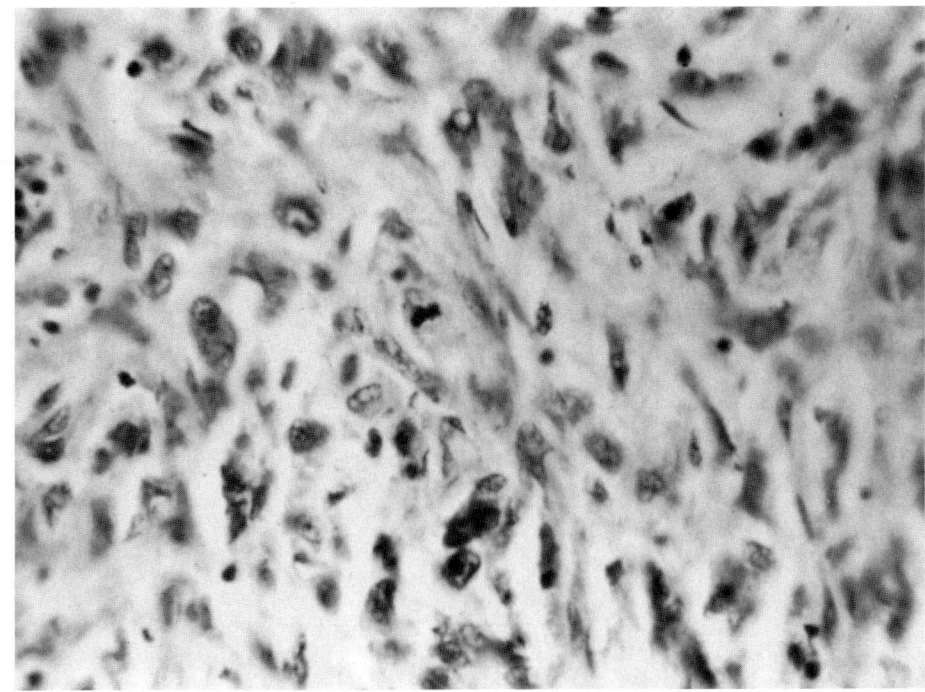

FIGURE 25-26. Malignant fibrous histiocytoma. Elongated cells with hyperchromatic nuclei and some mitotic figures. Some cells demonstrate large amounts of cytoplasm suggesting histiocytic origin. (Original magnification × 600; courtesy of Rudolf Garret, M.D.)

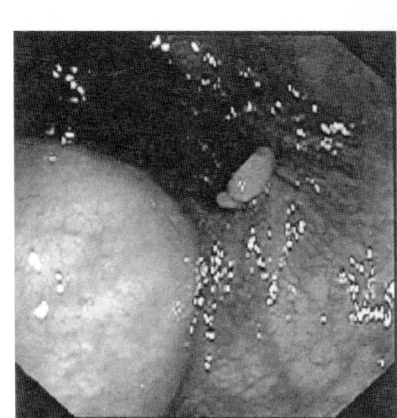
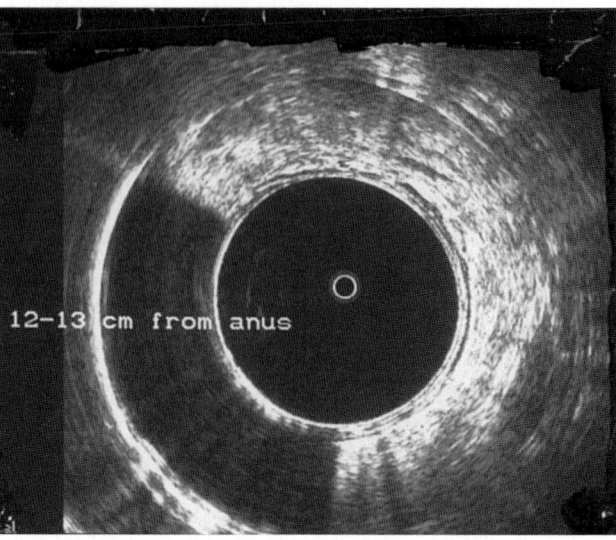

FIGURE 25-27. Malignant gastrointestinal stromal tumor (GIST). **(A)** Extrarectal mass *(arrows)* seen on retroflexion of colonoscope demonstrating mucosal preservation. **(B)** Endorectal ultrasound shows a posterior mass of mixed echogenicity *(arrows)* that upon excision proved to be a GIST. (See Color Fig. 25-27.)

people each year develop GISTs. Men and women are equally affected. GISTs are most often diagnosed in people 50 years of age or older, but they can occur in any age group. There appears to be an association with neurofibromatosis, and there have also been reports in which several family members are affected.

Symptoms

Often patients experience no symptoms from these tumors, but, when symptomatic, complaints include rectal bleeding (50%), abdominal pain (30% to 40%), vomiting (from obstruction), and fatigue (from anemia). About one half have metastatic disease at the time of presentation.[149]

Diagnosis and Tumor Behavior

The diagnosis of GIST is usually made on biopsy or, more commonly, at the time of exploratory laparotomy that was performed for an unknown mass. However, the diagnosis of GIST may be suggested by preoperative CT through the presence of a large mass *without* adenopathy.[98] An incidental extrarectal mass may be felt or seen at the time of routine digital examination, proctoscopy, or colonoscopy (Figure 25-27).

In GIST, a specific mutation in the DNA causes a tyrosine kinase enzyme, known as KIT, to be switched "on" all the time. KIT is responsible for sending growth and survival signals inside the cell. If it is on, the cell stays alive and grows or proliferates. The overactive mutant KIT enzyme triggers the uncontrolled growth of GIST tumor cells. KIT can be identified by looking for a portion of the enzyme, the CD117 antigen. The presence of CD117 is, in fact, a defining feature of GIST and is widely used to confirm the diagnosis.

Distinguishing benign from malignant tumors may be quite difficult. It is important to recognize that the current concept is that all GISTs are at risk for malignancy (Figure 25-28). The location of the tumor seems to affect behavior, but probably the most important prognostic factors for metastatic risk are tumor size at diagnosis and mitotic count. Still, a small GIST in the small intestine may grow more quickly and be more likely to spread than a large gastric tumor. When a GIST metastasizes, it usually spreads to the liver or peritoneal cavity but rarely spreads to the lymph nodes.

Treatment

Until recently, the only treatment for GIST had been wide surgical resection. However, surgery alone for larger GISTs or for GISTs that have spread yields disappointing results. Unfortunately, conventional chemotherapy or radiation after surgery has not been demonstrably effective. However, imatinib mesylate (formerly known to as ST1571) and manufactured as Gleevec in the United States and Glivac in Europe has been demonstrated to be an effective inhibitor of tyrosine kinases.[98] Preliminary reports have shown this drug to be the first effective systemic agent for metastatic and locally inoperable GIST.

Results

There is a very wide range in survival rates reported for these tumors, a fact that makes interpretation of published data quite difficult. As many as perhaps 90% of patients who have undergone resection for GIST develop re-

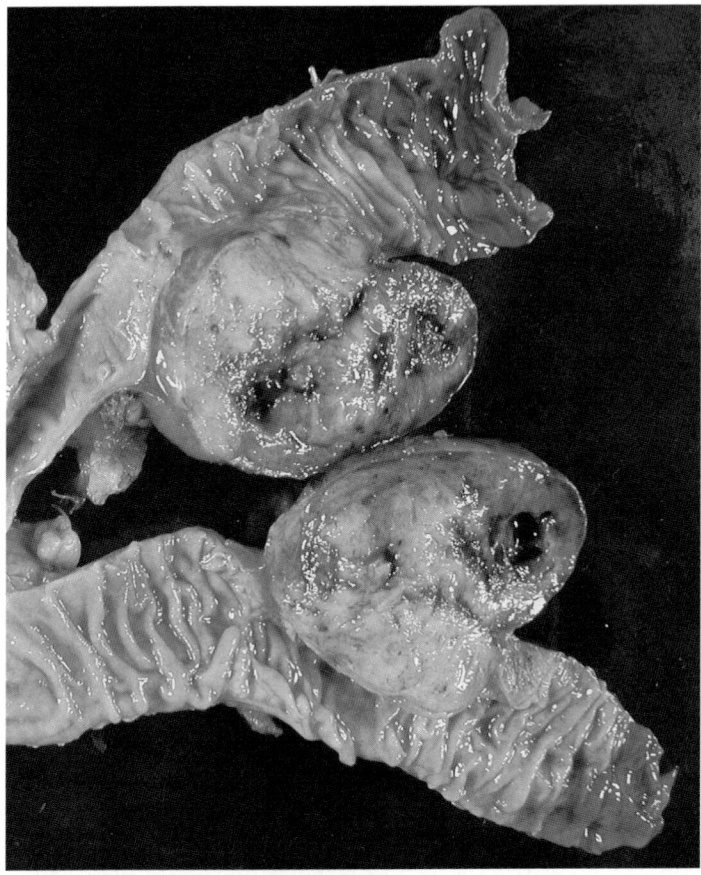

A

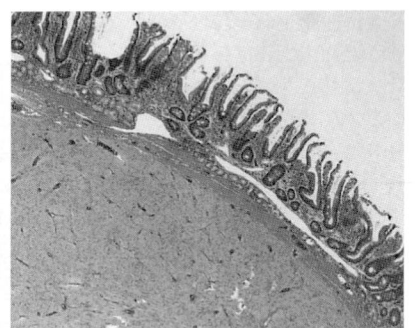

B

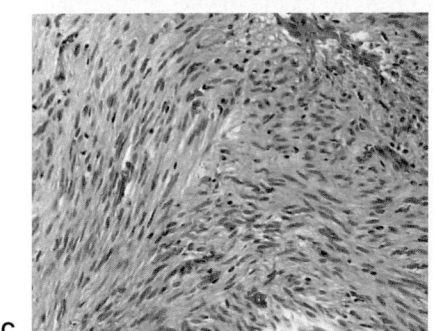

C

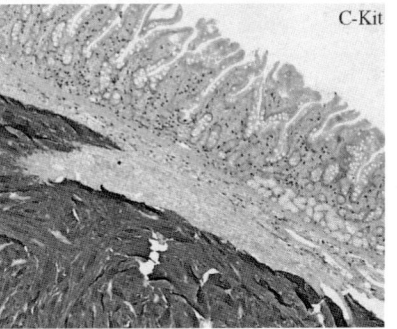

D

C-Kit

FIGURE 25-28. Gastrointestinal stromal tumor (GIST). **(A)** Cut section of tumor, located within the wall of the small bowel, with a pale, fleshy appearance. The overlying mucosa is intact. **(B)** Low-power photomicrograph demonstrates intact small bowel mucosa and muscularis mucosae overlying a well-circumscribed spindle cell neoplasm. **(C)** At high magnification, the uniform spindle-shaped cells with cigar-shaped nuclei bear a close resemblance to smooth muscle cells. **(D)** Positive immunohistochemical staining for the antigen CD117 (C-KIT) is diagnostic of a GIST tumor rather than a smooth muscle tumor. (Courtesy of Leonard Kahn, M.D.)

currence.[113] Connolly and co-workers performed a MEDLINE literature search and concluded that the 5-year survival rate after complete excision is approximately 50%.[98] Langer and colleagues reviewed their experience with GISTs in 39 patients.[284] As one would expect, failure to extirpate the tumor completely had an adverse consequence on survival when compared with those lesions that could be completely removed. Tumor size of 5 cm or greater, mitotic count of two or more, and proliferative activity greater than 10% were significantly associated with a shorter recurrence-free survival. These investigators also found that patients did better if the tumors demonstrated significantly fewer genetic alterations.

Smooth Muscle Origin

Colonic Leiomyoma

Smooth muscle tumors of the alimentary tract are rare, and benign smooth muscle tumors of the colon are exceedingly uncommon. Stout conducted a 50-year study in which he found 30 leiomyomas in 200 benign neoplasms.[469] In a 15-year study, Ferguson and Houston reported two leiomyomas from a total of 67 benign tumors.[143] Skardalakis and colleagues reviewed 59 cases of leiomyomas, and MacKenzie and co-workers collected reports of 19 cases from the literature and added eight of their own.[306,449]

Smooth muscle tumors are found in patients of all ages, with a gradual increase in frequency and malignant degeneration up to the sixth decade.[257] The tumor is classified according to its appearance and direction of growth. The intracolonic type may be pedunculated or sessile. The extracolonic type grows away from the lumen of the bowel and lies in the abdominal cavity attached to the wall. The dumbbell type grows into the lumen and

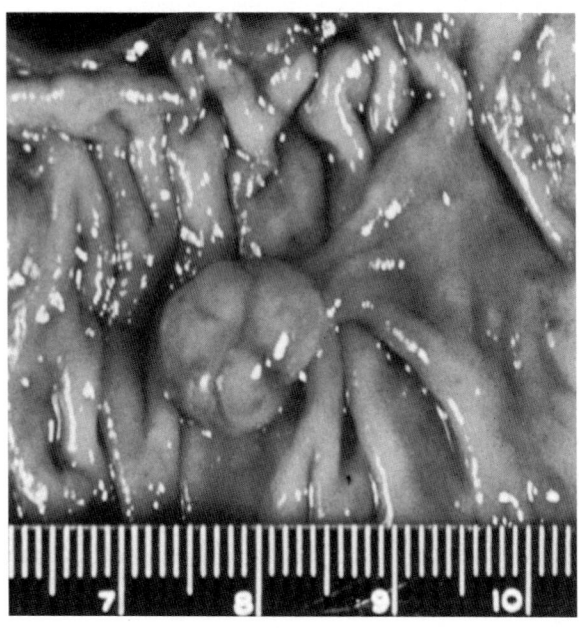

FIGURE 25-29. Pedunculated leiomyoma.

into the abdominal cavity simultaneously. This type of tumor accounts for 4% of all smooth muscle tumors of the GI tract. These usually reach a much larger size than those with unilateral spread. The constrictive type encircles a variable length of bowel. Lookanoff and Tsapralis observed that the sigmoid and transverse colon seemed to be the most common sites and that very few leiomyomas were found in the cecum.[297]

The tumor may be an incidental finding in an asymptomatic individual, or the patient may present with pain or a lump. Perforation, intestinal obstruction (secondary to the tumor itself or to intussusception), and hemorrhage have been reported.[349]

Macroscopically, the tumor appears well encapsulated. On cross-section, leiomyomas have a fleshy appearance; because the tumor is under pressure, it tends to protrude (Figs. 25-29 through 25-31).

Histologically, a typical spindle cell neoplasm can be observed (Figure 25-32). Most investigators believe that the mitotic rate is the single most important criterion for diagnosis of malignancy (Figure 25-33).[52,62,137,470] Other indicators are a variation in nuclear size and shape, hyperchromasia, frequent bizarre cells, and difficulty in identification of longitudinal myofibrils.[52,62,137] If the mitotic rate is high, if the growth is rapid, if an ulcer is present, or if the lesion is greater than 2.5 cm in diameter, malignant degeneration should be suspected. Smooth muscle tumors are usually locally invasive, but metastasis from a primary tumor in the GI tract has been described.[62]

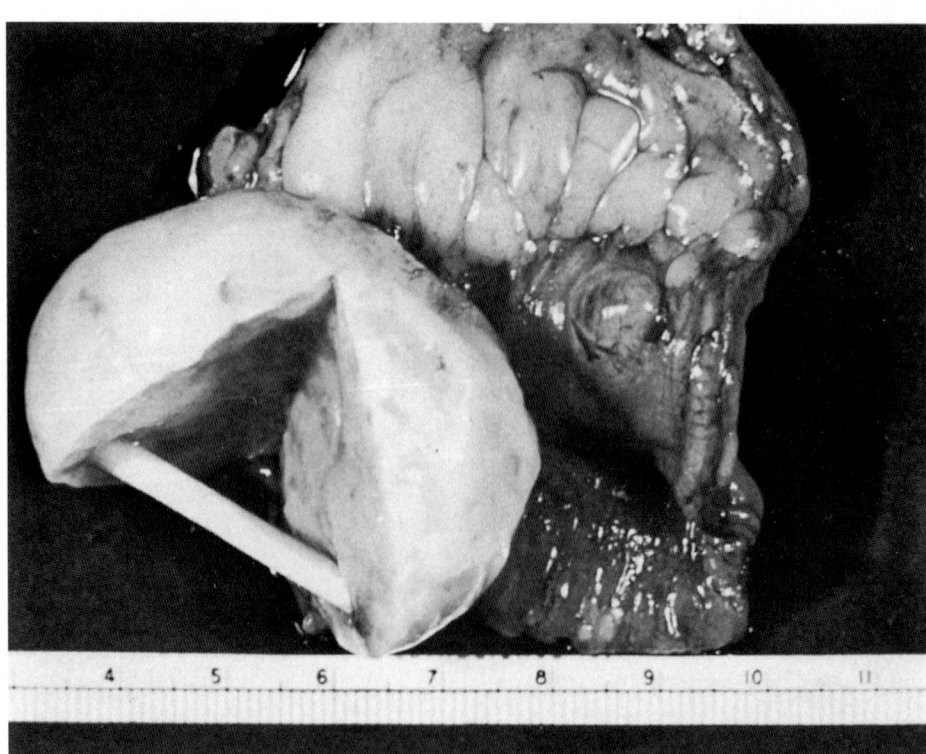

FIGURE 25-30. Leiomyoma. A well-encapsulated mass in the bowel wall. (Courtesy of Rudolf Garret, M.D.)

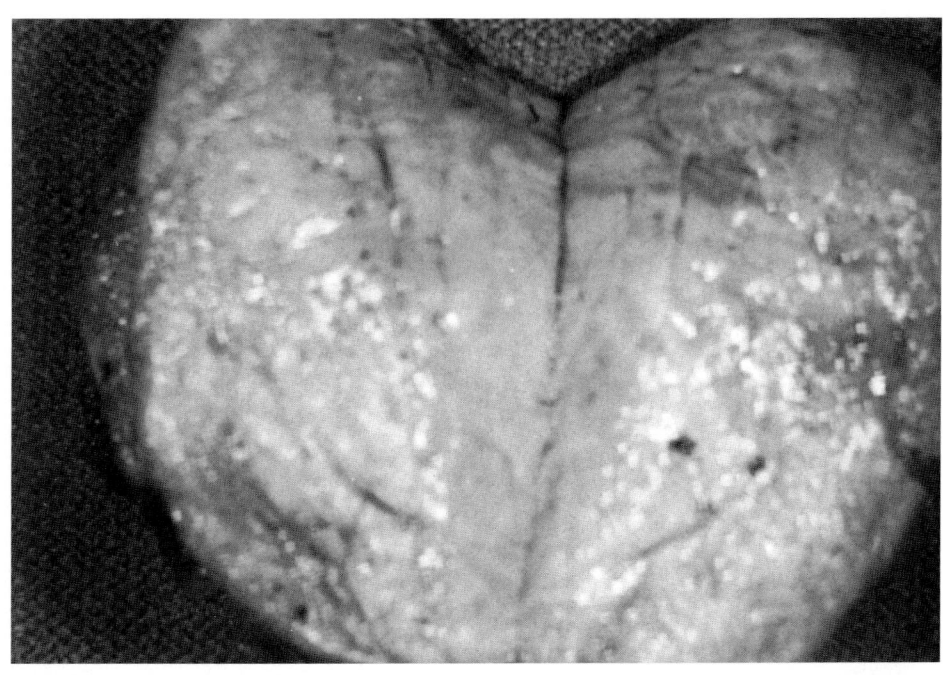

FIGURE 25-31. A leiomyoma removed from the hepatic flexure reveals a fleshy tumor on cross-section. (Courtesy of Rudolf Garret, M.D.)

Radiologic features vary depending on whether the tumor is intramural, submucosal, subserosal, or dumbbell shaped.[35]

Treatment

Surgical excision results in cure unless the tumor is extraperitoneal or rectal (see later). Complete removal should be attempted regardless of the radiologic appearance or of probable inoperability. Swerdlow and colleagues reported a case of an elderly individual with a benign leiomyoma of the cecum that had ulcerated and perforated the bowel wall.[478] The patient presented with an acute abdomen. Because it is generally not possible to distinguish benign from malignant lesions preoperatively, a standard cancer operation should be performed under such circumstances.

Rectal Leiomyoma

Only a few cases of rectal leiomyomas have been reported.[16,359,428,437] Vorobyov and colleagues reported their experience at the Research Institute of Proctology

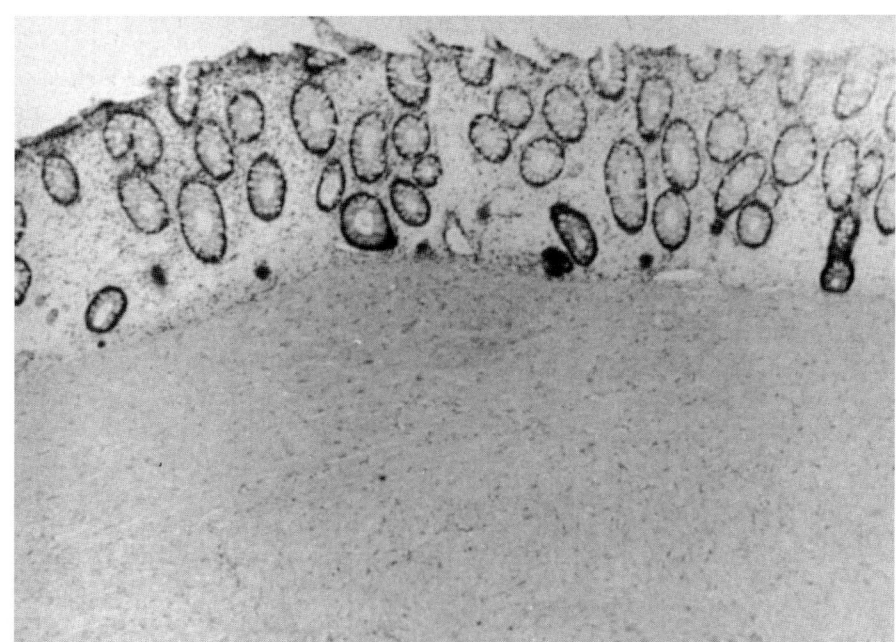

FIGURE 25-32. Leiomyoma of the colon. Spindle cell neoplasm filling the submucosa with thinning of the overlying mucosa. Nuclei are blunted at ends with surrounding vacuoles. There is no evidence of mitoses or pleiomorphism. (Original magnification × 100.)

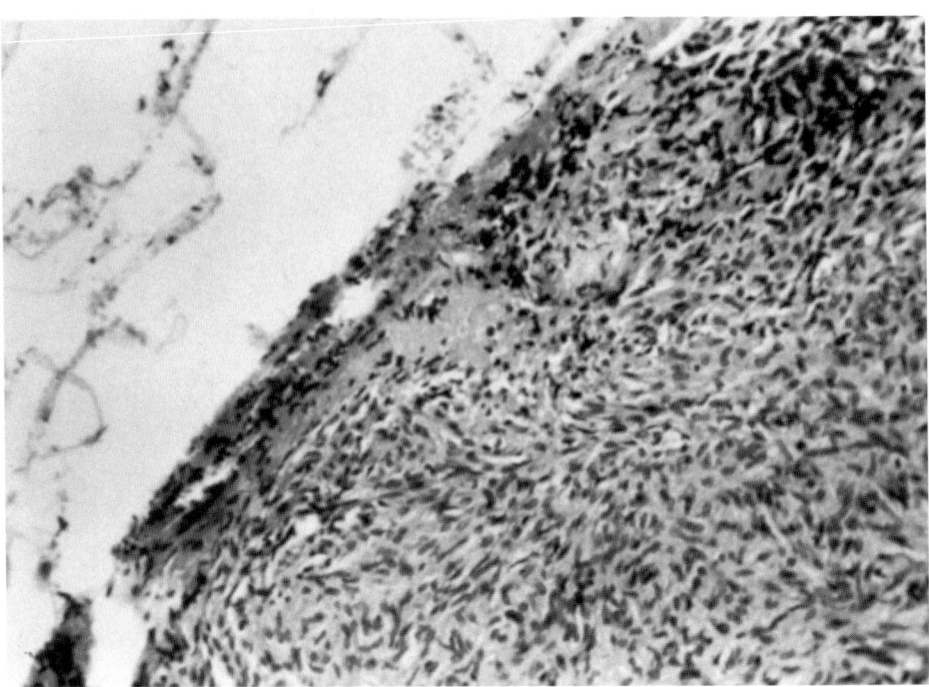

FIGURE 25-33. Interlacing bundles of smooth muscle surrounded by a fibrous capsule. No motoses are evident. (Original magnification × 260; courtesy of Rudolf Garret, M.D.)

in Moscow.[510] Thirty-six patients with benign leiomyoma of the rectum underwent surgery between the years 1972 and 1990. Approximately one third were male. In this experience, the tumors often tended to arise from the internal anal sphincter. Some investigators have found that endorectal ultrasound is helpful in determining the limits of the lesion.[437] A homogeneous hypoechoic tumor without invasion of the perirectal tissue may be noted.[223]

Smaller myomas usually cause no symptoms, can be found on routine rectal examination, and are usually removed with a diathermy snare or by transanal excision. Large lesions may cause interference with defecation, a sense of fullness in the rectum, and a frequent desire to defecate. Because of these distressing symptoms and the possibility of obstruction and malignant degeneration, removal of the growth is indicated.

When the tumor is essentially extrarectal, it is best to excise it by means of an extrarectal approach rather than transanally. Even large tumors may be treated by local excision, but if clinical suspicion of malignancy exists, such as ulceration, hemorrhage, or extrarectal fixation, radical surgical treatment by excision of the rectum is indicated. Biopsies may be difficult to interpret in such cases. In the experience of the group from the Research Institute of Proctology, one third (n = 12) of their patients harbored lesions less than 1 cm in diameter, and these lesions were all removed by means of transanal excision.[510] An additional ten patients with tumors from 2.5 to 5 cm also were treated by this approach. Six other individuals underwent excision by means of a perirectal operation,

whereas abdominoperineal resection or abdominoanal operations were performed in those with tumors measuring from 8 to 20 cm. Recurrence was found in nine patients, all of whom had local procedures. In seven, malignant transformation was the reason.

Leiomyosarcoma

Colon

Leiomyosarcoma of the large bowel is a very rare lesion. The total number of published cases is probably fewer than 150, although many would today probably be classified as GIST tumors (see earlier discussion).[21,30,35,71,87,221,398,409,435,465] No age predilection for this disease is apparent. It affects the genders equally and is more than twice as common in the rectum as it is in the rest of the colon.

Leiomyosarcoma arises from the smooth muscle of the bowel wall (Figure 25-34). A very insidious disease, it can remain asymptomatic for a long period. Weight loss is almost never recorded, but pain is a common symptom. Tarry stools and the sequelae of anemia are the most frequent presentations (Figure 25-35). A palpable tumor is almost always present when the lesion occurs in the rectum, and in some instances, obstruction is also seen.

Diagnosis of this lesion preoperatively is extremely difficult because it resembles carcinoma of the colon in its radiographic appearance. The tumor may project into the lumen of the bowel, grow outward, or present as a dumbbell-type tumor.[410] An interesting radiologic finding may be demonstrated when tracts of barium extend into a sub-

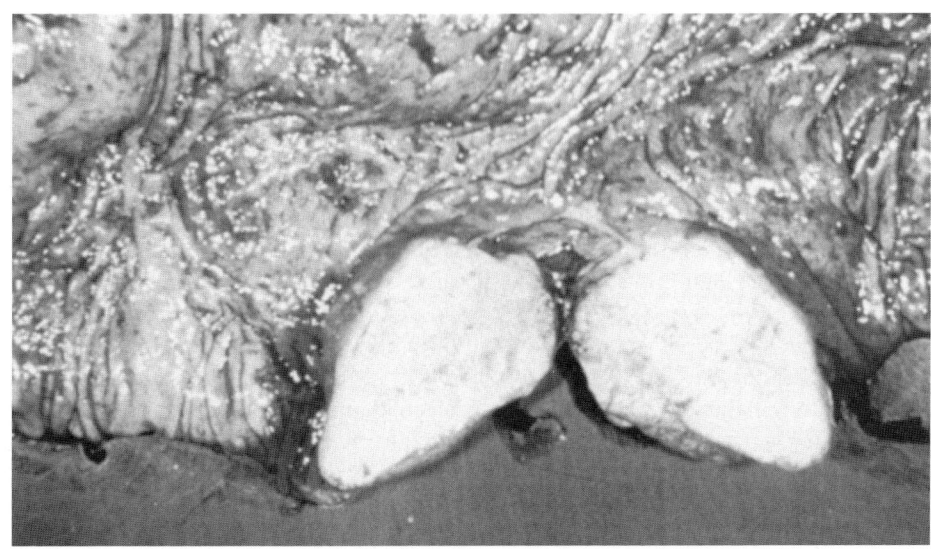

FIGURE 25-34. Leiomyosarcoma. This tumor of the bowel wall looks well encapsulated, but histologic examination revealed frequent mitotic figures. (From Corman ML, Veidenheimer MC, Swinton NW. *Diseases of the anus, rectum and colon. Part I: neoplasms.* New York: Medcom, 1972.)

serosal tumor.[71] Sonographic features may include a thick echogenic rim with central cavitation.[245] Colonoscopy and biopsy are useful in confirming the diagnosis.

An attempt to stage the disease for the sake of better management was reported by Astarjian and colleagues as follows:[21]

Stage I: tumor confined to the intestinal wall; no invasion, no ulceration
  A. Submucosal tumor
  B. Subserosal tumor
Stage II: tumor extending beyond the wall of the colon
  A. Intraluminal ulceration
  B. Infiltration into adjacent extracolonic tissues
Stage III: tumor with distant metastases

Based on this staging and on the slow-growing nature of colonic leiomyosarcoma, these investigators suggested that the prognosis for patients with this tumor is as follows:

Stage I-A and I-B: excellent
Stage II-A: excellent
Stage II-B: fair
Stage III: poor

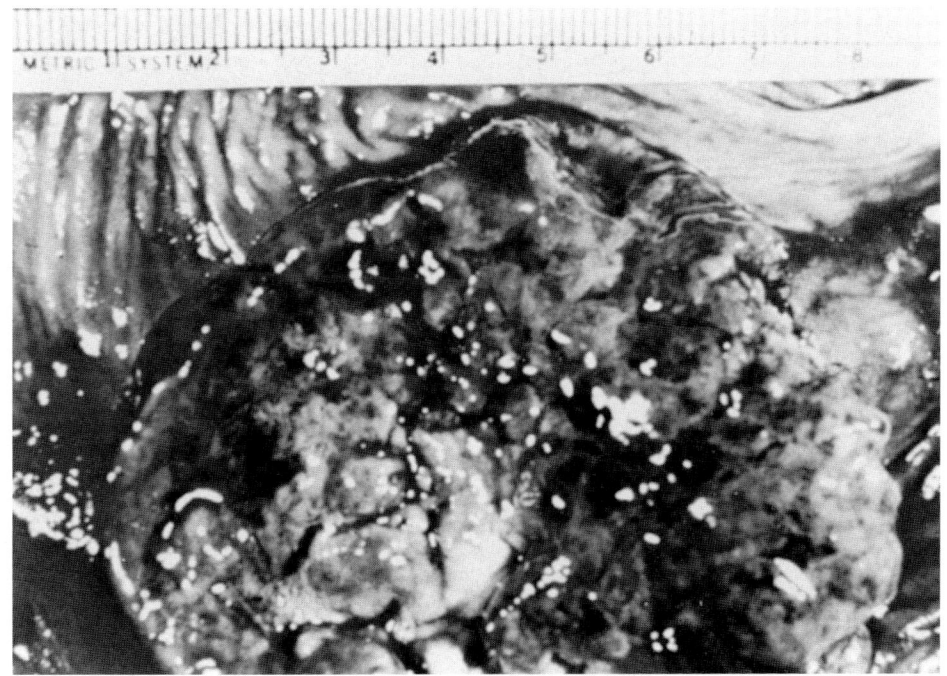

FIGURE 25-35. Ulcerating leiomyosarcoma producing hematochezia. The absence of infiltrating margins indicates that it is less likely to be an adenocarcinoma. (From Corman ML, Veidenheimer MC, Swinton NW. *Diseases of the anus, rectum and colon. Part I: neoplasms.* New York: Medcom, 1972.)

The accuracy of prognosis based upon the degree of differentiation has been described by the Mayo Clinic group.[7] Grade 1 tumors have a greater abundance of cells than leiomyomas; mitotic activity is minimal with no pleiomorphism or anaplasia. With grade 2 tumors, mitoses are noted in one of five high-power fields. In grade 3 leiomyosarcoma, a mitosis is seen in every high-power field. Grade 4 lesions demonstrate marked cellularity, pleomorphism, and three or more mitoses per high-power field.

Most of the reported cases have been managed by resection of the tumor-bearing portion of the colon. Leiomyosarcoma is usually a tumor of low-grade malignancy. Patients who have been treated by resection have lived many years despite residual tumor or metastases.[174] The lungs and regional lymph nodes are rarely involved, but the tumor does have a tendency to metastasize to the liver.

Rectum

More than 200 cases of rectal leiomyosarcoma have been recorded in the literature.[16,22,54,116,130,150,256,346,394,426,443,455,460,477,491,537,540] The tumor arises in the smooth muscle of the rectal wall. Most are seen in the lower one third of the rectum and are more commonly found in men than in women. The tumor may present as a nodular or protuberant swelling with some central ulceration that appears to arise in the deeper layers of the bowel wall. Most are large and consist microscopically of interlacing bands of smooth muscle fibers that are well differentiated and histologically of a low-grade malignancy (Figs. 25-36 and 25-37). Extensive direct spread into the perirectal tissue is a characteristic feature. This may make surgical removal so difficult that local recurrence even after excision of the rectum is not uncommon.

Smooth muscle sarcomas of the rectum do not usually metastasize to regional lymph nodes unless they are poorly differentiated. An exception was described by Thorlakson and Ross in a case with lymphatic spread to one hemorrhoidal lymph node and with venous involvement.[491]

As with colonic leiomyosarcoma, radical resection is generally the preferred approach. Local excision is liable to be followed by recurrence, even though this may be delayed for some years.[117,142,537] The tumor is not generally considered radiosensitive. Luna-Pérez and colleagues suggested that in rectal sarcoma, surgery plus radiotherapy may reduce the incidence of local recurrence and, in selected patients, allow for anal sphincter preservation.[302] Chemotherapy with vincristine, cyclophosphamide, actinomycin D, and doxorubicin (Adriamycin) has also been advocated.[18]

Results of Treatment of Leiomyosarcoma

Morson pointed out that although most leiomyosarcomas are of a low-grade malignancy, the ultimate prognosis is very poor.[346] This is essentially because of late diagnosis and extensive local spread by the time of surgery. In the experience of the Memorial Sloan-Kettering Cancer

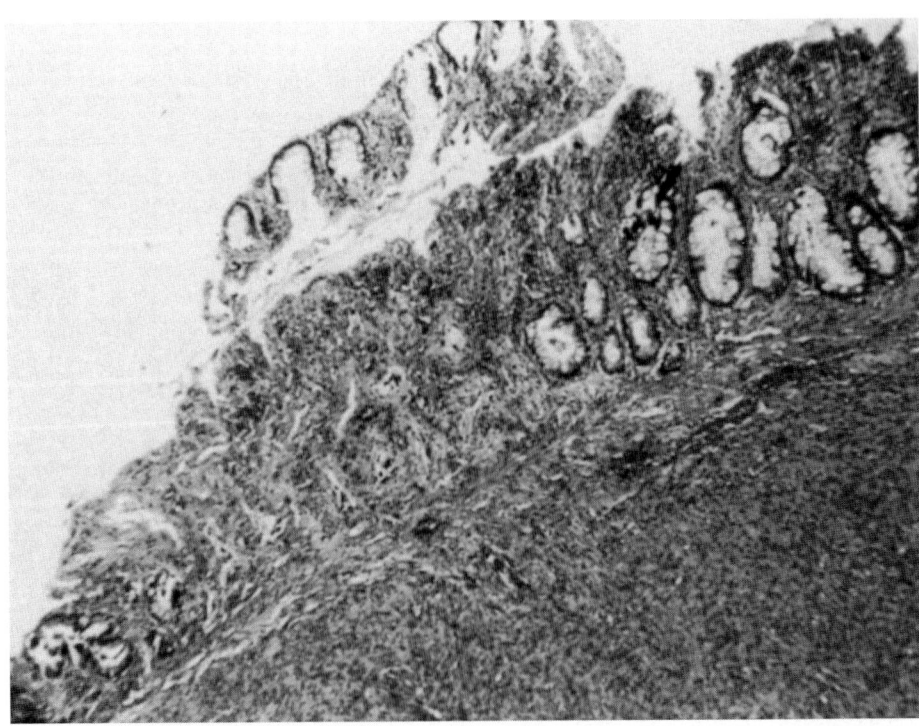

FIGURE 25-36. Leiomyosarcoma. A mass of cells consisting of smooth muscle fibers adjacent to the muscularis mucosae of the rectum. (Original magnification × 80; courtesy of Rudolf Garret, M.D.)

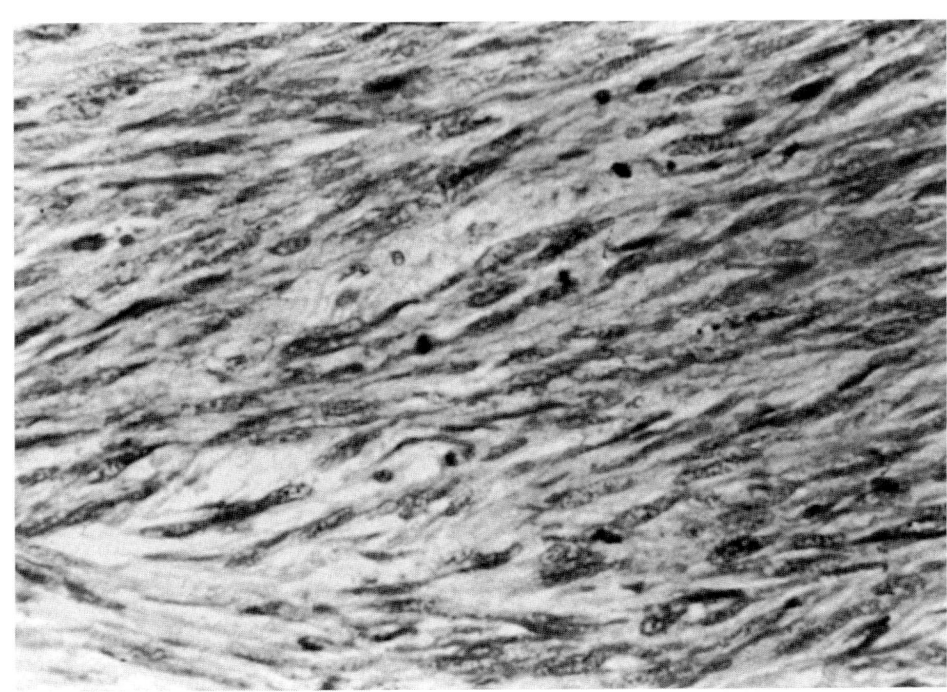

FIGURE 25-37. Leiomyosarcoma. Smooth muscle fibers showing at least six mitotic figures. (Original magnification × 600; from Corman ML, Veidenheimer MC, Swinton NW. *Diseases of the anus, rectum and colon. Part I: neoplasms.* New York: Medcom, 1972.)

Center, a high-grade tumor and, obviously, the presence of metastases were the two unfavorable characteristics that had independent prognostic value.[324] Rectal disease has been shown to have an overall survival rate of 20%.[130] In the experience of Yeh and associates in Taipei, Taiwan, involving 40 patients with rectal tumors, the 5-year, disease-free survival was 46%, but 75% were alive at that time.[537] In addition to high histologic grade, younger age was a significant poor prognostic factor. Apart from local recurrence, metastasis to the liver and lungs is the most common cause of death.

Many of these patients give a rather long history of symptoms before coming to treatment.[7] Their general clinical course confirms the histologic observation that these smooth muscle tumors are mostly well differentiated and of a low-grade malignancy.

Rhabdomyosarcoma

Rhabdomyosarcoma is the most common soft tissue sarcoma in children; it occurs most frequently in the head and neck, genitourinary tract, extremity, and trunk.[335] A few cases have been reported in the perirectal area.[334,430] Horn and Enterline classified rhabdomyosarcoma into four types: pleomorphic, alveolar, embryonal, and botryoid.[220] However, the histologic diagnosis may be confused with other mesenchymal lesions.[334]

The patient usually presents with a mass in the perianal area. Current therapy should include adequate local excision or resection followed by chemotherapy (vin-

cristine, actinomycin D, and cyclophosphamide).[334,430] Prognosis is generally poor.

Adipose Tissue Origin

Lipoma

Excluding hyperplastic polyps, lipoma is the second most common benign tumor of the colon (after adenomatous polyp) and the most common intramural tumor. However, it is still a relatively rare entity. Weinberg and Feldman reviewed more than 60,000 autopsy reports and found only 135 lipomas of the colon (0.2%).[518] Haller and Roberts found 11 lipomas in more than 3,400 autopsies (0.3%).[195]

Colonic lipomas are well-differentiated, benign fatty tumors arising from deposits of adipose connective tissue in the bowel wall. Malignant change has not been reported. Approximately 90% are submucosal and 10% subserosal. The submucosal lipoma is covered by mucosa and occasionally by muscularis mucosae and grows toward the intestinal lumen (Figs. 25-38 and 25-39). The mucosa covering the tumor may become atrophic, congested, ulcerated, or even necrotic, or it may retain its normal yellowish appearance. The subserosal type usually originates from the appendices epiploicae and grows toward the peritoneal cavity.

Colonic lipomas usually occur in patients between the ages of 50 and 70 years with about an equal gender distribution. The average age is similar to that of individuals with colonic carcinoma. Patients with colonic lipoma do not appear ill nor do they experience anorexia, weight

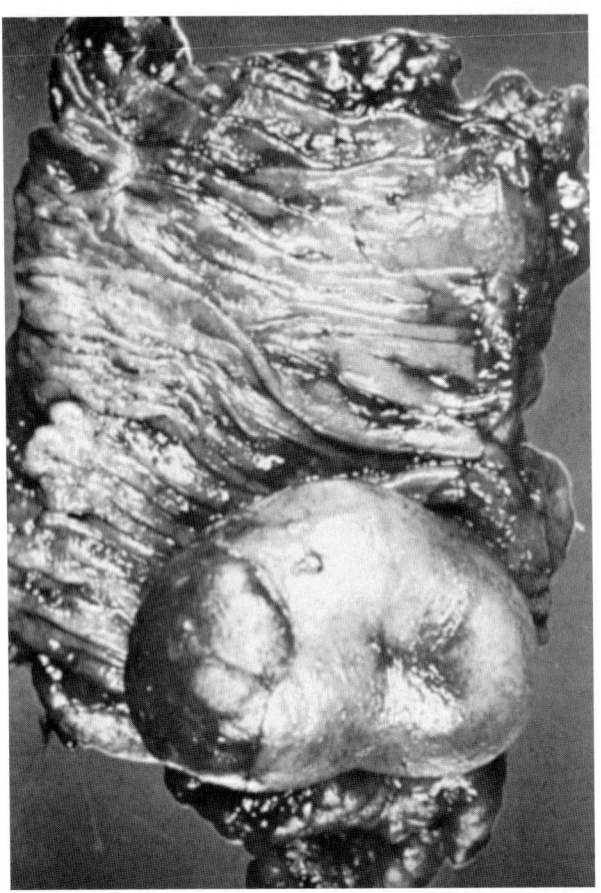

FIGURE 25-38. Submucosal lipoma in the region of the ileocecal valve. (From Corman ML, Veidenheimer MC, Swinton NW. *Diseases of the anus, rectum and colon. Part I: neoplasms.* New York: Medcom, 1972.)

loss, or anemia. Most colonic lipomas are asymptomatic and are found at autopsy or incidentally during an operation for some other problem. However, with size in excess of 2 cm, approximately one third will give rise to some symptom.[332] This may include constipation, diarrhea, abdominal pain, and rectal bleeding (Figure 25-40).[408] The presence of a palpable mass may be the lipoma itself, impaction of fecal material, or intussuscepted bowel.[332]

The most common sites for lipoma are the cecum, ascending colon, and sigmoid colon. Lipoma or lipomatosis of the ileocecal valve is characterized by diffuse submucosal adipose infiltration of the valve.[494] Pemberton and McCormack found 50 tumors in the right colon, 15 in the transverse colon, and 37 in the left colon and rectum.[379] Castro and Stearns reported 45 tumors, 31 of which were in the right colon (69%).[74] Eleven of their patients (26%) had two or more lipomas, and four had three or more. All multiple lipomas were found in the right half of the colon.

Barium enema examination can usually distinguish a lipoma from that of another type of tumor (Figs. 25-41 through 25-43). A water enema with low-kilovoltage technique may take advantage of the different absorption coefficients of fat and water: fat-containing lesions will appear relatively radiolucent.[314] The shape of the mass may be observed to change during fluoroscopic examination as a consequence of peristalsis or of manual pressure, the so-called "squeeze sign."[332] CT appearance is that of a homogeneous mass consistent with the density of fat.

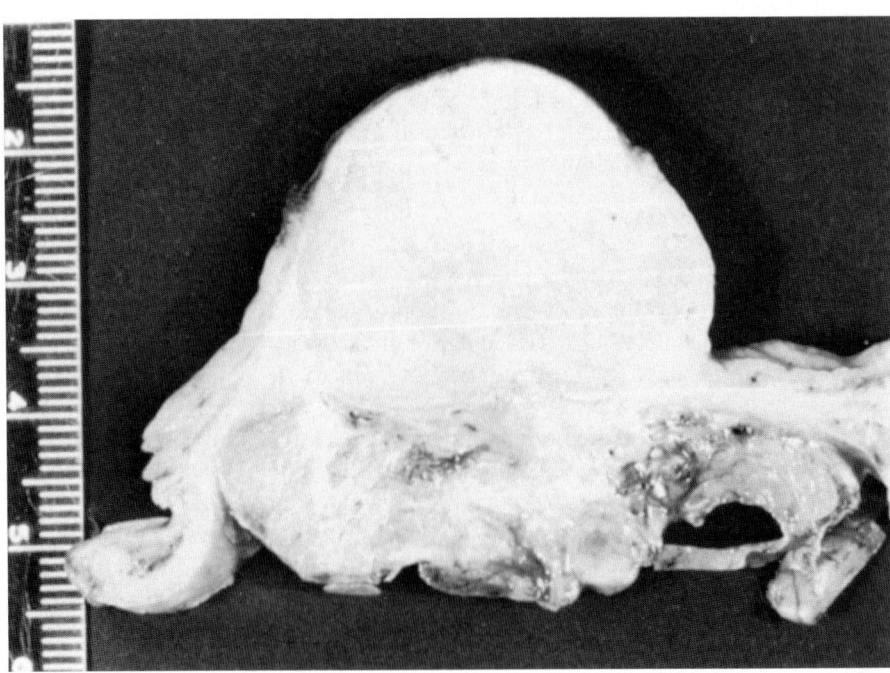

FIGURE 25-39. Lipoma. A formalin-fixed specimen of a well-circumscribed mass in the wall of the large bowel. (Courtesy of Rudolf Garret, M.D.)

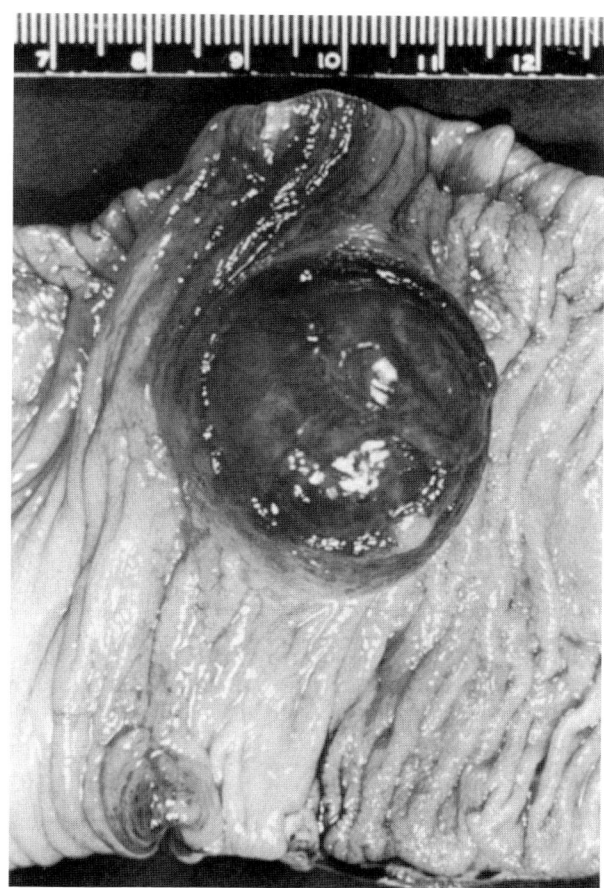

FIGURE 25-40. Submucosal lipoma of the transverse colon. Rectal bleeding is explained by the hemorrhagic appearance of the lesion. (Courtesy of Rudolf Garret, M.D.)

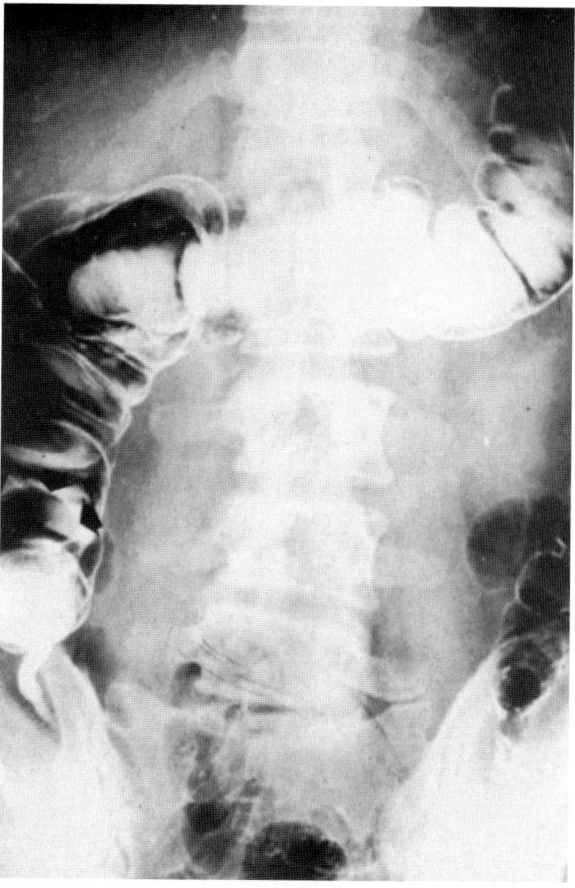

FIGURE 25-41. Barium enema demonstrates a characteristic filling defect in the proximal ascending colon *(arrows)*. The smooth, spherical outline is practically pathognomonic of this disease. (Corman ML, Veidenheimer MC, Swinton NW. *Diseases of the anus, rectum and colon. Part I: neoplasms.* New York: Medcom, 1972.)

Mucosal lipomas can also be diagnosed with the colonoscope (Figure 25-44).[112,494] Certain endoscopic features suggesting lipoma have been described, including the "cushion sign" (identification of the lipoma with pressure from a biopsy forceps), the "tenting sign" (elevation of the overlying mucosa with the biopsy forceps), and the "naked fat sign" (extrusion of fat following biopsy).[408] Not uncommonly, they may be removed by means of this instrument.[42,515] However, this approach is usually limited to symptomatic patients and those in whom the lesion is somewhat pedunculated (Figs. 25-45 and 25-46).

The microscopic appearance is that of mature adipose tissue surrounded by a fibrous capsule (Figure 25-47).

Colonic lipomas do not require treatment except when they ulcerate. Once the diagnosis has been established and carcinoma has been ruled out, the patient need only be reassured. However, in the symptomatic patient, a limited resection or colotomy and lipomectomy will usually be advised. Laparoscopic removal has also been reported.[418] The requirement for resection because of confusion with a malignant process should be a rare occur-

rence today, with the availability of colonoscopy and CT.[222,246,415]

Lipoma of the *rectum* is extremely rare. When it can be reached with the finger, it usually is felt as a soft, smooth, lobulated mass. Pedunculated lesions may prolapse and present a slight problem of differential diagnosis, especially if it is hemorrhagic or necrotic. Tenesmus may result when the growth is in the lower rectum and involves the internal sphincter. When situated in the rectum or the sigmoid, it may produce symptoms because of its size or when traumatized. If seen with the aid of a proctoscope, the yellow color of the fat of which it is composed is usually apparent through the mucosa.

The most frequent site in the rectal area is the perianal region, in which case the tumor develops from the subcutaneous tissue. A lipoma in this area or buttock usually causes no symptoms unless it becomes quite large, and the overlying skin becomes irritated.

Ligation of the base and removal may be performed when the tumor is pedunculated. Incision and enucle-

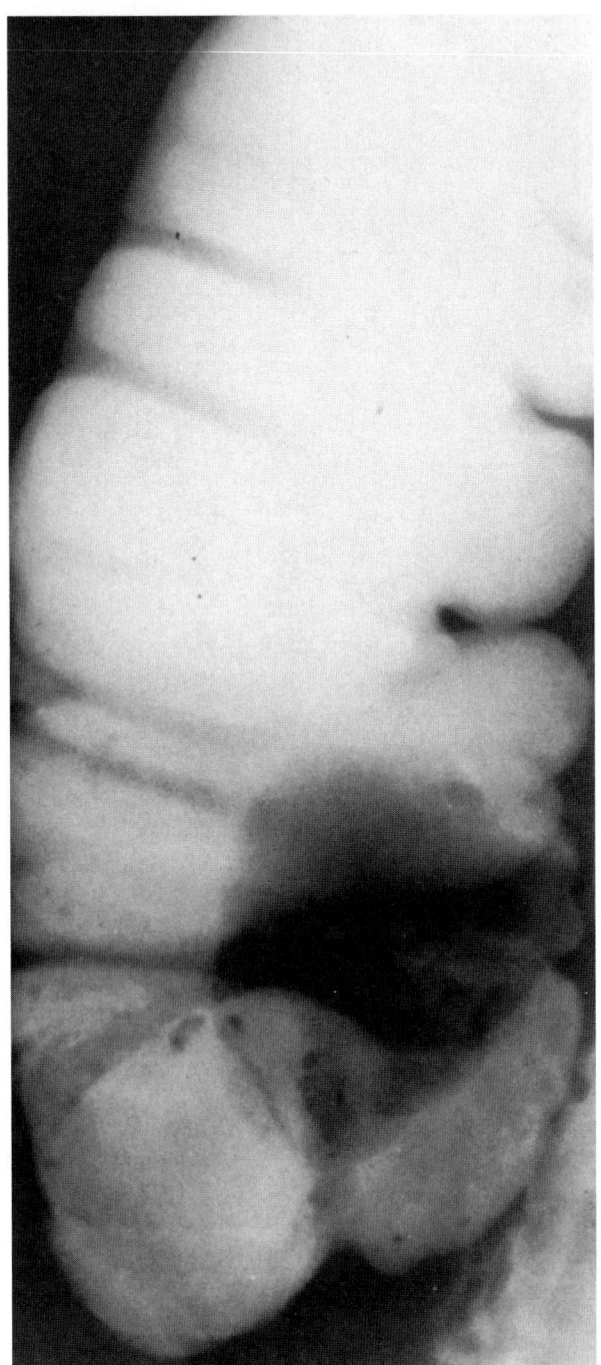

FIGURE 25-42. A lipoma of the ileocecal valve that produced abdominal pain and vomiting.

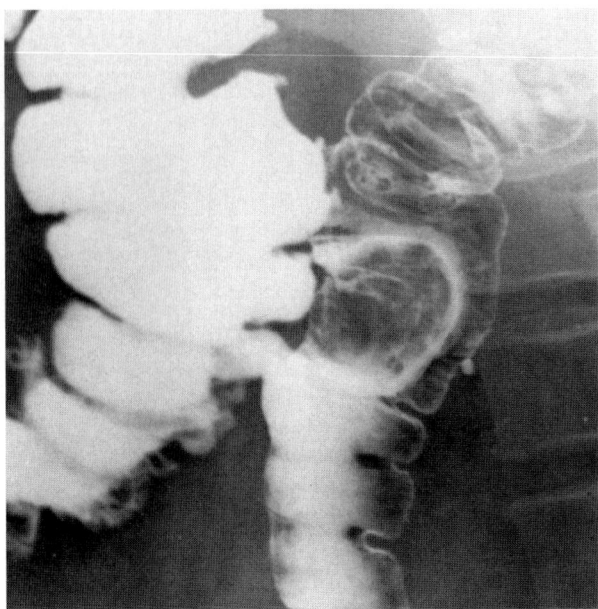

FIGURE 25-43. Lipoma of the descending colon. A submucosal polypoid mass without mucosal irregularity or destruction. The patient complained of left upper abdominal pain.

107 lipomas.[294,474] Radiographically, colonic lipomatosis must be differentiated from numerous benign and malignant conditions. These include familial polyposis,[315] juvenile polyposis,[446] Gardner syndrome,[542] Cronkhite-Canada syndrome,[106] Peutz-Jeghers syndrome,[173] nodular lymphoid hyperplasia,[154] inflammatory bowel disease with pseudopolyposis, lymphosarcoma,[529] ganglioneurofibromatosis,[65] malacoplakia,[417] pneumatosis coli, and colitis cystica profunda.[516]

In 1985, Snover and colleagues described 24 cases of mucosal "pseudolipomatosis."[458] The lesions were removed through the colonoscope, but the absence of adipocytes led the authors to conclude that the condition was due to entrapment of gas in the lamina propria.

ation may be employed if the lipoma is confined to the rectal wall.

Lipomatosis

Swain and co-workers reported a child with lipomatous polyposis throughout the entire colon, and Ling and associates resected the colon of a 60-year-old woman with

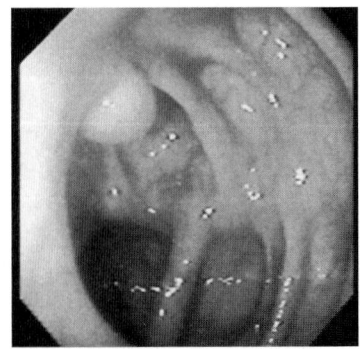

FIGURE 25-44. Lipoma of the ileocecal valve can be seen through the colonoscope. (See Color Fig. 25-44.)

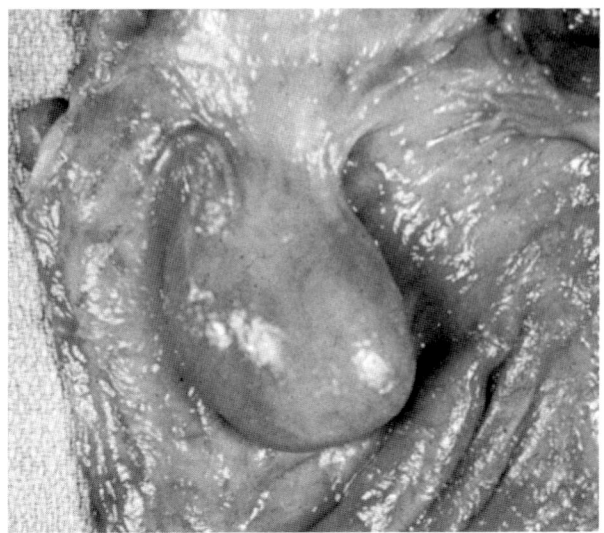

FIGURE 25-45. Pedunculated lipoma treated by bowel resection. (Courtesy of Rudolf Garret, M.D.)

TUMORS OF NEURAL ORIGIN

Neurofibroma

Neurofibromas are benign nerve-sheath tumors. Von Recklinghausen first described multiple subcutaneous neurofibromas (neurofibromatosis) in 1882.[509] The condition has since come to be known as von Recklinghausen's disease. Visceral involvement in disseminated neurofibromatosis is considered rare, yet reports appeared as early as 1930.[123] The possibility of this disease should be considered if GI bleeding or intestinal obstruction occurs in a patient known to have generalized neurofibromatosis.[43,184,289,312,387] It may, however, be seen in the alimentary tract and nowhere else.

The lesions in the intestinal tract arise in the submucosa or muscularis (Figs. 25-48 and 25-49).[168] As the tumor enlarges, the overlying mucosa becomes ulcerated and bleeds. Intussusception can produce intestinal obstruction, and sarcomatous degeneration is a recognized complication.[259,289] Three cases of solitary neurofibromas have been confirmed in the anal canal.[156]

Local excision is preferred unless a large cluster is noted in one segment. Under these circumstances, resection may be advisable.

Ganglioneuromatosis

Ganglioneuromas are neuroectodermal tumors that are rarely found in the colon. They are composed of nerve fibers, Schwann sheath elements, and ganglion cells (Figs. 25-50 through 25-52).[55] When solitary, they may resemble a carcinoma radiologically. Donnelly and colleagues reported a 9-year-old boy who underwent total

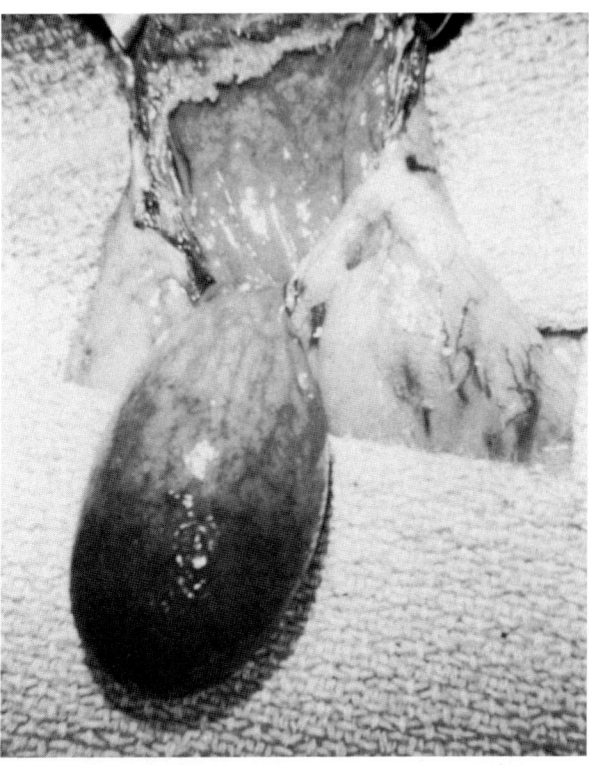

FIGURE 25-46. Pedunculated lipoma at laparotomy, treated by colotomy and lipomectomy. Attempt at colonoscopic removal was unsuccessful.

colectomy because of multiple colonic polyps that caused severe rectal bleeding.[120] Of the two kinds of polyps found, one was largely composed of groups of ganglion cells and nerve fibers in trunks and networks, and the other resembled retention polyps. Ganglion cells, nerve fiber networks, or both were also found in the nonpolypoid colonic mucosa and in the mucosa of the stalks of the retention polyps. These authors selected the term ganglioneuromatosis for its descriptive value and suggested that this lesion is probably akin to neurofibromatosis and should be distinguished from ganglioneuroma, although its precise relationship to the former is not definitely established. Normann and Otnes reported a case of diffuse intestinal ganglioneuromatosis in which severe diarrhea was the predominant symptom.[360] Kanter and colleagues described a 40-year-old man with the disease in association with a colorectal cancer.[247] They opined that ganglioneuromatous polyposis should be considered a premalignant condition.

Treatment is local excision or resection.

Neurilemoma or Schwannoma

Neurilemoma is a rare neoplasm that originates from Schwann cells. When it occurs in the GI tract the colon is the least likely site. Fewer than ten cases have appeared

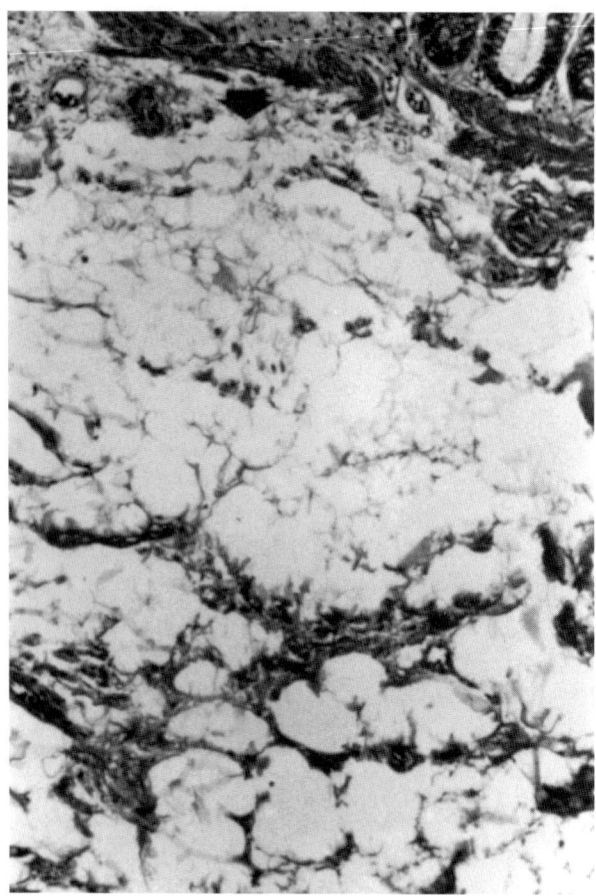

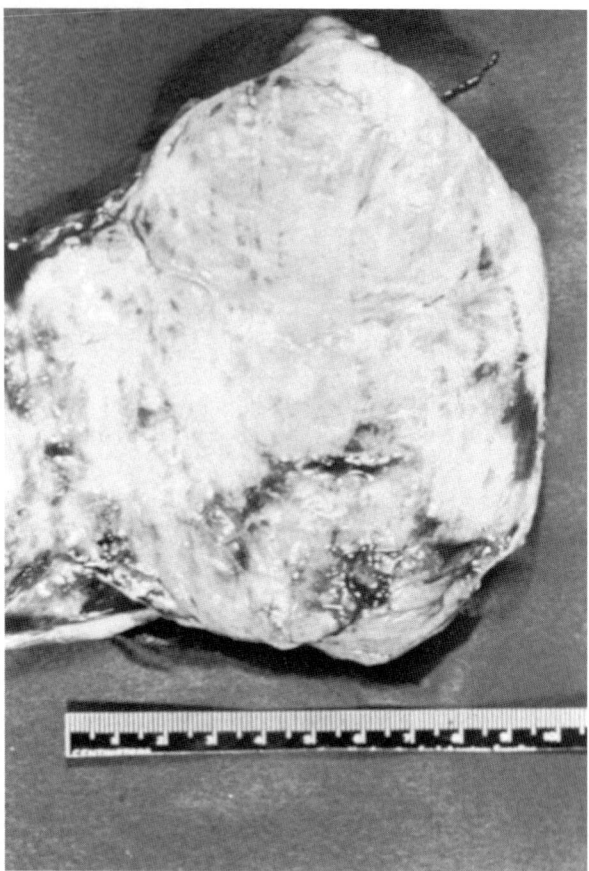

FIGURE 25-47. Lipoma. Well-differentiated, mature adipocytes (fat cells) in the submucosa of the bowel *(arrow)*. (Original magnification × 260.)

FIGURE 25-48. Neurofibroma. A firm, fleshy, whitish tumor attached to wall of the bowel. (Courtesy of Rudolf Garret, M.D.)

in the literature.[450] Neurogenic tumors have also been reported to be the cause of masses in the presacral space. They may be identified by palpation on rectal examination and confirmed by CT (Figure 25-53). Treatment is local excision or resection, usually by a transcoccygeal approach (Figure 25-54; see later). Kovalcik and colleagues removed a 13-cm neurilemoma by means of a combined abdominotranssacral approach.[272] Anorectal neurilemoma has been reported uncommonly and also should be adequately treated by excisional biopsy.[2]

Granular Cell Tumor

Granular cell tumor is an uncommon tumor of uncertain histogenesis. It was first described in 1926 by Abrikossoff, who named the tumor because of its resemblance to primitive myoblasts and its proximity to striated muscle.[4] He believed that neoplastic cells were formed from damaged adult muscle cells in the process of regeneration. Willis regarded the process as nonneoplastic and regenerative in nature.[526] However, Klinge suggested that the tumor could arise from heterotopic rests of myoblasts, a

theory that was later accepted by Abrikossoff and Murray.[5,262,351]

Fisher and Wechsler, using electron microscopy and histochemical studies, concluded that the tumor had a definite neural pattern most closely resembling a damaged Schwann cell.[147] They believed that it was not similar to muscular tissue and noted that the tumor had a more histiocytic than neoplastic nature (Figure 25-55). I have elected to place this tumor in the classification under neural origin for these reasons.

Usually the tumor involves the tongue (33%), skin and subcutaneous soft tissues (10%), and skeletal muscle (5%). About 50% of the tumors occur in the oral cavity and nasopharynx.[94] However, the lesion has also been reported in most other organ systems. Involvement of the GI tract is rare. Yanai-Inbar and associates, in their review of the literature, found 17 cases involving the large intestine, mainly in the proximal portion of the colon.[536] Only two tumors were identified in the rectum. Anal and perianal lesions have also been reported.[88,305,402,412,527]

In the colon, granular cell tumors appear as yellowish white submucosal nodules, usually less than 2 cm in diameter. Most are found incidentally, but abdominal pain and bleeding can occur. Malignant degeneration may re-

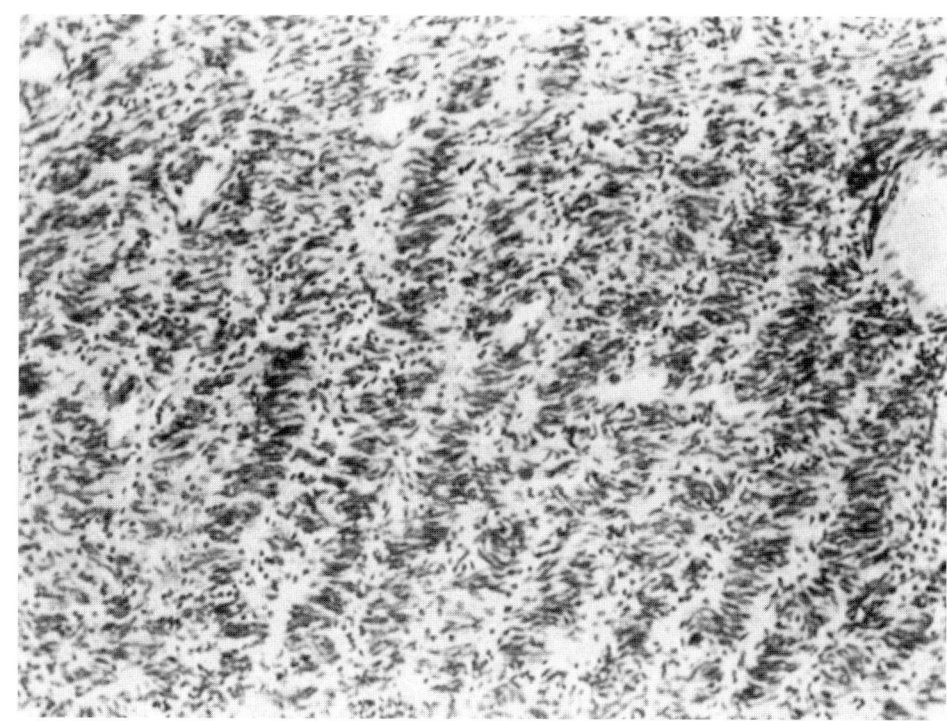

FIGURE 25-49. Neurofibroma, showing the herringbone appearance characteristic of nerve tissue tumor. (Original magnification × 260; courtesy of Rudolf Garret, M.D.)

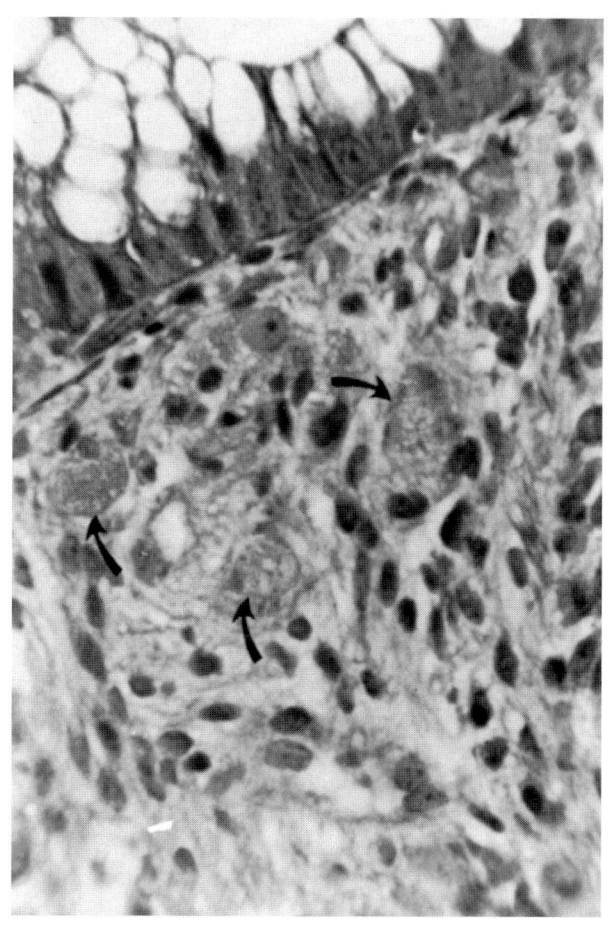

FIGURE 25-50. Ganglioneuroma. Interlacing bundles of nerve cells mixed with ganglion cells *(arrows)*. (Original magnification × 280; courtesy of Lauren M. Monda, M.D.)

sult, but this is unusual, and the possibility of such an association is still controversial.

Treatment is local excision when possible or resection. Success with colonoscopic removal may prove to be the optimal therapy for most lesions.[307]

VASCULAR LESIONS

Hemangioma

Vascular malformations of the GI tract have been reported since 1839 with Phillips' initial description of a lesion in the rectum.[384] The Armed Forces Institute of Pathology in Washington, DC, has included venous angiomas in its list of benign vascular malformations as well as arteriovenous angiomas (racemose aneurysms), plexiform angiomas, and several other variants of hemangiomas.[282]

For the purposes of this chapter, this section deals only with hemangiomas. The vascular lesion that has come to be known as an arteriovenous malformation or vascular ectasia is discussed in Chapter 28. Hemangiomas are found in virtually every organ of the body, with the skin a particularly common location. However, it is one of the rarest tumors found in the colon. Gentry and associates reviewed the world literature through 1945 and found reports of 283 benign vascular tumors of the GI tract.[167] Only 31 of these were hemangiomas of the colon. Rissier reviewed 18 cases in 1960.[403] Thirteen additional reports appeared in the literature between 1957 and 1971.[126,146,175,261,325,345,367,375,400,414,444,467,500]

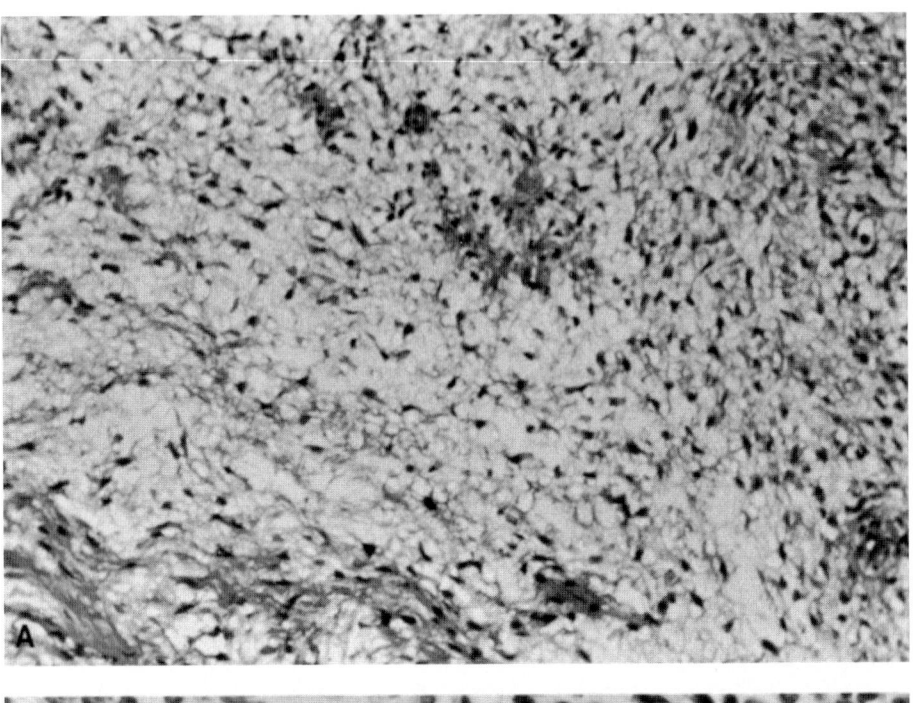

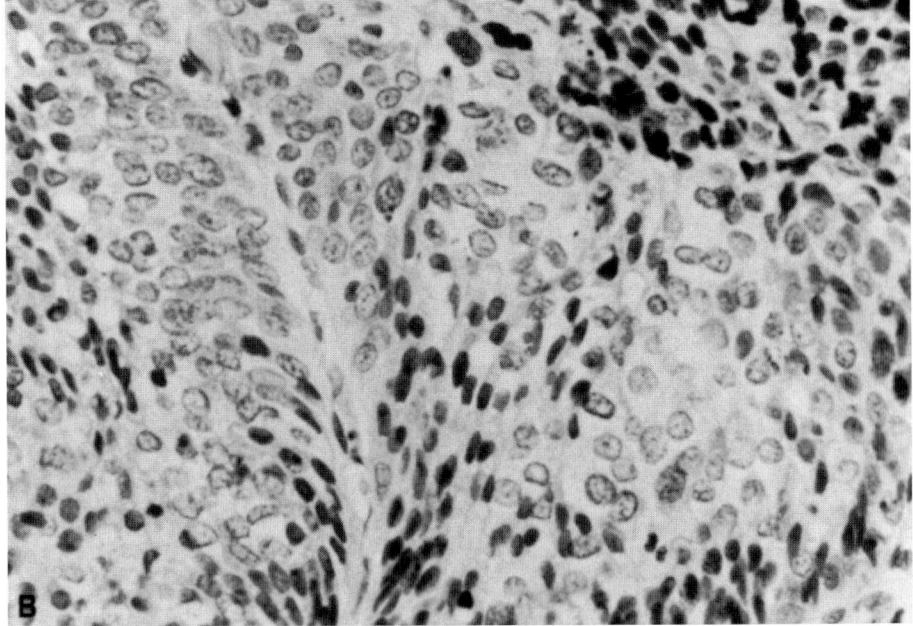

FIGURE 25-51. Neurilemoma. **(A)** Edematous cells (Antoni A pattern) characteristic of schwannoma. (Original magnification × 260; courtesy of Rudolf Garret, M.D.) **(B)** Section of a multinodular tumor characterized by bland spindle-shaped cells arranged in a palisading pattern (Antoni B). (Original magnification × 260.)

The pathogenesis of these tumors is not well defined. However, they are generally agreed to be congenital, with their origin in embryonic sequestrations of mesodermal tissue. Enlargement occurs by projection of budding endothelial cells. Whether these growths are neoplastic or congenital is a matter of some controversy.

The capillary hemangioma consists of small, thin-walled, closely packed vessels with a well differentiated, hyperplastic endothelial lining. These tumors are distributed equally throughout the GI tract. They represent 6%

of benign vascular tumors, arise from the submucosal vascular plexus, and are often encapsulated. Mucosal ulceration occurs in one half of these lesions.

The cavernous hemangioma is composed of large, thin-walled vessels that are much larger than those of the capillary hemangioma. The supporting stroma contains scant connective tissue and may contain smooth muscle fibers (Figs. 25-56 and 25-57). These lesions may be of the "multiple phlebectasia" type, characterized by a multitude of discrete tumors less than 1 cm in diameter. Al-

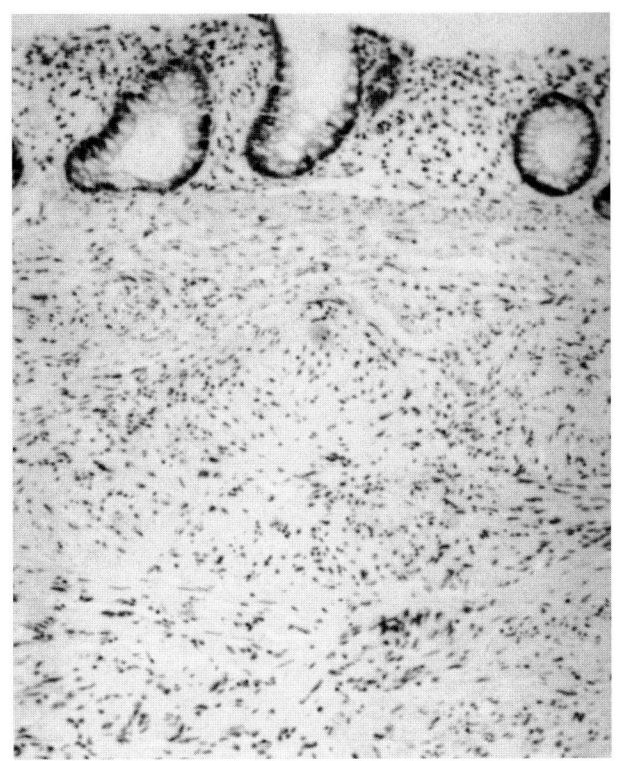

FIGURE 25-52. Schwannoma (perineural fibroblastoma). Well-delineated tumor replacing the submucosa. Interlacing bundles of cells with elongated nuclei of Antoni A pattern. (Original magnification × 80.)

though they represent one third of all the benign vascular tumors of the GI tract, they are frequently overlooked. The simple polypoid type of cavernous hemangioma constitutes 10% of benign vascular intestinal malformations and is usually of sufficient size to produce such symptoms as obstruction and hemorrhage. The diffuse, expansive type varies widely in shape and size, and often involves 20 to 30 cm of intestine, occasionally in multiple locations. Diffuse cavernous hemangiomas, which produce severe symptoms at a relatively early age, account for 20% of intestinal angiomas.

Venous angiomas are often confused with cavernous hemangiomas. Both are composed of large, thin-walled vessels with large lumens. However, the walls of venous angiomas contain varying amounts of smooth muscle and usually resemble veins. Many of these tumors are extensive, especially those found in the extremities. Thrombosis is common in venous as well as in cavernous hemangiomas, and calcification frequently occurs in these thrombi as well as in the surrounding interstitial tissue.

Enlarged hemangiomas may produce symptoms of obstruction or hemorrhage. The obstructive symptoms may be caused by the tumor, by volvulus, or by intussusception. Intussusception has most frequently been reported from eastern Europe. Additionally, invasion of adjacent structures has been described, including ureter and iliac vessels.[482]

The most common complication of hemangioma of the colon is bleeding (60% to 90%). Early onset and frequency of hemorrhage often lead to a diagnosis in adolescence or early adulthood. Characteristically, colonic hemangiomas bleed episodically, slowly, and persistently. Other symptoms include melena and the results of anemia: fatigue and weakness. Cavernous hemangiomas

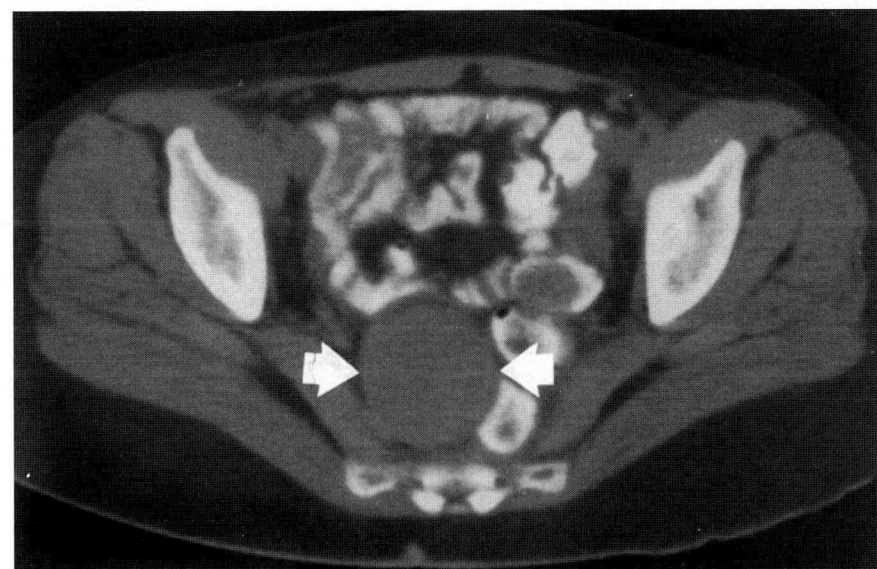

FIGURE 25-53. Computed tomography of the pelvis demonstrates a well-defined, presacral mass *(arrows),* which proved to be the lesion shown in Figure 25-54. (Courtesy of William G. Robertson, M.D.)

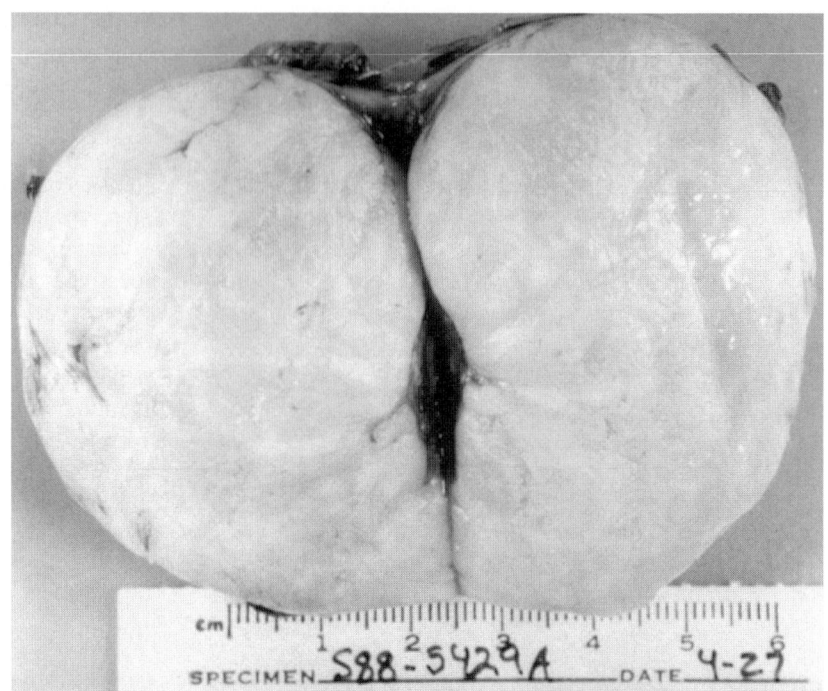

FIGURE 25-54. Schwannoma. Homogeneous encapsulated mass with gray-white stroma and with small cystic foci and focal gelatinous areas characteristic of this type of tumor. (Courtesy of William G. Robertson, M.D.)

tend to bleed massively much more frequently than capillary hemangiomas (Figure 25-58). Melena begins in childhood, is recurrent throughout adolescence, and results in intermittent symptomatic anemia. Bleeding tends to become more severe with each recurrent episode. Although early onset of bleeding with recurrence usually leads to a definitive diagnosis and treatment during adolescence, hemangiomas of the colon may be difficult to confirm before laparotomy. A positive family history may be helpful.

Physical examination is often unremarkable, but the presence of hemangiomas of the skin or mucous mem-

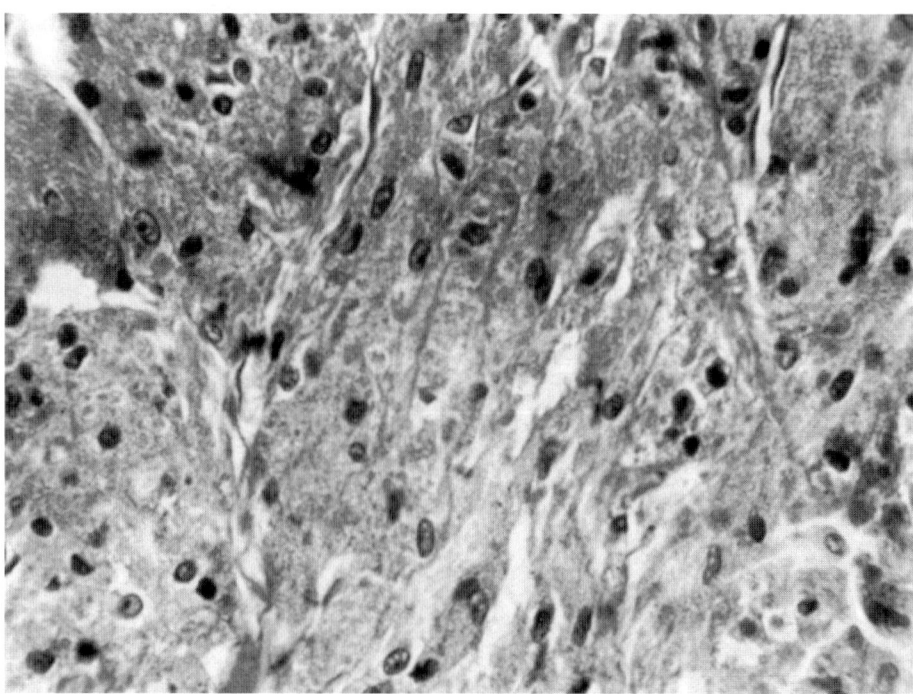

FIGURE 25-55. Granular cell tumor. Granular cells with uniform nuclei and granular cytoplasm. (Original magnification × 280; courtesy of Rudolf Garret, M.D.)

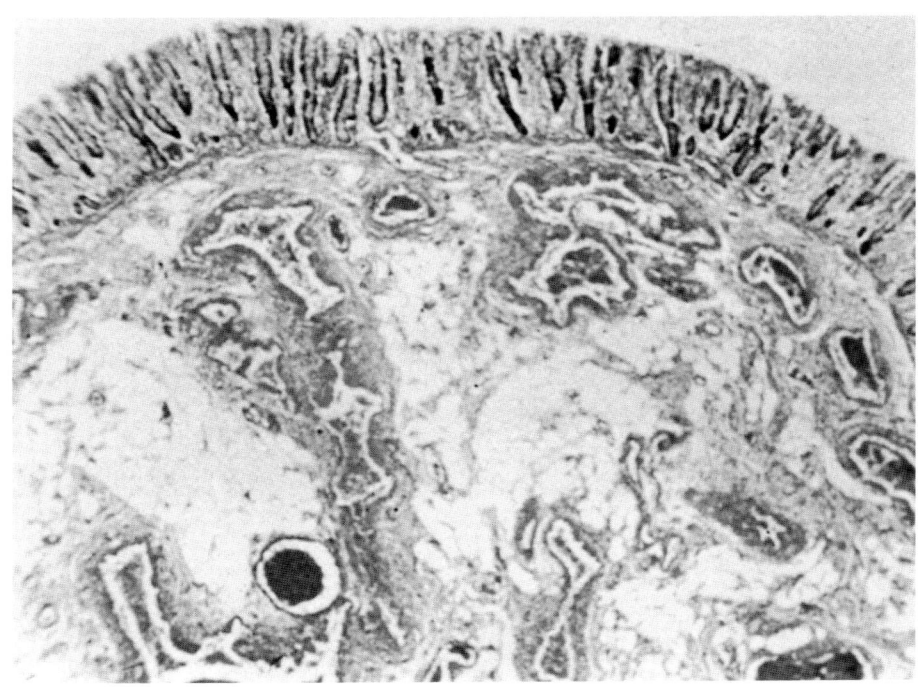

FIGURE 25-56. Hemangioma. Irregularly shaped arteries and veins in the areolar tissue of the submucosa. (From Corman ML, Veidenheimer MC, Swinton NW. *Diseases of the anus, rectum and colon. Part I: neoplasms.* New York: Medcom, 1972.)

brane should raise a suspicion that a similar lesion could be present in the colon.

Barium enema may reveal a filling defect, and phleboliths may be noted within the filling defect (Figure 25-59). Hollingsworth first documented the association of narrowing of the sigmoid colon on barium enema examination with an area of surrounding phleboliths.[217] The oc-

currence of multiple, calcified, well-circumscribed densities is probably related to thrombosis within the tumor and is seen particularly with cavernous hemangioma of the colon.[34,217,367] CT has been shown to demonstrate certain characteristic findings—a thickened mesentery containing large vacuoles and transmural thickening of the involved segment.[26] Selective angiography may also reveal a

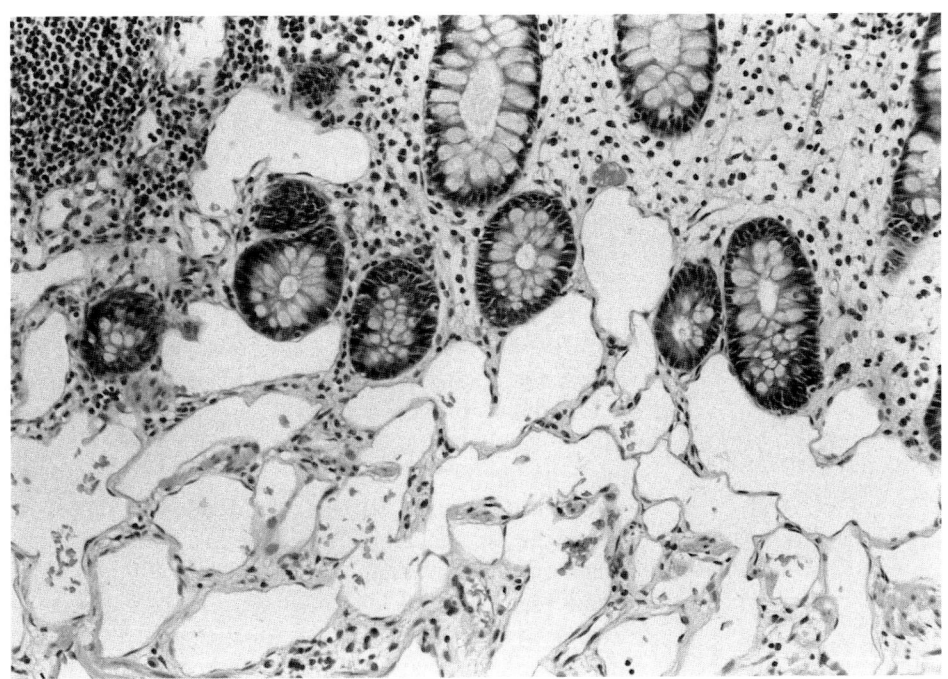

FIGURE 25-57. Cavernous hemangioma. Mucosa and submucosa contain multiple, dilated, benign vascular channels. (Original magnification × 600).

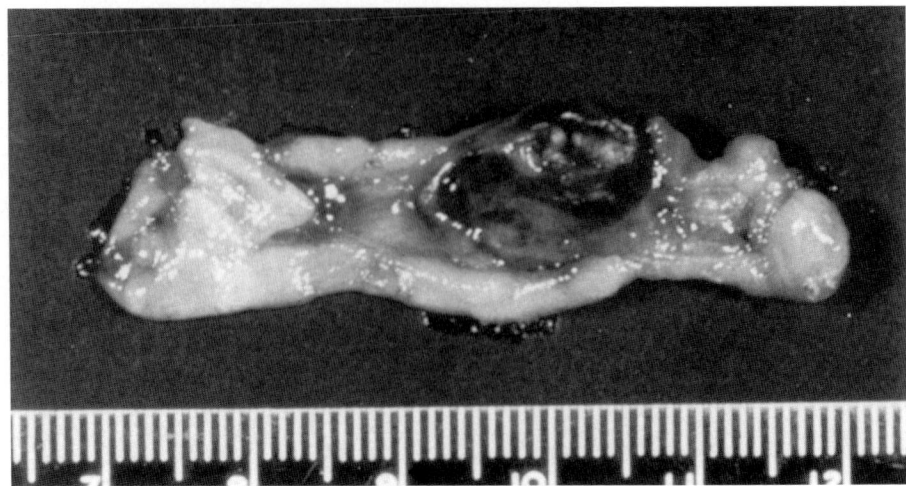

FIGURE 25-58. Cavernous hemangioma of the sigmoid colon with ulceration. Bleeding necessitated a resection. (Courtesy of Rudolf Garret, M.D.)

vascular malformation, particularly in the late vascular phase (see Figs. 28-14 and 28-15), although the differential diagnosis between angioma and arteriovenous malformation is often confusing. Injection of the resected specimen with contrast material may be useful for ensuring adequacy of the margins.[100]

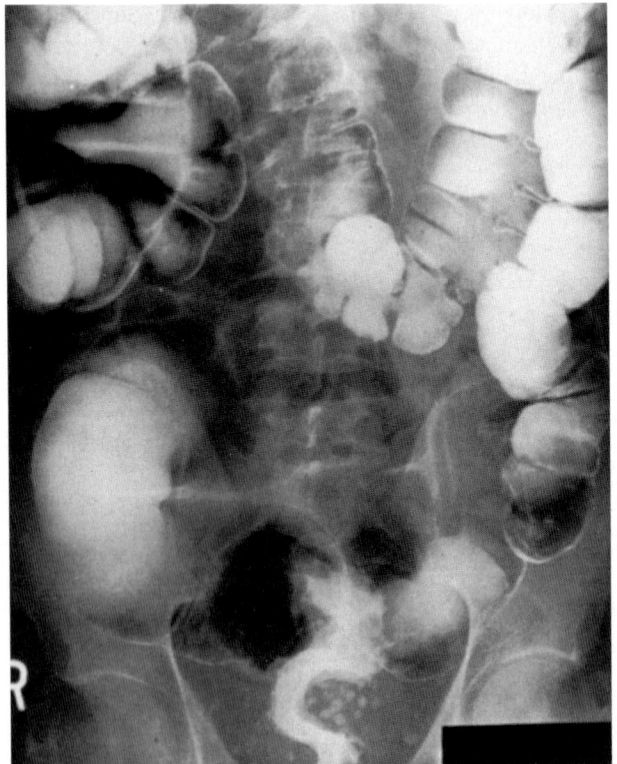

FIGURE 25-59. Hemangioma. Barium enema reveals extrinsic compression of the left wall of the rectum and irregularity of the rectosigmoid wall. The surrounding soft tissue mass contains multiple calcifications.

Skovgaard and Sorensen reported an 8-year-old boy with a hemangioma of the sigmoid colon whose tumor was diagnosed by colonoscopy.[451] These investigators believed that because hemangioma can be diagnosed radiographically only if it is large and can easily be overlooked at exploratory laparotomy, and colonoscopy should be used in evaluating all children with lower intestinal hemorrhage of unknown cause. Endoscopic diagnosis usually is not difficult; the tumor will appear deep red or purple. Hasegawa and colleagues performed colonoscopic polypectomy for a polypoid lesion, but their article was followed by an editorial comment cautioning the reader to be wary of the possibility of inducing uncontrolled hemorrhage.[200]

Resection of a bleeding colonic hemangioma is the optimal treatment.[100,303,388] If the benign nature of the tumor can be determined at laparotomy and confirmed by adequate frozen-section examination, local excision of the hemangioma is sufficient. If malignancy cannot be excluded, resection of the involved segment should be undertaken.

Only 75 cases of hemangioma of the rectum had been reported in the world literature before 1978.[233] Treatments that have been proposed include sclerosing agents,[128] ligation of the feeding vessels,[158] local excision,[203] abdominoperineal resection,[204] and resection with coloanal anastomosis.[230,296,513] It seems reasonable to attempt a sphincter-saving operation, if hemorrhage can be controlled and there is no evidence for malignant change.[26,109,401]

Because radiation has been reported to be a successful treatment for hemangiomas of the neck and face,[215,433] Chaimoff and Lurie applied this technique in a woman who presented with a low-lying perirectal hemangioma.[78] Nearly 2 years after treatment consisting of five successive sessions of 3 Gy each (for a total of 15 Gy), the patient was asymptomatic.

Lymphangioma

Lymphangioma of the GI tract is a very rare lesion, and the colon is the least frequent site involved. Fleming and Carlson reported on nine lymphatic cysts of the abdomen diagnosed at the Mayo Clinic between 1959 and 1968.[148] Of these, three arose submucosally in the GI tract, and one originated in the colon. Only a few other cases have been published.[13,20,170,183,213,264,276,277,364,390] However, with increasing use of endoscopy to visualize the GI tract, this submucosal lesion is being observed with increased frequency.[390]

The lesion originates in the lymphatic plexus within the submucosa into which the lacteals of the villi empty. In 1958, Willis noted the frequent association of lymphangioma with smooth muscle and believed that these cysts, like angiomas, are hamartomas rather than true tumors.[526]

Another theory considers lymphangiomas to be secondary to obstructed mesenteric lymph nodes, with subsequent stasis and dilatation caused by a rise in pressure in the nodes, a mechanism similar to the production of postoperative lymphocysts.[118] If this theory were valid, one would expect an increased incidence of such lymphangiomatous cysts after laparotomy and abdominal node dissection. This finding has not been reported.

Lymphangiomas of the colon may be submucosal or pedunculated. The small number of documented submucosal lymphangiomas of the GI tract does not permit satisfactory analysis of the radiologic characteristics. However, Kuramoto and colleagues suggested that it is possible to diagnose these lesions endoscopically.[276] Because the tumors are lustrous and smooth on the surface, pliable on compression, and frequently have a stalk or a "waist" at the base, these investigators suggested that lesions less than 20 mm in diameter can be safely removed via the colonoscope. On other occasions, however, the mucosa may appear quite nodular. The example shown in Figure 25-60 reveals such a nodular mucosa.

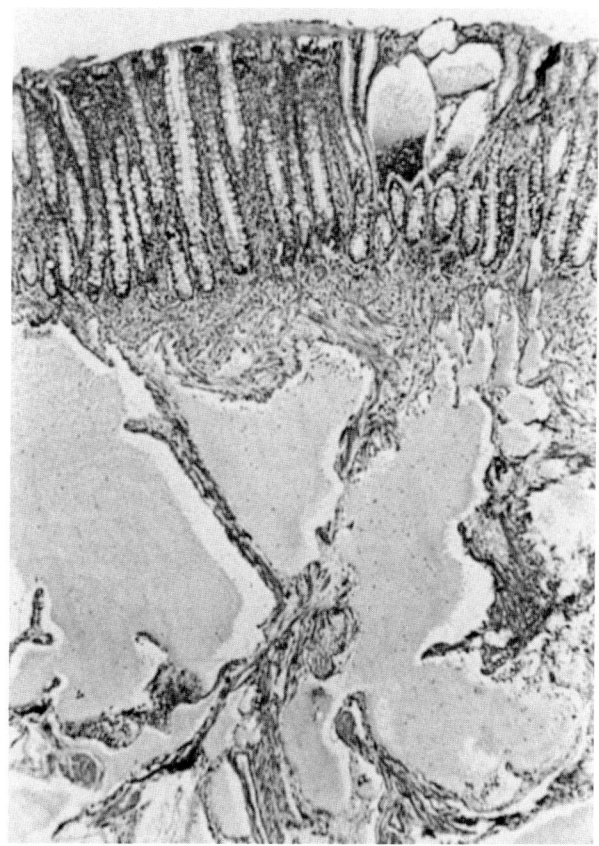

FIGURE 25-61. Lymphangioma. Endothelial-lined, irregular spaces in the submucosa of the bowel. (Original magnification × 80; from Corman ML, Veidenheimer MC, Swinton NW. *Diseases of the anus, rectum and colon. Part I: neoplasms.* New York: Medcom, 1972.)

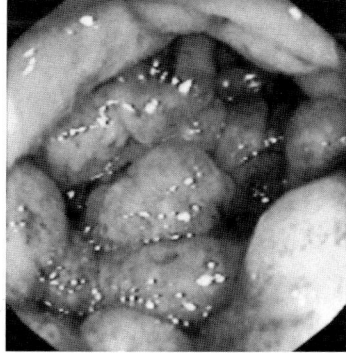

FIGURE 25-60. Submucosal cystic nodules were proven on biopsy to be lymphatic cysts. (See Color Fig. 25–60.)

The first report of lymphangioma of the rectum in an English-language journal was that of Chisholm and Hillkowitz in 1932.[86] In 1973, we reported the case of a woman with rectal bleeding who had previously undergone a hemorrhoidectomy for this complaint.[101] Proctosigmoidoscopy revealed numerous extramucosal cystic masses scattered from the anorectal ring to approximately 9 cm from the anal verge and appearing to contain clear fluid. After a GI investigation produced negative findings, the cystic masses were excised through the operating proctoscope. Pathologically, a noncapsulated, poorly circumscribed mass of cavernous, thin-walled vascular channels occupied the submucosa. These channels were irregular in size and shape. They had walls or septa formed of fibrous tissue and were lined by a single layer of flattened endothelium. Although the mucosal surface was intact throughout, focal discontinuities in the muscularis mucosa permitted some of the dilated lymphatic vessels to extend into the lamina propria. Homogeneous pink material, presumably lymph, filled most of the vessels (Figure 25-61). A few contained erythrocytes. Accu-

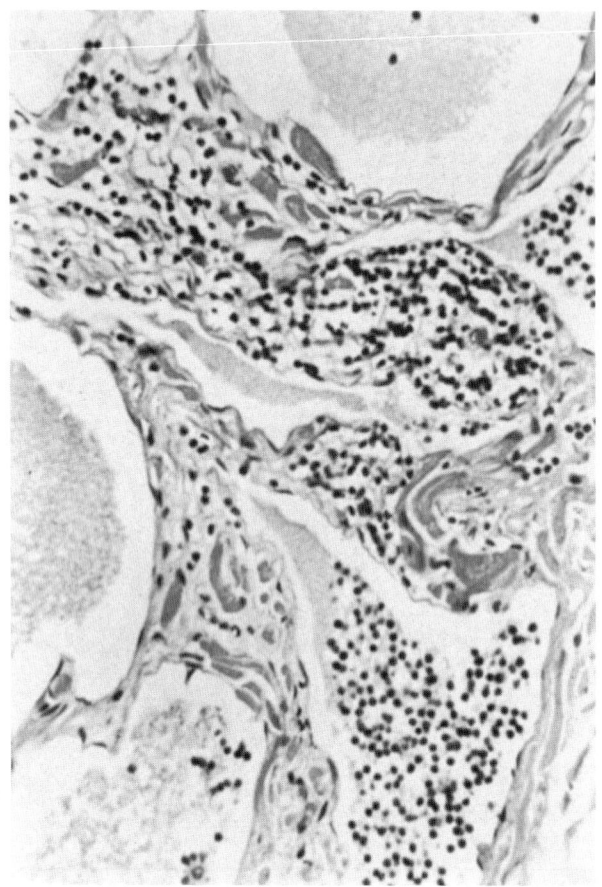

FIGURE 25-62. Lymphangioma. Endothelial-lined spaces, some of which contain lymphocytes. (Original magnification × 300; from Corman ML, Veidenheimer MC, Swinton NW. *Diseases of the anus, rectum and colon. Part I: neoplasms.* New York: Medcom, 1972.)[102]

(oleoma) may be more difficult to recognize. Gas cysts of recent origin may lack a lining. When they are chronic, they are lined by giant cells similar to those of the oil granuloma.

None of the reported lymphangiomas of the colon and rectum had infiltrated the muscularis propria. However, such infiltration did occur in a lymphangioma of the small bowel reported by Wood.[532]

Excision biopsy with careful visualization under suitable anesthesia is the recommended procedure for rectal lesions. Colonoscopy is a valuable adjunct in the diagnosis of more proximal lesions. A cystic lymphangioma of the colon has been diagnosed by means of catheter endosonography.[227] The typical image is that of an anechoic, septated lesion within the submucosa. Colonoscopic polypectomy for pedunculated lymphangiomas appears to be a satisfactory treatment, but a limited resection should be considered for all sessile or infiltrative tumors.

Hemangiopericytoma

Hemangiopericytoma is an extremely rare tumor that arises from pericytes and is usually found in the soft tissue of the trunk and extremities. Review of English-language publications revealed only two cases involving the colon, the small intestine being the most common GI site.[24,165] Abdominal pain, intestinal obstruction, intussusception, and rectal bleeding are associated with intestinal tumors. Malignant degeneration is usually based on the clinical course (recurrence or metastases) rather than the histologic picture. Microscopically, the tumor is characterized by multiple endothelial-lined capillaries or capillary buds (Figure 25-63). Resection is the preferred treatment.[165]

Malignant Vascular Tumors

Malignant vascular tumors include hemangioendothelioma, angiosarcoma, Kaposi's sarcoma, and benign metastasizing hemangioma. They represent approximately 13% of all vascular lesions of the colon and rectum, but with the epidemic of AIDS and the association of this condition with Kaposi's sarcoma, many more cases may be anticipated.[49,56,97,131,133,153,249,281,299,354,389,395,459,512,517,522]

Angiosarcoma

Angiosarcoma is a malignant tumor of the vascular endothelium that is thought to arise from an hemangioma. The histology is characterized by varying degrees of endothelial proliferation and the formation of anastomosing vascular channels. Fewer than a dozen of these tumors have

mulations of lymphocytes were present both within the lymphatic channels and in the thin septa between them. The diagnosis of lymphangioma was made because of the presence of lymphocytes within the vessel and septa, the scarcity of elastic tissue, and the predominance of lymphatic elements (Figure 25-62).

The presence of blood vessels within many lesions designated as lymphangiomas is well recognized and has been taken as evidence that these lesions actually represent vascular malformations or hamartomas rather than true neoplasms. Differentiation from hemangioma may be impossible in those lesions that lack abundant intraluminal and interstitial lymphocytes as evidence of their lymphatic origin.

Apart from lymphangioma, the histologic differential diagnosis includes lesions that may produce cystic spaces in the submucosal region of the bowel. The epithelial lining of colitis cystica profunda usually permits its easy recognition. However, the giant cell lining that remains behind after dissolution of the oils in an oil granuloma

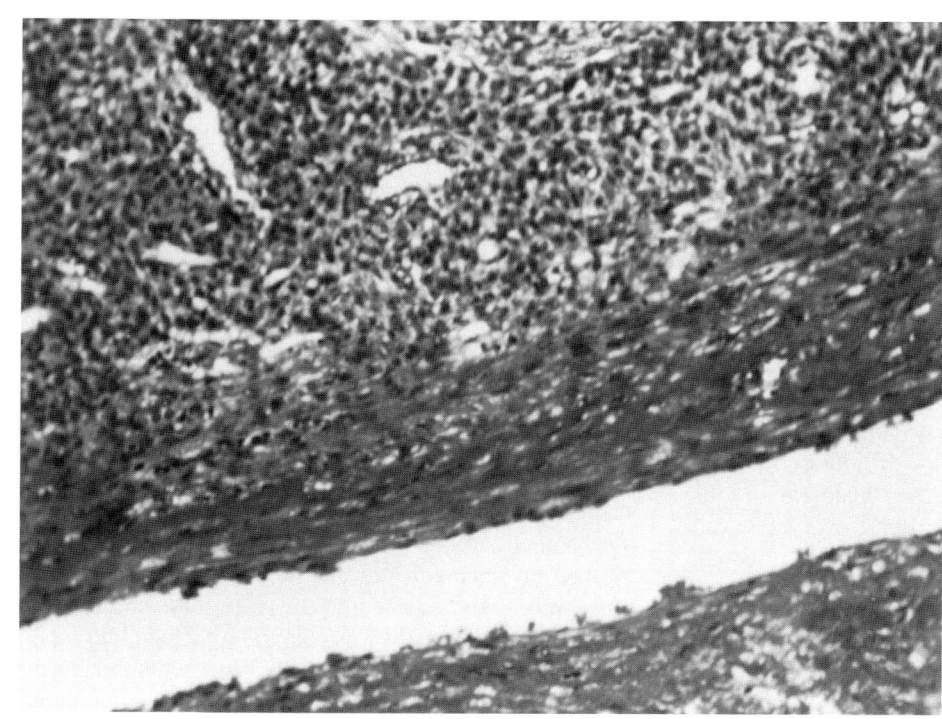

FIGURE 25-63. Hemangiopericytoma. Uniform cells deriving from Zimmerman's pericytes surrounding the vascular spaces. (Original magnification × 260; courtesy of Rudolf Garret, M.D.)

been described involving the colon and rectum.[456] Treatment is resection, but the prognosis is poor.

Kaposi's Sarcoma

See Chapter 20.

HETEROTOPIAS AND HAMARTOMAS

Endometriosis

Endometriosis is a disorder resulting from the presence of actively growing and functioning endometrial tissue, both glandular and stromal, in sites outside the uterus. In 1897, Pfannenstiel reported the case of a patient with aberrant endometrium that involved the rectovaginal septum.[383] In 1909, Meyer described the first instance of bowel endometriosis; the patient ultimately required resection.[329] In 1922, Blair-Bell, in noting a series of cases of aberrant endometrium, first used the terms endometriosis and endometrioma, the former for the disease, the latter for the individual cystic lesion.[58]

Pathogenesis

The pathogenesis of this common disorder is not clearly understood. Many theories have been proposed to explain the disease. Sampson believed that fragments of endometrium regurgitated with the menstrual blood through the oviducts in a retrograde fashion and im-

planted onto peritoneal surfaces and pelvic and abdominal structures.[425] These would then erode into the subserosal tissues with viable cells growing and functioning and would ultimately lead to further implantation. This is the theory of tubal reflux and implantation.

Another proposal is that of coelomic epithelial metaplasia. This assumes that dormant, immature cellular elements of müllerian origin are known to persist into adult life, particularly throughout the central region of the pelvis. After menarche, repeated cyclic ovarian stimulation of these elements, with their totipotential capacities for differentiation, could result in the metaplastic formation of functioning endometrial tissue in ectopic sites.

Other theories have been suggested, including lymphatic dissemination of endometrial cells and deportation of normal endometrium by way of venous channels. These do not seem to offer a satisfactory explanation for the pathologic features.

Incidence

Endometriosis occurs almost exclusively in women. In 75% the condition develops between the ages of 20 and 40 years, and in 25% up to the age of menopause. Isolated case reports of endometriosis in men with prostatic cancer who are receiving estrogen therapy have also appeared.[385] The incidence of intestinal endometriosis among patients known to have endometriosis has been reported to be 5.4%.[392]

Symptoms and Signs

The classic history is one of acquired or secondary dysmenorrhea. The pain is related to, but does not necessarily occur simultaneously with, each menstrual period. Pelvic discomfort associated with endometriosis is more likely to begin a day or two before the onset of menstrual flow, although its intensity may increase during the early days of menstruation. It tends to be a deep-seated ache or bearing-down pain in the lower part of the abdomen, posterior pelvis, vagina, or back, and it often radiates into the rectal and perineal areas with tenesmus and symptoms suggestive of an irritable bowel. When, as is often the case, an endometrioma of one or both ovaries is present, dull unilateral or bilateral lower abdominal pain, often with radiation to the thighs, may be noted.

The discomfort tends to abate after 2 or 3 days, subsiding completely toward the end of or just after the menstrual period. The patient will then be comfortable once more until a day or two before the onset of the next menstrual flow. However, as the disease progresses, pain tends to increase in severity and may last most of each cycle.

Not all patients with endometriosis have pain, however. Despite extensive disease that may be palpable on pelvic examination or found at laparotomy, 15% to 20% of patients report no discomfort whatsoever. They may harbor other manifestations of the pathologic process, notably infertility or the presence of a mass. Other symptoms include dyspareunia, cyclic bowel disturbances with painful defecation, rectal bleeding, and intestinal obstruction. Although rectal bleeding is an uncommon presenting symptom of endometriosis, colon endometriosis should be considered when bleeding is associated with the menses.

Leakage or rupture of an enlarging ovarian endometrioma may produce generalized peritonitis and an acute abdominal problem. Spillage of the contents of a "chocolate" endometrial cyst produces an intense local irritation and inflammatory response that results in chemical peritonitis.

A characteristic, almost diagnostic, physical finding is the hard, fixed, fibrotic nodule in the uterosacral ligaments, cul-de-sac, or posterior surface of the lower uterine wall and cervix. This nodularity is almost universally present in patients with endometriosis and is pathognomonic for the disease. In endometriosis of the rectovaginal septum, bidigital rectovaginal examination helps to define the pathologic condition.

Diagnostic Studies

If the history is characteristic but the physical findings are minimal or equivocal, laparoscopy or culdoscopy may prove valuable in establishing a definitive diagnosis.

When a trial of medical therapy is being considered, pelvic endoscopy using the laparoscope or culdoscope will usually provide a precise diagnosis before initiating treatment.

Other diagnostic tests include barium enema (Figs. 25-64 and 25-65), CT to determine the location and degree of obstruction (if involvement of the ureters or periureteral tissue is suspected), and cystoscopy (during the menstrual period) to reveal the characteristic bluish black, submucosal, cystic lesions if endometriosis of the bladder is suspected. Ileal endometriosis, especially, may present some confusion in differential diagnosis with Crohn's disease. Both conditions produce local inflammation and stricture.[72]

Schröder and colleagues evaluated 16 patients with suspected fixation of endometriomas to the rectal wall by means of endorectal ultrasound.[434] In six individuals, rectal wall involvement was diagnosed. In two, endometriomas were found adjacent to the rectal wall, and in eight, rectal wall involvement was able to be excluded. Preoperative diagnosis was confirmed in all patients during the operation. Laparotomy was limited to those individuals with preoperatively assessed rectal wall involvement, whereas the remaining patients were treated by means of laparoscopic excision.[434] The authors concluded that preoperative endorectal ultrasound is reliable for assessing rectal wall involvement, thereby determining the type of operative approach that would appear to be best for the individual. Others have confirmed the high sensitivity and specificity of endorectal ultrasound for rectal endometriosis as well as its impact on operative decision making.[119]

Often endometriosis is first discovered at the time laparotomy is performed for some other reason. In the experience of Keane and Peel, none of their patients with intestinal or abdominal wall endometriosis was helped by preoperative investigations.[253] However, these investigators did not have the benefit of endorectal ultrasound.

Histopathology

The three diagnostic histologic features of endometriosis are endometrial glands, endometrial stroma (Figure 25-66), and evidence of fresh hemorrhage (red cells and hemosiderin pigment) or old hemorrhage (hemosiderin-laden macrophages).

Because of its microscopic resemblance to normal endometrium and its known response to ovarian hormonal stimulation, the functioning epithelium of an endometrioma sometimes closely duplicates phases of the normal intrauterine endometrium, showing proliferative changes in the preovulatory or progestational phase. However, more often, the ectopic endometrial tissues are out of phase with the normal endometrium

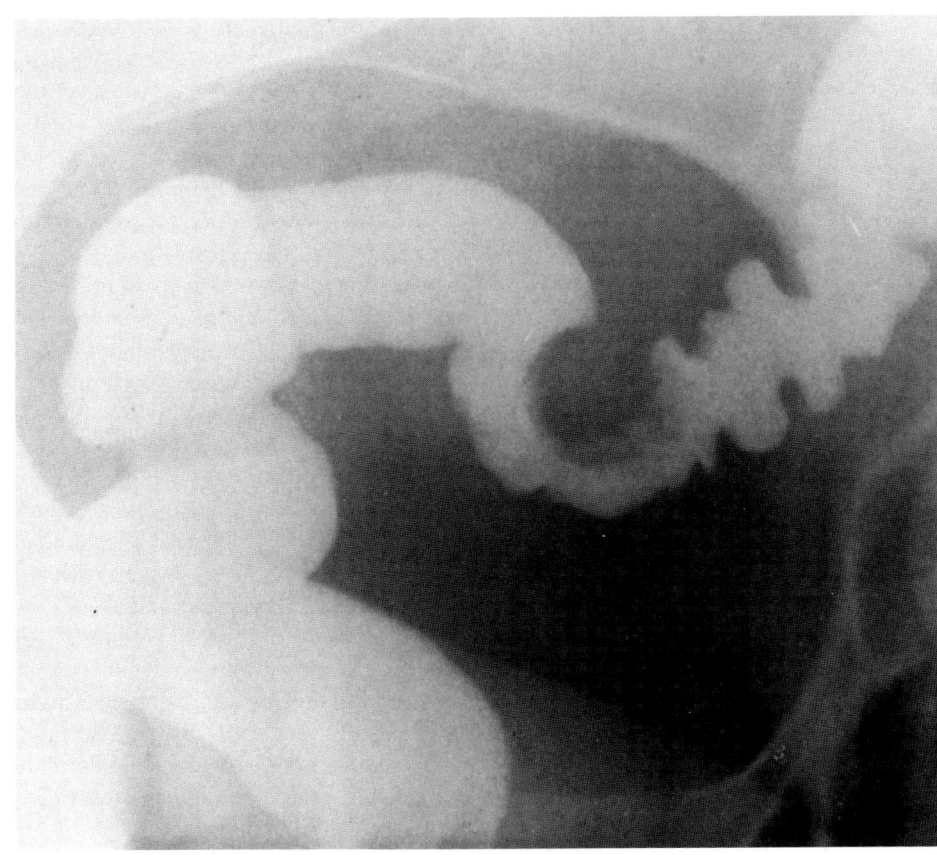

FIGURE 25-64. Endometrioma. Barium enema reveals a well-demarcated sigmoid mass. Confusion with carcinoma should not occur because the lesion demonstrated here has an intact overlying mucosa.

and are found in the proliferative stage even during the secretory phase of the normal menstrual cycle. This may result from the difference in blood supply and the effects of increasing tissue fibrosis surrounding the endometriosis. Malignant transformation to adenocarcinoma has been reported.[309]

In the ovary, the process is almost always bilateral. The tendency is for the formation of cystic structures varying from tiny bluish or dark brown blisters to large "chocolate" cysts. Usually present are considerable fibrosis and puckering of the ovarian surface in the region of the cyst and adherence to neighboring structures.

Treatment

Treatment of endometriosis is often based on the patient's age, severity of symptoms, hormonal status, and desire for childbearing.[392]

Medical Treatment

Kistner observed that endometrial implants disappear after administration of large doses of progestins and estrogen.[260] Riva and associates likewise reported the beneficial effects of these compounds as observed by culdoscopy but cautioned about the rapidity of recurrence

in some instances.[404] Gunning and Moyer, after using medroxyprogesterone acetate (Depo-Provera), demonstrated by culdoscopy and laparoscopy the shrinkage of endometrial tissue and confirmed microscopically that the endometriosis had disappeared.[191] The action of these therapies has not been completely elucidated. Endometriosis disappears, but follow-up studies have shown considerable variation in the rate of reappearance. The use of progestin alone or in combination with estrogen has become the standard method of hormonal treatment of endometriosis.

Another medication for the management of endometriosis is danazol (Danocrine).[182] Its efficacy is based on the fact that it creates a hypoestrogenic-hyperandrogenic state, which is detrimental to the growth and function of endometrial tissue.[40] In doses of 200 to 800 mg/day, studies have shown that the pituitary inhibiting action results in suppression of ovulation, abolition of the midcycle increase of luteinizing hormone, and amenorrhea. The recommended dosage schedule for danazol in the treatment of endometriosis is 200 mg four times a day for at least 6 months. A maintenance dose of 200 to 400 mg daily may control pain after the initial treatment. Menstruation ceases with the commencement of therapy and returns promptly after the treatment has been discontinued. The pain of endometriosis is usually relieved

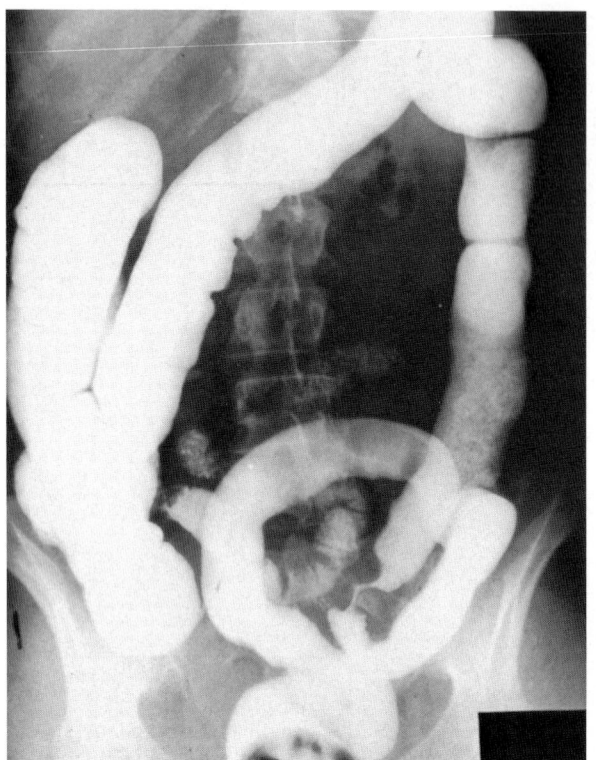

FIGURE 25-65. Endometrioma. Annular lesion of the proximal sigmoid. Because there is no mucosal abnormality, the lesion is either intramural or extrinsic.

in at least 80% of patients. Unfortunately, danazol has major side effects in approximately 85% of women treated with the drug.[40] These include weight gain, edema, acne, hirsutism, oily skin, deepening of the voice, clitoromegaly, and menometrorrhagia.

Most recently, the use of gonadotropin-releasing hormone (GRH) agonists has proved to be beneficial for the treatment of endometriosis. GRH is a hypothalamic decapeptide that controls pituitary secretion of luteinizing hormone and follicle-stimulating hormone.[40] Henzl and colleagues employed such a GRH agonist, nafarelin, to inhibit ovarian function reversibly and to induce hypoestrogenemia.[210] When administered by nasal spray (400 to 800 µg/day) and compared with danazol, the authors concluded that the drug was as effective as danazol and had fewer side effects, other than hypoestrogenism. As of this writing, the drug is offered only to women who cannot tolerate danazol therapy.

Surgical Treatment

When endometriosis involves the small or large bowel, it may be preferentially excised. Certainly, resection and anastomosis of the bowel is advisable for obstructing lesions or when malignancy cannot be excluded (Figure 25-67).[392] However, caution is suggested against extensive dissection beneath the peritoneal reflection, in the posterior

cul-de-sac, or in the rectovaginal septum. Fistula complicating low anterior resection for endometriosis is not an uncommon occurrence. Bailey and collegues reported 130 women who had undergone intestinal resection for endometriosis.[33] Most had undergone previous surgical procedures and hormonal therapy before their intestinal surgery. Operations included low anterior resection with anastomosis to the extraperitoneal rectum (n = 109), sigmoid resection (n = 10), disc excision of the rectum (n = 7), ileocecal resection (n = 2), and small bowel resection (n = 2). There were no clinically apparent anastomotic leaks. With respect to fertility, of those who tried to become pregnant following resection, almost 50% went on to successful delivery. After a mean follow-up of 60 months, 100% noted relief with respect to cyclic bleeding, and 91% were free of rectal pain. It is evident from these authors' experience that a resectional approach to all visible colorectal endometriosis is a reasonable option for women with advanced disease.[33] Urbach and co-workers undertook low anterior resection for all but 7% of their 29 patients.[501] All reported subjective improvement, but only 46% were "cured" on the basis of not requiring additional medical or surgical treatment. The only variable that was associated with "cure" was concomitantly performed total abdominal hysterectomy and bilateral salpingo-oophorectomy. Laparoscopic resection has also been described.[162,399]

If pelvic endometriosis is so extensive that complete resection or fulguration is impossible or inadvisable, and if childbearing has been completed, bilateral oophorectomy is curative, because recurrence or progression depends on cyclic ovarian hormone production. Natural menopause, if imminent, may also be relied on to cure the process.

After surgical castration for relief of endometriosis, estrogen replacement therapy to prevent menopausal symptoms should be considered. Medroxprogesterone acetate used for the first 6 to 9 months after operation alleviates menopausal symptoms and promotes further necrobiosis of any residual endometriosis.

Management to Maintain Reproductive Capacity

The most difficult therapeutic decisions arise when young women with extensive disease would like to retain reproductive capability. Reasonable efforts should be made to eradicate the disease surgically in these individuals. Postoperatively, patients should be advised to commence childbearing as soon as possible. Because pregnancy eliminates menstruation for a period of 9 months, some therapeutic benefit may be expected. When childbearing is completed, definitive surgical therapy is less traumatic.

If childbearing is not a practical alternative, the patient should be given hormone therapy designed to prevent menstruation. Oral contraceptive pills given in a cyclic manner to allow intermittent withdrawal bleeding

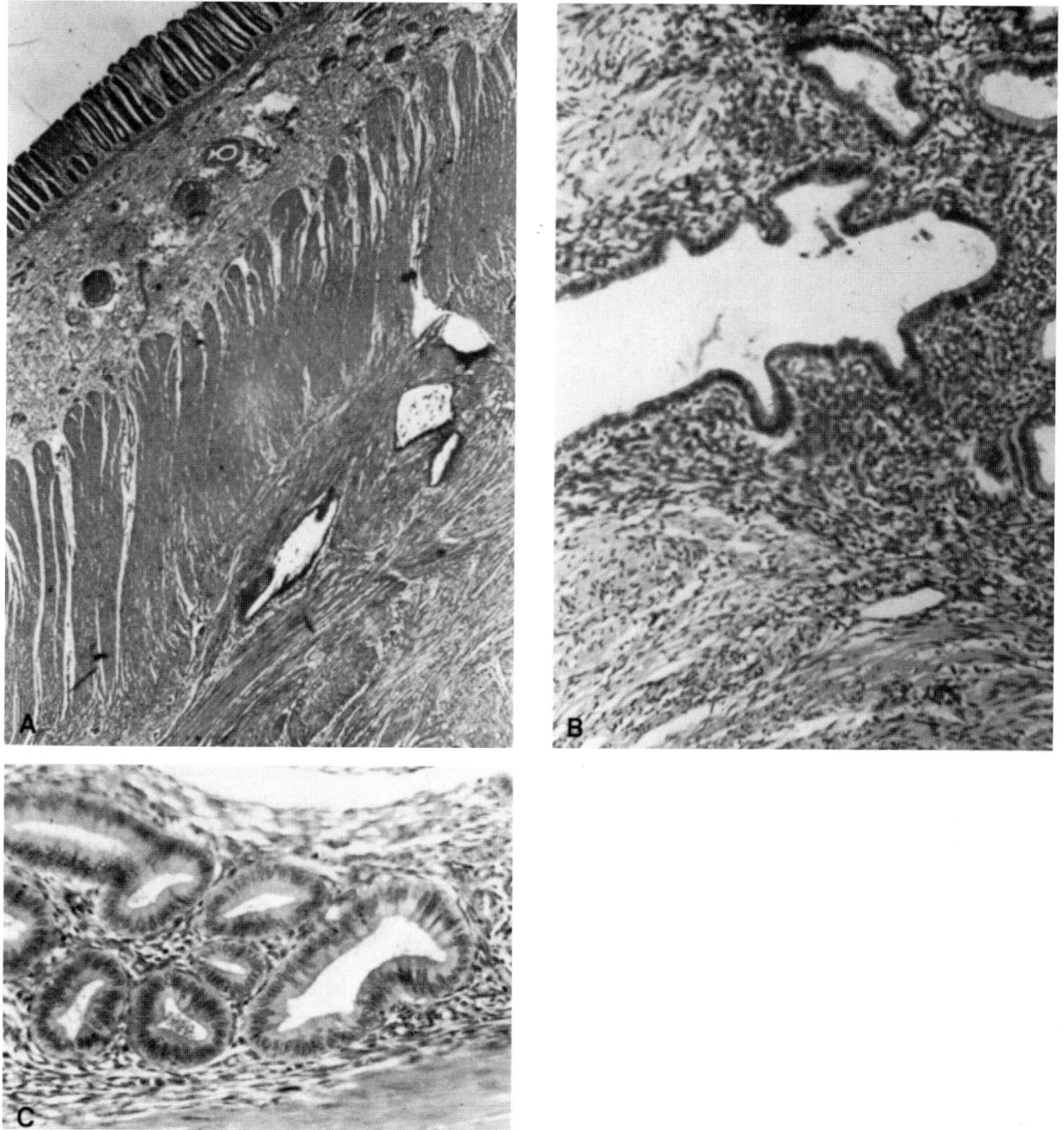

FIGURE 25-66. Endometrial glands and stroma within the wall of the bowel. **(A)** Original magnification × 80. **(B)** Original magnification × 260. **(C)** Original magnification × 400.

are not beneficial therapeutically. Birth control pills given daily and in sufficient potency to prevent breakthrough bleeding will result in softening, resorption, and necrobiosis of the endometrial glands. Medroxyprogesterone acetate, 100 to 150 mg, given by intramuscular injection every 2 to 3 months, will suppress menstruation. Its main disadvantages are occasional troublesome breakthrough bleeding requiring the addition of estrogen for control and, in a small percentage of women, permanent anovulation and resultant sterility. Medroxyproges-

terone acetate is not generally recommended in patients who are interested in further childbearing. Danazol is the treatment of choice.

In the experience of most physicians, hormone therapy does not always cure the process, but it gives the patient time to consider alternatives and to complete childbearing before progression of the disease or before increased symptoms and complications require the absolutely successful therapy: bilateral oophorectomy with hysterectomy.[93,107]

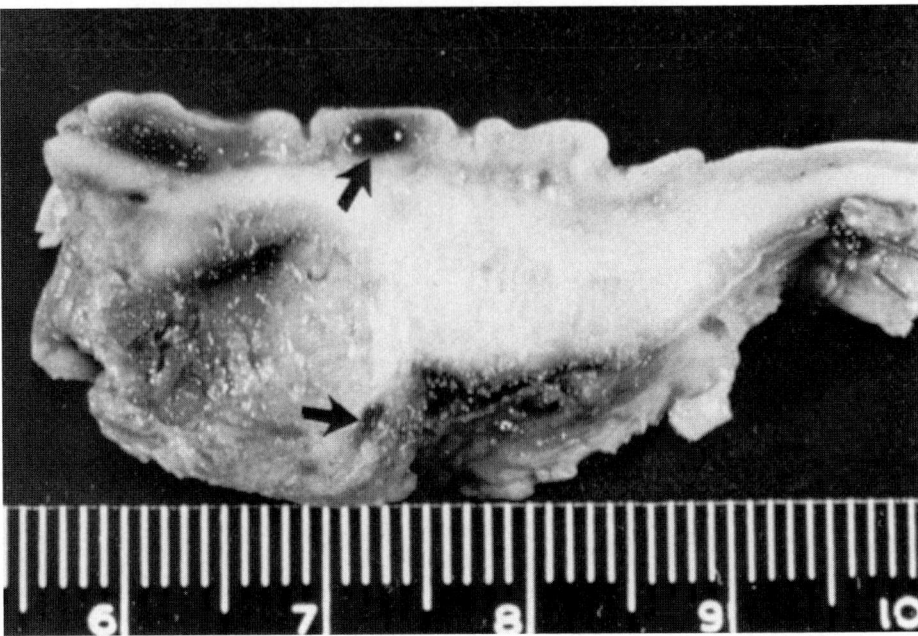

FIGURE 25-67. Endometriosis. Longitudinal section of the sigmoid colon showing blood-filled cysts *(arrows)*.

Perineal Endometrioma

Perineal endometrioma is a special situation in which implantation of viable endometrial cells occurs in episiotomy incisions. A tender nodule producing cyclic symptoms at the site of an episiotomy is highly suggestive of the diagnosis.[198] As with other benign and malignant conditions in the area, endoanal ultrasound has been employed for its assessment.[211] Local excision is the preferred treatment, although suppressive therapy may be employed. Patients harboring involvement of the anal sphincter have been managed successfully by wide excision and sphincteroplasty.[121,432]

Hamartoma

Albrecht introduced the term hamartoma to describe tumorlike malformations that result from inborn errors of tissue development.[9] These malformations are characterized by abnormal mixtures of mature tissue indigenous to that area. Hamartomas may be derived from any of the germinal layers, and any type of tissue may predominate.

According to Willis, the term hamartoma should be applied only to lesions for which evidence of a developmental anomaly is definite.[527] This includes either actual malformation with tissue excess present at birth or an inborn tissue anomaly that manifests itself by excessive growth continuing until puberty. The nomenclature depends on the tissue type that predominates: with vascular predominance, it is angiomatous; with fatty tissue, it is lipomatous; and with lymphoid tissue, it is lymphomatous.

Eichel and Hallberg differentiated hamartomas from teratomas and dermoids.[129] The term teratoma describes a spontaneous, autonomous new growth derived from pluripotential tissues. It is foreign to the region in which it occurs and is composed of elements of all three germinal layers. A dermoid tumor has the same histogenesis but differs in that it is usually cystic. Unlike a teratoma, it originates from only two germinal layers, the ectoderm and the mesoderm. Clinically, it is difficult to differentiate between teratomas, dermoids (especially when small), and hamartomas.

Suspicion of hamartoma may be aroused by a small but definite funnel-shaped dimple in the posterior midline at the anal margin or the midanal level. This anal dimple, associated with a higher lesion, has been reported only once, although it must have been encountered many times.[489]

Complete surgical removal is the only effective treatment for retrorectal cystic hamartoma. The surgical approach may be either through the anal canal or posteriorly, that is, transcoccygeally. However, when a large cyst lies at a very high level, an abdominal approach is indicated.

Dermoid Cyst and Teratoma

Dermoid cysts are tumors of epithelial origin believed to be caused by faulty inclusion of ectoderm when the embryo coalesces. They generally do not appear until adult life and are more common in women than in men.[229,357,479]

Galletly published a report in 1924 in which he stated: "Simple presacral cysts, lined by squamous or columnar epithelium, probably originate from cells of the neurenteric canal."[161] He included in his study 17 cases reported by Skutsch, all alleged to be dermoids.[452] Thomason reported one patient with a deep suppurating sinus extending from an anal dimple into the presacral region who required three operations.[489] Microscopic section showed a cyst lined with columnar epithelium and mucous glands in its wall. Robertson and Wride reported a patient who had a tumor with a draining sinus at the base of the spine with a foul-smelling discharge.[406] The sinus had a convoluted pattern, was anterior to the sacrum and coccyx, and was lined with columnar epithelium of a mucous type. Gius and Stout reported two patients, one of whom had three operations for multilocular lesions; the other underwent operation for an asymptomatic cystic tumor situated anterior to the coccyx.[171] Jackman and associates recognized the possibility that recurrent fistula may be associated with an infected dermoid cyst.[229] They believed that the cyst arose from remnants of the neurenteric canal. Landmann and Lewis reported a patient with a benign cystic ovarian teratoma who presented with a bleeding rectal lesion.[283] In a report from the Mayo Clinic, 49 congenital cystic lesions were identified: 15 epidermoid cysts, 16 mucus-secreting cysts, 15 teratomas, and three teratocarcinomas.[231] Others have also reported malignant changes in cysts.[38,108]

Currarino and colleagues described a syndrome of sacral agenesis and anorectal and presacral anomalies.[110] Others have confirmed the validity of this observation, the so-called "Currarino triad," observing a high incidence of presacral teratomas.[369] The most common sacral anomaly was believed to be meningocele. Thambidorai and associates identified 200 cases of Currarino triad from the literature, but in only 22 did the presacral mass contain both meningocele and teratoma.[488]

Patients may be asymptomatic but are usually found to have an extrarectal mass as an incidental finding on rectal examination. Endoscopic examination is usually unrewarding. As mentioned, a cyst may become infected and mimic an anorectal abscess or fistula. Cysts may also prove to be of anal duct or gland origin.[274] A plain abdominal radiograph may be helpful, but CT should be employed if there is any question of malignancy (e.g., chordoma). Preoperative biopsy is unnecessary and should not be performed.

Resection of the mass can frequently be accomplished by means of a posterior approach, with or without removal of the coccyx (see later).[3] An abdominal or abdominosacral operation may be required for a more extensive or more proximal lesion. Prognosis is excellent. Recurrence after surgery, however, is possible if the lesion is incompletely removed.

Dermoid cysts can also occur within the rectum, but this is even more unusual than the postanal or presacral locations. In this situation, intraluminal cysts may produce varied rectal symptoms, including hair protruding from the anus. Aldridge and colleagues identified only 12 such cases.[10] Their patient developed rectal bleeding and prolapse of the mass. With this type of presentation, transanal excision is the recommended approach. Endoscopic resection has also been described.[181]

Colitis Cystica Profunda or Enterogenous Cysts

Colitis cystica profunda is a rare, nonneoplastic condition characterized by the presence of mucous cysts deep to the muscularis mucosa and usually confined to the sigmoid colon and rectum. The most common symptoms are rectal bleeding, passage of mucus, diarrhea, and rectal pain.[41,316] The primary diagnosis from which it must be differentiated is mucus-producing adenocarinoma.

Wayte and Helwig categorized colitis cystica profunda into two groups: localized, in which the cysts are confined to a distinct area of the rectum; and diffuse, in which the cysts are located in extensive areas.[516] The histogenesis of this benign condition remains in dispute. Based on differences in the evaluation of clinical and pathologic findings, the following descriptive terms have been used at one time or another:

Colitis cystica profunda[134,516]
Solitary ulcer of the rectum (see Chapter 17)[201,230,308]
Syndrome of the descending perineum (see Chapter 17)[376]
Enterogenous cysts of the rectum[481]
Hamartomatous inverted polyp of the rectum[11]

Colitis cystica profunda of the localized type may protrude slightly into the lumen of the bowel as a polypoid mass and can thus mimic carcinoma of the rectum. Because it is usually located on the anterior rectal wall, the most common site for solitary ulcer, considerable confusion may exist.

The etiology of the condition is unknown. However, some patients give a history of prior rectal trauma, especially the removal of a large polyp. Madigan and Morson described the correlation between anorectal dysfunction and this disease.[308] Epstein and associates theorized that the most probable primary factor was a weakness or defect in the muscularis mucosa resulting in mucosal herniation.[134] Certainly, the fact that resolution has followed the successful management of internal procidentia and rectal prolapse implies a causative or an associative role with these conditions.[190] Peterkin and colleagues identified three patients with paraplegia

contraindicated, however, for this benign condition. Another option that has been described is mucosal sleeve excision with coloanal pull-through.[192] Reassurance and periodic proctosigmoidoscopy are suggested for those not amenable to complete removal of the lesion.

Ectopic Tissue

Besides ectopic gastric or pancreatic mucosa in a Meckel's diverticulum, ectopic tissue in the intestine or colon is very unusual. The two types that have been reported are gastric mucosal replacement of the rectal mucosa and salivary gland tissue in the submucosa.[298,358,442,473,519,530] It has been suggested that the cells lining the primitive gut have the capacity to differentiate into any epithelial type that would normally be present at another level. This would not, however, explain the presence of salivary gland tissue. Perhaps the presence of stem cells lining the cloacal zone may account for this rare observation.[442]

Testart and colleagues reviewed the literature on heterotopic gastric mucosa producing rectal "peptic" ulceration.[487] Analysis of 28 cases revealed the main features to be as follows:

All but one were diagnosed in infants or in adults younger than 26 years of age.
Rectal peptic ulceration was identified in only one half, but almost all exhibited rectal bleeding.
Rectal duplication was present in 21%.
Limited excision is generally successful.[487]

Protrusion of tissue may occur in a child, thus causing one to suspect the presence of a juvenile polyp. Patients may be asymptomatic or complain of mucous discharge, change in bowel habits, or rectal bleeding.

The true pathologic nature of the lesion is usually not suspected at the time of removal but is confirmed by histologic examination (Figure 25-70). Carlei and colleagues were able to show different types of endocrine cells in the rectal and heterotopic mucosa by means of immmunocytochemistry.[73] They could affirm that the heterotopic event also involved the differentiation of the endocrine elements into gastric-type endocrine cells. In their case, they were able to demonstrate that the activities of the heterotopic mucosa, such as endocrine system and mucin and acid production, were almost identical to those of the normal stomach.[73]

Transanal local excision is the appropriate treatment (Figure 25-71).

There has been a total of six documented cases of heterotopic gastric mucosa occurring in the large bowel, proximal to the rectum. Most have been managed by resection, because bleeding identified by means of angiography or radioisotope scan leads to surgery. It is only when the lesion has been submitted to histologic evalua-

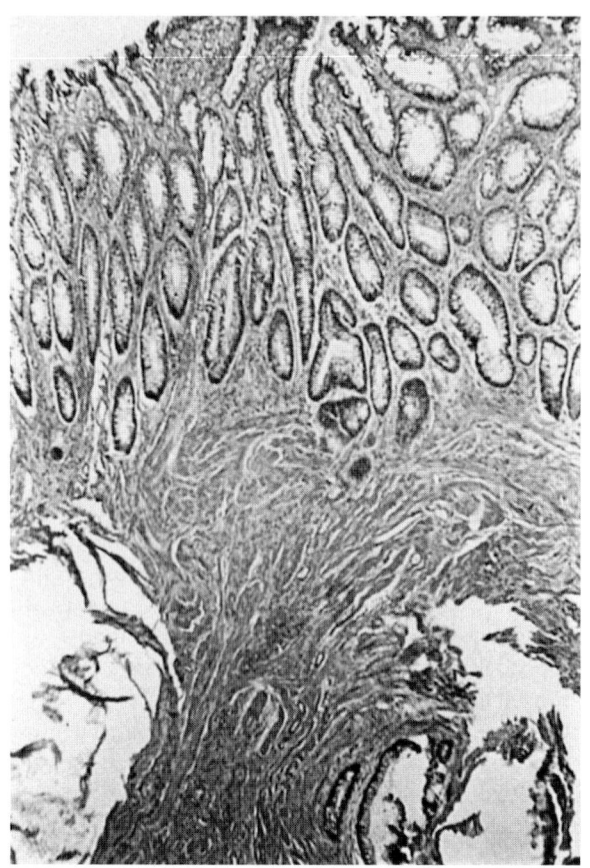

FIGURE 25-68. Colitis cystica profunda. Cystic structures in the wall of the bowel, one of which is lined by columnar epithelium *(arrow)*. The other cyst has lost epithelium. (Original magnification × 80; from Corman ML, Veidenheimer MC, Swinton NW. *Diseases of the anus, rectum and colon. Part I: neoplasms.* New York: Medcom, 1972.)

who developed proctitis cystica profunda.[381] This particular population may be at an increased risk because of digital stimulation applied to effect evacuation. One patient required a colostomy for recurrent symptoms.

Differentiation by biopsy may be difficult.[11] In order to establish the diagnosis with certainty adequate tissue must be obtained in order to reveal submucosal cyst formation.[185] In Madigan and Morson's series, 31 of 51 patients had lesions with histologic appearances suggestive of both solitary ulcer and colitis profunda (Figs. 25-68 and 25-69).[308]

Although successful medical management through the use of steroid enemas has been reported, transanal excision of the lesion is the optimal therapy if it can be accomplished. A transcoccygeal approach is another alternative. Martin and associates reviewed the Mayo Clinic experience of 66 patients with this condition.[316] Fewer than three fourths were asymptomatic after local excision. Not uncommonly, the lesion is unresectable except by radical abdominoperineal resection. Such treatment is

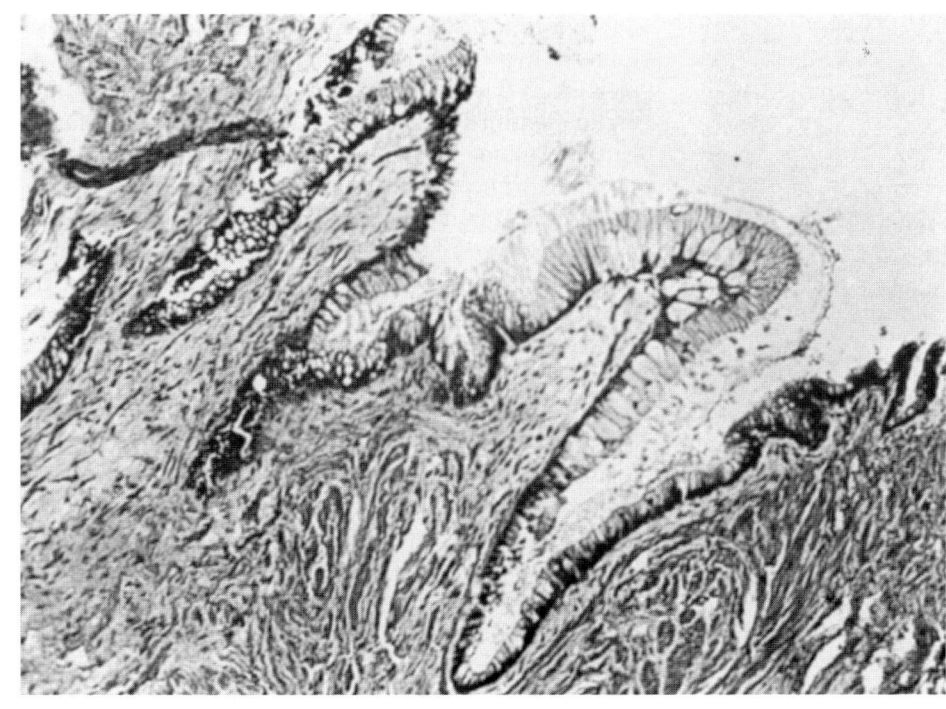

FIGURE 25-69. Colitis cystica profunda. The lining of the cyst shows columnar epithelium. (Original magnification × 260; from Corman ML, Veidenheimer MC, Swinton NW. *Diseases of the anus, rectum and colon. Part I: neoplasms.* New York: Medcom, 1972.)

tion that the true cause is confirmed. There are now reports of successful management in individuals by means of a histamine (H$_2$) antagonist.[73,350]

EXOGENOUS, EXTRINSIC, AND MISCELLANEOUS TUMORS

Extraskeletal Osteosarcoma

Extraskeletal osteosarcoma is a rare, malignant tumor arising from soft tissue *without* attachment to bone or to periosteum. A single case that was primary to the colon has been reported.[441]

Choriocarcinoma

Choriocarcinoma primary to the colon is an exceedingly rare tumor, with only seven cases reported in the literature according to a review by Le and colleagues.[285] The etiology has been thought by some to be dedifferentiation of an adenocarcinoma, but there is also the possibility that the lesion may arise *de novo*. Treatment is resection, but prognosis is poor.

Metastatic Tumor

Metastatic tumor to the colon and rectum can cause symptoms of abdominal pain, bleeding, and change in bowel habits. Life-threatening emergencies, in the form

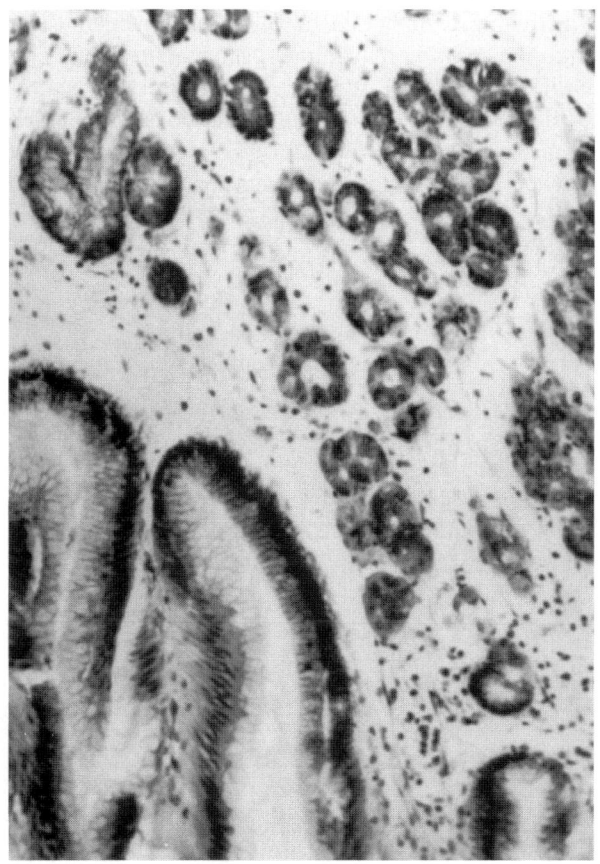

FIGURE 25-70. Heterotopic gastric mucosa in the rectum. Colonic mucosa on the left with gastric cells on the right. Special stains showed the presence of chief and parietal cells. (Original magnification × 260.)

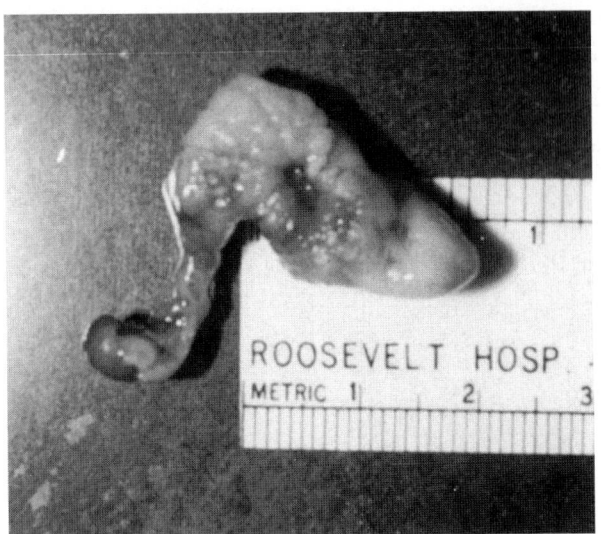

FIGURE 25-71. Heterotopic gastric mucosa in the rectum. Polypoid mass with 3-mm ulceration. The ulcer was found to contain the gastric glands seen in Figure 25-70.

of massive GI hemorrhage, obstruction, and perforation, have been reported.[457] Although usually it produces extrinsic compression of the bowel on barium enema examination, ulceration may mimic primary carcinoma of the colon (Figure 25-72). Tumors of adjacent organs that may invade the colon and rectum include prostate, uterus (Figs. 25-73 and 25-74), ovary (Figure 25-75), kidney, stomach, duodenum, and pancreas.

Metastatic disease to the colon can occur from breast tumors, hypernephroma, lung tumors, and malignant melanoma (Figure 25-72).[225,255,320,447,457] The Mayo Clinic group identified 24 patients treated for metastatic malignant melanoma.[486] The median interval between diagnosis of the primary lesion and the development of metastatic disease was more than 7 years. The most common presentation was bleeding. The 5-year survival for those who were resected was 21%. Palliative resection or bypass is usually advised for symptomatic tumors, but perforation or obstruction implies a poor prognosis.[225,255,486]

Barium Granuloma

A submucosal rectal nodule that can be confused with a neoplastic condition, especially a carcinoid, may be the result of a barium granuloma. Such lesions appear in the lower rectum, usually as submucosal white or yellowish plaques, and are frequently asymptomatic. A break in the continuity of the rectal mucosa is the probable initiating factor. Transanal excision is mandatory for diagnosis.

Rand studied the effects of injection of barium in the rectal wall of dogs.[397] He produced a granulomatous ulcer that healed spontaneously despite retained barium in the tissues. Histologically, the presence of barium produces a typical foreign body granulomatous reaction (Figure 25-76). The barium crystals lie in a pool in the submucosa in early lesions, but macrophages rapidly accumulate and phagocytose in the crystalline barium sulfate. Care in the introduction of the enema catheter and

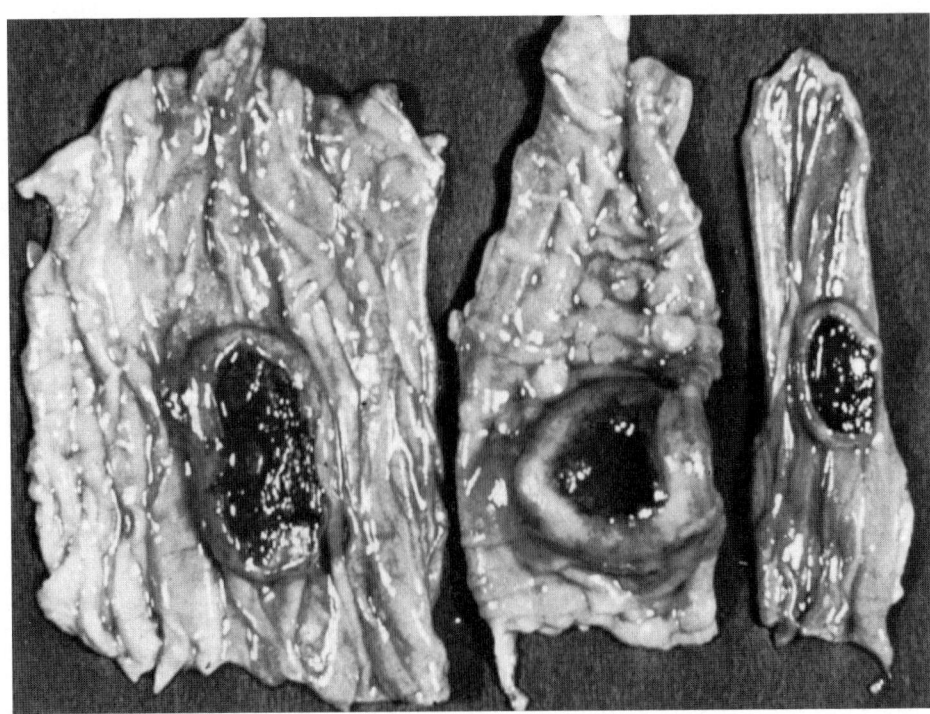

FIGURE 25-72. Multiple lesions of metastatic melanoma from the skin to the bowel mucosa; normal mucosa surrounds the deep ulcer in the center. (Courtesy of Rudolf Garret, M.D.)

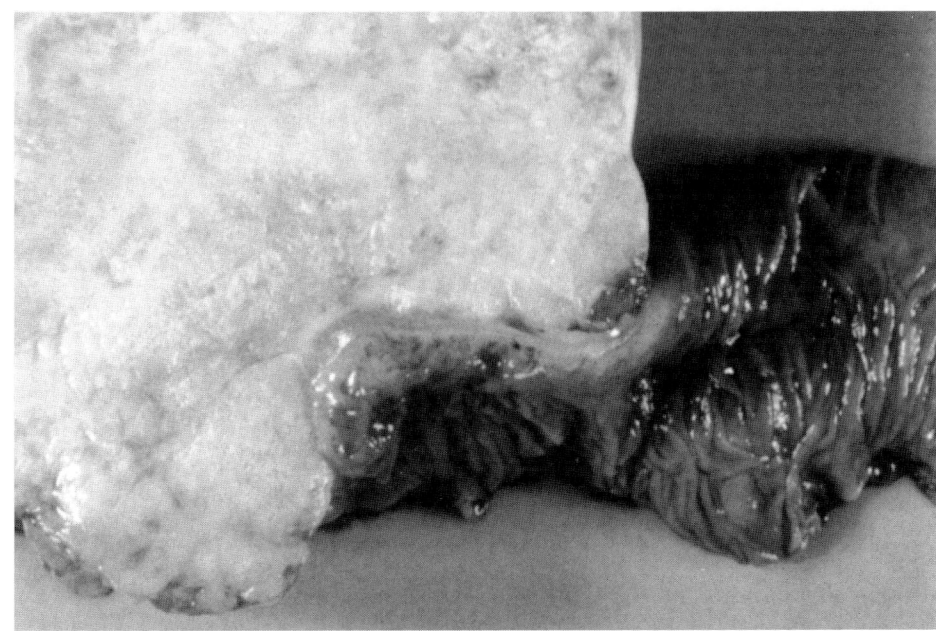

FIGURE 25-73. Tumor invading the serosa of the sigmoid colon from a uterine cancer.

caution with the use of the balloon tip are clearly indicated for prevention of barium granuloma.

Numerous cases of rupture of the bowel with barium peritonitis have been reported when barium enema examination has followed rectal biopsy.[208] Margulis and Burhenne stated that double-contrast examination of the colon should not be performed for at least 2 weeks after rectal biopsy.[313] Optimally, if a polyp excision or electrocoagulation is contemplated on an individual who is to have barium enema examination, the patient should complete the contrast study and then return for the other procedure (see Chapter 4). Barium granuloma of the more proximal colon is usually related to inflammatory bowel disease.[178]

Oleoma, Eleoma, Oil Granuloma, and Paraffinoma

Oleoma, also known as oleogranuloma or paraffinoma, is a rare entity that occurs in the GI tract or skin as a result of an injection of mineral oil (paraffin) for the treatment of hemorrhoids or enema or vegetable oil in the management of constipation. The lesion seen may be defined as an intramural pseudotumor that develops as a foreign body reaction. The "tumor" is occasionally cystic and may be termed an oleocyst. The differential diagnosis must be confirmed by biopsy to rule out other neoplastic and inflammation conditions.

The clinical manifestations may develop very rapidly or may not present for many years after oil enters the tissue. The injection site usually appears as one or more irregular, firm nodules. In the GI tract, oleomas are usually found proximal to the dentate line in the lower portion of the rectum.

An oleoma is usually localized to the submucosa. However, considerable inflammation of the mucosa and even the perianal skin may be present. The appearance of the lesion depends on the oil present. Vegetable oils produce the least reaction, animal oils a greater one, and mineral oils the most severe changes.[194]

Histologically, oleomas are typified by large mononuclear phagocytes, epithelioid cells, eosinophilic leukocytes, and multinucleated giant cells of the foreign body type, surrounding large, clear spaces that give the tissue a Swiss-cheese or spongiform appearance under low-power amplification. Histologic staining with oil red O verifies the presence of the lipid. The reaction usually remains localized to the submucosa, but not infrequently involves the lamina propria of the mucosa and may actually extend into the perirectal fat (Figure 25-77).[194]

Mazier and associates reported four cases of oleoma.[319] All patients recovered after simple excision of the lesion.

Sarcoidosis

Sarcoidosis is a generalized granulomatous disease with protean manifestations. The condition usually creates restrictive lung disease but can occasionally involve the GI tract. In the limited number of cases reported, patients usually do not have symptoms referable to the bowel.[267,495] Proctosigmoidoscopic examination may reveal mild inflammatory changes or a submucosal rectal nodule.

The characteristic noncaseating granuloma of sarcoidosis may be seen on biopsy or excision of a lesion (Figure 25-78). Histologic examination may confirm a granuloma composed primarily of histiocytes, but there is no evidence of caseous necrosis.

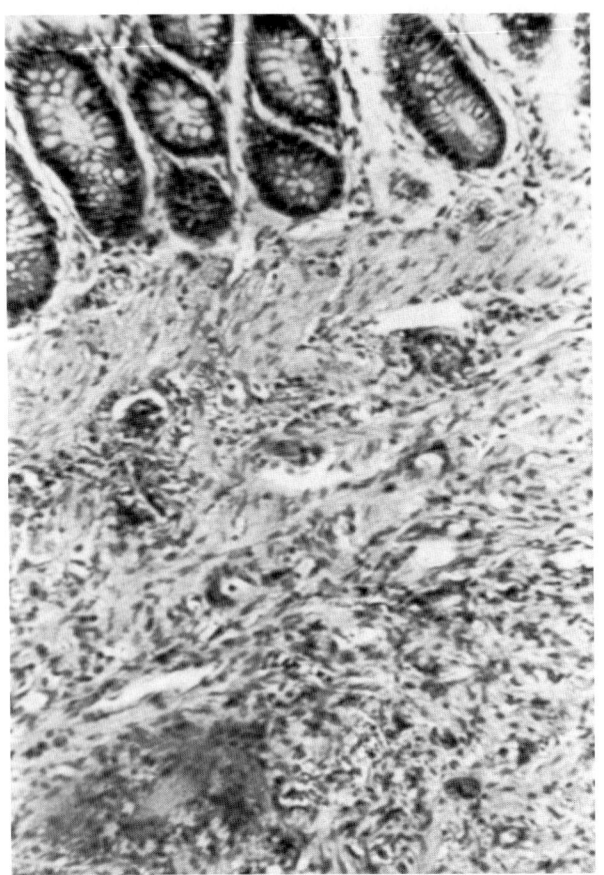

FIGURE 25-74. Metastatic adenocarcinoma from the uterine cervix. Note the normal overlying colonic epithelium. The wall is infiltrated by tumor cells forming small glandular structures. (Original magnification × 260; courtesy of Rudolf Garret, M.D.)

The clinical patterns produced by intestinal sarcoidosis are not well established, but anorexia, nausea, vomiting, abdominal pain, and GI bleeding have all been described.[194] Differential diagnosis must include Crohn's disease, but the presence of a lesion in the lung will usually clarify any possible confusion.

Wegener's Granulomatosis

Wegener's granulomatosis, a necrotizing vasculitis associated with granulomatous lesions of the upper and lower respiratory tract and the kidney, was reported in one instance to present as a perianal ulcer.[27] Treatment was by immunosuppressive therapy.

Amyloidosis

Amyloidosis is a pathologic condition caused by the deposition within tissues of a fibrillar protein known as amyloid.[483] Virchow misnamed the substance because he thought it resembled starch or cellulose. The Third International Symposium on Amyloidosis recommended the following classification:

Primary amyloidosis: no evidence of preceding or coexisting disease except multiple myeloma
Secondary amyloidosis: coexistence of other conditions
Localized amyloid: single organ rather than generalized involvement
Familial
Senile amyloid[234]

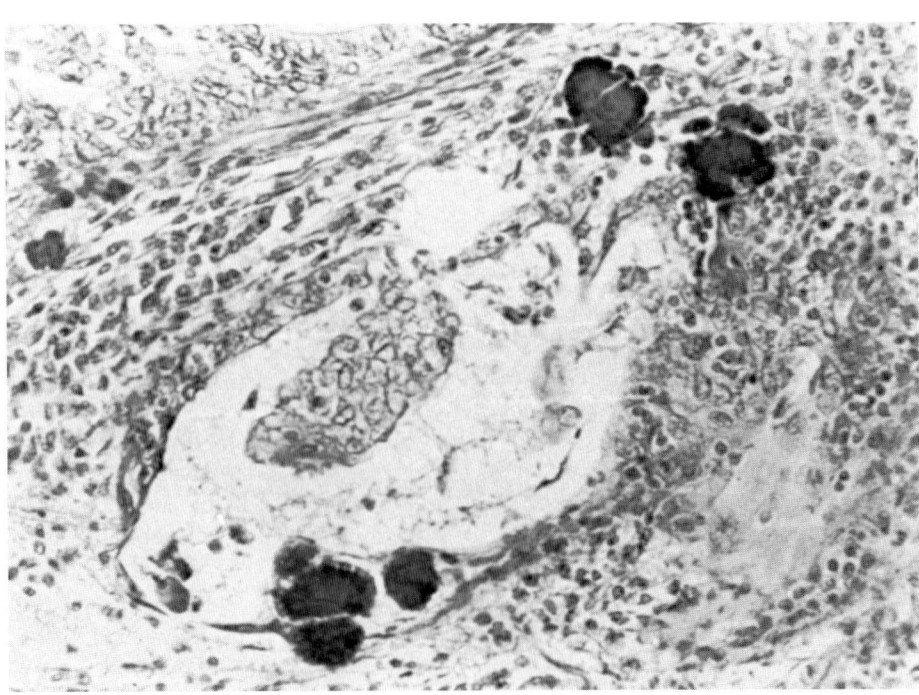

FIGURE 25-75. Metastatic tumor consisting of undifferentiated cells forming abortive glands with psammoma bodies. The tumor was metastatic from an ovary. (From Corman ML, Veidenheimer MC, Swinton NW. *Diseases of the anus, rectum and colon. Part I: neoplasms.* New York: Medcom, 1972.)

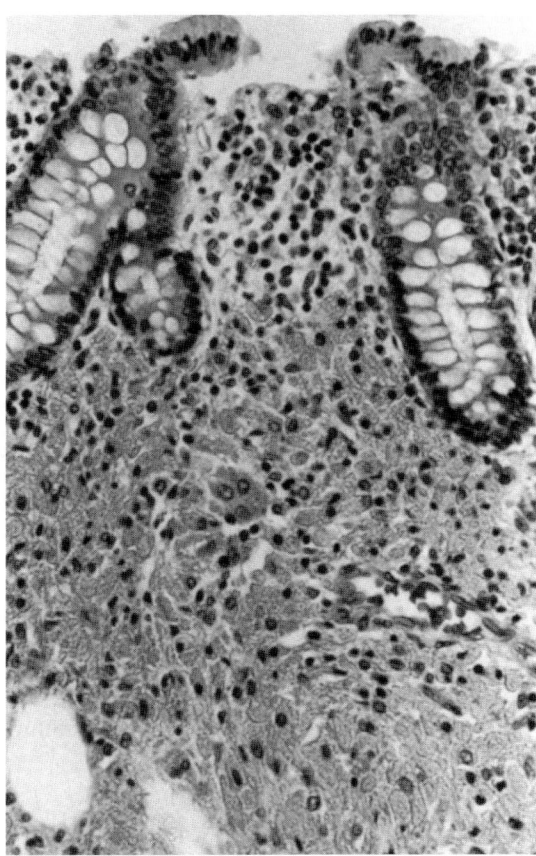

FIGURE 25-76. Barium granuloma. Normal glandular mucosa overlying plump, foamy histiocytes filled with refractile material when visualized under polarized light. (Original magnification × 80; courtesy of Rodger C. Haggitt, M.D.)

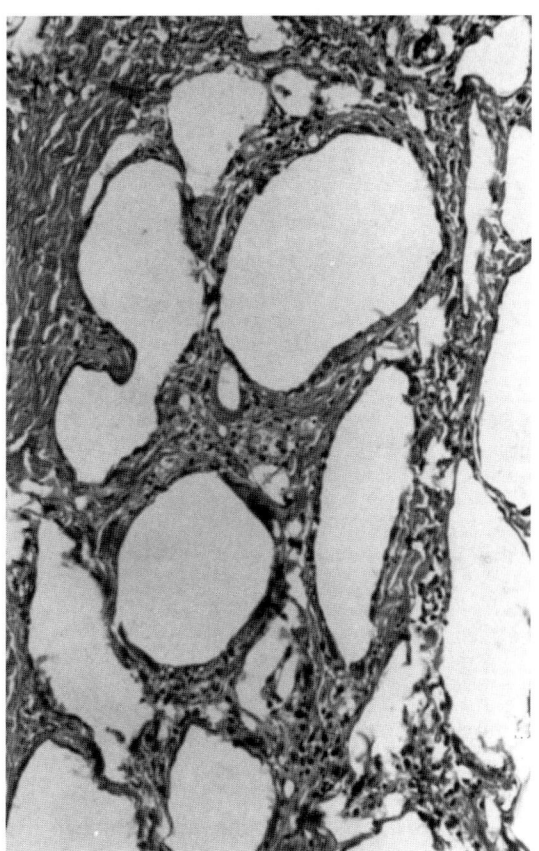

FIGURE 25-77. Oleogranuloma. Submucosal cysts of varied size with surrounding foreign body giant-cell reaction and granulomatous change. The diagnosis is confirmed with oil red O stain. (Original magnification × 50; courtesy of Rodger C. Haggitt, M.D.)

It is not within the purview of this text to undertake an assessment of the disease, itself. Under the circumstances, the reader is advised to seek out any of a number of comprehensive reviews on the subject.[278]

Involvement of the GI tract is reported in 70% of patients with primary amyloidosis and 55% of those with the secondary form.[234,237] Amyloidosis not uncommonly affects the colon in association with a number of systemic diseases, particularly pulmonary, renal, hematologic, and arthritic. Symptoms include malabsorption, diarrhea, bleeding, vomiting, abdominal pain, and, rarely, signs of peritonitis, but the condition is usually asymptomatic. Ischemic colitis as a consequence of vascular involvement of the bowel is a well-recognized complication of the disease.[405]

Rectal Biopsy

The value of rectal biopsy for establishing the diagnosis of systemic amyloid has been a matter of controversy. Biopsies of the liver, spleen, or oral tissue (particularly gingiva) have been suggested as alternative sites.[436] Von Dinges and

associates performed an autopsy study of 100 cases and took biopsy specimens of the rectum and gingiva.[508] In this unselected study there was a higher incidence of amyloid detected in the gingival and buccal mucosa than in the rectal mucosa. Three fourths of the biopsies taken from the mouth yielded positive results, as compared with one third of the rectal mucosal specimens. The authors concluded that in view of the frequently found extensive amyloid deposits present in the mouth, biopsy should be obtained from the rectal mucosa. The theory behind this recommendation is that amyloid found on gingival biopsy is of less significance than if it were found on rectal biopsy.

Gafni and Sohar performed rectal biopsy on 30 patients with known amyloidosis, and a positive result was found in 26.[159] Blum and Sohar found that rectal biopsy yielded a 75% positive result in those with amyloidosis.[60] This was exceeded only by renal biopsy (87% positive). Biopsy of the liver gave positive results in less than one half of the patients, and gingival biopsy in fewer than 20%.

In a study by Kyle and co-workers, 17 of 20 patients with primary systemic amyloidosis were found to have positive rectal biopsies for amyloid.[279] In two of the three

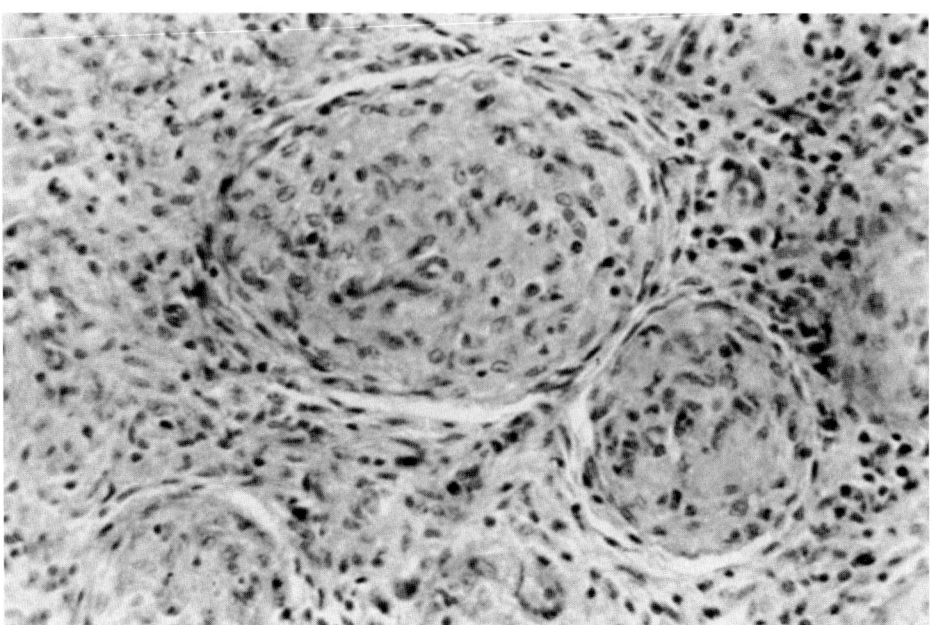

FIGURE 25-78. Sarcoidosis. Granuloma without caseous necrosis. Note the characteristic epithelioid cells. (Original magnification × 360; from Corman ML, Veidenheimer MC, Swinton NW. *Diseases of the anus, rectum and colon. Part I: neoplasms.* New York-Medcom, 1972.)

remaining individuals, the specimen did not contain submucosal tissue.

This is an important point. It is imperative that adequate submucosal tissue be obtained in order to confirm the diagnosis. Although some authors have advocated a suction biopsy forceps, my own preference is to employ the ordinary rectal biopsy instrument. Because one is not taking a sample of tissue from an exophytic lesion, the biopsy should be obtained from a valve of Houston or from the posterior rectal wall. If bleeding is encountered, pressure with an epinephrine-soaked cotton swab is advised. Electrocoagulation should be avoided because of the risk of perforating the bowel.

An interesting diagnostic point was made by Slagel and Lupton concerning the observation of "postproctoscopic periorbital purpura."[453] The hydrostatic forces imposed on the delicate periorbital vasculature when the patient is placed in the prone jackknife position for biopsy may precipitate rupture of the vessels whose walls are compromised by amyloid deposition.

Special stains are important for identification of amyloid. A homogeneous eosinophilic substance can be seen by means of Congo red stain. This material may be overlooked if the standard hematoxylin and eosin technique is used (Figure 25-79).

Response to Treatment

Another purpose of rectal biopsy is to evaluate the success of different modalities of treatment. Bacon and colleagues performed repeated rectal biopsies in a group of patients who underwent penicillamine therapy.[31] Improvement could be observed by serial histologic examinations. Melphalan and prednisone have been employed with limited benefit. The mechanism is to decrease immunoglobulin production and prevent progressive amyloid deposition.[483] Colchicine has also been reported to have some therapeutic value as well as autologous hematopoietic stem cell transplantation.

Amyloid Tumor

Localized amyloid tumors of the GI tract are extremely unusual. All reported cases involving the large bowel presented with lower GI bleeding.[234] A colonic perforation has also been observed.[177] Rarely, amyloidosis of the colon may produce a mass lesion or obstructive symptoms.[238,275] Resection should be considered for a symptomatic, well-defined tumor.

Malacoplakia

In 1902, Michaelis and Gutmann described malacoplakia as a rare chronic inflammatory disorder most commonly affecting the urinary bladder and other portions of the genitourinary tract.[329] In 1965, Terner and Lattes reported the first case of colonic involvement.[485] This was followed by the publication of reports of several other patients.[396]

Clinical presentation is varied, but rectal bleeding, diarrhea, and obstructive symptoms are most commonly described. The lesion may be observed as an incidental finding. There is a preponderance of women among patients with the genitourinary lesion, but this is not the case with those who have colonic involvement.

There are no characteristic radiologic changes of malacoplakia. The barium enema may be indistinguishable from carcinoma or from granulomatous colitis.[243]

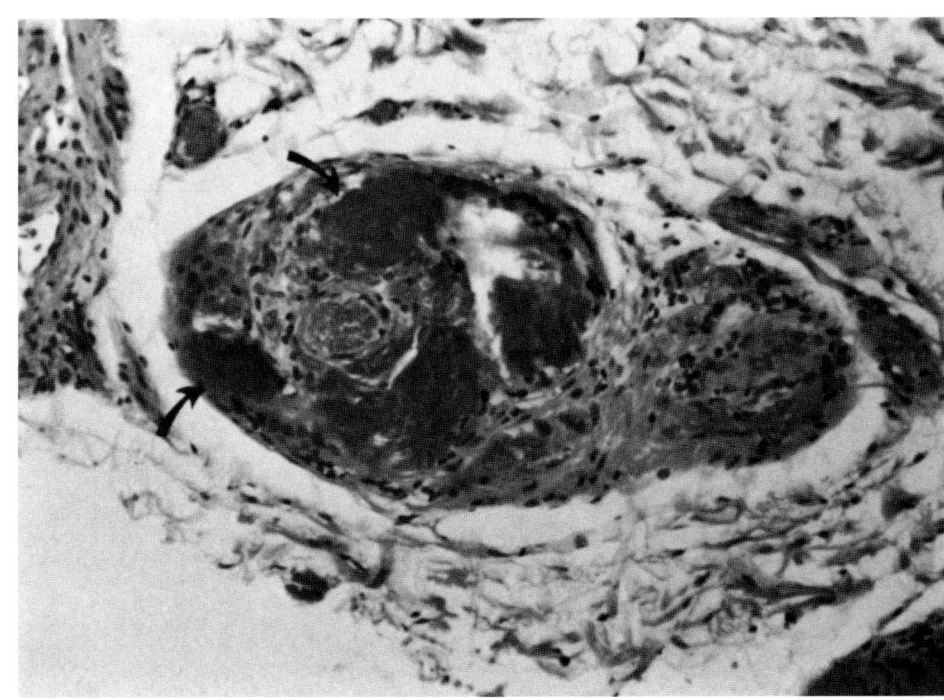

FIGURE 25-79. Amyloidosis. Congo red stain, which produces green color under polarized light, reveals homogeneous material *(arrows)* within the wall of an artery in the submucosa of the rectum. (Original magnification × 280.)

The macroscopic lesion appears as a mucosal thickening or plaque and may assume a polypoid configuration. Histologically, one observes a proliferation of eosinophilic, coarsely granular histiocytes (Hansemann's cells) of granular periodic acid–Schiff–positive inclusions often containing laminated calcific concretions, the so-called Michaelis-Gutmann bodies that are virtually pathognomonic of this entity (Figure 25-80).[318] The histiocytic proliferation is accompanied by a chronic inflammatory infiltrate and sometimes by fibrosis (Figure 25-81).

Although the pathogenesis is not fully understood, ultrastructural evidence suggests that altered heat response to certain species of gram-negative bacteria may be involved.[81,291] Abdou and colleagues have demonstrated a reversible lysosomal defect that could impair lysosomal bacterial killing in this disorder.[1] Sound ultrastructural evidence implies that the Michaelis-Gutmann body is a morphologic by-product of impaired lysosomal function.[300] There may be an immunologic association as well, because the condition has been identified in a patient with hypogammaglobulinemia.[337] A genetic predisposition has also been observed.[132]

In 1981, McClure reviewed the world literature of malacoplakia of the GI tract.[321] There were 34 recorded cases with 86 sites involved, most commonly in the rectum and colon.

Although the lesions are for the most part self-limited or responsive to antibiotic therapy, occasionally resection is necessary because of bleeding, the development of nonhealing fistulas, or localized anatomic complications.[243] Biopsy and histologic examination are necessary to differentiate this lesion from carcinoma, which it may resemble clinically. It is of interest that malacoplakia has been associated as an incidental finding with colonic carcinoma that may actually cause the surgeon to overestimate the extent of the invasion by tumor.[318,321,396]

Sacrococcygeal Chordoma

Sacrococcygeal chordoma, a rare tumor of the fetal notochord, is characterized by a slow but inexorably progressive growth that usually spans a period of years. It invades by direct extension. Irrespective of the method of treatment chosen, the prognosis is poor. This tumor, thought by many to remain a local disease, has been reported to demonstrate distant metastases in more than 40% of patients.[166,214] The usual sites of distribution of chordoma are sacrococcygeal (50%), sphenooccipital (35%), and vertebral (15%). There are rare examples of extranotochordal origin.[196]

Signs, Symptoms, and Findings

Symptoms are produced as the tumor proliferates; it often reaches considerable size before the diagnosis is made. Surrounding soft tissue and viscera are at first simply displaced, but eventually adjacent bone is gradually eroded (Figure 25-82). The most common initial symptom is pain. This is often so gradual in onset and of such indefinite character that patients with this complaint often experience a delay in diagnosis of months to years. Constipation is the second most common presenting complaint.[466]

The most significant physical finding is a firm, smooth, presacral mass with overlying intact rectal

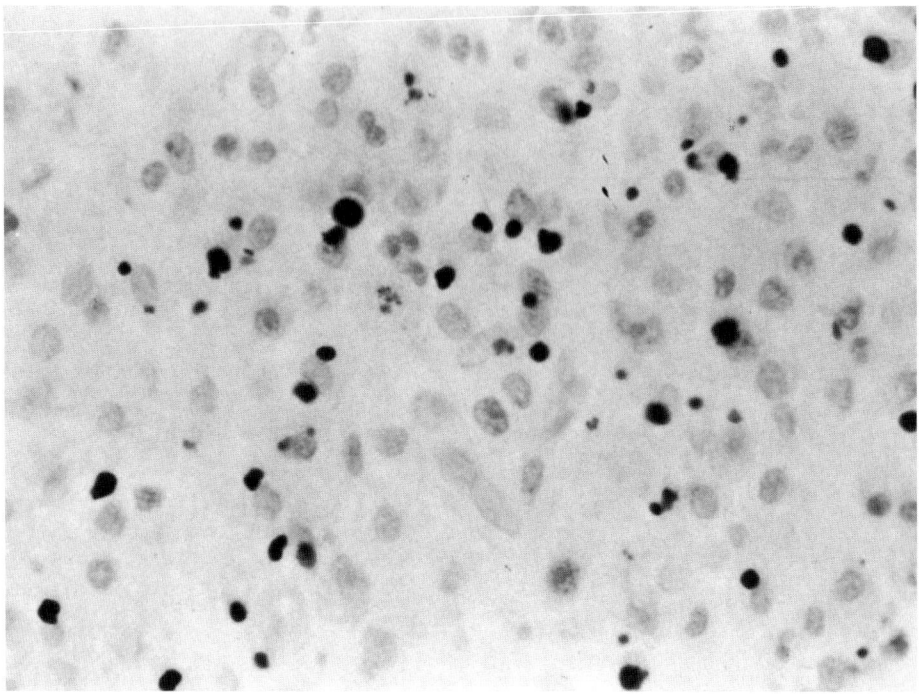

FIGURE 25-80. Malacoplakia. Von Kossa stain showing Michaelis-Gutmann bodies. (Original magnification × 600; Courtesy of Rudolf Garret, M.D.)

mucosa. There may be a history of prior treatment for a neurologic, orthopedic, or urologic disorder.

Evaluation

Bone destruction, a soft tissue mass, and anterior displacement of the rectum are the characteristic radiographic signs. These tumors often involve far more soft tissue than the osseous deformity would imply, and at operation bone destruction is likely to be more extensive than had been evident from the radiographic studies.[245]

Radiographic examination, including CT scan and MRI (Figure 25-83), is the only investigative procedure necessary for making the diagnosis of chordoma. Suga and colleagues evaluated four patients with primary sacrococcygeal chordoma by means of bone scintigraphy with technetium-99m hydroxymethylene diphos-

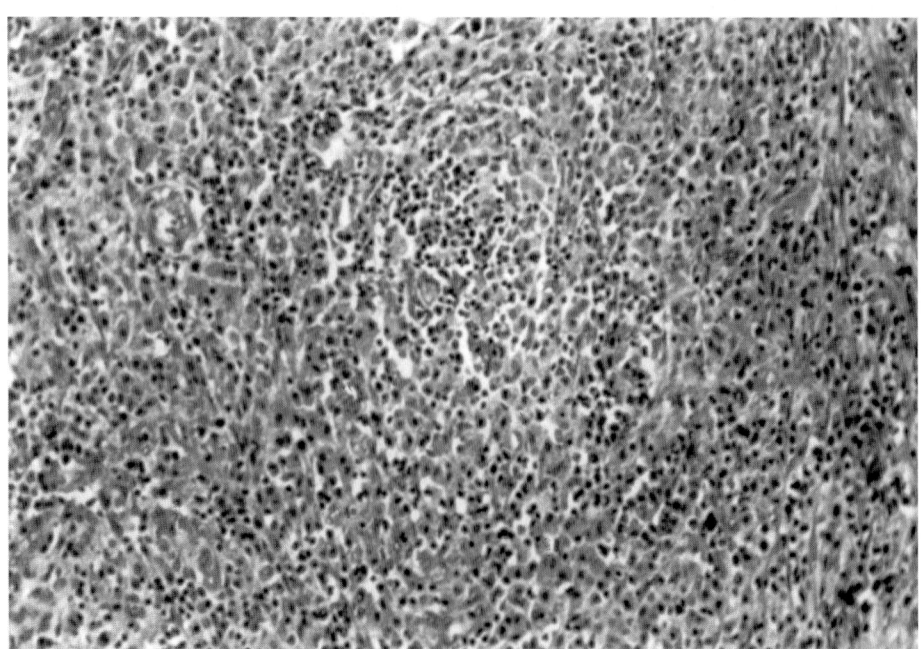

FIGURE 25-81. Malacoplakia. Many macrophages and lymphocytes are evident. (Original magnification × 260; courtesy of Rudolf Garret, M.D.)

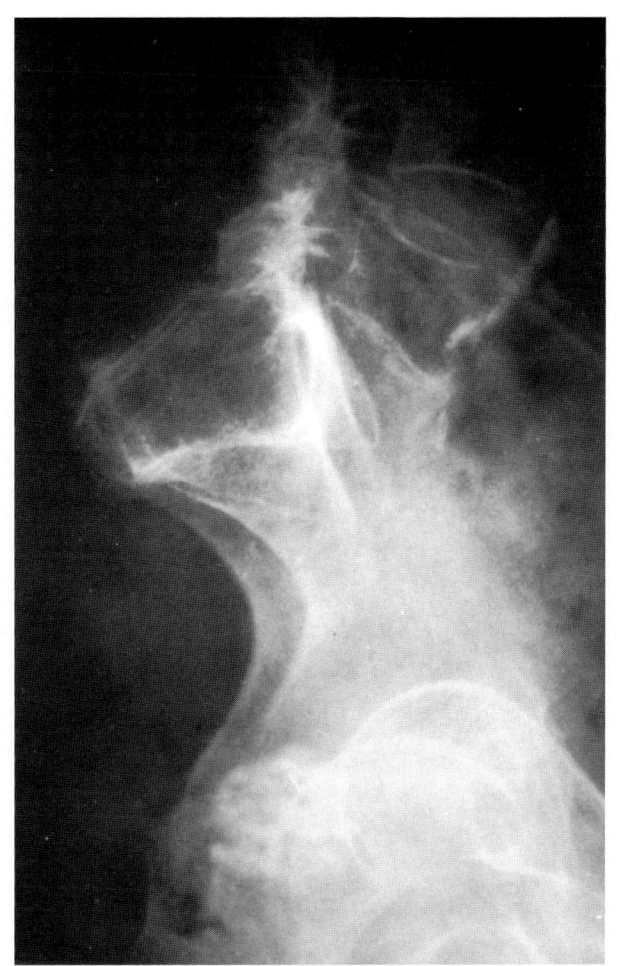

FIGURE 25-82. Sacrococcygeal chordoma. Invasion of the sacrum produces complete destruction, as seen on lateral projection.

phonate and gallium scintigraphy.[472] All demonstrated photon-deficient or cold lesions corresponding to the tumor on scintigraphy. The findings led the authors to conclude that a tumor consistent with a chordoma demonstrates a cold lesion on scintigraphy with no increased accumulation on gallium scan. This is much more consistent with a chordoma as opposed to a malignant neoplasm.[472] Needle biopsy is to be condemned because of the likelihood of implanting viable tumor cells (Figs. 25-84 and 25-85).

Treatment

Cure of sacrococcygeal chordoma depends on complete extirpation of the tumor, ideally by *en bloc* removal of the coccyx and the lower sacral segments with the lesion (Figs. 25-86 through 25-88). The limiting factor of the extent of resection performed is the need to preserve the S2 nerve roots, because their removal will lead to permanent neurologic damage and fecal and urinary incontinence.[19,352] However, a report of normal continence was observed in a patient with preservation of only one S2 root.[17] In addition to neurologic impairment, resections more extensive than the lower three sacral segments may result in instability and collapse of the pelvis and descent of the lumbar spine.[48,378]

The patient must understand that there is significant risk of impairment in spite of all precautions. Furthermore, it is strongly suggested that neurosurgical consultation be available in the operating room for all procedures involving the removal of a sacral chordoma.

Some surgeons favor a radical approach, including abdominosacral resection or even posterior exenteration and sacrectomy.[224,250,251,295] Exposure of the sciatic and pudendal nerves is required if one must extirpate a large growth that extends into the buttocks.[250] High sacral resections may be performed by dividing the fused sacral laminae with fine rongeurs, opening the sacral canal, exposing the dural sac and sacral roots, and dividing the sacral bodies with an osteotome.[250,252]

Radiation therapy is controversial, because the tumor has not been proved to be radiosensitive. It is often used, however, when surgical excision is impossible. No chemotherapeutic regimen has thus far proved beneficial.[29] If recurrence develops following resection, debulking may palliate pain symptoms. If radiotherapy has been employed, subsequent healing may be considerably delayed, or the wound may not heal at all. For unremitting pain, uncontrolled by medication, chordotomy may be necessary.

Results

Results of surgical treatment for chordoma are difficult to interpret because patients often live a long time, even with persistent localized or disseminated disease. Furthermore, many publications are based on small numbers, with only a few months of follow-up.[372,538] The overall 5-year survival in the Mayo Clinic series of 30 patients was 75%.[231] However, only 30% were considered cured. Chandawarkar reviewed a 50-year experience with 50 consecutive patients.[80] All underwent partial sacrococcygectomy. Postoperative complications included the following:

Urinary incontinence (14%)
Anal incontinence (6%)
Hemorrhage (4%)
Rectal injury (2%)[80]

In his reported experience, the average disease-free survival was 63 months.

Opinion

Because of the high likelihood of recurrence,[79,111,214,497] my own attitude is rather fatalistic. If the tumor cannot be excised by the posterior route alone, it is extremely unlikely that the disease will be controlled by any means.

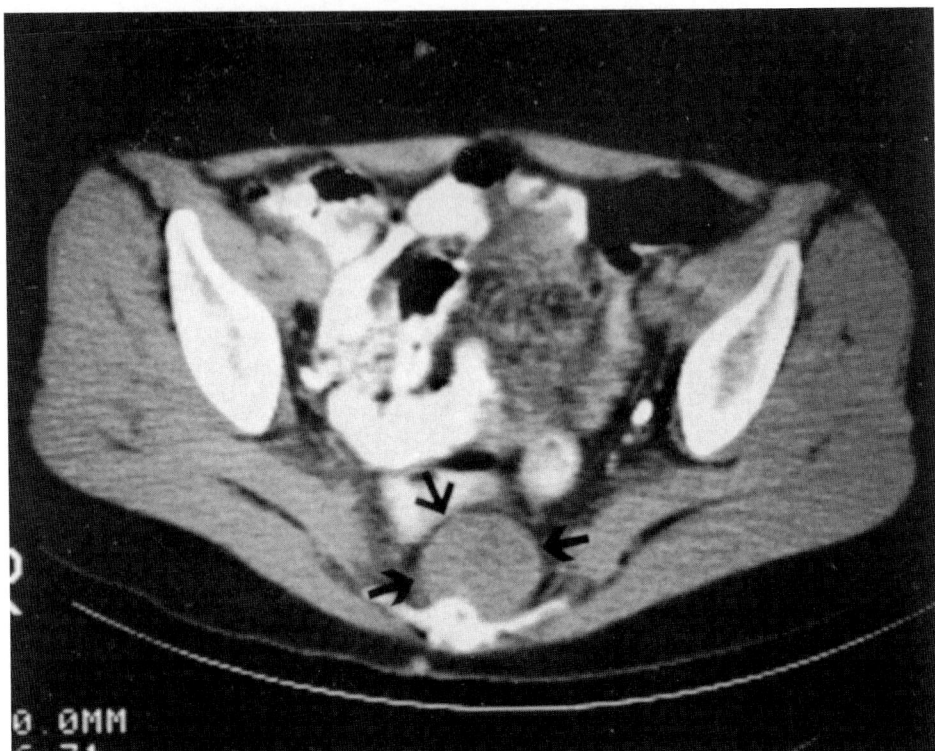

FIGURE 25-83. Sacrococcygeal chordoma. This computed tomography scan demonstrates a well-circumscribed mass invading the sacrum *(arrow)*.

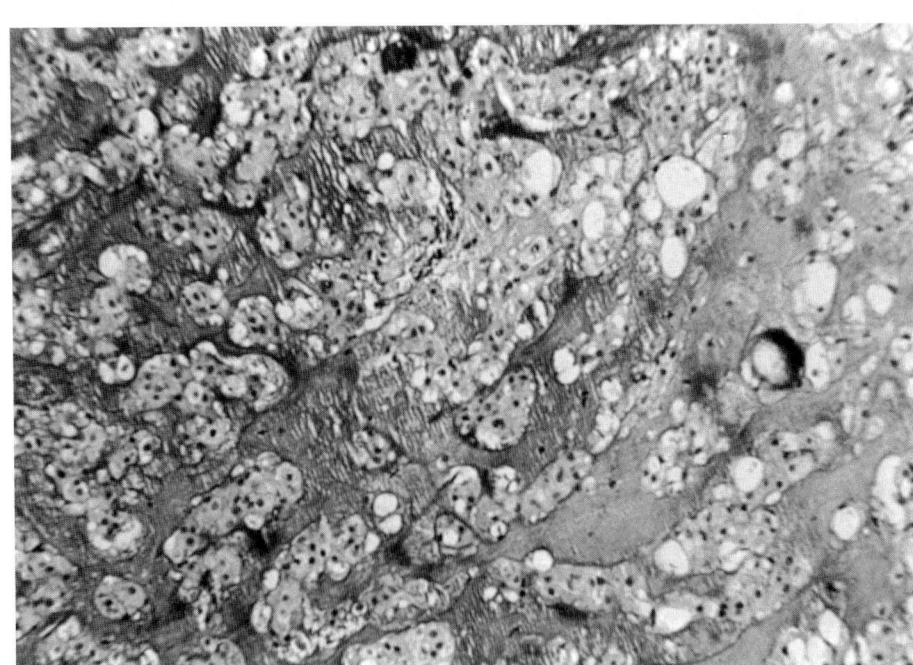

FIGURE 25-84. Sacrococcygeal chordoma. Cells with vacuolated cytoplasm resembling chondrocytes. (Original magnification × 280; courtesy of Rudolf Garret, M.D.)

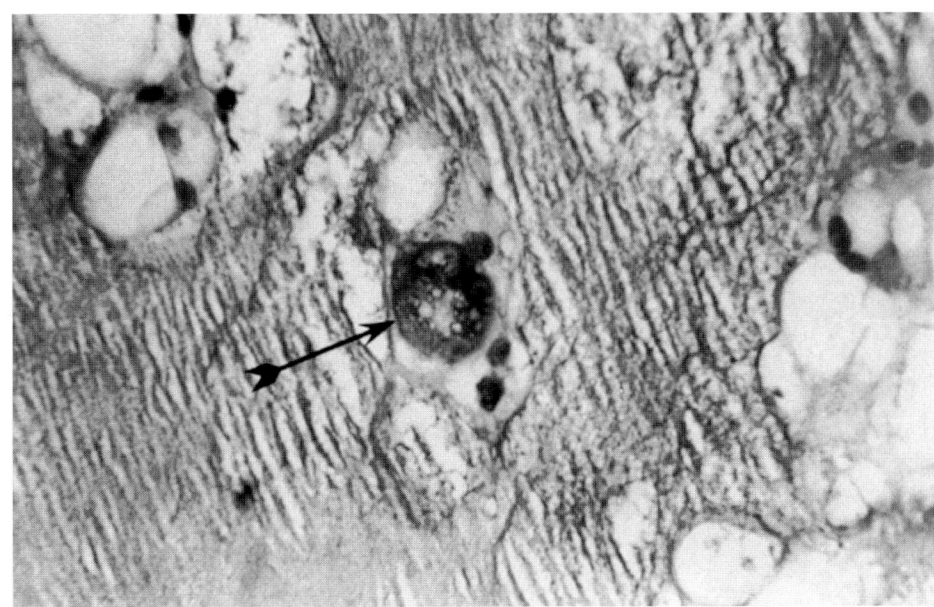

FIGURE 25-85. Sacrococcygeal chordoma. A physaliphorous cell *(arrow)*, a large cell with a lobulated, large nucleus, is evident in the chordoma. (Original magnification × 600; courtesy of Rudolf Garret, M.D.)

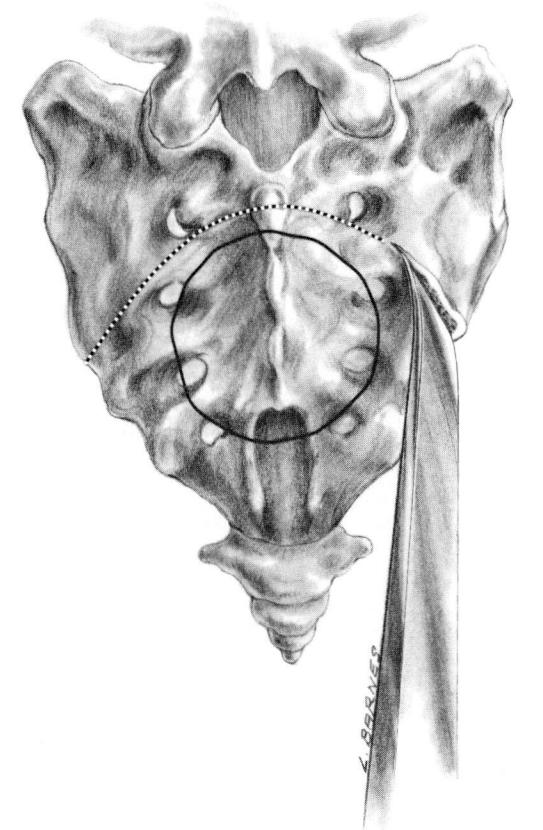

FIGURE 25-86. Technique of removing the sacrum with an osteotome.

Ependymoma

Ependymomas are the most common tumors of glial origin in the spinal cord, especially in the region of the cauda equina.[493] Clinically, a mass, thought to be a pilonidal cyst or sinus is a common presenting feature.[15] These lesions occur mainly in patients during the third decade of life and present either in the soft tissue posterior to the rectum or in the pelvis.[344] Those whose tumors are pelvic in location present with sphincter dysfunction attributable to sacral nerve involvement. The recognition of this entity has generally been attributed to Mallory in his 1902 presentation at the Harvard Medical School in Boston.[310]

Histologic examination reveals a papillary neoplasm with cells containing relatively regular nuclei without significant mitotic activity (Figure 25-89). Timmerman and Bubrick reviewed the literature and reported a patient with postsacral extraspinal ependymoma, the seventeenth such case.[493] in addition, there were 28 reports in a presacral location.[493] According to the authors, a postsacral tumor is most likely to present with an obvious mass, but in the presacral location the signs and symptoms are similar to those of chordoma. Conventional and CT studies may reveal erosion of the sacrum, and myelography will demonstrate an extradural mass indenting the thecal sac from below.[344]

Wide excision is the preferred treatment, but as with chordoma, recurrence is common. A combined posterior and anterior approach with the goal of complete tumor removal (as with chordoma) is ideal when possible.[344] If this is not feasible, radiation therapy should be considered as palliative treatment.[15] Because of the increased incidence of systemic metastases, the average postoperative survival is approximately 10 years.[209,344,503,531] In the

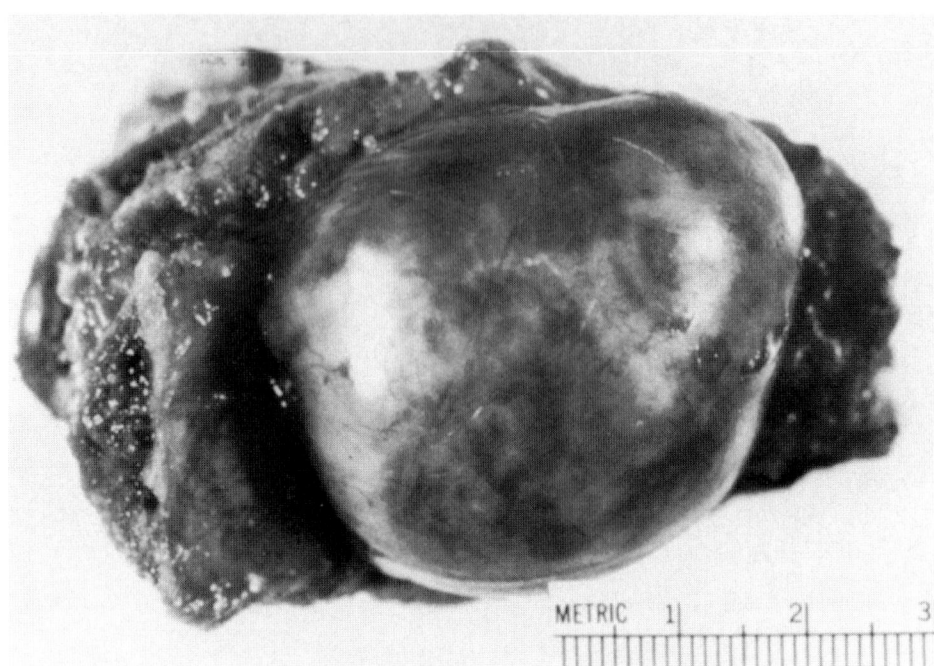

FIGURE 25-87. Sacrococcygeal chordoma. A well-encapsulated mass adherent to the sacrum.

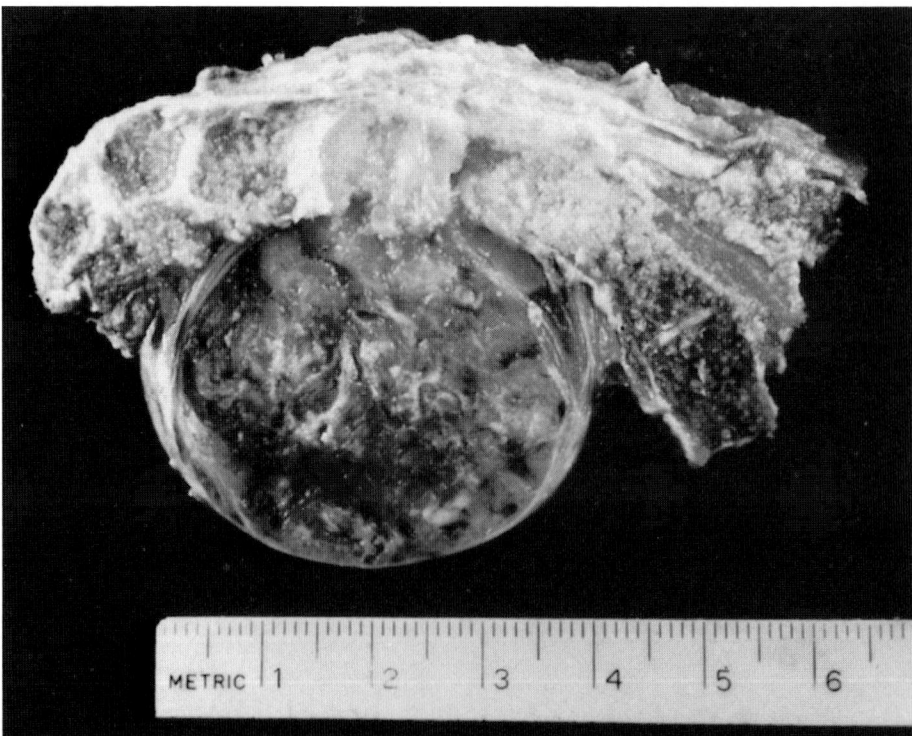

FIGURE 25-88. Sacrococcygeal chordoma. Cut section reveals the gelatinous appearance of the tumor.

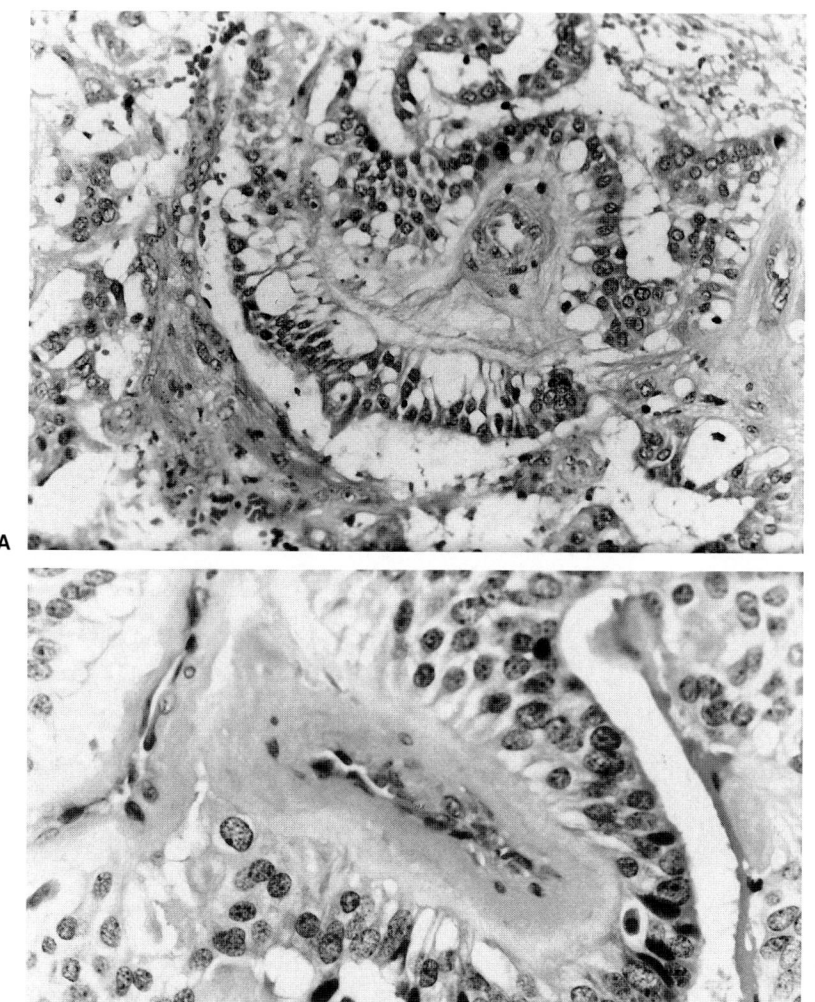

FIGURE 25-89. Malignant ependymoma. This tumor demonstrates papillary structures with fibrovascular cores lined by low epithelial cells displaying rather monotonous nuclei. Note the characteristic perivascular clearing. **(A)** Original magnification × 180. **(B)** Original magnification × 560. The patient subsequently developed pulmonary metastases. (Courtesy of David W. Kolegraff, M.D. and Peter L. Morris, M.D.)

experience of Helwig and Stern with 23 patients, six were followed for at least 15 years with metastases occurring in four (an incidence of 17%).[207]

Extramedullary (Extraadrenal Myelolipoma or Angiomyelolipoma)

Myelolipomas are usually found in the adrenal glands, but they rarely can be seen in other sites. These include intrathoracic, paravertebral, retroperitoneal, intracranial, and presacral locations as well as the liver, stomach, and iliac fossa. The most frequent extraadrenal sight is the presacral area.

Symptoms include low back pain, rectal fullness, pain on sitting, and urinary symptoms. Rectal examination may reveal an anterior sacral mass. Because of the benign nature of the disease, radiologic studies do not demonstrate bony invasion (Figure 25-90).

Myelolipoma is characterized histologically by the presence of active hematopoietic elements intermixed with fat (Figure 25-91).[125,535]

Treatment consists of a standard transcoccygeal approach. One can anticipate a complete cure for this benign process. Four cases of angiomyelolipoma affecting the colon have been described.[83] Treatment is with resection.

Anterior Sacral Meningocele

Anterior sacral meningocele is a congenital cystic structure that may appear as a presacral mass. Located in the presacral space, it communicates with the dural sac through a narrow neck that passes through a much larger, smooth, sacral bony defect.[271] Radiography of the pelvis may demonstrate the characteristic "scimitar sign."[271]

The treatment approach is via a posterior sacral laminectomy.

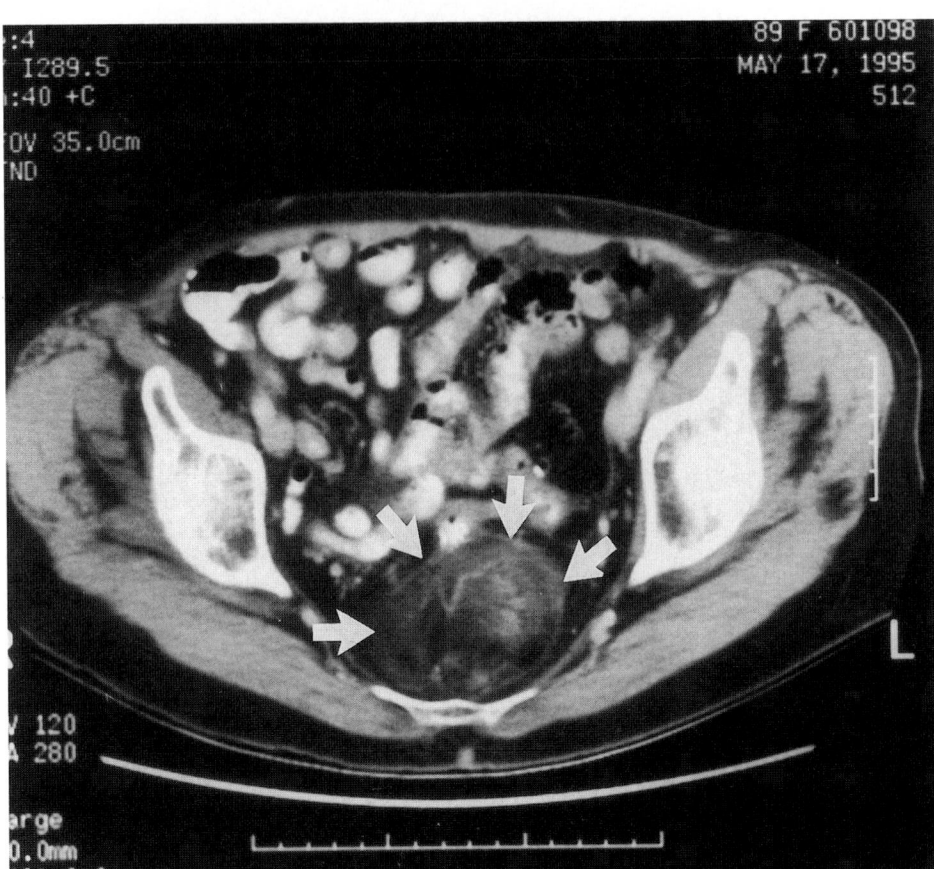

FIGURE 25-90. Extramedullary myelolipoma. Computed tomography scan demonstrates a presacral mass *(arrows)* without evident bony invasion.

Extramedullary Hematopoiesis

Another retrorectal (presacral) mass that has been described in a solitary case report is asymptomatic extramedullary hematopoiesis.[429] The diagnosis was established by CT-guided biopsy, which revealed hematopoietic marrow and fatty bone marrow. The patient was treated nonoperatively, with no change in the mass at 1 year.[429]

Pneumatosis Cystoides Intestinalis or Pneumatosis Coli

Pneumatosis cystoides intestinalis (pneumatosis coli, when the condition is confined to the colon) is a relatively uncommon disease of unknown etiology. It is characterized by the presence of gas-filled cysts within the wall of portions of the GI tract. Koss reported an extensive review of the condition and noted that it most commonly occurs in the jejunum and ileum, with only 6% of cases being seen in the colon.[269] The disease is noted usually in the older population, but it can occur at any age. Its relationship with other conditions has been well documented. The most frequently associated diseases are pulmonary (e.g., chronic obstructive lung disease), but it can also be seen with peptic ulcer, py-loric stenosis, collagen disease, acute gastroenteritis, nontropical sprue, intestinal obstruction, mesenteric occlusion, ischemic colitis, inflammatory bowel disease, carcinoma of the colon, following abdominal trauma, as a result of endoscopic maneuvers (especially colonoscopy), with steroid therapy, with exposure to organic solvents (e.g., trichloroethylene), following organ transplantation, and after surgical procedures on the bowel.[144,160,163,188,237,265,328,333,471,534]

Etiology

The reasons for the occurrence in association with such diverse entities are unclear. One possibility is that increased intraluminal pressure may force the gas into the wall of the bowel. This may account for its association with certain primary diseases of the GI tract. However, on close inspection of the bowel in such patients, it does not appear that the integrity of the mucosa is breached.

The theory for the condition's occurring in association with chronic obstructive pulmonary disease is that a pulmonary bleb ruptures and dissects retroperitoneally along the vessels, reaching the bowel wall. In support of

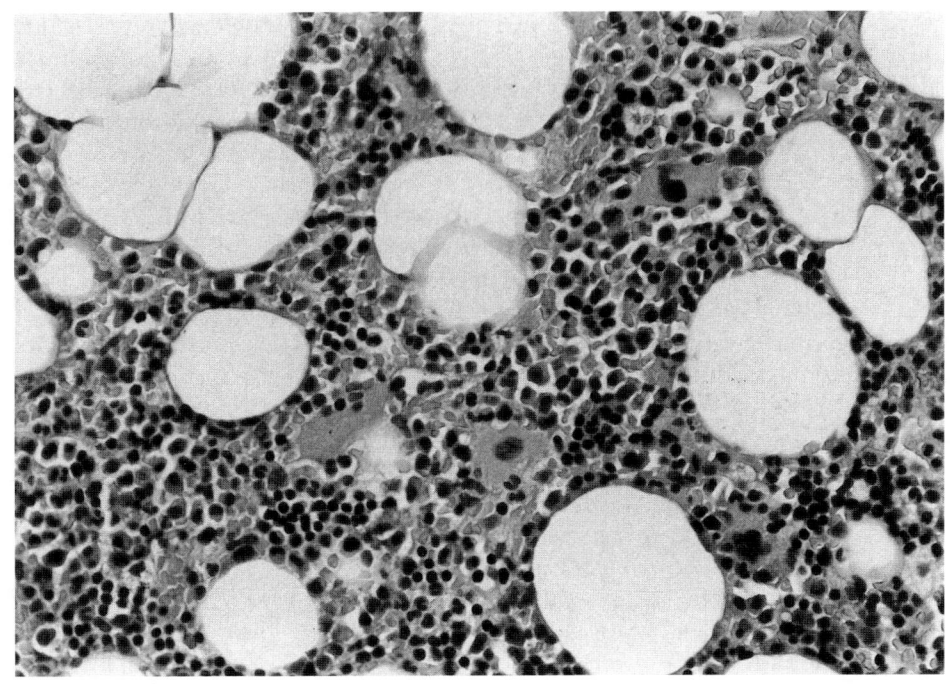

FIGURE 25-91. Extraadrenal myelolipoma. Maturing hematopoietic elements are scattered in the background of benign adipose tissue. (Original magnification × 600.) This is the histologic specimen obtained from the patient whose computed tomography scan is demonstrated in Figure 25-90. (Courtesy of James T. Dunn, M.D.)

this postulate is the fact that segmental distribution of the blebs usually is observed (Figure 25-92). A third theory, which may be more relevant in infants with severe gastroenteritis, speculates that gas-forming bacteria account for the formation of the cysts.[187]

Another possible implicating factor is the suggestion that the condition may result from abnormal hydrogen metabolism. Christl and colleagues measured hydrogen and methane levels in patients with pneumatosis cystoides intestinalis and found that these patients excrete more hydrogen than controls.[90] They further observed that the activity of methanogenic and sulfate-reducing bacteria is virtually absent in these individuals, possibly explaining the observed gas accumulation.

Symptoms and Findings

Many patients who harbor this condition do so without symptoms. The lesions may be noted on radiographic examination or at the time of endoscopy. When symptoms are present, they may be vague, or they may include abdominal pain, diarrhea, and the passage of mucus and blood in the stool.

Physical examination is usually unrewarding. Rarely is there abdominal tenderness or distension. Digital examination of the rectum may reveal the presence of an extramucosal mass if the cysts indeed extend into that area.

Barium enema examination will usually reveal well-demarcated, lucent wall defects of varying size, usually

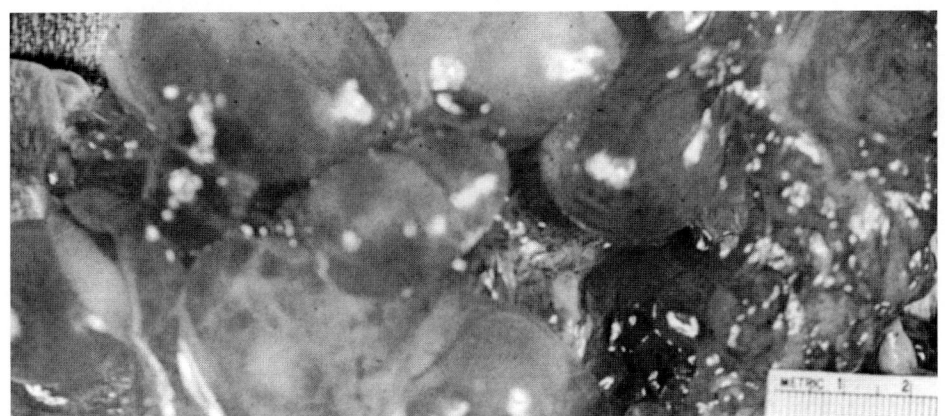

FIGURE 25-92. Pneumatosis coli. Cysts filled with gas, measuring up to 3 cm in diameter, occupy the sigmoid colon. (Courtesy of Rudolf Garret, M.D.)

grouped in clusters with an intact overlying mucosa (Figure 25-93).[59] The condition may be confused with inflammatory bowel disease, multiple polyposis, or carcinoma. Definitive diagnosis can be established by means of colonoscopy; some have advocated this technique for confirming the presence of the benign cysts (Figure 25-94).[114,151]

Pathology

Histologic examination of the biopsy specimen reveals normal mucosa beneath which cystic spaces are seen to be lined by endothelium (Figure 25-95).[178] There may be a mild inflammatory infiltrate. Multinucleated giant cells are noticed frequently (Figs. 25-96 and 25-97).

Treatment

It is important to recognize this entity and to differentiate it from neoplasms. Spigelman and colleagues suggested that needle deflation may be helpful if gross appearances are suggestive of cysts rather than of polyps.[461]

In 1973, Forgacs and colleagues proposed replacement of the gas (which consists mainly of nitrogen) with oxygen.[152] By administering oxygen at relatively high concentration, resorption of the gas in the cysts should occur. Although the re is no consistent recommendation about its administration, most authors believe that it is necessary to reach an arterial oxygen tension in excess of 300 mm Hg to achieve the desired results. A concentration of oxygen between 55% and 75% is generally used in the inhaled gas.[336] A minimum of 48 hours of therapy is recommended for up to 5 days. Holt and colleagues suggested a standardized regimen of intermittent high-flow oxygen therapy.[218] One must be concerned, however, about the possibility of oxygen toxicity. In these individuals, the ameliorative effect of oxygen therapy usually is apparent within 1 or 2 days. A report of successful treatment with metronidazole lends credence to the theory that anaerobic bacteria may in some manner be responsible.[232]

Surgery is usually reserved for those with localized disease and when hemorrhage, obstruction, or perforation supervenes.[263,506] Treatment of obstruction by means of endoscopic puncture and sclerotherapy of the cyst walls has been described.[236]

Management of Pneumoperitoneum

Pneumoperitoneum can supervene in a patient with pneumatosis. However, abdominal signs and symptoms are usually absent. If the patient has been known to harbor cysts, a trial of conservative therapy is advocated. Usually no communication with the GI tract exists. Therefore, one should not treat the radiographic finding. Expectant management will usually be followed by gradual disappearance of the free gas. If one embarks on an exploratory laparotomy for this presentation, it is probably better to close the abdomen, rather than to undertake a resection. In the rare situation in which the disease continues to cause symptoms and

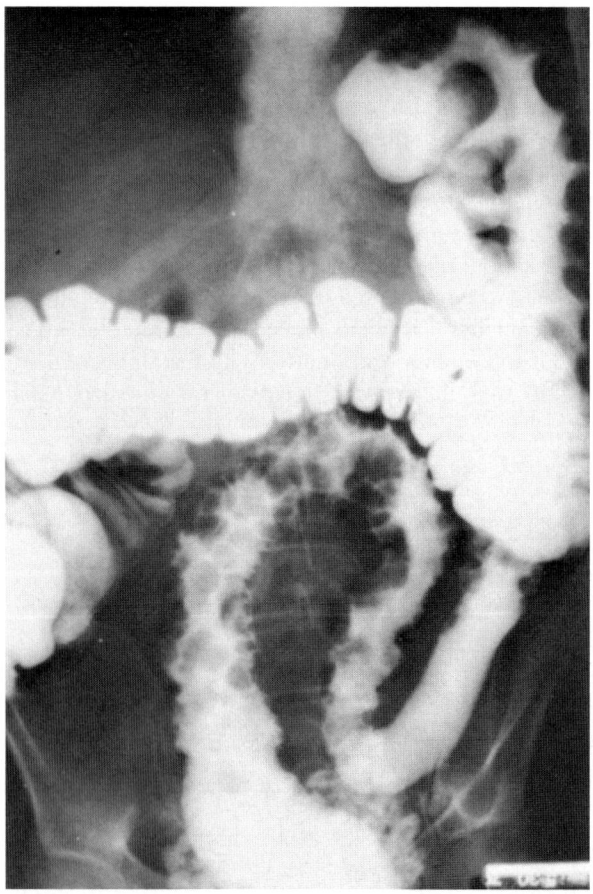

FIGURE 25-93. Pneumatosis coli. Multiple lucent cyst-like defects throughout the left colon.

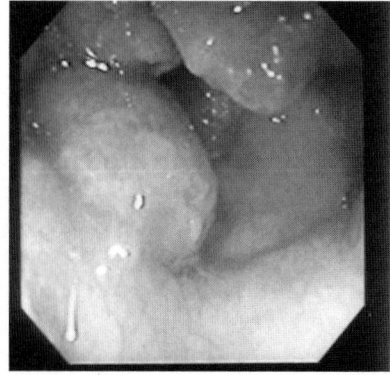

FIGURE 25-94. Pneumatosis cystoides intestinalis. Colonoscopy demonstrates cystic masses that pose a potential problem in differential diagnosis. Biopsy, however, revealed the histologic picture consistent with this condition. (See Color Fig. 25-94.)

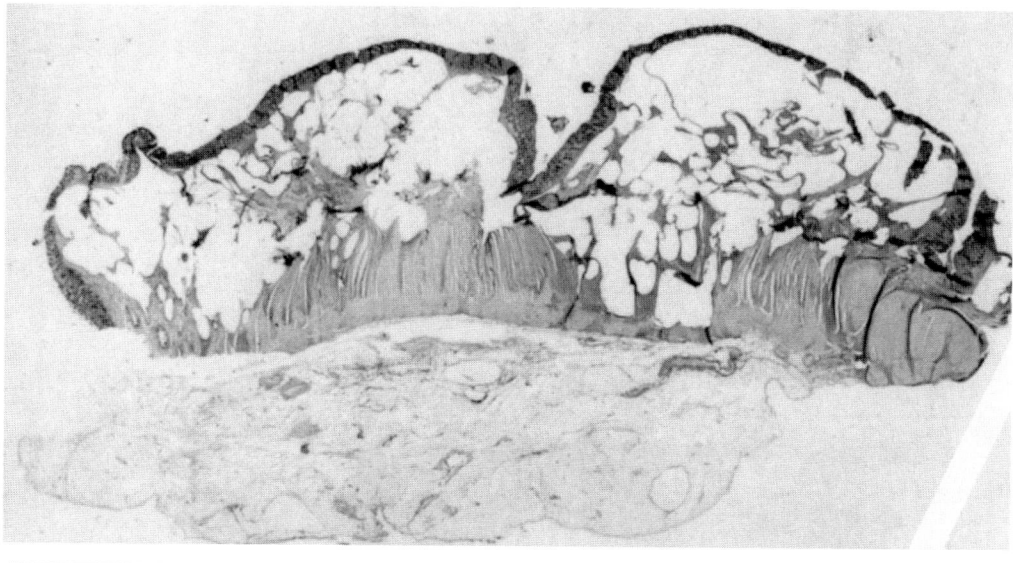

FIGURE 25-95. Pneumatosis cystoides intestinalis. Whole-mount specimen showing air-filled spaces in the submucosa of the colon. Some of the spaces are separating the bundles of the muscularis propria. (Courtesy of Rudolf Garret, M.D.)

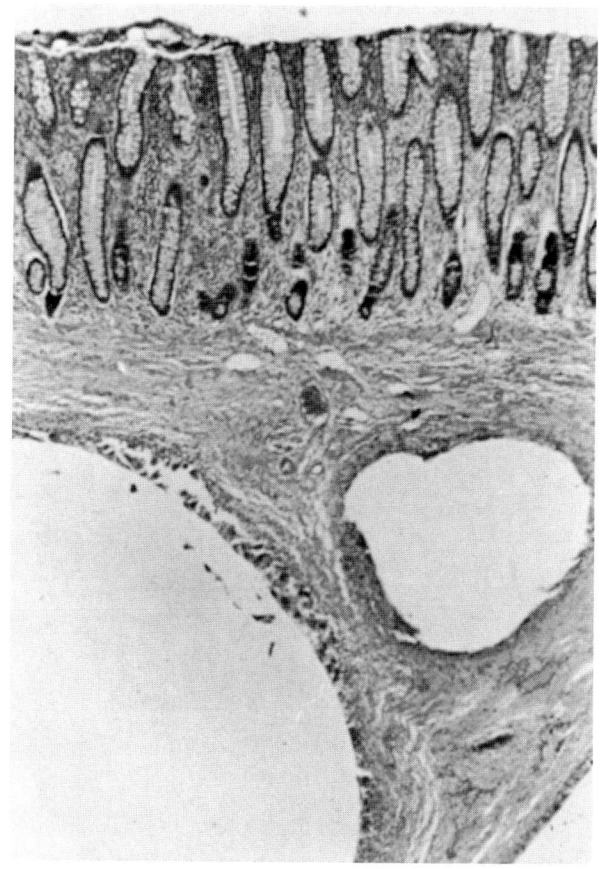

FIGURE 25-96. Pneumatosis coli. Cystic spaces occupy the submucosa. (Original magnification × 120; from Corman ML, Veidenheimer MC, Swinton NW. *Diseases of the anus, rectum and colon. Part I: neoplasms.* New York: Medcom, 1972.)

the cysts are localized to a limited segment of the bowel, resection should be considered. Unusual complications, such as volvulus, intestinal obstruction, or massive bleeding, will also necessitate operative intervention.

Duplication

Colon

Colonic duplication is an uncommon congenital anomaly that usually occurs during infancy or early childhood.[44] However, occasional cases can present in the older age groups. Obstruction and the presence of an abdominal mass are usually the signs and symptoms apparent in infancy. Progressive abdominal pain, bleeding, an abdominal mass, and rarely perforation are characteristic of childhood or adult onset.[416] Diarrhea, constipation, distension, and obstruction are additional symptoms, and an intussusception may sometimes be observed.

True intestinal duplications must be distinguished from enteric cysts. Characteristics of this anomaly include intimate attachment to some part of the alimentary tract, a smooth muscle coat, and a mucosal lining similar to that of the stomach, small bowel, or colon.[44] Four subtypes have been described:

A tubular duplication branching into the mesenteric leaves

A double-barreled, communicating structure (Figure 25-98)

A free-lying, cystic duplication connected to the alimentary tract by a thin mesenteric stalk

A cystic duplication attached to the bowel by a common wall[416]

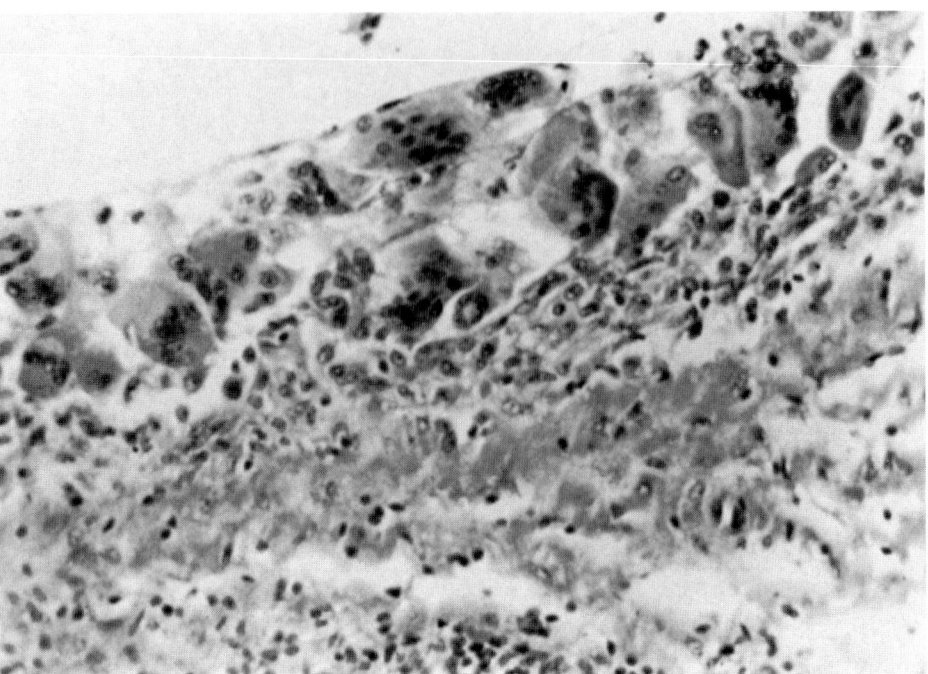

FIGURE 25-97. Pneumatosis coli. The cyst lining consists of multinucleated giant cells, which probably represent a reaction to the gaseous material trapped within the cyst. (From Corman ML, Veidenheimer MC, Swinton NW. *Diseases of the anus, rectum and colon. Part I: neoplasms.* New York: Medcom, 1972.)

Plain abdominal x-ray films may demonstrate a soft tissue mass, evidence of small or large bowel obstruction, and the presence of a gas-filled structure with an air-fluid level on the erect film.[44] Barium enema examination may demonstrate displacement of the bowel, compression by the mass, or, in the case of a communicating lesion, an irregular double lumen.[135] The condition is not uncommonly associated with other congenital anomalies, such as malrotation, Meckel's diverticulum, lumbosacral spine deformities (e.g., double vertebrae), and genitourinary abnormalities (double uterus, double vagina, double bladder, and double urethra).[541] CT and an intravenous pyelogram should be part of the evaluation of any individual found to harbor a colon or rectal duplication.

Treatment may involve excision of the mass with preservation of the normal colon (a communication is usually not demonstrable), although ischemia of the bowel wall and perforation are potential hazards if this approach is employed. Alternatively, an *en bloc* resection

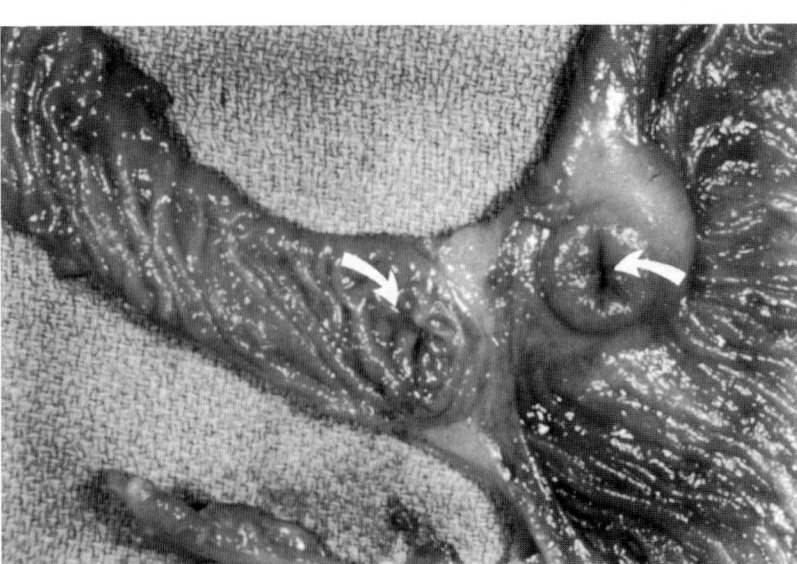

FIGURE 25-98. Colonic duplication. Note two distinct lumina *(arrows).* (Courtesy of Rudolf Garret, M.D.)

with anastomosis may be required when there is a double-barreled, communicating lesion.

Rectum

As suggested, all regions of the gut may be associated with a duplication, but the rectum is the least common location. Only about 70 cases have been reported.[343] It is likely that many patients remain asymptomatic, unless the situation is complicated by infection, bleeding, or malignant degeneration.[122] A painless buttock mass was described as the presenting manifestation in one report.[343] Numerous publications have addressed the issue of carcinoma arising in a rectal duplication, a finding suggesting that all such duplications should be treated by surgical excision, even if they appear benign.[122,169,523] The diagnosis can usually be made on the basis of examination of the rectum and confirmed on radiologic study, especially MRI, and by endosonography (Figure 25-99).[362] There is little diagnostic problem when there are two

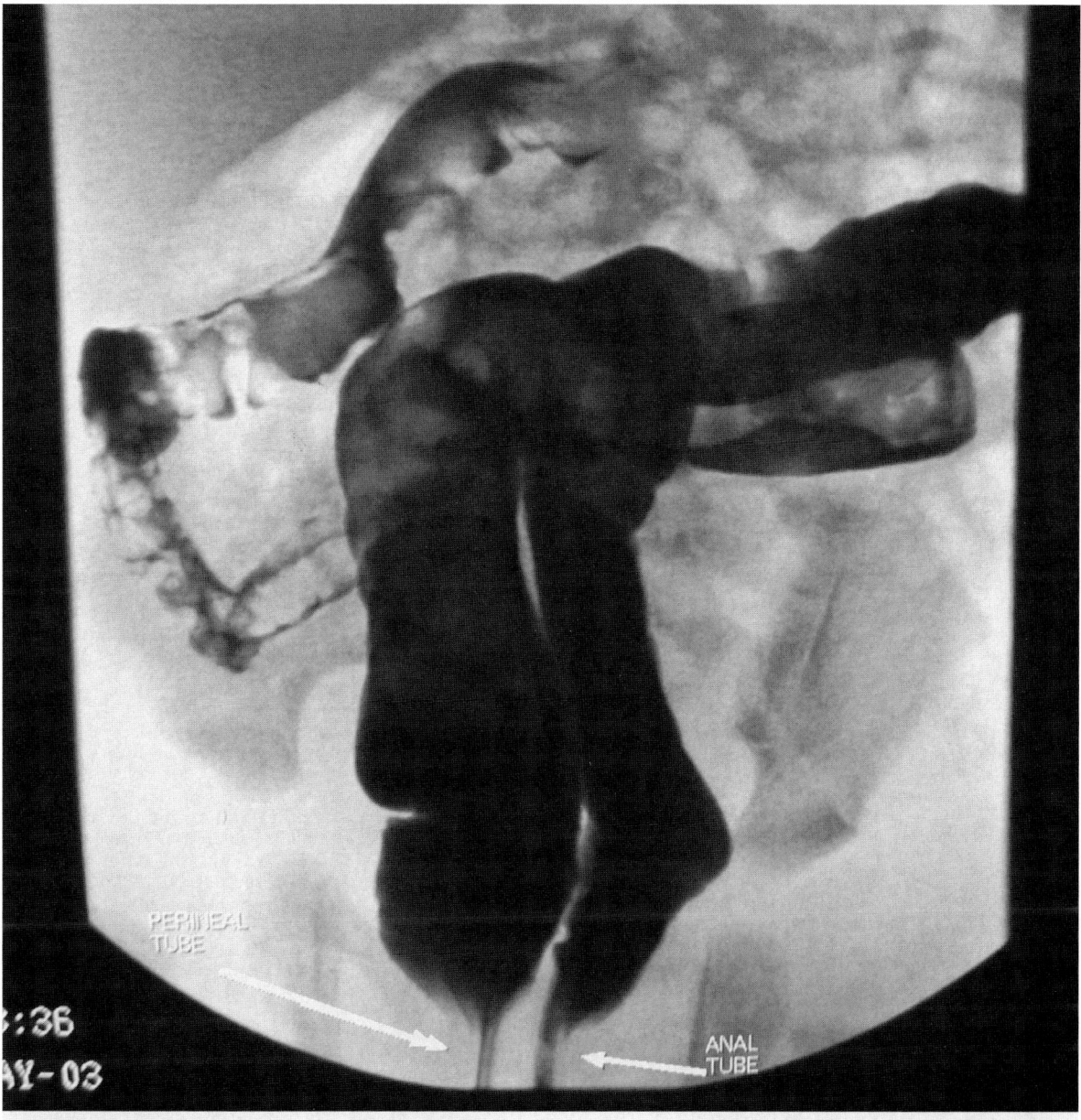

PERINEAL TUBE   **ANAL TUBE**

FIGURE 25-99. Rectal duplication. Barium study demonstrates two perineal openings communicating with two separate rectums that merge in the lower sigmoid colon. (Courtesy of Umut Sarpel, M.D.)

openings in the perineum or when a double-lumen appearance is noted on proctosigmoidoscopy. However, when there is no communication, the impression is that of a retrorectal mass compressing the rectum. Under these circumstances, the definitive diagnosis may not become evident until surgery.

Care must be taken to remove the duplication or cyst and still preserve integrity of the rectum, but the possibility of recurrence resulting from multiple satellites in the wall of the duplication should be recognized.[273]

REFERENCES

1. Abdou NI, Napombejara C, Sagawa A, et al. Malakoplakia: evidence for monocyte lysosomal abnormality correctable by cholinergic antagonist in vitro and in vivo. *N Engl J Med* 1977;297:1413.
2. Abel ME, Kingsley AE, Abcarian H, et al. Anorectal neurilemomas. *Dis Colon Rectum* 1985;28:960.
3. Abel ME, Nelson R, Prasad ML, et al. Parasacrococcygeal approach for the resection of retrorectal developmental cysts. *Dis Colon Rectum* 1985;28:855.
4. Abrikossoff AI. Über Myome, ausgehend von der quergestreiften willkürlichen Muskalatur. *Virchows Arch* 1926;260:215.
5. Abrikossoff AI. Weiter Untersuchunger über Myoblastenmyome. *Virchows Arch* 1931;280:723.
6. Aird I. *A companion in surgical studies*, 2nd ed. Edinburgh: E & S Livingstone, 1957.
7. Akawri OE, Dozois RR, Weiland LH, et al. Leiomyosarcoma of the small and large bowel. *Cancer* 1978;42:1375.
8. Albin J, Lewis E, Eftekhari F, et al. Computed tomography of rectal and perirectal disease in AIDS patients. *Gastrointest Radiol* 1987;12:67.
9. Albrecht E. Ueber Hamartome. *Verh Dtsch Ges Pathol* 1904;7:153.
10. Aldridge MC, Boylston AW, et al. Dermoid cyst of the rectum. *Dis Colon Rectum* 1983;26:333.
11. Allen MS Jr. Hamartomatous inverted polyps of the rectum. *Cancer* 1966;19:257.
12. Alvear DT. Localized lymphoid hyperplasia: an unusual cause of rectal bleeding. *Contemp Surg* 1984;25:29.
13. Alvich JP, Lepow HI. Cystic lymphangioma of hepatic flexure of colon: report of a case. *Ann Surg* 1960;152:880.
14. Anderson A, Bergdahl L. Carcinoid tumors of the appendix in children: a report of 25 cases. *Acta Chir Scand* 1977;143:173.
15. Anderson MS. Myxopapillary ependymomas presenting in the soft tissue over the sacrococcygeal region. *Cancer* 1996;19:585.
16. Anderson PA, Dockerty MB, Buie LA. Myomatous tumors of the rectum (leiomyomas and myosarcomas). *Surgery* 1950;28:642.
17. Andreoli F, Balloni F, Bigiotti A, et al. Anorectal continence and bladder function: effects of major sacral resection. *Dis Colon Rectum* 1986;29:647.
18. Angerpointner TA, Weitz H, Haas RJ, et al. Intestinal leiomyosarcoma in childhood-case report and review of the literature. *J Pediatr Surg* 1981;16:491.
19. Anson KM, Byrne PO, Robertson RW, et al. Radical excision of sacrococcygeal tumors. *Br J Surg* 1994;81:460.
20. Arnett NL, Friedman PS. Lymphangioma of the colon; roentgen aspects: a case report. *Radiology* 1956;67:881.
21. Astarjian NK, Tseng CH, Keating JA, et al. Leiomyosarcoma of the colon: report of a case. *Dis Colon Rectum* 1977;20:139.
22. Asuncion CM. Leiomyosarcoma of the rectum: report of two cases. *Dis Colon Rectum* 1969;12:281.
23. Atlay RD, Cuschieri A. Torsion of a colonic fibroma complicating pregnancy. *Aust NZ J Obstet Gynecol* 1969;9:262.
24. Ault GW, Smith RS, Castro CF. Hemangiopericytoma of the sigmoid colon: case report. *Surgery* 1951;30:523.
25. Avilés A, Neri N, Huerta-Guzmán J. Large bowel lymphoma: an analysis of prognostic factors and therapy in 53 patients. *J Surg Oncol* 2002;80:111.
26. Aylward CA, Orangio GR, Lucas GW, et al. Diffuse cavernous hemangioma of the rectosigmoid-CT scan, a new diagnostic modality, and surgical management using sphincter-saving procedures: report of three cases. *Dis Colon Rectum* 1988;31:797.
27. Aymard B, Bigard MA, Thompson H, et al. Perianal ulcer: an unusual presentation of Wegener's granulomatosis: report of a case. *Dis Colon Rectum* 1990;33:427.
28. Azizkhan RG, Tegtmeyer CJ, Wanebo HJ. Malignant rectal carcinoid: a sequential multidisciplinary approach for successful treatment of hepatic metastases. *Am J Surg* 1985;149:210.
29. Axxarelli A, Quagliuolo V, Serasoli S, et al. Chordoma: natural history and treatment results in 33 cases. *J Clin Oncol* 1988;37:185.
30. Bacon HE. *Cancer of the colon, rectum and anal canal.* Philadelphia: JB Lippincott, 1964.
31. Bacon PA, Tribe CR, Harrison P, et al. Rheumatoid disease, amyloidosis, and its treatment with penicillamine. *Arthritis Rheum* 1981;44:454(abst).
32. Bader TR, Semelka RC, Chiu VCY, et al. MRI of carcinoid tumors: spectrum of appearances in the gastrointestinal tract and liver. *J Magn Reson Imaging* 2001;14:261.
33. Bailey HR, Ott MT, Hartendorp P. Aggressive surgical management for advanced colorectal endometriosis. *Dis Colon Rectum* 1994;37:747.
34. Bailey JJ, Barrick CW, Jenkinson EL. Hemangioma of the colon. *JAMA* 1956;160:658.
35. Baker HL Jr, Good CA. Smooth-muscle tumors of the alimentary tract: their roentgen manifestations. *AJR Am J Roentgenol* 1955;74:246.
36. Ballantyne GH, Savoca PE, Flannery JT, et al. Incidence and mortality of carcinoids of the colon. *Cancer* 1992;69:2400.
37. Balfour TW. Does squamous carcinoma of the colon exist? *Br J Surg* 1972;59:410.
38. Ballantyne EN. Sacrococcygeal tumors: adenocarcinoma of a cystic congenital embryonal remnant. *Arch Pathol* 1932;14:1.
39. Baratz M. Ostrzega N, Michowitz M, et al. Primary inflammatory malignant fibrous histiocytoma of the colon. *Dis Colon Rectum* 1986;29:462.
40. Barbieri RL. New therapy for endometriosis. *N Engl J Med* 1988;318:512.
41. Barcia PJ, Washburn ME. Colitis cystica profunda: an unusual surgical problem. *Am Surg* 1979;45:61.
42. Bar-Meir S, Halla A, Baratz M. Endoscopic removal of colonic lipoma. *Endoscopy* 1981;13:135.
43. Barton AD, Inglis K. Neurofibromatosis with both cutaneous and visceral lesions. *J Coll Surg Australas* 1931;3:397.
44. Bass EM. Duplication of the colon. In: Greenbaum EI, ed. *Radiographic atlas of colon disease.* Chicago: Year Book, 1980:153.
45. Bassler A, Peter AG. Fibrosarcoma, an unusual complication of ulcerative colitis: report of a case. *Arch Surg* 1949;59:227.
46. Basson MD, Ahlman H, Wangberg B, Modlin IM. Biology and management of the mid-gut carcinoid. *Am J Surg* 1993;165:288.
47. Bates HR Jr. Carcinoid tumors of the rectum. *Dis Colon Rectum* 1962;5:270.
48. Beaugie JM, Mann CV, Butler EC. Sacrococcygeal chordoma. *Br J Surg* 1969;56:586.

49. Beral V, Peterman TA, Berkelman RL, et al. Kaposi's sarcoma among persons with AIDS: a sexually transmitted infection? *Lancet* 1990;335:123.

50. Berardi RD. Carcinoid tumors of the colon (exclusive of the rectum): review of the literature. *Dis Colon Rectum* 1972; 15:383.

51. Berardi RD, Chen HP, Lee SS. Squamous cell carcinoma of the colon and rectum. *Surg Gynecol Obstet* 1986;163:493.

52. Berg J, McNeer G. Leiomyosarcoma of the stomach: a clinical and pathological study. *Cancer* 1960;13:25.

53. Bernick PE, Klimstra DS, Shia J, et al. Neuroendocrine carcinomas of the colon and rectum. *Dis Colon Rectum* 2004;47:163.

54. Bhargava KS, Lahiri B, Gupta RC, et al. Leiomyosarcoma of the rectum. *J Indian Med* Assoc 1964;42:228.

55. Bibro MC, Houlihan RK, Sheahan DG. Colonic ganglioneuroma. *Arch Surg* 1980;115:75.

56. Biggs VA, Crowe SM, Lucas CR, et al. AIDS-related Kaposi's sarcoma presenting as ulcerative colitis and complicated by toxic megacolon. *Gut* 1987;28:1302.

57. Black WC III. Enterochromaffin cell types and corresponding carcinoid tumors. *Lab Invest* 1968;19:473.

58. Blair-Bell W. Endometrioma and endometriomyoma of ovary. *J Obstet Gynecol Br Emp* 1922;29:443.

59. Bloch C. The natural history of pneumatosis coli. *Radiology* 1977;123:311.

60. Blum A, Sohar E. The diagnosis of amyloidosis: ancillary procedures. *Lancet* 1962;1:721.

61. Bluth I. Gastrointestinal carcinoid tumors: roentgen features. *Radiology* 1960;74:573.

62. Botting AJ, Soule EH, Brown AL Jr. Smooth muscle tumors in children. *Cancer* 1965;18:711.

63. Box JC, Watne AL, Lucas GW. Small bowel carcinoid: review of a single institution experience and review of the literature. *Am Surg* 1996;62:280.

64. Braasch JW, Denbo HE. Tumors of the small intestine. *Surg Clin North Am* 1964;44:791.

65. Brodey PA, Hoover HC. Polypoid ganglioneurofibromatosis of the colon. *Br J Radiol* 1974;47:494.

66. Burgess PA, Lupton EW, Talbot IC. Squamous-cell carcinoma of the proximal colon: report of a case and review of the literature. *Dis Colon Rectum* 1979;22:241.

67. Burke M, Shepherd N, Mann CV. Carcinoid tumours of the anus and rectum. *Br J Surg* 1987;74:358.

68. Byrne WJ, Jiminez JF, Euler AR, et al. Lymphoid polyps (focal lymphoid hyperplasia) of the colon in children. *Pediatrics* 1982;69:598.

69. Cagir B, Nagy MW, Topham A, et al. Adenosquamous carcinoma of the colon, rectum and anus: epidemiology, distribution, and survival characteristics. *Dis Colon Rectum* 1999;42:258.

70. Caldarola VT, Jackman RJ, Moertel CG, et al. Carcinoid tumors of the rectum. *Am J Surg* 1964;107:844.

71. Calem SH, Keller RJ. Leiomyosarcoma of the sigmoid colon. *Mt Sinai J Med* 1973;40:818.

72. Capell MS, Friedman D, Mikhail N. Endometriosis of the terminal ileum simulating the clinical roentgenographic, and surgical findings in Crohn's disease. *Am J Gastroenterol* 1991;86:1057.

73. Carlei F, Pietroletti R, Lomanto D, et al. Heterotopic gastric mucosa of the rectum-characterization of endocrine and mucin-producing cells by immunochemistry and lectin histochemistry: report of a case. *Dis Colon Rectum* 1989; 32:159.

74. Castro EB, Stearns MW. Lipoma of the large intestine: a review of 45 cases. *Dis Colon Rectum* 1972;15:441.

75. Catalano MF, Levin B, Hart RS, et al. Granulocytic sarcoma of the colon. *Gastroenterology* 1991;100:555.

76. Cebrian J, Larach SW, Ferrara A, et al. Small-cell carcinoma of the rectum: report of two cases. *Dis Colon Rectum* 1999;42:274.

77. Cerezo L, Alverez M, Edwards O, Price G. Adenosquamous carcinoma of the colon. *Dis Colon Rectum* 1985;28:597.

78. Chaimoff C, Lurie H. Hemangioma of the rectum: clinical appearance and treatment. *Dis Colon Rectum* 1978;21:295.

79. Chambers PW, Schwinn CP. Chordoma: a clincopathologic study of metastasis. *Am J Clin Pathol* 1979;72:765.

80. Chandawarkar RY. Sacrococcygeal chordoma: review of 50 consecutive patients. *World J Surg* 1996;20:717.

81. Chaudhry AP, Saigal KP, Intengan M, et al. Malakoplakia of the large intestine found incidentally at necropsy: light and electron microscopic features. *Dis Colon Rectum* 1979;22:73.

82. Cheek RC, Wilson H. Carcinoid tumors. *Curr Probl Surg* 1970;Nov:4.

83. Chen J-S, Kuo L-J, Lin P-Y, et al. Angiomyolipoma of the colon: report of a case and review of the literature. *Dis Colon Rectum* 2003;46:547.

84. Cheng J-Y, Lin J-C, Yu D-S, et al. Flow cytometric DNA analysis of colorectal carcinoid. *Am J Surg* 1994;168:29.

85. Chevinsky AH, Berelowitz M, Hoover HC Jr. Adenosquamous carcinoma of the colon presenting with hypercalcemia. *Cancer* 1987;60:1111.

86. Chisholm AJ, Hillkowitz P. Lymphangioma of the rectum. *Am J Surg* 1932;17:281.

87. Cho KC, Smith TR. Multiple leiomyosarcoma of the transverse colon: report of a case and discussion. *Dis Colon Rectum* 1980;23:118.

88. Cohen MG, Greenwald ML, Garbus JE, et al. Granular cell tumor—a unique neoplasm of the internal anal sphincter: report of a case. *Dis Colon Rectum* 2000;43:1444.

89. Cohnheim J. Ein Fall von Pseudoleukämie. *Virchows Arch* 1865;33:451.

90. Christl SU, Gibson GR, Murgatroyd PR, et al. Impaired hydrogen metabolism in pneumatosis cystoides intestinalis. *Gastroenterology* 1993;104:392.

91. Chulia F, Camps C, Rodriguez A, et al. Epidermoid carcinoma of the colon: description of a lesion located in the hepatic flexure. *Dis Colon Rectum* 1986;29:665.

92. Clery AP, Dockerty MB, Waugh JM. Small-cell carcinoma of the colon and rectum: a clinicopathologic study. *Arch Surg* 1961;83:164.

93. Cobb CF. Endometriosis in the general surgery patient. *Surg Rounds* 1985;8:66.

94. Colberg JE. Granular cell myoblastoma. *Surg Gynecol Obstet* 1962;115:205.

95. Collins JO, Falk M, Guibone R. Benign lymphoid polyposis of the colon: a case report. *Pediatrics* 1966;38:897.

96. Comer TP, Beahrs OH, Dockerty MB. Primary squamous cell carcinoma and adenoacanthoma of the colon. *Cancer* 1971;28:1111.

97. Cone LA, Woodard DR, Potts BE, et al. An update on the acquired immunodeficiency syndrome (AIDS): associated disorders of the alimentary tract. *Dis Colon Rectum* 1986; 29:60.

98. Connolly EM, Gaffney E, Reynolds JV, et al. Gastrointestinal stromal tumours. *Br J Surg* 2003;90:1178.

99. Contreary K, Nance FC, Becker WF. Primary lymphoma of the gastrointestinal tract. *Ann Surg* 1980;191:593.

100. Coppa GF, Localio SA. Surgical management of diffuse cavernous hemangioma of the colon, rectum and anus. *Surg Gynecol Obstet* 1984;159:17.

101. Corman ML, Haggitt RC. Lymphangioma of the rectum: report of a case. *Dis Colon Rectum* 1973;16:524.

102. Corman ML, Veidenheimer MC, Swinton NW. *Diseases of the anus, rectum and colon. Part I: neoplasms.* New York: Medcom, 1972.

103. Cornes JS. Multiple lymphomatous polyposis of the gastrointestinal tract. *Cancer* 1961;14:249.

104. Cornes JS, Wallace MH, Morson BC. Benign lymphomas of the rectum and anal canal: a study of 100 cases. *J Pathol Bacteriol* 1961;82:371.

105. Cosens CG. Gastro-intestinal pseudoleukemia: a case report. *Ann Surg* 1958;148:129.

106. Cronkhite LW Jr, Canada WJ. Generalized gastrointestinal polyposis: unusual syndrome of polyposis, pigmentation, alopecia and onychotropia. *N Engl J Med* 1955;252:1011.

107. Croom RD III, Donovan ML, Schwesinger WH. Intestinal endometriosis. *Am J Surg* 1984;148:660.
108. Crowley LV, Page HG. Adenocarcinoma arising in presacral enterogenous cyst. *Arch Pathol* 1960;69:64.
109. Cunningham JA, Garcia VF, Quispe G. Diffuse cavernous rectal hemangioma-sphincter-sparing approach to therapy: report of a case. *Dis Colon Rectum* 1989;32:344.
110. Currarino G, Coln D, Votteler T. Triad of anorectal, sacral, and presacral anomalies. *AJR Am J Roentgenol* 1981;137:395.
111. Dahlin DC, MacCarty CS. Chordoma: a study of fifty-nine cases. *Cancer* 1952;5:1170.
112. DeBeer RA, Shinya H. Colonic lipomas: an endoscopic analysis. *Gastrointest Endosc* 1975;22:90.
113. DeMatteo RP, Lewis JJ, Leung D, et al. Two hundred gastrointestinal stromal tumours: recurrence patterns and prognostic factors for survival. *Ann Surg* 2000;231:51.
114. Desbaillets LG, Mangla JC. Pneumatosis cystoides intestinalis diagnosed by colonoscopy. *Gastrointest Endosc* 1974;20:126.
115. Devine RM, Beart RW Jr, Wolff BG. Malignant lymphoma of the rectum. *Dis Colon Rectum* 1986;29:821.
116. Diamante M, Bacon HE. Leiomyosarcoma of the rectum: report of a case. *Dis Colon Rectum* 1967;10:347.
117. Doak PB, Montgomerie JZ, North JD, et al. Reticulum cell sarcoma after renal homotransplantation and azathioprine and prednisone therapy. *BMJ* 1968;4:746.
118. Dodd GD, Rutledge R, Wallace S. Postoperative pelvic lymphocysts. *AJR Am J Roentgenol* 1970;108:312.
119. Doniec JM, Kahlke V, Peetz F, et al. Rectal endometriosis: high sensitivity and specificity of endorectal ultrasound with an impact for the operative management. *Dis Colon Rectum* 2003;46:1667.
120. Donnelly WH, Sieber WK, Yumis EJ. Polypoid ganglioneurofibromatosis of the large bowel. *Arch Pathol* 1969;87:537.
121. Dougherty LS, Hull T. Perineal endometriosis with anal sphincter involvement: report of a case. *Dis Colon Rectum* 2000;43:1157.
122. Downing R, Thompson H, Alexander-Williams J. Adenocarcinoma arising in a duplication of the rectum. *Br J Surg* 1978;65:572.
123. Dudley GS. Visceral neurofibroma. *Surg Clin North Am* 1930;10:539.
124. Dukes C, Bussey HJR. The number of lymphoid follicles of the human large intestine. *J Pathol Bacteriol* 1926;29:111.
125. Dusenbery D. Extra-adrenal myelolipoma. Intraoperative cytodiagnosis on touch preparations. *Acta Cytol* 1990;34:89.
126. Dzioba H, Kabza R. Naczyniaki jelita grubego. *Pol Tyg Lek* 1965;20:147.
127. Edelstein PS, Wong WD, La Valleur J, et al. Carcinoid tumor: an extremely unusual presacral lesion. *Dis Colon Rectum* 1996;39:938.
128. Edgerton MT. The treatment of hemangiomas: with special reference to the role of steroid therapy. *Ann Surg* 1976;183:517.
129. Eichel BS, Hallberg OE. Hamartoma of the middle ear and eustachian tube: report of a case. *Laryngoscope* 1966;76:1810.
130. Eitan N, Auslander L, Cohen Y. Leiomyosarcoma of the rectum: report of three cases. *Dis Colon Rectum* 1978;21:444.
131. Ell CH, Matek W, Gramatzki M, et al. Endoscopic findings in a case of Kaposi's sarcoma with involvement of the large and small bowel. *Endoscopy* 1985;17:161.
132. El-Mouzan MI, Satti MB, Al-Quorain AA, et al. Colonic malacoplakia: occurrence in a family. *Dis Colon Rectum* 1988;31:390.
133. Endean ED, Ross CW, Strodel WE. Kaposi's sarcoma appearing as a rectal ulcer. *Surgery* 1987;101:767.
134. Epstein SE, Ascari WQ, Ablow RC, et al. Colitis cystica profunda. *Am J Clin Pathol* 1966;45:186.
135. Espalieu P, Balique JG, Cuilleret J. Tubular colonic duplications: a case report and literature review. *Anat Clin* 1985;7:125.
136. Espinosa MH, Quan SHQ. Anal fibrosarcoma: report of a case and review of literature. *Dis Colon Rectum* 1975;18:522.
137. Evans N. Malignant myomas and related tumors of the uterus. (Report of seventy-two cases occurring in a series of 4000 operations for uterine fibromyomas.) *Coll Papers Mayo Clin* 1919;11:349.
138. Ewing J. *Neoplastic diseases: a treatise on tumors*, 4th ed. Philadelphia: WB Saunders, 1940.
139. Fahey JL. Cancer in the immunosuppressed patient. *Ann Intern Med* 1971;75:310.
140. Fan C-W, Changchien CR, Wang J-Y, et al. Primary colorectal lymphoma. *Dis Colon Rectum* 2000;43:1277.
141. Fayemi AO, Toker C. Gastrointestinal fibroma: a clinicopathological study. *Am J Gastroenterol* 1974;62:250.
142. Feldtman RW, Oram-Smith JC, Teears RJ, et al. Leiomyosarcoma of the rectum: the military experience. *Dis Colon Rectum* 1981;24:402.
143. Ferguson EF Jr, Houston CH. Benign and malignant tumors of the colon and rectum. *South Med J* 1972;65:1213.
144. Fernandes C, Bungay P, O'Driscoll BR, et al. Mixed connective tissue disease presenting with pneumonitis and pneumatosis intestinalis. *Arthritis Rheum* 2000;43:704.
145. Ferrarese R. Fibroma semplice del mesentere in sede ileocecale. *Arch Ostet Ginecol* 1968;73:94.
146. Figliolini FJ, Cutait DE, de Oliveria MR, et al. Rectosigmoidal hemangioma: report of two cases. *Dis Colon Rectum* 1961;4:349.
147. Fisher ER, Wechsler H. Granular cell myoblastoma—a misnomer: electron microscopic and histochemical evidence concerning its Schwann cell derivation and nature (granular cell schwannoma). *Cancer* 1962;15:936.
148. Fleming MP, Carlson HC. Submucosal lymphatic cysts of the gastrointestinal tract: a rare cause of submucosal mass lesion. *AJR Am J Roentgenol* 1970;110:842.
149. Fletcher CD, Berman JJ, Corless C, et al. Diagnosis of gastrointestinal stromal tumors: a consensus approach. *Hum Pathol* 2002;33:459.
150. Fontaine R, Suhler A, Babin S, et al. A propos de deux nouveaux cas de leiomyosarcome du rectum: revue de la littérature. *Ann Chir* 1965;19:1353.
151. Forde KA, Whitlock RT, Seaman WG. Pneumatosis cystoides intestinalis: report of a case and colonoscopic findings of inflammatory bowel disease. *Am J Gastroenterol* 1977;68:188.
152. Forgacs P, Wright PH, Wyatt AP. Treatment of intestinal gas cysts by oxygen breathing. *Lancet* 1973;1:579.
153. Frager DH, Frager JD, Brandt LJ, et al. Gastrointestinal complications of AIDS: radiologic features. *Radiology* 1986;158:597.
154. Franken EA Jr. Lymphoid hyperplasia of the colon. *Radiology* 1970;74:329.
155. Freeman FJ. Lymphoid hyperplasia and gastrointestinal bleeding in children. *Guthrie Clin Bull* 1964;33:175.
156. Frick EJJr, Lapos L, Vargas HD. Solitary neurofibroma of the anal canal: report of two cases. *Dis Colon Rectum* 2000;43:109.
157. Frizelle FA, Hobday KS, Batts KP, et al. Adenosquamous and squamous carcinoma of the colon and upper rectum: a clinical and histopathologic study. *Dis Colon Rectum* 2001;44:341.
158. Gabriel WB. *The principles and practice of rectal surgery*, 5th ed. Springfield, IL: Charles C Thomas, 1963.
159. Gafni J, Sohar E. Rectal biopsy for the diagnosis of amyloidosis. *Am J Med Sci* 1960;240:332.
160. Galanduik S, Fazio VA. Pneumatosis cystoides intestinalis: a review of the literature. *Dis Colon Rectum* 1986;29:358.
161. Galletly A. Presacral tumors of congenital origin. *Proc R Soc Med* 1924;17:105.

162. Garcha IS, Perloe M, Strawn EY, et al. Laparoscopic resection of sigmoid endometrioma. *Am Surg* 1996;62:274.

163. Gefter WB, Evers KA, Malet PF, et al. Nontropical sprue with pneumatosis coli. *AJR Am J Roentgenol* 1981;137:624.

164. Gelas T, Peyrat P, Francois Y, et al. Primary squamous-cell carcinoma of the rectum: report of six cases and review of the literature. *Dis Colon Rectum* 2002;45:1535.

165. Genter B, Mir R, Strauss R, et al. Hemangiopericytoma of the colon: report of a case and review of literature. *Dis Colon Rectum* 1982;25:149.

166. Gentil F, Coley BL. Sacrococcygeal chordoma. *Ann Surg* 1948;127:432.

167. Gentry RW, Dockerty MB, Clagett OT. Collective review: vascular malformations and vascular tumors of the gastrointestinal tract. *Surg Gynecol Obstet* 1949;88:281(abst).

168. Ghrist TD. Gastrointestinal involvement in neurofibromatosis. *Arch Intern Med* 1963;112:357.

169. Gibson TC, Edwards JM, Shafiq S. Carcinoma arising in a rectal duplication cyst. *Br J Surg* 1986;73:377.

170. Girdwood TG, Philip LD. Lymphatic cysts of the colon. *Gut* 1971;12:933.

171. Gius JA, Stout P. Perianal cysts of vestigial origin. *Arch Surg* 1938;37:268.

172. Gleason TH, Hammar SP. Plasmacytoma of the colon: case report with lambda light chain demonstrated by immunoperoxidase studies. *Cancer* 1982;50:130.

173. Godard JE, Dodds WF, Phillips JC, et al. Peutz-Jeghers syndrome: clinical and roentgenographic features. *AJR Am J Roentgenol* 1971;113:316.

174. Golden T, Stout AP. Smooth muscle tumors of the gastrointestinal tract and retroperitoneal tissues. *Surh Gynecol Obstet* 1941;73:784.

175. Goldlust D, Chalut J, Rault JJ, et al. L'hémangiomatose recto-sigmoidienne. *J Radiol Electrol Med Nucl* 1971;52:108.

176. Goldstein WB, Poker N. Multiple myeloma involving the gastrointestinal tract. *Gastroenterology* 1966;51:87.

177. González Sánchez JA, Martin Molinero R, Dominguez Sayans J, et al. Colonic perforation by amyloidosis: report of a case. *Dis Colon Rectum* 1989;32:437.

178. Goodall RJR. Pneumatosis coli: report of two cases. *Dis Colon Rectum* 1978;21:61.

179. Gouzi J-L, Laigneau P, Delalande J-P, et al. Indications for right hemicolectomy in carcinoid tumors of the appendix. *Surg Gynecol Obstet* 1993;176:543.

180. Granet E. Simple lymphoma of the sphincteric rectum in identical twins. *JAMA* 1949;141:990.

181. Green JB, Timmcke AE, Mitchell WT Jr. Endoscopic resection of primary rectal teratoma. *Am Surg* 1993;59:270.

182. Greenblatt RB, Dmowski WP, Mahesh VB, et al. Clinical studies with an antigonadotropin: Danazol. *Fertil Steril* 1971;22:102.

183. Greene EI, Kirshen MM, Greene JM. Lymphangioma of the transverse colon. *Am J Surg* 1962;103:723.

184. Grill J, Kuzma JF. Recklinghausen's disease with unusual symptoms from intestinal neurofibroma. *Arch Pathol* 1942;34:902.

185. Grotz RL, Macaulay WP. Colitis cystica profunda. *Contemp Surg* 1989;35:57.

186. Gruenberg J, Mackman S. Multiple lymphoid polyps in familial polyposis. *Ann Surg* 1972;175:552.

187. Gruenberg JC, Batra SK, Priest RJ. Treatment of pneumatosis cystoides intestinalis with oxygen. *Arch Surg* 1977;112:62.

188. Gruenberg JC, Grodsinksy C, Ponka JL. Pneumatosis intestinalis: a clinical classification. *Dis Colon Rectum* 1979;22:5.

189. Gruenwald P. Abnormal accumulation of lymph follicles in the digestive tract. *Am J Med Sci* 1942;203:823.

190. Guest CB, Reznick RK. Colitis cystica profunda: review of the literature. *Dis Colon Rectum* 1989;32:983.

191. Gunning JE, Moyer D. The effect of medroxyprogesterone acetate on endometriosis in the human female. *Fertil Steril* 1967;18:759.

192. Guy PJ, Hall M. Colitis cystica profuncda of the rectum treated by mucosal sleeve resection and colo-anal pull-through. *Br J Surg* 1988;75:289.

193. Habal N, Sims C, Bilchik AJ. Gastrointestinal carcinoid tumors and second primary malignancies. *J Surg Oncol* 2000;75:301.

194. Haggitt RC. Granulomatous diseases of the gastrointestinal tract. In: Ioachim HE, ed. *Pathology of granulomas.* New York: Raven, 1983:257.

195. Haller JD, Roberts TW. Lipomas of the colon: a clinicopathologic study of 20 cases. *Surgery* 1964;55:773.

196. Halls JM. Lymphomas of the large intestine. In: Greenbaum EI, ed. *Radiographic atlas of colon disease.* Chicago: Year Book, 1980:303.

197. Halpern J, Kopolovic J, Catane R. Malignant fibrous histiocytoma developing in irradiated sacral chordoma. *Cancer* 1984;53:2661.

198. Hambrick E, Abcarian H, Smith D. Perineal endometrioma in episiotomy incisions: clinical features and management. *Dis Colon Rectum* 1979;22:550.

199. Hampton JM, Gandy JR. Plasmacytoma of the gastrointestinal tract. *Ann Surg* 1957;145:415.

200. Hasegawa K, Lee W-Y, Noguchi T, et al. Colonoscopic removal of hemangiomas. *Dis Colon Rectum* 1981;24:85.

201. Haskell B, Rovner H. Solitary ulcer of the rectum. *Dis Colon Rectum* 1965;8:333.

202. Hayes HT, Burr HB. Benign lymphomas of the rectum. *Am J Surg* 1952;84:545.

203. Head HD, Baker JQ, Muir RW. Hemangioma of the colon. *Am J Surg* 1973;126:691.

204. Hellstrom J, Hultborn KA, Engstedt L. Diffuse cavernous hemangioma of the rectum. *Acta Chir Scand* 1955;109:277.

205. Hellwig CA. Extramedullary plasma cell tumors as observed in various locations. *Arch Pathol* 1943;36:95.

206. Helwig EB, Hansen J. Lymphoid polyps (benign lymphoma) and malignant lymphoma of the rectum and anus. *Surg Gynecol Obstet* 1951;92:233.

207. Helwig EB, Stern JB. Subcutaneous sacrococcygeal myxopapillary ependymoma. *Am J Clin Pathol* 1984;81:156.

208. Hemley SD, Kanick V. Perforation of the rectum: a complication of barium enema following rectal biopsy: report of 2 cases. *Am J Dig Dis* 1963;19:882.

209. Hendren TH, Hardin CA. Extradural metastatic ependymoma. *Surgery* 1963;54:880.

210. Henzl MR, Corson SL, Moghissi K, et al. Administration of nasal nafarelin as compared with oral danazol for endometriosis: a multicenter double-blind comparative clinical trial. *N Engl J Med* 1988;318:485.

211. Hernández-Magro PM, Sáenz EV, Fernández FA-T, et al. Endoanal sonography in the assessment of perianal endometriosis with external anal sphincter involvement. *J Clin Ultrasound* 2002;30:245.

212. Heule BV, Taylor CR, Terry R, et al. Presentation of malignant lymphoma in the rectum. *Cancer* 1982;49:2602.

213. Higgason JM. Lymphatic cyst of the transverse colon: report of a case. *AJR Am J Roentgenol* 1958;79:850.

214. Higinbotham NL, Phillips H, Farr W, et al. Chordoma: thirty-five year study at Memorial Hospital. *Cancer* 1967;20:1841.

215. Hoehn JG, Farrow GM, Devine KD, et al. Invasive hemangioma of the head and neck. *Am J Surg* 1970;120:495.

216. Hoehn JL, Hamilton GH, Beltaos E. Fibrosarcoma of the colon. *J Surg Oncol* 1980;13:223.

217. Hollingsworth G. Haemangiomatous lesions of the colon. *Br J Radiol* 1951;24:220.

218. Holt S, Gilmour HM, Buist TS, et al. High-flow oxygen therapy for pneumatosis coli. *Gut* 1979;20:493.

219. Holtz F, Schmidt LA III. Lymphoid polyps (benign lymphoma) of the rectum and anus. *Surg Gynecol Obstet* 1958;106:639.

220. Horn RC Jr, Enterline HT. Rhabdomyosarcoma: a clinico-pathological study and classification of 39 cases. *Cancer* 1958;11:181.

221. Horowitz J, Spellman JE Jr, Driscoll DL, et al. An institutional review of sarcomas of the large and small intestine. *J Am Coll Surg* 1995;180:465.

222. Howerton RA, Bonello JC. A lipoma simulating colon cancer. *Contemp Surg* 1989;35:20.

223. Hsieh J-S, Huang C-J, Wang J-Y, et al. Benefits of endorectal ultrasound for management of smooth-muscle tumor of the rectum: report of three cases. *Dis Colon Rectum* 1999;42:1085.

224. Huth JF, Dawson EG, Eilber FR. Abdominosacral resection for malignant tumors of the sacrum. *Am J Surg* 1984;148:157.

225. Ihde JK, Coit DG. Melanoma metastatic to stomach, small bowel, or colon. *Am J Surg* 1991;162:208.

226. Immunology and cancer [Annotation]. *Lancet* 1968;1:1298.

227. Irisawa A, Bhutani MS. Cystic lymphangioma of the colon: endosonographic diagnosis with through-the-scope catheter miniprobe and determination of further management: report of a case. *Dis Colon Rectum* 2001;44:1040.

228. Jackman RJ, Beahrs OH. *Tumors of the large bowel.* Philadelphia: WB Saunders, 1968.

229. Jackman RJ, Clark PL III, Smith ND. Retrorectal tumors. *JAMA* 1951;145:956.

230. Jalan KN, Brunt PW, Maclean N, et al. Benign solitary ulcer of the rectum-a report of 5 cases. *Scand J Gastroenterol* 1970;5:143.

231. Jao S-W, Beart RW Jr, Reiman HM, et al. Retrorectal tumors. *Dis Colon Rectum* 1985;28:644.

232. Jauhonen P, Lehtola J, Karttunen T. Treatment of pneumatosis coli with metronidazole: endoscopic follow-up of one case. *Dis Colon Rectum* 1987;30:800.

233. Jeffery PJ, Hawley PR, Parks AG. Colo-anal sleeve anastomosis in the treatment of diffuse cavernous haemangioma involving the rectum. *Br J Surg* 1976;63:678.

234. Jensen K, Raynor S, Rose SG, et al. Amyloid tumors of the gastrointestinal tract: a report of two cases and review of the literature. *Am J Gastroenterol* 1985;80:784.

235. Jetmore AB, Ray JE, Gathright JB Jr, et al. Rectal carcinoids: the most frequent carcinoid tumor. *Dis Colon Rectum* 1992;35:717.

236. Johansson K, Lindström E. Treatment of obstructive pneumatosis coli with endoscopic sclerotherapy: report of a case. *Dis Colon Rectum* 1991;34:94.

237. John A, Dickey K, Fenwick J, et al. Pneumatosis intestinalis in patients with Crohn's disease. *Dig Dis Sci* 1992;37:813.

238. Johnson DH, Guthrie TH, Tedesco FJ, et al. Amyloidosis masquerading as inflammatory bowel disease with a mass lesion simulating malignancy. *Am J Gastroenterol* 1982;77:141.

239. Johnson LA, Lavin P, Moertel CG, et al. Carcinoids: the association of histologic growth pattern and survival. *Cancer* 1983;51:882.

240. Johnson RC, Bleshman MH, DeFord JW. Benign lymphoid hyperplasia manifesting as a cecal mass. *Dis Colon Rectum* 1978;21:510.

241. Johnstone JM, Morson BC. Inflammatory fibroid polyp of the gastrointestinal tract. *Histopathology* 1978;2:349.

242. Jona JZ, Belin RP, Burke JA. Lymphoid hyperplasia of the bowel and its surgical significance in children. *J Pediatr Surg* 1976;11:997.

243. Joyeuse R, Lott JV, Michaelis M, et al. Malakoplakia of the colon and rectum: report of a case and review of the literature. *Surgery* 1977;81:189.

244. Juturi JV, Francis B, Koontz PW, et al. Squamous-cell carcinoma of the colon responsive to combination chemotherapy: report of two cases and review of the literature. *Dis Colon Rectum* 1999;42:102.

245. Kaftouri JK, Aharon M, Kleinhaus U. Sonographic features of gastrointestinal leiomyosarcoma. *J Clin Ultrasound* 1981;9:11.

246. Kang JY, Chan-Wilde C, Wee A, et al. Role of computed tomography and endoscopy in the management of alimentary tract lipomas. *Gut* 1990;31:550.

247. Kanter AS, Hyman NH, Li SC. Ganglioneuromatous polyposis: a premalignant condition: report of a case and review of the literature. *Dis Colon Rectum* 2001;44:591.

248. Kaplan LD, Abrams DI, Feigal E, et al. AIDS-associated non-Hodgkin's lymphoma in San Francisco. *JAMA* 1989;261:719.

249. Kaplan LD, Wofsy CB, Volberding PA. Treatment of patients with acquired immunodeficiency syndrome and associated manifestations. *JAMA* 1987;257:1367.

250. Karakousis CP. Sacral resection with preservation of continence. *Surg Gynecol Obstet* 1986;163:271.

251. Karakousis CP, Park JJ, Fleminger R, et al. Chordomas: diagnosis and management. *Am Surg* 1981;47:497.

252. Karakousis CP, Wabnitz RC. Tumor involving the sacrum. In: Karakousis CP, ed. *Atlas of operations for soft tissue tumors.* St. Louis: McGraw-Hill, 1985:301.

253. Keane TE, Peel ALG. Endometrioma: an intra-abdominal troublemaker. *Dis Colon Rectum* 1990;33:963.

254. Keeling WM, Beatty GL. Lymphoid polyps of the rectum: report of 3 cases in siblings. *Arch Surg* 1956;73:753.

255. Khadra MH, Thompson JF, Milton GW, et al. The justification for surgical treatment of metastatic melanoma of the gastrointestinal tract. *Surg Gynecol Obstet* 1990;171:413.

256. Khalifa AA, Bong WL, Rao VK, et al. Leiomyosarcoma of the rectum: report of a case and review of the literature. *Dis Colon Rectum* 1986;29:427.

257. Khanna KK, Chandra RK, Veliath AJ, et al. Leiomyoma of the cecum. *Am J Dis Child* 1968;116:675.

258. Kim HH, Williams TJ. Endometrioid carcinoma of the uterus and ovaries associated with immunosuppressive therapy and anticoagulation: report of a case. *Mayo Clin Proc* 1972;47:39.

259. Kim HR, Kim YJ. Neurofibromatosis of the colon and rectum combined with other manifestations of von Recklinghausen's disease: report of a case. *Dis Colon Rectum* 1998;41:1187.

260. Kistner RW. The use of newer progestins in the treatment of endometriosis. *Am J Obstet Gynecol* 1958;75:264.

261. Kitoraga NF. Hemangioma of the large intestine causing profuse hemorrhage. *Vestn Khir* 1962;88:125.

262. Klinge F. Ueber die sogenannten ureifen, nicht guergestreiften Myoblastenmyome. *Verh Dtsch Ges Pathol* 1928;23:376.

263. Knechtle SJ, Davidoff AM, Rice RP. Pneumatosis intestinalis: surgical management and clinical outcome. *Ann Surg* 1990;212:160.

264. Koenig RR, Claudon DB, Byrne RW. Lymphatic cyst of the transverse colon: report of a case radiographically simulating neoplastic polyp. *Arch Pathol* 1955;60:431.

265. Koep LJ, Peters TG, Starzl TE. Major colonic complications of hepatic transplantation. *Dis Colon Rectum* 1979;22:218.

266. Kölby L, Persson G, Franzén S, et al. Randomized clinical trial of the effect of interferon on survival in patients with disseminated midgut carcinoid tumours. *Br J Surg* 2003;90:687.

267. Konda J, Ruth M, Sassaris M, et al. Sarcoidosis of the stomach and rectum. *Am J Gastroenterol* 1980;73:516.

268. Kontozoglou TE, Moyana TN. Adenosquamous carcinoma of the colon—an immunocytochemical and ultrastructural study: report of two cases and review of the literature. *Dis Colon Rectum* 1989;32:716.

269. Koss LG. Abdominal gas cysts (pneumatosis cystoides intestinorum hominis): an analyis with a report of a case and a critical review of the literature. *Arch Pathol* 1952;53:523.

270. Koura AN, Giacco GG, Curley SA, et al. Carcinoid tumors of the rectum: effect of size, histopathology, and surgical treatment on metastasis free survival. *Cancer* 1997;79:1294.

271. Kovalcik PJ, Burke JB. Anterior sacral meningocele and the scimitar sign: report of a case. *Dis Colon Rectum* 1988; 31:806.

272. Kovalcik PJ, Simstein NL, Cross GH. Benign neurilemmoma manifesting as a presacral (retrorectal) mass: report of a case. *Dis Colon Rectum* 1978;21:199.

273. Kraft RO. Duplication anomalies of the rectum. *Ann Surg* 1962;55:230.

274. Kulaylat MN, Doerr RJ, Neuwirth M, et al. Anal duct/gland cyst: report of a case and review of the literature. *Dis Colon Rectum* 1998;41:103.

275. Kumar SS, Appavu SS, Abcarian H, et al. Amyloidosis of the colon: report of a case and review of the literature. *Dis Colon Rectum* 1983;26:541.

276. Kuramoto S, Sakai S, Tsuda K, et al. Lymphangioma of the large intestine: report of a case. *Dis Colon Rectum* 1988; 31:900.

277. Kuroda Y, Katoh H, Ohsato K. Cystic lymphangioma of the colon. *Dis Colon Rectum* 1984;27:679.

278. Kyle RA, Bayrd ED. Amyloidosis: review of 236 cases. *Medicine* 1975;54:271.

279. Kyle RA, Spence RJ, Dahlin DC. Value of rectal biopsy in the diagnosis of primary systemic amyloidosis. *Am J Med Sci* 1966;251:501.

280. Lafreniere R, Ketcham AS. Primary squamous carcinoma of the rectum: report of a case and review of the literature. *Dis Colon Rectum* 1985;28:967.

281. Laine L, Amerian J, Rarick M, et al. The response of symptomatic gastrointestinal Kaposi's sarcoma to chemotherapy: a prospective evaluation using an endoscopic method of disease quantification. *Am J Gastroenterol* 1990;85:959.

282. Landing BH, Farber S. Tumors of the cardiovascular system. In: *Atlas of tumor pathology,* 1st series. Sect. 3. Fasc. 7. Washington, DC: Armed Forces Institute of Pathology, 1956:45.

283. Landmann DD, Lewis RW. Benign cystic ovarian teratoma with colorectal involvement: report of a case and review of the literature. *Dis Colon Rectum* 1988;31:808.

284. Langer C, Gunawan B, Schüler P, et al. Prognostic factors influencing surgical management and outcome of gastrointestinal stromal tumours. *Br J Surg* 2003;90:332.

285. Le DT, Austin RC, Payne SNP, et al. Choriocarcinoma of the colon: report of a case and review of the literature. *Dis Colon Rectum* 2003;46:264.

286. Leach SD, Modlin IM, Goldstein L, et al. Laparoscopic local excision of a proximal rectal carcinoid. *J Laparosc Surg* 1994;4:65.

287. Lee MH, Waxman M, Gillooley JF. Primary malignant lymphoma of the anorectum in homosexual men. *Dis Colon Rectum* 1986;29:413.

288. Leong WL, Pasieka JL. Regression of metastic carcinoid tumors with octreotide therapy: two case reports and a review of the literature. *J Surg Oncol* 2002;79:180.

289. Levy D, Khatib R. Intestinal neurofibromatosis with malignant degeneration: report of a case. *Dis Colon Rectum* 1960;3:140.

290. Levy M, Stone AM, Platt N. Reticulum cell sarcoma of the cecum and macroglobulinemia: a case report. *J Surg Oncol* 1976;8:149.

291. Lewin KJ, Harell GS, Lee AS, et al. Malacoplakia—an electron-microscopic study: demonstration of bacilliform organisms in malacoplakic macrophages. *Gastroenterology* 1974;66:28.

292. Lewin KJ, Ranchod M, Dorfman RF. Lymphomas of the gastrointestinal tract: a study of 117 cases presenting with gastrointestinal disease. *Cancer* 1978;42:693.

293. Lifschitz O, Lew S, Witz M, et al. Inflammatory fibroid polyp of sigmoid colon. *Dis Colon Rectum* 1979;22:575.

294. Ling CS, Leagus C, Stahlgren LH. Intestinal lipomatosis. *Surgery* 1959;46:1054.

295. Localio SA, Francis KC, Rossaro PG. Abdominosacral resection of sacrococcygeal chordoma. *Ann Surg* 1967;166: 394.

296. Londono-Schimmer EE, Ritchie JK, Hawley PR. Coloanal sleeve anastomosis in the treatment of diffuse cavernous haemangioma of the rectum: long-term results. *Br J Surg* 1994;81:1235.

297. Lookanoff VA, Tsapralis PC. Smooth-muscle tumors of the colon: report of a case involving the cecum and ascending colon. *JAMA* 1966;198:206.

298. Lord PH, Tribe CR. Gastric tissue in the rectum. *Lancet* 1970;1:566.

299. Lorenz HP, Wilson W, Leigh B, et al. Kaposi's sarcoma of the rectum in patients with the acquired immunodeficiency syndrome. *Am J Surg* 1990;160:681.

300. Lou Ty, Teplitz C. Malacoplakia; pathogenesis and ultrastructural morphogenesis: a problem of altered macrophage (phagolysosomal) response. *Hum Pathol* 1974;5:191.

301. Lubarsch O. Ueber den primaren Krebs des Ileum, nebst Bemerhunge uber das gleichzeitge Vorkommen von Krebs und Tuberculose. *Virchows Arch* 1888;111:280.

302. Luna-Pérez P, Rodríguez DF, Luján L, et al. Colorectal sarcoma: analysis of failure patterns. *J Surg Oncol* 1998;69:36.

303. Lyon DT, Mantia AG. Large-bowel hemangiomas. *Dis Colon Rectum* 1984;27:404.

304. Lyttle JA. Primary squamous carcinoma of the proximal large bowel: report of a case and review of the literature. *Dis Colon Rectum* 1983;26:279.

305. Ma WH. Myoblastoma: report of a case with review of 287 cases collected from the literature. *Chin Med J* 1952;70:35.

306. MacKenzie DA, McDonald JR, Waugh JM. Leiomyoma and leiomyosarcoma of the colon. *Ann Surg* 1954;139:67.

307. Madiedo G, Komorowski RA Dhar GH. Granular cell tumor (myoblastoma) of the large intestine removed by colonoscopy. *Gastrointest Endosc* 1980;26:108.

308. Madigan MR, Morson BC. Solitary ulcer of the rectum. *Gut* 1969;10:871.

309. Magtibay PM, Heppell J, Leslie KO. Endometriosis-associated invasive adenocarcinoma involving the rectum in a postmenopausal female: report of a case. *Dis Colon Rectum* 2001;44:1530.

310. Mallory FB. Three gliomata of ependymal origin: two in the fourth ventricle, one subcutaneous over the coccyx. *J Med Res* 1902;8:1.

311. Mani S, Modlin IM, Ballantyne G, et al. Carcinoids of the rectum. *J Am Coll Surg* 1994;179:231.

312. Manley KA, Skyring AP. Some heritable causes of gastrointestinal disease: special reference to hemorrhage. *Arch Intern Med* 1961;107:182.

313. Margulis AR, Burhenne HJ, eds. *Alimentary tract roentgenology,* vol 2. St Louis, MO: CV Mosby, 1967.

314. Margulis AR, Jovanovich A. The roentgen diagnosis of submucous lipomas of the colon. *AJR Am J Roentgenol* 1960;84:1114.

315. Marshak RH, Moseley JE, Wolf BS. The roentgen findings in familial polyposis with special emphasis on differential diagnosis. *Radiology* 1963;80:374.

316. Martin JK Jr, Culp CE, Weiland LH. Colitis cystica profunda. *Dis Colon Rectum* 1980;23:488.

317. Maruyama M, Fukayama M, Koike M. A case of multiple carcinoid tumors of the rectum with extraglandular endocrine cell proliferation. *Cancer* 1988;6l:131.

318. Matter MJC, Gygi C, Gillet M, et al. Malacoplakia simulating organ invasion in a rectosigmoid adenocarcinoma: report of a case. *Dis Colon Rectum* 2001;44:1371.

319. Mazier WP, Sun KM, Robertson WG. Oil-induced granuloma (eleoma) of the rectum: report of four cases. *Dis Colon Rectum* 1978;21:292.

320. McClenathan JH. Metastatic melanoma involving the colon: report of a case. *Dis Colon Rectum* 1989;32:70.

321. McClure J. Malakoplakia of the gastrointestinal tract. *Postgrad Med J* 1981;57:95.

322. McGee HJ Jr. Inflammatory fibroid polyps of the ileum and cecum. *Arch Pathol* 1960;70:203.

323. McSwain B, Beal JM. Lymphosarcoma of the gastrointestinal tract: report of 20 cases. *Ann Surg* 1944;119:108.

324. Meijer S, Peretz T, Gaynor JJ, et al. Primary colorectal sarcoma: a retrospective review and prognostic factor study of 50 consecutive patients. *Arch Surg* 1990;125:1163.

325. Mendoza CC. Arteriovenous angioma of the colon. *South Med J* 1962;55:40.

326. Merkel IS, Rabinovitz M, Dekker A. Cecal inflammatory fibroid polyp presenting with chronic diarrhea: a case report and review of the literature. *Dig Dis Sci* 1992;37:133.

327. Meyer R. Ueber entzündliche heterotope Epithel vucherungen im weiblichen Genitalgebiete und ueber eine bis in die Wurzel des Mesocolon ausgedehnte benigne Wucherung des Darmepithels. *Virchows Arch* 1909;195:487.

328. Meyers MA, Ghahremani GG. Pneumatosis coli. In: Greenbaum EI, ed. *Radiographic atlas of colon disease.* Chicago: Year Book, 1980:389.

329. Michaelis L, Gutmann C. Ueber Einschlusse in Blasentumoren. *Klin Med (Mosk)* 1902;47:208.

330. Michelassi F, Mishlove LA, Stipa F, et al. Squamous-cell carcinoma of the colon: experience at the University of Chicago, review of the literature, report of two cases. *Dis Colon Rectum* 1988;31:228.

331. Michelassi F, Montag AG, Block GE. Adenosquamous-cell carcinoma in ulcerative colitis: report of a case. *Dis Colon Rectum* 1988;31:323.

332. Michowitz M, Lazebnik N, Noy S, et al. Lipoma of the colon: a report of 22 cases. *Am Surg* 1985;51:449.

333. Miercort RD, Merrill FG. Pneumatosis and pseudoobstruction in scleroderma. *Radiology* 1969;92:359.

334. Mihara S, Yano H, Matsumoto H, et al. Perianal alveolar rhabdomyosarcoma in a child: report of a long-term survival case. *Dis Colon Rectum* 1983;26:730.

335. Miller RW, Dalager NA. Fatal rhabdomyosarcoma among children in the United States, 1960–1969. *Cancer* 1974;34:1897.

336. Miralbés M, Honojosa J, Alonso J, et al. Oxygen therapy in pneumatosis coli: what is the minimum oxygen requirement? *Dis Colon Rectum* 1983;26:458.

337. Mir-Madjlessi SH, Tavassolie H, Kamalian N. Malakoplakia of the colon and recurrent colonic strictures in a patient with primary hypogammaglobulinemia: an association not previously described. *Dis Colon Rectum* 1982;25:723.

338. Modlin IM, Lye KD, Kidd M. A 5-decade analysis of 13,715 carcinoid tumors. *Cancer* 2003;97:934.

339. Moertel CG. Large bowel. In: Holland JF, Frei E III, eds. *Cancer medicine.* Philadelphia: Lea & Febiger, 1973:1597.

340. Moertel CG, Dockerty MB, Judd ES. Carcinoid tumors of the veriform appendix. *Cancer* 1968;21:270.

341. Moertel CG, Sauer WG, Dockerty MB, et al. Life history of the carcinoid tumor of the small intestine. *Cancer* 1961;14:901.

342. Moertel CG, Weiland LH, Nagorney DM, et al. Carcinoid tumor of the appendix: treatment and prognosis. *N Engl J Med* 1987;317:1699.

343. Monek O, Martin L, Heyd B, et al. Rectal duplication in an adult: unusual cause of a buttock mass: report of a case. *Dis Colon Rectum* 1999;42:816

344. Morantz RA, Kepes JJ, Batnitzky S, et al. Extraspinal ependymomas: report of three cases. *J Neurosurg* 1979;51:383.

345. Morl FK, Dortenmann J. Hämangiome des Dickdarms. *Med Welt* 1968;45:2483.

346. Morson BC. In: Dukes CE, ed. *Cancer of the rectum,* vol 3. Edinburgh: E & S Livingstone, 1960:92.

347. Morson BC. Pathology of carcinoid tumours. In: Jones FA, ed. *Modern trends in gastroenterology.* London: Butterworth, 1958:107.

348. Mourra N, Caplin S, Parc R, et al. Presacral neuroendocrine carcinoma developed in a tailgut cyst: report of a case. *Dis Colon Rectum* 2003;46:411.

349. Murphy B. Leiomyoma of intestine. *J Ir Med Assoc* 1973;66:153.

350. Murray FE, Lombard M, Dervan P, et al. Bleeding from multifocal heterotopic gastric mucosa in the colon controlled by an H_2 antagonist. *Gut* 1988;29:848.

351. Murray MR. Cultural characteristics of 3 granular-cell myoblastomas. *Cancer* 1951;4:857.

352. Nakahara S, Itoh H, Mibu R, et al. Anorectal function after high sacrectomy with bilateral resection of S2–S5 nerves: report of a case. *Dis Colon Rectum* 1986;29:271.

353. Neary PC, Redmond PH, Houghton T, et al. Carcinoid disease: review of the literature. *Dis Colon Rectum* 1997;40:349.

354. Neff R, Kremer S, Voutsinas L, et al. Primary Kaposi's sarcoma of the ileum presenting as massive rectal bleeding. *Am J Gastroenterol* 1987;82:276.

355. Nelson RL. The association of carcinoid tumors of the rectum with myelofibrosis: report of two cases. *Dis Colon Rectum* 1981;24:548.

356. Neoplasms. A complication of organ transplants? *JAMA* 1968;206:246.

357. Nigam R. A case of dermoid arising from the rectal wall. *Br J Surg* 1947;35:218.

358. Nigro ND, Hiratzka T. Aberrant gastric mucosa in the rectum: a case report. *Dis Colon Rectum* 1961;4:275.

359. Norbury L. Specimen of post-rectal fibro-leiomyoma. *Proc R Soc Med* 1934;27:930.

360. Normann T, Otnes B. Intestinal ganglioneuromatosis, diarrhoea and medullary thyroid carcinoma. *Scand J Gastroenterol* 1969;4:553.

361. Oberndorfer S. Karzinoide Tumoren des Dünndarms. *Frank Z Pathol* 1907;1:426.

362. Oberwalder M, Tschmelitsch J, Conrad F, et al. Endosonographic image of a retrorectal bowel duplication: report of a case. *Dis Colon Rectum* 1998;41:802

363. O'Brien JE, Stout AP. Malignant fibrous xanthomas. *Cancer* 1964;17:1445.

364. Ochsner SF, Ray JE, Clark WH Jr. Lymphangioma of the colon: a case report. *Radiology* 1959;72:423.

365. Ohri SK, Keane PF, Sackier JM, et al. Primary rectal lymphoma and malignant lymphomatous polyposis: two cases illustrating current methods in diagnosis and management. *Dis Colon Rectum* 1989;32:1071.

366. Okano H, Azar HA, Osserman EF. Plasmacytic reticulum cell sarcoma: case report with electron microscopic studies. *Am J Clin Pathol* 1966;46:546.

367. Olnick HM, Woodhall JP Jr, Clay CB Jr. Hemangioma of the colon. *J Med Assoc Ga* 1957;46:383.

368. Orda R, Bawnik JB, Wiznitzer T, et al. Fibroma of the cecum: report of a case. *Dis Colon Rectum* 1976;19:626.

369. O'Riordain DS, O'Connell PR, Kirwan WO. Hereditary sacral agenesis with presacral mass and anorectal stenosis: the Currarino triad. *Br J Surg* 1991;78:536.

370. Orloff MJ. Carcinoid tumors of the rectum. *Cancer* 1971;28:175.

371. O'Toole D, Ducreux M, Bommelaer G, et al. Treatment of carcinoid syndrome: a prospective crossover evaluation of lanreotide versus octreotide in terms of efficacy, patient acceptability, and tolerance. *Cancer* 2000;88:770.

372. Ozaki T, Hillmann A, Winkelmann W. Surgical treatment of sacrococcygeal chordoma. *J Surg Oncol* 1997;64:274.

373. Palvio DHB, Sorensen FB, Klove-Mogensen M. Stem cell carcinoma of the colon and rectum: report of two cases and review of the literature. *Dis Colon Rectum* 1985;28:440.

374. Pardo MV, Rodriquez TI. Eosinophilic granuloma of the colon. *Arch Hosp Univ Havana* 1952;4:248.

375. Paris J, Goudemand M, Leduc M, et al. Angiome isolé du colon droit avec hemorragies digestives repetées pendant 15 ans. *Lille Med* 1967;12:592.

376. Parks AG, Porter NH, Hardcastle J. The syndrome of the descending perineum. *Proc R Soc Med* 1966;59:477.

377. Paterson C, Musselman L, Chorneyko K, et al. Merkel cell (neuroendocrine) carcinoma of the anal canal: report of a case. *Dis Colon Rectum* 2003;46:676.

378. Pearlman AW, Friedman M. Radical radiation therapy of chordoma. *AJR Am J Roentgenol* 1970;108:332.

379. Pemberton J, McCormack CJ. Submucous lipomas of colon and rectum. *Am J Surg* 1937;37:205.

380. Penn I, Starzl TE. Immunosuppression and cancer. *Transplant Proc* 1973;5:943.

381. Peterkin GA III, Moroz K, Kondi ES. Proctitis cystica profunda in paraplegics: report of three cases. *Dis Colon Rectum* 1992;35:1174.

382. Petrelli NJ, Valle AA, Weber TK, et al. Adenosquamous carcinoma of the colon and rectum. *Dis Colon Rectum* 1996;39:1265.

383. Pfannenstiel J. Über die Adenomyome des Genitalstrangs. *Verh Dtsch Ges Gynaekol* 1897;7:195.

384. Phillips B. Lectures on the principles and practices of surgery. *London Med Gaz* 1839;1:608.

385. Pinkert TC, Catlow CE, Straus R. Endometriosis of the urinary bladder in a man with prostatic carcinoma. *Cancer* 1979;43:1562.

386. Pitchumoni CS, Dearani AC, Burke AV, et al. Eosinophilic granuloma of the gastrointestinal tract. *JAMA* 1970;211:1180.

387. Poate H, Inglis K. Ganglioneuromatosis of the alimentary tract. *Br J Surg* 1928;16:221.

388. Pontecorvo C, Lombardi S, Mottola L, et al. Hemangiomas of the large bowel: report of a case. *Dis Colon Rectum* 1983;26:818.

389. Port JH, Traube J, Winans CS. The visceral manifestations of Kaposi's sarcoma. *Gastrointest Endosc* 1982;28:179.

390. Poulos JE, Presti ME, Phillips N, et al. Presentation and management of lymphatic cyst of the colon. *Dis Colon Rectum* 1997;40:366.

391. Price AB. Benign lymphoid polyps and inflammatory polyps. In: Morson BC, ed. *The pathogenesis of colorectal cancer.* Philadelphia: WB Saunders, 1978:33.

392. Prystowsky JB, Stryker SJ, Ujiki GT, et al. Gastrointestinal endometriosis: incidence and indications for resection. *Arch Surg* 1988;123:855.

393. Quan SH, Bader G, Berg JW. Carcinoid tumors of the rectum. *Dis Colon Rectum* 1964;7:197.

394. Quan SH, Berg JW. Leiomyoma and leiomyosarcoma of the rectum. *Dis Colon Rectum* 1962;5:415.

395. Quinn TC. Gastrointestinal manifestations of AIDS. *Pract Gastroenterol* 1985;9:23.

396. Ranchod M, Kahn LB. Malacoplakia of the gastrointestinal tract. *Arch Pathol* 1972;94:90.

397. Rand AA. Barium granuloma of the rectum. *Dis Colon Rectum* 1966;9:20.

398. Rao BK, Kapur MM, Roy S. Leiomyosarcoma of the colon: a case report and review of literature. *Dis Colon Rectum* 1980;23:184.

399. Redwine DB, Koning M, Sharpe DR. Laparoscopically assisted transvaginal segmental resection of the rectosigmoid colon for endometriosis. *Fertil Steril* 1996;65:193.

400. Reiss H, Ryc K. Roxlegly naczyniak jelita grubego i odbytnicy o mieszanej budowie. *Pol Przegl Chir* 1971;43:115.

401. Richardson JD. Vascular lesions of the intestines. *Am J Surg* 1991;161:284.

402. Rickert RR, Larkey IG, Kantor EB. Granular-cell tumors (myoblastomas) of the anal region. *Dis Colon Rectum* 1978;2l:413.

403. Rissier HL Jr. Hemangiomatosis of the intestine: discussion, review of the literature and report of two new cases. *Gastroenterologia* 1960;93:357.

404. Riva HL, Kawasaki DM, Messinger AJ. Further experience with norethynodrel in treatment of endometriosis. *Obstet Gynecol* 1962;19:111.

405. Rives S, Pera M, Rosiñol L., et al. Primary systemic amyloidosis presenting as a colonic stricture: successful treatment with left hemicolectomy followed by autologous hematopoietic stem-cell transplantation: report of a case. *Dis Colon Rectum* 2002;45:1263.

406. Robertson FN, Wride GE. Case of persistent cyst of postanal gut origin in an adult. *Can Med Assoc J* 1934;31:535.

407. Robidoux A, Monte M, Heppel J, et al. Small-cell carcinoma of the rectum. *Dis Colon Rectum* 1984;28:594.

408. Rodriguez DI, Drehner DM, Beck DE, et al. Colonic lipoma as a source of massive hemorrhage: report of a case. *Dis Colon Rectum* 1990;33:977.

409. Roo T de. Leiomyosarcoma of the colon, a rare tumor: three case reports and review. *Radiol Clin Biol* 1974;43:187.

410. Roo T de, Vaas F. Leiomyosarcoma of the transverse and descending colon: two case reports and review. *Am J Gastroenterol* 1969;52:150.

411. Rose TF. True fibroma of the caecum. *Med J Aust* 1972;1:532.

412. Rosenberg I. Perianal granular cell myoblastoma: report of a case. *J Int Coll Surg* 1960;33:346.

413. Rosenberg JM, Welch JP. Carcinoid tumors of the colon: a study of 72 patients. *Am J Surg* 1985;149:775.

414. Ruiz-Moreno F. Hemangiomatosis of the colon: report of a case. *Dis Colon Rectum* 1962;5:453.

415. Ryan J, Martin JE, Pollock DJ. Fatty tumours of the large intestine: a clinicopathological review of 13 cases. *Br J Surg* 1989;76:793.

416. Ryckman FC, Glenn JD, Moazam F. Spontaneous perforation of a colonic duplication. *Dis Colon Rectum* 1983;26:287.

417. Rywlin AM, Ravel R, Hurwitz A. Malakoplakia of the colon. *Am J Dig Dis* 1969;14:491.

418. Saclarides TJ, Ko ST, Airan M, et al. Laparoscopic removal of a large colonic lipoma: report of a case. *Dis Colon Rectum* 1991;34:1027.

419. Saclarides TJ, Szeluga D, Staren ED. Neuroendocrine cancers of the colon and rectum. *Dis Colon Rectum* 1994;37:635.

420. Saegesser F, Gross M. Carcinoid syndrome and carcinoid tumors of the rectum. *Am J Proctol* 1969;20:27.

421. Safai B, Diaz B, Schwartz J. Malignant neoplasms associated with human immunodeficiency virus infection. *CA Cancer J Clin* 1992;42:74.

422. Sakanoue Y, Kusunoki M, Shoji Y, et al. Malignant histiocytosis of the intestine simulating Crohn's disease: report of a case. *Dis Colon Rectum* 1992;35:266.

423. Sallach S, Schmidt T, Pehl C, et al. Primary low-grade B cell non-Hodgkin's lymphoma of MALT type simultaneously arising in the colon and in the lung: report of a case. *Dis Colon Rectum* 2001;44:448.

424. Saltzstein SL. Extranodal malignant lymphomas and pseudolymphomas. *Pathol Annu* 1969;4:159.

425. Sampson JA. Intestinal adenomas of endometrial type. *Arch Surg* 1922;5:217.

426. Sanders RJ. Leiomyosarcoma of the rectum: report of six cases. *Ann Surg* 1961;154:150.

427. Sanders RJ, Axtell HK. Carcinoids of the gastrointestinal tract. *Surg Gynecol Obstet* 1964;119:369.

428. Sanger BJ, Leckie BD. Plain muscle tumours of the rectum. *Br J Surg* 1959;47:196.

429. Sarmiento JM, Wolff BG. A different type of presacral tumor: extramedullary hematopoiesis: report of a case. *Dis Colon Rectum* 2003;46:683.

430. Sasajima K, Okawa K, Sasamoto Y, et al. Pararectal rhabdomyosarcoma: report of a case. *Dis Colon Rectum* 1980;23:576.

431. Sauven P, Ridge JA, Quan SH, et al. Anorectal carcinoid tumors: is aggressive surgery warranted? *Ann Surg* 1990;211:67.

432. Sayfan J, Benosh L, Segal M, et al. Endometriosis in episiotomy scar with anal sphincter involvement: report of a case. *Dis Colon Rectum* 1991;34:713.

433. Schlernitzauer DA, Font RL. Sebaceous gland carcinoma of the eyelid following radiation therapy for cavernous hemangioma of the face. *Arch Ophthalmol* 1976;94:1523.

434. Schröder J, Löhnert M, Doniec JM, et al. Endoluminal ultrasound diagnosis and operative management of rectal endometriosis. *Dis Colon Rectum* 1997;40:614.

435. Schumann F. Leiomyosarcoma of the colon: report of a case and review of treatment and prognosis. *Dis Colon Rectum* 1972;15:211–216

436. Selikoff IJ, Robitzek EH. Gingival biopsy for the diagnosis of generalized amyloidosis. *Am J Pathol* 1947;23:1099.

437. Serra J, Ruiz M, Lloveras B, et al. Surgical outlook regarding leiomyoma of the rectum: report of three cases. *Dis Colon Rectum* 1989;32:884.

438. Sewell R, Levine BA, Harrison GK, et al. Primary malignant fibrous histiocytoma of the intestine: intussusception of a rare neoplasm. *Dis Colon Rectum* 1980;23:198.

439. Sharma S, Longo WE, Baniadam B, et al. Colorectal manifestations of endocrine disease. *Dis Colon Rectum* 1995; 38:318.

440. Sherlock P, Winawer SJ, Goldstein MJ, et al. Malignant lymphoma of the gastrointestinal tract. In: Glass GB, ed. *Progress in gastroenterology*, vol 2. New York: Grune & Stratton, 1970:367.

441. Shimazu K, Funata N, Yamamoto Y, et al. Primary osteosarcoma arising in the colon: report of a case. *Dis Colon Rectum* 2001;44:1367.

442. Shindo K, Bacon HE, Holmes EJ. Ectopic gastric mucosa and glandular tissue of a salivary type in the anal canal concomitant with a diverticulum in hemorrhoidal tissue: report of a case. *Dis Colon Rectum* 1972;15:57.

443. Shirouzu K, Isomoto H, Kakegawa T, et al. Treatment of rectal carcinoid tumors. *Am J Surg* 1990;160:262.

444. Shklovskii GS, Kadyrov FA. Gemangioma tolst oi kishki s invaginatsiei. *Vestn Khir* 1964;93:114.

445. Sidani MS, Campos MM, Joseph JI. Primary plasmacytomas of the colon. *Dis Colon Rectum* 1983;26:182.

446. Silverberg SG. "Juvenile" retention polyps of the colon and rectum. *Am J Dig Dis* 1970;15:617.

447. Silverman JM, Hamlin JA. Large melanoma metastases to the gastrointestinal tract. *Gut* 1989;30:1783.

448. Simon SR, Fox K. Neuroendocrine carcinoma of the colon: correct diagnosis is important. *J Clin Gastroenterol* 1993; 17:304.

449. Skardalakis JE, Gray SW, Shepard D, et al. *Smooth muscle tumors of the alimentary tract: leiomyomas and leiomyosarcomas—a review of 2525 cases.* Springfield, IL: Charles C Thomas, 1962:155.

450. Skopelitou AS, Mylonakis EP, Charchanti AV, et al. Cellular neurilemoma (schwannoma) of the descending colon mimicking carcinoma: report of a case. *Dis Colon Rectum* 1998; 41:1193

451. Skovgaard S, Sorensen FH. Bleeding hemangioma of the colon diagnosed by coloscopy. *J Pediatr Surg* 1976;11: 83.

452. Skutsch. Quoted in Galletly A. *Z Gebutschulfe Gunakol* 1899;11:353.

453. Slagel GA, Lupton GP. Postproctoscopic periorbital purpura. *Arch Dermatol* 1986;122:463.

454. Slooter GD, Mearadji A, Breeman WAP, et al. Somatostatin receptor imaging, therapy and new strategies in patients with neuroendocrine tumours. *Br J Surg* 2001;88:31.

455. Smith G. Leiomyosarcoma of the rectum. *Br J Surg* 1963;50:633.

456. Smith JA, Bhathal PS, Cuthbertson AM. Angiosarcoma of the colon: report of a case with long-term survival. *Dis Colon Rectum* 1990;33:330.

457. Smith JL, Painter RW, Berman MM. Breast carcinoma: colonic metastases with perforation—report of two cases. *Contemp Surg* 1989;35:47.

458. Snover DC, Sandstad J, Hutton S. Mucosal pseudolipomatosis of the colon. *Am J Clin Pathol* 1985;84:575.

459. Sohn N. Surgical conditions of the anus and rectum in male homosexuals. *Pract Gastroenterol* 1985;9:46.

460. Somervell JL, Mayer PF. Leiomyosarcoma of the rectum. *Br J Surg* 1971;58:144.

461. Spigelman AD, Williams CB, Ansell JK, et al. Pneumatosis coli: a source of diagnostic confusion. *Br J Surg* 1990;77: 155.

462. Spread C, Berkel H, Jewell L, et al. Colon carcinoid tumors: a population based study. *Dis Colon Rectum* 1994; 37:482.

463. Staren ED, Gould VE, Warren WH, et al. Neuroendocrine carcinomas of the colon and rectum: a clinicopathologic evaluation. *Surgery* 1988;104:1080.

464. Starr GF, Dockerty MB. Leiomyomas and leiomyosarcomas of the small intestine. *Cancer* 1955;8:101.

465. Stavorovsky M, Jaffa AJ, Papo J, et al. Leiomyosarcoma of the colon and rectum. *Dis Colon Rectum* 1980;23:249.

466. Steckler RM, Martin RG. Sacrococcygeal chordoma. *Am Surg* 1974;40:579.

467. Stening SG, Heptinstall DP. Diffuse cavernous haemangioma of the rectum and sigmoid colon. *Br J Surg* 1970; 57:186.

468. Stoller R, Weinstein JJ. Fibrosarcoma of the rectum: a review of the literature and the presentation of two additional cases. *Surgery* 1956;39:565.

469. Stout AP. Tumors of the colon and rectum (excluding carcinoma and adenoma). *Surg Clin North Am* 1955;35: 1283.

470. Stout AP, Hill WT. Leiomyosarcoma of the superficial soft tissues. *Cancer* 1958;11:844.

471. Stuart M. Pneumatosis coli complicating carcinoma of the colon: report of a case. *Dis Colon Rectum* 1984;27:257.

472. Suga K, Tanaka N, Nakanishi T, et al. Bone and gallium scintigraphy in sacral chordoma: report of four cases. *Clin Nucl Med* 1992;17:206.

473. Sugarman GI, Weitzman JJ, Isaacs H Jr, et al. Rectal bleeding from gastric tissue in the rectum. *Lancet* 1970;1:251.

474. Swain VA, Young WF, Pringle EM. Hypertrophy of the appendices epiploicae and lipomatous polyposis of the colon. *Gut* 1969;10:587.

475. Swanson MA, Schwartz RS. Immunosuppressive therapy: the relation between clinical response and immunologic competence. *N Engl J Med* 1967;277:163.

476. Swartley RN, Stayman JW Jr. Lymphoid hyperplasia of the intestinal tract requiring surgical intervention. *Ann Surg* 1962;155:238.

477. Swartzlander FC. *A clinico-pathological review of submucosal rectal nodules.* Thesis. Minneapolis, MN: University of Minnesota, 1955.

478. Swerdlow DB, Pecora C, Gardone F. Leiomyoma of the cecum presenting as an acute surgical abdomen: report of a case. *Dis Colon Rectum* 1975;18:438.

479. Swinton NW, Lehman G. Presacral tumors. *Surg Clin North Am* 1958;38:849.

480. Symmers D. Lymphoid disease: Hodgkin's granuloma, giant follicular lymphadenopathy, lymphoid leukemia, lymphosarcoma and gastrointestinal pseudoleukemia. *Arch Pathol* 1948;45:73.

481. Talerman A. Enterogenous cysts of the rectum (colitis cystica profunda). *Br J Surg* 1971;58:643.

482. Tan TCF, Wang JY, Cheung YC, et al. Diffuse cavernous hemangioma of the rectum complicated by invasion of pelvic structures: report of two cases. *Dis Colon Rectum* 1998; 41:1062.

483. Tarver R, Smith GF, Kukora JS. Intestinal amyloidosis. *Contemp Surg* 1985;26:69.

484. Taxy JB, Mendelsohn G, Gupta PK. Carcinoid tumors of the rectum: silver reactions, fluorescence, and serotonin content of the cytoplasmic granules. *Am J Clin Pathol* 1980;74:791.

485. Terner JY, Lattes R. Malakoplakia of colon and retroperitoneum: report of a case with a histochemical study of the Michaelis-Gutmann inclusion bodies. *Am J Clin Pathol* 1965;44:20.

486. Tessier DJ, McConnell EJ, Young-Fadok T, et al. Melanoma metastatic to the colon: case series and review of the literature with outcome analysis. *Dis Colon Rectum* 2003;46:441.

487. Testart J, Maupas JL, Metayer J, et al. Rectal peptic ulceration-a rare cause of rectal bleeding: report of a case. *Dis Colon Rectum* 1988;31:803.

488. Thambidorai CR, Muin I, Razman J, et al. Currarino triad with dual pathology in the presacral mass: report of a case. *Dis Colon Rectum* 2003;46:974.

489. Thomason TH. Cysts and sinuses of the sacrococcygeal region. *Ann Surg* 1934;99:585.

490. Thompson GB, van Heerden J, Martin JK Jr, et al. Carcinoid tumors of the gastrointestinal tract: presentation, management, and prognosis. *Surgery* 1985;98:1054.

491. Thorlakson RH, Ross HM. Leiomyosarcoma of the rectum. *Ann Surg* 1961;154:979.
492. Tichansky DS, Cagir B, Borrazzo E, et al. Risk of second cancers in patients with colorectal carcinoids. *Dis Colon Rectum* 2002;45:91.
493. Timmerman W, Bubrick MP. Presacral and postsacral extraspinal ependymoma: report of a case and review of the literature. *Dis Colon Rectum* 1984;27:114.
494. Tinkoff GH, Yum KY. Endoscopic diagnosis of lipomatosis of the ileocecal valve. *Contemp Surg* 1987;30:69.
495. Tobi M, Kobrin I, Ariel I. Rectal involvement in sarcoidosis. *Dis Colon Rectum* 1982;25:491.
496. Toti A, Tedeschi M. Fibroma cecale insorto su monocone appendicolare invaginato. *Minerva Chir* 1952;7:420.
497. Touran T, Frost DB, O'Connell TX. Sacral resection: operative technique and outcome. *Arch Surg* 1990;125:911.
498. Tsioulas G, Muto T, Kubota Y, et al. DNA ploidy pattern in rectal carcinoid tumors. *Dis Colon Rectum* 1991;34:31.
499. Turell R. *Diseases of the colon and anorectum,* 2nd ed. Philadelphia: WB Saunders, 1969.
500. Upson JF, Bunnell I, Kikkinopoulis E. Hemangioma of the cecum: diagnosis by angiography. *JAMA* 1971;217:1104.
501. Urbach DR, Reedijk M, Richard CS, et al. Bowel resection for intestinal endometriosis. *Dis Colon Rectum* 1998;41: 1158.
502. Usher FC. *Lymphosarcoma of the intestines.* Thesis. Minneapolis, MN: University of Minnesota, 1940.
503. Vagaiwala MR, Robinson JS, Galicich JH, et al. Metastasizing extradural ependymoma of the sacrococcygeal region. *Cancer* 1979;44:326.
504. Venkitachalam PS, Hirsch E, Elguezabal A, et al. Multiple lymphoid polyposis and familial polyposis of the colon: a genetic relationship. *Dis Colon Rectum* 1978;21:336.
505. Vezeridis MP, Herrera LO, Lopez GE, et al. Squamous-cell carcinoma of the colon and rectum. *Dis Colon Rectum* 1983;26:188.
506. Viamonte M III, Viamonte ME. Pneumatosis cystoides intestinalis: case presentation and review of the literature. *Contemp Surg* 1990;37:37.
507. Vitolo RE, Rachlin SA. Inflammatory fibroid polyp of large intestine: report of a case. *J Int Coll Surg* 1955;23:700.
508. Von Dinges HP, Werner R, Watzek G. The incidence and significance of amyloid deposits in gingival, buccal and rectal mucous membranes. *Wien Klin Wochenschr* 1978;90: 431.
509. Von Recklinhausen FH. *Ueber die multiplen Fibrome der Haut und ihre Beziehung zu den multiplen Neuromen.* Berlin: Festrschr Virchow, A Hirschwald, 1882.
510. Vorobyov GI, Odaryuk TS, Kapuller LL, et al. Surgical treatment of benign, myomatous rectal tumors. *Dis Colon Rectum* 1992;35:328.
511. Waldenström JG. Studies on conditions associated with disturbed gamma globulin formation (gammopathies). *Harvey Lect* 1960–1961;56:211.
512. Wall SD, Friedman SL, Margulis AR. Gastrointestinal Kaposi's sarcoma in AIDS: radiographic manifestations. *J Clin Gastroenterol* 1984;6:165.
513. Wang C-H. Sphincter-saving procedure for treatment of diffuse cavernous hemangioma of the rectum and sigmoid colon. *Dis Colon Rectum* 1985;28:604.
514. Waxman M, Faegenburg D, Waxman JS, et al. Malignant fibrous histiocytoma of the colon associated with diverticulitis. *Dis Colon Rectum* 1983;26:339.
515. Waye JD, Frankel A. Removal of pedunculated lipoma by colonoscopy. *Am J Gastroentrol* 1974;62:221.
516. Wayte DM, Helwig EB. Colitis cystica profunda. *Am J Clin Pathol* 1967;48:159.
517. Weber JN, Carmichael DJ, Boylston A, et al. Kaposi's sarcoma of the bowel-presenting as apparent ulcerative colitis. *Gut* 1985;26:295.
518. Weinberg T, Feldman M. Lipomas of the gastrointestinal tract. *Am J Clin Pathol* 1955;25:272.
519. Weitzner S. Ectopic salivary gland tissue in submucosa of rectum. *Dis Colon Rectum* 1983;26:814.
520. Welch CE, Hedberg SE. *Polypoid lesions of the gastrointestinal tract,* 2nd ed. Philadelphia: WB Saunders, 1975: 121.
521. Welch JP, Donaldson GA. Recent experience in the management of cancer of the colon and rectum. *Am J Surg* 1974;127:258.
522. Weprin L, Zollinger R, Clausen K, et al. Kaposi's sarcoma: endoscopic observations of gastric and colon involvement. *J Clin Gastroenterol* 1982;4:357.
523. Wexner SD, Breed JR. Carcinoma arising in a rectal duplication (enterocystoma). *Ann Surg* 1963;157:476.
524. Williams ED, Sandler M. The classification of carcinoid tumours. *Lancet* 1963;1:238.
525. Williams GT, Blackshaw AJ, Morson BC. Squamous carcinoma of the colorectum and its genesis. *J Pathol* 1979; 129:139.
526. Willis RA. *The borderland of embryology and pathology.* London: Butterworth, 1958.
527. Willis RA. *Pathology of tumours,* 3rd ed. London: Butterworth, 1960.
528. Wilson JAP. Richter's syndrome mimicking chronic colitis: a patient with diffuse histiocytic lymphoma complicating chronic lymphocytic leukemia. *Dis Colon Rectum* 1986; 29:191.
529. Wolf BS, Marshak RH. Roentgen features of diffuse lymphosarcoma of the colon. *Radiology* 1960;75:733.
530. Wolff M. Heterotopic gastric epithelium in the rectum: a report of three cases with a review of 87 cases of gastric heterotopia in the alimentary canal. *Am J Clin Pathol* 1971;55:604.
531. Wolff M, Santiago H, Duby MM. Delayed distant metastasis from a subcutaneous sacrococcygeal ependymoma. *Cancer* 1972;30:1046.
532. Wood DA. Tumors of the intestines. In: *Atlas of tumor pathology,* 2nd series. Sect. 6. Fasc. 22. Washington, DC: Armed Forces Institute of Pathology, 1967:52.
533. Wychulis AR, Beahrs OH, Woolner LB. Malignant lymphoma of the colon: a study of 69 cases. *Arch Surg* 1966; 93:215.
534. Yamaguchi K, Shirai T, Shimakura K, et al. Pneumatosis cystoides intestinalis and trichloroethylene exposure. *Am J Gastroenterol* 1985;80:753.
535. Yang GCH, Coleman B, Daly JM, et al. Presacral myelolipoma: report of a case with fine needle aspiration cytology and immunohistochemical and histochemical studies. *Acta Cytol* 1992;36:932.
536. Yani-Inbar I, Odes HS, Krugliak P, et al. Granular cell myoblastoma of the sigmoid colon. *Dig Dis Sci* 1981;26: 852.
537. Yeh C-Y, Chen H-H, Tang R, et al. Surgical outcome after curative resection of rectal leiomyosarcoma. *Dis Colon Rectum* 2000;43:1517.
538. Yonemoto T, Tatezaki S-I, Takenouchi T, et al. The surgical management of sacrococcygeal chordoma. *Cancer* 1999;85: 878.
539. Yoshida A, Yano M, Fujinaga Y, et al. Argentiffin carcinoid tumor of the rectum. *Cancer* 1981;48:2103.
540. Yoshikawa O. A case of leiomyosarcoma of the rectum. *Arch Jpn Chir* 1969;38:342.
541. Yousefzadeh DK, Bickers GH, Jackson JH, et al. Tubular colonic duplication-review of 1876–1981 literature. *Pediatr Radiol* 1983;13:65.
542. Ziter FMH Jr. Roentgenographic findings in Gardner's syndrome. *JAMA* 1965;192:1000.

Chapter 26

Diverticular Disease

Solitary Cecal Ulcer

Diet cures more than the lancet.

Spanish Proverb

Man shall not live by bread alone.

Matthew 4:4; Luke 4:4

Diverticular disease (diverticulitis and diverticulosis) was a rare condition before the end of the nineteenth century. Although the manifestations were described accurately by such renowned nineteenth-century surgeons and pathologists as Cruveilhier, Rokitansky, Cripps, and Virchow, the condition was regarded as a surgical curiosity.[182] However, the disease had become progressively more pervasive in the twentieth century and virtually epidemic in Western countries today. A person's risk for the development of diverticular disease by age 60 in the United States approximates 50%. By the age of 80 years, virtually all Americans have the condition. Yet, not more than 20% of persons with colonic diverticula have symptoms, and only a few of these ever require surgery.[185] Of the approximately 10% to 15% of persons with diverticulosis who go on to develop diverticulitis, 75% have uncomplicated cases. However, 25% manifest an abscess, obstruction, perforation, or fistula formation. Perforation itself is indeed an uncommon event, occurring at about the rate of four per 100,000 per year, with women having about half the incidence of men.

In the United States, diverticular disease accounts for approximately 450,000 annual hospitalizations, 2 million office visits, and 112,000 disability cases, and claims approximately 3,000 lives per year. Diverticulosis of the colon is most common in the sigmoid colon in United States, whereas the location is primarily right sided in Asian populations.

PATHOGENESIS

Diverticula occur in areas of the colon where there is relative weakness—most commonly where the blood vessels penetrate the wall (hence, the most frequent manifestation of a complication is a mesenteric phleg-

mon) and on the antimesenteric surface of the bowel, between the taeniae (Figs. 26-1 and 26-2). The tunnels formed by the blood vessels weaken the muscle, and presumably the diverticula become manifest as a result of high intracolonic pressure affecting these areas.[181] This is an important anatomic fact that may also be relevant to the complication of hemorrhage from diverticula (see Chapter 28).[168]

Pathophysiology

Study of the physiology of the normal colon by means of pressure tracings reveals that the principal waveform represents a slow change of pressure, waxing and waning during about 30 seconds.[55] Complete quiescence may normally be present for several hours. Usually, the waves are not transmitted to adjacent areas of the colon, but occasionally the transport of material through considerable distance does occur.[55] Radiologically, this is seen as a loss of haustration succeeded by movement of the contents through a number of centimeters. Motor studies in patients with diverticular disease reveal an exaggerated response to pharmacologic stimuli, increased intraluminal pressures, and faster frequency waves and rapid contractions (more than five per minute).[55] A comprehensive discussion of colonic motility can be found in Chapters 2 and 6.

Increased pressure is brought about through progressive colonic narrowing and segmentation. When contraction occurs in a segment that is relatively narrowed, considerable intraluminal pressure develops, causing the colon to hypertrophy. The pressure is related to the narrowness or spasticity of the involved segment. According to the law of Laplace, the tension in the wall of a hollow cylinder is proportional to its radius multiplied by the pressure within the cylinder. This implies that the intraluminal pressure is greater when the lumen is narrowed and explains the increased likelihood that diverticula will develop in the sigmoid colon, the narrowest segment.[55] The thickened colonic muscle becomes uneven, with resultant herniation through the weakened

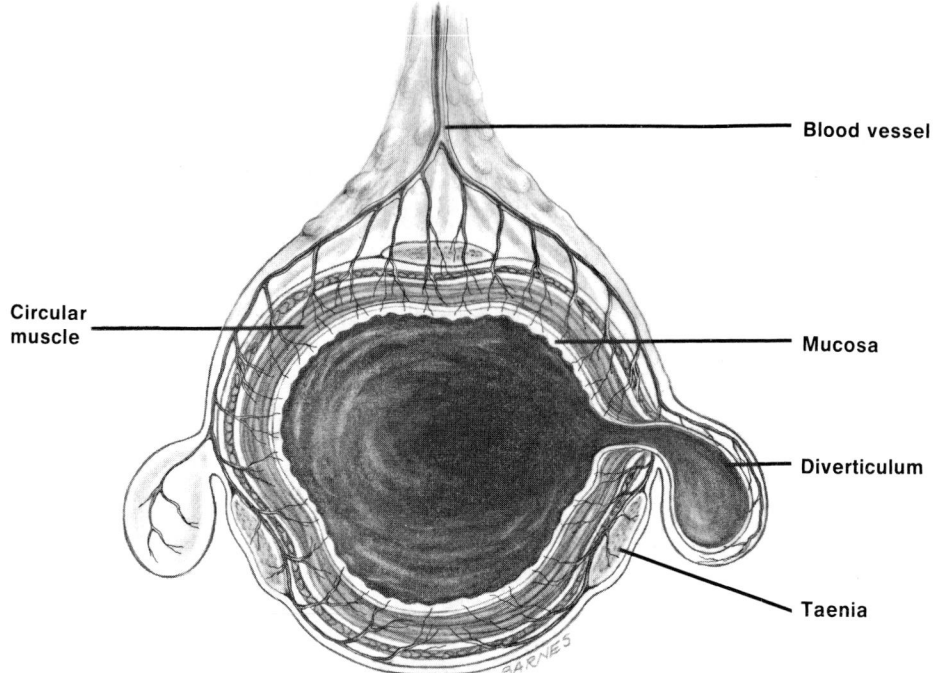

FIGURE 26-1. Cross-section of colon showing areas of weakness through which the diverticula become manifest.

parts of its wall (Figure 26-3).[181] The problem is exacerbated by the fact that the tensile strength and elasticity of the colon decline with age; this is most marked on the left side.[262] Additionally, the sigmoid must propel the most formed fecal material, which contributes further to the problem in this area (Figs. 26-4 and 26-5).[181] Cortesini and Pantalone performed colonic motility studies by means of pressure transducers introduced into the bowel lumen in individuals with diverticular disease.[57] High intraluminal pressure recordings were found in symptomatic subjects.

Histology

Microscopically, the diverticula are of the pulsion type, consisting only of mucous membrane and peritoneum. In the absence of complications, particularly inflammation,

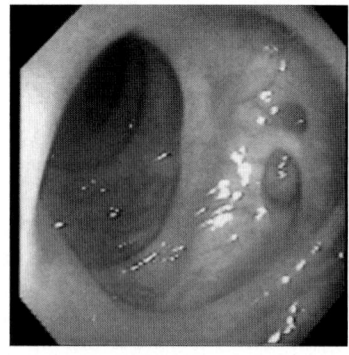

FIGURE 26-2. Colonoscopy reveals two diverticular openings in the region of the lower sigmoid colon. (See Color Fig. 26-2.)

the lining is entirely normal except for an increase in the size and number of lymphoid follicles.[168] The muscle shows thickening but no evidence of cellular hypertrophy or hyperplasia.[169] Antimesenteric diverticula have only a very thin layer of investing longitudinal muscle, mucous membrane, and muscularis mucosae separating the fecal contents of the bowel from the peritoneal cavity (Figure 26-6).[169]

ETIOLOGY, EPIDEMIOLOGY, AND DIET

Painter and Burkitt (see the biography in Chapter 22) are the two individuals most responsible for our current concepts of the etiology and epidemiology of diverticular disease.[41,42,179–182] Because the condition was extremely rare in the nineteenth century and began to be relatively commonly observed in Western countries only after 1920, the authors postulated that a change in the dietary habits in those countries was the incriminating factor. During the years 1870 and 1880, the grist mills for grinding wheat into whole-meal flour were replaced by the much more efficient roller mills. This new process succeeded in crushing the grain so effectively that a very pure white flour was produced. At about the same time, with the advent of effective refrigeration and canning, consumption of refined sugar, fat, and protein increased. The result was a critical decrease in the amount of fiber available in the diet. Fiber is the portion of the dietary intake that is not absorbed; this is usually in the form of cellulose.

Painter stated that the greatest change in our diet in the past 100 years has been a reduction in the amount of

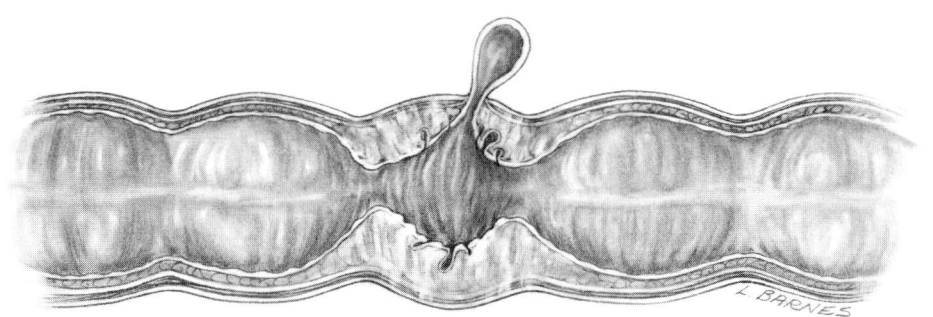

FIGURE 26-3. Mechanism of segmental contraction with elevated, localized intracolonic pressure and resultant diverticulum.

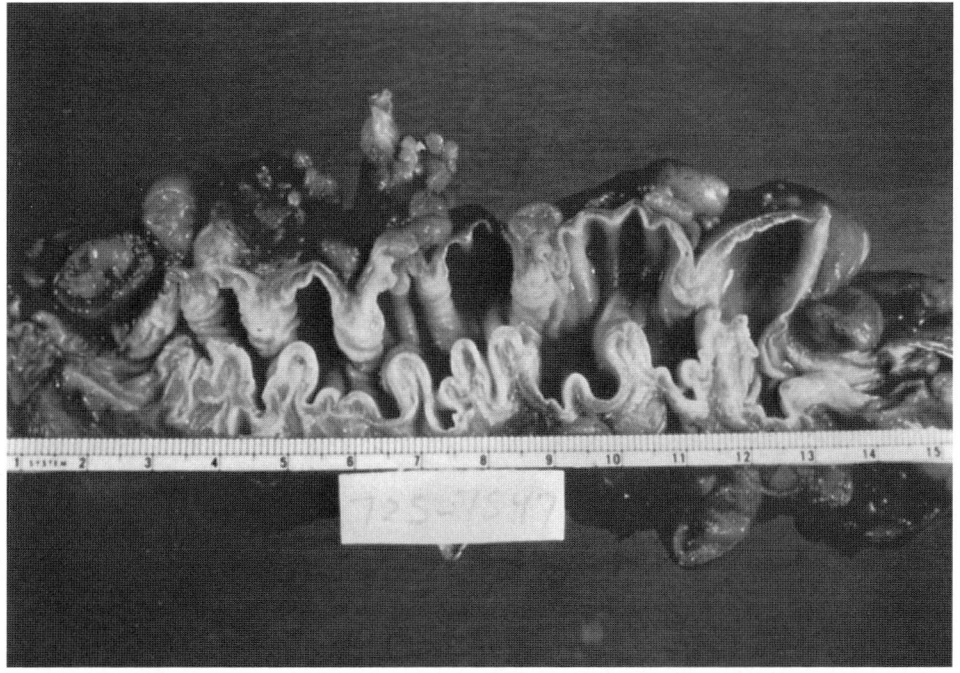

FIGURE 26-4. Resected portion of the sigmoid colon demonstrating multiple "little bladders" or "rooms" resulting from hypertrophy and segmentation.

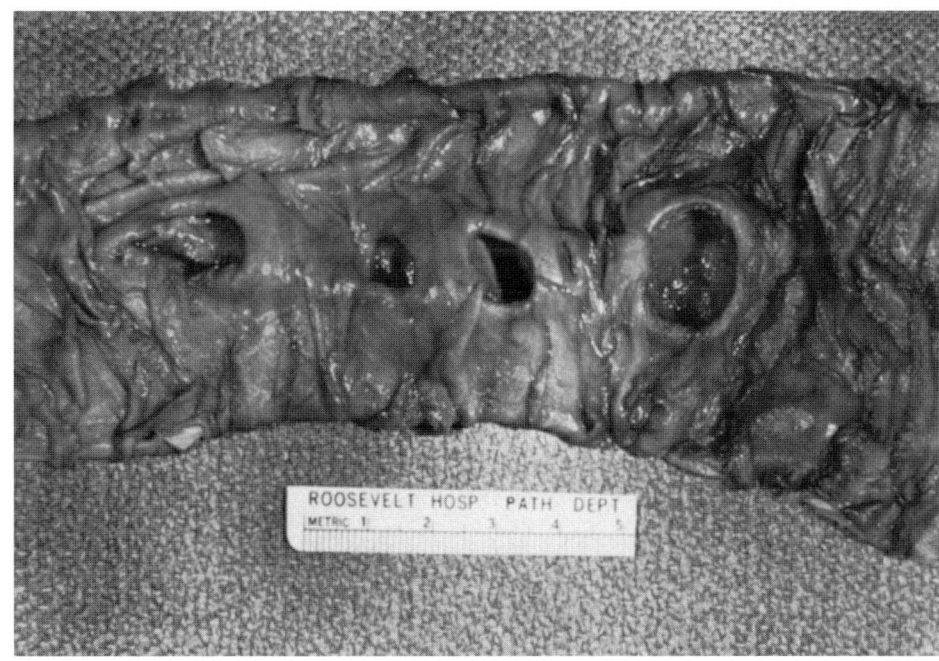

FIGURE 26-5. Portion of the sigmoid colon showing large-mouth diverticula. (Courtesy of Rudolf Garret, M.D.)

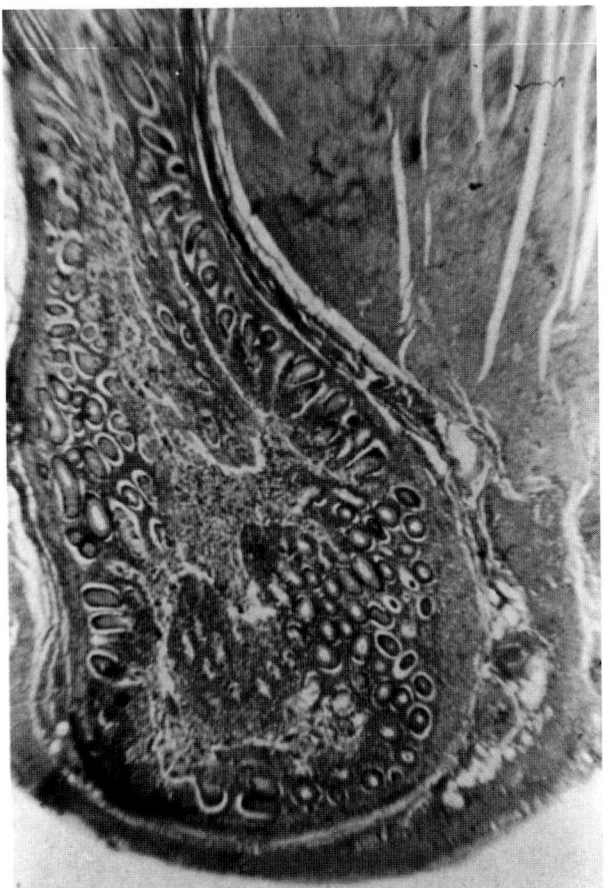

FIGURE 26-6. Diverticulum demonstrating only mucous membrane, muscularis mucosae, and peritoneum separating the lumen from the peritoneal cavity. (Original magnification × 80.)

cereal fiber consumption to as little as one tenth of that previously eaten.[181] Because of this very sudden change, within a matter of approximately 40 years diverticular disease has become epidemic.

Fiber increases stool weight, decreases whole-gut transit time, and lowers colonic intraluminal pressure.[58] A high-fiber diet produces a large, bulky stool that requires less "effort" by the bowel to propel the contents. Bran, for example, appears to increase the stool weight by virtue of its water-retentive properties. Bowel wall muscular hypertrophy does not occur, and segmentation is much less likely to develop. Transit time is considerably reduced, the consequences of which may in part explain the less frequent development of colon and rectal carcinoma in individuals who consume a high-fiber diet (see Chapter 22).

Burkitt and associates compared the transit times and stool weights of various ethnic groups.[42] They were particularly interested in the low incidence of colorectal disease in rural African natives. Ugandan villagers passed over 400 g of stool within 35 hours, whereas the shore-based United Kingdom naval personnel produced 100 g of constipated stool with a transit time of approximately 5 days.[180]

Gear and colleagues reported the results of barium enema examination in vegetarians and nonvegetarians.[85] The mean intake of dietary fiber was twice as great in the former group. Vegetarians were found to have a 12% incidence of diverticular disease, compared with a 33% incidence among nonvegetarians. Others have confirmed the importance of diet in the pathogenesis of diverticulosis.[100,152]

The evidence for the role of fiber in preventing diverticular disease is compelling. With economic development, affluence, and westernization of diet, an increased incidence of diverticular disease has been noted among native Africans.[253] Other studies have demonstrated an increased incidence in immigrants to Western countries from less developed nations in comparison with persons remaining in the country of origin. Finally, the addition of fiber has been shown to be effective in the treatment of many symptomatic patients with uncomplicated diverticular disease.[36,67,111,180,181]

The outer covering of any cereal grain, the bran, is a particularly rich source of fiber. Certain vegetables and fruits are also relatively high in fiber, whereas milk and milk products, chicken, fish, meat, eggs, fats, and beverages have no fiber. The vegetables highest in fiber content are the legumes. Enthusiasm for their consumption, however, is somewhat muted; daily consumption of beans can be rather tedious, and the troublesome consequence of flatulence is also a distinct disadvantage. Many people believe that by eating a salad each day they should be achieving adequate fiber intake. However, a whole head of lettuce is not quite the equivalent of one serving (one third of a cup) of a bran cereal in the amount of nonabsorbed fiber. Despite the availability of high-fiber foods, most people find them either unpalatable or intolerably repetitious.

An alternate approach is to employ one of a number of proprietary preparations, the so-called bulk laxatives. These are made from the outer covering of the psyllium grain or from sterculia- and ispaghula-derived hydrophilic colloids. There is, however, little proof correlating fiber values with their biologic effects. Over-the-counter preparations include Konsyl, Citrucel, FiberCon, Fiberall, and Metamucil. A daily whole-grain cereal or bran bread may become rather monotonous, but most people have a glass of juice in the morning. By adding one of the preparations to juice or a glass of water, once or twice daily, an effective fiber supplement to the diet may be achieved.

Age, Sex, and Heredity

Most studies report that diverticular disease is more common in women, the incidence increasing with advancing age.[184] Results of postmortem examinations usually place the frequency at about 50%.[184] However, the correlation between the incidence of the condition and the presence or duration of symptoms is less clear. For example, young men are more likely to require surgical intervention for complications than are elderly patients, some even during the initial attack.[80] Female patients tend to present about one half a decade after male patients with complications requiring surgery, according to the Mayo Clinic (Rochester, Minnesota) experience.[158] An inheritable tendency may also be a factor; resection has been performed for acute disease in identical twins.[81]

Relationship to Nonsteroidal Anti-inflammatory Drugs

Numerous studies have suggested an association between nonsteroidal anti-inflammatory drugs (NSAIDs) and the development of complications of diverticular disease.[43,166,269] Possible explanations include a direct effect on the bowel wall through inhibition of prostaglandin synthesis itself or the inhibitory effect of leukocyte function with failure of the immune system to localize the process. In case-control studies, it has been consistently found that more individuals with complicated diverticulitis were taking NSAIDs than were randomly selected other groups.[43,269] In addition to NSAIDs, opioid analgesics and corticosteroids are positively associated with the risk of complications in patients with diverticular disease.[166]

Immunocompromised State

An immunocompromised patient is predisposed to infection, and someone harboring diverticulosis is at an increased for the development of complicated diverticulitis. Such patients often mask typical symptoms and signs of an acute inflammatory processes of the abdomen. Patients with connective tissue disorders are often immunocompromised because of corticosteroids, but they appear to have an additional risk of complicated diverticulitis related to the underlying disorder (see later). Uncomplicated diverticular disease does not appear to be causally related to the immunocompromised condition.

Smoking and Alcohol

In a study reported by Papagrigoriadis and co-workers, smoking seemed to be an independent factor predisposing to the development of complications of diverticular disease.[183] This is counterintuitive in light of the fact that nicotine is a smooth muscle relaxant. It has also been shown that the risk of *diverticulitis* is significantly increased in patients with alcoholism.[251]

SYMPTOMS AND FINDINGS

Irritable Bowel Syndrome

The irritable bowel syndrome is estimated to affect up to one fourth of the population of Western countries. Unfortunately, the condition is not well understood, as implied in the discussion by Dr. Petrini in Chapter 3. Early writers on this subject shared three beliefs: first, the symptoms arise from the colon; second, the disorder is functional and not anatomically definable; and third, the basic abnormality lies within the nervous system.[48] It has been also found to be associated with depressive disorders, endocrine disease, food allergy, other neurologic disorders, and stress.

Most people who harbor diverticular disease do not have symptoms specifically related to the condition. This implies that surgical extirpation of the affected bowel will not necessarily ameliorate the patient's intestinal complaints. These individuals probably have the so-called irritable bowel syndrome. Other synonyms include functional gastrointestinal disorder, mucous colitis, psychophysiologic gastrointestinal disturbance, splenic flexure syndrome, and spastic colon. Persons with irritable bowel symptoms constitute the vast majority of patients seen by gastroenterologists. The condition is also the single most common reason for referral reported by major medical clinics. In England, one fifth of a sample from the general population had experienced abdominal pain more than six times in 1 year.[142] Approximately one fourth of a similar sample in the United States reported abdominal pain more than six times in that year.[142]

Fundamentally, the diagnosis of irritable bowel syndrome is a diagnosis of exclusion. Diagnostic criteria include the continuous or recurrent presence of the following symptoms for at least 3 months:[263]

- Abdominal pain relieved by defecation or associated with a change in frequency or consistency of stool
- Disturbed defecation at least 25% of the time and three or more of the following:
- Altered stool frequency
- Altered stool form
- Altered stool passage (straining, urgency, or tenesmus)
- Passage of mucus
- Abdominal distension

The term *irritable bowel syndrome* suggests that these patients have an abnormality in the intestine, but the symptoms can develop without any anatomic defect and certainly in the absence of diverticulosis. It is important to recognize the distinction between the two often concurrent conditions. The problem is to differentiate between those individuals who harbor diverticula and whose symptoms are related to the presence of this anatomic abnormality and those whose symptoms are unrelated (Figs. 26-7 and 26-8). In a study of 88 patients with irritable bowel syndrome, Havia and Manner found that colonic diverticula developed in 24%.[99] Ritchie found that a high proportion of patients with irritable bowel syndrome had a lower threshold for pain when the colon was distended with a balloon, similar to that observed in individuals who had diverticular disease.[213]

Patients with an irritable bowel syndrome may experience altered bowel function with or without abdominal pain. The pain often varies in severity and duration. It may be colicky in nature and related to defecation, to the passage of gas, or to a host of nonspecific gastrointestinal complaints (e.g., heartburn, indigestion, bloating, and nausea). Commonly, a history of stress is often noted. Conspicuous by their absence are fever, leukocytosis, and signs of peritoneal irritation. However, abdominal tenderness and even the suggestion of fullness or a mass in the left lower quadrant may be evident. Gastrointestinal evaluation by means of contrast studies and endoscopy may reveal no abnormality, but many patients are found to have diverticulosis coincidentally with or without evidence of "bowel spasm." The regimen for therapy often includes dietary modification, antidiarrheal medication (if appropriate), anticholinergics, and possibly antianxiety compounds.

Diverticulitis

Symptoms

Patients with diverticulitis complain primarily of abdominal pain. The pain is usually located in the left lower quadrant and tends to be constant rather than colicky in nature. The pain may radiate to the back, left flank, groin, and leg, although these observations may also be seen with an irritable bowel. The duration and severity of symptoms are quite variable, depending on whether the patient has a localized or diffuse process. Nausea and vomiting are uncommon complaints unless there is some element of intestinal obstruction. A change in bowel habits is frequently observed; there may be an absence of bowel movements or the patient may experience diarrhea.

Patients with acute diverticular disease often mention urinary problems (dysuria, urgency, frequency, nocturia), which may be attributable to impingement of the inflammatory mass on the wall of the bladder. A urinary tract infection may imply communication with the bowel (see later). Passage of gas in the urine or through the vagina is diagnostic of a fistula (see later).

Fever is also commonly observed in patients with acute diverticulitis. This is usually of a low grade, but if peritonitis develops or if an abscess is present, the temperature can be considerably elevated.

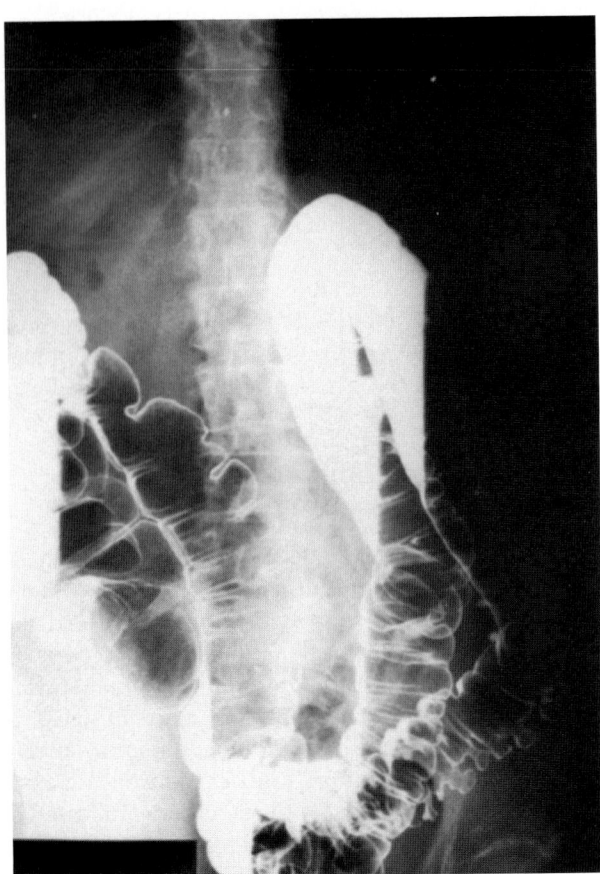

FIGURE 26-7. Air-contrast barium enema demonstrates extensive sigmoid diverticulosis without colonic narrowing. The patient's abdominal complaint is unlikely to be relieved by resection.

Rectal bleeding has been thought to be part of the symptom complex of diverticulosis, but there is confusion on this issue. Massive lower gastrointestinal bleeding in the presence of diverticular disease can be caused by a vascular malformation rather than diverticulosis, but there is evidence to suggest that some patients do bleed from diverticular disease.[33] Still, there is no inflammation or infection with this manifestation of the condition. This aspect of the presentation is discussed in Chapter 28.

Physical Examination

Physical examination may reveal tenderness, voluntary guarding, and, in the presence of peritonitis, absent bowel sounds, a boardlike abdomen, and all the signs and symptoms of an acute abdominal catastrophe. Tenderness and a mass in the pelvis from a sigmoid phlegmon may be noted on rectal or vaginal examination. An abdominal mass may be felt. Extraperitoneal infection can present with back, buttock, and hip and leg pain; a positive psoas sign; a lower extremity abscess;[44] perineal and

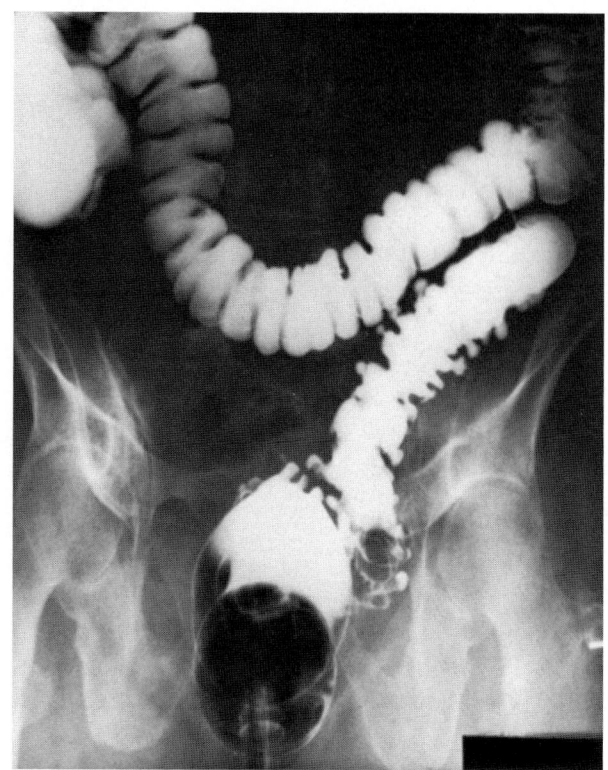

FIGURE 26-8. Extensive sigmoid diverticular disease with slight spasm but no stigmata of acute inflammation. In the absence of classic symptoms and signs of diverticulitis, surgery is not advised solely on the basis of this radiographic appearance.

scrotal pain and swelling; and subcutaneous, mediastinal, and cervical emphysema.[203] Perforation below the peritoneal reflection can lead to a buttock abscess and a consequent anorectal fistula (see Chapters 10 and 11).[65] Pathways of extraperitoneal pelvic abscess spread to the gluteal area are through the suprapiriformis and infrapiriformis fossae, to the external genitalia via the obturator canal, and to the ischiorectal fossa through the pelvic floor.[203]

Endoscopy

There is some controversy about whether endoscopy should be performed in the presence of acute inflammation (see Chapter 5). There is a risk of disturbing a walled-off perforation with the instrument itself or, more likely, by the insufflation of air. Proctosigmoidoscopic examination is usually quite limited because of tenderness and because of the presence of the mass. Negotiation of the rectosigmoid is usually impossible with a rigid instrument in the acute situation. Although rigid proctosigmoidoscopy can be carried out with minimal use of air, considerable caution should be exercised with air insufflation when the flexible instrument is em-

ployed. There is a far greater likelihood of injuring an acutely inflamed bowel with flexible sigmoidoscopy or colonoscopy. Alternatively, direct visualization may be helpful if one is to distinguish between diverticulitis and other pathologic conditions (e.g., ischemic colitis, carcinoma, inflammatory bowel disease; see later). As is often the case, the surgeon must weigh the risk of the procedure against the potential benefit of the information gleaned.

Contrast Studies

Despite the overwhelming propensity for physicians, especially gastroenterologists, to "throw" the colonoscope in anyone who harbors a large bowel, the most valuable study for evaluating patients with diverticular disease is the barium enema examination (see Figs. 26-9 through 26-19). Barium enema can demonstrate extrinsic compression, narrowing, redundancy, tethered mucosa, and, of course, the extent of diverticulosis and diverticulitis. Preservation of the mucosa is the single most important criterion for differentiating the condition from that of a malignant process. In the acute situation, however, this investigation should not be performed, at least not with barium. Should a perforation be present or should one be created by the instillation of barium, barium peritonitis, an often fatal complication, may result (see Chapter 4). If there is any concern about the presence of an acute process, a gentle, water-soluble enema (e.g., Gastrografin) should be used. The major limitation of a contrast enema is that an abscess itself is unlikely to be demonstrated. Obviously, no therapeutic possibility exists with this technique either. However, in a study of 71 patients admitted with left lower quadrant peritonitis, Wexner and Dailey reported that the early use of this study was the most accurate and the most cost-effective means for establishing the diagnosis.[266]

Computed Tomography

As mentioned earlier, the barium enema or air-contrast enema has been the standard radiographic study for establishing the diagnosis of colonic diverticular disease. However, numerous articles today stipulate that computed tomography (CT) should be the initial imaging technique, because of more accurate diagnosis, earlier identification of complications, the superior definition of bowel wall thickness, and the extent of extraluminal disease—that is, the question whether there is an abscess present (Figure 26-20).[11,35,110,115,144,167,195]

Labs and colleagues evaluated 42 patients by means of CT.[133] All those with abscesses at operation were diagnosed by CT through the triad of diverticula, a segmen-

(text continues on page 1182)

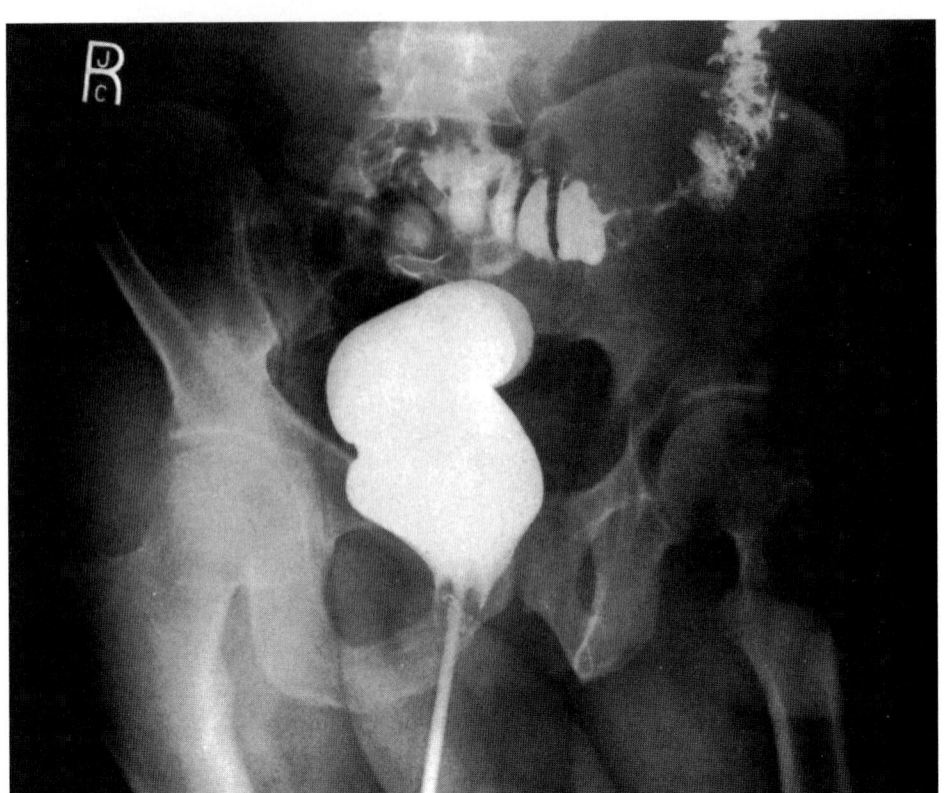

FIGURE 26-9. Sigmoid diverticulitis. Proximal sigmoid stricture with intact mucosa.

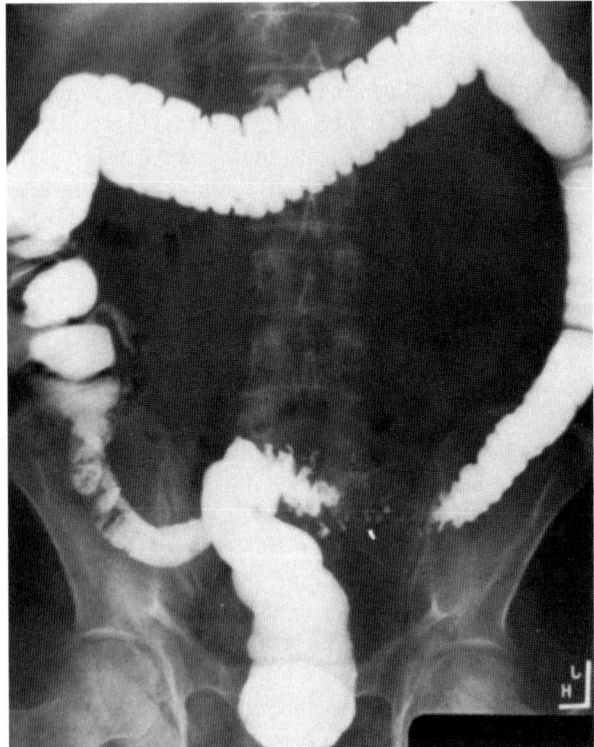

FIGURE 26-10. Sigmoid diverticulitis. A mass containing multiple diverticula with preservation of mucosa.

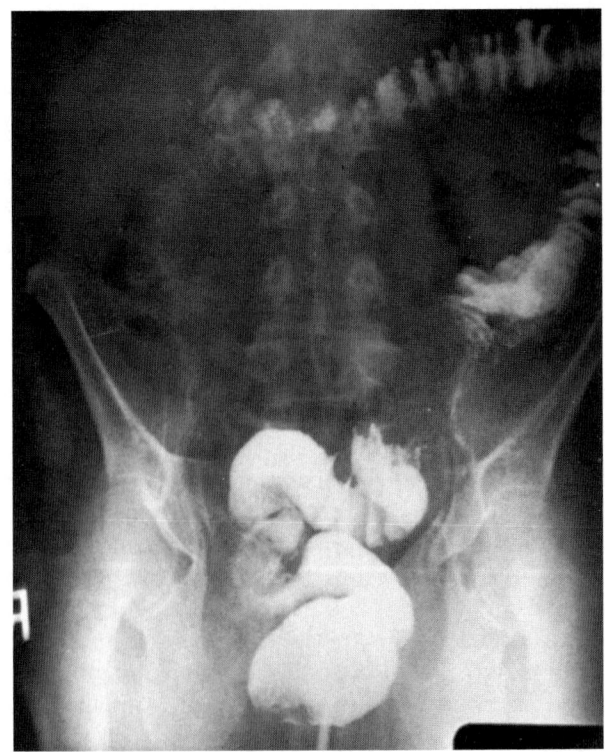

FIGURE 26-11. Sigmoid diverticulitis. A large mass with suggestive "overhanging" margins but with normal mucosa.

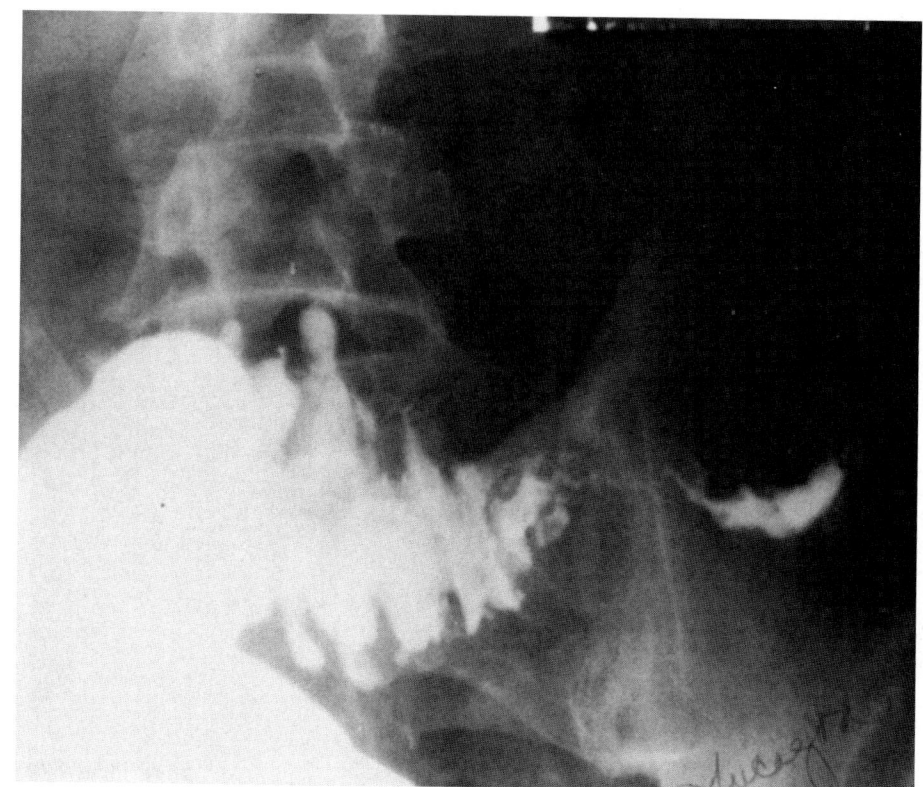

FIGURE 26-12. Sigmoid diverticulitis. Presumed mucosal preservation in an inadequately studied colon.

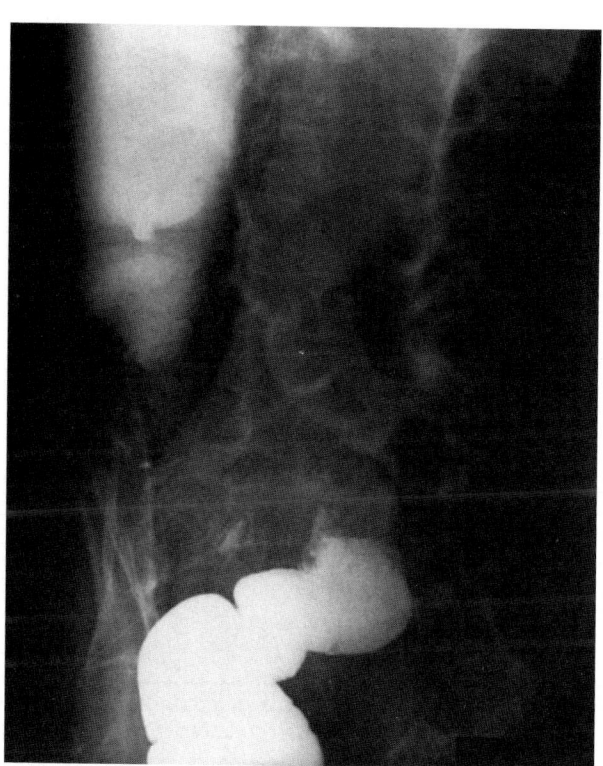

FIGURE 26-13. Sigmoid colon obstruction. Differential diagnosis between carcinoma and diverticulitis is impossible. The lesion eventually proved to be diverticulitis.

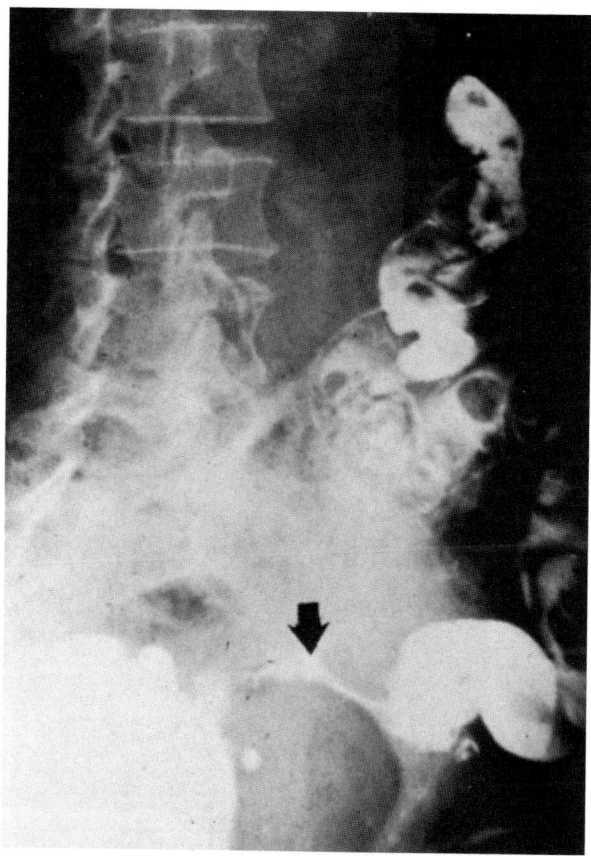

FIGURE 26-14. Sigmoid diverticulitis. The long stricture (arrow) is more consistent with inflammatory change than with neoplasm.

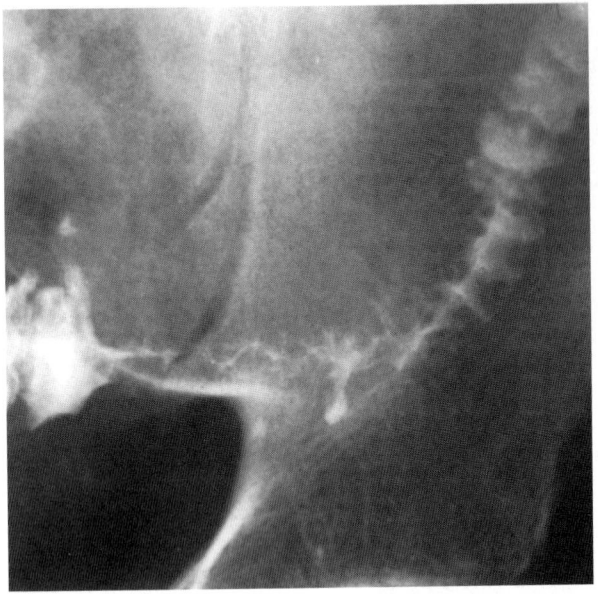

FIGURE 26-15. Typical long stricture of sigmoid colon with edematous mucosa, consistent with diverticulitis.

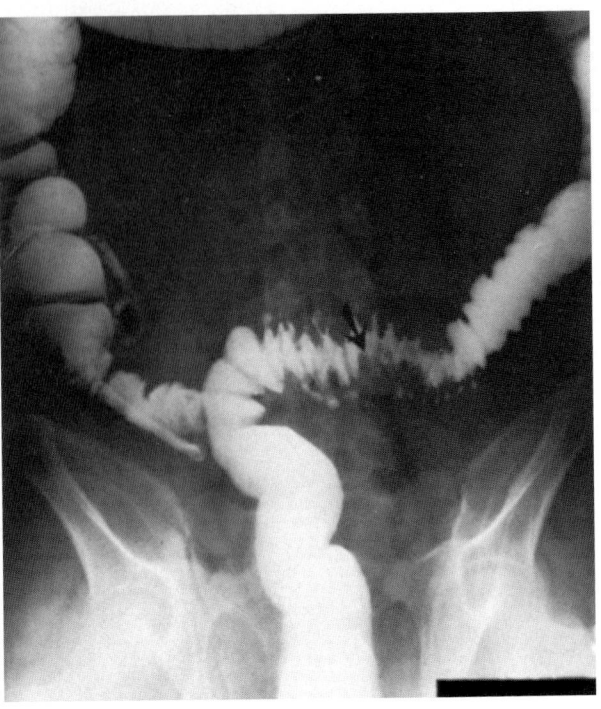

FIGURE 26-17. Sigmoid diverticulitis. An irregular mass in the wall of the bowel *(arrow)* with extensive associated diverticulosis and with mucosal preservation.

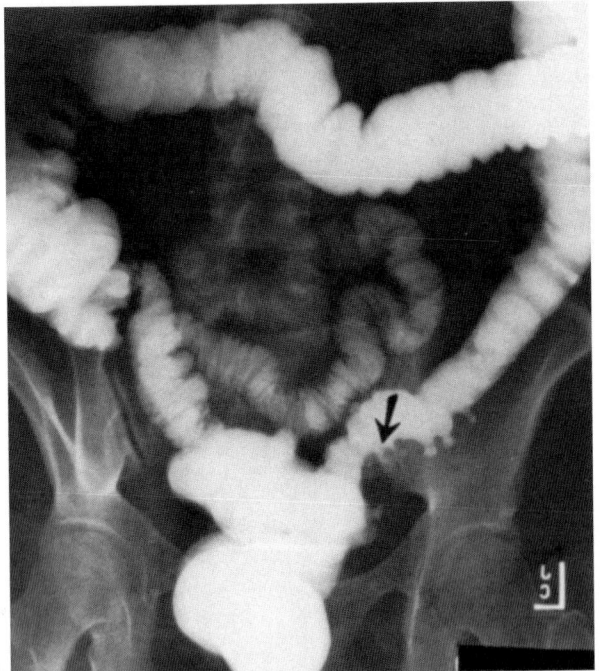

FIGURE 26-16. Sigmoid diverticulitis. Intramural abscess *(arrow)* of the proximal sigmoid with intact mucosa.

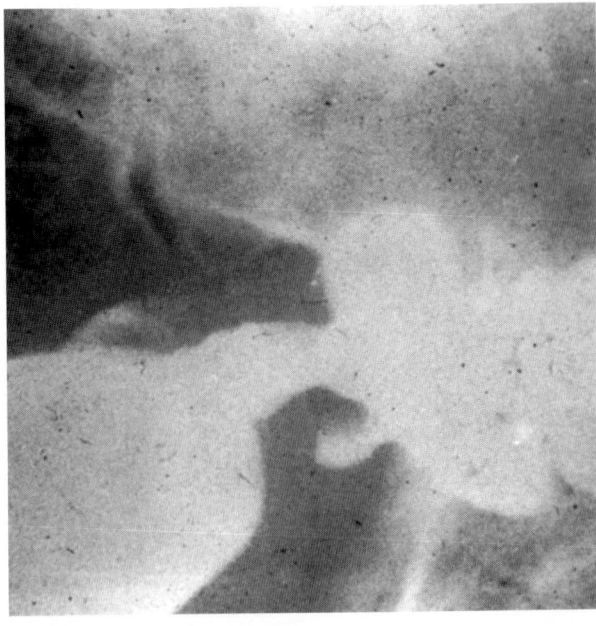

FIGURE 26-18. Carcinoma of the sigmoid. Pseudodiverticula or even true diverticula may be frequently associated with cancer of the sigmoid colon.

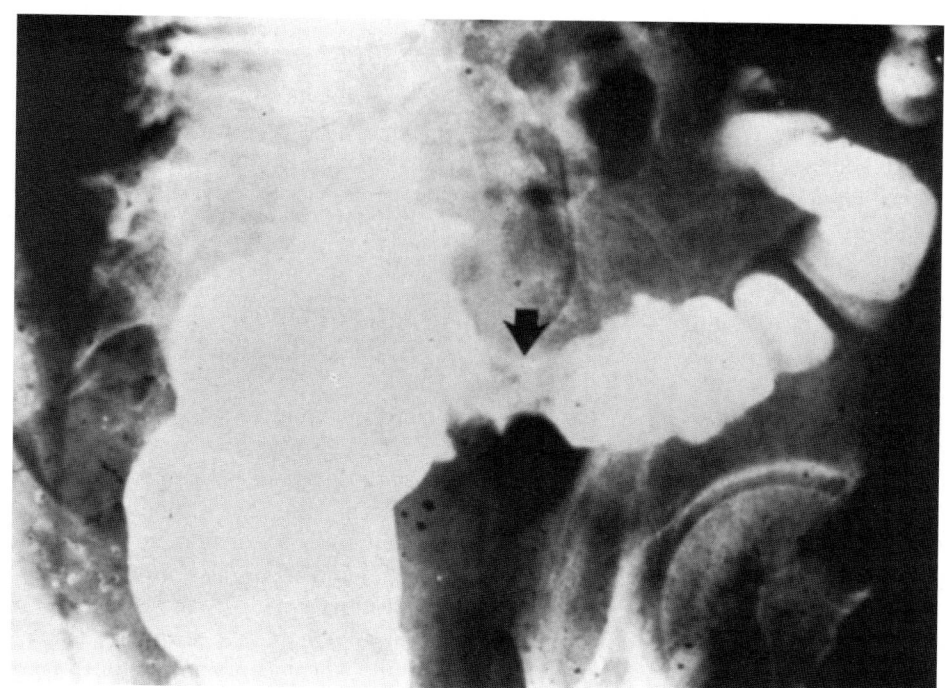

FIGURE 26-19. Sigmoid diverticulitis. An apparent "napkin ring" lesion, overhanging margins, and mucosal irregularity. The lesion proved to be benign.

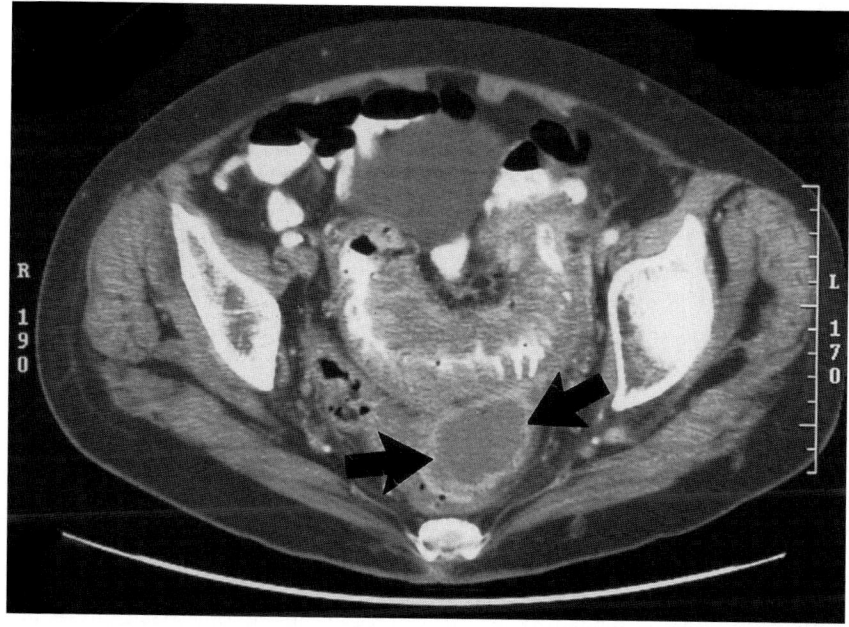

FIGURE 26-20. Computed tomography demonstrating classic findings of acute sigmoid diverticulitis with bowel wall thickening, extensive diverticular outpouchings, narrowing of the lumen, and an abscess *(arrows)*.

tally thickened colon, and extravisceral fluid collection. Only 25% of those studied by contrast enema were thought to have abscesses. Additionally, in 11 of 12 individuals, colovesical fistula was confirmed through CT by the identification of air in the bladder, thickened colon adjacent to an area of thickened bladder, and the presence of colonic diverticula. Contrast enema identified only three of eight cases. Raval and co-workers recommend that CT be performed with the administration of a rectal contrast medium to demonstrate the origin of the colonic inflammation, to assess pericolic extent, and to confirm the presence or absence of a colovesical fistula.[199] Ambrosetti and associates compared the performance of water-soluble contrast enema with CT in 420 patients who underwent both studies.[11] CT was significantly superior both in terms of sensitivity and evaluation of severity. For example, only 29% had indirect signs of an associated abscess when it had been demonstrated on CT. CT has also been thought to be particularly valuable in the diagnosis of right-sided diverticulitis.[60]

CT is obviously a useful study, not only as a diagnostic but also as a therapeutic modality, through the application of CT-guided drainage (see later). However, most clinicians and radiologists are of the opinion that in the elective situation especially, barium enema is more likely to yield a specific diagnosis.[115,235,236] Therefore, the contrast enema should probably remain the initial "routine" examination, and CT should be reserved for those individuals who should not or cannot undergo an adequate contrast enema examination, who are suspected of having an abdominal abscess, who are unresponsive to medical therapy, or who are potential candidates for percutaneous drainage.[115]

Ultrasonography

Schwerk and colleagues evaluated high-resolution real-time ultrasonography in the diagnosis of acute and complicated colonic diverticulitis in 130 patients.[230] The diagnosis was established with an overall accuracy of 97.7%, a sensitivity of 98.1%, and a specificity of 97.5%. The authors describe the echomorphologic features of acute diverticulitis as follows: hypoechogenic thickening of the bowel wall and a targetlike appearance in transverse view attributable to inflammatory changes and muscular thickening. They are of the opinion that sonography with compression is highly sensitive and specific for the imaging diagnosis of acute diverticulitis with or without abscess.[230] A hemispheric mass, the "dome sign," has also been described.[125] Unfortunately, the examination in the acutely tender patient is extremely uncomfortable and may not be possible. Zielke and co-workers prospectively observed 143 unselected consecutive patients with sus-

pected acute colonic diverticulitis, excluding those with generalized peritonitis.[273] Of those with proven diverticulitis, the diagnosis was made ultrasonographically in 88%, with an 84% sensitivity. The authors concluded that ultrasonography is especially helpful when the clinical findings are equivocal.

MEDICAL MANAGEMENT OF ACUTE DIVERTICULAR DISEASE

As has been discussed in prior chapters, the American Society of Colon and Rectal Surgeons established a Standards Task Force for the purpose of identifying guidelines in the management of a number of conditions. Such "parameters" have been produced for sigmoid diverticulitis.[241] I believe that the following discussion, for both the medical and surgical management of the condition, is consistent with these guidelines. The reader is encouraged to peruse the supporting documentation for the recommendations in accordance with the reference provided.[241]

Patients who present with tenderness and the suggestion of a sausage-like mass in the left lower quadrant can, in the absence of systemic signs and symptoms, be initially treated on an outpatient basis. A low-residue diet is suggested during the acute phase of the illness. It may be preferable to place the bowel at relative rest until such time as the inflammatory process has resolved. In the opinion of some physicians, outpatient treatment should consist of an even more restricted diet, allowing clear liquids only. Seven to 10 days of orally administered broad-spectrum antibiotics are recommended. This should cover aerobic and anaerobic organisms, such as *Bacteroides fragilis*, *Clostridium*, *Escherichia coli*, *Klebsiella*, *Proteus*, *Streptococcus*, and *Enterobacter*.

One popular antibiotic regimen is a combination of ciprofloxacin and metronidazole. If the symptoms continue to improve, elective evaluation is undertaken when the acute process has resolved. If the patient's symptoms fail to improve, inpatient therapy is recommended.

For a person who has more severe abdominal signs and symptoms, has pyrexia, is immunocompromised, or appears systemically ill, hospitalization is indicated. Medical management includes the usual supportive measures. No oral intake is advised unless the patient's symptoms fail to suggest the need for imminent operation. Under such circumstances, clear liquids are permitted. It is usually unnecessary to employ a nasogastric tube unless intestinal obstruction or vomiting is evident. In the inpatient setting, antibiotics are administered systemically. As the symptoms improve, a progressive diet is instituted, supplemented by a stool softener. Although the observed hypermotility of the sigmoid colon in many symptomatic patients with diverticular disease provides a rationale for the use of anticholinergic drugs, their efficacy has never been clearly documented.[9] Personally, I have not found them helpful; hence, I do not employ them in the medical management of the resolving acute inflammatory condition. With aggressive medical management, the patient's symptoms should improve considerably within 24 to 48 hours. As long as consistent improvement is observed, investigation may be deferred until the acute process has largely resolved, but it is the unusual situation today wherein one is admitted to the hospital with a presumptive diagnosis of acute diverticulitis who will not rapidly undergo CT.

Schechter and associates conducted a survey of fellows of the American Society of Colon and Rectal Surgeons to document medical treatment preferences for patients with uncomplicated acute diverticulitis.[226] There were 373 responders. The most common single antibiotic regimens were either a second generation cephalosporin (27%) or ampicillin/sulbactam (16%). The most frequently employed combination was ciprofloxacin/metronidazole (28%). Upon discharge, 74% prescribed oral antibiotics for 7 to 10 days. Interestingly, dietary recommendations included low residue (68%), regular (21%), and high residue (10%). Clearly, there is an enormous variation in the medical management of diverticulitis among colon and rectal surgeons in the United States.

The duration and nature of symptoms have an important bearing on the outcome of the disease. Parks noted that one half of the patients with diverticular disease of the colon were in good health until less than 1 month before hospitalization, and three fourths had symptoms for less than 1 year.[184] Individuals with some of the most serious complications were essentially asymptomatic until just before admission. One may therefore postulate on the basis of the patient's history what the likelihood of resolution will be with medical management.

DIFFERENTIAL DIAGNOSIS

Carcinoma

The most important aspect of the differential diagnosis, and the reason for examining the bowel, is the possible identification of a cancer as the cause of the patient's symptoms. If a carcinoma is present, surgical intervention will be required within a relatively short period of time, irrespective of the fact that the symptoms may not have completely resolved. Conversely, if one is satisfied that the patient's findings are a result of diverticulitis, surgery may be delayed for as long as the clinical condition improves. Unfortunately, differentiation between sigmoid diverticulitis and carcinoma is not always possible. In a study by Parks and co-workers, the traditional criteria employed for radiographic differential diagnosis were applied by three independent radiologists, assessing the studies of 40 patients.[187] All three agreed in only 15 instances.

The *sine qua non* for distinguishing the two conditions is the presence of intact colonic mucosa (Figs. 26-9 through 26-11). In my opinion, this is the most valuable radiologic finding for permitting differentiation. It is extremely important, therefore, to fill the bowel lumen on both sides of the stricture, but this may not always be possible if significant sigmoid narrowing is present. Whereas the radiograph shown in Figure 26-12 probably reveals a normal mucosa despite inadequate proximal filling, that shown in Figure 26-13 precludes the possibility of an accurate diagnosis.

The length of the narrowed segment has also been believed to be a helpful differential diagnostic radiologic finding. In patients with carcinoma, the stricture is usually quite short, whereas with diverticulitis, strictures usually tend to be longer (Figure 26-14). One should not, however, place a great deal of credence on the accuracy of this particular radiologic observation, although the combination of a long, narrowed segment with an intact mucosa is quite reassuring (Figure 26-15).

The presence of a mass in the wall of the bowel with the mucosa intact is a third diagnostic point consistent with diverticulitis. An intramural or mesenteric abscess is the most common complication of diverticular disease (Figs. 26-16 and 26-17).

The presence of associated diverticula within or around the segment of narrowing has also been thought to be reasonable circumstantial evidence for the presence of benign disease. However, because carcinoma of the colon and diverticular disease are frequently seen concurrently, too much emphasis should not be placed on this finding. Figure 26-18 illustrates a diverticulum within a segment of narrowing that proved to be a carcinoma. Pseudodiverticula can result from deformity produced by invasive cancer, and overhanging margins are highly suggestive. However, none of the observations described is infallible for establishing the diagnosis. For example, in Figure 26-19, overhanging edges and mucosal destruction are clearly apparent. Following resection, pathologic evaluation revealed this to be sigmoid diverticulitis.

As previously mentioned, flexible sigmoidoscopy and colonoscopy may be usefully employed to differentiate between diverticulitis and carcinoma. The problem, however, is to negotiate the sigmoid colon satisfactorily without causing a perforation in the acute situation. Even in the noninflamed bowel, the sigmoid colon may be quite narrow because of thickening of the muscularis propria. The surgeon can feel assured only if the entire mucosa has been visualized and appears intact. Erythema and edema of the bowel wall may be seen, and occasionally pus may be observed to exude from one of the orifices.

Numerous studies have been published advocating colonoscopy as an effective tool in the differentiation of carcinoma and diverticulitis.[62,77,154,268] However, the risk of injury from the instrument itself is only one problem. Less obvious is the hidden hazard of air pressure causing overt perforation through a thin-walled diverticulum or walled-off abscess.[268] For these reasons, only the most courageous or foolhardy of endoscopists would embark upon this procedure in an acutely ill patient. Examination under such circumstances is probably contraindicated, but as the individual's symptoms improve, endoscopic evaluation should be considered if the differential diagnosis is still in question.

Dean and Newell reported 36 patients in whom barium enema examination had suggested the possibility of carcinoma in a segment of diverticular disease.[62] All were examined at least 6 weeks following an acute exacerbation of the condition. The authors found that the procedure was particularly difficult to perform, having failed to visualize the diseased segment in approximately one half of the cases. However, they were able through colonoscopy to establish the diagnosis of carcinoma in four patients and to exclude it in five. Max and Knutson performed colonoscopic evaluation of 26 patients in whom radiologic examination disclosed an area of spasm or diverticulitis that raised a suspicion of carcinoma.[154] In 19, the questionable area was completely visualized, and in every individual successfully examined the diagnosis was proved correct. Another, albeit somewhat theoretical, concern is the development of adenocarcinoma within a colonic diverticulum. Such a presentation is extremely rare. Because of herniation of the mucosa through the muscular coat of the diverticulum, a cancer arising in this area may actually penetrate the serosa.[52] The obvious consequence is that medical attention may not be obtained until perforation has occurred. How one can make the diagnosis preoperatively in a relatively early lesion is problematic at best.

Contrast enema remains the primary diagnostic study for differentiating perforating carcinoma from diverticulitis, but what can CT accomplish in this regard? Signs of localized wall thickening, increased soft tissue density in the pericolic fat, and large soft tissue masses related to diverticulitis are helpful,[144,195] but perforated carcinoma may exhibit the same changes on CT. The latter study may be preferable for demonstrating the extent of the pericolic inflammation or mass, an issue that is generally underestimated with a contrast enema, but the critical question remains whether this is sufficiently diagnostic to exclude cancer. One would think not. Some investigators have confirmed the value of CT in identifying intraabdominal abscess and phlegmon, bladder wall thickening and edema, and extracolonic extension, as well as relatively subtle features suggestive of diverticulitis,[167,195] but the decision for or against surgical intervention will in all probability be based on clinical grounds. It is unlikely that a perforating cancer will respond to nonoperative management. However, even when surgery is undertaken, especially in this acute circumstance, it may not be possible to distinguish tumor from inflammation at the operating table (see later discussion).

Polyps

There has been some concern about the differential diagnosis between sigmoid diverticulosis and a concomitant polyp. The "bowler hat" sign is the well-known appearance of a colonic polyp seen *en face* at a certain degree of obliquity on a double-contrast barium enema study.[163] The bowler hat is produced by a ring of barium along the base of the polyp and a second curvilinear collection of barium along the dome of the polyp. Miller and colleagues described a principle for evaluating this sign in order to determine whether it is caused by a polyp or a diverticulum.[163] They stated that if the bowler hat points toward the center of the long axis of the bowel, it represents an intraluminal structure (i.e., a polyp). If, however, it points away from the center of the long axis of the bowel, it represents a diverticulum. My own feeling is that if there is no active inflammation, I would feel much more comfortable performing an endoscopy to be certain what the true nature of the lesion is.

Other Diseases

Without a doubt, the most important differential diagnostic concern, and the one that presents the most difficulty, is that of carcinoma. Other diseases, however, can demonstrate signs, symptoms, and findings that may mimic diverticulitis. These include Crohn's disease, ulcerative colitis, acute appendicitis, ischemic colitis, pelvic inflammatory disease, and conditions affecting the urinary tract (e.g., infection and nephrolithiasis).

Crohn's Disease

It is sometimes quite difficult to differentiate Crohn's disease from diverticulitis. There are several symptoms, however, that may lead the surgeon to suspect the possibility of the former, especially if the patient complains of diarrhea and rectal bleeding. The presence of anal inflammation (e.g., fissure or fistula) is also suggestive of Crohn's disease (see Chapters 11 and 30). Sigmoidoscopic examination reveals a normal rectum in diverticulitis, whereas with Crohn's disease, the rectum may or may not be spared. At the time of laparotomy, it may still be impossible to distinguish between the two conditions, even if the resected specimen is opened. Usually, however, with diverticulitis the mucosal surface, although edematous, is otherwise normal. Evidence of granularity or ulceration is indicative of inflammatory bowel disease. If a frozen-section examination is performed, the presence of granulomas does not necessarily indicate Crohn's disease, because foreign body giant cells as a reaction to pericolonic abscess can be seen with diverticulitis.[169]

We reported our experience with 25 patients who required colonic resection for "diverticulitis" a second time; all eventually proved to have Crohn's disease.[26] In many instances, the diagnosis of Crohn's colitis was suspected, but not until after a subsequent resection with histopathologic confirmation was provided. Symptoms and signs of recurrent illness were similar to those present when the patient was initially seen, that is, before the first operation. In these individuals, there was often a history of smoldering illness, in contrast to the more episodic nature of the symptoms in patients with diverticulitis. Age was not particularly helpful in distinguishing the two conditions, because, in the older age group especially, Crohn's disease often tends to involve the large rather than the small bowel. The presence of extracolonic manifestations (e.g., pyoderma, arthritis), unusual technical difficulty in performing the resection, and failure of decompression to result in resolution of the colonic inflammatory process should lead the surgeon to suspect Crohn's disease.

Ulcerative Colitis

The distinction between acute diverticulitis and a complication of ulcerative colitis should not be difficult. Proctosigmoidoscopic examination virtually always reveals disease in the rectum in patients with ulcerative colitis (see Chapter 29). However, the rectum is spared with diverticulitis. Although the two conditions can occasionally coexist, it is difficult to imagine how one may be able to distinguish acute diverticulitis superimposed on acute ulcerative colitis. The importance of performing even a limited sigmoidoscopic examination before embarking on surgery for acute diverticulitis cannot be overestimated. The presence of inflammatory changes in the rectum or a high index of suspicion of inflammatory bowel disease

would certainly dictate different medical management or an alternative operative approach.

Ischemic Colitis

Ischemic colitis may pose a problem in differential diagnosis. This is particularly true if the ischemic changes include the rectosigmoid. However, patients who have disease limited to this location usually present with frequent bowel movements and rectal bleeding. Abdominal pain is suggestive of a more fulminant manifestation and a more extensive one. The presence of thumbprinting on the plain abdominal film and involvement of the region of the splenic flexure in the process suggest ischemia (see Chapter 28).

COMPLICATIONS

Free Perforation

Free perforation with generalized peritonitis is an uncommon complication of diverticulitis. When it occurs, it can have catastrophic consequences. Patients are critically ill and demonstrate the usual signs and symptoms of septicemia. The history may be one of a rather sudden onset of abdominal pain, usually in the lower abdomen, progressing to generalized involvement. Marked abdominal distension may be noted, caused by pneumoperitoneum (Figure 26-21). Abdominal rigidity is usually observed. An upright film of the abdomen or a lateral decubitus x-ray film will reveal the presence of free gas (Figure 26-22). It has been suggested that the amount of gas present on the roentgenogram will help the surgeon to determine whether it is a colonic or gastroduodenal perforation: the more gas present, the greater the likelihood of a colonic perforation. This may be a useful distinguishing feature in determining the area where the incision should be made. CT may also demonstrate a perforation or free gas in the peritoneal cavity (Figs. 26-23 and 26-24).

Phlegmon or Abscess

The most common complication of sigmoid diverticulitis is a walled-off perforation or abscess; the acute inflammatory reaction usually involves the sigmoid colon and its mesentery. Signs and symptoms are most often confined to the left lower quadrant of the abdomen. Varying degrees of peritoneal irritation may be manifested. Contrast radiologic evaluation may reveal the changes previously described, but in addition there may be tracking of the barium into other areas. The barium may fill an ab-

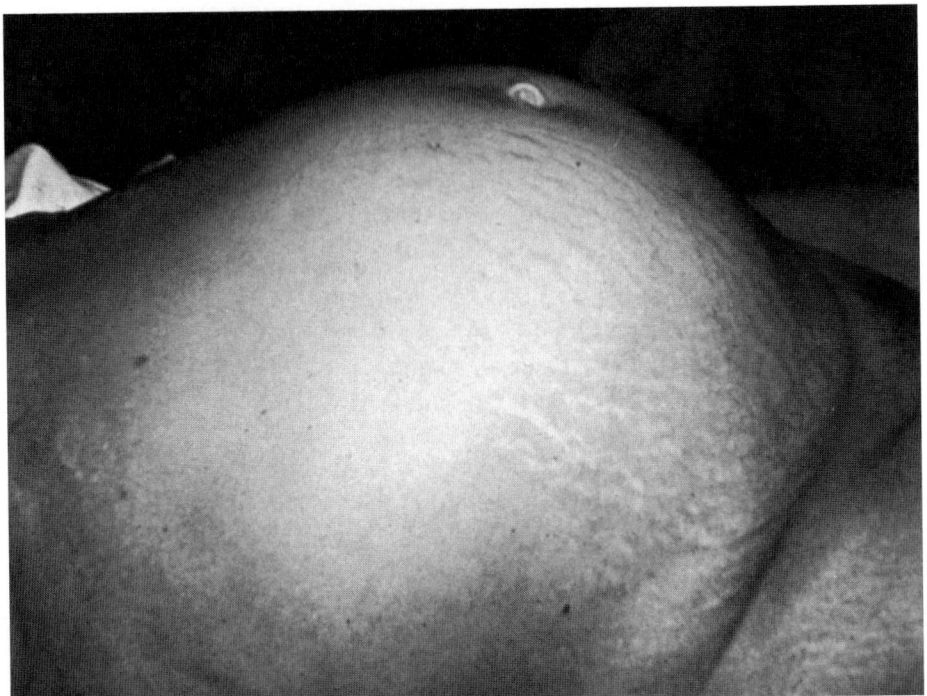

FIGURE 26-21. Free colonic perforation with pneumoperitoneum producing profound abdominal distension.

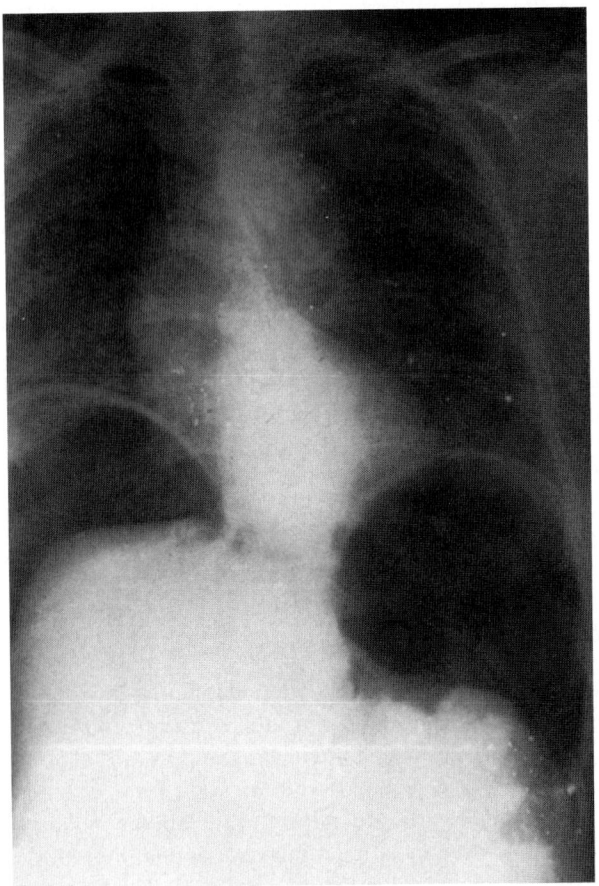

FIGURE 26-22. Upright abdominal roentgenogram reveals free gas under both hemidiaphragms. Perforation of the colon secondary to diverticulitis was found.

scess cavity adjacent to the perforation (Figure 26-25), track down into the pelvis to present as an ischiorectal abscess (Figure 26-26), lead to a pelvic abscess with consequent rectal narrowing and deviation (Figs. 26-27 and 26-28), perforate into the abdominal wall (Figure 26-29), or track into quite distant areas, such as the hip joints or thigh (Figure 26-30; see later). CT, however, is the "gold standard" radiologic study for evaluating patients with acute diverticulitis.

Whereas surgical intervention in a case of free perforation is mandatory and a decision easily reached, this is not necessarily true of the patient with an acute phlegmonous diverticulitis or localized abscess. The medical measures previously mentioned are usually instituted, but in patients who continue to have pain, fever, white blood cell count elevation, or failure to tolerate oral alimentation, the surgeon should suspect the presence of an abscess.

Computed Tomography–Guided Percutaneous Drainage

Patients who fail to respond despite vigorous medical management or who are found on the basis of contrast studies, ultrasonography, or CT to have a localized abscess, should be considered for CT-guided percutaneous drainage of the septic process.[71,92,170,174,219] Success depends on the ability to find a safe, direct route to the abscess cavity (Figure 26-31). Pelvic and intra-abdominal abscesses usually require a staged surgical

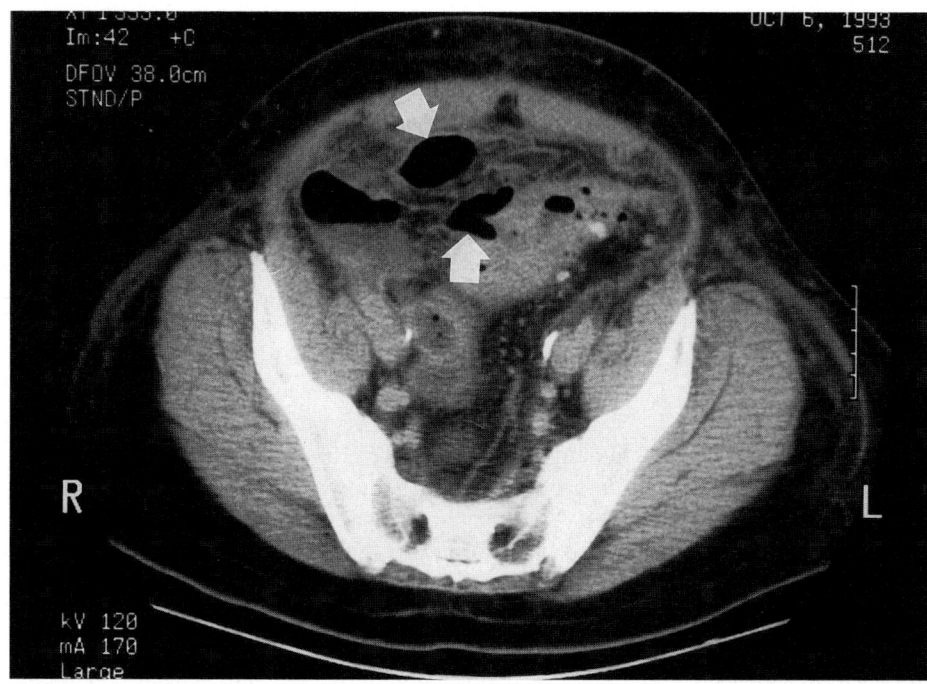

FIGURE 26-23. Computed tomography demonstrates perforated diverticulitis with extraluminal gas *(arrows)*.

procedure if initial percutaneous drainage cannot be performed successfully.

Mueller and colleagues reported that 14 of 24 patients who underwent such a drainage procedure proceeded to a single-stage resection within 10 days.[170] Brolin and associates suggest that patients with persistent leukocytosis or fever at 4 days after drainage should be reevaluated by CT or ultrasonography and considered for either re-

peated drainage (if appropriate) or laparotomy.[37] Stabile and co-workers reported the following follow-up statistics on their 19 patients who underwent drainage: complications (0%); persistent fever and leukocytosis (11%); colonic fistula on sinogram (47%); completed treatment with elective, one-stage colectomy (74%).[240] Ambrosetti and co-workers suggest that mesocolic abscesses can usually be managed without drainage.[12]

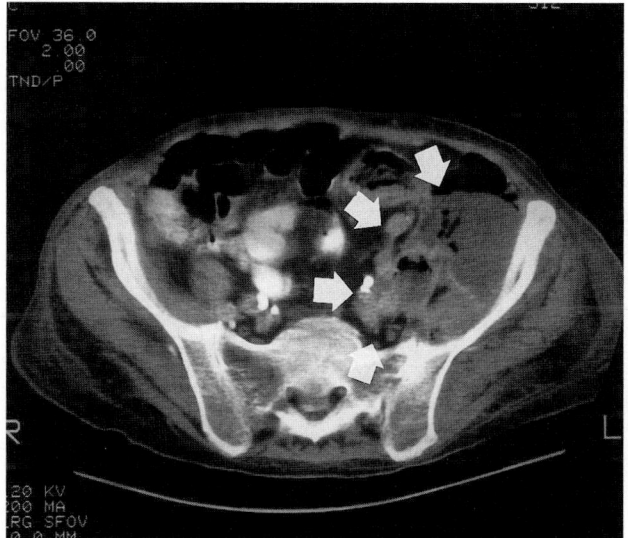

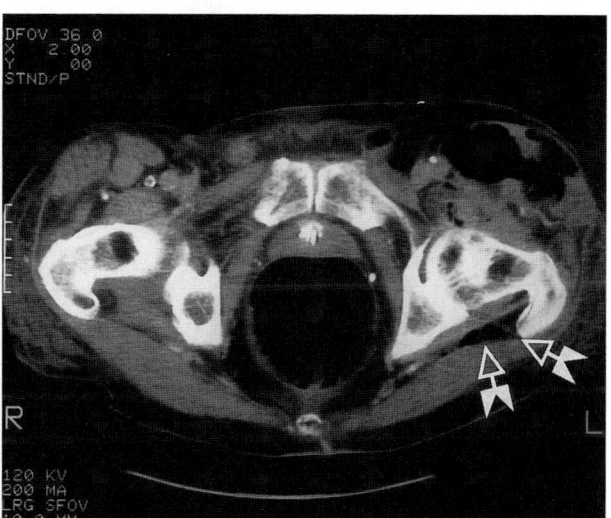

A   B

FIGURE 26-24. Perforated diverticulitis. Computed tomography demonstrates **(A)** a large fluid collection with gas involving the iliopsoas muscle *(arrows)*, representing a large abscess. **(B)** An inferior computed tomographic scan demonstrates extension of the abscess seen in **(A)** into the left groin. Note the gas in the buttock *(arrows)*.

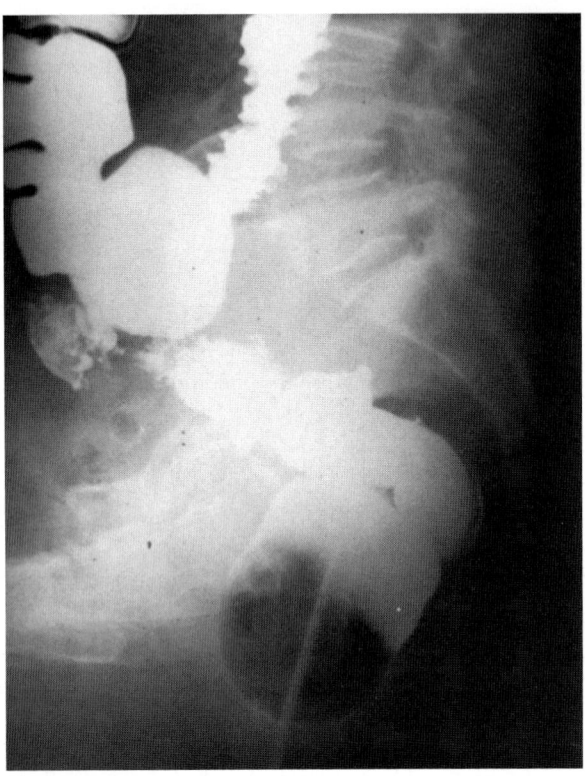

FIGURE 26-25. Diverticulitis with abscess seen on barium enema in the lateral projection.

Fistulas

Although a fistula is relatively infrequently seen, colovesical fistula is the most common internal fistula complicating diverticulitis. In the experience of Colcock and Stahmann, these accounted for one half of all fistulas secondary to this disease.[53] The second most common fistula was colocutaneous, followed by colovaginal, coloenteric, and other unusual manifestations (e.g., coloureteric, colouterine). The least common fistula is between the colon and the fallopian tube.[96]

In our experience, among the 55 patients found to have colovesical fistulas, diverticulitis was the cause in 30 cases (55%).[127] Other less frequent causes include malignant tumors from several organs, nonspecific inflammatory bowel disease (in particular, Crohn's disease), and the sequelae of radiation therapy. Rarely, injury to the urinary tract or kidney, nephrolithiasis, chronic suppurative processes, tuberculosis, and tumors of the kidney can lead to an enteric communication.[117]

Hool and colleagues reviewed more than 2,300 patients with diverticular disease, 80 of whom required operative treatment.[106] Four coloenteric fistulas were noted, an incidence of 5%. Pheils and colleagues noted that 25% of 80 patients for whom elective resection was performed had a fistula, a very high incidence.[193] In the series of Orebaugh and associates, 10% of the 144 patients who underwent resection for diverticular disease (elective and emergency operation) had a colonic fistula.[177]

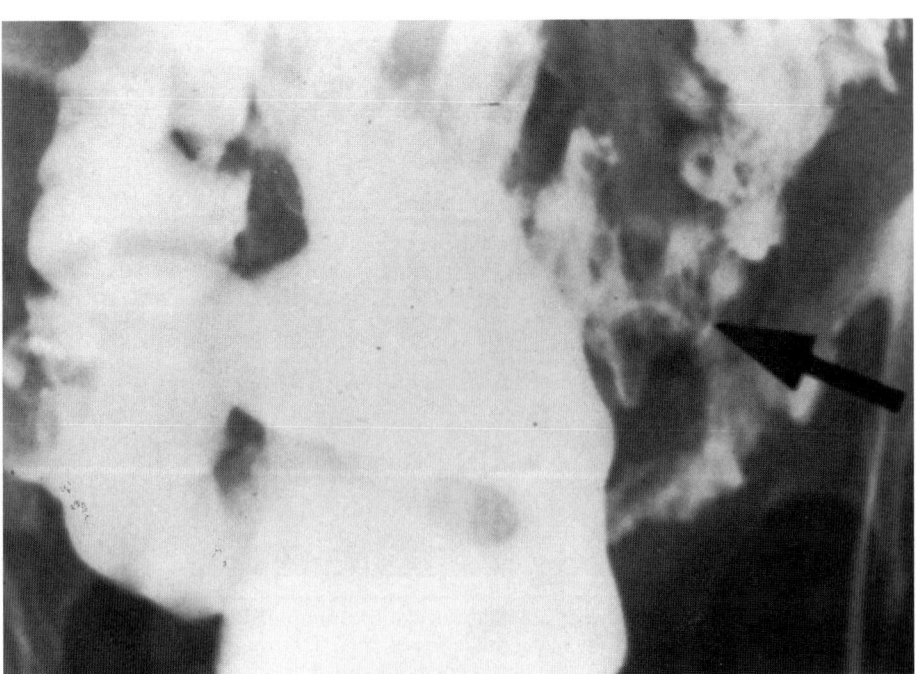

FIGURE 26-26. Perforated diverticulitis with tracking into the pelvis.

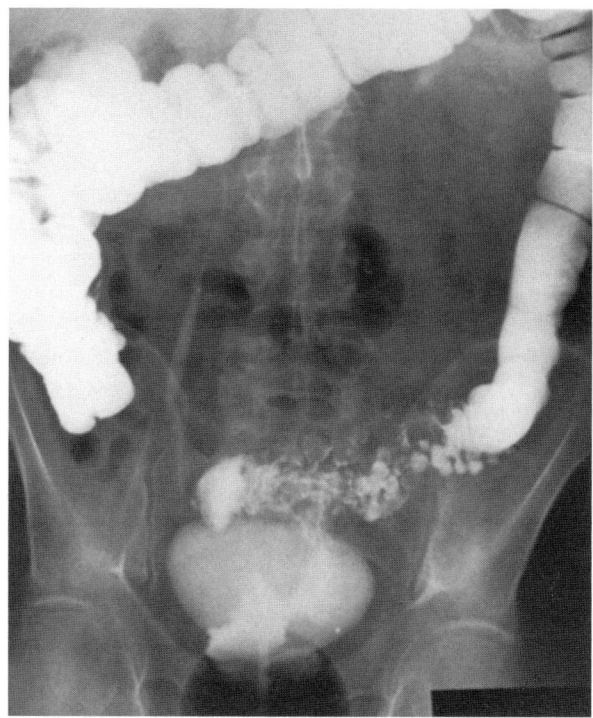

FIGURE 26-27. Perforated diverticulitis with a pelvic mass and rectal deviation.

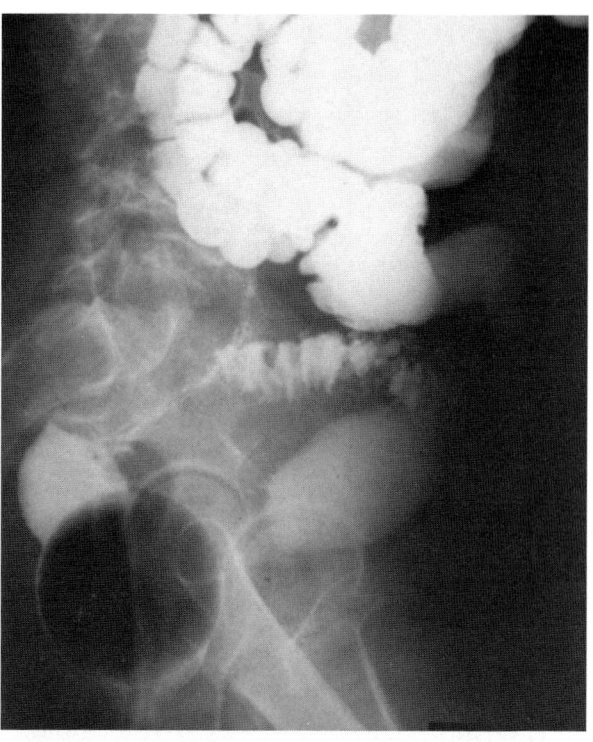

FIGURE 26-28. Pararectal and pelvic abscess secondary to diverticulitis producing rectal narrowing.

Colovesical Fistula

In our experience, 69% of patients presented with symptoms related to the urinary tract. Pneumaturia was the most frequent, followed by urinary frequency, dysuria, fecaluria, and hematuria. Complaints unrelated to the urinary tract included lower abdominal pain and fever; fewer than one fourth of the patients experienced these symptoms, however. Passage of urine through the rectum is exceedingly rare and is probably the result of concomitant bladder outflow obstruction.

The studies employed to evaluate patients suspected of having colovesical fistula include urinalysis, urine culture, barium enema, cystoscopy, cystography, CT, and endoscopy (Figure 26-32).[198] Occasionally, other techniques, such as rectal administration of methylene blue dye during cystoscopy, are used, as well as oral charcoal. CT scan confirms the existence of a colovesical fistula when there is air or oral contrast material in the bladder (Figure 26-33). It is believed to be diagnostic in more than 90% of patients. Sarr and colleagues demonstrated the pathognomonic finding of air within the bladder in 20 of 23 patients by CT, although the site of the fistula could not be shown by this means.[223] In terms of a specific abnormality found, however, it is the most accurate diagnostic tool for confirming that a communication exists between the urinary and gastrointestinal tracts.[15,113,257] Another benefit of CT is

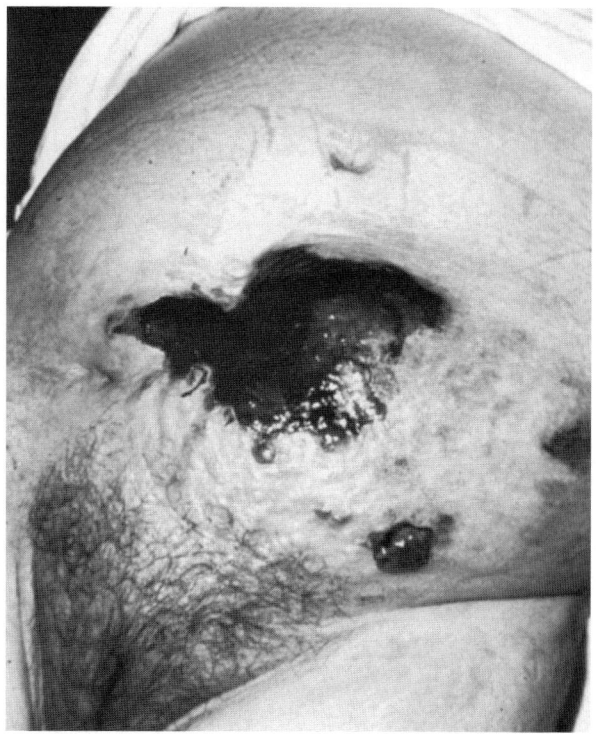

FIGURE 26-29. Gangrene of the abdominal wall from perforation of the underlying sigmoid colon.

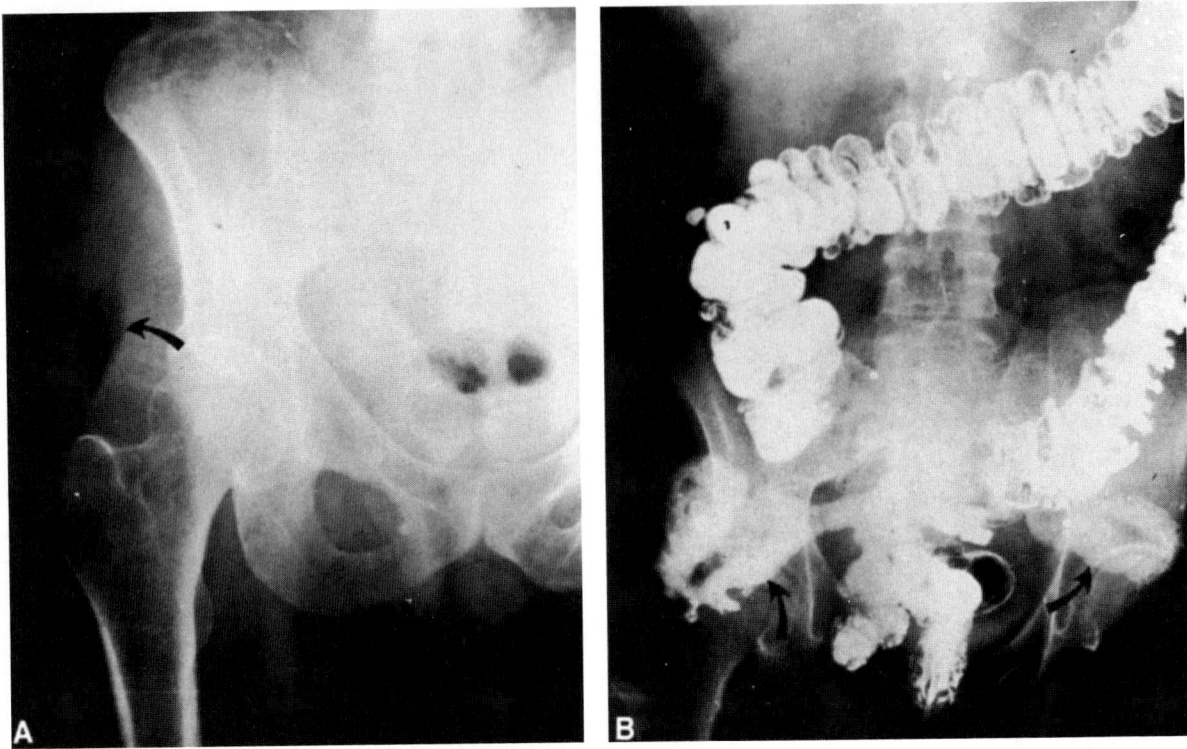

FIGURE 26-30. Perforated diverticulitis. **(A)** Gas shadow above the hip joint *(arrow)* in a patient with lower abdominal pain. **(B)** Subsequent barium enema reveals extravasation in both acetabula *(arrows)*.

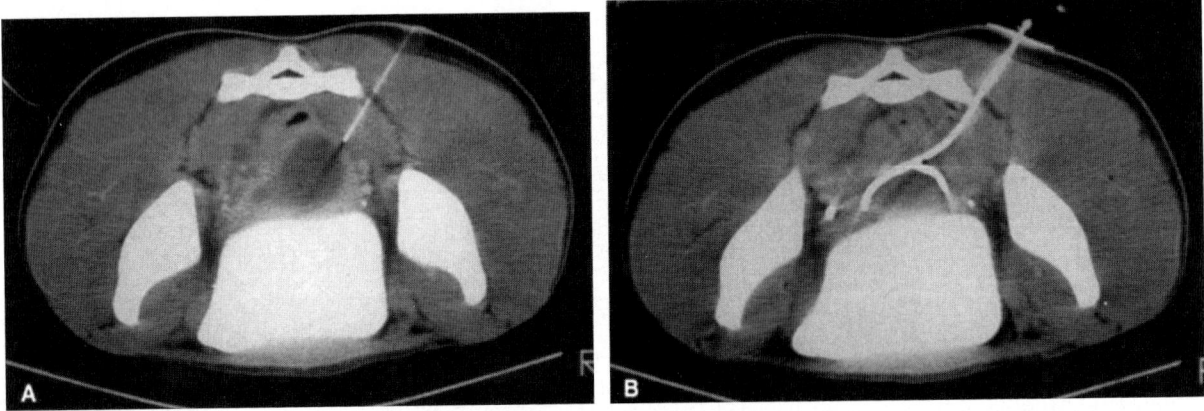

FIGURE 26-31. Pelvic abscess as a consequence of perforated diverticulitis. **(A)** Computed tomography–guided needle aspiration through a transgluteal approach confirms the location of the abscess cavity. **(B)** A catheter is inserted with the drainage complete; note the absence of gas.

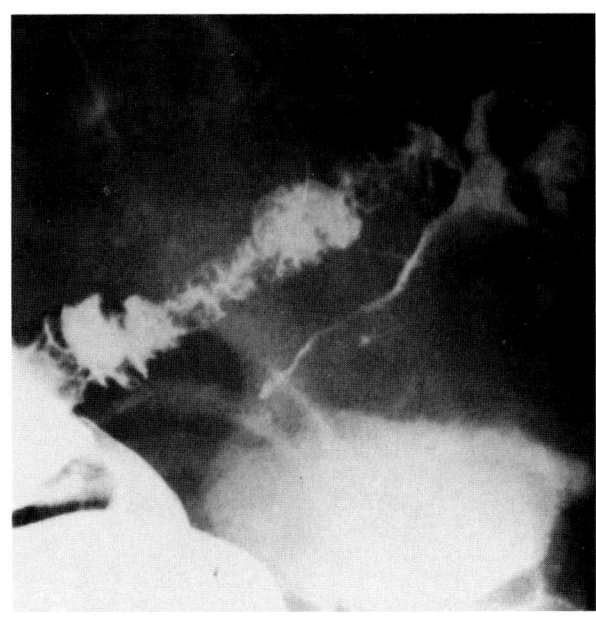

FIGURE 26-32. Colovesical fistula secondary to diverticulitis.

the detection of ureteral involvement, particularly by extrinsic compression (see Chapter 23).[175] Some believe that cystoscopy is most likely to identify the fistula,[162] but this is usually inferred by the visualization of an inflammatory reaction in the bladder mucosa. Although sigmoidoscopy may be helpful in evaluating the presence or absence of inflammatory bowel disease, in our experience, it failed to

disclose a single fistula. There have been no articles to support the concept of an increased yield with flexible sigmoidoscopy or colonoscopy.

Despite intensive radiologic and endoscopic studies, it may not be possible to identify a fistula with certainty. An operation can still be recommended, however, on the basis of clinical suspicion, without the requirement for such confirmation. The surgical management of acute diverticular disease is discussed later, but the unique features of colovesical and colovaginal fistulas are important to note.

Characteristically, at laparotomy the sigmoid colon is seen to be tethered in the pelvis, fixed to the bladder wall, or, in a woman whose uterus is surgically absent, adherent to the apex of the vagina (Figure 26-34). Usually, the fistula can be divided by blunt dissection, pinching the area between the colon and the bladder or vagina (Figure 26-35). Occasionally, when a long-standing fistula causes extensive fibrosis, sharp dissection and division of the communication are required. It is not necessary to close a vaginal opening. A drain may be placed through the vagina into the pelvis if the surgeon prefers, but this is not mandatory. It is not even necessary to close the bladder hole, but some like to suture the opening with interrupted absorbable sutures, often in two layers (Figure 26-36). Excision of a portion of the bladder wall, formally closing the organ in an area where there is no fibrosis, is an unnecessarily meddlesome technique (Figure 26-35, *inset*). A catheter should be left in place for 1 week. This is usually a sufficient period to permit healing of the

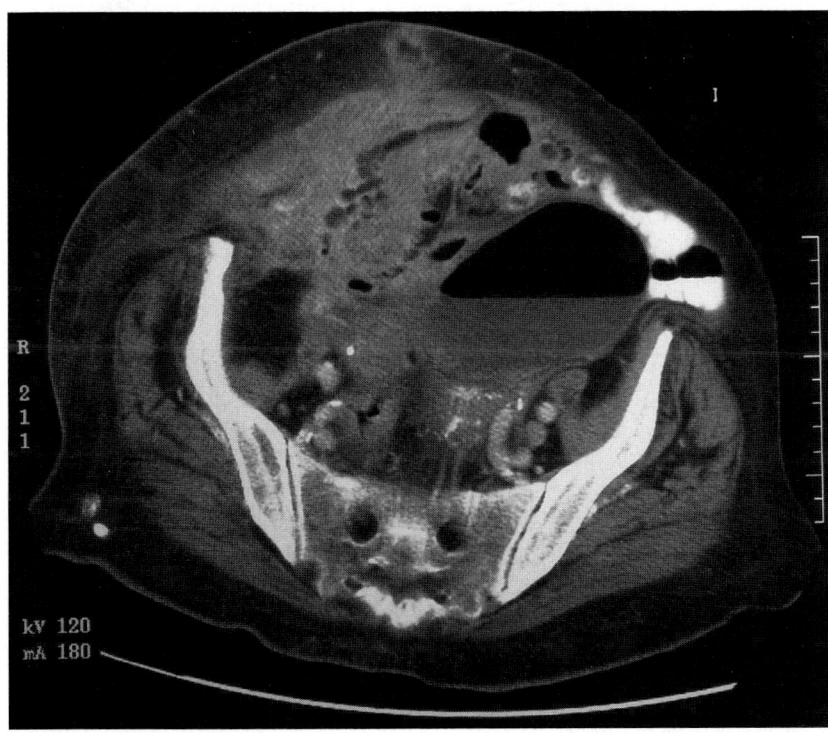

FIGURE 26-33. Computed tomography demonstrates an abnormal sigmoid colon with multiple diverticula and with a large amount of air within the bladder consistent with a colovesical fistula.

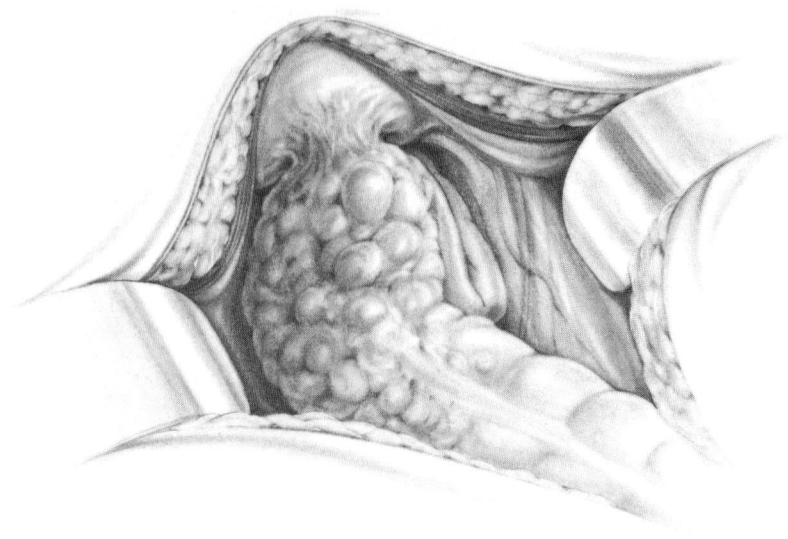

FIGURE 26-34. A colovesical fistula secondary to diverticulitis. A sigmoidal mass is fixed in the pelvis to the bladder.

bladder (Figure 26-37). The bowel is resected and a primary anastomosis is performed to the upper rectum. Fecal diversion is not advised.

Results

In our review of surgery for diverticular disease, 51 patients were operated on for colonic fistula.[102] There were three deaths (6%), as shown in Table 26-1. Woods and colleagues reported the Cleveland Clinic experience with internal fistulas.[271] There were three deaths (3.5%), a 21% incidence of wound infections, one enterocutaneous fistula, and a 5% incidence of anastomotic leaks. Other studies demonstrate the relative safety of one-stage resection.[162,198,221,247] Di Carlo and associates of McGill University in Montreal conducted an historical cohort study of patients who underwent surgery for fistula complicating diverticulitis and compared the results of general surgeons with that of colon and rectal surgeons.[61] They concluded that specialization in colon and rectal surgery contributed to an improved outcome, with a lower frequency of fecal diversion, a shorter hospital stay, and a lower complication rate.

Colovaginal Fistula

Colovaginal fistula may be a late consequence of acute diverticulitis, after abdominal signs and symptoms resolve, but this complication is very rare.[207] It virtually never occurs in a woman who still has her uterus. The presence of the uterus seems to protect against the development of a colovaginal fistula. Conversely, the most common cause of a high rectovaginal fistula is injury as a consequence of hysterectomy. Discharge of feces, blood, pus, mucus, or gas are the usual complaints. Pelvic examination usually reveals an opening or granular area at the apex of the

vagina, most commonly on the left side. Barium enema may identify the communication (see Figure 12-2), or another diagnostic method, as discussed in Chapter 12, may be used. This may include vaginography and tandem colovaginoscopy.[2,17,136] The former method involves the insertion of a Foley catheter with a 30-mL balloon into the vagina; the balloon is then inflated. The patient is instructed to keep her legs together, and water-soluble contrast material is inserted through the catheter to demonstrate any fistula. With the latter method, a colonoscope is passed transanally while a gastroscope is inserted into the vagina.[3] Transmission of light may be seen at the fistula orifice. A more obvious communication may permit the passage of a biopsy forceps, thereby allowing direct visualization of the instrument. As with colovesical fistula, one-stage resection is the preferred surgical approach.[54]

Ureterocolic Fistula

Ureterocolic fistula is extremely rare and is usually caused by urinary calculi. Cirocco and colleagues reviewed the literature of those patients whose condition was precipitated by diverticulitis.[50] They noted that urologic symptoms predominate, especially urinary tract infection (100%); fecaluria (75%) and abdominal (75%) or flank (50%) pain were the next in frequency. Barium enema is the most reliable diagnostic test for demonstrating the fistula. The left ureter is involved in approximately three fourths of the cases.

Thigh Abscess

As mentioned earlier, enteric infections on rare occasions can spread to the thigh. Rotstein and colleagues reviewed 46 reported cases and found that 39 arose from the colon

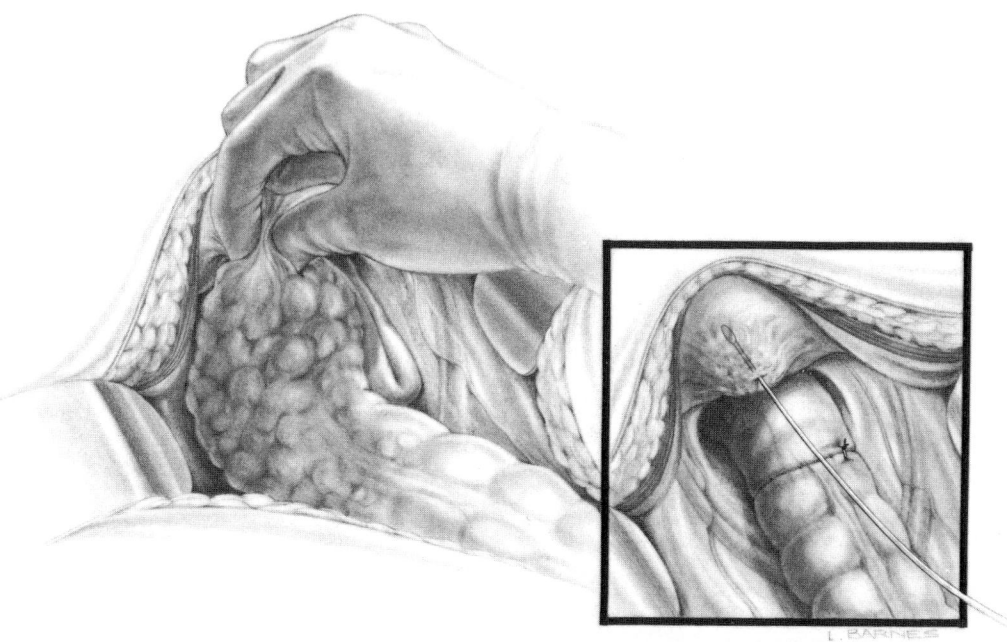

FIGURE 26-35. Using a pinching technique, one can separate the colon mass from the bladder. This minimizes the risk for bladder injury and avoids potential ureteral compromise if bowel fixation is posterior. Occasionally, the fibrosis is too dense for this maneuver, and sharp dissection is required. An opening in the bladder can be confirmed by inserting a probe **(inset)**.

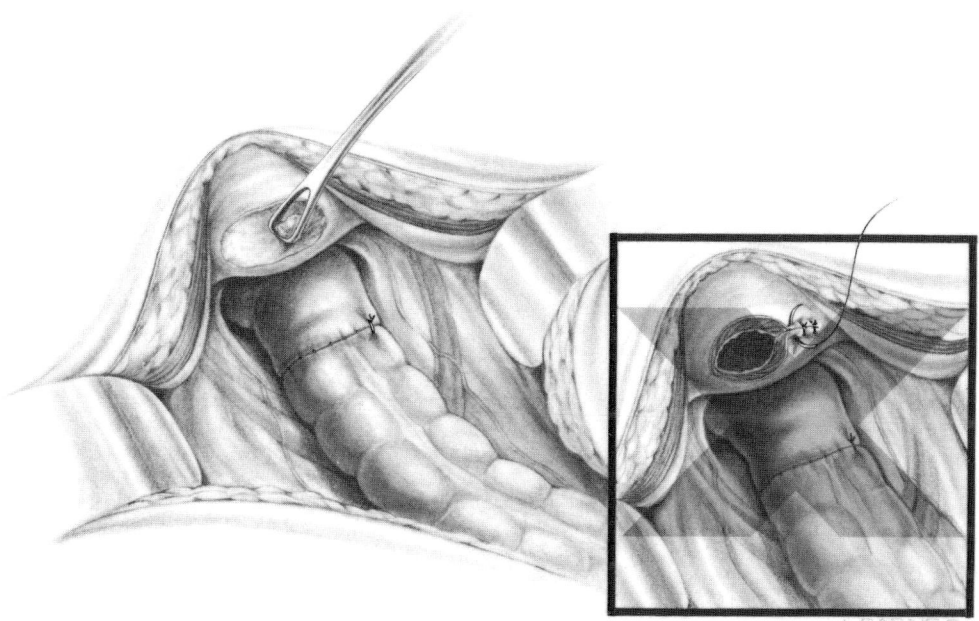

FIGURE 26-36. Curettage of granulation tissue may be all that is necessary for the bladder side of the fistula. The surgeon may wish to place one or two sutures to close the hole, but this is not a requisite, because catheter drainage inevitably results in healing. Formal bladder wall excision and closure are unnecessary and meddlesome **(inset)**.

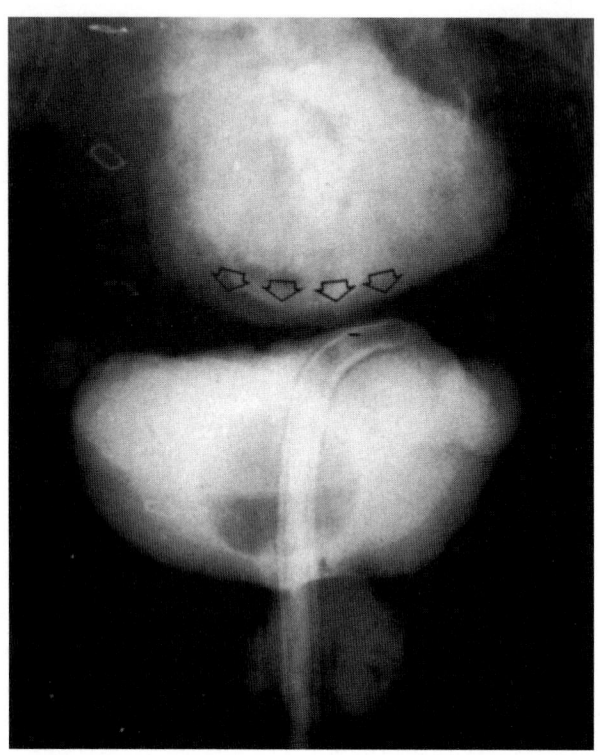

FIGURE 26-37. Bladder extravasation. Precipitous removal of the catheter resulted in leakage from a prior bladder fistula site *(arrows)*.

and rectum.[216] The most common routes by which the infection can develop in this area were as follows:

1. Via the neurovascular bundles that penetrate the muscle and fascia of the abdominal wall
2. Through the inguinal rings
3. Through the pelvic floor along the rectum.[216]

According to the authors, the underlying pathologic abnormality is usually a retroperitoneal perforation by tumor or by diverticulitis. One should be suspicious of the possibility of a colonic perforation if culture of a thigh abscess reveals enteric organisms.

Septic Thrombophlebitis

In very rare instances, inflammatory changes in the colon can result in a septic thrombophlebitis involving the mesenteric veins draining the area.[64] This can lead to demonstration of gas in the mesenteric and ultimately the portal venous system on CT imaging. The etiology is uncertain, but the possibility of gas-forming organisms entering the circulation is a reasonable theory. This complication is obviously an independent factor that mandates bowel resection.

Hemorrhage

Hemorrhage is not considered a presentation of diverticulitis. It can be, however, a complication of diverticulosis. The reader is referred to Chapter 28 for a discussion of this manifestation.

SURGICAL TREATMENT OF ACUTE DIVERTICULITIS

If the patient fails to respond to medical measures or if an individual's condition is deteriorating, urgent surgical intervention should be performed. Obviously, in someone with generalized peritonitis or a pneumoperitoneum, emergency operation is indicated.

There are numerous operations available for the treatment of acute sigmoid diverticulitis in the acute situation from the "peek and shriek" to the esoteric (Figure 26-38). All have potential benefits and disadvantages, depending on the presentation, the findings, and the technical capabilities of the surgeon. Understanding the relative indications for each option will help the surgeon make the

▌ **TABLE 26-1** Surgery for Diverticular Disease: Morbidity and Mortality

Presentation	Number of Patients	Number of Complications*	Number of Deaths	Percentage of Mortality (%)
Phlegmon	99	56	7	7
Fistula	51	44	3	6
Abscess	33	31	2	6
Obstruction	9	6	1	10
Perforation	7	9	1	14
Total	155	146	14	9

* Some patients had more than one complication.

From Helbraun MA, Corman ML, Coller JA, et al. Diverticular disease. Reported at the annual meeting of the American Society of Colon and Rectal Surgeons, 1979.

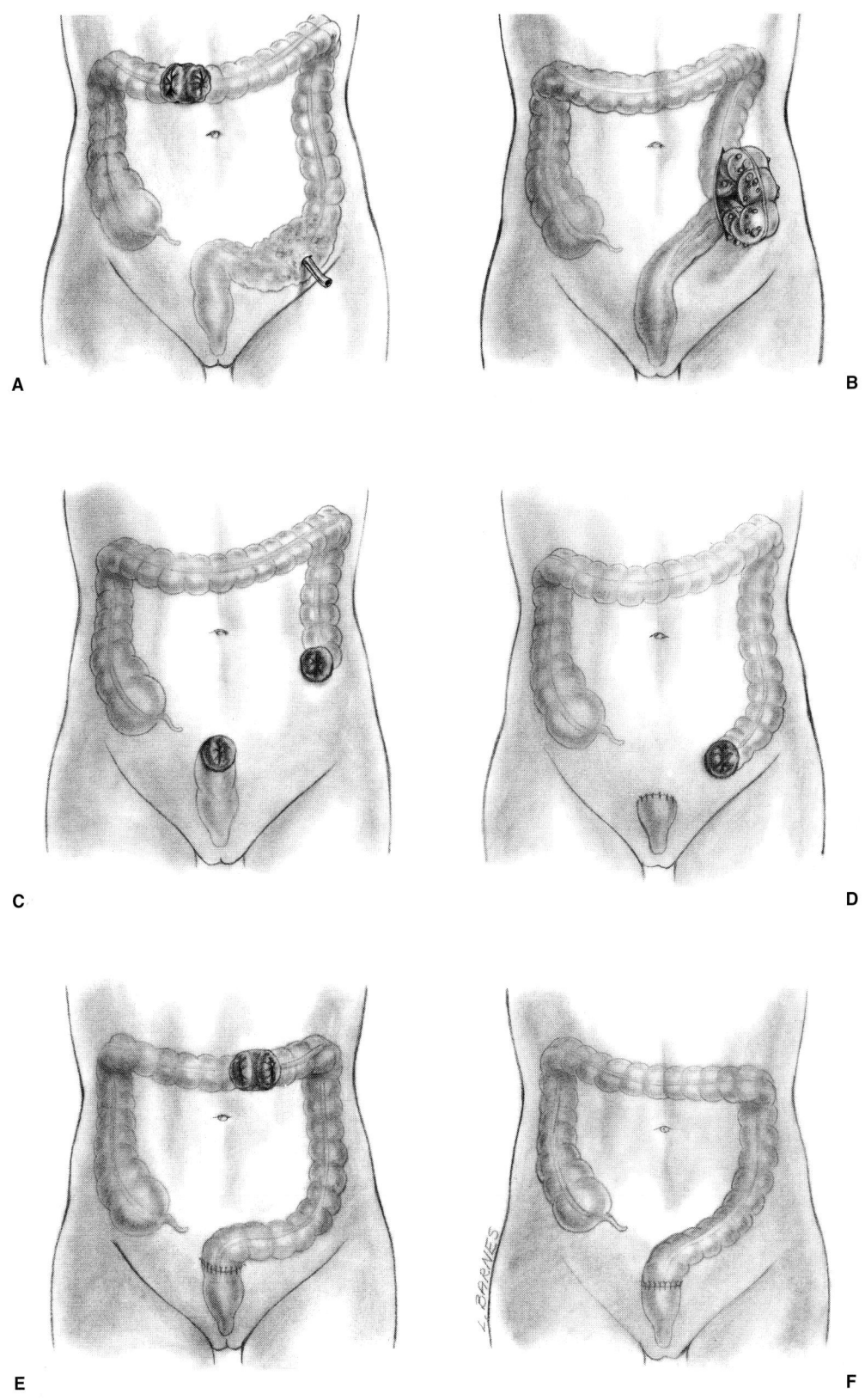

FIGURE 26-38. Alternative operations for acute sigmoid diverticulitis. **(A)** Loop transverse colostomy and drainage. **(B)** Exteriorization. **(C)** Resection, colostomy, and mucous fistula. **(D)** Resection, end colostomy, and rectal closure (Hartmann's). **(E)** Resection, anastomosis, and colostomy. **(F)** Resection and anastomosis (no stoma).

appropriate operative decision in a given situation. Although not an exhaustive list of every possibility, they include the following:

- Fecal diversion (ileostomy or colostomy) and drainage of the perforation
- Exteriorization of the involved segment (essentially historical only)
- Resection: sigmoid or descending colon colostomy and mucous fistula
- Resection: end-colostomy and closure of rectal stump (Hartmann's)
- Resection: primary anastomosis and fecal diversion
- Limited resection and primary anastomosis (no stoma)
- Limited resection and primary anastomosis with on-table lavage
- Limited resection and primary anastomosis with intra-luminal bypass (not available in the United States)
- Total colectomy with primary anastomosis

In 1978, Hinchey and colleagues proposed a method for identifying the clinical presentation of patients with acute diverticulitis that was designed to permit a comparison of the choices of operations and the results of surgery.[103] This has come to be known as the *Hinchey Classification* and is as follows:

Stage I. Pericolic abscess or phlegmon
Stage II. Pelvic, intraabdominal, or retroperitoneal abscess
Stage III. Generalized purulent peritonitis
Stage IV. Generalized fecal peritonitis

In principle, such a concept would seem laudable, but it this classification rarely used in colon and rectal surgery references. In the more than 25 years since the publication of the Hinchey classification, it has not proved to be helpful in guiding the surgeon toward improved operative decision-making nor in analyzing the comparative results of the diversity of procedures.

Fecal Diversion and Drainage

A three-stage operation had been recommended for the treatment of acute diverticulitis for many years and by many prominent authorities: Mayo in 1907, Rankin and Brown, and Smithwick.[156,206,237] The procedure consists of a diversionary colostomy and drainage, elective resection, and finally closure of the colostomy. Until relatively recently, intestinal diversion was believed to be the safest surgical procedure for carrying the patient through the critical phase of the illness. A transverse loop colostomy is performed, and drainage of the infected area is established (see Figure 26-38A). Alternatively, one may create an ileostomy for the same pur-

pose. The technique of stomal construction is described in Chapter 31.

Although this operation has been successful in the acute management of these individuals, morbidity and mortality for the three stages have been consistently high. The patient must contend for some time with a difficult stoma. In addition, the nidus of sepsis may persist for many weeks or even months. In essence, the entire left colon is available to drain through the perforation if the opening is still freely communicating with the peritoneal cavity. Furthermore, adequate external drainage may not have been established in the first instance. For example, simply placing a drain on top of an inflamed colon is not necessarily sufficient. If a mesenteric abscess is present, it will obviously remain untreated. When the surgeon decides to embark on a three-stage procedure, it is important for the inflammatory mass to be mobilized sufficiently to break up any loculations and to effect adequate drainage. One must differentiate between perforated diverticulitis with fecal peritonitis and a walled-off perforation or phlegmon in deciding whether to divert or to resect. Fecal diversion with drainage is rarely the optimal alternative, and it is a very poor choice indeed when a free perforation is present.

There is, however, no good reason for performing a right transverse colostomy, although when a subsequent resection is performed the stoma need not be taken down at that time. It is not technically easier to create than one on the left side, it is likely to be associated with prolapse of the efferent limb, and theoretically the effluent is more liquid. If a colostomy is to be performed, a left transverse colostomy is suggested when this operation is elected. At least it will be the proximal, functioning limb that will prolapse, and an appliance can be maintained in this situation. However, a still better diversion option is a loop ileostomy. Regardless, if the patient succeeds in recovering from the initial procedure, unless the stoma is synchronously closed or resected, at least two more operations can be anticipated. The diseased bowel is resected and an anastomosis performed. Closure of the colostomy or ileostomy is the final step in the three-stage approach. Each one of these procedures has its attendant morbidity and mortality.

Timing of Subsequent Resection

The question is often asked, "When should one intervene and resect the bowel after the fecal stream has been diverted?" My own preference is to wait approximately 6 to 8 weeks. I have not uncommonly found the dissection quite facile at this stage and do not believe that further delay simplifies the subsequent operation. In fact, I have been in the position of struggling to perform a resection 6 months or even 1 year following the initial acute episode and doubt whether further procrastination would alter the conditions.

Results

In 1980, Thompson stated in Maingot's *Abdominal Operations* that "any perforation should be sutured and covered with adjacent appendix epiploica and a transverse colostomy performed."[250] Alexander-Williams reviewed four series and noted a mean mortality rate of 45% following treatment of perforated diverticular disease by drainage and colostomy.[7] His own experience from the Birmingham General Hospital during the period from 1969 through 1973 (a total of 333 patients) revealed 68 deaths, a mortality rate of 22%. It was his opinion that this mortality rate was excessively high, implying that simple drainage and transverse colostomy is an inadequate operation for perforated diverticular disease, especially in the presence of generalized peritonitis or gross fecal contamination. Griffin cautions that although each patient should be individualized, the standard three-stage technique of right transverse colostomy, followed by resection of the involved colon and finally closure of the transverse colostomy, should be used rarely, if at all.[94]

Greif and associates reviewed more than 1,300 cases of acute perforated sigmoid diverticulitis from the literature, using 19 references from 1965 through 1979.[93] Criteria for selection of the cases included the presence of an abscess with localized or diffuse peritonitis. The surgery was performed during the acute illness, and the operative mortality was clearly stated. Among patients who had perforated diverticulitis with abscess and localized peritonitis (510 patients), those who initially underwent resection were found to have a 2% operative mortality, whereas those who underwent a proximal diverting colostomy (306 patients) had a 12% operative mortality. These differences were statistically significant. More than 800 patients with perforated diverticulitis and generalized peritonitis underwent emergency surgery. The combined operative mortality was 12% for patients undergoing resection initially, contrasted with 29% for those who underwent colostomy and drainage.

Classen and co-workers reported a retrospective review of a 10-year experience with the three-stage operation.[51] Only individuals with fecal or generalized peritonitis, or pelvic peritonitis with abscess, were included in the study. More than 200 patients were considered. The operative mortality after the first stage was 8.5%, at the second stage, 0.7%, and at the third stage, 4%, so that the overall mortality rate was 11%.

Wara and associates ascertained the outcome of staged operations for complicated sigmoid diverticulitis for the 10-year period ending in 1979.[260] Of the 83 patients in the study, only 58% subsequently underwent a resection of the diseased segment, and fewer (46%) eventually had their intestinal continuity restored. Eleven of 25 patients died of generalized peritonitis when managed by proximal colostomy and drainage only (one third of those with purulent peritonitis and more than 80% of those with fecal peritonitis).

Opinion

When presenting the results of the three-stage resection, it is inappropriate for an author to state that patients survive the initial insult and then compare mortality statistics with those of other operations that initially involve resection. The total morbidity and mortality of the three stages must be considered if one is to compare the various techniques fairly. Unfortunately, many studies fail to do this. All too often, staged operations with an initial colostomy are not carried through to the final procedure. Patients may be lost to follow-up, become too ill or be at too great a risk to undergo a secondary or tertiary procedure, refuse further surgery because they are relatively well, or have expired in the interim. In selecting this operation, the surgeon should consider the likelihood of eventually reestablishing intestinal continuity in the patient.

Colostomy with drainage is a reasonable alternative if the surgeon does not feel comfortable with colon resection even under elective circumstances. That is certainly not the time to embark on emergency colectomy. Another possible reason for deferring resection and performing a drainage and diversionary procedure initially is that the colon cannot be mobilized with reasonable safety, but this is more often a matter of experience and judgment. If the surgeon is faced with such a predicament, consideration should be given to the possibility that an underlying carcinoma is present or that the patient has Crohn's disease.

Another reason that has been expressed for embarking specifically on a three-stage approach rather than Hartmann's procedure is the difficulty of reestablishing intestinal continuity following the latter operation. However, I do not believe that this is a valid concern today with the availability of stapling alternatives (see later).

Exteriorization and Resection with Colostomy and Mucous Fistula

Colonic exteriorization has been advocated for cancer since the end of the nineteenth century (Figure 26-38*B*). Eponymous operations have been associated with Bloch, Paul, and von Mikulicz (see Historical Notes, Chapter 23).[30,161,188] Traditionally, resection was subsequently undertaken and anastomosis was effected, often with some form of spur-crushing clamp (Figure 26-39). This opera-

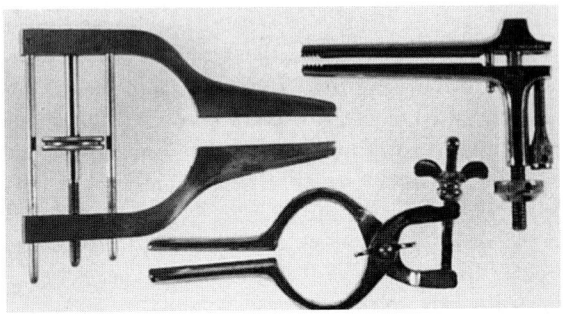

FIGURE 26-39. Spur-crushing clamps. (Courtesy of Thomas J. Anglem, M.D.)

tion succeeds in removing the nidus of sepsis from the peritoneal cavity, the single most important aim of surgery for complicated sigmoid diverticulitis. Today, however, it is considered neither appropriate nor necessary to delay resection until the peritoneal cavity has "sealed." The bowel is removed at the time of stomal construction (see Figure 26-38C).

A sigmoid colostomy is an eminently satisfactory stoma to manage. The stool is formed and can be handled with a conventional colostomy appliance; the patient may even elect to irrigate and to employ only a small dressing (see Chapter 32). If for one reason or another the colostomy must be permanent, the patient should not be significantly inconvenienced, at least not to the same extent as with a colostomy located in the transverse colon. Transverse colostomies have all the disadvantages not only of colostomy, but also of ileostomy: a relatively liquid and malodorous effluent. After a period of time, most loop transverse colostomies will prolapse. Even dividing the stoma is no guarantee of preventing the subsequent development of this complication.

An important advantage of colostomy and mucous fistula is the fact that the procedure requires only two stages to effect restoration of intestinal continuity. The second operation is relatively simple because the distal bowel can be easily identified. The difficulty with recommending this operation is that the disease rarely occurs at a sufficiently proximal location in the bowel to enable the distal colon to be delivered to the level of the skin. Far more commonly, the inflammatory reaction is confined to the sigmoid colon, usually almost to the level of the peritoneal reflection. Under these circumstances, it is impossible to bring the distal bowel out to the abdominal wall. Thus, although the concept of resection with colostomy and mucous fistula is a reasonable one, its application is quite limited.

Bell believed that every effort should be made to create a mucous fistula.[21] In order to permit sufficient length to enable the surgeon to effect this, he suggested that less sigmoid colon be resected, even if it means leaving behind some element of residual disease or inflammation. At the second stage, the remainder of the sig-

moid can be resected and anastomosis created in the normal rectum. Others have suggested a similar approach—that is, minimal resection of the distal segment.[22] I have had no experience with this technique, but in the situations with which I have been often confronted, the large phlegmon would not permit preservation of adequate colon to create a mucous fistula. As suggested, if one were to do this, in most cases it would be necessary to leave behind a potential source for sepsis. There is also a risk for perforation developing in the residual, diseased bowel before it can be subsequently removed, a particular concern if the patient is steroid dependent.[78] Probably my single greatest criticism is that one may have a tendency not to remove all of the distal sigmoid at the time of the second operation, re-establishing intestinal continuity in the "high-pressure zone" rather than into the rectum. This is a conceptual and technical error. In order to minimize the risk of developing recurrent diverticuliti, it is imperative that the anastomosis be effected in the non–tenia-bearing rectum.

Over the years, there have been a number of advocates of this procedure.[243,261,264] Its relatively limited usefulness, however, implies that other methods for the treatment of acute sigmoid diverticulitis must be sought if morbidity and mortality are to be decreased.

Resection with Sigmoid Colostomy and Closure of Rectal Stump (Hartmann's Procedure)

It is generally agreed that if the source of infection can be removed at the initial operation, this would be the most satisfactory operative approach. In 1923, Henri Hartmann published a two-paragraph observation of a procedure for the treatment of rectal cancer that succeeded in achieving for him eponymous immortality (see the biography and translation in Chapter 23).[98] Although the operation is only occasionally performed for cancer today, it has become the most commonly employed procedure for the treatment of acute diverticulitis in the United States (Figure 26-38D).

The operation involves resection of the inflamed bowel, and an end-sigmoid colostomy with closure of the rectal stump. The procedure effectively removes the source of sepsis from the peritoneal cavity, creates a most satisfactory stoma, and obviates the risk of anastomosis under septic conditions. It does, however, have one major disadvantage: the second stage of the operation, performed 6 or more weeks later, requires a major abdominal procedure. At that time, the colostomy must be excised and the proximal bowel liberated. This often necessitates mobilizing the splenic flexure, a procedure that poses some risk for splenic injury. The so-called Hartmann's pouch may be difficult to identify and may be considerably retracted, although it is no longer necessary to mobilize it to the extent that was previously required for conventional sutured anastomosis. However, there is still the risk for a complication related to the anastomosis itself. Because the operation is of some magnitude, many high-risk patients have been deprived of the opportunity of having intestinal continuity reestablished. Sometimes, therefore, Hartmann's operation results in a permanent stoma.

Technique

The technique of removing the acutely inflamed colon is worthy of amplification. When entering the peritoneal cavity, the surgeon is often confronted with what appears to be a "large, fixed, unresectable mass"(Figure 26-40). However, one should not be overwhelmed by first appearances. The acute inflammatory reaction can often be dealt with by careful blunt dissection without fear of injuring vital retroperitoneal structures, such as a ureter. Attempts at such mobilization at a later time may be impossible without sharp scissors dissection. In the latter circumstances, the ureter is much more likely to be injured. If one begins the dissection by gently passing the left hand lateral to the inflammatory mass and easing the bowel away from the parietal peritoneum, one may be pleasantly surprised at how readily the mass seems to come free. An occasional fibrous band may be snipped with the scissors, but virtually the entire dissection is carried out bluntly with the tips of the fingers, either pushing to identify the plane of dissection or pinching adherent areas.

Abcarian and Pearl make the point that the operation should be commenced proximal to the inflamed segment, dividing the bowel with a linear stapler at this location and developing the plane over Gerota's fascia.[1] A proximal-to-distal dissection is then undertaken, with the ureter identified at the cephalad aspect of the mobilization. When the bowel is delivered into the abdominal cavity, the surgeon can usually identify 1 or 2 cm of distal rectosigmoid that seems to be free of inflammatory reaction (Figure 26-41). This is an important point, because it is this sparing of the rectosigmoid that permits a relatively safe anastomosis, should one elect to perform it at this time. However, if the surgeon prefers Hartmann's operation, the bowel is resected, a colostomy is created, and the rectal stump is closed. Stump closure can be effected by conventional suture technique or more commonly by using a stapler.

Anastomosis Following Hartmann's Procedure

Numerous procedures have been devised to simplify subsequent reanastomosis of Hartmann's rectal pouch. Some suggest that the pouch be sutured to the promontory of the sacrum. Madure and Fiore advise the use of the linear stapling device as well as permanent marking of the two "corner" areas with 2–0 polypropylene (Prolene) sutures, leaving the ends trimmed to a length of 1 or 2 inches.[149] They found that these maneuvers permitted ready identification of the pouch in all 30 patients in whom the technique was used. Other methods for demonstrating the rectal stump include insertion of a Foley

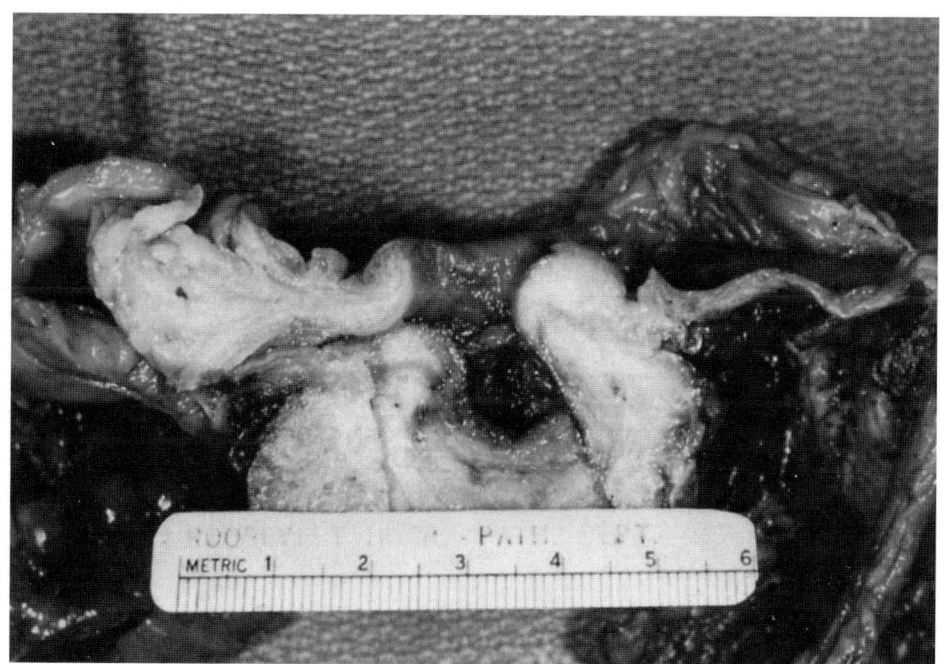

FIGURE 26-40. Acute and chronic diverticulitis with inflammatory mass. The diverticulum simulates ulcerating carcinoma. (Courtesy of Rudolf Garret, M.D.)

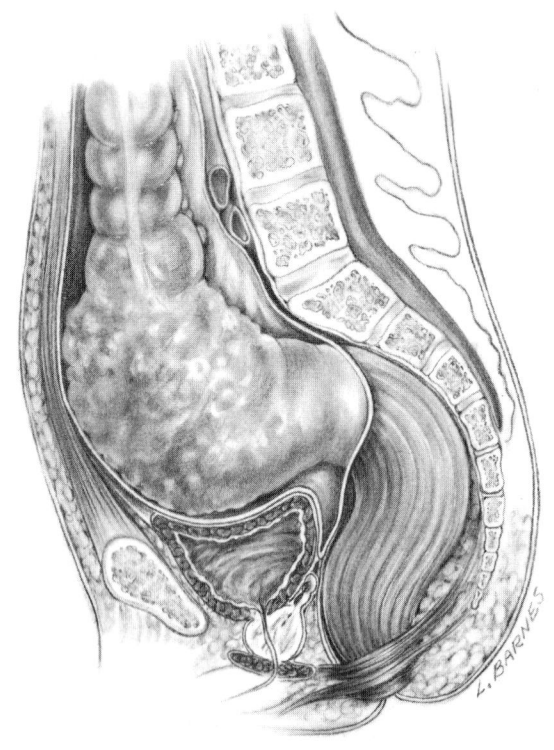

FIGURE 26-41. Sigmoid diverticulitis. The mass usually terminates distally in relatively normal, uninflamed bowel, just above the peritoneal reflection.

catheter into the rectum, distension of the pouch with saline solution, insertion of a firm rectal tube, application of the staple gun head sizers, and visualization of transmitted light from a fiberoptic sigmoidoscope.[59,88,192]

Instead of conventional suturing to effect a colorectal anastomosis, use of the circular stapling instrument is strongly advised. Ramirez and associates recommend initially inserting a rigid sigmoidoscope into the rectum with the distal end of the instrument pointed against the apex of the pouch.[197] The illuminated scope tip serves as the identification point for creating a small stab wound in the rectal wall, but with the trocar-tip instrument now being used this approach would seem unnecessary. A No. 18 French urethral catheter with beveled tip can be passed through the stab wound and out the rectum. The catheter is then attached to the center rod and trocar tip of the circular stapling device (Figure 26-42A). The instrument is then introduced into the rectum until the rod is passed through the opening that was created in the rectal pouch. No distal purse-string suture is required. After removal of the catheter, the proximal bowel segment is drawn over the anvil, and the previously applied proximal purse-string suture is tied. The parts of the instrument are then reconnected and the stapling gun is fired, creating an end-to-end anastomosis without rectal mobilization (Figure 26-42B). Others have used a variation of the catheter technique,[267] and Buchmann and Baumgart-

ner describe a special proctoscope that permits identification of the rectal stump and the atraumatic introduction of the stapling instrument without the anvil.[40]

The circular stapling instruments can simplify the above task considerably. The rectum need not be mobilized. The anvil can be removed so that the proximal limb can be inserted at a considerable distance from the pelvic pouch (see Chapter 23). Alternatively, if the surgeon prefers, the option is still available of performing the technique as described earlier. The center shaft can be reattached with a simple, snap-together maneuver. The anastomosis is then completed in the manner previously described.

Laparoscopic Closure

The laparoscopically assisted approach has been advocated for reestablishing intestinal continuity following Hartmann's procedure.[215,238] This technique is discussed in Chapter 27. Sosa and colleagues performed laparoscopically assisted reversal of Hartmann's procedure in 18 individuals and completed the operation in 14.[238] Basically, the results were comparable with those of the open procedure. Laparoscopic-assisted colectomy is discussed later in this chapter.

Reversal of Colostomy

It is usually unnecessary for one to study the rectal stump before closure of the colostomy, but this presupposes that one knows exactly what was accomplished at the time of Hartmann's operation. In other words, was the rectum preoperatively evaluated (as it should have been), and was the entire sigmoid colon removed! If the surgeon is not the one who performed the first operation or did not do what he or she should have done the first time, it is mandatory that a proctoscopic examination be performed in order to determine that there is no rectal pathology. Furthermore, it is prudent to perform a limited water-soluble contrast enema so that one may be certain that there is no remaining distal colon. If some sigmoid colon is identified, it must be resected at the time of Hartmann's closure. Conversely, if the surgeon is satisfied that there is only a rectal stump remaining, closure can be effected without mobilization and resection if the circular-stapled technique is being employed.

As it is with the timing of resection following diversion following three-stage resections, the question of timing of the reanastomosis following Hartmann's resection is a matter of some controversy. Roe and colleagues compared the morbidity and mortality of patients who underwent closure before and after 4 months, noting no significant difference.[214] In a similar study, Geoghegan and Rosenberg found that early colorectal anastomosis (1 month following the primary procedure) did not increase

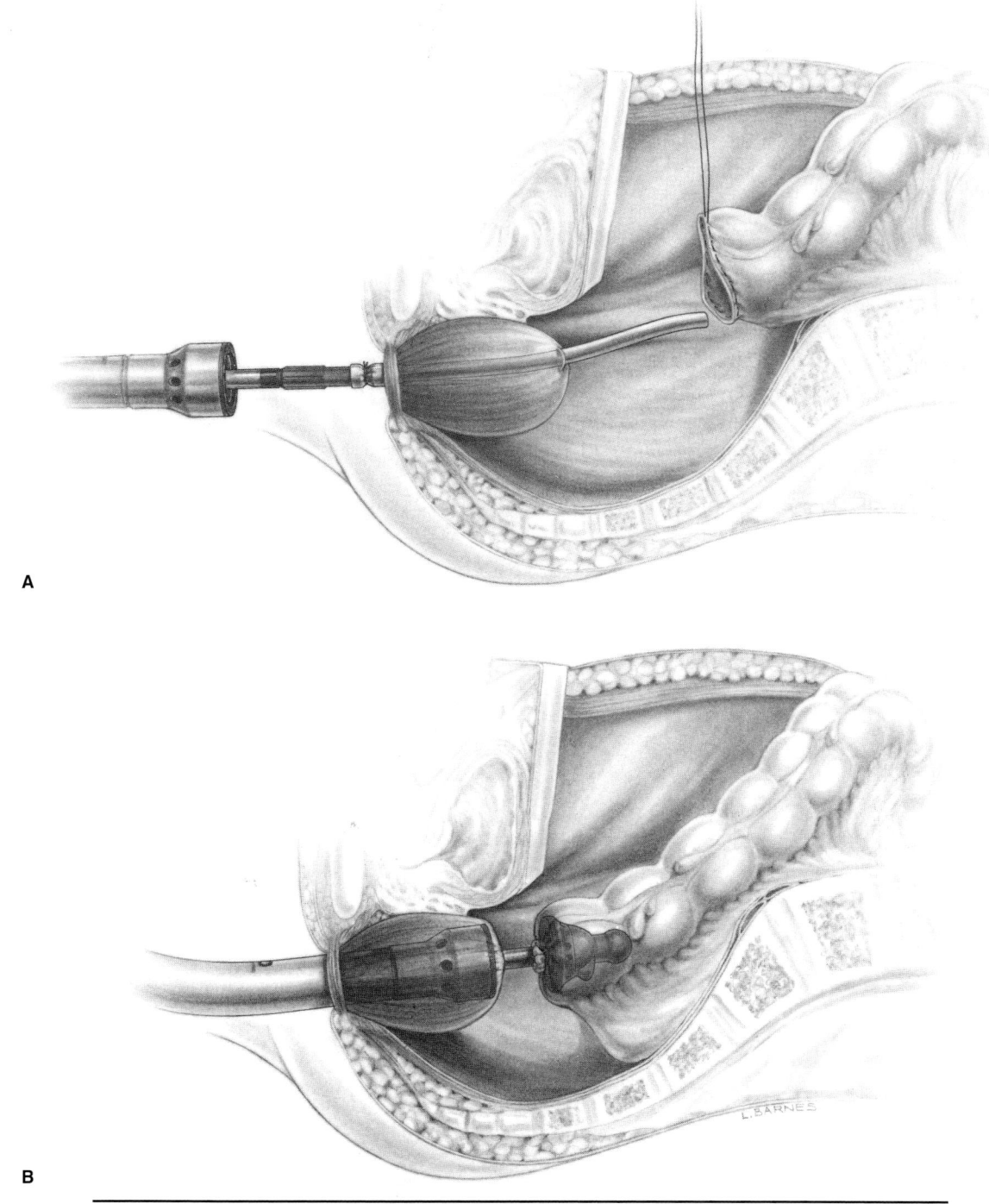

FIGURE 26-42. Circular staple technique for Hartmann's pouch anastomosis. **(A)** The stapler is introduced and guided by catheter (the anvil has been removed). **(B)** The proximal bowel is brought down to effect the anastomosis.

risk and may have been technically easier to perform when compared with later closure.[86]

Pierce and co-workers reported the outcome of 145 patients who underwent Hartmann's resection with respect to reversal of the colostomy.[189] Eighty patients proceeded to reanastomosis. Multifactorial analysis was undertaken to determine the risks and revealed the following: The interval between the primary and secondary operation was found to be the most important factor. There were no leaks if the reanastomosis was delayed for longer than 6 months, compared with a 50% incidence of leak when the interval was less than 3 months. Likewise, Keck and associates noted that the operative difficulty appears to be less after a delay of 15 weeks.[119]

Their mortality for reversal was 2%, their anastomotic leak rate was 4%, and the overall complication rate was 26%.[119] The complication rate in 19 individuals who underwent closure of Hartmann's colostomy procedure, according to the experience from the University of Minnesota group, was 23%, including an anastomotic leak rate of 2%.[23]

Use of Seprafilm

In order to minimize the extent of dissection and the attendant risks associated with reoperative surgery following Hartmann's resection, I believe it is especially prudent to use Seprafilm (Genzyme Corp., Cambridge, MA; *www.genzyme.com*) at the time of the initial operation. A sheet placed in the floor of the pelvis will minimize adhesion formation and permit ready exposure of the rectal stump, thereby avoiding the likelihood of an extensive pelvic dissection and adhesiolysis. Furthermore, by wrapping the colostomy before delivering the bowel through the defect in the abdominal wall, the subsequent takedown of the stoma will be greatly facilitated (Figure 26-43). The use of Seprafilm has been described in Chapter 22.

Results

In analyzing the results of Hartmann's resection for acute or perforated diverticular disease, it is inadequate to talk merely in terms of the first stage. In calculating the overall morbidity and mortality, one must consider the subsequent procedure or procedures. Unfortunately, much of the literature (which is voluminous) fails to deal with the entire spectrum of surgery required to effect complete resolution of the disease process, including reestablishment of intestinal continuity.

Nunes and colleagues performed Hartmann's resection on 25 patients for complications of acute diverticuli-

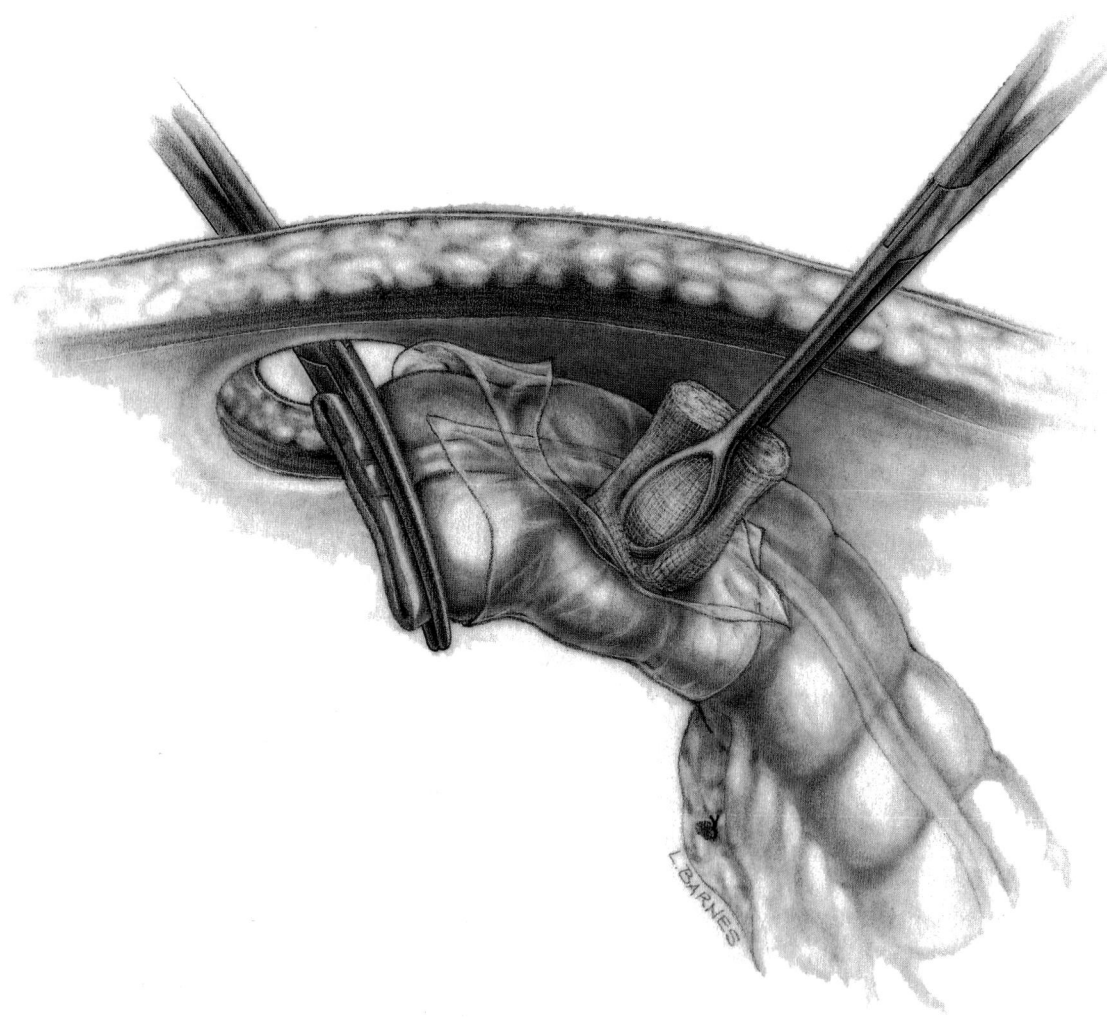

FIGURE 26-43. Wrapping the colostomy with Seprafilm (Genzyme Corp., Cambridge, MA; *www.genzyme.com*) before delivering it through the opening in the abdominal wall facilitates subsequent takedown.

tis.[176] Five failed to undergo a second-stage procedure (20%). There were two deaths after the first operation, a mortality rate of 8%. No deaths were reported after the second stage. However, three anastomotic leaks developed (15%), necessitating transverse colostomy. Approximately two thirds of the patients had essentially an uneventful postoperative course after the second operation. Labow and associates reported a complication rate of 67% in 15 patients treated by Hartmann's procedure, but there were no deaths.[132] Laimon reported only one death in 36 patients.[134]

Howe and colleagues compared their experience with the three-stage procedure and Hartmann's resection in patients with colon perforation secondary to diverticular disease.[108] An overall morbidity of 71% was noted after the three-stage operation, and of 37% after Hartmann's procedure. Wound infection comprised the major morbidity. The operative mortality in the former was 5%, versus approximately 6% in the latter. Only four additional surgical procedures were required in Hartmann's group, whereas 34 additional operations were required in the three-stage group. Others also have reported favorable results with Hartmann's operation for perforated diverticulitis.[28,70,130,131135,145,173,212,254]

Zeitoun and colleagues (France) undertook a randomized study involving 103 patients who were to undergo primary or secondary resection.[272] Random assignment was made in the operating room once the surgeon had opened the abdomen. If primary resection were selected the surgeon was free to choose Hartmann's operation, or restoration of continuity with or without diversion. After primary resection postoperative peritonitis occurred less often ($p < .01$), early reoperation was performed less often ($p < .02$), and a shorter hospital stay was required ($p < .05$). The opposite point of view was expressed by Kronborg in a prospective, randomized trial involving patients with diffuse peritonitis.[129] The mortality rate was significantly higher after resection than after colostomy and drainage. Furthermore, the mortality rate in patients with fecal peritonitis did not differ significantly between those who underwent colostomy alone and those who underwent resection. This observation is contrary to other publications dealing with this subject.

Resection and Primary Anastomosis

With Fecal Diversion

The primary disadvantages of the previously mentioned Hartmann's operation are the potential technical difficulties and the risks involved in subsequently reestablishing intestinal continuity. An alternative approach is to effect an anastomosis at the initial operation and protect it with a transverse colostomy or loop ileostomy (Figure 26-38E). The second-stage procedure is therefore simplified, although it too is not without morbidity (see Chapters 23

and 31). The resection and anastomosis can be performed in accordance with the principles outlined, with the recognition that there is almost always a rim of uninvolved proximal rectum that will permit a reasonably safe anastomosis.

Another advantage of performing colorectal anastomosis at the first stage is that adequate mobility can usually be achieved without taking down the splenic flexure. Because more bowel usually must be sacrificed at the second stage of Hartmann's resection, mobilization of the splenic flexure is not uncommonly required.

If a colostomy is used, it should, in my opinion, be placed on the left side of the transverse colon (Figure 26-38E). As previously mentioned, there is no advantage to a right-sided stoma. The stool is theoretically more liquid, and the location predisposes to efferent limb prolapse. A left transverse colostomy is performed as far to the left as is possible, so that the splenic flexure tethers the efferent limb. The colostomy should, however, be delivered through the split rectus muscle (see Chapter 31).

Should the colostomy be divided to accomplish complete diversion? In my opinion, the answer is no. A properly constructed loop-ostomy stoma should not retract and is therefore completely diverting. Stool does not appear from the proximal limb, look around, and disappear into the distal opening. However, the major criticism of a divided colostomy is that it requires a formal resection and anastomosis, compared with the possible option, at least, of simple closure of the anterior wall with the loop-ostomy.

My own preference for fecal diversion, should I elect to employ it under these circumstances, is a loop ileostomy. Regardless, fecal diversion should not be undertaken whimsically. Considerable morbidity is associated with stomal creation as well as closure (see Chapters 23 and 31). However, once the surgeon has embarked on this approach, the colostomy or ileostomy should remain at least 6 weeks. As with Hartmann's operation, the morbidity of closure before this time is excessively high, probably because of the degree of inflammatory reaction.

A particular concern about primary colorectal anastomosis with diversion is that an inordinate delay in colostomy closure has been associated with a high incidence of stricture, especially if a circular stapled anastomosis was initially undertaken. It is, therefore, probably wiser to use a conventional suture technique rather than stapling if the surgeon elects to perform this operation. There are always differences of opinion among surgeons. The issues of the method of diverting the fecal stream and the timing of the closure always seem to stimulate heated discussion at meetings.

Before colostomy closure, the anastomosis should be examined by means of the rigid proctosigmoidoscope or flexible instrument. The presence of pus suggests the possibility of a dehiscence. A water-soluble enema is also advised to ascertain whether the anastomosis is intact. Not

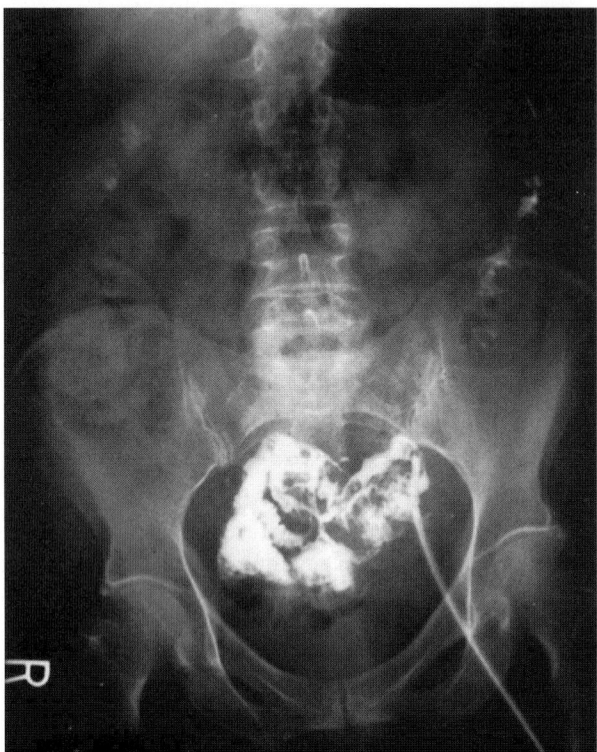

FIGURE 26-44. Status after anterior resection for perforated diverticulitis. A fistulogram through the abdominal wall reveals communication with the colon as well as the small bowel.

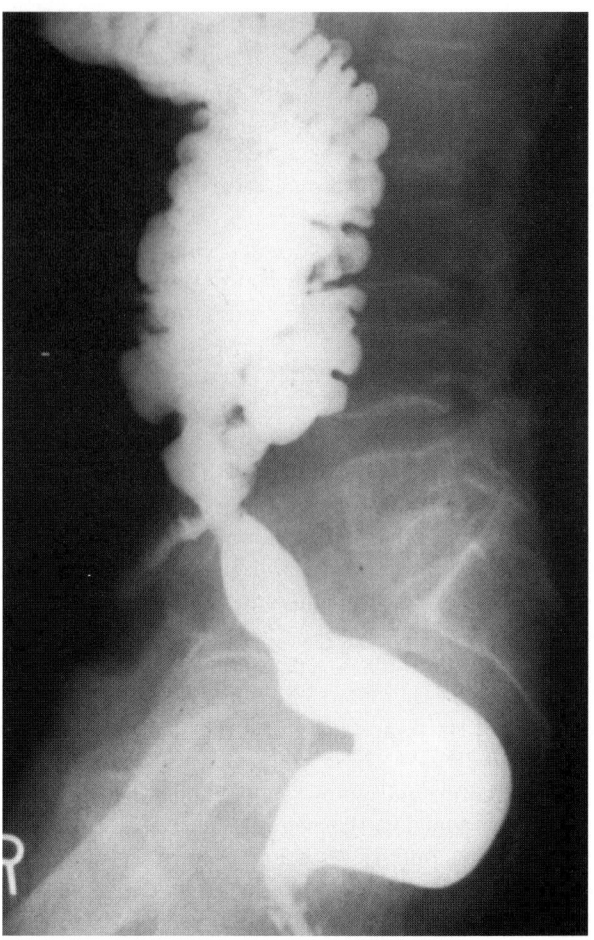

FIGURE 26-45. Leak following resection for diverticulitis. Note the anastomotic area above the sacral promontory with considerable residual sigmoid colon evident.

uncommonly, a short tract may be present, usually extending posteriorly. Rarely should this pose a problem, and colostomy closure can be performed safely. A long, blind tract may give the surgeon pause, but if it is unchanged after another month I believe one can safely close the ostomy. An obvious exception to this advice is made when a communication exists to the abdominal wall (Figure 26-44). In this situation, a colocutaneous fistula may be the consequence of an ill-advised colostomy closure. This complication may be attributed to the usual predisposing factors discussed in Chapter 23, but it also has been clearly shown to be related to inadequate resection of the diverticular disease, especially the failure to place the anastomosis into the rectum (Figure 26-45).[75] Repeated resection of the anastomosis may be required if healing does not take place within 3 or 4 months. However, no generalization can be made on this issue. Some will close spontaneously, others will heal following development of a fecal fistula, and still others will never become manifest, never become symptomatic.

Without Fecal Diversion

The treatment of perforated diverticulitis of the sigmoid colon by primary resection and anastomosis but with no colostomy was advocated by Madden (see the biography in Chapter 23) and Tan in 1961 (Figure 26-38F).[147] Although

stating that "treatment . . . is admittedly contrary to the generally accepted surgical principles," the authors believed that their results suggested that this could be the preferred approach. By 1966, however, Madden, although still adhering to the concept of resection at the first stage, believed that colostomy should be employed, particularly in cases of diffuse peritonitis, fecal loading, and gross contamination, and in situations in which the rectum was mobilized.[146]

Results

Evaluation of reported series is difficult. Some investigators use the term *primary resection* interchangeably with *primary anastomosis (no colostomy)*, *primary anastomosis (with colostomy)*, and *Hartmann's resection*. Many authors equate primary resection with staged resection, and the reader never is told whether fecal diversion was employed.

Farkouh and associates performed primary resection and anastomosis without colostomy on 15 patients with perforation and peritonitis.[73] The operation was restricted to those whose bowel demonstrated no obstruction, was empty of feces, and was minimally edematous. Further criteria included normal distal bowel above the peritoneal reflection, no fecal contamination, and good general health of the patient. One death and one anastomotic leak occurred. In reviewing a total of nine series with 73 patients so treated, these authors noted an operative mortality of 8.2%. Schilling and co-workers of Bern, Switzerland, evaluated 55 patients with perforated diverticulitis (Hinchey stage III and IV) who underwent emergency surgery.[227] Thirteen patients were submitted to Hartmann's operation, whereas the remainder received a primary anastomosis without fecal diversion, but this was not a prospectively randomized study. There were no anastomotic leaks, and there was no increased morbidity with the latter approach. However, there was a considerably increased cost associated with the requirement for a second operation. Furthermore, 22% of the patients never were submitted to colostomy closure due to their refusal, to medical problems or to interval death.

Gooszen and co-workers of Leiden University in the Netherlands prospectively evaluated 45 patients who underwent primary anastomosis for acute, complicated diverticulitis with respect to the Acute Physiology And Chronic Health Evaluation (APACHE) II score, the Mannheim Peritonitis Index (MPI), and the Hughes' peritonitis classification.[89] Neither anastomotic leakage (9%) nor death (6.7%) was related to higher scores. However, death, anastomotic leaks, wound infection, and the requirement for reoperation were observed more frequently when there was evidence of colonic obstruction.

Most surgeons agree that if the bowel is reasonably well prepared, such as is often the case when a patient has been in the hospital for several days before resection is undertaken, no stoma is required. It is also believed that concomitant fecal diversion is not mandatory in the presence of a pericolic abscess, a localized pelvic abscess, or a mesenteric phlegmon.[5,19] However, with generalized peritonitis, gross fecal contamination, fecal diversion is a requisite. Others advise that patients who are receiving steroids or who are immunocompromised (see later) should have a concomitant stoma created.[220]

The need for a large, prospective, randomized, controlled clinical trial in the management of acute diverticulitis has been expressed by many surgeons and investigators.[148]

Intracolonic Bypass

In 1984, Ger and Ravo presented an experimental technique whereby a safe colorectal anastomosis could be performed by means of implanting a latex (Silastic) sheeting within the lumen of the bowel, even in the presence of massive contamination.[87] The principle of the so-called intracolonic bypass involves suturing a specially prepared soft tube within the lumen of the proximal bowel. This device then conducts the fecal flow into the distal bowel without fecal contact of the anastomotic site. Their initial ten patients, for whom a colostomy would normally have been required, underwent this operation without significant morbidity or mortality.[201] They and others assert that the device, called Coloshield permits an anastomosis without a colostomy even in the presence of copious fecal loading, perforation, pus, or peritonitis.[205] On the basis of still another experimental study, Ravo and colleagues suggest that intraluminal contact caused by fecal loading at the anastomosis is a more important factor contributing to anastomotic complications than is peritonitis.[204]

Technique of Implantation

The technique involves the intraluminal placement of a soft, pliable tube, similar to a surgical glove. Following resection, with the use of four stay sutures, the proximal 3 cm of bowel are everted (Figure 26-46A). The Coloshield is removed from the package but should not be unfolded. The device is inserted into the proximal colon, and the reinforcing cuff is sutured to the mucosa and submucosa. A separate suture should be employed for each hemicircumference to eliminate the possibility of a purse-string effect. A continuous locking stitch is recommended with 2–0 long-term absorbable sutures, placed close together to create a watertight seal (Figure 26-46A). The stay sutures are then removed. The posterior wall of the anastomosis is then completed by conventional suture technique (Figure 26-46B). A rectal probe (catheter) is then attached onto the connector and the device unfolded. The probe is then passed into the rectum with the attached Coloshield and out through the anus (Figure 26-46C). The anterior wall of the anastomosis is then completed in the usual manner. At this point, the redundant device is excised outside the anal verge with the application of slight tension, so that it can lie within the rectum. If the anastomosis is very low, it can be left outside, secured to a collecting bag (Figure 26-46D). A modification of the anastomosis is also possible through the use of the circular stapler. The Coloshield passes spontaneously 2 to 4 weeks later.

Results

Ravo, Ger, and colleagues reported 29 patients who underwent this procedure with neither death nor anastomotic leak.[200,202,205] All except one passed the tube between the fifteenth and thirtieth postoperative days. In one individual, the tube became affected and required manual evacuation. As all were passed with intact sutures, it was presumed that expulsion is the method of separation from the bowel.

Sackier and Wood submitted 51 consecutive patients to low anterior resection, randomly allocating them to

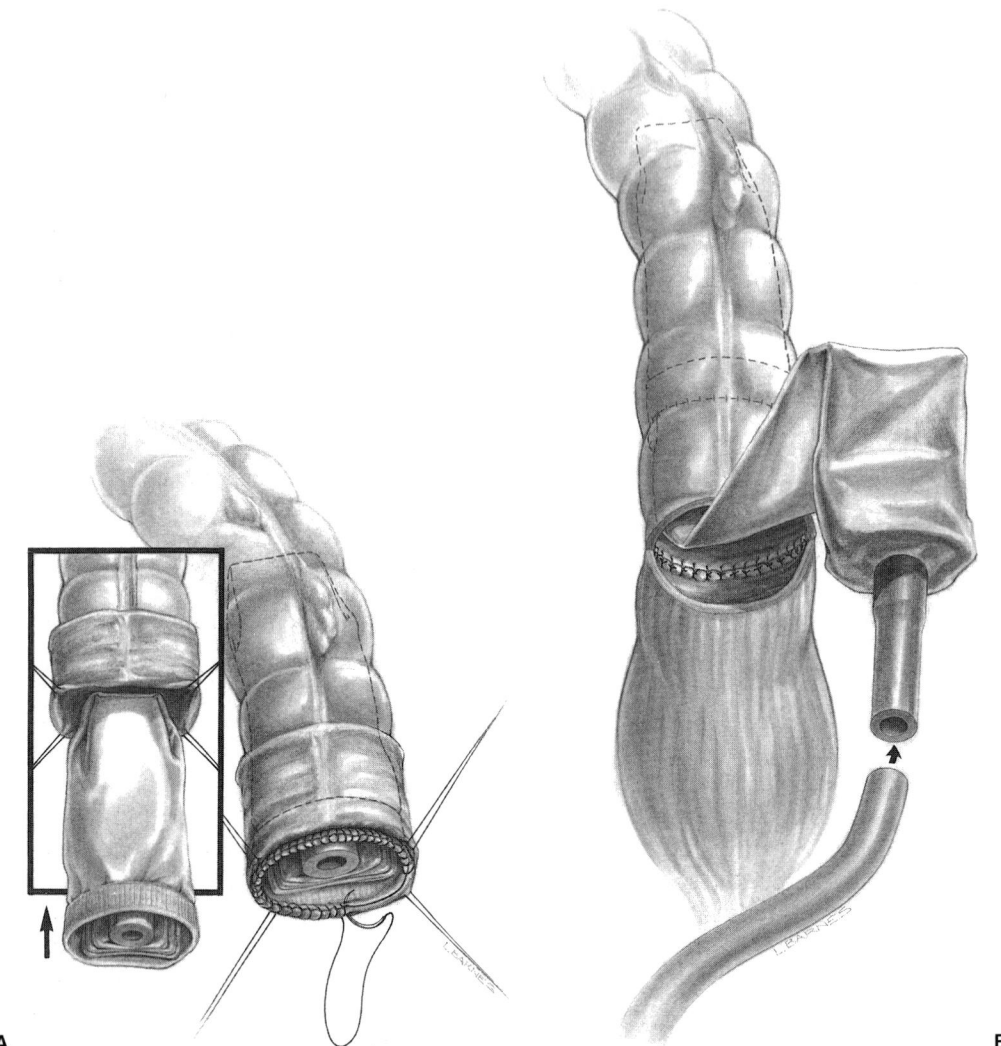

FIGURE 26-46. Anastomosis by means of the intracolonic bypass (Coloshield). **(A)** The proximal bowel is everted with stay sutures, and the device is secured into place with continuous, interlocking sutures of long-term absorbable material, incorporating the mucosa and submucosa. **(B)** The posterior wall of the anastomosis is completed, and the rectal probe is attached. **(C)** The Coloshield is unfolded and passed into the rectum and out the anus. **(D)** Final position with device lying outside the anus and with appliance attached, or cut short and lying within the rectum **(inset)**. *(CONTINUED)*

receive an anastomosis with or without the intraluminal bypass tube.[218] These individuals were not, however, ill with complicated diverticulitis. The tube was passed on average at 15 days. There were no clinical leaks and only one radiologic leak in the bypass group, whereas there were five clinical leaks and eight radiologic leaks in those submitted to conventional anastomosis. Keane and co-workers performed this operation on six patients with left-sided obstruction.[118] No mortality or clinical anastomotic leak occurred. However, colonic necrosis at the insertion of the device has been observed.[69] Others report satisfactory experiences,[217] but difficulty remains in honestly assessing the results, as it is not always clear whether patients truly qualify as candidates for urgent or emergency operation. In the United States, the point is moot, because the device has not been approved as of 2004.

Limited Resection, On-Table Lavage, and Primary Anastomosis

Colonic obstruction is not a common presentation of acute diverticulitis. Although it is much more frequently associated with left-sided colon cancer, the application of on-table lavage in order to perform a limited resection is theoretically as valid for acute sigmoid diverticulitis. The management by this technique is discussed in Chapter 22, but there is no "literature" on the results for diverticulitis.

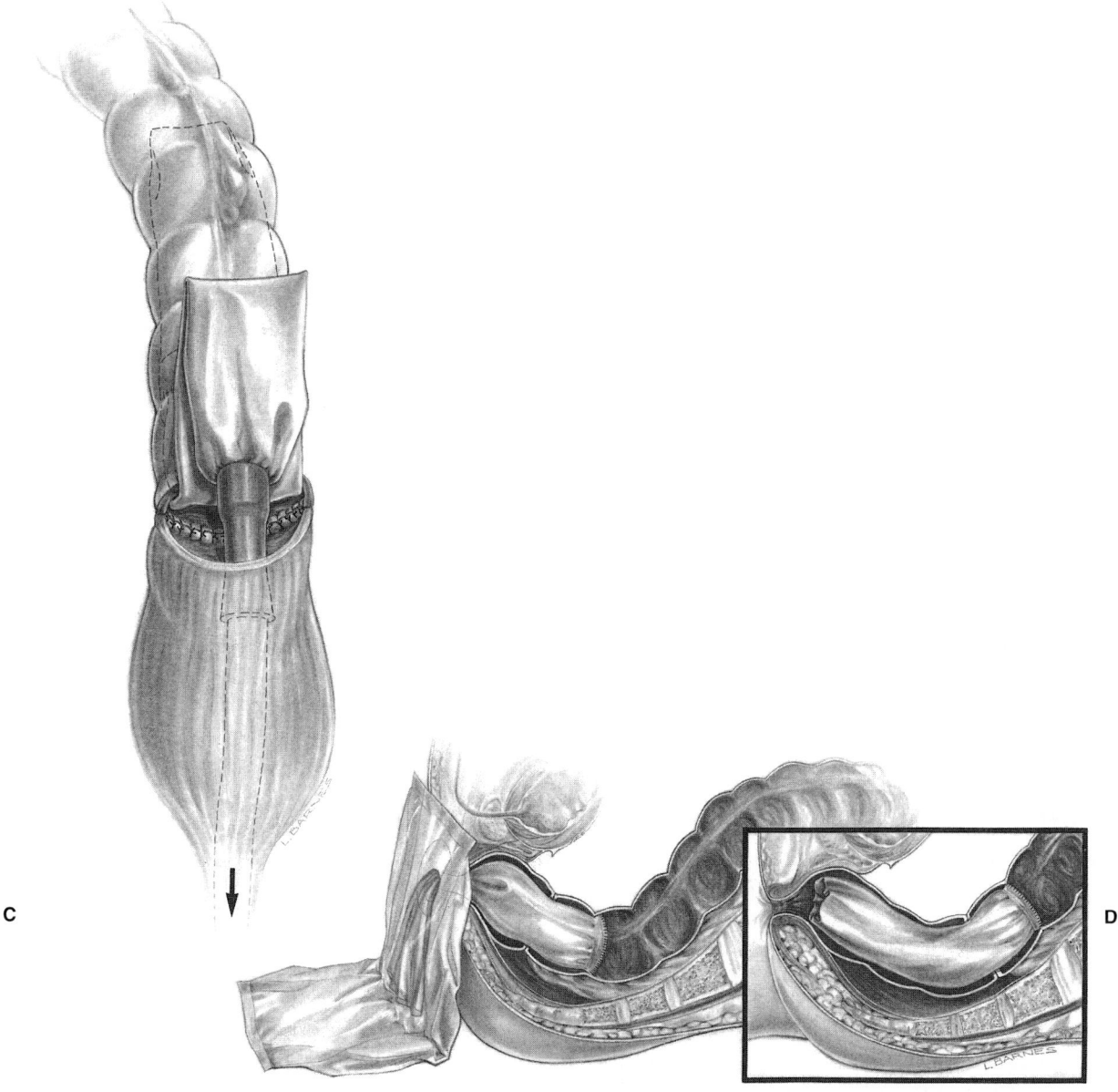

FIGURE 26-46. *(CONTINUED).*

Total Colectomy

Removing the entire colon for acute diverticulitis is an extraordinarily rare scenario. As mentioned earlier, colonic obstruction is an uncommon indication for surgery for this condition. Still, as with on-table lavage, it is a procedure that on may appropriately consider under the same circumstances as that for cancer (see Chapter 22). The main difference as an indication, however, is that one does not have the added concern of removing a

synchronous tumor with diverticulitis as one has with malignant obstruction.

Overview on the Emergency Surgical Management of Acute Diverticulitis

With rare exception, the intent of surgery for acute diverticular disease should be to remove the disease at the first operation. Ideally, an anastomosis may be effected at the initial procedure if conditions warrant. The surgeon may elect to perform a left transverse colostomy or loop ileostomy with resection and primary anastomosis based on his or her good clinical judgment. Hartmann's resection is recommended when there is generalized peritonitis, significant fecal contamination, a stool-laden bowel, obstruction, or diffuse (not localized) pus. Fecal diversion is usually not used if the bowel is relatively well prepared (a not uncommon situation when the patient has been hospitalized for a number of days before operation). If the perforation is into the mesentery or if the abscess is relatively small and localized, a colostomy is not a requisite.

Drainage is recommended if an abscess is present. Irrigation with large volumes of Ringer's lactate solution is advised for fecal peritonitis and should be continued for 48 hours following the procedure. Because anaerobes are usually the predominant organism (*Bacteroides* is almost always present), along with coliforms and enterococci, systemic antibiotic therapy is necessary. Rather than become repetitious my thoughts on the management of colonic obstruction can be found in Chapter 22.

ELECTIVE RESECTION

Natural History of Complicated Diverticular Disease

The decision whether to intervene surgically in a patient with uncomplicated sigmoid diverticulosis is a matter of considerable controversy and is always a cause of debate and conflict between internists and surgeons. Clearly, the presence of diverticular disease in and of itself is not sufficient justification for recommending an operation. In the absence of one of the aforementioned manifestations or complications, diverticulosis is unlikely to be the source of a patient's symptoms (i.e., bloating, cramps, abdominal pain, constipation). However, the antecedent history of a complication of diverticulitis somewhat simplifies the operative recommendation, but many patients who could benefit from resection do not have such a prior history.

How does one choose to offer surgery? Radiologic evaluation that reveals narrowing, deformity, or even partial obstruction may help decide in favor of a procedure, but one can never be certain that symptoms will resolve following resection unless acute disease is found at laparotomy. If colonoscopy reveals edema, stricture, or pus, resection at some point would seem indicated. Conversely, if colonoscopic evaluation is unremarkable, resection of the sigmoid colon is less likely to resolve the patient's complaints. Rennie and associates demonstrated a low operative complication rate in 88 patients who underwent elective resection for uncomplicated di-

verticular disease, but persistent symptoms were evident in 86%.[210]

If the patient recovers from an acute attack, the question of whether to perform an elective resection must be addressed. Unfortunately, there are few useful articles on the subject. In 1970, Parks and Connell reported the outcome of 455 patients who had been admitted to the hospital for treatment of diverticular disease.[186] Two thirds were suitable for medical management, and one third required an operation. One of four on long-term management required readmission (25%). Follow-up of medically treated patients revealed that 43% had persistent symptoms (severe in 5%), but evaluation following surgery demonstrated complaints in 33%.[186] Farmakis and co-workers reported the natural history of complicated diverticular disease on the basis of a questionnaire sent to 300 patients.[74] Of 120 responders, ten had died of recurrent complicated diverticular disease. Of the remaining 110, 40 were still symptomatic. These data generally support the recommendation for elective resection to prevent persistent symptoms and potentially lethal complications.[74]

Mäkelä and associates of Oulu, Finland, published their experience with 366 patients admitted with diverticulitis over a 10-year period.[151] Men under the age of 50 underwent more primary operations and developed more recurrences than did older individuals of either sex. Although not statistically meaningful, the authors recommend resection after two episodes of acute diverticulitis. Chautems and co-workers of Geneva followed 118 patients who were successfully managed nonoperatively (median follow up, 9.5 years).[45] Young age and "severe" diverticulitis were both statistically significant factors associated with a poor outcome. The authors recommend elective resection for these categories of individuals after one attack.

Age

Vignati and colleagues reviewed the records of 40 patients, ages 50 or younger, who were hospitalized with acute diverticulitis and followed for a minimum of 5 years.[258] Ten (25%) required surgery during the initial hospitalization. Of the remaining 30 individuals, one third underwent surgical resection, whereas two thirds continued to be managed nonoperatively. The authors concluded that surgery in this population after a single episode of diverticulitis that resolves is not recommended.[258] When reading their article, however, one can truly make the opposite conclusion. Ambrosetti and associates found that patients younger than 50 years were significantly more prone to recurrences and complications after conservative treatment of their diverticulitis, whereas older individuals required operation significantly more often during their initial hospitalization.[13,14] They further observed that abscess formation and extracolonic contrast or gas are findings indicative of failure of medical treatment during the initial admission. Moreover, the risk for secondary complications after initial successful management of acute diverticulitis is high.[10] Likewise, Konvolinka opines that any patient under age 40 should undergo resection following the first documented attack of acute diverticulitis.[124]

Spivak and colleagues of Beth Israel Medical Center, New York, evaluated 63 patients younger than 45 who were treated for acute diverticulitis at their institution.[239] The overwhelming majority had contained disease, Hinchey stage I (90%). Two thirds were treated successfully with antibiotics and bowel rest, whereas the remainder required an emergency operation. The authors point out that 20% of their patients were misdiagnosed with diverticulitis and at surgery were found to have acute appendicitis. They caution that it is critically important to assess the true nature of the pathology adequately when a young patient presents with signs, symptoms and findings suggestive of acute diverticulitis. Others conclude that young patients do not have a more virulent form of the disease nor is the risk of recurrence greater than older patients.[29] This is counterintuitive logic because one expects younger people to live longer.

Technique

The technical details of elective resection for diverticulitis are essentially the same as that for carcinoma of the sigmoid colon, with minor differences. The reader is referred to the illustrations and narrative in Chapter 22 for the surgical approach to management. Resection should be performed with the anastomosis placed into the rectum. Splenic flexure mobilization is not usually required, and attempt at removal of all diverticula is meddlesome and unnecessary.

Laparoscopically Assisted Resection

As of this writing (2004), perforation and peritonitis are contraindications to performing laparoscopic colon surgery. However, for certain operations, such as reestablishment of intestinal continuity following Hartmann's resection and elective resection for diverticular disease, a laparoscopic approach has been enthusiastically advocated by some surgeons.[39,79,121,140,228,231,246,256] In the experience at the Lahey Clinic Medical Center, Burlington, MA, elective laparoscopic resection was found to be as safe as the conventional, open operation and was associated with a shorter hospitalization and more rapid recovery.[38] However, the authors cautioned that the higher cost of operating room time may make it difficult to justify the procedure economically, but this becomes less of a concern with increased experience. In fact, the Cleveland Clinic (Ohio) group was able to show that laparoscopic colectomy is a "cost-effective means of electively managing sigmoid diverticular disease."[231]

Surgical experience and the presence of severe diverticular disease are the primary predictive factors for conversion to an open procedure.[140] Vargas and co-workers observed that the requirement for conversion appears to be associated with complicated diverticulitis, such as fistula and abscess, and opined that this manifestation would suggest that a better approach might be an open operation.[256] Bruch and co-workers of Lubeck, Germany, undertook 217 laparoscopic colectomies for diverticulitis with a conversion rate to the open procedure of 9.2%.[39] Overall morbidity was 20.8%, and the reoperation rate for complications was 7.1%. Two port-site hernias required late operation. Dwivedi and associates compared laparoscopic sigmoid colectomy with open colectomy for sigmoid diverticular disease in a retrospective fashion.[66] The mean estimated blood loss, time until a liquid diet was commenced, and length of hospital stay were all significantly less with the laparoscopic technique. The conversion rate to the open procedure was 19.7%. Outside of a very high frequency of hematuria, presumably because of the utilization of ureteral stents with the laparoscopic approach, there was no difference in the rate of complications. However, Stevenson and co-workers of Brisbane, Australia, noted that the complication rate following conversion was significantly greater than when the patient did not need an open operation (75% versus 16%).[246] Conversely, Le Moine and colleagues of France found that conversion did not increase the morbidity rate in their series of 168 patients.[140] The laparoscopically assisted technique is discussed in Chapter 27.

Results of Elective Surgery

Although there is no gainsaying the fact that patients who require surgery for complications of diverticulitis have their conditions ameliorated by operation, the questions remain whether individuals who have recovered should be submitted to elective operation and, if so, what the long-term results are. Moreover, there is considerable controversy as to the relative merit of operating on someone electively with sigmoid diverticular disease who has abdominal pain but who has never objectively demonstrated an acute attack of diverticulitis.

We reviewed our results of elective surgery for diverticular disease in 100 consecutive patients.[34] There were no operative deaths. Symptoms were ameliorated in 94%, whereas 6% still had major complaints (mostly pain that affected one's daily life). One could, however, identify preoperative factors that were associated with a higher likelihood of obtaining a favorable result. These included male sex, preoperative bowel complaints of less than 1 year's duration, abdominal pain localized to the left lower quadrant, and radiologic evidence of "diverticulitis" rather than "diverticulosis." A highly significant variable that was associated with resolution of symptoms was the presence of inflammatory changes in the resected specimen—that is, a histopathologic diagnosis of diverticulitis. Even in the elective situation, an unexpected abscess, phlegmon, fistula, or sealed perforation may be present. All patients with pathologic evidence of acute or chronic inflammation in the resected specimen were improved in our experience.[34] Of course, that information is obtained *ex post facto* and cannot be used to determine the relative merits of that factor preoperatively. Those in whom some or most of these indicators were absent may also benefit from the operation, but not with the high frequency of success anticipated in the former group. Two preoperative factors associated with more frequent postoperative complaints were the presence of bowel management problems for more than 1 year and abdominal pain not localized to the left lower quadrant.

As previously stated, diverticular disease and the irritable bowel syndrome are two common diseases that often have overlapping clinical features. With respect to the apparent difference between the sexes in the results of surgery, men are less likely to have functional bowel complaints. Hence, misinterpretation of symptoms is less of a problem, and the correlation with radiologic and clinical findings is usually self-evident. The Uppsala, Sweden group showed that individuals with functional symptoms or symptoms suggestive of an irritable bowel before surgery predicted a less successful result ($p < .05$).[252]

Emergency or urgent surgery for complicated diverticulitis is associated with high rates of morbidity and mortality. Therefore, rather than wait for another attack in someone who recovered initially, it seems prudent to offer a patient an interval operation. In our retrospective review, 133 patients underwent resection for diverticular disease as a planned, elective operation.[102] There were no deaths, and only ten complications were noted. During the same period, 155 patients underwent an operation for complicated diverticulitis. The overall operative mortality was 9% (Table 26-1). The complication rate was also extremely high.

Resection for diverticular disease is associated with a higher complication rate than is essentially the same operation for cancer, although the operative mortality is less.[32,72] Why this is true, even in the absence of sepsis, is somewhat difficult to explain. Incisional hernia is much more frequently observed (10% in our experience).[34] With respect to this complication alone, special precautions concerning the method of wound closure should be taken. Perhaps longevity permits the development of late complications; many individuals who undergo resection for colon carcinoma do not have a prolonged survival.

With careful selection of patients most likely to benefit from resection, excellent long-term results may be anticipated. Wolff and co-workers reviewed the Mayo Clinic experience with 505 elective resections for sigmoid diverticular disease between 1971 and 1976.[270] When the barium enema studies of 61 of these patients were reviewed between 5 and 9 years after resection, only nine (14.7%) showed progression of diverticula, and this was believed to be minimal in all cases. However, in seven patients (11.4%), signs and symptoms of recurrent diverticulitis developed. Although the authors believed that there was no benefit in resecting all of the diverticula-bearing colon, the results are somewhat disturbing. Because they described the operation as a "sigmoid resection," the explanation for their less-than-optimal results could be that the anastomosis was not placed into the rectum and that a zone of increased pressure was permitted to remain distal to the anastomosis. A later study from the same institution confirmed this observation. Recurrent diverticulitis developed in 12.5% of the patients in whom the sigmoid colon had been used for the distal anastomosis but in only 6.7% of whose in whom the rectum had been used ($p = .03$).[224] Reoperation was required in 3.4% of the patients in whom the sigmoid colon had been used as the distal anastomotic site and in 2.2% of those in whom the rectum had been used ($p < .05$).[24] The Cleveland Clinic Florida group concluded, on the basis of their 236 patients, that colorectal (rather than colosigmoid) anastomosis was the single predictor of lower recurrence rates after elective resection for uncomplicated diverticulitis.[248]

The Mayo Clinic group analyzed 930 patients with diverticular disease over a 10-year period.[107] The authors described what they call "smoldering diverticular disease" in 5%. These are individuals with chronic, debilitating, left lower quadrant abdominal pain as the only symptom, with no documented history of fever, elevated white count, or radiologic evidence of diverticulitis. These individuals were found to have complete resolution of symptoms in 76%, with 88% being pain free.

Opinion: Recommendation for Elective Resection

Based on the foregoing observations, elective resection is advised for patients who have had one or more attacks of left lower quadrant pain associated with fever, leukocytosis, and radiologic evidence of diverticulitis, especially if any of the following apply:

- The patient is less than 55 years of age.[46,178]
- There is radiologic evidence of leak.
- The patient has urinary tract symptoms (suggestive of impending fistula).
- There is evidence of obstruction.

If radiologic and endoscopic changes that cannot exclude cancer are present, resection is mandated.

MYOTOMY

Myotomy is mentioned here as an option, especially with a thickened bowel wall, but in reality, this procedure is more of historic interest. In 1964, Reilly recommended sigmoid myotomy in the treatment of diverticular disease.[208] In a later report, he stated that the primary indication for the procedure was long-standing, uncomplicated diverticular disease that did not respond to standard medical measures.[209] Such patients comprised 75% of his 104 cases. The remainder were those who exhibited complications of sigmoid diverticulitis and who underwent elective myotomy following resolution of the acute process, sometimes after colostomy and drainage.

The procedure involves division of the antimesenteric taenia and underlying circular muscle from the rectosigmoid junction for "whatever distance is necessary," sometimes as much as 60 cm. The mucosa is permitted to pout. If the lumen of the bowel is entered, Reilly recommended closure of the mucosa with catgut.

In 1973, Hodgson and colleagues proposed transverse taeniamyotomy in the treatment of diverticular disease.[104,105] The two antimesenteric taeniae are transversely incised at 2-cm intervals from the rectosigmoid junction proximally to the normal colon. A later report from Hodgson's group implied less enthusiasm for the technique.[155] The authors believed the procedure to be simpler than Reilly's, whereas Reilly stated that Hodgson's operation is less thorough. Decreased intraluminal pressure and decreased motility following natural and pharmacologic stimuli have been reported for transverse taeniamyotomy.[137] Modifications have been suggested, with favorable functional results.[56]

Comment

It is difficult to interpret Reilly's experience. In the uncomplicated group, it would appear that the procedure was in actuality being performed for irritable bowel complaints. Reilly in fact observed that the indications for application of the procedure seemed to be diminishing.[1209] He suggested that better medical treatment could be the reason.

The application of this technique for an irritable bowel, for the "prediverticular state," and for diverticulosis may prove useful and is worthy of further investigation. Physiologic evaluation (motility and pressure studies) may permit identification of patients who will benefit from this approach.

I have had no experience with myotomy in the management of diverticular disease. I am of the opinion, however, that careful and expeditious resection of the acute inflammatory disease will prove to be the best operation with respect to morbidity, mortality, and long-term results. Others must concur, because there seem to have been no further writings on this technique in the English language, peered journals for more than 25 years.

SPECIAL CONCERNS: THE IMMUNOCOMPROMISED PATIENT (e.g., STEROIDS, ORGAN TRANSPLANTATION, AND RENAL FAILURE)

Patients who have been receiving long-term steroid therapy (e.g., for rheumatoid arthritis), who are immunocompromised, who have renal failure, or who have undergone organ transplantation are prone to the development of a variety of colonic complications, including colonic dilatation, intestinal obstruction, ischemic colitis, necrotizing enterocolitis, ulceration, hemorrhage, and perforated diverticulitis.[4,27,49,95,112,116,122,123,165,211,224] The manifestation of *free* perforation is much more likely in renal transplant recipients, whereas mesenteric abscess or walled-off perforation is more common in individuals with diverticular disease who have not undergone transplantation (Figure 26-47). The use of immunosuppressive agents and steroids is believed to be responsible and can be of catastrophic consequence in these patients. Even when a person does not manifest systemic signs and symptoms, surgical intervention should be performed early and should always include a resection (Figure 26-48). These patients must have the nidus of sepsis removed. In other words, diversion and drainage are not acceptable options. Likewise, nonoperative treatment is unlikely to carry the patient through the hospitalization to discharge. Because of diminished host resistance, demonstrable perforation or abscess will not resolve with conservative therapy and will delay needed surgical intervention.[6,191]

The medical records were reviewed following 1,401 consecutive renal transplants performed between 1951 and 1995 at the Brigham and Women's Hospital in Boston.[244] Early diagnosis and intervention improved the prognosis, but still 22% of those operated on within 24 hours expired. However, this compared with 47% who died after a delay in surgical intervention. The incidence and outcome of colonic perforations following transplantation were associated with the intensity of immunosuppression.[244] Twenty-eight percent of the perforations occurred within the first month, and 47% were seen within 3 months. The masking effects of corticosteroids on symptoms and signs need to be considered.

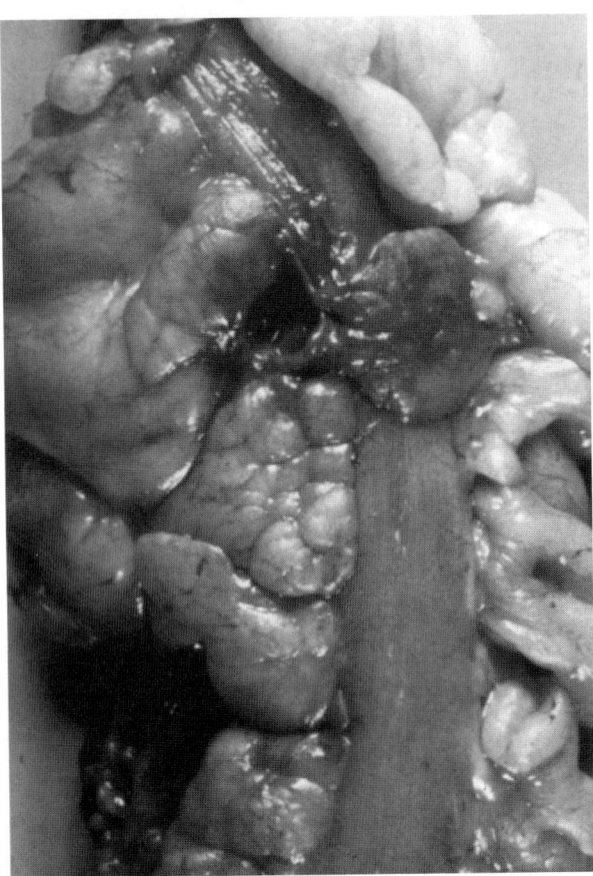

FIGURE 26-47. Perforated sigmoid colon in an immunosuppressed patient. Note the lack of inflammatory response.

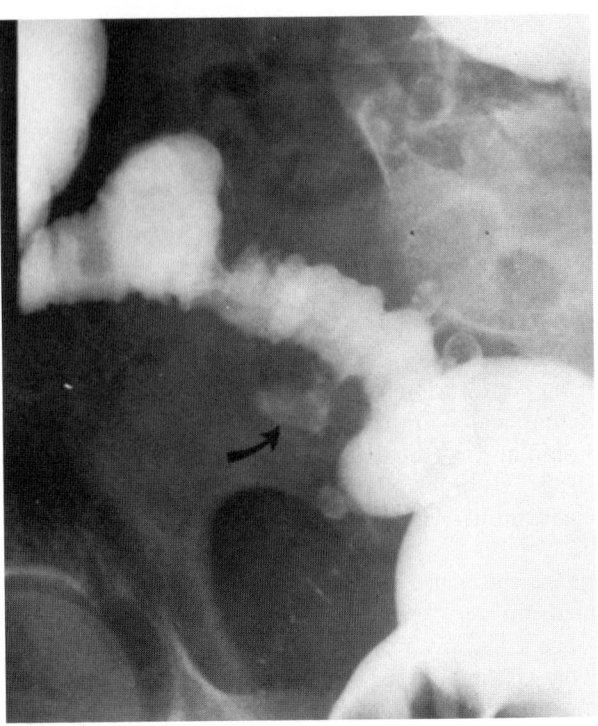

FIGURE 26-48. Perforation of diverticulum *(arrow)* in a renal transplant patient. No symptoms were apparent except that the patient felt a mass.

An increased incidence of colon perforation has been observed in individuals who have undergone lung transplantation.[20] Since the inception of the lung transplant program at the University of Colorado, 60 procedures had been performed by 1996, with four patients suffering spontaneous colonic perforation (7%).[20] Bowel perforation has been demonstrated to be a frequent cause of mortality after pediatric orthotopic liver transplantation. In the series from the University of California at Los Angeles, 24 bowel perforations occurred in 246 recipients (10%).[232] Most involved the small bowel, predominantly at the Roux-en-Y limb, but eight involved the transverse colon or terminal ileum.

Starnes and colleagues reported 25 patients with colonic diverticulitis complicating renal failure.[242] Most patients described acute abdominal pain. The overall mortality was 28%, with no correlation between survival rate and the type of operation performed. Koneru and co-workers noted that six of seven patients (86%) survived when surgery was performed within 24 hours of perforation, whereas only 25% survived when further delay was permitted.[123]

GIANT COLONIC DIVERTICULUM

Giant colonic diverticulum is a rare clinical entity, although more than 100 cases have been reported in the past 35 years.[8,83,101,120,128,153,160,225,265] The condition was originally described by Hughes and Greene and by Gabriel.[82,109] The disease most frequently involves the sigmoid colon, but there are reports of solitary giant diverticula found in other areas of the bowel. All described cases originated from the antimesenteric border of the colon, with the lesion representing a pseudodiverticulum with or without intact mucosa that becomes progressively enlarged. Still more rarely, one may encounter a giant diverticulum in which all layers of the bowel wall are observed—a giant true diverticulum. Choong and Frizelle believed that this condition should be defined by any diverticulum larger than 4 cm.[47] In their review of the literature, they classified the 103 reported cases as type I, a pseudodiverticulum (87%), and type II (13%), a true diverticulum.

Muhletaler and associates described the pathogenesis of giant diverticula.[171] They and others believed that the disease represents an unusual complication of diverticulitis. Theories include distension of a diverticulum by gas-forming organisms after the neck has been occluded and a ball-valve mechanism that causes trapping of gas in the abscess cavity when the intraluminal pressure of the

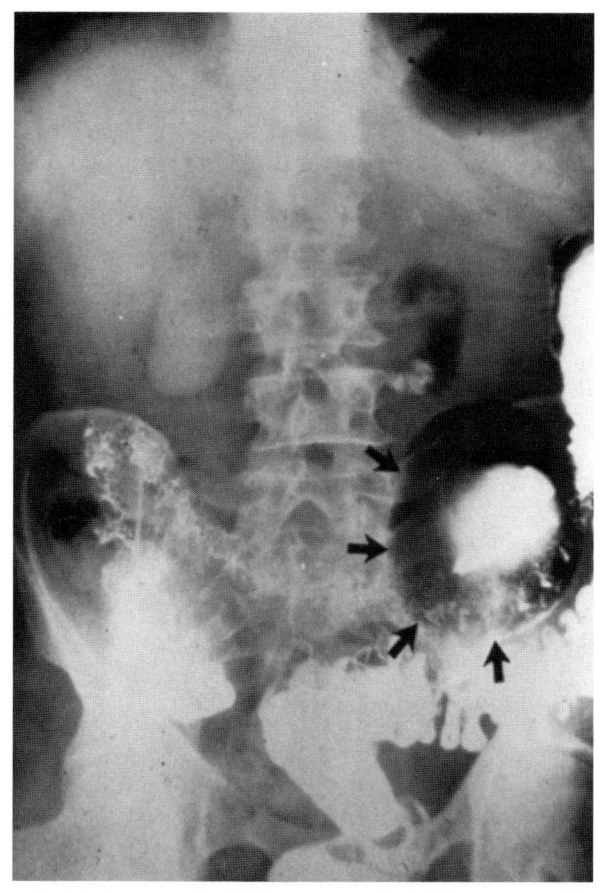

FIGURE 26-49. Giant sigmoid diverticulum. Barium fills part of the cavity; gas is also evident within the lumen *(arrows)*.

bowel increases. With few exceptions, reports have revealed that the diverticulum is not lined by mucosa or by muscularis mucosae. The wall of the cavity is usually composed of the components of a colonic inflammatory reaction.

Patients may present with perforation, sepsis, intestinal obstruction (resulting from compression by the mass), and rectal bleeding. Most complain of abdominal pain or the presence of a lump.[143] A plain abdominal x-ray film may reveal a gas-filled mass of considerable size. Differential diagnosis includes congenital duplication of the colon, colonic volvulus, emphysematous cholecystitis, infected pancreatic pseudocyst, pneumatosis cystoides intestinalis, giant duodenal diverticulum, intestinal obstruction, intraabdominal lipoma, and intraabdominal abscess.[83] Barium enema examination will usually confirm the diagnosis, because approximately two thirds of the time, the diverticulum will fill with contrast material (Figure 26-49). Presumably, compression by the mass under some circumstances may preclude visualization. CT will show an air-filled mass. Perhaps colonoscopy would be able to identify the communication, but as of

this writing no successful application of this technique has been reported.

Treatment by means of resection of the diverticulum in continuity with the sigmoid colon is advised, although there have been a few reports of diverticulectomy alone (Figure 26-50).[8,47,143,245] This is not usually advised, however, because it is believed that removal of the source of the complication—namely, the sigmoid diverticular disease—is important. The dissection is often quite difficult because of the inflammatory reaction induced by the mass.

DIVERTICULAR DISEASE OF THE RIGHT COLON

Diverticulitis of the cecum was first described by Potier in 1912.[196] Although the disease is uncommon, many reports and reviews have been published over the years.[16,18,76,84,91,126,138,150,159,222,229,255,259]

Pathophysiology and Epidemiology

Diverticula that involve the right colon may be solitary or multiple, but they should be distinguished from right-sided diverticula that exist concurrently with extensive diverticulosis throughout the colon. The former type of diverticulum traditionally has been thought to be congenital, and most were believed to be true diverticula—that is, containing all layers of the intestine. However, Murayama and colleagues measured the thickness of the right colon muscle in right-sided diverticular disease together with the number of haustra in the right colon.[172] They suggested that the etiology is the same as that of left-sided diverticular disease—abnormal thickening of the muscle in the wall of the colon. In support of the theory of a congenital origin, proponents have observed that the condition tends to occur at a much earlier age than does left-sided colitis. Characteristically, a solitary diverticulum has a shorter and wider neck than do multiple diverticula.[138]

Right-sided diverticular disease is more common in Asia than elsewhere. At least in this population, adoption of a Western diet may influence the prevalence of diverticular disease, but the site at which diverticula tend to occur is probably determined more by race or by genetic predisposition.[141]

Signs and Symptoms

The symptoms and signs of right-sided diverticulitis mimic those of appendicitis. Patients may complain of epigastric pain, nausea, and vomiting, with migration of the pain into the right iliac fossa. Depending on whether the process is localized or diffuse, low-grade fever, mod-

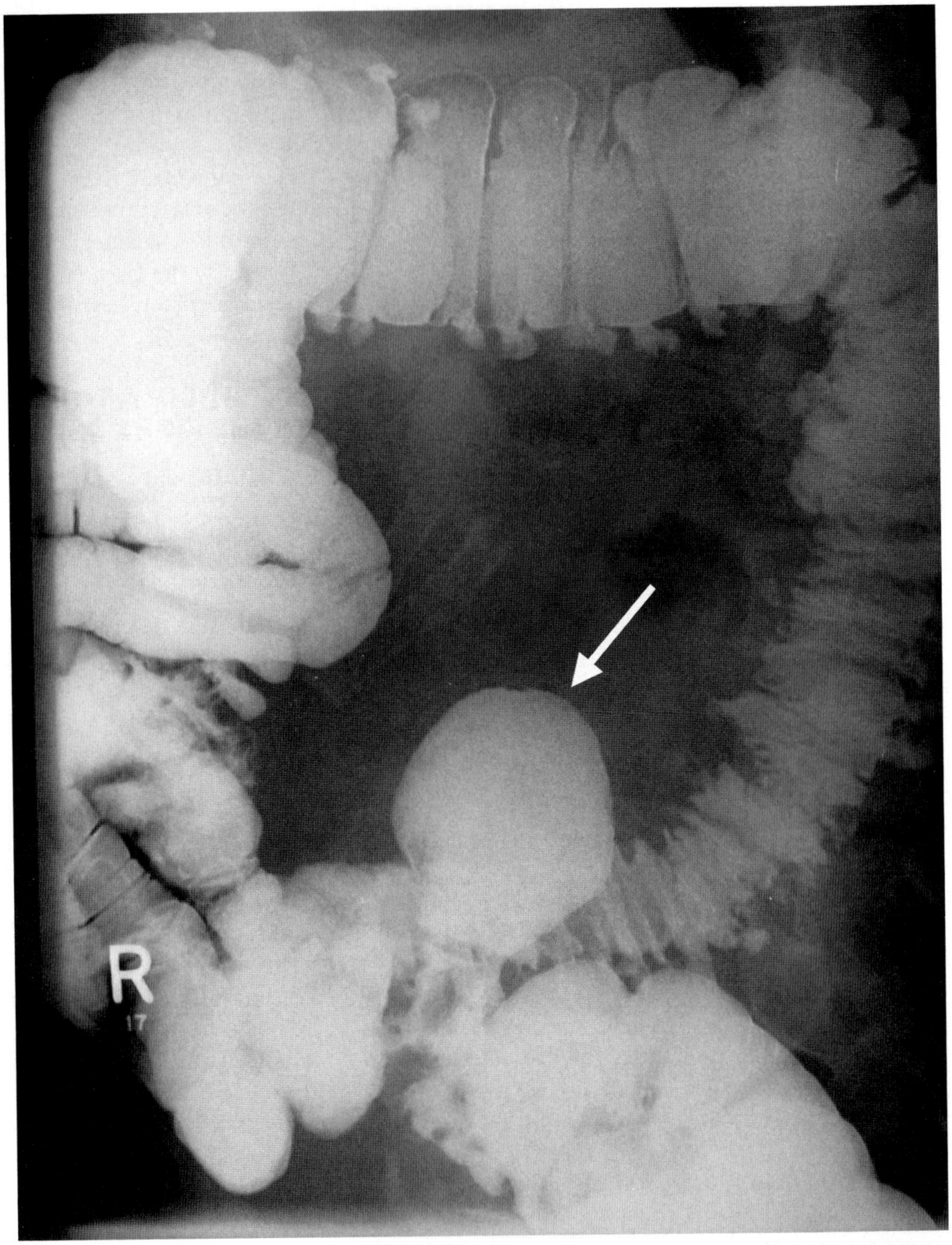

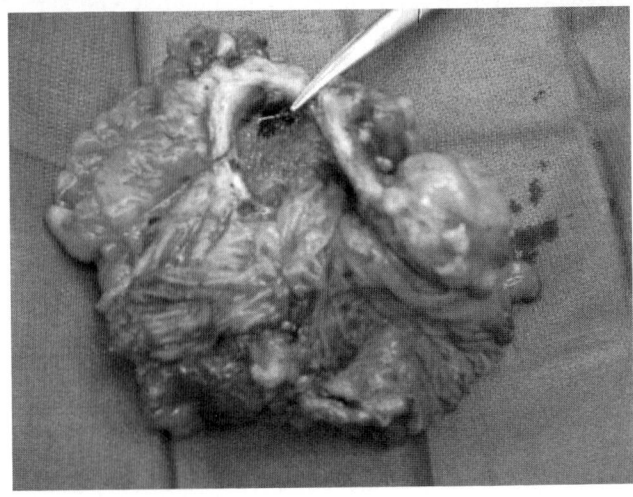

FIGURE 26-50. Giant sigmoid diverticulum. **(A)** Barium enema study with diverticulum *(arrow)*. **(B)** Resected specimen. (Courtesy of Keith P. Meslin, M.D.)

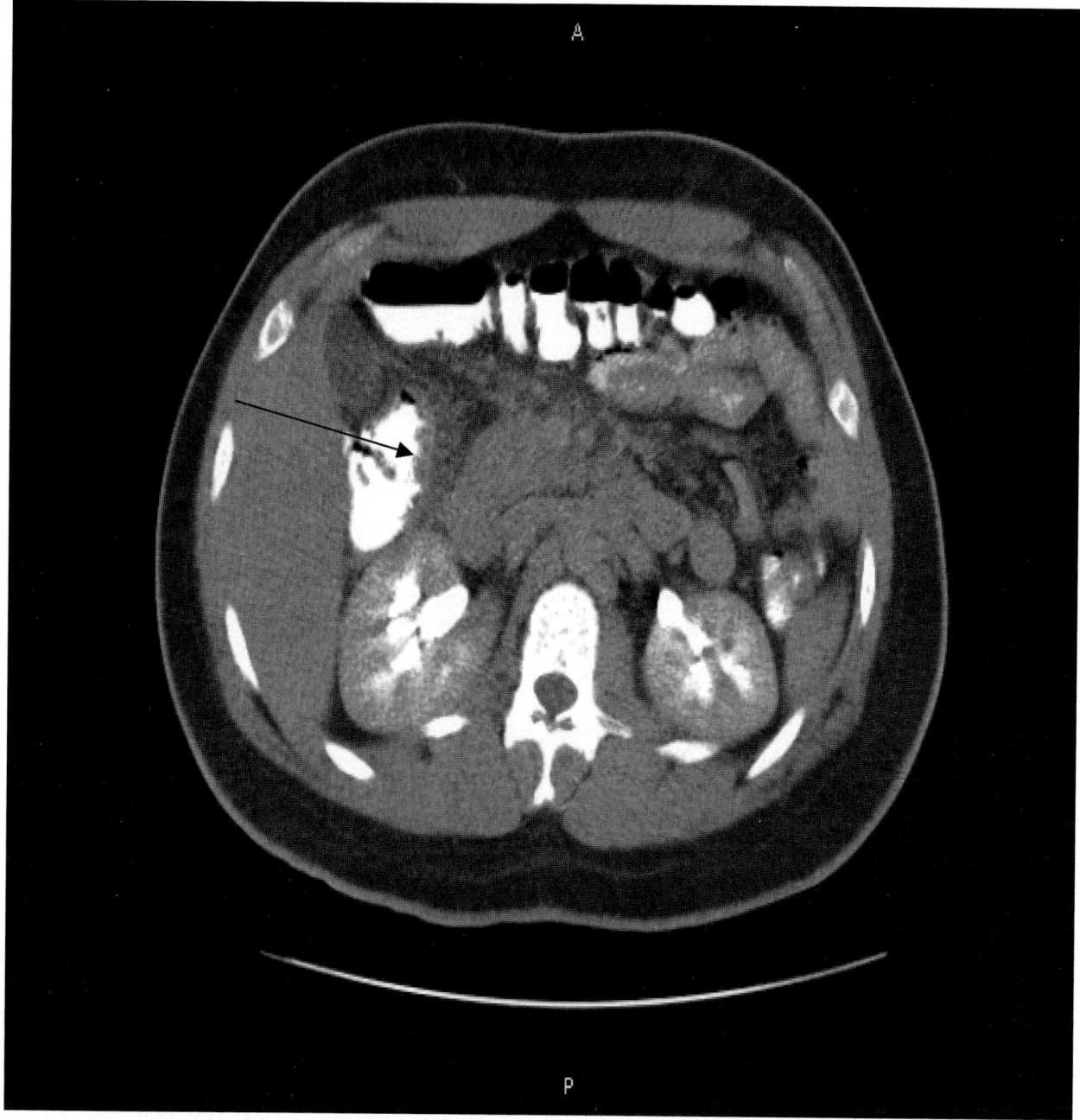

FIGURE 26-51. Right colon diverticulitis. Computed tomography demonstrates eccentric inflammation on the medial wall of the proximal ascending colon, with wall thickening *(arrow)* and with mucosal preservation consistent with diverticulitis. (Courtesy of Avraham Belizon, M.D.)

erate tenderness, guarding, and rebound may be noted. The leukocyte count is usually elevated.

Radiologic Studies

Radiologic findings consistent with right-sided diverticulitis include the presence of a paracolic mass, a calcified fecalith, and a distended loop of small bowel near the mass.[25] However, these findings are also found with acute appendicitis, so unless the patient has had the appendix previously removed, this triad of radiologic observations is not particularly helpful. On barium enema examination, an eccentric mural defect, a paracolic mass, or a fistula is highly suggestive of the presence of cecal diverticulitis (Figure 26-51).[25]

Crist and colleagues performed CT on seven patients with diverticulitis of the cecum and ascending colon.[60] Findings suggestive of acute diverticulitis included thickening of the bowel wall and pericolonic inflammation. Five patients were found to have an associated abscess. Because of the successful interpretation, one patient was managed nonoperatively with antibiotics. CT may be of value primarily for patients with atypical findings of acute appendicitis, especially in the older age group, and for those who have had prior appendectomy. The potential for CT-guided drainage further justifies selective application of this modality. However, the success of resection without special concern for a temporary stoma makes CT drainage a less attractive consideration.

Treatment

At the time of surgery, it may be difficult to distinguish the condition from acute appendicitis or even from sigmoid diverticulitis. In the latter situation, it is imperative to identify the source of the inflammation. A transverse colostomy for acute cecal diverticulitis is unlikely to ameliorate the condition. The preoperative diagnosis is rarely correct, so a high index of suspicion must be maintained, particularly in those who have undergone prior appendectomy or when rectal bleeding accompanies the abdominal signs and symptoms.

Ideally, a limited surgical approach would include simple excision of the involved diverticulum and closure of the bowel. However, because the inflammatory mass usually involves much of the cecum or right colon, resection is usually required. Moreover, partial colectomy is probably advisable whenever an inflammatory mass is present, because of the difficulty in distinguishing the lesion from a perforating carcinoma.

Results

Kovalcik and Sustarsic reported 11 patients who underwent surgical procedures for cecal diverticulitis during a 10-year period.[126] The average age was 49 years, considerably less than the average age for patients with left-sided diverticulitis. Without benefit of preoperative barium enema, nine patients underwent resection, all but one of whom had a primary anastomosis. No deaths or anastomotic leaks were reported. Two patients who underwent elective resection had a simple diverticulectomy. Gouge and colleagues reported 14 patients with diverticulitis of the right colon.[91] All were found to have an inflammatory mass medial and posterior to the ascending colon. Eight had perforation with an abscess, but neither free perforation nor generalized peritonitis was noted. All patients underwent resection with ileocolic anastomosis. There were no deaths and no leaks. These authors also found a younger age for patients with right-sided diverticulitis (51 years, compared with 62 years); they also observed an equal sex distribution. McFee and associates reported 18 patients with right-

sided diverticulitis with an average age of 46 years.[159] Barium enema examination was not helpful, and in only two cases was the preoperative diagnosis correct. All but one individual underwent resection with primary anastomosis. There were no deaths. Sardi and colleagues evaluated 30 cases.[222] The preoperative diagnosis was accurate in only 7%, and even at the time of surgery, the diagnosis was correct in fewer than 60%. The operative mortality was low (2.5%).

It appears, then, that the disease is rarely recognized preoperatively. There is also general agreement that resection with primary anastomosis is almost always the preferred treatment, with the anticipation of a low mortality rate.

DIVERTICULAR DISEASE OF THE TRANSVERSE COLON

Reports of acute diverticulitis of the transverse colon are extremely rare.[157,194,234,249] Peck and Villar identified 27 cases and added three of their own.[190] The mean age in the collected series was 53 years, and most of the patients (83%) were women. As with right colon diverticulitis, individuals tend to be younger and are most commonly thought to have acute appendicitis or cholecystitis. Other differential diagnostic concerns include perforated colon cancer, ischemic colitis, and Crohn's disease.

Evaluation by means of CT has identified the following findings on the basis of the four cases reported by Jasper and colleagues of Washington University, St. Louis, Missouri: stranding within the adjacent mesenteric fat, asymmetric wall thickening, and the presence of extraluminal gas or fluid (Figure 26-52).[114] These observations are not dissimilar to that observed in right-sided or sigmoid diverticulitis. Contrast enema is the study most likely to be diagnostic through the identification of mucosal preservation, but the correct diagnosis is usually made at the time of operation. Even then, the condition may be confused with carcinoma of the colon. As with sigmoid diverticulitis, in those who are unresponsive to bowel rest and antibiotics, resection is the preferred treatment.

SOLITARY CECAL ULCER

Solitary cecal ulcer is a condition of uncertain etiology. Numerous theories have been postulated to explain its occurrence, including drugs (especially corticosteroids), stasis with stercoral ulceration, diverticulitis, inflammatory bowel disease, foreign body, arteriovenous malformation, infection, ischemia, and a genetic predisposition.[31,233] In the more recent literature, solitary cecal ulcer seems to be quite frequently associated with end-stage renal disease.[139,164]

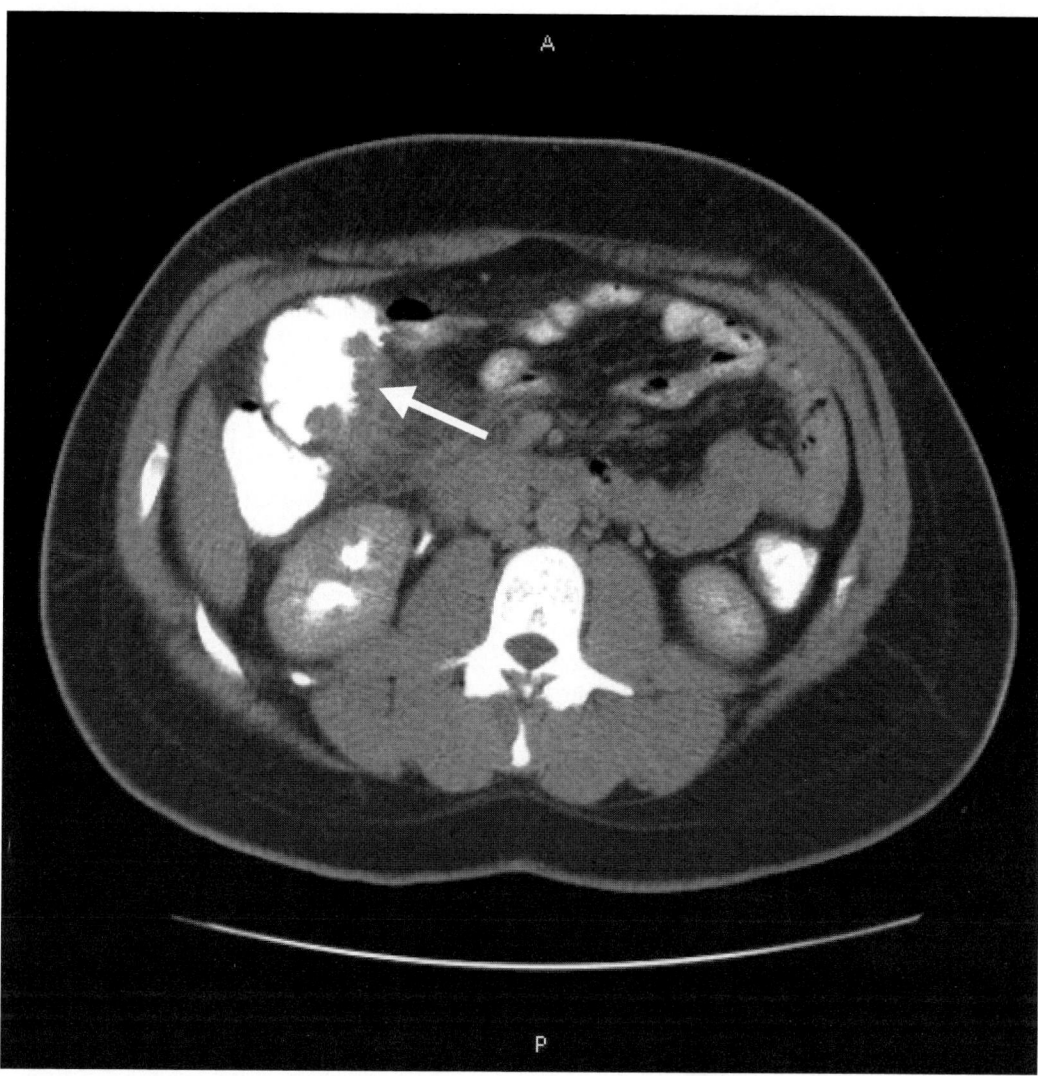

FIGURE 26-52. Diverticulitis of the proximal transverse colon. Computer tomography demonstrates eccentric inflammation on the inferior aspect of the bowel *(arrow)* and the suggestion of an inflammatory mass. (Courtesy of Avraham Belizon, M.D.)

Patients may present with signs and symptoms suggestive of acute appendicitis. Massive hemorrhage is not an uncommon consequence. The diagnosis may occasionally be made preoperatively by means of colonoscopy.

Macroscopically, the lesion resembles a peptic ulcer, ranging from 5 mm to 5 cm in diameter, usually located on the antimesenteric border, and generally quite well demarcated from the surrounding tissue.[233]

The surgical treatment for perforation requires a resection of the involved segment. In patients with hemorrhage, the protocol used in Chapter 28 should apply. However, because the lesion may actually be a result of ischemia, Last and Lavery suggested that the use of intraarterial vasopressin may precipitate a perforation.[139] Although conservative therapy should be considered, the differential diagnosis of a possible ulcerating carcinoma implies that at minimum a biopsy specimen should be obtained. Wedge excision may be undertaken for localized lesions that are clearly benign.

DIVERTICULAR DISEASE OF THE RECTUM

Rectal diverticular disease is a very unusual condition with only a handful of case reports having been published.[97] In the review by Piercy and colleagues, two theories for the low incidence in this area were proposed: the low pressure in the rectum and a lower peristaltic activity.[194] In contrast to the pseudodiverticula of sigmoid disease, rectal diverticula involve all layers of the bowel wall. Because of the usual absence of symptoms, no treatment is advised. However, inspissated fecal material leading to ischiorectal abscess formation with subsequent extrasphincteric fistula following incision and drainage has been observed. Another reported complication is rectal prolapse from an inverted diverticulum.[68]

DIVERTICULAR DISEASE OF THE SMALL BOWEL

Diverticular disease, excluding Meckel's diverticulum, can occur anywhere in the small intestinal but is quite uncommon. Most patients are asymptomatic, with the outpouching discovered incidentally during an abdominal exploration or seen in a small bowel series that had been performed for another indication. However, occasionally an individual may develop symptoms related to its presence. Small bowel diverticula may present with such complications as malabsorption, hemorrhage, obstruction, abscess, and fistula formation.[90] Complaints may include abdominal pain, nausea, bloating, vomiting, flatulence, weight loss, and diarrhea. Bleeding is usually the result of erosion of a mesenteric vessel and may be diagnosed by angiography (see Chapter 28). Bowel obstruction may be a consequence of adhesions, stricture, volvulus, intussusception, or the presence of an enterolith.[563] When inflammation ensues, the presentation is indistinguishable from that of peptic ulcer disease, colon diverticulitis, or appendicitis.[90] If the patient fails to respond to conservative measures, such as bowel rest, nasogastric tube, and antibiotics, or if someone presents with signs and symptoms of perforation, laparotomy with resection is advised.

REFERENCES

1. Abcarian H, Pearl R. A safe technique for resection of perforated sigmoid diverticulitis. *Dis Colon Rectum* 1990; 33:905.
2. Adachi A, Gold M. Vaginography for enterovaginal fistula. *Am J Obstet Gynecol* 1978;131:227.
3. Adams DB, Perry TG. Tandem colovaginoscopy in the diagnosis of colovaginal fistulas. *Dis Colon Rectum* 1988;31:653.
4. Aguilo JJ, Zincke H, Woods JE, et al. Intestinal perforation due to fecal impaction after renal transplantation. *J Urol* 1976;116:153.
5. Alanis A, Papanicolaou GK, Tadros RR, et al. Primary resection and anastomosis for treatment of acute diverticulitis. *Dis Colon Rectum* 1989;32:933.
6. Alexander P, Schuman E, Vetto RM. Perforation of the colon in the immunocompromised patient. *Am J Surg* 1986;151:557.
7. Alexander-Williams J. Management of the acute complications of diverticular disease: the dangers of colostomy. *Dis Colon Rectum* 1976;19:289.
8. Al-Jurf AS, Foucar E. Uncommon features of giant colonic diverticula. *Dis Colon Rectum* 1983;26:808.
9. Almy TP, Howell DA. Diverticular disease of the colon. *N Engl J Med* 1980;302:324.
10. Ambrosetti P, Grossholz M, Becker C, et al. Computed tomography in acute left diverticulitis. *Br J Surg* 1997;84:532.
11. Ambrosetti P, Jenny A, Becker C, et al. Acute left colonic diverticulitis—compared performance of computed tomography and water-soluble contrast enema: prospective evaluation of 420 patients. *Dis Colon Rectum* 2000;43:1363.
12. Ambrosetti P, Robert J, Witzig JA, et al. Incidence, outcome, and proposed management of isolated abscesses complicating acute left-sided colonic diverticulitis: a prospective study of 140 patients. *Dis Colon Rectum* 1992; 35:1072.
13. Ambrosetti P, Robert J, Witzig JA, et al. Prognostic factors from computed tomography in acute left colonic diverticulitis. *Br J Surg* 1992;79:117.
14. Ambrosetti P, Robert J, Witzig JA, et al. Acute left colonic diverticulitis: a prospective analysis of 226 consecutive cases. *Surgery* 1994;115:546.
15. Anderson GA, Goldman IL, Mulligan GW. 3-dimensional computerized tomographic reconstruction of colovesical fistulas. *J Urol* 1997;158:795.
16. Anderson L. Acute diverticulitis of cecum: study of 99 surgical cases. *Surgery* 1947;22:479.
17. Arnold MW, Aguilar PS, Stewart WRC. Vaginography: an easy and safe technique for diagnosis of colovaginal fistulas. *Dis Colon Rectum* 1990;33:344.
18. Asch MJ, Markowitz AM. Cecal diverticulitis: report of 16 cases and review of literature. *Surgery* 1969;65:906.
19. Auguste LJ, Wise L. Surgical management of perforated diverticulitis. *Am J Surg* 1981;141:122.
20. Beaver TM, Fullerton DA, Zamora MR, et al. Colon perforation after lung transplantation. *Ann Thorac Surg* 1996; 62:839.
21. Bell GA. Closure of colostomy following sigmoid colon resection for perforated diverticulitis. *Surg Gynecol Obstet* 1980;150:85.
22. Bell GA, Panton ONM. Hartmann resection for perforated sigmoid diverticulitis: a retrospective study of the Vancouver General Hospital experience. *Dis Colon Rectum* 1984; 27:253.
23. Belmonte C, Klas JV, Perez JJ, et al. The Hartmann procedure: first choice or last resort in diverticular disease? *Arch Surg* 1996;131:612.
24. Benn PL, Wolff BG, Ilstrup DM. Level of anastomosis and recurrent colonic diverticulitis. *Am J Surg* 1986;151:269.
25. Beranbaum SL. Diverticular disease of the right colon. In: Greenbaum EI, ed. *Radiographic atlas of colon disease*. Chicago: Year Book, 1980:125.
26. Berman IR, Corman ML, Coller JA, et al. Late-onset Crohn's disease in patients with colonic diverticulitis. *Dis Colon Rectum* 1979;22:524.
27. Bernstein WC, Nivatvongs S, Tallent MB. Colonic and rectal complications of kidney transplantation in man. *Dis Colon Rectum* 1973;16:255.
28. Berry AR, Turner WH, Mortensen NJMcC, et al. Emergency surgery for complicated diverticular disease: a five-year experience. *Dis Colon Rectum* 1989;32:849.
29. Biondo S, Parés D, Martí Ragué J. Acute colonic diverticulitis in young patients under 50 years of age. *Br J Surg* 2002;89:1137.
30. Bloch O. Om extra-abdominal behandlung af cancer intestinalis (rectum, derfra, untaget) foretagne operationer og deref resultater. *Nord Med Ark Stockh* 1982;2:1.
31. Blundell CR, Earnest DL. Idiopathic cecal ulcer: diagnosis by colonoscopy followed by nonoperative management. *Dig Dis Sci* 1980;25:494.
32. Bokey EL, Chapuis PH, Pheils MT. Elective resection for diverticular disease and carcinoma: comparison of postoperative morbidity and mortality. *Dis Colon Rectum* 1981; 24:181.

33. Bokhari M, Vernava AM, Ure T, et al. Diverticular hemorrhage in the elderly: is it well tolerated? *Dis Colon Rectum* 1996;39:191.

34. Breen RE, Corman ML, Robertson WG, et al. Are we really operating on diverticulitis? *Dis Colon Rectum* 1986;29:174.

35. Brengman ML, Otchy DP. Timing of computed tomography in acute diverticulitis. *Dis Colon Rectum* 1998;41:1023.

36. Brodribb AJM. Treatment of symptomatic diverticular disease with a high-fibre diet. *Lancet* 1977;1:664.

37. Brolin RE, Flancbaum L, Ercoli FR, et al. Limitations of percutaneous catheter drainage of abdominal abscesses. *Surg Gynecol Obstet* 1991;173:203.

38. Bruce CJ, Coller JA, Murray JJ, et al. Laparoscopic resection for diverticular disease. *Dis Colon Rectum* 1996;39:S1.

39. Bruch H, Schwandner O, Roblick U, et al. Laparoscopic colectomy for diverticulitis: prospective series of 217 patients. *Dis Colon Rectum* 2001;44:A5.

40. Buchmann P, Baumgartner D. A sigmoidoscope to facilitate reanastomosis following a Hartmann procedure. *Dis Colon Rectum* 1987;30:145.

41. Burkitt DP, Walker ARP, Painter NS. Effect of dietary fibre on stools and transit times, and its role in the causation of disease. *Lancet* 1972;2:1408.

42. Burkitt DP, Walker ARP, Painter NS. Dietary fibre and disease. *JAMA* 1974;229:1068.

43. Campbell K, Steele RJC. Non-steroidal anti-inflammatory drugs and complicated diverticular disease: a case-control study. *Br J Surg* 1991;78:190.

44. Chankowsky J, Dupuis P, Gordon PH. Sigmoid diverticulitis presenting as a lower extremity abscess. *Dis Colon Rectum* 2001;44:1711.

45. Chautems RC, Ambrosetti P, Ludwig A, et al. Long-term follow-up after first acute episode of sigmoid diverticulitis: is surgery mandatory? A prospective study of 118 patients. *Dis Colon Rectum* 2002 July;45:962.

46. Chodak GW, Rangel DM, Passaro E Jr. Colonic diverticulitis in patients under age 40: need for earlier diagnosis. *Am J Surg* 1981;141:699.

47. Choong CK, Frizelle FA. Giant colonic diverticulum: report of four cases and review of the literature. *Dis Colon Rectum* 1998;41:1178.

48. Christensen J. Pathophysiology of the irritable bowel syndrome. *Lancet* 1992;340:1444.

49. Church JM, Braun WE, Novick AC, et al. Perforation of the colon in renal homograft recipients: a report of 11 cases and a review of the literature. *Ann Surg* 1986;203:69.

50. Cirocco WC, Priolo SR, Golub RW. Spontaneous ureterocolic fistula: a rare complication of colonic diverticular disease. *Am Surg* 1994;60:832.

51. Classen JN, Bonardi R, O'Mara CS, et al. Surgical treatment of acute diverticulitis by staged procedures. *Ann Surg* 1976;184:582.

52. Cohn KH, Weimar JA, Fani K, et al. Adenocarcinoma arising within a colonic diverticulum: report of two cases and review of the literature. *Surgery* 1993;113:223.

53. Colcock BP, Stahmann FD. Fistulas complicating diverticular disease of the sigmoid colon. *Ann Surg* 1972;175:838.

54. Colonna JO II, Kang J, Jiuliano AE, et al. One-stage repair of colovaginal fistula complicating acute diverticulitis. *Am Surg* 1990;56:788.

55. Connell AM. Applied physiology of the colon: factors relevant to diverticular disease. *Clin Gastroenterol* 1975;4:23.

56. Correnti FS, Pappalardo G, Mobarhan S, et al. Follow-up results of a new colomyotomy in the treatment of diverticulosis. *Surg Gynecol Obstet* 1983;156:181.

57. Cortesini C, Pantalone D. Usefulness of colonic motility study in identifying patients at risk for complicated diverticular disease. *Dis Colon Rectum* 1991;39:339.

58. Cranston D, McWhinnie D, Collin J. Dietary fibre and gastrointestinal disease. *Br J Surg* 1988;75:508.

59. Criado FJ, Wilson TH Jr. Technique for re-establishing continuity after the Hartmann operation. *Am Surg* 1981;47:366.

60. Crist DW, Fishman EK, Scatarige JC, et al. Acute diverticulitis of the cecum and ascending colon diagnosed by computed tomography. *Surg Gynecol Obstet* 1988;166:99.

61. Di Carlo A, Andtbacka RHI, Shrier I, et al. The value of specialization: is there an outcome difference in the management of fistulas complicating diverticulitis? *Dis Colon Rectum* 2001;44:1456.

62. Dean ACB, Newell JP. Colonoscopy in the differential diagnosis of carcinoma from diverticulitis of the sigmoid colon. *Br J Surg* 1973;60:633.

63. de Bree E, Grammatikakis J, Christodoulakis M, et al. The clinical significance of acquired jejunoileal diverticula. *Am J Gastroenterol* 1998;93:2523.

64. Draghetti MJ, Salvo AF. Gas in the mesenteric veins as a nonfatal complication of diverticulitis: report of a case. *Dis Colon Rectum* 1999;42:1497.

65. Duffy FJ, Lowell JA, Tahan SR, et al. Rectal diverticulitis complicated by perforation and obstruction. *Contemp Surg* 1994;44:111.

66. Dwivedi A, Chahin F, Agrawal S, et al. Laparoscopic colectomy vs. open colectomy for sigmoid diverticular disease. *Dis Colon Rectum* 2002;45:1309.

67. Eastwood MA, Smith AN, Brydon WG, et al. Comparison of bran, ispaghula, and lactulose on colon function in diverticular disease. *Gut* 1978;19:1144.

68. Edwards VH, Chen MY, Ott DJ, et al. Rectal diverticulum appearing as a prolapsed rectum. *J Clin Gastroenterol* 1994; 18:254.

69. Egozi L, Sorrento JJ, Golub R, et al. Complication of the intracolonic bypass: report of a case. *Dis Colon Rectum* 1993;36:191.

70. Eng K, Rauson JHC, Localio SA. Resection of perforated segment: a significant advance in treatment of diverticulitis with free perforation or abscess. *Am J Surg* 1977; 133:67.

71. Ercoli FR, Milgrim LM, Nosher JL, et al. Percutaneous catheter drainage of abscesses associated with enteric fistulae. *Am Surg* 1988;54:45.

72. Failes D, Killingback M, Stuart M, et al. Elective resection for diverticular disease. *Aust NZ J Surg* 1979;49:66.

73. Farkouh E, Hellou G, Allard M, et al. Resection and primary anastomosis for diverticulitis with perforation and peritonitis. *Can J Surg* 1982;25:314.

74. Farmakis N, Tudor RG, Keighley MRB. The 5-year natural history of complicated diverticular disease. *Br J Surg* 1994; 81:733.

75. Fazio VW, Church JM, Jagelman DG, et al. Colocutaneous fistulas complicating diverticulitis. *Dis Colon Rectum* 1987;30:89.

76. Fischer MG, Farkas AM. Diverticulitis of the cecum and ascending colon. *Dis Colon Rectum* 1984;27:454.

77. Forde KA. Colonoscopy in complicated diverticular disease. *Gastrointest Endosc* 1977;23:192.

78. Fowler C, Aaland M, Johnson L, et al. Perforated diverticulitis in a Hartmann rectal pouch. *Dis Colon Rectum* 1986; 29:662.

79. Franklin ME, Dorman JP, Jacobs M, et al. Is laparoscopic surgery applicable to complicated colonic diverticular disease? *Surg Endosc* 1997;11:1025.

80. Freischlag J, Bennion RS, Thompson JE Jr. Complications of diverticular disease of the colon in young people. *Dis Colon Rectum* 1986;29:639.

81. Frieden JH, Morgenstern L. Sigmoid diverticulitis in identical twins. *Dig Dis Sci* 1985;30:182.

82. Gabriel WB. Diverticulitis of the pelvic colon with large solitary diverticulum. *Proc R Soc Med* 1953;46:416.

83. Gallagher JJ, Welch JP. Giant diverticula of the sigmoid colon: a review of differential diagnosis and operative management. *Arch Surg* 1979;114.1079.

84. Garner OP Jr, Bolin JA, LeSage MA, et al. Acute solitary cecal diverticulitis. *Am Surg* 1973;39:700.

85. Gear JSS, Ware A, Fursdon P, et al. Symptomless diverticular disease and intake of dietary fibre. *Lancet* 1979;1:511.

86. Geoghegan JG, Rosenberg IL. Experience with early anastomosis after the Hartmann procedure. *Ann R Coll Surg Engl* 1991;73:80.

87. Ger R, Ravo B. Prevention and treatment of intestinal dehiscence by an intraluminal bypass graft. *Br J Surg* 1984; 71:726.

88. Gervin AS, Fischer RP. Identification of the rectal pouch of Hartmann. *Surg Gynecol Obstet* 1987;164:177.

89. Gooszen AW, Tollenaar RAEM, Geelkerken RH, et al. Prospective study of primary anastomosis following sigmoid resection for suspected acute complicated diverticular disease. *Br J Surg* 2001;88:693.

90. Gross SA, Katz S. Small bowel diverticulosis: an overlooked entity. *Curr Treat Options Gastroenterol* 2003;6:3.

91. Gouge TH, Coppa GF, Eng K, et al. Management of diverticulitis of the ascending colon. *Am J Surg* 1983;145:387.

92. Greco RS, Kamath C, Nosher JL. Percutaneous drainage of peridiverticular abscess followed by primary sigmoidectomy. *Dis Colon Rectum* 1982;25:53.

93. Greif JM, Fried G, McSherry CK. Surgical treatment of perforated diverticulitis of the sigmoid colon. *Dis Colon Rectum* 1980;23:483.

94. Griffin WO Jr. Management of the acute complications of diverticular disease: acute perforation of colonic diverticula. *Dis Colon Rectum* 1976;19:293.

95. Hadjiyannakis EJ, Evans DB, Smellie WAB, et al. Gastrointestinal complications after renal transplantation. *Lancet* 1971;22:781.

96. Hain JM, Sherick DG, Cleary RK. Salpingocolonic fistula secondary to diverticulitis. *Am Surg* 1996;62:984.

97. Halpert RD, Crnkovich FM, Schreiber MH. Rectal diverticulosis: a case report and review of the literature. *Gastrointest Radiol* 1989;14:274.

98. Hartmann H. Nouveau procédé d'ablation des cancers de la partie terminale du colon pelvien. *Cong Franc Chir* 1923;30:411.

99. Havia T, Manner R. The irritable colon syndrome: a follow-up study with special reference to the development of diverticula. *Acta Chir Scand* 1971;137:569.

100. Heaton KW. Diet and diverticulosis: new leads. *Gut* 1985; 26:541.

101. Heimann T, Aufses AH Jr. Giant sigmoid diverticula. *Dis Colon Rectum* 1981;24:468.

102. Helbraun MA, Corman ML, Coller JA, et al. Diverticular disease. Reported at the annual meeting of the American Society of Colon and Rectal Surgeons, San Diego, CA, 1978.

103. Hinchey EJ, Schaal PG, Richards GK. Treatment of perforated diverticular disease of the colon. *Adv Surg* 1978;12: 85.

104. Hodgson WJB. Transverse teniamyotomy for diverticular disease. *Dis Colon Rectum* 1973;16:283.

105. Hodgson WJB, Schauzer H, Bakare S, et al. Transverse taenia myotomy in localized acute diverticulitis. *Am J Gastroenterol* 1979;71:61.

106. Hool GJ, Bokey EL, Pheils MT. Diverticular colo-enteric fistulae. *Aust NZ J Surg* 1981;51:358.

107. Horgan AF, McConnell EJ, Wolff BG, et al. Atypical diverticular disease: surgical results. *Dis Colon Rectum* 2001; 44:1315.

108. Howe HJ, Casali RE, Westbrook KC, et al. Acute perforations of the sigmoid colon secondary to diverticulitis. *Am J Surg* 1979;137:184.

109. Hughes WL, Greene RC. Solitary air cyst of the peritoneal cavity. *Arch Surg* 1953;67:931.

110. Hulnick DH, Megibow AJ, Balthazar EJ, et al. Computed tomography in the evaluation of diverticulitis. *Radiology* 1984;152:491.

111. Hyland JMP, Taylor I. Does a high-fibre diet prevent the complications of diverticular disease? *Br J Surg* 1980; 67:77.

112. Indudhara R, Kochhar R, Mehta SK, et al. Acute colitis in renal transplant recipients. *Am J Gastroenterol* 1990;85: 964.

113. Jarrett TW, Vaughan EDJr. Accuracy of computerized tomography in the diagnosis of colovesical fistula secondary to diverticular disease. *J Urol* 1995;153:44.

114. Jasper DR, Weinstock LB, Balfe DM, et al. Transverse colon diverticulitis: successful nonoperative management in four patients. Report of four cases. *Dis Colon Rectum* 1999;42: 955.

115. Johnson CD, Baker ME, Rice RP, et al. Diagnosis of acute colonic diverticulitis: comparison of barium enema and CT. *AJR Am J Roentgenol* 1987;148:541.

116. Julien PJ, Goldberg HI, Margulis AR, et al. Gastrointestinal complications following renal transplantation. *Radiology* 1975;117:37.

117. Karamchandani MC, Riether R, Sheets J, et al. Nephrocolic fistula. *Dis Colon Rectum* 1986;29:747.

118. Keane PF, Ohri SK, Wood CB, et al. Management of the obstructed left colon by the one-stage intracolonic bypass procedure. *Dis Colon Rectum* 1988;31:948.

119. Keck JO, Collopy BT, Ryan PJ, et al. Reversal of Hartmann's procedure: effect of timing and technique on ease and safety. *Dis Colon Rectum* 1994;37:243.

120. Kempczinski RF, Ferrucci JT Jr. Giant sigmoid diverticula: a review. *Ann Surg* 1974;180:864.

121. Kockerling F, Schneider C, Reymond MA, et al. Laparoscopic resection of sigmoid diverticulitis: results of a multicenter study. *Surg Endosc* 1999;13:567.

122. Koep LJ, Peters TG, Starzl TE. Major colonic complications of hepatic transplantation. *Dis Colon Rectum* 1979; 22:218.

123. Koneru B, Selby R, O'Hair DP, et al. Nonobstructing colonic dilatation and colon perforations following renal transplantation. *Arch Surg* 1990;125:610.

124. Konvolinka CW. Acute diverticulitis under age forty. *Am J Surg* 1994;167:562.

125. Kori T, Nemoto M, Maeda M, et al. Sonographic features of acute colonic diverticulitis: the "dome sign." *J Clin Ultrasound* 2000;28:340.

126. Kovalcik PJ, Sustarsic DL. Cecal diverticulitis. *Am Surg* 1981;47:72.

127. Kovalcik PJ, Veidenheimer MC, Corman ML, et al. Colovesical fistula. *Dis Colon Rectum* 1976;19:425.

128. Krishnan S, Hitti IF, Arya Y, et al. Giant sigmoid diverticulum. *Surg Rounds* 1987;10:124.

129. Kronborg O. Treatment of perforated sigmoid diverticulitis: a prospective randomized trial. *Br J Surg* 1993;80: 505.

130. Krukowski ZH, Koruth NM, Matheson NA. Evolving practice in acute diverticulitis. *Br J Surg* 1985;72:684.

131. Krukowski ZH, Matheson NA. Emergency surgery for diverticular disease complicated by generalized and faecal peritonitis: a review. *Br J Surg* 1984;71:921.

132. Labow SB, Salvati EP, Rubin RJ. The Hartmann procedure in the treatment of diverticular disease. *Dis Colon Rectum* 1973;16:392.

133. Labs JD, Sarr MG, Fishman EK, et al. Complications of acute diverticulitis of the colon: improved early diagnosis with computerized tomography. *Am J Surg* 1988;155:331.

134. Laimon H. Hartmann resection for acute diverticulitis. *Rev Surg* 1974;31:1.

135. Lambert ME, Knox RA, Schofield PF, et al. Management of the septic complications of diverticular disease. *Br J Surg* 1986;73:576.

136. Lambie RW, Rubin S, Dann DS. Demonstration of fistulas by vaginography. *Am J Roentgen Rad Ther Nucl Med* 1963;90:717.

137. Landi E, Fianchini A, Landa L, et al. Multiple transverse teniamyotomy for diverticular disease. *Surg Gynecol Obstet* 1979;148:221.

138. Langdon A. Solitary diverticulitis of the right colon. *Can J Surg* 1982;25:579.

139. Last MD, Lavery IC. Major hemorrhage and perforation due to a solitary cecal ulcer in a patient with end-stage renal failure. *Dis Colon Rectum* 1983;26:495.

140. Le Moine M-C, Fabre J-M, Vacher C, et al. Factors and consequences of conversion in laparoscopic sigmoidectomy for diverticular disease. *Br J Surg* 2003;90:232.

141. Lee Y-S. Diverticular disease of the large bowel in Singapore: an autopsy survey. *Dis Colon Rectum* 1986;29:330.

142. Lennard-Jones JE. Functional gastrointestinal disorders. *N Engl J Med* 1983;308:431.

143. Levi DM, Levi JU, Rogers AI, et al. Giant colonic diverticulum: an unusual manifestation of a common disease. *Am J Gastroenterol* 1993;88:139.

144. Lieberman JM, Haaga JR. Computed tomography of diverticulitis. *J Comput Assist Tomogr* 1983;7:431.

145. Lubbers E-JC, de Boer HHM. Inherent complications of Hartmann's operation. *Surg Gynecol Obstet* 1982;155:717.

146. Madden JL. Treatment of perforated lesions of the colon by primary resection and anastomosis. *Dis Colon Rectum* 1966;9:413.

147. Madden JL, Tan PY. Primary resection and anastomosis in the treatment of perforated lesions of the colon, with abscess or diffusing peritonitis. *Surg Gynecol Obstet* 1961; 113:646.

148. Maddern GJ, Nejjari Y, Dennison A, et al. Primary anastomosis with transverse colostomy as an alternative to Hartmann's procedure. *Br J Surg* 1995;82:170.

149. Madure JA, Fiore AC. Reanastomosis of a Hartmann rectal pouch. *Am J Surg* 1983;145:279.

150. Magness LJ, Sanfelippo PM, van Heerden JA, et al. Diverticular disease of the right colon. *Surg Gynecol Obstet* 1975; 140:30.

151. Mäkelä J, Vuolio S, Kiviniemi H, et al. Natural history of diverticular disease: when to operate? *Dis Colon Rectum* 1998;41:1523.

152. Manousos O, Day NE, Tzonou A, et al. Diet and other factors in the aetiology of diverticulosis: an epidemiological study in Greece. *Gut* 1985;26:544.

153. Maresca L, Maresca C, Erickson E. Giant sigmoid diverticulum: report of a case. *Dis Colon Rectum* 1981;24:191.

154. Max MH, Knutson CO. Colonoscopy in patients with inflammatory colonic strictures. *Surgery* 1978;84:551.

155. Mayefsky E, Sicular A, Hodgson WJB. Recurrent diverticulitis after conservative surgery. *Mt Sinai J Med* 1979;46: 556.

156. Mayo WJ. Acquired diverticulitis of the large intestine. *Surg Gynecol Obstet* 1907;5:8.

157. McClure ET, Welch JP. Acute diverticulitis of the transverse colon with perforation. *Arch Surg* 1979;114:1068.

158. McConnell EJ, Tessier DJ, Wolff BG. Population-based incidence of complicated diverticular disease of the sigmoid colon based on gender and age. *Dis Colon Rectum* 2003;46: 1110.

159. McFee AS, Sutton PG, Ramos R. Diverticulitis of the right colon. *Dis Colon Rectum* 1982;25:254.

160. McNutt R, Schmitt D, Schulte W. Giant colonic diverticula—three distinct entities: report of a case. *Dis Colon Rectum* 1988;31:624.

161. von Mikulicz J. Chirurgische Erfahrung über das Darmcarcinom. *Arch Clin Chir* 1903;69:28.

162. Mileski WJ, Joehl RJ, Rege RV, et al. One-stage resection and anastomosis in the management of colovesical fistula. *Am J Surg* 1987;153:75.

163. Miller WT, Levine MS, Rubesin SE, et al. Bowler-hat sign: a simple principle for differentiating polyps from diverticula. *Radiology* 1989;173:615.

164. Mills B, Zuckerman G, Sicard G. Discrete colon ulcers as a cause of lower gastrointestinal bleeding and perforation in end-stage renal disease. *Surgery* 1981;89:548.

165. Misra MK, Pinkus GS, Birtch AG, et al. Major colonic disease complicating renal transplantation. *Surgery* 1973;73: 942.

166. Morris CR, Harvey IM, Stebbings WSL, et al. Anti-inflammatory drugs, analgesics and the risk of perforated colonic diverticular disease. *Br J Surg* 2003;90:1267.

167. Morris J, Stellato TA, Haaga JR, et al. The utility of computed tomography in colonic diverticulitis. *Ann Surg* 1986; 204:128.

168. Morson BC. Pathology of diverticular disease of the colon. *Clin Gastroenterol* 1975;4:37.

169. Morson BC. Diverticular disease of the colon. *Acta Chir Belg* 1979;78:369.

170. Mueller PR, Saini S, Wittenburg J, et al. Sigmoid diverticular abscesses: percutaneous drainage as an adjunct to surgical resection in 24 cases. *Radiology* 1987;164:321.

171. Muhletaler CA, Berger JL, Robinette CL Jr. Pathogenesis of giant colonic diverticula. *Gastrointest Radiol* 1981;6:217.

172. Murayama N, Baba S, Susumu K, et al. An aetiological study of diverticulosis of the right colon. *Aust NZ J Surg* 1981;51:420.

173. Nagorney DM, Adson MA, Pemberton JH. Sigmoid diverticulitis with perforation and generalized peritonitis. *Dis Colon Rectum* 1985;28:71.

174. Neff CC, van Sonnenberg E, Casola G, et al. Diverticular abscesses: percutaneous drainage. *Radiology* 1987;163:15.

175. Ney C, Cruz FS Jr, Carvajal S, et al. Ureteral involvement secondary to diverticulitis of the colon. *Surg Gynecol Obstet* 1986;163:215.

176. Nunes GC, Robnett AH, Kremer RM, et al. The Hartmann procedure for complications of diverticulitis. *Arch Surg* 1979;114:425.

177. Orebaugh JE, McCris JA, Lee JF. Surgical treatment of diverticular disease of the colon. *Am Surg* 1978;44:712.

178. Ouriel K, Schwartz SI. Diverticular disease in the young patient. *Surg Gynecol Obstet* 1983;156:1.

179. Painter NS. Diverticular disease of the colon: a disease of this century. *Lancet* 1969;2:586.

180. Painter NS. The treatment of uncomplicated diverticular disease of the colon with a high-fibre diet. *Acta Chir Belg* 1979;78:359.

181. Painter NS. Diverticular disease of the colon: the first of the Western diseases shown to be due to a deficiency of dietary fibre. *South Afr Med J* 1982;61:1016.

182. Painter NS, Burkitt DP. Diverticular disease of the colon: a deficiency disease of Western civilization. *BMJ* 1971;1:450.

183. Papagrigoriadis S, Macey L, Bourantas N, Rennie JA. Smoking may be associated with complications in diverticular disease. *Br J Surg* 1999;86:923.

184. Parks TG. Natural history of diverticular disease of the colon. *Clin Gastroenterol* 1975;4:53.

185. Parks TG. The clinical significance of diverticular disease of the colon. *Practitioner* 1982;226:643.

186. Parks TG, Connell AM. The outcome in 455 patients admitted for treatment of diverticular disease of the colon. *Br J Surg* 1970;57:775.

187. Parks TG, Connell AM, Gough AD, et al. Limitations of radiology in the differentiation of diverticulitis and diverticulosis of the colon. *BMJ* 1970;2:136.

188. Paul FT. Colectomy. *Liverpool Med Chir J* 1895;15:374.

189. Pearce NW, Scott SD, Karran SJ. Timing and method of reversal of Hartmann's procedure. *Br J Surg* 1992;79:839.

190. Peck MD, Villar HV. Perforated diverticulitis of the transverse colon. *West J Med* 1987;147:81.

191. Perkins JD, Shield CF III, Chang FC, et al. Acute diverticulitis: comparison of treatment in immunocompromised and nonimmunocompromised patients. *Am J Surg* 1984; 148:745.

192. Perry EP, Peel ALG. The staple gun head sizers: an alternative use. *Br J Surg* 1985;72:883.

193. Pheils MT, Chapuis PH, Bokey EL, et al. Diverticular disease: a retrospective study of surgical management—1970–1980. *Aust NZ J Surg* 1982;52:53.

194. Piercy KT, Timaran C, Akin H. Rectal diverticula: report of a case and review of the literature. *Dis Colon Rectum* 2002;45:1116.

195. Pillari G, Greenspan B, Vernace FM, et al. Computed tomography of diverticulitis. *Gastrointest Radiol* 1984;9:263.

196. Potier F. Diverticulite et appendicite. *Bull Mem Soc Anat (Paris)* 1912;87:29.

197. Ramirez OM, Hernandez-Pombo J, Marupundi SR. New technique for anastomosis of the intestine after the Hart-

mann's procedure with the end-to-end anastomosis stapler. *Surg Gynecol Obstet* 1983;156:366.

198. Rao PN, Knox R, Barnard RJ, et al. Management of colovesical fistula. *Br J Surg* 1987;74:362.

199. Raval B, Lamki N, St. Ville E. Role of computed tomography in diverticulitis. *J Comput Tomogr* 1987;11:144.

200. Ravo B. Colorectal anastomotic healing and intracolonic bypass procedure. *Surg Clin North Am* 1988;68:1267.

201. Ravo B, Ger R. A preliminary report on the intracolonic bypass as an alternative to a temporary colostomy. *Surg Gynecol Obstet* 1984;159:541.

202. Ravo B, Ger R. Temporary colostomy: an outmoded procedure? *Dis Colon Rectum* 1985;28:904.

203. Ravo B, Khan SA, Ger R, et al. Unusual extraperitoneal presentations of diverticulitis. *Am J Gastroenterol* 1985; 80:346.

204. Ravo B, Metwally N, Casera P, et al. The importance of intraluminal anastomotic fecal contact and peritonitis in colonic anastomotic leakages: an experimental study. *Dis Colon Rectum* 1988;31:868.

205. Ravo B, Mishrick A, Addei K, et al. The treatment of perforated diverticulitis by one-stage intracolonic bypass procedure. *Surgery* 1987;102:771.

206. Rankin FW, Brown PW. Diverticulitis of colon. *Surg Gynecol Obstet* 1930;50:836.

207. Reeves KO, Young RL, Gordon AN, et al. Sigmoidovaginal fistula secondary to diverticular disease: a report of three cases. *J Reprod Med* 1988;33:313.

208. Reilly MCT. Sigmoid myotomy: a new operation. *Proc R Soc Med* 1964;57:556.

209. Reilly MCT. The place of sigmoid myotomy in diverticular disease. *Acta Chir Belg* 1979;78:387.

210. Rennie JA, Charnock MC, Wellwood JM, et al. Results of resection for diverticular disease and its complications. *Proc R Soc Med* 1975;68:575.

211. Rice RP, Thompson WM. Colon complications following renal transplantation. In: Greenbaum EI, ed. *Radiographic atlas of colon disease*. Chicago: Year Book, 1980:89.

212. Risholm L. Primary resection in perforating diverticulitis of the colon. *World J Surg* 1982;6:490.

213. Ritchie J. Pain from distension of the pelvic colon by inflating a balloon in the irritable colon syndrome. *Gut* 1973;14: 125.

214. Roe AM, Prabhu S, Ali A, et al. Reversal of Hartmann's procedure: timing and operative technique. *Br J Surg* 1991;78: 1167.

215. Rosenbaum J, Thabit M, Feinberg M. A simplified method of laparoscopic-assisted reversal of the Hartmann procedure. *Surg Rounds* 1995;18:January:17.

216. Rotstein OD, Pruett TL, Simmons RL. Thigh abscess: an uncommon presentation of intra-abdominal sepsis. *Am J Surg* 1986;151:414.

217. Rubio PA. The Coloshield intracolonic bypass procedure: initial experience in Houston. *Houston Med* 1989;5:17.

218. Sackier JM, Wood CB. Low anterior resection and the intraluminal bypass tube. *Br J Surg* 1988;75:1232.

219. Saini S, Mueller PR, Wittenberg J, et al. Percutaneous drainage of diverticular abscess: an adjunct to surgical therapy. *Arch Surg* 1986;121:475.

220. Sakai L, Daake J, Kaminski DL. Acute perforation of sigmoid diverticula. *Am J Surg* 1981;142:712.

221. Sankary HN, Eugene JH, Juler GL. Colovesical fistula: a comparison of the morbidity associated with staged surgical procedures. *Contemp Surg* 1988;32:28.

222. Sardi A, Gokli A, Singer JA. Diverticular disease of the cecum and ascending colon: a review of 881 cases. *Am Surg* 1987;53:41.

223. Sarr MG, Goldman SM, Cameron JL. Enterovesical fistula. *Surg Gynecol Obstet* 1987;164:41.

224. Sawyerr OI, Garvin PJ, Codd JE, et al. Colorectal complications of renal allograft transplantation. *Arch Surg* 1978; 113:84.

225. Scerpella PR, Bodensteiner JA. Giant sigmoid diverticula. *Arch Surg* 1989;124:1244.

226. Schechter S, Mulvey J, Eisenstat TE. Management of uncomplicated acute diverticulitis: results of a survey. *Dis Colon Rectum* 1999;42:470.

227. Schilling MK, Maurer CA, Kollman O, et al. Primary *vs.* secondary anastomosis after sigmoid colon resection for perforated diverticulitis (Hinchey stage III and IV): a prospective outcome and cost analysis. *Dis Colon Rectum* 2001;44:699.

228. Schlacta CM, Mamazza J, Poulin EC. Laparoscopic sigmoid resection for acute and chronic diverticulitis: a comparison with resection for nondiverticular disease. *Surg Endosc* 1999;13:649.

229. Schuler JG, Bayley J. Diverticulitis of the cecum. *Surg Gynecol Obstet* 1983;156:743.

230. Schwerk WB, Schwarz S, Rothmund M. Sonography in acute colonic diverticulitis: a prospective study. *Dis Colon Rectum* 1992;35:1077.

231. Senagore AJ, Duepree HJ, Delaney CP, et al. Cost structure of laparoscopic and open sigmoid colectomy for diverticular disease: similarities and differences. *Dis Colon Rectum* 2002;45:485.

232. Shaked A, Vargas J, Csete ME, et al. Diagnosis and treatment of bowel perforation following pediatric orthotopic liver transplantation. *Arch Surg* 1993;128:994.

233. Shallman RW, Kuehner M, Williams GH, et al. Benign cecal ulcers: spectrum of disease and selective management. *Dis Colon Rectum* 1985;28:732.

234. Shperber Y, Halevy A, Oland J, et al. Perforated diverticulitis of the transverse colon. *Dis Colon Rectum* 1986;29:466.

235. Shrier D, Skucas J, Weiss S. Diverticulitis: an evaluation by computed tomography and contrast enema. *Am J Gastroenterol* 1991;86:1466.

236. Smith TR, Cho KC, Morehouse HT, et al. Comparison of computed tomography and contrast enema evaluation of diverticulitis. *Dis Colon Rectum* 1990;33:1.

237. Smithwick RH. Experiences with surgical management of diverticulitis of the sigmoid. *Ann Surg* 1942;115:969.

238. Sosa JL, Sleeman D, Puente I, et al. Laparoscopic-assisted colostomy closure after Hartmann's procedure. *Dis Colon Rectum* 1994;37:149.

239. Spivak H, Weinrauch S, Harvey JC, et al. Acute colonic diverticulitis in the young. *Dis Colon Rectum* 1997;40:570.

240. Stabile BE, Puccio E, van Sonnenberg E, et al. Preoperative percutaneous drainage of diverticular abscesses. *Am J Surg* 1990;159:99.

241. Standards Task Force, American Society of Colon and Rectal Surgeons. Practice parameters for sigmoid diverticulitis. *Dis Colon Rectum* 1995;38:125.

242. Starnes HF Jr, Lazarus JM, Vineyard G. Surgery for diverticulitis in renal failure. *Dis Colon Rectum* 1985;28:827.

243. Staunton MD. Treatment of perforated diverticulitis coli. *BMJ* 1962;1:916.

244. Stelzner M, Vlahakos DV, Milford EL, et al. Colonic perforations after renal transplantation. *J Am Coll Surg* 1997; 184:63.

245. Stephenson BM, Wheeler MH. Unpredictable course of minimal diverticular disease. *Br J Surg* 1994;81:1050.

246. Stevenson ARL, Stitz RW, Lumley JW, et al. Laparoscopically assisted anterior resection for diverticular disease: follow-up of 100 consecutive patients. *Ann Surg* 1998;227: 335.

247. Suits GS, Knoepp LF. A community experience with entericovesical fistulas. *Am Surg* 1985;51:523.

248. Thaler K, Baig MK, Berho M, et al. Determinants of recurrence after sigmoid resection for uncomplicated diverticulitis. *Dis Colon Rectum* 2003;46:385.

249. Thompson GF, Fox PF. Perforated solitary diverticulum of the transverse colon: case report. *Am J Surg* 1944;66:280.

250. Thompson HR. Diverticulosis and diverticulitis of the colon. In: Maingot R, ed. *Abdominal operations*, 7th ed. New York: Appleton-Century-Crofts, 1980:1874.

251. Tønnesen H, Engholm G, Møller H. Association between alcoholism and diverticulitis. *Br J Surg* 1999;86:1067.
252. Thörn M, Graf W, Stefànsson T, et al. Clinical and functional results after elective colonic resection in 75 consecutive patients with diverticular disease. *Am J Surg* 2002;183:7.
253. Trowell HC, Burkitt DP. Diverticular disease in urban Kenyans. *BMJ* 1979;1:1795.
254. Underwood JW, Marks CG. The septic complications of sigmoid diverticular disease. *Br J Surg* 1984;71:209.
255. Vaughn AM, Narsete EM. Diverticulitis of the cecum. *Arch Surg* 1952;65:763.
256. Vargus HD, Ramirez RT, Hoffman GC, et al. Defining the role of laparoscopic-assisted sigmoid colectomy for diverticulitis. *Dis Colon Rectum* 2000;43:1726.
257. Vasilevsky CA, Belliveau P, Trudel JL, et al. Fistulas complicating diverticulitis. *Int J Colorectal Dis* 1998;13:57.
258. Vignati PV, Welch JP, Cohen JL. Long-term management of diverticulitis in young patients. *Dis Colon Rectum* 1995;38:627.
259. Wagner DE, Zollinger RW. Diverticulitis of the cecum and ascending colon. *Arch Surg* 1961;83:436.
260. Wara P, Sorensen K, Berg V, et al. The outcome of staged management of complicated diverticular disease of the sigmoid colon. *Acta Chir Scand* 1981;147:209.
261. Watkins GL, Oliver GA. Management of perforative sigmoid diverticulitis with diffusing peritonitis. *Arch Surg* 1966;92:928.
262. Watters DAK, Smith AN. Strength of the colon wall in diverticular disease. *Br J Surg* 1990;77:257.
263. Weber FH, McCallum RW. Clinical approaches to irritable bowel syndrome. *Lancet* 1992;340:1447.
264. Weckesser EC. Functional exteriorized colon for perforations due to diverticulitis. *Am J Surg* 1980;139:298.
265. Wetstein L, Camera A, Trillo RA, et al. Giant sigmoidal diverticulum: report of a case and review of the literature. *Dis Colon Rectum* 1978;21:110.
266. Wexner SD, Dailey TH. The initial management of left lower quadrant peritonitis. *Dis Colon Rectum* 1986;29:635.
267. Wiest JW, Kestenberg A, Becker JM. A technique for safe transanal passage of the circular end-to-end stapler for low anterior anastomosis of the colon. *Am J Surg* 1986;151:512.
268. Williams CB. Diverticular disease and strictures. In: Hunt RH, Waye JD, eds. *Colonoscopy: techniques, clinical practice and colour atlas.* London: Chapman & Hall, 1981:363.
269. Wilson RG, Smith AN, Macintyre IMC. Complications of diverticular disease and non-steroidal anti-inflammatory drugs: a prospective study. *Br J Surg* 1990;77:1103.
270. Wolff BG, Ready RL, MacCarty RL, et al. Effect of sigmoidal resection on progression of diverticulosis. *Dis Colon Rectum* 1984;27:645.
271. Woods RJ, Lavery IC, Fazio VW, et al. Internal fistulas in diverticular disease. *Dis Colon Rectum* 1988;31:591.
272. Zeitoun G, Laurent A, Rouffet F, et al. Multicentre, randomized clinical trial of primary versus secondary sigmoid resection in generalized peritonitis complicating sigmoid diverticulitis. *Br J Surg* 2000;87:1366.
273. Zielke A, Hasse C, Nies C, et al. Prospective evaluation of ultrasonography in acute colonic diverticulitis. *Br J Surg* 1997;84:385.

Laparoscopic-Assisted Colon and Rectal Surgery

I have asked Dr. Jonathan M. Sackier, Professor of Surgery at the George Washington University School of Medicine and Health Sciences, and Director, Washington Institute of Surgical Endoscopy, and Dr. Frank H. Chae, Assistant Professor of Surgery, University of Colorado Health Sciences Center to give their perspectives on this growing approach to the management of colorectal diseases. They have a large experience with laparoscopic bowel surgery and have written extensively on the subject of minimally invasive surgery.

MLC

> Now a surgeon should be youthful or at any rate
> nearer youth than age; with a strong and steady
> hand which never trembles, and ready to use
> the left hand as well as the right; with vision
> sharp and clear, and spirit undaunted.
>
> Celsus: *De Medicina, VIII, Prooemium*

The advent of videoendoscopy has stimulated a profound interest in the implementation of laparoscopy in the practice of the general surgeon and has facilitated an avalanche of technologic advances through the undertaking of major operative procedures by means of minimal incisions.[75] Published reports include techniques for diagnostic laparoscopy, appendectomy,[205,262] lysis of adhesions, colotomy and removal of a polyp and lipoma,[190] rectal suspension,[13,40,86,103] cecopexy,[21] creation of a loop colostomy and ileostomy,[114,226] cecostomy, removal of a foreign body,[167] repair of parastomal hernia,[116] resection for endometriosis,[164] restorative proctocolectomy,[112,123] and colectomy for other benign conditions as well as for cancer, including abdominoperineal resection and low anterior resection.[11,34,38,66,83,92,158,196,199,237,254,263] Because of the large numbers of colon operations that are performed, it seems natural that many of the recent laboratory and clinical efforts have been to develop the techniques for accomplishing bowel resection and even anastomosis, intracorporeally. Whether efforts to perform the procedures laparoscopically prove merely to be the situation of technology in advance of an application or truly represent a singular advance in the management of individuals with colorectal disease remains to be proven. The two primary sources for obtaining such data are the prospective COST (clinical outcomes of surgical therapy) and COLOR (colon carcinoma laparoscopic or open resection) study groups in which the results of laparoscopic versus open colectomy remain inconclusive. Short-term benefits were observed within the laparoscopy group, but the long-term cancer survival outcomes have yet to be established in both evaluations.[85,248]

Abcarian has remarked, "Laparoscopic colon resection is the perfect operation for the slow surgeon." However, a greater concern is the loss of one's tactile sense. Unless one employs a hand-assisted port, exploration is not comparable (Figs. 27-1, 27-2, and 27-3).[120] However, it is probably true that, with the availability of computed tomography, virtual colonoscopy, abdominal ultrasonography, and transcolorectal endosonography, complete preoperative assessment can be undertaken before surgery for a malignant process.[231] Still, the use of a hand port increases the cost of the procedure and theoretically may increase the length of hospitalization when compared with a procedure that is completed totally laparoscopically. No benefit for the patient was observed in bariatric surgery, for example, although a hand-assisted port may be used to supplement the skills necessary for the novice laparoscopic surgeon who is learning advanced techniques.[49]

In one seminar, concerns expressed by surgeons experienced with laparoscopic procedures are, perhaps, worth quoting:[95]

> "It is surgeon driven and industry-driven . . . We must be extremely careful."

> "I am very concerned about the problem of staging in cancer patients."

> "It is far too early to prove its validity."

> "We need to demonstrate that this way is better than the traditional open procedure."

> "Its uncontrolled expansion is the biggest unaudited free-for-all in the history of surgery."[39]

Conversely, on the more optimistic side were these views:[95]

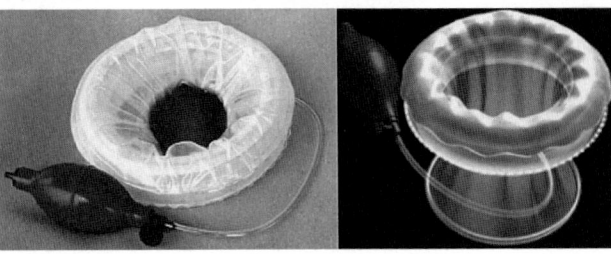

FIGURE 27-1. HandPort System. (Courtesy of Smith & Nephew, London, UK.)

"We are in an embryonic stage, just entering a new frontier . . . [Ultimately,] we'll be able to do everything from the inside, and it won't be long before all surgery is done this way."

In the ninetieth annual convention of the American Society of Colon and Rectal Surgeons (1991), a resolution was adopted by the Fellows of the Society. The following statement was the result of the consensus:

WHEREAS new technology is evolving to remove intra-abdominal organs with less invasive methods, and

WHEREAS the efficacy of this technology is unproven, and

WHEREAS the complications of the use of this technology, including morbidity, mortality, and inadequate treatment, are unknown and may exceed traditional therapies, and

WHEREAS it is important to encourage and foster the development of this technology, therefore be it

RESOLVED that the American Society of Colon and Rectal Surgeons regards laparoscopic colectomy as an unproven technology, and that it is only appropriate to perform laparoscopic intestinal resections in an environment designed to meaningfully evaluate patient safety and efficacy of this technique.

As a consequence of this action, the society established a registry for laparoscopic colon operations, the appropriate forms for which are available from the society's office

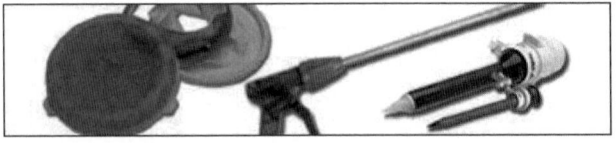

FIGURE 27-2. Gelport hand-access system. (Courtesy of Applied Medical, Rancho Santa Margarita, CA.)

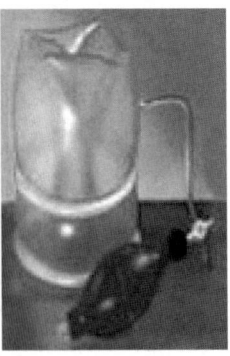

FIGURE 27-3. Omniport hand-assisted system. (Courtesy of Weck Closure Systems, Research Triangle Park, NC.)

(American Society of Colon and Rectal Surgeons, 85 West Algonquin Road, Suite 550, Arlington Heights, IL 60005).[85,248]

HISTORICAL PERSPECTIVE

It may seem to the casual observer that the laparoscope is a tool that has been developed specifically to enable the surgical revolution that attended the introduction of minimally invasive cholecystectomy in the late 1980s. Nothing could be further from the truth. It was Georg Kelling, a young German physician whose doctoral thesis had been entitled *On Measuring Stomach Capacity*, who was the originator of laparoscopy. What he succeeded in accomplishing was to apply the earlier work of Robert Simons of Bonn who, at the inspiration of Von Recklinghausen, had written a dissertation on the effects of pneumoperitoneum in 1870.[216] This phenomenon was originally called "abdominal emphysema" by Wegner,[249] but curiously was not seen to cause inflammation. The concept of pneumoperitoneum was instituted in 1882 by von Mosetig-Moorhof for the treatment of tuberculosis, with apparent cure.[240] This work was confirmed by another German physician, Willem Nolen. In 1901, Kelling established that an intraabdominal pressure of approximately 50 mm Hg could arrest intraabdominal hemorrhage. Over the ensuing years, he devoted himself to the development of equipment for this area of investigation. Although some of his experiments were successful, a number of the animals on whom he performed these procedures succumbed, presumably as a result of the high pressures used.[106]

On the basis of these experimental data, Kelling introduced a Nitze cystoscope to observe the effects that air tamponade produced on the abdominal viscera and presented his work to the seventy-third congress of German

Natural Scientists and Physicians in Hamburg in the year, 1902. That same year, Dimitri Ott, a German gynecologist, also succeeded in viewing the abdominal cavity, but he utilized an incision in the posterior fornix of the vagina.[143] He also succeeded in bringing light into the abdomen through the use of head mirrors.

The credit for the first true human celioscopy is usually given to Jacobaeus (1912), who promoted the procedure for the treatment of ascites.[96] The following year, Bernheim published his experience with *Organoscopy*,[17] and Kelling reported his initial laparoscopic series in 1923.[107] In 1929, another German physician, Heinz Kalk, published an article on the use of the laparo-thorascope with which he had performed 41 examinations on 36 patients.[104] He credited Jacobaeus for being the major contributor to the development of laparoscopy and believed that the technique held its primary application for that of the evaluation of liver disease. An Irish immigrant to the United States, John Ruddock, was another proponent of peritoneoscopy. In 1934, he also commented on the value of performing laparoscopy in patients with ascites.[168] Additionally, he introduced a number of instruments and developed the concept of retrieving biopsies under laparoscopic control.

Over the years, many surgeons have been advocates of the technique that has been variously called peritoneoscopy, celioscopy, ventroscopy, and laparoscopy. Names, such as Benedict of Boston,[8] Hamilton of Louisville, Kentucky,[81] Donaldson of Arkansas,[52] and later, Berci of Los Angeles,[10] are familiar to many surgeons performing laparoscopy. Additionally, in Europe, Cuschieri in Scotland[37] and Semm in Germany[203] have helped to bring laparoscopy into the modern era.

Over the past several decades, there have been important technologic advances in the management of colon and rectal diseases.[6] In the late 1960s and early 1970s, the development of the flexible endoscope resulted in the ability to manage colonic neoplastic disease noninvasively. Later in the 1970s, the advent of stapling devices radically altered the way surgeons reestablished intestinal continuity. Then, in the late 1980s and the beginning of the 1990s, we witnessed the development of videoendoscopy, a consequence of which has been the promulgation of laparoscopic surgery. Colonoscopy and stapling devices have, without question, improved operative morbidity and mortality and reduced the cost. This has been accomplished without sacrificing the long-term benefits of surgical treatment. Now one is confronted with the reality that laparoscopic colon surgery has been implemented in all medical centers.

The first application of laparoscopy to general surgery was that of appendectomy. This was initially performed by Semm in the early 1980s,[205] although DeKok had performed a laparoscopically assisted procedure in 1977.[44]

However, it was the introduction of video-assisted endoscopy that permitted the surgeon to share the intraoperative view with assistants, as well as the development of improved hand instrumentation, that led to the explosion in laparoscopic technology in the late 1980s.

The introduction of laparoscopic cholecystectomy in Europe[51,53,137,149] and in the United States[13,64,109,122,162,236] led to numerous other investigators employing the technique for virtually every operation. The laparoscope has been the eyes of surgeons for essentially every known colorectal procedure, in addition to that of the Nissen fundoplication,[37] vagotomy,[136] nephrectomy,[108] partial hepatectomy,[161] bariatric surgery,[48] Whipple's operation,[71] adrenalectomy,[157] and even resection of aortic aneurysm.[29] Clearly, human imagination appears to be the only limiting factor. Indeed, minimally invasive techniques have been developed and are now being evaluated for a variety of other procedures. It is rather like the concept, "If one is a hammer, the whole world looks like a nail." This philosophy of trying to minimize the effect of treatment through a limited entrance to the pathology had been applied in the past with the development of colonoscopy by Shinya,[211] Williams,[257] and Waye.[247] This philosophical approach has also been demonstrated through the introduction of transanal endoscopic microsurgery by Buess and others (see Chapter 23).[24,25,191] As seen later in this chapter, one must carefully evaluate whether these techniques are truly beneficial for the patient and not just an exercise that enhances the surgeon's ego.

TRAINING AND CREDENTIALING

Traditionally and ideally, a new technique in surgery is developed, evaluated, matured, and introduced into surgical residency training programs. Unfortunately, this is not an ideal world. Technology is too often driven by factors not necessarily in the best interest of the patient—demands from the media, demands from corporations, and of course, demands from the patient himself or herself. As a result of these pressures, the introduction of laparoscopic operations led to a dilemma for those providing care of the surgical patient as well as to those involved in the teaching of surgeons.[56]

There are numerous means through which a practicing physician can obtain training in performing laparoscopic procedures, even if they were not learned through a residency program. A good example may be seen in the field of bariatric surgery. The Society of American Gastrointestinal Endoscopic Surgeons (SAGES), in concordance with the American Society of Bariatric Surgery, is developing credentialing guidelines, teaching seminars, and preceptorship programs under the auspices of the American College of Surgeons for the rapidly growing field of laparoscopic bariatric surgery. Obviously, observation of a surgeon familiar with the technique, as well as assisting that surgeon, has some merit. This is not, however, the optimal method for developing the necessary skills for performing laparoscopic procedures. At best, one may develop familiarity with the techniques of pneumoperitoneum and tissue manipulation.[181] Attendance at a course is certainly beneficial. Specific guidelines have been established by SAGES for conducting and attending such programs.[219] However, attendance at a course, alone, should *not* be considered sufficient for one to apply his or her new-found knowledge in the clinical situation. One should expand this initial experience into that of a preceptorship. It is extremely helpful to work with a surgeon who has the skill and ability, as well as the experience in performing a large number of laparoscopic surgical procedures. Additionally, practicing is recommended in a skills laboratory where components of laparoscopic surgery, such as suturing and two-handed operating, can be refined under the guidance of an experienced laparoscopic surgeon.[178,179,215,260]

Although a great deal of focus has been directed to the use of animal models for teaching laparoscopic colorectal surgery, these models are not without problems. Quite apart from the moral and ethical issues of using laboratory animals for training, there are a number of practical concerns. The canine colon, for example, is extremely mobile and straight; thus, it does not present a particular challenge even to the least adept

endoscopic surgeon. Conversely, the porcine colon is spiral, densely adherent, and bears little similarity to that of the human. Furthermore, the rectum is long and the pelvis narrow. Considerable experience can be obtained through the use of training boxes that allow the surgeon to become more facile by manipulating instruments, suturing, and by improving hand-eye coordination (Figure 27-4).[184] It is likely that in the not too distant future, virtual reality training systems will be developed with sufficient realism to replace *in vivo* models entirely.[55,142,193,194]

Having completed this part of an individuals training, the surgeon must be aware of the credentialing requirements of his or her hospital. SAGES has recommended a set of criteria for determining training and competence.[178] These include a formal fellowship or residency in general surgery and/or colon and rectal surgery, demonstrated proficiency in the performance of laparoscopic procedures, and the clinical judgment obtained in a residency training program. For those who have completed the residency training program, the minimum requirements should be completion of an approved residency training in general surgery, credentialing in diagnostic laparoscopy, training in laparoscopic general surgery by a surgeon experienced in laparoscopic surgery, or completion of a university-sponsored or academic society–recognized didactic course with clinical experience and hands-on laboratory practice. Finally, observation of laparoscopic surgical procedures performed by a surgeon (or surgeons) experienced in the performance of such operations is necessary. Moni-

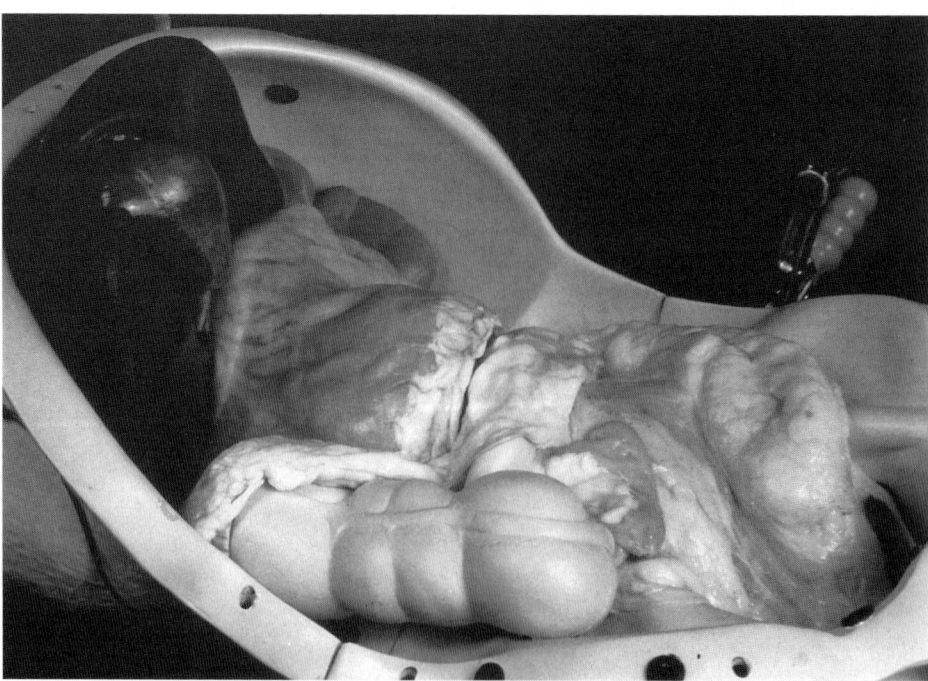

FIGURE 27-4. Model abdomen can be used to develop and to improve laparoscopic technique.

toring of the new surgeon for the first few cases should be mandatory, with implementation of an authorized approval leading to credentialing before allowing one to embark upon the operation independently. Finally, continuing medical education related to laparoscopic surgery should be required as part of the periodic renewal of privileges.[179] See and colleagues demonstrated that the rate of complications associated with the so-called clinical learning curve can be decreased by additional education following the initial course in laparoscopy.[202] Some of the recommendations in the United States have stemmed from the State of New York Department of Health memorandum recommendations on laparoscopic surgery.[224]

The requirement for proctoring a surgeon by one who has recognized skills in this area should be regarded not as an obstacle, but rather as an opportunity for confirmation of one's technical abilities. One must recognize the difference, however, between a preceptor assisting the surgeon and a proctor evaluating him or her. Probably, as important as all of the foregoing, it is for surgeons to inquire of themselves whether they have the necessary skills to ensure an optimal result for the patient through the use of minimally invasive surgery.

Because of the widespread popularity of laparoscopic surgery, most training institutions have at least one highly skilled laparoscopic surgeon who can impart his or her experience to the trainee. Although some have commented that younger residents and surgeons are more proficient at laparoscopy because they are members of the "Nintendo generation," we have not found this to be true. Many senior, experienced surgeons have adapted to the rigors of laparoscopy with ease, whereas other, young surgeons have demonstrated little talent for this new modality. In other words, one should not feel that he or she is beyond the capability of learning this technique simply because of lack of experience during residency days. Still, it is important for surgeons to have the humility and the self-awareness to understand fully whether this technique is suitable for themselves or for their patients.

LAPAROSCOPIC TEAM

Sir Charles Bell stated: "If it be a great operation, and especially if the assistants and nurses are not habituated, be careful to appoint them their places and their duties; for nothing tends more to the right performance of an operation of magnitude, than that composure and quietness which result from arrangement." (The Principles of Surgery, London, T. Cadell & EW Davis, 1826–1828.)

The foregoing comment was made in 1821, yet it is still extremely important to the contemporary operating room scene. There is no doubt that laparoscopic colorec-

tal procedures are "operations of magnitude." With so many distractions of equipment, individuals, often in unfamiliar circumstances, it is essential to consider all that is required to ensure quietness and composure.

Operating Room

Clearly, a dedicated room for the performance of laparoscopic surgery would be ideal, but especially today, most hospitals will have neither the requisite clinical material nor the financial resources to provide such a facility. The operating room needs to be large enough to accommodate all of the equipment necessary for undertaking complex procedures (Figure 27-5). Ideally, ceiling-suspended television mounts reduce the need for floor space to accommodate the monitors. The carts, themselves, which are necessary for supporting laparoscopic procedures, require a great deal of floor space. Ordinary operating rooms have insufficient electrical outlets. Thus, supplementary ones need to be created if a dedicated room is not available. Maintaining the optimal ambient room temperature is often challenging for a conventional open procedure, but when the patient's abdomen is continually being perfused by cooling gases, special attention needs to be paid to this issue. When one contemplates the development of a dedicated room, easy egress with this bulky equipment needs to be created. Furthermore, the use of a C-arm may be required, not to mention advanced robotic equipment.[46] This can lead to further difficulties with moving other pieces of equipment, unless the room has been dedicated to this purpose.

Anesthesia

It is important for the anesthesiologist to understand the special requirements of laparoscopic surgery. For example, it is often important to have the television monitor located at the head of the table, a situation that may have adverse implications concerning access to patients' airways. Operating room personnel may inadvertently plug power-draining equipment directly into the ventilator accessory outlets, thereby causing a short circuit of the respirator when the patient is under anesthesia. Cooperation between the operating team and the anesthesiologist is essential in order to provide optimal patient care.[104] The anesthesiologist must also understand potential complications of laparoscopy that are either unique to this procedure or are at an increased risk with this operation. These include gas embolism, cardiac dysrhythmia, carbon dioxide retention, and oxygen desaturation, as well as the potential for pneumothorax and pneumomediastinum. Careful attention to a host of

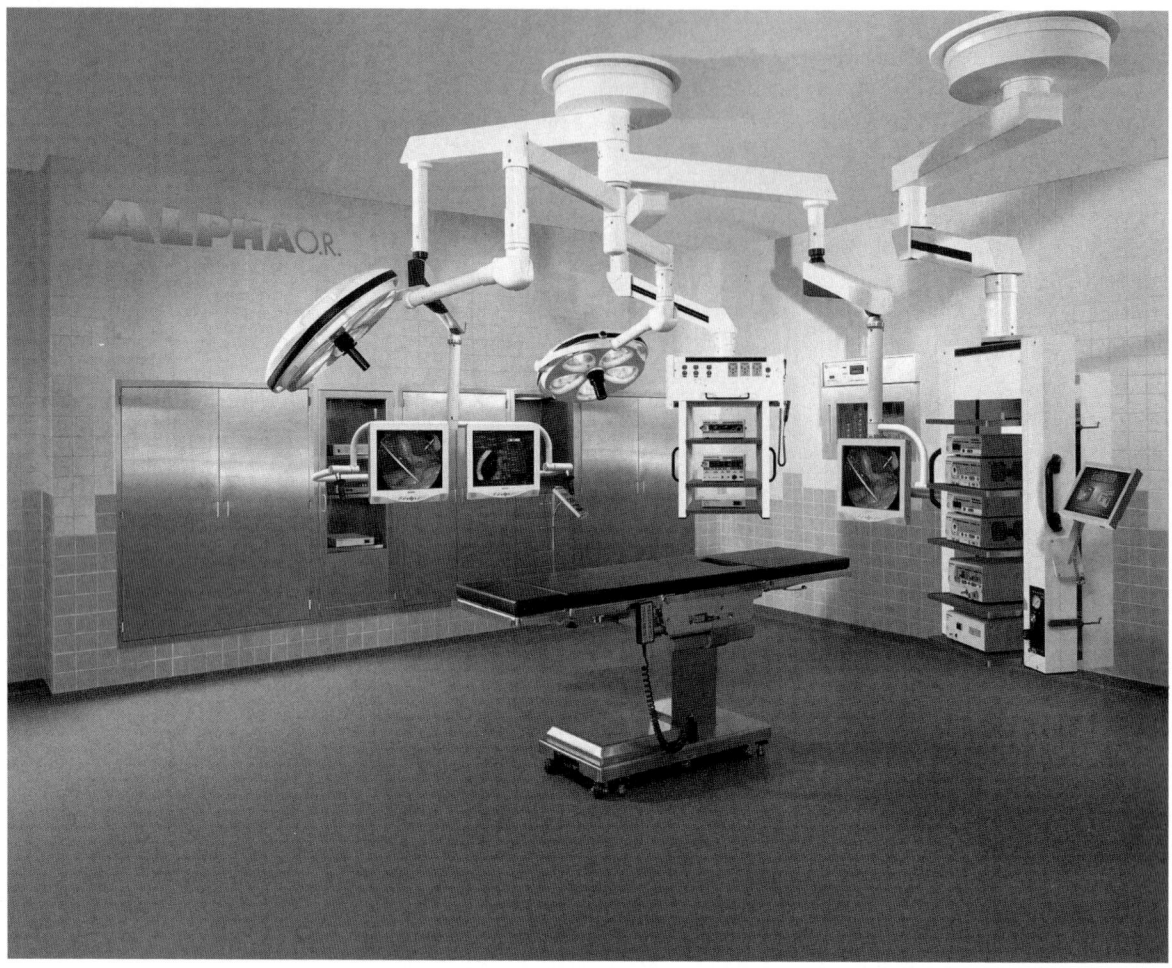

FIGURE 27-5. Alpha O.R. Olympus' fully integrated operating suite. (Courtesy of Olympus America, Inc., Melville, NY.)

physiologic parameters must be maintained during the course of the procedure. Another concern is the use of nitrous oxide, which can lead to intestinal distension. This complication may preclude adequate visualization and is truly the enemy of all laparoscopic surgeons, because it minimizes the space available to perform the operation.[26,51,147,258] Additionally, the requirement for changing the patient's position may interfere with venous return and oxygenation and may possibly increase intracranial pressure.[80,259]

At the completion of the operation, leakage of carbon dioxide into the preperitoneal or retroperitoneal spaces may result in profound subcutaneous emphysema. One must decide whether to keep the patient intubated in order to allow sufficient time for the carbon dioxide to be reabsorbed. Failure to do this may lead to carbon dioxide retention, which in the recently anesthetized patient may have dire consequences. Finally, as in all operations, care must be taken with patient positioning in order to avoid nerve compression injury. Special warming devices are

usually required, especially if one anticipates that the procedure may take a relatively long time. As mentioned, gas flow within the peritoneal cavity can lead to hypothermia, with profound pejorative effects upon a patient's metabolic balance.

Nursing

The training experience for a surgeon, as discussed previously, is just as applicable to the operating room nurse. Ideally, the nurse will join the surgeon in the training efforts so that the two can learn as a team. Alternatively, specific courses are available for operating room nurses that will educate them in a variety of procedures, the equipment required, the room setup, and the nurses' professional obligations and legal requirements. One nurse should be given the responsibility for all of the laparoscopic equipment. A checklist should be prepared before each operation, much like a pilot will use before takeoff. This includes such important issues as ensuring sufficient spare gas cylinders, bulbs for light sources, and tape roles for digital image capture units, for example. Obviously, the nurse must be assured that all equipment is functioning properly. Because the nurse is responsible for setting the room up with all the equipment in the appropriate position for each operation, any measure that will permit efficient and effective use is of critical import: complexity is counterproductive while simplicity is ideal. Finally, it is mandatory to have the required equipment available for conversion to an open procedure should the need arise. Usually, this consists of having a scalpel and laparotomy pads on the Mayo stand, as well as standard open surgical equipment in the room.

TECHNIQUE: GENERAL PRINCIPLES

Pneumoperitoneum

In order to obtain the space needed to perform surgery, gas must be introduced into the abdomen. This is usually accomplished by means of a Veress needle (Figure 27-6), which is introduced through a small puncture wound. The needle is available in either a reusable or disposable form. The benefits of reusable equipment are the reduced cost and the feel of a finely crafted surgical instrument. Conversely, disposable equipment is reliably clean, sterile, and sharp. However, it is often associated with increased cost. The Veress needle consists of a sharp outer trocar with a blunt, hollow, spring-loaded inner obturator.[238] When one inserts the needle, the obturator is pushed back into the trocar until the peritoneal cavity is entered. The obturator then springs back to prevent trauma to any underlying structures.

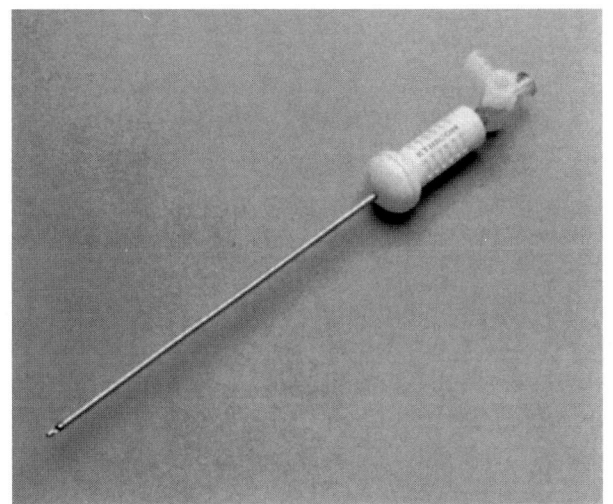

FIGURE 27-6. Verres-type disposable 120-mm pneumoperitoneum needle. (Courtesy of Ethicon Endosurgery, Inc., Cincinnati, Ohio.)

In order to avoid injury, the surgeon lifts up the abdominal wall and uses a second finger to prevent the inadvertent introduction of the needle too far and to avoid pointing the needle in the direction of a major vessel. Having entered the supposed peritoneal cavity, one should aspirate the needle with a syringe. If blood is obtained the needle should be repositioned. If a gush of blood is found, the surgeon must consider that the aorta, vena cava, or iliac vessel has been entered. There should be no hesitation in converting to an open laparotomy at this point.

If intestinal contents are noted in the syringe, one may reasonably continue with the planned laparoscopic surgery, subsequently evaluating the nature of the injury. This is most commonly a small hole in the bowel; this can usually be sutured satisfactorily. Having aspirated, the surgeon should then inject saline and aspirate again. If one is in the peritoneal cavity, fluid cannot be retrieved. Conversely, if one is in the preperitoneal space, the saline will be aspirated. Under these circumstances, the needle needs to be repositioned. Another useful test is the hanging drop technique. A drop of saline is placed at the open end of the needle while the surgeon lifts up the abdominal wall. If the peritoneal cavity has been entered, the fluid will disappear. Some suggest that if one opens the tap at the top of the needle while lifting the abdominal wall, an audible hiss will be heard. We have not found this test useful.

An alternative to the Veress technique for entering the abdomen was described initially by Hasson in 1978.[84] The abdominal cavity is entered through a small incision under direct visualization. This is most commonly accomplished under the umbilicus through the raised linea alba, entering the abdomen at the thinnest point of the anterior wall. The Hasson cannula has a blunt tip and wings to which stay sutures may be attached. Even this approach is not without risk, for if there are adhesions underneath the abdominal wall at this point, the bowel may be injured. Hasson's technique should be routinely employed if laparoscopic surgery is planned in an individual who has had prior abdominal surgery, who harbors an umbilical hernia, or if a Veress needle penetration has failed.

Having introduced either a needle or Hasson cannula, gas should then be pumped into the abdomen. A high-flow insufflator attached to a carbon dioxide cylinder is normally utilized. It is self-evident that there should be a spare gas cylinder and a wrench and gasket in the operating room before the operation commences. Concern has been expressed about whether a filter should be placed between the insufflator and the patient in order to avoid aspirating body fluids back into the insufflator at the end of the operation, thereby risking transmission to the next patient.[67,144,151] This concern is exaggerated, however, if one simply turns the gas flow off before desufflating the abdomen.

The gas should be introduced no faster than 1.5 L/min in order to prevent the potentially fatal complications of diaphragmatic rupture and/or dysrhythmia. Additionally, the pressure should not exceed 15 mm Hg in order to minimize the risk of impeding venous return, to avoid vagal stimulation by diaphragmatic stretching (leading to postoperative pain), and to limit the likelihood of pneumothorax and pneumomediastinum. Furthermore, the surgeon should be aware that pneumoperitoneum will cause acidosis from carbon dioxide absorption. Finally, the peritoneal surface may appear inflamed because of vascular dilation, which, in higher-risk patients, may lead to vascular collapse. Finally, if the needle is inadvertently introduced into a vessel or a solid organ, the potential exists for producing a carbon dioxide gas embolism. This may be recognized by drastic alterations in the patient's hemodynamic state and the production of the characteristic mill wheel cardiac murmur.[26,147,156,218,222]

Some have suggested that laparoscopic surgery can be performed without a pneumoperitoneum, by creating space through elevation of the abdominal wall.[104] Such gasless laparoscopy has yet to achieve popularity or, indeed, to be proven to have any benefit when compared with conventional open operations. Thus, it has gained few supporters.

Operative Ports

In common parlance, the words "trocar" and "cannula" have become interchangeable. The word "trocar" probably originates from *trochartor trois-quarts*, a three-sided sharp perforator within a metal cannula.[230] The original trocars for laparoscopy consisted of a hollow, three-sided, sharp blade with a metal sheath and a flap or button valve. If adequately maintained and frequently sharpened, they are still an effective means for performing laparoscopy. Various disposable trocar/cannula assemblies have been manufactured, with their proponents suggesting that less force is needed to achieve entry with resultant improved safety (Figure 27-7).[35] Additionally, these devices have safety shields meant to prevent injury to the abdominal contents or replaced entirely by blunted plastic trocar tips. Despite these methods for reassurance, the best way to ensure that no harm is caused is to judiciously introduce subsequent trocars under direct visualization. If a larger port is required than had previously been created, a dilating obturator can be inserted (Figure 27-8). The size of trocar one selects will be dictated by the instruments one must employ. Currently, trocars are available in a range of sizes from 2.7 to 33 mm. The largest size looks suspiciously like a small incision.

If after creating a pneumoperitoneum with the Veress needle the surgeon has any concerns about intraabdominal adhesions, a maneuver suggested by Palmer is advised.[145] By this test, one attaches a syringe with saline to the needle and sequentially injects and aspirates in a circumferential fashion. If there are any adhesions impeding the tip of the needle, it will be impossible to inject freely, and one will not be able to aspirate gas bubbles back into the syringe.

Port placement has become something of a pseudoscience. There are perhaps as many recommendations for

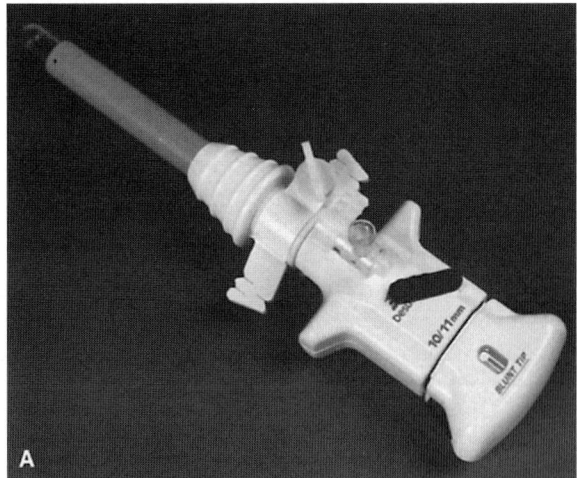
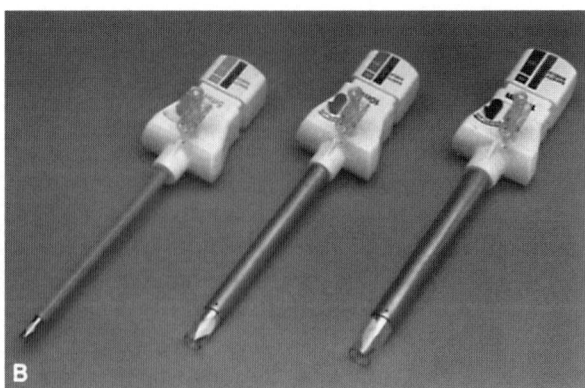

FIGURE 27-7. Abdominal trocars. **(A)** Endopath 10/11-mm blunt tip. (Courtesy of Ethicon, Inc., Cincinnati, OH.) **(B)** Surgiport 5-, 10-, and 12-mm trocars. (Courtesy of United States Surgical Corporation, Norwalk, CT.)

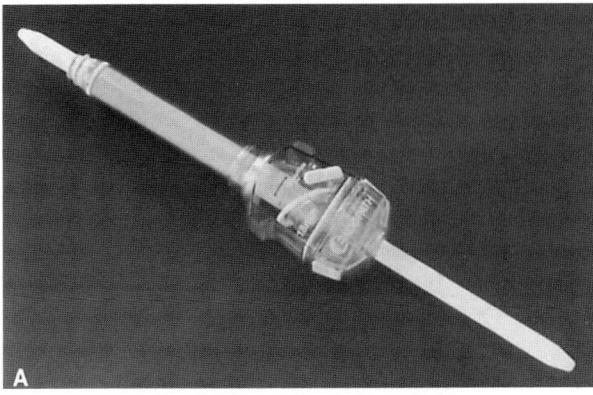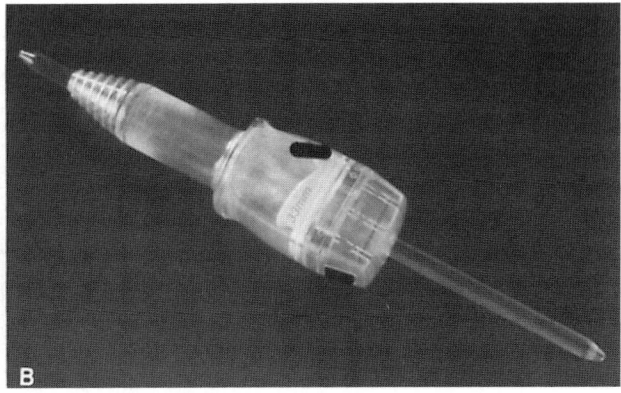

FIGURE 27-8. Disposable surgical transparent trocar sleeve with dilating obturator. **(A)** 18 mm. **(B)** 33 mm. (Courtesy of Ethicon Endosurgery, Inc., Cincinnati, OH.)

the placement of ports as there are surgeons who perform the procedures. Still, there are a few basic principles that need to be observed in order to obtain the most effective use of these ports and to facilitate the undertaking of the procedure. Because the pneumoperitoneum is usually created through the umbilicus, the first trocar is usually positioned at this site, and the camera introduced here. Subsequent ports should be placed in accordance with the following principles:

The instruments introduced through them must be able to reach the target organ.

The instrument tip should not point toward the camera. This will impede depth-of-field perception.

The tips of the instruments should not be working parallel with the line of sight. This will prevent visualization of the working mechanism.

The instruments should not be close together. This will lead to what has been termed "fencing."[171]

The cannulas should not rest directly on the iliac crest or costal margin. This will lead to postoperative pain.

The cannulas should not be inserted directly through visible vessels in the abdominal wall or the known location of the epigastric vessels.

Ideally, instruments should be brought in to 60 to 120 degrees from the line of sight (Figure 27-9).

Light Sources

Lighting of the abdomen is optimally achieved by means of a 300-watt xenon cold light source. However, if only a diagnostic laparotomy is intended, a 150-watt halogen source may be sufficient. Still, it is always better to have the option of more illumination. Furthermore, it may be necessary to have additional light sources available in the room should ancillary equipment be required, such as an illuminated ureteral stent. Because one is unable to pal-

pate the ureters laparoscopically and they are sometimes difficult to identify, it is often helpful to insert a ureteral stent preoperatively. At the appropriate point in the dissection, the laparoscopic light is reduced, and the light attached to the ureteral stent is increased.[180] An additional light source may be required if the surgeon intends to perform intraoperative colonoscopy in order to identify the location of a lesion, or if a gastroscope is required to view the duodenum when performing a right colectomy.

Visualization

A large range of laparoscopes is available, varying in size from 2.7 to 10 mm, in disposable or reusable forms, and with a variety of viewing lenses (Figure 27-10). A 0-degree optic provides a straight view and is easier to manipulate. However, angled telescopes with either a 30-degree or a 45-degree optic have the advantage of permitting the surgeon to view a structure from several perspectives (Figure 27-11). It is helpful for one to learn how to use the various instruments. Flexible-tip laparoscopes are also available (Figure 27-12).[192] A means of preventing fogging of the tip of the telescope is necessary. In fact, commercially available antifogging solutions are frequently employed. However, the simple expedient of using a flask containing hot water to clean and warm the telescope at the same time is a cost-effective alternative.[182] Some scopes have complex symptoms for intraabdominal cleaning and warming, a tribute to the ingenuity of endoscopic equipment manufacturers.

The older laparoscopes follow the Palmar-Jacobs design, wherein the beam is split to provide an offset viewing channel and with a lumen for introduction of instruments. Modern laparoscopes do not utilize this construction, and a television camera attaches directly to the eyepiece. The cameras are either one- or three-chip in-

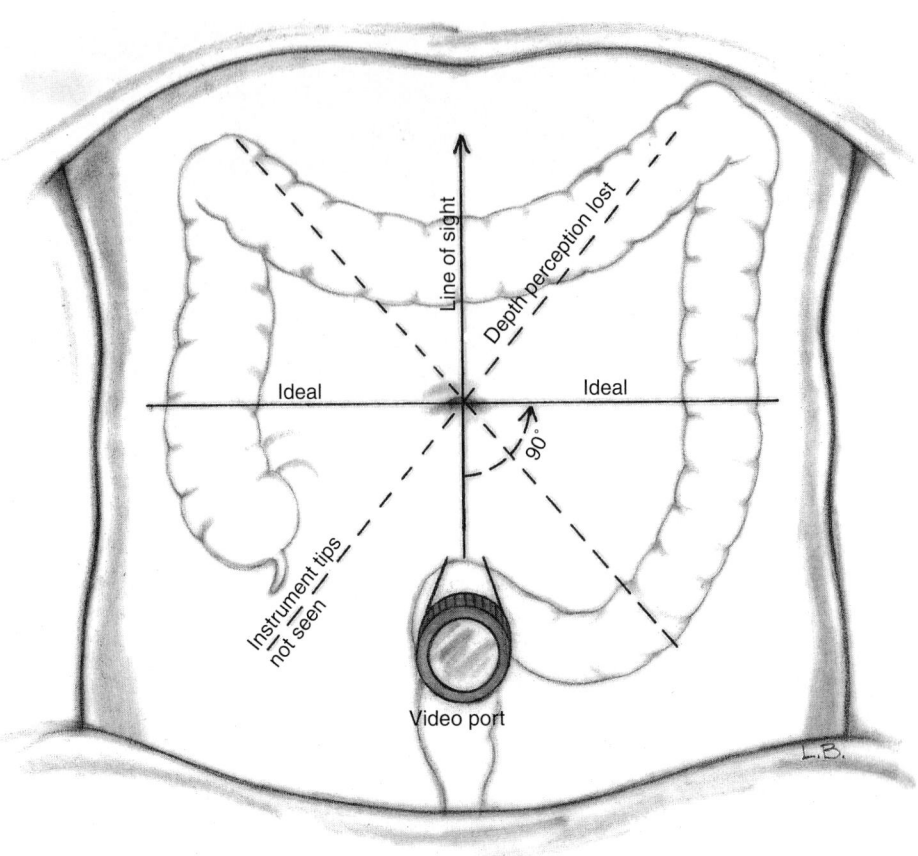

FIGURE 27-9. Schematic port selection. The line of sight dictates what angles of introduction will best serve the surgeon. Too acute, and the tips of the instruments will not be observed; too obtuse, and depth-of-field perception will be impaired.

struments. Although the latter provides better color definition, because conventional 420-line televisions are employed, the advantage is lost. With the introduction of high-definition television, plasma screen and projection television in the operating room (all with multipicture-in-picture function), the addition of digital enhancement technology may increase the popularity of the three-chip cameras.

Documentation

It is often useful for one to obtain a permanent record of the procedure to augment the patient's chart, to provide the surgeon with a mechanism for communicating operative findings to other physicians, and, regrettably, for medicolegal purposes (see Chapter 34). Capturing images on video is certainly feasible but has a number of practi-

cal drawbacks. First, the storage is costly. Second, there is the question of who is the legal owner. Third, whom does it benefit: the patient, the surgeon, or the legal community? For teaching purposes, however, video images are ideal. Super-VHS, CD-ROM, DVD, or digital hard drive are excellent formats and ideal for later editing. Hard-image capture with either digital or analog technology provides high-quality pictures that are well suited to teaching or to publication. Some systems enable images to be incorporated into the operative report much as those used by flexible endoscopists.[105,148]

Energy Sources

The word "laser" has become synonymous with "laparoscopy," but this is completely erroneous. Most laparoscopic procedures can be safely performed by means of

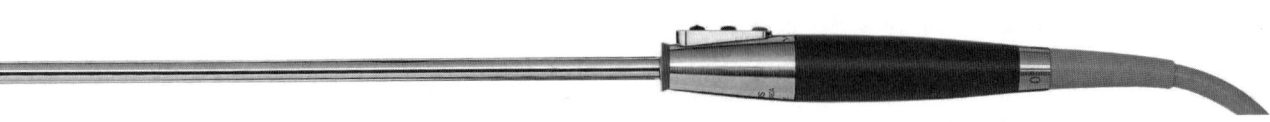

FIGURE 27-10. A 10-mm, 0-degree surgical videoscope. (Courtesy of Olympus America, Inc., Melville, NY.)

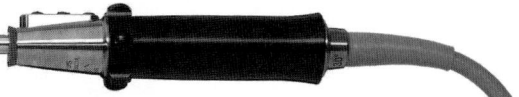

FIGURE 27-11. A 10-mm, 30-degree surgical videoscope. (Courtesy of Olympus America, Inc., Melville, NY.)

monopolar or bipolar electrosurgery, a modality with which most surgeons are familiar.[241] The generators for electrocoagulation and cutting are readily available and extremely efficient. Furthermore, many hand instruments now incorporate electrosurgery, some providing additional suction and irrigation, which eliminate the number of instrument changes required (Figure 27-13). Bipolar electrosurgery has the theoretical advantage of limiting energy spread, but it is certainly slower and more cumbersome.

A widely used alternative is the harmonic scalpel, an ultrasonic cutting and coagulating device that limits heat spread and has the capability of coagulating relatively large blood vessels (Figure 27-14).[113,134] It has been demonstrably effective for taking down the mesentery in laparoscopic colectomy.

Robotic Control

A major drawback to laparoscopic surgery is the requirement for someone to hold the camera. If the surgeon takes on this task, he or she is limited to the use of one hand for operating, truly an impossible situation if applied to open surgery. Therefore, most surgeons use another physician, nurse, technician, or medical student to hold the camera. Apart from being an unrewarding and boring experience, it is extremely frustrating for the surgeon to have to communicate visual commands to an individual who may have little knowledge of how to respond. The slightest tremor, physiologic or even as a consequence of the magnification produced by working close to a structure, can cause nausea for the entire operating team. Furthermore, the inability to follow the movement of every instrument into and out of the abdomen may lead to iatrogenic injury.

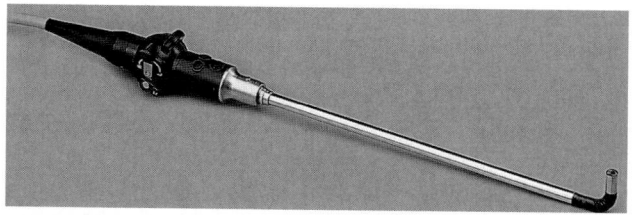

FIGURE 27-12. LTF-V3 deflectable-tip surgical videoscope. (Courtesy of Olympus America, Inc., Melville, NY.)

The development of the automated endoscopic system for optimal positioning (AESOP) robot has solved much of the problem.[189] The system, which provides effective and predictable camera control, has achieved widespread popularity. Numerous interfaces for controlling this device are available, including foot and hand control. More recently, a voice-activation system has been instituted.[176]

The next generation of robotic advances includes the ZEUS and DAVINCI units. These are designed to operate and perform complex tasks, such as anastomotic suturing. These units are ideally suited for microsurgery in cardiac surgery and neurosurgery. Whether they will have a dramatic impact on intestinal surgery remains to be seen. There have been a few reports of robotic-assisted bowel operations.[46,89,169]

Hand Instruments

Most laparoscopic instruments are clones of the standard open varieties and include most of the familiar patterns. Endoscopic grasping forceps, scissors, Babcock and Allis clamps, dissectors, retractors, cannulas, clip appliers, and a host of others are available (Figs. 27-15 and 27-16).[186] Special purse-string devices have been developed specifically for laparoscopic surgery,[170] as well as deployable bowel clamps to obviate the need for utilizing ports with every single instrument. Stapling devices are also available, analogous to the instruments for open surgery (Figure 27-17). The requirement for occluding vessels has led to the development of a wide range of clip appliers (Figure 27-18), pretied suture loops (Figure 27-15*E*), and sewing machines. It is necessary, however, for the serious laparoscopic surgeon to develop the necessary skills for performing intracorporal suturing and knotting. Specially designed needle holders and sutures are available for this purpose.[41,227] Laparoscopic instruments are, in fact, being applied to open abdominal operations and to transanal surgery. The added length and excellent construction provide particular advantages in certain situations.[70]

Intraoperative Ultrasound

The use of ultrasound has become a familiar part of the practice of many colon and rectal surgeons through its application transanally for the evaluation of rectal can-

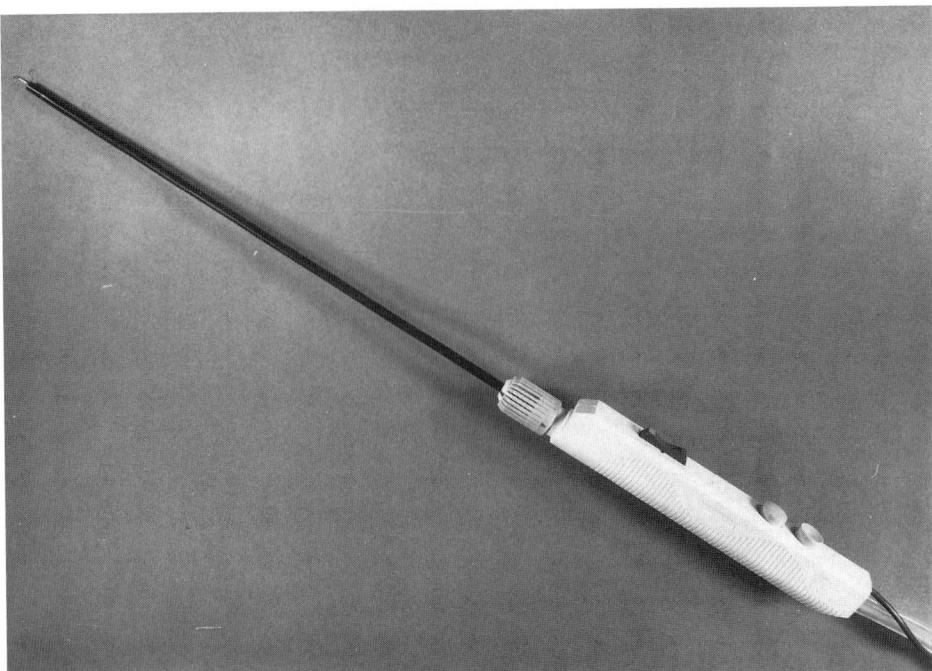

FIGURE 27-13. This device provides the surgeon with hand-controlled monopolar electrosurgery, suction, and irrigation.

cer. Ultrasound is also used in the emergency room for the triage of trauma patients.[2] With the development of the laparoscopic ultrasound probe (Figure 27-19), a whole host of indications has been proposed. It is of obvious importance to evaluate the liver in patients with malignancy, a task that is impossible in the absence of tactile sensation. Intraoperative ultrasound is an extremely important adjunct for assessing liver metastases in this situation. Furthermore, the use of Doppler signals assists in locating vessels within a fatty mesentery and can identify lymph nodes inside the peritoneal cavity.[20,138] Some investigators recommend that intraoperative ultrasound be a standard component for the evaluation of patients undergoing laparoscopic colorectal cancer surgery.[82,124,132]

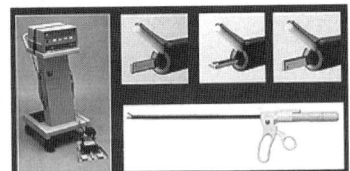

FIGURE 27-14. The Harmonic Scalpel system consists of a generator, a hand-piece with a connecting cable, a blade system, and a foot pedal. The Laparosonic Coagulating Shears (LCS) shown with three blade positions (blunt, flat, and shear). (Courtesy of Johnson & Johnson, Gateway, Piscataway, NJ.)

LAPAROSCOPIC-ASSISTED COLECTOMY

Background

There is no question that laparoscopic surgery has not attained the level of popularity in the management of colorectal disease as it is has for gallbladder surgery, antireflux surgery, or even bariatric surgery. Wexner and Weiss explained this on the basis of a number of factors:[255]

Laparoscopic colorectal surgery requires frequent movement of the surgeon, instruments, and television monitors. One may feel that the procedure is being undertaken in a less organized way when compared with the open procedure. Conversely, laparoscopic cholecystectomy requires the patient to be positioned in only one place for the entire operation.

In contrast to cholecystectomy or appendectomy, many large vessels require ligation. This is time-consuming and potentially hazardous.

Retrieving the specimen mandates laparotomy, essentially a defeat of the whole laparoscopic philosophy.

Having removed the specimen in laparoscopic cholecystectomy the operation is completed. With colon resection, an anastomosis must be fashioned, a technique quite awkward to accomplish intracorporeally.

The potential benefits of laparoscopic surgery—reduced pain, reduced length of hospitalization, earlier return to normal activity, and a better cosmetic result are insignificant if the primary concern is treating malignancy.

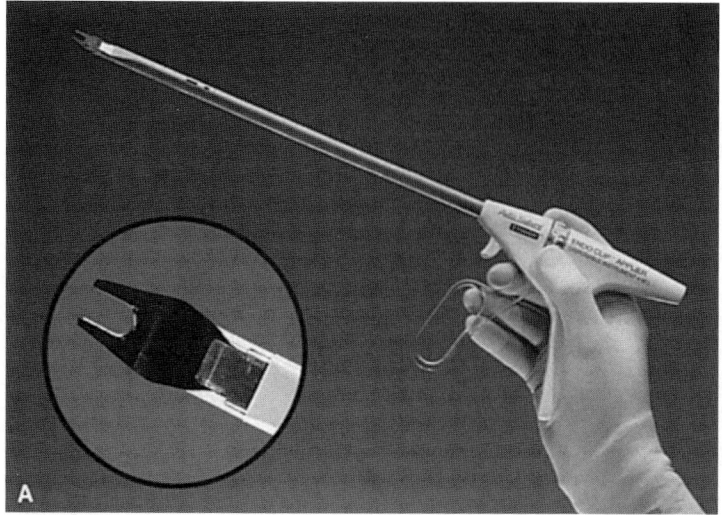
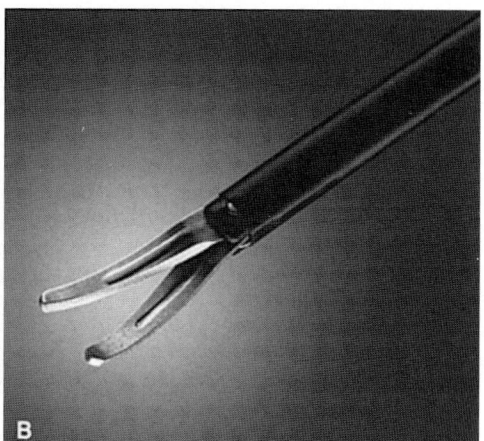
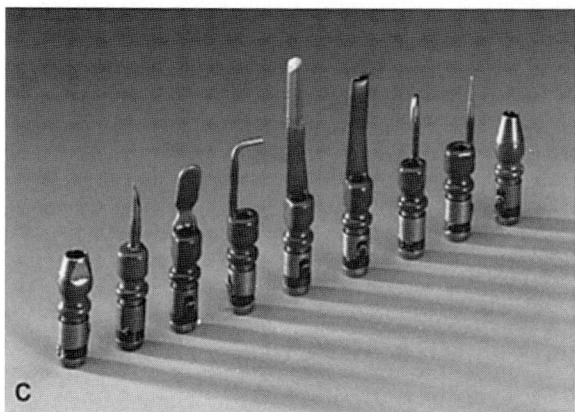
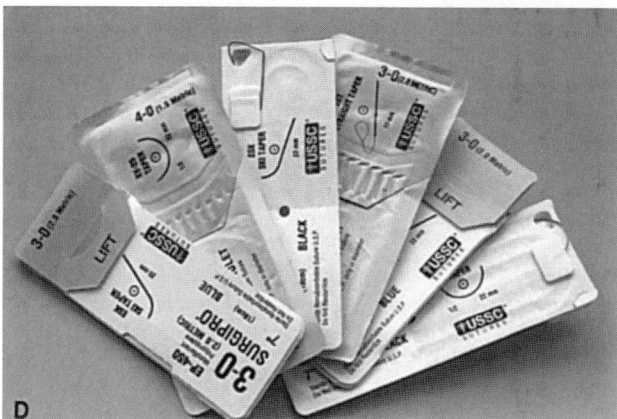
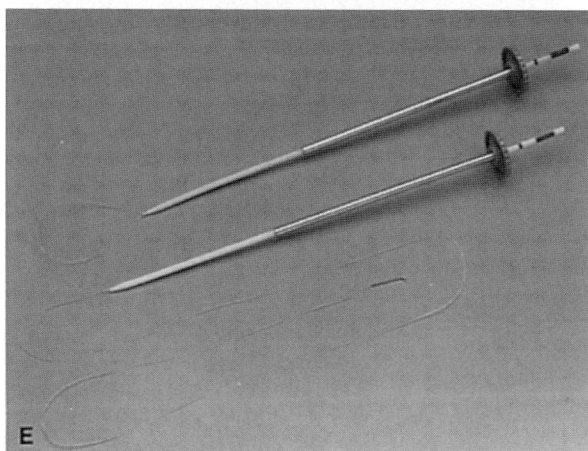
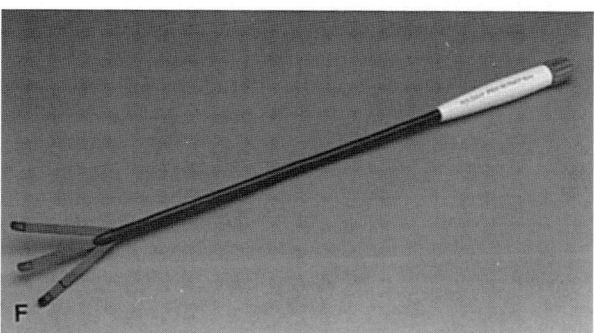

FIGURE 27-15. Assortment of laparoscopic instruments. (**A**) Clip applier. (**B**) Endo Shears. (**C**) Various dissectors, probes, and suction devices. (**D**) Laparoscopic sutures. (**E**) Surgitie disposable ligating loop (**top**) and Surgiwip disposable suture ligature (**bottom**). (**F**) Retractor. (Courtesy of United States Surgical Corporation, Norwalk, CT.)

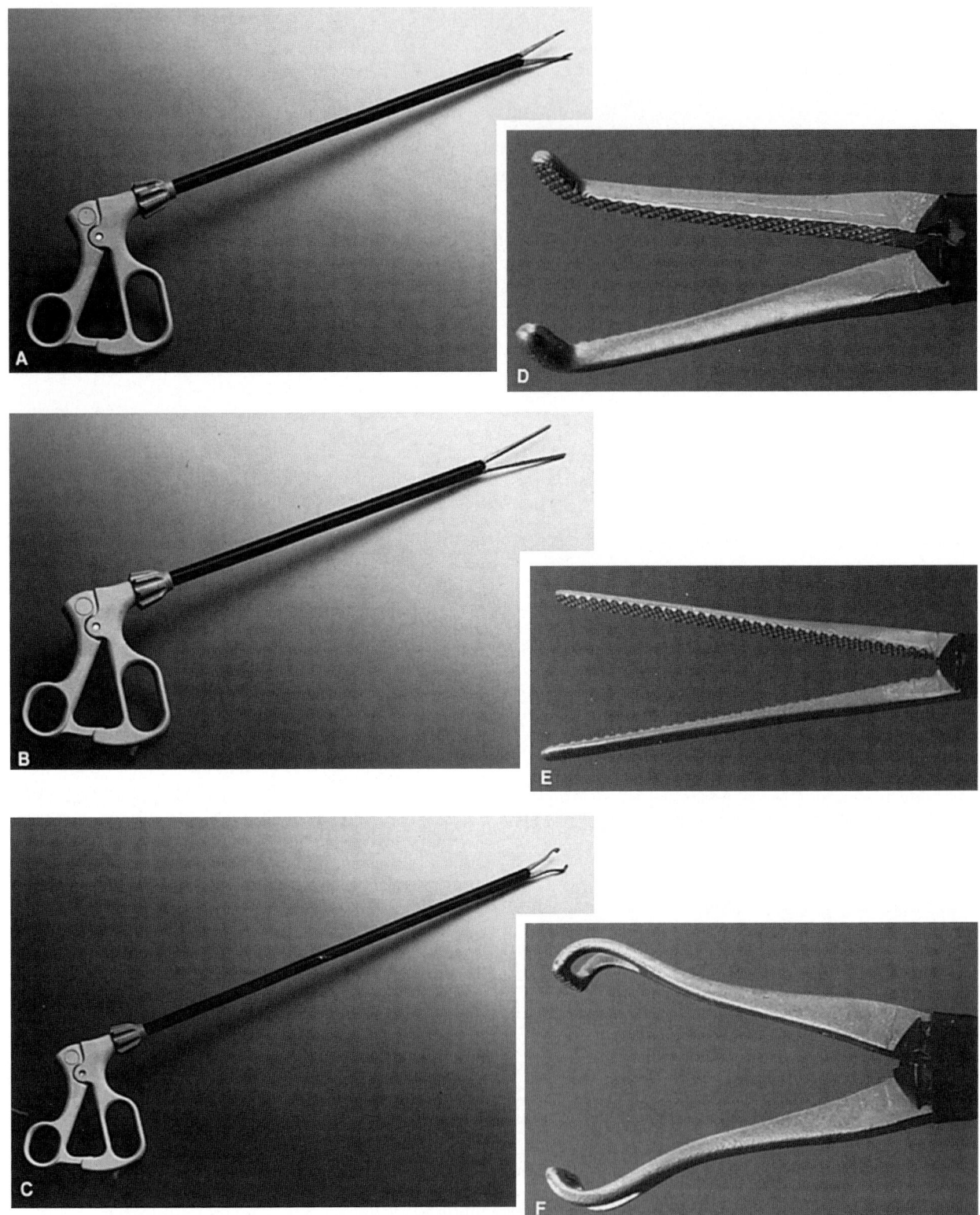

FIGURE 27-16. Laparoscopic bowel clamps. **(A)** Right angle **(inset, closeup)**. **(B)** Straight **(inset, closeup)**. **(C)** Babcock **(inset, closeup)**. (Courtesy of Ethicon Endosurgery, Inc., Cincinnati, OH.)

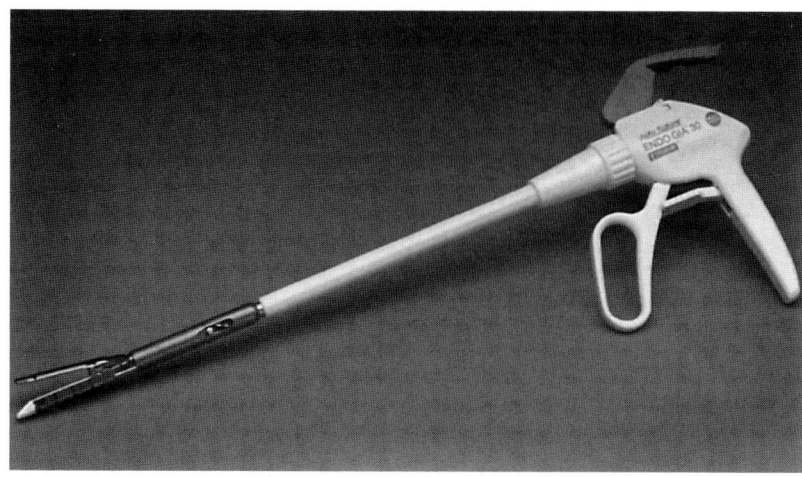

FIGURE 27-17. Linear stapler (Endo GIA 30) for laparoscopic vessel and bowel division. (Courtesy of United States Surgical Corporation, Norwalk, CT.)

With the fanfare . . . accompanied the introduction of laparoscopic cholecystectomy and laparoscopic bariatric surgery, and in spite of the foregoing concerns, laparoscopic-assisted colectomy . . . host of colorectal problems. Still, it is somewhat of a stepchild among colorectal surgeons. Until just a few years ago it had been virtually impossible to conduct a meaningful assessment of the true benefit. Numerous articles have been published, however, that attest to the reduced pain, the improved cosmetic result, the earlier discharge, and the earlier return to work in those individuals who underwent various laparoscopic procedures, ranging from appendectomy to gastric bypass, but some reports have called these results into question, commenting, for example, that small-incision cholecystectomy can accomplish the same results. One pos-sible benefit of laparoscopic surgery is a reduction in adhesion formation, an observation that has been described by gynecologists for a number of years. Theoretically, this would certainly limit readmissions for intestinal obstruction.[28] However, prospective data following laparoscopic-assisted colectomy concerning adhesion formation are, as of this writing, absent. Still, in a Cleveland Clinic (Ohio) retrospective cohort evaluation of 716 consecutive patients who underwent bowel resection (505, open and 211, laparoscopic), laparoscopic access significantly reduced the incidence of small bowel obstruction when compared with the open procedure.[54]

Even today, the safety and efficacy of laparoscopic surgery for colorectal cancer are still indeterminate, but preliminary data are encouraging.[195,263] The multicenter,

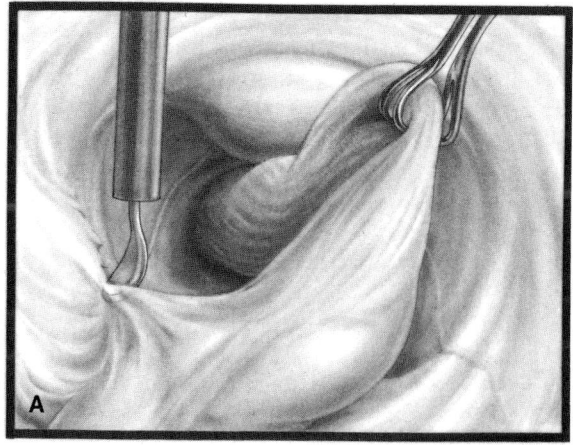 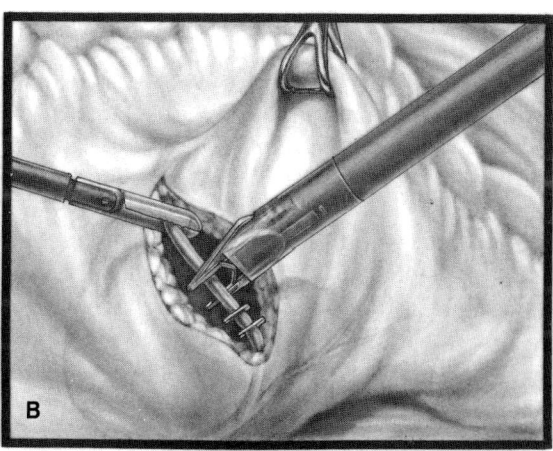

FIGURE 27-18. Laparoscopic-assisted colectomy. **(A)** Mobilization of the sigmoid colon by lifting the bowel with Babcock forceps and using either a scissors or electrocautery to incise the peritoneum. **(B)** Vessels are doubly clipped before division.

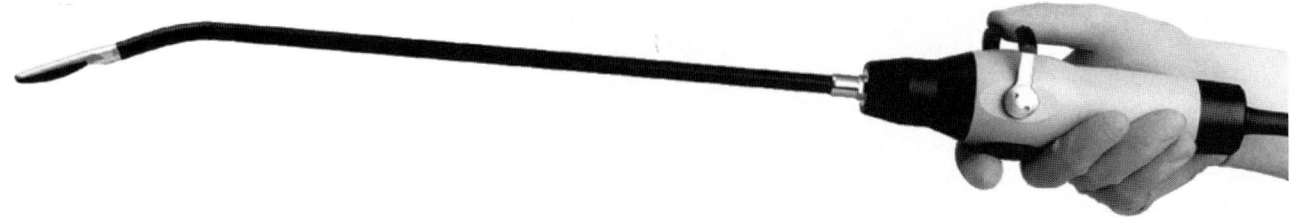

FIGURE 27-19. Laparoscopic ultrasound probe. Model 8566 4-way laparoscopic transducer. (Courtesy of B-K Medical Systems, Inc., Wilmington, MA.)

randomized controlled North American trial (COST) closed in 2004.[248] This study concluded that laparoscopic surgery for colon cancer is as effective as open colectomy in preventing recurrence and death from cancer. The European study group (COLOR) holds a similar point of view.[85]

The issue of cost with laparoscopy is extremely difficult to analyze. In the current health care environment within the United States, it is difficult to amortize cost across the broad spectrum of reimbursement plans—fee-for-service, contractual arrangements, and the indigent patient. What does seem likely, however, is that whatever savings are achieved through reduction in hospital stay will be more than eliminated by the increased operative time and the requirement for expensive equipment. One is uncertain that having patients return to the workplace sooner will outweigh the increased equipment cost.[139,152,153] However, in a study from the Cleveland Clinic, laparoscopic colectomy was compared with open colorectal surgery through the use of a matched, prospective database.[45] The former group was demonstrated to have significantly lower direct costs. Ideally, this question can be answered through a prospective, randomized trial.

Some investigators have attempted to address the benefits of laparoscopic surgery from the perspective of immune function. It has been shown in laparoscopic cholecystectomy that the acute-phase proteins are elevated far less than in open cholecystectomy.[79] Additionally, it has been demonstrated that cell-mediated immune function is preserved better after laparoscopic surgery than after open surgery.[19,47] This may have implications for postoperative infection and may indeed affect survival following resection for malignant disease.[60,155] It is well known that cell-mediated immunity is limited by surgical procedures—the more extensive the operation, the more profound the suppression.[90] In studies with mice undergoing laparoscopy, those undergoing laparotomy, and a control group with anesthesia, lower proliferation rates were noted in the laparotomy and control groups than in the laparoscopy group.[93] Ex-

periments of delayed-type hypersensitivity have also demonstrated that laparoscopic surgery causes less suppression than does open bowel surgery.[232] Others, however, have failed to demonstrate any difference in immune response with respect to a number of measured parameters when comparing laparoscopic with conventional bowel resection.[57,261]

Some studies with mouse mammary carcinoma cell lines have demonstrated reduced growth when laparoscopy had been performed as compared with open laparotomy.[160,234] Furthermore, work by Allendorf and colleagues demonstrated better preservation of immune function after laparoscopic-assisted bowel resection in a mouse model when compared with the open procedure.[3] Although the ultimate answer to the immunity issue will come from clinical studies, it seems logical that the diminished tissue destruction caused by laparoscopic wounds should lead to improved immune function.

Finally, the greatest concern that has been raised against the performance of laparoscopic colectomy for malignancy are the risks of seeding tumor at port sites and of spreading tumor as a consequence of increased intraabdominal pressure from the pneumoperitoneum. These fears were initiated by isolated case reports but have not been substantiated by the ongoing multicenter trial. Yet, the concern brought about through these anecdotal reports has led to an unwarranted reluctance for one to perform laparoscopy for cancer. However, numerous *in vivo* studies and human clinical trials have shown that there is no significant increased risk of tumor spread by the laparoscopic approach to cancer surgery.[85,126,214,248,265,266]

Patient Preparation

The preparation of a patient for laparoscopic colorectal procedures is essentially the same as that for conventional, open surgery (see Chapter 22).[100] There are, however, areas in which potential differences occur.

In addressing the patient's history, knowledge of prior surgical procedures will help the surgeon evaluate the likelihood of finding intraabdominal adhesions, which could render a laparoscopic operation difficult or impossible to accomplish with safety. A special note should be made of a history of bleeding tendency or likelihood of liver disease. For example, portal hypertension and varices can cause massive hemorrhage. The surgeon should be aware of the possibility of respiratory problems, because the use of carbon dioxide pneumoperitoneum can lead to impaired gas exchange. One may consider utilizing either a gasless laparoscopic approach or falling back on an open procedure. Knowledge that the patient harbors a hiatal hernia can pose a problem in and of itself. A large hernia filled with carbon dioxide may impair respiration.

Physical examination should note any evidence of inguinal hernias. Some surgeons recommend placing a truss perioperatively, in order to prevent massive distension of a hernia sac, a consequence of gas insufflation.[185]

The usual preoperative studies are undertaken, but the threshold for performing pulmonary function evaluation should be lower, especially in older patients undergoing laparoscopy. The use of ultrasound has also been recommended to map intraabdominal adhesions preoperatively.[213] This helps to determine whether the surgeon enters the abdomen with a Veress needle or by the Hasson cannula (see earlier discussion). This application of ultrasound for this indication requires the radiologist to be familiar with the visceral slide technique.

Consent

As with all operations, appropriate informed consent is mandatory. This communication should include a comprehensive discussion of the alternatives and the possibility of conversion to an open procedure. It is our opinion that it should include a discussion about the surgeon's experience with laparoscopic procedures. However, this is a matter between the surgeon and his or her own conscience. A discussion of the risks should include the possibility of needle or trocar injury, problems with insufflation, the possibility of postoperative subcutaneous emphysema, and the standard complications usually addressed when obtaining consent for the open procedure. Every consent form should carry the phrase, " . . . . laparoscopic . . ., possible open . . . ." We also believe that, when possible, this conversation should take place in the presence of the next of kin and that a detailed record be kept of this communication. For the American surgeon, in particular, these are especially litigious times (see Chapter

34). However, if one maintains clear and thorough documentation, there is reasonable expectation for averting such unpleasantry.

Indications

The indications for laparoscopic colectomy are essentially the same as that for conventional operations on the bowel. However, as of this writing (2004), for colorectal cancer, laparoscopic colectomy should not be offered until long-term data are announced by either the COST or COLOR study group and an endorsement is issued by either the American Society of Colon and Rectal Surgeons or the American College of Surgeons. For nonmalignant disease, it should be clearly understood, however, that the application of this modality in no way changes traditional surgical judgment, nor should it lead to a compromise in technique.[6] Initial experience suggests that the procedure may be more difficult to undertake if the patient has had prior abdominal surgery, with the usual attendant adhesion problem. Although theoretically any adhesion can be taken down by means of laparoscopy, the procedure may be so prolonged that the individual may be subjected to an unnecessarily increased risk. It is, therefore, incumbent upon the surgeon to use his or her good judgment in selecting individuals who are appropriate for this undertaking. This technology should be an alternative to traditional surgical techniques, but should not be viewed as an exclusive one.[6] The patient must not be subjected to a procedure that compromises the effectiveness of what could have been accomplished by conventional means, nor should there be an increased risk. If, during the course of the operation, the surgeon believes that efficacy or safety is being compromised, then it is appropriate, or even a requisite, to abandon laparoscopic surgery and return to one of the standard open methods.[6] As stated, the operation must not be unduly prolonged, nor should adequate resection be compromised. Conversion to an open procedure should never be viewed as a failure.

Diagnostic Laparoscopy

Elective

Cancer It is extremely useful for surgeons wishing to incorporate laparoscopy into their practices to use their oncologic experiences as a means for increasing familiarity with the laparoscopic perspective of the abdomen. Some have recommended the performance of a diagnostic laparotomy to evaluate the liver and peritoneal surfaces before undertaking a resection for colorectal cancer.[33,77] There is no denying that laparoscopic assessment is an extremely effective method for evaluating patients

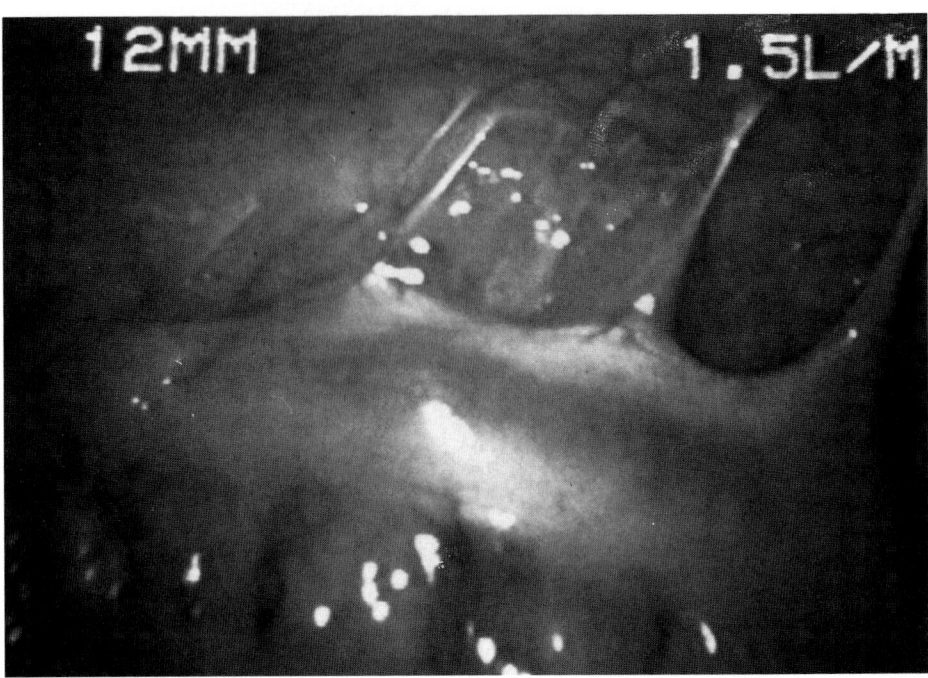

FIGURE 27-20. Congenital adhesions from the sigmoid colon to parietal peritoneum were thought to be the cause of pain in this patient. These bands were divided with resolution of symptoms.

following resection and with computed tomography or monoclonal scan evidence suggestive of recurrent disease (see Chapter 22). Biopsies may be taken from areas of the liver that are inaccessible to the percutaneous approach as well as from the serosal surface of the bowel, omentum, and peritoneum.[88,133,245] The concept of a second-look procedure has been employed for many years by gynecologists for follow-up evaluation of individuals who were diagnosed with ovarian cancer.

Pain The use of laparoscopy for the evaluation of an individual with abdominal pain has been well documented in the literature, both gynecologic and general surgical. A thorough evaluation of the abdominal contents can be achieved by this method. Ultimately, however, a diagnostic laparoscopy for pain often leads to the performance of an appendectomy or to lysis of adhesions with no objective expectation that this will resolve any complaints (Figure 27-20).

Inflammatory Bowel Disease In circumstances in which the diagnosis is in question, or in order to evaluate another aspect of the condition, such as concomitant liver disease, a laparoscopic approach may be useful.

Fever Occasionally, patients will present with fever of unknown origin in whom all other tests fail to locate a source. Laparoscopic evaluation may identify tuberculosis, brucellosis, inflammatory bowel disease, lymphoma, or abscess.

Emergency

Pain It is not uncommon for diagnostic confusion to arise in a patient with abdominal pain, especially in women of reproductive age. Although gynecologists have used laparoscopy for this indication for many years, general surgeons have begun to apply it with increased frequency for this indication.[32,146] If the diagnosis of appendicitis is made, the surgeon can proceed with appendectomy. It should be noted, however, that laparoscopy is not a substitute for clinical examination and good judgment. Other conditions, such as diverticulitis, may cause the surgeon either to continue the procedure with laparoscopic guidance or to convert to open surgery, depending on ones experience and the nature of the disease.

Obstruction Utilization of laparoscopic guidance in the patient with intestinal obstruction must be applied with particular caution, for obvious reasons. It is for this reason that assessment of the source and location of intestinal obstruction has not been widely practiced by this method. The distended bowel, as well as concern for creating additional trauma from trocar placement, has dissuaded many otherwise experienced laparoscopic surgeons from adopting this approach. However, it is possible that with judicious application of the technique, the cause of obstruction and the relief of the source may be undertaken laparoscopically. At the very least, it permits the surgeon to select an incision that is optimal for the condition and the patient.[68]

Ischemia Patients with mesenteric ischemia are most often elderly and have concomitant, significant disease. Such individuals tolerate major surgical procedures very poorly. A diagnostic laparoscopy, which may even be performed at the bedside in the intensive care unit or emergency room, can clarify any confusion about the diagnosis. If one identifies gangrene affecting a large segment of the bowel, no surgical intervention may be considered. If the bowel is viable, the surgeon may elect to maximize oxygen delivery and improve hemodynamic status by means of a cannula left *in situ*. Following completion of an open procedure for ischemia, the surgeon may leave a cannula in place with a purse-string tied around the fascia. The tip of the cannula can be buried in a pocket of peritoneum to enable bedside second-look laparoscopy.[7,36,121,177]

Diverticulitis Although the primary means of staging for diverticulitis is computerized tomography, laparoscopy may permit assessment of the disease and, in certain circumstances, assist in the placement of a drain.[187]

Trauma Laparoscopy has been effectively applied for triage of patients with blunt abdominal trauma. The procedure may be carried out in the emergency room in a similar manner to that of diagnostic peritoneal lavage. The limitation of diagnostic peritoneal lavage is that false-positive determinations are not uncommon. The consequence of an incorrect evaluation is to perform an unnecessary laparotomy, an occurrence in up to 25% of patients.[39,58,72] In the absence of multisystem injury, laparoscopy may be performed in the emergency room utilizing local anesthesia. Under these circumstances, one simply attempts to grade the pathologic findings.[12]

If intestinal contents are seen within the abdominal cavity, it is evident that bowel damage has occurred. A laparotomy is, therefore, mandatory. If blood is identified, one should consider the following categories:[14]

Minor: A small amount of blood is seen and may be irrigated away; it is not appear to re-accumulate. No source is identified. Such patients may have other injuries attended to and undergo reevaluation later.

Moderate: Blood is seen along the paracolic gutters or between loops of intestines. It is irrigated away, but reaccumulates. If a bleeding source is seen, the surgeon may decide whether it requires immediate attention or perhaps other injuries should be attended to first.

Major: Upon inserting the Veress needle, frank blood is obtained, or when inserting the laparoscope, the intestines are seen to float on a pool of blood. Such patients require immediate laparotomy.

Obviously, knowledge of the mechanism of injury is important. For example, deceleration accidents are much more likely to be associated with tears to the bowel or mesentery.

Penetrating trauma to the colon from knife wounds, not only to the abdomen, but also to the perineum, may be evaluated by means of laparoscopy. The skin entrance wound should be closed before the laparoscope is inserted. If no breach of the peritoneum is seen, then one may assume that there is no intraperitoneal injury. Conversely, if the peritoneum has been lacerated, one must search for an injury and ascertain whether the patient requires open surgery or simply further observation.[175] One may also consider the possibility of selectively utilizing laparoscopy to assess a gunshot wound, especially when the bullet seems to take an oblique course, or perhaps with injury as a consequence of a smaller-caliber weapons.[220,221] Obviously, a bullet wound of the colon must be treated by open surgery.

Therapeutic Laparoscopy

Appendectomy

Laparoscopic appendectomy was first described in 1983 by Semm, a gynecologist.[204] Many of the early reports of this operation involve primarily removing normal appendices in individuals with abdominal pain. Many now believe that laparoscopic appendectomy should be the standard of care for all patients presenting with appendicitis, be they women of reproductive age, children, or men.[141,154,235]

Technique The surgeon stands on the patient's left, the television is placed by the patient's right foot, and the operation is performed with the table tilted right side up and head down in order to permit abdominal contents to fall away from the right iliac fossa. The laparoscope is introduced through a port at the umbilicus, and two additional ports are placed, one in the right upper quadrant and one in the left iliac fossa (Figure 27-21). It is our preference to use only large ports, so that the telescope may be moved from position to position. The appendix is grasped, and if not clearly visible, the cecum is mobilized from its retroperitoneal attachments by the use of monopolar electrocautery. The blood supply should be divided by means of electrocautery (monopolar or bipolar), the harmonic scalpel, individual clips and scissors, or a stapling device. Ligatures can be utilized, but this tends to be rather time consuming. The junction of the appendix with the cecum is then clearly identified. The appendix is then removed following division at the base after roeder loops are applied, individual staples used, or a linear

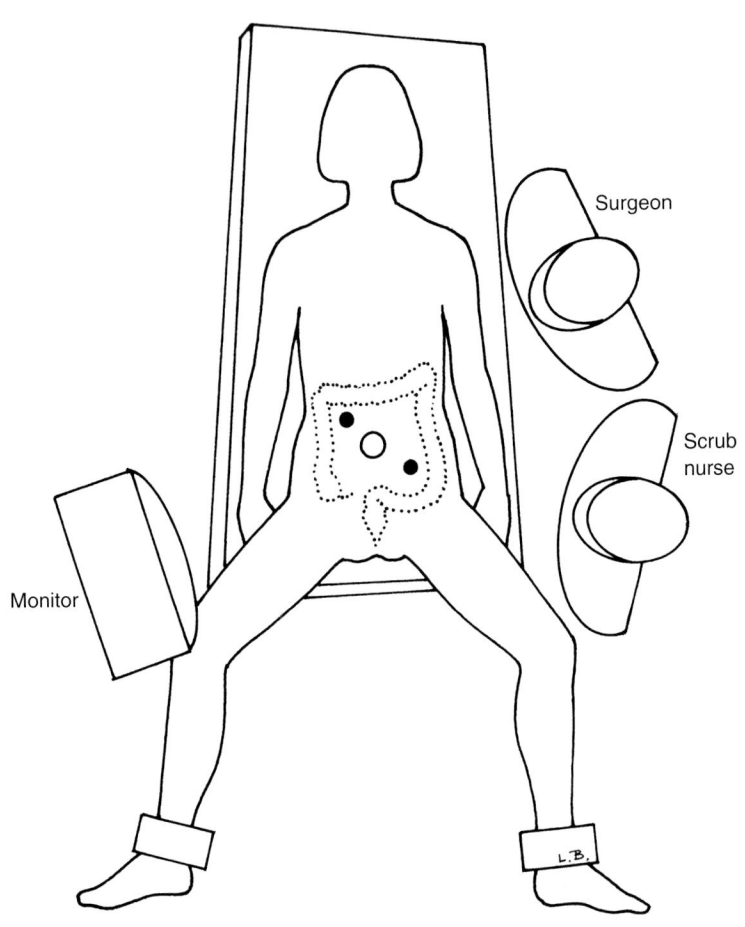

FIGURE 27-21. Trocar positions and room setup for laparoscopic appendectomy. Lithotomy stirrups allow access to the vagina for uterine manipulation.

stapler employed. The appendix is then placed in a bag or withdrawn through a metal reducer tube (according to the technique of Semm).[174]

Colon Resection

Indications

INFLAMMATORY BOWEL DISEASE. Because surgery for inflammatory bowel disease is often undertaken in young patients, the concern for a good cosmetic result has been suggested as an important reason to perform laparoscopically assisted colectomy. Furthermore, individuals with Crohn's disease often must undergo repeated operations because of complications and recurrence. These patients may benefit from a laparoscopic approach because reduction of adhesions seems to be associated with this method. Whether tissue handling with laparoscopic instruments is associated with a higher recurrence rate in Crohn's disease or a higher rate of complications has not been determined. However, studies suggest that laparoscopic surgery is an effective and reasonable alternative for such individuals.[15,118,131,135,166,246] In a prospective, randomized trial for ileal and ileocecal disease, Milsom and colleagues found that laparoscopic

resection was associated with a more rapid recovery and fewer complications.[131]

VOLVULUS. It has been previously mentioned that laparoscopy in the presence of an obstructed, distended colon is challenging and potentially hazardous. However, in a patient who has had successful reduction of a volvulus and who requires resection, the utilization of a aparoscopic approach is quite reasonable. The resection can be performed close to the bowel wall, thereby minimizing the risk of ureteral injury. Furthermore, one need not identify the major vessels to that segment of the colon, and often one has to do very little mobilization.[172]

DIVERTICULAR DISEASE. With respect to elective resection for diverticular disease, the same principle holds as has been mentioned with volvulus. With a benign process, one may stay close to the bowel wall, thus limiting the risk of injury to retroperitoneal structures and major blood vessels. However, the role of laparoscopic surgery in the treatment of acute diverticulitis is less clear. In the experience of Bruce and colleagues from the Lahey Clinic Medical Center in Boston, laparoscopic resection in patients who underwent elective surgery could be safely performed and was associated with faster recovery and shorter hospital stay when compared with conventional open surgery.[23] However, the higher cost of operating room usage time made this approach difficult to justify economically. Two clear benefits when compared with conventional, open surgery were the absence of incisional hernia and the absence of postoperative intestinal obstruction. However, only 25 patients underwent laparoscopic surgery, whereas 17 underwent the open technique.[23] Subsequent reports have shown benefit through decreased pain, reduced ileus, reduced length of hospital stay, shortened disability, cost-effectiveness, and improved cosmetic appearance.[59,207]

One of the concerns that has been expressed is the potential for adverse consequences associated with conversion from a laparoscopic to an open procedure. Le Moine and co-workers in Montpellier, France, analyzed this issue in 168 consecutive patients who underwent colectomy for sigmoid diverticular disease.[117] Not surprisingly, they identified three preoperative risk factors that were associated with a significantly higher risk of conversion: technical expertise, presence of a fistula, and the severity of inflammation on the basis of pathologic assessment. However, the morbidity of conversion was not significantly different from those procedures that were completed laparoscopically.[117] Conversely, Marusch and colleagues in Cottbus, Germany, found in their multicenter, prospective, observational study that conversion was associated with appreciably poorer results in terms of morbidity, mortality, requirement for blood transfusion, convalescence, and hospital stay.[125]

CANCER. As previously addressed, the appropriateness of performing laparoscopic surgery for malignant disease of the colon is the single greatest question facing surgeons utilizing this technique. Certainly, from the technical perspective, there is no doubt that laparoscopically guided colectomy is feasible for this indication. The real question is whether the theoretic reduction of days in the hospital, the apparent decreased pain, and the possibility of returning to work earlier are worthwhile objectives. However, many of these patients with cancer have retired from the work force, so the last advantage may be spurious. Wexner and Weiss posed a reasonable question: "In the absence of a scientifically valid answer, are the extra few meals and few days at home a fair trade for the possibility of increased risk of recurrence?"[255]

The American Society of Colon and Rectal Surgeons has made the following statement:

The absence of 5-year survival data makes it premature to endorse laparoscopic colon resection for can-

cer. If laparoscopic colon resection is performed, it is important to follow traditional surgical principles and standards. It is appropriate to continue to perform all laparoscopic resections in an environment where the outcomes can be meaningfully evaluated. The American Society of Colon and Rectal Surgeons encourages the development of randomized, prospective studies to evaluate the safety, efficacy, and benefits of this alternative.

The American Society of Colon and Rectal Surgeons, the Society of American Gastrointestinal Endoscopic Surgeons, and the American College of Surgeons Commission on Cancer jointly sponsored a registry to identify as early as possible the patterns of practice and acute complications of laparoscopic colectomy.[140] Indeed, the National Cancer Institute took up the challenge in 1994 by organizing a multicenter, randomized trial (COST study group) in which 449 consecutive patients with clinically resectable colon cancer were enlisted.[248] The study was closed in February of 1999, but it will not be for a few years that definitive conclusions may be drawn. A similar issue is pertinent to the European COLOR study group, which closed for patient enrollment in the year 2002.[85]

There is no question that potentially curative oncologic resections can be performed. Early outcomes are comparable to those of conventional therapy.[63] One may obtain appropriate resection margins,[69] harvest large numbers of lymph nodes,[119] and succeed in performing high ligation of blood vessels.[128] Milsom and colleagues evaluated lymph nodes obtained following laparoscopic proctosigmoidectomy on nine cadavers.[129] Only one had a node remaining on the inferior mesenteric artery pedicle. Numerous studies have been published that demonstrate comparable results in the treatment of colorectal cancer by a laparoscopic approach to that of the open technique.[61,70,223]

There are some studies that show less consistency with a laparoscopic approach than one would perhaps prefer. For example, there has been a concern about the variability in the distal margin that one obtains at laparoscopic resection.[69,229] There is also the possibility that adequate removal of the mesorectum for low rectal resections may not be as thorough, an important consideration, at least as expressed by some contributors (see Chapter 23).[87] Others believe that laparoscopic abdominoperineal resection can be performed according to oncologic principles with proximal vascular ligation of the inferior mesenteric artery, wide clearance of pelvic side walls, and complete removal of the mesorectum.[43,111] Inadequate circumferential margins in individuals undergoing laparoscopic abdominoperineal resection have also been reported.[42] The issue of the lack of tactile sensation for exploring the abdomen is also an expressed concern. In fact, Scott and Darzi developed a dexterity arm that allows the surgeon to place his or her hand and arm into the insufflated peritoneum through an incision and securing the arm with a sealed sleeve with a Velcro strap.[201,228] Although it is certainly true that one of the pitfalls of laparoscopic colectomy is missing significant intraabdominal pathology,[127] the concept of creating a wound sufficiently large for a surgeon to pass an arm into the abdomen is certainly against the concept of minimally invasive surgery.[228]

As has been mentioned, the concern for reports of port-site recurrence following laparoscopic-assisted colectomy has stimulated the writing of a number of papers on this subject.[99,115,250,252,256] Because of this issue, some have opined that except for controlled, clinical studies, laparoscopic colectomy for malignancy should be abandoned.[31] Still, the incidence is quite low.[159,242] With respect to conventional surgery, in one study on 1,711 patients only three developed a wound recurrence.[165]

When compared with the incidence of wound seeding with the open procedure, the statistics are no more meaningful than with laparoscopic surgery. There have been only two published series that addressed wound seeding before the laparoscopic era. Hughes and colleagues found 13 instances in 1,603 patients who underwent colectomy for carcinoma.[94] In one half of these, the recurrence was associated with carcinomatosis. The actual incidence of isolated wound recurrence was only 0.4%. An early report by Sistrunk, in 1928, presaged the concern about wound seeding by making the suggestion that it was inappropriate to bring a colon cancer through a small incision.[217] It is certainly clear from the literature for tumors other than the colon that port site recurrence has been a concern.[4,30,74,210,225,233,244] Laparoscopic cholecystectomy has been associated with port site recurrence when an unsuspected gallbladder cancer has been removed.[173] Although one may excuse wound recurrence in advanced cancers, a report of port site recurrence with a Dukes' A lesion is most disturbing.[115]

There have been experimental studies designed to evaluate the mechanism by which tumor implantation takes place, using a number of animal models. Jones and colleagues studied the effect of carbon dioxide pneumoperitoneum on the rate of tumor implantation at trocar sites in hamsters.[102] These investigators found that pneumoperitoneum increased implantation of free intraabdominal cancer cells at wound sites in the abdominal wall or within the abdominal cavity. The suggestion is that pneumoperitoneum, itself, increases the risk of tumor implantation. Other studies have confirmed this observation,[97] but still others were not able to demonstrate this phenomenon.[110]

The issue of port site recurrence has been resolved. The results from both the COST and COLOR study groups do not show increased port site tumor seeding or

tumor spreading.[85,248] Based on the data published to date, the concern for tumor spreading may have been excessive.[27,242,243]

POLYPECTOMY. Some have proposed that a laparoscopic approach is appropriate for the removal of large polyps.[4] One must be concerned, however, that this could represent a compromise of adequate cancer surgery. Certainly, most benign polyps can be removed colonoscopically, and those that are too large merit formal resection. In other words, if an abdominal approach is indicated, the same principles that are discussed in Chapter 21 concerning resection must be applied. Surgical principles must not be compromised merely to accommodate a laparoscopic approach.

COLONOSCOPIC PERFORATION. Minimally invasive surgery has been applied to the repair of colonoscopic perforations of colon. The approach is recommended on two fronts. Rather than observe the patient to see whether he or she develops signs and symptoms of peritonitis (see Chapter 5), the surgeon may consider laparoscopic exploration in order to determine whether there is actually a free perforation. Additionally, direct suture repair of colonic perforation has been reported.[163,198] The technique permits early direct assessment of the extent of injury and, theoretically, prevents delay in the identification of the source.

PULL-THROUGH PROCEDURES. Pull-through operations for Hirschsprung's disease have been described in the pediatric population.[73] This approach appears to be gaining popularity among pediatric surgeons, although perineal procedures are often replacing laparotomy for this indication (see Chapter 18).

Techniques

STOMAL CONSTRUCTION. In the usual manner, the telescope is introduced through the umbilicus. A site that has been preselected for the stoma is utilized for a large trocar opening. A 12-mm opening is ideal for an ileostomy, whereas a 15-mm is recommended for a colostomy. The loop that has been selected is held with graspers introduced through an appropriately positioned trocar site, and a window is made in an avascular portion of the mesentery. A Penrose drain is introduced into the abdomen, passed through the window, and grasped with a secure instrument placed through the cannula at the proposed stoma site (Figure 27-22). Some have recommended the use of cotton tapes to encircle the intestine in order to effect atraumatic traction.[130] The pneumoperitoneum is released, and the bowel is brought up through the incision. If one wishes, slow introduction of a pneu-

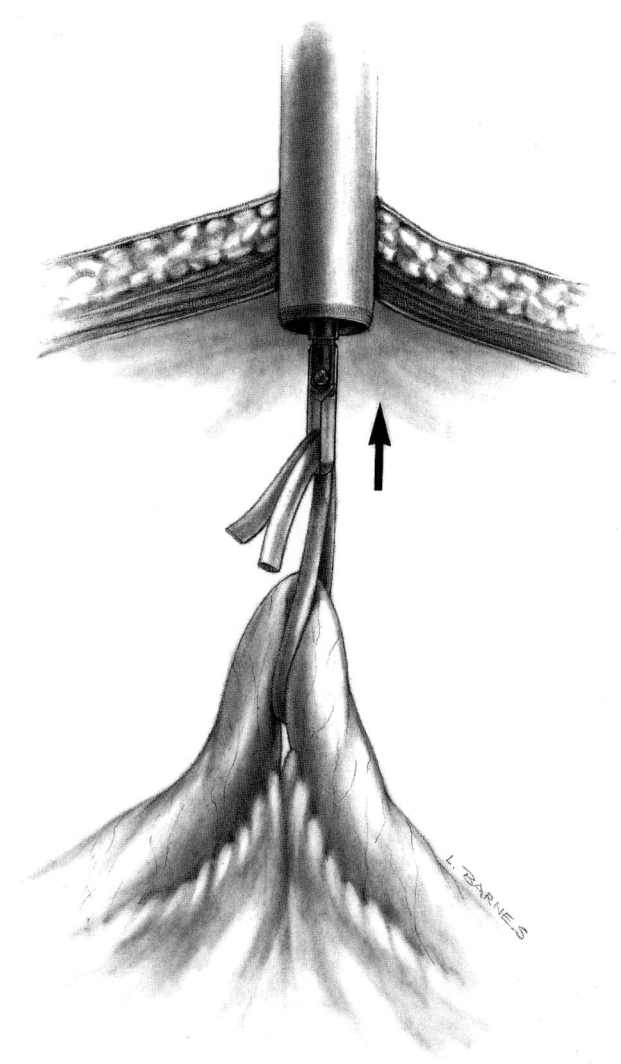

FIGURE 27-22. The chosen loop of bowel is isolated, and a Penrose drain is placed through an avascular mesenteric window. The drain is grasped via a cannula passed into the abdomen at the selected stoma site.

moperitoneum will allow the surgeon to secure the mesentery to the peritoneal surface by sutures. The cannulas are then withdrawn and the stoma matured in the usual fashion (Figure 27-23).

CLOSURE FOLLOWING HARTMANN'S OPERATION. Reestablishment of intestinal continuity can be achieved following Hartmann's procedure by laparoscopic means. The technique involves mobilization of the stoma with placement of the anvil into the proximal bowel with a purse-string suture by the usual method. The abdomen is then insufflated following closure of the stomal wound. The rectal stump is identified and an intracorporeal anastomosis created (Figure 27-24). Successful laparoscopic reestab-

lishment of intestinal continuity may be impeded, however, because of dense adhesions from the original inflammatory reaction.[76,239]

RECTOPEXY. Rectal prolapse is a condition that lends itself quite nicely to a laparoscopic approach.[103] Trocar sites are created at the umbilicus and in the left and right upper quadrants of the abdomen. If necessary, an additional trocar site may be placed in the substernal region if cephalad traction on the rectum is required. The patient is placed in a steep Trendelenburg position. An oblique-viewing laparoscope facilitates visualization for mobilizing the rectum. One may then employ a standard suture rectopexy (see Figure 17-47), or a mesh may be inserted.[40] If the latter is used, the tacking technique as suggested by Berman[16] is advised. This obviates the problems associated with a laborious and time-consuming suture method. Nevertheless, one must utilize a suture technique for securing the mesh to the rectum, itself.

CECOPEXY. The application of cecopexy for the treatment of cecal volvulus by conventional, open technique is discussed in Chapter 28. The benefits of this approach are problematic. The fact that one can perform the operation laparoscopically does not, in and of itself, suggest that it is an appropriate method, is a good operation for the indication, or increases the likelihood of success.[21,212] As previously stated, one should not use a laparoscopic approach for the treatment of the condition if it in any way compromises the likelihood of a successful result. However, if the indications are appropriate, two trocar sites are positioned in the midline, one above and one below the telescope insertion site. Additional traction may be supplied by a cannula positioned in the right upper quadrant. The patient is rolled with the right side up and head down in order to provide optimal access to the cecum. Sutures are then placed from the taenia of the right colon into the peritoneal surface.

LAPAROSCOPIC COLECTOMY. Some surgeons prefer to place the patient in the supine position on the operating table, but the perineolithotomy position is routinely suggested. This permits an assistant (or surgeon) to be placed between the patient's legs if necessary, but more importantly, enables one to perform synchronous colonoscopy should it be necessary to corroborate the area of disease. Hemodynamic monitoring is a requisite for all laparoscopic procedures, but with the generally longer period of time required for laparoscopic colectomy, this is an especially important issue. The measurement of arterial blood gases is necessary to limit the likelihood of complications resulting from acidosis, a particular concern in individuals with marginal cardiopulmonary status.[6]

Numerous operating room configurations are advised, but as one gains experience, it is common for each sur-

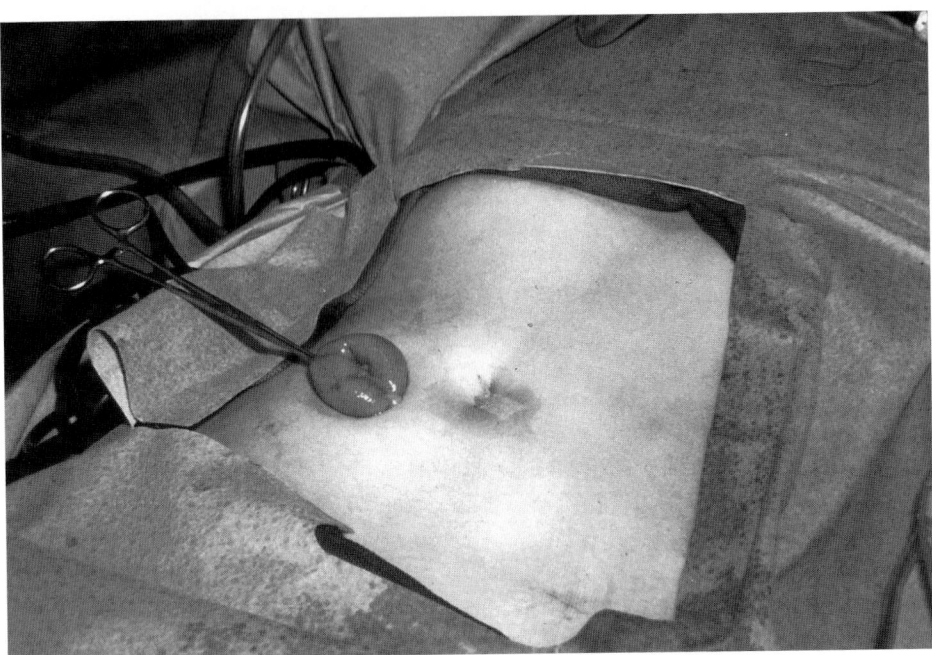

FIGURE 27-23. A loop of ileum is exteriorized laparoscopically in a patient with Crohn's disease.

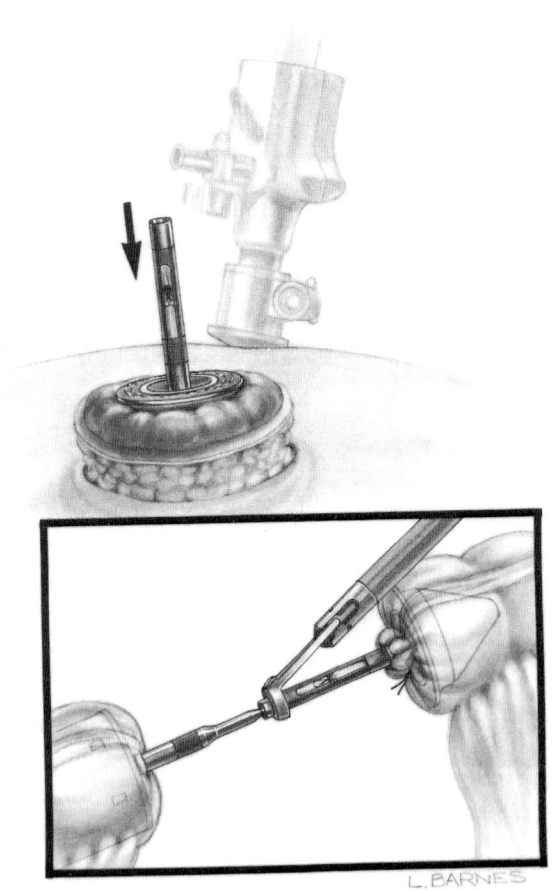

L.BARNES

FIGURE 27-24. Modification of colostomy closure, such as re-anastomosis following Hartmann's resection. Note specially designed grasping clamp to facilitate attachment of the two center rods.

geon to adopt an approach not only for the placement of the surgeon, assistant, camera operator, and nurse, but also for the locations of the various ports. Although many surgeons prefer to place the video camera in the patient's umbilicus, others do not believe that this is always optimal, because it fails to permit identification of all areas of the colon (see earlier discussion). Requisite principles are to be flexible, to be innovative, and to be willing to move the ports around or to create new ports as necessary.

Once the abdomen is entered and the abdominal cavity is visualized, additional ports can be placed. If a larger port is required than had previously been created, a dilating obturator can be inserted (Figure 27-8). At the site of the camera placement one uses 10- to 12-mm ports, but regardless of the planned application of the port site, smaller sizes than these should rarely be considered.[5] The upper portal permits visualization of the lower two thirds of the abdomen, but when it becomes necessary to visualize either the flexures or the transverse colon, the camera can be moved to one of the hypogastric ports. Generally, the operating surgeon uses the suprapubic port plus another port on the side of the abdomen opposite from which the bowel is being mobilized or resected. Conversely, the assistant employs the operative port on the same side that is being dissected, and an additional port is utilized if the assistant is capable of performing a two-handed technique. In contrast to laparoscopic cholecystectomy, the patient is placed in a steep Trendelenburg position and rotated away from side of the colon being resected, in order to move the small intestine out of the operative field.[6] The importance of patient po-

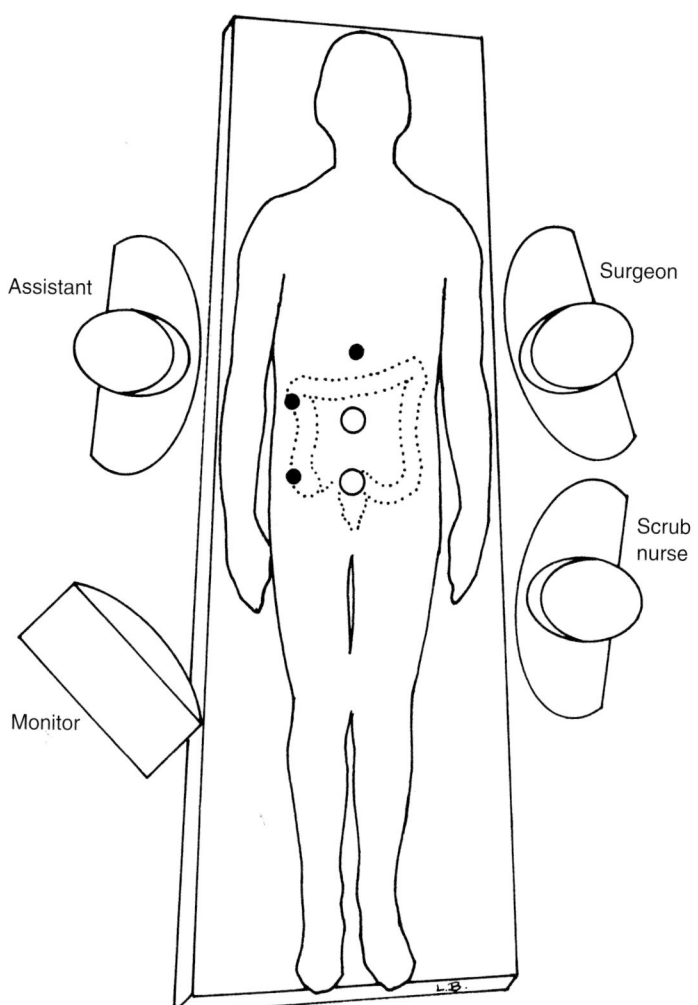

FIGURE 27-25. The position for trocars, personnel, and equipment in laparoscopic right hemicolectomy.

sition, with lateral rotation to either side, cannot be overestimated, because these maneuvers are essential for providing the optimum possible exposure. The dissection can now be commenced.

Right Hemicolectomy

Because one does not have the luxury of manually retracting the small bowel with ease during colon mobilization, patients undergoing right hemicolectomy are optimally positioned in the left lateral decubitus position.[101] Our own preference is to utilize the port positions described for cecopexy (Figure 27-25). Should conversion to open colectomy be necessary, either a midline incision joining the cannula insertion sites or a right transverse incision can be made. During the dissection of the ileocecal region, the patient is placed in the Trendelenburg position and in the reverse Trendelenburg position during the dissection of the hepatic flexure. The right colon is mobilized in the usual manner with the endoscopic electrocoagulation system. The right colic vessels are dissected and coagulated with electrocoagulation forceps

and are ligated with an endoclip applicator. The technique for resection and anastomosis is discussed in the following section. At the present time, there is no method for withdrawing the specimen without creating an incision. Therefore, it is appropriate to perform the mobilization intracorporeally with internal division of the vessels and then to exteriorize the specimen for resection and anastomosis.[264]

Left Hemicolectomy/Anterior Resection

Trocar positions are essentially the mirror image of those recommended for right hemicolectomy (Figure 27-26). The patient is rolled with the left side up and the head down. The small bowel is then gently teased toward the right upper quadrant. The colon is mobilized in a similar manner described previously and the vessels divided (Figure 27-18). The surgeon can then effect an anastomosis by one of several means, but the major differences are with respect to the performance of either an intracorporeal or an extracorporeal anastomosis.

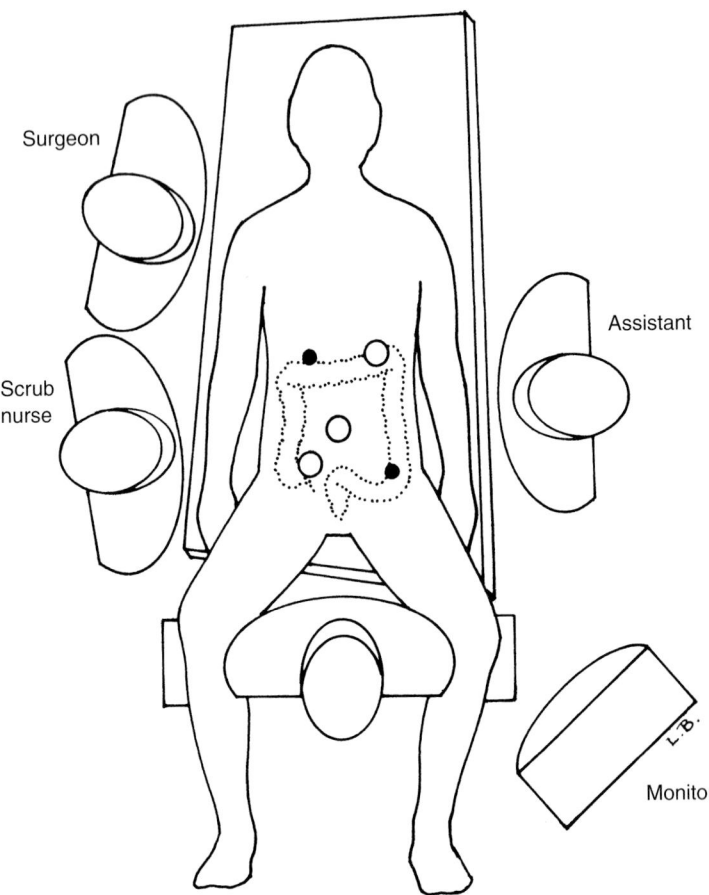

FIGURE 27-26. Preferred position for performing left hemicolectomy and anterior resection of the rectum.

EXTRACORPOREAL ANASTOMOSIS. It is usually unnecessary to skeletonize the bowel wall when an extracorporeal anastomosis is contemplated (Figure 27-27).[6] The bowel is exteriorized in continuity, resected, and anastomosed externally.[65] A major advantage of perfoming an extracorporeal anastomosis is that one can be certain that the diseased segment of bowel has been identified and eliminated. Conversely, if an intracorporeal anastomosis is contemplated, one must have available the option of intraoperative colonoscopy to make certain that the proper segment of bowel is being removed.

MODIFIED EXTRACORPOREAL TECHNIQUE. Once the mobilization has been completed, the bowel is grasped through the nearest operative port. For right colon surgery, this usually means a port in the right lower quadrant. For sigmoid lesions, this may mean the midline suprapubic port, and for left colon operations, the left lower quadrant port. A small incision is made adjacent to the site, and the bowel is visualized. It is then grasped and drawn into the wound. A 5-cm incision is usually adequate to accomplish the task, unless there is a larger mass present. A finger can be inserted through the incision and passed through the window in the mesentery. With appropriate traction, the mobilized bowel is drawn into the incision, and the mesentery is identified, clamped, and divided as required (Figure 27-27). The anastomosis is completed once the pathologic features have been confirmed. The bowel is then replaced in the abdomen and the incision closed. A pneumoperitoneum is then reinstituted and the abdomen carefully inspected for hemostasis. The cavity is copiously irrigated, and any clots are removed. The ports are withdrawn under direct visualization and the sites closed.

This method effects a compromise between a total extracorporeal resection and anastomosis and that of a total intracorporeal resection and anastomosis. The bowel is divided internally using a linear stapler/cutter (Figure 27-28; see also Figure 27-17) or with the application of bowel clamps. The colon is divided, and the proximal end brought out through a large trocar insertion site. One may then utilize a biofragmental anastomosis ring[188] or the anvil of the stapling gun or return the proximal end to the abdominal cavity after the resection has been completed in order to perform a sutured anastomosis. However, this last approach is challenging and time consuming.[98]

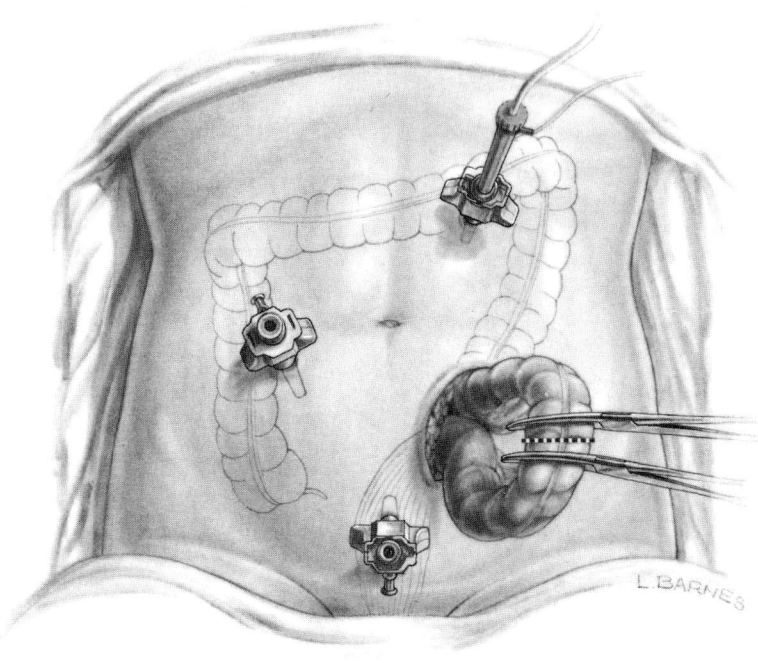

FIGURE 27-27. Laparoscopic-assisted sigmoid colectomy. Extracorporeal division of the bowel in preparation for resection and anastomosis.

INTRACORPOREAL ANASTOMOSIS. Although technically feasible, the completion of a total intracorporeal anastomosis is a highly advanced laparoscopic technical concept. It may be regarded as a less than satisfactory approach for reestablishing intestinal continuity for many patients and indeed for most surgeons familiar with laparoscopy. Still, there is validity for its application, and it is worth discussing the technical approaches to accomplish this. One obvious concern is the risk for fecal contamination when one divides the bowel.[6]

The generally recommended technique is as follows: The proximal resection margin is identified and divided with a linear stapler. My own preference is to leave the proximal bowel clamped but unstapled. The distal margin to be resected is then divided. A plastic bag is introduced through the rectum and the specimen retrieved and extracted transanally. Alternatively, the specimen may be removed through a small incision which is then closed before effecting an anastomosis (Figure 27-29C). One may now perform a sutured anastomosis with whatever technique the surgeon selects, or one may utilize a stapling technique.

If a stapling option is elected, the following is the approach: The anvil of the circular stapling device is detached from the stapling gun, and a suture is tied to the prong on the anvil and wrapped around it. It is then reattached to the

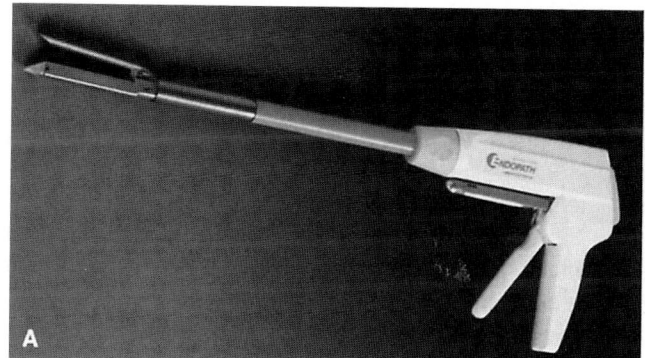

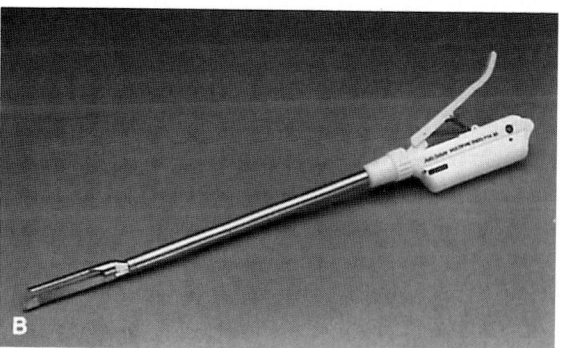

FIGURE 27-28. Endoscopic linear staplers, 60-mm, for intracorporeal bowel resection and anastomosis. **(A)** Endopath linear cutter. (Courtesy of Ethicon Endosurgery, Inc., Cincinnati, OH.) **(B)** Multifire powered Endo TA. (Courtesy of United States Surgical Corporation, Norwalk, CT.)

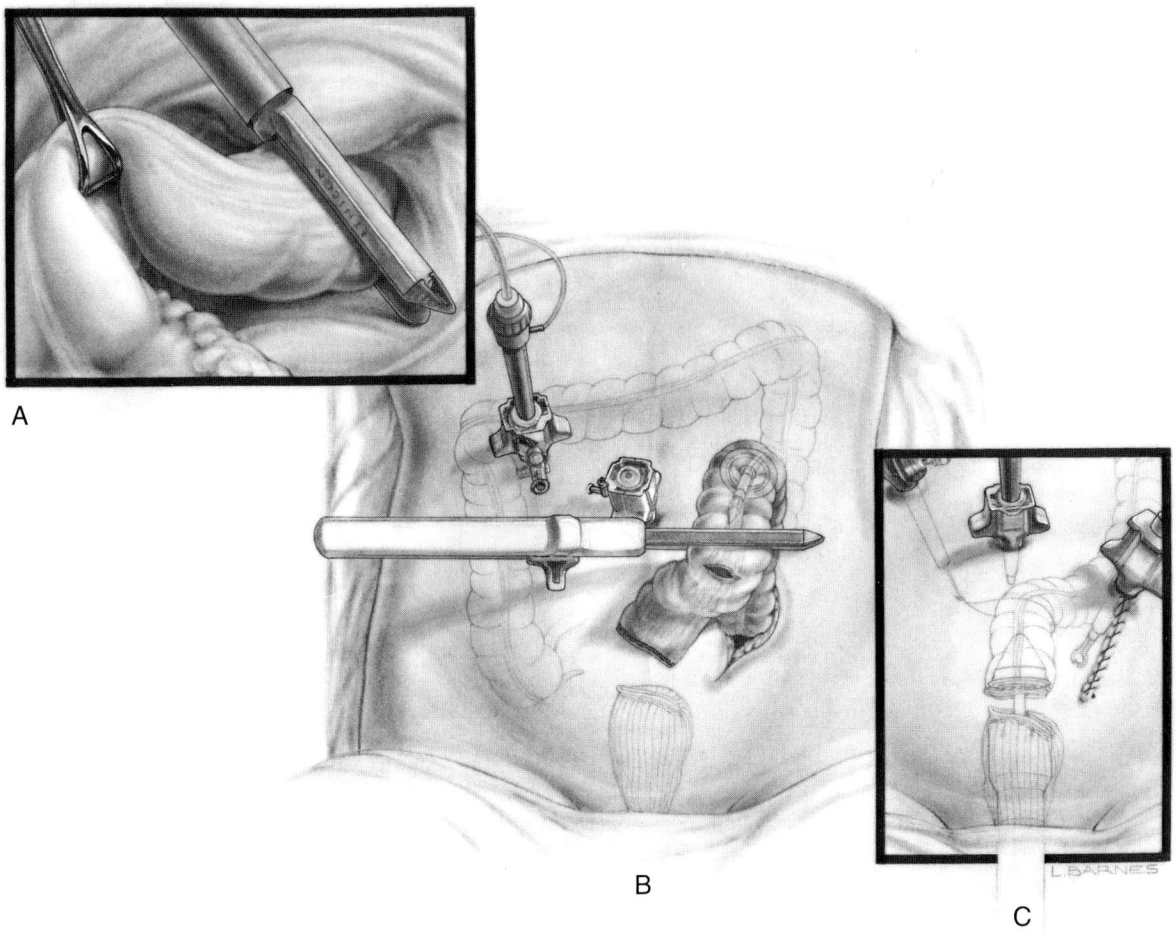

FIGURE 27-29. Bowel resection with intracorporeal anastomosis. **(A)** A Linear stapler divides the distal bowel at the level of the rectosigmoid. **(B)** The proximal bowel is brought out through an incision made at the left lower quadrant port. **(C)** Anastomosis is effected by means of a double-stapling technique. The proximal anvil had been placed extracorporeally (not shown).

gun, introduced into the anal canal, and the anvil retrieved within the abdominal cavity. The anvil is then placed inside the proximal colon, and the needle with the suture is brought out through a tenia, close to the edge of the bowel. The proximal colon is then stapled closed, thereby entrapping the anvil inside. A small incision is made at the staple line on the proximal bowel. Traction on the suture allows one to bring the center rod through this opening. The rectum is then closed with a linear stapler. An end-to-end circular stapled anastomosis is then effected in the usual double-stapled fashion as has been discussed in Chapter 23. Figure 27-30 illustrates the technique as described for performing a complete intracorporeal anastomosis. Other intracorporeal anastomotic options are illustrated in Figure 27-29 above, as well as in Figures 27-31 and 27-32.

Total Colectomy

Laparoscopic total colectomy obviously implies not only the mobilization and resection of the right and left colon, but removal of the transverse colon. This is undoubtedly the most difficult part of the operation, because it involves either separation of the omental attachments or inclusion of the omentum in the resected specimen. This is a much more cumbersome undertaking in that it is necessary to move the television monitors depending on the surgeon's position and the section of the colon which is being mobilized. As previously mentioned, when working on the patient's right, the surgeon stands on the left side, and the television is placed at the patient's right hip. The opposite is true if the left colon is being mobilized. If the ultimate goal is to perform an ileorectal anastomosis, such as in an operation for colonic inertia, the specimen may be extracted through the rectum and a sutured or stapled anastomosis in accordance with the principles previously discussed is accomplished. However, if the operation is being performed for inflammatory bowel disease and a reservoir-anal procedure is contemplated, an extracorporeal pouch construction is usually performed.[150,253]

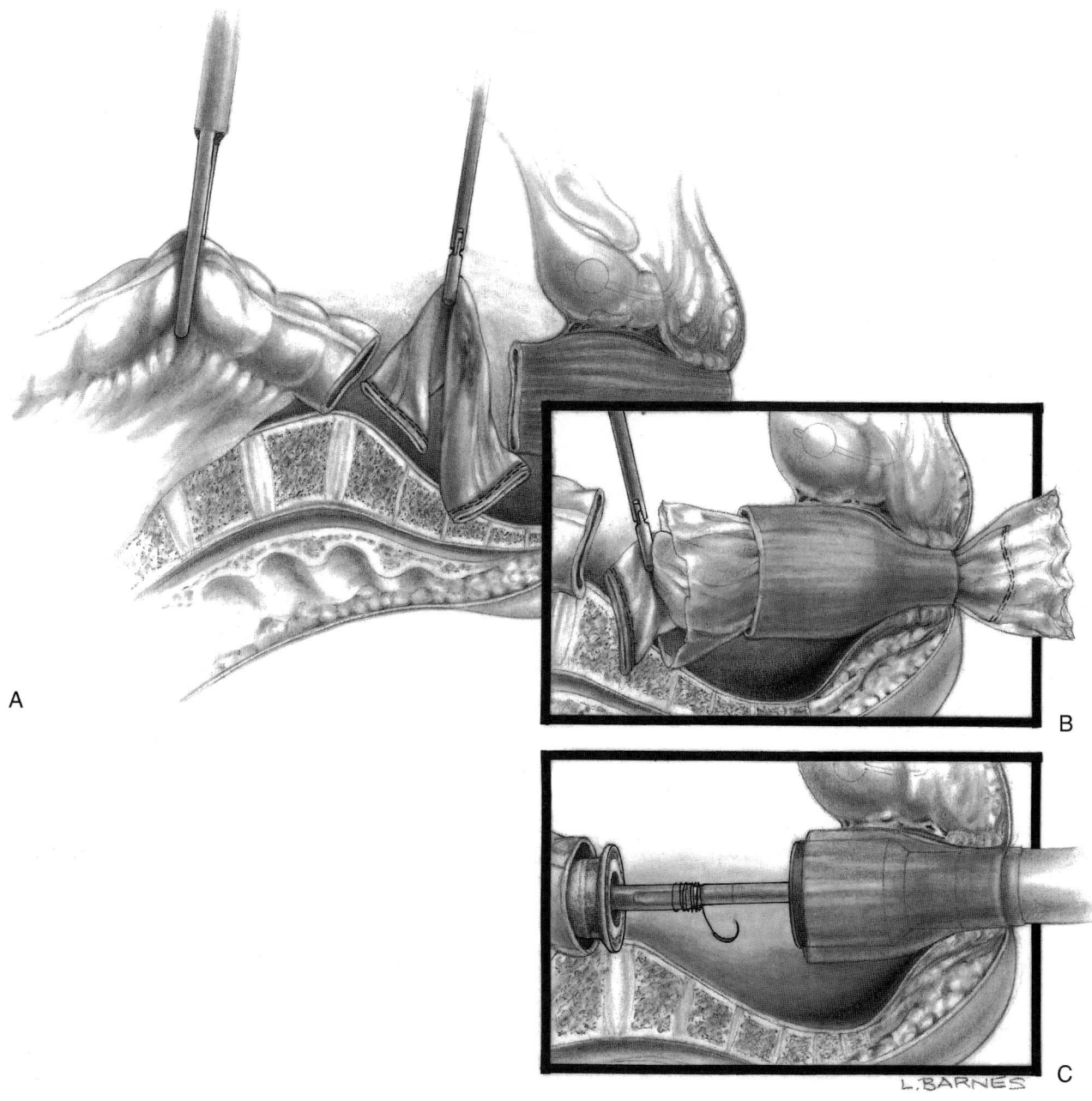

FIGURE 27-30. Intracorporeal anastomotic technique. **(A)** The proximal bowel is occluded, and the specimen stapled at both resection margins. **(B)** A plastic bag is introduced through the rectum. It is then opened to receive the specimen, which is then withdrawn. **(C)** The circular stapler is inserted into the rectum. A suture is secured to the anvil. (*CONTINUED*)

Abdominoperineal Resection

A laparoscopic approach to removing the colon with sigmoid colostomy was initially described for benign disease.[183] There have now been a number or reports of abdominoperineal resection for the treatment of rectal cancer.[43] Removing the specimen presents no problem because one merely needs to excise the rectum through the perineal incision. The laparoscopic approach is used to mobilize and divide the bowel as well as to create the colostomy.

The patient is placed in a steep Trendelenburg position, rotated to the right or left, depending on which side of the rectum is being dissected.[42] Following complete mobilization, the perineal dissection is carried out as described in Chapter 23. The rectum is then delivered and the perineal wound closed, with drainage

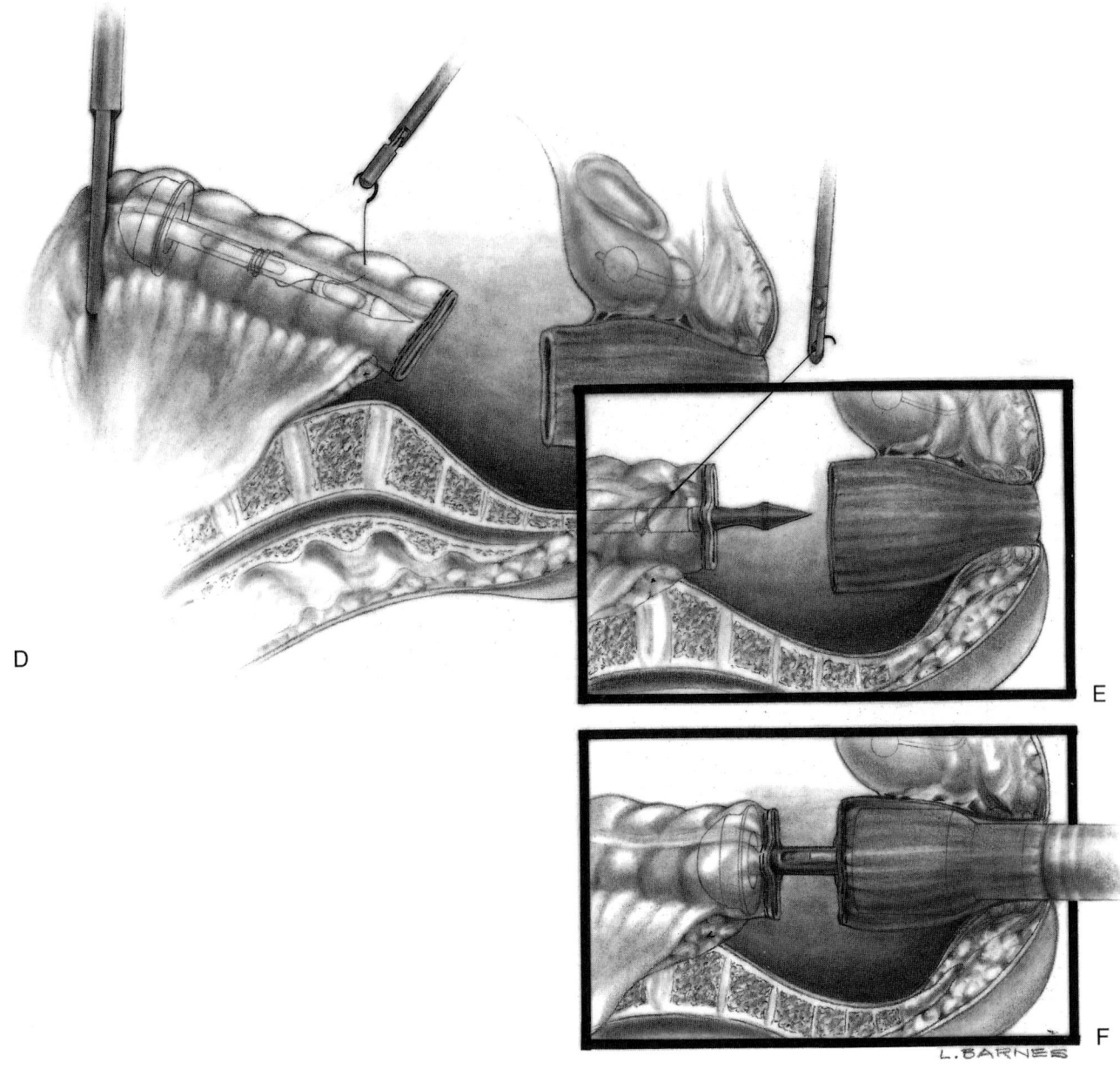

FIGURE 27-30. *(CONTINUED)* **(D)** The anvil is placed into the proximal colon, and the circular stapler is withdrawn from the anus. The suture is passed from within the bowel lumen to provide a "handle." The proximal bowel is stapled. **(E)** The anvil is controlled by means of the suture and brought through the staple line. The suture is then cut. **(F)** The rectum is then stapled across and the circular stapler inserted in accordance with the standard, "double-stapling" technique, such as is illustrated in Figure 23-101.

effected either through the perineum or through the abdomen.

Results of Laparoscopic Colon Operations

As of October 1995, 167 patients underwent laparoscopic colorectal procedures at the Cleveland Clinic Florida.[1] Many had the operation performed for inflammatory bowel disease (42%), whereas approximately one third underwent the operation for neoplastic conditions. The most significant variable affecting intraoperative laparoscopic complications was the surgical experience measured by the time it took to perform the procedure. The authors concluded that this learning curve appears to require more than 50 cases to achieve competence.[1] Others have also commented on the issue of the learning curve, but most of them believe that the number of cases re-

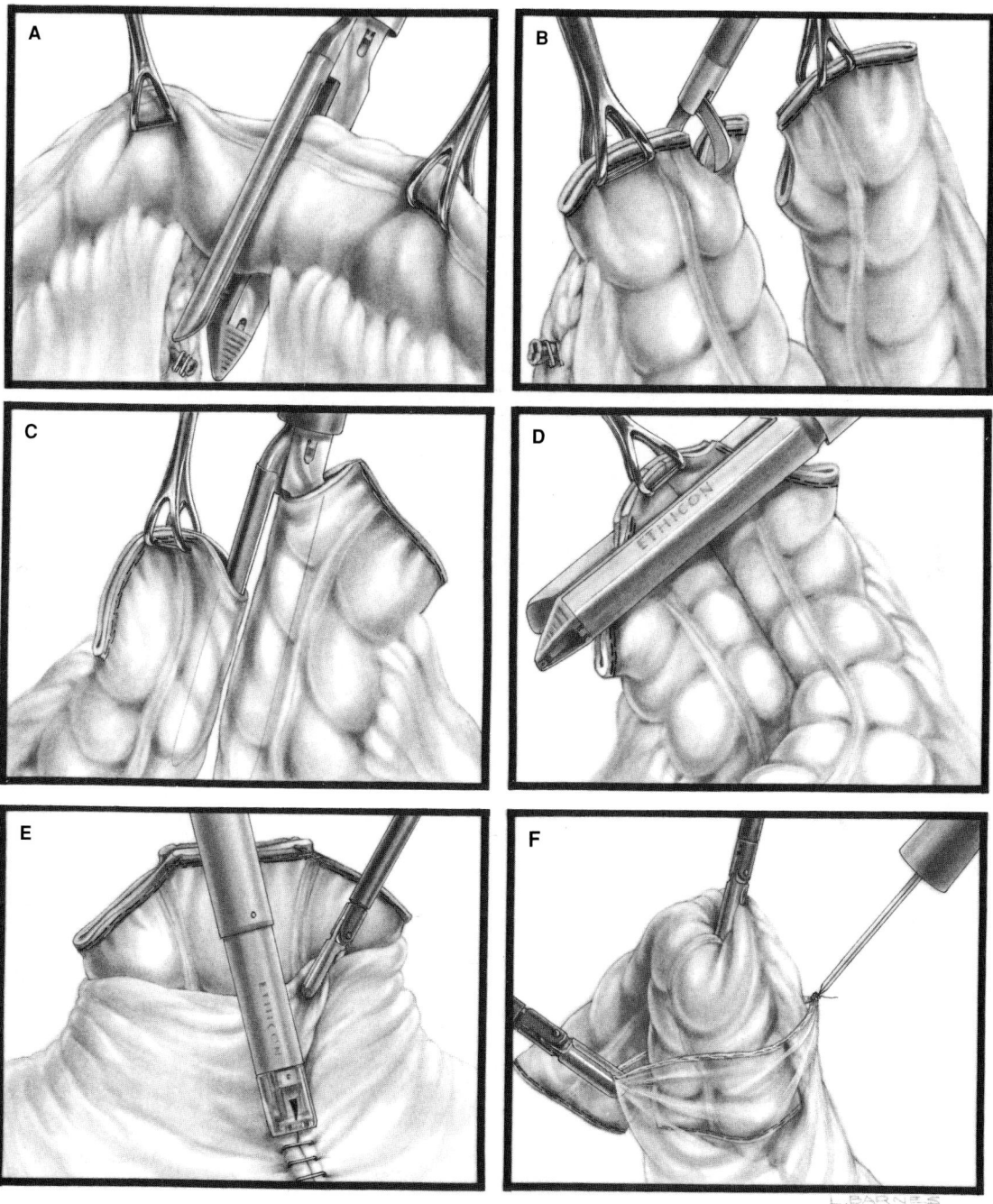

FIGURE 27-31. Intracorporeal segmental resection with functional end-to-end anastomosis. **(A)** Following mobilization and division of the blood supply, the bowel is divided by means of the linear stapler. **(B)** Corners of the closed bowel are incised or excised. **(C)** Through utilization of the same 60-mm linear stapler, a functional end-to-end anastomosis is created. **(D)** Closure of the common enterotomy is facilitated by the stapler. **(E)** The mesenteric defect is closed by a multifeed stapler. **(F)** The resected bowel can be placed in a special bag to minimize contamination. The specimen is then removed through a minilaparotomy at one of the trocar sites.

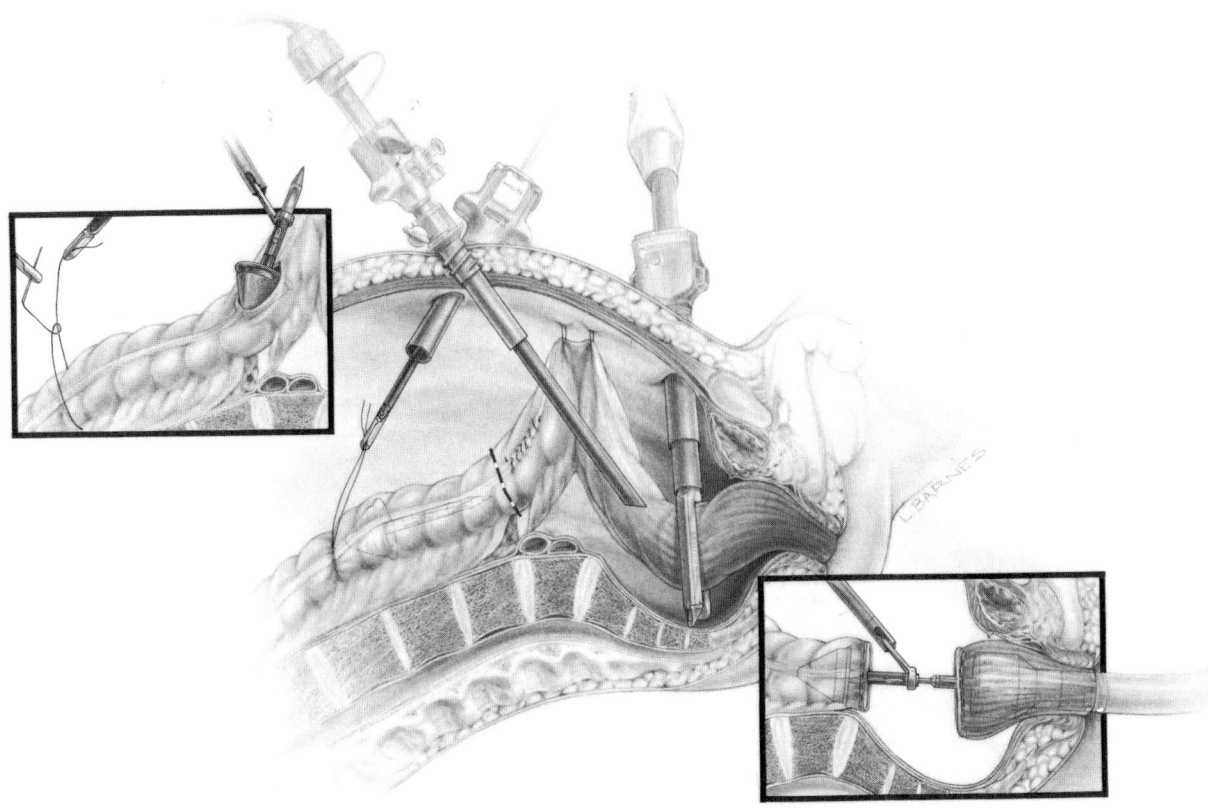

FIGURE 27-32. A plethora of intracorporeal resection/anastomotic options using some of the contemporary tools.

quired is probably fewer.[9,197,208] Dinçler and co-workers believed that the assessment of a learning curve should not be limited to measurement of a decrease in operative time but should also include the conversion and complication rates.[50] In their study, the "steady state" was reached after approximately 70 to 80 interventions.

The general consensus from the literature is that the procedure is safe, as effective as the open operation, and applicable to most of the standard colorectal procedures. All commented that this approach is generally associated with shorter hospitalization and less patient discomfort than the open alternative.[62,91,151,200,209] Others opined that there is no statistically significant difference with respect to morbidity and mortality and indeed, no benefit with respect to length of hospital stay or duration of postoperative ileus.[18,22] Wexner and colleagues demonstrated in a prospective trial comparing laparoscopic-assisted colon and rectal surgery with standard procedures that, specifically, operating time, length of ileus, and length of hospitalization were not improved.[251] Conversely, Tate and colleagues, in their prospective comparison, found that recovery following surgery was improved with a laparoscopic approach.[229] The COST study group noted only minimal short-term, quality of life, benefits with laparoscopic colectomy for colon cancer when compared with open colectomy.[248]

The Cleveland Clinic (Ohio) group compared the actual and predicted risk-adjusted morbidity and mortality for laparoscopic colectomy using both the Physiological and Operative Severity Score for the enUmeration of Mortality and morbidity (POSSUM) and Portsmouth POSSUM (P-POSSUM) scoring systems.[206] Consecutive operations (251) were performed by a single surgeon. The morbidity and mortality rates were significantly lower than predictable by these scoring systems, a finding suggesting that laparoscopic surgery may pose a lower risk for the patient. However, one must consider that the results from this obviously highly skilled and experienced surgeon may not be duplicated by others. A prospective, randomized trial would be more likely to resolve this issue.

The prospective, randomized, multicenter COST study group is now closed for accrual of patients, and its data are being analyzed for cancer survival. From September of 1994 through February of 1999, 449 patients with resectable colon cancer were enrolled in the study. Short-term better quality of life outcome, less pain, and fewer days required for analgesic use, were reported for the laparoscopic study group.[248] However, the safety and efficacy data are not yet available. In the COLOR European multicenter randomized trial that began in 1997, 1,200 patients have been enrolled.[85] Twenty-seven hospitals participated, including those from Sweden, the Netherlands, Germany, France, Italy, Spain, and the United Kingdom. The primary end point is cancer-free survival at 3 years. Although laparoscopic surgery appears to be of comparable value in the treatment of colon cancer, final results are still awaited as of this writing.

Comment

The introduction of laparoscopic techniques has been a recent phenomenon. The explosion in the technology and equipment has been remarkable, with proliferation of training opportunities enabling many surgeons to embark upon the various laparoscopic approaches to the treatment of colon and rectal disease. We may even be on the verge of newer vistas in the minimally invasive management of surgical problems through total endoluminal operations with advanced external imaging, flexible microinstrumentation, and the expanded use of robotics. Inevitably, improvement in visualization and tissue manipulation will permit an increased number of procedures to be performed by means of laparoscopy, but it is incumbent upon all of us to approach this new technology in a way that does not harm the patient. Although the issue of patient discomfort and perhaps earlier hospital discharge are worthy objectives, it will only be through carefully controlled trials that the complications and results will enable us to make reasoned, appropriate decisions on behalf of our patients.

REFERENCES

1. Agachan F, Joo JS, Weiss EG, et al. Intraoperative laparoscopic complications: are we getting better? *Dis Colon Rectum* 1996;39:S14.
2. Ali J, Rozycki GS, Campbell JP, et al. Trauma ultrasound workshop improves physician detection of peritoneal and pericardial fluid. *J Surg Res* 1996;63:275.
3. Allendorf JDF, Bessler M, Kaytun ML, et al. Tumor growth after laparotomy or laparoscopy. *Surg Endosc* 1995;9:49.
4. Andersen JR, Stoen K. Implantation metastases after laparoscopic biopsy of bladder cancer. *J Urol* 1995;153:1047.
5. Averbach M, Cohen RV, de-Barros MV, et al. Laparoscopy-assisted colonoscopic polypectomy. *Surg Laparosc Endosc* 1995;5:137.
6. Beart RW Jr. Laparoscopic-assisted colectomy. In: Corman ML, ed. *Colon and rectal surgery*, 3rd ed. Philadelphia: JB Lippincott, 1993:552–564.
7. Bender JS, Talamini MA. Diagnostic laparoscopy in critically ill intensive care unit patients. *Surg Endosc* 1992;6:302.
8. Benedict EB. Peritoneoscopy. *N Engl J Med* 1938;218:713.
9. Bennett CL, Stryker SJ, Ferreira MR, et al. The learning curve for laparoscopic colorectal surgery: preliminary results from a prospective analysis of 1194 laparoscopic-assisted colectomies. *Arch Surg* 1997;132:41.
10. Berci G. Laparoscopy in general surgery. In: Berci G, ed. *Endoscopy*. New York: Appleton-Century-Crofts, 1976:382–400.
11. Berci G, Cuschieri A. *Practical laparoscopy*. London: Bailliàre Tindall, 1986.
12. Berci G, Dunkelman D, Michel SL, et al. Emergency mini-laparoscopy in abdominal trauma: an update. *Am J Surg* 1983;146:261.
13. Berci G, Sackier JM, Paz-Partlow M. A new endoscopic treatment for symptomatic gallbladder disease. *Gastrointest Endosc Clin North Am* 1991;1:191.
14. Berci G, Sackier JM, Paz-Partlow M. Emergency laparoscopy. *Am J Surg* 1991;161:355.
15. Bergamaschi R, Pessaux, Arnaud J-P. Comparison of conventional and laparoscopic ileocolic resection for Crohn's disease. *Dis Colon Rectum* 2003;46:1129.
16. Berman IR. Sutureless laparoscopic rectopexy for procidentia: technique and implications. *Dis Colon Rectum* 1992;35:689.
17. Bernheim BM. Organoscopy. *Ann Surg* 1911;53:764.
18. Bernstein MA, Dawson JW, Reissman P, et al. Is complete laparoscopic colectomy superior to laparoscopic assisted colectomy? *Am Surg* 1996;62:507.
19. Bessler M, Whenlan RL, Halverson A, et al. Is immune function better preserved after laparoscopic versus open colon resection? *Surg Endosc* 1994;8:881.
20. Bezzi M, Merlino P, Orsi F, et al. Laparoscopic sonography during abdominal laparoscopic surgery: technique and imaging findings. *AJR Am J Roentgenol* 1995;165:1193.
21. Bhandarkar DS, Morgan WP. Laparoscopic cecopexy for cecal volvulus. *Br J Surg* 1995;82:323.
22. Bokey EL, Moore JWE, Chapuis PH, et al. Morbidity and mortality following laparoscopic-assisted right hemicolectomy for cancer. *Dis Colon Rectum* 1996;39:S24.
23. Bruce CJ, Coller JA, Murray JJ, et al. Laparoscopic resection for diverticular disease. *Dis Colon Rectum* 1996;39:S1.
24. Buess G, Lirici MM. Endoluminal therapy of rectal tumors: transanal endoscopic microsurgery. In: Hunter JG, Sackier JM, eds. *Minimally invasive surgery*. New York: McGraw-Hill, 1993:191–196.
25. Buess G, Thiess R, Gunther M, et al. Endoscopic operative procedure for the removal of rectal polyps. *Coloproctology* 1984;6:254.
26. Carlson MA, Frantzides CT. Complications of laparoscopic procedures. In: Frantzides CT, ed. *Laparoscopic and thoracoscopic surgery*. St. Louis: Mosby–Year Book, 1995:224–252.
27. Chae FH, Sackier JM. Laparoscopic cholecystectomy: lessons learned from gallbladder cancer. In: Geraghty JG, Sackier JM, Young H, et al, eds. *Minimal access surgery in oncology*. London: Greenwich Medical Media, 1997.
28. Chamberlain GVP, Carron-Brown JA. *Report of the working party of the confidential inquiry into gynaecological laparoscopy*. London: Royal College of Obstetricians and Gynaecologists, 1978.
29. Chen MHM, DAngelo AJ, Murphy EA, et al. Laparoscopically assisted abdominal aortic aneurysm repair. *Surg Endosc* 1996;10:1136.
30. Childers JM, Aqua KA, Surwit EA, et al. Abdominal wall tumor implantation after laparoscopy for malignant conditions. *Obstet Gynecol* 1994;84:765.
31. Cirocco WC, Schwartzman A, Golub RW. Abdominal wall recurrence after laparoscopic colectomy for colon cancer. *Surgery* 1994;116:842.
32. Clark PJ, Hands LJ, Gough MH. The use of laparoscopy in the management of right iliac fossa pain. *Ann R Coll Surg Engl* 1986;68:68.
33. Conlon KC, Dougherty E, Klimstra DS, et al. The value of minimal access surgery and the staging of patients with potentially resectable peripancreatic malignancy. *Ann Surg* 1996;223:143.
34. Cooperman AM, Katz V, Zimmon D, et al. Laparoscopic colon resection: a case report. *J Laparoendosc Surg* 1991;1:221.
35. Corson SL, Batzer FR, Gocial B, et al. Measurement of the force necessary for laparoscopic trocar entry. *J Reprod Med* 1989;44:282.
36. Cosgrove J, Korman J, Chen M, et al. Laparoscopy for the acute abdomen. *Semin Laparosc Surg* 1996;3:131.

37. Cuschieri AE. Hiatal hernia and reflux esophagitis. In: Hunter JG, Sackier JM, eds. *Minimally invasive surgery.* New York: McGraw-Hill, 1993:87–111.

38. Cuschieri AE. Whither minimal access surgery: tribulations and expectations. *Am J Surg* 1995;169:9.

39. Cuschieri AE, Hennessy T, Stephens R, et al. Diagnosis of significant abdominal trauma after road traffic accidents: preliminary results of a multicenter clinical trial comparing minilaparoscopy with peritoneal lavage. *Ann R Coll Surg Engl* 1988;70:153.

40. Cuschieri AE, Shimi SM, Vander-Velpen G, et al. Laparoscopic prosthetic fixation rectopexy for complete rectal prolapse. *Br J Surg* 1994;81:138.

41. Cuschieri A, Szabo Z. *Tissue approximation in endoscopic surgery.* Oxford: Isis Medical Media, 1995.

42. Darzi A, Lewis C, Menzies-Gow N, et al. Laparoscopic abdominoperineal resection of the rectum. *Surg Endosc* 1995; 9:414.

43. Decanini C, Milsom JW, Bohm B, et al. Laparoscopic oncologic abdominoperineal resection. *Dis Colon Rectum* 1994;37:552.

44. Dekok H. A new technique for resecting the non-inflamed not-adhesive appendix through a mini-laparotomy with the aid of the laparoscope. *Arch Chir Neerl* 1977;29:195.

45. Delaney CP, Kiran RP, Senagore AJ, et al. Case-matched comparison of clinical and financial outcome after laparoscopic or open colorectal surgery. *Ann Surg* 2003;238:67.

46. Delaney CP, Lynch AC, Senagore AJ, et al. Comparison of robotically performed and traditional laparoscopic colorectal surgery. *Dis Colon Rectum* 2003;46:1633.

47. Delgado S, Lacy AM, Filella X, et al. Acute phase response in laparoscopic and open colectomy in colon cancer: randomized study. *Dis Colon Rectum* 2001;44:638.

48. Demaria EJ, Sugerman HJ, et al. Results of 281 consecutive total laparoscopic Roux en Y gastric bypasses to treat morbid obesity. *Ann Surg* 2002;235:640.

49. Demaria EJ, Schweitzer MA, et al. Hand-assisted laparoscopic gastric bypass does not improve outcome and increases costs when compared to open gastric bypass for the surgical treatment of obesity. *Surg Endosc* 2002;16: 1452.

50. Dinçler S, Koller MT, Steurer J, et al. Multidimensional analysis of learning curves in laparoscopic sigmoid resection: eight-year results. *Dis Colon Rectum* 2003;46:1371.

51. Doctor HN, Hussain Z. Bilateral pneumothorax associated with laparoscopy: a case report of a rare hazard and review of the literature. *Anesthesiology* 1973;23:75.

52. Donaldson JK, Sanderlin JH, Harrell WB. A method of suspending the uterus without open abdominal incision: use of the peritoneoscope and a special needle. *Am J Surg* 1942; 55:537.

53. Dubois F, Berthelots G, Levard H. Cholecystectomy par coelioscopie. *Presse Med* 1989;18:980.

54. Duepree H-J, Senagore AJ, Delaney CP, et al. Does means of access affect the incidence of small bowel obstruction and ventral hernia after bowel resection? Laparoscopy versus laparotomy. *J Am Coll Surg* 2003;197:177.

55. Dumay ACM, Jense GJ. Endoscopic surgery simulation in a virtual environment. *Comput Biol Med* 1995;25:139.

56. Dunham R, Sackier JM. Is there a dilemma of adequately training surgeons in open and laparoscopic biliary surgery. *Surg Clin North Am* 1994;74:913.

57. Dunker MS, Ten Hove T, Bemelman WA, et al. Interleukin-6, C-reactive protein, and expression of human leukocyte antigen-DR on peripheral blood mononuclear cells in patients after laparoscopic vs. conventional bowel resection. *Dis Colon Rectum* 2003;46:1238.

58. Du Priest RW Jr, Rodriguez A, Khaneja SC, et al. Open diagnostic peritoneal lavage in blunt abdominal trauma victims. *Surg Gynecol Obstet* 1979;148:890.

59. Dwivedi A, Chahin F, Agrawal S, et al. Laparoscopic colectomy vs. open colectomy for diverticular disease. *Dis Colon Rectum* 2002;45:1309.

60. Eilber FR, Morton DL. Impaired immunologic reactivity and recurrence following cancer surgery. *Cancer* 1970;25: 362.

61. Falk PM, Beart RW Jr, Wexner SD, et al. Laparoscopic colectomy: a critical appraisal. *Dis Colon Rectum* 1993;36: 28.

62. Fleshman JW, Fry RD, Birnbaum EH, et al. Laparoscopic-assisted and minilaparotomy approaches to colorectal diseases are similar in early outcome. *Dis Colon Rectum* 1996; 39:15.

63. Fleshman JW, Nelson H, Peters WR, et al. Early results of laparoscopic surgery for colorectal cancer: retrospective analysis of 372 patients treated by clinical outcomes of surgical therapy (COST) study group. *Dis Colon Rectum* 1996; 39:S53.

64. Flowers JL, Bailey RW, Scovill WA, et al. The Baltimore experience with laparoscopic management of acute cholecystitis. *Am J Surg* 1991;161:388.

65. Fowler DL, White SA. Laparoscopy assisted sigmoid resection. *Surg Laparosc Endosc* 1991;1:183.

66. Francis DMA. Relationship between blood transfusion and tumour behavior. *Br J Surg* 1991;78:1420.

67. Frankel SM, Fitzgerald RL, Sackier JM. Utility of insufflation filters in laparoscopic surgery. *Surg Endosc* 1998;12: 1137.

68. Franklin ME Jr, Dorman JP, Pharand D. Laparoscopic surgery in acute small bowel obstruction. *Surg Laparosc Endosc* 1994;4:289.

69. Franklin ME Jr, Rosenthal D, Abrego-Medina D, et al. Prospective comparison of open vs. laparoscopic colon surgery for carcinoma: five-year results. *Dis Colon Rectum* 1996;39:535.

70. Frizelle FA, Cuschieri AE. Use of laparoscopic instruments in conventional mobilisation of the rectum [Letter]. *Ann R Coll Surg Engl* 1995;77:397.

71. Gagner M, Pomp A. Laparoscopic pylorus-preserving pancreatoduodenectomy. *Surg Endosc* 1994;8:408.

72. Gazzaniga AB, Slanton WW, Bartlett RH. Laparoscopy in the diagnosis of blunt and penetrating injuries to the abdomen. *Am J Surg* 1976;131:315.

73. Georgeson KE, Fuenfer MM, Hardin WD. Primary laparoscopic pull-through for Hirschsprung's disease in infants and children. *J Pediatr Surg* 1995;30:1017.

74. Gleeson NC, Nicosia SV, Mark JE, et al. Abdominal wall metastases from ovarian carcinoma after laparoscopy. *Am J Obstet Gynecol* 1993;169:522.

75. Gordon AG, Magos AL. The development of laparoscopic surgery. *Ballieres Clin Obstet Gynecol* 1989;3:429.

76. Gorey TF, OConnell PR, Waldrop D, et al. Laparoscopically assisted reversal of Hartmann's procedure. *Br J Surg* 1993; 80:109.

77. Greene FL. Laparoscopy in malignant disease. *Surg Clin North Am* 1992;72:1125.

78. Gurland BH, Wexner SD. Laparoscopic surgery for inflammatory bowel disease: results of the past decade. *Inflamm Bowel Dis* 2002;8:46.

79. Halevy A, Lin GP, Gold-Deutsch R, et al. Comparison of serum C-reactive protein concentrations for laparoscopic versus open cholecystectomy. *Surg Endosc* 1995;9:280.

80. Halverson A, Buchanan R, Jacobs L, et al. Evaluation of mechanism of increased intracranial pressure with insufflation. *Surg Endosc* 1998;12:266.

81. Hamilton JE. Peritoneoscopy in gunshot and stab wounds of the abdomen. *Surgery* 1940;7:582.

82. Hartley JE, Kumar H, Drew PJ, et al. Laparoscopic ultrasound for the detection of hepatic metastases during laparoscopic colorectal cancer surgery. *Dis Colon Rectum* 2000; 43:320.

83. Hartley JE, Mehigan BJ, Queshi AE, et al. Total mesorectal excision: assessment of the laparoscopic approach. *Dis Colon Rectum* 2001;44:315.

84. Hasson HM. Open laparoscopy versus closed laparoscopy: a comparison of complication rates. *Adv Planned Parenthood* 1978;13:41.

85. Hazebroek EJ et al. COLOR: a randomized clinical trial comparing laparoscopic and open resection for colon cancer. *Surg Endosc* 2002;16:949.

86. Heah SM, Hartley JE, Hurley J, et al. Laparoscopic suture rectopexy without resection is effective treatment for full-thickness rectal prolapse. *Dis Colon Rectum* 2000;43:638.

87. Heald RJ, Ryall RDH. Recurrence and survival after total mesorectal excision for rectal cancer. *Lancet* 1986;1:1479.

88. Hemming AW, Nagy AG, Scudamore CH, et al. Laparoscopic staging of intra-abdominal malignancy. *Surg Endosc* 1995;9:325.

89. Hildebrandt U, Plusczyk T, Kessler K, et al. Single-surgeon surgery in laparoscopic colonic resection. *Dis Colon Rectum* 2003;46:1640.

90. Hjortso NC, Kehlet H. Influence of surgery, age and serum albumin on delayed hypersensitivity. *Acta Chir Scand* 1986;152:175.

91. Hoffman GC, Baker JW, Fitchett CW, et al. Laparoscopic-assisted colectomy: initial experience. *Ann Surg* 1994;219:732.

92. Hong D, Tabet J, Anvari M. Laparoscopic vs. open resection for colorectal adenocarcinoma. *Dis Colon Rectum* 2001;44:10.

93. Horgan PG, Fitzpatrick M, Couse NF, et al. Laparoscopy is less immunotraumatic than laparotomy. *Minim Invasive Ther* 1992;1:241.

94. Hughes ES, McDermott FT, Poliglase AI, et al. Tumor recurrence in the abdominal wall scar after large bowel cancer surgery. *Dis Colon Rectum* 1983;36:571.

95. Hutman S. Operating at the cutting edge: nine surgeons speak out on laparoscopic-guided colon resection. *J Clin Laser Med Surg* 1991;9:Oct:313.

96. Jacobaeus HC. Uber Laparo und Thorakoskopie. *Beitr Klin Tuberk* 1912;25:185.

97. Jacobi CA, Ordemann J, Bohm B, et al. Increased tumor growth after laparoscopy with air vs. CO_2. *Surg Endosc* 1996;33:551(abst).

98. Jacobs M, Verdeja JC, Goldstein HS. Minimally invasive colon resection (laparoscopic colectomy). *Surg Laparosc Endosc* 1991;1:144.

99. Jacquet P, Averbach AM, Stephens AD, et al. Cancer recurrence following laparoscopic colectomy. *Dis Colon Rectum* 1995;38:1110.

100. Jagelman DG, Fabian TC, Nichols RL, et al. Single-dose cefotetan versus multiple-dose cefoxitin as prophylaxis in colorectal surgery. *Am J Surg* 1988;155:71.

101. Jager RM. Laparoscopic right hemicolectomy in left lateral decubitus position. *Surg Laparosc Endosc* 1994;4:348.

102. Jones DB, Guo L-W, Reinhard MK, et al. Impact of pneumoperitoneum on trocar site implantation of colon cancer in hamster model. *Dis Colon Rectum* 1995;38:1182.

103. Kairaluoma MV, Viljakka MT, Kellokumpu IH. Open vs. laparoscopic surgery for rectal prolapse: a case-controlled study assessing short-term outcome. *Dis Colon Rectum* 2003;46:353.

104. Kalk H. Erfahrungen mit der Laparoskopie (Zugleich mit Beschreibung eines neuen Instrumentes). *Z Klin Med* 1929;111:303.

105. Kanyrim K, Seidlitz HK, Hagnmullei F, et al. Color performance of video endoscopes: quantitative measurement of color reproduction. *Endoscopy* 1987;19:233.

106. Kelling G. Die Tamponade der Bauchhohle mit Luft zur Stillung lebensgefahrlicher Intestinalblutungen. *Munch Med Wochenschr* 1901;48:1480.

107. Kelling G. Zur Colioskopie und Gastroskopie. *Arch Klin Chir* 1923;126:226.

108. Reference cited in text; to be added here.

109. Kitano S, Tomikawa M, Iso Y, et al. A safe and simple method to maintain a clear field of vision during laparoscopic cholecystectomy. *Surg Endosc* 1992;6:197.

110. Kockerling F. Laparoscopy alone. Paper presented at SAGES Scientific Session, March 13–17, 1996.

111. Köckering F, Scheidbach H, Schneider C, et al. Laparoscopic abdominoperineal resection: early postoperative results of a prospective study involving 116 patients. *Dis Colon Rectum* 2000;43:1503.

112. Ky AJ, Sonoda T, Millsom JW. One-stage laparoscopic restorative proctocolectomy: an alternative to the conventional approach? *Dis Colon Rectum* 2002;45:207.

113. Lacock WS, Trus TL, Hunter JG. New technology for the division of short gastric vessels during laparoscopic Nissen fundoplication: a prospective randomized trial. *Surg Endosc* 1996;10:71.

114. Lange V, Meyer G, Schardey HM, et al. Laparoscopic creation of a loop colostomy. *J Laparoendosc Surg* 1991;1:307.

115. Lauroy J, Champault G, Risk N, et al. Metastatic recurrence at the cannula site: should digestive carcinomas still be managed by laparoscopy?. *Br J Surg* 1994;81:31(abst).

116. LeBlanc KA, Bellanger DE. Laparoscopic repair of paraostomy hernias: early results. *J Am Coll Surg* 2002;194:232.

117. Le Moine M-C, Fabre J-M, Vacher C, et al. Factors and consequences of conversion in laparoscopic sigmoidectomy for diverticular disease. *Br J Surg* 2003;90:232.

118. Liu CD, Rolandelli R, Ashley SW, et al. Laparoscopic surgery for inflammatory bowel disease. *Am Surg* 1995;61:1054.

119. Lord SA, Larach SW, Ferrara A, et al. Laparoscopic resections for colorectal carcinoma: a three year experience. *Dis Colon Rectum* 1996;39:148.

120. Lucarini L, Galleano R, Lombezzi R, et al. Laparoscopic-assisted Hartmann's reversal with the Dexterity^R Pneumo Sleeve™. *Dis Colon Rectum* 2000;43:1164.

121. MacSweeney STR, Postlethwaite JC. Second-look laparoscopy in the management of acute mesenteric ischemia. *Br J Surg* 1994;81:90.

122. Majeed AW, Troy G, Nicholl JP, et al. Randomized, prospective, single-blind comparison of laparoscopic versus small incision cholecystectomy. *Lancet*1996;347:989.

123. Marcello PW, Milsom JW, Wong SK, et al. Laparoscopic restorative proctocolectomy: case-matched comparative study with open restorative proctocolectomy. *Dis Colon Rectum* 2000;43:604.

124. Marchesa P, Milsom JW, Hale JC, et al. Intraoperative laparoscopic liver ultrasonography for staging of colorectal cancer: initial experience. *Dis Colon Rectum* 1996;39:S73.

125. Marusch F, Gastinger I, Schneider C, et al. Importance of conversion for results obtained with laparoscopic colorectal surgery. *Dis Colon Rectum* 2001;44:207.

126. Mavrantonis C, Wexner SD, Nogueras JJ, et al. Current attitudes in laparoscopic colorectal surgery. *Surg Endosc* 2002;16:1152.

127. McDermott JP, Devereaux DA, Caushaj PF. Pitfall of laparoscopic colectomy: an unrecognized synchronous cancer. *Dis Colon Rectum* 1994;37:602.

128. Meyer HJ, Ebert KH. Laparoscopic abdomino-perineal rectum excision with high dissection of the inferior mesenteric artery: simplification by intraoperative ventral fixation of the rectosigmoid. *Chirurg* 1994;65:1136.

129. Milsom JW, Bohm B, Deconini C, et al. Laparoscopic oncologic proctosigmoidectomy with low colorectal anastomosis in a cadaver model. *Surg Endosc* 1994;8:1117.

130. Milsom JW, Bohm B, Stolfi VM, et al. Use of cotton tapes in laparoscopic intestinal surgery. *Br J Surg* 1993;80:768.

131. Milsom JW, Hammerhofer KA, Böhm B, et al. Prospective, randomized trial comparing laparoscopic vs. conventional surgery for refractory ileocolic Crohn's disease. *Dis Colon Rectum* 2001; 44:1.

132. Milsom JW, Jerby BL, Kessler H, et al. Prospective, blinded comparison of laparoscopic ultrasonography vs. contrast-enhanced computerized tomography for liver assessment in patients undergoing colorectal carcinoma surgery. *Dis Colon Rectum* 2000;43:44.

133. Molloy RG, McCourtney JS, Anderson JR. Laparoscopy in the management of patients with cancer of the gastric cardia and oesophagus. *Br J Surg* 1995;82:352.

134. Msika S, Deroide G, Kianmanesh R, et al. Harmonic scalpel in laparoscopic surgery. *Dis Colon Rectum* 2001;44:432.

135. Msika S, Iannelli A, Deroide G, et al. Can laparoscopy reduce hospital stay in the treatment of Crohn's disease? *Dis Colon Rectum* 2001;44:1661.

136. Mouiel J, Katkhouda N. Laparoscopic vagotomy in the treatment of chronic duodenal ulcer disease. *Probl Gen Surg* 1991;8:358.

137. Muhe E. Laparoskopiesche Cholezystektomie: Spatergebnisse. Kongressbericht 1991. *Langenbecks Arch Chir* 1991; ??[Suppl]:416.

138. Murugiah M, Paterson-Brown S, Windsor JA, et al. Early experience of laparoscopic ultrasonography in the management of pancreatic carcinoma. *Surg Endosc* 1993;7:119.

139. Musser PJ, Boorse RC, Madera F, et al. Laparoscopic colectomy: at what cost? *Surg Laparosc Endosc* 1994;4:1.

140. Ortega AE, Beart RW Jr, Steele GD Jr, et al. Laparoscopic bowel surgery registry: preliminary results. *Dis Colon Rectum* 1995;38:681.

141. Ortega AE, Hunter JG, Peters JH, et al. A prospective, randomized comparison of laparoscopic appendectomy with open appendectomy. *Am J Surg* 1995;169:208.

142. Ota D, Loftin B, Sito T, et al. Virtual reality in surgical education. *Comput Biol Med* 1995;25:127.

143. Ott DO. Die Beleuchtung der Bauchhohle (Ventroskopie) als Methode bei vaginaler Koliotomie. *Centrbl Gynakol* 1902;26:817.

144. Ott DE. Contamination by gynecologic endoscopy insufflation. *J Gynecol Surg* 1989;5:205.

145. Palmer R. Security in laparoscopoy In: Phillips JM, Keith L. eds. *Gynecological laparoscopy: principles and techniques.* New York: Symposia Specialist Medical Books, 1974:17.

146. Patterson-Brown S, Eckersley JRT, Sim AJW, et al. Laparoscopy as an adjunct to decision making in the acute abdomen. *Br J Surg* 1986;73:1022.

147. Paw P, Sackier JM. Complications of laparoscopy and thoracoscopy. *J Intensive Care Med* 1994;9:290.

148. Paz-Partlow M. The importance of permanent documentation of endoscopic findings. *Probl Gen Surg* 1991;8:407.

149. Perissat J, Collet D, Belliard R. Gallstones: laparoscopic treatment. *Surg Endosc* 1990;4:1.

150. Peters WR. Laparoscopic total proctocolectomy with creation of ileostomy for ulcerative colitis. *J Laparoendosc Surg* 1992;2:175.

151. Peters WR, Bartels TL. Minimally invasive colectomy: are the potential benefits realized? *Dis Colon Rectum* 1993; 36:751.

152. Pfeifer J, Wexner SD, Reissman P, et al. Laparoscopic versus open colon surgery: cost and outcome. *Surg Endosc* 1995;9:1322.

153. Phillips EH, Franklin M, Carroll BJ, et al. Laparoscopic colectomy. *Ann Surg* 1993;216:703.

154. Pier A, Gotz F, Bacher C. Laparoscopic appendectomy in 625 cases: from innovation to routine. *Surg Laparosc Endosc* 1991;1:8.

155. Pietsch JB, Meakins JL, MacLean LD. The delayed hypersensitivity response: application in clinical surgery. *Surgery* 1977;82:349.

156. Rademaker BM, Bannenberg JJ, Kalkman CJ, et al. Effects of pneumoperitoneum with helium on hemodynamics and oxygen transport: a comparison with carbon dioxide. *J Laparoendosc Surg* 1995;5:15.

157. Raeburn CD, McIntyre RC Jr. Laparoscopic approach to adrenal and endocrine pancreatic tumors. *Surg Clin North Am* 2000;80:1427.

158. Ramos JM, Beart RW, Goes R, et al. Role of laparoscopy in colorectal surgery: a prospective evaluation of 200 cases. *Dis Colon Rectum* 1995;38:494.

159. Ramos JM, Gupta S, Anthone GJ, et al. Laparoscopy and colon cancer: is the port site at risk? A preliminary report. *Arch Surg* 1994;129:897.

160. Ratajczak HV, Lange RW, Sothern RB, et al. Surgical influence of murine immunity and tumor growth: relationship of body temperature and hormones with splenocytes. *Proc Soc Exp Biol Med* 1992;199:432.

161. Rau HG, Meyer G, Cohnert TU, et al. Laparoscopic liver resection with the water jet dissector. *Surg Endosc* 1995;9: 1009.

162. Reddick EJ, Olsen DO. Laparoscopic laser cholecystectomy. *Surg Endosc* 1989;3:131.

163. Regan MC, Boyle B, Stephens RB. Laparoscopic repair of colonic perforation occuring during colonoscopy. *Br J Surg* 1994;81:1073.

164. Reiertsen O, Bakka A, Tronnes S, et al. Routine double contrast barium enema and fiberoptic colonoscopy in the diagnosis of colorectal carcinoma. *Acta Chir Scand* 1988;154: 43.

165. Reilly WT, Nelson H, Schroeder G, et al. Wound recurrence following conventional treatment of colorectal cancer: a rare but perhaps underestimated problem. *Dis Colon Rectum* 1996;39:200.

166. Reissman P, Salky BA, Pfeiffer J, et al. Laparoscopic surgery in the management of inflammatory bowel disease. *Am J Surg* 1996;171:47.

167. Rispoli G, Esposito C, Monachese D, et al. Removal of a foreign body from the distal colon using a combined laparoscopic and endoanal approach: report of a case. *Dis Colon Rectum* 2000;43:1632.

168. Ruddock JC. Peritoneoscopy. *West J Surg* 1934;42:392.

169. Ruurda JP, Broeders IA. Robot-assisted laparoscopic intestinal anastomosis. *Surg Endosc* 2003;17:236.

170. Sackier JM. A purse string device for laparoscopic surgery [Letter]. *Surg Endosc* 1994;8:1252.

171. Sackier JM. Laparoscopic cholecystectomy. In: Hunter JG, Sackier JM, eds. *Minimally invasive surgery.* New York: McGraw-Hill, 1993:213–229.

172. Sackier JM. Laparoscopic colon and rectal surgery. In: Hunter JG, Sackier JM, eds. *Minimally invasive surgery.* New York: McGraw-Hill, 1993:179–189.

173. Sackier JM. Laparoscopic surgery comes of age [Editorial]. *Int Surg* 1994;79:186.

174. Sackier JM. Laparoscopy for acute appendicitis. *Semin Laparosc Surg* 1996;3:185.

175. Sackier JM. Laparoscopy in the emergency setting. *World J Surg* 1992;16:1083.

176. Sackier JM. Robotics, telepresence and virtual reality. In: Ashton D, ed. *New horizons in high technology medicine.* London: Royal Society of Medicine Press, 1997.

177. Sackier JM. Second look laparoscopy in the management of acute mesenteric ischemia [Letter]. *Br J Surg* 1994;81: 1546.

178. Sackier JM. Training for laparoscopic biliary surgery. In: Cuschieri AE, Berci G, eds. *Laparoscopic biliary surgery,* 2nd ed. London: Blackwell, 1992:1–13.

179. Sackier JM. Training for minimal access surgery. *Curr Pract Surg* 1992;4:227.

180. Sackier JM. Visualisation of the ureter during laparoscopic colon resection. *Br J Surg* 1993;80:1332.

181. Sackier JM, Berci G. Diagnostic and interventional laparoscopy for the general surgeon. *Contemp Surg* 1990; 37:15.

182. Sackier JM, Berci G. Maintaining a clear view in laparoscopic surgery. *Surg Endosc* 1994;8:824.

183. Sackier JM, Berci G, Hiatt JR, et al. Laparoscopic abdominoperineal resection of the rectum. *Br J Surg* 1992; 79:1207.

184. Sackier JM, Berci G, Paz-Partlow M. A new training device for laparoscopic surgery. *Surg Endosc* 1991;5:158.

185. Sackier JM, Berci G, Paz-Partlow M. Elective diagnostic laparoscopy. *Am J Surg* 1991;161:326.

186. Sackier JM. Halverson A, Jacobs LK, et al. A deployable bowel clamp for use in laparoscopic surgery. *Ital J Coloproctol* 1997;16: 59.

187. Sackier JM, Munson JL, Rossi R. Laparoscopic cholecystectomy. In: Braasch J, Sedgewick CE, Ellis FH, et al, eds. *Lahey Clinic atlas of surgery.* New York: Lippincott, 1990: 309–318.

188. Sackier JM, Slutzki S, Wood CB, et al. Laparoscopic endocorporeal mobilization followed by extracorporeal sutureless anastomosis for the treatment of carcinoma of the left colon. *Dis Colon Rectum* 1993;36:610.

189. Sackier JM, Wang, Y. Robotically assisted laparoscopic surgery: from concept to development. *Surg Endosc* 1994;8:63.

190. Saclarides TJ, Ko ST, Airan M, et al. Laparoscopic removal of a large colonic lipoma. Report of a case. *Dis Colon Rectum* 1991;34:1027.

191. Saclarides TJ, Smith L, Ko ST, et al. Transanal endoscopic microsurgery. *Dis Colon Rectum* 1992;35:1183.

192. Sanowski RA, Bellapravalu S. Initial experience with a flexible fiberoptic laparoscope. *Gastrointest Endosc* 1986;32:409.

193. Satava RM. Virtual reality and telepresence for military medicine. *Comput Biol Med* 1995;25:229.

194. Satava RM. Virtual reality surgical simulator: the first steps. *Surg Endosc* 1993;7:203.

195. Scheidbach H, Schneider C, Huegel O, et al. Laparoscopic sigmoid resection for cancer: curative resection and preliminary medium-term results. *Dis Colon Rectum* 2002;45:1641.

196. Schiedeck THK, Schwander O, Baca I, et al. Laparoscopic surgery for the cure of colorectal cancer: results of a German five-center study. *Dis Colon Rectum* 2000;43:1.

197. Schlachta CM, Mamazza J, Seshadri PA, et al. Defining a learning curve for laparoscopic colorectal resections. *Dis Colon Rectum* 2001;44:217.

198. Schlinkert RT, Rasmussen TE. Laparoscopic repair of colonoscopic perforations of the colon. *J Laparosc Surg* 1994;4:51.

199. Schutte B, Reynders MMJ, Wiggers T, et al. Retrospective analysis of the prognostic significance of DNA content and proliferative activity in large bowel carcinoma. *Cancer Res* 1987;47:5494.

200. Scoggin SD, Frazee RC, Snyder SK, et al. Laparoscopic-assisted bowel surgery. *Dis Colon Rectum* 1993;36:747.

201. Scott HJ, Darzi A. Tactile feedback in laparoscopic colonic surgery. *Br J Surg* 1997;84:1005.

202. See WA, Cooper CS, Fisher RJ. Predictors of laparoscopic complications after formal training in laparoscopic surgery. *JAMA* 1993;270:2689.

203. Semm K. Die laparoskopie in der Gynakologie. *Geburtshilfe Frauenheilkd* 1967;27:1029.

204. Semm K. Endoscopic appendicectomy. *Endoscopy* 1983;15:59.

205. Semm K, Freys I. Endoscopic appendectomy: technical operative steps. *Minim Invasive Ther* 1991;1:41.

206. Senagore AJ, Delaney CP, Duepree HJ, et al. Evaluation of POSSUM and P-POSSUM scoring systems in assessing outcome after laparoscopic colectomy. *Br J Surg* 2003;90:1280.

207. Senagore AJ, Duepree HJ, Delaney CP, et al. Cost structure of laparoscopic and open sigmoid colectomy for diverticular disease: similarities and differences. *Dis Colon Rectum* 2002;45:485.

208. Senagore AJ, Luchtefeld MA, Mackeigan JM. What is the learning curve for laparoscopic colectomy? *Am Surg* 1995;61:681.

209. Senagore AJ, Luchtefeld MA, Mackeigan JM, et al. Open colectomy versus laparoscopic colectomy: are there differences? *Am Surg* 1993;59:549.

210. Shepherd JH, Carter PG. Wound recurrence by implantation of a borderline ovarian tumor following laparoscopic removal. *Br J Obstet Gynecol* 1994;101:265.

211. Shinya H, Wolff WI. Morphology, anatomic distribution and cancer potential of colonic polyps: analysis of 7,000 polyps endoscopically removed. *Ann Surg* 1979;190:679.

212. Shoop SA, Sackier JM. Laparoscopic cecopexy for cecal volvulus. *Surg Endosc* 1993;7:450.

213. Sigel B, Golub RM, Loiacano L, et al. Technique of ultrasonic detection and mapping of abdominal wall adhesions. *Surg Endosc* 1991;5:161.

214. Silecchia G, Perrotta N, Giraudo G, et al. Abdominal wall recurrences after colorectal resection for cancer: results of the Italian registry of laparoscopic colorectal surgery. *Dis Colon Rectum* 2002;45:1172.

215. Simons AJ, Anthone GJ, Ortega AE, et al. Laparoscopic-assisted colectomy learning curve. *Dis Colon Rectum* 1995;38:600.

216. Simons R. Vorlaufige Mittheilungen über eine neue Genese der Temperaturerniedrigung. *Med Diss Bonn* 1870.

217. Sistrunk WE. Mikulicz operation for resection of the colon: its advantages and dangers. *Ann Surg* 1928;88:577.

218. Sobeck G. Insufflation devices subject laser patients to contaminants. *Clin Laser Monthly* 1993;10:64.

219. Society of American Gastrointestinal Endoscopic Surgeons. Granting of privileges for laparoscopic general surgery. *Am J Surg* 1991;161:324.

220. Sosa JL, Markley M, Sleeman D, et al. Laparoscopy in abdominal gunshot wounds. *Surg Laparosc Endosc* 1993;3:417.

221. Sosa JL, Sims D, Martin L, et al. Laparoscopic evaluation of tangential abdominal gunshot wounds. *Arch Surg* 1992;127:111.

222. Southern DA, Mapleson WW. Which insufflation gas for laparoscopy. *BMJ* 1993;307:1424.

223. Stage JG, Schulze S, Mller P, et al. Prospective randomized study of laparoscopic versus open colonic resection for adenocarcinoma. *Br J Surg* 1997;84:391.

224. State of New York. *Department of Health memorandum: laparoscopic surgery.* Health facilities series H-18 (series 92–20). Albany, NY: State of New York, 1992.

225. Stolla V, Ross D, Bladow F, et al. Subcutaneous metastases after coelioscopic lymphadenectomy for vesical urothelial carcinoma. *Eur Urol* 1994;36:342.

226. Swain BT, Ellis CN Jr. Laparoscopy-assisted loop ileostomy: an acceptable option for temporary fecal diversion after anorectal surgery. *Dis Colon Rectum* 2002;45:705.

227. Szabo Z, Hunter J, Berci G, et al. Analysis of surgical movements during suturing in laparoscopy. *Surg Endosc* 1994;2:55.

228. Targarona EM, Gracia E, et al. Hand-assisted laparoscopic surgery. *Arch Surg* 2003;138:133.

229. Tate JJT, Kwok S, Dawson JW, et al. Prospective comparison of laparoscopic and conventional anterior resection. *Br J Surg* 1993;80:1396.

230. Thompson CJ. *The history and evolution of surgical instruments.* New York: Schuman, 1942.

231. Tio TL, Coene PPLO, van Delden OM, et al. Colorectal carcinoma: preoperative TNM classification with endosonography. *Radiology* 1991;179:165.

232. Trokel MJ, Bessler M, Treat MR, et al. Preservation of immune response after laparoscopy. *Surg Endosc* 1994;8:1385.

233. Ugarte F. Laparoscopic cholecystectomy port seeding from a colon carcinoma. *Am J Surg* 1995;61:820.

234. Vaage J, Pepin K. Morphological observations during developing concomitant immunity against a C3H/HE mammary tumor. *Cancer Res* 1985;45:659.

235. Valla JS, Limonne B, Valla V, et al. Laparoscopic appendectomy in children: report of 465 cases. *Surg Laparosc Endosc* 1991;1:166.

236. Vanek VW, Rhodes R, Dallis DJ. Results of laparoscopic versus open cholecystectomy in a community hospital. *South Med J* 1995;88:555.

237. Vargas HD, Ramirez RT, Hoffman GC, et al. Defining the role of laparoscopic-assisted sigmoid colectomy for diverticulitis. *Dis Colon Rectum* 2000;43:1726.

238. Veress J. Neues Instrument zu Ausfuhrung von Brust Oder Bauchpunktionen. *Dtsch Med Wochenschr* 1938;41:1480.

239. Vernava AM III, Liebscher G, Longo WE. Laparoscopic restoration of intestinal continuity after Hartmann procedure. *Surg Laparosc Endosc* 1995;5:129.

240. Von Mosetig-Moorhof A. Zur Therapie der Peritonealtuberculose. *Wien Med Presse* 1893;34:1.

241. Voyles CR, Meena AL, Petro AB, et al. Electrocautery is superior to laser for laparoscopic cholecystectomy [Editorial]. *Am J Surg* 1990;160:457.
242. Vukasin P, Ortega AE, Greene FL, et al. Wound recurrence following laparoscopic colon cancer resection: results of the American Society of Colon and Rectal Surgeons Laparoscopic Registry. *Dis Colon Rectum* 1996;39:S20.
243. Wade TP, Comitalo JB, Andrus CH, et al. Laparoscopic cancer surgery: lessons from gallbladder carcinoma. *Surg Endosc* 1995;8:698.
244. Walsh GL, Nesfitt JC. Tumor implants after thoracoscopic resection of a metastatic sarcoma. *Ann Thorac Surg* 1995;59:215.
245. Warshaw AL, Tepper JE, Shipley WU. Laparoscopy in the staging and planning of therapy for pancreatic cancer. *Am J Surg* 1986;151:76.
246. Watanabe M, Hasegawa H, Yamamoto S, et al. Successful application of laparoscopic surgery to the treatment of Crohn's disease with fistulas. *Dis Colon Rectum* 2002;45: 1057.
247. Waye JD, Hunt RH. Colonoscopic diagnosis of inflammatory bowel disease. *Surg Clin North Am* 1982;62:905.
248. Weeks JC, Nelson H, Gelber S, et al. Short-term quality-of-life outcomes following laparoscopic-assisted colectomy vs open colectomy for colon cancer. *JAMA* 2002;287:321.
249. Wegner G. Chirurgische Bemerkungen über die Peritonealhohle, mit besonderer Berucksichtigung der Ovariotomie. *Arch Klin Chir* 1876;20:51.
250. Wexner SD, Cohen SM. Port site metastases after laparoscopic colorectal surgery for cure of malignancy. *Br J Surg* 1995;82:295.
251. Wexner SD, Cohen SM, Johansen OB, et al. Laparoscopic colorectal surgery: a prospective assessment and current perspective. *Br J Surg* 1993;80:1602.
252. Wexner SD, Cohen SM, Ulrich A, et al. Laparoscopic colorectal surgery–are we being honest with our patients? *Dis Colon Rectum* 1995;38:723.
253. Wexner SD, Johansen OB, Nogueras JJ, et al. Total abdominal colectomy: a prospective assessment. *Dis Colon Rectum* 1992;35:651.
254. Wexner SD, Moscovitz ID. Laparoscopic colectomy in diverticular and Crohn's disease. *Surg Clin North Am* 2000;80:1299.
255. Wexner SD, Weiss ES. Laparoscopic colectomy for carcinoma: addressing the concerns and benefits in minimal access surgery. In: Geraghty JG, Sackier JM, Young H, et al, eds. *Minimal access surgery in oncology.* London: Greenwich Medical Media, 1997.
256. Whelan RL, Sellers GJ, Allendorf JD, et al. Trocar site recurrence is unlikely to result from aerosolization of tumor cells. *Dis Colon Rectum* 1996;39:S7.
257. Williams C, Teague R. Colonoscopy. *Gut* 1973;14:990.
258. Windberger U, Siegl H, Woisetschlager R, et al. Hemodynamic changes during prolonged laparoscopic surgery. *Eur Surg Res* 1994;26:1.
259. Wittgen CM, Andrus CH, Fitzerald SD, et al. Analysis of the hemodynamic and ventilatory effects of laparoscopic cholecystectomy. *Arch Surg* 1991;126:997.
260. Wolfe BM, Szabo Z, Moran ME, et al. Training for minimally invasive surgery: need for surgical skills. *Surg Endosc* 1993;7:93.
261. Wu FPK, Sietses C, von Blomberg BME, et al. Systemic and peritoneal inflammatory response after laparoscopic or conventional colon resection in cancer patients: a prospective, randomized trial. *Dis Colon Rectum* 2003;46:147.
262. Wullstein C, Barkhausen S, Gross E. Results of laparoscopic vs. conventional appendectomy in complicated appendicitis. *Dis Colon Rectum* 2001;44:1700.
263. Yamamoto S, Watanabe M, Hasegawa H, et al. Prospective evaluation of laparoscopic surgery for rectosigmoidal and rectal carcinoma. *Dis Colon Rectum* 2002;45:1648.
264. Young-Fadok TM, Nelson H. Laparoscopic right colectomy: five-step procedure. *Dis Colon Rectum* 2000;43:267.
265. Ziprin P, Ridgway PF, Peck DH, et al. The theories and realities of port-site metastases: a critical appraisal. *J Am Coll Surg* 2002;195:395.
266. Zmora O, Weiss EG. Trocar site recurrence in laparoscopic surgery for colorectal cancer: myth or real concern? *Surg Oncol Clin North Am* 2001;10:625.

Vascular Diseases

Hemorrhage, Mesenteric Occlusive and Nonocclusive Disease, Ischemia, Radiation Enteritis, and Volvulus

The only weapon with which the unconscious patient can immediately retaliate on the incompetent surgeon is hemorrhage.

William Stewart Halsted

HEMORRHAGE

Gastrointestinal (GI) bleeding can be due to numerous causes. It is self-evident that conditions such as colorectal cancer, inflammatory bowel disease, hemorrhoids, infectious colitides, ischemia, radiation, Meckel's diverticulum, and virtually every disease that affects the mucosa of the intestinal tract can be associated, at some time, with bleeding.[185,239] Lower GI tract hemorrhage as a consequence of renal transplantation, presumably due to immunosuppression, has also been reported.[294] Uncommon conditions that can produce massive bleeding are coagulopathy, Osler-Weber-Rendu telangiectasia, Dieulafoy's disease, blue rubber nevus syndrome, Behçet's disease, aortoduodenal fistula, rupture of a splenic artery aneurysm, microaneurysm of the superior hemorrhoidal artery, rupture of a pancreatic pseudocyst into the colon, and angiosarcoma.[29,55,75,170,173,189,239,264] A rare cause of *lower* GI hemorrhage is variceal bleeding. This may be due to a congenital vascular abnormality, portal hypertension, obstruction of mesenteric venous circulation, splenic vein thrombosis, or a cardiac anomaly.[155,325] Those with AIDS can present with GI tract hemorrhage from a number of causes: colitis from cytomegalovirus, herpes simplex, or bacteria; lymphoma; idiopathic proctocolitis; and Kaposi's sarcoma.[75] For our purposes, five specific conditions will be discussed in this section: diverticulosis, angiodysplasia, colorectal varices, Dieulafoy's lesion, and Meckel's diverticulum.

Diverticulosis

Classically, massive lower GI bleeding has been generally attributed to diverticular disease, usually without any evidence of diverticulitis.[121,219,334] As discussed in Chapter 26, diverticular disease occurs where tunnels formed by the blood vessels weaken the muscle. Theoretically, the vasa rectum, through its proximity with the diverticulum, can rupture either at the apex or at the neck as the vessel proceeds into the submucosa of the colon (Figure 28-1). Baer demonstrated that 20 of 22 patients had a pathologically proved ruptured vasa rectum within a diverticulum as the source of lower GI hemorrhage (Figure 28-2).[27]

The problem, however, is that most lower GI hemorrhage comes from the right side of the colon, where there are few or no diverticula. Evidence suggests that unexplained vigorous lower intestinal bleeding, even in the presence of known diverticulosis, is most likely due to an arteriovenous malformation (vascular ectasia, angiodysplasia).[10,36,37,291] With the availability of angiography and scintigraphy, and the ability to identify preoperatively the site of bleeding, arteriovenous malformations have not uncommonly been observed in areas where diverticulosis is present.

Angiodysplasia or Vascular Ectasia

The contemporary attitude is that most lower GI bleeding originates from a vascular malformation. Since vascular ectasia is more commonly seen in the right colon and that is the most common site for lower GI hemorrhage, one can inferentially presume that this is the case.[28,48,132,138,207,287,293,299] However, Höchter and colleagues challenged this theory when they reported 59 patients with angiodysplasia to have a more uniform bowel distribution.[148] The sites of the lesions were as follows: cecum, 37%; ascending colon, 17%; transverse colon, 7%; descending colon, 7%; sigmoid, 18%; and rectum, 14%.[148]

Bleeding associated with ectasia is usually less severe than that from diverticular hemorrhage. It tends to be intermittent and is probably due to venous encroachment of the mucosa as compared with the ruptured vasa rectum of a bleeding diverticulum.

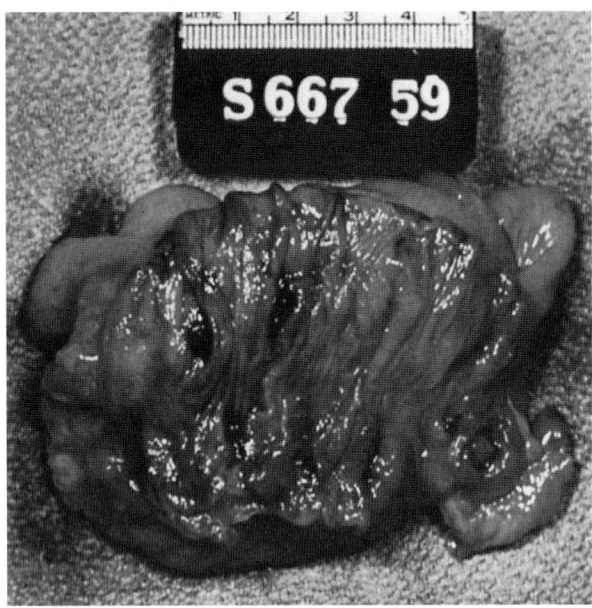

FIGURE 28-1. Portion of sigmoid colon removed for massive lower intestinal hemorrhage that was presumed due to diverticulosis reveals clot in several diverticula.

The etiology of the condition remains somewhat problematic. Boley and associates suggest that the vascular lesions are degenerative, from an acquired and progressive dilatation of previously normal blood vessels, the result of the aging process.[48,51] They propose that muscular contraction or increased intraluminal pressure produces obstruction of the perforating veins.[232] These submucosal structures become dilated and tortuous, with an associated arteriovenous communication (Figure 28-3). Others suggest a congenital etiology, some proposing an association with Meckel's diverticulum,[147] but this only serves to cause confusion. It is perhaps wiser to accept the concept that angiodysplasia is an acquired condition that should be distinguished from the blood vessel tumor, hemangioma (see Chapter 25).

Pathologically, angiodysplastic lesions appear to be ectasias, or dilatations of vascular structures. They represent collections of thin-walled, dilated vessels (either capillaries or veins) usually lying in the submucosa (Figs. 28-4 and 28-5). Rarely, the condition may be

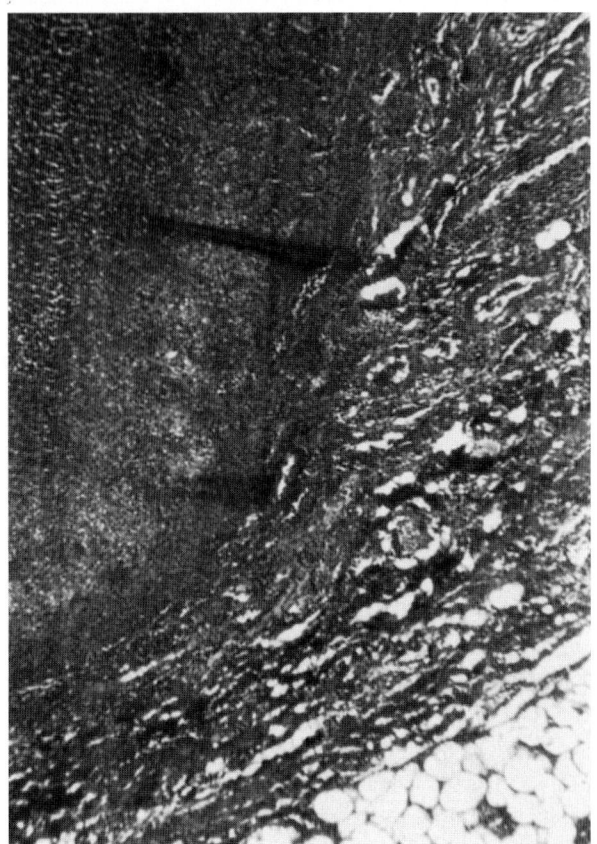

FIGURE 28-2. Diverticulum lined by hemorrhagic granulation tissue in a patient who had massive lower gastrointestinal hemorrhage. (Original magnification × 260.) (Courtesy of Rudolf Garret, M.D.)

associated with vascular malformations elsewhere in the GI tract (e.g., Osler-Weber-Rendu disease) (Figure 28-6).

There does not appear to be any gender predilection for vascular ectasias. However, two-thirds of the patients of Boley and Brandt were more than 70 years old.[48] Richardson and associates reported 39 patients with bleeding due to vascular malformations of the intestine.[250] There seemed to be a bimodal age distribution, with younger patients having no associated disease, whereas older people often had a cardiac lesion

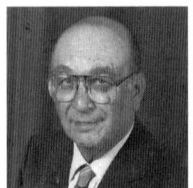

Scott J. Boley (1927–present) Scott Boley was born in Brooklyn, New York, June 1, 1927. He attended Wesleyan University in Connecticut and graduated from Jefferson Medical College in 1949. Following 11 years in private practice he made a commitment to an academic career at the Albert Einstein College of Medicine and the Montefiore Medical Center and is currently Professor of Surgery and Pediatrics. Boley has made numerous contributions to the field of colorectal surgery in particular. For example, he provided the initial description of the entity of noniatrogenic, noncatastrophic colonic ischemia (ischemic colitis) in 1963; he elucidated the cause of small bowel ulcers resulting from enteric-coated potassium diuretic tablets (1965); and he described the endorectal pull-through operation with primary anastomosis for Hirschsprung's disease (1964). He was the first to identify the nature and etiology of vascular ectasia (angiodysplasia) of the colon (1977) and advocated an aggressive approach to the management of acute mesenteric ischemia through the use of early angiography and intra-arterial vasodilators. He also performed the first operation for total aganglionosis of the colon. Boley has published more than 250 articles and book chapters and has edited several books and monographs. He continues in active practice as of this writing.

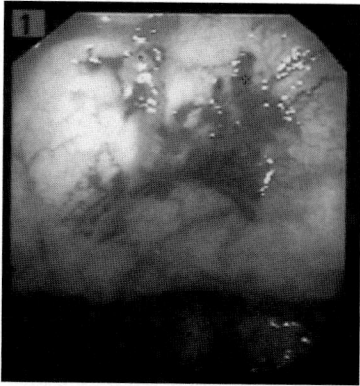

FIGURE 28-3. An angiodysplastic lesion, seen on colonoscopy, is characteristically a focal, submucosal, vasular ectasia. (See Color Fig. 28-3.)

(especially aortic stenosis [see later] and severe atherosclerotic disease). The most common site of bleeding was the cecum, with resection controlling the hemorrhage in the vast majority of patients. However, bleeding can occur from angioplastic lesions in more than one area of the colon.[287] Foutch and colleagues reviewed their experience with 964 patients diagnosed with angiodysplasia.[110] They concluded with the following:

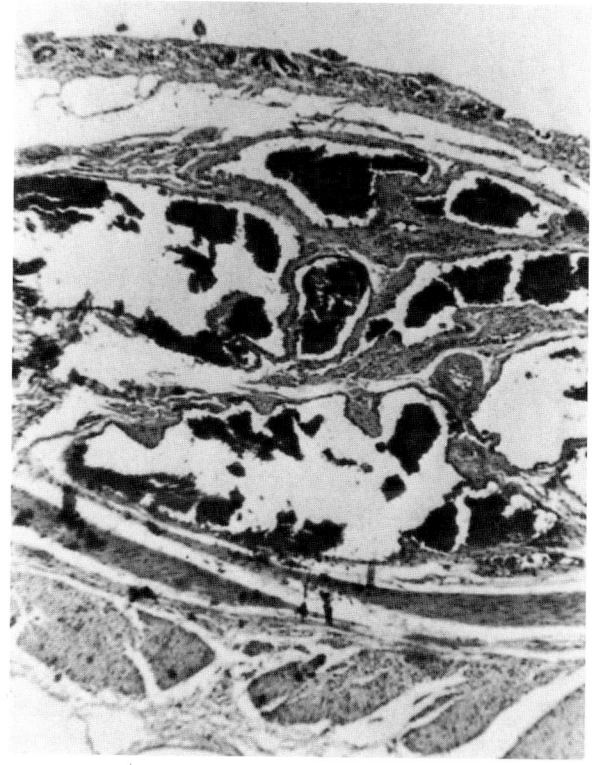

FIGURE 28-4. Angiodysplasia of the cecum. Note the irregular veins and arteries. (Original magnification × 120.) (Courtesy of Rudolf Garret, M.D.)

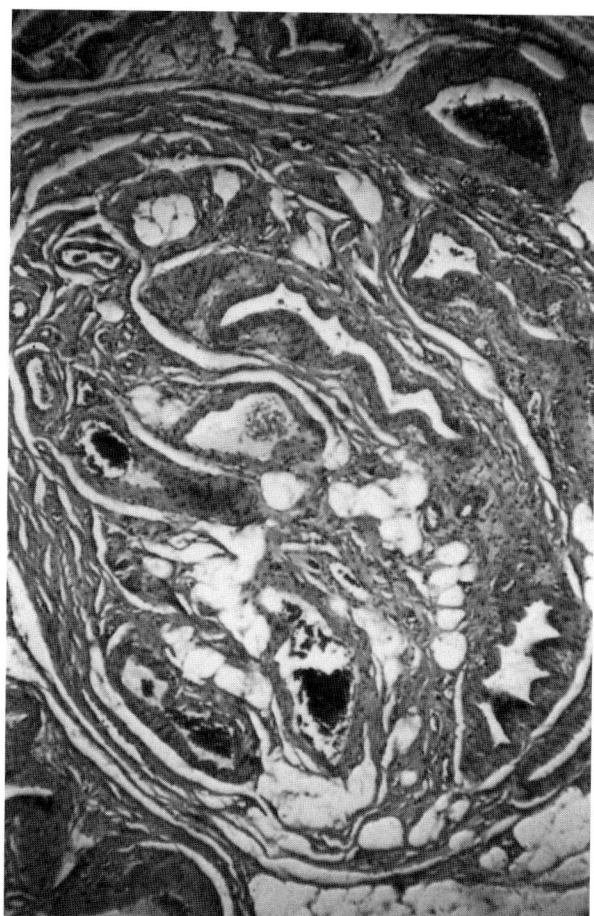

FIGURE 28-5. Vascular malformation showing thick-walled veins and arteries in an irregular distribution. (Original magnification × 250.) (Courtesy of Rudolf Garret, M.D.)

Colonic angiodysplasia is uncommon among healthy asymptomatic individuals (0.83%).

Lesions are usually small (<10 mm) and are located proximal to the hepatic flexure.

The natural history is benign, with the risk of bleeding over a 3-year period nonexistent.

Most opine that endoscopic treatment for nonbleeding lesions is unnecessary.

Relationship to Calcific Aortic Stenosis

Love identified the syndrome of calcific aortic stenosis and GI hemorrhage, suggesting treatment of the bleeding by aortic valve replacement.[182] Shbeeb and colleagues reviewed Love's experience and confirmed the association of calcific aortic stenosis and obscure GI bleeding in the elderly.[278] These authors and others believe that this operation not only corrects the cardiac hemodynamic instability but also stops the GI hemorrhage.[72,130]

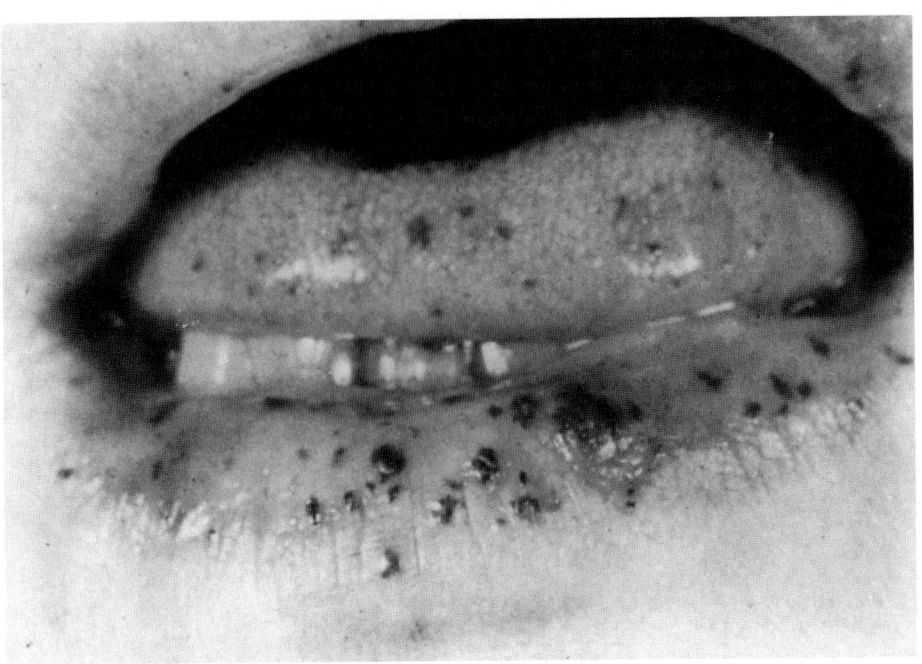

FIGURE 28-6. Telangiectasis of the lips in a patient with hereditary malformations and gastrointestinal hemorrhage. (Courtesy of Rudolf Garret, M.D.)

A mechanism for the association and the ameliorative response to cardiac surgery is not clear. It may be a consumption phenomenon or a qualitative alteration of platelet function produced by the roughened stenotic valve in the area of greatest pressure and velocity of the bloodstream.[182] This subtle coagulation defect combined with a thin-walled vascular lesion may tend to promote the hemorrhage. Another contributing factor may be the abnormal arterial inflow pulse wave.[130] A coagulation panel, including platelet function, should be part of the preoperative assessment of any patient suspected of bleeding from angiodysplasia.[287] One should be aware of this relationship so that earlier diagnosis may spare these patients from multiple hospitalizations and transfusions.

Dieulafoy's Lesion

Dieulafoy's lesion, also known as Dieulafoy's malformation, was originally described by Paul Georges Dieulafoy in 1898 as a gastric, submucosal aneurysm.[96] Significant, and often recurrent, hemorrhage occurs from a pinpoint nonulcerated arterial lesion, usually high in the gastric

fundus. However, the condition has also been described as an unusual cause of small bowel hemorrhage and even rarely the source of bleeding in the colon, rectum, and anal canal.[202]

The lesion has characteristically been described as a solitary, protuberant, serpiginous, and abnormally wide artery located in the submucosa that has the appearance of a submucosal tumor in an otherwise normal mucosa.[202] Endoscopic criteria for diagnosis include a less than a 3-mm mucosal defect in combination with any of the following:[25]

- A protruding 1- to 2-mm blood vessel
- Active arterial bleeding
- Fresh adherent clot with a narrow point of attachment
- Inactive lesion with associated intraluminal blood suggestive of recent hemorrhage

Microscopically, there is usually noted to be a thick-walled vessel without an associated inflammatory reaction.

Treatment may involve intraarterial vasopressin (see later, Evaluation of Hemorrhage), sclerotherapy, oversewing (if within reach of rectal instrumentation), or resection.

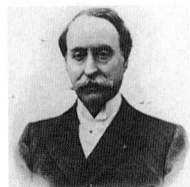

Paul Georges Dieulafoy (1839–1911)   Paul Dieulafoy was born in Toulouse, France, November 18, 1839. He studied in Paris and received his doctorate there in 1869. He ultimately became Professor of Medicine and Chief of Medical Services at the Hôtel-Dieu in Paris. Dieulafoy has been recognized as an innovative investigator and a keen observer who did seminal work on typhoid, Bright's disease, and appendicitis. Among his eponymously associated contributions were his *apparatus*—a suction pump to evacuate fluid from the chest cavity; his *erosion*—an erosion or ulcer-complicating pneumonia and causing upper gastrointestinal hemorrhage; his *pancreatic crisis*—symptoms of acute abdomen at the onset of hemorrhagic pancreatitis; his *triad*—a hypersensitivity of the skin, tenderness, and muscular contraction at McBurney's point in acute appendicitis; and, of course, his *lesion* or vascular malformation of the stomach. He wrote a manual on pathology and was elected President of the French Académie de Médecin in 1910. Dieulafoy died August 16, 1911, in Paris.

Meckel's Diverticulum

Meckel's diverticulum is generally acknowledged to be the most prevalent congenital anomaly of the GI tract.[190] Johann Meckel was not the first to recognize this entity, however. Fabricus Hildanus had reported this in 1598 as an unusual diverticulum of the small intestine, but it was Meckel who in 1809 published a meticulous description of its anatomy and embryonic origin.[200] The condition is present in 1% to 2% of autopsies. It represents a diverticulum of the ileum derived from the unobliterated yolk stalk; that is, the remnant of the vitelline duct. Generally, it is found more commonly in males in the ratio of 2:1. In almost 90% of cases the diverticulum arises on the antimesenteric border. When the remnant persists, it may result in a variety of intra-abdominal complications.

The rule of 2s is the classical description. It is located about 2 feet from the end of the small intestine, is often about 2 inches in length, occurs in about 2% of the population, is twice as common in males, and can contain two types of ectopic tissue—stomach or pancreas.

In the adult, the diverticulum is usually 1.5 to 2 inches long and occurs approximately 2 feet from the ileocecal valve (Figure 28-7). However, the distance is quite variable. The diverticulum contains all layers of the bowel wall, but in some cases it may harbor heterotopic gastric, pancreatic, biliary, or even colonic tissues (Figure 28-8).[60] The two most frequently observed complications are intestinal obstruction and hemorrhage (Figure 28-9). So-called Meckel's diverticulitis is a third presentation. Intussusception in young children may lead to intestinal obstruction and/or rectal bleeding. Serious hemorrhage from the rectum from a Meckel's diverticulum is usually due to peptic ulceration. This occurs most frequently in children between the ages of 10 and 15, but it is not unusual to observe this presentation in adults. The blood is usually dark red as opposed to the tarry stool of an upper GI source for the hemorrhage or bright red rectal bleeding from a more distal location.

Vane and colleagues reported 217 children with vitelline duct anomalies.[316] Forty-eight presented with rectal bleeding, and at the time of surgery all were found to have ectopic gastric mucosa. Yamaguchi and co-workers identified ectopic gastric mucosa in only 9.1% of their 596 cases.[341] In the experience of Mackey and Dineen, 25% of the individuals who were symptomatic presented with lower GI bleeding.[190] Those who were younger than 40 years were most likely to have symptoms develop.

Diagnostic Studies

Kusumoto and colleagues compared the various modalities of evaluation of bleeding from Meckel's diverticulum in 138 individuals.[167] All underwent any one or more of three examinations: 99mTc-scintigraphy, angiography, and barium enema study. Thirty-eight percent of patients had positive angiography. Forty-seven percent were diagnosed as having a Meckel's diverticulum on barium study, but scintigraphy had a diagnostic accuracy rate of 83%. The authors concluded that Tc99m-pertechnetate scintigraphy is the preferred test for evaluating bleeding when Meckel's diverticulum is suspected.[167] Schwartz and Lewis opined, however, that there is a relatively high false-positive and false-negative rate with scintigraphic imaging.[273] Based on their findings, it was suggested that the scanning be supplemented with small bowel infusion or arteriography or both to improve preoperative evaluation in adult patients when this diagnosis is entertained.

Treatment

Excision of the Meckel's diverticulum can usually be accomplished by simple diverticulectomy, although a small bowel resection may be necessary, particularly if the base of the diverticulum is quite broad. Closure can be effected by conventional suturing or by any number of techniques utilizing the stapling devices. A laparoscopically assisted approach to Meckel's diverticulectomy has also been described.[24] Essentially, this consists of the ap-

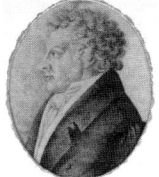

Johann Friedrich Meckel (1781–1833) Johann Meckel was born October 17, 1781, in Halle, Prussia. He is known as the Younger, having been born into a family of prominent physicians. His father, Philipp Friedrich Theodore Meckel, was Professor of Anatomy and Surgical Obstetrics at the University of Halle, and his grandfather, Johann Friedrich Meckel (the Elder), had occupied the same prestigious chair. Meckel's younger brother, August Albrecht Meckel, also inherited the family's academic attributes and became Professor of Anatomy and Forensic Medicine at the University of Bonn in 1821. The younger Meckel, however, as a child had an outspoken aversion to medicine in general and anatomy in particular, perhaps as a consequence of his having to help his father perform dissections. Despite this he ultimately became one of the greatest anatomists of his time. He began his medical studies at Halle and in 1801 moved to the University of Göttingen to expand his interest in comparative anatomy. He received his medical degree the following year in Halle. After several years of travel and study throughout Europe he ultimately collaborated with the brilliant French anatomist, Cuvier, and translated Cuvier's five-volume work into German, a task that he completed in 1810. Returning to his native Halle in 1806, he found that Napoleon himself had been using his home as temporary headquarters, an intrusion that may have aided in preserving the valuable anatomic collection of the Meckel family. In 1808, he was appointed Professor of Normal and Pathological Anatomy, Surgery and Obstetrics at Halle. Meckel attracted large numbers to his lectures at Halle, which was then the center of comparative anatomy in Germany. Among his lasting contributions was the study of the abnormalities occurring during embryologic development. Meckel's *Teratology* was the first comprehensive description of birth defects. Johann Meckel died October 31, 1833, in Halle. (Photograph courtesy of the Anatomical Institute of the University of Halle.)

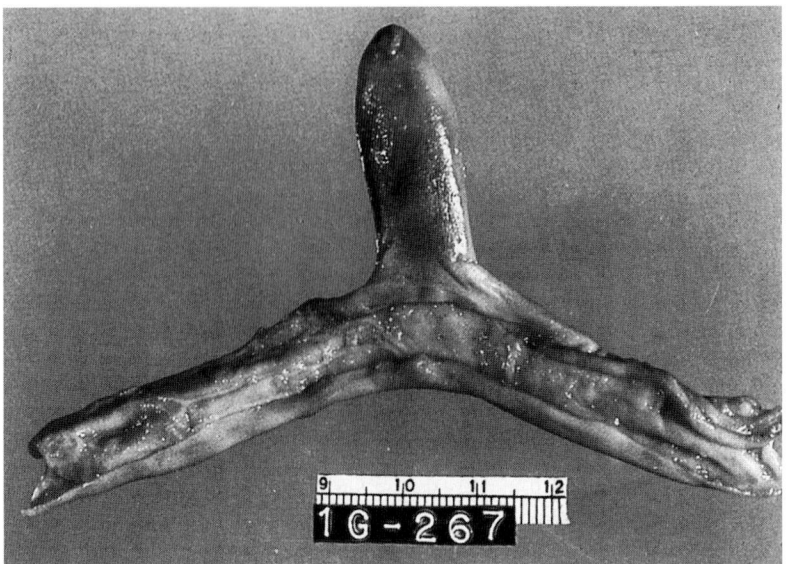

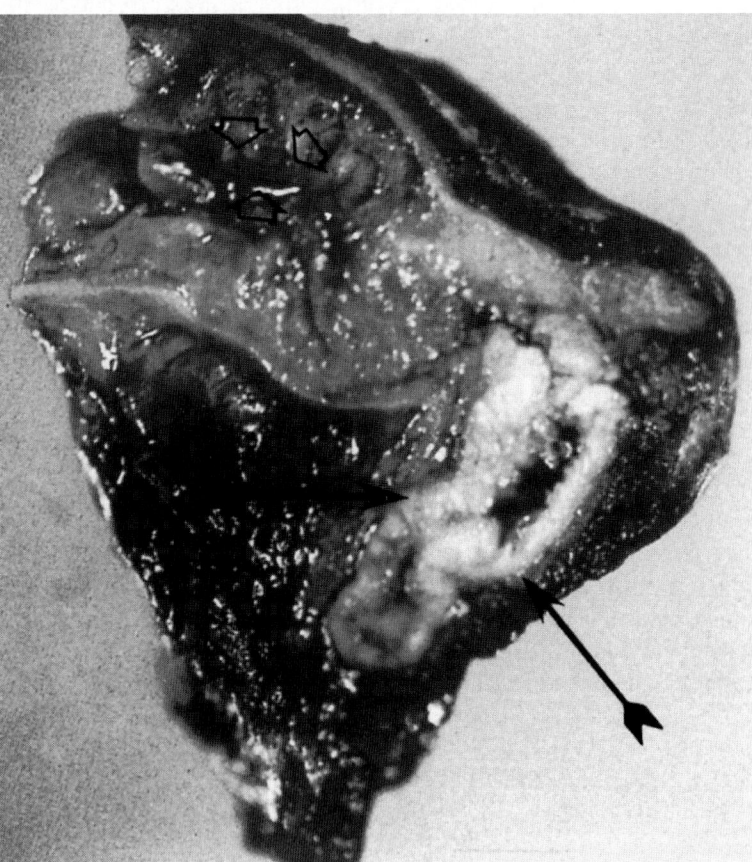

FIGURE 28-7. Meckel's diverticulum. **(A)** Typical long, sausagelike resected specimen. **(B)** Macroscopic appearance of the opened diverticulum revealing a thick, heterotopic mucosa (*closed arrows*) with an ulcer (*open arrows*) in the otherwise normal bowel. (Reproduced with permission from Lewin KJ, Riddell RH, Weinstein WM. *Gastrointestinal pathology and its clinical implications.* New York: Igaku-Shoin, 1992.)

plication of a stapling instrument across the base of the exteriorized diverticulum.

Incidental Removal

What of the natural history of Meckel's diverticulum? Should it be removed incidentally when identified?

Soltero and Bill studied 202 cases over a 15-year period to attempt an answer to this question.[290] Using the popu-

lation averages and the number of cases in each age group (assuming a 2% incidence of Meckel's diverticulum in the general population), they calculated the rates per year of a complication developing from a Meckel's diverticulum utilizing life-table techniques. They concluded that a Meckel's diverticulum has a 4.2% likelihood of causing symptoms during a lifetime, decreasing to zero with old age. They also concluded that it would be necessary to remove approximately 800 asymptomatic Meckel's divertic-

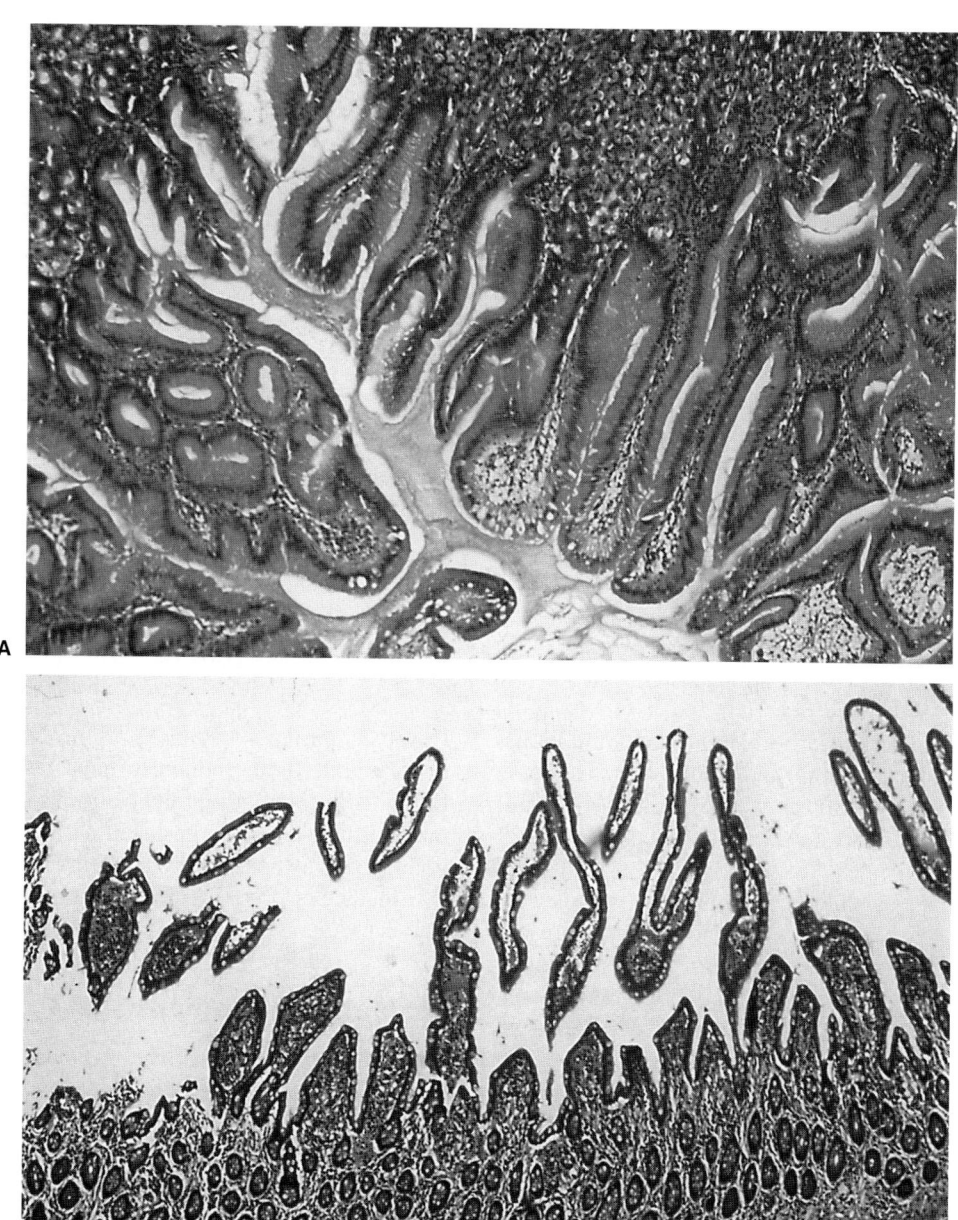

FIGURE 28-8. Meckel's diverticulum demonstrating the appearance of typical small bowel mucosa **(A)** and gastric heterotopia **(B)**. In the latter situation the mucosa has the appearance of gastric fundus with gastric glands. Occasional goblet cells are present. (Courtesy of Matthew Curran, M.D.)

ula in order to save one patient's life from the complications of their presence. The obvious recommendation was that the removal of an asymptomatic Meckel's diverticulum is rarely, if ever, justified.

Colorectal Varices

Since originally described in 1954, fewer than 100 cases of colonic varices have reported in the literature.[323] This rare cause of lower intestinal hemorrhage is almost always as-

sociated with cirrhosis, with resultant portal hypertension, or portal venous obstruction.[153] The condition has been reported in approximately 2.5% of those undergoing sclerotherapy for esophageal varices.[111] As few as 3.6% and as many 56% of cirrhotic patients have been demonstrated to have concomitant rectal varices. Parenthetically, it must be remembered that hemorrhoids are not rectal varices, and this misnomer should never be applied to that condition.

Another presentation of variceal bleeding that is of interest to the colon and rectal surgeon is also a conse-

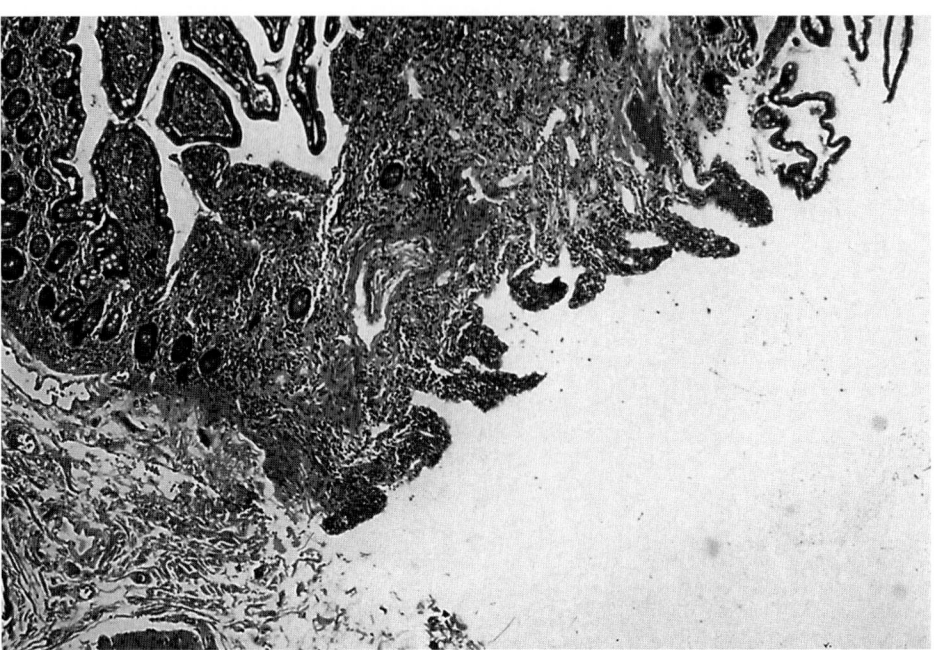

FIGURE 28-9. Meckel's diverticulum. Loss of surface mucosa in an ulcerating, bleeding lesion. (Courtesy of Matthew Curran, M.D.)

quence of portal hypertension—that of stomal and parastomal varices, especially in an individual with sclerosing cholangitis and biliary cirrhosis as an extraintestinal manifestation of inflammatory bowel disease (see Chapters 29 and 31).[139]

A still rarer cause of colonic varices is the so-called familial or idiopathic variety.[153] The condition may present at any age, including the first decade of life. To conclude that the condition truly represents idiopathic colonic varices, liver disease and portal venous obstruction must be excluded.

Contrast-enhanced three-dimensional magnetic resonance angiography has been recommended as uniquely helpful for visualizing ectopic varies, that is, colorectal and stomal varices.[139]

Management

Generally, if the bleeding is in the group of patients whose colonic varices are secondary to liver disease, treatment parallels that of the management of bleeding esophageal varices from portal hypertension.[279] Conversely, in those individuals whose colonic varices are attributed to a congenital etiology, favorable prognosis has been associated with colonic resection.[323] Transanal application of the circular stapling instrument for the treatment of bleeding rectal varices has also been described.[47]

Symptoms of Hemorrhage

The importance of obtaining an accurate history cannot be overemphasized. For example, knowledge of prior abdominal aorta surgery may be critical (Figure 28-10).

However, patients usually present with no antecedent history, and they frequently have no abdominal pain. Blood from the rectum may be bright red or maroon and may contain clots. If the bleeding is severe enough, hypotension may ensue, with the requirement for resuscitative measures. Usually, however, the individual's condition is relatively stable, permitting time for evaluation.

Evaluation of Hemorrhage

Physical examination of the bleeding patient is usually unrewarding. Additionally, even before one can begin investigations, the opportunity for identifying the source of bleeding may be lost, since spontaneous cessation is not uncommon. The therapeutic effect of the administration of an enema before endoscopic examination or of a barium enema study is well recognized,[3] but this may be simply coincidental. McGuire undertook a study to ascertain the course of bleeding in 78 individuals who were admitted a total of 106 times for this complaint with no specific cause other than colonic diverticula.[199] Bleeding stopped spontaneously in 75% of episodes and in 99% of patients requiring fewer than 4 units/day of transfusion.

A detailed history, clinical examination, and hematologic assessment are mandatory. One must also be wary and cognizant of an individual's consumption of herbal agents, since many of these products have anticoagulant properties. One should, obviously, perform a digital rectal examination and a limited rigid sigmoidoscopy initially. If the source is found, appropriate therapy can be implemented. One must remember that bleeding suggestive of a lower GI source may actually be originating from the upper GI tract. The simple expediency of the

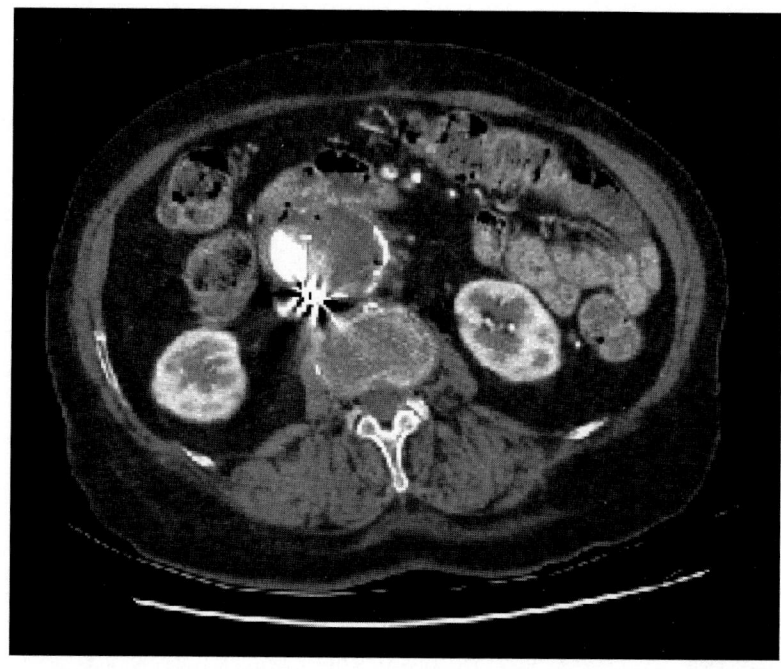

FIGURE 28-10. Aortoduodenal fistula. CT reveals bubbles of air within a mural thrombus. Patient underwent prior reconstruction for an abdominal aortic aneurysm. Note the overlying duodenum. (Courtesy of Allison Burkett, M.D.)

placement of a nasogastric tube can eliminate the stomach as a potential source, especially if clear bile is returned. If the aspirate is positive, one should then proceed with upper GI endoscopy. Employing the barium enema examination is not advisable at this time. A contrast study will preclude the possibility of performing an adequate angiographic examination for perhaps several days. Although barium enema may succeed in identifying a lesion, the presence of a diverticulum does not indicate that it is the source of the bleeding. For example, one would be hard pressed indeed to identify which diverticulum was the site of the hemorrhage in Figure 28-11, if bleeding were coming from one of them in the first place. An organized approach to the evaluation of the patient with hemorrhage of presumed colonic origin is suggested. An algorithm is presented in Figure 28-12 that provides an overview for carrying out the proper sequence of investigations in the bleeding patient.

Colonoscopy

Although the value of colonoscopy is undeniable in the investigation of a patient with undiagnosed rectal bleeding,[166,297] its use during an episode of massive colonic hemorrhage is limited. The instrument can, in fact, induce hemorrhage that may have ceased previously. The procedure is technically complex and should be performed only by the most experienced endoscopist. Instruments with large-bore suction channels, additional aspirating–irrigating equipment, and fluoroscopic control are strongly recommended.[321]

Examination within 24 to 36 hours of cessation of active bleeding enables the endoscopist to undertake the examination without a complete bowel preparation.[321] Forde reported the results of colonoscopy performed on 25 patients during or soon after an episode of active rectal bleeding, when the barium enema or mesenteric angiogram was not feasible or when the results were negative.[108] He advises frequent changing of the patient's position. By this technique, the instrument can be passed while the liquid blood is in a rather dependent portion of the bowel. Forde found five patients to be bleeding from diverticular disease, three from unsuspected carcinomas, and two each from polyps, ischemic colitis, and arteriovenous malformations. Results of five examinations were negative. There was one perforation that was recognized immediately. Although the author's results were impressive, he cautions that the technique is not particularly valuable when bleeding is active, but it is most usefully applied soon after the onset or the cessation of hemorrhage. He also emphasizes the requirement for more experience and skill than is usually necessary for routine colonoscopy.

The American Society for Gastrointestinal Endoscopy published a series of statements discussing the use of endoscopy in clinical situations, utilizing these guidelines to aid the physician in the appropriate use of this modality in various clinical situations.* It was concluded that emergency colonoscopy has the advantages of disclosing a bleeding lesion in 50% to 70% of patients examined and that definitive treatment of an identified lesion by snare cautery, fulguration, or laser photocoagulation may be

---

*American Society for Gastrointestinal Endoscopy, 13 Elm St., Manchester, MA 01944.

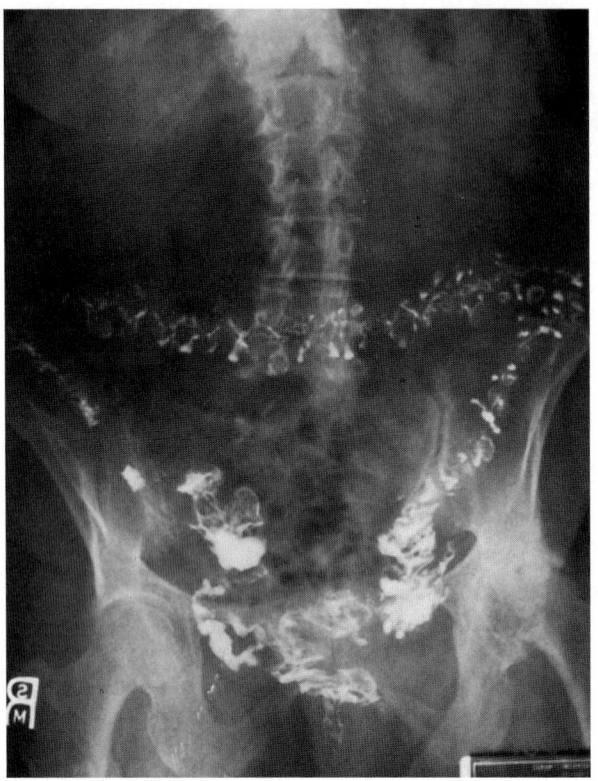

FIGURE 28-11. Postevacuation barium enema in a patient with massive intestinal hemorrhage shows extensive diverticulosis. Identification of the specific source of bleeding is impossible.

possible. Furthermore, massively bleeding lesions that have stopped may be more readily identifiable by colonoscopy than by other means, such as angiography. Disadvantages of colonoscopy under these circumstances include the following:

The need for available and skilled endoscopists
An increased risk of perforation
Delay to adequately prepare the bowel (1 to 3 hours)
The possibility of unsuccessful diagnosis or treatment because of technical problems

Jensen and Machicado evaluated the safety and efficacy of 80 consecutive urgent colonoscopic examinations in individuals with severe, ongoing hematochezia of unknown cause.[160] In the intensive care unit, each patient received a saline or sulfate purge administered orally or via a nasogastric tube. Four to 14 liters were instilled to clear the bowel over a period of 2 to 7 hours. The authors were able to identify lesions in all but 9%. Others confirm the safety and efficacy of this approach.[256]

With less vigorous bleeding, Max and associates identified an angiodysplastic lesion in 14 of 26 patients, confirming arteriographic findings in many.[196] Of interest is the fact that this was the only modality able to establish the diagnosis in three patients. Tedesco and colleagues, using colonoscopy, noted that in 11% of 46 patients with recurrent episodes of melena, vascular malformations were the cause.[304] Skibba and associates employed colonoscopy to

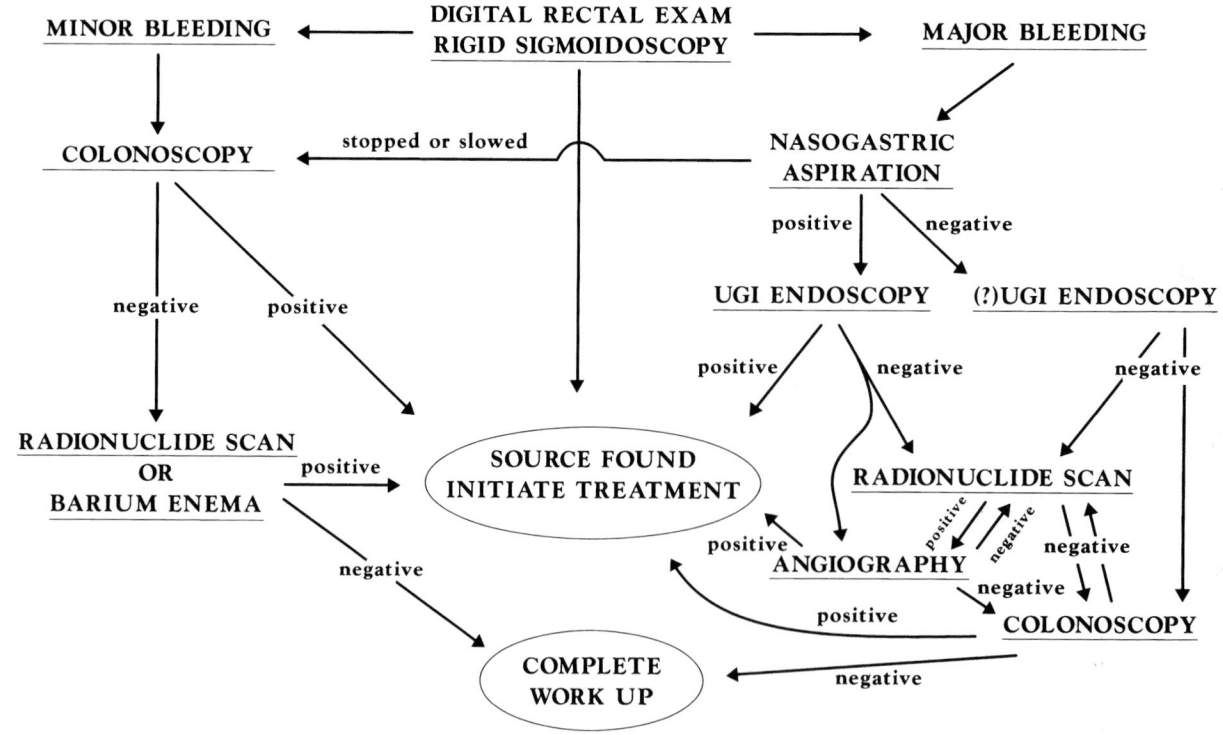

FIGURE 28-12. Recommended algorithm for the management of gastrointestinal bleeding.

establish the diagnosis of angiodysplasia of the cecum in an individual with GI bleeding of unknown origin.[285] Others have successfully used colonoscopy in the evaluation of nonactive bleeding from angiodysplasia and from hereditary hemorrhagic telangiectasis, an autosomal dominant disease.[135,289,303,306]

Irvine and colleagues prospectively evaluated 71 patients with overt rectal bleeding by means of flexible sigmoidoscopy, double-contrast barium enema, and colonoscopy.[154] Because of a higher predictive value, the authors believe that colonoscopy should be the first-line investigation in those individuals likely to require either biopsy or therapeutic intervention. Rex and co-workers found that initial flexible sigmoidoscopy plus air contrast barium enema was a more cost-effective study for the evaluation of nonemergency lower GI bleeding in younger people, but in those older than 55 years of age, initial colonoscopy was preferred.[248]

Therapeutic Colonoscopy

Specifically for the treatment of angiodysplastic lesions, sclerotherapy, electrocoagulation, and, more recently, endoscopic GI laser therapy have been successfully employed (see Chapter 4).[48,64,135,148,150,235,270,311] The recommended technique is to treat the periphery initially and the center last, in order to reduce the vascular supply to the lesion and to diminish the potential for later bleeding.[48]

Trudel and colleagues reported 71 patients with lower GI bleeding secondary to arteriovenous malformations, of whom 80% were diagnosed by colonoscopy.[311] The mean number of prior hemorrhages was 6.1. Of the 28 individuals treated by endoscopic coagulation, bleeding ceased in approximately two-thirds. A surgical procedure controlled the recurrent bleeding in six of seven cases where electrocoagulation had failed.

Computed-Tomographic (CT) Colonography

CT colonography is an alternative imaging modality that could, in theory, be effectively used before colonoscopy in selected patients.[302] Still, this technique is applicable primarily for those patients who have stopped bleeding and in whom the source of bleeding cannot be readily detected by other means. As with the earlier discussion on virtual colonoscopy (see Chapter 4), its primary advantage is for evaluating the colon in someone who has not been able to undergo a complete colonoscopy. A full-bowel preparation is required.

Angiography

If the source of bleeding has been identified by means of rectal examination, sigmoidoscopy, upper GI endoscopy, or colonoscopy (if attempted at all), therapy can be instituted. Unfortunately, in patients who bleed massively from the colon, these studies are usually not helpful except to eliminate another cause. The next investigative procedure that should be performed is either selective angiography or radionuclide scan. Unless angiography is not available at the hospital, the patient should not be taken to the operating room without this radiologic investigation. Unfortunately, there are no useful factors that will predict which patients are actively bleeding and who will benefit most from angiography, except perhaps an immediate blush on ^{99m}Tc-labeled red blood cell scintigraphy (see later).[216,233] Direct selective catheterization of the celiac, superior mesenteric, and inferior mesenteric arteries is accomplished by way of the groin using a modified Seldinger technique.[276] In suspected lower GI bleeding, the superior mesenteric artery is injected first, because of the higher incidence of colonic bleeding from the right side.[125] If the site of the bleeding is not found, the inferior mesenteric artery is studied. Finally, if no source is identified, a celiac injection should be made. As mentioned, on rare occasions upper GI bleeding may seem to be of colonic origin. Radiographic abnormalities include extravasation (Figs. 28-13 and 28-14), arteriovenous malformation (Figure 28-15), a delayed emptying vein, and an early-filling vein (Figure 28-16).

The standard sensitivity that most publications suggest to identify blood loss by means of angiography is 0.5 mL/min. This is probably an unrealistically low estimate, because it is based on the results of studies performed on the animal model. Bowel gas, the presence of fluid within the lumen, body habitus, and other variables may make it impossible for one to identify extravasation unless the rate of bleeding is as much as 5 mL/min (300 mL/hr).

The cecal branch of the ileocolic artery usually is the most likely site for a vascular malformation. The characteristic angiographic signs of angiodysplasia were described by Boley and colleagues and include a dense, slowly emptying vein (92%), a vascular tuft (68%), and an early-filling vein (56%).[52] Extravasation of the contrast material is the least frequently observed finding (8%). Many reports testify to the success of identifying a bleeding site by angiography. For example, Allison and colleagues ascertained the source in 87% of patients done as an emergency, and 74%, electively.[12]

Injection of the major blood vessel in the resected specimen with silicon rubber compound and clearing with methyl salicylate may reveal a vascular tuft or dilated blood vessels (Figure 28-17). The potential value of the technique is to permit the pathologist to identify the lesion macroscopically.[8]

Therapeutic Angiography

If the bleeding point is identified, it may be possible to control the hemorrhage by means of either an embolization technique (Figs. 28-18 and 28-19) or the infusion of Pitressin (vasopressin). Vasopressin causes contraction

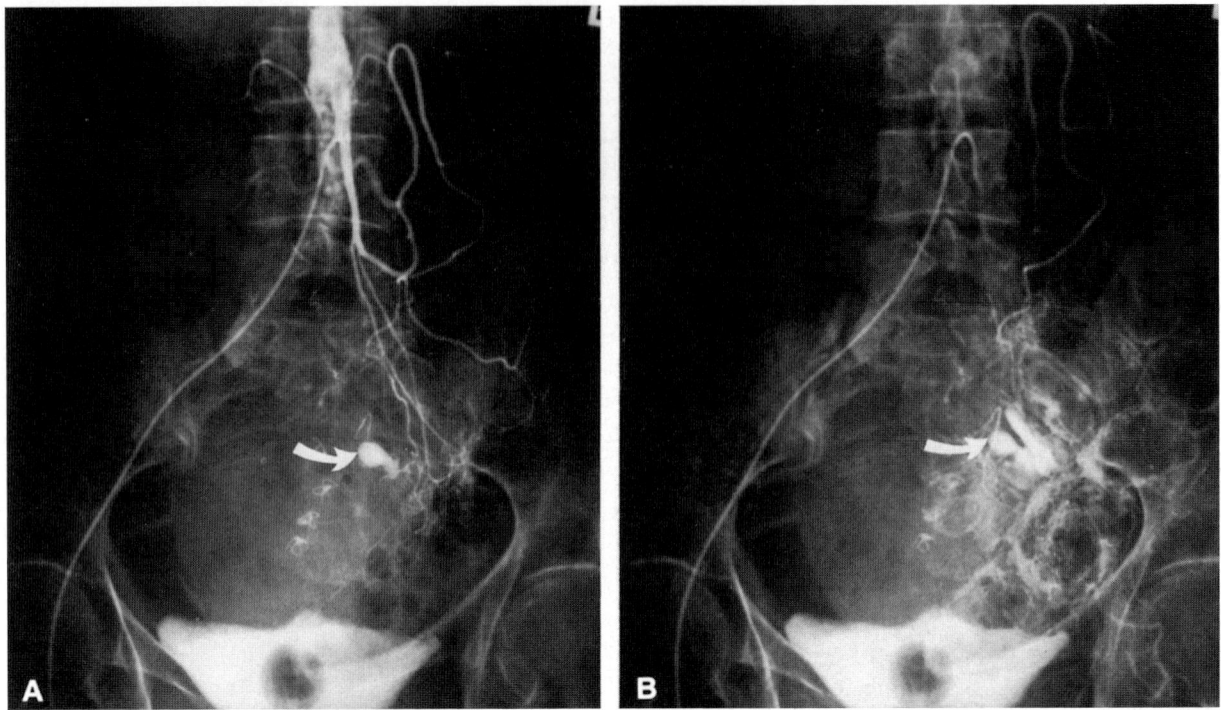

FIGURE 28-13. Bleeding from diverticulum. Early **(A)** and late **(B)** arterial phases of an inferior mesenteric arteriogram demonstrate an active bleeding site in the distal transverse colon (*arrow*).

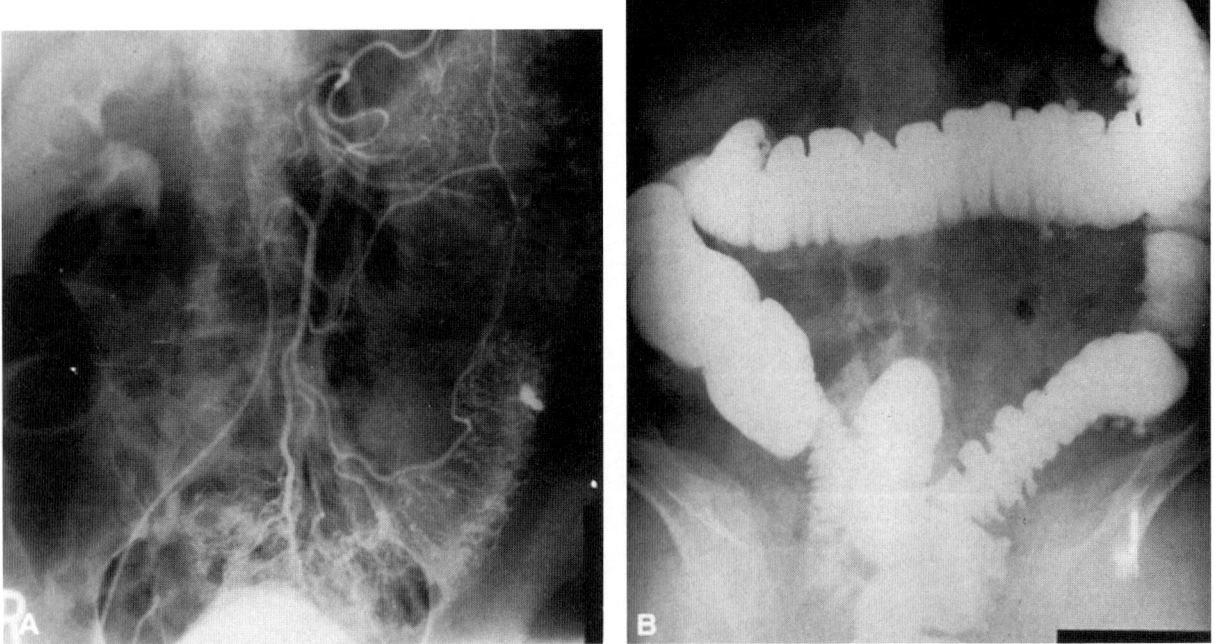

FIGURE 28-14. Bleeding from diverticulum. **(A)** Angiogram demonstrates extravasation in upper sigmoid. **(B)** Site of bleeding corresponds to larger diverticulum on barium enema.

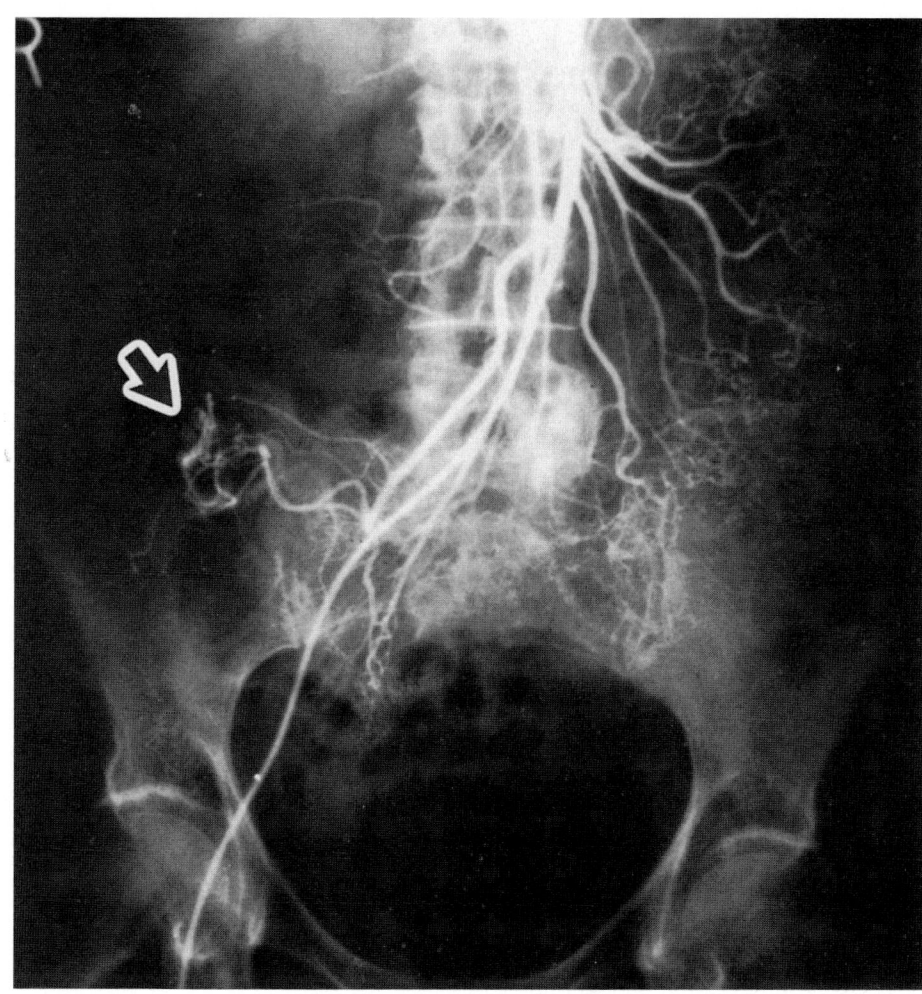

FIGURE 28-15. Arteriovenous malformation "vascular tuft" (*arrow*) demonstrated by SMA injection. (Courtesy of Brian R. Schnier, M.D.)

of smooth muscle, especially the capillaries, small arterioles, and venules, with less effect on the smooth musculature of the larger veins. Many papers have been published that deal with the efficacy of vasopressin in the treatment of GI hemorrhage.[38,55,99,245,312] But the use of vasopressin has several disadvantages. The drug itself has a number of side effects, including decreased cardiac output, hypertension, and arrhythmias.[125] Since many of these patients are elderly or perhaps have an unstable cardiovascular condition, it is important to carefully monitor the intake and output. Vasopressin has a profound antidiuretic effect. Additionally, there are potential concerns related to prolonged catheter use: embolism, hemorrhage around the puncture site, hematoma, and limitation of activity. An arterial pump is needed to administer the drug, and the position of the catheter has to be checked daily by means of a portable x-ray unit.

Embolization has been reported to be an acceptable alternative to infusing a vasoconstrictive substance.[88,90.126,184,195,204,254,255,288] In the experience of DeBarros and coworkers (Hartford, Connecticut), all 27 patients who had

an angiographically visualized source for colonic hemorrhage underwent successful embolization.[88] Six patients rebled (22%), five of whom required surgery. Two demonstrated ischemia (7.4%), one of whom required operation.

Diagnostic angiography can be followed by selective embolization with Gelfoam strips, by autologous clotted blood, or by a Gianturco coil using the same catheter. Since Gelfoam particles have a low coefficient of friction and can, therefore, readily pass through comparatively small catheters, injection can take place satisfactorily even through relatively small bleeding arterial branches.[195]

Transcatheter embolization will inevitably lead in some patients to postembolic colonic ischemia and possibly even to infarction.[255] Theoretically, the same segment of bowel would require removal, a procedure that might be performed under less urgent circumstances than hemorrhage. The incidence of ischemic complications may be reduced by using the least number of emboli required to control the hemorrhage.[255] Not every patient is suitable,

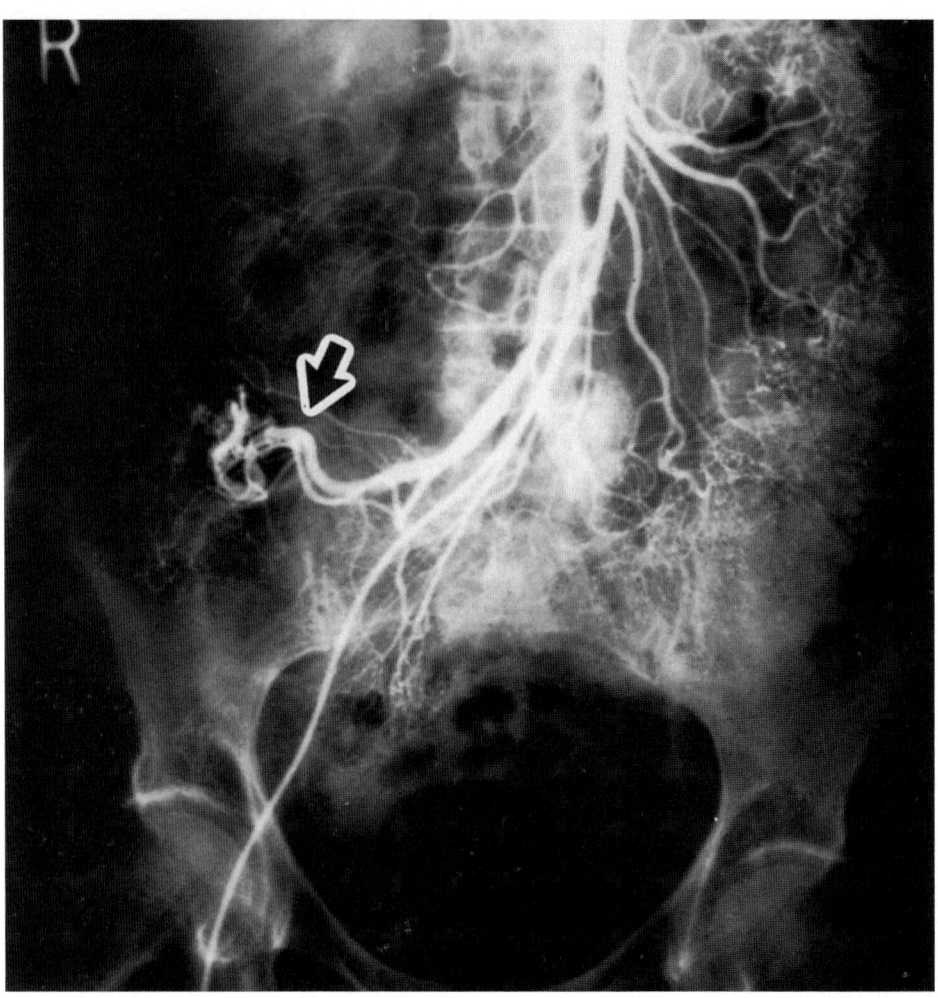

FIGURE 28-16. Early filling vein (*arrow*) draining from the arteriovenous malformation shown in Fig. 28-14. (Courtesy of Brian R. Schnier, M.D.)

nor is every lesion amenable to such therapy. However, for those deemed appropriate and who achieve a satisfactory response, operative intervention may be avoided or at least delayed so that it can be undertaken at an elective time.

Nuclear Medicine Techniques

Technetium Sulfur Colloid Scintigraphy

Localizing the site of acute GI hemorrhage has been attempted using technetium sulfur colloid scintigraphy (^{99m}Tc).[187,235,271224,282,324] The imaging agent used for conventional liver scans is injected into the venous circulation, and with the abdomen of the patient under the gamma camera, a radionuclide angiogram is obtained. The principle of the study is that the labeled colloid is rapidly cleared from the bloodstream by the reticuloendothelial system, but an active site of bleeding appears as a "hot spot," since the extravasated isotope is no longer recirculating and cannot be cleared by the system.[282,324]

A number of reports have confirmed the success of this approach.[6,7,216,282,335] Alavi and Ring evaluated 43 patients with lower GI bleeding.[7] In the 20 patients with negative scintigrams, arteriography also failed to demonstrate the site of bleeding. In the remaining individuals with positive scans, fewer than one-half had positive arteriograms. Orrecchia and colleagues reported 76 patients with lower GI bleeding.[225] Of the 16 who required an emergency operation, the site of bleeding was localized in all but one. However, of the 60 patients who did not require an operation, bleeding was localized in only 11. Others have demonstrated that the true positive rate, as well as the predictive value for a positive study, is 100%, but in this same series 69 of 82 examinations were negative.[335] Others have had a less satisfactory experience with the use of nuclear scintigraphy. Garofalo and Abdu performed a retrospective study involving 155 patients who underwent nuclear scintigraphic examinations because of GI bleeding.[118] This was compared with angiography and the actual site of GI bleeding as confirmed by surgery or by endoscopy. When strict criteria (i.e., exact location) were used, 39% were correct in localizing the bleeding source. They concluded that the routine use of nuclear scintigraphy cannot be justified because it is neither accurate nor cost-effective for diagnosing or localizing the site of GI bleeding.

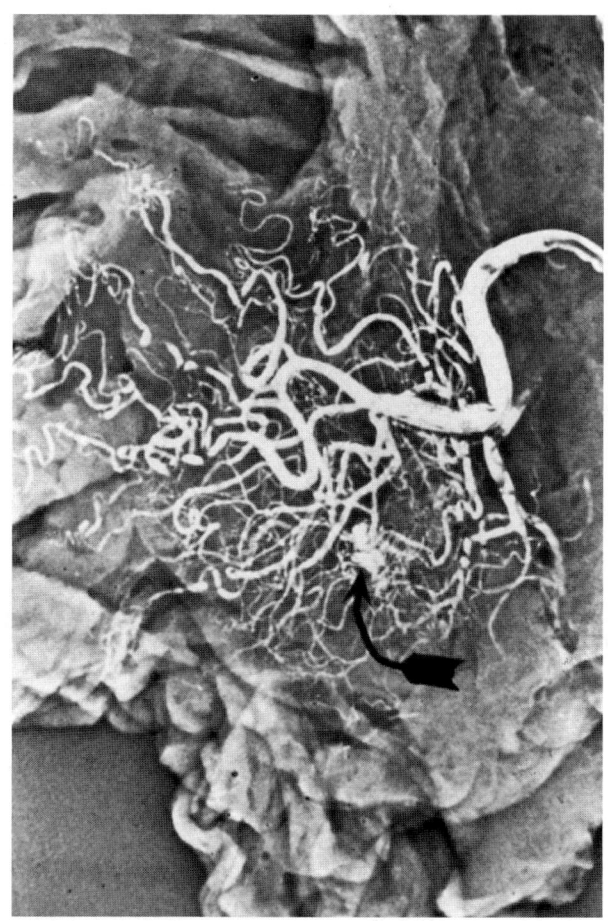

FIGURE 28-17. Angiodysplastic lesion (*arrow*) in an injected specimen following resection for cecal arteriovenous malformation.

The technique would, therefore, seem to be most valuable in the identification of the site of bleeding in a patient about to undergo emergency operation. The problem is that the isotope is cleared so rapidly that bleeding must be quite active to demonstrate a positive scan. Sulfur colloid, although theoretically advantageous in minimizing background activity and promoting the highest contrast ratios, has limited value because of this reduced sensitivity.[324]

Tagged Red Blood Cells

Another alternative is the use of technetium (Tc 99m) tagged red blood cells.[336,337] This technique permits identification of a bleeding point due to hemorrhage of a lesser magnitude. In contrast to technetium sulfur colloid scintigraphy, the labeled red cells are not cleared rapidly and are available to produce a positive scan through repeated periods of imaging even if the extravasation occurs over a number of days. Retention of this blood-pool radiotracer in the vascular compartment permits this possibility (Figs. 28-20 and 28-21). The disadvantage, of course, is that the radioactivity persists for a relatively long time. But the technique can be successful in detecting the presence of continuing hemorrhage with transfusion requirements as little as 500 mL within 24 hours, or 0.05 to 0.1 mL/minute.[337]

Bunker and colleagues, in their initial study, confirmed the site of bleeding in 10 of 11 patients by this method.[68] A later report of 100 individuals demonstrated clear superiority of ^{99m}Tc red blood cells over ^{99m}Tc sulfur colloid, with a sensitivity of 93%, a specificity of 95%,

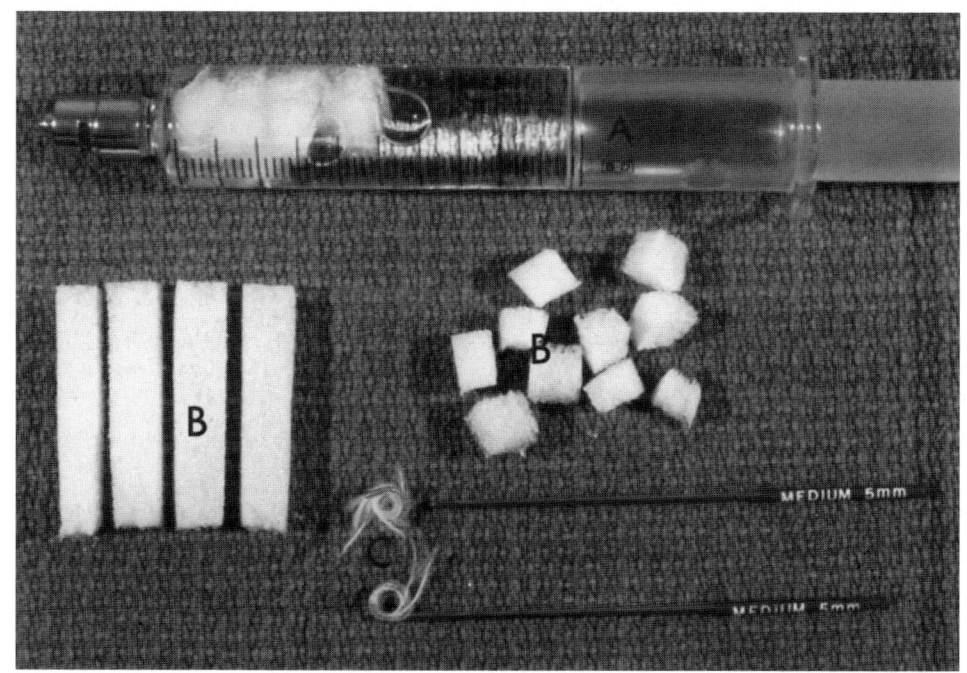

FIGURE 28-18. Thromboembolic devices. **(A)** Syringe with Gelfoam. **(B)** Gelfoam. **(C)** Gianturco coils for occluding medium-sized vessels. (Courtesy of John G. Mardiat, M.D.)

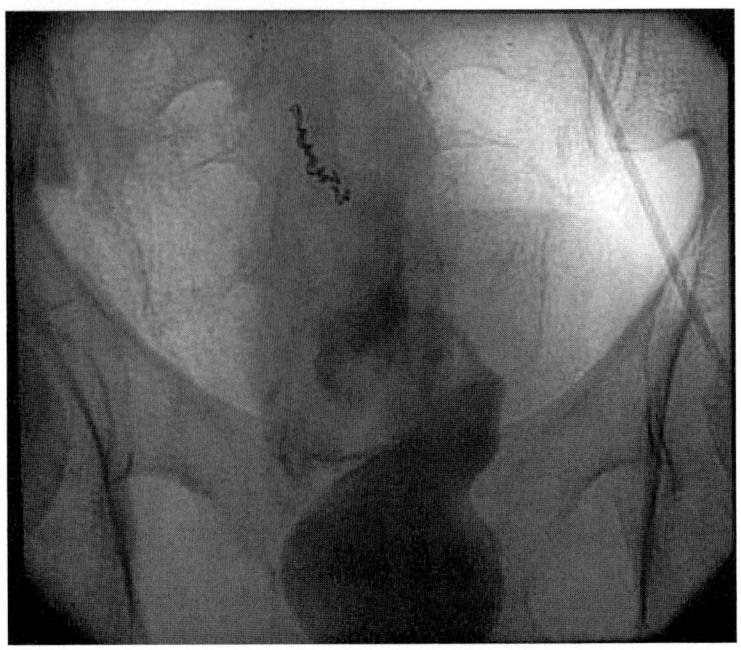

FIGURE 28-19. Embolization with Gianturco coil. Note position of the coil in the upper pelvis.

and an overall accuracy of 94% in detecting and localizing GI hemorrhage.[69] In 32 patients with documented hemorrhage reported by Winzelberg and colleagues, 29 had positive scintiscans (sensitivity, 91%; 5% false negatives).[336] The data of others support the concept of increasing application.[218] Baum has suggested that as radionuclide scans are more widely employed, angiography will eventually be performed only in those patients with positive scans.[35] Conversely, Bentley and Richardson noted that tagged scans accurately localized the site of bleeding in only 52% of cases and offered the opinion that it is a poor technique for identifying the source.[41] They further questioned its use as a screening tool before

angiography. Others also have expressed concern about the scan's ability to accurately localize the site of bleeding. Hunter and Pezim found that performing a surgical procedure that relies exclusively on this technique for localization will "produce an undesirable result in at least 42% of patients."[151]

A recent perspective concerning the place of labeled red blood cell scans in the investigation of GI bleeding was offered by the group at the University of Southern California Department of Surgery and Department of Nuclear Medicine.[100] Eighty patients underwent scanning over a 4-year period. Twenty-eight percent had positive scans with the site of bleeding confirmed by angiography.

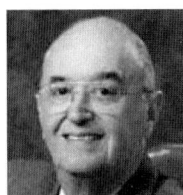

Stanley Baum (1929–present)   Stanley Baum was born in New York City, December 26, 1929. He received his medical degree in 1957 from the Faculty of Medicine at the University of Utrecht in Holland and completed an internship at Kings County Hospital Medical Center in New York City and a radiology residency at the University of Pennsylvania in Philadelphia. He became a National Cancer Institute trainee before completing a fellowship in cardiovascular radiology at Stanford University Medical Center. Following a brief time on the faculty at Stanford he returned to the University of Pennsylvania and advanced to the rank of Professor of Radiology. In 1971 he moved to Harvard as Professor of Radiology and Chief of Cardiovascular Radiology at Massachusetts General Hospital. In 1975, he returned to the University of Pennsylvania as Professor and Chairman of the Department of Radiology. Baum held that post for more than 20 years, during which time he became the Eugene P. Pendergrass Professor of Radiology. He contributed to early MR imaging development and made a significant impact on angiography by describing the roles of vasoconstrictors in controlling gastrointestinal bleeding and of angiography in assessing vascular bleeding. He was one of the first interventional radiologists in the United States and was the founder and first president of the Society of Cardiovascular and Interventional Radiology. He was also one of the first diagnostic radiologists elected to the Institute of Medicine. Despite these monumental achievements, some of Baum's most important work came after he stepped down as chairman. He was a founding member of the Academy of Radiology Research (ARR) and was ARR president when the bill to establish the National Institute of Biomedical Imaging and Bioengineering was introduced in the United States Senate. Among his numerous awards and honors are the Cannon Medal from the Society of Gastrointestinal Radiologists, and gold medals from the Association of University Radiologists, American Roentgen Ray Society, and Society of Cardiovascular and Interventional Radiology. In 2002, the University of Pennsylvania established the Stanley Baum Professorship in the Department of Radiology. (With appreciation to Arie Pelta, M.D.)

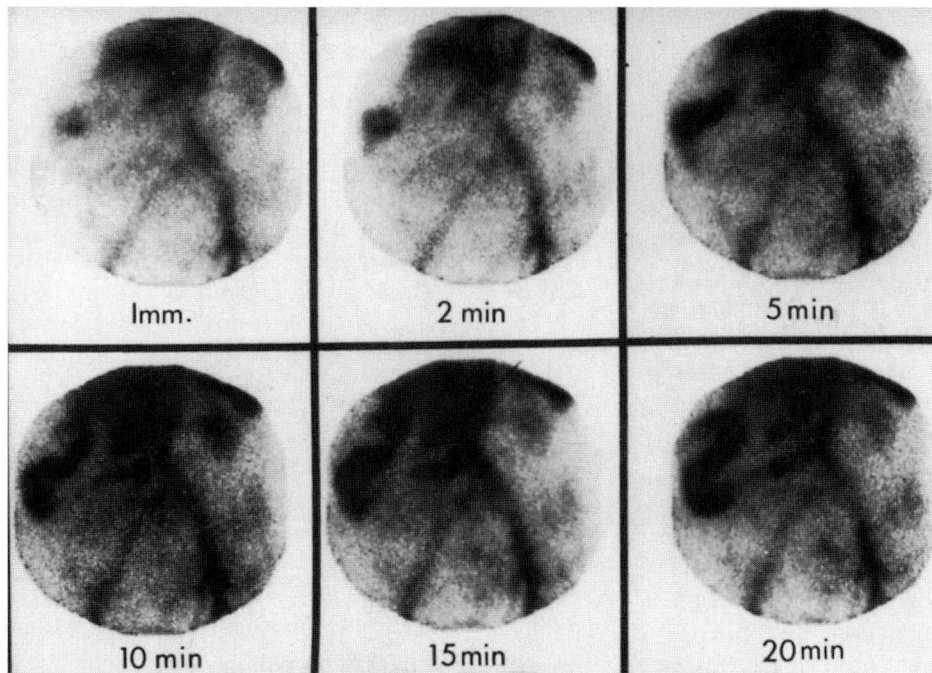

FIGURE 28-20. Scintiscan with ^{99m}Tc–labeled red blood cells. The bleeding site in the ascending colon is seen shortly following injection. The uptake from that site increases in intensity and moves along the bowel. Hemorrhage originated in the hepatic flexure. (Courtesy of Kenneth A. McKusick, M.D.)

The authors observed that failure to identify the site of bleeding is frequently due to an upper GI tract source, a conclusion that has been reached by a number of other investigators. At the University of Southern California, the protocol consisted of a continuous phase of imaging every 5 to 15 minutes during the first 2 hours.[100] They concluded that the accuracy of the scan can be extrapolated to the entire continuous imaging phase as long as

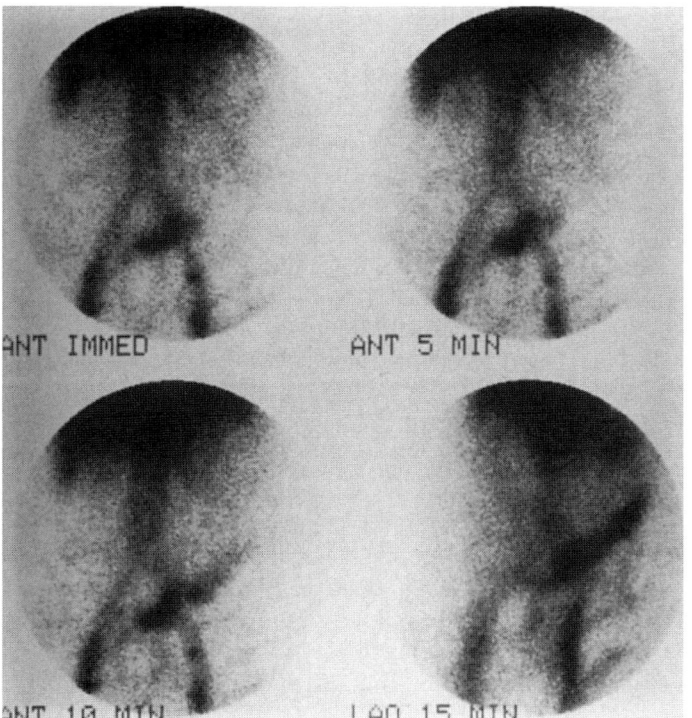

FIGURE 28-21. Labeled red blood cell study reveals prompt extravascular site of bleeding localized just below the bifurcation of the aorta. This is seen to progress transversely to the left upper quadrant. Later views showed the tracer to move down along the left side. This was interpreted to be bleeding that originated in the mid-transverse colon.

the images are taken at this frequency. Hence, maximum accuracy in correctly localizing the site of the bleeding can be achieved. Ng and co-workers (Ochsner Clinic, New Orleans, Louisiana) undertook a study to evaluate the time interval from injection of the radioactive red cells until the presence of a "blush" or positive scan as a potential indicator for management.[216] They found that those with a delayed blush have low angiographic yields and may be observed and evaluated electively with colonoscopy. Conversely, those with an immediate blush benefited from urgent angiography. It is well said that ^{99m}Tc-labeled red blood cell scintigraphy is of primary benefit in directing the patient's diagnostic rather than therapeutic management.[216]

Treatment

As implied from the foregoing, if the bleeding point is identified by means of angiography, tagged red cell scan, endoscopy, or barium enema examination, the appropriate therapy can be instituted: medical management, a local procedure or resection, depending on the nature of the lesion and the patient's clinical course.

Estrogen–Progesterone Therapy

A number of papers have appeared that indicate estrogen–progesterone therapy may be effective in controlling severe, recurrent bleeding from GI vascular malformations.[129,212,249,314] The mechanism of action of hormonal therapy to control bleeding with this condition is not clearly understood. Theories include an effect on coagulation, induction of stasis in the mesenteric microcirculation, and improvement in the integrity of the vascular endothelial lining.[212] Side effects are of some concern and include thromboembolic disease, an increased risk for the development of malignancies, nausea, vomiting, loss of libido, and gynecomastia. Still, hormonal therapy should be considered in situations when prolonged obscure GI bleeding thought to be due to angiodysplasia cannot adequately be managed by other means.[212] Richardson and Lordon present the typical patient who may be a candidate for this approach.[249] They describe three individuals with chronic renal failure who had GI bleeding caused by angiodysplasia that responded to this approach.

Obscure Bleeding

Thomas suggests the use of the expression "obscure bleeding" to describe the following situations:

■ The cause exists but has been difficult to diagnose or has been overlooked.

■ Bleeding results from multisystem disease.
■ Investigations have failed to localize the site of hemorrhage.[307]

The reality is, however, that it is only through an organized, algorithmic approach that one may hope to identify and treat the source of gastrointestinal bleeding. The small bowel, in particular, has been the most difficult area to assess, an area of special concern in an individual with obscure bleeding or bleeding from an unknown source. In the elective situation, a small bowel series, enteroclysis, or capsule endoscopy imaging (see Chapter 4) must be considered.

Operative Management

Self-expanding Stent

In addition to the previously discussed minimally invasive methods, we have successfully employed a self-expanding metallic stent to control lower gastrointestinal hemorrhage from metastatic tumor.[87] The expansion of the stent against the lesion presumably provides sufficient pressure to tamponade the bleeding area.

Resection

What is the proper treatment if the patient continues to bleed and the source has not been identified? In the past, individuals were submitted to exploratory laparotomy in the hope that a lesion could be found at the operating table. Multiple enterotomies were undertaken to identify the proximal limit of the bleeding and to perform operative colonoscopy. In someone at high risk, such a prolonged operative procedure exposes the patient to increased mortality as well as to the possibility of additional morbidity from infection. Alternatively, blind left colectomy has historically been advocated, and later, right colectomy. Most surgeons today, however, believe that subtotal colectomy is the preferred procedure when the source of bleeding has not been identified preoperatively or intraoperatively.

Operative Colonoscopy and Enteroscopy

Another option for operatively identifying the source of bleeding involves a combination of laparotomy and colonoscopy through the application of a two-team approach.[42] A rapid, intraoperative cleansing of the bowel may be effected through a small cecostomy if this is felt advisable.[274] This is analogous to the technique of on-table lavage (see Chapter 22). The abdominal surgeon can assist the colonoscopist in the passage of the instrument to make one final attempt to identify a discrete bleeding point.[321] If one is seen, it may be dealt with through the instrument, or it may be effectively treated by a less than total abdominal colectomy.

Intraoperative enteroscopy can be accomplished with the colonoscope passed per orum, guiding the instrument through the duodenum and into the small bowel. Segmental visualization can be accomplished, occluding the bowel at intervals to avoid overdistention.[91] The endoscopic appearance can be supplemented by simultaneous viewing from the serosal aspect of the transilluminated bowel. Although intraoperative enteroscopy with conventional gastroscopes or colonoscopes has been accomplished for many years, the Sonde enteroscope represents an additional advance in the technique of small bowel endoscopy.[179] The SIF-SW Sonde endoscope (Olympus Corporation of America, Orangeburg, NY) has an outer diameter of 5 mm, a working length of 279 cm, and a 120-degree field of view. It contains two channels, one for air insufflation or irrigation and the other for inflating a balloon located at the tip of the instrument. This balloon helps to manipulate the endoscope through the small intestine and into the colon. There is no tip-control mechanism, nor is there a therapeutic channel, so that it is not possible to perform such procedures as biopsy or electrocoagulation. The technique is well described in the article by Lopez and colleagues.[179] In their experience involving 16 patients with this instrument, all were examined for the entire small bowel length, and in 14 the site of bleeding was revealed.

Desa and colleagues identified the source in 10 of 12 cases of obscure bleeding by the method of operative enteroscopy using different equipment.[91] These individuals had previously undergone multiple surgical procedures as well as the usual specialized testing. Flickinger and associates found that this technique influenced the operation in 93% of cases.[107] When an angiodysplastic lesion is identified one can treat it by electrocoagulation, laser photoablation, or suturing.[1]

Operative Arteriography

Intraoperative localization of vascular ectasias may be accomplished by placing the bowel to be examined on a sterile cassette cover.[252] The segmental arterial branch feeding the area is isolated and injected with methylglucamine diatrizoate (Renografin 76). With the bowel exhibiting pallor and contracting, the film is exposed to identify the lesion. I have had no experience with this technique but would consider its applicability only for small bowel lesions. This method, though, has the potential advantage of a therapeutic option.

McDonald and associates described the use of highly selective angiographic catheter placement combined with intraoperative methylene blue dye injection to precisely identify the source of hemorrhage in three patients who had a small bowel source of bleeding confirmed.[198] At operation, 0.5 ml of methlyene blue dye (50 mg/mL) was injected into the catheter, which resulted in immediate demarcation of the small intestine over a length of approximately 20 cm with a brilliant blue color. This enabled the surgeons to resect a limited amount of small intestine.

Results of Surgery

Smith and colleagues identified 24 patients with lower GI hemorrhage due to angiodysplasia, 17 of whom required surgery.[287] With the bleeding point found preoperatively, no patient rebled following either a limited resection or a subtotal colectomy. But coagulopathy, specifically platelet disorders, contributed to a high mortality rate. Boley and Brandt accept a 20% rebleeding rate after right hemicolectomy for angiographically demonstrated ectasias and believe that the risk of subtotal colectomy is greater than the risk of rebleeding.[48] Bender and colleagues reported a mortality of 27% following total colectomy and opined that the procedure under these circumstances is associated with excessive morbidity and mortality.[40] Whether this is a valid criticism of the surgery or a reflection of multiple blood transfusions, age, and other factors was not analyzed. Irrespective of the type of surgery, Leitman and colleagues found that those who failed transcatheter treatment had a mortality of 36%.[173] Parkes and co-workers reviewed the records of 31 patients who underwent colon resection to determine the most effective surgical treatment for massive lower GI bleeding.[228] The rebleeding rate for subtotal colectomy with a mean follow-up of 1 year was nil. With a segmental resection, even with a positive angiogram, the rebleeding rate was 14%, and if the angiogram was negative, a segmental resection was associated with a rebleeding rate of 42%. This last group of patients was associated with the highest complication rate in the series (83%). This same group of patients had an extremely high mortality rate also (57%).

Comment

Fortunately, with the diagnostic studies available, the surgeon should rarely have to resort to blind resection. It is axiomatic that if a lesion is clearly demonstrated on angiography and cannot be controlled by minimally invasive means, a limited resection is appropriate. However, if there is not complete certainty about the source of the bleeding, the few minutes necessary to remove the remainder of the bowel should add very little risk. Furthermore, in the absence of blood in the small bowel, the maneuvers associated with operative colonoscopy and operative angiography truly prolong the surgical time with its attendant risks, and have the potential hazards of contamination with the former technique and toxicity with the latter.

MESENTERIC OCCLUSIVE AND NONOCCLUSIVE DISEASE

The gut receives 20% of resting and 35% of postprandial cardiac output, of which 70% supplies the mucosa.[54] In the fasting state, only one in five mesenteric capillaries is open. The bowel, as one can see, has therefore a remarkably resistant ability to withstand ischemia.[54] However, if the blood pressure falls below 70 mm Hg, intestinal perfusion may be compromised. Below 40 mm Hg this mechanism fails, and the bowel becomes progressively more ischemic, with anaerobic metabolism replacing aerobic.[54] The nature and rapidity of the ischemic process are affected by the collateral circulation and by disorders of splanchnic autoregulation.

Major occlusive disease is usually caused by mesenteric vascular obstruction by atheroma, thrombus, or embolus. Other etiologies include dissecting aneurysm, arteritis, sepsis, intestinal obstruction, and trauma. Acute mesenteric ischemia usually occurs in patients older than 50 years of age, particularly in those with arteriosclerotic heart disease or valvular involvement.[49] The characteristic person is an elderly man with prior heart disease and symptoms of peripheral atherosclerosis.[284] Hypercoagulable conditions and the use of oral contraceptives may also precipitate intestinal vascular thromboses, often involving the venous circulation. Other factors that predispose to ischemia include long-standing congestive heart failure, the prolonged use of diuretics, cardiac arrhythmias, recent myocardial infarction, hypovolemia, hypotension, burns, pancreatitis, and GI hemorrhage.[49,50] Most patients, in fact, who develop ischemic changes of the small and large bowel do not have a demonstrably significant vascular lesion but have so-called nonocclusive vascular disease.

Signs and Symptoms

The most frequent symptoms of mesenteric occlusion are abdominal pain and rectal bleeding (up to 98%). An early characteristic feature is the disparity between the severity of the pain and the paucity of significant abdominal findings.[49] In other words, the pain is generally out of proportion to the physical findings. Signs and symptoms of peritonitis rapidly ensue in the presence of intestinal infarction. Hypothermia is not uncommonly observed.[284] Other complaints include back pain, nausea, vomiting, and diarrhea. In patients with so-called abdominal angina, abdominal pain is also evident, usually developing 15 to 20 minutes following the ingestion of food.[112] Pain is characteristically epigastric or periumbilical, and weight loss and malnutrition may ensue.

Laboratory and Radiologic Studies

Laboratory investigations usually reveal an elevated white blood cell count (out of proportion to the physical findings) and evidence of hemoconcentration—nonspecific abnormalities to be sure, but consistent with the diagnosis of mesenteric ischemia. Metabolic acidosis frequently is noted in patients with intestinal infarction. This is due to tissue hypoxia, persistent hypotension, and the release of vasoactive materials. Determination of arterial blood gases confirms the base deficit and should serve to alert the physician to the severity of the illness.

Although a wide range of investigations is available for the assessment of mesenteric ischemia, with the exception of angiography and computed tomography (CT), none is particularly helpful.[54] However, magnetic resonance angiography has been recently advocated as a minimally invasive tool for diagnosing mesenteric and portal vascular disease.[26] Plain films of the abdomen may demonstrate thickened bowel loops, a ground-glass appearance from ascites, the classic "thumb-printing," and gas in the bowel wall, portal vein, or peritoneal cavity. However, one-fourth of patients with mesenteric infarction have a normal plain film of the abdomen.

Ultrasonography may be useful in excluding other diagnoses, and CT may demonstrate ascites, intestinal wall thickening, and additional findings, but experience with this modality in the management of patients with mesenteric ischemia is quite limited.

Evaluation and Treatment Protocol

Boley and his colleagues propose a comprehensive, algorithmic approach to the diagnosis and therapy of mesenteric occlusive and nonocclusive disease (Figure 28-22).[49,50,53] The protocol advocates initial treatment directed at correction of the predisposing or precipitating causes of the ischemia. Vasopressors and digitalis are discontinued if at all possible. After the initial supportive measures have been completed, radiologic studies are undertaken. A plain film of the abdomen is obtained to be certain that there is no other obvious cause for the abdominal signs and symptoms, such as a perforation or intestinal obstruction. Angiography is then performed. Following a flush aortogram, selective angiography is undertaken to detect emboli, thrombosis, or mesenteric vasoconstriction in the superior mesenteric artery or its branches (Figure 28-23).[53] Based on the angiographic findings and the presence or absence of peritoneal signs, the patient is then treated according to the protocol that these authors have established.

If the angiogram is normal and no peritoneal signs are found, observation is the treatment of choice. With a normal angiogram and the presence of peritoneal signs, exploratory laparotomy is undertaken. If an angiogram

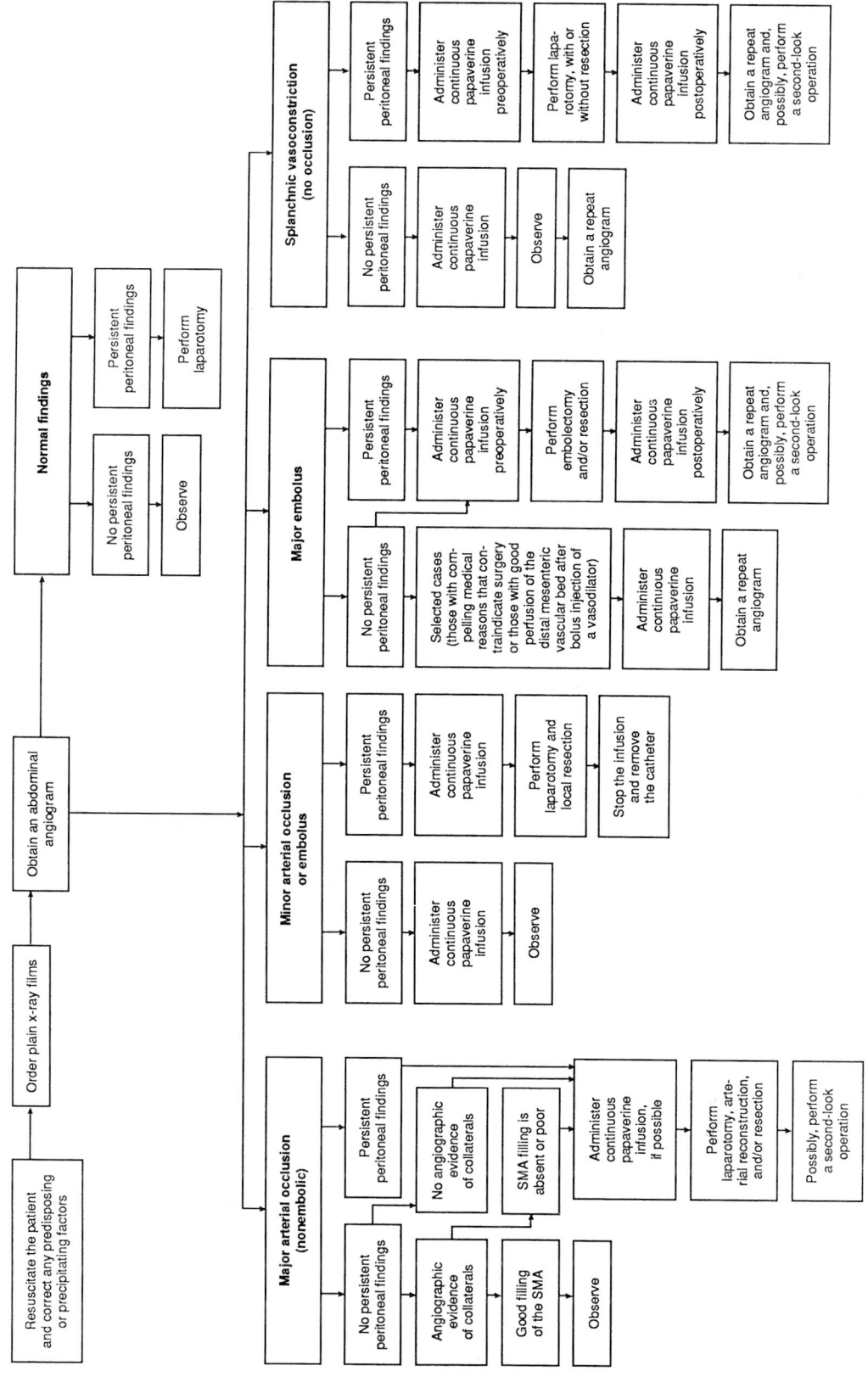

FIGURE 28-22. Managing acute mesenteric ischemia based on the angiographic findings. (Reproduced with permission from Border E, Boley SJ. Acute mesenteric ischemia: treat aggressively for best results. *J Crit Illness* 1986;1:54.)

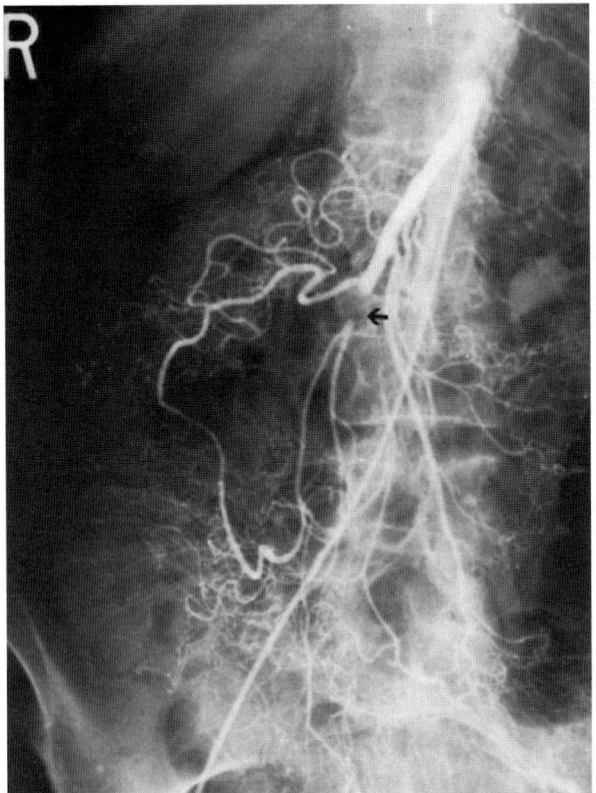

FIGURE 28-23. Superior mesenteric artery embolism (*arrow*). Note the collateral circulation through the meandering vessel.

demonstrates a major embolus, with or without peritoneal signs, preoperative papaverine infusion is begun, and an embolectomy is performed, with or without a bowel resection.

If a minor occlusion or embolus is noted, in the absence of peritoneal signs, papaverine can be considered and the patient can be observed. VanDeinse and colleagues report a case of high-grade stenosis of the superior mesenteric artery treated by percutaneous transluminal angioplasty.[315] With peritoneal signs, preoperative papaverine is infused and a laparotomy and limited resection are performed if indicated.

With a major nonembolic occlusion and peritoneal signs, papaverine may be infused and arterial reconstruction performed, with or without a resection if necessary. A second-look procedure may be considered subsequently, depending on the nature of the original pathology. If a major occlusion is not associated with peritoneal signs and the angiogram identifies a good collateral blood supply, observation is the treatment of choice. In the absence of collaterals and the presence of splanchnic vasoconstriction, papaverine is infused. A laparotomy with arterial reconstruction and possible resection is undertaken. In this situation, a second-look procedure may be indicated later.

If the angiogram fails to demonstrate an occlusion (splanchnic vasoconstriction only), in the absence of peritoneal signs papaverine is infused. The patient is observed and the angiogram is subsequently repeated. If peritoneal signs exist, preoperative papaverine is infused, and an exploratory laparotomy is performed. A resection is undertaken if indicated (Figure 28-24). A repeat angiogram and the possibility of a second-look operation should be considered.

The amount of intestine that should be removed is always a source of concern. Visual appreciation of bowel damage based on capillary bleeding, color, and contractility is often misleading and commonly induces the surgeon to remove more bowel than is truly necessary.[67] A number of authors have compared clinical judgment with other methods of determining intestinal viability. Clinical judgment was associated with a relatively high sensitivity, specificity, and overall accuracy, but had a low predictive value.[269] Bowel was incorrectly assessed to be nonviable in 46% of patients, leading to the removal of more bowel than was necessary. In an experimental study, Brolin and colleagues compared five methods for assessing intestinal viability: threshold stimulus level (TSL), the minimal electrical current necessary to produce a smooth muscle contractile response; intestinal color; peristalsis; Doppler ultrasound; and histologically evaluated resection margin.[59] The bowel color, the presence of peristalsis, and the histologic findings failed to correlate with the intestinal survival rate. Conversely, blood flow measured by Doppler ultrasound and the myoelectric parameters established through an electronic contractility meter were directly related to viability. Bulkley and co-workers compared clinical judgment at the time of the operation with Doppler ultrasound and with the use of fluorescein to determine bowel viability in a prospective, controlled study of patients with intestinal ischemia.[67] The fluorescein method was shown to be superior to the Doppler method.

Results

Boley and colleagues reported their experience with 47 patients with intestinal ischemia due to superior mesenteric artery emboli.[50] The overall mortality was 66%. Those with infarction of more than 50% of the small intestine did especially poorly (17 of 19 such patients died). A survival rate of 55% was obtained in patients managed according to the preceding protocol, whereas only 20% of those treated by traditional methods survived. The best results were obtained in patients who were diagnosed within 24 hours of the onset of pain.

Clavien and colleagues reported their experience of 81 individuals with mesenteric infarction documented by angiography.[79] Almost one-half were felt to have an inop-

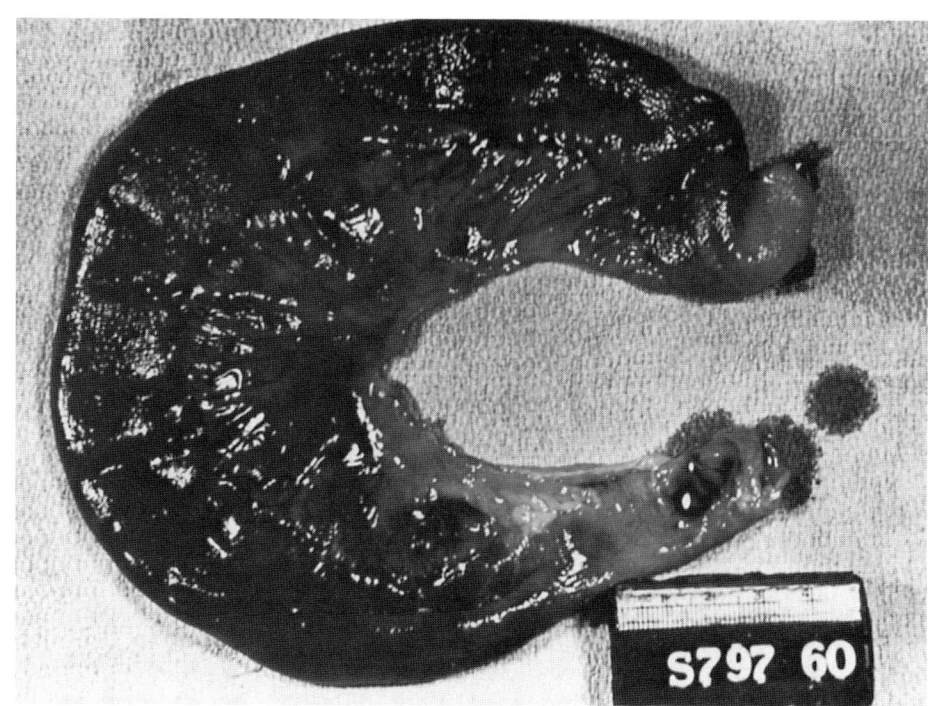

FIGURE 28-24. A resected segment of small bowel showing infarction from prolonged hypotension due to nonocclusive vascular disease. (Courtesy of Rudolf Garret, M.D.)

erable situation and were treated by supportive care only. Of those who underwent a laparotomy, 45% survived. Because of the high frequency of progressive infarction following resection (32%), the authors recommend preoperative perfusion of the superior mesenteric artery with vasodilators and postoperative anticoagulation. Sitges-Serra and colleagues identified 44 individuals who underwent massive small bowel resection (mean length of remaining bowel, 60 cm), noting a 46% mortality.[284] Levy and associates reported an overall mortality in 62 surgically treated patients of 40%.[175] They emphasize the importance of establishing double stomas whenever the viability of the remaining bowel is equivocal. Endean and co-workers assessed the University of Kentucky experience in 170 patients with acute intestinal ischemia.[101] Nonthrombotic patients represented 60%; thrombotic, 34%; and indeterminate, 6%. The survival rate for arterial embolism was 41% and for thrombosis, 38%. These results are indicative of an improvement when compared with earlier reports.

Schoots and associates analyzed the published data on survival following mesenteric ischemia over the past four decades.[272] Forty-five observational studies contained 3,692 patients. They made the following conclusions:

- Prognosis with acute mesenteric venous occlusion is better (see later).
- Prognosis after mesenteric artery embolism is better than following thrombosis or nonocclusive ischemia.
- The mortality rate following surgical treatment of arterial embolism and venous thrombosis (54% and 32%,

respectively) is less than that after surgery for arterial thrombosis and nonocclusive ischemia (77% and 73%, respectively).

- The overall survival has improved during this time.

Venous Mesenteric Ischemia

Venous thrombosis is a rare cause of mesenteric infarction, but the diagnosis is notoriously difficult to make. Causes may be primary, such as those conditions that increased viscosity of the blood or its tendency to coagulate (e.g., splenectomy, polycytemia ruba vera, sickle cell disease, platelet disorders, myeloproliferative disease, the use of contraceptive pills, pregnancy, and carcinomatosis).[54] A new disease entity, idiopathic mesenteric phlebosclerosis (i.e., nonthrombotic stenosis or occlusion of the mesenteric veins) has been described.[156] Secondary causes (60%) include portal hypertension, intra-abdominal sepsis, pancreatitis, intra-abdominal neoplasms, inflammatory bowel disease, abdominal trauma, and various gastroenterides. The condition is usually confined to a limited segment of the bowel and therefore carries with it a better prognosis than that of arterial occlusive or nonocclusive disease. Clavien and colleagues used contrast-enhanced CT to identify a triad of findings in this condition: hypodensity in the trunk of the superior mesenteric vein, thickening of the intestinal wall and valvulae conniventes localized in a jejunoileal segment, and considerable peritoneal fluid.[78]

Optimal treatment in those patients with reversible damage is anticoagulation. Intravenous heparin should be administered before operation.

ISCHEMIC COLITIS

Ischemic colitis is a term coined by Marston and associates to describe a syndrome due to occlusive or nonocclusive vascular disease as it affects the large bowel.[194] It is a condition that usually is found in the aging population, with an increased incidence in women,[229] although the disease has been associated with hemorrhagic shock even in young patients.[71] Abel and Russell reported that approximately 60% were 70 years of age or older; 78% were women.[2] Ischemic colitis can be a consequence of various resective procedures on the bowel, of operations performed on the aorta (see later), and of embolization for the treatment of colonic hemorrhage.[255] A number of conditions, some of which are included within this chapter, produce their pathologic manifestations at least in part on an ischemic basis. These include arteriosclerosis, emboli, myocardial infarction, vasculitis, colorectal neoplasms, portal hypertension, strangulated hernia, volvulus, diabetes mellitus, hypertension, chronic renal failure, periarteritis nodosa, systemic lupus erythematosus, rheumatoid arthritis, polycythemia vera, scleroderma, hemodialysis, anaphylactoid shock, strict dieting, methamphetamine abuse, and many others.[42,80C,233B,258,49,97,280,310] Frequent hypotensive episodes in response to fluid removal and an associated low-flow state are probably responsible for this complication in individuals undergoing hemodialysis.[157] In the experience of Longo and colleagues ischemic colitis commonly occurred during an unrelated hospital admission and following surgery.[178]

The blood supply to the colon is contributed through the meandering artery or anastomosis of Riolan (the vascular communication between the superior and inferior mesenteric arteries; see Chapter 1). The reduction of splanchnic blood flow through this vessel appears to have its greatest vulnerability in two watershed areas: Sudeck's* point and Griffiths'† point (see Chapter 1).[131,295] However, a number of factors, such as large and small vessel arterial disease, perfusion pressure, plasma viscosity, and adequacy of collateral circulation, may combine to produce even total colonic ischemia.[329]

Classification, Symptoms, Findings, and Diagnosis

Ischemic colitis has been classified on the basis of its three general manifestations:

- Gangrenous
- Strictured
- Transient or reversible

In the experience of West and colleagues, of 27 patients who had colonic ischemia, 12 had reversible or transient colitis, and 13 developed a stricture or gangrene that required surgery.[332] The sigmoid colon was the most frequent area of symptomatic stricture.

If gangrene of the colon develops, the patient may complain of severe abdominal pain, nausea, and vomiting. Bowel movements may be absent, or bloody diarrhea may be noted. Passage of a large bowel cast as a consequence of the ischemia has been described.[21] Physical examination will reveal evidence of peritonitis if the bowel is involved by transmural disease, and certainly if there is a perforation. Upright abdominal x-ray may demonstrate free gas under the diaphragm.

The development of an ischemic stricture probably is a consequence of an initial extensive inflammatory process, but not to the point of bowel perforation. This is a very rare manifestation of the ischemic process. Patients may have minimal symptoms, or nausea, vomiting, and abdominal distention may develop. Barium enema may reveal a lesion difficult to distinguish from carcinoma (Figure 28-25). According to Brandt and colleagues, approximately one-third of patients present with a colonic stricture or "chronic colitis."[56] Often the ischemic nature of the radiologic finding is not readily apparent, although colonoscopy and biopsy will inevitably fail to identify malignant cells. One can consider reevaluation at a later time, but if the patient has a symptomatic stricture and the diagnosis cannot be established with certainty, resection is indicated.

In patients who have reversible or transient ischemic disease, rectal bleeding may be the only complaint. Abdominal pain and tenderness on the left side are usually minimal or may not even be evident. Colonoscopic examination almost always will reveal rectal sparing, with inflammatory changes commencing usually at a level of approximately 15 cm (Figure 28-26). More florid manifestations of inflammatory changes in the mucosa from ischemic colonic disease can be seen in the colonoscopic appearance in Figure 28-26E. It would be essentially im-

---

*Sudeck's (critical) point: the region in the colon between the blood supply from the colic artery (i.e., the last sigmoid artery) and that from the superior hemorrhoidal artery.
†Griffiths' point: the potentially vulnerable area in the region of the splenic flexure, which, under some circumstances, may have an inadequate blood supply in the area served by the middle colic artery and the ascending branch of the left colic artery.

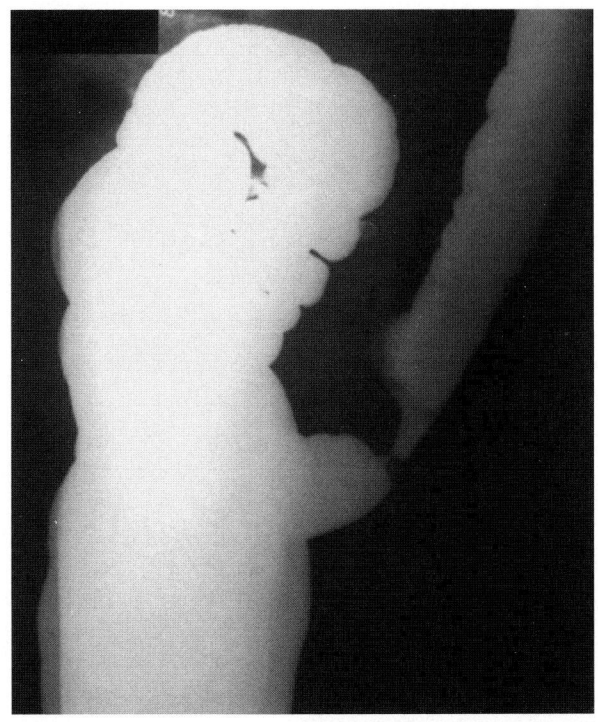

FIGURE 28-25. Ischemic stricture. Barium enema demonstrates profound narrowing at the level of the sigmoid–descending colon junction in an elderly, asymptomatic woman. Intact mucosa suggests a diagnosis other than carcinoma. Biopsy identified only chronic inflammatory cells.

possible to distinguish the changes observed here from those of nonspecific inflammatory bowel disease. The rectum is rarely involved in the ischemic process because of its abundant collateral blood supply,[215] although ischemic proctitis has been reported to be caused by adventitial fibromuscular dysplasia of the superior rectal artery and by myointimal hyperplasia of the mesenteric veins.[243,265] However, if the rectum is involved (see later), serious consideration should be given to another etiology (e.g., ulcerative colitis, antibiotic-associated colitis, or an infectious colitis). It may be very difficult to distinguish the condition from nonspecific inflammatory bowel disease, except that the age of the patient and the history are often helpful. Other endoscopic changes include pallor of the mucosa and hemorrhagic areas. The latter are more likely to be appreciated early in the evolution of the inflammatory reaction.

A plain film of the abdomen may reveal characteristic "thumb-printing," usually in the region of the splenic flexure. Depending on the severity of the process, dilated loops of small and large bowel may be seen. In more advanced cases one may note the presence of gas in the wall of the colon. Barium enema examination characteristically shows thumbprinting, edema of the bowel wall, and narrowing primarily in the areas of the splenic flexure,

the distal transverse colon, and the descending colon (Figs. 28-27 and 28-28). But with a patient who has a suspected bowel infarction, barium enema is contraindicated (Figure 28-29). An arteriogram may reveal helpful information even if only a flush study of the aorta is carried out (Figure 28-30). Occlusion of one of the major vessels or branches should lead the surgeon to suspect the cause of the patient's symptoms.

Pathologic changes of the colon may reveal disease limited to the mucosa and submucosa (Figure 28-31) because the rich blood supply makes this area more sensitive to ischemic changes. The muscularis propria is relatively resistant to the effects of decreased perfusion, but transmural involvement can occur (Figure 28-32).

Management

Medical management includes intravenous fluid replacement, nasogastric suction, broad-spectrum antibiotic therapy, and the usual supportive measures.[333] In most cases of colonic ischemia, signs and symptoms subside within a day or two, with resolution of the submucosal or intramural hemorrhage.[117] Surgical intervention is indicated for signs and symptoms of peritonitis and for obstruction.

The intraoperative diagnosis of the degree of colonic ischemia is often difficult to determine. Care must be taken at the time of resection to ensure adequacy of the blood supply. Partial colectomy for primary colonic ischemia is generally a poor alternative, but if undertaken should always be accompanied by fecal diversion, unless the quality of life with an ileostomy is felt to be unacceptable for that individual. Subtotal or total colectomy is the preferred approach if an anastomosis is contemplated, but even with a total colectomy resection with an ileostomy is undoubtedly safer.

Results

There are no meaningful statistics concerning the comparative results of the surgical options. Guttormson and Bubrick evaluated 39 individuals with this condition, confirming a close association between ischemic colitis and a number of systemic diseases.[137] The overall mortality rate was 53% for those treated both surgically and nonsurgically. Parish and colleagues observed an increased proportion of postoperative patients with this disease than had been previously noted, an indication, perhaps, that fewer spontaneous cases required hospitalization.[230] Their operative mortality was 62%, whereas those who did not require surgical intervention had a mortality of only 14%. Because of the high incidence of associated cardiovascular diseases, the authors emphasize the importance of early diagnosis, as well as careful monitoring, to

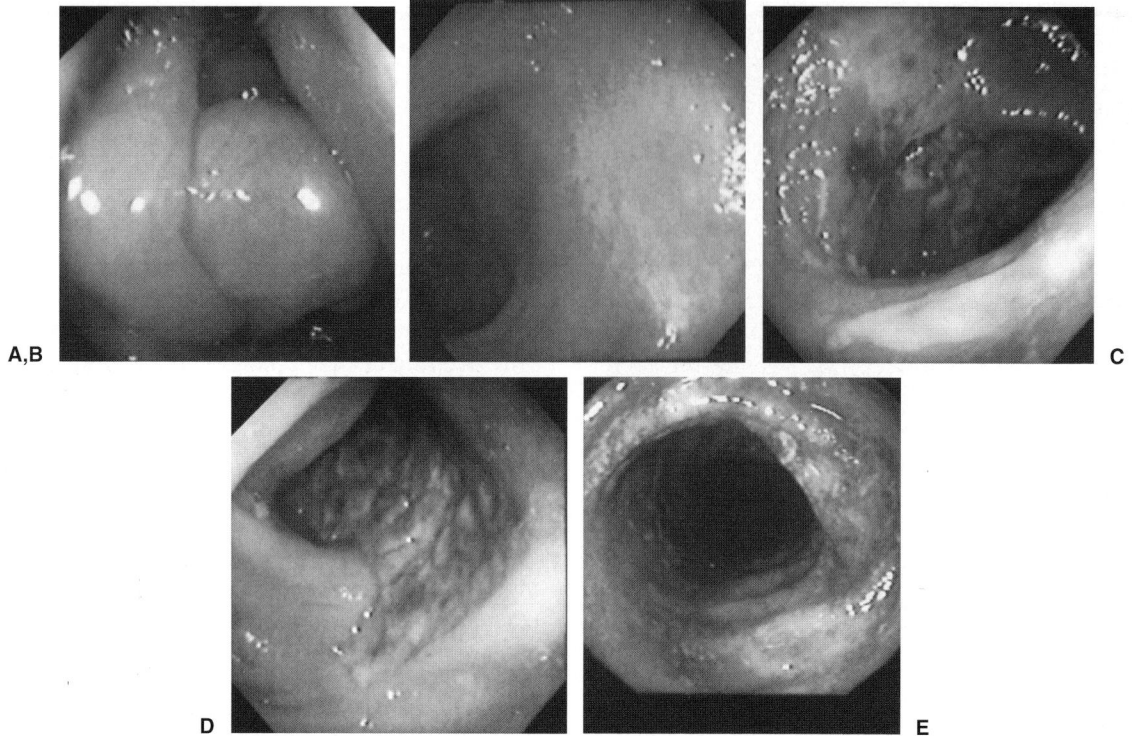

FIGURE 28-26. Colonoscopy reveals all of the characteristic changes of ischemic colitis in the region of the sigmoid colon of the same patient. **(A)** Edema. **(B)** Hyperemia. **(C)** Contact bleeding. **(D)** Mucosal pallor and necrosis. **(E)** Hemorrhagic, ulcerated mucosa. The condition is difficult to differentiate from inflammatory bowel disease. (See Color Fig. 28-26.)

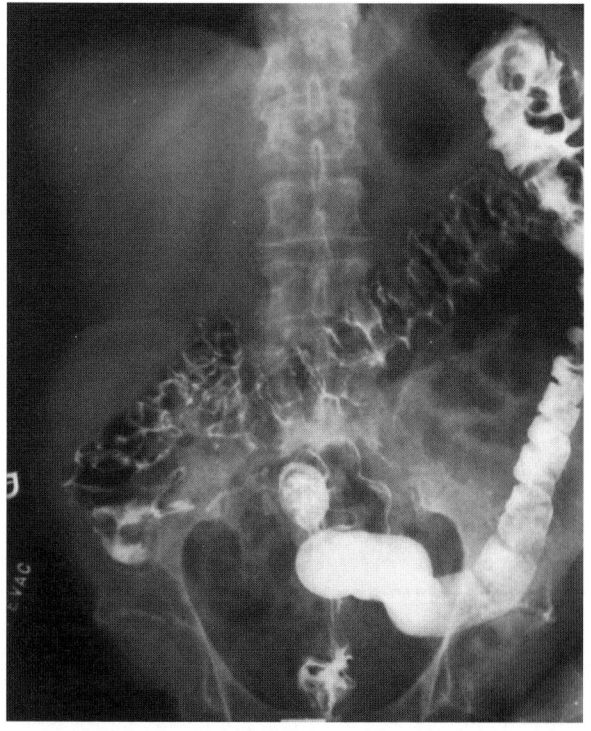

FIGURE 28-27. Ischemic colitis. Postevacuation barium enema showing characteristic thumbprinting from cecum to proximal descending colon.

improve the survival figures. Longo and co-workers identified 47 patients with nonocclusive ischemia of the large intestine over a 7-year period at Yale University School of Medicine.[177] Almost half of the patients had right colon involvement. Fifteen of 16 were successfully treated non-operatively with bowel rest and antibiotics, but one died. The remainder required bowel resection, of which almost one-half had their intestinal continuity reestablished. There was a 29% operative mortality. Others have observed that the right colon appears to be the most severely affected area in this condition. Landreneau and Fry expressed an opinion about the possibility of a "mesenteric steal" from more proximal branches of the superior mesenteric arterial circulation during periods of compromised perfusion as the reason for this distribution.[169] It is evident that if operative intervention is required for ischemic colitis, it is associated with a very high mortality rate, probably because of the fact that many patients are elderly and have multisystem diseases.[178,201]

Ischemic Colitis and Surgery of the Abdominal Aorta

Ischemic colitis may develop following resection of an abdominal aortic aneurysm.[57,109,140,163,171,330] The incidence of this complication has been variously reported

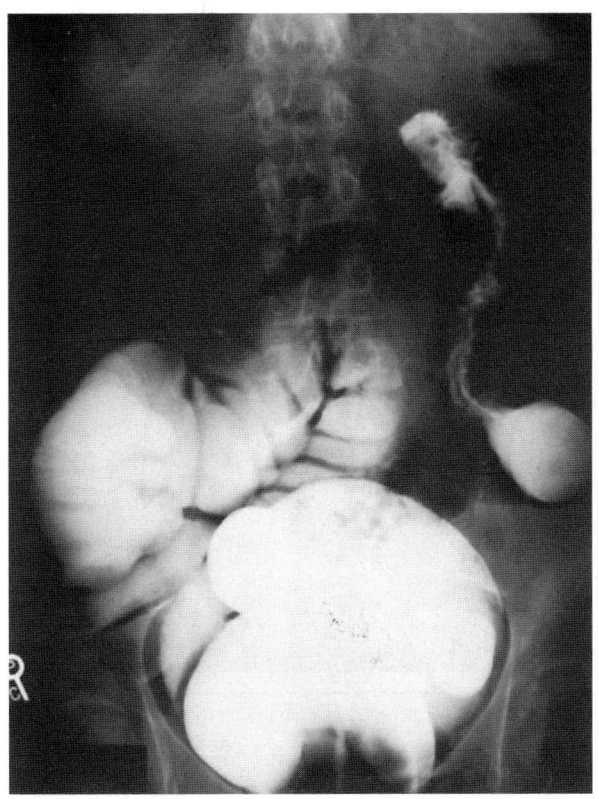

FIGURE 28-28. Ischemic colitis. Barium enema reveals thumbprinting of the splenic flexure, and edema and spasm of the descending colon. Note the preservation of mucosa.

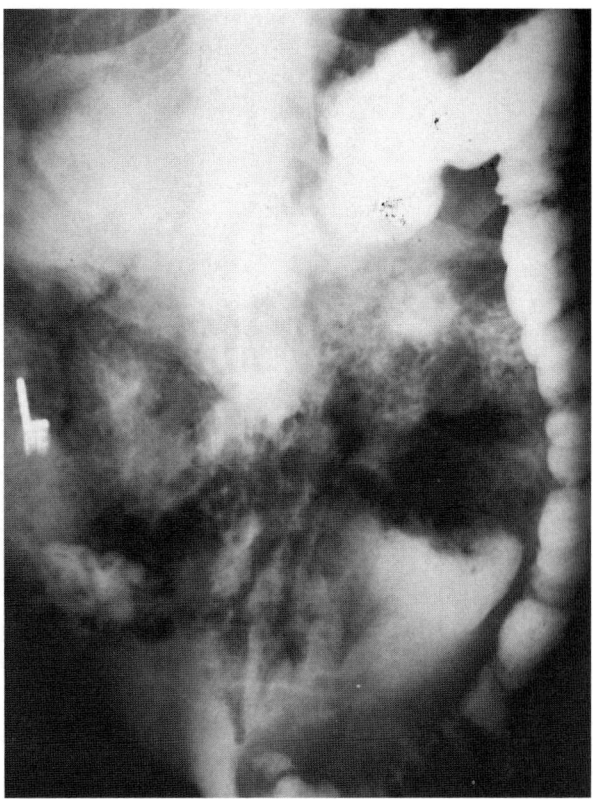

FIGURE 28-29. Ischemic colitis. Transverse colon perforation. Note the extravasation of barium into the peritoneal cavity. (The marker is on the wrong side.)

to be from less than 1% to more than 25%. The higher rates are usually associated with other factors, such as the prolonged hypotension that often accompanies the management of ruptured aneurysm. The changes may be reversible or, as with ischemic colitis not associated with aneurysmectomy, may subsequently lead to stricture, gangrene, or perforation. The combination of intraabdominal sepsis with a prosthetic vascular graft is potentially catastrophic. With a mortality rate of 75%, this complication may account for as many as one-fourth of the deaths following operations performed on the aorta.[271]

Diagnosis and Prevention

Recommendations for preventing this complication at the time of surgery have included reimplantation of the inferior mesenteric artery if it is large, measurement of the stump pressure, Doppler ultrasound, indirect measurement of pH in the wall of the sigmoid colon, and preservation of the first branch of the vessel.[105,266,271] Unfortunately, inferior mesenteric artery reimplantation does not guarantee colon viability in aortic surgery, im-

plying that other issues, such as intraoperative hypotension, may be an important factor.[205]

Rectal bleeding within the first 72 hours following aneurysmectomy is a characteristic symptom that mandates investigation. Forde and colleagues suggest that colonoscopy is a particularly useful technique for establishing the diagnosis of ischemic colitis in the postoperative period.[109] The findings are similar to those previously described: the rectum and distal sigmoid colon are often spared, with more proximal mucosal ulceration apparent. Dark blue or black nodular areas are suggestive of possible gangrene. The serum D-lactate level has also been shown to have predictive value as an early marker of bowel ischemia after ruptured abdominal aortic aneurysm repair.[238]

Ernst and associates undertook a prospective study on 50 patients to determine the incidence of this complication.[102] Colonoscopic examination was performed within 4 days of operation; three patients had evidence of ischemia (6%). Arteriographic evaluation of collateral circulation by the superior mesenteric artery revealed that colon ischemia did not develop when the collateral blood supply was identified. These authors suggest that despite the relative rarity of clinically significant colitis following

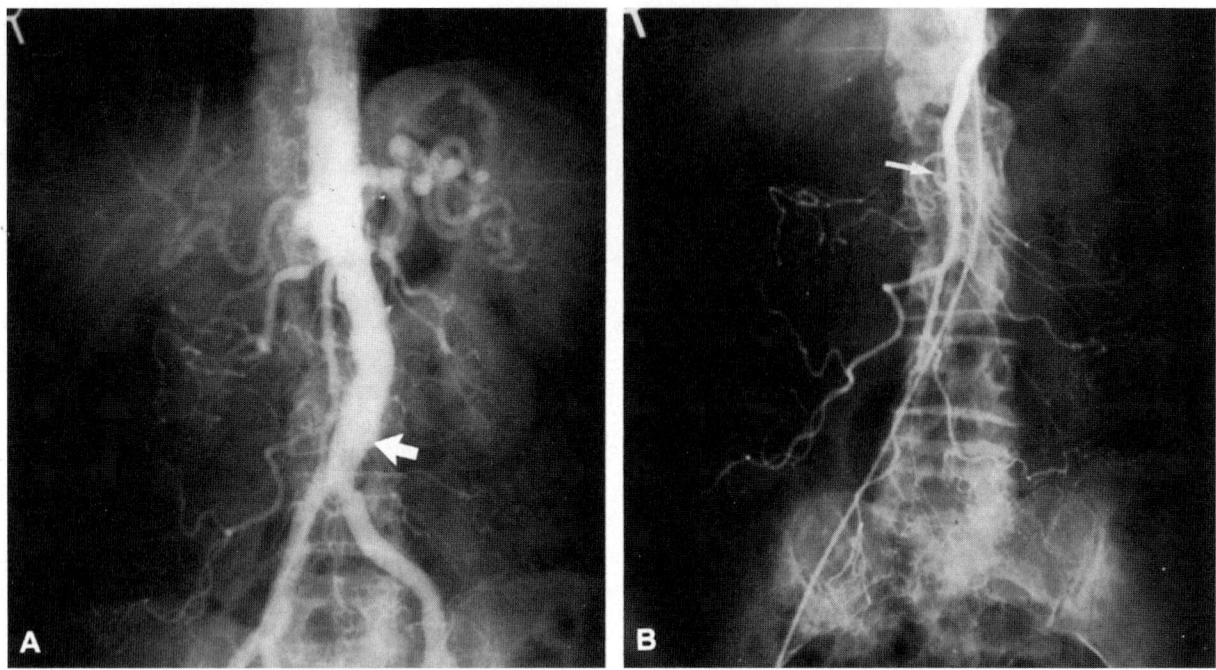

FIGURE 28-30. Ischemic colitis. **(A)** Aortogram shows occluded inferior mesenteric artery (*arrow*). **(B)** Superior mesenteric angiogram demonstrates occlusion of the middle colic artery (*arrow*).

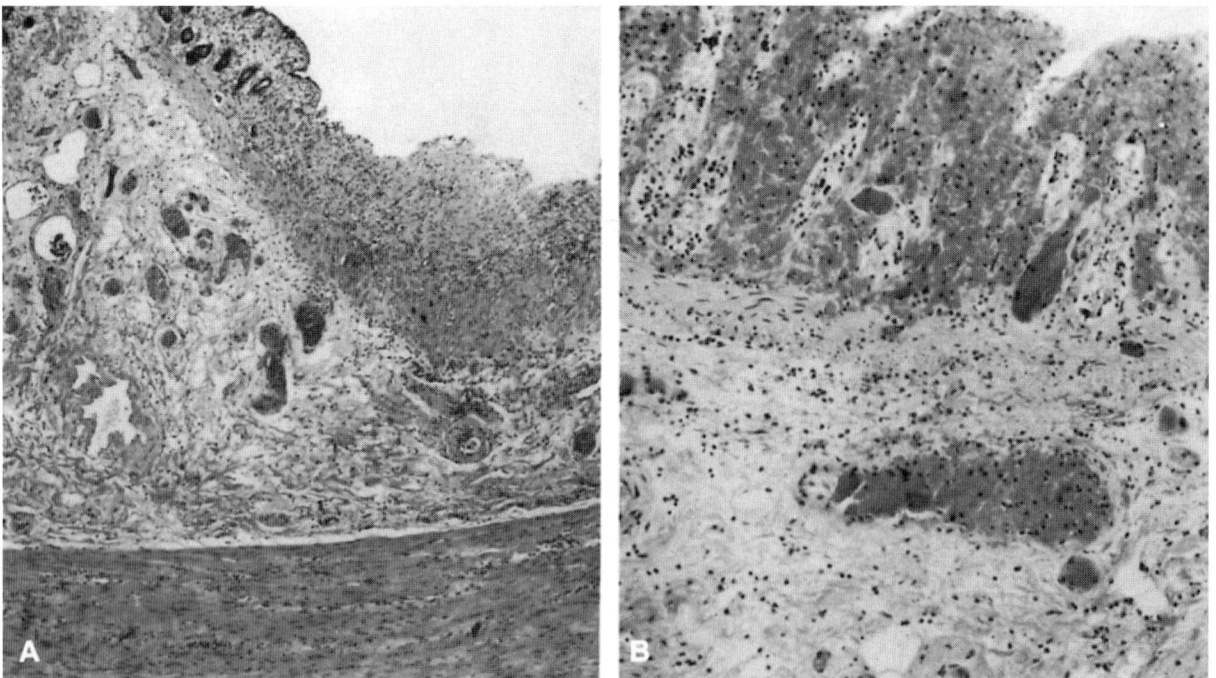

FIGURE 28-31. Ischemic colitis. **(A)** Superficial necrosis and ulceration of mucosa with congested submucosal blood vessels. Muscularis propria is viable. (Original magnification × 100.) **(B)** Necrosis of full thickness of mucosa with retention of ghost outline of epithelium. (Original magnification × 260.)

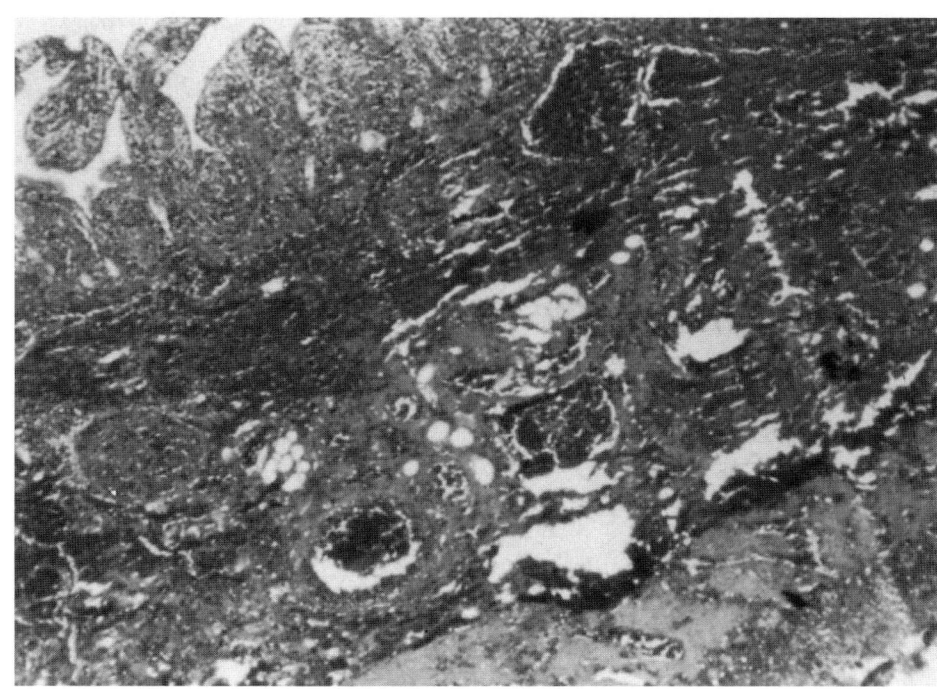

FIGURE 28-32. Ischemic colitis. Necrosis of full thickness of bowel wall. Note hemorrhage and dilated blood vessels. (Original magnification × 80.) (Courtesy of Rudolf Garret, M.D.)

aortic reconstruction, colonoscopy may be of value for early detection of possible ischemic changes so that therapy might, if necessary, be initiated sooner. In a study of postoperative colonoscopy following abdominal aortic reconstruction, Hagihara and colleagues determined that 11 of 163 patients who underwent reconstruction of the abdominal aorta demonstrated ischemic changes (7%).[140] These authors implied that the incidence might have been even higher if all patients surviving resection of ruptured abdominal aneurysms had undergone postoperative colonoscopy. In another prospective study by Welch and associates (Manchester Royal Infirmary), colonic ischemia was identified *histologically* in biopsies from 16 of 53 patients (30%) who underwent elective infrarenal aortic surgery.[328] In a retrospective review by Brewster and colleagues from the Massachusetts General Hospital, 0.9% of patients had overt ischemia.[57]

Kim and colleagues analyzed the risk factors for the development of ischemia of the colon following abdominal aortic resection for aneurysm.[163] Prolonged cross-clamp time, hypoxemia, rupture of the aneurysm, hypotension, and arrhythmia occurred with significantly greater frequency among the patients with ischemia than among control subjects. Schiedler and colleagues compared intramural pH measured through a silicone balloon placed in the lumen of the sigmoid colon with risk factor analysis and inferior mesenteric artery stump pressures as predictors of ischemic colitis in 34 patients undergoing elective or emergency operations on the abdominal aorta.[266] Logistic regression analysis demonstrated that aortic aneurysm, age, and stenosis of the superior mesenteric artery were the only risk factors that bore a statistical relationship to the development of ischemic colitis.[266]

Treatment

When colonic ischemia occurs as a consequence of surgery on the abdominal aorta, a high index of suspicion is required, and treatment must be initiated promptly and aggressively. As implied from the foregoing, when the condition is recognized intraoperatively, the problem can be handled in one of two ways. One option is to remove the inferior mesenteric artery from its origin, along with a cuff of aorta, and to reimplant it into the aortic prosthesis.[171] One can also consider the possibility of vascular reconstruction by means of endarterectomy and angioplasty. The other obvious alternative is to resect the diseased segment of bowel when the lack of viability becomes apparent.

Brewster and colleagues reviewed the experience with intestinal ischemia complicating abdominal aortic surgery at the Massachusetts General Hospital.[57] Of the more than 2,000 patients who underwent abdominal aortic reconstruction, 1.1% had overt intestinal ischemia documented by reoperation or by endoscopic findings. In the group of five individuals recognized to have colonic ischemia during surgery, three with a patent inferior mesenteric artery (IMA) on preoperative angiography underwent IMA reimplantation. Another underwent sigmoid resection with colostomy, and the fifth underwent repair of the marginal artery. All those in this category did well. Of the 14 patients with the diagnosis of ischemia made after the vascular procedure, one-half were managed nonoperatively. Three recovered without complication, and four developed colonic stricture. Half required resection for this complication. The remainder underwent resection for transmural infarction. The mortality rate on these individuals was 57%. Therefore, looking at the entire group, if reoperation was required, the mortality rate was 50%.[57]

It would therefore seem self-evident that every effort to determine the adequacy of the circulation to the colon during operations on the aorta remains the primary goal.

Ischemic Proctitis

As discussed earlier, generally the rectum is spared from ischemia because of the collateral blood supply. Fewer than 50 cases have been reported that extended to the level of the dentate line. The implication of this manifestation in such a distal location is inadequate collateral circulation.

Diagnosis is usually made by the characteristic appearance on proctosigmoidoscopy. In four of six patients identified with this acute ischemic proctitis by Nelson and colleagues, surgical interruption of splanchnic blood flow due to aortoiliac disease was the primary precipitating event.[214] When ischemia of the rectum occurs, the symptoms and pathologic changes are identical to that which has been described for the colon. Treatment usually involves correction of the underlying problem and expectant management, but a single case of hemorrhagic proctitis as a consequence of ischemia was satisfactorily treated with the topical installation of 4% formalin.[74]

Ischemic Colitis: Collagen Vascular Diseases

The collagen vascular diseases represent a collection of conditions that are believed to be due to pathologic alterations in the immune system. They can occur in any organ and may be associated with varied GI complaints. The conditions can affect the blood supply to the colon and produce ischemic changes either isolated to this organ or as part of the systemic process. These diseases included polyarteritis nodosa, cryoglobulinemia, Henoch-Schönlein purpura, Behçet's syndrome, systemic lupus erythematosus, polymyositis, and scleroderma (Figure 28-33).[187,188,226,246] Colonic ischemia in the setting of collagen vascular diseases is usually caused by a vasculitis or, less commonly, thrombosis.[128] Deposition of immune complexes in blood vessel walls is the most widely accepted pathogenic mechanism. This can lead

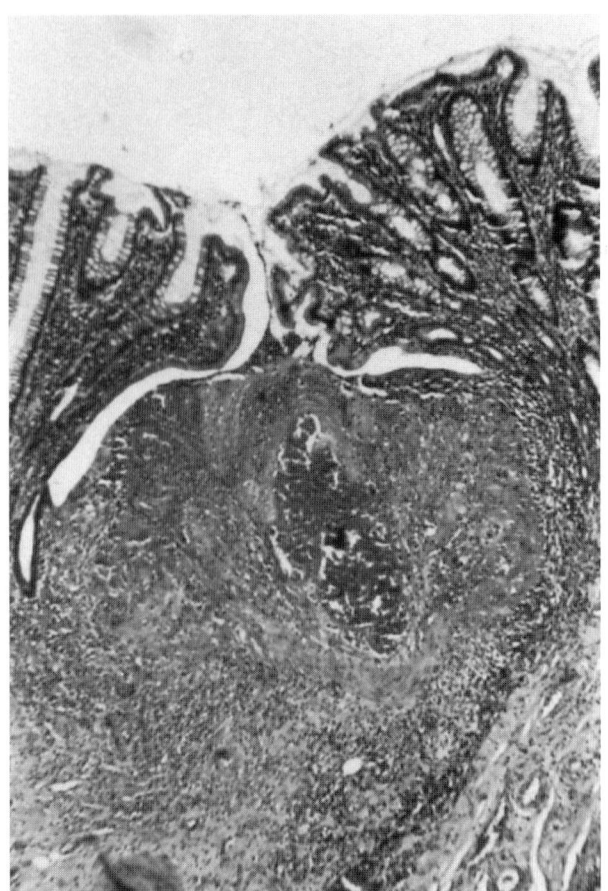

FIGURE 28-33. Polyarteritis nodosa. Blood vessel showing fibrinoid necrosis of the wall with surrounding exudate and superficial ulceration of overlying mucosa. (Original magnification × 120.) (Courtesy of Rudolf Garret, M.D.)

to hemorrhage, infarction with perforation, or problems with functional colonic disorders such as inertia (see Chapter 16).[176]

Medical management is usually the primary therapy, but on occasion a patient will require surgical intervention for hemorrhage, obstruction, necrosis, or perforation.

If surgery does become necessary for acute abdominal complications of polyarteritis nodosa, the prognosis is grim. Zizic and colleagues noted no survivors because of involvement by extensive segments of gangrenous bowel.[342] Approximately one-half of the patients with SLE who had acute abdomens died.

When GI manifestations are complications of Behçet's disease the prognosis is poor.[55] Patients may present with mesenteric ischemia and infarction because of large-vessel disease or with mucosal disease as a result of small-vessel involvement. The condition usually affects the right side of the colon. Hence, it must be differentiated from Crohn's disease. Iida and colleagues studied the postoperative course of intestinal Behçet's disease in nine individuals.[152] Eighty percent developed recurrence of intestinal ulcers. In most instances these were at or near the anastomotic site. But the mainstay of therapy is medical: corticosteroids, immunosuppressants, and anti-inflammatory medications.

RADIATION ENTERITIS

You have to operate your way in and then operate your way out.

Rubert B. Turnbull (commenting on surgery after radiation)

Radiation injuries to the GI tract are among the most difficult management problems facing the surgeon. It is not uncommon for the patient to suffer the deleterious effects of ionizing radiation long after the primary disease process for which the radiation was employed had been cured. Radiation is indeed a two-edged sword. Because of the serious consequences and the late complications (which are sometimes lethal), many surgeons have been reluctant to employ this modality if another alternative is felt to be reasonably efficacious.

Radiation damage is cumulative and progressive. A finite amount of radiation is tolerable, beyond which additional radiotherapy at any time following the initial treatment may precipitate complications. Certain conditions, such as diabetes mellitus, hypertension, and previous abdominal surgery, are believed to predispose the bowel to radiation injury.[20] Other factors that increase the risk include infection, single portal therapy, overlapping portals of therapy, poorly calibrated or uncalibrated dosimeters, inadequate vaginal packing during implants, the presence of intra-abdominal adhesions (by fixing loops of bowel), concomitant chemotherapy, and overlooking signals of distress or masking them by overmedication.[257,301]

It has been estimated that 50% of all cancer patients will receive radiotherapy at some stage during their illness.[103] That figure today may be conservative, in light of the increased application of combined therapy. The incidence of radiation enteritis may be increasing according to the experience of Galland and Spencer at the Hammersmith Hospital.[116] This, they believe, can be attributed to the combination of internal and external treatment, and to the technique of "afterloading." Virtually all who undergo radiation to the abdomen will develop early symptoms of radiation injury to the bowel, and 5% to 20% will have long-term sequelae of radiation enteritis.[83,103,210]

Patients receiving more than 50 Gy are most likely to develop this complication. All individuals are not equally susceptible to intestinal radiation injury, however. For example, children are more likely to have complications associated with radiation enteritis,[98] and people with light complexions are more sensitive than those with dark.[268]

Historically, cervical cancer has been the most commonly radiated lesion and thus is associated with the most radiation complications. Schmitz and colleagues reported that the original diseases in their 37 patients with radiation injuries were cervical carcinoma in 29 and endometrial carcinoma in eight.[268] Other primary diseases for which radiation therapy may subsequently produce problems include carcinoma of the endometrium, carcinoma of the bladder, carcinoma of the rectum or rectosigmoid, prostatic cancer, ovarian cancer, and carcinoma of the anal canal (Figure 28-34). In a review by Hayne and co-workers based on a literature search (Medline), more than three-fourths of patients receiving pelvic radiotherapy experience acute anorectal symptoms, and up to one-fifth suffer from late-phase radiation proctitis.[145] Approximately 5% develop other complications, such as fistula, stricture, and fecal incontinence.

Marks and Mohiudden reported that the most common area of injury was the ileum, followed by the rectum, rectosigmoid, cecum, sigmoid colon, and jejunum.[193] The most common lesion noted in the Cleveland Clinic experience was proctitis; other complications included ulceration, stricture, and fistula to the vagina, bladder, or both.[172] Others have reported that although the small bowel is more sensitive to irradiation, the most common site of injury is the rectum, owing to its fixity in the pelvis.[20,301] Since lymphoid tissue is extremely sensitive to the effects of radiation and there is a high concentration of lymphoid tissue in Peyer's patches, the explanation becomes evident for the frequency of terminal ileal damage despite its relative mobility.[301]

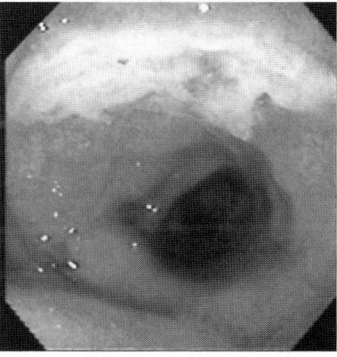

FIGURE 28-34. Endoscopy reveals a whitish area of scar surrounded by erythematous mucosa with evident stenosis characteristic of radiation proctitis. (See Color Fig. 28-34.)

Since radiotherapy has been only relatively recently advocated either as primary or as adjunctive therapy for carcinoma of the rectum, it is too soon to determine what the frequency of complications will be from its use. It is hoped that there will not be the incidence that has been seen hitherto for the treatment of carcinoma of the cervix and endometrium, primarily because of improved techniques of radiation administration. The use of multidirectional, sharply collimated, high-energy photon and electron beams allows concentration of the radiation to the tumor rather than to normal structures.[82] The treatment is facilitated by highly accurate computer-assisted dosimetric tumor localization systems, by individualized custom-blocking and visceral displacement techniques, and by progressively reducing the radiation field size during the treatment course.[82,251] Early onset of symptoms such as cramping or diarrhea and an objective confirmation of radiation changes on endoscopy or biopsy should alert the therapist to consider modification of the treatment plan by reducing the dose, increasing fractionation over longer periods of time, or temporarily interrupting the therapy.[210]

With respect to prevention, the techniques of administration of the radiation have already been mentioned. In addition, a number of substances may be given prophylactically that act as radioprotective agents. An elemental diet given during the course of the treatment has been demonstrated to be beneficial, but the mechanism of action of this is unclear.[116] Wiesmann and colleagues, in an experimental study on rats, documented the prevention of histologic changes with the use of an elemental diet, vitamin A, and sodium meclofenamate.[338] With respect to prevention in the patient being considered for postoperative radiation therapy, the surgeon should attempt to exclude the small intestine from the pelvis before closure of the abdomen (see Chapter 23).[92,93,251,296]

Symptoms

The symptoms of radiation injury depend on whether one is dealing with the acute process, usually occurring during the course of the treatment, or the result of therapy, weeks, months, or even years later. Nausea, vomiting, diarrhea, and cramping abdominal pain are seen in 75% of patients who undergo radiotherapy.[20] Because of complications of radiation to the small intestine, malabsorption, partial intestinal obstruction, and severe diarrhea may lead to malnutrition and fluid and electrolyte imbalance. Complete bowel obstruction may supervene. Depending on the site and type of radiation injury, patients may develop signs and symptoms of urinary fistula, vaginal fistula, anorectal ulcer, and many other manifestations.

One must also be wary of the asymptomatic patient who has undergone radiation therapy and who requires

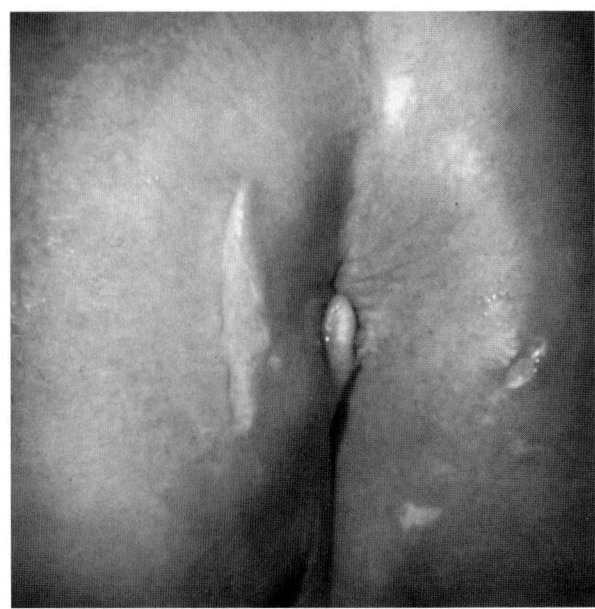

FIGURE 28-35. Erythema and linear ulcerations of the buttocks are evident in this patient who is undergoing radiation therapy for a carcinoma of the anal canal. Part of the lesion is apparent protuding from the anal verge. (See Color Fig. 28-35.)

an operation for another complaint. There is a serious risk of injuring previously irradiated bowel (see later). Even with the surgeon taking great care, the patient may develop a perforation while convalescing from an operation such as a lysis of adhesions.[114]

Evaluation

For disease involving the rectum or rectosigmoid, proctoscopic examination may reveal loss of vessel pattern, edema, contact bleeding, and telangiectasis (Figure 28-35). Ulceration and granularity may be noted. Later changes may include thickening of the rectal wall, stricture, or fistula into the vagina or into the bladder. Colonoscopy has been used for studying patients with presumed radiation colitis, particularly for bleeding and for inspection of a colonic stricture.[247] Endoscopic evidence of injury includes pallor of the mucosa, prominent submucosal telangiectatic vessels, friability, erythema, and granularity.

Radiologic studies performed during the course of therapy will usually not be helpful in identifying specific radiation changes. Increased irritability and motility of the small bowel are usually noted, and there may be some associated spasticity in the colon.[257] Months or years after the treatment, however, profound radiologic changes may be apparent on contrast study of the intestinal tract. Commonly involved areas include the sigmoid colon, rectum, and terminal ileum (Figure 28-36).

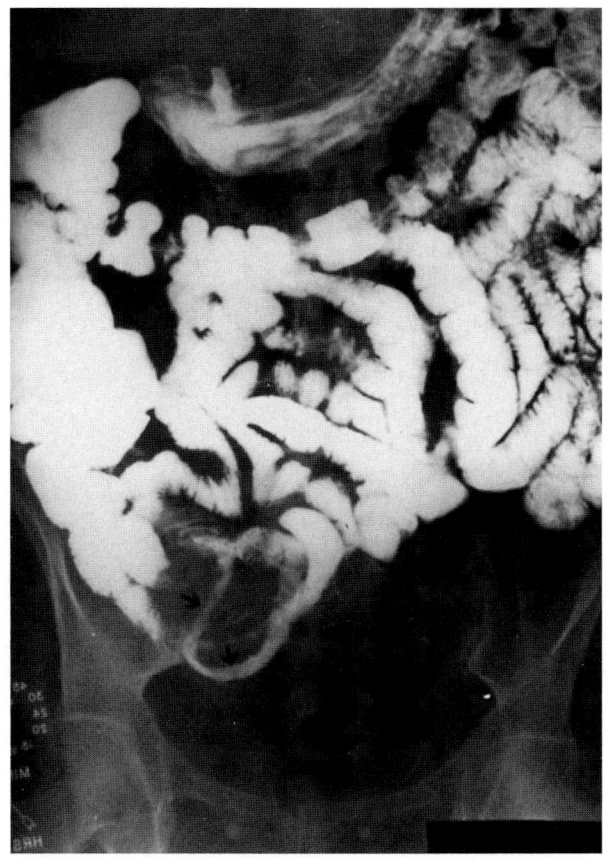

FIGURE 28-36. Radiation enteritis. Terminal ileal radiation changes include rigidity and edema of the bowel wall, apparent mass between loops (*arrows*), and destruction of the mucosal pattern.

Angiographic studies may reveal arterial and venous irregularity, beading and focal obstruction of the bowel wall vasculature, and crowding of vessels because of foreshortening of the intestine.[257]

Pathophysiology

Three phases of radiation effects have been identified: (a) acute, primarily affecting the mucosa; (b) subacute, with predominant effects in the submucosa; and (c) chronic, generally affecting all layers of the bowel wall.[193] Acute radiation enteritis is due to destruction of the rapidly dividing cells at the base of the crypts of the GI mucosa.[103] Destruction of cells that rapidly turn over and obliteration of blood vessels, combined with a fibroblastic response, are the events that produce the less acute and chronic manifestations.[73] Impaired regeneration of the irradiated mucosal epithelium may contribute to the erosions or ulcers, but progressive fibrosis and vascular lesions leading to ischemia are the most important factors.[44]

Depending on the phase, the changes may vary from a colitis with capillary dilatation, hemorrhage, edema, and inflammatory cell infiltration in the acute situation, to an ischemia from an obliterative endarteritis and fibrosis in the chronic (Figs. 28-37 through 28-39). The normal submucosal space may be altered by the deposition of dense hyaline material lacking the normal fibrillar structure of collagen.[165]

Recent studies in microbiology have been revealing with respect to the pathogenesis of radiation enteritis. By means of a literature search, Nguyen and colleagues attempted to identify factors that affect the disease process.[217] They observed that long-term complications are characterized by excessive stimulation of transforming growth factor (TGF-β1). They further suggest that interferon gamma (IFN-γ) inhibits the effects of TGF-β1 and may be ultimately clinically applicable in a treatment program for patients with radiation enteritis.

Surgical Treatment

Before operation it is important to evaluate the entire intestinal tract for the presence of associated radiation-induced abnormalities and for the possibility of recurrent primary disease. Upper GI x-ray, barium enema, and complete endoscopic examinations are necessary. Evaluation of the urinary tract is particularly important because of the high incidence of associated damage to the outflow tracts. The presence of ureteral obstruction necessitates cystoscopy and retrograde pyelography. Additionally, if a resection is attempted it is helpful to have ureteral catheters inserted at the time of operation (see Chapter 23). The presence of ureteral catheters does not, of course, guarantee that injury will be avoided, but it is reassuring to be able to palpate the catheters and know the locations of these important structures.

The most frequent indication for surgical intervention in a patient with radiation injury is the presence of a fistula to the vagina or to the bladder, but also to the skin and to other areas of the intestinal tract. Obstructive symptoms also often require surgical treatment.

The choice of procedure will depend on the level of the injury, the patient's prognosis, and the extent of radiation damage as determined at the time of exploration. There are five available options in the surgical management of radiation enteritis: primary closure (of a fistula), resection, bypass, exclusion, and diversionary stoma (ileostomy or colostomy) (Figure 28-40). A sixth alternative may be considered, that of strictureplasty. This has been described by the Cleveland Clinic Ohio Group in five patients with obstructing, diffuse radiation enteritis.[94] The technique is described in Chapter 30. It is generally agreed, however, that operations for radiation enteritis should be avoided except

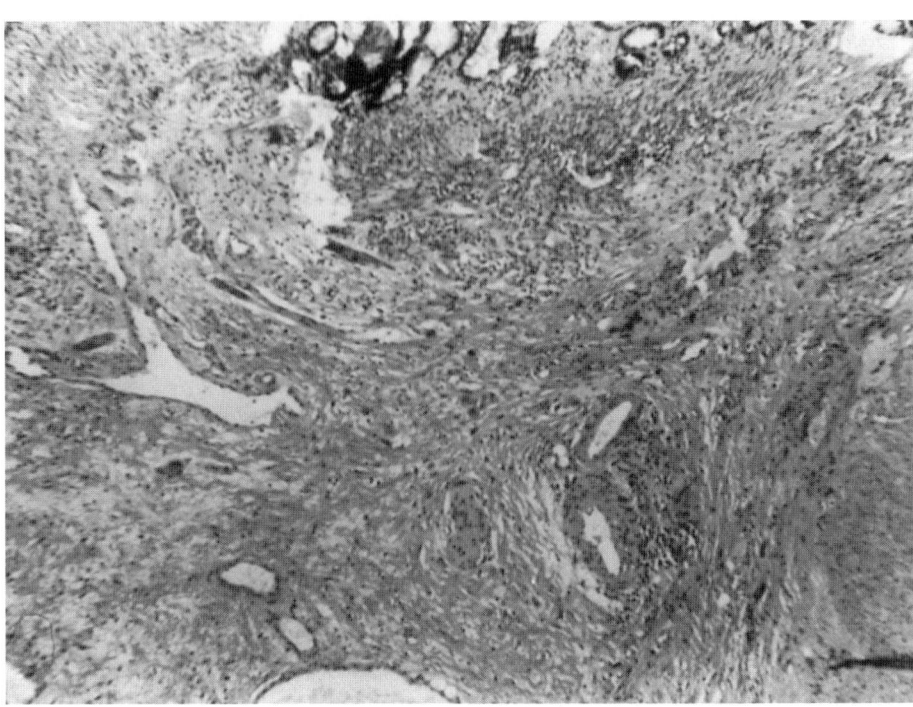

FIGURE 28-37. Radiation colitis. Subacute changes include fibrosis of the submucosa, sclerosis of blood vessels, and perivascular mononuclear cell infiltrate. (Original magnification × 240.) (Courtesy of Rudolf Garret, M.D.)

when complications develop. In fact, radiation enteropathy may be characterized by long, symptom-free intervals.[208] Morgenstern stressed a number of general principles that he thought should be employed, if possible, in the management of these patients; they are as follows[208]:

Avoid operation.
Achieve optimal preoperative nutritional status.

Use long intestinal tubes.
Use standard mechanical and antibiotic bowel preparation and postoperative systemic antibiotics.
Employ resection rather than bypass.
Resect rather than close fistulas.
Limit the amount of adhesiolysis.
Use meticulous anastomotic technique.
Identify the anastomosis with a radiopaque marker.

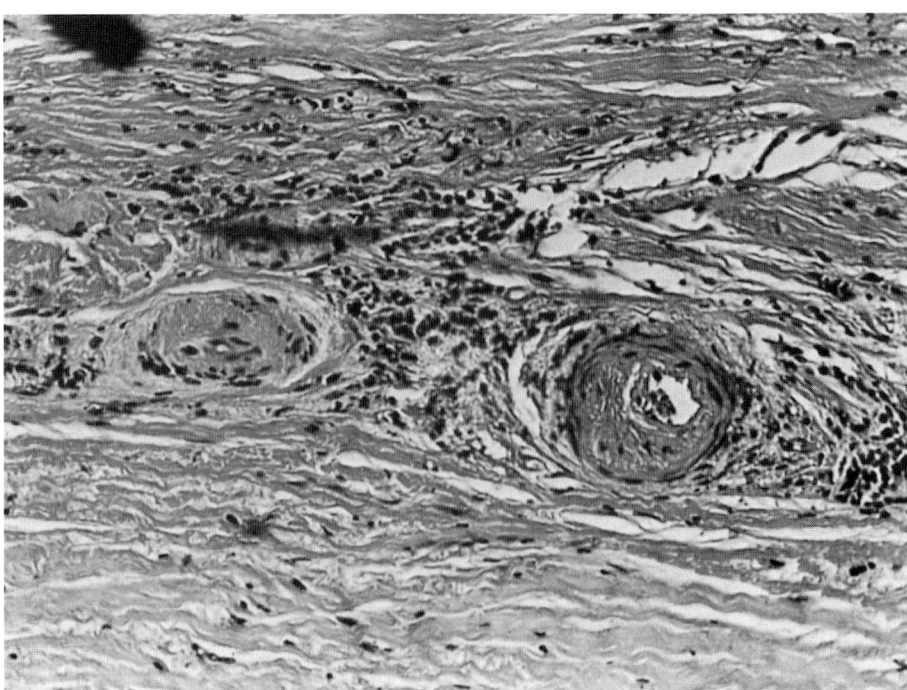

FIGURE 28-38. Radiation colitis. Chronic changes comprise fibrosis, dilatation of the lymphatics, and virtual obliteration of the blood vessels. (Original magnification × 280.) (Courtesy of Rudolf Garret, M.D.)

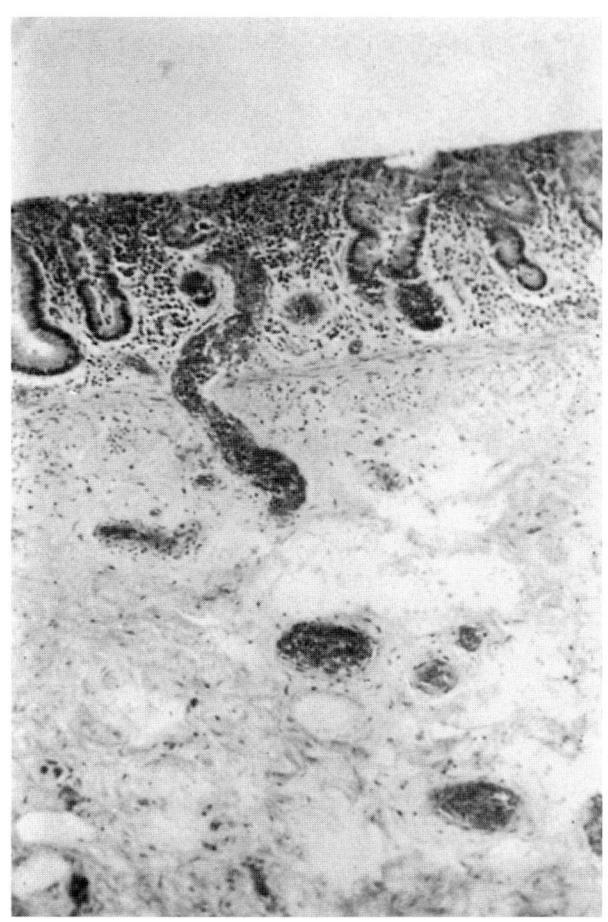

FIGURE 28-39. Radiation proctitis. Atrophy of the mucosa with fibrosis and telangiectasis of the submucosa. (Original magnification × 170.)

Delay postoperative oral alimentation; use prolonged long-tube decompression.
Avoid irradiated bowel for stomas.

Results

Characteristically, there is a tendency to underestimate the amount of damage produced by the radiation when examination of the serosal surface of the intestine is performed. If one is to anticipate a favorable result of the operation, all radiation-injured tissue must be adequately excised and an anastomosis effected in relatively normal bowel. Morgenstern and colleagues recommend, on the basis of their experience with 52 patients, if an anastomosis is required in the region of the terminal ileum, that it be performed in the colon in order to avoid a pelvic suture line.[209,210] Others have reported a lower incidence of leak with ileoileal anastomoses than with ileocolic, but it is impossible to evaluate the significance of this observation with small numbers of patients and with various clinical presentations.[144] Anastomotic leak rates are reported as high as 65%, with

mortality rates in excess of 50%, but there is general agreement today that if resection is performed, an ileocolonic anastomosis is preferred.[115,142]

Bypass operations often fail to relieve symptoms or are associated with recurrent problems.[115] Smith and DeCosse observed that 92% of individuals who harbored an enteric fistula and who underwent an exclusion procedure, without an extensive resection of small bowel, were successfully treated.[286] This compared with a success rate for resection of 67% and for bypass of 69%. Aitken and Elliot reported three patients who successfully underwent sigmoid exclusion for colovesical and colovaginal fistula.[5] The involved sigmoid colon was isolated on its mesentery, the ends closed, and a colorectal or coloanal anastomosis performed. By this technique a permanent stoma and a urinary conduit could be avoided.

Schmitt and Symmonds reported 93 patients with small bowel radiation enteritis.[267] More than two-thirds underwent intestinal resection, and 20 underwent bypass procedures. Adhesions were lysed in eight patients. Factors used to select the appropriate operative procedure included age and general medical condition; the location, extent, and degree of the radiation changes; and whether the procedure was carried out on an elective or an emergency basis. Anastomotic dehiscence occurred in 10 patients, and there were six operative deaths. Cram and associates reviewed their experience with 89 patients with radiation injury to the bowel, of whom 31 required surgical intervention.[83] These authors tended to perform a resection or a bypass for small bowel disease, and a colostomy for large bowel involvement. Although they conceded that the "conservative" approach to large bowel radiation injury is not universally accepted, they felt that the high rates of morbidity and mortality associated with resection, and the requirement for possibly multiple procedures, impelled them to adopt this particular approach.

Wellwood and Jackson reported their experience with 38 patients with intestinal complications after radiotherapy, noting a mortality rate of 37%.[331] These authors advise formation of a combined surgical–radiotherapy clinic to monitor and investigate those at risk. They also suggested that prompt radiologic investigation of the intestinal tract be performed if symptoms suggestive of radiation damage are elicited. Tests for malabsorption should also be performed. A number of papers attest to the high morbidity associated with surgical intervention and the need for liberal implementation of a diversionary stoma.[84,143,164,183,203]

Home parenteral nutrition has been advocated for the treatment of patients with severe radiation enteritis.[172] Five individuals were reported from the Cleveland Clinic who would have been unable to survive their severe state of malnutrition without this treatment. They were not considered candidates for surgical intervention because of extensive disease and their poor nutritional state. One

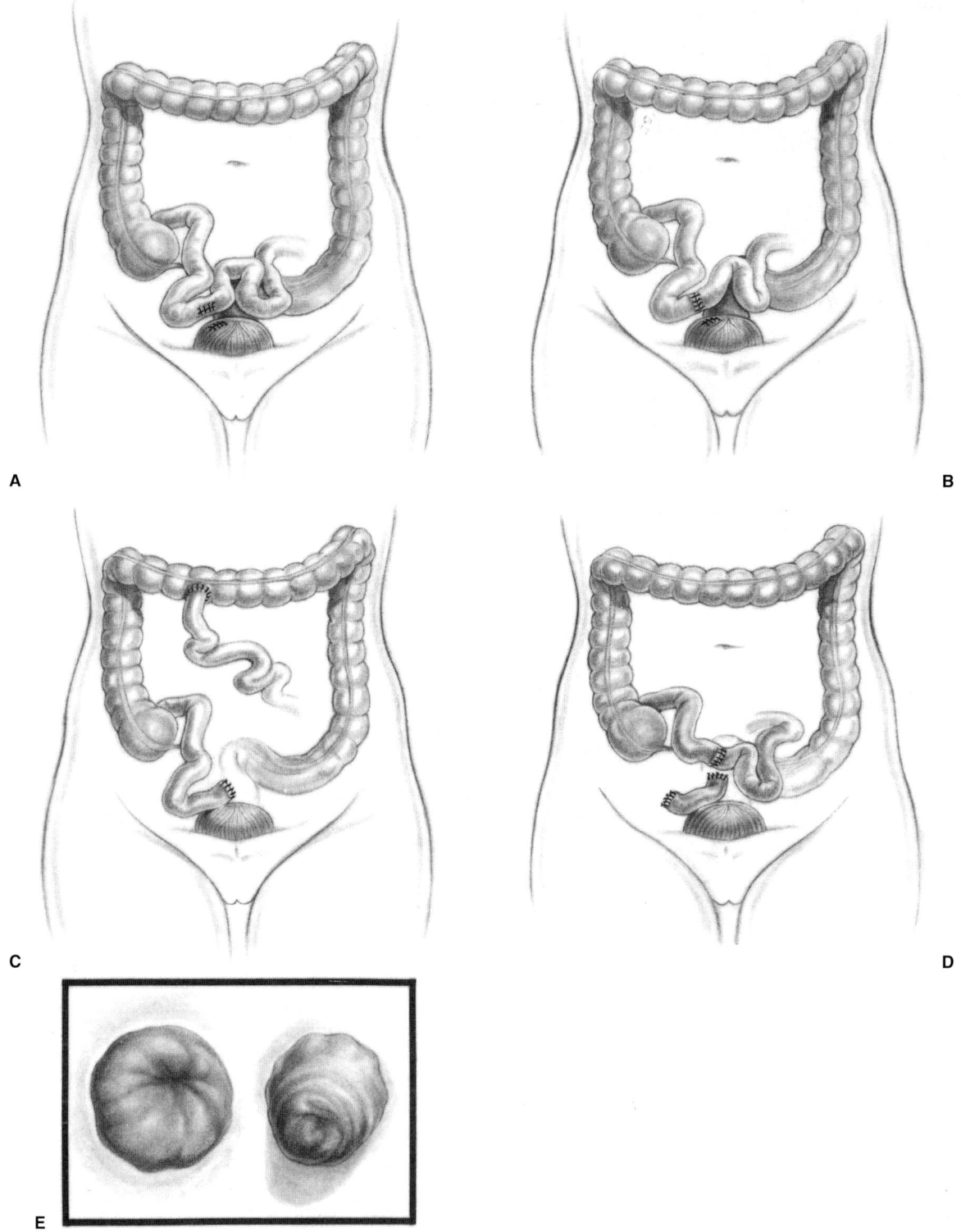

FIGURE 28-40. Options in the surgical management of radiation enteritis with vesical fistulous. **(A)** Closure of fistulous communication. **(B)** Resection. **(C)** Bypass. **(D)** Exclusion. **(E)** Colostomy or ileostomy.

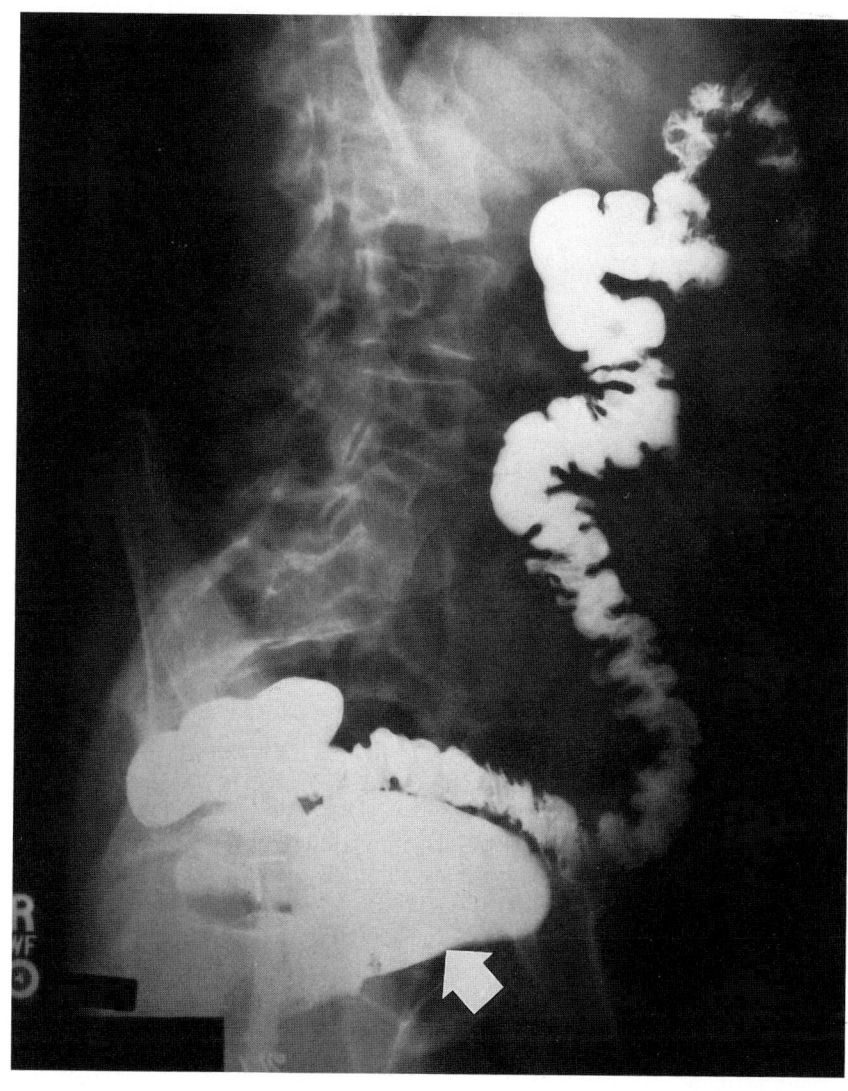

FIGURE 28-41. Recto-vesical fistula. Barium enema demonstrates contrast material filling the bladder (*arrow*) from a fistula located in the distal rectum. Patient had undergone intensive radiation therapy for prostatic cancer.

patient died of recurrent carcinoma after 14 months, and another died as a result of a pharmaceutical error after 30 months. The other three remained free of morbidity (attributed to the parenteral nutrition) at the time of the follow-up report.

RADIATION PROCTITIS

Because of its fixed position, the rectum is particularly vulnerable to the effects of radiation. Ulcerative proctitis secondary to radiation-induced injury may produce symptoms of rectal bleeding, abdominal pain, diarrhea, passage of mucus, rectal pain, incontinence, and tenesmus.[162] Stricture, obstruction, and fistula formation into the bladder, urethra, or vagina are potential consequences of chronic radiation injury (Figure 28-41). It is an extremely troublesome condition to treat.

Manometric studies confirm a significant reduction in the rectal volume at sensory threshold, suggesting that this reduction and poor compliance are responsible for the frequency and urgency.[319] Dysfunction of the internal anal sphincter from damage to the myenteric plexus can contribute further to the symptoms caused by abnormalities of rectal function.[320]

Treatment

Management is usually directed to dietary measures, the addition of "slowing" medications for diarrhea, bulk agents, stool softeners, iron replacement if anemia is a concern, and antispasmodics. Oral vitamin A therapy, 8,000 IU twice daily, has been successfully employed in one instance for an individual in the healing of a postradiation anal ulcer.[174]

The primary complaint that often demands attention, if not concern, is rectal bleeding. Retention enemas containing hydrocortisone have been recommended, but I have not found them particularly helpful. Approximately one-third of the patients treated by Allen-Mersh and colleagues with a similar regimen had their symptoms resolve within a period of 2 years.[11] Many individuals need only be reassured that they are not harboring a recurrent tumor and that bleeding may be a symptom with which they can and should live in peace.

A number of other topical approaches to the control of symptoms associated with radiation proctitis have been offered, including sulfasalazine, tranexamic acid, and sucralfate enemas, but the efficacy of these approaches has not been well documented.

Formalin

Topical formalin has been used successfully for a number of years to control intractable hemorrhagic cystitis. In recent years a number of publications have appeared that suggest that rectal bleeding may be controlled by the topical administration of this agent.[186,227,258,261,277] One approach consists of irrigation with a total of 2 liters of 3.6% formalin solution for 15 minutes, followed by irrigation with sodium chloride solution.[258] Another consists of the application of gauze soaked in 4% formalin, laid in contact with the hemorrhagic surface until the bleeding ceases.[277] Success was reported in seven of eight patients by this initial application according to Seow-Choen and colleagues.[277] Saclarides and associates instilled 500 mL of a 4% formalin solution in 50-mL aliquots in 16 patients.[261] Each aliquot was kept in contact with the rectal mucosa for approximately 30 seconds. Success was identified in 75%, but four developed significant postoperative anal pain. Parikh and co-workers reported 36 patients treated for bleeding from radiation proctitis with topical application of a cotton pledget soaked in 4% formalin.[227] There were no complications, with 88% reporting improvement or cessation of symptoms. Others report equally satisfactory results.[186]

Short-Chain Fatty Acid

Short-chain fatty acids have been described as having a pivotal role in the regulation of mucosal proliferation and providing more than half the energy requirements of the mucosa.[322] The application of this concept through the rectal instillation of butyrate enemas for radiation proctitis would seem to be a logical conclusion. Vernia and associates (Milan, Italy) undertook a randomized, cross-over, double-blind study involving 20 patients with radiation proctitis through the use of a 3-week course of sodium butyrate enemas (80 mmol/L).[322] A

statistically significant benefit was achieved with respect to symptoms, endoscopic appearance, and histology. Pinto and colleagues (Lisbon, Portugal) opined, also in a prospective, randomized, double-blind, controlled trial, that short-chain fatty acid enemas can accelerate the process of healing, but treatment must be continuous to obtain a sustained and complete response.[237] Still, at 6 months, no differences in the two groups were observed. However, Talley and co-workers (Sydney, Australia), in a randomized, double-blind, placebo-controlled, cross-over pilot trial with the use of a 2-week course of butyric acid enemas (40 mmol) twice a day, failed to demonstrate any benefit when compared with a placebo.[300]

Laser Photocoagulation

Those who fail to respond to noninvasive or minimally invasive treatment can be offered the possibility of laser therapy to control symptoms of bleeding caused by radiation proctitis.[9,43,65,66,222,298,308] The procedure can be performed via the flexible sigmoidoscope. Both the argon laser and the Nd-YAG laser have proved effective, but Buchi recommends the former, because it has a superficial penetration and is selectively absorbed by hemoglobin, thereby effectively coagulating the mucosal vascular lesions without injuring the underlying submucosa or bowel wall.[65]

Taïeb and co-workers (Grenoble, France) successfully managed 11 such individuals who failed to respond to less invasive measures (mean follow-up, 19 months).[298] Tjandra and Sengupta also noted significant reduction in the severity and frequency of the bleeding in their 12 patients (median follow-up, 11 months).[308] Dent and associates (Canberra, Australia) undertook a prospective Rectal Bleeding Quality of Life Scale patient-completed questionnaire in those who underwent laser or formalin therapy for radiation-induced rectal bleeding.[89] They found a significant improvement with respect to the quality of life reported by these individuals.

Hyperbaric Oxygen

Another option that has been offered in the approach to the management of radiation proctitis as well as radiation colitis is hyperbaric oxygenation. Nakada and colleagues employed this therapy, which consisted of 100% oxygen inhalation at two absolute atmospheric pressures for 90 minutes daily for 30 days.[213] Although the treatment succeeded in alleviating the hemorrhage problem and reversed the endoscopic changes, it is difficult to know whether such an occurrence would have taken place in the absence of this treatment. Others, however, have reported successful healing of anal ulcers that re-sisted conservation treatment.[39]

Operative Approaches

A number of operative approaches to the management of radiation injuries to the rectum have been suggested: clo-sure of a fistula by transrectal, transvaginal, transperi-neal, and transcoccygeal approaches (see Chapters 11 and 23); and resection with restoration of continuity by the abdominosacral procedure, by abdominoanal pull-through, and by coloendoanal anastomosis.[58,104]

Cuthbertson suggests that the pull-through resection with delayed anastomosis is the optimal procedure, but his experience is limited to that of four patients.[85] Jao and colleagues reported 720 patients from the Mayo Clinic with radiation-induced proctitis, 8.6% of whom re-quired surgical intervention.[159] These 62 individuals un-derwent a total of 143 operations with eight operative deaths (13%). The morbidity rate was lower after colostomy alone (44%) than after a more aggressive re-section (80%). An upper abdominal stoma was safer than a sigmoid colostomy.

Anseline and colleagues reported the Cleveland Clinic experience of 104 patients with radiation injuries to the rectum as a result of therapy for gynecologic or urologic malignancy.[20] Fifty were treated surgically, and 54 were treated conservatively. The authors concluded that diver-sion was the safest form of treatment for rectovaginal fis-tula, rectal stricture, and proctitis that had been unrespon-sive to medical measures. High rates of morbidity and mortality were recorded in those who underwent resection.

Marks recommends a combined abdominotranssacral reconstruction for the radiation-injured rectum (see Chap-ter 23).[192] He emphasizes the importance of excising all ra-diation-injured tissue, performing an anastomosis in nor-mal bowel, mobilizing the splenic flexure, use of ureteral catheters, and obligatory implementation of a diversionary procedure. The author also suggests avoiding retention su-tures if at all possible, and instead using delayed primary wound closure or permitting the skin to heal by second in-tention. He and Mohiudden reviewed their experience with more than 100 patients and noted a very low morbidity and mortality rate, considerably at variance with virtually all other published data.[193] There was not a single instance of a failed intraperitoneal anastomosis, and only four of 52 abdominotranssacral anastomoses developed a complica-tion.[193] Lucarotti and colleagues recommend using a coloanal J-reservoir to permit a safer anastomosis with op-timal functional results (see Chapter 23).[183]

Cooke and deMoor reported 37 patients with radiation damage to the rectum, 28 of whom had rectovaginal fis-tulas.[80] Treatment involved resection with restoration of continuity by means of coloanal anastomosis. They noted technical success in all but two individuals with no mor-tality. Although some patients had impairment of fecal continence, the overwhelming result was favorable. Con-tinued success was evident in a later presentation from the same institution with 59 patients.[81] Faucheron and co-workers (Paris, France) prefer Soave's procedure, hav-ing performed this operation in 30 patients with radia-tion-induced rectal lesions.[104] Others prefer mucosal proctectomy and coloanal anastomosis for radiation stricture, fistula, bleeding, and pain.[11,63,119,221,318]

Lopez and colleagues used a segment of nonirradiated colon for repair of postirradiation rectal stricture.[180] The normal proximal bowel was turned down and anasto-mosed to the side of the rectum below the site of the injury, creating an end-to-side anastomosis. A proximal anasto-mosis was effected between the upper colon and the apex of the U of the distally rotated bowel. The authors reported successful application of this technique in one patient. A number of papers have been published that attest to the high morbidity of surgery in these individuals as well as to what should be a low threshold on the part of the surgeon for performing fecal diversion.[84,143,164,203]

Comment

Intestinal complications of radiation therapy present dif-ficult management problems. My own attitude is to at-tempt resection for patients who are symptomatic when the disease involves primarily the small intestine. Con-versely, because of my lack of success with restorative op-erations for those who have radiation changes in the rec-tum, particularly with stricture or fistula, I prefer a proximal diversionary procedure. My tendency is to limit resective sphincter-saving operations to those individuals whose prognosis for long-term survival is good and in whom the gross disease is no lower than the mid-rectum. It must be remembered that it is not only the successful application of surgical technique for reestablishing in-testinal continuity that is important—the subsequent functional results are extremely relevant. The fact is that with a low anastomosis in this group of patients (who often have injury to the sphincter muscle, with attendant impairment for bowel control) the functional result may be far less salutary than is a colostomy or ileostomy.

VOLVULUS

Sigmoid Volvulus

Sigmoid volvulus is a relatively rare condition that has been recognized since antiquity. Ballantyne noted that the authors of the Ebers papyrus from ancient Egypt wrote that either the volvulus spontaneously reduced or the sigmoid colon rotted.[32] Detorsion was recognized even then as the requirement for ameliorating the condition. Whether this can be accomplished by medical or by surgical means has been the subject of a considerable body of literature.

In the United States, sigmoid volvulus is a relatively rare cause of intestinal obstruction, whereas in other areas of the world it is the single most common etiology. Ballantyne reported that 30% of intestinal obstructions were caused by sigmoid volvulus in Pakistan, 25% in Brazil, 20% in India, 17% in Poland, and 16% in Russia.[33] High altitude is said to play an important role, but the reason for this is unknown. For example, 230 cases were reported from the Andes region of Bolivia.[23] In the United States, however, the incidence is only approximately 5%. The overall distribution of volvulus at various sites indicates that the sigmoid colon is by far the most commonly involved location (1,400 cases) as compared with the cecum (400 cases), transverse colon (35 cases), and the splenic flexure (four cases) according to a 1982 publication.[33]

In Ballantyne's report, two different age patterns appear.[33] In countries where sigmoid volvulus is relatively prevalent, the disease is usually seen in middle-aged men. However, in English-speaking countries the average age is considerably older, and the condition is as likely to occur in either gender.

Pathogenesis

The pathogenesis of sigmoid volvulus is obscure. Most patients are elderly and have a high incidence of associated medical or psychiatric problems.[17] In this group, chronic constipation is thought to be an important factor.

The condition is associated with an extremely redundant colon, a finding that may be seen in a number of illnesses, such as Chagas' disease, Parkinson's disease, paralytic conditions, ischemic colitis, ulcer disease, and many others.[33] Neurologic problems in particular are frequently seen in association with volvulus. In fact, the high incidence of the condition in institutionalized patients may be more a reflection of the associated neurologic disease than of the fact that the patient happens to reside in such a facility.

An interesting observation is that volvulus is second only to adhesions as the most common cause of intestinal obstruction in pregnant women, presumably because a redundant colon is predisposed to torsion and twisting as the uterus raises out of the pelvis.[33,141,181] Mobilization of the colon coincident with other surgical procedures can predispose to volvulus. For example, this may occur following a sling procedure for rectal prolapse wherein the sigmoid colon may be quite redundant, with fixation at either end of the redundancy (see Chapter 17).

The greater incidence of volvulus in eastern Europe, India, and Africa is thought to be related to a high-residue diet. The anatomic conditions that predispose to sigmoid volvulus—a long, mobile sigmoid loop with close approximation of the afferent and efferent limbs, creating a short base of mesentery around which axis the volvulus occurs—is found in both Eastern and Western groups of patients.[317] A genetic predisposition has been identified within families and within certain tribes.[220,317]

Signs and Symptoms

Patients with sigmoid volvulus usually present with the characteristic signs and symptoms of colonic obstruction. These include absence of bowel movements, failure to pass flatus, crampy abdominal pain, nausea, and vomiting. Almog and colleagues reported a case of secretory diarrhea and hypokalemia due to intermittent sigmoid volvulus.[13]

Physical examination usually reveals a distended abdomen. Minimal to mild tenderness may be noted, but signs of peritoneal irritation are usually absent unless viability of the bowel is compromised. Rectal examination characteristically demonstrates an empty ampulla.

Investigations

The plain abdominal x-ray will usually reveal a markedly dilated sigmoid colon and proximal bowel, with relatively minimal gas noted in the rectum (Figure 28-42). Agrez and Cameron reviewed the radiologic findings in 20 patients diagnosed as having a sigmoid volvulus.[4] The standard radiographic feature was that of a distended ahaustral sigmoid loop, the bent inner-tube appearance. In analyzing the plain films of 18 individuals found to have sigmoid volvulus, an enlarged ahaustral loop was seen in 11 of them. In the remaining it was not possible to differentiate the distended loop from that of the transverse colon.

Contrast enema examination may demonstrate complete retrograde obstruction at the level of the torsion or may reveal an area of narrowing with proximal dilatation if the obstruction is incomplete or recently reduced (Figure 28-43). In the experience of Agrez and Cameron, 10 patients were submitted to barium enema study.[4] In three there was a probable torsion point; four were definitely diagnostic (e.g., bird's beak sign or mucosal spiral pattern), and three had markedly redundant sigmoid loops. None of the barium enema examinations relieved the volvulus.

Treatment

Ballantyne reviewed the evolution of nonoperative and operative treatment of sigmoid volvulus since the original description from Egyptian antiquity.[32] Suppositories,

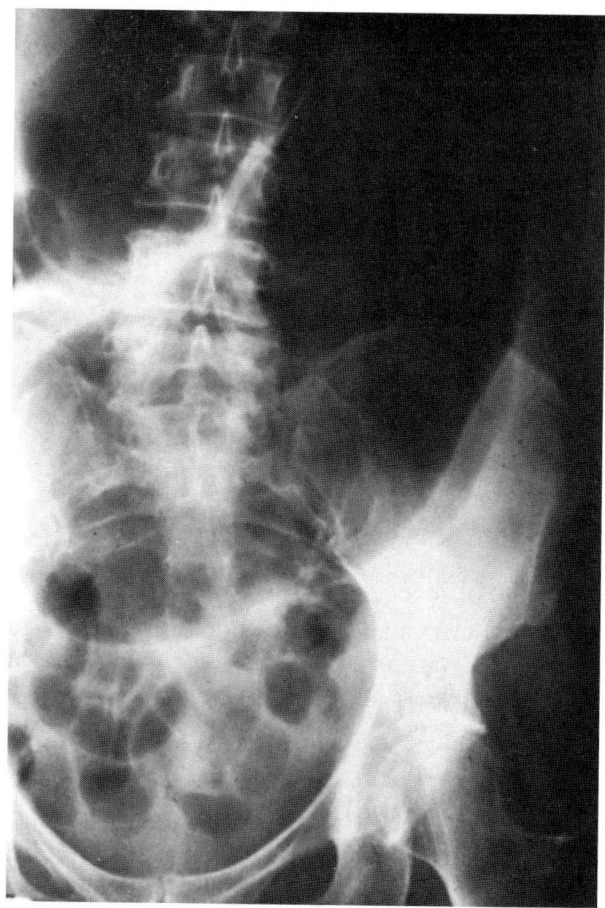

FIGURE 28-42. Sigmoid volvulus. Plain abdominal film reveals massive dilatation of the sigmoid and the so-called bent tire appearance. (Courtesy of Hector P. Rodriguez, M.D.)

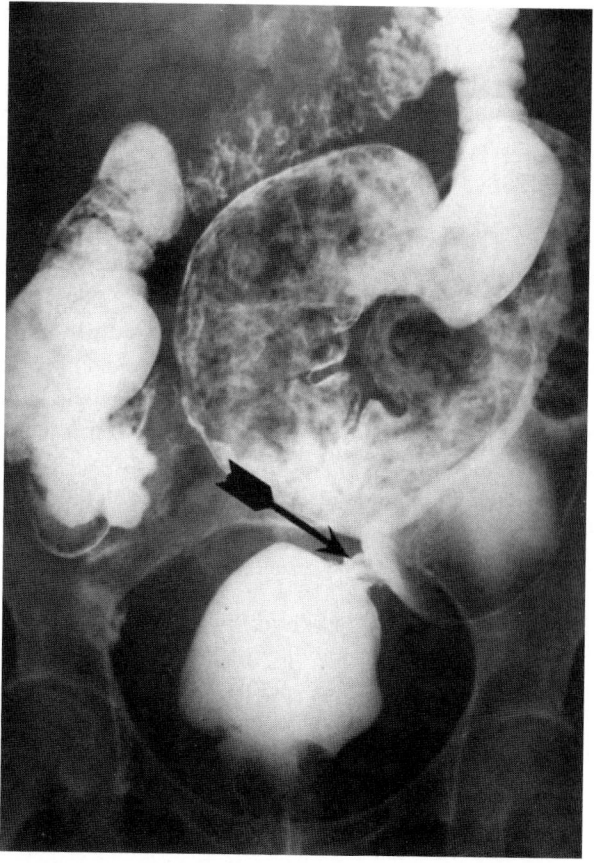

FIGURE 28-43. Sigmoid volvulus. Barium enema reveals a dilated sigmoid loop with a "corkscrew" appearance of the narrowed segment (*arrow*) at the rectosigmoid junction. (Courtesy of Hector P. Rodriguez, M.D.)

clysters, enemas, reduction by external manipulation, and a rectal tube have all had their advocates. It was not until the twentieth century, however, that laparotomy was employed for the treatment of this condition.

Nonoperative Treatment

Initial management depends on whether the surgeon believes that the bowel is viable or nonviable. In the former circumstance, attempt at reduction should be made by means of proctosigmoidoscopy and insertion of a rectal tube. If the volvulus can be reduced, an explosive discharge of gas and feces will occur. The rectal tube should be left in place, either taped or, ideally, sutured to the buttock for about 48 hours to avoid the possibility of immediate recurrence.

Flexible sigmoidoscopy and colonoscopy have also been successfully employed in the treatment of sigmoid volvulus.[22,122,241,263,292] The technique has the advantage of permitting evaluation of the viability of a greater area of colonic mucosa, but the procedure must be performed with limited manipulation and limited air to minimize the risk of perforation of the distended and edematous bowel.[225] Intraluminal stenting to prevent early recurrence can be accomplished through the use of flexible plastic tubing or a blunt-ended guide wire.[241,340] An attempt at colonoscopic reduction may be considered if proctosigmoidoscopic manipulation has been unsuccessful. Salim combined percutaneous deflation of the dilated bowel to successfully employ sigmoidoscopic decompression in 20 patients.[262]

If necrotic bowel is observed at the time of endoscopic examination, the surgeon should prepare the patient for an exploratory laparotomy. Proctosigmoidoscopic examination should be undertaken even if the patient has signs and symptoms of nonviable bowel in order to attempt to confirm the extent of involvement and perhaps to establish the diagnosis with certainty. The procedure should be performed, however, with great care to avoid perforating the bowel. The principle of evaluation of the rectum is a requisite before surgery for suspected colonic pathology because there is no way for one to evaluate the extraperitoneal rectum at the time of laparotomy.

In reviewing almost 600 patients, Ballantyne found that proctosigmoidoscopy and rectal tube insertion were successful in reducing the sigmoid volvulus in 40% of cases; proctosigmoidoscopy alone, in 19%; barium enema, in 5.4%; and other modalities, in approximately 6%.[33] Seventy percent of patients were successfully reduced by some means in the 19 series reviewed by that author. More recent studies generally indicate that if the bowel is viable, one may anticipate successful reduction of the volvulus at least 90% of the time. Arigbabu and colleagues decompressed 83 consecutive patients with viable bowel by means of colonoscopy.[22] In the United States Department of Veterans Affairs database, Grossman and co-workers found that 81% of the 189 patients underwent successful endoscopic decompression,[133] and Chung and associates (Singapore) noted success in 28 of their 29 patients.[76]

Recurrence Following Reduction

Although nonsurgical reduction of the volvulus allows one to avoid an emergency operation, the recurrence rate is very high. In a combined series of 149 patients who were followed after successful reduction, 43% developed a recurrence.[32] There was a mortality rate in excess of 10% in this group. Brothers and colleagues reported that 57% of patients initially treated by endoscopic decompression developed a recurrence.[61] Chung's group found that 12 of their 14 patients who refused operation developed recurrent volvulus at a median of 2.8 months later,[76] whereas the Veterans Administration study noted a 23% recurrence rate.[133] Therefore, if the patient can possibly undergo an elective operation, this should optimally be performed during the same hospitalization after the bowel has been adequately prepared.

Operative Management

If one has been unsuccessful in reducing the volvulus, laparotomy is indicated, assuming that the patient can tolerate a laparotomy. The choice of procedure depends on whether the viability of the bowel is compromised. Possible surgical alternatives include resection and anastomosis (total or partial colectomy with or without a proximal colostomy), Hartmann resection, exteriorization resection, detorsion alone, detorsion with colopexy, and most recently, percutaneous colostomy and percutaneous endoscopic sigmoidopexy.[86,236] Gurel and colleagues used the technique of intraoperative on-table lavage to perform resection and primary anastomosis of the obstructed bowel (see Chapter 23).[136] Others have employed a fixation technique, with or without mesh implantation.[146] Chung and co-workers opine that subtotal colectomy is the preferred approach in the presence of a megacolon or megarectum.[76]

Daniels and associates (Chichester, England) selectively utilized percutaneous endoscopic colostomy for 14 patients in whom conventional surgery was considered unsafe or inappropriate following successful endoscopic decompression.[86] The procedure is analogous to that of percutaneous endoscopic gastrostomy (PEG). The procedure was carried out under intravenous sedation with a local anesthetic. There were no deaths, but the volvulus recurred in three of eight patients when the tube was removed. Pinedo and Kirberg successfully performed percutaneous colonoscopic sigmoidopexy with the use of T-fasteners for the fixation in two individuals considered unfit for surgery.[236]

Obviously, if the colon is demonstrated to be nonviable, a resection is indicated. This is undertaken for the same reason and in the same manner that one would perform a resection of a perforated colon for any other condition (diverticulitis, carcinoma). The objective is to remove the focus of sepsis. Whether to perform an anastomosis, a Hartmann procedure, or one of the other surgical options available is a judgment that each individual surgeon must make. The pros and cons of the different operative approaches are discussed in Chapter 26.

Results

Ballantyne reviewed the experience of 25 American series that included more than 600 patients.[32] Delayed elective resection with primary anastomosis was associated with the lowest mortality rate (8%). Operative mortality, however, in those who underwent resection on an emergency basis was extremely high (at least 25%), irrespective of the method of treatment. When one combines the American experience with that of other countries it becomes clear that the prognosis of patients with sigmoid volvulus falls into two groups: those with viable bowel and those whose bowel is nonviable. Those with viable bowel had an overall 12.3% operative mortality as compared with an operative mortality of 53% in those with nonviable bowel.[32]

Ballantyne reported his personal experience of 12 patients with sigmoid volvulus.[31] The two patients who underwent emergency resection both expired, whereas mortality following elective resection was 25%. Pasch and Adams noted a 57% mortality for emergency resection and a 20% mortality rate for elective resection.[231] Bak and Boley, however, reported only a 6% mortality rate for elective resection.[30] Others have found that reduction alone is associated with a lower mortality than resection, but at the cost of a higher incidence of recurrence.[327]

Ryan reported 66 patients with sigmoid volvulus.[260] Emergency operation was required in almost one-half and was associated with a 22% operative mortality rate. The mortality rate with viable colon was twice as high when resection was carried out as when detorsion alone was performed. Because of this observation, Ryan recommends performing only detorsion unless gangrene or perforation require resection. In the report from the Veterans Affairs Medical Centers, the mortality rate was 24% for emergency operations and 6% for elective procedures.[133] Most papers confirm four factors contributing to an adverse outcome: older age, emergency surgery, nonviable bowel, and a history of prior volvulus.[120,123,168,234,313]

Anderson and Lee reported 134 patients with sigmoid volvulus.[16] Rectal decompression was effective in 85%. The best results in individuals who had a nonviable colon were obtained with a Hartmann resection, although the number in this group was small. Because of the general success of a resective procedure when viable bowel was found, these authors do not advise detorsion alone. However, they had a limited experience with this approach.

Morrissey and Deitch noted that little attention has been focused on the recurrence rate of sigmoid volvulus following surgical therapy.[211] The authors point out the importance of an associated megacolon with obstruction secondary to the volvulus. Surprisingly, the overall recurrence rate was 36%, higher than most would anticipate. This rate varied only slightly according to the operative procedure performed. The authors recommend that a subtotal colectomy should be considered the surgical procedure of choice in those individuals operated on for sigmoid volvulus who have an associated megacolon.[211]

Bhatnagar and Sharma (India) performed an extraperitoneal colostomy (without resection) in 84 patients with nongangrenous sigmoid volvulus.[46] The operative mortality was 9%. There were no recurrences in the 76 patients available for follow-up (median, 6 years).

Comment

My own preference is to perform a limited resection with or without a primary anastomosis, depending on the patient's condition and whether the operation is undertaken on an elective or an emergency basis and whether the bowel is viable or nonviable. I do not consider detorsion or sigmoidopexy adequate long-term therapy.

Sigmoid Volvulus in Children

Sigmoid volvulus has been infrequently reported in children, with fewer than 50 cases having been published in the English language.[197] Extremely rarely, the condition has been identified in association with Hirschsprung's disease or with imperforate anus.[158] Volvulus in children is difficult to diagnose, the course tends to be fulminant, passage of a rectal tube or endoscope may be difficult or impossible, and early operative intervention is more often advised than in adults.[275]

Ileosigmoid Knotting

Ileosigmoid knotting is unusual in Western countries but is relatively common in Africa, Asia, and the Middle East. The condition is initiated by a loop of ileum wrapping around the base of a redundant sigmoid colon.[14] The manifestation may be a variant of intestinal malrotation and mid-gut volvulus.[95] According to Alver and colleagues, as of 1993 the collected series represents 68 patients with this condition, constituting 8.8% of 773 cases of sigmoid volvulus.[14] The authors classified the condition into four types, according to the active component initiating the knot formation and the direction of rotatory movement. Approximately three-fourths of the patients developed gangrene of the bowel. Following resection the mortality rate was 30.9% in this series.

Cecal Volvulus

Cecal volvulus is less common than volvulus of the sigmoid colon, representing approximately 25% to 30% of patients with this condition. There is less correlation with geographic location than with sigmoid volvulus, although the two presentations have been known to occur simultaneously.[283] The sine qua non for developing this manifestation is a failure of fusion of the parietal peritoneum to the cecum and ascending colon. Abnormal mobility of the cecum and ascending colon has been estimated to occur in 10% to 20% of the population (Figure 28-44).[253] This predisposes the bowel to twist on its axis (Figure 28-45), to rotate and twist, or to fold upward (cecal bascule) (Figure 28-46). The resultant vascular compromise leads to gangrene and to perforation.

Volvulus of the cecum occurs more frequently in younger patients than does volvulus of the sigmoid. Precipitating causes include distal obstruction, meteorism occurring from unpressurized air travel, pregnancy, prior abdominal operations (adhesions), congenital bands, violent coughing, intermittent positive-pressure breathing, mesenteric adenitis, prolonged constipation, distal obstructing lesion, and colonic atony (adynamic ileus).[106,127,240] An association with jogging has also been reported.[242] The simultaneous occurrence of volvulus of the cecum and sigmoid colon has also been documented.[206]

Signs and Symptoms

Abdominal pain is usually the predominant complaint and may be relatively low-grade and colicky in nature. Frequently present is abdominal distention, which may be asymmetric, with a mass in the hypogastrium or on the right side. Bowel sounds are usually obstructive. Some patients have more chronic manifestations, with

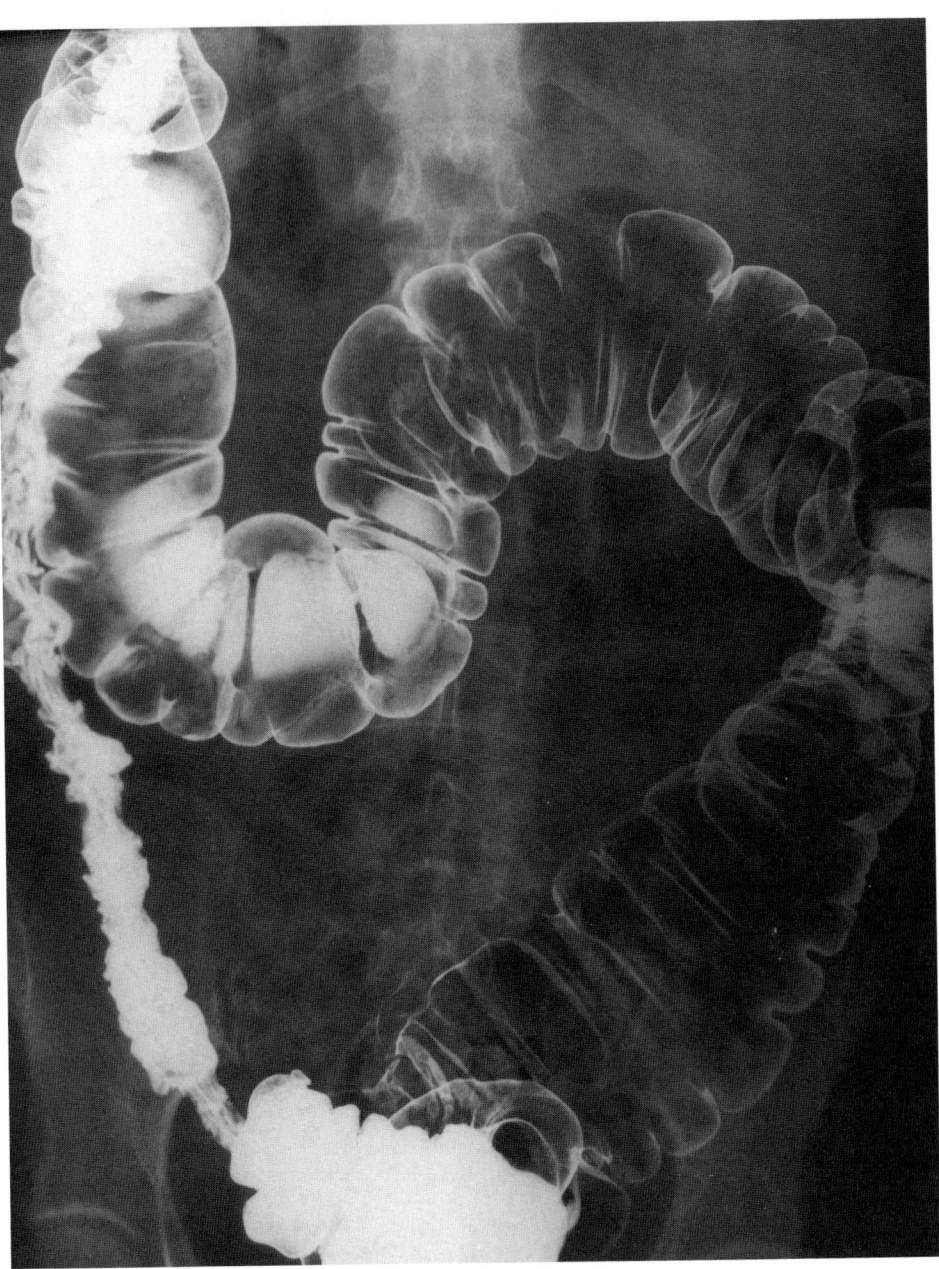

FIGURE 28-44. Mobile cecum and right colon is readily evident on this air-contrast barium enema.

intermittent cramping abdominal pain and distention that usually resolves spontaneously.

Radiologic Studies

Radiologic investigation usually reveals characteristic findings. The cecum and ascending colon can be found in any part of the abdomen, but the most common displacement is into the epigastrium and to the left upper quadrant.[106] An obliquely oriented cecum and ascending colon may be identified extending across the abdominal cavity (Figure 28-47). Classic x-ray findings include a "coffee-bean" shape and visible mucosal folds at the site of obstruction (Figure 28-48).[127] Usually, no gas can be seen distal to the point of obstruction. Multiple gas–fluid levels may be noted in the small intestine. Barium enema may reveal the classic bird's beak deformity due to obstruction in the region of the cecum (Figure 28-49).

Treatment

As with the management of sigmoid volvulus, colonoscopy has been successfully employed to reduce volvulus of the cecum. It is important to recognize, however, that unless the procedure is initiated early, persistent efforts are very likely to be more harmful than helpful.[18] Friedman and colleagues failed to successfully reduce any of their 10 patients with cecal volvulus by this means.[113]

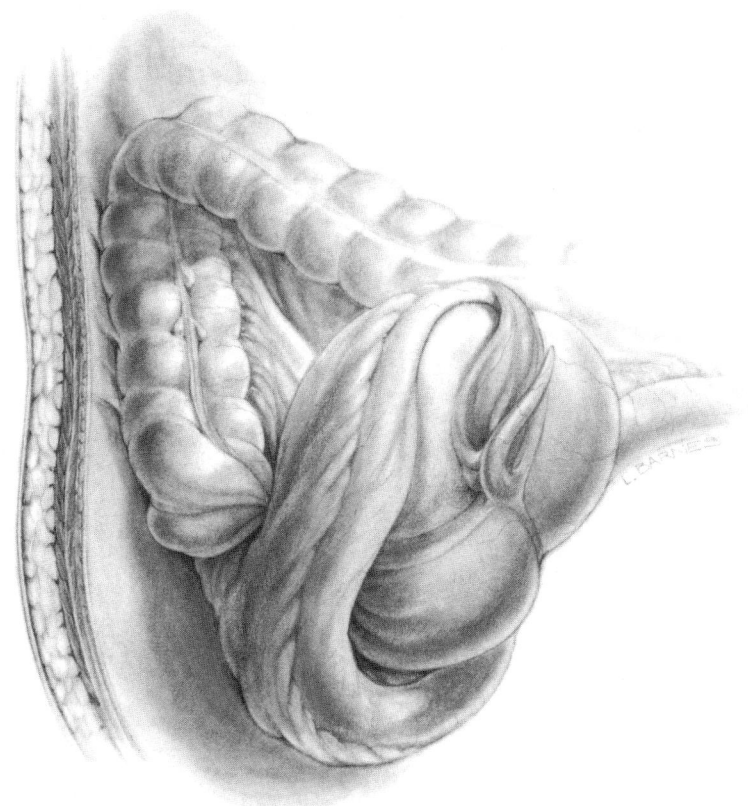

FIGURE 28-45. Cecal volvulus manifested by a twisting of the bowel, a consequence of lack of fixation and redundancy.

Choices of surgical procedures for cecal volvulus without perforation or gangrene include detorsion (with or without appendectomy—Figure 28-50), cecopexy, cecostomy (or a combination of the two), and resection (Figs. 28-51, 28-52 and 28-53). Ryan and colleagues suggest another option, that of cecopexy, with the placement of a long (Baker) tube via the rectum to decompress the bowel.[259] This has the theoretical advantages of providing postoperative colonic decompression, minimizing pressure from a full colon on the cecopexy suture line, and avoiding contamination. Laparoscopic cecopexy by placement of anchoring sutures has also been reported.[45,281] Obviously, if the viability of the bowel is compromised or if perforation is present, resection is required.

Results

Detorsion alone or with appendectomy is generally felt to be associated with a high recurrence rate and is not advocated in any of the contemporary articles on the subject.[70] Interpretation of the results of the other surgical alternatives is somewhat difficult, because most papers address mortality and recurrence, but not morbidity.

O'Mara and colleagues reported 50 patients who underwent surgery for cecal volvulus.[223] A variety of operations were performed in the 41 individuals who had no evidence of gangrenous bowel at the time. Four under-

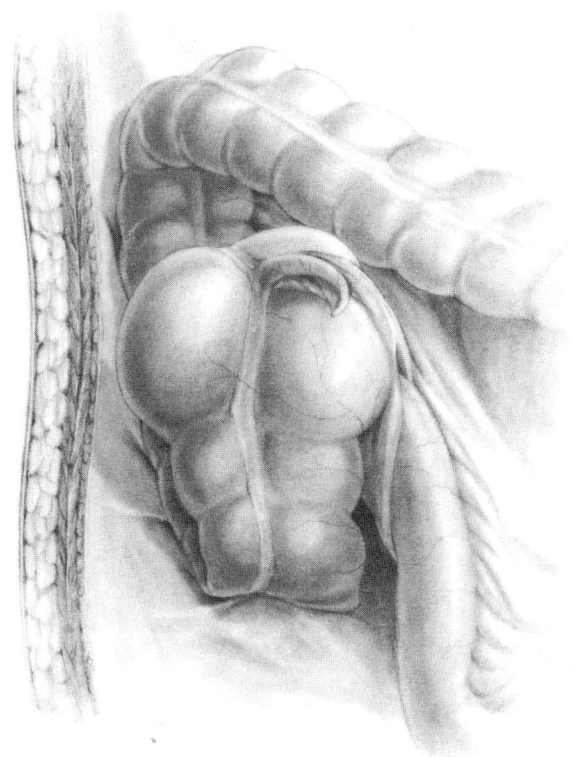

FIGURE 28-46. Cecal bascule. This is a type of volvulus-producing obstruction from a folding of the bowel on itself.

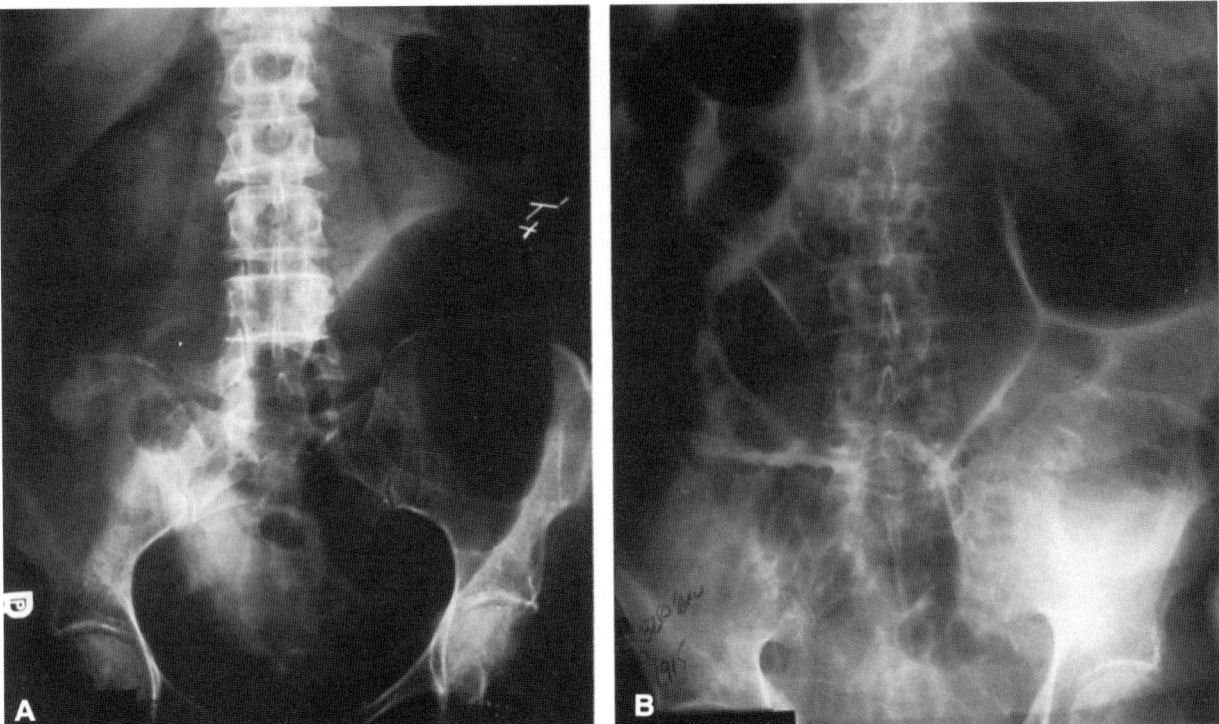

FIGURE 28-47. Cecal bascule. Plane abdominal film demonstrates markedly dilated loop of large bowel projecting to the left upper quadrant. There is no gas in the remainder of the colon. **(A)** Without small bowel obstruction. **(B)** With small bowel obstruction.

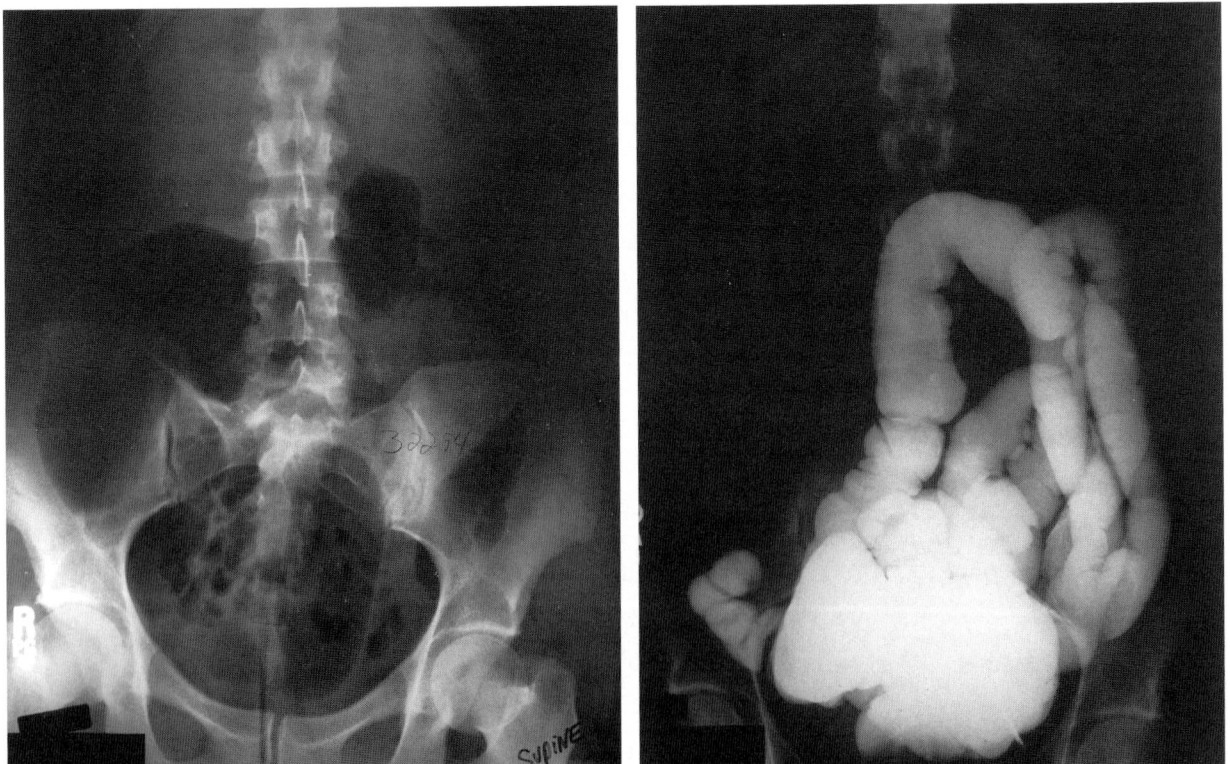

FIGURE 28-48. Cecal volvulus. **(A)** Note "coffee-bean" appearance on plain abdominal x-ray. **(B)** Barium enema shows markedly redundant colon with retrograde obstruction to the flow in the ascending colon.

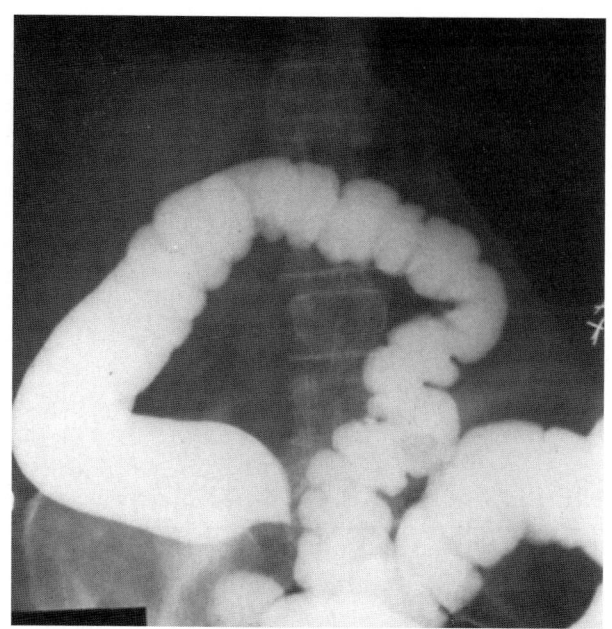

FIGURE 28-49. Cecal volvulus. Barium enema demonstrates obstruction in the proximal ascending colon with "bird's beak" deformity. (Courtesy of Hewitt R. Lang, M.D.)

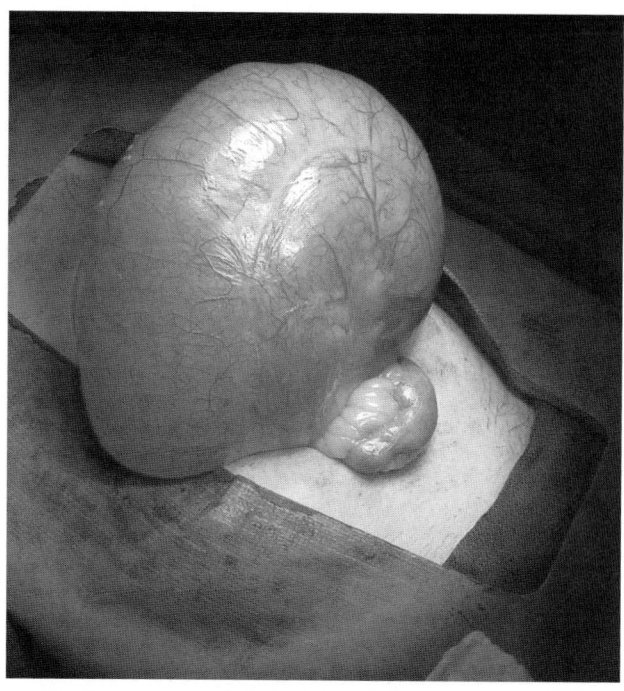

FIGURE 28-50. Intraoperative view of a cecal volvulus with demonstrably viable bowel. (Courtesy of Scott Fields, M.D.)

went tube cecostomy, with one death. Seven patients underwent resection and primary anastomosis, with no deaths, and 12 underwent detorsion alone, with two operative deaths. Cecopexy was performed on 18 patients, with no deaths. Nine had a gangrenous cecum at the time of surgery; of these individuals, there were three operative deaths (33%). Most series note a high mortality rate in the presence of gangrenous bowel (33% to 55%).[15,16,34]

Cecopexy has the advantage of avoiding potential contamination in unprepared bowel, but the question of recurrence must be addressed. Howard and Catto reported 16 patients with cecal volvulus, 14 of whom underwent a nonresective procedure.[149] In a follow-up averaging 5.6 years, no recurrence was demonstrable. These authors concluded that a resectional operation for viable bowel was unnecessary. Conversely, Todd and Forde, in a review of a number of series, noted that the recurrence rate for cecopexy alone was approximately 28%.[309] There were no recurrences following tube cecostomy, as well as no recurrences following resection, in their search of the literature. These authors, therefore, advocate tube cecostomy as the procedure of choice because it is less hazardous than resection. Depending on whom one reads, an advocate for detorsion alone, cecopexy alone, cecostomy alone, or resection can usually be found in contemporary publications.[244,305]

Anderson and Lee reported 41 cases of acute cecal volvulus.[16] They emphasize that prompt surgery is imperative. Cecopexy was associated with a 25% recurrence

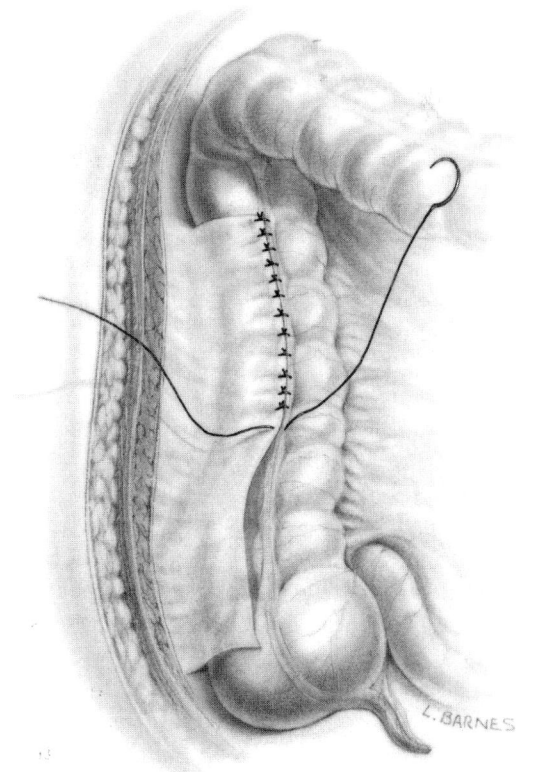

FIGURE 28-51. Cecopexy. An improved method for anchoring the colon is to employ a lateral peritoneal flap. (Adapted from Rogers RL, Harford FJ. Mobile cecum syndrome. *Dis Colon Rectum* 1984;27:399.)

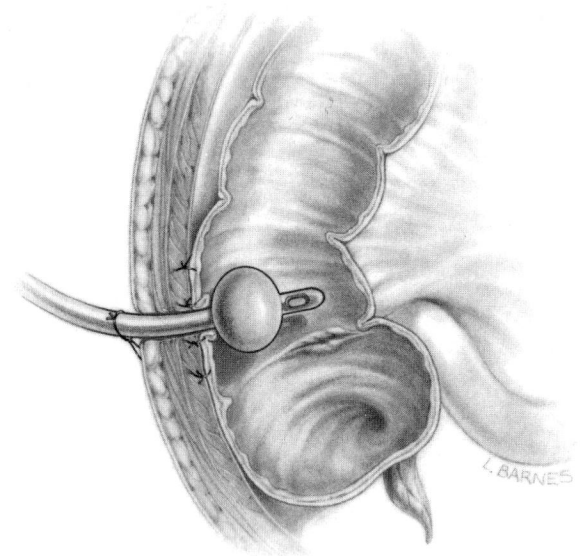

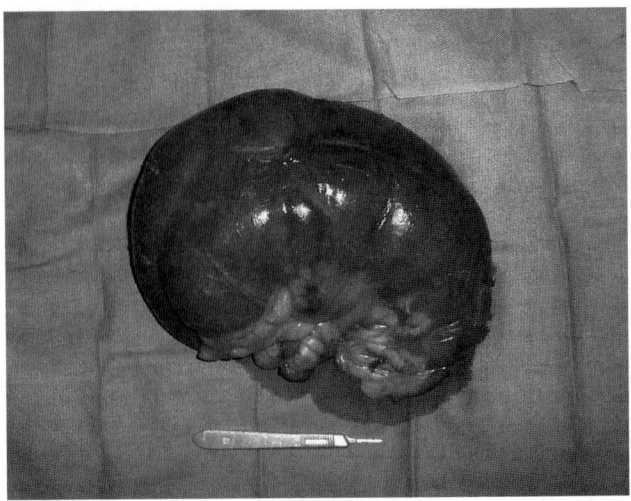

FIGURE 28-53. Resected specimen shown in Fig. 28-50.

FIGURE 28-52. Tube cecostomy. Cecum is pulled to abdominal wall and anchored with several sutures.

rate, but cecopexy with cecostomy was effective in preventing recurrence of symptoms. In the experience of Anderson and Welch with 49 patients having viable bowel, cecopexy alone was followed by a recurrence in 20%, whereas there were no recurrences with cecopexy and cecostomy.[17] The effectiveness of this procedure seems to be due to decompression or venting of the dilated segment, together with fixation in two planes at 90 degrees to each other.[15]

Madiba and Thomson concluded in their review of the subject that resection and anastomosis is the favored option for both gangrenous and viable bowel.[191] The decision of whether to restore intestinal continuity at the time is obviously a matter surgical judgment.

Opinion

I have had very few opportunities to perform operations for cecal volvulus. It is evident from the preceding discussion, however, that there is a relatively safe and effective method for the management of the condition when the bowel is viable—cecostomy and cecopexy. But tube cecostomy can be associated with serious potential complications. So I am still inclined to perform resection of the right colon, a procedure that has been demonstrably successful in individuals requiring an emergency operation for other pathologic entities. With respect to "laparoscopically hindered" cecopexy, I am able to contain my enthusiasm for an approach that is known to be suboptimal even when performed by an open technique.

Volvulus of the Transverse Colon

The transverse colon is the area of the colon in which volvulus least frequently occurs, representing less than 10% of all volvuli.[339] Usually, supporting tissues (e.g., gastrocolic omentum, lienocolic and phrenicocolic ligaments) are congenitally absent or may have been surgically removed.[124,326] Another predisposing factor may be an asthenic habitus that permits close approximation of the flexure attachments.[134] As with cecal volvulus, the condition may be associated with distal obstructing lesions, chronic constipation, prior abdominal surgery, or pregnancy. Anderson and colleagues identified 59 cases in the literature and added seven of their own.[18] The condition is usually not diagnosed preoperatively. The radiologic findings are not truly characteristic except for the demonstration of obvious colonic dilatation. Gangrene was noted in approximately 16% of the patients from the reported series.

In reviewing the literature, Anderson and associates noted that simple colopexy was followed by a high incidence of recurrence.[18] They therefore suggest that at least the transverse colon be resected. This is usually accomplished by means of an extended right hemicolectomy or a partial left colectomy, depending on the presentation. Successful decompression by means of the colonoscope has been described.[161]

Volvulus and Pregnancy

As previously mentioned, one of the predisposing factors for the development of volvuli of all types is pregnancy. Intestinal obstruction during pregnancy is extremely rare, with a reported incidence of one to three per 100,000 pregnancies.[141] However, in this group of patients, 25% of obstructions are caused by volvulus, almost the same incidence as that produced by adhesions.[141,240] The enlarging uterus is believed to create pressure on any redundant or abnormally mobile bowel. Because of the risk not only to the mother, but also to the fetus, urgent surgical intervention is demanded.

REFERENCES

1. Aalders GJ, Baeten CGMJ, Loffeld RJLF. Suturing angiodysplastic lesions of the small intestine. *Surg Gynecol Obstet* 1991;173:323.
2. Abel ME, Russell TR. Ischemic colitis: comparison of surgical and nonoperative management. *Dis Colon Rectum* 1983;26:113.
3. Adams JT. The barium enema as treatment for massive diverticular bleeding. *Dis Colon Rectum* 1974;17:439.
4. Agrez M, Cameron D. Radiology of sigmoid volvulus. *Dis Colon Rectum* 1981;24:510.
5. Aitken RJ, Elliot MS. Sigmoid exclusion: a new technique in the management of radiation-induced fistula. *Br J Surg* 1985;72:731.
6. Alavi A, Dann RW, Baum S, Biery DN. Scintigraphic detection of acute gastrointestinal bleeding. *Radiology* 1977;124:753.
7. Alavi A, Ring EJ. Localization of gastrointestinal bleeding: superiority of 99mTc sulfur colloid compared with angiography. *AJR* 1981;137:741.
8. Aldabagh SM, Trujillo YP, Taxy JB. Utility of specimen angiography in angiodysplasia of the colon. *Gastroenterology* 1986;91:725.
9. Alexander TJ, Dwyer RM. Endoscopic Nd/YAG laser treatment of severe radiation injury of the lower gastrointestinal tract: long-term follow-up. *Gastrointest Endosc* 1988;34:407.
10. Alfidi RJ, Esselstyn CD, Tarar R, et al. Recognition and angio-surgical detection of arteriovenous malformations of the bowel. *Ann Surg* 1971;174:573.
11. Allen-Mersh TG, Wilson EJ, Hope-Stone HF, et al. The management of late radiation-induced rectal injury after treatment of carcinoma of the uterus. *Surg Gynecol Obstet* 1987;164:521.
12. Allison DJ, Hemingway AP, Cunningham DA. Angiography in gastrointestinal bleeding. *Lancet* 1982;2:30.
13. Almog Y, Dranitzki-Elhahlel M, Lax E, et al. Sigmoid volvulus presenting as chronic secretory diarrhea responsive to octreotide. *Am J Gastroenterol* 1992;87:148.
14. Alver O, Oren D, Tireli M, et al. Ileosigmoid knotting in Turkey: review of 68 cases. *Dis Colon Rectum* 1993;36:1139.
15. Anderson Jr, Lee D. Acute caecal volvulus. *Br J Surg* 1980;67:39.
16. Anderson JR, Lee D. The management of acute sigmoid volvulus. *Br J Surg* 1981;68:117.
17. Anderson JR, Welch GH. Acute volvulus of the right colon: an analysis of 69 patients. *World J Surg* 1986;10.336.
18. Anderson JR, Lee D, Taylor TV, et al. Volvulus of the transverse colon. *Br J Surg* 1981;68:179.
19. Anderson MJ Sr, Okike N, Spencer RJ. The colonoscope in cecal volvulus: report of three cases. *Dis Colon Rectum* 1978;21:71.
20. Anseline PF, Lavery IC, Fazio VW, et al. Radiation injury of the rectum: evaluation of surgical treatment. *Ann Surg* 1981;194:716.
21. Ardigo GJ, Longstreth GF, Weston LA, et al. Passage of a large bowel cast caused by acute ischemia. Report of two cases. *Dis Colon Rectum* 1998;41:793.
22. Arigbabu AO, Badejo OA, Akinola DO. Colonoscopy in the emergency treatment of colonic volvulus in Nigeria. *Dis Colon Rectum* 1985;28:795.
23. Asbun HH, Castellanos H, Balderrama B, et al. Sigmoid volvulus in the high altitude of the Andes: review of 230 cases. *Dis Colon Rectum* 1992;35:350.
24. Attwood SEA, McGrath J, Hill ADK, et al. Laparoscopic approach to Meckel's diverticulectomy. *Br J Surg* 1992;79:211.
25. Azimuddin K, Stasik JJ, Rosen L, et al. Dieulafoy's lesion of the anal canal: a new clinical entity. *Dis Colon Rectum* 2000;43:423.
26. Baden JG, Racy DJ, Grist TM. Contrast-enhanced three-dimensional magnetic resonance angiography of the mesenteric vasculature. *Br J Surg* 1999;10:369.
27. Baer JW. Pathogenesis of bleeding colonic diverticulosis: new concepts. *Crit Rev Diagn Imaging* 1978;11:1.
28. Baer JW. Vascular ectasias. In: Greenbaum EI, ed. *Radiographic atlas of colon disease.* Chicago: Year Book, 1980:623.
29. Baig MK, Lewis M, Stebbing JF, et al. Multiple microaneurysms of the superior hemorrhoidal artery: unusual recurrent massive rectal bleeding: report of a case. *Dis Colon Rectum* 2003;46:978.
30. Bak MP, Boley SJ. Sigmoid volvulus in elderly patients. *Am J Surg* 1986;151:71.
31. Ballantyne GH. Sigmoid volvulus: high mortality in county hospital patients. *Dis Colon Rectum* 1981;24:515.
32. Ballantyne GH. Review of sigmoid volvulus: history and results of treatment. *Dis Colon Rectum* 1982;25:494.
33. Ballantyne GH. Review of sigmoid volvulus: clinical patterns and pathogenesis. *Dis Colon Rectum* 1982;25:823.
34. Ballantyne GH, Brandner MD, Beart RW Jr, et al. Volvulus of the colon: incidence and mortality. *Ann Surg* 1985;202:83.
35. Baum S. Angiography and the gastrointestinal bleeder. *Radiology* 1982;143:569.
36. Baum S, Athanasoulis CA, Waltman AC. Angiographic diagnosis and control of large-bowel bleeding. *Dis Colon Rectum* 1974;17:447.
37. Baum S, Athanasoulis CA, Waltman AC, et al. Angiodysplasia of the right colon: a cause of gastrointestinal bleeding. *Am J Roentgenol* 1977;129:789.
38. Baum S, Rösch J, Dotter CT, et al. Selective mesenteric arterial infusions in the management of massive diverticular hemorrhage. *N Engl J Med* 1973;288:1269.
39. Bem J, Bem S, Singh A. Use of hyperbaric oxygen chamber in the management of radiation-related complications of the anorectal region: report of two cases and review of the literature. *Dis Colon Rectum* 2000;43:1435.
40. Bender JS, Wiencek RG, Bouwman DL. Morbidity and mortality following total abdominal colectomy for massive lower gastrointestinal bleeding. *Am Surg* 1991;57:536.
41. Bentley DE, Richardson JD. The role of tagged red blood cell imaging in the localization of gastrointestinal bleeding. *Arch Surg* 1991;126:821.
42. Berken CA. Nd:YAG laser therapy for gastrointestinal bleeding due to radiation colitis. *Am J Gastroenterol* 1985;80:730.
43. Berry AR, Campbell WB, Kettlewell MGW. Management of major colonic haemorrhage. *Br J Surg* 1988;75:637.
44. Berthrong M. Pathologic changes secondary to radiation. *World J Surg* 1986;10:155.
45. Bhandarkar DS, Morgan WP. Laparoscopic caecopexy for caecal volvulus. *Br J Surg* 1995;82:323.
46. Bhatnagar BNS, Sharma CLN. Nonresective alternative for the cure of nongangrenous sigmoid volvulus. *Dis Colon Rectum* 1998;41:381.
47. Biswas S, George ML, Leather AJM. Stapled anopexy in the treatment of anal varices: report of a case. *Dis Colon Rectum* 2003;46:1284.
48. Boley SJ, Brandt LJ. Vascular ectasias of the colon—1986. *Dig Dis Sci* 1986;31:26S.

49. Boley SJ, Brandt LJ, Veith FJ. Ischemic disorders of the intestine. *Curr Probl Surg* 1978;15:1.
50. Boley SJ, Feinstein FR, Sammartano R, et al. New concepts in the management of emboli of the superior mesenteric artery. *Surg Gynecol Obstet* 1981;153:561.
51. Boley SJ, Sammartano R, Adams A, et al. On the nature and etiology of vascular ectasias of the colon. *Gastroenterology* 1977;72:650.
52. Boley SJ, Sprayregen S, Sammartano RJ, et al. The pathophysiologic basis for the angiographic signs of vascular ectasias of the colon. *Radiology* 1974;125:615.
53. Boley SJ, Sprayregen S, Siegelman SS, et al. Initial results from an aggressive roentgenological and surgical approach to acute mesenteric ischemia. *Surgery* 1977;82:848.
54. Bradbury AW, Brittenden J, McBride K, et al. Mesenteric ischaemia: a multidisciplinary approach. *Br J Surg* 1995;82:1446.
55. Bradbury AW, Milne AA, Murie JA. Surgical aspects of Behçet's disease. *Br J Surg* 1994;81:1712.
56. Brandt LJ, Katz HJ, Wolf EL, et al. Simulation of colonic carcinoma by ischemia. *Gastroenterology* 1985;88:1137.
57. Brewster DC, Franklin DP, Cambria RP, et al. Intestinal ischemia complicating abdominal aortic surgery. *Surgery* 1991;109:447.
58. Bricker EM, Kraybill WG, Lopez MJ. Functional results after postirradiation rectal reconstruction. *World J Surg* 1986;10:249.
59. Brolin RE, Semmlow JL, Sehonanda A, et al. Comparison of five methods of assessment of intestinal viability. *Surg Gynecol Obstet* 1989;168:6.
60. Brookes VS. Meckel's diverticulum in children. *Br J Surg* 1954;42:57.
61. Brothers TE, Strodel WE, Eckhauser FE. Endoscopy in colonic volvulus. *Ann Surg* 1987;206:1.
62. Browder W, Cerise EJ, Litwin MS. Impact of emergency angiography in massive lower gastrointestinal bleeding. *Ann Surg* 1986;204:530.
63. Browning GGP, Varma JS, Smith AN, et al. Late results of mucosal proctectomy and colo-anal sleeve anastomosis for chronic irradiation rectal injury. *Br J Surg* 1987;74:31.
64. Buchi KN. Endoscopic gastrointestinal laser therapy. *West J Med* 1985;143:751.
65. Buchi K. Radiation proctitis: therapy and prognosis. *JAMA* 1991;265.1180.
66. Buchi KN, Dixon JA. Argon laser treatment of hemorrhagic radiation proctitis. *Gastrointest Endosc* 1987;33:27.
67. Bulkley GB, Zuidema GD, Hamilton SR, et al. Intraoperative determination of small intestinal viability following ischemic injury. *Ann Surg* 1981;194:628.
68. Bunker SR, Brown JM, McAuley RJ, et al. Detection of gastrointestinal bleeding sites: use of *in vitro* technetium Tc 99m-labeled RBCs. *JAMA* 1982;247:789.
69. Bunker SR, Lull RJ, Tanasescu DE, et al. Scintigraphy of gastrointestinal hemorrhage: superiority of 99mTc red blood cells over 99mTc sulfur colloid. *AJR* 1984;143:543.
70. Burke JB, Ballantyne GH. Cecal volvulus: low mortality at a city hospital. *Dis Colon Rectum* 1984;27:737.
71. Byrd RL, Cunningham MW, Goldman LI. Nonocclusive ischemic colitis secondary to hemorrhagic shock. *Dis Colon Rectum* 1987;30:116.
72. Cappell MS, Lebwohl O. Cessation of recurrent bleeding from gastrointestinal angiodysplasias after aortic valve replacement. *Ann Intern Med* 1986;105:54.
73. Carr ND, Pullen BR, Hasleton PS, et al. Microvascular studies in human radiation bowel disease. *Gut* 1984;25: 448.
74. Cataldo PA, Zarka MA, Formalin instillation for ischemic proctitis with unrelenting hemorrhage: report of a case. *Dis Colon Rectum* 2000;43:261.
75. Cello JP, Wilcox CM. Evaluation and treatment of gastrointestinal tract hemorrhage in patients with AIDS. *Gastroenterol Clin North Am* 1988;17:639.
76. Chung YFA, Eu K-W, Nyam DCNK, et al. Minimizing recurrence after sigmoid volvulus. *Br J Surg* 1999;86:231.
77. Clavien P-A. Diagnosis and management of mesenteric infarction. *Br J Surg* 1990;77:601.
78. Clavien P-A, Huber O, Rohner A. Venous mesenteric ischaemia: conservative or surgical treatment? *Lancet* 1989; 2:48.
79. Clavien P-A, Muller C, Harder F. Treatment of mesenteric infarction. *Br J Surg* 1987;74:500.
80. Cooke SR, deMoor NG. The surgical treatment of the radiation-damaged rectum. *Br J Surg* 1981;68:488.
81. Cooke SAR, Wellsted MD. The radiation-damaged rectum: resection with coloanal anastomosis using the endoanal technique. *World J Surg* 1986;20:220.
82. Cox JD, Byhardt RW, Wilson JF, et al. Complications of radiation therapy and factors in their prevention. *World J Surg* 1986;10:171.
83. Cram AE, Pearlman NW, Jochimsen PR. Surgical management of complications of radiation-injured gut. *Am J Surg* 1977;133:551.
84. Cross MJ, Frazee RC. Surgical treatment of radiation enteritis. *Am Surg* 1992;58:132.
85. Cuthbertson AM. Resection and pull-through for rectovaginal fistula. *World J Surg* 1986;10:228.
86. Daniels IR, Lamparelli MJ, Chave H, et al. Recurrent sigmoid volvulus treated by percutaneous endoscopic colostomy. *Br J Surg* 2000;87:1419.
87. Dauphine CE, Tan PY, Beart RW Jr. Self-expanding metallic stents in the management of lower gastrointestinal hemorrhage. *J Laparoscop Adv Surg Tech* 2003;13:407.
88. DeBarros J, Rosas L, Cohen J, et al. The changing paradigm for the treatment of colonic hemorrhage: superselective angiographic embolization. *Dis Colon Rectum* 2002;45: 802.
89. Dent OF, Galt E, Chapuis PH, et al. Quality of life in patients undergoing treatment for chronic radiation-induced rectal bleeding. *Br J Surg* 1998;85:1251.
90. Derodra JK, Reidy JF, Jourdan MH. Embolization of superior haemorrhoidal artery in the management of life-threatening rectal bleeding. *Br J Surg* 1992;79:704.
91. Desa LA, Ohri SK, Hutton KAR, et al. Role of intraoperative enteroscopy in obscure gastrointestinal bleeding of small bowel origin. *Br J Surg* 1991;78:192.
92. Devereux DF. Protection from radiation-associated small bowel injury with the aid of an absorbable mesh. *Semin Surg Oncol* 1986;2:17.
93. Devereux DF, Thompson D, Sandhaus L, et al. Protection from radiation enteritis by an absorbable polyglycolic acid mesh sling. *Surgery* 1987;101:123.
94. Dietz DW, Remzi FH, Fazio VW. Strictureplasty for obstructing small-bowel lesions in diffuse radiation enteritis—successful outcome in five patients. *Dis Colon Rectum* 2001;44:1772.
95. Dietz DW, Walsh RM, Grundfest-Broniatowski S, et al. Intestinal malrotation: a rare but important cause of bowel obstruction in adults. *Dis Colon Rectum* 2002;45:1381.
96. Dieulafoy G. Exulcertio simplex. *Bull Acad Med* 1898;49: 49.
97. Dirkx CA, Gerscovich EO. Sonographic findings in methamphetamine-induced ischemic colitis. *J Clin Ultrasound* 1998;26:479.
98. Donaldson SS, Jundt S, Ricour C, et al. Radiation enteritis in children. *Cancer* 1975;35:1167.
99. Eisenberg H, Laufer I, Skillman J. Arteriographic diagnosis and management of suspected colonic diverticular hemorrhage. *Gastroenterology* 1973;64:1091.
100. Emslie JT, Zarnegar K, Siegel ME, et al. Technetium-99m-labeled red blood cell scans in the investigation of gastrointestinal bleeding. *Dis Colon Rectum* 1996;39:750.
101. Endean ED, Barnes SL, Kwolek CJ, et al. Surgical management of thrombotic acute intestinal ischemia. *Ann Surg* 2001;233:801.
102. Ernst CB, Hagihara PF, Daugherty ME, et al. Ischemic colitis incidence following abdominal aortic reconstruction: a prospective study. *Surgery* 1976;80:417.

103. Fabri PJ. Intestinal ischemia in radiation enteritis. In: Cooperman M, ed. *Intestinal ischemia.* Mount Kisco, NY: Futura, 1983:315.

104. Faucheron JL, Rosso R, Tiret E, et al. Soave's procedure: the final sphincter-saving solution for iatrogenic rectal lesions. *Br J Surg* 1998;85:962.

105. Fiddian-Green RG, Amelin PM, Herrmann JB, et al. Prediction of the development of sigmoid ischemia on the day of aortic operations: indirect measurements of intramural pH in the colon. *Arch Surg* 1986;121:654.

106. Figiel LS, Figiel SJ. Volvulus of the cecum and right colon. In: Greenbaum EI, ed. *Radiographic atlas of colon disease.* Chicago: Year Book, 1980:637.

107. Flickinger EG, Stanforth AC, Sinar DR, et al. Intraoperative video panendoscopy for diagnosing sites of chronic intestinal bleeding. *Am J Surg* 1989;157:137.

108. Forde KA. Colonoscopy in acute rectal bleeding. *Gastrointest Endosc* 1981;27:219.

109. Forde KA, Lebwohl O, Wolff M, et al. Reversible ischemic colitis: correlation of colonoscopic and pathologic changes. *Am J Gastroenterol* 1979;72:182.

110. Foutch PG, Rex DK, Lieberman DA. Prevalence and natural history of colonic angiodysplasia among healthy asymptomatic people. *Am J Gastroenterol* 1995;90:564.

111. Foutch PG, Sirak MV. Colonic variceal haemorrhage after endoscopic infection sclerosis of oesophageal varices: a report of three cases. *Am J Gastroenterol* 1984;79:756.

112. Friedman G, Sloan WC. Ischemic enteropathy. *Surg Clin North Am* 1972;52:1001.

113. Friedman JD, Odland MD, Bubrick MP. Experience with colonic volvulus. *Dis Colon Rectum* 1989;32:409.

114. Galland RB, Spencer J. Spontaneous postoperative perforation of previously asymptomatic irradiated bowel. *Br J Surg* 1985;72:285.

115. Galland RB, Spencer J. Surgical management of radiation enteritis. *Surgery* 1986;99:133.

116. Galland RB, Spencer J. Natural history and surgical management of radiation enteritis. *Br J Surg* 1987;74:742.

117. Gandhi SK, Hanson MM, Vernava AM, et al. Ischemic colitis. *Dis Colon Rectum* 1996;39:88.

118. Garofalo TE, Abdu RA. Accuracy and efficacy of nuclear scintigraphy for the detection of gastrointestinal bleeding. *Arch Surg* 1997;132:196.

119. Gazet J-C. Parks' coloanal pull-through anastomosis for severe, complicated radiation proctitis. *Dis Colon Rectum* 1985;28:110.

120. Geer DA, Arnaud G, Beitler A, et al. Colonic volvulus: the Army Medical Center experience, 1983–1987. *Am Surg* 1991;57:295.

121. Gennaro AR, Rosemond GP. Colonic diverticula and hemorrhage. *Dis Colon Rectum* 1973;16:409.

122. Ghazi A, Shinya H, Wolff WI. Treatment of volvulus of the colon by colonoscopy. *Ann Surg* 1976;183:263.

123. Gibney EJ. Volvulus of the sigmoid colon. *Surg Gynecol Obstet* 1991;173:243.

124. Goldberg M, Lernau OZ, Mogle P, et al. Volvulus of the splenic flexure of the colon. *Am J Gastroenterol* 1984;79: 693.

125. Goldberger LE. Diverticular disease of the colon: angiography in diverticular hemorrhage. In: Greenbaum EI, ed. *Radiographic atlas of colon disease.* Chicago: Year Book, 1980:113.

126. Goldberger LE, Bookstein JJ. Transcatheter embolization for treatment of diverticular hemorrhage. *Radiology* 1977; 122:613.

127. Goosenberg EB, Greenfield SM, Kasama RK. Cecal volvulus update. *Contemp Gastroenterol* 1991;4:11.

128. Gorfine SR. The colon in collagen vascular disease. Presented at the Annual Meeting American College of Surgeons, San Francisco, 1996.

129. Granieri R, Mazzula J, Yarborough G. Estrogen-progesterone therapy for recurrent gastrointestinal bleeding secondary to gastrointestinal angiodysplasia. *Am J Gastroenterol* 1988;83:556.

130. Greenstein RJ, McElhinney AJ, Reuben D, et al. Colonic vascular ectasias and aortic stenosis: coincidence or causal relationship? *Am J Surg* 1986;151:347.

131. Griffiths JD. Surgical anatomy of the blood supply of the distal colon. *Ann R Coll Surg Engl* 1956;19:241.

132. Groff WL. Angiodysplasia of the colon. *Dis Colon Rectum* 1983;26:64.

133. Grossmann EM, Longo WE, Stratton MD, et al. Sigmoid volvulus in Department of Veterans Affairs medical centers. *Dis Colon Rectum* 2000;43:414.

134. Gumbs MA, Kashan F, Shumofsky E, et al. Volvulus of the transverse colon: reports of cases and review of the literature. *Dis Colon Rectum* 1983;26:825.

135. Gupta N, Longo WE, Vernava AM III. Angiodysplasia of the lower gastrointestinal tract: an entity readily diagnosed by colonoscopy and primarily managed nonoperatively. *Dis Colon Rectum* 1995;38:979.

136. Gurel M, Alic B, Bac B, et al. Intraoperative colonic irrigation in the treatment of acute sigmoid volvulus. *Br J Surg* 1989;76:957.

137. Guttormson NL, Bubrick MP. Mortality from ischemic colitis. *Dis Colon Rectum* 1989;32:469.

138. Hagihara PF, Chuang VP, Griffen WO Jr. Arteriovenous malformations of the colon. *Am J Surg* 1977;133:681.

139. Handschin AE, Weber M, Weishaupt D, et al. Contrast-enhanced three-dimensional magnetic resonance angiography for visualization of ectopic varices. *Dis Colon Rectum* 2002;45:1541.

140. Hagihara PF, Ernst CB, Griffen WO Jr. Incidence of ischemic colitis following abdominal aortic reconstruction. *Surg Gynecol Obstet* 1979;149:571.

141. Harer WB Jr, Harer WB Sr. Volvulus complicating pregnancy and puerperium: report of three cases and review of literature. *Obstet Gynecol* 1958;12:399.

142. Harling H, Balslev I. Radical surgical approach to radiation injury of the small bowel. *Dis Colon Rectum* 1986;29: 371.

143. Harling H, Balslev I. Long-term prognosis of patients with severe radiation enteritis. *Am J Surg* 1988;155:517.

144. Hatcher PA, Thomson HJ, Ludgate SN, et al. Surgical aspects of intestinal injury due to pelvic radiotherapy. *Ann Surg* 1985;201:470.

145. Hayne D, Vaizey CJ, Boulos PB. Anorectal injury following pelvic radiotherapy. *Br J Surg* 2001;88:1037.

146. Hellman AA, Cramer WO. Mesh fixation of the mesentery for treatment of volvulus and recurrent stomal prolapse. *Surg Gynecol Obstet* 1988;167:249.

147. Hemingway AP, Allison DJ. Angiodysplasia and Meckel's diverticulum: a congenital association? *Br J Surg* 1982;69: 493.

148. Höchter W, Weingart J, Kühner W, et al. Angiodysplasia in the colon and rectum: endoscopic morphology, localisation and frequency. *Endoscopy* 1985;17:182.

149. Howard RS, Catto J. Cecal volvulus: a case for nonresectional therapy. *Arch Surg* 1980;115:273.

150. Hunter JG, Bowers JH, Burt RW, et al. Lasers in endoscopic gastrointestinal surgery. *Am J Surg* 1984;148:736.

151. Hunter JM, Pezim ME. Limited value of technetium 99m-labeled red cell scintigraphy in localization of lower gastrointestinal bleeding. *Am J Surg* 1990;159:504.

152. Iida M, Kobayashi H, Matsumoto T, et al. Postoperative recurrence in patients with intestinal Behçet's disease. *Dis Colon Rectum* 1994;37:16.

153. Iredale JP, Ridings P, McGinn FP, et al. Familial and idiopathic colonic varices: an unusual cause of lower gastrointestinal haemorrhage. *Gut* 1992;33:1285.

154. Irvine EJ, O'Connor J, Frost RA, et al. Prospective comparison of double contrast barium enema plus flexible sigmoidoscopy *v* colonoscopy in rectal bleeding: barium enema *v* colonoscopy in rectal bleeding. *Gut* 1988;29:1188.

155. Isbister WH, Pease CW, Delahunt B. Colonic varices: report of a case. *Dis Colon Rectum* 1989;32:524.

156. Iwashita A, Yao T, Schlemper RJ, et al. Mesenteric phlebosclerosis: a new disease entity causing ischemic colitis. *Dis Colon Rectum* 2003;46:209.

157. Jablonski M, Putzki H, Heymann H. Necrosis of the ascending colon in chronic hemodialysis patients: report of three cases. *Dis Colon Rectum* 1987;30:623.

158. Janik JS, Humphrey R, Nagaraj HS. Sigmoid volvulus in a neonate with imperforate anus. *J Pediatr Surg* 1983;18:636.

159. Jao S-W, Beart RW Jr, Gunderson LL. Surgical treatment of radiation injuries of the colon and rectum. *Am J Surg* 1986;151:272.

160. Jensen DM, Machicado GA. Diagnosis and treatment of severe hematochezia: the role of urgent colonoscopy after purge. *Gastroenterology* 1988;95:1569.

161. Joergensen K, Kronborg O. The colonoscope in volvulus of the transverse colon. *Dis Colon Rectum* 1980;23:357.

162. Johnston MJ, Robertson GM, Frizelle FA. Management of late complications of pelvic radiation in the rectum and anus: a review. *Dis Colon Rectum* 2003;46:247.

163. Kim MW, Hundahl SA, Dang CR, et al. Ischemic colitis after aortic aneurysmectomy. *Am J Surg* 1983;145:392.

164. Kimose H-H, Fischer L, Spjeldnaes N, et al. Late radiation injury of the colon and rectum. *Dis Colon Rectum* 1989; 32:684.

165. Kinsella TJ, Bloomer WD. Tolerance of the intestine to radiation therapy. *Surg Gynecol Obstet* 1980;151:273.

166. Knoepp LF Jr, McCulloch JH. Colonoscopy in the diagnosis of unexplained rectal bleeding. *Dis Colon Rectum* 1978; 21:590.

167. Kusumoto H, Motofumi Y, Takahashi I, et al. Complications and diagnosis of Meckel's diverticulum in 776 patients. *Am J Surg* 1992;164:382.

168. Kuzu MA, Aslar AK, Soran A, et al. Emergent resection for acute sigmoid volvulus. Results of 106 consecutive cases. *Dis Colon Rectum* 2002;45:1085.

169. Landreneau RJ, Fry WJ. The right colon as a target organ of nonocclusive mesenteric ischemia. *Arch Surg* 1990;125:591.

170. Lau WY, Yuen WK, Chu KW, et al. Obscure bleeding in the gastrointestinal tract originating in the small intestine. *Surg Gynecol Obstet* 1992;174:119.

171. Launer DP, Miscall BG, Beil AR Jr. Colorectal infarction following resection of abdominal aortic aneurysms. *Dis Colon Rectum* 1978;21:613.

172. Lavery IC, Steiger E, Fazio VW. Home parenteral nutrition in management of patients with severe radiation enteritis. *Dis Colon Rectum* 1980;23:91.

173. Leitman IM, Paull DE, Shires GT III. Evaluation and management of massive lower gastrointestinal hemorrhage. *Ann Surg* 1989;209:175.

174. Levitsky J, Hong JJ, Jani AB, et al. Oral vitamin A therapy for a patient with a severely symptomatic postradiation anal ulceration: report of a case. *Dis Colon Rectum* 2003; 46:679.

175. Levy PJ, Krausz MM, Manny J. Acute mesenteric ischemia: improved results—a retrospective analysis of ninety-two patients. *Surgery* 1990;107:372.

176. Lindsey I, Farmer CR, Cunningham IG. Subtotal colectomy and cecosigmoid anastomosis for colonic systemic sclerosis. Report of a case and review of the literature. *Dis Colon Rectum* 2003;46:1706.

177. Longo WE, Ballantyne GH, Gusberg RJ. Ischemic colitis: patterns and prognosis. *Dis Colon Rectum* 1992;35:726.

178. Longo WE, Ward D, Vernava AM III, et al. Outcome of patients with total colonic ischemia. *Dis Colon Rectum* 1997; 40:1448.

179. Lopez MJ, Cooley JS, Petros JG, et al. Complete intraoperative small-bowel endoscopy in the evaluation of occult gastrointestinal bleeding using the Sonde enteroscope. *Arch Surg* 1996;131:272.

180. Lopez MJ, Kraybill WG, Johnston WD, et al. Postirradiation reconstruction of the rectum in a male. *Surg Gynecol Obstet* 1982;55:67.

181. Lord SA, Boswell WC, Hungerpiller JC. Sigmoid volvulus in pregnancy. *Am Surg* 1996;62:380.

182. Love JW. The syndrome of calcific aortic stenosis and gastrointestinal bleeding. *J Thorac Cardiovasc Surg* 1982;83: 779.

183. Lucarotti ME, Mountford RA, Bartolo DCC. Surgical management of intestinal radiation injury. *Dis Colon Rectum* 1991;34:865.

184. Luchtefeld MA, Senagore AJ, Szomstein M, et al. Evaluation of transarterial embolization for lower gastrointestinal bleeding. *Dis Colon Rectum* 2000;43:532.

185. Lüdtke F-E, Mende V, Köhler H, et al. Incidence and frequency of complications and management of Meckel's diverticulum. *Surg Gynecol Obstet* 1989;169:537.

186. Luna-Pérez P, Rodríguez-Ramírez SE. Formalin instillation for refractory radiation-induced hemorrhagic proctitis. *J Surg Oncol* 2002;80:41

187. Luzar MJ. Systemic vasculitis. In: Cooperman M, ed. *Intestinal ischemia*. Mount Kisco, NY: Futura, 1983:355.

188. Luzar MJ. Connective tissue diseases. In: Cooperman M, ed. *Intestinal ischemia*. Mount Kisco, NY: Futura, 1983: 391.

189. Ma CK, Padda H, Pace EH, et al. Submucosal arterial malformation of the colon with massive hemorrhage: report of a case. *Dis Colon Rectum* 1989;32:149.

190. Mackey WC, Dineen P. A fifty year experience with Meckel's diverticulum. *Surg Gynecol Obstet* 1983;156:56.

191. Madiba TE, Thomson SR. The management of cecal volvulus. *Dis Colon Rectum* 2002;45:264.

192. Marks G. Combined abdominotranssacral reconstruction of the radiation-injured rectum. *Am J Surg* 1976;131:54.

193. Marks G, Mohiudden M. The surgical management of the radiation-injured intestine. *Surg Clin North Am* 1983;63:81.

194. Marston A, Pheils MT, Thomas ML, et al. Ischaemic colitis. *Gut* 1966;7:1.

195. Matolo NM, Link DP. Selective embolization for control of gastrointestinal hemorrhage. *Am J Surg* 1979;138:840.

196. Max MH, Richardson JD, Flint LM Jr, et al. Colonoscopic diagnosis of angiodysplasias of the gastrointestinal tract. *Surg Gynecol Obstet* 1981;152:195.

197. McCalla TH, Arensman RM, Falterman KW. Sigmoid volvulus in children. *Am Surg* 1985;51:514.

198. McDonald ML, Farnell MB, Stanson AW, et al. Preoperative highly selective catheter localization of occult small-intestinal hemorrhage with methylene blue dye. *Arch Surg* 1995;130:106.

199. McGuire HH Jr. Bleeding colonic diverticula: a reappraisal of natural history and management. *Ann Surg* 1994;220: 653.

200. Meckel J. Ueber die Divertikel am Darmkanal. *Arch die Physiol* 1809;9:421.

201. Medina C, Vilaseca J, Videla S, et al. Outcome of patients with ischemic colitis: review of fifty-three cases. *Dis Colon Rectum* 2004;47:180.

202. Metyas SK, Mithani VK, Tempera P. Dieulafoy's lesion, a rare cause of lower gastrointestinal hemorrhage. *Hosp Physician* 2001;September:41.

203. Miholi J, Schwarz C, Moeschi P. Surgical therapy of radiation-induced lesions of the colon and rectum. *Am J Surg* 1988;155:761.

204. Miller MD, Johnsrude IS, Jackson DC. Improved technique for transcatheter embolization of arteries. *Am J Roentgenol* 1978;180:183.

205. Mitchell KM, Valentine RJ. Inferior mesenteric artery reimplantation does not guarantee colon viability in aortic surgery. *J Am Coll Surg* 2002;194:151.

206. Moore JH, Cintron JR, Duarte B, et al. Synchronous cecal and sigmoid volvulus: report of a case. *Dis Colon Rectum* 1992;35:803.

207. Moore JD, Thompson NW, Appleman HD, et al. Arteriovenous malformations of the gastrointestinal tract. *Arch Surg* 1976;111:381.

208. Morgenstern L. Surgical aspects of radiation enteropathy. *Surg Rounds* 1985;8:60.

209. Morgenstern L, Hart M, Lugo D, et al. Changing aspects of radiation enteropathy. *Arch Surg* 1985;120:1225.

210. Morgenstern L, Thompson R, Friedman NB. The modern enigma of radiation enteropathy: sequelae and solutions. *Am J Surg* 1977;134:166.

211. Morrissey TB, Deitch EA. Recurrence of sigmoid volvulus after surgical intervention. *Am Surg* 1994;60:329.

212. Moshkowitz M, Arber N, Amir N, et al. Success of estrogen-progesterone therapy in long-standing bleeding gastrointestinal angiodysplasia: report of a case. *Dis Colon Rectum* 1993;36:194.

213. Nakada T, Kubota Y, Sasagawa I, et al. Therapeutic experience of hyperbaric oxygenation in radiation colitis: report of a case. *Dis Colon Rectum* 1993;36:962.

214. Nelson RL, Briley S, Schuler JJ, et al. Acute ischemia proctitis: report of six cases. *Dis Colon Rectum* 1992;35:375.

215. Nelson RL, Schuler JJ. Ischemic proctitis. *Surg Gynecol Obstet* 1982;154:27.

216. Ng DA, Opelka FG, Beck DE, et al. Predictive value of technetium Tc 99m-labeled red blood cell scintigraphy for positive angiogram in massive lower gastrointestinal hemorrhage. *Dis Colon Rectum* 1997;40:471.

217. Nguyen NP, Antoine JE, Dutta S, et al. Current concepts in radiation enteritis and implications for future clinical trials. *Cancer* 2002;95:1151.

218. Nicholson ML, Neoptolemos JP, Sharp JF, et al. Localization of lower gastrointestinal bleeding using *in vivo* technetium-99m-labelled red blood cell scintigraphy. *Br J Surg* 1989;76:358.

219. Noer R, Hamilton JE, Williams DJ, et al. Rectal hemorrhage: moderate and severe. *Ann Surg* 1962;155:794.

220. Northeast ADR, Dennison AR, Lee EG. Sigmoid volvulus: new thoughts on the epidemiology. *Dis Colon Rectum* 1984;27:260.

221. Nowacki MP, Szawlowski AW, Borkowski A. Parks' coloanal sleeve anastomosis for treatment of postirradiation rectovaginal fistula. *Dis Colon Rectum* 1986;29:817.

222. O'Connor JJ. Argon laser treatment of radiation enteritis. *Arch Surg* 1989;124:749.

223. O'Mara CS, Wilson TH Jr, Stonesifer GL, et al. Cecal volvulus: analysis of 50 patients with long-term follow-up. *Ann Surg* 1979;189:724.

224. Orchard JL, Mehta R, Khan AH. The use of colonoscopy in the treatment of colonic volvulus: three cases and review of the literature. *Am J Gastroenterol* 1984;79:864.

225. Orecchia PM, Hensley EK, McDonald PT, et al. Localization of lower gastrointestinal hemorrhage: experience with red blood cells labeled *in vitro* with technetium Tc 99m. *Arch Surg* 1985;120:621.

226. Papa MZ, Shiloni E, McDonald HD. Total colon necrosis: a catastrophic complication of systemic lupus erythematosus. *Dis Colon Rectum* 1986;29:576.

227. Parikh S, Hughes C, Salvati EP, et al. Treatment of hemorrhagic radiation proctitis with 4 percent formalin. *Dis Colon Rectum* 2003;46:596.

228. Parkes BM, Obeid FN, Sorensen VJ, et al. The management of massive lower gastrointestinal bleeding. *Am Surg* 1993;59:676.

229. Parks TG. Ischaemic disease of the colon. *Coloproctology* 1980;4:213.

230. Parish KL, Chapman WC, Williams LF Jr. Ischemic colitis: an ever-changing spectrum? *Am Surg* 1991;57:118.

231. Pasch AR, Adams JT. Acute volvulus of the sigmoid colon: current management. *Cont Surg* 1985;26:65.

232. Patel A, Boley SJ. Vascular ectasias of the colon. *Surg Rounds* 1990;7:25.

233. Pennoyer WP, Vignati PV, Cohen JL. Mesenteric angiography for lower gastrointestinal hemorrhage: are there predictors for a positive study? *Dis Colon Rectum* 1997;40:1014.

234. Peoples JB, McCafferty JC, Scher KS. Operative therapy for sigmoid volvulus: identification of risk factors affecting outcome. *Dis Colon Rectum* 1990;33:643.

235. Petrini JL. Endoscopic therapy for gastrointestinal bleeding. *Postgrad Med* 1988;84:239–244.

236. Pinedo G, Kirberg A. Percutaneous endoscopic sigmoidopexy in sigmoid volvulus with T-fasteners. *Dis Colon Rectum* 2001;44:1867.

237. Pinto A, Fidalgo P, Cravo M, et al. Short chain fatty acids are effective in short-term treatment of chronic radiation proctitis: randomized, double-blind, controlled trial. *Dis Colon Rectum* 1999;42:788.

238. Poeze M, Froon AHM, Greve JWM, et al. D-lactate as an early marker of intestinal ischaemia after ruptured abdominal aortic aneurysm repair. *Br J Surg* 1998;85:1221.

239. Potter GD, Sellin JH. Lower gastrointestinal bleeding. *Gastroenterol Clin North Am* 1988;17:341.

240. Pratt AT, Donaldson RC, Evertson LR, et al. Cecal volvulus in pregnancy. *Obstet Gynecol* 1981;57:37S.

241. Procaccino J, Labow SB. Transcolonoscopic decompression of sigmoid volvulus. *Dis Colon Rectum* 1989;32:349.

242. Pruett TL, Wilkins ME, Gamble WG. Cecal volvulus: a different twist for the serious runner. *N Engl J Med* 1985;312:1262.

243. Quirke P, Campbell I, Talbot IC. Ischaemic proctitis and adventitial fibromuscular dysplasia of the superior rectal artery. *Br J Surg* 1984;71:33.

244. Rabinovici R, Simansky DA, Kaplan O, et al. Cecal volvulus. *Dis Colon Rectum* 1990;33:765.

245. Ramanath H, Hinshaw JR. Management and mismanagement of bleeding colonic diverticula. *Arch Surg* 1971;103:311.

246. Regan PT, Weiland LH, Geall MG. Scleroderma and intestinal perforation. *Am J Gastroenterol* 1977;68:566.

247. Reichelderfer M, Morrissey JF. Colonoscopy in radiation colitis. *Gastrointest Endosc* 1980;26:41.

248. Rex DK, Weddle RA, Lehman GA, et al. Flexible sigmoidoscopy plus air contrast barium enema versus colonoscopy for suspected lower gastrointestinal bleeding. *Gastroenterology* 1990;98:855.

249. Richardson JD, Lordon RE. Gastrointestinal bleeding caused by angiodysplasia: a difficult problem in patients with chronic renal failure receiving hemodialysis therapy. *Am Surg* 1993;59:636.

250. Richardson JD, Mas MH, Flint LM Jr, et al. Bleeding vascular malformations of the intestine. *Surgery* 1978;84:430.

251. Ritter EF, Lee CG, Tyler D, et al. Advances in prevention of radiation damage to visceral and solid organs in patients requiring radiation therapy of the trunk. *J Surg Oncol* 1997;64:109.

252. Robertson HD, Gathright JB Jr. The technique of intraoperative segmental artery arteriography to localize vascular ectasias. *Dis Colon Rectum* 1985;28:274.

253. Rogers RL, Harford FJ. Mobile cecum syndrome. *Dis Colon Rectum* 1984;27:399.

254. Rösch J, Dotter CT, Brown MJ. Selective arterial embolization: a new method for control of acute gastrointestinal bleeding. *Radiology* 1972;102:303.

255. Rosenkrantz H, Bookstein JJ, Rosen RJ, et al. Postembolic colonic infarction. *Radiology* 1982;142:47.

256. Rossini FP, Ferrari A, Spandre M, et al. Emergency colonoscopy. *World J Surg* 1989;13:190.

257. Roswit B. Radiation injury of the colon and rectum. In: Greenbaum EI, ed. *Radiographic atlas of colon disease.* Chicago: Year Book, 1980:461.

258. Rubinstein E, Ibsen T, Rasmussen RB, et al. Formalin treatment of radiation-induced hemorrhagic proctitis. *Am J Gastroenterol* 1986;81:44.

259. Ryan JA Jr, Johnson MG, Baker JW. Operative treatment of cecal volvulus combining cecopexy with intestinal tube decompression. *Surg Gynecol Obstet* 1985;160:84.

260. Ryan P. Sigmoid volvulus with and without megacolon. *Dis Colon Rectum* 1982;25:673.

261. Saclarides TJ, King DG, Franklin JL, et al. Formalin instillation for refractory radiation-induced hemorrhagic proctitis: report of 16 patients. *Dis Colon Rectum* 1996;39:196.

262. Salim AS. Management of acute volvulus of the sigmoid colon: a new approach by percutaneous deflation and colopexy. *World J Surg* 1991;15:68.

263. Sanner CJ, Saltzman DA. Detorsion of sigmoid volvulus by colonoscopy. *Gastrointest Endosc* 1977;23:212.

264. Santos JCM Jr, Feres O, Rocha JJR, et al. Massive lower gastrointestinal hemorrhage caused by pseudocyst of the pancreas ruptured into the colon. *Dis Colon Rectum* 1992; 35:75.

265. Savoie LM, Abrams AV. Refractory proctosigmoiditis caused by myointimal hyperplasia of mesenteric veins: report of a case. *Dis Colon Rectum* 1999;42:1093.

266. Schiedler MG, Cutler BS, Fiddian-Green RG. Sigmoid intramural pH for prediction of ischemic colitis during aortic surgery: a comparison with risk factors and inferior mesenteric artery stump pressures. *Arch Surg* 1987;122: 881.

267. Schmitt EH, Symmonds RE. Surgical treatment of radiation induced injuries of the intestine. *Surg Gynecol Obstet* 1981;153:896.

268. Schmitz RL, Chao J-H, Bartolome JS Jr. Intestinal injuries incidental to irradiation of carcinoma of the cervix of the uterus. *Surg Gynecol Obstet* 1974;138:29.

269. Schneider TA, Longo WE, Ure T, et al. Mesenteric ischemia: acute arterial syndromes. *Dis Colon Rectum* 1994;37:1163.

270. Schrock TR. Colonoscopic diagnosis and treatment of lower gastrointestinal bleeding. *Surg Clin North Am* 1989; 69:1309.

271. Schroeder T, Christoffersen JK, Andersen J, et al. Ischemic colitis complicating reconstruction of the abdominal aorta. *Surg Gynecol Obstet* 1985;160:299.

272. Schoots IG, Koffeman GI, Legemate DA, et al. Systematic review of survival after acute mesenteric ischaemia according to disease aetiology. *Br J Surg* 2004;91:17.

273. Schwartz MJ, Lewis JH. Meckel's diverticulum: pitfalls in scintigraphic detection in the adult. *Am J Gastroenterol* 1984;79:611.

274. Scott HJ, Lane IF, Glynn MJ, et al. Colonic haemorrhage: a technique for rapid intra-operative bowel preparation and colonoscopy. *Br J Surg* 1986;73:390.

275. Seger DL, Middleton D. Childhood sigmoid volvulus. *Ann Emerg Med* 1984;13:133.

276. Seldinger SI. Catheter replacement of needle in percutaneous arteriography; new technique. *Acta Radiol (Stockh)* 1953;39:368.

277. Seow-Choen F, Goh H-S, Eu K-W, et al. A simple and effective treatment for hemorrhagic radiation proctitis using formalin. *Dis Colon Rectum* 1993;36:135.

278. Shbeeb I, Prager E, Love J. The aortic valve colonic axis. *Dis Colon Rectum* 1984;27:38.

279. Shibata D, Brophy DP, Gordon FD, et al. Transjugular intrahepatic portosystemic shunt for treatment of bleeding ectopic varices with portal hypertension. *Dis Colon Rectum* 1999;42:1581.

280. Shibata M, Nakamura H, Abe S, et al. Ischemic colitis caused by strict dieting in an 18-year-old female. Report of a case. *Dis Colon Rectum* 2002;45:425.

281. Shoop SA, Sackier JM. Laparoscopic cecopexy for cecal volvulus. *Surg Endosc* 1993;7:450.

282. Simpson AJ, Previti FW. Technetium sulfur colloid scintigraphy in the detection of lower gastrointestinal tract bleeding. *Surg Gynecol Obstet* 1982;155:33.

283. Singh G, Gupta SK, Gupta S. Simultaneous occurrence of sigmoid and cecal volvulus. *Dis Colon Rectum* 1985;28:115.

284. Sitges-Serra A, Mas X, Roqueta F, et al. Mesenteric infarction: an analysis of 83 patients with prognostic studies in 44 cases undergoing a massive small-bowel resection. *Br J Surg* 1988;75:544.

285. Skibba RM, Hartong WA, Mantz FA, et al. Angiodysplasia of the cecum: colonoscopic diagnosis. *Gastrointest Endosc* 1976;22:177.

286. Smith DH, DeCosse JJ. Radiation damage to the small intestine. *World J Surg* 1986;10:189.

287. Smith GF, Ellyson JH, Parks SN, et al. Angiodysplasia of the colon: a review of 17 cases. *Arch Surg* 1984;119:532.

288. Sniderman KW, Franklin J Jr, Sos T. Successful transcatheter Gelfoam embolization of a bleeding cecal vascular ectasia. *Am J Roentgenol* 1978;131:157.

289. Sogge MR, Dale JA, Butler ML. Detection of typical lesions of hereditary hemorrhagic telangiectasia by colonoscopy. *Gastrointest Endosc* 1980;26:52.

290. Soltero MJ, Bill AH. The natural history of Meckel's diverticulum and its relation to incidental removal. *Am J Surg* 1976;132:168.

291. Spencer J. Lower gastrointestinal bleeding. *Br J Surg* 1989; 76:3.

292. Starling JR. Initial treatment of sigmoid volvulus by colonoscopy. *Ann Surg* 1979;190:36.

293. Stewart WB, Gathright JB Jr, Ray JE. Vascular ectasias of the colon. *Surg Gynecol Obstet* 1979;148:670.

294. Stylianos S, Forde KA, Benvenisty AI, et al. Lower gastrointestinal hemorrhage in renal transplant recipients. *Arch Surg* 1988;123:739.

295. Sudek P. Über die Gefässversorgung des Mastdarmes in Hinsicht auf die operative Gangrän. *Münch Med Wochenschr* 1907;54:1314.

296. Sugarbaker PH. Intrapelvic prosthesis to prevent injury of the small intestine with high dosage pelvic irradiation. *Surg Gynecol Obstet* 1983;157:269.

297. Swarbrick ET, Fevre DI, Hunt RH, et al. Colonoscopy for unexplained rectal bleeding. *Br Med J* 1978;2:1685.

298. Taïeb S, Rolachon A, Cenni J-C. Effective use of argon plasma coagulation in the treatment of severe radiation proctitis. *Dis Colon Rectum* 2001;44:1766.

299. Talman EA, Dixon DS, Gutierrez FE. Role of arteriography in rectal hemorrhage due to arteriovenous malformations and diverticulosis. *Ann Surg* 1979;190:203.

300. Talley NA, Chen F, King D, et al. Short-chain fatty acids in the treatment of radiation proctitis: a randomized, double-blind, placebo-controlled, cross-over pilot trial. *Dis Colon Rectum* 1997;40:1046.

301. Tannenbaum GA, Forde KA. Radiation enteritis and colitis: general considerations in medical and surgical management. *Surg Rounds* 1986;9:42.

302. Taylor SA, Halligan S, Vance M, et al. Use of multidetector-row computer tomographic colonography before flexible sigmoidoscopy in the investigation of rectal bleeding. *Br J Surg* 2003;90:1163.

303. Tedesco FJ, Gottfried EB, Corless JK, et al. Prospective evaluation of hospitalized patients with nonactive lower intestinal bleeding: timing and role of barium enema and colonoscopy. *Gastrointest Endosc* 1984;30:281.

304. Tedesco FJ, Pickens CA, Griffin JW Jr, et al. Role of colonoscopy in patients with unexplained melena: analysis of 53 patients. *Gastrointest Endosc* 1981;27:221.

305. Tejler G, Jiborn H. Volvulus of the cecum: report of 26 cases and review of the literature. *Dis Colon Rectum* 1988; 31:445.

306. Thanik KD, Chey WY, Abbott J. Vascular dysplasia of the cecum as a repeated source of hemorrhage: role of colonoscopy in diagnosis. *Gastrointest Endosc* 1977;23: 167.

307. Thomas MG. Obscure lower gastrointestinal tract bleeding. *Br J Surg* 1999;86:579.

308. Tjandra JJ, Sengupta S. Argon plasma coagulation is an effective treatment for refractory hemorrhagic radiation proctitis. *Dis Colon Rectum* 2001;44:1759.

309. Todd GJ, Forde KA. Volvulus of the cecum: choice of operation. *Am J Surg* 1979;138:632.

310. Travis S, Davies DR, Creamer B. Acute colorectal ischaemia after anaphylactoid shock. *Gut* 1991;32:444.

311. Trudel JL, Fazio VW, Sivak MV. Colonoscopic diagnosis and treatment of arteriovenous malformations in chronic lower gastrointestinal bleeding: clinical accuracy and efficacy. *Dis Colon Rectum* 1988;31:107.

312. Uden P, Jiborn H, Jonsson K. Influence of selective mesenteric arteriography on the outcome of emergency surgery for massive, lower gastrointestinal hemorrhage: a 15-year experience. *Dis Colon Rectum* 1986;29:561.

313. Udezue NO. Sigmoid volvulus in Kaduna, Nigeria. *Dis Colon Rectum* 1990;33:647.

314. Van Custem E, Rutgeerts P, Vantrappen G. Treatment of bleeding gastrointestinal vascular malformations with oestrogen-progesterone. *Lancet* 1990;335:953.

315. VanDeinse WH, Zawacki JK, Phillips D. Treatment of acute mesenteric ischemia by percutaneous transluminal angioplasty. *Gastroenterology* 1986;91:475.

316. Vane DW, West KW, Grosfeld JL. Vitelline duct anomalies: experience with 217 childhood cases. *Arch Surg* 1987;122:542.

317. van Leeuwen JH. Sigmoid volvulus in a West African population. *Dis Colon Rectum* 1985;28:712.

318. Varma JS, Smith AN. Anorectal function following colo-anal sleeve anastomosis for chronic radiation injury to the rectum. *Br J Surg* 1986;73:285.

319. Varma JS, Smith AN, Busuttil A. Correlation of clinical and manometric abnormalities of rectal function following chronic radiation injury. *Br J Surg* 1985;72:875.

320. Varma JS, Smith AN, Busuttil A. Function of the anal sphincters after chronic radiation injury. *Gut* 1986;27:528.

321. Veidenheimer MC, Corman ML, Coller JA. Colonic hemorrhage. *Surg Clin North Am* 1978;58:581.

322. Vernia P, Fracasso PL, Casale V, et al. Topical butyrate for acute radiation proctitis: randomised, crossover trial. *Lancet* 2000;356:1232

323. Villarreal HA, Marts BC, Longo WE, et al. Congenital colonic varices in the adult. *Dis Colon Rectum* 1995;38: 990.

324. Waxman AD. Nuclear medicine techniques in the evaluation of gastrointestinal bleeding. *Curr Concepts Diagn Nucl Imaging* 1985;2:13.

325. Weingart J, Höchter W, Ottenjann R. Varices of the entire colon—an unusual cause of recurrent intestinal bleeding. *Endoscopy* 1982;14:69.

326. Welch GH, Anderson JR. Volvulus of the splenic flexure of the colon. *Dis Colon Rectum* 1985;28:592.

327. Welch GH, Anderson JR. Acute volvulus of the sigmoid colon. *World J Surg* 1987;11:258.

328. Welch M, Baguneid MS, McMahon RF, et al. Histological study of colonic ischaemia after aortic surgery. *Br J Surg* 1998;85:1095.

329. Welch GH, Shearer MG, Imrie CW, et al. Total colonic ischemia. *Dis Colon Rectum* 1986;29:410.

330. Welling RE, Roedersheimer R, Arbaugh JJ, et al. Ischemic colitis following repair of ruptured abdominal aortic aneurysm. *Arch Surg* 1985;120:1368.

331. Wellwood JM, Jackson BT. The intestinal complications of radiotherapy. *Br J Surg* 1973;60:814.

332. West BR, Ray JE, Gathright JB Jr. Comparison of transient ischemic colitis with that requiring treatment. *Surg Gynecol Obstet* 1980;151:366.

333. Williams LF, Wittenberg J. Ischemic colitis: an useful clinical diagnosis, but is it ischemic? *Ann Surg* 1975;182: 439.

334. Williams RA, Wilson SE. Current management of massive lower gastrointestinal bleeding. *Int Surg* 1980;2:157.

335. Winn M, Weissmann HS, Sprayregen S, et al. The radionuclide detection of lower gastrointestinal bleeding sites. *Clin Nucl Med* 1983;8:389.

336. Winzelberg GG, Froelich JW, McKusick KA, et al. Radionuclide localization of lower gastrointestinal hemorrhage. *Radiology* 1981;139:465–469

337. Winzelberg GG, McKusick KA, Waltman AC, et al. Evaluation of gastrointestinal bleeding by red blood cells labeled in vivo with technetium-99m. *J Nucl Med* 1979;20:1080.

338. Wiseman JS, Senagore AJ, Chaudry IH. Methods to prevent colonic injury in pelvic radiation. *Dis Colon Rectum* 1994;37:1090.

339. Wolf EL, Frager D, Beneventano TC. Volvulus of the transverse colon. *Am J Gastroenterol* 1984;79:797.

340. Wyman A, Zeiderman MR. Maintaining decompression of sigmoid volvulus. *Surg Gynecol Obstet* 1989;169:265.

341. Yamaguchi M, Takeuchi S, Awazu S. Meckel's diverticulum: investigation of 600 patients in Japanese literature. *Am J Surg* 1978;136:247.

342. Zizic TM, Classen JN, Stevens MB. Acute abdominal complications of systemic lupus erythematosus and polyarteritis nodosa. *Am J Med* 1982;73:525.

Chapter 29

Ulcerative Colitis

Five things are proper to the duty of a Chirurgian;
To take away that which is superfluous;
To restore to their places such things as are displaced;
To separate those things which are joined together;
To join those that are separated; and
To supply the defects of nature.

Ambroise Paré—*Works*, Book I, Chapter 2

The expression *nonspecific inflammatory bowel disease* (IBD) is used to describe two conditions of unknown etiology: ulcerative colitis and Crohn's disease. With respect to the differential diagnosis, the two diseases often have similar characteristics. The symptoms are frequently quite alike, radiologic investigation may pose confusion in differentiation, and even pathologic evaluation may reveal overlapping features, with an indeterminate colitis reported in as many as 15% of patients. Some have even reported that both conditions can coexist in the same individual.[743] Because of the often diverse approaches to management and the fact that a vulnerable age group is frequently affected (young persons in their late teens and early twenties), these diseases are among the most challenging confronting the physician today. Ulcerative colitis is discussed in this chapter; Crohn's disease and indeterminate colitis are presented in Chapter 30.

HISTORICAL PERSPECTIVE

It is difficult to know whether ulcerative colitis was truly recognized as a disease prior to the nineteenth century. Infectious and noninfectious diarrheas have existed since antiquity, but most of the descriptions are of a clinical syndrome—diarrhea and rectal bleeding, the so-called "bloody flux." Samuel Wilks is generally credited with coining the term *ulcerative colitis*.[745] In a letter to the editor of the *Medical Times and Gazette* published in 1859, he described the postmortem appearance of the intestine. Subsequently, the surgeon general of the Union army after the Civil War referred to th e disease, ulcerative colitis, and included photomicrographs of the condition.[218] Other detailed descriptions followed,[746] and by the early twentieth century more than 300 case reports of ulcerative colitis had been collected for presentation to the Royal Society of Medicine.[218]

EPIDEMIOLOGY (INCIDENCE, PREVALENCE) AND ETIOLOGY

As suggested, the nonspecific IBDs, especially Crohn's disease, have become pervasive worldwide, and the two conditions have thus emerged as one of the most important biomedical problems of our time.[351] Unfortunately, our understanding of their pathogenesis still remains obscure.

Evaluation of the epidemiology of the two conditions is made difficult by the plethora of diarrheal states found throughout the world that may be infectious or parasitic in nature and that present with symptoms not unlike those of nonspecific IBD.[351] Furthermore, because of international failure to classify the two diseases as distinct from the numerous specific inflammatory bowel problems, our ability to obtain meaningful data is compromised. Most of the information, therefore, has been accumulated from Western countries, where the diseases are relatively prevalent. In the United States, however, IBD is not a reportable condition.

Available evidence suggests considerable variation in the incidence rates—common in developed countries and unusual in Asia, Africa, and South America. Because a true surveillance of prevalence requires an exhaustive clinical, endoscopic, and radiologic evaluation of all members of a sample population, the true prevalence is based on inference rather than analysis of well-established data.[472] There even appears to be a seasonal variation, not only of onset, but also of relapse.[600] A statistically significant increase has been observed in the months of August to January.

The incidence of ulcerative colitis and Crohn's disease in England, the United States, and Scandinavia is reported to be from 4 to 6 cases per 100,000 white adults per year, with prevalence rates of between 40 and 100 cases per 100,000.[352] Most studies have demonstrated an increased incidence of Crohn's disease over the past 25 years.[54,64,148,376,457,486,526] The condition is more common in whites, among Jewish people, and among those of Western origin (especially northern Europe and the northern part of eastern Europe).[352] Other countries, such as South American nations, the former Soviet Union, and Japan, have a much lower incidence and prevalence.

As with carcinoma of the colon, the prevalence of IBD in many industrialized countries, and the development of the conditions among those from low-risk populations who emigrate to higher-risk areas, suggest an environmental cause.

Investigative efforts to identify the etiologic agent responsible for the nonspecific IBDs have thus far been unsuccessful. IBD that appears nonspecific in nature has been found in hamsters, horses, swine, and the canine population, but an experimental animal model for induction or transmission of the disease still eludes investigators. The three primary areas of investigation that continue to be pursued actively are genetics, immunology, and infection.

Genetics

Several studies have shown the existence of family aggregations with the disease, implying that genetic factors also must play a role.[5,120,152,350,353,381,738] For example, there is a high degree of concordance in monozygotic twins.[577] Although ulcerative colitis and Crohn's disease are not classic genetic disorders, the occurrence of IBD in family members born in widely separated areas or living apart for long periods, along with the increased incidence among Jews and the tendency toward familial aggregation of cases with ankylosing spondylitis in Crohn's disease, suggest a genetically mediated mechanism in the causation of the conditions.[152,352,544] Roth and colleagues, in a study of Ashkenazi Jews with IBD, calculated the true lifetime risk for the development of IBD in relatives to be 8.9% for offspring, 8.8% for siblings, and 3.5% for parents.[609] Although the possibility of a common environment may contribute to the increased risk of IBD, the shared genetic pool is much more likely to be the primary factor. A familial occurrence has been noted in 17.5% of more than 600 patients with IBD.[658] In a report from the Cleveland Clinic, Farmer and colleagues evaluated the family histories of more than 800 patients with an onset of IBD before the age of 21.[152] Twenty-nine percent of those with ulcerative colitis had a positive history, and 35% of those with Crohn's disease had a positive family history for IBD.

The first IBD susceptibility locus was found on chromosome 16 and identified as IBD1. This is apparently a purely Crohn's locus, however. Most of the current studies seem to demonstrate a consistent association with various genetic mutations and Crohn's disease, but not that of ulcerative colitis.

Satsangi and colleagues propose that the ethnic, familial, twin, disease association, and genetic marker studies of IBD are best explained by the concept that the conditions represent multifactorial diseases.[634] Environmental and genetic factors contribute to disease susceptibility. They conclude that it is possible for different susceptibility genes to underlie phenotypic differences between Crohn's disease and ulcerative colitis, leading to diverse manifestations of the two conditions as well as varied degrees of severity. Mendeloff believes that there is a deficiency in the investigation of these diseases because the mortality is low and the genetic determinants are multiple.[472] He suggests that in the future it will be necessary to develop a better fundamental means of acquiring and recording data, and that at least for the immediate present a concerted effort should be made to identify those families in which multiple cases of IBD exist and to investigate these people thoroughly. This would include genetic, psychological, and metabolic studies.

Autoimmunity

The idea of circulating antiepithelial antibodies combining with antigens on the intestinal cell surface and damaging the cells seems a reasonable theory to explain the etiology of IBD. This is the concept of autoimmunity. Snook clearly defines the criteria for the classification of a disease as autoimmune.[663] Such a condition ". . . requires the demonstration of autoreactive lymphocytes or autoantibodies, or both, which are specific for the disease concerned, present in all cases, and most important, capable of reproducing the disease on syngeneic transfer."[663] However, despite the demonstration of anticolon antibodies in both blood and tissue of patients with IBD, current evidence seems to militate against the likelihood that these play a primary pathogenetic role in the two conditions.[616]

Immune complex mediation of IBD has been thought by some to be a responsible factor, but studies have failed to corroborate a significantly increased frequency or concentration of these complexes regardless of disease activity.[616] Other immunologic mechanisms that have been investigated include abnormality and variability of circulating lymphocytes, lymphocyte cytotoxicity, defective cell-mediated immunity, immediate hypersensitivity, leukocyte chemotaxic impairment, and immunoregulatory cellular imbalance.[352,616] At the level of the immune response, a genetic influence is suggested by the association of ulcerative colitis with HLA-DR2 and by the occurrence of various autoantibodies in the unaffected relatives of patients with ulcerative colitis.[651]

Furthermore, studies of monozygotic twins have indicated that the altered mucosal production of immunoglobulin G1 (IgG1) and IgG2 in ulcerative colitis may be genetically determined.[651] James and colleagues suggest that the presence of circulating antigen-nonspecific suppressor T cells in patients with Crohn's disease in its early stages is the result of an immunoregulatory abnormality of antigen-specific helper and suppressor T cells.[311] A useful concept of the pathogenesis for IBD may involve an interaction between host responses, immunologic genetic influences, and external agents, but no definitive proof has yet been forthcoming.

Infection

With respect to infectious agents, ulcerative colitis in particular has been attributed to bacterial causes for more than 60 years. In 1928, Bargen reported that the condition was caused by a transmissible diplococcus.[25] He prepared a vaccine from this organism, an approach that was believed to be a valuable part of the treatment of the condition. In the article that introduced the technique of skin-grafted ileostomy for the surgical management of ulcerative colitis (see Chapter 31), Dragstedt and colleagues were persuaded that "bacterium necrophorum, together with other factors ... plays an etiologic role in the disease."[141] Crohn's disease specifically was often confused with tuberculosis. This observation led Crohn and coworkers to suggest that the disease might be caused by a mycobacterial agent.[113] Subsequent studies have failed to demonstrate conclusively an association with an infective agent, and, in fact, the incidence of IBD correlates inversely with that of the infectious dysenteries.[352] An exception is that of cytomegalovirus infection, which has been shown to complicate ulcerative colitis in immunocompromised patients, such as individuals with AIDS.[730]

The concept of a microbial infection as the offending agent has been resurrected with the recognition of new bacterial causes of enteritis and colitis (especially *Campylobacter jejuni* and *Clostridium difficile*).[60,378,512,710] Although several studies suggest the possibility of these two organisms contributing to relapse of IBD, Gurian and colleagues, in examination of stool specimens from 32 patients who had exacerbation of IBD, revealed no *C. difficile* cytotoxin and negative cultures for *C. jejuni*.[238] Other bacteriologic agents (*Shigella, Salmonella, Streptococcus faecalis, Pseudomonas* variant, *Chlamydia, Mycobacterium*, and many others) have been proposed, but their role has not been confirmed.[88,206,247,702] More recently it has been suggested that probiotics play an important role in preventing overgrowth of potentially pathogenic bacteria and in maintaining the integrity of the gut mucosal barrier.[726] Therefore, there may be a role for such agents in the treatment of IBD (see Medical Management).

There has been considerable interest in a possible viral etiology of ulcerative colitis and Crohn's disease. Transmission of granulomatous lesions has been successfully carried out in experimental animals.[97,135,694] Tissue culture and electron microscopic investigation have also suggested that a viral agent is present in tissue from patients with IBD.[12,207,744] However, considerable controversy continues concerning the specificity of these findings. Whether the evidence is sufficiently compelling to permit accurate identification of viral particles on electron microscopic examination of affected tissue remains unresolved.[616,757]

Diet

Dietary factors, especially cow's milk, have been implicated as possible causative agents for the development of IBD. Early studies seemed to demonstrate an elevated milk-protein antibody level in patients with ulcerative colitis in comparison with a control population. Subsequent studies in which milk was excluded from the diet failed to demonstrate an improvement in the clinical response, and later studies with milk and milk products failed to demonstrate any correlation. Other factors that have been under investigation include chemical food additives, mercury ingestion, inadequate fiber, excess intake of refined sugar, and even the increased consump-

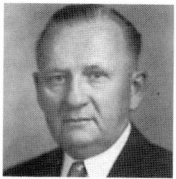

J. Arnold Bargen (1894–1976) Bargen was born at Mountain Lake, Minnesota. He attended Carleton College in Northfield, Minnesota, and received a bachelor of science degree from the University of Chicago in 1918. Following graduation from Rush Medical College, he completed an internship and a 1-year postgraduate fellowship in medicine at St. Luke's Hospital. He then joined the Mayo Clinic as an assistant in medicine and became a part of the clinic staff in 1926. He became head of a section of medicine in 1942, and in 1956, he undertook the chairmanship of four sections of medicine primarily concerned with gastroenterology. Bargen gained a national reputation for his work in diseases of the stomach and colon and was the author or co-author of four books as well as hundreds of published articles in these fields. Additionally, he served on the editorial board of the journal *Gastroenterology* and was a member or officer of numerous prestigious medical societies, including the American Gastroenterological Association, of which he was president, and the sections of gastroenterology of the American Medical Association and the World Congress of Gastroenterology, of which he was chairman. Bargen was one of the first to recognize the association of ulcerative colitis with carcinoma (1928),[24] but his early affirmation of the concept of a bacterial etiology for this condition was never corroborated. Following his retirement from the Mayo Clinic, he headed the department of gastroenterology at the Scott-White Clinic. He died in Sun City, Arizona, at the age of 82. (Photograph courtesy of the Mayo Clinic.)

tion of corn flakes.[456,616] Generally, articles dealing with diet and IBD are conflicting, confusing, and frequently unreliable. One can safely state that there is no clear consensus to suggest that dietary factors play a role in the etiology of either ulcerative colitis or Crohn's disease.

Oxidative Metabolism

Recent evidence suggests that abnormal oxidative metabolism may be of significance in the activity of IBD. Increased attention has been placed on the role of free radicals in both normal metabolism and defense against disease.[657] A free radical is defined as any species capable of independent existence that contains one or more unpaired electrons, an unpaired electron being defined as one that is alone in an orbital.[657] It appears that reactive oxygen metabolites are produced in excess in active IBD. The effects of specific antiinflammatory antioxidants, such as aminosalicylates, are compatible with the proposition that free radicals play a major role in the pathogenesis of IBD.[657]

Stool

Studies of the role of the fecal stream in causing an exacerbation of symptoms in Crohn's colitis have yielded confusing results. For example, Harper and colleagues evaluated the effects of introducing small-bowel effluent and a sterile ultrafiltrate of the effluent into the defunctionalized colon after a loop ileostomy had been created.[261] There was little response to the ultrafiltrate challenge, but there was a definite clinical exacerbation following introduction of the effluent. Conversely, Korelitz and colleagues reported that diverting the fecal stream had an adverse effect on the clinical course in four patients.[368] Following reestablishment of intestinal continuity, the bowel returned to normal.

Smoking

Two distinct patterns of cigarette smoking seem to be relevant in patients with IBD; those with ulcerative colitis are much less likely to smoke than those with Crohn's disease. Additionally, cigarette smoking has been found to have a negative correlation with ulcerative colitis.[73,123,262,316,708,728] In some cases, complete remission of symptoms was obtained through the use of nicotine-laced chewing gum. In other cases, exacerbation of the disease was noted when patients ceased smoking. Conversely, Crohn's disease is more common in smokers than in those who have never smoked.[331,708,728] The increased risk seems to be more apparent in women and may also be associated with a greater likelihood of recurrence.[685]

Oral Contraceptives

Both ulcerative colitis and Crohn's disease have been found to be more common among women using oral contraceptives than in those who do not.[728] A possible vascular (ischemic) basis for this observation has been suggested. There is no information to date on the effect of stopping the contraceptive pill on the activity of IBD.

Psychological Factors

The psychological aspects and the possible psychosomatic factors contributing to the onset and exacerbation of IBD, and of ulcerative colitis in particular, have been a subject of considerable debate since publication of the original article by Murray in 1930.[501] Karush and colleagues, in a book on psychotherapy in ulcerative colitis, state that susceptibility to the problem develops in colitic patients through "disruption and distortion of the relationship to the parents and to other significant persons as early as the second year of life."[330] They further contend that this results in exaggerated emotional manifestations, egocentricity, dependency conflicts, and poor mechanisms for coping with the stresses of life.[330] Frequent anxiety or depression, in the opinion of the authors, is also characteristic, and this predisposition, they believe, explains the relatively high incidence of schizophrenia in patients with ulcerative colitis. In their study of precipitating emotional factors, the authors reported that a well-defined event of powerful emotional impact preceded the onset of the disease by a few days or weeks. Subsequent recurrences were also heralded by such events.

Although many articles have been published to support this description of the susceptible personality, opponents of the psychosomatic theory point out that the concept is based on either anecdotal or uncontrolled studies.[616] Several publications have compared patients with ulcerative colitis with normal subjects and those with other illnesses and have found no evidence of an increased frequency of psychiatric illness.[45,142,273,473] Furthermore, those with ulcerative colitis who had a psychiatric illness did not appear to have more serious gastrointestinal involvement, nor did severity of the ulcerative colitis predict a more frequent or more severe psychiatric disorder.[273] Bercovitz noted that there are no long-term, prospective psychological studies available of any large group of people.[47] North and colleagues reviewed all known English-language articles at the time (138 studies) on the association between psychiatric factors and ulcerative colitis and found that most contained serious flaws in research design (e.g., absence of control subjects and lack of diagnostic criteria).[522] In the seven publications that truly represented meaningful, systematic, investigative efforts, no association was identified. Cunnien concluded that patients with ulcerative colitis have no universal unique personality characteristics and no documented increase in psychiatric illness when compared with medically ill and population controls.[116] He further observed that no demonstrable emotional precipitating factors have been uniformly identified, no symbolic emotional conflicts have been documented in controlled studies, and psychotherapy has not been effective in altering the disease course.

Comment

Serious illness during an extremely vulnerable period of emotional development, the need for hospitalization and psychotropic medications (e.g., corticosteroids), or the fear of surgery (especially the "mutilation" of an ileostomy) may induce considerable stress. In fact, it would be the remarkable patient indeed who was not emotionally troubled by the consequences of such illness. The importance of providing emotional support to the patient cannot be overestimated. Psychotherapy has been demonstrated to be of value, but an internist or a surgeon who understands the role of emotional conflicts and anxieties either as a cause or a result of the patient's illness can provide such counsel.

Appendectomy

As has been suggested, the current concept of the etiology of IBD in most patients is that the condition may be triggered by genetic predisposition to a variety of environmental factors. The association of one of these factors, appendectomy, has been the subject of numerous investigations. Koutroubakis and colleagues undertook a meta-analysis of 17 case-controlled studies and found that appendectomy was inversely associated with the development of ulcerative colitis ($p < .0001$).[372] The role of the appendix in the development of mucosal immunity is currently the subject of intensive study.

Age, Sex, and Race

Ulcerative colitis and Crohn's disease occur at any age but are most commonly seen in persons under the age of 30 years. The incidence is highest among teenagers, but a small secondary peak in the incidence of the two conditions occurs late in the sixth decade.[352] In most series, both sexes are equally affected. Farmer and colleagues noted, in a study covering 20 years ending in 1974, that 838 patients were 20 years old or younger at the time of diagnosis at the Cleveland Clinic.[152] Thirteen percent with ulcerative colitis and 5% with Crohn's disease were less than 11 years of age. Approximately one third of the patients in each group were between the ages of 11 and 15. There were 316 patients with ulcerative colitis, with a male-to-female ratio of almost 1:1, and 522 patients with

Crohn's disease, 57% of whom were male. In Goligher's experience, approximately one half of the patients were between 20 and 39 years of age when the disease was diagnosed, with a 4:3 predominance of female over male patients.[214] With Crohn's disease, Goligher reported that in his own personal series, female patients predominated in a 3:2 ratio.[216] There seemed to be a tendency for the disease to develop later than ulcerative colitis does, 70% of patients being between the ages of 20 and 49 years.

In our experience of 151 patients who underwent proctocolectomy, the mean age at surgery for both ulcerative colitis and Crohn's disease was 36 years.[107] Fifty-six percent of patients with ulcerative colitis were men, whereas 57% who had Crohn's colitis were women.

Goldman and colleagues suggest that Crohn's disease in black patients may be more common than is generally appreciated.[210] This group represented 11% of the patients in their experience during a 10-year period. The authors noted that extraintestinal manifestations developed in all patients. Furthermore, the disease generally appeared to be associated with more severe complications than had been observed in whites.

DIFFERENTIAL DIAGNOSIS: ULCERATIVE COLITIS VERSUS CROHN'S DISEASE

Ulcerative colitis and Crohn's disease can usually be distinguished on the basis of the clinical course, symptomatology, manifestations, and endoscopic findings. Ulcerative colitis is a disease characterized by exacerbations and remissions. In contrast, the individual with Crohn's disease has less clear-cut periods of flare-up and remission; the disease often tends to run a more smoldering course. Frequently, the patient is really not well and yet is not sufficiently ill to warrant hospitalization. Table 29-1 summarizes a number of the characteristic features that may help to differentiate between the two conditions.

Rectal bleeding is virtually a sine qua non for the diagnosis of ulcerative colitis. A physician might seriously question the accuracy of the diagnosis in the absence of this symptom. Bleeding is much less frequently seen in Crohn's colitis; in fact, 25% of patients with Crohn's disease never manifest bleeding. This should not be surprising, because ulcerative colitis is an inflammatory disease of the mucosa, whereas with Crohn's colitis, ulceration may be minimal. However, in rare instances, massive lower gastrointestinal bleeding may be associated with Crohn's disease.[462]

Ulcerative colitis is confined to the colon and rectum; Crohn's disease can occur anywhere in the digestive tract, from the mouth to the anus. Anorectal disease in particular (fissures, abscesses, and fistulas) is more commonly noted in patients with Crohn's disease than in those with

▶ **TABLE 29-1** Features of Nonspecific Inflammatory Bowel Disease

	Ulcerative Colitis	*Crohn's Disease*
Course	Exacerbations and Remissions	Smoldering
Bleeding	Virtually always	Uncommon
Abdominal pain	Uncommon	Common
Perianal disease	Rare	Up to 40%
Fistulas	Never	Occasional
Abdominal mass	Never	Occasional
Carcinoma	Increased association	Increased, but less than in ulcerative colitis
Extraintestinal manifestations	Not unusual	Not unusual
Radiologic and Endoscopic		
Distribution	In continuity with rectum	Skip areas often observed
	Uniform distribution	Often eccentric
	Rectal involvement always	Often rectal sparing
Small bowel	Spared (backwash only)	Often involved
Stricture	Rare, virtually always malignant	Frequent, virtually always benign
Mucosa	Contact bleeding; granularity; superficial ulcers; pseudopolyps	Longitudinal ulcers; fissuring; cobblestone appearance
Microscopic		
Extent	Mucosa and submucosa	Transmural
Granulomas	Never	Common
Dysplasia	Yes	Yes
Lymph nodes	Reactive	With granulomas
Crypt abscesses	Present	Present
Mucus production	Decreased	Increased

ulcerative colitis (see Chapters 9, 10, and 11). The diagnosis is often suspected on examination of the perianal skin (see Figure 30-1).

Proctosigmoidoscopic examination may be of value in differentiating between the two conditions (see later discussion). The rectum is always diseased during attacks of ulcerative colitis. Characteristic changes include contact bleeding, granularity, and ulceration. In Crohn's colitis, 40% of the patients have sparing of the rectum, irrespective of anal or perianal involvement. However, when the rectum is involved by Crohn's disease, differentiation between the two may be quite difficult.

Extracolonic manifestations had been presumed to be found only with ulcerative colitis, but it is now recognized that these can be observed in both conditions. They are discussed in Chapter 30.

It may not be possible to differentiate between the two diseases either by radiologic or clinical means. In approximately 10% to 15% of cases, distinction cannot be made even pathologically; these patients are thus placed into the so-called indeterminate category (see Chapter 30). The appropriateness of utilizing the ileal pouch-anal op-

eration as an alternative in this group of patients is discussed in Chapter 30.

Physical Examination

Physical examination is usually unrewarding in patients with ulcerative colitis who do not have fulminant disease. Abdominal tenderness is usually absent, and there is no abdominal distension. No masses are palpable. However, in the acutely ill person, abdominal distension may be associated with toxic megacolon. Diffuse tenderness may be apparent, and if perforation has ensued, all the usual signs and symptoms of an intraabdominal catastrophe may be noted.

Endoscopic Examination

Proctosigmoidoscopy, flexible sigmoidoscopy, and colonoscopy are important tools for evaluating the bowel and for confirming the presence or absence of IBD. Proctosigmoidoscopic examination is particularly useful in differentiating Crohn's disease from ulcerative colitis; the rectum is always diseased during attacks of ulcerative colitis. The earliest manifestation of inflammation is the loss of a normal vessel pattern, the result of edema of the bowel wall. Contact bleeding, granularity, and ulceration are more obvious signs of inflammatory disease. The rectum is spared in 40% of patients with Crohn's colitis, irrespective of anal or perianal involvement. However, when the rectum is involved by this condition, differentiation between the two diseases may be quite difficult.

In individuals with distal disease (i.e., ulcerative proctitis or proctosigmoiditis), complete endoscopic examination by means of the colonoscope is unnecessary at the time of presentation. The extent of disease can usually be determined with the rigid instrument or the flexible sigmoidoscope. The presence of diffuse, confluent, symmetric disease from the dentate line cephalad to the limit of the inflammatory reaction is consistent with ulcerative proctitis or proctosigmoiditis, depending on the extent of involvement (Figure 29-1). In individuals with *treated* ulcerative colitis, the finding of rectal sparing or patchiness should not necessarily alter the diagnosis to Crohn's disease.[50] If the patient's symptoms are appropriate to the endoscopic findings, treatment can be initiated without further contrast study or colonoscopy. Conversely, if the patient's disease extends beyond the limit of the endoscopic procedure performed, it will be necessary at some point to undertake total colonic evaluation.

Colonoscopy has virtually replaced barium enema examination for the evaluation of IBD. Generally, endoscopic examination will identify more proximal inflammatory changes than will the radiologic study. Furthermore, histologic examination of random biopsy specimens will often reveal more proximal disease than was suspected by endoscopic examination.[147,753] Das and colleagues reported 31 patients with idiopathic proctitis who underwent colonoscopy while they were asymptomatic.[119] Multiple biopsy samples were taken from throughout the colon and rectum. Although the obvious disease appeared limited to the distal 20 cm, microscopic abnormalities were seen commonly in more proximal locations. The authors postulated that the clinical course would be more consistent with distal disease when this indeed could be confirmed by biopsy, whereas more proximal involvement usually implied that the disease would be refractory to conventional management (e.g., topical steroids). A corollary to this observation is to perform biopsies distal to obvious inflammatory changes if the rectum appears to be spared, because one may discover that the rectum is not truly normal. This may cause the physician to reassess the accuracy of a diagnosis of Crohn's disease based on what was initially thought to be a lack of rectal involvement.

The place of colonoscopy in the evaluation and follow-up of IBD has been extensively reviewed by many authors. Teague and Waye recommend colonoscopy for five

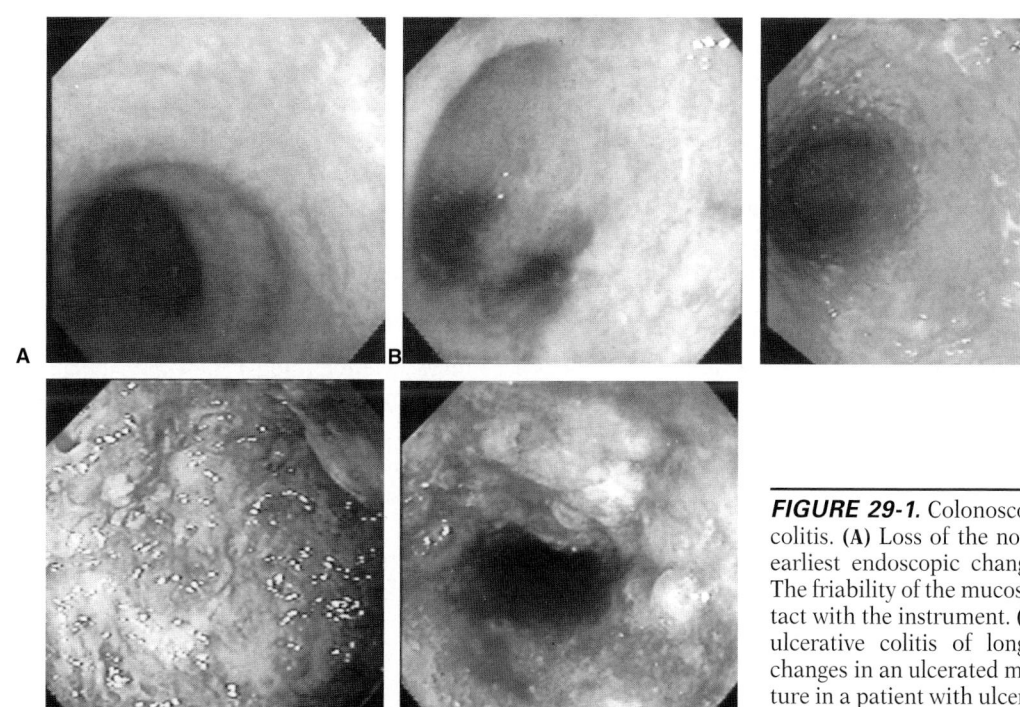

FIGURE 29-1. Colonoscopic changes in ulcerative colitis. **(A)** Loss of the normal vessel pattern is the earliest endoscopic change. **(B)** Contact bleeding. The friability of the mucosa is demonstrated by contact with the instrument. **(C)** Granularity appears in ulcerative colitis of longer duration. **(D)** Florid changes in an ulcerated mucosa. **(E)** A colonic stricture in a patient with ulcerative colitis proved on biopsy to be malignant. (See Color Fig. 29-1.)

indications: differential diagnosis, resolution of radiographic abnormalities (e.g., filling defects and strictures), preoperative and postoperative evaluation in Crohn's disease, examination of stomas, and screening for premalignant and malignant changes.[699]

Preparation

Often, colonoscopy can be performed without prior bowel cleansing in patients with mild to active IBD, with essentially the same comprehensive evaluation achieved as when a full preparation is used.[30] In the patient who has a history of IBD, the preparation for colonoscopy includes a modified diet. Clear liquids are suggested for 24 hours. Vigorous cleansing enemas such as those that may be used in the evaluation of an noninflamed colon are contraindicated. For someone with a relatively active colitis, no laxative is suggested. In more severe cases, a clear liquid diet as the sole modality for bowel preparation is probably the safer alternative. If the colitis is minimal or relatively inactive, a reduced dose of a laxative is suggested, although it is probably wiser to use a balanced electrolyte solution (e.g., Colyte, GoLytely).

Appearance

Ulcerative colitis and Crohn's disease are usually recognized endoscopically by excluding IBD due to specific cause, such as amebic colitis, ischemic colitis, pseudomembranous colitis, and so forth. The most common differential diagnostic problems are related to the numerous and varied infectious colitides (see Chapter 33). Other sources of confusion include radiation changes, the so-called solitary ulcer syndrome, and, of course, the differentiation between the two nonspecific IBD conditions, themselves—ulcerative colitis and Crohn's disease.[699] Biopsy may be helpful because histologic changes suggestive of Crohn's disease in particular may be apparent. Up to 20% of such patients may exhibit granulomas (see Figure 30-3). In patients with ulcerative colitis, rectal biopsy is extremely important for recognizing dysplasia, especially in those with long-standing disease (see Relationship to Carcinoma).

Waye has described a number of colonoscopic features in the differential diagnosis of IBD.[734] He suggests that patients with ulcerative colitis always have rectal involvement from the anal verge cephalad in continuity with whatever proximal involvement is present. Erythema of the colonic wall is one of the early manifestations. More obvious changes include granularity, friability, bleeding, edema with interhaustral septal thickening and blunting, ulceration, mucosal bridging, the presence of pseudopolyps, and the superimposition of carcinoma.

With granulomatous colitis, Waye observed the following major colonoscopic findings: a normal rectum (obviously this is not always the case), asymmetry or eccentricity of involvement, cobblestone appearance, normal vasculature (because friability is not usually encountered except in advanced disease), edema of the bowel wall (as seen in ulcerative colitis), normal mucosa intervening between areas of ulceration, serpiginous or rake ulcers (these may course for several centimeters), pseudopolyps (as in ulcerative colitis), and skip areas (lack of continuity of involvement).[734] He adds another observation, the presence of amyloidosis in the biopsy specimen.

Pera and colleagues undertook a prospective study by means of colonoscopy in 357 patients in order to obtain the best predictive information that would enable the authors to differentiate between the two conditions.[560] An "endoscopic score" was calculated by means of "likelihood ratios." Errors were more frequently noted when severe inflammation was encountered. The most useful endoscopic features in the differential diagnosis were discontinuous involvement, anal lesions, and cobblestone appearance of the mucosa for Crohn's disease, and erosions or microulcers and granularity for ulcerative colitis.[560]

Myren and colleagues performed routine and random histologic evaluation by means of colonoscopic biopsy in patients with and without IBD.[503] In 110 individuals, 278 biopsy specimens were obtained at different levels of the colon. Clinical information, including colonoscopic diagnosis, was available to the pathologist at the initial routine examination. Later, the sections were examined blindly and independently by two pathologists. Agreement was obtained in only two thirds of the patients. The authors concluded that the limiting factor in making reliable diagnoses was the small size of the tissue specimens available. Also, discrepancies may have been caused by the fact that biopsy specimens were not always representative of the process in the colonic mucosa.

Farmer and colleagues reviewed 100 patients who underwent colonoscopy for distal ulcerative colitis.[152] They classified their patients into two groups: those whose disease was confined to the distal 25 cm, and those whose mucosal changes extended above that level but not beyond the splenic flexure. Because flexible sigmoidoscopy or colonoscopy is not as accurate in defining disease in the rectum, whether it is inflammatory or neoplastic, there was a 5% disagreement about the presence of inflammation in that area of the bowel. Certainly, the rigid instrument is far more useful in evaluating the rectum than the colonoscope. Biopsy specimens were taken at multiple levels, and the retrospective review was performed during several years. It was determined that patients whose disease was initially limited to the rectum and sigmoid colon had a good prognosis—only 10% progressed to more extensive involvement. However, 25% of patients experienced recurrence. Prognosis was similar whether the disease was confined to the lower 25 cm or was distal to the splenic flexure.

Comment

Additional biopsy specimens for the evaluation of a patient with IBD should be obtained from an area that appears macroscopically, at least, to be relatively uninvolved. The true extent of the inflammation as well as the significance of the presence of granulomas (granulomas may be seen in patients with ulcerative colitis underlying an ulcer) can then be interpreted properly.

Colonoscopy Versus Barium Enema

In general, colonoscopy permits identification of segmental involvement and microulceration better than does barium enema. However, radiographic studies yield more information about haustrae, especially in the right colon.[197] One must remember, however, that the procedure is contraindicated in patients with acute exacerbation of the colitis and certainly in those who have a toxic megacolon. Myren and colleagues performed colonoscopic evaluation in 40 patients and compared the results with that of conventional barium enema.[502] Colonoscopic diagnosis and biopsy results were corroborating in 80% of the patients, whereas colonoscopic evaluation and radiologic survey revealed agreement in only 55%. The area in which radiology seemed to have an advantage was the decreased haustration that was more apparent by x-ray techniques. Erosions, mucosal edema, and vascular injection were not detected by barium enema. Others have confirmed the merits of colonoscopy in the evaluation of patients with nonspecific IBD.[188,695,735,747]

Radiographic Features

Plain Films

In any evaluation of a patient with IBD, the importance of a plain x-ray film of the abdomen (KUB) should not be underestimated. Without submitting patients to the rigors of a contrast study or colonoscopy, particularly when they may be acutely ill, the physician can obtain valuable information about the extent of disease (Figure 29-2).

The importance of a plain film of the abdomen is further increased in those who have toxic dilatation, a condition usually seen in the transverse colon (Figure 29-3). When the radiographic appearance of toxic dilatation is noted, a barium enema examination or colonoscopy is contraindicated, but serial abdominal films are clinically extremely valuable. The effectiveness of medical therapy can be evaluated by determin-

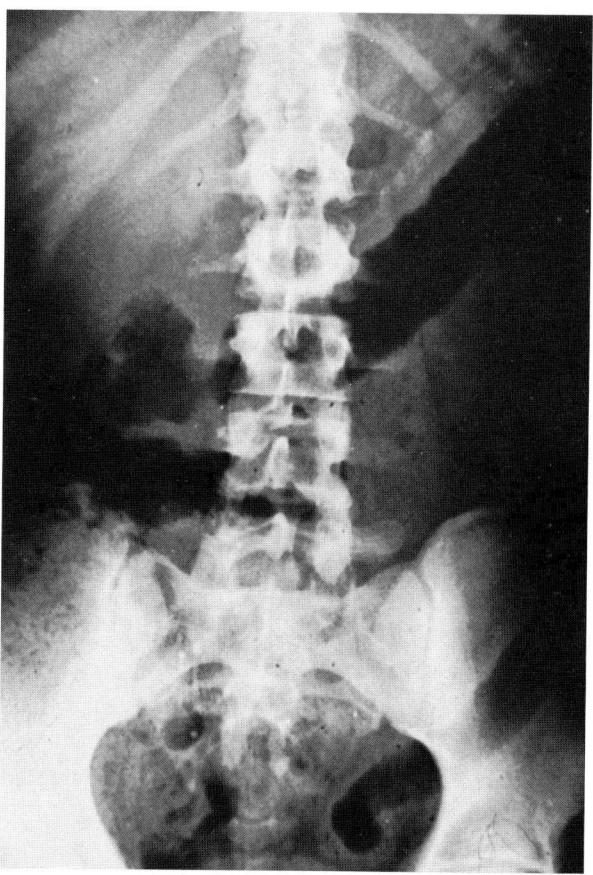

FIGURE 29-2. Ulcerative colitis. This plain abdominal film of an acutely ill patient reveals some thickening of the colonic wall, especially in the region of the sigmoid where it overlies the iliac crest, and loss of haustral markings throughout the left colon and transverse colon to the region of the hepatic flexure. Subsequent barium enema study demonstrated disease extending exactly to the point seen on the plain film. (From Corman ML, Veidenheimer MC, Nugent FW, et al. *Diseases of the anus, rectum and colon. Part II: nonspecific inflammatory bowel disease.* New York: Medcom, 1976.)

ing the increase or decrease in the degree of dilatation. The abdominal examination should not be relied on exclusively because the patient may frequently be confused or even obtunded. Furthermore, the high dose of steroids often used in the treatment of toxic megacolon may mask abdominal signs.

Barium Enema

The radiologic findings during the acute phase of ulcerative colitis include edema, ulceration, and changes in colonic motility. Edema may be apparent even on the plain film of the abdomen, such as is seen in Figure 29-3. Initially, ulceration may be minimal and difficult to identify. As the disease becomes fulminant, the ulceration becomes more obvious and may take on a "collar-button"

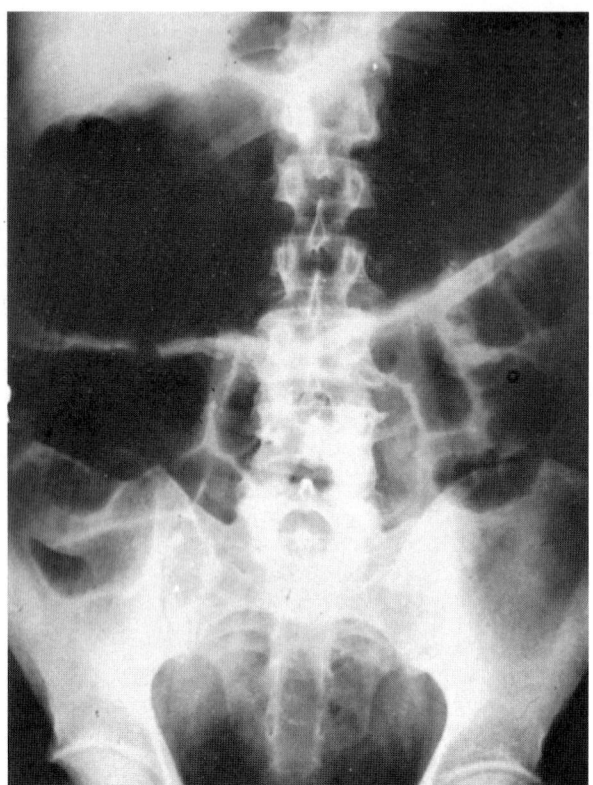

FIGURE 29-3. Ulcerative colitis. This plain abdominal x-ray film reveals marked dilatation of the transverse colon (toxic megacolon). (From Corman ML, Veidenheimer MC, Nugent FW, et al. *Diseases of the anus, rectum and colon. Part II: nonspecific inflammatory bowel disease.* New York: Medcom, 1976.)

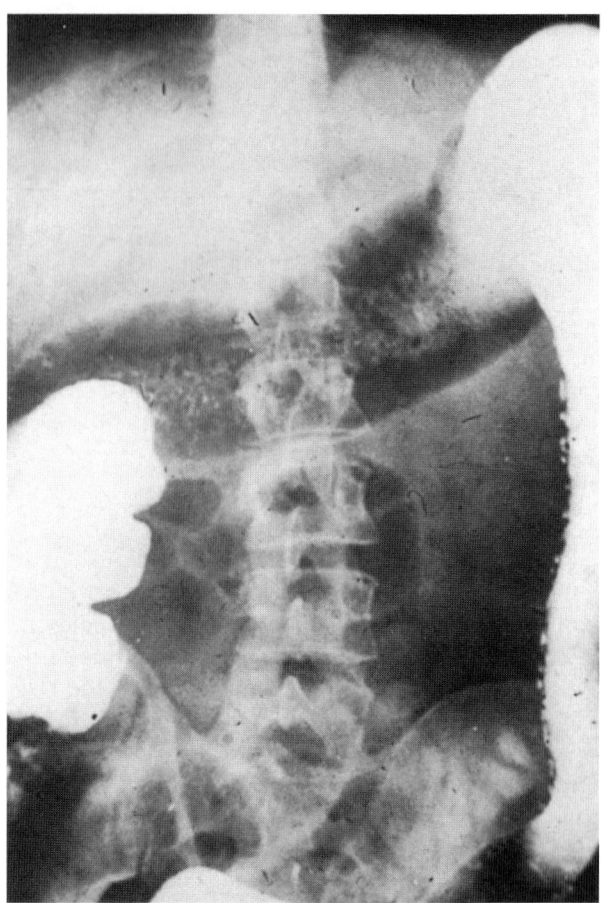

FIGURE 29-4. Acute ulcerative colitis. Note the loss of haustral markings up to and including the mid-ascending colon and numerous discrete ulcerations deep in the submucosa along the descending colon. (From Corman ML, Veidenheimer MC, Nugent FW, et al. *Diseases of the anus, rectum and colon. Part II: nonspecific inflammatory bowel disease.* New York: Medcom, 1976.)

appearance (Figure 29-4). Edema and inflammation of the mucosa may result in the radiologic appearance that has been called "thumb-printing," a phenomenon characteristically observed in patients with ischemic colitis (Figure 29-5).

When the disease enters a more chronic phase, other features are characteristic on the barium enema examination. These include fibrosis, which results in shortening of the bowel, depression of the flexures, pseudopolyposis, and stricture formation. The bowel wall is less distensible, and the motility pattern is disturbed. Diffuse, confluent, symmetric disease, beginning with the anorectal junction, are the hallmarks of the radiologic manifestations of chronic ulcerative colitis (Figs. 29-6 and 29-7). The presence of polypoid lesions throughout the entire colon may confuse the uninitiated with the radiologic picture seen in familial polyposis (Figure 29-8). Both diseases commonly present with rectal bleeding and diarrhea. In ulcerative colitis, however, foreshortening of the bowel may be evident, particularly at the flexures, and if the outline of the colon is carefully examined, numerous discrete ulcerations can usually be appreciated (Figure 29-9).

Benign strictures are extremely uncommon in ulcerative colitis. In fact, a stricture in this condition should be considered malignant until proved otherwise (see Relationship to Carcinoma).[382] Radiologic examination will usually reveal a smoothly outlined, concentric lumen with tapering margins (Figure 29-10). Areas of spasm are frequently seen in ulcerative colitis and may be difficult to differentiate from stricture. The administration of propantheline (10 mg of Pro-Banthine intravenously) or glucagon (2 mg intramuscularly) may eliminate the stricture caused by such spasm. If the lumen is concentric and the margins are smooth, the lesion may be benign. Conversely, if the lumen is eccentric and the margins are irregular, a carcinoma must be suspected.[449]

Another radiologic finding sometimes observed in patients with ulcerative colitis is "backwash ileitis." This is a very poor term because it implies that the ulcerative

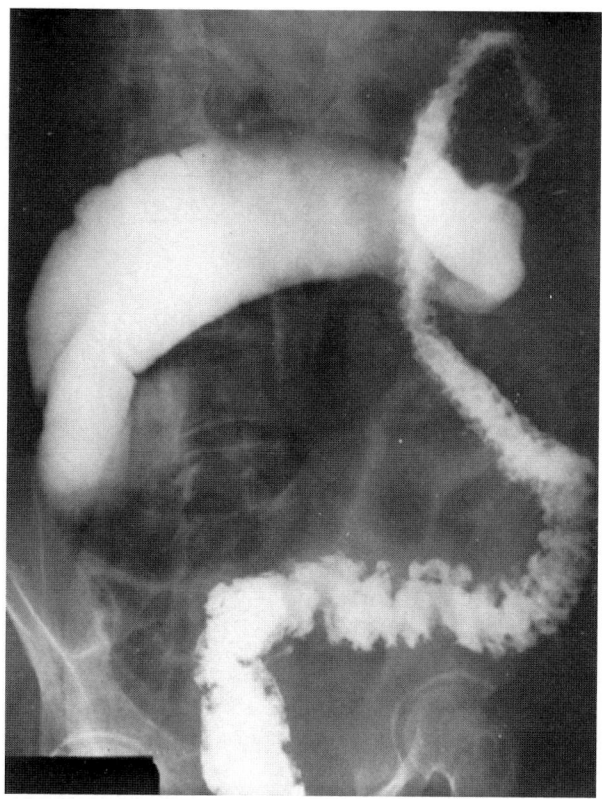

FIGURE 29-5. Edema of the bowel wall in acute ulcerative colitis; flocculation of barium caused by mucus (fuzzy appearance) and thumb-printing in the region of the splenic flexure.

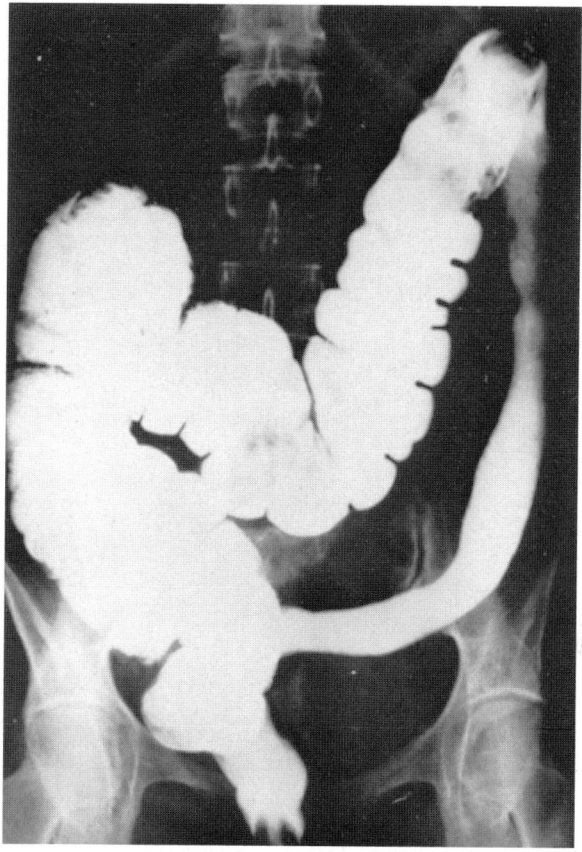

FIGURE 29-6. Chronic ulcerative colitis. Typical changes of left-sided disease include loss of haustral pattern, shortening of the sigmoid, and narrowing of the entire descending and sigmoid colon. (From Corman ML, Veidenheimer MC, Nugent FW, et al. *Diseases of the anus, rectum and colon. Part II: nonspecific inflammatory bowel disease.* New York: Medcom, 1976.)

colitis has somehow regurgitated through the ileocecal valve to cause the disease in the distal ileum. Marshak and Lindner were able to demonstrate the presence of this phenomenon in approximately 10% of patients with ulcerative colitis whom they had studied.[449] The changes may vary from lack of distensibility, as the head of pressure is increased when the barium is inserted, to ileal dilatation, narrowing, rigidity, and changes that may mimic those of regional enteritis (Figure 29-11).

Portal venous gas has been reported to be a benign, albeit unusual, consequence of air-contrast barium enema in patients with IBD. Although the implication of such an observation when made in other patients is that antibiotic treatment is required, it may not be necessary if the patient is without bacteremic symptoms.[332]

Computed Tomography

The advent of computed tomography (CT) has permitted direct visualization of the entire thickness of the bowel wall and mesentery, and determination of the presence or absence of fluid, fistula, or abscess.[430] With the exception of its unique application to abscess drainage, the role of this study in the diagnosis and management of patients

with IBD is controversial. One thing is certain, however; CT is of no value in assessing the extent of mucosal disease. Its advantages over contrast enema are primarily in delineating the presence and severity of pericolonic inflammation and in evaluating other organ disease. Although the place of CT in IBD is still a matter of conjecture, it is unlikely to prove to be of benefit in patients with ulcerative colitis. Because Crohn's disease is a transmural process, one may anticipate a greater application with this condition.

Ultrasonography

Hata and colleagues performed ultrasonographic examinations in individuals with ulcerative colitis and Crohn's disease and in 50 patients with no bowel disease.[266] Crohn's disease and ulcerative colitis could be detected by ultrasonography with a sensitivity of 86% and 89%, respectively. The primary benefit appeared to be in the

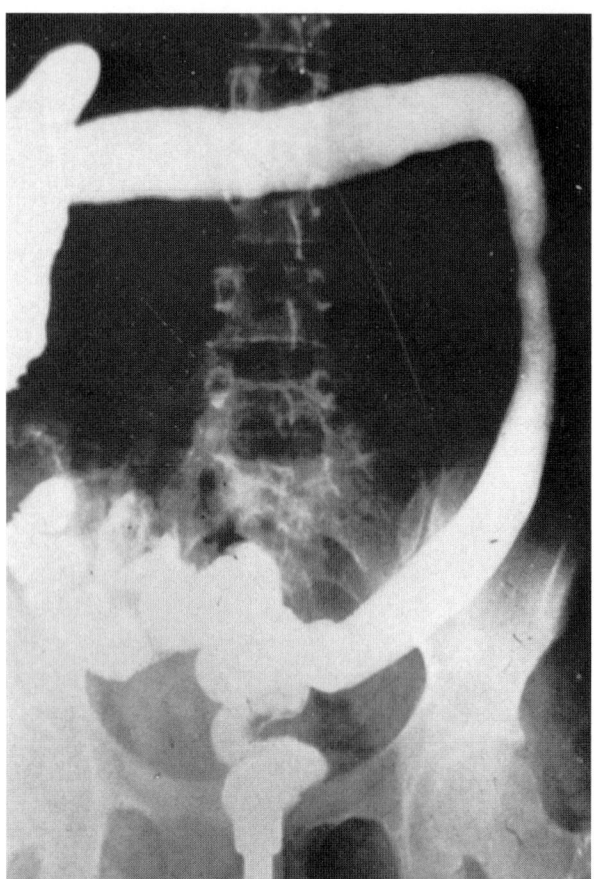

FIGURE 29-7. Chronic ulcerative colitis: a classic example of diffuse, symmetric, confluent disease. Characteristically, the left side is more involved than the right. Note that there is more foreshortening of the splenic flexure than of the hepatic flexure, and there is a suggestion of haustra on the right but not on the left. (From Corman ML, Veidenheimer MC, Nugent FW, et al. *Diseases of the anus, rectum and colon. Part II: nonspecific inflammatory bowel disease.* New York: Medcom, 1976.)

demonstration of thickening of the bowel wall. However, because the study is less invasive than other alternatives and can be done without preparation, it may be used to reduce the frequency of repeated colonoscopic or barium enema studies in patients already known to harbor IBD.[266]

Pathology

Macroscopic Appearance

Ulcerative colitis is a disease confined to the mucosa and submucosa of the bowel. The only exception to this occurs when transmural involvement produces so-called toxic megacolon. The bowel wall is not thickened, no granulomas are present (except a foreign body giant-cell reaction may occasionally be seen in an area of acute inflammation), and there are no skip areas. The rectum is

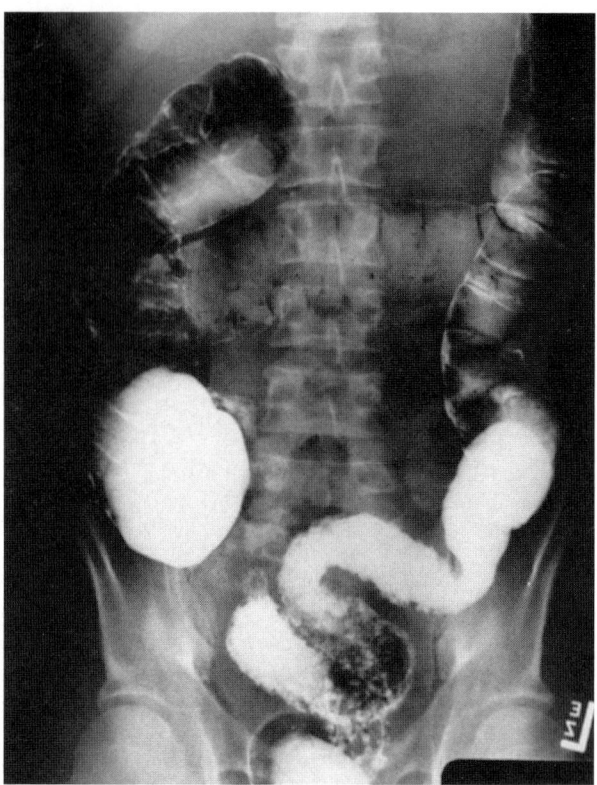

FIGURE 29-8. Ulcerative colitis. This barium enema study reveals extensive pseudopolyposis, especially in the region of the sigmoid colon. Close examination also reveals ulceration, so there should be no confusion with familial polyposis.

always involved, and the disease extends proximally for varying distances, but always with continuity of involvement to the proximal extent of the disease process (Figure 29-12). Characteristically, ulcerative colitis tends to involve the bowel more severely in a distal location than proximally. Despite extensive inflammatory reaction, the bowel wall retains its normal thickness (Figure 29-12). The results of the confluence of numerous ulcers are the longitudinal furrows of denuded mucosa that alternate with islands of heaped-up mucosa, the so-called pseudopolyps (Figs. 29-13 through 29-15). Pseudopolyps are inflammatory polyps, not neoplastic lesions. These are seen during a quiescent phase of ulcerative colitis and are a later manifestation of this condition. They may be confused with familial polyposis (see Chapter 21), but the absence of normal mucosa between these polyps suggests the correct diagnosis.

The entire colon, including the cecum and appendix, may be involved (Figure 29-16). Characteristically, however, the disease does not affect the ileum. In fact, if the small bowel is involved for more than a few centimeters, the diagnosis is not ulcerative colitis. One exception to this is the so-called backwash ileitis seen occasionally when the entire colon is affected. This reversible condi-

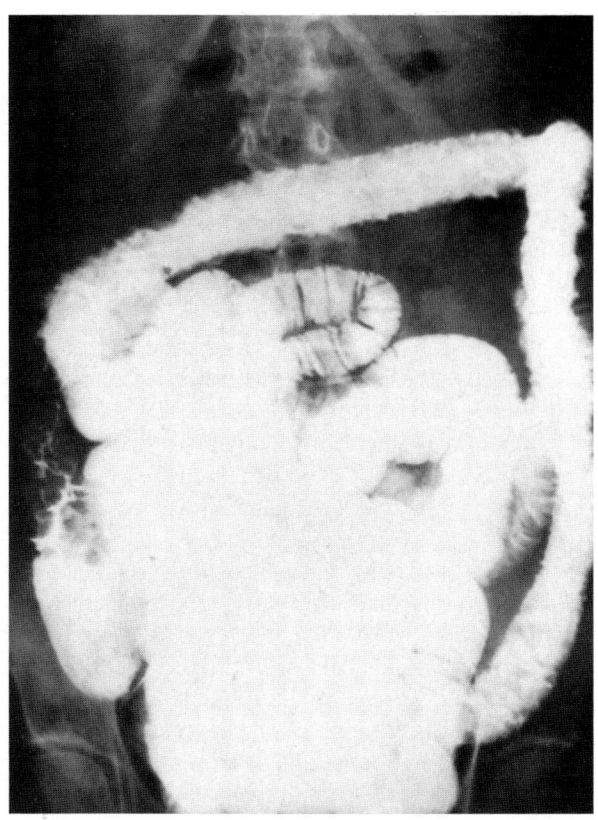

FIGURE 29-9. Ulcerative colitis. Extensive pseudopolyposis with foreshortening of the bowel. Note that the colon is outlined by ulcerations. (From Corman ML, Veidenheimer MC, Nugent FW, et al. *Diseases of the anus, rectum and colon. Part II: nonspecific inflammatory bowel disease.* New York: Medcom, 1976.)

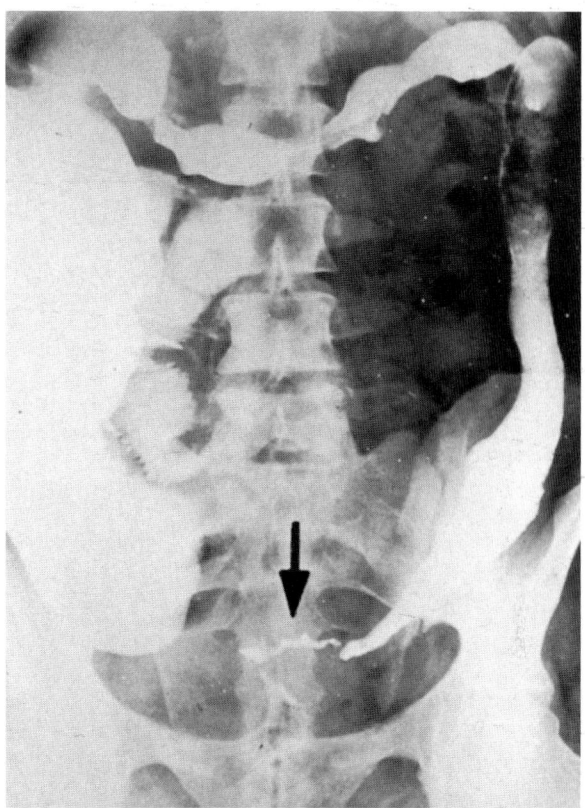

FIGURE 29-10. Ulcerative colitis with stricture. Inflammatory changes are noted to the hepatic flexure, with stricture in the distal sigmoid *(arrow)*. The patient subsequently underwent resection, and the lesion was found to be benign. (From Corman ML, Veidenheimer MC, Nugent FW, et al. *Diseases of the anus, rectum and colon. Part II: nonspecific inflammatory bowel disease.* New York: Medcom, 1976.)

tion, which may be demonstrated radiographically as edematous, thickened mucosal folds, is a nonspecific inflammatory reaction resulting from proximity of the ileum to the diseased colon.

The entire mucosa may be denuded in patients with long-standing, chronic ulcerative colitis (Figure 29-17). Under these circumstances, the physician may be lulled into a false sense of security, since the patient's symptoms are often minimal. It is unlikely that someone will experience discharge of mucus, diarrhea, or bleeding if no inflamed mucosa is present. It is this individual who is particularly susceptible to the development of carcinoma (see Relationship to Carcinoma).

Toxic megacolon is a condition in which an acute inflammatory reaction extends throughout the entire thickness of the bowel wall to the serosa. Gangrene and perforation can result (Figure 29-18). This is the only manifestation of ulcerative colitis that is not limited to the mucosa and submucosa. The term is a poor one, because it is not the colon that is toxic; it is obviously the patient.

Histologic Appearance

Ulcerative colitis is characterized histologically by an intense inflammation of the mucosa and submucosa, in addition to the presence of multiple crypt abscesses. Too much emphasis, however, should not be placed on the significance of crypt abscesses. Acute, self-limited colitis (in which cultures are negative) as well as infectious colitides (see Chapter 33) often have overlapping histopathologic features and must be distinguished from ulcerative colitis.[274,288] Marked vascular engorgement accounts for the propensity to rectal bleeding (Figure 29-19). There is an obvious decrease in production of mucus by the crypt epithelial cells (Figure 29-20). The decrease may be explained by injury to these cells.[351] Conversely, increased secretion of mucus is seen in patients with Crohn's disease.

If the bowel is cut longitudinally, it becomes apparent that the deeper parts of the colonic wall are spared. Confinement of the disease to the mucosa and submucosa is the most characteristic finding in ulcerative co-

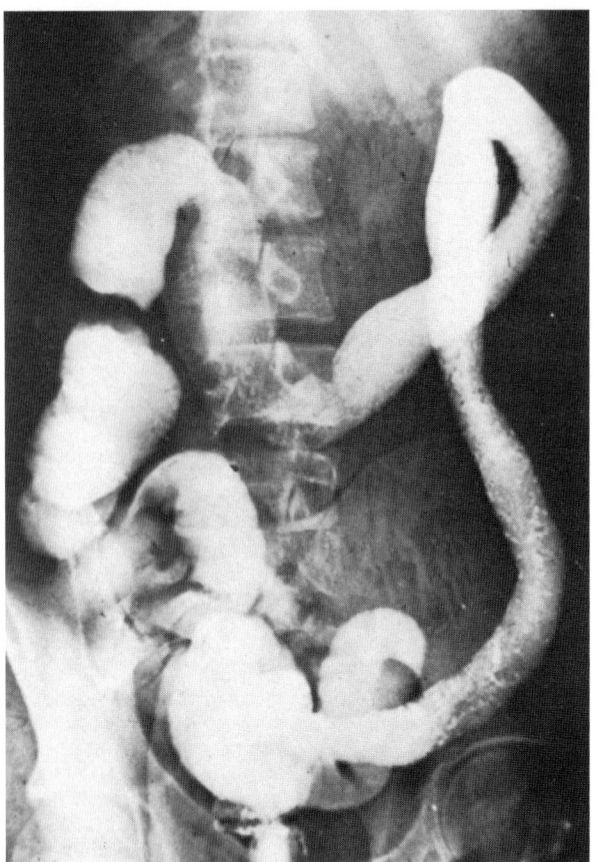

FIGURE 29-11. Extensive ulcerative colitis with loss of haustral markings and destruction of the normal mucosa throughout. Dilatation of the terminal ileum is evident, a characteristic observation in "backwash ileitis." (From Corman ML, Veidenheimer MC, Nugent FW, et al. *Diseases of the anus, rectum and colon. Part II: nonspecific inflammatory bowel disease.* New York: Medcom, 1976.)

litis (Figure 29-21). Abscesses may enlarge to undermine the mucosa, which may then be shed into the bowel lumen, leaving an ulcer behind. When multiple ulcers form, the remaining nonulcerated mucosa extends above the muscularis as polypoid projections, resulting in the well-known pseudopolyps of ulcerative colitis (Figs. 29-22 and 29-23). If ulceration continues, the entire mucosa may become denuded, and broad areas of the submucosa may be exposed to the fecal stream.

In toxic megacolon, there is full-thickness involvement of the bowel, necrosis, and friability, the histologic manifestation of which is shown in Figure 29-24.

Lymphoid hyperplasia involving the mucosa and submucosa occurs in up to 25% of patients with ulcerative colitis. This may be present beneath an area of relative inactivity (Figure 29-25).

Seldenrijk and colleagues prospectively performed blind evaluations of multiple colonic mucosal biopsy specimens in individuals with ulcerative colitis and Crohn's disease to identify reproducible histologic features that could be used to distinguish between the two conditions.[647] Three features—an excess of histiocytes in combination with a villous or irregular aspect of the mucosal surface and granulomas—had a high predictive value.

Watanabe and co-workers studied rectal biopsy specimens from patients with ulcerative colitis undergoing colonoscopic examinations for the presence of substance P–containing nerve fibers.[732] It is well-known that the bowel is rich in peptidergic innervation, which contributes to the mucosal immune responses. Because substance P has stimulatory effects on various immunocytes

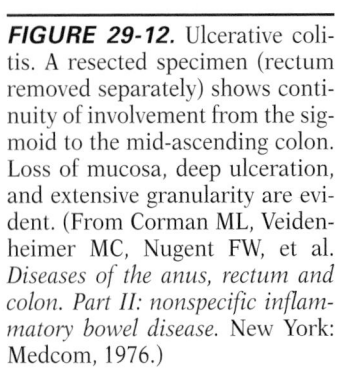

FIGURE 29-12. Ulcerative colitis. A resected specimen (rectum removed separately) shows continuity of involvement from the sigmoid to the mid-ascending colon. Loss of mucosa, deep ulceration, and extensive granularity are evident. (From Corman ML, Veidenheimer MC, Nugent FW, et al. *Diseases of the anus, rectum and colon. Part II: nonspecific inflammatory bowel disease.* New York: Medcom, 1976.)

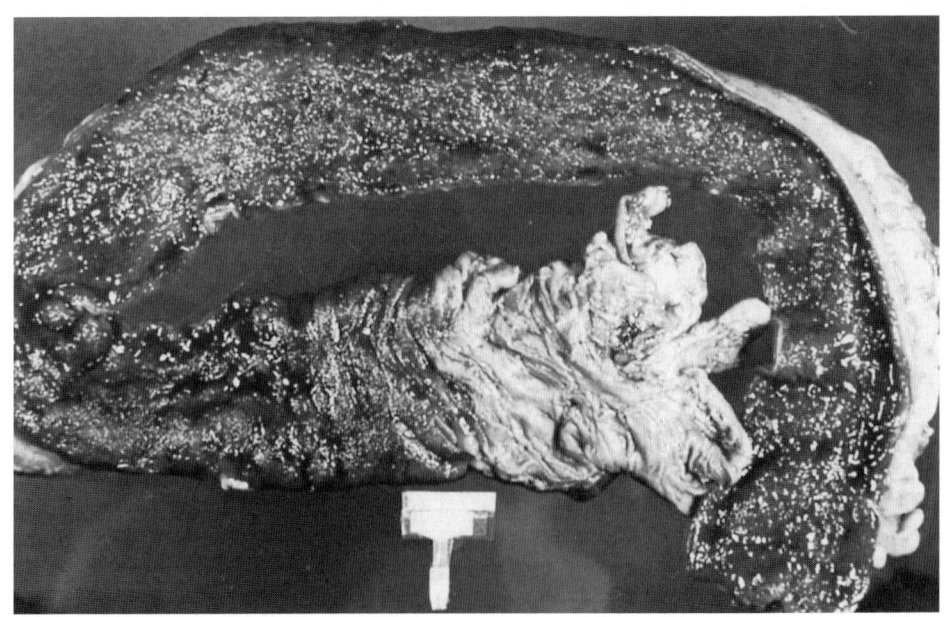

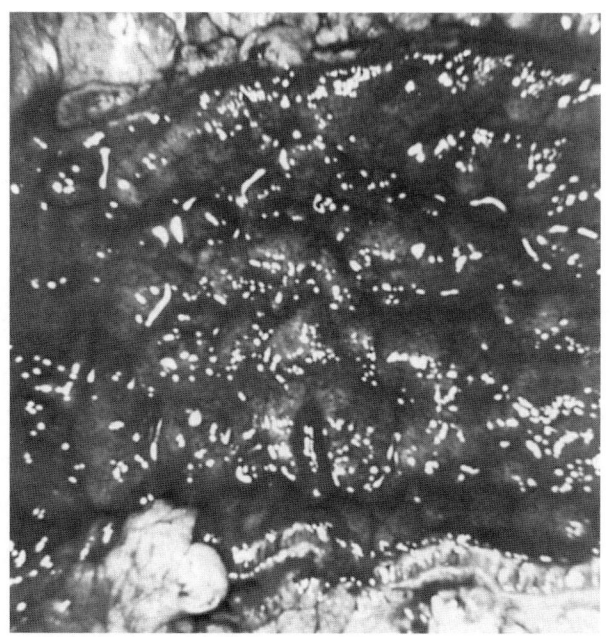

FIGURE 29-13. Ulcerative colitis. Longitudinal furrows of denuded mucosa alternate with islands of heaped-up mucosa, demonstrating how loss of mucosal integrity contributes to fluid and electrolyte depletion. (From Corman ML, Veidenheimer MC, Nugent FW, et al. *Diseases of the anus, rectum and colon. Part II: nonspecific inflammatory bowel disease.* New York: Medcom, 1976.)

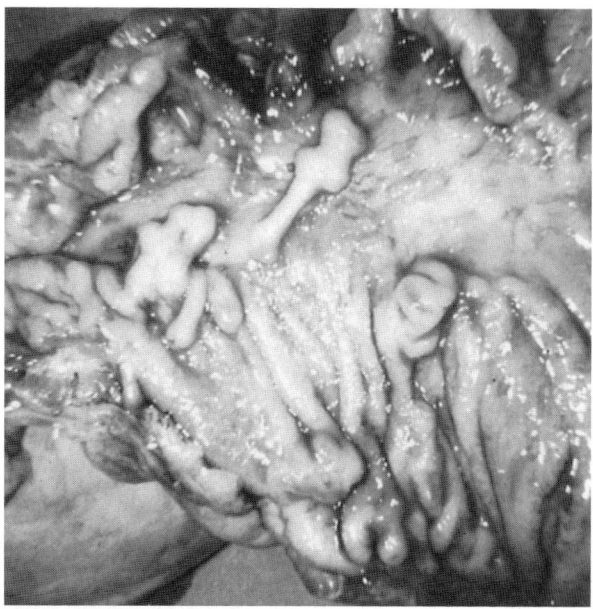

FIGURE 29-15. Ulcerative colitis. Islands of heaped-up mucosa and inflammatory polyps (pseudopolyps). (From Corman ML, Veidenheimer MC, Nugent FW, et al. *Diseases of the anus, rectum and colon. Part II: nonspecific inflammatory bowel disease.* New York: Medcom, 1976.)

in inflammatory diseases, its increased presence paralleling increased disease activity suggests that alterations play an important role in the pathogenesis of ulcerative colitis.[732]

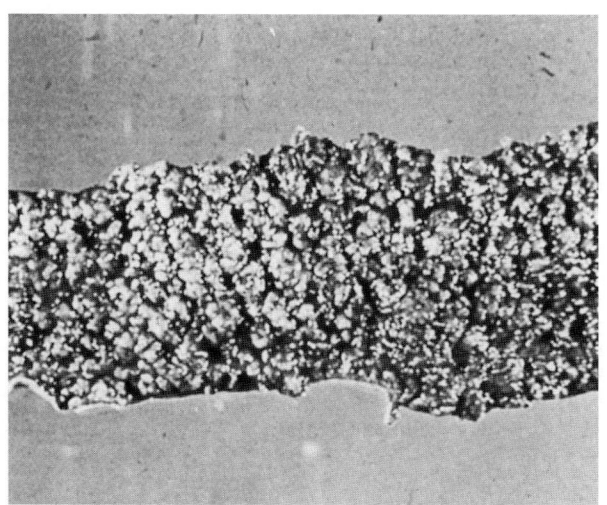

FIGURE 29-14. Extensive pseudopolyps in active ulcerative colitis. Note the relative uniformity of the polyps in comparison with the varied sizes seen in familial polyposis (see Chapter 21). (From Corman ML, Veidenheimer MC, Nugent FW, et al. *Diseases of the anus, rectum and colon. Part II: nonspecific inflammatory bowel disease.* New York: Medcom, 1976.)

Antineutrophil Cytoplasmic Antibody Determination

Various studies have shown that antineutrophil cytoplasmic antibodies (ANCAs) with a perinuclear staining pattern (pANCA) are present in up to 86% of patients with ulcerative colitis.[629] Theoretically, this autoimmunity may represent a possible pathogenetic mechanism for the development of ulcerative colitis. A set of marker antibodies is available for the screening and differential diagnosis of ulcerative colitis and Crohn's disease (Prometheus Laboratories, Inc., San Diego, CA). Proven applications of this new technology include the following:

- as an adjunct to clinical and tissue pathology in the differential diagnosis of IBD
- confirmation of the correct diagnosis before surgery
- identification of those patients with left-sided ulcerative colitis that may be resistant to treatment
- identification of those patients prone to the development of pouchitis following ileal pouch-anal anastomosis.

(text continues on page 1338)

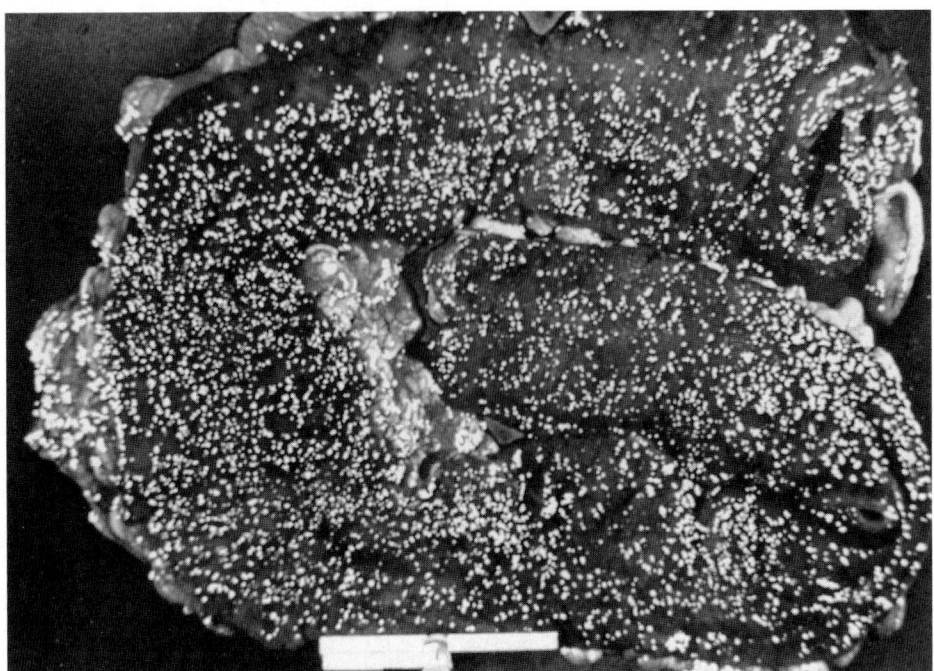

FIGURE 29-16. Ulcerative colitis. The entire colon is involved by inflammatory change, with sparing of the ileum *(arrow)*. (From Corman ML, Veidenheimer MC, Nugent FW, et al. *Diseases of the anus, rectum and colon. Part II: nonspecific inflammatory bowel disease.* New York: Medcom, 1976.)

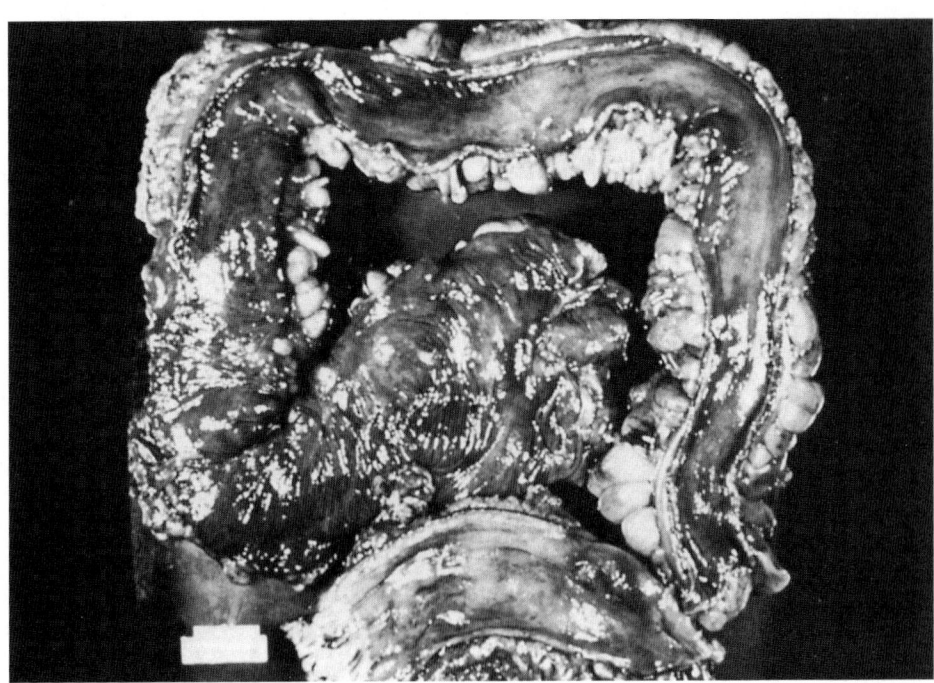

FIGURE 29-17. Ulcerative colitis. Complete desquamation of colonic mucosa. Note the normal bowel wall thickness. (From Corman ML, Veidenheimer MC, Nugent FW, et al. *Diseases of the anus, rectum and colon. Part II: nonspecific inflammatory bowel disease.* New York: Medcom, 1976.)

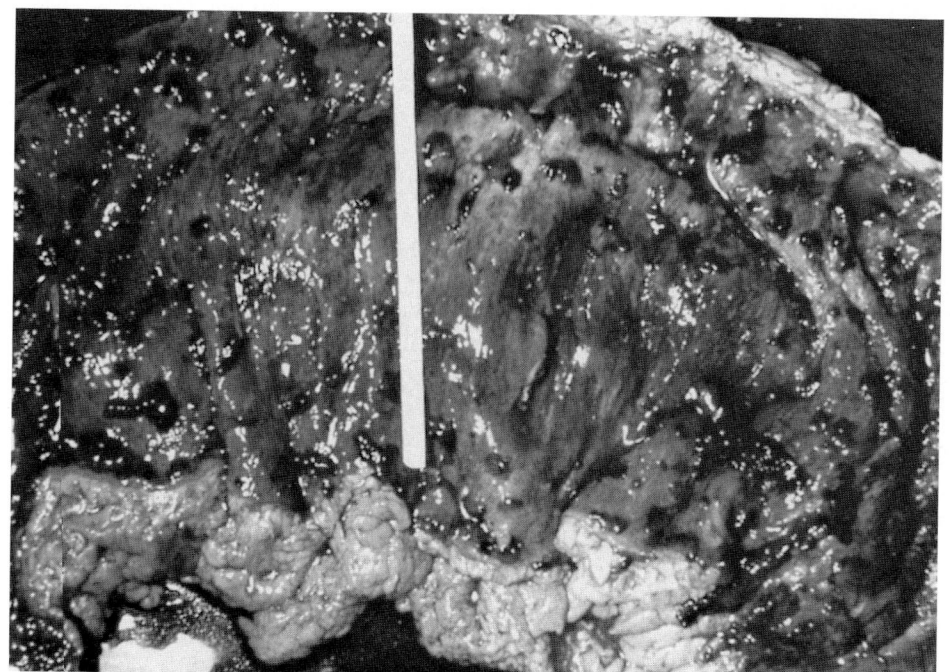

FIGURE 29-18. Ulcerative colitis. Portion of a resected transverse colon showing increased circumference of the bowel. There is practically no mucosa remaining, and circular muscle is exposed in some areas. (From Corman ML, Veidenheimer MC, Nugent FW, et al. *Diseases of the anus, rectum and colon. Part II: nonspecific inflammatory bowel disease.* New York: Medcom, 1976.)

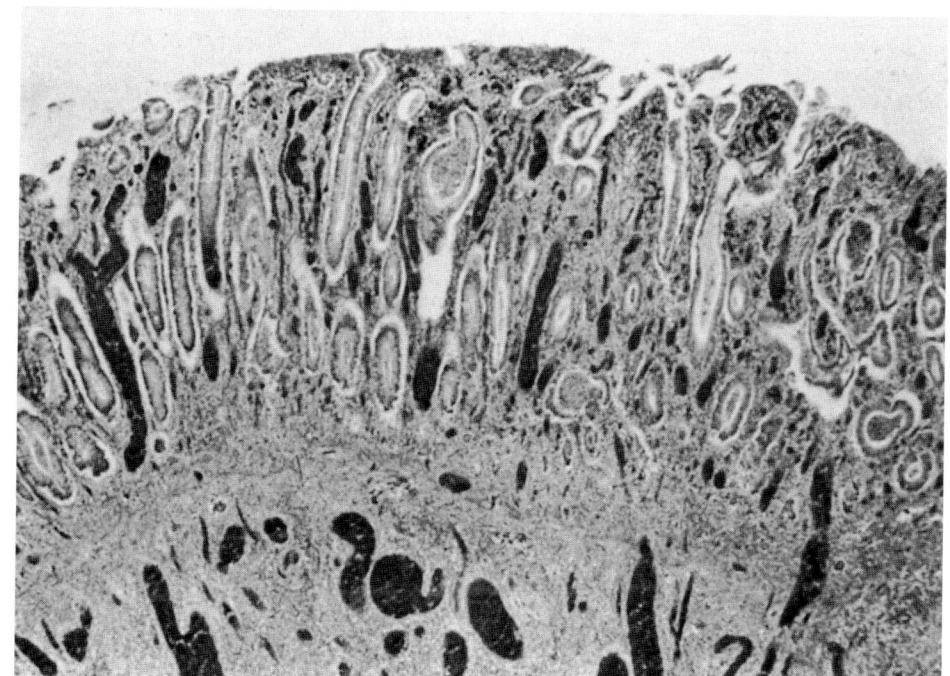

FIGURE 29-19. Ulcerative colitis. Intense inflammation of the mucosa with multiple crypt abscesses. (Original magnification × 80; from Corman ML, Veidenheimer MC, Nugent FW, et al. *Diseases of the anus, rectum and colon. Part II: nonspecific inflammatory bowel disease.* New York: Medcom, 1976.)

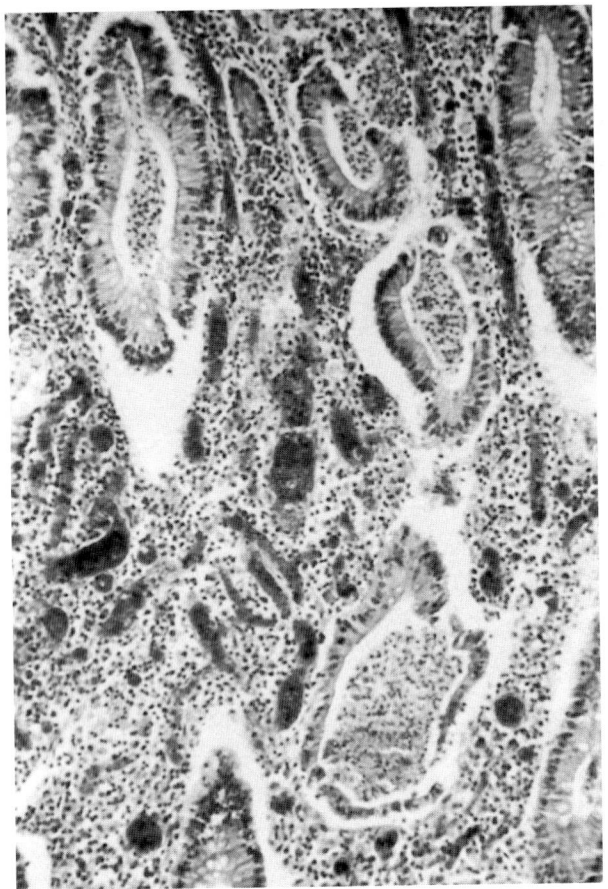

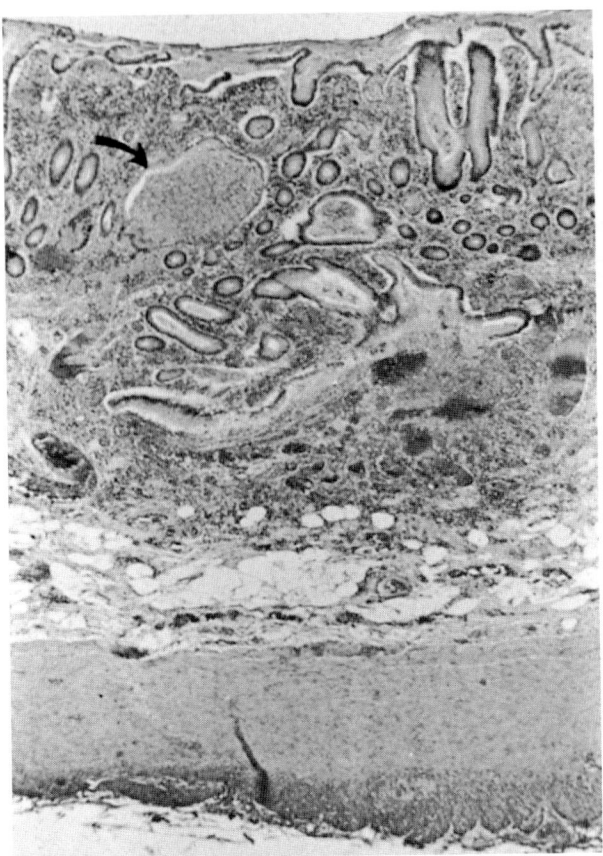

FIGURE 29-20. Ulcerative colitis. Crypt abscesses with degeneration of crypt epithelium and communication between the crypt lumina and lamina propria. Note vascular engorgement and decrease in mucus production by crypt epithelial cells. (Original magnification × 280; from Corman ML, Veidenheimer MC, Nugent FW, et al. *Diseases of the anus, rectum and colon. Part II: nonspecific inflammatory bowel disease.* New York: Medcom, 1976.)

FIGURE 29-21. Ulcerative colitis. Marked inflammation of the mucosa and submucosa. Note the large crypt abscess *(arrow)* that has penetrated into the submucosa and has been lined partially by epithelial cells growing down into the abscess cavity. (Original magnification × 80; from Corman ML, Veidenheimer MC, Nugent FW, et al. *Diseases of the anus, rectum and colon. Part II: nonspecific inflammatory bowel disease.* New York: Medcom, 1976.)

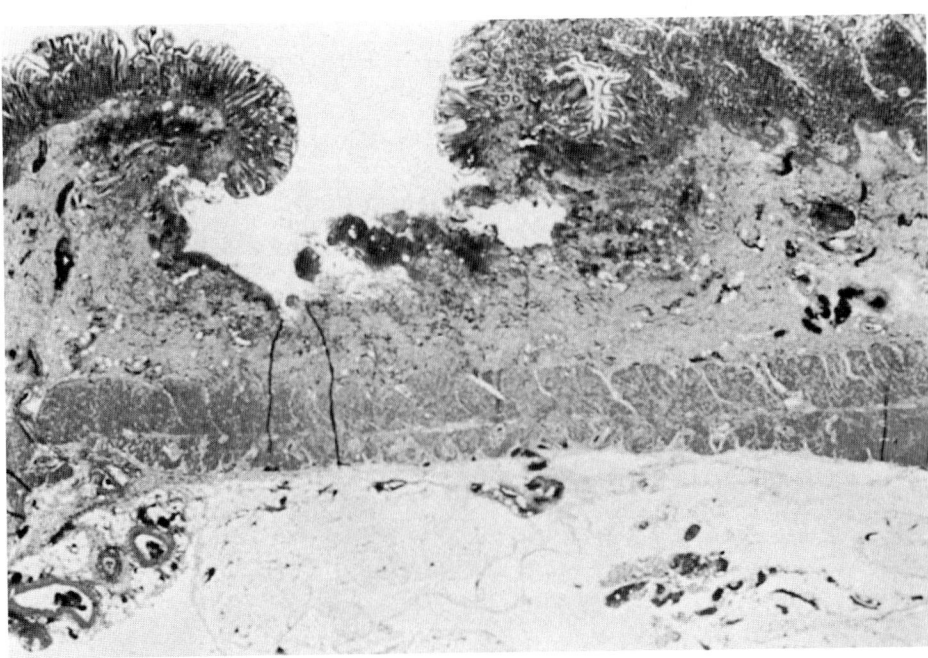

FIGURE 29-22. Ulcerative colitis. An enlarged abscess undermines the mucosa, leaving an ulcer. (Original magnification × 80; from Corman ML, Veidenheimer MC, Nugent FW, et al. *Diseases of the anus, rectum and colon. Part II: nonspecific inflammatory bowel disease.* New York: Medcom, 1976.)

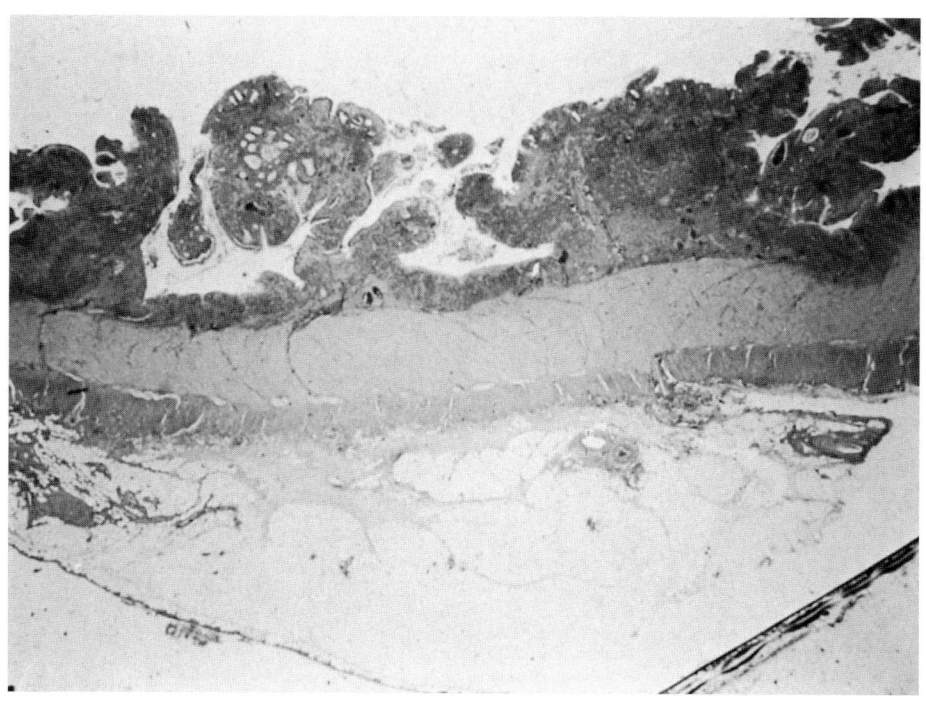

FIGURE 29-23. Ulcerative colitis. Confluence of ulcers results in pseudopolyps. (Original magnification × 80; from Corman ML, Veidenheimer MC, Nugent FW, et al. *Diseases of the anus, rectum and colon. Part II: nonspecific inflammatory bowel disease.* New York: Medcom, 1976.)

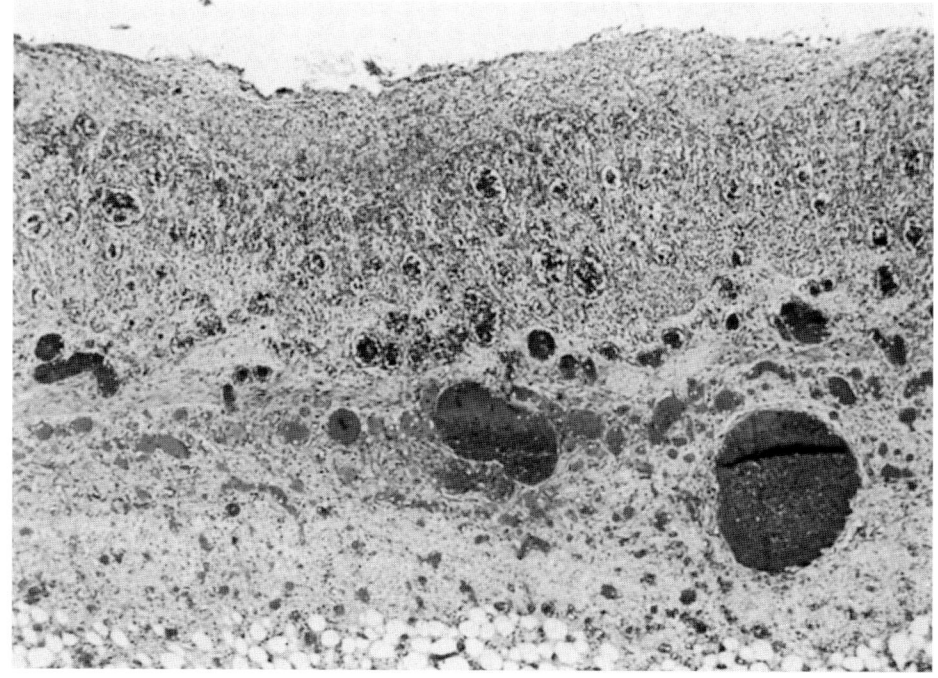

FIGURE 29-24. Ulcerative colitis. Toxic megacolon. Note the loss of epithelium, transmural necrosis, and hemorrhage. (Original magnification × 80; from Corman ML, Veidenheimer MC, Nugent FW, et al. *Diseases of the anus, rectum and colon. Part II: nonspecific inflammatory bowel disease.* New York: Medcom, 1976.)

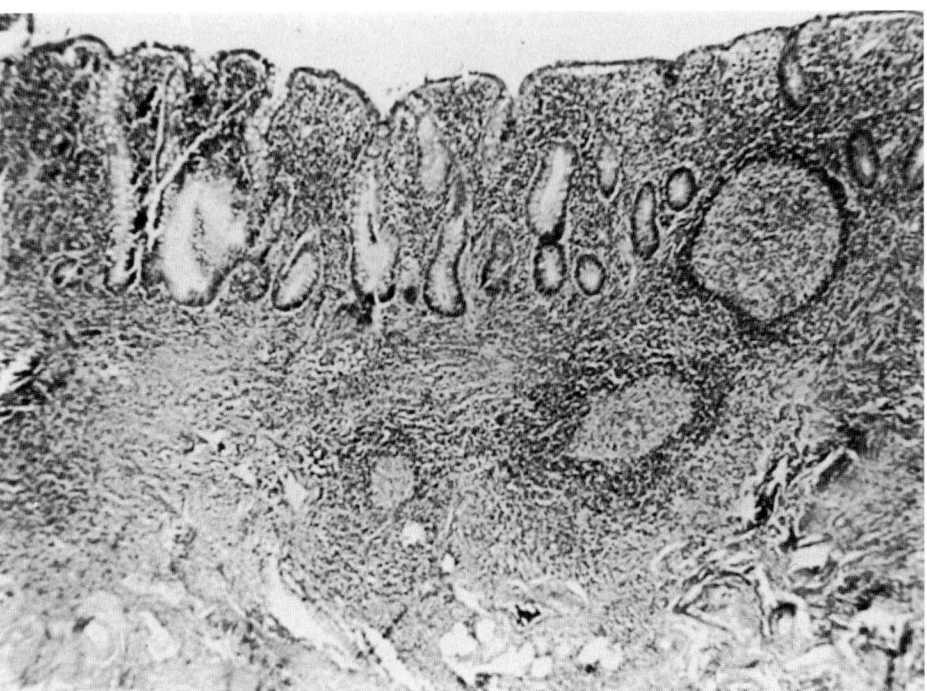

FIGURE 29-25. Lymphoid hyperplasia. Although mucosal disease is relatively inactive, lymphoid hyperplasia is pronounced. (Original magnification × 80; from Corman ML, Veidenheimer MC, Nugent FW, et al. *Diseases of the anus, rectum and colon. Part II: nonspecific inflammatory bowel disease.* New York: Medcom, 1976.)

Breath Pentane Analysis

As previously mentioned, neutrophils, macrophages, and other cells are capable of producing free oxygen radicals that can stimulate lipid peroxidation, especially during periods of active inflamm ation.[366] To assess the degree of inflammation in IBD, Kokoszka and colleagues quantitatively determined breath pentane and alkane generated by peroxidation of cellular fatty acids.[366] Individuals underwent indium-labeled granulocyte nuclear imaging to assess the presence and location of inflammation. The production of pentane, the product of the peroxidation of polyunsaturated fatty acids, can be quantified by measuring the content of exhaled breath. The investigators concluded that pentane analysis may be correlated with IBD activity.[366]

Leukocyte Scan

Abdominal scintigraphy by means of autologous-labeled leukocytes has been used to assess activity in IBD. Indium 111 (^{111}In) and technetium 99m (^{99m}Tc) have been the most helpful in this regard. Stählberg and colleagues undertook an evaluation using scintigraphy with ^{99m}Tc-labeled leukocytes to assess disease extent and activity in acute colitis.[551] With colonoscopy as the reference method, the maximum extent of colitis was correctly assessed by the scan in two-thirds of patients, but rectal involvement was not perceived in 19%. The intensity of inflammatory activity correlated significantly with the colonoscopic assessment. The authors concluded that the noninvasive nature of this particular approach makes it a reasonable al-

ternative to other investigations of the extent and activity of IBD.

SIGNS, SYMPTOMS, AND PRESENTATIONS

Patients with ulcerative colitis and Crohn's disease may present with very minimal symptoms and moderate complaints, or they may have fulminant manifestations. There is a considerable overlap in the symptomatology of the two conditions, but there are some differences in the presentation between the two. Rectal bleeding is always seen in patients with ulcerative colitis at some time during the course of the illness. It can be safely said that if the patient does not bleed, the diagnosis is not ulcerative colitis. Individuals with Crohn's disease also may bleed, but this is not as frequent a manifestation and may not be as severe. Abdominal pain may be mild or absent in patients with ulcerative colitis, but it is rarely severe except possibly when toxic megacolon supervenes. However, patients with Crohn's disease frequently have abdominal pain.[232] An abdominal mass is occasionally found on physical examination in a patient with Crohn's disease, but it is never seen in a patient with ulcerative colitis.

The presence of diarrhea and the passage of mucus are frequently observed in both conditions and do not serve as distinguishing characteristics. Diarrhea may be manifested as two or three loose stools a day or may be as severe as 20 or more bowel movements within a 24-hour period. Often, patients with ulcerative colitis are more troubled by the frequency of the bowel movements than are those with Crohn's disease. This is, perhaps, because distal disease tends to be associated with more urgency and, in some cases, tenesmus. Patients with Crohn's disease may have rectal sparing and are less likely to experience urgency.

Anal disease is much more commonly seen in Crohn's colitis than in ulcerative colitis. The presence of anal pain, swelling, and discharge may be a presenting feature of the former condition and may be the only abnormality observed on examination and subsequent investigation (see Chapters 11 and 30).

Fever is usually not a concern in patients with ulcerative colitis unless the patient is severely ill (toxic megacolon). However, in patients with Crohn's disease, a pyrexia is not uncommonly noted and is usually caused by an intraabdominal abscess or undrained septic focus. Nausea and vomiting are not frequently seen in either condition unless there is evidence of intestinal obstruction. Anorexia, weight loss, anemia, and general debility are associated with relatively long-standing or fulminant disease.

Disease in the Older Adult

The development of IBD in the older adult population has been a source of some confusion. Many older patients who have signs and symptoms suggestive of IBD

are thought to have ischemic colitis. Conversely, patients thought to have IBD subsequently have been proved to have ischemia as the cause of their symptoms. Brandt and colleagues reviewed 81 patients with colitis whose symptoms began after the age of 50 years.[65] In this retrospective review, one half of patients classified as having nonspecific IBD were really thought to have had ischemic colitis. In older persons, ulcerative colitis may have a sudden and fulminating onset progressing to a fatal outcome.

Disease in Children and Adolescents

Data from Edinburgh suggest that the rising incidence of IBD in young people is entirely a consequence of Crohn's disease, a condition now more common than ulcerative colitis in this age group.[645,646] When the condition occurs in children, there may be a more rapid onset and progression than when the disease occurs in young adults. Symptoms are the same as in adults, but toxic megacolon, bowel perforation, and massive hemorrhage are not uncommon sequelae. These youngsters often become chronically ill, have impaired growth and decreased mental acuity, and are less developed physically than their healthy peers (Figure 29-26).[121,122,484,700,718] Growth failure, especially, is the result of prolonged inadequate caloric intake.[343] It is because of these concerns that implementation of an elemental diet and parenteral nutrition are often part of

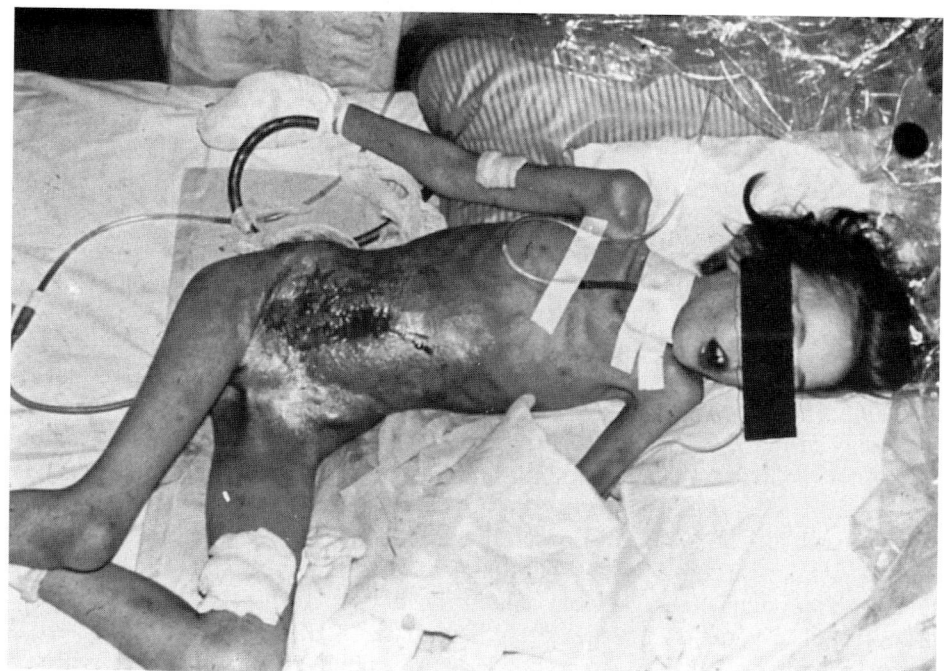

FIGURE 29-26. Crohn's disease. Severe wasting in a 17-year-old girl, who looks much younger. Note the external abdominal wall fistula. (From Corman ML, Veidenheimer MC, Nugent FW, et al. *Diseases of the anus, rectum and colon. Part II: nonspecific inflammatory bowel disease.* New York: Medcom, 1976.)

the management of patients in this age group (see Medical Management).[343,632] However, to be maximally effective, therapy must be initiated before puberty.[343] Furthermore, unless medical treatment can achieve a sustained remission, operative intervention may be the only appropriate method for addressing the problem of retarded development (see Surgical Management).[137] Particular emphasis should be placed on the assessment of growth and development as well as psychological support for both patient and family.[62,608,632] Close cooperation between the physician and the surgeon is perhaps even more than usually appropriate in the management of these vulnerable individuals.[602]

Disease in Pregnancy

Because IBD is common in patients of childbearing age, the possibility of becoming pregnant is often an issue in medical and surgical care. However, pregnancy is not that frequent an event in patients with IBD. The reason probably is related to the fact that these patients may suffer any number of hormonal imbalances as a result of acute and chronic illness, often severely impairing their ability to become pregnant.

However, ulcerative colitis and Crohn's disease do not adversely affect fertility, nor do they necessarily impede the progress of a pregnancy or the delivery of a normal, term infant. According to Zetzel, pregnancy in association with a preexisting colitis or complicated by the development of IBD is attended by the same prospect of a full-term delivery of a healthy child as is pregnancy in a healthy woman.[762] However, Schade and colleagues found a significantly greater incidence of low birth weight (less than 2,500 g) in infants of mothers with ulcerative colitis than in a control population.[636] Baird and colleagues found no evidence of an increased risk for pregnancy loss, but the likelihood of preterm birth was significantly greater.[18]

Levy and colleagues reviewed the *clinical course* of ulcerative colitis with respect to 60 pregnancies in 31 patients.[406] Twenty percent were improved, 18% deteriorated, and 62% demonstrated no change during the course of pregnancy. Fourteen percent of the pregnancies were ended by spontaneous abortion and two by artificial abortions. One premature birth was noted in 50 full-term deliveries. All the births produced healthy children. The authors concluded that pregnancy does not seem to exacerbate preexisting ulcerative colitis, nor does colitis interfere with the outcome of the pregnancy.

Crohn and colleagues reported 74 pregnancies in 47 women whose colitis was inactive at the time of conception.[114] All subsequent therapeutic and spontaneous abortions (including one stillbirth) occurred in patients in whom the colitis became activated. There was no difference in the incidence of abortion in patients who con-

ceived during an active phase of colitis in comparison with those who conceived during an inactive phase. These observations have been confirmed by others.[125]

What happens to the colitis in patients who are pregnant? Zetzel reviewed a number of reported series and found it helpful to group the patients into several categories.[762] Only 30% of patients who became pregnant during a quiescent phase of the colitis had an exacerbation of their disease, but a recrudescence developed in 60% when the pregnancy occurred during an active phase of the illness. In patients whose colitis developed initially during pregnancy or in the postpartum period, a particularly severe result was noted, with more than 60% having worsening of their symptoms. Khosla and colleagues noted that the infertility rate of patients with Crohn's disease was similar to that seen in the general population (12%).[345] Those whose condition was in remission at the time of conception had a normal pregnancy, with the disease remaining quiescent in most individuals. However, active disease at the time of conception tended to inhibit remission despite therapy.[345] In studies specifically in women with Crohn's disease, pregnancy entailed no increased risk for exacerbation of the bowel inflammation.[517,754] However, an increased risk for premature delivery and spontaneous abortion has been observed in those with active disease or in whom resection is required.

In the counseling of a colitis patient who is contemplating pregnancy, there is no justification for suggesting that attempts at conception be avoided, except when the possibility of teratogenic effects of a medication exists [e.g., the use of metronidazole (Flagyl)]. Certainly, immunosuppressive treatment should be avoided in a patient wishing to conceive.

Concerns are also expressed about the safety of drug therapy in men, which could damage sperm and theoretically be associated with teratogenicity. Infertility in men is commonly associated with sulfasalazine administration. Sperm analysis may be helpful in determining whether a problem in conception can be attributed to this cause.

As mentioned, women who have a quiescent form of the disease are unlikely to experience problems with pregnancy and delivery. Conversely, if the patient is experiencing an exacerbation of the colitis, the illness itself may preclude the possibility of pregnancy. If the disease is more than moderately active, Zetzel counsels a temporary waiting period and introduction of appropriate medical therapy to secure a remission.[762] However, even in this situation, the chances of a normal pregnancy and delivery approximate 50%.[762] Contraception need be considered only in those women whose disease is so severe that surgery is imminent.[761] Certainly, if the prospective parents wish to have a child, no benefit may be expected from a therapeutic abortion. Even in the severely ill pregnant woman, there is no evidence to suggest that the pregnancy cannot be brought to a successful conclusion with the birth of a healthy child.

If surgery becomes necessary during pregnancy, the method of treatment should be identical to that of a patient who is not pregnant. In other words, drug management (steroids, sulfasalazine) is not contraindicated. It has also been determined that azathioprine is safe and that termination of the pregnancy is not mandatory for those who conceive while taking the drug.[6] Similarly, if an operation becomes necessary, the procedure should be performed as if the patient were not pregnant, although one should probably defer the implementation of a major reconstructive procedure (see Surgical Management). Closer to term, the enlarged uterus may preclude the possibility of performing even a conventional proctectomy; a staged operation, sparing the rectum, is therefore appropriate.

A high fetal and maternal mortality has been reported if surgical intervention becomes necessary for fulminant colitis.[461,552] Bohe and colleagues noted two cases of fulminant disease during pregnancy that required subtotal colectomy and ileostomy in one, and proctocolectomy in the other.[58] These operations were undertaken in the thirty-second and thirty-third week of pregnancy, respectively. I have performed surgery in two women during pregnancy: one patient underwent a proctocolectomy at 3 months, and the other underwent a total abdominal colectomy and ileostomy at 5 months. Both proceeded to uneventful conclusions of their pregnancy and delivered normal, healthy infants. In my opinion, it is not in the interest of the mother or the fetus to delay surgery until the pregnancy can be terminated with a viable child. In other words, I do not advocate waiting until the thirty-second week to perform a cesarean section while the mother is forced to postpone needed surgery.

Lindhagen and colleagues assessed the fertility and outcome of pregnancy in 78 women who had previously undergone resection for Crohn's disease.[417] Neither the number of live births nor the frequency of abortions differed from that which would be expected in the general population. The major factor, again, appeared to be that the disease was in remission or, as in the above reference, removed.

Successful childbirth has been reported following *restorative proctocolectomy* with pelvic ileal reservoir (see later discussion in that section).[475,510,566] Twenty-eight patients carried 37 pregnancies to term after *continent (Kock) ileostomy*, according to a report from Göteborg, Sweden.[539] Problems encountered were an increased urge to empty the reservoir, especially in the last trimester, and some difficulties with intubation. In most patients, a vaginal delivery was successful, with cesarean section reserved for obstetric indications.

If pregnancy develops following *proctocolectomy and ileostomy*, the question arises as to whether the prospective mother should undergo a cesarean section or deliver vaginally. My own feeling is that if the pregnant woman has an adequate pelvis for a normal vaginal delivery, this should be attempted. A cesarean section is not mandatory simply because the patient has an ileostomy, but if an episiotomy is performed, there may be a delay in healing of the perineal wound. However, it has been my experience that the obstetrician almost invariably will opt for a cesarean section. A national registry of ostomates is being maintained; a 1985 United States published survey indicated that about 1,000 had become pregnant.[219]

Extraintestinal Manifestations

Extraintestinal manifestations were at one time thought to be primarily associated with Crohn's disease, but with several exceptions, they can be found in both conditions. These are discussed in Chapter 30.

COURSE AND PROGNOSIS

As with many diseases, the prognosis for ulcerative colitis today is very different from that of half a century ago. Generally, this is attributed to improved medications, advances in surgical technique, and associated support during major abdominal surgery. Nordenholtz and colleagues examined the causes of death in patients with Crohn's disease and ulcerative colitis through an analysis of death certificates in Rochester, New York.[520] Of the total of 1,358 patients with IBD followed from 1973 through 1989, 130 (59 with ulcerative colitis and 71 with Crohn's disease) were found to have recorded death certificates. Sixty-eight percent of patients with Crohn's disease and 78% of those with ulcerative colitis died of causes unrelated to their IBD.[520] Deaths caused by Crohn's disease decreased from 44% in the first 8-year period to 6% in the second. Colorectal cancer caused 14% of the deaths in patients with ulcerative colitis, three times more often than in persons with Crohn's disease. Excluding cancer, only two deaths were directly attributable to ulcerative colitis, both occurring within the first two years after diagnosis.[520]

With respect to course and prognosis, Langholz and associates at the University of Copenhagen examined 1,161 patients during a 25-year period.[379] The distribution of disease activity was remarkably constant each year, with about 50% of individuals in clinical remission. After 10 years, the colectomy rate was 24%. With 25 years of follow-up, the cumulative probability of a relapsing course was 90%.[379] The probability of maintaining working capacity up to 10 years was approximately 93%. The authors concluded that although ulcerative colitis is a troublesome condition, most patients can manage their lives with little interference.

Maunder conducted a Medline search for articles relating to ulcerative colitis and Crohn's disease published since 1981 to determine the quality of life.[453] Health-related quality of life is a quantitative measurement of the subjective perception of the state of one's health, including emotional and social aspects. The investigators determined that the articles published indicated a trend toward a higher quality of life during the period from 1984 to 1987 in comparison with the period from 1981 to 1984. Although one can certainly question the validity of such an investigative effort, it appears that the previous comment concerning the general improvement in our ability to treat these two conditions is supported.

RELATIONSHIP TO CARCINOMA

Carcinoma of the colon arising in a patient with ulcerative colitis was initially described by Crohn and Rosenberg in 1925. Since that time, numerous cases have been reported, so that there is uniform agreement with respect to the association between chronic ulcerative colitis and the subsequent development of adenocarcinoma. Primary malignant lymphoma complicating ulcerative colitis, although extremely rare, is nevertheless also thought to be associated with ulcerative colitis.[1] Unfortunately, the true incidence of carcinoma is often a matter of conjecture, depending on the referral nature of the institution from which the report emanates. For example, some population-based studies have shown a lower incidence of colorectal cancer than that reported from major medical centers.[203,579]

Predisposing Factors and Incidence

Various factors predispose a colitic patient to colon cancer. These include total colonic or pancolonic disease; prolonged duration of the illness (the earliest reported case is in a patient with the disease of 7 years' duration); continuous active disease, as opposed to intermittent symptoms; and possibly the severity of disease. An early age of onset probably poses no increased cancer risk save for the fact that cancer risk often parallels duration. The cumulative risk for cancer increases with the duration of colitis, reaching 25% to 30% at 25 years, 35% at 30 years, 45% at 35 years, and 65% at 40 years.[537] Sugita and colleagues observed a strong correlation between the age of onset of ulcerative colitis and the age of onset of cancer, a correlation found both in patients with extensive disease and in those with illness affecting the left side.[683] However, colitis and cancers developed in patients with left-sided colitis about a decade later than in those with extensive disease, although the mean duration of the colitis before the development of cancer was virtually the same in both groups (ap-

proximately 21 years), irrespective of the age at onset of the disease.[683] The incidence of cancer in patients with ulcerative colitis has been variously reported to be between 2% and 5%. Öhman reported the overall incidence to be 2.7%.[537] Johnson and co-workers noted long-term findings in more than 1,400 patients with ulcerative colitis and found that colorectal cancer developed in 63 (4.4%).[319] No statistically significant difference was observed in the probability of carcinoma of the colon and rectum developing following proctitis in comparison with total colitis. Patients with left-sided disease seemed to fare considerably better with respect to risk for the development of colorectal cancer. Greenstein reported that neoplasms developed in 11.2% of 267 patients with ulcerative colitis.[229] Colorectal cancers developed in 13% of patients with universal colitis, and malignant change developed in 5% with left-sided colitis. Cancer tended to develop in patients with left-sided disease at least a decade later than in those with universal colitis. The median duration from onset of colitis to diagnosis of cancer was 20 years for those with universal colitis and 32 years for individuals with left-sided colitis.[229] Cancer did not develop in any patient with left-sided colitis before the twenty-third year of disease. In a review of more than 1,200 patients seen at the Cleveland Clinic, the cumulative risk for colorectal cancer was significantly higher in those with extensive colitis than with left-sided disease.[489] Ekbom and colleagues reviewed more than 3,000 patients with ulcerative colitis and noted that the absolute risk for the development of colorectal cancer 35 years after diagnosis was 30%.[146]

In patients who undergo resective surgery for ulcerative colitis, the incidence of associated cancer is considerably higher. Van Heerden and Beart reported the Mayo Clinic experience with 726 patients who underwent surgical exploration for chronic ulcerative colitis between the years 1961 and 1975.[724] Seventy patients (9.6%) were found to have a carcinoma of the colon. These individuals represented 1.4% of all patients in whom chronic ulcerative colitis was diagnosed during the period of study.

Generally, the incidence of carcinoma is the same in both sexes. This is not surprising in light of the fact that ulcerative colitis affects each in approximately equal numbers. Welch and Hedberg reported a bimodal distribution of the incidence—one peak in the fourth decade and the other in the seventh.[737]

An increased risk of the development of colon carcinoma also appears to be evident in Crohn's disease, especially of the small bowel.[49] This is discussed in Chapter 30.

Characteristics

The distribution of tumors in patients having ulcerative colitis and carcinoma was reported by Öhman to demonstrate multicentricity much more commonly than in those having colorectal cancer without IBD.[537] He also noted

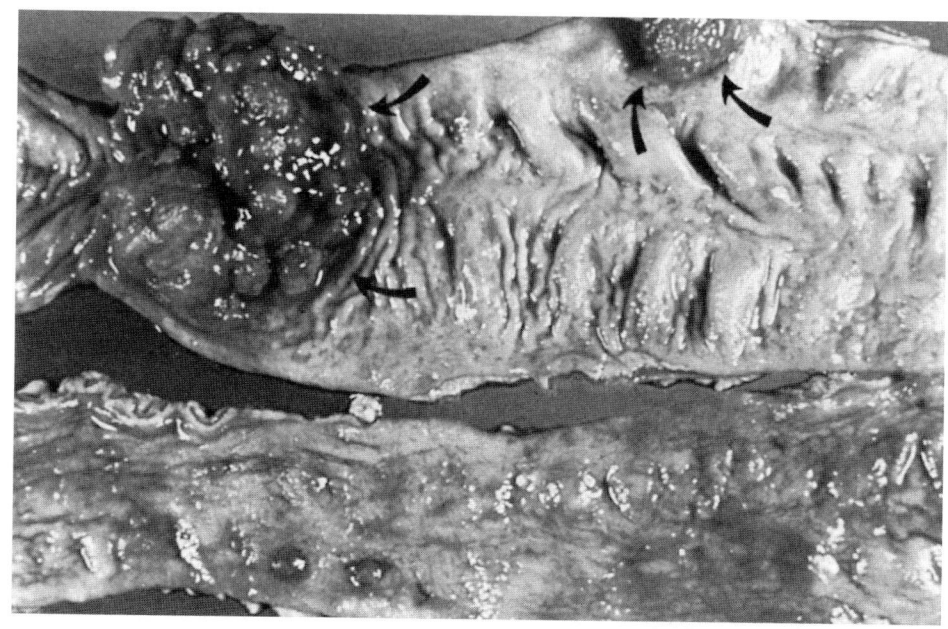

FIGURE 29-27. Carcinomas in ulcerative colitis *(arrows).* (From Corman ML, Veidenheimer MC, Nugent FW, et al. *Diseases of the anus, rectum and colon. Part II: nonspecific inflammatory bowel disease.* New York: Medcom, 1976.)

that 28% of patients had lesions of the transverse colon. Similarly, only 28% of patients had cancers involving the rectum and rectosigmoid, whereas patients with lesions of the sigmoid colon comprised 17% of the series. Conversely, Riddell and colleagues reported that the rectum was the most common site of involvement and that this was more noticeable in men than in women.[598] In their study, more than 40% of the cancers were found in the rectum, and approximately 25% of patients had multiple tumors. It is certainly clear that multicentricity of the cancers is a frequently reported phenomenon (Figure 29-27).

Another characteristic of colorectal cancer with ulcerative colitis is that very often the cancer tends to be infiltrative and scirrhous. Visible tumor involving the mucosa may not be observed even by careful endoscopic examination (Figure 29-28). Although such is the most common clinical presentation of cancer in this disease, it can also appear as a typical ulcerating or polypoid carcinoma (Figure 29-29).

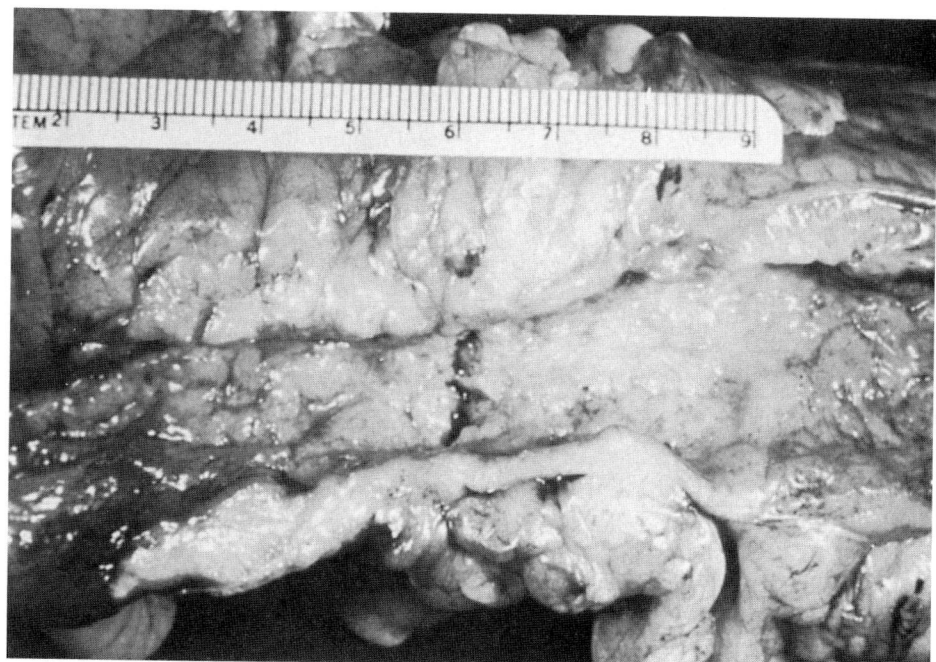

FIGURE 29-28. Carcinoma of the sigmoid in ulcerative colitis. Note the characteristic infiltration of the bowel wall, with an appearance resembling that of the linitis plastica type of carcinoma seen in the stomach. (From Corman ML, Veidenheimer MC, Nugent FW, et al. *Diseases of the anus, rectum and colon. Part II: nonspecific inflammatory bowel disease.* New York: Medcom, 1976.)

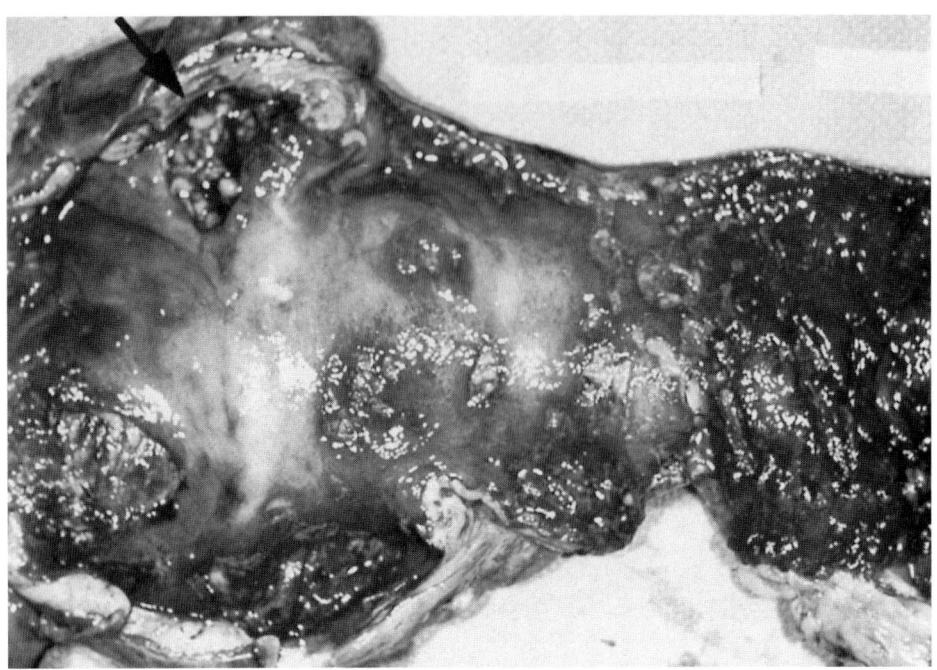

FIGURE 29-29. Ulcerative colitis with ulcerating carcinoma *(arrow)* in the hepatic flexure. (From Corman ML, Veidenheimer MC, Nugent FW, et al. *Diseases of the anus, rectum and colon. Part II: nonspecific inflammatory bowel disease.* New York: Medcom, 1976.)

Another pathologic feature of carcinoma arising in ulcerative colitis is the tendency of the lesion to be highly aggressive and poorly differentiated. More than half of young patients with ulcerative colitis and colorectal cancers have colloid carcinomas with histologically apparent mucus-secreting tumors of the signet-ring cell type[665] (Figure 29-30; see also Figure 22-21). The fact that there may be few or no symptoms tends to lull both patient and physician into a false sense of security. Witness the situation illustrated in Figure 29-17, in which the mucosa has been completely denuded. When no mucosa is present, bleeding does not occur and mucous discharge is no longer evident. This may cause the physician and the patient to believe the medical measures that have been implemented are effectively controlling the disease. It is in just this kind of situation, a patient with long-standing ulcerative colitis, that a carcinoma can supervene. As suggested, physical examination, barium enema, and even en-

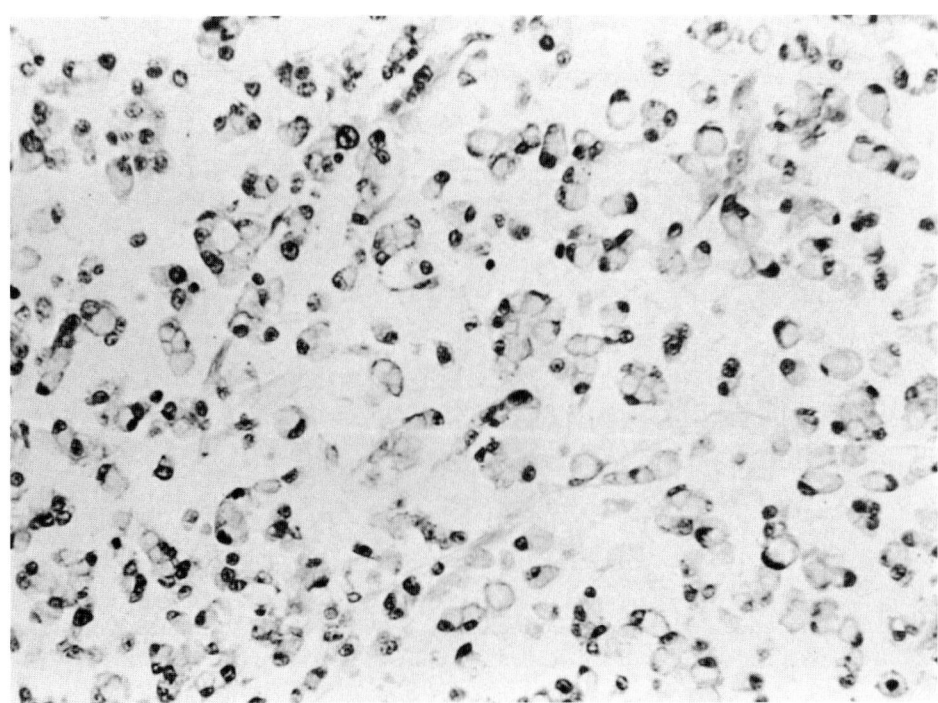

FIGURE 29-30. Signet-ring cell carcinoma in a patient with ulcerative colitis. (Original magnification × 600.)

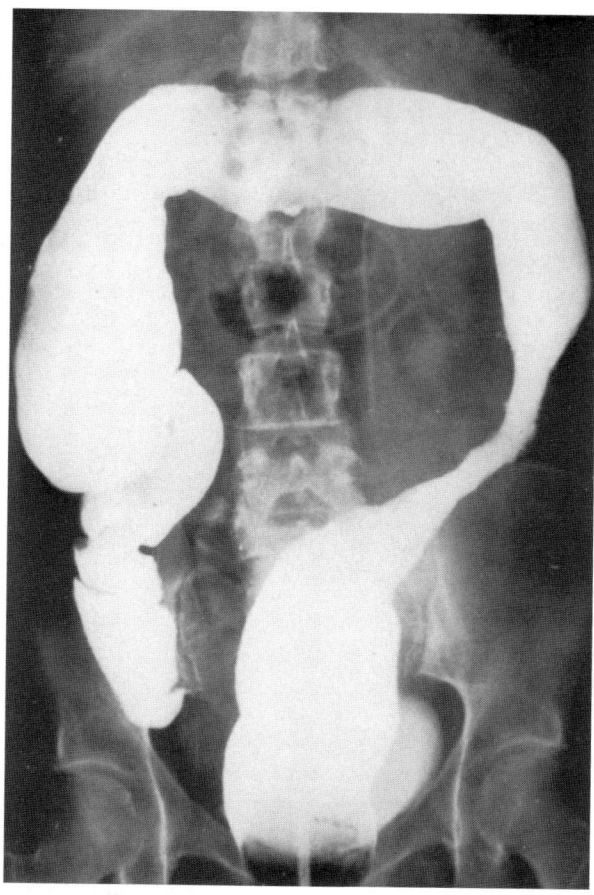

FIGURE 29-31. Stricture in ulcerative colitis. Foreshortening of the lower descending and sigmoid colon with stricture. Laparotomy revealed extensive carcinoma, hepatic metastases, and two additional unsuspected primary cancers in the resected specimen. (From Corman ML, Veidenheimer MC, Nugent FW, et al. *Diseases of the anus, rectum and colon. Part II: nonspecific inflammatory bowel disease.* New York: Medcom, 1976.)

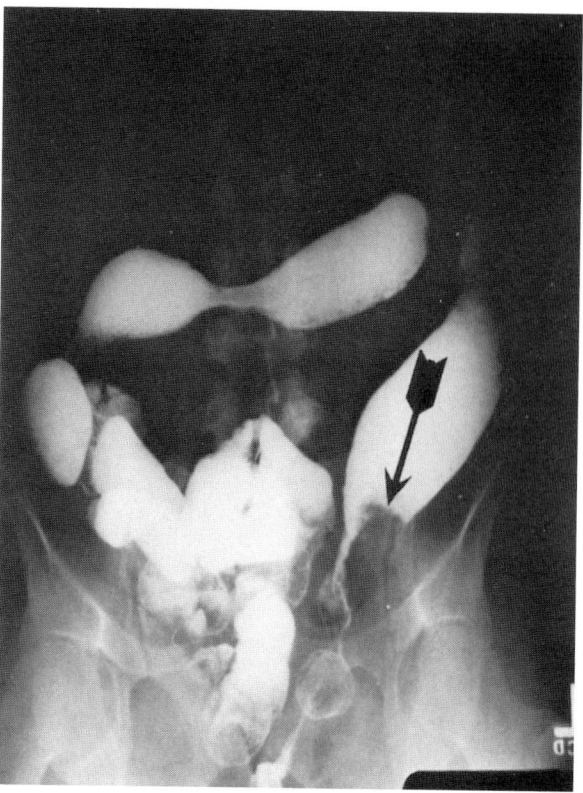

FIGURE 29-32. Carcinoma in ulcerative colitis. Note the loss of haustrations, marked shortening, and sigmoid stricture. The tumor extends cephalad from the stricture to appear as a polypoid filling defect *(arrow)*.

doscopic evaluation may fail to identify the lesion. But when stricture occurs, the patient must be presumed to have a carcinoma until it can be proved otherwise (Figs. 29-31 through 29-33). The presence of a stricture in a patient with ulcerative colitis is an indication for operative intervention. Lashner and colleagues demonstrated that of 15 patients with strictures, 11 had dysplasia and 2 were found to have cancer on colonoscopy/biopsy.[382] An additional 4 patients were found to have carcinomas at the stricture site at the time of colectomy.

Results of Surgery for Cancer Complicating Ulcerative Colitis

Ritchie and colleagues reviewed the St. Mark's Hospital (Harrow, United Kingdom) experience of carcinoma complicating ulcerative colitis between the years 1947 and 1980; 67 patients with carcinoma were identified.[603] In comparison with those who underwent surgery for carci-

noma of the colon and rectum in the same time period, it was felt that the colitic group had a higher proportion of inoperable and high-grade tumors, but the prognosis was found to be very similar in patients with and without colitis for the same stage of lesion. In the Mayo Clinic series, 40% of patients with carcinoma in chronic ulcerative colitis had a Dukes' A or B growth, in comparison with a 63% incidence if carcinoma arose in the absence of the disease.[724] Conversely, 60% with carcinoma and ulcerative colitis had Dukes' C and D lesions, in comparison with 37% who had carcinoma alone. The mean age of their patients at the onset of the colitis was 26 years, with a duration of disease of 17 years before the development of malignancy; 23% exhibited multicentric tumors. Those whose carcinoma was identified incidentally during prophylactic colectomy had a 5-year survival of 72%, whereas those with clinical or radiographic evidence suggestive of cancer had a much poorer survival rate (35%).

The advanced nature of the cancerous change is attested to by the report of Johnson and colleagues.[319] Only 57% of their patients underwent curative resection, and the overall survival rate in this group was 61%. In Öhman's experience, two thirds of those operated on for cure survived 5 years, a percentage virtually identical to the 69% of noncolitic patients.[537] All with Dukes' A

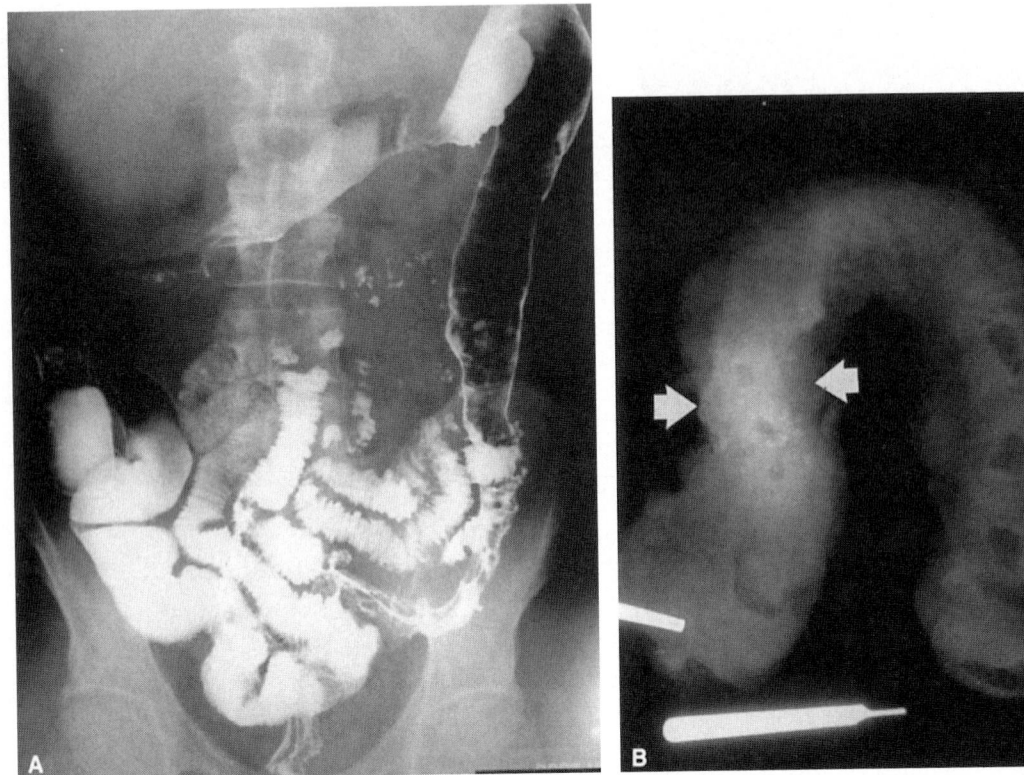

FIGURE 29-33. Carcinoma in ulcerative colitis involving the entire colon. **(A)** Barium enema study shows a long stricture in the proximal transverse colon, which proved to be malignant. The short stricture in the distal transverse colon was benign. Note also the dilated terminal ileum, a characteristic of backwash ileitis. **(B)** On x-ray film, resected specimen shows calcification *(arrows)* in the wall at the site of the stricture. This is seen with signet-ring malignant tumors and mucinous adenocarcinomas and is believed to be caused by inspissated mucin.

lesions survived 5 years. Lavery and colleagues reviewed the Cleveland Clinic experience with 79 patients found to have carcinoma arising in ulcerative colitis.[385] In comparing their survival statistics with those of patients with noncolitic cancer, they too noted no statistically significant difference in survival rates for the same stage of invasion. The poorer results were a consequence of the fact that a higher percentage of patients presented with more advanced or incurable disease at the time of surgery. All reports confirm that the prognosis for colitis-associated colorectal cancers, as for noncolitic cancers, is directly related to the degree of invasion (i.e., Dukes' stage).[101,682]

Dysplasia

In 1967, Morson and Pang described a phenomenon they called dysplasia, a frequent and widespread histologic change in patients with carcinoma complicating ulcerative colitis.[495] They suggested that biopsy of the rectum could detect this premalignant situation and possibly dictate the requirement for surgical intervention.

This appeared to be a singular advance in the management of patients with long-standing disease. Before the introduction of the concept of dysplasia, "prophylactic" proctocolectomy was advocated to protect patients from the development of malignancy. This was justified on the basis that although the patient might be asymptomatic, the cancer could be far advanced when discovered. Many individuals with few or no complaints related to the gastrointestinal tract were submitted to surgery because of this understandable concern. With the promulgation of this concept, one ideally can seek to identify those patients who on biopsy and histologic examination are found to harbor this dysplastic phenomenon.

Definition and Interpretation

Dysplasia may be interpreted to be mild, moderate, or severe, but the significance of these distinctions has become less important. Clearly, however, the correct interpretation of the biopsy results rests on the talent and experience of the pathologist. It is imperative, therefore,

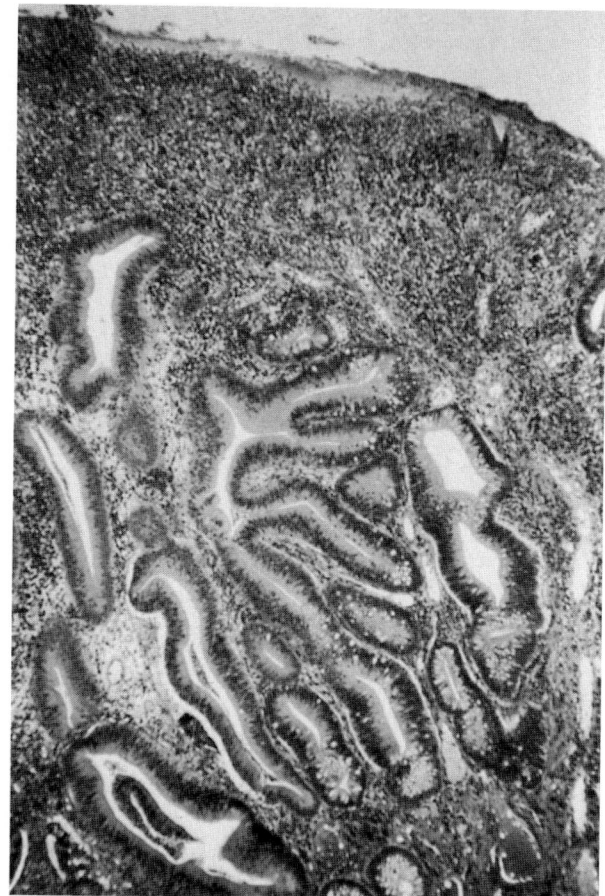

FIGURE 29-34. Moderate dysplasia in a patient with ulcerative colitis. Note the loss of polarity and decreased mucus production. (Original magnification × 80; courtesy of Rudolf Garret, M.D.)

to have available someone who is not only competent but also interested in this particular aspect of colon pathology.

The criteria for diagnosing dysplasia are problematic and vary from institution to institution. Dysplasia includes adenomatous and villous changes in the mucosa, irregular budding tubules beneath the muscularis mucosae, and cellular alterations consisting of a reduced number of goblet cells and the presence of hyperchromatic nuclei, stratified nucleoli, and coarse chromatin[351,613] (Figs. 29-34 through 29-36). The following criteria have been proposed by Nugent and colleagues:[524]

Mild dysplasia

- Preservation of crypt architecture
- Nuclear stratification, but not reaching the luminal surface
- Nuclear crowding and hyperchromasia
- Mitoses in upper portion of crypt
- Usually, moderate diminution of goblet cell mucin

Moderate dysplasia

- Distortion of crypt architecture with branching and lateral buds
- Nuclear abnormalities as in mild dysplasia, but stratification reaching luminal surface
- Usually, depletion of goblet cell mucin

Marked dysplasia

- More marked distortion of crypt architecture, frequently with villous configuration of surface epithelium
- Nuclear abnormalities as in moderate dysplasia, but with loss of polarity frequently present
- Frequently, presence of "back-to-back" glands

The last category includes all abnormalities short of invasive carcinoma and encompasses what some might designate as carcinoma-*in-situ*.

Results of Evaluation for Dysplasia

Nugent and colleagues reviewed the clinical and histologic data in a retrospective fashion of 23 patients with known colon carcinoma and chronic ulcerative colitis.[524] All but one were found to have dysplasia at a remote site from the cancer. On the basis of this experience, the authors enrolled 151 patients with more than 7 years of ulcerative colitis in an annual colonoscopy/biopsy surveillance program.[523] The number of specimens taken ranged from three to ten. Initial biopsies were positive for high-grade dysplasia in four patients, three of whom were found to harbor a carcinoma at the time of colectomy. Of 12 with low-grade dysplasia or high-grade dysplasia on initial biopsy, 11 had undergone colectomy; five cancers were found. Of ten patients in whom dysplasia developed on follow-up, nine underwent colectomy, and only one cancer was found. Carcinoma did not develop in any patient with left-sided disease. A later experience from the same group revealed that carcinoma subsequently developed in none of the 148 patients whose biopsy findings remained negative for dysplasia throughout the study.[525] In a still later review from the same institution, carcinoma associated with ulcerative colitis developed in 41 patients, 19 of whom were under colonoscopic surveillance and 22 of whom were not.[89] It seems then that carcinoma was detected at a significantly earlier Dukes' stage in the surveillance group. The 5-year survival rate was 77.2% for those surveyed, but only 36.3% for the no-surveillance group. The authors concluded that colonoscopic surveillance reduces colorectal carcinoma-related mortality by permitting the detection of carcinoma at an earlier Dukes' stage.[89]

Dickinson and colleagues surveyed 43 patients with long-standing ulcerative colitis extending proximal to the splenic flexure.[132] Dysplasia was found in nine patients in

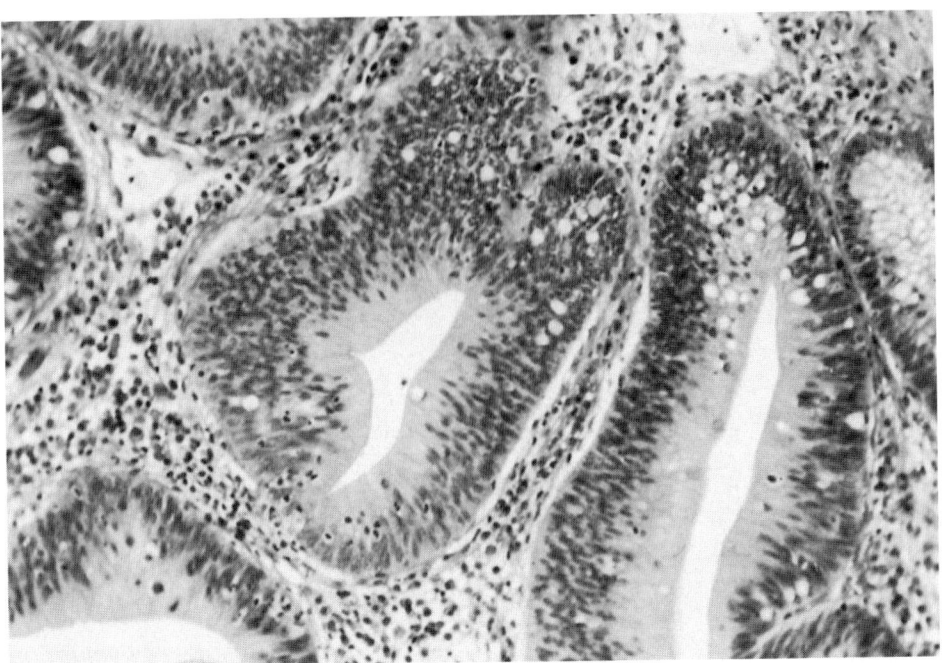

FIGURE 29-35. Moderate dysplasia in ulcerative colitis. Loss of polarity and proliferation of epithelial cells. (Original magnification × 260; courtesy of Rudolf Garret, M.D.)

one or more biopsy specimens (severe in two, moderate in one, and mild in six). The two patients with severe dysplasia were subsequently found to harbor carcinomas.

Blackstone and colleagues performed colonoscopy on 112 patients with long-standing ulcerative colitis during a 4-year period.[55] In 12 patients, the procedure revealed a polypoid mass that on biopsy exhibited dysplasia. Seven of these patients were subsequently found to have dyspla-

sia in the absence of a polypoid excrescence (i.e., a flat mucosa), and only one carcinoma was found later. The authors thought the identification of a single polypoid mass to be highly significant for the presence of concurrent invasive cancer. As such, this was strong evidence to support the need for colectomy.

Löfberg and colleagues studied 72 patients with total ulcerative colitis in a 15-year surveillance program.[422]

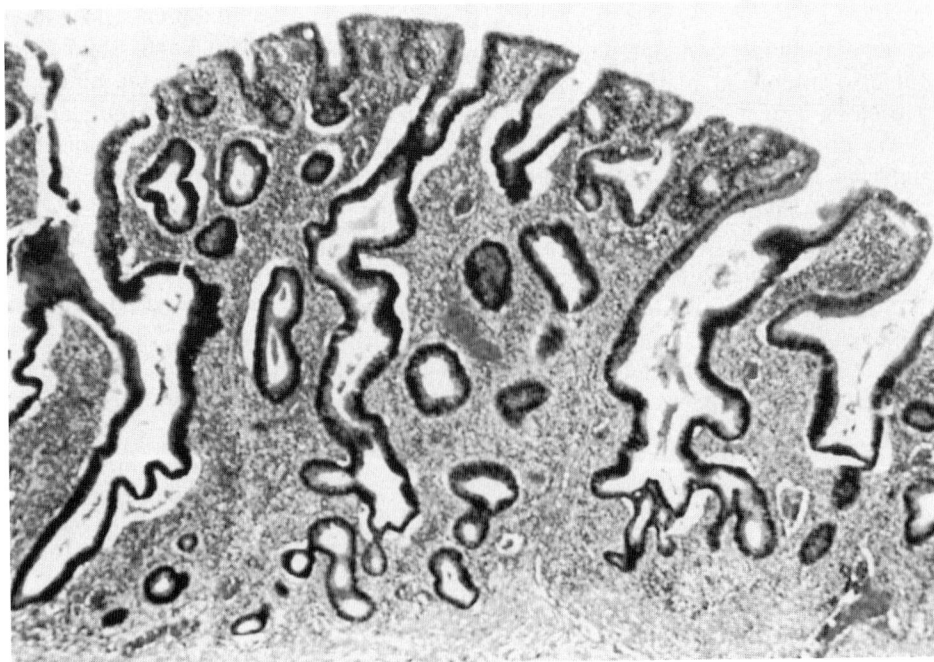

FIGURE 29-36. Severe dysplasia. Atypical hyperplasia with irregularly shaped crypts lined by crowded cells with hyperchromatic nuclei. (Original magnification × 80; from Corman ML, Veidenheimer MC, Nugent FW, et al. *Diseases of the anus, rectum and colon. Part II: nonspecific inflammatory bowel disease.* New York: Medcom, 1976.)

The cumulative risk for the development of at least low-grade dysplasia was found to be 14% after 25 years of disease. Others also recommend the use of surveillance colonoscopy in following patients with high-risk ulcerative colitis.[69,391,441,607,755] Furthermore, Lindberg and associates demonstrated in their 20-year surveillance program of 143 patients with ulcerative colitis that primary sclerosing cholangitis (see Chapter 30) is an independent risk factor for the development of dysplasia or cancer, especially in the proximal colon.[414]

Dysplasia Surveillance Limitations and Concerns

Although the increased risk for the development of colorectal cancer in individuals with long-standing ulcerative colitis is well-known and accepted, in recent years in particular there has been increased concern about the utility of surveillance colonoscopy.[115] For example, Jonsson and colleagues undertook a prospective study of 131 patients with ulcerative colitis and concluded that the surveillance program was resource-consuming, questioning the cost-to-benefit ratio.[324] Of greater concern, however, is the validity of the concept. Taylor and co-workers, reporting from the Mayo Clinic, evaluated the reliability of this premise by means of multiple random biopsies on resected specimens of patients with chronic ulcerative colitis, with and without cancer.[696] Using a standard technique of multiple random biopsies (see later discussion), they used ordinary colonoscopic biopsy forceps to obtain four biopsy specimens from mucosa that was not macroscopically suggestive of dysplasia or cancer in eight defined regions of each of 100 colon specimens obtained. Although an overall association between the presence of cancer and high-grade dysplasia was detected, the sensitivity and specificity to detect concomitant carcinoma were both 0.74. Their findings prompt concern that reliance on random biopsies obtained during colonoscopic surveillance may be inappropriate.[696]

Gorfine and associates reviewed 590 specimens for the presence of dysplasia and found that 77 (13.1%) contained at least one focus.[221] Cancers were significantly more common in those specimens with dysplastic changes than in those without such changes (33/77 versus 5/513; *p* < .001). Colonoscopically diagnosed dysplasia as a marker for synchronous cancer had a sensitivity of 81% and a specificity of 79%. The authors concluded that the concept of dysplasia is an unreliable marker for the detection of synchronous carcinoma, but when *any degree is discovered* colectomy is indicated.

Bernstein and co-workers summarized ten prospective studies to ascertain whether colonoscopic surveillance is the appropriate alternative to prophylactic colectomy.[51] First of all, the risk for progression to dysplasia was found to be only 2.4% for individuals whose initial evaluation was negative. Therefore, surveillance might perhaps be less frequently applied for those patients. Of a greater concern, however, is the fact that 32% of the patients with high-grade dysplasia were found to have invasive cancer. For this group, at least, the surveillance program failed to prevent the development of malignancy. However, when an unsuspected cancer is found at the time of surgery performed for dysplasia, it tends to be at a lower Dukes' stage than the cancer in patients in whom the diagnosis is made prior to surgery. In order for reasoned decisions to be made, therefore, it has been advised that patients be informed about the limitations of colonoscopic surveillance so that they can rationally take part in their management.[51] Unfortunately, a highly malignant carcinoma was reported to have developed in a patient without prior dysplasia or DNA aneuploidy who was enrolled in a colonoscopic surveillance program.[427]

An opposing viewpoint concerning the value of surveillance for dysplasia has been expressed by Collins and colleagues.[99] It is their contention that no compelling evidence proves that such follow-up evaluation is beneficial. Others have also expressed reservations.[380,396–398,580,597] This is especially true with respect to the significance of low-grade dysplasia. In the experience of Befrits and co-workers (Stockholm, Sweden) no progression to high-grade dysplasia was observed during 10 years of follow-up in 60 patients, leading to the conclusion that colectomy in cases with single or even repeated low-grade dysplasia is not justified.[42] Others opine that clinicians have to take not one but two giant leaps of faith to reject the null hypothesis and recommend surgery for low-grade dysplasia.[413] But today, most gastroenterologists are of the opinion that, because dysplasia implies concomitant neoplasia, individuals with even low-grade dysplasia should be counseled to undergo colectomy.[721]

The cost-effectiveness of surveillance colonoscopy has become a hotly debated issue, and as of this writing, accord with respect to the appropriate frequency of such examinations is still an unattained ideal (see the following section).[184,241] There is no controversy, however, with respect to those individuals who harbor a dysplasia-associated lesion or mass (DALM). These patients require colectomy.[42,413]

Surveillance Program

In a surveillance program, evaluation is advised for those who have had a minimum of 7 years of total or subtotal colonic disease. These persons are then submitted to total colonoscopy with biopsy of any demonstrable lesion. As suggested, the biopsy of a specific, elevated lesion will yield a much higher incidence of dysplasia. Multiple random biopsy samples should be taken throughout the colon. Although traditionally 10 such biopsies have been advised, in recent years some have suggested sampling 30 to 40 specimens. The examination should be performed every other year, or more often if dysplasia is identified. Whether one wishes to wait a year and repeat the study once dysplasia, irrespective of degree, has been identified is a subject of controversy (see earlier). It must be remembered, however, that colonoscopy in ulcerative colitis is not necessarily a benign procedure, and performing multiple biopsies may invite complications (Figure 29-37). Therefore, an experienced endoscopist should be selected to examine these patients. Preferably, biopsy specimens should be obtained in areas free from obvious inflammation.[523]

Comment

It is certainly true that cost-benefit analysis has not been determined, that incurable cancer may still supervene, that patient compliance is problematic, and that willingness of patients to commit themselves to a re-

section if the biopsy reveals dysplasia is doubtful. However, the alternative course is even less agreeable. Barium enema examination is useful only to demonstrate the macroscopic anatomy of the colon: loss of haustrations, shortening, and possible stricture. It is unlikely that this study will reveal a carcinoma earlier than will endoscopic examination with biopsy. Prophylactic colectomy after 8 to 10 years is one option; denial is another. However, until a better alternative is available, I shall continue to recommend the protocol as outlined, with the performance of flexible sigmoidoscopy in alternate years.

Aneuploidy

Another method for identifying precancerous changes is flow cytometry. Several studies have demonstrated that DNA aneuploidy correlates with the presence of dysplasia and, therefore, a high risk for developing cancer.[292,415,423,470,612,688] Suzuki and colleagues showed that 77% of dysplastic tissue demonstrated aneuploidy or polyploidy, whereas 94% of specimens of nondysplastic tissue exhibited diploidy.[688] Löfberg and colleagues found that 20% of 59 patients with long-standing total ulcerative colitis harbored an aneuploid DNA pattern on colonoscopy/biopsy, and that this correlated with the presence of dysplasia.[422] The frequency of aneuploidy is higher in patients with disease longer than 10 years and with a greater extent of involvement.[292]

As mentioned, one of the problems with the concept of dysplasia alone is interobserver and intraobserver variability.[423] Sampling error as well as total reliance on histologic information has its own inherent limitations. In the experience of Rubin and co-workers, a significant correlation between aneuploidy and severity of histologic abnormality was found in patients at high risk for cancer (negative, indefinite, dysplasia, or cancer).[612] In a prospective study from their institution of 25 high-risk individuals without dysplasia, 20% were found to have aneuploidy, and all of these patients progressed to dysplasia within 2.5 years. Conversely, all 19 individuals who failed to demonstrate aneuploidy did not progress to either aneuploidy or dysplasia within the limits of the study (up to 9 years). The authors concluded that patients who demonstrate aneuploidy should be submitted to more extensive and frequent colonoscopic surveillance, whereas those who do not require less frequent investigations.[612] Löfberg and colleagues confirmed that nuclear DNA content appears to be an earlier phenomenon than dysplasia in the malignant transformation of the colorectal mucosa, and that the use of flow cytometry in surveillance programs might be of particular value for selecting individuals at an increased risk for the development of cancer.[423]

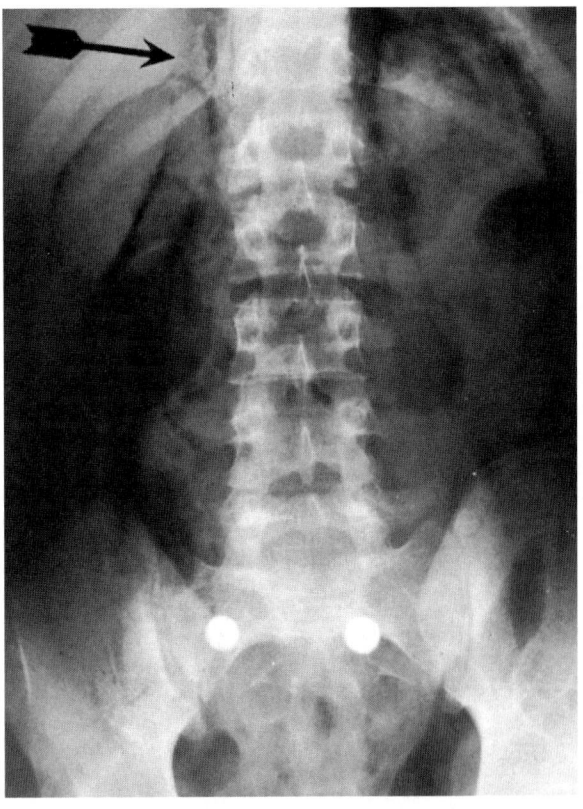

FIGURE 29-37. Retroperitoneal gas from a colon perforated during colonoscopic biopsy for dysplasia in a 19-year-old patient with ulcerative colitis. The renal outlines are clearly evident, as is the right adrenal gland *(arrow)*.

In summary, flow cytometry may be usefully applied to complement histologic examination when dysplasia is suspected.[404,470] However, there is no evidence to support the use of DNA aneuploidy as the sole indication for prophylactic cancer surgery in patients with ulcerative colitis.[415]

Treatment of Carcinoma

If a carcinoma is identified in the rectum of a patient with ulcerative colitis, proctocolectomy is the treatment of choice. No attempt should be made to preserve the rectal mucosa. Alternative operations may, however, include the continent ileostomy (Kock) and the ileoanal anastomosis with intervening pouch, provided that sphincter preservation does not compromise adequate tumor margins, and the risk for the requirement of postoperative radiation therapy is remote (see Surgical Management).

MEDICAL MANAGEMENT

I have asked a respected colleague, Seymour Katz, clinical professor of medicine at New York University School of Medicine and attending gastroenterologist, North Shore University Hospital-Long Island Jewish Medical Center to help me update this section. A prolific author and reviewer for numerous gastrointestinal journals, Dr. Katz is well-recognized as an authority on the medical management of IBD. (*MLC*)

The bewildering array of medications in the therapy of IBD often confounds the clinician in the choice of specific agents with respect to the balance between safety and efficacy. So many new and exciting drugs are now available that this can present a dilemma for the clinician in the choice of the most appropriate therapy. Moreover, the enthusiasm engendered by the availability of multiple therapies must be tempered by the practicalities of access and cost. Many drug programs are in clinical trials and are not available to the practitioner. Several agents may not be offered by managed care plans, even if approved by the United States Food and Drug Administration, or are too expensive for some patients, even with partial support by their insurance coverage.

In the year 2000, the American College of Gastroenterology established guidelines for the classification of ulcerative colitis based on severity of disease. It is as follows:

Mild

- Fewer than four stools daily with or without blood
- No systemic signs of toxicity
- Normal erythrocyte sedimentation rate

Moderate

- Greater than four stools daily
- Minimal toxicity

Severe

- Greater than six bloody stools daily
- Signs of toxicity, as shown by fever, tachycardia, anemia, or elevated erythrocyte sedimentation rate

The following approaches to medical therapy are presented in accordance with the severity of disease: mild to moderate, moderate to severe, and severe disease.

Mild to Moderate Disease

The activity of disease is usually assessed by clinical criteria as classically outlined by Truelove and Witts, with a modification for moderate disease.[711] Endoscopic activity may be evaluated concomitantly, but less reliance is placed on achieving a goal of complete healing and even less on the dependency of a histologic "cure".[354,599] Patients in this category average fewer than four loose bowel movements daily, which may contain blood, but lack systemic symptoms or an elevated erythrocyte sedimentation rate.

Aminosalicylates

The mainstays of therapy for mild to moderate ulcerative colitis have been the aminosalicylates. Sulfasalazine (Azulfidine, Salazopyrin) has for many years been the standard drug for preventing exacerbations of ulcerative colitis. Initially, it was thought that breakdown by bacteria in the bowel produced sulfapyridine, an antibiotic, and this was the basis for the therapeutic effect. It is now known, however, that there are multiple pharmacologically active roles (e.g., inhibition of prostaglandin synthesis, inhibition of proteolytic enzymes, and immunosuppression).

The oral dosage for sulfasalazine is usually begun at 2 g/day, up to a maximum of 4 g/day. Increasing the dosage further may lead to unpleasant side effects from the sulfapyridine moiety—skin rash, bone marrow depression, nausea, headache, and malaise; these may occur even at low doses (see Table 29-3). Folic acid deficiency may develop and go unrecognized. Therefore, daily supplements are recommended. Other side effects of greater consequence include hemolysis in patients with glucose-6-phosphate dehydrogenase deficiency, exfoliative skin disorders, and temporary infertility in men. Fertility problems, however, may be caused by other factors than drug effects.[75]

It has been shown that 5-aminosalicylic acid (5-ASA) is the most important active ingredient of sulfasalazine, at least with respect to its therapeutic effect if not its preventive role. The generic name for 5-ASA is mesalamine in the United States and mesalazine in the United Kingdom and Europe. Oral 5-ASA [olsalazine sodium (Dipentum); mesalamine (Pentasa, Asacol, Claversal, Salofalk)] requires the addition of an azo-bond or an acrylic resin coating to prevent absorption in the small intestine. Studies have shown that the drug is well tolerated and is effective for treating mild to moderately active ulcerative colitis and for maintaining remission.[242,305,642] The delivery depends either on the azoreductase capability of the colonic microflora or the time-release properties of the encapsulation. The most troublesome consequences appear to be nausea and diarrhea. Habal and Greenberg analyzed the rate of remission and incidence of side effects in patients treated for active ulcerative colitis in whom adverse reactions from sulfasalazine were sufficiently severe to warrant discontinuation of the drug.[242] Only those with mild or moderate disease responded to 5-ASA (64%). Of the 50 who were followed for 1 year, 78% remained in remission.

Balsalazide (BSA) is a dimer of 5-ASA in an azo-bond with an inert carrier. It has been claimed to achieve a greater remission rate—62% versus 37% with mesalamine—with a shorter median time to relief, a higher percentage of symptom-free days, and less treatment failure with fewer adverse events.[228,575] However, these results should be viewed with caution. In another trial there was no statistically significant difference when compared with a placebo with regard to stool frequency, blood in the stool, or sigmoidoscopy scores.[156,251] BSA is a large pill, which raises compliance concerns.[429] Moreover, it may interfere with metabolism of 6-mercaptopurine (6-MP), thus leading to the risk of toxic levels.[429] In general, no superiority of any one delivery system of 5-ASA has been demonstrated.

Induction of remission is best approached with aminosalicylates. In a meta-analysis of 19 studies, 5-ASA was superior to placebo but was not significantly more efficacious than sulfasalazine. There was no greater benefit for mesalamine. There is considerable cost savings when sulfasalazine is used, but not everyone can tolerate this drug.[686,687] Despite its proven value for maintaining remission, some believe that "on-demand" treatment may be as effective as continuous use for this purpose.[133]

The idiosyncratic and dose-dependent side effects of sulfasalazine are listed in Table 29-2. Of particular note is that sulfasalazine's deleterious effect on sperm motility and morphologic features, previously unrecognized, has led to medical-legal concerns with respect to fertility problems in these individuals.

The mesalamine experience in human pregnancy has been very promising. In a prospective controlled study of 165 patients, there was no significant difference in the maternal obstetric history of birth defects, miscarriage, pregnancy termination, ectopic pregnancy, fetal distress, or delivery problems. Therefore, aminosalicylates are not considered a major teratogenic risk when used at the recommended dosage.[131]

▶ **TABLE 29-2** **Adverse Effects of Sulfasalazine and 5-Aminosalicylate**

Sulfasalazine	Mesalamine
Dose-Dependent	
Nausea, anorexia, dyspepsia, alopecia, headaches, folate malabsorption, reversible sperm abnormalities	Headache, dyspepsia, diarrhea (olsalazine)
Idiosyncratic	
Hypersensitivity reaction (rash, lupus-like), hemolytic anemia (Heinz bodies), bone marrow suppression, hepatitis pancreatitis, pneumonitis, eosinophilia, fibrosing alveolitis, colitis	Hypersensitivity colitis, nephrotoxicity, myocarditis, pericarditis, pneumonitis, hepatitis, pancreatitis

The following summarizes the recommendations of the American College of Gastroenterology for managing mildly to moderately extensive ulcerative colitis:

Active disease

- Oral mesalamine, 2.0 to 4.8 g/day (first line)
- Oral olsalazine, 2 to 3 g/day (first line)
- Oral sulfasalazine, 4 to 6 g/day (first line)
- Oral prednisone, 40 to 60 mg/day, if refractory to above therapy
- 6-MP, or azathioprine, 1.5 to 2.5 mg/kg/day, if not responsive to oral prednisone and intravenous therapy not required
- Transdermal nicotine patch, 15 to 25 mg/day

Maintenance of remission

- Oral mesalamine
- Oral sulfasalazine, 2 to 4 g/day
- Oral olsalazine
- Oral balsalazide
- Chronic treatment with oral corticosteroids not recommended
- 6-MP or azathioprine recommended as corticosteroid-sparing agents or for corticosteroid- or 5-ASA-refractory patients

Management of Distal Disease

Treatment of nonspecific ulcerative proctitis and proctosigmoiditis can be problematic for a number of reasons: the uncertainty of the diagnosis, the empiric nature of the treatment, the difficulty in correlating the response to therapy (especially when spontaneous resolution is not uncommon), the variability of the duration of treatment, and the differences of opinion with respect to the relative merits of the diverse approaches.[151] Proximal extension occurs in approximately 10% of patients, almost always within 1 or at most 2 years of onset. However, in one group (between 15% and 30%), the course is characterized by multiple recurrences but without proximal extension.[151]

Campieri and colleagues were the first to employ 5-ASA as a retention enema, initially with patients who could not tolerate sulfasalazine.[80] They noted an 80% response rate. Since then, others have confirmed the effectiveness of this treatment for distal bowel disease.[52,53,117,684] Four grams of 5-ASA in a 100-mL retention enema has been demonstrably effective for colitis of the left side.[81] However, Guarino and colleagues noted that relapse is common as the frequency of enema administration is decreased.[236] Others have found that intermittent therapy with mesalazine enemas is more effective than continuous oral mesalazine for maintaining remission in patients with distal ulcerative colitis and proctitis.[442] Mesalamine (Rowasa, Pentasa, Claversal, Salofalk) has been recommended and approved as a rectal suspension enema containing 4 g in 60 mL. Rectal 5-ASA should not be tapered too soon or too quickly. Administration at 3-day intervals can be tolerated if need be, but daily dosage generally is more effective, although less convenient.

An isomer of 5-ASA, 4-ASA (para-aminosalicylic acid), has also been suggested as a retention enema for the treatment of distal colitis because of its stability in aqueous solution, its safety, and its low frequency of side effects.[194] Gandolfo and colleagues, in a controlled trial comparing this agent with a placebo, concluded that 4-ASA enemas in a dosage of 1 g twice daily were significantly more effective in the management of this condition.[194] Nagy and co-workers found that the response was favorable and comparable to that of sulfasalazine enemas.[504] Ginsberg and colleagues employed a placebo-controlled trial with oral 4-ASA in 40 patients with active ulcerative colitis for a period of 12 weeks.[204] Fifty-five percent of those who received 4-ASA showed improvement, in comparison with only 5% receiving the placebo.

Another application of 5-ASA is in suppository form. Campieri and colleagues treated 156 patients with mild or moderate disease by varying protocols.[79] This included a small number who used 400-mg suppositories of 5-ASA twice daily for up to 1 year. The remission rate was essentially the same as that observed in individuals treated with sulfasalazine. Others have confirmed the safety and relative efficacy.[118]

The rectal application of cortisone and hydrocortisone has been found to be beneficial in the management of patients with acute active distal disease. In a number of studies, steroids were more potent than sulfasalazine in active colitis, inducing faster clinical, endoscopic, and pathologic improvement.[248] Steroid retention enemas are often used initially and as the primary treatment for ul-

cerative proctitis. For a short time, a hydrocortisone enema is given once or twice daily. Enema kits containing 100 mg of hydrocortisone (Cortenema) or 40 mg of methylprednisolone acetate (Medrol Enpak) are convenient and effective for treating disease confined to the lower bowel. Very often, retention enemas containing cortisone administered over 2 weeks will resolve the patient's complaints. The rapidity of the clinical response and the lack of complications usually encountered with systemic steroid therapy are the primary advantages of this method of treatment. The rectal instillation of steroids is advantageous in that medication is applied directly to the involved mucosa, although it should be remembered that with persistent and frequent use, side effects of hyperadrenocorticism may ultimately develop. If this occurs, dosing should be reduced to alternate days so that within 2 or 3 weeks it can be discontinued. Some patients require longer treatment, and others have difficulty retaining the enema because of tenesmus or diarrhea. Studies have demonstrated not only the efficacy of the retention enema (reaching quite proximal areas of the colon) but also its favorable therapeutic benefit in comparison with low-dose oral steroids.[246,314]

Topical (i.e., rectal instillation) therapy plays a significant role in achieving remission and, in combination with oral therapy, is considered superior to oral or rectal treatment alone.[618] Rectal therapy produces a faster response when given with oral 5-ASA and actually has been shown to be superior to placebo or to corticosteroids topically.[251,328] A meta-analysis and overall review by a University of Chicago group confirms the superiority of mesalamine enemas over steroid enemas and the value of topical agents over oral therapies in achieving remission in left-sided disease. Similarly, for proctitis, 5-ASA had higher rates of remission than topical steroids. Mesalamine today remains the preferred drug in achieving and maintaining remission[96] (Table 29-2). Table 29-3 summarizes the position of the American College of Gastroenterology with respect to the management of distal disease.

Moderate to Severe Disease

Moderate to severe ulcerative colitis implies systemic toxicity and greater than four stools daily, often with blood and with more discomfort—that is, urgency, frequency, or cramping.

Corticosteroids

Most patients in this category require steroid therapy for induction of remission. The medication should, however, not be used for the treatment of diarrhea, but rather for patients who continue to bleed. A beginning dose of 20 mg of prednisone is suggested on a daily basis, which is then reduced by 5 mg after 1 week. Ideally, the medica-

▶ **TABLE 29-3** Recommendations for Managing Mild to Moderate Distal Ulcerative Colitis

Therapeutic Options for Achieving Remission
Oral mesalamine, 2.0–4.8 g/d
Oral olsalazine, 1.5–3.0 g/d
Oral sulfasalazine, 4–6 g/d
Topical mesalamine suppositories, 500 mg b.i.d., for patients with proctitis
Therapeutic Options for Maintaining Remission
Oral mesalamine, 1.5–4.0 g/d—can be increased up to 4.8 g/d
Oral sulfasalazine, 2–4 g/d
Mesalamine suppositories, 500 mg b.i.d., for patients with proctitis
Mesalamine enemas, 2–4 g every third night, for patients with distal colitis
Combination oral, 1.6 g/d, and topical (enema), 4 g twice weekly, mesalamine more effective than oral mesalamine alone

Reprinted with permission from Managing IBD at the Boundaries of Treatment Guidelines. Copyright © 2001, the University of Chicago.

tion is completely withdrawn in a period of 4 to 6 weeks. Higher doses of steroids may be used transiently but are not recommended for prolonged use. No benefit is seen with doses of prednisone exceeding 40 mg, and a once-daily dose is as effective as a divided dosage.[29,570] Corticotropin appears to be little used because of the inconvenience of injection, mineralocorticoid side-effects, occasional anaphylactic reaction, and the risk of adrenal infarction.[315] Every effort should be made to taper the level in a reasonable, nonprecipitous way.

To track corticosteroid dependence and resistance, 63 patients at the Mayo Clinic were given at least one course of corticosteroids and were followed.[143] Eighty-four percent achieved partial or complete remission at 30 days, and no response was seen in 16%. But at 1 year, only 49% maintained that response, 22% were steroid-dependent, and surgery was required in 29% of the initial responders. Lessons from this experience include the following: (a) only 34% of patients with ulcerative colitis ever require corticosteroids, indicating a relatively mild course of disease in this community-based study; (b) only 16% failed to respond to steroids; (c) steroid dependence and surgery were common, even among initial responders.

The need for steroids indicates a poorer prognosis and places the patient at a higher likelihood for requiring a colectomy. Note, however, that these conclusions were drawn from an experience that predated the use of immunomodulators [azathioprine (AZA), 6-mercaptopurine (6-MP), methotrexate, cyclosporine] and anti-tumor necrosis factor antibody therapy, which may be steroid-sparing or forestall the requirement for surgery (see later discussion).[143]

Budesonide is a 17-α substituted glucocorticoid with a strong receptor affinity and a 93% first-pass metabo-lism, thereby minimizing systemic side-effects. It appears to be a reasonable alternative to hydrocortisone enemas and has an efficacy comparable to that of 5-ASA.[252] An expanded experience with budesonide enemas in children demonstrates an efficacy similar to that of hydrocortisone.[150] Budesonide enema once daily was shown to have the same remission rate at 4 and 8 weeks as did twice daily instillations.[416] However, it has less efficacy and a lesser endoscopic response than does prednisone, but one has the benefit of reduced adrenal suppression. Oral budesonide is not as effective for distal disease; therefore, these patients will require topical therapy.[424] Oral budesonide's value in its present formulation is limited to Crohn's ileal and right-sided colonic disease. There is no long-term efficacy with budesonide or prednisone, and neither steroid preparation should be used for maintenance.

Another first pass metabolized steroid, *beclomethasone dipropionate* (BDP), has been shown in 177 patients to have a virtually identical clinical remission rate (63%) to that achieved by 5-ASA (62.5%).[78] Although a more favorable improvement in disease activity indices occurred in those with more extensive disease with BDP, the plasma cortisol levels were significantly reduced in the BDP group. This was not, however, a placebo-controlled trial.

One of the important aspects of education is to have the patient recognize that the condition may be relatively chronic and subject to exacerbations and remissions. In some individuals, bleeding persists for many months or even years. A common error is to augment the dose of prednisone or hydrocortisone in an attempt to eliminate every symptom. This inevitably eventuates in the varied, familiar, and potentially severe consequences of hyperadrenocorticism.

The toxic effects of corticosteroids are related to the dose and the duration of treatment. Complications of steroid management include the masking of an acute abdominal problem, such as intestinal perforation; osteonecrosis; metabolic bone disease; and growth retardation in children.[250] Corticosteroids can and have been used successfully during pregnancy without adverse side effects to the developing fetus.

Other Agents

Immunomodulators

Immunomodulatory drugs are now generally accepted as appropriate for long-term management in certain patients with IBD.[250,421] The rationale for their use is based on the observations concerning the implication of immune mechanisms in the pathogenesis of the disease.[446] The use of immunomodulators in ulcerative colitis is not well defined, without an established dose-response experience or documentation convincing the clinician to push for leukopenia. It is important, however, to consider their use early in therapy. There is no role, however, for their application in the acute setting, because studies of patients with Crohn's disease demonstrate that a mean response time of 3 months is necessary for efficacy.[571] One study reveals an earlier onset of action (i.e., 8 weeks) when a larger oral dose is used initially.[631]

Azathioprine and Mercaptopurine   Two agents that have been demonstrated to be effective are 6-mercaptopurine (6-MP) and its analogue, azathioprine (AZA). Azathioprine is rapidly absorbed and converted to mercaptopurine in red cells. Subsequent hepatic conversion produces active metabolites that inhibit purine ribonucleotide and, therefore, DNA synthesis.[250] The mechanism of action is believed to be inhibition of lymphocyte function, primarily that of T cells.

Thiopurine methyltransferase enzyme must be operable in order for a patient to metabolize the drug. Fortunately, 89% of patients have a normal level, that is, they are homozygous for high enzymatic activity, and they, therefore, are able to tolerate higher doses of AZA/6-MP. Eleven percent of patients are heterozygous—that is, they have intermediate enzymatic activity, and they require a lower dose of AZA/6-MP to achieve a therapeutic level to avoid leukopenia. It has been found that 0.3% of patients have no enzymatic activity and are at risk for life-threatening toxic reactions. Testing for thiopurine methyltransferase enzyme has been advised before embarking on an escalated drug schedule.

The largest experience with the use of these agents comes from the Lenox Hill Hospital and the Mount Sinai School of Medicine in New York City. During 18 years of observation from this unit, a total of 81 patients with resistant ulcerative colitis were treated with 6-MP.[2] All had failed therapy with sulfasalazine and steroids. The mean treatment period was 1.8 years, and the overall response rate was 61%. A low incidence of toxicity was encountered.[572]

One of the concerns with both of these agents is the development of pancreatitis, a complication that has been reported in up to 15% of patients. In addition, both cause bone marrow suppression, particularly neutropenia. Because this is dose-related and is essentially an ongoing concern, monitoring of blood counts should be performed at least four times a year.[250] Although in the past there has been concern about the carcinogenic and teratogenic potential of these agents, especially the development of lymphoma, controlled trials have failed to support this anxiety.

Gormet and colleagues studied the efficacy of AZA as a steroid-sparing and maintenance drug in ulcerative colitis in 131 patients.[224] Remission rates in those off steroids was 66% at 1 year and 41% at 3 years. This response fell to 23% if AZA was interrupted during remission. Colectomy rates were 57% at 3 years and 45% at 5 years, re-

spectively. Factors predicting AZA failure were short duration of disease, steroid resistance, and chronic active disease. It can be concluded from this retrospective multicenter study that remission rates with AZA in chronic ulcerative colitis are similar to that of Crohn's disease, but relapses on treatment are more frequent, with half of the patients requiring colectomy.

Mahadevin and co-workers undertook a study in which an intravenous loading dose of AZA was given to nine hospitalized patients with steroid-refractory ulcerative colitis.[436] Five were able to avoid colectomy. All five withdrew from steroids by week 12, and three entered clinical remission. Two other patients developed AZA toxicity, and although improved, did not enter remission.

Withdrawal of steroids prematurely often leads to failure of response and often requires both the use of steroids and immunomodulators simultaneously until a clinical and perhaps an endoscopic response is achieved.

Cyclosporine   The slow onset of action of azathioprine and mercaptopurine in patients with IBD has led to trials of more potent immunosuppressive drugs, such as cyclosporine.[250] The primary indications for the use of this agent are acute, severe ulcerative colitis and refractory Crohn's disease. The primary side effect is renal dysfunction. Other complications include neurotoxicity, seizures, and opportunistic infections.

Lichtiger and Present, in a preliminary report of 15 patients, noted intravenous cyclosporine to be an effective agent in the treatment of severe active ulcerative colitis not responding to steroids.[410] Seventy-three percent improved and avoided colectomy. A later report (1994) from the same group, now with 32 patients, supported the view that intravenous cyclosporine therapy is rapidly effective for individuals with severe, corticosteroid-resistant ulcerative colitis.[411] In children, Treem and colleagues found cyclosporine to be effective in achieving clinical remission in 80% of those with refractory, fulminant ulcerative colitis.[709] However, within 1 year, most initial responders required colectomy because of flare-up of the condition. They recommend that cyclosporine therapy be applied to ameliorate symptoms rapidly and prevent precipitous colectomy, to improve nutrition, and to allow psychological adaptation while reducing the steroid dose requirement.[709] Currently, cyclosporine is reserved for the treatment of severe, refractory disease when surgery is not appropriate or before other treatments have taken effect.[250]

Anti-Tumor Necrosis Factor-Alpha (Anti-TNF-α) Agent (Infliximab)

Tumor necrosis factor-α (TNF-α) is a protein secreted by lipopolysaccharide-stimulated macrophages that causes tumor necrosis *in vivo* when injected into tumor-bearing mice. Also known as cachectin, TNF-α is believed to mediate pathogenic shock and tissue injury associated with endotoxemia. Although it has little effect on many cultured normal human cells, TNF-α appears to be directly toxic to vascular endothelial cells. Other actions of TNF-α include stimulating growth of human fibroblasts and other cell lines, activating polymorphonuclear neutrophils and osteoclasts, and induction of interleukin 1, prostaglandin E2, and collagenase production.

Infliximab represents the first of a new class of "biological" medications, a "blocking" antibody that interferes with TNF, an important perpetuating signal of Crohn's disease inflammation. Given as an intravenous infusion, infliximab is used to treat Crohn's disease in corticosteroid-dependent or intractable patients, as well as those with chronic draining fistulas (see Chapter 30). Its use in ulcerative colitis, however, has been and is being explored.

Chey and co-workers reported initially that 16 of 17 patients improved after one to two 5 mg/kg infliximab infusions, and 7 of 8 colectomy candidates avoided surgery.[86] A more detailed analysis of a dramatic, 100% response of all 8 patients in a later report by the same group with the use of intravenous infliximab, 5 mg/kg, with no relapses at 5 months, must be viewed with caution, however.[87] This was an nonblinded, uncontrolled observation in a relatively older population. Five of eight patients had their disease for less than 6 years and also received intravenous corticosteroids, thereby clouding the interpretation of which drug was truly responsible for the improvement. "No relapse" may not be a tenable conclusion when the patients were receiving 5-ASA and 6-MP and still were on a tapering steroid schedule. Nevertheless, this experience with histologic improvement warranted further study.

Some important lessons can be learned from a pilot study from the University of Pennsylvania of 27 ulcerative colitis patients treated with single (52%) or multiple (48%) infliximab infusions.[681] Twelve individuals entered remission (44%), and six patients (22%) had a partial response. The median time to response was 4 days, and the median duration of response was 8 weeks. Five patients ultimately underwent colectomy. Interestingly, 9 of the 18 responders relapsed a total of 18 times, but all of these relapses successfully responded to repeat infusion. Steroid-refractory patients were uniquely less likely to respond to infliximab. Noteworthy was one death from line sepsis and subacute bacterial endocarditis, and one patient died with *Candida* sepsis.[681] Sandborn's review of seven open-label studies revealed a response in 60 of 83 patients (72%), but added an additional adverse event of one patient with *Staphylococcus aureus* sepsis, septic arthritis, and chronic osteomyelitis.[627]

Only two controlled trials of infliximab in ulcerative colitis have been conducted. Sands and colleagues reported a response in two of three patients who were given 5 mg/kg, one of three patients given 10 mg/kg, and two of two patients given 20 mg/kg, compared with none of three patients given a placebo.[633] However, of 42 steroid-resistant ulcerative colitis patients randomized to 5 mg/kg infliximab or placebo, clinical remission occurred in 36% of those who were treated as opposed to 30% of placebo patients. Moreover, no greater benefit was found in non-responders when treated with 10 mg/kg compared with similarly treated placebo patients (30% versus 33%). No conclusion is as yet possible regarding infliximab efficacy in chronic ulcerative colitis.[573]

Severe Ulcerative Colitis

The definition of severe ulcerative colitis invariably involves more than six bloody stools daily, pain, cramping, toxicity with fever, anemia, tachycardia, and elevated erythrocyte sedimentation rate. This manifestation always requires admission to the hospital for intravenous therapy and observation for the serious complications of megacolon and perforation.

Management

Patients with acute, fulminant, "toxic" megacolon may present with very minimal symptoms or may be critically ill. High fever, tachycardia, and abdominal pain are frequently noted. However, clinical signs and symptoms may be masked by the patient's medications, especially steroids. One must keep in mind the possibility of perforation, even in the absence of colonic dilatation. In the experience of Greenstein and colleagues, classic physical signs of peritonitis were absent in six of seven patients with free perforation.[231]

The usual supportive measures—intravenous fluid replacement, and blood, colloid, and steroid therapy—should be supplemented with broad-spectrum antibiotic coverage. The single most important guide in the management of a patient with acute toxic dilatation is the assessment obtained with plain abdominal x-ray studies. With serial abdominal films, the effectiveness of medical management can be evaluated (Figure 29-2). If the dilatation decreases, one may be reasonably assured that surgery can be deferred. Conversely, if colonic dilatation progresses or fails to improve during the period of maximum therapy, surgical intervention is advised.

Any medications that "slow" gastrointestinal activity, such as anticholinergics or opiates, are discontinued. A nasogastric tube is suggested, although some physicians prefer a long tube (e.g., Miller/Abbott) in the expectation of decompressing the colon. Placing the patient on the abdomen for a few minutes every 2 or 3 hours may help to distribute the gas, moving it into the rectum. Rectal tubes have also been advocated, but these are potentially dangerous in that they can cause a perforation of the sigmoid colon. Barium enema examination and colonoscopy are contraindicated; in fact, barium enema study has been reported to precipitate toxic megacolon. Interestingly, a case of successful decompression by means of colonoscopy has been reported in a patient who refused surgical intervention.[22]

The clinical course and ultimate outcome of toxic megacolon has been well documented by numerous investigators. A high incidence of recurrent toxic dilatation and perforation and the requirement for emergency or urgent operation have been reported.[226,276] This is in contrast to the group of patients with severe, acute colitis without dilatation, who can usually be effectively managed by nonsurgical means.[493] In the series reported by Fazio from the Cleveland Clinic, only 7 of 115 patients (6%) were successfully managed medically, and 5 of these came to colectomy in later years.[159]

For those who fail intravenous corticosteroid therapy, intravenous cyclosporine may be a reasonable approach, especially in those who refuse surgery. These usually are "first-episode" patients, those lacking a history of chronic debilitation or individuals whose comorbid conditions create a formidable surgical risk.

The cyclosporine experience has had a mixed response, with an initial 82% success rate, but falling to 59% at 6 months.[411] Review of more than 20 uncontrolled studies in 1998 demonstrated a 68% response in avoiding colectomy, but the long-term response was only 42%.[447] An international survey of practitioners (flawed perhaps in that two-thirds of responders had experience with fewer than five patients) reported "good" results in 29.5%, "acceptable" with recurrence in 58.6%, and "poor" in 14%.[480]

The University of Chicago study was most favorable, with 72% of initial responders avoiding colectomy after 5 years.[95] The important observation here was the value of concomitant 6-MP or AZA therapy. Of the patients receiving cyclosporine given these drugs, 80% avoided colectomy and maintained their initial response. Further analysis of a 5-year follow-up of 42 cyclosporine-treated patients at the University of Chicago initially receiving from 1 to 4 courses of intravenous cyclosporine revealed that 18 (43%) retained their colons after a median of 6.7 years.[91] It is interesting to note that only 1 of 8 patients receiving more than one course of cyclosporine avoided colectomy. These investigators concluded that short-term cyclosporine followed by 6-MP/AZA permits more than 50% of steroid-resistant patients to avoid colectomy. However, re-treatment with cyclosporine is rarely successful.[91]

Some reports confirm the efficacy of cyclosporine in the management of severe colitis.[304,459] Although many initial responders subsequently relapse, a substantial minority remain in long-term remission.[459] Moreover, there appears to be no increased incidence of perioperative complications associated with its use, provided the treatment is for a defined period, and needed surgery is not delayed.[304] It is, however, doubtful if cyclosporine can be considered in the realm of a truly long-term, effective therapy.[585]

The following are the Guidelines of the American College of Gastroenterology with respect to managing severe ulcerative colitis:

- Hospitalization
- Intravenous corticosteroids, 300 mg/day hydrocortisone, 48 mg/day methylprednisolone, or adrenocorticotropic hormone, for 7 to 10 days, if refractory to maximum doses of oral prednisone, 5-ASAs, and topical agents or if presenting with toxicity
- If no improvement after 7 to 10 days, administer intravenous cyclosporine, 4 mg/kg/day, or refer for surgery
- Adding 6-MP enhances long-term remission

Parenteral Nutrition

Neither an elemental diet nor total parental nutrition decreases the inflammation associated with ulcerative colitis.[250] However, evidence suggests that patients frequently are hospitalized with varying states of malnutrition. As a consequence, hyperalimentation, either parenteral or oral, has been recommended in a supportive role for patients with IBD. Specifically, elemental diets and total parenteral nutrition with bowel rest improved the symptoms, inflammatory sequelae, and nutritional status in individuals with Crohn's disease more readily than in those with ulcerative colitis (see Chapter 30). It has been demonstrated by some authors that patients who have lost more than 20% of their usual weight before undergoing abdominal surgery have higher rates of morbidity and mortality than those who have not exhibited weight loss. Conversely, in a study by Higgens and colleagues, preoperative weight loss did not adversely affect the postoperative outcome in those undergoing elective resection.[286] There is currently an extensive, often confusing literature on nutritional data, diet, and intravenous hyperalimentation.[93,196,269,323,370,401,402,593]

With IBD, the rationale for implementing intravenous hyperalimentation is that the bowel is "put to rest". If this were attempted without supplementary intravenous caloric intake, the patient's nutritional status would rapidly deteriorate. Intravenous hyperalimentation, therefore, permits the patient with IBD to be managed with bowel rest while simultaneously providing adequate amino acids and calories for anabolism.[134,263] If surgery is believed to be inevitable, however, the Veterans Administration Cooperative Study of 395 malnourished patients revealed that total parenteral nutrition should be limited to those who are severely malnourished unless there are other specific indications for this treatment.[729]

Comment (MLC)

My own attitude is to use total parenteral nutrition only in those patients for whom surgery should be avoided, or in whom the nutritional status is so poor that one may anticipate a very high rate of morbidity and mortality. The concept of short-term intravenous hyperalimentation in preparation for bowel surgery may have certain theoretical advantages, but expeditiously performed surgery should allow an earlier commencement of oral intake, a much preferred method of supplying calories. Furthermore, one cannot dispute the facts that intravenous hyperalimentation is costly and not without morbidity.

Other Agents and Approaches to the Management of the Ulcerative Colitis Patient

Sucralfate Enema

Sucralfate, a basic aluminum salt of sucrose octasulfate, has been demonstrated to be an effective drug in the management of peptic ulcer disease. It achieves its therapeutic effectiveness by adhering to mucosal surfaces, increasing prostaglandin levels, increasing mucosal blood flow, and stimulating secretion of mucus. In experimental studies of chemically produced colitis in rats, encouraging results were observed.[759] Kochhar and colleagues noted clinical and sigmoidoscopic improvement in most of their patients, but the study was quite preliminary and uncontrolled.[358] Further trials are awaited.

Butyrate Enema

Short-chain fatty acid irrigation has been demonstrated to be of benefit in the management of individuals with so-called diversion colitis (see Chapter 33). Scheppach and colleagues demonstrated the effect of butyrate enemas on the colonic mucosa in 10 individuals with distal ulcerative colitis who had been unresponsive to or intolerant of standard therapy for 2 months.[637] They showed that butyrate, as an end-product of bacterial fermentation in the large bowel, profoundly affects the colonic epithelium in ulcerative colitis. A statistically significant decreased frequency of bowel action was observed, in addition to a marked reduction in bleeding. The authors concluded that butyrate deficiency may actually play a role in the pathogenesis of distal ulcerative colitis and recommended the use of butyrate irrigation as part of a treatment protocol.[637]

Probiotics

Theoretically beneficial bacteria, such as *Lactobacillus acidophilus* and *Bifidobacterium bifidum*, are called probiotics. They are present in fermented dairy foods, especially live culture yogurt, and have been used as a folk remedy for hundreds of years. Probiotic bacteria have been espoused to alter the intestinal microflora, inhibit the growth of harmful bacteria, promote good digestion, improve immune function, and increase resistance to infection. They are important in recolonizing the bowel during and after antibiotic use.

Most physicians associate lactobacilli with *L. acidophilus*, the most popular species in this group of probiotic bacteria. However, other *Lactobacillus* species may be beneficial as well. For example, *L. rhamnosus* and *L. plantarum* appear to be involved in the production of short-chain fatty acids, as well as the amino acids arginine, cysteine, and glutamine. One probiotic, *Saccharomyces boulardii*, has been shown to prevent diarrhea in several clinical trials.

Probiotics have gained increasing popularity when used to replace or supplant the flora in IBD with so-called "kinder and gentler" species that may prevent an overgrowth of pathogenic bacteria and maintain the integrity of the mucosal barrier. The Italian experience with VSL#3, a mixture of four strains of lactobacilli, three strains of *Bifidobacteria*, and one *Streptococcus salivarius* subspecies, thermophilus, appeared to assist 15 of 20 patients into remission after 12 months.[727] Furthermore, VSL#3 was successful in treating 30 patients with active mild to moderate ulcerative colitis treated for 6 weeks. Nineteen achieved remission (63%) and seven responded (23%). Four had no response, and one patient worsened. No adverse events were reported. This very promising result awaits clinical trials if the marketing process of VSL#3 does not preclude such an attempt.[166] A Japanese study reported a reduction in the number of exacerbations for 3 of 11 patients with ulcerative colitis (27%) treated with a preparation of bifidobacterium-enhanced fermented milk, compared with 9 of 10 patients with ulcerative colitis who were given a placebo.[307]

Nicotine

In addition to what follows here, the reader should also refer to Smoking earlier in the chapter.

As the search for the cause of IBD continues, the association between cigarette smoking and a more favorable clinical course in ulcerative colitis remains the sole epidemiologic feature that distinguishes it from Crohn's disease.[249] Pullan and colleagues reported the results of a randomized, double-blind, controlled trial of transdermal nicotine in patients with active ulcerative colitis.[576] Seventy-two patients were managed with either nicotine patches or placebo patches for a period of 6 weeks. A statistically significant improvement with respect to remission was demonstrated in the treated group in comparison with the placebo group. The most common complaints attributed to the nicotine included nausea, lightheadedness, headache, and sleep disturbance.[576] The authors concluded that the addition of transdermal nicotine to conventional maintenance therapy improved symptoms in persons with active ulcerative colitis.

Nicotine, in two uncontrolled and six controlled trials, appeared to benefit 75% of ex-smokers but did not benefit nonsmokers. Low dosage with gradual escalation was needed for induction of remission, but low-dose transdermal nicotine was not effective for maintenance of remission. The anticipated side-effects of tachycardia, increased blood pressure, nausea, and lightheadedness were noted but appeared less frequently when given as nicotine tartrate in rectal enema with a similar 73% response rate. The fears of nicotine addiction, cardiovascular compromise, cancer, and osteoporosis have not been borne out, but drug interactions have been recorded.

Clearly, ulcerative colitis affects nonsmokers. Ex-smokers and some nonsmokers may enter remission with resumption of nicotine, but side-effects and intolerance are common.[168,626] Others question the validity of the effect of nicotine, because its slight physiologic effects may have improved patients expectations of benefit and altered their reporting of symptoms.[249] The mechanism for the effect of nicotine is unknown.

Antidiarrheal Agents

The addition of "slowing" medications may be appropriate for the patient having frequent bowel movements out of proportion to the degree of inflammatory involvement of the rectum. Products such as diphenoxylate (Lomotil), loperamide (Imodium), codeine, and deodorized tincture of opium, individually or in combination, can be quite helpful. If an individual harbors an active colitis, "slowing" medications should be avoided because they can precipitate a toxic megacolon.[272] In patients who have ileal disease or who have undergone ileal resection, cholestyramine (Questran) also causes a reduction in diarrhea by adsorbing and combining with bile acids in the intestine to form an insoluble compound that is excreted in the feces.[309]

Dietary Measures

Additional medical measures include dietary restrictions. This usually involves the omission of all foods that tend to produce increased frequency of bowel movements [e.g., fruits, milk products (especially if the patient has a lactose intolerance) and fiber]. However, there can be no hard-and-fast rule about complete restriction of these products for every patient. Some individuals may be more tolerant than others. For example, the addition of a bulk agent, such as one of the psyllium-containing products, may be of benefit in giving some form to the stool.

Counseling

The possible value of psychiatric counseling has been discussed earlier. Although the disease may not be of psychogenic origin, there is sufficient evidence to suggest that stress and emotions may play a role in exacerbation or remission of the condition. In addition to the medication and dietary measures presented, it is often helpful to supplement these conventional medical approaches with psychotherapy and other supportive care.

Maintenance of Remission

Therapy must be individualized to the patient's dose-response experience, the extent of the disease, prior relapse history, and whether therapy or "no therapy" has been of value previously. Clearly, most patients will benefit from some form of maintenance treatment. The concept of inducing a *complete remission* must be emphasized before considering changing or reducing an effective treatment program to a maintenance schedule. Prematurely tapering steroids prior to achieving complete remission is a frequent error, but of equal importance is the fact that steroids are ineffective in maintaining remission. Their value is in short-term use or in induction therapy.[250]

The mainstay in this effort is 5-ASA. If left untreated, 80% of patients will relapse. Numerous studies have shown that treated patients will remain in remission longer than those given a placebo.[145,481,490] A multicenter trial comparing oral, topical, and oral with topical mesalamine in maintaining remission in distal ulcerative colitis showed equal efficacy of all three therapies in the prevention of relapse.[287]

Common Errors in Management

Sachar, at the Mount Sinai School of Medicine, presented a personal essay on common errors in the management of IBD which I (*MLC*) thought worthy of reproducing here. They are as follows:

Over-Treating the Irritable Bowel Component

Recall that IBD patients have the same risk (15%) of having symptoms due to an irritable bowel as those individuals without inflammation. Bloating, gas, fullness, and so forth, are not, in and of themselves, indications for one to reach for the steroid bottle.

Under-Treating with Aminosalicylates

Since the efficacy of these agents is dose-related, more may be lost than gained in an effort to give a lower dosage. One should also consider the value of topical treatment for distal disease and encourage the patient to use an enema or suppository once or twice a week to maintain remission.

Over-Treating with Steroids

These drugs are, simply stated, *overused*. Steroids are neither safe nor effective for:

- repeated or frequent relapses
- prolonged, fruitless attempts at tapering
- maintenance of remission

Under-Treating with Antimetabolites

This problem is manifested in three ways:

1. delaying introduction
2. underdosing
3. early suspension or discontinuance

Misusing Infliximab

Sachar summarizes the failings in the use of this agent as follows:

- giving it to people who do not need it
- giving it to people who cannot benefit from it (bowel obstruction and internal fistulas)
- failure to have an exit strategy (the need to administer antimetabolites concomitantly)

Misusing Cyclosporine

Using this drug requires a satisfactory answer to three questions:

1. Does one have the luxury of time, such as with fulminating or hemorrhagic disease?
2. Is the colon really worth saving?
3. Where does one go after its use? This drug must be used as a bridge to other, safer regimens.

Misunderstanding Toxic Colitis

When the syndrome of toxic colitis (not toxic megacolon) persists beyond a few days, an immediate decision must be made either to try cyclosporine or infliximab, or to proceed directly to colectomy.

Choosing the Wrong Goals of Therapy

Coming from an internationally recognized gastroenterologist, Sachar's thoughts on this subject are worth quoting verbatim, even though I suspect in this text he would be truly preaching to the choir:

> We too readily accept as a criterion of success the ability to keep our patients from surgery. Somehow the internist tends to view surgery as a "last resort" or as an indication of "failure" of medical therapy. In adopting such an attitude, we render our patients a terrible disservice. The object of treatment should not be simply "the avoidance of surgery," but rather to make our patients well. To be sure, if we can accomplish this purpose with our panoply of pills, powders, and potions, well and good. But if we can restore patients to good health and wellbeing more swiftly, safely, and surely with surgery, then we should not hesitate to do so. Making people better is, after all, the name of the game.

And it is obviously the name of the game for every one of us—internist, gastroenterologist, and surgeon (*MLC*).

Conclusions

Kornbluth and colleagues conducted a Medline literature search, using the term *severe ulcerative colitis*, to determine the efficacy of current medical therapies.[371] They identified seven studies that comprised 319 treatment episodes in 306 patients. Clinical remission was achieved on average in 62%, whereas 38% came to early colectomy. Remission was maintained in 38% to 71% of patients who achieved success during an acute management episode.[371] The authors concluded that although current medical treatment has improved the outlook for severe ulcerative colitis, one cannot predict with certainty the likelihood of response to any specific therapy based on the clinical features or prior presentations of the disease.[371]

The cornucopia of medications available to clinicians can be overwhelming in deciding which therapy or therapies is appropriate. The key is to design an individualized program geared to that patient's specific needs. There is no "one size" or even "one dose" that fits all. The practitioner must evaluate the patient's response to treatment with each visit, weighing the risks of drug toxicity, cancer surveillance, long-term debility, and surgical candidacy.

SURGICAL MANAGEMENT

Indications

The indications for surgery in ulcerative colitis include toxic megacolon, toxic colitis, perforation, hemorrhage, intolerable extracolonic manifestations, and the concern for malignancy. In addition, because proctocolectomy is curative, resection may be advised for intractable symptoms, even in the absence of a complication. This is the most common indication for surgery today. Conversely, operative treatment for Crohn's disease is advised primarily for complications.

Emergency Surgery

Perforation usually occurs in the patient who exhibits toxic dilatation of the colon and in whom delay in proceeding to surgery has occurred. Diagnosis can usually be made quite readily on the basis of physical examination and a lateral decubitus film of the abdomen. A walled-off perforation may become evident at the time of laparotomy and may be converted to a free perforation as the bowel is mobilized. Although it is well recognized that ulcerative colitis can be associated with toxic megacolon and perforation, Crohn's disease can be as well. These complications tend to occur early in the course of the illness, before thickening of the bowel wall develops.

Hemorrhage

Hemorrhage is occasionally an indication for surgery in ulcerative colitis, but it is very unusual in Crohn's disease (Figure 29-38). Usually, even massive hemorrhage can be controlled by medical means. It should be remembered, however, that a subtotal or total colectomy without proctectomy may not succeed in arresting the bleeding if that is the indication for surgery. It may be necessary to perform a proctectomy in the immediate postoperative period in order to control hemorrhage. In a report from the Mount Sinai Medical Center, there was a 12% risk for continued rectal hemorrhage when subtotal colectomy had been performed for this indication.[604] Pesce and Ceccarino have used rectal washouts with adrenaline chloride in saline solution at 4° to 6°C with some success in controlling bleeding.[565]

Intractability

Intractability is by far the most common indication for surgery in ulcerative colitis. These patients usually harbor total or nearly total colonic disease. Even those individuals with lesser involvement may come to elective surgery, especially in the older age group (more than 60 years). These people seem to tolerate their bowel problems less satisfactorily. It has been said that, ideally, one

should be sick enough for long enough to "earn" an ileostomy—that is, a person should feel that the physical and psychological burden of caring for a stoma is indeed justified. Today, with the available alternative of a sphincter-saving approach, there may be a tendency to intervene surgically sooner. Irrespective of the choice of operation, there is no justification for deferring an operation until a patient is virtually moribund or has been reduced to a skeletal appearance. Regrettably, referral to the surgeon after such procrastination results in the physician's self-fulfilling prophesy: high morbidity and mortality.

Malignancy

The presence of cancer or the risk for malignant change as an indication for surgery has been previously discussed. Colonoscopic monitoring is still the preferred alternative, with operation reserved for those patients found to have dysplasia. It has been almost 20 years since cancer prevention as an indication for colectomy has been replaced by a cancer surveillance program.[395]

Extracolonic Manifestations

Other indications for surgery include growth retardation and extraintestinal manifestations, such as pyoderma gangrenosum, erythema nodosum, liver function abnormalities, eye complications, and joint disturbances (see Chapter 30).

Preparation of the Patient

Preparation of the patient for elective surgery is not significantly different whether the procedure is resection for IBD or surgery for cancer. It is a wise idea, however, to

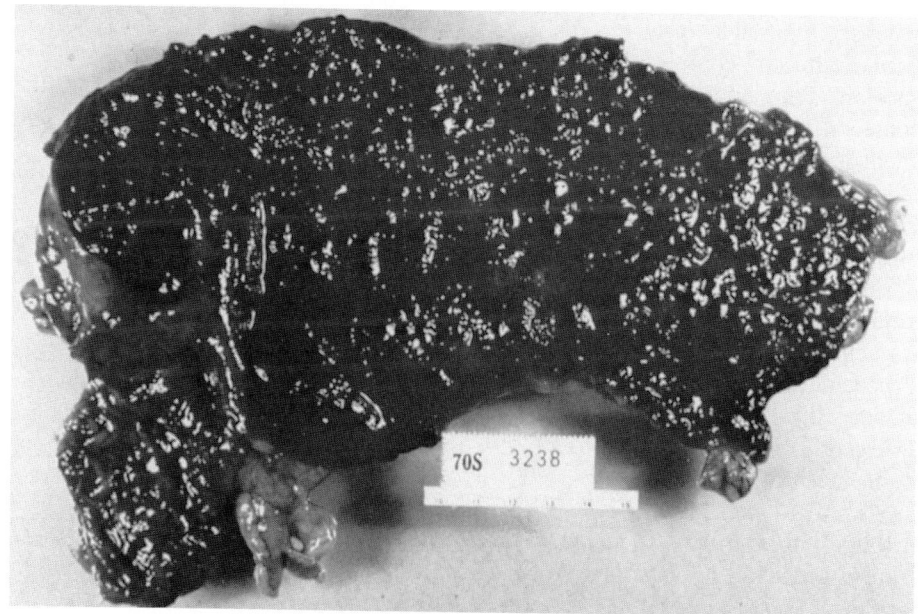

FIGURE 29-38. Ulcerative colitis. A blood clot in the cecum of a patient who underwent emergency proctocolectomy for hemorrhage. (From Corman ML, Veidenheimer MC, Nugent FW, et al. *Diseases of the anus, rectum and colon. Part II: nonspecific inflammatory bowel disease.* New York: Medcom, 1976.)

limit the amount of laxative administered. In fact, if a patient is troubled by diarrhea, a preoperative cathartic should be avoided. On the morning of surgery, an enema may be carefully administered until the returns are clear. This is the only mechanical preparation advised for patients with severe bowel frequency problems. Those who are to undergo small-bowel resection for Crohn's disease do not require a mechanical preparation unless the possibility of colonic resection also exists. The antibiotic preparation should be the same as that described in Chapter 22.

Because most individuals who are to undergo an operation for IBD have been on steroids for varying periods of time, it is imperative that adequate perioperative "coverage" be maintained to prevent the complications of adrenal insufficiency. Unless the person had been on short-term prednisone therapy many months before the operation, steroid protection should be afforded even if corticosteroids were withdrawn up to 2 years previously. The following protocol is one of many that would be considered acceptable:

- Evening before surgery, 9:00 PM: cortisone acetate, 100 mg intramuscularly
- Day of surgery, 6:00 AM: cortisone acetate, 100 mg intramuscularly
- Day of surgery, postoperatively: cortisone acetate, 100 mg intramuscularly, three times daily
- First postoperative day: cortisone acetate, 100 mg intramuscularly, three times daily (a tapering schedule is advised after the third postoperative day, depending on the condition of the patient)

A regimen including intravenous hydrocortisone must be appropriately undertaken to minimize the risk for inadequate replacement of the suppressed pituitary-adrenal response. This method requires either continuous infusion or administration every 4 hours. Adequate blood levels are more difficult to maintain if doses are given less often.

In an emergency situation, it is obviously impossible to prepare the bowel adequately, particularly for the complications of toxic colitis or megacolon. Preoperative preparation includes the correction of any fluid and electrolyte abnormalities, blood replacement as necessary, the placement of a nasogastric tube, the insertion of a Foley catheter (adequate urine output must be established), and the usual large-bore intravenous lines and monitors required for a very ill and potentially unstable patient.

In the elective situation, besides the ample literature available for the patient, it is always helpful to have an ostomate pay a visit. Someone who has achieved success, is of the same sex and age, and ideally of a similar socioeconomic status is preferred. If the surgeon is unable to suggest such a person, the local ostomy association will provide this counsel at no cost. I have always found my patients to be most appreciative of this input. The services of an enterostomal therapist are a great asset in preparing the patient, even if one anticipates employing a stoma on a temporary basis only.

Preoperative stoma marking should be accomplished for everyone who is to undergo surgery for IBD, and it is absolutely imperative if an ileostomy is contemplated. Although preoperative marking is strongly advised for those who are to undergo abdominoperineal resection for cancer, the consequences of a poorly placed stoma are not as profound as they are in patients who are to have an ileostomy. It must be remembered that to the patient the stoma is the most important feature of the operation. An improperly located stoma, one that does not permit convenient management, may cause a patient to become significantly disabled and reclusive. The surgeon should put as much effort into creating a satisfactory stoma, in terms of both preoperative location and technique of construction, as to securing adequate hemostasis. The techniques of stomal construction are discussed in Chapter 31, as are the complications of ileostomy and colostomy.

The optimal site is selected with the patient sitting, supine, and standing. It should be away from bony promontories, scars, and the umbilicus. In the elective situation, it may be helpful to have the patient wear the appliance for a day to be certain that the location is satisfactory (e.g., not interfering with the belt line). Often, one should mark two sites in the hypogastrium, one on each side; should it be impossible to create the stoma in one position, an alternative will then be available. The ileostomy should always be brought through the split thickness of the rectus muscle (Figure 29-39). My own

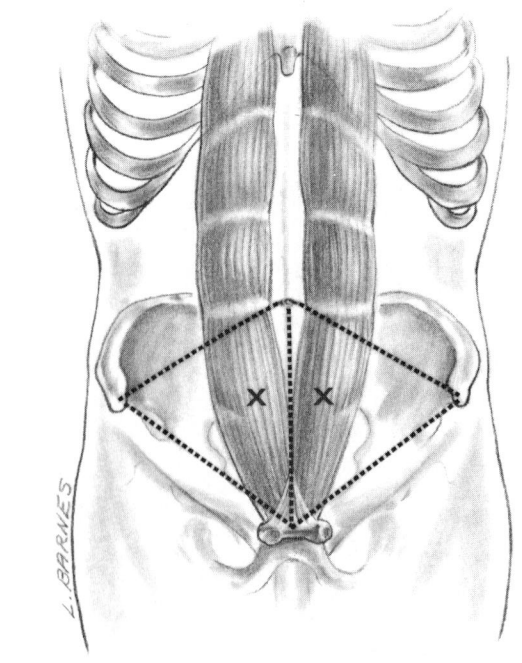

FIGURE 29-39. When a site for ileostomy is chosen, scars, bony prominences, and the umbilicus must be avoided.

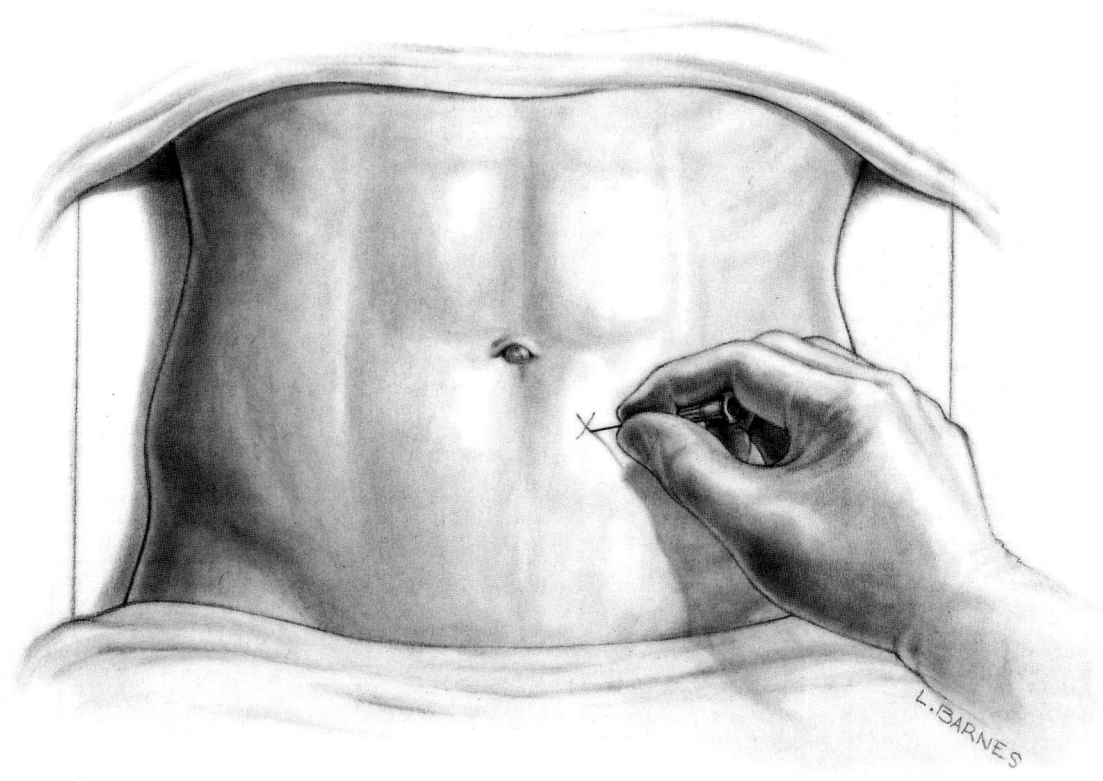

FIGURE 29-40. Stomal marking by scratching the skin with a hypodermic needle. This is easily visualized for 48 to 72 hours.

preference is to mark the site with a scratch from a hypodermic needle (Figure 29-40). Using a pen or India ink is not a good idea in my opinion. Even the best of dyes cannot be maintained with most skin preparations. It is not necessary to tattoo the scratch, because if the patient does not require a stoma, or it must be placed in another location, the tattoo will remain permanently. The scratch itself can easily be identified for several days until it heals.

In an emergency situation, it may not be possible to mark the site adequately preoperatively, particularly if a perforation precipitates the need for surgical intervention. Even under these circumstances, however, an effort should be made to mark the site. Attempts to do this during the operation, with the abdominal wall open, will often result in the stoma being in a less-than-satisfactory location. Before the incision is made, a site may be selected with some degree of assurance through the use of a flange that corresponds to the diameter of the faceplate of an appliance (Figure 29-41). Although the patient under these circumstances can be examined in the supine position only, it is a better alternative than a mere guess. The flange can be sterilized, so that one can still benefit from an intelligent effort to locate the optimal site even when the requirement for an ileostomy has not been anticipated.

The Operation

Alternatives

There are five basic operations for the surgical treatment of ulcerative colitis:

- proctocolectomy and conventional ileostomy
- total or subtotal colectomy with rectal preservation (ileorectal anastomosis, mucous fistula, or closure of rectal stump)
- total proctocolectomy with straight ileoanal anastomosis
- proctocolectomy with reservoir ileostomy (Kock, Barnett)
- total abdominal proctocolectomy with ileoanal (reservoir-anal) anastomosis and intervening pouch (Parks, Utsunomiya, Peck)

In patients with toxic megacolon, a sixth option is a diverting loop ileostomy with a decompressive skin-level ("blowhole") colostomy.

Incision and Exploration

The issue of the nature of the incision has become a heated subject, in light of the development of the minimally invasive approach to bowel resection, including

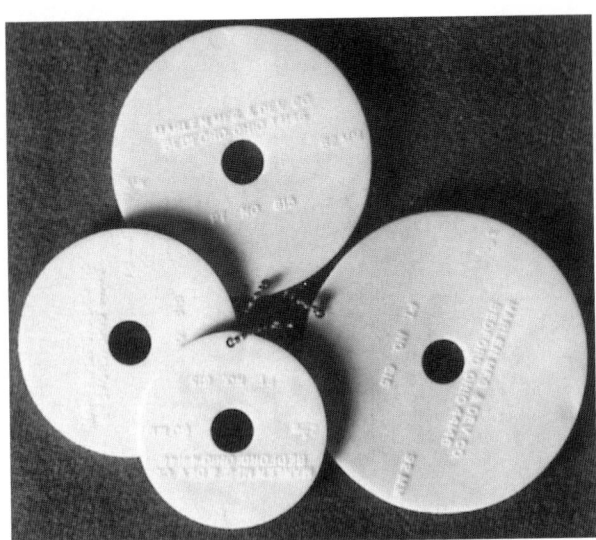

FIGURE 29-41. Variable-diameter faceplate templates for stomal marking. (Courtesy of Marlen Manufacturing and Development Co., Bedford, OH.)

some of the most complicated of colorectal operations. Although I no longer feel strongly, I have opined that the incision for all colon resections, including operations for IBD, always should be in the midline. The reasons for this have been discussed previously and include rapid and facile entry into the peritoneal cavity, good exposure of all areas within the abdomen, and, most importantly, accessibility of both sides of the abdomen for possible stomal placement. If a paramedian incision is used, that side of the abdomen is excluded for possible location of an ileostomy. This may not seem very important at the time of the procedure, particularly if the surgeon contemplates locating the stoma on the opposite side, but if the ileostomy ever requires relocation, unless the scar is flat, it may be extremely difficult to find a satisfactory alternative site. Placing the stoma in a pararectus location is inappropriate (see Chapter 31).

Generally, if a total abdominal colectomy or proctocolectomy is contemplated, the incision is made in the hypogastrium with supraumbilical extension for varying distances. Incision to the level of the xiphoid may be required if splenic flexure mobilization is difficult. In patients with long-standing ulcerative colitis, however, when foreshortening of the bowel may be present, one should begin the incision in the hypogastrium, ascertain the height of the flexures, and extend the incision cephalad if further exposure is required. When operating for toxic megacolon, it is imperative that one have adequate exposure to avoid possible injury to the colon or spleen.

However, as discussed in Chapter 22, I have been employing a Maylard incision (suprapubic, transverse, muscle-dividing) for many colon procedures, including restorative proctocolectomy as a so-called "minilaparo-

tomy." Generally, exposure is adequate and favorably "competes" with minimally invasive surgery on the issues of cosmetics and comfort. If additional exposure is required, the incision may be extended laterally and cephalad on either side to the costal margins, if necessary. Furthermore, any stoma is quite some distance from the incision. In a study by Brown and co-workers, wherein laparoscopic-assisted surgery was compared with minilaparotomy by means of a suprapubic incision in restorative proctocolectomies, there was no difference in postoperative recovery.[71] The only advantage was the slightly smaller wound with laparoscopy.

Exploration of the abdomen will usually reveal the extent of pathology in patients with Crohn's disease because this is a transmural inflammatory process and the serosa is virtually always involved. However, in patients with ulcerative colitis, one may be singularly unimpressed with the extent of disease as it appears from the serosal aspect. The surgeon may appreciate only tortuosity of the vessels, a pallor on the serosal aspect, and, of course, in the case of long-standing, chronic ulcerative colitis, bowel shortening.

When operating for ulcerative colitis, one should have a preconceived plan of the surgery that is to be performed. That is to say, almost irrespective of the operative findings, the entire colon should be removed. Whether one wishes to contemplate a more esoteric operation is a decision that should be made preoperatively. One must depend on the preoperative evaluation, history, endoscopic findings, and radiologic studies—not on the operative findings—to determine the extent of resection for ulcerative colitis. Conversely, in patients with Crohn's disease, it is not uncommon to discover that involvement is more extensive than might have been appreciated by preoperative evaluation. In both conditions one must inspect the entire small bowel for the possibility of other lesions. The small intestine should be carefully examined even in patients with presumed ulcerative colitis, because occasionally one may discover a lesion in the proximal bowel consistent with Crohn's disease. Obviously, this might compel the surgeon to perform a different operation.

Proctocolectomy with Ileostomy

Proctocolectomy with ileostomy is the conventional operative approach to the treatment of patients with ulcerative colitis and for most individuals with granulomatous colitis in which the rectum or anus is involved. However, it is interesting to note that there have been very few reports on the management of IBD by this operation in the past 25 years. This phenomenon is initially attributed to the development of the continent, reservoir ileostomy (Kock) and then to restorative proctocolectomy. Currently, the overwhelming number of publications on surgery for ulcerative colitis address the techniques, complications, and results of the various pouch-anal alternatives (see later discussion). However, proctocolectomy and conventional ileostomy should be considered the benchmark procedure with which all other operations must be compared. This approach has been established as relatively safe, curative, and permits the patient to live a virtually normal lifestyle.

The operation has evolved in a sequential way, beginning initially with appendicostomy as a decompressive procedure, then ileostomy, and then staged operations to effect removal of the colon and rectum.[70,83,84,104,377,437,465] During the era of staged procedures, which included staged thyroidectomy, esophageal diverticulectomy, abdominoperineal resection, and pancreatectomy, it was considered perfectly reasonable to perform four operations before completely extirpating the bowel for ulcerative colitis (ileostomy, right hemicolectomy, left hemicolectomy, and then abdominoperineal resection). With advances in anesthesia, blood transfusion, and antibiotics, as well as improved surgical techniques, the staged procedure was reduced to two operations (total abdominal colectomy followed by proctectomy), and inevitably to one-stage total proctocolectomy.[68,111,195,211]

The technique of proctocolectomy essentially combines the operations previously discussed in Chapters 22 and 23: total abdominal colectomy with proctectomy, using either the classic Miles approach or the perineolithotomy position (synchronous combined). There are some minor differences, however, that are important to consider. First, this is not a cancer operation. Hence, it is not necessary to remove a large area of mesentery containing the lymphatic structures. Furthermore, it is not appropriate for the surgeon to excise the parietal peritoneum widely, as one often does for carcinoma of the rectum. The peritoneal cut may be made directly on the bowel wall, thereby expediting and facilitating the dissection.

Another difference in surgical technique when removing the colon and rectum for IBD, as opposed to removing them for cancer, is rectal mobilization. Because of the potential for injury to sympathetic and parasympathetic nerves, it has been suggested that the posterior rectal dissection for this disease be performed between the rectal wall and the mesentery, or at least through the mesorectum. This maneuver is more likely to avoid injury to the presacral nerves, the sympathetic innervation to the pelvic viscera. However, the dissection is tedious and often quite conducive to hemorrhage. Furthermore, the technique fails to protect the parasympathetic innervation, which is usually of greater concern, especially in men. Erection is a parasympathetically mediated response that is transmitted through the nervi erigentes. These nerves arise from the second, third, and fourth sacral roots. Parasympathetic nerve injury can result in impotence, whereas injury to the presacral (sympathetic) nerves interferes with ejaculation. The presacral nerves originate from the tho-

racic and lumbar segments of the spinal cord and can be identified if the surgeon makes a modicum of effort to do so. Because there is a ready plain of dissection between the investing fascia of the mesentery of the rectum and the sacrum, I prefer to visualize the presacral nerves directly, displace them posteriorly, and proceed in this plain, in the same manner one does with proctectomy for carcinoma. To accomplish this safely, it is important to begin the dissection sharply with a scissors in the hollow of the sacrum rather than to initiate mobilization of the rectum from the promontory bluntly by means of the hand. After the dissection has proceeded well below the sacral promontory, it is then reasonable to complete the mobilization by blunt dissection, but I still prefer to use sharp dissection as far as it can be technically achieved. With a proper retractor and an able assistant one can directly visualize the entire posterior dissection to the level of the levatores most of the time.

An organized approach to the operation minimizes morbidity and mortality. Having ascertained the extent of the disease, the surgeon proceeds with mobilization of the sigmoid colon and rectum. At this time, the perineal surgeon commences that part of the operation. After completion of the proctectomy, the rectum is delivered to the abdominal operator and wrapped in a towel, and the rest of the colectomy is completed while the perineal surgeon closes the bottom end wound. Alternatively, the abdominal surgeon may elect to perform a total colectomy initially, calling the perineal surgeon in at the appropriate stage of the operation to complete the proctectomy.

If two teams are not available, the patient may be placed either in the perineolithotomy or in the supine position on the operating table, and the total abdominal colectomy is carried out. The rectum is divided and secured in a glove (see Figure 23-27), the abdomen closed, the ileostomy created, and the perineal dissection undertaken with the patient either in the left lateral position or in the lithotomy position as described for the one-team approach for carcinoma of the rectum.

In contradistinction to what is done in a proctectomy for carcinoma, the floor of the pelvis is not reconstituted. If one closes the floor with parietal peritoneum, a diaphragm-like effect is created. This results in a dead space that predisposes to the subsequent development of an abscess, perineal sinus, and delayed healing. One must endeavor, in essence, to lower the pelvic floor. Because it is not necessary to excise the levator muscle widely as is often done for cancer, it is always possible to reapproximate this and the external sphincter. It is the external sphincter and levatores, then, that form the floor of the pelvis in patients who undergo proctectomy for IBD.

The perineal dissection is undertaken in a manner somewhat different from that for carcinoma. The technique that I prefer is the intersphincteric dissection advocated by Lyttle and Parks[431] (Figure 29-42). This permits

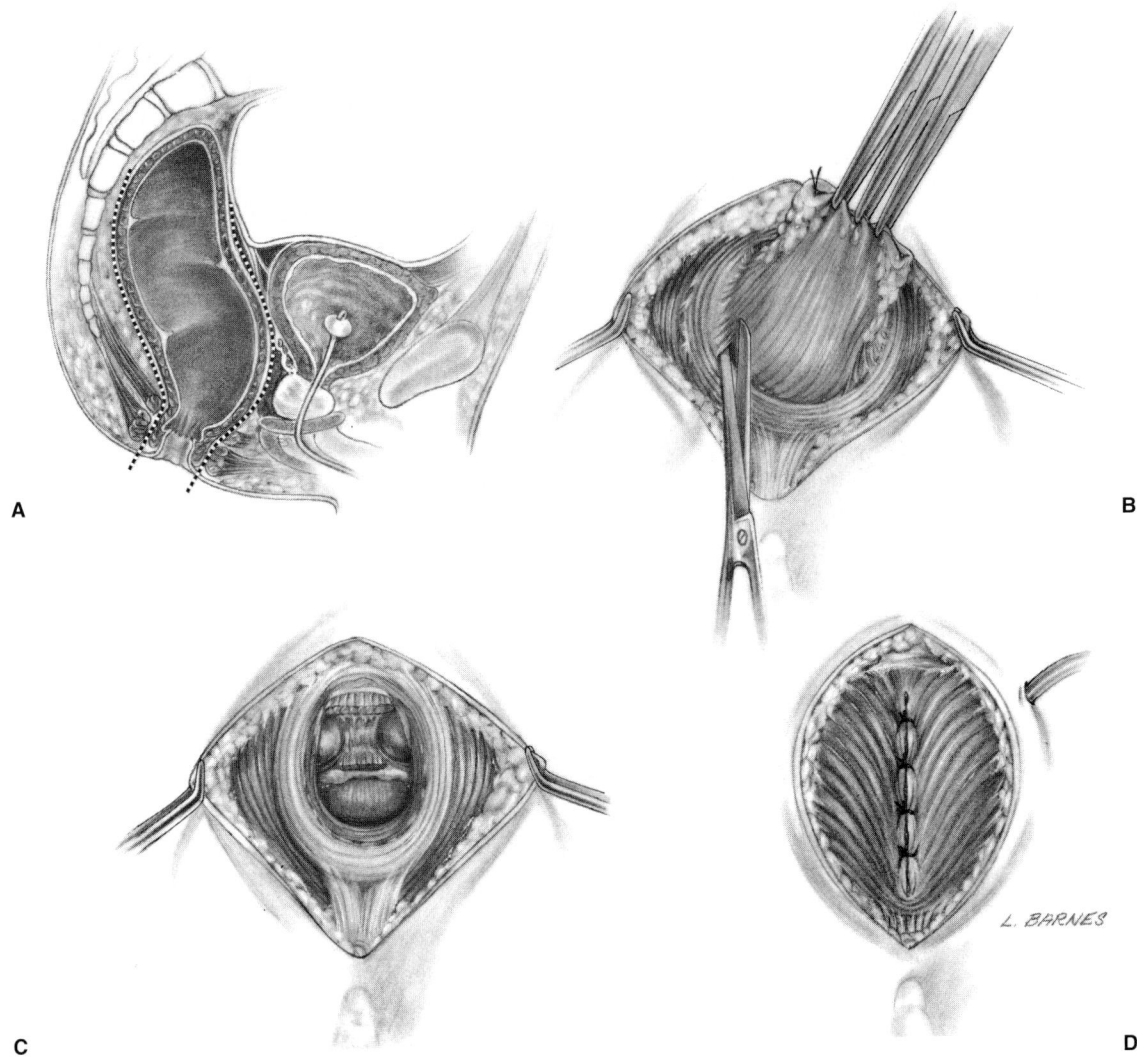

FIGURE 29-42. Technique of intersphincteric proctectomy. **(A)** Outline of the area removed. **(B)** Dissection proceeds in the intersphincteric plane. **(C)** Intact external sphincter and levatores following rectal removal. **(D)** Closure of levatores with drainage.

a much smaller perineal wound. In fact, the diameter of the incision is such that it is impossible to insert a Lace retractor, my preferred instrument for facilitating the perineal portion of the dissection for cancer of the rectum (see Figure 23-33). The procedure is carried out in the intersphincteric plain, between the internal and external anal sphincters. When the levator ani muscle is encountered, it is divided close to the rectum. The dissection is completed anteriorly in a manner identical to that for carcinoma of the rectum. A Silastic drain is placed into the pelvis, brought out through a stab wound in the buttock, and connected to continuous suction (Figure 29-42D; Figure 29-43). Alternatively, a suprapubic suction drain can be employed. The levator ani muscle and external sphincter are then approximated and the skin closed.

The drain is usually removed at 72 hours, depending on the amount collected.

Another method for performing an intersphincteric proctectomy is an endoanal mucosal stripping, such as is undertaken in conjunction with the ileal pouch-anal procedure (see later discussion).[157] This leaves yet a smaller wound, but the operation may be associated with delayed healing, is tedious to accomplish, and has the theoretical disadvantage of incomplete removal of the mucosa, thereby posing a potential risk for cancer and persistent perineal sinus.[278,546]

Resection of the distal small bowel is sometimes necessary when proctocolectomy is undertaken for Crohn's disease, depending on whether the intestine is involved by the inflammatory process. Conversely, the small intes-

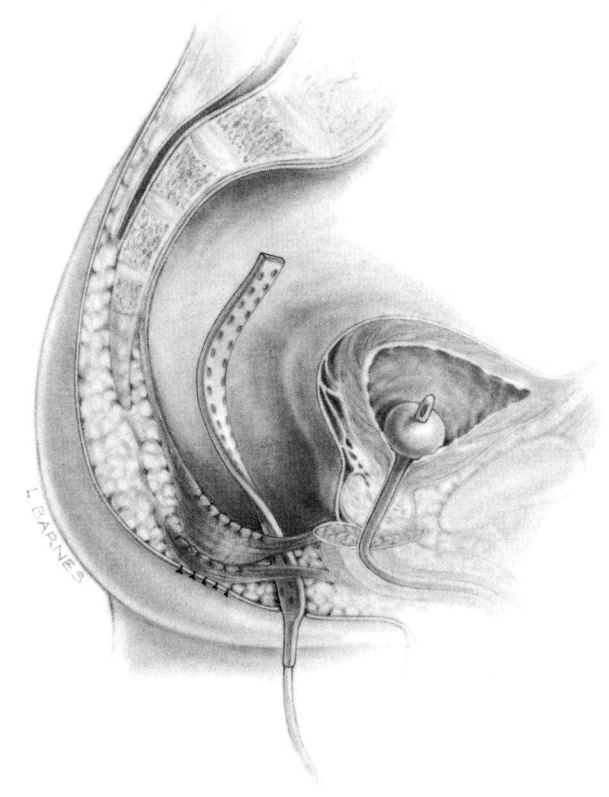

FIGURE 29-43. Lateral view of pelvis following proctectomy for ulcerative colitis. The peritoneal floor is open; the levatores, external sphincter, and skin are closed, and a drain is placed into the pelvis through a stab wound.

tine is spared when the operation is performed for ulcerative colitis. Every effort should be made to preserve the full length of the small bowel. Even modest resection of the distal ileum may lead to malabsorption of nutrients as well as to loss of water and electrolytes.[509]

The distal small bowel may be divided with crushing clamps and delivered through the abdominal opening in a manner similar to that described for colostomy after abdominoperineal resection (see Figure 23-26). Another option is to use a gastrointestinal anastomosis (GIA) stapling device, a Zachary Cope enterostomy clamp, or even paired umbilical clamps.[245] In creating the ileostomy for patients with ulcerative colitis, I prefer an extraperitoneal approach. This technique permits total obliteration of the paraileostomy gutter, thereby avoiding the potential for herniation. It also facilitates subsequent entrance into the abdominal cavity without the risk for injuring the mesentery to the small bowel. Kocher clamps are placed on the cut edge of the parietal peritoneum. The peritoneum is then gently elevated and stripped off the abdominal wall to the point where the ileostomy site is located. An abdominal wall opening is then created (see Figure 23-24), and the end of the ileum is delivered

through the defect (Figure 29-44A). The cut edge of the mesentery is then secured to the peritoneum that has been mobilized (Figure 29-44B). Following closure of the abdomen, the ileostomy is matured (see Figs. 31-46 through 31-48).

An intraperitoneal ileostomy is the commonly used alternative for most surgeons but is particularly recommended in patients who undergo proctocolectomy for granulomatous colitis, in those who have already had a portion of the terminal ileum removed, and in those for whom "stripping" of the parietal peritoneum is technically impossible. The technique for creation of an intraperitoneal ileostomy and obliteration of the lateral space is illustrated in Figure 29-45. As suggested, the disadvantages are the technical difficulties associated with complete obliteration of the right lateral gutter (the inferior aspect of the distal ileum does not lend itself to closure in a satisfactory fashion), and entrance into the abdominal cavity from the right upper quadrant is impeded. This cautionary note is best illustrated by the example of the patient who undergoes an open cholecystectomy several years after intraperitoneal obliteration of the lateral gutter. The surgeon usually elects a subcostal incision to avoid the ileostomy, but when the peritoneal cavity is entered, the mesentery to the small intestine can be divided, with resultant necrosis of the stoma. Even with a laparoscopic approach, placement of the ports may pose a risk of injury to the terminal ileal mesentery.

Another option is to leave the lateral gutter open because, as with sigmoid colostomy, it is better to have a very large opening than a small one. Some anchoring is nonetheless still required to avoid torsion of the distal ileum on itself (windlassing). A few sutures placed from the serosa of the ileum and its mesentery to the parietal peritoneum will usually prevent this complication (Figure 29-46).

Complications

Most complications following proctocolectomy are not unique to the operation: wound infection, intraabdominal sepsis, wound dehiscence, ureteral and splenic injury, and urinary, pulmonary, and cardiovascular problems. These are discussed in Chapters 22 and 23. Complications attributed more specifically to this operation include stomal problems, intestinal obstruction, sexual dysfunction, and perineal wound difficulties.

Stomal Problems. Stomal complications and their management are discussed in Chapters 31 and 32. Complications with respect to recurrent Crohn's disease are discussed in Chapter 30.

Intestinal Obstruction. This is a common complication of all operations in which a stoma is placed. The incidence has been reported to be as high as 25%, most oc-

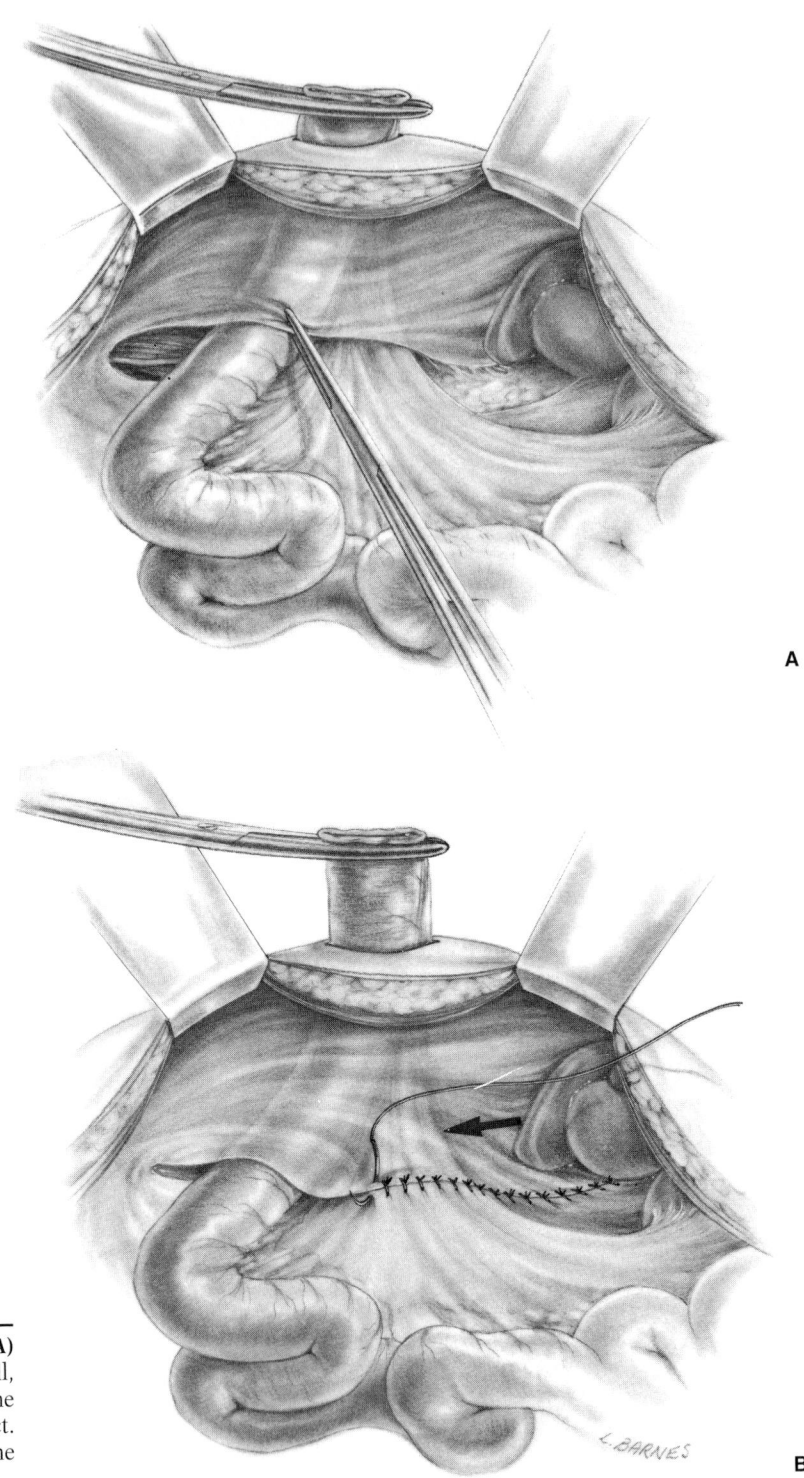

FIGURE 29-44. Extraperitoneal ileostomy. **(A)** Mobilized peritoneum from the abdominal wall, with delivery of the terminal ileum through the ileostomy site and closure of the mesenteric defect. **(B)** The peritoneum overlies the cut edge of the mesentery *(arrow)*.

curring within the first year. Turnbull reported that small-bowel obstruction developed in 6% of 261 patients who underwent proctocolectomy and ileostomy for ulcerative colitis and who underwent laparotomy.[719]

In patients in whom intestinal obstruction develops following ileostomy, consideration must be given to a para-

ileostomy hernia as the cause of the problem. Initial conservative management includes nasogastric intubation and possibly an attempt to relieve the obstruction by irrigating the stoma. Occasionally, the obstruction may be caused by inspissated fecal material or undigested food. As long as the patient is passing flatus, it is usually possi-

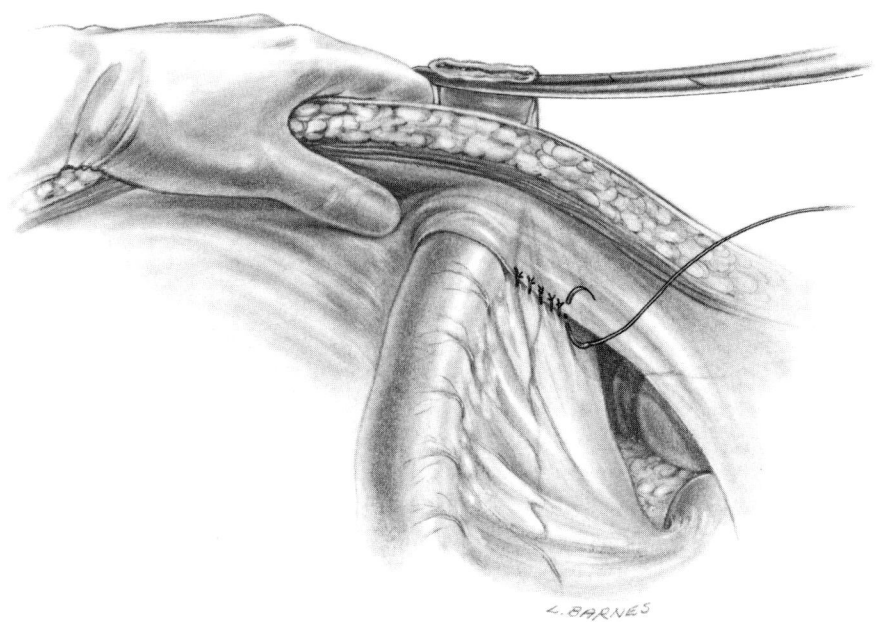

L. BARNES

FIGURE 29-45. Intraperitoneal fixation. The falciform ligament is the limit of closure cephalad. The cut edge of the mesentery is sutured to the parietal peritoneum.

ble to delay surgical intervention. However, if a complete intestinal obstruction is present, early operation may be imperative. The cause of the problem is often a simple adhesion, but if a paraileostomy hernia with entrapment of the small intestine is the cause, the small bowel must be reduced and the defect closed.

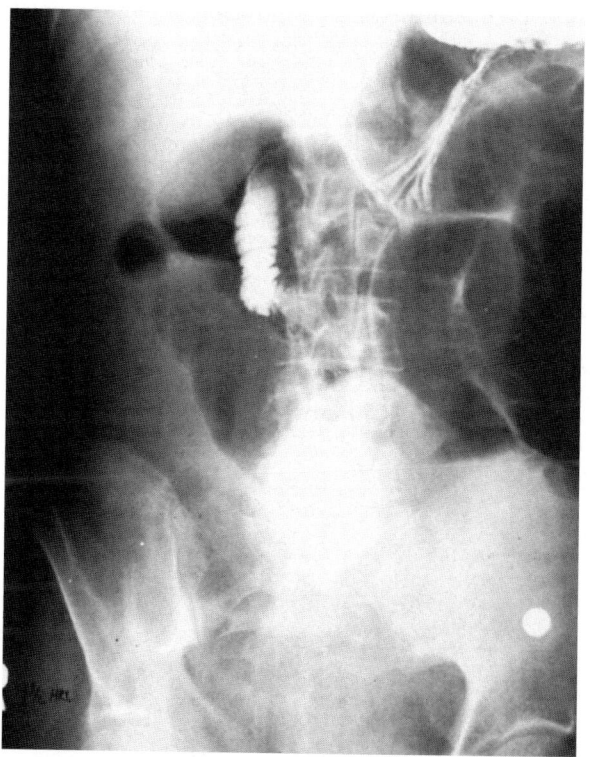

FIGURE 29-46. Small-bowel obstruction secondary to torsion of the ileum on its mesentery. Barium study reveals complete obstruction proximal to the ileostomy.

Ileal Necrosis. The presence of a nonviable stoma is usually a consequence of torsion. Obviously, if the stoma itself is necrotic, the preoperative diagnosis is self-evident and resection of the stoma and nonviable bowel is necessary. However, if the blood supply to the ileostomy is preserved, the surgeon may be tempted to resect the nonviable bowel and perform an anastomosis a few inches from the end of the ileostomy. Such a concept is a dangerous undertaking. Unless the area of nonviability is at least 25 cm from the ileostomy, no anastomotic attempt should be made. The stoma should be resected in continuity with the nonviable bowel and a new ileostomy created. This usually requires relocation to the left lower quadrant. Even though this means sacrificing additional intestine, the risk for an anastomotic leak is so great that preservation of this small segment is not justified.

Sexual Dysfunction. Sexual dysfunction (retrograde ejaculation and impotence) is well recognized as an unfortunate sequela of proctectomy. It is this complication that causes some surgeons to be unwilling to remove the rectum at the time of the initial procedure, preferring to perform proctectomy at a later date, when it is hoped that the patient will have achieved all procreative ambitions. It is doubtful, however, that a young man in his thirties, with perhaps a sufficient number of children, is particularly grateful for sexual dysfunction at his age any more than he might have been 10 years previously.

To delay operation, however, is not without consequences. The patient must contend with another major operation, with its implications of time lost from work, family hardship, and changes in lifestyle. Many patients who feel well are reluctant to submit to an operation that will make them, at least for a time, unwell.

Some are lost to follow-up, and some refuse operation. Finally, the risk for malignancy developing is a very real concern. Many surgeons have witnessed the tragedy of incurable carcinoma arising in the long forgotten, retained rectum. The concern about sexual dysfunction and the potential risk for malignancy in the retained rectum have become secondary issues in recent years, however, as the pouch-anal procedure is undertaken ideally as a primary procedure.

Impotence after abdominoperineal resection for carcinoma of the rectum is not an uncommon problem, but one questions whether preservation of the rectum in IBD is justified solely because of this risk. We reviewed our experience with 76 post-pubescent male patients who underwent proctocolectomy between the years 1964 and 1973.[106] The mean age of the patients at proctectomy was 36 years (range, 14 to 71). One person was found to have transient impairment of the ability to achieve an erection, but normal sexual function subsequently returned. After 6 years of follow-up, his function in this area was normal.

Table 29-4 summarizes the reports of other series on impotence following proctectomy for IBD. Although that of Watts and colleagues found a high incidence of impotence, patients in their series were older than those in most others.[733] In fact, five of seven patients with impotence were in their late fifties or sixties. When this series is excluded from the overall figures, the rate of impotence is 2.7%. The vast majority in all series who are impotent are in the older age groups.

Retrograde ejaculation occurs because of injury to the sympathetic nerves, a complication that has been variously reported to develop in up to 10% of male patients. More recent statistics suggest that, as with the problem of impotence, the complication is much less frequent in younger people. Fewer than 1% of the patients reported

by Bauer and colleagues exhibited this difficulty.[31] As previously stated, visualization and avoidance of the presacral nerves should make this complication a very rare occurrence indeed.

Sexual function in women has been less well surveyed than in men, probably because there is no concern about impotence. Metcalf and colleagues, in a review of 100 women who underwent proctocolectomy (with either a Kock pouch or an ileoanal anastomosis), noted that the majority experienced enhanced sexual function.[477] This was attributed to improved health. Those with a pouch had a significantly higher incidence of dyspareunia than those with an ileoanal anastomosis, presumably because of scarring or deformity associated with complete proctectomy (see later discussion).

Other concerns about sexual dysfunction are related primarily to the concept of an ileostomy itself—the need for an external appliance and the possibility of leakage—and its impact on sexuality and body image. These aspects are discussed in Chapters 31 and 32.

Comment. In my opinion, impotence appears to be less the result of the type of operative approach than of the age of the patient. It seems difficult to believe that careful attention to dissection close to the bowel wall is the reason for a low incidence of impotence whereas the "radical" operation for cancer produces a high incidence. Although one cannot gainsay meticulous surgical technique, preoperative libido is probably a more important factor. A report from the Mayo Clinic seems to concur with this opinion.[756]

Persistent Perineal Sinus. Persistent perineal sinus is one of the most troubling sequelae of proctectomy for IBD (Figs. 29-47 and 29-48). We reviewed our experience

▶ **TABLE 29-4 Impotence after Proctectomy for Inflammatory Bowel Disease**

Reference	Number of Patients	Impotence	
		Number	Percent
Bacon et al.[16]	39	1	2.8
Burnham et al.[76]	118	6	5.1
Donovan and O'Hara[136]	21	1	4.8
May[455]	47	3	6.4
Stahlgren and Ferguson[668]	25	0	0.0
Van Prohaska and Siderius[725]	79	0	0.0
Watts et al.[733]	41	7	17.1
Corman et al.[106]	76	0	0.0
Total of reported series	446	18	4.0

From Corman ML, Veidenheimer MC, Coller JA. Impotence after proctectomy for inflammatory disease of the bowel. *Dis Colon Rectum* 1978;21:418.

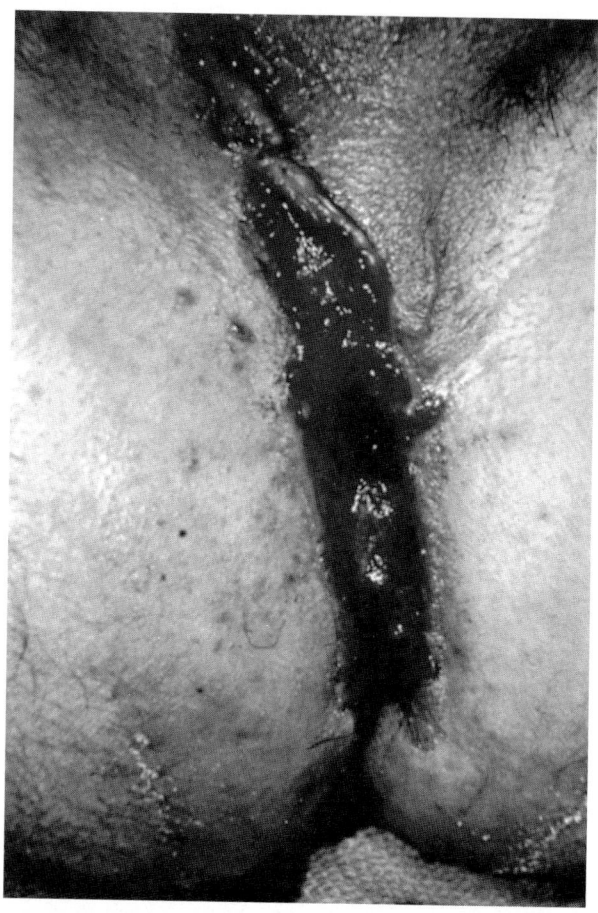

FIGURE 29-47. Persistent perineal sinus following proctectomy for inflammatory bowel disease. A chronic, indolent draining wound.

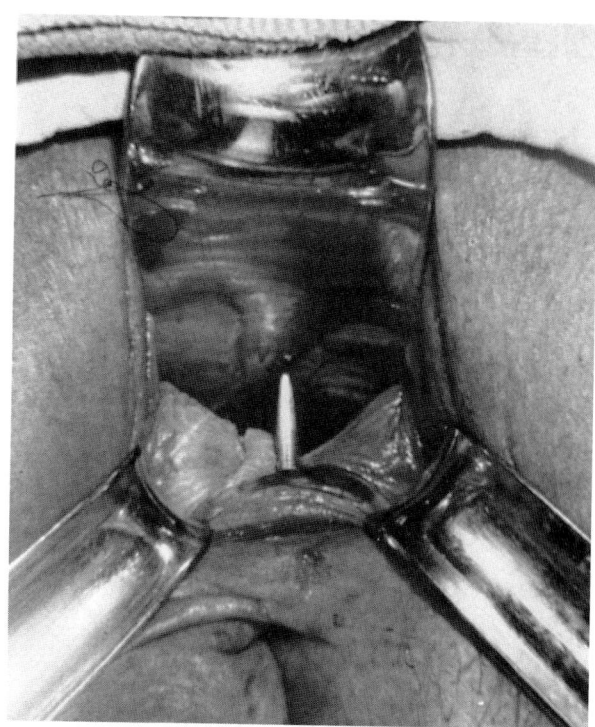

FIGURE 29-48. Perineovaginal fistula following proctectomy. Treatment requires fistulotomy. Pregnancy is unlikely to occur in this situation.

with 160 patients who underwent proctectomy for this condition.[107] The mean ages of the patients with ulcerative colitis and with Crohn's disease were the same (36 years). The sex incidence was also the same, but more men than women were given a diagnosis of ulcerative colitis and more women than men were diagnosed with Crohn's colitis. The perineal wounds in 75% of patients with ulcerative colitis were healed by the end of the follow-up period without reoperation, whereas only 51% of wounds in those with Crohn's colitis were healed. By the end of the follow-up study, the wounds of only 11% of patients with ulcerative colitis were not healed, but the wounds of more than one-third of the patients with Crohn's colitis had not healed.

Some authors have demonstrated that packing the perineal wound is associated with delayed healing.[310,611] In a retrospective review from the Cleveland Clinic, a highly significant difference was appreciated between packing versus levator closure with transabdominal drainage—31% were unhealed at 1 year or required further surgery in the former group, whereas only 9% were unhealed in the latter group.[529] Others have confirmed

the value of intersphincteric proctectomy in reducing the incidence of delayed perineal wound healing.[31,390,760] Cripps and colleagues even suggest that a proctectomy can be undertaken by preserving the internal sphincter, stripping out only the mucosa, thus leading to more rapid and improved perineal wound healing.[112]

Other factors may be associated with the development of this complication. In our experience, age was thought to be a relevant consideration. All patients with ulcerative colitis who were more than 50 years of age and all with Crohn's colitis who were more than 60 years of age had healed perineal wounds. With respect to sex, women with ulcerative colitis were more likely to have the perineal wound heal per primum (97.5%), whereas only 82% of men achieved such healing. However, no statistically significant difference in rates of healing was seen when sex distributions in patients with Crohn's disease were compared.

Evaluation of the presence or absence of a stoma before proctectomy revealed that in patients with ulcerative colitis, diversion implied an excellent chance for healing. Interestingly, the opposite was true for those with Crohn's colitis.

Perineal disease, specifically fistula-in-ano (present at the time of proctectomy), was not a statistically significant factor in nonhealing, although the numbers were small. The rates of nonhealing were almost the same in

▶ **TABLE 29-5 Healing after Proctectomy**

	Ulcerative Colitis			Crohn's Colitis		
	Healed	*Not Healed*	*Percent Healed*	*Healed*	*Not Healed*	*Percent Healed*
Age in Years						
<20	10	4	71.4	0	2	0.0
20–29	17	2	89.5	14	7	66.7
30–39	21	2	91.3	9	5	64.3
40–49	15	2	88.2	8	5	61.6
50–59	9	0	100.0	6	2	75.0
60–69	7	0	100.0	2	0	100.0
>69	1	0	100.0	1	0	100.0
Sex						
Men	41	9	82.0	17	9	65.4
Women	39	1	97.5	23	12	65.7
Stoma						
Yes	50	1	98.0	25	18	58.1
No	30	9	76.9	15	3	83.3
Fistula						
Yes	4	2	66.7	25	16	61.0
No	76	8	90.5	15	5	75.0

From Corman ML, Veidenheimer MC, Coller JA, Ross VH. Perineal wound healing after proctectomy for inflammatory bowel disease. *Dis Colon Rectum* 1978;21:155.

patients with ulcerative colitis and in those with Crohn's colitis when a fistula was present. However, in the absence of a perianal fistula, a patient with Crohn's colitis did not heal as well as one with ulcerative colitis. These factors are summarized in Table 29-5.

The number of prior operations, extent of disease, the emergent, urgent, or elective nature of the surgical procedure, contamination of the wound, presence or absence and duration of steroid therapy, level of serum albumin, and nutritional state of the patient were all analyzed and found to have no significant role in prolonging perineal wound healing.

A few studies have been summarized in Table 29-6, which serve to indicate the magnitude of the problem. In a report of 112 patients who underwent proctectomy for Crohn's disease, healing was delayed longer than 1 year in almost 20%.[635]

The failure of perineal wounds to heal readily has stimulated considerable discussion and has served as an impetus for the development of a number of operative approaches to deal with the problem.[10,67,300,438,601,614,623,654] Once a perineal sinus has developed, vigorous curettage, creating a pyramidal defect, should be undertaken at 6-month intervals until healing is achieved. Other methods that have been advocated include a gracilis or inferior gluteal myocutaneous flap,[17,63,615] semimembranosus muscle graft,[439] rectus abdominis flap,[660,758] use of an omental graft,[614] skin grafting,[10] and the application of a fibrin adhesive.[7,349] In a report from the General Hospital of Birmingham, England, 13 patients were submitted to treatment by means of this sealant, but only 5 were completely healed at the time of publication.[7]

Perineal Pain and Phantom Sensations. Phantom sensations of the "need to have a bowel movement" are not unusual after proctectomy. This difficulty is analogous to that which may occur following amputation of an extremity. The cerebral pathway still exists, so that an indeterminate stimulus to the perineum or pelvis may trigger this perception. Treatment is reassurance.

A more troublesome complaint is perineal pain. In contrast to pain that develops following proctectomy for rectal cancer, such pain is obviously not caused by recurrent malignancy, and it is possible to reassure the patient accordingly. Usually, the discomfort can be attributed to a neuroma. If the usual supportive measures (heat, rest, foam rubber cushion, antispasmotics, and nonnarcotic analgesic medications) fail to relieve the symptoms, one should consider excising the perineal fat pad. Almost invariably, the pathologist (if asked) will cooperate and succeed in identifying a neuroma, but the clinical significance and long-term benefits are problematic. Relief can be immediate, but recurrence may develop, presumably because the nerve regenerates. Fortunately, if this occurs, the pain is usually not as severe as initially reported.

▶ **TABLE 29-6** Perineal Wound Healing: Summary of Literature

Author, Year	Diagnosis	Healed, Months	Number Healed	Number Not Healed	Percent Healed
Hughes, 1965[295]	Ulcerative colitis	Not stated	58	13	81.7
Watts et al., 1966[733]	Ulcerative colitis	6	70	23	75.3
Jalan et al., 1969[310]	Ulcerative colitis	6	48	58	45.3
	Crohn's colitis	12	67	39	63.2
Roy et al., 1970[611]	Ulcerative colitis	3	Not stated	Not stated	81.6
	Crohn's colitis	3	Not stated	Not stated	76.3
Oates and Williams, 1970[532]	Both	Not stated	41	12	77.4
de Dombal et al., 1971[124]	Crohn's colitis	6	39	29	57.4
Ritchie, 1971[601]	Ulcerative colitis	6	121	101	54.5
	Crohn's colitis	6	4	15	21.1
Broader et al., 1974[67]	Ulcerative colitis	6	33	8	80.5
	Crohn's colitis	12	11	2	84.6
Irvin and Goligher, 1975[306]	Ulcerative colitis	6	23	10	69.7
	Crohn's colitis	6	12	7	63.2
Corman et al., 1978[107]	Crohn's colitis	6	17	44	27.9
	Ulcerative colitis	6	40	50	44.4

From Corman ML, Veidenheimer MC, Coller JA, Ross VH. Perineal wound healing after proctectomy for inflammatory bowel disease. *Dis Colon Rectum* 1978;21:155.

Results of Conventional Proctocolectomy and Ileostomy

Proctocolectomy and ileostomy today can be carried out with minimal morbidity and mortality. Mavroudis and Schrock reported an operative mortality of 2% in 100 patients who underwent total abdominal colectomy, proctectomy, or both.[454] In the experience of Goligher, 10 operative deaths were noted in 113 patients who underwent proctocolectomy and ileostomy for Crohn's disease, a rate of 9%.[212] In his personal experience in the management of 504 patients with ulcerative colitis, there were 34 operative deaths, an operative mortality of 6.7%.[215] Elective, urgent, and emergency operations revealed a mortality rate of 3%, 10.7%, and almost 25%, respectively. Other reports suggest that the overall operative mortality for proctocolectomy and ileostomy is between 7% and 10%. In my personal experience of more than 300 elective proctocolectomies, there has been one operative death, the consequence of a pulmonary embolism.

Ileostomy-Colostomy for the Treatment of Toxic Megacolon

Toxic megacolon has become a progressively rare manifestation of ulcerative colitis over the past 20 years. Because of the high mortality rate associated with the surgical treatment of toxic megacolon by colectomy (in some series, in excess of 30%), Turnbull and colleagues in 1971

advocated what they considered a lesser-risk procedure.[720] This consisted of a diversionary loop ileostomy and two decompressive colostomies, one in the transverse colon and the other in the sigmoid. The colostomies were created at the skin level and were designed to vent the dilated colon as a "blowhole." The major impetus for suggesting this operative approach was to avoid inadvertent fecal soiling of the peritoneal cavity when a walled-off perforation had been liberated by mobilization of the bowel. This usually occurs in the region of the splenic flexure, an area that is predisposed to bowel wall necrosis. Considerable contamination can result when the dilated colon is decompressed through this inadvertent opening. It was the opinion of the Cleveland Clinic group that diversion and decompression avoided this very serious consequence. This technique has also been successfully utilized in two women with toxic ulcerative colitis who were pregnant.[452]

The technique consists of making a small midline incision and identifying a loop of distal ileum. This is brought out through a previously marked site in the right lower quadrant, usually over a small rod (Figure 29-49). Ideally, the proximal limb is placed inferiorly and the distal limb superiorly, so that subsequent colon resection will not necessitate a change in the fixation of the distal ileum. Exploration of the right upper quadrant of the abdomen identifies the point of maximal dilatation of the transverse colon, and a small incision is made in the skin, fascia, and rectus muscle. If the sigmoid colon is dilated, it too can be decompressed by making a small incision in

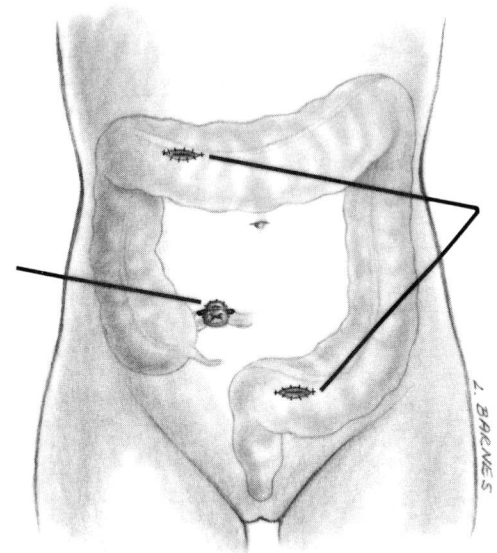

FIGURE 29-49. Diverting ileostomy and decompression colostomies for toxic megacolon. (Adapted from Turnbull RB Jr, Hawk WA, Weakley FL. Surgical treatment of toxic megacolon: ileostomy and colostomy to prepare patients for colectomy. *Am J Surg* 1971;122:325.)

the left iliac fossa, permitting the bowel to bulge into the incision. In later reports from the Cleveland Clinic, however, this second blowhole has rarely been thought to be necessary. The abdomen is then closed, and the loop ileostomy is matured, emphasizing the proximal limb (see Figs. 31-67 through 31-69).

Attention is then turned to the dilated transverse colon. Seromuscular sutures are placed into the colon and the peritoneum and rectus fascia with interrupted fine catgut. A second row of seromuscular sutures is placed between the bowel and the subcutaneous fat. The colon is then opened and the contents evacuated. With successful decompression, sutures may now be placed between the cut edge of the bowel and the skin. The same procedure can be used for the sigmoid colon if an opening is necessary in this area.

Although he, too, is relatively supportive of the occasional use of this particular approach, Fazio points out several potential disadvantages.[159] These include the necessity for further major abdominal surgery and possible continued bleeding if hemorrhage was a presenting problem (approximately one fourth of these patients will continue to bleed postoperatively). Also, if a septic focus persists, earlier surgical intervention than was first anticipated may be required.

The Cleveland Clinic group points out that the procedure should not be performed in cases of free perforation but only when obvious acute colonic dilatation exists without peritonitis. They further opine in a later publication that in carefully selected, hemodynamically stable patients with fulminant colitis and without megacolon, restorative proctocolectomy with ileal pouch-anal anastomosis can be safely performed (see later discussion).[763]

Results

Fazio reported the Cleveland Clinic experience of 115 patients seen from 1961 to 1967 with toxic megacolon.[159] Only seven were discharged following medical management. Of interest is the fact that five of the seven required subsequent colectomy. Subtotal colectomy with ileostomy was performed in 26 patients and decompression and diversion in the remaining 83. The mortality rate following subtotal colectomy was 11.5%. Three patients died after decompression and diversion, a mortality rate of 3.6%. However, two additional patients succumbed following elective colectomy, bringing the overall mortality to 6% for the decompression and diversion group. Among the 17 patients found to have free perforations, 5 deaths were reported, a mortality rate of almost 30%.

Fazio is reluctant to draw dogmatic conclusions about the value of diversion and decompression. The mortality rate appears to be lower when patients are treated by this technique, but the series is uncontrolled, and it appears that many of the patients who were treated initially by colectomy actually had free perforations, thus constituting a much higher-risk group.

Heppell and colleagues reviewed their experience with 65 patients who were treated for toxic megacolon.[276] The mortality rate following surgery was 27% when colectomy was undertaken for a free or sealed perforation. When toxic megacolon was associated with massive hemorrhage, the mortality was 33%. In the experience of Greenstein and Aufses, the incidence of perforation in toxic megacolon was three times greater for patients with ulcerative colitis than for those with Crohn's colitis.[230] In the absence of toxic megacolon, however, Crohn's disease was as likely to be associated with a perforation as was ulcerative colitis. Interestingly, mortality rates were lower if the perforation occurred in a patient with Crohn's disease.

Comment

I am able to restrain my enthusiasm for the decompression and diversion technique in the treatment of toxic megacolon, primarily for the reasons alluded to by Fazio. It is a troublesome concept to commit the patient to at least one other operation when the procedure can be accomplished in one stage, removing the source of sepsis and liberating the patient from contending with at least two abdominal orifices. Fecal drainage from upper and lower abdominal wounds may be a justifiable, albeit unaesthetic, experience if one is convinced that it is the only life-saving measure available. However, I believe that an expeditious, well-conceived resection can accomplish the optimal goal. To deal with a sealed perforation, it is suggested that the transverse colon be decompressed by simple needle aspiration before the splenic flexure is "attacked." Another alternative is to mobilize the sigmoid, descending, and transverse colon, to divide the bowel at the point of planned resection, and to exteriorize the segment, so that minimal contamination will result if a sealed perforation is encountered. Finally, there is a certain impracticality when one advises a "blowhole" colostomy for decompression. In my experience, attempting to suture a profoundly dilated, possibly necrotic transverse colon is more than a frustrating experience; it is impossible. Passing a suture into the bowel, itself, is likely to cause a perforation. The procedure is like attempting to sew wet toilet paper. In an admittedly small personal experience of 18 patients with toxic megacolon, I have applied resection as the modality of therapy, with no deaths.

Total Colectomy with Rectal Preservation

Total abdominal colectomy with ileorectal or ileosigmoid anastomosis for ulcerative colitis has been advocated by a number of authors, but it has been especially championed by Aylett.[13-15] At the Gordon Hospital in London, Aylett developed an interest in the surgical management of IBD. As discussed previously, the standard surgical treatment was removal of the diseased bowel and the creation of a permanent stoma. Aylett thought that the rectum could usually be retained and a stoma avoided. The surgical establishment was outraged by his practice. Critics claimed that the patient would have intractable diarrhea and the risk of cancer developing in the retained bowel. Aylett was pilloried in the medical press and at national meetings. Heated debates ensued, but Aylett consistently showed good results. Although he recognized that cancer was indeed a risk, he believed that with regular follow-up it could be identified and adequately treated. The surgical establishment failed to match Aylett's results, and it was suggested that with his charisma and charm he was able to seduce his patients into minimizing their problems after surgery. In the beginning of the 21st century, we are seeing his concept applied to selected patients with ulcerative colitis, especially if the rectum is relatively spared, is beneficial, when an individual is motivated and cooperative, and in those in the older age group.

The technical aspect of total colectomy is identical to the surgical approach described in Chapter 22. Laparoscopic total colectomy has also been advocated as a safe option in the elective case or even in acute, nonfulminant colitis.[443] Patients may be offered the option of reestablishment of intestinal continuity if the rectum is relatively free of disease. Under these circumstances, however, one must always recognize the possibility that the diagnosis may be somewhat in question. Still, if the patient subsequently is proved to have Crohn's disease, selection of this procedure might actually have been preferable. The relative merit of the ileorectal anastomosis for ulcerative colitis has diminished considerably, having been virtually replaced by the ileal pouch-anal procedures (see later discussion).

Alternatives to an ileorectal anastomosis are to either oversew the rectum or to bring out the rectosigmoid as a mucous fistula. My own preference is to close the rectal stump so that the patient will not have to contend with the profuse mucus discharge and blood that is frequently associated with a second opening on the abdominal wall. Many patients find this drainage to be more cumbersome to manage than the stoma, itself. There is the risk, however, of the stump blowing out and leaking contents into the peritoneal cavity. This is especially true when the residual bowel is severely inflamed. A reasonable compromise under the circumstances is to close the bowel in the subcutaneous tissue. If a leak occurs it can usually be addressed by simple incision and drainage on the abdominal wall. Carter and colleagues comment that exteriorization of the *closed rectal stump* is preferred to an open mucous fistula or a standard Hartmann closure.[82] It is associated with fewer pelvic septic complications, facili-

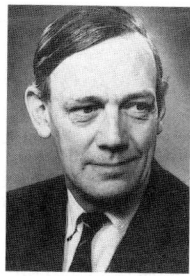

Stanley O. Aylett (1911–2003)   Stanley Aylett, the second son of a building contractor, was born in Islington, England, on July 8, 1911. He was educated at King's College, London. In 1929, he accepted a scholarship at King's College Hospital, at which institution he received a number of awards—including the prizes for anatomy, physiology, midwifery and gynecology, surgery, and surgical pathology. In 1932, he received a bachelor of science degree in physiology with first-class honors. In 1936, he was admitted to fellowship in the Royal College of Surgeons. Aylett joined the Royal Army Medical Corps during World War II and became attached to a casualty clearing station in France, treating the wounded. He was evacuated with the British Expeditionary Force from the beaches at Dunkerque. Subsequently, he served in forward field surgical units in North Africa. In 1944, he returned to England to train and command a field surgical unit in preparation for the impending invasion of Europe. He landed on D-Day plus three, attached to various casualty clearing stations, and was assigned to the relief of the Sandbostel concentration camp. He was awarded the Croix d'Honneur for services rendered to French prisoners at this camp, and in 1945 he was made a member of the Order of the British Empire for his indefatigable contributions to the care of the sick and wounded. From 1947 until his retirement, he was a consultant surgeon on the staff of the Gordon Hospital. In 1960, he was awarded a Hunterian professorship from the Royal College of Surgeons for his historic presentation on ileorectal anastomosis for ulcerative colitis. Aylett wrote numerous articles on many aspects of colon and rectal surgery, especially surgery for ulcerative colitis. In addition, he is the author of two books, *Surgery of the Rectum and Colon* and *Surgeon at War*. Many awards and honors had been bestowed on him by his colleagues all over the world, including an honorary fellowship in the American Society of Colon and Rectal Surgeons. Stanley Aylett died on January 7, 2003.

tates subsequent pelvic dissection, and is not associated with an increased activity in the retained rectum.

Another option is to perform a total abdominal proctocolectomy, removing the entire diseased bowel to the level of the levators. This then eliminates the requirement for rectal dissection at the time of the second procedure—that is, reservoir-anal anastomosis. This approach is probably not a good alternative in the emergency situation, however, when the patient is septic. One prefers not to open the extraperitoneal plains under these circumstances. Regardless, one should always divide the superior hemorrhoidal vessels in order to permit ready access to the presacral space at the subsequent operation.

Talbot and colleagues reviewed the St. Mark's Hospital experience with so-called conservative proctocolectomy.[692] This is the modification about which I just wrote, in which total abdominal proctocolectomy is performed with anal preservation. Besides the advantages of preserving the sphincters and facilitating the second operation, it does provide the opportunity to obtain a complete pathologic specimen for analysis, an important issue if Crohn's disease cannot be excluded or when there is concern for concomitant malignancy. Performing pelvic radiation in the presence of a pouch is not recommended.

Results

What is the risk for the development of cancer in the retained rectum? Aylett reported the single largest experience with ileorectal anastomosis for ulcerative colitis.[13–15] More than 400 patients underwent this operation, only 8% of whom had to undergo conversion to an ileostomy. Twelve subsequently underwent proctectomy because of carcinoma in the retained rectum.

Johnson and colleagues reported their experience with rectal preservation in patients with ulcerative colitis.[318] Of the 172 individuals who underwent subtotal colectomy and mucous fistula, more than one-half subsequently required rectal excision. In 27% the rectum remained as a mucous fistula. An additional 101 patients underwent an initial primary ileorectal anastomosis. Of the 273 at risk for rectal cancer, a malignant lesion subsequently developed in 10 (3.6%). Unfortunately, more than one half had disseminated disease at the time of rectal removal, and there were no Dukes' A lesions. The authors estimated that the cumulative probability of a cancer developing in the rectum following subtotal colectomy was 17% at 27 years from the onset of disease. Although the experience of the authors was reasonably favorable, careful endoscopic follow-up is a requisite. Others have also expressed their concern about the retained rectum after colectomy for ulcerative colitis.[369,373,386,458]

Grundfest and colleagues reviewed the Cleveland Clinic experience with 89 patients who underwent total abdominal colectomy and ileorectal anastomosis for ulcerative colitis.[235] Twenty-one percent required subsequent proctectomy, with the overall incidence of carcinoma being 4.8%. The cumulative risk for development of a rectal cancer was 12.9% (±8.3%) after 25 years, considerably less than when the colon is left intact. The authors caution that preexisting colonic cancer with severe dysplasia is a relative contraindication to rectal preservation. They also strongly recommend frequent proctosigmoidoscopy and rectal biopsy to look for dysplasia.

Khubchandani and co-workers performed a prospective study to evaluate dysplasia in 34 patients who had previously undergone colectomy and ileorectal anastomosis for IBD.[347] One patient with 23 years of disease demonstrated severe dysplasia, and subsequent proctectomy revealed carcinoma-*in-situ*. The authors recommended multiple biopsy examinations of the rectum, ideally from relatively free areas, every 6 months. If a biopsy demonstrates severe dysplasia, a repeated examination is suggested 3 months later. If sequential biopsy demonstrates severe dysplasia, excision of the rectum is recommended.

Evaluation of the rectum by means of proctosigmoidoscopy or flexible sigmoidoscopy can usually be performed relatively easily in a patient whose rectum is in continuity with the intestinal tract. However, if someone has a mucous fistula or an oversewn rectal stump, it may be impossible to pass an instrument in the disused rectum after a time. These individuals are at great risk for the development of malignancy. If continuity has not been reestablished within 2 years following colectomy, serious consideration should be given to removing the rectum. However, even after a considerable period of time following ileostomy, a restorative proctectomy may be offered. I have reestablished intestinal continuity by means of an ileal pouch-anal procedure in one patient 11 years following colectomy and ileostomy, with a satisfactory functional result.

It is difficult to comment on the relative merits of proctocolectomy and total colectomy with rectal preservation with respect to morbidity and mortality. For example, in most series experience with the latter operation suggests a much higher mortality, but these patients are often submitted to an emergency operation.[392] Farnell and colleagues reported the Mayo Clinic experience with rectal preservation in nonspecific IBD.[153] Sixty-three patients with ulcerative colitis underwent colectomy and ileorectal or ileosigmoid anastomosis. Follow-up was a minimum of 5 years, up to a maximum of 17 years. Preoperative proctoscopic examination revealed a normal rectum in slightly more than one-half of the patients. Moderate disease was present in 38%. During this interval carcinoma did not develop in the residual rectum in any patient. The requirement for subsequent proctectomy was quite similar for patients with ulcerative colitis and those with Crohn's disease (24% versus 29%, respectively). The quality of life was believed to be satisfactory in more than one-half of the patients with ulcerative colitis, but only approximately one-third of the patients with Crohn's disease were content. Early age of onset of ulcerative colitis was demonstrated to be a poor prognostic factor for subsequent rectal preservation. Conversely, patients in whom the disease developed later in life were more likely to avoid a subsequent proctectomy. Interestingly enough, the presence of moderate rectal mucosal disease did not increase the likelihood of subsequent proctectomy.

Hawley evaluated the St. Mark's Hospital experience with 125 ulcerative colitis patients who underwent colectomy and ileorectal anastomosis.[267] Subsequent excision was required in 33 (26%). A reduction in frequency of bowel movements to 6 or fewer within 24 hours was noted in 83%. Oakley and colleagues reported the Cleveland Clinic experience of 159 patients with this operation.[530,531] Subsequent proctectomy became necessary for 55%, and rectal cancer developed in 9 patients. Leijonmarck and colleagues found that 16% of their 43 patients experienced complications, with a 4% operative mortality.[394] Forty-three percent had their ileorectal anastomosis functioning at follow-up (mean observation time, 13 years). The functional outcome was better than that quoted in the literature for the pouch-anal procedures (see later discussion). Löfberg and colleagues reviewed the 46 patients who underwent this operation in Stockholm County.[425] Twenty-two (49%) subsequently underwent proctectomy for intractable symptoms and three (7%) for dysplasia. All of the remaining patients had no evidence of dysplasia, carcinoma, or DNA aneuploidy. Others have also been relatively enthusiastic in recommending ileorectal anastomosis for selected patients with IBD, but the importance of cancer surveillance must be emphasized.[296,317,322,346,387]

Comment

With ileorectal anastomosis for ulcerative colitis, I reiterate what I stated previously, that the possibility of carcinoma arising in the residual rectum is a source of great concern. If the patient truly understands this risk and is willing to submit to frequent follow-up examinations, I believe that ileorectal anastomosis should be considered for those in whom the rectum is not severely involved by inflammatory disease. However, if concern for possible development of carcinoma is sufficiently great, conventional proctocolectomy or a pouch-anal procedure should be considered.

Limited Resection

Other operations for ulcerative colitis that attempt to maintain intestinal continuity by a limited resection are poor alternatives. Segmental resection of the sigmoid colon, right colon, and so forth will result uniformly in a 100% recurrence rate that will necessitate further resection. The only exception to the admonition against this is the patient who has severe proctitis or proctosigmoiditis. In an individual incapacitated as a consequence of urgency, tenesmus, incontinence, or bleeding, an abdominoperineal resection might be considered. It is understood, however, that palliation of symptoms may not necessarily preclude the possibility of subsequent proximal disease recurrence.

Varma and colleagues reported four patients with symptomatic left-sided ulcerative colitis who were treated by resection, mucosal proctectomy, and coloanal anastomosis.[726] Within one year, recurrence developed in all, and three of them required proctocolectomy.

Ileoanal Anastomosis

Total colectomy and proctectomy, but with preservation of the anal canal and sphincter muscles, was described by Ravitch and Sabiston in 1947.[583,584] The procedure fell into disrepute primarily because of the difficulties associated

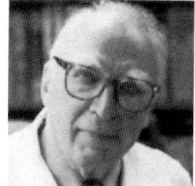

Mark M. Ravitch (1910–1989) Mark Ravitch was born in New York City, of Russian immigrant parents. He attended the University of Oklahoma and achieved a bachelor of arts degree in zoology in 1930. He spent 13 years at Johns Hopkins, first as a medical student and later as an intern and surgical resident. It was there that his extraordinary productivity in research and writing developed. He remained on the staff until 1952, at which time he assumed the position of director of surgery at the Mount Sinai Hospital in New York. He returned to Johns Hopkins, attaining the rank of professor of surgery and surgeon-in-chief at the Baltimore City Hospitals; then, in 1969, he assumed a professorship of surgery at the University of Pittsburgh. Ravitch's analysis of intussusception in infants and children led to the development of a nonoperative treatment for the disease—the use of hydrostatic pressure reduction through barium enema. In addition to the concept of ileoanal anastomosis, he suggested the technique of mucosal stripping to limit the likelihood of recurrent disease. Another of his outstanding contributions to colon and rectal surgery was the introduction and development of mechanical stapling devices in the United States. This came about as a result of his excursions to the Soviet Union; his fluency in the Russian language was in no small measure responsible for his success. Ravitch was the author or co-author of more than 450 articles and editorials, as well as 100 chapters in texts. The list of his honors and contributions encompasses a curriculum vitae of 51 pages. He died of complications related to carcinoma of the colon and prostate. (Photograph courtesy of the Department of Surgery, Montefiore Hospital, Pittsburgh, Pennsylvania.)

with frequent bowel movements and fecal incontinence. In 1977, Martin and colleagues described a procedure in children whereby the entire colon was removed in the usual manner, but the mucosa was stripped from its rectal muscular sleeve and an anastomosis effected between the ileum and the anal canal.[451] By this means, intestinal continuity was reestablished, and all the potential disease-bearing area was extirpated. This procedure is theoretically suitable for patients with ulcerative colitis and those with familial polyposis and is a popular option in the pediatric population. However, patients with Crohn's disease should not be considered for this alternative.

Operative Technique

Total colectomy is undertaken in the usual manner, and the bowel is resected in the most distal rectum. It was initially suggested that a mucosal stripping be performed and commenced at the level of the sacral promontory in order to preserve a long muscular sleeve (Figure 29-50). The dissection is facilitated, according to Ut-

sunomiya and colleagues, by the use of a balloon catheter as a rectal internal stent (Figure 29-50C).[722] Theoretically, it was believed that by preserving this sleeve the anastomosis would be protected. However, the development of complications such as "sleeve abscess," as well as the tedious dissection required, have convinced virtually all surgeons to abandon this particular approach. In current practice, one endeavors to amputate the rectum as low as is possible, removing any residual mucosa transanally. The procedure may be facilitated by infiltrating the submucosa with a dilute epinephrine solution. Because separation of the rectal mucosa may be difficult to accomplish in some patients, either because of friability or scarring, some surgeons advocate ultrasonic fragmentation and aspiration.[270,271] Others prefer to evert the anorectal remnant, exposing the mucosa and excising the stump from the dentate line to the cut edge of the rectum[217] (Figure 29-51). Other options for performing rectal mucosectomy are illustrated in Figures 29–52 and 29–53. Another preferred alternative is to employ one of

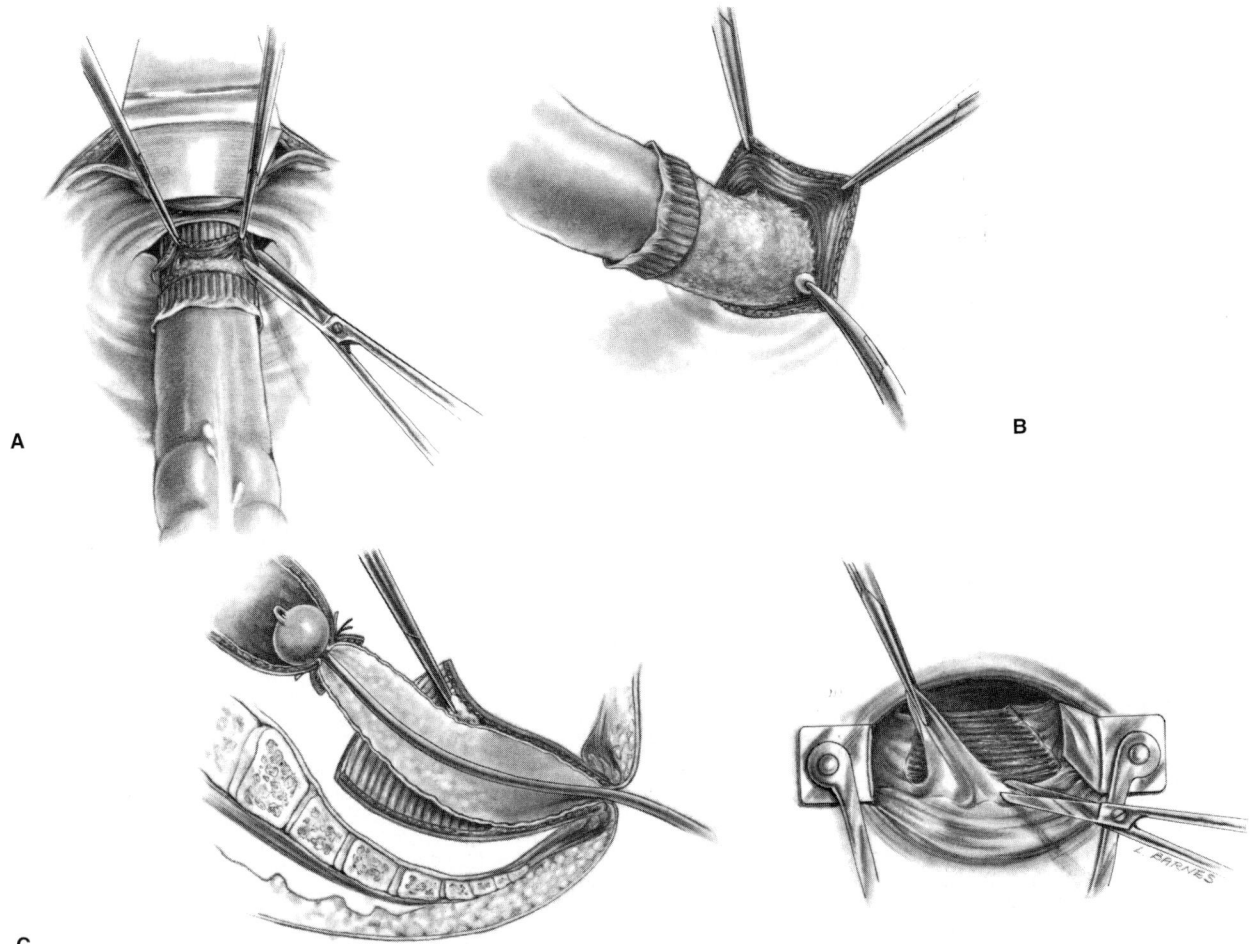

FIGURE 29-50. Classic rectal mucosal stripping. **(A)** Beginning at the top of the rectum, **(B)** completed from above, and **(C)** facilitated by internal stent. **(D)** By perineal route.

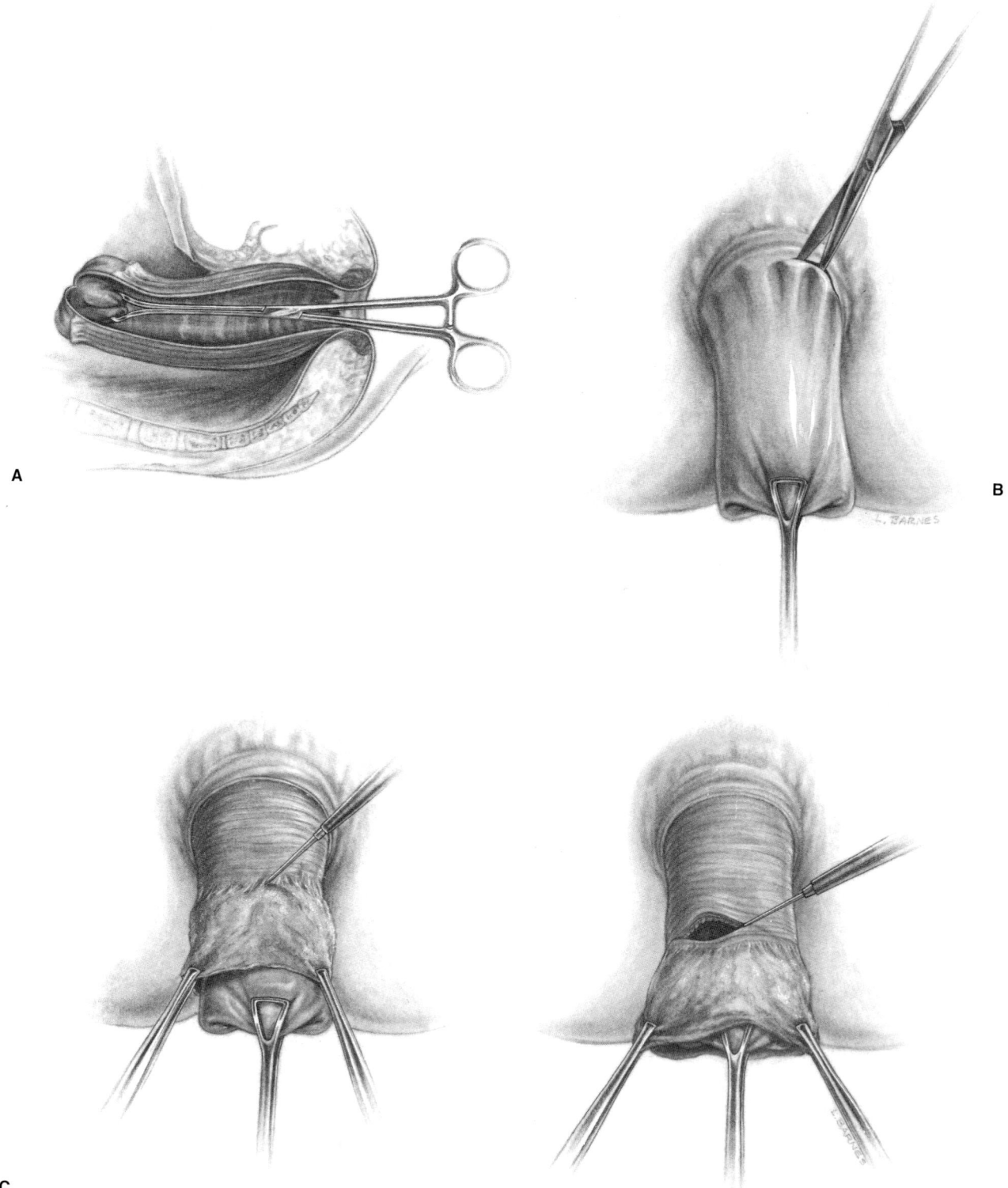

FIGURE 29-51. Technique of eversion mucosectomy. **(A)** The rectal stump is everted by placing a clamp on the proximal end. **(B)** Mucosal stripping is begun from the dentate line. **(C)** Mucosa is stripped using diathermy cautery or by scissors dissection. **(D)** The mucosa and redundant muscular sleeve are excised.

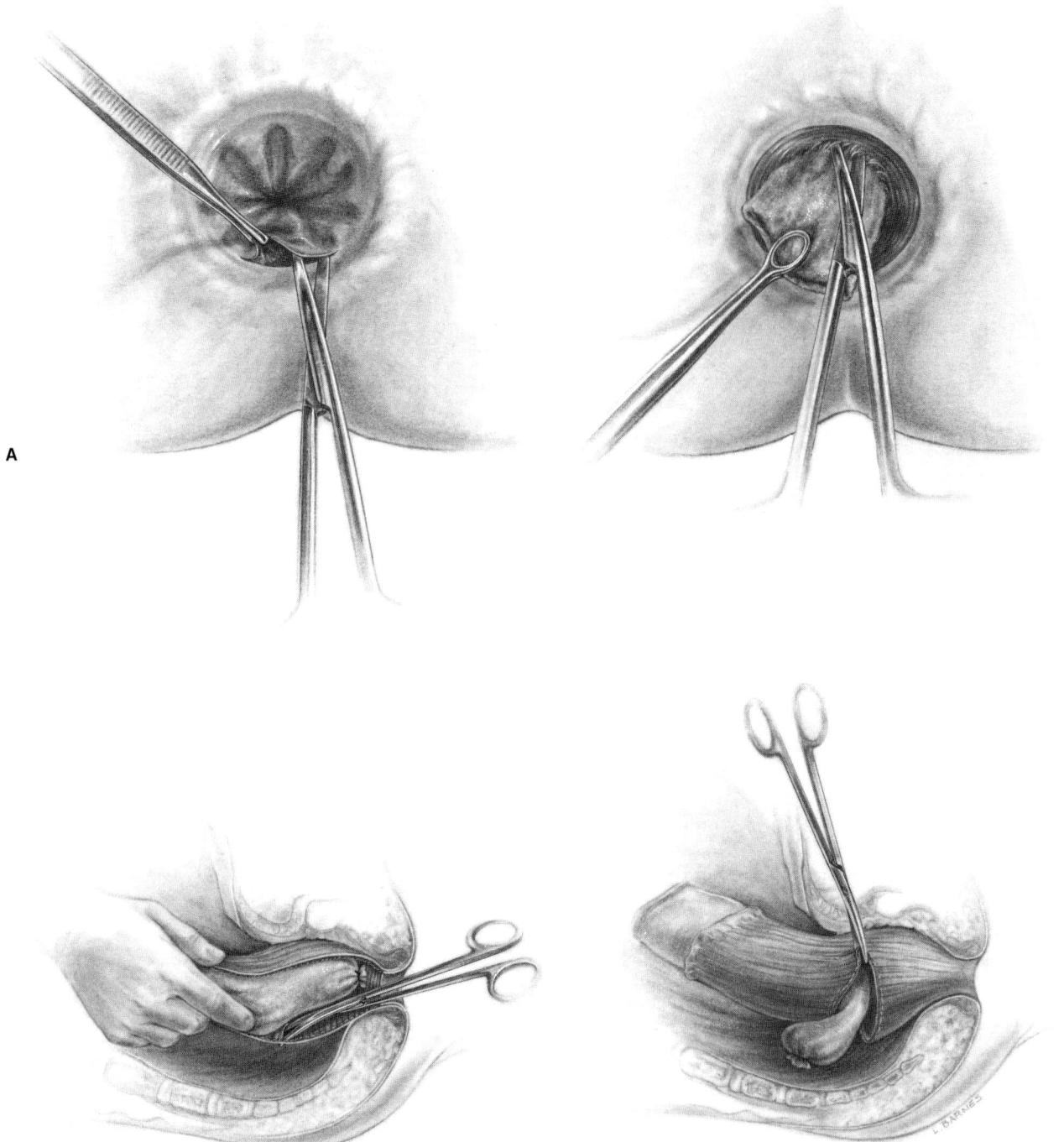

FIGURE 29-52. Rectal mucosectomy. **(A)** Circumferential incision at the level of the dentate line. **(B)** Elevation of mucosa and submucosa from the underlying internal sphincter. **(C)** Division of the muscular sleeve by the perineal surgeon. **(D)** Bowel and stripped mucosa are resected.

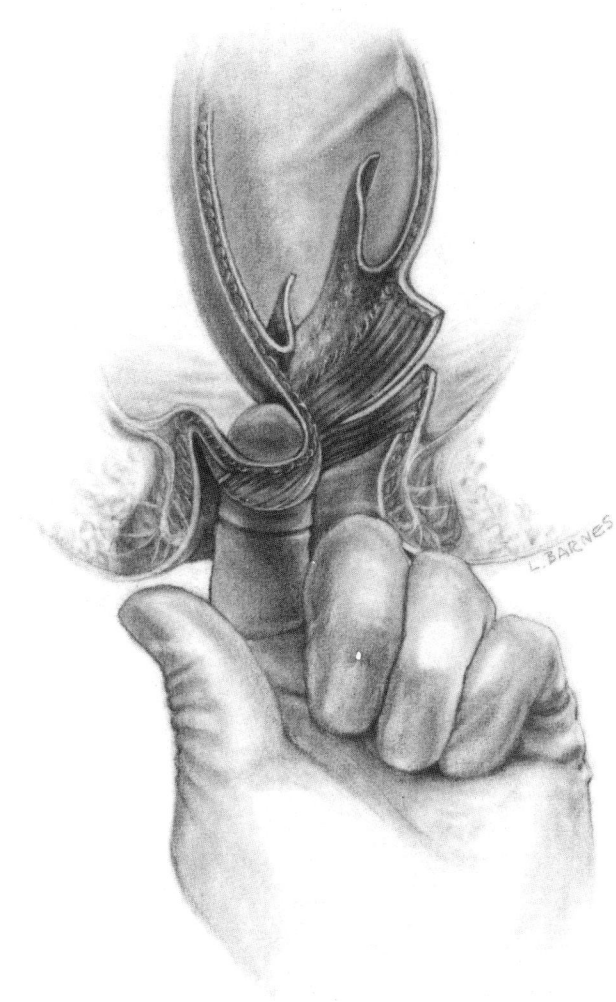

FIGURE 29-53. Rectal mucosectomy. Lateral rectal attachments are divided by the perineal surgeon.

the modifications of the double-stapling technique (see later discussion).

The ileal anastomosis is effected at the level of the dentate line using paired Gelpi retractors or an anal retractor (e.g., Parks, Lone Star; see Figs. 29-84 and 29-85) for exposure. Interrupted 3–0 long-term absorbable sutures are suggested, to anchor the end of the ileum to the anal canal and underlying internal sphincter (Figure 29-54). A loop ileostomy is virtually always advised (see Figs. 31-67 through 31-69).

Results

Very little current data are available for a straight ileoanal anastomosis, because the modification that incorporates an intervening pouch has made this operation practically obsolete except in children (see later discussion).[103,547,701] Utsunomiya and colleagues reported a few patients who underwent the procedure, but in the same article they describe a technique with an intervening pouch.[722] It is difficult to interpret the results because of the multiplicity of techniques used.

Beart and colleagues reported the Mayo Clinic experience with 50 patients who underwent total abdominal colectomy, excision of the rectal mucosa, and ileoanal anastomosis.[34] Forty-one were operated on for chronic ulcerative colitis; familial polyposis was the diagnosis in seven patients, and Crohn's disease in two. The authors emphasized the importance of meticulous hemostasis, preservation of the anoderm, careful stripping of all the rectal mucosa, and avoidance of tension on the suture line. A number of these patients had an intervening reservoir. Forty-two individuals had reestablishment of intestinal continuity by closure of the ileostomy, and no deaths occurred in the series. Two had anastomotic strictures requiring conversion to an ileostomy. Nine additional patients were dissatisfied because of intolerable stool frequency and were converted to either a continent ileostomy (Kock pouch—see later discussion) or a conventional ileostomy. In the remaining 30 individuals, stool frequency averaged 8 per day, and most required "slowing" medications.

Heppell and colleagues reviewed 12 of these patients at least 4 months after the procedure by means of physiologic studies.[277] Anal sphincter resting pressure and squeeze pressure of those who underwent the procedure were similar to that of healthy controls, although the rectal inhibitory reflex was absent. The greater the capacity of the new rectum, the fewer the number of bowel movements. Although the operation did indeed preserve the anal sphincter, the decreased capacity and compliance of the distal bowel impaired continence.

Coran reported the procedure in 36 children and adults with ulcerative colitis and familial polyposis.[102] Four patients were subsequently converted to an ileostomy. The median stool frequency was 7 per 24 hours. This was interpreted by the author to be an encouraging result. A later report by the same author of 100 patients (79 with ulcerative colitis) revealed comparable functional results (7.7 within 24 hours).[103] Interestingly, there was no statistically significant difference in stool frequency when the age of the patients was compared. Five required conversion to a conventional ileostomy. Morgan and colleagues evaluated 60 individuals with ulcerative colitis and multiple polyposis who had undergone endoanal anastomosis following total proctocolectomy.[494] Stool frequency after 3 years of follow-up was in excess of 8 per 24 hours. Data in children from the Mayo Clinic demonstrate that clinical results with respect to stool frequency and especially nighttime soiling are better with a J-pouch than with a straight ileoanal anastomosis.[547,701]

Nelson and colleagues describe converting the straight ileoanal procedure to a reservoir by means of a long, side-to-side ileal anastomosis, somewhat like that described

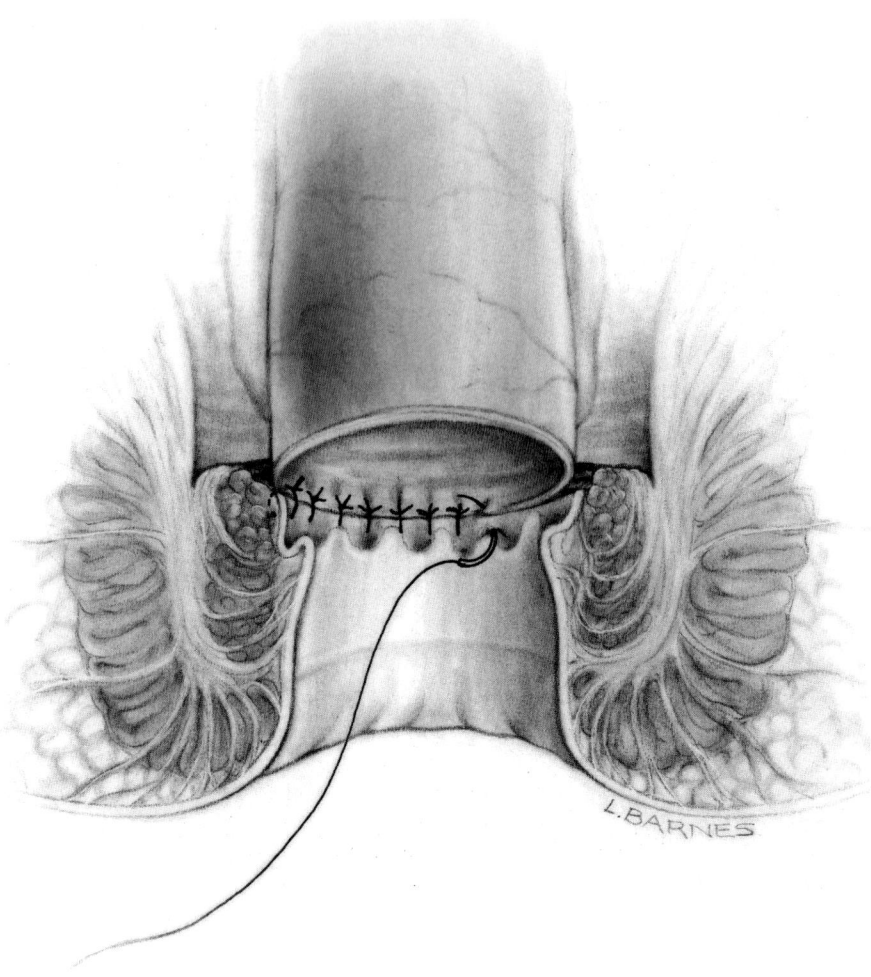

FIGURE 29-54. Endoanal, hand-sewn anastomotic technique. Paired Gelpi, Lone Star, or Parks retractors facilitate the exposure.

by Fonkalsrud (see Figure 29-100).[511] The distal ileum is folded over itself so that the point of division reaches down into the pelvis. The authors reported a favorable experience with three patients.

Comment

The straight ileoanal anastomosis permits reestablishment of intestinal continuity, but with the distinct disadvantage of frequent bowel movements. It requires great motivation indeed on the part of the patient to avoid an ileostomy and be willing to accept seven or more bowel movements per day. One wonders how many bowel movements the patient had preoperatively! In any event, further discussion appears moot. Witness the Mayo Clinic experience and their concern about the decreased reservoir function of the rectum. They have abandoned this procedure in favor of the ileoanal anastomosis with intervening pouch.

Continent Ileostomy or Kock Pouch Procedure

It is self-evident that many patients are dissatisfied with the encumbrance and emotional burden of wearing an ileostomy appliance. In 1969, Kock described a method

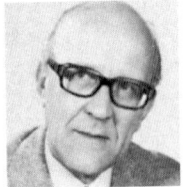

Nils G. Kock (1924–present) Nils Kock was born in Jacobstad, Finland. Following military service with the Finnish army during World War II, he entered the University of Helsinki medical school, graduating in 1951. He began his surgical residency in Finland and then spent 5 years in surgical training at the University of Göteborg in Sweden, the institution with which he remained affiliated for his entire professional career. In 1959, he earned a Ph.D. from the University of Göteborg and assumed the position of assistant professor of surgery. A series of promotions followed that culminated in his appointment in 1974 as a professor of surgery at Göteborg and chairman of the department of surgery of Sahlgren Hospital. In 1969, Kock published an article based on extensive laboratory and clinical work: a method for achieving fecal "continence" by means of an intraabdominal reservoir. For this he attained what many surgeons consider the pinnacle of success—an operation is eponymously associated with his name. In retirement, he continues to maintain a busy animal laboratory, developing techniques for dealing with a host of problems—including that of bowel and urinary conduits.

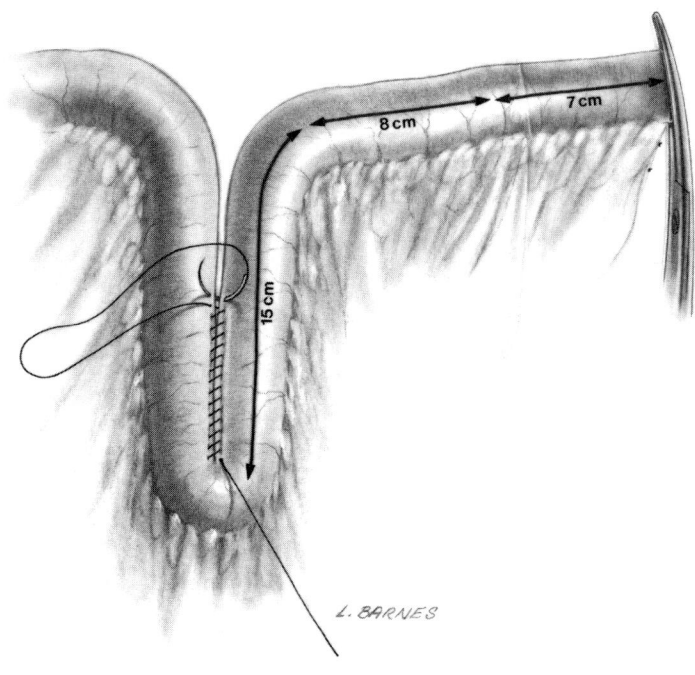

FIGURE 29-55. Continent ileostomy. Apposition of the bowel.

of creating a reservoir from the terminal ileum and subsequently modified it to create an intestinal obstruction by means of an intussuscepted portion of distal ileum, the so-called nipple valve.[359-361] Because no appliance is required, the stoma can be placed quite low on the abdominal wall and essentially flush with the skin. The procedure had been enthusiastically received, but in recent years it has been applied primarily in those for whom pouch-anal operations have failed or are inappropriate, or the rare individual who had previously undergone proctocolectomy and conventional ileostomy and wishes to have the stoma revised.

Technique

Traditional. There are two basic techniques that may be employed for constructing the reservoir. One is analogous to the *S*-shaped reservoir, such as is described for the Parks procedure (see Figs. 29-82 and 29-83). This method uses approximately 10 cm of ileum for each segment (three in all to create the pouch). An additional 18 to 20 cm is required to create the nipple valve and the conduit.

The Kock technique involves preparation of approximately a 50-cm segment of terminal ileum. A 30-cm segment is used to create the pouch and the remainder to make the valve and the external conduit. Figures 29-55 through 29-63 illustrate the procedure for preparing the continent (reservoir) ileostomy. An alternative to the conventional suturing method is to staple the pouch. This approach is illustrated in Figures 29-64

through 29-66. Another modification is shown later in Figure 29-102.

Before the ileostomy is "matured," the competence of the nipple valve should be tested by occluding the afferent limb with a rubber-shod clamp. A catheter is then inserted through the nipple valve into the reservoir, and the pouch is inflated with air. If the air fails to escape following catheter removal, one may assume that the valve is competent. The catheter is then replaced into the reservoir, and the air should dissipate. The completed reservoir is shown in Figure 29-67.

Modifications. The major problem with the Kock procedure is to maintain the position of the nipple. Slippage is attributed to traction forces on the mesentery of the nipple during filling of the reservoir.[144] Modifications have been proposed to address this complication, including implantation of Mersilene mesh to reinforce the nipple,[32] magnetic closure using the Maclet device,[625] stripping of the serosa, and even creation of a protecting loop ileostomy above the reservoir.[298] Bokey and Fazio have suggested the use of a fascial sling threaded through the mesentery.[59] Gerber and colleagues and others recommend encircling the ileal outlet with a 1-cm strip of Marlex mesh or Teflon (passed through the mesentery of the reservoir and outlet), although this can cause other problems (e.g., a fistula).[202,690,702] A combination of triangular stripping of the mesenteric fat, serosal scarification, and rotation of the nipple valve segments has been demonstrably safe and quite

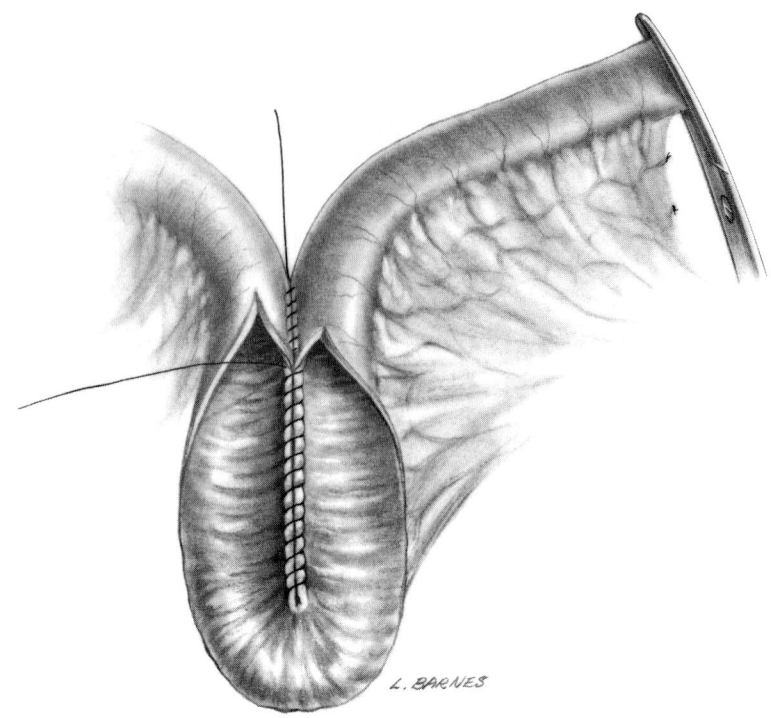

FIGURE 29-56. Continent ileostomy. Bowel opened and posterior row completed.

effective for preventing nipple desusception according to some surgeons.[301] Harford suggests the use of the Cavitational Ultrasonic Surgical Aspirator (CUSA, Valleylab Inc., Boulder, Colorado) to strip the mesentery and remove the fat.[255] Ecker and co-workers used the approach of ultrasonic mucosectomy in the area of the attached mesentery of the nipple and posterior wall of

the pouch.[144] Additionally, two continuous sutures of nylon are employed, through all the layers of the bowel on both sides of the main mesenteric vessels. Fazio and Tjandra describe a technique that the Cleveland Clinic group now prefers.[163] This involves anchoring the nipple valve to the anterior pouch wall by stapling. A 2-cm

(text continues on page 1391)

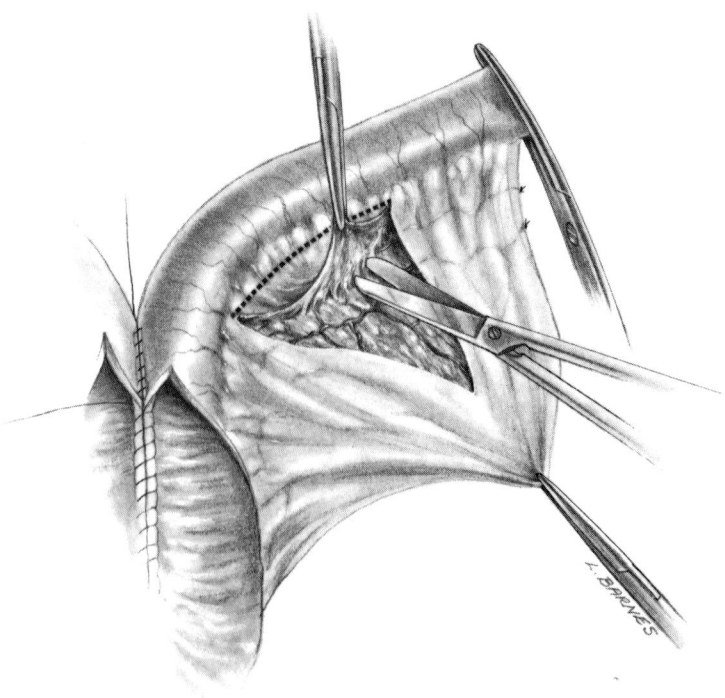

FIGURE 29-57. Continent ileostomy. Excision of peritoneal leaves and defatting of mesentery.

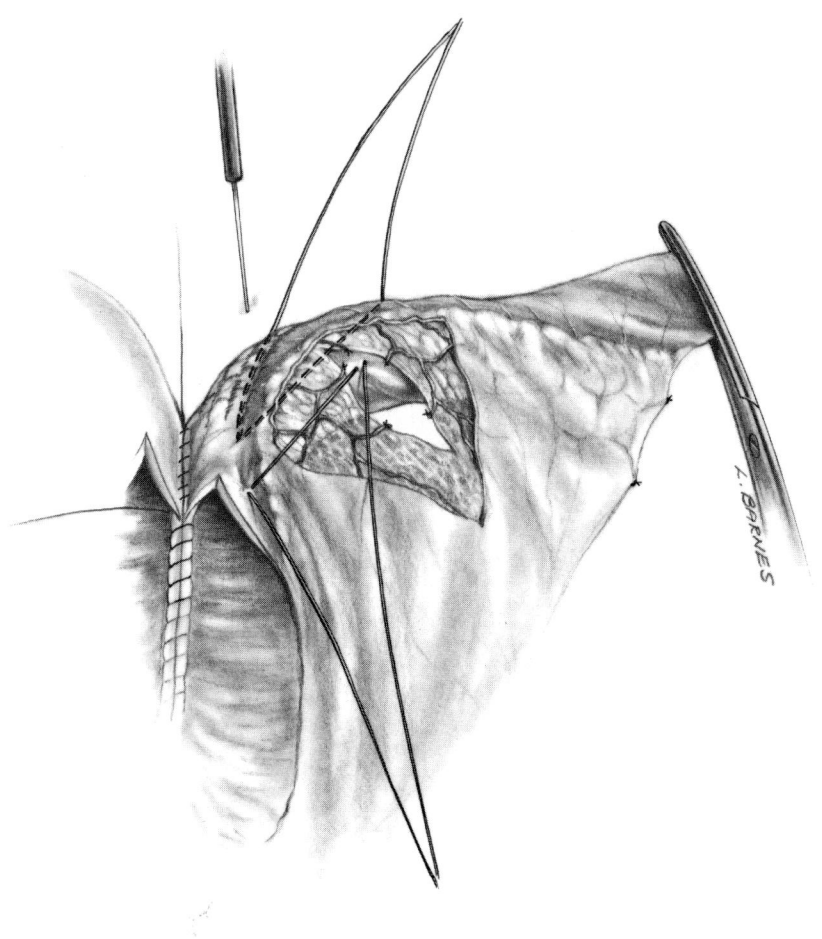

FIGURE 29-58. Continent ileostomy. Cauterization or stripping of the ileal serosa and placement of sutures to rotate the mesentery 90 degrees.

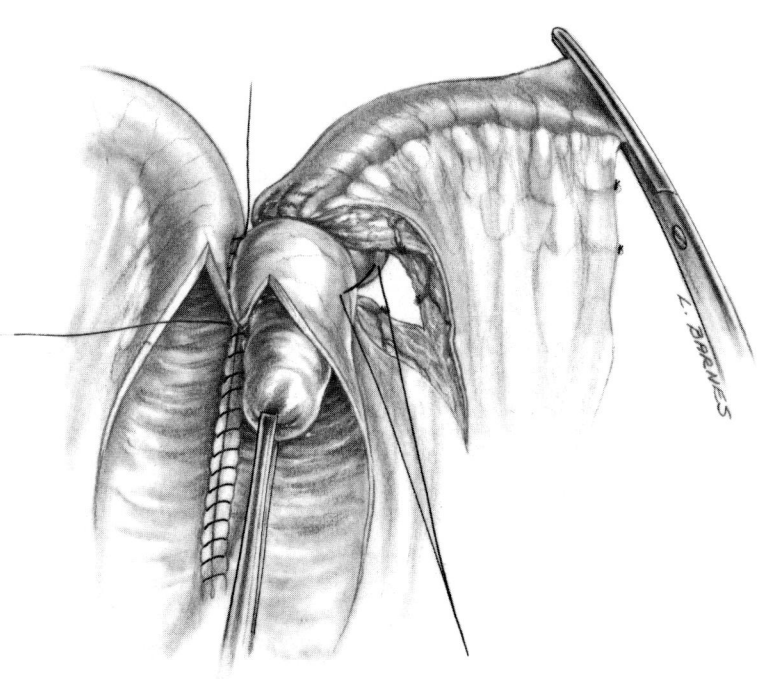

FIGURE 29-59. Continent ileostomy. A nipple is created and sutures are secured.

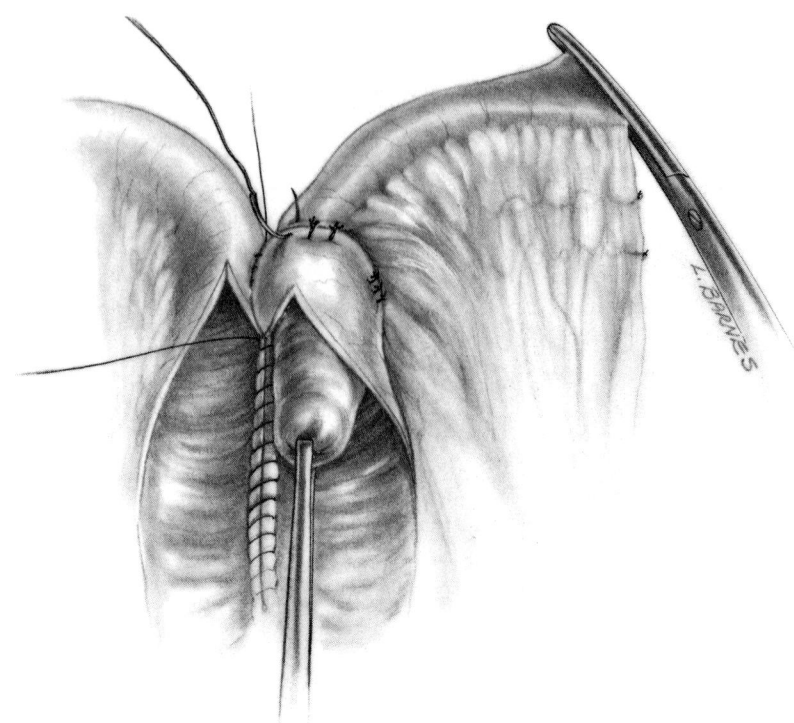

FIGURE 29-60. Continent ileostomy. Silk sutures are placed from conduit to reservoir.

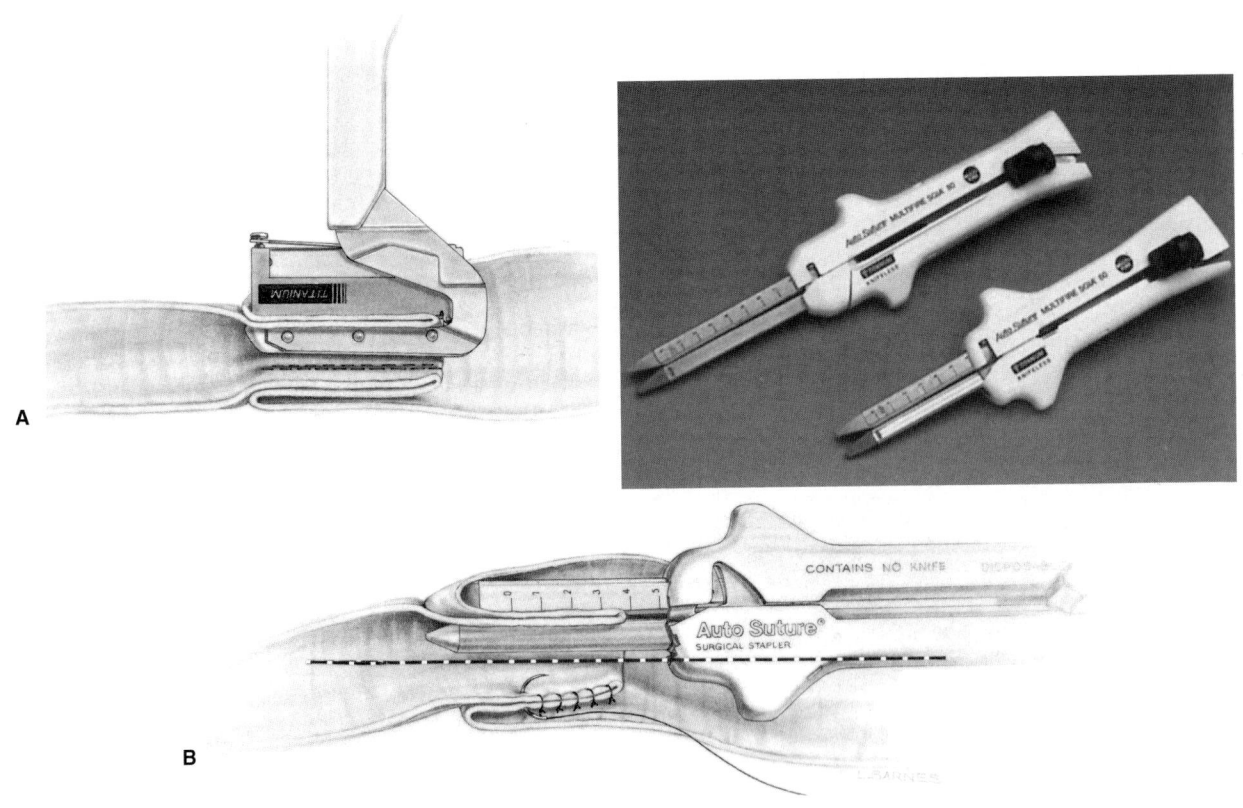

FIGURE 29-61. Continent ileostomy. **(A)** Application of the linear stapler to three areas in the nipple
valve to prevent desussception. **(B)** Alternatively, one may use an SGIA-60 stapler (without the blade)
or simple sutures. The instruments without the knife are available in two sizes **(inset)**. (Courtesy of
United States Surgical Corp., Norwalk, CT.)

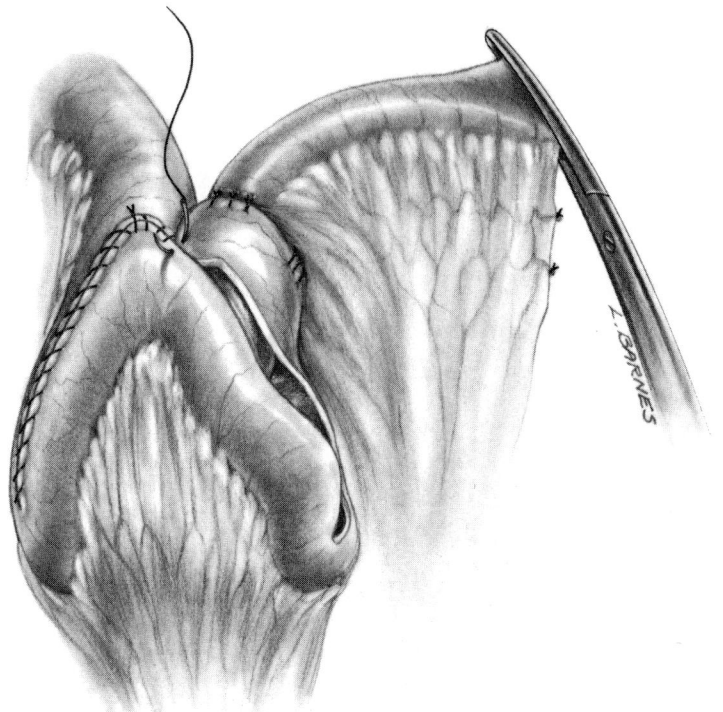

FIGURE 29-62. Continent ileostomy. The reservoir is closed by folding over.

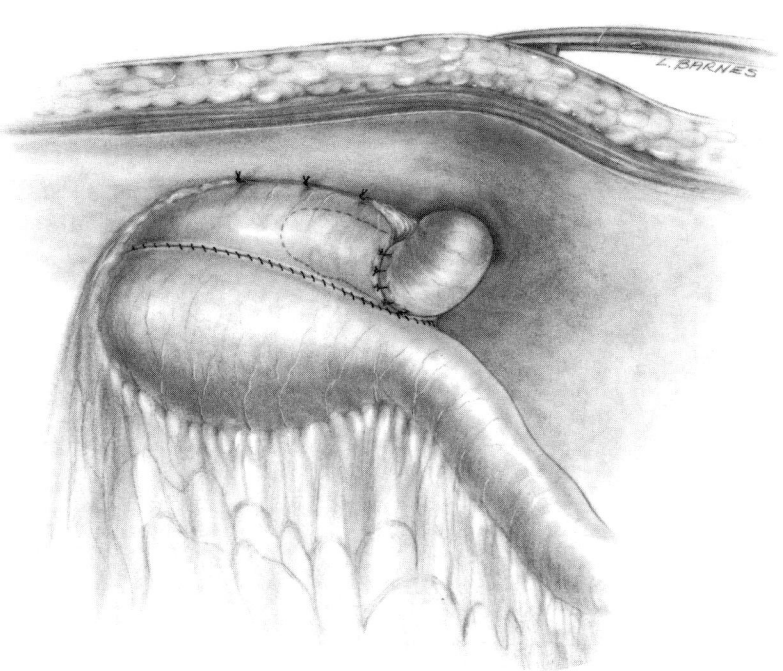

FIGURE 29-63. Continent ileostomy. The reservoir is anchored to the abdominal wall after the conduit has been brought through the opening. The ileostomy opening is usually placed low in the abdomen.

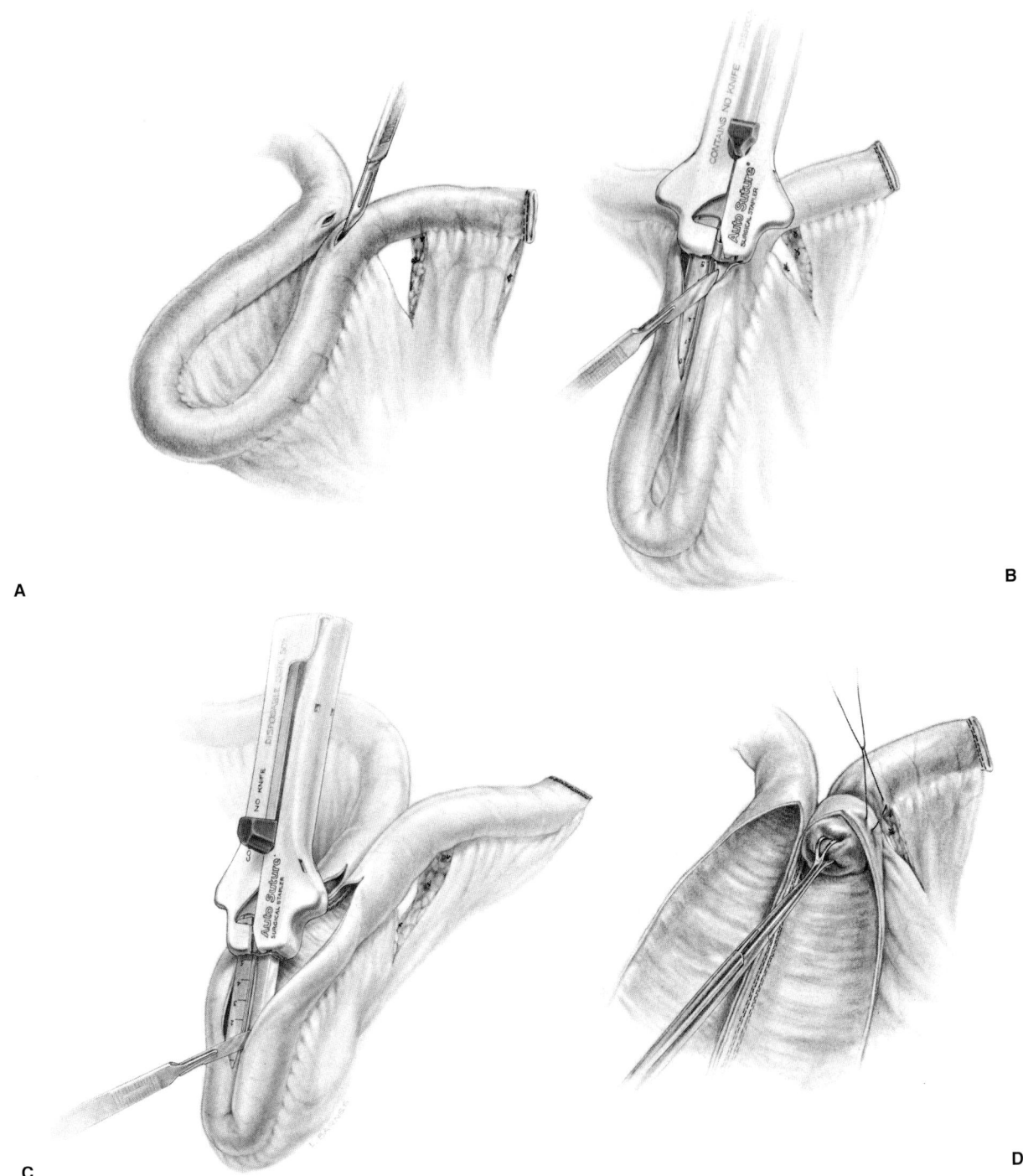

A

B

C

D

FIGURE 29-64. Stapled continent ileostomy (Kock). **(A)** Two enterotomies are created. **(B)** Insertion of SGIA stapler (without the knife blade). Bowel is incised on the instrument. **(C)** Second passage of SGIA stapler with incision of the bowel (third insertion may be required). **(D)** Distal ileum is intussuscepted.

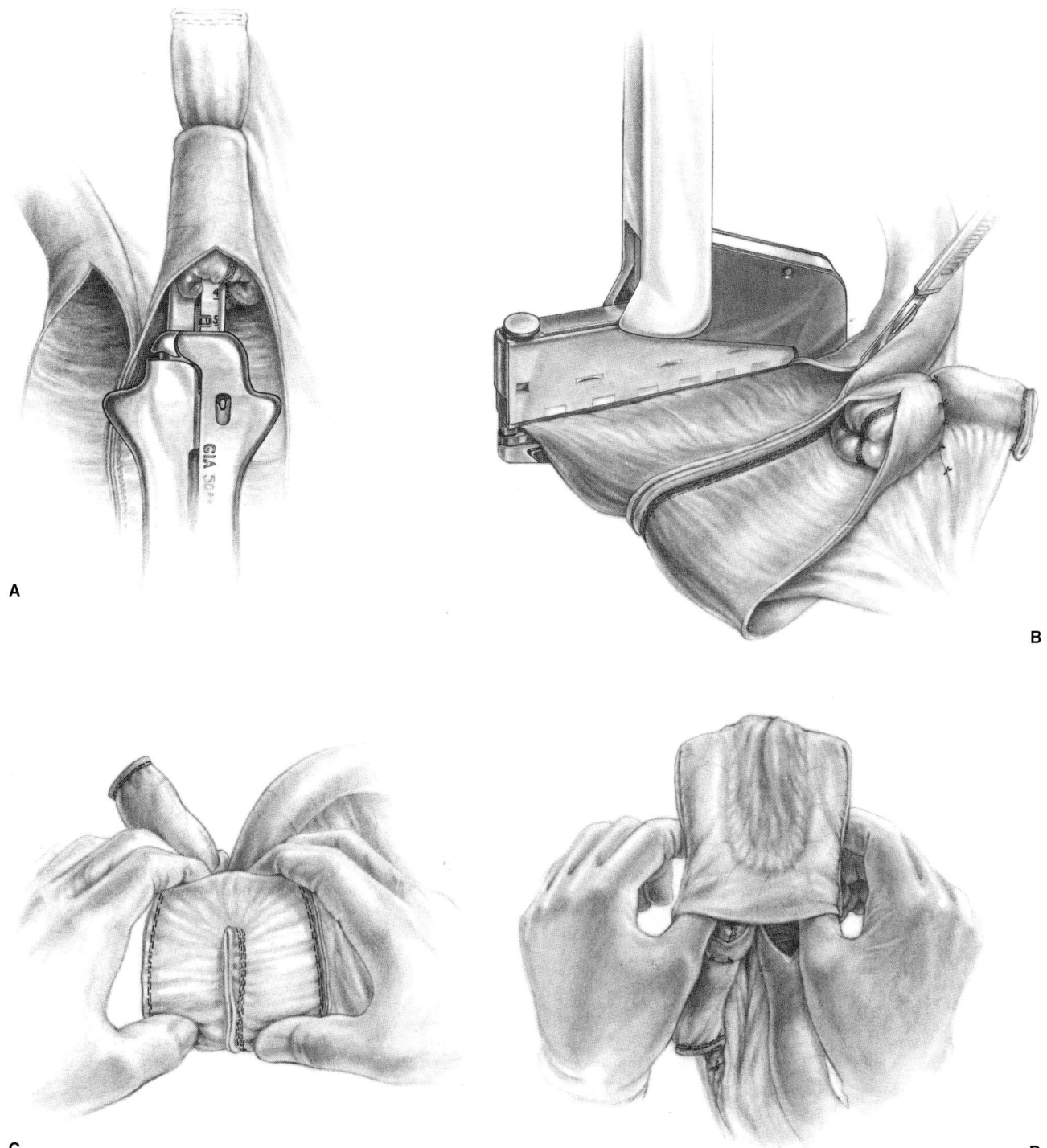

FIGURE 29-65. Stapled continent ileostomy (Kock). **(A)** Nipple valve stapled. **(B)** Long linear stapler (TA-90) secures opposing walls of the bowel. Staple lines are within the pouch. **(C,D)** Pouch is reinverted.

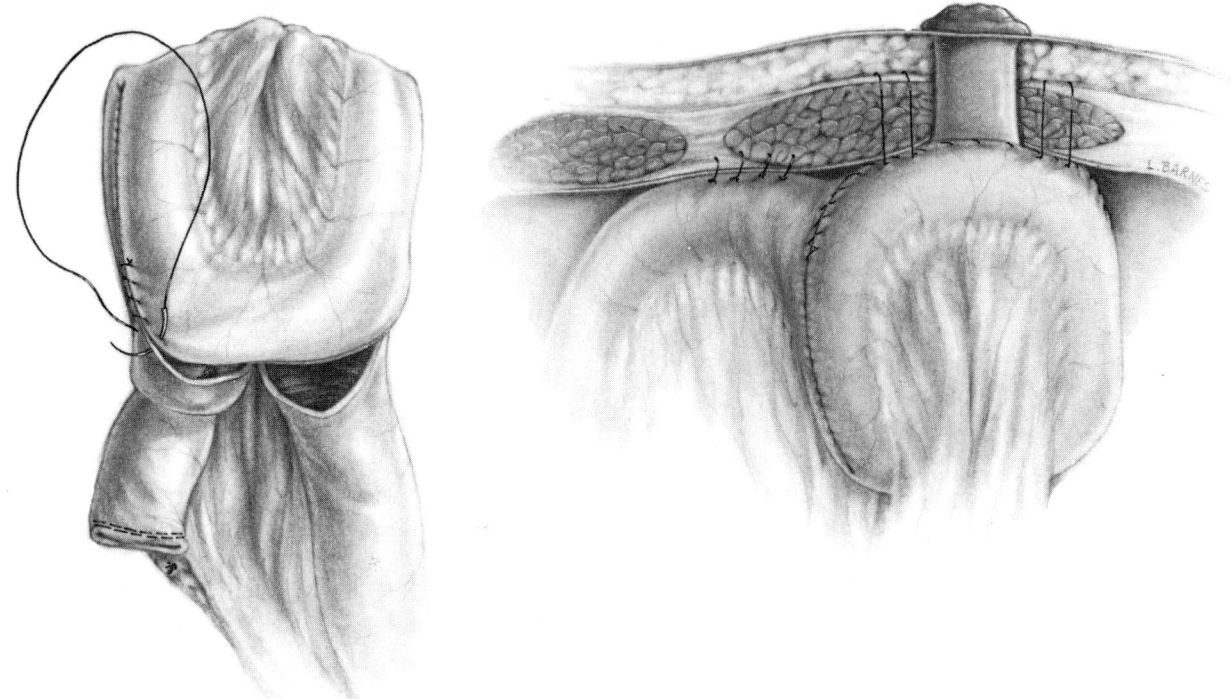

A

B

FIGURE 29-66. Stapled continent ileostomy (Kock). **(A)** Manual suture closure of defect. **(B)** Completed pouch.

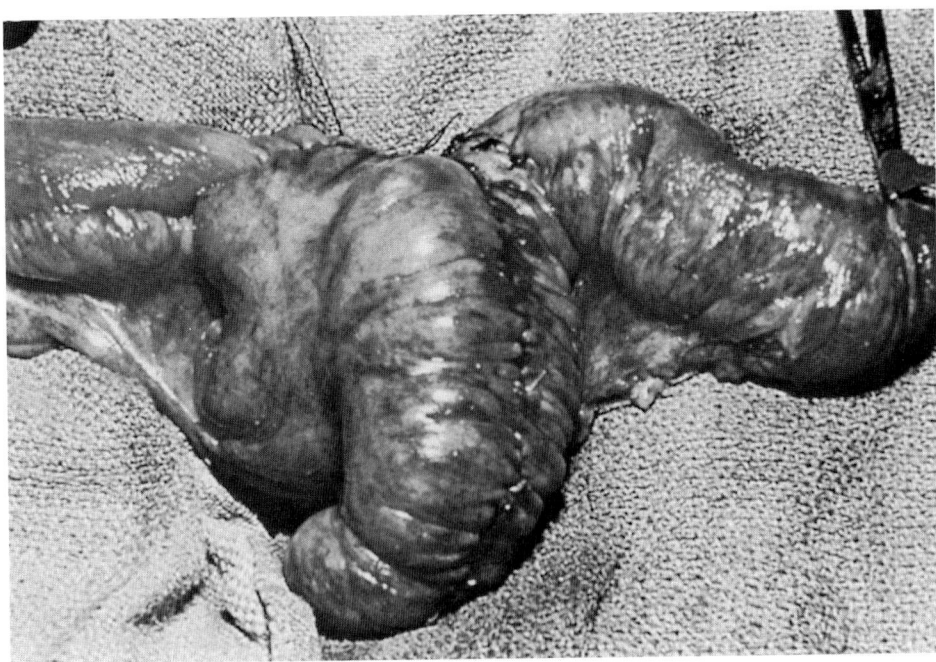

FIGURE 29-67. Continent ileostomy. Completed reservoir and nipple.

transverse enterotomy is made in the anterior pouch wall just below the point where the intussuscepted nipple lies. The valve is then aligned with the anterior pouch wall away from the primary anterior suture line, and a single application of the linear stapler is used to anchor the nipple valve to the anterior pouch wall. The anvil of the stapler is brought through the transverse enterotomy from outside the pouch to pass along the inside of the nipple valve, thereby effecting a stapled anchorage.[163] The anterior pouch wall and the enterotomy are then closed.

Barnett. Barnett undertook a modification for preventing desusception that uses an adjacent segment of intestine to encircle the base of the valve as a "collar," a maneuver analogous to that of a Nissen gastric fundoplication.[27] The lumen of the intestinal "collar" communicates with the pouch itself, allowing gas and fecal contents to enter. This acts to buttress the nipple valve and conduit, providing a greater degree of security against leakage. The technique is briefly described in Figure 29-68.

T-Pouch. Because of the high revision rate for valve failure and the oft requirement for frequent operations, even when applied to urologic conduits, a new type of pouch was developed in 1998 by Stein and associates as a neobladder (University of Southern California), the T-pouch.[672] It does not rely on an intussuscepted valve, which means it cannot come apart. Kaiser and colleagues, in their preliminary report involving six patients, have described their technique with this design as a continent ileostomy.[327] The procedure is illustrated in Figure 29-69.

Postoperative Care

Before leaving the operating room, the surgeon places a heavy silk suture around a Silastic catheter (Weber and Judd, Barlow Plaza, Rochester, Minnesota.) that has been inserted into the pouch. This is secured to the skin, and a dressing is applied in such a manner that the catheter exits upward and gently curves into a drainage tube, and then into a drainable bag. The straight exit of the catheter minimizes the risk for necrosis of the conduit should the catheter be under tension on one side. The dressing is left in place for 72 hours before the stoma is examined. An alternative is to use a Marlen continent ileostomy drainage system (Figure 29-70). The catheter can also be held in place by passing it through one of the perforations in a latex band, the type that is often used as a leg strap for a urine or

bile bag.[240] The Cleveland Clinic method is illustrated in Figure 32-3.

Usually, there will be only serosanguineous drainage for the first several days, but eventually this becomes bile-stained and then feculent. The patient is then started on a progressive schedule of oral intake, although a low-residue diet is suggested to avoid plugging of the catheter. The drainage tube remains in place for 3 weeks, after which the patient is advised to clamp it for 10 to 15 minutes every 3 or 4 hours. During the night, it is left to drain continuously. After 1 month intermittent catheterization is advised, initially every 3 or 4 hours, and usually once during the night. After approximately 1 week of this regimen, nightly intubations are omitted and the interval for catheterization during the day is extended. Ultimately, the patient develops a time frequency based on convenience and the feeling of fullness that compels one to drain the reservoir. However, because radiologic studies reveal that reflux into the afferent limb increases with sensations of fullness and abdominal pressure, the patient should probably empty the reservoir at regular intervals.[48]

Some continent ileostomy catheters are shown in Figure 29-71. Occasionally, formed fecal material and high-residue items (e.g., popcorn, mushrooms) require irrigation by means of a syringe, but this is usually unnecessary. A simple dressing is placed over the flush stoma, or one of the commercially available security pouches may be used.

Complications

Anastomotic Leak. The greatest concern in the postoperative period is the possibility of leakage from one of the reservoir suture lines. Obviously, this can be of catastrophic consequence, requiring emergency surgical intervention. Initially, this complication was reported very commonly. The reduced incidence can be attributed to the improved techniques of reservoir construction and the careful selection of patients who undergo this procedure.

If surgical intervention becomes necessary in the immediate postoperative period for presumed suture-line leakage, every attempt should be made to preserve the ileal reservoir. This can usually be accomplished by a diverting proximal loop ileostomy and appropriate surgical drainage with or without closure of the leak. Subsequent radiologic investigation may reveal that the fistula spontaneously closed even without repair.

However, if it appears that the reservoir is beyond salvation, it must be resected and a neoileostomy created. If the patient has undergone a procedure for what subsequently proves to be Crohn's disease, a suture-line leak

(text continues on page 1395)

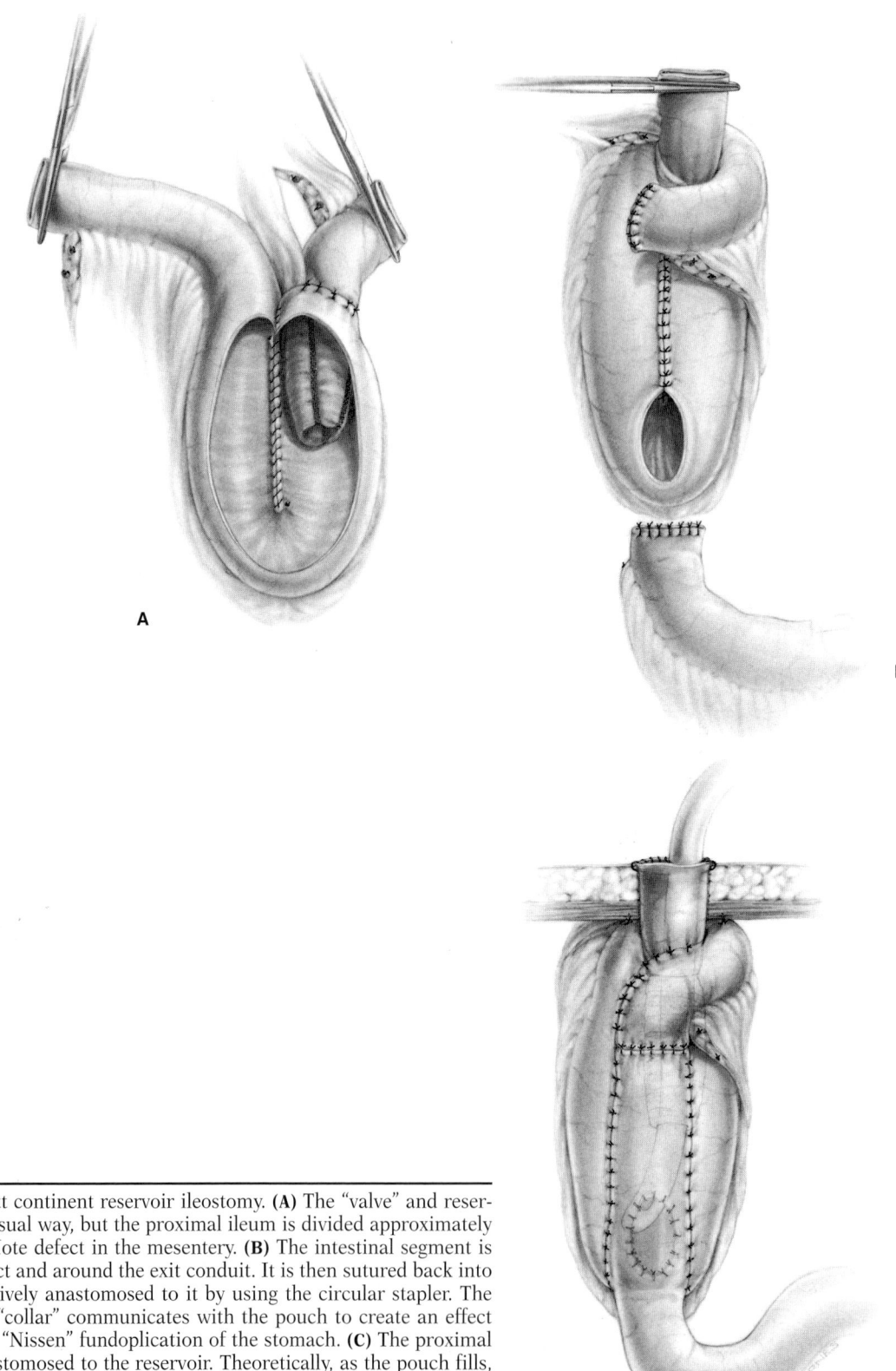

FIGURE 29-68. Barnett continent reservoir ileostomy. **(A)** The "valve" and reservoir are created in the usual way, but the proximal ileum is divided approximately 8 cm from the pouch. Note defect in the mesentery. **(B)** The intestinal segment is passed through the defect and around the exit conduit. It is then sutured back into the reservoir or alternatively anastomosed to it by using the circular stapler. The lumen of the intestinal "collar" communicates with the pouch to create an effect analogous to that of the "Nissen" fundoplication of the stomach. **(C)** The proximal small bowel is then anastomosed to the reservoir. Theoretically, as the pouch fills, the "collar" tenses with intestinal contents, and a greater degree of continence is achieved.

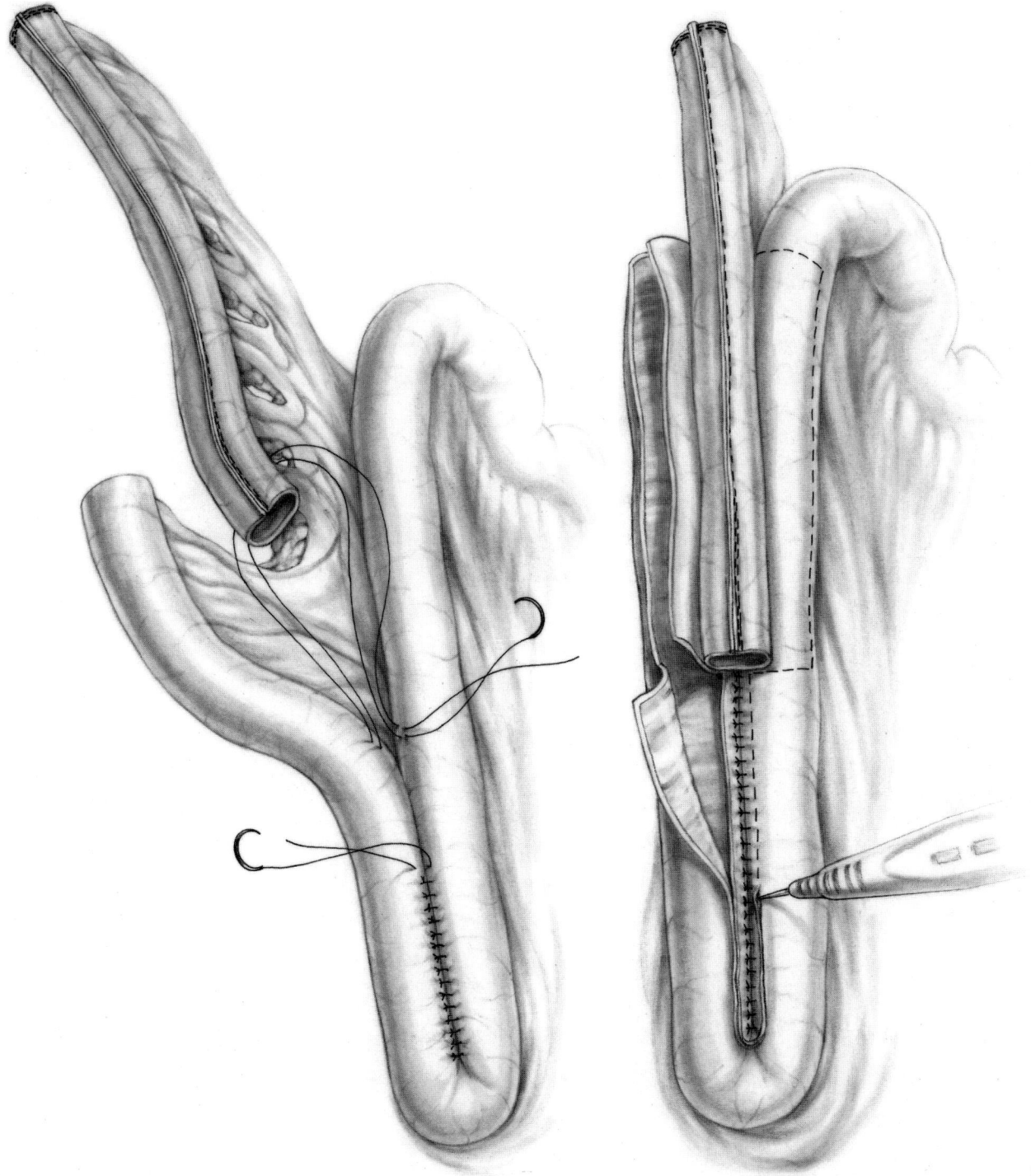

A
B

FIGURE 29-69. T-pouch. **(A)** Creation of the valve's back wall. The vascular arcades of the valve segment are preserved, but in between, the avascular mesenteric windows are opened **(inset)**. The whole segment is tapered on its antimesenteric side by means of a multifire gastrointestinal anastomosis (GIA) instrument. A series of interrupted seromuscular sutures approximate the serosa of the two adjacent segments of the **U** by passing through the previously opened avascular windows. The remaining base portion of the ileal **U** is closed with a running suture. **(B)** Preparation of the valve segment. The two limbs of the bowel **U** are opened along the seromuscular suture line on their mesenteric side up to the inner valve ostium, and then extending laterally to the antimesenteric border to provide wide flaps. *(continued)*

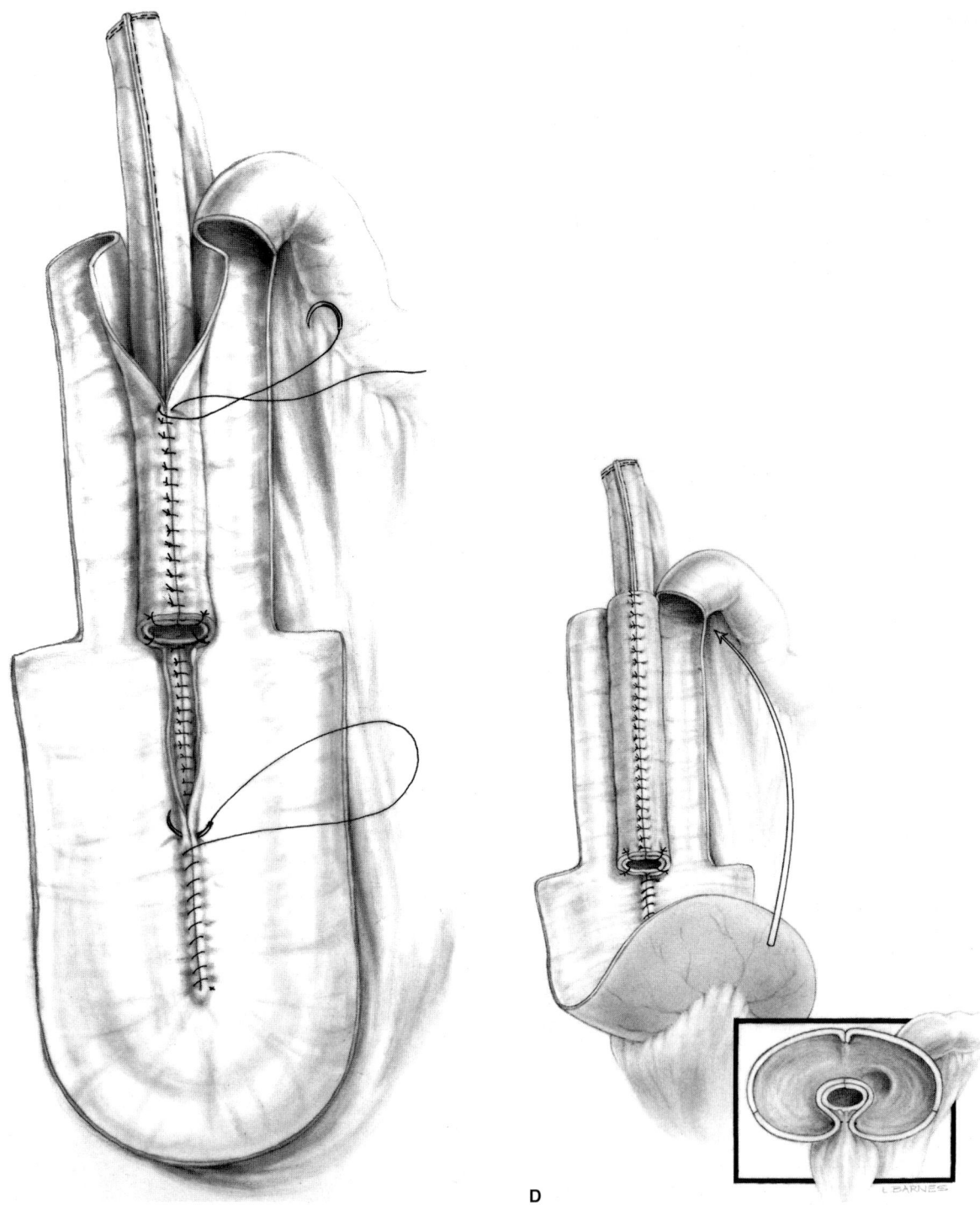

C   **D**   **E**

FIGURE 29-69. *(continued)* **(C)** Completion of the antireflux valve. The two flaps are brought over the interposed ileal segment to create the antireflux mechanism. The inner valve ostium is matured with interrupted sutures, and running sutures are used to accomplish a mucosal continuity between the two bowel areas. **(D)** Formation of the pouch reservoir. The ileal **U** is folded in half and its apex is approximated to the base of the pouch where the valve originates. The pouch construction is completed by closing both sides with running sutures. **(E)** Cross-section through completed T-pouch demonstrates the antireflux mechanism, with the isolated valve segment and maintained blood supply lying within a serosa-lined tunnel of the pouch reservoir that results in a flap-valve mechanism. (After Kaiser AM, Stein JP, Beart RW Jr. T-Pouch: a new valve design for a continent ileostomy. *Dis Colon Rectum* 2002;45:411.)

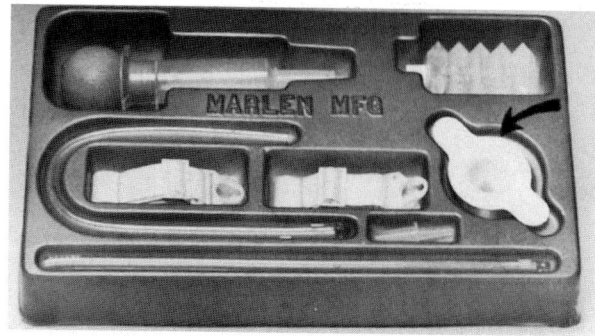

FIGURE 29-70. The continent ostomy set includes catheters, lubricant, belts, irrigating syringe, and a device for immediate postoperative support of the catheter *(arrow)*. (Courtesy of Marlen Manufacturing and Development Co., Bedford, OH.)

has an ominous prognosis indeed. Under such circumstances, it is probably the wiser course to remove the pouch and to create a new ileostomy.

Late complications of the continent ileostomy procedure are numerous and include fecal incontinence resulting from reduction of the nipple valve, ileitis ("pouchitis"), recurrent Crohn's disease, catheter perforation, pouch fistula, detachment of the pouch from the abdominal wall, volvulus of the reservoir, urolithiasis, obstruction from inspissated material, stomal stenosis, and intestinal obstruction from a lost catheter (Figs. 29-72 and 29-73).

Nipple Valve Complications—Slippage and Incontinence, Outlet Obstruction, Fistula. As previously stated, the complication associated with reduction of the nipple valve and resultant incontinence is the most troublesome and most frequently observed late management problem (Fig. 29-74). Difficulty with intubation of the reservoir is suggestive of desusception. The kinking of the intraabdominal portion of the distal ileum may in itself create a partial small-bowel obstruction. Usually, however, under these circumstances the patient is incontinent but not obstructed.

Physiologic studies of the nipple valve and pouch reveal that electric and motor patterns of the undistended ileum are similar with both types of ileostomy, but the anatomic and motor properties of the pouch allow it to accept far larger intraluminal volumes both during fasting and after feeding.[4] Pressure studies on the pouch, nipple valve, and outlet demonstrate the presence of a high-pressure zone in the nipple valve relative to the pouch.[521] Distension of the pouch with air causes a tonic contraction that travels from the pouch along the intestinal layers of the intussuscepted nipple valve and the outlet.[521] It is postulated that this is the mechanism for desusception of the nipple valve, a complication that may possibly be avoided by frequent intubation of the pouch. Other studies have demonstrated the functions of the mucosa and smooth muscle of the continent ileal pouch to be similar to those of normal ileum.[190]

The diagnosis of nipple valve slippage can usually be made clinically. However, it is valuable to confirm the

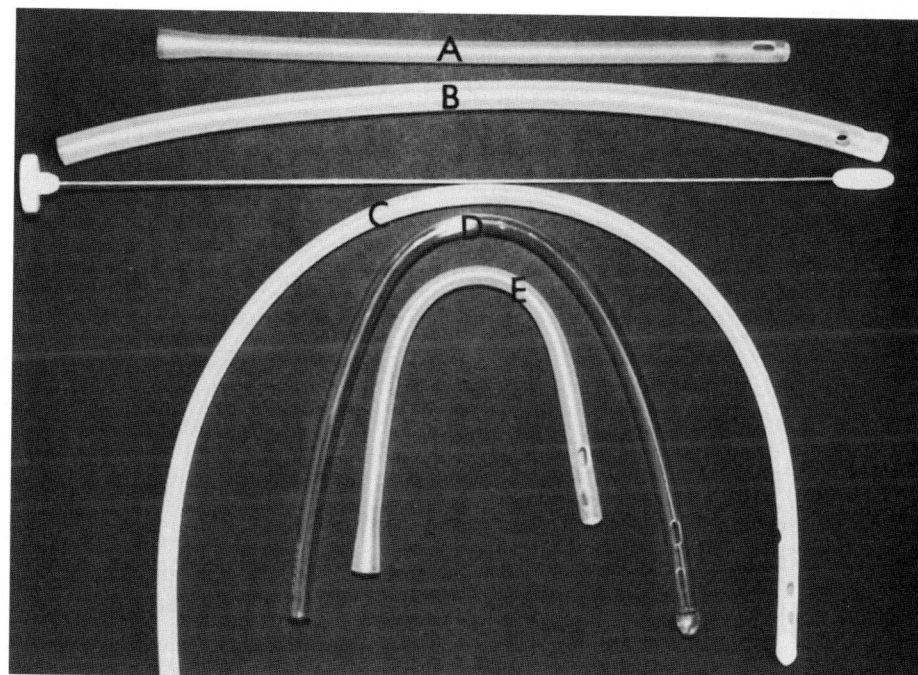

FIGURE 29-71. Continent ileostomy catheters. **(A)** Medena, straight (Göteborg, Sweden). **(B)** Heyer-Schulte, with introducer (Goleta, CA). **(C)** Waters (Rochester, MN). **(D)** Marlen (Bedford, OH). **(E)** Medena, curved.

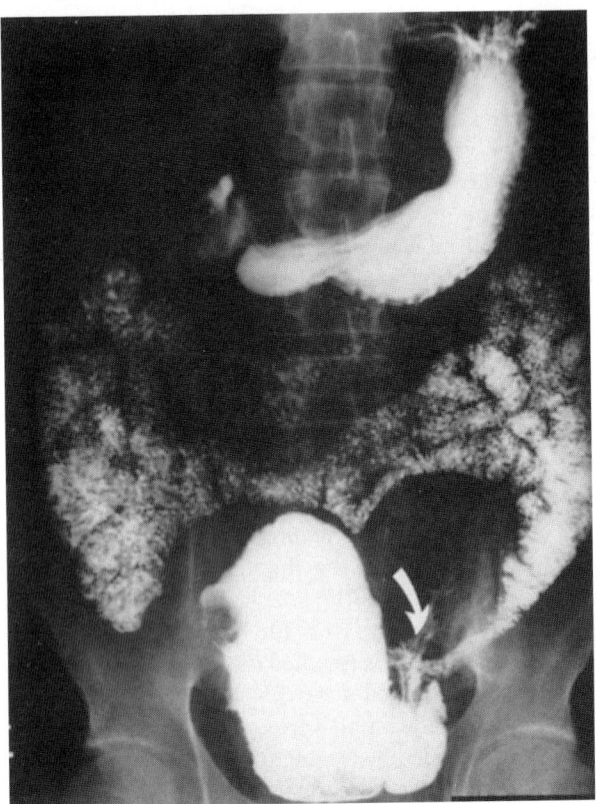

FIGURE 29-72. Continent ileostomy with leakage from pouch *(arrow)*. Nipple valve can be clearly seen.

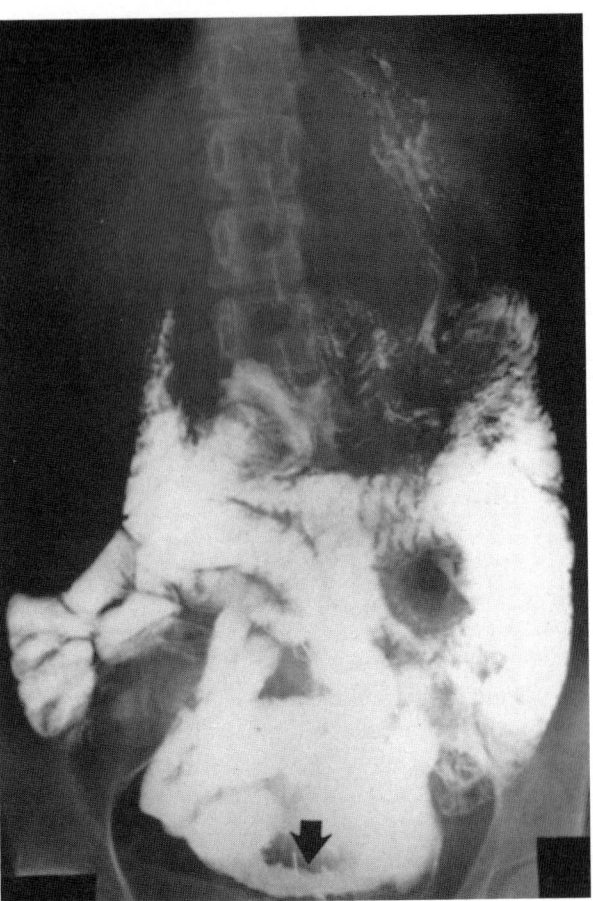

FIGURE 29-73. Recurrent Crohn's disease in terminal ileum *(arrow)* following continent ileostomy.

position of the nipple radiographically. This can be accomplished by a barium enema study through the stoma or by means of upper gastrointestinal roentgenography (Figure 29-75). The radiographic feature of a normal continent ileostomy on a plain abdominal film is the presence of a lobulated, gas-filled structure in the middle or right lower abdomen. With contrast material, the terminal, invaginated ileal segment resembles an inverted nipple protruding into the pouch.[492,647] Barium enema examination can reveal the size of the reservoir, the effluent can be measured and the adequacy of the emptying confirmed. Other complications of continent ileostomy may also be confirmed radiographically (e.g., small-bowel obstruction, anastomotic leakage, intraabdominal abscess, fistula formation, failure of the reservoir to dilate, and the presence of recurrent Crohn's disease).[492,703]

Obstruction at the level of the reservoir is usually caused by reduction of the nipple valve and kinking of the conduit. Outlet obstruction has also been described as a consequence of an implanted sling that had penetrated through the nipple valve into the reservoir.[355] Revision is required to relieve these problems. Although the purpose of the operation, of course, is to create an intestinal ob-

struction, one of the distinct disadvantages is the need to have a catheter readily available. If a patient loses it and is unable to obtain one conveniently (e.g., while on a camping trip), a serious problem ensues. Relief of the obstruction cannot be obtained unless proper equipment is available. Patients who enjoy outings away from civilization are well advised to secure the catheter on their person with great care.

Nipple Valve Revision. Reconstruction of the nipple may be accomplished by performing an enterotomy in the reservoir, re-intussuscepting the distal ileum, and re-securing it. However, it may not be possible to accomplish this maneuver because of necrosis of the ileum, inadequate length of the conduit, or bowel injury during the process of mobilization. Under these circumstances, a new nipple may be created without sacrificing the reservoir. This is achieved by using the afferent limb, oversewing the old efferent conduit opening, and performing an anastomosis of the proximal ileum to another part of the reservoir (Figure 29-76).

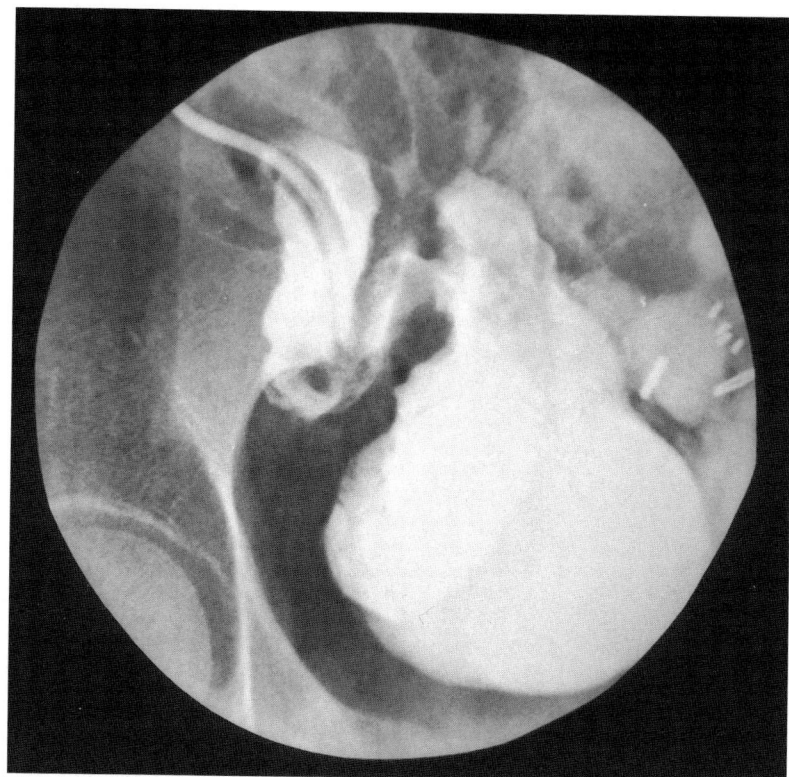

FIGURE 29-74. Desusscepted nipple can be readily appreciated on this "pouchogram." Acute angulation precludes catheterization even if there is no leakage.

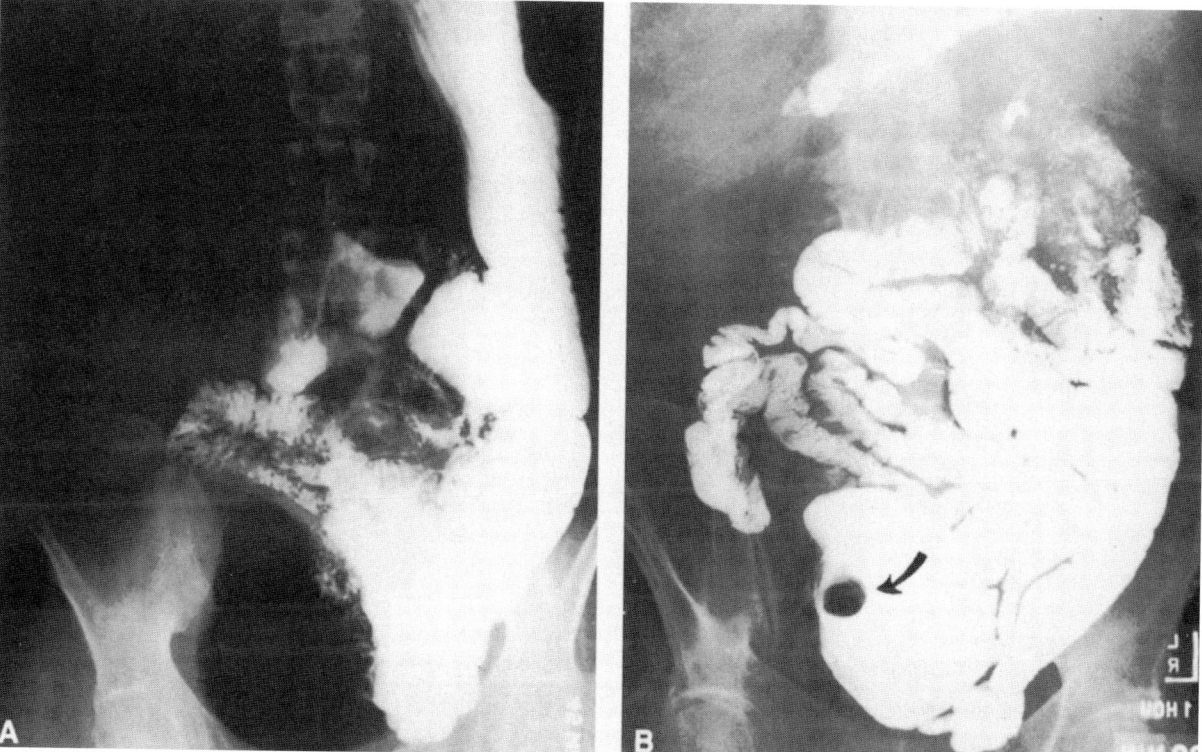

FIGURE 29-75. Continent ileostomy. Small-bowel series. **(A)** Normal pouch filling the pelvis on the right side. **(B)** Normal reservoir and nipple valve *(arrow)*.

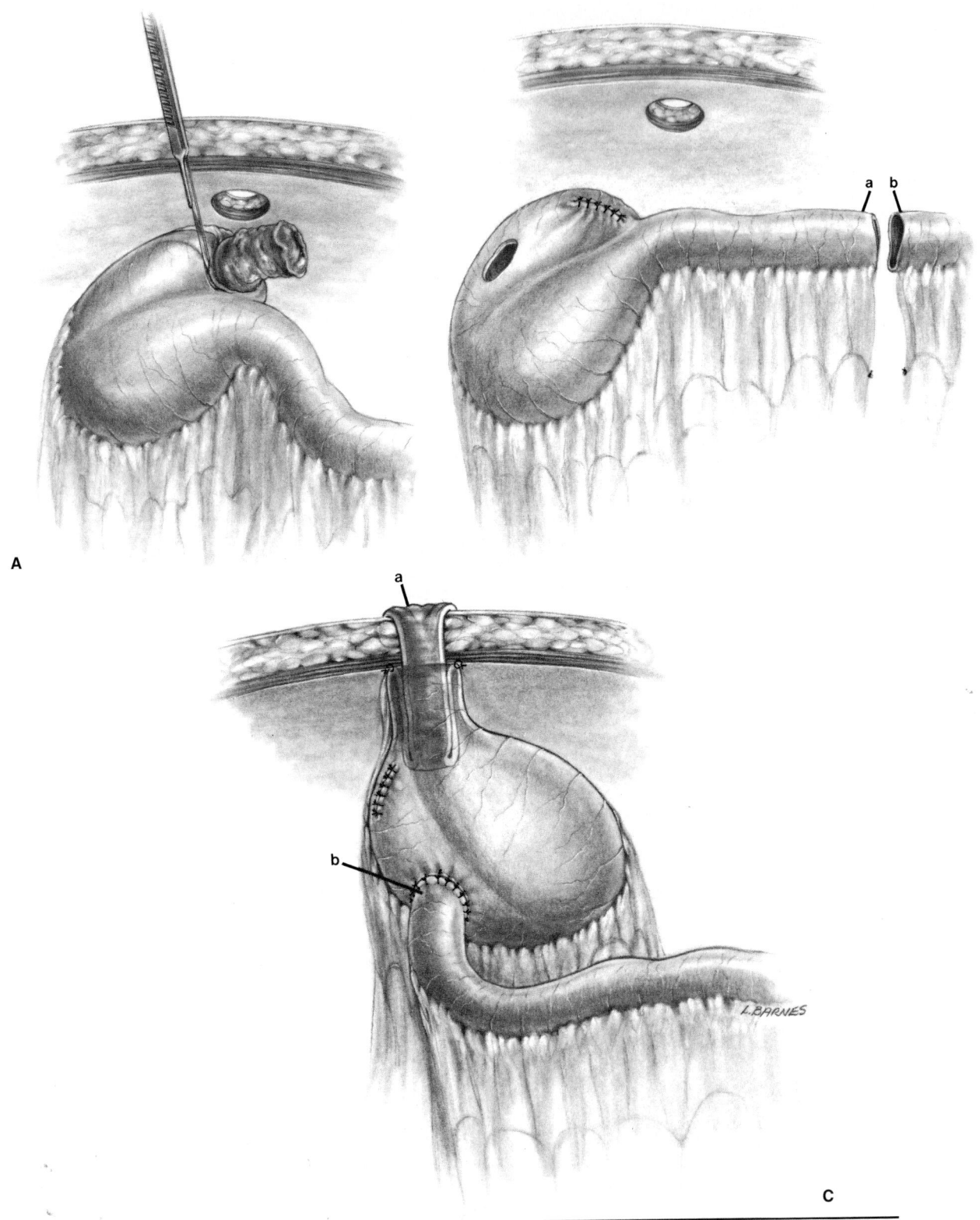

A

B

C

FIGURE 29-76. Construction of a new nipple valve. **(A)** Resection of the old conduit. **(B)** Division of the proximal (afferent) limb for the creation of a new nipple. **(C)** Final position of reservoir and conduit.

This is the method usually required to convert a reservoir-ileoanal anastomosis (Parks) to a continent ileostomy (Kock). In the former operation, there is usually none or an insufficient length of terminal ileum remaining (that had been anastomosed to the anal canal) to create a nipple valve and conduit. By oversewing the efferent end and using the proximal bowel to create a new nipple and conduit, the reservoir can be maintained. Conversely, if the sphincter muscles have been preserved, it may be possible to convert a Kock pouch to a reservoir-anal anastomosis. Hultén and colleagues suggest that if a short mesentery precludes the possibility of constructing a pelvic pouch, a temporary continent ileostomy can be performed with the expectation that the expanded reservoir may subsequently permit conversion.[299]

Gottlieb and Handelsman describe a number of outflow tract problems associated with the Kock pouch, offering various approaches to management.[225] Noninvasive means for maintaining continence after the valve has desuscepted include insertion of various balloon tubes (e.g., an endotracheal tube) or, my own preference, a Prager balloon plug (Figure 29-77). Unfortunately, it may not be possible to intubate the reservoir in the situation portrayed in Figure 29-77A.

Pouchitis. Pouch ileitis or "pouchitis" occurs at some time in 7% to 43% of patients with a continent ileostomy.[61,160] Manifestations include a flulike syndrome, fever, diarrhea, bleeding, abdominal pain, generalized toxicity, and severe ileitis. Increased ileostomy output re-

quiring more frequent intubation is a common presentation. The condition is believed to be caused by a change in the flora of the pouch, particularly an overgrowth of anaerobic organisms. Interestingly, this complication is quite rare in patients who undergo the procedure for familial polyposis. Barium enema study is usually not helpful, although thickening of the mucosal folds may be apparent. Endoscopic examination will usually reveal contact bleeding, friability, and an erythematous, ulcerated mucosa. Oral metronidazole (Flagyl) is the recommended treatment.[467] Additionally, many of these patients respond rapidly to steroids. Continuous drainage of the reservoir may have an ameliorative effect, but in the rare situation, removal of the pouch may be necessary. Recurrence is not uncommon, and under these circumstances consideration should be given to the possibility of Crohn's disease. The condition is also seen in those who have undergone restorative proctocolectomy with an ileal reservoir (see further discussion of pouchitis in that section).

Other Complications. Other unusual complications of the reservoir and nipple valve have been reported. These include the development of an enormous ileal pouch (the result of chronic outlet obstruction)[265,731] and *volvulus* with obstruction leading to perforation.[3] A case of invasive *adenocarcinoma* in a reservoir that had been in place for 17 years has also been reported,[109] but Hultén and co-workers found no incident of high-grade dysplasia or invasive carcinoma after a mean follow-up of 30 years in 40 patients, leading them to conclude that it is very

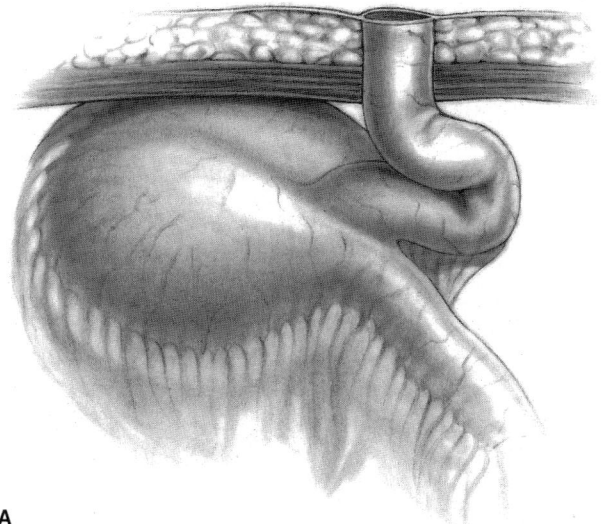

A

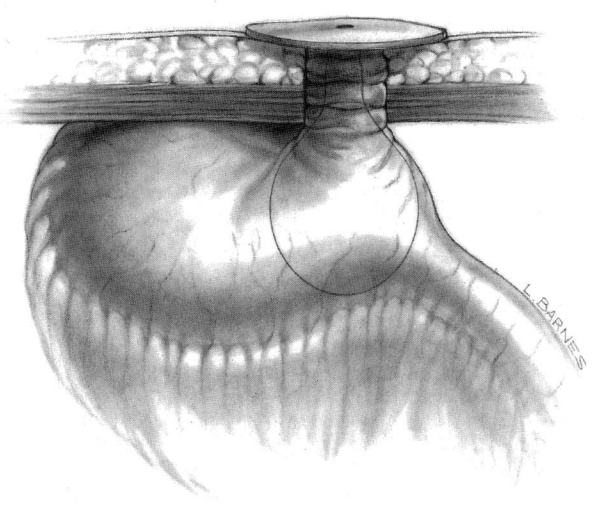

B

FIGURE 29-77. **(A)** Desusscepted nipple valve. **(B)** This is treated by the insertion of a balloon plug (see Chapter 13).

unlikely for invasive carcinoma to be a complication of this surgery.[302]

Hemorrhage from the nipple valve or reservoir has also been reported. This may be caused by trauma during insertion of the catheter (perforation of the pouch can actually occur), but it is usually associated with non-specific inflammation of the mucosa, in other words, pouchitis.

Detachment of the pouch from the anterior abdominal wall has been reported to produce angulation of the efferent limb and difficulty intubating the pouch.[736] Operative correction is required.

Urolithiasis is a well-known associated complication in patients who have undergone conventional ileostomy. Stern and colleagues evaluated the problem in patients who had undergone Kock ileostomies and compared them with nine matched patients who had undergone the conventional operation.[675] Both ileostomy groups demonstrated reduced urinary volume, with the Kock procedure group having the lower volume. There was no significant reduction in urinary pH or elevation in urine uric acid concentration in the continent ileostomy group. The results seemed to suggest no additional risk for uric acid stone formation in pouch patients.

Malabsorption has been suggested as a possible concern because of intestinal stasis and bacterial overgrowth. Kelly and colleagues studied the nature and frequency of malabsorption in 42 pouch patients and in 19 who had undergone conventional ileostomy.[340] Almost one-third with the reservoir were found to have excess fecal volumes accompanied by increased fecal loss of electrolytes, nitrogen, and fat, and by decreased vitamin B_{12} uptake. The remaining patients had fecal and urinary outputs similar to that of patients with conventional ileostomies. Gadacz and colleagues performed absorptive studies and motor function analysis of the pouch in eight patients.[190] The pouch absorbed vitamin B_{12} that was instilled together with intrinsic factor. Other studies of patients who had documented malabsorption or symptoms of a malfunctioning pouch revealed that the number of jejunal and ileal anaerobic bacteria decreased during treatment with metronidazole, implicating overgrowth of anaerobic bacterial flora in the pathogenesis of the syndrome.[341]

Kay and colleagues determined bile acid and neutral steroid excretion in 15 patients: 5 with conventional ileostomy, 5 with continent ileostomy, and 5 with continent ileostomy and an ileal resection.[333] Bile acid excretion rates were significantly increased in those with a continent ileostomy and an ileal resection. Also, continent ileostomy was associated with a significantly increased percentage of water content and a reduction in the pH of the ileal effluent. We have observed multiple cholesterol stones in the pouch of one patient (Figure 29-78).

Results

Cranley reviewed the development of the operation and reported that anastomotic leaks occurred in 8.8% of cases.[110] In the experience of Goligher with 62 reservoir operations, leakage occurred in 7 patients, with the development of diffuse peritonitis in 3 and of a localized abscess in 4.[213] An additional 2 patients required a proximal loop ileostomy for presumed leakage, although no defect in the reservoir could be identified at the time of surgery. Goligher humbly commented that his complications seemed to be observed more frequently than those of other surgeons.

The report by Kock and colleagues in 1981 revealed 7 deaths in 314 patients (2.2%).[363] All the operative deaths occurred prior to 1975, with no deaths recorded in the succeeding 152 patients. Early complications developed in 24% of those operated on between 1967 and 1974 and in 7% of patients in the latter period. Anastomotic leak or fistula occurred in 19 in the earlier group, but in only 1 from the latter. Results in 36 patients from Kock's unit who were followed for 16 to 20 years revealed no increased risk for gallstone formation or urinary stone development.[538] Interestingly, although 11 of the patients had reservoirs constructed without a valve, 92% of the series were continent.

Palmu and Sivula reported an experience of 51 patients.[549] There were 2 perforations of the reservoir (1 death), 4 fecal fistulas, and 8 intestinal obstructions. Gelernt and colleagues evaluated their experience of 54 patients and noted a fecal fistula in 6, with hemorrhage from the ileal reservoir in 5.[199] In a study by Halvorsen and colleagues, of the 36 patients who underwent a reservoir ileostomy, 3 died of septic complications.[244] Of the 150 individuals reported from the Mayo Clinic, 16 required excision of the pouch, but only 1 because of a fistula.[33]

Schrock reported a 15% incidence of immediate postoperative complications in 39 patients.[641] Factors that contributed to the complications included older age (greater than 40 years), obesity, and the presence of Crohn's disease. By far the most common problem was spontaneous reduction of the nipple valve, usually occurring within 3 months. This was observed by the author in one-third of his patients. A much higher incidence of nipple valve failure was noted in those who underwent a secondary operation rather than a primary procedure (proctocolectomy and continent ileostomy at the same time). Forty-six percent of secondarily operated patients had nipple failures, in comparison with 13% of primary surgery patients. Increased weight gain may have been a con-

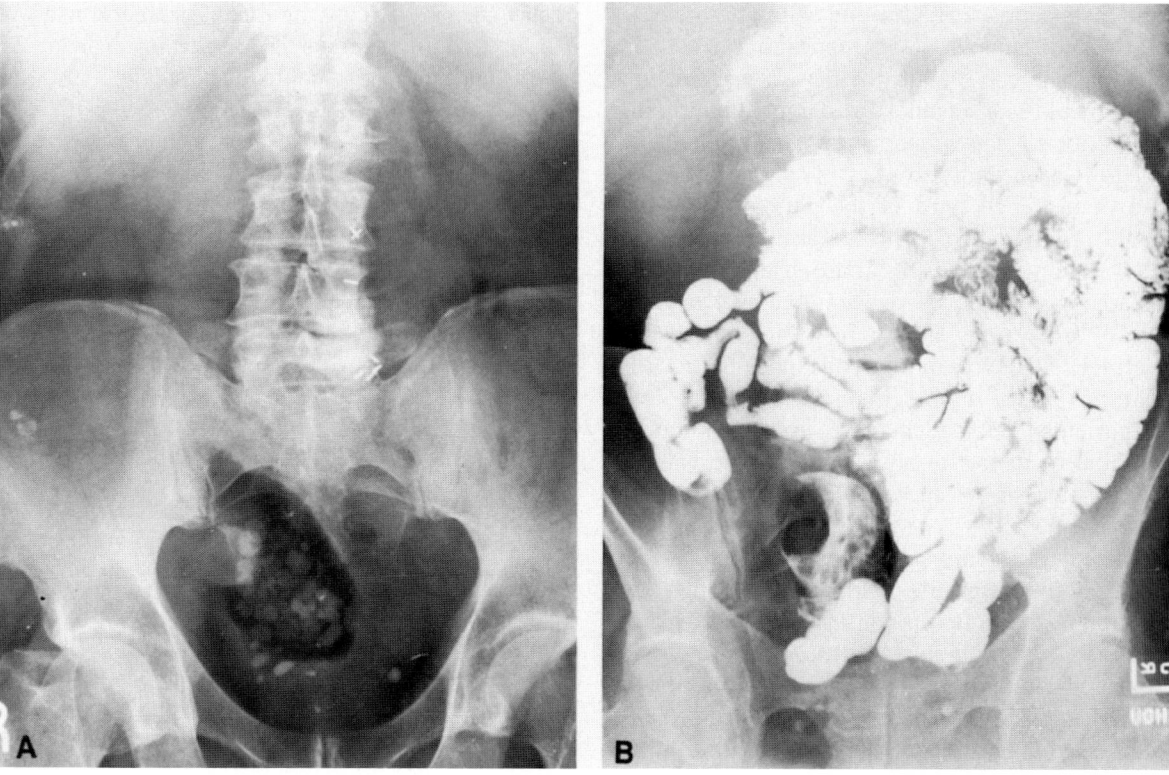

FIGURE 29-78. Continent ileostomy. **(A)** Plane abdominal film reveals radiopaque objects in the reservoir (note air shadow). **(B)** A small bowel series confirms the presence of "stones" in the pouch.

tributing factor since the patients were generally well and had a much more fatty mesentery when operated on the second time.

Dozois and colleagues reported the factors that affected the revision rate in the Mayo Clinic experience.[139] Among the nearly 300 patients who underwent continent ileostomy and were followed for at least 1 year, revision was required less often in women, in younger patients, and in those with a primary proctocolectomy and continent ileostomy. This was the same experience that Schrock reported. The authors advised that if a malfunctioning valve develops, it ideally should be revised rather than a new one created. Revision was believed to be technically simpler, and the long-term results were comparable.

Gerber and colleagues reported a 19% incidence of nipple valve slippage in their first 48 patients.[202] In the next 48, the incidence of this complication was only 4%. The authors attributed their success to stapling the valve rather than suturing and to the placement of a Marlex mesh sleeve around the conduit. They also reported success in patients with Crohn's colitis, but their experience with ileocolitis, even with removal of the

entire diseased bowel, was associated with a prohibitively high incidence of postoperative complications (see Chapter 30). Others suggest that the Kock continent ileostomy may be considered in patients with Crohn's disease, provided that there has been no evidence of recurrence for 5 years.[56]

Flake and colleagues reported their initial experience on 11 patients, three-fourths of whom required further surgery.[172] Four underwent a new Kock ileostomy, two required stomal revision, and two underwent revision of the valve with removal of the reservoir. Subsequently, two patients were converted to a conventional ileostomy.

At the Mayo Clinic, the results from the first 149 patients were compared with those from the last 150 patients.[138] There were no operative deaths. Fifteen pouches were excised in the early group, as opposed to only five in the later group. Furthermore, the requirement for revision of the valve at 1 year was 43% in the early group but only 22% in the later group. Long-term follow-up demonstrated complete continence in 60% of the patients in the early group and 75% in the later group.

The initial experience of Kock and colleagues revealed a 50% incidence of nipple valve complications necessitating revisional surgery.[363] With the newer modifications their subsequent report demonstrated a malfunction rate of 6%. As with all newer operations, it is evident that there is indeed a learning curve.

Approximately one third of the patients of Palmu and Sivula required revision for nipple insufficiency, but Gelernt and colleagues, in an experience of 54 patients, stated that no nipple revision had ever been required.[199,549] Only three patients reported some degree of incontinence. Halvorsen and colleagues noted "disinvagination" of the nipple in more than one-third of their patients.[244] Telander and co-workers reported a 20% requirement for revision of the nipple valve in those under 19 years of age who underwent this procedure.[700]

Nilsson and colleagues performed morphologic and histochemical studies on the continent ileostomy reservoir for up to 10 years after its construction.[519] No alarming changes in terms of dysplasia, fibrosis, or progressive atrophy were found. Histochemical investigation of the mucosa revealed largely unchanged, strong enzymatic activity involved in both oxidative metabolism and secretory functions.[519]

Several studies have been published on the long-term results of this operation. Järvinen and colleagues evaluated 76 such patients 9 years following surgery.[313] Late complications occurred in 54 (72%): 2 (2.7%) pouch-related deaths, 30 (41%) nipple desusceptions, 22 (30%) cases of pouchitis, and 12 (16%) cases of stomal stricture. Additional complications included ventral hernia, nipple valve fistula, intraabdominal abscess, and foreign body in the reservoir. Two thirds of the patients required re-operation and revision. However, despite the high complication rate, a good functional result was achieved in 83%, and only 4 reservoirs were removed. This study and those of others confirm a high level of patient satisfaction even though the complication rate is high. McLeod and Fazio noted that 97% of their patients would undergo revisional surgery rather than have the continent ileostomy removed.[466] Of 152 patients alive with a pouch from the Cleveland Clinic, 91% were continent.[160]

Lepistö and Järvinen reported their experience with 96 continent ileostomy patients from Helsinki, Finland.[399] Twenty-four percent required conversion to a conventional stoma. Fifty-nine percent underwent valve reconstruction. When compared with restorative proctocolectomy there was an overall statistically significantly lower success rate ($p < .01$).

Barnett reported 71 patients who underwent his particular modification, 54 of whom were revised from a conventional ileostomy.[28] The overall operative revision rate for valve and pouch problems was 7%. Mullen and colleagues reviewed a multicenter experie nce with the Barnett continent intestinal reservoir, involving 510 patients with ulcerative colitis or familial polyposis.[499] Follow-up time ranged from 1 to 5 years, with 92% still maintaining the reservoir. Replacement with a conventional ileostomy was required for 6.5%. This excision rate is certainly no worse than those of other series using more conventional approaches to creating the Kock pouch. Excluding pouch removal, the re-operation rate for major pouch-related complications was 12.8%.[499] Their pouch fistula problems and other surgery-related complications are higher than have generally been reported with the standard operation.

Comment

Most observers who are experienced with the continent ileostomy believe that the operation offers a reasonably satisfactory alternative to the conventional procedure.[33,160,213,390,518] The encumbrance of an appliance, the occasional "accidents" with appliance management, the unaesthetic proboscis on the abdominal wall, sexual inhibition, and psychological embarrassment have stimulated many patients to seek an alternative procedure. Unfortunately, however, the operation is no panacea. Despite the many improvements in surgical technique, the procedure is still fraught with numerous complications. The Kock pouch is also not for everyone. It is, in my opinion, contraindicated for patients with Crohn's disease, and the results in older people and those who are somewhat obese are quite poor. The patient should request this operation. It must not be "sold" by the surgeon. However, the quality of life for individuals who have elected the continent ileostomy is unquestionably improved in the vast majority of cases. But as previously stated, this discussion appears to be somewhat academic, because with the exception of conversion of a failed restorative proctocolectomy, the operation has been virtually replaced by the pouch-anal procedure.

Restorative Proctocolectomy [Total Proctocolectomy and Ileoanal Anastomosis with Intervening Pouch (Parks Procedure); Pouch-Anal Procedure; Ileal Pouch-Anal Procedure]

As previously discussed, total abdominal proctocolectomy with ileoanal anastomosis is associated with frequent bowel movements, urgency, and fecal incontinence in a high percentage of cases. To address this problem, the application of an intervening pouch with an ileoanal anastomosis was described in experimental animals as early as 1955 by Valiente and Bacon and in 1964 by Peck and Hallenbeck.[557,723] With the success of the ileal reservoir as developed by Kock (see previous discussion), Parks and Nicholls in 1978 reported an operation combining the application of an ileal pouch that eliminated propulsive activity and acted as a storage organ with preservation of the entire sphincter mechanism.[550] Others also proposed similar operations.[170,555] The procedure has also been reported, with various modifications, as a means of restoring intestinal activity after conventional proctocolectomy, sometimes after many years.[105,554] In the past 25 years, the preponderance of publications on the surgical management of ulcerative colitis have addressed variations on this procedure, the morbidity, the physiologic effects, and the functional results.

Several controversial issues with respect to this operation are known and are important to discuss. They include the following and will be addressed in this section:

- the type of pouch (J, S,W, Q, and now T)
- mucosectomy versus double-stapling
- loop ileostomy versus no protective stoma
- the significance of dysplasia and the risk of malignancy

S-Pouch

The patient is placed in the perineolithotomy position as if for an abdominoperineal resection. Following completion of the colectomy and excision of the rectum as far distally as is possible (see previous section), an ileal reservoir is created. The distal ileum is transected with the GIA stapler as close to the cecum as is possible (Figure 29-79).

Tension on the ileal mesentery is a potential problem because the bowel must be brought virtually to the perianal skin. Complete mobilization of the mesentery up to the level of the duodenum is imperative (Figure 29-80). The ileal artery may be divided to achieve additional length, and the parietal peritoneum of the distal ileum may be incised (Figure 29-81). Some believe that com-

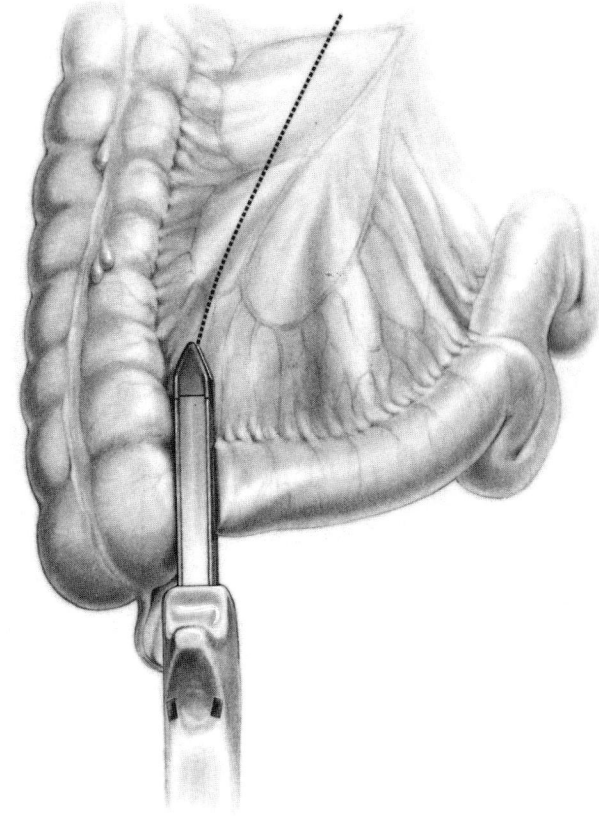

FIGURE 29-79. Ileum is divided as close to the cecum as possible. (Adapted from Burnstein MJ, Schoetz DJ Jr, Coller JA, Veidenheimer MC. Technique of mesenteric lengthening in ileal reservoir-anal anastomosis. *Dis Colon Rectum* 1987; 30:863.)

plete dissection of the root of the mesentery is a poor lengthening technique and that division of the ileocecal artery is the safest and most effective method for obtaining maximum length.[85] Goes and colleagues recommend preservation of the marginal vascular arcade of the right side of the colon to permit ligation of more

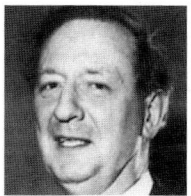

Alan Guyatt Parks (1920–1982)   Alan Parks, after attending Epsom College, proceeded to Brasenose, Oxford, and received his bachelor of arts degree in 1943. That same year, he was awarded a Rockefeller fellowship to attend Johns Hopkins University to complete his medical training and medical internship. He returned to Guy's Hospital, London, and in 1949 passed the examination for fellowship in the Royal College of Surgeons. After a period in the National Service in the Far East, Parks came back to Guy's to continue his research on the anatomy of the anal canal. Numerous publications followed, which provide an extraordinary testament to his dedication as a scientist and his ability as a creative writer. Parks was appointed consultant surgeon to the staff of St. Mark's Hospital in 1959 and to the London Hospital the same year. His practice attracted many surgeons from throughout the world who came to train and observe. In 1954, Parks was made a master of surgery for his work leading to a special operation for hemorrhoids (see Chapter 8). Through the years, the name of Alan Parks has been associated with innovation in the field of colon and rectal surgery. His contributions include the development of a number of surgical instruments, studies on the etiology and classification of anal fistula (see Chapter 11) and on the physiology and anatomy of the pelvic floor, the treatment of anal incontinence (see Chapter 13), and the application of the ileal reservoir with ileoanal anastomosis in the surgical management of ulcerative colitis and familial polyposis. Parks' honors have been numerous: presidency of the section of proctology of the Royal Society of Medicine, fellowship in the Royal College of Physicians, and honorary fellowships awarded by the American, Australasian, Canadian, Edinburgh, and Glasgow Colleges of Surgeons. His achievements were further recognized when he was granted a knighthood by the British Government.

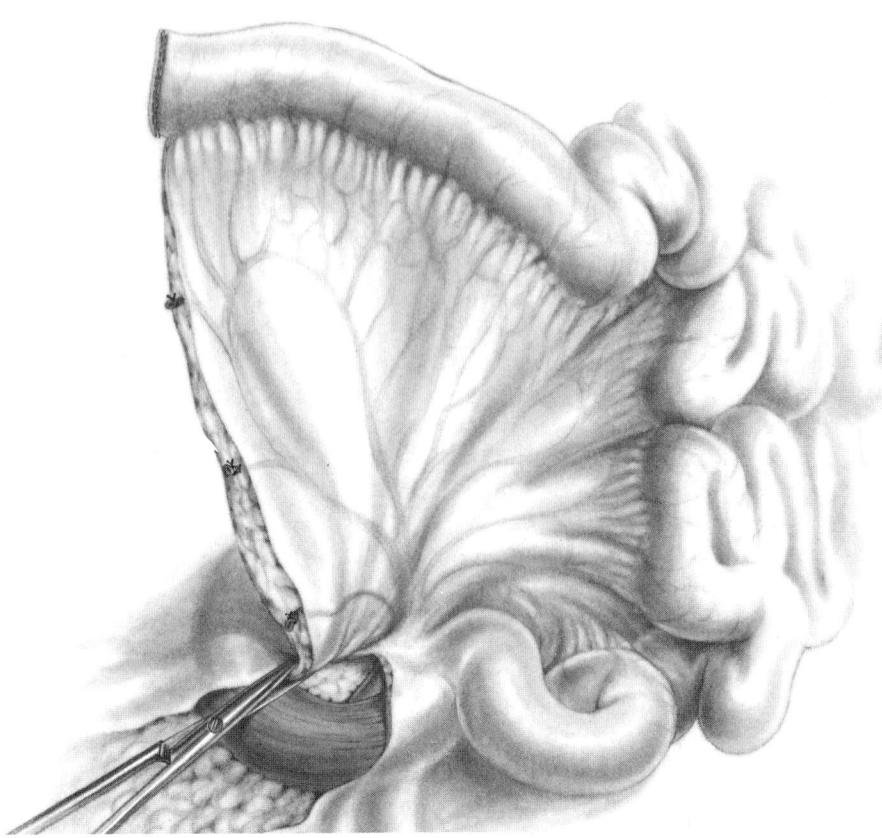

FIGURE 29-80. Dissection is carried out to the root of the mesentery. (Adapted from Burnstein MJ, Schoetz DJ Jr, Coller JA, Veidenheimer MC. Technique of mesenteric lengthening in ileal reservoir-anal anastomosis. *Dis Colon Rectum* 1987;30:863.)

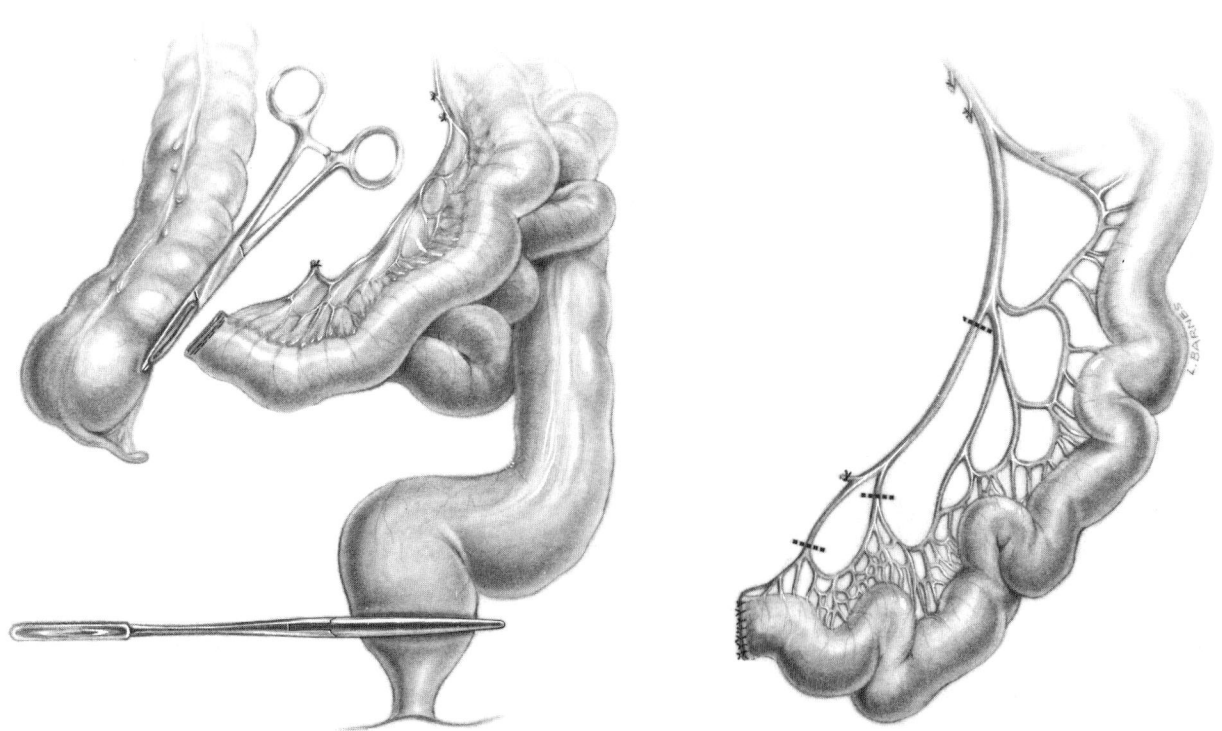

A   B

FIGURE 29-81. Preservation of the ileal blood supply. **(A)** Transection of the distal ileum as close to the cecum as possible. **(B)** Preservation of the blood supply by careful dissection with the aid of transillumination. The *dashed lines* indicate possible sites of division in order to obtain additional length.

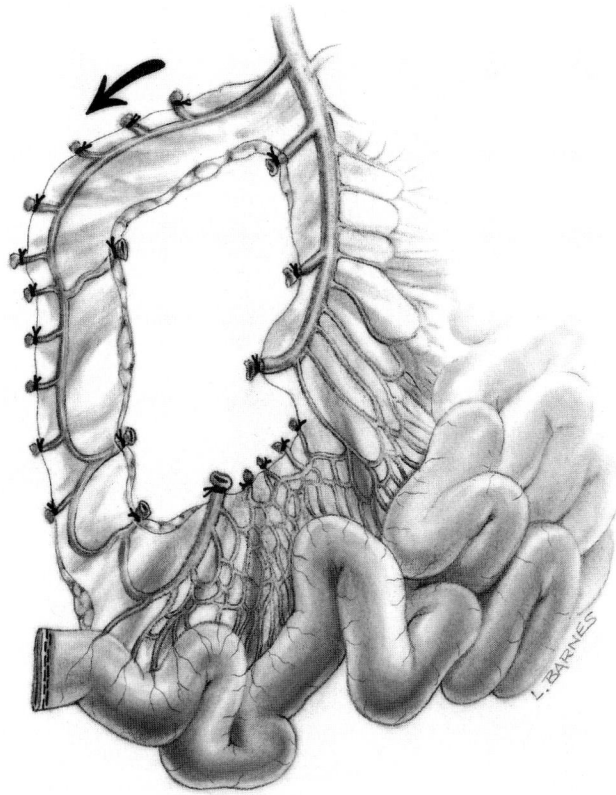

FIGURE 29-82. Schematic representation of the mesenteric vascular arcade with preservation of the blood supply that supplied the right colon. (After Goes RN, Nguyen P, Huang D, Beart RW Jr. Lengthening of the mesentery using the marginal vascular arcade of the right colon as the blood supply to the ileal pouch. *Dis Colon Rectum* 1995;38:893.)

mesenteric vessels and to increase the mesenteric length[209] (Figure 29-82). In a series of cadaver studies, Smith and co-workers observed that if the tip of the conduit (or pouch) reaches 6 cm below the pubic symphysis, the dentate line will be satisfactorily reached.[662] Martel and colleagues found that in fresh cadavers, the increase in mesenteric length was greater after dividing the superior mesenteric pedicle (mean, 6.5 cm) as compared with the ileocolic pedicle (mean, 3.0 cm), but if a pouch-anal anastomosis is to be performed, a short segment of terminal ileum must be removed.[450] Regardless of the lengthening technique, the most dependent part of the terminal ileum for effecting the anastomosis should be selected, not a specific, measured distance from the cut end of the ileum.

Parks and Nicholls suggested that an S-type reservoir be created[550] (Figure 29-83). In this modification, the terminal 50 cm of ileum is measured and then folded twice to give three segments of bowel, the proximal two of which are 15 cm long and the distal segment 20 cm long (Figure 29-83A). A 5-cm length of ileum projects

beyond the pouch, which is the area to be used for the anastomosis. The ileum is opened on its antimesenteric border (Figure 29-83B), and the adjacent loops are sutured (Figure 29-83C). An interrupted technique may be used, but a continuous suture of 3–0 long-term absorbable material is more expeditious. The two outer edges are then folded across to complete the pouch, with the closure effected using the same suture material (Figure 29-83D).

Another alternative for pouch construction is to employ a stapling technique (see later discussion). This is a much more rapid approach, but it has the theoretical disadvantage of more tissue inversion, and therefore decreased reservoir capacity.[674]

As previously mentioned, the anastomosis is performed via the transanal approach by using an anal retractor (e.g., Parks), paired Gelpi retractors placed at right angles, or a self-retaining Lone Star retractor[605,617] (Lone Star Medical Products, Inc., Houston, Texas; Figs. 29-84 and 29-85). In contrast to earlier suggestions, most surgeons today make no attempt to preserve a muscular sleeve (see Ileoanal Anastomosis, Operative Technique).[290] The full thickness of the ileum is sutured to the anal canal at the level of the dentate line, incorporating the underlying internal anal sphincter muscle (see Figure 29-54). Alternatively, an anastomosis can be performed in the anal canal by using the circular stapling device, with or without a double-stapling approach, but care must be taken to avoid placing the staple line too low (see later discussion).[268,556,748]

Ambroze and colleagues (Mayo Clinic) have emphasized that retention of the omentum reduces the incidence of sepsis without affecting the frequency of postoperative bowel obstruction.[9] With respect to drains, Parks and colleagues advised draining the pelvis through the intersphincteric plane, but some surgeons prefer either no drain or a suprapubic suction drain.[551] An alternative would be to place the drain in the pelvis and bring it out through the levatores and buttock. My personal preference is to use a closed suction drain, placed in the pelvis and brought out through a stab wound in the left lower quadrant. It is removed when the drainage is less than 100 mL in 24 hours.

Comment

It has been said that the S-pouch can permit an anastomosis lower in the pelvis than that of a J-pouch. In other words, it may be used in the circumstance when the application of a J-pouch cannot permit restoration of intestinal continuity. Such occasions must be rare indeed, however. Moreover, there are problems unique to the S-pouch, most especially emptying difficulties if the efferent limb is too long (see Complications of the Pouch Pro-

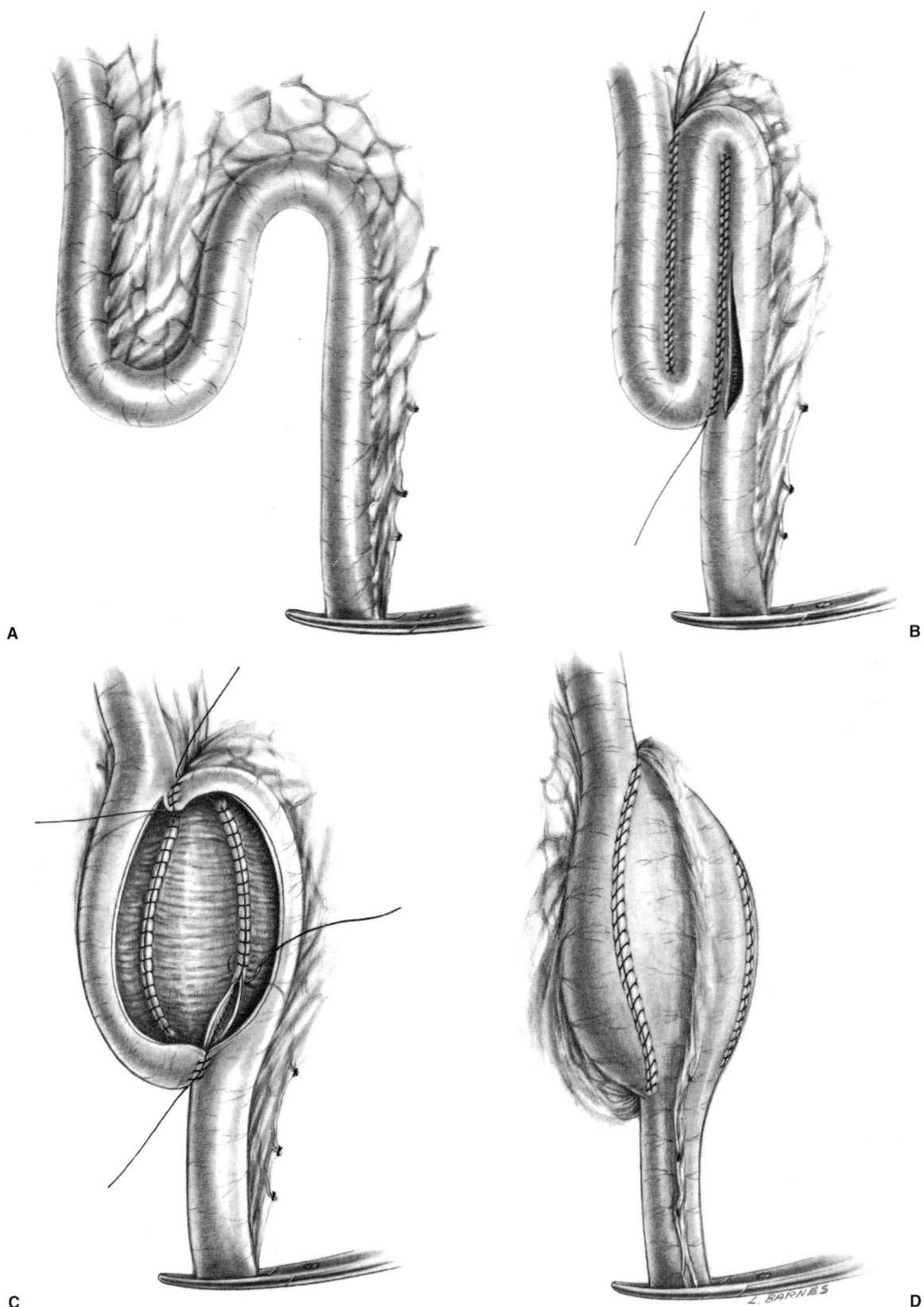

FIGURE 29-83. S-type (Parks) ileal reservoir. **(A)** The bowel is aligned. **(B)** The antimesenteric aspect is opened after serosal apposition. **(C)** Suturing of the adjacent walls. **(D)** The reservoir is completed with an ileoanal anastomosis.

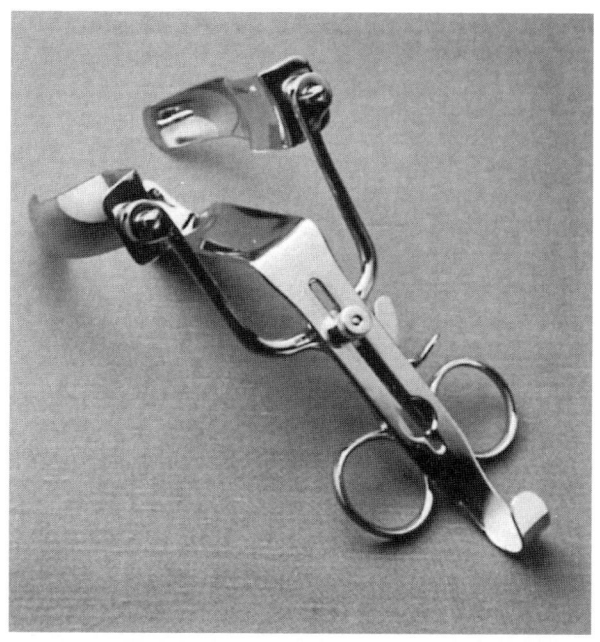

FIGURE 29-84. Parks three-bladed anal retractor for facilitating endoanal anastomoses. (Courtesy of Seward Medical Ltd., London, UK.)

cedures). The ease of construction of the J-reservoir and the comparable results with respect to bowel function (see next section) cause most surgeons to use the following technique.

J-Pouch

Another option, the so-called J-pouch, was initially suggested by Utsunomiya and colleagues.[722] This type of pouch is prepared by selecting the point at which the ileal loop reaches the lowest level in the pelvis, usually about 20 to 30 cm from the end of the ileum (Figure 29-86). The length of the pouch is variable but generally is approximately 20 cm.

As previously noted, one of the critical concerns in the performance of the reservoir-anal techniques is the creation of an anastomosis that is free of tension. Burnstein and colleagues at the Lahey Clinic have outlined a series of steps that they believe offer the optimal approach to mesenteric lengthening.[77] This consists of division of the terminal ileum as close to the cecum as is possible (Figure 29-79), mobilization of the mesentery of the small bowel to the third portion of the duodenum (Figure 29-80), and selection of the apex of the J-reservoir with the objective of its extension 6 cm beyond the pubic symphysis (Figure 29-86).[77] Mesenteric lengthening can be achieved through a number of possible maneuvers. In the first instance, care should be

taken to divide the mesentery as close to the right colon as possible to preserve the branches of the ileocolic artery. If incisions along the mesenteric peritoneum produce inadequate length and a window must be created, blood supply to the pouch can still be preserved (Figure 29-87).

Apposition of the loop can be performed by using a continuous double-layer suture technique, thereby creating a long, side-to-side anastomosis (Figure 29-88). Most surgeons today prefer to employ the GIA stapling device or equivalent to create the reservoir. An early approach was to use the conventional 5-cm instrument, inserting it by means of enterotomies 5 cm proximal to the point selected as the apex of the pouch (Figure 29-89A). The GIA stapler is then inserted toward the apex and fired. The pouch is turned around and two additional staple cartridges are fired in the opposite direction through the same enterotomies. With a total of three staple cartridges fired, a 15-cm pouch is created. The terminal septum must be inverted and divided either sharply or by another passage of the stapler (Figure 29-89B,C). The enterotomies are closed longitudinally, and the apex of the pouch is delivered to the anal area (Figure 29-89D). A small enterotomy is made in the pouch, and an anastomosis is effected between the full thickness of bowel and the anal canal in the manner described previously.

Current stapling instruments permit a simpler pouch construction, such as a long (9-cm) GIA (Figure 29-90). The stapler can be inserted in the middle of each limb (Figure 29-91) or optimally through the apex. Care must be taken to pull the mesentery away from the bowel to avoid its incorporation in the line of staples (Figs. 29-92 and 29-93). This opening can then be used for insertion of the proximal anvil (Figure 29-94). With this technique it may be necessary to pass the instrument cephalad once or twice more, using an intussuscepting maneuver (Figure 29-95). Nduka and colleagues suggest the use of an endoscopic stapler (Endo-GIA) to create the J-reservoir.[508] The length of this instrument allows the device to be applied multiple times without the problem of intussuscepting the intestine. Others have suggested performing the operation laparoscopically.[375,590]

Effecting the Anastomosis

Technique. With the apical purse-string suture in place, Peck initially described completing the anastomosis by means of the circular stapling instrument.[556] Another purse-string suture is placed at the top of the anal canal, incorporating the internal sphincter. The sutures are then secured, and the instrument is fired (Figure 29-96). By means of this alternative, Peck and others are

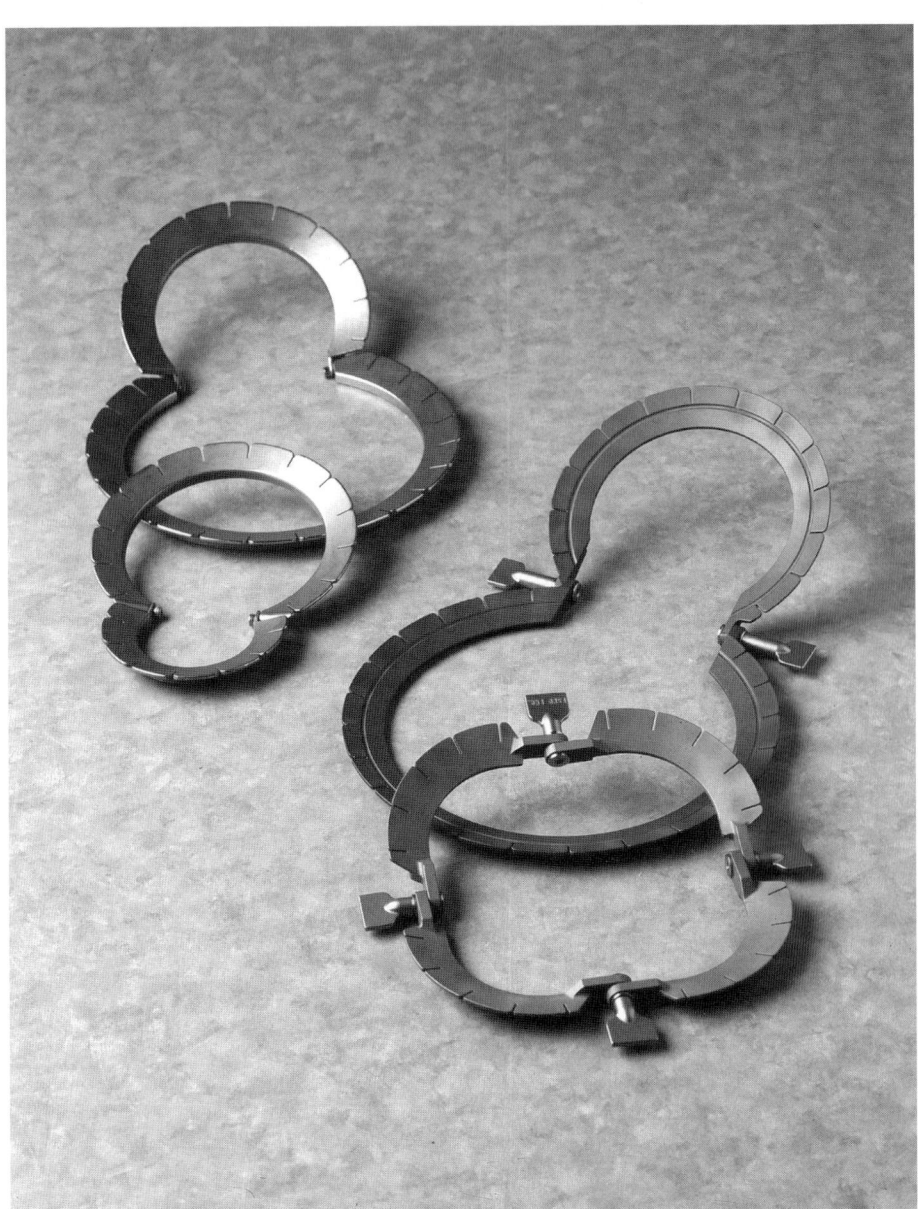

A

more likely to abjure a protecting ileostomy (see later discussion).[556] Of course, one can use a suture technique, as has been previously described, to complete the pouch-anal anastomosis.

Another method for completing the anastomosis is to employ the double-stapling technique. This is analogous to the method used for effecting a low anastomosis for cancer of the rectum (see Chapter 23). The pouch construction is the same as described previously, but linear closure of the rectal stump is performed instead of a purse string being used (Figure 29-97). Not uncommonly, however, it is not possible to place the linear stapling device sufficiently low onto the rectal

stump. Under these circumstances, Schoetz and Coller advocate serial placement of the 30-mm instrument in two or three applications until the bowel is divided (DJ Schoetz Jr and JA Coller, personal communication; Figure 29-98), although a single firing of the 30-mm device can often accomplish the task in this distal location.

Another technique is to perform a transanal application with a purse-string suture. This is often a tedious maneuver and risks excessive dilatation and stretching of the sphincter mechanism. A possible option is to perform eversion of the rectum to accomplish reestablishment of intestinal continuity, and to facilitate a muco-

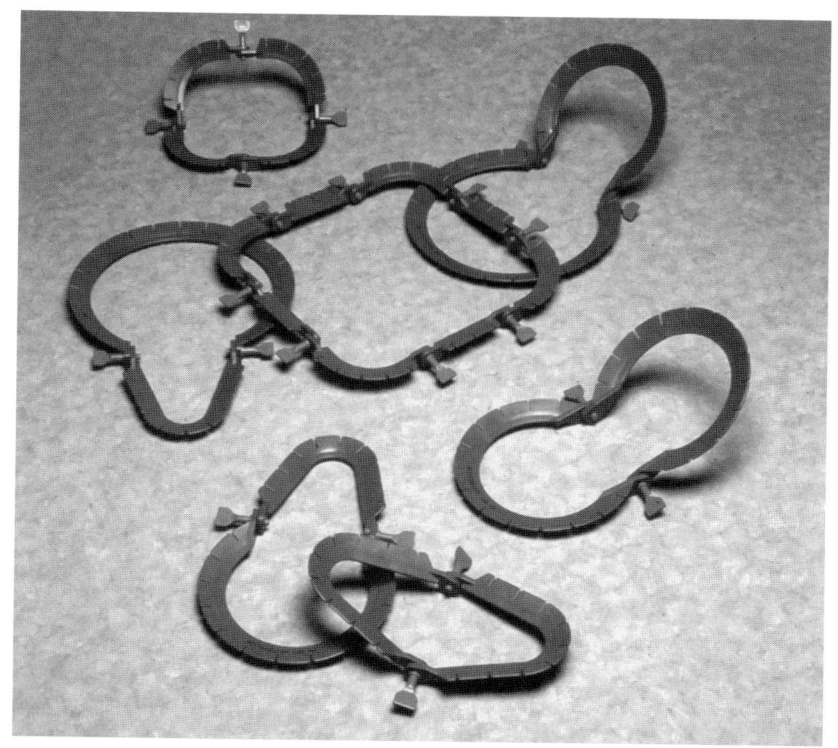

B

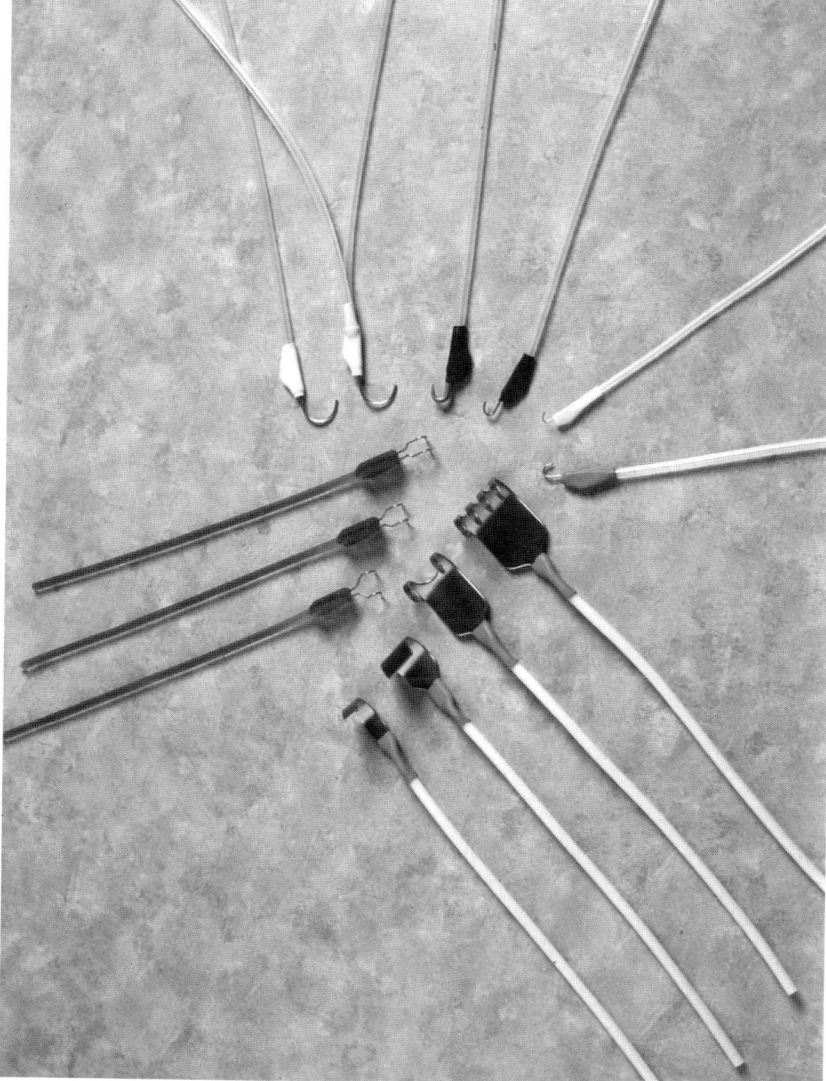

C

FIGURE 29-85. (continued)

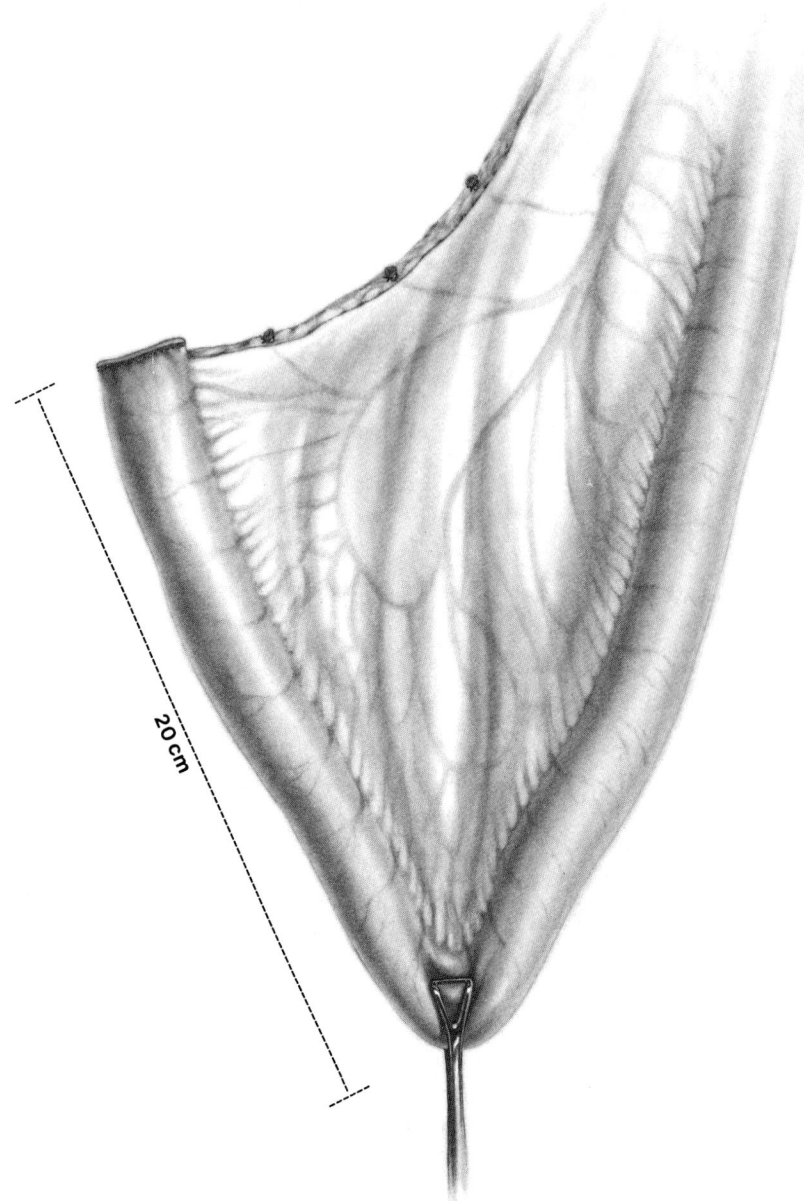

FIGURE 29-86. Maximum length of J-pouch is usually achieved with apex approximately 20 cm proximal to ileocecal valve. (Adapted from Burnstein MJ, Schoetz DJ Jr, Coller JA, Veidenheimer MC. Technique of mesenteric lengthening in ileal reservoir-anal anastomosis. *Dis Colon Rectum* 1987;30: 863.)

sectomy if one wishes to consider this[496] (Figure 29-99). By using this approach, Régimbeau and colleagues were able to perform a hand-sewn anal anastomosis on the dentate line, thereby avoiding an incomplete mucosectomy.[587] Another technique has been described through the stapling of a drain to the rectal stump and then pulling it through to evert the rectum.[644] The problem, as alluded to earlier, is that eversion is not associated with as good a functional outcome when compared with a stapled anastomosis prepared without eversion.[485,749]

The stapling technique has permitted relatively effortless pouch construction and anastomosis. As such, it is preferred by the overwhelming majority of surgeons.[127, 297,356,664,764] But there are consequences! Figure 29-100 demonstrates the radiographic appearance of a satisfactorily completed J-pouch.

Where to Place the Anastomosis

Where to place the anastomosis is a matter of controversy. Although there is some difference of opinion, most agree that a reservoir anastomosis at the level of the dentate line is associated with suboptimal functional results compared with an anastomosis at the top of the anal canal (see Results).[320,356,556,638,648] However,

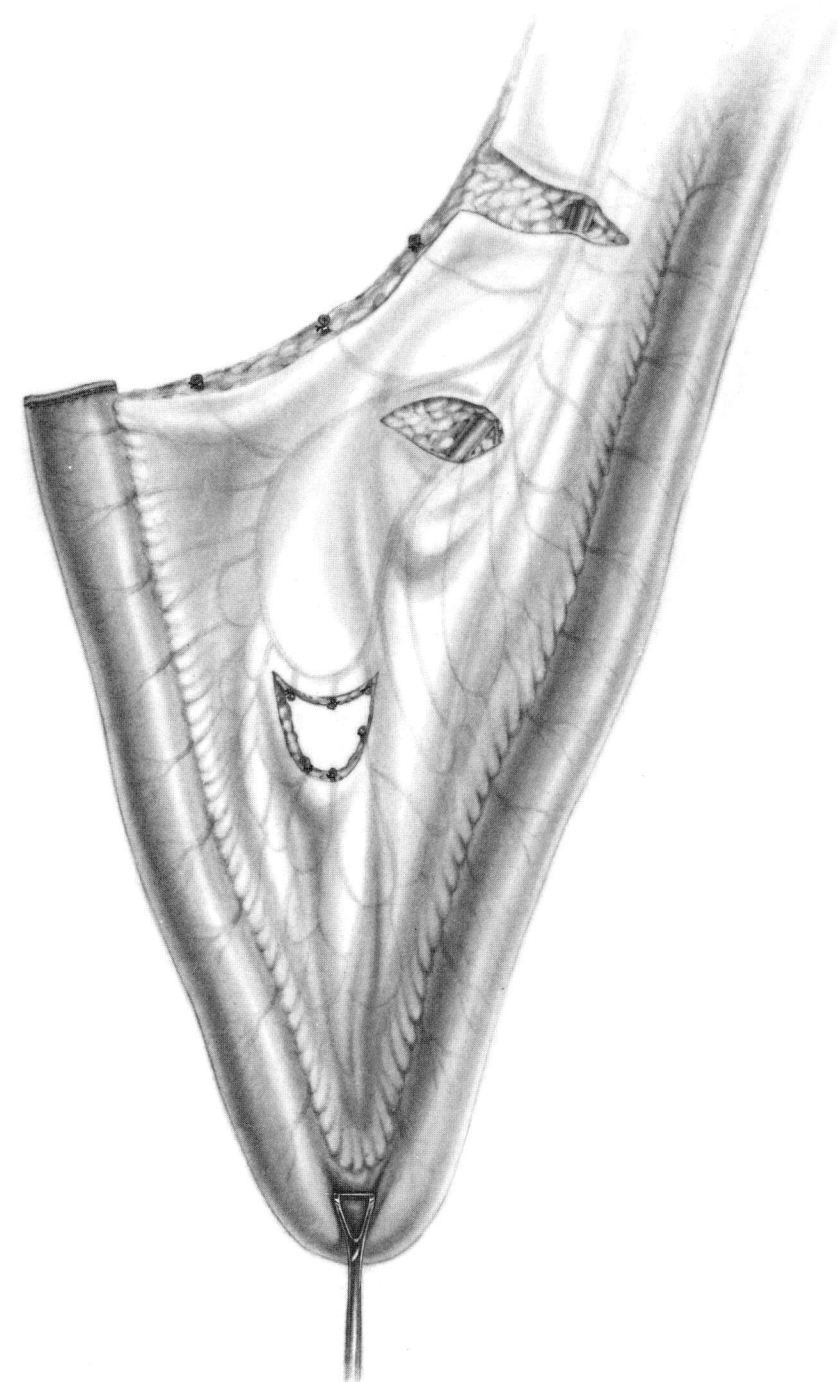

FIGURE 29-87. Incising the peritoneum of the mesentery and creating a window aid in achieving increased length. (Adapted from Burnstein MJ, Schoetz DJ Jr, Coller JA, Veidenheimer MC. Technique of mesenteric lengthening in ileal reservoir-anal anastomosis. *Dis Colon Rectum* 1987;30: 863.)

there is legitimate concern about leaving behind residual viable epithelium, and there is valid objection to unnecessary manipulation of the sphincter mechanism. How to reconcile the two mutually exclusive intentions has precipitated considerable debate. It is self-evident that the more one maneuvers and stretches the anal canal, the more likely one is to impact adversely on bowel control.

Some have criticized the double-stapling technique as inadequate for removing the rectal mucosa. The fear of the possibility of malignancy arising in the remaining glandular epithelium as well as the concern for symptoms from residual inflammation is quite real (see next section). Deen and colleagues opine that high anal transection and pouch-anal anastomosis should be the preferred option in

(text continues on page 1415)

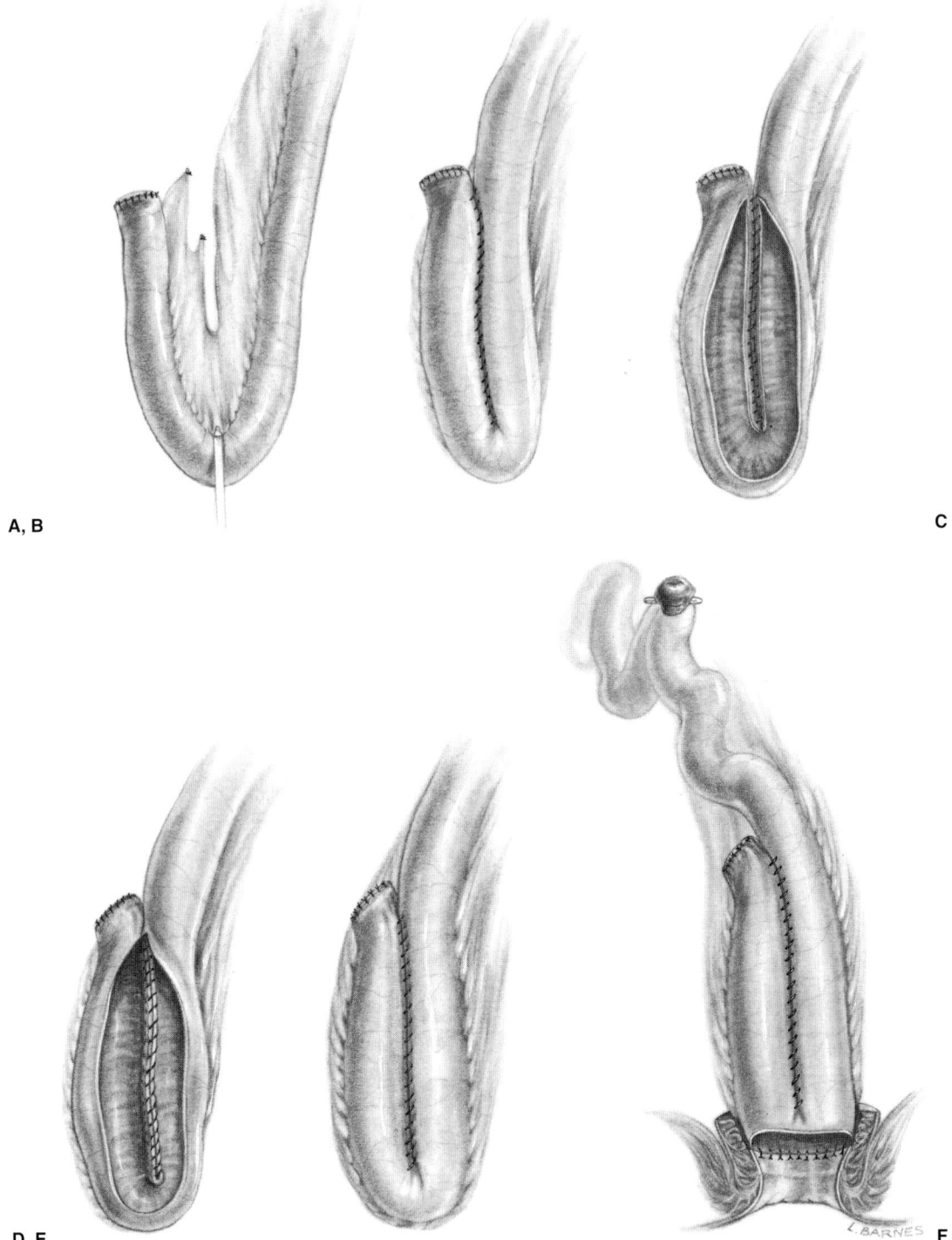

A, B

C

D, E

F

FIGURE 29-88. Pouch-anal procedure (J type). **(A)** Limbs identified with distal ileum closed. **(B)** Seromuscular apposition. **(C)** Long enterotomy. **(D)** Closure of posterior wall. **(E)** Closure of anterior wall. **(F)** Completed anastomosis of pouch to anus with protecting loop ileostomy.

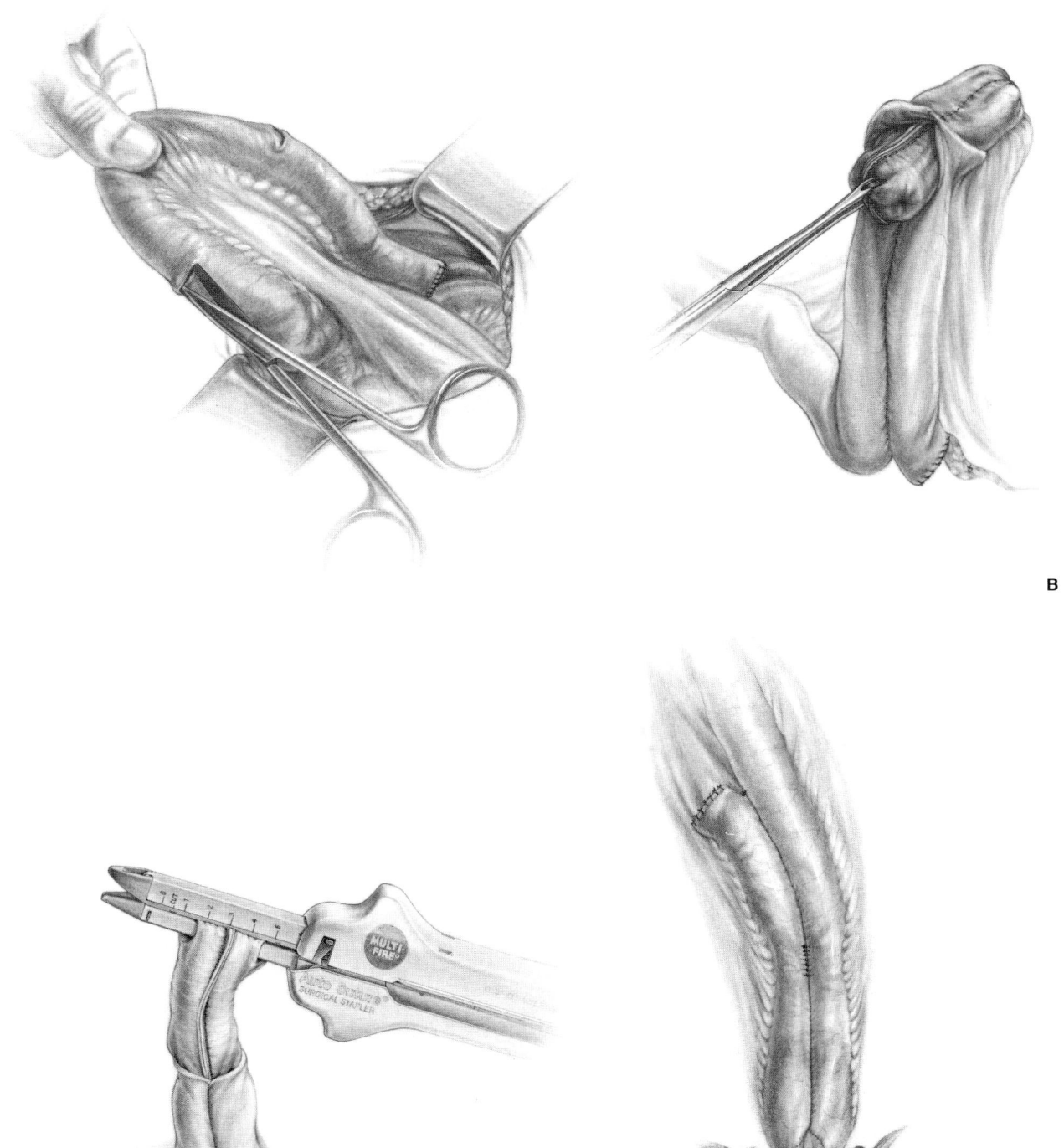

A

B

C

D

FIGURE 29-89. Stapled J-pouch procedure. **(A)** Two enterotomies are created and the GIA instrument is inserted in each limb in both directions. **(B)** Apical septum is inverted. **(C)** Septum is divided by GIA instrument. **(D)** Enterotomy is closed longitudinally and anastomosis of pouch to anus is effected.

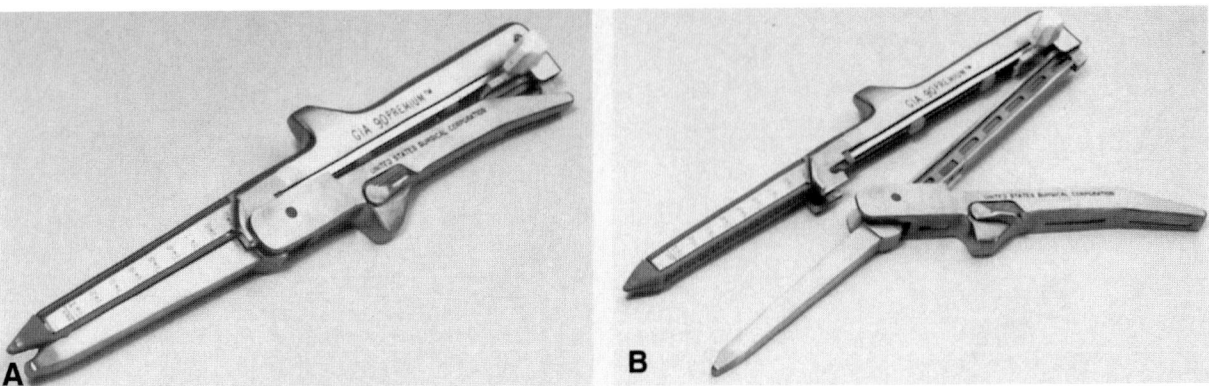

FIGURE 29-90. Long (9-cm) GIA stapler. **(A)** Closed position. **(B)** Open position. (Courtesy of United States Surgical Corp., Norwalk, CT.)

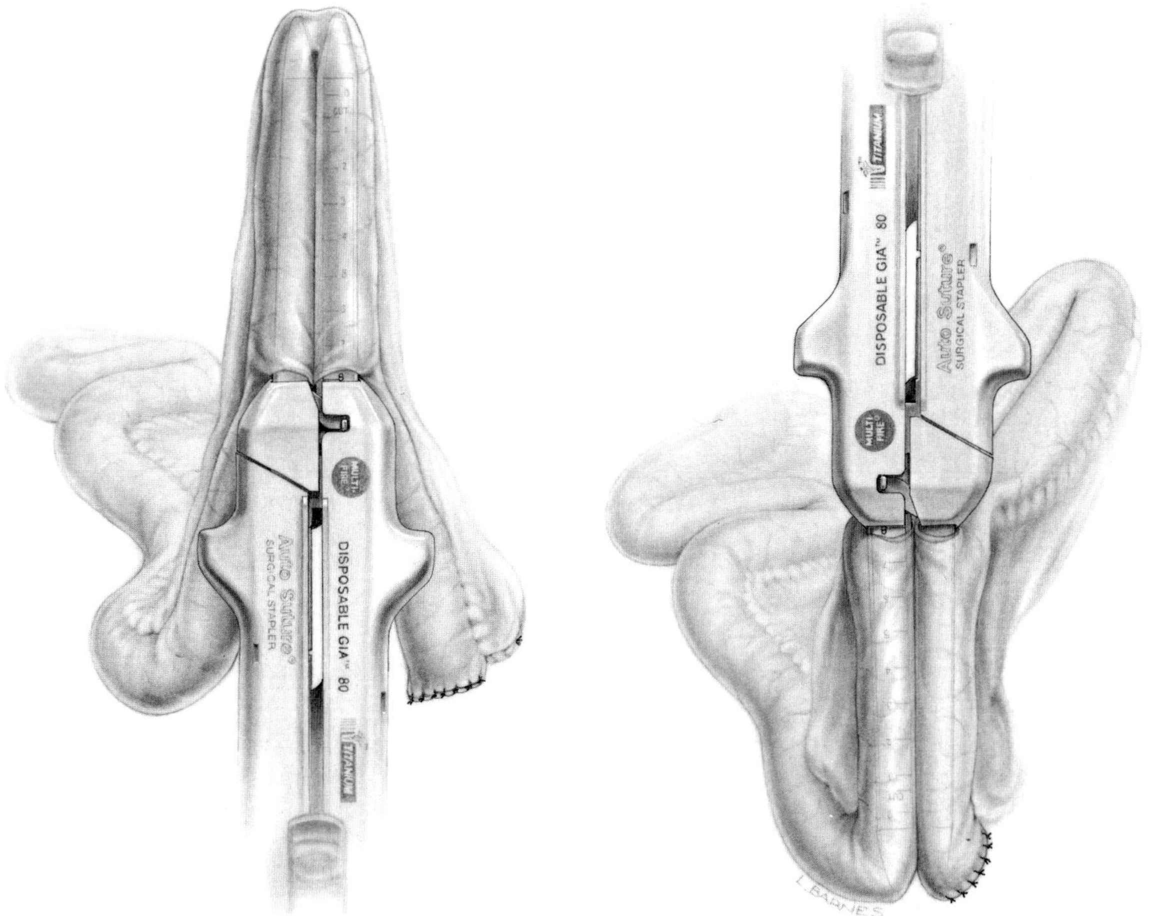

A

B

FIGURE 29-91. Construction of J-pouch with long (8-cm) GIA stapler. **(A)** Enterotomies with passage toward apex. **(B)** Passage cephalad in direction of ileal closure.

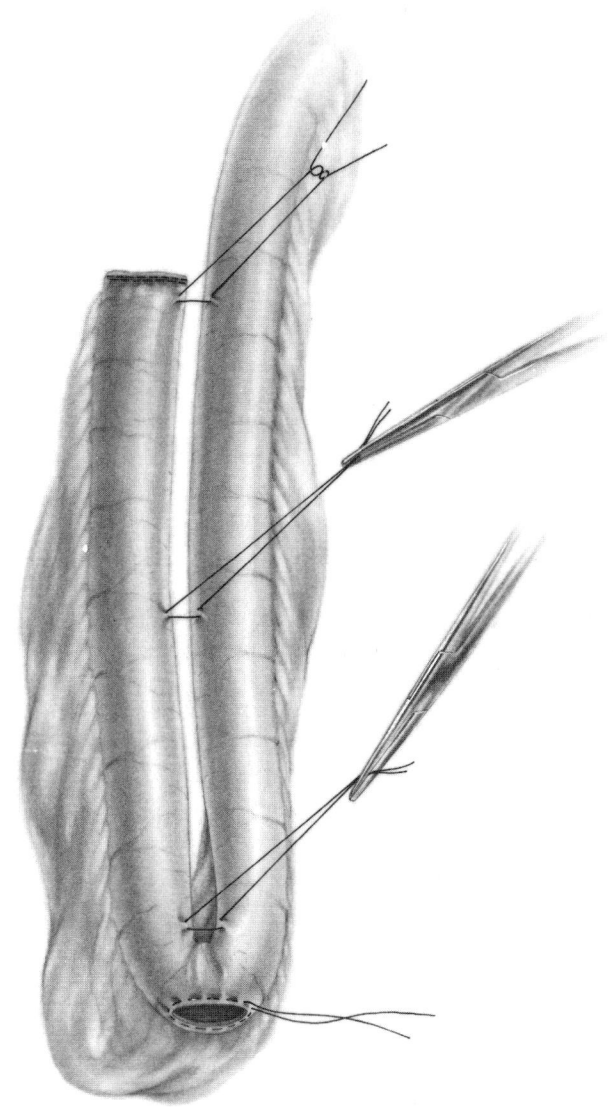

FIGURE 29-92. Lining up the two limbs in constructing the J pouch. (Adapted from Burnstein MJ, Schoetz DJ Jr, Coller JA, Veidenheimer MC. Technique of mesenteric lengthening in ileal reservoir-anal anastomosis. *Dis Colon Rectum* 1987; 30:863.)

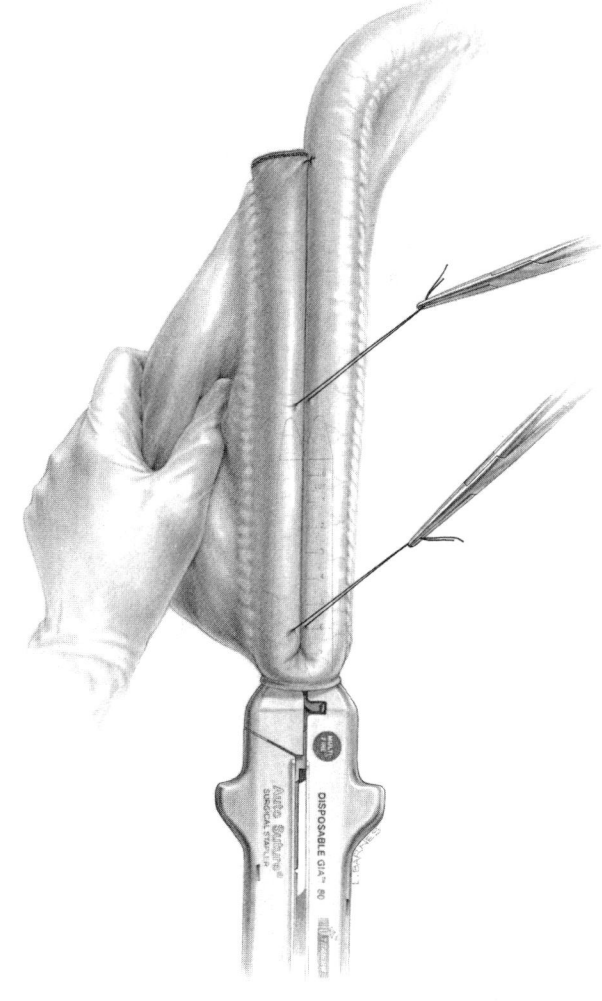

FIGURE 29-93. Tension on bowel mesentery prevents injury from stapler.

restorative proctocolectomy, because a dentate line anastomosis may not fully eliminate columnar epithelium.[126] Moreover, Thompson-Fawcett and co-workers have demonstrated that the anal transitional zone is shorter than most people have recognized, and that after double-stapled restorative proctocolectomy there remains a 1.5 to 2.0 cm cuff of diseased columnar epithelium, an important consideration for long-term follow-up.[705] Preservation of the anal transitional zone may actually preserve disease.[8] A particular concern arises if restorative proctocolectomy is performed with preservation of the anal transition zone in individuals who harbor high-grade dysplasia or carci-

noma (see Dysplasia and Malignancy).[764] Some of the criticism may be addressed if one understands that there is further distal rectum removed in the tissue ring when the circular stapler is applied, but there has now developed a considerable literature on the problems associated with residual, viable epithelium.

Mucosectomy (Yes or No!)

Keighley evaluated the functional results following J-pouch construction by comparing endoanal mucosectomy and abdominal mucosectomy.[334] He noted a statistically significant decrease in resting anal canal pressure after the endoanal procedure, but this was not observed with the abdominal approach. The author attributed the increased incidence of soiling with the former technique to the prolonged duration and extent of anal retraction that is required. Gemlo and co-

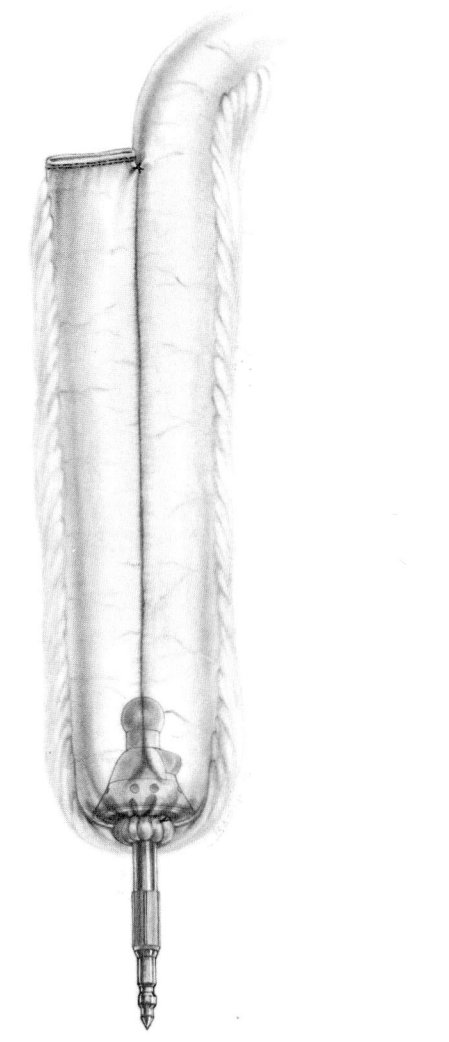

FIGURE 29-94. Anvil head is placed in the apex of the reservoir at the site of insertion of the long GIA stapler. The pursestring suture is then secured.

workers conclude that avoidance of mucosectomy does not influence stool frequency but does significantly improve fecal continence and, in their opinion, introduces an undetectable morbidity associated with the retained rectal mucosa.[200] Becker and associates found that the loss of resting pressure of the internal anal sphincter could be correlated with the extent of smooth-muscle resection during rectal mucosectomy, and that these factors correlate with increased stool frequency and a greater likelihood of nocturnal stool leakage (see Bowel Frequency and Continence).[39] Others have concluded that a stapled pouch-anal anastomosis, preserving the mucosa of the anal transitional zone, confers no apparent early advantage in terms of decreased stool frequency or fewer episodes of fecal incontinence compared with hand-sewn anastomosis, excising the mu-

cosa.[588] However, they observed that the stapled group had higher resting pressures and less nighttime incontinence.[588]

Dysplasia and Malignancy

One of the concerns expressed when one performs restorative proctocolectomy is the risk for the development of carcinoma if there is residual rectal mucosa present. Stern and colleagues reported the first such experience, a patient who had undergone a "classic" mucosectomy.[676] Since then several cases have been described.[23,44,384,578,610] Ståhlberg and co-workers opine that this risk may be greater in individuals with concomitant sclerosing cholangitis.[667] Invasive adenocarcinoma has also been described in the pouch, itself,[46,308] but it is unclear as to whether these arose from the ileal mucosa or from residual rectal epithelium. Heppell and co-workers obtained pathologic specimens of the ileoanal anastomoses from eight patients who required take-down.[278] Re-epithelialization of the rectal sleeve did not occur, although a few isolated rectal mucosal cells were seen. In a similar study of 29 patients, O'Connell and co-workers found that the rectal muscle cuff was bound to ileal serosa by dense fibrous tissue.[535] Active rectal mucosal disease, dysplasia, or re-epithelialization was not observed.

With less attention to mucosectomy and with no attempt to preserve a muscular sleeve, the concern for the subsequent development of malignancy should be minimal. However, Löfberg and colleagues identified a patient who underwent an S-pouch procedure and who was found 4 years later to harbor low-grade dysplasia and DNA aneuploidy on random biopsy.[426] In an evaluation from the Cleveland Clinic (Florida) of 109 patients who underwent restorative proctocolectomy with non-mucosectomy and a double-stapled reservoir anastomosis, the risk for malignant transformation in the strip of retained anorectal mucosa was found to be slight and did not increase appreciably in the first few years after operation.[254] According to a further report from the Cleveland Clinic, if there is symptomatic proctitis from the residual mucosa, delayed mucosectomy via a perineal approach can be successfully accomplished, provided that the stapled anastomosis is within 3 or 4 cm of the dentate line.[164]

The principle discussed earlier in this chapter concerning the significance of *dysplasia* in ulcerative colitis has been applied to surveillance of those individuals who have undergone restorative proctocolectomy. Coull and co-workers, at the Glasgow Royal Infirmary, analyzed 135 patients by means of cuff surveillance biopsy.[108] There was no evidence of either dysplasia or carcinoma in any of the patients. They concluded that cuff surveillance in the first decade after this operation,

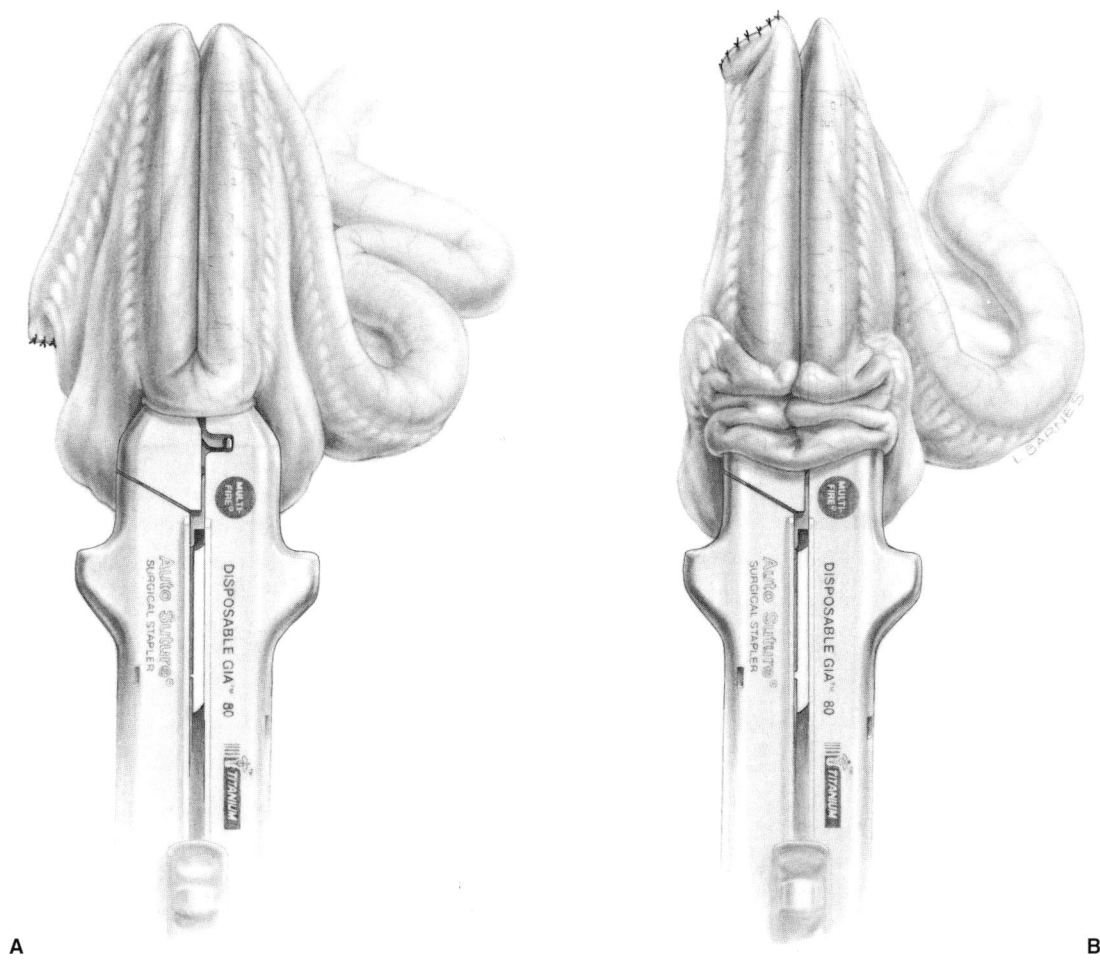

A   **B**

FIGURE 29-95. Construction of J-pouch with long (8-cm) GIA stapler. **(A)** Apex entry. **(B)** Intussusception after single firing of instrument from apical position.

in the absence of dysplasia or carcinoma in the original colectomy specimen, is unnecessary. Others confirm the rarity of such changes, but there appears to be a consensus among those most familiar with this operation that an *annual surveillance program* is suggested for all individuals who have undergone restorative proctocolectomy.[545,592,704] However, as with the Kock pouch, routine biopsy of the reservoir itself does not appear to be indicated.[280]

Two reports of patients in whom a lymphoma developed in the pouch following this operation have been described.[187,528]

Appropriateness of Restorative Proctocolectomy with Concomitant Cancer

With respect to whether restorative proctocolectomy is appropriate for patients found to harbor a carcinoma with ulcerative colitis or polyposis, Wiltz and colleagues suggest that it is probably prudent to delay the

pouch construction until a later date because of the potential difficulty of intraoperative staging and the possible requirement for adjuvant therapy.[751] Radiation of the ileal reservoir is poorly tolerated and will inevitably be associated with suboptimal functional results. It would seem self-evident that these individuals should undergo complete mucosectomy and be followed closely.

Management of Residual Symptomatic Mucosa or Dysplasia

If a patient develops bothersome symptoms of rectal bleeding from residual rectal epithelium or is found to harbor dysplasia, mucosectomy with pouch advancement is indicated. This can usually be accomplished without adversely affecting bowel function (continence and frequency) but may not be easy to accomplish because of scarring. At the very least, the mucosa can and

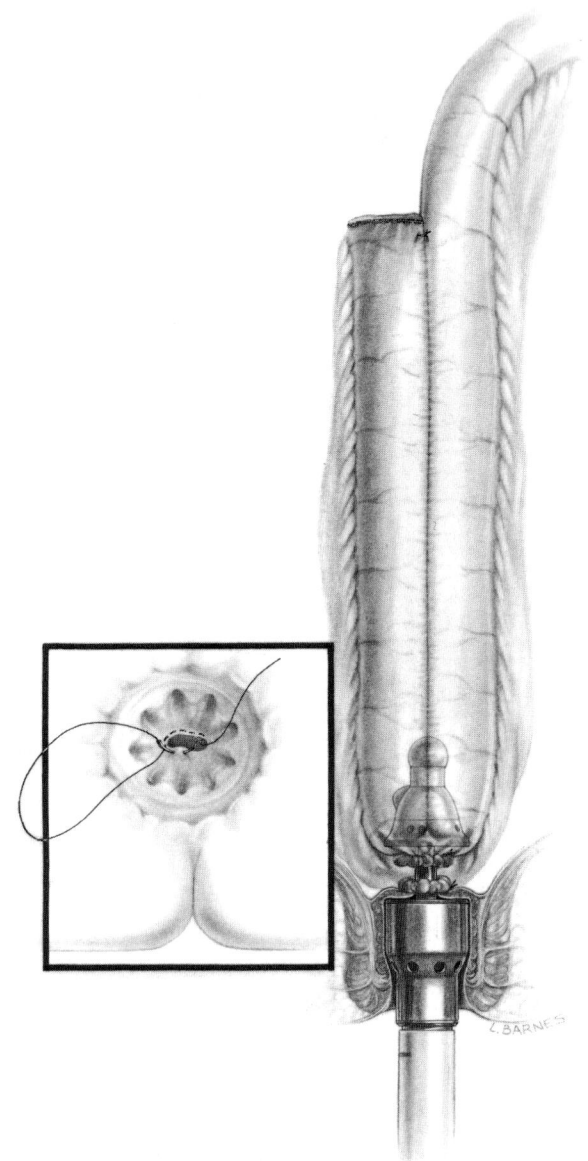

FIGURE 29-96. Pouch-anal anastomosis by means of circular stapler. Insertion of purse-string suture in the anal canal **(inset)**.

should be ablated. Close follow-up surveillance is, of course, required.

Lateral Ileal Pouch

Fonkalsrud has been an advocate of another type of ileoanal-pouch, the lateral ileal reservoir.[175–177] This is accomplished by dividing and oversewing the proximal end of the ileum approximately 25 to 30 cm above the peritoneal reflection. In the opinion of the author, an ileal reservoir of 14 to 16 cm in length appears to provide optimal function.[673] A temporary end-ileostomy is then used for diversion (Figure 29-101A). A lateral reservoir is con-

structed over the entire length of the original segment at a subsequent operation (Figure 29-101B). Fonkalsrud's approach seems to be used essentially by him alone and has never achieved the popularity of the other alternatives. In fact, Fonkalsrud ultimately adopted the less controversial J-pouch technique prior to his retirement.

W-Pouch

One of the concerns about the S-reservoir is the fact that many patients require catheterization of the pouch to effect evacuation. Conversely, the J-pouch, although eliminating the requirement for catheterization, has been thought to be associated with increased stool frequency because of a smaller reservoir capacity (see later discussion). To address these problems, another modification has been proposed, the so-called quadruple-loop or W-reservoir.[516] The terminal 50 cm of small bowel are folded into four loops, each 12 cm long, forming a W-shaped configuration (Figure 29-102). The W-pouch can also be constructed with the stapling instruments (Figure 29-103). Like the J-pouch, the reservoir itself may be anastomosed to the anal canal.

Pouch with "Nipple"

Harms and colleagues have suggested a modification whereby the apex of the second loop is positioned 3 to 4 cm short of the apex of the first to create a "nipple" on the end of the pouch, making the area for the anastomosis somewhat narrower.[260] Peck adopts an isoperistaltic nipple valve with the J-pouch in the hope of (a) preventing reflux, (b) effecting more complete emptying of the reservoir, (c) minimizing perianal irritation, and (d) slowing intestinal transit[566] (Figure 29-104). There has been no further data on this approach since its initial publication.

Ileal Kock Pouch

Kock and colleagues reported the application of the standard, double-folded ileal reservoir (Kock pouch) as a pouch-anal alternative.[362] Six patients underwent interposition of the pouch between the ileum and the anus following colectomy and mucosal proctectomy. After the ileostomy was closed, the range of bowel evacuations was three to five per 24-hour period. The large reservoir capacity and the low pressure were believed to explain the excellent functional results. Further experience with this approach seems warranted, but has not been evident in the literature.

Concomitant Ileostomy

Irrespective of the type of pouch undertaken, a loop ileostomy is usually advised to protect the anastomosis[344] (Figure 29-105; see Figs. 31-67 through 31-69), but some surgeons have selectively performed the procedure without a diversionary stoma.[452] The construc-

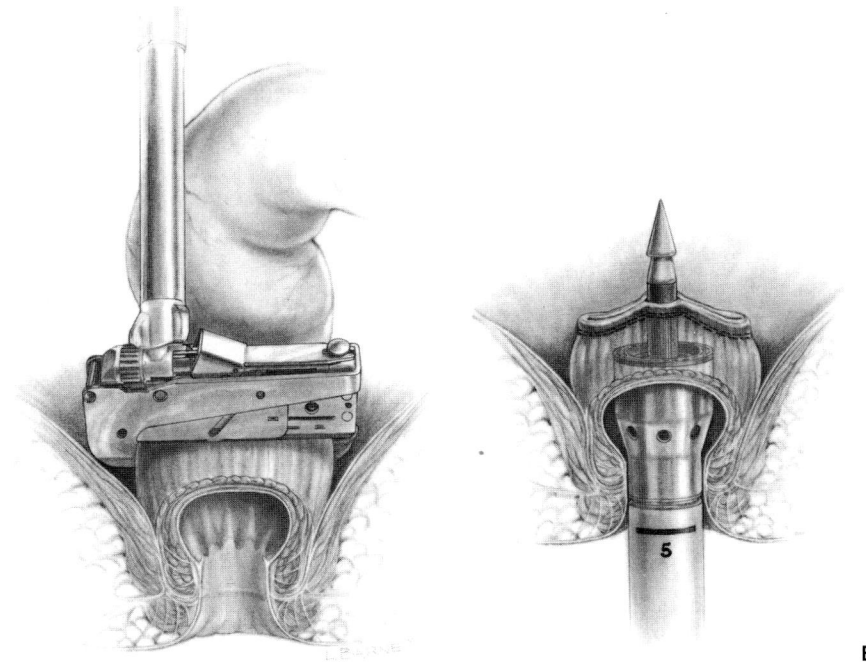

FIGURE 29-97. Pouch-anal anastomosis by double-stapling technique. **(A)** Roticulator facilitates linear closure of rectal remnant. **(B)** The trocar tip of the circular, end-to-end (CEEA) instrument effects anastomosis to the reservoir. (Courtesy of United States Surgical Corp., Norwalk, CT.)

A

B

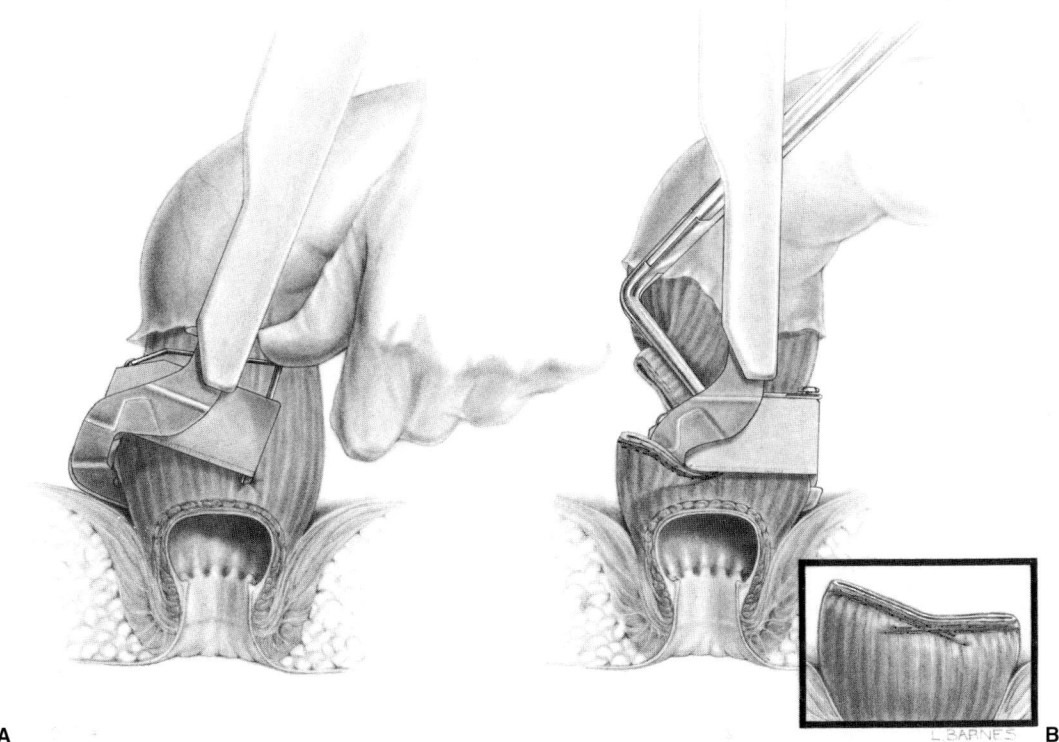

A

B

FIGURE 29-98. An alternative method of accomplishing pouch-anal anastomosis by double-stapling technique with narrow pelvis. **(A)** Linear stapler (30 mm) is applied across a portion of the rectum. Note that the pin must be pressed through the bowel wall for the instrument to fire. **(B)** Overlapping staple lines are created with a second application of the 30-mm linear stapler. The anastomosis is then completed in the manner described in Figure 29-97.

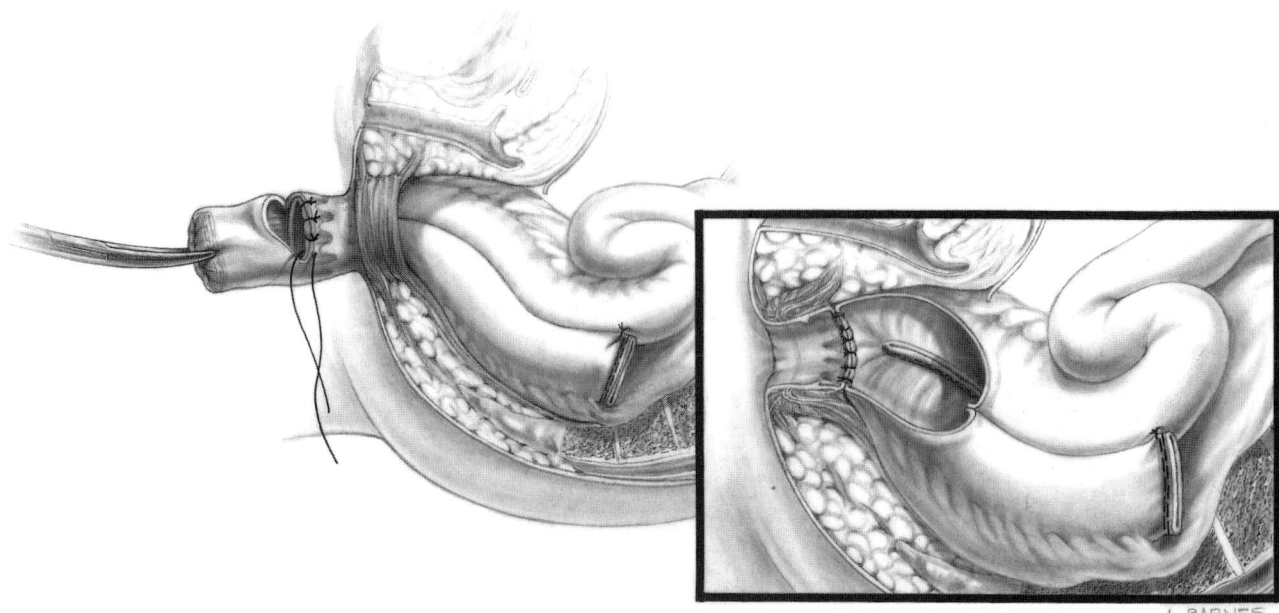

L. BARNES

A   B

FIGURE 29-99. J-pouch "Swenson" procedure. **(A)** The rectum is transected by quadrants just above the dentate line, allowing the ileal J-pouch anastomosis to be undertaken in a controlled manner. **(B)** Completed anastomosis. (After Motta JC, Ricketts RR. The J-pouch Swenson procedure for ulcerative colitis and familial polyposis. *Am Surg* 1992;58:613).

tion and closure of an ileostomy is not without morbidity (see Chapter 31) and may actually increase the risk for postoperative bowel obstruction. Winslet and colleagues observed that formation and closure of a loop ileostomy were associated with 41% and 30% complication rates, respectively, in a prospective evaluation of 34 patients.[752] Others have reported a statistically significant reduction in total hospital stay, reduced complication rates, fewer episodes of intestinal obstruction, and a shorter operating time in individuals not submitted to ileostomy at the time of pouch construction.[223,233,283,293,312,497,498,620]

Galandiuk and colleagues related the Mayo Clinic experience of 37 patients who underwent an ileal J-pouch procedure without ileostomy.[193] When they were compared with a matched group of patients having a protecting stoma, a higher incidence of postoperative complications was noted (22% versus 11%). However, subsequent functional results were comparable. According to the authors, suggested criteria for considering this option are absolute lack of tension on the anastomosis, good blood supply to the terminal ileum, good general health, and absence of recent steroids. Similarly Heuschen and co-workers undertook a matched-pair control study in which the one-stage and two-stage operations were compared.[283] The authors found that the proportion of patients *without* complications was significantly higher, and the frequency of late complications

was significantly lower in the one-stage group. Furthermore, the percentage of individuals who developed an anastomotic stricture was significantly higher with the two-stage operation. There were no other significant differences between the two groups with respect to a number of variables: early complications, pouch-related septic complications, pouchitis, duration of surgery, blood loss, and median hospital stay. The critical recommendation in this nonprospective study is, "*if there is a choice* [italics, mine] . . . the one stage operation is clearly superior."

Launer and Sackier offer another method for avoiding a protecting ileostomy with this operation, that of the intraluminal bypass tube (Coloshield; Figure 29-106; see Chapter 26).[383] The technique is similar to that described in Figure 26-46. The authors reported no anastomotic complications or morbidity related to the bypass tube in eight patients, but the device is not available in the United States.

Several reports have expressed caution with respect to the failure to employ temporary ileostomy when a reservoir-anal procedure is performed. Williamson and associates observed that life-threatening complications were more common among patients who did not have a defunctioning ileostomy.[750] Others observe that restorative proctocolectomy without diversion is not as safe as when it is performed with an ileostomy, especially in persons taking in excess of 20 mg of prednisone per day.[707]

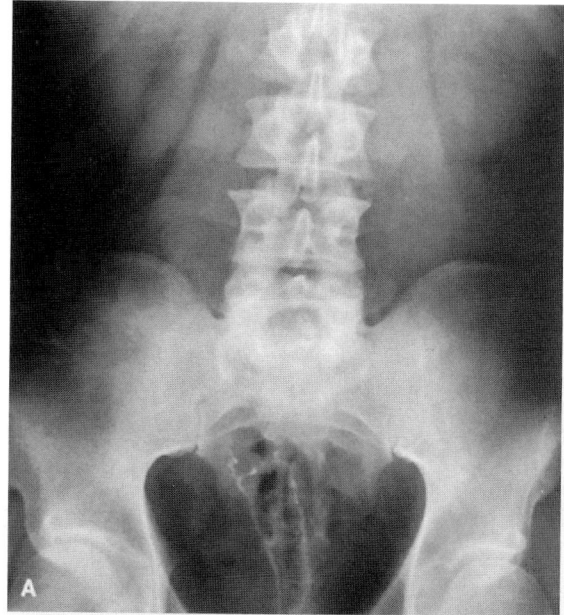

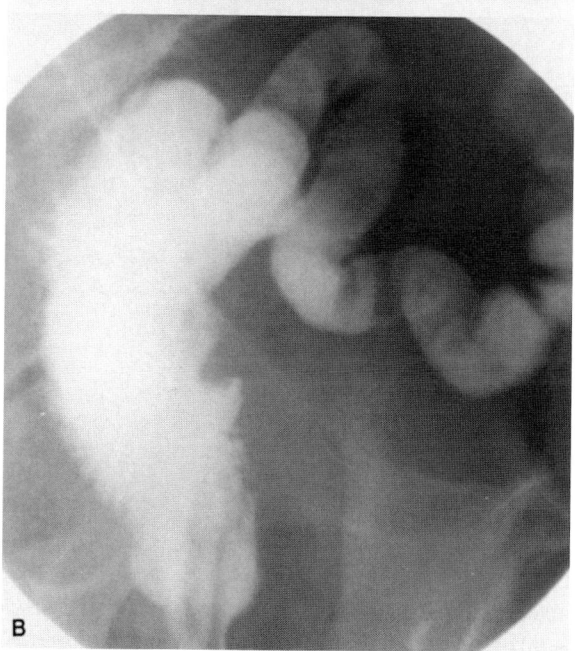

FIGURE 29-100. J-pouch–anal anastomosis by stapling technique. **(A)** Plain abdominal film demonstrates double line of staples forming the reservoir. **(B)** Barium study before ileostomy closure reveals an intact pouch.

Opinion

Caution would seem to dictate that an ileostomy is a requisite if there is the suggestion of tension on the suture line or if the procedure is performed for fulminant disease. A host of the usual relative contraindications should be considered (e.g., nutritional status, high-dose steroids). If I elect to abjure fecal diversion concomitant with a restorative proctocolectomy, it should have been a technically flawless and uncomplicated operation, with a perfect anastomosis, with no steroid side-effects, and with the patient in a good nutritional state. I recognize that there are a number of qualified surgeons who would not be as restrictive. However, I have sufficient chevrons on my sleeve to categorically state that if I do not have to deal with the consequences of another anastomotic leak for the remainder of my operating days I will not be chagrined. One needs to remember, however, that a defunctionalized, stapled anastomosis tends to stricture. My own preference, therefore, is to perform gentle, finger dilatation on a biweekly basis until the stoma has been closed.

Laparoscopic Approach

Although I do not consider the subject of laparoscopically hindered restorative proctocolectomy controversial (at least not in my mind), there is no denying the fact that highly qualified, respected surgeons are applying minimally invasive principles to this operation. Many use the technique primarily for taking down the flexures and performing a hypogastric transverse incision for the resection, pouch creation and anastomosis, but some surgeons complete virtually the entire procedure by laparoscopic means. As discussed earlier in this chapter, the concept of mini-laparotomy has addressed all of the issues for me that theoretically allow any advantage to laparoscopy. Therefore, it is unlikely that I shall be motivated to change. Regardless, even in the hands of "experts," the functional outcome and the quality of life of laparoscopic-assisted restorative proctocolectomy is not different from that of the conventionally performed surgery.[143] Even the cosmetic result may not be as satisfactory—after all, there are no port site scars with mini-laparotomy.

Postoperative Management

Following one-stage surgery or closure of the ileostomy, patients inevitably are troubled by frequent bowel movements and perhaps problems with continence. It is, therefore, important to prepare the patient emotionally for these consequences and to offer management alternatives. As with ostomates, an enterostomal therapist is an invaluable resource for counseling patients.[253] Certain food may increase or decrease stool output and frequency. Those that have been demonstrated to exacerbate gastrointestinal disturbances are apple juice, raw fruits, raw vegetables, popcorn, seeds, nuts, beans, corn, beer, caffeine, chocolate, milk and milk products, and spicy foods. The diet may be supplemented by one of the liquid nutrition products (e.g., Ensure). Ample fluid intake is strongly encouraged to avoid dehydration. Dehydration requiring readmission

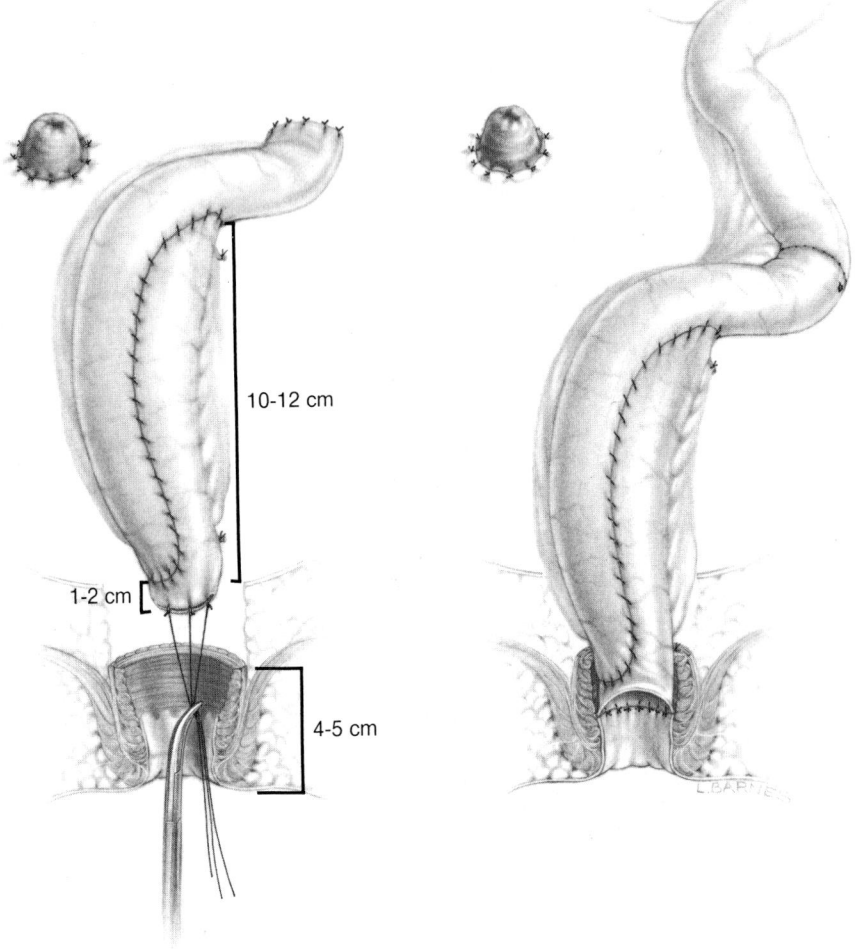

FIGURE 29-101. Lateral ileal reservoir (Fonkalsrud). **(A)** Ileal reservoir is created using a side-to-side technique, either by hand sewing or with the long GIA instrument. **(B)** The ileal spout is drawn through the rectal muscle cuff to the anus and the ileoanal anastomosis is effected. Note that Fonkalsrud prefers to use an end-ileostomy. (Adapted from Fonkalsrud EW, Phillips JD. Reconstruction of malfunctioning ileoanal pouch procedures as an alternative to permanent ileostomy. *Am J Surg* 1990;160:245.)

to the hospital occurred in 20% of the patients in the University of Toronto experience.[167] Supplementary medication in the form of "slowing" agents is often helpful [e.g., loperamide (Imodium), diphenoxylate (Lomotil), deodorized tincture of opium, paregoric, and codeine]. A bulking agent, such as one containing psyllium, may be added, and cholestyramine (Questran) may be ameliorative for some individuals, even without a colon. Topical agents for perianal irritation may be required. An aggressive approach to the medical management of these patients is necessary in order to give them confidence until time permits bowel function to become relatively stabilized.

Complications of the Pouch Procedures

Despite the magnitude of the operation, operative mortality has been remarkably low—virtually anecdotal.[569] In a review from the Mayo Clinic involving 1,603 patients who underwent proctocolectomy with pouch-

anal reconstruction, three deaths occurred postoperatively (0.2%).[367] Pulmonary embolism, perforated gastric ulcer, and subarachnoid hemorrhage were the reasons. Late deaths occurred in 29 patients (1.8%).[367] These were primarily related to malignancy and to extracolonic manifestations of underlying or unrelated coexisting diseases and events.[367] However, all published reports recognize that ileoanal-reservoir operations are associated with a high frequency of complications, often well in excess of 50%. These include pouchitis, anal stenosis, intestinal obstruction, "cuff abscess," stomal problems, ileus, fistulas, sepsis, hemorrhage, ischemia, bowel management problems, and others.[183,336,448,468,563,569,742] Generally, complications are more frequent in the early experience with the operation than in the later. Despite what may appear to be indomitable problems, every effort should be made to preserve the pouch. The success with various salvage operations has been reported by a number of investigators (see later discussion).[182,192,511,640,706]

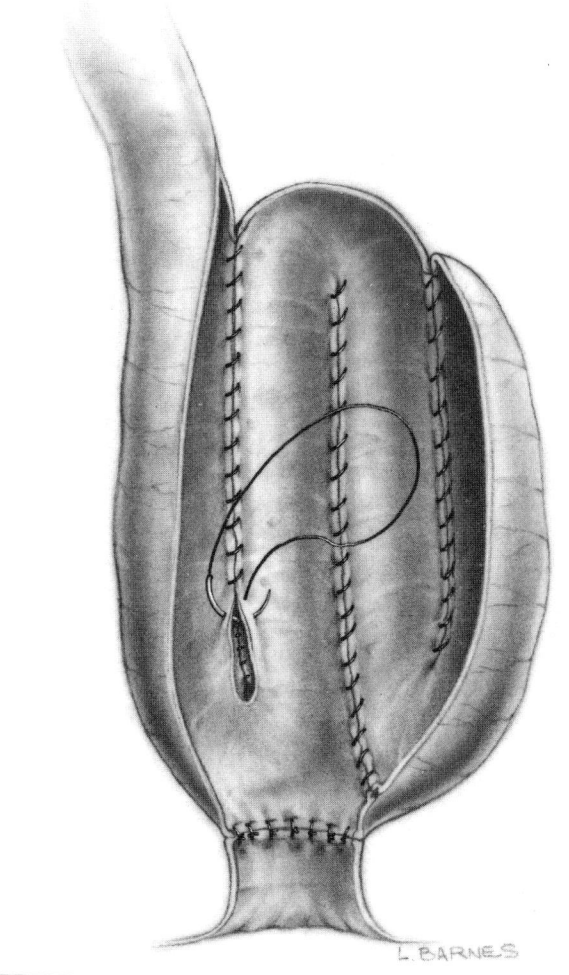

FIGURE 29-102. Quadruple reservoir—hand-sewn.

Anastomotic Leak. Anastomotic leak is inevitably caused by one or more of the usual suspects (tension on the suture line, ischemia, pelvic hematoma, or sepsis) and is often associated with the subsequent development of an anal stricture. It is because of the risk for this complication that a protecting ileostomy is usually advised. Fleshman and colleagues reported a 10% anal anastomotic leak rate in 179 patients.[173] The Mayo Clinic group revealed that radiologic or clinical leaks from the pouch or ileoanal anastomosis occurred in 14%.[698] However, because most centers have adopted a stapling technique, very little has been reported with respect to this particular complication in later years. Whether this is because of the application of an ileostomy by most surgeons or the failure to pursue appropriate investigation of patients within the first few weeks after operation is not known. Still, according to the University of Toronto group, although the leak rate has remained relatively stable, leaks following a stapled anastomosis seem to have a better prognosis than those that occur following handsewn anastomosis.[433]

It is generally agreed that the major causes for pouch failure are poor functional results, pelvic sepsis, and unsuspected Crohn's disease, as opposed to the other complications, including pouchitis and anastomotic leak.[201]

Cuff Abscess. Pelvic abscess was observed in 11% of patients in the earlier Mayo Clinic series.[478] As mentioned previously, Ambroze and colleagues favor preservation of the omentum to limit the risk for septic complications.[9] Keighley and colleagues observed a significant association between satisfactory functional results and pelvic sepsis.[336] Cuff abscess, specifically, results from the creation of a long muscular sleeve, was a frequently recognized problem when this technique was popularized. Because all surgeons now seem to avoid the creation of a muscular sleeve, this complication has disappeared, at least from the literature.

Intestinal Obstruction. Intestinal obstruction is one of the most frequently encountered problems after this operation. In the experience of Fleshman and colleagues, it developed in 19% of patients,[173] whereas McMullen and co-workers noted a 16% incidence.[468] Initial reports from the Mayo Clinic revealed that small-bowel obstruction was noted in 22%, almost one-half of whom required surgical intervention.[478,558] A later assessment found the incidence to be 17%.[186] The obstruction may be caused by adhesions, internal hernia, reservoir angulation, or outlet problems, or it may be related to the loop ileostomy.[173,178,179]

As has been discussed in Chapter 22, the frequency of abdominal adhesions leading to intestinal obstruction pre-

Perforation. With the techniques currently applied for creation of the reservoir, perforation of the pouch itself has become relatively unusual. The rate from Cohen's group at the Toronto General Hospital has been constant at approximately 4%, but the requirement for reservoir excision as a consequence of this complication has decreased as experience has been gained.[98,173] Other centers report rates of 1% to 2%. Perforation of the terminal ileal appendage of the J-pouch has also been noted[567] (Figure 29-107). To avoid this complication, it is probably wise to secure the distal ileum to the reservoir or to amputate any terminal ileal appendage after pouch construction. Parenthetically, perforation of the pouch as a consequence of blunt trauma to the abdomen has also been noted,[294] and one instance has been recorded of a perforation in a woman at 27 weeks' gestation, which was believed to be due to adhesions from the posterior wall of the uterus to the pouch.[11]

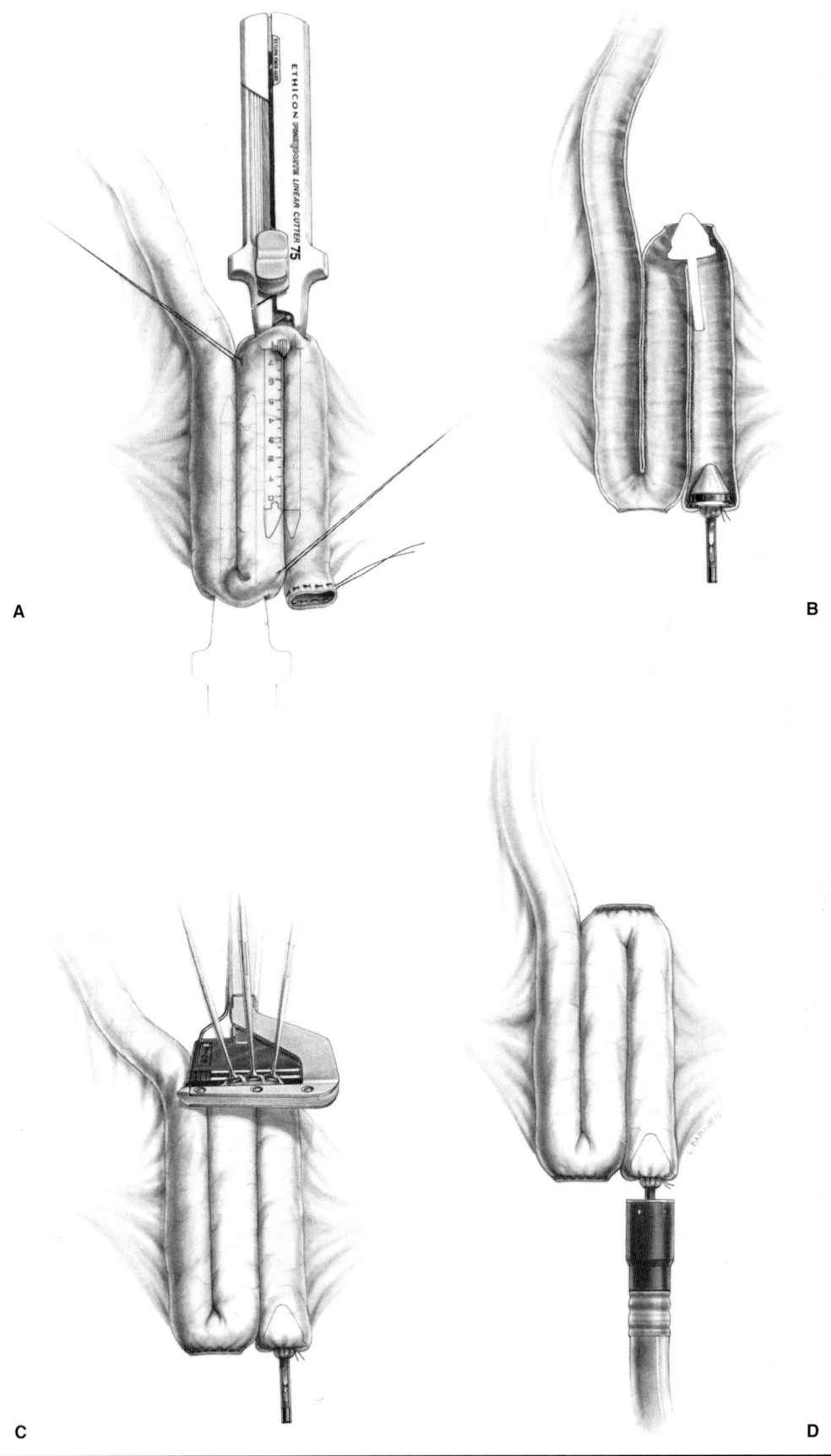

FIGURE 29-103. S-reservoir–anal anastomosis by stapling method. **(A)** Long GIA stapler is passed twice (in opposite directions). **(B)** The detachable anvil head is passed through one of the GIA stapler openings into the most distal limb. Alternatively, linear closure of the other areas can be effected and the proximal limb used. **(C)** Linear stapler closure is completed. **(D)** The anastomosis to the anal area (not shown) is accomplished in the usual way.

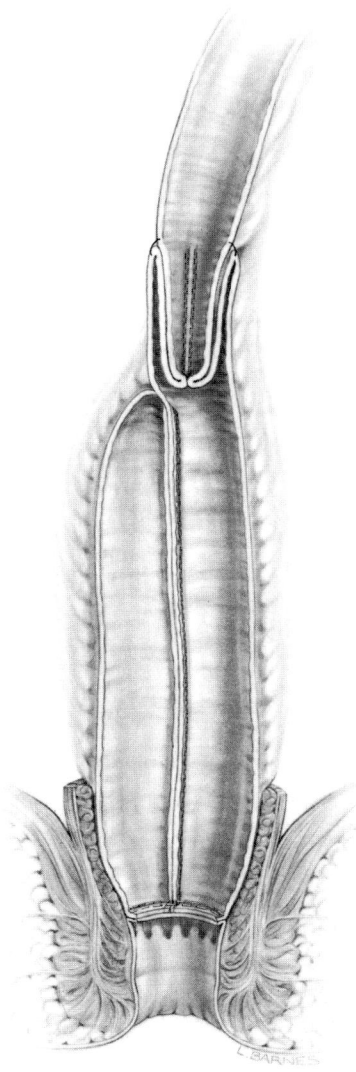

FIGURE 29-104. J-pouch–anal procedure with isoperistaltic valve, as suggested by Peck.

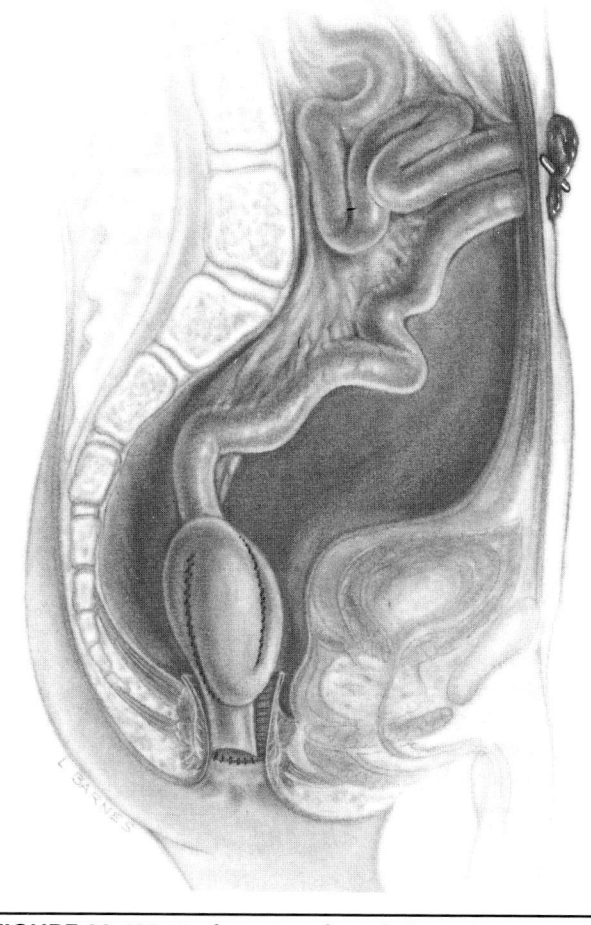

FIGURE 29-105. Final position of pouch-ileoanal anastomosis (S type) with protecting loop ileostomy.

cipitated a prospective, randomized trial with the use of a sodium hyaluronate-based bioresorbable membrane.[37] By means of direct, standardized peritoneal visualization before closure of the ileostomy, this membrane was demonstrated to be safe, and it also significantly reduced the incidence, extent, and severity of postoperative abdominal adhesions.[37]

In the experience of the Lahey Clinic surgeons, the most common point of obstruction was at closure of the ileostomy (52%).[445] The authors caution that the ileostomy should not be rotated to facilitate emptying, since this seems to predispose to subsequent obstruction in a number of patients. In another report from the same institution, small-bowel obstruction was often attributed to acute angulation of the afferent limb at the pouch inlet.[586] The authors offered the suggestion that bypass of the obstructed segment from the distal ileum to the pouch was not only possible but also constituted safe and effective management.

At least three cases of duodenal obstruction resulting from arteriomesenteric obstruction (superior mesenteric artery syndrome) have been reported.[20,90,208]

Stomal Complications. Ileostomy complications, such as stomal retraction, high ileostomy output, and parastomal hernia, are at least as frequent as the problems encountered relative to the pouch or the anastomosis. Stomal management problems are discussed in Chapters 31 and 32. In a report from the Mayo Clinic of 180 patients who underwent temporary ileostomy, transient bowel obstruction developed in 13% following take-down of the stoma.[476] More than one-half had problems with appliance management with retraction being seen in 16%. Other complications included prolapse, fistula, and abscess; ileostomy dysfunction alone was noted in 9%.[478] As discussed earlier, there have been suggestions by some experienced surgeons that a temporary ileostomy can be

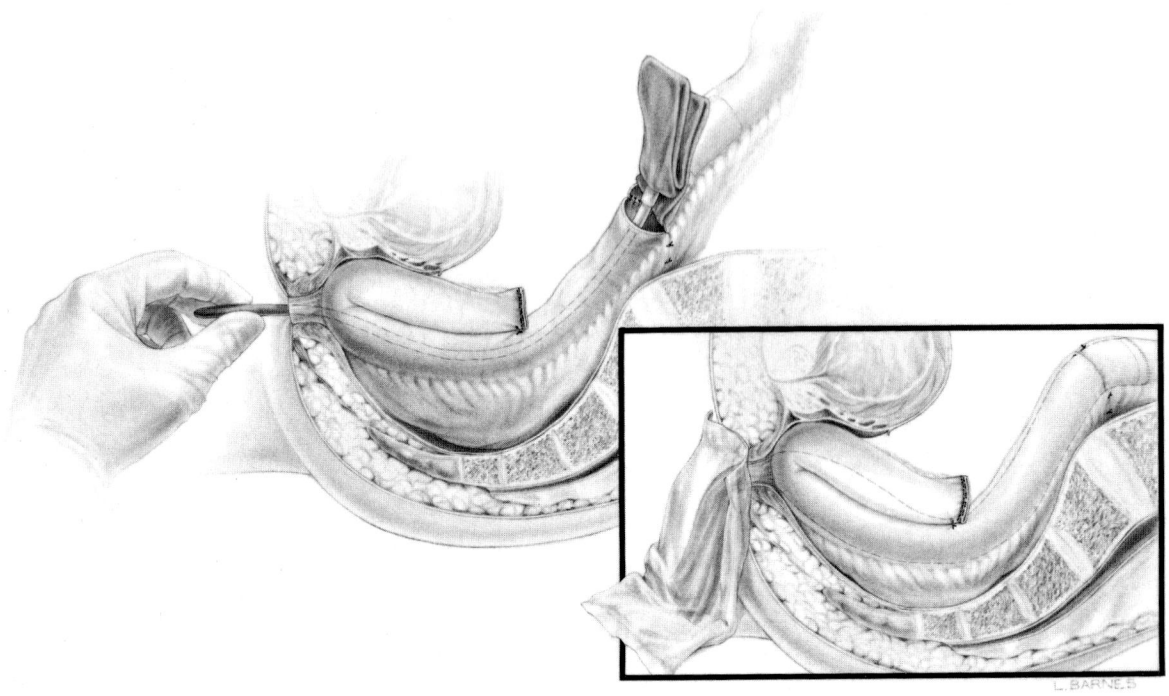

FIGURE 29-106. Ileal J-pouch–anal anastomosis using the Coloshield to avoid a temporary ileostomy. The technique for placing the device is shown in Figure 26-46. (Adapted from Launer DP, Sackier JM. Pouch-anal anastomosis without diverting ileostomy. *Dis Colon Rectum* 1991;34:193.)

avoided in selected patients.[479] However, it has been demonstrated that patients with incomplete fecal diversion have a significantly higher incidence of pouch-anal anastomotic complications (44%) than those who have had complete diversion (14%).[476]

Pouch-Anal Sinus. Anastomotic breakdown usually occurs posteriorly and may ultimately lead to a sinus. If this is recognized prior to ileostomy closure continued diversion is suggested. Otherwise, there is a risk of developing a pelvic abscess. But there comes a times when one must make a decision as to how to proceed. Probably it is wiser to create a larger opening and curette out the tract in order to permit adequate drainage. Removing a part of the back wall of the reservoir may be indicated in order to accomplish this adequately. Conversely, if the patient develops pelvic sepsis following ileostomy closure or if a stoma had not been performed in the first instance, an ileostomy must be established.

Swain and Ellis report successful treatment of pouch-anal anastomotic sinuses with fibrin glue.[689]

Pouch-Vaginal Fistula and Pouch-Perineal Fistula. Fistula between the pouch and the vagina is an uncommon complication following the pouch-anal operations, but is significantly more frequently observed when the operation is performed for ulcerative colitis than for familial adenomatous polyposis.[284] Although there is no clear documentation for the cause, it is likely due to trauma during the anterior dissection, either at the time of mobilization of the rectum through the abdomen, or when a transanal dissection is undertaken. It is suspected that in the latter situation, a woman with an ectopic anus (anterior displacement) is most vulnerable (see Chapter 13). Another consideration is the possibility that the patient has Crohn's disease.

Wexner and colleagues reviewed the experience from a number of centers (304 women) and noted an incidence of 6.9% with this complication.[741] The group from the University of Minnesota noted fistulas from the ileoanal reservoir to the perianal skin in 5%, and fistulas from the reservoir or anastomotic line to other sites in an additional 4%.[742]

Treatment options are essentially those that have been previously described for the management of this condition when it is not associated with a pouch procedure (see Chapters 12 and 13). These include transanal, transabdominal, and transvaginal closure; endoanal advancement flap; seton division; fecal diversion; and gracilis muscle interposition.[74,220,335,448,741] Most surgeons prefer endovaginal or endoileal flap advancement.[540] It is probably prudent, however, to consider temporary ileostomy concomitant with any repair.

The Cleveland Clinic group achieved success in the treatment of fistulas from pelvic pouches in more than 60%

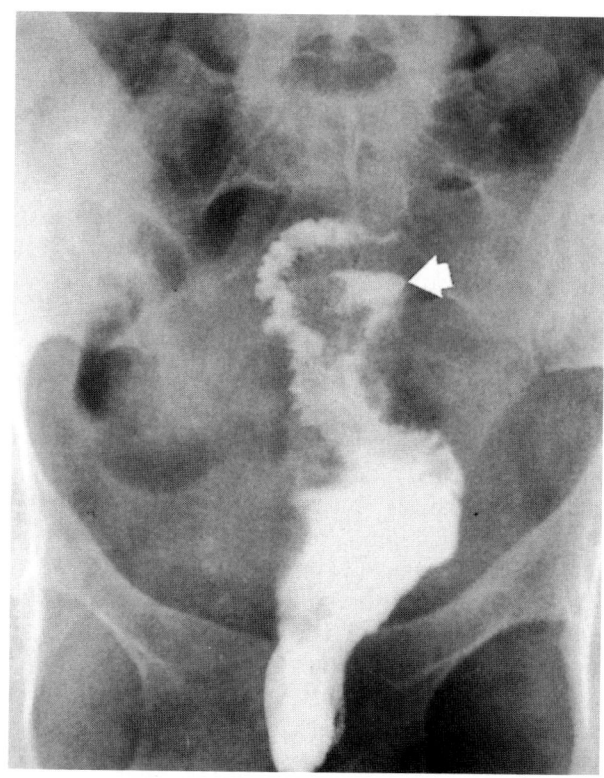

FIGURE 29-107. Pouch leakage. The distal pouch-anal anastomosis is intact. However, contrast is collecting adjacent to the proximal staple line *(arrow)*. This proved to be caused by breakdown of the closed end of the reservoir.

of their patients.[548,650] However, they observed that multiple procedures may be needed for a successful outcome, and ultimately 32% had their pouches excised. Heuschen and colleagues found that the incidence of requiring permanent defunctioning or excision of the pouch in 131 patients with septic complications was 23.7% and 6.1%, respectively.[281] Moreover, the estimated 3-, 5- and 10-year rate of pouch failure in those with septic complications was 9.6%, 31.1%, and 39.2%, respectively. In the Lahey Clinic experience, pouches complicated by fistulas not associated with Crohn's disease could be salvaged with temporary rediversion.[174] Others observe that the prognosis appears to be worse when pouch-vaginal fistula occurs after ileostomy closure.[234] Late presentation of a vaginal fistula is more frequently associated with Crohn's disease and is unlikely to result in pouch salvage.[198,389,553,650]

Impairment of bowel control following conventional fistula surgery in women is the rule rather than the exception. The likelihood of keeping one's ileoanal reservoir with this complication is therefore problematic.

Epidural Abscess. Murr and Metcalf have described recurrent epidural abscesses from an enteroepidural fistula arising from a J-pouch.[500]

Anal (Anastomotic) Stricture. Considerable variation is evident in the reported incidence of anastomotic stricture following restorative proctocolectomy. This may be attributed to whether a hand-sewn or a stapled technique was employed and whether the procedure was undertaken in one or two stages. Furthermore, most papers do not stratify strictures in the absence of sepsis, sinus, or fistula from that which is seen as a consequence of septic complications. In the experience of the Mayo Clinic group, strictures were observed in 213 of 1,884 patients (11.2%), somewhat less than in their earlier reports.[476,574] This group found that nonfibrotic strictures responded well to anal dilatation, whereas fibrotic strictures were more likely due to septic problems and required more extensive revision and perhaps salvage pouch surgery. Anastomotic stricture occurred in approximately 8% of patients in the Toronto experience.[173] Overweight males and those with blood loss in excess of 1,000 mL have been found to have an increased incidence.[173] According to Fleshman and colleagues, the presence of an anal stricture was the most significant factor contributing to a less-than-satisfactory functional result.[173]

Treatment consists usually of dilatation, but persistent symptoms may require an anoplasty (see Chapter 8) or a pouch advancement and neoileoanal anastomosis.[162] In the experience of the group from the General Infirmary in Leeds, England, the eventual clinical, functional outcome after dilatation of a stricture (39 patients) was as good as the outcome in the 63 patients in whom a stricture did not develop.[407]

Pouchitis. Pouchitis, a term coined by Kock to describe the reservoir ileitis seen with the continent ileostomy, is a well-recognized complication of all pouch procedures, and is seen about as frequently as that of small-bowel obstruction (see earlier discussion). The condition is usually manifested by increased output of liquid stool, sometimes with blood, a low-grade fever, weakness, and malaise. Endoscopic findings include a granular, easily traumatized, edematous mucosa with ulceration and histologic presence of polymorphonuclear leukocyte infiltration with ulceration. This is superimposed on the expected chronic inflammatory cell presence with crypt hyperplasia and villous atrophy.[630] Solitary pouch ulceration has also been described.[173,185,639]

In the Mayo Clinic experience with 734 patients followed for a mean of 41 months, pouchitis developed in 31% of those with ulcerative colitis and 6% with familial polyposis.[428] In the experience of Becker and Raymond, pouchitis was the most common late complication (18%).[41] The Minnesota group noted an incidence of 27%.[742] Ståhlberg and co-workers noted that the risk for pouchitis was highest during the initial 6-month period following pelvic pouch construction.[666] This leveled off after

2 years but was still considerable at 4 years (51%). However, only 2 patients (1.3%) had their pouches removed because of this complication in the experience of this group.[666] Others have also demonstrated that the incidence is approximately 50%, with two thirds of patients having multiple episodes.[303]

The most commonly used comparative diagnostic instrument is the Pouchitis Disease Activity Index, but it has been primarily a research tool. Still, it is helpful in developing an algorithm for diagnosis, classification, and management of this condition.[282] The Index was created in 1994 by Sandborn and associates of the Mayo Clinic group.[630] It is an 18-point instrument that consists of three principal component scores: symptoms, endoscopy, and histology (Table 29-7). The severity of the pouchitis has also been measured using another scoring system, the Heidelberg Pouchitis Activity Score.[282] A modified, somewhat simplified index has seen suggested by the Cleveland Clinic group.[653]

ETIOLOGY AND ASSOCIATED CONDITIONS. Pouchitis is believed to be caused by stasis of feces in the pouch with overgrowth of anaerobic organisms. There is the general impression that pouchitis occurs rarely when the various reservoir procedures have been performed for familial polyposis.[434] It has, therefore, been suggested that the likely etiology is related somehow to that of ulcerative colitis.[643]

Gustavsson and colleagues assessed whether the presence of "backwash ileitis" predisposed to the subsequent development of this problem.[239] Because pouchitis subsequently developed in 13% of patients with backwash ileitis and 16% without ileitis, the authors concluded that there was no relationship. The Mayo Clinic group reported that patients with preoperative and postoperative extraintestinal manifestations had significantly higher rates of pouchitis than did those without such manifestations.[428]

The etiology of the condition has been investigated at a number of centers. Levin and colleagues support a role for mucosal ischemia and production of oxygen free radicals.[403] They employed allopurinol, a xanthine oxidase inhibitor, and found that this agent either terminated an episode of acute pouchitis or prevented pouchitis from recurring in 50% of their patients.[403] Others have observed that smokers have significantly fewer episodes of pouchitis when compared with nonsmokers and former smokers.[474] Finally, the finding that antinuclear cytoplasmic antibodies (pANCA) occur more frequently in patients with chronic pouchitis suggests the possibility that this antibody may mark a genetically distinct subset of patients with ulcerative colitis who are predisposed to the subsequent development of pouchitis.[628] *Clostridium difficile* infection as a cause of refractory pouchitis has also been reported.[440]

The Lahey Clinic group has recognized two apparently distinct patterns of presentation based on the clinical course: those with two or fewer episodes and those with more than two.[581] Those in the former group responded generally to anti-anaerobic organism therapy, whereas only 25% in the latter group did so. The authors also identified a subset of patients with so-called short-segment pouchitis. They attributed this to retained rectal mucosa and have treated the problem successfully with topical steroid preparations.

MANAGEMENT. Therapy is medical, provided that mechanical outlet obstruction has been ruled out. Treatment usually consists of oral metronidazole, the mainstay of antibiotic therapy,[435] or enemas containing steroids or salicylate derivatives, but recurrence is not uncommon (see earlier discussion). Recourse to ciprofloxacin and amoxicillin/clavulinic acid has been successful if metronidazole's side effects become troublesome or if the drug is no longer effective.[630] A small, randomized trial from the Cleveland Clinic revealed a greater reduction of the Pouch Disease Activity Index in 6 patients on ciprofloxacin, 500 mg twice daily over 2 weeks, when compared with 9 patients on metronidazole (20 mg/kg).[655] The latter group demonstrated a 33% adverse event rate (emesis, dysgeusia, and peripheral neuropathy). In contrast, dual therapy of active pouchitis with ciprofloxacin and metronidazole over 4 weeks resulted in an 82% remission rate (36 of 44 patients) with 8 additional patients improved.[488]

Other agents include antiinflammatory drugs, such as 5-ASA and sulfasalazine; immunomodulators, such as budesonide/hydrocortisone enemas and AZA/6-MP/oral steroid combinations; probiotics (VSL#3[205] and lactobacillus GG); nutritional supplements (e.g., glutamine); and butyrate suppositories.

Recurrent or intractable disease should alert the physician to the possibility of Crohn's disease involvement. What recourse is available to those patients who are found to have Crohn's disease after ileoanal pouch surgery? The initial Mayo series with *infliximab* showed a response in six of seven patients after failure of conventional therapy.[594] This experience has been expanded at the Mayo Clinic to 29 patients with Crohn's disease of the pouch, 69% of whom had perianal pouch-vaginal fistulas.[100,595] Half of the patients had a long-term response but required maintenance infliximab therapy (see Chapter 30, Medical Management). There is no effective surgical salvage for pouchitis.[715]

Skin Irritation. Severe perianal skin irritation is reported to occur in up to 10% of patients. This may be attributed to frequent bowel action and incontinence. Bowel management programs, including bulking agents and diphenoxylate hydrochloride (Lomotil) or loperamide

▶ **TABLE 29-7 Pouchitis Disease Activity Index**

Criteria	Score
Clinical	
Stool frequency	
Usual postoperative stool frequency	0
1–2 stools/d > postoperative usual	1
3 or more stools/d > postoperative usual	2
Rectal bleeding	
None or rare	0
Present daily	1
Fecal urgency or abdominal cramps	
None	0
Occasional	1
Usual	2
Fever (temperature >37.8°C)	
Absent	0
Present	1
Endoscopic Inflammation	
Edema	1
Granularity	1
Friability	1
Loss of vascular pattern	1
Mucous exudates	1
Ulceration	1
Acute Histologic Inflammation	
Polymorphic nuclear leukocyte infiltration	
Mild	1
Moderate + crypt abscess	2
Severe + crypt abscess	3
Ulceration per low-power field (mean)	
>25%	1
25%–50%	2
>50%	3

From Sandborn WJ, Tremaine WJ, Batts KP, et al. Pouchitis after ileal pouch anal anastomosis: a pouchitis disease activity index. *Mayo Clin Proc* 1994;69:409–415.

(Imodium), have usually been advised. Topical application of 5% cholestyramine ointment in polyethylene glycol base has been reported to be helpful.[491] There is concern that patients with presumed ulcerative colitis and significant perianal disease may in fact have Crohn's disease.[596] However, a pelvic pouch procedure still may be an acceptable surgical alternative in those patients known to have ulcerative colitis but with perianal disease, because the overall pouch failure rate has not been demonstrated to be significantly increased.[596]

Recurrent Disease. The development of Crohn's disease following restorative proctocolectomy or Kock pouch implies an initial error in diagnosis (see earlier discussion). The concern about the performance of reservoir proce-

dures for Crohn's disease has been previously discussed and is further addressed in Chapter 30 (see also Management, above).

Evacuation Problems (Outlet Obstruction). Failure to evacuate adequately is usually associated with a long efferent limb, a particular concern with the S-pouch procedure (Figure 29-108; see Results).[412] It is because of this complication that every effort should be made to place the reservoir as close to the anal canal as is reasonably possible. Silvis and colleagues recommend dynamic defecography for determining which reparative approach is most appropriate in those who have problems with impaired evacuation.[656]

Treatment of this complication requires take-down of the anastomosis and shortening of the efferent limb. In the experience from the group at St. Mark's Hospital, combined abdominal-anal salvage surgery for outlet mechanical obstruction was successful in avoiding an ileostomy in 13 of 16 patients, and significantly improved pouch function in 12 of 15.[279]

Impotence and Infertility. As with conventional proctocolectomy and ileostomy, impotence does not seem to be a critical issue (unless you are the patient who experiences this complication), primarily because of the young age of most individuals. In the experience of Lindsey and colleagues the impotence rate was 3.8%, all in the 50- to 70-year age group.[420] As expected, there was no statistically significant difference in the rate of complete or partial impotence between close rectal and so-called mesorectal dissection. None of the patients experienced difficulty with ejaculation. However, in the Mayo Clinic experience, 9% of men were found to have retrograde ejaculation.[342] No impairment of bladder function was identified in patients of either sex. In a double-blind, placebo-controlled trial, Lindsey and co-workers found that sildenafil (Viagra) satisfactorily improved erectile dysfunction in 79% of those so afflicted.[419]

Other Complications. The usual complications experienced with any major abdominal procedure have been reported following the various pouch-anal procedures. These include adrenal insufficiency, hepatitis, pneumothorax, gastrointestinal bleeding, pancreatitis, cholecystitis, deep vein thrombosis, mesenteric vein thrombosis, and brachial palsy, as well as, of course, wound infection.[171,742] Whether the incidence is higher in comparison with other gastrointestinal operations is problematic.

Pregnancy, Delivery, and Fertility Successful childbirth has been reported following restorative proctocolectomy with pelvic ileal reservoir.[475,510,566] According to the Mayo Clinic experience, 20 women had had at least one successful pregnancy and delivery following an ileal pouch-anal procedure by 1989.[510] Neither vaginal delivery nor cesarean section affected pouch functional outcome, but the frequency of nocturnal stools increased during the pregnancy and for 3 months thereafter. A later report of 43 women who had a successful pregnancy and delivery following ileal pouch-anal anastomosis at the Mayo Clinic was reviewed.[326] Stool frequency, incontinence, and pad usage were significantly increased during pregnancy, but postpartum function was the same as before pregnancy. The incidence of pouch-related complications compared favorably with that of conventional ileostomy and Kock pouch. The incidence of cesarean section, however, was higher. The University of Toronto experience reflects 29 patients with 49 deliveries.[582] There were 25 vaginal deliveries and 24 cesarean sections. Two pouch-related complications were noted during the pregnancies, and four were postpartum. All were treated "conservatively." The consensus is that the type of delivery should be influenced by obstetric concerns only, not by issues relative to the restorative proctocolectomy.[326,582]

In a review from Sweden and Denmark of 258 consecutive women, comparing fertility prior to restorative proctocolectomy and after surgery with that of the na-

tional population, Olsen and co-workers found that there was a considerable reduction in postoperative fertility.[541]

Salvage Surgery Complications of restorative proctocolectomy are frequent and varied with the consequences of poor function and a diminished quality of life.[766] Ideally, the preferred initial methods of dealing with problems, such as outlet obstruction, fistula, stricture, and so forth are those that are nonoperative or require limited surgery. When these methods fail, salvage surgery must be considered. There are, in essence, five options:

- perineal operation (e.g., pouch advancement)
- remove, repair, and preserve the pouch, restoring continuity
- resect the pouch and redo the restorative proctocolectomy
- remove and preserve the pouch, and convert to a continent ileostomy
- resect the pouch, and convert to a conventional or continent ileostomy

Obviously, resecting the pouch is not exactly "salvage surgery." It salvages the patient, to be sure, but not the reservoir. A moderate literature on the experience has developed from a number of centers with respect to the results of salvage surgery. Tan and co-workers noted that of nine patients who had their pouches removed and were converted to an end-ileostomy, all experienced a higher stomal output, as would be expected, but the other measured parameters (systemic symptoms, functional, social and emotional impairment) did not differ significantly from that of individuals who had initially undergone a conventional proctocolectomy and ileostomy.[693] Behrens and associates converted 42 failed operations to the Barnett modification of a Kock pouch.[43] All but two have a functioning continent ileostomy.

Teulchinsky and colleagues (St. Mark's Hospital) successfully performed major revisional surgery for symptomatic *retained rectal stump* in 15 of 22 patients, noting that the results were worse than in those who underwent first-time restorative proctocolectomy.[717] Without doubt, poor function after pelvic pouch surgery offsets any advantage in body image when compared with a well-functioning ileostomy.[553,716]

The Cleveland Clinic (Florida) group identified 32 patients who underwent reoperative ileoanal pouch surgery.[766] Pouch salvage was attempted in 25 and pouch excision in 10 (3 patients were included in both groups). Five patients (20%) had pouch reconstruction; one was successful. The overall success rate of pouch salvage was 84% (all methods) with approximately two thirds of patients having acceptable function. Of interest is the fact that four of the ten patients who underwent pouch excision were ultimately diagnosed with Crohn's disease.[766]

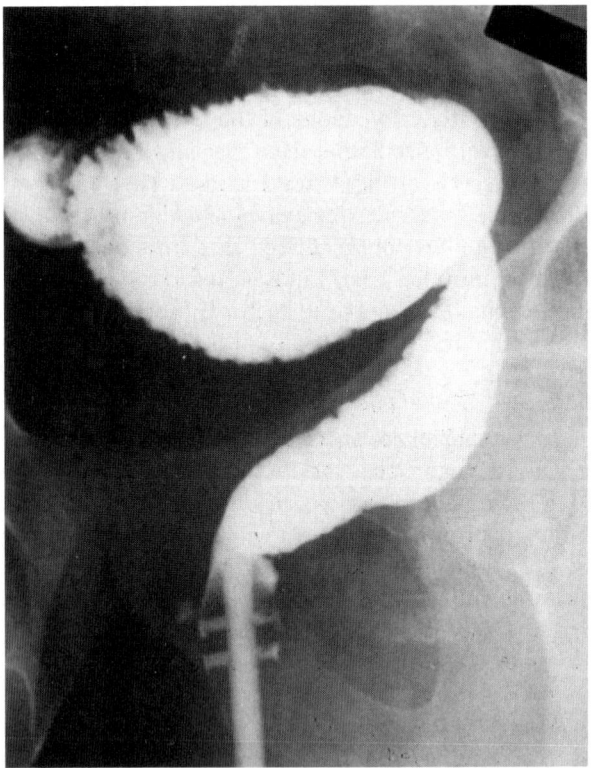

FIGURE 29-108. Long efferent limb of pouch-ileoanal procedure predisposes to difficulties in evacuation. Pouchogram demonstrates part of the reservoir to be inferior to the pouch outlet.

Gorfine and colleagues reported 51 patients who developed sinus or fistula tracts.[222] Eighty-nine salvage operations were performed. One-third required pouch excision, 9.8% had persistent fistulas and remained diverted, and 15.7% had persistent fistulas and were not diverted. The pouch was retained in 56.9%.

The Cleveland Clinic (Ohio) group identified 101 patients who underwent repeat restorative proctocolectomy.[19] Indications were as follows:

- chronic anastomotic fistula—27
- perineal or pouch-vaginal fistula—47
- anastomotic stricture—22
- dysfunction/long efferent limb of S-pouch—36

Some patients had more than one indication for reconstruction. Of these, 82% have a functioning pouch (median follow-up, 32 months). Thirteen percent underwent pouch excision. They note that although pouch failure occurs more commonly after a second attempt, patient satisfaction and quality of life remained high. The University of Toronto experience (2002) comprises 63 reconstructive procedures in 57 patients.[432] Forty-two (73.6%) maintained a functioning pouch with a mean follow-up of 60 months. More than 80% rated their physical and psychological health as being good to excellent. In a review of the literature on this subject, Tulchinsky and associates noted that failure of the surgery occurs indefinitely during the follow-up to a cumulative rate of about 15% at 10 to 15 years, with sepsis accounting for more than 50%.[715] Abdominal salvage surgery is successful in 20% to more than 80% of the reports, but the variable length of follow-up is probably responsible for this marked discrepancy in their opinion. The Mayo Clinic group has shown that increased experience decreases the risk of pouch-related complications and that with time the functional results remain stable, but the failure rate increases.[469]

Results

Physiologic Studies and Laboratory Evaluation

Anal Manometry; Rectoanal Inhibitory Reflex (RAIR); Determination of Reservoir Capacity; Compliance. Sharp and colleagues do not believe that clinical estimation of sphincter resting tone is a good predictor of postoperative function and advise manometric evaluation.[652] They found a significant decrease in the resting and maximal contraction pressures postoperatively. Grant and colleagues studied anal manometry in S-pouch patients with long rectal cuffs and with short cuffs, matching them for age, sex, and stool frequency.[227] Although functional results and manometric findings were similar, no patient demonstrated a normal rectoanal inhibitory reflex. Postoperative complications were significantly greater in those with long rectal cuffs.

The rectoanal inhibitory reflex is recognized as an important contributor to fecal continence through sampling and discrimination of contents. Preservation of the rectoanal inhibitory reflex has been shown to correlate with a decrease in the incidence of nocturnal soiling after restorative proctocolectomy.[624]

In a study of 34 patients with a J-pouch or with a straight ileoanal anastomosis, Beart and colleagues reported that both groups had satisfactory anal sphincter resting pressures and neorectal capacities, and that all could discriminate stool from gas.[35] It was their opinion that with normal sphincter function, continence correlates with reservoir capacity and compliance as well as with the frequency and strength of intrinsic bowel contractions. Others have demonstrated that the integrity of the sphincter mechanism can be satisfactorily maintained following ileoanal-reservoir operations.[564]

Church and co-workers (Cleveland Clinic, Ohio) used manometry to investigate the effects of ileal pouch-anal (n = 134) and ileal pouch-coloanal (n = 16) anastomosis on resting anal canal pressures in 150 patients.[92] Manometric measurements were taken preoperatively and 6 weeks following ileostomy closure. The authors reported a mean fall in pressure of 25 mm Hg for both ileal pouch-anal and ileal pouch-coloanal anastomoses, with no difference between hand-sewn or stapled techniques. However, analysis revealed a significant relationship between preoperative pressure and change in pressure. The authors reported that patients with high preoperative pressures are at risk for precipitous fall after surgery and, as a consequence, may have a suboptimal result. Paradoxically, patients with low preoperative pressures may actually demonstrate an increase in pressure following surgery. Those who are continent preoperatively are likely to remain continent postoperatively. Therefore, the authors stress that individuals with low preoperative resting pressures should not be denied an anastomosis to the anus based on this study alone. A later report from the same institution in which 1,439 patients had their data collected prospectively, revealed that there was a statistically significant association between seepage and degree of incontinence with quality of health, quality of life, energy level, and level of satisfaction with surgery.[243] Perioperative anal sphincter resting pressures greater than 40 mm Hg were associated with significantly better function and quality of life. Still, the authors conclude that a low preoperative resting pressure does not preclude a successful outcome.[243]

To study motor determinants of incontinence after ileal pouch-anal anastomosis, Ferrara and colleagues placed microtransducer catheters in 8 continent and 8 incontinent patients 15 months following surgery to record 24-hour ambulatory motor activity.[169] The investigators found that incontinent patients had lower resting pressures, extended anal canal relaxation, higher-amplitude high-pressure waves, and a nonresponsive anal canal, all indicating a reversal of the anal-canal pressure gradient. The authors concluded that incontinence is most likely a consequence of several factors, including a weak and less responsive anal canal, strong pouch motor activity, and dysfunctional coordination between pouch and anal canal.

Becker and colleagues assessed functional results by means of radiography and manometry.[36,38] The mean maximal anal sphincter resting pressure decreased from 87.1 mm Hg preoperatively to 68.1 mm Hg 8 weeks following surgery, but at 1 year it rose to 72.3 mm Hg. The change in sphincter pressure with voluntary squeeze was greater 8 weeks after the procedure than before the operation. Keighley and associates and others have confirmed that median resting anal canal pressure and maximum squeeze pressure are significantly lower in pouch patients when compared with a control population.[66,339,418] However, better results can be achieved with respect to voluntary control if the surgeon limits the potential for injury to the internal sphincter by avoiding anal dilatation and mucosectomy.[388,714] As has been discussed earlier, this must be balanced with the concern for residual mucosa predisposing to the development of dysplasia and carcinoma.[348]

Wexner and colleagues prospectively analyzed 15 patients who underwent construction of a reservoir anastomosis by the double-stapling technique.[739] There was no significant difference between preoperative values and those obtained 1 year following surgery when mean and maximal squeeze pressures were compared, although the length of the high-pressure zone decreased.

Nasmyth and colleagues as well as others found that the frequency of defecation was inversely correlated to both the capacity and the compliance of the pouch.[505,543] Patients who could postpone defecation for more than 30 minutes had higher anal squeeze pressures and emptied their pouches more completely than those who experienced leakage. The best clinical results were associated with a high anal pressure and with a large volume, high compliance, and complete emptying of the pouch. Harms and colleagues failed to demonstrate a difference in the mean pressure at normal evacuation volume between S- and W-reservoirs 2 and 12 months postoperatively.[259] Scott and Phillips noted that a low pouch compliance prior to ileostomy closure was associated with an increased frequency of nocturnal stooling, but anal canal length, anal sphincter squeeze pressure, and pouch capacity failed to predict functional outcome.[643] Steens and co-workers found no difference in pouch compliance and sensitivity in patients with uniform pouch design who had normal versus high stool frequency.[670] However, *postprandial pouch tone* was increased significantly in those with a high stool frequency. In another report from the same group, compliance was found to increase significantly during the first year after surgery to values of that in the range of rectal compliance.[671]

Holdsworth and colleagues used continuous ambulatory manometry to evaluate the function of the internal anal sphincter in 35 patients who underwent restorative proctocolectomy and 19 normal healthy volunteers.[291] Of the 35 individuals who underwent restorative proctocolectomy, 13 underwent mucosal proctectomy with endoanal ileoanal anastomosis and 22 patients had an end-to-end ileoanal anastomosis. The authors found that whereas only 38% of the patients who underwent mucosal proctectomy with sutured endoanal anastomosis showed evidence of basal internal sphincter activity, all patients with a stapled end-to-end anastomosis and all control subjects showed this baseline activity. The authors concluded that these data suggest mucosal proctectomy and endoanal anastomosis result in damage to the internal anal sphincter. In contrast, restorative proctectomy with stapled, end-to-end anastomosis was demonstrated to preserve internal anal sphincter function.

Jorge and colleagues used manometry and a questionnaire-based incontinence score to investigate the recovery of anal sphincter function after the double-stapled ileoanal reservoir procedure in 22 patients more than 50 years of age.[325] Manometric measurements were taken preoperatively and postoperatively (before and after ileostomy closure). Results were compared with those of a group of 50 patients with a median age of 32 years. The authors reported that no differences were found relative to preoperative pressures or clinical outcome. However, mean and high resting pressures were significantly lower in the over-50 group when they were examined before ileostomy closure. Although impairment of the internal anal sphincter was more severe after ileoanal reservoir, function had completely recovered after ileostomy closure. The authors concluded that the effect of the ileoanal reservoir on anal sphincters in persons over the age of 50 years is similar to that noted in younger patients.

Electromyography. Stryker and colleagues used electromyography (EMG) to evaluate the external anal sphincter in 27 patients.[679] Abnormal motor unit potentials were identified in 9 patients, a finding that usually correlates with poor bowel control. All patients over the age of 40 years had abnormal EMG results.

Farouk and co-workers employed preoperative and postoperative EMG and manometry in 66 patients to determine the role of the internal anal sphincter in the return of continence following restorative proctocolectomy.[154] At 18 months' follow-up, neither EMG measurements nor resting anal pressure measurements of internal anal sphincter function had fully returned to preoperative values. However, the authors concluded that recovery of internal sphincter EMG activity and resting anal pressure is progressive and associated with a gradual decrease in stool frequency. Eleven patients reported leakage in the follow-up period, with nocturnal incontinence the primary complaint, a problem that the authors attribute to poor pouch compliance during filling.

Motility. Pescatori studied electric and motor activity of the terminal ileum in seven patients who underwent this operation.[561] Recordings were carried out with an intraluminal probe, and observations were also made of the electric activity of the rectal sleeve and sphincter muscle. He observed that most of the electric and motor properties of the terminal ileum are retained after surgery, but that pouch motility is reduced. Others have found that jejunoileal motility is not greatly altered by the procedure.[678]

Patients who have poor functional results—incontinence and stool frequency—often have rapid pouch filling and an inability to evacuate completely.[680] O'Connell and colleagues evaluated ileal pouch motility in 23 patients 2 years following the operation by means of an intraluminal bag and pressure-sensitive catheters.[534] Pouch emptying was determined scintigraphically and by stool collection. The authors observed that ileal pouch motility and stool output were major determinants of stool frequency.

Kusunoki and colleagues attempted to determine the mechanism of anal canal motility with the use of various neuroreceptor agents.[374] Their results suggest that the neorectum has hybrid characteristics of both rectum and ileum.

Pouchography and Scintigraphy. Tsao and co-workers studied 463 patients undergoing a pouchogram (Gastrografin) enema before ileostomy closure following ileal pouch-anal anastomosis.[712] The purpose of their investigation was to determine the usefulness of a pouchogram in detecting complications and predicting clinical outcome. Normal pouchograms were reported in 389 (84%) patients, whereas pouchograms of 74 (16%) patients revealed pouch leaks and other abnormal findings. The authors found that abnormal pouchograms identified patients needing surgical intervention before closure as well as those patients who would likely benefit from a delay in ileostomy closure. In addition, the authors reported that abnormal pouchograms were associated with an overall long-term failure rate of 23%, in comparison with a 6% long-term failure rate for patients with normal findings. They concluded that pouchograms have a long-term clinical predictive value.

Pescatori and colleagues further evaluated 34 patients who underwent restorative proctocolectomy with an S-pouch by "evacuation pouchography."[562] The purpose was to determine why some patients could evacuate spontaneously and others had to insert a catheter several times a day to empty the pouch. The 50% who were able to have a spontaneous evacuation had a significantly shorter distal segment (mean, 8 ± 3 cm) than those who had to use a catheter to empty the pouch (mean distal segment length, 11 ± 4 cm). The authors believed that the longer the distal segment, the more likely it was to be angulated. Short segments were demonstrated to fill on straining, in contrast with the longer segments, which often failed to fill under such circumstances.

Heppell and colleagues compared the functional results of J-reservoirs and S-reservoirs by means of a radionuclide enema, measuring emptying following instillation of a semisolid medium labeled with 1.0 mCi of technetium-99m (^{99m}Tc)-sulfur colloid.[275] Ileal pouch counts were determined by using a scintillation camera and computer before and after spontaneous evacuation. Functional results were found to be similar in the two groups, but those who emptied less than 30% were improved by intermittent intubation. The authors believed that a semisolid radionuclide enema could be usefully applied to identify those who would benefit from such intubation.

Barkel and colleagues (Mayo Clinic) used a scintigraphic technique to determine whether the anorectal angle is preserved after ileal pouch-anal anastomosis.[26] They found that changes in the anorectal angle during defecation and during squeeze were similar to that of controls, but that the pelvic floor movements were impaired. Kmiot and co-workers assessed evacuation by means of videoproctography and observed anal stricture to be the only factor consistently associated with poor pouch emptying.[357]

Anal Sensation. Keighley and colleagues assessed anal sensation in control subjects and in patients with ulcerative colitis by means of a constant-current stimulator following restorative proctocolectomy.[337] Excision of the anal transition zone did not eliminate the ability to discriminate, and therefore did not increase the risk for control problems following this procedure. Conversely, Holdsworth and Johnston, in assessing the rectoanal inhibitory reflex and the ability of the patient to discriminate between flatus and feces, found that anal sensation and discriminatory function were significantly better without mucosal proctectomy.[289] Others have demonstrated improved sensation to be associated with preservation of the anal transition zone, but correlation with the actual functional results was not obtained.[487]

Bacteriology. O'Connell and colleagues studied the enteric bacteriology of 20 patients in an attempt to relate changes in the functional results of the operation.[536] They observed that jejunal bacterial overgrowth was associated with an increased stool output, azotorrhea, and a poor clinical result. Pouch ileitis did not appear to be caused simply by pouch stasis and bacterial overgrowth within the pouch.

Absorption. One of the concerns that has been expressed with respect to the various pouch-anal alternatives is the problem of absorptive capacity and consequent nutritional disturbance. Nasmyth and colleagues assessed bile acid absorption by using selenium-66 (^{66}Se) taurohomocholate and noted no statistically significant difference between patients with a conventional ileostomy and those with a pouch-anal procedure.[506] However, bacterial metabolism of primary conjugated bile acids was greater in those with a pouch. Others have observed that almost all postcolectomy patients have supersaturated bile with cholesterol crystals, findings that are usually seen in persons with cholesterol gallstones.[264]

Bowel Frequency and Continence

Interpretation of the results and the relative merits of the varied approaches to the assessment of ileoanal pouch function is obviously quite difficult. For example, one is not always certain how much or if any "slowing" medications are employed to achieve the median frequency of bowel action that is reported. The four characteristics generally evaluated include spontaneity of defecation, ability to defer defecation, continence, and stool frequency.[405] I have elected to summarize the experience of the largest published series.

St. Mark's Hospital. Parks and colleagues reported their early experience of 21 patients from St. Mark's Hospital with the S-pouch, 17 of whom had ulcerative colitis and 4 with polyposis.[551] All were observed to be completely continent of feces during the day, but one patient was incontinent at night. The average frequency of bowel evacuation was approximately 4 times in 24 hours. Approximately one-half of the patients needed a catheter to facilitate defecation. Two required medications to reduce the frequency of bowel actions. A later report from the same center, comprising 55 patients, revealed a mean daily stool frequency of 3.7 (20% required antidiarrheal medications).[514] Spontaneous defecation occurred in 40%, whereas 53% used a catheter to aid evacuation. Continence was "normal" in approximately two-thirds, and minor leakage was reported by 29%, with 5.4% noting soiling. Setti-Carraro and co-workers, reporting from the same institution, reviewed the first 10 years of experience with restorative proctocolectomy.[649] Long-term function was assessed in 80 patients, with a mean follow-up of 99.3 months after ileostomy closure. There were 24 patients with an S-pouch, 24 with a J-pouch, 31 with a W-pouch, and one with a pelvic Kock pouch. Sixty-six patients did not use a catheter, with an average diurnal minimum and maximum frequency of 3.8 and 4.9, respectively. Overall, the average minimum 24-hour frequency in these 66 patients was 4.1 and the maximum was 5.7. Forty-nine patients were completely continent. Of the remaining 31, 30 had minor mucous or fecal leaks. In a related study from the same center, Melville and colleagues showed that during a 15-year period (1976 through 1990), the number of elective surgeries for ulcerative colitis increased.[471]

Nicholls and Pezim compared three different designs of reservoirs in 104 patients (triple loop, double loop, and quadruple loop).[516] Frequency of defecation was significantly greater with the double loop and was associated with a much higher incidence of nighttime evacuation. All patients with double- or quadruple-loop reservoirs defecated spontaneously, whereas only 41% with triple-loop pouches did so. The authors concluded that a quadruple reservoir directly connected to the anal canal preserved spontaneous evacuation and was comparable with the triple loop in preserving adequate retentive ability. A report from the same unit involving functional assessment of 51 patients with the four-loop, W-reservoir revealed the frequency of defecation per day to be 3.3 (range, 1 to 8).[515] Nighttime evacuation occurred in 14%. Harms and colleagues noted a 24-hour stool frequency of 4.8 at 1 year with this type of pouch.[257]

Utsunomiya (Japan). Utsunomiya and colleagues reported their early experience with the J-pouch.[722] They believed that this type of pouch is superior because the reservoir is located in the lowest part of the pelvic area, similar to the normal rectal ampulla.

Mayo Clinic. Taylor and colleagues reported the initial Mayo Clinic experience with 74 patients who underwent ileal pouch-anal anastomosis with a J-reservoir.[697] In comparing their patients with those who underwent a straight ileoanal anastomosis, the authors noted that stool frequency with the pouch was less (mean, 7 per 24 hours, compared with 11 stools per 24 hours in the straight ileoanal group). Major nocturnal incontinence was also less in the pouch group (0% versus 20%). A later report of 157 patients assessed at least 60 days after ileostomy closure following the J-pouch procedure revealed that all evacuated the neorectum spontaneously.[478,558] Stool frequency was on average 6.0 daily and 1.2 nightly. Seepage was noted in 25% during the day and in 47% at night. Women had more spotting than men, and patients over 50 years had more stools per day than those 50 years or younger.[558] McIntyre and colleagues published a more recent report from the same institution.[464] They compared functional results 1 year and 10 years after ileal pouch-anal anastomosis for chronic ulcerative colitis.[464] Sixty-one consecutive subjects were identified who underwent a J-pouch procedure, and functional results were recorded 1 year and 10 years following ileostomy closure. At both follow-up times, the median stool frequency was 7 in a 24-hour period. At the 10-year follow-up, 70% had excellent daytime control, 23% had occasional soiling, and 7% reported poor control. Nighttime incontinence was a problem for 23 patients at 1 year, with only 5 reporting improvement at 10 years. Overall, 52% complained of nighttime soiling at the 10-year mark.

Köhler and co-workers, also from the Mayo Clinic, employed a written questionnaire assessing bowel habits, overall quality of life, and several performance-related activities to examine the long-term functional results of persons undergoing an ileal J-pouch–anal anastomosis.[364] A group of patients who had undergone cholecystectomy served as the control group. The authors reported that the ileoanal patients had a median of 6 stools per day and that 68% of the 240 participating individuals experienced episodes of fecal spotting. Bowel habits remained steady during the 8-year follow-up. Overall, 90% of ileoanal patients reported an excellent overall quality of life, with results closely paralleling those of the control group.

The Mayo Clinic experience with restorative proctocolectomy is commanding. Of the 1,386 patients who were reported in 2000 (median length of follow-up, 8 years), they found that functional outcomes were comparable between men and women, and daytime and nocturnal incontinence was more frequently observed in older individuals.[155]

Cleveland Clinic (Ohio). A nonrandomized report from the Cleveland Clinic compared the J-pouch with the S-pouch as performed by the same surgeon.[713] There was no statistically significant difference between the two with respect to the mean maximum resting and squeeze pressures and the maximum tolerated volume. However, a significant difference was noted in mean compliance, the incidence of daytime and nocturnal leakage, and the frequency of bowel action, the S-pouch being superior. In another report from the same institution, Fazio and co-workers retrospectively reviewed 1,005 patients who underwent ileal pouch-anal anastomoses from 1983 to 1993.[165] The J-pouch design was performed in two-thirds, with one-third having undergone an S-pouch. Two thirds of patients had stapled anastomoses, whereas the anastomoses of one-third were hand-sewn. Among the 812 patients who underwent the operation for ulcerative colitis, the median frequency of bowel movements per 24-hour period was 6 (range, 1 to 20). Nighttime seepage was reported in 29%, and 17% experienced day and night seepage. Forty-seven percent sometimes used antidiarrheal medications, and 15% indicated constant use.

More recent papers from the same institution now involve data from almost 2,000 patients. Pouch failure requiring pouch excision or permanent ileostomy was noted in 4.1%.[129] Fourteen percent experienced social, sexual, or work restrictions, and the functional outcome was not as good in older patients.[128] However, their compatriots at the Cleveland Clinic (Florida) note that while anorectal function is transiently impaired after restorative proctocolectomy, that impairment is not an age-related phenomenon.[691] Risk factors that have been found to be independent predictors of pouch survival included: patient diagnosis, prior anal pathology, abnormal anal manometry, patient comorbidity, pouch-perineal or pouch vaginal fistula, pelvic sepsis, anastomotic stricture, and separation.[161]

Lahey Clinic. Marcello and colleagues prospectively assessed long-term results in 460 patients between 1980 and 1991.[444] A J-pouch was constructed in 94%. With a follow-up greater than 60 months after ileostomy closure, the mean number of bowel movements per 24-hour period was 5.8. After 5 years, 50% of patients did not have nightly bowel movements, and 75% passed flatus independently. After 1 year, the frequency of seepage was 10%, occurring

on average 3 days per week. The authors reported that the rate of use of medications regulating gut function remained between 39% and 44% during the follow-up period.

Fonkalsrud (University of California, Los Angeles). Fonkalsrud reported his initial experience with the lateral ileal reservoir in 21 patients (mean age, approximately 17 years) with ulcerative colitis or polyposis.[175,-177] He initially thought that the results of the procedure were superior to the results obtained with an S-pouch. A mean of 4 continent bowel movements per 24 hours was achieved within 4 weeks in patients with lateral reservoirs. A later update comprised a total of 83 patients.[667] Late obstruction of the ileal reservoir developed in 19. In 9 patients, the obstruction was caused by a long rectal muscular cuff and a longer distance from the lower end of the reservoir to the anus than is optimal. He recommended that the length be from 10 to 15 cm for children and from 18 to 22 cm for adults. It was also suggested that the pouch be no farther than 5 cm from the ileoanal anastomosis. A still later report involving 127 patients who underwent a lateral reservoir revealed a significantly lower morbidity in comparison with that of patients undergoing the other pouch alternatives.[180] As mentioned earlier, Fonkalsrud is the only surgeon who has extensive experience with this approach. He has also reviewed the long-term results after colectomy and ileoanal pull-through procedure in 116 children 18 years of age or younger.[181] Ninety-four had ulcerative colitis, 17 had familial polyposis coli, and 5 had Hirschsprung's disease. Sixty-two patients had a lateral pouch, 47 a J-pouch, and 7 a straight pull-through. An average of 5.6 bowel movements per 24 hours was found at 3 months, which decreased to 3.9 at 6 months. By 3 months, fewer than 10% of patients experienced daytime soiling, whereas nocturnal soiling was present in 18% at 3 months. However, at the 6-month mark, the incidence had fallen to 6%. Prior to his retirement, Fonkalsrud recommended a J-pouch because of the ease of construction and paucity of long-term complications. He reserved the lateral pouch for patients with a short ileal mesentery and inadequate length for a J-pouch to extend to the anus without tension.

Other Investigators. Becker and Raymond reported their experience with 100 patients who underwent the J-pouch procedure.[41] Stool frequency at 1, 3, 6, 12, and 24 months was 7.5, 6.5, 6.2, 5.4, and 5.4, respectively. No patient was incontinent during the day. By 1 year, 25% noted nocturnal leakage. In contrast to other investigators, the authors did not believe that age was a factor in determining stool frequency. Smith noted that 14 of his 19 patients had 6 or fewer bowel movements per day.[661] Bodzin and colleagues reported that their 19 patients had 3 to 9 bowel movements per day, and nearly all wore a sanitary pad for unpredictable leakage.[57]

Nasmyth and co-workers noted no significant differences between the S-pouches and J-pouches with respect to continence or frequency of defecation at 6 months.[507] However, at 1 year, those with the S-reservoir had a lower stool frequency than those with a J-pouch. Conversely, McHugh and colleagues found that patients with S-pouches appeared to have better early functional results, but no differences were appreciated at 1 year following ileostomy closure.[463]

Reissman and colleagues studied the functional results of the double-stapled ileoanal reservoir in 124 patients at a mean follow-up of 24 months.[589] They reported a mean of 5.4 (range, 2 to 13) bowel movements during the day and a mean of 1.2 (range, 0 to 4) at night. Ninety-five percent of patients reported perfect or almost perfect continence during the day, and 92% during the night. The same authors studied the functional results of the double-stapled ileoanal reservoir in patients over 60 years of age. They found this operation to be safe and the functional and physiologic results to be comparable with those in younger patients.[591] Keighley and colleagues compared the stapled J-pouch with the sutured W-pouch, observing that the functional results were identical.[338] They concluded that the excessive time required to construct the W-reservoir would not seem to be justified.

A plethora of articles on the functional results of the pouch-anal procedures can be found.[40,72,94,130,189,191,237,258,][329,365,392,400,409,460,482,483,539,568,606,619,621] The general consensus is that this operation, with its various modifications, offers the best quality of life when compared with the alternatives. Tables 29-8 and 29-9 summarize the experiences from a number of institutions that address the issues of bowel frequency and bowel control following restorative proctocolectomy.

Comparison of Reservoir Designs

Much effort has been directed to comparing the functional outcome of patients who have undergone restorative proctocolectomy with creation of a variety of pelvic ileal reservoirs. Although the choice of reservoir is largely a function of the surgeon's personal preference, options are available, including the duplicated-J, triplicated-S, quadruplicated-W, and lateral, as well as modified versions of these.[622] Lewis and colleagues investigated the factors that are important in the creation of an ideal pelvic pouch for achievement of perfect anal continence.[408] The authors found four factors that correlate significantly with an optimal functional result. These are maximum resting anal pressure, sensory threshold in the upper and middle anal canal, compliance of the ileal reservoir, and the presence of a pouch-anal inhibitory reflex. They concluded that the quality of anal continence depends on a compliant ileal reservoir and a strong, sensitive anal sphincter.[408] Various studies have been conducted to investigate the advantages and drawbacks of each design.

Harms and co-workers examined the appropriateness of the W-reservoir in the treatment of ulcerative colitis

and familial polyposis in 109 individuals.[256] Stool frequency over a 24-hour period decreased from 7.3 at 2 months to 4.9 at 12 months of follow-up. Ninety-six percent reported continence during the day at 12 months, whereas 10% experienced episodes of nighttime seepage. In addition, compliance increased from 12.7 mL/mm Hg to 14.3 mL/mm Hg between 2 and 12 months of follow-up. The authors concluded that W-ileal reservoirs exhibit optimal function and compliance properties when compared with lower-capacity designs.

Johnston and colleagues performed a prospective, randomized trial to elucidate what influence pelvic pouch design has on functional outcome.[321] Sixty patients received either a J- or a W-reservoir, constructed with either 30 or 40 cm of ileum. The authors found that median bowel frequency in 24 hours did not differ significantly in patients with J-reservoirs from that of patients with W-pouches. Similarly, the size (30 or 40 cm) of the reservoir did not produce a significant difference in bowel frequency. The authors concluded that their findings support the use of a small, duplicated ileal reservoir, which is simple to construct by means of linear stapling techniques. Others have confirmed this finding.[285]

Commentary on Restorative Proctocolectomy

The ileal reservoir with endoanal anastomosis has become relatively standardized, at least with respect to the value of the procedure in the surgical management of individuals with ulcerative colitis and the polyposis syndromes. There is no question that most patients are satisfied with the functional results and to some extent serve as their own controls (because most have a protecting ileostomy for a time). However, these so-called control patients may have a less-than-satisfactory loop ileostomy. Moreover, it is more proximally located than a conventional end-stoma, and the effluent is therefore more liquid. Furthermore, despite meticulous attention to creating a loop ileostomy, surgeons often find that a consistently salutary stoma is an unachieved ideal. Thus said, however, a report from the Mayo Clinic compares the quality of life after conventional (Brooke) ileostomy with that after the pouch-anal procedure.[559] After adjusting for age, diagnosis, and reoperation rate, logistic regression analysis of performance scores in seven different categories were used to discriminate between operations. The authors concluded that patients experience significant advantages with respect to their daily activities and quality of life with the pouch-anal procedure in comparison with the standard end-ileostomy.

One must also consider the obvious fact that despite many surgeons' increased experience with the technique, the procedure continues to have a high morbidity, albeit much lower than the initial reports indicated. Mortality, however, is quite low, primarily because an ileostomy is usually accomplished until the restorative anastomoses have healed.

▶ **TABLE 29-8** Bowel Frequency Following Pouch-Anal Procedures

Institution	Year	Number of Patients	Primary Pouch	Daily Evacuations Total (Mean)	Night (Mean)	Day (Mean)
Mayo Clinic[464]	1994	1,400	J	6	0–1	5–6
St. Mark's Hospital[649]	1994	110	J, S	6	0–1	5
Cleveland Clinic[165]	1995	521	J	6	NS	NS
Cleveland Clinic (FL)[589]	1995	107	J	6.6	1.2	5.4
University of Wisconsin[256]	1992	109	W	4.9	NS	NS
Lahey Clinic[444]	1993	382	J	7	1	6
University of Chicago[483]	1993	50	J	6	NS	NS
Radcliffe Hospital[606]	1997	177	J	5	0–1	4.5
Uppsala, Sweden[329]	2000	155	J	NS	5 (74%)	NS
University of Minnesota[7]	2002	136	J	7	5	2
University of Chicago[482]	2003	234	J	8.5	2.5	6

NS, not stated.

Analysis of the numerous reports in the literature reveals a considerable variability in operative technique between surgeons and institutions. Furthermore, with rare exception, the failure to randomize patients also inhibits accurate assessment of the relative merits and risks of the plethora of approaches. Still, a number of appropriate conclusions may be drawn. Before the surgeon agrees to undertake this procedure as an alternative to conventional ileostomy, the patient should be highly motivated to accept the consequences: frequent bowel movements (a minimum of four to six stools per day and the possible requirement for intubation if an S-pouch is elected) as well as the risk for soilage and incontinence. It may take upward of 1 year for a patient to achieve reasonable stability with respect to bowel function and frequency.

A number of factors may make restorative proctocolectomy technically difficult or impossible to accomplish. For example, obesity tends to be associated with a shortened mesentery which may preclude the possibility of bringing the ileum down to effect an anastomosis. One may not be able to position the reservoir in the pelvis if there is consid-

erable fat or if there is narrowing of the inlet. Some surgeons believe that the terminal ileum reaches the dentate line more readily with the S-pouch than when the J-reservoir is used. The patient must, therefore, understand that technical factors or unanticipated pathology may necessitate an alternative surgical approach.

Because of the risk of recurrence, this operation should not be performed in patients with Crohn's disease in my opinion (see Chapter 30). Toxic megacolon is also a contraindication for embarking on this procedure at the time of emergency intervention. The wiser course in the latter situation is to perform a total colectomy and conventional ileostomy with rectal preservation, returning later to perform the restorative procedure. Older age is in itself not a contraindication, but most agree that because the aging process has a pejorative effect on sphincter muscle function, the procedure should probably be limited to patients younger than 70 years, although this is by no means a requirement.

With respect to the type of pouch, a trade-off seems to have evolved: the possible requirement of intubation with

▶ **TABLE 29-9** Bowel Control Following Pouch-Anal Procedures

Institution	Year	Number of Patients	Primary Pouch	Excellent or Good (%)	Impaired (%)
Mayo Clinic[464]	1994	1,400	J	48	52
St. Mark's Hospital[649]	1994	110	J, S	45	55
Cleveland Clinic[165]	1995	521	J	71	29
Cleveland Clinic (FL)[589]	1995	107	J	87	13
University of Wisconsin[256]	1992	109	W	61	39
Lahey Clinic[444]	1993	382	J	90	10
University of Chicago[483]	1993	50	J	54	46
Uppsala, Sweden[329]	2000	155	J	76	24
University of Minnesota[72]	2002	136	J	83	17
University of Chicago[482]	2003	234	J	70	30

an the S-pouch versus the theoretically lowered capacity (and therefore increased frequency of defecation) of the J-reservoir. Conversely, many reports suggest that the size of the reservoir may be of limited importance.

Preoperative physiologic studies that evaluate anal squeeze pressure or at least subjectively assess the effectiveness of the sphincter mechanism should be considered before an ileal reservoir anastomosis is performed. The real questions are whether preoperative physiologic studies help to predict the functional results following restorative proctocolectomy or even affect the decision-making process. Still, older patients, and those with a poor resting tone or suboptimal maximum squeeze pressure, might be forewarned that continence could be less than satisfactory.

We have more than reached the point wherein restorative proctocolectomy deserves complete legitimacy for the surgical management of ulcerative colitis. Soldiers on active duty, for example, can anticipate continuation of their military careers after such surgery.[21] Until relatively recently, I had been concerned that the complexity of the operation mandated that it be performed only by surgeons with a sufficiently large number of patients in order to gain adequate experience with the technique. However, with the stapled J-pouch and the application of the double-stapling technique for effecting the anastomosis, the technical aspects of the surgery are relatively well standardized and can be performed by most general surgeons. Yet, the admonition concerning who should perform these restorative procedures has validity. The major problem now is not so much the surgical technique (although this is critically important) as is the requirement for an obsessive, competently applied, follow-up program, as well as the obvious commitment of the surgeon to such a regimen. In my opinion, it is unconscionable for a surgeon to embark on this or any other procedure unless he or she is prepared to adequately communicate the risks and alternatives and to have the knowledge and commitment to appropriately treat the myriad complications and consequences. It appears today, then, that conventional ileostomy will be used primarily for patients with Crohn's disease, for older patients or those doomed to be incontinent, for those with failed pouch procedures, and for those who are not motivated to assume the potential burdens of the pouch alternative.

REFERENCES

1. Abulafi AM, Fiddian RV. Malignant lymphoma in ulcerative colitis. *Dis Colon Rectum* 1990;33:615.
2. Adler DJ, Korelitz BI. The therapeutic efficacy of 6-mercaptopurine in refractory ulcerative colitis. *Am J Gastroenterol* 1990;85:717.
3. Agrez MV, Dozois RR, Beahrs OH. Volvulus of the Kock pouch with obstruction and perforation: a case report. *Aust N Z J Surg* 1981;51:311.
4. Akwari OE, Kelly KA, Phillips SF. Myoelectric and motor patterns of continent pouch and conventional ileostomy. *Surg Gynecol Obstet* 1980;150:363.
5. Almy TP, Sherlock P. Genetic aspects of ulcerative colitis and regional enteritis. *Gastroenterology* 1966;51:757.
6. Alstead EM, Ritchie JK, Lennard-Jones JE, et al. Safety of azathioprine in pregnancy in inflammatory bowel disease. *Gastroenterology* 1990;99:443.
7. Ambrose NS, Alexander-Williams J. Appraisal of a tissue glue in the treatment of persistent perineal sinus. *Br J Surg* 1988;75:484.
8. Ambroze WL, Pemberton JH, Dozois RR, et al. The histological pattern and pathological involvement of the anal transition zone in patients with ulcerative colitis. *Gastroenterology* 1993;104:514.
9. Ambroze WL Jr, Wolff BG, Kelly KA, et al. Let sleeping dogs lie: role of the omentum in the ileal pouch-anal anastomosis procedure. *Dis Colon Rectum* 1991;34:563.
10. Anderson R, Turnbull RB Jr. Grafting the unhealed perineal wound after coloproctectomy for Crohn's disease. *Arch Surg* 1976;111:335.
11. Aouthmany A, Horattas MC. Ileal pouch perforation in pregnancy: report of a case and review of the literature. *Dis Colon Rectum* 2004;47:243.
12. Aronson MD, Phillips CA, Beeken WL, Forsyth BR. Isolation and characterization of a viral agent from intestinal tissue of patients with Crohn's disease and other intestinal disorders. *Prog Med Virol* 1975;21:165.
13. Aylett SO. Diffuse ulcerative colitis and its treatment by ileorectal anastomosis. *Ann R Coll Surg Engl* 1960;27:260.
14. Aylett SO. Three hundred cases of diffuse ulcerative colitis treated by total colectomy and ileo-rectal anastomosis. *Br Med J* 1966;1:1001.
15. Aylett SO. Rectal conservation in the surgical treatment of ulcerative colitis. *Arch Mal App Dig* 1974;63:585.
16. Bacon HE, Bralow SP, Berkley JL. Rehabilitation and long-term survival after colectomy for ulcerative colitis. *JAMA* 1960;172:324.
17. Baek S-M, Greenstein A, McElhinney AJ, Aufses AH Jr. The gracilis myocutaneous flap for persistent perineal sinus after proctocolectomy. *Surg Gynecol Obstet* 1981;153:713.
18. Baird DD, Narendranathan M, Sandler RS. Increased risk of preterm birth for women with inflammatory bowel disease. *Gastroenterology* 1990;99:987.
19. Baixauli J, Delaney CP, Wu JS, et al. Functional outcome and quality of life after repeat ileal pouch-anal anastomosis for complications of ileoanal surgery. *Dis Colon Rectum* 2004;47:2.
20. Ballantyne GH, Graham SM, Hammers L, Modlin IM. Superior mesenteric artery syndrome following ileal J-pouch anal anastomosis: an iatrogenic cause of early postoperative obstruction. *Dis Colon Rectum* 1987;30:472.
21. Bamberger PK, Otchy DP. Ileoanal pouch in the active duty population: effect on military career. *Dis Colon Rectum* 1997;40:60.
22. Banez AV, Yamanishi F, Crans CA. Endoscopic colonic decompression of toxic megacolon, placement of colonic tube, and steroid colon clysis. *Am J Gastroenterol* 1987;82:692.
23. Baratsis S, Hadjidimitriou F, Christodoulou M, Lariou K. Adenocarcinoma in the anal canal after ileal pouch-anal anastomosis for ulcerative colitis using a double stapling technique: report of a case. *Dis Colon Rectum* 2002;45:687.
24. Bargen JA. Chronic ulcerative colitis associated with malignant disease. *Arch Surg* 1928;17:561.
25. Bargen JA. Chronic ulcerative colitis: bacteriologic studies and specific therapy. *Trans Am Proctol Soc* 1928;28:93.
26. Barkel DC, Pemberton JH, Pezim ME, et al. Scintigraphic assessment of the anorectal angle in health and after ileal pouch-anal anastomosis. *Ann Surg* 1988;208:42.
27. Barnett WO. New approaches for continent ostomy construction. *J Miss State Med Assoc* 1987;28:1.
28. Barnett WO. Current experiences with the continent intestinal reservoir. *Surg Gynecol Obstet* 1989;168:1.
29. Baron JH, Connell AM, Kanaghinis TG, et al. Outpatient treatment of ulcerative colitis: comparison between three doses of oral prednisone. *Br Med J* 1962;2:441.

30. Bat L, Pines A, Ron E, et al. Colonoscopy without prior preparation in mild to moderate active ulcerative colitis. *J Clin Gastroenterol* 1991;13:46.

31. Bauer JJ, Gelernt IM, Salk BA, Kreel I. Proctectomy for inflammatory bowel disease. *Am J Surg* 1986;151:157.

32. Bayer I, Feller N, Chaimoff CH. A new approach to the nipple in Kock's reservoir ileostomy using Mersilene mesh. *Dis Colon Rectum* 1981;24:428.

33. Beart RW Jr, Beahrs OH, Kelly KA, et al. Continent ileostomy: a viable alternative. *Mayo Clin Proc* 1979;54:643.

34. Beart RW Jr, Dozois RR, Kelly KA. Ileoanal anastomosis in the adult. *Surg Gynecol Obstet* 1982;154:826.

35. Beart RW Jr, Dozois RR, Wolff BG, Pemberton JH. Mechanisms of rectal continence: lessons from the ileoanal procedure. *Am J Surg* 1985;149:31.

36. Becker JM. Anal sphincter function after colectomy, mucosal proctectomy, and endorectal ileoanal pull-through. *Arch Surg* 1984;119:526.

37. Becker JM, Dayton MT, Fazio VW, et al. Prevention of postoperative abdominal adhesions by a sodium hyaluronate-based bioresorbable membrane: a prospective, randomized, double-blind multicenter study. *J Am Coll Surg* 1996;183:297.

38. Becker JM, Hillard AE, Mann FA, et al. Functional assessment after colectomy, mucosal proctectomy and endorectal ileoanal pull-through. *World J Surg* 1985;9:598.

39. Becker JM, LaMorte W, St. Marie G, Ferzoco S. Extent of smooth muscle resection during mucosectomy and ileal pouch-anal anastomosis affects anorectal physiology and functional outcome. *Dis Colon Rectum* 1997;40:653.

40. Becker JM, McGrath KM, Meagher MP, et al. Late functional adaptation after colectomy, mucosal proctectomy, and ileal pouch-anal anastomosis. *Surgery* 1991;110:718.

41. Becker JM, Raymond JL. Ileal pouch-anal anastomosis: a single surgeon's experience with 100 consecutive cases. *Ann Surg* 1986;204:375.

42. Befrits R, Ljung T, Jaramillo E, Rubio C. Low-grade dysplasia in extensive, long-standing inflammatory bowel disease. A follow-up study. *Dis Colon Rectum* 2002;45:615.

43. Behrens DT, Paris M, Luttrell JN. Conversion of failed ileal pouch-anal anastomosis to continent ileostomy. *Dis Colon Rectum* 1999;42:490.

44. Bell SW, Parry B, Neill M. Adenocarcinoma in the anal transitional zone after ileal pouch for ulcerative colitis: report of a case. *Dis Colon Rectum* 2003;46:1134.

45. Bellini M, Tansella M. Obsessional scores and subjective general psychiatric complaints of patients with duodenal ulcer or ulcerative colitis. *Psychol Med* 1976;6:461.

46. Bentrem DJ, Wang KL, Stryker SJ, Adenocarcinoma in an ileal pouch occurring 14 years after restorative proctocolectomy. *Dis Colon Rectum* 2003;46:544.

47. Bercovitz ZT. Etiology and pathogenesis. In: Bercovitz ZT, Kirsner JB, Lindner AE, et al, eds. *Ulcerative and granulomatous colitis*. Springfield, IL: Charles C Thomas, 1973:180.

48. Berglund B, Asztély, Kock NG, Myrvold HE. Reflux from the continent ileostomy reservoir: a radiologic evaluation combined with pressure recording. *Dis Colon Rectum* 1985;28:502.

49. Bernstein CN, Blanchard JF, Kliewer E, Wajda A. Cancer risk in patients with inflammatory bowel disease. *Cancer* 2001;91:854.

50. Bernstein CN, Shanahan F, Anton PA, Weinstein WM. Patchiness of mucosal inflammation in treated ulcerative colitis: a prospective study. *Gastrointest Endosc* 1995;42:232.

51. Bernstein CN, Shanahan F, Weinstein WM. Are we telling patients the truth about surveillance colonoscopy in ulcerative colitis? *Lancet* 1994;343:71.

52. Biddle WL, Greenberger NJ, Swan JT, et al. 5-Aminosalicylic acid enemas: effective agent in maintaining remission in left-sided ulcerative colitis. *Gastroenterology* 1988;94:1075.

53. Biddle WL, Miner PB Jr. Long-term use of mesalamine enemas to induce remission in ulcerative colitis. *Gastroenterology* 1990;99:113.

54. Binder V, Both H, Hansen PK, et al. Incidence and prevalence of ulcerative colitis and Crohn's disease in the county of Copenhagen, 1962 to 1978. *Gastroenterology* 1982;83:563.

55. Blackstone MO, Riddell RH, Rogers BHG, Levin B. Dysplasia-associated lesion or mass (DALM) detected by colonoscopy in long-standing ulcerative colitis: an indication for colectomy. *Gastroenterology* 1981;80:366.

56. Bloom RJ, Larsen CP, Watt R, Oberhelman HA Jr. A reappraisal of the Kock continent ileostomy in patients with Crohn's disease. *Surg Gynecol Obstet* 1986;162:105.

57. Bodzin JH, Kestenberg W, Kaufmann R, Dean K. Mucosal proctectomy and ileoanal pull-through technique and functional results in 23 consecutive patients. *Am Surg* 1987;53:363.

58. Bohe MG, Ekelund GR, Genell SN, et al. Surgery for fulminating colitis during pregnancy. *Dis Colon Rectum* 1983;26:119.

59. Bokey LE, Fazio VW. The mesenteric sling technique. A new method of constructing an intestinal nipple valve for the continent ileostomy. *Cleve Clin Q* 1978;45:231.

60. Bolton RP, Sherrif RJ, Read AE. *Clostridium difficile*-associated diarrhoea: a role in inflammatory bowel disease? *Lancet* 1980;1:383.

61. Bonello JC, Thow GB, Manson RR. Mucosal enteritis: a complication of the continent ileostomy. *Dis Colon Rectum* 1981;24:37.

62. Booth IW, Harries JT. Inflammatory bowel disease in childhood. *Gut* 1984;25:188.

63. Bostwick J III, Moore J, McGarity WC. Inferior gluteal musculocutaneous flap for the obliteration of acute and chronic proctocolectomy defects. *Surg Gynecol Obstet* 1988;166:169.

64. Brahme F. Crohn's disease in a defined population. *Gastroenterology* 1975;69:342.

65. Brandt L, Boley S, Goldberg L, et al. Colitis in the elderly. *Am J Gastroenterol* 1981;76:239.

66. Braun J, Treutner KH, Harder M, et al. Anal sphincter function after intersphincteric resection and ileal pouch-anal anastomosis. *Dis Colon Rectum* 1991;34:8.

67. Broader JH, Masselink BA, Oates GD, et al. Management of the pelvic space after proctectomy. *Br J Surg* 1974;61:94.

68. Brooke BN. The outcome of surgery for ulcerative colitis. *Lancet* 1956;2:532.

69. Broström O, Löfberg R, Öst A, Reichard H. Cancer surveillance of patients with long-standing ulcerative colitis: a clinical, endoscopical, and histological study. *Gut* 1986;27:1408.

70. Brown JY. Value of complete physiological rest of large bowel in ulcerative and obstructive lesions. *Surg Gynecol Obstet* 1913;16:610.

71. Brown SR, Eu KW, Seow-Choen F. Consecutive series of laparoscopic-assisted *vs.* minilaparotomy restorative proctocolectomies. *Dis Colon Rectum* 2001;44:397.

72. Bullard KM, Madoff RD, Gemlo BT. Is ileoanal pouch function stable with time? Results of a prospective audit. *Dis Colon Rectum* 2002;45:299.

73. Bures J, Fixa B, Komárková O, Fingerland A. Nonsmoking: a feature of ulcerative colitis. *Br Med J* 1982;285:440.

74. Burke D, van Laarhoven CJHM, Herbst F, Nicholls RJ. Transvaginal repair of pouch-vaginal fistula. *Br J Surg* 2001;88:241.

75. Burnell D, Mayberry J, Calcraft BJ, et al. Male fertility in Crohn's disease. *Postgrad Med J* 1986;62:269.

76. Burnham WR, Lennard-Jones JE, Brooke BN. The incidence and nature of sexual problems among married ileostomists. *Gut* 1976;17:391(abst).

77. Burnstein MJ, Schoetz DJ Jr, Coller JA, Veidenheimer MC. Technique of mesenteric lengthening in ileal reservoir-anal anastomosis. *Dis Colon Rectum* 1987;30:863.

78. Campieri M, Adamo S, Valpiani D, et al. Oral beclomethasone dipropionate in the treatment of extensive and left-sided active ulcerative colitis: a multicentre randomized study. *Aliment Pharmacol Ther* 2003;17:1471.

79. Campieri M, Gionchetti P, Belluzzi A, et al. 5-Aminosalicylic acid suppositories in the management of ulcerative colitis. *Dis Colon Rectum* 1989;32:398.

80. Campieri M, Lanfranchi GA, Bazzocchi G, et al. Treatment of ulcerative colitis with high-dose 5-aminosalicylic acid enemas. *Lancet* 1981;2:270.

81. Campieri M, Lanfranchi GA, Brignola C, et al. Retrograde spread of 5-aminosalicylic acid enemas in patients with active ulcerative colitis. *Dis Colon Rectum* 1986;29:108.

82. Carter FM, McLeod RS, Cohen Z. Subtotal colectomy for ulcerative colitis: complications related to the rectal remnant. *Dis Colon Rectum* 1991;34:1005.

83. Cattell RB. The surgical treatment of ulcerative colitis. *JAMA* 1935;104:104.

84. Cave HW. The surgical management of chronic intractable ulcerative colitis. *Am J Surg* 1939;46:79.

85. Cherqui D, Valleur P, Perniceni T, Hautefeuille P. Inferior reach of ileal reservoir in ileoanal anastomosis: experimental anatomic and angiographic study. *Dis Colon Rectum* 1987;30:365.

86. Chey WY, Hussain A, Ryan C, et al. Infliximab is an effective therapeutic agent for ulcerative colitis. *Am J Gastroenterol* 2000;95:A2530.

87. Chey WY, Hussain A, Ryan C, et al. Infliximab for refractory ulcerative colitis. *Am J Gastroenterol* 2001;96:2373.

88. Chiodini RJ, Van Kruiningen HJ, Thayer WR, et al. Possible role of mycobacteria in inflammatory bowel disease. I: An unclassified *Mycobacterium* species isolated from patients with Crohn's disease. *Dig Dis Sci* 1984;29:1073.

89. Choi PM, Nugent FW, Schoetz DJ Jr, et al. Colonoscopic surveillance reduces mortality from colorectal cancer in ulcerative colitis. *Gastroenterology* 1993;105:418.

90. Christie PM, Schroeder D, Hill GL. Persisting superior mesenteric artery syndrome following ileo-anal J-pouch construction. *Br J Surg* 1988;75:1036.

91. Chung PY, Cohen RD, Kirschner BS, et al. Intravenous cyclosporin in ulcerative colitis: long-term follow-up of the University of Chicago experience. Paper presented at the American College of Gastroenterology; October 15, 2003.

92. Church JM, Saad R, Schroeder T, et al. Predicting the functional result of anastomoses to the anus: the paradox of preoperative anal resting pressure. *Dis Colon Rectum* 1993; 36:895.

93. Clark ML. Role of nutrition in inflammatory bowel disease: an overview. *Gut* 1986;27:72.

94. Coffey JC, Winter DC, Neary P, et al. Quality of life after ileal pouch-anal anastomosis: an evaluation of diet and other factors using the Cleveland global quality of life instrument. *Dis Colon Rectum* 2002;45:30.

95. Cohen R, Stern R, Hanauer SB. Intravenous cyclosporin in ulcerative colitis: a five-year experience. *Am J Gastroenterol* 1999;94:1587.

96. Cohen RD, Woseth DM, Thisted RA, et al. A meta-analysis and overview of the literature on treatment options for left-sided ulcerative colitis and ulcerative proctitis. *Am J Gastroenterol* 2000;95:1263.

97. Cohen Z, Cook MG, Festenstein H. The transmission of human Crohn's disease in inbred strains of mice. *Ann R Coll Phys Surg Can* 1978;2:51(abst).

98. Cohen Z, McLeod RS, Stephen W, et al. Continuing evolution of the pelvic pouch procedure. *Ann Surg* 1992;216:506.

99. Collins RH Jr, Feldman M, Fordtran JS. Colon cancer, dysplasia, and surveillance in patients with ulcerative colitis: a critical review. *N Engl J Med* 1987;316:1654.

100. Columbel JF, Ricart E, Loftus EV, et al. Management of Crohn's disease (CD) of the ileoanal pouch with infliximab. *Gastroenterology* 2003;124[Suppl 1]:A519.

101. Connell WR, Talbot IC, Harpaz N, et al. Clinicopathological characteristics of colorectal carcinoma complicating ulcerative colitis. *Gut* 1994;35:1419.

102. Coran AG. The ileal endorectal pull-through procedure. *Surg Rounds* 1982;(Nov):40.

103. Coran AG. A personal experience with 100 consecutive total colectomies and straight ileoanal endorectal pull-throughs for benign disease of the colon and rectum in children and adults. *Ann Surg* 1990;212:242.

104. Corbett RS. Discussion on the surgical treatment of idiopathic ulcerative colitis and its surgical sequelae. *Proc R Soc Med* 1940;33:647.

105. Corman ML. Total anal reconstruction to restore intestinal continuity after conventional proctocolectomy: report of a case. *Colorectal Dis* 2003;5:595.

106. Corman ML, Veidenheimer MC, Coller JA. Impotence after proctectomy for inflammatory disease of the bowel. *Dis Colon Rectum* 1978;21:418.

107. Corman ML, Veidenheimer MC, Coller JA, Ross VH. Perineal wound healing after proctectomy for inflammatory bowel disease. *Dis Colon Rectum* 1978;21:155.

108. Coull DB, Lee FD, Henderson AP, et al. Risk of dysplasia in the columnar cuff after stapled restorative proctocolectomy. *Br J Surg* 2003;90:72.

109. Cox CL, Butts DR, Roberts MP, et al. Development of invasive adenocarcinoma in a long-standing Kock continent ileostomy: report of a case. *Dis Colon Rectum* 1997;40:500.

110. Cranley B. The Kock reservoir ileostomy: a review of its development, problems and role in modern surgical practice. *Br J Surg* 1983;70:94.

111. Crile G Jr, Thomas CY Jr. Treatment of acute toxic ulcerative colitis by ileostomy and simultaneous colectomy. *Gastroenterology* 1951;19:58.

112. Cripps NPJ, Senapati A, Thompson MR. Improved perineal healing after internal sphincter-preserving proctectomy in ulcerative colitis. *Br J Surg* 1999;86:1344.

113. Crohn BB, Ginzburg L, Oppenheimer GD. Regional ileitis: a pathologic and clinical entity. *JAMA* 1932;99:1323.

114. Crohn BB, Yarnis H, Walter RI, et al. Ulcerative colitis as affected by pregnancy. *N Y State J Med* 1956;56:2651.

115. Crowson TD, Ferrante WF, Gathright JB Jr. Colonoscopy: inefficacy for early carcinoma detection in patients with ulcerative colitis. *JAMA* 1976;236:2651.

116. Cunnien AJ. Psychiatric aspects of chronic ulcerative colitis. *Semin Colon Rectal Surg* 1990;1:158.

117. Danish 5-ASA Group. Topical 5-aminosalicylic acid versus prednisolone in ulcerative proctosigmoiditis: a randomized, double-blind multicenter trial. *Dig Dis Sci* 1987;6:598.

118. D'Arienzo A, Panarese A, D'Armiento FP, et al. 5-Aminosalicylic acid suppositories in the maintenance of remission in idiopathic proctitis or proctosigmoiditis: a double-blind placebo-controlled clinical trial. *Am J Gastroenterol* 1990; 85:1079.

119. Das KM, Morecki R, Nair P, Berkowitz JM. Idiopathic proctitis: I. The morphology of proximal colonic mucosa and its clinical significance. *Am J Dig Dis* 1977;22:524.

120. Dassei PM. A familial pattern in inflammatory disease of the bowel (Crohn's disease and ulcerative colitis). *Dis Colon Rectum* 1977;20:669.

121. Daum F, Alperstein G. Inflammatory bowel disease in children and adolescents. *Pediatr Gastroenterol* 1982;6:26.

122. Davidson M. Juvenile ulcerative colitis. *N Engl J Med* 1967; 277:1408.

123. de Castella H. Non-smoking: a feature of ulcerative colitis. *Br Med J* 1982;284:1706.

124. de Dombal FT, Burton I, Goligher JC. The early and late results of surgical treatment for Crohn's disease. *Br J Surg* 1971;58:805.

125. de Dombal FT, Watts JM, Watkinson G, Goligher JC. Ulcerative colitis and pregnancy. *Lancet* 1965;2:599.

126. Deen KI, Hubscher S, Bain I, et al. Histological assessment of the distal doughnut in patients undergoing stapled restorative proctocolectomy with high or low anal transection. *Br J Surg* 1994;81:900.

127. Deen KI, Williams JG, Grant EA, et al. Randomized trial to determine the optimum level of pouch-anal anastomosis in stapled restorative proctocolectomy. *Dis Colon Rectum* 1995;38:133.

128. Delaney CP, Dadvand B, Remzi FH, et al. Functional outcome, quality of life, and complications after ileal pouch-anal anastomosis in selected septuagenarians. *Dis Colon Rectum* 2002;45:890.

129. Delaney CP, Fazio VW, Remzi FH, et al. Prospective, age-related analysis of surgical results, functional outcome, and quality of life after ileal pouch-anal anastomosis. *Ann Surg* 2003;238:221.

130. de Silva HJ, de Angelis CP, Soper N, et al. Clinical and functional outcome after restorative proctocolectomy. *Br J Surg* 1991;78:1039.

131. Diav-Citrin O, Park YH, Veerasunthram G, et al. Safety of mesalamine in human pregnancy: prospective controlled study. *Gastroenterology* 1998;114:23.

132. Dickinson RJ, Dixon MF, Axon ATR. Colonoscopy and the detection of dysplasia in patients with long-standing ulcerative colitis. *Lancet* 1980;2:620.

133. Dickinson RJ, King A, Wight DGD, et al. Is continuous sulfasalazine necessary in the management of patients with ulcerative colitis? Results of a preliminary study. *Dis Colon Rectum* 1985;28:929.

134. Diehl JT, Steiger E, Hooley R. The role of intravenous hyperalimentation in intestinal diseases. *Surg Clin North Am* 1983;63:11.

135. Donnelly BJ, Delaney PV, Healy TM. Evidence for a transmissible factor in Crohn's disease. *Gut* 1977;18:360.

136. Donovan MJ, O'Hara ET. Sexual function following surgery for ulcerative colitis. *N Engl J Med* 1960;262:719.

137. Doyle PJ, McKay AJ, Browne MK. Failure to thrive in adolescence due to inflammatory bowel disease. *Practitioner* 1979;222:253.

138. Dozois RR, Kelly KA, Beart RW Jr, Beahrs OH. Improved results with continent ileostomy. *Ann Surg* 1980;192:319.

139. Dozois RR, Kelly KA, Ilstrup D, et al. Factors affecting revision rate after continent ileostomy. *Arch Surg* 1981;116:610.

140. Dozois RR, Kelly KA, Welling DR, et al. Ileal pouch-anal anastomosis: comparison of results in familial adenomatous polyposis and chronic ulcerative colitis. *Ann Surg* 1989;210:268.

141. Dragstedt LR, Dack GM, Kirsner JB. Chronic ulcerative colitis: a summary of evidence implicating bacterium necrophorum as an etiologic agent. *Ann Surg* 1941;114:653.

142. Drossman DA. Psychosocial factors in inflammatory bowel disease. *Pract Gastroenterol* 1992;16:24N.

143. Dunker MS, Bemelman WA, Slors JFM, et al. Functional outcome, quality of life, body image, and cosmesis in patients after laparoscopic-assisted and conventional restorative proctocolectomy. *Dis Colon Rectum* 2001;44:1800.

144. Ecker KW, Hildebrandt U, Haberer M, Feifel G. Biomechanical stabilization of the nipple valve in continent ileostomy. *Br J Surg* 1996;83:1582.

145. Edwards F, Truelove SC. The course and prognosis of ulcerative colitis. Short-term prognosis. *Gut* 1963;4:299.

146. Ekbom A, Helmick C, Zack M, Adami H-O. Ulcerative colitis and colorectal cancer: a population-based study. *N Engl J Med* 1990;323:1228.

147. Emmanouilidis A, Manoussos O, Nicolaou A, et al. Colonoscopy in ulcerative colitis. *Am J Proctol Gastroenterol Colon Rectal Surg* 1983;34:5.

148. Evans JG, Acheson ED. An epidemiological study of ulcerative colitis and regional enteritis in the Oxford area. *Gut* 1965;6:311.

149. Everett WG. Experience of restorative proctocolectomy with ileal reservoir. *Br J Surg* 1989;76:77.

150. Eydenham J, Browaldh L, Johansson L, et al. Is budesonide enema effective in children? *Gastroenterology* 2000;118:A778(abst).

151. Farmer RG. Nonspecific ulcerative proctitis. *Gastroenterol Clin North Am* 1987;16:157.

152. Farmer RG, Michener WM, Mortimer EA. Studies of family history among patients with inflammatory bowel disease. *Clin Gastroenterol* 1980;9:271.

153. Farnell MB, Van Heerden JA, Beart RW Jr, Weiland LH. Rectal preservation in nonspecific inflammatory disease of the colon. *Ann Surg* 1980;192:249.

154. Farouk R, Duthie GS, Bartolo DCC. Recovery of the internal anal sphincter and continence after restorative proctocolectomy. *Br J Surg* 1994;81:1065.

155. Farouk R, Pemberton JH, Wolff BG, et al. Functional outcomes after ileal pouch-anal anastomosis for chronic ulcerative colitis. *Ann Surg* 2000;231:919.

156. Farrell RT, Peppercorn MA. Equimolar doses of balsalazide and mesalamine: are we comparing apples and oranges? *Am J Gastroenterol* 2002;98:1283.

157. Fasth S, Öresland T, Ahrén C, Hultén L. Mucosal proctectomy and ileostomy as an alternative to conventional proctectomy. *Dis Colon Rectum* 1985;28:31.

158. Faubion NA Jr, Loftus EV, Harmsen WS, et al. The natural history of corticosteroid therapy for inflammatory bowel disease: a population study. *Gastroenterology* 2001;121:255.

159. Fazio VW. Toxic megacolon in ulcerative colitis and Crohn's colitis. *Clin Gastroenterol* 1980;9:389.

160. Fazio VW, Church JM. Complications and function of the continent ileostomy at the Cleveland Clinic. *World J Surg* 1988;12:148.

161. Fazio VW, Tekkis PP, Remzi F, et al. Quantification of risk for pouch failure after ileal pouch anal anastomosis surgery. *Ann Surg* 2003;238:605.

162. Fazio VW, Tjandra JJ. Pouch advancement and neoileoanal anastomosis for anastomotic stricture and anovaginal fistula complicating restorative proctocolectomy. *Br J Surg* 1992;79:694.

163. Fazio VW, Tjandra JJ. Technique for nipple valve fixation to prevent valve slippage in continent ileostomy. *Dis Colon Rectum* 1992;35:1177.

164. Fazio VW, Tjandra JJ. Transanal mucosectomy: ileal pouch advancement for anorectal dysplasia or inflammation after restorative proctocolectomy. *Dis Colon Rectum* 1994;37:1008.

165. Fazio VW, Ziv Y, Church JM, et al. Ileal pouch-anal anastomoses: complications and function in 1005 patients. *Ann Surg* 1995;222:120.

166. Fedorak RN, Gionchetti P, Campieti M, et al. VSL#3 probiotic mixture induces remission in patients with active ulcerative colitis. *Gastroenterology* 2003;124:A377(M1582).

167. Feinberg SM, McLeod RS, Cohen Z. Complications of loop ileostomy. *Am J Surg* 1987;153:102.

168. Fergani H, Fardy J. Smoking and inflammatory bowel disease: an effect of disease or disease location: a meta-analysis. *Gastroenterology* 2002;122:A604.

169. Ferrara A, Pemberton JH, Grotz RL, Hanson RB. Motor determinants of incontinence after ileal pouch-anal anastomosis. *Br J Surg* 1994;81:285.

170. Ferrari BT, Fonkalsrud EW. Endorectal ileal pullthrough operation with ileal reservoir after total colectomy. *Am J Surg* 1978;136:113.

171. Fichera A, Cicchiello LA, Mendelson DS, et al. Superior mesenteric vein thrombosis after colectomy for inflammatory bowel disease: a not uncommon cause of postoperative acute abdominal pain. *Dis Colon Rectum* 2003;46:643.

172. Flake WK, Altman MS, Cartmill AM, Gilsdorf RB. Problems encountered with the Kock ileostomy. *Am J Surg* 1979;138:851.

173. Fleshman JW, Cohen Z, McLeod RS, et al. The ileal reservoir and ileoanal anastomosis procedure: factors affecting

technical and functional outcome. *Dis Colon Rectum* 1988; 31:10.

174. Foley EF, Schoetz DJ Jr, Roberts PL, et al. Rediversion after ileal pouch-anal anastomosis: causes of failures and predictors of subsequent pouch salvage. *Dis Colon Rectum* 1995;38:793.

175. Fonkalsrud EW. Total colectomy and endorectal ileal pullthrough with internal ileal reservoir for ulcerative colitis. *Surg Gynecol Obstet* 1980;150:1.

176. Fonkalsrud EW. Endorectal ileal pullthrough with lateral ileal reservoir for benign colorectal disease. *Ann Surg* 1981;194:761.

177. Fonkalsrud EW. Endorectal pullthrough with ileal reservoir for ulcerative colitis and polyposis. *Am J Surg* 1982; 144:81.

178. Fonkalsrud EW. Endorectal ileoanal anastomosis with isoperistaltic ileal reservoir after colectomy and mucosal proctectomy. *Ann Surg* 1984;199:151.

179. Fonkalsrud EW. Endorectal ileal pullthrough with isoperistaltic ileal reservoir for colitis and polyposis. *Ann Surg* 1985;202:145.

180. Fonkalsrud EW. Update on clinical experience with different surgical techniques on the endorectal pullthrough operation for colitis and polyposis. *Surg Gynecol Obstet* 1987; 165:309.

181. Fonkalsrud EW. Long-term results after colectomy and ileoanal pull-through procedure in children. *Arch Surg* 1996;131:881.

182. Fonkalsrud EW, Phillips JD. Reconstruction of malfunctioning ileoanal pouch procedures as an alternative to permanent ileostomy. *Am J Surg* 1990;160:245.

183. Fonkalsrud EW, Stelzner M, McDonald N. Experience with the endorectal ileal pullthrough with lateral reservoir for ulcerative colitis and polyposis. *Arch Surg* 1988;123:1053.

184. Fozard JBJ, Dixon MF. Colonoscopic surveillance in ulcerative colitis—dysplasia through the looking glass. *Gut* 1989;30:285.

185. Franceschi D, Chen PF, Yuh J-N. Solitary J-pouch ulcer causing pouchitis-like syndrome. *Dis Colon Rectum* 1986; 29:515.

186. Francois Y, Dozois RR, Kelly KA, et al. Small intestinal obstruction complicating ileal pouch-anal anastomosis. *Ann Surg* 1989;209:46.

187. Frizzi JD, Rivera DE, Harris JA, Hamill RL. Lymphoma arising in an S-pouch after total proctocolectomy for ulcerative colitis: report of a case. *Dis Colon Rectum* 2000;43: 540.

188. Frümorgen P. Diagnosis of inflammatory disease of the colon by colonoscopy. *Acta Gastroenterol* 1974;37:154.

189. Fujita S, Kusunoki M, Shoji Y, et al. Quality of life after total proctocolectomy and ileal J-pouch-anal anastomosis. *Dis Colon Rectum* 1992;35:1030.

190. Gadacz TR, Kelly KA, Phillips SF. The continent ileal pouch: absorptive and motor features. *Gastroenterology* 1977;72: 1287.

191. Galandiuk S, Pemberton JH, Tsao J, et al. Delayed ileal pouch-anal anastomosis: complications and functional results. *Dis Colon Rectum* 1991;34:755.

192. Galandiuk S, Scott NA, Dozois RR, et al. Ileal pouch-anal anastomosis. *Ann Surg* 1990;212:446.

193. Galandiuk S, Wolff BG, Dozois RR, Beart RW Jr. Ileal pouch-anal anastomosis without ileostomy. *Dis Colon Rectum* 1991;34:870.

194. Gandolfo J, Farthing M, Powers G, et al. 4-Aminosalicylic acid retention enemas in treatment of distal colitis. *Dig Dis Sci* 1987;32:700.

195. Gardner C, Miller GG. Total colectomy for ulcerative colitis. *Arch Surg* 1951;63:370.

196. Gassull MA, Abad A, Cabré E, et al. Enteral nutrition in inflammatory bowel disease. *Gut* 1986;27:76.

197. Geboes K, Vantrappen G. The value of colonoscopy in the diagnosis of Crohn's disease. *Gastrointest Endosc* 1975; 22:18.

198. Gecim IE, Wolff BG, Pemberton JH, et al. Does technique of anastomosis play any role in developing late perianal abscess or fistula? *Dis Colon Rectum* 2000;43:1241.

199. Gelernt IM, Bauer JJ, Kreel I. The reservoir ileostomy: early experience with 54 patients. *Ann Surg* 1977;185:179.

200. Gemlo BT, Belmonte C, Wiltz O, Madoff RD. Functional assessment of ileal pouch-anal anastomotic techniques. *Am J Surg* 1995;169:137.

201. Gemlo BT, Wong WD, Rothenberger DA, Goldberg SM. Ileal pouch-anal anastomosis: patterns of failure. *Arch Surg* 1992;127:784.

202. Gerber A, Apt MK, Craig PH. The Kock continent ileostomy. *Surg Gynecol Obstet* 1983;156:345.

203. Gilat T, Fireman Z, Grossman A, et al. Colorectal cancer in patients with ulcerative colitis: a population study in central Israel. *Gastroenterology* 1988;94:870.

204. Ginsberg AL, Davis ND, Nochomovitz LE. Placebo-controlled trial of ulcerative colitis with oral 4-aminosalicylic acid. *Gastroenterology* 1992;102:448.

205. Gionchetti P, Rizzello F, Venturi A, et al. Oral bacteriotherapy as maintenance treatment in patients with chronic pouchitis: a double-blind, placebo-controlled trial. *Gastroenterology* 2000;119:305.

206. Gitnick G. Is Crohn's disease a mycobacterial disease after all? *Dig Dis Sci* 1984;29:1086.

207. Gitnick GL, Rosen VJ, Arthur MH, Hertweck SA. Evidence for the isolation of a new virus from ulcerative proctitis patients: comparison with virus derived from Crohn's disease. *Dig Dis Sci* 1979;24:609.

208. Goes RN, Coy CSR, Amaral CA, et al. Superior mesenteric artery syndrome as a complication of ileal pouch-anal anastomosis: report of a case. *Dis Colon Rectum* 1995;38: 543.

209. Goes RN, Nguyen P, Huang D, Beart RW Jr. Lengthening of the mesentery using the marginal vascular arcade of the right colon as the blood supply to the ileal pouch. *Dis Colon Rectum* 1995;38:893.

210. Goldman CD, Kodner IJ, Fry RD, MacDermott RP. Clinical and operative experience with non-Caucasian patients with Crohn's disease. *Dis Colon Rectum* 1986;29:317.

211. Goligher JC. Primary excisional surgery in treatment of ulcerative colitis. *Ann R Coll Surg Engl* 1954;15:316.

212. Goligher JC. Inflammatory disease of the bowel [Symposium]: results of resection for Crohn's disease. *Dis Colon Rectum* 1976;19:584.

213. Goligher JC. Continent ileostomy: commentary. *World J Surg* 1980;4:147.

214. Goligher JC. *Surgery of the anus, rectum and colon*, 4th ed. London: Bailliére Tindall, 1980:689.

215. Goligher JC. *Surgery of the anus, rectum and colon*, 4th ed. London: Bailliére Tindall, 1980:793.

216. Goligher JC. *Surgery of the anus, rectum and colon*, 4th ed. London: Bailliére Tindall, 1980:828.

217. Goligher JC. Eversion technique for distal mucosal proctectomy in ulcerative colitis: a preliminary report. *Br J Surg* 1984;71:26.

218. Goligher JC, de Dombal FT, Watts J McK, Watkinson G. *Ulcerative colitis*. London: Bailliére, Tindall and Cassell, 1968:2.

219. Gopal KA, Amshel AL, Shonberg IL, et al. Ostomy and pregnancy. *Dis Colon Rectum* 1985;28:912.

220. Gorenstein L, Boyd JB, Ross TM. Gracilis muscle repair of rectovaginal fistula after restorative proctocolectomy: report of two cases. *Dis Colon Rectum* 1988;31:730.

221. Gorfine SR, Bauer JJ, Harris MT, Kreel I. Dysplasia complicating chronic ulcerative colitis. *Dis Colon Rectum* 2000; 43:1575.

222. Gorfine SR, Fichera A, Harris MT, Bauer JJ. Long-term results of salvage surgery for septic complications after restorative proctocolectomy: does fecal diversion improve outcome? *Dis Colon Rectum* 2003;46:1339.

223. Gorfine SR, Gelernt IM, Bauer JJ, et al. Restorative proctocolectomy without diverting ileostomy. *Dis Colon Rectum* 1995;38:188.

224. Gormet JM, Lemann M, Cosnes J, et al. Azathioprine (AZA) for ulcerative colitis: a retrospective multicenter study of 131 patients. *Gastroenterology* 2001;120:625(A3174)(abst).

225. Gottlieb LM, Handelsman JC. Treatment of outflow tract problems associated with continent ileostomy (Kock pouch): report of six cases. *Dis Colon Rectum* 1991;34:936.

226. Grant CS, Dozois RR. Toxic megacolon: ultimate fate of patients after successful medical management. *Am J Surg* 1984;147:106.

227. Grant D, Cohen Z, McHugh S, et al. Restorative proctocolectomy: clinical results and manometric findings with long and short rectal cuffs. *Dis Colon Rectum* 1986;29:27.

228. Green JEB, Lobo AJ, Holdsworth RT, et al. Balsalazide is more effective and better tolerated than mesalamine in ulcerative colitis. *Gastroenterology* 1998;114:15.

229. Greenstein A. Cancer in inflammatory bowel disease. *Surg Rounds* 1982;(Oct):44.

230. Greenstein AJ, Aufses AH Jr. Differences in pathogenesis, incidence and outcome of perforation in inflammatory bowel disease. *Surg Gynecol Obstet* 1985;160:63.

231. Greenstein AJ, Barth JA, Sachar DB, Aufses AH Jr. Free colonic perforation without dilatation in ulcerative colitis. *Am J Surg* 1986;152:272.

232. Greenstein AJ, Mann D, Heimann T, et al. Spontaneous free perforation and perforated abscess in 30 patients with Crohn's disease. *Ann Surg* 1987;205:72.

233. Grobier SP, Hosie KB, Keighley MRB. Randomized trial of loop ileostomy in restorative proctocolectomy. *Br J Surg* 1992;79:903.

234. Groom JS, Nicholls RJ, Hawley PR, Phillips RKS. Pouch-vaginal fistula. *Br J Surg* 1993;80:936.

235. Grundfest SF, Fazio V, Weiss RA, et al. The risk of cancer following colectomy and ileorectal anastomosis for extensive mucosal ulcerative colitis. *Ann Surg* 1981;193:9.

236. Guarino J, Chatzinoff M, Berk T, Friedman LS. 5-Aminosalicylic acid enema in refractory distal ulcerative colitis: long-term results. *Am J Gastroenterol* 1987;82:732.

237. Guillemot F, Leroy J, Boniface M, et al. Functional assessment of coloanal anastomosis with reservoir and excision of the anal transition zone. *Dis Colon Rectum* 1991;34:967.

238. Gurian L, Klein K, Ward TT. Role of *Clostridium difficile* and *Campylobacter jejuni* in relapses of inflammatory bowel disease. *West J Med* 1983;138:359.

239. Gustavsson S, Weiland LH, Kelly KA. Relationship of backwash ileitis to ileal pouchitis after ileal pouch-anal anastomosis. *Dis Colon Rectum* 1987;30:25.

240. Gutierrez P, Stahlgren LH. A technique for catheter fixation for continent ileostomy. *Surg Gynecol Obstet* 1983;156:808.

241. Gyde S. Screening for colorectal cancer in ulcerative colitis: dubious benefits and high costs. *Gut* 1990;31:1089.

242. Habal FM, Greenberg GR. Treatment of ulcerative colitis with oral 5-aminosalicylic acid including patients with adverse reactions to sulfasalazine. *Am J Gastroenterol* 1988;83:15.

243. Halverson AL, Hull TL, Remzi F, et al. Perioperative resting pressure predicts long-term postoperative function after ileal pouch-anal anastomosis. *J Gastrointest Surg* 2002;6:316.

244. Halvorsen JF, Heimann P, Hoel R, Nygaard K. The continent reservoir ileostomy: review of a collective series of 36 patients from three surgical departments. *Surgery* 1978;83:252.

245. Ham RJ, Ball A. A convenient alternative to the Zachary Cope enterostomy clamp. *Ann R Coll Surg Engl* 1985;67:82.

246. Hamilton I, Pinder IF, Dickinson RJ, et al. A comparison of prednisolone enemas with low-dose oral prednisolone in the treatment of acute distal ulcerative colitis. *Dis Colon Rectum* 1984;27:701.

247. Hampson SJ, McFadden JJ, Hermon-Taylor J. Mycobacteria and Crohn's disease. Gut 1988;29:1017.

248. Hanauer SB. Medical therapy of ulcerative colitis. *Lancet* 1993;342:412.

249. Hanauer SB. Nicotine for colitis—the smoke has not yet cleared. *N Engl J Med* 1994;330:856.

250. Hanauer SB. Inflammatory bowel disease. *N Engl J Med* 1996;334:841.

251. Hanauer S. Commentary. *Gut* 1999;44:455.

252. Hanauer S, Robinson M, Pruitt R, et al. Budesonide enema for treatment of active distal ulcerative colitis and proctitis: a dose ranging study. *Gastroenterology* 1998;115:525.

253. Hanson PA. Diet for control of an ileoanal reservoir. *Ostomy/Wound Management* 1990;28(May/June):24.

254. Haray PN, Amarnath B, Weiss EG, et al. Low malignant potential of the double-stapled ileal pouch-anal anastomosis. *Br J Surg* 1996;83:1406.

255. Harford FJ Jr. Use of the ultrasonic aspirator to strip the mesentery in construction of the continent ileostomy. *Dis Colon Rectum* 1987;30:736.

256. Harms BA, Andersen AB, Starling JR. The W ileal reservoir: long-term assessment after proctocolectomy for ulcerative colitis and familial polyposis. *Surgery* 1992;112:638.

257. Harms BA, Hamilton JW, Yamamoto DT, Starling JR. Quadruple-loop (W) ileal pouch reconstruction after proctocolectomy. *Surgery* 1987;102:561.

258. Harms BA, Myers GA, Rosenfeld DJ, Starling JR. Management of fulminant ulcerative colitis by primary restorative proctocolectomy. *Dis Colon Rectum* 1994;37:971.

259. Harms BA, Pahl AC, Starling JR. Comparison of clinical and compliance characteristics between S and W ileal reservoirs. *Am J Surg* 1990;159:34.

260. Harms BA, Pellett JR, Starling JR. Modified quadruple-loop (W) ileal reservoir for restorative proctocolectomy. *Surgery* 1987;101:234.

261. Harper PH, Lee ECG, Kettlewell MGW, et al. Role of the faecal stream in the maintenance of Crohn's colitis. *Gut* 1985;26:279.

262. Harries AD, Baird A, Rhodes J. Non-smoking: a feature of ulcerative colitis. *Br Med J* 1982;284:706.

263. Harries AD, Danis VA, Heatley RV. Influence of nutritional status on immune functions in patients with Crohn's disease. *Gut* 1984;25:465.

264. Harvey PRC, McLeod RS, Cohen Z, Strasberg SM. Effect of colectomy on bile consumption, cholesterol crystal formation, and gallstones in patients with ulcerative colitis. *Ann Surg* 1991;214:396.

265. Hashimoto L, Seidner D, Steiger E, et al. Recurrent small bowel obstruction secondary to a dilated Kock pouch: a case report. *Am Surg* 1995;61:334.

266. Hata J, Haruma K, Suenaga K, et al. Ultrasonographic assessment of inflammatory bowel disease. *Am J Gastroenterol* 1992;87:443.

267. Hawley PR. Ileorectal anastomosis. *Br J Surg* 1985;72 [Suppl]: S75.

268. Heald RJ, Allen DR. Stapled ileo-anal anastomosis: a technique to avoid mucosal proctectomy in the ileal pouch operation. *Br J Surg* 1986;73:571.

269. Heimann TM, Greenstein AJ, Mechanic L, Aufses AH Jr. Early complications following surgical treatment for Crohn's disease. *Ann Surg* 1985;201:494.

270. Heimann TM, Kurtz RJ, Aufses AH Jr. Ultrasonic fragmentation: a new technique for mucosal proctectomy. *Arch Surg* 1985;120:1200.

271. Heimann TM, Slater G, Kurtz RJ, et al. Ultrasonic mucosal proctectomy in patients with ulcerative colitis. *Ann Surg* 1989;210:787.

272. Heit HA. Use of antidiarrheals in ulcerative colitis [Letter and Reply]. *Gastroenterology* 1988;94:1520.

273. Helzer JE, Stillings WA, Chammas S, et al. A controlled study of the association between ulcerative colitis and psychiatric diagnosis. *Dig Dis Sci* 1982;27:513.

274. Hensley GT. Interpretation of colonic mucosal biopsy in IBD: potential pitfalls. *Pract Gastroenterol* 1987;11(3):15.

275. Heppell J, Belliveau P, Taillefer R, et al. Quantitative assessment of pelvic ileal reservoir emptying with a semisolid ra-

dionuclide enema: a correlation with clinical outcome. *Dis Colon Rectum* 1987;30:81.

276. Heppell J, Farkouh E, Dubé S, et al. Toxic megacolon: an analysis of 70 cases. *Dis Colon Rectum* 1986;29:789.

277. Heppell J, Kelly KA, Phillips SF, et al. Physiologic aspects of continence after colectomy, mucosal proctectomy, and endorectal ileo-anal anastomosis. *Ann Surg* 1982;195: 435.

278. Heppell J, Weiland LH, Perrault J, et al. Fate of the rectal mucosa after rectal mucosectomy and ileoanal anastomosis. *Dis Colon Rectum* 1983;26:768.

279. Herbst F, Sielezneff I, Nicholls RJ. Salvage surgery for ileal pouch outlet obstruction. *Br J Surg* 1996;83:368.

280. Herline AJ, Meisinger LL, Rusin LC, et al. Is routine pouch surveillance for dysplasia indicated for ileoanal pouches? *Dis Colon Rectum* 2003;46:156.

281. Heuschen UA, Allemeyer EH, Hinz U, et al. Outcome after septic complications in J pouch procedures. *Br J Surg* 2002;89:194.

282. Heuschen UA, Autschbach F, Allemeyer EH, et al. Long-term follow-up after ileoanal pouch procedure: algorithm for diagnosis, classification, and management of pouchitis. *Dis Colon Rectum* 2001;44:487.

283. Heuschen UA, Hinz U, Allemeyer EH, et al. One- or two-stage procedure for restorative proctocolectomy: rationale for a surgical strategy in ulcerative colitis. *Ann Surg* 2001;234:788.

284. Heuschen UA, Hinz U, Allemeyer EH, et al. Risk factors for ileoanal J pouch-related septic complications in ulcerative colitis and familial adenomatous polyposis. *Ann Surg* 2002; 235:207.

285. Hewett PJ, Stitz R, Hewett MK. Comparison of the functional results of restorative proctocolectomy for ulcerative colitis between the J and W configuration ileal pouches with sutured ileoanal anastomosis. *Dis Colon Rectum* 1995;38:567.

286. Higgens CS, Keighley MRB, Allan RN. Impact of preoperative weight loss and body composition changes on postoperative outcome in surgery for inflammatory bowel disease. *Gut* 1984;25:732.

287. Hinojosa J, Aad A, Panes J, et al. Multicenter, randomized trial comparing oral, topic and oral plus topic mesalazine in prevention of relapse in distal ulcerative colitis (DUC). *Gastroenterology* 2001;120:A12(abst).

288. Holdsworth CD. Acute self-limited colitis [Editorial]. *Br Med J* 1984;289:270.

289. Holdsworth PJ, Johnston D. Anal sensation after restorative proctocolectomy for ulcerative colitis. *Br J Surg* 1988;75:993.

290. Holdsworth PJ, Johnston D. Use of the end-to-end anastomosis without mucosal stripping diminishes morbidity and time in hospital after restorative proctocolectomy. *Br J Surg* 1988;75:1232.

291. Holdsworth PJ, Sagar PM, Lewis WG, et al. Internal anal sphincter activity after restorative proctocolectomy for ulcerative colitis: a study using continuous ambulatory manometry. *Dis Colon Rectum* 1994;37:32.

292. Holzmann K, Klump B, Borchard F, et al. Flow cytometric and histologic evaluation in a large cohort of patients with ulcerative colitis: correlation with clinical characteristics and impact on surveillance. *Dis Colon Rectum* 2001;44: 1446.

293. Hosie KB, Grobler SP, Keighley MRB. Temporary loop ileostomy following restorative proctocolectomy. *Br J Surg* 1992;79:33.

294. Hsu T-C. Traumatic perforation of ileal pouch: report of a case. *Dis Colon Rectum* 1989;32:64.

295. Hughes ESR. The treatment of ulcerative colitis. *Ann R Coll Surg Engl* 1965;37:191.

296. Hughes ESR, McDermott FT, Masterton JP. Ileorectal anastomosis for inflammatory bowel disease: 15-year follow-up. *Dis Colon Rectum* 1979;22:399.

297. Hughes JP, Bauer AR Jr, Bauer CM. Stapling techniques for easy construction of an ileal J-pouch. *Am J Surg* 1988;155: 783.

298. Hultén L, Fasth S. Loop ileostomy for protection of the newly constructed ileostomy reservoir. *Br J Surg* 1981;68: 11.

299. Hultén L, Fasth S, Nordgren S, Öresland T. Kock's pouch converted to a pelvic pouch: report of a case. *Dis Colon Rectum* 1988;31:457.

300. Hultén L, Kewenter J, Knutsson U, et al. Primary closure of perineal wound after proctocolectomy or rectal excision. *Acta Chir Scand* 1971;137:467.

301. Hultén L, Svaninger G. Facts about the Kock continent ileostomy. *Dis Colon Rectum* 1984;27:553.

302. Hultén L, Willén R, Nilsson O, et al. Mucosal assessment for dysplasia and cancer in the ileal pouch mucosa in patients operated on for ulcerative colitis: a 30-year follow-up study. *Dis Colon Rectum* 2002;45:448.

303. Hurst RD, Molinari M, Chung TP, et al. Prospective study of the incidence, timing, and treatment of pouchitis in 104 consecutive patients after restorative proctocolectomy. *Arch Surg* 1996;131:497.

304. Hyde GM, Jewell DP, Kettlewell MGW, Mortensen NJMcC. Cyclosporin for severe ulcerative colitis does not increase the rate of perioperative complications. *Dis Colon Rectum* 2001;44:1436.

305. Ireland A, Mason CH, Jewell DP. Controlled trial comparing olsalazine and sulphasalazine for the maintenance treatment of ulcerative colitis. *Gut* 1988;29:835.

306. Irvin TT, Goligher JC. A controlled clinical trial of three different methods of perineal wound management following excision of the rectum. *Br J Surg* 1975;62:287.

307. Ishikawa A, Lamoke A, Umesaki Y, et al. Randomized controlled trial of the effect of bifidobacterium-fermented milk on ulcerative colitis. *Gastroenterology* 2000; 128: A778 (abst).

308. Iwama T, Kamikawa J, Higuchi T, et al. Development of invasive adenocarcinoma in a long-standing diverted J-pouch for ulcerative colitis: report of a case. *Dis Colon Rectum* 2000;43:101.

309. Jacobsen O, Hojgaard L, Moller EH, et al. Effect of enterocoated cholestyramine on bowel habit after ileal resection: a double-blind crossover study. *Br Med J* 1985;290:1315.

310. Jalan KN, Smith AN, Ruckley CV, et al. Perineal wound healing in ulcerative colitis. *Br J Surg* 1969;56:749.

311. James SP, Strober W, Quinn TC, Danovitch SH. Crohn's disease: new concepts of pathogenesis and current approaches to treatment. *Dig Dis Sci* 1987;32:1297.

312. Jörvinen HJ, Luukkonen P. Comparison of restorative proctocolectomy with and without covering ileostomy in ulcerative colitis. *Br J Surg* 1991;78:199.

313. Jörvinen HJ, Mökitie A, Sivula A. Long-term results of continent ileostomy. *Int J Colorect Dis* 1986;1:40.

314. Jay M, Digenis GA, Foster TS, Antonow DR. Retrograde spreading of hydrocortisone enema in inflammatory bowel disease. *Dig Dis Sci* 1986;31:139.

315. Jewell DP. Corticosteroids for the management of ulcerative colitis and Crohn's disease. *Gastroenterol Clin North Am* 1989;18:21.

316. Jick H, Walker AM. Cigarette smoking and ulcerative colitis. *N Engl J Med* 1983;308:261.

317. Johnson WR, Hughes ESR, McDermott FT, Katrivessis H. The outcome of patients with ulcerative colitis managed by subtotal colectomy. *Surg Gynecol Obstet* 1986;162:421.

318. Johnson WR, McDermott FT, Hughes ESR, et al. The risk of rectal carcinoma following colectomy in ulcerative colitis. *Dis Colon Rectum* 1983;26:44.

319. Johnson WR, McDermott FT, Hughes ESR, et al. Carcinoma of the colon and rectum in inflammatory disease of the intestine. *Surg Gynecol Obstet* 1983;156:193.

320. Johnston D, Holdsworth PJ, Nasmyth DG, et al. Preservation of the entire anal canal in conservative proctocolectomy for ulcerative colitis: a pilot study comparing end-to-end ileo-anal anastomosis without mucosal resection with mucosal proctectomy and endo-anal anastomosis. *Br J Surg* 1987;74:940.

321. Johnston D, Williamson MER, Lewis WG, et al. Prospective controlled trial of duplicated (J) versus quadruplicated (W)

pelvic ileal reservoirs in restorative proctocolectomy for ulcerative colitis. *Gut* 1996;39:242.

322. Jones PF, Bevan PG, Hawley PR. Ileostomy or ileorectal anastomosis for ulcerative colitis. *Br Med J* 1978;1:1459.

323. Jones VA, Dickinson RJ, Workman E, et al. Crohn's disease: maintenance of remission by diet. *Lancet* 1985;2:177.

324. Jonsson B, Åhsgren L, Andersson LO, et al. Colorectal cancer surveillance in patients with ulcerative colitis. *Br J Surg* 1994;81:689.

325. Jorge JMN, Wesner SD, James K, et al. Recovery of anal sphincter function after the ileoanal reservoir procedure in patients over the age of 50. *Dis Colon Rectum* 1994;37:1002.

326. Juhasz ES, Fozard B, Dozois RR, et al. Ileal pouch-anal anastomosis function following childbirth: an extended evaluation. *Dis Colon Rectum* 1995;38:159.

327. Kaiser AM, Stein JP, Beart RWJr. T-pouch: a new valve design for a continent ileostomy. *Dis Colon Rectum* 2002;45: 411.

328. Kam L, Cohen H, Dooley C, et al. A comparison of mesalamine suspension enema and oral sulfasalazine for treatment of active distal ulcerative colitis in adults. *Am J Gastroenterol* 1996;91:1138.

329. Karlbom U, Raab Y, Ejerblad S, et al. Factors influencing the functional outcome of restorative proctocolectomy in ulcerative colitis. *Br J Surg* 2000;87:1401.

330. Karush A, Daniels GE, Flood C, O'Connor JF. *Psychotherapy in chronic ulcerative colitis.* Philadelphia: WB Saunders, 1977:148.

331. Katschinski B, Logan RFA, Edmond M, Langman MJS. Smoking and sugar intake are separate but interactive risk factors in Crohn's disease. *Gut* 1988;29:1202.

332. Katz BH, Schwartz SS, Vender RJ. Portal venous gas following a barium enema in a patient with Crohn's colitis: a benign finding. *Dis Colon Rectum* 1986;29:49.

333. Kay RM, Cohen Z, Siu KP, et al. Ileal excretion and bacterial modification of bile acids and cholesterol in patients with continent ileostomy. *Gut* 1979;21:128.

334. Keighley MRB. Abdominal mucosectomy reduces the incidence of soiling and sphincter damage after restorative proctocolectomy and J-pouch. *Dis Colon Rectum* 1987;30: 386.

335. Keighley MRB, Grobler SP. Fistula complicating restorative proctocolectomy. *Br J Surg* 1993;80:1065.

336. Keighley MRB, Winslet MC, Flinn R, Kmiot W. Multivariate analysis of factors influencing the results of restorative proctocolectomy. *Br J Surg* 1989;76:740.

337. Keighley MRB, Winslet MC, Yoshioka K, Lightwood R. Discrimination is not impaired by excision of the anal transition zone after restorative proctocolectomy. *Br J Surg* 1987;74:1118.

338. Keighley MRB, Yoshioka K, Kmiot W. Prospective randomized trial to compare the stapled double-lumen pouch and the sutured quadruple pouch for restorative proctocolectomy. *Br J Surg* 1988;75:1008.

339. Keighley MRB, Yoshioka K, Kmiot W, Heyen F. Physiological parameters influencing function in restorative proctocolectomy and ileo-pouch-anal anastomosis. *Br J Surg* 1988;75:997.

340. Kelly DG, Branon ME, Phillips SF, Kelly KA. Diarrhoea after continent ileostomy. *Gut* 1980;21:711.

341. Kelly DG, Phillips SF, Kelly KA, et al. Dysfunction of the continent ileostomy: clinical features and bacteriology. *Gut* 1983;24:193.

342. Kelly KA. Ileal pouch-anal anastomosis after proctocolectomy. *Surg Rounds* 1985;8(Jan):48.

343. Kelts DG, Grand RJ, Shen G, et al. Nutritional basis of growth failure in children and adolescents with Crohn's disease. *Gastroenterology* 1979;76:720.

344. Khoo REH, Cohen MM, Chapman GM, et al. Loop ileostomy for temporary fecal diversion. *Am J Surg* 1994; 167:519.

345. Khosla R, Willoughby CP, Jewell DP. Crohn's disease and pregnancy. *Gut* 1984;25:52.

346. Khubchandani IT, Sandfort MR, Rosen L, et al. Current status of ileorectal anastomosis for inflammatory bowel disease. *Dis Colon Rectum* 1989;32:400.

347. Khubchandani IT, Stasik JJ Jr, Nedwich A. Prospective surveillance by rectal biopsy following ileorectal anastomosis for inflammatory disease. *Dis Colon Rectum* 1982; 25:343.

348. King DW, Lubowski DZ, Cook TA. Anal canal mucosa in restorative proctocolectomy for ulcerative colitis. *Br J Surg* 1989;78:970.

349. Kirkegaard P, Madsen PV. Perineal sinus after removal of the rectum: occlusion with fibrin adhesive. *Am J Surg* 1983;145:791.

350. Kirsner JB. Genetic aspects of inflammatory bowel disease. *Clin Gastroenterol* 1973;2:557.

351. Kirsner JB, Shorter RG. Recent developments in "nonspecific" inflammatory bowel disease, part I. *N Engl J Med* 1982;306:775.

352. Kirsner JB, Shorter RG. Recent developments in nonspecific inflammatory bowel disease, part II. *N Engl J Med* 1982;306:837.

353. Kirsner JB, Spencer JA. Family occurrences of ulcerative colitis, regional enteritis, and ileocolitis. *Ann Intern Med* 1963;59:133.

354. Kjeldsen J, Schaffalitzky DE, Muckadell OB. Assessment of disease activity and severity in inflammatory bowel disease. *Scand J Gastroenterol* 1993;28:1.

355. Klingler PJ, Neuhauser B, Peer R, et al. Nipple complication caused by a mesenteric GORE-TEX® sling reinforcement in a Kock ileal reservoir: report of a case. *Dis Colon Rectum* 2001;44:128.

356. Kmiot WA, Keighley MRB. Totally stapled abdominal restorative proctocolectomy. *Br J Surg* 1989;76:961.

357. Kmiot WA, Yoshioka K, Pinho M, Keighley MRB. Videoproctographic assessment after restorative proctocolectomy. *Dis Colon Rectum* 1990;33:566.

358. Kochhar R, Mehta SK, Aggarwal R, et al. Sucralfate enema in ulcerative rectosigmoid lesions. *Dis Colon Rectum* 1990; 33:49.

359. Kock NG. Intra-abdominal "reservoir" in patients with permanent ileostomy: preliminary observations on a procedure resulting in fecal "continence" in five ileostomy patients. *Arch Surg* 1969;99:223.

360. Kock NG, Darle N, Hultén L, et al. Ileostomy. *Curr Probl Surg* 1977;14:1.

361. Kock NG, Darle N, Kewenter J, et al. The quality of life after proctocolectomy and ileostomy: a study of patients with conventional ileostomies converted to continent ileostomies. *Dis Colon Rectum* 1974;17:287.

362. Kock NG, Hultén L, Myrvold HE. Ileoanal anastomosis with interposition of the ileal "Kock pouch"—preliminary results. *Dis Colon Rectum* 1989;32:1050.

363. Kock NG, Myrvold HE, Nilsson LO, Philipson BM. Continent ileostomy: an account of 314 patients. *Acta Chir Scand* 1981;147:67.

364. Köhler LW, Pemberton JH, Hodge DO, et al. Long-term functional results and quality of life after ileal pouch-anal anastomosis and cholecystectomy. *World J Surg* 1992;16:1126.

365. Köhler LW, Pemberton JH, Zinmeister AR, Kelly KA. Quality of life after proctocolectomy: a comparison of Brooke ileostomy, Kock pouch, and ileal pouch-anal anastomosis. *Gastroenterology* 1991;101:679.

366. Kokoszka J, Nelson RL, Swedler WI, et al. Determination of inflammatory bowel disease activity by breath pentane analysis. *Dis Colon Rectum* 1993;36:597.

367. Kollmorgen CF, Nivatvongs S, Dean PA, Dozois RR. Long-term causes of death following ileal pouch-anal anastomosis. *Dis Colon Rectum* 1996;39:525.

368. Korelitz BI, Cheskin LJ, Sohn N, Sommers SC. Proctitis after fecal diversion in Crohn's disease and its elimination with reanastomosis: implications for surgical management. Report of four cases. *Gastroenterology* 1984;87: 710.

369. Korelitz BI, Dyck WP, Klion FM. Fate of the rectum and distal colon after subtotal colectomy for ulcerative colitis. *Gut* 1969;10:198.

370. Koretz RL. Nutritional support: how much for how much? *Gut* 1986;27:85.

371. Kornbluth A, Marion JF, Salomon P, Janowitz HD. How effective is current medical therapy for severe ulcerative and Crohn's colitis? An analytic review of selected trials. *J Clin Gastroenterol* 1995;20:280.

372. Koutroubakis IE, Vlachonikolis IG, Kouroumalis EA. Role of appendicitis and appendectomy in the pathogenesis of ulcerative colitis: a critical review. *Inflamm Bowel Dis* 2002; 8:277.

373. Kurtz LM, Flint GW, Platt N, Wise L. Carcinoma in the retained rectum after colectomy for ulcerative colitis. *Dis Colon Rectum* 1980;23:346.

374. Kusunoki M, Shoji Y, Fujita S, et al. Characteristics of anal canal motility after ileoanal anastomosis. *Surg Gynecol Obstet* 1992;174:22.

375. Ky AJ, Sonoda T, Milsom JW. One-stage laparoscopic restorative proctocolectomy: an alternative to the conventional approach. *Dis Colon Rectum* 2002;45:207.

376. Kyle J. An epidemiological study of Crohn's disease in northeast Scotland. *Gastroenterology* 1971;61:826.

377. Lahey FH. Ulcerative colitis. *N Y State J Med* 1941;41:475.

378. La Mont JT, Trnka YM. Therapeutic implications of *Clostridium difficile* toxin during relapse of chronic inflammatory bowel disease. *Lancet* 1980;1:381.

379. Langholz E, Munkholm P, Davidsen M, Binder V. Course of ulcerative colitis: analysis of changes in disease activity over years. *Gastroenterology* 1994;107:3.

380. Lashner BA. Recommendations for colorectal cancer screening in ulcerative colitis: a review of research from a single university-based surveillance program. *Am J Gastroenterol* 1992;87:168.

381. Lashner BA, Evans AA, Kirsner JB, Hanauer SB. Prevalence and incidence of inflammatory bowel disease in family members. *Gastroenterology* 1986;91:1396.

382. Lashner BA, Turner BC, Bostwick DG, et al. Dysplasia and cancer complicating strictures in ulcerative colitis. *Dig Dis Sci* 1990;35:349.

383. Launer DP, Sackier JM. Pouch-anal anastomosis without diverting ileostomy. *Dis Colon Rectum* 1991;34:993.

384. Laureti S, Ugolini F, D'Errico A, et al. Adenocarcinoma below ileoanal anastomosis for ulcerative colitis: report of a case and review of the literature. *Dis Colon Rectum* 2002;45:418.

385. Lavery IC, Chiulli RA, Jagelman DG, et al. Survival with carcinoma arising in mucosal ulcerative colitis. *Ann Surg* 1982;195:508.

386. Lavery IC, Jagelman DG. Cancer in the excluded rectum following surgery for inflammatory bowel disease. *Dis Colon Rectum* 1982;25:522.

387. Lavery IC, Michener WM, Jagelman DG. Ileorectal anastomosis for inflammatory bowel disease in children and adolescents. *Surg Gynecol Obstet* 1983;157:553.

388. Lavery IC, Tuckson WB, Easley KA. Internal anal sphincter after total abdominal colectomy and stapled ileal pouch-anal anastomosis without mucosal proctectomy. *Dis Colon Rectum* 1989;32:950.

389. Lee PY, Fazio VW, Church JM, et al. Vaginal fistula following restorative proctocolectomy. *Dis Colon Rectum* 1997;40:752.

390. Leicester RJ, Ritchie JK, Wadsworth J, et al. Sexual function and perineal wound healing after intersphincteric excision of the rectum for inflammatory bowel disease. *Dis Colon Rectum* 1984;27:244.

391. Leidenius M, Kellokumpu I, Husa A, et al. Dysplasia and carcinoma in long-standing ulcerative colitis: an endoscopic and histological surveillance programme. *Gut* 1991;32:1521.

392. Leijonmarck C-E, Broström O, Monsen U, Hellers G. Surgical treatment of ulcerative colitis in Stockholm County, 1955 to 1984. *Dis Colon Rectum* 1989;32:918.

393. Leijonmarck C-E, Liljeqvist L, Poppen B, Hellers G. Surgery after colectomy for ulcerative colitis. *Dis Colon Rectum* 1992;35:495.

394. Leijonmarck C-E, Löfberg R, Öst A, Hellers G. Long-term results of ileorectal anastomosis in ulcerative colitis in Stockholm County. *Dis Colon Rectum* 1990;33:195.

395. Leijonmarck C-E, Persson PG, Hellers G. Factors affecting colectomy rate in ulcerative colitis: an epidemiologic study. *Gut* 1990;31:329.

396. Lennard-Jones JE. Cancer risk in ulcerative colitis: surveillance or surgery. *Br J Surg* 1985;72[Suppl]:S84.

397. Lennard-Jones JE. Compliance, cost, and common sense limit cancer control in colitis. *Gut* 1986;27:1403.

398. Lennard-Jones JE, Melville DM, Morson BC, et al. Precancer and cancer in extensive ulcerative colitis: findings among 401 patients over 22 years. *Gut* 1990;31:800.

399. Lepistö AH, Järvinen HJ. Durability of Kock continent ileostomy. *Dis Colon Rectum* 2003;46:925.

400. Lepistö AH, Luukkonen P, Järvinen HJ. Cumulative failure rate of ileal pouch-anal anastomosis and quality of life after failure. *Dis Colon Rectum* 2002;45:1289.

401. Levenstein S, Prantera C, Luzi C, D'Ubaldi A. Low residue or normal diet in Crohn's disease: a prospective controlled study in Italian patients. *Gut* 1985;26:989.

402. Levi AJ. Diet in the management of Crohn's disease. *Gut* 1985;26:985.

403. Levin KE, Pemberton JH, Phillips SF, et al. Role of oxygen free radicals in the etiology of pouchitis. *Dis Colon Rectum* 1992;35:452.

404. Levine DS, Rabinovitch PS, Haggitt RC, et al. Distribution of aneuploid cell populations in ulcerative colitis with dysplasia or cancer. *Gastroenterology* 1991;101:1198.

405. Levitt MD, Lewis AAM. Determinants of ileoanal pouch function. *Gut* 1991;32:126.

406. Levy N, Roisman I, Teodor I. Ulcerative colitis in pregnancy in Israel. *Dis Colon Rectum* 1981;24:351.

407. Lewis WG, Kuzu A, Sagar PM, et al. Stricture at the pouch-anal anastomosis after restorative proctocolectomy. *Dis Colon Rectum* 1994;37:120.

408. Lewis WG, Miller AS, Williamson MER, et al. The perfect pelvic pouch—what makes the difference? *Gut* 1995;37: 552.

409. Lewis WG, Sagar PM, Holdsworth PJ, et al. Restorative proctocolectomy with end-to-end pouch-anal anastomosis in patients over the age of 50. *Gut* 1993;34:948.

410. Lichtiger S, Present DH. Preliminary report: cyclosporin in treatment of severe ulcerative colitis. *Lancet* 1990;336:16.

411. Lichtiger S, Present DH, Kornbluth A, et al. Cyclosporine in severe ulcerative colitis refractory to steroid therapy. *N Engl J Med* 1994;330:1841.

412. Liljeqvist L, Lindquist K. A reconstructive operation on malfunctioning S-shaped pelvic reservoirs. *Dis Colon Rectum* 1985;28:506.

413. Lim CH, Axon ATR. Low-grade dysplasia: nonsurgical treatment. *Inflamm Bowel Dis* 2003;9:270.

414. Lindberg BU, Broomé U, Persson B. Proximal colorectal dysplasia or cancer in ulcerative colitis. The impact of primary sclerosing cholangitis and sulfasalazine. Results from a 20-year surveillance study. *Dis Colon Rectum* 2001; 44:77.

415. Lindberg JÖ, Stenling RB, Rutegard JN. DNA aneuploidy as a marker of premalignancy in surveillance of patients with ulcerative colitis. *Br J Surg* 1999;86:947.

416. Lindgren S, Suhr OB, Persson T, et al. Budesonide enema once daily shows similar efficacy as budesonide enema twice daily for treatment of active distal ulcerative colitis. *Gastroenterology* 2001;120:A748.

417. Lindhagen T, Bohe M, Ekelund G, Valentin L. Fertility and outcome of pregnancy in patients operated on for Crohn's disease. *Int J Colorectal Dis* 1986;1:25.

418. Lindquist K. Anal manometry with microtransducer technique before and after restorative proctocolectomy. *Dis Colon Rectum* 1990;33:91.

419. Lindsey I, George B, Kettlewell M, Mortensen N. Randomized, double-blind, placebo-controlled trial of sildenafil (Viagra®) for erectile dysfunction after rectal excision for cancer and inflammatory bowel disease. *Dis Colon Rectum* 2002;45:727.

420. Lindsey I, George B, Kettlewell M, Mortensen N. Impotence after mesorectal and close rectal dissection for in-

flammatory bowel disease. *Dis Colon Rectum* 2001;44: 831.

421. Lobo AJ, Foster PN, Burke DA, et al. The role of azathioprine in the management of ulcerative colitis. *Dis Colon Rectum* 1990;33:374.

422. Löfberg R, Broström O, Karlén P, et al. Colonoscopic surveillance in long-standing total ulcerative colitis—a 15-year follow-up study. *Gastroenterology* 1990;99:1021.

423. Löfberg R, Broström O, Karlén P, et al. DNA aneuploidy in ulcerative colitis: reproducibility, topographic distribution, and relation to dysplasia. *Gastroenterology* 1992;102:1149.

424. Löfberg R, Danielsson A, Sohr O, et al. Oral budesonide versus prednisolone in patients with active extensive and left sided colitis. *Gastroenterology* 1996;110:1713.

425. Löfberg R, Leijonmarck C-E, Broström O, et al. Mucosal dysplasia and DNA content in ulcerative colitis patients with ileorectal anastomosis. *Dis Colon Rectum* 1991;34: 566.

426. Löfberg R, Liljeqvist L, Lindquist K, et al. Dysplasia and DNA aneuploidy in a pelvic pouch. *Dis Colon Rectum* 1991;34:280.

427. Löfberg R, Lindquist K, Veress B, Tribukait B. Highly malignant carcinoma in chronic ulcerative colitis without preceding dysplasia or DNA aneuploidy: report of a case. *Dis Colon Rectum* 1992;35:82.

428. Lohmuller JL, Pemberton JH, Dozois RR, et al. Pouchitis and extraintestinal manifestations of inflammatory bowel disease after ileal pouch-anal anastomosis. *Ann Surg* 1990; 211:622.

429. Lowry AW, Franklin DL, Weaver AL, et al. Leukopenia resulting from drug interaction between azathioprine or 6-mercaptopurine and mesalamine, sulfasalazine or balsalazide. *Gut* 2001;49:656.

430. Lubat E, Balthazar EJ. The current role of computerized tomography in inflammatory disease of the bowel. *Am J Gastroenterol* 1988;83:107.

431. Lyttle JA, Parks AG. Intersphincteric excision of the rectum. *Br J Surg* 1977;64:413.

432. MacLean AR, O'Connor B, Parkes R, et al. Reconstructive surgery for failed ileal pouch-anal anastomosis: a viable surgical option with acceptable results. *Dis Colon Rectum* 2002;45:880.

433. MacRae HM, McLeod RS, Cohen Z, et al. Risk factors for pelvic pouch failure. *Dis Colon Rectum* 1997;40:257.

434. Madden MV, Farthing MJG, Nicholls RJ. Inflammation in ileal reservoirs: "pouchitis." *Gut* 1990;31:247.

435. Madden MV, McIntyre AS, Nicholls RJ. Double blind crossover trial of metronidazole vs. placebo in chronic unremitting pouchitis. *Dig Dis Sci* 1994;39:1193.

436. Mahadevin V, Tremaine WJ, Johnson T, et al. Intravenous azathioprine in severe ulcerative colitis. A Pilot Study. *Am J Gastroenterol* 2000;95:3463.

437. Maingot R. Terminal ileostomy in ulcerative colitis. *Lancet* 1942;2:121.

438. Manjoney DL, Koplewitz MJ, Abrams JS. Factors influencing perineal wound healing. *Am J Surg* 1983;145:183.

439. Mann CV, Springall R. Use of a muscle graft for unhealed perineal sinus. *Br J Surg* 1986;73:1000.

440. Mann SD, Pitt J, Springall RG, Thillainayagam AV. *Clostridium difficile* infection—an unusual cause of refractory pouchitis: report of a case. *Dis Colon Rectum* 2003;46:267.

441. Manning AP, Bulgim OR, Dixon MF, Axon ATR. Screening by colonoscopy for colonic epithelial dysplasia in inflammatory bowel disease. *Gut* 1987;28:1489.

442. Mantzaris GJ, Hatzis A, Petraki K, et al. Intermittent therapy with high-dose 5-aminosalicylic acid enemas maintains remission in ulcerative proctitis and proctosigmoiditis. *Dis Colon Rectum* 1994;37:58.

443. Marcello PW, Milsom JW, Wong SK, et al. Laparoscopic total colectomy for acute colitis: a case-control study. *Dis Colon Rectum* 2001;44:1441.

444. Marcello PW, Roberts PL, Schoetz DJ Jr, et al. Long-term results of the ileoanal pouch procedure. *Arch Surg* 1993; 128:500.

445. Marcello PW, Roberts PL, Schoetz DJ Jr, et al. Obstruction after ileal pouch-anal anastomosis: a preventable complication? *Dis Colon Rectum* 1993;36:1105.

446. Margolin ML, Krumholz MP, Fochios SE, Korelitz BI. Clinical trials in ulcerative colitis: II. Historical review. *Am J Gastroenterol* 1988;83:227.

447. Marion JF, Present DH. Modern medical management of acute severe ulcerative colitis. *Eur J Gastroenterol Hepatol* 1997;9:831.

448. Markham NI, Watson GM, Lock MR. Rectovaginal fistulae after ileoanal pouches. *Lancet* 1991;337:1295.

449. Marshak RH, Lindner AE. Radiologic diagnosis of chronic ulcerative colitis and Crohn's disease of the colon. In: Kirsner JB, Shorter RG, eds. *Inflammatory bowel disease.* Philadelphia: Lea & Febiger, 1975:241.

450. Martel P, Blanc P, Bothereau H, et al. Comparative anatomical study of division of the ileocolic pedicle or the superior mesenteric pedicle for mesenteric lengthening. *Br J Surg* 2002;89:775.

451. Martin LW, LeCoultre C, Schubert WK. Total colectomy and mucosal proctectomy with preservation of continence in ulcerative colitis. *Ann Surg* 1977;186:477.

452. Matikainen M, Santavirta J, Hiltunen K-M. Ileoanal anastomosis without covering ileostomy. *Dis Colon Rectum* 1990; 33:384.

453. Maunder RG, Cohen Z, McLeod RS, Greenberg GR. Effect of intervention in inflammatory bowel disease on health-related quality of life: a critical review. *Dis Colon Rectum* 1995;38:1147.

454. Mavroudis C, Schrock TR. The dilemma of preservation of the rectum: retention of the rectum in colectomy for inflammatory disease of the bowel. *Dis Colon Rectum* 1977; 20:644.

455. May RE. Sexual dysfunction following rectal excision for ulcerative colitis. *Br J Surg* 1966;53:29.

456. Mayberry JF, Rhodes J. Epidemiological aspects of Crohn's disease: a review of the literature. *Gut* 1984;25:886.

457. Mayberry J, Rhodes J, Hughes LE. Incidence of Crohn's disease in Cardiff between 1934 and 1977. *Gut* 1979;20: 602.

458. Mayo CW, Fly OA Jr, Connelly ME. Fate of the remaining segment after subtotal colectomy for ulcerative colitis. *Ann Surg* 1956;144:753.

459. McCormack G, McCormick PA, Hyland JM, O'Donoghue DP. Cyclosporin therapy in severe ulcerative colitis: is it worth the effort? *Dis Colon Rectum* 2002:45:1200.

460. McCourtney JS, Finlay IG. Totally stapled restorative proctocolectomy. *Br J Surg* 1997;84:808.

461. McEwan HP. Ulcerative colitis in pregnancy. *Proc R Soc Med* 1972;65:279.

462. McGarrity TJ, Manasse JS, Koch KL, Weidner WA. Crohn's disease and massive lower gastrointestinal bleeding: angiographic appearance and two case reports. *Am J Gastroenterol* 1987;82:1096.

463. McHugh SM, Diamant NE, McLeod R, Cohen Z. S-pouches versus J-pouches. A comparison of functional outcomes. *Dis Colon Rectum* 1987;30:671.

464. McIntyre PB, Pemberton JH, Wolff BG, et al. Comparing functional results 1 year and 10 years after ileal pouch-anal anastomosis for chronic ulcerative colitis. *Dis Colon Rectum* 1994;37:303.

465. McKittrick LS, Miller RH. Idiopathic ulcerative colitis: a review of 149 cases with particular reference to the value of, and indications for, surgical treatment. *Ann Surg* 1935; 102:656.

466. McLeod RS, Fazio VW. Quality of life with the continent ileostomy. *World J Surg* 1984;8:90.

467. McLeod RS, Taylor DW, Cohen Z, Cullen JB. Single patient randomised clinical trial: use in determining optimum treatment for patient with inflammation of Kock continent ileostomy reservoir. *Lancet* 1986;1:726.

468. McMullen K, Hicks TC, Ray JE, et al. Complications associated with ileal pouch-anal anastomosis. *World J Surg* 1991; 15:763.

469. Meagher AP, Farouk R, Dozois RR, et al. J ileal pouch-anal anastomosis for chronic ulcerative colitis: complications and long-term outcome in 1310 patients. *Br J Surg* 1998; 85:800.

470. Melville DM, Jass JR, Shepherd NA, et al. Dysplasia and deoxyribonucleic acid aneuploidy in the assessment of precancerous changes in chronic ulcerative colitis. *Gastroenterology* 1988;95:668.

471. Melville DM, Ritchie JK, Nicholls RJ, Hawley PR. Surgery for ulcerative colitis in the era of the pouch: the St Mark's Hospital experience. *Gut* 1994;35:1076.

472. Mendeloff AI. The epidemiology of idiopathic inflammatory bowel disease. In: Kirsner JB, Shorter RG, eds. *Inflammatory bowel disease*, 2nd ed. Philadelphia: Lea & Febiger, 1980:5.

473. Mendeloff AI, Monk M, Siegel CI, Lilienfeld A. Illness experience and life stresses in patients with irritable colon and ulcerative colitis: an epidemiologic study of ulcerative colitis and regional enteritis in Baltimore, 1960–1964. *N Engl J Med* 1970;282:14.

474. Merrett MN, Mortensen N, Kettlewell M, Jewell DO. Smoking may prevent pouchitis in patients with restorative proctocolectomy for ulcerative colitis. *Gut* 1996;38:362.

475. Metcalf A, Dozois RR, Beart RW Jr, Wolff BG. Pregnancy following ileal pouch-anal anastomosis. *Dis Colon Rectum* 1985;28:859.

476. Metcalf AM, Dozois RR, Beart RW Jr, et al. Temporary ileostomy for ileal pouch-anal anastomosis: function and complications. *Dis Colon Rectum* 1986;29:300.

477. Metcalf AM, Dozois RR, Kelly KA. Sexual function in women after proctocolectomy. *Ann Surg* 1986;204:624.

478. Metcalf AM, Dozois RR, Kelly KA, et al. Ileal "J" pouch-anal anastomosis: clinical outcome. *Ann Surg* 1985;202: 735.

479. Metcalf AM, Dozois RR, Kelly KA, Wolff BG. Ileal pouch-anal anastomosis without temporary diverting ileostomy. *Dis Colon Rectum* 1986;29:33.

480. Meuwissen SGM, Ewe K, Gassull MA, et al. I.O.I.B.D., questionnaire on the clinical use of azathioprine, 6-mercaptopurine, cyclosporin and methotrexate in the treatment of I.B.D. *Gut* 1996;39:A242(abst).

481. Meyer S, Janowitz HD. The "natural history" of ulcerative colitis: an analysis of the placebo response. *J Clin Gastroenterol* 1989;11:33.

482. Michelassi F, Lee J, Rubin M, et al. Long-term functional results after ileal pouch anal restorative proctocolectomy for ulcerative colitis: a prospective observational study. *Ann Surg* 2003;238:433.

483. Michelassi F, Stella M, Block GE. Prospective assessment of functional results after ileal J pouch-anal restorative proctocolectomy. *Arch Surg* 1993;128:889.

484. Michener WM. Ulcerative colitis in children. *Pediatr Clin North Am* 1967;94:159.

485. Miller AS, Lewis WG, Williamson MER, et al. Does eversion of the anorectum during restorative proctocolectomy influence functional outcome? *Dis Colon Rectum* 1996;39: 489.

486. Miller DS, Keighley AC, Langman MJS. Changing patterns in epidemiology of Crohn's disease. *Lancet* 1974;2:691.

487. Miller R, Bartolo DCC, Orrom WJ, et al. Improvement of anal sensation with preservation of the anal transition zone after ileoanal anastomosis for ulcerative colitis. *Dis Colon Rectum* 1990;33:414.

488. Mimura T, Rizzello F, Gionchetti P, et al. Four-week treatment of metronidazole and ciprofloxacin markedly decreases refractory pouchitis and improves the quality of life. *Gastroenterology* 2001;120:A453(abst).

489. Mir-Madjlessi SH, Farmer RG, Easley KA, Beck GJ. Colorectal and extracolonic malignancy in ulcerative colitis. *Cancer* 1986;58:1569.

490. Misciewicz JJ, Lennard-Jones JE, Connell AM, et al. Controlled trial of sulfasalazine in maintenance therapy for ulcerative colitis. *Lancet* 1965;1:185.

491. Moller P, Lohmann M, Brynitz S. Cholestyramine ointment in the treatment of perianal skin irritation following ileoanal anastomosis. *Dis Colon Rectum* 1987;30:106.

492. Montagne J-P, Kressel HY, Moss AA, Schrock TR. Radiologic evaluation of the continent (Kock) ileostomy. *Radiology* 1978;127:325.

493. Morel P, Hawker PC, Allan RN, et al. Management of acute colitis in inflammatory bowel disease. *World J Surg* 1986; 10:814.

494. Morgan RA, Manning PB, Coran AG. Experience with the straight endorectal pullthrough for the management of ulcerative colitis and familial polyposis in children and adults. *Ann Surg* 1987;206:595.

495. Morson BC, Pang LSC. Rectal biopsy as an aid to cancer control in ulcerative colitis. *Gut* 1967;8:423.

496. Motta JC, Ricketts RR. The J-pouch Swenson procedure for ulcerative colitis and familial polyposis. *Am Surg* 1992; 58:613.

497. Mowschenson PM, Critchlow JF. Outcome of early surgical complications following ileoanal pouch operation without diverting ileostomy. *Am J Surg* 1995;169:143.

498. Mowschenson PM, Critchlow JF, Rosenberg SJ, Peppercorn MA. Factors favoring continence, the avoidance of a diverting ileostomy and small intestinal conservation in the ileoanal pouch operation. *Surg Gynecol Obstet* 1993; 177:17.

499. Mullen P, Behrens D, Chalmers T, et al. Barnett continent intestinal reservoir: multicenter experience with an alternative to the Brooke ileostomy. *Dis Colon Rectum* 1995;38: 573.

500. Murr MM, Metcalf AM. Spinal epidural abscess complicating an ileal J-pouch-anal anastomosis. *Dis Colon Rectum* 1993;36:293.

501. Murray CB. Psychogenic factors in the etiology of ulcerative colitis and bloody diarrhea. *Am J Med Sci* 1930;180: 239.

502. Myren J, Eie H, Serck-Hanssen A. The diagnosis of colitis by colonoscopy with biopsy and x-ray examination. A blind comparative study. *Scand J Gastroenterol* 1976;11:141.

503. Myren J, Serck-Hanssen A, Solberg L. Routine and blind histological diagnosis on colonoscopic biopsies compared to clinical-colonoscopic observations in patients without and with colitis. *Scand J Gastroenterol* 1976;11:135.

504. Nagy F, Karacsony G, Varro V. Experience with topical administration of 4-aminosalicylic acid in ulcerative colitis. *Dis Colon Rectum* 1989;32:134.

505. Nasmyth DG, Johnston D, Godwin PGR, et al. Factors influencing bowel function after ileal pouch-anal anastomosis. *Br J Surg* 1986;73:469.

506. Nasmyth DG, Johnston D, Williams NS, et al. Changes in the absorption of bile acids after total colectomy in patients with an ileostomy or pouch-anal anastomosis. *Dis Colon Rectum* 1989;32:230.

507. Nasmyth DG, Williams NS, Johnston D. Comparison of the function of triplicated and duplicated pelvic ileal reservoirs after mucosal proctectomy and ileo-anal anastomosis for ulcerative colitis and adenomatous polyposis. *Br J Surg* 1986;73:361.

508. Nduka CC, Menzies-Gow N, Darzi A. Simple ileal J-pouch construction using an endoscopic stapler. *Dis Colon Rectum* 1995;38:98.

509. Neal DE, Williams NS, Barker MCJ, King RFGJ. The effect of resection of the distal ileum on gastric emptying, small bowel transit and absorption after proctocolectomy. *Br J Surg* 1984;71:666.

510. Nelson H, Dozois RR, Kelly KA, et al. The effect of pregnancy and delivery on the ileal-pouch-anal anastomosis functions. *Dis Colon Rectum* 1989;32:384.

511. Nelson RL, Prasad ML, Pearl RK, Abcarian H. Inverted U-pouch construction for restoration of function in patients with failed straight ileoanal pull-throughs. *Dis Colon Rectum* 1991;34:1040.

512. Newman A, Lambert JR. *Campylobacter jejuni* causing flare-up in inflammatory bowel disease [Letter]. *Lancet* 1980;2:919.

513. Nicholls RJ, Gilbert JM. Surgical correction of the efferent ileal limb for disordered defaecation following restorative proctocolectomy with the S ileal reservoir. *Br J Surg* 1990; 77:152.

514. Nicholls J, Pescatori M, Motson RW, Pezim ME. Restorative proctocolectomy with a three-loop ileal reservoir for ulcerative colitis and familial adenomatous polyposis. *Ann Surg* 1984;199:383.

515. Nicholls RJ, Lubowski DZ. Restorative proctocolectomy: the four loop (W) reservoir. *Br J Surg* 1987;74:564.

516. Nicholls RJ, Pezim ME. Restorative proctocolectomy with ileal reservoir for ulcerative colitis and familial adenomatous polyposis: a comparison of three reservoir designs. *Br J Surg* 1985;72:470.

517. Nielsen OH, Andreasson B, Bondesen S, et al. Pregnancy in Crohn's disease. *Scand J Gastroenterol* 1984;19:724.

518. Nilsson LO, Kock NG, Kylberg F, et al. Sexual adjustment in ileostomy patients before and after conversion to continent ileostomy. *Dis Colon Rectum* 1981;24:287.

519. Nilsson LO, Kock NG, Lindgren I, et al. Morphological and histochemical changes in the mucosa of the continent ileostomy reservoir 6–10 years after its construction. *Scand J Gastroenterol* 1980;15:737.

520. Nordenholtz KE, Stowe SP, Stormont JM, et al. The cause of death in inflammatory bowel disease: a comparison of death certificates and hospital charts in Rochester, New York. *Am J Gastroenterol* 1995;90:927.

521. Nordgren S, Cohen Z, Greig PD, Diamant NE. Pressure studies on the continent reservoir ileostomy. *Surg Gynecol Obstet* 1982;155:646.

522. North CS, Clouse RE, Spitznagel EL, Alpers DH. The relation of ulcerative colitis to psychiatric factors: a review of findings and methods. *Am J Psychiatry* 1990;147:974.

523. Nugent FW, Haggitt RC. Results of a long-term prospective surveillance program for dysplasia in ulcerative colitis. *Gastroenterology* 1984;86:1197.

524. Nugent FW, Haggitt RC, Colcher H, Kutteruf GC. Malignant potential of chronic ulcerative colitis. *Gastroenterology* 1979;76:1.

525. Nugent FW, Haggitt RD, Gilpin PA. Cancer surveillance in ulcerative colitis. *Gastroenterology* 1991;100:1241.

526. Nunes GC, Ahlquist RE. Increasing incidence of Crohn's disease. *Am J Surg* 1983;145:578.

527. Nyam DC, Pemberton JH, Sandborn WJ, Savcenko M. Lymphoma of the pouch after ileal pouch-anal anastomosis: report of a case. *Dis Colon Rectum* 1997;40:971.

528. Nyam DCNK, Wolff BG, Dozois RR, et al. Does the presence of a pre-ileostomy closure asymptomatic pouch-anastomotic sinus tract affect the success of ileal pouch-anal anastomosis? *J Gastrointest Surg* 1997;1:274.

529. Oakley JR, Fazio VW, Jagelman DG, et al. Management of the perineal wound after rectal excision for ulcerative colitis. *Dis Colon Rectum* 1985;28:885.

530. Oakley JR, Jagelman DG, Fazio VW, et al. Complications and quality of life after ileorectal anastomosis for ulcerative colitis. *Am J Surg* 1985;149:23.

531. Oakley JR, Lavery IC, Fazio VW, et al. The fate of the rectal stump after subtotal colectomy for ulcerative colitis. *Dis Colon Rectum* 1985;28:394.

532. Oates GD, Williams JA. Primary closure of the perineal wound in excision of the rectum. *Proc R Soc Med* 1970;63[Suppl]:128.

533. O'Bichere A, Wilkinson K, Rumbles S, et al. Functional outcome after restorative proctocolectomy for ulcerative colitis decreases an otherwise enhanced quality of life. *Br J Surg* 2000;87:802.

534. O'Connell PR, Pemberton JH, Brown ML, Kelly KA. Determinants of stool frequency after ileal pouch-anal anastomosis. *Am J Surg* 1987;153:157.

535. O'Connell PR, Pemberton JH, Weiland LH, et al. Does rectal mucosa regenerate after ileoanal anastomosis? *Dis Colon Rectum* 1987;30:1.

536. O'Connell PR, Rankin DR, Weiland LH, Kelly KA. Enteric bacteriology, absorption, morphology and emptying after ileal pouch-anal anastomosis. *Br J Surg* 1986;73:909.

537. Öhman U. Colorectal carcinoma in patients with ulcerative colitis. *Am J Surg* 1982;344.

538. Öjerskog B, Kock NG, Nilsson LO, et al. Long-term follow-up of patients with continent ileostomies. *Dis Colon Rectum* 1990;33:184.

539. Öjerskog B, Kock NG, Philipson BM, Philipson M. Pregnancy and delivery in patients with a continent ileostomy. *Surg Gynecol Obstet* 1988;167:61.

540. O'Kelly TJ, Merrett M, Mortensen NJ, et al. Pouch-vaginal fistula after restorative proctocolectomy: aetiology and management. *Br J Surg* 1994;81:1374.

541. Olsen KØ, Joelsson M, Laurberg S, Öresland T. Fertility after ileal pouch-anal anastomosis in women with ulcerative colitis. *Br J Surg* 1999;86:493.

542. Ooi BS, Remzi FH, Fazio VW. Turnbull-blowhole colostomy for toxic ulcerative colitis in pregnancy: report of two cases. *Dis Colon Rectum* 2003;46:111.

543. Öresland T, Fasth S, Nordgren S, et al. Pouch size: the important functional determinant after restorative proctocolectomy. *Br J Surg* 1990;77:265.

544. Orholm M, Munkholm P, Langholz E, et al. Familial occurrence of inflammatory bowel disease. *N Engl J Med* 1991;324:84.

545. O'Riordain MG, Fazio VW, Lavery IC, et al. Incidence and natural history of dysplasia of the anal transitional zone after ileal pouch-anal anastomosis. *Dis Colon Rectum* 2000;43:1660.

546. Orkin BA, Soper NJ, Kelly KA, Dent J. Influence of sleep on anal sphincteric pressure in health and after ileal pouch-anal anastomosis. *Dis Colon Rectum* 1992;35:137.

547. Orkin BA, Telander RL, Wolff BG, et al.. The surgical management of children with ulcerative colitis: the old versus the new. *Dis Colon Rectum* 1990;33:947.

548. Ozuner G, Hull T, Lee P, Fazio VW. What happens to a pelvic pouch when a fistula develops? *Dis Colon Rectum* 1997;40:543.

549. Palmu A, Sivula A. Kock's continent ileostomy: results of 51 operations and experiences with correction of nipple-valve insufficiency. *Br J Surg* 1978;65:645.

550. Parks AG, Nicholls RJ. Proctocolectomy without ileostomy for ulcerative colitis. *Br Med J* 1978;2:85.

551. Parks AG, Nicholls RJ, Belliveau P. Proctocolectomy with ileal reservoir and anal anastomosis. *Br J Surg* 1980;67:533.

552. Patterson M, Eytinge EJ. Chronic ulcerative colitis and pregnancy. *N Engl J Med* 1952;246:691.

553. Paye F, Penna C, Chiche L, et al. Pouch-related fistula following restorative proctocolectomy. *Br J Surg* 1996;83: 1574.

554. Pearl RK, Nelson RL, Prasad ML, et al. Ileoanal anastomosis 24 years after total proctocolectomy for ulcerative colitis. *Dis Colon Rectum* 1985;28:180.

555. Peck DA. Rectal mucosal replacement. *Ann Surg* 1980;191:294.

556. Peck DA. Stapled ileal reservoir to anal anastomosis. *Surg Gynecol Obstet* 1988;166:562.

557. Peck DA, Hallenbeck GA. Fecal continence in the dog after replacement of rectal mucosa with ileal mucosa. Surg Gynecol Obstet 1964;119:1312.

558. Pemberton JH, Kelly KA, Beart RW Jr, et al. Ileal pouch-anal anastomosis for chronic ulcerative colitis: long-term results. *Ann Surg* 1987;206:504.

559. Pemberton JH, Philips SF, Ready RR, et al. Quality of life after Brooke ileostomy and ileal pouch-anal anastomosis. *Ann Surg* 1989;209:620.

560. Pera A, Bellando P, Caldera D, et al. Colonoscopy in inflammatory bowel disease: diagnostic accuracy and proposal of an endoscopic score. *Gastroenterology* 1987;92:181.

561. Pescatori M. Myoelectric and motor activity of the terminal ileum after pelvic pouch for ulcerative colitis. *Dis Colon Rectum* 1985;28:246.

562. Pescatori M, Manhire A, Bartram CI. Evacuation pouchography in the evaluation of ileoanal reservoir function. *Dis Colon Rectum* 1983;26:365.

563. Pescatori M, Mattana C, Castagneto M. Clinical and functional results after restorative proctocolectomy. *Br J Surg* 1988;75:321.

564. Pescatori M, Parks AG. The sphincteric and sensory components of preserved continence after ileoanal reservoir. *Surg Gynecol Obstet* 1984;158:517.

565. Pesce G, Ceccarino R. Treatment of severe hemorrhage from a defunctionalized rectum with adrenaline chloride in ulcerative colitis. *Dis Colon Rectum* 1991;34:1139.

566. Pezim ME. Successful childbirth after restorative proctocolectomy with pelvic ileal reservoir. *Br J Surg* 1984;71:292.

567. Pezim ME, Taylor BA, Davis CJ, Beart RW Jr. Perforation of terminal ileal appendage of J-pelvic ileal reservoir. *Dis Colon Rectum* 1987;30:161.

568. Phillips RKS. Pelvic pouches. *Br J Surg* 1991;78:1025.

569. Poppen B, Svenberg T, Bark T, et al. Colectomy-proctomucosectomy with S-pouch: operative procedures, complications, and functional outcome in 69 consecutive patients. *Dis Colon Rectum* 1992;35:40.

570. Powell-Tuck J, Brown RL, Lennard-Jones JE. A comparison of oral prednisolone given as a single or multiple daily doses for active proctocolitis. *Scand J Gastroenterol* 1970; 13:833.

571. Present DH, Korelitz BI, Wosch N, et al. Treatment of Crohn's disease with 6-mercaptopurine: a long term randomized double blind study. *N Engl J Med* 1980;302:981.

572. Present DH, Meltzer SJ, Krumholz MP, et al. 6-Mercaptopurine in the management of inflammatory bowel disease: short- and long-term toxicity. *Ann Intern Med* 1989;111: 641.

573. Probert SJL, Herring SD, Schreiber S, et al. Infliximab in steroid resistant ulcerative colitis: a randomized controlled trial. *Gastroenterology* 2002;122:499.

574. Prudhomme M, Dozois RR, Godlewski G, et al. Anal canal strictures after ileal pouch-anal anastomosis. *Dis Colon Rectum* 2003;46:20.

575. Pruitt R, Hanson J, Safdi M, et al. Balsalazide is superior to mesalamine in the time to improvement of signs and symptoms of acute ulcerative colitis. *Gastroenterology* 2000;118: A120(abst).

576. Pullan RD, Rhodes J, Ganesh S, et al. Transdermal nicotine for active ulcerative colitis. *N Engl J Med* 1994;330:811.

577. Purrmann J, Bertrams J, Borchard F, et al. Monozygotic triplets with Crohn's disease of the colon. *Gastroenterology* 1986;91:1553.

578. Puthu D, Rajan N, Rao R, et al. Carcinoma of the rectal pouch following restorative proctocolectomy. *Dis Colon Rectum* 1992;35:257.

579. Ransohoff DF. Colon cancer in ulcerative colitis. *Gastroenterology* 1988;94:1089.

580. Ransohoff DF, Riddell RH, Levin B. Ulcerative colitis and colonic cancer: problems in assessing the diagnostic usefulness of mucosal dysplasia. *Dis Colon Rectum* 1985;28: 383.

581. Rauh SM, Schoetz DJ Jr, Roberts PL, et al. Pouchitis—is it a wastebasket diagnosis? *Dis Colon Rectum* 1991;34:685.

582. Ravid A, Richard CS, Spencer LM, et al. Pregnancy, delivery, and pouch function after ileal pouch-anal anastomosis for ulcerative colitis. *Dis Colon Rectum* 2002;45:1283.

583. Ravitch MM. Anal ileostomy with sphincter preservation in patients requiring total colectomy for benign conditions. *Surgery* 1948;24:170.

584. Ravitch MM, Sabiston DC Jr. Anal ileostomy with preservation of the sphincter: a proposed operation in patients requiring total colectomy for benign lesions. *Surg Gynecol Obstet* 1947;84:1095.

585. Rayner CK, McCormack G, Emmanuel AV, et al. Long-term results of low-dose intravenous cyclosporin for acute severe ulcerative colitis. *Aliment Pharmacol Ther* 2003;18: 303.

586. Read TE, Schoetz DJ Jr, Marcello PW, et al. Afferent limb obstruction complicating ileal pouch-anal anastomosis. *Dis Colon Rectum* 1997;40:566.

587. Régimbeau JM, Panis Y, Pocard M, et al. Handsewn ileal pouch-anal anastomosis on the dentate line after total proctectomy: technique to avoid incomplete mucosectomy and the need for long-term follow-up of the anal transition zone. *Dis Colon Rectum* 2001;44:43.

588. Reilly WT, Pemberton JH, Wolff BG, et al. Randomized prospective trial comparing ileal pouch-anal anastomosis performed by excising the anal mucosa to ileal pouch-anal anastomosis performed by preserving the anal mucosa. *Ann Surg* 1997;225:666.

589. Reissman P, Piccirillo M, Ulrich A, et al. Functional results of the double-stapled ileoanal reservoir. *J Am Coll Surg* 1995;181:444.

590. Reissman P, Salky BA, Pfeifer J, et al. Laparoscopic surgery in the management of inflammatory bowel disease. *Am J Surg* 1996;171:47.

591. Reissman P, Teoh T-A, Weiss EG, et al. Functional outcome of the double-stapled ileoanal reservoir in patients more than 60 years of age. *Am Surg* 1996;62:178.

592. Remzi FH, Fazio VW, Delaney CP, et al. Dysplasia of the anal transitional zone after ileal pouch-anal anastomosis: results of prospective evaluation after a minimum of ten years. *Dis Colon Rectum* 2003;46:6.

593. Rhodes J, Rose J. Does food affect acute inflammatory bowel disease? The role of parenteral nutrition, elemental and exclusion diets. *Gut* 1986;27:471.

594. Ricart E, Panaccione R, Loftus EV, et al. Successful management of Crohn's disease of the ileoanal pouch with infliximab: a case report of seven patients. *Am J Gastroenterol* 1998;94:2648.

595. Ricart E, Panaccione R, Loftus EV, et al. Successful management of Crohn's disease of the ileoanal pouch with infliximab. *Gastroenterology* 1999;117:429–32.

596. Richard CS, Cohen Z, Stern HS, McLeod RS. Outcome of the pelvic pouch procedure in patients with prior perianal disease. *Dis Colon Rectum* 1997;40:647.

597. Riddell RH. Dysplasia and cancer in inflammatory bowel disease. *Br J Surg* 1985;72[Suppl]:S83.

598. Riddell RH, Shove DC, Ritchie JK, et al. Precancer in ulcerative colitis. In: Morson BC, ed. *The pathogenesis of colorectal cancer*. Philadelphia: WB Saunders, 1978:95.

599. Riley SAS, Mani V, Goodman MJ, et al. Microscopic activity in ulcerative colitis. What does it mean? *Gut* 1991;32: 174.

600. Riley SA, Mani V, Goodman MJ, Lucas S. Why do patients with ulcerative colitis relapse? *Gut* 1990;31:179.

601. Ritchie JK. Ileostomy and excisional surgery for chronic inflammatory disease of the colon: a survey of one hospital region. *Gut* 1971;12:528.

602. Ritchie JK. Crohn's disease in young people. *Br J Surg* 1985;72[Suppl]:S90.

603. Ritchie JK, Hawley PR, Lennard-Jones JE. Prognosis of carcinoma in ulcerative colitis. *Gut* 1981;22:752.

604. Robert JH, Sachar DB, Aufses AH Jr, Greenstein AJ. Management of severe hemorrhage in ulcerative colitis. *Am J Surg* 1990;159:550.

605. Roberts PL, Schoetz DJ Jr, Murray JJ, et al. Use of new retractor to facilitate mucosal proctectomy. *Dis Colon Rectum* 1990;33:1063.

606. Romanos J, Samarasekera DN, Stebbing JF, et al. Outcome of 200 restorative proctocolectomy operations: the John Radcliffe Hospital experience. *Br J Surg* 1997;84:814.

607. Rosenstock E, Farmer RG, Petras R, et al. Surveillance for colonic carcinoma in ulcerative colitis. *Gastroenterology* 1985;89:1342.

608. Rosenthal SR, Snyder JD, Hendricks KM, Walker WA. Growth failure and inflammatory bowel disease: approach to treatment of a complicated adolescent problem. *Pediatrics* 1983;72:481.

609. Roth M-P, Petersen GM, McElree C, et al. Familial empiric risk estimates of inflammatory bowel disease in Ashkenazi Jews. *Gastroenterology* 1989;96:1016.

610. Rotholtz NA, Pikarsky AJ, Singh JJ, Wexner SD. Adenocarcinoma arising from along the rectal stump after double-stapled ileorectal J-pouch in a patient with ulcerative colitis: the need to perform a distal anastomosis. *Dis Colon Rectum* 2001;44:1214.

611. Roy PH, Sauer WG, Beahrs OH, Farrow GM. Experience with ileostomies: evaluation of long-term rehabilitation in 497 patients. *Am J Surg* 1970;119:77.

612. Rubin CE, Haggitt RC, Burmer GC, et al. DNA aneuploidy in colonic biopsies predicts future development of dysplasia in ulcerative colitis. *Gastroenterology* 1992;103:1611.

613. Rubio CA, Johansson C, Slezak P, et al. Villous dysplasia: an ominous histologic sign in colitic patients. *Dis Colon Rectum* 1984;27:283.

614. Ruckley CV, Smith AN, Balfour TW. Perineal closure by omental graft. *Surg Gynecol Obstet* 1970;131:300.

615. Ryan JA Jr. Gracilis muscle flap for the persistent perineal sinus of inflammatory bowel disease. *Am J Surg* 1984;148:64.

616. Sachar DB, Auslander MO, Walfish JS. Aetiological theories of inflammatory bowel disease. *Clin Gastroenterol* 1980;9:231.

617. Sachs T, Applebaum H, Touran T. An effective self-retaining retractor for anorectal procedures. *J Pediatr Surg* 1991;26:90.

618. Safdi M, DeMicco M, Sninsky C, et al. A double blind comparison of oral versus rectal mesalamine versus combination therapy in the treatment of distal ulcerative colitis. *Am J Gastroenterol* 1997;92:1867.

619. Sagar PM, Holdsworth PJ, Godwin PGR, et al. Comparison of triplicated (S) and quadruplicated (W) pelvic ileal reservoirs: studies on manovolumetry, fecal bacteriology, fecal volatile fatty acids, mucosal morphology, and functional results. *Gastroenterology* 1992;102:520.

620. Sagar PM, Lewis W, Holdsworth PJ, Johnston D. One-stage restorative proctocolectomy without temporary defunctioning ileostomy. *Dis Colon Rectum* 1992;35:582.

621. Sagar PM, Lewis W, Holdsworth PJ, et al. Quality of life after restorative proctocolectomy with a pelvic ileal reservoir compares favorably with that of patients with medically treated colitis. *Dis Colon Rectum* 1993;36:584.

622. Sagar PM, Taylor BA. Pelvic ileal reservoirs: the options. *Br J Surg* 1994;81:325.

623. Saha SK, Robinson AF. A study of perineal wound healing after abdominoperineal resection. *Br J Surg* 1976;63:555.

624. Saigusa N, Belin BM, Choi H-J, et al. Recovery of the rectoanal inhibitory reflex after restorative proctocolectomy: does it correlate with nocturnal continence? *Dis Colon Rectum* 2003;46:168.

625. Salmon R, Bloch P, Loygue J. Magnetic closure of a reservoir ileostomy. *Dis Colon Rectum* 1980;23:242.

626. Sandborn WJ. Nicotine therapy for ulcerative colitis: a review of rationale, mechanisms, pharmacology, and clinical results. *Am J Gastroenterol* 1995;90:220.

627. Sandborn WJ. Advances in IBD symposium. December 7, 2002; New York, NY.

628. Sandborn WJ, Landers CJ, Tremaine WJ, Targan SR. Antineutrophil cytoplasmic antibody correlates with chronic pouchitis after ileal pouch-anal anastomosis. *Am J Gastroenterol* 1995;90:740.

629. Sandborn WJ, Landers CJ, Tremaine WJ, Targan SR. Association of antineutrophil cytoplasmic antibodies with resistance to treatment of left-sided ulcerative colitis: results of a pilot study. *Mayo Clin Proc* 1996;71:431.

630. Sandborn WJ, Tremaine WJ, Batts KP, et al. Pouchitis after ileal pouch anal anastomosis: a pouchitis disease activity index. *Mayo Clin Proc* 1994;69:409.

631. Sandborn WJ, Tremaine WJ, Wolf BG, et al. A randomized double blind placebo controlled multicenter trial of IV azathioprine loading to decrease the time to response in refractory Crohn's disease. *Am J Gastroenterol* 1998;93:A356.

632. Sanderson IR, Walker-Smith JA. Crohn's disease in childhood. *Br J Surg* 1985;72[Suppl]:S87.

633. Sands BE, Tremaine WJ, Sandborn WJ, et al. Infliximab in the treatment of severe steroid refractory ulcerative colitis: a pilot study. *Inflamm Bowel Dis* 2001;7:83.

634. Satsangi J, Jewell DP, Rosenberg WMC, Bell JI. Genetics of inflammatory bowel disease. *Gut* 1994;35:696.

635. Scammell BE, Keighley MRB. Delayed perineal wound healing after proctectomy for Crohn's colitis. *Br J Surg* 1986;73:150.

636. Schade RR, Van Thiel DH, Gavaler JS. Chronic idiopathic ulcerative colitis: pregnancy and fetal outcome. *Dig Dis Sci* 1984;29:614.

637. Scheppach W, Sommer H, Kirchner T, et al. Effect of butyrate enemas on the colonic mucosa in distal ulcerative colitis. *Gastroenterology* 1992;103:51.

638. Schmitt SL, Wexner SD, Lucas FV, et al. Retained mucosa after double-stapled ileal reservoir and ileoanal anastomosis. *Dis Colon Rectum* 1992;35:1051.

639. Schoetz DJ Jr, Coller JA, Veidenheimer MC. Ileoanal reservoir for ulcerative colitis and familial polyposis. *Arch Surg* 1986;121:404.

640. Schoetz DJ Jr, Coller JA, Veidenheimer MC. Can the pouch be saved? *Dis Colon Rectum* 1988;31:671.

641. Schrock TR. Complications of continent ileostomy. *Am J Surg* 1979;138:162.

642. Schroeder KW, Tremaine WJ, Ilstrup DM. Coated oral 5-aminosalicylic acid therapy for mildly to moderately active ulcerative colitis. *N Engl J Med* 1987;317:1625.

643. Scott AD, Phillips RKS. Ileitis and pouchitis after colectomy for ulcerative colitis. *Br J Surg* 1989;76:668.

644. Scotté M, Téniére P, Planet M, et al. Eversion of the rectum: a simplified technical approach to ileoanal anastomosis. *Dis Colon Rectum* 1995;38:96.

645. Sedgwick DM, Barton JR, Hamer-Hodges DW, et al. Population-based study of surgery in juvenile-onset Crohn's disease. *Br J Surg* 1991;78:171.

646. Sedgwick DM, Barton JR, Hamer-Hodges DW, et al. Population-based study of surgery in juvenile-onset ulcerative colitis. *Br J Surg* 1991;78:176.

647. Seldenrijk CA, Morson BC, Meuwissen SGM, et al. Histopathological evaluation of colonic mucosal biopsy specimens in chronic inflammatory bowel disease: diagnostic implications. *Gut* 1991;32:1514.

648. Seow-Choen, Tsunoda A, Nicholls RJ. Prospective randomized trial comparing anal function after hand-sewn ileoanal anastomosis with mucosectomy versus stapled ileoanal anastomosis without mucosectomy in restorative proctocolectomy. *Br J Surg* 1991;78:430.

649. Setti-Carraro P, Ritchie JK, Wilkinson KH, et al. The first 10 years' experience of restorative proctocolectomy for ulcerative colitis. *Gut* 1994;35:1070.

650. Shah NS, Remzi F, Massmann A, et al. Management and treatment outcome of pouch-vaginal fistulas following restorative proctocolectomy. *Dis Colon Rectum* 2003;46:911.

651. Shanahan F. Pathogenesis of ulcerative colitis. *Lancet* 1993;342:407.

652. Sharp FR, Bell GA, Seal AM, Atkinson KG. Investigations of the anal sphincter before and after restorative proctocolectomy. *Am J Surg* 1987;153:469.

653. Shen B, Achkar J-P, Connor JT, et al. Modified pouchitis disease activity index: a simplified approach to the diagnosis of pouchitis. *Dis Colon Rectum* 2003;46:748.

654. Silen W, Glotzer DJ. The prevention and treatment of the persistent perineal sinus. *Surgery* 1974;75:535.

655. Shen B, Achkar JP, Lashner BA, et al. A randomized clinical trial of ciprofloxacin and metronidazole to treat acute pouchitis. *Inflamm Bowel Dis* 2001;7:301.

656. Silvis R, Delemarre JBVM, Gooszen HG. Surgical treatment and role of dynamic defecography in impaired evacuation after ileal pouch-anal anastomosis: technical solutions to a difficult problem. *Dis Colon Rectum* 1997;40:84.

657. Simmonds NJ, Rampton DS. Inflammatory bowel disease: a radical view. *Gut* 1993;34:865.

658. Singer HC, Anderson JGD, Frischer H, et al. Familial aspects of inflammatory bowel disease. *Gastroenterology* 1971;61:423.

659. Skarsgard ED, Atkison KG, Bell GA, et al. Function and quality of life results after ileal pouch surgery for chronic ulcerative colitis and familial polyposis. *Am J Surg* 1989;157:467.

660. Skene AI, Gault DT, Woodhouse CRJ, et al. Perineal, vulval and vaginoperineal reconstruction using rectus abdominis myocutaneous flap. *Br J Surg* 1990;77:635.

661. Smith LE. A review of 21 rectal mucosectomy and ileal pouch pull-through procedures. *Am Surg* 1986;52:182.

662. Smith L, Friend WG, Medwell SJ. The superior mesenteric artery: the critical factor in the pouch pull-through procedure. *Dis Colon Rectum* 1984;27:741.

663. Snook J. Are the inflammatory bowel diseases autoimmune disorders? *Gut* 1990;31:961.

664. Soper NJ, Becker JM. A stapled technique for construction of ileal J pouches. *Surg Gynecol Obstet* 1988;166:557.

665. Stahl D, Tyler G, Fischer JE. Inflammatory bowel disease—relationship to carcinoma. In: *Current problems in cancer*. Chicago: Year Book Medical Publishers, 1981:5.

666. Ståhlberg D, Gullberg K, Liljeqvist L, et al. Pouchitis following pelvic pouch operation for ulcerative colitis. *Dis Colon Rectum* 1996;39:1012.

667. Ståhlberg D, Veress B, Tribukait B, Broomé U. Atrophy and neoplastic transformation of the ileal pouch mucosa in patients with ulcerative colitis and primary sclerosing cholangitis: a case control study. *Dis Colon Rectum* 2003;46: 770.

668. Stahlgren LH, Ferguson LK. Effects of abdominoperineal resection on sexual function in 60 patients with ulcerative colitis. *Arch Surg* 1959;78:604.

669. Standertskjöld-Nordenstam C-G, Palmu A, Sivula A. Radiologic assessment of nipple-valve insufficiency in Kock's continent reservoir ileostomy. *Br J Surg* 1979;66:269.

670. Steens J, Bemelman WA, Meijerink WJHJ, et al. Ileoanal pouch function is related to postprandial pouch tone. *Br J Surg* 2001;88:1492.

671. Steens J, Penning C, Brussee J, et al. Prospective evaluation of ileoanal pouch characteristics measured by barostat. *Dis Colon Rectum* 2002;45:1295.

672. Stein JP, Lieskovsky G, Ginsberg DA, et al. The T-pouch: an orthotopic ileal neobladder incorporating a serosal lined ileal antireflux technique. *J Urol* 1998;159:1836.

673. Stelzner M, Fonkalsrud EW. Significance of reservoir length in the endorectal ileal pullthrough with ileal reservoir. *Arch Surg* 1988;123:1265.

674. Stern H, Bernstein M, Killam S, et al. A stapled S-shaped ileoanal reservoir. *Dis Colon Rectum* 1987;30:214.

675. Stern H, Cohen Z, Wilson DR, Mickle DAG. Urolithiasis risk factors in continent reservoir ileostomy patients. *Dis Colon Rectum* 1980;23:556.

676. Stern H, Walfisch S, Mullen B, et al. Cancer in ileoanal reservoir: a new late complication? *Gut* 1990;31:473.

677. Stone MM, Lewin K, Fonkalsrud EW. Late obstruction of the lateral ileal reservoir after colectomy and endorectal ileal pullthrough procedures. *Surg Gynecol Obstet* 1986; 162:411.

678. Stryker SJ, Borody TJ, Phillips SF, et al. Motility of the small intestine after proctocolectomy and ileal pouch-anal anastomosis. *Ann Surg* 1985;201:351.

679. Stryker SJ, Daube JR, Kelly KA, et al. Anal sphincter electromyography after colectomy, mucosal rectectomy, and ileoanal anastomosis. *Arch Surg* 1985;120:713.

680. Stryker SJ, Phillips SF, Dozois RR, et al. Anal and neorectal function after ileal pouch-anal anastomosis. *Ann Surg* 1986;203:55.

681. Su CG, Salzberg BA, Lewis JD, et al. Efficacy of anti-tumor necrosis factor therapy in patients with ulcerative colitis. *Am J Gastroenterology* 2001;96:S310(A531)(abst).

682. Sugita A, Greenstein AJ, Ribeiro MB, et al. Survival with colorectal cancer in ulcerative colitis: a study of 102 cases. *Ann Surg* 1993;218:189.

683. Sugita A, Sachar DB, Bodian C, et al. Colorectal cancer in ulcerative colitis. Influence of anatomical extent and age at onset on colitis-cancer survival. *Gut* 1991;32:167.

684. Sutherland LR, Martin F, Greer S, et al. 5-Aminosalicylic acid enema in the treatment of distal ulcerative colitis, proctosigmoiditis, and proctitis. *Gastroenterology* 1987;92: 1894.

685. Sutherland LR, Ramcharan S, Bryant H, Fick G. Effect of cigarette smoking on recurrence of Crohn's disease. *Gastroenterology* 1990;98:1123.

686. Sutherland LR, Robinson M, Onstad G, et al. A double blind placebo controlled multicenter study of the efficacy of 5-amino-salicylic acid tablets in the treatment of ulcerative colitis. *Can J Gastroenterol* 1990;4:463.

687. Sutherland LR, Roth DE, Beck PL. Alternatives to sulfasalazine: a meta-analysis of 5-ASA in the treatment of ulcerative colitis. *Inflamm Bowel Dis* 1997;3:65.

688. Suzuki K, Muto T, Masaki T, Morioka Y. Microspectrophotometric DNA analysis in ulcerative colitis with special reference to its application in diagnosis of carcinoma and dysplasia. *Gut* 1990;31:1266.

689. Swain BT, Ellis CN. Fibrin glue treatment of low rectal and pouch-anal anastomotic sinuses. *Dis Colon Rectum* 2004; 47:253.

690. Taha AM, Shah RS. A modified technique for Kock ileostomy. *Surg Gynecol Obstet* 1986;163:376.

691. Takao Y, Gilliland R, Nogueras JJ, et al. Is age relevant to functional outcome after restorative proctocolectomy for ulcerative colitis? Prospective assessment of 122 cases. *Ann Surg* 1998;227:187.

692. Talbot RW, Ritchie JK, Northover JMA. Conservative proctocolectomy: a dubious option in ulcerative colitis. *Br J Surg* 1989;76:738.

693. Tan HT, Morton D, Connolly AB, et al. Quality of life after pouch excision. *Br J Surg* 1998;85:249.

694. Taub RN, Sachar D, Janowitz HD, Siltzbach LE. Induction of granulomas in mice by inoculation of tissue homogenates from patients with inflammatory bowel disease and sarcoidosis. *Ann N Y Acad Sci* 1976;278:560.

695. Tawile NT, Priest RJ, Schuman BM. Colonoscopy in inflammatory bowel disease. *Gastrointest Endosc* 1975;22:11.

696. Taylor BA, Pemberton JH, Carpenter HA, et al. Dysplasia in chronic ulcerative colitis: implications for colonoscopic surveillance. *Dis Colon Rectum* 1992;35:950.

697. Taylor BM, Beart RW Jr, Dozois RR, et al. Straight ileoanal anastomosis versus ileal pouch-anal anastomosis after colectomy and mucosal proctectomy. *Arch Surg* 1983;118: 696.

698. Taylor BM, Beart RW Jr, Dozois RR, et al. The endorectal ileal pouch-anal anastomosis. *Dis Colon Rectum* 1984; 27:347.

699. Teague RH, Waye JD. Inflammatory bowel disease. In: Hunt RH, Waye JD, eds. *Colonoscopy: techniques, clinical practice and colour atlas*. London: Chapman & Hall, 1981: 343.

700. Telander RL, Smith SL, Marcinek HM, et al. Surgical treatment of ulcerative colitis in children. *Surgery* 1981;90:787.

701. Telander RL, Spencer M, Perrault, et al. Long-term follow-up of the ileoanal anastomosis in children and young adults. *Surgery* 1990;108:717.

702. Thayer WR, Coutu JA, Chiodini RJ, et al. Possible role of mycobacteria in inflammatory bowel disease. II. Mycobacterial antibodies in Crohn's disease. *Dig Dis Sci* 1984;29: 1080.

703. Thompson JS, Williams SM. Fistula following continent ileostomy. *Dis Colon Rectum* 1984;27:193.

704. Thompson-Fawcett MW, Rust NA, Warren BF, Mortensen NJM. Aneuploidy and columnar cuff surveillance after stapled ileal pouch-anal anastomosis in ulcerative colitis. *Dis Colon Rectum* 2000;43:408.

705. Thompson-Fawcett MW, Warren BF, Mortensen NJMcC. A new look at the anal transitional zone with reference to restorative proctocolectomy and the columnar cuff. *Br J Surg* 1998;85:1517.

706. Thomson WHF, O'Kelly TJ. Ileal salvage from failed pouches. *Br J Surg* 1988;75:1227.

707. Tjandra JJ, Fazio VW, Milsom JW, et al. Omission of temporary diversion in restorative proctocolectomy: is it safe? *Dis Colon Rectum* 1993;36:1007.

708. Tobin MV, Logan RFA, Langman MJS, et al. Cigarette smoking and inflammatory bowel disease. *Gastroenterology* 1987;93:316.

709. Treem WR, Cohen J, Davis PM, et al. Cyclosporine for the treatment of fulminant ulcerative colitis in children: imme-

diate response, long-term results, and impact on surgery. *Dis Colon Rectum* 1995;38:474.

710. Trnka YM, LaMont JT. Association of *Clostridium difficile* toxin with symptomatic relapse of chronic inflammatory bowel disease. *Gastroenterology* 1981;80:693.

711. Truelove SC, Witts LJ. Cortisone in ulcerative colitis: final report on a therapeutic trial. *Br Med J* 1955;2:18.

712. Tsao JI, Galandiuk S, Pemberton JH. Pouchogram: predictor of clinical outcome following ileal pouch-anal anastomosis. *Dis Colon Rectum* 1992;35:547.

713. Tuckson WB, Fazio VW. Functional comparison between double and triple ileal loop pouches. *Dis Colon Rectum* 1991;34:17.

714. Tuckson W, Lavery I, Fazio V, et al. Manometric and functional comparison of ileal pouch-anal anastomosis with and without anal manipulation. *Am J Surg* 1991;161:90.

715. Tulchinsky H, Cohen CRG, Nicholls RJ. Salvage surgery after restorative proctocolectomy. *Br J Surg* 2003;90:909.

716. Tulchinsky H, Hawley PR, Nicholls J. Long-term failure after restorative proctocolectomy for ulcerative colitis. *Ann Surg* 2003;238:229.

717. Tulchinsky H, McCourtney JS, Subba Rao KV, et al. Salvage abdominal surgery in patients with a retained rectal stump after restorative proctocolectomy and stapled anastomosis. *Br J Surg* 2001;88:1602.

718. Tumen HJ, Valdes-Dapena A, Haddad H. Indications for surgical intervention in ulcerative colitis in children. *Am J Dis Child* 1968;116:641.

719. Turnbull RB Jr. The surgical approach to the treatment of inflammatory bowel disease (IBD): a personal view of techniques and prognosis. In: Kirsner JB, Shorter RG, eds. *Inflammatory bowel disease*. Philadelphia: Lea & Febiger, 1975:338.

720. Turnbull RB Jr, Hawk WA, Weakley FL. Surgical treatment of toxic megacolon: ileostomy and colostomy to prepare patients for colectomy. *Am J Surg* 1971;122:325.

721. Ullman TA. Patients with low-grade dysplasia should be advised to undergo colectomy. *Inflamm Bowel Dis* 2003; 9:267.

722. Utsunomiya J, Iwama T, Imajo M, et al. Total colectomy, mucosal proctectomy, and ileoanal anastomosis. *Dis Colon Rectum* 1980;23:459.

723. Valiente MA, Bacon HE. Construction of pouch using "pantaloon" technique for pull-through of ileum following total colectomy: report of experimental work and results. *Am J Surg* 1955;90:742.

724. Van Heerden JA, Beart RW Jr. Carcinoma of the colon and rectum complicating chronic ulcerative colitis. *Dis Colon Rectum* 1980;23:155.

725. Van Prohaska J, Siderius NJ. The surgical rehabilitation of patients with chronic ulcerative colitis. *Am J Surg* 1962; 103:42.

726. Varma JS, Browning GGP, Smith AN, et al. Mucosal proctectomy and colo-anal anastomosis for distal ulcerative proctocolitis. *Br J Surg* 1987;74:381.

727. Venturi A, Gionchetti P, Rizzello F, et al. Impact on the composition of the faecal flora by a new probiotic preparation: preliminary data on maintenance treatment of patients with ulcerative colitis. *Aliment Pharmacol Ther* 1999;13:1103.

728. Vessey M, Jewell D, Smith A, et al. Chronic inflammatory bowel disease, cigarette smoking, and use of oral contraceptives: findings in a large cohort study of women of childbearing age. *Br Med J* 1986;292:1101.

729. The Veterans Affairs Total Parenteral Nutrition Cooperative Study Group. Perioperative total parenteral nutrition in surgical patients. *N Engl J Med* 1991;325:525.

730. Wada Y, Matsui T, Matake H, et al. Intractable ulcerative colitis caused by cytomegalovirus infection. A prospective study on prevalence, diagnosis and treatment. *Dis Colon Rectum* 2003;46[Suppl]:S59.

731. Wapnick S, Grosberg S, Farman J, et al. Volvulus of the Kock reservoir. *Dis Colon Rectum* 1979;22:55.

732. Watanabe T, Kubota Y, Muto T. Substance P-containing nerve fibers in rectal mucosa of ulcerative colitis. *Dis Colon Rectum* 1997;40:718.

733. Watts JM, de Dombal FT, Goligher JC. Long-term complications and prognosis following major surgery for ulcerative colitis. *Br J Surg* 1966;53:1014.

734. Waye JD. The role of colonoscopy in the differential diagnosis of inflammatory bowel disease. *Gastrointest Endosc* 1977;23:150.

735. Waye JD. Endoscopy in inflammatory bowel disease. *Clin Gastroenterol* 1980;9:279.

736. Weinstein M, Rubin RJ, Salvati EP. Detachment of the continent ileostomy pouch from the anterior abdominal wall: report of two unusual cases. *Dis Colon Rectum* 1976;19:705.

737. Welch CE, Hedberg SE. Colonic cancer in ulcerative colitis and idiopathic colonic cancer. *JAMA* 1965;191:815.

738. Weterman IT, Peña AS. Familial incidence of Crohn's disease in the Netherlands and a review of the literature. *Gastroenterology* 1984;86:449.

739. Wexner SD, James K, Jagelman DG. The double-stapled ileal reservoir and ileoanal anastomosis: a prospective review of sphincter function and clinical outcome. *Dis Colon Rectum* 1991;34:487.

740. Wexner SD, Jensen L, Rothenberger DA, et al. Long-term functional analysis of the ileoanal reservoir. *Dis Colon Rectum* 1989;32:275.

741. Wexner SD, Rothenberger DA, Jensen L, et al. Ileal pouch vaginal fistulas: incidence, etiology, and management. *Dis Colon Rectum* 1989;32:460.

742. Wexner SD, Wong WD, Rothenberger DA, Goldberg SM. The ileoanal reservoir. *Am J Surg* 1990;159:178.

743. White CL III, Hamilton SR, Diamond MP, Cameron JL. Crohn's disease and ulcerative colitis in the same patient. *Gut* 1983;24:857.

744. Whorwell PJ, Phillips CA, Beeken WL, et al. Isolation of reovirus-like agents from patients with Crohn's disease. *Lancet* 1977;1:1169.

745. Wilks S. The morbid appearances in the intestines of Miss Bankes. *Med Times Gaz* 1859;2:264.

746. Wilks S, Moxon W. *Lectures on pathological anatomy*, 2nd ed. London: J & A Churchill, 1875:408,672.

747. Williams CB, Waye JD. Colonoscopy in inflammatory bowel disease. *Clin Gastroenterol* 1978;7:701.

748. Williams NS, Marzouk DEMM, Hallan RI, Waldron DJ. Function after ileal pouch and stapled pouch-anal anastomosis for ulcerative colitis. *Br J Surg* 1989;76:1168.

749. Williamson MER, Lewis WG, Miller AS, et al. Clinical and physiological evaluation of anorectal eversion during restorative proctocolectomy. *Br J Surg* 1995;82:1391.

750. Williamson MER, Lewis WG, Sagar PM, et al. One-stage restorative proctocolectomy without temporary ileostomy for ulcerative colitis: a note of caution. *Dis Colon Rectum* 1997;40:1019.

751. Wiltz O, Hashmi HF, Schoetz DJ Jr, et al. Carcinoma and the ileal pouch-anal anastomosis. *Dis Colon Rectum* 1991; 34:805.

752. Winslet MC, Barsoum G, Pringle W, et al. Loop ileostomy after ileal pouch-anal anastomosis—is it necessary? *Dis Colon Rectum* 1991;34:267.

753. Wolff WI, Shinya H, Geffen A, et al. Comparison of colonoscopy and the contrast enema in 500 patients with colorectal disease. *Am J Surg* 1975;129:181.

754. Woolfson K, Cohen Z, McLeod RS. Crohn's disease and pregnancy. *Dis Colon Rectum* 1990;33:869.

755. Woolrich AJ, DaSilva MD, Korelitz BI. Surveillance in the routine management of ulcerative colitis: the predictive value of low-grade dysplasia. *Gastroenterology* 1992;103: 431.

756. Yeager ES, Van Heerden JA. Sexual dysfunction following proctocolectomy and abdominoperineal resection. *Ann Surg* 1980;191:169.

757. Yoshimura HH, Estes MK, Graham DY. Search for evidence of a viral aetiology for inflammatory bowel disease. *Gut* 1984;25:347.

758. Young MRA, Small JO, Leonard AG, McKelvey STD. Rectus abdominis flap for persistent perineal sinus. *Br J Surg* 1988;75:1228.

759. Zahavi I, Avidor I, Marcus H, et al. Effect of sucralfate on experimental colitis in the rat. *Dis Colon Rectum* 1989; 32:95.

760. Zeitels JR, Fiddian-Green RG, Dent TL. Intersphincteric proctectomy. *Surgery* 1984;96:617.

761. Zeldis JB. Pregnancy and inflammatory bowel disease. *West J Med* 1989;151:168.

762. Zetzel L. Fertility, pregnancy, and idiopathic inflammatory bowel disease. In: Kirsner JB, Shorter RG, eds. *Inflammatory bowel disease.* Philadelphia: Lea & Febiger, 1975:146.

763. Ziv Y, Fazio VW, Church JM, et al. Safety of urgent restorative proctocolectomy with ileal pouch-anal anastomosis for fulminant colitis. *Dis Colon Rectum* 1995;38:345.

764. Ziv Y, Fazio VW, Church JM, et al. Stapled ileal pouch-anal anastomoses are safer than hand-sewn anastomoses in patients with ulcerative colitis. *Am J Surg* 1996;171:320.

765. Ziv Y, Fazio VW, Sirimarco MT, et al. Incidence, risk factors, and treatment of dysplasia in the anal transitional zone after ileal pouch-anal anastomosis. *Dis Colon Rectum* 1994;37:1281.

766. Zmora O, Efron JE, Nogueras JJ, et al. Reoperative abdominal and perineal surgery in ileoanal pouch patients. *Dis Colon Rectum* 2001;44:1310.

Crohn's Disease and Indeterminate Colitis

The knife cannot always have fresh fields for conquest; and although methods of practice may be modified and varied, and even improved to some extent, it must be within a certain limit.

Sir John Erichsen (*Lancet* 1873;2:489)

CROHN'S DISEASE

Crohn's disease of the bowel was initially described by Crohn, Ginzburg, and Oppenheimer in 1932, at which time they noted a transmural inflammatory condition of the terminal ileum.[88] The authors apparently listed their names in alphabetical order for the purpose of publication. It would certainly appear that if one is concerned about eponymous immortality, it is helpful to have a name occurring early in the alphabet. Interestingly, many of the cases were based on the large patient experience of Berg.[305] Had Dr. Berg wished to include his name on the paper, the condition today would probably be termed *Berg's disease*. Ginzburg reflected on the myths and misunderstandings concerning the evolution of the concept of Crohn's disease in his interesting paper "The Road to Regional Enteritis."[160] A number of publications followed from the experience of Crohn and his associates, confirming the location in the small bowel, but also noting that in a number of cases the colon was to some extent involved.

Another interesting historical footnote was suggested by Goligher[169]: that Crohn's disease was actually initially described in 1907 by Lord Moynihan when Moynihan

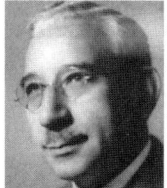

Burrill Bernard Crohn (1884–1983)   Burrill Crohn was born in New York City, June 13, 1884. He graduated from the City College of New York in 1902, and received his medical degree from Columbia University College of Physicians and Surgeons in 1907. Crohn began his internship at Mount Sinai Hospital, the institution with which he was affiliated for his entire professional life. In 1920, he was named the first head of the Department of Gastroenterology. Henry Janowitz wrote that the "eponym [of Crohn's disease] is deserved not because of a fortuitous alphabetical listing, but because for many years Crohn alone called attention to this enigmatic inflammation of the bowel, by carefully collecting cases and by publishing his clinical observations." Janowitz further stated that although not displeased with the honor and the name recognition, Crohn was always modest with respect to his role in the original description. Crohn himself expressed the feeling that the name *Crohn's disease* was inappropriate despite its virtually universal use, preferring instead the term *regional enteritis*. In 1956, when President Dwight D. Eisenhower required surgery for ileitis, it was Crohn who was called to the White House to act as spokesman to explain the disease and the prognosis to the American people. Crohn authored three texts and more than 100 scientific papers. Among his numerous awards were the Townsend Harris Medal by the City College of New York, the Julius Friedenthal Medal of the American Gastroenterological Association, and the Mount Sinai Hospital's Jacobi Medal. He was also elected President of the American Gastroenterological Association. Crohn died in New Milford, Connecticut, at the age of 99.

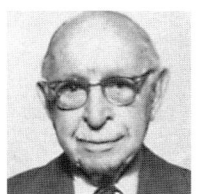

Leon Ginzburg (1899–1988)   Leon Ginzburg was born in Bayonne, New Jersey. He completed his undergraduate studies at Columbia University in 1920 and went on to accomplish his surgical training at the Mt. Sinai Hospital. Following a tour of the major European institutions he returned to become A. A. Berg's House Surgeon at Mt. Sinai. For the ensuing 5 years he was an adjunct on Berg's ward service and his assistant in the private practice of surgery. The association with Mt. Sinai lasted for 40 years, with Ginzburg achieving the rank of Clinical Professor. From 1947 to 1967, he was Director of Surgery at the Beth Israel Hospital, as the medical center was then known. The recognition of ileitis was accomplished by examining surgically excised specimens, which led in 1927 to his first description. There was a well-recognized controversy between Ginzburg and Crohn concerning each individual's respective role in the early observations. As both physicians neared their 90s, Ginzburg compared the discovery of regional ileitis to the controversy over the naming of the United States after Amerigo Vespucci rather than after Christopher Columbus. He likened the former map maker to Crohn, who spent considerable time and effort traveling, lecturing, and spreading knowledge about the disease, while he credited himself with the original description. Leon Ginzburg was active in practice at Beth Israel Medical Center until his death in 1988 at the age of 89. (With special appreciation to Lester Rosen, M.D.)

presented his experience with six patients who harbored benign lesions that mimicked carcinoma.[329] In 1913, Dalziel reported an obscure tuberculosis-like condition that he called "chronic interstitial enteritis" but which must have been Crohn's disease.[89] In 1923, Moschowitz and Wilensky described four patients with a granulomatous disease of the intestine and the amelioration of the condition by intestinal bypass.[327]

In 1951, Marshak noted the radiologic findings of what he felt was granulomatous disease of the *colon,* a clinical entity distinct from that of ulcerative colitis.[305] This view was not generally accepted until 1959, when Morson and Lockhart-Mummery described the charac-

teristic pathologic features of granulomatous colitis.[325] It can be appreciated, therefore, that our concepts of disease involvement in this area are less than one-half century old.

Incidence, Epidemiology, Etiology, and Pathogenesis

The incidence, epidemiology, and theories concerning the etiology and pathogenesis of both Crohn's disease and ulcerative colitis are discussed in Chapter 29. IBD remains a complex polygenic disorder interacting with environmental factors that trigger abnormal responses in

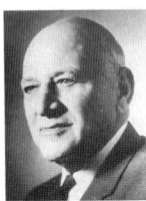

Gordon David Oppenheimer (1900–1974) Gordon Oppenheimer was born on June 30, 1900, in New York City and received his baccalaureate from Columbia College in 1919, and his medical degree from Columbia College of Physicians and Surgeons in 1922. He then became a house officer at the Mount Sinai Hospital, eventually entering the pathology laboratory where he collaborated with Ginzburg in his work on the study of inflammatory lesions of the terminal ileum. Oppenheimer ultimately became a urologist, rising to the position of Chief of Urology at Mt. Sinai Hospital, a post he occupied from 1947 to 1963. He authored 69 papers, including a monograph he published with Leon Ginzburg, *Urological Complications of Regional Ileitis.* In addition to his responsibilities as chairman of the department and director of the residency program, Oppenheimer found time to serve for 14 years as a medical officer with the New York City Fire Department. During World War II he acted as Second in Command of the General Surgical Service at Mount Sinai Hospital. He is remembered as a kind, gentle, and humble man, an especially humane physician who was much sought after as a consultant urologist. He died of cardiac failure, December 9, 1974, at the age of 74.

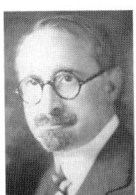

Albert Ashton Berg (1872–1950) It might seem incongruous that I have elected to include A.A. Berg as an individual to be recognized with a biographic sketch in this text. But he represents for me a special person—someone who could afford the "luxury of integrity." Berg declined to add his name to the alphabetical listing of coauthors because, even though the publication was based on his surgical patients, he did not contribute to the writing. He was born in New York City, August 10, 1872, and attended City College of New York, graduating from the College of Physicians and Surgeons at Columbia University in 1894. After his surgical training at the Mt. Sinai Hospital he joined the staff. In his early years he was an assistant to Arpad Gerster, the man who introduced Listerian principles to the United States. Berg developed an enormous clinical practice, arguably the largest in the city of New York, having been recognized as a phenomenal technician. He is credited with having performed the first gastrectomy for ulcer disease in the United States. In 1930, he published his experiences with more than 500 patients on the morbidity and mortality of subtotal gastrectomy in the management of gastric and duodenal ulcer. In 1905 he published a text, *Surgical Diagnosis: A Manual for Students and Practitioners.* In 1934, when he retired from the teaching service at Mt. Sinai, the hospital published *The Surgical Technique of Dr. A.A. Berg: A Tribute to 40 Years of Service at the Mt. Sinai Hospital.* The chapters were written by his students, including contributions on the small bowel and colon by Leon Ginzburg. Along with his brother (an internist) he amassed a library of 50,000 rare volumes of English and American literature, bequeathing the collection to New York University, Mt. Sinai Hospital, and the New York Public Library. Today there exists at Mt. Sinai a Berg Laboratory Building and an Institute for Research, and at the New York Public Library, a Berg Room, where the collection is housed. Albert Berg died following kidney surgery on July 1, 1959, at the age of 77.

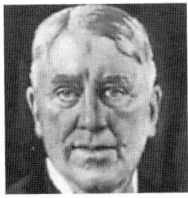

Berkeley George Andrew Moynihan (1865–1936) Berkeley Moynihan was born on the island of Malta, the only son of a distinguished army captain. He received his premedical education at the Royal Naval School and his medical training at the Leeds Medical School (1885) and at the University of London (1887). In 1893 he was awarded a gold medal in the examination for Master of Surgery. In 1895 he married the daughter of T. R. Jessop, the man who preceded him as surgeon to the Leeds General Infirmary. Moynihan was a masterful surgeon, particularly for surgery of the abdomen. He served as Professor of Surgery from 1902, becoming Emeritus Professor in 1926. In 1905 he published his outstanding book, *Abdominal Operations,* which ran through four editions. Among his numerous contributions and distinctions were founder and editor of the *British Journal of Surgery,* President of the Royal College of Surgeons, Hunterian Professor, and successively, knight, baronet, and baron.

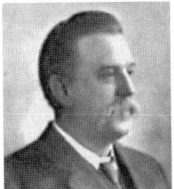

Thomas Kennedy Dalziel (1861–1924) T. Kennedy Dalziel (pronounced "dee-yell") was born in Scotland at Merkland, Penpont, Dumfriesshire. He received his early education at a private school in Dumfries and studied medicine at Edinburgh University, graduating in 1883. He continued his medical studies in Berlin and Vienna, where he specialized in experimental surgery and pathology. In 1885 he began his practice in Glasgow, and in 1889 he joined the staff of the Royal Hospital for Sick Children. For his services in World War I to the Advisory Council of the Royal Army Medical Corps, the king conferred on him the honor of knighthood. His successes and the public position he attained were the result of an unusual combination of qualities—charm, kindliness, extraordinary teaching skills, and marvelous manipulative dexterity. He was considered the best technical surgeon in the West of Scotland. His contributions to the medical literature were considerable, dealing primarily with that of abdominal surgery.

genetically susceptible individuals.[352] The coincidence of IBD development in identical twins is 60% in Crohn's but only 15% in ulcerative colitis.[421] Subclinical intestinal inflammation has been documented in symptomatic first-degree relatives of Crohn's disease patients.

It is interesting to note that *Mycobacterium paratuberculosis* DNA has been found in Crohn's diseased tissue.[420] The concept of a bacterial cause for inflammatory bowel disease (IBD) was discussed in Chapter 29, a concept that has generally been refuted. In one study, however, *M. paratuberculosis* was identified in 65% of specimens in indiviudals with Crohn's disease but in only 4.3% of those with ulcerative colitis.[420] The control tissues were found to have this DNA element in 12.5%. It was concluded that these observations are consistent with an etiologic role for *M. paratuberculosis* in Crohn's disease. A statistically significant association between the onset of Crohn's disease and prior antibiotic use has been demonstrated.[67] This suggests that a change in the bacterial environment within the intestinal tract in a susceptible host may be responsible for triggering the disease in some patients. Smokers are also overrepresented in Crohn's patients and underrepresented in ulcerative colitis, and they have an increased risk of recurrence after surgery when compared with nonsmokers.[515,520]

Another observation involves the identification of genes associated with IBD. Pokorny and associates identified a genetic and clinical association between the DNA repair gene, *MLH1*, and both ulcerative colitis and Crohn's disease (see Chapter 29).[366] Most exciting is the identification of the NOD2 gene (now renamed CARD15) as the IBD1 gene in the pericentromeric region of chromosome 16 which signals the opening of a vast arena of genetic research to provide a basic understanding of IBD.[195,224,348] NOD2 is involved in the activation of nuclear factor-kappa B (NF-κB) transcription factor that plays a significant role in Crohn's disease. NOD2 encodes a protein homologous to plant-disease resistance genes that are involved in the immune response to infectious organisms, particularly the leucine-rich region that binds to bacterial lipopolysaccharides. Ten percent of Crohn's patients have a frameshift mutation (via a cytosine insertion) that fails to induce NF-κB in the presence of bacterial lipopolysaccharide, suggesting a common link to the failure of immune response to bacterial components and thereby possibly explaining the role of antibiotics or the value of probiotics in the therapy of Crohn's. Certainly, Crohn's disease appears to be influenced by a wide range of genetic and environmental factors.[450]

Signs, Symptoms, and Presentations

Patients with Crohn's disease may present with very minimal symptoms and moderate complaints, or they may have fulminant manifestations. The considerable overlap in the presentations of ulcerative colitis and Crohn's disease is addressed in Chapter 29. For example, individuals with Crohn's disease may bleed, but this is not as frequent a presentation and may not be as severe.[313] However, life-threatening hemorrhage has been reported.[77] Abdominal pain may be mild or absent in patients with ulcerative colitis, but those with Crohn's disease frequently complain of pain. This may be colicky in nature and may be associated with intestinal obstruction, or it may be continual and related to the presence of a septic process within the abdomen. An abdominal mass is not uncommonly found on physical examination in a patient with Crohn's disease, but it is never seen in a patient with ulcerative colitis.

Diarrhea is usually a more troublesome concern in patients with ulcerative colitis. This may be because distal disease tends to be associated with more urgency, and in some cases, tenesmus. Patients with Crohn's disease may have rectal sparing and are less likely to experience this urgency. Conversely, with rectal involvement, Crohn's patients experience symptoms similar to those with ulcerative colitis. It is important to consider also the possibility of opportunistic infections and concomitant neoplasms, including cytomegaloviral infection and Kaposi's sarcoma, especially in individuals with prolonged immunosuppressive therapy for this disease (see later, Medical Management).[81]

Anal disease is much more commonly seen in patients with Crohn's colitis than in those with ulcerative colitis. The presence of anal pain, swelling, and discharge may be a presenting feature of the former condition and may be the only abnormality observed on examination and on subsequent investigation. In our reported experience with anal complications in patients with Crohn's disease, 22% of 1,098 were so afflicted.[503] Anal fissure was diagnosed in 29% of patients who had anal manifestations; a fistula was found in 28%, an abscess in 23%, and multiple presentations in 20%. Crohn's colitis was much more frequently associated with an anal lesion than was Crohn's disease of the small bowel (52% versus 14%). Within 1 year following the anal manifestation, Crohn's disease presented elsewhere in 59% of patients. All the remaining developed gastrointestinal disease within 5 years. In the St. Mark's Hospital experience, 34% of patients with small bowel Crohn's disease had anal lesions, whereas 58% of those with colon disease were found to have anal involvement.[288] Of 126 consecutive patients with perianal Crohn's disease seen regularly in one outpatient clinic, 48% were diagnosed as having an abscess.[298]

A high level of suspicion should exist if the examiner notes characteristic edematous tags, blue discoloration of the skin, an eccentrically located fissure, a broad-based ulcer, a rigid or strictured canal, or an anal fistula, especially if the patient reports gastrointestinal symptoms. A clinical classification of perianal Crohn's disease has been proposed by Hughes.[221] The reader is referred to Chapters 10 and 11 for a discussion of the management of anal complications.

Fever is usually not a concern in patients with ulcerative colitis unless the patient is severely ill (e.g., toxic megacolon). However, in those with Crohn's disease, a pyrexia is not uncommonly noted, and is usually due to the presence of an intraabdominal abscess or undrained septic focus. Nausea and vomiting are not frequently noted in either condition unless there is evidence of intestinal obstruction. Anorexia, weight loss, anemia, and general debility are associated with relatively long-standing or fulminant disease.

Disease in Children and Adolescents

When the condition occurs in children, there may be a more rapid onset and progression than when the disease occurs in young adults. These youngsters often become chronically ill, have growth impairment, have decreased mental acuity, and are less developed physically than their healthy peers (see Figure 29-26). It is because of these concerns that implementation of either an elemental diet or parenteral nutrition is an especially important part of the management in this age group (see Medical Management).[238,419] However, in order to be maximally effective, therapy must be initiated before puberty.[238] Furthermore, unless medical treatment can achieve a sustained remission, operative intervention may be the only effective means for addressing the problem of retarded development (see later).[106]

Elliott and colleagues reported the prognosis of 57 patients with Crohn's disease of the large bowel seen within 6 months of the onset of symptoms during 1969 to 1978 and followed until 1984 at St. Mark's Hospital.[119] The cumulative probability of an operation was 35% at 5 years and 39% at 10 years. They concluded that about one-half of all such patients can be treated successfully without abdominal surgery. However, children and adolescents with colonic disease are much more likely to require resection, often after a relatively short period of illness.[151,384] Growth retardation as an indication for surgery may be one of the reasons for this difference.

As with adults, the efficacy of surgery for Crohn's disease in children seems to depend mainly on disease location and perhaps the choice of surgical procedure itself.[91] Assessment of growth and development, psychological support for both the patient and the family, and close cooperation between the physician and the surgeon are important concepts in the management of these young people.[394,400,419]

Disease in Pregnancy

For a discussion of disease in pregnancy see Chapter 29.

Physical Examination

In contrast to individuals with ulcerative colitis, even in the absence of toxic megacolon a patient with Crohn's disease may demonstrate obvious findings on physical examination. As mentioned, although it is true that anorectal disease can occur with ulcerative colitis, it is much more common in those with Crohn's disease. The diagnosis is often suspected on examination of the perianal skin (Figure 30-1). Simple inspection will often show the edematous tags, fissures, abscess, or fistulas characteristically seen in this condition. The anal canal may be stenotic, fibrotic, and thickened on digital examination. If an anal fissure is apparent, severe pain is noted (Figure 30-2). Pelvic examination in a woman may reveal a rectovaginal fistula, and bimanual examination may show the presence of a pelvic mass. A biopsy of a sinus tract or an abscess cavity may demonstrate the granulomas characteristic of Crohn's colitis (Figure 30-3).

Abdominal findings are more common in patients with Crohn's disease than in those with ulcerative colitis. A mass may be felt in the right iliac fossa, a common observation when regional enteritis involves the terminal ileum. A large, mesenteric abscess can often be palpated.

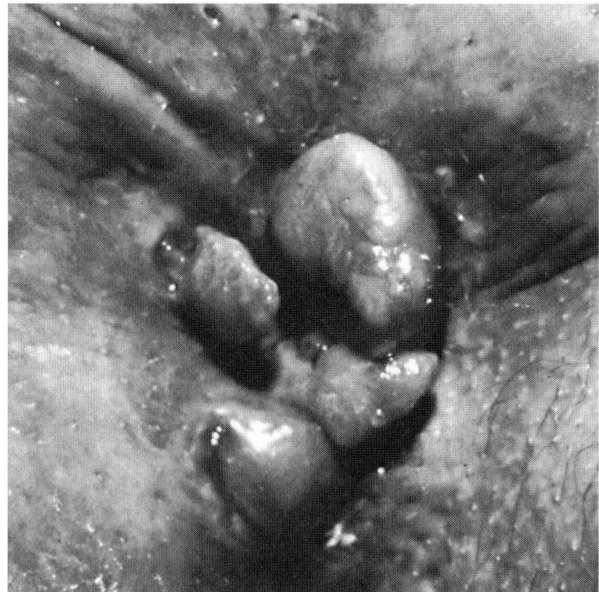

FIGURE 30-1. Anal Crohn's disease. Note the thickened, edematous tags with furrowing and fissuring of the skin. (From Corman ML, Veidenheimer MC, Nugent FW, et al. *Diseases of the anus, rectum and colon. Part II: Non-specific inflammatory bowel disease.* New York: Medcom, 1976.)

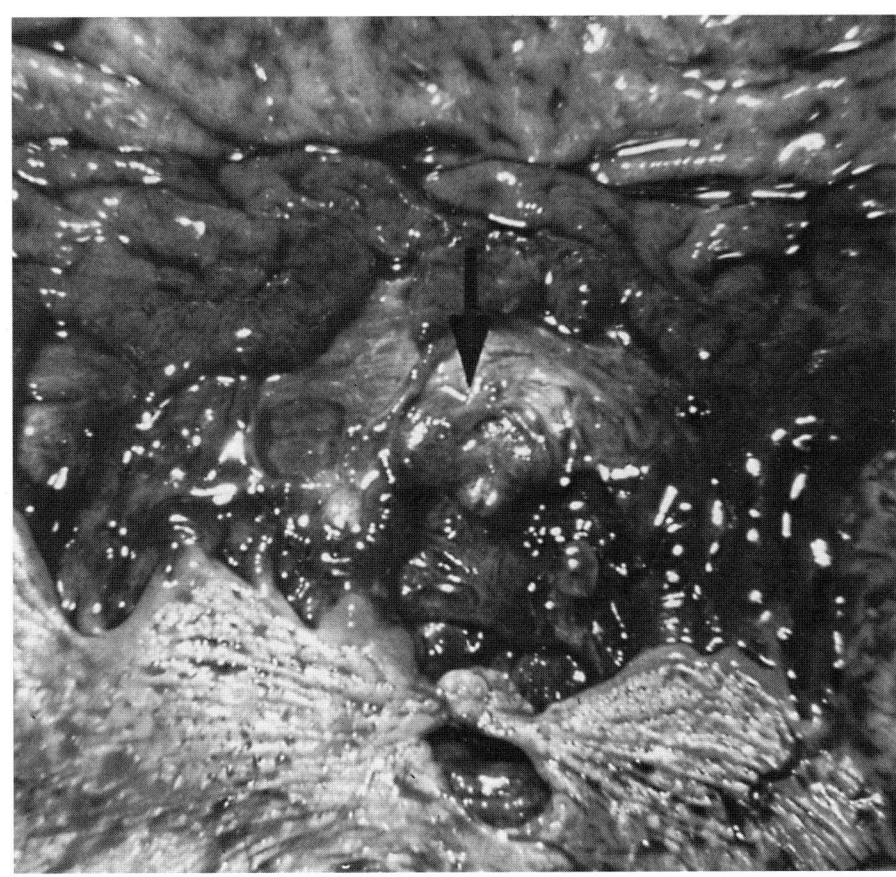

FIGURE 30-2. Crohn's disease. Proctectomy specimen with a broad-based anal fissure (*arrow*). Just distal to the dentate line, an external opening of a fistula is evident. (From Corman ML, Veidenheimer MC, Nugent FW, et al. *Diseases of the anus, rectum and colon. Part II: Non-specific inflammatory bowel disease.* New York: Medcom, 1976.)

Crohn's colitis, however, usually is not associated with clinically demonstrable abdominal abnormalities.

Endoscopic Examination

Proctosigmoidoscopic examination is often helpful in differentiating between ulcerative colitis and Crohn's disease. The rectum is always diseased during attacks of ulcerative colitis, whereas with Crohn's colitis, 40% of patients have sparing of the rectum, irrespective of anal or perianal involvement (see Chapter 29). But when the rectum is involved by Crohn's disease, differentiation between the two may be quite difficult.

A corollary to this observation is to perform biopsies distal to obvious inflammatory changes if the rectum appears to be spared, because one may discover that the rectum is not truly normal. This may cause the physician to reassess the accuracy of a diagnosis of Crohn's disease for what was initially thought to be lack of rectal involvement. Biopsy may be helpful because histologic changes suggestive of Crohn's disease in particular may be apparent. Up to 20% of such patients may exhibit granulomata.

The place of colonoscopy in the evaluation and follow-up of IBD has been extensively reviewed by many authors. Teague and Waye recommend colonoscopy for five indications: differential diagnosis, resolution of radiographic abnormalities (e.g., filling defects and strictures), preoperative and postoperative evaluation in Crohn's disease, examination of stomas, and screening for premalignant and malignant changes.[469] With granulomatous colitis, Waye observed the following major colonoscopic findings: a normal rectum (obviously this is not always the case), asymmetry or eccentricity of involvement, cobblestone appearance, normal vasculature, edema of the bowel wall (as seen in ulcerative colitis), normal mucosa intervening between areas of ulceration, serpiginous ulcers (these may course for several centimeters), pseudopolyps (as in ulcerative colitis), and skip areas (lack of continuity of involvement).[296] He adds another observation, the presence of amyloidosis in the biopsy specimen. An endoscopic index for determining the severity of colonic Crohn's disease has also been proposed.[308] Figure 30-4 illustrates some of the characteristic changes.

Unfortunately, there are frequent difficulties in the interpretation of the biopsies obtained by means of proctosigmoidoscopy or colonoscopy. In a prospective study that Geboes and Vantrappen performed over an 18-

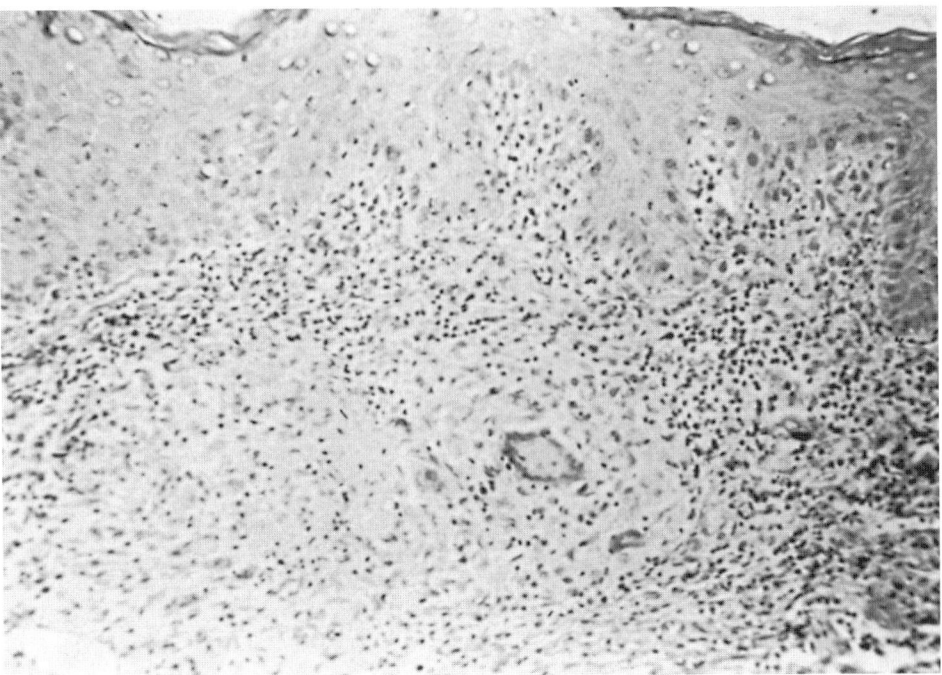

FIGURE 30-3. This section from a macroscopically normal anus reveals a submucosal granuloma. The patient subsequently proved to have Crohn's disease. (Original magnification × 80.) (From Corman ML, Veidenheimer MC, Nugent FW, et al. *Diseases of the anus, rectum and colon. Part II: Non-specific inflammatory bowel disease.* New York: Medcom, 1976.)

month period, 71 colonoscopies were undertaken on 59 patients with Crohn's disease.[152] In comparison with barium enema examination, the segmental nature of the involvement was more apparent by means of colonoscopy. Microulceration was also more evident than by radiologic means. Radiographs yielded more information about the haustra, especially in the right colon. Colonoscopy permitted a histologic diagnosis in 24% of patients, but granulomas were found in only 19 of 321 specimens (6%). In more than one-fourth of the patients, the entire colon could not be examined, and no complications occurred. Hogan and colleagues observed that inconsisten-

cies are often noted between macroscopic observations by the endoscopist and histologic interpretation of the biopsy specimen by the pathologist.[219] They felt that the reason for this problem is the overlapping of the histologic features of the two conditions, ulcerative colitis and Crohn's disease.

Changes in patients with ulcerative colitis are truly nonspecific, unless atypia or frank carcinoma supervenes. The most useful lesion found on colonoscopic mucosal biopsy of patients with Crohn's disease is a granuloma. The limiting factor in establishing the correct diagnosis by means of biopsy, however, is the small size of the spec-

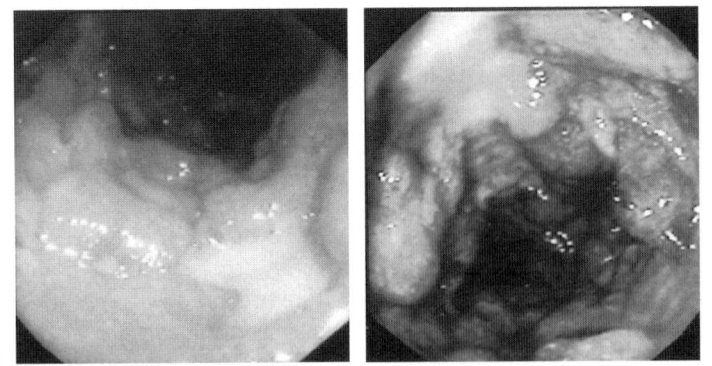

FIGURE 30-4. Colonoscopic changes in Crohn's disease. **A:** Deep ulceration with pus can be seen; the colon is relatively spared more distally. **B:** Florid inflammatory changes with longitudinal furrows (i.e., rake ulcers) constitute the characteristic appearance of granulomatous colitis. (See Figure 30-1.)

imen. Hence, the physician or surgeon, having the benefit of clinical evaluation and the history, is often in the better position to make the correct diagnosis.

Distribution

The primary locations of the disease have been categorized by Bernell and co-workers as follows[34]:

- Orojejunal (oral to the ligament of Treitz)
- Small bowel (excluding terminal 30 cm of ileum)
- Ileocecal (distal 30 cm of ileum with or without cecal involvement)
- Continuous ileocolic (continuous ileocolic involvement))
- Discontinuous ileocolic (both small and large bowel involvement, but without continuous inflammation in the ileocecal region)
- Colorectal (confined to the colon or rectum or both only)

Radiographic Features

As previously mentioned, Crohn's disease can occur anywhere in the alimentary tract. The disease tends to be segmental and asymmetric. Radiologic findings include skip lesions, contour defects, longitudinal ulcers, transverse fissures, eccentric involvement, pseudodiverticula, narrowing or stricture formation, pseudopolypoid changes that may be cobblestone-like, sinus tracts, and fistulas.[306]

A plain film of the abdomen may be quite useful in the early stages of Crohn's colitis. Although toxic megacolon is much less common in Crohn's disease than it is in ulcerative colitis, acute toxic dilatation may occur before any firm cicatrix has formed in the bowel wall (Figure 30-5).

Colon

The postevacuation film is most useful in identifying numerous discrete ulcers (Figure 30-6). Small ulcerations may combine to produce large, longitudinal ulcers (Figure 30-7), and when the longitudinal ulcers combine with transverse fissures, they produce the cob-

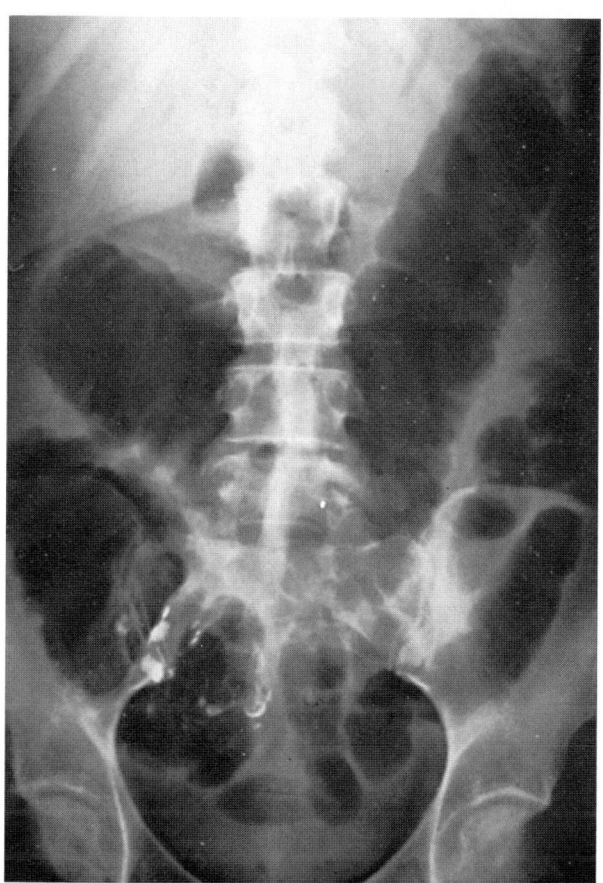

FIGURE 30-5. Crohn's colitis. This plain abdominal film demonstrates marked colonic dilatation. Toxic megacolon may be recognized during the initial attack, before fibrosis and thickening develop. (From Corman ML, Veidenheimer MC, Nugent FW, et al. *Diseases of the anus, rectum and colon. Part II: Non-specific inflammatory bowel disease.* New York: Medcom, 1976.)

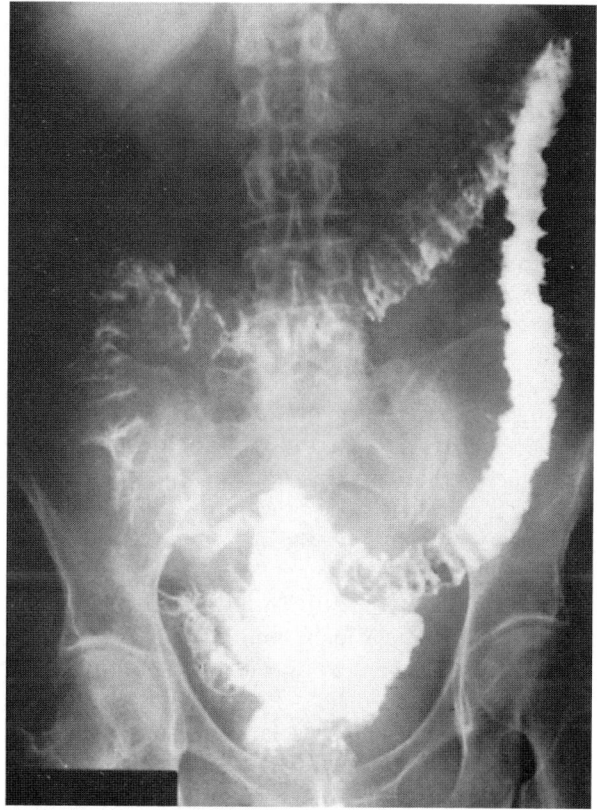

FIGURE 30-6. Crohn's colitis. Extensive loss of the normal mucosal pattern with multiple tiny marginal ulcers along the left colon border. Deeper ulcers are evident on the inferior margin of the distal transverse colon.

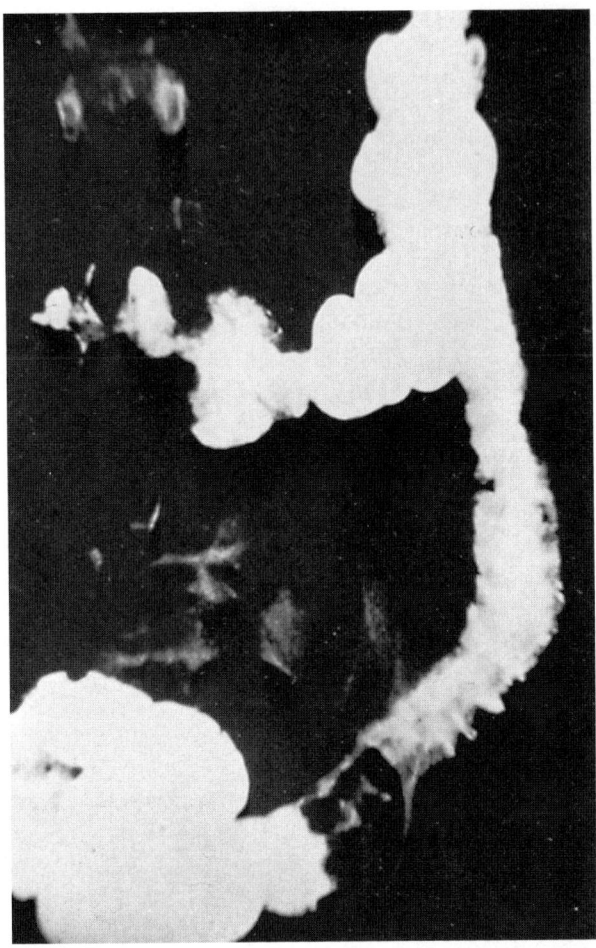

FIGURE 30-7. Crohn's colitis. Extensive longitudinal and transverse ulcers are evident in the descending and sigmoid colon. (From Corman ML, Veidenheimer MC, Nugent FW, et al. *Diseases of the anus, rectum and colon. Part II: Non-specific inflammatory bowel disease.* New York: Medcom, 1976.)

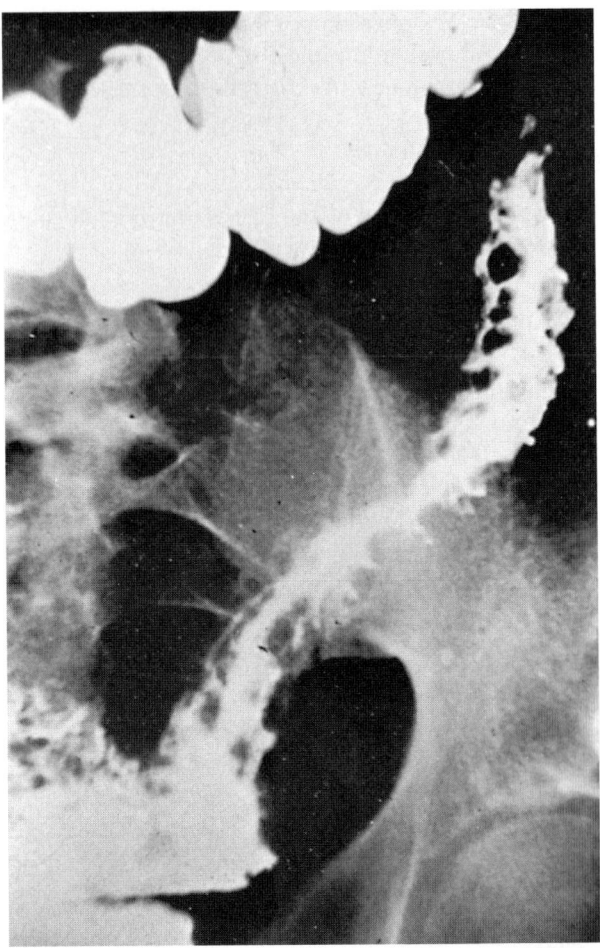

FIGURE 30-8. Crohn's colitis. Coarse cobblestoning of the left colon with intramural fistula traversing longitudinally along the bowel wall. (From Corman ML, Veidenheimer MC, Nugent FW, et al. *Diseases of the anus, rectum and colon. Part II: Non-specific inflammatory bowel disease.* New York: Medcom, 1976.)

blestone appearance seen radiologically (Figure 30-8). Intramural fistulas can result from the coalescing of the numerous longitudinal ulcers, which in turn may produce a double-lumen appearance (Figure 30-9). Ulcerations may penetrate beyond the contour of the bowel and present as numerous long spicules or as sinus tracts (Figure 30-10). These deep fissures may be confused with diverticula, but with experience the physician should be readily able to differentiate them. If one examines the whole-mount specimen shown in Figure 30-42, one can appreciate how such a radiologic picture can evolve.

Although the standard barium enema examination has been routinely employed in the past for evaluating IBD, contemporary evidence suggests that the air-contrast technique is preferred. Radiologists have prided themselves on their ability to identify somewhat unusual radiographic features of IBD. These include mucosal bridg-

ing and aphthoid ulcers.[40,194,417,441] Although these findings are helpful in the evaluation of patients with IBD, their ready documentation by means of colonoscopy would diminish the value of the radiologic observation.

Superficial mucosal abnormalities are not uncommonly seen in the distal part of the ileum, and concern is often expressed as to the likelihood of such a patient developing clinically recognizable Crohn's disease. Ekberg and colleagues identified mucosal abnormalities in the distal ileum of 21 patients by means of air-contrast enemas.[117] From 4 to 7 years later neither Crohn's disease nor any other progressive condition of the small bowel developed.

Figure 30-11 demonstrates a number of the classical changes that one may see in the radiographic appearance of Crohn's colitis. These include segmental distribution with sparing of the rectum, stenosis, thickening of the bowel wall, ulceration, and a suggestion of a double-lumen appearance.

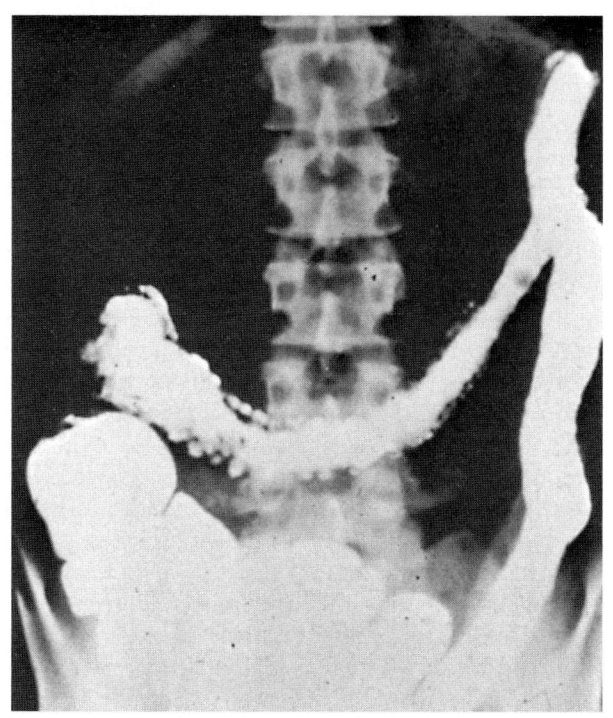

FIGURE 30-9. Crohn's colitis. Longitudinal intramural fistulas are evident in the proximal transverse colon and splenic flexure. (From Corman ML, Veidenheimer MC, Nugent FW, et al. *Diseases of the anus, rectum and colon. Part II: Non-specific inflammatory bowel disease.* New York: Medcom, 1976.)

Strictures are of variable lengths and may be quite extensive indeed (Figs. 30-12 and 30-13). When a stricture occurs in Crohn's disease it does not imply a malignant association, such as when it is seen in a patient with ulcerative colitis. However, individuals with Crohn's disease have been shown to have an increased risk for the development of malignancy (see Relationship to Carcinoma). Differential diagnosis between a Crohn's stricture and that of a carcinoma is usually not difficult. Close inspection often reveals that the bowel in adjacent areas is ulcerated (Figure 30-14). Contrast this x-ray with that of Figure 30-15. Although a scirrhous carcinoma must always be considered in the differential diagnosis, the lack of associated ulceration or inflammatory changes elsewhere in the colon usually clarifies the dilemma. Still, one must be wary of the possibility (see Figure 30-13).

A most difficult problem is to differentiate radiographically Crohn's disease from tuberculosis (see Chapter 33). When the condition is confined to the ileocecal region, it is virtually impossible to distinguish between the two diseases.

Barium enema has been used to evaluate the anal canal in patients with Crohn's disease.[107] While direct visual examination is more accurate, there are characteristic changes that may be identified by means of careful radiologic examination of the area. The hallmark of a radiologically normal anal canal is the presence of straight, smooth lines of barium between the folds, whereas an abnormal anal canal may show distortion of the folds, ulcers, fissures, sinus tracts, and

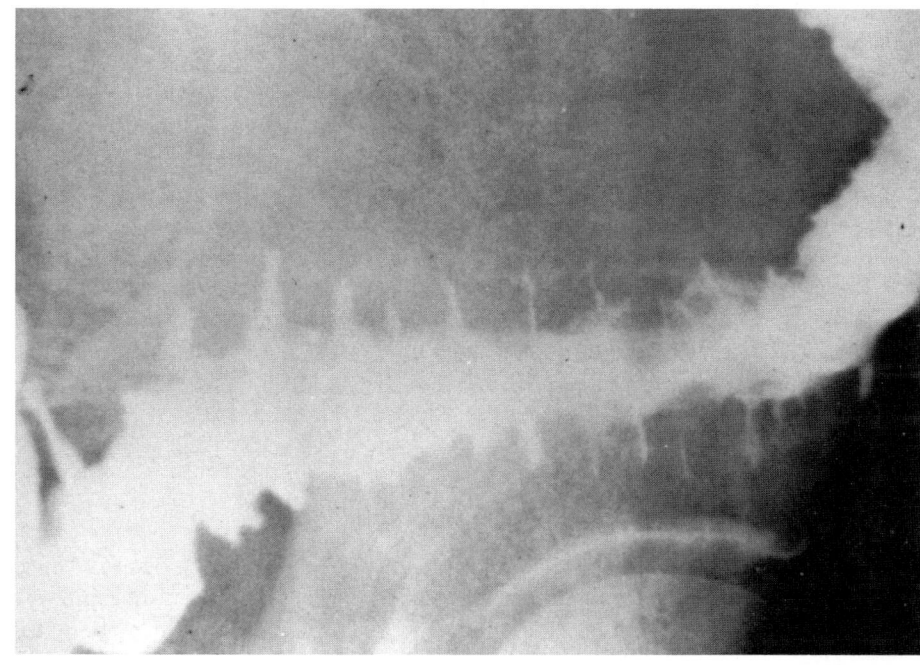

FIGURE 30-10. Crohn's colitis. Deep fissuring of the bowel wall in the sigmoid colon giving a thornlike appearance. (From Corman ML, Veidenheimer MC, Nugent FW, et al. *Diseases of the anus, rectum and colon. Part II: Non-specific inflammatory bowel disease.* New York: Medcom, 1976.)

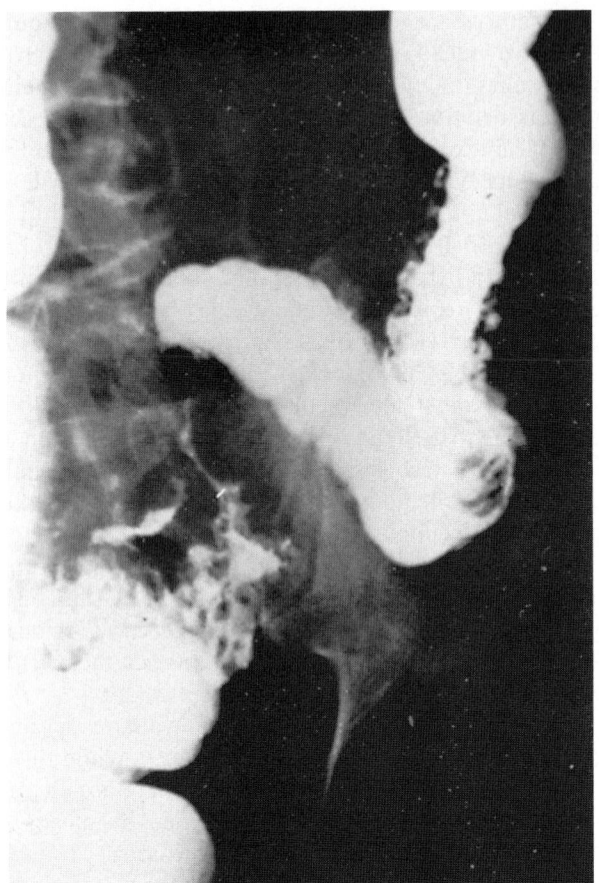

FIGURE 30-11. Crohn's colitis. Typical segmental involvement with a normal rectum, markedly stenotic lower sigmoid, relatively normal midsigmoid area, and then a further area of involvement of the upper sigmoid just distal to an uninvolved descending colon. Thickening of the bowel wall is seen in the upper sigmoid. (From Corman ML, Veidenheimer MC, Nugent FW, et al. *Diseases of the anus, rectum and colon. Part II: Non-specific inflammatory bowel disease.* New York: Medcom, 1976.)

fistulas.[107] However, if one requires the assistance of a radiologist to make the diagnosis of anal Crohn's disease, that physician must be considered diagnostically destitute.

Small Bowel

Upper gastrointestinal and small bowel x-ray films are quite helpful for evaluating IBD in this area of the alimentary tract, especially since there is no truly adequate nonoperative endoscopic examination of the small intestine, except for the very distal ileum. Radiologically, evaluation of the terminal ileum is best obtained by reflux on barium enema examination, but unfortunately, as many as 20% of patients will not demonstrate this phenomenon. Alternatively, a small bowel follow-through study or an enteroclysis with good spot films can be used.

Crohn's disease of the terminal ileum has a characteristic appearance. Thickening of the bowel wall narrows the lumen, resulting in a degree of obstruction in some patients. This is the most frequent cause of abdominal pain in individuals with Crohn's disease. The radiologic appearance of the terminal ileum has been described as having a "string sign" (Figure 30-16). Involvement of the terminal ileum may be seen as an isolated finding or may be associated with multiple diseased areas throughout the small intestine (Figure 30-17). In contrast to radiologic evaluation of the colon for Crohn's disease, it is virtually impossible to differentiate a benign from a malignant stricture in the small intestine (Figure 30-18). As with carcinoma of the small bowel in an individual without Crohn's disease, the prognosis is extremely poor.

Fistulous complications are frequently seen in patients with Crohn's disease. Communication between the ileum and colon is not uncommon (Figure 30-19), but other types of fistulas have been observed, including coloduodenal (Figure 30-20), and those to pelvic organs (Figure 30-21).

Ultrasound

Ultrasound examination is of quite limited value in patients with IBD because of the presence of considerable artifact associated with the loops of bowel. The presence of air or fluid in the intestine and adhesed loops may simulate a septic focus. That stated, Sonnenberg and colleagues performed a prospective clinical trial comparing 51 patients with Crohn's disease with 124 controlled subjects by means of gray scale ultrasound.[454] Diagnosis by ultrasound reflected primarily the thickening of the gastrointestinal wall itself, perceived as a characteristic "target" appearance. The study demonstrated that there were very few false negatives. The occasional false-positive phenomenon was usually attributed to the presence of a gastrointestinal tumor.

Van Outryve and colleagues studied transrectal ultrasound in individuals with Crohn's disease and in control subjects.[489] The authors observed that the procedure sharply delineates the rectal wall and may detect unsuspected abscesses and fistulas in the pararectal and paraanal tissues (see Chapters 4 and 6).

Computed Tomography

Computed tomography (CT) is able to demonstrate thickening of the colon, nodularity, adenopathy, and intraabdominal abscess (Figure 30-22). The presence of any fis-

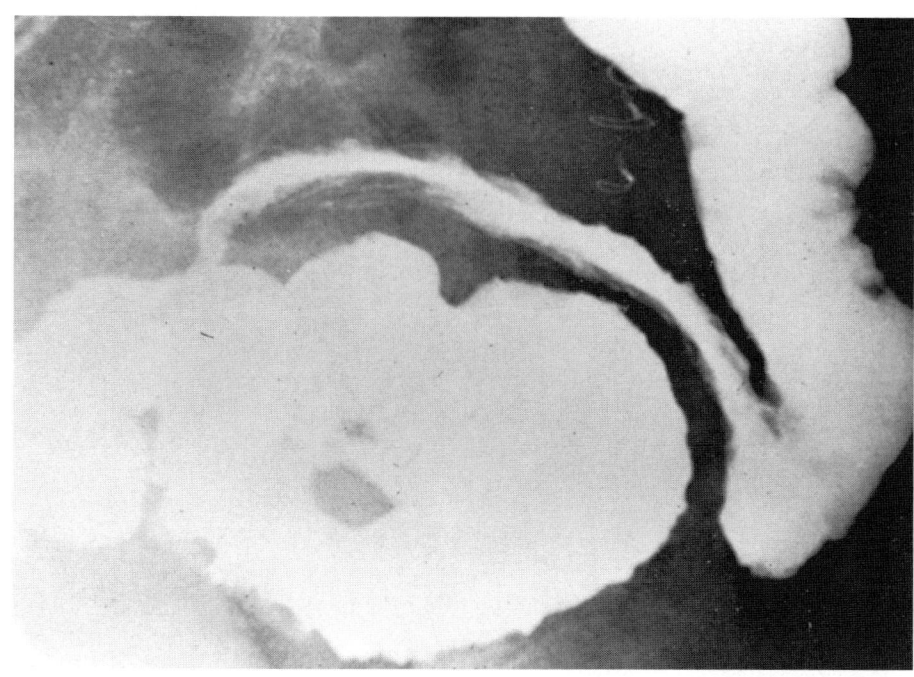

FIGURE 30-12. Crohn's colitis. Long sigmoid stricture with ulceration distally. (From Corman ML, Veidenheimer MC, Nugent FW, et al. *Diseases of the anus, rectum and colon. Part II: Non-specific inflammatory bowel disease.* New York: Medcom, 1976.)

tula, especially an enterocutaneous communication, is often demonstrable by means of CT scan with oral or rectal contrast. In most cases, however, adequate evaluation of intraabdominal pathology can be obtained by means of endoscopic examination and by standard contrast techniques.

Yousem and colleagues studied CT scans of 200 consecutive patients with Crohn's disease in order to determine the frequency and patterns of perirectal and perianal involvement.[524] They observed inflammation of fat planes (73%), bowel wall thickening (30%), fistulas or sinus tracts (22%), and abscesses (14%). Since more than one-third had abnormal CT manifestations below the symphysis pubis, the authors emphasize the importance of scanning sequences to the perineum in individuals with Crohn's disease.

Gore and colleagues attempted to provide the perspective of CT criteria in the evaluation of ulcerative, granulomatous and indeterminate colitis.[171] Unfortunately, features were often overlapping, and CT did not alter the original diagnosis in any patient.

Capsule Endoscopy

The application of capsule endoscopy for evaluating the small bowel has been discussed in Chapter 4. Several studies have been published that attest to its value in assessing the small bowel in individuals with Crohn's disease.[118,143,213] However, although it may be useful for identifying an occult source of bleeding, the reality is that the overwhelming majority of patients can have their disease identified by simpler, less expensive means. Furthermore, there is a real risk of precipitating a small bowel obstruction if the capsule cannot pass a strictured area. Still, in a limited number of individuals, capsule endoscopy may be a useful diagnostic tool for this condition.

Angiography

Another method for identifying the site of small bowel bleeding in an individual with Crohn's disease has been described, that of the combined use of preoperative angiography and highly selective methylene blue injection.[389] It was felt that this technique may aid the surgeon in the preoperative and intraoperative localization of occult bleeding sites in this condition.

The Significance of Special Laboratory Studies

A number of specialized laboratory studies have been advised, primarily for evaluation of Crohn's disease. Some have suggested the use of an indium-labeled leukocyte scan to distinguish patients for whom medical therapy may be preferable from those who may be optimally treated by surgery.[446] For example, in active Crohn's disease, labeled leukocytes are excreted into the bowel lumen from the inflamed mucosa. Patients with positive scans, therefore, have higher values of indices of disease activity. In a study by Slaton and colleagues, a negative indium leukocyte scan suggested a fibrotic

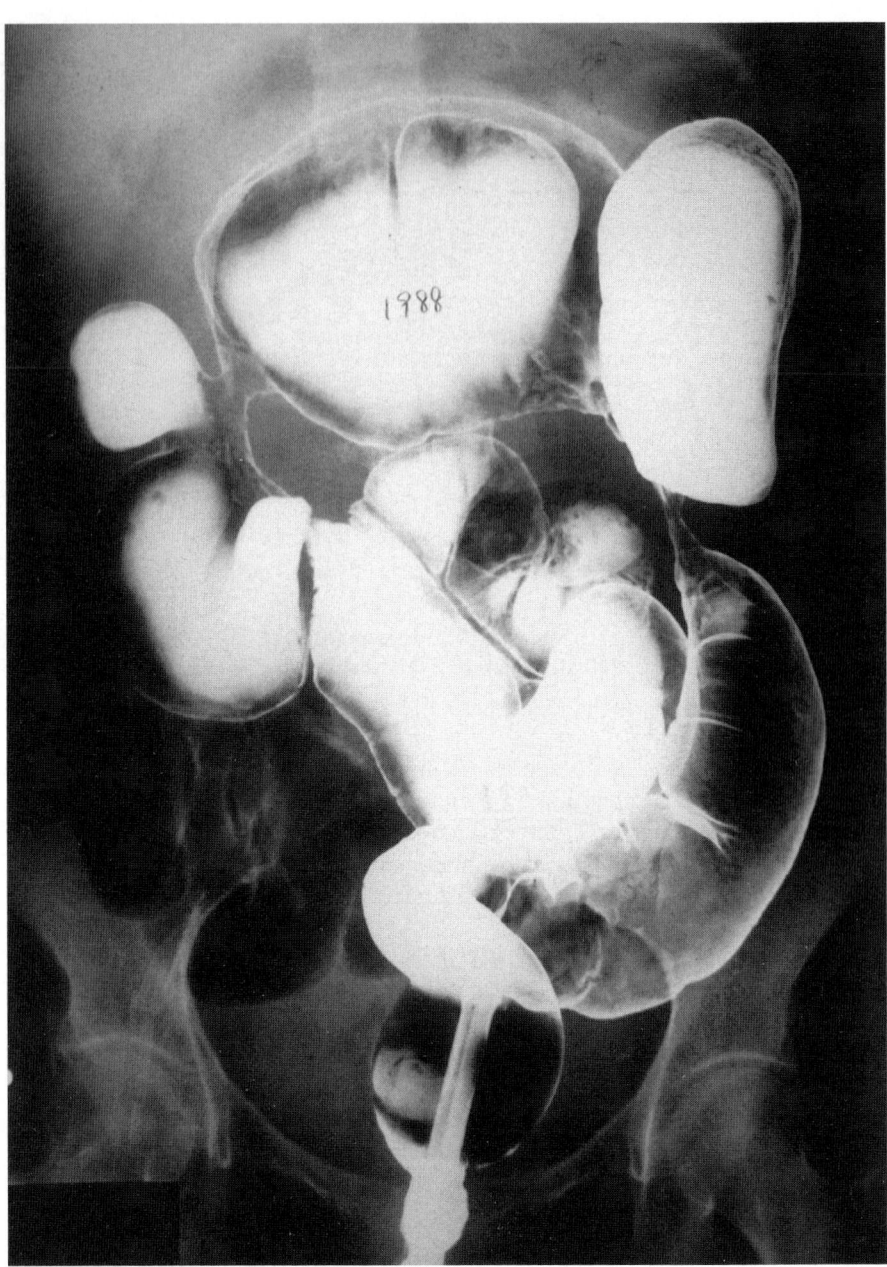

FIGURE 30-13. Air-contrast barium enema reveals multiple strictures in the colon in an individual with Crohn's disease. At the time of surgery, these all proved to be benign.

ileal stricture and the advisability of surgical intervention.[446] As an anatomic indicator of acute granulocytic infiltration of the intestinal mucosa and submucosa, Nelson and colleagues found that this scan had a 97% rate of sensitivity and a 100% specificity.[336] The study may be best applied in individuals with fulminant disease, especially those who cannot safely be put through the rigors of endoscopy or barium contrast radiologic evaluation.

Brignola and colleagues studied various laboratory indices to determine whether any had predictive value for recurrence of Crohn's disease.[52] There was a signifi-cant correlation with recurrence and alteration of acid 1-glycoprotein, 2-globulin, and erythrocyte sedimentation rate in comparison with the patients who remained in remission. Also, it has been demonstrated that patients with Crohn's disease requiring operative treatment often have a severe peripheral lymphopenia.[210] Mahida and colleagues have been able to detect interleukin-6 in seven out of eight peripheral and mesenteric samples from patients with Crohn's disease.[297] Heimann and Aufses showed that individuals who developed recurrences had significantly lower preoperative lymphocyte counts than those who were free of disease 3 years following resec-

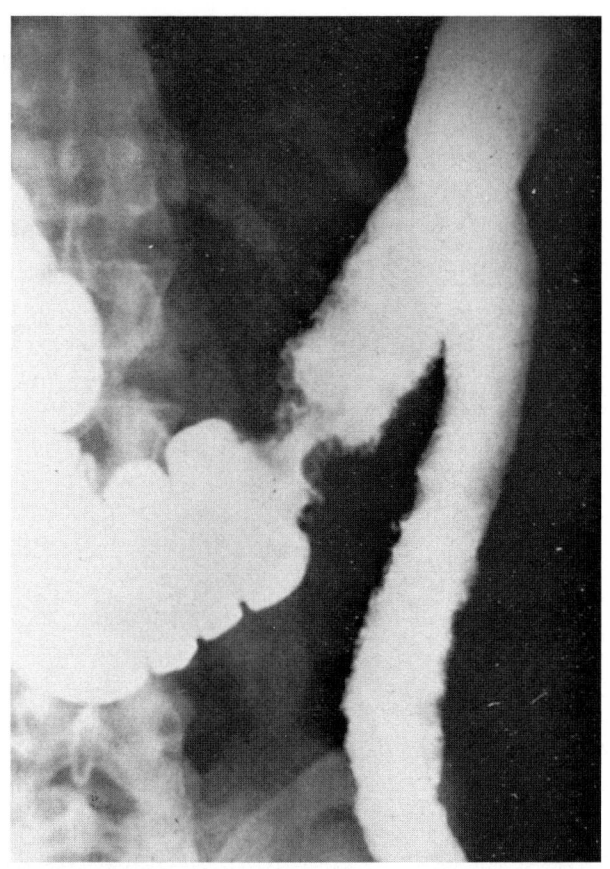

FIGURE 30-14. Crohn's colitis with transverse colon stricture, an "apple core" lesion suggestive of carcinoma. Note, however, that the distal bowel is ulcerated. (From Corman ML, Veidenheimer MC, Nugent FW, et al. *Diseases of the anus, rectum and colon. Part II: Non-specific inflammatory bowel disease.* New York: Medcom, 1976.)

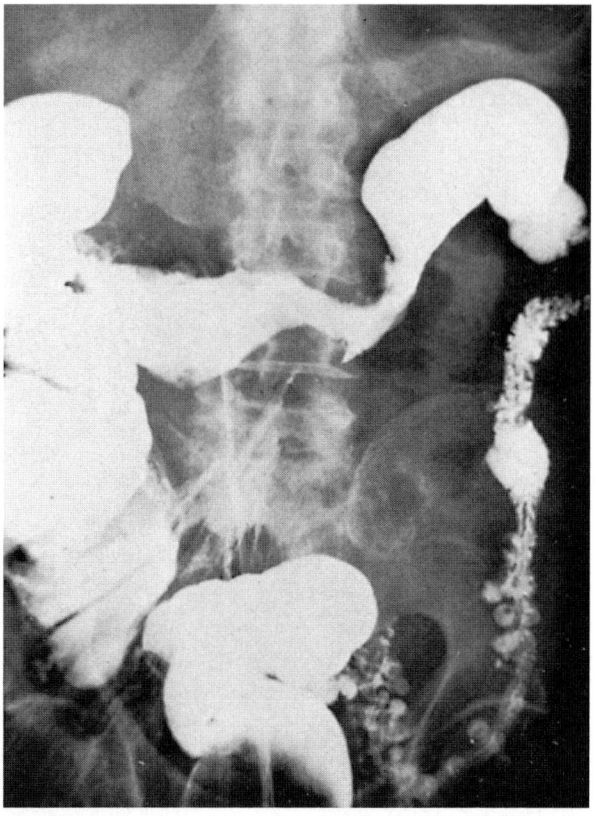

FIGURE 30-15. Scirrhous carcinoma of the transverse colon. Contrast the absence of adjacent mucosal abnormality with the previous figure. (From Corman ML, Veidenheimer MC, Nugent FW, et al. *Diseases of the anus, rectum and colon. Part II: Non-specific inflammatory bowel disease.* New York: Medcom, 1976.)

tion.[209] As more information becomes available, it is possible that these and other studies will help the physician and surgeon determine which patients are at increased risk and perhaps influence the timing and the type of therapy.

Pathology

Macroscopic Appearance

Crohn's disease may have protean clinical and pathologic manifestations. The condition can be confined to the colon alone or may involve only the anal canal. Fistulas, segmental involvement, rectal sparing, perianal disease, and abscess formation are all characteristic of granulomatous colitis.

Some of the earliest changes in the serosal aspect of the small intestine involved by Crohn's disease may be immediately recognizable if the patient is submitted to surgery. Subserosal extension of fat around the surface of the bowel ("fat-wrapping") and a prominent vascular pattern in the serosa are characteristic of the disease (Figure 30-23). The serosal surface may be granular and bleed easily on any intraoperative abrasion. It has been demonstrated that fat-wrapping correlates best with transmural inflammation and represents part of the connective-tissue changes that accompany intestinal Crohn's disease.[435]

The disease frequently affects the bowel in a segmental fashion. This may produce extensive skip areas (Figs. 30-24 and 30-25), limited involvement to an area of the bowel (Figure 30-26), or even a focal, isolated stricture (Figure 30-27).

Classically, Crohn's colitis involves the intestine in an asymmetric fashion. Areas of the bowel may demonstrate disease on the mucosal aspect with sparing of adjacent sites, leaving islands of somewhat edematous but otherwise nonulcerated mucosa (Figs. 30-28 through

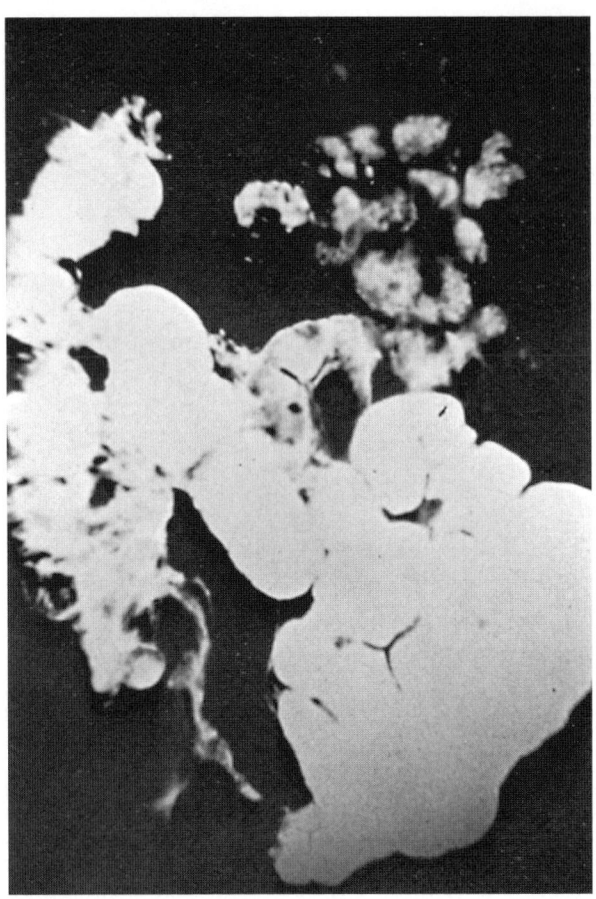

FIGURE 30-16. Distal ileal Crohn's disease. Edema and thickening of the bowel wall produce the characteristic "string sign." (From Corman ML, Veidenheimer MC, Nugent FW, et al. *Diseases of the anus, rectum and colon. Part II: Non-specific inflammatory bowel disease.* New York: Medcom, 1976.)

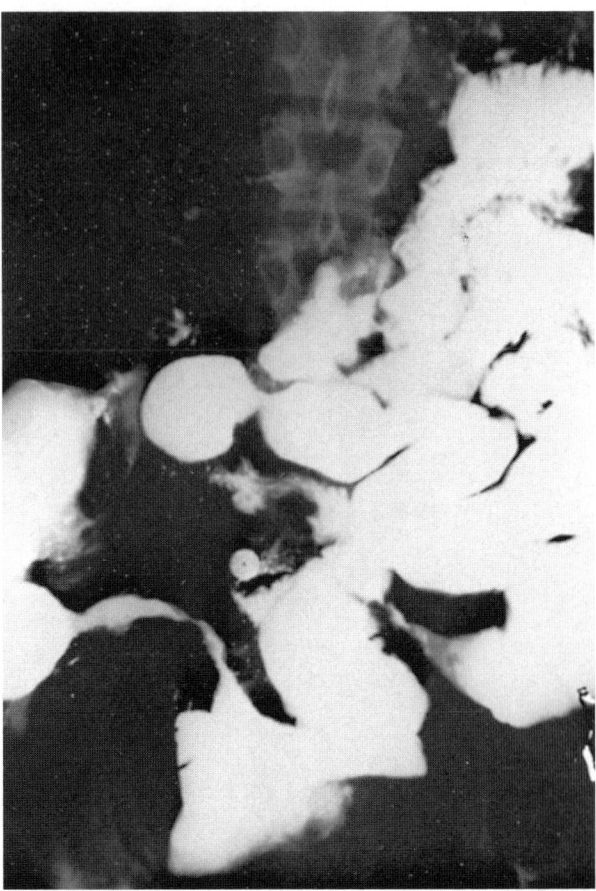

FIGURE 30-17. Small bowel Crohn's disease. Terminal ileal disease in addition to multiple skip areas. (From Corman ML, Veidenheimer MC, Nugent FW, et al. *Diseases of the anus, rectum and colon. Part II: Non-specific inflammatory bowel disease.* New York: Medcom, 1976.)

30-30). Ulceration in an irregular fashion with large areas of uninvolved mucosa interspersed between broad, twisting lesions is quite characteristic. The relative sparing between ulcers is not seen in ulcerative colitis. Another characteristic feature of the macroscopic appearance of Crohn's disease is the thickening of the bowel wall. Involvement through all the layers, along with the cobblestone appearance of the mucosa, has been described as "stones in a running brook" (Figure 30-31).

Crohn's colitis frequently involves the colon and ileum in continuity. Conversely, cecal ulceration can be seen with primarily ileal disease (Figure 30-32). Occasionally, the ileal disease may terminate abruptly at the ileocecal valve, sparing the large bowel (Figure 30-33). Thickening of the bowel wall may produce sufficient narrowing to precipitate intestinal obstruction or to impede the passage of swallowed seeds or nuts (Figure

30-34). Gallstone ileus has even been reported to produce obstruction at a point of stenosis caused by Crohn's disease.[431]

A common manifestation of Crohn's disease is fistula formation. Fistulas may occur into any adjacent organ, such as the small or large bowel, bladder, vagina, uterus, ureter, or skin. Burrowing of the fissures deep into the bowel wall predisposes to fistula formation. Fistulas occur more commonly in the mesocolic aspect of the bowel than on the antimesocolic border (Figure 30-35).

Occasionally, diffuse mucosal disease may produce a pseudopolypoid pattern similar to that of chronic ulcerative colitis. Giant pseudopolyps may actually mimic neoplasms endoscopically and radiographically. The condition is most likely the result of fusion of numerous fingerlike pseudopolyps.[186] A number of reports and reviews of this manifestation have been published.[101,186,235]

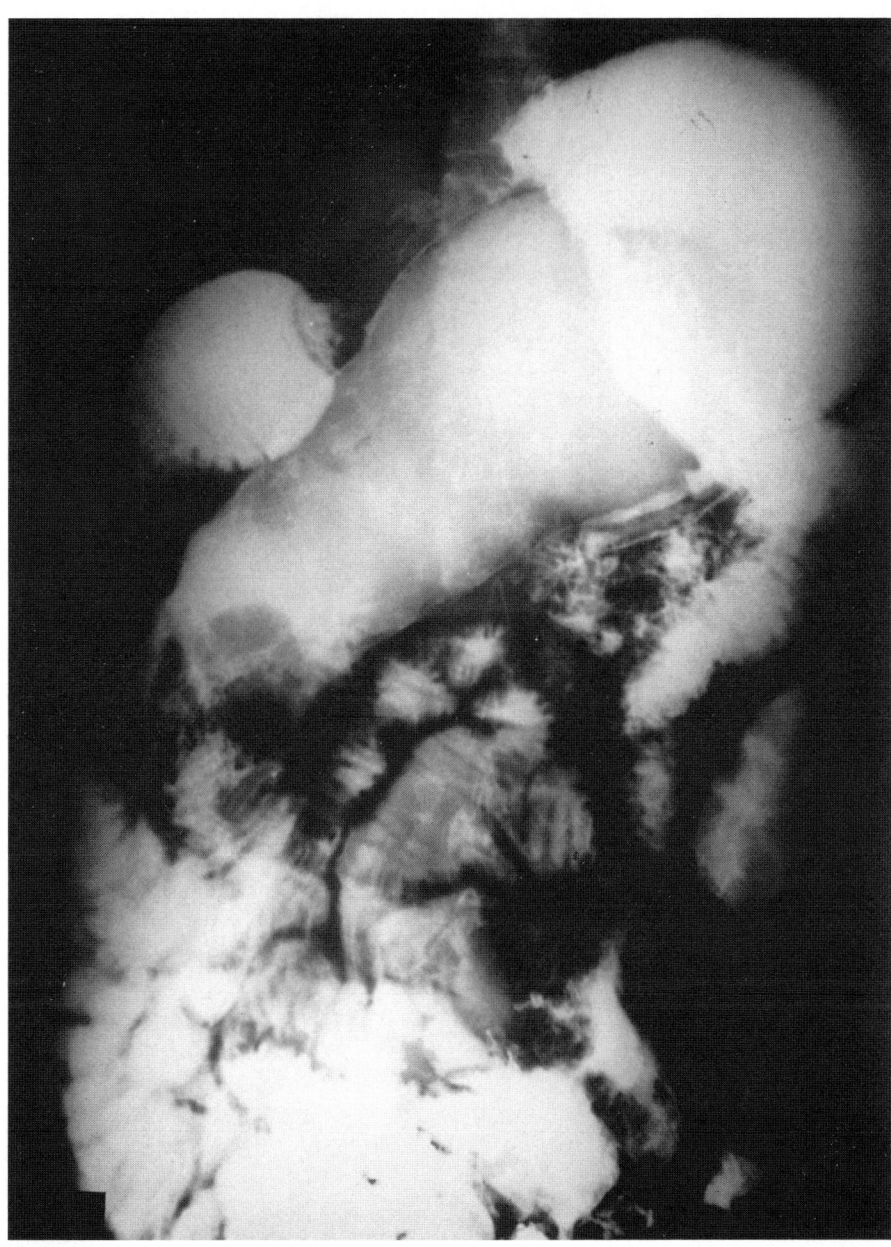

FIGURE 30-18. Small bowel series demonstrates proximal obstruction secondary to a stricture that proved to be malignant. Additional benign strictures from Crohn's disease are also evident on this radiologic study.

Histologic Appearance

The three primary histopathologic findings in patients with Crohn's colitis are transmural inflammation and fibrosis, granulomas, and narrow, deeply penetrating ulcers or "fissures" (Figure 30-36). The mucosal inflammation of Crohn's disease differs from that of ulcerative colitis in that typically there are fewer crypt abscesses, there is less congestion, and there is better preservation of the goblet cell population (Figure 30-37).

Granulomas may occur in any part of the bowel wall and are usually identified in approximately two thirds of all patients with Crohn's colitis. If a biopsy is performed in an attempt to differentiate between the two inflammatory conditions, the material should be obtained from a noninflamed area if possible (Figure 30-38). A granuloma, albeit a foreign-body type, may actually be seen even with ulcerative colitis in an area of acute inflammation. Multiple biopsy specimens are suggested because submucosal lesions tend to be very small (microgranulomas).[258] The microscopic appearance of the granuloma is not diagnostic, and the possibility of an infectious agent should always be considered (Figure 30-39). Granulomas can also occur in the liver (Figure 30-40) and in the omentum (Figure 30-41) as well as in other sites.

(text continues on page 1475)

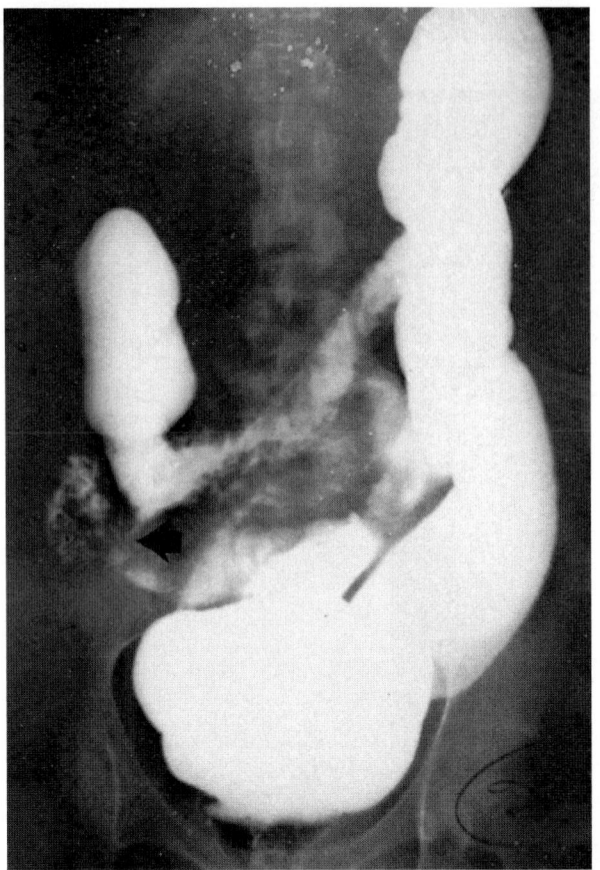

FIGURE 30-19. Ileocolic fistula (*arrow*). Extensive transverse colon disease with fistulous communication to the ileum. (From Corman ML, Veidenheimer MC, Nugent FW, et al. *Diseases of the anus, rectum and colon. Part II: Non-specific inflammatory bowel disease.* New York: Medcom, 1976.)

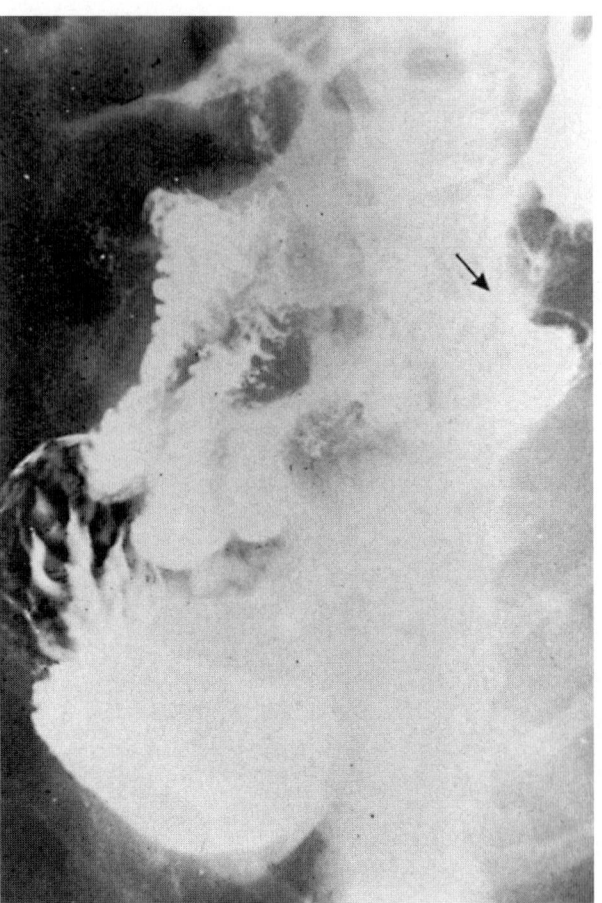

FIGURE 30-20. An upper gastrointestinal series demonstrates fistula (*arrow*) between the duodenum and the ascending colon. (From Corman ML, Veidenheimer MC, Nugent FW, et al. *Diseases of the anus, rectum and colon. Part II: Non-specific inflammatory bowel disease.* New York: Medcom, 1976.)

FIGURE 30-21. A fistula between the colon and the fallopian tube is an unusual complication of Crohn's colitis. Note that a second fistula passes into an abscess and out to the skin (*arrow*). (From Corman ML, Veidenheimer MC, Nugent FW, et al. *Diseases of the anus, rectum and colon. Part II: Non-specific inflammatory bowel disease.* New York: Medcom, 1976.)

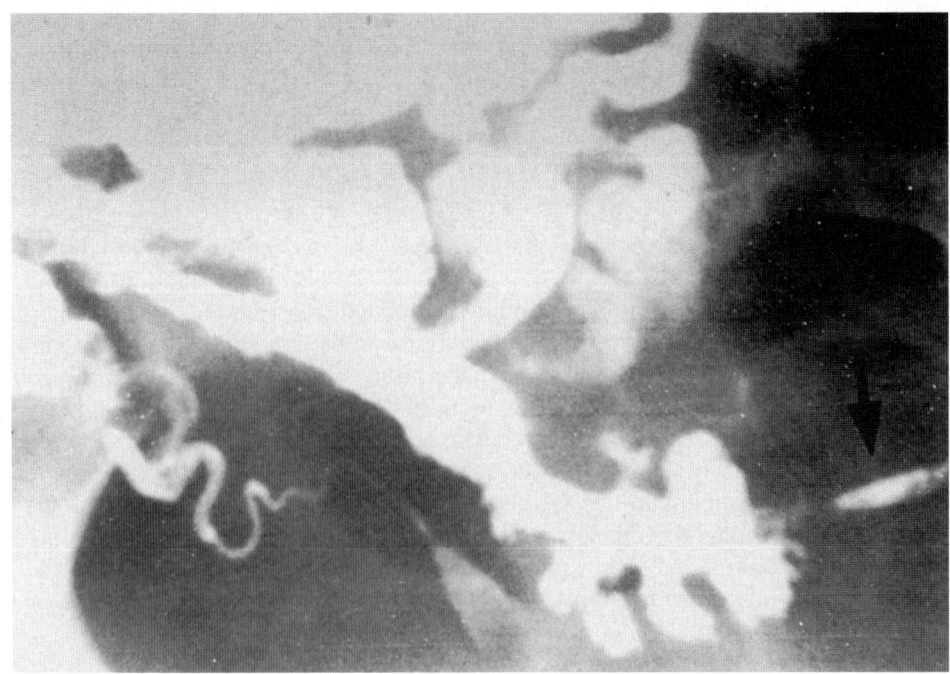

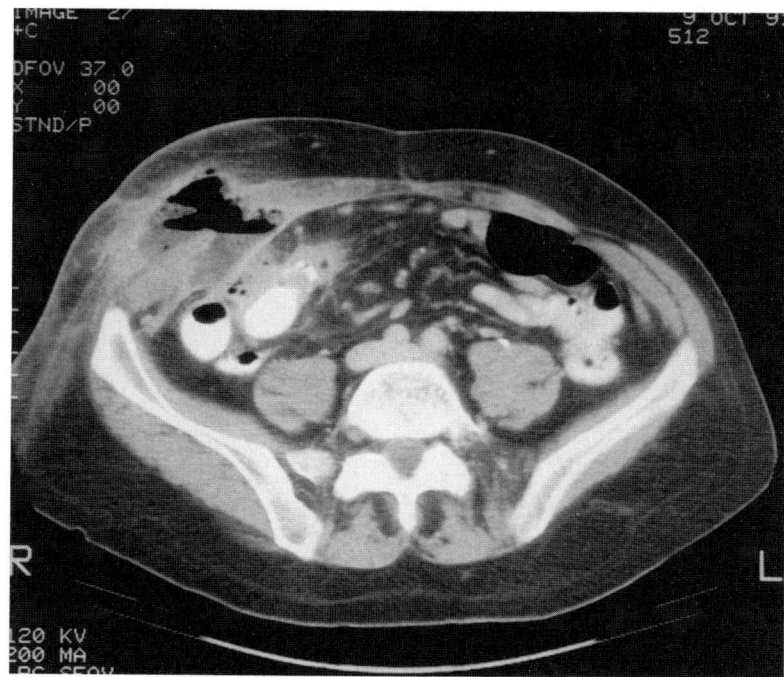

FIGURE 30-22. Computed tomography demonstrates abdominal wall abscess on the right side. This was secondary to a perforating ileocolic Crohn's inflammation.

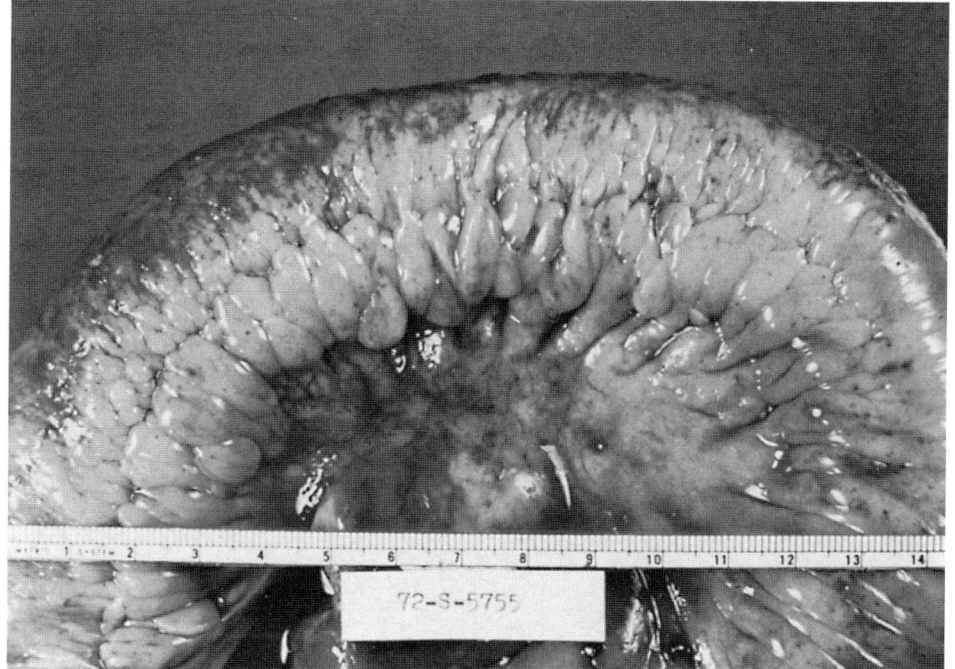

FIGURE 30-23. Ileal Crohn's disease. Subserosal inflammation and "fat-wrapping" are evident. (From Corman ML, Veidenheimer MC, Nugent FW, et al. *Diseases of the anus, rectum and colon. Part II: Non-specific inflammatory bowel disease.* New York: Medcom, 1976.)

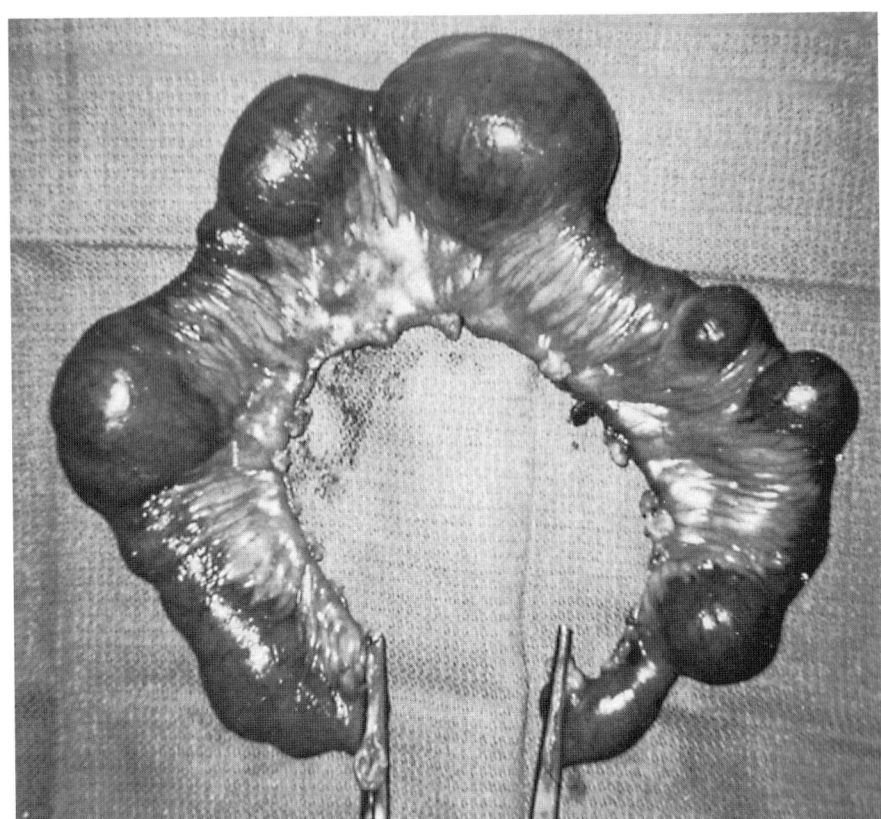

FIGURE 30-24. Crohn's disease. Segmental constrictions of small bowel with dilated bowel between each stenotic area. (From Corman ML, Veidenheimer MC, Nugent FW, et al. *Diseases of the anus, rectum and colon. Part II: Non-specific inflammatory bowel disease.* New York: Medcom, 1976.)

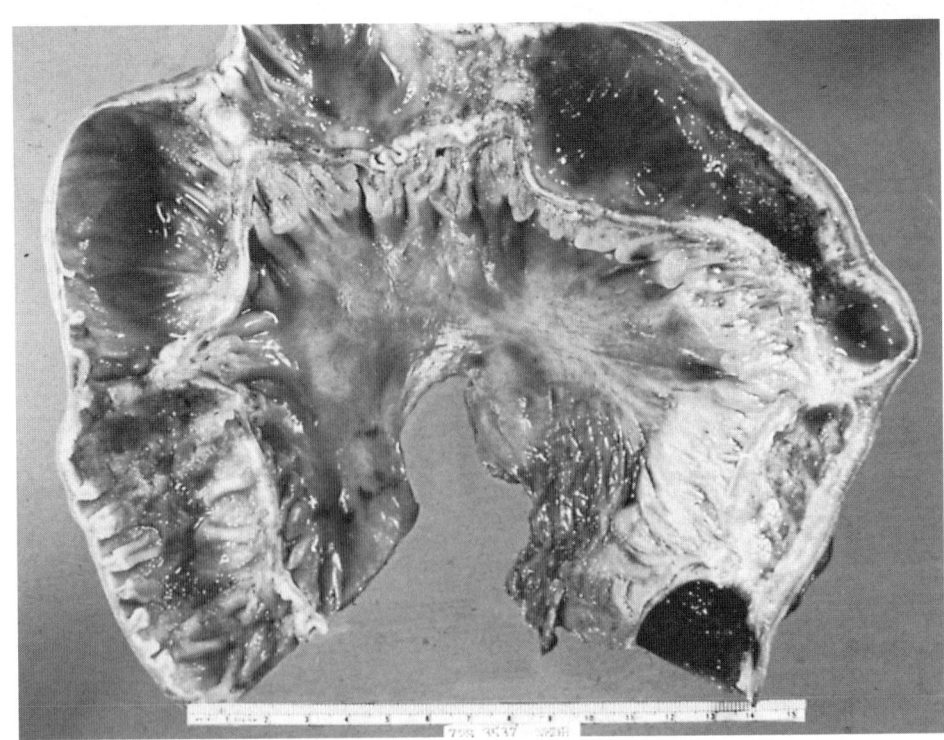

FIGURE 30-25. Crohn's disease. This opened specimen from Fig. 30-24 reveals the segmental nature of the disease. Thickening of the mesentery is a prominent feature. (From Corman ML, Veidenheimer MC, Nugent FW, et al. *Diseases of the anus, rectum and colon. Part II: Non-specific inflammatory bowel disease.* New York: Medcom, 1976.)

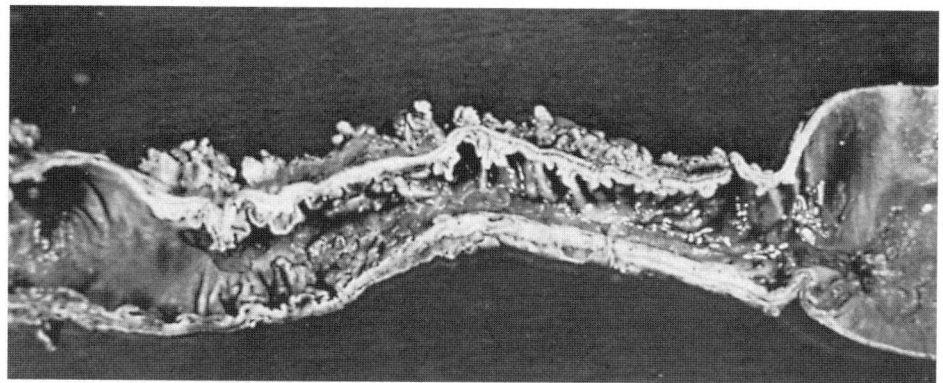

FIGURE 30-26. Crohn's colitis. Segmental involvement of the sigmoid with marked narrowing of the midportion. Thickening of all layers of bowel is evident. At each end, the bowel is less involved and more distensible. (From Corman ML, Veidenheimer MC, Nugent FW, et al. *Diseases of the anus, rectum and colon. Part II: Non-specific inflammatory bowel disease.* New York: Medcom, 1976.)

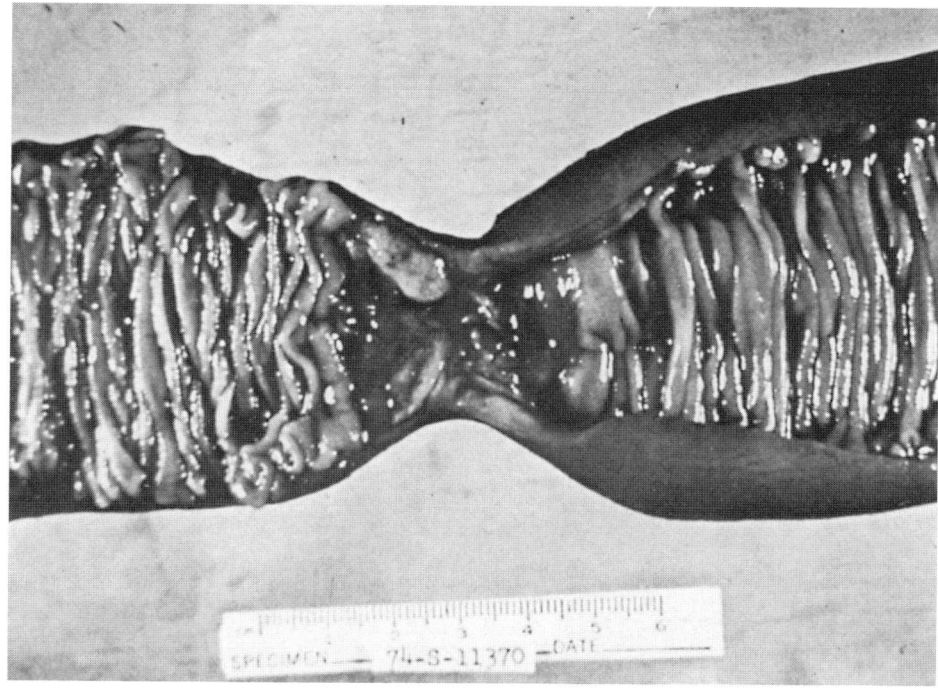

FIGURE 30-27. Crohn's disease. Short segment of constriction. Note edematous mucosa and evidence of bowel dilatation on the right side, produced by partial obstruction. (From Corman ML, Veidenheimer MC, Nugent FW, et al. *Diseases of the anus, rectum and colon. Part II: Non-specific inflammatory bowel disease.* New York: Medcom, 1976.)

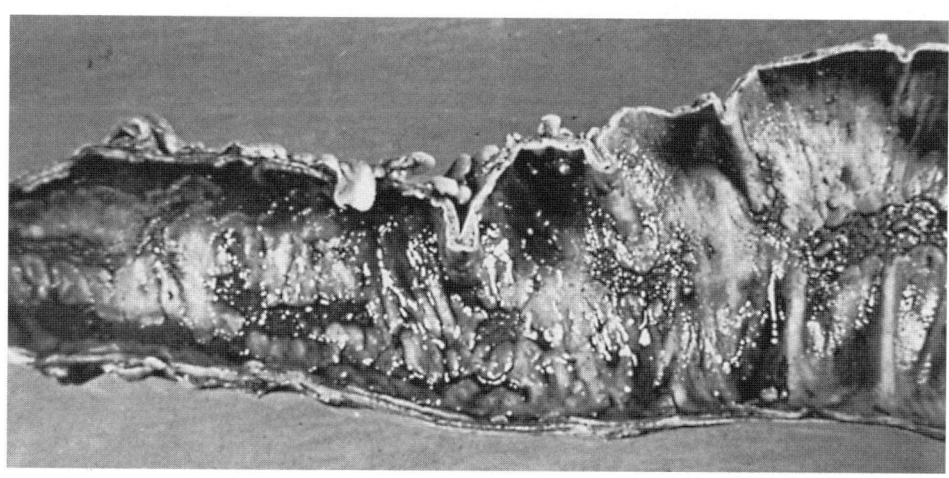

FIGURE 30-28. Crohn's colitis. Irregularly ulcerated mucosa with sparing between ulcers. (From Corman ML, Veidenheimer MC, Nugent FW, et al. *Diseases of the anus, rectum and colon. Part II: Non-specific inflammatory bowel disease.* New York: Medcom, 1976.)

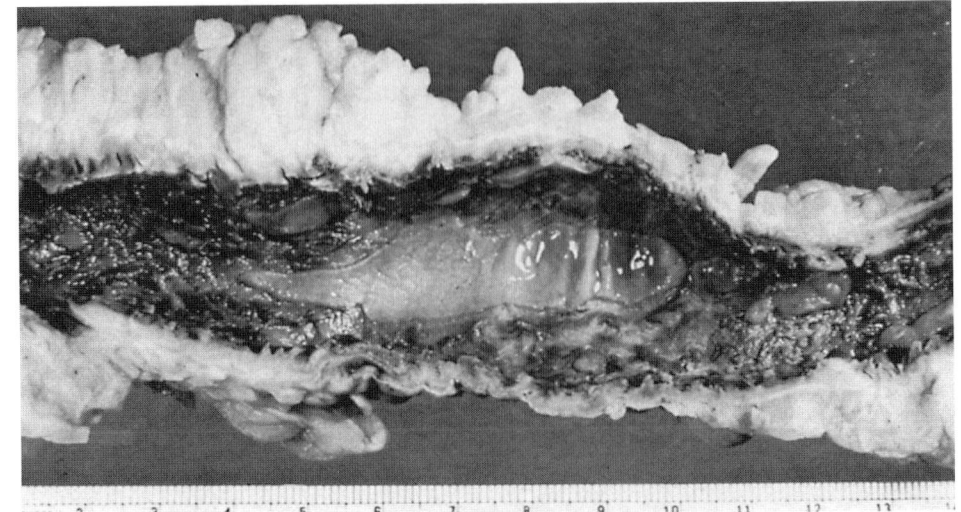

FIGURE 30-29. Crohn's colitis. An island of normal mucosa lies in the middle of the specimen, with largely denuded, ulcerated mucosa on either side. (From Corman ML, Veidenheimer MC, Nugent FW, et al. *Diseases of the anus, rectum and colon. Part II: Non-specific inflammatory bowel disease.* New York: Medcom, 1976.)

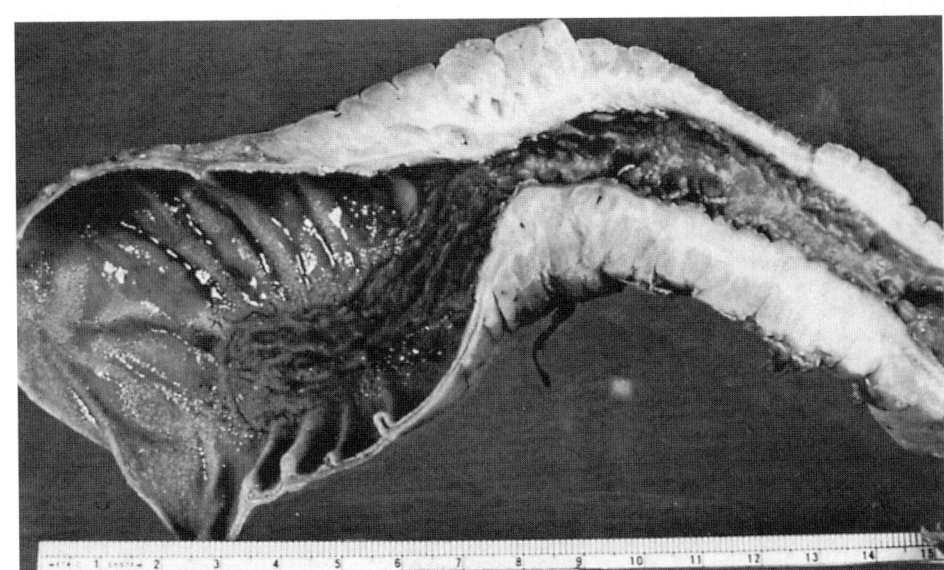

FIGURE 30-30. Crohn's colitis. Severe stenosis on the right and ulceration surrounded by normal mucosa on the left, a typical feature of this disease. (From Corman ML, Veidenheimer MC, Nugent FW, et al. *Diseases of the anus, rectum and colon. Part II: Non-specific inflammatory bowel disease.* New York: Medcom, 1976.)

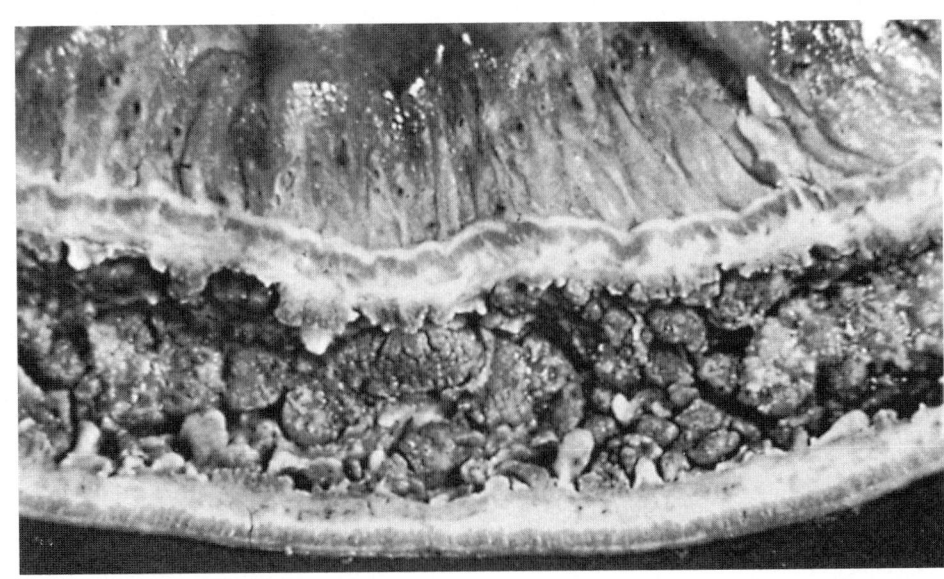

FIGURE 30-31. Crohn's ileitis. The cobblestone appearance of the mucosa is produced by transverse and longitudinal intersecting ulcerations. Note the thickened bowel wall. (From Corman ML, Veidenheimer MC, Nugent FW, et al. *Diseases of the anus, rectum and colon. Part II: Non-specific inflammatory bowel disease.* New York: Medcom, 1976.)

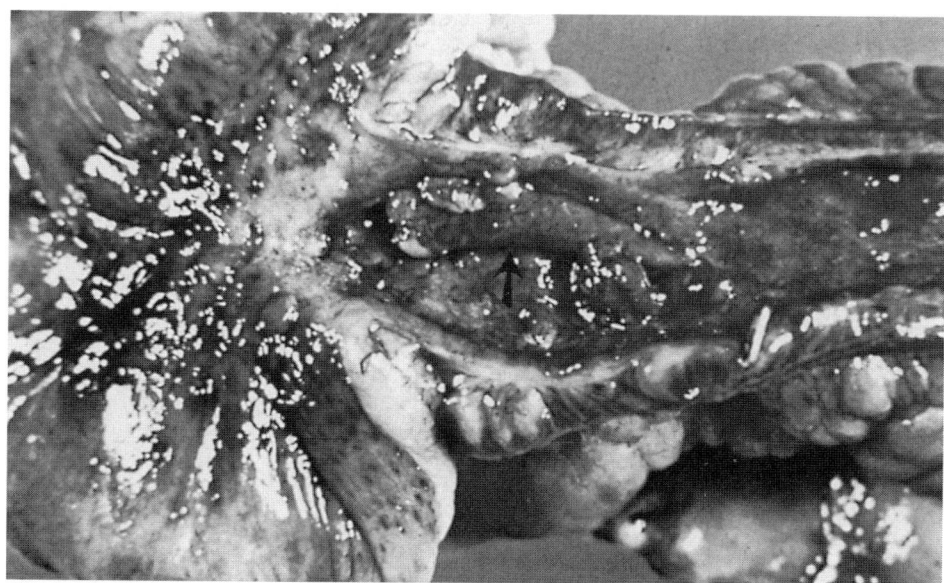

FIGURE 30-32. Crohn's disease. Cecal ulceration and ileal disease with involvement of the ileocecal valve. Note the large ileal mucosal tag (*arrow*). (From Corman ML, Veidenheimer MC, Nugent FW, et al. *Diseases of the anus, rectum and colon. Part II: Non-specific inflammatory bowel disease.* New York: Medcom, 1976.)

Narrow, deeply penetrating ulcers or "fissures" are the third characteristic feature of Crohn's disease. The fissures may penetrate through the inner circular layer of the muscularis and are visible on the radiographs after a barium enema as spicules. A sinus tract present in the fat adjacent to the bowel wall indicates that one of the fissures has penetrated through the wall (Figure 30-42). When this occurs a sinus may burrow into another organ to produce a fistula (Figure 30-43).

Information about the pathology of IBD has been further gleaned by means of *electron microscopy*. Early epithelial changes can be identified using this modality in areas that appear to be uninvolved. These include necrosis of individual columnar epithelial cells; budding of the tips of microvilli; thickening, shortening, irregularity, and fusion of intestinal villi; numerous Paneth's cells; hyperplasia of goblet cells; and augmented mucous secretion.[241] Other studies, such as tissue-enzyme analysis, jejunal-surface pH, and differences in sodium flux and mucosal potential, imply that the disease often is far more extensive than is recognized by other, more conventional means, and certainly much more extensive than is usually apparent at the time of surgery.

Another observation is the increased secretion of mucus by the bowel in Crohn's disease as compared with decreased colonic mucus in ulcerative colitis. The decrease may be explained by destruction of the epithelial cells.[241] A number of biochemical changes have also been observed.

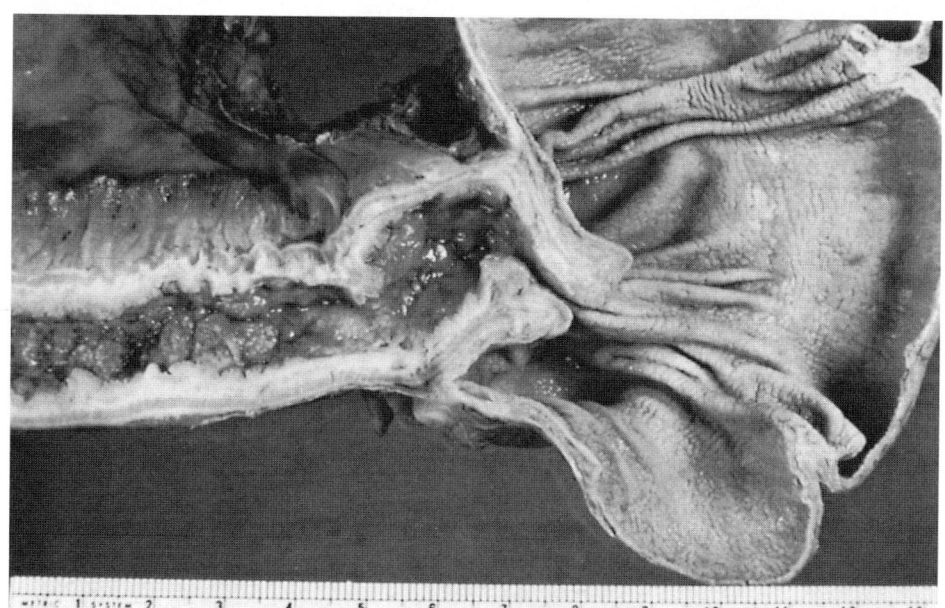

FIGURE 30-33. Crohn's ileitis. Ileal involvement with sparing of the large bowel. Note the abrupt cessation of the disease at the ileocecal valve. (From Corman ML, Veidenheimer MC, Nugent FW, et al. *Diseases of the anus, rectum and colon. Part II: Non-specific inflammatory bowel disease.* New York: Medcom, 1976.)

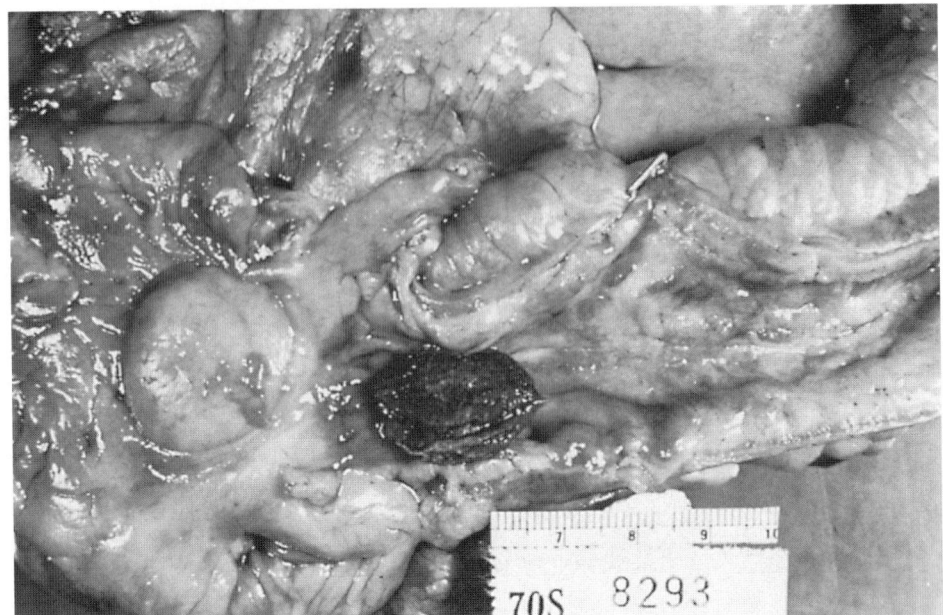

FIGURE 30-34. Crohn's ileitis. This unusual specimen demonstrates a prune pit trapped in a narrowed segment of terminal ileum, precipitating intestinal obstruction. (From Corman ML, Veidenheimer MC, Nugent FW, et al. *Diseases of the anus, rectum and colon. Part II: Non-specific inflammatory bowel disease.* New York: Medcom, 1976.)

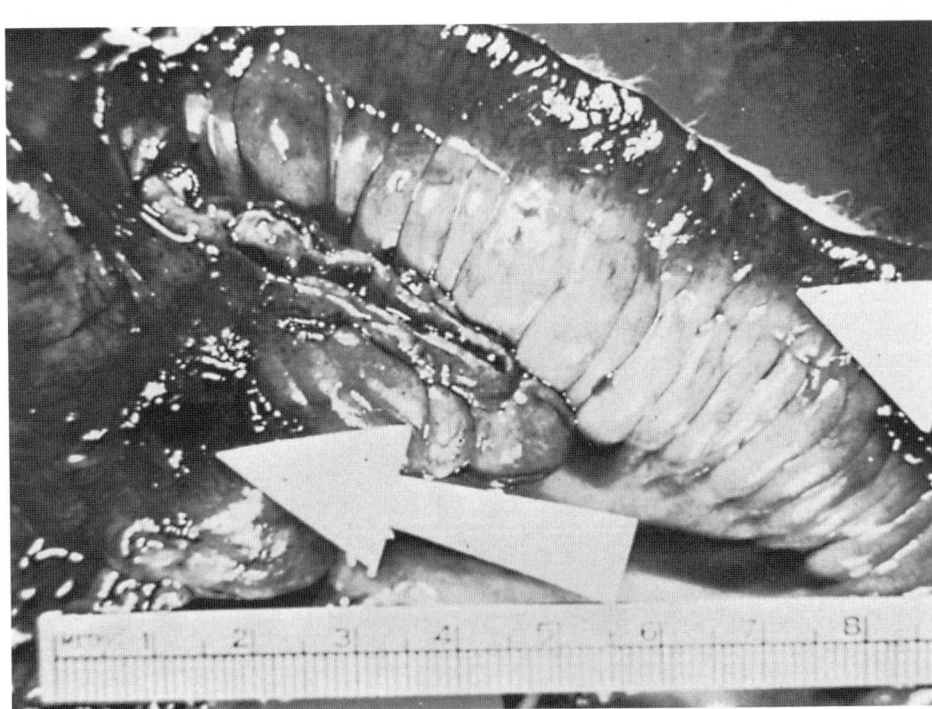

FIGURE 30-35. Crohn's disease. A fistula (*arrow*) has passed through the mesocolon and into an adjacent structure at some distance from the point of origin in the bowel. The characteristic small bowel fat wrapping is marked at right (*arrowhead*). (From Corman ML, Veidenheimer MC, Nugent FW, et al. *Diseases of the anus, rectum and colon. Part II: Non-specific inflammatory bowel disease.* New York: Medcom, 1976.)

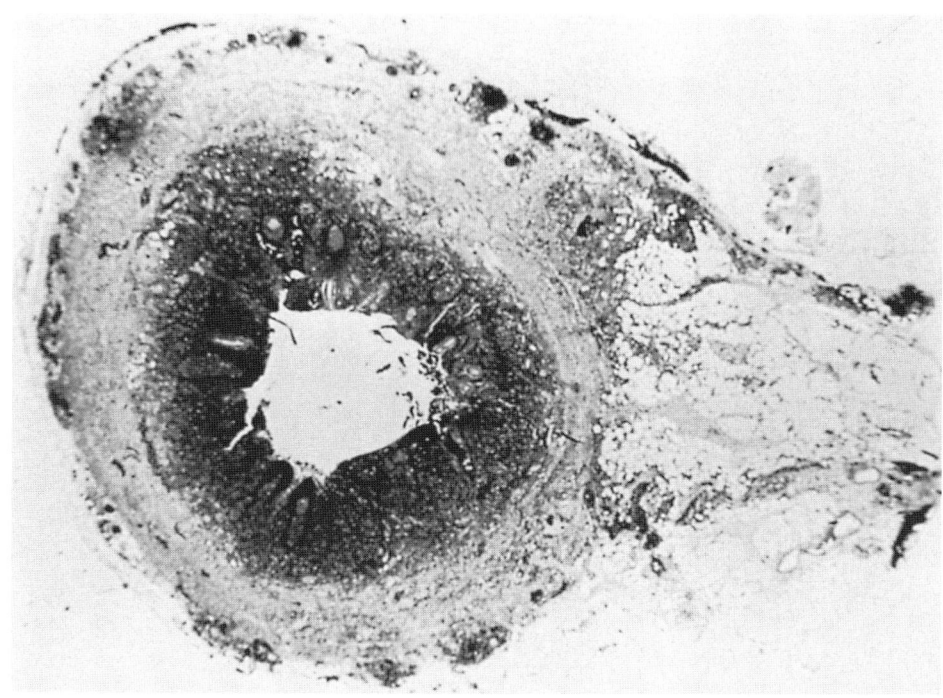

FIGURE 30-36. Crohn's disease of the appendix. Cross-section demonstrates inflammatory changes at all levels: mucosa, muscularis, and serosa. (Original magnification × 80.) (From Corman ML, Veidenheimer MC, Nugent FW, et al. *Diseases of the anus, rectum and colon. Part II: Non-specific inflammatory bowel disease.* New York: Medcom, 1976.)

Extra-intestinal Manifestations

For convenience and in order to avoid duplication I have elected to place the discussion of extra-intestinal manifestations in this chapter. Moreover, since so many of the manifestations in other areas of the body are exclusively seen in Crohn's disease, the discussion is placed within this chapter, although many such problems may be seen in both ulcerative colitis and Crohn's disease. Increasing evidence supports the statement that inflammatory disease of the intestine is a systemic problem rather than one localized to the small or large bowel. In a population-based study from Sweden of 1,274 patients with ulcerative colitis, the overall prevalence of extra-colonic diagnoses was 21%.[324] As discussed in Chapter 29, many etiologic concepts have been considered, but regardless of the sequence of pathologic changes in the colon, there is little question

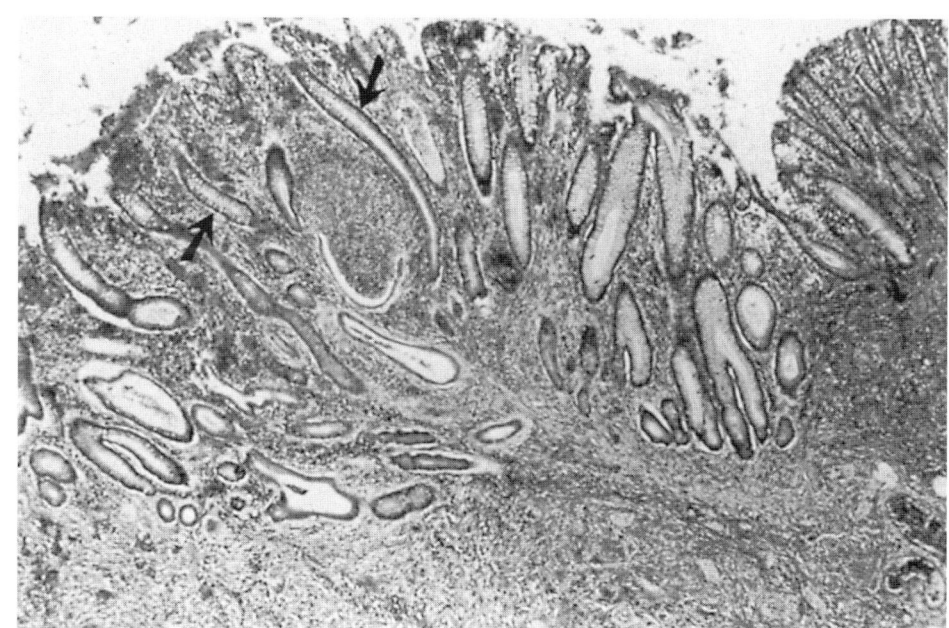

FIGURE 30-37. Crohn's disease. Note the crypts (*arrows*) on either side of the crypt abscess contain an almost normal complement of globlet cells. (Original magnification × 80.) (From Corman ML, Veidenheimer MC, Nugent FW, et al. *Diseases of the anus, rectum and colon. Part II: Non-specific inflammatory bowel disease.* New York: Medcom, 1976.)

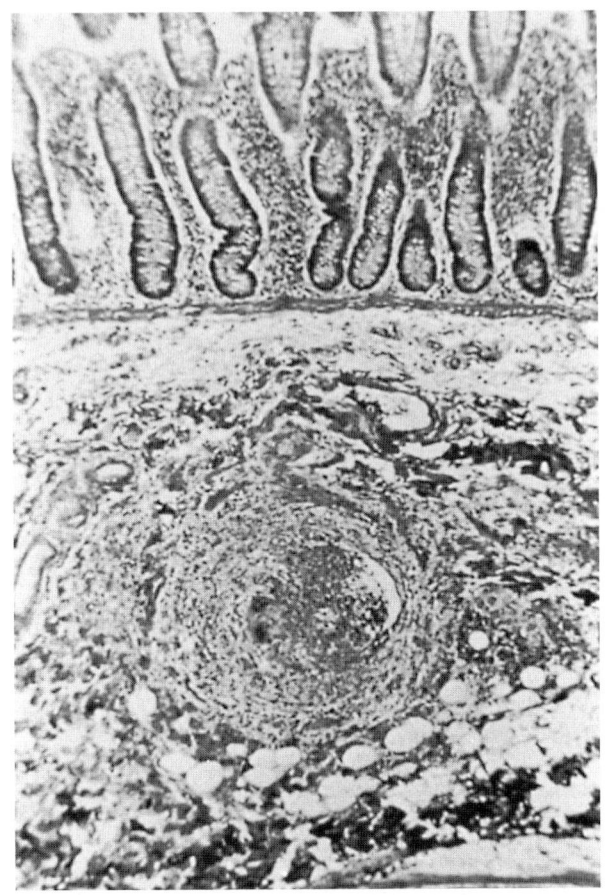

FIGURE 30-38. Crohn's disease. Submucosal granuloma. Note that the overlying mucosa has inflammatory cells in the lamina propria but no crypt abscess or ulceration. (Original magnification × 80.) (From Corman ML, Veidenheimer MC, Nugent FW, et al. *Diseases of the anus, rectum and colon. Part II: Non-specific inflammatory bowel disease.* New York: Medcom, 1976.)

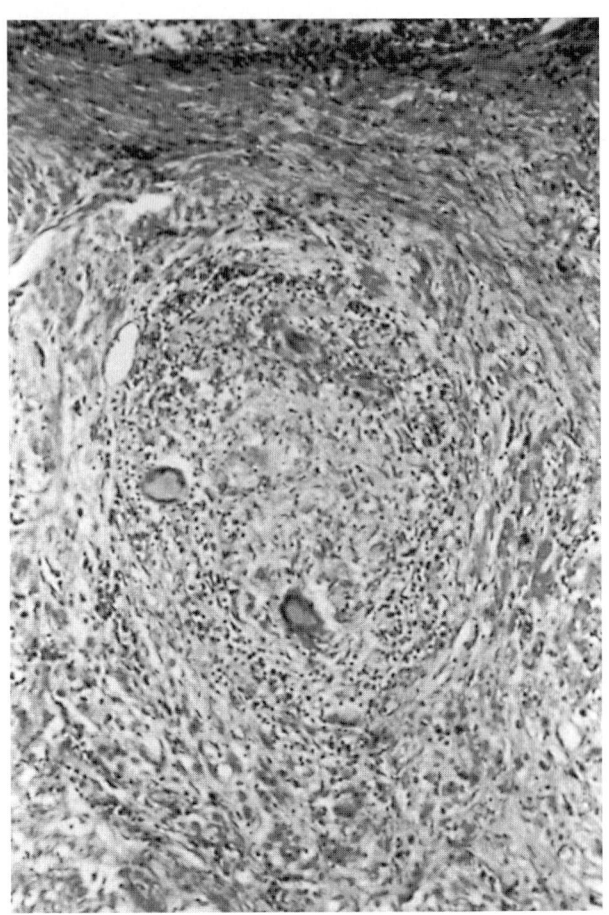

FIGURE 30-39. Crohn's disease. Granuloma within muscularis propria. (Original magnification × 280.) (From Corman ML, Veidenheimer MC, Nugent FW, et al. *Diseases of the anus, rectum and colon. Part II: Non-specific inflammatory bowel disease.* New York: Medcom, 1976.)

FIGURE 30-40. Crohn's disease. Granuloma of the liver in a patient with Crohn's colitis. (Original magnification × 260.) (From Corman ML, Veidenheimer MC, Nugent FW, et al. *Diseases of the anus, rectum and colon. Part II: Non-specific inflammatory bowel disease.* New York: Medcom, 1976.)

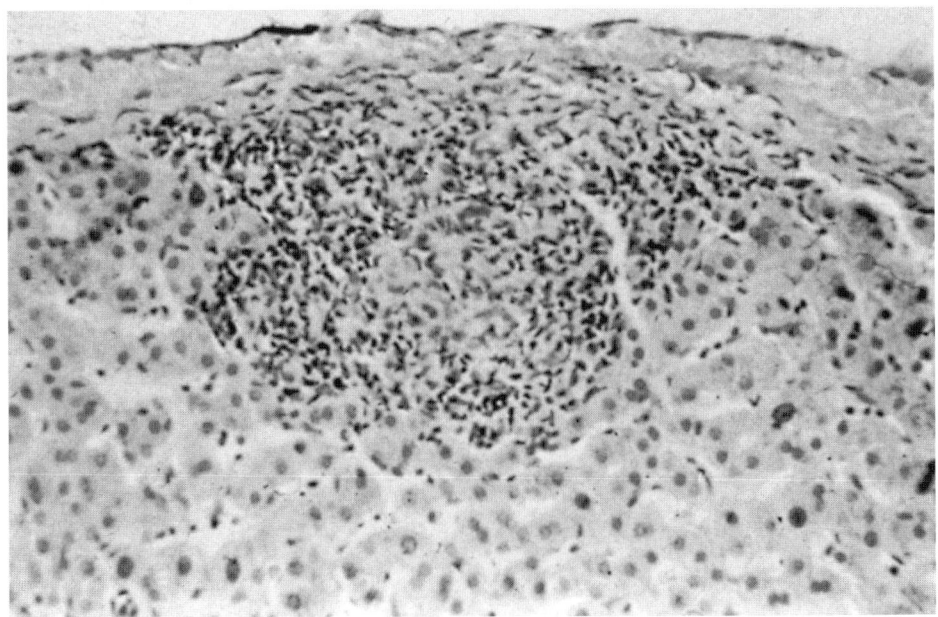

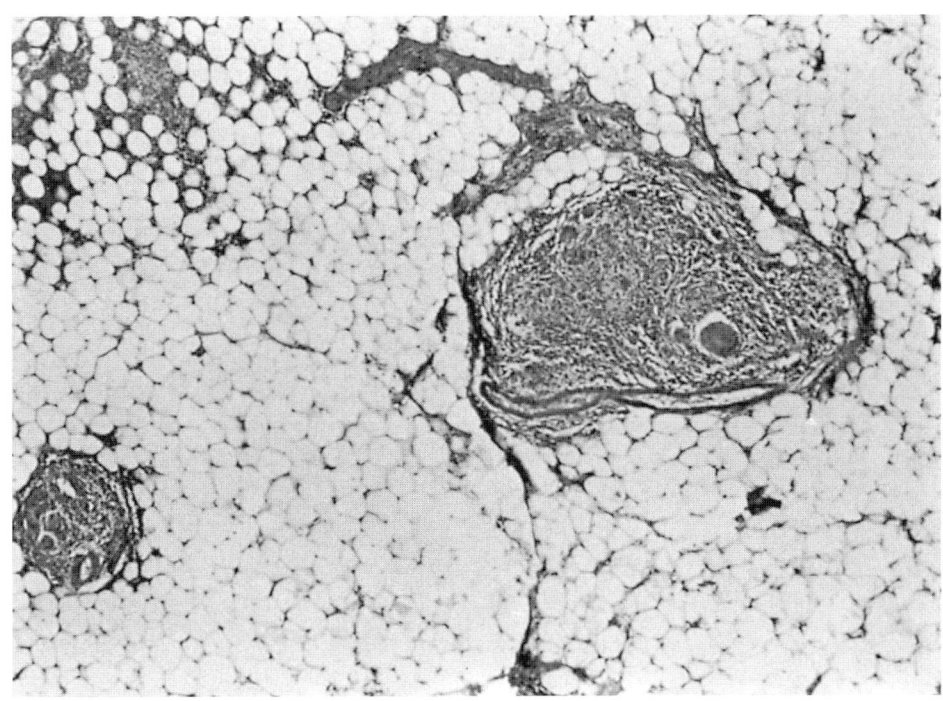

FIGURE 30-41. Crohn's colitis. Two omental granulomas are seen in a patient with Crohn's colitis. (Original magnification × 80.) (From Corman ML, Veidenheimer MC, Nugent FW, et al. *Diseases of the anus, rectum and colon. Part II: Non-specific inflammatory bowel disease.* New York: Medcom, 1976.)

about the presence of related events, at times profound, in distant areas of the body. The joints, skin, liver, kidneys, eyes, mouth, blood, nervous system, and, of course, other areas of the alimentary tract may be sites of lesions that, at least in the extra-intestinal manifestations, often seem dependent on the presence of diseased bowel. So broad indeed is the spectrum of Crohn's disease that specialists in dentistry, otorhinolaryngology,

ophthalmology, and dermatology must be prepared to recognize its manifestations.

Oral Manifestations

Oral lesions were first identified in Crohn's disease by Dudeney and Todd in 1969.[108] Since then a number of papers have been published on the subject.[38,41,449,492] In-

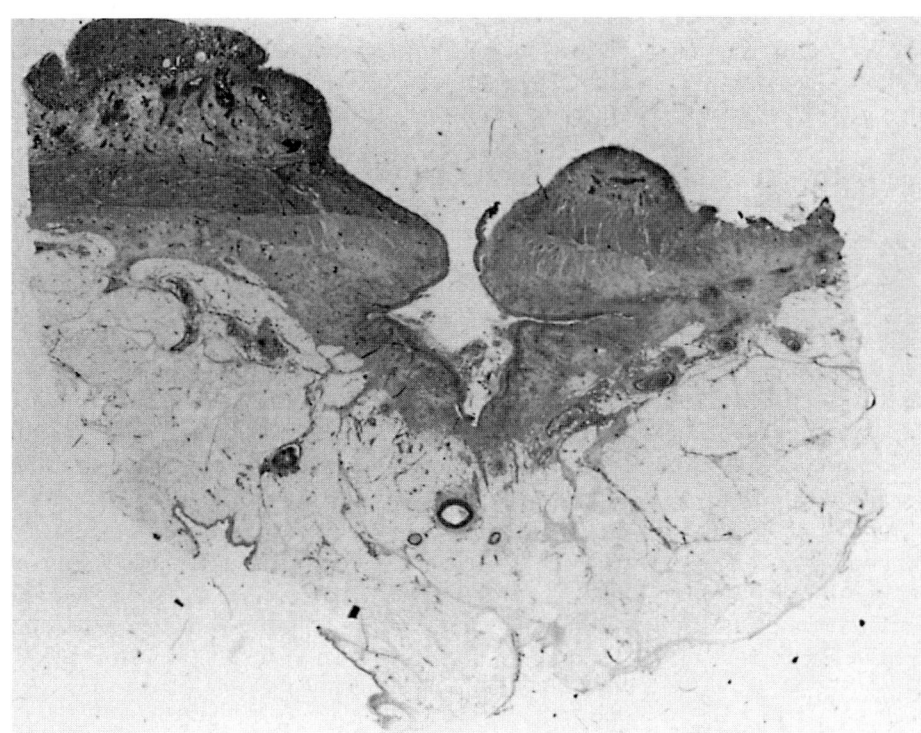

FIGURE 30-42. Crohn's disease: a whole-mount specimen demonstrates a fissure extending through the colon wall and into the pericolonic fat. This is the origin of a fistula. (From Corman ML, Veidenheimer MC, Nugent FW, et al. *Diseases of the anus, rectum and colon. Part II: Non-specific inflammatory bowel disease.* New York: Medcom, 1976.)

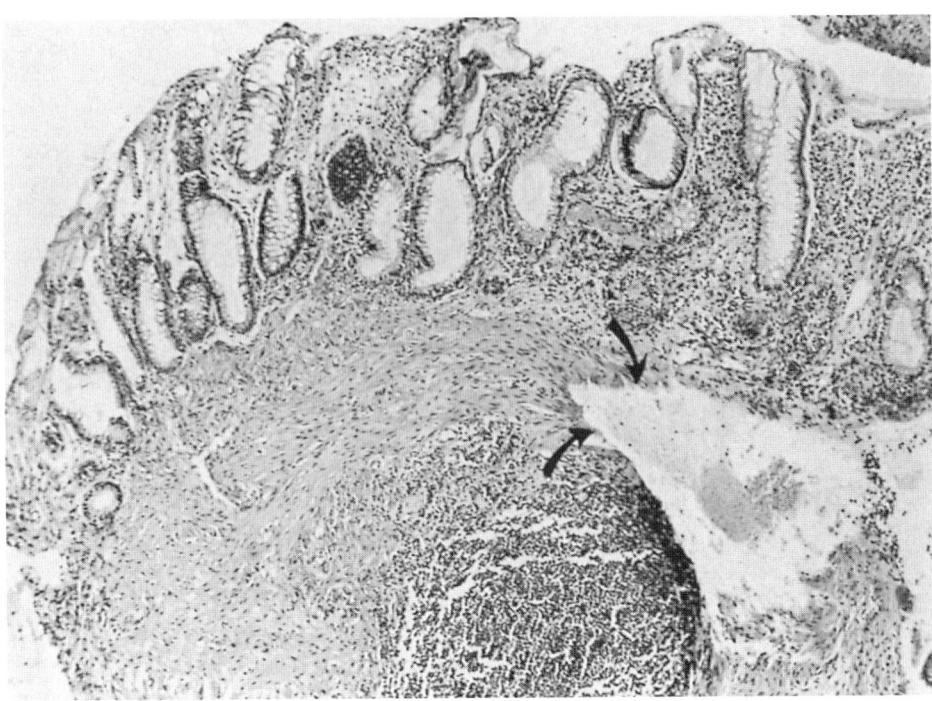

FIGURE 30-43. Crohn's colitis with fistula. A sharply defined early fistula in the submucosa (*arrows*). (Original magnification × 80.) (Courtesy of Rudolf Garret, M.D.)

flammatory changes in the mouth may even be the initial site of involvement.[79] Basu and Asquith reviewed the oral manifestations of IBD, describing a number of lesions.[28] These included recurrent aphthous ulcers, pyoderma gangrenosum, pyostomatitis vegetans, hemorrhagic ulceration, glossitis, macroglossia, and moniliasis. The authors reported that the incidence is not as uncommon as one might expect, with up to 20% having been described as having oral lesions. The most frequently affected areas and their respective appearances are the buccal mucosa (a cobblestone pattern), the vestibule (linear, hyperplastic folds), and the lips (diffusely swollen and indurated).[39]

Aphthous ulcers usually parallel the course or activity of the IBD: the more active the disease, the more likely one is to develop this complication. Biopsy usually shows a chronic inflammatory reaction.

Pyostomatitis vegetans is an unusual manifestation of IBD. Papillary projections of mucous membrane can be seen separated by small areas of ulceration (Figure 30-44). Biopsy may reveal suprabasal separation of the oral epithelium and infiltration with eosinophils.

The recognition of the specific oral granuloma is important, since it may be the first manifestation of Crohn's disease.[449] Scully and colleagues reported 19 patients with clinical evidence of oral Crohn's disease but no intestinal symptoms.[430] More than one-third were demonstrated either on rectal biopsy or by contrast gastrointestinal x-ray films to have IBD, even in the absence of symptoms.

Treatment

Since the lesions are resistant to local therapy, general measures for soothing the oral discomfort are advised. The symptoms and clinical findings of oral problems are often ameliorated with appropriate treatment of the intestinal disease.

Esophageal Involvement

Patients with Crohn's disease of the esophagus will present with symptoms not unlike those associated with other lesions of that organ, such as carcinoma. Substernal discomfort, dysphagia, epigastric pain, weight loss, nausea, and vomiting are all part of the clinical spectrum. Other gastrointestinal symptoms are usually due to the presence of disease elsewhere in the alimentary tract.[112,154,208] It must be remembered that dysphagia and the demonstration of an esophageal ulcer or esophagitis in a patient with known Crohn's disease can be due to reflux esophagitis, certain drugs or corrosive agents, pressure from a nasogastric tube, infectious agents, sarcoidosis, or Behçet's disease.[339] In point of fact, many published reports of esophageal Crohn's disease cannot be supported by critical review.

Physical examination is usually unrewarding with respect to esophageal involvement. Diagnosis is usually made by a high index of suspicion and radiologic investigation, which obviously would include a barium swallow (Figure 30-45). This study may reveal thickened mucosal folds, multiple ulcerations, or, most com-

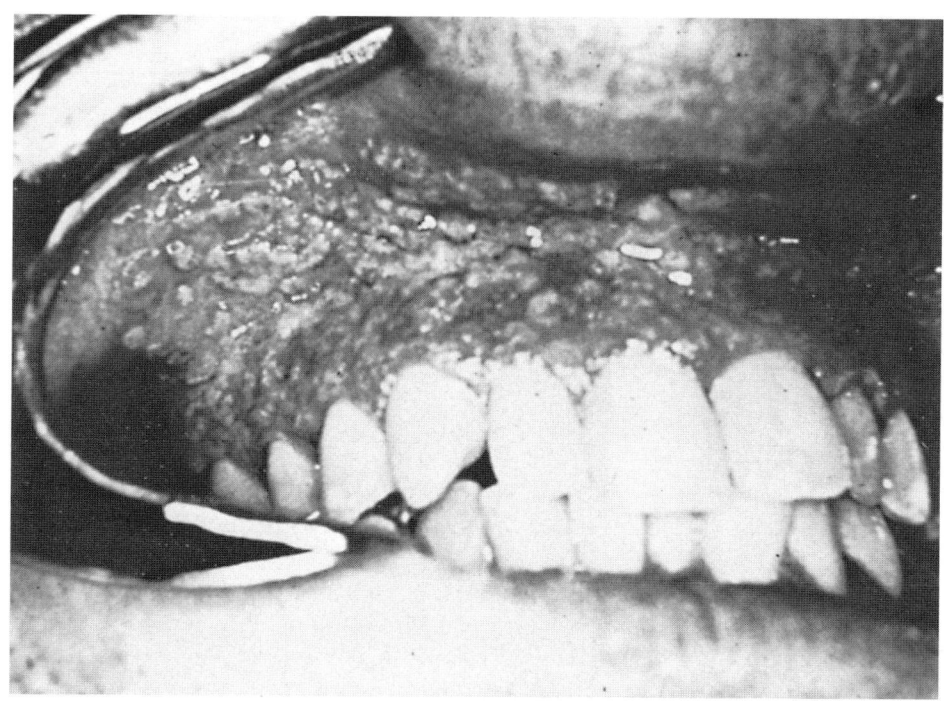

FIGURE 30-44. Pyostomatitis vegetans. Involvement of the gingival mucosa by papillary projections. (From Corman ML, Veidenheimer MC, Nugent FW, et al. *Diseases of the anus, rectum and colon. Part II: Non-specific inflammatory bowel disease.* New York: Medcom, 1976.)

monly, a stricture. This last finding makes differentiation from carcinoma quite difficult, except that the presence of disease elsewhere or the relatively young age of the patient should lead one to suspect an inflammatory process.

Endoscopic examination will usually reveal hyperemia with possibly either an ulcerated mucosa or the presence of an inflammatory stricture. Biopsies usually show an inflammatory reaction, but the absence of granulomata does not exclude the diagnosis of Crohn's disease.[112]

Treatment usually consists of the standard medical management appropriate for Crohn's disease of the small or large bowel (see Chapter 29 and Medical Management). Resection is rarely indicated.

Gastroduodenal Crohn's Disease

Crohn's disease involving the stomach and duodenum may not be as rare as originally suspected. Since the original description in 1937 by Gottlieb and Alpert of the condition in the duodenum, a number of cases have been reported.[172] In 1981 Korelitz and colleagues performed random endoscopic biopsies of the stomach and duodenal mucosa in patients with Crohn's disease, frequently demonstrating the presence of microscopic alterations consistent with this inflammatory process in the upper gastrointestinal tract.[251] Clinically, evident IBD of the gastroduodenal area is believed to occur in approximately 2% or 3% of all patients with Crohn's dis-

ease. The condition can occur without involvement elsewhere in the gastrointestinal tract, but this is extremely uncommon.

Patients usually present with epigastric abdominal symptoms exacerbated by eating—nausea, vomiting, and weight loss. Symptoms may resemble those of ulcer disease. Obstruction, perforation, fistula, and hemorrhage can occur. A fistula into the stomach characteristically produces symptoms of feculent vomiting, eructation, and odor. Duodenocolic fistula is a recognized complication of duodenal disease, but in evaluation of patients with this finding it is important to ascertain whether the fistula arose from inflammatory disease of the intestinal tract outside of the duodenum or from the duodenum, itself (see Figure 30-20). Most observers agree that gastroenteric and duodenoenteric fistulas are almost always due to intestinal disease.

Radiologic investigation may reveal the findings summarized by Cohen.[83] These include antral inflammation, contiguous disease in the duodenum, cobblestone mucosal appearance with thickened folds, reduced distensibility or stricture, and ulceration (Figure 30-46). Barium enema examination is the preferred study for identifying a fistula between the upper gastrointestinal tract and the colon.

Endoscopic examination may reveal ulceration, cobblestoning, or stricture. As with esophageal disease, the absence of granulomata does not necessarily mean that the patient does not have Crohn's. Nugent and Roy found granulomas in 37 of 76 individuals (49%).[344]

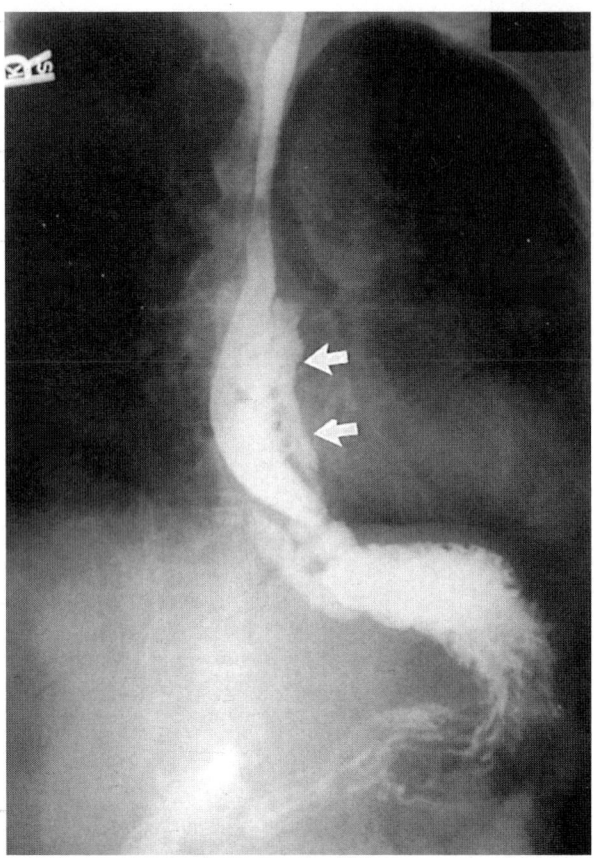

FIGURE 30-45. Esophageal Crohn's disease in patient with known, extensive small bowel involvement. Large ulcerating lesion involving the distal third of the esophagus extending to the gastroesophageal junction, with possible involvement of the cardia. There are irregular superior and inferior margins and a suggestion of two intramural tracts or double-lumen appearance (*arrows*).

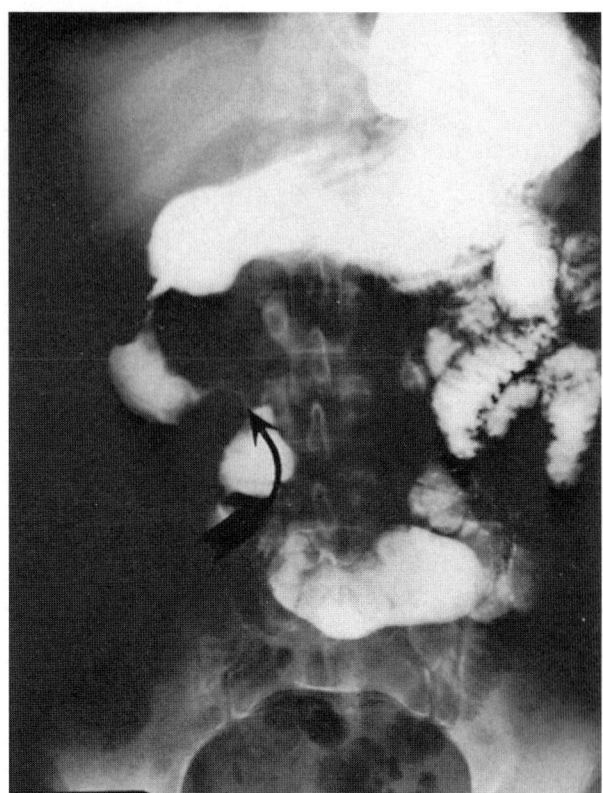

FIGURE 30-46. Duodenal Crohn's disease. This film from an upper GI series demonstrates stricture of the second portion of the duodenum with a fistula from the third portion to the small bowel (*arrow*).

Treatment usually consists of antacids and proton pump inhibitors or H_2 receptor blockers (an antiulcer program), the medical regimens discussed later, hyperalimentation, and possibly surgical intervention. The primary indications for operation are the presence of a fistula and obstruction (see later). If hemorrhage cannot be controlled by medical means, either resectional surgery or oversewing the bleeding point is the treatment of choice. Usually, however, surgery for primary gastroduodenal Crohn's disease can be avoided.

Management of Duodenal Stricture

The most commonly performed operative procedure for duodenal Crohn's disease is gastrojejunostomy, but complications such as bile reflux gastritis, stomal ulceration, blind loop syndrome, and the potential need for a vagotomy are real concerns. Strictureplasty has also been applied for duodenal disease, but in the findings of the Birmingham, England, group, it is associated with a high incidence of postoperative complications, the need for reoperative surgery, and a likelihood of restricture.[519] However, the Cleveland Clinic group undertook duodenal strictureplasty on 13 patients and found that it is a safe and effective operation that should be considered when technically feasible.[514]

A number of cases and reviews have been published on the evaluation and management of the condition as it affects this area.[85,90,125,145,227,413,510] Nugent and colleagues reported 18 patients from the Lahey Clinic who were relieved of obstruction by means of gastrojejunostomy.[343] This was their preferred treatment for those with this duodenal complication. The authors did not advise vagotomy because of the risk of diarrhea and the fact that there was no difference in results between the vagotomized and nonvagotomized groups. A later report from the same institution involved 25 patients who required operation.[332] That study revealed that one-third who underwent bypass required reoperation, usually for marginal ulceration or for gastroduodenal obstruction. Although the authors did not feel that the addition of vagotomy protected against the subsequent development of marginal ulceration, they now recommend that a vagotomy be performed. Shepherd and Alexander-Williams have lent additional support to the concept of vagus nerve interruption when they reported a patient who developed a stomal ulcer 8 weeks following gastroenterostomy without vagotomy.[436]

Management of Gastric and Duodenal Fistulas

When a fistula develops as a consequence of intestinal disease, simple closure of the stomach or duodenum is all that is usually required, along with resection of the involved bowel segment. Gastric fistulas are always due to disease in the intestine. Treatment of the gastric opening is wedge excision. Occasionally, the opening in the duodenum may occur in an area that is difficult to close, such as adjacent to the pancreas. In this situation and when a large defect is created, an omental or jejunal patch, or the creation of a duodenojejunostomy may be necessary. Lee and Schraut reported one death due to a duodenal leakage in 11 patients with fistulas.[267] Greenstein and colleagues noted only nine instances of gastric fistula in a review of 1,480 individuals with Crohn's disease.[180]

Results

Ross and associates reviewed the long-term results of surgery for duodenal Crohn's disease that had been initially reported by Farmer and colleagues.[125,401] Of the 11 patients, seven required a total of 10 further operations; the mean follow-up was approximately 14 years. Indications for subsequent surgery included marginal ulceration, recurrence producing obstruction at the enteroenterostomy, and duodenal fistula. Eight of the 11 also required surgery for Crohn's disease elsewhere in the intestinal tract. The authors concluded that bypass surgery alone was unsatisfactory in the long term and suggested that vagotomy be added at the time of operation. Functional results were felt to be better, particularly if reoperative surgery were done in an expeditious and timely manner.

The Lahey Clinic experience now comprises 89 patients.[344] Their investigators conclude that irrespective of medical or surgical treatment, duodenal Crohn's disease follows a more benign course than when it affects the small bowel or colon.

Pancreatic Manifestations

Pancreatitis or pancreatic insufficiency has occasionally been reported with IBD, but this had been felt to be coincidental. One must be aware, however, of the risk of pancreatitis that may be associated with the administration of mercaptopurine (Purinethol). Seyrig and colleagues identified six patients who were thought to have a non-

fortuitous association.[432] They noted the following, possibly important, clinical distinctions:

- Abdominal pain was absent or moderate, and probably due to bowel involvement.
- Pancreatic calcifications were absent.
- Those patients with pancreatic insufficiency had essentially normal pancreatograms.
- More information will be necessary before one can establish with certainty whether pancreatic disease is truly an extra-intestinal manifestation of IBD.

Hepatobiliary Disease

Liver function studies and liver biopsy often demonstrate abnormal results in both ulcerative colitis and Crohn's disease patients. Cohen and associates performed a prospective study of liver function in 50 consecutive patients with regional enteritis.[82] Thirty percent had abnormal results, most commonly an elevation of the serum alkaline phosphatase, but none had significant liver disease. Fifteen patients of the 19 who underwent liver biopsy had evidence of chronic pericholangitis. Others reported an even higher associated incidence of liver abnormalities.[93,105] The reasons for the association between hepatobiliary disease and IBD are not known, but a number of studies have postulated that recurrent cholangitis is due to a portal bacteremia from the interrupted intestinal mucosa, in addition to a probable genetic predisposition.[74] Hepatoportal venous gas has been seen in patients with known Crohn's disease.[12]

Gallbladder

Cholelithiasis has been reported in up to one-third of patients with IBD, especially in those with Crohn's ileitis.[82] The explanation for this association is believed to involve the enterohepatic circulation. Disease or resection of the terminal ileum leads to loss or malabsorption of bile acids. Since the solubility of cholesterol depends on bile acids, excessive loss may precipitate this substance. This, in turn, may result in stone formation. Another explanation may be the colonization of the terminal ileum by anaerobic bacteria that deconjugate the bile acids to less-well-absorbed substances. It is not clear, however, that there is a higher incidence of gallstones in patients with Crohn's disease than in individuals with ulcerative colitis. Lorusso and colleagues demonstrated an increased risk of gallstones in both conditions, but it was highest in those with Crohn's disease involving the distal ileum.[293] Because of the high prevalence of cholelithiasis in the population, gallbladder imaging has been recommended preoperatively and in the follow-up of IBD patients.[259]

A different perspective was expressed by Chew and colleagues.[73] They retrospectively studied 134 of their patients who had undergone ileocolic resection for Crohn's disease by means of a questionnaire, using a control group matched for age and gender. There was no significant difference between the groups with respect to prevalence of cholecystectomy. However, those who had more than 30 cm of ileum removed were more likely to have undergone a cholecystectomy. The investigators concluded that synchronous prophylactic cholecystectomy with ileocolic resection cannot be justified on the basis of their data.[73]

Fatty Degeneration

Fatty degeneration is probably the most frequently encountered microscopic abnormality (Figure 30-47). The incidence has been reported to be as high as 80% and to be due to the relatively poor nutritional state of many colitic patients.[74] Occasionally, a granuloma may be seen (Figure 30-48). Treatment is directed toward correction of the malnutrition.

Pericholangitis

Another common histologic manifestation of liver disease is pericholangitis (Figure 30-48). A more accurate term is *portal triaditis,* because of involvement of bile ductules, portal venules, lymphatics, and hepatic parenchyma.[74] The condition may present with jaundice, abdominal pain, fever, and pruritus. Many patients, however, are asymptomatic. Bacterial infection and an autoimmune process have been implicated as possible causative factors. There is no specific treatment for this condition.

Hepatitis

Chronic active hepatitis occurs in only 1% of patients with IBD. Conversely, the incidence of IBD in patients with chronic active hepatitis varies from 4% to 30%.[74] Patients have been reported to improve following removal of diseased bowel.

Sclerosing Cholangitis

One of the most serious, albeit rare, consequences of IBD that occurs as a complication of both ulcerative colitis and Crohn's disease is primary sclerosing cholangitis. Olsson and associates diagnosed this condition in 3.7% of individuals with ulcerative colitis.[350] La Russo and colleagues reported that 70% of their patients with primary sclerosing cholangitis had IBD.[262] Broomé and co-workers determined in their evaluation of 76 patients with primary sclerosing cholangitis that histologic changes within the bowel itself may be observed and may actually precede development of clinical symptoms by as much as 7 years.[54] The importance of identifying such individuals cannot be overestimated. It has been suggested that even the preclinical manifestations of IBD may subject that individual to an increased risk for the development of malignancy.

Primary sclerosing cholangitis has been much more common in patients with ulcerative colitis than in those with Crohn's disease. The cause is unknown, but toxins, infectious agents, altered immunity, and a genetic predisposition have been suggested.[262] To establish this diagnosis there must be no prior history of biliary surgery or gallstones, no diffuse involvement of the extra-hepatic biliary ducts, and the absence of subsequent development of cholangiocarcinoma.[494] Symptoms include right upper quadrant abdominal pain, vomiting, jaundice, and

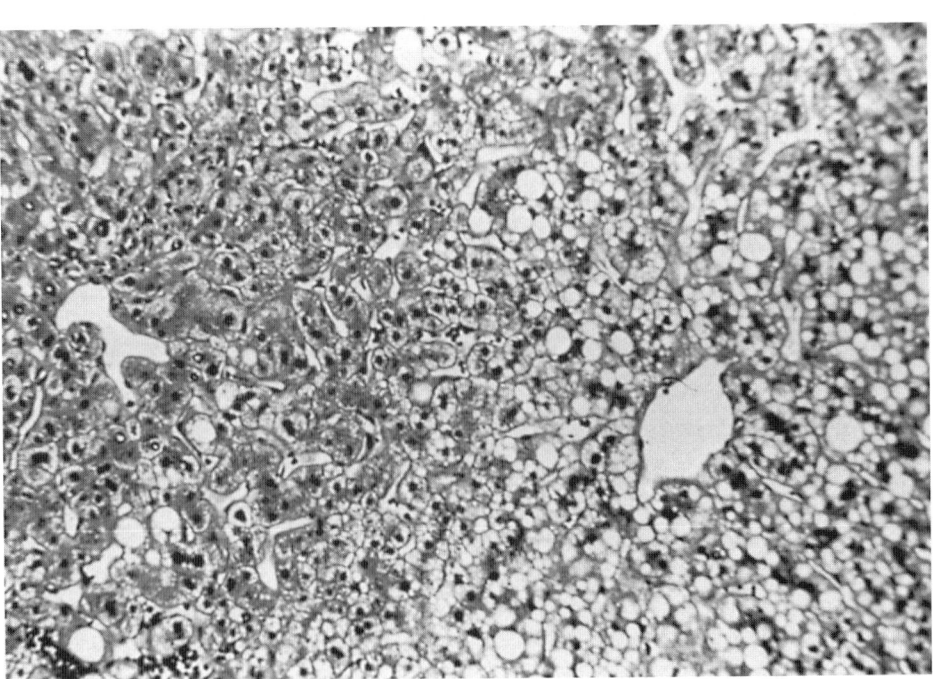

FIGURE 30-47. Fatty degeneration of the liver. Note the fat globules in the liver parenchyma. (Original magnification × 260.) (From Corman ML, Veidenheimer MC, Nugent FW, et al. *Diseases of the anus, rectum and colon. Part II: Non-specific inflammatory bowel disease.* New York: Medcom, 1976.)

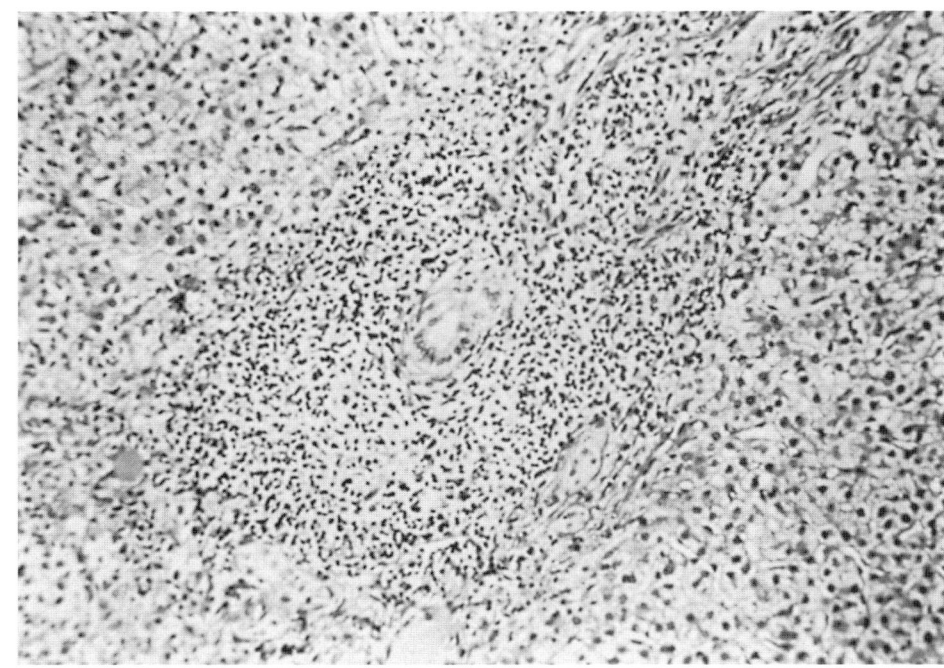

FIGURE 30-48. Pericholangitis. An inflammatory infiltrate within the portal areas surrounds the bile ducts and may result in cirrhosis through a process of progressive fibrosis. (Original magnification × 260.) (From Corman ML, Veidenheimer MC, Nugent FW, et al. *Diseases of the anus, rectum and colon. Part II: Nonspecific inflammatory bowel disease.* New York: Medcom, 1976.)

pruritus. Laboratory studies demonstrate the usual changes suggestive of an obstructive jaundice. Cholangiogram reveals a strictured bile duct (Figure 30-49). In contrast to other extra-intestinal manifestations of IBD, when the sclerosing cholangitis has been established, removal of the diseased colon *does not reverse the condition*.

The disease is progressive and ultimately fatal, except if a liver transplantation is performed. Shaked and co-workers reported their experience with 36 patients who underwent orthotopic liver transplantation for primary sclerosing cholangitis, utilizing immunosuppression with cyclosporine, azathioprine, and steroids.[434] Of these individuals, 29 were known to have chronic ulcerative colitis. The investigators demonstrated that liver replacement and immunosuppression in those suffering from sclerosing cholangitis and ulcerative colitis do not alter the course of the colonic disease. Bleday and colleagues have demonstrated that there appears to be a group of patients who have undergone liver transplant who rapidly develop colorectal malignancy.[43] These individuals require frequent, long-term surveillance following transplant. This suggests that the immunosuppressive agents employed for managing patients who have undergone orthotopic liver transplantation may have a pejorative effect on the colon through increased predisposition for the development of malignancy. But there is no evidence to suggest an association between sclerosing cholangitis itself and colorectal carcinoma in patients with IBD.[341] However, a number of cases of carcinoma of the gallbladder have been described in individuals with sclerosing cholangitis and ulcerative colitis.[106]

Interestingly, despite massive immunosuppression associated with transplanting small intestine, histologically confirmed recurrent Crohn's disease has been demonstrated in the transplanted bowel.[463]

Cangemi and colleagues prospectively compared the progression of clinical, biochemical, cholangiographic, and hepatic histologic features in 45 patients with both primary sclerosing cholangitis and ulcerative colitis, 20 of whom underwent proctocolectomy and 25 of whom had not.[65] No beneficial effect was seen as a consequence of the operation. Because of the profoundly serious consequences of progressive cholangitis, a case may be made for "prophylactic" removal of the inflammatory bowel process if early changes in the biliary tract are observed. This has been suggested even when the gastrointestinal manifestations are quite minimal, but there is no evidence to support implementation of this concept. Still, if surgical treatment is needed for the IBD itself, those with well-controlled primary sclerosing cholangitis can undergo such operations as restorative proctocolectomy safely (for ulcerative colitis).[367]

Cirrhosis

Although cirrhosis is an uncommon complication of IBD, it has, in the past at least, been felt to cause 10% of deaths.[74] When it occurs it is usually a consequence of sclerosing cholangitis. Patients may develop the characteristic stigmata of portal hypertension, including bleeding esophageal varices, and ileostomy hemorrhage (see Chapter 31).

Carcinoma of the Bile Duct

Carcinoma of the bile duct arising in a patient with ulcerative colitis is a rare complication. The association was originally described by Parker and Kendall in 1954.[358] In 1974, Ritchie and colleagues identified 67 cases.[395] The

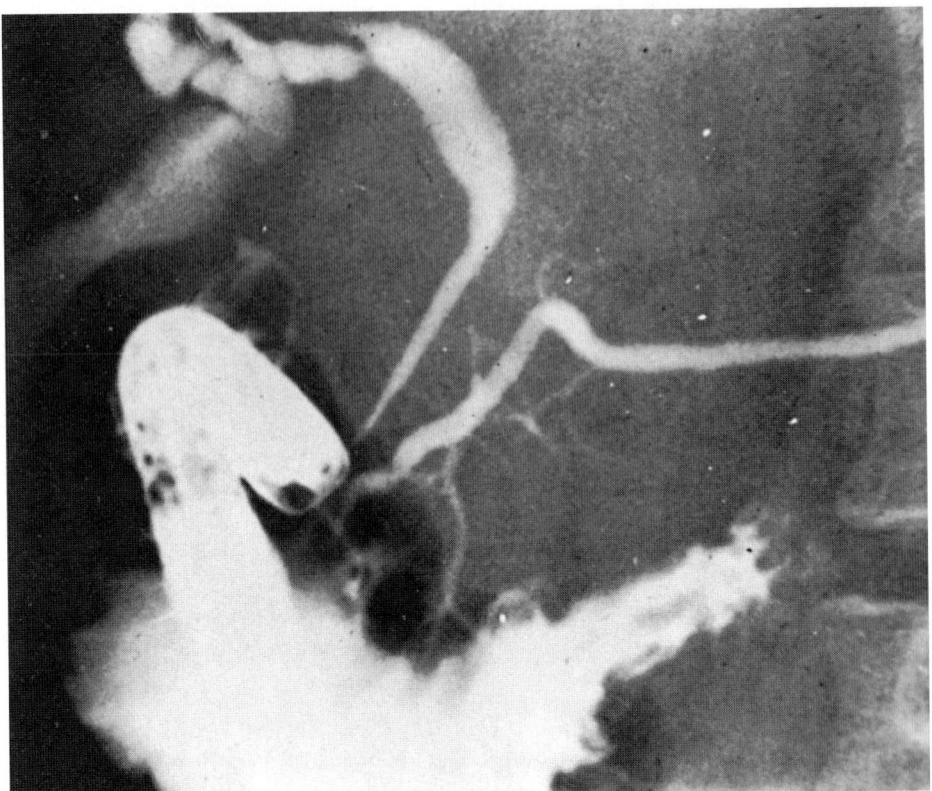

FIGURE 30-49. Sclerosing cholangitis endoscopic retrograde cholangiopancreatography (ERCP) demonstrates narrowing of the distal common bile duct with complete obstruction at the level of the common hepatic duct. (From Corman ML, Veidenheimer MC, Nugent FW, et al. *Diseases of the anus, rectum and colon. Part II: Non-specific inflammatory bowel disease.* New York: Medcom, 1976.)

condition is more common in men and is usually seen in patients who have had a prolonged history of colitis. Patients give a history of typical biliary obstruction with painless jaundice, weight loss, and pruritic symptoms. Diagnosis is usually confirmed by ultrasound demonstration of dilated intrahepatic ducts and by endoscopic retrograde cholangiography. Prognosis is poor, with biliary diversion the usual surgical approach.[505]

Cutaneous Manifestations

Pyoderma Gangrenosum

Pyoderma gangrenosum is a condition found exclusively in individuals with IBD but is fortunately uncommon, occurring in no more than 2% of patients.[323] Schoetz and associates identified eight of 961 with Crohn's disease (an incidence of 0.8%).[427] The vast majority of patients have active intestinal disease at the time the pyoderma develops, although in rare cases the skin lesions may antedate apparent bowel involvement.[323] Clinically, the lesion appears as a spreading, undermining ulceration that has a characteristic violaceous border (Figs. 30-50 and 30-51). It is usually found on the extremities, the most common location being the anterior tibial area.[371] However, the ulcers can occur on the trunk, buttocks, and other places. Usually, there are only one or two lesions, but these can be of considerable size.

Biopsy shows no definite characteristics that would identify the ulcer as being specific for a complication associated with IBD. A vasculitis has been suggested as a possible etiology.

Treatment consists of administration of systemic steroids and occasionally intralesional steroids, and, of course, the management of the colitis.[166] Successful response to topical disodium cromoglycate (DSG) has been reported.[69] Since it is known that DSG prevents the release of histamine from mast cells, an allergic component may be involved in the mechanism for its efficacy. Topical measures also should include appropriate antibiotics if culture suggests the value of such treatment or if lymphangitis or cellulitis is present. As with so many other extra-intestinal manifestations, the course of the pyoderma parallels the clinical progress of the intestinal disease.

Rarely does the skin condition assume such significance that colectomy must be performed for this indication alone. I have experienced a situation in which a total colectomy with preservation of the rectum resulted in 90% healing of the pyoderma, but the residual skin problem failed to clear until proctectomy was subsequently performed (Figure 30-52).

Polyarteritis Nodosa

Polyarteritis nodosa is a rare cutaneous manifestation of Crohn's disease. Kahn and colleagues reviewed 11 cases in the literature and added one of their own.[283] The

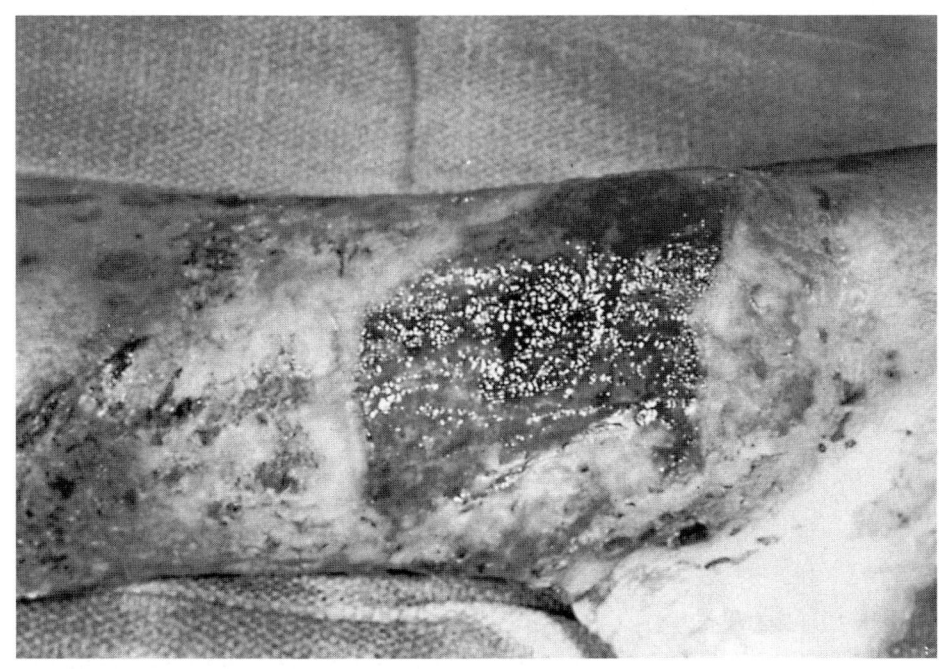

FIGURE 30-50. Pyoderma gangrenosum. Irregularly outlined, sharply defined ulceration with edematous edges and pyodermatous base in a patient with ulcerative colitis. (Courtesy of Rudolf Garret, M.D.)

presence of erythematous, tender nodules in the extremities should lead one to suspect the diagnosis. Biopsy or excision may reveal an arteritis with luminal narrowing by fibrinous thrombus.

The relationship of the cutaneous manifestation to systemic polyarteritis nodosa is controversial, but in the case reported by the authors, when subsequent resection of the bowel was carried out, there was no evidence of such an arteritis. The condition should be distinguished from other cutaneous manifestations, such as those in the following discussion.

Erythema Nodosum

Erythema nodosum is another cutaneous manifestation that is relatively uncommonly seen with IBD with up to 5% of patients reported to be afflicted.[231] In a report

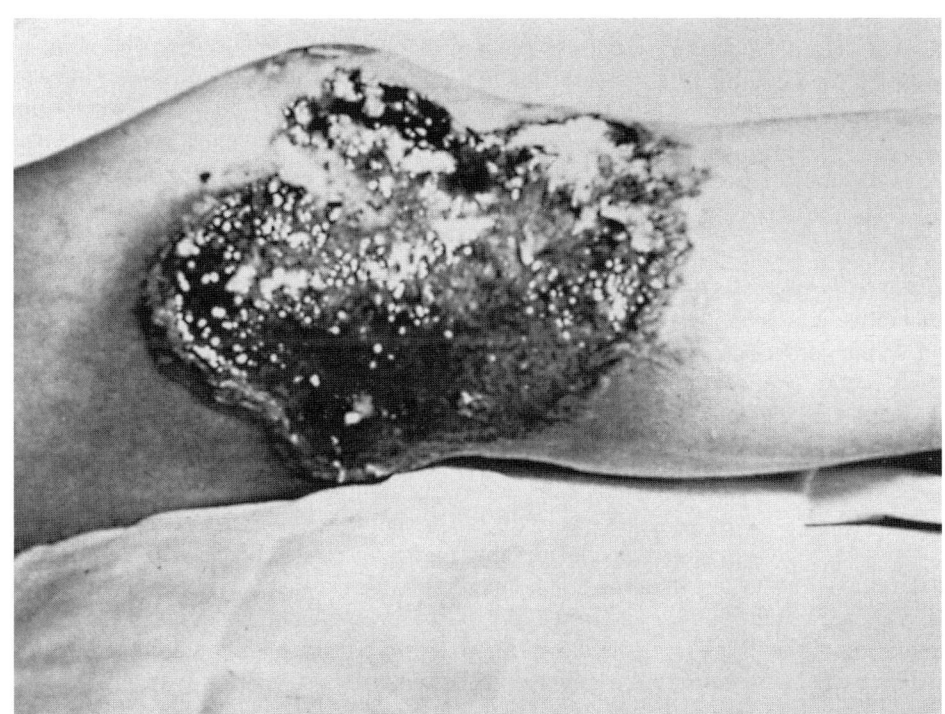

FIGURE 30-51. Pyoderma gangrenosum. An undermined ulcer with a violaceous border. (From Corman ML, Veidenheimer MC, Nugent FW, et al. *Diseases of the anus, rectum and colon. Part II: Non-specific inflammatory bowel disease.* New York: Medcom, 1976.)

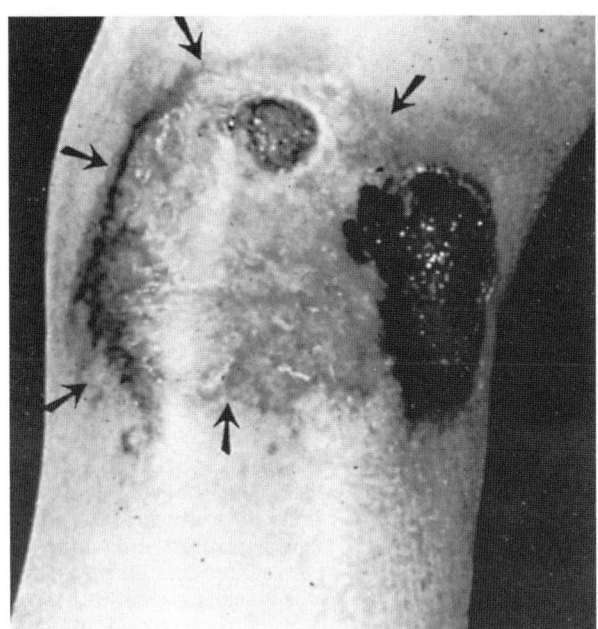

FIGURE 30-52. Pyoderma gangrenosum. In this photograph taken 1 month following a protocolectomy, a much smaller ulcer is evident. Compare this with the original lesion (outlined by *arrows*). (From Corman ML, Veidenheimer MC, Nugent FW, et al. *Diseases of the anus, rectum and colon. Part II: Nonspecific inflammatory bowel disease.* New York: Medcom, 1976.)

from the Cleveland Clinic, 90% had active bowel disease at the time skin lesions developed.[323] In their experience, erythema nodosum typically occurred as a single episode and lasted for several days, associated with active bowel disease and joint symptoms. Tender, subcutaneous nodules are usually seen on the pretibial aspects of the legs. As with other extra-colonic manifestations, the clinical course usually parallels that of the intestinal disease.

Psoriasis

There appears to be an increased risk for the development of psoriasis in patients with IBD.[223,399] In a report by Yates and colleagues, the prevalence of psoriasis in Crohn's disease (11.2%) and in ulcerative colitis (5.7%) was significantly greater than that of the control group (1.5%).[522] The increased association of the two conditions as well as the higher rate of psoriasis in first-degree relatives of Crohn's patients implies the possibility of a genetic link.[266]

Cutaneous Crohn's Disease

Crohn's disease of the skin can develop with the characteristic histologic feature of the bowel condition—specifically, granulomatous inflammation of the dermis. When this occurs other than by direct extension from the gastrointestinal tract, it has been given what I consider to be a poor but now accepted term, *metastatic cu-*

taneous Crohn's disease. Fewer than 50 cases have been reported.[188,278,444,465,484] The condition has a variable macroscopic appearance, including ulceration, erythema, and nodularity. Biopsy is required to establish the diagnosis, with differentiation from sarcoidosis a potential problem, since the two diseases have similar cutaneous findings.[314] Treatment by means of intralesional steroid therapy has been attempted with usually transient improvement. Therapeutic benefit has also been achieved with oral metronidazole (Flagyl).[46,428]

Arthritis and Rheumatologic Conditions

Depending on the interpretation of what truly constitutes arthritic or rheumatologic conditions associated with IBD, there are perhaps as many as four clinical patterns: a peripheral joint synovitis that is closely related to the activity of the bowel disease (15% to 20% of patients); second, ankylosing spondylitis (3% to 6%), in which the relationship with the bowel disorder is less clearly defined; third, a bilateral symmetric sacroiliitis (5% to 15%); and a fourth category, which includes rheumatic complications, such as granulomas of bones and joints, clubbing, periostitis, osteomalacia, osteoporosis, septic arthritis, and complications of corticosteroid therapy.[173,338]

Colitic Arthritis

Colitic arthritis or enteropathic arthritis is the most common joint manifestation of IBD and is seen more frequently with Crohn's disease than with ulcerative colitis. The large joints are primarily involved (knees, ankles, elbows, and wrists). They may be swollen, warm, and red (Figure 30-53). The appearance may not be dissimilar to that of rheumatoid arthritis, but it is nondeforming and seronegative: that is, rheumatoid factor is absent from the blood. Although any joint may be attacked, small joints are less frequently affected (Figure 30-54).

Symptoms of the arthritis usually develop after the IBD has been diagnosed and tend to parallel the course of the intestinal disease. The inflammation is usually adequately controlled by means of antiinflammatory agents or by the use of steroids. The arthritis completely resolves after colectomy.

Rheumatoid Spondylitis

As stated, other joint disorders that may be encountered are severe arthralgias and rheumatoid spondylitis.[1,173,228,312,528] The incidence of rheumatoid spondylitis is considerably higher in patients with IBD than in the general population, with estimates ranging in excess of 20 times. The well-known gender incidence (4:1 ratio of men to women) is reversed when rheumatoid spondylitis complicates IBD. A genetic association between the two diseases has been demonstrated. In contradistinction to most other extra-colonic manifestations, spondylitis does

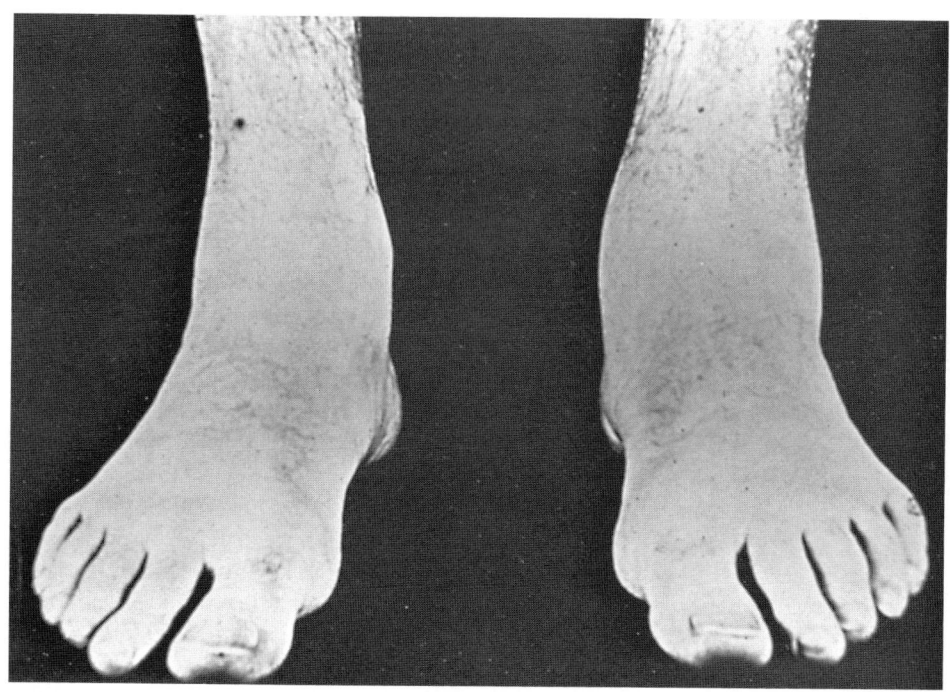

not parallel the activity of the bowel disease. The incidence is similar in Crohn's disease and ulcerative colitis.

The patient initially develops pain in the lumbosacral region, but the discomfort may rapidly progress to involve the thoracic and cervical spine. As ankylosis progresses, the patient exhibits the characteristic dorsal kyphosis (Figure 30-55). Interestingly, isolated asymptomatic sacroiliitis occurs more often than does spinal involvement (4% to 18%).[173]

Treatment consists of physiotherapy, antiinflammatory agents, and steroids. Colectomy is not indicated for the treatment of the arthritic manifestations.

Hypertrophic Osteoarthropathy or Finger Clubbing

Finger clubbing has also been reported in association with IBD. It may regress after resection of the involved bowel segment and usually correlates with disease activity.[142]

Polymyositis

Polymyositis has been reported on rare occasions to be a condition associated with IBD, especially ulcerative colitis.[75] As with other unusual extra-intestinal manifestations, one must always be concerned about the possibility that the condition may be simply coincidental. Still, because of the possible autoimmune etiology of the two diseases, a causal link may be considered plausible.

Bronchopulmonary Disease

Pulmonary manifestations have been said to be associated with IBD, including bronchiectasis, granulomatous lung disease, interstitial fibrosis, and sulfasalazine pneumonitis.[14,272] Storch and co-workers reported more than 400 instances, categorizing the cases by disease mechanism into drug-induced disease, anatomic disease, overlap syndromes, autoimmune disease, physiologic conse-

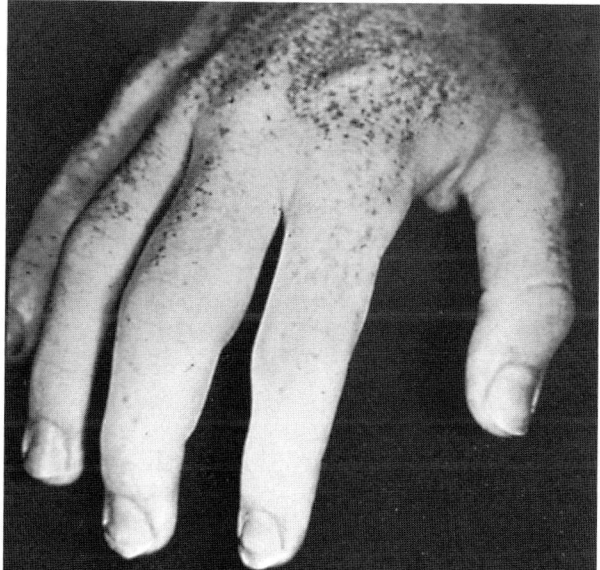

FIGURE 30-54. Colitic arthritis. Proximal interphalangeal joint involvement in a 20-year-old man with acute ulcerative colitis. (From Corman ML, Veidenheimer MC, Nugent FW, et al. *Diseases of the anus, rectum and colon. Part II: Non-specific inflammatory bowel disease.* New York: Medcom, 1976.)

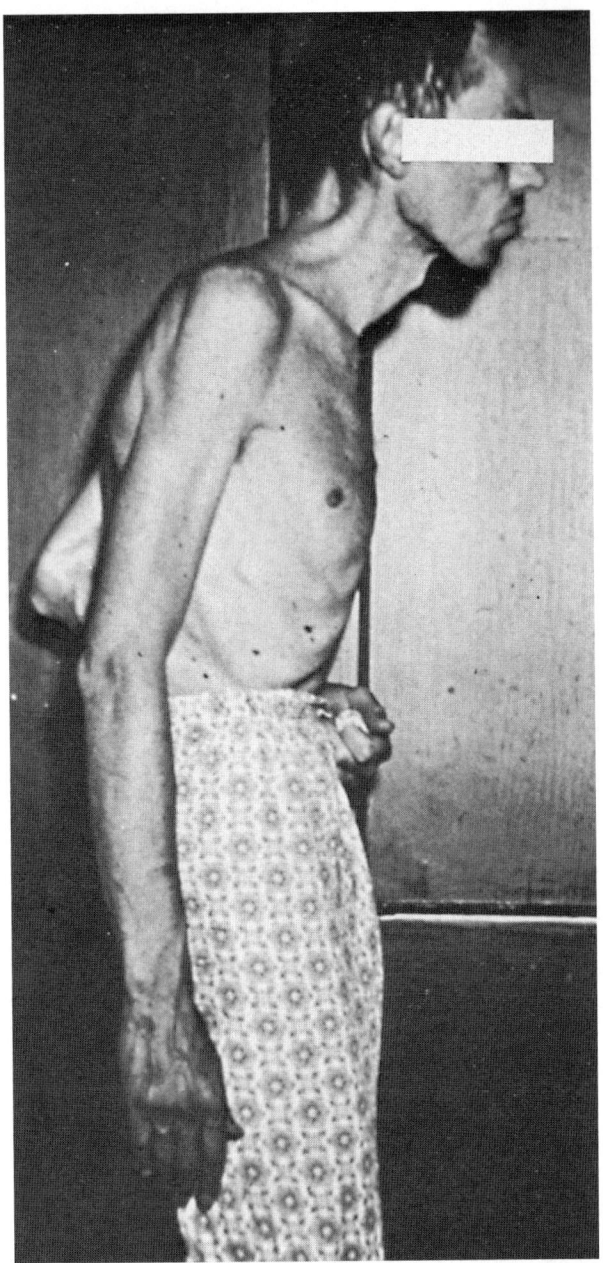

FIGURE 30-55. Rheumatoid spondylitis. Note the kyphosis in this patient with chronic ulcerative colitis. (From Corman ML, Veidenheimer MC, Nugent FW, et al. *Diseases of the anus, rectum and colon. Part II: Non-specific inflammatory bowel disease.* New York: Medcom, 1976.)

quences of IBD, pulmonary function test abnormalities, and nonspecific lung disease.[461] The authors conclude that manifestations of IBD in the lung vary and often present a confounding diagnostic problem, necessitating a complex work-up.[461] Investigation of respiratory factors in patients with Crohn's disease free of clinical pulmonary symptoms and with normal chest roentgenograms was studied by Bonniere and colleagues.[48] This included serum angiotensin-converting enzyme, pulmonary func-

tion tests, bronchoalveolar lavage, and pulmonary scanning. Results suggest that most patients with Crohn's disease have a much higher frequency of latent lung abnormalities than would be expected in a control population.

Ocular Manifestations

Ocular disease, including orbital congestion, uveitis, conjunctivitis, iritis, and keratitis, are found in up to 10% of patients with IBD. The most common ocular lesion is episcleritis, an inflammation overlying the sclera, under the conjunctiva. A thickened, deep red appearance is usually noted in one segment of the eye (Figure 30-56). Burning, itching, and pain are the primary symptoms, but the patient often seeks medical attention because of the appearance. Steroids and antiinflammatory agents are the treatments of choice. Episcleritis is often associated with exacerbations of the underlying IBD but is unrelated to extent or severity.[14] Because of the complications that may lead to a chorioretinitis, ophthalmologic consultation is advised.

Uveitis usually produces ocular pain, blurred vision, and headache, and may occur whether the underlying disease is symptomatic or in remission.[14] The diagnosis is established by slit-lamp examination. Treatment consists of pupillary dilatation to relieve spasm, an eye patch, and the application of topical corticosteroids.

Amyloidosis

Secondary amyloidosis was initially described in 1949 by Cohen and Fishman in a patient with IBD and is still a rare reported finding.[80] When recognized, it occurs almost exclusively with Crohn's disease. The diagnosis has been made usually at postmortem examination, although confirmation has been established in a few patients who presented with renal failure and who underwent renal biopsy.[14] In the absence of kidney dysfunction, a search for secondary amyloidosis is probably not justified.[294] The application of rectal biopsy for establishing the diagnosis is discussed in Chapter 25. Regression of proteinuria and other manifestations of renal as well as hepatic dysfunction has been reported following bowel resection.[114,144,161]

Urologic Complications

Urologic complications are commonly seen in association with IBD. These include chronic interstitial nephritis, chronic pyelonephritis, acute tubular necrosis, urinary fistulas, ureteral obstruction, and nephrolithiasis.

Ureteral Obstruction

Ureteral obstruction is much more frequently identified in association with Crohn's disease than with ulcerative colitis (Figure 30-57). The incidence has been reported to be as high as 50% in this group of patients. An inflammatory mass involving the terminal ileum and oc-

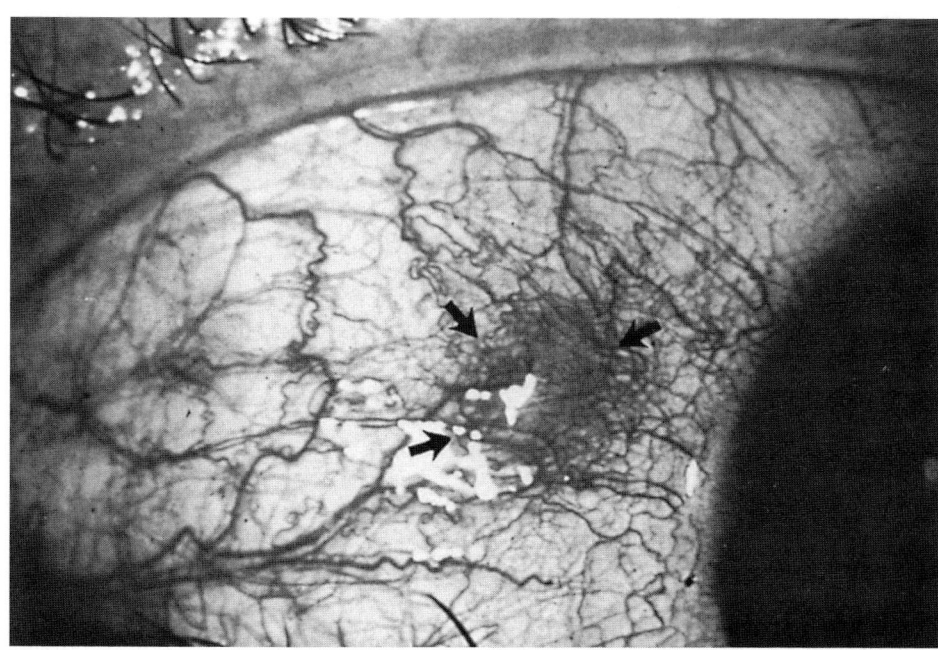

FIGURE 30-56. Episcleritis. Note the nodular, focal, erythematous lesion (*arrows*). (From Corman ML, Veidenheimer MC, Nugent FW, et al. *Diseases of the anus, rectum and colon. Part II: Non-specific inflammatory bowel disease.* New York: Medcom, 1976.)

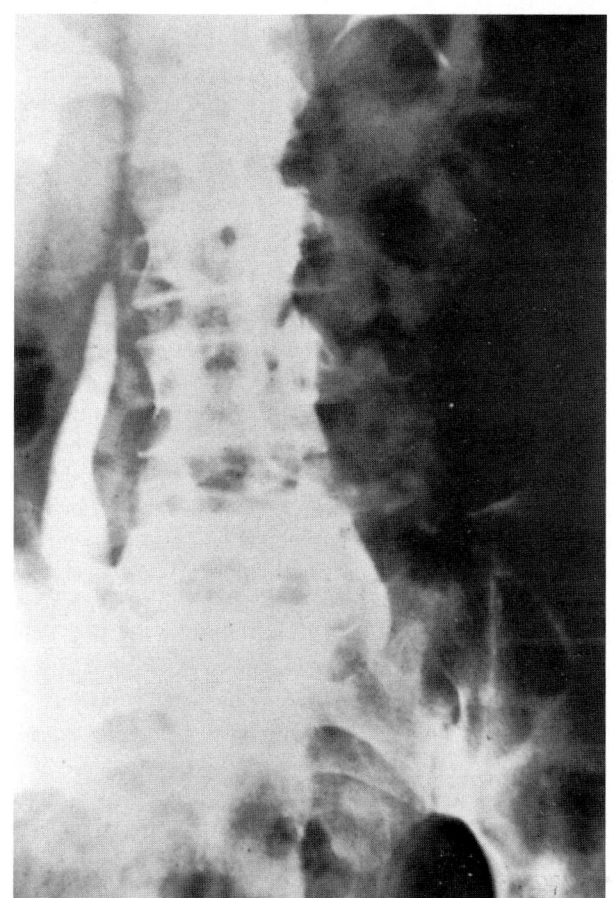

FIGURE 30-57. Ureteral obstruction in a patient with distal ileitis and pelvic abscess. Note the dilated right collecting system and the right ureter. (From Corman ML, Veidenheimer MC, Nugent FW, et al. *Diseases of the anus, rectum and colon. Part II: Non-specific inflammatory bowel disease.* New York: Medcom, 1976.)

casionally the sigmoid colon can produce extrinsic compression of the distal ureters, with the right more frequently involved than the left. The result is hydroureter, hydronephrosis, and possibly, caliectasis. Symptoms related to the urinary tract may be minimal, and if present may actually be due to compression of the bladder by an inflammatory mass rather than to the obstruction of a ureter. Flank pain is suggestive of ureteral obstruction.

Treatment involves removal of the mass that is causing the compression. Complete resolution may be expected, assuming that the obstruction has not produced irreversible renal damage. Preoperative identification of ureteral dilatation should warn the surgeon that a meticulous dissection may be required to avoid ureteral injury (see Chapter 23). The preoperative placement of ureteral catheters should be considered.

Nephrolithiasis and Bladder Calculi

Nephrolithiasis and bladder calculi are seen in at least 5% of individuals with IBD. Following proctocolectomy and ileostomy, patients are still at risk for the development of nephrolithiasis. Many factors contribute to the development of calculi in chronic IBD: decreased urine volume, increased crystalloid concentration, urinary electrolyte and pH changes, and recurrent urinary tract infections. The more acid urine favors precipitation of urates, and, as a result, uric acid calculi are more common in patients with IBD than in the "normal" population of stone formers. Intestinal absorption of oxalate is increased when ileal disease is present, and this is a further reason for formation of stones. Figure 30-58 demonstrates numerous bladder calculi that developed in a 60-year-old man who had extensive Crohn's disease of the small intestine for more than 20 years.

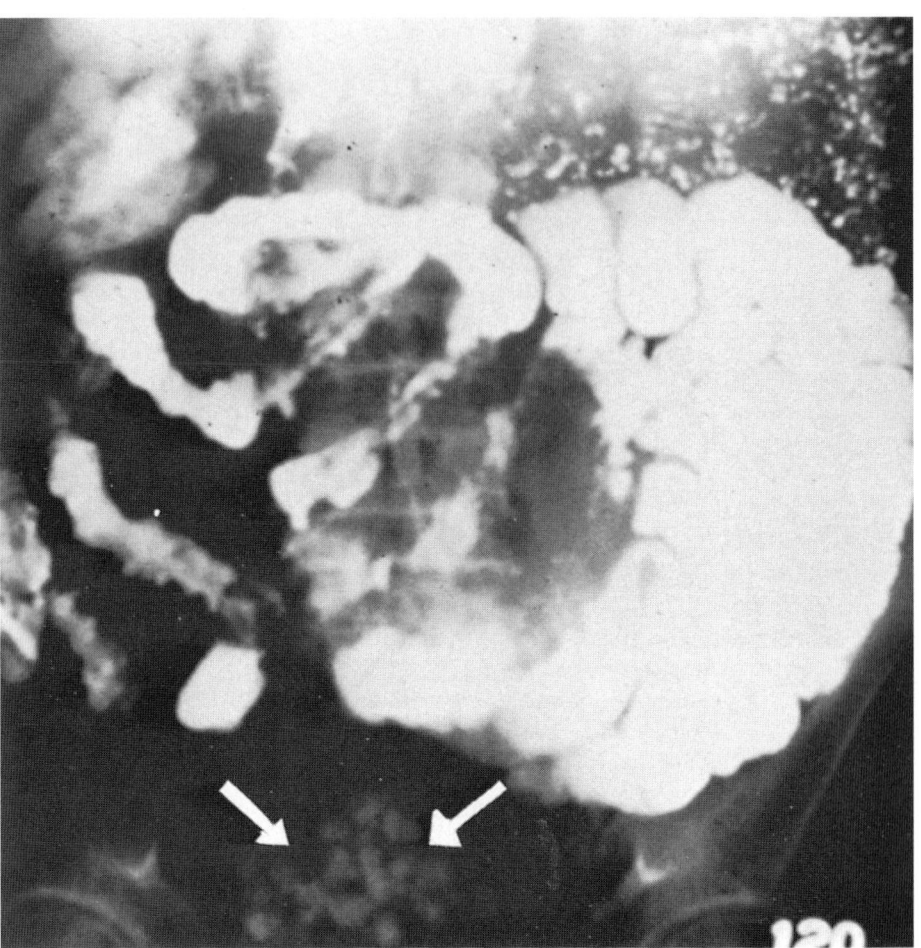

FIGURE 30-58. Bladder calculi (*arrows*) in a patient with long-standing Crohn's disease. (From Corman ML, Veidenheimer MC, Nugent FW, et al. *Diseases of the anus, rectum and colon. Part II: Non-specific inflammatory bowel disease.* New York: Medcom, 1976.)

Bambach and associates reported that 10% of patients who underwent resection for IBD gave a history of urinary stone formation after surgery.[25] Ileostomy patients were demonstrated to have a significantly lowered urinary pH and volume, and a higher concentration of calcium, oxalate, and uric acid. The authors advise close follow-up of patients with ileostomies and with small bowel resections in particular, in order to assess fecal losses and urinary composition. Ideally, patients who are at an increased risk for the formation of urinary stones could then be identified.

An adequate urinary volume should be maintained by encouraging the patient to consume sufficient water to increase urinary volume without increasing ileostomy output, by alkalinization in selected patients, by a diet low in oxalate and fat, and by "slowing" medications to reduce the ileostomy volume.[25]

Psoas Abscess

Psoas abscess has long been recognized as a complication of Crohn's disease, but it has also been found, albeit rarely, with ulcerative colitis.[4,490] In the experience of the Cleveland Clinic group, 73% of individuals presenting with this manifestation had regional enteritis.[383] When seen as a consequence of Crohn's disease it may be the result of a fistula or abscess from the terminal ileum on the right side or of disease of the jejunum or sigmoid on the left.[275] Pain in the iliac fossa, abdomen, groin, or hip is the usual symptom. Chills and fever, abdominal or flank mass, and an associated cutaneous fistula may be apparent. Drainage of the abscess with appropriate bowel resection is the preferred treatment, in addition to adequate, prolonged antibiotic coverage. Extension of the septic process with establishment of a spinal extradural abscess requiring emergency laminectomy has been reported.[6]

Cardiac Complications

Cardiac complications in association with IBD are extremely unusual, with pericarditis being the most frequently described. Ballinger and Farthing postulate that heart block may, in some individuals, be a complication of ulcerative colitis and not a coincidental association.[24] Others opine that IBD may be considered an independent risk factor for the development of bacterial endocarditis.[257] Therefore, endocarditis prophylaxis should be considered, according to some investigators, even in the absence of predisposing primary cardiac factors for the development of bacterial endocarditis.[257]

Other Manifestations

A number of other conditions have been suggested to be associated with nonspecific IBD. Evidence of Crohn's disease has been found in voluntary muscle, the larynx, and the ovary. Whether these and other manifestations, such as hyperthyroidism, hyperparathyroidism, and hematologic problems are coincidental has not been clearly established.

Relationship to Carcinoma

For many years it was felt that there was no increased risk for the development of carcinoma in patients who had Crohn's disease. However, an accumulation of published reports beginning in the 1960s seems to indicate an exponential increase in the frequency of this observation.[404] Some have suggested that the observations are merely coincidental. Most investigators, however, accept the thesis that such a relationship does indeed exist.[15,37,51,86,158,175,192,253,261,390,423,455,521] This association is not equivalent to that which has been observed in long-standing, chronic ulcerative colitis, however.

In 1980, Zinkin and Brandwein identified 43 patients with adenocarcinoma arising in a segment of Crohn's colitis and added one of their own.[527] Hawker and associates reviewed the literature on Crohn's disease of the small intestine and identified 61 cases, including their own experience.[207] There were 41 tumors of the ileum, 18 of the jejunum, one in the duodenum and ileum, and one in the ileum and colon. Eighteen occurred in bypassed intestinal loops. More recently, Rubio and colleagues found 174 small and large bowel cancers occurring in Crohn's disease in their literature review. Stahl and co-workers identified 22 patients with malignancies at the Lahey Clinic.[455] The median age at diagnosis of Crohn's disease was 37 years and at diagnosis of carcinoma was 54 years.

It is very difficult to assess the true incidence of Crohn's disease and carcinoma in the small intestine because small bowel carcinoma is such a rare condition. However, the association appears genuine and is based on several observations. There is a different distribution of small bowel cancer in Crohn's disease when compared with cancer of the small intestine that occurs in the absence of this inflammatory condition. In Crohn's disease, two-thirds of the small bowel cancers occur in the ileum, whereas no more than 30% develop in this area when it is not involved by disease.[207] In the large intestine, Crohn's disease with cancer is usually found on the right side of the colon, as compared with the usual more distal bowel

involvement in the general population. In a study from Birmingham, England, Gyde and colleagues demonstrated a significant excess of tumors in both the upper and lower gastrointestinal tract in patients with Crohn's disease.[191] They further demonstrated that the whole tract may be at an increased risk and that this risk is not confined to areas of obvious inflammatory involvement. Additional features of carcinoma in Crohn's disease include multifocal lesions and metachronous intestinal and extraintestinal cancers. Patients who develop carcinoma in Crohn's disease are usually relatively young, and more than one-half with colonic cancer are under the age of 40 years.[448] A long duration of illness also appears to be an underlying factor, and there is perhaps a 10-fold greater risk of developing colon cancer in this circumstance than in the general population.[393]

The likelihood of the development of carcinoma is greatly enhanced in patients who have undergone intestinal bypass.[182,192,207] This is particularly true when chronic inflammatory disease persists for many years. Lavery and Jagelman identified two cases of carcinoma that developed in the out-of-circuit rectum after subtotal colectomy and ileostomy for Crohn's disease.[263] The mortality rate from patients who develop cancer in excluded bowel is extremely high (>80%), probably because recognition is very late in the progression of the disease.[175] Even without an exclusion or bypass procedure having been performed, survival is poor with small bowel cancer. In the experience of Michelassi and co-workers the mean survival rate was only 6 months compared with 65 months for those with large bowel cancer.[320] The observation of new signs and symptoms after a prolonged period of quiescence, particularly with long-standing disease, and especially if the patient had previously undergone an exclusion or bypass procedure, should be vigorously evaluated for the possible presence of a malignancy.

This change in symptoms after a period of quiescence is of critical concern also with respect to prior strictureplasty (see later). Ribeiro and colleagues recommend that all strictures be widely opened and carefully examined prior to strictureplasty, with frozen section biopsies of all suspicious areas.[390] Although the risk of adenocarcinoma developing at the site of a strictureplasty is quite remote, several such instances have been reported.[229,302]

Anal Crohn's disease also appears to be associated with an increased risk for the development of anal carcinoma.[51,261,445,451] Malignant changes may be inapparent, especially when the tumor arises in a fistula. Pain, stricture and induration often preclude the performance of an adequate examination.[261] Deterioration of an individual's perianal symptoms and clinical findings warrants investigation and possible biopsy.[51] There also seems to be a relationship with intestinal–cutaneous fistulas, although there is always the question of whether the fistula may be secondary to an underlying malignancy in the intestine.[78]

Whether the anal or abdominal fistula causes malignant change to occur by "irritation" or by a stimulus to mucosal regeneration is a matter for conjecture.

Although carcinoma arising at the stomal site in patients with polyposis or ulcerative colitis has been described (see Chapter 31), it was only recently that the complication has been reported in Crohn's disease.[438] In both of the cases dysplasia was identified in adjacent tissue.

Specific symptoms suggestive of malignancy are rarely identified. However, the important issue, as stated, is that any change, especially following a period of quiescence, demands investigation. Cancer should also be considered when complete obstruction fails to resolve with adequate decompression.[390]

Dysplasia

As with carcinoma in ulcerative colitis, radiologic diagnosis of malignant change in patients with Crohn's disease is virtually impossible. Endoscopic examination likewise is of very little benefit in establishing the diagnosis. However, dysplasia, if present, probably is as significant a finding as it is with ulcerative colitis.[165,192,363] The dysplasia that is recognized is essentially identical to that described in patients with ulcerative colitis (see Chapter 29).[159,248,391,393,403,404] Unfortunately, with the exception of the very distal ileum, the small intestine does not lend itself to investigation by means of biopsy, especially if the segment is excluded. It is probably a reasonable precaution to recall all patients who have undergone a bypass or an exclusion procedure and evaluate them for resection.

Korelitz and colleagues analyzed 356 patients with Crohn's disease by means of rectal biopsy in order to study epithelial dysplasia.[248] Eighteen (5%) exhibited this finding, including those with a normal-appearing mucosa. Colorectal carcinoma was found in 11% of these individuals. Four patients developed carcinoma who did not have dysplasia on rectal biopsy. Löfberg and colleagues evaluated 24 patients with long-standing colonic Crohn's disease by means of colonoscopic biopsy at 10 predetermined sites.[289] Although none had definite dysplasia, three demonstrated DNA aneuploidy, one of whom subsequently developed a carcinoma. The authors believe that dysplasia is rare in Crohn's disease but that DNA aneuploidy needs to be carefully assessed. Obviously, further studies are needed. Richards and associates suggest that surveillance of the colon should commence after 10 years of disease.[393] How frequently this should be undertaken is still not determined, but the issues and concerns expressed in Chapter 29 should be well heeded.

Comment

As was discussed in Chapter 29, the concept of surveillance to identify dysplasia before malignancy supervenes has been subjected to a more critical analysis in recent years. The same should be true for the concept in the management of patients with Crohn's disease. A statement made by Sachar is worth quoting completely, because it reflects my own views on this subject.

> The most rationale position, therefore, in view of the equivalent risks, might be to adopt equivalent policies for the two diseases. In other words, debate the pros and cons of surveillance programs to your heart's content; but in the end, whatever you choose to do for your patients with ulcerative colitis, do no differently for those with Crohn's colitis of similar duration and extent.[414]

Other Malignancies

The issue of extra-intestinal malignancies with IBD is a matter of some controversy. Whether the association is valid or merely coincidental is still unresolved. Concomitant malignant melanoma and lymphoma have been suggested to be more than mere coincidence, perhaps related to immunosuppression from the disease itself or from medical treatment.[133,137179,183]

Medical Management

The reader is directed to Chapter 29 for a comprehensive discussion of the medical management of ulcerative colitis. However, I have again asked Dr. Seymour Katz, Clinical Professor of Medicine at the New York University School of Medicine and Attending Gastroenterologist at North Shore University Hospital-Long Island Jewish Health Systems, to provide his input specifically with respect to the contemporary opinions on the medical management of Crohn's disease.—MLC

The management of Crohn's disease is dependent on the assessment of the disease location, the severity, the exclusion of abscess, and the elimination of extra-luminal factors, such as cigarette smoking, nonsteroidal antiinflammatory drugs, *Clostridium difficile*, acute self-limited infections, or irritable bowel-like symptoms that might better respond to conventional therapy.[197] Confounding factors, of course, include undetected but coexistent carcinoma and AIDS. Dietary problems referable to sorbitol or lactose may obscure the initial concern that this is actually Crohn's disease. Approaches to the management of patients include lifestyle, diet, and pharmaceuticals, each of which may independently aid in the management of the asymptomatic individual with Crohn's disease.[218] The therapeutic goals are to induce a clinical remission, to maintain that remission, and to prevent postoperative relapse.

The plethora of information regarding pathogenetic mechanisms in the understanding of Crohn's disease has led to a number of imaginative and innovative treatment approaches. Kornbluth and colleagues undertook a study to determine the efficacy of various medical therapies in the treatment of severe IBD on the basis of a Medline computer-assisted literature search.[252] They determined that clinical remission was achieved on average in 65% of individuals with Crohn's disease. They concluded that current medical therapy for severe Crohn's colitis seems to spare many patients early colectomy. The Crohn's Disease Activity Index, which consists of the clinical variables correlated with the physician's assessment of the patient's well-being, although validated, has been criticized because of its subjectivity and interobserver variability.[196]

Mild to Moderate Disease

In mild to moderate disease, the initial drug of choice is 5-ASA in a form targeted to the inflammatory site, using higher doses than that which is required for ulcerative colitis. It is anticipated that there will be a 40% to 60% response rate.[443] Metronidazole and ciprofloxacin regimens can produce results similar to those of 5-ASA, particularly in Crohn's ileocolitis and in perianal disease.[373,464] However, these observations have been challenged for induction of remission with either high-dose 5-ASA or antibiotics and certainly are not as impressive as those with immunomodulator therapy.[199]

Moderate to Severe Disease

Moderate to severe disease almost always requires steroids initially, but only for short-term use. No long-term benefit has been proven. However, there is an 80% relapse rate when steroids are terminated prematurely. The concern, of course, is that 35% of patients may become steroid-dependent in 1 year, but 20% remain in remission.[330] There is no value in low-dose steroids in preventing relapse.

Severe Disease

In severe Crohn's disease, patients are admitted into the hospital and treated with intravenous medications only (Figure 30-59). There have been no unequivocal data that intravenous cyclosporine has a therapeutic advantage over intravenous corticosteroids, nor has a sustained benefit been demonstrated in Crohn's disease.[138] This has been particularly true with the low dose and the oral route. Drainage of abscess is, of course, mandatory.

Maintenance of Remission

In maintaining remission, the maintenance dose of 5-ASA is the inductive dose—that is, the dose that prevents relapse or recurrence after surgery. However, it may be less effective if steroids, 6-MP, or azathiaprine (AZA) induced that remission. If steroids did induce the remission there is a better chance of maintaining that remission with 6-MP and AZA (or possibly methotrexate) than with continued use of 5-ASA.[197]

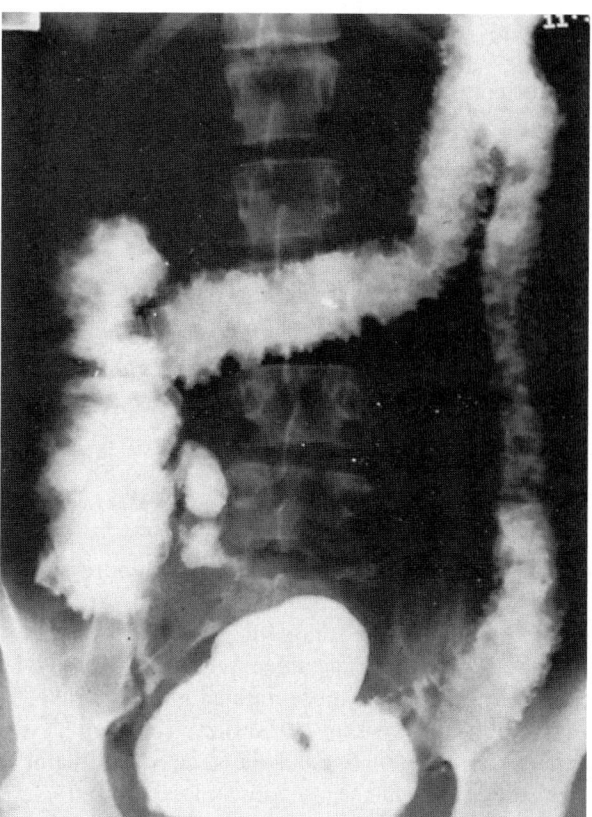

FIGURE 30-59. Fulminant acute Crohn's colitis. Barium enema reveals total colonic ulceration and bowel wall edema.

Postoperative Recurrence

The maintenance of remission following resection for Crohn's disease continues to be a topic of concern among internists, gastroenterologists, and surgeons. Symptomatic relapses occur at a rate of 40% to 70% in most series within 2 years following operation.[155] Endoscopic recurrence actually increases that rate to 80%. In the natural course of the disease, the inflammatory process may tend to extend distally, but rarely proximally. However, once the patient undergoes surgery, proximal involvement is more likely to develop, usually at and just above the anastomosis.

Korelitz believed that sulfasalazine is more effective in preventing recurrence in Crohn's disease than it is with ulcerative colitis.[244] However, the initial enthusiasm for the value of 5-ASA in reducing the likelihood of postoperative recurrence has not been supported by later investigations.[53] The European Cooperative Crohn's Disease Study showed no significant reduction in the clinical relapse rate.[285] Yet a metaanalysis of the 5-ASA experience did show an effect on reducing recurrence postoperatively.[2]

There is, however, value to the postoperative use of immunomodulators and some short-term improvement with metronidazole if side-effects can be tolerated.[247] Further study of 55 postoperative Crohn's patients randomized to 6-MP or control showed *no* difference in time to relapse, but the postoperative endoscopic score of disease activity was significantly lower in the 6-MP patients.[42]

Aminosalicylates

The primary drugs that have been traditionally employed for the treatment of Crohn's disease are sulfasalazine and steroids (see Chapter 29). Aminosalicylates can delay recurrence, but concern has been expressed about the clinical efficacy of 5-ASA and antibiotics in Crohn's disease.[199] For example, sulfasalazine has been shown to have a minimal effect on inducing remission in active Crohn's disease when compared with a placebo.[462] Moreover, convincing evidence is lacking that mesalamine is effective for treatment of active Crohn's disease. Gendre and colleagues employed a placebo-controlled study with the use of oral mesalamine (Pentasa) for maintenance therapy and found a statistically significant difference in the maintenance of quiescence in the treated group.[155] Likewise, Brignola and co-workers performed a controlled study with mesalamine and found a statistically significant difference in the incidence of endoscopic lesions and severity in the treated group compared with the placebo.[53] A similar favorable result was observed in individuals who were treated with oral 5-ASA (Asacol).[374]

Sandborn and Feagan suggest an alternative treatment algorithm as a result of their analysis of randomized controlled trials for mild to moderate Crohn's disease.[418] Their evidence-based conclusions are as follows:

1. Colonic disease.
2. Sulfasalazine for colonic Crohn's induction of remission with budesonide 9 mg/day for ileal or right disease.
3. Conventional steroids for more severe disease activity, budesonide failures, and patients allergic to or intolerant of sulfasalazine.

Mesalamine has limited value in preventing relapse after a medically induced remission, especially if it has been steroid-induced, or in maintaining remission postoperatively.[62,285] The question of mesalamine's role in preventing postoperative recurrence of Crohn's disease has been revisited by Caprilli and co-workers, who found no clinically significant advantage between 84 patients receiving 4.0 g/day (12%) versus 81 patients given 2.4 g/day (14%).[66]

Steroids

A dramatic response is often observed when intravenous steroids are administered. A mass may rapidly disappear, or a patient's acute abdominal symptoms may resolve. The natural history of corticosteroid use in IBD was reviewed in 173 patients treated in Olmstead County, Minnesota, a community-based experience rather than a study of patients referred to a tertiary medical center.[131] Of 74 individuals (43%) treated with corticosteroids, 43 (58%) entered complete remission, 19 (26%) had a partial remission, and 12 (16%) had no response. At 1 year, however, only 24 (32%) still had a prolonged response, yet 21 (28%) were steroid dependent, and 38 required surgery (38%). Thus, of 84% initial responders, only 32% maintained that response free of steroids and without surgery. It should be noted that only 38% of Crohn's patients in this population needed steroids, thus speaking for mild disease. A second lesson learned was that the need for steroids in this group suggested a poorer prognosis and a higher likelihood that surgery would be required.

A double-blind study of the effectiveness of sulfasalazine compared with 6-methylprednisolone in patients with Crohn's disease revealed that the addition of the former drug offered no advantage.[300]

Budesonide (Entocort) in ileocolonic Crohn's disease produced a 45% improvement in 8 weeks in the Canadian experience, with no significant long-term steroid side effects, and with a remission rate at 8 weeks comparable to that of prednisone, with less adrenal suppression.[64] Both prednisone and budesonide induced remission in approximately 60% of patients, with fewer side effects with budesonide in the Italian and Israeli experience.[26,63,353,412] Short-term use of budesonide appeared superior to that of mesalamine (5-ASA) in preventing relapse at 1 year in steroid-dependent patients who were intolerant to AZA/6-MP.[156]

Budesonide may be a reasonable alternative as replacement therapy in glucocorticoid-dependent patients. Cortot and colleagues described 118 individuals with inactive Crohn's disease who were randomized to budesonide, 6 mg, or placebo, while tapering prednisolone.[87] At 13 weeks 68% of budesonide patients were in remission vs. 35% of placebo patients. There was a demonstrable reduction of glucocorticoid side effects, that is, moon face, acne, insomnia, and mood swings, in both the budesonide and the placebo groups.

In a metaanalysis, budesonide was less likely to induce remission in active Crohn's disease than conventional corticosteroids but was better than mesalamine or placebo over 8 weeks and with fewer steroid adverse events.[354] There appears to be a role for budesonide as pulse therapy for quickly inducing a remission for a Crohn's flare and using it as bridge therapy until AZA/6-MP can "kick in."

Antibiotics (Metronidazole [Flagyl] and Ciprofloxacin [Cipro])

Metronidazole was initially introduced for the treatment of *Trichomonas vaginalis* infections but was subsequently demonstrated to be a very effective antibiotic against anaerobic organisms. It was also found to have activity against gram-positive and gram-negative bacteria. The drug is a substituted imidazole that is rapidly absorbed orally and rectally and can be given intravenously to the acutely ill patient. A number of theories suggesting the mechanism of its action have been proposed: immunosuppression, an effect on wound healing, stimulation of leukocyte chemotaxis, and, of course, its antimicrobial effect.

A controlled clinical trial from Sweden compared the efficacy of metronidazole with sulfasalazine in the treatment of patients with active Crohn's disease.[398,485] Seventy-eight participated in the study during two 4-month periods. Metronidazole was demonstrated to be slightly more effective than sulfasalazine. Although metronidazole may be beneficial for some patients with intestinal disease, some have shown that it does not appear to have therapeutic potential for preventing relapse of Crohn's disease.[17] In other studies metronidazole appears to be of modest value in preventing postoperative recurrence or maintaining remission, but it is limited by bacterial resistance and drug intolerance, particularly the neuropathic side effects and lack of response at the 3-year mark.[50,411] When it has been added to ciprofloxacin there has been an improvement through the reduction of the Crohn's disease activity index (CDAI). Forty-five percent of patients went into remission in both the Italians' and the Canadians' experiences, with better results noted with colonic or ileocolonic disease as opposed to ileal disease alone.[174,376] Patients undergoing prolonged treatment need to be closely monitored for the development of peripheral neuropathy.[111]

Prolonged antibiotic therapy (i.e., 6 months) appears to be of value in cipro-treated patients by reducing their CDAI compared with placebo.[22] It is not surprising since many clinicians maintain patients on antibiotics for years with ileocolonic Crohn's.

Conclusions regarding clinical trials of antibiotics support a role for metronidazole–imidazoles, cipro, and possibly clarithromycin in Crohn's colitis and ileocolitis, and less so for ileitis. Better data are still needed with respect to efficacy, recognition of the toxicity of metronidazole, and the expense of other medications.

Metronidazole has been suggested as being particularly useful in the management of *anal and perianal Crohn's disease* (see Chapters 10 and 11).[38,50,116] Bernstein and associates demonstrated that drainage, erythema, and induration diminished dramatically in all 21 patients so treated, with complete healing obtained in more than one-half of those who were maintained on therapy.[38] Eisenberg compared surgery alone in the management of complicated anal Crohn's disease with surgery plus metronidazole.[116] The patients were randomly allocated, but it was not a double-blind study. An intravenous loading dose of 15 mg/kg (usually 1 g) was given, with mainte-

nance therapy of 500 mg intravenously every 6 hours for 5 days. Outpatient treatment was continued at the dosage of 250 mg, three times daily, for 4 weeks or until complete healing occurred. Twelve of 14 patients (86%) receiving metronidazole treatment had a satisfactory response—complete healing of anorectal–perineal disease without relapse during a follow-up period of 1 to 5 years. In the control group, 11 of 17 patients (65%) treated by surgery alone had satisfactory healing.

In a follow-up study of long-term administration of metronidazole, Brandt and colleagues evaluated whether the drug could be reduced or stopped in these patients without creating an exacerbation.[50] They reported that dosage reduction was associated with recurrent disease activity in all patients but that healing occurred promptly when the full dose of metronidazole was reinstituted.

It appears, then, that definitive anal surgery can be undertaken even in the presence of anal Crohn's disease with some reasonable expectation of success if supplementary metronidazole therapy is administered.

Antituberculous Chemotherapy

As has been discussed in Chapter 29 concerning etiology, Crohn's disease had been thought to resemble tuberculosis in many respects, and multiple attempts to isolate microbacteria have been made, albeit unsuccessfully. A controlled trial of antituberculous chemotherapy was performed through the Department of Gastroenterology at the University of Wales at Cardiff.[466] In a double-blind, randomized program involving rifampin, isoniazid, and ethambutol, or placebo, no tangible benefit from these agents was identified.[466]

Immunosuppressive Agents

Azathiaprine and 6-Mercaptopurine

Because of the supposition that IBD is an autoimmune condition, treatment with immunosuppressive drugs has been recommended.[246,377,509] The two agents that have been used extensively are 6-mercaptopurine (6-MP) and its analog, azathioprine (AZA). Although immunosuppressive drugs have been shown to be effective in both ulcerative colitis and Crohn's disease, and with few exceptions the complications have been reversible, many physicians, perhaps inappropriately, fear to employ this modality in the management of their patients.

Korelitz uses immunosuppressive drugs when other treatment modalities fail, when there is no indication for operative intervention, and as an option offered to the patient as an alternative to surgery.[245] Present and colleagues performed a double-blind study on 83 patients and noted a 67% response with 6-mercaptopurine as compared with a modest 8% improvement with a placebo.[377]

Azathioprine and 6-mercaptopurine have been successful in maintaining remission, with a 5% recurrence rate using azathioprine versus a 41% rate of recurrence with placebo at 1 year.[347] Long-term follow-up in the 6-MP experience in 120 patients revealed that those on 6-MP had a relapse of 47% at 5 years, whereas those who discontinued 6-MP had a 97% relapse rate. This was higher in younger patients who had discontinued the drug for "other reasons than a relapse."[240] The question, "Why do patients stop AZA and what happens to them?" was answered in a study of 266 patients.[104] Twenty-five percent discontinued the AZA for blood count abnormalities, and of those who stopped, 60% needed surgery or became steroid-dependent.

The use of 6-MP and AZA as medical therapy for enterovesical fistula seems to have been supported by the Mt. Sinai Hospital experience with 31 patients.[500] Wheeler and colleagues demonstrated a 58% clinical response to 5-ASA, antibiotics, and AZA. The fistulas closed in 13 of 31 patients (42%), with two-thirds medically successfully managed over 8 years.

There appears to be no greater risk of malignancy with 6-MP or AZA in the experience involving 626 patients treated for a mean of 27 months and mean follow-up of 13.7 years in the United Kingdom.[146] Their overall rates of colorectal cancer or dysplasia was 0.4% at 10 years, 1.3% at 20 years, 9% at 30 years, and 15.5% at 40 years. The study from the Lenox Hill Hospital in New York involving 410 patients followed between 1980 to 1999 revealed that 6-MP and AZA are safe drugs for long-term use.[493] However, there is concern regarding the predisposition to lymphoma with long-term use of 6-MP in some series.[128,309]

Ewe and colleagues performed a randomized, prospective study comparing AZA in combination with prednisolone versus prednisolone alone in the treatment of active Crohn's disease.[124] They found that the combination regimen was superior to that of treatment with prednisolone alone, in that more frequent remissions were observed and with lower doses of prednisolone.[124] Most studies have demonstrated efficacy in approximately two-thirds of patients. The drugs are not felt to be effective in the treatment of fulminant disease but should be used in those individuals who can tolerate the relatively slow response to treatment (commonly, at least 6 months). They have been recommended for the treatment of perianal disease, small bowel obstruction (when surgery is contraindicated), and fistula complications, and for the management of children.[249] In the experience of Lecomte and colleagues (Paris, France), one third of patients with perianal lesions improved.[264] Prophylaxis after two surgical resections is another possible indication.

Complications include bone marrow suppression, liver abnormalities (including liver necrosis), pancreatitis, and hair loss. Present and colleagues assessed the toxicity of 6-MP in 396 patients (276 with Crohn's dis-

ease).[379] Pancreatitis was seen in 3.3%, bone marrow depression in 2%, and allergic reactions in 2%. All were reversible. Markowitz and colleagues identified no serious complications with treatment of 36 adolescents by means of 6-MP in dosages of 1.5 mg/kg to a maximum of 75 mg/day.[303] Follow-up after 1 year demonstrated continued remission in 77%. Others have also confirmed the effectiveness and relative safety of these drugs.[346] The steroid-sparing effects are felt to be of particular benefit in this group of patients.

Methotrexate

In addition to the preceding, methotrexate (MTX), a folic acid antagonist, has been used in the treatment of IBD. In an open-label pilot study, Kozarek and colleagues used this drug in ulcerative colitis and Crohn's disease patients who had failed conventional medical therapy.[256] Preliminary results were encouraging. Feagan and colleagues, with the North American Crohn's Study Group Investigators, conducted a double-blind, placebo-controlled multicenter study of weekly injections of MTX in patients who had chronically active Crohn's disease despite a minimum of 3 months of prednisone therapy.[140] They were randomly assigned to treatment with methotrexate or a placebo for a period of 16 weeks. A statistically significant improvement was observed in the methotrexate group with respect to symptoms and the reduction of requirement for prednisone.[140]

Forty-one of 49 French patients entered clinical remission and were then maintained on MTX for a median of 18 months.[273] Relapse rates were 29% at 1 year, 41% at 2 years, and 48% at 3 years, with a greater relapse rate in women and in ileocolitis patients. A randomized 16-week single-blind comparison of 15 or 25 mg of MTX in 32 Crohn's patients at the Mayo Clinic showed the same efficacy of remission (17%) and response rate (45%) with both doses.[115] The experience in 76 refractory Crohn's patients at the University of Chicago resulted in 63% improvement at 9 weeks.[70] In another study, an impressive 65% of MTX-treated patients (26/40), as the only therapy, remained in remission from 16 to 24 weeks, compared with 39% of the controls.[139] There appears to be a role for MTX in maintaining remission *if* MTX induced that remission. Its success in causing remission may be facilitated by the concomitant use of corticosteroids.

Cyclosporine

Cyclosporine, a drug that has been widely used in organ transplantation, has been subjected to extensive evaluation in the management of Crohn's disease. The cyclosporine story, however, has not been favorable. In one study, a 52% relapse rate occurred during its acute use.[270] However, in a randomly assigned, placebo-controlled, double-blind study of a group of patients who were resistant to or intolerant of steroids, Brynskov and colleagues found a significant improvement in the Crohn's Disease Activity

Index.[55] Elson suggested that the rapidity of response may give it some role in the acutely ill individual.[121]

Cyclosporine's value with perianal Crohn's disease seems more impressive, with 10 of 14 patients (71%) achieving relief of fistulous drainage.[271] Hanauer and Smith employed cyclosporine in the management of five patients with chronic draining fistulas that had been unresponsive to prior surgery, steroids, antibiotics, total parenteral nutrition (TPN), and other immunosuppressives.[198] All fistulas responded to this infusion through decreased drainage and with improvement of both inflammatory reaction and patient comfort. However, cyclosporine has not been shown to be of value for maintaining remission, and its toxicity precludes its long-term use.

Antibody Therapy

Tumor necrosis factor-α (TNF-α) has been shown to have an important role in the pathogenesis of Crohn's disease. Stack and co-workers performed a double-blind, placebo-controlled study, utilizing a genetically engineered human antibody to TNF-α, CDP571, to determine whether disease activity could be modified.[454] A significant fall in the median Crohn's Disease Activity Index was identified in the treatment group. These data suggest that antibody neutralization of TNF-α is a potentially effective strategy in the management of Crohn's disease.

In a short-term study using a single infusion of a chimeric monoclonal antibody to tumor necrosis factor, 65% of the patients improved versus 17% with the placebo.[467] Clinical remission was achieved at 4 weeks in 33% of the patients treated versus 4% of those treated with a placebo. A majority maintained that response at 12 weeks. Additional experience demonstrated that fistulas closed in 62% of the patients versus 26% in the placebo group.[378] In another report, however, despite the fact that infliximab (Remicade) was associated with a 61% complete or partial response rate, the drug did not supplant the requirement for surgery.[368] Seventy-three percent either ultimately needed surgery or had persistent fistulas, although the drug was much more effective in controlling perianal disease. Others have found that selective seton placement, combined with infliximab infusion and maintenance immunosuppressives, resulted in complete healing of two-thirds of perianal fistulas.[480]

The continued experience with anti-TNF has shown that there is considerable endoscopic healing in resistant, active Crohn's disease. In the Amsterdam report involving 108 patients, 65% showed improvement when treated with infliximab.[100] The clinical postmarketing experience with more than 170,000 patients so managed appears to mirror the results achieved in the initial trials. Two thirds of patients responded, and one-third entered remission.

The first 100 patients treated at Beth Israel Hospital in Boston and Brown University with infliximab demonstrated a 60% response rate, and 36% went into remission.[129] The mean time to response was 6.5 days, but the mean duration of response was only 12 weeks. The Mayo Clinic's experience with the first 100 patients was compartmentalized into those with complete, partial, or no response and by disease activity.[392] Inflammatory Crohn's patients had the best response (52.5%), whereas fistula patients had a 34.6% complete response. Fistulas healed completely in 46% and partially in 23%, with a mean duration of response of 10 weeks.

Short-term infliximab has been shown to be well tolerated, but the incidence of serious adverse events (serum sickness, sepsis, autoimmune phenomena, and opportunistic infections) requires careful surveillance.[84] Additionally, caution is required in individuals with stricture.[98,481,498] A decreased (i.e., worsened) response occurred in 57 stricture patients compared with the nonstricture population in a University of Pennsylvania report.[433] Yet infliximab itself has not been shown to cause intestinal stricture or obstruction.[280]

Rectovaginal fistula in Crohn's disease represents one of the most challenging problems. Remarkably, five of six such patients responded to a three-infusion regimen and four continued to improve with an 8-week infusion cycle while on immunomodulators.[406] Four of six became asymptomatic, with a range of remission from 4 to 7 weeks. Another report involved 28 patients with rectovaginal fistula.[422] A 57% response rate was noted with a three-dose induction regimen. Although fistulas appear to respond to treatment longer than for those with luminal disease following three doses of infliximab, evaluation by MRI or endorectal sonography may still demonstrate clinically unapparent abscesses or persistent fistulas.[5,30,487] A parameter that may predict responsiveness to infliximab is endoscopic healing, which significantly correlates with a more prolonged time to relapse.[408] Results of responses to an IBD questionnaire reveal that infliximab significantly improved the quality of life in those with active disease, thereby increasing ability to work and to participate in leisure activities while decreasing feelings of fatigue, depression, and anger.[279]

Because of the increased risk of tuberculosis in patients given infliximab, it is now advised that patients be skin tested and a chest x-ray be obtained.[328] Any evidence of active TB mandates treatment before initiating infliximab therapy.

Enteric-Coated Fish Oil

Belluzzi and associates performed a 1-year, double-blind, placebo-controlled study to investigate the effects of a fish oil preparation on the maintenance of remission in 78 patients with Crohn's disease.[31] A statistically significant difference was achieved with the use of this preparation when compared with the placebo group with respect to reduction of relapses. The antiinflammatory effect of fish oil has been well documented to reduce production of a number of agents, such as leukotriene B_4 and thromboxane A_2, which have been observed in the inflamed intestinal mucosa of patients with Crohn's disease. Inhibition of the synthesis of cytokines and tumor necrosis factor has also been demonstrated with fish oil.

Withdrawal of Smoking

Smoking has been shown to have a pejorative effect on the clinical course of individuals with Crohn's disease. Lindberg and associates demonstrated a statistically significantly increased risk of the requirement for surgery in those who smoke more than one half pack of cigarettes a day.[283] Irrespective of how the course of Crohn's disease is analyzed, it is much less favorable for those who smoke, especially if they are heavy smokers. As part of the therapeutic regimen, therefore, patients with Crohn's disease should be dissuaded from smoking.[283]

Oral contraceptives together with smoking are additive risk factors for relapse in Crohn's disease, with some 40% of patients relapsing with unfavorable outcomes. Prior smoking, however, has not been shown to be an increased risk, but prior oral contraceptives were used more frequently in relapsed patients in one study.[476]

Nutritional Therapy

Parenteral Hyperalimentation

As discussed in Chapter 29, hyperalimentation, either parenteral (TPN) or oral (enteral), has been recommended in a supportive role for patients with Crohn's disease.[205,212,232,276,277,439] The rationale is to replenish nutritional deficits, to allow bowel rest for healing and "repair," and to provide perioperative support for healing in an attempt to reduce morbidity and mortality.[439] Fazio and colleagues reported the Cleveland Clinic's experience of 81 courses of TPN in the treatment of Crohn's disease.[134] Two groups of patients were treated, one by definitive therapy and a second for adjunctive treatment. Indications in the former group included diffuse small intestinal disease, short bowel syndrome, acute ileitis or colitis (in which there was inadequate response to alternative medical treatment), poor nutrition, and enteric fistulas. A subsequent report revealed 23 patients in the primary therapy group.[201] A remission occurred in approximately two-thirds, while the remaining eight patients required an operation during the hospitalization. In the adjunctive group, 58 patients were treated, of whom almost one-fourth entered remission, obviating the need for surgical intervention during that hospitalization. These patients, in fact, satisfied the criteria for pri-

mary therapy, although this was not the design in that group of patients. The course of treatment ranged from 10 to 264 days. The average treatment course was almost 3 weeks.

Of the 21 patients with Crohn's disease who were treated with TPN as primary therapy, there were only four (19%) who did not eventually require surgery. Three of the five patients with ulcerative colitis who were so treated responded well enough to medical therapy to have deferred surgery for an average of 2 years. The authors concluded that there appeared to be no lasting benefit for hyperalimentation as a primary method of therapy for patients with IBD, particularly for those with Crohn's disease. However, if the purpose of the treatment is to defer surgical intervention so that it can be pursued on an elective basis, hyperalimentation should be considered.

Shiloni and Freund studied the effect of TPN on 19 patients suffering from active Crohn's disease.[440] Although only approximately one-third did not require surgery during the follow-up (up to 3 years), the authors felt that the treatment was highly effective as supportive therapy, enabling a patient to undergo uneventful major surgery. Others have recommended preoperative TPN for at least 5 days in patients with IBD who have severe protein depletion.[397] However, McIntyre and colleagues, in a controlled trial of 47 severe, acute colitis patients, noted that bowel rest did not affect the outcome.[316] An extensive review by Payne-James and Silk can be summarized by the statement, "Evidence at present indicates that TPN in Crohn's disease should be restricted to a supportive role, rather than employed as primary therapy."[360] In a more general sense, a cooperative Veterans Administration study of 395 malnourished patients who required laparotomy or noncardiac thoracotomy, concluded that the use of preoperative TPN should be limited to those who are severely malnourished.[491]

Home Hyperalimentation

One additional application of hyperalimentation needs to be addressed—home parenteral nutrition—for the patient who has a short bowel syndrome, a potential consequence of multiple or extensive resections for Crohn's disease.[109,185,269,310,456] The growth of the home intravenous therapy market in the United states has been truly exponential. In 1990 alone, TPN represented one-third ($937 million) of the home intravenous market (according to Total Pharmaceutical Care, Inc., Santa Barbara, CA). In 1983, the Oley Foundation was established as a nonprofit organization affiliated with the Clinical Nutrition Division of the Albany Medical College to address the special needs of those involved in home parenteral and enteral nutrition (PEN) (The Oley Foundation, 214 Hun Memorial, A-28, Albany Medical Center, Albany, NY 12208). The foundation maintains a national patient registry known as OASIS, a cooperative project undertaken with the American Society of Parenteral and Enteral Nutrition. As of January 1991, more than 6,000 patients were registered. Such a registry has also been created in the United Kingdom and in Ireland.[459]

Almost all patients who require rehospitalization do so because of problems with the catheter, and in the experience of the Cleveland Clinic, mortality is usually due to the underlying disease process rather than to the therapy.[456] Dudrick and colleagues have accumulated more than 100 patient-years' experience with home TPN.[109] Catheter-related sepsis occurred seven times, equivalent to one episode per three catheter-years. The Cleveland Clinic group has also accumulated more than 100 years of patient experience.[149] Greater than one-half had at least one or more hyperalimentation-related complications—catheter sepsis, blocked or damaged catheters, and dehydration or electrolyte imbalance. Analysis seems to indicate that the only valued nutritional parameters in monitoring patient well-being are body weight and serum albumin.[459] Although this therapeutic modality is extremely tedious for the patient, it does permit an improvement in the quality of life.

Oral or Enteral Nutrition

The place of an elemental diet in the management of Crohn's disease has been evaluated. Teahon and colleagues reported success in inducing remission in 85% of 113 patients.[470] Some suggest that the remission rate may be comparable to that achieved with steroids.[16,351] Failure to tolerate the diet is, of course, one potential problem. Lochs and associates showed that enteral nutrition was less effective than a combination of 6-MP and sulfasalazine in treating active Crohn's disease.[286] Obviously, if the patient fulfills the same criteria for treatment as those selected for ambulatory hyperalimentation, it would seem that the preferred alternative is oral management, if indeed it can be adequately achieved.

However, drug therapy remains the primary approach, with no good evidence to suggest that nutritional therapy alone alters the clinical course of Crohn's disease or of ulcerative colitis.[361,482] TPN may play an adjunctive role in achieving remission in steroid-refractory Crohn's disease individuals who are unable to maintain the enteral route. There is little difference in efficacy with the type of TPN or enteral support regarding healing of fistulas or delaying surgery, and there is no superiority of elemental diets over so-called polymeric diets.

Comment

I state again, as I did in Chapter 29, that I do not defer needed surgery in order to employ TPN. The concept of short-term intravenous hyperalimentation may have certain theoretical advantages, but an expeditiously performed operation should allow an earlier resumption of oral intake, a much preferred method of administrating calories. If the patient is severely malnourished and can be placed in a more favorable nutritional state by such treatment, I obviously would have no objections. But there is no question in my mind that hyperalimentation, as the sole modality of therapy, cannot be justified.

Somatostatin

Somatostatin, a tetradecapeptide growth-hormone-release inhibiting factor, has been found to have a powerful inhibitory action on gastrointestinal endocrine and exocrine secretions.[103,243,342] As a consequence of its ability to profoundly decrease the volume and the enzyme content of the gastrointestinal tract, the drug has been used in the management of intestinal fistulas. It therefore has particular merit for the treatment of patients with Crohn's disease, especially those individuals who have fistula complications.[453] Continuous intravenous infusion of somatostatin (250 µg/hr) has been demonstrated to result in reduced output and in some cases, spontaneous fistula closure.[153] The synthetic analog, SMS 901–225 (Sandostatin), has been developed to provide a longer half-life with less influence on insulin secretion.[342] It has also been shown to prolong gastrointestinal transit time and to improve water and electrolyte absorption. The drug is supplied in 1-mL ampoules containing 100 µg and is administered subcutaneously at a dose of 1 mL every 8 hours. I have had considerable success with a limited number of fistula patients who have been submitted to this treatment.

Probiotics

Probiotics are microbial supplements presumed to antagonize the effect of more noxious or pathogenic gut microorganisms. These microbial "cocktails" include *Lactobacillus* bifidobacteria, *Streptococcus salivarius,* and enterococci, as well as yeasts, such as sacchomonocytes, *Aspergillus,* or *Torulopsis*.[298]

The presumption is that the "good bugs" will replace the "bad bugs." These "good bugs" then will produce nutrients essential to gut integrity, prevent overgrowth of the more pathogenic organisms, stimulate the intestinal immune systems, and eliminate intestinal toxins. However, the experience in Crohn's is more limited than that which has been reported for ulcerative colitis (see Chapter 29). The discouraging news of the failure of lactobacillus GG to prevent endoscopic recurrence or reduce the severity of recurrent lesions has dampened the initial enthusiasm.[375]

Growth Hormone, Glutamine, and Diet

There have been several papers from the Brigham and Women's Hospital of Harvard Medical School by Wilmore and colleagues that report a new method of treatment for individuals with short bowel syndrome through the administration of growth hormone, glutamine, and a specialized diet.[59,60,506] With this regimen, the investigators were able to reduce parenteral nutrition requirements in 80% of the more than 125 patients they treated. Furthermore, more than 40% were relieved of the TPN requirement completely. The theory concerning the efficacy of treatment is based on the fact that intestinal growth and adaptation are mediated in part by factors extrinsic to the gastrointestinal tract, such as growth hormone and thyroxine.[59] Furthermore, the amino acid glutamine is a primary energy source for the gastrointestinal tract by exerting trophic effects on the bowel and through stimulation of nutrient absorption.[59,60] The authors emphasize that such a bowel rehabilitation program offers patients a reduction in risk that is normally associated with TPN while improving an individual's lifestyle.[506]

Conclusion—Medical Management

The task of caring for the patient with Crohn's disease can be daunting. There is no "one size fits all" therapy. Each individual's condition and treatment response is unique. The challenge for the clinician is to continually remain informed as to the varied and evolving options in order to find the "right fit" for that person.

Operative Management

Indications

Operative treatment for Crohn's disease is advised primarily for complications (abscess, fistula, perforation, obstruction; see Figure 29-26), since surgical intervention may not cure the patient. Severe inanition, extraintestinal manifestations, and the presence or risk of malignancy are uncommon indications for surgery in this condition. It is well established that ulcerative colitis can produce toxic megacolon and perforation, but it is important to recognize that early in the course of the illness, Crohn's disease can also.[58]

Free perforation of the small bowel in Crohn's disease has been reported to occur in fewer than 1% of hospitalized patients.[177,178] *Hemorrhage* is rarely an indication for surgery with Crohn's disease, although the approach to surgical intervention tends to be somewhat more conservative than that with ulcerative colitis. Since the latter condition can be cured with resection, there is less tendency to procrastinate if hemorrhage is profuse. A more circumspect attitude generally pervades with Crohn's disease. Robert and colleagues identified 21 patients from the Mount Sinai Hospital who were admitted with severe lower intestinal hemorrhage.[396] Their data suggested that removal of diseased bowel with the initial episode

of hemorrhage was probably the better option, since 30% who were treated conservatively subsequently bled massively.

The presence of an *abscess* or *fistula* virtually excludes the diagnosis of ulcerative colitis. Internal and external fistulas associated with Crohn's disease are usually indications for surgical intervention.[162,167,177,226,260,488] As previously stated, TPN may succeed in effecting temporary closure, and the place of somatostatin has likewise been addressed.[153] However, patients almost invariably develop symptoms severe enough to justify surgical intervention. In the experience of Greenstein and colleagues, 36 of 38 patients (95%) eventually required operation.[184] Glass and colleagues suggest that an internal fistula is not an absolute indication for surgery and that severity of the symptoms should dictate the treatment.[163,164] Even if the fistula involves the bladder, the authors believe that urinary tract infection may respond to antibiotics, and spontaneous closure may occur, although this surely must represent a minority opinion.

Greenstein and colleagues identified 770 patients who underwent intestinal surgery for Crohn's disease during a 24-year period.[177] They felt that the disease presents essentially in two clinical patterns—perforating and nonperforating. Operations for perforating indications were followed by the requirement for reoperation approximately twice as often as those patients who underwent surgery for the other indication.

Abscess formation is usually a consequence of fistula in Crohn's disease.[181,458] Greenstein and colleagues reported that 20% of 230 patients with Crohn's colitis and ileocolitis underwent surgery for intraabdominal abscess.[181] The most frequent site of origin was the terminal ileum, with the abscess located in the right lower quadrant.

Stricture is a common feature of Crohn's disease and a frequent indication for surgery. A number of reports suggest that abnormalities of collagen metabolism may be important in the pathogenesis of both fistulas and strictures, and in fact may predate gross pathologic changes.[7]

Appendiceal Crohn's Disease

Crohn's disease confined to the appendix is a very unusual entity. In 1990, Ruiz and colleagues identified 85 cases limited to the appendix in the literature.[407] The disease was found most commonly in the second and third decades. The signs and symptoms mimicked those of acute appendicitis, with 27% having a palpable mass. The authors suggest that a protracted preoperative history of symptoms should alert the surgeon to this possibility. Lindhagen and associates identified 50 cases and added 12 of their own.[284] The indications for surgery in their patients were appendicitis in eight, appendiceal abscess in two, suspected pyosalpinx in one, and ovarian cyst in one. All but two of the eight appendicitis patients underwent appendectomy, while the others underwent a more extensive resection. There was no incident of subsequent fecal fistula. With a median follow-up of almost 14 years, and with no further manifestation of the disease, the authors concluded that when Crohn's disease is confined to the appendix the prognosis is very favorable.

Acute Ileitis Masquerading As Acute Appendicitis

Occasionally, a patient is submitted to a laparotomy for presumed appendicitis and found to have distal ileal Crohn's disease (acute ileitis). There is some controversy about the appropriate management under these circumstances, the critical issue being whether one removes the appendix.[255,307,442] Simonowitz and associates reviewed the records of 20 patients who underwent incidental appendectomy and made the following recommendations: if the patient has abdominal pain for less than 1 week, appendectomy is followed by minimal complications.[442] For those who have symptoms longer than this period, incidental appendectomy is followed by an 83% incidence of fistula or sinus tract arising *not* from the appendiceal stump but from the terminal ileum. Most surgeons agree that the fistula arises from the ileum unless the cecum is involved with the disease. Weston and associates, reporting from the Lahey Clinic Medical Center, identified 36 patients who had laparotomy for presumed appendicitis and who were found to have Crohn's disease of the terminal ileum.[499] After initial ileocolic resection, one-half required no further resection, with a mean follow-up of more than 12 years. Conversely, 92% of those who did not undergo resection required ileocolic resection for intractability or complications of Crohn's disease. The authors concluded that most patients who are found to have Crohn's disease at laparotomy for appendicitis require an early ileocolic resection.[499] They opine that perhaps the traditional concept of nonresectional surgery for these individuals should be reevaluated.

My own preference is to perform an appendectomy if I am convinced that the cecum is normal. It simplifies the differential diagnosis in the subsequent evaluation of abdominal pain. In reality, however, right lower quadrant abdominal pain with the finding of peritoneal signs not related to the known Crohn's disease must be virtually unheard of.[387] And if it does occur, it is very likely to be associated with a long delay before one initiates surgical treatment.

The surgeon should exercise caution if terminal ileitis is identified at the time of operation for what was presumed to be acute appendicitis. It may be easier to advise than to perform, but the surgeon should not attempt to "break up" adhesions to the abdominal wall under these circumstances, because of the risk of precipitating an abscess or a fecal fistula.

One must always be aware of the differential diagnosis in the presence of terminal ileitis. A self-limited process due to *Yersinia enterocolitica* should be considered, as should the diagnosis of *Campylobacter* (see Chapter 33).

Anal Manifestations

Anorectal abscess and anal fistula are frequent complications of Crohn's disease, especially when the condition involves the colon or rectum. If the disease is confined to the small intestine, however, anal manifestations are less common. In the absence of other areas of involvement, anorectal disease itself is rarely an indication for surgical intervention outside of the anus and perineum. However, in those patients with fecal incontinence, or in whom a rectovaginal or anovaginal fistula develops, radical surgery may be indicated for these complications alone.[215] Under these circumstances, a permanent ileostomy or colostomy is usually required, but a temporary diversionary procedure may permit the surgeon to perform a reconstruction on selected patients. Linares and colleagues evaluated 44 patients with anorectal strictures complicating Crohn's disease to determine the natural history and outcome of surgical treatment.[281] Almost all had demonstrable proctitis. Approximately one-half required either a proctectomy or a diversion, whereas the remainder could be managed by means of periodic dilatations.

Definitive surgery has been recommended and has been successfully performed in patients with anal fistulas in Crohn's disease (see Chapter 11).[8,141,148,217,304] The success that these authors have had is, I am certain, due to careful patient selection. One must make the distinction between anal Crohn's disease and a fistula-in-ano arising in the patient who has IBD without anal involvement. In this latter group, definitive anal surgery may be undertaken with reasonable expectation of healing. This is particularly true if the involved bowel segment either has been resected or is quiescent. Conversely, healing of wounds in a patient with anal Crohn's disease or with active disease elsewhere in the gastrointestinal tract will often lead to chronic, draining, indolent, painful ulcers, which create more problems in management than did the original complaint (see Figure 11-43). To assess adequately the extent of disease, examination under anesthesia may be required. Endoscopic and/or radiologic evaluation of the entire gastrointestinal tract is a requisite before one considers definitive surgery in a patient with known or suspected anal Crohn's disease.

In a report from the Mayo Clinic of 86 patients with anorectal involvement, only those whose active proximal disease was removed benefited from conservative management.[513] On the basis of experience with 109 patients with perianal disease, Alexander-Williams and Buchmann recommend a conservative policy.[10] It is self-evident that the optimal form of therapy for anal Crohn's is medical management (see earlier) and simple drainage of an abscess when it occurs (see Chapters 10 and 11).[381] Long-term catheter or seton drainage may offer the best palliation for recurrent suppuration (see Figs. 11-45 through 11-47). Treatment by local depot methylprednisolone injection (Depomedrone, 40 to 80 mg) has been attempted with some success in alleviating severe anal pain.[222]

Preparation of the Patient

For a discussion of preparing the patient see Chapter 29.

Operative Approaches

Regardless of the choice of operation and irrespective of how radical the extirpation, surgery for Crohn's disease is primarily palliative, not curative. Therefore, operative intervention is recommended essentially for the complications that have been previously discussed. For individuals requiring surgery for disease involving the colon and rectum, proctocolectomy with ileostomy is considered the optimal operation, although preservation of the rectum may be contemplated if this area is relatively spared and/or compliant. When Crohn's disease affects other segments of the gastrointestinal tract, the choice of operation will depend on the location and the extent of disease. Most surgeons are of the opinion that restorative proctocolectomy and the continent ileostomy are contraindicated in individuals with granulomatous colitis, but some are selectively applying these alternative (see later).

General Principles of Intraoperative Evaluation and Decision Making

Exploration of the abdomen will usually reveal the extent of pathology in those with Crohn's disease, since this is a transmural inflammatory process, and the serosa is virtually always involved. In fact, it is not uncommon to discover that the disease is more extensive than can be appreciated by preoperative evaluation. Conversely, with ulcerative colitis, one is usually unimpressed with the severity of inflammation as perceived from the serosal aspect.

The small intestine should be carefully examined and the areas of disease identified and marked with sutures, if necessary. This is a particularly important principle if more than one segment is surgically treated. Measurement of the length of residual normal and diseased bowel (if left behind) is very helpful if further surgery is to be considered later.

Some surgeons had at one time thought it prudent to remove enlarged lymph nodes, believing that the nodes harbor a factor that predisposes the individual to recurrent disease. There is no evidence to suggest that this is the case, and the surgeon is not advised to pursue a more radical excision in an effort to eliminate this tissue.

An intraabdominal abscess is not uncommonly encountered during the course of a laparotomy for Crohn's disease. Obviously, one would have preferred to have had the abscess drained preoperatively by means of a CT-guided approach. However, when an abscess is encountered at surgery, this does not necessarily mean that a stoma must be performed. Generally, the procedure should be undertaken as planned. In the St. Mark's Hospital experience of 28 patients who were found to have an abscess at surgery, only four required a stoma, but the complication rate was 43%.[230] Risk factors for intraabdominal sepsis after surgery for Crohn's disease include preoperative low albumin level, steroid use, and the presence of an abscess or fistula.[517]

In patients with Crohn's disease, retroperitoneal inflammation may pose some risk for ureteral injury during mobilization of the right colon or the rectosigmoid. Care should be taken during this maneuver to identify the ureter and to keep it out of harm's way (see Chapter 23). Similarly, the duodenum is vulnerable to injury, particularly if transmural involvement by Crohn's disease causes fixation of the bowel to the second and third portions. Careful dissection between these structures must be performed by dropping the duodenum posteriorly until it is well out of the area of dissection. Shortening and thickening of the mesentery of the right colon and proximal transverse colon also predisposes the duodenum to possible injury. By clamping the blood vessels on one side only, dividing the mesentery on the bowel side, one is less likely to incorporate the side wall of the duodenum. Back-bleeding can then be addressed with the bowel delivered away from the area of potential injury. This maneuver is analogous to that which one may perform when dividing the lateral ligaments of the rectum (see Figs. 23-22 and 23-23). One may even employ a finger-fracture technique in the dissection of the small and large bowel mesentery, similar to that described for hepatic resection, identifying the vessels after the mesentery has been separated (Figure 30-60).[92] This is a particularly valuable technique when the mesentery is extremely thick.

Proctocolectomy

Proctocolectomy with ileostomy is the conventional operative approach for the treatment of ulcerative colitis and for most patients with Crohn's colitis in which the rectum or anus is involved. The technique is described in detail in the preceding chapter. Resection of the distal small bowel is sometimes necessary when proctocolectomy is undertaken for Crohn's disease, depending on whether the small bowel is involved by the

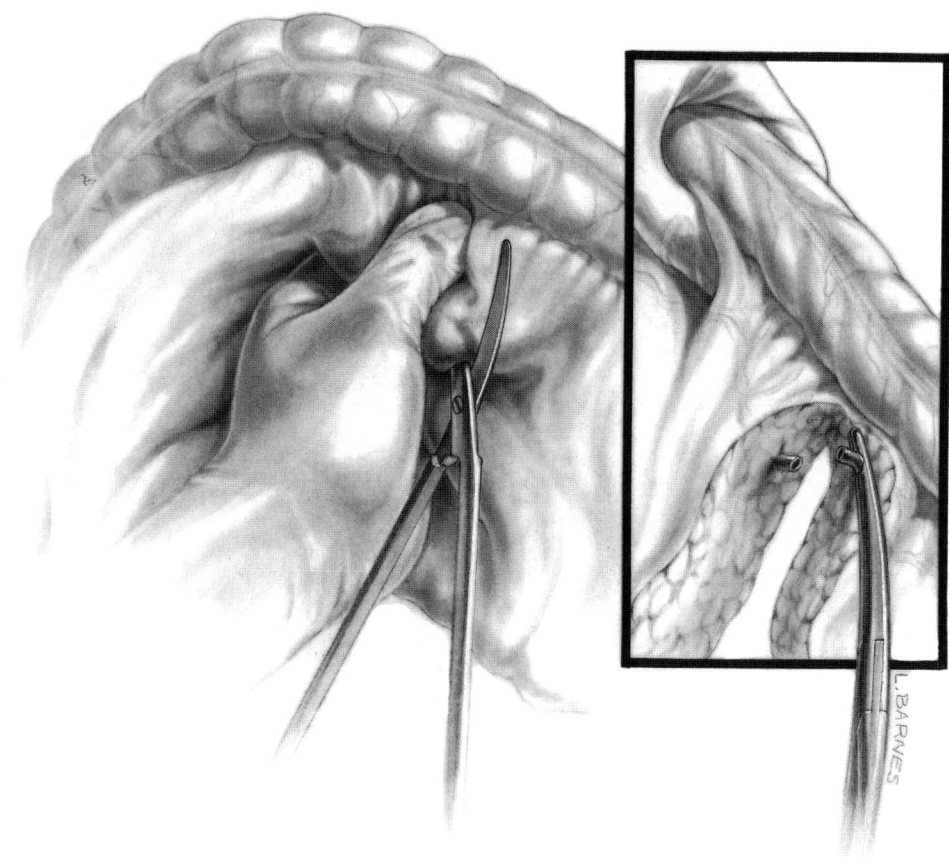

FIGURE 30-60. Division of thickened mesentery in a patient with Crohn's disease by finger-fracture technique. Inset: Illustrates identification of the individual vessel for clamping.

inflammatory process. Even modest resection of the distal ileum may lead to rapid small bowel transit and malabsorption of nutrients, as well as water and electrolyte loss.[335] The surgeon should not remove any normal small bowel and should limit the resection of ileum to the minimum length necessary for extirpation of macroscopic disease (see Management of Small Bowel Crohn's Disease).

An intraperitoneal ileostomy is the recommended technique for stomal creation in a patient with Crohn's colitis, in those who have already had a portion of the terminal ileum removed, and in those for whom "stripping" of the parietal peritoneum is technically impossible. The technique for creating an intraperitoneal ileostomy and obliteration of the lateral space is illustrated in Figure 29-45. The relative disadvantages of this procedure when compared with the extraperitoneal approach are mitigated by the occasional requirement for revision as a consequence of recurrent disease. This is easier to accomplish with an intraperitoneal ileostomy. Since recurrence is not a concern with ulcerative colitis, I favor an extraperitoneal stoma when performed for this condition.

Complications Most complications of proctocolectomy are not specific for this operation and are discussed in Chapters 22, 23, and 29. However, proctocolectomy for Crohn's disease is associated with a high incidence of complications, especially delayed perineal wound healing.[516,518] Sexual dysfunction, intestinal obstruction, and perineal difficulties are addressed in Chapter 29.

STOMAL PROBLEMS Stomal problems and their management are discussed in Chapters 31 and 32. A special concern is recurrence in the ileum or in the ileostomy following proctocolectomy for Crohn's disease (Figure 30-61). Although proctocolectomy is usually curative when Crohn's colitis is confined to the colon, rectum, and anus, between 10% and 20% of patients will develop a proximal recurrence, usually at or just above the ileostomy. The development of a paraileostomy abscess in a patient who has undergone resection for Crohn's disease implies recurrence until proved otherwise. Evaluation may include endoscopic examination of the ileostomy, radiologic investigation by means of a barium enema through the stoma, or both (Figure 30-62).

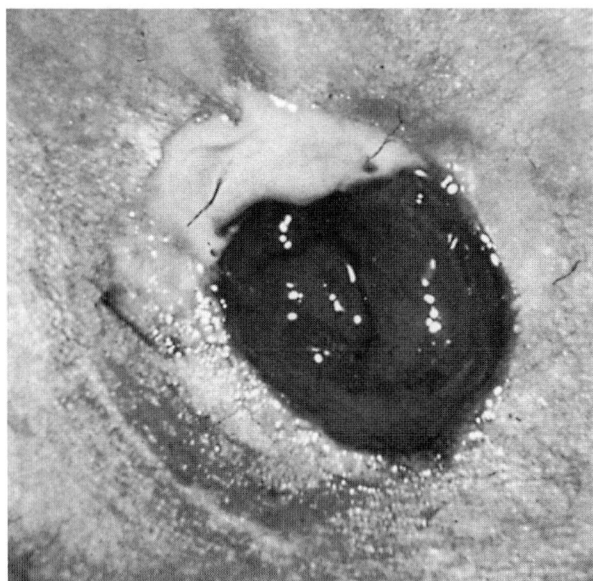

FIGURE 30-61. Paraileostomy abscess following protocolectomy and ileostomy for Crohn's disease. The patient was demonstrated to have terminal ileal recurrence.

Treatment almost always requires resection of the involved ileum and ileostomy with relocation of the stoma to another site. In the acute situation it may be possible to drain the abscess by inserting a clamp at the mucocutaneous junction and liberating the pus. This, then, can be incorporated in the ileostomy appliance with a drain left in the cavity. Alternatively, if the abscess "points" at some distance from the ileostomy, drainage should be effected outside of the faceplate of the appliance. Every attempt should be made to avoid draining the abscess directly under the faceplate, because such a maneuver will inevitably make management of the ileostomy effluent most difficult.

RECURRENT CROHN'S DISEASE Recurrent Crohn's disease can develop at any time following resection for the condition, even as early as a few days postoperatively. On two occasions I have had to reoperate on patients who underwent proctocolectomy and ileostomy whose entire small bowel was felt to be normal at the time of resection. Because of acute peritoneal signs the patients were submitted to reexploration within 1 week of the surgery and were found to have fulminant IBD involving extensive areas of the ileum and jejunum.

Results In the experience of Goligher, 10 operative deaths were noted in 113 patients who underwent this operation for Crohn's disease, a rate of 9%.[168] Today this would be considered an unacceptably high rate. In the experience of the Birmingham, England, group, the operative mortality was 2% in the 103 patients who underwent this procedure.[516] Today proctocolectomy and ileos-

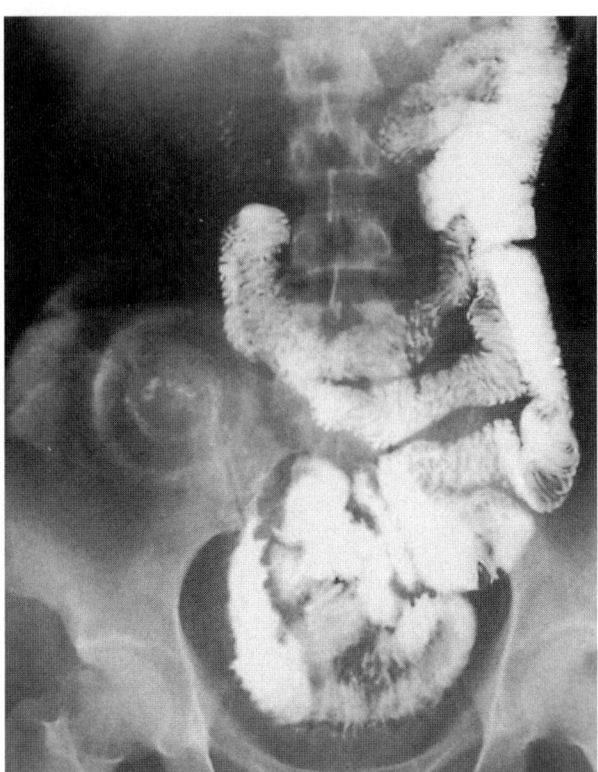

FIGURE 30-62. Recurrent Crohn's disease in distal ileum following proctocolectomy and ileostomy.

tomy can be carried out with minimal morbidity and mortality.

Recurrence following proctocolectomy for Crohn's disease, when the disease is confined to the colon has been reported to be between 10% and 25%, depending on the length of the follow-up.[20,168,250,457,516] Of Goligher's 162 patients treated by ileostomy and colectomy or proctocolectomy and followed for a mean of 15 years, 14.8% developed a recurrence.[170] Scammell and colleagues reported a cumulative reoperation rate at 5 and 10 years of 19% and 24%, respectively.[425] Male patients had a significantly higher incidence of recurrence than females in one study.[516] The prognosis appears to be better if total proctocolectomy is performed as compared with restoration of intestinal continuity.[345] The recurrence rates following restorative surgery in the small and large bowel are discussed later.

Ileostomy

Although ileostomy (without resection) for the management of toxic megacolon in patients with ulcerative colitis is generally appreciated, it may also be usefully applied to those whose disease fails to respond to medical therapy or who have specific problems (e.g., perianal sepsis).[113,130] Zelas and Jagelman reported loop ileostomy as the sole initial procedure in 79 patients who were severely debilitated with Crohn's colitis, 91% of whom improved.[526] Definitive resection was then undertaken at a later stage without an operative death. They recommended loop ileostomy in certain severely ill patients with this disease. Likewise, Harper and associates discussed the value of ileostomy alone for IBD.[204] In 102 patients with Crohn's colitis, there was an immediate clinical improvement in 95, with sustained remission of symptoms for considerable lengths of time. It was possible to restore intestinal continuity subsequently in a number of patients who might otherwise have been treated by proctocolectomy. Winslet and colleagues found that 70% of their 44 patients who underwent fecal diversion for colonic Crohn's disease maintained a sustained period of remission.[507] Furthermore, diversion was associated with a significant reduction of steroid requirements and a significant improvement in the blood count as well as the serum albumin. They concluded with a statement that restoration of intestinal continuity for these individuals is quite problematic. Others have found that fecal diversion alone is associated with acute rapid clinical remission in the majority of patients with Crohn's colitis and severe perianal disease, but sustained benefit occurs less often.[113]

In the experience of Greenstein and Aufses, the incidence of perforation in toxic megacolon was three times higher for ulcerative colitis patients than for those with Crohn's colitis.[176] Without toxic megacolon, however, Crohn's disease was as likely to be associated with a perforation as was ulcerative colitis. Interestingly, mortality rates were better if the perforation occurred in a patient with Crohn's disease.

Harper and colleagues found that instillation of ileostomy effluent into the efferent limb of a divided or loop ileostomy may cause exacerbation of the IBD.[203] Others have attempted to use this information to determine selectively which patients could have the stoma closed without resection, but the results correlate poorly.[130,508]

The indications and technique for ileostomy with and without so-called blowhole colostomy are discussed in Chapter 29.

Colectomy with Ileorectal Anastomosis

For patients with colonic Crohn's disease and rectal sparing, colectomy and ileorectal anastomosis constitute the optimal procedure. This procedure offers the best functional results for an individual who wishes to maintain intestinal continuity. Whether one is an appropriate candidate for this operation depends on the presence (or absence) of the following favorable criteria:

- Rectal sparing or relative rectal sparing
- Compliant rectum
- Absence of anal or perianal disease
- Normal, intact small bowel

- Absence of extra-intestinal manifestations
- Individual motivated to avoid a stoma
- Individual motivated to be followed up closely
- Older age (?)

The technique is described in Chapter 22.

Results   Interpretation of the results of colonic resection is often difficult, because some authors combine limited, segmental resection of the colon with that of total colectomy.[20,290] Farnell and colleagues reported the Mayo Clinic experience with rectal preservation in nonspecific IBD.[127] Eighty patients with Crohn's disease underwent colectomy and ileorectal or ileosigmoid anastomosis. Follow-up was a minimum of 5 years up to a maximum of 17 years. The rectum was felt to be uninvolved in 70%, and moderate disease was present in 19%. During this interval no patient developed carcinoma in the residual rectum. The requirement for subsequent proctectomy was quite similar for both ulcerative colitis and Crohn's disease patients (24% versus 29%, respectively). Whereas the quality of life was felt to be satisfactory in more than one-half of the patients with ulcerative colitis, only one third of those with Crohn's disease were content.

Buchmann and colleagues reported 105 patients treated with colectomy and ileorectal anastomosis for Crohn's disease.[56] The mean follow-up was approximately 7.5 years. The presence or absence of ileal disease or perianal disease at the time of the anastomosis did not affect the prognosis, but patients with sigmoidoscopic evidence of inflammatory disease in the rectum appeared to do less well. The need for reoperation due to recurrence was calculated actuarially to be 50% after 16 to 20 years. The authors felt that the anastomotic procedure as described was a reasonable alternative for most patients with Crohn's colitis who do not have severe involvement of the rectum.

From the same unit, Keighley and associates performed balloon distention of the rectum and barium enema examination to assess rectal capacity.[237] They determined that a severely contracted rectum was associated with the need for a stoma in six of seven patients, compared with only two of 13 patients who did not have radiologic signs of narrowing. A later study with a longer follow-up confirms the predictive value of maximum tolerated volume with respect to function of an ileorectal anastomosis.[497]

Ambrose and colleagues evaluated 63 patients with Crohn's disease treated by colectomy and ileorectal anastomosis.[18] At 10 years, the cumulative reoperation rate was 48%, and the cumulative recurrence rate was 64%. Even after resection for proximal recurrence, intestinal continuity could often be preserved. With a mean follow-up time of 10 years, two thirds of the patients had an intact anastomosis. Goligher followed

45 patients treated by colectomy and ileorectal anastomosis for a mean period of 15 years and noted a recurrence rate of 71%.[170] Nineteen (42%) proceeded to rectal excision and ileostomy.

Mortensen and colleagues evaluated 18 patients who underwent emergency colectomy, 17 of whom were initially spared excision of the rectum, with subsequent proctectomy required in 10 individuals.[326] This result suggested to the authors that acute colonic Crohn's disease requiring surgery is less likely than ulcerative colitis to be amenable to restorative surgery despite a policy of rectal preservation.

In the experience of the Cleveland Clinic group, 131 patients underwent ileorectal anastomosis for Crohn's colitis.[291] After a mean follow-up of 9.5 years, 61% retained a functioning anastomosis, with 61% being free of disease. The mean stool frequency was 4.7/day. Cartan and colleagues (Paris, France) noted that 63% of their 144 patients who underwent total colectomy had a functional ileorectal anastomosis 10 years following surgery.[68] Moreover, they observed that absence of extraintestinal manifestations and prophylactic treatment with 5-ASA were felt to be important facts associated with long-term rectal preservation. Others confirm that total colon resection without proctectomy can in selected individuals with limited rectal disease delay or avoid the necessity of a permanent stoma.[45,72,122,292,359,372]

Comment Ileorectal anastomosis for Crohn's colitis is the procedure of choice when the rectum is relatively spared and when the patient does not have significant anal disease. With the passage of time, approximately one-third will develop symptoms severe enough to require either proctectomy or diversion. Even those who must undergo a second procedure can be relatively well served by temporarily avoiding an ileostomy. The problem, of course, is to select the appropriate patients, an exceedingly difficult task. One is often surprised at the degree of inflammatory reaction a patient may harbor in the rectum or indeed in the anal region and still have for a time a relatively salutary result following a restorative operation. However, patients who demonstrate pelvic sepsis, an intraabdominal abscess, or a fistula to the rectum should probably undergo a diverting loop ileostomy to protect the anastomosis. This is obviously a surgical decision, and each patient must be treated on an individual basis. Preoperative decision making can be facilitated by a determination of rectal capacity and compliance. These physiologic studies are discussed in Chapters 4 and 6.

Those who are troubled by frequent bowel movements can often be helped by the addition of a bulk agent containing psyllium, as well as "slowing" medications such as codeine, deodorized tincture of opium, and diphenoxylate or loperamide. If resection of the distal ileum were performed, cholestyramine (Questran) may be helpful in controlling diarrhea.

Segmental Colon Resection

With Crohn's disease, restoration of intestinal continuity is certainly a viable option under many circumstances, depending on the location and the extent of involvement. Because the condition can occur anywhere in the gastrointestinal tract, it is difficult to discuss the operative choices as they pertain solely to the colon and rectum. However, it is probably appropriate to perform one of only three sphincter-saving operations for colonic disease: right hemicolectomy (for ileocolonic and right-sided involvement), total or subtotal colectomy (for disease involving at least one-half of the colon), and sigmoid colectomy or anterior resection (in the unusual situation when the disease is limited to this area). One may add abdominoperineal resection with sigmoid colostomy as another limited-resectional option for patients whose disease is limited to the anorectum and in whom the complications were unable to be controlled by local measures or fecal diversion alone.

Results Results of segmental resection suggest that recurrence rates and requirement for reoperation are similar to those of total colectomy with restoration of continuity. Olaison and associates noted that lesions appear endoscopically soon after ileocolic resection, implicating new inflammation rather than residual disease or incomplete anastomotic healing.[349] Their data further suggest that despite clinical remission after complete extirpation of disease, the bowel is "permanently inflamed" in this condition. Longo and colleagues reported a recurrence rate of 62% in those treated by segmental resection and 67% managed by total colectomy.[290] In spite of these suboptimal statistics, more than 80% of patients were able to preserve bowel continuity. Andrews and colleagues noted cumulative reoperation rates at 5 and 10 years after right hemicolectomy to be 26% and 46%, respectively; after total colectomy and ileorectal anastomosis it was 46% and 60%.[20] Allan and associates, reporting a very limited experience with segmental colon resection (colo-colonic anastomosis), implied that there is no difference in complication and recurrence rates when the procedure is compared with total colectomy and ileorectal anastomosis.[13] I question the validity of their observations, and I counsel against any anastomotic procedure in the colon except those previously mentioned. Still, Andersson and co-workers (Linköping, Sweden) opine that resection with colo-colic anastomosis should be considered in limited Crohn's colitis,[19] However, their numbers were few, and in the absence of a prospective study I shall continue to stand by my opinion.

The perioperative morbidity associated with the performance of intestinal anastomoses in this condition has been prospectively reviewed in 429 patients from the University of Heidelberg.[269] Postoperative complications and mortality were observed in 9.7% and 0.5%, respectively. Besides the presence of sepsis at the time of operation, long-term corticosteroid therapy was the only variable found to significantly affect morbidity. No statistically significant association was observed with respect to age, gender, duration of disease, prior surgery, nutritional status, extent of disease, type, number and location of anastomoses, or presence of disease at the margin of resection.[369]

An interesting technical variation designed to reduce the incidence of recurrent disease was suggested by the Mayo Clinic group.[331] They performed a case-control comparative analysis of 138 patients, half of whom underwent conventional sutured end-to-end anastomosis; the other half received a wide-lumen stapled (side-to-side, function end-to-end) anastomosis. They found that the cumulative reoperation rate for anastomotic recurrence was significantly lower (*p* = .017) for the wide-lumen anastomosis group. It would therefore seem prudent to perform as large an anastomosis as is reasonable when the patient undergoes a colectomy for this indication.

Laparoscopic Resection

As with virtually all operations on the intestinal tract, laparoscopic techniques have been applied for resection in patients with Crohn's disease. The hypothetical and actual advantages, such as earlier return of bowel function, reduced length of stay, less discomfort, faster recovery of pulmonary function, and more cosmetic incisions, have been discussed elsewhere in this book (see Chapter 27). The greater benefit of this approach for this condition is the likelihood of the requirement for reoperation. Conversely, the disadvantage of the lack of tactile ability (unless a hand-port is used), in an operation wherein careful inspection and even palpation of the entire small bowel must be performed, requires consideration. One must be mindful that surgery for Crohn's disease often involves hand dissection and specifically a finger-fracture technique.

There is a rapidly expanding literature on the experience of laparoscopic resection for this condition.[20,32,110,123,206,295,322,426,495] Preliminary results suggest comparable recurrence rates. There may even be a reduced incidence of small bowel obstruction, a critically important issue in differential diagnosis and therapy with these patients.[32] Still, this can be a technically demanding approach—it is not for the novice laparoscopist, especially in the presence of a phlegmon, fistula, or abscess.[123]

Resection with Exclusion of Rectum (Hartmann Procedure)

As previously suggested, resection of the colon without reestablishment of intestinal continuity is a reasonable option in the management of Crohn's colitis. Guillem

and colleagues reviewed the Lahey Clinic experience of such surgery to determine the factors relating to the fate of the rectal segment.[189] At a median follow-up time of 6 years, 70% had developed disease in the excluded rectum. Approximately one-half of the total series had undergone proctectomy by 2.4 years. Nineteen percent retained the rectum with disease. Neither initial involvement of the terminal ileum nor endoscopic inflammatory changes seen in the rectum predicted eventual disease of the excluded rectal segment. However, initial perianal disease was predictive of persistent rectal segment involvement, often requiring subsequent proctectomy. The authors suggest that early completion proctectomy or primary total proctocolectomy should be seriously considered in this group of patients. Harling and associates observed a 5-year cumulative ileal resection rate with an out-of-circuit rectum of 29%.[202] The 10-year risk of subsequent proctectomy was 50%.

Sher and associates noted that a Hartmann resection affords excellent palliation in individuals with severe anorectal disease.[437] Although none of their 25 patients subsequently underwent reestablishment of intestinal continuity, the authors felt that the problem of an unhealed perineal wound can be averted when elective resection is undertaken with quiescent anorectal and perianal disease.

Management of Small Bowel Crohn's Disease

The indications for surgery for regional enteritis include inanition, intraabdominal sepsis, intestinal obstruction, fistulas, urologic complications, and extra-intestinal manifestations. In our reported experience with the long-term follow-up of small intestinal Crohn's disease, the most common indication for surgical treatment was chronic obstruction (35%), followed by internal fistulas (30%), intractability (22%), and abscess formation (11%).[460] Types of operation include limited small bowel resection, multiple small bowel resections (with enteroenterostomy and/or diversion), bypass, strictureplasty, balloon dilatation, and resection of small bowel in continuity with cecum, or right colon, or most or all of the colon, and rectum.

Acute Ileitis

As previously discussed, occasionally a patient is submitted to laparotomy with a presumed diagnosis of acute appendicitis. The appendix may be safely removed if there is no evidence of cecal disease. Conversely, if the cecum appears to be involved by the inflammatory process, appendectomy may result in a fecal fistula. Laparotomy alone may lead to a fistula through handling of the diseased bowel, presumably from disrupting microperforations of the distal ileum.[132] In any event, resection of the ileum is not advised under these circumstances. In an extensive review of the incidence of progression of regional enteritis involving only the distal ileum, Gump and associates reported that fewer than 10% of patients developed subsequent identifiable ileitis.[190]

Small Bowel Resection

When an operation is indicated for other than acute ileitis, resection of the involved segment is usually performed. The choice of operative procedure depends on the intraabdominal findings—including the length of segment or segments involved, the location within the intestinal tract, whether there is concomitant colonic involvement, the presence of a fistula or abscess, whether bowel had been resected previously, how much one is removing and how much would remain. It is not usually difficult to identify the area of involvement because of the macroscopic appearance of the serosal surface of the bowel—fat wrapping, inflammatory changes, stricture, and so on. Still, it is discouraging to note that in a study

by Lescut and co-workers, 65% of patients operated on for Crohn's disease had lesions of the small intestine undetected by the surgeon but which were identified by means of perioperative endoscopy of the whole small bowel.[274] It appears then that recurrence may not truly represent recurrence in every instance, but may represent persistent disease.

Small bowel resection is usually a rather straightforward procedure, an operation that is familiar to all general surgeons. A special concern is the often remarkable thickness of the mesentery. It is sometimes helpful to simply divide the mesentery without the use of clamps, maintaining pressure on the blood supply with the fingers, and then performing suture ligation of the cut ends of the vessels (see Figure 30-60). This will certainly expedite what can be a tedious dissection, one that can lead to significant blood loss and a large mesenteric hematoma. The finger fracture technique has been mentioned earlier.[92] Transillumination of the mesentery is another method for identifying the blood supply to the bowel (Figure 30-63). It is a particularly useful method when creating an ileostomy or performing a pouch pro-

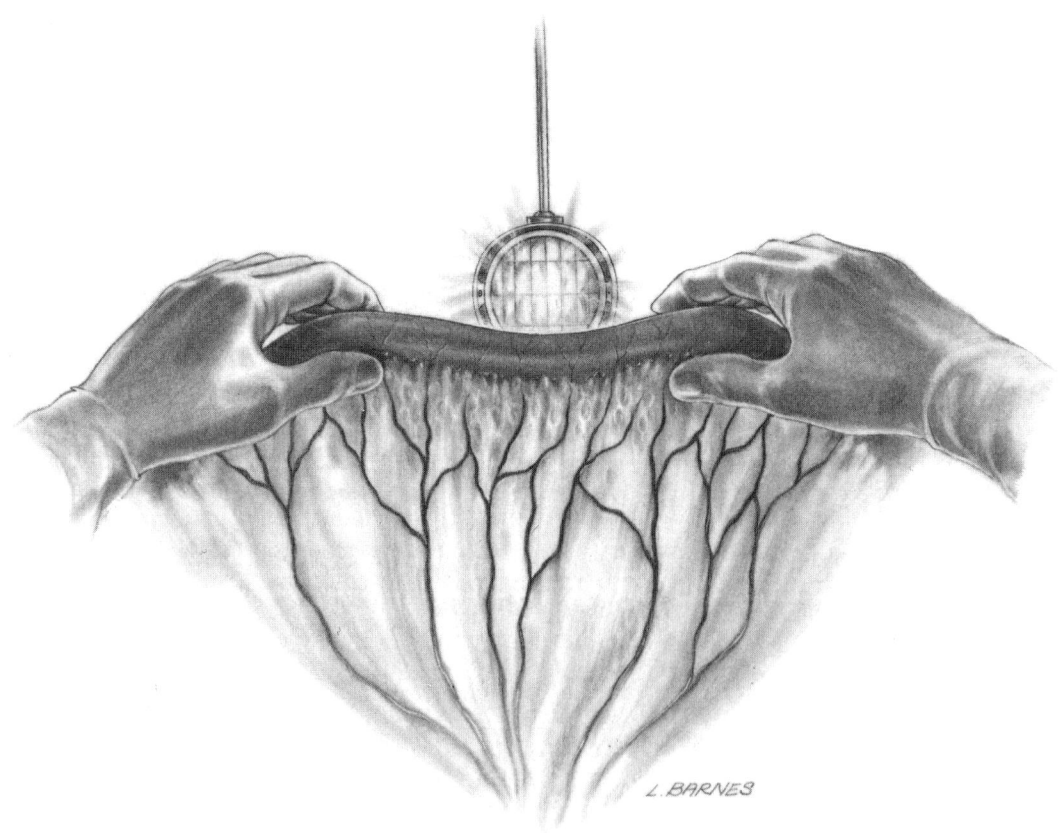

FIGURE 30-63. Transillumination is a useful technique for identifying the mesenteric blood supply. When tailoring the distal ileum in preparation for an ileostomy or the creation of a pouch, this approach can be invaluable.

cedure. To ensure adequacy of the blood supply to the area, the overhead light is lowered or, preferably, a portable lamp is used. (Goligher took great pride in mounting a Rolls Royce headlamp on a pole in the operating room. The concept was that if you could see the back-country road surface on a foggy night in Yorkshire, this light should permit you to visualize the blood supply to the small bowel.)

The intestine is elevated to reveal the vascular structures. If one uses a sharply pointed forceps and paired straight clamps, the mesentery can be divided much more expeditiously than with the familiar curved clamp "poke-through and hunt for the opening" method (Figure 30-64). Although it has been said that the small bowel can be safely reapproximated with chewing gum and baling wire, an interrupted single-layer technique or stapling method is suggested (Figs. 30-65 and 30-66).

Resection is usually undertaken leaving a minimum normal bowel margin of 5 or 6 cm. If multiple "skip" areas are present, one endeavors to remove or bypass only the most constricting portions that may be causing the symptoms. If two segments are involved in relative proximity (e.g., <30 cm), it is probably safer to perform an en bloc resection of both segments rather than to perform two anastomoses.

Smedh and colleagues have suggested an innovative concept to prevent coloileal reflux after ileocecal resection.[447] They suggest that reflux of intestinal contents may be responsible for recurrence at and just proximal to the anastomosis. The technique is shown in Figure 30-67. The authors observed that there was a suggestion of radiologically demonstrable preserved nipple function and remission of disease when compared with patients who underwent conventional anastomosis and those who had no visible nipple on follow-up examination. Further information on this unique concept is certainly warranted.

Strictureplasty

Radical excision of the small bowel in an attempt to remove all obvious disease may result in profound disturbances in fluid and electrolytes as well as severe malnutrition (Figure 30-68). In recent years, strictureplasty has been suggested as an alternative in this situation.[9,49,57, 102,133,136,296,355,357,468,475,478,479,514] The procedure was originally advocated by Katariya and colleagues for the treatment of tubercular strictures but was successfully applied to the management of extensive Crohn's disease by Lee and Papaioannou.[234,265] The primary indications are the presence of multiple, relatively short strictures, and the need to conserve intestinal length because of extensive disease or prior resection. The procedures advocated for pyloroplasty (either Heineke-Mikulicz for short strictures or Finney for long ones) may be utilized (Figs. 30-69 and 30-

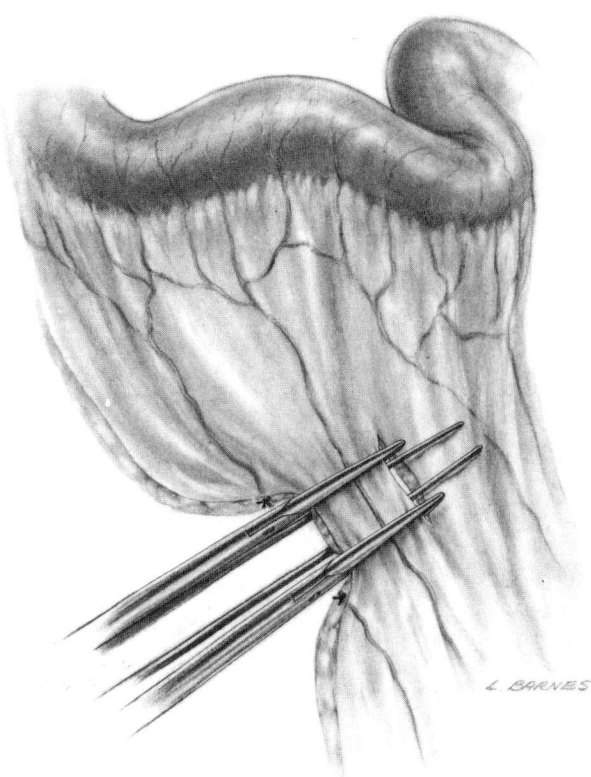

FIGURE 30-64. Small bowel resection using sharply pointed forceps and paired straight clamps.

70). An interrupted single-layer technique is less likely to cause luminal narrowing, and patching the suture line to the serosa of the adjacent bowel may help prevent leakage.[471] Taschieri and co-workers offer a number of bowel-sparing techniques for the management of long strictures due to Crohn's disease (Figs. 30-71 through 30-73).[468] As with all operations designed to coapt intestine, a stapler modification may also be used, but the presence of thickened bowel may preclude the application of this instrument (Figs. 30-74 and 30-75).[57,97,236] Kendall and colleagues suggest the use of a 2-cm bougie to identify all areas of significant narrowing.[239] Alexander-Williams prefers to use a Foley catheter,[9] whereas García-Granero and co-workers recommend a 2.5 cm medical plastic sphere.[150] One may combine strictureplasty with limited small bowel resection and bypass, all within the same individual, depending on the operative findings.

One of the concerns that has been expressed is the possibility of performing strictureplasty in the presence of cancer arising in Crohn's disease. It is therefore prudent to perform a small biopsy of the full thickness of the bowel before completing the procedure, obtaining frozen sections to confirm the absence of malignant

(text continues on page 1515)

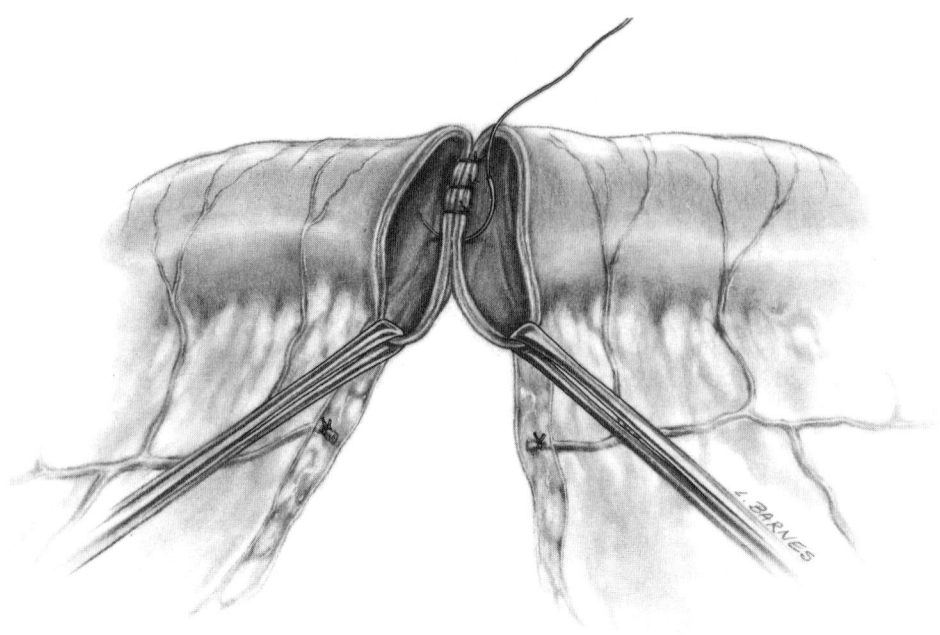

FIGURE 30-65. Small bowel resection. Anastomosis by conventional, interrupted, inverting, single-layer suture.

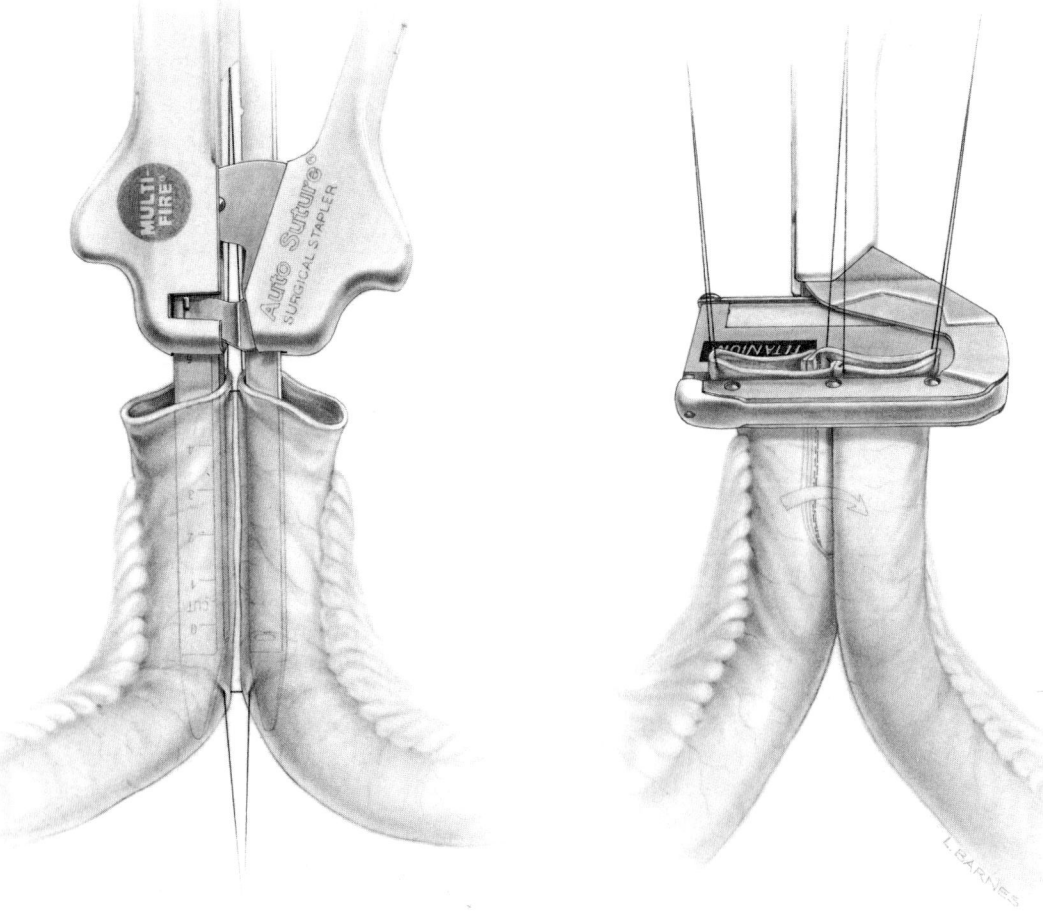

A   B

FIGURE 30-66. Functional end-to-end small bowel anastomosis. **(A)** The GIA stapler is inserted. **(B)** Linear closure is effected with the TA-55 stapling device.

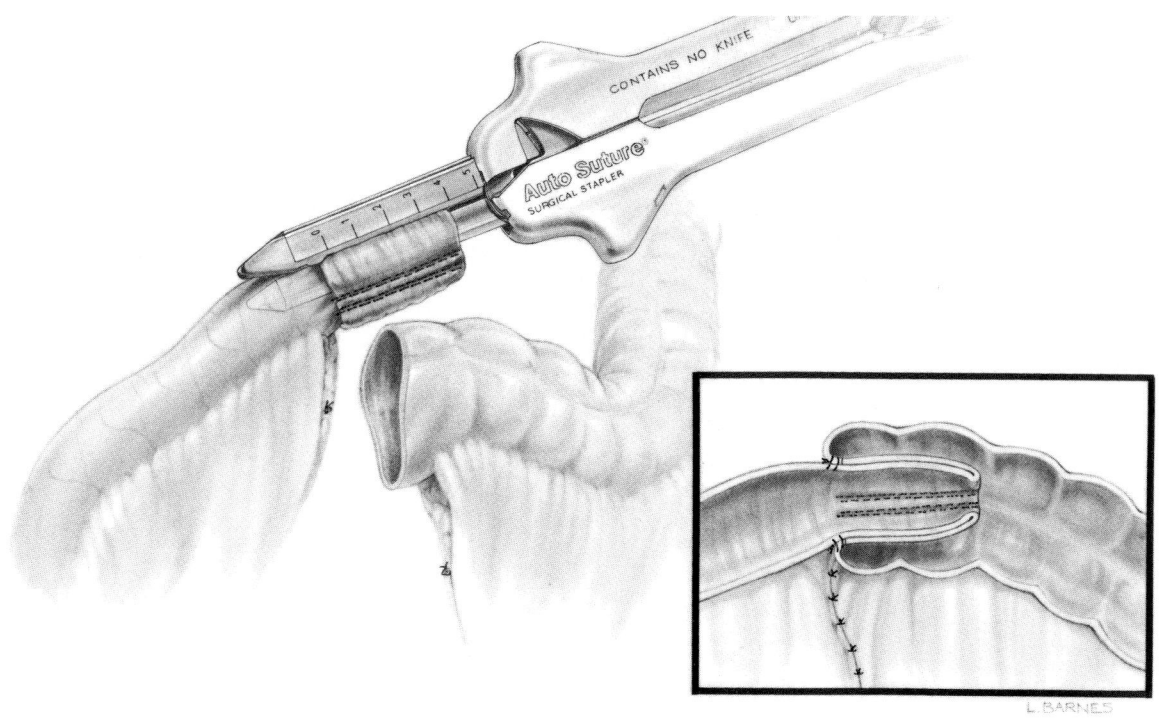

FIGURE 30-67. Construction of ileocecal nipple anastomosis as advocated by Smedh and associates.[447]

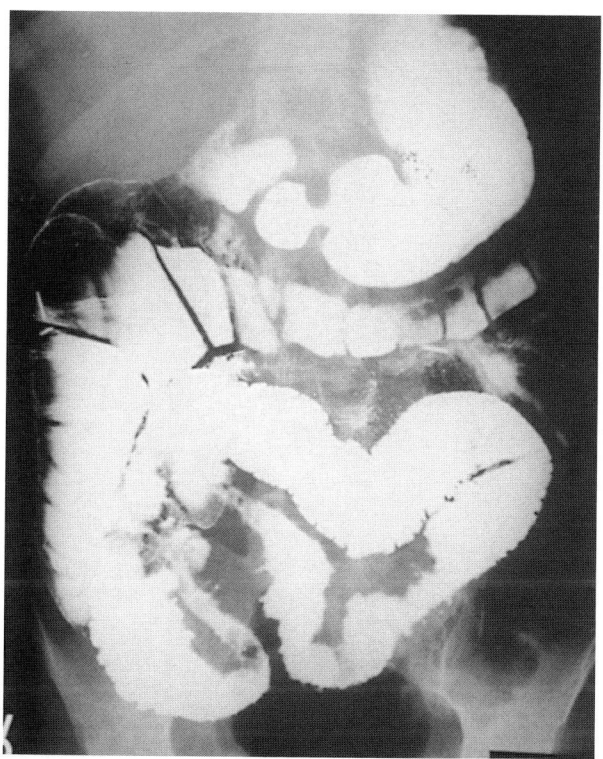

FIGURE 30-68. Upper gastrointestinal small bowel series demonstrates only a limited amount of small bowel remaining in an individual who had previously undergone several resections. Note that the small intestine which remains is extensively involved by recurrent Crohn's disease. Parenthetically, the colon appears spared.

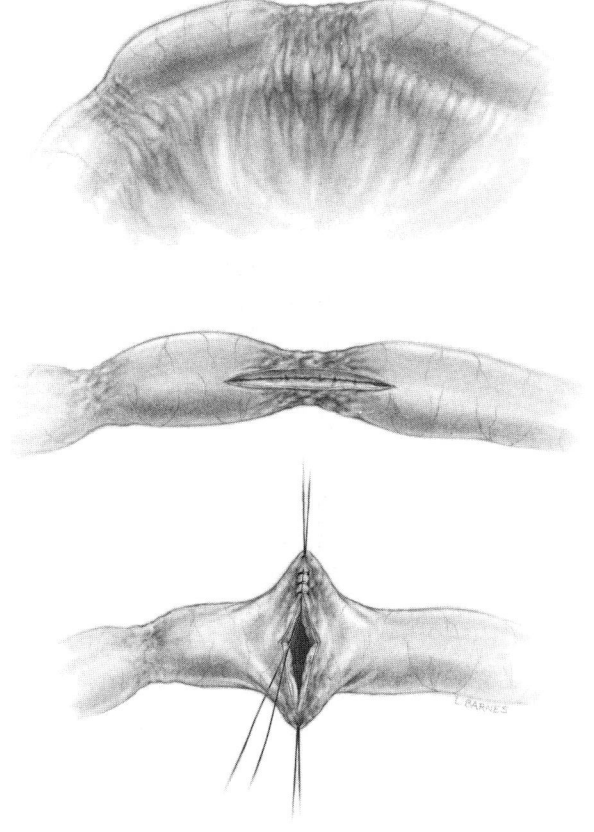

FIGURE 30-69. Strictureplasty for Crohn's disease. Short stricture treated by the technique analogous to Heineke-Mikulicz pyloroplasty. Longitudinal enterotomy is closed transversely using interrupted #3–0 long-term absorbable sutures.

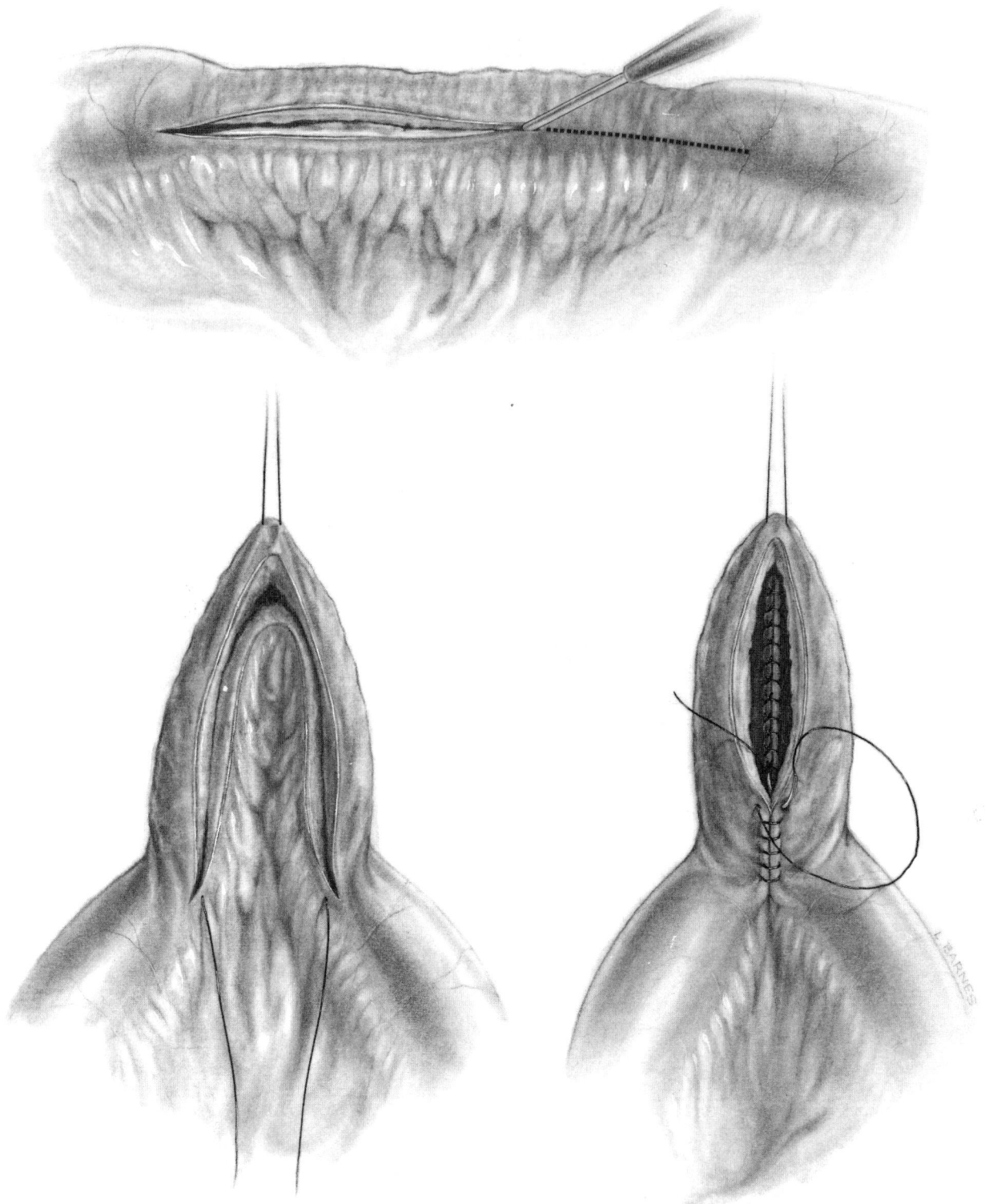

FIGURE 30-70. Strictureplasty for Crohn's disease. Long stricture treated by equivalent of Finney "pyloroplasty" technique. A long antimesenteric incision is made over the stricture site and carried into the normal bowel.

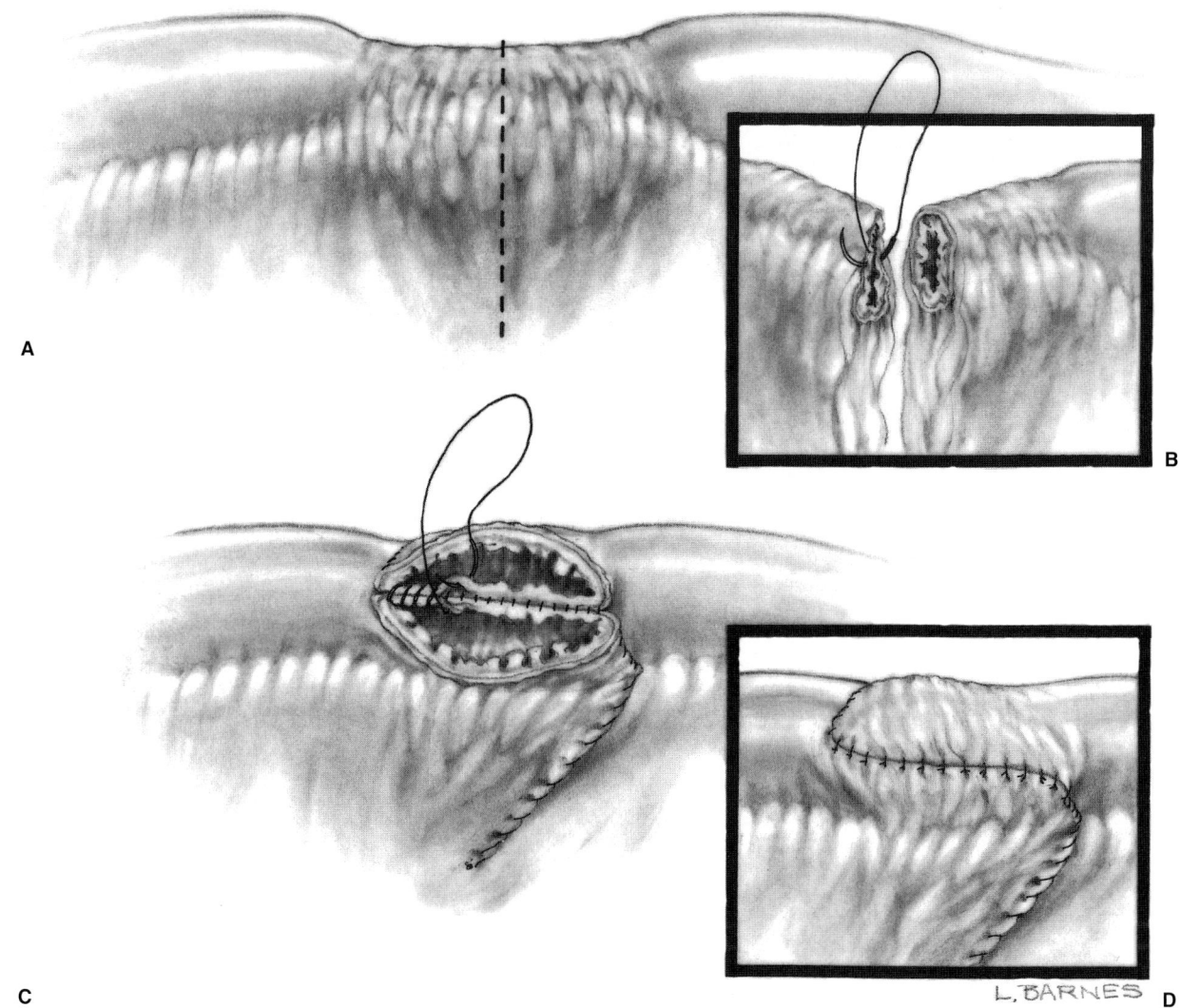

A

B

C

D

L. BARNES

FIGURE 30-71. Crohn's stricture. **(A)** Severe narrowing of a long segment of small bowel. **(B)** The bowel is transected. **(C)** Suturing of the two ends by means of a two-layer, hand-sewn running suture. Approximation of the two segments in a parallel fashion. **(D)** Completion of side-to-side ileal-ileal anastomosis. The original lumen has been doubled, thus sparing half the length of the intestine. (After Taschieri AM, Cristaldi M, Elli M, et al. Description of new bowel-sparing techniques for long strictures of Crohn's disease. *Am J Surg* 1997;173:509.)

change. The Cleveland Clinic group also recommends that the site(s) of the strictureplasty(ies) be marked with a titanium clip for subsequent radiologic and possible operative localization.

Results

Alexander-Williams reviewed 146 procedures performed on 57 patients without a death.[9] There were four anastomotic leaks, and eight required reoperation 6 months to 3 years later. Kendall and colleagues treated seven patients by a total of 45 strictureplasties.[239] Two developed enterocutaneous fistulas; recurrent symptoms were noted in six, four of whom required surgery.

The Cleveland Clinic Group has reported what is inarguably the world's largest experience with strictureplasty.[356] The latest publication involves 162 patients who underwent a total of 698 strictureplasties (Heineke-Mikulicz, 617; Finney, 81). The mean number performed for each individual was three. There were no deaths. The cumulative 5-year incidence of reoperation for recurrence was 28%, with a mean follow-up of 42 months. Symptoms of obstruction were relieved in 98% of the patients. Reoperative rates were comparable to that of resection.[356] For patients treated by strictureplasty alone the cumulative reoperation rate at 5 years was 31%, whereas for those who underwent concomitant bowel resection it was 27%.

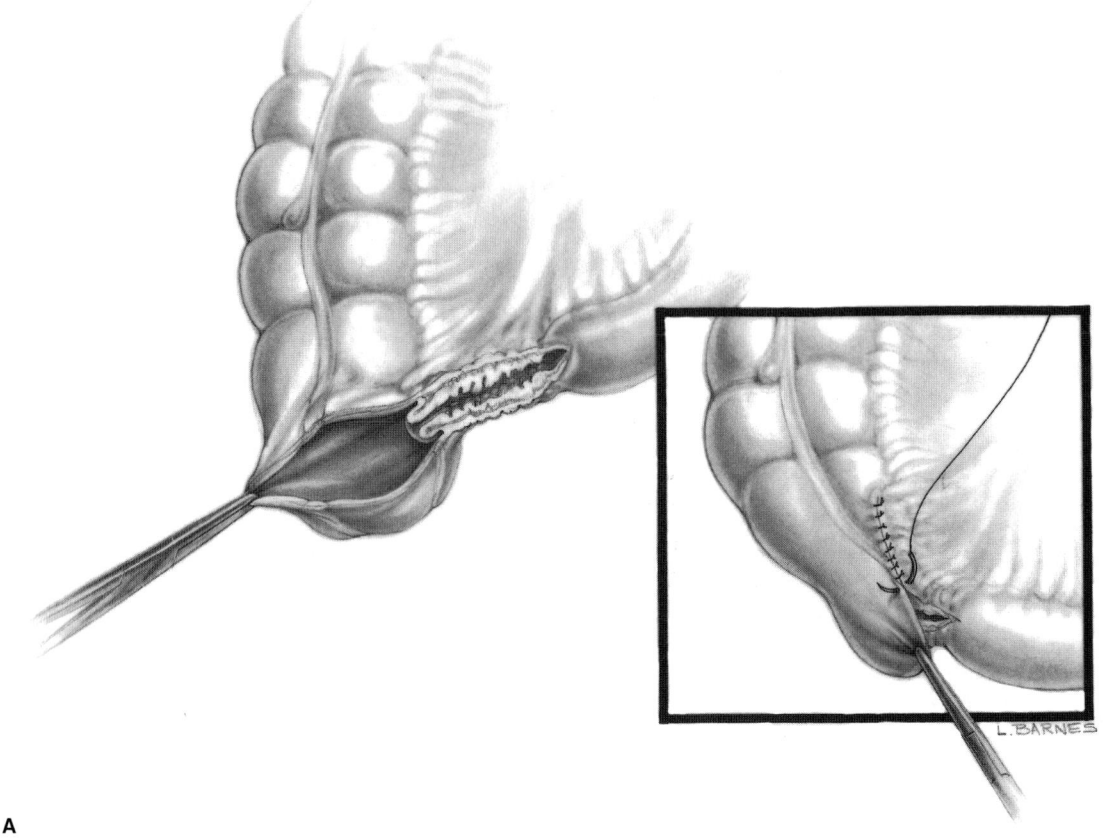

A   B

FIGURE 30-72. Terminal ileal Crohn's disease. **(A)** Severe disease with extensive narrowing at the level of the ileocecal valve. **(B)** Side-to-side ileocolic anastomosis. (After Taschieri AM, Cristaldi M, Elli M, et al. Description of new bowel-sparing techniques for long strictures of Crohn's disease. *Am J Surg* 1997;173:509.)

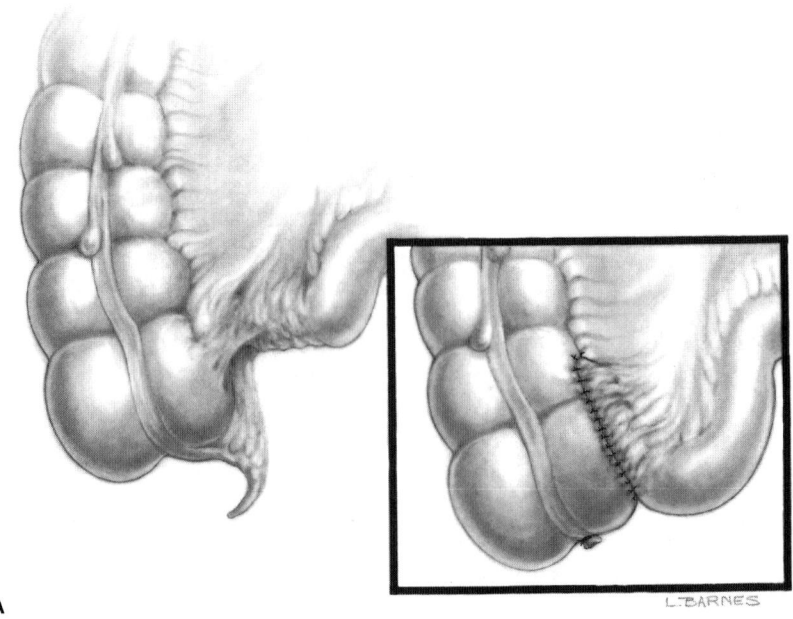

FIGURE 30-73. (A) Marked narrowing of the terminal ileum with associated narrowing at the level of the ileocecal valve. **(B)** Side-to-side ileocolic anastomosis. (After Taschieri AM, Cristaldi M, Elli M, et al. Description of new bowel-sparing techniques for long strictures of Crohn's disease. *Am J Surg* 1997;173:509.)

A   B

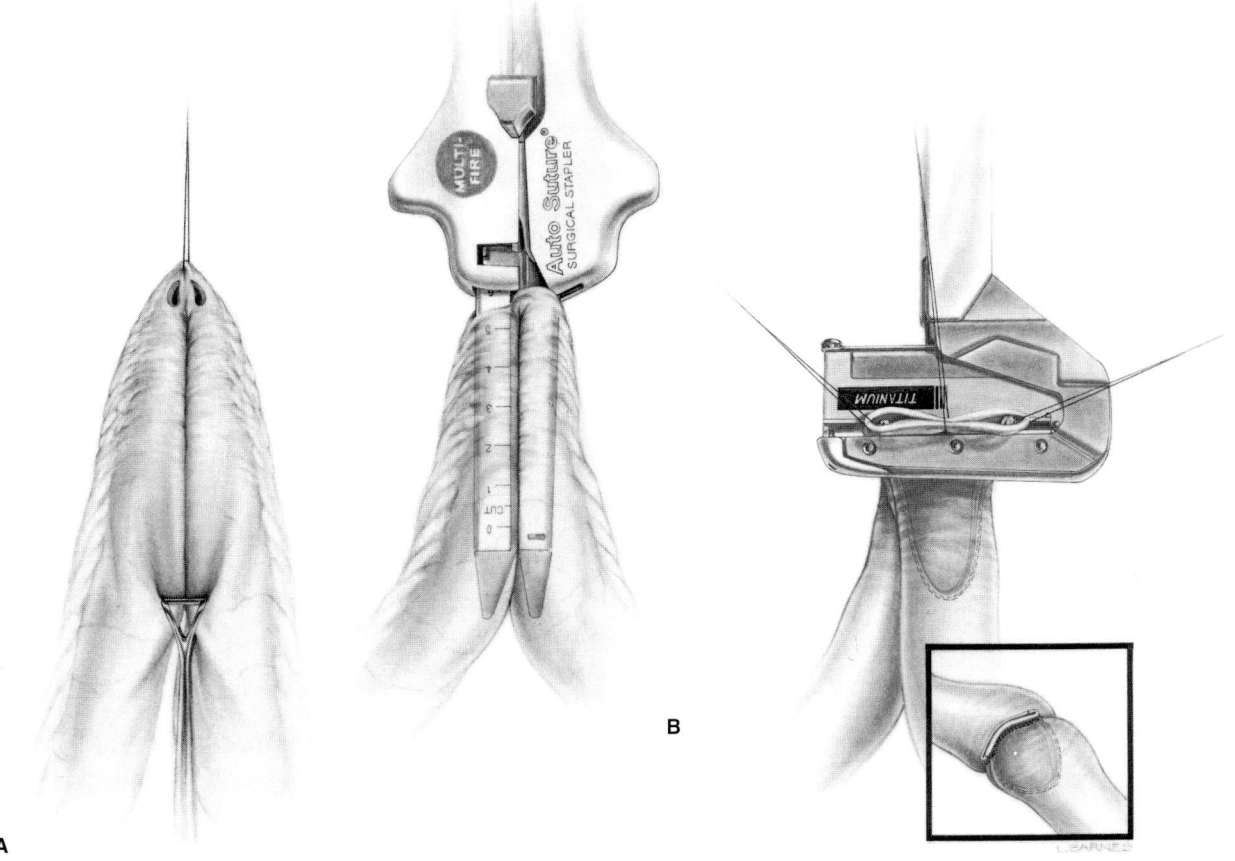

FIGURE 30-74. Stapled strictureplasty for Crohn's disease. **(A)** The midpoint of the stricture becomes the apex; the bowel is held in position by means of a suture or a Babcock clamp. Two small enterotomies are created. **(B)** The two limbs of the stapler are inserted and fired. The stapler instrument size may be changed to accommodate the length of the stricture. **(C)** The linear stapler is fired. A biopsy specimen may be obtained by trimming the residual tissue **(inset)**.

In another report from the same institution with longer follow-up, the investigators conclude that strictureplasty is a safe and durable alternative to resection for diffuse Crohn's jejunoileitis, but those with a short duration of disease and reduced interval since the last surgery are at an increased risk of accelerated recurrence.[102]

Saylan and colleagues studied the need for reoperation following this procedure.[424] The results were also not significantly different from those individuals treated by resection. Others have confirmed the comparative safety and effectiveness of this operation.[9,49,57,94,357,468,478] Moreover, there is ample radiologic, endoscopic, histopathologic, and operative evidence that active Crohn's disease regresses at the site of the strictureplasty, especially when a large anastomosis (i.e., Finney-type) has been performed.[318,475,479] For example, with the use of abdominal ultrasound, Maconi and colleagues found that the thickening of diseased bowel wall may improve after conservative surgery, a favorable prognostic factor.[296]

The Cleveland Clinic group has also performed strictureplasty for recurrent disease at the ileocolic anastomosis.[477] In 22 individuals so treated, there was no mortality or major septic complication. This method is therefore recommended to preserve small bowel length and as a reasonable alternative to re-resection.[477]

Balloon Dilatation

Another alternative to the management of colonic strictures is balloon dilatation. This technique has been performed successfully via the colonoscope with the use of the Riglex TTS dilating balloons.[337] Williams and Palmer have undertaken the procedure in seven patients without complication.[502] Two were unsuccessful, but five exhibited sustained improvement for up to 2 years. Alexander-Williams has used operative balloon dilatation of strictures between 20 and 25 mm in diameter, whereas Neufeld and colleagues noted that endoscopic application of the

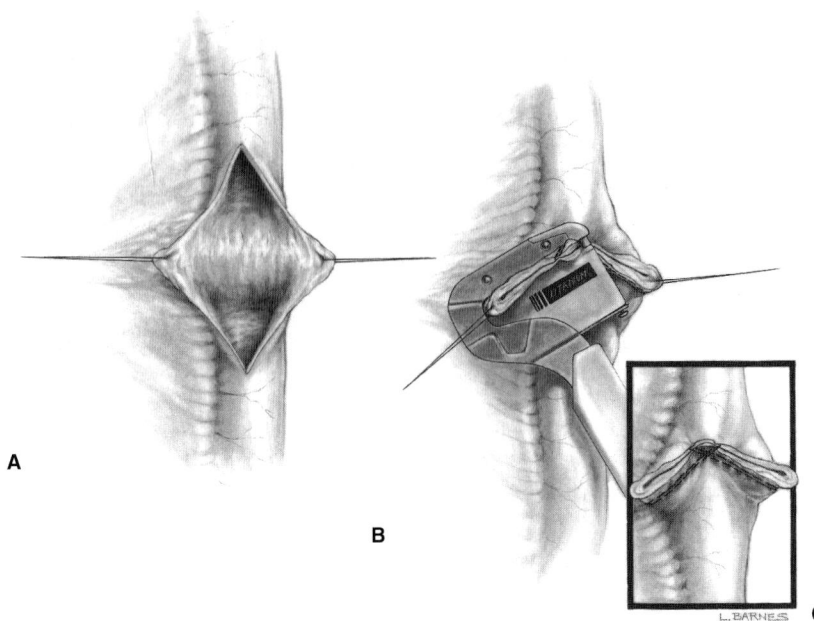

FIGURE 30-75. Stapled stricture-plasty. **(A)** The bowel is opened in a longitudinal fashion. **(B,C)** Utilizing a linear stapler and overlapping staple lines, the stricture-plasty is performed.

electrosurgical sphincterotome can be applied to fibrotic strictures.[11,337]

Management of Enteric Fistulas

Approximately 30% of patients with Crohn's disease will develop a fistula; one third of these will be external. An external fistula may be the manifestation by which the patient presents initially, but it is obviously much more commonly recognized as a postoperative complication. The nonsurgical approach to this problem has been discussed previously (see Medical Management). Hill and colleagues reported the principles of surgical and metabolic management in accordance with a standard protocol[216]:

- Drainage of the septic process
- Correction of any metabolic deficits
- Identification of anatomy and the pathologic process
- Resection

In a group of 85 patients, 69 (82%) achieved successful closure (approximately one-half surgically and one-half spontaneously). The authors distinguish between two groups of individuals—those whose fistulas are unrelated to Crohn's disease and those with known residual IBD. They contend that enterocutaneous fistulas arising from diseased small intestine all require surgery.

When an enteroenteric fistula is identified, it is important to try to ascertain whether the bowel is primarily or secondarily involved by Crohn's disease (Figure 30-76). For example, in the latter situation, resection of the segment of intestine that is not actually diseased can often

be avoided. Such a circumstance arises when the involved terminal ileum creates an ileosigmoid fistula. Resection of the ileum is undertaken with division of the fistulous communication to the sigmoid colon. Whether resection of the sigmoid is appropriate depends on the degree of inflammatory reaction; if the opening can simply be sutured, no resection is advised.

Saint-Marc and colleagues reviewed their experience with 74 patients who harbored 100 internal fistulas.[416] Closure of the defect of the so-called victim organ was achieved by resection in 41 instances and sutured in 59. In the Mayo Clinic experience involving 90 patients with ileosigmoid fistula secondary to Crohn's disease, repair rather than resection did not increase the risk of complications, provided that standard surgical principles were applied.[523] Others confirm that the procedure can be accomplished with minimal morbidity and mortality.[319]

If a *vesical fistula* develops, management of the bladder is essentially the same as that described when the communication is a consequence of radiation injury (see Figure 28-41). Since there is no disease affecting the bladder itself, no specific measures aside from urinary drainage are indicated. Cystoscopy is the most accurate investigative procedure for identifying such a fistula.[317]

Bypass or Exclusion

A bypass or exclusion procedure has in the past been advocated for distal ileal and cecal Crohn's disease. These operations are open to criticism because of the high incidence of persistent septic problems and the association with the subsequent development of carcinoma (see ear-

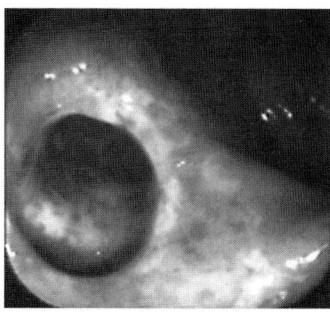

FIGURE 30-76. Colonoscopy demonstrates the opening of a fistula into the small intestine with acute and chronic inflammatory reaction. The proximal lumen of the colon can be seen in the upper right. (See Figure 30-2.)

lier). Therefore, they should only be undertaken if the inflammatory process cannot be removed for technical reasons or because of co-morbid conditions.

One exception to the caution of applying bypass is in patients with duodenal Crohn's. A gastroenterostomy is often advised in this circumstance, but a strictureplasty should definitely be considered (see earlier discussion).

Continent or Kock Ileostomy

As stated earlier, the application of the continent ileostomy in the management of Crohn's colitis is contraindicated. The technique is described in Chapter 29. Myrvold and Kock reported 52 patients with Crohn's disease who underwent continent ileostomy.[334] Most were performed in the mistaken belief that the patient had ulcerative colitis. Recurrence in the reservoir and/or distal ileum occurred in 53%. While the functional results were in general reasonably satisfactory, the incidence of postoperative and late complications was significantly higher than that which was observed in those who underwent the procedure for ulcerative colitis.

There are "courageous surgeons" (I prefer the phrase "courageous patients"), however, who believe that the procedure can be applied selectively to some individuals with this disease. The usual circumstance is the patient who underwent proctocolectomy and conventional ileostomy a number of years previously, with no evidence of recurrence in the interim. With this scenario, one may be willing to accept the risks of high morbidity and recurrent disease, and with appropriate patient consent proceed to a continent ileostomy. However, one must remember the issues and concerns expressed earlier in this chapter. I refer to the support for the concept of creating a large anastomosis or a wide-open strictureplasty. By producing a distal obstruction one changes the environment to the extent that it is quite likely that the risk of recurrence will be considerably increased.

Bloom and colleagues reported the clinical course of seven patients who were submitted to this procedure.[44] All were women, with a mean disease-free interval before conversion of nearly 8 years (minimum, 5 years). The postoperative complication rate and revision rate of 28% was comparable to that which is observed when the operation is performed for ulcerative colitis or multiple polyposis (see Chapter 29). No patient underwent conversion to a conventional ileostomy. Gerber and associates also reported success in patients with Crohn's colitis, but their experience with ileocolitis, even with removal of the entire diseased bowel, was associated with a prohibitively high incidence of postoperative complications.[157] Handelsman and co-workers reported their experience from The Johns Hopkins University Hospital with eight patients diagnosed with Crohn's disease or colitis of indeterminate origin who underwent a continent ileostomy.[200] All required removal of the pouch or continued medical management for recurrent disease. In their opinion and in mine, Crohn's disease is an absolute contraindication for performing this operation.

Barnett utilized a continent jejunal reservoir in three patients with colonic Crohn's disease, theorizing that there should be a reduced risk of recurrence in a pouch constructed at such a proximal level.[27] The new pouch and valve are transplanted and anastomosed to the terminal ileum. This concept proved to be disastrous for all concerned.

Restorative Proctocolectomy (Ileo-Pouch-Anal Procedure)

The experience with the restorative proctocolectomy in this condition is based primarily on those who underwent the operation for presumed ulcerative colitis only to discover after pathologic assessment of the surgical specimen that the diagnosis was in error. Another group of patients who have undergone this procedure are those who subsequently develop Crohn's disease even though retrospective analysis of the specimen fails to confirm the diagnosis. The third and smallest group represents those known to have Crohn's disease confined to the colon and rectum, with no small bowel or anal involvement.

Results Following Restorative Proctocolectomy

Results according to the Cleveland Clinic experience suggest that there are two distinct categories of patients: those with preoperative stigmata of Crohn's disease and those whose Crohn's disease was not suspected but only discovered on the basis of the histologic evaluation.[225] Patients in whom there is any preoperative suggestion of Crohn's disease, clinically or pathologically, had very poor results following this operation. Conversely, in the short term at least, if the clinical diagnosis of ulcerative colitis seems assured, early results following restorative proctocolectomy are significantly better with postoperative, histologically proven Crohn's disease than when Crohn's disease is suspected preoperatively. In a preliminary report, 15 of 16 patients in the former group maintained their pouches, compared with only one of nine in the latter in the Cleveland Clinic experience.[225]

On the basis of the poor results observed in most of the nine patients found to have Crohn's disease postoperatively, the Toronto General Hospital Group counsel that the pelvic pouch procedure should not knowingly be performed in these individuals.[96] A total of 37 patients was identified in the Mayo Clinic experience who inadvertently underwent restorative proctocolectomy and were subsequently proven to have Crohn's disease.[415] Approximately one-third developed complex fistulas. Recurrent Crohn's disease developed in 100%. However, after a mean of 10 years (range, 3 to 14 years), the pouch remained in place in 20 individuals, but in seven a diversion was performed. The overall failure rate was interpreted to be 45%.[415] In the report of Regimbeau and co-workers (Clichy, France), 41 patients with Crohn's disease underwent ileal-pouch anastomotic surgery.[388] In 26 the diagnosis was established preoperatively or in the pathologic report, whereas 15 subsequently developed Crohn's disease-related complications. Twenty patients were followed for more than 10 years. The rates of Crohn's disease-related complications and pouch excision were 35% and 10%, respectively. These results led the investigators to conclude that it is reasonable to propose restorative proctocolectomy in selected patients with limited colorectal Crohn's disease.

The Birmingham, United Kingdom, group performed restorative proctocolectomy in 23 patients with Crohn's disease, 12 of whom had disease evidence at the time of the operation.[333] At a mean follow-up of 10.2 years almost 50% underwent pouch excision. In a comparison with ileoproctostomy the investigators concluded that restorative proctocolectomy was inferior, but the functional results of those with a successful outcome were comparable. Others confirm that the short- to medium-term functional results are acceptable if the pouch can be retained.[187]

Comment

The concept of offering restorative proctocolectomy to individuals with Crohn's disease in which the small bowel and anal areas are spared is based on the understanding that any operation for this condition will not guarantee cure, and even proctocolectomy and ileostomy in such a patient is associated with a recurrence rate of approximately 20%. Therefore, why not consider restoration of intestinal continuity and provide such a person with the benefits of that operation? Now that one has longer-term follow-up, it appears that the rate of pouch excision may be only slightly greater than when the operation is per-

formed for ulcerative colitis in these selected patients. Members of the panel at a meeting of the American Society of Colon and Rectal Surgeons in 1990 opined that they would refuse to perform reservoir procedures in patients with Crohn's disease, even when the disease has been limited to the colon, and despite no evidence of small bowel recurrence with long-term follow-up.[402] Clearly, that attitude can no longer be considered the standard of care. Many of these same individuals have altered their position, but there is no disagreement that the patient must have a full and complete understanding of the risks associated with this alternative.

Recurrence

A number of factors have been at some time suggested to contribute to an increased risk for recurrence after resection: site of involvement, age at onset of disease, age at first resection, gender, prior resection, extent of resection, presence or absence of gross/microscopic disease at resection margin, presence of perianal disease, immunologic factors (T-cell and total lymphocyte counts), blood transfusion, choice of operation, pathologic variables, and probably others.[504]

Following the Patient

The protocol for following the patient who has undergone resection in order to identify early recurrence has never been clearly established, nor is it without controversy. A variety of approaches include regular follow-up visits, periodic endoscopic evaluation, and radiologic and laboratory investigations, as well as issues involving long-term drug therapy. The fecal excretion of 1-antitrypsin has been felt to be a reliable marker of intestinal protein loss. It has therefore been evaluated for its efficacy as an early indicator for recurrence in Crohn's disease.[47] Boirivant and colleagues believe that it is indeed a sensitive, noninvasive, inexpensive marker for those who undergo regular supervision after surgery.[47]

Stoma vs. Anastomosis

Ileostomy itself seems to be associated with a significantly lower early recurrence risk than those individuals who have undergone colon anastomoses.[211] Others suggest that the fecal stream and reflux of colonic contents are important factors in determining the pattern of recurrence.[61] However, more recently surgeons have been exploring the concept of a wide side-to-side anastomosis of the ileum to the colon and also in the small bowel as a means for delaying the time interval for recurrence.[511] Prospective, randomized trials are currently being conducted on this variation in technique.

Trnka and colleagues reviewed 113 patients with Crohn's disease whose initial procedure involved an anastomosis.[483] The recurrence rate was 29% at 5 years, 52% at 10 years, and 84% at 25 years. There was no relationship between the incidence of recurrence and the age of the patient, the gender, the duration of disease, the presence or absence of granulomas, the length of the resected specimen, and the presence or absence of disease at the proximal resection margin. Patients with colon disease who underwent an anastomosis had a much higher incidence of recurrence than those who had small bowel involvement.

Location

The Cleveland Clinic has been associated with more papers, with greater numbers of patients, than any other institution. Results of a study involving 615 consecutive patients seen at that institution revealed the following primary clinical patterns: ileocolic, 41%; small intestine, 28.6%; colon, 27%; anorectal, 3.4%.[137] At 10 years, more than 90% of patients with ileocolitis underwent surgery, and nearly 70% of patients with ileal or colonic disease required operation. Those with ileocolic disease had the highest rate of recurrence requiring another operation (53%), compared with 45% for colonic and 44% for small intestinal patterns.[137] Fazio and Wu conclude with the following main characteristics of patients with Crohn's disease:

- Most undergo surgery at some point.
- Reoperation is always a possibility.
- Prognosis with respect to recurrence differs based on the initial pattern of presentation. [137]

Whelan and colleagues reviewed the Cleveland Clinic experience with 592 patients followed for a mean of 13 years.[501] Those with ileocolic disease had the highest rate of recurrence: 53%, compared with 45% for colonic and 44% for small intestinal involvement. The estimated median time for recurrence was similar for all three groups, but the presence of an internal fistula or perianal disease was associated with an increased risk. Lock and colleagues reported the Cleveland Clinic's experience of 127 patients with Crohn's disease of the large bowel who underwent excisional surgery.[287] Initial involvement of the terminal ileum as well as the large bowel was associated with a significantly higher incidence of overall recurrence and earlier postoperative recurrence when compared with patients who had ileal sparing.

Another report from the same institution analyzed perforating and nonperforating Crohn's disease to see if these two expressions are reflected in a difference in the incidence of subsequent recurrence.[311] No such relationship was observed.

Chardavoyne and colleagues reviewed the records of 187 patients who underwent resection for Crohn's disease.[71] Age, gender, age at onset of the disease and at time of resection, family history, presence of granulomata, and microscopic involvement at the line of resection did not affect the rate of recurrence. Patients with predominantly large bowel disease were found to have a higher rate of re-resection (45%) than those with small intestinal involvement (32%). Lind and colleagues noted that the cumulative reoperation rate at 10 years was 71% for ileocolonic disease, 47% for colonic, and 58% for small bowel.[282] The crude reoperation rate for patients who had one resection in the experience of Valviulis and Currie was 37%.[486] Frikker and Segall reported that patients with small bowel disease had a better prognosis than did individuals with ileocolic involvement.[147]

In the experience of the group from Huddinge, Sweden, the cumulative 10-year risk of a symptomatic recurrence was 58% after colectomy and ileorectal anastomosis and 47% after segmental colonic resection.[36] Their resection rates for ileocecal disease were 61%, 77%, and 83% at 1, 5, and 10 years, respectively.[35] They conclude that three of four patients with Crohn's disease will undergo a bowel resection, half of whom will ultimately relapse.[34]

Homan and Dineen compared the results of resection, bypass, and exclusion for ileocecal Crohn's disease.[220] In a total of 161 patients, resection was performed in 115, bypass with exclusion in 25, and bypass alone in 21. Recurrence rates were 25% for resection, 63% for bypass with exclusion, and 75% for bypass alone. With 15 years of follow-up, bypass was seen to be associated with a 94% recurrence rate. The authors concluded that resection can be performed with morbidity and mortality equivalent to either of the bypass procedures and that the recurrence rate following resection is significantly lower than that for either bypass or exclusion. Others confirm that bypass and diversion procedures increase the likelihood of the need for further surgery.[120]

In our experience of resection for small bowel disease, 85% underwent excision of the terminal ileum and cecum with an anastomosis performed between the distal ileum and the ascending colon.[460] No frozen-section biopsies of the proximal margin were performed, and subsequent histologic examination revealed two instances (3%) in which the surgeon did not suspect involvement. Recurrent Crohn's disease developed after the initial bowel resection in 51 patients (69%). Of these, 28 (55%) required a second operation. Of these individuals, 18 had further recurrence of the disease, but in none did additional operative intervention prevent subsequent recurrence. Some patients even required a third and fourth procedure because of disease-related complications. In other words, no patient was cured if he or she required a third operation (Figure 30-77).

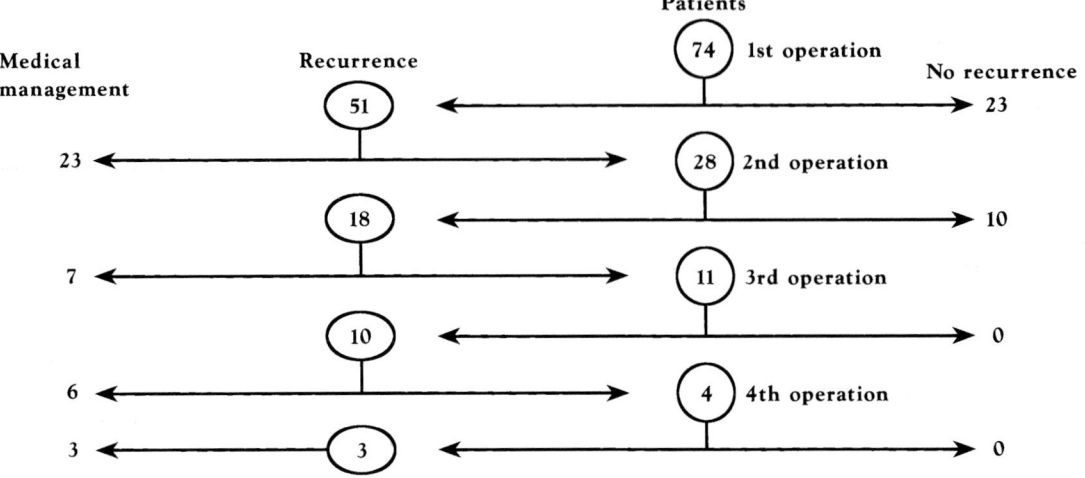

FIGURE 30-77. Pattern of recurrence in patients who underwent resection for small bowel Crohn's disease. (Adapted from Stone W, Veidenheimer MC, Corman ML, et al. The dilemma of Crohn's disease: long-term follow-up of Crohn's disease of the small intestine. *Dis Colon Rectum* 1977;20:372.)

Margin

A number of studies have demonstrated that the risk of recurrence is unaffected by the width of the macroscopically normal margin of resection.[135,511] Furthermore, recurrence rates are generally felt not to be increased when microscopic Crohn's disease is present at the resection margins, although there is difference of opinion. Some have opined that the presence of granulomas is associated with a statistically significant increased risk of recurrence.[21] There appears to be a close correlation between the duration of postoperative recurrence and the extent of presurgical disease.[99] Others confirm that disease extent has prognostic value with respect to the risk of symptomatic recurrence, whereas the length of resection margins does not appear to influence this risk.[385] All these papers reaffirm the importance of a conservative approach to resection margin in individuals with Crohn's disease.[370]

Adloff and colleagues reviewed 58 patients who underwent resection for Crohn's disease and found no statistically significant difference in recurrence rates between individuals with and without involved margins.[3] Wolff and associates reported the Mayo Clinic experience of more than 700 patients who underwent surgery for Crohn's disease with an anastomosis.[512] Those who were demonstrated to have microscopic involvement of the resection margin were found to have a recurrence rate of more than 90% within the follow-up period of 8 years. Those patients who did not have such involvement had a 55% incidence of recurrence at 10 years. The authors concluded that clear margins should be obtained in resections for Crohn's disease if this is at all possible. Conversely, others have demonstrated that microscopic involvement does not seem to increase the rate of recurrence.[214,254]

Hamilton and colleagues analyzed 79 patients who underwent resection and ileocolonic anastomosis.[193] In approximately one-half, the margin was determined by frozen section, and in the other group by visual inspection alone. In spite of negative initial microscopic evaluation, one-third was demonstrated to have involvement on final section. There was no statistically significant difference in the outcome of the two groups. The authors' findings support the concept of visual examination of the margins of resection, especially since one is usually able to preserve additional bowel by this approach. I believe that this is the correct position for a surgeon to take.

Rutgeerts and colleagues performed endoscopy and biopsy on 114 patients who underwent "curative" resection of the terminal ileum and part of the colon.[409] The recurrence rate within 1 year of the operation was 72%. A later report from the same group revealed that the endoscopic recurrence rate had increased to 85% at 3 years.[410] When patients were stratified for preoperative disease activity, the severity of lesions found at endoscopy remained a strong predictive factor for symptomatic recurrence.

Blood Transfusion

Because blood transfusion has been demonstrated to suppress the immune system (see Chapter 22), Peters and colleagues reviewed the records of 79 patients to determine whether perioperative blood transfusion affects recurrence rates.[362] A decreased rate of recurrence in those who received multiple transfusions was noted. However, an opposite conclusion was reached in a review of 197 patients from St. Mark's Hospital; there appeared to be no such association.[429] Although no one is suggesting a prospective clinical trial for obvious reasons, it would be ideal if this issue could be resolved.

Recurrent "Diverticulitis"

As mentioned in Chapter 26, patients who require re-resection after a procedure for what was initially thought to have been sigmoid diverticulitis should be presumed to have Crohn's colitis until proved otherwise. A high index of suspicion should be apparent if the illness is characterized by the requirement for multiple operations, if a diversionary procedure fails to control the distal disease, or if one of the following is noted: anorectal disease, rectal bleeding, or fistula. In our experience with 25 patients requiring resection for "diverticulitis" a second time, all pathologic specimens were diagnosed as Crohn's disease.[33]

Mortality

Probert and colleagues studied the mortality among 610 people with Crohn's disease that were identified in a population-based study from 1972 to 1989.[382] The overall mortality was not increased. Nordgren and associates studied the long-term follow-up in 136 patients from Göteborg, Sweden.[340] In a follow-up of 16.6 years, 18 patients had died, three from Crohn's disease. In the Cleveland Clinic series of 592 patients observed for a mean of 13 years, 12.7% died from all causes, but 6% of the deaths were directly related to Crohn's disease.[126] General opinion is that Crohn's disease does not significantly increase long-term mortality, a factor that needs to be conveyed to actuaries, insurers, and those individuals who advise employers.[382]

Surgical Management of Short Bowel Syndrome

For the sake of completeness it is worth mentioning that there are surgical approaches to the treatment of patients with the short bowel syndrome. Some are considered somewhat experimental, such as intestinal transplantation and the growing of new intestinal mucosa by means of serosal patching.[78,321,472,474] Other options include intestinal tapering and lengthening, creating of intestinal valves and sphincters, constructing antiperistaltic intestinal segments, intestinal pacing, and implementation of recirculating intestinal loops.[365] It is not within the purview of this text to detail all the potential options. Thompson has very nicely outlined the range of possibilities and appends a useful bibliography from which the reader may begin his or her exploration.[473]

INDETERMINATE COLITIS

The differential diagnosis between ulcerative colitis and Crohn's colitis can usually be made on the basis of clinical, radiologic, endoscopic, and pathologic criteria. However, up to 15% of patients develop nonspecific IBD of a type that cannot clearly be labeled as one or the other, often because of overlapping features. These individuals therefore have been classified as having an indeterminate colitis.

Indeterminate colitis is essentially a pathologic diagnosis; that is to say, there are often equivocal or contradictory histologic observations. In a review from St. Mark's Hospital of 30 such cases, nearly all patients had undergone urgent surgery.[380] As a consequence, these individuals had histologic features of incipient or established fulminant disease. This clinical presentation is probably the reason for the confusing histologic picture, since the pathology of Crohn's disease and that of ulcerative colitis in the acute phase have much in common.[380] There is insufficient opportunity—clinically, radiologically, or endoscopically—to clarify the nature of the disease. It follows, then, that the disease activity affects the evaluation of morphologic features and that, given the opportunity, repeat evaluation during a quiescent phase may clarify any confusion.

The diagnosis of Crohn's colitis is made by either the clinician (preoperatively or intraoperatively) or the pathologist. It is the latter who is responsible for creating the diagnosis of indeterminate colitis. Typical features in patients otherwise thought to have ulcerative colitis include "intermittent" ulceration, relative rectal sparing, preservation of goblet-cell population, and deep fissuring. Absence of granulomas in certain patients with presumed Crohn's disease also may place the patient in an indeterminate category. Lee and colleagues suggest the additional criteria of extensive mucosal and submucosal ulceration separated by normal colonic mucosa, nonaggregate full-thickness inflammation, increased vascularity in the base of the ulceration, and absence of both crypt abscesses and transmural lymphoid aggregates.[268]

Surgical Options

If the accuracy of the clinical (endoscopic, radiologic) and pathologic diagnosis is problematic, the surgeon would be wise to stage the procedure and not to embark on restorative proctocolectomy. Unfortunately, this admonition is only helpful when there is indeed a heightened suspicion as to the potential for error in diagnosis. By definition, patients with indeterminate colitis never have the diagnosis truly clarified, or Crohn's disease is demonstrated in the resected specimen, or Crohn's disease develops subsequently. One may also consider performing a total abdominal proctocolectomy, leaving only the anus and sphincters. This important technical consideration, resecting the rectum as low as is possible, facilitates the subsequent procedure—either completion proctectomy or a restorative operation. A particularly compelling caution against performing restorative proctocolectomy is the presence of an anal fistula or perineal disease.

Results of Restorative Proctocolectomy

Pezim and colleagues reviewed the Mayo Clinic experience with 25 patients who underwent restorative proctocolectomy for indeterminate colitis.[364] There were no significant differences in complication rates, pouch function, incidence of "pouchitis," or requirement for pouch excision, when comparing these individuals with those who underwent the operation for ulcerative colitis. However, the experience from the Lahey Clinic was quite different.[242] In a retrospective review of 18 patients so identified, 50% experienced complications. This compares with a complication rate of only 3% when the procedure was performed for ulcerative colitis. Furthermore, the requirement for subsequent ileostomy was much greater in individuals with indeterminate colitis. In another paper from the same institution, the authors suggest that "pouchitis" will usually respond to metronidazole and is less likely to recur if the patient truly harbored ulcerative colitis initially.[386] Conversely individuals with indeterminate colitis were less likely to respond to metronidazole, required sulfasalazine and/or steroids, and had more frequent exacerbations. In a still later paper from the Lahey Clinic Medical Center, now involving 42 patients with indeterminate colitis, the preceding concerns still persisted—that is, increased risk of pouch-related complications, eventual pouch failure, and the discovery of Crohn's disease subsequently.[301]

The Cleveland Clinic experience with indeterminate colitis consists of 115 individuals.[95] Functional results and incidence of some complications were comparable to that of the ulcerative colitis patients. The incidence of pouch failure was identical also, 3.4%. However, indeterminate colitis patients were more likely to develop minor perineal fistulas, pelvic abscess, and, of course, Crohn's disease.

A report from the Mayo Clinic involved 71 patients who underwent ileal pouch-anal anastomosis for what proved to be indeterminate colitis.[315] At a mean of nearly 5 years following surgery, failure occurred more frequently in those with indeterminate colitis that in those diagnosed with ulcerative colitis. Still, more than 80% were felt to have long-term functional results identical

to those of patients with ulcerative colitis.[315] In a later report from the same institution involving 82 patients, with a median follow-up of 83 months, the investigators concluded that those who underwent restorative proctocolectomy who did not subsequently develop Crohn's disease had nearly identical results as those who underwent the surgery for ulcerative colitis.[525] Conversely, those who developed Crohn's disease had significantly poorer results. The experience of Atkinson and colleagues was similar.[23] In their 16 patients diagnosed with indeterminate colitis, the success rate for restorative proctocolectomy was 81%, compared with 95% for ulcerative colitis. Others opine that it is reasonable to offer restorative proctocolectomy to those with indeterminate colitis despite the increased incidence of fistulas.[405] Until further data become available, utilization of the pouch procedure in these individuals requires circumspection.

CONCLUSION

The results of surgery for Crohn's disease are less than satisfactory. The concept that repeated resections will ultimately cure the patient is obviously erroneous. It is evident that as additional operations are required, the likelihood of recurrence is actually increased. One must, therefore, limit surgical intervention to those patients who have complications severe enough to justify an operation. Long-standing disease is not yet a surgical indication, as it classically has been for ulcerative colitis. Since it is not clear what the actual prognostic validity of the concept of dysplasia is in patients with Crohn's colitis, and since the incidence of malignant change is low, long duration of disease is not itself an indication for surgical intervention. However, recent opinions suggest that when dysplastic changes are identified, resection should be advised. Bypass procedures and exclusion operations should not be performed except under unusual circumstances. If carried out, definitive resection should be undertaken at the earliest possible time. Strictureplasty should be applied for those in whom a resection would result in the potential for significant disability. Creating a large anastomosis whenever one is performed is probably prudent, even without level-one evidence to support the concept. Since important endoscopic lesions may be present without clinical symptoms, periodic colonoscopy should be part of the follow-up evaluation of all patients who have undergone an anastomosis in the colon for Crohn's disease.

The future is very hopeful. There are a number of new and exciting nonoperative treatments. It is hoped that within the next few years successful medical management can be anticipated and that surgery for this condition will be relegated to that of a historical curiosity.

REFERENCES

1. Acheson ED. An association between ulcerative colitis, regional enteritis, and ankylosing spondylitis. *Q J Med* 1960; 29:489.
2. Achkar JP, Hanauer SB. Medical therapy to reduce postoperative Crohn's disease recurrence. *Am J Gastroenterol* 2000;95:1139.
3. Adloff M, Arnaud J-P, Ollier J-C. Does the histologic appearance at the margin of resection affect the postoperative recurrence of Crohn's disease? *Am Surg* 1987;53:543.
4. Agha FP, Woolsey EJ, Amendola MA. Psoas abscess in inflammatory bowel disease. *Am J Gastroenterol* 1985;80:924.
5. Agnholt J, Dahlerup J, Lyhne-Nielsen S, et al. Treatment of fistulizing Crohn's disease with infliximab: one year follow by MR scan, ultrasound and clinical examination. *Gastroenterology* 2002;122:A612.
6. Aitken RJ, Wright JP, Bok A, et al. Crohn's disease precipitating a spinal extradural abscess and paraplegia. *Br J Surg* 1986;73:1004.
7. Alexander AC, Irving MH. Accumulation and pepsin solubility of collagens in the bowel of patients with Crohn's disease. *Dis Colon Rectum* 1990;33:956.
8. Alexander-Williams J. Perianal Crohn's disease. *World J Surg* 1980;4:203.
9. Alexander-Williams J. The technique of intestinal strictureplasty. *Int J Colorect Dis* 1986;1:54.
10. Alexander-Williams J, Buchmann P. Perianal Crohn's disease. *World J Surg* 1980;4:203.
11. Alexander-Williams J, Haynes IG. Conservative operations for Crohn's disease of the small bowel. *World J Surg* 1985; 9:945.
12. Al-Jahdali H, Thompson WG, Matzinger FR. Non-fatal portal pyaemia complicating Crohn's disease of the terminal ileum. *Gut* 1994;35:560.
13. Allan A, Andrews H, Hilton CJ, et al. Segmental colonic resection is an appropriate operation for skip lesions due to Crohn's disease in the colon. *World J Surg* 1989;13:611.
14. Allan RN. Extra-intestinal manifestations of inflammatory bowel disease. *Clin Gastroenterol* 1983;12:617.
15. Allen DC, Hughes DF, Calvert CH. Carcinoma in Crohn's disease of the colon. *Dis Colon Rectum* 1986;29:760.
16. Alum Jones V. Comparison of total parenteral nutrition and elemental diet in induction of remission of Crohn's disease. *Dig Dis Sci* 1986;32:100.
17. Ambrose NS, Allan RN, Keighley MRB, et al. Antibiotic therapy for treatment in relapse of intestinal Crohn's disease: a prospective randomized study. *Dis Colon Rectum* 1985;28:81.
18. Ambrose NS, Keighley MRB, Alexander-Williams J, et al. Clinical impact of colectomy and ileorectal anastomosis in the management of Crohn's disease. *Gut* 1984;25:223.
19. Andersson P, Olaison G, Hallbök O, et al. Segmental resection or subtotal colectomy in Crohn's colitis? *Dis Colon Rectum* 2002;45:47.
20. Andrews HA, Lewis P, Allan RN. Prognosis after surgery for colonic Crohn's disease. *Br J Surg* 1989;76:1184.
21. Anseline PF, Wlodarczyk J, Murugasu R. Presence of granulomas is associated with recurrence after surgery for Crohn's disease: experience of a surgical unit. *Br J Surg* 1997;84:78.
22. Arnold GL, Beaves MR, Pryjdun VO, et al. Preliminary study of ciprofloxacin in active Crohn's disease. *Inflamm Bowel Dis* 2002;8:10.
23. Atkinson KG, Owen DA, Wankling G. Restorative proctocolectomy and indeterminate colitis. *Am J Surg* 1994;167:516.
24. Ballinger A, Farthing MJG. Ulcerative colitis complicated by Wenckebach atrioventricular block. *Gut* 1992;33:1427.
25. Bambach CP, Robertson WG, Peacock M, et al. Effect of intestinal surgery on the risk of urinary stone formation. *Gut* 1981;22:257.
26. Bar-Meir S, Chowers Y, Lavy A, et al. Budesonide vs. prednisone in the treatment of active Crohn's disease. *Gastroenterology* 1998;115:835.
27. Barnett WO. The continent jejunal reservoir in Crohn's colitis. *J Miss State Med Assoc* 1986;27:119.
28. Basu MK, Asquith P. Oral manifestations of inflammatory bowel disease. *Clin Gastroenterol* 1980;9:307.
29. Bauer JJ, Harris MT, Grumbach NM, et al. Laparoscopic-assisted intestinal resection for Crohn's disease. *Dis Colon Rectum* 1995;38:712.
30. Bell SJ, Halligan S, Windsor A, et al. Value of MRI in assessing the response of fistulating Crohn's disease to treatment with infliximab. *Gastroenterology* 2002;122:A617.
31. Belluzzi A, Brignola C, Campieri M, et al. Effect of an enteric-coated fish-oil preparation on relapses in Crohn's disease. *N Engl J Med* 1996;334:1557.
32. Bergamaschi R, Pessaux, Arnaud J-P. Comparison of conventional and laparoscopic ileocolic resection for Crohn's disease. *Dis Colon Rectum* 2003;46:1129.
33. Berman IR, Corman ML, Coller JA, et al. Late onset Crohn's disease in patients with colonic diverticulitis. *Dis Colon Rectum* 1979;22:524.
34. Bernell O, Lapidus A, Hellers G. Risk factors for surgery and postoperative recurrence in Crohn's disease. *Ann Surg* 2000;231:38.
35. Bernell O, Lapidus A, Hellers G. Risk factors for surgery and recurrence in 907 patients with primary ileocaecal Crohn's disease. *Br J Surg* 2000;87:1697.
36. Bernell O, Lapidus A, Hellers G. Recurrence after colectomy in Crohn's colitis. *Dis Colon Rectum* 2001;44:647.
37. Bernstein CN, Blanchard JF, Kliewer E, et al. Cancer risk in patients with inflammatory bowel disease: a population-based study. *Cancer* 2001;91:854.
38. Bernstein LH, Frank MS, Brandt LJ, et al. Healing of perineal Crohn's disease with metronidazole. *Gastroenterology* 1980;79:357.
39. Bernstein ML, McDonald JS. Oral lesions in Crohn's disease: report of two cases and update of the literature. *Oral Surg* 1978;46:234.
40. Beubige EJ, Bagless TM, Milligan FD. Mucosal bridging in Crohn's disease of the colon. *Gastrointest Endosc* 1975;21:189.
41. Bishop RP, Brewster AC, Antonioli DA. Crohn's disease of the mouth. *Gastroenterology* 1972;62:302.
42. Blank A, Korelitz BI. Efficacy of 6-MP in prevention of endoscopic recurrence at anastomotic site after ileo-colic resection for Crohn's disease. *Am J Gastroenterol* 2002;97: S255.
43. Bleday R, Lee E, Jessurun J, et al. Increased risk of early colorectal neoplasms after hepatic transplant in patients with inflammatory bowel disease. *Dis Colon Rectum* 1993; 36:908.
44. Bloom RJ, Larsen CP, Watt R, et al. A reappraisal of the Kock continent ileostomy in patients with Crohn's disease. *Surg Gynecol Obstet* 1986;162:105.
45. Bodzin JH, Klein SN, Priest SG. Ileoproctostomy is preferred over ileoanal pull-through in patients with indeterminate colitis. *Am Surg* 1995;61:590.
46. Boerr LA, Bai JC, Olivares L, et al. Cutaneous metastatic Crohn's disease: treatment with metronidazole. *Am J Gastroenterol* 1987;82:1326.
47. Boirivant M, Pallone F, Ciaco A, et al. Usefulness of fecal α_1-antitrypsin clearance and fecal concentration as early indicator of postoperative asymptomatic recurrence in Crohn's disease. *Dig Dis Sci* 1991;36:347.
48. Bonniere P, Wallaert B, Cortot A, et al. Latent pulmonary involvement in Crohn's disease: biological, functional, bronchoalveolar lavage and scintigraphic studies. *Gut* 1986;27:919.

49. Borley NR, Mortensen NJMcC, Chaudry MA, et al. Recurrence after abdominal surgery for Crohn's disease. *Dis Colon Rectum* 2002;45:377.

50. Brandt LJ, Bernstein LH, Boley SJ, et al. Metronidazole therapy for perineal Crohn's disease: a follow-up study. *Gastroenterology* 1982;83:383.

51. Brenner A, Lavery I, Church J, et al. Perianal Crohn's disease and associated carcinoma. *Dis Colon Rectum* 2001;44: A27.

52. Brignola C, Campieri M, Bazzocchi G, et al. A laboratory index for predicting relapse in asymptomatic patients with Crohn's disease. *Gastroenterology* 1986;91:1490.

53. Brignola C, Cottone M, Pera A, et al. Mesalamine in the prevention of endoscopic recurrence after intestinal resection for Crohn's disease. *Gastroenterology* 1995;108:345.

54. Broomé U, Löfberg R, Lundqvist K, et al. Subclinical time span of inflammatory bowel disease in patients with primary sclerosing cholangitis. *Dis Colon Rectum* 1995;38: 1301.

55. Brynskov J, Freund L, Rasmussen SN, et al. A placebo-controlled, double-blind, randomized trial of cyclosporine therapy in active chronic Crohn's disease. *N Engl J Med* 1989;321:845.

56. Buchmann P, Weterman IT, Keighley MRB, et al. The prognosis of ileorectal anastomosis in Crohn's disease. *Br J Surg* 1981;68:7.

57. Bufo AJ, Feldman S, Daniels GA, et al. Stapled stricturoplasty for Crohn's disease: a new technique. *Dis Colon Rectum* 1995;38:664.

58. Bundred NJ, Dixon JM, Lumsden AB, et al. Free perforation in Crohn's colitis: a ten-year review. *Dis Colon Rectum* 1985;28:35.

59. Byrne TA, Morrissey TB, Nattakom TV, et al. Growth hormone, glutamine, and a modified diet enhance nutrient absorption in patients with severe short bowel syndrome. *J Parenteral Enteral Nutr* 1995;19:296.

60. Byrne TA, Persinger RL, Young LS, et al. A new treatment for patients with short-bowel syndrome: growth hormone, glutamine, and a modified diet. *Ann Surg* 1995;222:243.

61. Cameron JL, Hamilton SR, Coleman J, et al. Patterns of ileal recurrence in Crohn's disease: a prospective randomized study. *Ann Surg* 1992;215:546.

62. Camma C, Giuta M, Rosselli M, et al. Mesalamine in the maintenance and treatment of Crohn's disease: a meta-analysis adjusted for confounding variables. *Gastroenterology* 1997;113:1465.

63. Campieri M, Ferguson A, Doe W, et al. Oral budesonide is as effective as oral prednisone in active Crohn's disease. The global budesonide study group. *Gut* 1997;41:209.

64. Canadian Inflammatory Bowel Disease Study Group. Oral budesonide in active Crohn's disease: interim report of a placebo-controlled randomized trial. *Gastroenterology* 1993; 104:A175.

65. Cangemi JR, Wiesner RH, Beaver SJ, et al. Effect of proctocolectomy for chronic ulcerative colitis on the natural history of primary sclerosing cholangitis. *Gastroenterology* 1989;96:790.

66. Caprilli R, Areoli A, Capurso L, et al. Oral mesalamine (5-aminosalicylic acid; Asacol) for the prevention of post-operative recurrence of Crohn's disease. *Aliment Pharmacol Ther* 1994;8:35.

67. Card T, Logan RFA, Rodrigues LC, et al. Antibiotic use and the development of Crohn's disease. *Gut* 2004;53:246.

68. Cattan P, Bonhomme N, Panis Y, et al. Fate of the rectum in patients undergoing total colectomy for Crohn's disease. *Br J Surg* 2002;89:454.

69. Cave DR, Burakoff R. Pyoderma gangrenosum associated with ulcerative colitis: treatment with disodium cromoglycate. *Am J Gastroenterol* 1987;82:802.

70. Chang RY, Hanauer SB, Cohen RD, et al. Parenteral methotrexate in refractory Crohn's disease. *Aliment Pharmacol Ther* 2001;15:15.

71. Chardavoyne R, Flint GW, Pollack S, et al. Factors affecting recurrence following resection for Crohn's disease. *Dis Colon Rectum* 1986;29:495.

72. Chevalier JM, Jones DJ, Ratelle R, et al. Colectomy and ileorectal anastomosis in patients with Crohn's disease. *Br J Surg* 1994;81:1379.

73. Chew SSB, Douglas PR, Newstead GL, et al. Cholecystectomy in patients with Crohn's ileitis. *Dis Colon Rectum* 2003;46:1484.

74. Christophi C, Hughes ER. Hepatobiliary disorders in inflammatory bowel disease. *Surg Gynecol Obstet* 1985;160: 187.

75. Chugh S, Dilawari JB, Sawhney IMS, et al. Polymyositis associated with ulcerative colitis. *Gut* 1993;34:567.

76. Church JM, Weakley FL, Fazio VW, et al. The relationship between fistulas in Crohn's disease and associated carcinoma. *Dis Colon Rectum* 1985;28:361.

77. Cirocco WC, Reilly JC, Rusin LC. Life-threatening hemorrhage and exsanguination from Crohn's disease. *Dis Colon Rectum* 1995;38:85.

78. Clark CLI, Lear PA, Wood S, et al. Potential candidates for small bowel transplantation. *Br J Surg* 1992;79:676.

79. Coenen C, Börsch G, Müller K-M, et al. Oral inflammatory changes as an initial manifestation of Crohn's disease antedating abdominal diagnosis. *Dis Colon Rectum* 1988;31: 548.

80. Cohen H, Fishman AP. Regional enteritis and amyloidosis. *Gastroenterology* 1949;12:502.

81. Cohen RL, Tepper RE, Urmacher C, et al. Kaposi's sarcoma and cytomegaloviral ileocolitis complicating long-standing Crohn's disease in an HIV-negative patient. *Am J Gastroenterol* 2001;96:3029.

82. Cohen S, Kaplan M, Gottlieb L, et al. Liver disease and gallstones in regional enteritis. *Gastroenterology* 1971;60:237.

83. Cohen WN. Gastric involvement in Crohn's disease. *Am J Roentgenol* 1967;101:425.

84. Colombel JF, Loftus EV Jr, Tremaine WJ, et al. The safety profile of infliximab for Crohn's disease in clinical practice: the Mayo Clinic experience in 500 patients. *Gastroenterology* 2004;126:19.

85. Comfort MW, Weber HM, Baggenstoss AH, et al. Nonspecific granulomatous inflammation of the stomach and duodenum: its relation to regional enteritis. *Am J Med Sci* 1950;220:616.

86. Connell WR, Sheffield JP, Kamm MA, et al. Lower gastrointestinal malignancy in Crohn's disease. *Gut* 1994;35:347.

87. Cortot A, Colombel J-F, Rutgeerts P, et al. Switch from systemic steroids to budesonide in steroid dependent patients with inactive Crohn's disease. *Gut* 2001;48:186–190.

88. Crohn BB, Ginzburg L, Oppenheimer GD. Regional ileitis: a pathologic and clinical entity. *JAMA* 1932;99:1323.

89. Dalziel TK. Chronic interstitial enteritis. *Br Med J* 1913; 2:1068.

90. Danzi JT, Farmer RG, Sullivan BH Jr, et al. Endoscopic features of gastroduodenal Crohn's disease. *Gastroenterology* 1976;70:9.

91. Davies G, Evans CM, Shand WS, et al. Surgery for Crohn's disease in childhood: influence of site of disease and operative procedure on outcome. *Br J Surg* 1990;77:891.

92. Decker GAG, Schein M. The finger fracture technique in the fat laden mesentery. *Surg Gynecol Obstet* 1988;166: 369.

93. de Dombal FT, Goldie W, Watts J, et al. Hepatic histological changes in ulcerative colitis: a series of 58 consecutive operative liver biopsies. *Scand J Gastroenterol* 1966;1:220.

94. Dehn TCB, Kettlewell MGW, Mortensen NJMcC, et al. Ten-year experience of strictureplasty for obstructive Crohn's disease. *Br J Surg* 1989;76:339.

95. Delaney CP, Remzi FH, Gramlich T, et al. Equivalent function, quality of life and pouch survival rates after ileal pouch-anal anastomosis for indeterminate and ulcerative colitis. *Ann Surg* 2002;236:43.

96. Deutsch AA, McLeod RS, Cullen J, et al. The results of the pelvic pouch procedure in patients with Crohn's disease. *Dis Colon Rectum* 1991;34:475.

97. Deutsch AA, Stern HS. Stapler strictureplasty for Crohn's disease. *Surg Gynecol Obstet* 1989;169:458.

98. Devang NP, Saeian K, Kim J, et al. Symptomatic luminal strictures underlies infliximab non-response in Crohn's disease. *Gastroenterology* 2002;A100 (A777).

99. D'Haens GR, Gasparaitis AE, Hanauer SB. Duration of recurrent ileitis after ileocolonic resection correlates with presurgical extent of Crohn's disease. *Gut* 1995;36:715.

100. D'Haens GR, van Deventer SJH, Van Hogezand R, et al. Anti-TNFa monoclonal antibody (cA2) produces endoscopic healing in patients with treatment-resistant, active Crohn's disease. *Am J Gastroenterol* 1998;114:A964.

101. Di Febo G, Gizzi G, Cappelo IP. Unusual case of colonic sub-obstruction by giant pseudopolyposis in Crohn's colitis. *Endoscopy* 1981;13:90.

102. Dietz DW, Fazio VW, Laureti S, et al. Strictureplasty in diffuse Crohn's jejunoileitis: safe and durable. *Dis Colon Rectum* 2002;45:764.

103. Dollinger HC, Raptis S, Pfeiffer EF. Effects of somatostatin on exocrine and endocrine pancreatic function stimulated by intestinal hormones in man. *Horm Metab Res* 1976;8:74.

104. Donnelly MT, Davies DR, Carter MJ, et al. Why do patients with inflammatory bowel disease stop azathioprine and what happens to them? *Am J Gastroenterol* 1998;114:A968.

105. Dordal E, Glagov S, Kirsner JB. Hepatic lesions in chronic inflammatory bowel disease. *Gastroenterology* 1967;52:239.

106. Dorudi S, Chapman RW, Kettlewell MGW. Carcinoma of the gallbladder in ulcerative colitis and primary sclerosing cholangitis. *Dis Colon Rectum* 1991;34:827.

107. DuBrow RA, Frank PH. Barium evaluation of anal canal in patients with inflammatory bowel disease. *AJR* 1983;140:1151.

108. Dudeney TP, Todd IP. Crohn's disease of the mouth. *Proc R Soc Med* 1969;62:1237.

109. Dudrick SJ, O'Donnell JJ, Englert DM, et al. 100 patient-years of ambulatory home: total parenteral nutrition. *Ann Surg* 1984;199:770.

110. Duepree H-J, Senagore AJ, Delaney CP, et al. Advantages of laparoscopic resection for ileocecal Crohn's disease. *Dis Colon Rectum* 2002;45:605.

111. Duffy LF, Daum F, Fisher SE, et al. Peripheral neuropathy in Crohn's disease patients treated with metronidazole. *Gastroenterology* 1985;88:681.

112. Dyer NH, Cook PL, Kemp-Harper RA. Oesophageal stricture associated with Crohn's disease. *Gut* 1969;10:549.

113. Edwards CM, George BD, Jewell DP, et al. Role of a defunctioning stoma in the management of large bowel Crohn's disease. *Br J Surg* 2000;87:1063.

114. Edwards P, Cooper DA, Turner J, et al. Resolution of amyloidosis (AA type) complicating chronic ulcerative colitis. *Gastroenterology* 1988;95:810.

115. Egan LJ, Sandborn WJ, Tremaine WJ, et al. A randomized dose-response and pharmacokinetic study of methotrexate for refractory inflammatory Crohn's disease and ulcerative colitis. *Aliment Pharmacol Ther* 1999;13:1597.

116. Eisenberg HW. Combined metronidazole and surgery in the management of complicated Crohn's disease. *Contemp Surg* 1982;21:95.

117. Ekberg O, Baath L, Sjöström B, et al. Are superficial lesions of the distal part of the ileum early indicators of Crohn's disease in adult patients with abdominal pain? A clinical and radiologic long term investigation. *Gut* 1984;25:341.

118. Eliakim R, Fischer D, Suissa L, et al. Wireless capsule video endoscopy is a superior diagnostic tool in comparison to barium follow-through and computerized tomography in patients with suspected Crohn's disease. *Eur J Gastroenterol Hepatol* 2003;15:363.

119. Elliott PR, Ritchie JK, Lennard-Jones JE. Prognosis of colonic Crohn's disease. *BMJ* 1985;291:178.

120. Ellis L, Calhoun P, Kaiser DL, et al. Postoperative recurrence in Crohn's disease: the effect of the initial length of bowel resection and operative procedure. *Ann Surg* 1984;199:340.

121. Elson CO. Cyclosporine in Crohn's disease—low doses won't do it. *Gastroenterology* 1990;98:1383.

122. Elton C, Makin G, Hitos K, et al. Mortality, morbidity and functional outcome after ileorectal anastomosis. *Br J Surg* 2003;90:59.

123. Evans J, Poritz L, MacRae H. Influence of experience on laparoscopic ileocolic resection for Crohn's disease. *Dis Colon Rectum* 2002;45:1595.

124. Ewe K, Press AG, Singe CC, et al. Azathioprine combined with prednisone or monotherapy with prednisone in active Crohn's disease. *Gastroenterology* 1993;105:367.

125. Farmer RG, Hawk WA, Turnbull RB Jr. Crohn's disease of the duodenum (transmural duodenitis): clinical manifestations: report of 11 cases. *Am J Dig Dis* 1972;17:191.

126. Farmer RG, Whelan G, Fazio VW. Long-term follow-up of patients with Crohn's disease. Relationship between the clinical pattern and prognosis. *Gastroenterology* 1985;88: 1818.

127. Farnell MB, Van Heerden JA, Beart RW Jr, et al. Rectal preservation in nonspecific inflammatory disease of the colon. *Ann Surg* 1980;192:249.

128. Farrell RJ, Ang Y, Kileen P, et al. Increased incidence of non-Hodgkin's lymphoma in inflammatory bowel disease patients or immunosuppressive therapy but overall risk is low. *Gut* 2000;47:514.

129. Farrell FJ, Shah SA, Lodhavia PJ, et al. Infliximab therapy in 100 Crohn's disease patients: Adverse events and clinical efficacy. *Am J Gastroenterol* 2000;95:3490.

130. Fasoli R, Kettlewell MGW, Mortensen N, et al. Response to faecal challenge in defunctioned colonic Crohn's disease: prediction of long-term course. *Br J Surg* 1990;77:616.

131. Faubion WA Jr, Loftus EV Jr, Harmsen WS, et al. The natural history of corticosteroid therapy for inflammatory bowel disease: a population-based study. *Gastroenterology* 2001;121:255.

132. Fazio VW. Regional enteritis (Crohn's disease): indications for surgery and operative strategy. *Surg Clin North Am* 1983;63:27.

133. Fazio VW, Galandiuk S, Jagelman DG, et al. Strictureplasty for Crohn's disease. *Ann Surg* 1989;210:621.

134. Fazio VW, Kodner I, Jagelman DG, et al. Inflammatory disease of the bowel: parenteral nutrition as primary or adjunctive treatment (symposium). *Dis Colon Rectum* 1976; 19:574.

135. Fazio VW, Marchetti F, Church JM, et al. Effect of resection margins on the recurrence of Crohn's disease in the small bowel: a randomized controlled trial. *Ann Surg* 1996;224: 563.

136. Fazio VW, Tjandra JJ, Lavery IC, et al. Long-term follow-up of strictureplasty in Crohn's disease. *Dis Colon Rectum* 1993;36:355.

137. Fazio VW, Wu JS. Surgical therapy for Crohn's disease of the colon and rectum. *Surg Clin North Am* 1997;77:197.

138. Feagan BG. Cyclosporine has no proven role as therapy in Crohn's disease. *Inflamm Bowel Dis* 1995;1:335–339.

139. Feagan BG, Fedorak RN, Irvine EJ, et al. A comparison of methotrexate with placebo for the maintenance of remission in Crohn's disease. *New Engl J Med* 2000;342:1627.

140. Feagan BG, Rochon J, Fedorak RN, et al. Methotrexate for the treatment of Crohn's disease. *N Engl J Med* 1995;332: 292.

141. Fielding JF. Perianal lesions in Crohn's disease. *J R Coll Surg Edinb* 1972;17:32.

142. Fielding JF, Cooke WT. Finger clubbing in regional enteritis. *Gut* 1971;12:442.

143. Fireman Z, Mahajna E, Broide E, et al. Diagnosing small bowel Crohn's disease with wireless capdule endoscopy. *Gut* 2003;52:390.

144. Fitchen JH. Amyloidosis and granulomatous colitis: regression after surgical removal of the involved bowel. *N Engl J Med* 1975;292:352.

145. Fitzgibbons TJ, Green G, Silberman H, et al. Management of Crohn's disease involving the duodenum, including duodenal cutaneous fistula. *Arch Surg* 1980;115:1022.

146. Fraser AG, Orchard TR, Robinson EM, et al. Long-term risk of malignancy after treatment of inflammatory bowel disease with azathioprine. *Aliment Pharmacol Ther* 2002; 16:1225.

147. Frikker MJ, Segall MM. The resectional reoperation rate for Crohn's disease in a general community hospital. *Dis Colon Rectum* 1983;26:305.

148. Fry RD, Shemesh EI, Kodner IJ, et al. Techniques and results in the management of anal and perianal Crohn's disease. *Surg Gynecol Obstet* 1989;168:42.

149. Galandiuk S, O'Neill M, McDonald P, et al. A century of home parenteral nutrition for Crohn's disease. *Am J Surg* 1990;159:540.

150. García-Granero E, Esclápez P, García-Armengol J, et al. Simple technique for the intraoperative detection of Crohn's strictures with a calibration sphere. *Dis Colon Rectum* 2000;43:1168.

151. Gazzard B. Long term prognosis of Crohn's disease with onset in childhood and adolescence. *Gut* 1984;25:325.

152. Geboes K, Vantrappen G. The value of colonoscopy in the diagnosis of Crohn's disease. *Gastrointest Endosc* 1975; 22:18.

153. Geerdsen JP, Pedersen VM, Kjaergard HK. Small bowel fistulas treated with somatostatin: preliminary results. *Surgery* 1986;100:811.

154. Gelfand MD, Krone CL. Dysphagia and esophageal ulceration in Crohn's disease. *Gastroenterology* 1968;55:510.

155. Gendre J-P, Mary J-Y, Florent C, et al. Oral mesalamine (pentasa) as maintenance treatment in Crohn's disease: a multicenter placebo-controlled study. *Gastroenterology* 1993; 104:435.

156. Gerassimos J, Mantzaris GJ, Petraki K, et al. Budesonide is superior to mesalazine in maintaining disease remission for patients with steroid-dependent Crohn's disease. *Gastroenterology* 2000;118, 780 (A4174).

157. Gerber A, Apt MK, Craig PH. The Kock continent ileostomy. *Surg Gynecol Obstet* 1983;156:345.

158. Gillen CD, Andrews HA, Prior P, et al. Crohn's disease and colorectal cancer. *Gut* 1994;35:651.

159. Gillen CD, Walmsley RS, Prior P, et al. Ulcerative colitis and Crohn's disease: a comparison of the colorectal cancer risk in extensive colitis. *Gut* 1994;35:1590.

160. Ginzburg L. The road to regional enteritis. *Mt Sinai J Med* 1974;41:272.

161. Gitkind MJ, Wright SC. Amyloidosis complicating inflammatory bowel disease: a case report and review of the literature. *Dig Dis Sci* 1990;35:906.

162. Givel J-C, Hawker P, Allan RN, et al. Enterovaginal fistulas associated with Crohn's disease. *Surg Gynecol Obstet* 1982; 155:494.

163. Glass RE. The management of internal fistulae in Crohn's disease. *Br J Surg* 1985;72:S93.

164. Glass RE, Ritchie JK, Lennard-Jones JE, et al. Internal fistulas in Crohn's disease. *Dis Colon Rectum* 1985;28:557.

165. Glotzer DJ. The risk of cancer in Crohn's disease. *Gastroenterology* 1985;89:438.

166. Goldstein F, Krain R, Thornton JJ. Intralesional steroid therapy of pyoderma gangrenosum. *J Clin Gastroenterol* 1985;7:499.

167. Goldwasser B, Mazor A, Wiznitzer T. Enteroduodenal fistulas in Crohn's disease. *Dis Colon Rectum* 1981;24:485.

168. Goligher JC. Inflammatory disease of the bowel: results of resection for Crohn's disease (symposium). *Dis Colon Rectum* 1976;19:584.

169. Goligher JC. *Surgery of the anus, rectum and colon*, 5th ed. London: Balliére Tindall, 1984:971.

170. Goligher JC. The long-term results of excisional surgery for primary and recurrent Crohn's disease of the large intestine. *Dis Colon Rectum* 1985;28:51.

171. Gore RM, Marn CS, Kirby DF, et al. CT findings in ulcerative, granulomatous, and indeterminate colitis. *AJR* 1984; 143:279.

172. Gottlieb C, Alpert S. Regional jejunitis. *AJR* 1937;38:881.

173. Gravallese EM, Kantrowitz FG. Arthritic manifestations of inflammatory bowel disease. *Am J Gastroenterol* 1988;83: 703.

174. Greenbloom SL, Steinhart AH, Greenberg GR, et al. Ciprofloxacin and metronidazole: combination antibiotic therapy for ileocolonic Crohn's disease. *Gastroenterology* 1995; 108:A827.

175. Greenstein A. Cancer in inflammatory bowel disease. *Surg Rounds* 1982;Oct:44.

176. Greenstein AJ, Aufses AH Jr. Differences in pathogenesis, incidence and outcome of perforation in inflammatory bowel disease. *Surg Gynecol Obstet* 1985;160:63.

177. Greenstein AJ, Lachman P, Sachar DB, et al. Perforating and non-perforating indications for repeated operations in Crohn's disease: evidence for two clinical forms. *Gut* 1988; 29:588.

178. Greenstein AJ, Mann D, Sachar DB, et al. Free perforation in Crohn's disease: I. A survey of 99 cases. *Am J Gastroenterol* 1985;80:682.

179. Greenstein AJ, Mullin GE, Strauchen JA, et al. Lymphoma in inflammatory bowel disease. *Cancer* 1992;69:1119.

180. Greenstein AJ, Present DH, Sachar DB, et al. Gastric fistulas in Crohn's disease: report of a case. *Dis Colon Rectum* 1989;32:888.

181. Greenstein AJ, Sachar DB, Greenstein RJ, et al. Intraabdominal abscess in Crohn's (ileo) colitis. *Am J Surg* 1982; 143:727.

182. Greenstein AJ, Sachar D, Pucillo A, et al. Cancer in Crohn's disease after diversionary surgery: a report of seven carcinomas occurring in excluded bowel. *Am J Surg* 1978; 135:86.

183. Greenstein AJ, Sachar DB, Shafir M, et al. Malignant melanoma in inflammatory bowel disease. *Am J Gastroenterol* 1992;87:317.

184. Greenstein AJ, Sachar DB, Tzakis A, et al. Course of enterovesical fistulas in Crohn's disease. *Am J Surg* 1984; 147:178.

185. Grundfest S, Steiger E. Home parenteral nutrition. *JAMA* 1980;244:1701.

186. Grüner OPN, Refsum S, Fausa O, et al. Giant pseudopolyposis causing colonic obstruction: report of a case seemingly associated with Crohn's disease of the colon. *Scand J Gastroenterol* 1978;13:65.

187. Grobler SP, Hosie KB, Affie E, et al. Outcome of restorative proctocolectomy when the diagnosis is suggestive of Crohn's disease. *Gut* 1993;34:1384.

188. Guest GD, Fink RLW. Metastatic Crohn's disease. *Dis Colon Rectum* 2000;43:1764.

189. Guillem JG, Roberts PL, Murray JJ, et al. Factors predictive of persistent or recurrent Crohn's disease in excluded rectal segment. *Dis Colon Rectum* 1992;35:768.

190. Gump FE, Lepore M, Barker HG. A revised concept of acute regional enteritis. *Ann Surg* 1967;166:942.

191. Gyde SN, Prior P, Macartney JC, et al. Malignancy in Crohn's disease. *Gut* 1980;21:1024.

192. Hamilton SR. Colorectal carcinoma in patients with Crohn's disease. *Gastroenterology* 1985;89:398.

193. Hamilton SR, Reese J, Pennington L, et al. The role of resection margin frozen section in the surgical management of Crohn's disease. *Surg Gynecol Obstet* 1985;160:57.

194. Hammerman AM, Shatz BA, Susman N. Radiographic characteristics of colonic "mucosal bridges": sequelae of inflammatory bowel disease. *Radiology* 1978;47:611.

195. Hampe J, Cuthbert A, Crouchrer PJ, et al. Association between insertion mutation in NOD2 gene and Crohn's disease in German and British populations. *Lancet* 2001;357: 1925.

196. Hanauer SB. Inflammatory bowel disease. *N Engl J Med* 1996;334:841.

197. Hanauer SB, Meyers S. Management of Crohn's disease in adults. *Am J Gastroenterol* 1997;92:559.

198. Hanauer SB, Smith MB. Rapid closure of Crohn's disease fistulas with continuous intravenous cyclosporin A. *Am J Gastroenterol* 1993;88:646.

199. Hanauer SB, Stromberg V. Efficacy of oral piñatas 4 gm in treatment of active Crohn's disease: a meta-analysis double-blind placebo controlled trial. *Gastroenterology* 2001; 120 (suppl.I):A453

200. Handelsman JC, Gottlieb LM, Hamilton SR. Crohn's disease as a contraindication to Kock pouch (continent ileostomy). *Dis Colon Rectum* 1993;36:840.

201. Harford FJ Jr, Fazio VW. Total parenteral nutrition as primary therapy for inflammatory disease of the bowel. *Dis Colon Rectum* 1978;21:555.

202. Harling H, Hegnj J, Rasmussen TN, et al. Fate of the rectum after colectomy and ileostomy for Crohn's colitis. *Dis Colon Rectum* 1991;34:931.

203. Harper PH, Lee ECG, Kettlewell MGW, et al. Role of the faecal stream in the maintenance of Crohn's colitis. *Gut* 1985;26:279.

204. Harper PH, Truelove SC, Lee ECG, et al. Split ileostomy and ileocolostomy for Crohn's disease of the colon and ulcerative colitis: a 20 year survey. *Gut* 1983;24:106.

205. Harries AD, Danis VA, Heatley RV. Influence of nutritional status on immune functions in patients with Crohn's disease. *Gut* 1984;25:465.

206. Hasegawa H, Watanabe M, Nishibori H, et al. Laparoscopic surgery for recurrent Crohn's disease. *Br J Surg* 2003;90:970.

207. Hawker PC, Gyde SN, Thompson H, et al. Adenocarcinoma of the small intestine complicating Crohn's disease. *Gut* 1982;23:188.

208. Heffernon EW, Kepkay PH. Segmental esophagitis gastritis and enteritis. *Gastroenterology* 1954;26:83.

209. Heimann TM, Aufses AH Jr. The role of peripheral lymphocytes in the prediction of recurrence in Crohn's disease. *Surg Gynecol Obstet* 1985;160:295.

210. Heimann TM, Bolnick K, Aufses AH Jr. Prognostic significance of severe preoperative lymphopenia in patients with Crohn's disease. *Ann Surg* 1986;203:132.

211. Heimann TM, Greenstein AJ, Lewis B, et al. Prediction of early symptomatic recurrence after intestinal resection in Crohn's disease. *Ann Surg* 1993;218:294.

212. Heimann TM, Greenstein AJ, Mechanic L, et al. Early complications following surgical treatment for Crohn's disease. *Ann Surg* 1985;201:494.

213. Herrerías JM, Caunedo A, Rodríguez-Téllez M, et al. Capsule endoscopy in patients with suspected Crohn's disease and negative endoscopy. *Endoscopy* 2003;35:564.

214. Heuman R, Boeryd B, Bolin T, et al. The influence of disease at the margin of resection on the outcome of Crohn's disease. *Br J Surg* 1983;70:519.

215. Heyen F, Winslet MC, Andrews H, et al. Vaginal fistulas in Crohn's disease. *Dis Colon Rectum* 1989;32:379.

216. Hill GL, Bourchier RG, Witney GB. Surgical and metabolic management of patients with external fistulas of the small intestine associated with Crohn's disease. *World J Surg* 1988;12:191.

217. Hobbis JH, Schofield PF. Management of perianal Crohn's disease. *J R Soc Med* 1982;75:414.

218. Hodgson HH. Keeping Crohn's disease quiet. *N Engl J Med* 1996;334:1599.

219. Hogan WJ, Hensley GT, Geenen JE. Endoscopic evaluation of inflammatory bowel disease. *Med Clin North Am* 1980;64:1083.

220. Homan WP, Dineen P. Comparison of the results of resection, bypass, and bypass with exclusion for ileocecal Crohn's disease. *Ann Surg* 1978;187:530.

221. Hughes LE. A clinical classification of perianal Crohn's disease. *Dis Colon Rectum* 1992;35:928.

222. Hughes LE, Donalson DR, Williams JG, et al. Local depot methylprednisolone injection for painful anal Crohn's disease. *Gastroenterology* 1988;94:709.

223. Hughes S, Williams SE, Turnberg LA. Crohn's disease and psoriasis. *N Engl J Med* 1983;308:101.

224. Hugot JP, Charmaillard M, Zonali H, et al. Association of NOD2 leucine rich repeat variants with susceptibility to Crohn's disease. *Nature* 2001;411:599.

225. Hyman NH, Fazio VW, Tuckson WB, et al. Consequences of ileal pouch-anal anastomosis for Crohn's colitis. *Dis Colon Rectum* 1991;34:653.

226. Irving M. Assessment and management of external fistulas in Crohn's disease. *Br J Surg* 1983;70:233.

227. Jacobson IM, Schapiro RH, Warshaw AL. Gastric and duodenal fistulas in Crohn's disease. *Gastroenterology* 1985;89:1347.

228. Jalan KN, Prescott RJ, Walker RJ, et al. Arthropathy, ankylosing spondylitis, and clubbing of fingers in ulcerative colitis. *Gut* 1970;11:748.

229. Jaskowiak NT, Michelassi F. Adenocarcinoma at a strictureplasty site in Crohn's disease: report of a case. *Dis Colon Rectum* 2001;44:284.

230. Jawhari A, Kamm MA, Ong C, et al. Intra-abdominal and pelvic abscess in Crohn's disease: results of non-invasive and surgical management. *Br J Surg* 1998;85:367.

231. Johnson ML, Wilson HT. Skin lesions in ulcerative colitis. *Gut* 1969;10:255.

232. Jones VA, Dickinson RJ, Workman E, et al. Crohn's disease: maintenance of remission by diet. *Lancet* 1985;2:177.

233. Kahn EI, Daum F, Aiges HW, et al. Cutaneous polyarteritis nodosa associated with Crohn's disease. *Dis Colon Rectum* 1980;23:258.

234. Katariya RN, Sood S, Rao PG, et al. Stricture-plasty for tubercular strictures of the gastro-intestinal tract. *Br J Surg* 1977;64:496.

235. Katz S, Rosenberg RF, Katzka I. Giant pseudopolyps in Crohn's colitis. *Am J Gastroenterol* 1981;76:267.

236. Keighley MRB. Stapled strictureplasty for Crohn's disease. *Dis Colon Rectum* 1991;34:945.

237. Keighley MRB, Buchmann P, Lee JR. Assessment of anorectal function in selection of patients for ileorectal anastomosis in Crohn's colitis. *Gut* 1982;23:102.

238. Kelts DG, Grand RJ, Shen G, et al. Nutritional basis of growth failure in children and adolescents with Crohn's disease. *Gastroenterology* 1979;76:720.

239. Kendall GPN, Hawley PR, Nicholls RJ, et al. Strictureplasty: a good operation for small bowel Crohn's disease? *Dis Colon Rectum* 1986;29:312.

240. Kim PS, Zlatanic J, Gleim GM, et al. Long-term follow-up of 6MP-treated Crohn's disease patients. *Am J Gastroenterol* 1997;92:A310 (1661).

241. Kirsner JB, Shorter RG. Recent developments in "nonspecific" inflammatory bowel disease, Part I. *N Engl J Med* 1982;306:775.

242. Koltun WA, Schoetz DJ Jr, Roberts PL, et al. Indeterminate colitis predisposes to perineal complications after ileal pouch-anal anastomosis. *Dis Colon Rectum* 1991;34:857.

243. Konturek SJ. Somatostatin and the gastrointestinal secretions. *Scand J Gastroenterol* 1976;11:1.

244. Korelitz BI. Therapy of inflammatory bowel disease, including use of immunosuppressive agents. *Clin Gastroenterol* 1980;9:331.

245. Korelitz BI. The treatment of ulcerative colitis with "immunosuppressive" drugs. *Am J Gastroenterol* 1981;76:297.

246. Korelitz BI, Glass JL, Wisch N. Long-term immunosuppressive therapy of ulcerative colitis. *Am J Dig Dis* 1973;18:317.

247. Korelitz B, Hanauer S, Rutgeerts P, et al. Post-operative prophylaxis with 6MP, 5-ASA or placebo in Crohn's disease: A 2-year multicenter trial (abstract) *Gastroenterology* 1998;114:A1011.

248. Korelitz BI, Lauwers GY, Sommers SC. Rectal mucosal dysplasia in Crohn's disease. *Gut* 1990;31:1382.

249. Korelitz BI, Present DH. Favorable effect of 6-mercaptopurine on fistulae of Crohn's disease. *Dig Dis Sci* 1985;30:58.

250. Korelitz BI, Present DH, Alpert LI, et al. Recurrent regional ileitis after ileostomy and colectomy for granulomatous colitis. *N Engl J Med* 1972;287:110.

251. Korelitz BI, Waye JD, Kreuning J, et al. Crohn's disease in endoscopic biopsies of the gastric antrum and duodenum. *Am J Gastroenterol* 1981;76:103.

252. Kornbluth A, Marion JF, Salomon P, et al. How effective is current medical therapy for severe ulcerative and Crohn's

colitis? An analytic review of selected trials. *J Clin Gastroenterol* 1995;20:280.

253. Kotanagi H, Kon H, Iida M, et al. Adenocarcinoma at the site of ileoanal anastomosis in Crohn's disease. Report of a case. *Dis Colon Rectum* 2001;44:1210.

254. Kotanagi H, Kramer K, Fazio VW, et al. Do microscopic abnormalities at resection margins correlate with increased anastomotic recurrence in Crohn's disease? A prospective analysis of 100 cases. *Dis Colon Rectum* 1991;34:909.

255. Kovalcik P, Simstein L, Weiss M, et al. The dilemma of Crohn's disease: Crohn's disease and appendectomy. *Dis Colon Rectum* 1977;20:377.

256. Kozarek RA, Patterson DJ, Gelfand MD. Methotrexate induces clinical and histologic remission in patients with refractory inflammatory bowel disease. *Ann Intern Med* 1989; 110:353.

257. Kreuzpaintner G, Horstkotte D, Heyll A, et al. Increased risk of bacterial endocarditis in inflammatory bowel disease. *Am J Med* 1992;92:391.

258. Kuramoto S, Oohara T, Ihara O, et al. Granulomas of the gut in Crohn's disease: a step sectioning study. *Dis Colon Rectum* 1987;30:6.

259. Kurchin A, Ray JE, Bluth EI, et al. Cholelithiasis in ileostomy patients. *Dis Colon Rectum* 1984;27:585.

260. Kurtz RS, Heimann TM, Aufses AH. The management of intestinal fistulas. *Am J Gastroenterol* 1981;76:377.

261. Ko A, Sohn N, Weinstein MA, et al. Carcinoma arising in anorectal fistulas of Crohn's disease. *Dis Colon Rectum* 1998;41:992.

262. LaRusso NF, Wiesner RH, Ludwig J, et al. Primary sclerosing cholangitis. *N Engl J Med* 1984;310:899.

263. Lavery IC, Jagelman DG. Cancer in the excluded rectum following surgery for inflammatory bowel disease. *Dis Colon Rectum* 1982;25:522.

264. Lecomte T, Contou J-F, Beaugerie L, et al. Predictive factors of response of perianal Crohn's disease to azathiaprine or 6-mercaptopurine. *Dis Colon Rectum* 2003;46:1469.

265. Lee ECG, Papaioannou N. Minimal surgery for chronic obstruction in patients with extensive or universal Crohn's disease. *Ann R Coll Surg Engl* 1982;64:229.

266. Lee FI, Bellary SV, Francis C. Increased occurrence of psoriasis in patients with Crohn's disease and their relatives. *Am J Gastroenterol* 1990;85:962.

267. Lee KKW, Schraut WH. Diagnosis and treatment of duodenoenteric fistulas complicating Crohn's disease. *Arch Surg* 1989;124:712.

268. Lee KS, Medline A, Shockey S. Indeterminate colitis in the spectrum of inflammatory bowel disease. *Arch Pathol Lab Med* 1979;103:173.

269. Lees CD, Steiger E, Hooley RA, et al. Home parenteral nutrition. *Acta Chir Scand* 1981;507:113.

270. Lemann M, Gerard de La Valussiere F, Bouhnik Y, et al. Intravenous cyclosporine for refractory attacks of Crohn's disease (CD): long-term follow-up of patients. *Am J Gastroenterol* 1998;114:A1020.

271. Lemann M, Gerard de La Valussiere F, Carbonnel F, et al. Intravenous cyclosporine for perianal Crohn's disease (CD). *Gastroenterology* 1998;114:A1020.

272. Lemann M, Messing B, D'Agay F, et al. Crohn's disease with respiratory tract involvement. *Gut* 1987;28:1669.

273. Lemann M, Zenjari T, Bouhnik Y, et al. Methotrexate in Crohn's disease: long-term efficacy and toxicity. *Am J Gastroenterol* 2000;95:1619.

274. Lescut D, Vanco D, Bonniére P, et al. Perioperative endoscopy of the whole small bowel in Crohn's disease. *Gut* 1993;34:647.

275. Leu S-Y, Leonard MB, Beart RW Jr, et al. Psoas abscess: changing patterns of diagnosis and etiology. *Dis Colon Rectum* 1986;29:694.

276. Levenstein S, Prantera C, Luzi C, D'Ubaldi A. Low residue or normal diet in Crohn's disease: a prospective controlled study in Italian patients. *Gut* 1985;26:989.

277. Levi AJ. Diet in the management of Crohn's disease. *Gut* 1985;26:985.

278. Levine N, Bangert J. Cutaneous granulomatosis in Crohn's disease. *Arch Dermatol* 1982;118:1006.

279. Lichtenstein GR, Bala M, Han C, et al. Infliximab improves quality of life in patients with Crohn's disease. *Inflamm Bowel Dis* 2002;8:237.

280. Lichtenstein GR, Olson A, Bao W, et al. Infliximab treatment does not result in an increased risk of intestinal strictures or obstruction in Crohn's disease patients: Accent 1 Study Results. *Am J Gastroenterol* 2002;97:S255.

281. Linares L, Moreira LF, Andrews H, et al. Natural history and treatment of anorectal strictures complicating Crohn's disease. *Br J Surg* 1988;75:653.

282. Lind E, Fausa O, Gjone E, et al. Crohn's disease: treatment and outcome. *Scand J Gastroenterol* 1985;20:1014.

283. Lindberg E, Jäärnerot G, Huitfeldt B. Smoking in Crohn's disease: effect on localisation and clinical course. *Gut* 1992;33:779.

284. Lindhagen T, Ekelund G, Leandoer L, et al. Crohn's disease confined to the appendix. *Dis Colon Rectum* 1982; 25:805.

285. Lochs H, Mayer M, Fleig WE, et al. Prophylaxis of postoperative relapse in Crohn's disease with mesalamine. *Gastroenterology* 2000;118:264.

286. Lochs H, Steinhardt HJ, Klaus-Wentz B, et al. Comparison of enteral nutrition and drug treatment in active Crohn's disease. *Gastroenterology* 1991;101:881.

287. Lock MR, Fazio VW, Farmer RG, et al. Proximal recurrence and the fate of the rectum following excisional surgery for Crohn's disease of the large bowel. *Ann Surg* 1981;194:754.

288. Lockhart-Mummery HE. Anal lesions in Crohn's disease. *Br J Surg* 1985;72:S95.

289. Löfberg R, Broström O, Karlén P, et al. Carcinoma and DNA aneuploidy in Crohn's colitis—a histological and flow cytometric study. *Gut* 1991;32:900.

290. Longo WE, Ballantyne GH, Cahow E. Treatment of Crohn's colitis. *Arch Surg* 1988;123:588.

291. Longo WE, Oakley JR, Lavery IC, et al. The outcome of ileorectal anastomosis for Crohn's disease. *Dis Colon Rectum* (in press).

292. Longo WE, Oakley JR, Lavery IC, et al. Outcome of ileorectal anastomosis for Crohn's colitis. *Dis Colon Rectum* 1992; 35:1066.

293. Lorusso D, Leo S, Mossa A, et al. Cholelithiasis in inflammatory bowel disease: a case-control study. *Dis Colon Rectum* 1990;33:791.

294. Lowdell CP, Shousha S, Parkins RA. The incidence of amyloidosis complicating inflammatory bowel disease: a prospective survey of 177 patients. *Dis Colon Rectum* 1986; 29:351.

295. Ludwig KA, Milsom JW, Church JM, et al. Preliminary experience with laparoscopic intestinal surgery for Crohn's disease. *Am J Surg* 1996;171:52.

296. Maconi G, Sampietro GM, Cristaldi M, et al. Preoperative characteristics and postoperative behavior of bowel wall on risk of recurrence after conservative surgery in Crohn's disease: a prospective study. *Ann Surg* 2001;233:345.

297. Mahida YR, Kurlac Gallagher A, et al. High circulating concentrations of interleukin-6 in active Crohn's disease but not ulcerative colitis. *Gut* 1991;32:1531.

298. Makowiec F, Jehle EC, Becker H-D, et al. Perianal abscess in Crohn's disease. *Dis Colon Rectum* 1997;40:443.

299. Malchow HA. Crohn's disease and *Escherichia coli:* a new approach to therapy to maintain remission of colonic Crohn's disease. *J Clin Gastroenterol* 1997;25:653.

300. Malchow H, Ewe K, Brandes JW, et al. European cooperative Crohn's disease study (ECCDS): results of drug treatment. *Gastroenterology* 1984;86:249.

301. Marcello PW, Schoetz DJ Jr, Roberts PL, et al. Evolutionary changes in the pathologic diagnosis after the ileoanal pouch procedure. *Dis Colon Rectum* 1997;40:263.

302. Marchetti F, Fazio VW, Ozuner G. Adenocarcinoma arising from a strictureplasty site in Crohn's disease. *Dis Colon Rectum* 1996;39:1315.

303. Markowitz J, Rosa J, Grancher K, et al. Long-term 6mercaptopurine treatment in adolescents with Crohn's disease. *Gastroenterology* 1990;99:1347.

304. Marks CG, Ritchie JK, Lockhart-Mummery HE. Anal fistulas in Crohn's disease. *Br J Surg* 1981;68:525.

305. Marshak RH, Lindner AE. Chronic inflammatory disease of the colon: historical perspective. In: Bercovitz ZT, Kirsner JB, Lindner AE, et al, eds. *Ulcerative and granulomatous colitis.* Springfield, MO: Charles C Thomas, 1973: xvii.

306. Marshak RH, Lindner AE. Radiologic diagnosis of chronic ulcerative colitis and Crohn's disease of the colon. In: Kirsner JB, Shorter RG, eds. *Inflammatory bowel disease.* Philadelphia: Lea & Febiger, 1975:241.

307. Marx FW Jr. Incidental appendectomy with regional enteritis. *Arch Surg* 1964;88:546.

308. Mary JY, Modigliani R. Development and validation of an endoscopic index of severity for Crohn's disease: a prospective multicentre study. *Gut* 1989;30:983.

309. Massell SC, Hanauer SB. Increased association of lymphoma and inflammatory bowel disease. *Gastroenterology* 2000;118:A119.

310. Matuchansky C. Parenteral nutrition in inflammatory bowel disease. *Gut* 1986;27:81.

311. McDonald PJ, Fazio VW, Farmer RG, et al. Perforating and nonperforating Crohn's disease: an unpredictable guide to recurrence after surgery. *Dis Colon Rectum* 1989; 32:117.

312. McEwen C, Di Tata D, Lingg C, et al. Ankylosing spondylitis and spondylitis accompanying ulcerative colitis, regional enteritis, psoriasis and Reiter's disease: a comparative study. *Arthritis Rheum* 1971;14:291.

313. McGarrity TJ, Manasse JS, Koch KL, et al. Crohn's disease and massive lower gastrointestinal bleeding: angiographic appearance and two case reports. *Am J Gastroenterol* 1987; 82:1096.

314. McGillis ST, Huntley AC. Metastatic Crohn's disease. *West J Med* 1989;151:203.

315. McIntyre PB, Pemberton JH, Wolff BG, et al. Indeterminate colitis: long-term outcome in patients after ileal pouch-anal anastomosis. *Dis Colon Rectum* 1995;38:51.

316. McIntyre PB, Powell-Tuck J, Wood SR, et al. Controlled trial of bowel rest in the treatment of severe acute colitis. *Gut* 1986;27:481.

317. McNamara MJ, Fazio VW, Lavery IC, et al. Surgical treatment of enterovesical fistulas in Crohn's disease. *Dis Colon Rectum* 1990;33:272.

318. Michelassi F, Hurst RD, Melis M, et al. Side-to-side isoperistaltic strictureplasty in extensive Crohn's disease: a prospective longitudinal study. *Ann Surg* 2000;232:401.

319. Michelassi F, Stella M, Balestracci T, et al. Incidence, diagnosis, and treatment of enteric and colorectal fistulae in patients with Crohn's disease. *Ann Surg* 1993;218:660.

320. Michelassi F, Testa G, Pomidor WJ, et al. Adenocarcinoma complicating Crohn's disease. *Dis Colon Rectum* 1993;36: 654.

321. Middleton SJ, Pollard S, Friend PJ, et al. Adult small intestinal transplantation in England and Wales. *Br J Surg* 2003;90:723.

322. Milsom JW, Hammerhofer KA, Böhm B, et al. Prospective, randomized trial comparing laparoscopic *vs.* conventional surgery for refractory ileocolic disease. *Dis Colon Rectum* 2001;44:1.

323. Mir-Madjlessi SH, Taylor JS, Farmer RG. Clinical course and evolution of erythema nodosum and pyoderma gangrenosum in chronic ulcerative colitis: a study of 42 patients. *Am J Gastroenterol* 1985;80:615.

324. Monsén U, Sorstad J, Hellers G, et al. Extracolonic diagnoses in ulcerative colitis: an epidemiological study. *Am J Gastroenterol* 1990;85:711.

325. Morson BC, Lockhart-Mummery HE. Crohn's disease of the colon. *Gastroenterologia* 1959;92:168.

326. Mortensen NJMcC, Ritchie JK, Hawley PR, et al. Surgery for acute Crohn's colitis: results and long term follow-up. *Br J Surg* 1984;71:783.

327. Moschowitz E, Wilensky AO. Non-specific granulomata of the intestine. *Am J Med Sci* 1923;166:48.

328. Mow WS, Abreu MT, Papadakis KA, et al. High incidence of anergy limits the usefulness of PPD screening for tuberculosis prior to Remicade in inflammatory bowel disease. *Gastroenterology* 2002;122:A100.

329. Moynihan BGA. The mimicry of malignant disease in the large intestine. *Edinburgh Med J* 1907;21:228.

330. Munkholm P, Langholz E, Davidsen M, et al. Frequency of glucocorticoid resistance and dependency in Crohn's disease. *Gut* 1994;35:360.

331. Muñoz-Juárez M, Yamamoto T, Wolff BG, et al. Wide-lumen stapled anastomosis *vs.* conventional end-to-end anastomosis in the treatment of Crohn's disease. *Dis Colon Rectum* 2001;44:20.

332. Murray JJ, Schoetz DJ Jr, Nugent FW, et al. Surgical management of Crohn's disease involving the duodenum. *Am J Surg* 1984;147:58.

333. Mylonakis E, Allan RN, Keighley MRB. How does pouch construction for a final diagnosis of Crohn's disease compare with ileoproctostomy for established Crohn's proctocolitis? *Dis Colon Rectum* 2001;44:1137.

334. Myrvold HE, Kock NG. Continent ileostomy in patients with Crohn's disease. *Gastroenterology* 1981;80:1237.

335. Neal DE, Williams NS, Barker MCJ, et al. The effect of resection of the distal ileum on gastric emptying, small bowel transit and absorption after proctocolectomy. *Br J Surg* 1984;71:666.

336. Nelson RL, Subramanian K, Gasparaitis A, et al. Indium 111-labeled granulocyte scan in the diagnosis and management of acute inflammatory bowel disease. *Dis Colon Rectum* 1990;33:451.

337. Neufeld DM, Shemesh EI, Kodner IJ, et al. Endoscopic management of anastomotic colon strictures with electrocautery and balloon dilation. *Gastrointest Endosc* 1987; 33:24.

338. Neumann V, Wright V. Arthritis associated with bowel disease. *Clin Gastroenterol* 1983;12:767.

339. Niv Y. Esophageal involvement in Crohn's disease. *Am J Gastroenterol* 1988;83:205.

340. Nordgren SR, Fasth SB, Öresland TO, et al. Long-term follow-up in Crohn's disease: mortality, morbidity, and functional status. In: Schölmerich J, Goebell H, Kruis W, et al., eds. *Inflammatory bowel disease: pathophysiology as basis of treatment.* Dordrecht: Kluwer Academic Publishers, 1992:334.

341. Nuako KW, Ahlquist DA, Sandborn WJ, et al. Primary sclerosing cholangitis and colorectal carcinoma in patients with chronic ulcerative colitis. *Cancer* 1998;82:822.

342. Nubiola P, Badia JM, Martinez-Rodenas F, et al. Treatment of 27 postoperative enterocutaneous fistulas with the long half-life somatostatin analogue SMS 201–995. *Ann Surg* 1989;210:56.

343. Nugent FW, Richmond M, Park SK. Crohn's disease of the duodenum. *Gut* 1977;18:115.

344. Nugent FW, Roy MA. Duodenal Crohn's disease: an analysis of 89 cases. *Am J Gastroenterol* 1989;84:249.

345. Nugent FW, Veidenheimer MC, Meissner WA, et al. Prognosis after colonic resection for Crohn's disease of the colon. *Gastroenterology* 1973;65:398.

346. O'Brien JJ, Bayless TM, Bayless JA. Use of azathioprine or 6-mercaptopurine in the treatment of Crohn's disease. *Gastroenterology* 1991;101:39.

347. O'Donoghue DP, Dawson AM, Powell-Tuck J, et al. Double-blind withdrawal trial of azathioprine as maintenance treatment for Crohn's disease. *Lancet* 1978;2:955.

348. Ogura Y, Bonen DK, Inohara N, et al. A frameshift mutation in NOD2 associated with susceptibility to Crohn's disease. *Nature* 2001;411:603.

349. Olaison, G, Smedh K, Sjödahl R. Natural course of Crohn's disease after ileocolic resection: endoscopically visualized ileal ulcers preceding symptoms. *Gut* 1992;33:331.

350. Olsson R, Danielsson Å, Jäärnerot G, et al. Prevalence of primary sclerosing cholangitis in patients with ulcerative colitis. *Gastroenterology* 1991;100:1319.

351. O'Morain C, Segal AW, Levi AJ. Elemental diet as primary treatment of acute Crohn's disease: a controlled trial. *BMJ* 1984;288:1859.
352. Orholm M, Binder V, Sorensen TL, et al. Concordance of inflammatory bowel disease among Danish twins. Results of a nationwide study. *Scand J Gastroenterol* 2000;35:1075.
353. Ostergaard-Thomsen O, Cortot A, Lewell D, et al. A comparison of budesonide and mesalamine for active Crohn's disease. *N Engl J Med* 1998;339:370–375.
354. Otley A, Thomson AB, Modigiliani R, et al. Budesonide for the induction of remission in Crohn's disease: meta-analysis of randomized controlled trials. *Gastroenterology* 2003;124:A378.
355. Ozuner G, Fazio VW, Lavery IC, et al. How safe is strictureplasty in the management of Crohn's disease? *Am J Surg* 1996;171:57.
356. Ozuner G, Fazio VW, Lavery IC, et al. Reoperative rates for Crohn's disease following strictureplasty. *Dis Colon Rectum* 1996;39:1199.
357. Pace BW, Bank S, Wise L. Strictureplasty: an alternative in the surgical treatment of Crohn's disease. *Arch Surg* 1984;119:861.
358. Parker RGF, Kendall EJC. Liver in ulcerative colitis. *BMJ* 1954;2:1030.
359. Pastore RLO, Wolff BG, Hodge D. Total abdominal colectomy and ileorectal anastomosis for inflammatory bowel disease. *Dis Colon Rectum* 1997;40:1455.
360. Payne-James JJ, Silk DBA. Total parenteral nutrition as primary treatment in Crohn's disease—RIP? *Gut* 1988;29:1304.
361. Pearson M, Teahor K, Levi AJ, et al. Food intolerance and Crohn's disease. *Gut* 1993;34:783.
362. Peters WR, Fry RD, Fleshman JW, et al. Multiple blood transfusions reduce the recurrence rate of Crohn's disease. *Dis Colon Rectum* 1989;32:749.
363. Petras RE, Mir-Madjlessi SH, Farmer RG. Crohn's disease and intestinal carcinoma: a report of 11 cases with emphasis on associated epithelial dysplasia. *Gastroenterology* 1987;93:1307.
364. Pezim ME, Pemberton, JH, Beart RW Jr, et al. Outcome of "indeterminant" colitis following ileal pouch anal anastomosis. *Dis Colon Rectum* 1989;32:653.
365. Pokorny WJ, Fowler CL. Isoperistaltic intestinal lengthening for short bowel syndrome. *Surg Gynecol Obstet* 1991;172:39.
366. Pokorny RM, Hofmeister A, Galandiuk S, et al. Crohn's disease and ulcerative colitis are associated with the DNA repair gene *MLH1*. *Ann Surg* 1997;225:718.
367. Poritz LS, Koltun WA. Surgical management of ulcerative colitis in the presence of primary sclerosing cholangitis. *Dis Colon Rectum* 2003;46:173.
368. Poritz LS, Rowe WA, Kolyun WA. Remicade does not abolish the need for surgery in fistulizing Crohn's disease. *Dis Colon Rectum* 2002;45:771.
369. Post S, Betzler M, von Ditfurth B, et al. Risks of intestinal anastomoses in Crohn's disease. *Ann Surg* 1991;213:37.
370. Post S, Herfarth C, Böhm E, et al. The impact of disease pattern, surgical management, and individual surgeons on the risk for relaparotomy for recurrent Crohn's disease. *Ann Surg* 1996;223:253.
371. Powell FC, Schroeter AL, Su WPD, et al. Pyoderma gangrenosum: a review of 86 patients. *Q J Med* 1985;55:173.
372. Prabhakar LP, Laramee C, Nelson H, et al. Avoiding a stoma: role for segmental or abdominal colectomy in Crohn's colitis. *Dis Colon Rectum* 1997;40:71.
373. Prantera C, Kohn A, Zannari F, et al. Metronidazole plus ciprofloxacin in the treatment of active refractory Crohn's disease: results of an open study. *J Clin Gastroenterol* 1994;19:79.
374. Prantera C, Pallone F, Brunetti G, et al. Oral 5-aminosalicylic acid (Asacol) in the maintenance treatment of Crohn's disease. *Gastroenterology* 1992;103:363.
375. Prantera C, Scrihano ML, Falasco G, et al. Ineffectiveness of probiotics in preventing recurrence after "curative" resection for Crohn's disease: a randomized controlled trial with lactobacillus GG. *Gut* 2002;51:405.
376. Prantera C, Zannoni F, Scriband ML, et al. An antibiotic regimen for the treatment of active Crohn's disease: a randomized controlled clinical trial of metronidazole plus ciprofloxacin. *Am J Gastroenterol* 1996;91:A328.
377. Present DH, Korelitz BI, Wisch N, et al. Treatment of Crohn's disease with 6-mercaptopurine: a long-term randomized, double-blind study. *N Engl J Med* 1980;302:981.
378. Present DH, Mayer L, van Deventer SJH. Anti-TNF alpha chimeric antibody (cA2) is effective in the treatment of fistulae of Crohn's disease: a multi-center, randomized, double-blind, placebo-controlled study. *Am J Gastroenterol* 1997;92:A648 (1746).
379. Present DH, Meltzer SJ, Krumholz MP, et al. 6-mercaptopurine in the management of inflammatory bowel disease: short- and long-term toxicity. *Ann Intern Med* 1989;111:641.
380. Price AB. Overlap in the spectrum of non-specific inflammatory bowel disease-colitis indeterminate. *J Clin Pathol* 1978;31:567.
381. Pritchard TJ, Schoetz DJ, Roberts PL, et al. Perirectal abscess in Crohn's disease: drainage and outcome. *Dis Colon Rectum* 1990;33:933.
382. Probert CSJ, Jayanthi V, Wicks ACB, et al. Mortality from Crohn's disease in Leicestershire, 1972–1989: an epidemiological community based study. *Gut* 1992;33:1226.
383. Procaccino JA, Lavery IA, Fazio VW, et al. Psoas abscess: difficulties encountered. *Dis Colon Rectum* 1991;34:784.
384. Puntis J, McNeish AS, Allan RN. Long term prognosis of Crohn's disease with onset in childhood and adolescence. *Gastroenterology* 1984;25:329.
385. Raab Y, Bergström R, Ejerblad S, et al. Factors influencing recurrence in Crohn's disease: an analysis of a consecutive series of 353 patients treated with primary surgery. *Dis Colon Rectum* 1996;39:918.
386. Rauh SM, Schoetz DJ Jr, Roberts PL, et al. Pouchitis: is it a wastebasket diagnosis? *Dis Colon Rectum* 1991;34:685.
387. Rawlinson J, Hughes RG. Acute suppurative appendicitis: a rare associate of Crohn's disease. *Dis Colon Rectum* 1985;28:608.
388. Regimbeau JM, Panis Y, Pocard M, et al. Long-term results of ileal pouch-anal anastomosis for colorectal Crohn's disease. *Dis Colon Rectum* 2001;44:769.
389. Remzi FH, Dietz DW, Unal E, et al. Combined use of preoperative provocative angiography and highly selective methylene blue injection to localize an occult small-bowel bleeding site in a patient with Crohn's disease: report of a case. *Dis Colon Rectum* 2003;46:260.
390. Ribeiro MB, Greenstein AJ, Heimann TM, et al. Adenocarcinoma of the small intestine in Crohn's disease. *Surg Gynecol Obstet* 1991;173:343.
391. Ribeiro MB, Greenstein AJ, Sachar DB, et al. Colorectal adenocarcinoma in Crohn's disease. *Ann Surg* 1996;223:186.
392. Ricart E, Panaccione R, Loftus EV, et al. Infliximab for Crohn's disease in clinical practice at the Mayo Clinic: The first 100 patients. *Gastroenterology* 2000;118:568 (A2967).
393. Richards ME, Rickert RR, Nance FC. Crohn's disease associated carcinoma: a poorly recognized complication of inflammatory bowel disease. *Ann Surg* 1989;209:764.
394. Ritchie JK. Crohn's disease in young people. *Br J Surg* 1985;72:S90.
395. Ritchie JK, Allan RN, Macartney J, et al. Biliary tract carcinoma associated with ulcerative colitis. *Q J Med* 1974;43:263.
396. Robert JR, Sachar DB, Greenstein AJ. Severe gastrointestinal hemorrhage in Crohn's disease. *Ann Surg* 1991;213:207.
397. Rombeau JL, Barot LR, Williamson CE, et al. Preoperative total parenteral nutrition and surgical outcome in patients with inflammatory bowel disease. *Am J Surg* 1982;143:139.
398. Rosén A, Ursing B, Alm T, et al. A comparative study of metronidazole and sulfasalazine for active Crohn's disease:

the cooperative Crohn's disease study in Sweden. I. Design and methodologic considerations. *Gastroenterology* 1982; 83:541.

399. Rosenberg EW, Spitzer RE, Marley, et al. Inflammatory bowel disease, psoriasis, and complement. *N Engl J Med* 1982;307:685.

400. Rosenthal SR, Snyder JD, Hendricks KM, et al. Growth failure and inflammatory bowel disease: approach to treatment of a complicated adolescent problem. *Pediatrics* 1983;72:481.

401. Ross TM, Fazio VW, Farmer RG. Long-term results of surgical treatment for Crohn's disease of the duodenum. *Ann Surg* 1983;197:399.

402. Rothenberger DA (moderator), Fazio VW, Cohen Z, et al. Symposium on ileoanal anastomosis in Crohn's disease: is it feasible? Presented at 89th Convention of the American Society of Colon and Rectal Surgeons, St. Louis, April 29 to May 4, 1990.

403. Rubio CA, Befrits R. Colorectal adenocarcinoma in Crohn's disease: a retrospective histologic study. *Dis Colon Rectum* 1997;40:1072.

404. Rubio CA, Befritz R, Poppen B, et al. Crohn's disease and adenocarcinoma of the intestinal tract. *Dis Colon Rectum* 1991;34:174.

405. Rudolph WG, Uthoff SMS, McAuliffe TL, et al. Indeterminate colitis: the real story. *Dis Colon Rectum* 2002;45:1528.

406. Rusche M, O'Brian J. Infliximab in the management of recto-vaginal fistulous Crohn's disease. *Am J Gastroenterol* 2001;95:S306.

407. Ruiz V, Unger SW, Morgan J, et al. Crohn's disease of the appendix. *Surgery* 1990;107:113.

408. Rutgeerts P, Colombel JF, van Deventer S, et al. Endoscopic healing induced by infliximab maintenance therapy correlates with long-term clinical response in patients with active Crohn's disease. Results of endoscopic substudy of Accent I. *Am J Gastroenterol* 2002;97:S260.

409. Rutgeerts P, Geboes K, Vantrappen G, et al. Natural history of recurrent Crohn's disease at the ileocolonic anastomosis after curative surgery. *Gut* 1984;25:665.

410. Rutgeerts P, Geboes K, Vantrappen G, et al. Predictability of the postoperative course of Crohn's disease. *Gastroenterology* 1990;99:956.

411. Rutgeerts P, Hiele M, Gelives K, et al. Controlled trial of metronidazole treatment for prevention of Crohn's recurrence after ileal resection. *Gastroenterology* 1995;108:1617.

412. Rutgeerts P, Lofberg R, Melchow H, et al. Budesonide versus prednisone for the treatment of active ileocecal Crohn's disease: a European, multi-center trial. *Gastroenterology* 1993;104:A772.

413. Rutgeerts P, Onette E, Vantrappen G, et al. Crohn's disease of the stomach and duodenum: a clinical study with emphasis on the value of endoscopy and endoscopic biopsies. *Endoscopy* 1980;12:288.

414. Sachar DB. Cancer in Crohn's disease: dispelling the myths. *Gut* 1994;35:1507.

415. Sagar PM, Dozois RR, Wolff BG. Long-term results of ileal pouch-anal anastomosis in patients with Crohn's disease. *Dis Colon Rectum* 1996;39:893.

416. Saint-Marc O, Tiret E, Vaillant J-C, et al. Surgical management of internal fistulas in Crohn's disease. *J Am Coll Surg* 1996;183:97.

417. Samach M, Train J. Demonstration of mucosal bridging in Crohn's colitis. *Am J Gastroenterol* 1980;74:50.

418. Sandborn WJ, Feagan BG. Review article: mild to moderate Crohn's disease: defining the basis for a new treatment algorithm. *Aliment Pharmacol Ther* 2003.18:263.

419. Sanderson IR, Walker-Smith JA. Crohn's disease in childhood. *Br J Surg* 1985;72:S87.

420. Sanderson JD, Moss MT, Tizard MLV, et al. *Mycobacterium paratuberculosis* DNA in Crohn's disease tissue. *Gut* 1992; 33:890.

421. Sands BE. Therapy of inflammatory bowel disease. *Gastroenterology* 2000;118 (Suppl 1):S68.

422. Sands B, Blank M, Masters P, et al. Long-term treatment of rectovaginal fistulas in Crohn's disease: response to infliximab in the Accent II trial. *Gastroenterology* 2003;124:A380.

423. Savoca PE, Ballantyne GH, Cahow CE. Gastrointestinal malignancies in Crohn's disease: a 20-year experience. *Dis Colon Rectum* 1990;33:7.

424. Saylan J, Wilson DAL, Allan A, et al. Recurrence after strictureplasty or resection for Crohn's disease. *Br J Surg* 1989; 76:335.

425. Scammell BE, Andrews H, Allan RN, et al. Results of proctocolectomy of Crohn's disease. *Br J Surg* 1987;74:671.

426. Schmidt CM, Talamini MA, Kaufman HS, et al. Laparoscopic surgery for Crohn's disease: reasons for conversion. *Ann Surg* 2001;233:733.

427. Schoetz DJ Jr, Coller JA, Veidenheimer MC. Pyoderma gangrenosum and Crohn's disease: eight cases and a review of the literature. *Dis Colon Rectum* 1983;26:155.

428. Schulman D, Beck LS, Roberts IM, et al. Crohn's disease of the vulva. *Am J Gastroenterol* 1987;82:1328.

429. Scott ADN, Ritchie JK, Phillips RKS. Blood transfusion and recurrent Crohn's disease. *Br J Surg* 1991;78:455.

430. Scully C, Cochran KM, Russell RI, et al. Crohn's disease of the mouth: an indicator of intestinal involvement. *Gut* 1982;23:198.

431. Senofsky GM, Stabile BE. Gallstone ileus associated with Crohn's disease. *Sugrery* 1990;108:114.

432. Seyrig J-A, Jian R, Modigliani R, et al. Idiopathic pancreatitis associated with inflammatory bowel disease. *Dig Dis Sci* 1985;30:1121.

433. Shah SA, Fefferman DS, Farrell RJ, et al. Efficacy and safety of infliximab in 221 Crohn's disease patients. *Am J Gastroenterol* 2000;95:2640(A787).

434. Shaked A, Colonna JO, Goldstein L, et al. The interrelation between sclerosing cholangitis and ulcerative colitis in patients undergoing liver transplantation. *Ann Surg* 1992;215: 598.

435. Sheehan AL, Warren BF, Gear MWL, et al. Fat-wrapping in Crohn's disease: pathological basis and relevance to surgical practice. *Br J Surg* 1992;79:955.

436. Shepherd AFI, Alexander-Williams J. Stomal ulcer complicating bypass for duodenal Crohn's disease. *World J Surg* 1986;10:146.

437. Sher ME, Bauer JJ, Gorphine S, et al. Low Hartmann procedure for severe anorectal Crohn's disease. *Dis Colon Rectum* 1992;35.

438. Sherlock DJ, Suarez V, Gray JG. Stomal adenocarcinoma in Crohn's disease. *Gut* 1990;31:1329.

439. Shiloni E, Coronado E, Freund HR. Role of total parenteral nutrition in the treatment of Crohn's disease. *Am J Surg* 1989;157:180.

440. Shiloni E, Freund HR. Total parenteral nutrition in Crohn's disease: is it a primary or supportive mode of therapy? *Dis Colon Rectum* 1983;26:275.

441. Simkins KC. Aphthoid ulcers in Crohn's colitis. *Clin Radiol* 1977;28:601.

442. Simonowitz DA, Rusch VW, Stevenson JK. Natural history of incidental appendectomy in patients with Crohn's disease who required subsequent bowel resection. *Am J Surg* 1982;143:171.

443. Singleton JW, Hanauer SB, Gitnick GL, et al. Mesalamine capsules for the treatment of active Crohn's disease: results of a 16-week trial. *Gastroenterology* 1993;104:1293.

444. Slaney G, Muller S, Clay J, et al. Crohn's disease involving the penis. *Gut* 1986;27:329.

445. Slater G, Greenstein A, Aufses AH Jr. Anal carcinoma in patients with Crohn's disease. *Ann Surg* 1984;199:348.

446. Slaton GD, Navab F, Boyd CM, et al. Role of delayed indium-111 labeled leukocyte scan in the management of Crohn's disease. *Am J Gastroenterol* 1985;80:790.

447. Smedh K, Olaison G, Sjödahl R. Ileocolic nipple valve anastomosis for preventing recurrence of surgically treated Crohn's disease: long-term follow-up in six patients. *Dis Colon Rectum* 1990;33:987.

448. Smith TR, Conradi H, Bernstein R, et al. Adenocarcinoma arising in Crohn's disease: report of two cases. *Dis Colon Rectum* 1980;23:498.

449. Snyder MB, Cawson RA. Oral changes in Crohn's disease. *J Oral Surg* 1976;34:59.

450. Sofaer J. Crohn's disease: the genetic contribution. *Gut* 1993;34:869.

451. Somerville KW, Langman MJS, Da Cruz DJ, et al. Malignant transformation of anal skin tags in Crohn's disease. *Gut* 1984;25:1124.

452. Sonnenberg A, Erckenbrecht J, Peter P, et al. Detection of Crohn's disease by ultrasound. *Gastroenterology* 1982;83:430.

453. Spiliotis J, Briand D, Gouttebel M-C, et al. Treatment of fistulas of the gastrointestinal tract with total parenteral nutrition and octeotide in patients with carcinoma. *Surg Gynecol Obstet* 993;176:575.

454. Stack WA, Mann SD, Roy AJ, et al. Randomised controlled trial of CDP571 antibody to tumour necrosis factor-á in Crohn's disease. *Lancet* 1997;349:521.

455. Stahl TJ, Schoetz DJ Jr, Roberts PL, et al. Crohn's disease and carcinoma: increasing justification for surveillance? *Dis Colon Rectum* 1992;35:850.

456. Steiger E, Srp F. Morbidity and mortality related to home parenteral nutrition in patients with gut failure. *Am J Surg* 1983;145:102.

457. Steinberg DM, Allan RN, Thompson H, et al. Excisional surgery with ileostomy for Crohn's colitis with particular reference to factors affecting recurrence. *Gut* 1974;15:845.

458. Steinberg DM, Cooke WT, Alexander-Williams J. Abscess and fistulae in Crohn's disease. *Gut* 1973;14:865.

459. Stokes MA, Irving MH. How do patients with Crohn's disease fare on home parenteral nutrition? *Dis Colon Rectum* 1988;31:454.

460. Stone W, Veidenheimer MC, Corman ML, et al. The dilemma of Crohn's disease: long-term follow-up of Crohn's disease of the small intestine. *Dis Colon Rectum* 1977;20:372.

461. Storch I, Sachar D, Katz S. Pulmonary manifestations of inflammatory bowel disease. *Inflamm Bowel Dis* 2003;9:104.

462. Summers RW, Switz DM, Sessions JTJr, et al. National Cooperative Crohn's Disease Study: results of drug treatment. *Gastroenterology* 1979;77:847.

463. Sustento-Reodica N, Ruiz P, Rogers A, et al. Recurrent Crohn's disease in transplanted bowel. *Lancet* 1997;349:688.

464. Sutherland L, Singleton J, Sessions J, et al. Double-blind, placebo-controlled trial of metronidazole in Crohn's disease. *Gut* 1991;32:1071.

465. Sutphen JL, Cooper PH, Mackel SE, et al. Metastatic cutaneous Crohn's disease. *Gastroenterology* 1984;86:941.

466. Swift GL, Srivastava ED, Stone R, et al. Controlled trial of anti-tuberculous chemotherapy for two years in Crohn's disease. *Gut* 1994;35:363.

467. Targan SR, Hanauer SB, van Deventer SJH, et al. A short-term study of chimeric monoclonal antibody cA2 to tumor necrosis factor alpha for Crohn's disease. Crohn's Disease cA2 Study Group. *N Engl J Med* 1997;337:1029.

468. Taschieri AM, Cristaldi M, Elli M, et al. Description of new bowel-sparing techniques for long strictures of Crohn's disease. *Am J Surg* 1997;173:509.

469. Teague RH, Waye JD. Inflammatory bowel disease. In: Hunt RH, Waye JD, eds. *Colonoscopy: techniques, clinical practice and colour atlas.* London: Chapman & Hall, 1981:343.

470. Teahon K, Bjarnson I, Pearson M, et al. Ten years' experience with an elemental diet in the management of Crohn's disease. *Gut* 1990;31:1133.

471. Thompson JS. Strategies for preserving intestinal length in the short-bowel syndrome. *Dis Colon Rectum* 1987;30:208.

472. Thompson JS. Surgical management of short bowel syndrome. *Surgery* 1993;113:4.

473. Thompson JS. The current status of surgical therapy for the short bowel syndrome. *Contemp Surg* 1988;33:27.

474. Thompson S, Langnas AN, Pinch LW, et al. Surgical approach to short-bowel syndrome: experience in a population of 160 patients. *Ann Surg* 1995;222:600.

475. Tichansky D, Cagir B, Yoo E, et al. Strictureplasty for Crohn's disease: meta-analysis. *Dis Colon Rectum* 2000;43:911.

476. Timmer A, Sutherland L, Martin F. Oral contraceptive use and smoking are risk factors for relapse in Crohn's disease. *Gastroenterology* 1998;114:1143.

477. Tjandra JJ, Fazio VW. Strictureplasty for ileocolic anastomotic strictures in Crohn's disease. *Dis Colon Rectum* 1993;36:1099.

478. Tjandra JJ, Fazio VW. Strictureplasty without concomitant resection for small bowel obstruction in Crohn's disease. *Br J Surg* 1994;81:561.

479. Tonelli F, Fedi M, Paroli GM, et al. Indications and results of side-to-side isoperistaltic strictureplasty in Crohn's disease. *Dis Colon Rectum* 2004;47:494.

480. Topstad DR, Panaccione R, Heine JA, et al. Combined seton placement, infliximab infusion, and maintenance immunosuppressives improve healing rate in fistulizing anorectal Crohn's disease: a single center experience. *Dis Colon Rectum* 2003;46:577.

481. Toy LS, Scherl EJ, Kornbluth A, et al. Complete bowel obstruction following initial response to infliximab therapy for Crohn's disease: a series of a newly described complication. *Gastroenterology* 2000;118:569 (A2974).

482. Tremaine WJ. Maintenance therapy in IBD. *Inflamm Bowel Dis* 1998;44:292.

483. Trnka YM, Glotzer DJ, Kasdon EJ, et al. The long-term outcome of restorative operation in Crohn's disease: influence of location, prognostic factors and surgical guidelines. *Ann Surg* 1982;196:345.

484. Tweedie JH, McCann BG. Metastatic Crohn's disease of thigh and forearm. *Gut* 1984;25:213.

485. Ursing B, Alm T, Bárány F, et al. A comparative study of metronidazole and sulfasalazine for active Crohn's disease: the cooperative Crohn's disease study in Sweden. II. Result. *Gastroenterology* 1982;83:550.

486. Valiulis A, Currie DJ. A surgical experience with Crohn's disease. *Surg Gynecol Obstet* 1987;164:27.

487. van Bodegraven AA, Sloots CEJ, Felt-Bersma RJF, et al. Endosonographic evidence of persistence of Crohn's disease-associated fistulas after infliximab treatment, irrespective of clinical response. *Dis Colon Rectum* 2002;45:39.

488. van Dongen LM, Lubbers E-JC. Fistulas of the bladder in Crohn's disease. *Surg Gynecol Obstet* 1984;158:308.

489. van Outryve MJ, Pelckmans PA, Michielsen PP, et al. Value of transrectal ultrasonography in Crohn's disease. *Gastroenterology* 1991;101:1171.

490. Van Patter WN, Bargen JA, Dockerty MB, et al. Regional enteritis. *Gastroenterology* 1954;26:347.

491. The Veteran Affairs Total Parenteral Nutrition Cooperative Study Group. Perioperative total parenteral nutrition in surgical patients. *N Engl J Med* 1991;325:525.

492. Ward CS, Dunphy EP, Jagoe WS, et al. Crohn's disease limited to the mouth and anus. *J Clin Gastroenterol* 1985;7:516.

493. Warman JI, Korelitz BI, Fleisher MR, et al. Cumulative experience with short and long-term toxicity in 6-mercaptopurine in the treatment of Crohn's disease and ulcerative colitis. *J Clin Gastroenterol* 2003;37:220.

494. Warren KW, Athanassiades S, Monge JI. Primary sclerosing cholangitis. *Am J Surg* 1966;3:23.

495. Watanabe M, Hasegawa H, Yamamoto S, et al. Successful application of laparoscopic surgery to the treatment of Crohn's disease with fistulas. *Dis Colon Rectum* 2002;45:1057.

496. Waye JD. The role of colonoscopy in the differential diagnosis of inflammatory bowel disease. *Gastrointest Endosc* 1977;23:150.

497. Weaver RM, Keighley MRB. Measurement of rectal capacity in the assessment of patients for colectomy and ileorectal anastomosis in Crohn's colitis. *Dis Colon Rectum* 1986; 29:443.

498. Weinberg AM, Lewis JD, Su C, et al. Response to infliximab in Crohn's disease: do strictures make a difference? *Am J Gastroenterol* 2001;96:S312

499. Weston LA, Roberts PL, Schoetz DJ Jr, et al. Ileocolic resection for acute presentation of Crohn's disease in the ileum. *Dis Colon Rectum* 1996;39:841.

500. Wheeler SC, Marion JF, Present DH. Medical therapy, not surgery, is the appropriate first line treatment for Crohn's enterovesical fistula. *Am J Gastroenterol* 1998;114:A1113.

501. Whelan G, Farmer RG, Fazio VW, et al. Recurrence after surgery in Crohn's disease: relationship to location of disease (clinical pattern) and surgical indication. *Gastroenterology* 1985;88:1826.

502. Williams AJK, Palmer KR. Endoscopic balloon dilatation as a therapeutic option in the management of intestinal strictures resulting from Crohn's disease. *Br J Surg* 1991; 78:453.

503. Williams DR, Coller JA, Corman ML, et al. Anal complications in Crohn's disease. *Dis Colon Rectum* 1981;24:22.

504. Williams JG, Wong WD, Rothenberger DA, et al. Recurrence of Crohn's disease after resection. *Br J Surg* 1991; 78:10.

505. Williams SM, Harned RK. Bile duct carcinoma associated with chronic ulcerative colitis. *Dis Colon Rectum* 1981;24:42.

506. Wilmore DW, Lacey JM, Soultanakis RP, et al. Factors predicting a successful outcome after pharmacologic bowel compensation. *Ann Surg* 1997;226:288.

507. Winslet MC, Andrews H, Allan RN, et al. Fecal diversion in the management of Crohn's disease of the colon. *Dis Colon Rectum* 1993;36:757.

508. Winslet MC, Keighley MRB. Faecal challenge as a predictor of the effect of restoring intestinal continuity in defunctionalized Crohn's colitis. *Gut* 1988;29:1475.

509. Wisch N, Korelitz BI. Immunosuppressive therapy for ulcerative colitis, ileitis, and granulomatous colitis. *Surg Clin North Am* 1972;52:961.

510. Wise L, Kyriakos M, McCown A, et al. Crohn's disease of the duodenum: a report and analysis of eleven new cases. *Am J Surg* 1971;121:184.

511. Wolff BG. Resection margins in Crohn's disease. *Br J Surg* 2001;88:771.

512. Wolff BG, Beart RW Jr, Frydenberg HB, et al. The importance of disease-free margins in resection for Crohn's disease. *Dis Colon Rectum* 1983;26:239.

513. Wolff BG, Culp CE, Beart RW Jr, et al. Anorectal Crohn's disease: a long-term prospective. *Dis Colon Rectum* 1985; 28:709.

514. Worsey MJ, Hull T, Ryland L, et al. Strictureplasty is an effective option in the operative management of duodenal Crohn's disease. *Dis Colon Rectum* 1999;42:596.

515. Yamamoto T, Allan RN, Keighley MRB. Smoking is a predictive factor for outcome after colectomy and ileorectal anastomosis in patients with Crohn's disease. *Br J Surg* 1999;86:1069.

516. Yamamoto T, Allan RN, Keighley MRB. Audit of single-stage proctocolectomy for Crohn's disease: postoperative complications and recurrence. *Dis Colon Rectum* 2000; 43:249.

517. Yamamoto T, Allan RN, Keighley MRB. Risk factors for intra-abdominal sepsis after surgery in Crohn's disease. *Dis Colon Rectum* 2000;43:1141.

518. Yamamoto T, Allan RN, Keighley MRB. Persistent perineal sinus after proctocolectomy for Crohn's disease. *Dis Colon Rectum* 1999;42:96.

519. Yamamoto T, Bain IM, Connolly AB, et al. Outcome of strictureplasty for duodenal Crohn's disease. *Br J Surg* 1999; 86:259.

520. Yamamoto T, Keighley MRB. Smoking and disease recurrence after operation for Crohn's disease. *Br J Surg* 2000; 78:398.

521. Yamazaki Y, Ribeiro MB, Sachar DB, et al. Malignant colorectal strictures in Crohn's disease. *Am J Gastroenterol* 1991;86:882.

522. Yates VM, Watkinson G, Kelman A. Further evidence for an association between psoriasis, Crohn's disease and ulcerative colitis. *Br J Dermatol* 1982;106:323.

523. Young-Fadok TM, Wolff BG, Meagher A, et al. Surgical management of ileosigmoid fistulas in Crohn's disease. *Dis Colon Rectum* 1997;40:558.

524. Yousem DM, Fishman EK, Jones B. Crohn disease: perirectal and perianal findings at CT. *Radiology* 1988;167:331.

525. Yu CS, Pemberton JH, Larson D. Ileal pouch-anal anastomosis in patients with indeterminate colitis. *Dis Colon Rectum* 2000;43:1487.

526. Zelas P, Jagelman DG. Loop ileostomy in the management of Crohn's colitis in the debilitated patient. *Ann Surg* 1980;191:164.

527. Zinkin LD, Brandwein C. Adenocarcinoma in Crohn's colitis. *Dis Colon Rectum* 1980;23:115.

528. Zvaifler NJ, Martel W. Spondylitis in chronic ulcerative colitis. *Arthritis Rheum* 1960;3:76.

Intestinal Stomas

Th' incurable cut off, the rest reforme.
Ben Jonson—Cynthia's Revels 5.11

The applications of colostomy and ileostomy have been discussed in detail in Chapters 23, 29, and 30. The purpose of this chapter is to amplify on the methods of creating a satisfactory stoma, methods of closure, results with these procedures, and complications and their management.

PREPARING THE PATIENT

Overcoming ignorance and fear is often the most important issue that must be addressed by the surgeon in preparing an individual for a stoma. Some patients have had unpleasant associations with ostomies through experiences and jeremiads of family and friends. Myths and misunderstandings further prejudice the patient. The surgeon must confront one's fear of the disease itself, the potential for complications, and, indeed, possible mortality. These issues must be addressed as part of a comprehensive rehabilitative program. It is usually very helpful to provide literature concerning the nature of the surgery and the reasonableness of living with a colostomy or an ileostomy. In addition, it is often helpful to have an individual of similar age, gender, and socioeconomic position serve to acquaint a patient with the concept of living and functioning normally with a stoma. Whenever possible, the enterostomal therapist should be involved with the preoperative counseling, not necessarily to provide detailed stomal care at that time, but to supply information about the wide variety of ostomy products available.[1] Bass and colleagues evaluated their stoma registry, consisting of 1,790 patients, for early and late complications with respect to whether they underwent stomal marking (see later) and education by the enterostomal therapist.[17] The difference in the total number of complications between the two groups was found to be statistically significant, confirming that preoperative evaluation by an enterostomal therapist, marking of the skin site, and providing patient education contribute to reduction of adverse outcomes. Nu-

gent and coworkers (Southampton, United Kingdom) concluded in their questionnaire involving 391 patients that improved preoperative assessment and counseling with longer follow-up by the stoma department would be helpful in the management of these patients and probably would contribute to improvement in the quality of their lives."[159] With this, the fifth edition of this text, I consider this area to be so crucial that I have separated enterostomal therapy into a separate chapter (see Chapter 32).

Stomal Marking

The location of the stoma has a direct bearing on subsequent ostomy management. Establishment of the stomal site prior to surgery is usually the responsibility of the surgeon, but in many instances may be delegated to a trained enterostomal therapist. Proper location of the colostomy or ileostomy can often prevent complications such as prolapse, hernia, and skin problems.[49,107]

The groin, the waistline, the costal margins, the umbilicus, skin folds, and scars frequently interfere with appliance management. It is advisable to leave a 5-cm margin of smooth skin around the stoma. The stoma should always be placed at the summit of the infraumbilical bulge and within the rectus muscle. When the site is being marked, it is helpful to have the patient lie in the supine position and tense the abdominal muscles. This allows one to feel the lateral border of the rectus muscle. A triangle is formed by drawing an imaginary line from the umbilicus to the pubis, one from the umbilicus to the anterosuperior iliac spine, and another from the pubis to the anterosuperior iliac spine (the inguinal ligament; see Figure 29-39). The stoma usually should be in the center. The faceplate should be taped over the site and the patient should stand, sit, and bend with the faceplate in place. Slight adjustments may be required because of interference from skin creases and adiposity.

Another factor to consider is the patient's preference for clothing style, especially where the belt is worn, because stomas must be placed below the waist and preferably below the belt line. Should an individual require two stomas, the new opening must be placed either above or below the existing one. Occasionally, it may be necessary to keep a faceplate in place for 24 hours to ensure the patient's subsequent comfort and ease of movement. This is especially true when the abdomen contains multiple scars. My own preference is simply to scratch a mark onto the proposed location (see Figure 29-40). The use of a pen is not advised, since such marks are often obliterated during the abdominal preparation.

If a site is not selected until the patient is in the operating room, what is perceived to be an ideal location may subsequently present a difficult management problem. The outer margin of the faceplate may appear at the waistline or in the groin, or the stoma may be found on the undersurface of the infraumbilical bulge, making it impossible for the patient to fit the skin barrier properly and to center the pouch. At the very least, a flange can be used that corresponds to the diameter of the faceplate of an appliance in order to identify the site and to give some degree of assurance.

The above considerations are applicable to all intestinal stomas—ileostomy, sigmoid colostomy, transverse colostomy, and urinary conduit. However, it is unfortunate that what we surgeons strive for may be difficult to achieve—namely, preoperative determination of the proper site for the stoma. Because patients are commonly admitted the day of surgery in the United States, preoperative counseling and stomal location often are relegated to a secondary role because of other, important concerns, such as anesthetic clearance, operative consent, site verification, confirmation of the presence of a myriad of legal and medical paperwork on the chart—the list seems endless. This is why every effort should be made to accomplish this task at a time when one is not attempting to respond to the demands and concerns that are inherent to the preoperative preparation process.

LAPAROSCOPIC-ASSISTED STOMAL CREATION

One of the primary indications for minimally invasive surgery, that is, laparoscopic intestinal surgery, is the creation and closure of intestinal stomas (see Chapter 27). A number of papers have been published that attest to the fact that this approach is well tolerated and can be performed safely and effectively.[72,97,105,135,182,210,214] Obvious advantages include the avoidance of a laparotomy while still maintaining the ability to precisely identify and orient the pertinent bowel segment. The technical approach to performing this technique is discussed in Chapter 27.

COLONOSCOPIC-ASSISTED STOMAL CREATION

Another minimally invasive approach to the creation of a colostomy is to insert a colonoscope in order to identify the site in the colon that could permit by means of transillumination the appropriate site for creating the stoma.[137,156] Of course, one may still do the entire stomal construction through the same opening from which the subsequent colostomy or ileostomy will be created, especially in someone with a favorable body habit.

PERCUTANEOUS ENDOSCOPIC COLOSTOMY

A modification of colonoscopic-assisted colostomy or cecostomy is analogous to that of percutaneous gastrostomy, that of percutaneous endoscopic colostomy. A colonoscope is passed, and a percutaneous colostomy tube is inserted into the bowel lumen. One must be concerned about the risk of fecal contamination or rupture of the thin colon wall, a potentially catastrophic consequence when there is no ready means available to limit the amount of spillage. Furthermore, with this minimally invasive alternative, the fecal stream is not diverted; therefore, this application is very limited. Heriot and colleagues employed this approach as an alternative to a conventional colostomy in a single patient with obstructed defecation.[99] It has also been used for the management of sigmoid volvulus[54] and for colonic pseudo-obstruction.[31,168]

SIGMOID COLOSTOMY

The most common indication for performing a *permanent* sigmoid colostomy is carcinoma of the rectum. Other possible indications for either a permanent or a temporary stoma include diverticulitis, Crohn's disease, congenital anomalies, anal incontinence, and colorectal trauma. Certainly, the most common reason for performing a sigmoid colostomy today is the Hartmann procedure for sigmoid diverticulitis, although the stoma is generally intended to be temporary.

The historical aspects of the evolution of colostomy are discussed in Chapters 22 and 23. See also comprehensive reviews on the subject by Cromar,[52] Dinnick,[55] and McGarity.[140] The technique for creating a satisfactory end sigmoid colostomy has been described previously as it pertains to the abdominoperineal resection for carcinoma of the rectum (see Figs. 23-24 through 23-29). As

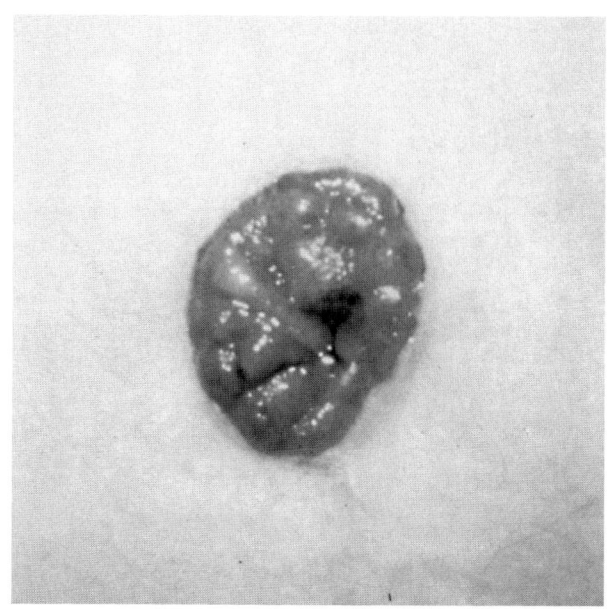

FIGURE 31-1. Normal-appearing end-sigmoid colostomy.

has been repeatedly emphasized, it is important that the colon be brought through the split rectus muscle and sutured to the skin without tension. Ideally, redundant colon should be excised in order to permit a satisfactory irrigation should the patient so elect. Some surgeons perform a paramedian incision and then must create the stoma either in a pararectus location or bring the colostomy through the wound. Neither of these methods is in my opinion acceptable. A pararectus colostomy predisposes to peristomal hernia (see later).

A "flush" colostomy can be performed with reasonable safety because the colostomy effluent is non-corrosive, but this technique is not advised. With the patient's possible weight gain, the stoma tends to retract. This makes appliance management more difficult. Hence, the stoma should be permitted to pout slightly, but not to the extent of a conventional ileostomy (Figure 31-1).

When the colostomy has been created, a transparent drainable bag is placed before the patient leaves the operating room (see Figure 32-5). This permits visualization of the stoma during the immediate postoperative period, and the viability of the bowel can be determined on a continual basis. Usually, when the colostomy begins to function (after 2 or 3 days), the bag is removed and the stoma and skin are carefully inspected.

Complications

The principles of proper stomal construction have already been outlined. The bowel must be drawn through the abdominal wall without tension; it must be brought

through the split rectus muscle; it must be sutured primarily to the skin; and the viability of the end of the colon must be clearly demonstrated.[229] Although no method guarantees that subsequent complications will be avoided, attention to the above principles will minimize the risks. But the fact of the matter is that most colostomy complications are preventable.

Ischemia and Stomal Necrosis

Ischemia and stomal necrosis are obviously due to inadequate blood supply. This is more likely to develop if the ascending branch of the left colic artery is not preserved, a consequence of high ligation of the inferior mesenteric artery (on the aorta). Another possible source for compromise of the blood supply occurs if the meandering artery of Drummond has been divided or if collateral circulation from the middle colic vessels is inadequate.

Recognition of stomal ischemia should not be difficult. If the mucosa looks blue, it probably is ischemic. Occasionally, after a difficult abdominoperineal resection, one may be less compulsive in creating the colostomy or perhaps somewhat less concerned about the possible nonviability of the stoma. It is better to reopen the abdomen to free a further length in order to effect a satisfactory stoma at the time of the resection than to have to return the patient to the operating room several days or weeks later. The philosophy expressed by the statement, "It looks a bit dark, but it will probably be all right," is delusional. If the stoma is nonviable, the bowel may retract into the peritoneal cavity. Peritonitis can ensue and necessitate emergency surgical intervention. Less critical, but almost as unpleasant a consequence, is the situation illustrated in Figure 31-2. The sigmoid colostomy has retracted and the stool presents in the lower portion of the abdominal incision, tracking subcutaneously from the original opening in the rectus fascia. In a less ominous consequence, the stoma may separate from the skin at the area of nonviability, with a resultant stricture (Figure 31-3).

Management

If the patient cannot cope with the retraction or stenosis, revision is required. Dilatation alone of a skin-level stenosis is not recommended. The trauma from manipulation may cause hemorrhage and further inflammatory reaction, and may actually worsen the condition.

A formal laparotomy with colostomy resection and the creation of a new stoma are necessary if adequate length cannot be established by a limited approach. However, an attempt should be made to circumcise the colostomy, to free up the bowel, and to re-suture it (Figure 31-4).

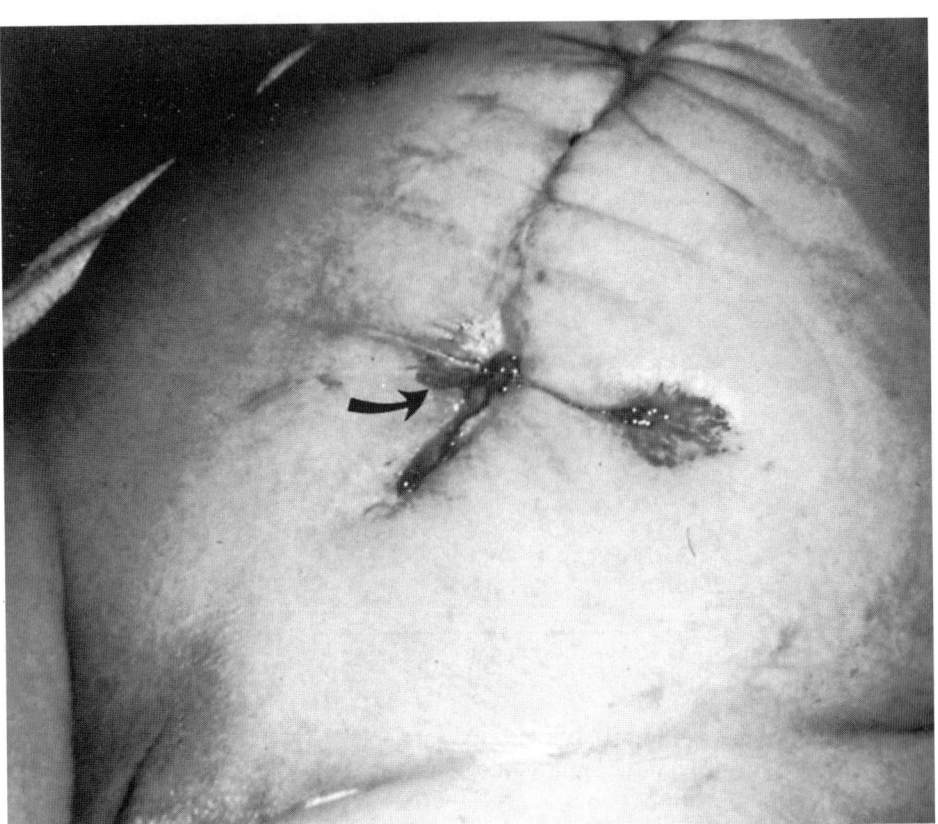

FIGURE 31-2. Sigmoid colostomy. Retraction with feces draining entirely from the abdominal wound (*arrow*).

Rarely, the stenosis occurs at the fascial level. This is usually due to an inadequate opening in the fascia itself or to vascular compromise. Treatment will require mobilization of the bowel, enlargement of the opening in the fascia, and re-suturing of the colon.

Results

Only a limited number of recent papers are available. Allen-Mersh and Thomson reviewed their experience with the surgical treatment of colostomy complications, identifying 65 patients who underwent revision due to stenosis.[9] This represented 53% of the operative stomal problems. Local excision of the scar tissue at the mucocutaneous junction was associated with a 61% success rate for relief of the stenosis.

Paracolostomy Abscess and Perforation

Paracolostomy abscess is an unusual postoperative complication. It should be a particularly unlikely event if the stoma is placed outside of the abdominal incision. The problem is more likely to be seen after an ileostomy when sutures may be placed too deeply and penetrate the bowel lumen at the time of eversion. Another possible cause of a parastomal abscess in a patient who has undergone an ileostomy is recurrent Crohn's disease.

If the colostomy retracts and there is fecal contamination in the subcutaneous tissue, an abscess can result. However, by far the most common reason for paracolostomy abscess is the application of an improper irrigation technique (see Chapter 32). Either the irrigating fluid or the device used for insertion into the stoma perforates the bowel.

Symptoms include an unrewarding irrigation, which is often associated with immediate abdominal pain.[108] Obvious sepsis may supervene with evidence of cellulitis of the abdominal wall. If the process dissects into the peritoneal cavity or had started within the abdomen, it can lead to generalized peritonitis. Predisposing factors for the development of this complication include the presence of a pericolostomy hernia, alcoholism, psychological disturbance (e.g., self-mutilation), and, of course, carelessness. A case of burn and stricture of the ostomy has been reported due to the accidental insertion of boiling water for irrigation.[80]

Management

Treatment usually requires laparotomy and relocation of the colostomy, but Reynolds and colleagues reported satisfactory management by means of adequate surgical drainage and intravenous hyperalimentation or an elemental diet.[178] No proximal diversion was undertaken. However, in my experience with this complication, usu-

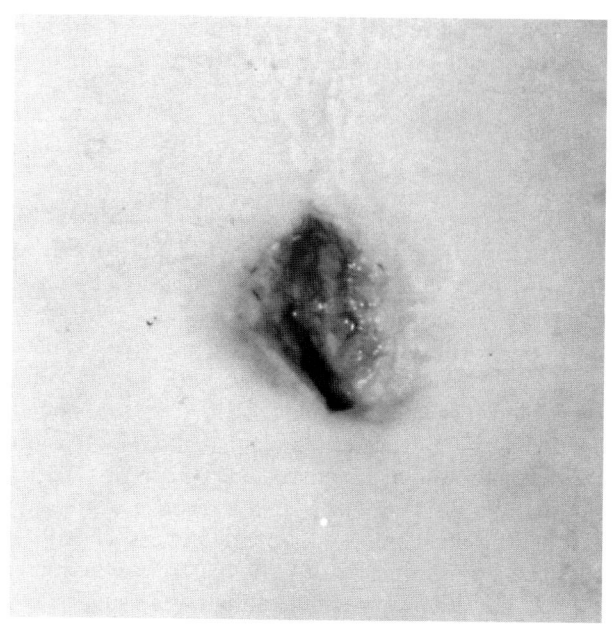

FIGURE 31-3. Retracted sigmoid colostomy. Only granulation tissue evident.

ally in patients who develop a bowel perforation secondary to irrigation, this is a major septic problem requiring an urgent operation and extensive debridement, drainage, stomal relocation, and, in some situations, a proximal colostomy or ileostomy. Gomez and Rosenthal recommended a semi-synthetic biologic dressing (Bio-

brane) as a skin substitute when colostomy perforation caused massive abdominal wall tissue loss.[87]

Results

Isa and Quan reviewed the Memorial Sloan-Kettering experience with colostomy perforation.[108] This was observed ten times in a 10-year period ending in 1975. In nine cases, the cause of the perforation was irrigation of the colostomy, and in one instance a barium enema examination. Barium enema perforation can usually be avoided by the use of a cone tip (see Figure 4-21B) or other device.[194] As previously discussed, the use of a balloon catheter should be vigorously condemned.

Hemorrhage

Colostomy hemorrhage is extremely unusual in the immediate postoperative period. However, in the event of underlying portal hypertension from cirrhosis secondary to alcohol ingestion or sclerosing cholangitis, the mucosa of the exposed bowel is predisposed to the possibility of considerable bleeding (Figure 31-5). This rare complication is more commonly seen in someone with an ileostomy, usually because of the association between inflammatory bowel disease (IBD) and sclerosing cholangitis (see Figure 31-64 below). Roberts and colleagues identified 12 patients from the Lahey Clinic who had bleeding from stomal varices; all but one had ulcerative colitis.[180]

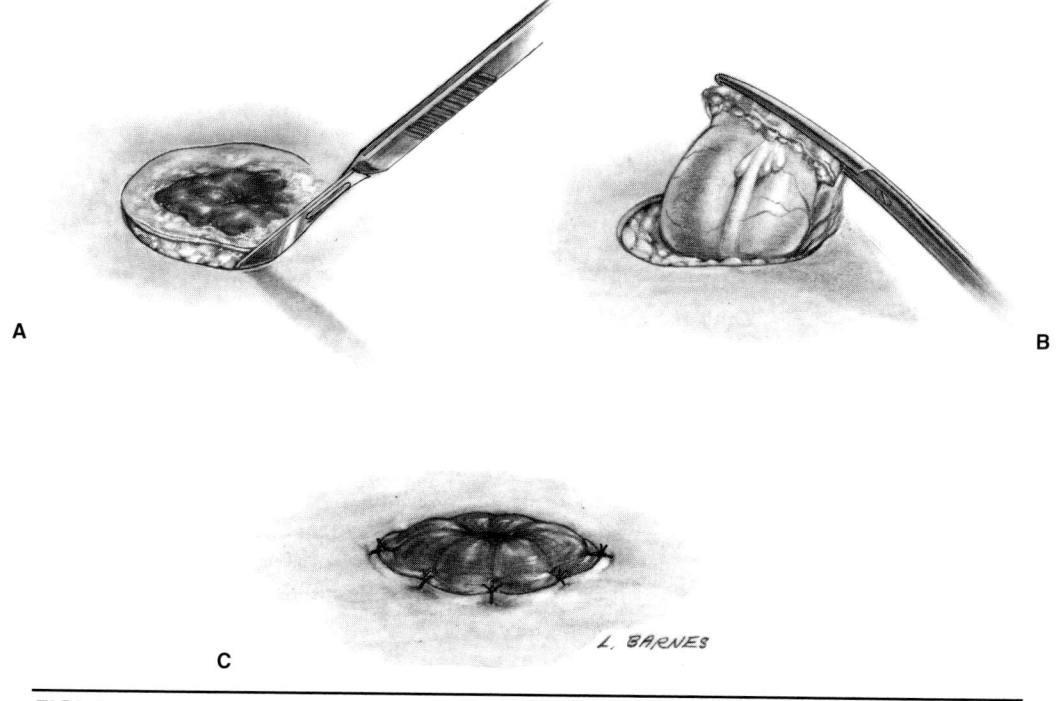

A

B

L. BARNES

C

FIGURE 31-4. Revision of retracted or stenotic colostomy. **(A)** Skin is incised. **(B)** Bowel is mobilized. **(C)** New stoma is matured.

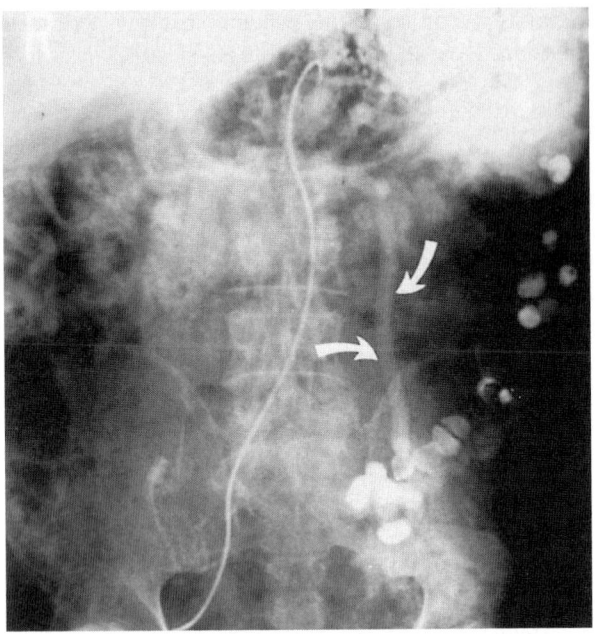

FIGURE 31-5. Hemorrhage from colostomy in patient with portal hypertension. Angiogram demonstrates delayed emptying of inferior mesenteric vein (*arrows*).

The bleeding originates from enterostomal varices located at the level of the mucocutaneous junction, a consequence of communication with the high-pressure venous network of the superior and inferior mesenteric veins.[46,180] Erosion of the varix or trauma can exacerbate the hemorrhage.

Handschin and co-workers (Zurich, Switzerland) reported a man with portal hypertension and recurrent bleeding from varices in a sigmoid colon stoma.[94] They localized the bleeding source through contrast-enhanced three-dimensional magnetic resonance angiography. The bleeding was subsequently controlled by means of the implantation of a transjugular intrahepatic shunt.

Treatment

Direct pressure is usually the initial approach. Other alternatives, such as suture ligation of the bleeding areas, beta blockade, and injection sclerotherapy (by means of polidocanol, phenol [5%] in almond oil, or tetradecyl sulfate) have all been tried with varying degrees of success.[65,100,152] Goldstein and colleagues concluded in their review that control of major stomal hemorrhage by local measures is often ineffective and that portasystemic shunting may be required.[85]

Beck and colleagues performed mucocutaneous disconnections in 9 of their 11 patients who failed with one or more of the lesser options.[19] The dissection is carried down to the level of the fascia, and the varix is divided and ligated. With a follow-up of up to 4.6 years, two indi-

viduals required re-operation for hemorrhage. The alternative approach employed by this group was stomal relocation (two patients, one failure).

Prolapse

Colostomy prolapse is an uncommon complication following abdominoperineal resection. Chandler and Evans identified only two patients of 217 who underwent the procedure (less than 1%).[41] The problem occurs much more frequently in those who have undergone a loop colostomy (see later) than in those with an end stoma. The etiology of the problem may be an oversized opening in the abdominal wall, a redundant sigmoid loop leading to the stoma, sudden increased abdominal pressure (e.g., straining or coughing), or a rigid appliance worn with a tight belt.[125] The condition is frequently associated with a pericolostomy hernia. Adequate fixation of the mesentery and bowel to the peritoneum has been suggested as a means for preventing this complication, but I do not agree with this view. In my experience, those who develop end-sigmoid colostomy "prolapse" usually have a stoma that was initially created too long (Figure 31-6). This technical error, in combination with several other predisposing factors, such as the presence of a redundant loop of sigmoid colon, an asthenic patient, or an individual with chronic obstructive lung disease, tends to create the problem.

Treatment

In the absence of an associated hernia, treatment of a prolapse usually does not require a laparotomy. If the prolapse occurs relatively soon after it has been constructed, the colostomy is circumcised at the mucocutaneous junction and the bowel liberated, resected, and resutured (Figure 31-7). If the prolapse occurs several months after the initial operation, the incision should be made *into the mucosa* rather than into the skin (Figure 31-8A). The blood supply from the adjacent skin will be sufficient to maintain viability of the stoma, and an anastomosis is actually effected between the distal colon and the residual mucosa (Figure 31-8C). This technical detail is an important concept to remember, because if the skin is incised too large an opening will be created when the stoma is subsequently matured (Figure 31-8D). It is important to liberate as much intra-abdominal colon as possible and to resect it in order to avoid recurrent prolapse. With a particularly mobile colon, one may actually create an end transverse colostomy in the left iliac fossa.

Abulafi and colleagues offer a unique approach to the management of colostomy prolapse, a modification of the Delorme procedure (see Chapter 17).[5] The submucosa is infiltrated with a dilute adrenaline solution, and a mucosal incision is made 10 to 15 mm from the mucocu-

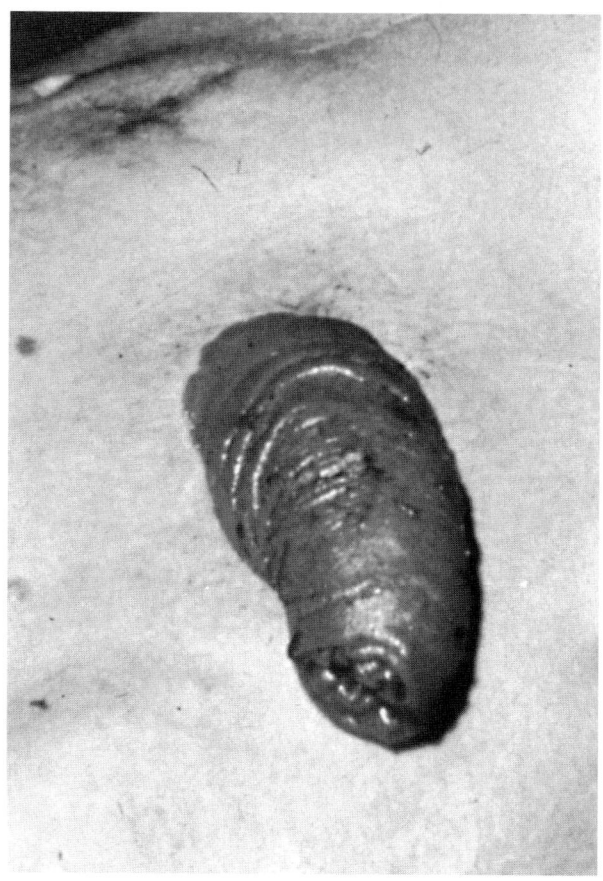

FIGURE 31-6. This sigmoid colostomy prolapse developed 1 month following operation after a bout of coughing. At the time of the initial procedure, considerable redundant sigmoid colon had been permitted to remain.

taneous junction (Figure 31-9*A*). Following separation of the mucosa for the full length of the prolapse, six to eight plicating sutures are placed in the muscular wall from the mucocutaneous junction to the apex (Figure 31-9*B,C*). The redundant mucosa is excised and the mucosa resutured (Figure 31-9*D*).

Acute stomal prolapse is uncommon and requires immediate attention to reduce it. This is usually accomplished by gentle pressure such as has been described in the chapter on rectal prolapse (see Chapter 17). As with osmotic therapy through the use of sugar applied to the prolapse, the same treatment has been demonstrated to be effective for acute, irreducible stomal prolapse.[68]

Rarely, sigmoid colostomy prolapse may produce compromise of the blood supply to the bowel and gangrene of the stoma (Figure 31-10). Depending on the level of involvement, resection of the necrotic bowel may be accomplished without a laparotomy, or alternatively an intra-abdominal procedure may be required. If a prolapse is associated with a pericolostomy hernia, relocation of the stoma may be necessary (see the following).

Results

The previously mentioned report of Allen-Mersh and Thomson identified 16 individuals who underwent surgery for colostomy prolapse.[9] This represented 13% of the stomal complications requiring operation. Local fixation procedures failed to prevent recurrent prolapse in two-thirds.

Peristomal Hernia

Peristomal hernia is the most common late complication of abdominoperineal resection. As mentioned earlier, the usual reason for this difficulty is the placement of the stoma in a pararectus location. Sjödahl and colleagues studied the location of the stoma in relation to the rectus abdominis muscle, noting that the prevalence of parastomal hernia was 2.8% in those brought through the muscle and 21.6% in those placed laterally, a highly significant difference.[203] Other possible causes of peristomal hernia include locating the stoma in the incision itself and the creation of too large an opening in the abdominal wall (Figs. 31-11 through 31-13). Some surgeons are sufficiently nihilistic that they believe this complication is inevitable if the patient survives long enough—a theory impossible to dispute. Certainly, weight gain, the effects of the aging process, other systemic diseases, nutritional problems, and many other factors may predispose to the development of this problem. Because of this concern, Bayer and colleagues and Light insert a mesh on a prophylactic basis to "strengthen the colostomy outlet" at the time of stomal construction.[18,133]

The St. Mark's Hospital group studied the long-term complication rate of end-sigmoid colostomy, and found that the crude and actuarially corrected risks of pericolostomy complications in 203 patients at 13 years were 51.2% and 58.1%, respectively.[134] They concluded that siting the stoma through the rectus muscle did not reduce the risk of hernia. However, an extraperitoneal course was associated with a significantly lower risk of herniation when compared with a transperitoneal course. The authors opined that peristomal hernia is technically avoidable.[134]

Treatment

The choices of operative approaches to the repair of a peristomal hernia are usually dictated by its size. Relatively small defects can be repaired by direct suture, circumcising the colostomy, repairing the abdominal wall, and re-maturing the stoma (Figure 31-14). This technique, suggested by Thorlakson,[224] should be employed only if the colostomy has been created in the proper location, that is, through the split rectus muscle, and is a small defect. If a small hernia is present in conjunction

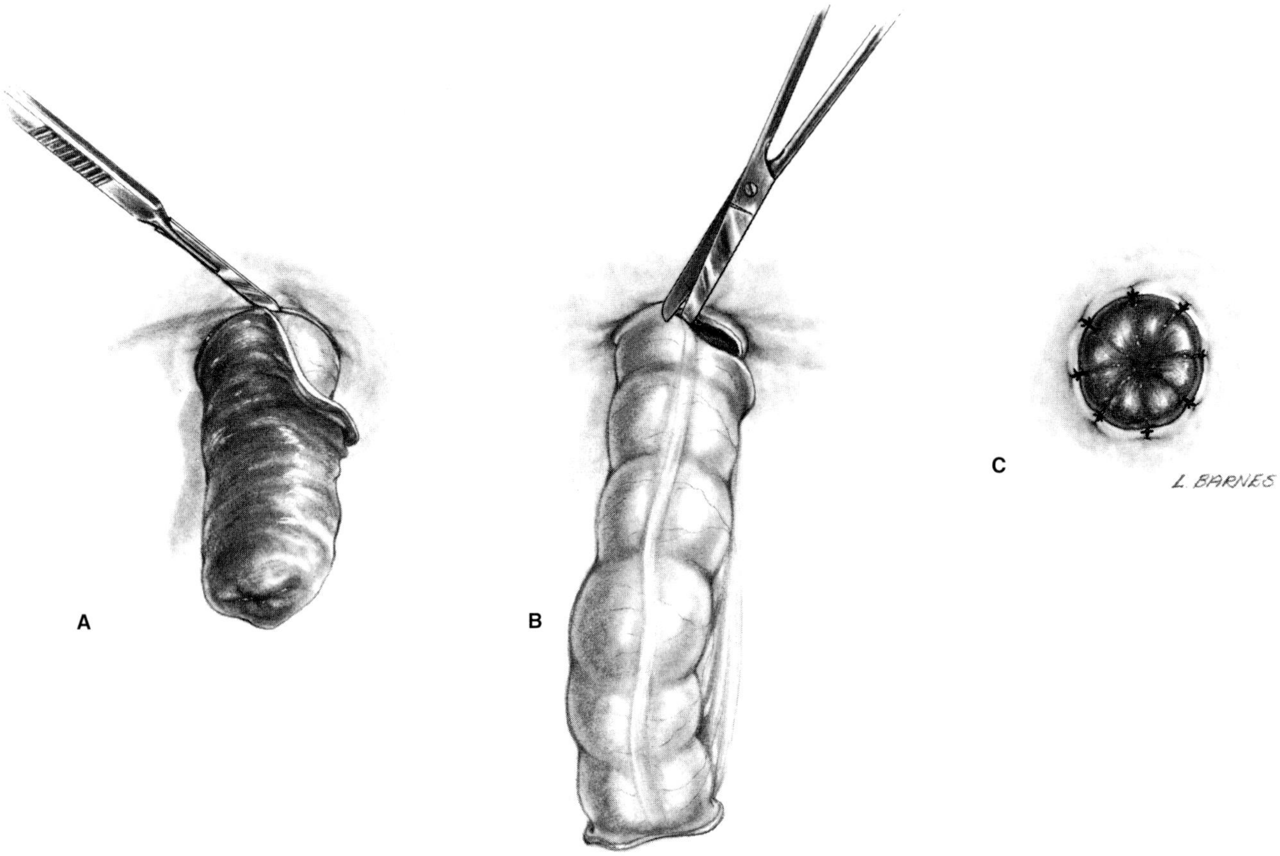

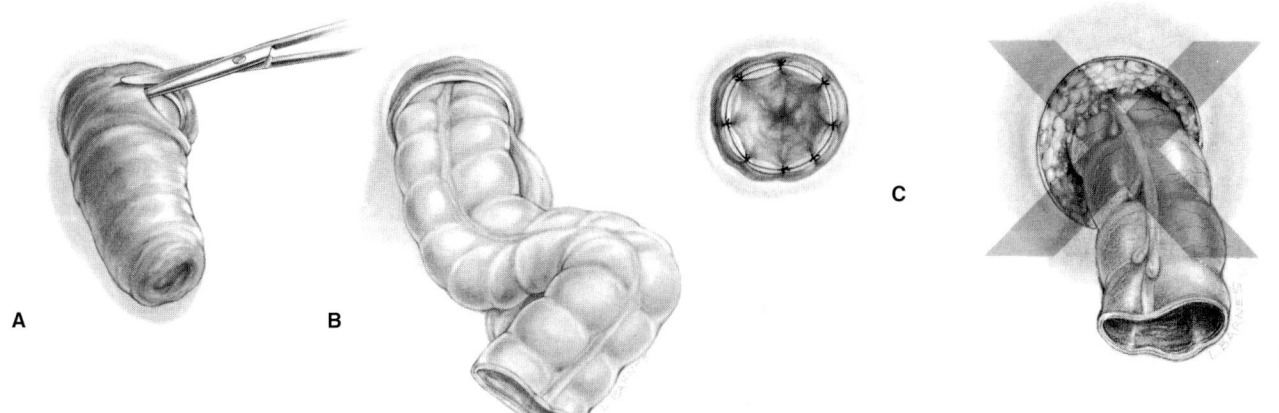

FIGURE 31-7. Revision of sigmoid colostomy prolapse that took place relatively soon after surgery. **(A)** Incision at the mucocutaneous junction. **(B)** Delivery and resection of redundant bowel. **(C)** Colostomy matured in the usual manner.

FIGURE 31-8. Revision of prolapsed sigmoid colostomy (after several months). **(A)** Incision into mucosa itself rather than at mucocutaneous junction. **(B)** The redundant bowel is exteriorized and resected. **(C)** Final maturation is obtained by mucosa-to-mucosa suturing. **(D)** Incorrect incision in the skin creates a too-large opening.

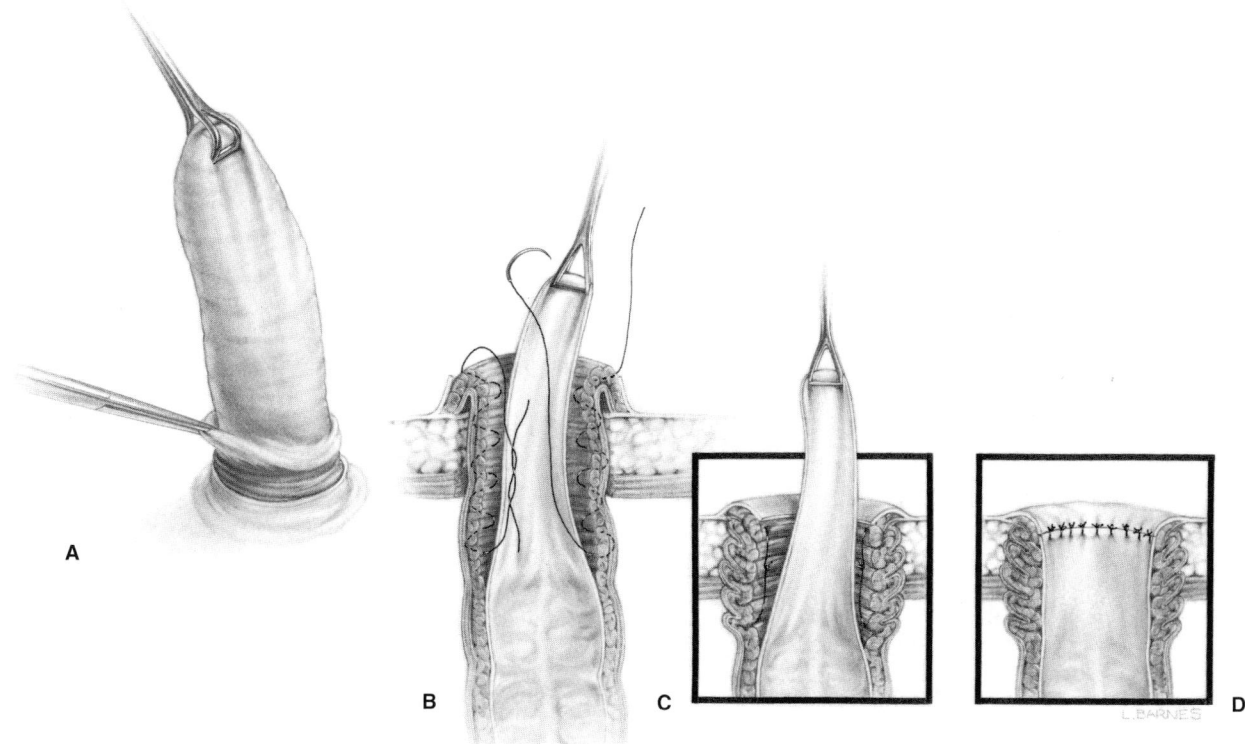

FIGURE 31-9. Repair of colostomy prolapse by Delorme modification. **(A)** Incision into the mucosa is made proximal to the mucocutaneous junction. **(B)** Plicating sutures of an absorbable material are taken in the muscularis from the apex of the prolapse to the most distal point. **(C)** The sutures are then tied and the redundant mucosa excised. **(D)** Mucosa-to-mucosa apposition takes place with interrupted, simple, absorbable sutures.

with an improperly located stoma, the colostomy should probably be relocated. Such relocation can usually be accomplished by an intraperitoneal tunnel method, closing the defect at the original site by primary suture (Figure 31-15). If the rectus location is still available, this is the optimal site. If this is not considered appropriate, one has essentially two recourses: to use the opposite side of the abdomen or to place the stoma at the umbilicus.

The use of the umbilical site is not a unique concept. Some surgeons prefer to create the colostomy in the umbilicus initially. Raza and colleagues evaluated 101 patients in whom they performed such a stoma.[176] They strongly supported the concept of this location because of their low incidence of complications: only four patients required re-operation. There were no peristomal hernias and no prolapses in their experience. If an umbilical colostomy is created, the technique of construction is essentially the same, but it is important to remove all of the skin that tends to turn inward. Turnbull (see Biography) commented that this is why the Almighty created the umbilicus—namely, as a back-up resource for the placement of a stoma.

It is always better to use the patient's own tissue for repair if one can achieve a successful result, but reconstruction of larger or massive hernias usually requires insertion of a synthetic material, such as Marlex mesh or Gore-Tex.[2,35,115,151,175,187,212,219] In the repair of the hernia, some surgeons prefer to maintain the stoma at the original location, using the mesh around the colostomy. Others bring the bowel through the middle of the material (Figure 31-16). I had always preferred to use Marlex mesh to effect the repair if foreign material was required, relocating the stoma elsewhere (Figure 31-17). While there is always the concern about the possibility of sepsis if prosthetic material is placed in a contaminated field, this is rarely a concern. Now I use Sepramesh, since this material minimizes the risk of adhesion formation.

A number of modifications for the placement of mesh have been offered. Tekkis and colleagues use a Thorlakson method at the site of the stoma, incorporating an incomplete circumferential mesh.[219] Sugarbaker suggests a peritoneal approach to insertion, avoiding contamination by securing the exiting bowel lateral to the prosthesis.[213] Despite the author's success with six patients, I believe that

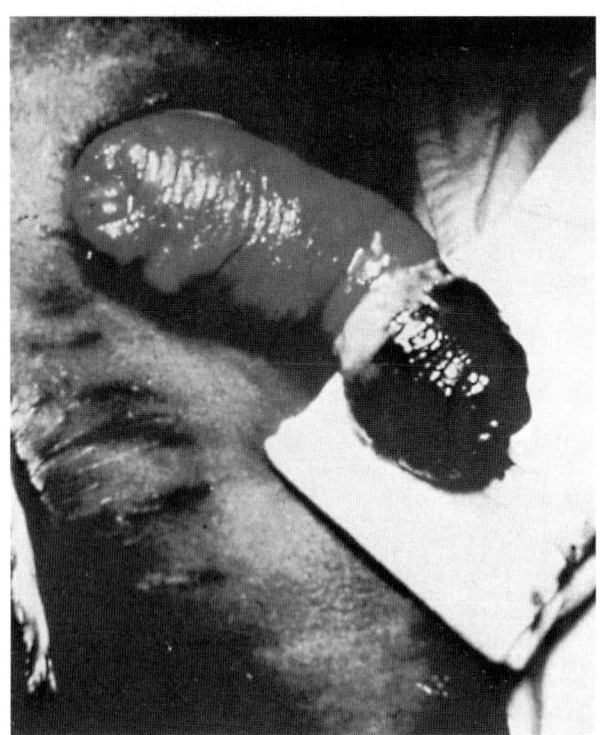

FIGURE 31-10. Gangrene at the end of a prolapsed colostomy. Obviously, a resection is mandated.

the advantage of direct visualization and secure repair far outweigh the theoretical potential benefit of this alternative. In recent years, there has been an interest in effecting repair by means of a laparoscopic technique.[25,170,236] LeBlanc and Bellanger recommend the PTFE patch method (DualMesh Plus prosthesis) as an intraperitoneal covering of the hernial defect.[131]

Moisidis and co-workers simulated the "stresses" imposed on the Marlex mesh and found that the hole tends to enlarge and to become distorted.[151] They suggest that the cut margins should be reinforced with a polypropylene pursestring suture in order to stabilize the opening. Hofstetter and co-workers (University of Southern California) describe a technique using PTFE mesh in 13 patients, wherein the stoma is fully mobilized, but the mucocutaneous anastomosis is not disrupted.[104] The abdominal wall repair is reinforced with a 10-cm × 12-cm sheet, with the mesh incised and wrapped around the bowel. The hole that is created in the mesh is described as having an eight-pointed, star-shaped configuration.

Results

Allen-Mersh and Thomson identified 42 individuals who underwent repair of paracolostomy hernia, an incidence of 34% of all operative stomal complications.[9] Local repair failed in 47%, but re-siting the stoma to the umbilicus or to right side of the abdomen was more successful (57%). Re-siting to the same (left) side was associated with a failure rate of 86%.

Alexandre and Bouillot utilized a Dacron prosthesis in ten patients with pericolostomy hernia.[8] There were no

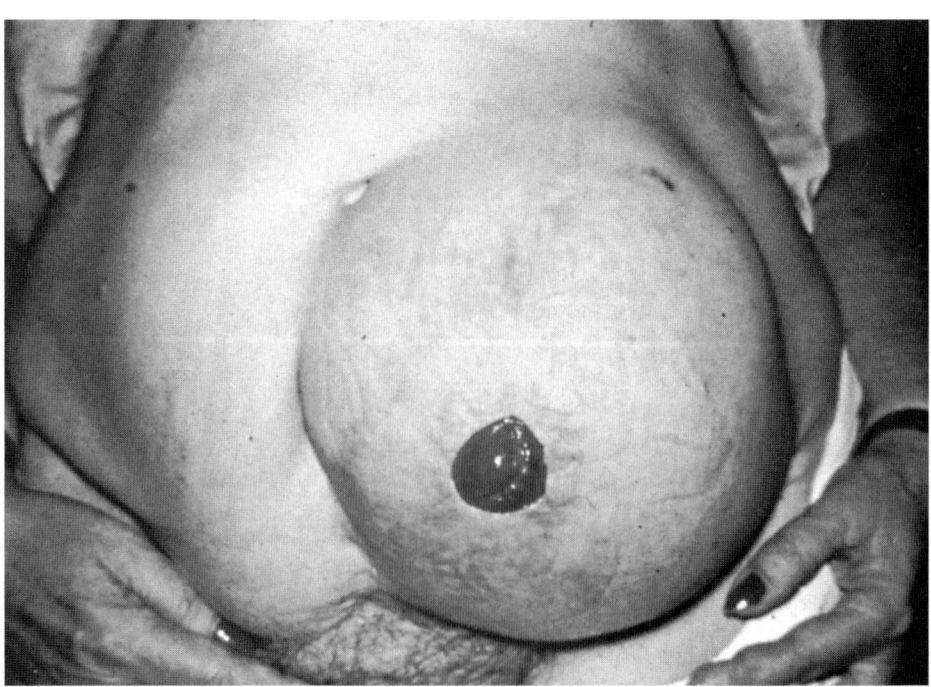

FIGURE 31-11. Massive pericolostomy hernia. Note that the stoma has been brought through the left paramedian incision.

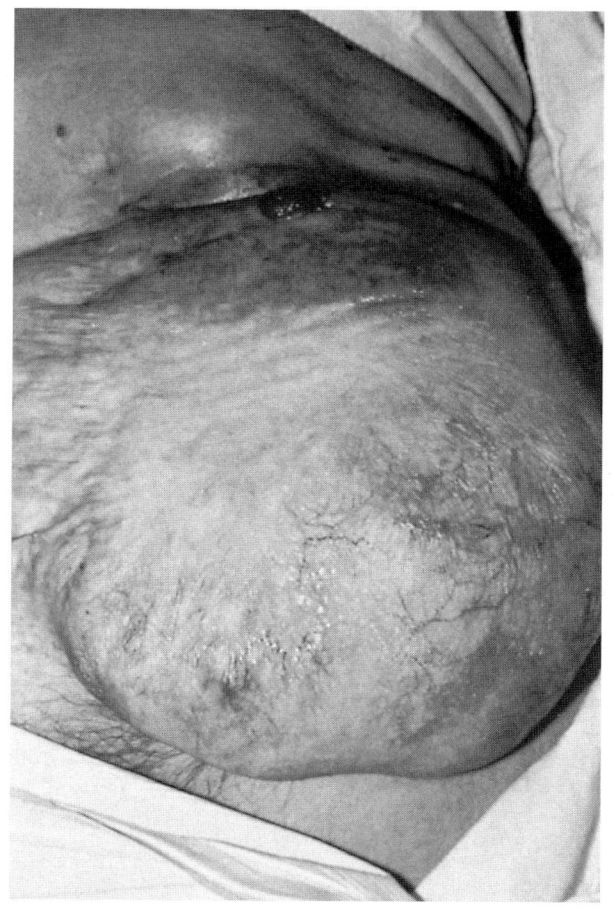

FIGURE 31-12. Pericolostomy hernia. Atrophic skin is the only covering of the abdominal cavity. The stoma is at the proximal aspect of the defect.

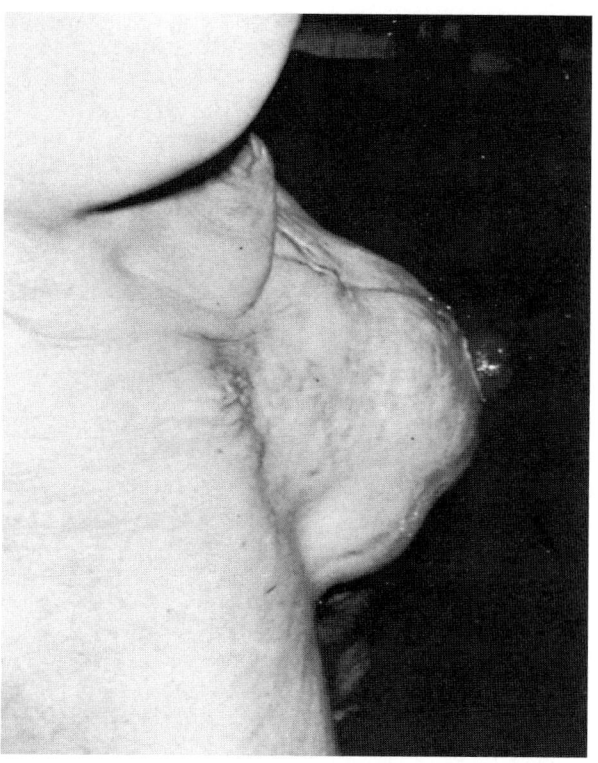

FIGURE 31-13. Typical pericolostomy hernia with the stoma at the center of the defect.

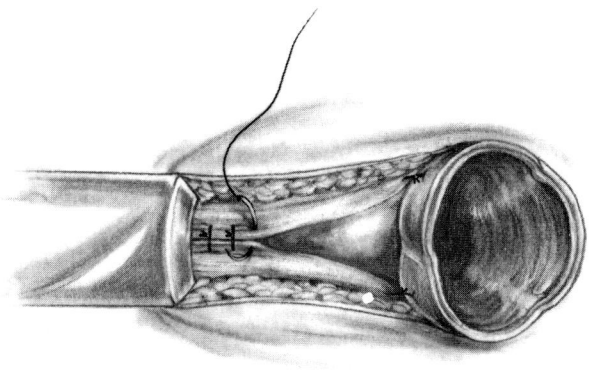
A

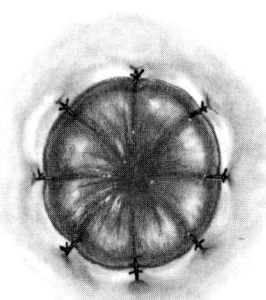
L. BARNES B

FIGURE 31-14. Pericolostomy hernia repair for a small defect at the correctly located site. **(A)** Direct repair with fascial closure (note serosa to fascia sutures). **(B)** Mucocutaneous sutures are placed in the usual way.

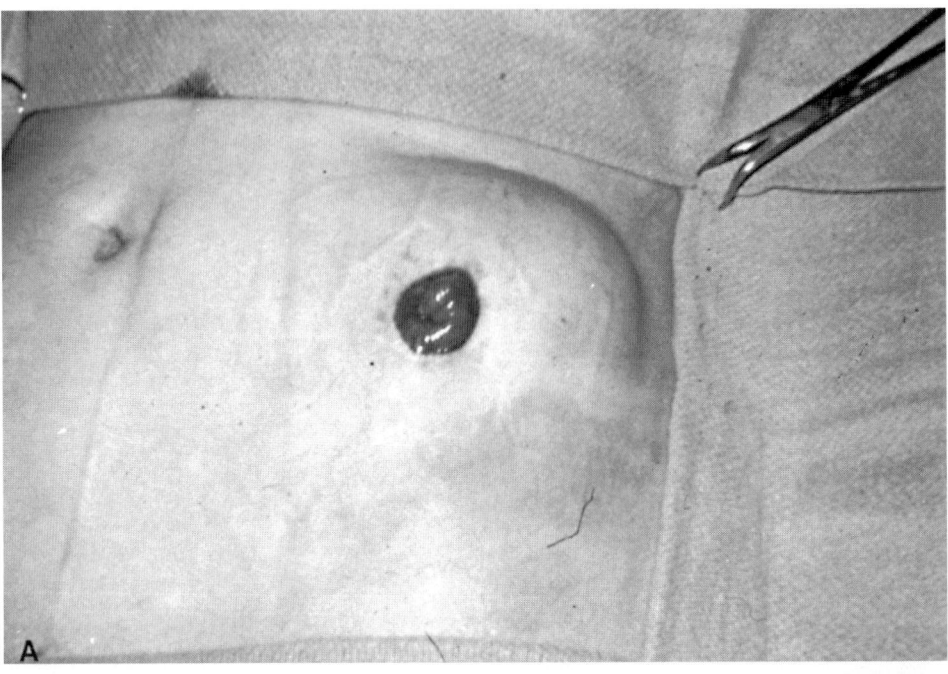

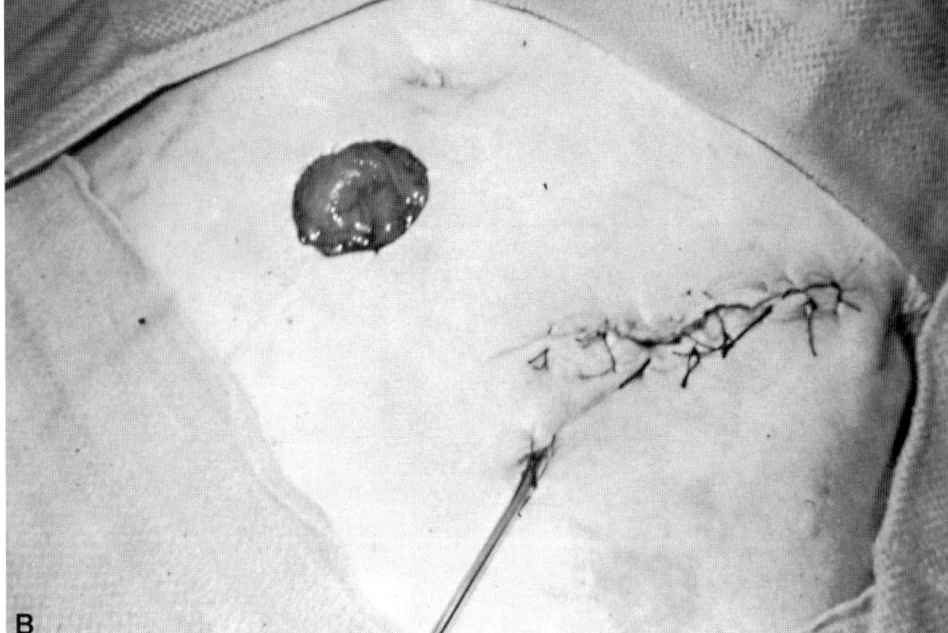

FIGURE 31-15. Pericolostomy hernia repair for small defects in the pararectus location. **(A)** The stoma has been relocated after intraperitoneal tunneling and the defect repaired. **(B)** The wound probably should be closed secondarily, not by the primary closure and drainage method, which is shown.

infections and no mortality, but there was one recurrence. In a retrospective review by Rubin and colleagues involving 80 patients who underwent peristomal hernia repairs, the investigators concluded that stomal relocation is superior to direct fascial repair.[189] Furthermore, for those that recur, they found that the use of prosthetic material is the most successful method for effecting cure. Cheung and associates (Hong Kong) retrospectively reviewed their 43 patients who underwent repair of peristomal hernia.[42] The overall recurrence rate was 40%. Stelzner and co-workers (Dresden, Germany) reviewed 20

patients who underwent PTFE repair for large stomal hernias.[209] There were no infections and three recurrences (mean follow-up, 3.5 years). In a literature review on the use of mesh repairs for parastomal hernias, Tekkis and colleagues were able to identify 72 cases.[219] The overall failure rate due to recurrence or mesh-related sepsis was 8.3%. Carne and co-workers conducted a search using the Medline database and concluded that no technical factors related to construction have been shown to prevent herniation.[37] However, Jänes and colleagues
(text continues on page 1552)

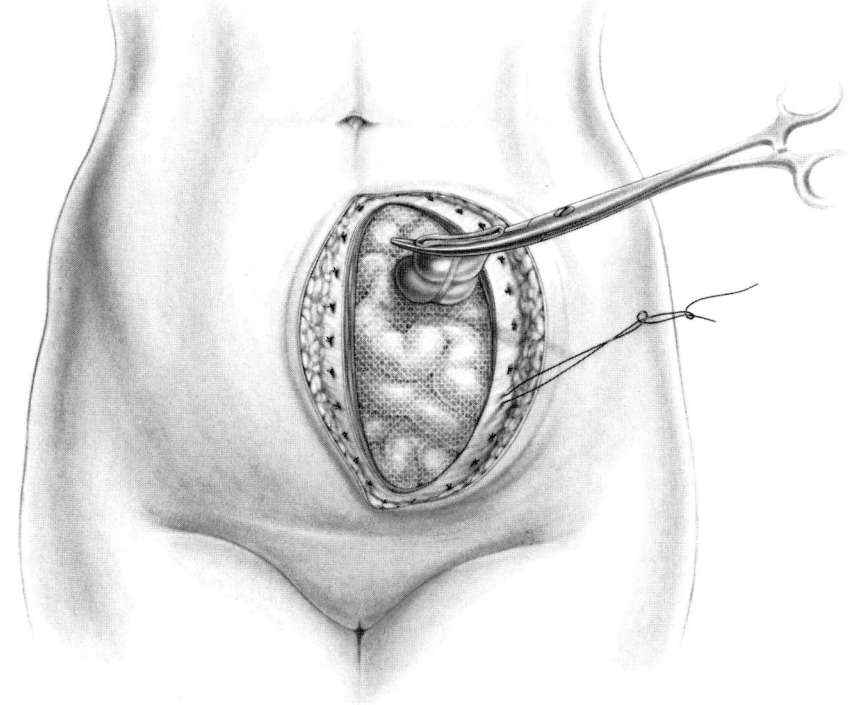

A

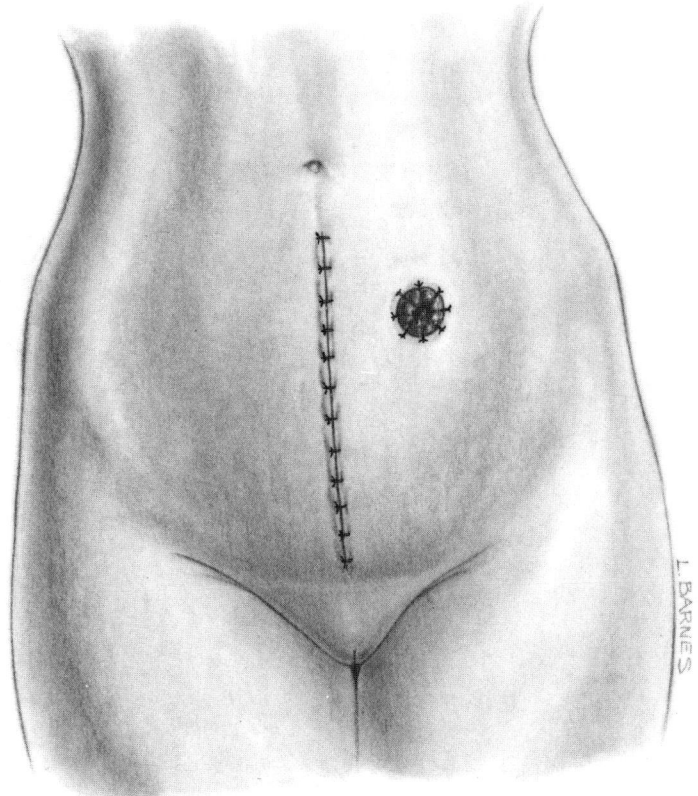

B

FIGURE 31-16. Repair of large parastomal hernial defect with Marlex mesh, without relocating stoma. **(A)** The stoma is brought through the mesh, and the mesh anchored to the fascia with monofilament nonabsorbable sutures by an interrupted mattress technique placed through the abdominal wall muscle and fascia. **(B)** Stoma is matured at the original location.

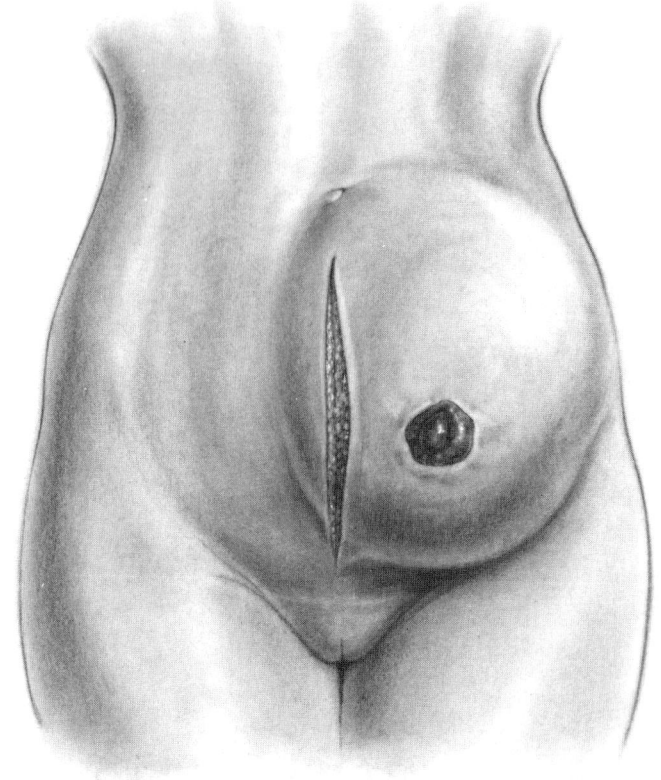

A

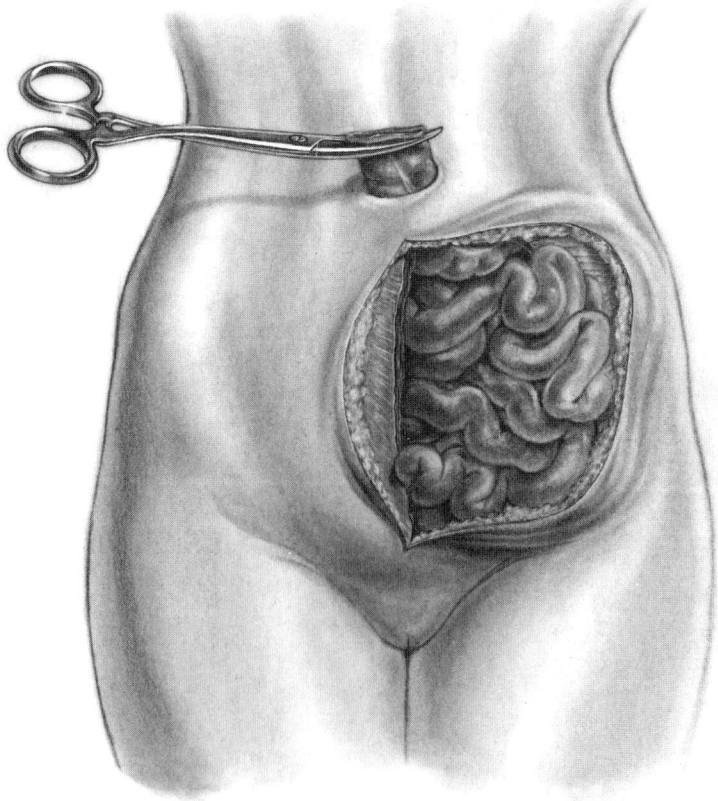

FIGURE 31-17. Repair of large parastomal hernial defect with Marlex mesh, transplanting stoma. **(A)** Incision. **(B)** Relocation of stoma to the umbilicus. **(C)** Placement of Marlex mesh, anchoring it to the undersurface of the abdominal wall with interrupted, monofilament, nonabsorbable sutures. **(D)** Wound closure and maturation of stoma. *(continued)*

B

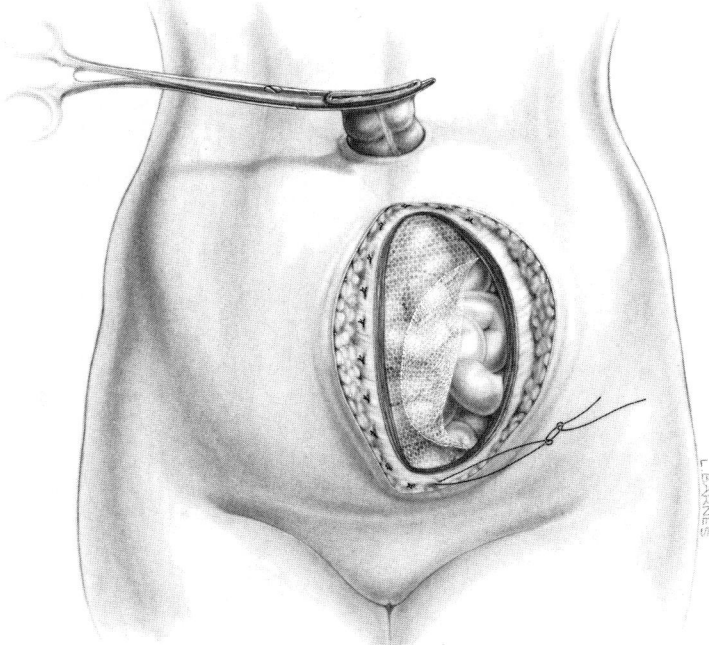

C

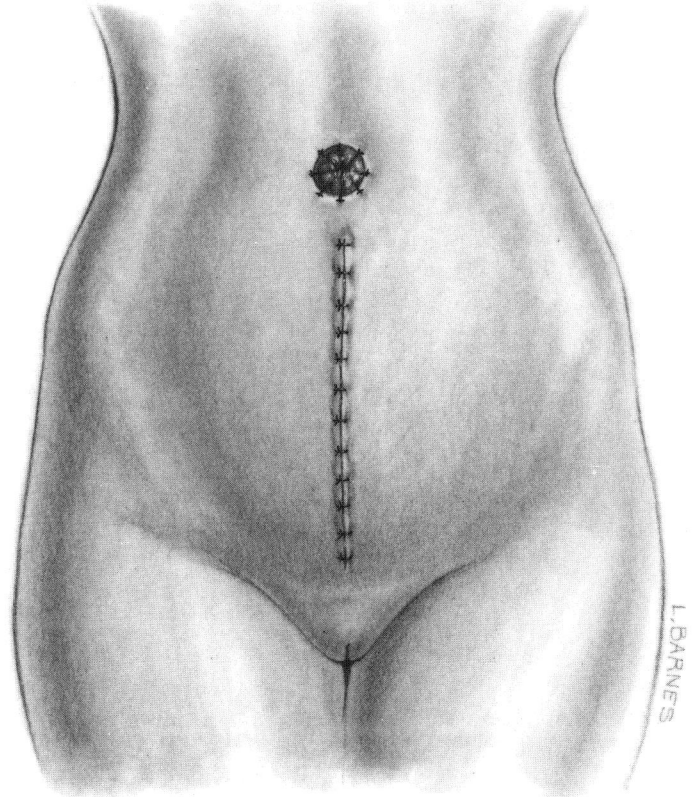

D

FIGURE 31-17. *(continued)*

undertook a prospective clinical trial in which 54 individuals undergoing permanent colostomy were randomized to have a conventional stoma or a mesh placed in a sublay position.[109] No infection or fistula was observed. At the 12-month follow-up, peristomal hernia was present in 8 of 18 without a mesh and none of 16 patients in whom the mesh was used.[109]

Unfortunately, many of colostomy patients are elderly or represent a high risk for a major abdominal operation, and relocation and mesh implant indeed comprise a major procedure. There may be no recourse for some except to use some form of abdominal support. Fortunately, most individuals are relatively asymptomatic[164]; hence, operative intervention is not necessarily a requisite.

Recurrent Disease

Recurrence of the primary condition may develop at the site of the stoma. This is usually seen in patients who have undergone abdominoperineal resection or a diversionary colostomy for IBD (ulcerative colitis or Crohn's disease). The mucosa appears edematous and friable, bleeds easily, and may be granular or ulcerated. Medical management of the underlying disease process may resolve the inflammation and ameliorate the patient's complaints. However, because of diarrhea and the inability to maintain an appliance satisfactorily, a more extensive bowel resection and possible ileostomy may be required (see Ileostomy Complications).

Recurrent malignancy may occur at the site of the colostomy, and is a rare and potentially fatal complication (Figure 31-18). This may be due to tumor implantation at the time of the resection or due to an inadequate margin of resection. Another possibility is that it may actually represent a second primary lesion. Epidermoid carcinoma of the parastomal skin has also been reported.[79] Radical resection of the involved area, including part of the abdominal wall with relocation of the stoma, is the recommended treatment.

Results of Colostomy Creation

Whittaker and Goligher reviewed their experience with colostomy following abdominoperineal resection of the rectum in 251 patients who survived for at least 2 years.[241] Upon comparison of extraperitoneal and intraperitoneal colostomy, it appeared that the complication rate was higher with the latter technique (see Figs. 29-44 and 29-45). The difference, however, was not statistically significant. Table 31-1 demonstrates the results of this study. It can be appreciated that colostomy construction is associated with a high incidence of complications. Almost 50% of the patients in this series (those who survived for at least 2 years) developed a stomal problem. One can only conjecture that had the patients been followed for a

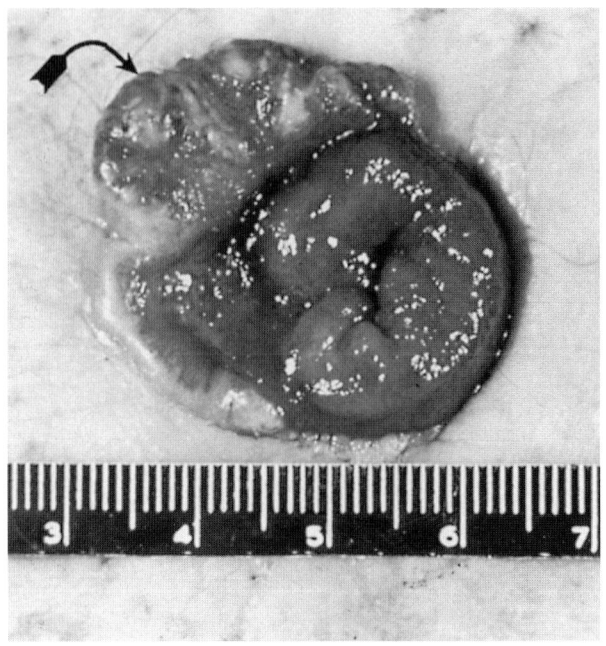

FIGURE 31-18. Recurrent carcinoma adjacent to the stoma (*arrow*). (Courtesy of Rudolf Garret, M.D.)

longer period of time, the complication rate would be higher.

Porter and colleagues reviewed their experience with 130 end-colostomies, followed for an average of 35 months.[169] There were 69 complications in 55 patients (44%). These included 11 strictures, 9 wound infections, 14 hernias, 9 small bowel obstructions, 4 prolapses, 2 abscesses, and 1 peristomal fistula. Mealy and associates reviewed 120 patients who underwent colostomy both on an elective and an emergency basis.[143] Colostomy-related morbidity included stenosis, retraction, prolapse, and hernia formation. These were observed in 19.2% of their 120 patients. There was no difference in incidence between the emergency and elective groups.

Marks and Ritchie reviewed their experience with complications following abdominoperineal resection for carcinoma of the rectum during the period 1968 through 1972 at St. Mark's Hospital.[136] Of the 227 patients who formed the basis of this study, three died in the postoperative period. By far the most common stomal problem encountered was hernia, which occurred in 23 patients, approximately 10%. It was felt that the cumulative risk of developing a pericolostomy hernia in the 6th postoperative year was approximately 33%. The authors believed that extraperitoneal colostomy seemed to offer some protection against herniation. The other reported complications included retraction, stenosis, abscess, and prolapse. The cumulative incidence of all these stomal complications was approximately 7%. This report and others con-

(251 Patients)

Complication	Number of Cases	Percent of Series
Infection	34	14
Mucocutaneous separation	24	10
Pericolostomy hernia	36	14
Prolapse	12	5
Recession (retraction)	1	0.4
Stenosis	9	4
Fistula	1	0.4

Adapted from Whittaker M, Goligher JC. A comparison of the results of extraperitoneal and intraperitoneal techniques for construction of terminal iliac colostomies. *Dis Colon Rectum* 1976;19:342.

firm that most colostomy hernias seem to develop in the first few years.[126]

Alternative Techniques for Sigmoid Colostomy Creation and Management

Maturation by Stapling

In addition to the conventional maturation technique for sigmoid colostomy, the circular stapling device has been advocated for performing end colostomies.[43,124,177] This permits a geometrically perfect opening that can be theoretically calibrated to be optimal for a particular bowel diameter. However, the factors that predispose to the subsequent development of stoma complications are related to ischemia, tension, and improper location, issues that are not avoided merely by creating a perfectly circular aperture.

Technique

Instead of a disk of skin being excised from the abdominal wall, a small opening is created just large enough to pass the center rod without the anvil. A purse string is created of the distal colon in the usual manner and the anvil inserted into the bowel. The cartridge and anvil are approximated, and the instrument is fired. One tissue "doughnut" consists of the skin, and the other is made up of the bowel. In effect, it is a colocutaneous anastomosis by means of the circular stapling device.

Another application of a stapler is the use of ordinary skin staples for maturing the stoma.[11] They are then removed on the 10th postoperative day.

Opinion

Although the former procedure does have some theoretical appeal, it would certainly make the subcutaneous dissection and rectus splitting much more tedious. Furthermore, it is more likely that the inferior epigastric vessels will be injured during the course of the dissection. As

for the use of skin staplers to mature the stoma, one may reasonably ask what the advantage is when an additional effort must be made to remove them.

Primary Insertion of Mesh Implant

As mentioned earlier, it has been suggested that a mesh implant be performed prophylactically in order to limit the likelihood of the patient developing a peristomal hernia.[16,109,133] The prosthetic mesh is appropriately tailored and a window created of adequate size to permit the colon to pass through. The mesh is secured to the peritoneum and posterior fascia. The Bayer group reported 43 patients with no evidence of hernia after a 4-year follow-up.

I cannot recommend this approach, believing instead that a properly located and matured stoma is unlikely to pose a subsequent problem.

Continent Colostomy

The search for continence in a colostomy has stimulated many attempts to control bowel movements by means of prosthetic devices. Tenney and colleagues reviewed the various approaches that have been attempted or proposed.[220] The authors considered the concepts according to four categories: external devices, surgical technique alone, surgical technique with passive implanted devices, and surgical technique with active implanted devices.

Kock Continent Colostomy

Kock and associates proposed a method, analogous to that of the continent ileostomy, through the use of the descending colon to create a nipple valve.[120] In five patients, the end sigmoidostomy was provided with such a valve, but evacuation by irrigation through a catheter was laborious, and the procedure has since been abandoned.[121] Some success was noted, however, with a continent cecostomy (see later).

Inflatable Cuff

A simple inflatable cuff has been attempted by the Mayo Clinic group, using the cuff end of a tracheostomy tube. The procedure was performed initially in animals and then in patients who had failed nipple valves following a Kock continent ileostomy. It was also considered for patients with conventional ileostomies who had not undergone a reservoir procedure.

Colostomy Plug

In 1986, Burcharth and colleagues reported the use of a colostomy plug (Conseal, Coloplast, Inc., Tampa, FL) on 53 patients.[33] The device is a two-piece system consisting of an adhesive baseplate and a disposable plug attachable to the plate (Figure 31-19). It is packed and compressed in

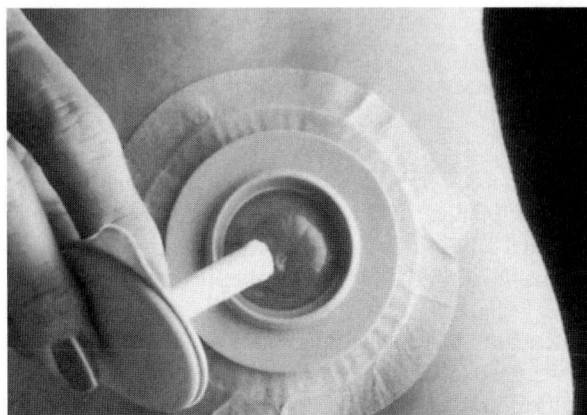

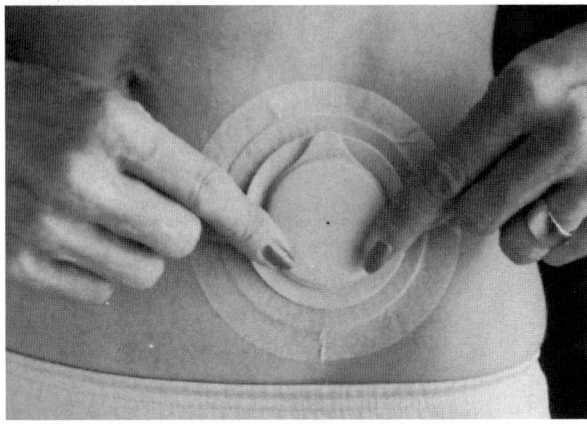

FIGURE 31-19. Conseal continent colostomy system. (Courtesy of Coloplast, Inc.)

a water-soluble film that disintegrates after insertion, allowing the plug to expand and prevent the passage of feces. Fecal continence and the passage of flatus without noise or odor were achieved in 90% of individuals.[33] Patients were able to effectively utilize the device for a median application time of 8 hours. Potential advantages include the elimination of noise, the filtering of odor, the elimination of a pouch, and the lack of obtrusiveness.

Clague and Heald used this device in 100 individuals.[44] Analysis of patient evaluations indicated that the plug restored continence and improved lifestyle in more than one-third of the ostomates who used it. Others have also reported a favorable experience with this device.[39,206]

Cerdán and colleagues describe a new one-piece disposable plug composed of a soft, flexible cylinder of open-celled polyurethane foam.[40] The device is supplied in a compressed form, enclosed in a water-soluble, lubricated, polyvinyl alcohol film. This is analogous to the plug illustrated in Figure 13-15 for the management of anal incontinence. The authors used the device in 20 patients with sigmoid colostomies. All but three found it comfortable and that it contributed to an improved quality of life. There were no complications associated with its use.

Artificial Sphincter

Szinicz described an implantable hydraulic sphincter prosthesis that consists of a compressible driving and control system together with a sleeve that is implanted around the bowel.[216] The sleeve is connected to the compliance chamber by means of a connecting tube. The author reported his experience in animal experiments and in seven patients. Heiblum and Cordoba implanted an inflatable plastic balloon in the subcutaneous tissue around the stoma in order to achieve fecal continence.[96] The connecting tube was tunneled subcutaneously from the balloon and brought out through a small wound at some distance from the stoma. The authors reported their experience in six patients, all but one of whom underwent the prosthesis insertion secondarily. Complete continence to feces and gas was obtained. One device had to be removed because it eroded the skin, and subcutaneous infection was a problem in three individuals.

Muscle Transplantation

Intestinal smooth muscle has been used to construct a continent colostomy.[195] Freely transplanted a 10- to 15-cm–long segment of large intestinal muscle (usually the sigmoid), devoid of mucosa and mesenteric fat. The seromuscular sleeve is incised longitudinally through one of the taeniae, soaked in an antibiotic solution, and sutured to the serosa of the bowel approximately 2 or 3 cm proximal to the site for the creation of the stoma. Sutures are placed so that the transplant is imbricated. This creates a length of about 6 cm, which in effect increases the muscular mass. The author emphasizes that, after securing one edge of the graft, the muscle must be stretched maximally, and the graft wrapped around the bowel and secured. The mesenteric vessels are incorporated by the graft.

Schmidt reported his experience with this technique in more than 500 patients, 231 of whom underwent surgery in his own unit.[195] Approximately 80% did not require an appliance, there was no mortality, and only five required removal of the surgical implant. Apparently the transplants are nourished by means of secondary vascularization, and an irrigation technique facilitates defecation. In most patients who underwent the procedure secondarily, "nearly all viewed their postoperative situation as markedly improved."

Kostov and coworkers used a modified smooth muscle "sphincteroplasty" for increasing intraluminal pressure in the colon proximal to the stoma in 72 rectal cancer patients.[122] Their technique involves resection and transplantation of a 4-cm–long portion of sigmoid colon muscularis. This is then passed around the colon through a defect in the mesentery, fixing it to the taenia. The procedure is combined with colonic irrigation to produce some level of bowel control and regularity. In an experience involving 72 patients, the weekly spontaneous stools were felt to be three to five times less frequent than in controls.

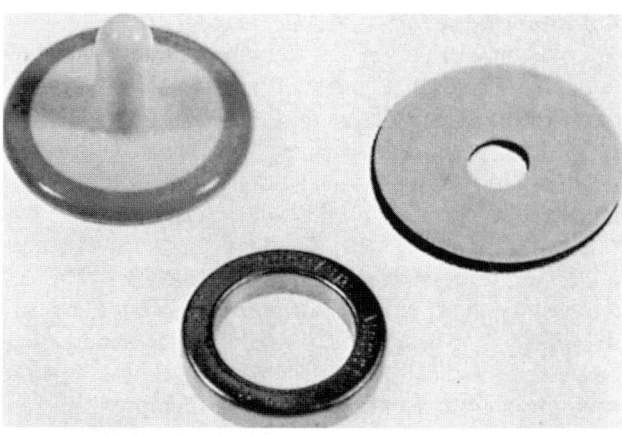

FIGURE 31-20. Magnetic ring, cap, and disposable charcoal filter. (From Khubchandani IT, Trimpi HD, Sheets JA, et al. The magnetic stoma device: a continent colostomy. *Dis Colon Rectum* 1981;24:344.)

Magnetic Colostomy

In 1975, Feustel and Hennig of Erlangen, Germany, described a device to create continence in patients who underwent conventional sigmoid colostomy: a magnetic ring implant (Figure 31-20).[63] A ring of samarium cobalt encased in plastic is buried in the subcutaneous tissue around the colon. The colostomy is matured in the usual manner and, when the wound has completely healed (usually several weeks later), an external cap containing a ring magnet in the top and a core magnet in the center pin is inserted to create a plug.

Results of the magnetic continent colostomy device were initially quite favorable, although subsequent results have been less optimistic.[86] Khubchandani and associates reported their experience in 14 patients, one-half of whom had good results.[119] There was no morbidity attributable to insertion of the ring, and there was no incident of wound infection. However, other problems developed, including the triggering of security monitors at airports, disturbances of television reception if one is sitting close, malfunctioning of wrist watches, and adherence of the patient to anything metallic (e.g., a kitchen sink). The authors further emphasized that one must be physically and mentally able to cope with the magnetic device.

Alexander-Williams and associates reviewed their experience with 61 patients: 55 primary and six secondary implants.[7] One individual died, possibly as a consequence of sepsis at the site of the implant. Twelve (20%) required removal of the ring because of failure of healing or late skin necrosis. Approximately one-half of the remaining patients were not using the magnetic cap at all at the time of the review. The reason for this failure was the fact that the device did not afford complete continence. Of the 21 patients who used the cap regularly, 15 were continent. In these authors' experience, therefore,

only one-fourth of the patients who underwent the operation were completely continent.

Kewenter reported 21 patients who underwent magnetic colostomy, all but three of whom had the procedure performed at the time of the primary resection.[117] Three died soon after operation (unrelated to the surgery). Eight were considered a success in that the cap was used under all circumstances, and two patients were considered partial successes. If one groups these two categories together, excluding the patients who expired, the rate of success with the procedure in Kewenter's experience was 44%.

Comment It appears that implantation of the magnetic stoma device is not a very forgiving technique. It requires meticulous dissection and careful patient selection. Complete control is successful in no more than 50% of patients. The matter now, however, is academic, since the device has been taken from the market and is no longer available. As a consequence, I no longer include a description of the operative technique or the illustrations in this text, but I do wish to remind the reader that the concept of an implanted device to create a continent colostomy should not be resurrected. The following is another.

Implantable Ring and Balloon Plug

In 1983, Prager described a device for control of feces following abdominoperineal resection and sigmoid colostomy.[171] It is composed of two parts, a silicone ring, which is produced in three different internal diameters with a flange on the upper surface reinforced with Dacron mesh, and a silicone balloon, which is made in varying lengths. The balloon is inflated and deflated by means of a 30-ml syringe. The ring is implanted within the peritoneal cavity and sewn onto the undersurface of the abdominal wall where the opening has been made for the stoma to be delivered. The abdominal incision is then closed and the colostomy matured in the usual manner. Beginning approximately 1 week after the operation, the patient begins to use the plug.

Results A multi-center study was undertaken to evaluate the safety and efficacy of the device.[172] Seventy-four patients underwent insertion of the ring.[172] Three were removed because of encapsulation of the ring. This is a complication common to all medical-grade implantable silicon, and appears to be an insoluble dilemma. Two patients had the rings removed because of bowel necrosis or fistulization (Figure 31-21). Many individuals elected not to use the plug, preferring instead to employ a conventional appliance or irrigation. Generally, younger patients have found the device to be more satisfactory.

Comment As with the magnetic ring colostomy device, the Prager implantable ring and balloon plug are no longer available because of the complications of erosion

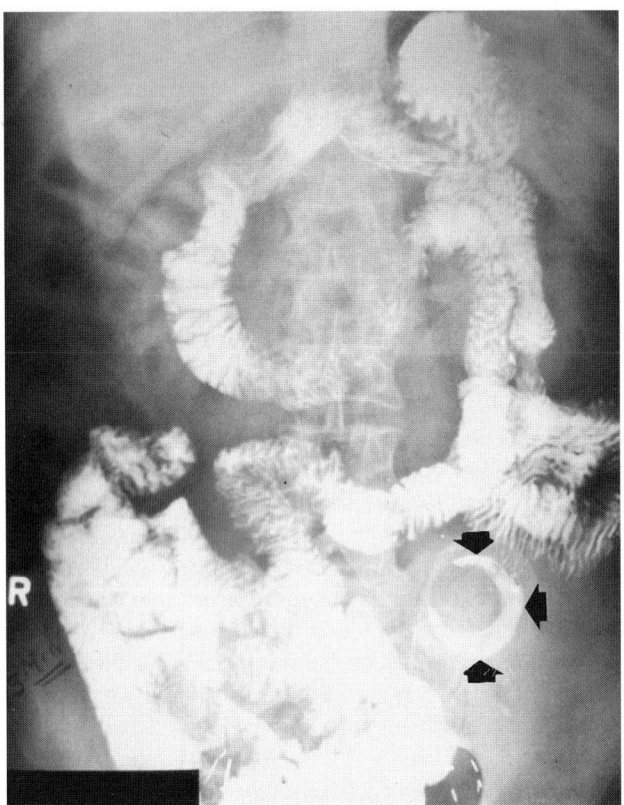

FIGURE 31-21. Small-bowel barium study demonstrates a halo of extravasated contrast material (*arrows*) at the site of the implantable ring. It is because of this complication that the implantable ring and balloon plug are no longer considered appropriate for patients with a sigmoid colostomy.

and necrosis of the stoma or bowel. Hence, I have removed most of the technical details and artwork from this edition. There may be a place for the balloon, however, in the treatment of individuals with fecal incontinence. This is discussed in Chapter 13.

Tampon Occlusion

Fischer and Gervin described the use of a tampon to occlude the colostomy stoma following abdominoperineal resection.[66] With this noninvasive device, the authors concluded that tampon occlusion can prevent contamination during laparotomy when a colostomy is present.

Opinion Leakage of stool during the course of an abdominal operation is really not much of a concern to me, personally. However, I was attracted to this article because it might possibly represent another alternative for creating continence for patients who wish to be relieved of the burden and responsibility of an appliance.

Colostomy Irrigation

Colostomy irrigation is a method of bowel control offered to selected patients with sigmoid or descending colon colostomies. Success depends on personal interest, bowel habits before surgery, manual dexterity, available toilet facilities, and lifestyle. Gawron suggests the following selection criteria for colostomy irrigation[77]:

- Permanent descending or sigmoid colostomy
- Physically and mentally capable of performing self-care
- Motivated to learn the procedure and adhere to a schedule
- No prior history of IBD, radiation therapy (to the abdomen or pelvis), or other major intestinal resection
- A history of regular bowel pattern or constipation
- Availability of bathroom facilities, including running water

Irrigation techniques are often taught on the 5th or 6th postoperative day, and for some individuals, a few months following the operation. Again, because of cost-containment and the possibility of delaying discharge, some patients may require instruction a few weeks later.

Most individuals tend to return to the bowel habits they had prior to operation, usually within 6 to 12 weeks after surgery. In other words, if one defecated every morning after breakfast, the colostomy will probably function on that schedule. Under these circumstances, irrigating may be unnecessary, and such patients can frequently avoid an appliance for the rest of the day or merely use a small dressing or Stoma Cap. A closed-ended "security pouch" can also be employed.

Conversely, if a patient had irregular bowel function preoperatively, the colostomy will probably act irregularly postoperatively. Such a person may be more content by irrigating. However, under no circumstances should one insist that the stoma be irrigated. It may be advisable to learn the technique, but the decision as to whether to actually use irrigation should be personal.

Method A nipple, cone, or catheter is inserted into the stoma. The cone tip is now being used more frequently for colostomy irrigation than the catheter, not only because there is less risk of perforating the bowel, but also because it provides a dam to prevent backflow. If a catheter is selected it should be inserted no farther than 3". A rubber nipple with a hole enlarged to accommodate the catheter tip acts as a flange and temporary dam while fluid is running in. Several companies manufacture irrigation kits (Figure 31-22).

The colon does not need to be washed out; the bowel is merely stimulated with the irrigant to produce evacuation. The bottom of the bag for irrigation is usually placed at shoulder height when the patient is seated. However, the height of the bag should be adjusted to permit a steady

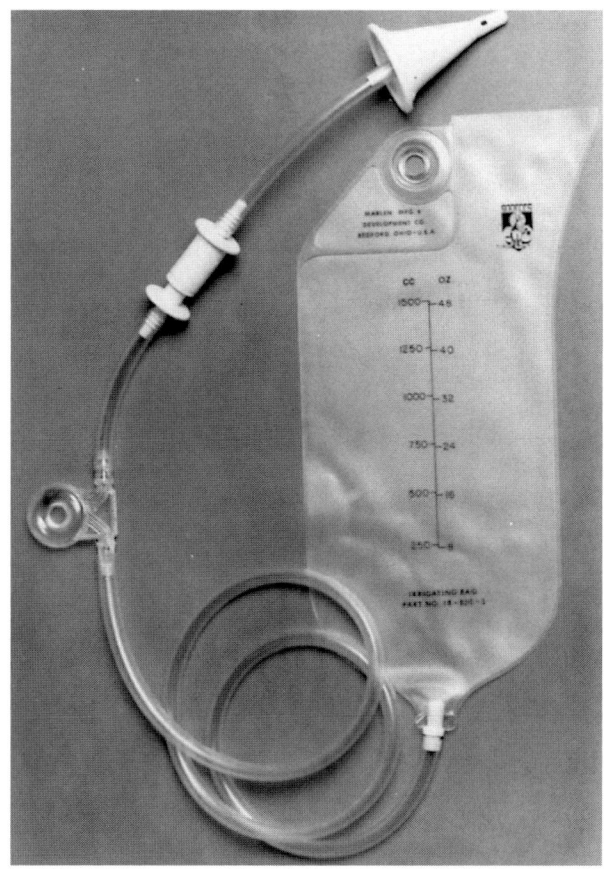

FIGURE 31-22. Colostomy irrigating system. This unit has a soft-tipped cone. (Courtesy of Marlen Manufacturing and Development Co.)

flow into the stoma.[67] An alternative technique has been suggested by Schwemmle and coworkers; a specially constructed basin is used at stoma level when the patient is standing.[197] Obviously, this requires a unique plumbing arrangement in the patient's bathroom.

Tepid water (750 to 1,000 ml) is slowly instilled over a 5- to 10-minute period. After waiting approximately 1 minute, the patient removes the cone, and the water and stool are permitted to pass through the irrigation sleeve into the toilet bowl. Most of the returns are usually collected within 15 minutes. The collecting sleeve can then be closed while one tends to other activities. After about 45 minutes, the irrigant usually will have been expelled. With time the patient may require irrigations only every 48 hours or even every 72 hours. Some, however, may never be able to irrigate satisfactorily and may require a pouch all of the time. Under these circumstances, it is difficult to justify the time and effort expended to perform this task.

Results Meyerhoff and colleagues performed a randomized study, comparing the effects of irrigating with different volumes: 250, 500, and 1,000 ml.[146] A double-isotope technique was developed to evaluate colonic emptying of irrigation fluid and feces. This was accomplished through radioactive labeling of the fecal contents by the ingestion of 10 MBq ^{69}Cr-EDTA 24 hours before scintigraphic investigation. The authors discovered that the general recommendation of 1,000 ml is not optimal for all patients. In many instances, a volume of 500 ml was preferred because of reduced inflow time, complete colonic emptying of more consistent fecal contents, and minimal retention of irrigant. It appears, therefore, that one should experiment with different irrigation volumes in order to determine the most efficacious program for the individual.

Watt categorized those patients who probably are not candidates for controlling bowel elimination by irrigation as follows: those with irritable bowel syndrome, individuals who underwent irradiation therapy and sustained radiation enteritis, and the terminally ill. Stomal management problems such as hernia and stenosis, poor eyesight, impaired dexterity, fear of the irrigation procedure, and resentment of the time necessary militate against irrigating.[238]

Terranova and colleagues evaluated irrigation and compared the technique with natural evacuation in 340 patients.[221] They concluded that because of the feeling of security gained by relative continence, cleanliness, and the avoidance of an appliance, the vast majority of patients preferred irrigating. Williams and Johnston performed a prospective randomized study using colostomy irrigation and natural evacuation in 30 selected patients.[244] The mean time spent managing the stoma was 45 minutes/day in the spontaneous group versus 53 minutes when irrigation was performed. Because of reduction of odor and flatus, the lack of requirement for medication, and the ability of many to avoid an appliance, irrigation seemed to offer an improved lifestyle. In a questionnaire response of 223 patients from the Mayo Clinic, 60% were "continent" with irrigation, 22% were "incontinent" with irrigation, and 18% had discontinued the technique for various reasons.[110] Doran and Hardcastle performed a controlled trial of colostomy management by natural evacuation, by irrigation, and by means of a foam enema.[57] By evaluating 20 patients who used each technique for 2 months, the authors concluded that almost all felt that irrigation or the foam enema improved their quality of life. Furthermore, they opted to continue with irrigation on completion of the study.

The St. Mark's Hospital group attempted to shorten the time it takes to complete a satisfactory irrigation through the use of glyceryl trinitrate solution.[160] They had demonstrated that this agent, through the induction of gastrointestinal smooth muscle relaxation, accelerates stool expulsion. In a study involving 15 colostomy patients, each with more than 3 years of experience with irrigation, a significant reduction in colostomy irrigating time was noted when compared with tap water. However, there was an extremely high incidence of cramping and headaches with the glyceryl trinitrate solution.

Venturini and colleagues evaluated colostomy irrigation in the elderly, noting that age is no restriction on the ability to achieve successful irrigation and to improve the quality of life.[234]

TRANSVERSE COLOSTOMY

The history of colostomy is in Chapters 22 and 23. The first documented transverse colon stoma was performed by Fine in 1797 in Geneva.[64] He successfully decompressed an obstruction from carcinoma of the rectum by drawing out a loop of bowel and securing the mesentery to the skin. Maydl (1888) was the first to suggest an external apparatus to accomplish stomal support for minimizing retraction and for facilitating spur formation.[138] However, it was not until 1951 that Patey advised that a transverse colostomy should be opened and matured at the time of the initial procedure.[163] See Corman and Odenheimer's review of the evolution of methods used for creating a loop colostomy.[47]

Numerous alternatives have been offered to accomplish adequate diversion, such as a deep retention suture with retained polyethylene sleeve, the application of a skin bridge, suturing of the fascia between the leaves of the mesentery, and various support devices (goose quill, harelip pin, rods, tubes, drains, and catheters) from the ingenious to the absurd (Figure 31-23).[14,23,32,67,83,111, 127,184,235] One may elect to simply use a no. 14 French red rubber catheter to support the spur of the loop, and sew a no. 24 French catheter onto each end. Any tubing or drain has the advantage of flexibility, permitting relative ease in changing the appliance. Alternatively, one may employ a commercially prepared system such as that made by Hollister (Figure 31-24) or by ConvaTec (Figure 31-25).

For many years, the ritual of "unveiling the stoma" had been a standard part of the postoperative management of patients who underwent a diverting loop colostomy. A large plastic or glass rod was placed beneath the bowel and a rubber hose was attached to both ends to keep it from slipping out of place. A bulky dressing was then applied. Approximately 48 hours later, the dressing was removed, and at the bedside, a cautery or soldering iron was employed to open the colon. The bloody, feculent scene that resulted might have been reminiscent of the battle of Sebastopol: assistants rushing to find hemostats, feces on the floor, on the bedclothes, and on the walls (Figure 31-26). Ultimately, a temporary appliance was draped around the large rod and changed frequently, because the apparatus was certain to leak. Not uncommonly, additional problems included ischemia or gangrene of the stoma when hidden from view by the dressing, and retraction of the colostomy into the peritoneal cavity if the rod slipped out.

Few surgeons today are reluctant to open the colostomy at the initial operation. There are three reasons why opening the colostomy at the time is important:

1. For patients with obstruction, it affords an immediate opportunity to decompress the bowel.
2. It obviates the necessity for a subsequent tedious bedside procedure.
3. It provides the physician and the nursing staff with an opportunity to inspect the viability of the stoma at frequent intervals.

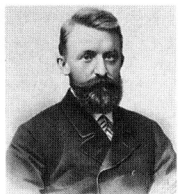

Karl Maydl (1853–1903)   Karl Maydl was born March 10, 1853, in Rokitnic, Czechoslovakia, and entered medical school in Prague. He undertook his doctoral thesis in 1876 and began his surgical residency under the direction of Heine. Following a teaching position at Innsbruck and Vienna he entered the Military Medical School in Belgrade, and in 1886 became a surgical professor and chief of the surgical unit of the General Ambulance in Vienna. In 1891, Maydl became head of surgery at the University of Prague where he had great impact on Czechoslovakian surgery. The so-called Maydl technique concerned visceral ectopy, and his artificial anus method was a well-recognized and important achievement. He is the individual who perfected the concept of a loop colostomy, accomplished initially through the use of gauze passed through the mesocolon, but he also suggested that a rod may be created using rubber (vulcanite) or a goose feather. He was also one of the first to perform a laminectomy and to remove a tumor of the central nervous system. Karl Maydl died August 8, 1903, in Dobrichovic, Czechoslovakia. (Biography, Courtesy of Oliver Pfaar, M.D.)

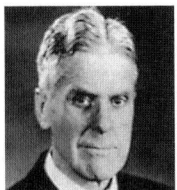

David Howard Patey (1899–1977)   David Patey was born in Monmouthshire, Wales, the eldest of three children. In 1916, he entered Middlesex Hospital Medical School for his preclinical and clinical work, an institution with which he maintained affiliation for the remainder of his life. Following interruption for military service during World War I, he returned to Middlesex and won the hospital's highest undergraduate award. He passed the final M.B. of London University in 1923 with the gold medal, and with honors in surgery and in obstetrics and gynecology. In 1930, after a period as a research fellow in the department of anatomy, Patey was appointed to the staff of the Middlesex Hospital. That same year he won the Jacksonian Prize of the Royal College of Surgeons and was Streatfield Scholar of the Royal College of Physicians. The following year he was named Hunterian Professor, receiving the honor again in 1964. Patey was recognized for his work and publications primarily on salivary gland tumors, breast cancer, and interestingly, pilonidal sinus. Perhaps his most important contribution was founding the Surgical Research Society of Great Britain, for which he later became president. A true scholar with a fluent knowledge of Russian and French, Patey was recognized for his unshakable integrity, unassuming modesty, and clear thinking. He died in his 78th- year. (Photograph courtesy of Professor Michael Hobsley, David Patey Professor, Department of Surgery, University College and Middlesex School of Medicine, London, United Kingdom.)

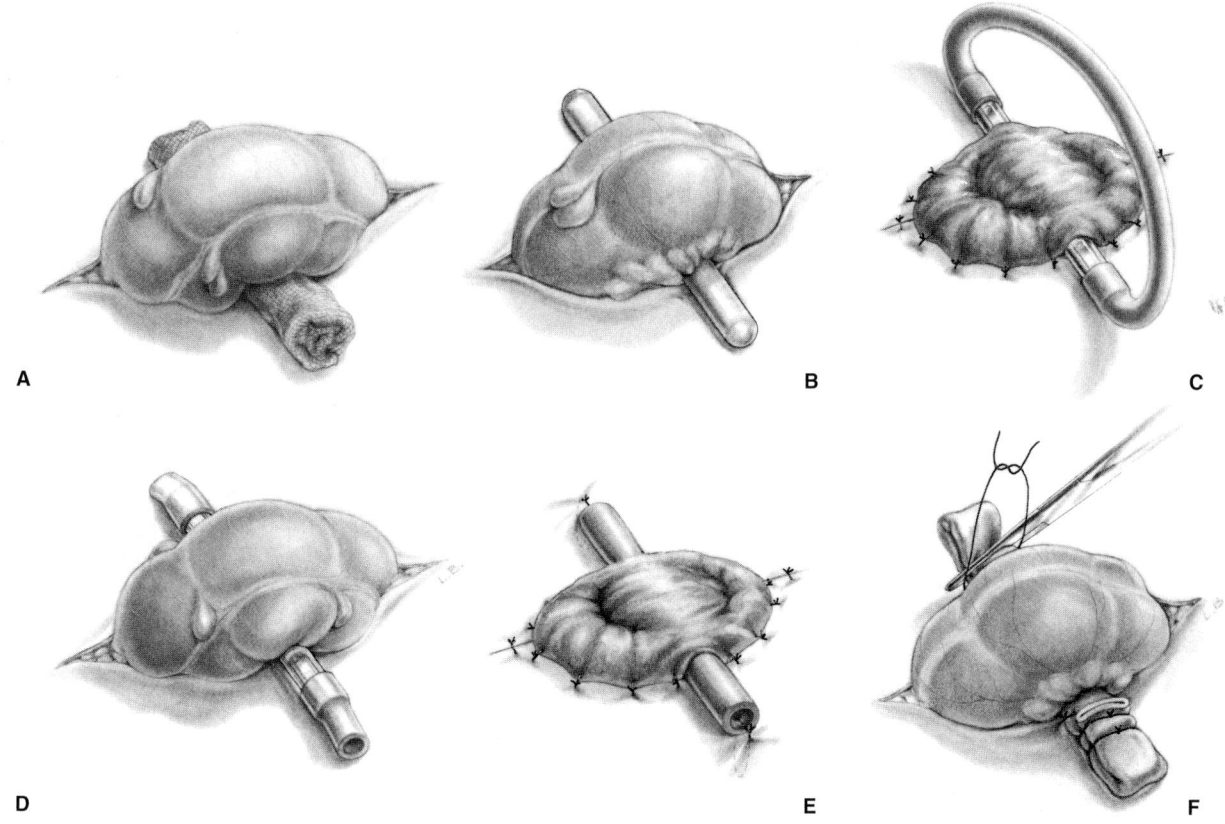

A **B** **C**

D **E** **F**

FIGURE 31-23. Alternatives for securing the loop of colon. **(A)** Rolled gauze. **(B)** Glass rod. **(C)** Glass rod with rubber loop. **(D)** Glass rod with rubber sleeves. **(E)** Rubber tubing. **(F)** Folded tubing or drain. (From Corman JM, Odenheimer DB. Securing the loop—historical review of the methods used for creating a loop colostomy. *Dis Colon Rectum* 1991;34:1014.)

A dressing tends to dissuade anyone from examining the site and precludes any possibility of identifying nonviable bowel.[48]

Indications

Transverse colostomy is a procedure often employed on a temporary basis for a number of indications: obstructing or perforating lesions of the colon, trauma, anastomotic leak, congenital anomalies, fecal incontinence, and to protect the anastomosis. With improvement of suturing and stapling techniques, however, this last indication has become less applicable.

Technique

Loop Colostomy

As has been suggested in Chapter 26, if a transverse colostomy is undertaken in an emergency situation, it should be accompanied by a full exploratory laparotomy, identifying the nature of the pathology. Ideally, the colostomy should be created as distally as possible and, if

performed in the transverse colon, should be accomplished on the left side. This is an important point, because if a transverse colostomy is maintained for a sufficient time, the efferent limb will tend to prolapse. By placing the opening in the left transverse colon, the splenic flexure tethers the bowel and limits the risk of this complication. Another reason for performing the colostomy in the distal transverse colon is that the stool is theoretically somewhat more formed than it would be in a more proximal location. There is simply no practical or theoretical advantage for using the right transverse colon as the stomal site.

As with sigmoid colostomy and ileostomy, the transverse colostomy should be brought through the split rectus muscle (Figure 31-27). The omentum is freed from the colon for a sufficient distance to permit exteriorization without tension. A tape or Penrose drain is passed through the leaves of the mesentery and the bowel delivered through the abdominal wound. A rod or bridge is passed through the same plane as the drain (Figs. 31-23 and 31-28 through 31-30).[198] The colostomy is then "matured" by opening it longitudinally and suturing the bowel edge to the skin (Figure 31-31). An appliance is

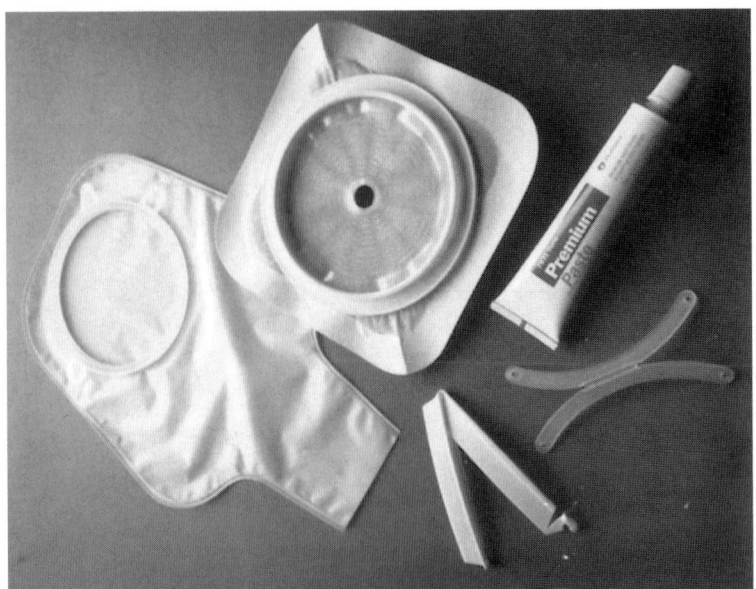

FIGURE 31-24. Two-piece loop ostomy system with bridge. (Courtesy of Hollister, Inc.)

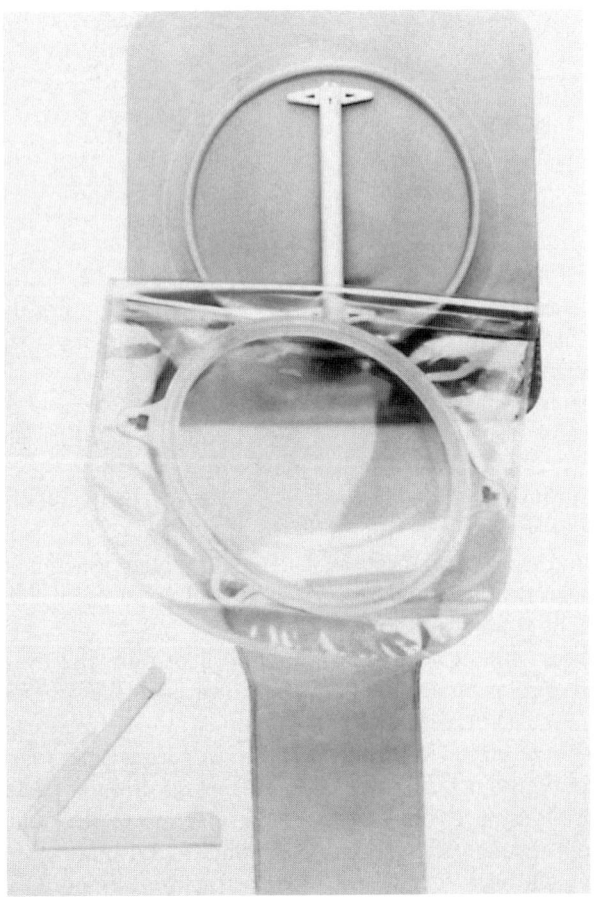

FIGURE 31-25. Gentle-Touch loop ostomy system. (Courtesy of ConvaTec, a division of E.R. Squibb and Sons, Inc.)

then used (Figure 31-32). A number of authors have expressed concern about the difficulty in managing an appliance with a rod in place. Some suggest the interposition of a tongue-shaped skin flap, while others offer a subcutaneous modification of a bridging approach (Figure 31-33).[14,21]

Adequacy of Diversion

A properly constructed loop transverse colostomy should be fully diverting, relatively easy to manage, and not offensive (Figure 31-34). Stool does not have eyes. It cannot enter the bag, look around and disappear into the distal limb. There is no such event as the fecal jumping distance. Conversely, if the proximal limb retracts, stool may flow into the distal bowel. The bridge or rod can be removed as soon as sufficient edema is present to maintain exteriorization of the colon. It is not necessary to leave the rod or tube in place for an arbitrary 1 week, as has been sometimes advised, because very often the rod itself will cause an element of obstruction that impedes the patient's recovery. Conversely, if the colostomy seems to be functioning well with the rod in place, and very little edema is evident, the bridge may be maintained for a longer period of time.

Rombeau and colleagues performed a barium swallow in 25 patients following loop transverse colostomy.[185] Follow-up films were obtained up to 4 days later, and barium was not visible in the distal colon in any of the patients. This same study performed *4 weeks* following diverting colostomy failed to show barium in the distal colon segment. Others attest to the adequacy of diversion if a loop colostomy is properly constructed.[154] However, while intra-abdominal or skin-level colostomies without a bridge,

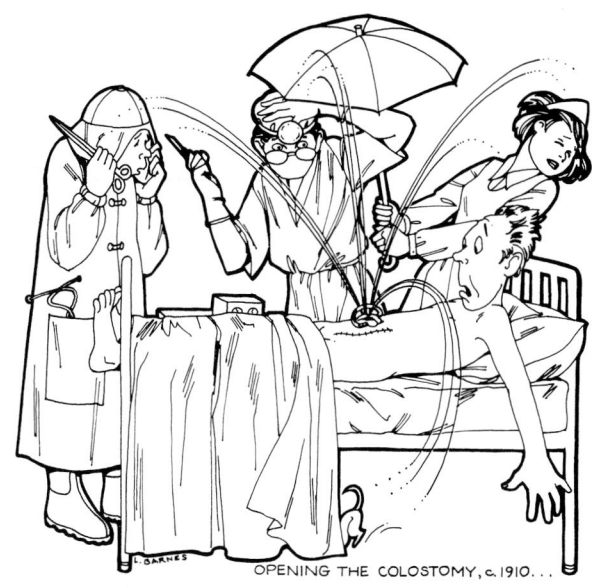

FIGURE 31-26. Cartoonist's perception of the ritual of opening the colostomy at the bedside.

rod, drain, or tube may succeed in venting the colon adequately, they are not truly diverting.[60,215]

Fontes and colleagues identified three factors that are usually responsible for the failure of loop colostomies to be fully diverting[69]:

- Retraction
- Reduction of a prolapsed loop colostomy (invariably associated with retraction)
- Improper technique

Divided Colostomy

The theoretical concern about inadequate diversion can be addressed by "stapling" the distal end,[155,190] or by dividing the colon, creating an end-transverse colostomy and performing a side-to-side colon anastomosis of the distal segment.[129] This last method, an alternative to the concept of a "double-barreled" stoma, is time-consuming to create and may require a laparotomy to close.

The so-called "end-loop colostomy" is another option. The proximal limb and the anti-mesenteric corner of the distal limb are drawn through the abdominal wall following stapled division of the bowel.[173,202,230] In an obese patient, it is sometimes impossible to deliver the transverse colon out as a loop. Accordingly, the bowel is divided and the distal end oversewn. The colostomy is then created using the end of the transverse colon, maturing it in a similar manner to that of a conventional sigmoid colostomy (Figure 31-35). Another alternative in an obese individual is to perform a loop ileostomy (see later).

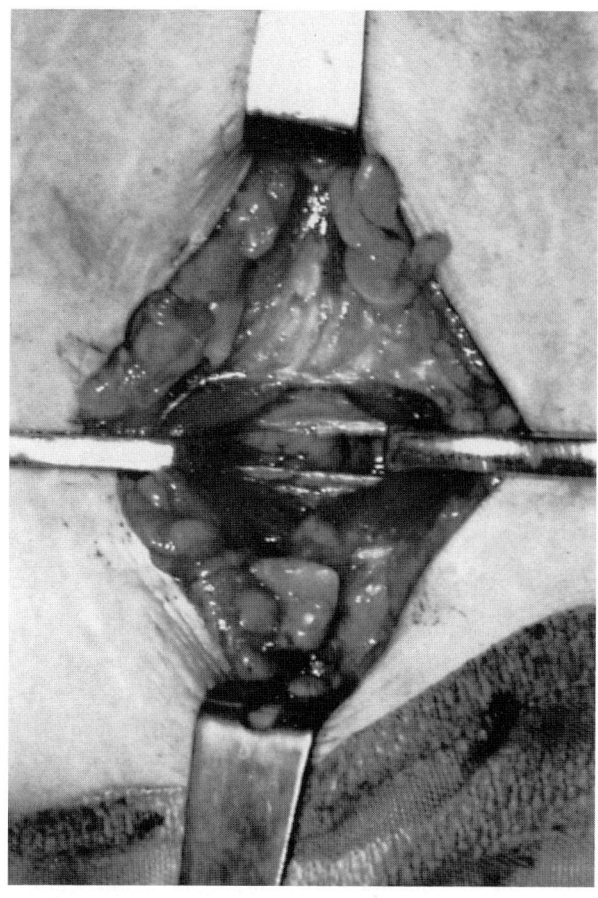

FIGURE 31-27. Creation of a transverse colostomy. The rectus muscle is split.

Results of Loop Colostomy Construction

Numerous modifications have been proposed to simplify the creation of a loop colostomy stoma, to facilitate appliance management, and to expedite closure with a decreased morbidity.[14,32,60,101,129,158,184,185,190,215] My associates and I reviewed our experience with complications of colostomy construction and closure.[149] In 162 patients who underwent a loop colostomy, 12 (7.4%) developed a prolapse, 6 (3.7%) were noted to have retracted stomas, and 4 (2.5%) had abscesses. In the series, almost 14% developed a complication related to the colostomy construction alone. This does not, of course, take into consideration the morbidity associated with closure of a colostomy (see Colostomy Closure section).

Embarking upon a transverse colostomy cannot be considered a whimsical undertaking. As has been discussed in Chapter 22, one must be able to justify the indications for the procedure and to ensure that it is not being performed because it makes the surgeon "feel better." Abrams and colleagues reported an overall complication rate of 41% in 248 patients who underwent a colostomy.[4] A hospital death rate of 24% was also noted. However, many of the

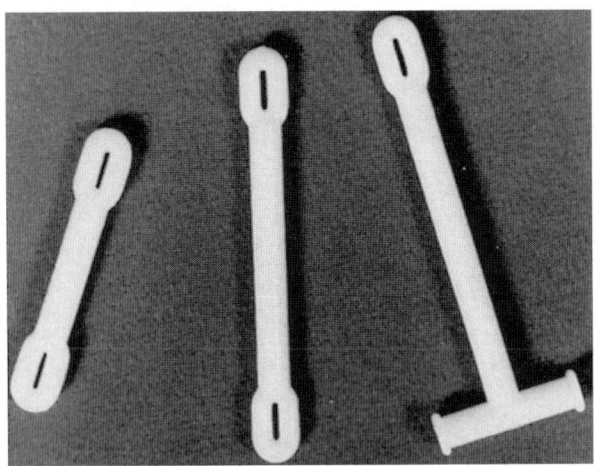

FIGURE 31-28. Marlen plastic loop ostomy rods. (Courtesy of Marlen Manufacturing and Development Co.)

patients had other serious illnesses, so that one cannot blame the colostomy exclusively for the high rates of morbidity and mortality. Wara and -coworkers reviewed 250 patients who underwent transverse colostomy for fecal diversion, with a morbidity rate of 28%.[237] The two most important factors affecting the morbidity were emergency procedures and colostomies in infants. The overall incidence of specific colostomy complications was 26% in adults and 50% in children. Excluding infection, the most common complication was prolapse, followed by retraction, peristomal hernia, and stomal necrosis. Miles and

Greene noted a complication rate related to stomal construction of 11% in almost 200 patients, and Smit and Walt reported almost a 10% incidence of complications related to creation of the stoma.[147,205]

The methods for preventing complications of transverse colostomy are quite similar to that of sigmoid colostomy. The size of the opening must be adequate in order to avoid edema, stricture, and obstruction. Ideally, the appropriate site should be selected before the operation, but this is not always possible if the colostomy construction was unanticipated. If the colostomy is created with the bowel under tension, it is likely to retract or to necrose (Figure 31-36). But a more common complication is colostomy prolapse, inevitably of the efferent (nonfunctioning) limb (Figure 31-37) see earlier discussion). If a colostomy is brought through the abdominal incision, it will always prolapse (Figure 31-38).

Chandler and Evans reported that 40% of adult loop colostomies involving the right side of the transverse colon prolapsed, a statistically significant increased incidence exceeding the rate for loop colostomies in more distal sites.[41] They further observed that the presence of obstruction at the time the colostomy was created seemed to predispose to the subsequent development of prolapse. Thirty-eight percent of all stomas originally made for obstruction prolapsed, compared with only 7% of those placed in unobstructed bowel. The proposed mechanism for this appeared to be a disproportion between the size of the fascial defect and the smaller diameter of the bowel following decompression.

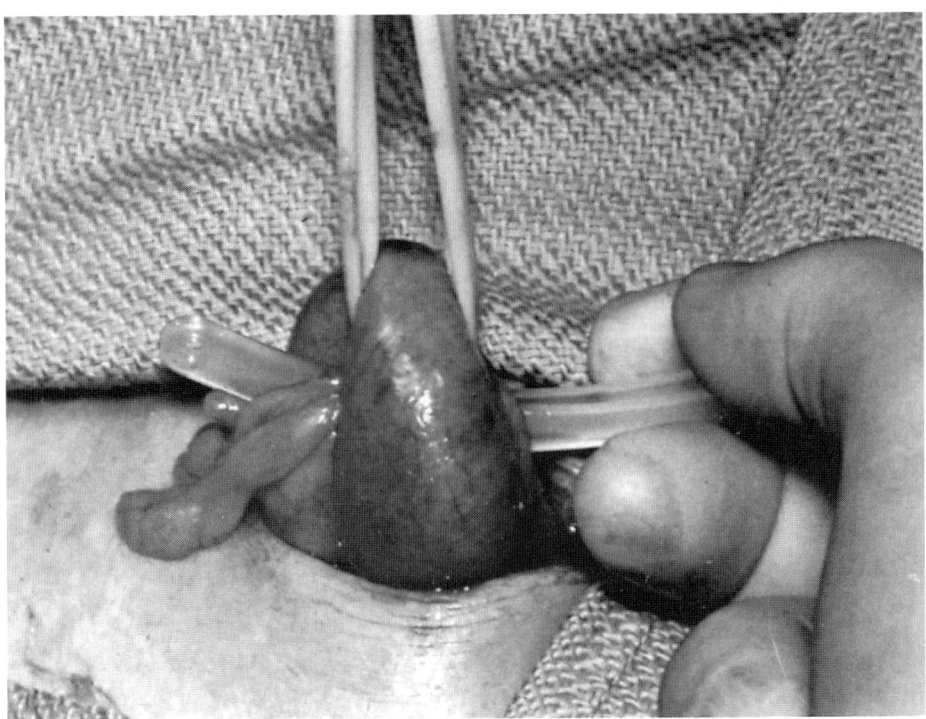

FIGURE 31-29. Creation of a transverse colostomy. A Hollister bridge is passed through the mesentery. Traction on the Penrose drain delivers the bowel.

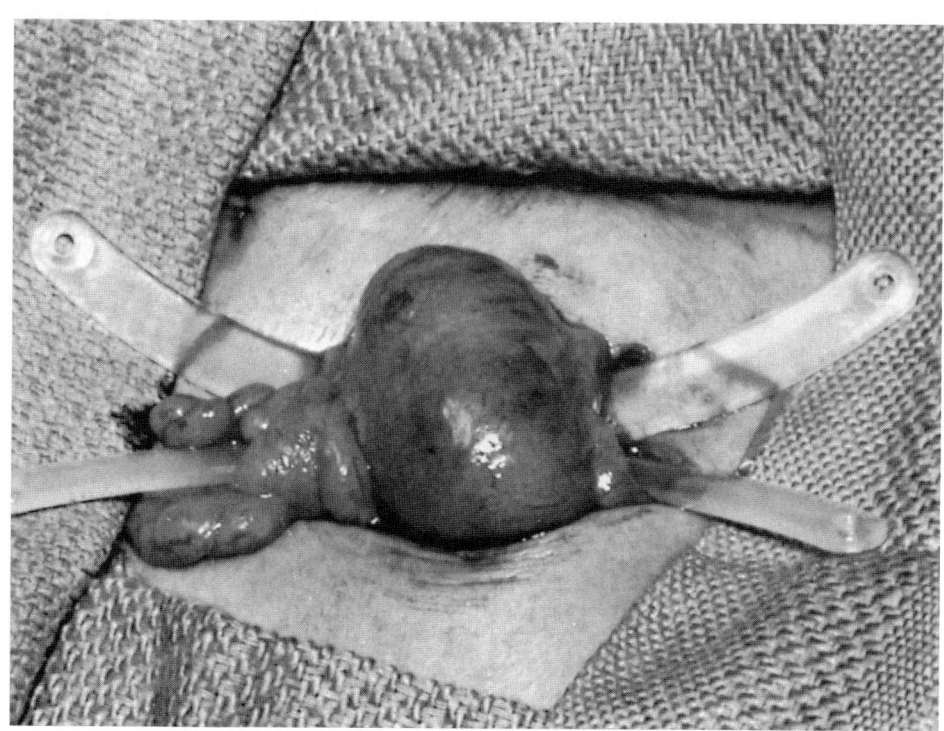

FIGURE 31-30. Creation of a transverse colostomy. Bridge in place.

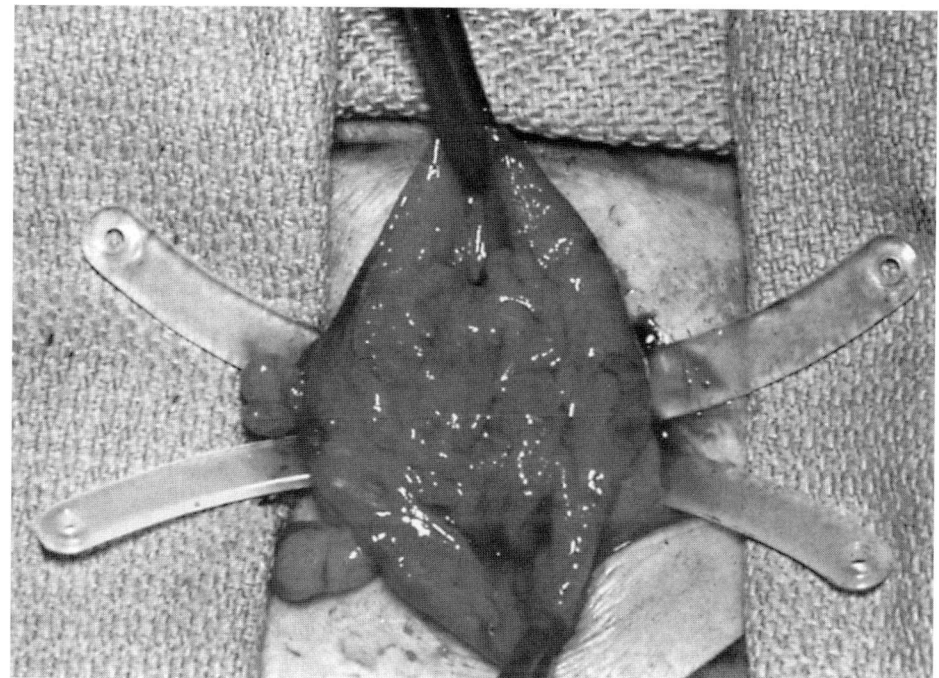

FIGURE 31-31. Creation of a transverse colostomy. Colostomy is matured.

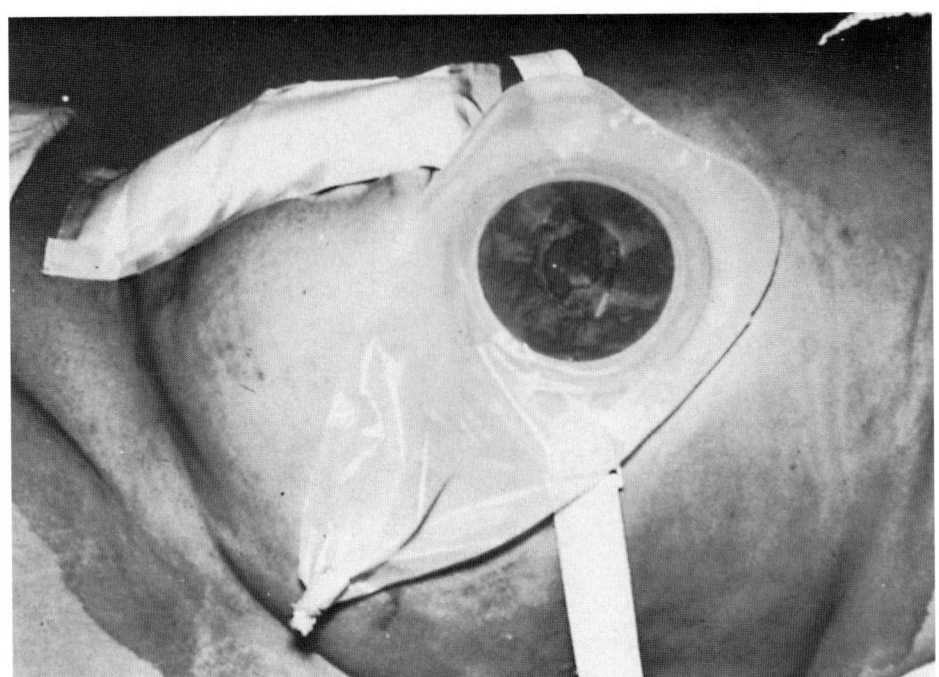

FIGURE 31-32. Creation of a transverse colostomy. Appliance is secured.

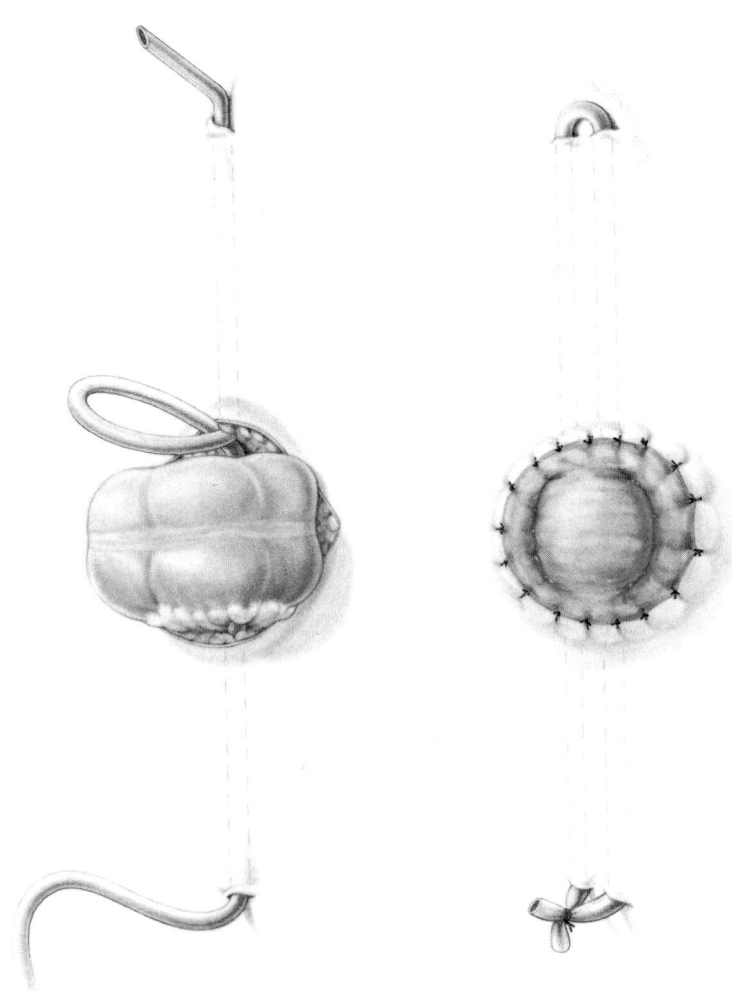

FIGURE 31-33. Technique of colostomy bridging by means of a plastic tubing and trocar. **(A)** The catheter is secured quite laterally. **(B)** The stoma is matured in the usual way. (Adapted from Bergren CT, Laws HL. Modified technique of colostomy bridging. *Surg Gynecol Obstet* 1990;170:453.)

A

B

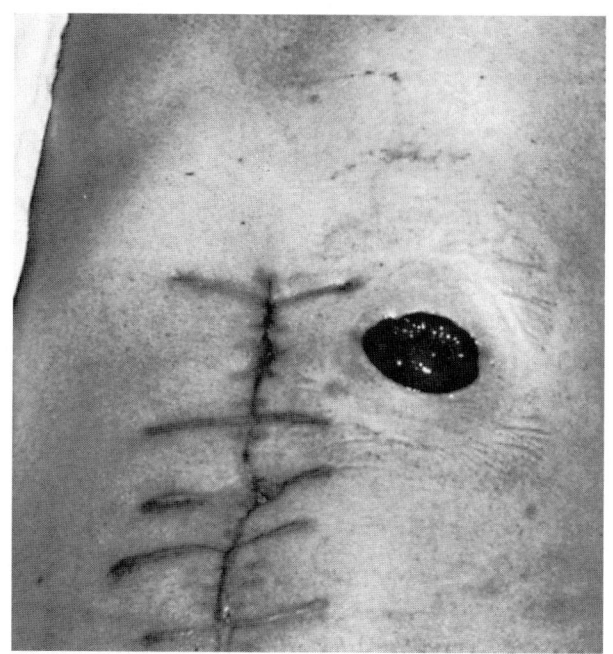

FIGURE 31-34. Loop transverse colostomy. The patient is shown 1 month following perforated diverticulitis with a well-functioning, fully diverting stoma.

Schofield and colleagues recommend rotating the colostomy 90 degrees so that the proximal end is in a dependent position.[196] The authors contend that not only is the stool less likely to flow into the distal loop, but they suggest that this method avoids colostomy prolapse and hernia. It is difficult for me to understand why this would be so, since the predisposing factors for these complications are still present. Furthermore, as previously mentioned, with a properly constructed standard loop colostomy, overflow into the distal limb should not occur.

Unti and colleagues reported their experience with the end-loop colostomy as performed on 135 patients.[230] The authors also included 70 ileocolostomies and 24 ileostomies, so it is impossible to state what the exact complication rate is with the colon alone. The overall complication rate was as follows: leakage (3.5%), retraction (3.5%), partial necrosis (2.6%), and peristomal sepsis (1.8%).

Treatment of Loop Colostomy Prolapse

A number of methods have been devised to treat colostomy prolapse. Zinkin and Rosin modified the technique originally described by Mayo and have adapted it to an office procedure.[139,250] A smooth-backed button is placed on the abdominal wall, and a non-absorbable suture is passed through the buttonhole, skin, fascia, and intestine. A finger in the lumen of the intestine helps to reduce the prolapse and to direct the entrance of the needle through the bowel. The result is to fix the reduced intestine firmly against the anterior abdominal wall, preventing further intussusception.

Krasna uses a purse-string suture to narrow the colostomy orifice, whereas Colmer and Foxx describe an external prolapse control device that consists of attaching the base of a Gellhorn pessary to the faceplate of a colostomy appliance.[45,123] The device is held in place by a colostomy bag belt. Since the "cork" is not completely obstructing, the stool passes around it, but the prolapse remains reduced.

Another option for treating prolapse is to circumcise the distal limb, divide the bowel, oversew it, and re-suture the end colostomy stoma (Figure 31-39). This can often be accomplished with a local anesthetic.

Comment

Winkler and Volpe advise that loop transverse colostomy is a holdover from the past, and that it is all too often permanent rather than temporary.[246] They suggest that all colostomies should be created as end stomas. Although their proposal emphasizes the magnitude of the problem, I prefer a loop stoma because of the relative ease of subsequent closure, but I hate loop transverse colostomy.

Fortunately, most patients who have undergone a transverse colostomy are inconvenienced for a relatively short period of time. When the colostomy is performed for terminal disease, however, many individuals live long enough to develop severe management problems with the stoma. This is particularly true when abdominal distention as a result of liver enlargement or ascites produces a peristomal hernia or an irreducible prolapse. In fact, the problems associated with stomal management may be a source of greater disability than all other aspects of the care of the terminally ill patient. Therefore, one should endeavor to avoid if at all possible a permanent loop transverse colostomy.

Occasionally, a so-called temporary colostomy may inevitably become permanent. This is usually because a distal anastomosis has failed to heal or the patient has developed other serious medical problems that preclude further surgical intervention. If such a problem arises, the surgeon might consider one of the methods described to control prolapse of the efferent limb. The complication of diversion colitis and its management are discussed in Chapter 33.[91]

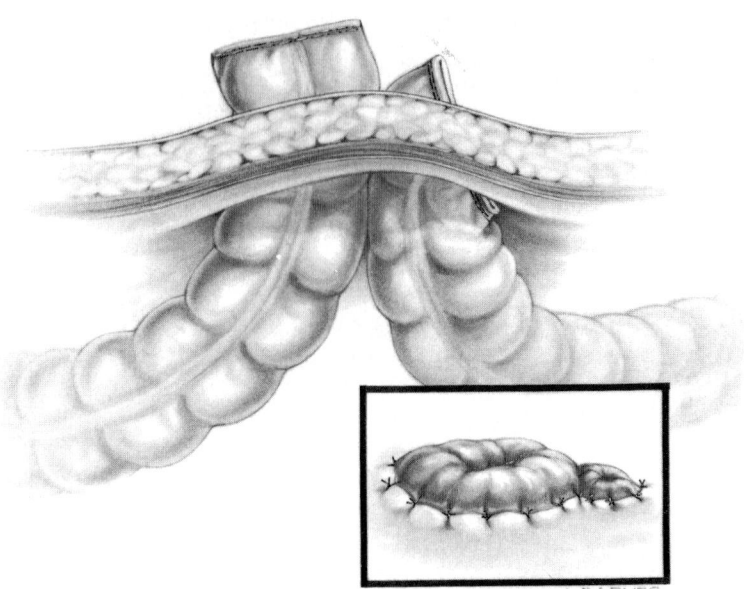

FIGURE 31-35. Divided colostomy (end-loop colostomy). The functioning end is matured and the distal end deemphasized.

Colostomy Closure

Because of the high rate of morbidity associated with colostomy closure, a voluminous literature has accumulated addressing the factors that predispose to complications. Attempts have been made to proselytize colleagues

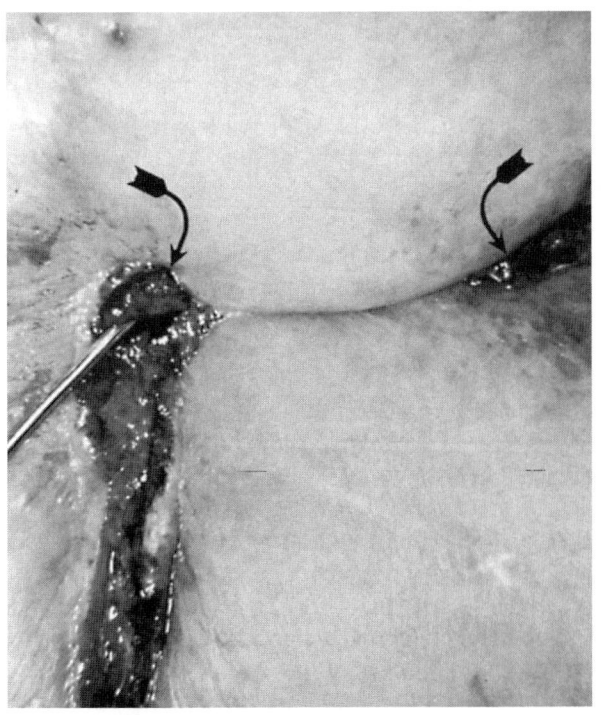

FIGURE 31-36. Retracted transverse loop colostomy, the result of mesenteric tension in an obese patient. Only two fecal fistulas remain (*arrows*).

in an effort to convince the skeptic of the optimal method for reestablishing intestinal continuity, but notably infrequent are controlled studies. Controversy still exists over the relative merits of intra-abdominal versus extra-abdominal closure, closure with resection versus closure without resection, and primary wound closure versus delayed.

Yajko and colleagues reported a 28% incidence of complications associated with colostomy closure in 100 patients.[249] Wound infection was noted in 10% and fecal fistula in 4%. These authors advocated an open, two-layer anastomosis with delayed wound closure.

Beck and Conklin analyzed the records of 77 Vietnam War casualties who underwent loop colostomy closure.[20] The postoperative complication rate was 9% with simple loop closure as compared with 24% with resection and anastomosis. These authors felt that closure without resection was technically easier and associated with a lower morbidity than resection of the stoma with re-anastomosis.

Wara and associates noted a morbidity rate of 57% (a leakage rate of 10%) and a mortality rate of 1.7% in 105 patients.[237] There was a significantly increased incidence of fecal fistula and incisional hernia when closure was performed as a single procedure subsequent to a definitive resection. They believed that the difference might be explained by better accessibility when the colostomy was performed at the same time as the definitive resection.

Smit and Walt reported a complication rate of 30% in 167 patients who underwent colostomy closure.[205] Wound infection was seen in more than 17%. These authors felt that the optimal period for closure was from two to three months after colostomy construction. They further noted that there was a higher incidence of complications in pa-

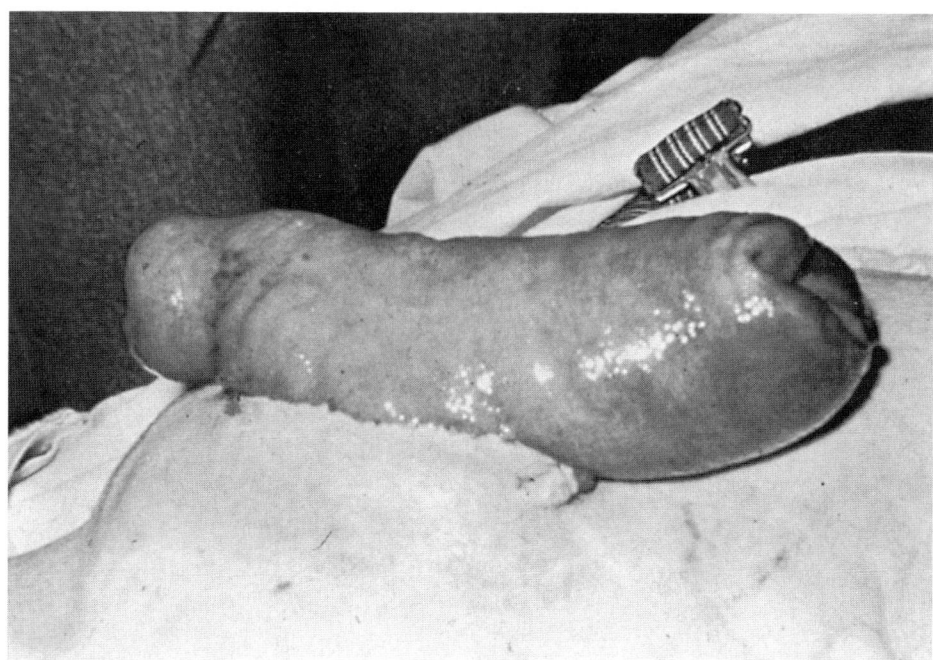

FIGURE 31-37. Loop transverse colostomy with prolapse.

tients who did not undergo a full bowel preparation or who were not on antibiotics.

Todd and colleagues reviewed their experience in a retrospective fashion of 206 colostomy closures.[226] They found that the method employed did not significantly influence the postoperative morbidity or mortality, and that there was no evidence that the timing of the colostomy closure was a critical factor for the subsequent development of anastomotic complications. Varnell and Pemberton found that the time interval between colostomy creation and closure did not affect morbidity, nor did intraoperative wound management, the use of systemic antibiotics alone, and the location of the loop colostomy.[232] Their morbidity rate was 44%. Aston and Everett also felt that early closure of a loop colostomy could be undertaken relatively safely.[12] Pittman and Smith observed that complications were not related to the time interval between creation and closure, and that no significant difference was found in the anastomotic leak rates between sutured and stapled techniques.[167]

Conversely, Freund and colleagues felt that the two major factors determining subsequent complications were timing and method of closure.[71] Simple closure was associated with fewer complications than resection, and colostomies closed sooner than 12 weeks after their construction had twice the incidence of complications than those which were closed after that time. Oluwole and associates also concur that colostomy closure three months following construction is preferred.[162] Other factors associated with a lower incidence of complications in their experience included mechanical and antibiotic bowel

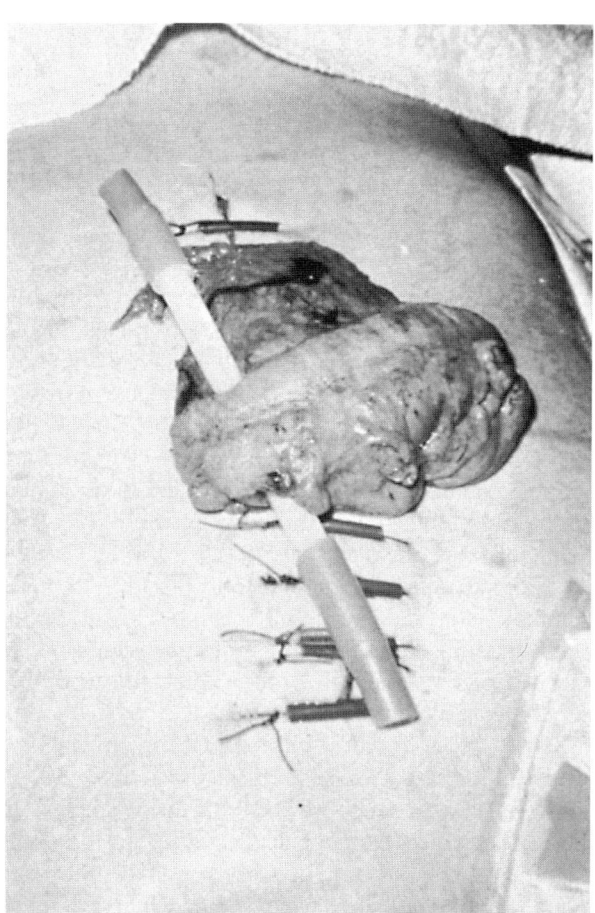

FIGURE 31-38. Prolapsed loop colostomy. This developed immediately following the operation, a consequence of bringing the colon through the abdominal incision.

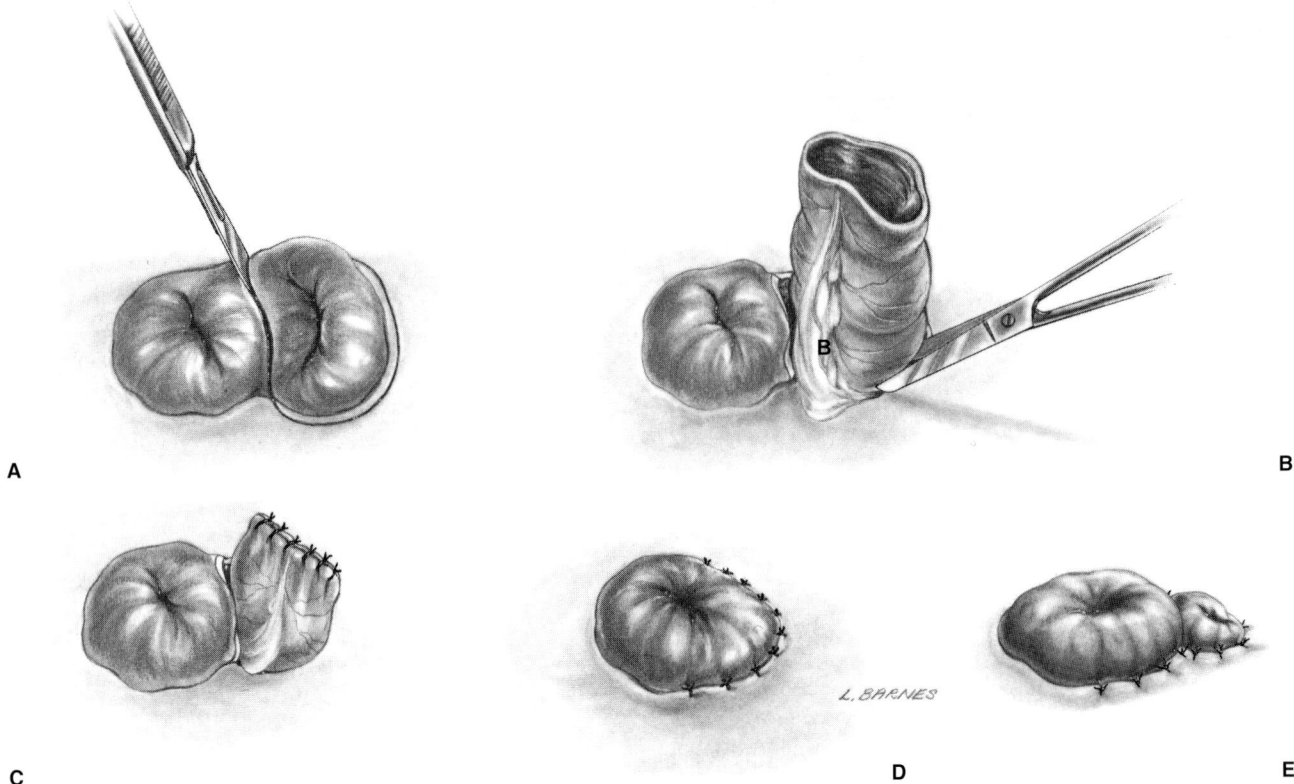

A

B

C

D

E

FIGURE 31-39. Surgical treatment of loop colostomy prolapse. **(A)** The distal mucosal rim is circumcised. **(B)** The bowel is divided. **(C)** The distal bowel is oversewn or stapled. **(D)** Final maturation as an end stoma. **(E)** Alternatively, the distal end can be opened as previously described.

preparation, intraperitoneal closure, resection of the anastomosis, and delayed (secondary) skin closure. Rosen and Friedman, however, noted that the incidence of wound infection was not significantly improved by the use of systemic or non-absorbable intestinal antibiotics.[186] Furthermore, intraperitoneal drainage alone or in combination with subcutaneous drainage resulted in the highest rate of wound infection in their experience.

Billings and colleagues suggest that the high rate of morbidity associated with colostomy closure may be attributable to an inadequate blood supply.[26] They recommend that consideration be given to performing weekly laser Doppler flowmetry of the stoma until an optimal blood flow is achieved.

Berne and colleagues performed a prospective randomized study of three different methods of wound closure: primary, primary with subcutaneous drainage, and delayed primary.[24] No statistically significant difference in frequency of wound infections was demonstrated (overall wound infection rate, 4.8%). Banerjee uses a purse-string closure of the skin that permits drainage of hematoma or exudate through the gap.[16]

Rickwood and colleagues reported a study of 100 consecutive colostomy closures in infants and children; they used a resection technique with intraperitoneal closure.[179] Wound infection was noted in 43 patients, a fecal fistula in 5, and other major complications in 8 instances. The overall morbidity, therefore, was in excess of 50%.

In addition to the studies already referred to, 11 selected reports from the literature on the results of colostomy closure revealed a mean morbidity rate of 24% (range, 14% to 38%).[10,28,56,74,98,102,148,150,169,192,240]

We reviewed our experience with colostomy closure at the Lahey Clinic from 1963 to 1974.[149] The results were most unsatisfactory, perhaps because much of the period covered during the study antedated contemporary techniques. The combined early and late morbidity was 49%, with wound infections found in about 25%. A fecal fistula occurred in 9.3%. Closure of the colostomy without resection was associated with the lowest incidence of complications (6.8%) when compared with other types of closure. Superficial subcutaneous drains did not prevent wound infections, and patients with intra-abdominal drains had an even higher incidence. Analysis of the intervals between creation and closure of the colostomies demonstrated that individuals whose stomas were closed within 3 months after creation had a morbidity rate of more than 50% (Table 31-2). This decreased to

▶ **TABLE 31-2** Interval Between Colostomy and Closure

Interval (Months)	Number of Patients	Number with Complications	Percent with Complications
0–3	41	21	51.2
4–6	35	12	34.3
7–12	26	9	34.6
>12	16	3	18.8
Total	118	45	—

From Mirelman D, Corman ML, Veidenheimer MC, et al. Colostomies: indications and contraindications: Lahey Clinic experience, 1963–1974. *Dis Colon Rectum* 1978;21:172.)

approximately 34% for closure after at least a 4-month interval.

Late complications occurred in 28 patients, with incisional hernia, suture sinus, and intestinal obstruction being the most frequently seen (Table 31-3). As previously mentioned, with a complication rate such has been reported in most series, particularly with respect to closure of the colostomy, the surgeon should be circumspect in the initial selection of patients for a diversionary procedure.

One must recognize that the results of many published studies would not tolerate the scrupulous assessment of statistical analysis, and that indeed the picture is not as discouraging as the literature often implies. Subjectively at least, most surgeons have noted a decreased incidence of complications in all aspects of bowel surgery, including that of colostomy closure. For example, Foster and colleagues compared the first and second 4-year periods of colostomy closure in their evaluation of 113 patients.[70] Improvement was noted in the rate of wound infection (24% versus 51%) and in the frequency of anastomotic leak (10% versus 30%).

Two reports demonstrate a remarkably low incidence of problems associated with colostomy closure. Salley and colleagues reported a complication rate of 7.8% in 166 patients operated on from 1974 to 1981.[191] The infec-

tion rate was extremely low—only 2.4%. The authors attributed their success to a vigorous mechanical bowel preparation and the use of luminal and parenteral antibiotics. With respect to operative technique, the bowel was sutured both by resection and by simple closure, and the wounds were closed by four different methods. Garnjobst and associates reviewed their experience of 125 consecutive colostomy closures, noting a complication rate of 5.6% in the early phase, and a later complication rate of 4% (primarily due to incisional hernia).[75] The authors credited their low rates of morbidity to simple closure rather than to resection of the bowel (no local complications in 63 patients), antibiotic wound irrigation, and primary wound closure.

Comment

If, after reading the above outlined review, the surgeon is not confused about the optimal means for avoiding complications following colostomy closure, one should be greatly surprised. If a thread of consistency can be extracted from the data, it is that early closure of the colostomy is associated with a high rate of morbidity and that resection of the bowel, in the experience of most surgeons, is more hazardous than simple closure. Wound infection is by far the most common complication. Delayed wound closure should obviate that concern, however. The following technique is the procedure I prefer.

Technique

The patient is placed on a full bowel preparation as if for colon resection. Irrigation of both limbs of the colostomy and of the rectum is performed the morning of surgery until the returns are clear. Antibiotics are administered in the operating room prior to initiating the surgery, that is, the same protocol employed for bowel resection.

The colostomy is circumcised by means of a diathermy cautery, leaving an attached cuff of skin (Figure 31-40A). No attempt is made to pack the lumen with sterile dressings or to suture the edges closed. Four Kocher clamps

▶ **TABLE 31-3** Late Complications of Colostomy Closure

Complication	Number of Patients	Percent of Series
Incisional hernia	19	16.4
Suture sinus	3	2.6
Intestinal obstruction	2	1.7
More than one of the above	4	3.7
Total	28	24.4

From Mirelman D, Corman ML, Veidenheimer MC, et al. Colostomies: indications and contraindications: Lahey Clinic experience, 1963–1974. *Dis Colon Rectum* 1978;21:172.

are placed on the skin around the colostomy, and four triple hooks (Lahey) are placed on the surrounding skin to act as retractors (Figure 31-40B). The Kocher clamps are held by the surgeon and serve as a handle while the assistant uses the hooks as retractors. The peritoneal cavity is entered, clamps are placed on the fascia, and the bowel is liberated (Figure 31-40C).

With the colostomy now separated from the abdominal wall, the skin and any remaining fibrous tissue are excised (Figure 31-41A). Closure of the anterior wall of the bowel is then effected in a transverse fashion with interrupted long-term absorbable sutures in the same manner that the anterior row of a colon anastomosis is completed (Figure 31-41B). Alternatively, if edema and fibrosis prevent safe closure, the bowel is resected and an anastomosis performed as with any colon resection. The fascia is then approximated with interrupted, heavy, long-term

absorbable sutures (Figure 31-41C). An alternative, simpler approach is to effect closure by means of a stapling technique (Figure 31-42).

Because of the high risk of infection, the wound is left open for delayed primary closure. This is accomplished by placing skin sutures in loosely and securing them onto a tongue depressor (Figure 31-43A). The wound is packed either with iodoform gauze or a Betadine-soaked sponge, and the wound is secondarily closed 3 or 4 days later (Figure 31-43B). The incision is closed completely by pulling on the tongue depressor, and the assistant merely cuts each suture in turn while the surgeon ties it. With this technique no anesthetic is required, and the tension produced by individually pulling and tying the sutures is avoided.

Postoperatively, the patient is maintained on intravenous fluids until oral intake can be tolerated. No nasogastric tube is advised.

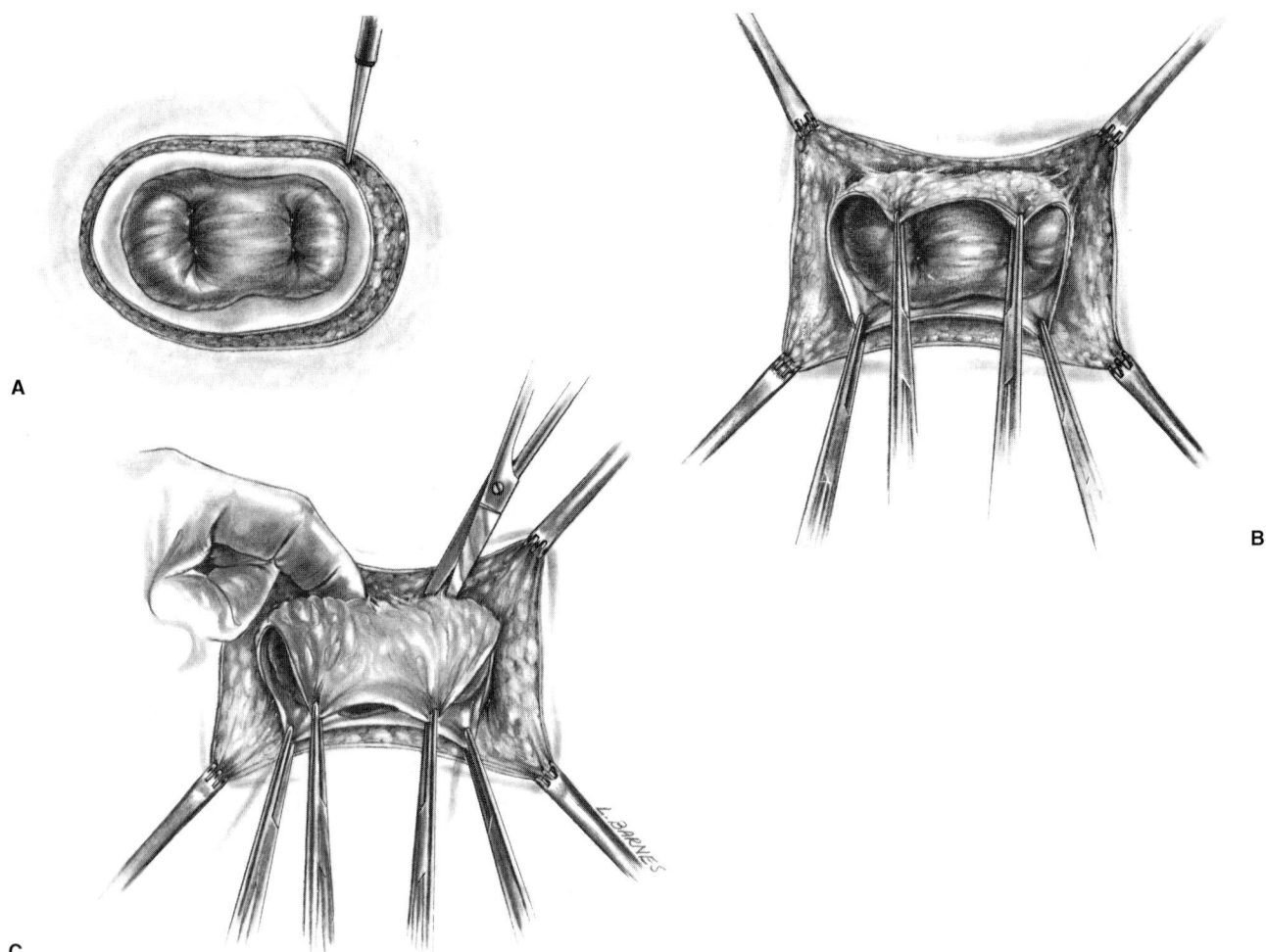

FIGURE 31-40. Technique of loop colostomy closure. **(A)** The colostomy is circumcised. **(B)** Kocher clamps on the skin around the stoma serve as a handle, and triple hooks are used as retractors. **(C)** The peritoneal cavity is entered, and the colostomy is dissected from the abdominal incision.

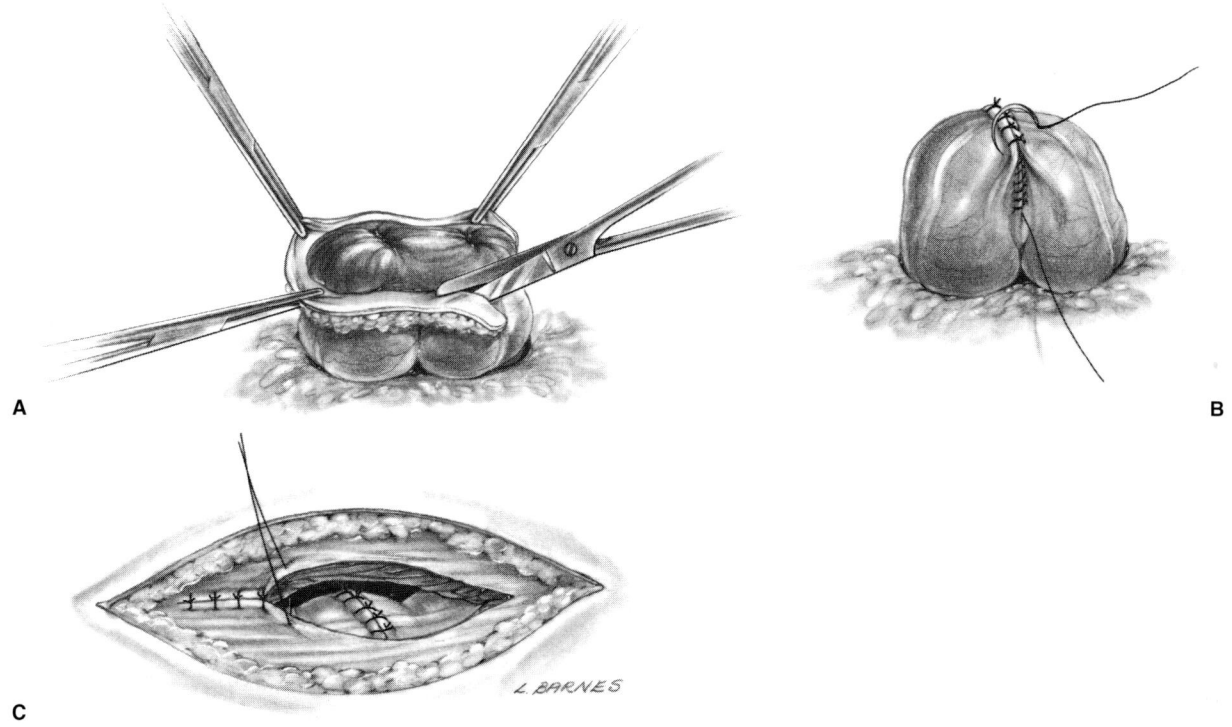

L. BARNES

FIGURE 31-41. Technique of loop colostomy closure. (**A**) Excision of the skin and eschar. (**B**) The anterior bowel wall is closed transversely. (**C**) The fascia is closed.

CECOSTOMY

The procedure of cecostomy could be removed from our surgical armamentarium with very little consequence to the quality of health care delivery. In fact, because the operation is often used for the wrong indications, it probably is responsible for adverse results more often than it ameliorates a condition. The procedure has been advocated to "protect" a left-sided anastomosis, in the treatment of large bowel obstruction, for cecal perforation, and in the management of cecal volvulus.[22,84,103,222,248] In my opinion, the only possible valid indications for performing cecostomy are cecal volvulus (see Chapter 28) and colonic ileus (Ogilvie's syndrome; see Chapter 16). But even with these conditions, the applicability is extremely limited. Simply stated, in my opinion cecostomy is anathema to quality in colorectal surgery.

A cecostomy is a decompressive procedure and, as such, produces essentially a venting of the bowel. *It does not divert the fecal stream.* Therefore, if a diversion is required, a loop ileostomy (see later) or transverse colostomy should be considered. In a study by Thomson and coworkers (Gloucester, United Kingdom), 226 patients underwent restorative rectal resection with on-table lavage and tube cecostomy.[223] Clinical anastomotic leak rates occurred in 25 patients (11.1%). The authors concluded

that not only does tube cecostomy fail to protect an anastomosis, but complications are common and may indeed be life threatening under the circumstances.

A loop ileostomy is an eminently satisfactory procedure not only for diversion, but also for permitting reasonable appliance management. Cecostomy virtually always commits the patient to continued hospitalization until such time as the opening is surgically closed. An exception to this is if a so-called tube cecostomy is employed (see Figure 28-45). Other problems may still develop, however. For example, the tube may obstruct, or the cecum may become detached from the abdominal wall, leading to an intra-abdominal abscess or even generalized peritonitis. Ultimately, the fistula may still require surgical closure.

With the limited indications mentioned, cecostomy should optimally be accomplished by the exteriorization technique. If it is to be performed as a "blind" procedure for acute cecal dilatation, a small incision is made in the right lower quadrant in a manner similar to the approach used for appendectomy. However, instead of the muscle being split, the external and internal oblique and transversus abdominis are divided. The peritoneum is exposed and carefully incised. The cecum will tend to pout into the open wound, but if it is so distended that it cannot be delivered through the incision, it can be decompressed by

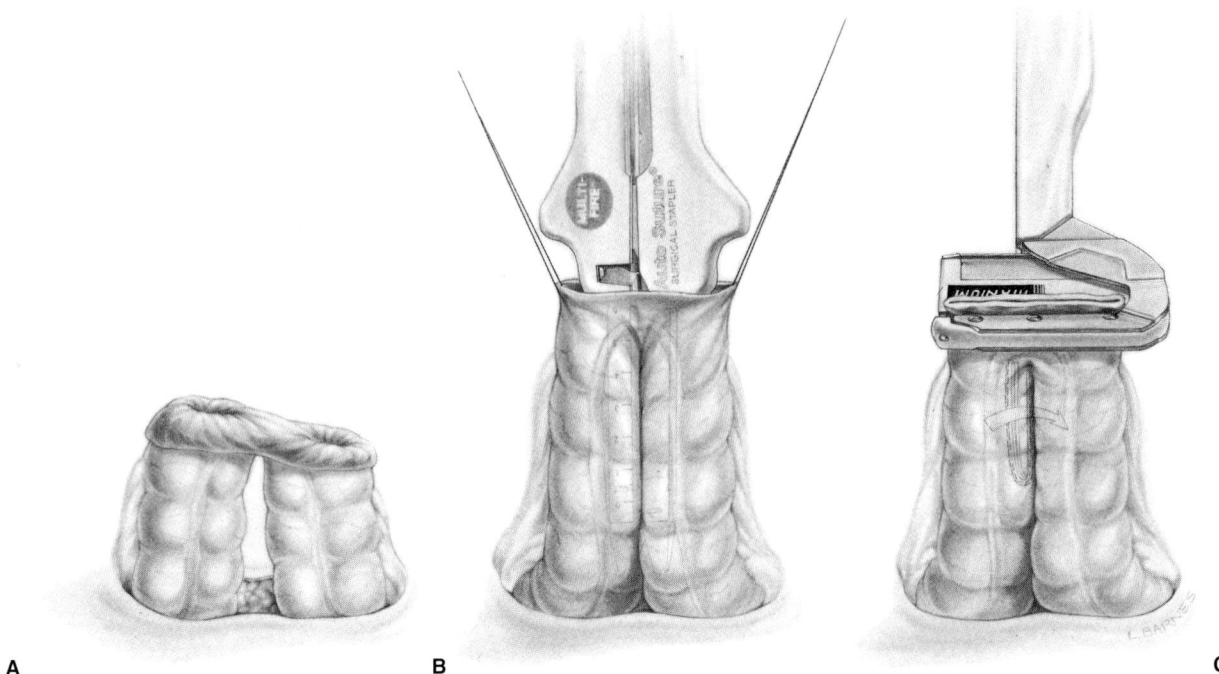

FIGURE 31-42. Closure of loop colostomy by stapling technique. **(A)** The colostomy is circumcised in the usual manner. **(B)** The GIA stapler effects a functional end-to-end anastomosis. **(C)** Closure of the bowel is accomplished with the linear stapler.

needle or trocar aspiration. The seromuscular surface of the cecum is sutured to the abdominal wall with interrupted long-term absorbable sutures (Figure 31-44). After the peritoneal cavity is walled off in this manner, the cecum is opened and the cut edge of the bowel is sutured to the full thickness of the skin in a manner similar to that used when one matures a conventional colostomy.

Even when this technique is applied properly, appliance management can be extremely cumbersome. The effluent is corrosive and liquid. But since the cecostomy does not truly divert, drainage may actually be quite minimal. It may consist mostly of gas, hence its primary benefit for decompressing an acutely dilated cecum. At least with the procedure mentioned, the cecum is unlikely to

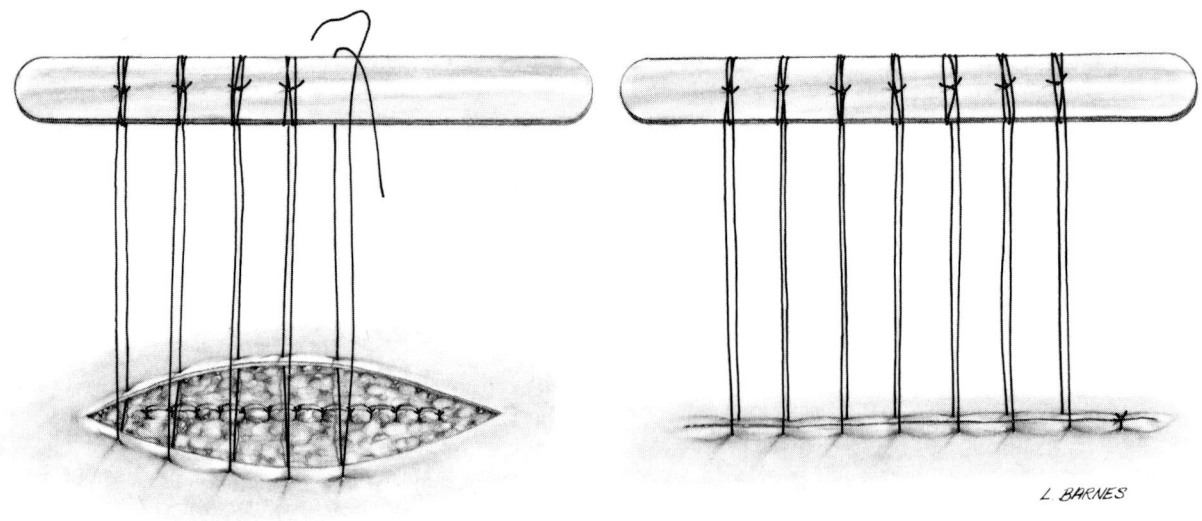

FIGURE 31-43. Delayed wound closure. **(A)** Sutures are placed and taped onto a tongue depressor. **(B)** The wound is pulled closed and the sutures tied.

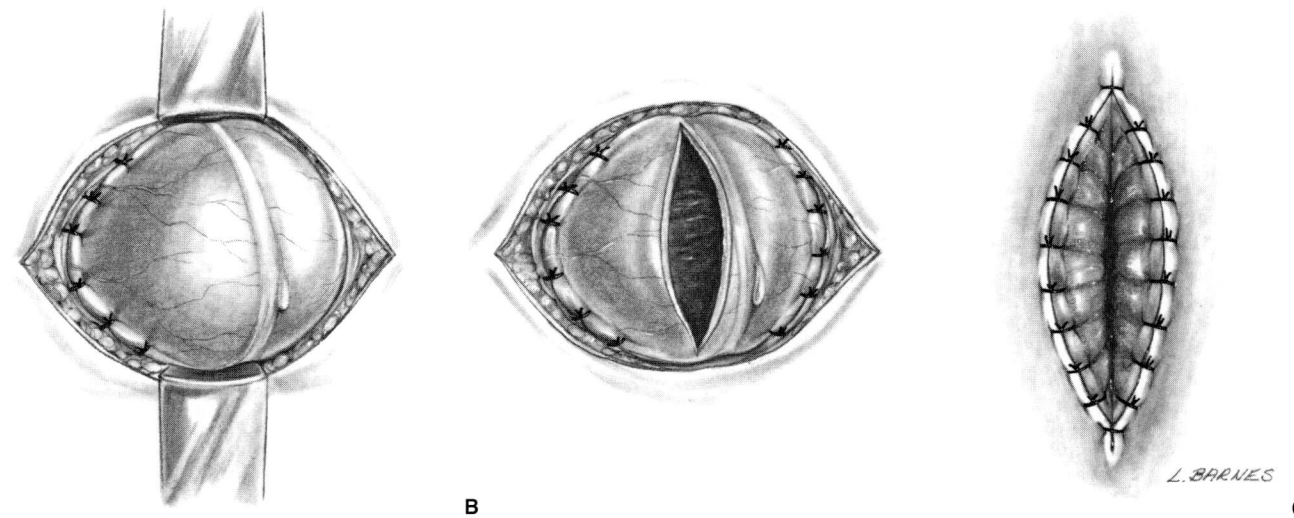

FIGURE 31-44. Technique of cecostomy. **(A)** Obliteration of the peritoneal opening by suture of the bowel wall to the fascia. **(B)** Opening of the cecum. **(C)** Primary maturation to the skin.

become detached or to retract into the peritoneal cavity, leading to a possibly life-threatening situation.

The paucity of recent literature on the subject is a testament to its lack of applicability and to its replacement by alternative diversionary procedures.

Continent Cecostomy

Kock and colleagues performed a continent cecostomy on 30 patients by isolating the cecum from the remainder of the colon and providing the distal end with an intussuscepted valve constructed from an isolated segment of ileum.[121] Eight were later given continent ileostomies, two were converted to conventional sigmoid colostomies, and one had continuity reestablished. The complication rate was 23%, with two thirds of the patients requiring revision of the intussuscepted valve. When comparing the functional results of the continent cecostomy with that of continent ileostomy, it becomes obvious that the latter is superior.

ILEOSTOMY

An ileostomy is usually advised for IBD (ulcerative colitis or Crohn's disease). Other indications include familial polyposis, carcinomatosis, trauma, and congenital anomalies. Ideally, the patient should be well informed about the need for an ileostomy long before the operation is required. It is usually of great benefit to acquaint the patient with someone of comparable age, gender, and socioeconomic status who has an ileostomy and is well adjusted to it, so that the individual can be assured

of a normal lifestyle. Unfortunately, some patients do not receive adequate preoperative counseling, either because the physician fails to mention the possibility of an ileostomy during the course of treatment of the condition, or because the patient requires urgent surgical intervention, such as may be necessary for hemorrhage, toxic megacolon, perforation, or sepsis. Under these circumstances, one may always believe that the operation was performed too precipitously and that, perhaps with more vigorous medical management, surgery might have been avoided or at least deferred until a later time.

As has been previously discussed, preoperative consideration of the placement of the stoma is mandatory. The patient may actually wear the appliance prior to the operation and note areas where subsequent appliance management may become difficult: an area of skin folds, the waist line, and the usual position of pants or belt. One should not delay the determination of the site of the stoma until the patient is on the operating table, because abdominal skin folds may not be apparent when someone is lying down.

Historic Perspective

Prior to the 1940s, for a patient to be confronted with an ileostomy was a traumatic event indeed. The colectomy itself was a high-risk procedure, often performed in stages—an initial ileostomy, then a right hemicolectomy, followed by a left hemicolectomy. The fourth stage was the proctectomy. There were no appliances as we now appreciate them, so the ileum was brought out several inches to drain with a decompression tube

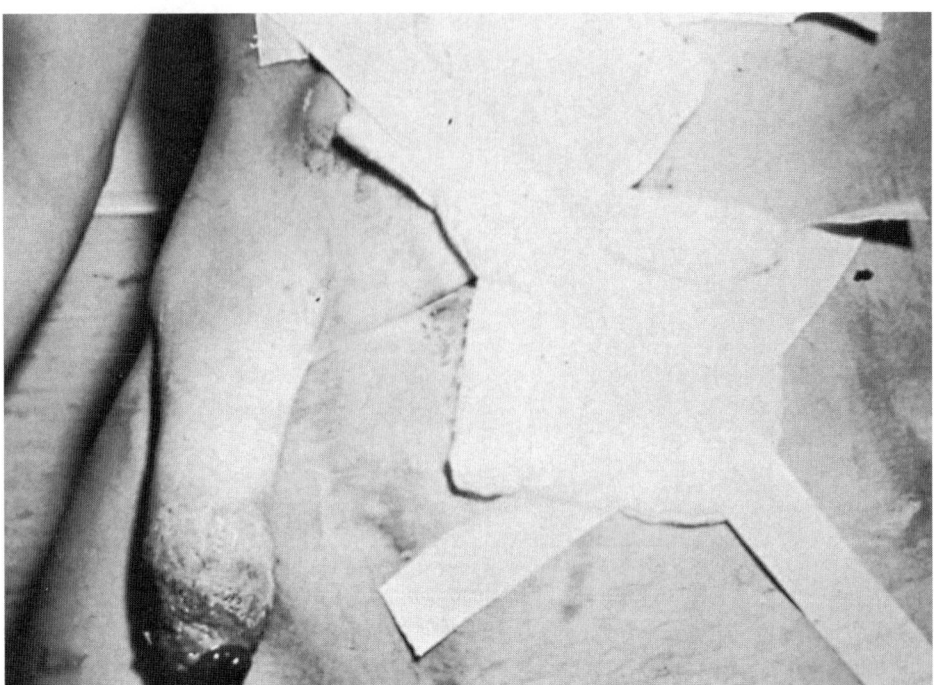

FIGURE 31-45. Dragstedt skin-grafted ileostomy created before the development of effective adhesives and the current maturation techniques. (From Corman ML, Veidenheimer MC, Coller JA. Ileostomy complications: prevention and treatment. *Contemp Surg* 1976;8:36.)

inserted. This technique is generally attributed to Cattell.[38] In 1941, grafting of skin onto the end of the ileum was suggested in order for the corrosive effluent to be able to pass into some kind of appliance, the so-called "Dragstedt ileostomy" (Figure 31-45).[58] In 1948, Sanders commented that "the therapeutic efficacy of ileostomy is antagonized by the morale-destroying elaborateness and messiness of the dressing care needed to reduce or avoid skin excoriation."[193] He felt that the Dragstedt skin-grafted ileostomy, was the most satisfactory method for addressing these shortcomings. In 1951, Warren and McKittrick of Boston, coined the

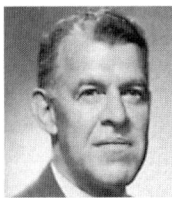

Richard B. Cattell (1900–1964) Richard Cattell was born in Martin's Ferry, Ohio. At the age of 17, he served in France as a private in a U.S. Army Evacuation Hospital. After the war, he received his A.B. from Mount Union College in Alliance, Ohio, and graduated from Harvard Medical School in 1925. Following internship at St. Luke's Hospital in New York, he joined the Lahey Clinic in 1927, demonstrating his surgical skills in many fields. Like Lahey, he acquired special experience and competence in surgery of the thyroid. He also became particularly interested in surgery of the biliary tract and pancreas and was considered the world authority on reconstruction of biliary stricture. Upon the death of Lahey in 1953, he succeeded as director of the Lahey Clinic. Cattell was largely responsible for developing the Ciné Clinics film program, one of the most popular features of the Annual Clinical Congress of the American College of Surgeons. One of the first films produced (1950) was his performance of an abdominoperineal resection. Those who worked with him remember the smooth, unhurried grace of movement, which was the outstanding characteristic of his surgical technique. His Miles resection was called "the hour of charm." Cattell became a member of the Board of Governors of the American College of Surgeons and received numerous honors and recognitions throughout the world. His vast clinical experience has been documented in a total of 252 publications. Cattell died in Boston 2 years after failing health compelled him to retire from professional activities. (Photograph courtesy of Fabian Bachrach.)

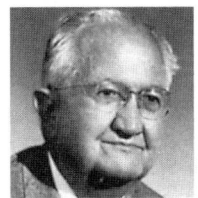

Lester R. Dragstedt (1893–1975) Lester Dragstedt was born in Anaconda, Montana, the son of Swedish immigrant parents. His entire college and professional education was taken at the University of Chicago where he received the B.S. degree in 1915, a master's degree in physiology in 1916, a Ph.D. in physiology in 1920, and the M.D. degree in 1921. His first academic appointment was as a physiologist at the State University of Iowa. In 1925, Dragstedt was recruited by Dallas B. Phemister to help design the new University Hospital research facilities on the campus of the University of Chicago. Following completion of this responsibility, Phemister appointed Dragstedt to serve as associate professor of surgery, stating, "I can teach surgery to a physiologist; I am interested in teaching physiology to surgeons." In 1947, Dragstedt succeeded Phemister as chair, a post he occupied until his retirement in 1959. Dragstedt was particularly recognized for his contributions as physiologist–surgeon to the treatment of diseases of the pancreas, parathyroids, and especially diseases of the stomach. In 1943, he performed a transthoracic vagotomy on a patient with a duodenal ulcer who refused to accept the standard operation, subtotal gastrectomy. Dragstedt was the originator of the skin-grafted ileostomy in the treatment of ulcerative colitis. He described a complete "take" of the split-thickness graft in four patients, although he perceived that the "resulting ileostomy looked somewhat like a penis." Dragstedt's competence as a basic scientist was illustrated by his election to the National Academy of Sciences. Following his Chicago retirement he became again a full-time physiologist with appointments as research professor at the University of Florida College of Medicine. Active until the end, he died at his summer home on Elk Lake, Michigan.

term "ileostomy dysfunction" to describe functional obstruction of the stoma.[144] In an evaluation based on 240 ileostomy patients, the authors recognized a syndrome of watery discharge, abdominal cramps, and hypovolemia as signs of intestinal obstruction attributed to edema of the non-everted, non-matured stoma. To overcome what they thought was contracting scar when the serosa of the ileum is exposed to the air, they recommended longitudinal incisions through the indurated seromuscular layers, performing this operation more than 100 times.[144] In 1952, a signal advance was made in ileostomy construction through Brooke's publication, which stated rather non-dramatically, "A more simple device is to evaginate the ileal end at the time of the operation and suture the mucosa to the skin; no complications have accrued from this."[29] This author further observed that the ileostomy did not retract, but stood out in conical form; furthermore, prolapse was not encountered.

At about the same time, Turnbull suggested that so-called ileostomy dysfunction could be prevented by covering the serosa of the newly constructed ileostomy with mucosa.[228] He advised a technique whereby the seromuscular coat of the distal one-half of the exteriorized ileostomy was removed, and the residual mucosal tube was pulled down over the ileostomy as a viable sliding graft. Subsequently, Crile and Turnbull confirmed Warren and McKittrick's concept of ileostomy dysfunction, a violation of the basic surgical principle of exposing an unprotected surface.[51] This exposure leads to serositis with fibrinopurulent exudate by the 3rd or 4th postoperative day; in essence, peritonitis of the protruding seg-

ment. It is on the basis of the writings of Brooke, Crile, and Turnbull that our current concepts of primary ileostomy maturation have developed.

Principles and Concerns

Despite the advances in operative technique, the creation of a satisfactory ileal stoma and the proper management of ileostomy complications are often unachieved ideals. This is not difficult to comprehend for a number of reasons.

First, most busy general surgeons perform perhaps only two or three ileostomies in a given year. Second, when the procedure is performed on an emergency basis, the surgeon's main concern is saving the patient's life, and sufficient care may not be given to creating the stoma. For example, during a colectomy and ileostomy for toxic megacolon, the colon must be removed as expeditiously as possible. In addition, the patient's cardiac, renal, and pulmonary functions may be severely compromised. With these pressing concerns, the surgeon may not be as meticulous as he or she should in performing the ileostomy.

Another reason for difficulties with ileostomy management may be the surgeon's lack of familiarity with techniques for properly locating and maturing the stoma. Besides problems with the appliance itself, the primary causes of encumbrance following an ileostomy are improper placement and incorrect construction of the stoma.

Unfortunately, a mystique surrounds stomal management. Surgeons who can successfully treat gangrene of the abdominal wall are confounded by a peristomal der-

---

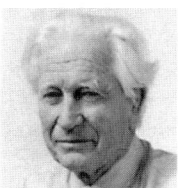

Bryan N. Brooke (b. 1915) Bryan Brooke graduated from Cambridge and St. Bartholomew's Hospital in 1940, achieving his F.R.C.S. in 1942 and masters in surgery in 1944. After military service in World War II, he was appointed senior lecturer in Aberdeen in 1946 and reader in surgery at the University of Birmingham in 1947. In 1963, he was offered the chair in surgery at St. George's Hospital in London, a position he occupied until 1976. Many of Brooke's important writings were in the field of colon and rectal surgery, including that of ulcerative colitis and Crohn's disease. As a consequence of his unique contributions to the development of improved surgical techniques for stomal construction, he was motivated to become founder and president of the Ileostomy Association of Great Britain and Ireland, a post he held for 26 years. A recipient of many awards, he was recognized by Corpus Christi College of Cambridge University through the Copeman Medal for scientific research. Additionally, he received the A.B. Graham award of the American Proctologic Society in 1961 and is an honorary fellow of many international organizations. Brooke has been described as an individual with a great zest for life, coupled with a wonderful sense of humor. He has held numerous one-man exhibitions of his paintings, many of which currently reside at prominent public institutions throughout the world. Professor Brooke resides in London, retired from the active practice of surgery, but not from painting or writing.

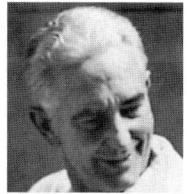

Rupert Beach Turnbull, Jr. (1913–1981) Rupert Turnbull was born in Pasadena, California. An outstanding athlete, he represented the United States in the 1932 Olympics in Italy, and won the cup for outboard hydroplane racing. He attended Pomona College, graduating in 1936, and achieved his medical degree from McGill University in 1940. During World War II, he served in the South Pacific as a field surgeon and then in China as hospital commander. Following the war, he elected to continue his surgical training at the Cleveland Clinic and ultimately joined the staff. Turnbull began to develop an interest in colon and rectal surgery, especially after he "inherited" the ostomy patients of his late chief, Tom Jones. Many of his earlier writings, in particular, were on stomal problems and their management. He serendipitously discovered the value of karaya as a skin protector and co-designed the first postoperative pouch for ostomy patients. Through his encouragement, the nursing specialty of enterostomal therapy was initiated. In 1962, during a convention held in Cleveland, Turbull was a principal in founding the United Ostomy Association. Turnbull contributed extensively to the literature, primarily in the treatment of inflammatory bowel disease and cancer. With his colleague, Frank L. Weakley, he wrote the definitive *Atlas of Intestinal Stomas*. Turnbull achieved numerous honors and distinctions throughout his career. He is remembered as a master surgeon and an innovative thinker. (Photo courtesy of the Cleveland Clinic.)

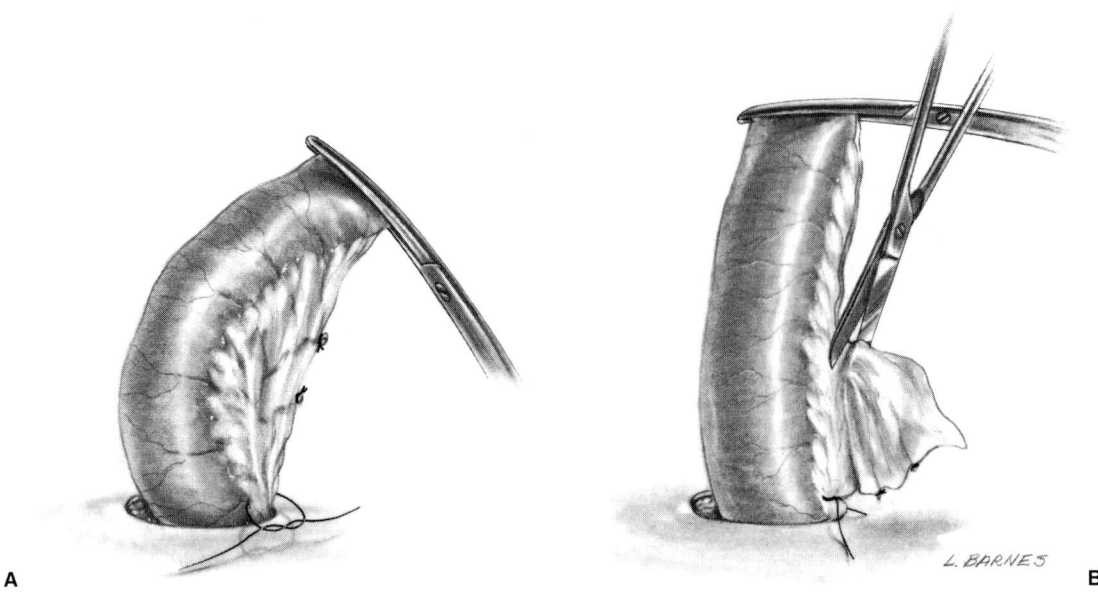

FIGURE 31-46. Maturation of ileostomy stoma by excising the mesentery. **(A)** Ligation of the mesentery at the skin level. **(B)** Trimming of the mesentery to remove the "chordee." (Adapted from Turnbull RB, Weakley FL. *Atlas of intestinal stomas*. St. Louis: Mosby, 1967.)

matitis. In the past, patients themselves had to search for answers amidst ignorance and superstition. It was because of this lack of support that ostomy associations were formed. Today patients with stoma problems are most often referred to these groups. Enterostomal therapy is designed to meet the needs of such individuals, but the person's own physician can assist greatly by learning how to apply a few, simple principles.

Technique

A disk of skin is excised from a previously marked site on the abdominal wall. Because a subcuticular technique is used instead of sutures through full-thickness skin, it is preferable to cut the skin obliquely, such as shown in Figure 23-22A. This emphasizes the subcuticular aspect for easy suturing. The ileum is brought through the split rectus muscle protruding for a distance of approximately 4 or 5 cm. There is no reason to create a stoma that when everted is longer than 2 cm, because the appliances that are now available are so satisfactory that a phallus-like ileostomy is truly unnecessary. Following extraperitoneal or intraperitoneal fixation (see Figs. 29-44 and 29-45), the mesentery to the distal ileum is trimmed (Figure 31-46).

Turnbull and Weakley have advised passing an absorbable suture around the mesentery at skin level and excising the mesenteric fat from the distal ileum to overcome the bowing effect (Figure 31-46).[229] The submucosal vascular supply can nourish at least 6 cm of ileum after the mesentery has been divided. While this may be a safe maneuver in patients with ulcerative colitis, those

with Crohn's disease who may have a thickened mesentery or in whom the bowel is partially obstructed do not tolerate mesenteric stripping for such a length. One should exercise caution in carrying out this maneuver under such circumstances. At this point, any redundant ileum should be amputated leading to a final ileostomy length of approximately 2 cm.

Three sutures are then placed, one on the anti-mesenteric aspect and one each on either side of the mesentery (Figure 31-47). A triangulation technique is recommended. This consists of a full-thickness suturing of the end of the bowel, the seromuscular aspect of the ileum (at the skin level), and the subcuticular skin. The seromuscular bite aids in the subsequent eversion of the bowel. Some surgeons criticize this method because of the risk of possible fistula formation should the suture be placed too deeply. Obviously, care is required if one is to perform this maneuver properly and avoid this complication. Babcock clamps placed within the bowel lumen and at the end facilitate eversion. With proper length and appropriate eversion, the stoma is primarily matured (Figure 31-48). Interrupted sutures of no. 4–0 chromic catgut complete the construction.

Complications: Prevention and Treatment

Complications following an ileostomy may be due to a technical error on the part of the surgeon, such as improper location or a faulty maturation technique. Second, disease may be a cause for subsequent stomal problems.

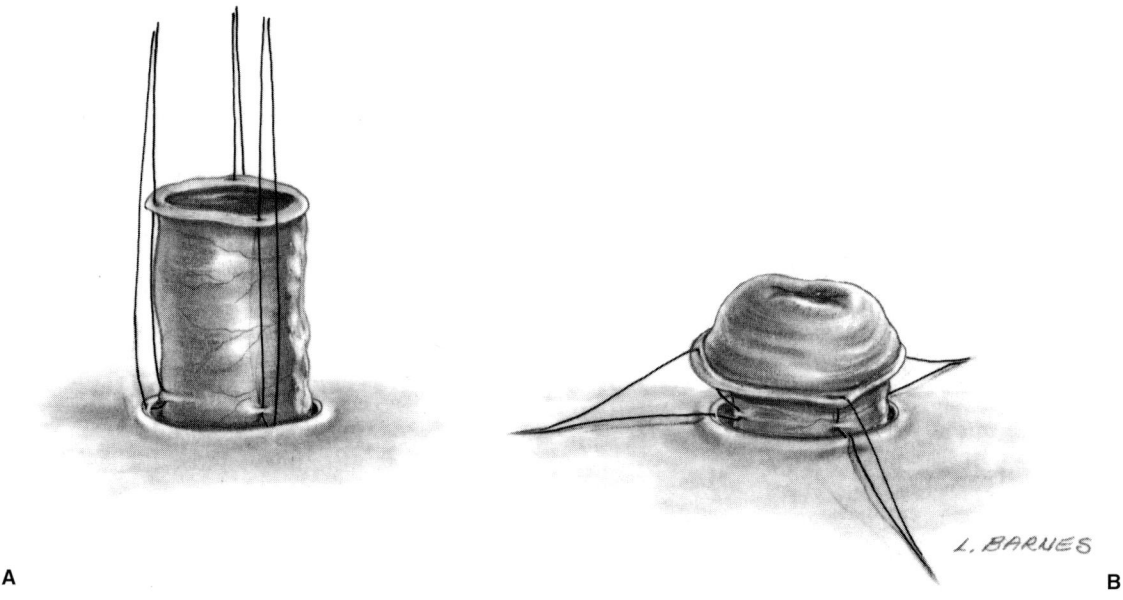

A   B

FIGURE 31-47. Maturation of ileostomy stoma. **(A)** Three sutures are placed, incorporating the sero-muscular layer to facilitate eversion. **(B)** The sutures are secured, everting the bowel.

Third, the patient, either through inadequate education, neglect, or misuse, can precipitate stomal problems that may actually necessitate surgical intervention.

Complications Due to Improper Maturation Technique

Stenosis and Retraction

Stenosis and retraction are the most common indications for revising an ileostomy in our experience.[82] My colleagues and I noted that 30% of revisions were performed for these reasons. Speakman and colleagues estimated an incidence of 18.5% from the literature.[207] As has been mentioned with respect to colostomy, the primary causes are inadequate initial stomal length, vascular compromise, and improper skin excision (Figure 31-49). With respect to the issue of blood supply, the attitude that the stoma may be a little purple or perhaps a bit blue, but it will probably be all right, is usually an unrealized prophecy. It is far preferable to reopen the abdomen and create an adequate length of viable bowel, prolonging the operation for whatever time is necessary, than to return on a subsequent occasion or to relegate the patient to a disability because of difficulty in managing the appliance. In addition to one of these factors (Figure 31-50), weight gain may also be responsible (Figure 31-51). It is not inconceivable that a patient can triple his or her weight within a period of 1 year following proctocolectomy.

Handelsman and Fishbein recommend that retraction or prolapse can be prevented by placing a ribbon of fascia obtained from the abdominal wall through the mesentery adjacent to the bowel between the vessels.[93] It is neither wrapped around the intestine nor sutured to it. The authors believe that this technique will secure the position of the ileostomy without risking a possible fistula from suturing the bowel wall. I personally doubt the need for such a procedure.

Treatment Ideally, revision of a stenosis or retraction may be accomplished without a formal abdominal operation. Unfortunately, retraction is a complication that may sometimes require a laparotomy in order to obtain the desired length of ileum necessary to create a satisfactory stoma. Therefore, it is prudent to warn the patient that this may be an eventuality.

Correction of the retraction or stenosis requires (1) excision of sufficient skin to create a proper-sized opening, and (2) mobilization of the bowel as much as is necessary to prepare a stoma of adequate length. Intraperitoneal freeing of the ileum is carried out as far as possible, and the stoma is matured in the usual manner. Truedson and Press suggest the implantation of three strips of polyglactin 910 (Vicryl) mesh, longitudinally fixed to the serosa prior to eversion, in order to prevent subsequent retraction.[227]

Winslet and colleagues describe a method of stabilization to prevent recurrence of retraction by means of a GIA stapling device without the blade.[247] This can be accomplished without an anesthetic, but only if the retraction is not of the fixed type. That is, the ileostomy protrudes for an appropriate length but intermittently falls back to produce a flush or retracted stoma. Three

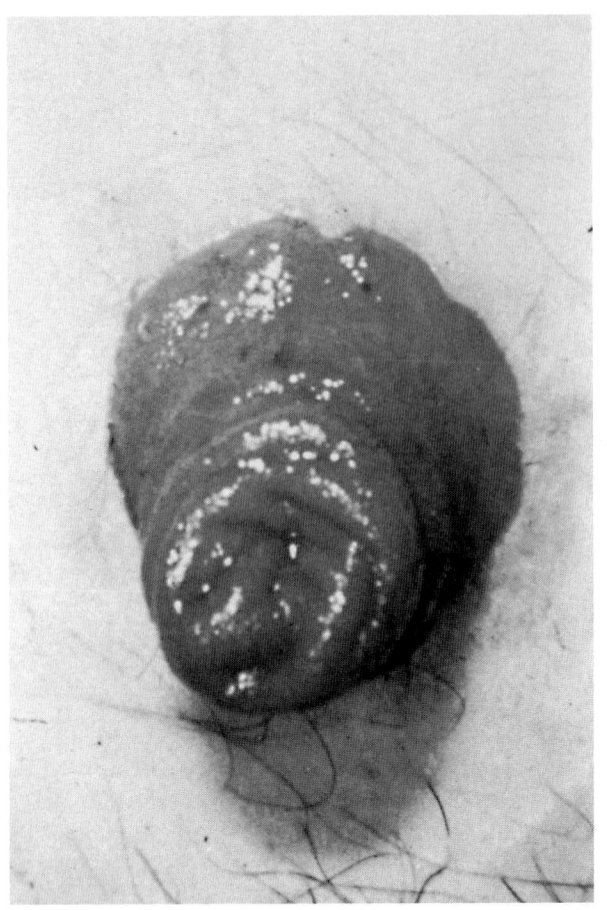

FIGURE 31-48. Normal ileostomy of optimal length.

rows of the stapler are fired the length of the ileostomy. One may also elect to use a linear stapler for the same purpose, thereby facilitating the maintenance of an everted position. The authors comment that initially the stoma is unsightly, but after 6 weeks the staples are no longer evident. Speakman and associates reported the St. Mark's Hospital experience with this method in ten patients.[207] There were four failures requiring additional surgery (40%: two re-retractions, one sepsis, one abscess).

A particularly difficult problem arises when an individual subsequently becomes obese, and the stoma disappears into the fat. This can be addressed by performing a panniculectomy and abdominoplasty, with relocation of the stoma into the new, flattened abdominal wall. Such an operative undertaking does not necessarily require the expertise of a plastic surgeon. As a matter of fact, plastic surgeons are often reluctant to embark upon a major reconstruction when there is risk of contamination from stool or the presence of a stoma. However, we who muck around in the bowels all day have no such fear. Besides, the principles of skin flap elevation and advancement are quite familiar to colon and rectal surgeons (see Anoplasty section, Chapter 8). One does not require advanced reconstructive surgical credentialing to perform this relatively straightforward operation. Figure 31-52 illustrates the technique for accomplishing a revision under these circumstances. Evans and colleagues performed abdominal wall re-contouring and stomal revision on eight patients using a similar technique.[61] All experienced improvement in appliance management and body image.

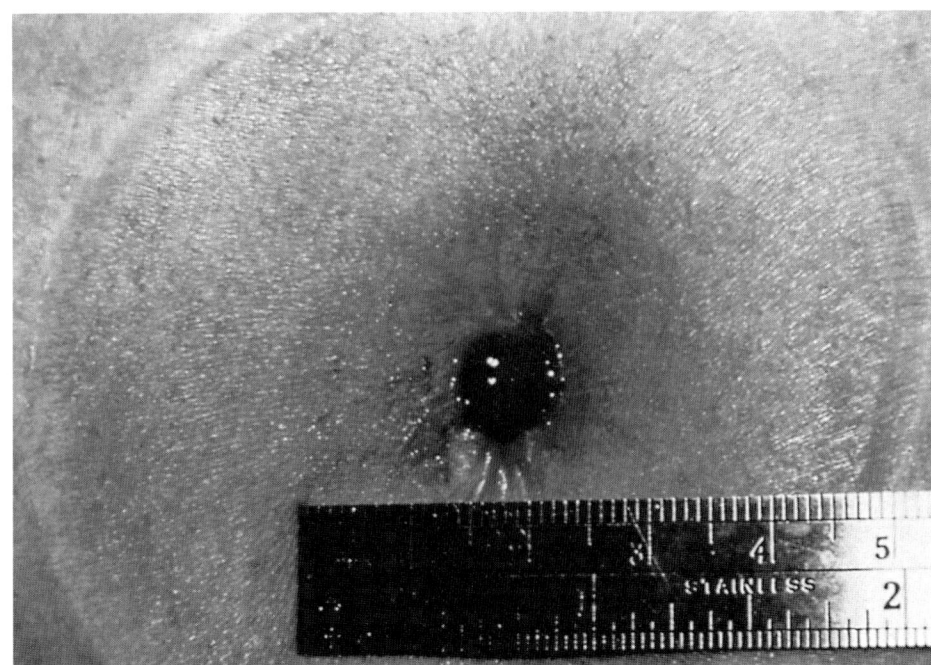

FIGURE 31-49. Stenotic ileostomy due to inadequate skin excision and necrosis of the end of the ileum.

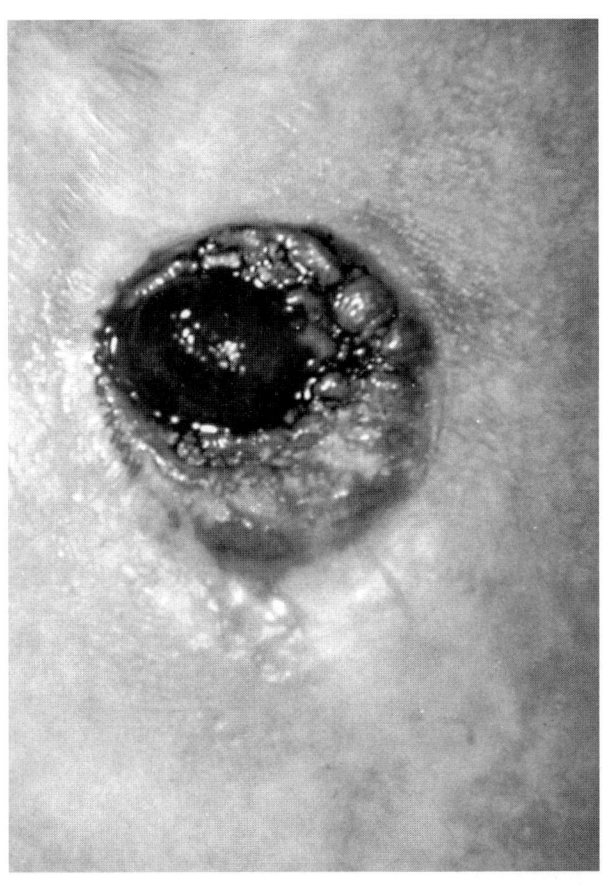

FIGURE 31-50. Retracted ileostomy with stricture due to inadequate length of the initially created stoma. (From Corman ML, Veidenheimer MC, Coller JA. Ileostomy complications: prevention and treatment. *Contemp Surg* 1976;8:36.)

Prolapse

Prolapse may be of two types: fixed (irreducible) or sliding. In my experience, the fixed type always occurs without any prior history of stomal revision. Conversely, the sliding type is seen with the second or later revision. This implies inadequate abdominal fixation and indicates that mobilizing an ileostomy when performing a revision predisposes to subsequent problems with the sliding type of prolapse (Figure 31-53). Prolapse is usually not associated with skin problems if it is of the fixed type, but if it retracts and becomes flush, leakage can occur. Too long a stoma is prone to trauma from contact with the appliance and may lead to psychological problems as well (Figure 31-54).

Treatment If the stomal protrusion is not a true prolapse, but simply an ileostomy that was created too long initially, treatment is relatively simple. The ileal mucosa is incised, preserving the mucocutaneous junction, and the stoma is inverted (Figure 31-55). Redundant ileum is resected, and the stoma is matured in the usual manner. This maneuver is identical to that shown earlier for colostomy prolapse, remembering that the incision must be made into the bowel itself, not into the skin. This will maintain the proper-sized opening in the abdominal wall.

One should not attempt to perform an intra-abdominal dissection so that the intraperitoneal fixation is not disrupted. Occasionally, however, with a sliding type of prolapse, so much small bowel is delivered that some form of intraperitoneal fixation is required. Reduction of

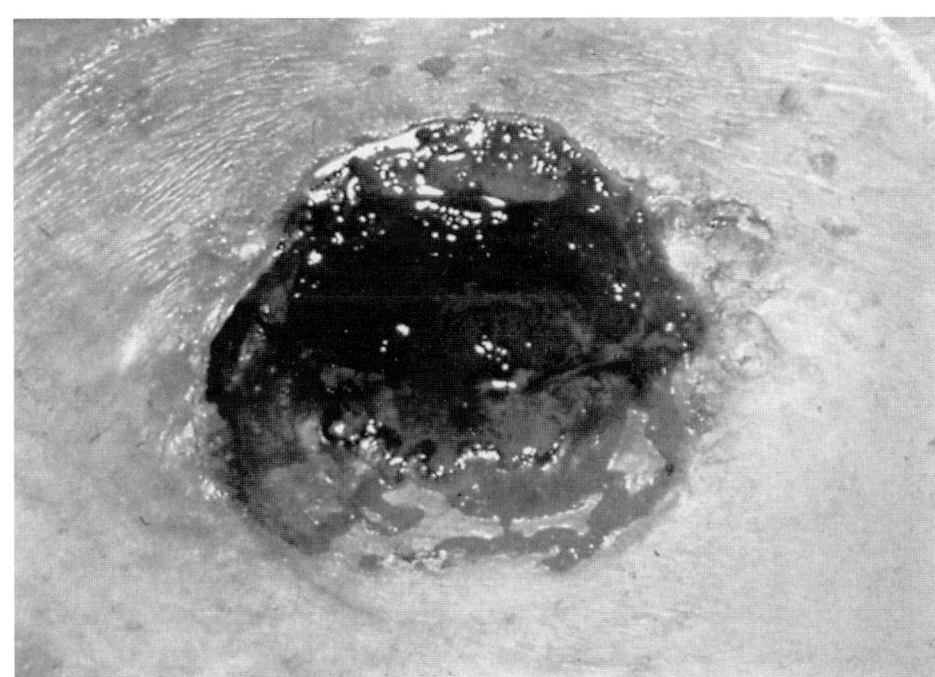

FIGURE 31-51. Retracted ileostomy with skin excoriation secondary to weight gain. (From Corman ML, Veidenheimer MC, Coller JA. Ileostomy complications: prevention and treatment. *Contemp Surg* 1976;8:36.)

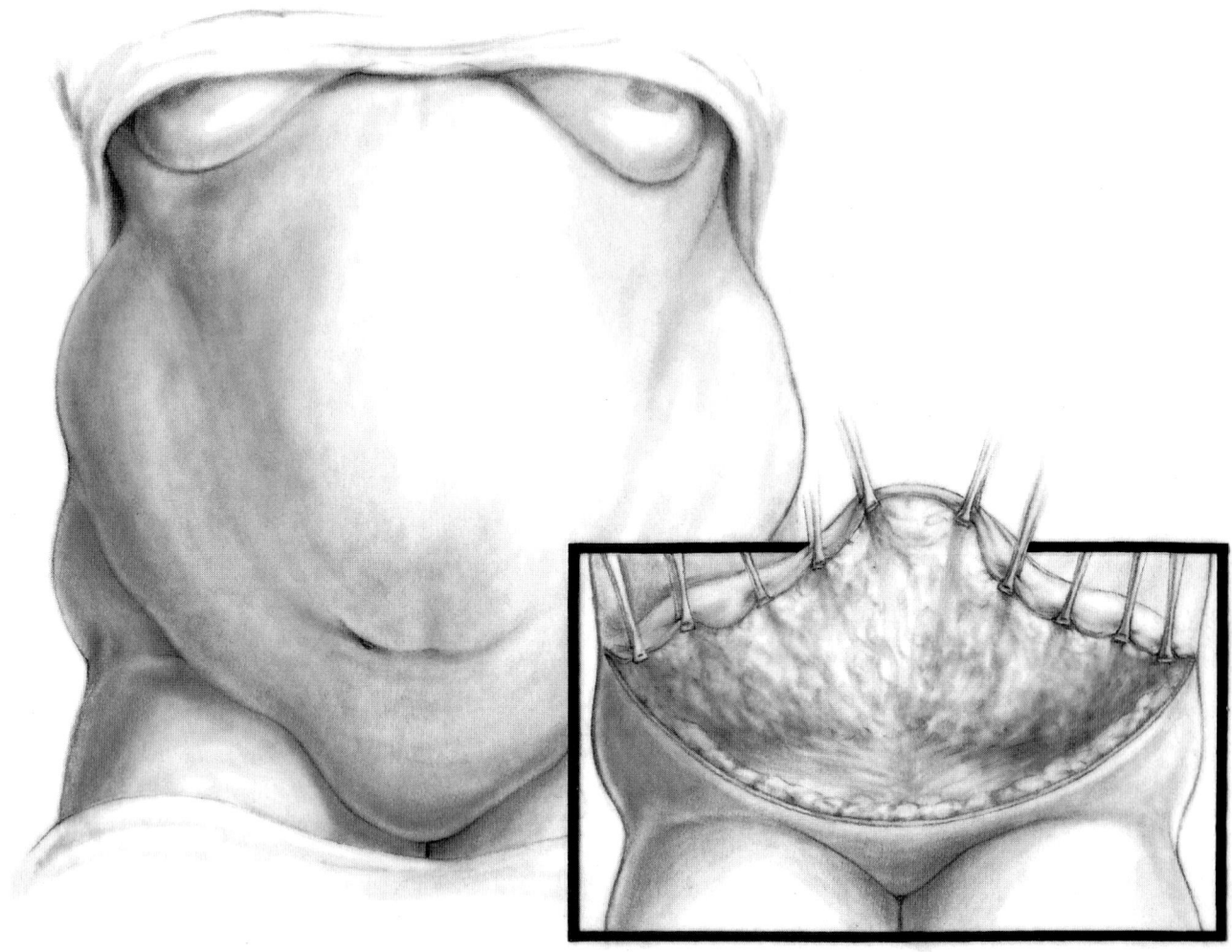

A   B

FIGURE 31-52. Technique for revision of an ileostomy due to weight gain (panniculectomy and abdominoplasty). **(A)** Ileostomy is retracted into fold of panniculus. **(B)** Long, transverse, suprapubic incision deepened to expose the fascia. *(continued)*

the ileum is usually technically difficult to accomplish and may result in recurrence of the prolapse, but resection of a long segment of intestine is not justified. Intraperitoneal fixation may necessitate a laparotomy to manage the complication adequately. Alternatively, one may consider the linear stapling method of fixation mentioned in the previous section.

Fistula

Fistula is not an uncommon reason for ileostomy revision in that 15% are performed for this indication. The most frequent cause of fistula is recurrent Crohn's disease. Erosion of the stoma by the faceplate of an appliance or from deep placement of a suture (Figure 31-56) are other possible etiologies. This complication presents a much more difficult management problem than does prolapse. Closure of the fistula may be attempted if no in-

flammatory disease is present, but subsequent breakdown is quite likely. If the fistula is resected, a laparotomy may be required in order to obtain sufficient length of ileum for adequate maturation.

Greatorex suggested a simplified method for closing a fistula, the insertion of a pipe cleaner soaked in 6% aqueous phenol.[89] Immediate cessation of leakage with subsequent healing occurred in two of three patients.

Greenstein and colleagues identified 15 of 214 patients with an ileostomy constructed for Crohn's disease who developed a paraileostomy fistula.[90] In every case, this was due to recurrent disease. All required resection and reconstruction of the stoma.

If the skin at the original stomal site has been injured by the ileal effluent or if additional small bowel must be resected, the stoma should be created in an alternative location, usually in the left lower quadrant.

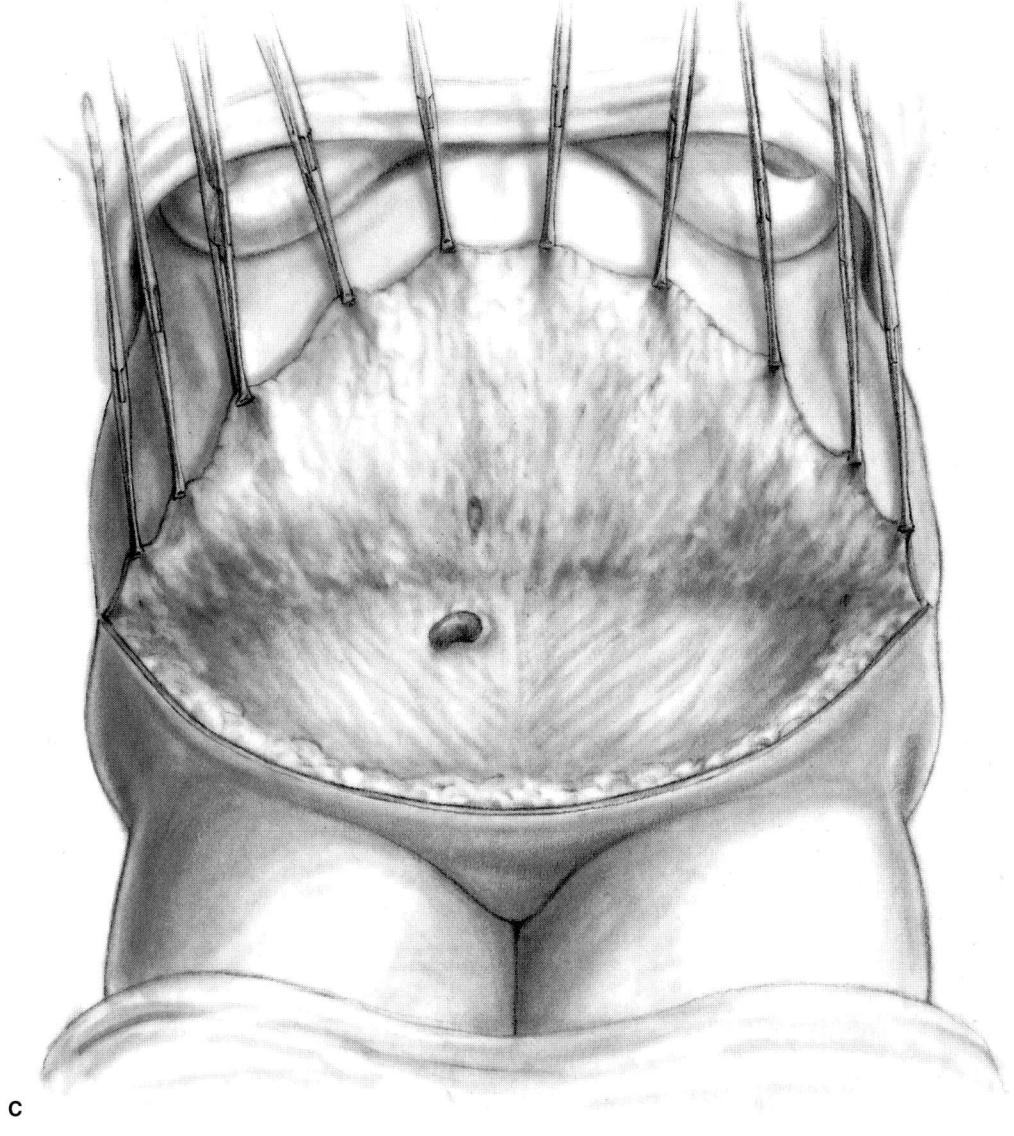

c

FIGURE 31-52. *(continued)* **(C)** The skin and subcutaneous tissue are elevated to the costal margin, detaching the stoma.

Seeding

Seeding of viable ileal mucosa can develop along the suture line if subcuticular sutures for maturation are not employed (Figure 31-57). Such seeding can lead to persistent secretion and, consequently, to problems in fitting the appliance (Figure 31-58).

Management For what might seem to be a rather trivial concern, treatment is quite difficult. Attempts at cauterizing of the ectopically located mucosa are fruitless. The only effective management is excision, and even with this procedure the viable ileal mucosal cells may grow again to the surface from a deeply implanted location. A plastic surgical procedure, rotating a skin flap to cover the defect, may be attempted successfully, but more often relocation of the stoma may be required.

This is a totally preventable complication if one uses a subcuticular suturing technique.

Complications Due to Improper Placement

The above complications were due to errors in ileostomy maturation technique. Another cause of difficulty after stomal construction is the initial improper location of the stoma. As discussed previously, the site chosen should be free of eschar, especially if the scar is irregular rather than flat. The stoma should not be near any bony promontory, such as the iliac crest (Figure 31-59) or the rib margin (Fig-

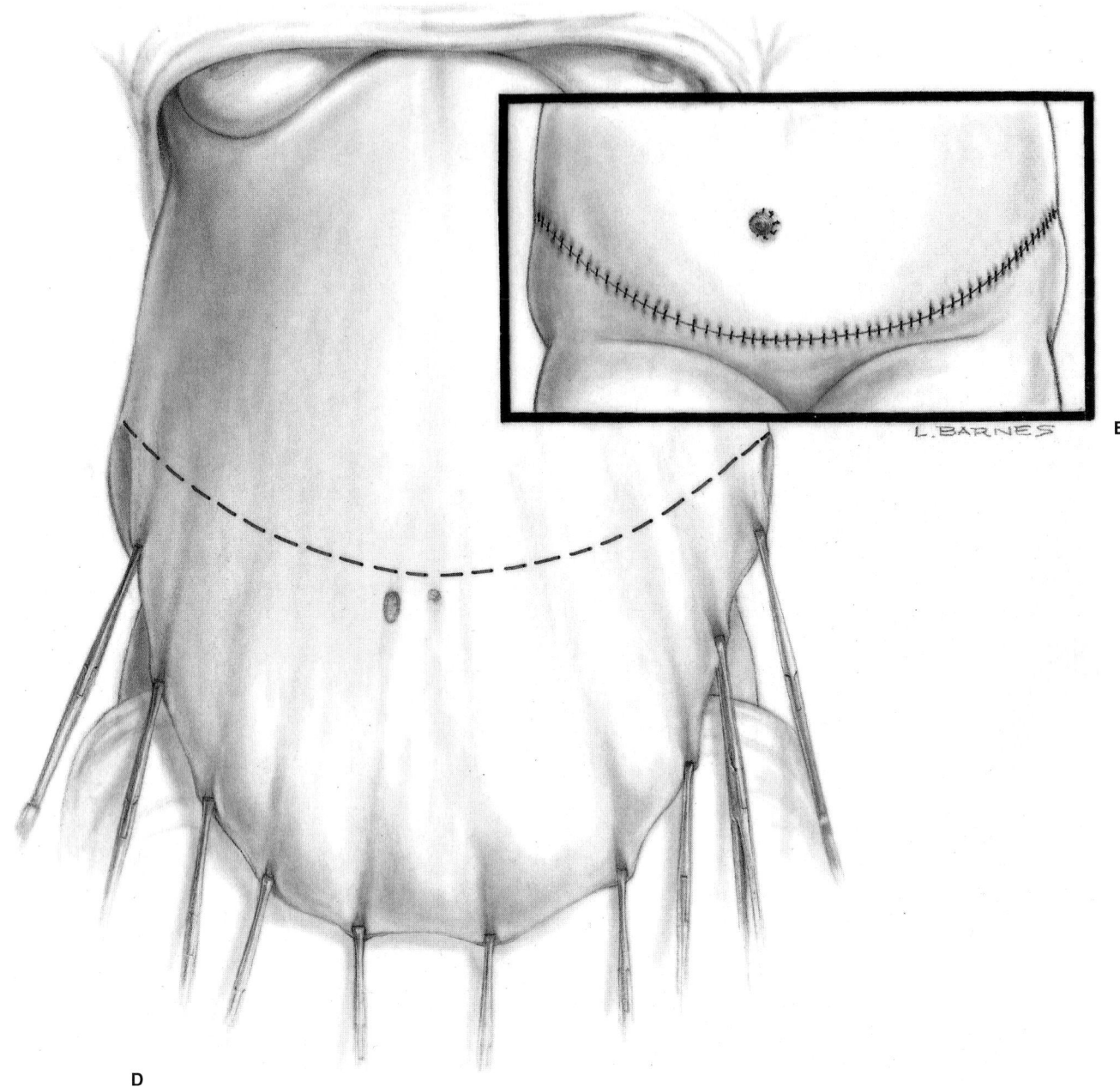

D

FIGURE 31-52. *(continued)* **(D)** The panniculus is advanced and the redundant tissue excised (usually just above the umbilicus). **(E)** The new opening is created for the ileostomy, and the stoma is matured in the usual way. Closed-suction, subcutaneous drains (not shown) are advised. If a hernia is present, mesh may be used for the repair. If further intestinal length or relocation of the stoma is necessary, the abdomen may be opened.

ure 31-60), and should be placed in such a way that the intestine can be pulled through the split rectus muscle. Failure to do so often results in peristomal herniation (Figure 31-61). Bringing the stoma through the incision is contraindicated with an ileostomy, not only because of the risk of hernia, but also because of the difficulties in maintaining an appliance and the delay in wound healing created by spilling of the effluent onto the skin (Figure 31-62). The

stoma must be placed in an area where the patient can care for it properly, wearing the appliance with confidence, without the fear of leakage (Figure 31-63).

Treatment

If the stoma is improperly located and appliance management is unsatisfactory, relocation is necessary. This usually involves a laparotomy with its attendant morbid-

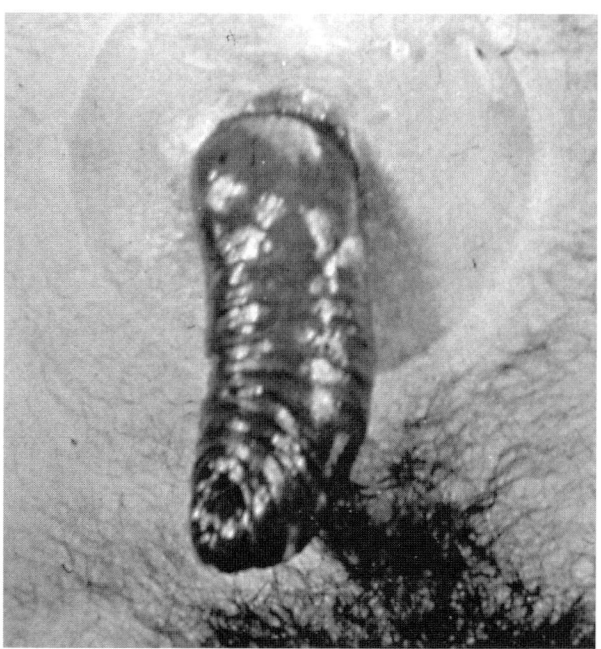

FIGURE 31-53. Ileostomy "prolapse" in this patient was due to creating a too-long stoma initially.

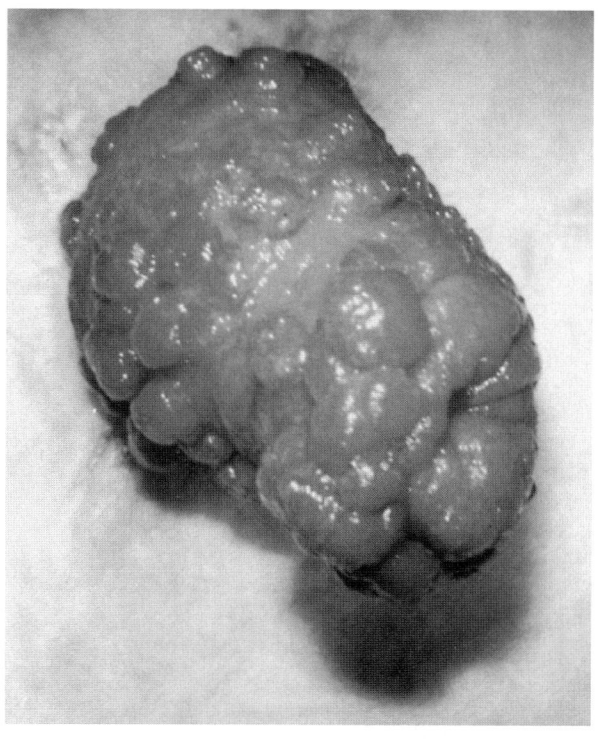

FIGURE 31-54. A prolapse of ileostomy causing irritative trauma from the appliance. This produces so-called pseudo-epitheliomatous hyperplasia.

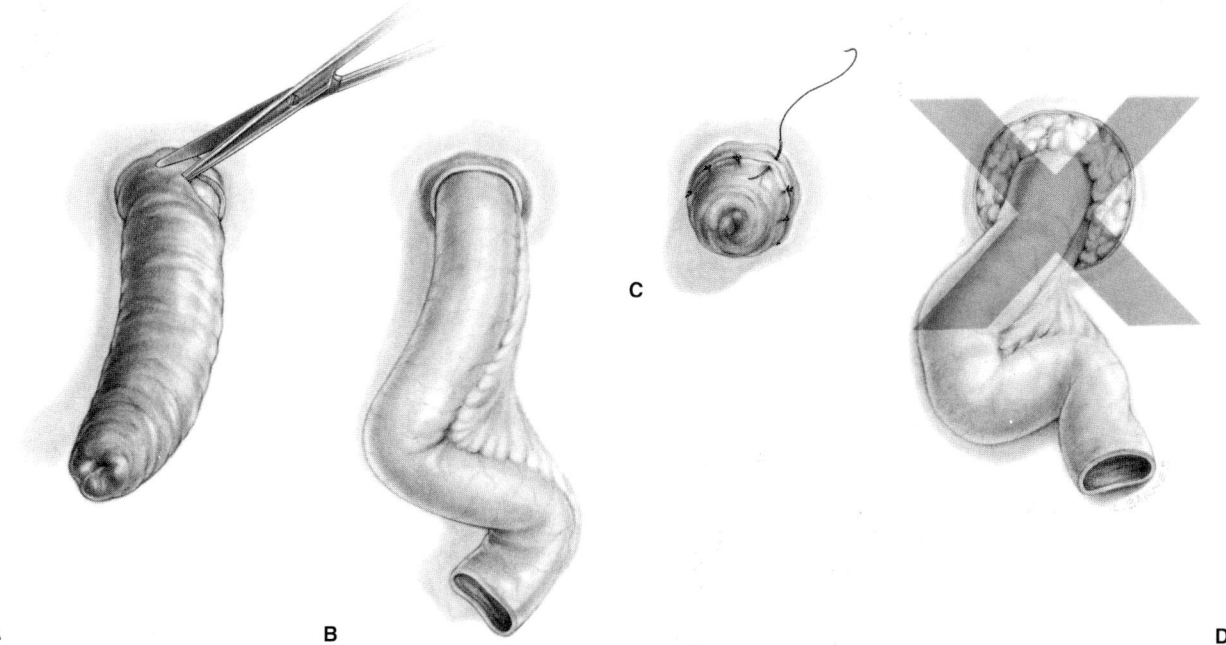

FIGURE 31-55. Revision of ileostomy prolapse. **(A)** Incision is made into the ileostomy, not at the mucocutaneous junction. A large skin opening should be avoided. **(B)** The redundant bowel is delivered. **(C)** The ileostomy is then "matured" in the usual way. **(D)** A large defect would be produced if the incision had initially been made in the skin.

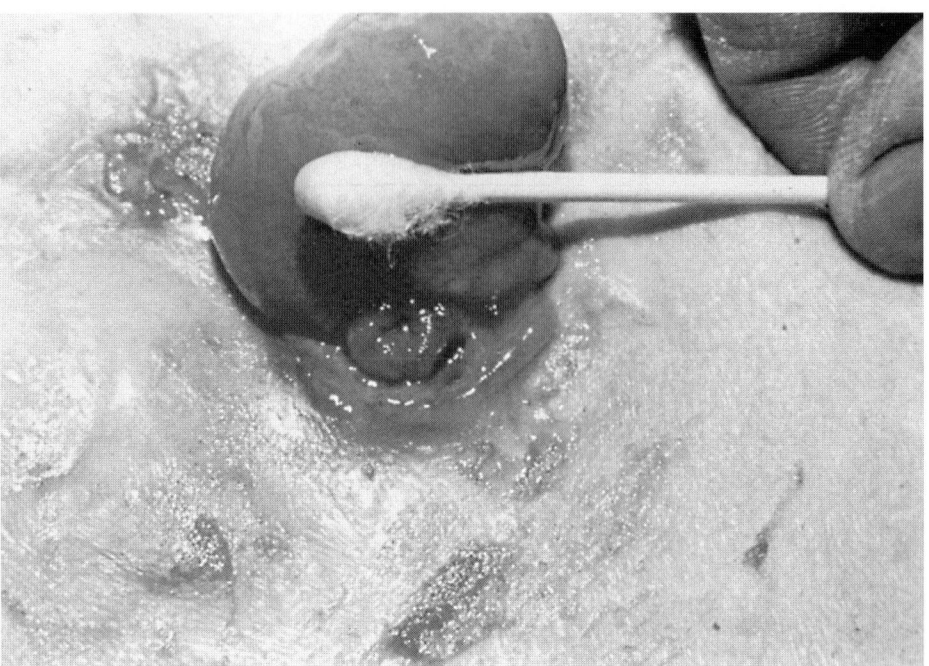

FIGURE 31-56. Ileostomy fistula presumed secondary to a deeply placed seromuscular anchoring suture. (From Corman ML, Veidenheimer MC, Coller JA. Ileostomy complications: prevention and treatment. *Contemp Surg* 1976;8:36.)

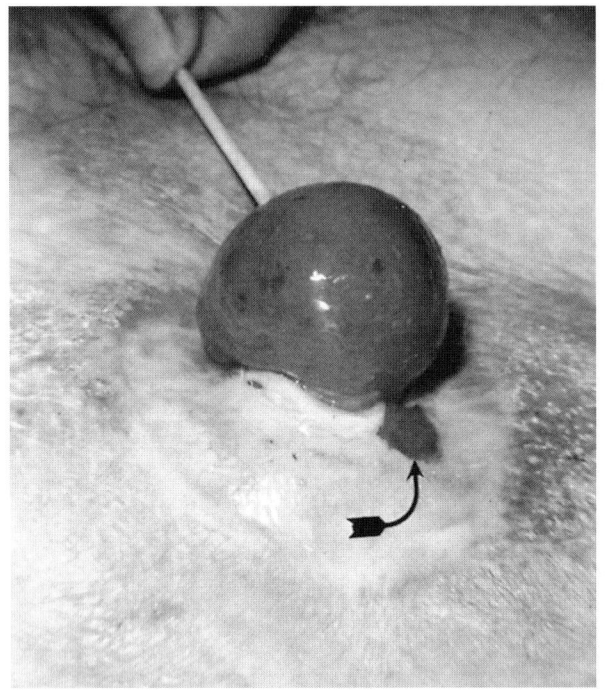

FIGURE 31-57. Mucosal "seeding" (*arrow*) due to improper suturing of the ileum to the subcuticular skin.

ity, although it is possible to perform a revision and relocation of the stoma by a tunneling method, without a complete abdominal exploration.[218] As usual, the site selection is carefully determined preoperatively. The ileal stoma is mobilized by a circumstomal incision into the peritoneal cavity. The distal segment is delivered if possible and resected. The bowel is returned to the peritoneal cavity after closure of the distal end. Long sutures are left outside the abdomen should retrieval be necessary. By blunt dissection from the original abdominal wall opening, a space is created to tunnel the distal ileum to the new site. A disk of skin is excised, the rectus is split, and the peritoneal cavity is entered at the new location. The ileum is pulled through by means of the long sutures that had been left attached, and the new stoma is constructed.

Comment

Although one can avoid a larger incision by this technique, I do not believe that it is a quantum advance in the treatment of ileostomy complications requiring revision. The fact of the matter is that stomal location errors are completely preventable problems.

Paraileostomy Hernia

Williams and colleagues reviewed 46 patients who had undergone an end ileostomy for ulcerative colitis or Crohn's disease for evidence of paraileostomy hernia.[243] This complication was observed in 13 individuals (28%). The authors found that computed tomography was helpful in confirming the presence of the defect.

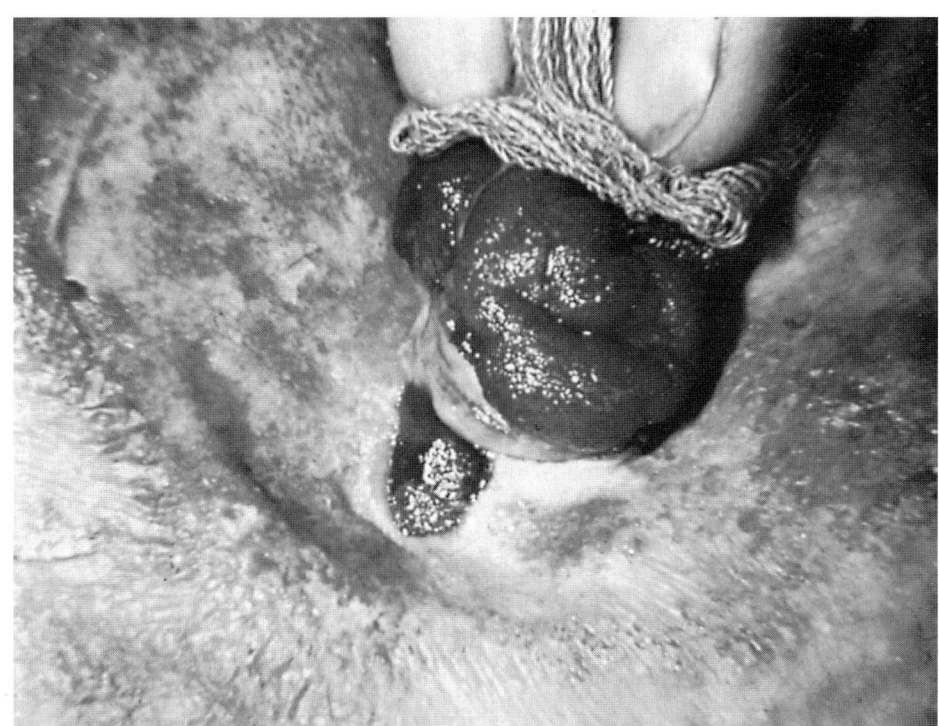

FIGURE 31-58. Mucosal seeding leading to inability to maintain the appliance. Note the severe skin changes. (From Corman ML, Veidenheimer MC, Coller JA. Ileostomy complications: prevention and treatment. *Contemp Surg* 1976; 8:36.)

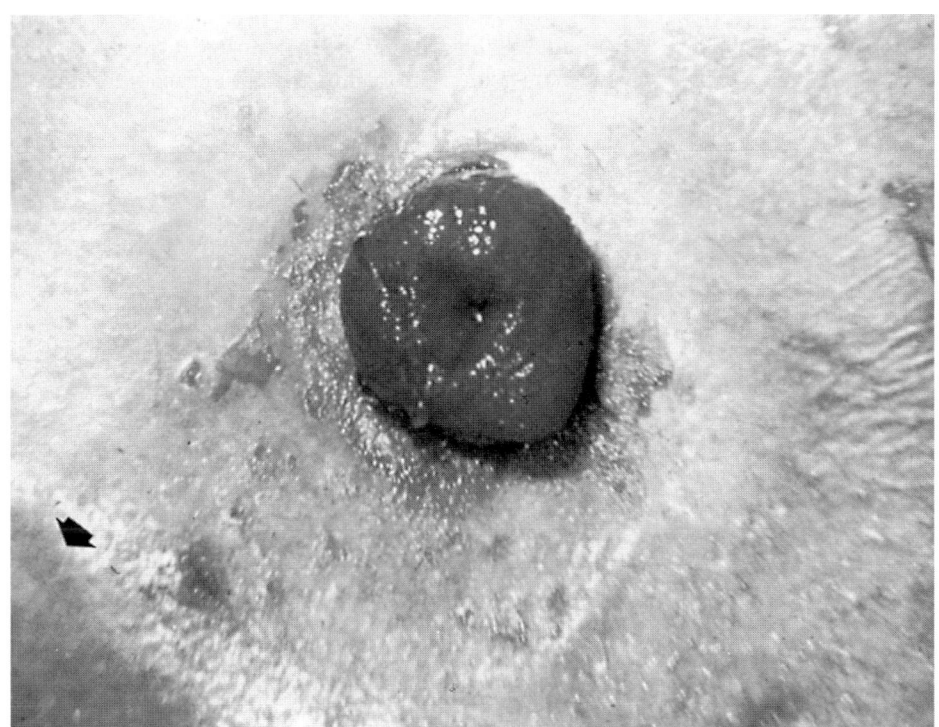

FIGURE 31-59. Positioning the stoma too close to the iliac crest causes an inability to maintain the appliance. Note the parastomal dermatitis. *Arrow* indicates the anterior superior iliac spine. (From Corman ML, Veidenheimer MC, Coller JA. Ileostomy complications: prevention and treatment. *Contemp Surg* 1976;8:36.)

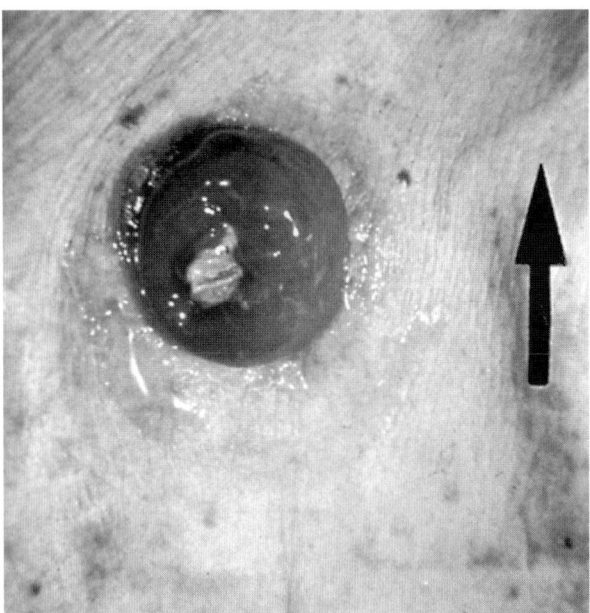

FIGURE 31-60. Ileostomy too close to the rib margin (*arrow*). (From Corman ML, Veidenheimer MC, Coller JA. Ileostomy complications: prevention and treatment. *Contemp Surg* 1976;8:36.)

Treatment As with colostomy hernia, this complication is usually due to an error in the location of the stoma. Repair is effected in a similar manner to that which has been previously described for colostomy hernia with or without mesh (see Figs. 31-14 through 31-17 above).[76]

Unfortunately, most such complications usually require relocation of the ileostomy.

Even in the absence of a parastomal hernia, additional pouch support may be achieved by the use of a belt, especially during lifting or exercise (Figure 31-64). For nonsurgical management of a hernia, the device is available up to 9" wide.

Other Complications

Recurrent Crohn's Disease and Other Manifestations of Inflammatory Bowel Disease at the Ileostomy

It is self-evident that Crohn's disease can recur in the stoma or in the small bowel proximal to the ileostomy. Management of this problem is discussed in Chapter 30. Additionally, paraileostomy skin ulceration may be a consequence of IBD. Pyoderma gangrenosum is an associated condition with IBD (see Chapter 30). The variable clinical outcome of parastomal pyoderma gangrenosum may be related to the activity of the underlying IBD and, in fact, may not be successfully treated until the residual disease has been extirpated (see Chapter 30).[225] A vigorous program involving an enterostomal therapist is usually required (see Chapter 32). Any disseminated skin condition when it occurs adjacent to or near the stoma can present severe management problems. For example, pemphigus vulgaris has been reported to cause severe skin management problems in a patient who harbored a stoma (see Chapter 19).[95] A case of bullous pemphigoid at the ostomy site has also been reported.[231]

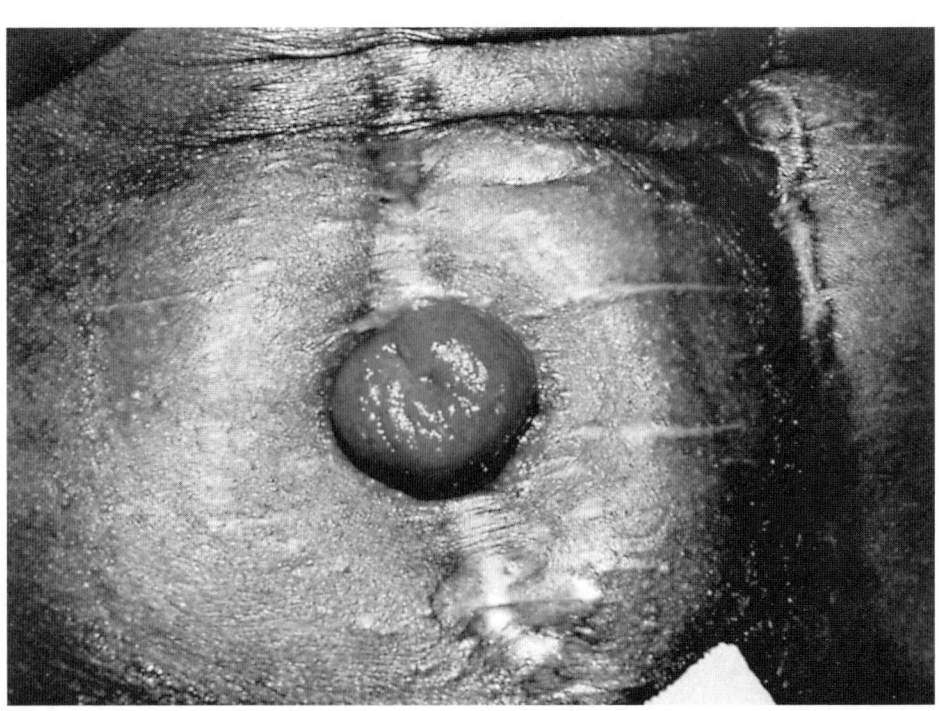

FIGURE 31-61. Ileostomy brought through an abdominal incision creates difficulty in appliance management. Note hernia.

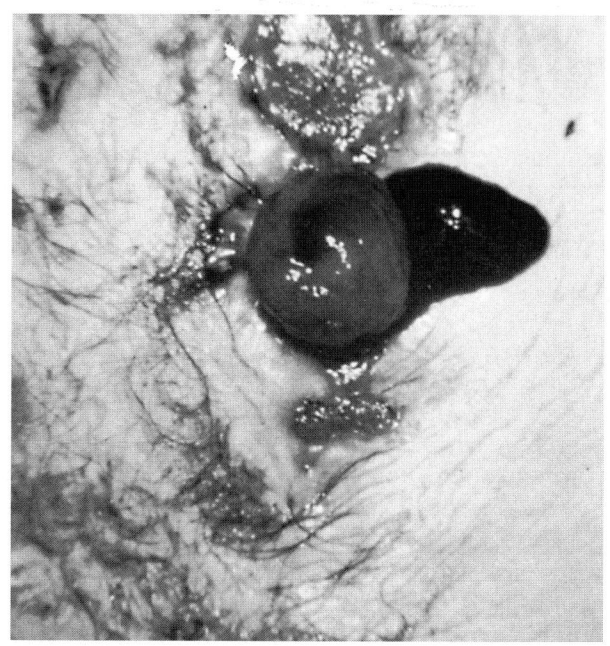

FIGURE 31-62. Open, indolent, draining incision due to the fact that the ileostomy was brought through the wound.

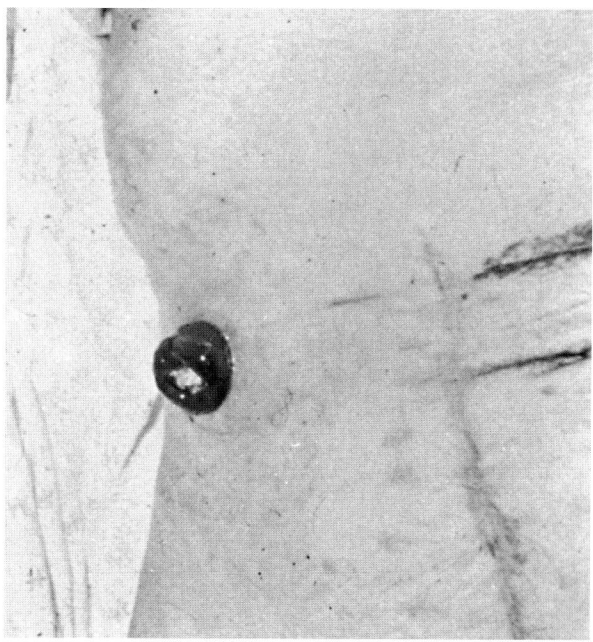

FIGURE 31-63. Appliance management is a challenge when the stoma is placed on the hip. (From Corman ML, Veidenheimer MC, Coller JA. Ileostomy complications: prevention and treatment. *Contemp Surg* 1976;8:36.)

Last and colleagues reported 17 patients with Crohn's disease who developed parastomal ulcers.[128] Conservative management included debridement, curettage, unroofing, and pouching of the stoma with Telfa strips placed in the ulcer base with a conventional appliance or a Perry Model no. 51 device. Most were healed by 3 months. When medical therapy fails, surgical revision with possible relocation is necessary.[141] Rotation or advancement skin grafts have also been employed with some success.

Infectious Enteritides

Campylobacter jejuni has been reported to cause profound ulceration of the stoma in association with an acute ileitis.[145] This case report emphasizes the importance of obtaining a stool culture in the evaluation of a patient with suspected recurrent IBD.

Carcinoma at the Ileostomy

Inflammatory Bowel Disease A number of instances of carcinoma arising in an ileostomy following proctocolectomy have been reported, possibly due to seeding viable tumor cells at the time of the original procedure, but more likely a consequence of a late-developing dysplastic phenomenon.[21,27, 53,73,113,181,201,204,233] Sherlock and colleagues have reported the first two instances of stomal adenocarcinoma in Crohn's disease.[200] Most publications note that this complication develops many years following the construction of the stoma.[73]

The most common presenting signs and symptoms include bleeding, ulceration, and the presence of a friable mass at the ileostomy site.[233]

The pathogenesis is largely speculative, but Roberts and colleagues observed that with one exception, all individuals in their study had antecedent backwash ileitis or dysplasia.[181] Although this should not necessarily be considered a preventable complication, particular attention should be given to the application of proper cancer technique if a tumor is present at the time of stomal construc-

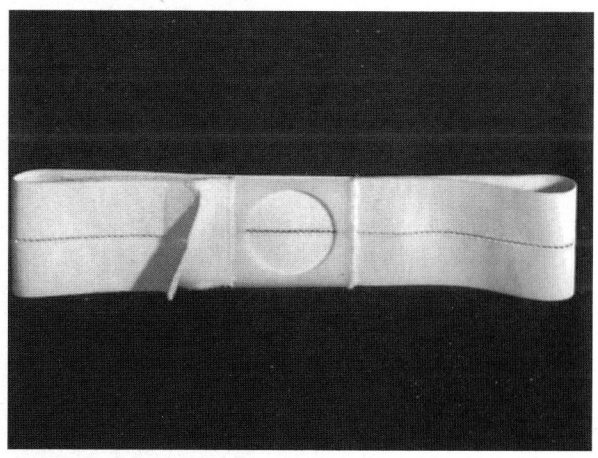

FIGURE 31-64. Support belt for ostomy. (Courtesy of Nu-Hope Laboratories, Inc.)

tion. Certainly, if the tumor appears to have seeded the abdomen or has breached the seromuscular surface of the bowel wall, perhaps at least a change of gloves is in order at the time of the maturation of the ileostomy. Treatment requires en bloc resection of the stoma, adjacent mesentery, and abdominal wall, and the creation of a new ileostomy.[63] Screening of asymptomatic patients with ileostomies of long standing by means of biopsy, looking for dysplastic or neoplastic changes, may be appropriate.[63,200,204]

A single case of primary squamous cell carcinoma of a skin-grafted ileostomy has been described[161] as has squamous cell carcinoma of the peristomal skin.[36]

Familial Adenomatous Polyposis

As discussed in Chapter 21, familial adenomatous polyposis (FAP) may be associated with tumors and tumor-like conditions throughout the gastrointestinal tract. While most lesions in the small bowel are areas of lymphoid hyperplasia, Nakahara and colleagues found adenomas to be present in 20% of the ileums studied.[157] Such tumors may be evident on the stoma. Adenocarcinoma has also been reported.[78] In light of the fact that the potential for malignant change has not been clearly defined, careful follow-up with ileoscopy and biopsy is recommended.

Hemorrhage

Patients who have undergone an ileostomy for chronic ulcerative colitis or Crohn's disease may develop cirrhosis and portal hypertension. The problem is relatively common in those with sclerosing cholangitis. These individuals have the potential for shunts developing within adhesions between the ileal (portal) veins and the anterior abdominal wall (systemic) veins.[165] This may lead to ileostomy hemorrhage from parastomal varices (Figure 31-65).[46,180] Of interest is the fact that colectomy probably limits the likelihood of the development of encephalopathy.

Sclerotherapy may be expected to afford only temporary benefit (see earlier discussion with respect to colostomy). Successful shunting directed at relieving the portal hypertension should prevent subsequent hemorrhage, but the procedure may accelerate liver failure.[165]

Adson and Fulton identified 19 cirrhotic patients who bled repeatedly from the mucocutaneous junction of the ileal or colonic stomas and added three of their own.[6] These individuals were treated by portasystemic shunting with no evidence of recurrent bleeding. The authors advised ileostomy revision to control hemorrhage, but when stomal and esophageal varix bleeding coexist, a portasystemic shunt procedure was felt to be justified. Others also have concluded that a shunt procedure offers the best opportunity for controlling the bleeding.[46,180]

Trauma

Trauma to the ileostomy can be accidental or deliberate (Figure 31-66). Wilkinson and Humphreys reported a patient who suffered a laceration of the ileostomy as a re-

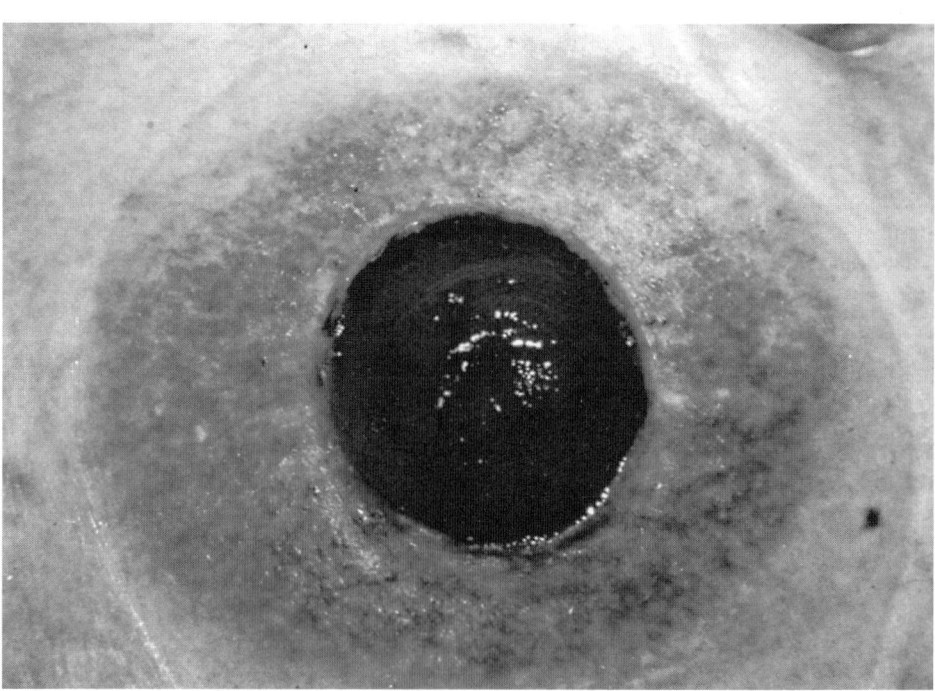

FIGURE 31-65. Peristomal varices in a patient with portal hypertension.

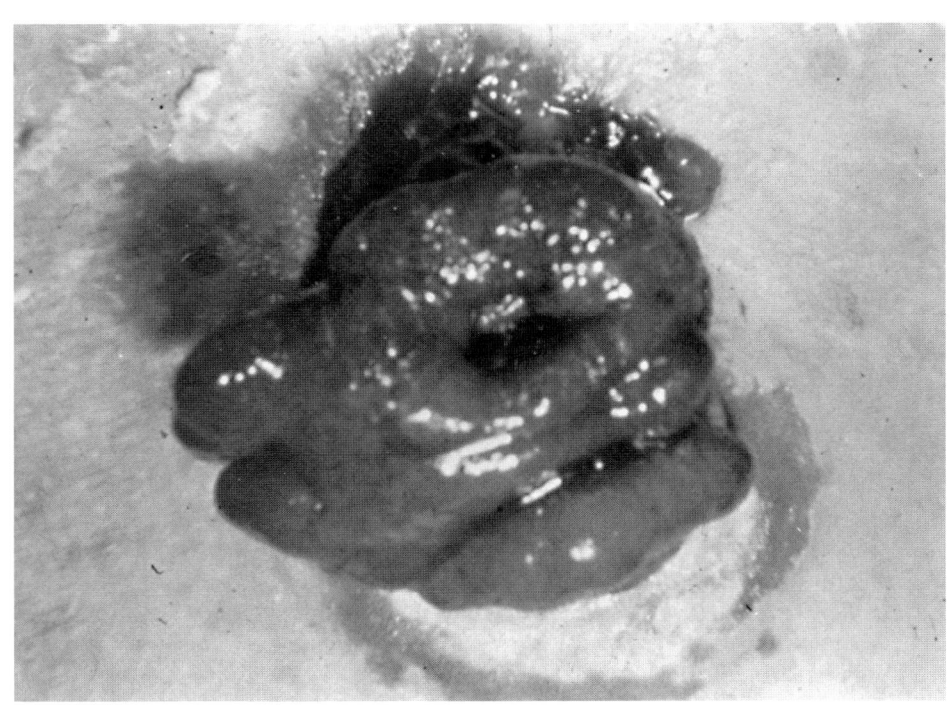

FIGURE 31-66. Macerated ileostomy with multiple fistulas in a psychotic patient who attempted to "destroy" the stoma.

sult of a seatbelt injury.[242] Following satisfactory repair, the individual was admitted to another hospital at a later time with total avulsion of his stoma as a result of direct trauma during a brawl. While these types of injuries are not necessarily preventable, and although one should create the stoma of sufficient prominence to satisfactorily maintain an appliance, a longer length not only is unsightly but also increases susceptibility to injury.

Results As recently as 35 years ago, the complication rate for ileostomy alone approached 100%. In 1981, Morowitz and Kirsner observed that at least one-fourth of their patients required ileostomy revision.[153] Re-operation for bowel obstruction was performed in more than 10%, and diarrhea and nephrolithiasis were frequent problems. Medication was necessary for 20%.

My colleagues and I reviewed our experience with ileostomy complications requiring revision during a 10-year period ending in 1973.[72] Eighty-four revisions were performed on 50 individuals. The reasons for revision are summarized in Table 31-4. Thirty-one patients underwent only one revision, and subsequent stomal operations were required in 19. Nine of these underwent a third revision, four a fourth, and two a fifth. Ileostomy complications requiring revision were more frequent in those who had Crohn's disease.[72] Roy and colleagues noted that 9.7% of their patients with ulcerative colitis needed revisions, as compared with 26.5% with Crohn's disease.[188] Steinberg

and co-workers found a similar incidence.[208] Leong and associates reported the St. Mark's Hospital experience with ileostomy complications actuarially analyzing 150 permanent stomas constructed over a 10-year period.[132] By 20 years, the incidence of stomal complications approached 76% in those with ulcerative colitis and 59% in those with Crohn's disease. These differences were statis-

▶ **TABLE 31-4 Reasons for Ileostomy Revision**

Complication	Number	Percent
Stenosis	20	23.8
Fistula	12	14.2
Prolapse	10	11.9
Retraction	10	11.9
Recurrent disease	8	9.5
Small bowel obstruction	8	9.5
Poor placement	5	6.0
Stomal bleeding	3	3.6
Dermatitis	2	2.4
Necrosis	2	2.4
Stomal pain	2	2.4
Paraileostomy hernia	1	1.2
Paraileostomy abscess	1	1.2
Total	84	100.0

From Goldblatt MS, Corman ML, Haggitt RC, et al. Ileostomy complications requiring revision: Lahey Clinic experience, 1964–1973. *Dis Colon Rectum* 1977;20:209.

tically significant and essentially the opposite ratio of that reported in the three papers mentioned above. Revisional rates were also higher in individuals with ulcerative colitis. The four commonest complications were skin problems (cumulative probability, 34%), intestinal obstruction (23%), retraction (17%), and peristomal herniation (16%).[132] Interestingly, the incidence of peristomal herniation was not reduced by siting through the rectus muscle (21%) when compared with those that were created outside of the muscle (7%). While the differences were not statistically significant, they are certainly opposite from what one would have predicted, and which I have repeatedly advised throughout this chapter.

Ileostomy in the Elderly

Advanced age does not appear to be a contraindication to ileostomy. My colleagues and I reviewed our experience with ileostomy in patients aged more than 60 years.[3] The median age was 64 at the time of surgery, and there was no mortality. All accepted and managed their stomas in much the same manner as younger people; no specialized nursing care was necessary. Four of ten required ileostomy revisions. Although this was a small series, the incidence is not significantly greater than in younger people. Stryker and colleagues surveyed 67 patients older than 60 from the Mayo Clinic.[211] They found that although lifestyle did not appear to be altered more in the elderly than in younger individuals, older patients experienced a greater frequency of appliance management difficulties.

CONTINENT ILEOSTOMY DEVICE

Pemberton and colleagues have described the Mayo Clinic use of a continent ileostomy device in four individuals with conventional ileostomies.[166] The apparatus consists of a modified endotracheal tube. Through the application of intermittent balloon inflation an obstruction is created, dilatation of the ileum is produced, and a simulated reservoir results. The authors concluded that chronic intermittent occlusion with an indwelling stomal device achieves enteric continence without impairing intestinal function. However, no subsequent reports have been forthcoming.

PATIENT EVALUATION OF RESULTS: LIFESTYLE AND SEXUAL FUNCTION

Morowitz and Kirsner reported their experience using a questionnaire of almost 2,000 patients who had undergone ileostomy for ulcerative colitis.[153] Satisfaction with the ileostomy was certainly improved when compared

with preoperative status. This was substantiated by the dramatic decrease in the number of colitis patients under the care of a physician after the operation. Furthermore, the ileostomy seemed to have an ameliorative effect on marital status, and there appeared to be no significant adverse effect on childbearing. A relatively low number of unemployed persons was noted in their experience. Conversely, Halevy and colleagues reported a survey from the Israel Ostomy Association and found a low rate of rehabilitation as measured by failure to return to previous occupation and problems with sexual and social adjustment.[92]

Many studies have addressed the psychological and sexual aspects of patients who have undergone an operation resulting in an ileostomy or colostomy.[30,34,81,142,183] Problems expressed include impotence, dyspareunia, decreased physical attractiveness, concern for odor, fear of injuring the stoma, fear of leakage, and fear of rejection by the sexual partner. In a survey performed by McLeod and colleagues of 322 ileostomies from the Cleveland Clinic, 22% reported psychological problems because of "poor body image" and 12% noted sterility or impotence.[142] Skin irritation (49%), offensive noise and odor (42%), and detection of the appliance (29%) were some of the problems encountered.[142] Awad and co-workers conducted a postal questionnaire of 113 patients with a permanent ileostomy.[13] They analyzed the quality of life as well as the psychological morbidity, including whether the patient would prefer to have an ileoanal pouch. A total of 93% of the respondents were content with the ileostomy and appeared to have a normal lifestyle. Furthermore, approximately 87% stated that they would keep the ileostomy rather than be submitted to a major operation for reestablishment of intestinal continuity. Significant psychological morbidity was observed in only 5% of patients.[13]

These reviews uniformly suggest that the surgeon and/or enterostomal therapist should discuss these concerns with patients prior to performing permanent ostomy surgery. Brouillette and colleagues observed that many problems were resolved by the patients themselves, but the authors strongly advocate that an understanding surgeon as well as a knowledgeable enterostomal therapist and site visitor can create a climate in which the patient can feel at ease in asking for guidance on sexual matters (see Chapter 32).[30]

LOOP ILEOSTOMY

Loop ileostomy was originally described by Turnbull and Weakley as a procedure to divert the fecal stream primarily for the treatment of toxic megacolon (see

Chapter 29).[229] It is also a technique that is effective for the management of colonic obstruction (much preferred to a cecostomy) and to protect an ileorectal anastomosis, especially when performed for IBD. More recently, it has been routinely applied to protect the ileoanal anastomosis concomitant with restorative proctocolectomy.

An indication for loop ileostomy that is not generally appreciated is when an end ileal stoma is technically difficult to create. Such a problem arises with obese patients, in whom the mesentery may be shortened and thickened, and it can also be encountered when the distal ileum has been previously resected.[50] In the latter situation the blood supply often enters radially, with little collateral circulation between the arcade vessels.

Every surgeon has been confronted with the problem of insufficient bowel length to create an adequate stoma. This necessitates trimming the mesentery, which in turn may result in devascularization of the distal ileum. When the devitalized bowel is excised, a satisfactory length is unavailable, and the mesenteric vessels are again divided with the same viability problem. Finally, the surgeon may compromise and accept a less-than-optimal stomal protrusion or construct an ileostomy of sufficient length but

of questionable viability. This problem can be avoided by using a loop ileostomy.

Construction Technique

After the colectomy has been performed, the distal end of the small intestine is oversewn. A disk of skin is excised in the same manner and at the same location as if for a conventional ileostomy. A point is selected 10 cm proximal to the closed ileum (a more proximal site is chosen in a grossly obese patient), and a Penrose drain is placed around the intestine. The loop of small bowel is brought through the split rectus muscle (Figure 31-67). A rod or catheter supports the loop, and the bowel is opened at the level of the skin on the distal, nonfunctioning side. The stoma is created by eversion with interrupted mucosubcuticular sutures of fine catgut (Figure 31-68). Eversion may be facilitated by means of Babcock clamps. The technique that has been illustrated is an alternative to an end -stoma, but it is essentially the same approach if used in continuity with the distal ileum and the colon or a reservoir. It is extremely useful to place Seprafilm around the small bowel before it is passed through the abdominal wall (see Fig. 26-43). This greatly facilitates the subse-

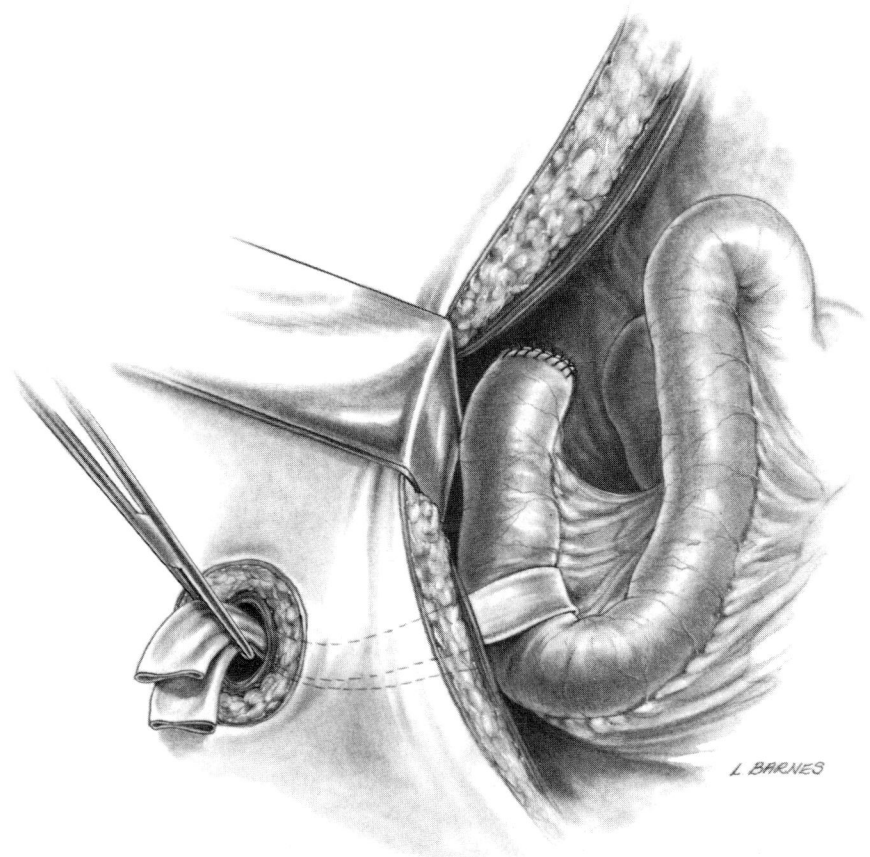

FIGURE 31-67. Loop ileostomy. The distal ileum is closed and the loop prepared for exteriorization.

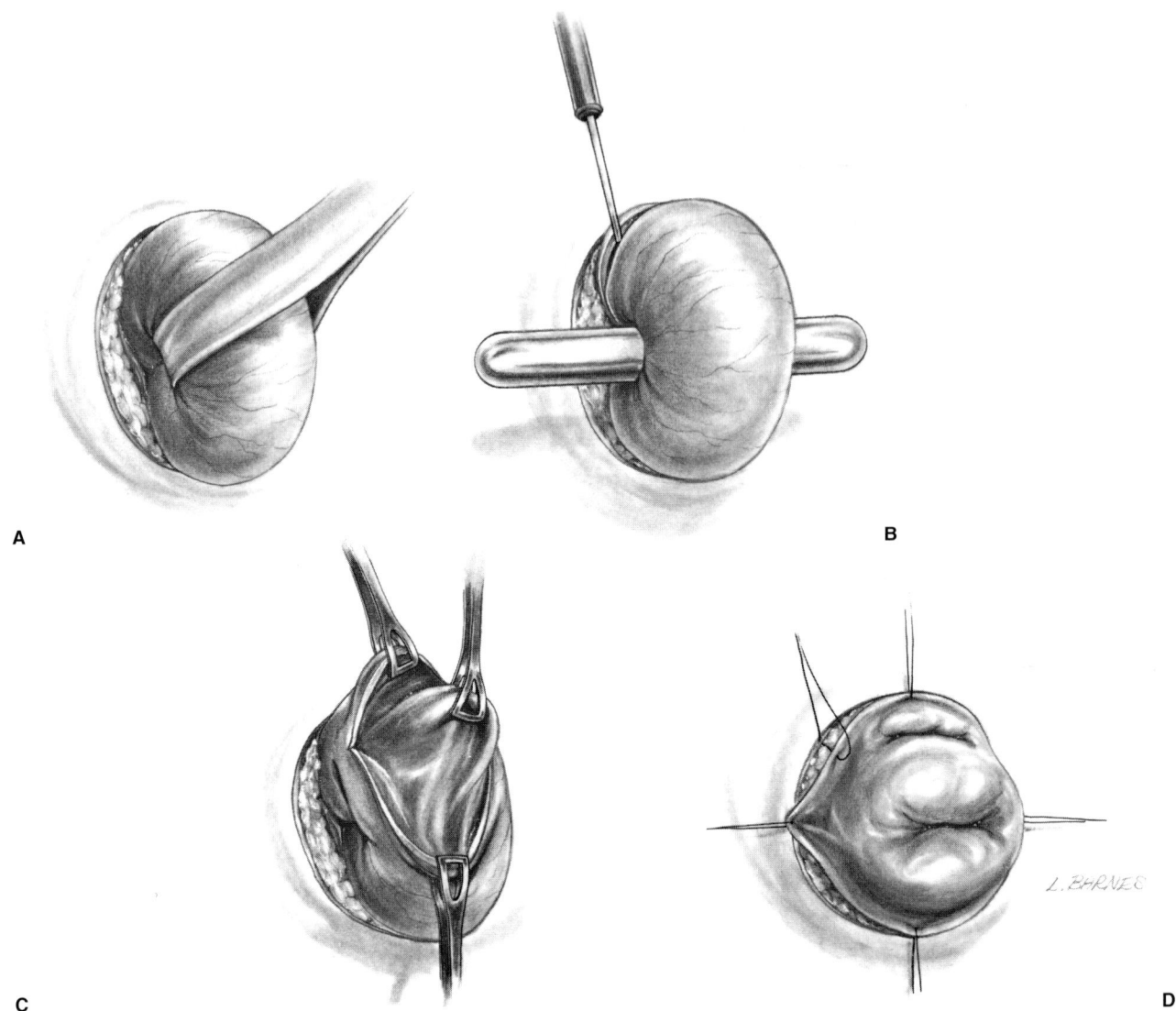

FIGURE 31-68. Loop ileostomy. **(A)** Exteriorization. **(B)** The distal limb is incised from mesentery to mesentery at skin level. Care must be taken to make certain which side is proximal. **(C)** Eversion. **(D)** Maturation. The rod has been omitted for simplicity of illustration.

quent takedown of the stoma. Moreover, the use of this material has been shown to facilitate early closure.[217]

The rod or catheter is usually removed in 3 to 5 days. Eventually, the distal end completely retracts, and the general appearance and the functional results are virtually identical to that obtained by conventional end ileostomy (Figure 31-69).

Prasad and colleagues believe that the small bowel can be transected, the mesentery incised, and the proximal and distal ends brought out together, with the distal segment deemphasized.[174] This is analogous to that of the previously mentioned end-loop colostomy (see Figure 31-35 above). While this may often be accomplished with safety, there is the potential risk of compromise to the

blood supply. The procedure has also been described laparoscopically (see Chapter 27).[112,118]

Results

The place of loop ileostomy on a temporary basis as associated with restorative proctocolectomy has been discussed in Chapter 29. As was mentioned, there are indeed complications associated with the creation of the ileostomy itself, and they must be considered when a temporary stoma of this nature is considered. Senapati and colleagues reviewed the experience from the St. Mark's Hospital with 296 patients over a 15-year period.[199] Ileostomy-related complications prior to closure occurred in

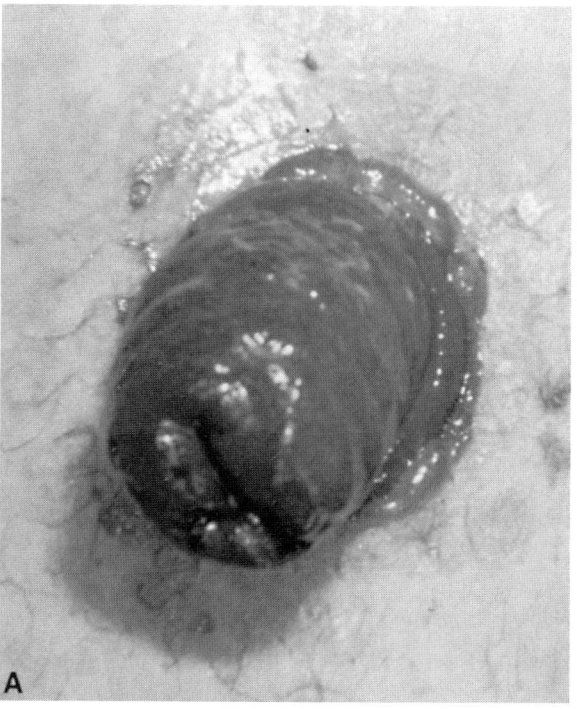
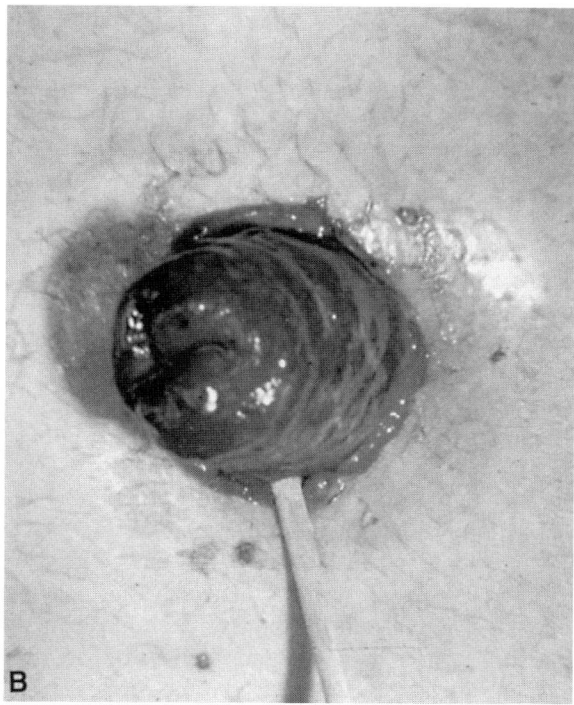

FIGURE 31-69. Loop ileostomy several weeks following construction. **(A)** On inspection, simulates an end stoma. **(B)** A cotton-tip applicator disappears into the distal limb.

5.7%. Laparotomy for obstruction was required in 2.4%, retraction requiring revision occurred in 1%, and a peristomal abscess occurred in one patient (0.3%). Appliance management problems were seen in 2.4%. These are actually fewer complications than have been reported from other series.

Wexner and associates reported the Cleveland Clinic (Florida) experience in a prospective fashion on 83 consecutive patients who required temporary loop ileostomy for anastomoses associated with various operative procedures.[239] Four patients developed dehydration and electrolyte abnormalities secondary to high stomal output. One stomal retraction following rod removal. Specifically, there was no instance of stomal ischemia, hemorrhage, prolapse, or mortality.[239]

Williams and colleagues performed a prospective trial of patients who were undergoing colorectal surgery, randomly allocating 24 to a loop colostomy and 23 to a loop ileostomy.[245] While both procedures adequately diverted the fecal stream, loop ileostomy was associated with significantly less odor, required fewer appliance changes, and had a lower incidence of complications when closed. Similarly, Edwards and associates (Basingstoke, United Kingdom) performed a prospective, randomized trial of the two diversion methods concomitant with low colorectal and coloanal anastomoses.[59] The higher frequency of herniation with colostomy supported their preference for loop ileostomy. Others—including me—also advocate

loop ileostomy as being superior to transverse colostomy for temporary fecal diversion.[62]

A contrary view has been expressed by Law and co-workers (Hong Kong) who randomized patients following low anterior resection to loop ileostomy or loop transverse colostomy.[130] Intestinal obstruction and ileus were more common after loop ileostomy. They, therefore, recommend loop transverse colostomy as the preferred method of proximal diversion following this operation. In another randomized study of these two alternatives applied to those who underwent left-sided colon anastomoses, Gooszer and co-workers (Netherlands) concluded that both types of stomas have a high complication rate.[88] They too prefer transverse colostomy because construction, as well as closure of a loop ileostomy, was associated with more frequent and more serious complications.

Technique for Closure

Closure of a loop ileostomy may involve a resection or no resection. The procedure can be undertaken without a complete laparotomy, circumcising the ileostomy as if for a revision. The proximal and distal bowel is mobilized, and the intestine is either resected or the skin and mucosa are debrided prior to simple closure. A conventional single-layer, interrupted anastomosis may be performed, and the bowel is returned to the peritoneal cavity. Along with others, I prefer, whenever possible, to employ a stapling technique, performing a side-to-side (functional end-to-end) anastomosis with the GIA stapler.[116] This has the theoretical advantage of creating a much larger luminal diameter and is generally simple to accomplish. Closure with the linear stapler completes the anastomosis in a manner similar to that described in Figure 31-42 (as applied to loop colostomy). However, resection and/or a sutured anastomosis may be necessary when there is bowel thickening or edema or when intraperitoneal adhesions limit one's ability to deliver an adequate length in order to use the side-to-side stapling instrument.

Results

As mentioned above, the Cleveland Clinic (Florida) experience was reported by Wexner and colleagues in a prospective study involving 83 consecutive patients who underwent loop ileostomy for various indications.[239] Of the 67 who had re-establishment of intestinal continuity, three required a full laparotomy. A side-to-side stapled anastomosis was effected in approximately three-quarters of the patients. All skin wounds were left open, and the mean hospital stay was 5 days. Two developed anastomotic leaks that spontaneously healed without re-operation. One wound infection was observed, but with the skin wounds left open, this should be a rare complication indeed. As a matter of fact, I now do a subcuticular closure of the skin with an ileostomy closure.

Hull and associates evaluated the Cleveland Clinic's (Ohio) experience with hand-sewn versus stapled loop ileostomy closure.[106] This was undertaken in a randomized, prospective fashion. The procedure was performed in a statistically significant shorter time in the stapled group, but the incidence of complications were similar and infrequent when the two were compared.[106]

When a patient is re-admitted to the hospital for a problem related to the stoma or with intestinal obstruction, it is reasonable to study the patient with respect to the feasibility of earlier closure of the ileostomy. If the anastomosis is intact, the operation can be undertaken with relative ease and safety, especially if Seprafilm had been initially employed.[15,217] Kalady and colleagues (Duke University) have even established a protocol for 23-hour hospitalization after loop ileostomy closure, noting no increased complications or hospital readmissions in 28 patients.[114]

REFERENCES

1. Abcarian H, Pearl RK. Stomas. *Surg Clin North Am* 1988; 68:1205.
2. Abdu RA. Repair of paracolostomy hernias with Marlex mesh. *Dis Colon Rectum* 1982;25:529.
3. Abrams AV, Corman ML, Veidenheimer MC. Ileostomy in the elderly. *Dis Colon Rectum* 1975;18:115.
4. Abrams BL, Alsikafi FH, Waterman NG. Colostomy: a new look at morbidity and mortality. *Am Surg* 1979;45:462.
5. Abulafi AM, Sherman IW, Fiddian RV. Delorme operation for prolapsed colostomy. *Br J Surg* 1989;76:1321.
6. Adson MA, Fulton RE. The ileal stoma and portal hypertension: an uncommon site of variceal bleeding. *Arch Surg* 1977;112:501.
7. Alexander-Williams J, Amery AH, Devlin HB, et al. Magnetic continent colostomy device. *BMJ* 1977;1:1269.
8. Alexandre JH, Bouillot JL. Paracolostomal hernia: repair with use of a dacron prosthesis. *World J Surg* 1993;17:680.
9. Allen-Mersh TG, Thomson JPS. Surgical treatment of colostomy complications. *Br J Surg* 1988;75:416.
10. Anderson E, Carey LC, Cooperman M. Colostomy closure: a simple procedure? *Dis Colon Rectum* 1979;22:466.
11. Antrum RM, Price JJ. Use of skin staples for fashioning colostomies. *Br J Surg* 1988;75:736.
12. Aston CM, Everett WG. Comparison of early and late closure of transverse loop colostomies. *Ann R Coll Surg Engl* 1984;66:331.
13. Awad RW, El-Gohary TM, Skilton JS, et al. Life quality and psychological morbidity with an ileostomy. *Br J Surg* 1993;80:252.
14. Baker FS. The "rodless" loop colostomy. *Dis Colon Rectum* 1975;18:528.
15. Bakx R, Busch ORC, van Geldere D, et al. Feasibility of early closure of loop ileostomies. *Dis Colon Rectum* 2003; 46:1680.
16. Banerjee A. Pursestring skin closure after stoma reversal. *Dis Colon Rectum* 1997;40:993.
17. Bass EM, Del Pino A, Tan A, et al. Does preoperative stoma marking and education by the enterostomal therapist affect outcome? *Dis Colon Rectum* 1997;40:440.
18. Bayer I, Kyzer S, Chaimoff CH. A new approach to primary strengthening of colostomy with Marlex mesh to prevent paracolostomy hernia. *Surg Gynecol Obstet* 1986; 163:579.
19. Beck DE, Fazio VW, Grundfest-Broniatowski S. Surgical management of bleeding stomal varices. *Dis Colon Rectum* 1988;31:343.
20. Beck PH, Conklin HB. Closure of colostomy. *Ann Surg* 1975;181:795.
21. Bedetti CD, DeRisio VJ. Primary adenocarcinoma arising at an ileostomy site: an unusual complication after colectomy for ulcerative colitis. *Dis Colon Rectum* 1986;29:572.
22. Benacci JC, Wolff BG. Cecostomy: therapeutic indications and results. *Dis Colon Rectum* 1995;38:530.
23. Bergren CT, Laws HL. Modified technique of colostomy bridging. *Surg Gynecol Obstet* 1990;170:453.
24. Berne TV, Griffith CN, Hill J, et al. Colostomy wound closure. *Arch Surg* 1985;120:957.
25. Bickel A, Shinharevsky E, Eitan A. Laparoscopic repair of paracolostomy hernia. *J Laparoendosc Adv Surg Tech* 1999; 9:353.
26. Billings PJ, Leaper DJ. Laser Doppler velocimetry and the measurement of colostomy blood flow. *Dis Colon Rectum* 1987;30:376.
27. Blake DP, Scheithauer BW, van Heerden JA. Metastasis to a Brooke ileostomy: an unusual cause of stomal dysfunction. *Dis Colon Rectum* 1981;24:644.
28. Bozzetti F, Nava M, Bufalino R, et al. Early local complications following colostomy closure in cancer patients. *Dis Colon Rectum* 1983;26:25.
29. Brooke BN. The management of an ileostomy including its complications. *Lancet* 1952;2:102.
30. Brouillette JN, Pryor E, Fox TA Jr. Evaluation of sexual dysfunction in the female following rectal resection and intestinal stoma. *Dis Colon Rectum* 1981;24:96.
31. Brown S, Holloway B, Hosie K. Percutaneous endoscopic colostomy: an alternative treatment of acute colonic pseudo-obstruction. *Colorectal Dis* 2000;2:367.
32. Browning GGP, Parks AG. A method and the results of loop colostomy. *Dis Colon Rectum* 1983;26:223.

33. Burcharth F, Ballan A, Kylberg F, et al. The colostomy plug: a new disposable device for a continent colostomy. *Lancet* 1986;2:1062.

34. Burnham WR, Lennard-Jones JE, Brooke BN. Sexual problems among married ileostomists: survey conducted by the Ileostomy Association of Great Britain and Ireland. *Gut* 1977;18:673.

35. Byers JM, Steinberg JB, Postier RG. Repair of parastomal hernias using polypropylene mesh. *Arch Surg* 1992;127: 1246.

36. Carne PWG, Farmer KCR. Squamous-cell carcinoma developing in an ileostomy stoma: report of a case. *Dis Colon Rectum* 2001;44:594.

37. Carne PWG, Robertson GM, Frizelle FA. Parastomal hernia. *Br J Surg* 2003;90:784.

38. Cattell RB. A new type of ileostomy for chronic ulcerative colitis. *Surg Clin North Am* 1939;19:629.

39. Cazador AC, Piñol M, Rague JM, et al. Multicentre study of a continent colostomy plug. *Br J Surg* 1993;80:930.

40. Cerdán FJ, Díez M, Campo J, et al. Continent colostomy by means of a new one-piece disposable device. *Dis Colon Rectum* 1991;34:886.

41. Chandler JG, Evans BP. Colostomy prolapse. *Surgery* 1978; 84:577.

42. Cheun M-T, Chia N-H, Chiu W-Y. Surgical treatment of parastomal hernia complicating sigmoid colostomies. *Dis Colon Rectum* 2001;44:266.

43. Chung RS. End colostomy and Brooke's ileostomy constructed by surgical stapler. *Surg Gynecol Obstet* 1986;162: 63.

44. Clague MB, Heald RJ. Achievement of stomal continence in one-third of colostomies by use of a new disposable plug. *Surg Gynecol Obstet* 1990;170:390.

45. Colmer ML, Foxx MJ. A device for the control of colostomy prolapse. *Surg Gynecol Obstet* 1981;152:827.

46. Conte JV, Arcomano TA, Naficy MA, et al. Treatment of bleeding stomal varices: report of a case and review of the literature. *Dis Colon Rectum* 1990;33:308.

47. Corman JM, Odenheimer DB. Securing the loop—historic review of the methods used for creating a loop colostomy. *Dis Colon Rectum* 1991;34:1014.

48. Corman ML, Veidenheimer MC, Coller JA. An appliance for management of the diverting loop colostomy. *Arch Surg* 1974;108:742.

49. Corman ML, Veidenheimer MC, Coller JA. Ileostomy complications: prevention and treatment. *Contemp Surg* 1976; 8:36.

50. Corman ML, Veidenheimer MC, Coller JA. Loop ileostomy as an alternative to end stoma. *Surg Gynecol Obstet* 1979; 149:585.

51. Crile G Jr, Turnbull RB Jr. The mechanism and prevention of ileostomy dysfunction. *Ann Surg* 1954;140:459.

52. Cromar CDL. The evolution of colostomy. *Dis Colon Rectum* 1968;11:256,367,423.

53. Cuesta MA, Donner R. Adenocarcinoma arising at an ileostomy site: report of a case. *Cancer* 1976;37:949.

54. Daniels I, Lamparelli M, Chave H, et al. Recurrent sigmoid volvulus treated by percutaneous endoscopic colostomy. *Br J Surg* 2000;87:1419.

55. Dinnick T. The origins and evolution of colostomy. *Br J Surg* 1934–35;22:142.

56. Dolan PA, Caldwell FT, Thompson CH, et al. Problems of colostomy closure. *Am J Surg* 1979;137:188.

57. Doran J, Hardcastle JD. A controlled trial of colostomy management by natural evacuation, irrigation, and foam enema. *Br J Surg* 1981;68:731.

58. Dragstedt LR, Dack GM, Kirsner JB. Chronic ulcerative colitis: a summary of evidence implicating *Bacterium necrophorum* as an etiologic agent. *Ann Surg* 1941;114: 653.

59. Edwards DP, Leppington-Clarke A, Sexton R, et al. Stoma-related complications are more frequent after transverse colostomy than loop ileostomy: a prospective randomized clinical trial. *Br J Surg* 2001;88:360.

60. Eng K, Localio A. Simplified complementary transverse colostomy for low colorectal anastomosis. *Surg Gynecol Obstet* 1981;153:734.

61. Evans JP, Brown MH, Wilkes GH, et al. Revising the troublesome stoma: combines abdominal wall recontouring and revision of stomas. *Dis Colon Rectum* 2003;46:122.

62. Fasth S, Hultén L. Loop ileostomy: a superior diverting stoma in colorectal surgery. *World J Surg* 1984;8:401.

63. Feustel H, Hennig G. Kontinent kolostomie durch magnetverschluss. *Dtsch Med Wochenschr* 1975;100:1063.

64. Fine P. *Am de la Soc de Montpelier* 1797;6:34.

65. Finemore RG. Repeated haemorrhage from a terminal colostomy due to mucocutaneous varices with coexisting hepatic metastatic rectal adenocarcinoma: a case report. *Br J Surg* 1979;66:806.

66. Fischer RP, Gervin AS. Tampon occlusion of colostomy stoma during laparotomy. *Am Surg* 1994;60:709.

67. Fitzgibbons RJ Jr, Schmitz GD, Bailey RT Jr. A simple technique for constructing a loop enterostomy which allows immediate placement of an ostomy appliance. *Surg Gynecol Obstet* 1987;164:79.

68. Fligelstone LJ, Wanendeya N, Palmer BV. Osmotic therapy for acute irreducible stoma prolapse. *Br J Surg* 1997;84: 390.

69. Fontes B, Fontes W, Utiyama EM, et al. The efficacy of loop colostomy for complete fecal diversion. *Dis Colon Rectum* 1988;31:298.

70. Foster ME, Leaper DJ, Williamson RCN. Changing patterns in colostomy closure: the Bristol experience 1975–1982. *Br J Surg* 1985;72:142.

71. Freund HR, Raniel J, Muggia-Sulam M. Factors affecting the morbidity of colostomy closure: a retrospective study. *Dis Colon Rectum* 1982;25:712.

72. Fuhrman GM, Ota DM. Laparoscopic intestinal stomas. *Dis Colon Rectum* 1994;37:444.

73. Gadacz TR, McFadden DW, Gabrielson EW, et al. Adenocarcinoma of the ileostomy: the latent risk of cancer after colectomy for ulcerative colitis and familial polyposis. *Surgery* 1990;107:698.

74. Garber HI, Morris DM, Eisenstat TE, et al. Factors influencing the morbidity of colostomy closure. *Dis Colon Rectum* 1982;25:464.

75. Garnjobst W, Leaverton GH, Sullivan ES. Safety of colostomy closure. *Am J Surg* 1978;136:85.

76. Garnjobst W, Sullivan ES. Repair of paraileostomy hernia with polypropylene mesh reinforcement. *Dis Colon Rectum* 1984;27:268.

77. Gawron CL. Colostomy irrigations: mechanism guidelines. *Ostomy/Wound Management* 1990;28:56.

78. Gilson TP, Sollenberger LL. Adenocarcinoma of an ileostomy in a patient with familial adenomatous polyposis: report of a case. *Dis Colon Rectum* 1992;35:261.

79. Gingold BS, Januzzi JL. Paracolostomy carcinoma. *Am J Proctol Gastroenterol Colon Rectal Surg* 1984;35:9.

80. Giunchi F, Cacciaguerra G, Drudi G. Burn and stricture of the ostomy due to colostomy irrigation: report of a case. *Dis Colon Rectum* 1985;28:873.

81. Gloeckner MR, Starling JR. Providing sexual information to ostomy patients. *Dis Colon Rectum* 1982;25:575.

82. Goldblatt MS, Corman ML, Haggitt RC, et al. Ileostomy complications requiring revision: Lahey Clinic experience, 1964–1973. *Dis Colon Rectum* 1977;20:209.

83. Goldstein S, Sohn N, Weinstein MA, et al. Simplified loop ostomy fixation using rubber tubing. *Surg Gynecol Obstet* 1984;158:375.

84. Goldstein SD, Salvati EP, Rubin RJ, et al. Tube cecostomy with cecal extraperitonealization in the management of obstructing left-sided carcinoma of the large intestine. *Surg Gynecol Obstet* 1986;162:379.

85. Goldstein WZ, Edoga J, Crystal R. Management of colostomal hemorrhage resulting from portal hypertension. *Dis Colon Rectum* 1980;23:86.

86. Goligher JC, Lee PWR, McMahon MJ, et al. The Erlangen magnetic colostomy control device: technique of use and results in 22 patients. *Br J Surg* 1977;64:501.

87. Gomez ER, Rosenthal D. Management of a subcutaneous colostomy perforation: the role a new synthetic skin. *Dis Colon Rectum* 1984;27:651.

88. Gooszen AW, Geelkerken RH, Hermans J, et al. Temporary decompression after colorectal surgery: randomized comparison of loop ileostomy and loop colostomy. *Br J Surg* 1998;85:76.

89. Greatorex RA. Simple method of closing a paraileostomy fistula. *Br J Surg* 1988;75:543.

90. Greenstein AJ, Dicker A, Meyers S, et al. Periileostomy fistulae in Crohn's disease. *Ann Surg* 1983;197:179.

91. Guillemot F, Colombel JF, Neut C, et al. Treatment of diversion colitis by short-chain fatty acids. Prospective and double-blind study. *Dis Colon Rectum* 1991;34:861.

92. Halevy A, Adam Y, Eshchar J. Ileostomates in Israel. *Dis Colon Rectum* 1977;20:482.

93. Handelsman JC, Fishbein RH. Stabilization of ileostomy position with fascia. *Surgery* 1983;93:88.

94. Handschin AE, Weber M, Weinhaupt D, et al. Contrast-enhanced three-dimensional magnetic resonance angiography for visualization of ectopic varices. *Dis Colon Rectum* 2002;45:1541.

95. Harries K, Owen C, Mills C, et al. Acute stomal contact dermatitis or pemphigus. *Br J Surg* 1997;84:685.

96. Heiblum M, Cordoba A. An artificial sphincter: a preliminary report. *Dis Colon Rectum* 1978;21:562.

97. Hellinger MD, Martinez SA, Parra-Davila E, et al. Gasless laparoscopic-assisted stoma creation through a single incision. *Dis Colon Rectum* 1999;42:1228.

98. Henry MM, Everett WG. Loop colostomy closure. *Br J Surg* 1979;66:275.

99. Heriot AG, Tilney HS, Simson JNL. The application of percutaneous endoscopic colostomy to the management of obstructed defecation. *Dis Colon Rectum* 2002;45:700.

100. Hesterberg R, Stahlknecht CD, Röher HD. Sclerotherapy for massive enterostomy bleeding resulting from portal hypertension. *Dis Colon Rectum* 1986;29:275.

101. Hines JR. A method of transverse loop colostomy. *Surg Gynecol Obstet* 1975;141:426.

102. Hines JR, Harris GD. Colostomy and colostomy closure. *Surg Clin North Am* 1983;57:1379.

103. Hoffmann J, Jensen H-E. Tube cecostomy and staged resection for obstructing carcinoma of the colon. *Dis Colon Rectum* 1984;27:24.

104. Hofstetter WL, Vukasin P, Ortega AE, et al. New technique for mesh repair of paracolostomy hernias. *Dis Colon Rectum* 1998;41:1054.

105. Hollyoak MA, Lumley J, Stitz RW. Laparoscopic stoma formation for faecal diversion. *Br J Surg* 1998;85:226

106. Hull TL, Kobe I, Fazio VW. Comparison of handsewn with stapled loop ileostomy closures. *Dis Colon Rectum* 1996;39:1086.

107. Hunt N, Corman ML. Enterostomal therapy. *Contemp Educ* 1982;April:79.

108. Isa S, Quan SHQ. Colostomy perforation. *Dis Colon Rectum* 1978;21:92.

109. Jänes A, Cengiz Y, Israelsson LA. Randomized clinical trial of the use of a prosthetic mesh to prevent parastomal hernia. *Br J Surg* 2004;91:280.

110. Jao S-W, Beart RW Jr, Wendorf LJ, et al. Irrigation management of sigmoid colostomy. *Arch Surg* 1985;120:916.

111. Jarpa S. Transverse or sigmoid loop colostomy fixed by skin flaps. *Surg Gynecol Obstet* 1986;163:373.

112. Jess P, Christiansen J. Laparoscopic loop ileostomy for fecal diversion. *Dis Colon Rectum* 1994;37:721.

113. Johnson WR, McDermott FT, Pihl E, et al. Adenocarcinoma of an ileostomy in a patient with ulcerative colitis. *Dis Colon Rectum* 1980;23:351.

114. Kalady MF, Fields RC, Klein S, et al. Loop ileostomy closure at an ambulatory surgery facility: a safe and cost-effective alternative to routine hospitalization. *Dis Colon Rectum* 2003;46:486.

115. Kald A, Landin S, Masreliez C, et al. Mesh repair of parastomal hernias: new aspects of the onlay technique. *Tech Coloproctol* 2001;5:169.

116. Kestenberg A, Becker JM. A new technique of loop ileostomy closure after endorectal ileoanal anastomosis. *Surgery* 1985;98:109.

117. Kewenter J. Continent colostomy with the aid of a magnetic closing system: a preliminary report. *Dis Colon Rectum* 1978;21:46.

118. Khoo REH, Montrey J, Cohen MM. Laproscopic loop ileostomy for temporary fecal diversion. *Dis Colon Rectum* 1993;36:966.

119. Khubchandani IT, Trimpi HD, Sheets JA, et al. The magnetic stoma device: a continent colostomy. *Dis Colon Rectum* 1981;24:344.

120. Kock NG, Geroulantos S, Hahnloser P, et al. Continent colostomy: an experimental study in dogs. *Dis Colon Rectum* 1974;17:727.

121. Kock NG, Myrvold HE, Philipson BM, et al. Continent cecostomy: an account of 30 patients. *Dis Colon Rectum* 1985;28:705.

122. Kostov DV, Temelkov TD, Dragnev NA, et al. Smooth muscle sphincteroplasty in colostomy. *Dis Colon Rectum* 2004;47:486.

123. Krasna IH. A simple purse string suture technique for treatment of colostomy prolapse and intussusception. *J Pediatr Surg* 1979;14:801.

124. Krause R, Freund HR, Fischer JE. A new technique for performing end enterostomies using a stapling device. *Am J Surg* 1979;138:461.

125. Kretschmer KP. *The intestinal stomas: indications, operative methods, care, rehabilitation.* Philadelphia: WB Saunders, 1978.

126. Kronborg O, Kramhöft J, Backer O, et al. Late complications following operations for cancer of the rectum and anus. *Dis Colon Rectum* 1974;17:750.

127. Lafreniere R, Ketcham AS. The Penrose drain: a safe, atraumatic colostomy bridge. *Am J Surg* 1985;149:288.

128. Last M, Fazio V, Lavery I, et al. Conservative management of paraileostomy ulcers in patients with Crohn's disease. *Dis Colon Rectum* 1984;27:779.

129. Lau JTK. Proximal end transverse colostomy in children: a method to avoid colostomy prolapse in Hirschsprung's disease. *Dis Colon Rectum* 1983;26:221.

130. Law WL, Chu KW, Choi HK. Randomized clinical trial comparing loop ileostomy and loop transverse colostomy for faecal diversion following total mesorectal excision. *Br J Surg* 2002;89:704.

131. LeBlanc KA, Bellanger DE. Laparoscopic repair of paraostomy hernias: early results. *J Am Coll Surg* 2002;194:232.

132. Leong APK, Londono-Schimmer EE, Phillips RKS. Life-table analysis of stomal complications following ileostomy. *Br J Surg* 1994;81:727.

133. Light HG. A secure end colostomy technique. *Surg Gynecol Obstet* 1992;174:67.

134. Londono-Schimmer EE, Leong APK, Phillips RKS. Life table analysis of stomal complications following colostomy. *Dis Colon Rectum* 1994;37:916.

135. Ludwig KA, Milsom JW, Garcia-Ruiz A, et al. Laparoscopic techniques for fecal diversion. *Dis Colon Rectum* 1996;39:285.

136. Marks CG, Ritchie JK. The complications of synchronous combined excision for adenocarcinoma of the rectum at St. Mark's Hospital. *Br J Surg* 1975;62:901.

137. Mattingly M, Wasvary H, Sacksner J, et al. Minimally invasive, endoscopically assisted colostomy can be performed without general anesthesia or laparotomy. *Dis Colon Rectum* 2003;46:271.

138. Maydl K. Zur technik der kolostomie. *Centralbl Chir* 1888;24:433.

139. Mayo CW. Button colopexy for prolapse of colon through colonic stoma. *Mayo Clin Proc* 1939;14:439.
140. McGarity WC. The evolution of continence following total colectomy. *Am Surg* 1992;58:1.
141. McGarity WC, Robertson DB, McKeown PP, et al. Pyoderma gangrenosum at the parastomal site in patients with Crohn's disease. *Arch Surg* 1984;119:1186.
142. McLeod RS, Lavery IC, Leatherman JR, et al. Patient evaluation of the conventional ileostomy. *Dis Colon Rectum* 1985;28:152.
143. Mealy K, O'Broin E, Donohue J, et al. Reversible colostomy—what is the outcome? *Dis Colon Rectum* 1996;39:1227.
144. Warren R, McKittrick LS. Ileostomy for ulcerative colitis: technique, complications, and management. *Surg Gynecol Obstet* 1951;93:555.
145. Meuwissen SM, Bakker PJM, Rietra PJGM. Acute ulceration of ileal stoma due to *Campylobacter fetus* subspecies *jejuni*. *BMJ* 1981;282:1362.
146. Meyerhoff HH, Andersen B, Nielsen SL. Colostomy irrigation: a clinical and scintigraphic comparison between three different irrigation volumes. *Br J Surg* 1990;77:1185.
147. Miles RM, Greene RS. Review of colostomy in a community hospital. *Am Surg* 1983;49:182.
148. Mileski WJ, Rege RV, Joehl RJ, et al. Rates of morbidity and mortality after closure of loop and end colostomy. *Surg Gynecol Obstet* 1990;171:17.
149. Mirelman D, Corman ML, Veidenheimer MC, et al. Colostomies: indications and contraindications. Lahey Clinic experience, 1963–1974. *Dis Colon Rectum* 1978;21:172.
150. Mitchell WH, Kovalcik PJ, Cross GH. Complications of colostomy closure. *Dis Colon Rectum* 1978;21:180.
151. Moisidis E, Curiskis JI, Brooke-Cowden GL. Improving the reinforcement of parastomal tissues with Marlex[R] mesh: laboratory study identifying solutions to stomal aperture distortion. *Dis Colon Rectum* 2000;43:55.
152. Morgan TR, Feldshon SD, Tripp MR. Recurrent stomal variceal bleeding: successful treatment using injection sclerotherapy. *Dis Colon Rectum* 1986;29:269.
153. Morowitz DA, Kirsner JB. Ileostomy in ulcerative colitis: a questionnaire study of 1803 patients. *Am J Surg* 1981;141:370.
154. Morris DM, Rayburn D. Loop colostomies are totally diverting in adults. *Am J Surg* 1991;161:668.
155. Moseson MD, Labow SB, Hoexter B. Technique for totally diverting loop transverse colostomy. *Dis Colon Rectum* 1983;26:195.
156. Mukherjee A, Parikh VA, Aguilar PS. Colonoscopic-assisted colostomy—an alternative to laparotomy: report of two cases. *Dis Colon Rectum* 1998;41:1458.
157. Nakahara S, Itoh H, Iida M, et al. Ileal adenomas in familial polyposis coli: differences before and after colectomy. *Dis Colon Rectum* 1985;28:875.
158. Narasimharao KL, Chatterjee H. A new technique of prolapse-free transverse colostomy. *Surg Gynecol Obstet* 1984;158:283.
159. Nugent KP, Daniels P, Stewart B, et al. Quality of life in stoma patients. *Dis Colon Rectum* 1999;42:1569.
160. O'Bichere A, Bossom C, Gangoli S, et al. Chemical colostomy irrigation with glyceryl trinitrate solution. *Dis Colon Rectum* 2001;44:1324.
161. O'Connell PR, Dozois RR, Irons GB, et al. Squamous cell carcinoma occurring in a skin-grafted ileostomy stoma: report of a case. *Dis Colon Rectum* 1987;30:475.
162. Oluwole SF, Freeham HP, Davis K. Morbidity of closure of colostomy. *Dis Colon Rectum* 1982;25:422.
163. Patey DH. Primary epithelial apposition in colostomy. *Proc R Soc Med* 1951;44:423.
164. Pearl RK. Parastomal hernia. *World J Surg* 1989;13:569.
165. Peck JJ, Boyden AM. Exigent ileostomy hemorrhage: a complication of proctocolectomy in patients with chronic ulcerative colitis and primary sclerosing cholangitis. *Am J Surg* 1985;150:153.
166. Pemberton JH, Van Heerden JA, Beart RW Jr, et al. A continent ileostomy device. *Ann Surg* 1983;197:618.
167. Pittman DM, Smith LE. Complications of colostomy closure. *Dis Colon Rectum* 1985;28:836.
168. Ponsky JL, Aszodi A, Perse D. Percutaneous endoscopic cecostomy: a new approach to nonobstructive colonic dilation. *Gastrointest Endosc* 1986;32:108.
169. Porter JA, Salvati EP, Rubin RJ, et al. Complications of colostomies. *Dis Colon Rectum* 1989;32:299.
170. Porcheron J, Payan B, Balique JG. Mesh repair of parastomal hernia by laparoscopy. *Surg Endosc* 1998;12:1281.
171. Prager E. The continent colostomy. *Dis Colon Rectum* 1984;27:235.
172. Prager E, Gall F. A new method of stoma control. *Contemp Surg* 1985;26:81.
173. Prasad ML, Pearl RK, Abcarian H. End-loop colostomy. *Surg Gynecol Obstet* 1984;158:380.
174. Prasad ML, Pearl RK, Orsay CP, et al. Rodless ileostomy: a modified loop ileostomy. *Dis Colon Rectum* 1984;27:270.
175. Prian GW, Sawyer RB, Sawyer KC. Repair of peristomal colostomy hernias. *Am J Surg* 1975;130:694.
176. Raza SD, Portin BA, Bernhoft WH. Umbilical colostomy: a better intestinal stoma. *Dis Colon Rectum* 1977;20:223.
177. Resnick S. New method of bowel stoma formation. *Am J Surg* 1986;152:545.
178. Reynolds HM Jr, Frazier TG, Copeland EM III. Treatment of paracolostomy abscess without proximal diverting colostomy: report of two cases. *Dis Colon Rectum* 1976;19:458.
179. Rickwood AMK, Hemalatha V, Brooman P. Closure of colostomy in infants and children. *Br J Surg* 1979;66:273.
180. Roberts PL, Martin FM, Schoetz DJ Jr, et al. Bleeding stomal varices: the role of local treatment. *Dis Colon Rectum* 1990;33:547.
181. Roberts PL, Veidenheimer MC, Cassidy S, et al. Adenocarcinoma arising in an ileostomy. *Arch Surg* 1989;124:497.
182. Roe AM, Barlow AP, Durdey P, et al. Indications for laparoscopic formation of intestinal stomas. *Surg Laparosc Endosc* 1994;4:345.
183. Rolstad BS, Wilson W, Rothenberger DA. Sexual concerns in the patient with an ileostomy. *Dis Colon Rectum* 1983;26:170.
184. Rombeau JL, Turnbull RB Jr. Hidden-loop colostomy. *Dis Colon Rectum* 1978;21:177.
185. Rombeau JL, Wilk PJ, Turnbull RB Jr, et al. Total fecal diversion by the temporary skin-level loop transverse colostomy. *Dis Colon Rectum* 1978;21:223.
186. Rosen L, Friedman IH. Morbidity and mortality following intraperitoneal closure of transverse loop colostomy. *Dis Colon Rectum* 1980;23:508.
187. Rosin JD, Bonardi RA. Paracolostomy hernia repair with Marlex mesh: a new technique. *Dis Colon Rectum* 1977;20:299.
188. Roy PH, Saver WG, Beahrs OH, et al. Experience with ileostomies: evaluation of long-term rehabilitation in 497 patients. *Am J Surg* 1970;119:77.
189. Rubin MS, Schoetz DJ Jr, Matthews JB. Parastomal hernia: is stoma relocation superior to fascial repair? *Arch Surg* 1994;129:413.
190. Sachatello CR, Maull KI. Rapid totally diverting loop sigmoid colostomy with noncontaminating rectal irrigation. *Am J Surg* 1977;134:300.
191. Salley RK, Bucher RM, Rodning CB. Colostomy closure: morbidity reduction employing a semistandardized protocol. *Dis Colon Rectum* 1983;26:319.
192. Samhouri F, Grodsinsky C. The morbidity and mortality of colostomy closure. *Dis Colon Rectum* 1979;22:312.
193. Sanders GB. Experiences with the Dragstedt skin-covered ileostomy. *Arch Surg* 1948;57:487.
194. Sarashina H, Ozaki A, Fukao K, et al. A new device for barium-enema examination following colostomy. *Radiology* 1979;133:241.
195. Schmidt E. The continent colostomy. *World J Surg* 1982;6:805.

196. Schofield PF, Cade D, Lambert M. Dependent proximal loop colostomy: does it defunction the distal colon? *Br J Surg* 1980;67:201.
197. Schwemmle K, Kunze H-H, Padberg W. Management of the colostomy. *World J Surg* 1982;6:554.
198. Senapati A, Nicholls RJ. Formation of a loop stoma. *Br J Surg* 1991;78:23.
199. Senapati A, Nicholls RJ, Ritchie JK, et al. Temporary loop ileostomy for restorative proctocolectomy. *Br J Surg* 1993; 80:628.
200. Sherlock DJ, Suarez V, Gray JG. Stomal adenocarcinoma in Crohn's disease. *Gut* 1990;31:1329.
201. Sigler L, Jedd FL. Adenocarcinoma of the ileostomy occurring after colectomy for ulcerative colitis: report of a case. *Dis Colon Rectum* 1969;12:45.
202. Sigurdson E, Myers E, Stern H. A modification of the transverse loop colostomy. *Dis Colon Rectum* 1986;29:65.
203. Sjödahl R, Anderberg B, Bolin T. Parastomal hernia in relation to site of the abdominal stoma. *Br J Surg* 1988;75:339.
204. Smart PJ, Sastry S, Wells S. Primary mucinous adenocarcinoma developing in an ileostomy stoma. *Gut* 1988;29:1607.
205. Smit R, Walt AJ. The morbidity and cost of the temporary colostomy. *Dis Colon Rectum* 1978;21:558.
206. Soliani P, Carbognani P, Piccolo P, et al. Colostomy plug devices: a possible new approach to the problem of incontinence. *Dis Colon Rectum* 1992;35:969.
207. Speakman CTM, Parker MC, Northover JMA. Outcome of stapled revision of retracted ileostomy. *Br J Surg* 1991;78: 935.
208. Steinberg DM, Allan RN, Brooke BN, et al. Sequelae of colectomy and ileostomy: comparison between Crohn's colitis and ulcerative colitis. *Gastroenterology* 1975;68:33.
209. Stelzner S, Hellmich G, Ludwig K. Repair of paracolostomy hernias with a prosthetic mesh in the intraperitoneal onlay position: modified Sugarbaker technique. *Dis Colon Rectum* 2004;47:185.
210. Stephenson ER Jr, Ilahi O, Koltun WA. Stoma creation through the stoma site: a rapid, safe technique. *Dis Colon Rectum* 1997;40:112.
211. Stryker SJ, Pemberton JH, Zinsmeister AR. Long-term results of ileostomy in older patients. *Dis Colon Rectum* 1985; 28:844.
212. Sugarbaker PH. Prosthetic mesh repair of large hernias at the site of colonic stomas. *Surg Gynecol Obstet* 1980;150: 577.
213. Sugarbaker PH. Peritoneal approach to prosthetic mesh repair of paraostomy hernias. *Ann Surg* 1985;201:344.
214. Swain BT, Ellis CN Jr. Laparoscopy-assisted loop ileostomy: an acceptable option for temporary fecal diversion after anorectal surgery. *Dis Colon Rectum* 2002;45: 705.
215. Sykes FR. Transcutaneous defunctioning colostomy. *Br J Surg* 1979;66:505.
216. Szinicz G. A new implantable sphincter prosthesis for artificial anus. *Int J Artif Organs* 1980;3:358.
217. Tang C-L, Seow-Choen F, Fook-Chong S, et al. Bioresorbable adhesion barrier facilitates early closure of the defunctioning ileostomy after rectal excision: a prospective, randomized trial. *Dis Colon Rectum* 2003;46:1200.
218. Taylor RL, Rombeau JL, Turnbull RB Jr. Transperitoneal relocation of the ileal stoma without formal laparotomy. *Surg Gynecol Obstet* 1978;146:953.
219. Tekkis PP, Kocher HM, Payne JG. Parastomal hernia repair: modified Thorlakson technique, reinforced by polypropylene mesh. *Dis Colon Rectum* 1999;42:1505.
220. Tenney JB, Eng M, Graney MJ. The quest for continence: a morphologic survey of approaches to a continent colostomy. *Dis Colon Rectum* 1978;21:522.
221. Terranova O, Sandei F, Rebuffat C, et al. Irrigation vs. natural evacuation of left colostomy: a comparative study of 340 patients. *Dis Colon Rectum* 1979;22:31.
222. Thomson JPS. Caecostomy and colostomy. Part I: surgical procedures and complications. *Clin Gastroenterol* 1982;11: 285.
223. Thomson WHF, White S, O'Leary DP. Tube caecostomy to protect rectal anastomoses. *Br J Surg* 1998;85:1533.
224. Thorlakson RH. Technique of repair of herniations associated with colonic stomas. *Surg Gynecol Obstet* 1965;120:347.
225. Tjandra JJ, Hughes LE. Parastomal pyoderma gangrenosum in inflammatory bowel disease. *Dis Colon Rectum* 1994;37:938.
226. Todd GJ, Kutcher LM, Markowitz AM. Factors influencing the complications of colostomy closure. *Am J Surg* 1979;137:749.
227. Truedson H, Press V. A new method of stomal reconstruction in patients with retraction of conventional ileostomy. *Surg Gynecol Obstet* 1986;162:60.
228. Turnbull RB Jr. Management of ileostomy. *Am J Surg* 1953;86:617.
229. Turnbull RB, Weakley FL. *Atlas of intestinal stomas*. St. Louis: CV Mosby, 1967:207.
230. Unti JA, Abcarian H, Pearl RK, et al. Rodless end-loop stomas: seven-year experience. *Dis Colon Rectum* 1991;34: 999.
231. Vande Maele DM, Reilly JC. Bullous pemphigoid at colostomy site: report of a case. *Dis Colon Rectum* 1997;40: 370.
232. Varnell J, Pemberton LB. Risk factors in colostomy closure. *Surgery* 1981;89:683.
233. Vasilevsky C-A, Gordon PH. Adenocarcinoma arising at the ileocutaneous junction occurring after proctocolectomy for ulcerative colitis. *Br J Surg* 1986;73:378.
234. Venturini M, Bertelli G, Forno G, et al. Colostomy irrigation in the elderly. Effective recovery regardless of age. *Dis Colon Rectum* 1990;33:1031.
235. Vogel SL, Maher JW. An improved method for construction of loop colostomy. *Surg Gynecol Obstet* 1986;162:377.
236. Voitk A. Simple technique for laparoscopic paracolostomy hernia repair. *Dis Colon Rectum* 2000;43:1451.
237. Wara P, Sorensen K, Berg V. Proximal fecal diversion: review of ten years' experience. *Dis Colon Rectum* 1981;24: 114.
238. Watt RC. Colostomy irrigation: yes or no? *Am J Nurs* 1977;77:442.
239. Wexner SD, Taranow DA, Johansen OB, et al. Loop ileostomy is a safe option for fecal diversion. *Dis Colon Rectum* 1993;36:349.
240. Wheeler MH, Barker J. Closure of colostomy: a safe procedure? *Dis Colon Rectum* 1977;20:29.
241. Whittaker M, Goligher JC. A comparison of the results of extraperitoneal and intraperitoneal techniques for construction of terminal iliac colostomies. *Dis Colon Rectum* 1976;19:342.
242. Wilkinson AJ, Humphreys WG. Seat-belt injury to ileostomy. *BMJ* 1978;1:1249.
243. Williams JG, Etherington R, Hayward MWJ, et al. Para-ileostomy hernia: a clinical and radiological study. *Br J Surg* 1990;77:1355.
244. Williams NS, Johnston D. Prospective controlled trial comparing colostomy irrigation with "spontaneousaction" method. *BMJ* 1980;281:107.
245. Williams NS, Nasmyth DG, Jones D, et al. Defunctioning stomas: a prospective controlled trial comparing loop ileostomy with loop transverse colostomy. *Br J Surg* 1986; 73:566.
246. Winkler MJ, Volpe PA. Loop transverse colostomy: the case against. *Dis Colon Rectum* 1982;25:321.
247. Winslet MC, Alexander-Williams J, Keighley MRB. Ileostomy revision with a GIA stapler under intravenous sedation. *Br J Surg* 1990;77:647.
248. Yagüe S. A new technique for temporary transparietocecal ileal diversion in the prevention of anastomotic leakage in colonic operations. *Surg Gynecol Obstet* 1986;162:381.
249. Yajko RD, Norton LW, Bioemendal L, et al. Morbidity of colostomy closure. *Am J Surg* 1976;132:304.
250. Zinkin LD, Rosin JD. Button colopexy for colostomy prolapse. *Surg Gynecol Obstet* 1981;152:89.

Chapter 32

Enterostomal Therapy

I asked Dr. Victor W. Fazio and Paula Erwin-Toth of the Cleveland Clinic Foundation to contribute this chapter to the fourth edition of this text. With the fifth edition, I also asked a clinical nurse specialist, Susan Feldman, to correct any errors and discrepancies and to update equipment and supplies. She was kind enough to proof this chapter and make the appropriate changes. She is a certified enterostomal therapist at the Long Island Jewish Medical Center.

The Department of Colon and Rectal Surgery at the Cleveland Clinic has a long and illustrious history in the field of colon and rectal surgery through the initial efforts of Rupert Turnbull (see biography, Chapter 31). Dr. Fazio needs no introduction to readers of the literature in colon and rectal surgery. He has contributed voluminously to the field and is chair of the Department of Colon and Rectal Surgery at the Cleveland Clinic Foundation. He is also editor-in-chief of the journal *Diseases of the Colon and Rectum*. He is past president of both the American Board of Colon and Rectal Surgery and the American Society of Colon and Rectal Surgeons.

Paula Erwin-Toth is a certified enterostomal therapy nurse and is manager of enterostomal therapy nursing at the Cleveland Clinic Foundation. Furthermore, she is director of the Enterostomal Therapy Education Program at that institution. She is the ideal person to contribute her thoughts and her experiences to this text. I consider it a personal honor that these three superb individuals were willing to take the time to supplement my writings in Chapter 31.—MLC

> It is necessary hoe hym that is sycke to have
> two or three good keepers.
> Andrew Boorde (1490–1549)—*The Dyetary of Helth XL*

The care of the patient who will undergo or who has undergone ostomy surgery involves close cooperation among the surgeon, the wound, ostomy, continence (WOC)/ enterostomal therapy (ET) nurse, and the patient in order to achieve optimal rehabilitation. As discussed in Chapter 31, the technique for fashioning an ostomy falls within the purview of the surgeon. However, much of the physical, emotional, and educational aspects of the rehabilitation process usually fall within the domain of the WOC/ET nurse.[6,14] Still, if an WOC/ET nurse is not available, responsibility for stoma assessment, fitting, and rehabilitation still properly rests with the surgeon.[6]

PREOPERATIVE CARE

As stated in Chapter 31, optimal postoperative stomal management begins with preoperative preparation.[8] The patient and family members ideally should receive comprehensive information concerning overall ostomy rehabilitation, plans, and management. This includes activity,

diet, clothing, and sexual concerns. The patient should be reassured that self-care may, at first, seem awkward, but all can be mastered by almost any patient at any age in a relatively short time.[8] Contact with an ostomy visitor may be especially beneficial. A confident, fully rehabilitated ostomy/site visitor can provide hope and improve morale for the apprehensive patient.

As discussed in Chapter 31, the site should ideally fall below the umbilicus in the left or right lower quadrant, on the superior aspect of the infraumbilical fat mound, and should lie within the surface marking of the rectus sheath (see Figs. 29-39 and 29-40).[7,14] It is important to avoid scars, creases, and bony prominences in order to provide a smooth pouching surface postoperatively (Figure 32-1). It is also imperative for the individual to see the site. To accomplish this, the patient is evaluated while he or she is supine, sitting, and standing, since positional changes can materially alter the abdominal configuration (Figure 32-2). A patient with a protuberant abdomen or someone requiring long-term use of a wheelchair may be better served with a stoma located in the upper abdomen.[7] It is axiomatic that self-care will be rendered difficult or impossible if the patient is unable to see the stoma. While stoma site selection is truly the responsibility of the surgeon, it is appropriate and reasonable to delegate this task to an WOC/ET nurse.[14] Preoperatively, utilizing a surgical marking pen or a fine-gauge needle (see Figure 29-40) provides a guide to the ideal location so that intraoperative guessing is eliminated. Even those patients who undergo emergency or temporary stomas should optimally have preoperative stomal marking.[7,14]

Independence in ostomy care requires integration of the stoma into the patient's everyday life. In addition to site selection, stoma construction, itself, can have a profound influence on the effectiveness of a pouching system (see Chapters 29 and 31). A budded stoma in a preselected location offers the best chance for successful ostomy management. A patient who is offered a comprehensive preoperative educational program is much more likely to be an active participant in postoperative activities. Even those individuals in whom there is only the possibility of a stoma or in whom the stoma is to be temporary should be marked and offered counseling preop-

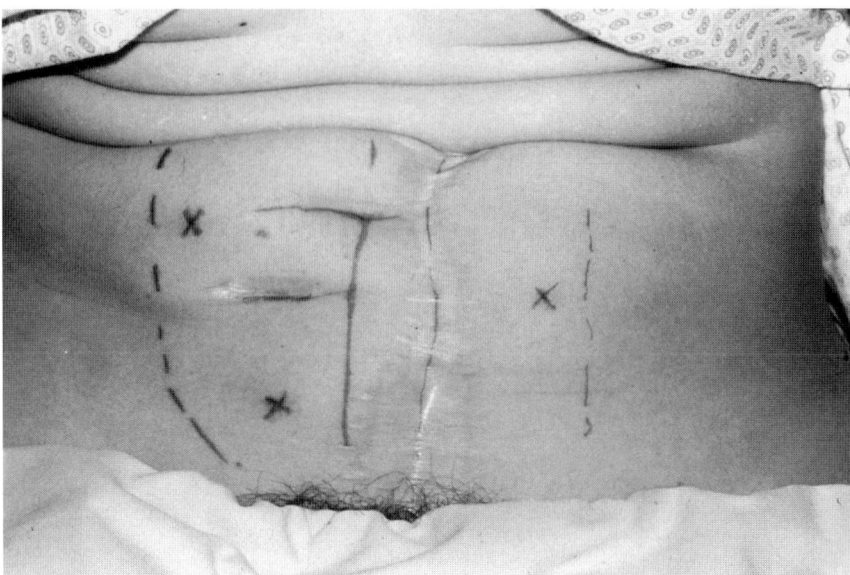

FIGURE 32-1. Selection of potential stomal sites is particularly difficult in this obese patient with a left paramedian incision. Also, note the scar from a prior stoma in the right lower quadrant. The dashed lines represent the outer border of the rectus muscles. The optimal site in this individual is the one marked on the left side.

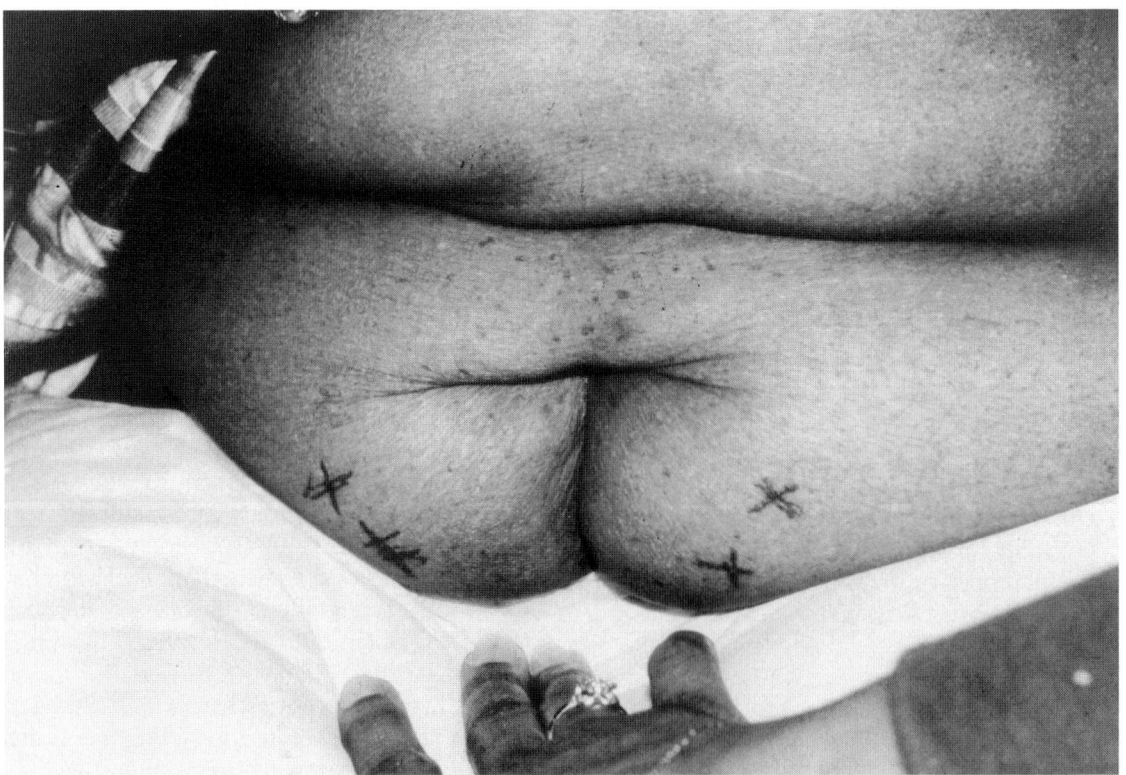

FIGURE 32-2. Site selection was inappropriately marked on both sides with the patient supine. The X's in the superior aspect were elected since the inferior ones would have fallen below the fat bulge.

eratively by the surgeon and/or the WOC/ET nurse.[8] National guidelines for enterostomal patient education have been established by the Standards Development Committee of the United Ostomy Association, with the assistance of Prospect Associates.[2]

STOMAL FUNCTION AND CARE

Fecal and urinary diversion may be performed in patients for a variety of clinical indications and situations. A brief overview of these various stomas follows.

Gastrointestinal Stomas

Jejunostomy

Jejunostomy function usually begins within the first 48 hours after surgery. Initially, the effluent is watery, clear, and dark green. Because the volume of output may approach 2,400 ml in 24 hours, the patient must be monitored closely for electrolyte imbalance. Since the absorption of nutrients, fluids, and electrolytes may be deficient in a patient with a jejunostomy, total parenteral nutrition or fluid/electrolyte support may be required.[14] In order to minimize the inconvenience associated with the need for frequent pouch emptying, connection to gravity drainage is advisable.

Ileostomy

An ileostomy generally begins to function within the first 48 to 72 hours after surgery, although those undergoing laparoscopic construction may evidence an effluent within 24 hours. The initial appearance may be viscous and green, but such an output does not necessarily indicate the return of peristalsis. Rather, it may represent the elimination of secretions that have collected in the distal small bowel. Once peristalsis has returned, the patient may enter a period of high-volume output known as the adaptation phase. Output during this time exceeds 1,000 ml/day, frequently reaching 1,500 to 1,800 ml/day. The physiological basis for this high-output phase is the loss of the colonic absorptive surface, coupled, theoretically, with the loss of the ileocecal valve. During this period, the patient should be monitored for signs and symptoms of fluid and electrolyte imbalance.

A loop ileostomy–supporting rod is removed by the 3rd to 5th postoperative day, depending on the amount of edema of the stoma itself. The greater the swelling, the earlier the rod may be removed. The less tissue reaction present, the longer the rod should be maintained. Edema itself tends to prevent the stoma from retracting, and the rod may actually intensify and prolong the duration of the edematous reaction. Patients with a loop ileostomy proximal to a pelvic pouch will experience a higher output and have an increased risk for fluid and electrolyte management problems. Readmission may be necessary for these individuals, and early stomal closure may be required for this indication. As with jejunostomy, connection of the pouch to gravity drainage will prevent overdistension of the appliance. If the stool thickens but output remains high, use of anesthesia tubing and a plastic bottle can be adapted. This is especially convenient if one utilizes a two-piece pouching system. While ambulating, the patient can wear a standard pouch and closure clamp, but a second pouch secured to the gravity drainage system can be attached while one is resting.

Over a period of days to weeks, the proximal small bowel increases fluid absorption. Gradually the volume of output decreases and the stool thickens to toothpaste-like consistency. Initially, the output from an ileostomy can vary from 500 to 1,500 ml in a 24-hour period. But, after adaptation, the average output decreases to between 500 and 800 ml/day.[14]

Continent Ileostomy

Since the advent of the pelvic pouch procedure (see Chapter 29), the continent ileostomy today is primarily performed for the indications of an elective conversion in those with a permanent, conventional (Brooke) ileostomy, for those with a failed reservoir-anal procedure, and for patients with anal incontinence. One of the important concerns is to stabilize the defunctioning drainage catheter that is placed in the pouch (see Figs. 29-70 and 29-71). This may be achieved through a variety of methods, including a stomal plate, ostomy appliance belt, or a baby nipple (Figure 32-3). A sterile gauze dressing around the stoma will absorb mucous and moisture as well as afford protection.[9,18]

To minimize tube blockage, gentle irrigation with 20 to 30 ml of normal saline is recommended, commencing in the recovery unit and continuing every 2 to 3 hours for the next few days.[9,18] Intervals between irrigations can be increased based on how well the tube is draining. It is extremely important to avoid over-distention of the pouch for the first few weeks following surgery in order to limit the likelihood of desussception. A bedside drainage bag or leg bag must be used to maintain constant drainage.

Colostomy

The initial output from a colostomy varies depending on the location of the stoma within the colon. Because the colon absorbs all but approximately 100 ml of the 1,000

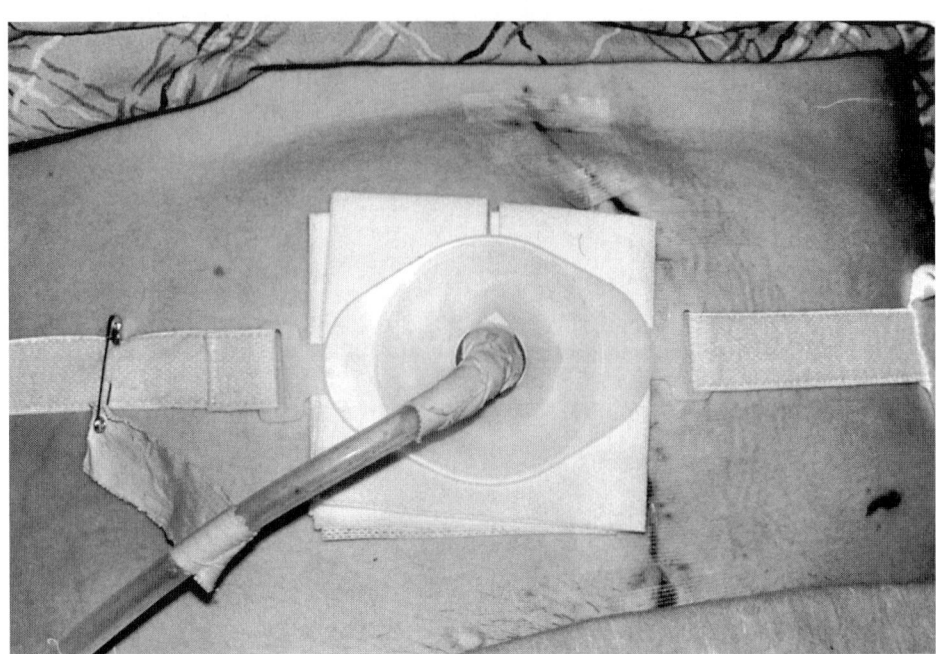

FIGURE 32-3. Continent ileostomy stoma plate. Baby bottle nipple anchors catheter device.

ml of contents that passes through the ileocecal valve daily, the output from distal colonic stomas has a thicker consistency and smaller volume than that of proximal colonic stomas.

Cecostomy

A cecostomy usually begins to function by the 3rd postoperative day. The output may be projectile (because of close proximity to the ileocecal valve), and it is initially liquid. The place of cecostomy in colon and rectal surgery has been discussed in the previous chapter and in Chapters 16 and 31. A cecostomy may be either skin level or tubal (see Figs. 28-52 and 31-44). As has already been discussed in this text, the location, output characteristics, and construction combine to make this a difficult stoma with which to deal. The tube cecostomy poses a special management problem, because stool tends to flow both through and around the tube. Furthermore, tube cecostomies are also associated with a greater risk of intra-abdominal spillage.

Transverse Colostomy

A transverse colostomy usually begins to function on postoperative day three or four. Output, which varies from pasty to soft, usually occurs after meals and at intervals throughout the day. For a loop colostomy, a supporting device (e.g., rod or bridge) placed during surgery is removed 3 to 5 days later (see Chapter 31). Corman and Odenheimer have described numerous methods for cre-

ating a loop colostomy in order to maintain stomal support.[5]

Descending/Sigmoid Colostomy

A descending or sigmoid colostomy requires the longest time to regain normal function, perhaps not until postoperative day 5. After this period, one logically should be concerned with issues that may cause delay in colonic function—ileus, administration of narcotics, obstruction, and so on. One may consider the option of stimulating colonic evacuation by means of a no. 20 French Foley catheter gently advanced into the stoma. A warmed solution of 500 ml of normal saline can be instilled via gravity drainage and allowed to return.[6,8,14] This procedure initiates a reflex contraction, stimulating peristalsis and providing relief of gaseous distention. Since many patients with a colostomy are discharged as early as the 4th postoperative day, self-care instruction may not be adequate because of the lack of output. Another alternative is to utilize a stool substitute placed in the pouch to assist in teaching pouch-emptying techniques. Instruction is continued following hospital discharge in the patient's home or in the out-patient department.

Once normal bowel function has returned, the output from a descending or sigmoid colostomy usually is a soft, formed stool. Elimination patterns generally are the same as that experienced by the patient before he or she became ill. Colostomy irrigation with a cone may also be performed as a management option to avoid an appliance in selected patients or in preparation for diagnostic

▶ TABLE 32-1 Colostomy Irrigation With a Cone

1. Apply the irrigation sleeve securely around the stoma to prevent leakage.
2. Close the shutoff valve. Fill the irrigation bag with 500 to 100 ml of tepid water and hang the irrigation bag on a hook.
3. Remove air from the tubing by opening the shutoff valve until the water runs out of the cone. Close the shutoff valve and lubricate the end of the cone with water-soluble lubricant.
4. Sit up straight on a chair or toilet with irrigating sleeve just touching the water level in the toilet bowl.
5. Open the shutoff valve until the water flows slowly. Insert the lubricated cone into the stoma until the water enters without leakage. Increase the flow rate as tolerated. If a cramp develops, stop or decrease the water flow until the cramp passes and then resume the water flow.
6. When the 500 to 1000 ml of water has entered the colon, remove the cone and close the top of the irrigation sleeve. The bottom of the irrigation sleeve should remain in the toilet bowl for no less than *15 minutes*. By then, the majority of the stool and water will have returned.
7. Rinse the inside of the irrigation sleeve with water to remove the waste material. Remove the irrigation sleeve from the bowl. Dry and clip the bottom of the irrigation sleeve to the top of the sleeve. It may take up to *45 minutes* for the rest of the water and stool to return.

testing (Fig. 31-22). The technique for colostomy irrigation has been discussed in Chapter 31. However, instructions for the patient appear in Tables 32-1 and 32-2.

Urinary Stomas

Vesicostomy

Drainage is provided by a Foley catheter placed in the anterior dome of the bladder. Should pouching be requested, the suprapubic location can make obtaining a secure seal problematic. Shaving the pubic hair is helpful in order to facilitate pouch adherence and removal.

Ureterostomy

Creation of unilateral or bilateral ureteral openings to the skin is uncommonly employed. The flush or retracted stoma associated with ureterostomies can pose a real pouching challenge. If the stoma is located in the flank, self-care may be impossible. Therefore, a family member

▶ TABLE 32-2 Colostomy Irrigation Helpful Hints

Spray the inside of the irrigation sleeve with any liquid soap or detergent before the enema so that the stool will drain easily, the sleeve will clean faster, and less odor will be retained.

***During* the enema, if you experience**
CRAMPING:
May indicate constipation; recall firmness of prior evacuation.
• Slow or stop the flow of water, relax and deep breathe.
• Re-check the rate of water flow; flow rate should be around 10 minutes for 1,000 ml of water; 5 to 7 minutes for 500 ml.
• Check the height of enema bag; should be approximately 12 to 20 inches (30 to 50 cm) above shoulder level when you are seated.
SLUGGISH/NO RETURNS:
May indicate constipation; recall firmness of prior evacuation.
• Look at diet; may need to increase bulk, such as bran, fresh fruits, and vegetables.
May indicate dehydration; increase oral fluid intake to *8 glasses* of liquid per day.
• Increase physical activity.

***After* the enema, if you experience**
SPILLAGE:
May indicate constipation; recall firmness of prior evacuation.
• Look at the volume of water inserted during the enema; most individuals require 1,000 ml.
• Do not use more than 1,000 ml without physician's permission.
• Check that the enema solution does not escape around the cone or shield.
EXCESSIVE GAS OR FLATUS:
• Avoid gas-forming foods.
• Eat regular meals; chew food well.
• Avoid air swallowing, that is, mouth breathing, gum chewing, smoking, straws, carbonated beverages, alcohol.

or other home caregiver should be instructed on how to manage this ostomy.[8]

Nephrostomy

Generally, nephrostomies are managed by means of a closed drainage system. A skin-barrier wafer is usually placed on the skin around the tube to protect the skin and to anchor the tube to prevent accidental dislodgement.[8]

Conduits

Ileal, jejunal, and colonic conduits are frequently employed methods for effecting urinary diversion. Preoperative stoma sighting and construction of a properly budded stoma will improve the potential for obtaining a secure pouch seal.

Continent Urinary Diversion

A variety of forms of continent urinary diversion are performed. Pre- and post-operative management techniques for these types of diversion are similar to that of continent ileostomy.

The ileocecal reservoir, commonly known as an Indiana pouch, utilizes a variety of tubes and drains. Drainage of the newly created urinary reservoir is accomplished by means of a cecostomy tube, bilateral urinary stents, and a catheter placed into the plicated exit conduit (Figure 32-4).[1,9,18] Depending on the surgeon's preference, gentle irrigation of the cecostomy tube with 20 to 30 ml of normal saline is performed every 2 to 3 hours.[9] As with the continent ileostomy, the goal is to maintain the patency of the catheter and to prevent over-distension of the newly created reservoir. It is not uncommon to cap the catheter into the exit conduit to avoid disruption of the newly plicated ileal segment.

Stabilization of the tubes and drains can be achieved by a variety of tube anchoring devices. Use of constant drainage by means of a bedside drainage bag or leg bag is recommended for the first few weeks after surgery.[9,18]

OSTOMY MANAGEMENT

Immediate Postoperative Period

Proper application of a pouching system should begin in the operating room. The appliance is fixed to clean, dry skin in order to protect the incision and the peristomal skin, and to contain stomal discharge. While it is true that most fecal stomas will not begin to function for a few days, mucosal secretions are ideally collected with a pouch. Conversely, urinary stomas will function immedi-

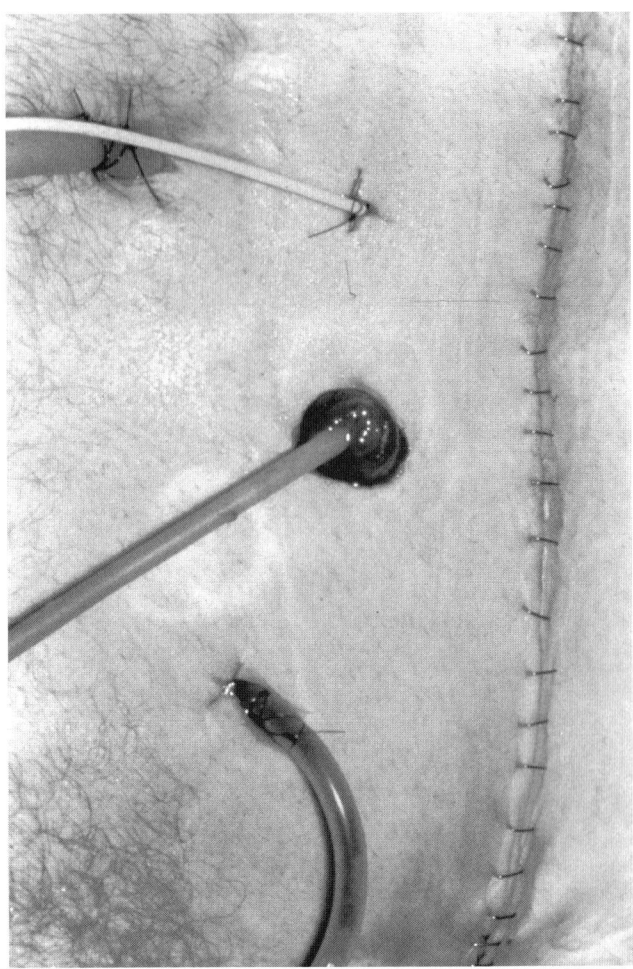

FIGURE 32-4. Multiple tubes are shown as described in a patient who underwent a so-called Indiana reservoir.

ately unless anastomotic disruption of the urinary-bowel connection has occurred. Pouch application coupled with connection to gravity drainage is indicated for urinary stomas.

A variety of one-piece or two-piece, disposable, odorproof, pouching systems may be used (Figure 32-5 and Table 32-3). By using a disposable measuring guide, and by sizing the aperture of the pouch within one-eighth inch (3 mm) of the base of the stomal mucosa, one can protect the peristomal skin and prevent mucosal trauma (Figure 32-6). Removal of the release paper and gentle pressure to the abdomen following pouch application will enhance pouch adherence. A transparent, drainable pouch will permit the clinician to assess stoma viability as well as output. A closure clamp or tubing device is then securely applied (Figure 32-7).

A healthy, viable stoma appears moist, beefy red, and often edematous. However, a continent ileostomy stoma may have a darker, bruised appearance due to mesenteric

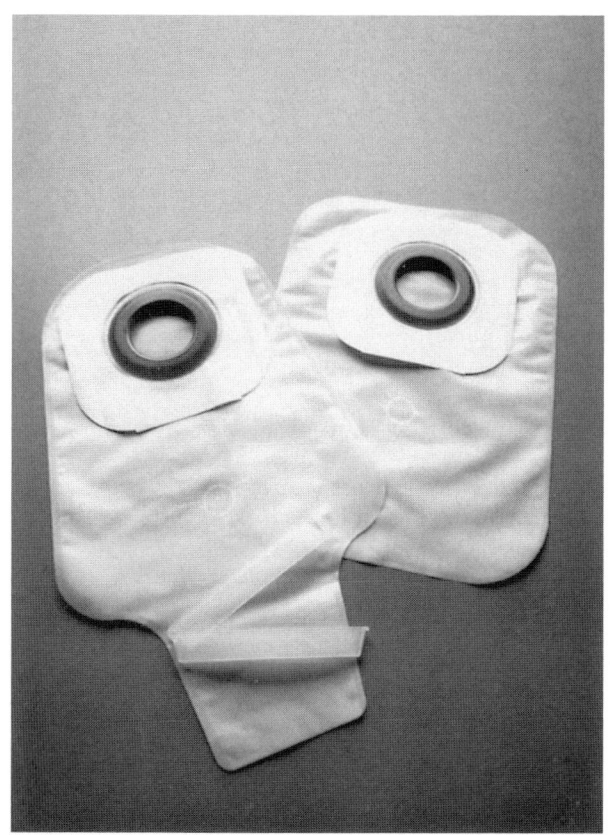

FIGURE 32-5. Drainable and closed pouches with karaya seal and adhesive. (Courtesy of Hollister, Inc.)

venous compression. Some individuals with a history of using senna-containing laxatives may demonstrate melanosis coli in the mucosa of their colostomy. This stoma may appear moist and gray to brown or even black in appearance due to staining of the bowel mucosa (see Color Figure 16-11).

Assessment of the mucosa is evaluated with each pouch change. Viability and function can be assessed daily by the surgeon and WOC/ET nurse and by each shift of the nursing staff.

Principles of Fitting

In order to provide some appreciation for the alternative methods of managing ostomies, it is important to have an understanding of ostomy collection devices. It is not important for a surgeon to be familiar with every company and every product in the field. It is merely necessary to be aware of the general principles for using the various devices and to have, perhaps, one or two alternatives from which to choose should the need arise.

Three primary parts—skin barrier, faceplate, and pouch—are necessary for an effective collecting system, but there are a variety of additional accessories.[11] The

newer generation of appliances incorporates these parts into a single disposable or reusable system.

Skin Protective Agent

A skin protective agent, such as Skin Prep or Skin Gel, provides a clear dressing that coats the skin. Generally, protective agents are used when tape-like products (e.g., double-faced disks) or cement contact the skin, in order to limit the likelihood of irritation. They also augment adherence of an appliance and facilitate adhesive removal from reusable faceplates.[19] These protective agents are available as gels, sprays, wipes, paint-on solutions, or pastes. Distinction must be made between a skin barrier and a protecting agent; individuals with ileostomies should never use a protective agent in place of a skin barrier.

Skin Barrier

A skin barrier is an adherent porous material that offers protection from the contents of the colon or ileum (e.g., karaya). Preserving the integrity of the skin is of great concern in the immediate postoperative period. Moist, weeping, oily, eroded skin will lead to leakage, odor, and loss of appliance adhesion. Meticulous attention to skin care must begin in the operating or recovery room with the first application of the skin barrier and placement of the pouch. The most commonly employed skin barriers are discussed in the following sections.

Karaya Products

Karaya is a resin that forms a protective base when combined with glycerin, thus inhibiting the corrosive effects of ileal contents. It is relatively insoluble and quite hydroscopic. It is refined and marketed in different forms, including powders, washers, wafers, and blankets, and mixed with natural clays. It is also manufactured in paste form, which provides an excellent means for filling in crevices created by abdominal folds near the stoma. Karaya stretches, and when it is used as a washer, it should measure about one-fourth inch smaller than the base of the stoma in order to fit it snugly. Specially prepared hole-cutter tools are available from several ostomy manufacturers (Figure 32-8).

Karaya is non-allergenic, although the ingredients in some products may cause some sensitivity. If this is a problem, a change to a karaya product manufactured by another company may be all that is required.

One disadvantage of karaya products is the tendency to break down in the presence of urine. Therefore, they should never be used with urinary diversions. Karaya melts easily in heat or even when the patient has an elevated temperature. Thus, for ostomates who live in warm

▶ **TABLE 32-3 Pouching Systems**

Type	Features/Varieties
One-piece drainable, closed-end urostomy	Flexible, semi-flexible, firm, with or without skin barrier attached.
	Flat and with convexity ranging from shallow to very deep pre-cut and cut to fit.
Two-piece	With or without adhesive tape collar.
	Pre-cut and cut-to-fit varieties.
	Built-in convexity or option of convex insert.
	Adult/pediatric sizes.
	Pouch removable without disturbing flange.
	Clear and opaque pouches.
	Variety of size and shapes of pouches, irrigation sleeves, and stoma caps.
	Belt hooks for optional belt use. Provides sense of security especially for very active ostomates.
Pouching tips	Peel off all backing paper.
	Size properly—decrease aperture as stoma edema decreases.
	Assess need for convexity.
	Close pouch properly.
	Be alert for candidiasis.
	Snap on pouch securely to flange in two-piece system.

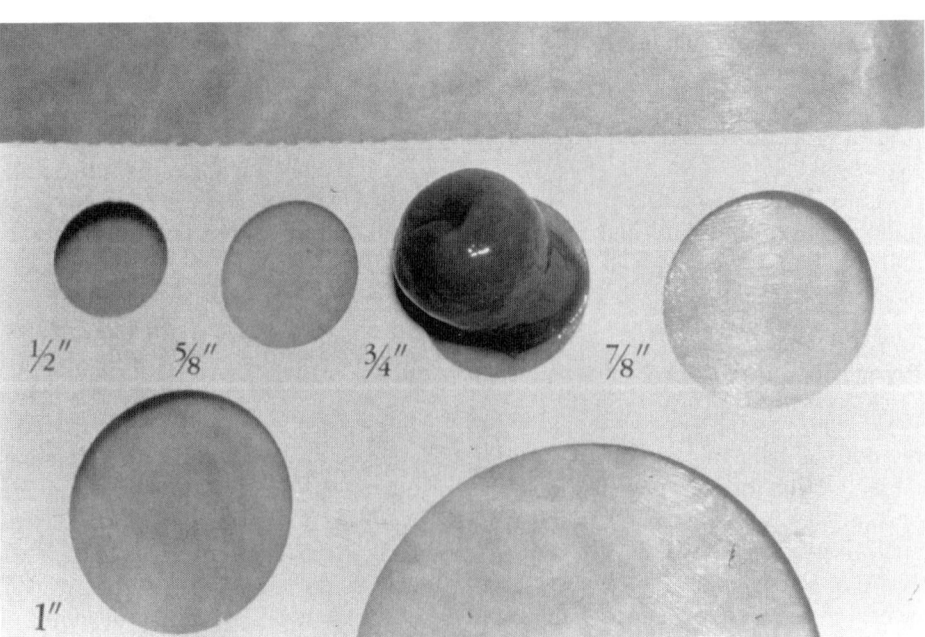

FIGURE 32-6. Disposable measuring guide permits use of properly sized faceplate.

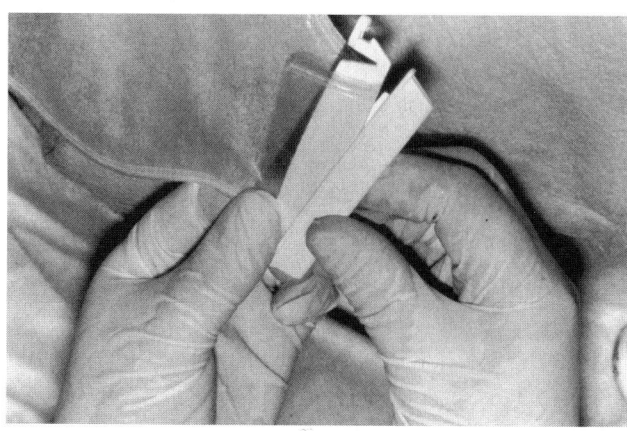

FIGURE 32-7. Applying closure clamp to drainable pouch.

climates, a different skin barrier should be used (e.g., Stomahesive or Hollihesive). Generally, the use of karaya is advised less often than the products subsequently discussed.

Colly-Seel

Colly-Seel is another, more solid form of karaya. Natural clays have been added, which cause it to be less vulnerable to heat; thus, it is a suitable barrier for both urinary and ileostomy effluents. Colly-Seel is available

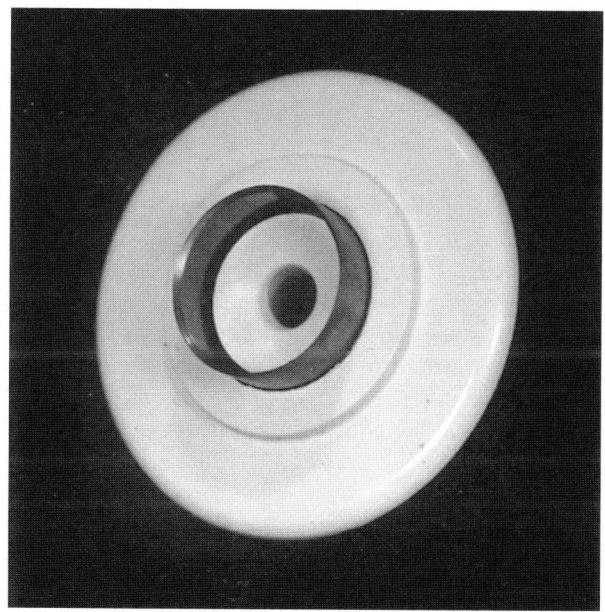

FIGURE 32-8. Hole cutter tool. A steel blade is mounted in a plastic handle. This can be prepared by request for various diameters. (Courtesy of Nu-Hope Laboratories.)

in varying thicknesses as well as in washer, wafer, and sheet form. It does not stretch, and so the inner diameter should be cut approximately the same size or one-sixteenth inch larger than the diameter of the stomal base. It must be moistened slightly before application. Colly-Seel is sometimes recommended for a patient with a soft or flabby abdominal wall or when considerable scarring is present. However, it is used less often today, having been replaced by more flexible products. It should be placed on the abdomen while it is still sticky.

Gelatin–Pectin Skin Barriers

Generally, the gelatin–pectin skin barriers have an advantage over the karaya products because they are more water resistant, and therefore permit a longer interval between appliance changes.[19]

Stomahesive

Stomahesive is composed of gelatin, pectin, carboxymethylcellulose sodium, and polyisobutylene. It is non-allergenic and looks like a piece of American cheese. Its shiny surface is affixed to the appliance, and the sticky side is secured to the skin. It should be cut to fit around the stoma leaving a 2- or 3-mm clearance, and it may be used as a washer or as a whole wafer. The product is also available in a powder or a paste, which many WOC/ET nurses and patients prefer to karaya. Stomahesive can be applied directly onto excoriated skin and provides an excellent means for filling in crevices created by abdominal folds near the stoma.

A skin barrier such as Stomahesive is appropriate for intestinal as well as urinary tract diversions and should be placed on the skin immediately after the operation. The inner diameter should be cut to fit around the base of the stoma. The outer aspect should be rounded and made slightly smaller than the adhesive portion of a soft-backed disposable clear pouch. The skin must be completely dry before applying Stomahesive or any other skin barrier.

Durahesive

Durahesive is similar to Stomahesive, but it has specific hydrophilic properties that absorb fluid from the effluent. This causes the product to swell or "turtleneck" around the stoma. It is a particularly advantageous barrier for urinary ostomies. It has been reported that some patients may achieve up to 14 days without leakage when this product is employed.

Hollihesive

Hollihesive is similar to Stomahesive, except that it is a bit more flexible and stickier to the touch. It, too, is available as a paste. Another product from the same manufacturer is called Premium Barrier. It is allegedly more resistant to breakdown.

Reliaseal

Reliaseal is similar in composition to Stomahesive. It is available in a round or oval disc with pre-cut inner diameter sizes at one-eighth-inch intervals. It has two adhesive sides, one covered with white paper and the other with blue. The white paper is peeled off and that side is placed directly on the skin; then the blue paper covering is removed, and that side is placed directly on the faceplate of the pouch. "Blue to the sky" is a helpful memory device to teach patients how to use this barrier. Reliaseal is also an effective washer for an ileal conduit. When using Stomahesive or Reliaseal, many patients choose to add a small karaya or Stomahesive washer before applying the barrier for an added peristomal seal.

Crixiline

Crixiline is an extremely sticky silicone-like barrier that comes in rings and sheets. This material also is available attached to a disposable, soft-backed, open- or closed-ended pouch called "Stomaplast-plus" with a micropore tape backing. This product is very useful around drains. To achieve good adhesion, the skin must be dry.

Other Barriers

United's Soft-Guard XL is very pliable, and is resistant to breakdown. Coloplast manufactures Comfeel, and Nu-Hope has skin barrier wafers, pre-cut round and oval washers, and paste strips for flexibility. Eakin Cohesive Seals can be used as an ostomy seal or an external packing agent around stomas. They are moldable, pectin-based rings that absorb moisture and act as a physical and waterproof barrier. They are marketed in the United States by ConvaTec.

Faceplate

The faceplate or mounting area is that part of the appliance that supports the pouch and attaches it to the body.[11] It may be made of rubber, metal, paper, adhesive, or plastic. It can be flexible or hard; convex, flat, or concave.

Adhesives

Adhesives are of two types: liquids (cements) and disks. Adhesive cements are generally made of acrylic or rubber but are usually unnecessary.[19] If used, they should be applied lightly and evenly as a single coat to the skin or to the barrier. Those who seem to prefer this method usually have had their appliance for many years. Cement is occasionally recommended for a patient with a difficult abdominal contour or in whom a satisfactory seal cannot be established by another means.

The most popular method of adhering a reusable appliance is by a double-faced adhesive cloth disk. This must exactly measure the inner diameter of the faceplate. Before a new disk is applied, the faceplate should be cleansed of any residual adhesive.

Pouch

There are numerous disposable and reusable pouch systems available (Table 32-3 and Figs. 32-9 through 32-12). Selection will depend on a variety of physical and psychosocial factors affecting the patient. The pouch can be made of synthetic material or of rubber. Some disposal pouches come with an adhesive or microporous tape backing and, in some instances, with a soft plastic faceplate and belt tabs (Figs. 32-5 and 32-9). A number of such commonly used products include the Hollister, Sur-Fit (ConvaTec), United, Marlen, Coloplast, Bard, and Nu-Hope pouches. They are lightweight, easy to apply, and very effective choices for the firm abdomen that does not require a more rigid faceplate for peristomal support. In addition, no assembly is required.

Two-piece disposable appliances have become quite popular. They consist of a skin barrier with a plastic ring (Figure 32-10). A pouch with a ring snaps onto the barrier-ring, much like the Tupperware product. Variations on this concept are made by ConvaTec (Squibb), Hollister, United, and Coloplast.

The disadvantages of the disposable system include the possibility of a shorter wearing time, increased cost, and limitation to certain body configurations. A faceplate with a firm base provides better peristomal support, particularly in a patient with a "flabby" abdomen. A disposal pouch always requires a skin barrier to enhance the wearing time and to provide adequate skin protection.

Reusable or "permanent" appliances are available in one or two pieces, depending on whether the faceplate is detachable (Figs. 32-11 and 32-12). A faceplate for any appliance must always have a means of securing it to the body regardless of the type of skin barrier used. Attachment is usually accomplished through the use of pre-cut, double-faced adhesive seals or disks. The inner diameter

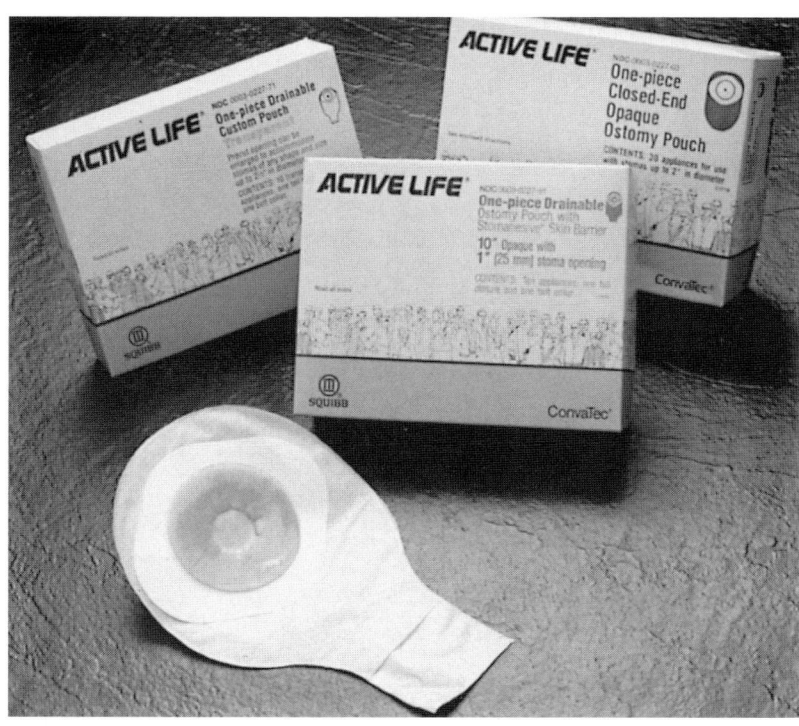

FIGURE 32-9. Drainable and closed-end pouches. Sur-Fit system with Stomahesive wafer and flange. (Courtesy of ConvaTec, a division of Bristol-Myers Squibb.)

of an adhesive disk must exactly equal the inner diameter of the faceplate.

A one-piece appliance may be preferred by patients with arthritis affecting the hands, those who have poor eyesight or who are blind, active youngsters who need a secure pouch construction with ease of application, patients with a neurologic deficit, and those with flush stomas. Disposable one-piece equipment often is available pre-cut, so that one merely peels off the protective paper and affixes the appliance (e.g., Squibb Active Life; Hollister First-Choice). However, the selection of a one-piece appliance may also be simply personal preference.

The main advantages of the two-piece system are cost-effectiveness and durability. An elastic ring around the neck of the pouch holds the appliance to the faceplate. The attachment of a double-faced adhesive disk to the back of the faceplate is the same as that with the one-piece appliance. Generally, the firmer the abdomen, the softer and flatter the faceplate should be. For example, a pregnant woman will require a soft, flat faceplate, but a corpulent person will need a firm, convex one to lend sufficient peristomal support in order to prevent undermining of the seal. Most patients, with the exception of those who are very slender or who have firm abdomens, will need a slightly convex faceplate. In addition to the reusable system, many individuals maintain a supply of disposable pouches for an "emergency," for rapid change, or for camping and traveling. Although it is valuable for

everyone to be aware of the availability of both systems, the overwhelming majority of patients select disposable equipment.

Even though commercially manufactured equipment is preferred, an adequate "homemade" appliance can be constructed if one has limited financial resources or if there is lack of access to manufactured products.[17] Meier and Tarpley, working in Ogbomoso, Nigeria, write of an appliance made from a tin can, a piece of rubber from an inner tube, household twine, and disposable plastic bags.[16]

Belt and Tape

Many patients feel secure when wearing a belt, but this device is not meant to hold the appliance in place. It is intended merely to support the weight of the pouch. Belts may ride up on the hip and cause detachment of the appliance, which may then lead to stomal injury. Some patients wear the belt too tightly and cause deep marks on the skin or even ulceration. With few exceptions (e.g., active children or problem stomas where revision is not advisable), the use of belts should be discouraged.

An alternative to a belt, such as framing the faceplate or adhesive area with paper tape, is much the preferred approach. For swimming or bathing, many types of waterproof tapes are available.

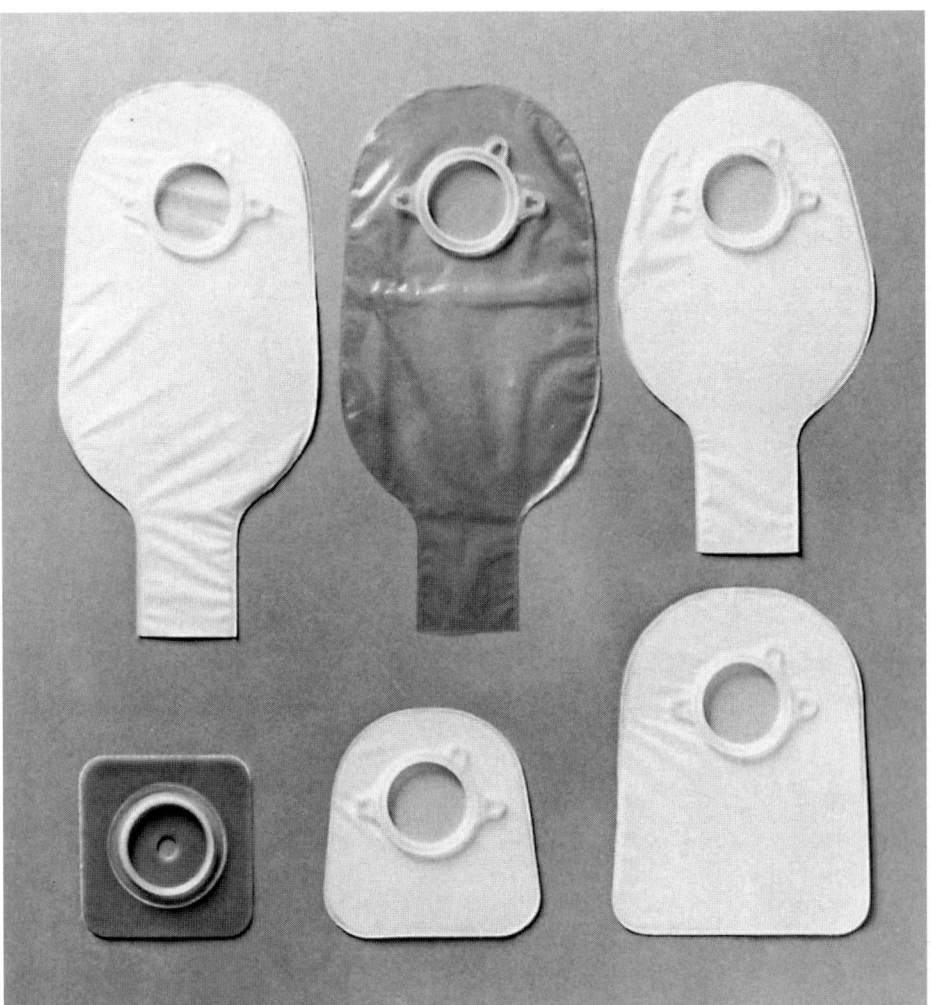

FIGURE 32-10. Drainable and closed-end pouches. Sur-Fit system with Stomahesive wafer and flange. (Courtesy of ConvaTec, a division of Bristol-Myers Squibb.)

Appliance Management

Establishment of the optimum frequency for a pouch change requires individual adjustment and experimentation. In the immediate postoperative period the pouch is changed more frequently than is required at a later time in order to permit stomal assessment and to provide instruction in self-care procedures. After discharge the patient is encouraged to gradually extend the interval between pouch changes until optimum frequency can be determined. This frequency then becomes the basis for routine pouch changes. The patient is also taught to recognize the signs of undermining and impending leakage (i.e., itching or burning of the peristomal skin, odor noted when the pouch is closed, or visible meltdown of the skin barrier), and to change the pouch promptly whenever any of these signs are present. The goal is to change the pouch before leakage or skin irritation occurs.

There is no correct frequency for pouch change. The goal is to establish a routine schedule that prevents leakage and provides the individual with control. The stoma that is appropriately sited and well constructed usually can be managed with a pouch change every 5 to 7 days. The presence of a rigid rod will require the use of a flexible barrier that will mold over the rod. Use of a barrier under a rod is usually not recommended due to potential stoma damage from pressure or from traumatic removal.

The selection criteria for a pouching system include the type of effluent and the size, shape, and location of the stoma. Contour of the patient's abdomen and any special psychomotor challenges are also considerations. Patients with ileostomies, jejunostomies, and urostomies are often optimally managed with extended-wear barriers that do not readily erode in a high-output, liquid environment.[6,8]

Initially, cut-to-fit barriers are preferred in order to adapt to decreasing stomal edema. After 6 to 8 weeks, the patient may elect to use a presized pouch if the stoma size has stabilized. Individuals with oval stomas may still be best served with cut-to-fit systems. Some pouches can be custom cut at the factory to accommodate a special need.[8]

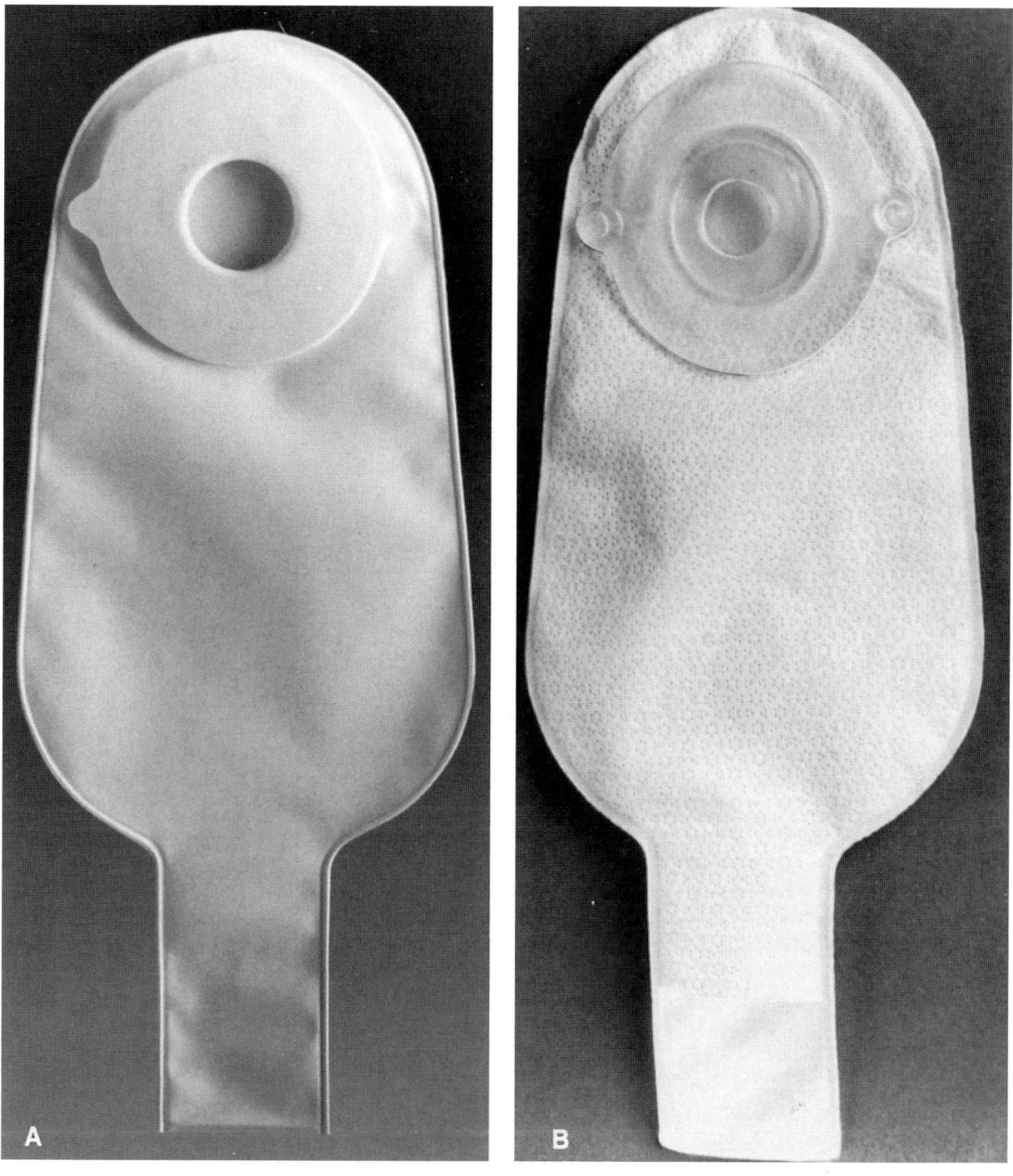

FIGURE 32-11. Reusable ileostomy appliances. **(A)** One-piece standard appliance ("odor ban"). **(B)** One-piece lightweight ("solo") limited reusable appliance. (Courtesy of Marlen Manufacturing and Development Co.)

As mentioned, patients who have a soft abdomen, with a flush or retracted stoma, may require a semi-flexible system or one with shallow to medium convexity. A budded stoma, which is preferable from a fitting standpoint, may be pouched with a flat or semi-flexible system or may require shallow convexity. Convexity, which can make a significant contribution to preventing leakage, adds varying degrees of pressure around the base of the stoma to aid in securing a seal.

Shallow convexity can be achieved through a convex insert, either added to or built into a one- or two-piece pouching system. A patient with a very soft abdomen

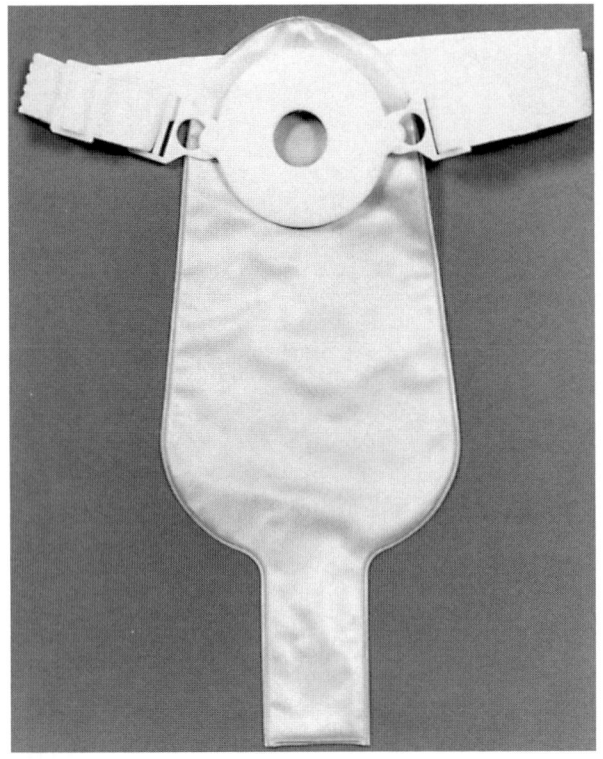

FIGURE 32-12. Examples of one-piece, precut convex pouches.

may require a firm system with deep to very deep convexity (Figure 32-13).[6,8] The WOC/ET nurse can determine the amount of convexity needed by assessing the presence and depth of skin creases, as well as by applying gentle pressure around the base of the flush stoma, to determine how much pressure is required to help the stoma bud out. Even deep convex systems can be modi-

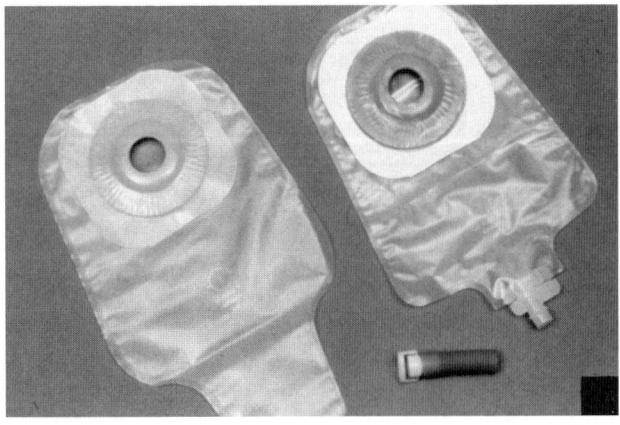

FIGURE 32-13. Examples of one-piece, precut convex pouches.

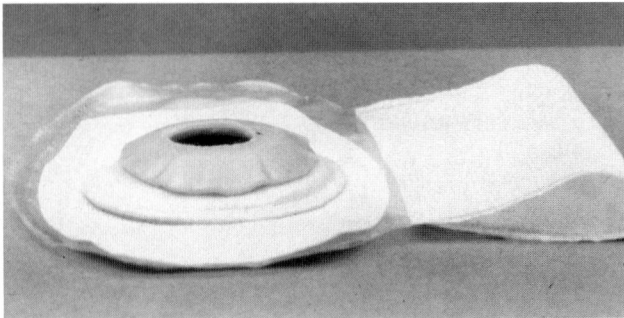

FIGURE 32-14. One-piece, precut, deep convex pouch with skin barrier washer added to deepen convexity.

fied to increase convexity by the addition of a skin barrier washer (Figure 32-14). Accessories such as skin barrier pastes, powders, and belts, applied with gentle tension, can all improve pouching success (see previous discussion and Tables 32-4 and 32-5). In the presence of severe peristomal skin erosion, modifications of pouching equipment systems can be made to create a nonadherent system. This approach is not highly secure, but the advantages are ready access to the stoma site and containment of the effluent.

The major difference between an ileostomy and a colostomy appliance is that some form of protective ring must be used around the ileostomy stoma because of the corrosive nature of the effluent. During the first 6 to 8 days after surgery, a disposable, soft-backed pouch will be required in addition to an appropriate skin barrier. By the 7th or 8th day, the stoma should be re-measured, because the edema will usually have resolved, although it usually takes from 4 to 6 weeks for the stoma to shrink to its smallest size. Therefore, opening changes will be required during this initial period.

Figure 32-15 outlines the procedure for application of a conventional reusable appliance. With a well-positioned stoma of adequate length, a properly applied reusable pouch should remain in place without leakage and without skin injury for 4 to 7 days. One may also shower or bathe with the pouch in place.

When removing the pouch, if a protective skin shield was used, the appliance may be pulled directly away from the skin. However, if adhesive cement has been employed, it may be necessary to drip a solvent with a pipette between the skin and the faceplate as it is lifted off. Adhesive-remover wipes are also available. All of the solvent should then be thoroughly washed off the skin.

Before limitations imposed on hospitals and physicians concerning acceptable duration of hospital stay for a given illness, the patient was able to remain until adequate appliance training had been achieved. However,

▌TABLE 32-4 **Skin Products**

Product	Form	Composition
Skin sealants	Wipes, sprays, gels, liquids	Contain plasticized ethylcellulose & alcohol. Some are water soluble.
Skin barriers	Wafers, rings, washers, paste, strips, powders	May be made from karaya gum, pectin, carboxymethyl cellulose, gelatin, co-polymers.
Skin adhesives/cement	Liquids, sprays, tubes	Silicone or latex based.
Skin solvents	Wipes, liquids	Primary ingredient: trichlor-ethane, a liquid petroleum.
Skin cleansers	Liquids, wipes, sprays, foams	May contain water, lanolin, urea, propylene glycol, fragrance, and artificial colors. Rinsing may be required to remove residue of cleanser before pouching.
Skin lotions	Wipes, creams	May contain lanolin, fragrance, water. Some contain topical steroids and antifungal ingredients. Apply sparingly and remove residue before applying pouching system.

because of so-called cost -containment, individuals are now sent home much sooner.

The following factors are essential to a properly fitting appliance:

- It must not leak contents nor cause odor.
- It must not cause skin or stomal irritation.
- It must be comfortable for all levels of activity.
- It must not require a wardrobe change.
- It must be unobtrusive.

With knowledge of a few basic principles, a satisfactory management protocol can be developed. What may seem complex in the beginning will be routine in a brief

▌TABLE 32-5 **Accessories**

Types	Description and Comments
Belts	Some are company specific, others interchangeable. Sizes, small, medium, large, extra large, and pediatric. Support belts 2" to 6" with or without prolapse support can be special ordered to accommodate specific needs.
Convex inserts	Can be added to selected two-piece systems. Some systems can accommodate two inserts for additional convexity. Insert should be 1/8" larger than stoma.
Bedside drainage system for urinary stomas	Can be secured to bed frame, mattress, or put on floor. Available as bags or bottles. Can be attached to pouch with use of adapter.
Pouch covers	Prevent allergic rash of skin to pouch. Provide moisture barriers between pouch/skin. Custom fit or already made. Adult and pediatric sizes. May enhance feelings of attractiveness.
Underwear/swimwear	Provide support to pouching system. Adult and pediatric sizes. May enhance feelings of attractiveness.
Closure clamps	Available from numerous manufacturers. Some not interchangeable from one manufacturer to another.
Stoma guide strips	Made from rice paper. Can be inserted in opening of pouching system to aid patient when centering during application. Strip will dissolve when moistened.
Tapes	Most are hypoallergenic. May be waterproof. Available in many sizes and types from variety of manufacturers.

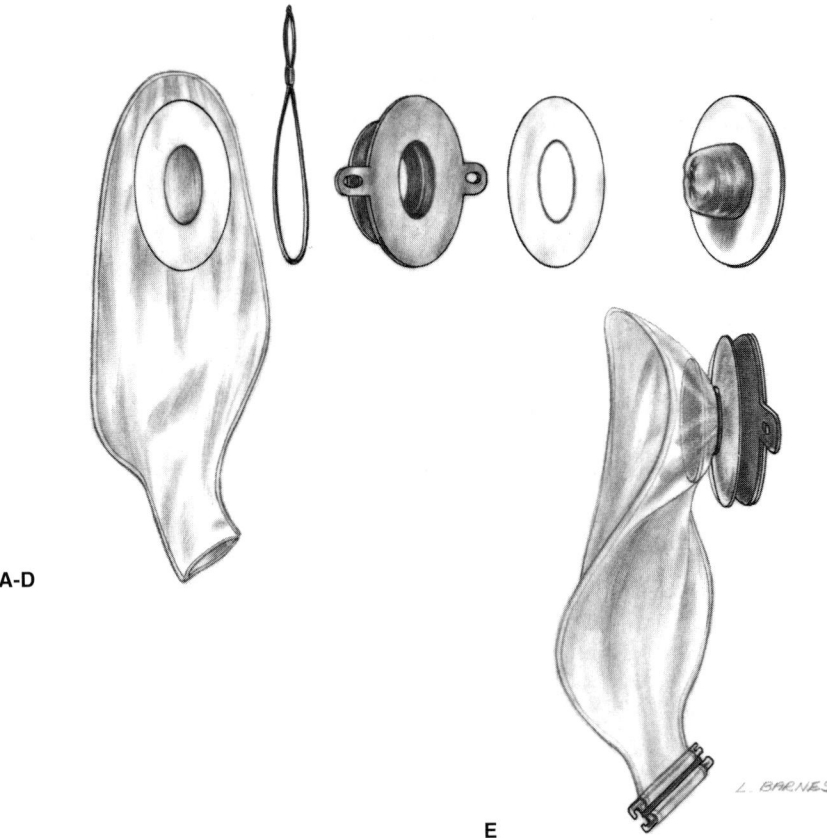

A-D

E

FIGURE 32-15. Application of a reusable appliance. (**A, B**) Mount the faceplate on the pouch (if using a two-piece appliance) and apply the elastic O-ring. (**C**) Apply the double-faced adhesive to the back of the faceplate. (**D**) After the skin is prepared, place the skin protector around the stoma. (**E**) After exposure of the other side of the adhesive disk, the appliance is seated with the aid of a guide strip.

time as the patient gains confidence that the system will not leak and will enable him or her to return to productive activity.

Patient/Family Education

Ideally, the timing of instruction should be based on learner readiness. However, as mentioned, shorter hospital lengths of stay often accelerate the teaching process, but unfortunately, learning may not be enhanced.[8,20] Support from family, friends, and home care nurses will ease the transition to home self-care. It is important that these support services build on the patient's previous knowledge in order to avoid fostering dependence.[15] Lessons should be conducted when the patient is alert and rested. Early in morning, right after breakfast, is the optimal time for effective teaching.

If the patient's activity tolerance and space permit, self-care lessons should be conducted in the bathroom. This encourages the patient and the family to relate ostomy care to toilet activities, rather than to a medical, nursing procedure.[8]

Ostomy self-care instructions ideally take place at least 3 to 4 consecutive days prior to discharge. The first lesson may consist of a detailed demonstration of the entire pouch-changing procedure. The patient is instructed on pouch emptying, the use of the closure clamp or spout, and ostomy system removal. Soiled pouches should be placed in a plastic bag or similar container and disposed of promptly. Examples of patient instruction sheets distributed at the Cleveland Clinic Foundation are reproduced in Tables 32-6 and 32-7.

The peristomal skin is cleansed using a non-oily cleanser or non-lotion, non-deodorant soap, and then rinsed and patted dry. Use of lotions or ointments on the peristomal skin is discouraged because these products may prevent the ability of the skin barrier or adhesive to adhere to the skin. If hair growth in the peristomal area is a problem, it can be removed with an electric razor or scissors. Use of a disposable blade is discouraged since it may result in stripping the epithelial surface of the skin and in predisposing the patient to folliculitis.[8,13] The skin should be cleansed from the outside in towards the stoma since this will prevent mucus and effluent from re-soiling the skin. Because the stoma is highly vascular, slight bleeding during cleansing is not unusual.[8,13] For reasons of cost, patients are encouraged to use washcloths or soft paper towels at home instead of the gauze commonly used in hospitals. After discharge, many individuals elect

▌ **TABLE 32-6** How to Change Your Disposable, One-Piece, Cut-to-Fit Pouch with Attached Skin Barrier

Gather the following supplies:
Washcloths or paper towels
Nonoily soap (Ivory and Dial are recommended brands)
Scissors
Plastic bag or newspaper
New pouch
Accessory products
Prepare the new pouch:
Trace the pattern (sized to fit within $$" of stoma) onto the cover paper of the skin barrier.
Cut out the skin barrier. Be careful not to cut through the front of the pouch.
Remove the covers from the skin barrier and the adhesive surface of the pouch.
Set the pouch aside, sticky side up.
Remove the worn pouch:
Holding the pouch upright, remove the clip from the end of the pouch.
Empty the waste from the pouch into the toilet.
Remove the worn pouch by:
• Applying light pressure on the skin with one hand.
• Gently pulling the pouch from the skin with the other hand.
• Wrap the worn pouch in newspaper, or place in a plastic bag and discard.
Cleanse the skin around the stoma:
Wash the area around the stoma with nonoily soap and warm water.
Rinse the area thoroughly with warm water.
Pat the skin dry with a washcloth or paper towel.
Apply the new pouch:
Center the pouch opening over the stoma and press into place.
Smooth the sticky surface of the pouch onto the skin.
Hold the pouch firmly in place for a few moments.
Close the pouch end securely
Fasten the pouch end securely with the clip.

▌ **TABLE 32-7** How to Change Your Disposable, Two-Piece Pouch with Cut-to-Fit Skin Barrier Flange

Gather the following supplies:
Washcloths or paper towels
Nonoily soap (Ivory and Dial are recommended brands)
Scissors
Plastic bag or newspaper
New pouch
Skin barrier flange
Accessory products
Prepare the new pouch:
Trace the pattern (sized to fit within $$" of stoma) on the cover paper of the skin barrier flange.
Cut out the skin barrier flange.
Remove the cover papers from the skin barrier and the adhesive surface of the flange.
Set the skin barrier flange aside, sticky side up.
Set the pouch next to the flange.
Remove the worn pouch:
Holding the pouch upright, remove the clip from the end of the pouch.
Empty the waste from the pouch into the toilet.
Remove the worn pouch and skin barrier by:
—Applying light pressure on the skin with one hand.
—Gently pulling the pouch from the skin with the other hand.
Wrap the worn pouch in newspaper, or place in a plastic bag and discard.
Cleanse the skin around the stoma:
Wash the area around the stoma with nonoily soap and warm water.
Rinse the area thoroughly with warm water.
Pat the skin dry with a washcloth or paper towel.
Apply the prepared pouch:
Center the skin barrier flange opening over the stoma and press into place.
Smooth the sticky surface of the skin barrier flange onto the skin.
Snap the pouch securely onto the skin barrier flange.
Hold the pouch firmly in place for a few moments.
Close the pouch end securely:
Fasten the pouch end securely with the clip.

to shower before or after they have removed their pouches. It is important to remind patients that it is not necessary to remove the pouch every time they bathe. Those with colostomies or ileostomies will wish to time their pouch changes to coincide with intestinal activity. Since urinary stomas function at will, the timing of the pouch change and showering is best undertaken prior to ingestion of liquids.

Patients and families need to be supplied with a discharge folder that includes step-by-step written instructions specific for their type of ostomy and pouching system, along with stock numbers and ordering information, a list of dealers and manufacturers, referral phone numbers, and discharge instructions (Table 32-8). Information related to the advantages of wearing a medical

condition identification tag is advisable. If the patient is ever in an accident or unconscious, the nature of the ostomy can be communicated to emergency medical personnel. This is especially important for patients with continent diversions or pelvic pouches.

Prior to discharge those with continent diversions are instructed in catheter irrigation, stoma and skin care, and management of leg and bedside drainage bags. Once the internal reservoir is safely healed, intubation instruction is generally conducted in the outpatient department or office by the WOC/ET nurse 3 to 4 weeks following discharge. A patch or gauze is then applied

▶ **TABLE 32-8 Colostomy Manufacturers and Products**

Company	Products	Company	Products
CR Bard, Inc. 111 Spring Street Murray Hill, NJ 07974	Disposable pouches; ReliaSeal; skin care cream and cleanser	Nu-Hope Laboratories, Inc. 12640 Branford St. Pacoima, CA 91331	Appliances; adhesive foam pads; accessories; support belts; appliance covers; hole cutter tool; skin barriers
Blanchard Ostomy Products 1510 Raymond Ave. Glendale, CA 91201	Karaya wafers and powder; pouches; faceplates; accessories	Palex Medical, Inc. 8807 Northwest 23rd St. Miami, FL 33172	Ostomy products
Chattem, Inc. 1715 W. 38th Street Chattanooga, TN 37409	Nullo deodorant	Partheneon Co., Inc. 3311 W. 2400 South Salt Lake City, UT 84119	Devrom chewable tablets
Coloplast Corp. 1955 West Oak Circle Marietta, GA 30062	Disposable appliances; two-piece system; conseal continent colostomy system; Comfeel; Skin creams and ointments; Peri-Wash	Perma-Type Co., Inc. 83 Northwest Drive Farmington Industrial Park Plainville, CT 06062	Reusable appliances; accessories; Fresh Tabs (deodorant)
ConvaTec, Bristol-Myers/ Squibb P.O. Box 5254 Princeton, NJ 08543–5254 www.convatec.com	Sur-Fit System; DuoDERM; Kenalog spray; Mycostatin powder; Stomahesive; Durahesive; Active life; pediatric pouches	HW Rutzen and Son 345 W Irving Park Road Chicago, IL 60618	Reusable appliances; accessories
Cymed Ostomy Co. 1440C Fourth St. Berkeley, CA 94710 www.cymed-ostomy.com	Disposable appliances	Rystan Co., Inc. 47 Center Street, P.O. Box 214 Little Falls, NJ 07424	Derifil tablets and powder
Hollister, Inc. 2000 Hollister Drive Libertyville, IL 60048 www.hollister.com	Disposable appliances; Hollihesive; irrigation equipment; karaya paste; Skin Gel; incontinence devices; accessories	Schilling and Morris Marketing, Ltd. 215 Tremond St. Rochester, NY 14614	Ostobon deodorant
Incutech, Inc. 307-A, S. Westgate Drive Greensboro, NC 27407	Disposable pouches; skin barriers; skin lotion; irrigation equipment accessories	Richard C. Shelton Co. 1525 Wayne Avenue Dayton, OH 45409	Osto-Zyme (spray deodorant)
Marlen Manufacturing and Development Co. 5150 Richmond Road Bedford, OH 44146	Reusable appliances; accessories; stoma paper guide strips; loop ostomy rods; irrigation equipment; stoma location disks	Smith and Nephew United, Inc. P.O. Box 1970 Largo, FL 34649	Appliances; accessories; adhesive foam pads; Banish; Skin Prep; irrigation educational material and teaching aids; Soft-Guard XL skin barrier
Mason Laboratories, Inc. P.O. Box 334 Horsham, PA 19044	Colly-Seel$$; Skin Tac; appliances; M-9 deodorant drops	Torbot Co. 1185 Jefferson Blvd. Warwick, RI 12886	Reusable appliances; accessories; rigid faceplates
Mentor Corporation 600 Pine Avenue Santa Barbara, CA 93117	Appliances; accessories; irrigation equipment; Stomapaper guide strips; Skin Shields	VPI—A Cook Group Co. P.O. Box 266 Spencer, IN 47460	Nonadhesive ostomy systems
3M Medical Products 3M Center St. Paul, MN 55101	Double-faced adhesives; adhesive foam pads; micropore paper tape; Stomaseal		

over the stoma to absorb mucous.[9,18] Frequency of intubation is initially every 2 hours for the first week, increasing the interval by 1 hour the following weeks. Eventually, most patients will intubate approximately every 4 hours. During the night they are advised to set an alarm or connect the catheter to constant drainage. Prevention of over-distension of the pouch must be emphasized.

Prevention and Treatment of Skin Irritation

As previously discussed, the corrosive effluent from an ileostomy demands careful appliance management. Additionally, mechanical irritation, allergic and non-allergic dermatitis, and various infections may predispose the ostomate to the risk of injury in spite of fastidious care and a properly fitting appliance. To prevent complications from developing, it is important for the patient to return annually for a stomal inspection. This provides the physician (or WOC/ET nurse) with an opportunity to re-measure the stoma and to evaluate the integrity of the peristomal skin. In addition, the patient can be informed about any new developments in equipment.

Weight gain or loss has major implications for stomal management (Figure 32-16). Appliance size and convexity may require a change (Figure 32-17), and skin sensitivity may develop to products even after many years of use (Figs. 32-18 and 32-19). A number of skin complications and treatments are discussed in Table 32-9.

Mild Irritation

Even mild skin irritation must be treated promptly to prevent serious consequences. Mild or moderate dermatitis may be treated by gently washing the peristomal skin with warm water. Standard soaps should not be used; several companies make special ones for ostomy care only (e.g., Sween Peri-Wash; United Uniwash). The area should be permitted to dry thoroughly. A hair dryer (on the coolest setting) held approximately 1 foot away from the skin can be used. Karaya or Stomahesive powder should be dusted on the area, and the excess brushed off. After a skin protective agent is applied and permitted to dry, a skin barrier is used with a clean appliance.

Severe Irritation

Severe irritation may be caused by improper fitting of the faceplate, leakage, allergy to the adhesive product, or yeast infection (Figs. 32-19 through 32-22). Cleansing the area with an antacid usually relieves the irritation. This is done by decanting the antacid (e.g., Amphojel, Maalox, Milk of Magnesia) and spreading it thinly over the skin. The alkaline application may be soothing initially, but may decrease the skin acid mantle and predispose the patient to bacterial proliferation. After drying, a skin protective agent is applied, followed by a skin barrier and a clean pouch. Occasionally, a small piece of Telfa may be placed over a draining area to prevent undermining of the skin barrier and to allow drainage to take place. This appliance must be changed daily until the problem resolves.

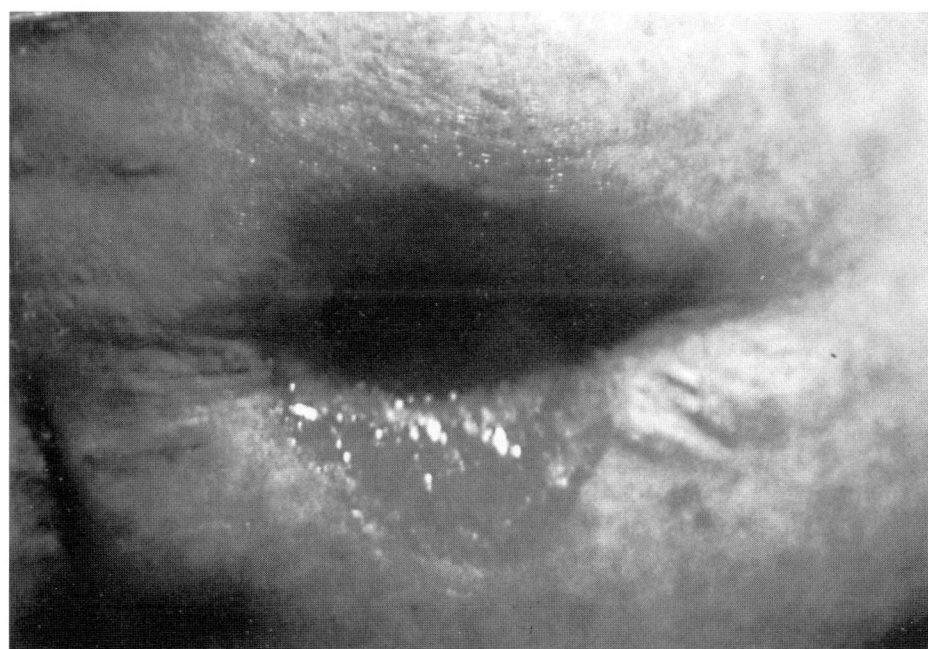

FIGURE 32-16. Weight gain and poor colostomy location in a skin fold result in a stoma that cannot be managed by conventional means. Note dermatitis inferior to the retracted osteotomy opening.

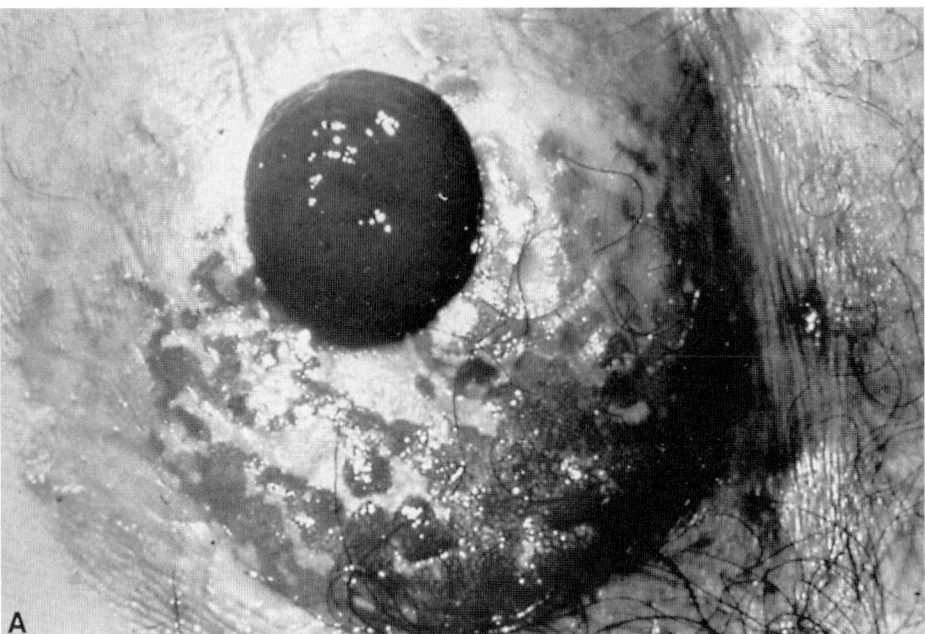

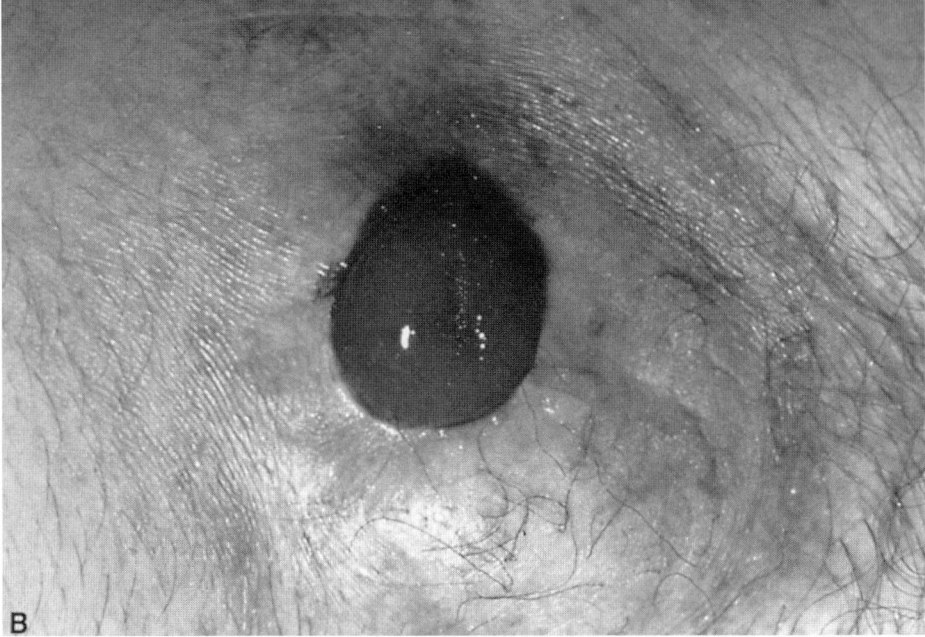

FIGURE 32-17. Improper fitting faceplate. (**A**) Severe peristomal dermatitis from the faceplate being too large. (**B**) Resolution following use of a proper-fitting appliance. (From Corman ML, Veidenheimer MC, Coller JA. Ileostomy complications: prevention and treatment. *Contemp Surg* 1976;8:36.)

Yeast and Fungal Infections

Problems with yeast or fungal infections often occur during warm weather or whenever moisture accumulates under the appliance (Figure 32-23). The area should be cleansed and dried gently, and a small amount of Kenalog may be sprayed on the affected area. (Use of Kenalog is not always used initially with a fungal infection. The response to a topical anti-fungal agent alone is generally effective.) After the excess is wiped off, the area should be dusted lightly with Mycostatin powder. The skin barrier should follow, and then the pouch. Depending on the severity of the infection, this unit may be left in place for 48 hours and the process repeated once or twice more if necessary.

Diet

Dietary modifications in patients with fecal and urinary diversions may be advisable. Generally, a low residue diet is suggested for the first 6 to 8 weeks following surgery. Patients with ileostomies may find it difficult to tolerate poorly digested foods, such as corn, nuts, and raw fruits and vegetables. These products may result in a food bolus obstruction at the ileostomy. Certain foods such as apple-

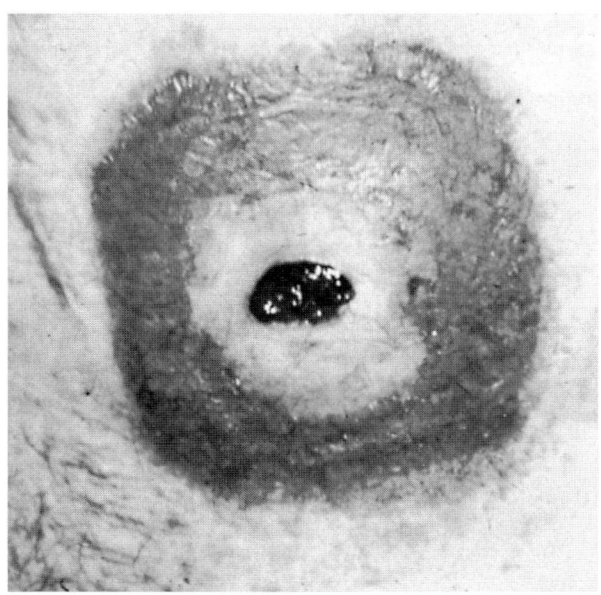

FIGURE 32-18. Pericolostomy dermatitis from an allergy to adhesive. Note the halo of protected skin around the stoma from the karaya ring.

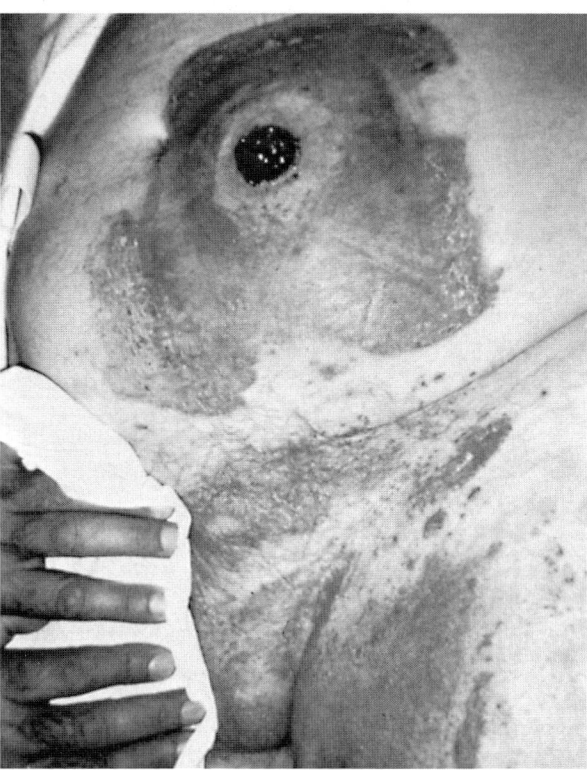

FIGURE 32-19. Severe allergy to adhesive and to the pouch itself. The bag hung in the groin, hence the inflammation in that area. Skin testing with a piece of pouch plastic yielded a positive response.

sauce, rice, and bananas can decrease bowel frequency. Conversely, caffeine, fiber, spicy foods, and raw fruits and vegetables may increase function. Individuals with continent ileostomies will need to keep the stool fairly liquid in order to allow passage of the effluent through the catheter. Six or 8 ounces of prune juice daily may adequately thin the stool for this purpose. All patients with small bowel stomas are advised to avoid the use of laxatives.

After the initial postoperative period, individuals with urostomies have no dietary restrictions. However, patients may find that fish and asparagus can cause a strong, offensive odor. Use of ascorbic acid, cranberry supplements, and prophylactic antibiotic therapy is controversial. When concerned, a patient should be referred to a urologist.

Odor Control

Diet and personal hygiene probably are the most effective means for decreasing odor.[4] Gazzard and associates studied 50 ileostomy patients and 50 colostomy patients in an attempt to ascertain which foods upset stomal function.[12] Only a small variety of foodstuffs produced symptoms in a significant number of patients. Individuals with colostomies found flatulence to be more of a problem than odor, particularly after eating vegetables or fruit. Items in this study that tended to be associated with an increased odor differed for ileostomy patients when compared with those who had a colostomy. Fish, eggs, cheese, and onions, in that order, were a greater problem for ileostomy patients, and green vegetables were the pri-

mary agents in patients with a colostomy. Yogurt, buttermilk, and parsley have been said to decrease odor in colostomy patients.[4]

A number of products are available that help to reduce odor (Table 32-10). Liquid deodorants are generally more successful than tablets for use in pouches, because tablets do not dissolve quickly enough. Recommended items include Banish, Greer Guard, M-9, Dignity, Osto-Zyme, and Nil-Odor. Approximately six drops are placed inside the pouch after each emptying.

If these are not adequate for control, several oral preparations are very effective. Derifil (chlorophyllin), one to three tablets daily taken orally, has been demonstrated to be an effective agent for eliminating or reducing odors of fecal and urinary drainage. Devrom (bismuth subgallate), a chewable tablet taken one-half hour before meals, two or three times daily, is also an effective odor-reduction agent. It also tends to thicken and darken the stool. Bismuth subcarbonate has a similar effect.

Sexual Concerns

Patients may or may not express concerns about sexuality during their hospitalization. In collaboration with the surgeon, the WOC nurse should address this topic as part

▶ **TABLE 32-9 Important Peristomal Skin Conditions**

Condition	Characteristics	Treatment
Allergic contact dermatitis (Figs. 32-18 and 32-19)	Allergic response generated by patient sensitivity to a particular product. Skin appears erythematous, edematous, eroded, weepy or bleeding. Generally corresponds to the exposed area.	Remove the allergen, avoid other irritants, protect the skin. Patch test with other products as needed.
Candidiasis (Fig. 32-23)	Warm, moist environment creates milieu for proliferation of *Candida albicans.* Generally diffuse erythematous papules. Can form plaques with characteristic advancing border and satellite lesions. Severe pruritus common.	Topical antifungal powder. Assess pouching system for leakage or undermining of seal.
Caput medusa (peristomal varices) (Figs. 31-65 and 32-24)	In patients with portal hypertension, the pressure at the portal systemic shunt in the mucocutaneous junction increases, creating venous engorgement. With trauma profuse bleeding can occur.	Direct pressure or use of hemostatic agents, *e.g.*, silver nitrate. Cautery or surgical ligation may be necessary. Careful pouch removal. Avoid aggressive skin barriers and skin sealants. If stoma is relocated varices will eventually recur around the new stoma.
Folliculitis (Fig. 32-25)	Traumatic removal of hair during pouch changes results in inflammation and infection of hair follicles. Lesions are painful and moist.	Topical antimicrobial powder, cover large lesions with non-adherent gauze. Once healed, patient should carefully shave area. Use of adhesive remover and skin sealant is advised.
Irritant dermatitis (Fig. 32-26)	Chemical destruction of the skin caused by topical products or leakage. Area appears erythematous, moist and painful. May be localized to a specific area of pouch undermining or leakage.	Review patients product usage and techniques to determine cause. Correct as needed.
Mechanical trauma (Figs. 32-22 and 32-27)	External item or force causing damage to the stoma and/or skin from pressure, laceration, friction or shear.	Assess equipment and pouching technique. Modify equipment and accessories to prevent re-injury.
Peristomal ulcer or abscess (Fig. 32-28)	Presents with one or more open, painful lesions surrounded by a halo of erythema. Not uncommon in patients with active Crohn's disease in distal bowel.	Unroofing of ulcer by surgeon. Management depends on size. Options include nonadherent gauze, hydrogel, astringent solution, or hydrocolloid wafer. A nonadherent pouching system can be fashioned with a one-piece pouch with belt tabs and an extra gasket.
Pseudoverrucous lesions (Figs. 31-54 and 32-29)	Overgrowth of tissue caused by overexposure to moisture. Appears as raised, moist lesions with wart-like appearance. Lesions are often painful.	Assess equipment for proper aperture and fit. Resize as needed. In severe cases, sharp debridement may be required.
Pyoderma gangrenosum (Fig. 32-30)	Associated with IBD, arthritis, leukemia, polycythemia vera, and multiple myeloma. Red open lesions become raised with irregular purplish margins.	Systemic treatment of underlying disease, local ulcer treatment. Curettage is generally not advised. Topical therapy and pouching same as with abscess.
Radiation injury	Red, thinned skin. Easily traumatized by removal of skin adhesives.	Gently cleanse skin with cool water. Select pouching system with barrier that is easy to remove. Be cautious in use of solvents or skin sealants due to frequent sensitivities.
Parastomal abscess (Fig. 30-61)	Mucocutaneous sepsis. Infected parastomal hematoma. Occult fistula. Extraperitoneal perforated colostomy. Recurrent Crohn's disease	Incision and drainage. May be done well lateral to stoma so skin barrier can still be applied or drainage catheter can be used at site of mucocutaneous separation and incorporated into pouch.

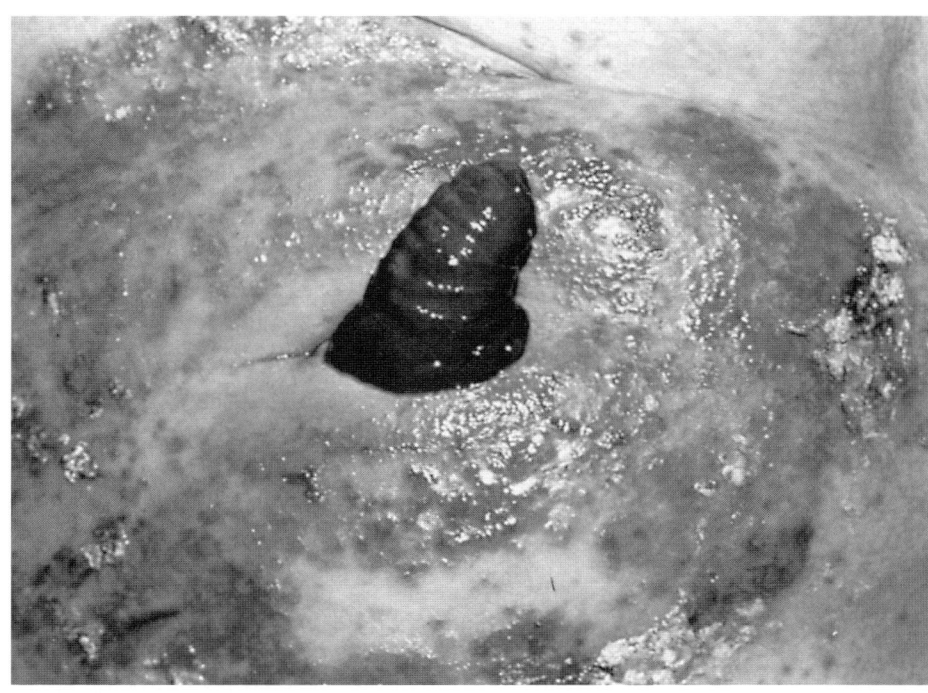

FIGURE 32-20. Severe dermatitis with a yeast infection in a patient whose appliance management was poor, with frequent leakage.

of the patient's preoperative and postoperative counseling. Concerns about reproduction, sexual function, and interpersonal relationships are common. Teenagers may be especially reluctant to talk about dating, sex, and reproduction in front of their families. Women with pelvic pouches or perineal incisions often experience vaginal dryness. Use of a water-soluble lubricant during sexual intercourse may therefore be indicated.[3] Support for gay or lesbian patients with ostomies can be obtained from the gay/lesbian support group (GLO) of the United Ostomy Association. Initially, most individuals are often more concerned with the practical aspects of managing

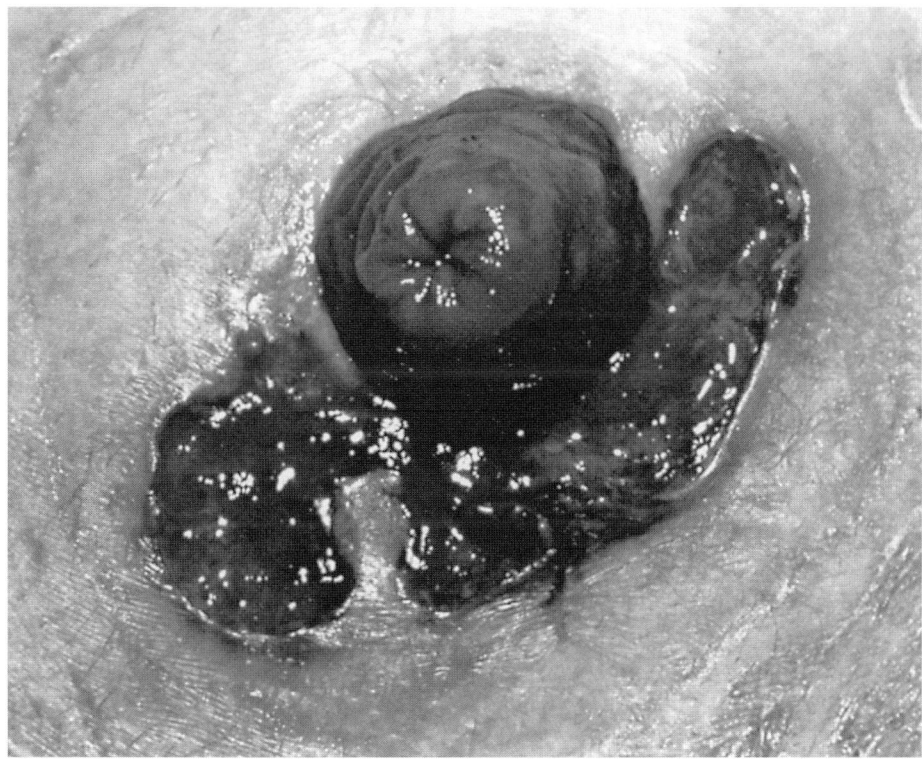

FIGURE 32-21. Ulcerating areas around an ileostomy are due to a neglected leakage problem.

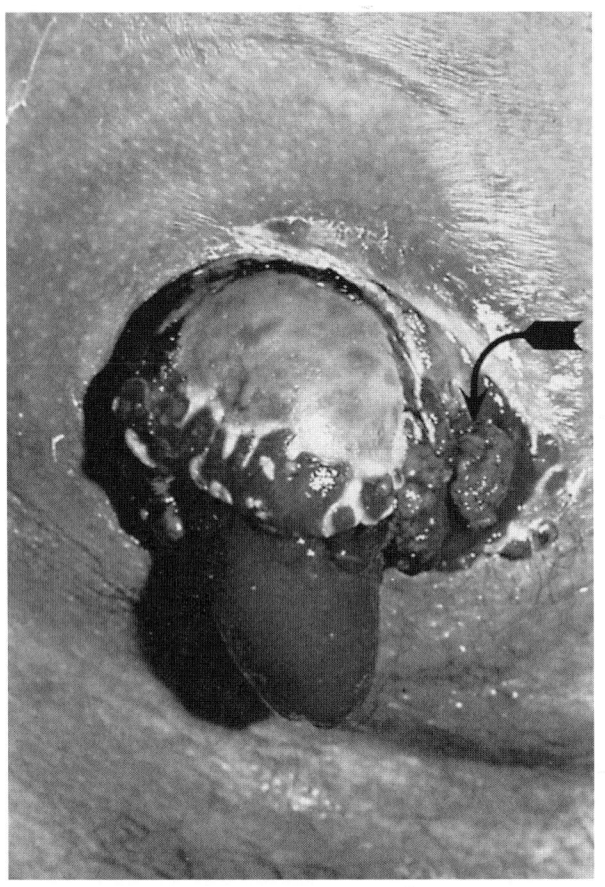

FIGURE 32-22. Fecal fistula (*arrow*) secondary to erosion from an improperly fitted appliance.

their ostomies than with psychosexual concerns. It is for this reason that post-discharge follow-up by a WOC/ET nurse is beneficial.

Discharge Planning

Discharge planning should begin at the time of admission to the hospital.[10] Active communication among the surgeon, nurse providing ostomy care, staff nurses, social worker, case manager, discharge planner, and the patient and family will ease the transition to life at home.[6,8,10] If placement in a subacute unit or extended care facility is contemplated, the nurse or social worker will contact the institution to promote continuity of care.[21] If a home care referral is initiated, contact between the hospital-based nurse providing ostomy care and the staff nurse at the home care agency is essential. For an especially complex pouching system, it is helpful for the hospital nurse and the home care or extended care facility nurse to make a joint visit prior to the patient's discharge from the hospital.[21] Long-term follow-up will be based on the patient's underlying condition. It is recommended that the WOC/ET nurse or surgeon evaluate the stoma, pouching, skin, and overall rehabilitation at least once a year.

Activity

Once recuperation from surgery is complete, patients should be encouraged to enjoy a full and active life. Heavy lifting and contact sports are best avoided because of the risk for hernia or stomal trauma. Otherwise, there

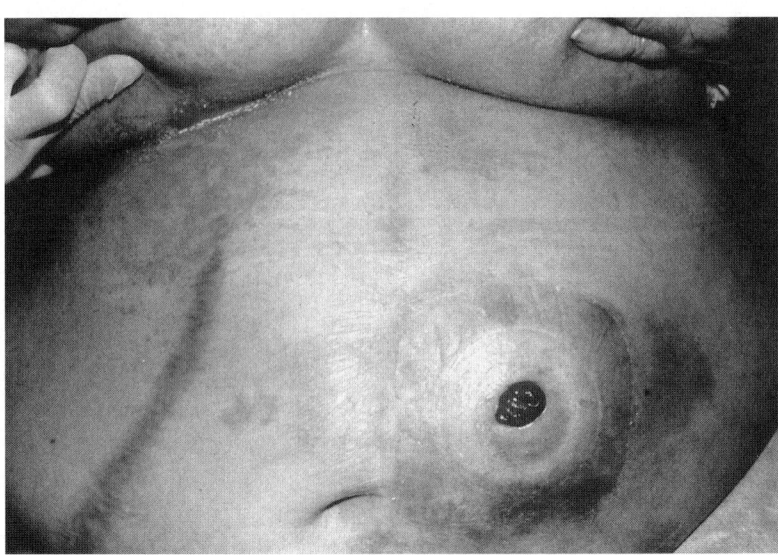

FIGURE 32-23. Candidiasis. Peristomal involvement is seen as well as involvement beneath the breast.

▌**TABLE 32-10** **Products to Control Odor**

Internal	Form	Side Effects
Activated Charcoal	Capsules	Large dose can interfere with absorption of vitamins. Darkens stool.
Chlorophyllin copper complex	Tablets	Absorbs some gas. Turns stool dark green.
Bismuth subgallate	Tablets	Can cause toxicity if taken in large doses.
Bismuth subcarbonate	Tablets	Constipation.
External	**Form**	**Description**
Pouch deodorizing agents	Liquids, powder, tablets	May contain a combination of water, zinc ricinoleate, propylene glycol. Some contain silver nitrate, organic acids, urea, and fragrance.
Air deodorizing agents	Aerosol, pump spray, liquids, solids	May contain water, ethanol, fragrance, and artificial colors.
Pouch cleaning/deodorizing agents		Used to clean and deodorize reusable stoma plates and pouches. May contain water, detergent, surfactants, liquid petroleum. Must rinse well.
Gas filters	Stick to one- to two-piece drainable pouches	Charcoal filter incorporated to deodorize gas. Some plastic pouches may not permit a secure seal of the adhesive. Not suitable for use with watery effluent.

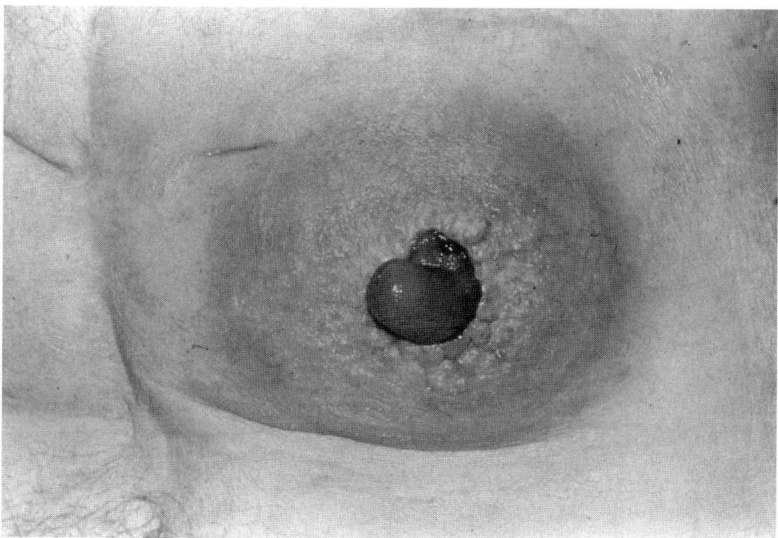

FIGURE 32-24. Caput medusa.

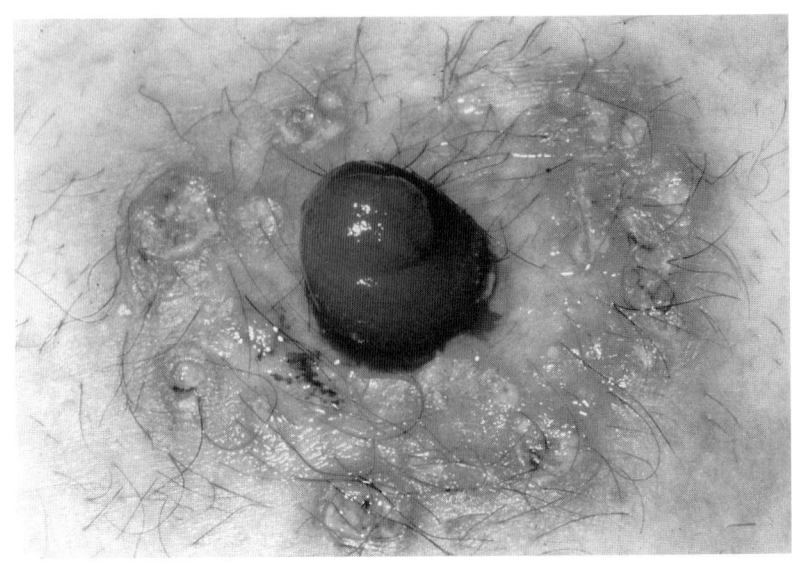

FIGURE 32-25. Folliculitis.

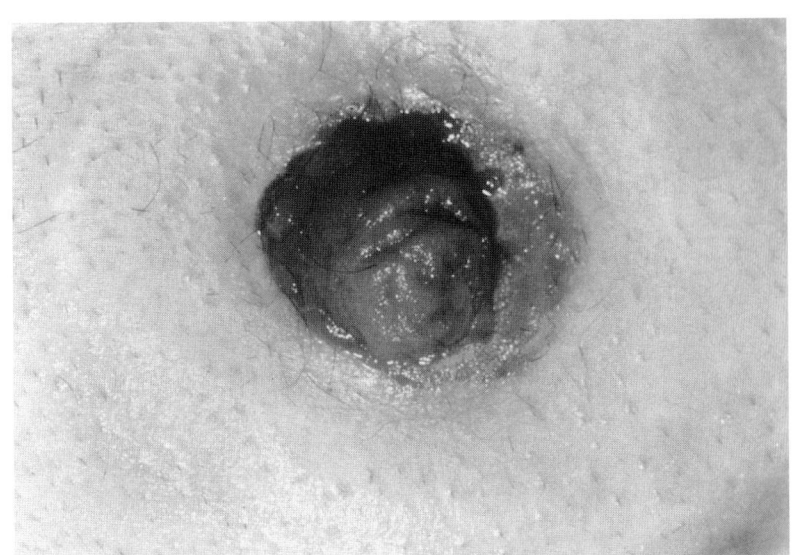

FIGURE 32-26. Ileostomy with chemical destruction of skin.

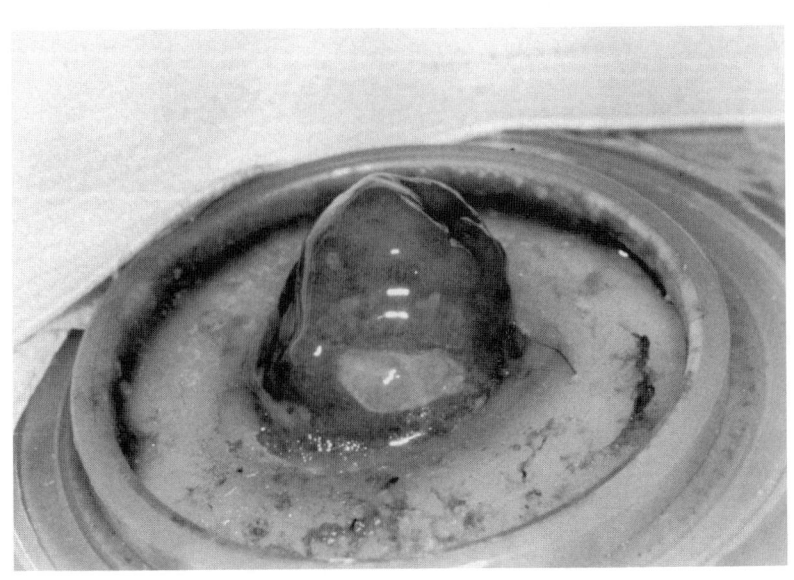

FIGURE 32-27. Mechanical trauma. Stomal laceration.

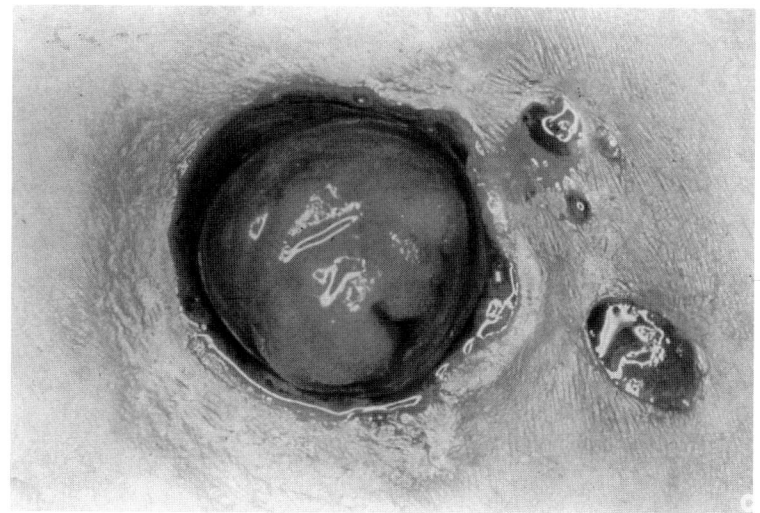

A

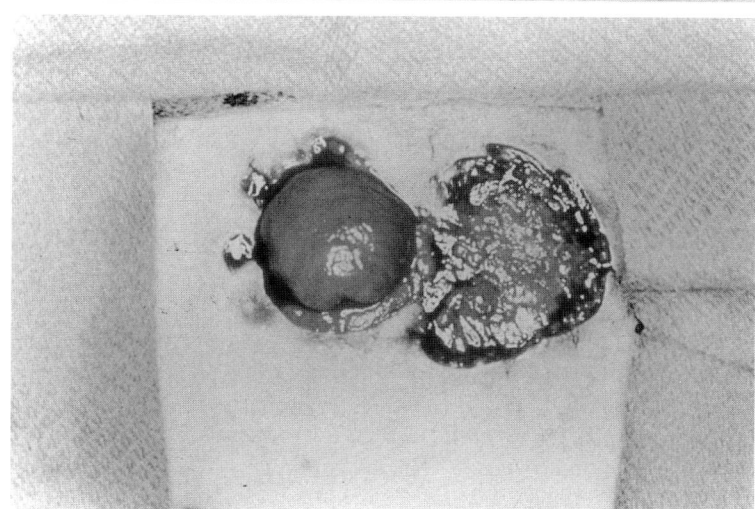

B

FIGURE 32-28. (A) Peristomal ulcer. (B) Peristomal ulcer after unroofing.

are no physical restrictions associated with fecal or urinary diversions.

Additional Considerations

Insurance coverage is an important concern. In the United States, patients with Medicare are afforded protection included under "prosthetic devices." This will provide coverage for much of the appliance expense. The usual cost for equipment is $500 to $1,000 a year.

As part of a comprehensive rehabilitative planning program, it is helpful to provide other resources for information. The local chapter of the American Cancer Society and the United Ostomy Association make available a number of booklets and brochures that the patient will usually find quite helpful (see the following).

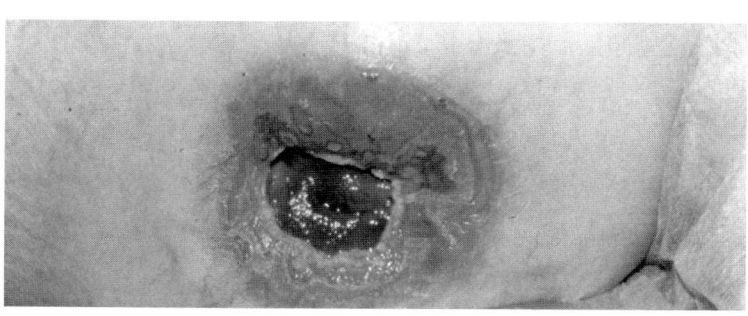

FIGURE 32-29. Pseudoverrucous lesions (formerly known as pseudoepitheliomatous hyperplasia).

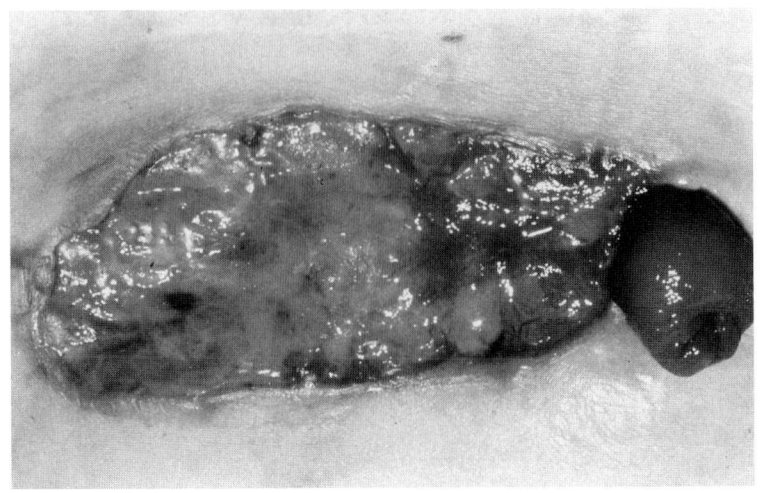

FIGURE 32-30. Peristomal pyoderma gangrenosum.

ADDITIONAL INFORMATION RESOURCES

American Cancer Society
1599 Clifton Rd. NE
Atlanta, GA 30329
Phone: (404) 320–3333
For information and support for people with cancer. Also contact local chapter of the American Cancer Society.

United Ostomy Association
19772 MacArthur Blvd.
Irvine, CA 92612–2405
Phone: (714) 660–8624 or (800) 826–0826
Website: *www.uoa.org*
For emotional support from others who have undergone the same or similar surgeries, including access to the following publications: *Ileostomy: a guide*; *Urinary ostomies—a guide for patients*; *Colostomies: a guide*; *Sex and the female ostomate*; *Pregnancy and the female ostomate*; *Sex, courtship and the single ostomate*; *Sex and the male ostomate*; *All about Jimmy and his friend* (an ostomy coloring storybook); *Handicapped ostomate*; *Transverse colostomies—a guide*; *The continent ileostomy*; *My child has an ostomy*; and *The ostomy handbook*.

International Association for Enterostomal Therapy
27241 La Paz Rd., Ste. 121
Laguna Niguel, CA 92656
Phone: (714) 476–0268

Wound, Ostomy and Continence Nurses Society
2755 Bristol St., Ste. 110
Costa Mesa, CA 92626
and
4700 W. Lake Ave.
Glenview, IL 60025

Phone: (714) 476–0268 or (800) 228–4238 (888–224-WOCN)
Referral to a local WOC/ET nurse for support and advice regarding skin care, pouching, or adjustment difficulties.

Crohn's and Colitis Foundation of America
444 Park Ave. South
New York, NY 10016
Phone: (212) 685–3440
For information on and support for people with Crohn's disease or ulcerative colitis.

The Cleveland Clinic Foundation
Enterostomal Therapy Nursing
9500 Euclid Ave.
Cleveland, OH 44195
Phone: (216) 444–6677 or (800) 223–2273, ext. 46677
Fax: (216) 445–6343
For ET nursing support and advice regarding pouch management or adjustment difficulties.

Patient Education Press
417 Cleveland Ave.
Plainfield, NJ 07060
For the following publications: *Ostomy care for children, Colostomy care, Ileostomy care, Urinary diversion,* and *Ostomy dietary guidelines*.

Other Publications

Broadwell DC, Jackson BS, eds. *Principles of ostomy care*. St. Louis: Mosby, 1982.
Cox BG, Wentworth AE. *The ileal pouch procedure*. Rochester: Mayo Comprehensive Cancer Center, 1977.
Hampton B, ed. *Ostomies and continent diversions*. St. Louis: Mosby–Year Book, 1992.
Hill GL. *Ileostomy: surgery, physiology, and management*. New York: Grune and Stratton, 1976.
Jeter KF. *These special children*. Palo Alto, CA: Bull Publishing, 1982.

Journal of Enterostomal Therapy. Official publication of the International Association of Enterostomal Therapists, published quarterly by Mosby (St. Louis).

Mullen BD, McGinn DA. *The ostomy book*. Palo Alto, CA: Bull Publishing, 1980. Lliving comfortably with colostomies, ileostomies, and urostomies.

Ostomy Quarterly. a publication of the United Ostomy Association, published quarterly.

Steiner P, Banks PA, Present DH, eds. *People not patients: a source book for living with inflammatory bowel disease*. New York: National Foundation for Ileitis and Colitis, 1985.

Walker FC, ed. *Modern stoma care*. London: Churchill-Livingstone, 1976.

REFERENCES

1. Ahlering TE, Weinbert AC, Razor B. Modified Indiana Pouch. *J Urol* 1991;145:1156.
2. Aukett LK, Bonsaint R, Corbin C, et al. National guidelines for enterostomal patient education. *Dis Colon Rectum* 1994;37:559.
3. Bambrick M, Fazio V, Hull T. Sexual function following restorative proctocolectomy in women. *Dis Colon Rectum* 1996;39:610.
4. Boston A, Litman L, Rush A, et al. Controlling colostomy odor. *Am J Nurs* 1977;77:444.
5. Corman JM, Odenheimer DB. Securing the loop: historic review of the methods used for creating a loop colostomy. *Dis Colon Rectum* 1991;34:1014.
6. Erwin-Toth P. Advances in enterostomal therapy. *Perspect Colon Rectal Surg* 1995;8:227.
7. Erwin-Toth P, Barrett P. Stoma site marking: a primer. *Ostomy/Wound Management* 1997;43:18.
8. Erwin-Toth P, Doughty D. Principles and procedures of stomal management. In: Hampton B, Bryant R, eds. *Ostomies and continent diversions: nursing management*. St. Louis: Mosby, 1992.
9. Erwin-Toth P, Floruta C. Nursing management of continent ostomy diversions. *Progressions* 1993;5:3.
10. Ewing G. The nursing preparations of stoma patients for self-care. *J Adv Nurs* 1989;14:411.
11. Felice P. The many parts of ostomy collection systems: what are your options? *Ostomy/Wound Management* 1985;9:31.
12. Gazzard BG, Saunders B, Dawson AM. Diets and stoma function. *Br J Surg* 1978;65:642.
13. Kodner I. Stoma complications. In: Fazio V, ed. *Current therapy in colon and rectal surgery*. Philadelphia: BC Decker, 1990.
14. Lavery I, Erwin-Toth P. Stoma therapy. In: MacKeigan J, Cataldo P, eds. *Intestinal stomas: principles, techniques, and management*. St. Louis: Quality Medical Publishing, 1993:60.
15. Lewis C. *Aging: the health care challenge*. Philadelphia: FA Davis, 1990.
16. Meier DE, Tarpley JL. Improvisation in the developing world. *Surg Gynecol Obstet* 1991;173:404.
17. Rodriguez R, Wiener I. A home-made colostomy bag. *Surg Gynecol Obstet* 1986;163:277.
18. Rolstad BS, Hoyman K. Continent diversions and reservoirs, ostomies and continent diversions. *Nurse Manager* 1992;145:55.
19. Rothstein MS. Prevention and treatment of peristomal skin problems. *Ostomy/Wound Management* 1985;9:6.
20. Ruzicki D. Realistically meeting the educational needs of hospitalized acute and short stay patients: cross-cultural perceptions on patient teaching. *Nurs Clin North Am* 1989;24:3.
21. Zarle N. Continuity of care: balancing care of elders between health care settings. *Nurs Clin North Am* 1989;24:3.

Miscellaneous Colitides

With T. Cristina Sardinha

I have asked Dr. Cristina Sardinha, a superb surgical resident with whom I had worked and who at the time of this writing was a resident in Colon and Rectal Surgery at the Cleveland Clinic Florida, to extensively revise and update this chapter for the 5th edition. Dr. Sardinha, as has already been noted, has contributed much to this text. I truly value her diligence, her dedication and her commitment to the highest ideals of a surgeon/investigator. I am deeply appreciative of her and am confident the reader will feel similarly.—MLC

This chapter addresses a number of inflammatory conditions of the bowel that, in general, are either infectious or noninfectious. The two conditions that have been discussed in previous chapters, ulcerative colitis and Crohn's disease, have been excluded. The common denominator for all of these diseases is an association with the symptom of diarrhea. The great majority of colitides are infectious in nature and are frequently the result of ingestion of contaminated food or water. Colitis can also be sexually transmitted, particularly through anal intercourse. This is a particular issue in immunosuppressed and HIV patients (see Chapter 20).

While diarrheal disease is still one of the leading causes of morbidity and mortality, especially among children in the developing world, it is not an insignificant source for morbidity in Western countries. In the United States, adults experience an average of 1.5 to 2 episodes per year. Certainly, in elderly individuals or those who are immunocompromised, the potential for mortality is increased. While it is indeed true that most diarrheal conditions are self-limiting, the surgeon must always be alert to the fact that even an acute onset of diarrheal disease may be the initial presentation of an underlying disorder that mandates thorough gastrointestinal investigation.[284]

NONINFECTIOUS COLITIDES

I am poured out like water, and all my bones are out of joint; my heart is like wax; it is melted in the midst of my bowels.

Psalm 22:14

Eosinophilic Gastroenteritis or Eosinophilic Colitis

Primary eosinophilic gastroenteritis is a disorder that selectively affects the gastrointestinal tract. It is characterized by an eosinophil-predominant chronic inflammatory process of unknown etiology. The eosinophilia is present not only in the peripheral blood but also in the intestinal tissue.[242] Initial publications suggested an allergic association, but this has not been proved.[190] However, it is known that the expansion and tissue distribution of eosinophils are regulated by IL-5 and eotaxin 1.[230] Furthermore, eosinophilic gastroenteritis has strong genetic and allergic components and presents immunopathogenic features similar to those of other allergic disorders, such as asthma.

The three major clinical patterns are as follows: primary mucosal disease with enteric protein loss and malabsorption, predominant muscle layer disease with obstructive symptoms, and primary subserosal disease with eosinophilic ascites.[150]

The gastric antrum and the proximal small intestine are most frequently involved, while the colon is a rare location for the condition. Perianal disease has also been reported.[156]

The most common presenting symptoms are abdominal pain and change in bowel habits. Nausea, vomiting, weight loss, and rectal bleeding are also frequently noted. If mucosal disease predominates, gastrointestinal bleeding, protein-losing enteropathy, diarrhea, and malabsorption are the most common complaints.[201] Serosal involvement may be manifested as eosinophilic ascites. Large bowel obstruction secondary to a colocolonic intussusception has also been described.[29]

Tissue eosinophilia is a common feature of eosinophilic gastroenteritis. Although eosinophiles are a recognized manifestation in numerous gastrointestinal conditions, especially Crohn's disease and ulcerative colitis, there is no comparison with the massive infiltration present in eosinophilic gastroenteritis and colitis.[190] When the condition occurs in the colon, it may radiologically mimic tuberculosis, amebiasis, or Crohn's dis-

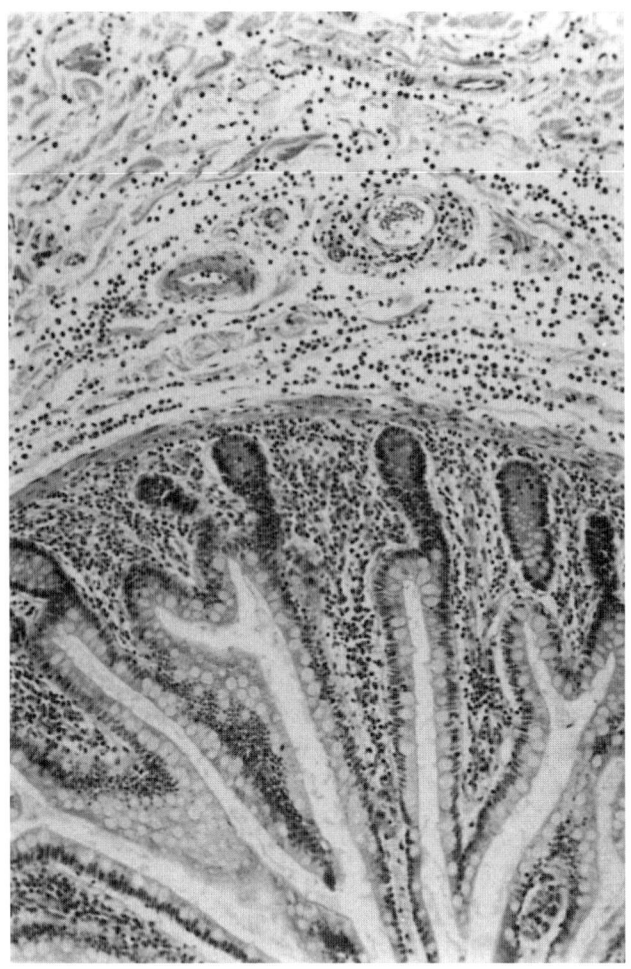

FIGURE 33-1. Eosinophilic enteritis. Intense inflammatory infiltration by eosinophils is seen within the mucosa and submucosa of the small bowel. (Original magnification ×330.)

ease.[242] Based on the few cases reported thus far, the proximal colon seems to have a greater predilection for involvement. Colonoscopic evaluation may reveal changes from erythema and friability, to granularity and narrowing.[201] Tedesco and colleagues suggested that eosinophilic ileocolitis may be more common than originally thought, and postulated that biopsy and counting of high-power microscopic fields for eosinophils may be a useful means for distinguishing eosinophilic colitis from that of Crohn's disease (Figure 33-1).[268] In addition to inflammatory bowel disease, the differential diagnosis should include infectious colitides, such as helminthiasis and amebiasis (see later), systemic hypereosinophilia syndrome, milk protein colitis, vasculitis, and allergic gastroenteropathy.[29] Evaluation of IgE levels may help in determining the possibility of allergen involvement. Moreover, immunohistochemical analysis of intestinal eosinophil activation in patients with

eosinophilic gastroenteritis suggests that the eosinophil cationic protein stored in eosinophil granules and secreted by activated eosinophils may be a tissue marker for eosinophilic gastroenteritis.[21] However, the combination of histologic and clinical patterns is the mainstay for the diagnosis of inflammatory conditions of the colon.[40]

Prognosis is generally good, with clinical, hematologic, roentgenographic, and histologic improvement occurring spontaneously or on steroid therapy.[109] Moreover, new therapeutic approaches in the management of eosinophilic gastroenteritis are currently being assessed, including treatment with anti–IL-5 (mepolizumab).[90] However, resection of the involved bowel may be required for unremitting symptoms or to exclude another diagnosis.[190]

Microscopic Colitis

Microscopic colitis is a condition initially described by Kingham and colleagues in which a number of patients with severe, watery diarrhea were found to have no detectable abnormality of the bowel except by microscopic examination of biopsy specimens.[138] This chronic diarrheal condition is characterized by colonic intraepithelial lymphocytosis and is manifested by watery diarrhea, normal endoscopic findings, and characteristic histologic features. Collagenous colitis and lymphocytic colitis present with similar symptoms but may differ through the presence of subepithelial collagen deposition.[263]

The actual incidence of microscopic colitis is unknown since it is a poorly reported condition. A study from Sweden by Olesen and colleagues[193] reported an increasing incidence of microscopic colitis over the past decades from 1.8/100,000 to 6/100,000 inhabitants. The authors concluded that the incidence of microscopic colitis is higher than previously described, and is currently as common as Crohn's disease in Orebro, Sweden. Microscopic colitis was diagnosed in 10% of patients with non-bloody diarrhea and up to 20% of those individuals who were over age 70 years. There is no association of microscopic colitis with an increased risk of colorectal cancer.[165]

The clinical course of this disease is benign, with spontaneous remission of symptoms within a few years of onset. There is no evidence to suggest an infectious agent, ischemia, dietary predisposition, or endocrine abnormality. Surreptitious laxative or diuretic use has been vigorously sought for but never discovered.[137] Anemia, increased erythrocyte sedimentation rate, hypokalemia, and hypoalbuminemia are common findings. These patients are usually middle-aged or elderly women, and all have watery diarrhea of lengthy duration as the predomi-

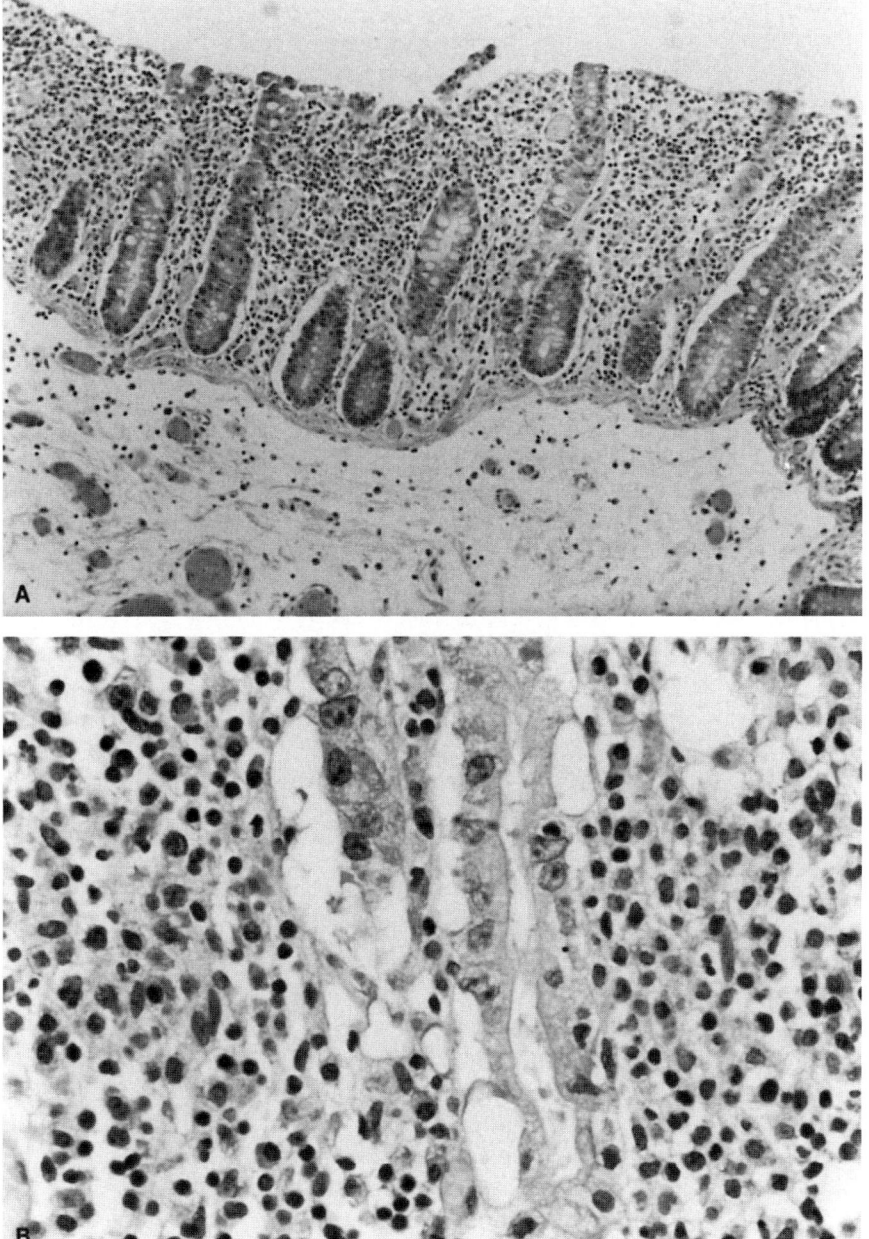

FIGURE 33-2. Microscopic colitis. **(A)** Heavy lymphocytic infiltration confined to the mucosa and filling the lamina propria. There is a decrease in glandular mucus content as well as cryptoglandular distortion, but there is no suggestion of crypt abscess. (Original magnification ×330.) **(B)** Higher magnification (×400) reveals infiltration of glands by lymphocytes.

nant symptom, associated with frequent problems of anal incontinence.[137]

The diagnosis is based on histologic evaluation of rectal and colonic biopsy. The changes consist of a pancolonic, diffuse, acute, and chronic inflammation of the lamina propria with preserved crypt architecture (Figure 33-2). The inflammation is found to be remarkably uniform, indicative of a total colitis. Sandmeier and Bouzourene[237] described a rare histopathologic subtype of microscopic colitis characterized by the presence of subepithelial multinucleated giant cells. The authors considered this factor to be an important diagnostic criterion

in the differential diagnosis of granulomatous infections and Crohn's disease. Moreover, it seems that this subtype of microscopic colitis has a more favorable prognosis and a better response to corticosteroid therapy.

There has been some debate as to whether microscopic and collagenous colitis represent variants of the same condition.[137] Sylwestrowicz and colleagues argued that the histologic variability of collagenization and inflammation during the course of both conditions, as well as the clinical feature of watery diarrhea, suggest that the two entities should be grouped together as "the watery diarrhea–colitis syndrome."[262]

The severe reduction of colonic fluid absorption probably contributes to the development of the chronic diarrhea.[26] Others have suggested a pathophysiological role for bile salt malabsorption, since cholestyramine has been demonstrably effective.[215] This condition may also be responsive to anti-inflammatory agents.

Collagenous Colitis

Collagenous colitis is a disease characterized clinically by profuse watery diarrhea, and histologically by marked thickening of the colonic subepithelial basement membrane.[196] It has also been reported to involve the terminal ileum.[160] As with microscopic colitis, patients are predominantly middle-aged to elderly women who are essentially well except for the diarrhea and abdominal pain.[139] Only rarely is the severity of the diarrhea sufficient to cause dehydration.[283] Clinical symptoms often become manifest before a fully developed histologic pattern can be appreciated.[246]

In a multi-institutional review from Sweden, 163 histopathologically verified cases were reported.[25] Of these, 85% followed a chronic, intermittent course. Nocturnal diarrhea was noted in 27%, abdominal pain in 41%, and weight loss in 42%. Forty percent had one or more associated diseases.

Endoscopic examination and radiologic studies have demonstrated a normal appearing mucosa in the majority of individuals. However, edema, friability, pinpoint mucosal hemorrhages, and hyperemia have been occasionally seen.[216] As the disease progresses, the collagen may gradually increase and possibly act as a diffusion barrier that may further exacerbate diarrheal symptoms (Figure 33-3).[216] Tanaka and associates investigated the distribution of the collagen band in 33 patients in order to estimate the likelihood of the disease being diagnosed through biopsy specimens from the left side of the colon, such as are usually obtained by means of flexible sigmoidoscopy.[265] They concluded that this limited examination is not necessarily adequate to exclude collagenous colitis when based solely on the presence of a thickened collagen band, and that total colonoscopy with multiple biopsy specimens may be required.

The pathogenesis of the condition and the subepithelial fibrosis characterizing the disease remain uncertain, although two instances of its development in a setting of nonsteroidal anti-inflammatory agents have been reported.[94] The thickening of the subepithelial collagen layer may be a response to chronic inflammation or a local abnormality of collagen synthesis.[254] It has been postulated that the disease may be attributable to reduced cell turnover, allowing fibrocytes to remain longer in the mature phase, hence producing more collagen

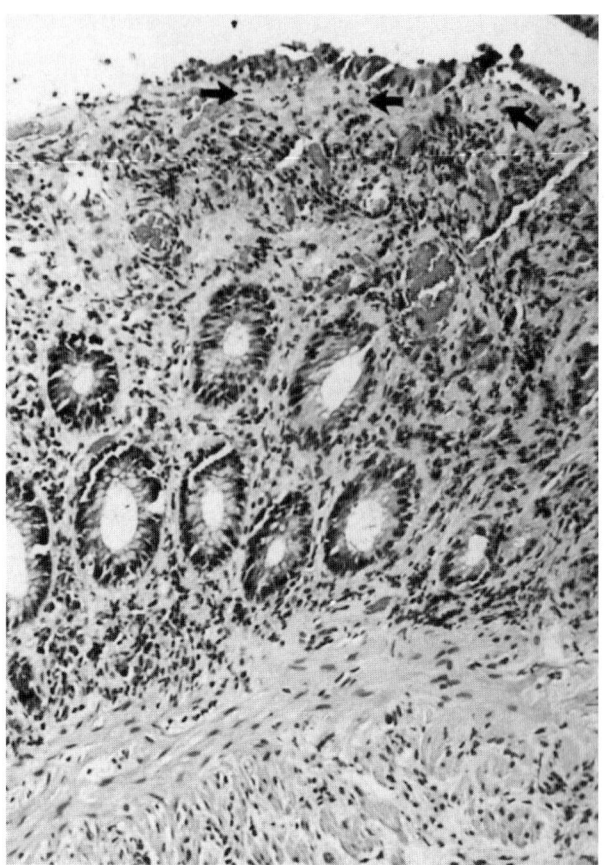

FIGURE 33-3. Collagenous colitis. Note the deposit of collagen in the upper lamina propria (*arrows*) underneath the slightly denuded superficial epithelium. (Original magnification ×100; courtesy of Lauren M. Monda, M.D.)

and a thicker collagen plate.[139] The possibility of this being another of the autoimmune conditions has also been suggested.[12,93] The association of collagenous colitis with other autoimmune diseases, such as polyarteritis nodosa may support this statement.[209]

Recommended treatments have included sulfasalazine, antibiotics, pentoxifylline, octreotide, bile salt-binding agents, bismuth subsalicylate, aminosalicylates, budesonide, and corticosteroids.[168] Nonspecific anti-diarrheal agents, such as loperamide and diphenoxylate, appear to be ineffective in this patient population. In the Swedish experience, prednisolone was most effective, with a response rate of 82%. However, the required dose was often quite high, and the effect was not maintained following withdrawal of the medication.[25] The response rate for antibiotics, cholestyramine, and loperamide were 63%, 59%, and 71%, respectively. Conversely, spontaneous resolution may occur. A publication by the Cochrane Database based on a review of five randomized trials, identified three treatment options for collagenous colitis.[44] Budesonide was found to be an effective agent for the management of this disease; however, there was weak evidence to support the value of bismuth subsalicylate and prednisolone.[44]

Rare refractory cases may benefit from operative management, but the role of surgery in this condition is extremely limited.[110] Fecal diversion, subtotal colectomy,[168] and restorative proctocolectomy with ileo-pouch anal anastomosis have all been suggested as therapeutic options.[278] As previously stated, it is not inconceivable that microscopic colitis and collagenous colitis represent different manifestations of a single disease entity.[15,278]

Neutropenic Enterocolitis, Ileocecal Syndrome, and Typhlitis

Neutropenic enterocolitis, ileocecal syndrome, and typhlitis describe a syndrome associated with bowel wall necrosis that can occur during treatment of hematologic malignancies, especially leukemia, lymphoma, and aplastic anemia.[151] Neutropenic enterocolitis has also been reported as a complication of other therapeutic modalities, such as anti-thyroid therapy,[46] chemotherapy for lung adenocarcinoma,[80] or as the presenting complication of acute lymphoblastic leukemia.[212] It has also been described as a complication of cyclic neutropenia, a rare benign hematologic disorder.[192] Profound neutropenia secondary to chemotherapy has been considered the hallmark of the disease and the major etiologic factor in its development.[186] This is a condition characterized by regular oscillations in blood neutrophil counts, in which sporadic disappearance of these cells from the circulation occurs. Involvement of the process is most commonly seen in the terminal ileum, cecum, and right colon, possibly because of the higher concentration of lymphatic tissue in these areas.

Patients exhibit symptoms of diarrhea, abdominal pain, sepsis, and findings typical of acute appendicitis. Even when the pain is localized to the right lower quadrant, the rapidity of the appearance of toxicity, with tachycardia, fever, and delirium, can be extremely dramatic. Koea and Shaw reported three individuals with leukemia who presented with fever, abdominal pain, and signs of peritonitis localized to the right iliac fossa.[146] Each patient was found to have a nonviable cecum. Although the precise pathogenic mechanism is not well understood, current evidence suggests that neutropenic ulceration of the bowel wall facilitates invasion and propagation of *Clostridium septicum*, resulting in bowel necrosis and septicemia.[158]

The diagnosis is based on clinical presentation and a low neutrophil count. The finding of radiologic abnormalities, however, may aid in the differential. For example, Kirkpatrick and Greenberg described pneumatosis intestinalis as the most common computed tomographic observation suggestive of neutropenic enterocolitis (21% of patients).[140] Thickened bowel wall, mesenteric stranding, bowel dilatation, mucosal enhancing, and ascites are also frequently reported.[140]

With obvious peritoneal signs, surgical resection is mandatory. A high operative mortality rate must be anticipated due to the patient's underlying disease. However, the majority of individuals with neutropenic enterocolitis have minimal, if any, abdominal symptoms and do not progress to develop necrosis, perforation, or peritonitis.[186]

Diversion Colitis, Disuse Colitis, and Starvation Colitis

Diverting the fecal stream and defunctionalizing the bowel can produce a noninfectious colitis, an observation made by Glotzer and colleagues in 1981.[98] Generally, patients are asymptomatic, although mucus discharge and bleeding may be noted. Fenton and Siegel have shown that 70% of their ostomy patients had gross or microscopic findings of diversion colitis despite the absence of symptoms.[79] Roe and colleagues reported that all of their 12 patients who had undergone a Hartmann procedure demonstrated histologic abnormalities consistent with diversion colitis by 3 months.[220] An association of microcarcinoids with diversion colitis has also been reported.[104] This occurrence has been attributed to neurogenic hyperplasia, which represents proliferation of a separate, neuron-associated, extraglandular population of endocrine cells.[103]

Proctosigmoidoscopic findings are essentially that of a mild inflammatory bowel disease suggestive of ulcerative colitis. Microscopic alterations, however, tend to be rather focal and include crypt abscesses, epithelial cell degeneration, acute and chronic inflammation in the lamina propria, and regenerative changes in the crypts (Figure 33-4).[98] The crypt cell production rate has been determined to be less than half that of controls. Additionally, crypt length and width are lower.[8] However, the histologic picture with the condition is quite variable. Pathologic evaluation of more severely diseased, resected specimens may demonstrate diffuse nodularity caused by lymphoid hyperplasia and an inflammatory process confined to the mucosa and submucosa.[187]

The mucosa of the intestinal tract is unique in that it draws nutrients not only from the vasculature, but also from the bowel lumen.[221] It is not difficult to appreciate how this entity can develop when examining the radiologic picture shown in Figure 33-5. Nutrition of the

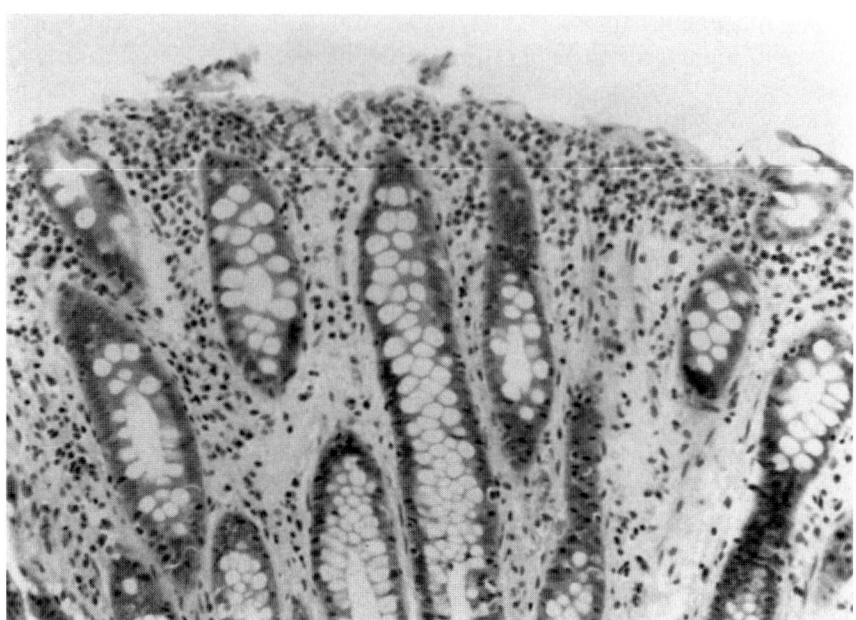

FIGURE 33-4. Diversion colitis. A 37-year-old woman underwent a Hartmann resection for perforated diverticulitis. Because of the complaint of mucus discharge, a biopsy was taken. Edematous colonic mucosa with focal surface erosion is seen, in addition to a mild increase of chronic inflammatory cells in the lamina propria and into the glandular epithelium. The changes are consistent with diversion colitis. (Original magnification ×280.)

colonic epithelial cells is mainly from short-chain fatty acids produced by bacterial fermentation in the colonic lumen.[221] Deficiency in these substances initially leads to mucosal hypoplasia and subsequently to a more typical picture of nonspecific inflammatory bowel disease. Harig and colleagues have shown that negligible amounts of short-chain fatty acids can be identified in a segment of excluded rectosigmoid.[113] They further demonstrated that installation of a solution containing short-chain fatty acids twice daily resulted in the disappearance of symptoms and in the inflammatory changes observed at endoscopy within a period of 6 weeks. Short-chain fatty acids have also been used for the management of diversion colitis in children.[135] Others have shown that the condition may be successfully treated with the use of 5-aminosalicylic acid enemas.[272] However, the only curative approach is stoma reversal or rectal excision.

The affected bowel rapidly returns to a normal appearance following reestablishment of intestinal continuity. Orsay prospectively evaluated 34 patients who were scheduled to undergo colostomy closure and who were demonstrated to have diversion colitis.[194] There was no increased infection rate or any other complications following colostomy closure.

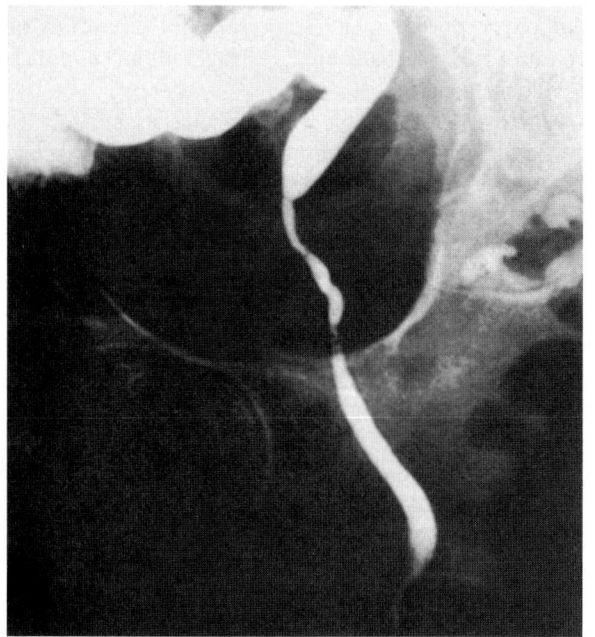

FIGURE 33-5. Barium study reveals an atrophic rectum, a consequence of disuse for many years following the creation of a colostomy.

Disinfectant Colitis (Pseudolipomatosis)

Ryan and Potter have emphasized the poorly recognized entity of disinfectant colitis (or pseudolipomatosis) in colonic mucosa, thus creating a unique form of colitis.[233] Commercially available endoscope disinfecting solutions, such as glutaraldehyde and hydrogen peroxide can injure the crypt epithelium or mucosal stroma with resultant tissue necrosis if there has been contact with the colonic mucosa. Patients may experience signs and symptoms of

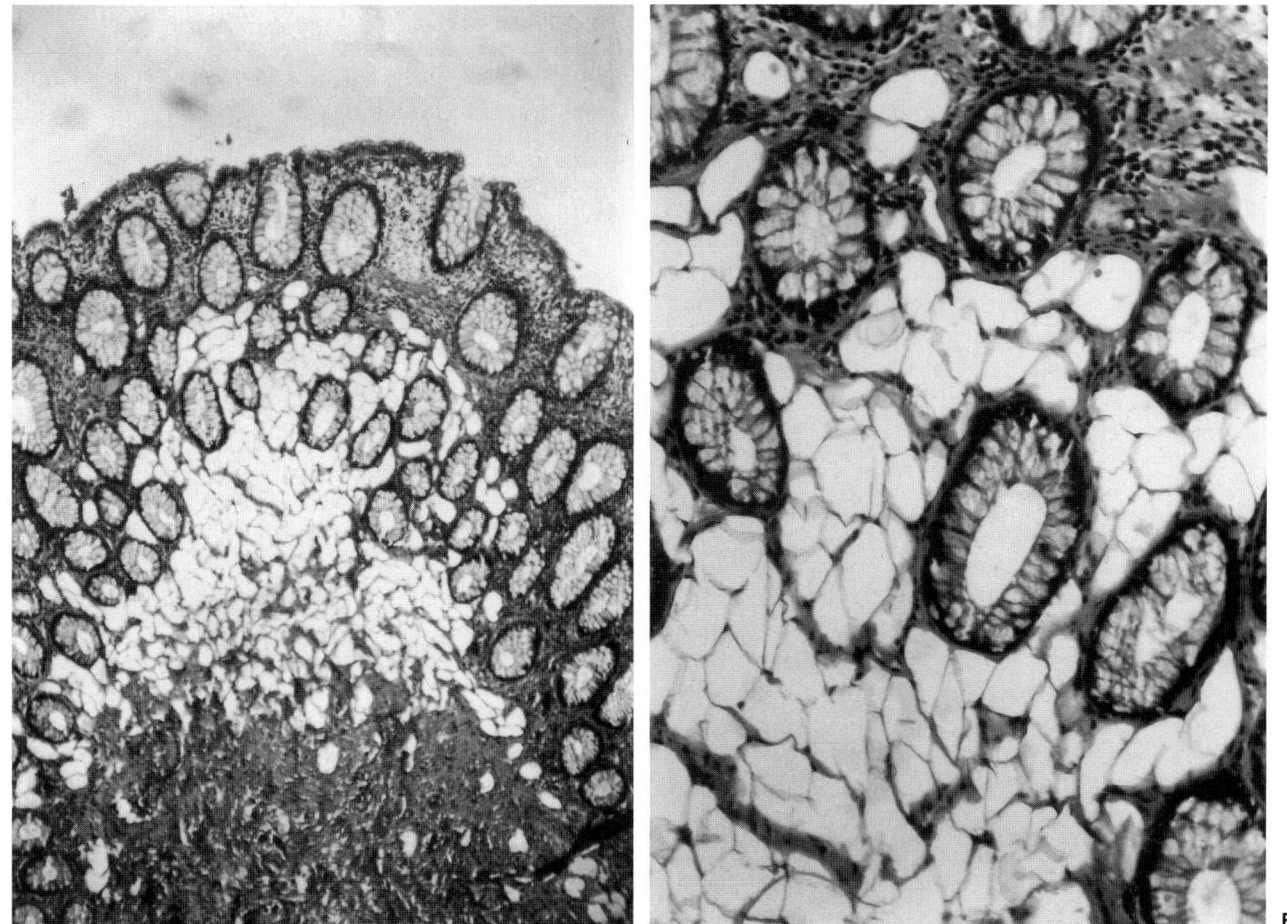

FIGURE 33-6. Disinfectant colitis (pseudolipomatosis). **(A)** Colonic mucosa demonstrating spaces devoid of epithelial lining in the lamina propria. Note the similarity to pneumatosis coli (see Fig. 25-96). (Original magnification ×280.) **(B)** Note the absence of nuclei. These are empty spaces, not lipocytes. (Original magnification ×560.)

abdominal pain, fever, and bloody diarrhea.[87,280] This usually commences 12 to 48 hours following endoscopy. While controversial, this entity may become visible as opaque plaques or pseudomembranes, even when the colonoscopy is in progress.[233]

Based on experimental studies it is felt that hydrogen peroxide alone is responsible for the unique form of colitis that has been termed by pathologists as pseudolipomatosis (Figure 33-6).

While it is certainly important to be concerned about the serious implications of communicable diseases, and strict attention must be paid to the appropriate disinfecting of endoscopes, adequate rinsing and thorough air-drying should prevent this complication. Another suggestion for prevention is the use of a disposable endoscope sheath that is replaced with each procedure, thereby obviating the requirement for a disinfecting agent.[239] Recognition of this entity, especially when the endoscopist notes the sudden appearance of abnormal pseudomembranous-like plaques during a procedure should help avoid confusion as to the diagnosis.

Corrosive Colitis

Oral administration of a host of corrosives is a well-recognized entity for which surgical intervention is often required. Less well recognized, however, is the installation of various toxic or corrosive materials by means of an enema. Cappell and Simon reviewed the literature on the reported intra-rectally administered toxic agents and found that the most common was hydrogen peroxide.[38] Other agents included detergent enemas, herbal medicines, acetic acid, ethyl alcohol, sodium hydroxide, and hydrofluoric acid. Pikarsky and colleagues presented a case of severe formalin-induced colitis 5 days after rectal instillation of formalin for radiation proctitis.[203] Drugs such as ergotamine can also be associated with inflammatory reaction and toxicity. Toxic exposure may result from conventional medical therapy, unconventional medical therapy, radiographic examination, colonoscopic examination (see previous discussion), deliberate self-mutilation, or accidental self-administration.[38]

Rectal bleeding, diarrhea, and abdominal pain are frequent symptoms. Endoscopic examination usually reveals nonspecific changes consistent with inflammatory bowel disease, including erythema, ulceration, granularity, friability, and purulent exudate. A history of medication use or exposure to toxic agents is obviously helpful.

Treatment is generally supportive care, although emergency laparotomy and bowel resection may be required for fulminant acute colitis, stricture, or perforation (see also Chapter 14).

NSAID-Induced Colitis

Adverse effects of nonsteroidal anti-inflammatory drugs (NSAIDs) on the upper gastrointestinal tract and small intestine are well recognized.[63] Since the initial description of NSAID-induced colonic injury by Debenham,[65] a growing number of reports have associated the use of NSAIDs and salicylates with colonic complications. However, the true incidence of NSAID-induced colitis is unknown. A study from Jersey (United Kingdom) estimated that approximately 1:1200 NSAID-users may develop colitis.[97]

The clinical presentation of NSAID-induced colitis is based on the development of an acute, non-specific inflammatory process involving the colonic mucosa.[84] Symptoms include bloody diarrhea, sporadic melanotic stool leading to iron-deficiency anemia, weight loss, fatigue, anorexia, and even to fatality. The pathogenesis of NSAID-induced colitis may be related to the inhibition of prostaglandin synthesis.[63] In addition to the oral route, NSAID-induced suppository toxicity has been recognized.

Colonoscopy may demonstrate diffuse inflammation, with erosions or ulcerations. The presence of diaphragmatic-like strictures or webs, most commonly in the right colon, has been described as a pathognomonic sign of NSAID-induced colitis.[133] However, the most common finding is a solitary or limited number of cecal ulcerations, or they may be scattered throughout the colon and rectum.[208] The condition may be difficult to differentiate from that of ulcerative colitis in its early presentation.

NSAID ingestion should certainly be considered in the differential diagnosis of colitis. The use of NSAIDs in the form of suppositories may induce rectal bleeding and proctitis due to the high concentration of the drug in direct contact with the rectal mucosa.[96,159] Moreover, the severity of rectal symptoms may be dose dependent. It has been estimated that up to 30% of patients using NSAID-containing suppositories may develop rectal symptoms such as pain, inflammation, bleeding, ulcerations, and stricture.[63]

One would certainly expect an ameliorative response of the bowel to the discontinuation of the medication.

Additionally, the use of sulfasalazine and metronidazole has proven to be somewhat beneficial.[74] Surgical treatment is reserved for cases of life-threatening complications or refractory colitis.

Toxic Epidermal Necrolysis

Toxic epidermal necrolysis is a rare and severe reaction to certain drugs that results in full-thickness epidermal skin necrosis.[41] Other mucosal surfaces have been implicated, including the large bowel. The most common drugs associated with this condition include sulfonamides, penicillin, NSAIDs (see previous discussion), phenytoin anticonvulsants, and barbiturates.[41]

Symptoms include abdominal pain and bloody diarrhea, usually concomitant with the development of the skin lesions. Several cases of colonic necrosis complicating this condition have been reported.[41]

INFECTIOUS COLITIDES

Tis now the very witching time of night,
when churchyards yawn and hell itself
breathes out contagion to this world.
                    William Shakespeare—*Hamlet, III, 2*

Viruses, bacteria, fungi, as well as a host of parasites, may cause infections of the gastrointestinal tract. The upper intestine tends to be attacked by organisms that produce toxins (e.g., *Vibrio cholerae*), whereas in general, colon infection is associated with organisms that produce dysentery (e.g., *Shigella*). In the former situation, infection tends to leave the mucosa uninvolved, whereas in the latter, the intestinal mucosa is often ulcerated or destroyed. Upper intestinal organisms tend to produce diarrhea with severe dehydration. However, there is usually no septicemia. Those that affect the large bowel often produce severe abdominal pain, tenesmus, and signs and symptoms of generalized infection (e.g., malaise, pyrexia). A rapid onset is often due to the presence of a toxin produced by a bacterium rather than to the bacterium itself. This type of syndrome is occasionally associated with certain restaurant foods. Gorbach stated that the incubation period from a toxin is so brief that the symptoms occur either when one is paying the check or when on the way to the parking lot.[102]

Most episodic diarrheas are caused by an infection acquired by ingesting fecally contaminated food or beverages. *Escherichia coli* is the most common pathogen, although many other bacteria, viruses, and protozoa have been implicated.[56] The "immunologically naive traveler" to developing areas is the individual most susceptible to the bacterial and protozoal indigenous organisms.[107] Prevention can be best described by the adage, "cook it, boil it, peel it, or forget it."[107]

Recommended antimicrobial therapy for severe cases of diarrhea includes trimethoprim/sulfamethoxazole, trimethoprim alone, quinolones (e.g., ciprofloxacin [Cipro], norfloxacin [Noroxin]), metronidazole (Flagyl), or doxycycline, but the majority of infectious diarrheas represent little more than a self-limited nuisance. In 1990, a National Institutes of Health panel of experts recommended that antibiotics not be used as routine prophylaxis for traveler's diarrhea because of adverse drug reactions and increasing world-wide bacterial resistance.[78] Instead, the conference endorsed the use of two tablets of bismuth subsalicylate three to four times daily for this purpose.

Comprehensive microbiologic testing and thorough gastrointestinal studies for every individual with the complaint of diarrhea is impractical and very expensive.[114,295] No investigations, except perhaps a rigid or flexible sigmoidoscopy and biopsy, are required for younger patients if weight is stable and the stool is free of occult blood.[114] But the fact is that a few individuals do require a more extensive evaluation, a decision that must rest with the physician's clinical judgment. Appropriate precautions, however, are mandatory if one is to prevent the spread of infectious diarrhea in the hospital environment.[86]

In this section the various diarrheas of potential interest to the surgeon are discussed: presentation, diagnosis, and therapy.

Bacterial Infections

Antibiotic-Associated Colitis, Pseudomembranous Colitis, and *Clostridium difficile* Colitis

The first reported case of pseudomembranous colitis actually antedated the antibiotic era and is generally attributed to Finney of Johns Hopkins.[82] His patient developed bloody diarrhea, perhaps as a consequence of enema feedings following a gastric procedure. The discussants of his paper presented what were than a "who's who" of American medicine prior to the turn of the 20th century—Halstead, Osler, Thayer, and Flexner.

Epidemiology, Etiology, and Incidence

Clostridium difficile is a gram-positive, anaerobic, spore-forming bacillus, first described in 1935 as a component of normal newborn fecal flora.[111] However, the role of *C. difficile* in the pathogenesis of antibiotic-associated colitis was not reported until the late 1970s.[259] The rising incidence of *C. difficile* colitis in hospitalized patients has become a matter of concern among physicians, especially surgeons. Recent reports have shown that 20% to 25% of hospitalized individuals will acquire *C. difficile*. Moreover, one third of these patients will develop diarrhea.[105] Therefore, *C. difficile* colitis, previously considered an uncommon infectious colonic disease as stated in prior editions of this text, is currently thought to be one of the most common nosocomial infections. Generally, this has been attributed to a heightened awareness of the condition, better diagnostic methods, the more wide-spread use of broad-spectrum antibiotics, and the increasing number of elderly or immunocompromised patients.[30,163,170]

Any patient who develops diarrhea either during or after receiving antibiotic therapy must be considered at risk for this complication until proven otherwise, although it is certainly possible that colitis may not be associated with antibiotic therapy.[68] Antibiotic-associated diarrhea is often mild and self-limited, demonstrating rapid improvement with discontinuance or change of the antibiotic. Although almost one third of cases of antibiotic-associated diarrhea are due to *C. difficile*, 2% to 3% are secondary to other infectious organisms, such as *Clostridium perfringens*, *Staphylococcus aureus*, and *Candida albicans*.[121] *Clostridium difficile*–associated diarrhea may commence within 48 hours after the administration of the drug. However, the condition can develop after 6 to 10 weeks following stoppage of the antibiotic, an observation noted in 25% to 40% of patients.[105]

The pathophysiology of *Clostridium difficile* colitis is related to the breakdown of normal colonic microflora, followed by colonization with *C. difficile* and the production of invasive toxins leading to mucosal inflammation. Contamination occurs via the oral-fecal route. *Clostridium difficile* produces two toxins in the intestinal lumen, known as A (enterotoxin) and B (cytotoxin), which ad-

---

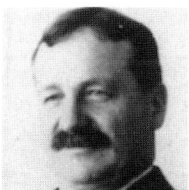

John Miller Turpin Finney (1863–1942) Finney was born in Natchez, Mississippi, the son and grandson of Presbyterian ministers. He grew up in Bel Air, Maryland, where his father assumed a church position. Finney attended Princeton University, receiving his bachelor's degree in 1884, and graduated from Harvard Medical School in 1889. He then spent 18 months at the Massachusetts General Hospital before accepting a faculty position at the Johns Hopkins Medical School. He became head of the surgical dispensary and ultimately rose to become professor of clinical surgery and surgeon-in-chief. In 1910, he rejected an offer to become president of Princeton University when Woodrow Wilson left to enter politics. While developing one of the largest practices of surgery in the United States, he was one of the key figures in establishing the Hopkins surgical residency training program. When the American College of Surgeons was formed in 1913, Finney was named its first president. He subsequently served as president of the American Surgical Association. With the entrance of the United States into World War I, Finney went to France as director of a base hospital. He was elevated to brigadier general and assumed the responsibility of chief consultant for the Allied Expeditionary Forces. For his services to the armies, he was awarded the Distinguished Service Medal and the French Legion of Honor. Finney devoted his last years to numerous charitable activities and to serving on the boards of a number of schools and universities. (Photo courtesy of the Alan Mason Chesney Medical Archives of the Johns Hopkins Medical Institutions, Baltimore, MD.)

here to the surface of the epithelial layer and produce an inflammatory reaction. Toxin A causes actin disaggregation and intracellular release of calcium. Toxin B is a necrotizing enterotoxin significantly more potent than toxin A. Both toxins, however, cause colonic mucosal damage and diarrhea. Nonetheless, *C. difficile* rarely produces colonic injury by direct invasion of the mucosa.[72] The severity of co-morbid conditions and low serum levels of IgG antibody to toxin A have been related to a higher probability of acquiring symptomatic *C. difficile* colitis.[152]

As previously stated, the incidence of *C. difficile*–associated colitis has increased considerably. Current reports cite up to 3 million cases of *C. difficile* diarrhea and colitis each year in the United States alone.[188] Two to three percent of healthy individuals are asymptomatic carriers. However, more than 80% of neonates and up to 70% of infants and young children harbor *C. difficile* in fecal flora without any intestinal manifestations.[105,121] This number declines, however, as children approach adulthood.[188,250] In a prospective analysis from the Department of Surgery at the New York Hospital–Cornell University Medical Center, the incidence of diarrhea in surgery patients was 6.1%, and the incidence of *Clostridium difficile*–associated diarrhea was found to be 2%.[170]

The most common antibiotics associated with *C. difficile* colitis are cephalosporin, clindamycin, ampicillin, and amoxicillin. However, virtually all antibiotics, including metronidazole and vancomycin, have been suggested to cause this syndrome. In the Mayo Clinic experience, 70% of their cases were associated with a cephalosporin.[264] The significance of this observation is somewhat diminished by the fact that this is the class of antibiotics most often administered in hospitals.[227] In addition to antibiotics, *C. difficile* colitis has also been reported in patients receiving anti-neoplastic agents, such as cisplatin, doxorubicin, methotrexate, teicoplanin, and tacrolimus.[188] The condition has also been reported as a complication of sulfasalazine therapy in a patient with inflammatory bowel disease.[205] The occurrence of this particular complication poses a considerable challenge in the differential diagnosis since the symptoms of the two diseases are very similar.

Those who appear to be at increased risk are individuals who are somewhat immunocompromised (e.g., with cystic fibrosis, neurologic disease, liver or renal disease, malnutrition, diabetes mellitus and hematologic disorders).[227,250] Other factors associated with an increased risk of infection include advanced age, malignancy, chronic pulmonary disease, prolonged hospitalization (more than 4 weeks), nursing home residents, transfer from another hospital, antibiotic course of more than 7 days, treatment with more than one antibiotic, immunosuppressive medication, chemotherapy, anti-peristaltic medica-

tions, antacid therapy, an intensive care unit location, non–single-room accommodation, and those conditions in which the intestinal motility is altered.[30] With respect to pathogenesis and prevention, a number of authors have emphasized that education of the hospital staff is mandatory if one is to reduce the incidence of this common and costly colitis.[147] For example, McFarland and colleagues found that the infection is frequently transmitted among hospitalized patients and that the organism is often present on the hands of hospital personnel caring for these individuals.[171] The American College of Gastroenterology and the Society for Healthcare Epidemiology of America have developed practice guidelines for the prevention and control of *Clostridium difficile* infection (Table 33-1).[125]

Clinical Manifestations

The clinical presentation of *C. difficile* colitis varies from one extreme, the asymptomatic carrier, to a fulminant illness that may result in death. The mortality rate has been reported to be from 10% to 30%.[105,188] Mild disease presents with diarrhea, crampy abdominal pain, and diffuse patchy, nonspecific colitis on endoscopic examination. Moderate cases are often associated with fever, nausea, anorexia, abdominal distention and cramps, in addition to profuse diarrhea. Those patients with severe *C. difficile* colitis appear toxic, dehydrated, and with signs of peritonitis on physical examination. These individuals in particular may go on to manifest a fulminant colitis, develop a colonic perforation, and succumb to the complications of their disease.

Evaluation

The initial assessment of a patient with possible *C. difficile*–associated diarrhea and colitis includes a complete history and physical examination as well as laboratory evaluation of electrolytes, white blood cell count, nutritional status, and stool testing to rule out other sources of diarrhea. Dehydration, electrolyte imbalance, leukocytosis, and hypoalbuminemia may often accompany severe disease. Stool examination reveals the presence of leukocytes in one-half of the cases. The hemoccult test may be positive in severe colitis, but grossly bloody diarrhea is unusual.

The *stool cytotoxin assay* is the preferred diagnostic test because of its high specificity and sensitivity, 99% and 100% respectively.[105,188] Filtering the stool and adding to cultured fibroblasts will demonstrate a cytopathic effect of toxin B that is neutralized by the specific antiserum. This will confirm a positive or negative test, since it detects as little as 10 picograms of the toxin in the stool.[188] The disadvantages are that it is expensive and re-

▶ **TABLE 33-1** Practice Guidelines for Prevention and Control of *Clostridium difficile* Infection

American College of Gastroenterology Recommendations	Society for Healthcare Epidemiology of America Recommendations
1. Limit the use of antimicrobial drugs.	1. Antimicrobial use restriction is indicated if a specific antimicrobial, particularly clindamycin is identified as a risk for CDAD.
2. Wash hands between contact with all patients.	2. Handwashing with either an antimicrobial agent or soap is recommended after contact with patients, their body substances, or environmental surfaces.
3. Use enteric (stool) isolation precautions for patients with *C. difficile* diarrhea.	3. Isolation of patients with CDAD in private rooms is recommended if private rooms are available; priority should be given to patients unable to maintain bowel continence and good hand-washing hygiene.
4. Wear gloves when in contact with patients who have *C. difficile* diarrhea/colitis, or with their environment.	4. Glove use by personnel for the handling of body substances of all patients is recommended to reduce the rate of CDAD.
5. Disinfect objects contaminated with *C. difficile* with sodium hypochlorite, alkaline glutaraldehyde, or ethylene oxide.	5. Replacement of electronic thermometers with disposable thermometers is recommended if CDAD rates are high.
6. Educate the medical, nursing, and other appropriate staff members about the disease and its epidemiology.	

CDAD, *Clostridium difficile*–associated diarrhea.
From Johnson S, Gerding D. Clostridium difficile–associated diarrhea. *Clin Infect Dis* 1998;26:1027, with permission.

quires overnight incubation in a tissue culture facility. *Enzyme-linked immunosorbent assay (ELISA)* detects 100 to 1,000 picograms of toxin A and/or B in the stool.[105] This test is less expensive and quicker. However, due to its lower sensitivity and specificity (87% to 98% and 71% to 99%, respectively), repeating the study may be necessary in up to one-third of cases wherein there is a high clinical suspicion.[105] The *latex agglutination test* detects the presence of glutamate dehydrogenase produced by *C. difficile*. However, this test is often not recommended because of the low sensitivity (48% to 59%) and specificity (95%).[105] *Stool culture* is difficult and time consuming (Figure 33-7). Moreover, non-toxigenic strains of *C. difficile* may grow in the culture media.

Endoscopic evaluation will demonstrate edema and mucosal inflammation. Pseudomembranes are present in 14% to 25% of patients with mild disease and 87% of those with severe colitis.[104] The disease often involves the entire colon. Therefore, colonoscopy is preferable to that of flexible sigmoidoscopy since 10% of patients present with pseudomembranes beyond the reach of the sigmoidoscope (Figure 33-8). Seppälä and associates also stressed the importance of colonoscopy in the diagnosis of this condition.[245] In a review of 16 patients with histologically proven antibiotic-associated pseudomembranous colitis, only 31% were confirmed by sigmoidoscopy, as compared with 85% in whom colonoscopy was performed. Others have noted the importance of total colonoscopy as the preferred means for establishing the diagnosis, particularly since there is not uncommonly right-sided involvement and a relatively normal distal

bowel.[34,61,232,236,267] Tedesco showed that five of six patients with tissue-culture evidence of a clostridial toxin in the stool had either a normal or merely an edematous distal rectal mucosa.[267] Thus, proctosigmoidoscopy would have failed to identify the abnormality.

Biopsy of the lesion is not mandatory for confirming the diagnosis. However, if there is any question as to the etiology of the inflammatory change, tissue should be obtained (Figs. 33-9 and 33-10). Histopathologic examination of the pseudomembranous plaque shows a mix of mucinous fibrinous exudate and polymorphonuclear neutrophils.

Radiographic imaging studies may reveal a paralytic ileus and pancolonic dilatation. Differential diagnosis must include Ogilvie's syndrome (colonic ileus), ischemia, and volvulus.[271] Pneumoperitoneum due to colonic perforation in severe or toxic colitis can also be found on plain abdominal radiography. Computerized tomography may show a diffusely thickened and edematous colonic wall.[188] Barium enema examination may demonstrate "thumbprinting," which is due to bowel wall edema. In more advanced stages, severe ulceration may be present (Figure 33-11). The procedure, however, is contraindicated in the acutely ill patient because of the risk of precipitating toxic megacolon or a perforation.[54,77,250]

Treatment

Despite the high mortality rate in critically ill individuals, most patients with mild *C. difficile* colitis will recover even without specific treatment. Adequate antibiotic therapy

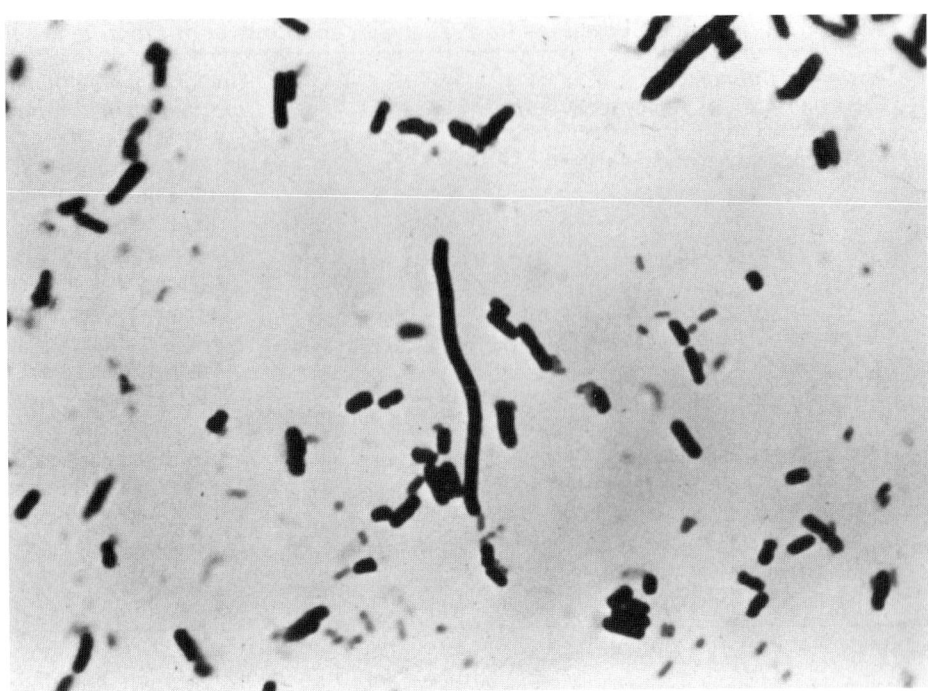

FIGURE 33-7. Clostridium difficile. Gram stain of stool reveals gram-positive rods. (Original magnification ×800.)

with metronidazole or vancomycin leads to symptomatic improvement in the overwhelming majority within the first 24 to 72 hours, with complete resolution in one or two weeks.

Treatment of *C. difficile* colitis includes cessation of the causative antibiotic. Adequate fluid and electrolyte replacement is also essential to overall patient management. Asymptomatic carriers do not require treatment. Conversely, fulminant colitis frequently requires intensive care monitoring and emergency surgery. More than 95% of patients respond to therapy with oral or intravenous metronidazole or oral vancomycin.[105,188] Metronidazole is the treatment of choice, however, because of the high fecal concentration, thus leading to a 99.9% reduction in organisms. Moreover, metronidazole provides a 95% to 100% response rate and is more cost-effective

than vancomycin.[105] The recommended dose is 250 mg, orally, twice daily or 500 mg, orally or intravenously, three times daily, for a total of 10 to 14 days. The intravenous route is used in patients who are intolerant of oral intake.

Vancomycin is equally as effective as metronidazole when taken orally, because the poor intestinal absorption promotes a high luminal concentration. Its mechanism of action is the inhibition of bacterial wall synthesis. In addition to the high cost, the major disadvantage of this drug is the emergence of vancomycin-resistant enterococci. Furthermore, unlike metronidazole, intravenous vancomycin is not excreted into the gastrointestinal tract. The recommended dose is 125 mg, orally, four times daily for 10 to 14 days and 40 mg/kg/day, divided three or four times a day for 7 to 10 days in pedi-

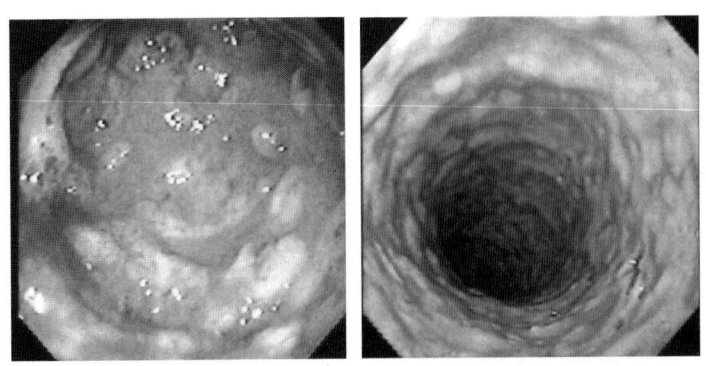

FIGURE 33-8. **(A, B)** Colonoscopy clearly demonstrates the patterns of yellow and yellow white adherent plaques in pseudomembranous colitis. (See Color Fig. 33-8.)

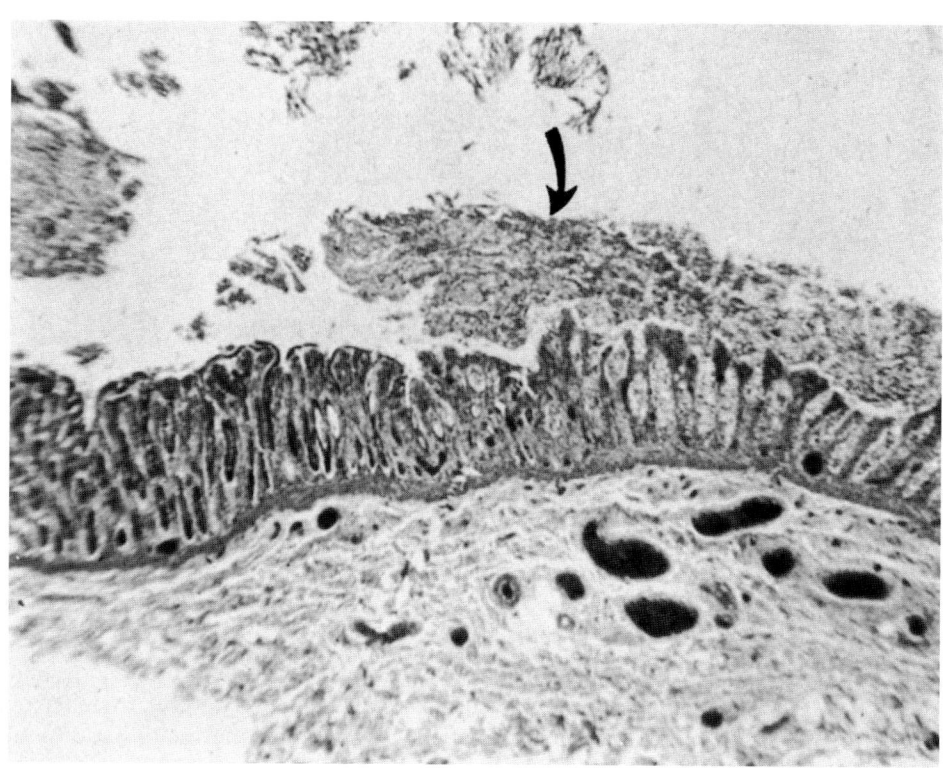

FIGURE 33-9. Pseudomembranous colitis. Superficial necrosis (*arrow*) with acute inflammatory mucosal exudate. (Original magnification ×80.)

atric patients.[105] Vancomycin enemas can be used in patients with *C. difficile* proctosigmoiditis or in those who have undergone emergency subtotal colectomy with an end-ileostomy. Under these circumstances, with a diseased rectum topical vancomycin is a very good treatment option.

Anion exchange resins, such as cholestyramine (Questran) will bind to the *C. difficile* toxin, forming a non-absorbable complex with bile acids in the intestinal lumen. Cholestyramine will also bind to vancomycin. Therefore, both medications should not be used in combination. This drug is less efficacious than metronidazole

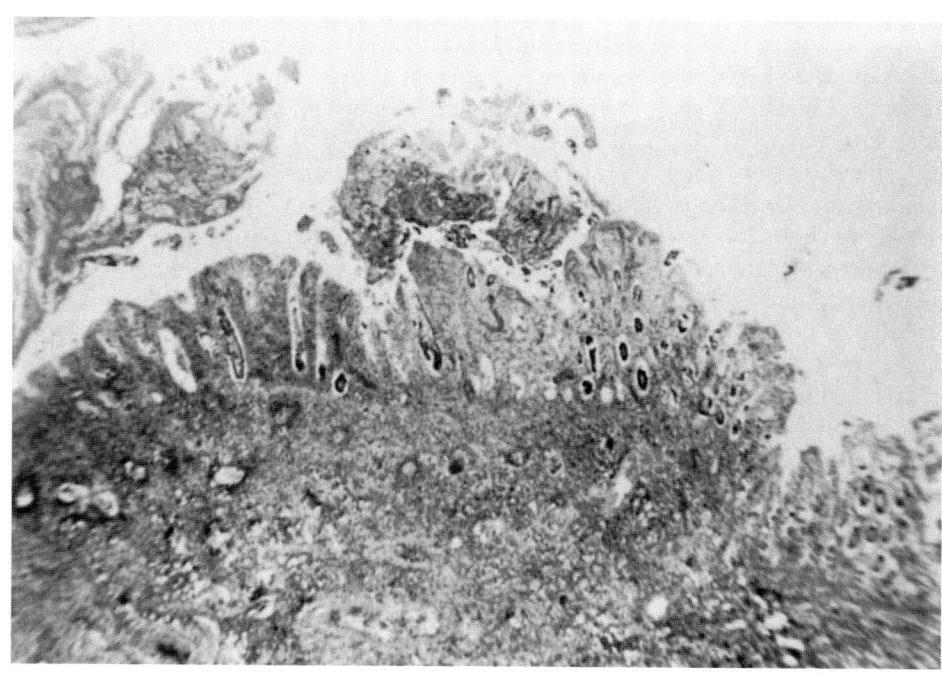

FIGURE 33-10. Pseudomembranous colitis. Total necrosis of the mucosa with inflammatory exudate in the submucosa. (Original magnification ×80.)

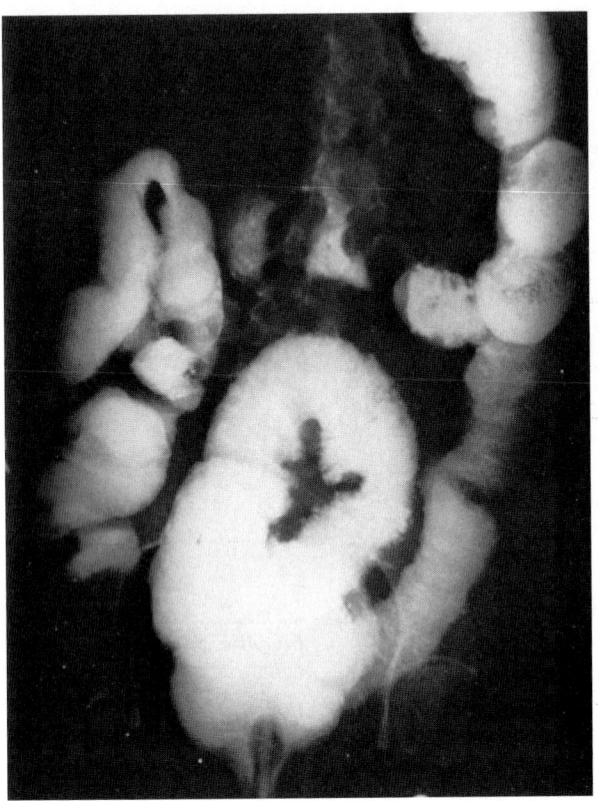

FIGURE 33-11. Pseudomembranous colitis. Barium enema demonstrates extensive ulceration. Note the collar-button appearance of the ulcers extending into the bowel wall.

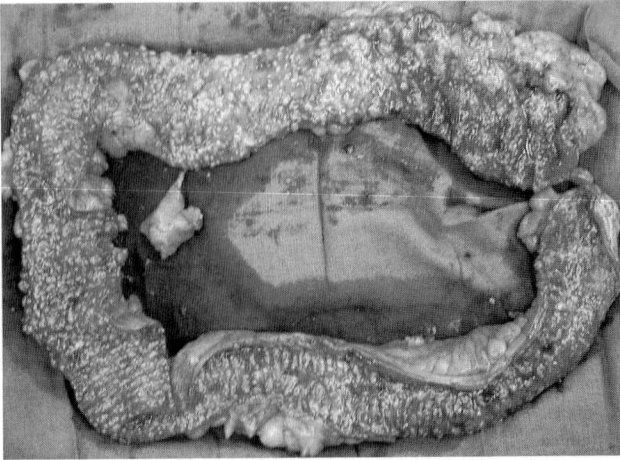

FIGURE 33-12. Pseudomembranous colitis. Opened total colectomy specimen demonstrates the classic mucosal findings of this disease. (Courtesy of T. Cristina Sardinha, M.D.)

or vancomycin, but it may have a role in patients with relapsing disease. The suggested dose is 4g orally, three times daily for 10 to 14 days.[72,105] Since *C. difficile* is a transferable enteric pathogen, stool precautions for the duration of the illness are advised.[10]

Medications that slow peristalsis should be avoided, since elimination of the toxin is inhibited.[77] In fact, some have suggested that reduced colonic motility as seen with colonic obstruction, sepsis, uremia, generalized debilitating conditions, burns, and other illnesses, may contribute to the development of pseudomembranous colitis.[51]

The most frequent indication for operative intervention is perforation, although pseudomembranous colitis may be a terminal complication in patients with a malignancy. Figures 33-12 and 33-13 demonstrate the appearance of the mucosa in such individuals. Acute abdominal signs and symptoms may, in fact, be the initial presenting manifestations.[271] Total colectomy with ileostomy, preserving the rectum, is the preferred treatment for a perforation or for fulminant disease.[163,173,184,185,273] It must be remembered that at laparotomy the external colonic appearance may be deceptively normal. This finding should not influence the surgical procedure–that is, total colectomy.[163] With sepsis or a dilated bowel, and in the ab-

sence of necrosis or perforation, an ileostomy, alone, may be adequate surgical management. However, there are no meaningful statistics concerning the relative merits of this option.

Lipsett and colleagues reported an overall mortality rate in their series of 38%, with a 100% mortality in those who underwent partial colectomy and a 14% mortality for those who underwent subtotal colectomy.[163] Others report a high mortality rate for this disease, especially if a less than subtotal colectomy is performed.[173,184,273]

Recurrence

One of the concerns with this disease is the possibility of relapse following therapy, a frequency which has been reported to be from 10% to 30%.[105] This often occurs within 1 to 3 weeks following completed therapy and is likely due to the original *C. difficile* strain. However a new strain may be found, especially if the patient remains in the same high-risk environment. The number of relapses increases exponentially after the second episode to greater than 65%.[105] Walters and colleagues reported relapse of antibiotic-associated colitis while the patient was maintained on vancomycin therapy.[282] Eight of 15 individuals so treated demonstrated a clinical relapse after therapy was discontinued. These results suggest that stool evaluation should be performed during and after treatment to indicate whether the antibiotic therapy should be maintained or re-instituted, or that alternative therapeutic approaches be considered.

Recurrence due to antibiotic resistance has yet to be proven, but it seems that persistent *C. difficile* spores in the colon may lead ultimately to clinical disease. It has also been proposed that the absence of Bacteroides species

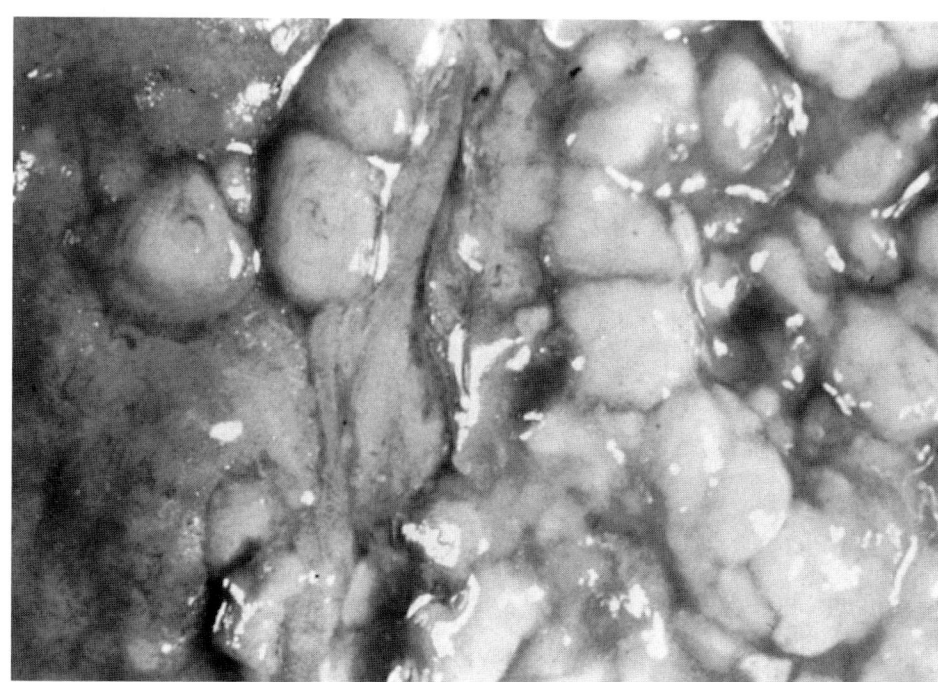

FIGURE 33-13. Pseudomembranous colitis. Whitish plaques of pseudomembrane cannot be wiped off. The patient expired of acute leukemia.

predisposes to recrudescence. Attempts have been made to identify risk factors for recurrence, including those with prior *C. difficile* infection, chronic renal failure, prolonged antibiotic therapy, patients with community-acquired *C. difficile*, significant leukocytosis, and particular strains of *C. difficile*.[76,188]

Management in this situation is quite challenging, with no uniform treatment having been accepted. The first relapse after successful treatment of *C. difficile* colitis may be treated with a repeat course of metronidazole or vancomycin for a total of 10 to 14 days.[188] This regimen is effective in 95% of cases. However, a small number of patients will go on to develop multiple episodes of recurrence. For this population a 4 to 6 week tapering course of metronidazole or vancomycin has been effective. The combination of vancomycin and rifampin (600 mg, orally, twice daily) may have some efficacy for those with recurrence. *Saccharomyces boulardii*, in combination with standard antibiotic therapy, is also an option for refractory disease, but this is not available in the United States.[105,125] *Saccharomyces cerevisiae* (brewer's yeast) is more widely available and has been successfully used in patients with refractory *C. difficile* colitis.[125] Successful treatments with rectal installation of homologous feces as well as a mixture of ten different facultative aerobic and anaerobic bacteria have been reported—so-called biotherapy.[274]

Campylobacter Enteritis

Campylobacter jejuni and *Campylobacter coli* are leading causes of infectious enterocolitis worldwide. In fact, *Campylobacter* has become one of the major causes of infectious diarrhea in the United States. Post-infectious sequelae, such as arthritis, Reiter's syndrome, and Guillain-Barré syndrome are potential consequences of this disease.[16] The organism is a curved or "gull-wing" microaerophilic, gram-positive rod. Transmission occurs by way of the fecal-oral route through contaminated fruit and water or by direct contact with infected animals or persons.[23] Epidemiologic studies have demonstrated an association with the handling and consumption of poultry and beef. The risk of contamination is higher with raw meats, especially at barbecues. This is believed to be due to the ready transfer of the bacteria to other foods and then to the mouth.[36] This bacterium is also found in shellfish and dairy products and has also been diagnosed in hospitalized patients. *Campylobacter* is vulnerable to temperature extremes as well as to oxygen in atmospheric concentrations. In contrast to that of *Salmonella*, *Campylobacter* does not survive pelleted meals, egg powder, and spices.

Symptoms and findings may be difficult to differentiate from those of other diseases affecting the intestinal tract, particularly nonspecific inflammatory bowel disease.[211] In fact, *Campylobacter* enteritis must be considered in the differential diagnosis of any patient who presents with rectal bleeding and diarrhea. Abdominal pain, fever, nausea, and vomiting may also be associated complaints. Toxic megacolon, necessitating total colectomy, has been reported.[7]

Proctosigmoidoscopic examination usually reveals an edematous, inflamed mucosa. Histologic examination of biopsy specimens is nonspecific. A double-contrast barium enema may demonstrate aphthoid ulcers and a stippled appearance.[270]

A high index of suspicion must be maintained if one is to establish the diagnosis and to initiate therapy promptly. Examination of the fecal specimen within 2 hours of passage by dark-field or phase-contrast microscopy may identify the organism.[23] The presence of polymorphonuclear leukocytes in the fecal stream is not uncommon but is not pathognomonic for the condition.

The infection is usually self-limited, but relapses are frequent. In severe cases, hospitalization and fluid and electrolyte replacement may be necessary. Ciprofloxacin (250 to 500 mg orally, four times a day for 7 days) is the recommended treatment, although erythromycin, tetracycline, doxycycline, gentamicin, and clindamycin may also be used. Appropriate stool precautions (particularly for hospitalized patients) are indicated, with proper disposal of contaminated linens and washing of hands. With respect to prevention, avoiding raw meats, particularly poultry, is recommended.

Currently, research is focusing on the identification and eradication of bacterial reservoirs. Additionally, molecular studies, leading to a better understanding of *Campylobacter*-associated diseases, are being conducted in order to improve prevention techniques and to offer alternative therapeutic approaches.[162]

Yersinia Enterocolitis

Yersinia enterocolitica is a relatively recently recognized cause of enteric infection. *Yersinia* enterocolitis is of particular interest to the surgeon because of its prevalence and its occasional confusion with regional enteritis. A former name for the causative organism was *Pasteurella pseudotuberculosis*, again implying confusion with another bacterial infection that tends to involve the ileocecal region. Epidemics due to contamination of food, water, and milk have been reported.[22] *Yersinia* most commonly affects infants, young children, and young adults.

The disease is caused by a facultative anaerobic gram-negative coccoid bacillus resembling nonlactose-fermenting *Escherichia coli*.[58,277] It grows optimally in cold temperatures. The diagnosis is established by isolation of the bacteria from the stool. However, *Yersinia* culture is not standard in most clinical laboratories and must be specifically requested.[277] Biotyping and serotyping according to O antigens have been the most helpful of the epidemiologic techniques.[58]

The organism usually produces signs and symptoms of an acute gastroenteritis as a consequence of invasion of epithelial cells and the penetration of the intestinal mucosa. Bloody diarrhea is frequently observed in addition to abdominal pain.[235] Joint pain may also be a manifestation of this disease. Drainage of the bacteria into regional lymph nodes accounts for the systemic complications. A syndrome simulating appendicitis is seen in 40% of patients—fever, leukocytosis, right lower-quadrant abdominal tenderness, and pain.[58,235] However, a small number of patients with *Yersinia* will actually develop true appendicitis as a manifestation of the disease.[247] The condition may produce generalized septicemia and "metastatic" abscesses in other organs. It can also present as a colonic abscess or as toxic megacolon.[238,260] Sometimes the disease may pursue a chronic course for many weeks, particularly if not treated with appropriate antibiotics. Post-infection manifestations include erythema nodosum and reactive arthritis.[58] Predisposing factors to the development of the infection follow:

- cirrhosis
- hemochromatosis
- acute iron poisoning
- transfusion-dependent blood dyscrasias
- immunosuppression
- diabetes mellitus
- malnutrition[58]

Results of radiologic examination were evaluated in a review by Vantrappen and colleagues.[277] A coarse, irregular, nodular mucosal pattern was seen in the terminal ileum; ulcerations were also noted. In contrast to Crohn's disease, infection of the terminal ileum is usually confined to the mucosa and submucosa, and the characteristic "string sign" is absent. Endoscopic examination demonstrates signs of inflammatory disease in approximately one half of the patients.

Recommended treatment includes anti-pseudomonal aminoglycosides, trimethoprim/sulfamethoxazole, ceftizoxime, or ceftriaxone, but antimicrobial therapy has not been proven essential or necessarily efficacious in the uncomplicated situation.[58] However, when systemic illness supervenes or when the patient is immunocompromised, doxycycline or trimethoprim/sulfamethoxazole is advisable. *Yersinia* is generally resistant to penicillin.

Prevention of yersiniosis includes adequate treatment and handling of raw poultry, beef, and pork as potential sources of infection. Consumption of raw milk should be avoided and hand washing after using the toilet or diaper changes as well as after handling pets and animals is mandatory.[191]

Salmonellosis and Typhoid Fever

The food-borne bacillus, *Salmonella typhi*, is the causative agent of typhoid fever. This infectious enterocolitis affects approximately 16 million people worldwide each year. However, due to a lack of culturing facilities and poor performance of the Widal test, salmonellosis is often under-diagnosed and frequently unconfirmed. Surveillance for febrile illnesses in developing countries may assist in the identification and treatment of food-borne infections, such as salmonellosis. This method has been utilized in Egypt and has succeeded in identifying 13/100,000 persons per year with typhoid fever.[60] An increased incidence has been noted in places with higher temperatures. This issue raises the possibility of a greater health problem with continued global warming.[60] In 1999, the Centers for Disease Control and Prevention reported a nationwide outbreak of *Salmonella enterica* related to consumption of contaminated mangoes due to hot water treatment as the possible point of contamination.[251]

The recently completed *Salmonella enterica* serovar typhi genome sequence has led researchers to new avenues of investigation into the biology of this pathogen. *Salmonella typhi* produces extensive epithelial invasion along the small bowel and colon without destruction of the intestinal mucosa.[27] The bacteria breach the mucosa and submucosa in areas of an inflammatory reaction, and an endotoxin is produced upon autolysis of the bacterial cell. Since the condition is endemic in many underdeveloped countries, the diagnosis is usually suspected when symptoms occur in such areas. However, in Western countries it is rarely considered. Humans are the only known reservoir, with transmission effected by the fecal-oral route, usually through contamination of drinking water. Stool culture may reveal the organism or, in the case of typhoid sepsis, blood culture may identify *Salmonella*. *Salmonella* bacteremia, involving many serotypes including *typhi*, has been recognized as an emerging concern in AIDS (see Chapter 20).[83]

If the organism enters the bloodstream, severe septicemia may result. Characteristics of this illness include fever, headache, delirium, splenic enlargement, abdominal pain, maculopapular rash, and leukopenia.[182] Generalized hyperplasia of the entire reticuloendothelial system occurs, particularly in the Peyer's patches of the ileum and solitary lymph follicles of the cecum.[182]

Of interest to the surgeon is the fact that acute cholecystitis may occur, which may progress to gangrene and perforation. Toxic megacolon and intestinal perforation can also complicate the disease, and on rare occasion, massive lower gastrointestinal hemorrhage can develop.[95,100,182,219,291] The process is usually limited to the terminal 70 cm of ileum and proximal colon.

Abdominal examination may reveal mild tenderness or signs suggestive of generalized peritonitis if a perforation has ensued. Obviously a laparotomy is required if perforation supervenes. The choice of operation, however, is open to some debate. Meier and colleagues reported their operative experience from Nigeria with 108 consecutive patients who developed perforated typhoid enteritis.[174] Multiple perforations were found in 19%. De-

bridement of the perforations with closure was effected in 93% of these individuals, with an operative mortality of 32%. In an experience from Ghana involving 195 patients, the overall mortality rate of 31% was worsened by extremes of age, generalized peritonitis, lower white blood cell count, increased numbers of perforations, and the presence of a postoperative enterocutaneous fistula.[179] However, the mortality rate was reduced to 8% if patients received a combination antibiotic regimen that included chloramphenicol, gentamicin, and metronidazole. If the surgeon has the benefit of Western surgical facilities, resection and/or diversion usually offers better results.

Medical management includes the use of parenteral or enteral nutrition and antibiotics (amoxicillin [1 g orally, three times a day for 3 to 14 days], ciprofloxacin, chloramphenicol, or trimethoprim/sulfamethoxazole). However, resistance to chloramphenicol, ampicillin, and trimethoprim/sulfamethoxazole has been a major problem in Asia and some countries in Africa. Fluoroquinolones, third-generation cephalosporins, and azithromycin are effective antibiotics for the management of salmonellosis.[200] Vaccines have also been developed, but they are not currently used in endemic areas due to public health restrictions.

Tuberculosis

Tuberculosis involving the intestinal tract may be due to either *Mycobacterium tuberculosis* or *Mycobacterium bovis*. In the former situation, the disease is primary to the lungs and is carried to the intestinal tract by swallowing of sputum. The latter organism produces the infection in association with swallowing non-pasteurized milk. This condition is extremely unusual in most Western countries since pasteurization of milk is standardized. However, it has more recently increased in countries such as the United Kingdom and the United States, a fact which has been attributable to the large number of Asian immigrants.[1,129] In fact, Guth and Kim suggest that there are two distinctly identifiable patient populations with this disease—the aforementioned immigrants and individuals infected with HIV.[108] Compared with immunocompetent patients, the proportion of extrapulmonary tuberculosis is much higher in patients with AIDS, hence the increased frequency of published reports of intestinal tuberculosis in these individuals.[112] The fact is that fewer than 200 cases of abdominal tuberculosis were reported in the United States from 1950 to 1980, but the incidence, especially in urban areas, has been increasing steadily for the past 20 years.[120] Peritoneal tuberculosis is presently the sixth most common site of extrapulmonary tuberculosis in the United States, followed by lymphatic, genitourinary, bone and joint, miliary, and meningeal involvement.[164]

When the disease does affect the intestinal tract it is usually caused by the pulmonary strain and most commonly is localized to the ileocecal region (for discussion of anorectal tuberculosis, see Chapter 19). The reasons for this distribution are believed to be the presence of abundant lymphoid tissue in the area, an increased physiologic stasis, and an increased rate of absorption in the proximal bowel.[130] Although the condition is most commonly seen in the proximal colon and ileum, segmental bowel involvement has occasionally been observed.[33]

Symptoms and Findings

The most common presenting complaints are abdominal pain, weight loss, and fever. Pain is usually confined to the hypogastrium and frequently localized to the right lower quadrant. Other symptoms include anorexia, fever, and weight loss. Bowel obstruction may also be a presentation of intestinal tuberculosis.[32] Tuberculous peritonitis, however, usually presents as an acute abdomen that mimics appendicitis and is seen mainly in young children or adolescents.[2] Ascites, with abdominal pain and disten-

tion, may be the first indication of this complication. In the experience of Lisehora and colleagues from the Tripler Army Medical Center in Honolulu, Hawaii, most individuals presented with a chronic wasting illness, mild abdominal pain, and fever.[164]

Physical examination may reveal the presence of a mass, usually in the right lower quadrant. In the rare situation when tuberculosis involves the rectum or anus, a stricture may be apparent. Depending on whether the lesion produces ulceration or stricture, it can simulate carcinoma. In fact, in the absence of a pulmonary lesion, it is not unlikely that the surgeon would perform a cancer operation for this disease.[136]

Evaluation

The diagnosis requires a high index of suspicion. Obviously, when a pulmonary lesion is present, intestinal tuberculosis should be considered. However, in a report from Britain the chest x-ray was abnormal in a minority of patients.[197] Acid-fast bacilli will rarely be identified in the stool (Figure 33-14). Although a positive tuberculin test result may be useful, it does not establish the diagnosis with certainty.

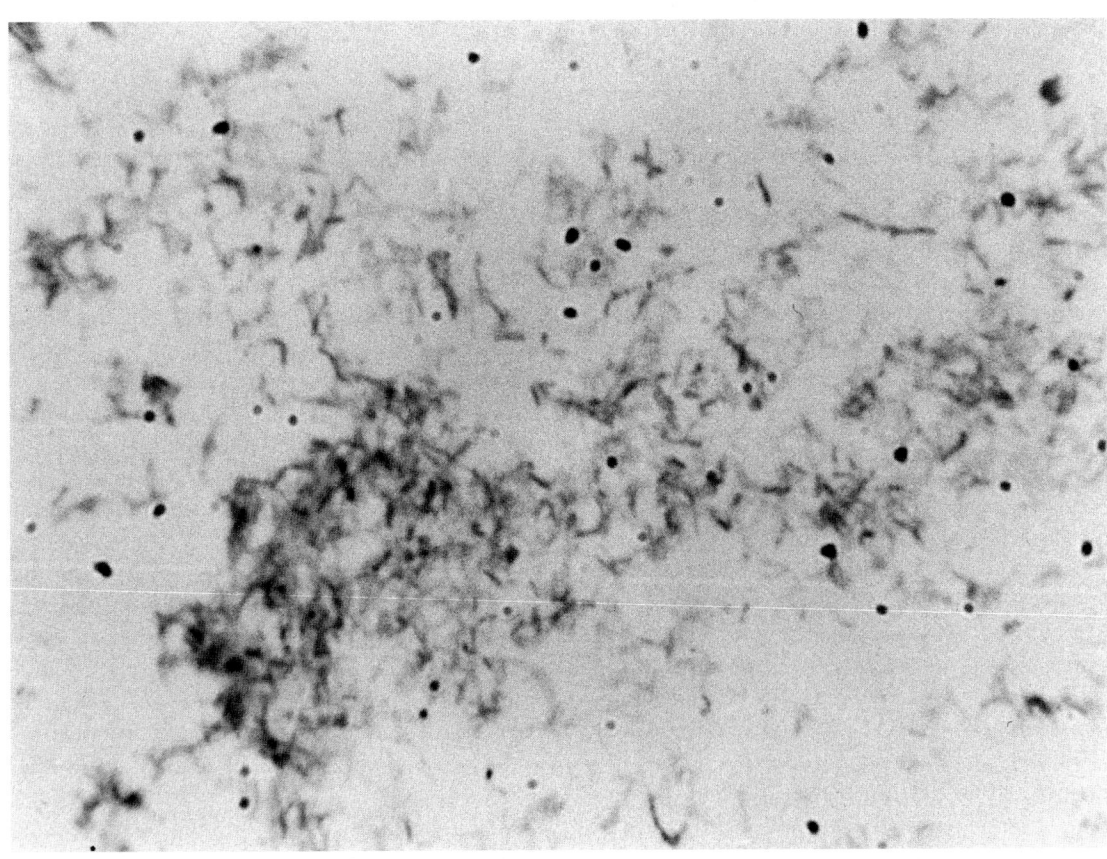

FIGURE 33-14. Pleiomorphic red-staining bacilli that are acid-fast because they retain carbol fuchsin and resist decolorization with acid alcohol. (Original magnification ×1,060). (See Color Fig. 33-14.)

Radiologic investigation is helpful but not necessarily diagnostic of the condition. A plain abdominal x-ray film in a patient with intestinal obstruction secondary to a stricture or mass may reveal the absence of gas shadows in the right iliac fossa or distortion of the cecum and ascending colon by a mass.[45] Free perforation with pneumoperitoneum is extremely rare. Barium enema study may reveal retrograde obstruction, stricture, or a "conical cecum." The terminal ileum may be normal, dilated, ulcerated, or strictured. Han and colleagues reviewed double-contrast barium enema examinations in 25 patients in an attempt to identify characteristic findings of tuberculous colitis.[112] They found that involvement was asymmetric in 12, with skip lesions noted in 13. They concluded that ulcers aligned in a transverse or circumferential pattern, involvement at the right colon, and deformity of the ileocecal valve suggest a diagnosis of tuberculous colitis.[112]

A nonspecific ultrasonic finding, the "pseudokidney sign," has also been identified in association with ileal tuberculosis.[24] This is a pattern that consists of a strong echogenic center surrounded by a sonolucent rim, the common factor being bowel wall thickening. Computed tomographic (CT) evaluation may provide more insight into the disease process by identification of subclinical ascites, adenopathy, abscess, and thickening of the bowel wall.[108,164] Yilmaz and -coworkers also identified nonspecific CT changes in abdominal tuberculosis, such as ascites, intra- and extraperitoneal lymphadenopathy, ileocecal wall thickening, and thickening and calcifications on peritoneal surfaces.[294] However, these findings can only be relevant if abdominal tuberculosis is suspected, a consideration that usually involves high-risk populations.

The distinction between tuberculosis and Crohn's disease may not be possible radiologically or endoscopically, although colonoscopy with biopsy has been suggested as a useful tool.[33,85,118,149] Kochtrar and colleagues were able to use colonoscopic fine needle aspiration cytology in two patients in order to identify acid-fast bacilli and establish the diagnosis of ileocecal tuberculosis.[145] Most recently, Gan and associates suggested the use of polymerase chain reaction (PCR) in the differential diagnosis of Crohn's disease and intestinal tuberculosis.[89] PCR was performed on endoscopic biopsy samples of patients with intestinal tuberculosis and on those with Crohn's disease. Positivity rates of 64.1% and 0%, respectively, were reported.

Laparoscopy has been found to be useful procedure for the diagnosis of tuberculous peritonitis. Bhargava and colleagues reported the laparoscopic findings in 38 cases of peritoneal tuberculosis.[20] They classified the laparoscopic appearances according to three types: thickened peritoneum with miliary, yellowish white tubercles, with or without adhesions (n = 25), thickened peritoneum only, with or without adhesions (n = 8), and a fibroadhesive pattern (n = 5); visual diagnosis was accurate in 95% of patients. The authors concluded that while

target biopsy is an effective method of obtaining an early diagnosis of peritoneal tuberculosis, they believe that chemotherapy may be initiated on the basis of the visual laparoscopic appearance alone.[20]

Histopathology

Generally, the macroscopic appearance of the cecum is indistinguishable from that of Crohn's disease, but the diagnosis may be established by histologic examination.[197] According to Radhakrishnan and colleagues, the yield of biopsy-proved granulomas in tuberculous lesions was 100%, although acid-fast bacilli could not be recovered.[214]

Examination of the resected specimen may reveal thickening of the bowel wall, mucosal ulceration, localized segmental disease, or skip lesions. The mucosal appearance may demonstrate characteristic transverse ulcers (Figure 33-15). The classical histologic criteria include the presence of submucosal or serosal Langhans giant cells and the presence of caseous necrosis (Figure 33-16). The organism may be demonstrated in the specimen or may be grown by guinea pig culture.

Treatment

Conventional antituberculous agents are recommended in the uncomplicated case. Approximately one half of the patients with colonic or ileocolonic tuberculosis may be adequately treated with medical therapy alone.[62] Possible regimens include a combination of isoniazid with ethambutol or rifampin. Others prefer pyrazinamide to ethambutol because of the lower incidence of side effects.[197] During treatment the patient must be carefully monitored since all of the drugs can produce hepatic dysfunction, although this is relatively uncommon.[241] Patients with ulcerating lesions are more likely to respond to medical management than are those with the hypertrophic form of the disease. Anand and colleagues undertook a prospective clinical trial of 39 patients with bowel obstruction and evidence of intestinal stricture secondary to tuberculosis.[6] All were treated with conventional antituberculous drugs (streptomycin, rifampin, and isoniazid); only three were unresponsive and underwent surgery. Complete resolution of the radiologic abnormality was noted in 70%.[6]

As has been implied, abdominal tuberculosis can be cured medically if recognized early, but the nonspecific presentation that is often observed tends to delay the diagnosis in many instances.[143]

Surgical treatment should be limited to those patients with symptomatic localized disease (Figure 33-17).[120] Obviously, if the distinction cannot be made between tuberculosis and carcinoma by endoscopic means, a resection

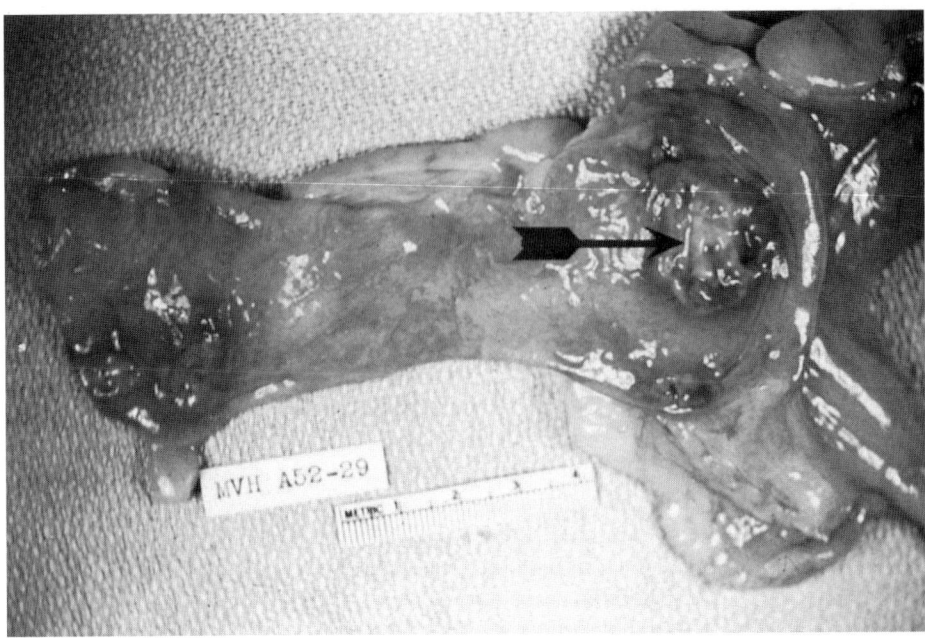

FIGURE 33-15. Cecal tuberculosis. Note the transverse ulcer (*arrow*). (Courtesy of Rudolf Garret, M.D.)

is indicated. Tubercular involvement of the rectum, although uncommon, is an important cause of rectal strictures in India.[210] Even in this area, response to antitubercular chemotherapy is quite good, and surgery is seldom required for these individuals.

Gonococcal Proctitis

Gonorrhea is a common sexually transmitted acute infectious disease of the mucous membranes affecting the urethra, vagina, and cervix. Rectal gonorrhea, however, has been relatively recently recognized. Most physicians, in fact, did not appreciate the concept of rectal coitus in men prior to Kinsey's report in 1948, which discussed the widespread incidence of male homosexuality.[195]

The disease is caused by the bacterium, *Neisseria gonorrhoeae* (the gonococcus), a gram-negative coccus occurring in pairs or clumps. Characteristically, the organism appears on smears as intracellular gram-negative diplococci (Figure 33-18). In order to confirm the presence of the organism by culture, rectal swabs are inoculated on a selective chocolate agar (Thayer Martin) and sent to the

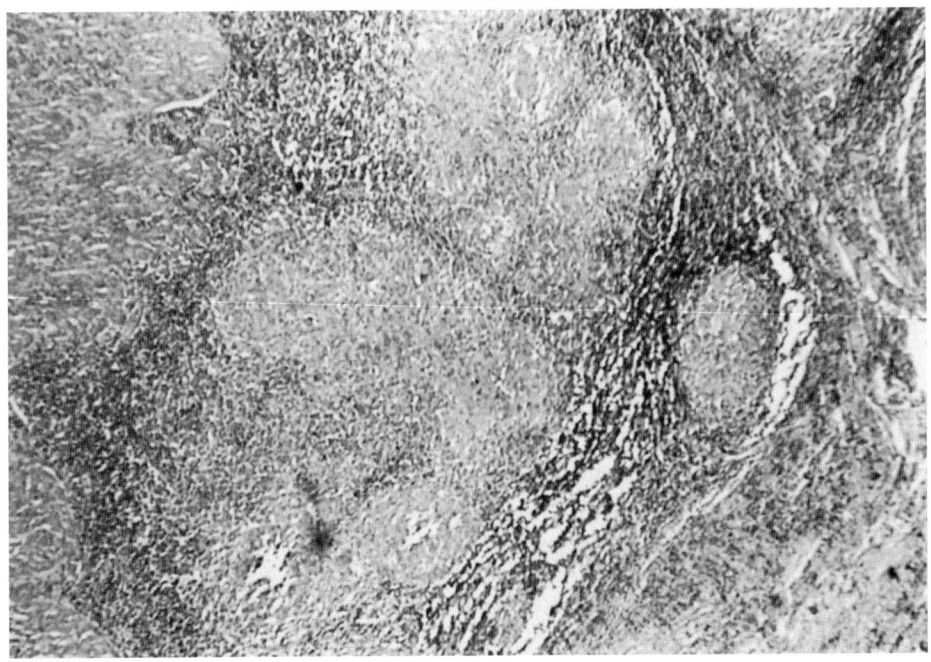

FIGURE 33-16. Tuberculous granulomas (note caseous necrosis) in a mesenteric lymph node. (Original magnification ×180; courtesy of Rudolf Garret, M.D.)

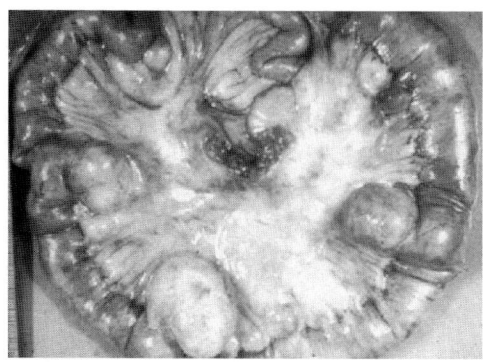

FIGURE 33-17. Tuberculosis of the small bowel. Resected specimen demonstrates typical caseating masses of the adjacent mesentery. (Courtesy of T. Cristina Sardinha, M.D.)

laboratory without delay, where they are placed in a carbon dioxide jar and incubated.

In men, the disease is most commonly associated with the homosexual population and is transmitted by anal intercourse (see Chapter 20). However, in women the disease is usually transferred to the rectum by discharge from the vagina, presumably when the rectal mucosa is everted during defecation.[42] Usually, only the lower rectum is involved.

Asymptomatic gonococcal proctitis has been proven to be a misconception. However, the incidence has been declining due to better patient education with respect to safe sex practices. Symptoms usually start 5 to 7 days after exposure and include pruritus, mucous or pus-like discharge, rectal bleeding, diarrhea, and concerns referable to either gonorrhea or syphilis in other sites. Disseminated disease may occur (septicemia), as well as pericarditis, endocarditis, meningitis, perihepatitis, and gonococcal arthritis. Characteristically, the arthritis produces an acute purulent effusion of a single joint.[42]

Proctosigmoidoscopic examination usually reveals edematous, friable mucosa with occasional areas of ulceration. Biopsy may show degeneration of the epithelium, capillary engorgement, and infiltration with inflammatory cells.[195] However, in many individuals no identifiable lesion will be noted.

Quinn and colleagues reviewed their experience with anorectal infections in 52 homosexual men.[213] They reported that the gram stain of the rectal exudate was insensitive for the diagnosis of rectal gonorrhea, with up to 50% of missed culture-positive cases. The authors further observed that due to the reportedly high prevalence of asymptomatic anorectal gonorrhea and the frequency of mixed infections, the isolation of the organism from a homosexual male with anorectal symptoms did not prove that the gonococcus was responsible for the symptoms. Lebedeff and Hochman showed, in a study of 1,262 patients who had rectal symptoms, that 554 had culture-proven rectal gonorrhea.[155] Of the individuals who had demonstrated organisms, 82% were symptomatic, one fourth had a history of contact, and 10% had a history of a prior positive culture. Of those who reported symptoms, 71% complained of mucus in the stool and 62% reported rectal discomfort.

Janda and associates studied the prevalence and pathogenicity of *Neisseria* in 815 homosexual men.[124] Interestingly, *Neisseria meningitidis* was isolated from more

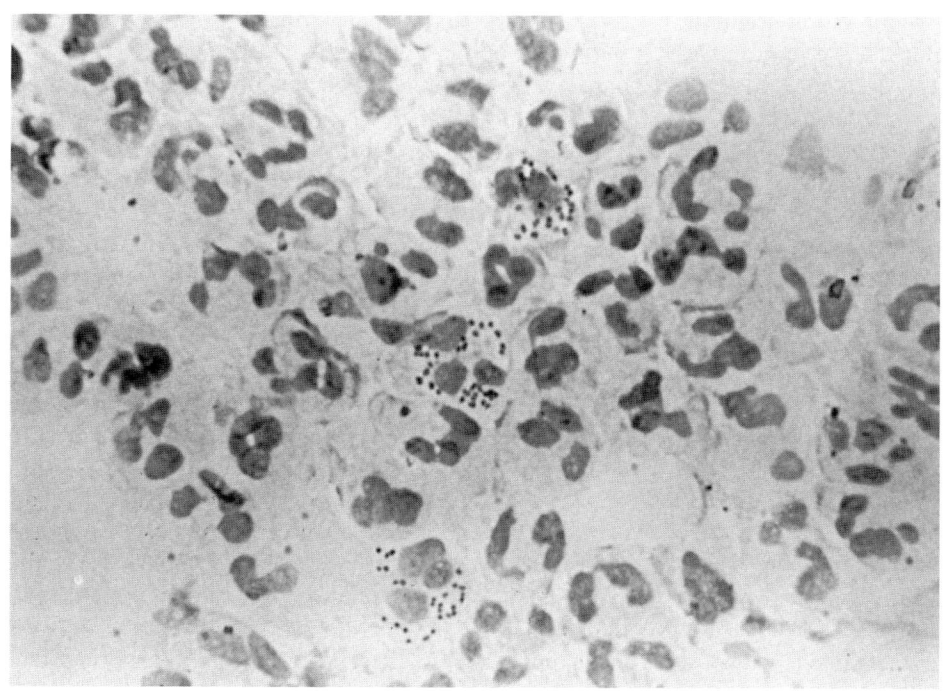

FIGURE 33-18. Gonorrhea. Smear reveals gram-negative intracellular diplococci in the cytoplasm of polymorphonuclear cells. (Original magnification ×1,000.)

patients than *N. gonorrhoeae*. When the organism occurred in the rectum, it was usually not associated with clinical illness.

Stansfield evaluated anorectal gonorrhea in women.[256] In a retrospective assessment of 159 patients who had undergone proctosigmoidoscopy, 127 (80%) had known contacts with infected patients. One half of these individuals harbored the organism. Of these, the vast majority had the organism in the rectum as well as in the urethra and cervix; only four (6.3%) had the organism confined to the rectum. Gram-stain smears demonstrated positive results in less than one half of the patients with rectal gonorrhea.

DNA assays are currently used for the diagnosis of urogenital gonococcal infection; however, this has not been extensively studied for gonococcal proctitis. Lewis and -coworkers reported 100% sensitivity for detecting gonococcal proctitis through the application of the PACE-2 DNA probe assay (Gen-Probe, San Diego, CA) in a population where the prevalence of gonococcal proctitis was 4.7%.[161]

Treatment

The therapy of *N. gonorrhoeae* proctitis consists of single-dose regimens of drugs effective against β-lactamase–producing strains. A single dose of ceftriaxone, 125 mg, intramuscularly, cures 99.1% of uncomplicated anorectal and urogenital gonorrhoeae.[244] Other effective therapeutic options include single oral-dose fluoroquinolones, such as ciprofloxacin (500 mg), or ofloxacin (400 mg). This has been shown to result in cure rates of 99.8% and 98.4%, respectively.[183] Many other drugs have been successfully used to treat *N. gonorrhoeae* infections, such as ceftizoxime, 500 mg intramuscularly; cefotaxime, 500 mg intramuscularly; cefotetan, 1 g intramuscularly; cefoxitin, 2 g intramuscularly; and probenecid, 1 g orally. However, none offer any benefit over ceftriaxone. In addition, ceftriaxone is also effective in the treatment of incubating syphilis, in contrast to the fluoroquinolones.[42,83,195,223] The importance of close follow-up examination with culture, in order to assess the adequacy of the therapy cannot be overestimated.

Syphilis of the Rectum or Syphilitic Proctitis

Syphilis of the anal canal and perianal skin is a well-recognized clinical entity (see Chapter 19), but the manifestation of syphilitic proctitis is less familiar to most physicians. The condition occurs almost exclusively in the gay male population.

Symptoms include mucus discharge, bleeding, tenesmus, and change in bowel habits. During the first stage of the disease, a single painless ulcer with raised borders is often found at the site of sexual contact. This is known as

a sore or chancre. In addition, enlarged, firm, and rubbery inguinal lymph nodes can also be palpable. In the second phase, syphilitic anal and rectal wart-like growths are seen. The late or third stage of the disease manifests with cardiovascular and neurologic involvement.[253]

Anorectal lesions have been divided into four categories[3]:

- anal ulceration
- rectal ulceration
- granulomatous (hyperplastic)
- miscellaneous (fixed, tumor-like)

Endoscopic examination may reveal a mass or an ulcerating lesion that is suggestive of carcinoma.[11] However, biopsies fail to reveal tumor.

While the diagnosis can be confirmed by means of dark-field examination of the exudate (see Figure 19-40), disclosing the presence of the treponemal organisms, this does require a high index of suspicion.[3] Treatment is that which has been described in Chapter 19.

Shigellosis

Shigellosis, also known as bacillary dysentery, is an infectious enterocolitis caused by one of four species of the genus, *Shigella*. These include *Shigella dysenteriae*, *Shigella flexneri*, *Shigella boydii*, and *Shigella sonnei*. This non–spore-forming, gram-negative rod is divided into 40 serotypes (Figure 33-19). According to the World Health Organization, shigellosis is a worldwide endemic disease that affects 163.2 million people in developing countries and 1.5 million in industrialized countries. Estimated yearly mortality is 1.1 million.[92,289] Transmission is via the fecal-oral route from patients or carriers even if a very small number of organisms are ingested. Contaminated water and milk are also major sources of infectious transmission.

Shigellosis is a communicable disease during the acute infectious phase, and while the infectious agent is in the stool, this may last up to 4 weeks. *S. sonnei* is the most common subtype causing colitis, while *S. boydii*, *S. dysenteriae*, and *S. flexneri* occur more frequently in developing countries, but travelers can obviously import the organism.

Shigellosis may present acutely with fever, diarrhea, nausea, vomiting, abdominal cramps, and severe dehydration. The patient may actually seek emergency care with severe toxemia.[115] Nonetheless, asymptomatic infections can occur. Most commonly patients present with diarrhea that contains blood, mucous, and pus. This illness is frequently self-limited, averaging 4 to 7 days. While the symptoms are usually related to the mucosal manifestation, intestinal obstruction and toxic megacolon have been reported.[15] In the experience of Bennish and col-

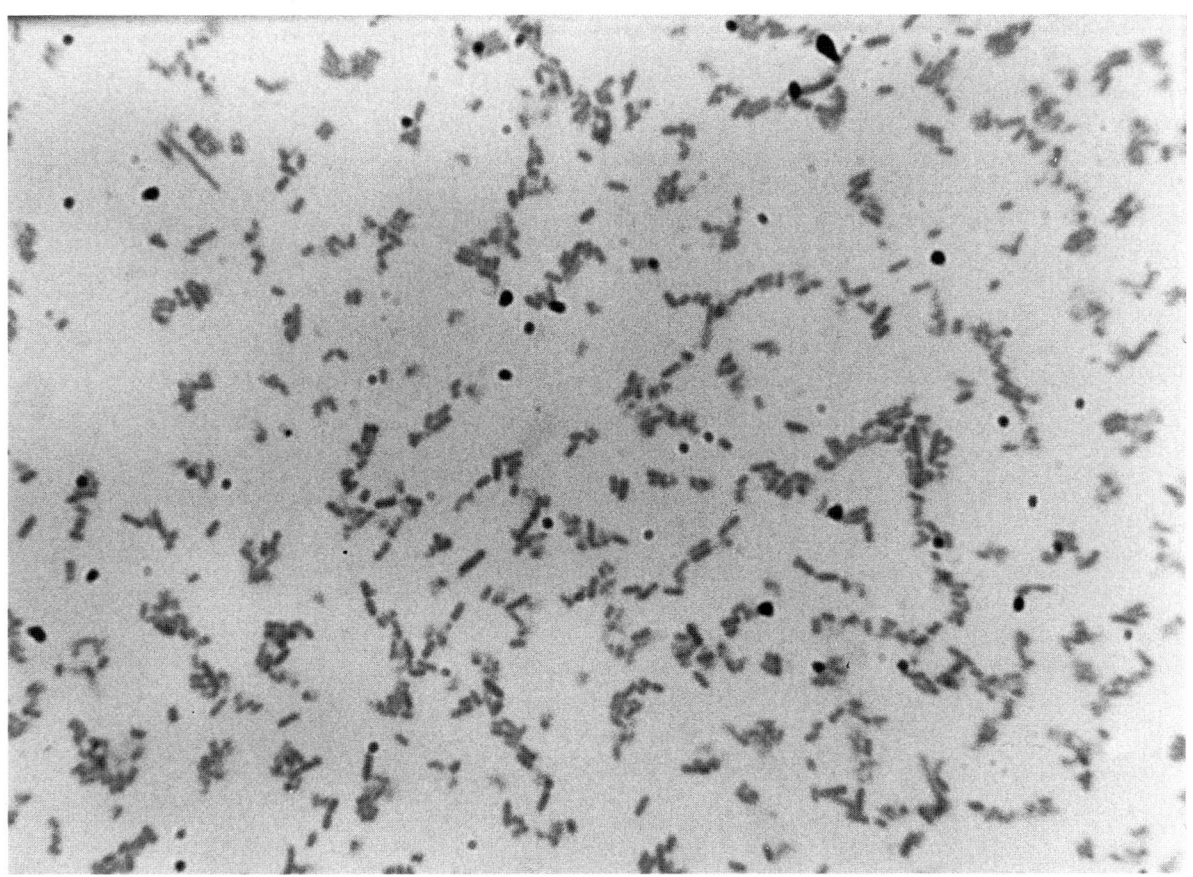

FIGURE 33-19. Shigella. Gram-negative bacillae, which, on biochemical and serological testing, reveal *Shigella*. (See Color Fig. 33-19.) (Original magnification ×1,060.)

leagues, 9% of those treated in Bangladesh developed obstruction, one third of whom died.[15]

The severity of the disease depends on the *Shigella* serotype as well as the patient's age and nutritional status. Infection caused by *S. dysenteriae* is often severe and associated with a high fatality rate, as opposed to *S. sonnei* that usually presents with a short clinical course and has a low fatality rate. Two thirds of cases and most deaths are in children under 10 years of age.

Shigellosis is another disease that is virtually epidemic in the male homosexual population and in those individuals with AIDS (see Chapter 20). Bovee and colleagues demonstrated that *S. sonnei* is the usual infective agent in homosexual patients.[28] In the experience of Heller with this population, the clinical presentation may be one of subacute or chronic abdominal distress without fever and/or diarrhea.[115] Alternatively, the organism may persist in the stool of untreated patients for prolonged periods in a "carrier state."[115] Obviously, this presents an epidemiologic problem. The author states that, unlike the heterosexual population in which the need for antibiotic therapy may not be indicated, all homosexual men with *Shigella* cultures should be treated.

The hallmark of the inflammatory reaction is invasion and destruction of the intestinal mucosa.[27] Watery diarrhea is succeeded by severe abdominal pain, tenesmus, and rectal bleeding. The small-bowel phase of the symptoms may be determined by an enterotoxin, whereas the invasive phase is typical of the large bowel.[27]

Sigmoidoscopic examination may reveal the typical changes of a proctitis, with edema, friability, and ulceration. The appearance may be indistinguishable from that of nonspecific inflammatory bowel disease. The most satisfactory means for establishing the diagnosis is culture obtained by swabbing any ulcerating lesion during endoscopy; alternatively, mucus or fecal material may be used for culture.[62] Because the organism is somewhat labile, the plates should be inoculated as soon as possible.

Treatment

As suggested, because of the usually self-limited nature of the condition, supportive measures may be the only treatment required, although some believe that all patients should undergo antibiotic therapy irrespective of the severity of symptoms.

The treatment of choice is ciprofloxacin, 500 mg orally, twice daily for 3 to 5 days. A 5-day course of ciprofloxacin was highly effective in the treatment of the *S. dysenteriae* serotype 1 outbreak in West Africa in 1999. This therapy reduced the case fatality rate from 3.1% to 0.9% in high-risk patients.[106] Ceftriaxone, ampicillin, or trimethoprim-sulfamethoxazole can also be used to treat the disease.

As with other infectious colitides, it is important to reevaluate the stool to be certain that the bacterium has been eliminated. Moreover, epidemic measures should also be employed to investigate food, water, and milk supplies. Specific attention must be given to hand washing after toilet using.

Brucellosis

Brucellosis is a zoonosis, that is, a disease transmitted from animals to humans. There are six main species of *Brucella*, named after the animal source or feature of the infection. Four of the species cause infection in humans; these are *Brucella suis* (from pigs, highly infective), *Brucella melitensis* (from sheep with the highest pathogenicity), *Brucella abortus* (from cattle), and *Brucella canis* (from dogs). *Brucella* is an aerobic gram-negative coccobacilli. The disease is caused by the ingestion of unpasteurized milk, direct contact with an infected animal, or inhalation of aerosols. However, the most common routes of contamination in the United States are via needlestick, conjunctival exposure through eye splash, and inhalation.[167,257] While relatively common in developing countries, it is rarely seen in the West. However, the potential for long-lasting infection and the easy transmission through aerosols and inhalation makes *Brucella* species an appealing choice for a terrorist. *Brucella* spreads through the lymphatic system and can affect any organ in the body.

Rarely, brucellosis can also cause a severe colitis.[126,257] The symptoms and endoscopic findings are essentially the same as that for other inflammatory bowel conditions. Antibody testing is the most reliable method of diagnosing brucellosis.[281] Doxycycline is the preferred treatment for a simple infection. However, more severe involvement requires combination therapy, including doxycycline and streptomycin, rifampin, or gentamycin.[167]

Actinomycosis

Actinomycosis is a suppurative, granulomatous disease that tends to form draining sinus tracts, discharging granules (see Figure 19-29 and Chapter 19 for discussion of perirectal actinomycosis). The organism, *Actinomyces israelii*, an anaerobic, gram-positive bacterium, is a normal inhabitant of the mouth, lungs, and intestinal tract.[269]

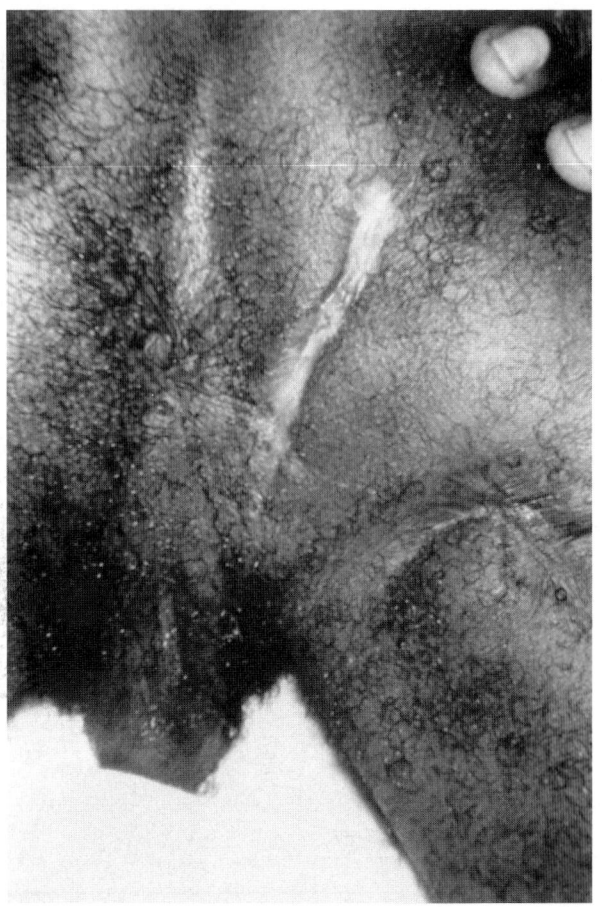

FIGURE 33-20. Actinomycotic fistula. (Courtesy of Daniel Rosenthal, M.D.)

When the disease involves the colon or rectum, it usually presents with an abdominal mass, a fistula, or a sinus (Figure 33-20). While ileocecal involvement is the most common intestinal manifestation, rectal stricture has also been reported.[217] Differentiating actinomycosis from a neoplasm may be quite difficult.

Weese and Smith reviewed their experience of 57 patients who were subsequently proven to have this condition.[287] In only four cases was the disease diagnosed correctly on admission. Udagawa and associates reported two patients with primary actinomycotic infections involving the colon and rectum.[275] The diagnosis was established by histologic examination and by bacteriologic culture. In one patient, the presence of an abdominal mass was noted by the patient herself. Back pain, weight loss, and night sweats were also prominent complaints. Barium enema examination revealed segmental involvement of the descending colon by a stricture, and resection was undertaken. In the second patient, proctologic examination revealed a mass in the perianal area. This is a much more frequent finding in those who present with actinomycosis, and is more likely to lead one to suspect the diagnosis. Others have pointed out that the lesion usually masquerades as an abdominal neoplasm.[269] Hence, unless material is available for histologic study, the disease is usually not diagnosed until resection has been performed.

Cintron and colleagues confirmed that radiologic studies have not generally been useful in the preoperative assessment.[52] However, CT, in their experience, seemed to be quite helpful, demonstrating a solid mass with focal areas of attenuation, or a cystic mass with a thickened wall that enhances with infusion. They further opined that CT scanning in conjunction with fine needle aspiration may not only be diagnostic but therapeutic.[52]

The treatment of actinomycosis consists of abscess drainage and high doses of penicillin. Tetracycline, erythromycin, or clindamycin may be options, especially in patients allergic to penicillin. Antibiotics should be taken for 6 to 12 months to prevent relapse.[70] For actinomycosis confined to the colon, resection is the optimal treatment, in addition to that of antibiotic therapy.

VIRAL INFECTIONS

Viral infections that specifically attack the rectum or colon are extremely rare. However, there are three areas that merit attention in a book on colon and rectal surgery—AIDS, herpes simplex proctitis, and cytomegalovirus infection.[249,253] HIV is important to address, because so many of the complications and manifestations of the disease affect the anus, rectum, and colon. The reason for this is the fact that the gastrointestinal tract is the largest lymphoid organ in the body, and as such is an enormous potential reservoir for HIV.[252] The adverse consequences upon the cellular and humoral defense mechanisms lead to a plethora of viral, bacterial, fungal, and protozoal infestations.

AIDS is discussed in Chapter 20. Cytomegalovirus infection is also discussed in Chapter 20. The one remaining area is herpes simplex proctitis that is addressed, to some extent, in Chapter 19. The following discussion, however, is limited to that of the inflammatory change in the rectum.

Herpes Simplex Proctitis

Herpes simplex virus (HSV) proctitis has been stated to be the most common cause of non-gonococcal proctitis in sexually active male homosexuals (see Chapter 19).[213] Klausner and colleagues reported a 16% incidence among homosexual men.[141] HSV-2 is the most common type of herpes virus that causes proctitis, but HSV-1 can also produce genital infections and proctitis. Anorectal herpes can be acquired via anal intercourse or anal-oral sex.

Herpes proctitis appears to be a distinctive condition that can often be clinically distinguished from other infectious proctitises. Initially, the infection may involve the perianal skin and anal canal and progress into the rectum. Herpes infections in AIDS patients may also develop an ulcerative proctitis which remains confined to the rectum.[55] In a report by Goodell and associates, the virus was detected in approximately 20% of 102 male homosexuals who presented with anorectal pain, discharge, tenesmus, or rectal bleeding, as compared with three of 75 homosexual men without intestinal symptoms.[101] The likelihood of having a proctitis that is due to the herpes virus is greater if the patient has tenesmus, anorectal pain, constipation, and perianal ulceration. Difficulty in urinating, S4-S5 dysesthesias, sacral paresthesias, temporary impotence, and diffuse ulceration of the distal rectal mucosa also suggest the nature of the condition. Anorectal incontinence may also occur during the acute phase, with resolution after treatment of the HSV infection.[127] Intestinal perforation associated with intestinal herpes simplex infection in an immunocompromised patient has been reported.[285]

Examination of the perianal area reveals typical herpetic vesicles, pustules, and ulcerations. The most severe cases present with edema and erythema that can be confused with a yeast infection. Digital examination and anoscopy are very painful.

Sigmoidoscopic examination reveals an acute proctitis. The mucosa is often edematous friable and ulcerated. The infection is usually confined to the rectum in immunocompetent individuals and rarely extends beyond 15 cm.[223] A high index of suspicion as to the etiology may be based on the fact that an individual is a homosexually active male. The diagnosis is established by immunoassay of the antibody to the virus or by immunofluorescent staining. In addition, herpes simplex virus may be isolated by culture from rectal swabs or biopsy specimens.

As discussed in Chapter 19, acyclovir has been demonstrated to eradicate perirectal herpes simplex virus infection.[176] An evaluation of oral therapy (400 mg, five times daily for 10 days) in the treatment of proctitis was undertaken by Rompalo and colleagues.[224,225] In one analysis of 24 patients, in a double-blind, placebo-controlled study, a significant decrease in mean viral shedding time, duration of anal pain, rectal discomfort, and tenesmus was appreciated in the treated group. In another trial from the same institution, it was demonstrated that daily administration of 2 g of oral acyclovir for 10 days alleviated some of the clinical signs of herpes simplex rectal infection.[224] In still another report from the same institution, individuals with acute proctitis were submitted to an empirical regimen of penicillin and probenecid, followed by doxycycline.[226] Since 25% failed to respond, the authors recommended appropriate pretreatment diagnostic tests and the empirical regimen for the initial management of acute proctitis in homosexual men with no clinical evidence of AIDS or AIDS-related complex.[226]

Severe infection in AIDS patients, regardless of the site, should be treated with intra-venous acyclovir at 5 to 10 mg/kg every 8 hours until clinical resolution. Moreover, suppressive therapy is also recommended to decrease relapses. Schacker and coworkers reported, in a prospective, placebo-controlled, crossover trial of oral famciclovir (500 mg twice daily) versus placebo for a total of 8 weeks, a significant reduction in HSV infection symptoms.[240] In addition, there was a significant reduction in HSV shedding among symptomatic and asymptomatic HIV-positive patients. This regimen also decreased the percentage of genital lesions from 13.8% to 4.9%. All recurrent anogenital lesions were due to HSV-2.

FUNGAL INFECTIONS

Candidiasis or Moniliasis

Severe fungal infections of the gastrointestinal tract are extremely rare in the healthy person. However, fungemia can be lethal in debilitated and immunosuppressed individuals. For example, diffuse fungal infections are common causes of death in those with terminal cancer. Asymptomatic oropharyngeal colonization can be found in 30% to 55% of healthy adults, and *Candida* species may be present in 40% to 65% of normal fecal flora.[119] *Candida* species are the most common fungal pathogens causing mucosal and systemic infections. Associated risk factors include parental hyperalimentation, granulocytopenia, indwelling catheters, prolonged use of broad-spectrum antibiotics, malignancy, recent trauma or major gastrointestinal surgery, prolonged hospitalization, burns, and HIV/AIDS. All of the above factors may lead to immunosuppression and are also associated with increased candidal colonization of mucocutaneous surfaces.

The most frequent segment of the gastrointestinal tract affected by *Candida* is the oropharynx and esophagus, followed by the stomach and small bowel. The frequency of large bowel infection by *Candida* is approximately 20%.[119] Symptoms of gastrointestinal candidiasis include epigastric or abdominal pain, nausea, vomiting, fever, and the presence of an abdominal mass. Internal fistulas may develop. *Candida* peritonitis may occur as a consequence of gastrointestinal surgery, perforated viscus, or peritoneal dialysis. Fifteen percent of patients with *Candida* peritonitis will develop candidemia.

The diagnosis of *Candida* infection is based on clinical suspicion, culture, and endoscopic findings. Because approximately 20% to 25% of the population is colonized by *Candida* species, culture alone should not be the sole diagnostic criterion.[116] Endoscopic examination reveals small, creamy-white, curd-like patches on the mucosal surface. In addition, the mucosa also appears edematous and inflamed. Biopsies should be taken for histologic identification of yeast cells, hyphae, or pseudohyphae (Figure 33-21). Infection of the perianal skin is discussed in Chapter 19.

Over 100 different species of *Candida* have been described. However, only a few are clinically significant, including *Candida albicans* (50% to 60%), *Candida glabrata* (15% to 20%) *Candida parapsilosis* (10% to 20%), *Candida tropicalis* (6% to 12%), *Candida crusei* (1% to 3%),

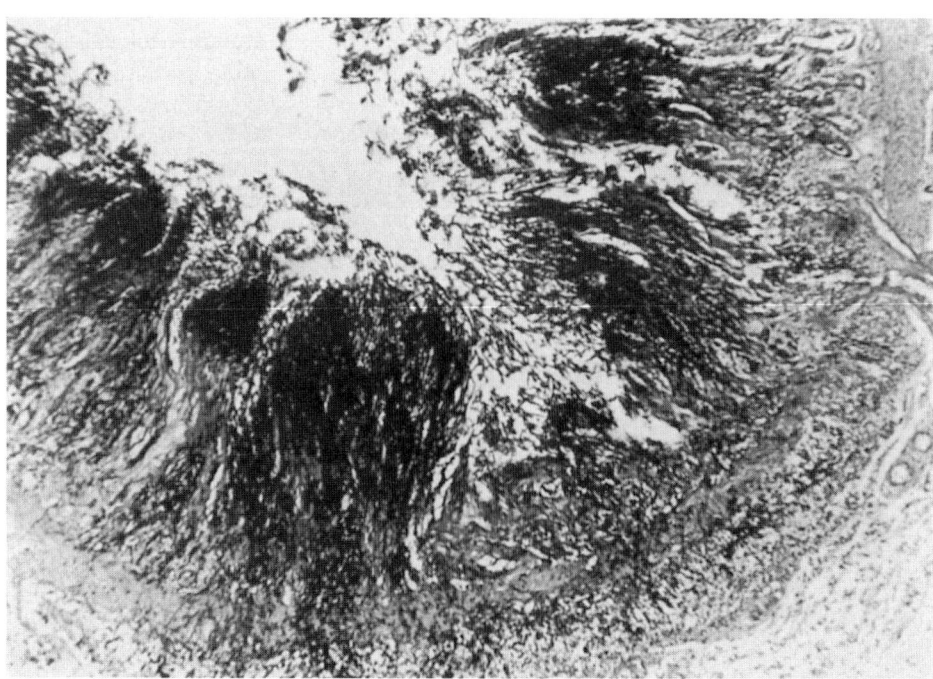

FIGURE 33-21. Intestinal candidiasis (moniliasis). Postmortem biopsy demonstrates characteristic pseudohyphae replacing mucosa. (Original magnification ×180; courtesy of Rudolf Garret, M.D.)

Candida lusitaniae (<5%), and *Candida dubliniensis* (primarily in HIV patients).[119]

The management of gastrointestinal candidiasis requires systemic antifungal therapy with fluconazole, 200 mg daily for at least 14 days. Alternatively, itraconazole can also be used. Severe *Candida* infection and candidemia are treated with fluconazole, with a loading dose of 800 mg, followed by a maintenance dose of 400 mg daily for at least 2 weeks.[116] Amphotericin B is reserved for fluconazole-resistant *Candida* sepsis. Liposomal preparations of amphotericin B may also be an option for patients with infections refractory to fluconazole, infusion toxicity, or renal insufficiency. The most recently approved therapy for systemic fungal infection is caspofungin.[119] A 70-mg loading dose is given, followed by 50 mg, intravenously, daily for a minimum of 14 days. Prophylactic antifungal therapy is recommended for high-risk patients, such as those undergoing bone marrow or solid-organ transplants, and recurrent symptomatic candidiasis in HIV patients.

Histoplasmosis

Histoplasmosis is caused by the dimorphic fungus, *Histoplasma capsulatum*, principally an intracellular mycosis of the reticuloendothelial system.[157] It is endemic to areas of the Midwest, especially in the fertile river valleys.[53] It is usually a subclinical infection in otherwise healthy individuals, but in immunocompromised persons (e.g., those with AIDS) disseminated disease can ensue.[53,66] While the lung is by far the most common organ involved, the condition may affect the entire gastrointestinal tract, especially the terminal ileum and proximal colon.[261] When it involves this area, ulceration with bleeding, stricture, and even perforation have been reported.[117,157] The condition may sometimes be confused with colon carcinoma.[134] Isolated colonic histoplasmosis in immunosuppressed patient has also been reported.[123]

Endoscopic examination may reveal skip areas of inflammation, with plaques, ulcers, and pseudopolyps.[53] While biopsy may demonstrate the characteristic intracellular oval budding yeasts within the mucosa, serologic complement-fixation titers of 1:8 or greater are suggestive of the disease. Fungal culture of biopsy specimens will also confirm the diagnosis. If pathologic changes are correlated with the roentgenographic features, six patterns of gastrointestinal involvement have been described by Lee and Lin[157]:

- malabsorptive (edema, diffuse inflammatory infiltrates)
- ulcerative
- polypoid (nodular hyperplasia of lymphoid follicles)
- granulomatous (diffuse infiltrates)
- tumefactive (large granulomas)
- compressive (enlarged lymph nodes)

Common physical findings are peripheral lymphadenopathy and hepatosplenomegaly.[37]

Most healthy individuals with a normal immune system do not require treatment for histoplasmosis, because in the majority of cases the disease will subside within a few weeks without long-term sequelae. However, more severe cases require treatment with amphotericin B. Itraconazole is also an option for long-term therapy in order to prevent relapse, especially in HIV and immunosuppressed patients.[57] Diversion or resection of strictures may be indicated, in addition to aggressive long-term amphotericin B therapy for those afflicted with AIDS.[103]

PARASITIC INFECTIONS

Parasitoses are infectious diseases that afflict humans through the fecal-oral route. The ingestion of food or water contaminated by the feces of infected animals or humans is often the result of poor sanitation measures. Parasitic infections have a worldwide distribution. However, parasites are more frequently found in developing countries. The disease or asymptomatic carrier is more common among native individuals and travelers. Parasitic infections affecting immunocompromised individuals are often more severe and difficult to eradicate. Individuals chronically infected are commonly debilitated, often malnourished, and may manifest organ system involvement other than the gastrointestinal tract.

The diagnosis of a particular parasitic infection may be difficult due to the similarity of symptoms occurring in patients with parasitoses and other infectious and non-infectious diarrheas. The identification of the infective organism in the stool will confirm the clinical suspicion. The management of parasitoses is also controversial both in terms of the choice of treatment and the effectiveness. Nonetheless, there is no doubt that preventive measures are the mainstay in controlling this profound health care problem.

Amebiasis

While amebiasis is a worldwide disease that is most commonly found in the tropics, it is the most frequent parasitic condition encountered by surgeons in the United States.[69] Additionally, it has been deemed by some as the most frequently "diagnosed" cause of traveler's diarrhea, although giardiasis must be at least a close second. A patient will often believe that he or she has "amebiasis" based on a travel experience or contact with persons who are known to harbor the organism. However, Gorbach espouses that even in the tropics, the conferring of this impression is the "refuge of the diagnostically destitute," and that, in fact, the patient's symptoms are rarely due to this cause.[102]

An outbreak of amebiasis was reported to have occurred in a chiropractic clinic in patients who received colonic irrigation therapy.[122] But the largest reservoir for *Entamoeba histolytica* infection is the male homosexual population.[35,172] In a report by Allason-Jones and colleagues, 20% of men attending a clinic in London for the treatment of sexually transmitted diseases were infected with *E. histolytica*.[5]

Amebiasis is transmitted via the fecal-oral route. The risk factors for transmission of the disease in industrialized countries include recent travel to or from endemic areas, residents from mental institutions, and sexually active homosexual males (now primarily infected by *Entamoeba dispar*).

Pathogenesis

E. histolytica is caused by a protozoan that exists in the colon as either a trophozoite, the invasive form of the parasite (Figure 33-22), or as a cyst. The cytoplasm of the organism usually is quite granular owing to ingestion of many bacteria, red blood cells, and other cellular debris (Figure 33-23). Transmission occurs either through water or food contaminated by carriers of the cysts. The swallowed cysts pass into the small intestine where the trophozoites are released. These burrow into the mucosa and result in the characteristic flask-shaped ulcer (Figure 33-24). Ulcers are usually identified in the cecum and ascending colon, but the process may be diffuse throughout the bowel. It is rare for the small intestine to be involved.

Symptoms and Findings

The manifestations commence after an incubation period of 7 to 21 days.[131] Symptoms of amebiasis may be minimal, or the disease may be acute and fulminant. For example, acute intestinal amebiasis is often ushered in abruptly by cramping abdominal pain, tenesmus, and bloody stools.[266] The most common complaint is diarrhea, which may be bloody and contain mucus. Bowel movements can be frequent, in excess of ten per day. The most severe presentation of amebic colitis is fulminant necrotizing colitis. This is associated with a greater than 50% mortality rate and is more common in children, pregnant women, and patients on corticosteroids or who are immunosuppressed.[131] Amebiasis can also cause peritonitis, toxic megacolon, and extraintestinal manifestations, such as cutaneous amebiasis, ameboma, liver abscess, brain abscess, empyema, and pericarditis, as well as brain and skin involvement (see Chapter 19).

Liver abscess is the most common extraintestinal manifestation of amebiasis. Patients usually present with fever, right upper-quadrant pain, hepatomegaly, weight loss, and abnormal liver function tests. Most of the time this disease complication occurs in young male, Hispanic immigrants.[131] Misra and colleagues reported symptomatic

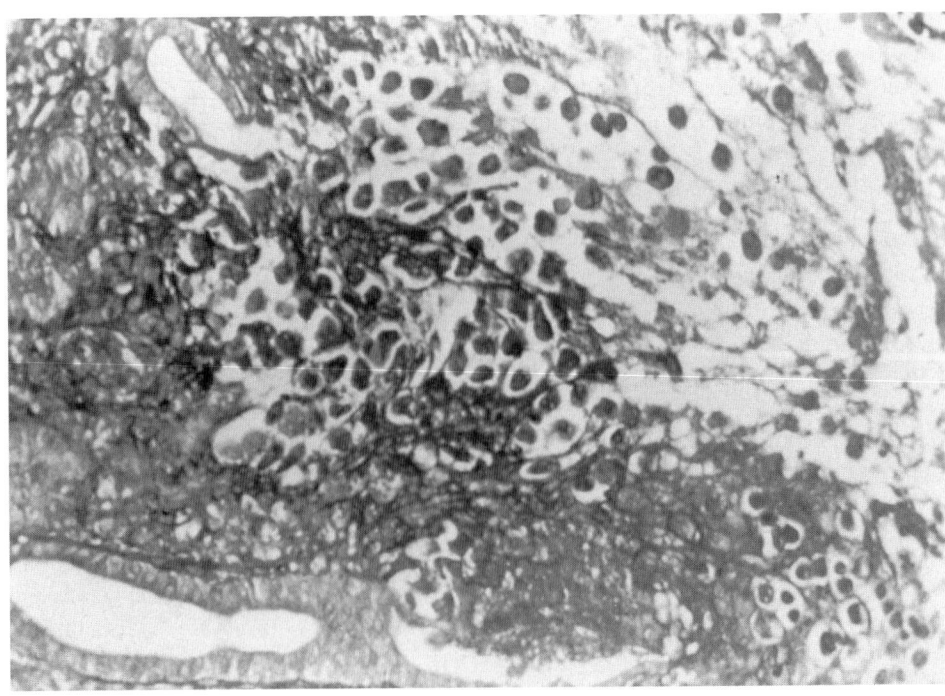

FIGURE 33-22. Entamoeba histolytica. Trophozoites in a colon ulcer. (Original magnification ×280; courtesy of Rudolf Garret, M.D.)

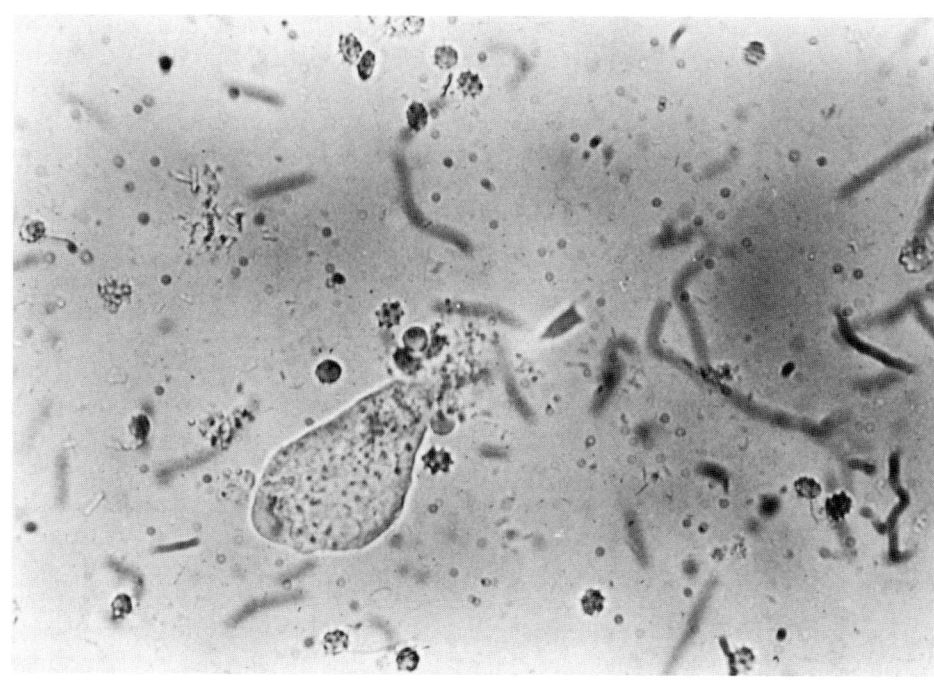

FIGURE 33-23. *Entamoeba histolytica* ingesting red blood cells. (Wet preparation, original magnification ×360; courtesy of Rudolf Garret, M.D.)

colonic involvement in more than half of patients who presented with amebic liver abscess.[178]

Diagnosis

The diagnosis is established by microscopic examination of fresh stool specimens for the trophozoites. Ninety percent of patients with symptomatic disease will demonstrate this finding.[62] It is important that stool examination be undertaken before any barium investigation. Moreover, the use of mineral oil and broad-spectrum antibiotics also impede the ability to identify the protozoan.[62] In addition to stool culture and at least three stool examinations for ova and parasites, amebic titer by indirect hemagglutination technique may establish the diagnosis. The sensitivity of the indirect hemagglutination assay is 99% for amebic

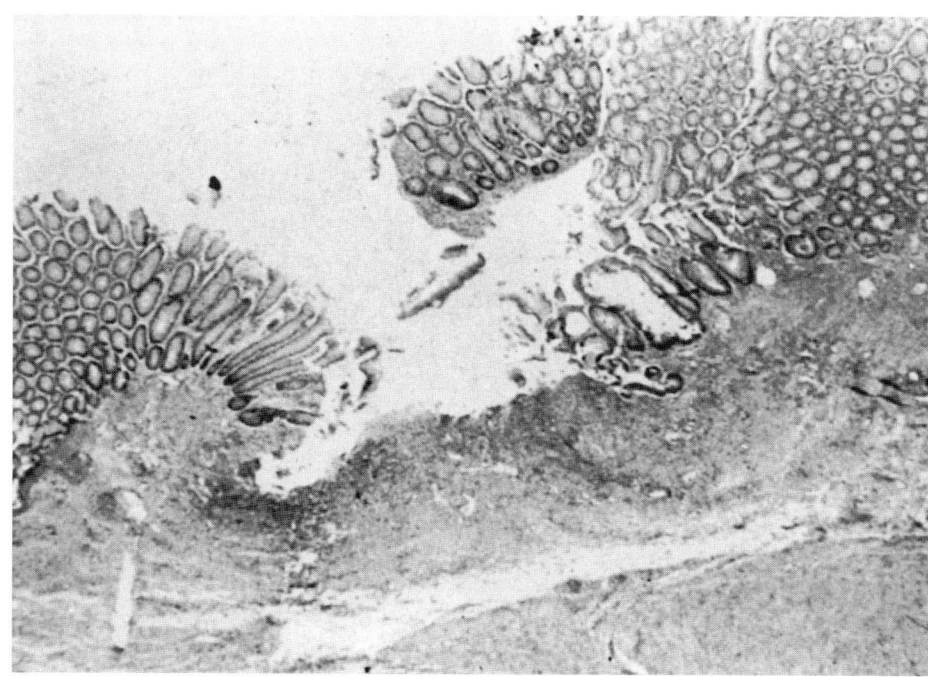

FIGURE 33-24. Amebic ulcer. Note the characteristic flask shape. (Original magnification ×80.)

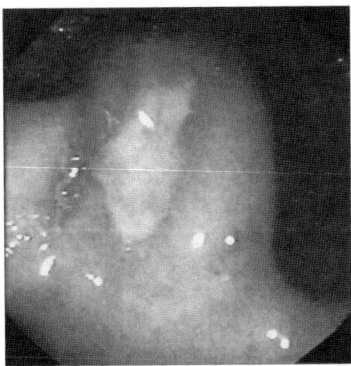

FIGURE 33-25. Colonoscopy demonstrates an exudative amebic ulcer that appears flask-shaped, even in this projection. Overhanging mucosa and undermining margins are present. Microscopic examination of the stool was positive for the trophozoites. (See Color Fig. 33-25.)

liver abscess and 88% for amebic colitis.[131] An amebic titer by this means should be obtained if examination reveals colonic inflammation, and if the results of stool examination and cultures are negative.[175] Although stool culture is more sensitive than microscopy, it takes approximately 1 week to obtain the results.

Sigmoidoscopic examination is a valuable method for diagnosis since ulcerations are visible in the rectum in up to 85% of the cases.[128] However, because the disease occurs more frequently in a proximal location than it does distally, a negative proctosigmoidoscopy does not rule out the diagnosis. Colonoscopy has been felt to be a useful technique for this reason (Figure 33-25).[214] Crowson and Hines reported identification of the disease by means of colonoscopy in an individual whose sigmoidoscopy was normal.[59] In the two patients of Rozen and colleagues, the symptom of rectal bleeding caused the authors to perform multiple colonoscopic biopsies that identified the nature of the condition.[231] Although the histologic appearance is usually indistinguishable from nonspecific inflammatory bowel disease, the overhanging mucosa, undermining margins, or flask shape, along with the appropriate history, suggest amebic colitis (Figure 33-26).

Occasionally a granulomatous reaction may lead to the formation of a mass, the so-called *ameboma*. When this clinical picture is present, it may be difficult to differentiate it from Crohn's colitis or carcinoma. Ameboma can be found in 1.5% of patients with amebiasis,[258] and has been reported to involve the rectum.[222]

Barium enema examination may reveal a multitude of changes in a patient with amebic colitis. As mentioned, toxic dilatation can occur, a contraindication to the performance of the study. Characteristic changes include the so-called collar-button ulcer, a cobblestone appearance, thumbprinting, and the signs of nonspecific inflammatory bowel disease. Amebiasis is almost always multifocal, so that a careful search throughout the length of the colon for other areas of infection is an important aspect of differential diagnosis.[198] The presence of a stricture or tumor-like ameboma may confuse the interpretation (Figure 33-27).

Management

The cornerstone for the management of amebiasis is metronidazole. This is the only nitroimidazole derivative available in the United States. The recommended dose is

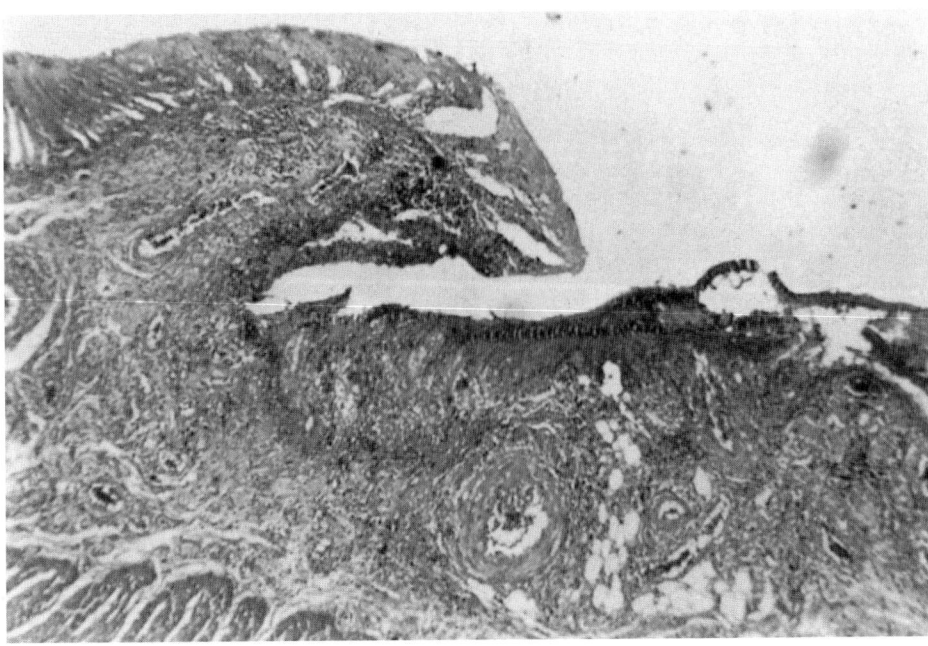

FIGURE 33-26. Amebic ulcer. Note the undermined margin. (Original magnification ×180; courtesy of Rudolf Garret, M.D.)

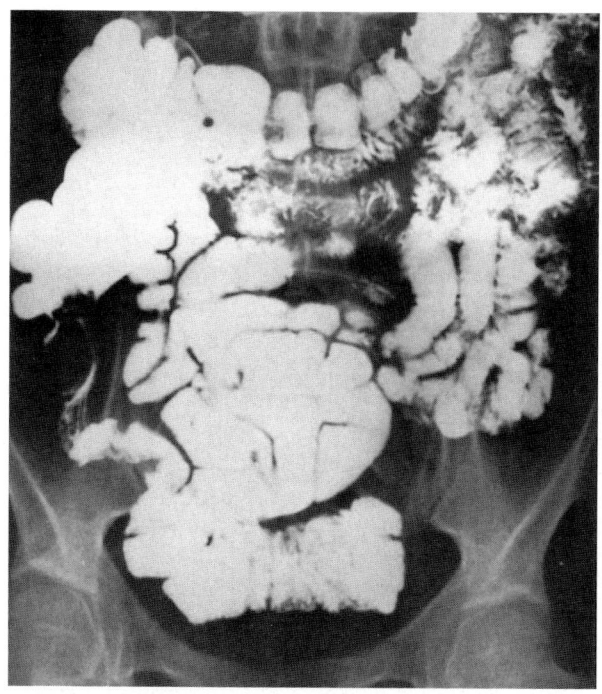

FIGURE 33-27. Cecal ameboma. Barium enema demonstrates extrinsic compression of the cecum and terminal ileum with marked narrowing. The mucosa appears intact.

750 mg, three times daily, either orally or intravenously for 5 to 10 days. This dose is effective not only for colitis but also for liver abscess. In cases of amebic colitis, a luminal agent, such as paromomycin, iodoquinol, or diloxanide may be required to eradicate colonization.[255] Amebic liver abscess can be treated with metronidazole alone in most instances. Surgical drainage of uncomplicated liver abscess should be avoided. The role of percutaneous drainage of amebic liver abscess is also controversial. However, in cases of large liver abscess, percutaneous aspiration may decrease the length of hospitalization and improve the overall clinical status of the patient.[62,127,255]

If the patient requires surgical intervention for hemorrhage or for perforation, resection of the involved bowel must be performed. Indications include the following:

- Free extraperitoneal perforation, impending perforation, or perforation during antiamebic chemotherapy
- Failure of perforation with a localized abscess to respond to antiamebic drugs
- Persistence of or the development of abdominal distention, and abdominal tenderness in patients undergoing treatment
- Persistence of severe diarrhea after 5 days of chemotherapy
- Symptoms of postamebic colitis with unremitting anemia and hypoproteinemia[153]

Total colectomy may be required if multiple areas of perforation are identified. Due to the high risk of anastomotic leak some suggest exteriorization, or at least, a concomitant diversionary procedure.[9,248] Luvuno advises that an ileostomy be performed in addition to colonic lavage rather than risk opening a walled-off perforation and further contaminating the abdominal cavity.[166] Even in patients for whom an operation is considered, aggressive medical treatment is recommended because it may obviate the need for surgery, or improve the likelihood of survival following resection in this high-risk situation.[50,199]

Balantidiasis

Balantidiasis is caused by a protozoan, *Balantidium coli*, a ciliate that is the only member of the subphylum *Ciliophora* known to affect humans.[49] Locomotion is by means of longitudinal rows of cilia that cover the body and propel it forward with a spiral motion.[142] It is believed that the worldwide prevalence is approximately 1%. However, infections are more frequent in Latin America, Southeast Asia, and New Guinea. Pigs are the known primary reservoir for *B. coli*.[49] The condition is found where sanitation is a problem.

The infection is acquired through ingestion of infective cysts. The cyst then passes into the small intestine where it excysts, and the trophozoite then migrates into the colon where it penetrates the intestinal epithelium.[49] Ulcerations are produced, not dissimilar to those seen with amebic colitis.[62,142] In fact, it is not uncommon for the two conditions to coexist. The trophozoite resides in the intestinal lumen, is quite large, and may occasionally be seen with the naked eye (Figure 33-28). A cyst develops when the organism is passed in the feces and is the source for dissemination of the disease.

Most patients will present with asymptomatic infections. However, common symptoms include watery diarrhea (a loose, offensive, pale stool) associated with nausea, vomiting, abdominal pain and distention, flatulence, dehydration, anorexia, and weight loss.[142] Diarrhea may be associated with blood and mucous with alternating periods of constipation.[181] Immunosuppressed and HIV patients may develop more profound manifestations of *B. coli* infection.[43,141]

The diagnosis can be made by examining wet smears of stool samples or scrapings from mucosal ulcers. The trophozoite can be recognized by the large size, short ciliary covering, and a spiraling motility. Colonoscopic evaluation with biopsies from the periphery of the ulcers will aid in the diagnosis of balantidiasis.[99] The endoscopic findings can mimic amebiasis. An additional method for confirmation is to obtain the trophozoites by means of duodenal aspiration or by the use of a recoverable nylon yarn swallowed in a weighted capsule.[142]

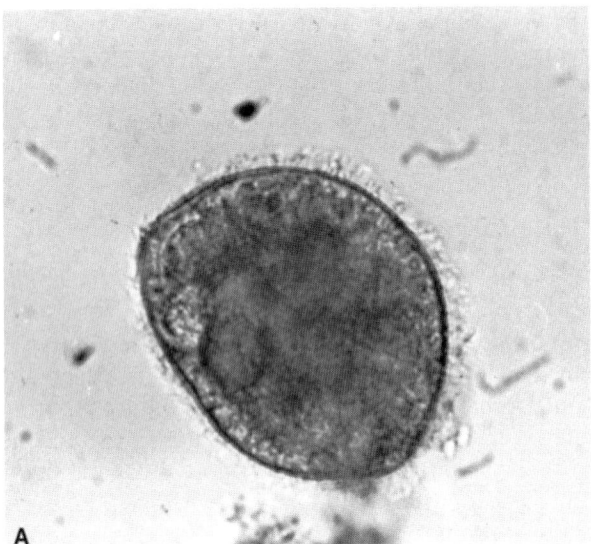
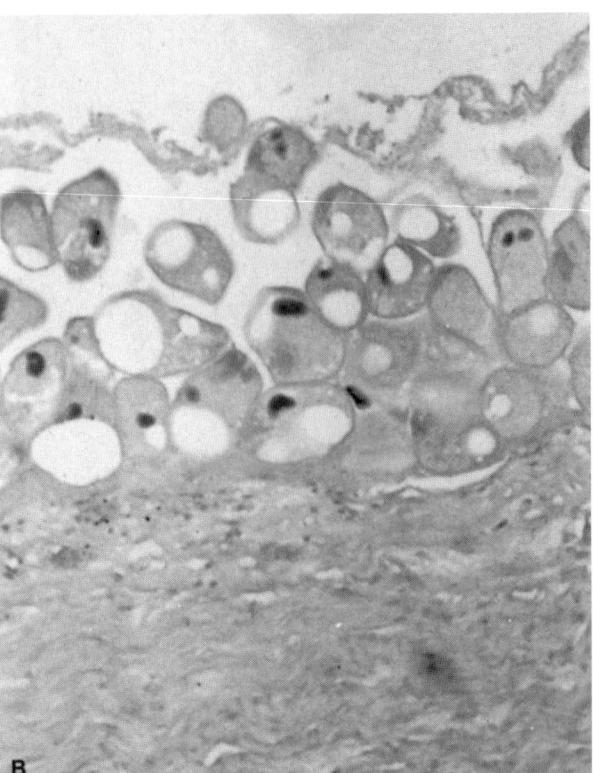

FIGURE 33-28. *Balantidium coli.* **(A)** Trophozoite. Note the cilia. **(B)** Surface of the colonic mucosa replaced by trophozoites of *B. coli*. (Original magnification ×280; courtesy of Rudolf Garret, M.D.)

A number of drugs are effective in the treatment of balantidiasis. However, tetracycline is preferred, with metronidazole considered a secondary option.[142] Iodoquinol is also considered an effective medication. Followup with a repeat stool test is required to ensure eradication of the parasite. Treatment should be directed toward the asymptomatic carrier, as well as to the patient with acute or chronic illness, in order to eliminate the organism and to prevent its spread.[62]

Cryptosporidiosis

Human cryptosporidiosis is caused by *Cryptosporidium parvum*, and is often a self-limited diarrheal infection in healthy individuals, mostly children. However, the disease has been recognized as an important opportunistic infection in immunocompromised patients, usually those with AIDS.[293] The main source of endemic cryptosporidiosis is human-to-human fecal-oral transmission. This is a very important concern in the hospital setting. Additionally, animal-to-human (especially cats) and waterborne transmission is also common.[266] There is also a high rate of infection among children in day-care facilities and among persons arriving from developing countries.[266] *C. parvum* is the most frequent pathogen in HIV-positive patients who have symptoms of diarrhea. In fact,

the diagnosis of AIDS can be made if the infection lasts longer than 3 weeks.[91] Nonetheless, the prevalence of cryptosporidiosis has decreased significantly since the introduction of highly effective antiretroviral therapy (HAART) in the management of HIV/AIDS.

The gastrointestinal tract is predominantly affected, with the production of severe, watery, debilitating, chronic diarrhea. Malabsorption, wasting, and weight loss may be evident. Systemic manifestations, such as fever, loss of appetite, malaise, nausea, and vomiting may also be present, but abdominal pain is unusual. However, extraintestinal manifestations, such as pancreatitis and biliary infection, are common in AIDS patients.

Cryptosporidiosis should be considered in all patients with chronic diarrhea, especially in those who are immunocompromised or have AIDS. The risk of *C. parvum* diarrhea in AIDS patients is higher when the CD4 count is 200 cells/mm³ or fewer.[293] The modified acid-fast staining of the organism or Kinyoun stain is the "gold standard" and simplest diagnostic method for identifying cryptosporidiosis (Figure 33-29).[154] The protozoan appears to attach to the mucosa and may be surrounded by a host cell membrane, but there is no evidence of invasion or tissue reaction.[91]

Currently, there is no effective antibiotic or chemotherapeutic regimen to eradicate *Cryptosporidium*. How-

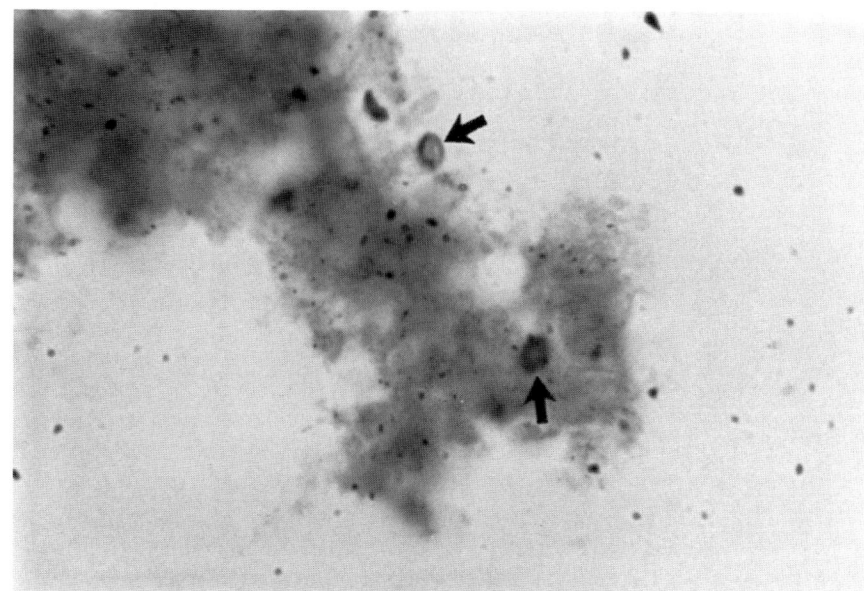

FIGURE 33-29. Cryptosporidiosis. Small round to oval-shaped forms (*arrows*) usually seen by acid-fast stain or fluorescent staining techniques. (Original magnification ×1,000.)

ever, there are drugs that can suppress the symptoms of cryptosporidiosis. The use of HAART, reconstituting the immune system in AIDS patients, is associated with resolution of cryptosporidiosis in most cases. In addition, supportive care through hydration and correction of electrolyte imbalance is important, since there is considerable loss of fluid and disturbance of electrolytes as a consequence of the diarrhea. If HAART does not improve the diarrhea, combination therapy with antimicrobial and antidiarrheal agents is still considered a good therapeutic option. Paromomycin, azithromycin, and most recently, nitazoxanide are frequently used to treat *C. parvum* diarrhea.[47,229] However, these antiparasitic drugs are only moderately effective. Spiromycin may shorten the duration of oocyst excretion and diarrhea in children.[56,207]

Giardiasis

Giardiasis is a disease caused by a flagellated protozoan, *Giardia lamblia*. It is a worldwide condition, with the vast majority of patients being asymptomatic. So-called traveler's diarrhea is commonly attributed to this protozoan. Hikers and backpackers drinking untreated water from mountain lakes and streams, where animals serve as a reservoir for the parasite, are at risk. It is probably the most common water-borne disease in the United States. Estimates based on the Centers for Disease Control and Prevention state surveillance data indicate an incidence of 2.5 million cases of giardiasis yearly.[88] The carrier rate is 30% to 60% among children in daycare centers, institutionalized individuals, and Native Americans living on reservations.[204] This disease, however, is much more prevalent in developing countries.

As with balantidiasis, the protozoan exists both as a cyst and as a trophozoite. Infection results from inges-

tion of the cyst, which excysts in the small intestine. The ingestion of 25 cysts will lead to a 100% infection rate.[204] This may lead to a variety of histologic changes, ranging from minimal cellular infiltration of the lamina propria, reduction in the height and the number of villi, loss of the brush border, and an increase in epithelial cell mitosis.[266]

Symptoms

Giardiasis causes explosive, watery diarrhea, associated with abdominal cramps and foul flatus. The mechanism for the diarrhea is poorly understood. Vomiting, fever, malaise, weight loss, and dehydration may also be experienced. The symptoms usually last 3 to 4 days before evolving into a subacute phase. However, the majority of patients will present with a more insidious onset of recurrent or resistant symptoms. Diarrhea may alternate with soft stool or even constipation. Since giardiasis is not a form of dysentery, stool does not contain blood or pus.

Giardiasis can also present with upper intestinal manifestations exacerbated by eating. These include epigastric pain, nausea, early satiety, bloating, sulfurous belching, substernal burning, and acid indigestion. Such symptoms can be confused with gastroesophageal reflux or peptic ulcer disease. Chronic disease in adults causes a long-standing malabsorption syndrome and, in children, a failure to thrive. While on rare occasions the disease can pursue a fulminating course, most infected individuals are asymptomatic carriers.

Evaluation

There are several commercially available tests to detect *G. lamblia*. These include the use of immunofluorescent antibody or enzyme-linked immunosorbent assay against

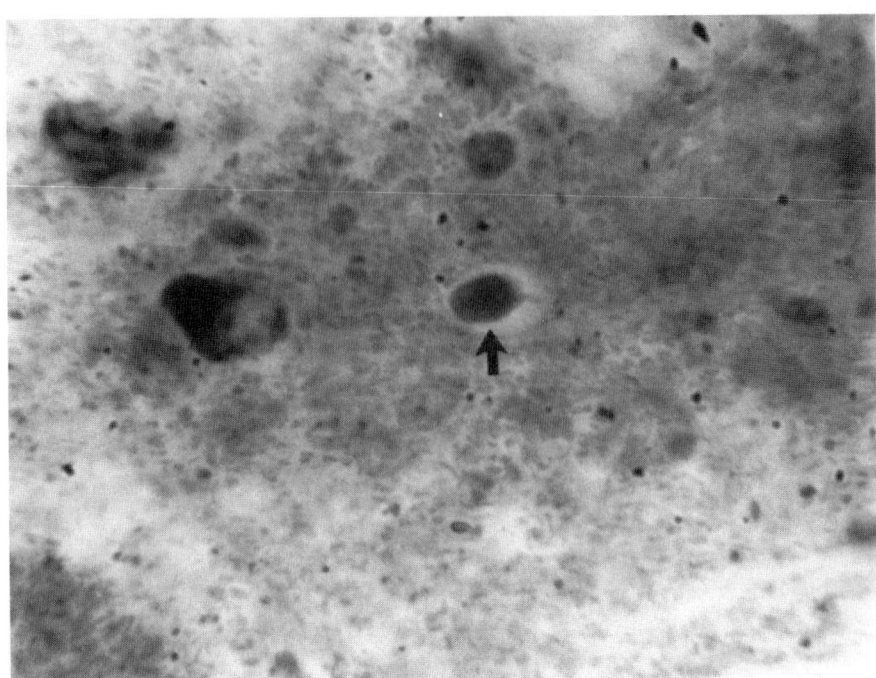

FIGURE 33-30. Giardiasis. Oval-shaped parasite demonstrating retraction from cyst wall (*arrow*). Two nuclei can be appreciated. (Original magnification ×1,000.)

the cyst or trophozoite antigens. Stool cultures are not useful because the organism does not reliably grow in the patient's stool samples. The trichrome stain is a useful test to identify the cysts and trophozoites.

Proctosigmoidoscopic examination may reveal changes impossible to differentiate from those of amebiasis. The diagnosis can also be made by examination of scrapings of the base of the ulcer for the trophozoites.[62] Loose stool contains only the trophozoites, but in formed stool there may be cysts as well (Figure 33-30).[142] The trophozoites disintegrate rapidly and may be undetectable unless fresh, semi-formed to formed stool is examined. Therefore, if not immediately examined, the stool sample should be preserved in polyvinyl, in alcohol, or in a formalin preparation. Rectal biopsy may also be helpful in identifying the organism. A negative stool examination, however, does not exclude the diagnosis. Therefore, at least three stool samples taken at 2-day intervals should be tested.

A more accurate determination of the etiology can be made by microscopic examination of the duodenal fluid or by a "string test." Most recently, a commercially available test, the ProSpecT/Giardia enzyme-linked immunosorbent assay (ELISA, Alexon, Inc., Mountain View, CA) has been found to be 96% to 98% sensitive and 100% specific.[169] This test is less expensive than the conventional ova and parasite series, it is 30% more sensitive, and the results are more readily available. Rosoff and colleagues demonstrated that the immunoassay was easy to run and to interpret and offered a simple, accurate alternative to the traditional difficulties encountered with attempting to diagnose Giardia infection.[228]

Treatment

Metronidazole is the first-line therapy for giardiasis. The suggested dose is 250 mg orally, three times daily for 5 to 7 days (the pediatric dose is 5 mg/kg, three times daily for 5 to 7 days). Paromomycin (25 to 30 mg/kg, three times daily for 7 to 10 days) may be considered for severe infection in pregnant women. Furazolidone, available in a liquid suspension, may be an alternative in children. Tinidazole appears to be a suitable therapeutic option for symptomatic individuals.[296]

The treatment of patients with refractory giardiasis is not well established, but combination therapy may be required, especially in AIDS patients. The association of quinacrine and metronidazole has been reported to be an effective option for this patient population.[48,189] Treatment of the asymptomatic carrier is somewhat controversial, but prudence would seem to dictate that both the asymptomatic person and the acute or chronically ill patient should undergo therapy in order to prevent spread of the disease. There is no chemoprophylactic agent available. However, patient education, especially directed to hikers and travelers, to avoid ingestion of potentially contaminated water, as well as strict personal hygiene and hand washing, will help to control the disease. In ad-

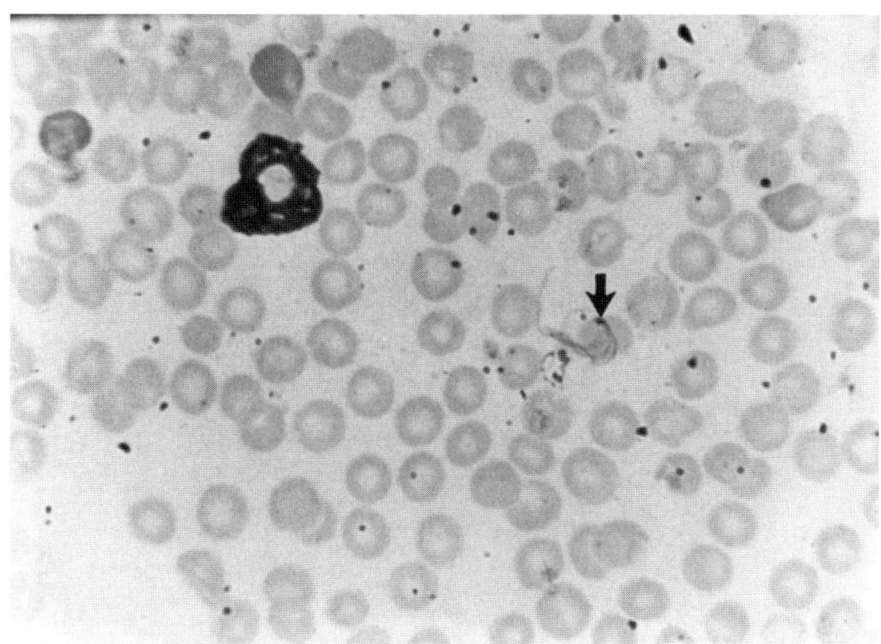

FIGURE 33-31. Trypanosomiasis. C-shaped configuration found in human blood. Organism has prominent terminal kinetoplast (*arrow*). Intercellular location is typical of trypanosomes. (Original magnification ×1,000.)

dition, patients should be advised to avoid oral-anal and oral-genital sex.

Trypanosomiasis or Chagas Disease

The disease reported in 1909 by the Brazilian physician, Carlos Chagas, is caused by the *Trypanosoma cruzi*. Chagas disease is frequently transmitted by a *Triatominae* known as the "kissing bug," because of its nocturnal habits and because it frequently bites the individual in the face while sleeping.[13,39] The trypanosomes are deposited from the feces of the bug when it is taking a blood meal. Phagocytosis of the invading organisms is performed by histiocytes in the skin, fat, and muscle; this is the so-called leishmanial form of the disease. Rupture of the cell causes escape of a large number of the trypanosomal forms into the circulation (Figure 33-31). Transmission through blood transfusion has becoming a growing problem in developing countries.[243] Vertical transmission through birth is also reported as well as through organ transplantation.[297]

Chagas disease is endemic in developing countries, especially in Central and South America. However, due to immigration, the disease has been reported in several states in the United States, especially Texas.[13] The destruction of rain forests has also contributed to the spread of the disease.[276] According to the World Health Organization, 300,000 new cases of Chagas disease are diagnosed annually. Moreover, 2 to 3 million individuals live with chronic complications of Chagas disease, thus leading to a enormous disease burden.[39,243,297]

Gastrointestinal manifestations occur from 2 to 20 years or more following initial infection.[181] The release of the toxin destroys the submucosal and myenteric plexi, with the colon and the esophagus most frequently involved, although the stomach, small bowel, bladder, and ureters can be affected. Involvement of the myocardium and central nervous system can also develop. In the intestine, the parasympathetic intramural denervation is dispersed irregularly, but the manifestations are primarily in the esophagus and the colon, especially the sigmoid. The

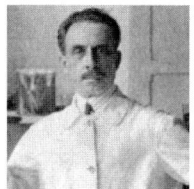

Carlos J. R. Chagas (1879–1933) Carlos Chagas was born in the town of Oliveira, Brazil, to an upper-class family of coffee growers. Chagas did not follow his mother's dream of his becoming a mining engineer, choosing instead a medical career. He firmly believed that the growth and evolution of Brazil depended upon the eradication of endemic diseases, such as yellow fever, smallpox, syphilis, malaria, and bubonic plague. Chagas went on to write his thesis at the Oswaldo Cruz Institute under the guidance of the renowned parasitologist Oswaldo Cruz. However, he refused Cruz's invitation to continue his work on malarial research and entered the practice of family medicine. Chagas, being of an inquisitive mind, was innovative and experimental. He studied parasites and insects in their natural habitat and evaluated epidemics in order to broaden his background. In 1908, Chagas set up a simple laboratory to study a disease that was taking the lives of immigrant railroad workers in central Brazil. By 1909, he not only identified the insect carrying the flagellate that transmitted the disease, but also described the complete cycle of the *Trypanosome cruzi*, which he named after his mentor. Through his extensive investigations, Chagas reported the acute clinical presentation as well as the diverse chronic manifestations of the disease that bears his name. Unfortunately, following his death in 1933, very few additional contributions have been made in the study of Chagas disease. (Courtesy of T. Cristina Sardinha, M.D.)

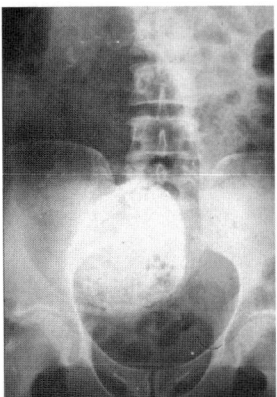

FIGURE 33-32. Abdominal x-ray showing fecaloma in a patient with Chagas disease. (Courtesy of T. Cristina Sardinha, M.D.)

bowel presents a functional peristaltic alteration leading to progressive dilatation and elongation of the affected segment which slows down the transit time The patient may be severely constipated as the bowel becomes progressively dilated because of the neurologic abnormality and the presence of inspissated feces (Figure 33-32). While obstipation may necessitate the frequent use of enemas, often the patient compensates and is able to pursue a fairly normal existence.[181] Volvulus, however, is a potential complication (Figs. 33-33 and 33-34). In those individuals with chagasic megacolon, clinical signs and symptoms include severe pain and progressive abdominal distention, accompanied by fever, severe toxemia, and shock.[144]

The diagnosis of Chagas disease is based on clinical presentation and immunologic tests such as indirect hemaglutination, immunofluorescence, and enzyme immunosorbent assay. PCR has also been described as a diagnostic modality, as well as hemoculture.[39]

Radiologic examination may reveal an enormously dilated and elongated colon (Fig 33-35). In contradistinction to other forms of megacolon, the distribution may be segmental (Figure 33-36).[181]

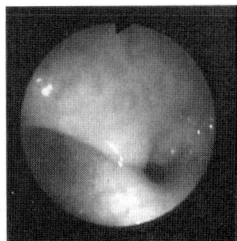

FIGURE 33-33. Proctosigmoidoscopic appearance of classic narrowing as a consequence of a sigmoid volvulus in a patient with Chagas disease. (Courtesy of T. Cristina Sardinha, M.D.) (See Color Fig. 33-33.)

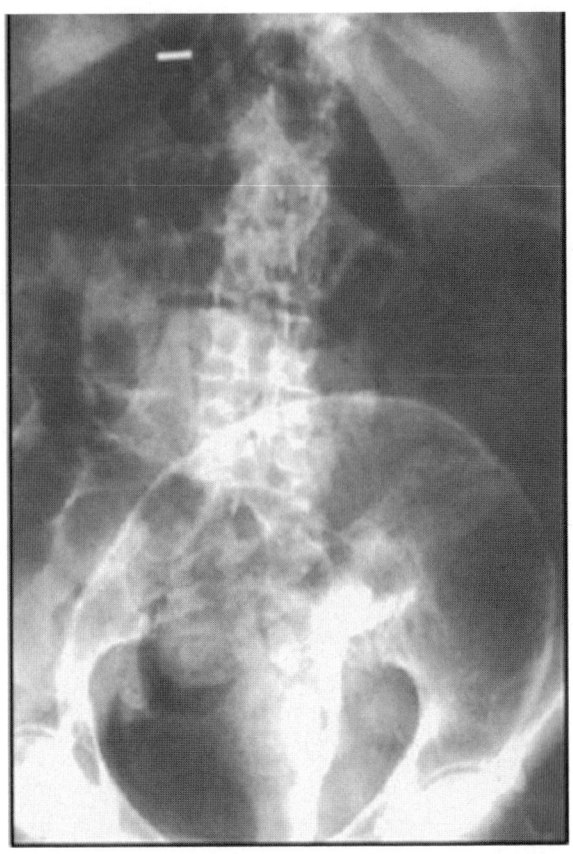

FIGURE 33-34. Plain abdominal x-ray showing sigmoid volvulus in a patient with Chagas disease. (Courtesy of T. Cristina Sardinha, M.D.)

Patients with achalasia caused by the disease may undergo treatment with pneumatic dilatation of the esophagus or possibly esophagomyotomy.[62] Resection of the aperistaltic esophagus or colon may be necessary if symptoms warrant (Fig 33-37). A variety of procedures have been proposed, including Duhamel–Haddad, sigmoidectomy, low anterior resection, left hemicolectomy, and subtotal colectomy. The rectal wall is also often thickened and hypertrophied in addition to the dilatation in the proximal rectum. This may result in difficulty with a stapled anastomosis and lead to an increased recurrence rate. Therefore, one is advised to perform a low anterior resection with distal colorectal anastomosis.[39] Total colectomy with ileostomy is suggested if toxic megacolon is the indication for the operation.

Currently, there is no effective treatment to eradicate Chagas disease. Surgical resection of the affected segment of bowel is the mainstay of therapy. Drugs such as benznidazole and nifurtimox have been successfully used in patients with early presentation. However, once the neurologic and anatomical damage has been established there is no possibility for cure.[39]

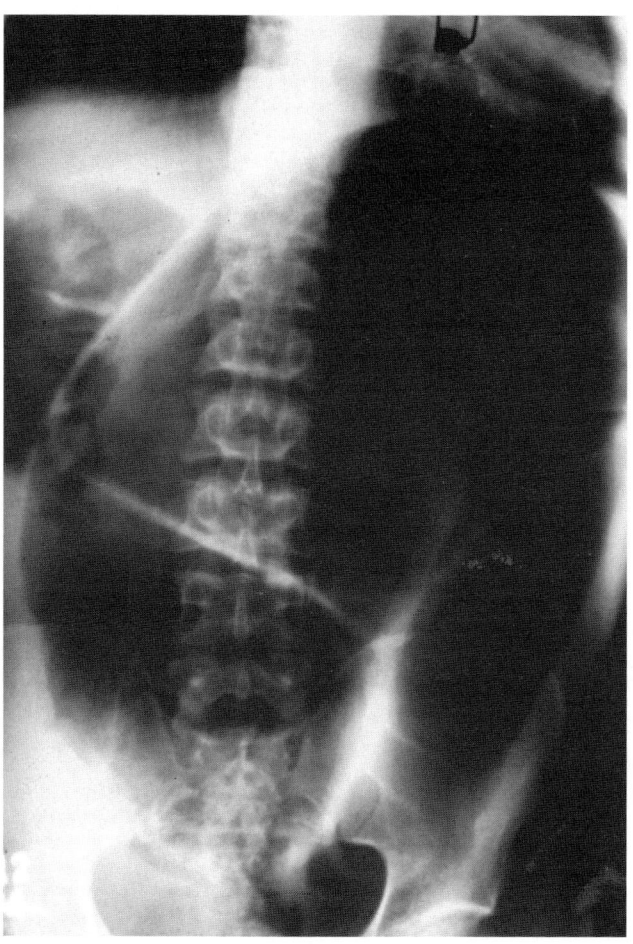

FIGURE 33-35. Chagasic megacolon. Plain abdominal x-ray reveals typical profound colonic dilatation.

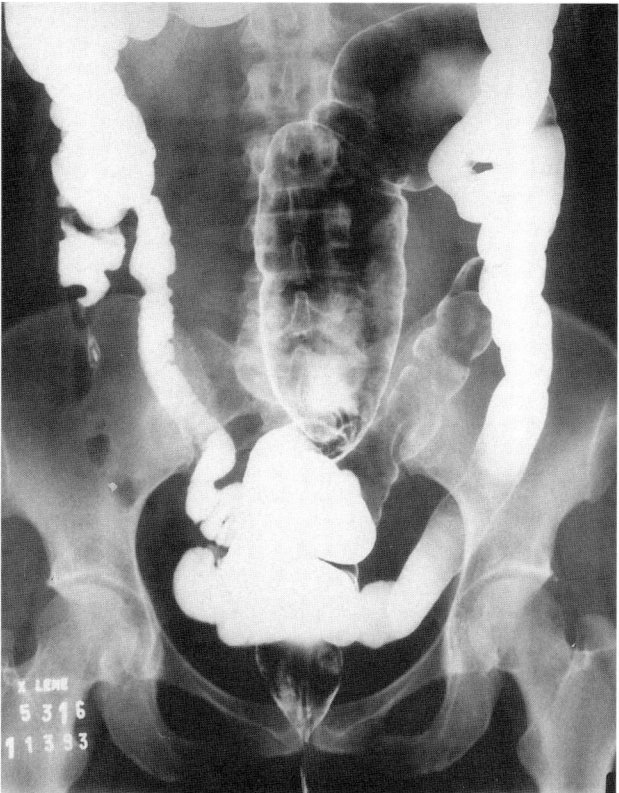

FIGURE 33-36. Chagas disease. Barium enema demonstrates segmental nature of the dilated colon.

Schistosomiasis or Bilharziosis

Schistosomiasis is a worldwide condition affecting more than 200 million people. The disease is caused by a trematode, a blood fluke that is seen in three forms: *Schistosoma mansoni, Schistosoma japonicum,* and *Schistosoma haematobium.* A snail host is required to complete the life cycle. The disease is frequently seen in tropical and subtropical climates.

Pathogenesis

The life cycle of the organism is of some interest. The infection is acquired by exposure to contaminated water containing the cercarial form (Figure 33-38).[62] The cercaria invades the skin, loses its tail, and enters the host's subcutaneous veins. From there it spreads to the heart and lungs and may produce a transient pneumonitis. Ultimately reaching the portal circulation, it grows, feeds, and differentiates into a male or a female form (Figure 33-39). Following fertilization, the worms migrate together into the terminal mesenteric venules. There, the female de-

posits the fertilized eggs. The egg secretes a lytic substance that permits it to migrate through the surrounding tissue, into the intestinal lumen, and into the stool.[62]

The three forms of the infestation are differentiated on the basis of the appearance of the *Schistosoma* ova (Figs. 33-40 and 33-41). The *S. mansoni* ovum has a prominent lateral spine, the *S. haematobium* has a projecting terminal spine, and the *S. japonicum* has no definite spine. *S. japonicum* preferentially invades the superior mesenteric veins, thus involving the small intestine and ascending colon, *S. mansoni* usually invades the inferior mesenteric veins, perforating through the descending colon, and *S. haematobium* tends to invade the bladder vessels, thus producing symptoms in the bladder, pelvic organs, and rectum.[62]

Signs and Symptoms

Symptoms are initially related to the cercarial dermatitis. This is a pruritic rash due to the cercaria penetrating the skin (see Chapter 19). The most common acute symptoms are fever, lethargy, and myalgia. Other complaints include cough, headache, lower abdominal pain, diarrhea, and anorexia. Usually the patient reports recent exposure to fresh water. Chronic manifestations of the dis-

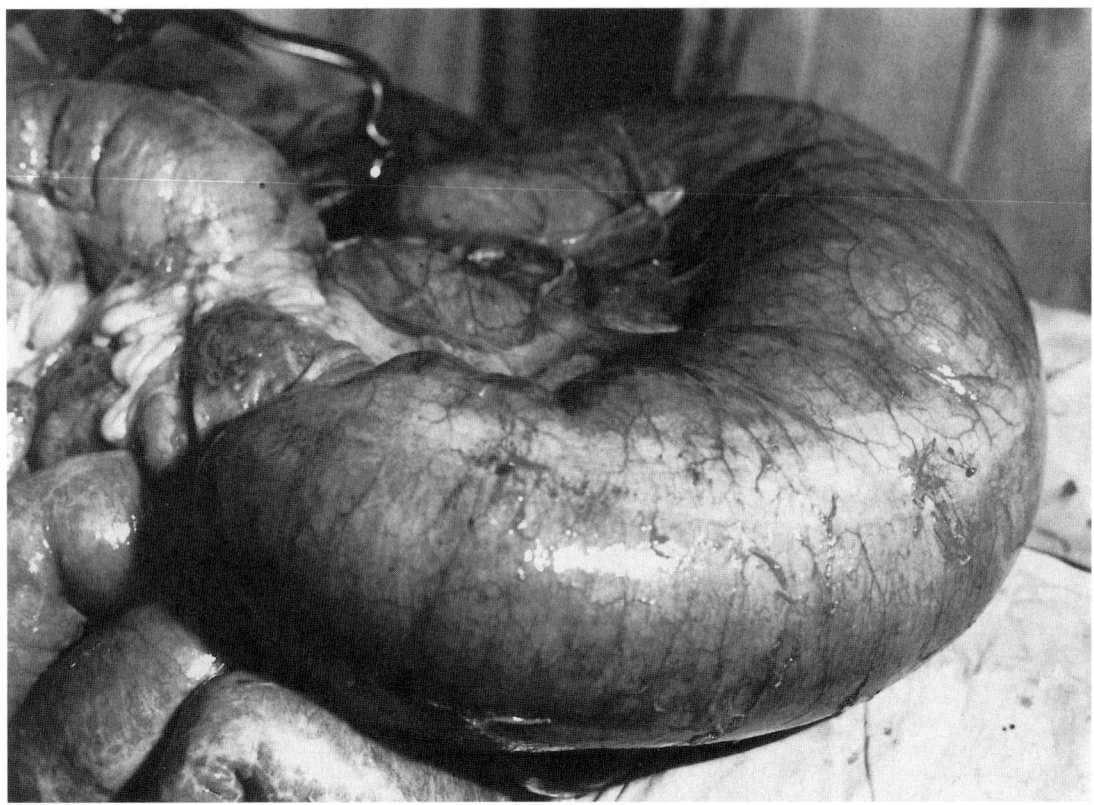

FIGURE 33-37. Resection of profoundly dilated Chagasic colon. (Courtesy of Fernando Jorge de Souza, M.D.)

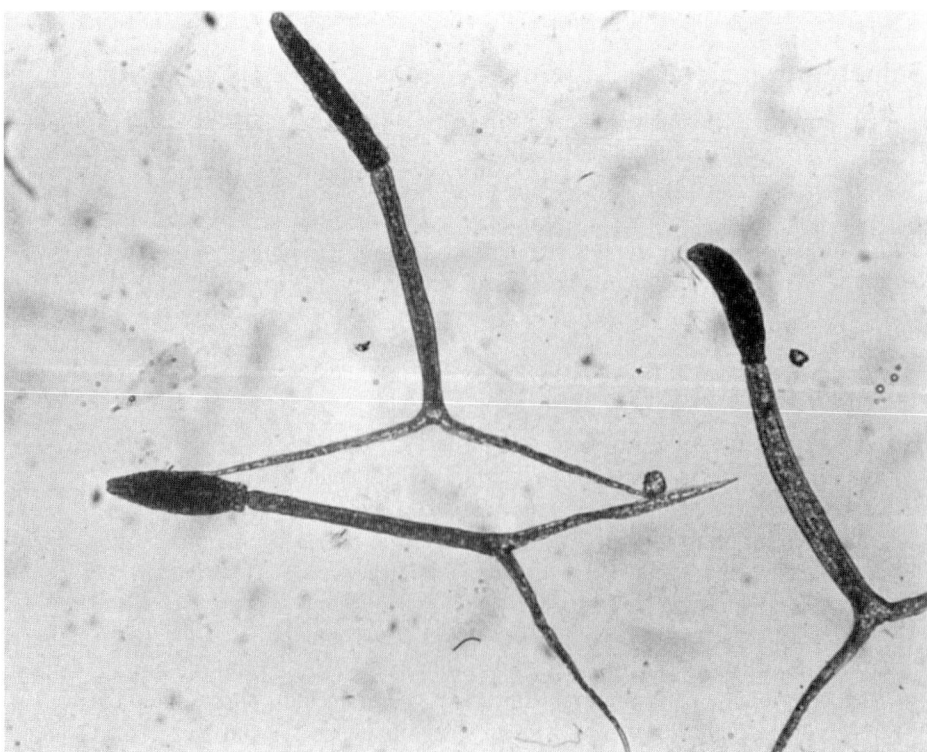

FIGURE 33-38. *Schistosoma*, fork-tailed cercaria. (Courtesy of Rudolf Garret, M.D.)

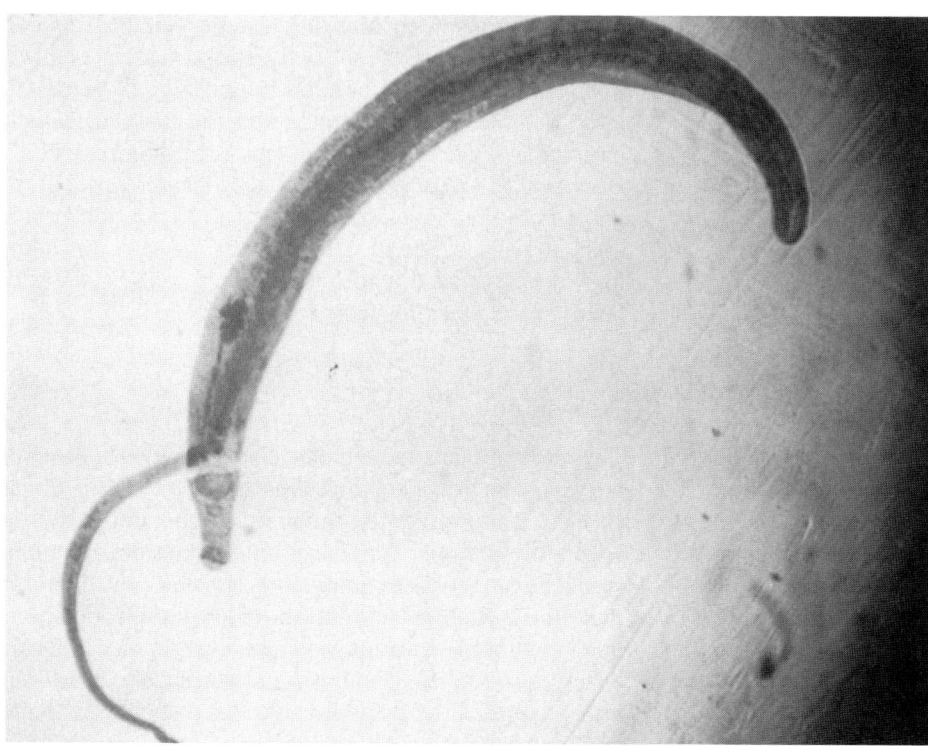

FIGURE 33-39. *Schistosoma mansoni*, adult male and female. The female occupies the male's genital groove. (Courtesy of Rudolf Garret, M.D.)

ease depend on which type is responsible for the infection. Bessa and associates reported 40 patients with colonic schistosomiasis due to *S. mansoni*, a common health problem in Egypt.[18] The primary complaint was severe diarrhea; three developed intestinal obstruction due to rectal or sigmoid stricture. Three fourths of the patients had a palpable mass.

Children are particularly susceptible to acute dysentery.[62,148] Fibrosis and thickening may result, and polyp formation may also occur. Other complications include intussusception and rectal prolapse. Portal involvement may produce granulomas, hepatosplenomegaly, and portal hypertension. Central nervous system complications can also develop.

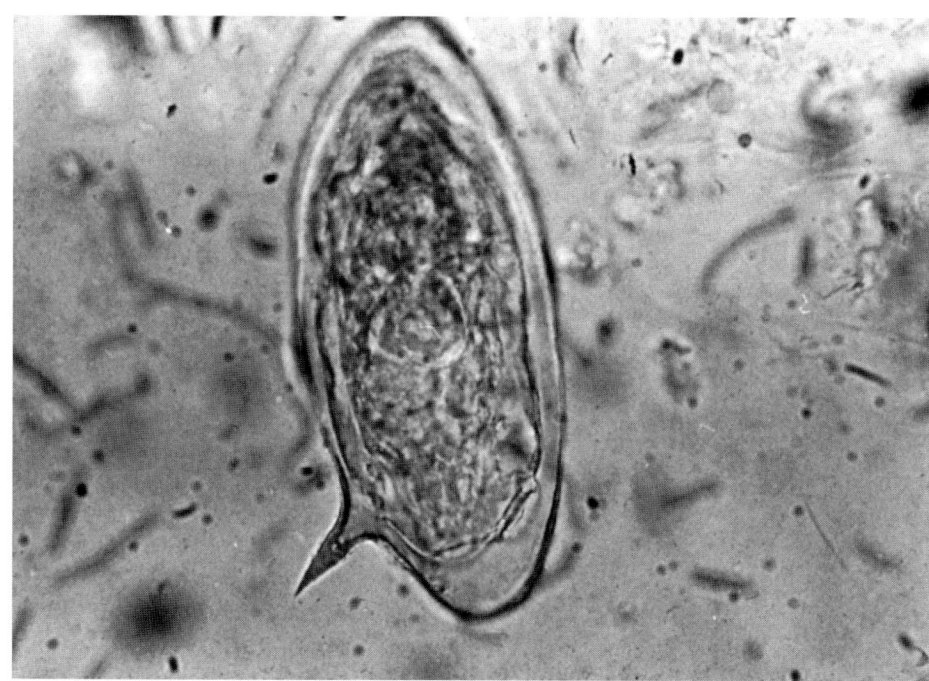

FIGURE 33-40. *S. mansoni* ovum. Note the lateral spine. (Courtesy of Rudolf Garret, M.D.)

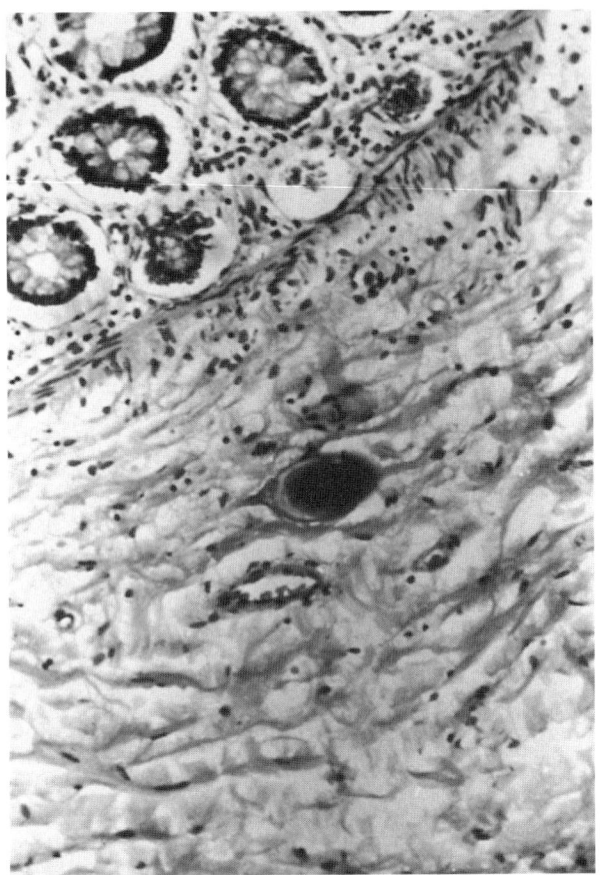

FIGURE 33-41. *S. haematobium* ovum in the rectal wall. Note the terminal spine. (Original magnification ×180; courtesy of Rudolf Garret, M.D.)

Diagnosis

The diagnosis is usually made by identification of the ova in fresh stool specimens. Rectal biopsy frequently reveals the presence of eggs in the mucosa or submucosa (Figs. 33-42 and 33-43). The diagnosis may also be made by means of a wet preparation; the biopsy specimen is compressed between two cover slips and examined for the ova (Figure 33-44). The urinary excretion of the eggs (usually *S. hematobium*) is more frequently found between 10 AM and 2 PM.[148] The urine or stool quantitative evaluation of the eggs suggests the severity of the infection.[148] Fewer than 100 eggs/g is a mild infection; more than 400 eggs/g is considered a heavy infection. The acute infection is often associated with an eosinophilia.

Serologic evaluation is a useful epidemiologic tool. However, it cannot differentiate past infection. The Falcon assay test (FAST), enzyme-linked immunoassay, and immunoblot assays are all highly specific for all species of schistosoma.[148] A skin test and numerous serologic tests are also available for the diagnosis; the complement fixation test and indirect hemagglutination test may be quite valuable.[62]

Colonoscopy with biopsy has been demonstrated to confirm the diagnosis, especially when ova are present.[214] Polyps are not uncommon, and since large or pedunculated ones tend not to regress but to cause persistent bleeding, colonoscopy–polypectomy is recommended.[17,180] However, one must expect that additional polyps will regrow since the mucosa does not revert to normal. Rectocolic and urinary tract calcifications, as seen on radiologic studies, are felt to be associated with a clinically latent or mild form of schistosomiasis.[73]

Treatment

The medical management of schistosomiasis is not without risk. The drugs employed differ, depending on which species is involved. A number of chemotherapeutic agents are variously effective and include praziquantel, metriphonate, oxamniquine (not currently available in the United States), sodium antimony dimercaptosuccinate (Astiban), antimony potassium tartrate (Tartar emetic), stibophen (Fuadin), and niridazole. However, praziquantel is the drug of choice.[148] It should be made available and affordable in endemic areas in order to control and ultimately to eradicate this disease.

Treatment of the colonic complications involves a variety of resective and diversionary procedures. Anastomosis without a colostomy appears to be associated with a prohibitively high incidence of leakage.[18]

Relationship to Carcinoma

The risk of cancer in patients with schistosomiasis is well-known, especially in those infected with *S. haematobium*. The malignancy with this type often occurs in the urinary bladder. This concern is especially evident in the Middle East and parts of Africa where there is a high incidence of schistosomiasis.[14] However, patients with long-standing schistosomal colitis are at an increased risk for the development of carcinoma, although this applies primarily to *S. japonicum*.[180] Ming-Chai and colleagues reported a retrospective study of 60 patients with schistosomal granulomatous disease of the large intestine without obvious evidence of carcinoma and noted that 36 had mild to severe dysplasia.[177] The authors regarded the changes as presumptive evidence for the premalignant potential of schistosomal colitis, and felt that the findings were analogous to those observed in patients with long-standing chronic ulcerative colitis. Although as of this writing there are no published studies of the use of colonoscopy in the diagnosis of premalignant change and the performance of prophylactic colectomy on the basis of such change, it may be anticipated that such a protocol will ultimately appear.

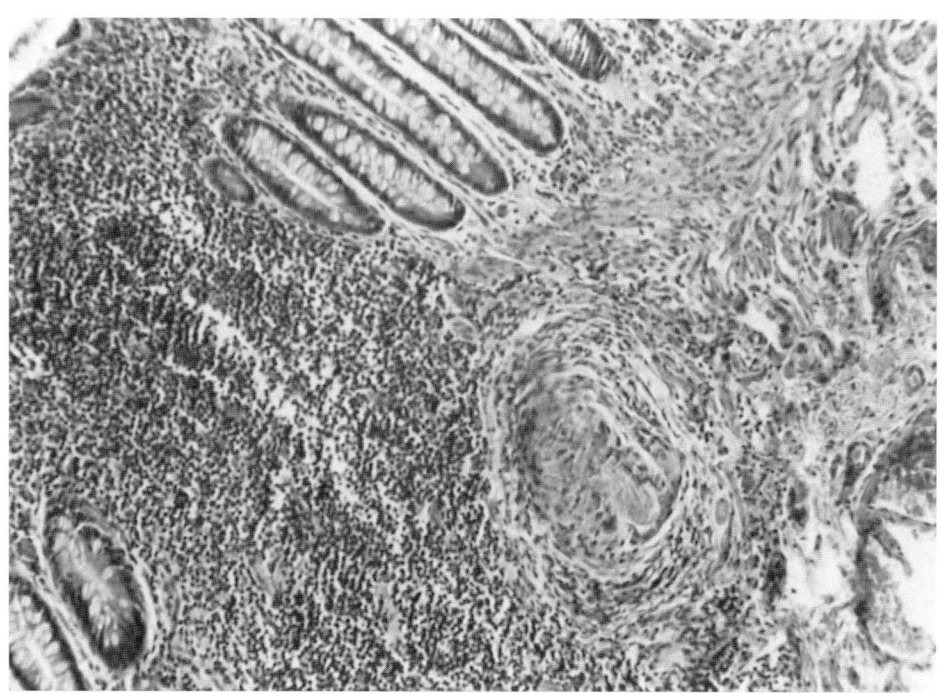

FIGURE 33-42. *S. mansoni* in the wall of the rectum. (Original magnification ×250; courtesy of Rudolf Garret, M.D.)

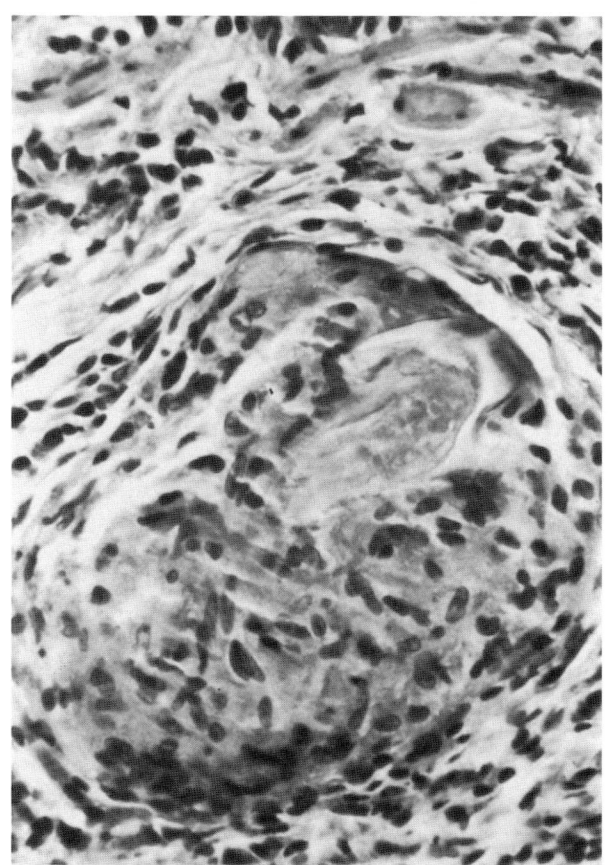

FIGURE 33-43. *S. mansoni* in the wall of the rectum surrounded by epithelioid cells. (Original magnification ×600; courtesy of Rudolf Garret, M.D.)

Relationship to Portal Hypertension

Cirrhosis with portal hypertension may produce massive hemorrhage from varices that requires emergency therapy. The initial management includes endoscopic ligation or sclerosis of the bleeding variceal vein.[19] However, failure of endoscopic control requires the placement of a transjugular intrahepatic portosystemic shunt. Long-term management of portal hypertension includes repeated endoscopic treatment, long-term β-blockers,[234] surgical shunt, and liver transplantation. The use of octreotide has also been reported as an effective measure for the management of bleeding.[71]

An approach has been suggested that involves cannulation of the portal vein, followed by trapping of the adult worms in a filter system (Figure 33-45). Administration of antimony potassium tartrate has been demonstrated to increase the yield of the worms removed by stimulating migration into the portal circulation.

Ascariasis

Ascariasis is caused by a large round worm, *Ascaris lumbricoides* (Figure 33-46). The disease is an enormous problem, with an estimated 25% of the world's population affected.[202] The condition is endemic in tropical and subtropical areas, but epidemics have been reported in Europe and even in small, focal areas of the United States. It is estimated that approximately 4 million people in the United States are infected with this worm.

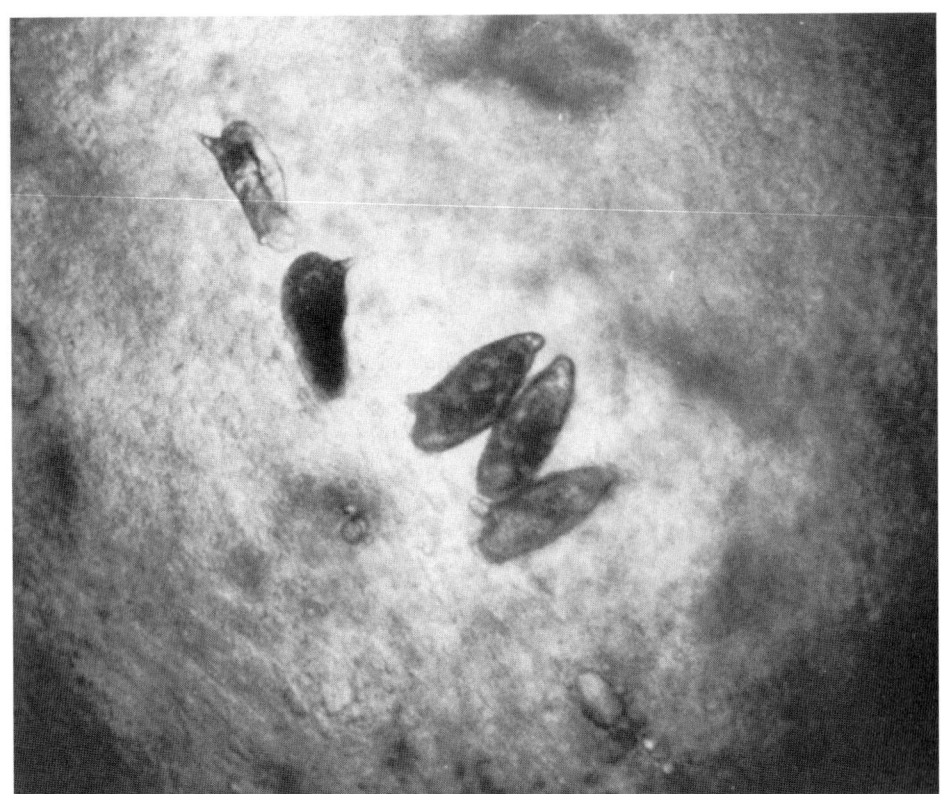

FIGURE 33-44. *S. mansoni* ova, wet preparation. (Courtesy of Rudolf Garret, M.D.)

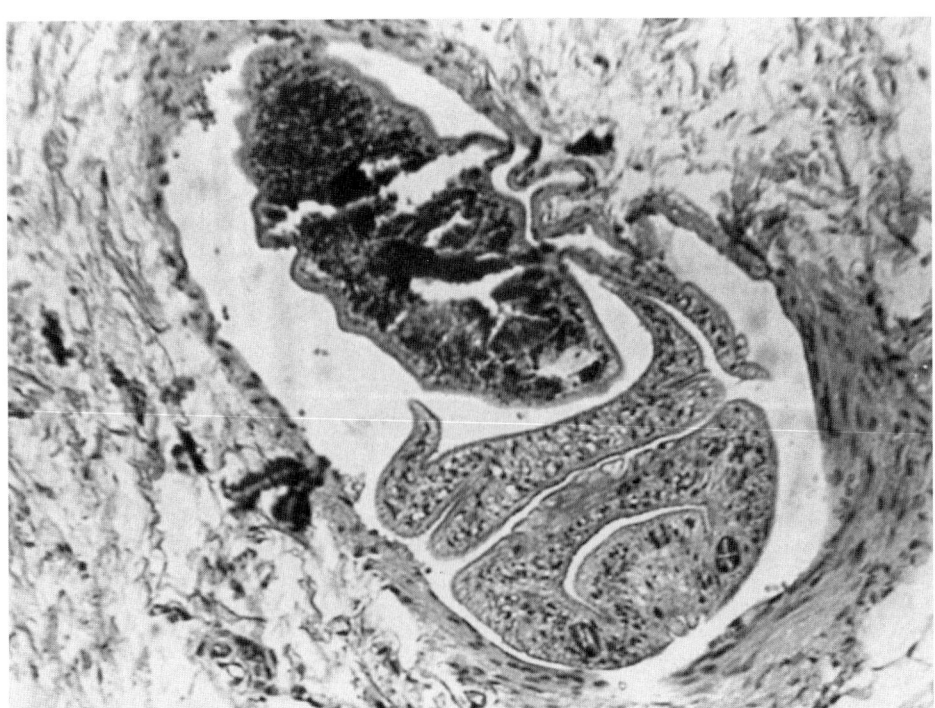

FIGURE 33-45. *S. mansoni* adult in a mesenteric vein. (Original magnification ×133; courtesy of Rudolf Garret, M.D.)

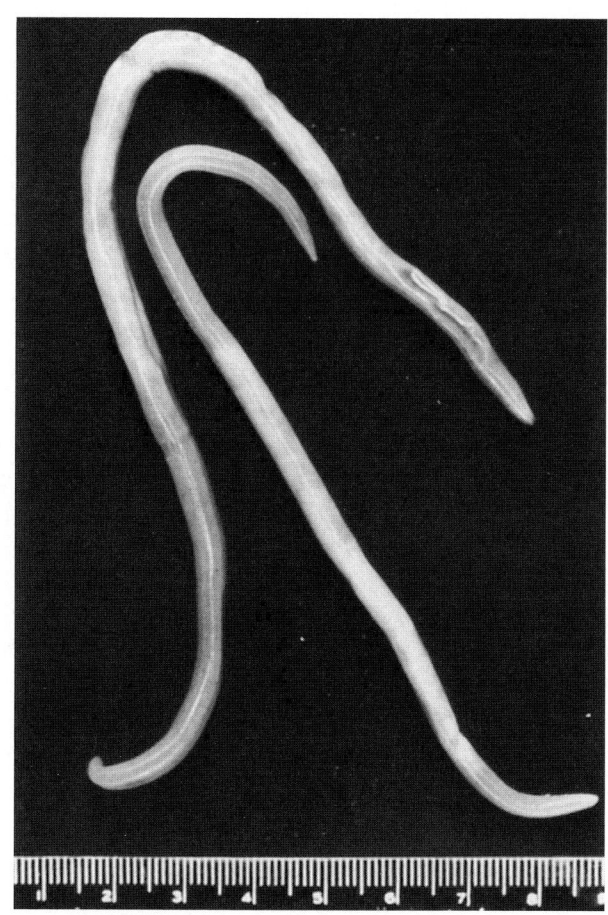

FIGURE 33-46. *Ascaris lumbricoides*, adult worms. (Courtesy of Rudolf Garret, M.D.)

Pathophysiology

Infection occurs from ingestion of the eggs in contaminated food and drink (Figure 33-47). Following ingestion, the larvae emerge from the ovum and migrate through the wall of the small intestine into the portal venous system, passing through the liver and into the lungs.[31] Ultimately the larvae migrate through the capillaries, into the alveoli and the bronchioles, and are coughed up and swallowed. In the small intestine they develop into the adult worm.

Symptoms and Signs

Most individuals infected with *A. lumbricoides* are asymptomatic. Early symptoms (4 to 16 days after ingestion of the egg) are related to the tissue-migratory phase and include fever, cough, and wheezing. During the late phase (6 to 8 weeks after contamination) patients present with gastrointestinal symptoms resulting from mechanical irritation of the adult parasite. Vague abdominal complaints, such as cramping, nausea, and vomiting are common. The migration of the worm can lead to pancreatitis, cholecystitis, biliary obstruction, bowel obstruction, and even appendicitis. The patient occasionally eliminates the parasite through the anus or through the mouth and nose, a particularly unpleasant event in children.[132,202] Bowel perforation is unlikely to be due to this condition, unless there is an associated ulceration of the intestine such as is seen with amebiasis or typhoid.[67] Small bowel volvulus can also occur.[289] Additionally, allergic reactions (asthma, urticaria, and conjunctivitis) may be the result of absorption of toxins from the worm.[31]

Physical examination may reveal minimal signs, but obviously in the presence of intestinal obstruction, abdominal distention and diffuse tenderness may be noted. Occasionally, perforation can ensue, and the patient will present with signs of peritonitis.

Diagnosis

The diagnosis of ascariasis is made by locating the eggs, larvae, or adult worms. It usually takes approximately 2 months from the time of infection before the eggs appear in the stool. The worms may also be recovered from the sputum and occasionally from emesis.[31] Laboratory studies are usually of no value, since the only significant abnormality is the presence of an eosinophilia.

Small bowel x-ray films may reveal the presence of the worms in the distal ileum. Characteristically, the gastrointestinal tract of the worm may be identified because it is filled with the contrast material (Figure 33-48). Ultrasonography has been found to be useful in the diagnosis of intestinal obstruction secondary to ascariasis. Characteristic sonographic features of railway track sign and bulls-eye appearance are helpful in making the diagnosis.[286]

Treatment

The treatment of ascariasis includes mebendazole (100 mg orally, twice daily, for three days), albendazole (400 mg, single oral dose, repeated in 3 weeks if not cured), and piperazine citrate (3.5 g orally, daily, for 2 days). Follow-up care is suggested to confirm cure.[288]

If an operation is required, and perforation has not occurred, it is best to attempt manipulation of the worms through the ileum into the cecum rather than to open the bowel. Resection is advised if required, as opposed to enterotomy and extraction of the worms (Figure 33-49). The instillation of intraluminal vermifuge intraoperatively has been reported to minimize the risk of postoperative worm migration through suture lines and anastomoses.[290] Early clinical diagnosis together with prompt surgery for ob-

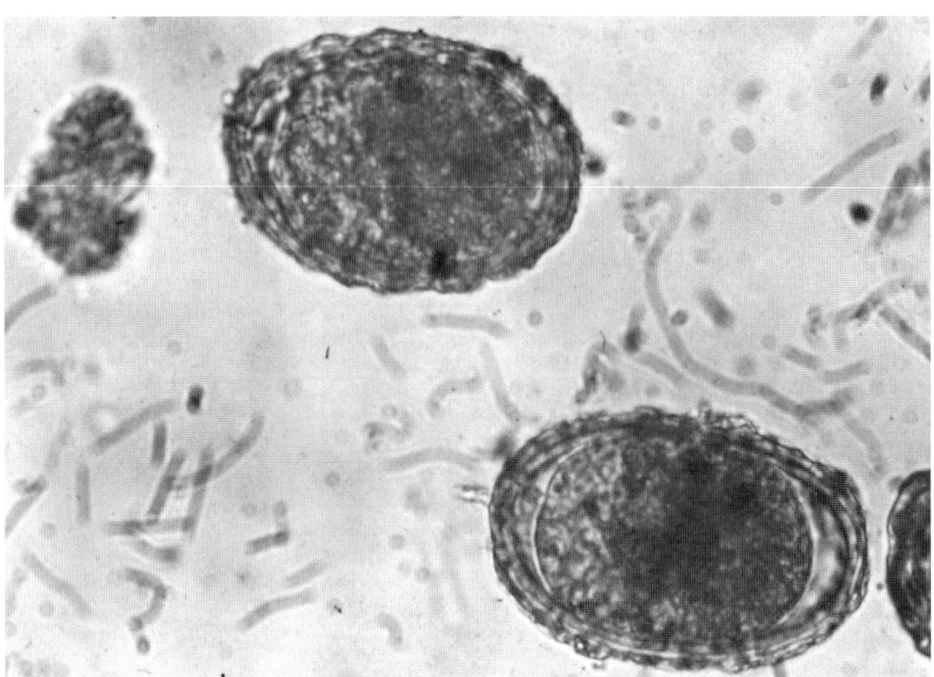

FIGURE 33-47. *A. lumbricoides,* ova. (Courtesy of Rudolf Garret, M.D.)

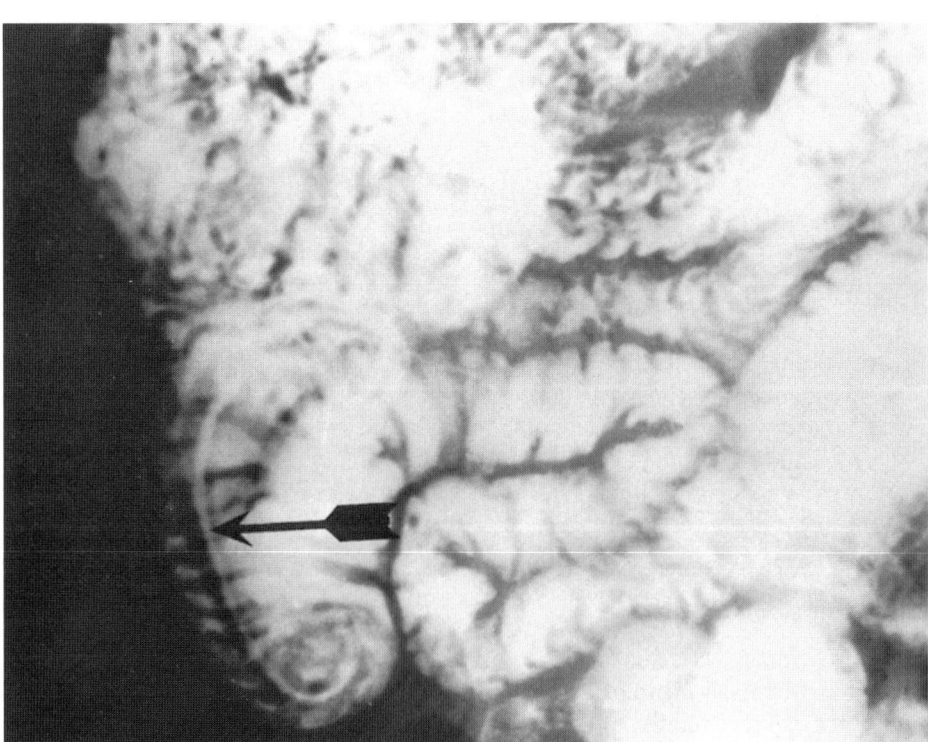

FIGURE 33-48. Ascariasis. Small bowel x-ray demonstrates *Ascaris.* The gastrointestinal tract of the worm can be identified (*arrow*).

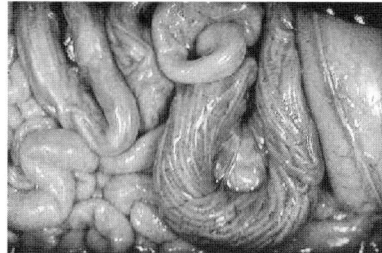

FIGURE 33-49. Multiple loops of small bowel containing innumerable, large round worms. (Courtesy of T. Cristina Sardinha, M.D.)

struction are important in reducing a high mortality rate in this potentially devastating condition.[4,286]

Strongyloidiasis

Strongyloidiasis is a parasitic disease often seen in tropical climates and caused by another roundworm, *Strongyloides stercoralis*. The condition usually occurs in the small bowel, but the colon may occasionally be the site of involvement. Somewhat similar to hookworm, the larvae penetrate the skin and are carried by way of the circulation to the lungs. They then rupture into the alveoli and develop into adolescent worms.[31] The swallowed female invades the small intestinal mucosa where it remains, depositing eggs (Figure 33-50).

Symptoms referable to the intestinal tract may be minimal, or the patient may complain of diarrhea, nausea, vomiting, and abdominal pain. Rectal pain and tenesmus have been reported in association with involvement in that area, and a proctitis may be present on sigmoidoscopy.[218] The clinical syndrome of hyperinfection with this parasite (overwhelming proliferation of the worms) may be seen in immunocompromised patients and is characterized by profound abdominal symptoms and signs and by secondary infection.[293] Those with lymphomas and leukemia are at greatest risk.

The diagnosis is established by examination of duodenal secretions; suction biopsy of the duodenum is a poor way of finding the parasite.[31] Additionally, strongyloidiasis can be diagnosed by finding the larvae in the feces; this is the only intestinal nematode from which larvae rather than eggs are identified in the stool.

In the severe form of the disease, mortality is usually due to dehydration and electrolyte imbalance; the result of vomiting and diarrhea.[81] Strongyloidiasis can be effectively treated in the acute and chronic phases with ivermectin (200 µg/kg/day, orally, for 2 days). Albendazole is the second-line therapy, and thiabendazole is used for disseminated illness or mixed helminthic infections.[206]

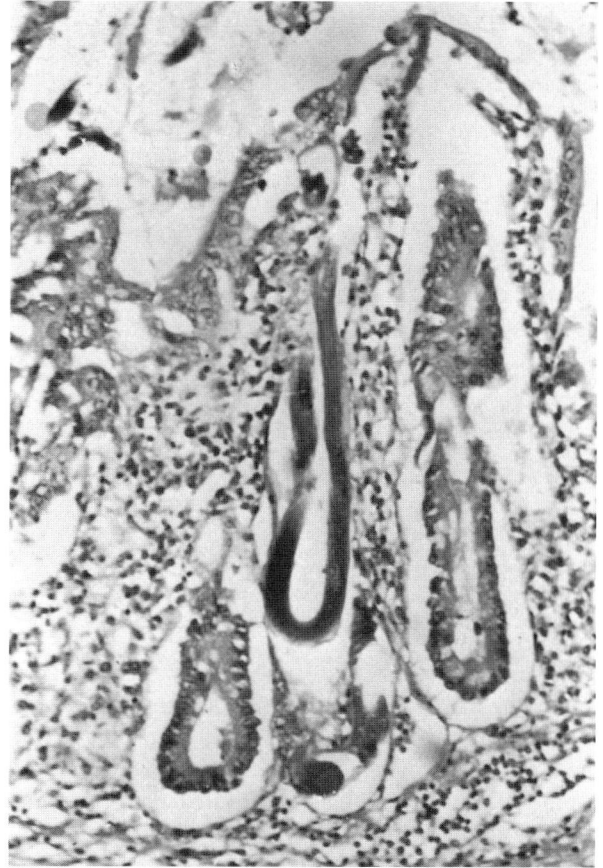

FIGURE 33-50. *Strongyloides stercoralis.* Larvae and eggs in intestinal mucosa. (Original magnification ×280; courtesy of Rudolf Garret, M.D.)

Trichuriasis

Trichuriasis is caused by the roundworm *Trichuris trichiura*, the so-called whipworm. Its common name is misleading because the whip or tail is actually its head (Figure 33-51). In some areas of the world, up to 90% of the population is infected. It may, in fact, be the most commonly recognized intestinal helminth in people returning from tropical areas.[292]

The egg has a characteristic barrel shape with a nonstaining prominence at each end (Figure 33-52). Ingestion of food or water containing the eggs is the method of contamination. In the intestinal tract the eggs are digested, releasing larvae into the small intestine. The larvae reside in the mucosa for several days, and then relocate to the cecal area where they mature (Figure 33-53).[31]

Patients may be virtually asymptomatic or have moderate or severe infective symptoms, depending on the extent of involvement. Lower abdominal pain, diarrhea, and rectal bleeding may be reported. Nausea, vomiting, flatulence, abdominal distention, headache, and weight loss are also noted.[292]

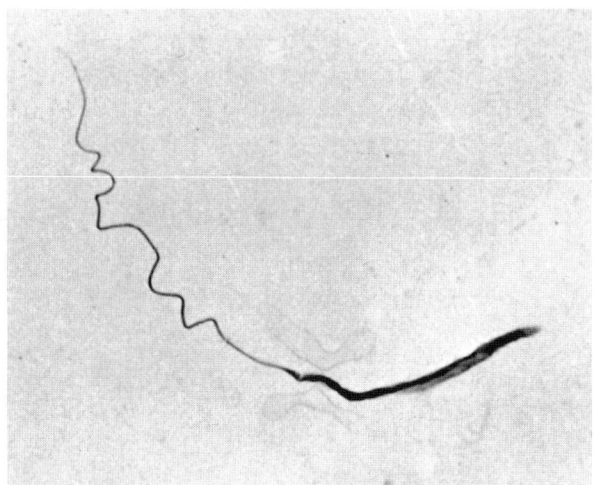

FIGURE 33-51. Adult *Trichuris trichiura*. Note the slender neck, which gives the worm its common name, whipworm. (Courtesy of Rudolf Garret, M.D.)

Appendicitis and rectal prolapse may be a consequence of whipworm infection.[31] A number of worms together, creating blockage of the appendiceal lumen, accounts for the signs and symptoms of appendicitis. Rectal prolapse is thought to result from straining at defecation due to the massive number of worms in the rectum.[292] *T. trichiura* eggs have also been identified in a patient with an anal abscess.[75] Furthermore, the worm

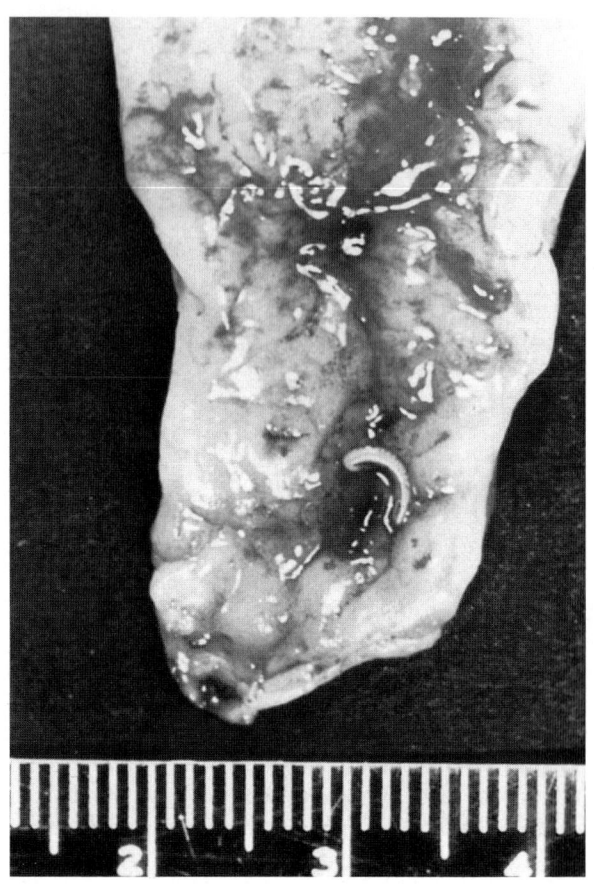

FIGURE 33-53. *T. trichiura* (whipworm) in the lumen of the appendix. (Courtesy of Rudolf Garret, M.D.)

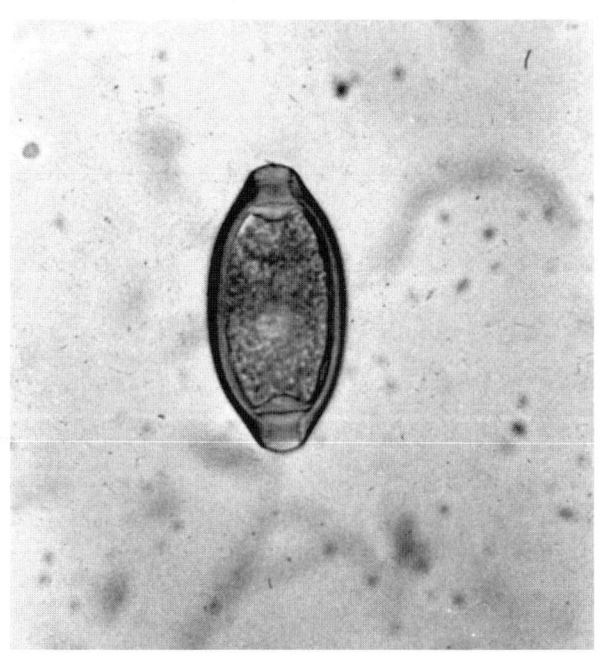

FIGURE 33-52. *T. trichiura* ovum. Note the characteristic barrel shape with a "plug" at either end. (Courtesy of Rudolf Garret, M.D.)

has been demonstrated to suck blood from the colon, and it is estimated that 0.005 mL may be lost per day per worm.[292] Hence, severe infestation may cause anemia. However, significant blood loss in the adult has only rarely been recognized.

The diagnosis is made by the identification of the characteristic eggs in the stool. Egg counts are useful in determining the degree of infection and for evaluating the efficacy of treatment.[292] Barium enema examination may reveal evidence of the worms on air-contrast study.

Treatment with mebendazole (Vermox) has been found to be highly effective against *Trichuris* as well as against other worms.[31] Albendazole is an alternative therapeutic option.

Anisakiasis

Anisakiasis or herring worm disease is caused by species of the marine roundworm, *Anisakidae*. The adult nematodes are intestinal parasites of marine mammals, such as seals and dolphins. When inadequately prepared fish is eaten, the larvae penetrate the mucosa of the stomach,

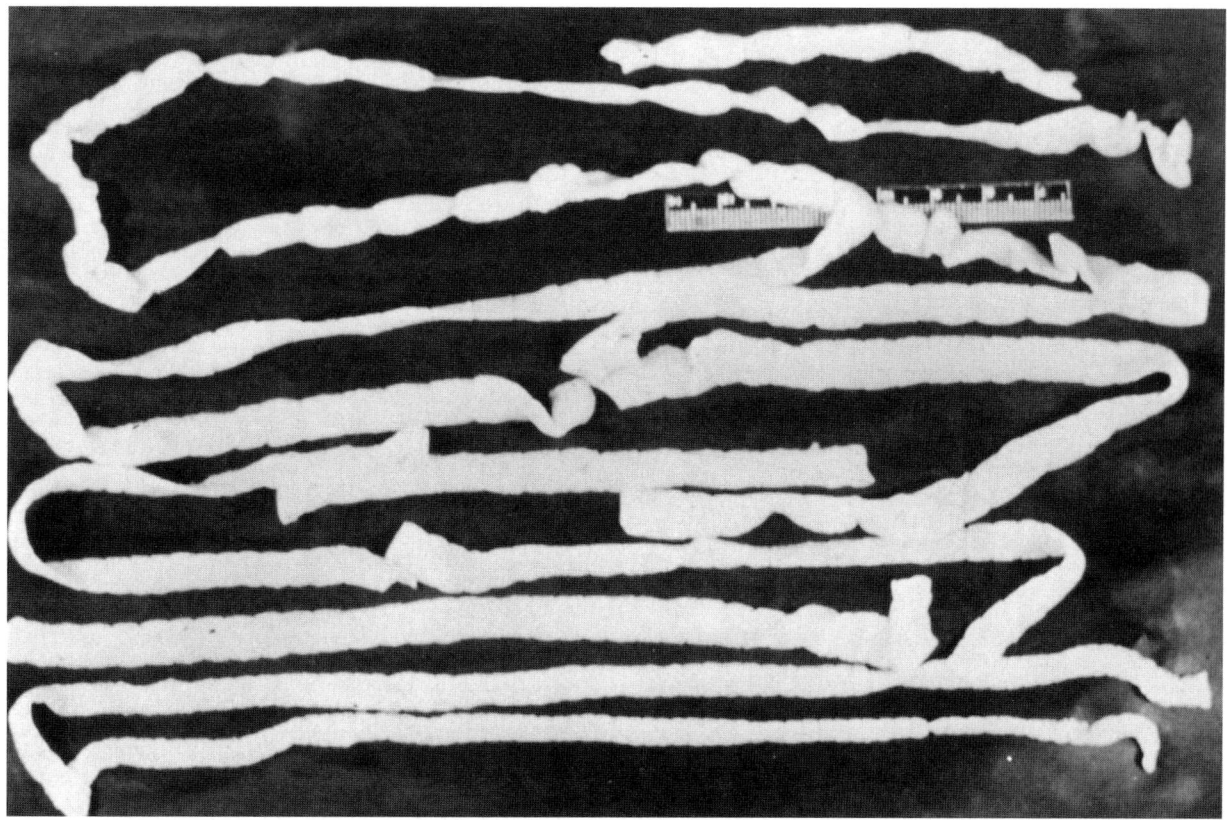

FIGURE 33-54. *Taenia saginata*. Beef tapeworm adult. (Courtesy of Rudolf Garret, M.D.)

the small intestine, or even the colon.[279] Patients present with acute abdominal pain together with an intestinal obstruction or appendicitis-like syndrome. Findings can mimic those of regional enteritis.

Verhamme and Ramboer suggest that a high index of suspicion must be maintained, requiring a carefully obtained history, if one is to avoid emergency laparotomy and bowel resection.[279] Most symptoms of infection with this parasite will resolve spontaneously.

Tapeworm (*Taenia saginata*)

The beef tapeworm is by far the most common taeniid in humans. It is found throughout the world except where meat is prohibited for religious reasons.[181] The adult, an hermaphroditic cestode, can achieve several meters in length (Figure 33-54). The eggs are spherical in shape and cannot be distinguished from those of the pork tapeworm (Figure 33-55).

Abdominal discomfort, nausea, vomiting, cutaneous sensitivity, headache, and malaise are reported symptoms, but most infections are asymptomatic.[181] Because of the large size of the worm obstructive symptoms can

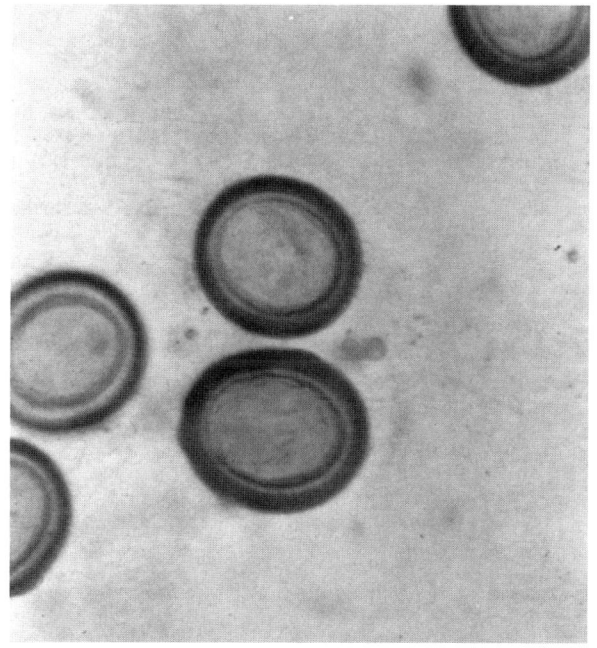

FIGURE 33-55. *T. saginata* eggs. (Courtesy of Rudolf Garret, M.D.)

occasionally develop. The recommended treatment for taeniasis is praziquantel.

REFERENCES

1. Abel ME, Chiu YS, Russell TR, et al. Gastrointestinal tuberculosis: report of four cases. *Dis Colon Rectum* 1990;33: 886.
2. Addison NV. Abdominal tuberculosis—a disease revived. *Ann R Coll Surg Engl* 1983;65:105.
3. Akdamar K, Martin RJ, Ichinose H. Syphilitic proctitis. *Dig Dis* 1977;22:701.
4. Akgun Y. Intestinal obstruction caused by *Ascaris lumbricoides*. *Dis Colon Rectum* 1996;39:1159.
5. Allason-Jones E, Mindel A, Sargeaunt P, et al. *Entamoeba histolytica* as a commensal intestinal parasite in homosexual men. *N Engl J Med* 1986;315:353.
6. Anand BS, Nanda R, Sachdev GK. Response of tuberculous stricture to antituberculous treatment. *Gut* 1988;29:62.
7. Anderson JB, Tanner AH, Brodribb AJM. Toxic megacolon due to *Campylobacter* colitis. *Int J Colorect Dis* 1986;1:58.
8. Appleton GVN, Williamson RCN. Hypoplasia of defunctioned rectum. *Br J Surg* 1989;76:787.
9. Babb RR, Trollope ML. Acute fulminating amoebic colitis: survival after total colectomy. *Gut* 1985;26:301.
10. Bartlett JG. Treatment of *Clostridium difficile* colitis. *Gastroenterology* 1985;89:1192.
11. Bassi O, Cosa G, Colavolpe A, et al. Primary syphilis of the rectum—endoscopic and clinical features: report of a case. *Dis Colon Rectum* 1991;34:1024.
12. Bayless TM, Giardello FM, Lazenby A, et al. Collagenous colitis [Editorial]. *Mayo Clin Proc* 1987;62:740.
13. Beard CB, Pye G, Steurer FJ, et al. Chagas disease in a domestic transmission cycle, southern Texas, USA, 2003. Available at: *www.cdc.gov/ncidod/EID/vol9no1/02–0217.htm.* Accessed 2004.
14. Bedwani R, Renganathan E, El Kwhsky F, et al. Schistosomiasis and the risk of bladder cancer in Alexandria, Egypt. *Br J Cancer* 1998;77:1186.
15. Bennish ML, Azad AK, Yousefzadeh D. Intestinal obstruction during shigellosis: incidence, clinical features, risk factors, and outcome. *Gastroenterology* 1991;101:626.
16. Bereswill S, Kist M. Recent development in *Campylobacter* pathogenesis. *Curr Opin Infect Dis* 2003;16:487.
17. Bessa SM, Helmy I, El-Kharadly Y. Colorectal schistosomiasis: endoscopic polypectomy. *Dis Colon Rectum* 1983;26: 772.
18. Bessa SM, Helmy I, Mekky F, et al. Colorectal schistosomiasis: clinicopathologic study and management. *Dis Colon Rectum* 1979;22:390.
19. Besson I, Ingrand P, Person B, et al. Sclerotherapy with or without octreotide for acute variceal bleeding. *N Engl J Med* 1995;333:555.
20. Bhargava DK, Shriniwas, Chopra P, et al. Peritoneal tuberculosis: laparoscopic patterns and its diagnostic accuracy. *Am J Gastroenterol* 1992;87:109.
21. Bischoff SC, Mayer J, Nguyen QT, et al. Immunohistological assessment of intestinal eosinophile activation in patients with eosinophilic gastroenteritis and inflammatory bowel disease. *Am J Gastroenterol* 1999;94:3521.
22. Black RE, Jackson RJ, Tsai T, et al. Epidemic *Yersinia enterocolitica* infection due to contaminated chocolate milk. *N Engl J Med* 1978;298:76.
23. Blaser MJ, Reller LB. *Campylobacter* enteritis. *N Engl J Med* 1981;305:1444.
24. Bluth EI, McVay LV III, Gathright JB Jr. Ultrasonic characteristics of ileal tuberculosis. *Dis Colon Rectum* 1985;28: 613.
25. Bohr J, Tysk C, Eriksson S, et al. Collagenous colitis: a retrospective study of clinical presentation and treatment in 163 patients. *Gut* 1996;39:846.
26. Bo-Linn GW, Vendrell DD, Lee E, et al. An evaluation of the significance of microscopic colitis in patients with chronic diarrhea. *J Clin Invest* 1985;75:1559.
27. Bottone EJ, Keush GT. Bacterial agents of diarrheal diseases. *API Species* 1981;5:29.
28. Bovee LP, Peerbooms PG, van den Hoek JA. Shigellosis, a sexually transmitted disease in homosexual men. *Ned Tijdschr Geneeskd* 2003;147:2438.
29. Box JC, Tucker J, Watne AL, et al. Eosinophilic colitis presenting as a left-sided colocolonic intussusception with secondary large bowel obstruction: an uncommon entity with a rare presentation. *Am Surg* 1997;63:741.
30. Bradbury AW, Barrett S. Surgical aspects of *Clostridium difficile* colitis. *Br J Surg* 1997;84:150.
31. Brandborg LL. Parasitic diseases. In: Sleisenger MH, Fordtran JS, eds. *Gastrointestinal disease*, 2nd ed. Philadelphia: WB Saunders, 1978:1154.
32. Brandt MM, Bogner PN, Franklin GA. Intestinal tuberculosis presenting as a bowel obstruction. *Am J Surg* 2002; 183:290.
33. Breiter JR, Hajjar J-J. Segmental tuberculosis of the colon diagnosed by colonoscopy. *Am J Gastroenterol* 1981;76: 369.
34. Burbige EJ, Radigan JJ. Antibiotic-associated colitis with normal appearing rectum. *Dis Colon Rectum* 1981;24:198.
35. Burnham WR, Reeve RS, Finch RG. *Entamoeba histolytica* infection in male homosexuals. *Gut* 1980;21:1097.
36. Butzler JP, Oosterom J. *Campylobacter*: pathogenicity and significance in foods. *Int J Food Microbiol* 1991;12:1.
37. Cappell MS, Mandell W, Grimes MM, et al. Gastrointestinal histoplasmosis. *Dig Dis Sci* 1988;33:353.
38. Cappell MS, Simon T. Fulminant acute colitis following a self-administered hydrofluoric acid enema. *Am J Gastroenterol* 1993;88:122.
39. Carlier Y, Luquetti AO, Dias JCP, et al. Chagas disease (American trypanosomiasis), 2004. Available at: *www.emedicine.com/MED/topic327.htm.*
40. Carpenter HA, Talley NJ. The importance of clinicopathological correlation in the diagnosis of inflammatory conditions of the colon: histological patterns with clinical implications. *Am J Gastroenterol* 2000;95:878.
41. Carter FM, Mitchell CK. Toxic epidermal necrolysis—an unusual cause of colonic perforation. *Dis Colon Rectum* 1993;36:773.
42. Catterall RD. Sexually transmitted diseases of the anus and rectum. *Clin Gastroenterol* 1975;4:659.
43. Cermeno JR, Hernandez de Cuesta I, Uzcategui O, et al. *Balantidium coli* in an HIV-infected patient with chronic diarrhea. *AIDS* 2003;17:941.
44. Chande N, McDonald J, MacDonald J. Interventions for treating collagenous colitis. *Cochrane Database Syst Rev* 2004;1:CD003575.
45. Chawla S. Tuberculosis of the colon. In: Greenbaum EI, ed. *Radiographic atlas of colon disease*. Chicago: Year Book Medical Publishers, 1980:557.
46. Chen DF, Chao IM, Huang SH. Neutropenic colitis with cecal perforation during anti-thyroid therapy. *J Formos Med Assoc* 2003;102:644.
47. Chen X-M, Keithly JS, Paya CV, et al. Cryptosporidiosis. *N Engl J Med* 2002;346:1723.
48. Chester AC, MacMurray FG, Restifo MD, et al. Giardiasis as a chronic disease. *Dig Dis Sci* 1985;30:215.
49. Chijide VM, Woeltje KF. Balantidiasis, 2004. Available at: *http://emedicine.com/med/topic203.htm.*
50. Chun D, Chandrasoma P, Kiyabu M. Fulminant amebic colitis: a morphologic study of four cases. *Dis Colon Rectum* 1994;37:535.
51. Church JM, Fazio VW. A role for colonic stasis in the pathogenesis of disease related to *Clostridium difficile*. *Dis Colon Rectum* 1986;29:804.
52. Cintron JR, Del Pino A, Duarte B, et al. Abdominal actinomycosis: report of two cases and review of the literature. *Dis Colon Rectum* 1996;39:105.

53. Clarkston WK, Bonacini M, Peterson I. Colitis due to *Histoplasma capsulatum* in the acquired immune deficiency syndrome. *Am J Gastroenterol* 1991;86:913.
54. Cone JB, Wetzel W. Toxic megacolon secondary to pseudomembranous colitis. *Dis Colon Rectum* 1982;25: 478.
55. Cone LA, Woodard DR, Potts BE, et al. An update on the acquired immunodeficiency syndrome (AIDS): associated disorders of the alimentary tract. *Dis Colon Rectum* 1986; 29:60.
56. Connolly GM, Dryden MS, Shanson DC, et al. Cryptosporidial diarrhoea in AIDS and its treatment. *Gut* 1988;29:593.
57. Couppie P, Sobesky M, Aznar C, et al. Histoplasmosis and acquired immunodeficiency syndrome: a study of prognostic factors. *Clin Infect Dis* 2004;38:134–138.
58. Cover TL, Aber RC. *Yersinia enterocolitica. N Engl J Med* 1989;321:16.
59. Crowson TD, Hines C Jr. Amebiasis diagnosed by colonoscopy. *Gastrointest Endosc* 1978;24:254.
60. Crump JA, Youssef FG, Luby SP, et al. Estimating the incidence of typhoid fever and other febrile illnesses in developing countries. *Emerg Infect Dis* 2003;9:539.
61. Cumming JA, McCann BG, Ralphs DNL. Fulminant pseudomembranous colitis with left hemicolon and rectal sparing. *Br J Surg* 1988;75:341.
62. Curtis KJ, Sleisenger MH. Infectious and parasitic diseases. In: Sleisenger MH, Fordtran JS, eds. *Gastrointestinal disease*, 2nd ed. Philadelphia: WB Saunders, 1978: 1679.
63. Davies NM. Toxicity of nonsteroidal anti-inflammatory drugs in the large intestine. *Dis Colon Rectum* 1995;38: 1311.
64. D'Souza RM, Becker NG, Hall G, et al. Does ambient temperature affect foodborne disease? *Epidemiology* 2004;15: 86.
65. Debenham GP. Ulcer of the cecum during oxyphenbutazone (Tandaril) therapy. *CAMJ* 1966;94:1182.
66. Demar M, Louvel D, Pradinaud R, et al. Histoplamosis and acquired immunodeficiency syndrome: a study of prognostic factors. *Clin Infect Dis* 2004;38:134.
67. Efem SEE. *Ascaris lumbricoides* and intestinal perforation. *Br J Surg* 1987;74:643.
68. Ellis ME, Watson BM, Milewski PJ, et al. *Clostridium difficile* colitis unassociated with antibiotic therapy. *Br J Surg* 1983;70:242.
69. Ellyson JH, Bezmalinovic Z, Parks SN, et al. Necrotizing amebic colitis: a frequently fatal complication. *Am J Surg* 1986;152:21.
70. Medical Network Inc. Encyclopedia Index A. Actinomycosis, 2003. Available at: *http://healthatoz.com/healthatoz/Atoz/ency/actinomycosis.html*. Accessed 2004.
71. Erstad BL. Octreotide for acute variceal bleeding. *Ann Pharmacother* 2001;35:618–626.
72. Fakety R. Guidelines for the diagnosis and management of *Clostridium difficile*–associated diarrhea and colitis. *Am J Gastroenterol* 1997;92:739.
73. Fataar S, Jacob GS, Bassiony H, et al. Rectocolonic calcification due to schistosomiasis: a clinicoradiologic study. *Dis Colon Rectum* 1984;27:164.
74. Faucheron JL, Parc R. Non-steroidal anti-inflammatory drug-induced colitis. *Int J Colorectal Dis* 1996;11:99.
75. Feigen GM. Suppurative anal cryptitis associated with *Trichuris trichiura*: report of a case. *Dis Colon Rectum* 1987;30:620.
76. Fekety R, McFarland LV, Surawicz CM, et al. Recurrent *Clostridium difficile* diarrhea: characteristics of risk factors for patients in a prospective, randomized, double-blinded trial. *Clin Infect Dis*.1997;24:324.
77. Fekety R, Quintiliani R. Current approach to the treatment of antibiotic-associated diarrhea. *Infect Surg* 1982; 1:13.
78. Fenton BW. Infectious diarrheas: to treat or not to treat. *Contemp Gastroenterol* 1990;July/Aug:9.
79. Fenton CM, Siegel RJ. A prospective evaluation of diversion colitis. *Am Surg* 1991;57:46.
80. Ferrazzi E, Toso S, Zanotti M, et al. Typhlitis (neutropenic enterocolitis) after a single dose of vinorelbine. *Cancer Chemother Pharmacol* 2001;47:277.
81. Filho EC. Strongyloidiasis. *Clin Gastroenterol* 1978;7:179.
82. Finney JMT. Gastroenterostomy for cicatrizing ulcer of the pylorus. *Johns Hopkins Hosp Bull* 1893;4:53.
83. Fischl MA, Dickinson GM, Sinave C, et al. *Salmonella* bacteremia as manifestation of acquired immunodeficiency syndrome. *Arch Intern Med* 1986;146:113.
84. Foucheron J. Toxicity of non-steroidal anti-inflammatory drugs in the large bowel. *Eur J Gastroenterol Hepatol* 1999; 11:389.
85. Franklin GO, Mohapatra M, Perrillo RP. Colonic tuberculosis diagnosed by colonoscopic biopsy. *Gastroenterology* 1979;76:362.
86. Fry RD. Infectious enteritis: a collective review. *Dis Colon Rectum* 1990;33:520.
87. Fukunaga K, Khatibi A. Glutaraldehyde colitis: a complication of screening flexible sigmoidoscopy in the primary care setting. *Arch Intern Med* 2000;133:315.
88. Furness BW, Beach MJ, Roberts JM. Giardiasis surveillance—United States, 1992–1997. *MMWR Morb Mortal Wkly Rep* 2000;49:1–13. Available at: *www.cdc.gov/epo/mmwr/preview/mmwrhtml/ss4907a1.htm*. Accessed 2004.
89. Gan HT, Chen YQ, Ouyang Q, et al. Differentiation between intestinal tuberculosis and Crohn's disease in endoscopic biopsy specimens by polymerase chain reaction. *Am J Gastroenterol* 2002;97:1446.
90. Garret JK, Jameson SC, Thompson B, et al. Anti–IL-5 (mepolizumab) therapy for hypereosinophilic syndromes. *J Allergy Clin Immunol* 2004;113:115.
91. Gazzard BG. HIV disease and the gastroenterologist. *Gut* 1988;29:1497.
92. Generic protocol to estimate burden of *Shigella* diarrhea and dysenteric mortality, 2003. Available at: *www.who.int/child-adolescence-health/publications/pubIMCI.htm*. Accessed 2004.
93. Giardiello FM, Bayless TM, Jesurun J, et al. Collagenous colitis: physiologic and histopathologic studies in seven patients. *Arch Intern Med* 1987;106:46.
94. Giardiello FM, Hansen FCIII, Lazenby AJ, et al. Collagenous colitis in setting of nonsteroidal anti-inflammatory drugs and antibiotics. *Dig Dis Sci* 1990;35:257.
95. Gill KP, Feeley TM, Keane FBV. Toxic megacolon and perforation caused by *Salmonella*. *Br J Surg* 1989;76:796.
96. Gizzi G, Villani V, Brandi G, et al. Anorectal lesions in patients taking suppositories containing non-steroidal anti-inflammatory drugs (NSAID). *Endoscopy* 1990;22:146–148.
97. Gleeson MH, Davis JM. Non-steroidal anti-inflammatory drugs, aspirin and newly diagnosed colitis: a case-control study. *Aliment Pharmacol Ther* 2003;17:817.
98. Glotzer DJ, Glick ME, Goldman H. Proctitis and colitis following diversion of the fecal stream. *Gastroenterology* 1981;80:438.
99. Gonzalez de Canales SP, del Olmo Martinez L, Cortejoso Hernandez A, et al. Colonic balantidiasis. *Gastroenterol Hepatol* 2000;23:129.
100. Gonzalez A, Vargas V, Guarner L, et al. Toxic megacolon in typhoid fever. *Arch Intern Med* 1985;145:2120.
101. Goodell SE, Quinn TC, Mkrtichian E, et al. Herpes simplex virus proctitis in homosexual men. *N Engl J Med* 1983; 201:868.
102. Gorbach SL. Infectious diarrheas. Paper presented at annual meeting, American Society of Colon and Rectal Surgeons, Boston, MA, 1983.
103. Graham BD, McKinsey DS, Driks MR, et al. Colonic histoplasmosis in acquired immunodeficiency syndrome. *Dis Colon Rectum* 1991;34:185.
104. Griffiths AP, Dixon MF. Microcarcinoids and diversion colitis in a colon defunction for 18 years: report of a case. *Dis Colon Rectum* 1992;35:685.

105. Gronczewski CA, Katz JP. *Clostridium difficile* colitis, 2003. Available at: *www.emedicine.com/med/topic3412.htm*. Accessed 2004.

106. Guerin PJ, Brasher C, Baron E, et al. *Shigella* dysenteriae serotype 1 in West Africa: intervention strategy for an outbreak in Sierra Leone. *Lancet* 2003;362:705.

107. Guerrant RL, Bobak DA. Bacterial and protozoal gastroenteritis. *N Engl J Med* 1991;325:327.

108. Guth AA, Kim U. The reappearance of abdominal tuberculosis. *Surg Gynecol Obstet* 1991;172:432.

109. Haberkern CM, Christie DL, Haas JE. Eosinophilic gastroenteritis presenting as ileocolitis. *Gastroenterology* 1978; 74:896.

110. Halaby IA, Rantis PC, Vernava AM III, et al. Collagenous colitis: pathogenesis and management. *Dis Colon Rectum* 1996;39:573.

111. Hall IC, O'Toole E. Intestinal flora in newborn infants with a description of a new pathogenic anaerobe, *Bacillus difficilis*. *Am J Dis Child* 1935;49:390.

112. Han JK, Kim SH, Choi BI, et al. Tuberculous colitis: findings at double-contrast barium enema examination. *Dis Colon Rectum* 1996;39:1204.

113. Harig JM, Soergel KH, Komorowski RA, et al. Treatment of diversion colitis with short-chain fatty acid irrigation. *N Engl J Med* 1989;320:23.

114. Heaton KW. Functional diarrhoea: the acid test. *BMJ* 1985; 290:1298.

115. Heller M. The gay bowel syndrome: a common problem of homosexual patients in the emergency department. *Ann Emerg Med* 1980;9:487.

116. Henderson SO. Candidiasis, 2002. Available at: *www.emedicine.com/emerg/topic76.htm*. Accessed 2004.

117. Heneghan SJ, Li J, Petrossian E, et al. Intestinal perforation from gastrointestinal histoplasmosis in acquired immunodeficiency syndrome: case report and review of the literature. *Arch Surg* 1993;128:464.

118. Hiatt GA. Miliary tuberculosis with ileocecal involvement diagnosed by colonoscopy. *JAMA* 1978;240:561.

119. Hidalgo JA, Vazquez JA. Candidiasis, 2002. Available at: *www.emedicine.com/med/topic264.htm*.

120. Horvath KD, Whelan RL, Weinstein S, et al. Isolated sigmoid tuberculosis: report of a case. *Dis Colon Rectum* 1995;38:1327.

121. Hurley BW, Nguyen CC. The spectrum of pseudomembranous enterocolitis and antibiotic-associated diarrhea. *Arch Intern Med* 2002;162:2177.

122. Istre GR, Kreiss K, Hopkins RS, et al. An outbreak of amebiasis spread by colonic irrigation at a chiropractic clinic. *N Engl J Med* 1982;307:339.

123. Jain S, Koirala J, Castro-Paiva F. Isolated gastrointestinal histoplasmosis: case report and review of the literature. *South Med J* 2004;97:172.

124. Janda WM, Bohnhoff M, Morello JA, et al. Prevalence and site-pathogen studies of *Neisseria meningitidis* and *N. gonorrhoeae* in homosexual men. *JAMA* 1980;244:2060.

125. Johnson S, Gerding D. *Clostridium difficile*–associated diarrhea. *Clin Infect Dis* 1998;26:1027.

126. Jorens PG, Michielsen PP, Van den Enden EJ, et al. A rare cause of colitis—*Brucella melitensis*: report of a case. *Dis Colon Rectum* 1991;34:194.

127. Joseph D, Jin H, Ryan C, et al. Resolution of anorectal incontinence in herpes proctitis confirmed by anorectal manometry. *Gastrointest Endoscopy* 1997;45:429.

128. Juniper K. Amoebiasis. *Clin Gastroenterol* 1978;7:3.

129. Kapoor VK, Sharma LK. Abdominal tuberculosis. *Br J Surg* 1988;75:2.

130. Kasulke RJ, Anderson WJ, Gupta SK, et al. Primary tuberculous enterocolitis: report of three cases and review of the literature. *Arch Surg* 1981;116:110.

131. Katz DE, Taylor DN. Parasitic infections of the gastrintestinal tract. *Gastroenterol Clin* 2001;30:1–13.

132. Katz Y, Varsano D, Siegal B, et al. Intestinal obstruction due to *Ascaris lumbricoides* mimicking intussusception. *Dis Colon Rectum* 1985;28:267.

133. Kaufman HL, Fisher Ah, Carroll M, et al. Colonic ulceration associated with nonsteroidal anti-inflammatory drugs. *Dis Colon Rectum* 1996;39:705–710.

134. Khalil M, Iwatt AR, Gugnani HC. African histoplasmosis masquerading as carcinoma of the colon: report of a case and review of literature. *Dis Colon Rectum* 1989;32:518.

135. Kiely EM, Ajayi NA, Wheeler RA, et al. Diversion proctocolitis: response to treatment with short-chain fatty acids. *J Pediatr Surg* 2001;36:1514.

136. King HC, Voss EC Jr. Tuberculosis of the cecum simulating carcinoma. *Dis Colon Rectum* 1980;23:49.

137. Kingham JGC. Microscopic colitis. *Gut* 1991;32:234.

138. Kingham JGC, Levison DA, Ball JA, et al. Microscopic colitis—a cause of chronic watery diarrhoea. *BMJ* 1982;285:1601.

139. Kingham JGC, Levison DA, Morson BC, et al. Collagenous colitis. *Gut* 1986;27:570.

140. Kirkpatrick ID, Greenberg HM. Gastrointestinal complications in the neutropenic patient: characterization and differentiation with abdominal CT. *Radiology* 2003;226:668.

141. Klausner JD, Kohn R, Kent C. Etiology of clinical proctitis among men who have sex with men. *Clin Infect Dis* 2004;38:300.

142. Knight R. Giardiasis, isosporiasis, and balantidiasis. *Clin Gastroenterol* 1978;7:31.

143. Ko CY, Schmit PJ, Petrie B, et al. Abdominal tuberculosis: the surgical perspective. *Am Surg* 1996;62:865.

144. Kobayasi S, Mendes EF, Rodrigues MAM, et al. Toxic dilatation of the colon in Chagas' disease. *Br J Surg* 1992; 79:1202.

145. Kochtrar R, Rajwanshi A, Goenka MK, et al. Colonoscopic fine needle aspiration cytology in the diagnosis of ileocecal tuberculosis. *Am J Gastroenterol* 1991;86:102.

146. Koea JB, Shaw JHF. Surgical management of neutropenic enterocolitis. *Br J Surg* 1989;76:821.

147. Kofsky P, Rosen L, Reed J, et al. *Clostridium difficile*—a common and costly colitis. *Dis Colon Rectum* 1991;34:244.

148. Kogulam P, Lucey DR. Schistosomiasis, 2002. Available at: *http://emedicine.com/med/topic2071.htm*. Accessed 2004.

149. Koo J, Ho J, Ong GB. The value of colonoscopy in the diagnosis of ileocecal tuberculosis. *Endoscopy* 1982;14:48.

150. Kraft SC, Kirsner JB. Immunology in gastroenterology. In: Berk JE, ed. *Bockus gastroenterology*, 4th ed. Philadelphia: WB Saunders, 1985:4507.

151. Kunkel JM, Rosenthal D. Management of the ileocecal syndrome: neutropenic enterocolitis. *Dis Colon Rectum* 1986; 29:196.

152. Kyne L, Warny M, Qamar A, et al. Asymptomatic carriage of *Clostridium difficile* and serum levels of IgG antibody against toxin A. *N Engl J Med* 2000;342:390.

153. Latimer RG. Discussion. In: Ellyson JH, Bezmalinovic Z, Parks SN, et al., eds. Necrotizing amebic colitis: a frequently fatal complication. *Am J Surg* 1986;152:21.

154. Leav BA, Mackay M, Ward HD. Cryptosporidium species: new insights and old challenges. *Clin Infect Dis* 2003; 36:903.

155. Lebedeff DA, Hochman EB. Rectal gonorrhea in men: diagnosis and treatment. *Arch Intern Med* 1980;92:463.

156. Lee FI, Costello FT, Cowley DJ, et al. Eosinophilic colitis with perianal disease. *Am J Gastroenterol* 1983;78:164.

157. Lee KR, Lin F. Gastrointestinal histoplasmosis, roentgenographic, clinical and pathological correlation. *Am J Gastroenterol* 1975;63:255.

158. Lev R, Sweeney KG. Neutropenic enterocolitis. Two unususal cases with review of the literature. *Arch Pathol Lab Med* 1993;117:524–527.

159. Levy N, Gasper E. Rectal bleeding and indomethacin suppositories [Letter]. *Lancet* 1975;305:577.

160. Lewis FW, Warren GH, Goff JS. Collagenous colitis with involvement of terminal ileum. *Dig Dis Sci* 1991;36:1161.

161. Lewis JS, Fakile O, Foss E, et al. Direct DNA probe assay for *Neisseria gonorrhoeae* in pharyngeal and rectal specimens. *J Clin Microbiol* 1993;31:2783.

162. Lindmark H, Harbom B, Thebo L, et al. Genetic characterization and antibiotic resistance of *Campylobacter* jejuni isolated from meats, water, and humans in Sweden. *J Clin Microbiol* 2004;42:700.

163. Lipsett PA, Samantaray DK, Tam ML, et al. Pseudomembranous colitis: a surgical disease? *Surgery* 1994;116:491.

164. Lisehora GB, Peters CC, Lee YTM, et al. Tuberculous peritonitis—do not miss it. *Dis Colon Rectum* 1996;39:394.

165. Loftus EV. Microscopic colitis: epidemiology and treatment. *Am J Gastroenterol* 2003;98[Suppl 12]:S31.

166. Luvuno FM. Role of intraoperative prograde colonic lavage and a decompressive loop ileostomy in the management of transmural amoebic colitis. *Br J Surg* 1990;77:156.

167. Maloney JR GE. CBRNE. Brucellosis, 2001. Available at: *www.emedicine.com/emerg/topic883.htm*. Accessed 2004.

168. Marshall JK, Irvine EJ. Lymphocytic and collagenous colitis: medical management. *Curr Treat Options Gastroenterol* 1999;2:127.

169. Mathews H, Addiss D, Stewart J, et al. Evaluation of a commercially available ELISA test for Giardia antigen in stool. Paper presented at 90th annual meeting of the American Society for Microbiology, New Orleans, LA 1990(abst).

170. McCarter MD, Abularrage C, Velasco FT, et al. Diarrhea and *Clostridium difficile*–associated diarrhea on a surgical service. *Arch Surg* 1996;131:1333.

171. McFarland LV, Mulligan ME, Kwok RYY, et al. Nosocomial acquisition of *Clostridium difficile* infections. *N Engl J Med* 1989;320:204.

172. McMillan A, Gilmour HM, McNeillage G, et al. Amoebiasis in homosexual men. *Gut* 1984;25:356.

173. Medich DS, Lee KKW, Simmons RL, et al. Laparotomy for fulminant pseudomembranous colitis. *Arch Surg* 1992;127:847.

174. Meier DE, Imediegwu OO, Tarpley JL. Perforated typhoid enteritis: operative experience with 108 cases. *Am J Surg* 1989;157:423.

175. Merritt RJ, Coughlin E, Thomas DW, et al. Spectrum of amebiasis in children. *Am J Dis Child* 1982;136:785.

176. Mildvan D, Mathur U, Enlow RW, et al. Opportunistic infections and immune deficiency in homosexual men. *Arch Intern Med* 1982;96:700.

177. Ming-Chai C, Chi-Yuan C, Fu-Pan W, et al. Colorectal cancer and schistosomiasis. *Lancet* 1981;1:971.

178. Misra SP, Misra V, Dwivedi M, et al. Factors influencing colonic involvement in patients with amebic liver abscess. *Gastrointest Endosc* 2004;59:512.

179. Mock CN, Amaral J, Visser LE. Improvement in survival from typhoid ileal perforation: results of 221 operative cases. *Ann Surg* 1992;215:244.

180. Mohamed ARE-S, Karawi MAA, Yasawy MI. Schistosomal colonic disease. *Gut* 1990;31:439.

181. Monroe LS. Gastrointestinal parasites. In: Berk JE, ed. *Bockus gastroenterology*, 4th ed. Philadelphia: WB Saunders, 1985:4250.

182. Montefusco PP, Geiss AC, Randall S. Typhoid fever and massive intestinal hemorrhage. *Contemp Surg* 1984;24:61.

183. Moran JS, Levine WC. Drugs of choice for the treatment of uncomplicated gonococcal infections. *Clin Infect Dis* 1995;20[Suppl]:S47.

184. Morris LL, Villalba MR, Glover JL. Management of pseudomembranous colitis. *Am Surg* 1994;60:548.

185. Morris JB, Zollinger RM Jr, Stellato TA. Role of surgery in antibiotic-induced pseudomembranous colitis. *Am J Surg* 1990;160:535.

186. Mower WJ, Hawkins JA, Nelson EW. Neutropenic enterocolitis in adults with acute leukemia. *Arch Surg* 1986;121:571.

187. Murray FE, O'Brien M, Birkett DH, et al. Diversion colitis: pathologic findings in a resected sigmoid colon and rectum. *Gastroenterology* 1987;93:1404.

188. Mylonakis E, Ryan ET, Calderwood SB. *Clostridium difficile*-associated diarrhea: A review. *Arch Intern Med* 2001;161:525.

189. Nash TE, Ohl CA, Thomas E, et al. Treatment of patients with refractory giardiasis. *Clin Infect Dis* 2001;33:22.

190. Naylor AR, Pollet JE. Eosinophilic colitis. *Dis Colon Rectum* 1985;28:615.

191. New York City Department of Health and Mental Hygiene Bureau of Communicable Disease. 2003. Available at: *www.nyc.gov/html/doh/html/cd/cdyer.html*. Accessed 2004.

192. O'Hanrahan T, Dark P, Irving MH. Cyclic neutropenia—unusual cause of acute abdomen. Report of a case. *Dis Colon Rectum* 1991;34:1125.

193. Olesen M, Eriksson S, Bohr J, et al. Microscopic colitis: a common diarrhoeal disease. An epidemiological study in Orebro, Sweden, 1993–1998. *Gut* 2004;53:346.

194. Orsay CP, Kim DO, Pearl RK, et al. Diversion colitis in patients scheduled for colostomy closure. *Dis Colon Rectum* 1993;36:366.

195. Owen RL. Rectal gonorrhea. In: Sleisenger MH, Fordtran JS, eds. *Gastrointestinal disease*, 2nd ed. Philadelphia: WB Saunders, 1978:1692.

196. Palmer KR, Berry H, Wheeler PJ, et al. Collagenous colitis—a relapsing and remitting disease. *Gut* 1986;27:578.

197. Palmer KR, Patil DH, Basran GS, et al. Abdominal tuberculosis in urban Britain—a common disease. *Gut* 1985;26:1296.

198. Palmer PES. Amebiasis and tropical diseases of the colon. In: Greenbaum EI, ed. *Radiographic atlas of colon disease*. Chicago: Year Book Medical Publishers, 1980:9.

199. Pangan JC. Severe amebic colitis with hemorrhage and perforation. *Contemp Surg* 1986;28:73.

200. Parry CM. Typhoid fever. *Curr Infect Dis Rep* 2004;6:27.

201. Partyka EK, Sanowski RA, Kozarek RA. Colonoscopic features of eosinophilic gastroenteritis. *Dis Colon Rectum* 1980;23:353.

202. Pawlowski ZS. Ascariasis. *Clin Gastroenterol* 1978;7:157.

203. Pikarsky AJ, Belin B, Efron J, et al. Complications following formalin instillation in the treatment of radiation induced proctitis. *Int J Colorect Dis* 2000;115:96.

204. Pennardt A. Giardiasis, 2002. Available at: *www.emedicine.com/emerg/topic215.htm*. Accessed 2004.

205. Pokorney BH, Nichols TW Jr. Pseudomembranous colitis: a complication of sulfasalazine therapy in a patient with Crohn's colitis. *Am J Gastroenterol* 1981;76:374.

206. Polenakovik H, Polenakovik S. Strongyloidiasis, 2004. Available at: *www.emedicine.com/med/topic2189.htm*. Accessed 2004.

207. Portnoy D, Whiteside ME, Buckley E III, et al. Treatment of intestinal cryptosporidiosis with spiramycin. *Arch Intern Med* 1984;101:202.

208. Price AB. Pathology of drug-associated gastrointestinal disease. *Br J Clin Pharmacol* 2003;56:477.

209. Procopiou M, Egger JF, De Torrente A. Collagenous colitis and cutaneous polyarteritis nodosa in the same patient. *Scand J Gastroenterol* 2004;39:89.

210. Puri AS, Vij JC, Chaudhary A, et al. Diagnosis and outcome of isolated rectal tuberculosis. *Dis Colon Rectum* 1996;39:1126.

211. Quondamcarlo C, Valentini G, Ruggeri M, et al. *Campylobacter* jejuni enterocolitis presenting as inflammatory bowel disease. *Tech Coloproctol* 2003;7:173.

212. Quigly MM, Bethel K, Nowacki M, et al. Neutropenic enterocolitis: a rare presenting complication of acute leukemia. *Am J Hematol* 2001;66:213.

213. Quinn TC, Corey L, Chaffee RG, et al. The etiology of anorectal infections in homosexual men. *Am J Med* 1981;72:395.

214. Radhakrishnan S, Al Nakib B, Shaikh H, et al. The value of colonoscopy in schistosomal, tuberculous, and amebic colitis: two-year experience. *Dis Colon Rectum* 1986;29:891.

215. Rampton DS, Baithun SI. Is microscopic colitis due to bile salt malabsorption? *Dis Colon Rectum* 1987;30:950.

216. Rams H, Rogers AI, Ghandur-Mnaymneh L. Collagenous colitis. *Arch Intern Med* 1987;106:108.

217. Ratliff DA, Carr N, Cochrane JPS. Rectal stricture due to actinomycosis. *Br J Surg* 1986;73:589.

218. Reddy KR, Thomas E. Proctitis: an unusual presentation of *Strongyloides stercoralis* infestation. *Am J Proctol Gastroenterol Colon Rectal Surg* 1983;34:11.

219. Reyes E, Hernandez J, Gonzalez A. Typhoid colitis with massive lower gastrointestinal bleeding: an unexpected behavior of *Salmonella typhi*. *Dis Colon Rectum* 1986;29:511.

220. Roe AM, Warren BF, Brodribb AJM, et al. Diversion colitis and involution of the defunctioned anorectum. *Gut* 1993;34:382.

221. Roediger WEW. The starved colon—diminished mucosal nutrition, diminished absorption, and colitis. *Dis Colon Rectum* 1990;33:858.

222. Rominger JM, Shah AN. Ameboma of the rectum. *Gastrointest Endosc* 1979;25:71.

223. Rompalo AM. Diagnosis and treatment of sexually acquired proctitis and proctocolitis: An update. *Clin Infect Dis* 1999;28[Suppl 1]:S84.

224. Rompalo AM, Mertz GJ, Davis LG, et al. Oral acyclovir for treatment of first-episode herpes simplex virus proctitis. *JAMA* 1988;259:2879.

225. Rompalo AM, Mertz GJ, Mkrtichian EE, et al. Oral acyclovir vs placebo for treatment of herpes simplex virus proctitis in homosexual men. *Clin Res* 1985;33:58A.

226. Rompalo AM, Roberts P, Johnson K, et al. Empirical therapy for the management of acute proctitis in homosexual men. *JAMA* 1988;260:348.

227. Rosenberg JM, Walker M, Welch JP, et al. *Clostridium difficile* colitis in surgical patients. *Am J Surg* 1984;147:486.

228. Rosoff JD, Sanders CA, Sonnad SS, et al. Stool diagnosis of giardiasis using a commercially available enzyme immunoassay to detect *Giardia*-specific antigen 65 (GSA 65). *J Clin Microbiol* 1989;27:1997.

229. Rossignol J-FA, Ayoub A, Ayers MC. Treatment of diarrhea caused by cryptosporidium parvum: a prospective, randomized, double-blind, placebo-controlled study of nitazoxanide. *J Infect Dis* 2001;184:103.

230. Rothenberger ME. Eosinophilic gastrointestinal disorders (EGID). *J Allergy Clin Immunol* 2004;113:11.

231. Rozen P, Baratz M, Rattan J. Rectal bleeding due to amebic colitis diagnosed by multiple endoscopic biopsies: report of two cases. *Dis Colon Rectum* 1981;24:127.

232. Russo A, Cirino E, Sanfilippo G, et al. Ampicillin-associated colitis. *Endoscopy* 1980;12:97.

233. Ryan CK, Potter GD. Editorial: disinfectant colitis: rinse as well as you wash. J *Clin Gastroenterol* 1995;21:6.

234. Saab S, DeRosa V, Nieto J, et al. Cost and clinical outcomes of primary prophylaxis of variceal bleeding in patients with hepatic cirrhosis: a decision analytic model. *Am J Gastroenterol* 2003;98:763.

235. Saeb A, Lassen J. Acute and chronic gastrointestinal manifestations associated with *Yersinia enterocolitica* infection: a Norwegian 10-year follow-up study on 458 hospitalized patients. *Ann Surg* 1992;215:250.

236. Sakurai Y, Tsuchiya H, Ikegama F, et al. Acute right-sided hemorrhagic colitis associated with oral administration of ampicillin. *Dig Dis Sci* 1979;24:910.

237. Sandmeier D, Bouzourene H. Microscopic colitis with giant cells: a rare new histopathologic subtype? *Int J Surg Pathol* 2004;12:45.

238. Sanford AH. *Yersinia enterocolitica* abscess of the transverse colon: report of a case. *Dis Colon Rectum* 1990;33:985.

239. Sardinha TC, Wexner SD, Gilliland J, et al. Efficiency and productivity of a sheathed fiberoptic sigmoidoscope compared with conventional sigmoidoscope. *Dis Colon Rectum* 1997;40:1228.

240. Schacker T, Hu H, Koelle DM, et al. Famciclovir for the suppression of symptomatic and asymptomatic herpes simplex virus reactivation in HIV-infected persons. *Arch Intern Med* 1998;128:21.

241. Schofield PF, ed. Abdominal tuberculosis. *Gut* 1985;26: 1275.

242. Schulze K, Mitros FA. Eosinophilic gastroenteritis involving the ileocecal area. *Dis Colon Rectum* 1979;22:47.

243. Schmunis GA, Zicker F, Pinheiro F, et al. Risk for transfusion-transmitted infectious diseases in Central and South America, 1998. Available at: *www.cdc.gov/ncidod/eid/vol4no1/scmunis.htm.* Accessed 2004.

244. Schwebke JR, Whittington W, Rice RJ, et al. Trends in susceptibility of *Neisseria gonorrhoeae* to ceftriaxone from 1985 through 1991. *Antimicrob Agents Chemother* 1995;39:917–920.

245. Seppälä K, Hjelt L, Sipponen P. Colonoscopy in the diagnosis of antibiotic-associated colitis: a prospective study. *Scand J Gastroenterol* 1981;16:465.

246. Shaz BH, Reddy SI, Ayata G, et al. Sequential clinical and histopathological changes in collageneous and lymphocytic colitis over time. *Mod Pathol* 2004;17:395–401.

247. Shorter NA, Thompsom MD, Mooney DP, et al. Surgical aspects of an outbreak of *Yersinia* enterocolitis. *Pediatr Surg Int* 1998;13:2.

248. Shukla VK, Roy SK, Vaidya MP, et al. Fulminant amebic colitis. *Dis Colon Rectum* 1986;29:398.

249. Siegal FP, Lopez C, Hammer GS, et al. Severe acquired immunodeficiency in male homosexuals, manifested by chronic perianal ulcerative herpes simplex lesions. *N Engl J Med* 1981;305:1439.

250. Silva J Jr. Update on pseudomembranous colitis. *West J Med* 1989;151:644.

251. Sivapalasingam S, Barrett E, Kimura A, et al. A multistate outbreak of *Salmonella enterica* serotype Newport infection linked to mango consumption: impact of water-dip disinfection technology. *Clin Infect Dis* 2003;37:1585.

252. Smith PD, Quinn TC, Strober W, et al. Gastrointestinal infections in AIDS. *Arch Intern Med* 1992;116:63.

253. Soni HC, Hardin E. Proctitis, 2001. Available at: *http://emedicine.com/aaem/topic368.htm.* Accessed 2004.

254. Stampfl DA, Friedman LS. Collagenous colitis: pathophysiologic considerations. *Dig Dis Sci* 1991;36:705.

255. Stanley Jr SL. Amoebiasis. *Lancet* 2003;361:1025–1034.

256. Stansfield VA. Diagnosis and management of anorectal gonorrhoea in women. *Br J Vener Dis* 1980;56:319.

257. Stermer E, Levy N, Potasman I, et al. Brucellosis as a cause of severe colitis. *Am J Gastroenterol* 1991;86:917.

258. Stockinger AT. Colonic ameboma: its appearance on CT: report of a case. *Dis Colon Rectum* 2004;47:527–529.

259. Stoddart B, Wilcox MH. *Clostridium difficile. Curr Opin Infect Dis* 2002;15:513–518.

260. Stuart RC, Leahy AL, Cafferkey MT, et al. *Yersinia enterocolitica* infection and toxic megacolon. *Br J Surg* 1986;73:590.

261. Sturim HS, Kouchoukos NT, Ahlvin RC. Gastrointestinal manifestations of disseminated histoplasmosis. *Am J Surg* 1965;110:435.

262. Sylwestrowicz T, Kelly JK, Hwang WS, et al. Collagenous colitis and microscopic colitis: the watery diarrhea-colitis syndrome. *Am J Gastroenterol* 1989;84:763.

263. Tagkalidis P, Bhathal P, Gibson P. Microscopic colitis. *J Gastroenterol Hepatol* 2002;17:236.

264. Talbot RW, Walker RC, Beart RW Jr. Changing epidemiology, diagnosis and treatment of *Clostridium difficile* toxin-associated colitis. *Br J Surg* 1986;73:457.

265. Tanaka M, Mazzoleni G, Riddell RH. Distribution of collagenous colitis: utility of flexible sigmoidoscopy. *Gut* 1992;33:65.

266. Tanowitz HB, Weiss LM, Wittner M. Diagnosis and treatment of protozoan diarrheas. *Am J Gastroenterol* 1988;83:339.

267. Tedesco FJ. Antibiotic associated pseudomembranous colitis with negative proctosigmoidoscopy examination. *Gastroenterology* 1979;77:295.

268. Tedesco FJ, Huckaby CB, Hamby-Allen M, et al. Eosinophilic ileocolitis: expanding spectrum of eosinophilic gastroenteritis. *Dig Dis Sci* 1981;26:943.

269. Thompson JR, Watts R Jr, Thompson WC. Actinomyce-toma masquerading as an abdominal neoplasm. *Dis Colon Rectum* 1982;25:368.

270. Tielbeek AV, Rosenbusch G, Muytjens HL, et al. Roentgeno-logic changes of the colon in *Campylobacter* infection. *Gastrointest Radiol* 1985;10:358.

271. Triadafilopoulos G, Hallston AE. Acute abdomen as the first presentation of pseudomembranous colitis. *Gastroenterology* 1991;101:685–891.

272. Tripodi J, Gorcey S, Burakoff R. A case of diversion colitis treated with 5-aminosalicylic acid enemas. *Am J Gastroenterol* 1992;87:645.

273. Trudel JL, Deschênes M, Mayrand S, et al. Toxic megacolon complicating pseudomembranous enterocolitis. *Dis Colon Rectum* 1995;38:1033.

274. Tvede M, Rask-Madsen J. Bacteriotherapy for chronic relapsing clostridium difficile diarrhoea in six patients. *Lancet* 1989;1:1156.

275. Udagawa SM, Portin BA, Bernhoft WH. Actinomycosis of the colon and rectum: report of two cases. *Dis Colon Rectum* 1974;17:687.

276. van der Kaay HJ. Human diseases in relation to the degradation of tropical rainforests, 1998. Available at: *www.xs4all.nl/ ~rainmed/bulletin/disdeg-e.html*. Accessed 2004.

277. Vantrappen G, Agg HO, Ponette E, et al. *Yersinia* enteritis and enterocolitis: gastroenterological aspects. *Gastroenterology* 1977;72:220.

278. Varghese L, Galandiuk S, Tremaine WJ, et al. Lymphocytic colitis treated with proctocolectomy and ileal J-pouch anastomosis: report of a case. *Dis Colon Rectum* 2002;45: 123–126.

279. Verhamme MAM, Ramboer CHR. Anisakiasis caused by herring in vinegar: a little known medical problem. *Gut* 1988;29:843.

280. Vila V, Brullet E, Montserrat A, et al. Glutaraldehyde-in-duced iatrogenic rectocolitis. *Gastroenterol Hepatol* 2001; 24:409.

281. Vrioni G, Gartzonika C, Kostoula A, et al. Application of a polymerase chain reaction enzyme immunoassay in peripheral whole blood and serum specimens for diagnosis of acute human brucellosis. *Eur J Clin Microbiol Infect Dis* 2004;23:194.

282. Walters BAJ, Roberts R, Stafford R, et al. Relapse of antibiotic associated colitis: endogenous persistence of *Clostridium difficile* during vancomycin therapy. *Gut* 1983; 24:206.

283. Wang KK, Perrault J, Carpenter HA, et al. Collagenous colitis: a clinicopathologic correlation. *Mayo Clin Proc* 1987; 62:665.

284. Wanke CA. Practical approach to diarrheal illness. *Mediguide Infect Dis* 1997;17:1.

285. Wasselle JA, Sedgwick JH, Dawson PJ, et al. Intestinal herpes simplex infection presenting with intestinal perforation. *Am J Gastroenterol* 1992;87:1475.

286. Wasadikar PP, Kulkarni AB. Intestinal obstruction due to ascariasis. *Br J Surg* 1997;84:410.

287. Weese WC, Smith IM. A study of 57 cases of actinomycosis over a 36-year period: a diagnostic "failure" with good prognosis after treatment. *Arch Intern Med* 1975;135:1562.

288. Weiss EL. *Ascaris lumbricoides*, 2003. Available at: *www. emedicine.com/emerg/topic840.htm*. Accessed 2004.

289. WHO Diarrheal Diseases Steering Committee. Montreaux, Switzerland: World Health Organization, September 10–11, 2003.

290. Wiersma R, Hadley GP. Small bowel volvulus complicating intestinal ascariasis in children. *Br J Surg* 1988;75:86.

291. Wig JD, Malik AK, Khanna SK, et al. Massive lower gastrointestinal bleeding in patients with typhoid fever. *Am J Gastroenterol* 1981;75:445.

292. Wolfe MS. Oxyuris, trichostrongylus and trichuris. *Clin Gastroenterol* 1978;7:201.

293. Wong B. Parasitic diseases in immunocompromised hosts. *Am J Med* 1984;76:479.

294. Yilmaz T, Sever A, Gur S, et al. CT findings of abdominal tuberculosis in 12 patients. *Comp Med Imag Graph* 2002; 26:321.

295. Yungbluth PM. Practical approach to the use of the laboratory in infectious enteritis. *Practical Gastroenterol* 1987; 11:35.

296. Zaat JOM, Mank T, Assendelft WJJ. Drugs for treating giardiasis. *Cochrane Database Syst Rev* 2004;1:1.

297. Zayas CF, Perlino C, Caliendo A, et al. Chagas disease after organ transplantation—United States, 2001 (2002). Available at: *www.cdc.gov/mmwr.preview/mmwrhtml/mm5110a3.htm*. Accessed 2004.

Chapter 34

Medicolegal Aspects of Colon and Rectal Surgery

In the United States, the issue of alleged medical negligence has reached crisis proportions in many jurisdictions. While no field of medicine is exempt from this concern, colon and rectal surgery has its own, unique areas of potential vulnerability. Practice patterns and self-education demand continuous reevaluation in order to provide the optimal care for our patents while protecting ourselves from the vicissitudes of the legal arena. For these reasons, I have asked Dr. Alan V. Abrams to contribute this new chapter to the fifth edition of this text. Dr. Abrams is the former director of the residency program in colon and rectal surgery and head of the Division of Colon and Rectal Surgery at Greater Baltimore Medical Center. He is currently clinical assistant professor of surgery at Weill Cornell Medical College in New York City. He has extensive experience as an expert witness in medical negligence cases involving colon and rectal surgery. He is retired from clinical practice and resides in New York City.

MLC

If he [the surgeon] caused loss of life or limb, he lost his hands . . .

Babylonian law[5]

The penalty for medical malpractice in contemporary society is thankfully less severe than that demanded by Babylonian law, but the ordeal of a malpractice suit can exact a heavy emotional, and sometimes financial toll on the surgeon. Although practicing "good medicine" is the best defense against claims of negligence, this is not always sufficient to avoid lawsuits. In fact, malpractice actions commonly arise in situations in which medical management has, by all objective criteria, conformed to

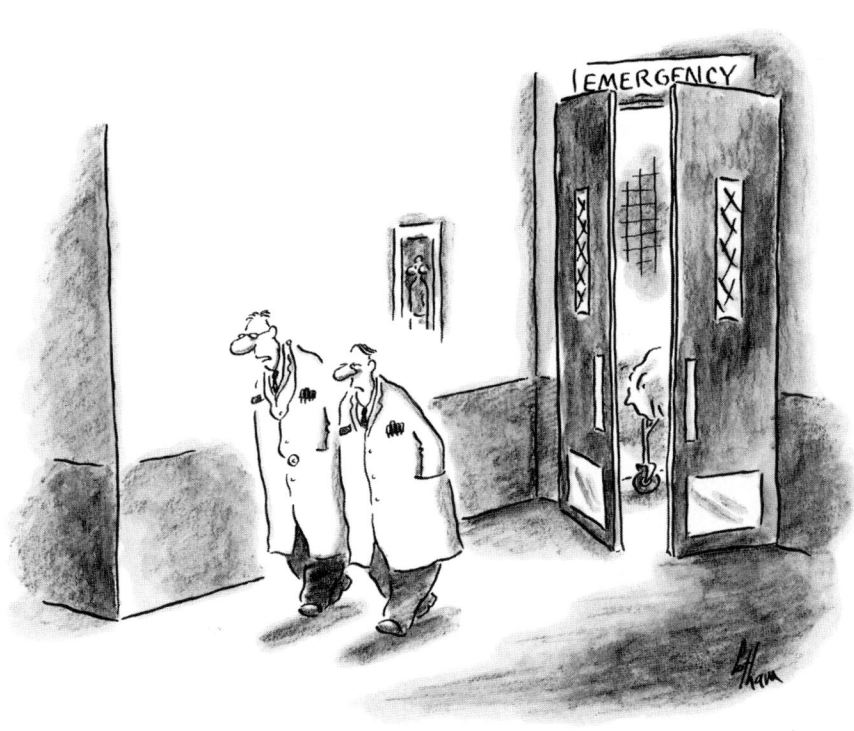

"I don't feel quite as fulfilled when I've saved a lawyer."

the standard of care. Conversely, although many patients incur injuries during the course of treatment, studies have shown that only one in ten individuals who sustain such injuries actually sue. Even in cases in which peer review evaluation concludes that negligence occurred, a patient rarely sues his or her physicians.[4] It is clear that in addition to the quality of care, other factors play a role in determining whether an injured patient will commence a legal action. Consequently, the surgeon must not only understand the law as it applies to medical malpractice, but must also be aware of the issues in order to minimize the likelihood of litigation when such an injury occurs.

HISTORICAL BACKGROUND

The concept of assessing penalty for negligence resulting in injury dates back to Babylonian times, when individuals and sometimes even their families were held directly accountable. Under Hammurabi's code of justice (c. 1750 B.C.), if a builder constructed a house so poorly that it collapsed and killed the son of the owner, the law allowed for the execution of the builder's son. As judged by the quotation above, physicians were held to a similarly harsh standard. After their Babylonian captivity, the Hebrews adopted many aspects of Babylonian law but limited penalties to the practitioner himself.[4] Greek civilization did not recognize professions as such, so the conceptual basis for professional negligence was lacking. Under Roman law, however, negligent infliction of personal injury could result in compensation for the patient's medical expenses and lost wages.

Licensing of physicians, which first occurred in the late Middle Ages, marked a major development in the evolution of personal injury law by identifying physicians as a class, separate from the rest of society by virtue of their possessing special knowledge and skill, and holding them responsible in the exercise of that skill.[2]

The first recorded suit for medical malpractice in English common law occurred in 1374. The United States, which adopted English common law, recorded its first case in 1794.[3]

THE WRITTEN LAW

Medical malpractice is not a separate branch of law, but rather is a subdivision of personal injury law. In order for the plaintiff (the patient) to prevail over the defendant (the physician) in a suit for malpractice, the law requires that four elements be proven: duty, breach of duty, causation, and damages.

Duty

The surgeon has a responsibility to the patient to conform to the standard of care—that is, to exercise the skill and

provide a level of medical care equivalent to that which is generally employed by the profession under similar circumstances. The duty element is usually not at issue in medical malpractice cases, because once the physician–patient relationship is established, the physician is obligated to provide competent care. The matter may be contested, however, if there is a question as to whether a valid physician–patient relationship existed.

Breach of Duty

The physician, either by omission or commission, did not conform to the standard of care. The central issue in most malpractice cases is determining what the standard of care should have been in a particular clinical setting, a matter usually argued by expert witnesses for each side. The law does not require that the physician's care be equivalent to the best available nationally or even locally—only that it meet an accepted, usually national, standard. If, as is often the case, there is more than one acceptable treatment for a condition, the physician cannot be held liable solely because the treatment mode selected results in an adverse outcome.

Causation

The physician's failure to conform to the standard of care directly caused or contributed to the patient's injury, a matter that is also usually the subject of expert witness testimony.

Damages

As a direct result of the physician's failure to meet the standard of care, the patient suffered an injury that, in a civil court, is compensable by awarding of monetary damages. Conversely, if the patient did not sustain an injury, he cannot recover anything, no matter what the level of care.

Unlike a criminal trial, in which the prosecution must prove its case beyond a reasonable doubt, a malpractice suit requires only that the plaintiff prove that his or her version of events is more likely than not, a standard commonly referred to as *proof to a reasonable degree of medical probability (or certainty)*. The burden of proof for all of these elements lies with the plaintiff, however, and if proof of any one element is lacking, the plaintiff's complaint of negligence cannot be sustained.

THE UNWRITTEN LAWS

The most important rule to which a surgeon must adhere in order to prevent malpractice suits is to practice high-quality medicine. Because of the complexity of medical decision making, the law allows physicians considerable latitude in their practice by defining the standard of care as *what a reasonable*, rather than what the most expert practitioner would do under similar circumstances and conditions. Nevertheless, it is essential that surgeons maintain and continually update their knowledge and skills by conscientiously keeping abreast of the medical literature and by regular attendance at meaningful educational conferences. Before undertaking a new procedure independently, the surgeon should receive adequate training and be mentored by someone competent in performing the technique. Aside from maintaining a high level of competence, however, there are many other factors that a surgeon must take into consideration to reduce the likelihood of being sued.

Patient Selection

One need not have extensive psychiatric training to realize that there are patients who, for a variety of reasons, seek to have surgery when none is indicated. Because the indications for many colorectal procedures (surgery for hemorrhoids, abdominal pain/diverticular disease, and constipation/colonic inertia) are, in part, subjective, such an issue is not infrequent. If there is any question about an individual's emotional stability or motivation, the surgeon must meticulously evaluate the patient to be certain that objectively verifiable indications for surgery exist, that the patient has realistic expectations about possible outcomes, including negative ones and complications, and that all of the above is documented in the medical record. Second opinions in these situations are also valuable.

Documentation

In combination with high-quality care, good documentation is the surgeon's strongest line of defense in malpractice litigation. Creating a medical record offers surgeons the opportunity to present their version of events contemporaneous with their occurrence. Such documentation has much more credibility in a legal setting than after-the-fact explanations and rationalizations.

Office notes should document not only the medical history, physical findings, and differential diagnosis, but also treatment alternatives, recommendations, and possible complications. Plans for follow-up should document the party to whom the discharge instructions were given, the plan of care, and the need for any additional testing. Missed appointments or other indicators of possible patient noncompliance should be noted. All telephone communications with the patient, including complaints, instructions, and recommendations, should be documented in the office records.

In both the operative consent and in a separate progress note, the surgeon should document that she or he

has informed the patient (or other responsible party) of the purpose and extent of the planned procedure, of possible treatment alternatives, and of the major risks and complications specific to the proposed procedure. The patient should be made aware of the possibility that the procedure may not achieve its intended goal. Guarantees of a successful outcome, whether stated or implied, are to be avoided. The risk of death, brain damage, and paralysis should be included in the consent form of any patient undergoing general anesthesia.

All too many operative reports devote an inordinate amount of attention to descriptions of opening and closing the wound, placing sutures, and firing staplers. Such "cookie cutter" notes offer little legal protection for the surgeon. An operative report should describe not only the technical aspects of the procedure, but also the findings and the decision-making process that flowed from them, leading the surgeon to do what was done.

Progress notes should be written at least daily on recent postoperative or severely ill patients. In addition to the date, the notes should record the time at which they were written. The notes should be factual. Impressions and tentative diagnoses, if included at all, should be clearly labeled as such. Inclusion of vital signs, physical findings, and laboratory and imaging results in the notes not only facilitates reconstruction of events long after they have occurred, but also documents the surgeon's awareness of them and may, at a later date, provide support in explaining why a particular course of action was adopted. Like operative reports, progress notes should describe not only the facts, but also the surgeon's reasoning in making his or her decisions.

Relations with Patient and Family

The surgeon's personal relationship with the patient and his family is often as important as the quality of care in determining whether an action for malpractice is brought. The key to that relationship is communication. The surgeon must remain accessible and communicative to the patient and family at all times, particularly if postoperative complications develop. Although the situation may be frustrating and emotionally draining for the surgeon, he or she must maintain a professional demeanor and avoid the appearance of antagonism, anger, or hostility.

During the preoperative period, the surgeon should explain the rationale and goals of treatment in terms readily comprehensible to the layperson. If the surgeon encounters an unexpected finding intraoperatively and is considering a significant deviation from the planned procedure, he or she is advised to leave the operating room, with the patient adequately monitored and supervised, to discuss the findings and possible courses of action with the responsible family member or health care proxy.

If significant postoperative complications develop, the surgeon should communicate on a regular, preferably daily, basis with the family to explain the nature of the problems, and what she is doing to investigate their causes and treat them. Patients and their families will often accept major complications, and even death, if they believe that the physician is sympathetic to their plight and that of their relative and that everything possible is being done to correct the problems. Conversely, even the best medical care may not avoid a lawsuit if accompanied by a perceived attitude of indifference or avoidance.

SPECIAL SITUATIONS IN COLON AND RECTAL SURGERY

Although the following guidelines are not intended to be either medically or legally definitive or exhaustive, they are offered in the hope that they may prove useful in managing common conditions that form the basis for much malpractice litigation in the field of colorectal surgery.

Anal Conditions

Hemorrhoids and fissures have two common features: their symptoms can often be ameliorated or cured by nonsurgical means, and they are not life threatening. Therefore, surgery should usually not be the first option for either condition. Instead, the surgeon should initially offer the patient a trial of nonoperative management, and only after this has failed should surgery be considered. Exceptions are the excruciatingly painful fissure that significantly impairs the patient's quality of life, and massively prolapsed, thrombosed hemorrhoids, situations in which surgery is often the most expeditious and humane means of alleviating the patient's pain and correcting the underlying pathology. Even in these settings, however, the surgeon should document that he has discussed possible nonoperative management alternatives with the patient, that surgery is recommended because of the severity of the clinical situation, and that the patient understands these considerations and accepts the recommendation.

Informed consent prior to elective anal surgery should include a discussion of the possibility of postoperative impairment of continence and of recurrence of symptoms. Exact figures regarding the incidence of these two complications should not be given unless specifically requested by the patient, but one must recognize, despite the low incidence, there is a possibility that either may occur postoperatively.

When performing a hemorrhoidectomy, the surgeon should refrain from undertaking a concomitant sphincterotomy unless a fissure is present and informed consent for this additional procedure has been granted. Should the surgeon ignore this guideline, any degree of postoperative incontinence experienced by the patient, even if physiologically unrelated to the sphincterotomy, may be attributed to it in a legal proceeding, serving as the basis of a lawsuit on the grounds that the sphincterotomy exceeded the scope of the patient's consent.

Similarly, when performing a sphincterotomy, hemorrhoids, except for sentinel tags and hemorrhoidal tissue adjacent to the fissure that may interfere with healing, should not be removed without the patient's prior approval.

Rectal Bleeding

Failure to conduct a thorough evaluation for rectal bleeding may result in a delayed diagnosis of cancer, which is one of the most common causes of malpractice litigation in colorectal surgery.[1] It is both impractical and unethical to recommend colonoscopy to every patient with rectal bleeding. At a minimum, however, patients with this complaint should have anoscopy or preferably rigid or flexible sigmoidoscopy. If a nonneoplastic source of bleeding is found within the anorectum, the surgeon may offer a course of nonoperative management and should arrange for follow-up, either office visit or telephone call, to document that the bleeding has resolved.

No matter what means of follow-up is selected, however, the surgeon should instruct the patient to establish contact within a stated time period if the bleeding persists, and document this recommendation in the record. Failure to adopt this simple measure has often resulted in a weakened defense in lawsuits charging delayed diagnosis of cancer, since the patient may deny or not remember ever having been informed of the requirement for follow-up. Written documentation of the surgeon's admonition avoids the dilemma that a jury may face in having to decide between the word of the patient and that of the surgeon.

If the bleeding persists despite adequate nonoperative or surgical treatment or if no source of bleeding is found on initial endoscopic examination in a patient who, either due to age or some other factor, is at increased risk for colorectal cancer, either a full colonoscopy, or less optimally, flexible sigmoidoscopy with barium enema, is indicated. Even if benign anorectal disease was the true source of bleeding, a colonic neoplasm may become manifest some time in the future, and the patient may claim delayed diagnosis on the basis of an incomplete evaluation of the colon in the face of ongoing rectal bleeding.

Anastomotic Leak

No matter how experienced or technically adept, every surgeon will encounter an anastomotic leak. Because anastomotic leak is recognized as a risk inherent in colon surgery, however, its occurrence is not, per se, evidence of substandard care. Instead, malpractice litigation in this setting is usually the result of the surgeon's failure to diagnose and treat the leak in a timely fashion. Because of their frequency and the serious consequences associated with this complication, the possibility of an anastomotic leak should be discussed preoperatively with the patient as part of the informed consent.

Most leaks become clinically apparent between the 5th and 10th postoperative days, presenting with tachycardia, fever, ileus, abdominal pain and distension, and leukocytosis. Although identical clinical findings may result from processes unrelated to the anastomosis, it is incumbent upon the surgeon, when confronted with this constellation of findings, to promptly establish whether an anastomotic leak exists. Appropriate tools for this purpose are CT scan of the abdomen and pelvis or a low-pressure contrast study of the anastomosis, preferably from below, using water-soluble contrast material.

If an anastomotic leak is diagnosed promptly and managed properly, the most serious sequelae of ongoing sepsis (acute respiratory distress syndrome, renal and hepatic failure) can often be avoided. Litigation commonly arises when the surgeon fails to consider the possibility of an anastomotic leak, often resulting in an extended period of untreated fecal peritonitis and its devastating consequences.

Colonoscopic Perforation

Perforation of the colon as the result of diagnostic or therapeutic colonoscopy has much in common with anastomotic leak. It is a risk inherent in the procedure, and this possibility should be mentioned in the informed consent. From a medico-legal perspective, litigation is often the result of delay in diagnosis.

The development of abdominal pain and distention within a few hours of completion of colonoscopy should suggest the possibility of mechanical injury to the colon. These symptoms are often relayed to the physician by the patient or his relative by telephone, since by this time the patient has usually been discharged from the endoscopy unit. If there is any question as to the significance or validity of the complaints, the patient should be examined by a qualified observer and imaging stud-

ies performed in order to endeavor to detect free intraperitoneal air. Upright chest x-rays and flat plate and upright abdominal films are usually sufficient, but if these studies are inconclusive CT scan of the abdomen may reveal small amounts of free air not readily identified on plain films.

Similar symptoms may develop following biopsy, fulguration, or removal of polyps or other lesions, although their onset in these settings may be delayed for a day or more because of the more gradual progression of the transmural injury. Again, direct physical examination and appropriate imaging studies should be undertaken to establish the diagnosis.

As with anastomotic leak, the occurrence of a colonoscopic perforation does not, in itself, constitute malpractice, whereas failure to recognize and treat it does. By giving credence to the patient's complaints, promptly performing the necessary examinations, and instituting the appropriate treatment, the surgeon will not only conform to good medical practice but also provide herself with the best protection against a malpractice claim.

IF YOU'RE SUED

Often the surgeon's first indication that a suit is being considered is receipt of a letter from an attorney requesting the medical record of a patient who has suffered a complication or incurred some other unfavorable outcome. Although receipt of such a request may alarm the surgeon, he must restrain the natural impulse to contact the patient, the family, or the attorney in order to discuss the case or to inquire what, if any, action may be contemplated. Instead the surgeon is advised to notify his liability insurance carrier or other responsible risk manager of the request and then comply with the request, provided that it is accompanied by a valid "release of information" form signed by the patient or designated medical power of attorney or, if the patient is deceased, by the next of kin. In complying with the request, the surgeon should send only a copy of the record, retaining the original. If a hospital chart is involved, it should be secured so that no outside parties have access to it. It is also recommended that the surgeon keep a second copy in a location remote from other office records to avoid the problems that would ensue if the original were to be damaged, lost, or stolen. If the patient has been hospitalized, the surgeon should acquire a copy of the complete hospital record, even if the latter is voluminous and expensive to duplicate. These copies of the office and hospital records will serve as "working" documents that can be marked and highlighted by the surgeon and her attorney in preparing the defense. It cannot be emphasized too strongly, however, that the original documents must not be altered in any way. Such after-the-fact changes, even if reflective of the true course of events, are easily detected and may be subsequently used to impugn the surgeon's integrity. Moreover, if the changes are fabrications, they may serve as the basis for criminal prosecution.

A sensitive situation arises if the patient, having enlisted an attorney to review the medical records, seeks ongoing care from the surgeon. In doing so the patient may be motivated by a genuine desire for treatment, or he or she may be attempting to elicit an expression of guilt or responsibility from the surgeon. If the surgeon is willing to continue treatment, parameters for the scope of physician–patient discussions should be developed with the assistance of the insurance carrier or risk manager. If the surgeon does not wish to continue treating the patient, she must follow established ethical and legal guidelines for terminating care. Failure to do so may result in a claim of abandonment.

In order to formally initiate a malpractice suit, the patient's attorney must file a complaint in state or federal court. The complaint may be specific as to its allegations, or it may only vaguely stipulate that the surgeon deviated from the standard of care and that injury resulted. The plaintiff's attorney must also issue a summons to the surgeon, specifying a time period in which to file a response to the complaint. Upon receipt of formal notification that a suit has been filed, the surgeon must notify the insurance carrier or risk manager promptly if this has not already been done. Otherwise, one risks denial of coverage! The insurance carrier will then appoint an attorney to defend the surgeon. Although reimbursed by the insurance carrier, the defense attorney's primary responsibility is to the surgeon, and if, for any reason, one is dissatisfied with the appointed attorney's performance, he or she has the right to request that an alternate be provided. Once the attorney–surgeon relationship has been established, the surgeon should not only fully cooperate with one's attorney, but also actively participate in the defense by supplying documents and conferring with the attorney as requested. The surgeon should refrain, however, from discussing the case with any other parties. In most situations, the defense attorney will also solicit opinions from physicians with appropriate expertise to evaluate the case. To assist in this process, the defendant may suggest the names of experts with whom he is familiar, but one should not include individuals with whom he has a professional, financial, or social relationship.

The next stage in formal proceedings is that of discovery, during which the plaintiff's attorney will issue a set of written questions (interrogatories) about the care rendered and to which the defendant must respond. The interrogatories are likely to be more detailed than the formal complaint with regard to specific claims of negligence, and will identify the plaintiff's expert witnesses as well as shed light on their opinions. Statements under oath (depositions) will then be taken from the patient, the surgeon, the expert witnesses, and any other relevant individuals, the purpose of which is to discover what the various parties are prepared to testify about at trial. Finally, in most jurisdictions, unless the case is settled, the action will proceed to trial, which is almost always conducted before a jury or arbitrating tribunal.

As the case proceeds along its legal pathway, the surgeon will be called upon to give testimony in depositions and at trial, proceedings for which she should adopt differing strategies. At deposition, the plaintiff's attorney will attempt to discover what factual testimony the surgeon will give at trial and to evaluate the surgeon's strengths and weaknesses as a witness before a jury. In this situation, the surgeon should answer questions precisely and honestly, but should not volunteer information not encompassed within the scope of the question, nor should explanations be offered of the medical technicalities unless specifically requested to do so.

In contrast, at trial the surgeon will be attempting to explain and justify to the jury the care that was rendered. In doing so the surgeon should conform to the testimony given at deposition, but should now feel free to expand on the answers in order to instruct the jury and explain the rationale and justification for one's actions. Despite competing demands for the surgeon's time, he or she should remain in attendance throughout the trial, not only to serve as a medical advisor to his or her attorney, but also to avoid giving the jury the impression of indifference as to the outcome.

At both deposition and trial, the surgeon, despite genuine feelings of concern as to the patient's problems, must remain firm in the conviction of the rightness of one's position and should avoid making admissions based on retrospective analysis or in speculating as to what she or he might have done differently in response to "knowing-what-you-know-now" questions. The surgeon can also favorably influence the jury by dressing conservatively without ostentatious jewelry, by remaining composed and polite, by not losing one's temper, and by not appearing arrogant or condescending. In presenting an image of competence, forthrightness, and professionalism, the surgeon will conform to the jury's image of what every patient would like to see in a physician and will thereby maximize the likelihood of a favorable outcome in what is inevitably a stressful and emotionally charged experience.

CONCLUSION

The guidelines contained in this chapter are intended to protect the surgeon from becoming the subject of a malpractice suit. Unfortunately, given the litigious atmosphere in which American surgeons practice, such claims are likely to arise during the course of a surgical career. Adherence to the principles of providing high quality care, documenting discussions and events clearly and comprehensively, and maintaining strong lines of communication with the patient and his or her family, however, will serve as the basis for a strong defense in the event of such an eventuality.

REFERENCES

1. Kern KA. Medical malpractice involving colon and rectal disease: a 20 year review of United States civil court litigation. *Dis Colon Rectum* 1993;36;531.
2. Moore TA. *Medical malpractice discovery and trial*, 7th ed. New York: Practising Law Institute Press, 2002.
3. Nora PF, ed. *Professional liability/risk management: a manual for surgeons*. Chicago: American College of Surgeons, 1991.
4. Sloan FA, et al. *Suing for medical malpractice*. Chicago: University of Chicago Press, 1993. (As quoted in Moore.)
5. Zane JM. *The story of law*, 2nd ed. Indianapolis: Liberty Fund, 1998 (1927). (As quoted in Moore).

history of, 91
in HIV infection, 675
in hyperplastic (metaplastic) polyps, 702
indications for, 99–101
instrument cleansing after, 113–114
instrumentation for, 93–94, 99*f*–100*f*
in intestinal pseudo-obstruction, 488
intraoperative, in colonic resection, 829
patient preparation for, 101–103
pediatric, 122
perforation during, malpractice and, 1687
in polyp follow-up, 744–745
in polypoid disease, 718–721, 720*f*
privileging and credentialing in, 101
rectal prolapse and, 503
sedation and monitoring for, 103–104
in stomal creation, 1538
techniques for
anorectal intubation, 108
approach to, 106–107
principles of, 104–106
rectal examination, 108
sigmoid-descending colon intubation, 108–109
sigmoid intubation, 108
therapeutic, 114–118
biopsy in, 114
complications of, 118–122
equipment for, 114–115
for foreign-body removal, 122
indications for, 115
intraoperative use of, 122
for polyp removal, 734–741
results of, 118
for sigmoid volvulus, 122
snare polypectomy in, 114
technique for, 115–117, 116*f*–118*f*
in ulcerative colitis, 1324–1327, 1325*f*
vesrs barium enema, 1327
virtual, 80, 81*f*, 82
versus virtual colonoscopy, 122–123
Colonoscopy-polypectomy, in polypoid disease, 718–721, 731–732, 731*f*
Coloplasty, coloanal anastomosis with, 1014, 1015*f*
COLOR (colon carcinoma laparoscopic or open resection) study, 1225, 1240, 1246, 1256
Colorectal anastomosis, rectal stricture at, 1002–1004
Colorectal cancer. *See also* Hereditary nonpolyposis colorectal cancer
anatomic distribution of, 723
de novo, versus polyp-cancer sequence, 724
development of
genetic alterations in, 728–730, 730*f*
molecular changes leading to, 728
distribution of, right-to-left shift in, 720
Dukes' classification of, 800*t*
epidemiology of, 745
familial adenomatous polyposis and, 746, 756
familial syndromes of, genetics of, 728–730
family history and, 723
genetics of, 725–730, 746–747
geographic distribution of, 723
melanosis coli and, 470, 471*f*

metachronous, with polypectomy, 722–723
multistep carcinogenesis in, 726–727
and natural selection, 726
polyp-cancer sequence and, 721–730
prevention of
antioxidant vitamins and, 741–742
diet and, 741–742
sex distribution of, 723
synchronous, with adenomas, 721–722, 722*f*
with ulcerative colitis
after resective surgery, 1342
age and, 1342
characteristics of, 1342–1345
dysplasia and, 1346–1350
gender and, 1342
incidence of, 1342
pathologic features of, 1343*f*–1346*f*, 1344–1345
predisposing factors, 1342
treatment of, 1351
results of, 1345–1346
Colorectal disease
anal incontinence caused by, 350
laparoscopic-assisted surgery for, and other diseases compared, 1236, 1239
Colorectal function, physiology laboratory tests of, 129
anorectal sensation, 160
biofeedback, 160–161
defecography, 139–144
electromyography, 154–158
emptying studies, 144–145
endoluminal ultrasound, 145–149
magnetic resonance imaging, 149–150
manometry, 130–138
manovolumetry, 138–139
motility studies, 150–154
perineography, 145
perineometry, 145, 145*f*
pudendal nerve terminal motor latency, 158–159
transit studies
colonic, 150–152
small bowel, 152–153
Colorectal trauma. *See* Trauma, colorectal
Colorectal varices, 1269–1270
Colostogram, distal, with anorectal malformations, 580, 1538
Colostomy
for anal incontinence, 414*f*–415*f*, 415–416
for anorectal malformations, 580, 580*f*
postoperative care for, 583–584
technique for, 580, 582*f*
for anorectal trauma, 444, 444*f*
for colorectal trauma, 433, 434, 435*t*, 436*t*
concomitant, in low anterior resection for rectal cancer, 988, 990, 993
in diverticular disease
exteriorization and resection with, 1195*f*, 1197–1198, 1198*f*
transverse, 1195*f*, 1196–1197
for Fournier's gangrene, 632
versus ileostomy, in rectal cancer management, 965–966
irrigating system for, 1556–1558, 1557*f*
magnetic, 1555, 1555*f*
manufacturers and products for, 1616*t*

necrotic, after abdominoperineal resection, 952–953
for obstructed right colon, 850, 853*f*
in patient with fecal incontinence, 414*f*–415*f*, 415–416
continent colonic conduit in, 416*f*
continet colonic conduit in, 416, 416*f*
when to close, 416, 416*f*
percutaneous endoscopic, 1538
for preliminary decompression in Hirschsprung's disease, 561
in radiation enteritis, 1295, 1298*f*
reversal of, in diverticular disease, 1200–1202
of sigmoid colon, in abdominoperineal resection, 924, 924*f*
Colostomy closure
after Hartmann operation, 1247, 1248*f*
after low anterior resection for rectal cancer, 996*t*, 999
and complications relationship, 993, 996*t*
in loop colostomy, 1566–1570, 1569*t*
interval between colostomy and closure, 1568–1569, 1569*t*
late complications of, 1569, 1569*t*
technique for, 1569–1570
Colostomy irrigation, 1556–1558, 1557*f*
with a cone, 1603*t*
helpful hints, 1603*t*
Colostomy plug, 1553–1554, 1554*f*
Colostomy stoma, 1601–1602
descending/sigmoid, 1602–1603, 1603*t*
transverse, 1602
Colotomy, and polypectomy, for pedunculated lesions, 734, 735*f*
Colovaginal fistula, in diverticular disease, 1192
Colovesical fistula, in diverticular disease, 1189, 1191–1192, 1191*f*–1194*f*
Colpocystodefecography, 508
Colporectopexy, for syndrome of the descending perineum, 513*f*
Columns, rectal, 10
Colyte. *See* Polyethylene glycol
Combination chemotherapy, for metastatic disease, 877
Combined modality therapy
for anal canal carcinomas, 1075–1076
salvage surgery following, 1076–1077
Comfeel, in ostomy management, 1608
Commode, for defecography, 139–140, 140*f*
Competence, criteria for, 101
Compliance
in manometry, 138
pouch, evaluation after Parks procedure, 1432
Computed tomography
in abdominal trauma
blunt, 431, 432
penetrating, 429
with arterial portography, in colon cancer recurrence evaluation, 872–873
in bowel evaluation, 78
of bowel obstruction after abdominoperineal resection, 953, 953*f*
in colon cancer evaluation, 786–788, 788*f*–790*f*

idiopathic AIDS-related ulcers and, 689
malignancy and, 691
Hill-Ferguson rectal retractor, 58, 59f
in anoplasty, 237, 239
Hilton, anocutaneous line of, 11
Hindgut
carcinoid tumor of, 1093t
embryology of, 1–2, 2f
mesenteric circulation and, 20
Hindgut inertia, bowel transit study in, 464, 465f
Hirschman anoscope, 57, 58f
Hirschman proctoscope, 58f
Hirschsprung's disease. See also Aganglionosis
adult, 478–482
aganglionic segment in, 556, 557f
anorectal malformations and, 557–558
anorectal manometry in, 559–560
barium enema in, 559, 560f
clinical manifestations of, 558–559
and constipation, 558
diagnosis of, 478, 479f, 480, 559–561
differential diagnosis of, 559
Down syndrome and, 558
embryology of, 556–557
genetic defects associated with, 558
historical perspective on, 555–556
incidence of, 557–558
inheritance patterns of, 557
late-onset, 478–482
malformations associated with, 557–558
management of, 561–569
medical therapy for, 561
megabowels as consequence of, 482
pathophysiology of, 556–557, 558f
radiologic studies in, 559
rectal biopsy in, 478, 479f, 560
surgical therapy for, 480, 481, 481f, 482, 556, 561–564
colostomy for preliminary bowel decompression, 561
definitive operations in, 561–566
Duhamel's procedure for, 480, 562–563, 563f, 564
one-stage repair in, 561
pull-through procedures, 1246
results of, 480, 482
Soave's procedure for, 563–564, 564–565, 565f, 566f
Swenson's procedure for, 561–562, 562f, 564
transanal approach to, 563–564, 567f–568f
two-stage repair in, 561
Histiocytoma, malignant fibrous, 1110, 1111f
of anal canal, 1083
Histoplasma capsulatum, 679, 1655
Histoplasmosis, 635
in HIV-infected patients, 679
intestinal, 1655
HIV. See Human immunodeficiency virus
HNPCC. See Hereditary nonpolyposis colorectal cancer
Hollihesive, in ostomy management, 1608
Home hyperalimentation, for short bowel syndrome, 1500–1501
Honey, topical application for Fournier's gangrene, 633

Hooded anus. See Perineal fistula
Hookworm, 636
Hopkins Symptom Checklist (SCL-90-R), in constipated patient evaluation, 467
Hormone therapy, for gastrointestinal bleeding, 1280
Horseshoe anal fistula
classification of, 296, 307
surgical treatment of, 307–308, 308f–309f
results of, 324
House advancement flap, for anal stenosis repair, 237, 240f
Houston, valves of
in rectal biopsy, 63
in rectal examination, 61, 62f
HPMPC (cidofovir), for condylomata acuminata, 650
HPV. See Human papillomavirus
HPZ. See High-pressure zone
HSSCC. See Hereditary site-specific nonpolyposis colonic cancer
HSV. See Herpes simplex virus
Human chorionic gonadotropin, tumor growth and spread and, 795
Human immunodeficiency virus
characteristics of, 671
intestinal and anorectal immunology and, 672–673
replication mechanism of, 671
transmission of
anorectal immunology and, 672–673
protection of surgeon against, 691, 693
Human immunodeficiency virus infection. See also Acquired immunodeficiency syndrome
anal lesions in, 274, 275
anorectal diease in, 682–691
AIDS-specific, 689–691, 689f–692f
examination and diagnostic principles, 682–683, 682f
malignancy, 691, 693f
nonsexually transmitted, 683–684, 683f
sexually transmitted, 684–689
colonic manifestations of, 675–682
diarrheal conditions, 675–678
histoplasmosis, 679
Kaposi's sarcoma, 680–682
non-Hodgkin's lymphoma, 679
hemorrhoidectomy in, 247–248
skin infections in, 653
Human papillomavirus infection, 647, 673. See also Anal intraepithelial neoplasia; Condyloma acuminatum
subtypes of, 686
Human papillomavirus vaccine, 688–689
Hydrocortisone therapy, before surgery in ulcerative colitis, 1362
Hydration, before colonic resection, 809
Hydrocodone (Vicodin), after hemorrhoidectomy, 229
Hydrocolpos, 579
bilateral, 588
persistent cloaca with, 591f
Hydrocortisone
for pouchitis, 1428
in ulcerative colitis management, 1353
Hydrogen peroxide injection, for anal fistula identification, 301
Hydromorphone

patient-controlled analgesia with, 171
potency of, 170t
Hydrophilic substances, for constipation, 44
Hydroxyzine hydrochloride, for colonoscopic examination, 103
Hyperalimentation
before colonic resection, 809–810
parenteral, for Crohn's disease, 1500
Hyperbaric oxygen therapy
for anal fissure, 260–261
for radiation proctitis, 1300–1301
for rectourethral fistula, 345
Hyperplasia
lymphoid, 1101–1102, 1102f–1104f
histologic appearance in, 1332, 1338f
symptoms of, 1101–1102
treatment of, 1102
mucosal, polypoid carcinoma of the colon with, 796f
Hyperplastic polyposis, 703–704
Hyperplastic polyps. See Polyp(s), hyperplastic (metaplastic)
Hypersensitivity, 611
Hyperthermochemoradiotherapy, for rectal cancer, 1041
Hypertrophic osteoarthropathy, in Crohn's disease, 1489
Hypertrophied anal papilla
in hemorrhoid differential diagnosis, 182, 182f
stapled hemorrhoidopexy and, 224
Hypokalemia, with villous adenomas, 713
Hypotension
ischemic colitis and, 1289
nonocclusive vascular disease and, 1285f
Hypothermia, colorectal trauma and, 436–437
Hysterectomy
concomitant with abdominoperineal resection, 940–941, 942f
rectovaginal fistula after, 335f

I

IAS. See Internal anal sphincter
IBD. See Inflammatory bowel disease
IBS. See Irritable bowel syndrome
Ice paks, in treatment of gangrenous, prolapsed or edematous hemorrhoids, 208
Idiopathic AIDS-related ulcer, 689–691, 689f–691f
Idiopathic incontinence, 351
Idiopathic perforation, single-contrast barium enema examination and, 76
IFL regimen, for metastatic disease, 875, 876, 877t
IFN-γ (interferon gamma), radiation enteritis and, 1295
Ileal conduits, for urinary diversion, 1604
Ileal Crohn's disease, 1468, 1471f
Ileal interposition, for ureteral injury repair, 949
Ileal pouch, in ulcerative colitis surgery
double-folded (Kock pouch), 1418
lateral, 1418, 1422f
Ileal pouch—anal anastomosis, 1402–1421. See also Parks procedure

Malignant fibrous histiocytoma, 1110, 1111*f*
 of anal canal, 1083
Malignant lymphoma, 1102–1106
 classification of, 1105–1106
 endoscopy and radiology in, 1104–1105, 1105*f*–1106*f*
 histopathology of, 1105, 1107*f*–1108*f*
 pathogenesis of, 1104
 signs and symptoms of, 1103–1104
 treatment of, 1106
Malignant melanoma, of anal canal, 1079–1081, 1080*f*–1082*f*
 histology of, 1080, 1081*f*–1082*f*
 physical findings in, 1079–1080, 1080*f*
 symptoms of, 1079
 treatment and results of, 1080–1081
Malignant polyps, removal at colonoscopy, 117
Malignant vascular tumors, 1132–1133. *See also* Kaposi's sarcoma
Malnutrition, and rectal prolapse in children, 542
Malone's procedure, in bowel management programs, 596
Malpractice
 in colon and rectal surgery, 1686–1687
 litigation process in, 1687–1688
 penalties for
  assessing, historical background on, 1684
  historical and contemporary, 1683–1684
 unwritten laws and, 1684–1686
 written laws and, 1684
Mannitol, before colonoscopy, 102
Manometry, anorectal. *See* Anorectal manometry
Manuvolumetry, 138–139
 equipment for, 138–139, 138*f*
 procedure for, 139
Marginal artery of Drummond, 20, 21
Marlen plastic loop ostomy rods, 1559, 1562*f*
Marlex mesh, for peristomal hernia repair, 1545, 1546, 1549*f*–1551*f*
Marlex sling repair, for rectal prolapse, 530, 531*f*–533*f*, 534
 postoperative management of, 535
 presacral hemorrhage management in, 534*f*
 results of, 535–536, 535*t*
Mass(es)
 anal and perianal, evaluation of, 54
 in colon cancer, 776
 inflammatory, acute and chronic diverticulitis with, 1199, 1199*f*
Maturation techniques
 in ileostomy stoma, 1575, 1576*f*
  improper, complications due to, 1577–1581, 1578*f*–1585*f*
 in sigmoid colostomy, 1553
Maximum resting anal pressure, 358, 359, 360
 after artificial spincter implantation, 413
 after Parks postanal pelvic floor repair, 392
Maximum squeeze pressure, 358, 359, 360
 after Parks postanal pelvic floor repair, 392
Maylard incision, in colonic resection, 810–811, 811*f*

disposable wound retractor through, 812*f*
MCC (mutated in colon carcinoma) gene, in colorectal cancer, 728
McGivney hemorrhoid ligator, 189*f*
McGown hemorrhoid ligator, 190*f*
Mebendazole
 for ascariasis, 1671
 for pinworm infestation, 637
 for trichuriasis, 1674
Meckel's diverticulectomy, with colonic resection, 857
Meckel's diverticulum, 1267–1270, 1268*f*–1270*f*
 diagnostic studies in, 1267
 incidental removal of, 1268–1269
 treatment of, 1267–1268
Meconium ileus, 559
Meconium-plug syndrome, 559
Medicaolegal issues. *See* Malpractice
Medroxyprogesterone acetate
 for desmoid tumors with familial polyposis, 756
 for endometriosis, 1135
Megacolon
 Chagasic, 1665*f*
 congenital, 555–569
 idiopathic, 482
 toxic. *See* Toxic megacolon
Megarectum
 differential diagnosis of, 559
 idiopathic, 482
Meissner's corpuscles, of anal canal, 27
Melanoma. *See* Malignant melanoma
Melanosis coli, 469–470, 469*f*–470*f*
 and colorectal cancer, 470, 471*f*
Melena, cavernous hemangiomas and, 1127, 1130*f*
Men. *See* Males
Meningocele, anterior sacral, 1153
Meperidine
 for colonoscopic examination, 103
 for pain control after colon resection, 858
 patient-controlled analgesia with, 171
 potency of, 170*t*
 pseudoseizure induced by, 170
 for sedation in colonoscopy, 108
Mercaptopurine
 for Crohn's disease, 1497–1498
 for pouchitis, 1428
 for ulcerative colitis, 1355
Merkel cell carcinoma, of anal canal, 1083
Mersilene tape, for Thiersch repair, 515, 515*f*, 516*f*
Mesalamine (mesalazine)
 for pouchitis, 1428
 for ulcerative colitis, 1351–1353, 1354*t*
  adverse effects of, 1352*t*
Mesenchymal tumors, 1089, 1107–1123
 of adipose tissue origin, 1119–1123
  lipoma, 1119–1122, 1120*f*–1124*f*
 of fibrous tissue origin, 1107–1110
  eosinophilic granuloma, 1108–1109, 1110*f*
  fibroma, 1107–1108
  fibrosarcoma, 1109–1110, 1110*f*, 1111*f*
  inflammatory fibroid polyp, 1108–1109, 1110*f*
  malignant fibrous histiocytoma, 1110, 1111*f*
 of smooth muscle origin, 1113–1119

leiomyoma, 1113–1116, 1114*f*–1115*f*
 leiomyosarcoma, 1116–1119, 1117*f*–1119*f*
 rhabdomyosarcoma, 1119
 of stromal origin, 1111–1113
Mesenteric arteries, 18–20, 19*f*
 collateral circulation between, 20–21
Mesenteric occlusive disease, 1282–1286
 emergency laparoscopy in, 1243
 evaluation of, 1282, 1283*f*, 1284, 1284*f*
 laboratory and radiologic studies in, 1282
 management of
  protocol for, 1282, 1283*f*, 1284
  results of, 1284–1285
 signs and symptoms of, 1282
 venous ischemia in, 1285–1286
  emergency laparoscopy and, 1243
Mesh implantation
 for pelvic floor reconstruction, 943, 944*f*–945*f*
 for sigmoid colostomy creation, 1553
Mesocolon, anatomy of, 3*f*
Mesorectum, 7
 male, lateral view of, 8*f*
Messenger RNA coding, for tumor-specific antigen L6, 866
Metaplastic polyps. *See* Polyp(s), hyperplastic (metaplastic)
Metastases
 implantation type, tumoricidal agents to prevent, 811
 inguinal node, with rectal cancer, 938
Metastasis suppressor gene, 729
Metastatic disease
 after colonic resection, treatment of cerebral, 874
  chemotherapeutic regimens in, 874–878, 877*t*
  liver, 872–874
  osseous, 874
  ovarian, 872
  penile, 875
  pulmonary, 871–872
 of liver, management during colonic resection, 854–855, 855*f*
 rectal cancer patient and, 920
Methadone, potency of, 170*t*
Methotrexate
 for Crohn's disease, 1498
 for dermatomyositis, 614
Methylene blue
 for anal fistula identification, 300
 for pruritus ani, 607
Methylprednisolone acetate, in ulcerative colitis management, 1353
Metoclopramide, for constipation, 46, 472
Metronidazole
 after hemorrhoidectomy, 229
 for amebiasis, 1658–1659
 for Crohn's disease, 1496–1497
  with perianal disease, 325
 for pouchitis, 51, 1428
 for trichomoniasis, 635
Miconazole
 for candidiasis, 634
 for tinea cruris, 634
Microgranulomas, in Crohn's disease, 1469
Microsatellite instability, in HNPCC diagnosis, 772
Microscopic colitis, 1630–1632, 1631*f*